VETERINARY MEDICINE

EDITION 11

A Textbook of the Diseases of Cattle, Horses, Sheep, Pigs, and Goats

VOLUME TWO

PETER D. CONSTABLE
KENNETH W. HINCHCLIFF
STANLEY H. DONE
WALTER GRÜNBERG

ELSEVIER

ELSEVIER

3251 Riverport Lane
St. Louis, Missouri 63043

VETERINARY MEDICINE: A TEXTBOOK OF THE DISEASES OF CATTLE, HORSES, SHEEP, PIGS, AND GOATS, ELEVENTH EDITION

Main ISBN: 9780702052460
Volume 2 ISBN: 978-0-7020-7056-3

Content Strategist: Penny Rudolph
Content Development Specialist: Laura Klein
Content Development Manager: Jolynn Gower
Publishing Services Manager: Hemamalini Rajendrababu
Senior Project Manager: Kamatchi Madhavan
Design Direction: Renee Duenow

Printed in Great Britain

Last digit is the print number: 9 8 7 6 5 4 3

Contents

Diseases of the Urinary System

13

Introduction

Diseases of the bladder and urethra are more common and more important than diseases of the kidneys in farm animals. Occasionally, renal insufficiency develops as a sequel to diseases such as pyelonephritis, embolic nephritis, amyloidosis, and nephrosis. Knowledge of the physiology of urinary secretion and excretion is required to properly understand disease processes in the urinary tract. The principles of renal insufficiency presented here are primarily extrapolated from research in other species, particularly human medicine. Although generally these principles probably apply to farm animals, the details of renal function and renal failure in farm animals have just started to be studied in depth.

PRINCIPLES OF RENAL INSUFFICIENCY

The kidneys excrete the end products of tissue metabolism (except for carbon dioxide), and maintain fluid, electrolyte, and acid-base balance, by varying the volume of water and the concentration of solutes in the urine. For conceptual purposes it is helpful to think of the kidney as composed of many similar nephrons, which are the basic functional units of the kidney. Each nephron is composed of blood vessels, the glomerulus, and a tubular system that consists of the proximal tubule, the loop of Henle, the distal tubule, and the collecting duct.

The glomerulus is a semipermeable filter that allows easy passage of water and low molecular weight solutes, such as electrolytes, glucose, and keto acids, but restricts passage of high molecular weight substances, such as plasma proteins. Glomerular filtrate is derived from plasma by simple passive filtration driven by arterial blood pressure. Glomerular filtrate is identical to plasma except that it contains little protein or lipids. The volume of filtrate, and therefore its content of metabolic end products, depends on the hydrostatic pressure and the plasma oncotic pressure in the glomerular capillaries and on the proportion of glomeruli, which are functional. Because these factors are only partially controlled by the kidney, in the absence of disease, the rate of filtration through the glomeruli is relatively constant.

Epithelial cells in the renal tubules actively and selectively reabsorb substances from the glomerular filtrate while permitting the excretion of waste products. Proximal tubular cells are therefore metabolically very active and, consequently, are susceptible to injury from ischemia (decreased blood blood) or hypoxia. Glucose is reabsorbed entirely, within the normal range of plasma concentration; phosphate is reabsorbed in varying amounts depending on the needs of the body for phosphorus conservation; other substances, such as inorganic sulfates and creatinine, are not reabsorbed in appreciable amounts. The tubules also actively secrete substances, particularly electrolytes, as they function to regulate acid-base balance. As a result of the balance between resorption and secretion, the concentration of solutes in the urine varies widely when the kidneys are functioning normally.

The principal mechanism that regulates water reabsorption by the renal tubules is antidiuretic hormone (ADH). Tissue dehydration and an increase in serum osmolality stimulate the secretion of ADH from the posterior pituitary gland. The renal tubules respond to ADH by conserving water and returning serum osmolality to normal, producing concentrated urine.

Diseases of the kidneys, and in some instances of the ureters, bladder, and urethra, reduce the efficiency of the kidney's functions, resulting in disturbances in protein, acid-base, electrolyte, and water homeostasis and in the excretion of metabolic end products. A partial loss of function is described as **renal insufficiency**. When the kidneys can no longer regulate body fluid and solute composition, **renal failure** occurs.

RENAL INSUFFICIENCY AND RENAL FAILURE

Renal function depends on the number and functionality of the individual nephrons. Renal insufficiency can occur from abnormalities in the

- Rate of renal blood flow
- Glomerular filtration rate
- Efficiency of tubular reabsorption.

Of these three abnormalities, the latter two are intrinsic functions of the kidney, whereas the first depends largely on vasomotor control, which is markedly affected by circulatory emergencies such as shock, dehydration, and hemorrhage. Circulatory emergencies may lead to a marked reduction in glomerular filtration, but they are extrarenal in origin and cannot be considered as true causes of renal insufficiency. However, prolonged circulatory disruption can cause renal ischemia and ultimately renal insufficiency.

Glomerular filtration and tubular reabsorption can be affected independently in disease states, and every attempt should be made to clinically differentiate glomerular disease from tubular disease. This is because the clinical and clinicopathologic signs of renal dysfunction depend on the anatomic location of the lesion and the imbalance in function between glomeruli and tubules. Renal dysfunction tends to be a dynamic process so the degree of dysfunction varies with time. If renal dysfunction is so severe that the animal's continued existence is not possible, it is said to be in a state of renal failure, and the clinical syndrome of uremia will be present.

CAUSES OF RENAL INSUFFICIENCY AND UREMIA

The causes of renal insufficiency, and therefore of renal failure and uremia, can be divided into prerenal, renal, and postrenal groups.

Prerenal causes include congestive heart failure and acute circulatory failure, either cardiac or peripheral, in which acute renal ischemia occurs in response to a decrease in renal blood flow. Proximal tubular function is affected by renal ischemia to a much greater extent than the glomerulus or distal tubules; this is because of the high metabolic demands of the proximal tubules. However, those parts of the tubules within the medulla are particularly susceptible to hypoxic damage because of the low oxygen tension in this tissue, the dependency of blood flow on glomerular blood flow, and the high metabolic rate of this tissue. Renal medullary necrosis is a direct consequence of these factors.

Renal causes include glomerulonephritis, amyloidosis, pyelonephritis, embolic nephritis, and interstitial nephritis. Acute renal failure can be produced in any of the farm animal species by administration of a variety of toxins (see the section Toxic Nephrosis). The disease is also secondary to sepsis and hemorrhagic shock. Experimental uremia has also been induced by surgical removal of both kidneys but the results, especially in ruminants, are quite different from those in naturally occurring renal failure. The clinical pathology is similar, but there is a prolonged period of normality after the surgery.

Postrenal uremia may also occur, specifically complete obstruction of the urinary tract by vesical or urethral calculus, or more rarely by bilateral urethral obstruction by transitional cell carcinoma located in the trigone region of the bladder. Internal rupture of any part of the urinary tract, such as the bladder, ureters, or urethra, will also cause postrenal uremia.

PATHOGENESIS OF RENAL INSUFFICIENCY AND RENAL FAILURE

Damage to the glomerular epithelium destroys its selective permeability and permits the passage of plasma proteins into the glomerular filtrate. The predominant protein is initially albumin, because of its negative charge and a lower molecular weight than globulins; however, with advanced glomerulonephritis (such as renal amyloidosis) all plasma proteins are lost. Glomerular filtration may cease completely when there is extensive damage to glomeruli, particularly if there is acute swelling of the kidney, but it is thought that anuria in the terminal stages of acute renal disease is caused by back diffusion of all glomerular filtrate through the damaged tubular epithelium rather than failure of filtration. When renal damage is less severe, the remaining nephrons compensate to maintain total glomerular filtration by increasing their filtration rates. When this occurs, the volume of glomerular filtrate may exceed the capacity of the tubular epithelium to reabsorb fluid and solutes. The tubules may be unable to achieve normal urine concentration. As a result, an increased volume of urine with a constant specific gravity is produced and solute diuresis occurs. This is exacerbated if the tubular function of the compensating nephrons is also impaired. The inability to concentrate urine is clinically evident as polyuria and is characteristic of developing renal insufficiency.

Decreased glomerular filtration also results in retention of metabolic waste products such as urea and creatinine. Although marked increases in serum urea concentration are probably not responsible for the production of clinical signs, because urea readily crosses cell membranes and therefore is an ineffective osmole, the serum urea nitrogen (SUN) concentration can be used to monitor glomerular filtration rate. However, the utility of SUN concentration as a measure of glomerular filtration rate is reduced because serum urea concentrations are influenced by the amount of protein in the diet, by hydration, and by gastrointestinal metabolism of urea. Serum urea concentrations are substantially higher in animals on high-protein diets, and dehydration increases serum urea concentration by increasing resorption of urea in the loop of Henle, which is independent of effects of hydration of the glomerular filtration rate. Urea is excreted into saliva of ruminants and metabolized by ruminal bacteria. In contrast, creatinine is excreted almost entirely by the kidney, creatinine originates from the breakdown of creatine phosphate in muscle, and serum concentrations of creatinine are a useful marker of glomerular filtration rate. The relationship between serum creatinine concentration and glomerular filtration rate is hyperbolic (a reduction in glomerular filtration rate by half results in a doubling of the serum creatinine concentration). Phosphate and sulfate retention also occurs when total glomerular filtration is reduced and sulfate retention contributes to metabolic acidosis in renal insufficiency. Phosphate retention also causes a secondary hypocalcemia, due in part to an increase in calcium excretion in the urine. In horses, the kidneys are an important route of calcium excretion; thus the decreased glomerular filtration rate present in horses with chronic renal failure usually results in hypercalcemia. Variations in serum potassium concentrations also occur and appear to depend on potassium intake. Hyperkalemia is not usually a serious complication of renal insufficiency in ruminants because affected animals often have decreased appetites and therefore reduced potassium intakes, and excess saliva can be excreted by the salivary glands and ultimately the feces.

Loss of tubular resorptive function is evidenced by a continued loss of sodium and chloride; hyponatremia and hypochloremia eventually occur in all cases of renal failure. The continuous loss of large quantities of fluid from solute diuresis can cause clinical dehydration. More often it makes the animal particularly susceptible to dehydration when there is an interruption in water availability or when there is a sudden increase in body water loss by another route, as in diarrhea.

The terminal stage of renal insufficiency, renal failure, is the result of the cumulative effects of impaired renal excretory and homeostatic functions. Sustained excretion of large volumes of dilute urine results in dehydration. If other circulatory emergencies arise, acute renal ischemia might result, leading to acute renal failure. Prolonged hypoproteinemia results in rapid loss of body condition and muscle weakness. Acidemia secondary to metabolic acidosis and hyponatremia can also be a contributing factor to muscle weakness and mental attitude. All these factors play some part in the production of clinical signs of renal failure, which are typically manifested as weakness, lethargy, inappetence and, with extensive glomerular lesions, dependent edema caused by hypoproteinemia. However, the clinical syndrome is variable and rarely diagnostic for renal failure. Bleeding diathesis can also be present in severely uremic animals and has been associated with a lack of antithrombin (a small protein readily lost through the damaged glomerulus), platelet factor 3, platelet dysfunction, or disseminated intravascular coagulation.

Renal failure is seen as the clinical state of uremia. Uremic animals exhibit clinical signs of disease, which should be compared with azotemic animals that have an increase in the plasma or serum concentrations of urea and creatinine and retention of other solutes as described earlier, but do not necessarily have clinical signs of disease.

Clinical Features of Urinary Tract Disease

The major clinical manifestations of urinary tract disease are

- Abnormal constituents of urine
- Variations in daily urine flow
- Abdominal pain, painful urination (dysuria), and difficult urination (dysuria and stranguria)
- Abnormal sized kidneys
- Abnormalities of the bladder and urethra
- Acute and chronic renal failure

ABNORMAL CONSTITUENTS OF THE URINE

Laboratory analysis of urine is initially done using dipstick and refractometry on a voided or catheterized urine sample and microscopic examination of the sediment from a centrifuged urine sample. Urine dipsticks and refractometry (optical and digital) provide excellent low-cost point-of-care tests for evaluation of the urinary system. Widely available urine dipsticks typically measure 1 factor (acetoacetate), 5 factors (blood, glucose, acetoacetate, pH, and protein) or 10 factors (blood, glucose, bilirubin, acetoacetate, pH, protein, specific gravity, urobilinogen, nitrite, and leukocytes). Specific information regarding tests of renal function and injury conducted on urine, such as specific gravity and osmolality, enzymuria, and quantitative proteinuria and glycosuria, are discussed later in this chapter.

VARIATIONS IN DAILY URINE FLOW

An increase or decrease in urine flow is often described in animals, but accuracy demands physical measurement of the amount of urine voided over a 24-hour period. This is not usually practicable in large-animal practice, and it is often necessary to guess whether the flow is increased or decreased. Accurate measurement of the amount of water consumed is often easier and is usually used to estimate 24-hour urine production. Care should be taken to differentiate increased daily urine flow from increased frequency in urination without increased daily flow. The latter is much more common. Decreased urine output rarely, if ever, presents as a clinical problem in agricultural animals.

Normal urine production is highly variable in large animals and is dependent to a large extent on diet, watering systems, and the palatability of the water. Pregnant mares housed in tie stalls consume approximately 53 ± 6 mL of water per kilogram body weight (BW) per day, of which 50 ± 8 mL/kg is from drinking water with the remainder being water in feed. However, most of this water is excreted in the feces, with fecal and urinary water excretion being 34 ± 8 (mL/kg)/day and 8 ± 2 (mL/kg)/day, respectively. Neonatal foals produce urine at an average rate of 150 (mL/kg)/day.

Polyuria

Polyuria occurs when there is an increase in the volume of urine produced over a 24-hour period. Polyuria can result from extrarenal causes, such as when horses habitually drink excessive quantities of water (**psychogenic polydipsia**) and, much less common, in **central diabetes insipidus**, when there is inappropriate secretion of ADH from the pituitary, or when there is failure of the tubules to respond to ADH (**nephrogenic diabetes insipidus**). Polyuria occurs in horses with tumors of the pars intermedia of the pituitary gland. Although the cause of the polyuria is not known, it might be secondary to osmotic diuresis associated with the glucosuria or to central diabetes insipidus. Central diabetes insipidus is reported in sibling colts but is extremely rare in other species with isolated reports in a ram and a cow. Another extrarenal cause is administration of diuretic drugs, including corticosteroids.

Kidney disease results in polyuria when the resorptive capacity of the remaining tubules is exceeded. Polyuria can also occur when the osmotic gradient in the renal medulla is not adequate to produce concentrated urine. Nephrogenic diabetes insipidus causes polyuria because the tubules fail to respond to ADH.

When polyuria is suspected, a urine sample should be collected to determine specific gravity or osmolality. If urine is isosthenuric with a constant specific gravity of 1.008 to 1.012 (the specific gravity of plasma), then the presence of renal disease should be strongly considered. Serum urea and creatinine concentrations should be determined to evaluate glomerular filtration. If serum urea and creatinine concentrations are within normal limits, a water deprivation test can be performed to assess the animal's ability to produce concentrated urine.

Oliguria and Anuria

Reduction in the daily output of urine (**oliguria**) and complete absence of urine (**anuria**) occur under the same conditions and vary only in degree. In dehydrated animals, urine flow naturally decreases in an effort to conserve water as plasma osmolality increases. Congestive heart failure and peripheral circulatory failure may cause a reduction in renal blood flow that oliguria follows. Complete anuria is most common in urethral obstruction, although it can also result from acute tubular nephrosis. Oliguria occurs in the terminal stages of all forms of nephritis. Anuria and polyuria lead to retention of solutes and disturbances of the acid-base balance that contribute to the pathogenesis of uremia.

Pollakiuria

This is an increase in the daily number of postures for urination and is usually accompanied by a decreased volume of urine. Pollakiuria may occur with or without an increase in the volume of urine excreted and is commonly associated with disease of the lower urinary tract such as cystitis, the presence of calculi in the bladder, urethritis, and partial obstruction of the urethra. Other causes of pollakiuria include equine herpesvirus infection, sorghum cystitis, neuritis of the cauda equina in horses, neoplasia, obstructive lesions and trauma to the urethra, abnormal vaginal conformation, and urachal infection.

Dribbling is a steady, intermittent passage of small volumes of urine, sometimes precipitated by a change in posture or increase in intraabdominal pressure, reflecting inadequate or lack of sphincter control. Dribbling occurs in large animals with incomplete obstructive urolithiasis and from persistent urachus.

Persistent urachus is also called pervious or patent urachus. Failure of the urachus to obliterate at birth in foals causes urine to dribble from the urachus continuously. Urine may also pass from the urethra. Retrograde infection from omphalitis is common, resulting in cystitis. Persistent urachus is extremely rare in calves, lambs, and kids.

Abnormalities of micturition are classified as neurogenic or nonneurogenic. Micturition is mediated principally by the pelvic and pudendal nerves through lumbosacral spinal cord segments under the involuntary control of centers in the brainstem and voluntary control of the cerebrum and cerebellum. Reported neurogenic causes of urinary incontinence in horses include cauda equine neuritis, herpesvirus-1 myelitis, Sudan grass toxicosis, sorghum poisoning, trauma, and neoplasia. Nonneurogenic causes of urinary incontinence in horses include ectopic ureter, cystitis, urolithiasis, hypoestrogenism, and abnormal vaginal conformation.

ABDOMINAL PAIN AND PAINFUL AND DIFFICULT URINATION (DYSURIA AND STRANGURIA)

Abdominal pain and painful urination (**dysuria**) and difficult and slow urination (**stranguria**) are manifestations of discomfort caused by disease of the urinary tract. Acute abdominal pain from urinary tract disease occurs only rarely and is usually associated with sudden distension of the renal pelvis or ureter, or infarction of the kidney. None of these conditions is common in animals, but occasionally cattle affected with pyelonephritis may have short episodes of acute abdominal pain caused by either renal infarction or obstruction of the pelvis by necrotic debris. During these acute attacks of pain, the cow may exhibit downward arching of the back, paddling with the hind feet, rolling, and bellowing. Abdominal pain from urethral obstruction and distension of the bladder is manifested by tail switching, kicking at the belly, and repeated straining efforts at urination accompanied by grunting. Horses with acute tubular nephrosis following vitamin K3 administration might show renal colic with arching of the back, backing into corners, and rubbing of the perineum and tail head.

Dysuria or **painful/difficult urination** occurs in cystitis, vesical calculus, urethritis, and is caused by the presence of periurethral masses such as pelvic lymphoma.[1] Dysuria is manifested by the frequent passage of small amounts of urine. Grunting may occur with painful urination, and the animal may remain in the typical posture after urination is completed. Differentiating pain caused by urinary disease from pain caused by other causes depends largely on the presence of other signs indicating urinary tract involvement.

Stranguria is slow and painful urination associated with disease of the lower urinary tract including cystitis, vesical calculus, urethral obstruction, and urethritis. The animal strains to pass each drop of urine. Groaning and straining may precede and accompany urination when there is urethral obstruction. In urethritis, groaning and straining occur immediately after urination has ceased and gradually disappear and do not recur until urination has been repeated.

Urine scalding of the perineum or urinary burn is caused by frequent wetting of the skin with urine. It may be the result of urinary incontinence or the animal's inability to assume normal posture when urinating.

MORPHOLOGIC ABNORMALITIES OF KIDNEYS AND URETERS

Enlarged or decreased size of kidneys may be palpable on rectal examination or detected by ultrasonography. In cattle, gross enlargement of the posterior aspect of the left kidney may be palpable in the right upper flank. Abnormalities of the kidneys, such as hydronephrosis in cattle, may also be palpable on rectal examination. Increases in the size of the ureter may be palpable on rectal examination and indicate ureteritis or hydroureter.

PALPABLE ABNORMALITIES OF THE BLADDER AND URETHRA

Abnormalities of the bladder that may be palpable by rectal examination include gross enlargement of the bladder, rupture of the bladder, a shrunken bladder following rupture, and palpable abnormalities in the bladder such as cystic calculi. Abnormalities of the urethra include enlargement and pain of the pelvic urethra and its external aspects in male cattle with obstructive urolithiasis and obstruction of the urethral process of male sheep with obstructive urolithiasis.

ACUTE AND CHRONIC RENAL FAILURE

The clinical findings of urinary tract disease vary with the rate of development and stage of the disease. In most cases, the clinical signs are those of the initiating cause. In horses, depression, colic, and diarrhea are common with oliguria or polyuria. Clinical signs in cattle with uremia are similar and in addition are frequently recumbent, and in severe and terminal cases cattle may have a bleeding diathesis. In chronic renal disease of all species, there is a severe loss of BW, weakness, anorexia, polyuria, polydipsia, and ventral edema.

UREMIA

Uremia is the systemic state that occurs in the terminal stages of renal insufficiency. Anuria or oliguria may occur with uremia. Oliguria is more common unless there is complete obstruction of the urinary tract. Chronic renal disease is usually manifested by polyuria, but oliguria appears in the terminal stages when clinical uremia develops. The uremic animal is depressed and anorexic with muscular weakness and tremor. In chronic uremia, the body condition is poor, probably as a result of continued loss of protein in the urine, dehydration, and anorexia. The respiration is usually increased in rate and depth but is not dyspneic; in the terminal stages it may become periodic in character. The heart rate is markedly increased because of terminal dehydration, but the rectal temperature remains normal except in infectious processes and some cases of acute tubular nephrosis. An ammoniacal or uriniferous smell on the breath is often described in textbooks but is rarely clinically detectable. **Uremic encephalopathy** occurs in a small proportion of cattle, goats, and horses with chronic renal failure that involves an unknown metabolic pathway. It is associated with seizures, tremors, abnormal behavior, and muscle weakness, and histologic evidence of myelin vacuolation may be present.[1]

The animal becomes recumbent and comatose in the terminal stages of uremia. The temperature falls to below normal and death occurs quietly; the whole course of the disease is one of gradual intoxication. Necropsy findings, apart from those of the primary disease, are nonspecific and include degeneration of parenchymatous organs, sometimes accompanied by emaciation and moderate gastroenteritis.

Uremia has been produced experimentally in cattle by bilateral nephrectomy and urethral ligation. There is a progressive increase in serum urea concentration (mean daily increase of 53 mg/dL), serum creatinine concentration (mean daily increase of approximately 3.5 mg/dL), and serum uric acid concentration. Similar findings are reported in prerenal uremia in cattle. Interestingly, serum phosphate and potassium concentrations were for the most part unchanged because of increased salivary secretion of both factors, and acidemia and metabolic acidosis were not evident. Serum potassium concentrations were mildly increased after 5 to 7 days of bilateral nephrectomy.

Special Examination of the Urinary System

Lack of accessibility limits the value of physical examination of the urinary tract in farm animals. Palpation per rectum can be performed on horses and cattle and is described in Chapter's 7 and 8. In small ruminants and calves the urinary system is largely inaccessible to physical examination, although the kidneys may be palpated transabdominally and the urethra palpated digitally with the finger for periodic contractions that are common in male sheep and goats with obstructive urolithiasis. Urinalysis and determination of the serum or plasma concentration of urea nitrogen or creatinine is a required component of any examination of the urinary system.

TESTS OF RENAL FUNCTION AND DETECTION OF RENAL INJURY

The simplest and most important test of urinary function is the determination of whether or not urine is being voided. This can be accomplished in large animals by keeping them on a clean, dry floor that is examined periodically. Placing an absorbent cloth under recumbent foals and calves will also help determine whether urine is being passed.

Renal function tests evaluate the functional capability of the kidney and generally assess blood flow to the kidneys, glomerular filtration, and tubular function. These tests depend on whether they are based on the examination of **serum/plasma**, **urine,** or both, and assess either **function** or the presence of **injury**. The most practical screening tests for the presence of decreased renal function are determination of serum creatinine concentration and urine specific gravity. Determination of both factors assists differentiation of renal azotemia from prerenal azotemia. In prerenal azotemia, tubular function remains intact and renal conservation of water is optimized, resulting in the production of concentrated urine. Animals with prerenal azotemia therefore have increased serum concentrations of creatinine and urea and increased urine specific gravity. For comparison, animals with some degree of renal azotemia have increased serum concentrations of creatinine and urea and a lower than expected value for urine specific gravity. Determination of urine specific gravity should therefore be routinely performed in all dehydrated animals before the initiation of treatment, because oral or intravenous (IV) fluid therapy will directly change urine specific gravity.

COLLECTION OF URINE SAMPLES

Collection of urine samples can be difficult. Free-flow and catheterized samples are equally useful for routine urinalysis. Urine samples for analysis should be collected by midstream voiding, or cystocentesis in small male ruminants, preferably with ultrasonographic guidance. Bethanechol (0.075 mg/kg subcutaneously) has occasionally been used to produce urine in reluctant individuals, but a spontaneously voided sample is preferred for initial screening, which is routinely done using urine dipsticks.

Horses will often urinate shortly after they are walked into a freshly bedded box stall. Cows urinate if they are relaxed and have their perineum and vulval tip massaged upward very gently, without touching the tail. Success rates in obtaining a urine sample can approach 100% if cows are recumbent and quietly encouraged to stand before attempting perineal stimulation to induce urination. Steers and bulls may urinate if the preputial orifice is massaged and splashed with warm water. Ewes often urinate immediately after rising if they have been recumbent for some time. Occluding their nostrils and threatening asphyxia may also induce urination just as they are released and allowed to breathe again; however, this is a stressful procedure and should not be performed in sick or debilitated sheep. An IV injection of furosemide (0.5–1.0 mg/kg BW) produces urination in most animals in about 20 minutes. The sample is useful for microbiologic examination but its composition has been drastically altered by the diuretic. Diuretics should be used with extreme caution in dehydrated animals.

Urine samples obtained by **bladder catheterization** using a urethral catheter are preferred for microbiologic examination, provided aseptic technique is applied, including bandaging the tail of female horses or holding the tail of cattle out of the way. The perineal region should then be cleaned with dilute povidone iodine or chlorhexidine to minimize urinary tract contamination, and there should be routine use of sterile surgical gloves and lubrication. Rams, boars, and young calves usually cannot be catheterized without fluoroscopy because of the presence of a suburethral diverticulum and the small diameter of the urethra. A precurved catheter and fluoroscopic guidance can be used to facilitate catheterization of rams and bucks. Ewes and sows can be catheterized, but their vulvas are often too small relative to hand size to allow access to the urethra. Cows can be catheterized relatively simply provided that a fairly rigid, small-diameter (0.5-cm) catheter is used, such as an artificial insemination pipette. A finger can be inserted into the suburethral diverticulum on the ventral aspect to direct the tip of the catheter over the diverticulum and into the external urethral orifice (Fig. 13-1). For longer term catheterization of adult cattle (3 days), 24- to 28-French Foley catheters are placed into the bladder using the same insertion method; however, insertion of Foley catheters is facilitated by application of sterile lube on the outside of the catheter and placement of an insemination pipette into the catheter lumen to increase rigidity. Retention of Foley catheters in cows is facilitated by using a balloon volume of 60 to 75 mL; use of smaller balloon volumes permits the catheter to move into the urethra, leading to pollakiuria,

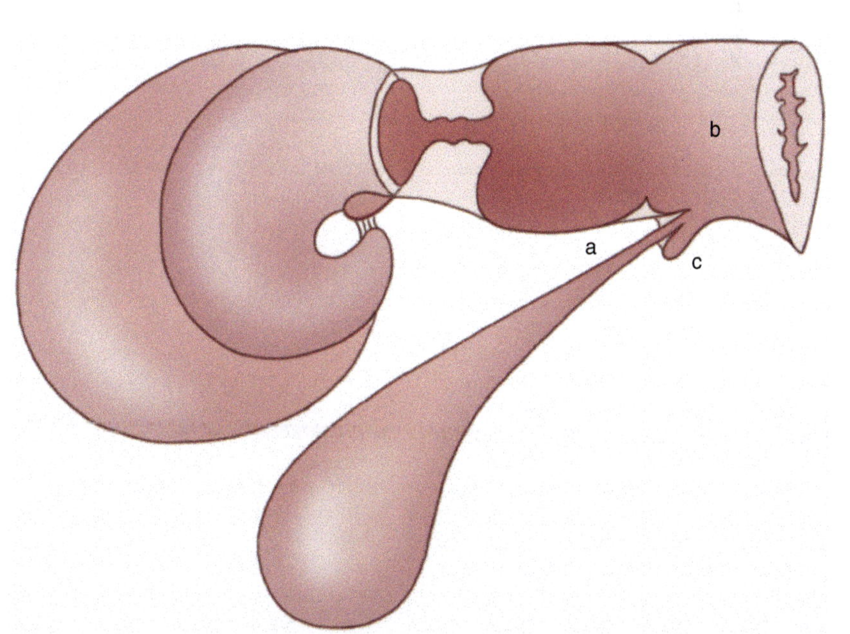

Fig. 13-1 Lateral view of the urethra (*a*), vagina (*b*), and suburethral diverticulum (*c*) in adult female cattle as viewed from the left. A finger is inserted into the suburethral diverticulum on the ventral aspect to direct the tip of the catheter over the diverticulum and into the external urethral orifice. (Reprinted with permission from Rosenberger G. *Clinical examination of cattle*. Berlin: Parey; 1979; 453.)

stranguria, and potential catheter extrusion. The incidence of urinary tract infection with indwelling Foley catheters in dairy cows is 3% per catheterized day;[2] the urine should therefore be periodically examined for evidence of cystitis and antimicrobial treatment instituted whenever indicated. Mares can be catheterized easily, either by blindly passing a rigid catheter into the external urethral orifice or by using a finger as a guide for a flexible catheter. Long-term catheterization of the bladder of the mare requires a similar technique to that described for cows.

Male horses can also be catheterized easily if the penis is relaxed. When urethral obstruction is present, the penis is usually relaxed, but administration of an ataractic drug (acepromazine is often used) makes manipulation of the penis easier and often results in its complete relaxation. Because of the long urethra, the catheter must be well lubricated. The catheter should be rigid enough to pass through the long urethra but flexible enough to pass around the ischial arch. In all species, catheterization overcomes the natural defense mechanisms that prevent infectious organisms from ascending the urinary tract. As a result, attention to hygiene during catheterization is essential.

TESTS OF URINE SAMPLES

Urinalysis is an essential component of the examination of the urinary system. The reader is referred to a textbook of veterinary clinical pathology for details of the biochemical and microscopic examination of the urine. Cytologic examination of urine should take place as soon after collection as possible because casts (cylindrically shaped molds that indicate tubular injury) are fragile and can rapidly disintegrate. The common abnormalities of urine are discussed later.

The urine sample should be centrifuged; the supernatant should be used for laboratory analysis and the sediment and remaining supernatant for routine urine analysis.

Specific Gravity

Specific gravity of urine is the simplest test to measure the capacity of renal tubules to conserve fluid and excrete solute. For most species, the normal specific gravity range is 1.015 to 1.035, and in azotemic animals, specific gravity should be greater than 1.020 if the azotemia is prerenal in origin. In chronic renal disease the urine specific gravity decreases to 1.008 to 1.012 and is not appreciably altered by either deprivation of water for 24 hours or the administration of large quantities of water by stomach tube. It is important to recognize that a specific gravity of less than 1.008 indicates that the kidney can produce dilute urine and, if sustained, indicates better renal function than a fixed urine specific gravity of 1.008 to 1.012.

Specific gravity can be inaccurate when other refractive particles are present in urine, such as glucose or protein. Urine specific gravity should therefore be used with caution in animals with proteinuria or glucosuria. As an alternative to specific gravity, osmolality of a fluid directly measures the concentration of solute in the fluid. Urine osmolality therefore provides a more accurate assessment of the tubule's ability to conserve or excrete solute than urine specific gravity and is the preferred test of urine concentrating ability for research studies. However, urine specific gravity is sufficiently accurate for clinical use in animals without proteinuria or glucosuria, because there is a linear relationship between urine specific gravity and osmolality and urine specific gravity explains 52% of the variation in urine osmolality. The 95% confidence interval for predicting osmolality from the specific gravity measurement is ±157 mOsmol/kg.

pH

The pH of urine can be measured using pH papers calibrated in 0.2 to 0.3 pH units or urine dipstick point-of-care tests that are calibrated in 0.5 pH units. The physiologic range of urine pH is 4.5 to 9.0, with herbivore urine typically being between 7.0 and 8.5. Cattle on high-grain diets may have slight aciduria (pH 6.0–7.0), and ruminants and horses ingesting an acidogenic diet will have aciduria, with urine pH as low as 5.0. Urine pH on free-catch samples is typically 0.1 to 0.2 pH units lower than anaerobically collected samples; the difference is most likely caused by the loss of CO_2 from urine during voided, which is accompanied by an increase in pH. It is for this reason that some research studies collect urine using a Foley catheter into a glass jar with mineral oil on the surface. For clinical use, it is sufficient to completely fill a screw top container with urine and minimize the air at the top of the container before urine pH is measured.

An interesting and consistent finding is that aciduria is always accompanied by increased urine excretion of calcium. Low luminal pH in the distal convoluted tubule and connecting tubule decreases the number of epithelial Ca channels (transient receptor potential vanilloid member 5 [TRPV5]); the TRPV5 channel is considered to be the primary gatekeeper of active calcium reabsorption in the distal region of the urinary tract. Low luminal pH also decreases the pore size of the TRPV5 channel, resulting in decreased calcium uptake from the tubular lumen into the epithelial cell. The low luminal pH-induced decrease in TRPV5 number and activity result in decreased calcium absorption in the distal convoluted tubule and connecting tubule, directly resulting in hypercalciuria.

Net Acid Excretion

The kidney plays a central role in acid-base homeostasis by adjusting urine electrolyte excretion to maintain constant blood pH. Measurement of urinary net acid excretion (NAE) provides a sensitive and clinically useful method for evaluating acid-base balance. This is because NAE provides an estimate of endogenous acid production and the magnitude of dietary acidification when an acidogenic diet is fed. The term NAE is commonly used in studies of renal physiology in humans, other omnivores, and carnivores, in which urine pH is typically acidic, compared with plasma pH in a healthy animal (7.40). The term net base excretion (NBE) is more appropriate in cattle and other herbivores because urine pH is usually alkaline. It should be recognized that NBE = −NAE, with both measured in milliequivalents per liter.[3]

Urinary NAE is the most sensitive index of acid-base status and is clinically underutilized. The Jørgensen method is often used to measure NAE and involves laboratory titration of urine to a standardized endpoint in which the temperature is 37°C, P_{CO_2} is 0 mm Hg, and pH is 7.40 (equivalent to plasma pH in a clinically normal animal). The method involves acidification of the urine sample to pH <4.0 to convert all HCO_3^- to CO_2 and dissolve the phosphate sediment, heating to a boil, cooling, and alkalinization back to pH 7.40 to determine measured titratable acidity (TA).[3] Measured TA is defined as the number of milliequivalents of OH^- (as NaOH) that must be added to a bicarbonate-free urine sample to increase the pH to 7.40. Formaldehyde is then added to the urine sample (which decreases the urine pH to below 7.40) and the sample titrated with NaOH back to pH 7.40 to determine the ammonium concentration ($[NH_4^+]$). NAE is then calculated as NAE = TA + $[NH_4^+]$. Accurate results are obtained with the Jørgensen method if urine is anaerobically stored at −20°C for up to 30 days and thawed at room temperature (20°C) for 2 hours, or anaerobically stored at 4°C for <3 days.

NAE for healthy pasture-fed or silage-fed cattle is usually less than −210 to −90 mEq/L, but is usually expressed as the negative of NAE, which is called NBE, where NBE = −NAE (i.e., NBE is usually +90 to +210 mEq/L). Mean NAE for grain-fed cattle with subclinical rumen acidosis (mean rumen pH 5.8–6.0) ranged from +80 to +140 mEq/L (i.e., NBE = −80 to −140 mEq/L). Urine pH and −NAE are related in herbivores, where $pH \approx 6.1 + \log_{10}(NBE + [NH_4^+])$, with NBE expressed in mEq/L and the urine ammonium ion concentration ($[NH_4^+]$) expressed in mEq/L (Fig. 13-2).[3]

Hematuria

Hematuria can be from prerenal causes when vascular damage occurs, such as trauma to the kidney, septicemia, and purpura hemorrhagica. Renal causes include acute glomerulonephritis, renal infarction, embolism of the renal artery, tubular damage from toxic insult, and pyelonephritis. Postrenal

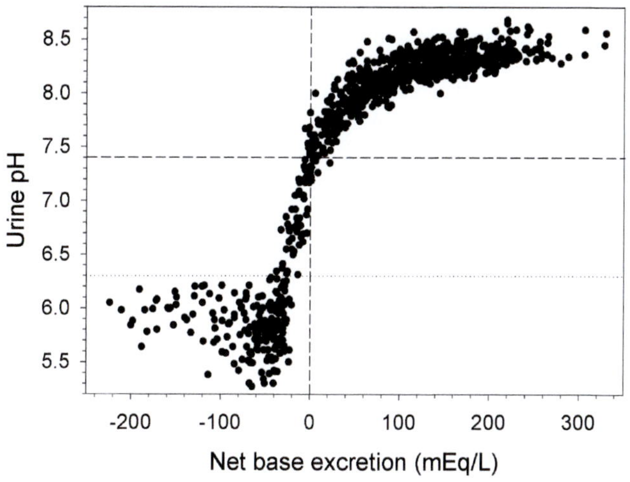

Fig. 13-2 Relationship between urine pH and net base excretion (equivalent to the negative value for net acid excretion) for cows fed diets of different dietary cation-anion difference. The dashed lines indicate that net base excretion = 0 mEq/L (by definition) when pH 7.40. Notice that urine pH is poorly associated with net base excretion at pH <6.3 (dotted line); at this urine pH renal ammonium ion concentration ($[NH_4^+]$) becomes markedly increased. (Reproduced with permission from Constable PD, Gelfert CC, Fürll M et al. *Am J Vet Res* 2009; 70(7):915-925.)

hematuria occurs particularly in urolithiasis and cystitis. A special instance of hematuria is enzootic hematuria of cattle when hemorrhage originates from tumors of the urinary bladder. In affected cattle, the strength of the urine dipstick reaction for blood is associated with the number and severity of tumor nodules (hemangiomas).[4] Hematomas of the bladder wall (cystic hematoma) cause hematuria in neonatal foals.[5] Treatment of foals with cystic hematoma can include medical and surgical approaches based on the degree of urinary tract obstruction and other signs.

Typically, lesions of the kidney, bladder, and proximal urethra cause hemorrhage throughout or toward the end of urination, whereas lesions of the middle and distal urethra are responsible for bleeding at the beginning of urination. In severe cases of hematuria, blood may be voided as grossly visible clots, but more often hematuria causes a deep red to brown coloration of the urine. Less severe cases may show only cloudiness that settles to form a red deposit on standing. The hematuria may be so slight that it is detectable only on microscopic examination of the sediment from a centrifuged urine sample. In females, free-flow urine samples may be contaminated by blood from the reproductive tract, and it may be necessary to collect a sample by urethral catheterization to avoid the chance of contamination of the urine occurring in the vagina.

Blood in urine is always positive on biochemical tests for hemoglobin and myoglobin. Because red blood cells can be lysed in dilute urine, red-colored urine should be examined microscopically for the presence of erythrocytes. The presence of a heavy brown deposit is not sufficient for a diagnosis of hematuria, because this may also occur in hemoglobinuria. If the bladder or urethra is involved in the process that causes hematuria, abnormalities may be detectable on physical examination.

Gross hematuria persisting for long periods may result in severe blood loss anemia. Severe urinary tract hemorrhage of undetermined origin in aged mares has been recorded. The syndrome is widely recognized, although not well documented, in Arabian mares. Endoscopic examination reveals hemorrhage in one ureter, but ultrasonographic examination of the kidneys does not reveal any significant abnormalities. Surgical removal of the affected kidney is not recommended, because the hemorrhage sometimes recurs in the remaining kidney. Treatment is nonspecific. Severe hematuria can also occur in horses with pyelonephritis.

Hemoglobinuria

False hemoglobinuria can be seen in hematuria when erythrocytes are lysed and release their hemoglobin. In this case erythrocytes can be detected only by microscopically examining urine sediment for cellular debris.

True hemoglobinuria causes a deep red to brown coloration of urine and gives a positive reaction to biochemical tests for hemoglobin. There is no erythrocyte debris in sediment. Dipstick tests for proteinuria may not be positive unless the concentration of hemoglobin is very high. There are many causes of intravascular hemolysis, which is the source of hemoglobinuria. The specific causes are listed later.

Normally, hemoglobin liberated from circulating erythrocytes is converted to bile pigments in the cells of the reticuloendothelial system. If hemolysis exceeds the capacity of this system to remove the hemoglobin, it accumulates in the blood until it exceeds a certain renal threshold and then passes into the urine. Some hemoglobin is reabsorbed from the glomerular filtrate by the tubular epithelium but probably not in sufficient amounts to appreciably affect the hemoglobin content of the urine. Hemoglobinuria will only be present when the plasma concentration exceeds the renal threshold. Consequently, hemoglobin is grossly visible in plasma by the time hemoglobinuria is visible. Hemoglobin precipitates to form casts in the tubules, especially if the urine is acidic, resulting in some plugging of tubules, but the chief cause of uremia in hemolytic anemia is ischemic tubular nephrosis.

Myoglobinuria

The presence of myoglobin (myohemoglobin) in the urine is evidence of severe muscle damage. The only notable occurrence in animals is azoturia of horses. Myoglobinuria is not common in enzootic muscular dystrophy, possibly because there is insufficient myoglobin in the muscles of young animals. The myoglobin molecule (molecular weight 16,500 g) is much smaller than hemoglobin (molecular weight 64,000 g) and passes the glomerulus much more readily, so a detectable dark brown staining of the urine occurs without very high plasma levels of myoglobin. There is no detectable discoloration of the serum as seen in hemoglobinemia. Inherited congenital porphyria is the other disease that causes a red-brown discoloration of urine. In porphyria, the plasma is also normal in color, but it is differentiated from myoglobinuria based on a negative reaction to the guaiac test and the characteristic spectrograph. The porphyrins in inherited congenital porphyria are the only pigments that fluoresce under ultraviolet light.

The presence and type of pigment in the urine can be determined accurately by spectrographic examination, but this is rarely clinically available. Myoglobinuria is usually accompanied by clinical signs and clinical biochemistry abnormalities of acute myopathy, and clinical differentiation of myoglobinuria from hemoglobinuria is usually made on the basis of the clinical signs and serum biochemical findings, including measurement of muscle-derived enzymes such as creatine kinase. As with hemoglobin, myoglobin can precipitate in tubules and may contribute to uremia.

Ketonuria

Ketonuria is a common finding in sick ruminants and is seen in starvation; acetonemia of lactating dairy cattle; and pregnancy toxemia of ewes, does, and beef cattle. A small amount of ketonuria is normally present in dairy cows in early lactation. As a result, it is important that the assay method used to demonstrate ketonuria is appropriate for urine, because there may be a risk for false-positive reactions on some tests. The standard test is **sodium nitroprusside**, which turns an intense purple color in the presence of **acetoacetate**, one of the three keto acids.

Glucosuria

Glucosuria occurs in acute tubular nephrosis as a result of failure of tubular resorption, and is one of the most sensitive indices for the presence of a proximal tubule. Glucosuria is occasionally detected in severely ill ruminants, particularly those with abomasal volvulus or a small intestinal obstruction. Glucosuria in combination with ketonuria occurs only in diabetes mellitus, an extremely rare disease in ruminants. Glucosuria might be seen in ruminants in association with enterotoxemia caused by *Clostridium perfringens* type D and can occur after parenteral treatment with dextrose solutions, adrenocorticotropic hormones, or glucocorticoid analogs. Horses with tumor of the pars intermedia of the pituitary gland often have glucosuria.

Glucose is freely filtered by the glomerulus and reabsorbed from the filtrate in the proximal tubules, with the renal threshold approximating 150 mg/dL in horses and cattle. Glucosuria in the face of a normal serum glucose concentration therefore indicates the presence of abnormal proximal tubular function. Glucosuria occurs early in the development of aminoglycoside-induced proximal tubule nephropathy and provides a useful inexpensive and practical screening test for nephrotoxicity in animals without hyperglycemia.

Proteinuria

Proteinuria can be prerenal, renal, or postrenal in origin, and it is clinically helpful to identify the anatomic source of protein loss. **Prerenal proteinuria** is caused by an abnormal plasma content of proteins that traverse glomerular capillary walls, and the proteins have normal permselectivity properties (such as hemoglobin, myoglobin, and immunoglobulin light chains). **Renal proteinuria** is caused by abnormal renal handling of normal plasma proteins and is functional or pathologic. **Functional renal proteinuria** is mild and transient as a result of altered renal physiology during or in response to a transient phenomenon, such as high-intensity exercise or fever. **Pathologic renal proteinuria** is caused by structural or functional lesions within the kidney, regardless of their magnitude or duration. There are three subcategories of pathologic renal proteinuria: glomerular, which is caused by lesions altering the permselectivity properties of the glomerular capillary wall; tubular, which is caused by lesions that impair tubular recovery of plasma proteins that ordinarily traverse glomerular capillary walls that have normal permselectivity properties (typically low molecular weight proteins); and interstitial, which is caused by inflammatory lesions or disease processes (such as acute interstitial nephritis) that result in exudation of proteins from the peritubular capillaries into the urine. **Postrenal proteinuria** is caused by entry of protein into the urine after it enters the renal pelvis and is urinary or extraurinary. **Urinary postrenal proteinuria** is caused by the entry of proteins derived from hemorrhagic or exudative processes affecting the renal pelvis, ureter, urinary bladder, and urethra. **Extraurinary postrenal proteinuria** is caused by entry of proteins derived from the genital tract or external genitalia during voiding or in the process of collecting urine for analysis.

Constituents in glomerular filtrate depend on the size, shape, and charge of the filtered particles, with most plasma constituents (such as electrolytes and glucose) readily filtered by the glomerulus; consequently, glomerular filtrate concentrations are usually similar to that of plasma. Proteins with molecular (formula) weights less than 60 kilodaltons (kDa = 60,000 g) pass through the glomerulus to some extent, but albumin (molecular weight 65 kDa) is usually not present in glomerular filtrate. Hemoglobin and myoglobin are small pigmented proteins (17 kDa) that are freely filtered and present in the glomerular filtrate; ultimately they are visible as hemoglobinuria or myoglobinuria. **Tamm-Horsfall protein** is a glycoprotein produced by tubular cells in the loop of Henle. The urine concentration of Tamm-Horsfall protein is usually low but may be increased in inflammatory diseases of the kidney, and the glycoprotein can be incorporated into urinary casts.

Normal urine contains only small amounts of protein that are insufficient to be detected using standard dipstick tests. It should be noted that the highly alkaline urine produced by herbivores always produces a false-positive reaction (trace or 1+) for protein on urine dipstick tests. Prerenal proteinuria may be detected using standard dipstick tests in animals with hemoglobinuria and myoglobinuria, because both compounds are proteins. Functional renal proteinuria is observed in normal foals, calves, kids, and lambs in the first 40 hours after they receive colostrum. Pathologic renal or postrenal proteinuria and hematuria may be present when urinary tract infections are present. Postparturient cows usually have protein present in a free-catch urine sample as a result of washout of uterine fluids that are expelled during urination or traces remain in the caudal vagina; this is a classic example of extraurinary postrenal proteinuria. Demonstration that proteinuria originates in the kidney is easier if abnormal elements that form in the kidney, such as tubular casts, are also present in the urine, or morphologic abnormalities of the kidneys are palpable per rectum or identified ultrasonographically.

Proteinuria is most accurately quantified by determining the amount of protein passed in a 24-hour period, but this is impractical in clinical cases. Proteinuria is more easily quantified by indexing the protein concentration to creatinine concentration in a single urine sample; this has been shown to provide an accurate representation of 24-hour protein loss in the urine.

Chronic pathologic renal proteinuria may cause hypoproteinemia as in chronic glomerulonephritis and acute tubular nephrosis in horses and in amyloidosis of cattle. When proteinuria originates from pyelonephritis or cystitis, other clinical and clinicopathologic evidence of these diseases is usually present.

Urine protein concentrations in animals without lower urinary tract disease or hematuria are normally much lower than serum protein concentrations and similar to cerebrospinal fluid (CSF) protein concentration. Glomerular filtrate normally contains low concentrations of low molecular weight proteins such as β_2-microglobulin (molecular weight 11,800 g) and lysozyme (molecular weight 14,400 g). This is because the healthy glomerulus excludes high molecular weight proteins such as albumin (molecular weight, 65,000 g) and globulins from the glomerular filtrate; normally functioning proximal tubules reabsorb these low molecular weight proteins, leading to very low urine protein concentrations. Alterations in tubular function can therefore lead to proteinuria, but typically glomerular injury produces much larger increases in urine protein concentration than those produced by altered proximal tubule function. A transient and marked proteinuria is reported in foals for the first 2 days of life after ingestion of colostrum; the proteinuria is attributed to the presence of low molecular weight proteins in colostrum that, after active absorption by small intestinal epithelial cells, end up in the glomerular filtrate.

Determination of urine protein concentrations requires a sensitive analytical test, such as the Coomassie brilliant blue method. Urinary protein concentrations may be indexed to the urine creatinine concentration to account for denominator effects of changes in urine volume. Dividing the urinary protein concentration (mg/dL) by the creatinine concentration (mg/dL) produces a unitless ratio, which provides a sensitive and reliable diagnostic method for the detection and quantification of proteinuria and is well correlated with 24-hour protein excretion in urine samples without evidence of blood.

The normal urinary protein to creatinine ratio in the horse appears to be less than 1.0,[6] and small increases in the ratio (from 0.1–0.4) are observed in horses during the developmental stage of experimentally induced laminitis in horses.[7] In animals with massive proteinuria, a urinary protein to creatinine concentration ratio of less than 13 is considered to be more indicative of tubular than glomerular proteinuria. Generally, increased urinary concentrations of albumin and β_2-microglobulin indicate **glomerular proteinuria** and **tubular proteinuria,** respectively. Proteinuria is massive and sustained in cattle and sheep with advanced renal amyloidosis and animals with advanced glomerulonephritis (glomerular proteinuria) but is mild in animals without glomerular disease but with proximal tubular injury (tubular proteinuria). Microalbuminuria does not appear to have been evaluated as an early and sensitive test of glomerular disease in large animals, but increases in urine albumin concentration would be expected in animals with glomerular disease.

Casts

Casts are organized, tubular structures that vary in appearance depending on their composition. They occur only when the kidney is involved in the disease process. Casts are present as an indication of inflammatory or degenerative changes in the kidney, where they form by agglomeration of desquamated cells and **Tamm–Horsfall proteins**. Casts may not form in all cases of renal disease. In addition, casts readily dissolve in alkaline urine and are best detected in fresh urine samples.

Cells and Pyuria

Leukocytes, erythrocytes, and epithelial cells in urine may originate in any part of the urinary tract. Leukocytes or pus in urine (pyuria) indicates inflammatory exudation at some point in the urinary tract, usually the renal pelvis or bladder. Pyuria may occur as grossly visible clots or shreds, but is often detectable only by microscopic examination of urine sediment. Individual cells and leukocytic casts may be present. Pyuria is usually accompanied by the presence of bacteria in urine.

Bacteriuria

Diagnosis of a urinary tract infection is based on finding a clinically relevant bacteriuria in urine collected by free catch (midstream collection into a sterile container), catheterization, or cystocentesis. In horses and adult cattle, collection of urine is limited to free catch and transurethral catheterization of the bladder, because the size of the animal and intrapelvic position of the bladder prevents cystocentesis. In contrast, cystocentesis can be performed under ultrasonographic guidance in calves, small ruminants, and pigs. When culturing a urine sample obtained by catheterization, the first 20 mL or so should be discarded because of the potential for contamination from vaginal or distal urethral flora.

Marked bacteriuria suggestive of bacterial infection is usually defined as more than 30,000 colony forming units (cfu)/mL from free-catch specimens (some laboratories use 10,000 or 100,000 cfu/mL), and more than 1000 cfu/mL from catheterized specimens. It is important to quantify the number of bacteria in urine samples, because the number of cfus is usually associated with disease severity in animals with bacterial cystitis or pyelonephritis. For example, 13% of urine samples obtained directly from the bladder of slaughtered male and female cattle using a sterile needle and syringe were positive for bacteria associated with urinary tract infection in cattle; however, gross or histologic evidence of infection was not identified in any animal.[8]

Rapid detection of urinary tract infection can be accomplished using the Uriscreen test, which is a solution of 10% H_2O_2 and a coloring agent. It provides a low-cost point-of-care test that detects catalase activity in a fluid sample placed in a tube by the development of a ring of foam within the tube within 2 minutes. The Uriscreen test has been used successfully to identify bacteriuria in septic calves[9] and has the potential for wider use in the detection of bacteriuria in other large animals.

Crystalluria

Crystalluria should not be overinterpreted in farm animals. Crystals in the urine of herbivorous animals have no special significance unless they occur in very large numbers and are associated with clinical signs of irritation of the urinary tract. Calcium carbonate and triple phosphate crystals are common in normal urine. If they occur in large numbers, it may suggest that the urine is concentrated and indicate the possible future development of urolithiasis. The presence of calcium carbonate crystals in the peritoneal fluid of a neonatal foal has been used to confirm a diagnosis of ruptured bladder.

The ventral aspect of the equine bladder may contain a calcium carbonate–rich sediment (called **sabulous material**), especially when horses are fed alfalfa hay. This sediment is observed toward the end of urination when the bladder is fully contracted, as evidenced by a change in urine clarity from clear to opaque.

Enzymuria

A clinically useful index of proximal tubular injury is determining the γ-glutamyl transferase (GGT) activity in urine.[10] Most enzymes present in serum and plasma have a molecular weight greater than that of albumin (i.e., >65,000 g) and are normally not detectable in the glomerular filtrate; the presence of high molecular weight enzymes in urine such as GGT (molecular weight 330,000 g) is called **parenchymatous enzymuria**. For comparison, the presence of low molecular weight enzymes (such as lysozyme) in urine is called **tubular enzymuria** because damage to the proximal tubule impairs its ability to reabsorb enzymes from the glomerular filtrate.

Most of the GGT activity in urine originates from the luminal brush border of the proximal tubular epithelial cells of the kidney. High levels of GGT activity in the urine result from an increase in the rate of proximal tubular epithelial cell destruction, and GGT is released into the urine during the active phase of tissue destruction; an increase in urine GGT activity therefore reflects parenchymatous enzymuria. The activity of GGT (or other high molecular weight enzymes such as β-*N*-acetylglucosaminidase, β-glucuronidase, and *N*-acetyl-β-glucosaminidase [NAD]) in urine can therefore be used to detect the presence of proximal renal tubular epithelial cell damage before the onset of renal dysfunction. GGT is the preferred enzyme for identifying the presence of parenchymatous enzymuria, because the assay is inexpensive and widely available and the kidney has the highest content of GGT of any organ in the body, increasing the sensitivity of the test.

Urine GGT activity is frequently indexed to an indicator of urine concentration, such as urine creatinine concentration, to correct for denominator effects induced by changes in urine volume, and a GGT to creatinine ratio higher than 25 IU/g creatinine is considered abnormal in the horse. However, it may be more appropriate to calculate the fractional clearance of GGT (which compares the extent of tubular damage with the amount of functioning kidney mass) instead of the urinary GGT to creatinine ratio (which compares the amount of tubular damage with muscle mass). Indexing serum/plasma GGT activity to serum/plasma creatinine concentration is not physiologically valid, because enzymes present in urine are not normally filtered through the glomerulus; using the urine GGT activity alone therefore appears to be more appropriate. Interestingly, urine GGT activity appears more sensitive as an index of tubular injury than the urine GGT to creatinine ratio in horses and sheep and appears to be the most sensitive indicator of tubular injury in animals treated with aminoglycosides.

Other enzymes, such as alkaline phosphatase, lactate dehydrogenase, NAD, matrix metalloproteinase (gelatinases localized to renal tubules, such as MMP-2), and membrane-associated carbonic anhydrase VI[11] have been examined in urine as potential indicators of tubular injury.[12] None of these enzymes have consistently proven superior to urine GGT activity in detecting tubular injury, and a systematic review of acute renal injury in humans identified urine GGT activity (indexed to urine creatinine concentration) as the preferred test.

TESTS OF SERUM

These tests depend on either the accumulation, in cases of renal insufficiency, of metabolites normally excreted by the kidney or the excretion of endogenous substances by the kidney.

Serum Urea Nitrogen and Creatinine Concentration

Determination of SUN and creatinine concentration is an essential component of any evaluation of the urinary system. These serum indices of function are simple estimates of glomerular filtration because urea and creatinine are freely filtered by the glomerulus. Serum concentrations of urea and creatinine do not rise appreciably above the normal range until 60% to 75% of nephrons are destroyed.

Serum urea and creatinine concentrations are influenced by blood flow to the kidneys and may be increased in prerenal uremia. They also suffer from the disadvantage that their serum concentrations can vary with the rate of protein catabolism (and protein intake in the case of serum urea concentration) and are not dependent only on renal function. In cattle, for example, serum urea concentrations caused by prerenal lesions may be higher than those resulting from renal disease, because salivary secretion of urea, rumen metabolism of urea, and decreased feed intake (and therefore decreased protein intake) may lower serum urea concentration in chronic disease. Urea is usually expressed in terms of urea nitrogen, but the term blood urea nitrogen (BUN) should no longer be used when analysis is performed on serum (SUN). The units for urea are reported as mg/dL or mmol/L and different when expressed in terms of urea nitrogen or urea, and are most commonly expressed as urea nitrogen, where 1 mg/dL = 0.357 mmol/L.

Creatinine in herbivores is essentially totally derived from endogenous creatine. Creatine is produced by the liver from amino acids and circulates in the plasma before being taken up by skeletal muscle, in which it stores energy in the form of phosphocreatine. Creatine is converted to creatinine by a nonenzymatic irreversible process and is distributed throughout the body water. Creatinine is therefore released from skeletal muscle at a constant rate in animals without myonecrosis and is therefore an indirect index of muscle mass; this is the reason why serum creatinine concentrations are highest in intact males, intermediate in adult females, and lowest in neonates and cachectic animals. Serum creatinine concentrations are constant within an animal because they reflect muscle mass, which does not change rapidly; an increase in serum creatinine concentration of more than 0.3 g/dL should be considered to be clinically significant. The units for creatinine are reported as mg/dL or μmol/L, where 1 mg/dL = 88.4 μmol/L.

Serum creatinine concentration is routinely measured using the Jaffe reaction, in which a colored product is formed from creatinine and picrate in an alkaline solution. However, the alkaline picrate reaction has poor specificity, because it also detects a number of noncreatinine chromogens in serum, which do not appear to be present in urine. In other words, the creatinine concentration may be overestimated in serum but is accurately measured in urine. The former induces some error in the calculation of fractional clearance of electrolytes. The progression of renal failure may be monitored by plotting the reciprocal of serum creatinine concentration against time. Extrapolation of the resultant linear relationship to the *x*-axis intercept provided some clinically useful prognostic information in a horse with advanced renal failure.

Glomerular Filtration Rate

The accepted gold standard measurement for renal function is measurement of the glomerular filtration rate using **inulin clearance**. Inulin, a metabolically inert carbohydrate, crosses freely across the glomerulus and is neither absorbed nor secreted by renal tubules. **Endogenous creatinine clearance** has also been used to estimate glomerular filtration rate; however, this test suffers from inaccuracies related to the presence of noncreatinine chromogens in plasma and the tubular secretion of creatinine in some species. **Exogenous creatinine clearance** minimizes the errors induced by noncreatinine chromogens in plasma but requires the IV injection of creatinine and is therefore complicated and expensive. Although the renal clearances of inulin or creatinine are the preferred research methods for measuring renal excretory function, these techniques are impractical in clinical patients and male ruminants because they require urethral catheterization, rinsing and removal of the bladder contents, and timed urine collections.

Renal excretory function is more practically assessed in clinical patients by measuring the **plasma clearance** of water-soluble, nonmetabolized compounds of exogenous origin that have low plasma protein binding (such as **iohexol**, **iodixanol**, **phenolsulfonphthalein,** or **sodium sulfanilate**), because these techniques do not require urine collection. A practical test to determine glomerular filtration rate is the IV injection of the radiologic contrast agent iohexol at 150 mg/kg, followed by collection of serum samples at 3 and 4 hours, or 4 and 6 hours, postinjection. An alternative test protocol used in calves is the IV injection of the radiologic contrast agent iodixanol at 40 mg/kg, followed by collection of serum samples at 1, 2, and 3 hours postinjection.[13] Plasma clearance of technetium-diethyleneaminopentaacetic acid or technetium-mercaptoacetyltriglycine has also been evaluated in horses, but the technique requires measurement by a gamma camera and is therefore not suitable for use in the field. Plasma clearance tests have been evaluated in cattle, goats, sheep, and horses and provide a useful clinical test to monitor renal function in an individual animal over time, particularly iohexol clearance. Iohexol has become the most popular of these tests because iohexol is freely filtered at the glomerulus, neither secreted nor absorbed by the kidneys, has a low degree of protein binding, and is not toxic, but is widely available, relatively inexpensive, and easily assayed.[14] However, the accuracy of plasma clearance techniques of exogenously administered compounds may not be sufficiently adequate for research studies.

TESTS OF URINE AND SERUM

Urine Osmolality to Serum Osmolality Ratio

A urine to plasma osmolality ratio of 1 indicates isoosmotic clearance of materials by the kidney. A ratio less than 1 indicates that the kidneys are diluting the urine, and a ratio more than 1 indicates that the urine is being concentrated. Because the plasma osmolality is much more constant than urine osmolality, the important clinical factor is whether urine osmolality is less than, equal to, or greater than, 300 mOsm/kg. Measurement of urine osmolality requires a dedicated laboratory unit and is rarely indicated in the clinical management of renal disease because of the widespread availability of handheld refractometers; measurement of urine osmolality is needed only in research studies.

Water Deprivation Test

This can be used to assess renal concentrating ability in animals that have isosthenuria with urine specific gravity of 1.008 to 1.012 but do not have azotemia. Water deprivation tests should not be performed on animals that are already azotemic and should be undertaken with extreme caution and frequent (hourly to every 2 hours) monitoring in animals that are polyuric but not azotemic. Animals that are unable to conserve water because of renal disease can rapidly become dehydrated and develop prerenal uremia as a result.

In brief, the water deprivation test monitors the animal's ability to detect an increase in serum osmolality, release ADH, and produce a concentrated urine as a result of the action of ADH on the kidney. The test usually requires documentation that the animal has polyuria and polydipsia, with water consumption greater than cohorts of the same age, lactation stage, and diet, when housed under the same conditions. Before conducting the water deprivation test, the animal is weighed and a Foley catheter is placed in the bladder (females), or the animal is housed in a dry stall (males). Access to water is prevented and the urine and serum are tested every 1 to 2 hours or when voided in males. The test should be stopped when the urine specific gravity increases to more than 1.015 to 1.020, when there is an increase in serum/plasma creatinine concentration of 0.3 g/dL or greater, or when there has been a decrease in BW of 5% or more.

Animals that concentrate their urine after water deprivation are diagnosed with **psychogenic polydipsia** and their water availability is gradually decreased. Animals that fail to concentrate their urine after water deprivation are diagnosed with diabetes insipidus; **nephrogenic diabetes insipidus** can be ruled out if the animal produces concentrated urine within a few hours of an intramuscular (IM) injection of exogenous vasopressin (0.15–0.30 U/kg BW). In the latter case, the diagnosis is **neurogenic diabetes insipidus** as a result of inadequate release of ADH. Such cases are extremely rare in large animals and have been attributed to pituitary neoplasia (particularly pituitary adenoma in horses) or encephalitis. Determination of plasma vasopressin concentrations using a radioimmunoassay may assist in differentiation of nephrogenic from neurogenic diabetes insipidus; in the former the plasma vasopressin concentration increases during the water deprivation test. However, because the assay for plasma vasopressin concentration is not widely available and has not been validated for all large animals, the response to exogenous vasopressin is the preferred clinical test for differentiating nephrogenic from neurogenic diabetes insipidus. Two related horses have been diagnosed with nephrogenic diabetes insipidus, suggesting that this may be inherited as an X-linked disorder.

Water deprivation tests are not needed if urine specific gravity is below 1.008, because the presence of hyposthenuria indicates that tubular function is acting to conserve solute and produce dilute urine. In other words, a specific gravity below 1.008 is a better clinical sign than a constant specific gravity of 1.008 to 1.012, because a low specific gravity indicates the presence of some tubular function. Low specific gravity may occur in diabetes insipidus, following excessive water intake or fluid administration, or following diuretic administration. Neonatal animals on fluid diets and dairy cows in early lactation often produce dilute urine.

Renal Clearance Studies

In animals with renal disease, serum/plasma creatinine and urea nitrogen concentrations are insensitive indicators of renal dysfunction and exceed the upper limit of the reference range only after extensive loss of nephron function. Increases in serum concentrations of creatinine or urea nitrogen cannot be used to distinguish between prerenal, renal, and postrenal azotemia. Urine specific gravity can be used to differentiate prerenal from renal azotemia. However, results of urinalysis do not reflect the magnitude of the disease and they are not specific for specific renal disease.

Calculation of renal clearance of creatinine, urea nitrogen, and electrolytes, along with measurement of specific enzyme activity in the urine, is a more sensitive indicator of damage to the tubules than serum biochemical analysis. Urinary diagnostic indices have been used to evaluate renal function and to detect and estimate the extent of renal damage in agricultural animals. For example, it can be clinically useful to determine the urine to serum concentration, the ratio of urinary creatinine to urea nitrogen, the renal clearance of creatinine and urea nitrogen, the urine to serum osmolality ratio, the urine protein concentration or urine protein to creatinine ratio, the fractional clearances of electrolytes, and urine enzyme activity. Early diagnosis of renal injury facilitates initiation of appropriate treatment and reduces the incidence of irreversible renal failure. Sequential measurement of these indices can aid in the determination of prognosis and allows monitoring and evaluation of the extent of recovery of renal function.

The tests require simultaneous sampling of blood and urine. Samples can also be collected daily for several days and weekly to determine any age-related changes. Analytical methods can have a large impact on measured values for urinary electrolytes. Urine samples need to be acidified (usually with HCl) to accurately measure urine calcium concentration[15]; however, this can be problematic if measurement of urine chloride concentration is required. Accurate measurement of urine sodium and potassium concentrations using ion-selective potentiometry requires at least 20-fold dilution to minimize salt type binding in urine. Occasionally such dilution is not sufficient to provide accurate potassium measurements because of the formation of zwitterion complexes. Accurate measurement of urine chloride concentration by ion-selective potentiometry because the electrode used is also sensitive to bicarbonate concentration, which is abundant in herbivore urine. As a consequence, urine chloride concentrations measured by potentiometry should be assumed to be an undermeasurement when performed in alkaline urine.

Fractional Clearance

The fractional clearance from plasma of a given substance is calculated by comparing the amount of the substance excreted in the urine with the amount filtered through the glomerulus. The formula used to calculate fractional clearance of substance X (FC_X) is

$$FC_X(\%) = ([U_X]/[S_X]) \times 100/([U_{creatinine}]/[S_{creatinine}])$$

where $[U_X]$ and $[S_X]$ are the urine and serum (or plasma) concentrations of X, respectively, and $[U_{creatinine}]$ and $[S_{creatinine}]$ are the urine and serum (or plasma) concentrations of creatinine, respectively. The fractional clearance provides information regarding the action of tubular transport mechanisms on the filtered substances; a value below 100% indicates net reabsorption, whereas a ratio above 100% indicates net secretion. Fractional clearance has been erroneously called fractional excretion; the latter term is confusing, inappropriate, and has no scientific basis.

Sodium and inorganic phosphate are reabsorbed from the glomerular filtrate by the renal tubules; therefore, the fractional clearance of sodium and phosphate provide clinically useful indices of tubular function and both can be accurately measured. Sodium retention is an important proximal tubular function, and the fractional clearance of Na is usually less than 1% for animals (and often <0.2%) unless they have a high oral or IV sodium intake, when fractional clearance values can be increased to 4%. Renal phosphorus excretion is affected by acid-base status and body calcium and phosphate status and is therefore a less specific indicator of tubular function than fractional clearance of sodium. Values for the fractional clearance of phosphorus normally vary from 0.1% to 0.4%, although higher values may be seen in ruminants with high phosphate intakes. Typically, tubular function can be adequately characterized by determining the fractional clearance of sodium alone, or sodium and phosphorus; the fractional clearance of chloride rarely adds useful information in clinical cases because it is highly correlated to the fractional clearance of sodium, and determination of the fractional clearance of potassium is hampered by methodologic limitations associated with zwitterion formation in urine. Determination of the fractional clearance of calcium can be useful when dietary intake and metabolism of calcium are evaluated. Substantial variations in fractional clearance values are present in horses over a 24-hour period as a result of the electrolyte load ingested with feed. Some standardization of the time of urine collection in relation to feeding is therefore needed in research studies but is clearly impractical in clinical cases.

Fractional clearance values for a number of electrolytes have been determined for horses, foals, cattle, and sheep. The urinary excretion of endogenous substances and other urinary diagnostic indices of renal function have been measured in healthy neonatal foals. The urine volume of neonatal foals is proportionately greater than that of calves, and the normal neonatal foal produces dilute urine. Compared with normal values in adult horses, fractional clearance of electrolytes was similar for sodium but higher for potassium, phosphorus, and calcium. Renal function in newborn calves is similar to adult cattle within 2 to 3 days of birth, and calves can excrete large load volumes in response to water overload and conserve water in response to water deprivation as efficiently as adult cattle.

Animals with acute renal azotemia have a low urinary creatinine to serum creatinine and urine nitrogen to serum nitrogen; animals with acute prerenal azotemia have a normal to high urinary creatinine to serum creatinine ratio and urinary nitrogen to serum nitrogen ratio. However, animals with acute renal azotemia also have a low urine specific gravity relative to the serum creatinine concentration, and it remains to be determined whether measurement of urinary creatinine and urea concentrations and serum urea concentrations provide any more information in clinical cases than that provided by urine specific gravity and serum creatinine concentration.

Summary of Renal Function Tests

In summary, the serum (or plasma) creatinine or urea nitrogen concentration provides a useful screening test for the presence of urinary tract disease, with an increase in serum creatinine concentration of 0.3 mg/dL or more over baseline providing a useful clinical test for the presence of nephrotoxicosis in normally hydrated animals treated with potentially nephrotoxic agents. Azotemia can be prerenal, renal, or postrenal in origin; the cause is most practically differentiated in azotemic animals by measuring the specific gravity of urine before any treatment has been administered. In animals suspected of having urinary tract disease, the urinary protein concentration and protein to creatinine ratio provide clinically useful indices of glomerular and tubular function and injury, the urine specific gravity and fractional clearance of sodium and phosphorus provide clinically useful indices of tubular function in animals not on IV or oral fluids and consuming a normal diet, and determination of urine GGT activity and analysis of urine for the presence of casts provide clinically useful and sensitive indices of tubular injury. The results of most other laboratory tests rarely provide additional information in an animal suspected to have urinary tract disease and are not currently recommended for routine clinical use. A summary table for indices of renal function in the horse is presented in Table 13-1.

Table 13-1 Indices of renal function in healthy adult horses and foals less than 30 days of age

Factor	Adult	Foal <30 days of age
Serum urea nitrogen (mg/dL)	12–25	4–15
Serum creatinine (mg/dL)	0.8–2.2	0.7–1.2
Urine specific gravity	>1.020	<1.008
Urine osmolality (mOsm/kg)	700–1500	<250
Fractional clearance sodium (%)	0.01–1.0	0.01–0.2
Fractional clearance phosphorus (%)	0.0–0.5	0.5–5.0
Urine pH	7.0–9.0	5.5–7.0
Urine production ([mL/kg BW]/h)	0.7–1.5	4.0–8.0

Adapted from Toribio RE. Vet Clin North Am Equine Pract *2007; 23:533.*

DIAGNOSTIC EXAMINATION TECHNIQUES

Ultrasonography

Transcutaneous and transrectal ultrasonography is commonly used to detect and characterize anatomic abnormalities of the kidneys, ureters, bladder, and urethra in horses, cattle, and small ruminants. Ultrasonography is an effective screening test for diagnosing obstructive conditions of the urinary tract, including hydronephrosis, hydroureter, and bladder distension and can be used to visualize the kidney and guide the biopsy needle during renal biopsy. Removal of the hair coat and the use of an ultrasonographic coupling gel assist in obtaining acceptable acoustic coupling, whereas saturation of a foal's hair coat with alcohol or coupling gel may be adequate when clipping is not desirable. Ultrasonography should be performed before endoscopy, because the latter introduces air into the bladder and urethra, which interferes markedly with ultrasonographic images.

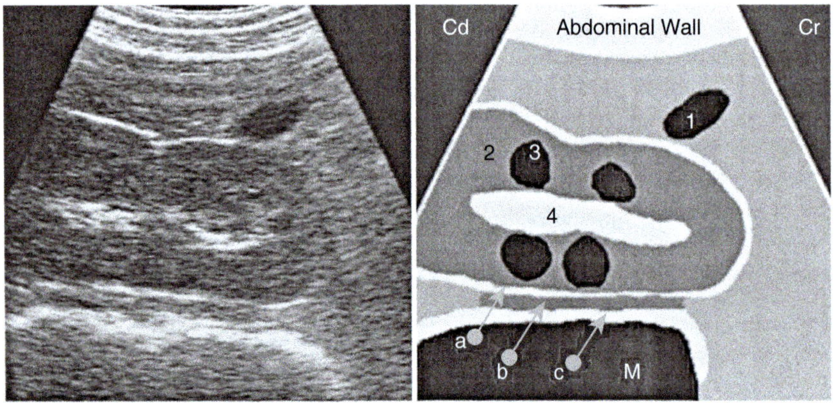

Fig. 13-3 Ultrasonographic image (*left*) and drawing (*right*) that illustrates a bovine left kidney imaged from the right paralumbar fossa obtained by placing the transducer parallel to the longitudinal axis of the cow just below the transverse processes of the lumbar vertebrae 3 to 5. The kidney is moved toward the right paralumbar fossa by palpation per rectum. *1,* caudal vena cava; *2,* renal cortex; *3,* medullary pyramid; *4,* renal sinus; *a,* hyperechoic line representing the perirenal fat; *b,* hypoechoic line representing the medial wall of the rumen; *c,* hyperechoic line (internal reverberation artifact) reflecting from the tissue-gas interphase superimposed on the image of the medial wall of the rumen; *Cr,* cranial; *Cd,* caudal; *M,* medial. (Reproduced with permission from Imran S, Sharma S. *Veterinarni Medicina* 2014; 59:29-32.)

Techniques for ultrasonographic evaluation of the urinary system of the horse have been described,[16] and extensive information is available that documents age-related changes in renal dimensions. Generally, a 5- to 10-MHz linear probe is used transrectally to image the left kidney and a 2.5- to 3-MHz sector transducer used transcutaneously to image the right kidney in adult horses. The right kidney is easy to visualize through the dorsolateral aspect of the last two to three right intercostal spaces. The left kidney is harder to visualize transcutaneously and is usually located medial to the spleen in the paralumbar region between horizontal lines drawn from the tuber coxae and tuber ischii. A translumbar approach using a 3.5-mHz transducer has also been used for ultrasonography in adult horses.[17] Kidneys are imaged in both cross-sectional and axial planes and are usually <18 cm long. Ureteral tears have been identified using transrectal ultrasonography. Uroperitoneum is readily diagnosed in foals by ultrasonographic examination of the ventral abdomen, as is the underlying lesion in the bladder or urachus. Ultrasonography has been used to visualize the renal changes in foals following administration of phenylbutazone.

In cattle, the right kidney is easily accessible to ultrasonography from the body surface. Generally, a 5- to 10-MHz linear probe is used transrectally and a 2.5- to 3.5-MHz sector transducer used transcutaneously in adult cattle. Images of the right kidney are visualized best using a transcutaneous approach with the transducer placed in the lumbar or paralumbar region,[18] whereas images of the left kidney are best obtained using a transrectal approach. A report of a transcutaneous approach for imaging the left kidney is available (Fig. 13-3).[19] Ultrasonographic changes in the cow with pyelonephritis include a dilated renal collecting system, renal or ureteral calculi, echogenic material within the renal collecting system, and subjective enlargement of the kidney with acute disease or a small irregular kidney with chronic disease. Cattle with enzootic bovine hematuria caused by chronic bracken fern ingestion have a thickened bladder wall (normally <2 mm) on transrectal ultrasonography and irregular sessile masses (transitional cell papilloma) extending into the bladder lumen. A complete description of the ultrasonographic examination of the bovine urinary tract is available.[20]

Techniques for ultrasonographic evaluation of the urinary system of the sheep and more recently the goat[21] have been described using a 5-MHz linear transducer. Kidneys were most easily detected from the 12th intercostal space on the right side and dorsal right flank. The right kidney was 8.0 ± 0.7 cm long (mean ± SD) and the left kidney was 8.4 ± 0.6 cm long. The bladder was 5.1 ± 1.4 cm in length, and the largest cross-sectional diameter was 2.6 ± 1.1 cm. The ureters could not be identified, but the urethra could be identified in most goats as echogenic lines with no visible lumen.

Endoscopy

Transurethral endoscopy can be easily performed in mares, stallions, geldings, and cows to examine the urethra and bladder and flow of urine from both ureters. Horses and cows are sedated and adequately restrained for the procedure, using a flexible endoscope of 12 mm or less outer diameter and a minimum length of 1 m for stallions and geldings. The tail of female horses and cattle should be bandaged or held out of the way and the perineal region cleaned with dilute povidone iodine or chlorhexidine to minimize urinary tract contamination. The endoscope should be disinfected using a glutaraldehyde-based product, including the accessory channel, and rinsed with sterile water.

The endoscope should pass easily along the urethra into the bladder. Air insufflation of the bladder is needed for adequate visualization. Biopsy of diseased tissue or mechanical disruption of calculi can be attempted under endoscopic guidance. Identification of an ectopic ureter may be assisted by IM administration of azosulfamide (2 mg/kg BW, provides a red color) or IV administration of sodium fluorescein (10 mg/kg BW, provides a green color), phenolsulfonphthalein (1 mg/kg BW, provides a red color), or indigo carmine (0.25 mg/kg BW, provides a purple blue color) to color the urine being produced, 5 to 20 minutes before endoscopy, which assists visualization of the urine stream. The ureters are identified at 10 and 2 o'clock and empty periodically in spurts; separate urine samples can be collected from each ureter to evaluate left and right kidney function.

Venous embolism has been reported during urinary tract endoscopy of a standing gelding.[22] Routine sedation and endoscopic procedures were used with the bladder and urethra distended to 20 mm Hg. The horse collapsed 30 minutes after the start of the procedure, exhibiting ataxia, generalized muscle twitching, and horizontal nystagmus. The horse recovered after an additional 30 minutes, and ultrasonographic examination the next day revealed the presence of gas in both ureters and the renal pelvis of both kidneys. Venous air embolism is reportedly more likely to occur in humans when the operative site is more than 5 cm above the right atrium, which was the case in this gelding.

Renal Biopsy

Percutaneous renal biopsy can be performed in sedated and adequately restrained cows and horses. A coagulation profile should be run before renal biopsy is attempted in animals with severe and chronic renal disease or those animals suspected to have a coagulopathy. Renal biopsy is contraindicated in animals with documented pyelonephritis because of the risk of perirenal abscessation after the biopsy procedure.

The left kidney is usually biopsied because it is more accessible. In cows, the left kidney is moved to the right paralumbar fossa and fixed in position by rectal manipulation. In horses, the left kidney is identified using transabdominal ultrasonography and fixed in position by palpation per rectum. The skin over the biopsy site is aseptically prepared and 5 to 10 mL of local anesthetic is infiltrated along the proposed track for the biopsy needle. A small stab incision is made in the skin with a scalpel, and a renal biopsy sample is collected by introducing a biopsy needle through the abdominal wall and manipulating it into the caudal pole of the kidney. The depth of insertion is typically 3 cm for the right kidney and approximately 7 cm for the left kidney (depth is more variable). The renal biopsy is fixed in 10% formalin and submitted for examination and histologic diagnosis. Biopsy of the caudal pole is thought to minimize the risk of trauma to the renal pelvis, renal artery, and renal vein, but a biopsy location effect has not been demonstrated in large animals. Laparoscopic biopsy of the kidneys, with or without the development of pneumoperitoneum, with the horse in a standing position has been reported.[23] Clear advantages of laparoscopic biopsy over an ultrasound-guided percutaneous biopsy method have not been identified.

Possible complications of renal biopsy are hemorrhage and bowel penetration in all animals and abscessation in animals with pyelonephritis. Hemorrhage after renal biopsy can be extensive, is usually perirenal, and can be life-threatening, with fatality rates reported of 2.1% (1/48)[24] in cattle using laparoscopic biopsy, 0% (0/82) in cattle using nonultrasound-guided biopsy[25] and 0% (0/25) in cattle using percutaneous ultrasound-guided biopsy of the right kidney,[18] and 0.7% (1/151)[26] in horses using percutaneous biopsy. These fatality rates should be compared with a fatality rate of 0.2% in humans undergoing renal biopsy. Occasionally, severe hematuria is present for hours after the biopsy procedure but usually resolves within a few days. Because of the potential for life-threatening sequelae, renal biopsy should only be performed when the etiology is uncertain and histologic examination will direct treatment or when an early and accurate prognosis is desired. In animals with acute tubular injury, electron microscopic examination of the basement membrane is required to provide an accurate prognosis on return to normal function.

Test of Uroperitoneum and Bladder Rupture

Ultrasonographic examination of the abdomen is most useful in detecting the presence of excessive fluid, and this examination frequently allows visualization of the lesion in the bladder or urachus. Further testing is sometimes needed to confirm that the fluid is urine. Generally, in uroperitoneum, substantial quantities of fluid can be easily obtained by abdominocentesis. Warming the fluid may facilitate detection of the urine odor, although this is a subjective and poorly sensitive diagnostic test. If there is doubt that the fluid is urine, its creatinine concentration can be compared with that in serum. If creatinine in the fluid is at least twice the serum value, the fluid is confirmed as urine, although ruptured bladder should be suspected whenever the abdominal fluid creatinine concentration exceeds that of serum. In animals with uroabdomen or suspected to have uroabdomen, the administration of 30 mL of sterile 1% methylene blue into the bladder via a urethral catheter or cystocentesis has been used to confirm that the bladder is the site of urine leakage. Abdominal paracentesis is performed some minutes after administration and the fluid examined visually for the presence of a blue tinge. Absence of a blue color suggests the presence of ureteral or renal rupture.

Radiography

Radiographic examination has limited value for the diagnosis of urinary tract disease in farm animals with the potential exception of radiolucent particles in the bladder of ruminants with urolithiasis. Contrast studies may be used to examine the lower urinary tract in neonatal animals. With the widespread availability of ultrasonography and endoscopy, the indications for radiography have become more limited. A positive-contrast urethrogram was of value in diagnosing urethral recess dilatation in a bull calf, and IV urography was successful in diagnosing a dilated ureter in a 4-month-old heifer calf. Historically, excretory urography, positive contrast cystography, and urethrography have been used, particularly in foals, but these tests are expensive, not widely available, and time-consuming. Radiography is currently being performed on animals with equivocal results using other cheaper, faster, and more widely available tests such as ultrasonography.

Cystometry and Urethral Pressure Profile

Urodynamic tests in the mare permit comparison of the normal micturition reflex with that of the incontinent patient. **Cystometry** involves measurement of luminal pressure during inflation of the bladder with measured volumes of 0.9% NaCl or carbon dioxide. The pressure–volume relationship during filling with fluid or gas provides information on bladder capacity, maximal luminal pressure during the detrusor reflex, and stiffness of the bladder wall. The **urethral pressure profile** involves measurement of pressure along the urethra while withdrawing a fluid-filled or gas-filled catheter at constant rate. The catheter tip pressure is graphed against distance, and the **maximum urethral closure pressure** is determined as the maximum urethral pressure minus bladder luminal pressure. The **functional urethral length** is defined as the length of the urethra in which urethral pressure exceeds bladder luminal pressure.

The test can be performed in restrained mares with or without xylazine sedation (1.1 mg/kg BW, intravenously), but sedation is recommended. Values for cystometry and urethral pressure profiles in female horses and pony mares are available.

Computed Tomography

Computed tomography (CT) is considered the method of choice in human medicine for the imaging diagnosis of pyelonephritis, renal tumors, and renal trauma. CT urography is also the preferred technique for evaluating urinary tract disorders in humans.[27] Consequently, there is interest in applying CT to urinary tract diseases of large animals, such as obstructive urolithiasis in goats and sheep. A CT study of 28 healthy female Saanen goats indicated that CT was a useful imaging modality that provided visualization of the kidneys, ureters, and urinary bladder.[27] The clinical utility of CT in obstructive urethral conditions of large animals remains to be determined.

Principles of Treatment of Urinary Tract Disease

Fluid and Electrolytes

Treatment of acute renal failure in all species is aimed at removing the primary cause and restoring normal fluid balance by correcting dehydration, acid-base disorders, and electrolyte abnormalities. The prognosis for acute renal failure will depend on the initiating cause and severity of the lesion. If the acute disease process can be stopped, the animal may be able to survive on its remaining functional renal tissue. When toxic nephrosis is suspected, an attempt should be made to identify and remove the initiating cause or to move the animal from the suspect environment.

Ruminants with chronic renal failure typically have mild to marked **hyponatremia** and **hypochloremia**; the serum calcium and potassium concentrations may be decreased because of inappetence, serum magnesium concentration may be normal or increased, and serum phosphate concentration may be normal or increased, because urine provides a route of excretion of magnesium and phosphorus. The acid-base status is characterized by acidemia and **metabolic acidosis** in severely affected cases to metabolic alkalosis in mildly affected cases. Ruminants with acute renal failure have similar clinicopathologic changes, although the serum phosphorus concentration is usually markedly elevated in acute renal failure, because many cases are initiated by decreased renal blood flow.

Horses with acute or chronic renal failure have similar electrolyte changes to those in ruminants, with the marked difference being the presence of **hypercalcemia** and **hypophosphatemia** in some horses. Hypercalcemia in horses with renal disease is attributed to poorly regulated intestinal calcium absorption, with urine being the predominant route of calcium excretion. Decreases in the function of nephrons in the horse will therefore decrease the urinary loss of calcium and result in hypercalcemia. The hypercalcemia is marked and is thought to result directly in hypophosphatemia in horses with renal failure.

Balanced electrolyte solutions or isotonic (0.9% NaCl) saline supplemented with potassium (if hyperkalemia is not present) and calcium (if hypercalcemia is not present) can be used to correct fluid and electrolyte deficits. The required volume of replacement fluid can be determined on the basis of clinical signs as outlined in Chapter 5. As the fluid deficit is corrected, the patient should be observed for urination. The healthy horse produces 15 to 30 mL urine/kg BW each day, which is equivalent to 7.5 to 15.0 L/day for a 500-kg horse. If anuria or oliguria is present, the rate of fluid administration should be monitored to prevent overhydration. If the patient has anuria or oliguria after the fluid volume deficit is corrected, a diuretic should be administered to help restore urine flow. **Furosemide** (1–2 mg/kg BW IV or IM every 2–6 hours) or **mannitol** (0.25–2.0 g/kg BW in a 20% solution administered IV over 15–20 minutes) may be used, but furosemide is preferred because of its much lower cost and ease of administration. Mannitol administration has not been proven to be effective in humans and is no longer recommended for treatment of oliguric acute renal failure in humans. Diuretics should not be used until dehydration has been corrected and furosemide administration should be used with caution in horses with acute renal failure caused by aminoglycoside toxicity, because furosemide may augment the nephrotoxicity. After urine flow is restored, the resulting diuresis will increase the maintenance fluid requirement. **B vitamins** should be frequently administered because their rate of loss in the urine is anticipated to be higher than normal in animals with renal failure.

Animals nonresponsive to fluid loading and diuretics could be administered low-dose ("renal dose") **dopamine** as a continuous IV infusion (3–5 µg/kg BW/min) with dopamine diluted in 0.9% NaCl, 5% dextrose, or lactated Ringer's solution. Dopamine is an α_1, β_1, β_2, DA_1, and DA_2 agonist and therefore has a complex pharmacodynamic profile that is dependent on species, organ, and cardiovascular status. Dopamine is theoretically the preferred pharmacologic agent to selectively increase renal blood flow and therefore glomerular filtration rate in animals with renal failure, although low-dose dopamine infusion does not alter creatinine clearance (an index of glomerular filtration rate) in healthy adult horses and has not been shown to be of benefit in treating renal failure in humans. Dopamine acts primarily as an inotropic agent at low doses (<5 µg/kg BW/min) and primarily as a vasopressor at higher doses. The mean arterial blood pressure and electrocardiogram should therefore be monitored during dopamine administration to ensure that dopamine infusion does not lead to hypertension or clinically significant cardiac arrhythmias. Although there are good theoretical grounds for use of dopamine in animals with renal failure, this is no longer the practice in human medicine because of the lack of efficacy of the drug in preventing or treating acute renal failure. Fenoldopam mesylate, a dopamine-1 receptor agonist, at 0.04 µg/kg BW/min may have a role in the treatment of anuria and oliguria in sick foals, because this rate of infusion increased urine output without altering systemic hemodynamics and cardiac output in healthy foals.[27] IV infusion of norepinephrine (0.1 µg/kg BW/min), with or without dobutamine (5 µg/kg BW/min), does not alter urine output, endogenous creatinine clearance, or fractional clearance of electrolytes in neonatal foals,[28] suggesting minimal therapeutic effects in foals with anuria or oliguria. Animals that remain anuric after IV fluid administration of furosemide/mannitol and dopamine have a grave prognosis and can only be managed with peritoneal dialysis or hemodialysis.

Intermittent-flow peritoneal dialysis has been used successfully in a foal with a ruptured urinary bladder. A urinary catheter was placed in the bladder and secured to the perineal region. An area of the ventral midline was clipped and prepared for aseptic surgery. Local anesthetic was infused, and a stab incision was made in the skin with a scalpel blade. An 11-French peritoneal dialysis catheter was placed in the stab incision then forced into the abdomen. The rigid stylet was removed, the catheter was secured to the skin, and the stab incision site was bandaged. Peritoneal fluid was allowed to drain; dialysis was then accomplished by infusing 2 L of a hypertonic dialysis solution, clamping the catheter for 1 hour, then opening the catheter and allowing drainage to occur for 2 to 3 hours. Dialysis was repeated 9 times over a 36-hour period. Intermittent-flow peritoneal dialysis has also been used in 4 adult horses with acute renal failure using a similar catheterization technique (24-French de Pezzer or 28-French catheter secured using a purse-string suture followed by a Chinese finger trap suture pattern) and periodic infusion of 10 to 15 L of warmed, sterile, acetated Ringer's or lactated Ringer's solution.[29] The fluid was left for 0.5 to 1 hour and then allowed to drain back into the fluid bag from which it was delivered. Not all of the infused fluid is usually recovered; attachment of a Heimlich valve to the catheter for several hours permits drainage of additional fluid.

Continuous-flow peritoneal dialysis has been used successfully in an adult horse with azotemia refractory to IV fluids, furosemide, dopamine infusion, and intermittent-flow peritoneal dialysis. A 28-French indwelling thoracic tube was placed in the ventral abdomen and a 2.2-mm diameter, 15-cm long spiral fenestrated catheter was placed in the left flank via peritoneoscopy to allow for inflow of dialysate (Fig. 13-4).[30] Acetated Ringer's with 1.5% glucose was continuously infused through the catheter in the left flank at approximately 3 L/h, with abdominal fluid collected into a sterile closed collection system from the catheter in the ventral midline of the abdomen. The quantity of intraabdominal fluid was controlled by positioning the collection bags relative to the level of the withers to maintain a constant and modest intraperitoneal pressure.

Hemodialysis (renal replacement therapy) has been used successfully to treat a foal with presumed oxytetracycline nephrotoxicosis. Venovenous hemodialysis was performed under isoflurane anesthesia after surgical placement of a Teflon/Silastic arteriovenous shunt in the median artery and vein using a dialysis delivery system, a hollow-fiber artificial kidney, and acetate-base dialysate. Anticoagulation during dialysis was accomplished with a loading dose of heparin (100 U/kg BW IV) and then hourly boluses of 20 U/kg BW or a continuous rate infusion of 50 IU/kg each hour to prolong the activated clotting time. Three dialysis treatments, lasting 4 to 6 hours, were administered over a 4-day period, resulting in a marked reduction in azotemia. The safety and efficacy of venovenous hemodialysis has been investigated in five adult horses.[31] Renal replacement therapy is more efficient than intermittent or continuous-flow peritoneal dialysis and requires shorter treatment intervals but does require vascular access, anticoagulation treatment, sterile filters and tubing, a peristaltic pump, and potentially a method for warming the fluids to core body temperature immediately before IV infusion.

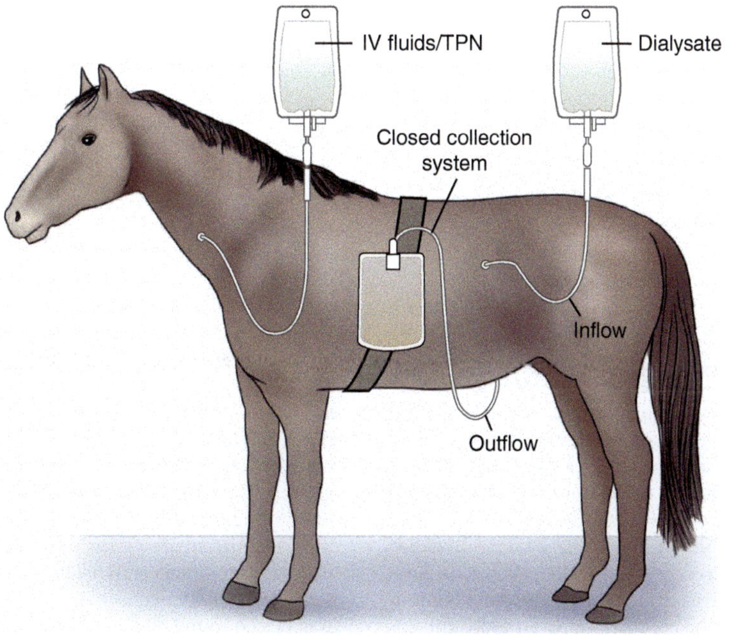

Fig. 13-4 Drawing of the system for continuous-flow peritoneal dialysis in an adult horse. *TPN*, total parenteral nutrition. (Reproduced with permission from Gallatin LL et al. *J Am Vet Med Assoc* 2005; 226:756-759.)

The treatment of chronic renal failure will depend on the stage of disease and the value of the animal. In chronic failure, therapy is aimed at prolonging life. In food-producing animals, emergency slaughter is not recommended because the carcass is usually unsuitable for human consumption. Animals in chronic failure should have free access to water and salt, unless edema is present. Stresses such as sudden environmental and dietary changes should be avoided. The ration should be high in energy-giving food and properly balanced for protein. Acute renal failure may occur in patients in chronic failure and can be treated like other cases of acute renal failure.

Antimicrobial Agents

Selection of antimicrobial agents for the treatment of urinary tract infections should be based on quantitative urine culture of a catheterized urine sample. A clinically relevant bacterial concentration indicative of cystitis or pyelonephritis is 1000 cfu/mL or 30,000 cfu/mL of urine from a catheterized or midstream free-catch sample, respectively.

The ideal antimicrobial for treatment of urinary tract infections should meet several criteria. It should

- **Be active against the causal bacteria**
- **Be excreted and concentrated in the kidney and urine**
- **Be active at the pH of urine**
- **Have low toxicity, particularly nephrotoxicity**
- **Be easily administered**
- **Be low in cost**
- **Have no harmful interactions with other concurrently administered drugs**

Appropriate first-line antimicrobials include penicillin, ampicillin, amoxicillin, ceftiofur, and cefquinome in ruminants and trimethoprim-sulfonamides and ceftiofur in horses. Antimicrobial therapy for lower urinary tract infections should continue for at least 7 days; for upper urinary tract infections 2 to 4 weeks of treatment is often necessary. Success of therapy can be evaluated by repeating the urine culture 7 to 10 days after the last treatment.

Manipulation of urine pH should be considered as part of the treatment of bacterial urinary tract infections. Generally, *Escherichia coli* attach best to urinary epithelial cells at pH 6.0, whereas *Corynebacterium renale* attaches best in alkaline urine. In other words, when treating an *E. coli* pyelonephritis or cystitis, the diet should be altered to ensure an alkaline urine pH. Likewise, urine pH should be acidic when treating urinary tract infections caused by *C. renale*.

FURTHER READING

Anon. European urinalysis guidelines. *Scand J Clin Lab Invest*. 2000;60:1-96.

Geor RJ. Acute renal failure in horses. *Vet Clin North Am Equine Pract*. 2007;23:577-591.

McKenzie EC. Polyuria and polydipsia in horses. *Vet Clin North Am Equine Pract*. 2007;23:641-653.

Menzies-Gow N. Diagnostic endoscopy of the urinary tract of the horse. *In Pract.* 2007;29:208-213.

Mueller K. Urinary tract disease in cattle. *UK Vet.* 2007;12:1-10.

Savage CJ. Urinary clinical pathologic findings and glomerular filtration rate in the horse. *Vet Clin North Am Equine Pract.* 2008;24:387-404.

Schott HC. Chronic renal failure in horses. *Vet Clin North Am Equine Pract.* 2007;23:593-612.

Schumacher J. Hematuria and pigmenturia of horses. *Vet Clin North Am Equine Pract.* 2007;23:655-675.

Toribio RE. Essentials of equine renal and urinary tract physiology. *Vet Clin North Am Equine Pract.* 2007;23:533-561.

Wilson ME. Examination of the urinary tract in the horse. *Vet Clin North Am Equine Pract.* 2007;23: 563-575.

REFERENCES

1. Montgomery JB, et al. *Can Vet J.* 2009;50:751.
2. Tamura T, et al. *J Vet Med Sci.* 2014;76:819.
3. Constable PD, et al. *Am J Vet Res.* 2009;70:915.
4. Pavelski M, et al. *Semina Ciências Agrárias, Londrina.* 2014;35:1369.
5. Arnold CE, et al. *J Am Vet Med Assoc.* 2005;227:778.
6. Uberti B, et al. *Am J Vet Res.* 2009;70:1551.
7. Uberti B, et al. *Am J Vet Res.* 2010;71:1462.
8. Hajikolaei MRH, et al. *Comp Clin Pathol.* 2015;24: 251.
9. Raboisson D, et al. *J Vet Intern Med.* 2010;24:1532.
10. Mathur S, et al. *Toxicol Sci.* 2001;60:385.
11. Nishita T, et al. *Vet J.* 2014;202:378.
12. Raekallio MR, et al. *Am J Vet Res.* 2010;71:1246.
13. Imai K, et al. *Vet J.* 2012;193:174.
14. Wilson KE, et al. *Am J Vet Res.* 2009;70:1545.
15. O'Connor CI, Nielsen BD. *J Anim Vet Adv.* 2006;5:165.
16. Diaz OS, et al. *Vet Radiol Ultrasound.* 2007;48:560.
17. Habershon-Butcher J, et al. *Vet Radiol Ultrasound.* 2014;55:323.
18. Mohamed T, Oikawa S. *J Vet Med Sci.* 2008;70:175.
19. Imran S, Sharma S. *Vet Med (Praha).* 2014;59:29.
20. Floeck M. *Vet Clin North Am Food Anim Pract.* 2009;25:651.
21. Steininger K, Braun U. *Schweiz Arch Tierheilkd.* 2012;154:67.
22. Romagnoli N, et al. *Equine Vet Ed.* 2014;26:134.
23. Kassem MM, et al. *Int J Morphol.* 2014;32:1234.
24. Braun U, et al. *Schweiz Arch Tierheilkd.* 2011;153: 321.
25. Chiesa OA, et al. *Can J Vet Res.* 2006;70:87.
26. Tyner GA, et al. *J Vet Intern Med.* 2011;25:532.
27. Hollis AR, et al. *J Vet Intern Med.* 2006;20:595.
28. Hollis AR, et al. *J Vet Intern Med.* 2006;20:1437.
29. Han JH, McKenzie HC. *Equine Vet Educ.* 2008;20:256.
30. Gallatin LL, et al. *J Am Vet Med Assoc.* 2005;226:756.
31. Wong DM, et al. *J Vet Intern Med.* 2013;27:308-316.

Diseases of the Kidney

GLOMERULONEPHRITIS

Glomerulonephritis can occur as a primary disease or as a component of diseases affecting several body systems, such as equine infectious anemia and chronic swine fever. In primary glomerulonephritis, the disease involves only the kidney, predominantly affecting the glomeruli, although the inflammatory process extends to affect the surrounding interstitial tissue and blood vessels. Primary and secondary glomerulonephritis are rare causes of clinical disease in farm animals. The disease is sometimes associated with other chronic, systemic illness such as in cows with Johne's disease, bovine virus diarrhea, fascioliasis,[1] or leptospirosis; pigs with hog cholera or African swine fever; and horses with equine infectious anemia. Proliferative glomerulonephritis is reported as an incidental finding in normal sheep, cattle, goats, and pigs. Clinical disease from glomerulonephritis is rare in these species but has been reported in cattle and as a congenital condition in sheep, as described later. Proliferative glomerulonephritis can cause chronic renal failure in horses. Glomerulonephritis is present is animals with amyloidosis, which is a generalized deposition of antibody–antigen complexes. Amyloidosis is discussed in detail in Chapter 11.

The immune system plays a major role in the pathogenesis of glomerular lesions. Glomerular injury can be initiated by an immune response in which antibodies are directed against intrinsic glomerular antigens or by foreign antigens planted in the glomerulus. Alternatively, and more commonly, circulating antigen–antibody complexes may be deposited in the glomerulus. As the complexes accumulate, they stimulate an inflammatory response that damages the glomerular filtration system. Inflammatory damage to the glomerulus alters the selective permeability of the filtration system allowing plasma protein, particularly albumin, to pass into the glomerular filtrate. In horses, the glomerular lesion is thought to be caused by the deposition of circulating antigen–antibody complexes, but the origin of these complexes is unknown. Infections with streptococci and equine infectious anemia virus may be involved but are not likely to be involved in all cases.

Glomerulonephritis is a common cause of chronic renal failure in horses. Several forms of glomerulonephritis are recognized in horses: membranous glomerulonephritis, poststreptococcal glomerulonephritis, membranoproliferative glomerulonephritis, and focal glomerulosclerosis. As discussed earlier, most are probably immune mediated and associated with circulating antibody–antigen complexes. Over 80% of horses with equine infectious anemia have glomerular lesions, and viral antigen–antibody complexes are present in the glomerular basement membrane. Purpura hemorrhagica is associated with glomerulonephritis.

The **nephrotic syndrome** is seen in some advanced cases of glomerulonephritis and is a clinical syndrome characterized by proteinuria, hypoproteinemia leading to generalized edema, and hypercholesterolemia. Nephrotic syndrome is rarely diagnosed in large animals for unknown reasons, relative to the dog and human, but is most common in cattle with advanced renal amyloidosis. Hypercholesterolemia is attributed to increased hepatic synthesis of proteins in response to chronic proteinuria, but appears to be an inconsistent finding in cattle.[1] **Dermatitis–nephropathy syndrome** is a systemic necrotizing vasculitis and glomerulonephritis syndrome of growing pigs in the UK and Canada. The cause is unknown, but an immune-mediated pathogenesis is suspected. Growing pigs are affected with a morbidity ranging from 1% to 3%. The skin is affected with a papular dermatopathy with a characteristic distribution of bluish red spots at least 1 cm in diameter beginning first in the perineal region and then extending to the pelvic limbs and along the ventral body wall to the neck and ears. In the glomeruli, there are extensive granular complement deposits with scattered immunoglobulins.

Porcine dense deposit disease, porcine membranoproliferative glomerulonephritis type II, is a common cause of early loss of newborn piglets in the Norwegian Yorkshire breed. The disease is associated with extensive complement activation caused by a deficiency of factor H, a plasma protein that regulates complement. Affected piglets are clinically normal at birth and for the first few weeks of life. Thereafter they become unthrifty and die of renal failure within 72 days of birth. In the kidneys there is extensive glomerular proliferation and marked thickening of the glomerular capillary wall. Large amounts of dense deposits are consistently found within the glomerular basement membrane. This disease is inherited with a simple autosomal recessive pattern and complete penetrance. A pathogenetic mechanism of a defective or missing complement regulation protein is hypothesized. A spontaneous glomerulonephritis of unknown etiology and unrelated to any breed has been recorded in pigs. A necrotizing glomerulonephritis is listed as occurring in pigs fed a waste product from an industrial plant producing a proteolytic enzyme. Glomerulonephritis has also been recorded in pigs in the absence of clinical illness, although an association with the "thin sow" syndrome is suggested.

In **Finnish Landrace lambs** less than 4 months of age there is an apparently inherited mesangiocapillary glomerulonephritis that is remarkably similar to forms of human glomerulonephritis. Affected lambs appear to absorb an agent from colostrum that induces an immunologic response, followed by the granular deposition of immune complexes and complement within the glomerular capillary walls; this initiates a fatal mesangiocapillary glomerulitis. Many affected lambs are asymptomatic until found dead. Some have signs of tachycardia, edema of the conjunctiva, nystagmus, walking in circles, and convulsions. The kidneys are enlarged and tender. There is severe proteinuria and low plasma albumin. SUN concentration is markedly increased with hyperphosphatemia and hypocalcemia. At necropsy the kidneys are large and pale and have multifocal pinpoint yellow and red spots throughout the cortex. On histopathologic examination, there are severe vascular lesions in the choroid plexuses and the lateral ventricles of the brain. The disease is thought to be conditioned in its occurrence by inheritance and to be limited to the Finnish Landrace breed; however, cases have also occurred in crossbred lambs.

Glomerulopathy and peripheral neuropathy in Gelbvieh calves is a familial and probably heritable disease causing illness in calves of this breed of less than 13 months of age. The initial physical abnormality is posterior ataxia that progresses to generalized paresis and recumbency. The neurologic deficits include loss of conscious proprioception and diminished or absent peripheral reflexes but maintained consciousness. Affected animals continue to eat and drink normally. Serum creatinine and urea concentrations are markedly elevated. Necropsy examination reveals neuropathy, myelopathy, and glomerulopathy. The disease is terminal.

REFERENCE

1. Murray GM, Sharpe AE. *Vet Rec.* 2009;164:179.

PYELONEPHRITIS

Pyelonephritis usually develops by ascending infection from the lower urinary tract. Clinically pyelonephritis is characterized by pyuria, hematuria, cystitis, ureteritis, and suppurative nephritis.

ETIOLOGY

Pyelonephritis may develop in a number of ways:

- Secondary to bacterial infections of the lower urinary tract
- Spread from embolic nephritis of hematologic origin such as septicemia in cattle associated with *Pseudomonas aeruginosa*
- Specific pyelonephritis associated with *C. renale, C. pilosum* (formerly *C. renale* type 2), and *C. cystitidis* (formerly *C. renale* type 3) in cattle and *C. suis* in pigs
- Secondary to anatomic abnormalities of the kidneys or distal structures permitted ascending infection of the kidney
- In association with nephroliths, although whether the nephrolith or the pyelonephritis occurred first is uncertain

PATHOGENESIS

Pyelonephritis develops when bacteria from the lower urinary tract ascend the ureters and become established in the renal pelvis and medulla. Bacteria are assisted in ascending the ureters by urine stasis and reflux of urine from the bladder. Urine stasis can occur as a result of blocking of the ureters by inflammatory swelling or debris, by pressure from the uterus in pregnant females, and by obstructive urolithiasis. Initially the renal pelvis and medulla are affected because they are relatively more hypoxic, and localized tissue hypertonicity depresses the phagocytic function of leukocytes. Infection in advanced cases may extend to the cortex. Pyelonephritis causes systemic signs of toxemia and fever and, if renal involvement is bilateral and sufficiently extensive, uremia develops. Pyelonephritis is always accompanied by pyuria and hematuria because of the inflammatory lesions of the ureters and bladder.

Pyelonephritis in cattle caused by *C. renale* used to be very common, but clinical disease has decreased markedly, with the majority of pyelonephritis cases in cattle now caused by *E. coli.* The reason for the decrease in *C. renale* isolation from clinical cases is unclear but is probably related to a change in diet toward concentrates with an associated decrease in urine pH. Other potential reasons could be the widespread use of β-lactam antibiotics and the marked decrease in urethral catheterization to obtain a urine sample in cows suspected to be ketotic. Transmission of *C. suis* in pigs may occur after mating with infected boars, because many boars carry *C. suis* in their preputial sac fluid. Field observations suggest that slight trauma at breeding, especially in small gilts, may be an important factor in transmission.

CLINICAL FINDINGS

The clinical findings in pyelonephritis vary between species. In sows there may be an initial period during which a vaginal discharge is noted, but most affected animals die without premonitory illness. Characteristically, affected pigs will lose weight and eventually become emaciated. The disease in cattle usually has a protracted course and is characterized by fever, pyuria or hematuria, and intermittent episodes of abdominal pain (see previous section Bovine Pyelonephritis).

The disease in horses is often chronic, although acute disease occurs. Gross hematuria is recognized in some horses with pyelonephritis, although this is not a common finding. Ultrasonographic examination of the kidneys can confirm the diagnosis, based on the presence of abnormally shaped kidneys with loss of the corticomedullary gradient, hypoechoic or hyperechoic abnormalities in the renal cortex, and increased echogenicity. These findings should prompt examination of the urine for leukocytes, casts, protein, and bacteria.

CLINICAL PATHOLOGY

Erythrocytes, leukocytes, and cell debris are present in the urine on microscopic examination and may be grossly evident in severe cases, particularly in horses. Quantitative urine culture is necessary to determine the causative bacteria.

NECROPSY FINDINGS

The kidney is usually enlarged, and lesions in the parenchyma are in varying stages of development. Characteristic lesions are necrosis and ulceration of the pelvis and papillae. The pelvis is usually dilated and contains clots of pus and turbid urine. Streaks of gray, necrotic material radiate out through the medulla and may extend to the cortex. Affected areas of parenchyma are necrotic and may be separated by apparently normal tissue. Healed lesions appear as contracted scar tissue. Infarction of lobules may also be present, especially in cattle. Histologically the lesions are similar to those of embolic nephritis except that there is extensive necrosis of the apices of the papillae. Necrotic, suppurative lesions are usually present in the bladder and ureters.

TREATMENT

General principles of treatment of urinary tract infections were presented earlier. A specific treatment for severe asymmetric pyelonephritis is unilateral nephrectomy, but this should only be done in nonazotemic animals. An overlooked component of treatment is alteration in urinary pH, which will affect the ability of the bacteria to attach to epithelial cells. As a generalization, *C. renale* attaches best in alkaline urine and *E. coli* attaches best in acidic urine.

DIFFERENTIAL DIAGNOSIS

The presence of pus and blood in the urine may suggest cystitis or embolic nephritis as well as pyelonephritis. It may be difficult to distinguish between these diseases, but renal enlargement or pain on rectal palpation of the kidney indicates renal involvement. Ultrasonographic changes associated with pyelonephritis include a dilated renal collecting system, renal or ureteral calculi, increased echogenicity, loss of corticomedullary echogenicity, and subjective enlargement of the kidney with acute disease or a small irregular kidney with chronic disease.[1] Parenchymal hyperechogenicity can be caused by tubular degeneration and replacement fibrosis.

REFERENCE

1. Braun U, et al. *Vet J.* 2008;175:240.

NEPHROSIS

Nephrosis includes degenerative and inflammatory lesions primarily affecting the renal tubules, particularly the proximal convoluted tubules. Nephrosis is classified into two main groups: (1) tubular injury caused by ischemic insult and (2) cell death or damage to the tubules caused by nephrotoxins (toxic agents that preferentially damage renal tubular epithelial cells). Nephrosis is the most common cause of acute kidney failure and often multiple animals are affected if there is exposure to nephrotoxins, such as plant toxicities. Uremia from nephrosis may develop acutely or may occur in the terminal stages of chronic renal disease.

ISCHEMIC NEPHROSIS

Reduced blood flow through the kidneys usually is caused by general circulatory failure. There is transitory oliguria followed by anuria and uremia if the circulatory failure is not corrected.

ETIOLOGY

Any condition that predisposes the animal to marked hypotension and release of endogenous pressor agents potentially can initiate hemodynamically mediated acute renal ischemia and renal failure. Ischemia may be acute or chronic.

Acute Renal Ischemia

- General circulatory emergencies such as shock, dehydration, acute hemorrhagic anemia, and acute heart failure; renal failure secondary to calf diarrhea has been described
- Embolism of renal artery, recorded in horses
- Extreme ruminal distension in cattle

Chronic Renal Ischemia

- Chronic circulatory insufficiency such as congestive heart failure

PATHOGENESIS

Acute ischemia of the kidneys occurs when compensatory vasoconstriction affects the renal blood vessels in response to a sudden reduction in cardiac output. As mean arterial blood pressure decreases below 60 mm Hg (the lower limit for autoregulation of renal blood flow), glomerular filtration decreases, and metabolites that are normally excreted accumulate in the bloodstream. The concentration of urea nitrogen in plasma or serum increases, giving rise to the name prerenal uremia. As glomerular filtration falls, tubular resorption increases, causing reduced urine flow. Up to a certain stage, the degenerative changes are reversible by restoration of renal blood flow, but if ischemia is severe enough and of sufficient duration, the renal damage is permanent. Proximal tubules are highly sensitive to ischemia because they are one of the energetically most active cells in the body. Acute circulatory disturbances are more likely to be followed by degenerative lesions than chronic congestive heart failure.

The parenchymatous lesions vary from tubular necrosis to diffuse cortical necrosis in which both tubules and glomeruli are affected. The nephrosis of hemoglobinuria appears to be caused by the vasoconstriction of renal vessels rather than a direct toxic effect of hemoglobin on renal tubules. Uremia in acute hemolytic anemia and in acute muscular dystrophy with myoglobinuria may be exacerbated by plugging of the tubules with casts of coagulated protein, but ischemia is also an important factor.

CLINICAL FINDINGS

Renal ischemia does not appear as a distinct disease, and its signs are masked by the clinical signs of the primary disease. Oliguria and azotemia will go unnoticed in most cases if the circulatory defect is corrected in the early stages. However, renal insufficiency may cause a poor response to treatment with transfusion or the infusion of other fluids in hemorrhagic or hemolytic anemia, in shock or dehydration. In these cases, unexplained depression or a poor response to therapy indicates that renal involvement should be investigated. The general clinical picture is one of acute renal failure and is described under uremia.

CLINICAL PATHOLOGY

Laboratory tests can be used to evaluate renal function once the circulatory condition has been corrected. Urinalysis as well as SUN and creatinine concentrations are common indices. Serum biochemistry on serially collected samples may also be used to monitor the response to therapy. On urinalysis, proteinuria is an early indication of damage to the renal parenchyma. The passage of large volumes of urine of low specific gravity after a period of oliguria is usually a good indication of a return of normal glomerular and tubular function.

NECROPSY FINDINGS

Lesions of renal ischemia are present primarily in the cortex, which is pale and swollen. There may be a distinct line of necrosis visible at the corticomedullary junction. Histologically there is necrosis of tubular epithelium and, in severe cases, of the glomeruli. In hemoglobinuria and myoglobinuria hyaline casts are present in the tubules. Severe ischemic injury can disrupt the basement membranes of the proximal tubules.

TREATMENT

Treatment must be directed at correcting fluid, electrolyte, and acid-base disturbance as soon as possible. If renal damage has occurred, supportive treatment as suggested for the treatment of acute renal failure should be instituted.

DIFFERENTIAL DIAGNOSIS

Evidence of oliguria and azotemia in the presence of circulatory failure suggests renal ischemia and the possibility of permanent renal damage. It is important to attempt to differentiate the early reversible prerenal stage from the stage in which degeneration of renal parenchyma has occurred. When ischemic renal lesions are present, urinalysis may be helpful in diagnosis, particularly if the urine is not appropriately concentrated in a dehydrated patient. After irreversible ischemic changes have occurred, it is impossible to differentiate clinically between ischemia and other primary renal diseases such as glomerulonephritis and toxic nephrosis. History and clinical signs of chronic disease will help determine whether the acute syndrome is superimposed on chronic renal disease.

TOXIC NEPHROSIS

The kidneys are particularly vulnerable to endogenous and exogenous toxins because they receive a large proportion of the total cardiac output (typically 20%) and because substances are concentrated in the kidney for excretion.

ETIOLOGY

Most cases of nephrosis are caused by the direct action of toxins, but hemodynamic changes may contribute to the pathogenesis.

Toxins

- Metals: mercury, arsenic, cadmium, selenium, and organic copper compounds; nephrosis can be reproduced experimentally in horses by the oral administration of potassium dichromate and mercuric chloride, including topical blistering agents containing mercuric chloride
- Antimicrobials, such as aminoglycosides, and overdosing with neomycin and gentamicin in the treatment of calves; treatment with tetracycline preparations accidentally contaminated by tetracycline degradation compounds and repeated daily dosing with long-acting oxytetracycline preparations may induce toxicity; treatment with sulfonamides
- Horses treated with vitamin K3 (menadione sodium bisulfite) administered by IM or IV injection
- Horses treated with vitamin D2 (ergocalciferol) and cholecalciferol (D3)
- Treatment of horses with nonsteroidal antiinflammatory drugs (NSAIDs), including phenylbutazone and flunixin meglumine; dose rates of more than 8.8 mg/kg BW of phenylbutazone per day for 4 days are likely to cause nephrosis; doses of 4.4 mg/kg BW are considered to be safe, but toxicity is enhanced by water. The usual presentation of NSAID toxicosis in horses is gastrointestinal ulceration, including right dorsal colitis
- Ketoprofen in sheep at 30 mg/kg IV, once[2]; renal toxicity may be facilitated

by concomitant activation of the alternative complement pathway
- Benzimidazole compounds used as anthelmintics; only some of them but including thiabendazole
- Monensin in ruminants
- Low-level aldrin poisoning in goats
- Highly chlorinated naphthalenes
- Oxalate in plants
- Oxalate in fungi, e.g., *Penicillium* spp. and mushrooms
- Oxalate in ethylene glycol or ascorbic acid, which is a metabolic precursor to oxalate
- Primary hyperoxaluria caused by an inherited metabolic defect in Beefmaster calves
- Tannins in the foliage of oak trees and acorns
- Unidentified toxin in *Amaranthus retroflexus* in pigs, cattle, and lambs,[2] in *Narthecium asiaticum* fed to cattle and *Isotropis forrestii* in ruminants
- Mycotoxins, such as ochratoxins and citrinins, fumonisins in ruminants
- Ingestion of *Lophyrotoma interrupta* (sawfly) larvae by cattle
- Cantharidin in horses following ingestion of dead blister beetles in alfalfa hay and hay products
- Most nonspecific endogenous or exogenous toxemias cause some degree of temporary nephrosis

PATHOGENESIS

In acute nephrosis there is obstruction to the flow of glomerular filtrate through the tubules caused by interstitial edema and intraluminal casts. If there is sufficient tubular damage, there may be back leakage of glomerular filtrate into the interstitium. There may also be a direct toxic effect on glomeruli, which decreases glomerular filtration. The combined effect is oliguria and uremia. In subacute cases, impaired tubular resorption of solutes and fluids may lead to polyuria.

CLINICAL FINDINGS

Clinical signs may not be referable to the urinary system. In peracute cases, such as those caused by vitamin K3 administered by injection, there may be colic and stranguria. In acute nephrosis there is oliguria and proteinuria with clinical signs of uremia in the terminal stages. These signs include depression, dehydration, anorexia, hypothermia, a slow or an elevated heart rate, and weak pulse. Diarrhea may be present that is sufficiently intense to cause severe clinical dehydration. In cattle there is a continuous mild hypocalcemia with signs reminiscent of that disease, which responds, in a limited way, to treatment with calcium. Cattle with advanced and severe nephrosis may exhibit a bleeding diathesis. Polyuria is present in chronic cases.

Many systemic diseases such as septicemia cause temporary tubular nephrosis. The degree of renal epithelial loss is not sufficient to cause complete renal failure and, provided the degree of renal damage is small, complete function is regained.

CLINICAL PATHOLOGY

In acute tubular nephrosis, urinalysis abnormalities are usually present before serum or plasma urea and creatinine concentrations are increased. Proteinuria, glucosuria, enzymuria, and hematuria are initial changes on urinalysis in experimental toxic nephrosis. The earliest indication of tubular epithelial damage in experimentally induced nephrosis is the detection of the proximal tubule enzyme GGT in urine. Hypoproteinemia may be present. In acute renal disease of horses, hypercalcemia and hypophosphatemia can be present, although this is not the usual finding. In the chronic stages the urine is isosthenuric and may or may not contain protein. Azotemia occurs when uremia is present. Ultrasonographically, renal changes are seen in foals receiving high daily doses of phenylbutazone.

NECROPSY FINDINGS

In acute cases the kidney is swollen and wet on the cut surface and edema, especially of perirenal tissues, may be apparent. Histologically there is necrosis and desquamation of tubular epithelium, and hyaline casts are present in the dilated tubules. In phenylbutazone poisoning the renal lesion is specifically a renal medullary necrosis. There may also be ulcers in all or any part of the alimentary tract from the mouth to the colon if phenylbutazone was administered orally.

TREATMENT

Treatment should be directed at general supportive care for acute renal disease as outlined earlier. If the toxin can be identified, it should be removed. Treatment for specific toxins may be available, as described elsewhere in the text. Hemodialysis was used successfully to treat a foal with presumed oxytetracycline nephrotoxicosis.

DIFFERENTIAL DIAGNOSIS

Clinical differentiation from acute glomerulonephritis is difficult, but clinical signs of involvement of other organs in the toxic process may be present.

- A combination of polyuria and glycosuria is an uncommon finding in large animals and is usually caused by nephrosis.
- Diabetes mellitus is rare in horses and extremely rare in ruminants.
- Cushing's syndrome (chronic hyperadrenocorticism pituitary pars intermedia dysfunction) is more common in horses and includes characteristic signs of polyuria, glycosuria, debilitation, hirsutism, polyphagia, and hyperglycemia.
- Diarrhea in terminal stages of uremia in a horse can be confused with the other causes of acute diarrhea. It requires a blood urea and creatinine estimation and a urinalysis for differentiation.

FURTHER READING

Schmitz DG. Toxins affecting the urinary system. *Vet Clin North Am Equine Pract.* 2007;23:677-690.

REFERENCES

1. Palviainen MJ, et al. *Acta Vet Scand.* 2015;57:15.
2. Kessell AE, et al. *Aust Vet J.* 2015;93:208.

RENAL TUBULAR ACIDOSIS

Renal tubular acidosis (RTA) is a rare disease of large animals that is characterized by normal glomerular function but abnormal tubular function. RTA should be suspected whenever there is a hyperchloremic strong ion (metabolic) acidosis and normal anion gap with no discernible extrarenal cause[1]; it is important to note that a common extrarenal cause of hyperchloremic strong ion acidosis is aggressive IV administration of 0.9% NaCl. This means that extreme caution needs to be exercised when attempting to diagnose RTA in sick animals receiving IV fluids.

Four major types of tubular functional defect exist in humans: (1) **nephrogenic diabetes insipidus**, in which the collection ducts do not respond to ADH (vasopressin); (2) **distal RTA (type I)**, which is a defect in the ability to secrete hydrogen ions in the distal convoluted tubules against a concentration gradient (in humans, type III is now considered a variant of type I); and (3) **proximal RTA (type II)**, which is characterized by decreased bicarbonate reabsorption in the proximal convoluted tubules. A variant of proximal RTA that does not appear to have been reported in large animals is Fanconi's syndrome, which is a genetic defect in humans related to the tubular resorption of glucose, various amino acids, urate, and phosphate. (4) **hyperkalemic distal RTA (type IV)** is caused by the resistance of distal nephron cells to aldosterone, resulting in hyperkalemia, natriuresis, and the inability to concentrate urine. Type IV RTA has not been reported in domestic animals.

Only a small number of RTA cases have been documented in horses, and these have been predominantly distal RTA (type I). Differentiating between RTA type I and type II is difficult and unreliable in horses,[1] and a report exists of a horse that may have both types.[2] The urine of humans with proximal RTA (type II) is acidic, whereas the urine of humans with distal RTA (type I) is very alkaline, regardless of the serum bicarbonate concentration, but aciduria is rarely present in herbivores suspected to have proximal RTA (type II). There is one report of RTA in a lethargic 3-month-old calf with *Salmonella enterica* serovar Agona that was more consistent with RTA type I than type II. The calf responded to IV sodium bicarbonate.[3]

Nephrogenic Diabetes Insipidus

This is a very rare condition with reports in three colts, of which two were related.[1] Clinical signs are chronic and extreme polydipsia and polyuria, poor body condition, and growth rate. Diagnosis in nonazotemic normally hydrated animals includes the inability to concentrate urine in response to IV hypertonic saline (7.5% NaCl, 1–2 mL/kg BW), which increases plasma osmolality and triggers released of ADH. Another diagnostic test is the administration of exogenous aqueous vasopressin (0.25–0.5 U/kg BW, IM) or desmopressin acetate (0.05 µg/kg, IV), a potent synthetic analog of vasopressin. An increase in urine specific gravity to greater than 1.025 within 2 hours is supportive of a diagnosis of central diabetes insipidus, and the failure to concentrate urine is supportive of a diagnosis of nephrogenic diabetes insipidus or medullary washout. Water deprivation can also be used, because it is expected to increase plasma vasopressin concentration.[4] Water deprivation typically rapidly dehydrates animals with nephrogenic diabetes insipidus, and their hydration status, BW, and urine specific gravity and volume should be monitored frequently.

Specific treatment protocols in horses with nephrogenic diabetes insipidus have not been identified but should focus on restricted water and sodium intake and the long-term administration of thiazide diuretics.

Distal Renal Tubular Acidosis (Type I)

Horses with distal RTA (type I) have a profound strong ion acidosis caused by hyperchloremia (normal anion gap metabolic acidosis), hypokalemia, an alkaline urine pH (typically >8.0), and increased fractional clearance of sodium. A practical diagnostic test for distal RTA (type I) involves examining the ability of the distal convoluted tubules to excrete hydrogen ions by the oral administration of ammonium chloride (0.1 g/kg BW in 6 L of water via nasogastric tube).[1,5] Inability to achieve an acidic urine (pH <6.5) after oral ammonium chloride administration is consistent with a diagnosis of distal RTA (type I).

Treatment of horses and a calf with distal RTA (type I) has been symptomatic and focuses on oral or IV administration of sodium bicarbonate.[3,5] Spontaneous recovery has been reported in horses.

Proximal Renal Tubular Acidosis (Type II)

The classic explanation for this disorder is a failure to reabsorb bicarbonate in the proximal tubules, resulting in excessive loss of bicarbonate in the urine and metabolic acidosis (decreased plasma bicarbonate concentration) but variable urine pH. Because the molecular basis for this defect has not been identified, it has been proposed that proximal RTA (type II) may result from channel dysfunctions of strong electrolytes in proximal renal tubule cells.[1] Reabsorption of bicarbonate requires energy, therefore, disease processes that lead to proximal tubular damage have the potential to result in proximal RTA (type II).

A practical diagnostic test for proximal RTA (type II) in humans is measuring the change in urine P_{CO_2} during oral or IV sodium bicarbonate administration, but this test does not appear to have been performed in horses. Normally, urine and plasma P_{CO_2} are similar but, during bicarbonate diuresis, urine P_{CO_2} becomes greater than plasma P_{CO_2}. The urine to plasma P_{CO_2} gradient during IV sodium bicarbonate administration is therefore measured; one horse with proximal RTA developed a urine to plasma P_{CO_2} gradient of 29 mm Hg during bicarbonate loading. Treatment of horses with proximal RTA (type II) is uncertain.

FURTHER READING

McKenzie EC. Polyuria and polydipsia in horses. *Vet Clin North Am Equine Pract.* 2007;23:641-653.

REFERENCES

1. Arroyo LG, Stampfli HR. *Vet Clin North Am Equine Pract.* 2007;23:631.
2. van der Kolk JH, et al. *J Vet Intern Med.* 2007;21:1121.
3. Hardefeldt LY, et al. *Vet Clin Pathol.* 2011;40:253.
4. Brashier M. *Vet Clin North Am Equine Pract.* 2006;22:219.
5. Gull T. *Vet Clin North Am Equine Pract.* 2006;22:229.

HEMOLYTIC UREMIC–LIKE SYNDROME

Glomerular and tubulointerstitial disease, consistent with profound microangiopathy and glomerular degeneration in humans with hemolytic–uremic syndrome, has been diagnosed in two horses. Both horses were in oliguric renal failure and had clinicopathologic evidence of intravascular hemolysis and morphologic evidence of arteriolar microangiopathy and intravascular coagulation. The mortality rate is expected to be extremely high. The pathogenesis in horses is unclear, although hemolytic–uremic syndrome in humans is caused by toxins produced by *E. coli* O157:H7.

HYDRONEPHROSIS

Hydronephrosis is a dilatation of the renal pelvis with progressive atrophy of the renal parenchyma. It occurs as a congenital or an acquired condition following obstruction of the urinary tract. Any urinary tract obstruction can lead to hydronephrosis, but the extent and duration of the obstruction are important in determining the severity of the renal lesion. Urinary tract obstructions that are chronic, unilateral, and incomplete are more likely to lead to hydronephrosis. Acute obstructions of bladder or urethra that are corrected promptly are not usually associated with significant kidney damage. As a result, recurrence of the obstruction rather than renal failure is the major sequel to urolithiasis in ruminants. In cases of acute complete obstruction the clinical picture is dominated by signs of anuria, dysuria, or stranguria.

Chronic or partial obstructions cause progressive distension of the renal pelvis and pressure atrophy of the renal parenchyma. If the obstruction is unilateral, the unaffected kidney can compensate fully for the loss of function and the obstruction may not cause kidney failure. Unilateral obstruction may be detectable on palpation per rectum of a grossly distended kidney. Chronic bilateral obstructions, although they are rare in large animals, can cause chronic kidney failure. Hydronephrosis and chronic renal failure have been recorded in a steer suffering from chronic partial obstruction of the penile urethra by a urolith. Partial obstruction of the ureters by papillomas of the urinary bladder has been recorded in a series of cows. Compression by neoplastic tissue in cases of enzootic bovine leukosis may also cause hydronephrosis. Ultrasonography can be used as an aid to diagnosis.

INTERSTITIAL NEPHRITIS

Interstitial nephritis is rarely recognized as a cause of clinical disease in farm animals, although it is a frequent postmortem finding in some species. Interstitial nephritis may be diffuse or have a focal distribution. In calves, focal interstitial nephritis (white-spotted kidney) is a common incidental finding at necropsy but does not present as a clinical urinary tract disease. Focal interstitial nephritis of cattle is not associated with leptospirosis or active bacterial infection. In pigs, diffuse interstitial nephritis is observed following infection by *Leptospira* sp. and is important clinically because of the resultant destruction of nephrons that occurs. The kidney is an important reservoir for *Leptospira* spp. in other species, particularly cattle, but renal disease is not a common clinical problem in carrier animals.

Chronic interstitial fibrosis is a common postmortem finding in horses suffering from chronic renal failure. This is thought to represent an end-stage condition rather than primary interstitial disease. The initiating cause of the renal disease is usually not evident, but most cases are thought to begin with acute tubular nephrosis. Horses with chronic interstitial nephritis have the clinical syndrome of chronic renal failure with uremia.

Chronic interstitial nephritis with diffuse zonal fibrosis (CINF) occurs in Japanese Black cattle (Wagyu) as an autosomal recessive disorder leading to death before puberty. Clinically there is growth retardation between 3 and 5 months of age. A genome-wide scan using microsatellite markers in a Wagyu pedigree segregated for CINF mapped the CINF locus to bovine chromosome 1.

EMBOLIC NEPHRITIS

Embolic lesions in the kidney do not cause clinical signs unless they are very extensive, in which case septicemia may be followed by uremia. Even though embolic nephritis may not be clinically evident, transient proteinuria and pyuria may be observed if urine samples are examined at frequent intervals.

ETIOLOGY

Embolic suppurative nephritis or renal abscess may occur after any septicemia or bacteremia when bacteria lodge in renal tissue.

Emboli may originate from localized septic processes such as

- Valvular endocarditis, in all species
- Suppurative lesions in uterus, udder, navel, and peritoneal cavity in cattle or be associated with systemic infections such as:
  - Septicemia in neonatal animals, including *Actinobacillus equuli* infection in foals and *E. coli* septicemia in calves
  - Erysipelas in pigs and *C. pseudotuberculosis* in sheep and goats
  - Septicemic or bacteremic *Streptococcus equi* infection in horses

PATHOGENESIS

Bacterial emboli localize in renal tissue and cause the development of focal suppurative lesions. Emboli can block larger vessels and cause infarction of portions of kidney, with the size varying with the caliber of the occluded vessel. Infarcts are not usually so large that the residual renal tissue cannot compensate fully and they usually cause no clinical signs. If the urine is checked repeatedly, the sudden appearance of proteinuria, casts, and microscopic hematuria, without other signs of renal disease, suggests the occurrence of a renal infarct. The gradual enlargement of focal embolic lesions leads to the development of toxemia and gradual loss of renal function. Clinical signs usually develop only when multiple emboli destroy much of the renal parenchyma, or when there are one or more large infected infarcts.

CLINICAL FINDINGS

Usually there is insufficient renal damage to cause signs of renal disease. Signs of toxemia and the primary disease are usually present. The kidney may be enlarged on rectal examination. Repeated showers of emboli or gradual spread from several large, suppurative infarcts may cause fatal uremia. Spread to the renal pelvis may cause signs similar to pyelonephritis. Large infarcts may cause bouts of transient abdominal pain.

CLINICAL PATHOLOGY

Hematuria and pyuria are present in embolic nephritis, but microscopic examination may be necessary to detect these abnormalities when the lesions are minor. Proteinuria is present but is also normally present in neonatal animals in the first 30 to 40 hours of life. Culture of urine at the time when proteinuria occurs may reveal the identity of the bacteria infecting the embolus. Hematology usually reveals evidence of an acute or chronic inflammatory process.

NECROPSY FINDINGS

In animals that die of intercurrent disease, the early lesions are seen as small gray spots in the cortex. In later stages these lesions may have developed into large abscesses, which may be confluent and in some cases extend into the pelvis. Fibrous tissue may surround long-standing lesions, and healed lesions consist of areas of scar tissue in the cortex. These areas have depressed surfaces and indicate that destruction of cortical tissue has occurred. Extensive scarring may cause an obvious irregular reduction in the size of the kidney.

TREATMENT

General information on treatment of urinary tract infections was presented earlier. Antimicrobials should be selected on the basis of quantitative urine culture and susceptibility testing. In treating septicemic neonatal animals, particular care must be taken to avoid the use of potentially nephrotoxic drugs. Antimicrobial treatment should be continued for a fairly lengthy period (7–14 days). In embolic nephritis, the primary disease and the renal disease must be controlled to prevent recurrence of the embolic lesions. In neonatal animals this may involve treatment for septic shock. The urine culture should be repeated at intervals after treatment is completed to ensure that the infection has been completely controlled.

DIFFERENTIAL DIAGNOSIS

Differentiation from pyelonephritis is difficult unless the latter is accompanied by signs of lower urinary tract infection such as cystitis or urethritis. The kidney is enlarged in both conditions, and the findings on urinalysis are the same when embolic nephritis invades the renal pelvis. Many cases of embolic nephritis go unrecognized clinically because of the absence of overt signs of renal involvement.

Severely dehydrated neonatal animals may experience prerenal uremia and are susceptible to ischemic tubular nephrosis. The presence of other signs of sepsis should increase suspicion of the presence of embolic nephritis.

The sudden occurrence of bouts of acute abdominal pain in some cases of renal infarction may suggest acute intestinal obstruction, but defecation is usually unaffected and rectal examination of the intestines is negative.

Infectious Diseases of the Kidney

LEPTOSPIROSIS

SYNOPSIS

Etiology *Leptospira interrogans* (many distinct serovars) and *L. borgpetersenii* (many distinct serovars) are found.

Epidemiology Worldwide distribution, most commonly in warm, wet climates. Occurs in cattle, sheep and goats, pigs, and horses. Host-adapted (maintenance or reservoir) and non–host-adapted (accidental or incidental) leptospirosis is dependent on the response of each species to particular serovars. Prevalence of infection is greater than incidence of clinical disease. Transmission by urine of infected animals; some wildlife species may transmit to cattle. Ground surface moisture is the most important factor for persistence of the organism; major zoonosis.

Signs Acute, subacute, and chronic forms; there is fever, acute hemolytic anemia, changes in milk, stillbirths, abortion in all species (especially pigs), weak neonates, infertility, milk drop syndrome, and periodic ophthalmia (recurrent uveitis in horse).

Clinical pathology Demonstration and/or culture of organism in blood, urine, cervicovaginal mucus, body fluids, and tissues. Serologic tests, primarily macroscopic agglutination test, and ELISA and DNA probes are done.

Lesions Anemia, jaundice, hemoglobinuria, serous hemorrhages, autolysis of aborted fetuses, fetal hepatitis, and nephritis are observed.

Diagnostic confirmation Culture or demonstrate organism in body fluids or tissues, and there are high serum titers.

Treatment Antimicrobials used to treat acute infection and eliminate leptospiruria.

Control Antimicrobials are used to eliminate carriers; vaccination is done with vaccines containing serovars that are causing the disease in that geographic area.

ETIOLOGY

Leptospires, which are spirochetes pertaining to the family Leptospiraceae are the causative agents of leptospirosis. They are motile, gram-negative, obligate aerobe microorganisms with an optimal growth temperature of 28°C to 30°C (82.4°F–86°F). The organism is characterized by its distinctive hooked ends. The genus *Leptospira* was initially divided into two species: *L. interrogans* sensu lato, which comprised the pathogenic strains, and *L. biflexa* sensu lato, comprising all saprophytic strains of the organism.[1] Within the two *Leptospira* spp., different serovars are differentiated based on **the cross-agglutination absorption test (CAAT).** For this classification two strains are considered different if, after cross-absorption with adequate amounts of heterologous antigen, 10% or more of the heterologous titer regularly remains in either of the two antisera. The serovar is considered the basic systematic unit for *Leptospira* spp., and antigenically related serovars are grouped into serogroups. Currently over 250 pathogenic serovars and 24 pathogenic serogroups are recognized.[1] However, the CAAT is cumbersome and time-consuming to perform and few diagnostic laboratories are able to perform it. Isolated strains are therefore not routinely identified at the serovar but only at the serogroup level, which can be determined by means of the microagglutination test (MAT). Serogroups have no taxonomic status, but are convenient for application such as diagnosis and epidemiology.

With molecular typing techniques becoming more available the taxonomy of *Leptospira* spp. has been reorganized based on genomic DNA-DNA hybridization, and the pathogenic strains previously comprised in the *Leptospira interrogans* sensu lato complex are now divided into 13 different species based on DNA hybridization studies. These are *L. alexanderi, L. alstonii, L. borgpetersenii, L. inadai, L. interrogans (sensu stricto), L. fainei, L. kirschneri, L. licerasiae, L. noguchi, L. santarosai, L. terpstrae, L. weilii,* and *L. wolffii.* However, the correlation between the serologic and the genotypic classification is poor, which makes the taxonomy of *Leptospira* spp. confusing. Not only can pathogenic and saprophytic strains be part of the same genotypic species, but a single serovar and serogroup can also pertain to different genotypic species. So are the antigenically similar serovars *Hardjo-bovis* and *Hardjo-prajitno* (serogroup Hardjo) now classified into two different genotypic species, which are *L. borgpetersenii* (for serovar *Hardjo-bovis*) and *L. interrogans* (sensu stricto, for serovar *Hardjo-prajitno*). The novel molecular classification is often conceived as impractical by clinical microbiologists, which is the reason the serologic taxonomy is still widely used.[2]

EPIDEMIOLOGY

Risk Factors

Animal Risk Factors

Serovars and Species Susceptibility

The epidemiology of leptospirosis is most easily understood by classifying the disease into two broad categories: **host-adapted** and **non–host-adapted** leptospirosis. An animal infected with a host-adapted species of the organism, is a **"maintenance"** or **"reservoir"** host. Exposure of susceptible animals to non–host-adapted serovars results in **accidental** or **incidental disease**. Each *Leptospira* species is adapted to one or a few particular **maintenance host(s)**, although it may cause disease in any mammalian species. The organism is maintained in nature by chronic infection of renal tubules of maintenance hosts.[2]

A specific species behaves differently within its maintenance host species than it does in other, incidental or accidental hosts. A **maintenance host** is characterized by

- A high susceptibility to infection
- Endemic transmission within the host species through direct contact
- Relatively low pathogenicity for its host
- A tendency to cause chronic rather than acute disease, producing insidious economic loss through reproductive losses
- Persistence of the strain in the kidney and sometimes the genital tract with chronic excretion of the pathogen in urine
- Prevalence of chronic excretion in urine increases with age
- A low antibody response to infection, with difficulties in diagnosis

Examples of this relationship are serovar Bratislava in swine, and serovar Hardjo-Bovis in cattle. In contrast, an **incidental host** is characterized by

- Relatively low susceptibility to infection but high pathogenicity for the host
- A tendency to cause acute, severe rather than chronic disease
- Sporadic transmission within the host species and acquisition of infection from other species, sometimes in epidemic form
- A short kidney phase
- A marked antibody response to infection, making for ease of diagnosis
- An example of this relationship is serovar Pomona (*kennewicki*) infection in cattle.

Some common leptospiral serovars and their maintenance hosts are seen in Box 13-9.

Serovar	Maintenance hosts
Hardjo:	Cattle
Bratislava:	Pig, horse
Pomona (kennewicki):	Pig, cattle, skunk, raccoon, opossum
Grippotyphosa:	Raccoon, opossum, squirrel, vole
Icterohaemorrhagiae:	Rat
Canicola:	Dog

Some common leptospiral serovars and their accidental hosts are seen in Box 13-10.

Serovar	Accidental hosts
Hardjo:	Sheep, man
Grippotyphosa:	Sheep, cattle, pig
Bratislava:	Horse
Icterohaemorrhagiae:	Cattle, pig, horse

Calves and lambs are highly susceptible to infection, and septicemia is likely to occur.

Pathogen Risk Factors

The mechanisms through which leptospires cause host tissue damage and disease are currently not well understood. Virulent strains were found to adhere to cultured renal tubular epithelial cells, and adhesion is enhanced by subagglutinating concentrations of homologous antibody because they are commonly found in infected maintenance hosts. The corresponding **adhesin** allowing this attachment has not been identified.[3] Leptospires are phagocytosed by macrophages and neutrophils in the presence of specific antibody and complement but are resistant to complement and killing in nonimmune hosts. Virulent strains were found to attach to neutrophils without being killed, suggesting that the outer membrane of such strains may possess an antiphagocytic component.[2]

There is no unequivocal evidence for a classical exotoxin that would be secreted by *Leptospira* spp., but the outer membrane of the organism contains a **lipopolysaccharide (LPS** or endotoxin) that resembles the standard gram-negative LPS chemically and immunogenically. However leptospiral LPS was found to be considerably less potent than LPS from gram-negative bacteria in standard tests for endotoxin activity such as the rabbit pyrogenicity or the mouse lethality test.[3] Leptospiral LPS possesses an antiphagocytic component and stimulates adherence of neutrophils to endothelial cells and platelets causing aggregation and suggesting a role in the development of thrombocytopenia.[2] In mice, apoptosis of lymphocytes is elicited by LPS via induction of tumor necrosis factor-α (TNF-α).[2]

Along with LPS, the leptospiral outer cell membrane contains several **outer membrane proteins (OMPs)** that are highly immunogenic. Indeed an inverse association between the expression of OMPs and virulence has been demonstrated for the serovar grippotyphosa. Downregulation of the expression of OMPs reduces the humoral immune response, facilitating the evasion from the host's immune system.

Some virulent strains were found to produce either cell-associated or extracellular sphingomyelinases, a class of substances that functions as **hemolysin**. Furthermore, these strains exhibit chemotaxis toward hemoglobin. The presence of a specific antibody prevents hemolysis.

Environmental and Management Risk Factors

The prevalence of a specific leptospiral serovar depends on the availability of a maintenance host species, which can be a domestic or wildlife species.

The occurrence of indirect disease transmission through contaminated soil, water, or other fomites is determined by a number of environmental factors. *Leptospira* spp. can survive for prolonged periods in a moist environment at warm temperatures (optimal around 28°C (82°C) and neutral or mildly stagnant water. In contrast, survival is impaired at temperatures below 10°C (50°F) or above 35°C (95°F) or on dry soil. **Ground surface moisture and water** is the most important factor governing the persistence of the organism in bedding or soil; it can persist for as long as 183 days in water-saturated soil but survives for only 30 minutes when the soil is air dried. In soil, under average conditions, survival is likely to be at least 42 days for *L.* Pomona. It survives in free, surface water for long periods; the survival period is longer in stagnant than in flowing water, although persistence in the latter for as long as 15 days has been recorded. Contamination of the environment and capacity of the organism to survive for long periods under favorable conditions of dampness may result in a high incidence of the disease on heavily irrigated pastures, in areas with high rainfall and temperate climate, in fields with drinking water supplies in the form of easily contaminated surface ponds, and in marshy fields and muddy paddocks or feedlots. Numerous outbreaks of leptospirosis have occurred following heavy rainfall events and floods.[4] Stagnant waters have been incriminated as a possible source of infection in pastured animals in tropical regions.[5] Exposure of humans, pets, or livestock to rodents and rats that are adapted hosts for certain serovars (e.g., Icterohaemorrhagiae or Grippotyphosa) has been shown to be an important risk factor for infection in many species.[4]

Certain management factors have been identified that pose risks of *L.* Hardjo infection being introduced into dairy herds:

- Purchase of infected cattle
- Cograzing or common grazing with infected cattle or sheep
- Purchase or loan of an infected bull
- Access of cattle to contaminated water supplies such as streams, rivers, flood, or drainage water

Occurrence and Prevalence of Infection

Leptospirosis is a disease affecting most animal species, including humans, and has a worldwide occurrence. It is considered the most common bacterial zoonosis worldwide with increasing incidence in industrialized and developing countries and has been classified as a reemerging infectious disease of humans, particularly in tropical and subtropical regions.[6] Leptospirosis has a higher prevalence in tropical and subtropical regions with seasonal occurrence. Peaks in disease incidence are observed during the warm months of the year in temperate climates and during the rainy season in the tropics.[4] Although more than 250 pathogenic serovars have been identified, generally few serovars prevail in a particular region, which largely depends on the presence of an adapted host species. Most leptospiral infections are subclinical, and infection is more common than clinical disease.

Numerous infection prevalence studies have been published for different species in different geographic regions. Reported values are, unfortunately, not easy to compare because some studies are based on serology, whereas others determine the occurrence of bacterial DNA in urine or renal tissue. Furthermore, there is no consensus on the criteria for positive or negative serology, and cutoff values for seropositivity differ between studies. It is generally assumed that serologic studies tend to underestimate the infection prevalence because isolation of bacterial DNA from seronegative individuals was commonly reported in different animal species.[7-9] The occurrence and infection prevalence of leptospirosis will be discussed for different animal species.

Serologic surveys of cattle in the African continent reveal evidence of antibodies against numerous leptospiral serovars and some previously not described strains of serovars. In West Africa, serosurveys of dairy herds revealed 45% of cattle were positive to one or more serovars, which probably represented natural infection because vaccination had not been practiced.

Leptospirosis is common in farm animals in Portugal. Outbreaks of clinical disease have been recorded in cattle and pigs, in sheep and goats and, to a lesser extent, in horses. In Italy, serologic surveys indicate that sheep, horses, pigs, and dogs have the highest number of positive responses.

Cattle

Serovars of *Leptospira* spp. of major importance in cattle include *L.* Hardjo and *L.* Pomona. Depending on the geographic region other serovars such as Icterohaemorrhagiae, Grippotyphosa, and Bratislava may occur with considerable prevalence. The serovar ***L.* Hardjo** is adapted to cattle, and **cattle are the only maintenance host** for this serovar. The serovar Hardjo of which two types, Hardjo-bovis and Hardjo-prajitno, are recognized has been split into two separate genospecies. Serovar Hardjo type Hardjo-bovis is now classified in the genospecies *L. borgpetersenii* serovar Hardjo, and serovar Hardjo, type Hardjo-prajitno now belongs to the genospecies *L. interrogans* serovar Hardjo. *L. borgpetersenii* serovar Hardjo (formerly serovar Hardjo-bovis) occurs worldwide, whereas *L. interrogans* serovar Hardjo (formerly Hardjo-prajitno) has been isolated primarily from cattle in the UK.

Hardjo and Pomona are the most prevalent serovars in the cattle population of North and South America, Australia, and New Zealand; in Europe, Hardjo is the most prevalent serovar in cattle.[10] Seroprevalences among cattle in the United States were estimated with 29% for serovar Hardjo, 23% for serovar Pomona, 19% for serovar Icterohaemorrhagiae, and 11% for serovar Canicola.[10] Seroprevalence surveys in Ontario found Hardjo was most common in beef cattle, whereas Pomona was most common in dairy cattle. In Prince Edward Island, 14% of dairy cows were serologically positive for serovar Hardjo. Serologic surveys of cattle farms in Alberta found infection with Hardjo was widespread across the province, and the prevalence has increased. In contrast, Pomona reactors were found usually on single premises within a locality compared with the clustering of Hardjo reactor herds. Surprisingly, the seroprevalence of unvaccinated beef cattle kept on community pastures in western Canada was 9.6% for serovar Pomona, 6.7% for serovar Grippotyphosa, 6.1% for serovar Icterohaemorrhagiae, and 5.2% for serovar Canicola but only 0.2% for serovar Hardjo.[11]

In beef cattle in Queensland, Australia, the major serovars in order of decreasing crude seroprevalence were Hardjo (15.8%), Tarassovi (13.9%), Pomona (4.0%), and Szwajizak (2%). Vaccinates were not included in the Hardjo and Pomona seroprevalence; and the seroprevalence for Hardjo and Pomona tended to increase with the age of the animals. The data indicate that serovars other than Hardjo, Pomona, and Tarassovi are unlikely to have a significant role in bovine infertility, and cattle are unlikely to be a source of human infection in central Queensland. In New Zealand, a seroprevalence rate in beef cattle of 40% for serovar Hardjo and 7% for serovar Pomona has been reported.[12]

The morbidity rate for clinical disease may vary from 10% to 30%, depending on the clinical manifestation of infection, and the case–fatality rate is usually low at about 5%. The case–fatality rate in calves is much higher than in adult cattle. A high rate of abortions (up to 30%) and loss of milk production are the major causes of loss, but deaths in calves may also be significant.

Recent serologic studies from Europe revealed comparatively low seroprevalence rates in dairy cattle below 1.6 % in dairy cattle in Sweden and Bosnia-Herzegovina.[13,14] The most prevalent serovars in Bosnia-Herzegovina were Pomona, followed by Hardjo and Grippotyphosa; in Sweden cattle were found to be free of serovar Hardjo. In a serologic survey of dairy cows conducted in herds with suboptimal reproductive efficiency in a region in Spain, *L.* Bratislava and *L.* Grippotyphosa were the most prevalent serovars. The risk of seroconversion against *L.* Grippotyphosa was higher during the spring season, whereas *L.* Bratislava did not differ among seasons. The prevalence of *L.* Hardjo was low, which indicates that the reproductive inefficiency was unassociated with Hardjo. In surveys of dairy and beef cattle in Spain, *L.* Bratislava is the most frequently detected serovar, whereas Hardjo is at a relatively low seroprevalence compared with similar studies in western European countries.

In Spain, serovars Grippotyphosa, Tarassovi, and Copenhageni are more frequent in dairy herds, probably related to management practices and geographic location of these herds, which facilitate the contact with maintenance hosts for these serovars.

In Turkey, *L.* Hardjo is the dominant serovar identified in serologic surveys of cattle, but *L.* Grippotyphosa is the dominant serovar causing clinical disease in cattle, the disease is uncommon in sheep.

In South Africa a seroprevalence of leptospirosis in cattle originating from communal grazing areas of 19.4% has been reported. Although serovar Pomona was most prevalent (22%), a wide variety of other serovars including Tarassovi (19%), Bratislava (15%), Canicola (13%), Hardjo (13%), Icterohaemorrhagiae (12%), Szwajizak (4%), and Grippotyphosa (2%) were common.[15]

Farmed Deer

Leptospirosis is a well-established clinical disease in farmed deer in New Zealand. Slaughterhouse surveys of farmed deer in New Zealand found serologic evidence of serovar Hardjo in 73.6%, Pomona in 41.5%, Copenhageni in 11.3%, and Tarassovi in 15.1% of farms.

A more recent study reported a herd seroprevalence of 42% for serovar Hardjo alone, 7% for serovar Pomona alone, and 23% for serovars Hardjo and Pomona combined. The individual animal seroprevalence was reported with 21% tested for serovar Hardjo alone, 9% for serovar Pomona alone, and 4% for both serovars.[12] Because of the high prevalence of serovar Hardjo in farmed deer in New Zealand, it has been proposed that farmed deer may function as maintenance hosts for this serovar.[16]

Sheep and Goats

The disease in sheep and goats has been reported in many countries. Reported prevalences range from 5% to 42%. Predominant serovars isolated in Australia and Italy included Castellonis, Poi, Sejroe, Hardjo, Copenhageni, and Cynopteri.[17,18] In Guyana, serovars Pomona, Grippotyphosa, Hardjo, and Bratislava, and in Trinidad serovars Copenhageni and Autumnalis were predominant.[19,20] Infection with *L.* Hardjo occurs but is unlikely to be a source of infection for cattle herds. Sheep are not natural maintenance hosts for pomona or hardjo and are likely to have infections of relatively short duration, producing severe pathologic effects. However, persistent leptospiruria caused by Hardjo in sheep in which no contact with cattle has occurred suggests that sheep may be a maintenance host for this serovar. This could complicate control of Hardjo infection in cattle, which are free of this serovar, and infected sheep are a potential zoonotic risk to abattoir workers, sheep farmers, and shearers, which previously had not been considered. Infection with serovar Hardjo is widespread in Merino stud rams in South Australia.

Seroprevalences reported for goats range among 2.1% in northern Italy, over 13.1% in Nigeria, and 20.8% in Brazil,[17,21,22] which involved Icterohaemorrhagiae and Copenhageni serovars.

Pigs

Leptospira serovars most common in pigs are Bratislava, for which this species is the maintenance host, and Pomona, and grippotyphosa; less common serovars include Icterohaemorrhagiae, Canicola, and Hardjo. In infected herds the prevalence of positive serologic reactors is high, and in large infected pig populations it is about 20%. In Iowa, 38% of sera from National Animal Health Monitoring System herds were positive for 1 or more of 12 serovars. The most common serovar antibodies found in pigs in Prince Edward Island swine herds were *L.* Icterohaemorrhagiae, *L.* Bratislava, *L.* Autumnalis, and *L.* Pomona. In Trinidad an individual animal seroprevalence of 5% with a farm prevalence of 33.3% has been reported. Predominant serovars were Bratislava of the Australis serogroup (2.0%) and members of the Icterohaemorrhagiae serogroup (2.5%).[19]

The Australis serogroup of leptospires is now important because of an increasing awareness that antibodies to Bratislava are widespread in the pig populations of many countries, the recovery of Lora, Muenchen, and Bratislava from pigs, and the involvement of Bratislava and Muenchen in reproductive problems of swine herds. All of the pig isolates of the Australis serogroup have been identified as either Bratislava or Muenchen, and there are also differences at the subserovar level, which may be important in understanding the epidemiology of the Australis serogroup, the development of efficacious vaccines, and the pathogenesis of disease. Economic losses are about equally divided between abortions and deaths of weak and unthrifty newborn pigs. Infection of pigs at slaughter is associated with multifocal interstitial nephritis, which results in condemnation of kidneys.

Swine are affected by several leptospiral serovars, and the clinical signs often associated with these infections include poor reproductive performance. Seropositive sows have a greater risk of weak newborn pigs and have more weak newborn piglets per litter. In some areas suboptimal reproductive performance was associated with certain serovars, such as Grippotyphosa, and not others, such as Autumnalis, Bratislava, Pomona, and Icterohaemorrhagiae.

Pigs in intensive housing present a different problem from those in more conventional housing or at pasture. In large pig units the possibility for cross-infection is high because of high population density. The movement of pigs from pen to pen and access to effluent from other pens are the critical means of spread in these circumstances. The spread of infection within piggeries is encouraged by mixing infected pigs with uninfected pigs, which results in epidemics within the pens. Transmission from infected to susceptible grower pigs occurs continuously in grower houses, with a constant proportion of pigs becoming infected each week. Introduction onto a farm may be via an imported boar; boars are frequently found to harbor leptospires in the genital tract. Leptospira were found commonly in the kidneys of slaughter fattening pigs in Vietnam but are not considered to be the cause of the white-spotted kidneys of pigs.

Horses

Although the precise prevalence of infection in horse populations of different geographic regions is not known, serologic evidence suggests leptospiral infection is common in horses. Predominant serovars occurring in this species include the serovars Bratislava, Pomona, Icterohaemorrhagiae, and Grippotyphosa. Because of the relatively frequent occurrence of *L.* Bratislava, horses are thought to be maintenance hosts for this serovar.

Serologic surveys of Thoroughbred and Standardbred horses in Ontario revealed a higher prevalence of Bratislava, which increased with age. In a survey of horses in Alberta, titers to *L.* Icterohaemorrhagiae, Bratislava, Copenhageni, and Autumnalis were common (94.6, 56.6, 46.5, and 43.5%, respectively). The prevalence to other serovars ranged from 0.8% to 27.2%. The probability of being seropositive increased by approximately 10% with each year of life. Horses managed as individuals (e.g., racetrack horses) were about half as likely to be seropositive as those managed in groups (e.g., rodeo horses).

A Swedish study determined a seroprevalence of 16.6% for Bratislava, 8.3% for Icterohaemorrhagiae, 1.2% for Sejroe, 0.5% for Pomona, and 0.4% for Grippotyphosa. An increase of the seroprevalence with age was found for serovars Bratislava and Icterohaemorrhagiae.[23] A bacteriologic survey of kidneys from abattoir horses in Portugal found serogroups *L. australis* and *L. pomona*, which were identified as *L.* Bratislava, and *L. kirschneri* serovar Tsaratsovo, respectively.

Rodent exposure was associated with risk of exposure to all serovars. Management was associated positively with the risk of exposure to serovars Pomona and Bratislava, but not with risk of exposure to Autumnalis. Soil and water had a positive association with risk of exposure to Pomona and Autumnalis but not to Bratislava. The wildlife index value and the population density of horses turned out together were associated with risk of exposure to Autumnalis. For the serovar Bratislava a Swedish study reported highest seroprevalences from April to June and from October to December and for serovar Icterohaemorrhagiae from October to December.[23]

Economic Importance

Leptospirosis is not only considered the most important bacterial zoonosis worldwide but also presents a major cause of economic loss in farm animals. The majority of leptospiral infections are subclinical and associated with fetal infections causing abortions, stillbirths, and the birth of weak neonates with a high death rate in cattle, sheep, horses, and pigs. In cattle, epidemics of abortions, infertility, and increased culling rate cause major economic losses. Epidemics of agalactia in dairy herds (the **milk drop syndrome**) are associated with infection with *L.* hardjo.

Zoonotic Implications

Leptospirosis is probably the most prevalent zoonotic disease in the world predominantly affecting tropical and subtropical regions. It is now recognized as an emerging, potentially epidemic disease associated with excess rainfall in tropical settings, representing a significant public health hazard. Most recent outbreaks were reported from Nicaragua in 2007, Sri Lanka in 2008, and the Philippines in 2009).[24]

Annual incidences of clinical leptospirosis vary greatly with highest rates on the Seychelles (43.2/100,000 population), Trinidad and Tobago (12/100,000), Barbados (10/100,000), Jamaica (7.8/100,000), and Costa Rica (6.7/100,000).[25] In the United States the Centers for Disease Control and Prevention estimate that between 100 and 200 clinical cases are diagnosed every year (0.1/100,000), half of which are in Hawaii. In Europe, the highest incidence rates have been reported from Croatia (1.7/100,000), Portugal (0.7/100,000), Denmark (0.6/100,000), and Slovenia (0.5/100,000).

Although most cases of leptospiral infection are asymptomatic or only associated with mild clinical disease, mortality in humans remains significant, particularly in developing countries because of delays in diagnosis caused by lack of diagnostic infrastructure and adequate clinical suspicion when patients are presented for medical diagnosis and care. The overall case–fatality rate ranges between 1% and 5%, depending on the clinical presentation and the age of the patient. The icteric form of the disease, which occurs in 5% to 10% of all patients, has an overall mortality of 5% to 15%, whereas mortality rates of over 50% have been reported in cases with myocardial involvement. Mortality is higher in the elderly.[26]

Leptospirosis can be prevented through appropriate hygiene, sanitation, and animal husbandry. It is essential to educate people working with animals or animal tissues about measures for reducing the risk of exposure to such zoonotic pathogens as leptospira.

Humans are considered to be purely incidental hosts for leptospirae and have rarely been implicated in spreading the disease.[27] Leptospirosis is an important zoonosis and is an occupational hazard to butchers, farmers, hunters, pet traders, rodent catchers, veterinarians, and sewer workers. In recent decades the epidemiology has undergone major changes, with a shift away from the traditional occupational disease in developed countries to a disease associated with recreational exposures. Human infection is most likely to occur by contamination with infected urine or uterine contents. Veterinarians may become infected by handling the tissues and urine of sows that have aborted from pomona infection. Although leptospirae may be present in cow's milk for a few days at the peak of fever in acute cases, the bacteria do not survive for long in the milk and are destroyed by pasteurization. However, farm workers who milk cows are highly susceptible to *L. interrogans* serovar Hardjo infection, and one New Zealand survey found 34% of milkers were seropositive, mostly to *L. interrogans* serovar Hardjo, but a high proportion were also positive to *L. interrogans* serovar Pomona. This has aroused alarm, and leptospirosis became known as "New Zealand's No.1 dairy occupational disease." A campaign of vaccination of dairy cattle across the country resulted in a marked decrease in the incidence of the disease in humans. In most situations, dogs, cats, and horses are unlikely to contribute to human infection.

The epidemiology of leptospirosis in New Zealand has been changing. The annual incidence of human leptospirosis in New Zealand from 1990 to 1998 was 4.4 per 100,000. Incidence was highest among meat-processing workers (163/100,000), livestock farm workers (91/100,000). and forestry-related workers (24/100,000). The most commonly detected serovar was ballum (11.9%). The annual incidence of leptospirosis declined from 5.7/100,000 from 1990 to 1992 to 2.9/100,000 from 1995 to 1998. The incidence of serovar Hardjo and serovar Pomona infection declined, whereas the incidence of serovar Ballum infection increased. The increasing incidence of serovar Ballum suggests changing transmission patterns via direct or indirect exposure to contaminated water.

Veterinary students may be exposed to leptospirosis by taking courses in food inspection and technology, on-farm clinical work experiences, contact with pets (especially carnivores), and contact with animal traders. In a 1-year period, the seroprevalence of leptospirosis in veterinary students in a veterinary school in Spain increased from 8.1% to 11.4%. The incidence of the disease during the study was 0.039.

Methods of Transmission

The source of infection is an infected animal that contaminates pasture, drinking water, and feed by infective urine, aborted fetuses, and uterine discharges. All of the leptospiral types are transmitted within and between species in this way. A viable infected neonate can harbor the infection for several weeks after birth. The semen of an infected bull may contain leptospirae, and transmission by natural breeding or artificial insemination can occur but is uncommon. In rams, the semen is likely to be infective for only a few days during the period of leptospiremia; in boars there is no evidence of coital transmission. *L. interrogans* serovar Hardjo is excreted from the genital tract of aborting cows for as long as 8 days after abortion or calving and is detectable in the oviducts and uterus for up to 90 days after experimental infection and in naturally infected cows. It may also be present in the genital tract of bulls, and venereal spread of the infection is possible. Young pigs may act as carriers for 1 year and adult sows for 2 months. Because of the high intensity and long duration of the infection in pigs, they play an important role in the epidemiology of leptospirosis.

Leptospiruria

Urine is the chief source of contamination because animals, even after clinical recovery, may shed leptospirae in the urine for long periods. All animals that have recovered from infection may intermittently shed organisms in the urine and act as "carriers." In cattle, leptospiruria may persist for a mean period of 36 days (10–118 days) with the highest excretion rate in the first half of this period. Sheep and horses are not common sources of infection because of low-grade and intermittent leptospiruria. In any species, the leptospirae may persist in the kidney for much longer periods than they can be recovered from the urine by routine laboratory methods. Urine drinking by calves is not an uncommon form of pica in some dairy herds and is a means of transmission.

Wildlife as Source of Infection

Although surveys of the incidence of leptospirosis in wildlife have been conducted and the pathogenic effects of *L.* Pomona on some species (particularly deer and skunks) have been determined, the significance of wildlife as a source of infection for domestic animals is uncertain. Variable rates of seroprevalence to leptospires have been documented in white-tailed deer, mule deer, pronghorns, moose, red deer, and elk. There is a high prevalence of infection in feral pigs, and in wild brown rats trapped on farms in the UK the prevalence of *L. icterohaemorrhagiae* and Bratislava was about 14%. *L.* Canicola is known to spread from domestic dogs and jackals to cattle and, when hygiene is poor, even from humans to cattle. The serovar Bratislava has been associated with severe interstitial nephritis in raccoons in a recreational area in Quebec, which were also serologically positive to Pomona, Hardjo, and Grippotyphosa.

The expanding wild boar population in urban and suburban areas has been incriminated as a possible source of infection for humans, domestic animals, and livestock in some countries. Infection prevalence rates in wild boars have been reported from Japan and Germany with 15.2% (positive polymerase chain reaction [PCR] on kidney tissue) and 18% (serology), respectively.[26,27] The most prevalent serovars in the German study were Pomona and Bratislava; in the Japanese study the predominant genospecies were *L. interrogans* and *L. borgpetersenii.*

Portal of Entry of Organism

Entrance of the organism into the body occurs most probably through cutaneous or mucosal abrasions. Transplacental transmission is uncommon, but neonatal infection in utero has occurred. Oral dosing is an unsatisfactory method for experimental transmission compared with injection and installation into the nasal cavities, conjunctival sac, and vagina.

PATHOGENESIS

Leptospirosis manifests itself as a disease in several different ways. Leptospires invade the host across mucosal surfaces or softened skin. They have the ability to bind to epithelial cells and attach to the constituents of the extracellular matrix through an active process involving surface proteins. Pathogenic leptospires are found extracellularly between cells of the liver and kidney. Release of lymphokines such as TNF-α from monocytes through the endotoxic activity of the leptospiral LPS may be an important virulence mechanism. Induction of TNF-α release may help explain the damage to endothelial cells with resultant hemorrhage seen in severe leptospirosis.

Leptospirosis can occur as an acute and severe disease caused by septicemia with evidence of endotoxemia such as hemorrhages, hepatitis, nephritis, meningitis; as a subacute moderately severe disease with nephritis, hepatitis, agalactia, and meningitis; or as a chronic disease characterized by abortion, stillbirth, and infertility. In the occult form, there is no clinical illness. The form of the disease depends largely on the species of the host as set out in Table 13-2. Variations between serotypes of *L. interrogans* in their pathogenicity also affect the nature of the signs that appear. For example, in *L.* Pomona infections, intravascular hemolysis and interstitial nephritis are important parts of the disease. However, *L.* Hardjo does not produce hemolysin and does not cause interstitial nephritis, but it does cause clinical infection in sexually mature, lactating or pregnant females. Thus infection occurs in the pregnant uterus and lactating mammary gland resulting in septicemia, abortion, and mastitis. The pathogenesis of the disease associated with *L.* Pomona is set out as follows.

Table 13-2 Forms of leptospirosis in the animal species

VetMed10	Acute form	Subacute form	Chronic form
Cattle	+ (Calves only)	+	+ (Abortion)
Sheep and goat	+ (Includes abortion)	–	–
Pig	+ (Rarely and only in piglets)	–	+ (Abortion)
Horse	–	+	+ (Abortion and periodic ophthalmia)

Acute Form

After penetration of the skin or mucosa, the organisms multiply in the liver and migrate to, and can be isolated from, the peripheral blood for several days until the accompanying fever subsides. At this time, serum antibodies begin to appear and organisms can be found in the urine.

Septicemia, Capillary Damage, Hemolysis, and Interstitial Nephritis

During the early period of septicemia, sufficient hemolysin may be produced to cause overt hemoglobinuria as a result of extensive intravascular hemolysis. This is an unlikely event in adult cattle but is common in young calves. If the animal survives this phase of the disease, localization of the infection may occur in the kidney. Hemolysis depends on the presence of a serovar that produces hemolysin. Capillary damage is common to all serovars and during the septicemic phase petechial hemorrhages in mucosae are common. Vascular injury also occurs in the kidney and if the hemolysis is severe, anemic anoxia and hemoglobinuric nephrosis may occur. There is some evidence that the leptospiral LPS may exacerbate the vascular lesions. The infection localizes in the renal parenchyma, causing an interstitial nephritis, and persistence of the leptospirae in these lesions results in prolonged leptospiruria. The renal lesion develops because the infection persists there long after it has been cleared from other tissue sites. In the acute phase of the disease, the animal may die of septicemia or hemolytic anemia or both. Subsequently, the animal may die of uremia caused by interstitial nephritis.

Focal chronic interstitial nephritis, also called white-spotted kidney, is a common finding in clinically healthy cattle at slaughter and has frequently been assumed to be related to current or prior infection with *Leptospira* spp. However, studies of white-spotted kidney in cattle at the abattoir indicate that neither *Leptospira* spp. nor active infection by other bacteria are associated with the lesions.

Abortion

Following systemic invasion, abortion may occur because of fetal death, with or without placental degeneration. Abortion usually occurs several weeks after septicemia because of the time required to produce the changes in the fetus, which is usually autolyzed at birth. Abortion occurs most often in the second half of pregnancy, probably because of the greater ease of invasion of the placenta at this stage, but may occur at any time from 4 months on. Although abortion often occurs in both cattle and horses after either the acute or the subacute form of the disease, abortion without prior clinical illness is also common. This is particularly the case in sows and occurs to a lesser extent in cows and mares; this may be from degenerative changes in the placental epithelium. Leptospirae are rarely present in the aborted fetuses; however, if the aborted fetus has survived the infection long enough to produce antibodies, these may be detectable.

Experimental infection of serologically negative pregnant cattle with a north Queensland strain of *L. borgpetersenii* serovar Hardjo resulted in seroconversion and shedding of the organism in the urine. Elective cesarean sections were done 6 weeks after challenge. There was no evidence of *L.* Hardjo infection of the fetuses. Some of the fetuses had histopathologic lesions consistent with *Neospora* sp. infection.

Encephalitis

Localization of leptospirae in nervous tissue is common in sheep and goats and may result in the appearance of signs of encephalitis.

Subacute and Occult Forms

In the subacute form, the pathogenesis is similar to that of the acute septicemic form, except that the reaction is less severe. It occurs in all species, but the common form is found in adult cattle and horses. Occult cases, with no clinical illness but with rising antibody titers, are common in all animals. These are difficult to explain but may be associated with strains of varying pathogenicity, but with leptospirosis, characteristically, differences between groups may be associated with prior immune status, environmental conditions, or number of carriers in relation to severity of exposure.

Periodic Ophthalmia (Recurrent Uveitis) in the Horse

There is some evidence of a causal relationship between leptospiral infection and periodic ophthalmia in the horse. The incidence of serologically positive reactors is higher in groups of horses affected with periodic ophthalmia than in normal animals. Agglutinins are present in the aqueous humor in greater concentration than in the serum. Serologic surveys indicate that leptospira infection is not a major factor in the etiology of equine anterior uveitis in the UK, but serologic evidence of Pomona is associated with uveitis in horses in the United States. The opacity in both cornea and lens is a consequence of the antigenic relationship between leptospires and components of the ocular tissues and does not require the presence of living bacteria. A 52-kDa protein appears to be involved in the antigenic relationship between the leptospires and equine ocular tissues and is located inside the bacterium. The uveitis alters the composition of the aqueous humor and impedes the nutrition of the ocular structures, leaving sequelae such as iris atrophy, synechiae, and corneal opacity.

Retinal immunopathology in horses with uveitis has been described and may be a primary immunologic event in equine uveitis, providing evidence that leptospira-associated uveitis may be a distinct subset of equine uveitis.

Pulmonary Hemorrhage

Respiratory manifestation of leptospirosis associated with severe respiratory distress, pulmonary hemorrhage, and high case fatality has been described in humans, dogs, and horses.[28-30] The pathogenesis of this clinical presentation only occurs in a small subset of infected patients and is poorly understood. Endothelial damage of small pulmonary blood vessels and fibrin deposition along alveolar walls have been reported as consistent findings. Furthermore, lung lesions were found to be associated with the expression of TNF and endothelial nitric oxide synthase in experimentally induced leptospirosis in hamsters, suggesting a role of local or systemic inflammatory mechanism in the pathogenesis of this pulmonary form of the disease.[33] Immune-mediated mechanisms have also been proposed as a possible cause for pulmonary hemorrhage, but corroborating evidence is not yet available.

Immune Mechanisms

Following infection, specific antibodies are induced that opsonize leptospires, facilitating their elimination from most parts of the body. However, leptospires that reach the proximal renal tubules, genital tract, and mammary glands appear to be protected from circulating antibodies. They persist and multiply in these sites and may be excreted and transmitted to susceptible, in-contact animals, primarily by urine. Furthermore, and of major importance, the level of serum antibody commonly declines to undetectable levels in animals that are persistently infected.

The first serologic response with *L.* Hardjo infection is the production of immunoglobulin M (IgM) antibodies. These rise rapidly but usually decline to undetectable concentrations by 4 weeks after infection. Within 1 to 2 weeks of infection, IgG_1 antibodies appear, and at 3 months they represent 80% of antibodies detected in the MAT. The MAT titer peaks 11 to 21 days after infection but may vary from 1:3200 to an undetectable concentration. It declines gradually over 11 months, but the persistence is variable. Vaccination induces antibodies that are mainly of the IgG class with levels peaking at 2 weeks after a two-dose vaccination but decreasing rapidly to levels lower than those after natural infection. Approximately 95% of vaccinated heifers do not have MAT antibodies 20 weeks after the second of two vaccinations given 4 weeks apart, but the absence of titers is not necessarily an indication that protection has waned. Vaccinated animals are protected from natural challenge for many months after their MAT titers become undetectable. The serologic response of calves vaccinated at 3 months of age is lower than those vaccinated at 6 months of age because of the presence of maternal antibody. Transfer of passive immunity antibodies to newborn calves occurs via the colostrum, and the antibodies persist in the calves for 2 to 6 months.

Although antibodies against leptospiral LPS give passive protection in some animal models, cattle vaccinated against serovar hardjo with pentavalent vaccines are vulnerable to infection with serovar hardjo despite the presence of high titers of anti-LPS antibody. It is now known that peripheral blood mononuclear cells (PBMCs) from cattle vaccinated with an *L. interrogans* serovar Hardjo vaccine, which protects against serovar Hardjo, proliferated in vitro in response to Hardjo antigens. Thus a cell-mediated immune response to serovar Hardjo is probably necessary for protection. A protective killed vaccine against serovar Hardjo induces a strong antigen-specific proliferative response by PBMC from vaccinated cattle 2 months after the first dose of vaccine. This response was absent from unvaccinated cattle. The mean response peaked by 2 months after completion of the two-dose vaccination regimen, and substantial proliferation was measurable in in vitro cultures throughout 7 months of the study period. Up to one-third of the PBMCs from vaccinated animals produced interferon gamma (IFN-γ) after 7 days in culture with antigen. One-third of the IFN-γ-producing cells were gamma delta lymphocytes, with the remainder cells being CD4+ T cells. Thus a very potent Th1-type immune response was induced and sustained following vaccination with a killed bacterial vaccine adjuvanted with aluminum hydroxide and the involvement of gamma delta T cells in the response. The induction of this Th1-type **cellular immune response** is associated with the protection afforded by the bovine leptospiral vaccine against *L. borgpetersenii* serovar Hardjo.

The immune response of naive and vaccinated cattle following challenge with a virulent strain of *L. borgpetersenii* serovar Hardjo has been examined. Beginning at 2 weeks after challenge, IFN-γ was measured in antigen-stimulated PBMC cultures from nonvaccinated animals, although the amount produced was always less than that in cultures of PBMC from vaccinated animals. IFN-γ^+ cells were also evident in antigen-stimulated cultures of PBMC from vaccinated but not from nonvaccinated animals throughout the postchallenge period. Naive and vaccinated animals had similar levels of antigen-specific IgG_1 following challenge; vaccinated animals had twofold more IgG_2. It is evident that although infection may induce a type 1 response, it is too weak to prevent establishment of chronic infection.

CLINICAL FINDINGS

The clinical findings in leptospirosis are similar in each animal species and do not vary greatly with the species of *Leptospira,* except that infection with *icterohaemorrhagiae* usually causes a severe septicemia. For convenience the various forms of the disease are described as they occur in cattle, and comparisons are made with the disease in other species. In all animals the incubation period is 3 to 7 days.

Cattle

Leptospirosis in cattle may be subclinical, acute, subacute, or chronic and is most often associated with serovars hardjo or pomona.

Acute Leptospirosis Associated With pomona

Calves up to 1 month old are most susceptible to the acute leptospirosis. The disease is manifested by septicemia, with high fever (40.5–41.5°C; 105–107°F), anorexia, petechiation of mucosae, depression, acute intravascular hemolysis with hemoglobinuria, jaundice, and pallor of the mucosae. Because of the ensuing anemia, tachycardia, loud heart sounds, and a more readily palpable apex beat are present; dyspnea is also prominent. The case–fatality rate is high, and if recovery occurs then convalescence is prolonged. In adult cattle, abortion caused by the systemic reaction may occur at the acute stage of the disease. Milk production is markedly decreased, and the secretion is thickened, red-colored, or may contain blood clots. The mammary gland is limp and soft. Mastitis as part of leptospirosis has often been described in cattle and a high somatic cell count in grossly abnormal milk suggests mastitis, but these changes are caused by a general vascular lesion rather than local injury to mammary tissue. Severe lameness caused by synovitis is recorded in some animals and a necrotic dermatitis, probably caused by photosensitization, is recorded in others.

Subacute Leptospirosis Associated With *L. pomona*

The subacute form of leptospirosis differs from the acute form only in degree. Similar clinical findings are observed in a number of affected animals, but not all of the findings are present in the same animal. The fever is milder (39–40.5°C; 102–105°F), and depression, anorexia, dyspnea, and hemoglobinuria are common, but jaundice may or may not be present. Abortion usually occurs 3 to 4 weeks later. One of the characteristic findings is the marked drop in milk production and the appearance of bloodstained or yellow-orange, thick milk in all four quarters without apparent physical change in the udder.

Chronic Leptospirosis Associated With *L. pomona*

The clinical findings in the chronic form of leptospirosis are mild and may be restricted to abortion. Severe "storms" of abortions occur most often in groups of cattle that are at the same stage of pregnancy when they are exposed to infection. The abortions usually occur during the last trimester of pregnancy. Apart from the abortion, there is no depression of reproductive efficiency in cattle affected by leptospirosis. Many animals in the group develop positive MATs without clinical illness.

There are occasional reports of leptospiral meningitis in cattle. In coordination, excessive salivation, conjunctivitis, and muscular rigidity are the common signs.

Leptospirosis Associated With *L. hardjo*

Infertility and milk drop syndrome occurs only in pregnant or lactating cows because the organism is restricted to proliferation in the pregnant uterus and the lactating mammary gland. There is a sudden onset of fever, anorexia, immobility, and agalactia. The milk is yellow to orange and may contain clots. The udder is flabby, there is no heat or pain, and all four quarters are equally affected. The sudden drop in milk production may affect up to 50% of cows at one time and cause a precipitate fall in the herd's milk yield. The decline may last for up to 8 weeks but an individual cow's milk production will return to normal within 10 to 14 days. The milk may have a high leukocyte count, which subsides over a period of about 14 days as milk production returns. In some cases, there is no evidence of mastitis, no change in the consistency of the milk, and no changes in the udders of affected cows, but leptospiruria may be present in up to 30% of affected cows.

The herd fertility status incorporating the first service conception rate, the number of services per conception for cows conceiving, the calving-to-conception interval, and the culling rate usually reveals a low reproductive performance, especially during the year of the diagnosis. The effect is also temporary and not easily detected. Exposure of nonvaccinated dairy cows to *L.* Hardjo can be associated with a subsequent reduction in fertility, as indicated by a greater time from calving to conception and a higher number of breeding times per conception.

Abortion may occur **several weeks after the initial infection** and may also occur as the only evidence of the disease; in some areas or circumstances it is the principal clinical manifestation of leptospirosis caused by serovar Hardjo and the principal cause of abortion in cattle. In others it is thought to be an uncommon cause of abortion. This may be related to different strains of the serotype or to the degree to which the disease has become enzootic. Thus outbreaks of milk yield drop and systemic illness appears to be the characteristic clinical picture when the disease first appears in an area. However, as natural immunity develops in adult cows only heifers become newly infected, and the only sign is abortion. Furthermore, many cows have subclinical infections with hardjo in which only a fall in milk yield may be detectable.

Pigs

Leptospira serovars Pomona and Bratislava are the most common causes of infection, and chronic leptospirosis is the most common form of the disease in pigs. Pigs are the maintenance host for serovar Bratislava, which generally does not cause clinical disease other than reproductive failure, including occasional abortions and stillbirths. Serovar Pomona is of intermediate pathogenicity for pigs and is characterized by abortion and a high incidence of stillbirths. Acute disease may be observed in young pigs infected with serovar Pomona. Clinical signs include fever, anorexia, hemolytic anemia with hemoglobinuria, and jaundice. In an infected herd, the rearing rate may fall as low as 10% to 30%. An abortion "storm" may occur when the disease first appears in a herd, but abortions diminish as herd immunity develops. Most abortions occur 2 to 4 weeks before term. Piglets produced at term may be dead or weak and die soon after birth. Serovar Hardjo may be a sporadic cause of reproductive disease. There was no association between infertility and antibodies to serovars autumnalis and icterohaemorrhagiae. Icterohaemorrhagiae infection causes septicemic leptospirosis with a high mortality rate.

Sheep and Goats

The disease is rare in sheep and goats so that good descriptions of the naturally occurring disease in them are lacking; most affected animals are found dead, apparently from septicemia. Affected animals are febrile, dyspneic, snuffle, and hang their heads down. Some have hemoglobinuria, pallor of mucosae, and jaundice and die within 12 hours. Lambs, especially those in poor condition, are most susceptible. The chronic form may occur and is manifested by loss of bodily condition, but abortion seems to be almost entirely a manifestation of the acute form when the infection is pomona. With Hardjo, abortion has been recorded as the only clinical sign, and oligolactia and agalactia, similar to the bovine milk drop syndrome, have been observed in lactating ewes.

Horses

Although clinical leptospirosis in horses is uncommon, serologic surveys suggest that subclinical infection frequently occurs. These serologic studies revealed that bratislava is among the most prevalent serovars in the horse population in many countries, and it has been proposed that horses are the reservoir host for this serovar, which is rarely associated with clinical disease. Clinical leptospirosis is in most cases caused by serovars Pomona and Grippotyphosa and is associated with abortions, stillbirths, severe systemic disease in foals, intravascular hemolysis, renal and liver disease, and recurrent uveitis.

Abortion

L. interrogans serovar Pomona is a major cause of abortions and stillbirths in the equine population. The gestational ages at which abortion occurs ranges from 140 days to full-term mean (250 days) and typically follows 2 to 3 weeks after an episode of mild clinical illness with fever, anorexia, and in rare instances with jaundice.

Periodic Ophthalmia

Recurrent uveitis in horses (**periodic ophthalmia, moon blindness, or recurrent iridocyclitis**) is a late complication of systemic leptospirosis in horses with signs beginning months to years after naturally acquired or experimentally induced infection. It is often associated with infection with *L. interrogans* serovar Pomona. Clinically there are recurrent episodes of ocular disease including photophobia, lacrimation, conjunctivitis, keratitis, a pericorneal corona of blood vessels, hypopyon, and iridocyclitis. Recurrent attacks usually terminate in blindness in both eyes. There is a strong relationship between uveitis and leptospiral seroactivity in horses. Seropositive horses with uveitis are at increased risk of losing vision, compared with seronegative horses with uveitis, and Appaloosas are at an increased risk of developing uveitis and associated blindness, compared with that in non-Appaloosas. The disease has been produced experimentally by producing infection with Pomona. Infection with pomona in foals has been observed in association with *Rhodococcus equi* to cause a very heavy mortality rate. The foals died of a combination of interstitial nephritis and uremia and pulmonary abscessation and chronic enteritis. Leptospirosis has been suspected as a cause of renal dysfunction in a horse and hematuria and leptospiruria described in a foal.

Nonulcerative keratouveitis associated with leptospiral infection has been described in horses. Photophobia, epiphora, and blepharospasm are common. Hyperemia of the bulbar conjunctiva, edema of the paralimbal cornea, pupillary block, and iris bombe are also present. As the disease progresses, there may be hyphema, hypopyon, and organized fibrin in the anterior chamber, miosis, and dyscoria caused by posterior synechiae, and the cornea may become opaque and vascularized. The cornea retains no fluorescein dye.

Neonatal Foal Disease

Acute leptospirosis in foals is the most severe form of the disease in horses characterized by vasculitis with petechial hemorrhages and intravascular hemolysis with hemoglobinuria, jaundice, and anemia. Renal failure, severe hepatopathy, and severe pulmonary hemorrhage have been reported in some instances.[32]

CLINICAL PATHOLOGY

General Considerations

Laboratory procedures used in the diagnosis of leptospirosis include culture or detection of leptospires or leptospiral DNA in blood or body fluids and detection and measurement of antibody in blood and body fluids such as urine, CSF, and cervicovaginal mucus. Culture of leptospires is laborious and can take up to 13 weeks. Serologic and microbiologic detection of chronically infected animals is difficult, as is the confirmation of leptospirosis as a direct cause of reproductive losses in a herd. A positive diagnosis of leptospirosis in individual animals is often difficult because of the variation in the nature of the disease, the rapidity with which the organism dies in specimens once they are collected, and their transient appearance in various tissues. During the septicemic stage, leptospirae are present only in the blood and there may be laboratory evidence of acute hemolytic anemia and increased erythrocyte fragility and often hemoglobinuria. A leukopenia has been observed in cattle, and in other species there is a mild leukocytosis. However, the only positive diagnostic measure at this stage of the disease is culture of the blood. If abortion occurs, the kidney, lung, and pleural fluid of the aborted fetuses should be examined for the presence of the organism. Serologic testing at the time of abortion is often unreliable because the acute titers have already peaked and are declining. In the stage immediately after the subsidence of the fever, antibodies begin to develop and the leptospirae disappear from the blood and appear in the urine. The leptospiruria is accompanied by albuminuria of varying degrees and persists for varying lengths of time in the different species.

The diagnosis of leptospirosis is much easier on a herd basis than in a single animal, because in an infected herd some animals are certain to have high titers and the chances of demonstrating or isolating the organism in urine or milk are increased with samples being taken from many animals. On the other hand, in a single animal, depending on when the infection occurred, the titer may have declined to a low level and be difficult to interpret. This becomes particularly important for the clinician confronted with a diagnosis of abortion caused by leptospirosis in which the infection may have occurred several weeks previously and the serum may be negative or the titers too low for an accurate interpretation. Examination of the urine may be useful in these cases, but intermittent shedding of the pathogen by chronically infected animals must be taken into account.

Serologic and Related Tests

Acute and convalescent sera taken 7 to 10 days apart should be submitted from each clinically affected animal, or from those with a history of abortion, and sera should also be taken from 15% to 25% of apparently normal animals. Ten blood samples should be taken from each of the yearlings, the first-calf dams, the second-calf dams, and the mature age group to determine the infection status across the herd. If possible, wildlife or rodents known to inhabit the farm and use nearby water supplies should be captured and laboratory examinations of their tissues and blood performed and the results compared with those obtained in the farm animals.

MAT is the most common serologic test for the diagnosis of leptospirosis. It is the reference test against which all other serologic tests are evaluated and is the prescribed diagnostic test for international trade.[32] It is a serogroup-specific test, and a serovar representative of each expected serogroup in the region should be tested. Although the MAT does not usually cross-react with antibodies against other bacteria, there is significant cross-reactivity between serovars and serogroups of *Leptospira*. Therefore, MAT cannot be used to definitively identify a serovar causing infection.[32]

In animals that survive infection, acute leptospirosis can readily be diagnosed on the basis of demonstrating a rising antibody titer against specific serovars in acute and convalescent sera. MAT is particularly useful in diagnosis of disease associated with incidental, non–host-adapted serovars or acute disease associated with host-adapted serovars. It is less useful in the diagnosis of chronic disease in maintenance hosts, because antibody response to infection may be negligible in chronic infections or may persist from subclinical infections. In pigs, MAT has an adequate sensitivity for some serovars, such as pomona, but is insensitive to infection associated with bratislava. The herd serologic response to infection is often more helpful than the individual's response in chronic infections in maintenance hosts.

A major concern is the failure of the MAT to differentiate between titers after vaccination and those after natural infection because the titers may be of similar magnitude; however, titers after infection are generally higher and persist longer than vaccination titers. In any case, the vaccination history must be taken into account when interpreting positive MAT results.[34] MAT is not a measure of immunity to infection because vaccination results primarily in an IgG response, with low (1 : 100–1 : 400) and transient (1–4 months) titers, but immunity is common in vaccinated animals long after MAT titers are negative. There is no consensus on the appropriate cutoff value for seropositivity; a MAT titer of ≥1 : 100 is frequently considered positive, and a fourfold rise in titer on a paired sample taken 2 weeks apart is diagnostic. In abortion associated with incidental serovars, MAT titers against pomona and other incidental serovars are high, often ≥1 : 3000. Paired sera are of limited value in chronic infections or in cases of aborting cattle because abortion occurs after infection and titers are static or declining. If several aborting cows have high titers (≥1 : 300), this is evidence for the diagnosis of leptospirosis in unvaccinated herds.

The antibody enzyme-linked immunosorbent assay **(ELISA) test** is sensitive but lacks the serovar specificity of the MAT.[34] It has convenient technical features including automation and can be used efficiently as a screening test for large numbers of serum samples. ELISA can be useful for detection of recent infection (IgM) before agglutinating antibodies (IgG) are present, but it is of limited use in regions where vaccination with leptospiral vaccine is common practice.[34] Specific ELISAs for IgM or IgG antibodies are available. A positive IgM-specific ELISA result can therefore indicate that infection occurred within the previous month. For a diagnosis of leptospiral abortion in cattle, a titer of 1 : 3000 is proposed as the threshold for Pomona, but no similar critical figure is available for Hardjo. ELISAs have also been developed for the use in milk of individual cows or in bulk milk to detect antibodies against serovar Hardjo.

An **indirect ELISA** has been developed for the detection of bovine antibodies to multiple *Leptospira* serovars including Canicola, Copenhageni, Grippotyphosa, Hardjo, Pomona, and Sejroe.

An **antibody capture ELISA** is available to detect antibodies to a protective LPS fraction of *L. borgpetersenii* serovar Hardjo in cattle.

An ELISA has been used to detect a specific antibody to *L.* Hardjo in the cervicovaginal mucus as early as 2 weeks after natural or experimental infection and may reach high levels after 8 weeks. This may show some promise in diagnosis but has not yet been evaluated.

A commercially available **ELISA** and the **ImmunoComb Leptospirosis Kit,** which detect *L.* hardjo antibodies, have been compared with the MAT. The ImmunoComb and ELISA tests both exceeded the positive results obtained with the MAT. The ImmunoComb is very simple and quick, requiring no sophisticated equipment.

Aqueous Humor Antibody

Measurement of aqueous humor antibody titers against leptospires in horses offers a more accurate means of establishing a diagnosis of leptospiral-associated uveitis than serology alone.

Demonstration or Culture of Organism

A number of tests are available to detect leptospires or leptospiral DNA in tissues or body fluids.

Culture of Urine

Of all the laboratory diagnostic tests for leptospirosis, the examination of urine samples for the organism probably offers the best opportunity to demonstrate the presence of infection. Failure to demonstrate the presence of *Leptospira* in a urine sample does not rule out chronic infection because intermittent shedding is common. In individual animals, negative tests on three consecutive weekly urine samples has been considered to be good evidence that the animal is not a chronic renal carrier.[34] Collection of urine following treatment with a diuretic such as furosemide was found to increase the chances of detecting the organism in voided urine.[34] Treatment with antimicrobials in the recent past decreases the chances to recover the pathogen from urine of a chronically infected patient. For maximum efficiency, one-half of each urine sample should be submitted with added formalin (1 drop to 20–30 mL of urine) and the other half submitted in the fresh state. The formalin prevents bacterial overgrowth, and the fresh urine sample may be used for culture. A liquid culture medium of 1% bovine serum albumin solution containing 5-fluorouracil at 100 to 200 µg/mL should be used as transport medium.[34] *Leptospira* are fastidious and slow growing and culture requires incubation on special growth media for at least 16 and preferably 26 weeks.[34] The time required for detection varies with the serovar and the number of organisms present in the sample.

Examination of urine using **dark-field microscopy or fluorescent antibody test** are useful tests. The fluorescent antibody test is more sensitive than dark-field microscopy, detects degenerated as well as intact leptospires, and may be serovar specific.

Leptospira in tissue can be identified by a variety of **immunochemical staining** techniques, such immunofluorescence, or by various immunohistochemical techniques. These immunostain techniques are rapid and can be performed on material unsuitable for culture but require a minimum amount of bacterial antigen. Because the number of *Leptospira* present in tissue of chronically infected animals is low and often localized these methods are less suitable to identify chronic carrier states.[34]

PCR-based assays provide rapid and sensitive diagnostic techniques for detection or leptospiral DNA in body fluids and tissues. A variety of primers are used, some of which are only specific for the genus *Leptospira* and others designated to identify only pathogenic species. These PCR assays do not identify the infecting serovar, although it is possible to identify a specific species by sequencing the PCR amplicons.[34] Detection of leptospiral DNA with PCR-based assays in urine was found to be highly sensitive and specific to identify chronically infected and shedding cattle and horses. Several studies reported a considerable number of seronegative individuals that were *Leptospira* positive by urine PCR.[7-9] A multiplex PCR is highly sensitive for detection of the organism in aborted bovine fetuses. Using a *Leptospira* PCR assay, *L. kirschneri* has been identified as a potential cause of abortion in a fetal foal born on a farm with a history of repeated abortions. Further confirmation of *L. kirschneri* was done by DNA sequence analyses of the PCR-amplified DNA fragment.

Using PCR to detect the presence of *Leptospira* DNA, 70% of horses with uveitis were positive for *Leptospira* DNA, and 28% were culture positive for leptospires from the aqueous humor; only 6% of horses free of uveitis used as controls were positive. The serologic results did not correlate well with the presence of *Leptospira* DNA or organisms in the aqueous humor.

NECROPSY FINDINGS

Acute bovine leptospirosis is characterized by anemia, jaundice, hemoglobinuria, and subserosal hemorrhages. There may be ulcers and hemorrhages in the abomasal mucosa. Pulmonary edema and emphysema are also common in this species. Histologically, there is focal or diffuse interstitial nephritis and centrilobular hepatic necrosis and in some cases, there are vascular lesions in the meninges and brain in subacute to chronic infections. Leptospirae may be visible in silver-stained sections, especially in the proximal convoluted tubules of the kidney. In acute infections, there may be minimal inflammation, with only hemoglobin-filled renal tubules and centrilobular hepatic necrosis evident microscopically.

In the later stages, the characteristic finding is a progressive interstitial nephritis manifested by small, white, cortical foci that are initially raised but become slightly depressed as the lesion ages. Many clinically normal cattle presented to abattoirs have these lesions, which may represent sequela to episodes of bacteremia from a variety of pathogens and should not be considered pathognomonic for leptospirosis.

Aborted bovine fetuses are usually autolyzed to the point where no lesions or bacteria can be demonstrated. Even in a fresh fetus the positive identification of leptospirae in lesions is not an easy task. Culture of these organisms is difficult, and *L. interrogans* serovar Hardjo is particularly fastidious in its cultural requirements. The use of a fluorescent antibody technique assists in the demonstration of organisms, but false positives are common unless the test is interpreted by an experienced diagnostician. Dark-field microscopy may be attempted but is not well suited to tissues collected at necropsy. PCR techniques show considerable promise, although sample processing requirements are stringent, and the use of multiple primer sequences may be required in some cases. Immunoperoxidase techniques are highly useful in the demonstration of leptospirae in formalin-fixed tissues, although this test is not serovar specific. Traditional silver-based staining of fixed material is also successful in a few cases. Antibodies to leptospirae are detectable in the serum of some aborted fetuses.

Gross placental lesions in cases of equine abortion and stillbirth associated with leptospirosis include nodular cystic allantoic masses, diffuse edema, and areas of necrosis with a mucoid exudate on the chorionic surface. The liver is enlarged, mottled, and pale-red to yellow. The kidneys are swollen and edematous with pale, radiating streaks in both cortex and medulla. Microscopic changes may include a suppurative and nonsuppurative nephritis, dissociation of hepatocytes, a mixed leukocytic infiltration of portal triads, a giant cell hepatopathy, pneumonia, and myocarditis. Thrombosis, vasculitis, and a mixed population of inflammatory cells are evident in the placenta. A variety of tests, as described for cattle, are available to try to confirm the diagnosis.

Aborted piglets are usually severely autolytic, with bloodstained fluid in the subcutis and filling the body cavities. Multiple necrotic foci, 1 to 4 mm in diameter and irregular in outline, are found in the liver of approximately 40% of aborted fetuses. Microscopic inflammatory changes may also be found in the kidneys. The fetal membranes are thick and edematous. Leptospirae can be demonstrated using the battery of tests already mentioned for cattle.

Samples for Confirmation of Diagnosis

- **Bacteriology:** chilled kidney, liver, placenta [CULT (has special growth requirements), fluorescent antibody test [FAT], PCR]
- **Histology:** formalin-fixed kidney, liver, brain, heart, lung, placenta (LM, immunohistochemistry [IHC])
- **Serology:** heart-blood serum or pericardial fluid from fetus (MAT, ELISA).

The zoonotic potential of this organism should be noted when handling carcasses and submitting specimens.

DIFFERENTIAL DIAGNOSIS

The differential clinical diagnosis of the common forms of leptospirosis in each species is as follows.

Cattle

- Acute leptospirosis: Must be differentiated from those diseases causing hemolytic anemia with or without hemoglobinuria (Table 13-3), which include babesiosis, anaplasmosis, rape and kale poisoning postparturient hemoglobinuria, and bacillary hemoglobinuria.
- Chronic leptospirosis causing abortion: Must be differentiated from all other causes of abortion in cattle; most diagnostic surveys reveal that a specific cause is identifiable in only about 30% of fetuses submitted to a diagnostic laboratory. The vaccination history of the aborting cattle is a crucial part of the history since, for example, outbreaks of abortions caused by infectious bovine rhinotracheitis occur primarily in unvaccinated cows. The specific causes of abortion in cattle vary depending on geographic location. Other common causes of abortion in cattle include infectious bovine rhinotracheitis and protozoal abortion (*Sarcocystis* sp., *Toxoplasma gondii*, and *Neospora caninum*). Less common causes are brucellosis, bovine viral diarrhea, pine needle abortion, mycotic placentitis, campylobacter, ureaplasma, and possibly mycoplasma.
- Milk drop syndrome: Characterized by a sudden drop in milk yield in up to 30%-50% of the cows within several days. Must be differentiated from other causes of a decline in milk production of the herd including (1) change of feed, (2) change of management, and (3) epidemic of infectious disease such as bovine respiratory disease.

Sheep and goats

Chronic copper poisoning and poisoning caused by rape in sheep may present a clinical picture similar to that in leptospirosis, but there will be no febrile reaction. Anaplasmosis associated with *Anaplasma ovis* may be accompanied by fever and hemoglobinuria but is more commonly a chronic, emaciating disease.

Horses

- Abortion, stillbirths, and perinatal deaths of foals: Causes include *Streptococcus zooepidemicus, Salmonella abortivoequina, Escherichia coli, and Actinobacillus equuli.* Other bacterial infections include equine herpes virus, equine viral arteritis, and fungal infections. Diagnosis depends on laboratory examination of fetal tissues and fluids including bacterial culture, direct fluorescent antibody test for equine herpes virus and leptospires, serologic examination of fetal fluids for leptospiral antibodies using the microagglutinin test, and special stains to demonstrate leptospires in fetal tissues.
- Isoimmune hemolytic anemia: Within 36 hours after birth, there is weakness, hemoglobinuria, pallor, failure to suck, tachycardia, high case–fatality rate, and cross-matching blood tests.
- Infectious equine anemia: Symptoms include chronic relapsing fever, anemia, weakness, jaundice, edema, oral mucous membrane hemorrhages, and a Coggins serologic test is used for diagnosis.
- Exertional rhabdomyolysis: Symptoms include acute onset of stiff gait, weakness, sweating, distress, myoglobinuria, and creatine kinase test is used for diagnosis.
- Periodic ophthalmia: Differentiate from other causes of iridocyclitis of horses, and conjunctivitis, keratitis, and hypopyon, which may occur in equine viral arthritis.

Pigs

Abortion in the last trimester: The common manifestation of leptospirosis in pigs must be differentiated from all other causes of abortion, mummification, and stillbirths in swine. Other common causes of abortion in swine are parvovirus and porcine reproductive respiratory syndrome. Less common causes are brucellosis; pseudorabies; and the stillbirth, mummification, embryonic death, infertility virus.

TREATMENT

Treatment objectives can be to treat individuals with clinical disease or to treat chronically infected animals that may be clinically normally but chronically or intermittently shedding leptospires in urine.

Antimicrobial Therapy

In vitro studies indicate that leptospires are highly susceptible to ampicillin, amoxicillin, penicillin G, cefotaxime, erythromycin, and fluoroquinolone ciprofloxacin and have a good susceptibility to streptomycin, tylosin, and tetracyclines.

For infections caused by pomona, dihydrostreptomycin (12 mg/kg IM twice daily for 3 days) is effective in the treatment of the systemic infection. For the elimination of leptospiruria in cattle and pigs, a single dose of dihydrostreptomycin (25 mg/kg IM) has been recommended. In an outbreak in cattle, the simultaneous treatment of all animals with dihydrostreptomycin (25 mg/kg IM as single dose) and vaccination has been successful in preventing new cases and abortion when pregnant cattle are involved. A similar approach is recommended for outbreaks in swine. **Annual revaccination** and **regular serologic testing** for new infections, combined with controlling the source of new infections, will usually successfully control further outbreaks. A surveillance system in the area is necessary; however, to detect the introduction of new serotypes. The use of streptomycin/dihydrostreptomycin in food-producing animals has been discouraged because their administration, even at label dose, had the potential to lead to residue violations, and these substances are no longer available for the use in food-producing animals in some countries.[35] Oxytetracycline, amoxicillin, tilmicosin, and ceftiofur are also effective for resolving leptospirosis in cattle.

Dihydrostreptomycin G (25 mg/kg IM for 1 day, 3 days, or 5 days), or oxytetracycline (40 mg/kg IM daily for 3 days or 5 days), tylosin (44 mg/kg IM daily for 5 days), or erythromycin (25 mg/kg IM daily for 5 days) are all effective for treatment of persistent leptospirosis caused by Pomona in swine, although these dose protocols exceed label recommendations. In groups of pigs, the feeding of oxytetracycline (800 g/t of feed for 8–11 days) is claimed to eliminate carriers. Antimicrobial feeding should begin 1 month before farrowing to avoid the occurrence of abortion.

For outbreaks of **leptospiral abortion in horses**, treatment of pregnant mares with dihydrostreptomycin (50 mg/kg) IM daily for 3 to 5 days can minimize further abortions; this treatment regimen, however, has not been extensively evaluated.

For **equine periodic ophthalmia**, most recommended treatments have little effect on the course of the disease. A course of a suitable antibiotic systemically, and the administration of a corticosteroid, either parenterally in an acute episode or subconjunctivally in a chronic case, is most likely to be satisfactory. Nonulcerative keratouveitis requires long-term and intensive medication and recurs with tapering of treatment. Topical and subconjunctival corticosteroids are recommended in controlling nonulcerative keratouveitis. Intravitreal implantation of cyclosporine is effective. Atropine eye ointment is also usually applied three times daily to maintain dilatation of the pupil.

Blood Transfusions

Blood transfusions (5–10 L/450 kg BW) are indicated as treatment for the hemolytic anemia in acute leptospirosis in cattle. The clinical indications for a blood transfusion include obvious pallor of the mucous membranes, weakness, and tachycardia.

Table 13-3 Differential diagnosis of diseases of cattle characterized by acute hemolytic anemia with or without hemoglobinuria

Disease	Epidemiology	Clinical findings	Laboratory findings
Leptospirosis	All ages, cattle on pasture	Acute fever, red-colored milk Hemoglobinuria abortion; may die in 24–48 hours	Leptospira titers
Postparturient hemoglobinuria	High-producing lactating cows 4–6 weeks postpartum	Acute; no changes in milk; no fever; die in 12–48 hours; marked hemoglobinuria	Hypophosphatemia
Bacillary hemoglobinuria	Usually mature cattle on summer pasture in enzootic area	Acute fever, abdominal pain; may die in 2–4 days; hemoglobinuria	Leukopenia or leukocytosis
Babesiosis	Enzootic areas, tick borne, young animals	Acute fever, jaundice, abortion, course of 2–3 weeks; marked hemoglobinuria	Blood smear, complement fixation test, transmission tests
Anaplasmosis	Yearling and mature cattle, common in summer, insect borne, common in feedlots	*No* hemoglobinuria, jaundice common, fever	Anaplasms on blood smear, complement fixation test
Chronic copper poisoning	Follows long-term oral administration of medicines or feeds containing copper	Severe jaundice; no fever Hemoglobinuria	Toxic levels of copper in blood, liver, and feces
Cold-water hemolytic anemia of calves	Following consumption of large quantities of cold water after period of limited intake	Sudden onset within 1 hour after ingestion; no fever; may die in a few hours; hemoglobinuria	Acute hemolytic anemia
Rape and kale poisoning	All ages of cattle on rape crop grown for fodder in fall	Peracute hemolytic anemia, may die in a few hours after onset; no fever Hemoglobinuria	Acute hemolytic anemia
Drug induced	Some drug preparations when given IV	Mild hemoglobinuria; no hemolytic anemia	Nil
Blood transfusion reaction	Using blood from same donor more than 1 week after initial transfusion	Sudden onset, dyspnea, hiccoughs, trembling, responds to adrenalin	Nil

The common causes of hematuria in cattle are pyelonephritis and cystitis caused by Corynebacterium renale*, nonspecific cystitis, and enzootic hematuria. Myoglobinuria occurs occasionally in young cattle affected with enzootic-nutritional muscular dystrophy and may be confused with hemoglobinuria.*

Treatment and Control

Cattle

Dihydrostreptomycin (25 mg/kg IM every 24 hours for 3–5 days) (R-2)

Oxytetracycline (20 mg/kg IM every 24 hours for 3–5 days) (R-2)

Oxytetracycline, long acting (20 mg/kg IM as a single or repeated dose) (R-2)

Tilmicosin (20 mg/kg SC as a single dose) (R-2)

Tulathromycin (2.5 mg/kg SC as single dose) (R-2)

Tylosin (18 mg/kg every 24 hours for 3–5 days) (R-2)

Erythromycin 8 mg/kg IM every 24 hours for 5 days (R-2)

Horses (abortion)

Dihydrostreptomycin (50 mg/kg IM every 24 hours for 3–5 days) (R-2)

Swine

Dihydrostreptomycin (25 mg/kg IM every 24 hours for 3–5 days) (R-2)

Oxytetracycline[a] (40 mg/kg IM every 24 hours for 3–5 days) (R-2)

Tylosin[a] (44 mg/kg every 24 hours IM for 5 days) (R-2)

Erythromycin[a] (25 mg/kg IM for 5 days) (R-2)

Control

Dihydrostreptomycin (25 mg/kg IM as a single dose) to all positive reactors (R-2)

Oxytetracycline, long acting (20 mg/kg IM as a single dose to all positive reactors) (R-2)

Tilmicosin (20 mg/kg SC as a single dose to all positive reactors) (R-2)

Tulathromycin (2.5 mg/kg SC as single dose to all positive reactors) (R-2)

Vaccination with multivalent vaccines[b] of exposed animals in an infected herd (R-2)

Vaccination with multivalent vaccines[b] of replacement heifers within 4–6 months of age (R-2)

[a]Dosage protocol exceeds label recommendations.
[b]Limited efficacy against infection with serovar hardjo.
IM, intramuscular; SC, subcutaneous.

CONTROL

Biosecurity and Biocontainment

The first step in control is to identify the source of the original source of infection and to interrupt transmission. Sources of infection include clinically affected animals, aborted fetuses, placentas, carrier animals, wildlife, dogs and cats, and environmental sources such as water supplies. Education about leptospirosis is an effective method for reducing its incidence and its effects. Intensive well-directed education and publicity campaigns in New Zealand, used in conjunction with a campaign for immunization of cattle, reduced the incidence of leptospirosis. Groups to which educational efforts should be directed include professionals in human and veterinary medicine and public health, primary human and animal health care practitioners, wildlife and conservation scientists, water and sewage engineers and planners, health administrators and educators, and last but not least, the public at risk.

Three main considerations are important when assessing the risks and likely financial implications of the disease to dairy producers:

1. Likelihood of a herd being infected
2. Likely effects of the disease on the dairy enterprise, both physically and financially, following the initial infection compared with a leptospirosis-free herd
3. Likely longer term effects of the disease

The probability of infection of cattle by *L.* Hardjo is increased by **four factors**:

1. Purchase of infected cattle
2. Cograzing or common grazing with infected cattle or sheep
3. Use of natural service with an infected bull
4. Access of cattle to contaminated water such as streams, rivers, flood, or drainage water

Assessment of the risks facing different types of herds suffering losses from *L.* hardjo can then be used to help support decisions concerning control of the disease.

Producers with one or more of the main risk factors should consider strategies that

(1) directly remove or diminish those risk factors or (2) indirectly diminish their importance for the herd, for example, by vaccination. Strategies that successfully diminish one or more of the risk factors but leave one other will yield little benefit because of the importance of each of the identified risk factors.

Vaccination is one strategy that can diminish all of the risk factors and provide some degree of assurance against potentially high and costly disease losses. Producers with high-risk herds are likely to choose vaccination. If a herd continues to have any of the risk factors, then whole-herd vaccination is likely to be the preferred option; otherwise the disease could easily be reintroduced. Decision tree analysis of leptospirosis vaccination in beef cattle in Australia indicates that the beneficial economic effects of vaccination depend on the value of the calf and the probability of calf loss caused by leptospirosis.

Eradication

Detection and elimination of carrier animals presents some difficulties. Positive reactors to the MAT do not necessarily void infective urine continuously, and chronically infected animals may shed leptospires while being serologically negative.[7-9] Repeated examination of the urine for the organism, either by culture or PCR, may be necessary to identify carrier animals. For practical purposes, serologically suspicious and positive reactors should be considered carriers and culled or treated as described previously.

In groups of pigs, it should be assumed that infection is herdwide and all pigs should be treated as though they were carriers. In these circumstances, the feeding of antimicrobials provides some protection, although it is not guaranteed to eliminate the carrier state. Leptospirosis has been eradicated from commercial pig herds by treating all pigs with dihydrostreptomycin at 25 mg/kg IM at one time. However, if the pigs have been exposed to heavy infection, not all of them are completely cleared of leptospiruria, and further treatment will be necessary.

In cattle herds, if the bulls are infected then they should not be used naturally or for artificial insemination even though the antimicrobials in the semen diluent is sufficient to ensure that no spread occurs. Elimination of infection can be difficult, especially in large commercial herds in an endemic area in which replacement cows and bulls are introduced from saleyards and cattle mingle with other herds on the range. Eradication of **Hardjo** is a possibility in purebred herds in which intensive measures are economically feasible, and owners should be urged to undertake a program to eliminate leptospirosis from the herd and to prevent its entry. **The following measures** can be taken to eliminate hardjo infection:

1. Judicious combination of group serologic testing
2. Segregation of age classes
3. Selective vaccination
4. Possibly artificial insemination
5. Isolation of the herd from outside sources of infection.

Bulls suspected of spreading infection should be treated to reduce the level of urinary shedding regardless of subsequent vaccination. Exposure of cattle to herds, heavily infected with leptospirosis, for example, on communal grazing pastures should be avoided. The herd should be monitored periodically, coincident with other serologic testing. In endemic areas, all cattle over 6 to 9 months of age should be vaccinated, and vaccination should be continued for up to 5 years to minimize the number of susceptible cattle until no long-term shedders remain in the herd.

Simple management procedures to limit the infection in beef cows until their second calves are born and the culling of older carriers can greatly decrease and possibly eradicate the infection from a herd. Virgin yearling bulls are used on virgin yearling heifers, and young cows are segregated from older cows until 38 to 39 months of age when they go to pasture after being bred with their second calf. This delays direct exposure of heifers to infected cattle until their third breeding. These practices must be combined by monitoring infection by serologic and other laboratory methods.

If eradication is attempted and completed, introduced animals should be required to pass a serologic test on two occasions at least 2 weeks apart before allowing them to enter the herd. Urine examination for leptospirae should be performed if practicable.

Hygiene

Control of the source of the organism is achieved by appropriate hygienic strategies. If the environmental sources of infection are identifiable, in the form of yards, marshes, and damp calf pens, every attempt must be made to avoid animal contact with these infective surroundings. Wet areas should be drained or fenced and pens disinfected after use by infected animals. The possibility that rats and other wild animals may act as a source of infection suggests that contact between them and farm animals should be controlled.

Vaccination

Vaccination against leptospirosis in cattle and swine is in general use and an effective method for control of the disease. In New Zealand, a publicity campaign to promote the widespread vaccination of cattle resulted in a marked reduction in the incidence of human leptospirosis. Most of the vaccines are formalin-inactivated bacterins containing one or more serotypes. Vaccines containing Freund's complete adjuvant induce higher serologic responses but not necessarily superior protection. The immune response is serotype specific and protection is dependent on the use of bacterins containing serotypes prevalent in the area. The bacterins induce a low titer to the MAT, which appears early and declines after several weeks; however, protective immunity against the disease and renal infection persists for at least 12 months in cattle. Regular serologic testing in herds vaccinated annually can be used to monitor new infections because these will induce a titer to the MAT. However, neither the ELISA nor the MAT can reliably differentiate serologic responses in cattle after leptospiral vaccination from those following natural infections.

Cattle

The difficulty of keeping purebred herds free of Hardjo infection increases as the reservoir of infection increases. Several control measures can be applied, especially in large herds that are at high risk. In endemic areas, transmission in commercial herds can be suppressed by annual vaccination of bulls, replacement heifers, and 2- and 3-year-old females a few weeks before release of the bulls. Potential replacement heifer calves should be handled and raised in segregation from the adult herd after weaning and vaccinated a month before exposure to older cattle. Herd sires should be purchased from uninfected herds or at least purchased subject to a negative serologic test.

Vaccination as part of a herd health program should start with the calves at 4 to 6 months of age, followed by revaccination annually. Such programs should provide significant rises in calving rates, but have little or no effect on perinatal or postnatal losses.

Bovine Leptospiral Vaccines and Their Efficacy

Current bovine multivalent leptospiral bacterins are inactivated whole-cell vaccines containing *L. interrogans* serovar Hardjo, Canicola, Pomona, and Icterohaemorrhagiae and *L. kirschneri* serovar Grippotyphosa and generally induce protective immunity against infection with non–host-adapted strains. In contrast, protection against the host-adapted serovar Hardjo is more elusive with conflicting evidence about vaccine efficacy. Vaccination of cattle with a pentavalent leptospiral vaccine containing either Hardjo-bovis or Hardjo-prajitno failed to protect cattle from experimental infection with hardjo-bovis 6 months after vaccination. They also failed to prevent abortion, stillbirth, and vertical transmission of infection when vaccinated cows were challenged with *L. borgpetersenii* serovar Hardjo during pregnancy, and the infection rates for control and vaccinated cattle did not differ. The Hardjo-bovis vaccine is more antigenic than the hardjo-prajitno as measured by higher antibody titers in vaccinated animals. Calves as young as 4 weeks of age, vaccinated in the presence of maternally derived antibody, can be fully protected against homologous virulent challenge.[36] However, monovalent vaccines with a field isolate of *L. borgpetersenii* serovar Hardjo and another with *L. interrogans* serovar Hardjo found these vaccines prevented infection and colonization following challenge with *L. borgpetersenii* serovar Hardjo strains from the United States and Europe.

A protective killed vaccine against serovar hardjo induced a strong, sustained Th1 or cell-mediated response. The vaccine is composed of a whole-cell bovine isolate of *L. borgpetersenii* serovar Hardjo and aluminum hydroxide and is given as two doses subcutaneously 4 weeks apart. Following vaccination, a Th1 cell-mediated response occurred characterized by the production of IFN-γ cells including CD4+ and WC1 gamma delta T cells.

A monovalent *L. borgpetersenii* serovar Hardjo (type Hardjo-bovis) vaccine commercially available in Australia, New Zealand, Ireland, and the UK, given as two doses, 4 weeks apart, protected heifers against renal colonization and urinary shedding when challenged with *L. borgpetersenii* serovar Hardjo strain 203, 4 months after vaccination. None of the animals shed leptospires in their urine or kidneys at necropsy. In contrast, all nonvaccinated control heifers became infected with serovar Hardjo and shed organisms in their urine. A pentavalent leptospiral vaccine with serovar Hardjo (type Hardjo-bovis) also containing BHV1, BVDV, PI-3, and BRSV fractions against important viral respiratory pathogens was found to protect heifers vaccinated at 1 month of age from colonization of the kidney and to reduce leptospiral shedding with urine in experimentally challenged animals for at least 1 year.[37]

Two monovalent hardjo vaccines provided protection from infection against *L. borgpetersenii* serovar Hardjo, whereas a pentavalent vaccine containing the Hardjo organisms did not. The protective monovalent vaccines produced strong cell-mediated immune responses in vaccinated cattle as demonstrated by proliferation of lymphocytes and production of IFN-γ by their PBMCs in response to culture with serovar hardjo antigens. This response is generally much lower or absent in antigen-stimulated cultures of PBMC from cattle vaccinated with the pentavalent vaccine and nonvaccinated cattle.

In conclusion, protective immunity to serovar Hardjo correlates with induction of a substantial immune response that is characterized by antigen-specific IFN-γ-producing T cells. There is no cross-immunity between *L.* Pomona and Hardjo, and in areas where both diseases occur, a bivalent vaccine is used routinely. If separate vaccines are used the *L.* Pomona vaccine should be administered at least once annually, but the *L.* Hardjo vaccine provides some protection against *L.* szwajizak.

Swine

Vaccination of sows and gilts before breeding with a bivalent vaccine, containing pomona and tarassovi, protects them against infection and the development of leptospiruria and is widely practiced, especially in large intensive piggeries. In the United-States, vaccination of gilts and sows with two doses of a bacterin containing five or six leptospiral serovars, one of which contained Bratislava, before the first breeding and thereafter before each breeding improves reproductive performance. *L.* Bratislava is an important cause of abortions in sows in North America and Europe, and vaccination is effective. Vaccination of pregnant gilts and sows can provide protection to the piglets for the first several weeks after birth.

Vaccination and Antimicrobial Strategies

Whether or not to vaccinate depends on the cost of the procedure relative to the losses that can be anticipated. If the disease is spreading rapidly, as evidenced by the frequent appearance of clinical cases with a high range of titers or rising titers in a number of animals, then (1) all clinical cases and positive reactors should be treated, (2) the negative animals vaccinated, and (3) the herd should be moved on the first day of treatment to a clean field. Retesting a group to determine the rate of spread would be an informative procedure, but active measures must usually be commenced before this information is available. Another variation of this program, and a highly practical one, is the vaccination of all cattle in the herd and the treatment with one dose of dihydrostreptomycin (25 mg/kg IM) of all pregnant cows to eliminate renal infection and leptospiruria. However, antimicrobial therapy is not highly efficacious, especially in cattle infected with Hardjo.

A successful control strategy has been described for Hardjo infection in a large, closed beef herd. All animals were treated with dihydrostreptomycin once followed by removal to a clean pasture to prevent new cases and annual vaccination of the whole herd for 5 years. All cattle introduced into the herd were treated with the antimicrobial and quarantined; at the end of the trial the entire herd was treated prophylactically with the antimicrobial to minimize the risk of residual infection. By the end of the trial all young stock entering the breeding program were seronegative. There was serologic evidence of a high level of control, and bacteriologic monitoring at the end of the trial indicated that Hardjo had been eliminated from the herd.

Vaccination is also recommended to protect animals continuously exposed to infection from wildlife, other domestic species, and rodents. The serologic status of these groups can also be determined as necessary before a decision is made to vaccinate.

If only sporadic cases occur, it may be more profitable to attempt to dispose of reactors or treat them to ensure that they no longer act as carriers. A degree of immunity is likely to occur in pigs after natural infection, and when the disease is endemic "herd immunity" may significantly decrease incidence of clinical disease.

One of the theoretical disadvantages of vaccination is the possible development of renal carrier animals that are sufficiently immune to resist systemic invasion but not colonization of the kidney, which leads to the development of a carrier animal with transient leptospiruria. This may occur but not frequently enough to invalidate vaccination.

FURTHER READING

Adler B. *History of Leptospirosis and Leptospira. Leptospira and Leptospirosis.* Berlin: Springer; 2015:1-9.
Adler B. Pathogenesis of leptospirosis: cellular and molecular aspects. *Vet Microbiol.* 2014;172:353-358.
Adler B, Pena-Moctezuma de la A. Leptospira. In: Gyles CL, Prescott JF, Songer JG, Thoen CO, eds. *Pathogenesis of Bacterial Infections in Animals.* 3rd ed. Oxford, UK: Blackwell; 2004:385-396.
Bharti AR, Nally JE, Ricaldi JN, et al. Leptospirosis: a zoonotic disease of global importance. *Lancet Infect Dis.* 2003;3:757-771.
Ellis WA. Leptospirosis as a cause of reproductive failure. Diagnosis of abortion. *Vet Clin North Am Food Anim Pract.* 1994;10:463-478.
Faine SB, Adler CA, Bolin CA, Perolat P. *Leptospira and Leptospirosis.* 2nd ed. Melbourne: MedSci Press; 1999.

REFERENCES

1. Cerqueira GM, Picardeau M. *Infect Genet Evol.* 2009;9:760.
2. Levett PN. *Clin Microbiol Rev.* 2001;14:296.
3. Adler B, de la Peña-Moctezuma A. *Vet Microbiol.* 2010;140:287.
4. Lau CL, et al. *Trans R Soc Trop Med Hyg.* 2010;104:631.
5. Martins G, et al. *Vet Rec.* 2010;167:629.
6. Jansen A, et al. *Emerg Infect Dis.* 2005;11:1048.
7. Otaka DY, et al. *Vet Rec.* 2012;170:338.
8. Hammond C, et al. *Vet Rec.* 2012;171:105.
9. Hernández-Rodríguez P, et al. *J Microbiol Methods.* 2011;84:1.
10. Bolin CA. *Proc North Am Vet Conf.* 2005.
11. Van de Weyer LM, et al. *Can Vet J.* 2011;52:619.
12. Subharat S, et al. *New Zeal Vet J.* 2012;60:215.
13. Lindahl E, et al. *Acta Vet Scand.* 2011;53:53.
14. Rifatbegovic M, Maksimocic Z. *Turk J Vet Anim Sci.* 2011;35:459.
15. Heesterber UW, et al. *J S Afr Vet Assoc.* 2009;80:45.
16. Ayanegui-Alcerreca MA, et al. *New Zeal Vet J.* 2007;55:102.
17. Ciceroni L, et al. *J Vet Med B.* 2000;47:217.
18. Ellis GR, et al. *Aust Vet J.* 2008;71:203.
19. Suepaul SM, et al. *Trop Anim Health Prod.* 2011;43:367.
20. Motte A, Myers DM. *Trop Anim Health Prod.* 2006;18:113.
21. Agunloye CA. *Israel J Vet Med.* 2002;57:2.
22. Lilienbaum W, et al. *Res Vet Sci.* 2008;84:14.
23. Baverud V, et al. *Acta Vet Scand.* 2009;51:15.
24. Hartskeerl RA, et al. *Clin Microbiol Infect.* 2011;17:494.
25. Pappas G, et al. *Int J Infect Dis.* 2008;12:351.

26. The Center of Food Security and Public Health. At <http://www.cfsph.iastate.edu/Factsheets/pdfs/leptospirosis.pdf>; 2005 Accessed 15.02.04.
27. Monahan AM, et al. *J Appl Microbiol.* 2009;107:707.
28. Jansen A, et al. *Emerg Infect Dis.* 2007;13:739.
29. Koizumi N, et al. *J Vet Med Sci.* 2009;71:797.
30. Marchiori E, et al. *Lung.* 2011;115:155.
31. Kohn B, et al. *J Vet Intern Med.* 2010;24:1277.
32. Broux B, et al. *J Vet Intern Med.* 2012;26:684.
33. Marinho M, et al. *Am J Trop Med Hyg.* 2009;80:832.
34. OIE terrestrial manual. At <http://www.oie.int/fileadmin/Home/eng/Health_standards/tahm/2.01.09_LEPTO.pdf>; 2008 Accessed 21.06.15.
35. Australian pesticides and veterinary medicine authority. At <http://apvma.gov.au/node/15006>; 2005 Accessed 21.06.15.
36. Zuerner RL, et al. *Clin Vacc Immunol.* 2011;18:684.
37. Zimmernan AD, et al. *J Am Vet Med Assoc.* 2013;242:1573.

BOVINE PYELONEPHRITIS

SYNOPSIS

Etiology *Corynebacterium renale* and *Escherichia coli* are the most common causative agents.

Epidemiology There is incidental disease with worldwide occurrence. Organisms pertain to normal flora of the lower urogenital tract. Ascending infection is most common in adult cows within weeks after calving, occasionally in calves as a complication of omphalourachitis. Predisposing factors are vaginal/uterine infection or immunosuppression.

Clinical findings Periodic episodes of hematuria, pyuria, colic, straining to urinate, fever, loss of condition, and drop in milk production are observed. Palpable abnormality of kidney, ureters, and bladder on rectal examination. Cystitis is determined by endoscopic examination and pyelonephritis by ultrasound examination.

Clinical pathology Cloudy urine with hematuria, proteinuria; on microscopic examination there is increased cellularity of sediment with bacteria. Elevated serum total protein, globulin and fibrinogen, and low serum albumin. Cases with markedly elevated serum creatinine and urea nitrogen concentrations have poor prognosis.

Necropsy findings Cystitis and pyelonephritis are found.

Diagnostic confirmation Gross changes in urine, together with palpable abnormalities in the urinary tract, and the presence of bacteria in the urine are seen.

Treatment Prognosis is fair at best, prolonged course of antimicrobial therapy, and nephrectomy in unresponsive cases.

Control Avoidance of urinary catheterization and artificial insemination.

ETIOLOGY

Pyelonephritis is an inflammation of the renal pelvis and renal parenchyma resulting from an ascending bacterial urinary tract infection. *C. renale* and *E. coli* are the pathogens most commonly isolated from cattle with pyelonephritis. Other bacteria that have been associated with bovine pyelonephritis include *C. pilosum, C. cystitidis, Trueperella* (formerly *Arcanobacterium) pyogenes, Proteus* spp., α-hemolytic *Streptococcus* spp., and *Staphylococcus.*[1,2] *C. pilosum* and *C. cystitidis* are commonly isolated in conjunction with *C. renale* but are considered part of the normal flora of the vulva.

Infection with *C. renale* may stimulate production of an antibody that causes cross-reactions with the complement-fixing test for Johne's disease.

EPIDEMIOLOGY

Occurrence

Although the disease is widespread in Europe, North America, Australia, Africa, Japan, and Israel and probably occurs all over the world, it seldom constitutes an important problem in any herd or area. As a rule, clinical cases are **sporadic**, even in herds found to harbor a significant number of carriers. Differences in disease prevalence can probably be explained by differences in predisposing management factors. One study in 7 herds found an annual incidence that varied from 0.5% to 1.5% and in one herd was 16%. A slaughterhouse survey conducted in the United States estimated the prevalence of pyelonephritis in the dairy cattle population with less than 1%.[3] Subclinical infection may be more frequent than first recognized, and 13% of adult cattle have bacteria associated with pyelonephritis in their bladder at slaughter, in the absence of gross or histologic evidence of pyelonephritis or cystitis.[4] Chronic cystitis and pyelonephritis (etiology unstated) have been found in 5.3% and 0.2% of cattle at slaughter.

Although pyelonephritis is considered to be a predominantly a bovine disease, sheep are occasionally affected.

Source of Infection and Transmission

Both *C. renale* and *E. coli* pertain to the resident flora of the lower urogenital tract of cattle. *C. renale* can be isolated from urine of affected or **carrier** animals and in Japan has been isolated from the vagina or vaginal vestibule of approximately 6% of healthy cows. Clinically and subclinically infected cattle can shed *C. renale* with urine for prolonged periods into the environment, in which it can survive for over 50 days. The incidence of cows excreting *C. renale* in their urine is higher in herds where the disease occurs than in herds where the disease is unknown.

In cattle, infection can be **transmitted** by direct contact, by the use of contaminated brushes, or by the careless use of **catheters.**

Venereal transmission of *C. renale* infection has also been proposed. This is suggested by the occasional occurrence of a series of cases in a herd, usually related to the use of a particular bull, and the cessation of cases when artificial insemination is used. The organism can often be isolated from the prepuce, urethra, and semen of bulls that have no detectable lesions in the prepuce. *C. renale* can be a cause of balanoposthitis in bulls.

Ascending infection of the urinary tract with *E.coli* has generally attributed to fecal contamination of the urinary tract, frequently in association with impaired urinary tract defense.[1]

Risk Factors

Animal Risk Factors

Pyelonephritis is most common in adult cows in the weeks to months following parturition. In young calves pyelonephritis can often be traced back to an ascending umbilical infection.[2] Female cattle are more susceptible to ascending urinary tract infections than males presumably because of a shorter and wider urethra. In bulls and steers pyelonephritis may occur as a complication of a urinary tract obstruction.

Approximately 75% of clinical cases occur in postparturient cows following abortion, dystocia, or puerperal infection, suggesting that inflammation and infection of the lower urogenital tract presents as an important predisposing factor.[2]

Pathogen Risk Factors

C. renale and *E.coli* are normal inhabitants of the lower urogenital tract of ruminants, but certain strains possess pili, a virulence factor facilitating the colonization of the mucosa of the urinary tract and the progression of the infection. Piliated strains of both bacteria occur and have a greatly enhanced ability to adhere to epithelial cells of the urinary tract.

Environmental Risk Factors

An increase in clinical cases is usually found in the colder seasons of the year and heavily fed, high-producing dairy herds appear to show an increased susceptibility.

The systematic use of urinary catheters to collect urine from cows in early lactation with suspect ketosis has been associated with increased occurrence rates of pyelonephritis. Although not intentionally produced, the disease occurred in 10% of a group of cattle used to teach veterinary students the technique of urinary catheterization.

In Israel, the ingestion of rock rose (*Cistus salvifolius*) is reported to produce urinary retention and predisposes cattle to pyelonephritis.

Economic Importance

Unless appropriate treatment is instituted early, the disease is highly fatal and economic loss is mainly caused by the deaths of affected animals.

PATHOGENESIS

Pyelonephritis usually develops as an **ascending urinary tract infection** involving successively the bladder, ureters, and kidneys. Trauma to the urethra, urine stasis, or a patent urachus in calves may facilitate ascending infection. The destruction of renal tissue and obstruction of urinary outflow ultimately result in uremia and the death of the animal.

Piliated and nonpiliated forms of *C. renale* are present in infected animals, but their relative importance to the pathogenesis of the disease is uncertain. Piliated forms of *C. renale* and *E. coli* have a greater ability to attach to urinary tract epithelium, are more resistant to phagocytosis, and are probably important to the carriage of the organism and to the initial ascending infection. However, in the course of an infection there is a shift from piliated to nonpiliated forms, which may reflect a response to the development of antipilus antibodies.

CLINICAL FINDINGS

Early signs vary considerably from case to case. The first sign observed may be the passage of **bloodstained or cloudy urine** in an otherwise normal cow. In other cases, the first sign may be an attack of acute **colic**, manifested by swishing of the tail, treading of the feet and kicking at the abdomen, and straining to urinate. The attack passes off in a few hours. Such attacks are caused by obstruction of a ureter or renal calyx by pus or tissue debris and may be confused with acute intestinal obstruction. More often the onset is gradual with a **fluctuating temperature** (about 39.5°C; 103°F), **capricious appetite**, loss of condition, and **drop in milk yield** over a period of weeks. Other than this, there is little systemic reaction, and the diagnostic signs are associated with the urinary tract.

The most **obvious sign** is the presence of **blood, pus, mucus, and tissue debris in urine**, particularly in the last portion voided (Fig. 13-5). Urination is frequent, may occur in a dribble rather than a stream, and may be painful. Periods during which the urine is abnormal may be followed by apparent recovery with later remissions.

In the early stages, **rectal examination** may be unremarkable, but later there is usually detectable thickening and contraction of the bladder wall and enlargement of one or both ureters. These are not normally palpable, but in chronic cases they may be felt in their course from the renal pelvis of the left kidney to the bladder. The terminal portion of the ureters may also be palpated through the floor of the vagina over the neck of the bladder. The palpable left kidney may show enlargement, absence of lobulation, and pain on palpation; the right kidney may be palpable in small ruminants if it is significantly enlarged. In many cases there are no distinct clinical signs referable to the urinary tract, and the history and clinical signs may be weight loss and suspected gastrointestinal disease. In these cases, examination of the urine is essential to diagnosis. The course is usually several weeks or even months and the terminal signs are those of uremia.

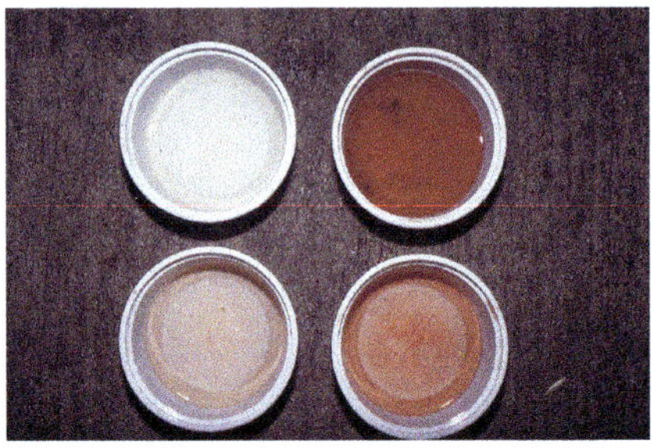

Fig. 13-5 Change in urine appearance during voiding in a Holstein-Friesian cow with chronic cystitis. Top left is from the initial urine stream, followed by the bottom left, and bottom right, and the top right is the last urine voided. Notice the presence of blood clots in the last urine sample.

Endoscopic examination of the urethra and bladder can be diagnostic. **Ultrasound** examination shows cystic changes in the affected kidney, a reduction in renal pelvis diameter, a reduction in renal parenchyma, a widened ureter, and a hyperechoic bladder wall.[5]

CLINICAL PATHOLOGY

Urine analysis reveals proteinuria and hematuria, and the latter is grossly apparent in most cases. Urine pH is greater than 8.5 in most but not all cases, whereas the specific gravity has been recorded between 1.008 and 1.021.[2] Microscopic examination will show pyuria. The presence of bacteria in suspected urine can be confirmed by culture, specific immunofluorescence, or direct microscopic examination.

Hematologic and blood biochemical examination reveals hypoalbuminemia and hypergammaglobulinemia in advanced cases. Neutrophilia may be present but is not constant in all cases. Serum creatinine and BUN are elevated in advanced and severe cases, but these parameters are not reliable indicators for the presence of pyelonephritis in mild or early cases.[2] Serum creatinine and BUN concentrations above 1.5 and 100 mg/dL, respectively, carry a grave prognosis.

Ultrasonography was found useful to confirm the diagnosis and determine the extent of the disease. In particular this allows examination of the right kidney, which is not accessible by rectal examination. Ultrasonography may demonstrate cystic changes in the affected kidney, dilated renal sinuses and ureters, and a thickened echogenic bladder.[2,5]

NECROPSY FINDINGS

With pyelonephritis, the kidneys are usually enlarged and the lobulation less evident than normal (Fig. 13-6). The renal calyces and grossly enlarged ureters contain blood, pus, and mucus. Light-colored necrotic areas may be observed on the kidney surface. Changes visible on the cut surface include excavation of papillae, abscessation, and wedge-shaped areas of necrosis that extend from the distal medulla into the cortex. The bladder and urethra are thick walled and their mucous membranes are hemorrhagic, edematous, and eroded (Fig. 13-7). Histologically, the renal lesions are a confusing mixture of acute suppurative changes and various degrees of fibrosis with mononuclear cell infiltration.

Samples for Confirmation of Diagnosis

- Bacteriology: kidney; culture swab from ureter (CULT)
- Histology: formalin-fixed kidney, ureter, bladder (LM)

DIFFERENTIAL DIAGNOSIS

Cases characterized by acute colic
- Acute intestinal obstruction
- Urinary tract obstruction in bulls and steers

Chronic cases
- Traumatic reticulitis

Blood in urine
- Cystitis
- Urolithiasis
- Enzootic hematuria
- Postparturient hemoglobinuria
- Anaplasmosis/babesiosis
- Leptospirosis

TREATMENT

Treatment recommendations for pyelonephritis reported in the literature are empirical, and unfortunately strong data supporting their clinical efficacy are not available. Common wisdom holds that pyelonephritis caused by *C. renale* is best treated with penicillin administered parenterally daily for at least 2 to 3 weeks. For cases of suspected or confirmed infection with *E. coli* a broad-spectrum antimicrobial should be chosen. A number of antimicrobials, including ampicillin, amoxicillin, tetracycline, trimethoprim-sulfas, ceftiofur, and gentamycin have been proposed.

In early cases where little structural damage has occurred, permanent recovery can be expected following such a course of treatment. Generally, a good prognosis is suggested by an improvement in condition, appetite, and milk yield and clearing of the urine. However, in well-established cases with extensive tissue destruction the prognosis is fair at best, relief is only transient, and relapses are common. For valuable animals, in which ultrasound has established the diagnosis and confirmed that the contralateral kidney is unaffected, unilateral nephrectomy may be an alternative with reasonable prognosis.[6] The surgical technique

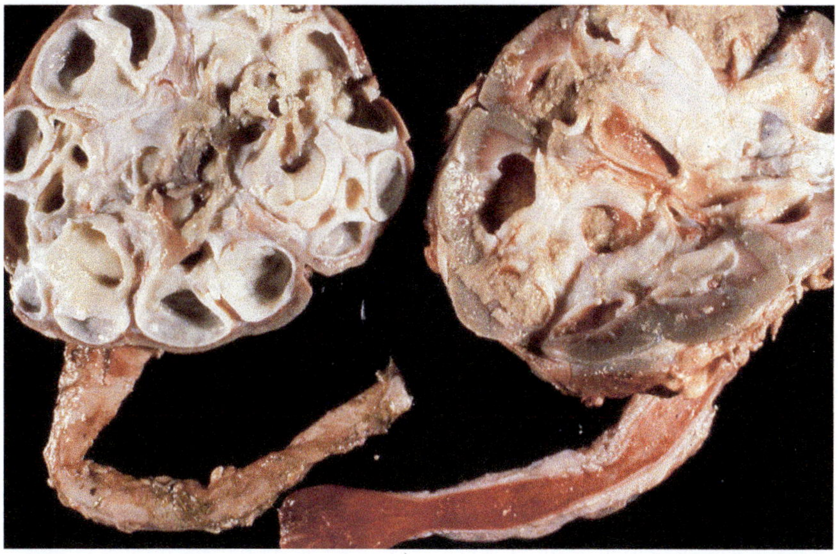

Fig. 13-6 Bilateral, severe, chronic pyelonephritis and ureteritis in an old Holstein-Friesian cow with profound azotemia and severe renal failure. Notice the extensive cortical thinning in response to hydronephrosis, particularly in the left kidney (*left*). (Photograph graciously provided by Dr. D. Michael Rings, United States.)

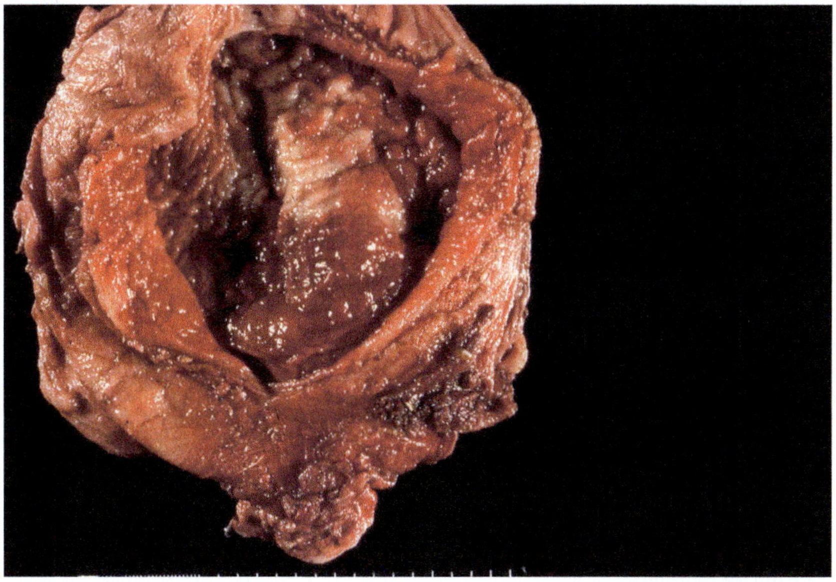

Fig. 13-7 Severe chronic cystitis in the same animal. The bladder is opened and focal areas of cystitis are evident. (Photograph graciously provided by Dr. D. Michael Rings, United States.)

has been described, and the surgery can be performed in the standing animal under local anesthesia.[7]

TREATMENT AND CONTROL

Treatment

Procaine penicillin (22,000 IU/kg IM every 12 hours or 44,000 IU/kg IM every 24 hours for 2–3 weeks) (R-2)

Ampicillin (10 mg/kg IM every 24 hours for 2–3 weeks) (R-2)

Amoxicillin (10 mg/kg IM every 24 hours for 2–3 weeks) (R-2)

Oxytetracycline (10 mg/kg IM every 24 hours for 2–3 weeks) (R-2)

Trimethoprim-sulfadoxine (16 mg combined per kg slow IV injection or IM every 12 hours for 2–3 weeks) (R-2)

Ceftiofur sodium (1.2–2.2 mg/kg IM or SC every 24 hours for 2–3 weeks) (R-2)

Control

Adhere to aseptic technique when catheterizing the bladder of the cow. (R-1)

Consider changing to artificial insemination in herd outbreaks of pyelonephritis with bull breeding. (R-2)

IM, intramuscular; SC, subcutaneous.

CONTROL

One specific control measure usually practiced is isolation of affected animals. Procedures such as urinary catheterization should be avoided, and routine vaginal examinations should be conducted with proper hygienic precautions. Where natural breeding is practiced, some reduction in occurrence may be achieved by the introduction of artificial insemination.

REFERENCES

1. Yeruhma I, et al. *Vet J.* 2006;171:172.
2. Braun U, et al. *Vet J.* 2008;175:240.
3. Rosenbaum A, et al. *Vet Rec.* 2005;157:652.
4. Hajikolaei M, et al. *Comp Clin Pathol.* 2015;24:251.
5. Floeck M. *Vet Clin North Am Food Anim Pract.* 2009;25:651.
6. Vogel SR, et al. *Vet Surg.* 2011;40:233.
7. Miesner M, Anderson DE. *Vet Clin North Am Food Anim Pract.* 2008;24:497.

URINARY DISEASE IN SWINE

Glomerulonephritis

In pigs, glomerulonephritis occurs sporadically and may be associated with immunologic, thrombotic, toxic, or unknown mechanisms. It has been seen as a sporadic event following infectious diseases such as African swine fever, classical swine fever, streptococcal infections, and cytomegalic virus infections. There is also a specific condition of glomerulonephritis in Yorkshire pigs in Norway. The condition of porcine dermatitis and nephropathy syndrome is a specific condition seen in many countries after the advent of porcine circovirus 2 infections but reaching its most severe in the UK. It is immune mediated, possibly through a type III hypersensitivity reaction, and is discussed in more detail in relation to porcine circovirus.

Nephrosis

Acute tubular necrosis (nephrosis) is a feature of a number of pig disorders including pig weed toxicity, nephrotoxins, and antibiotic use.

Embolic Nephritis

It is important to remember that the pig kidney has a wide range of congenital deformities, such as cystic kidneys, which persist into adult life. Most importantly it has a nephrogenic zone, which gives rise to new glomerular units in the 3 months after birth, and these are readily visible under the capsule of the kidney. They are readily involved in kidney lesions associated with septicemia and thrombosis, and involvement of these pathologic processes in the occurrence of the "Turkey egg" kidney has now been associated with over 30 different etiologic agents. The most important of these conditions are *Actinobacillus suis, Streptococcus. suis,* streptococci, staphylococci, *E.coli, Erysipelothrix. rhusiopathiae,* and *T. pyogenes.*

Interstitial Nephritis

One of the common causes of interstitial nephritis is leptospirosis and another is PCV2 infection. They may only be visible on histologic examination.

Other Conditions

These include urolithiasis, which is found in pigs that are sometimes on unusual diets or where there is a shortage of water. The bladder of sows sometimes also contains some sediment and there may be infection-induced calculi. Uric acid and urates are sometimes found in the kidneys of piglets. The kidney worm (*Stephanurus*) is a cause of kidney problems in some parts of the world, and mineralization of the kidneys in vitamin D toxicosis may also be seen very occasionally. Chronic salt intoxication has recently been seen in growing pigs and is characteristically seen as diffuse bilateral interstitial fibrosis.[1]

PORCINE CYSTITIS AND PYELONEPHRITIS

SYNOPSIS

Etiology *Actinobaculum suis* is the specific cause, but a range of other bacteria (principally *Escherichia coli*) may also cause the condition.

Epidemiology Infection of male pigs causes the disease in sows. The organism is in the prepuce and environment. Transmission is venereal and through dirty farrowing houses. Trauma to the urogenital tract of females predisposes to disease.

Clinical findings Unexpected death in acute cases. There is pain on urination, bloodstained, turbid urine accompanied by vaginal discharge; often after service; cystitis on endoscopic examination.

Clinical pathology Hematuria, pyuria, proteinuria, bacteremia are seen. Urine pH >8.5. Demonstration of organism by culture or immunofluorescence; azotemia, increased concentrations of urea and creatinine, hyperkalemia, and hyponatremia.

Necropsy findings Purulent cystitis and pyelonephritis.

Diagnostic confirmation Urinalysis, endoscopic examination, and demonstration of *A. suis*.

Treatment Unrewarding unless early in the course of the disease—antimicrobials and supportive therapy; humane destruction of cases.

Control Antimicrobials by injection, in water, or in feed; ensure adequate water supply for lactating sows to aid urination and improve postfarrowing hygiene.

ETIOLOGY

Cystitis and pyelonephritis are associated with a variety of agents including *E. coli* and others (*Pseudomonas aeruginosa*, staphylococci, streptococci, *Proteus* spp., *Klebsiella* spp., enterococci, and *A. pyogenes*). Infections with most of these organisms result in catarrhal/purulent cystitis.

The genotypic and phenotypic characterization of *E. coli* strains associated with porcine pyelonephritis has been described.[2] The specific disease is most commonly associated with *Actinobaculum suis*. This was formerly known as *Eubacterium suis* and before that as *Corynebacterium suis*. This organism is a large gram-positive rod that is difficult and slow to grow and requires special culture media.

EPIDEMIOLOGY

All these organisms causing cystitis and pyelonephritis are thought to produce the condition as a result of ascending infection. The disease is a particular problem when sows are in stalls or tethered. The condition may not be so serious when associated with all the species other than *A. suis* and in these cases may be seen as frequent urination, the presence of blood or pus in the urine, and a progressive loss of condition. It is in postpubertal sows that have bred.

Occurrence

The infection may be common but the disease is better viewed as sporadic. The disease is probably worldwide in outdoor and indoor units. There are no details of prevalence, although it has been described as the most important cause of sow deaths, with up to 25% associated with urinary tract infection. It probably occurs more frequently than is recognized because there is a considerable subclinical infection rate. In a recent study in the United States, *A. suis* was isolated from 4.7% of the bladders of sows collected at random at a slaughterhouse.

In small herds, the disease tends to occur in small outbreaks when a small number of sows become infected after being mated to a single boar. Often, the clinical outbreak may be 2 to 3 weeks after the use of the suspected boar. More serious outbreaks can occur in large, intensive piggeries. The disease can also occur sporadically and be a normal feature of sow mortality.

In a recent study of 1745 pregnant sows, 28.3% were found to have urinary infections and *A. suis* was found in 20.6% of these. It was less prevalent (13.7%) in the sows with urinary infections than in those without (23.1%). In an abattoir survey in the Netherlands, the prevalence of cystitis in slaughtered sows was 11%, with a variation depending on group from 0% to 35%. In this study of 114 bladders, *A. suis* was not isolated, but *E. coli* was the most commonly isolated together with *S. dysgalactiae*, *A. pyogenes*, *Aerococcus viridans*, and *S. suis*.

Source of Infection and Transmission

A. suis is a normal inhabitant of the porcine prepuce and can be isolated from the preputial diverticulum of boars of various ages. The prevalence of the infection in adult males may be as high as 90%, and the organism can be isolated from the floor of the pens containing infected boars.

Infection and colonization of the preputial diverticulum may occur in pigs as early as 5 weeks of age if they are housed with older pigs. Frequently, this infection may occur from pen floor contamination because of poor hygiene. Piglets can also become infected, at an early age, from sows that have chronic cystitis and pyelonephritis, and the infection can spread rapidly to other male pigs when they are grouped at weaning. Although infection is common in the male pig, cystitis and pyelonephritis is extremely uncommon in females. *A. suis* is rarely isolated from the urogenital tract of the healthy female pig.

Clinical disease is almost entirely restricted to the female pig that has bred. Venereal transmission is thought to be the primary if not the sole method of infection of the sow. Trauma to the vagina may be an important predisposing factor allowing infection to establish, and trauma at parturition with infection from the environment may also be important.

There is no doubt that, where the conditions in stall houses are rife with fecal contamination and poor drainage from the rear half of the stall, perineal and vulval contamination is much greater.

Risk Factors

Clinical signs may occur at any age but are common at 3 to 4 weeks postservice. The disease is more common in sows kept in intensive confinement conditions than in those that are kept in open lots, pens, or pasture, but it does occur in these systems if the hygiene is poor. Differences in feeding patterns and exercise that occur in the different management systems can influence the frequency and volume of water intake. This in turn has an important effect on the frequency of urination and the residual volume of urine in the bladder following micturition, which is one of the factors that may predispose to the establishment of urinary tract infection. Because many lactating sows will only stand when they are fed, usually twice a day, they will also only urinate and drink twice a day. If they cannot take in enough water from either a trough or a tap during this period at the correct flow rate, they may be suffering from an inadequate water intake. It has also been shown that crystalluria may well damage the mucosa and aid the formation of cystitis and that the crystals also support infection of the bladder, particularly where there is an insufficient water supply.

Economic Importance

In one of the best studies of sow mortality in the UK it was reported that the principal cause of death in up to 25% of the sows was urinary tract infection. If the sow mortality is below 5% then cystitis/pyelonephritis is unlikely to be an important problem in the herd.

Cystitis and pyelonephritis is of great importance because it is a major cause of death (annual death rate may be in excess of 5%) in sows in both Great Britain and the United States and, even more important, a cause of serious culling; the recommendation is to cull affected sows because they will always be a source of infection. Considerable prevention, treatment, and hygiene costs will also ensue.

PATHOGENESIS

The organism is widespread in the prepuce of boars, is introduced into the sow at service, but it usually rapidly dies out. In healthy sows, *A. suis* can be isolated from the vagina, but not from the bladder, for a short period after an infected service. In experimental infections of normal sows, it rapidly dies out. The factors that allow it to establish in the urogenital tract are unknown, but trauma to the vagina and urethral opening and service into the bladder are supposed factors. The other organisms listed may also act synergistically to damage the mucosa and facilitate colonization by *A. suis*. This may be true, because *A. suis* possesses two sorts of pili by which it attaches to damaged bladder epithelium. Cystitis results in damage to the ureterovesical junction facilitating ascending infection from the bladder to the kidneys. In infected sows, tortuosity and blockage of the ureters is fairly common. This and the changes in the kidney may lead to chronic renal failure and the inability to retain sodium with potassium retention in the blood and sudden death and even acute renal failure if the blockage is complete and bilateral.

CLINICAL FINDINGS

Mildly affected sows may only show transient inappetence, and other animals are recognized because they are uremic. In the more severely affected groups, the presentation is either as an acute case, usually postservice, or as a chronic one, which can occur at any time.

Most commonly sows present as acute renal failure and sudden death. Sows are suddenly severely ill, unwilling to rise, show profound depression and circulatory collapse, and die within 12 hours. In one series of cases, 40% of the affected sows presented as unexpected deaths, and in the remainder the mean interval between presenting signs and death was 1.6 days and the longest interval was 5 days. The condition may occur in older sows (fourth parity sows and above).

Where the surveillance is good, the sows are observed to be depressed, anorectic, mildly febrile (normal to 39.5°C; 103°F), and sometimes show arching of the back, twitching of the tail, and painful urination. There is frequent passage of bloodstained, turbid urine accompanied by vaginal discharge. Examination with a vaginal speculum will confirm the bladder as the source of the bloody discharge.

The case–fatality rate is high. Sows that survive the acute disease develop chronic renal failure with weight loss and polydipsia and polyuria. They are usually culled for poor performance.

Endoscopic examination of the bladder in acute cases may show little other than mild inflammation, but in more serious cases there are ulcerative and erosive bladder lesions. In sows large enough to allow rectal examination, it may be possible to feel the large and thickened bladder and dilated tortuous ureters in chronic cases. Boars are usually unaffected clinically but intermittent, hematuric episodes lasting several days have been recorded.

The condition can be seen as a sequel to any locomotor, particularly central brain or spinal, condition in which there is an inability to stand to drink or micturate, e.g., organophosphorus poisoning.

CLINICAL PATHOLOGY

Sows' urine is frequently turbid (83.1%) and usually this can be associated with the presence of crystals (96.1%).

Urinalysis usually shows hematuria, pyuria, proteinuria, and a pronounced bacteriuria (usually in excess of 10^5cfu/mL of urine). A Gram stain on a smear of the urine or pus may show the organisms. The urine is alkaline with a pH of more than 8.5 and usually approaching 9 as a result of the urease, which cleaves urea to produce ammonia. Midstream urine contains 10^5 cfu/mL or more. A number of species of bacteria may be found as suggested in the introduction, but *A. suis* requires special culture media. It is now possible to use immunofluorescence for a more rapid and specific diagnosis. Examination of blood shows a pronounced azotemia, with increased concentrations of urea and creatinine and also hyperkalemia and hyponatremia. NAD concentrations are elevated, indicating proximal renal tubular damage.

NECROPSY FINDINGS

A very varied pathology may be visible in these cases. In some sows, there may be an extensive purulent nephritis and pyelitis with similar changes in the dilated ureters and the bladder. In others there may be severely hemorrhagic kidneys and blood in the pelvis.

In acute cases, the bladder wall is swollen, edematous, and hyperemic and may be covered by a gritty, mucinous material. In other cases, the bladder wall may just be thickened, inflamed, and covered by extensive thick mucus. In some of these cases, the ureterovesical valves may have been completely destroyed by necrosis. There may be minimal gross changes in the kidneys in acute cases but there may be microscopic changes of a diffuse tubular and interstitial nephritis. In the chronic case, there are ulcerative and erosive lesions in the bladder wall and there may be pus in the bladder, thick-walled ureters, and an obvious pyelonephritis.

Samples for the Confirmation of Diagnosis

- Bacteriology: kidney, bladder, and ureter for aerobic and anaerobic culture and special media for *A. suis*. A special urea-enriched medium with polymixin or nalidixic acid is necessary in which dry colonies of *A. suis*, about 2 to 3 mm in diameter, grow after 2 days' incubation
- Histology: formalin-fixed bladder, ureter, and kidney

DIAGNOSIS

Diagnosis is based on high mortality; clinical findings; history of service; and clinical pathology, particularly bacteriology, immunofluorescence for specific bacteria, or isolation by culture have a similar sensitivity and specificity.

DIFFERENTIAL DIAGNOSIS

- Other causes of sudden and unexpected deaths
- Hematuria
- *Stephanurus dentatus* (where it occurs)
- The separation of the condition associated with *Actinobaculum suis* from those associated with other bacteria can only be achieved by bacterial culture and other laboratory techniques.

TREATMENT

Early treatment with antibiotics is recommended, but if there is acute renal failure then the case–fatality rate is high. Penicillin given at 15,000 IU/kg IM daily for 7 to 10 days has been successful in early cases. The IM injection of streptomycin at 10 mg/kg has also been used successfully. The isolation of other organisms may indicate the need for other broad-spectrum antibiotics. A recent outbreak of cystitis and endometritis associated with a falling conception rate from 88% to 75% and thought to be caused by *E. coli* (together with staphylococci and streptococci) was successfully treated with an ammonium chloride urinary acidifier, whereas the amoxicillin used previously was without effect. Enrofloxacin at the rate of 10 mg/kg BW in the feed for a period of 10 days has also proved effective, as has 2.5 mg/kg in the food for at least 20 days.

The response can be monitored by the reduction in the urine pH. Treated sows should be loose housed with access to plenty of water. The treatment should be continued for at least 2 to 3 weeks after the outbreak has appeared to finish clinically. Oral electrolyte therapy is also beneficial. In chronic cases, the lesions are well advanced and the organisms may be contained in the calculi and then therapy is not successful and relapses may occur. In many cases, humane destruction is the best option, especially because it is not possible, except in very early cases, to eliminate the organism. Preputial washing on a regular basis may prevent the carriage of organisms by boars, especially because it has been shown that semen may be frequently contaminated by *A. suis,* and up to 50% of boars in some studs may be affected.

CONTROL

Routine prophylactic administration of antibiotics has proved of little value in the long-term control of the disease. A temporary solution has been the use of sow treatment with oxytetracycline followed by in-feed medication with 400 g/t for 21 days. It is not possible to eradicate the infection from the prepuce of a boar, although daily infusions may help reduce the infection. Artificial insemination with the semen treated with antibiotics is a further option.

Trauma to the vagina at mating should be reduced by boar management and the supervision of mating. There should be nonslip floors in the service areas. Animals showing distress, pain, or bleeding after mating should be treated.

The service areas should have very good hygiene with regular cleaning and disinfection after every use. The perineal region of each sow should be cleaned before mating. Farrowing accommodation and crates should also be properly cleaned and disinfected and allowed to dry before sows are introduced. The major organism (*A. suis*) will persist on bad floors but is susceptible to phenolic, quaternary ammonium, and formalin-based products.

Other control procedures involve the provision of an adequate water intake. This should preferably be from the mains without impurities or toxins or bacterial contamination. Loose housing and twice-a-day feeding will encourage the consumption of water. The provision of adequate numbers of drinkers for the stage of the breeding cycle and providing the necessary flow rate for each age of pig is essential (at least 1.5 L/min for gestating sows and 2.2 L/min for lactating sows). A simple check on water supply can be to check appetite: if the sows are not consuming 10 kg of food on day 18 of lactation then there is probably something wrong with water provision. Similarly, troughs must contain at least a reasonable supply of water. In the welfare codes, all animals have to be provided with a fresh supply of high-quality water.

FURTHER READING

Done SH, Carr JC. The urinary tract. In: Sims LD, Glastonbury JRW, eds. *Pathology of the Pig.* Victoria, Australia: Agriculture Victoria; 1996:359-384.

REFERENCES

1. Alonso C, et al. *Proc Cong Int Pig Vet Soc.* 2010;21(1):98.
2. Krag L, et al. *Vet Microbiol.* 2009;134:318.

KIDNEY WORM DISEASE IN PIGS CAUSED BY *STEPHANURUS DENTATUS*

ETIOLOGY

Stephanurosis is a disease of swine caused by the migration of larvae and young adults of the nematode parasite *Stephanurus dentatus* through the body.

SYNOPSIS

Etiology The nematode parasite *Stephanurus dentatus.*

Epidemiology Eggs are shed in urine; infective larvae enter pig when swallowed or by skin penetration; earthworms can act as transport hosts; prepatent period is at least 6 months.

Signs Poor growth; emaciation in severe cases with stiffness of gait.

Clinical pathology Eggs in urine; eosinophilia.

LIFE CYCLE

S. dentatus are large (2- to 5-cm) thick roundworms that inhabit the perirenal tissues and less often inhabit the other abdominal organs and spinal canal of the pig. Adult worms lie in cysts around the renal pelvis and the wall of the ureter. The cysts communicate with the urinary passages, and the eggs are passed out into the urine of the host. They are very prolific egg layers; an infective adult sow may void as many as a million eggs in a day. Under suitable environmental conditions the eggs hatch and, after undergoing two molts, the larvae develop to the infective third stage in about 4 days. The eggs and larvae are very sensitive to cold and desiccation; eggs in a dry situation die within an hour. Exposure to temperatures below 10°C (50°F) is damaging and 4°C (40°F) is lethal. Most larvae in optimum conditions of moisture, warmth, and shelter from sunlight survive for about 3 months and some for as long as 5 months. Larvae may survive for long periods as facultative parasites in earthworms, and this may enable the larvae to survive even when the soil microclimate is adverse.

Larvae may penetrate the skin or be ingested. Larvae that are ingested cross the wall of the stomach, or more commonly the small intestine, and reach the liver via the portal vessels; from the skin the larvae reach the systemic circulation and pass to the liver via the lungs in 1 to 6 weeks. In the liver the larvae migrate from the blood vessels through the parenchyma and eventually, about 3 months after infestation, having undergone a fourth molt, penetrate the capsule of the liver and reach the perirenal tissues to establish themselves as adults. Egg laying usually commences about 6 months after infestation, but the prepatent period may be very much longer and individual worms appear to live as long as 2 years.

During their migration the larvae often follow an erratic path and cause the development of atypical lesions and clinical signs. These larvae often reach maturity in these aberrant sites, and prenatal infection can occur in this way.

EPIDEMIOLOGY

Kidney worms are common in most tropical and subtropical countries such as Africa, the East and West Indies, Brazil, Hawaii, the Philippines, the southern United States, and Australia, where the climate is sufficiently mild to permit the survival of eggs and larvae.

PATHOGENESIS

The principal effect of these worms is the damage caused by the migrating larvae and young adults. The migrating worms cause a great deal of necrosis, fibrosis, and occasional abscess formation along the path of their migration. This is most marked in the perirenal tissues and the liver. *S. dentatus* have been observed rarely in cattle. Experimentally dosed calves develop severe hepatic injury similar to that which occurs in pigs, but the life cycle is not completed and no perirenal lesions develop.

CLINICAL FINDINGS

The mortality rate is not high; production losses and condemnation of parts or all of the infested carcass are of greatest economic significance. Poor growth in spite of a good appetite may be the only sign in mild cases. Badly affected animals become emaciated and develop ascites. In the early stages, nodules in the skin of the belly wall and enlargement and soreness of the peripheral lymph nodes may be evident. Many apparently unrelated clinical signs are produced by aberrant larvae. For example, thrombi may be induced in blood vessels, such as the portal veins, hepatic artery, and posterior vena cava, and paralysis may result if larvae invade the spinal cord. Involvement of the psoas muscles causes local pain and stiffness of gait. The passage of larvae through the peritoneum and pleura gives rise to adhesions. Larvae may also become encysted in the lung. Weakness and eventual paralysis of the hindlegs occur in a number of cases. Passage through the peritoneum and pleura causes the formation of adhesions, and many larvae become encysted in the lung.

CLINICAL PATHOLOGY

Large, thin-walled, embryonated eggs are present in the urine when adult worms are present in the ureter wall. An eosinophilia is seen 2 to 3 weeks after infection, peaking at 6 to 7 weeks and still elevated at 20 weeks. However, this has little specific diagnostic significance. Anemia does not occur. Only a transient rise in aspartate aminotransferase is seen, and serum enzymes seem to be of little value in diagnosis.

NECROPSY FINDINGS

The common findings include fibrosis and abscess formation in perirenal tissues with large adult worms present and occasionally in the pelvis of the kidney and ureter; infarcts and scars in the kidney; and enlargement and scarring of the liver, sometimes accompanied by ascites. The hepatic lesions include irregular whitish tracks in the parenchyma, extensive fibrosis, hemorrhage, and eosinophilic abscess formation. The liver may be covered with a diphtheritic membrane. Larvae may also be present in peripheral lymph nodes and cutaneous nodules, in small abscesses in the lung and pancreas, and in thrombi of blood vessels, particularly in the liver and lungs. Pleurisy and peritonitis, if they are present, are usually manifested by adhesions.

DIAGNOSTIC CONFIRMATION

A definite diagnosis of stephanurosis may be made by finding eggs in the urine or by necropsy. Young pigs with a heavy infestation of larvae may present a problem in diagnosis because adult worms and characteristic renal lesions may not yet be present. An ELISA test can detect infection from 2 weeks after infection, but serologic tests are not likely to become a routine diagnostic procedure.

DIFFERENTIAL DIAGNOSIS

- Other causes of poor growth and emaciation in pigs, e.g., poor nutrition and chronic bacterial diseases such as necrotic enteritis and swine dysentery, but these are accompanied by intermittent diarrhea.
- Other parasitic diseases such as ascariasis and hyostrongylosis.
- Other causes of posterior weakness in pigs such as vitamin A deficiency, osteodystrophia, sometimes fracture of a lumbar vertebra, brucellosis, erysipelas when intervertebral joints are involved, or by spinal cord abscess or lymphoma.

TREATMENT

Single doses of ivermectin (SC) or doramectin (IM) at 0.3 mg/kg, or fenbendazole at 3 mg/kg in the feed for 3 days, are effective against migrating and adult stages, whereas levamisole at 8 mg/kg removes the adults only, preventing egg output for at least 4 weeks.

CONTROL

Regular anthelmintic treatment of all pigs with fenbendazole or ivermectin at 4-month intervals should prevent further contamination of the environment with eggs. The free-living stages should then eventually die out, but this may take some time as infected earthworms may survive for at least 1 year.

Management techniques may also be used for controlling kidney worm. Because the prepatent period of *S. dentatus* is at least 6 months, one method is to breed entirely from gilts until the transmission cycle is broken. Under this system the gilts are raised, allowed to farrow, and sent to market as soon as the litter is weaned and before any eggs are shed. Boars are confined on concrete to prevent contamination of the soil by eggs in their urine. This technique has the advantage of maintaining a fully stocked farm while control is achieved, but it has obvious economic penalties.

Other management techniques depend on the provision of dry ground in which eggs and larvae are less likely to survive. Sleeping shelters should be placed on high ground, preferably bare of vegetation. Because pigs in yards commonly urinate against fences, a 2- to 3-m strip of earth inside the boundary should be kept free of herbage. Muddy spots and water holes should be filled in and drainage provided. Water and feed troughs should be on a concrete apron. Young animals should be segregated from adults and fields rested for 3 to 6 months after the adults are removed. Such programs are rewarding if performed diligently and intelligently, but the extra work involved has militated against general acceptance of this approach. Because of the importance of mature animals as sources of infestation, early replacement of breeding stock is recommended in problem herds.

Toxic Agents Affecting the Kidney

CITRININ TOXICOSIS

Citrinin (CTN or CIT) is most widely known as a nephrotoxin produced by *Penicillium citrinum, P. verrucosum, Monascus ruber, Aspergillus ochraceus,* and *A. terreus.*[1-3] It is commonly found in combination with ochratoxin A (OTA) as a contaminant in human and animal feeds,[2,4,5] and the concentration of CTN often exceeds that of OTA.[6] When present as cocontaminants the effects of OTA and CTN are generally additive; at higher concentrations, the effects may be more than additive.[1]

The signs and lesions associated with poisoning by OTA and CTN are generally similar. The target organ is the kidney, but the liver and bone marrow have been implicated as well.[2] In mice and rats, CTN is embryocidal, fetotoxic, and has an adverse effect on reproduction.[2,7] An increase in testicular and preputial weight, abnormal sperm, and decreased numbers of live sperm were noted in mice treated with CTN.[7] Females mated to CTN-treated mice had a lower pregnancy rate. Information on carcinogenicity is rare, with benign renal tumors reported in mice receiving CTN for 60 to 80 weeks.[1]

CTN is rapidly absorbed and distributed, in particular to the liver and kidney.[1] In humans it is metabolized to dihydrocitrinone (DH-CIT), which may be the primary method of detoxification. Excretion is through the urine and feces. The presence of CTN in human and animal food and food products can be identified by several methods[5,8] and in human urine and plasma by liquid chromatography mass spectrometry (LC-MS/MS).[3]

CTN may play a different role in the pyrexia-pruritus-hemorrhagic syndrome in cattle.[9] Serious outbreaks of this idiopathic disease have been recorded in the UK since 1977 and may be related to CTN in moldy citrus pulp cubes. Clinical signs in affected cows include pruritus, hair loss, papular dermatitis, variable appetite with roughage being taken but not concentrates, fever (40–41.5°C; 104–106.7°F), and mucosal petechiation. Dermatitis is widespread, exudative, initially papular, and itchy. It occurs principally on the head, neck, perineum, and udder. Pruritus is variable in degree, but is often so marked that the skin becomes raw and bleeds. The dermatitis subsides but the fever persists, and over a period of 4 to 7 weeks the animal becomes so unthrifty that it is usually sent for slaughter. The morbidity rate is usually 10%, but may be as high as 100%. Seriously affected animals die. A similar but more severe syndrome occurs in which there is petechiation in all tissues, especially subserosally. In these cases, there are multiple hemorrhages in all mucosae and free blood at the anus and other orifices.

Postmortem examination shows petechiation in all organs and tissues, although it is absent altogether in some cases. Histologic findings include low-grade, long-standing interstitial nephritis and very little else of significance. Hematology, blood chemistry, and serum enzymes are similarly normal. Antibody reactivity to some components of ruminal contents may be elevated but not apparently significantly.

FURTHER READING

Krogh P, Hald B, Pederson EJ. Occurrence of ochratoxin A and citrinin in cereals associated with mycotoxic porcine nephropathy. *Acta Pathol Microbiol Scand [B] Microbiol Immunol.* 1973;81(6):689-695.

Radostits O, et al. *Citrinin. Veterinary Medicine: A Textbook of the Disease of Cattle, Horses, Sheep, Goats and Pigs.* 10th ed. London: W.B. Saunders; 2007:1901.

Saunders GK, Blodgett DJ, Hutchins TA, et al. Suspected citrus pulp toxicosis in dairy cattle. *J Vet Diagn Invest.* 2000;23:269-271.

REFERENCES

1. Föllmann W, et al. *Arch Toxicol.* 2014;88:1097.
2. Flajs D, et al. *Arch Ind Hyg Toxicol.* 2009;60:457.
3. Blaszkewicz M, et al. *Arch Toxicol.* 2013;87:1087.
4. Bragulat MR, et al. *Int J Food Microbiol.* 2008;126:43.
5. Xu B, et al. *Food Control.* 2006;17:271.
6. Kononenko GP, et al. *Agric Sci.* 2013;4:34.
7. Qingqing H, et al. *Exp Toxicol Pathol.* 2012;64:465.
8. Ramesh J, et al. *Int J Curr Microbiol App Sci.* 2013;2:350.
9. Fink-Gremmels J. *Vet J.* 2008;176:84.

ETHYLENE GLYCOL TOXICOSIS

Accidental poisoning with ethylene glycol may occur in swine, goats, cattle, and horses.[1,2] Although the most common source is antifreeze or windshield deicers, ethylene glycol is also found in paints, solvents, detergents, and some pharmaceuticals.[1] The toxic dose rates determined experimentally for cattle are 5 to 10 mL/kg BW in adults and 2 mL/kg in nonruminant calves.[1]

The pathogenesis of the disease is dependent on the development of acidosis and oxalate nephrosis. In swine this is manifested by ascites, hydrothorax and hydropericardium, depression, weakness, and posterior paresis. In cattle there is dyspnea, incoordination, paraparesis, recumbency, and death.

Metabolic acidosis, hypocalcemia, and uremia are hallmarks of intoxication. Calcium oxalate crystals are present in large numbers in the kidney (renotubular) and vasculature. Signs of acute renal failure are seen within the first 24 hours.[1] The treatment recommended for companion animals, ethanol or more often 4-methylpyrazole (fomepizole), is worth considering, especially in small pet ruminants.[2]

A variety of diagnostic tests are available including quantitation in serum. The presence of the chemical in tissue can be detected by chromatography. Kidney cortex (5–10 g) should be frozen in a Whirl-Pak before submission.[3]

FURTHER READING

Osweiler GD, Eness PG. Ethylene glycol poisoning in swine. *J Am Vet Med Assoc*. 1972;160:746-749.

REFERENCES

1. Barigye R, et al. *Can Vet J*. 2008;49:1018.
2. Van Metre DC. *Proc Central Vet Conf*. 2010.
3. Varga A, et al. *Vet Med*. 2012;3:111.

OCHRATOXINS (OCHRATOXICOSIS)

SYNOPSIS

Etiology Ochratoxin A produced primarily by *Aspergillus ochraceus* and *Penicillium verrucosum*.

Epidemiology Worldwide distribution; pigs and chickens are commonly affected.

Clinical pathology Increased serum concentrations of creatinine and urea nitrogen; glucosuria and proteinuria; decreased urine specific gravity.

Lesions Renal toxicity with damage to epithelial cells of proximal tubules.

Diagnostic confirmation High-performance liquid chromatography or liquid chromatography mass spectrometry on tissues (kidney, liver, and muscle).

Treatment Remove contaminated feed.

Control Nonspecific other than attention to harvesting and storage procedures.

ETIOLOGY

Ochratoxins are a group of isocoumarin derivative mycotoxins (A, B, and C) produced primarily by *Aspergillus ochraceus* and *Penicillium verrucosum* and less often by several other species of *Aspergillus* and *P. nordicum*.[1-3] Ochratoxin A (OTA) is the most toxic member of the group; ochratoxin B (OTB) and ochratoxin C (OTC) are less toxic and rarely occur.[3] OTA is a well-known nephrotoxin with neurotoxic, carcinogenic, genotoxic, immunotoxic, and teratogenic properties.[2,4]

EPIDEMIOLOGY

Occurrence

Cereal and cereal products are most often contaminated, but OTA can be found in a variety of other products including beer, chocolate, pork and pork products, poultry, raisins, and wine.[4,5] Feed contamination by OTA occurs worldwide from temperate to tropical climates with the incidence in the Northern Hemisphere considerably higher than the Southern Hemisphere.[6] *Aspergillus* spp. are present in the more tropical regions of the world and *Penicillium* spp. in temperate regions.[4] *P. verrucosum*-contaminated cereals are found more frequently in northern European countries as opposed to those in southern Europe.[5]

Risk Factors

Animal Risk Factors

Swine, dogs, other monogastric animals, and chickens are most often affected from ingestion of OTA-contaminated feeds.[4,7] Ruminant animals are more resistant to OTA toxicosis with goats the possible exception.[3,7] The oral LD_{50} of acute OTA toxicity in pigs is 1 mg/kg BW, that of cockerel chicks 3.3 to 3.9 mg/kg BW, and that of turkeys 5.9 mg/kg BW.[7]

Environmental Factors

The amount of OTA in feeds and thus residual in body organs varies from year to year depending on climate conditions, harvesting, and storage.

Human Risk Factors

Ochratoxin residues have been detected as a carryover in pigs and poultry meats and have significance for persons eating contaminated pork. Information regarding the presence of OTA in cow's milk is scarce, but the carryover is estimated to be less than 1%.[1,4,8]

Farm or Premise Risk Factors

The fungus grows primarily on stored barley or corn. Raw animal feed, especially unprocessed feeds, contain much higher levels of OTA than foods for human consumption. Experimentally, pigs fed diets containing OTA in concentrations as low as 25 µm/kg feed developed decreased feed efficiency and weight loss.[4]

PATHOGENESIS

In pigs, OTA is rapidly absorbed, highly protein bound (99%), undergoes enterohepatic recirculation, and is distributed to kidney, liver and muscle, and fat.[3,8,9] It is metabolized in the liver by carboxypeptidase and trypsins to a less toxic ochratoxin-α (OTα).[1,3] Elimination is slow, primarily because of high protein binding and renal reabsorption. Excretion is biliary and renal. The serum half-life in pigs is very long (72–150 hours).[3]

Ruminant resistance to OTA toxicity may be caused by decreased absorption and degradation of OTA to less toxic OTα by rumen protozoa and microbes.[1,3,7,8]

Nephrotoxicity from OTA involves several different mechanisms. The principal lesion is a degenerative change in the epithelial cells in the proximal convoluted tubules with impairment of tubular function and fibrosis.[1,6] Several other mechanisms such as inhibition of RNA synthesis, disruption of renal and hepatic mitochondria, and impairment of antioxidant enzymes also may be involved.[3,10,11]

CLINICAL FINDINGS

Affected pigs show a reduced daily weight gain, decreased feed efficiency, lower final BWs, polyuria, and polydipsia.[4,6,10] Ochratoxin is associated with poor sperm quality in boars, and is thought to be associated with fetal death and resorption, and thus abortion.[7]

CLINICAL PATHOLOGY

Creatinine and BUN levels are elevated, glucosuria and proteinuria are evident, and urine specific gravity is low.[7,8]

NECROPSY FINDINGS

The most obvious abnormalities are found in the kidneys with renal enlargement, fibrosis, and necrosis of renal tubular epithelium. Microscopic lesions in the proximal tubules included cloudy swelling, granular or vacuolar degeneration, and desquamation of the epithelial cells.[10] Poisoning by ochratoxin in pigs resembles Balkan endemic nephropathy, a naturally occurring disease of humans.[8]

DIAGNOSIS

Assessment of OTA levels in tissue is performed with a variety of methods including immunoassay and spectrometry.[12,13] LC-MS/MS has been demonstrated to be more sensitive and specific for OTA in pig tissues than high-performance liquid chromatography.[13]

DIFFERENTIAL DIAGNOSIS

Differential diagnosis list:
Citrinin toxicosis
Hereditary glomerular disease(s)
Melamine toxicosis
Polycystic kidney disease
Porcine dermatitis and nephropathy syndrome

TREATMENT

There is no specific treatment other than removing pigs from the contaminated feed and providing clean, mycotoxin-free food. Residues in the tissue persist for a long period of time, and it may take several months for them to decrease to an acceptable level.

CONTROL

Animal feeds should not be used unless they have levels of OTA less than 10 parts per billion. Several different gastrointestinal adsorbents (activated charcoal, bentonite, and cholestyramine) have been evaluated, but no single product has been effective against most mycotoxins.[4] Strategies should be used to decrease fungal growth (and thus OTA production) during harvesting and storage.

FURTHER READING

Galtier P, Alvinerie M, Charpenteau JL. The pharmacokinetic profiles of ochratoxin A in pigs, rabbits and chickens. *Food Cosm Toxicol.* 1981;19:735-738.

Petzinger E, Weidenbach A. Mycotoxins in the food chain: the role of ochratoxins. *Livestock Prod Sci.* 2002;76:245-250.

Radostits O, et al. *Ochratoxin. Veterinary Medicine: A Textbook of the Disease of Cattle, Horses, Sheep, Goats and Pigs.* 10th ed. London: W.B. Saunders; 2007:1906.

REFERENCES

1. Fink-Gremmels J. *Vet J.* 2008;176:84.
2. Cabanes FJ, et al. *Toxins (Basel).* 2010;2:1111.
3. Ringot D, et al. *Chem Biol Interact.* 2006;159:18.
4. Muzaffer D, et al. *Toxins (Basel).* 2010;2:1065.
5. Bragulat MR, et al. *Int J Food Microbiol.* 2008;126:43.
6. Freitas BV, et al. *J Anim Prod Adv.* 2012;2:174.
7. Duarte SC, et al. *Vet Microbiol.* 2011;143:1.
8. Pfohl-Leszkowicz A, et al. *Mol Nutr Food Res.* 2007;51:61.
9. Milićević DR, et al. *Arch Oncol.* 2009;17:59.
10. Stoev SD, et al. *Exp Toxicol Pathol.* 2012;64:733.
11. Boesch-Saadatmandi C, et al. *Food Chem Toxicol.* 2008;46:2665.
12. Matrella R. *Food Control.* 2006;17:114.
13. Milićević DR, et al. *J Environ Sci Heal B.* 2009;44:781.

PLANT POISONINGS CAUSED BY KNOWN TOXINS

IFORRESTINE

Iforrestine, a heterocyclic nephrotoxin, is present in six species of *Isotropis.* Lamb poison or Bloom poison, e.g., *I. forrestii, I. atropurpurea,* and *I. cuneifolia,* is associated with severe renal damage and uremia in cattle and sheep. Clinical signs include anorexia, depression, diarrhea, oliguria, anuria, recumbency, and death. Proteinuria and glycosuria are constant, and there is severe renal tubular necrosis.

PLANT POISONINGS FROM UNIDENTIFIED TOXINS

UREMIA, NEPHROSIS—WITH HIGH BLOOD UREA NITROGEN

- *Amaranthus* spp.
- *Anagallis arvensis*
- *Azadirachta indica*
- *Cassine buchanani*
- *Catha edulis* (khat)
- *Dimorphandra gardneriana*
- *Lythrum hyssopifolia*
- *Petiveria alliacea* (anamu)
- *Psilostrophe* spp. (paperflowers)
- *Sapium sebiferum* (Chinese tallow tree)
- *Sarcolobus globosus*
- *Sartwellia flaveriae*

POLYDIPSIA, POLYURIA

- *Orobanche minor* (broom rape).

RED URINE CAUSED BY A PIGMENTED SUBSTANCE FROM THE PLANT

- *Haloragis odontocarpa* (raspwort)
- *Swartzia madagascariensis*
- *Trifolium pratense* (red clover); in deer
- *Xanthorrhoea minor*; in cattle; probably associated with plant resins.

CYSTITIS

- *Gyrostemon* (= *Didymotheca*) *cupressiformis* (double-seeded emu bush).

FUNGI LACKING IDENTIFIED TOXINS

Grain infected with *Tilletia tritici* (wheat smut) fungus should not be included in rations for pigs because it is thought to be associated with glomerulonephritis and failure to gain weight. Estimates of the maximum safe content of infected grain that can be fed in the ration vary from 5% to 30%.

FURTHER READING

Colegate SM, Dorling PR, Huxtable CR, et al. Iforrestine: a novel heterocyclic nephrotoxin from *Isotropis forrestii. Aust J Chem.* 1989;42:1249-1255.

Gardiner MR, Royce RD. Poisoning of sheep and cattle in Western Australia due to species of *Isotropis* (Papilionaceae). *Crop Pasture Sci.* 1967;18:505-513.

Renal Neoplasia

Primary tumors of the kidney are rare. Renal carcinomas occur in cattle and horses and nephroblastomas occur in pigs. Enlargement of the kidney is the characteristic sign; in cattle and horses neoplasms should be considered in the differential diagnosis of renal enlargement. In pigs, nephroblastomas may be so big they cause visible abdominal enlargement. Renal adenocarcinomas are very slow growing but are not usually diagnosed until the disease is well advanced. The gross and histologic description of a series of primary renal cell tumors in slaughter cattle has been recorded.

In horses, the most common signs are weight loss, reduced appetite, hematuria, and intermittent bouts of abdominal pain.[1,2] Some affected horses have massive ascites and hemoperitoneum. Metastasis of the tumor to the axial skeleton can result in lameness, which can be the clinical abnormality that is recognized first. The tumor can also metastasize to the lungs and mouth. Masses on the left kidney of horses are usually readily palpable on rectal examination. Horses with renal carcinoma can have clinically apparent periods of hypoglycemia, which is confirmed by measurement of serum glucose concentration and is attributable to production of insulin-like growth factor by the neoplastic tissue. Ultrasonographic examination of the kidney and renal biopsy confirm the diagnosis. Unilateral nephrectomy was successful in the treatment of an 11-year-old female alpaca with hematuria caused by a transitional cell papilloma in the renal pelvis.[3]

Metastatic neoplasms are fairly common in the kidney, particularly in enzootic bovine leukosis, but they do not cause clinical renal disease. Tumor masses may be palpable as discrete enlargements in the kidneys of cattle or may involve the kidney diffusely, causing generalized enlargement of the kidney.

REFERENCES

1. Wise LN, et al. *J Vet Intern Med.* 2009;23:913.
2. Swain JM, et al. *J Vet Intern Med.* 2005;19:613.
3. Gerspach C, et al. *J Am Vet Med Assoc.* 2008;232:1206.

Congenital and Inherited Renal Diseases

RENAL HYPOPLASIA

Developmental abnormalities of the kidneys are classified as renal agenesis, hypoplasia, and dysplasia, with agenesis and hypoplasia representing different degrees of the same condition. Renal hypoplasia is defined as a decrease in total renal parenchyma of one-third or more, with a proportionately greater loss of medullary than cortical tissue. The diagnosis of renal hypoplasia is straightforward in neonates but can be difficult to differentiate from renal dysplasia in adults.

Renal agenesis results from failure of the ureteral bud to contact the metanephric blastema during organogenesis and has been reported to occur in cattle and alpacas.[1] Bilateral renal agenesis is fatal shortly after birth, but unilateral renal agenesis may be clinically undetectable except for compensatory hypertrophy of the remaining kidney.

Bilateral renal hypoplasia with or without agenesis is recorded in Large White piglets; the piglets die at birth or die in the first 3 months of life. Clinical signs exhibited by older pigs included lethargy, shivering, anorexia, diarrhea, and a slow rate of growth. The disease was suspected to be inherited in a simple autosomal recessive manner, and the basic defect appeared to be failure of development of mesonephric mesenchyme.

Cases of bilateral renal hypoplasia have been recorded in four horses 1 day to 3 years of age that had common histories of stunting, poor growth rate, anorexia, depression, and lethargy. Evidence of chronic renal failure was present on clinicopathologic examination. Transrectal and transabdominal ultrasonography revealed small kidneys and small renal medulla and pelves and was considered a useful diagnostic test.

Renal hypoplasia is part of a congenital multisystem disorder of Poll Merino/Merino sheep that has been named **brachygnathia, cardiomegaly, and renal hypoplasia syndrome (BCRHS)**.[2,3] The abnormalities are described in detail in Chapter 21.

REFERENCES

1. Sugiyama A, et al. *J Comp Pathol*. 2007;137:71.
2. Shariflou MR, et al. *Aust Vet J*. 2011;89:254.
3. Shariflou MR, et al. *Anim Genet*. 2012;44:231.

POLYCYSTIC KIDNEYS

In most species this is a common congenital defect. If it is extensive and bilateral the affected animal is usually stillborn or dies soon after birth. In some cases, bilateral defects are compatible with life, and clinical signs may not present until the residual nephron mass is gradually exhausted and the animal is adult. If it is unilateral no clinical signs appear because of compensatory activity in the other kidney, but in an adult the enormously enlarged kidney may be encountered during rectal examination.

In adult horses, polycystic disease may also be acquired rather than congenital. The disease is rare, but affected animals present in varying stages of chronic renal failure.

A high incidence of renal defects has been recorded in sucking pigs from sows vaccinated during early pregnancy with attenuated hog cholera virus; bilateral renal hypoplasia has been observed as a probably inherited defect in Large White pigs. Most polycystic kidneys in pigs appear to be inherited in a polygenic manner and have no effect on the pig's health or renal function. However, there is a record of the defect in newborn pigs in one herd in which it caused gross abdominal distension caused by moderate ascites and gross cystic distension of the kidneys and tract. There was no evidence that the disease was inherited in this instance, and a toxic origin was surmised.

Isolated cysts occur in the kidneys of all species and are of no clinical significance. The increased availability of ultrasonographic examination of the kidneys of animals facilitates antemortem identification of these cysts. The cysts are usually solitary and unilateral.

Congenital polycystic kidney disease of lambs occurs as an autosomal recessive trait.[1] The disease is recognized in Romney, Perendale, and Coopworth sheep in New Zealand and most likely originated in the Romney breed 50 years ago. Lambs die at or shortly after birth and there is no apparent sex predisposition. Necropsy examination reveals an abdomen distended by the enlarged kidneys (3.5–14 cm in length), which contain large numbers of fluid-filled 1- to 5-mm cysts. There are gross and histologic abnormalities of the liver and pancreas, and dysplastic changes and associated cyst formation are observed in bile ductal, pancreatic, and epididymal tissues. A likely candidate gene for the disorder is polycystic kidney hepatic disease 1. A pathologically similar disease is reported in a Nubian goat.

REFERENCE

1. Johnstone AC, et al. *New Zeal Vet J*. 2005;53:307.

RENAL DYSPLASIA

Renal dysplasia is defined as disorganized development of the renal parenchyma caused by anomalous differentiation. Each kidney is formed from separate metanephric and uteric buds, and an appropriate interaction between these buds is required for the development of normal renal architecture.[1] Histologically, renal dysplasia is characterized by persistence of abnormal mesenchymal structures, including undifferentiated cells, cartilage, immature collecting ductules, and abnormal lobar organization, and the lack of normal nephrons and collecting ducts. Affected kidneys do not function normally and azotemia develops.

Renal dysplasia is very rare in horses with isolated reports in several breeds. It is most commonly identified in foals but less severely affected animals can survive to adulthood. Clinicopathologic findings include azotemia, oliguria, and increased serum phosphorus and potassium concentrations in affected foals.[1] Renal dysplasia can occur as an apparent spontaneous disease in foals and in foals born to mares treated with sulfadimidine, pyrimethamine, and folic acid during pregnancy. Renal dysplasia has been diagnosed in a 4-month-old foal with benign ureteropelvic polyps associated with hydronephrosis. Renal dysplasia has also been diagnosed in two adult horses with weight loss, azotemia, hypercalcemia, and increased fractional clearance of sodium. Ultrasonographic examination of the kidneys revealed a poor distinction between the cortex and medulla caused by a hyperechoic medulla, which was caused by fibrosis. Histologic changes in both horses were indicative of interruption of nephrogenesis after the initiation, but before the complete differentiation, of the metanephric blastema. There is one report of **multiple renal cysts** being present in a 9-day-old Thoroughbred filly with renal dysplasia.[2]

Inherited cystic renal dysplasia has been identified in lambs sired by carrier Suffolk rams out of mixed ewes. Signs include recumbency and coma by days 2 to 3. Abortions and stillbirths occurred in the flocks at the same time. The kidneys are enlarged and cystic. The condition may have been caused by an autosomal dominant gene.

Congenital renal dysplasia has been recorded in two successive years in a Leicester sheep flock crossbred with Suffolk and Swaledale rams. Affected lambs were born alive, were reluctant to stand or move, sucked poorly, and had wet coats. Lambs improved with nursing and provision of warmth, but none with clinical signs at birth survived beyond 5 days after birth. At necropsy, the kidneys were bilaterally small with fine intracortical cysts and distinct cortical and medullary zones. An inherited dominant trait with complete penetrance is suspected.

Renal tubular dysplasia has been diagnosed in Japanese Black cattle (Wagyu) with renal failure, poor growth, and long hooves. Calves were undersized at birth and had repeated episodes of diarrhea during the neonatal period. They began to show signs of growth retardation from 2 to 5 months of age but had a normal appetite. Clinicopathologic findings included azotemia, increased serum phosphorus concentrations, and oliguria. At necropsy, the main lesion was dysplasia of the proximal tubule epithelial cells, with secondary interstitial fibrosis with a reduction in the numbers of glomeruli and tubules in older cattle. An autosomal recessive mode of inheritance has been determined associated with a deletion of the paracellin-1 gene on chromosome 1,[3] which has been renamed the claudin-16 (CL-16) gene. Bovine CL-16 deficiency is classified as type 1 or type 2 depending on the site of the gene mutation.[4] The CL-16 gene encodes a protein that is part of the tight junction of renal epithelial cells that restricts diffusion of solutes through the paracellular pathway. Deletion of the CL-16 gene is considered to be the cause for the renal tubular dysplasia, and a DNA-specific test for this mutation has been developed. Heterozygotes are usually clinically normal and have normal renal function, although one report indicated that some heterozygotes have histologic renal lesions.[4] Renal dysplasia with nephrosclerosis appears to be a different condition in cattle and has been reported in six calves with poor growth rates aged 3 to 6 months.[5] Renal dysplasia has also been diagnosed in Japanese Black cattle that are of normal gene type,[6] suggesting that although the renal lesions may be associated with a homozygous deletion of the CL-16 gene, there may be accompanying defects that have not been characterized.

REFERENCES

1. Philbey AW, et al. *Vet Rec.* 2009;165:626.
2. Medina-Torres CE, et al. *Can Vet J.* 2014;55:141.
3. Hardefeldt LY, et al. *Aust Vet J.* 2007;85:185.
4. Naylor RJ, et al. *Equine Vet Educ.* 2009;21:358.
5. Ohba Y, et al. *Genomics.* 2000;68:229.
6. Sugiyama A, et al. *J Comp Pathol.* 2007;137:71.

RENAL LIPOFUCINOSIS OF CATTLE

Dark brown or black discolored kidneys ("black kidneys") have been reported as incidental findings in slaughter cattle for more than 100 years,[1] and has been termed **renal lipofuscinosis** of Danish cattle. A pigment with characteristics similar to those lipofuscin is present in secondary liposomes in epithelial cells of the proximal tubules. Cases occurred only in Holstein cattle or the Red Danish Dairy Breed and mainly in animals aged 3 years or older. The prevalences of the abnormality were 0.3–0.4% and 1.3–2.5%, respectively in Holstein and Red Danish Dairy breeds.[2] Affected animals produce slightly less milk than similarly aged animals without renal lipofuscinosis. Epidemiologic, genealogic, and genotype analyses indicate an autosomal recessive inheritance on chromosome 17, with incomplete penetrance of the genotype in Danish Holsteins.[2]

REFERENCES

1. Rude H, et al. *J Comp Pathol.* 2005;132:303.
2. Agerholm J, et al. *Acta Vet Scand.* 2009;51:7.

EQUINE RENAL CORTICAL TUBULAR ECTASIA

A 16-year-old Thoroughbred pregnant mare with hemoabdomen, laminitis, and unilateral epistaxis was examined. Her physical condition deteriorated rapidly and the horse was euthanized. A ruptured ovarian artery was found to be the cause of the hemoabdomen, and variably sized, firm, light brown nodular cortical masses that did not extend past the corticomedullary junction were an incidental finding in both kidneys. Histologically, the masses were diagnosed as renal cortical tubular ectasia,[1] which has some similarities to medullary sponge kidney (Cacchi–Ricci syndrome) in humans. The renal cortical masses are thought to represent disruption at the "ureteric bud-metanephric mesenchyme" interface.

REFERENCE

1. Jackson C. *J Equine Vet Sci.* 2015;35:80.

Diseases of the Ureters, Bladder, and Urethra

ECTOPIC URETER AND URETERAL DEFECTS

Ectopic ureter has been recorded in cattle and horses. The condition may be unilateral or bilateral with **urinary incontinence** present since birth as the major clinical manifestation. Reported neurogenic causes of urinary incontinence in horses include cauda equine neuritis, herpesvirus-1 myelitis, Sudan grass toxicosis, sorghum poisoning, trauma, and neoplasia. Nonneurogenic causes of urinary incontinence in horses include ectopic ureter, cystitis, urolithiasis, hypoestrogenism, and abnormal vaginal conformation.

The ectopic ureter opens into the urogenital tract at a place other than the bladder such as the cervix, urethra, or vagina. The condition is often complicated by ascending infections, hydronephrosis, and dilatation of the ureter. Definite diagnosis requires excretory urography or endoscopy; visualization of the ureteral openings during endoscopy can be assisted by IV administration of phenolsulfonphthalein (0.01 mg/kg BW) or indigo carmine (0.25 mg/kg BW) to impart a red or blue color, respectively, to the urine being produced. Surgical treatment involving ureterovesical anastomosis or unilateral nephrectomy has been successful.

Unilateral and bilateral **ureteral defects** have been reported in newborn foals. The clinical presentation is similar to rupture of the urinary bladder, but ureteral defects may be more common in filly foals than in colts.

PARALYSIS OF THE BLADDER AND OVERFLOW INCONTINENCE

Paralysis of the bladder is uncommon in large animals. It usually occurs as a result of neurologic diseases affecting the lumbosacral spinal cord such as equine herpes myelopathy and cauda equina syndrome, and particularly ascending spinal meningitis in lambs after tail docking. In all species, compression of the lumbar spinal cord by neoplasia (lymphosarcoma and melanoma) or infected tissue (vertebral osteomyelitis) can cause paralysis of the bladder. Excessive tension on the tail, such as by application of tail ropes or use of the tail for restraint in cattle, can injure the cauda equina and result in bladder paralysis. In horses, spinal cord degeneration following consumption of sorghum can lead to bladder paralysis and posterior ataxia. Iatrogenic bladder paralysis occurs in horses in which there has been epidural injection of an excessive quantity of alcohol. Equine protozoal myeloencephalitis and equine polyneuritis can cause signs of cauda equina dysfunction in horses. In some horses, idiopathic bladder paralysis and overflow incontinence may occur sporadically in the absence of other neurologic or systemic signs. When the bladder is markedly distended from a urinary tract obstruction, it may take several days after removal of the obstruction before normal bladder tone returns.

When bladder paralysis arises from spinal cord disease, other upper or lower motor neuron signs are usually present. Bladder involvement is indicated by incontinence with constant or intermittent dribbling of urine. Urine flow is often increased during exercise. The bladder is enlarged on examination per rectum, and urine can be easily expressed by manual compression. In horses, chronic distension of the atonic or hypotonic bladder leads to accumulation of a sludge of calcium carbonate crystals called **sabulous urolithiasis.**[1] Urine stasis produces ideal conditions for bacterial growth, and cystitis is a common sequel. Treatment is supportive and aimed at relieving bladder distension by regular catheterization and lavage. During catheterization, care must be taken to avoid introducing infection. Manual or pharmacologically induced emptying of the bladder is incomplete so there is a constant risk of cystitis. Pharmacologic enhancement of bladder emptying can sometimes be achieved by administration of parasympathomimetic agents such as bethanechol (parasympathetic stimulation via the pelvic nerve stimulates detrusor contraction; 0.2 to 0.4 mg/kg every 6 to 8 hours, orally) and sympatholytics such as prazosin and phenoxybenzamine (sympathetic stimulation via the hypogastric nerve causes detrusor relaxation and internal sphincter contraction). The administration of antimicrobial agents as a prophylaxis against the development of cystitis is advisable. The prognosis for paralysis associated with spinal cord disease depends on the prognosis for the primary disease. Paralysis in the absence of spinal cord disease has a poor prognosis.

Cattle ingesting *Cistus salvifolius,* a shrub found in the Mediterranean region, had urinary retention as the primary clinical sign. Cattle had decreased appetites and rumen motility, weight loss, and persistent elevation of the tail head and difficulty in urination. A greatly distended urinary bladder was always detected on palpation per rectum. The mortality rate in advanced cases was high, and affected animals have severe cystitis, pyelonephritis, and a marked increase in bladder wall thickness. No evidence of neurologic injury was present, and it is likely that urine retention was secondary to severe cystitis and swelling of the bladder wall that prevented normal urination.

REFERENCE

1. Saulez MN, et al. *J Am Vet Med Assoc.* 2005;226:246.

EVERSION OF THE BLADDER

Bladder eversion through the urethra into the vagina and through the vulva occurs very rarely in mares and cows, and is most common immediately after parturition. Eversion is secondary to severe straining in the periparturient period, an increase in intraabdominal pressure, and the presence of a short wide urethra in mares or concomitant hypocalcemia in cows. Bladder eversion observed immediately after parturition must be differentiated from uterine prolapse. There is a report of bladder eversion in a nonpregnant mare secondary to chronic cystitis.[1] Treatment is administration of an epidural or sedation, aseptic cleaning of the perineal region and exposed tissue, examination of the prolapsed tissue to ensure lacerations or full thickness necrotic sections are not present, application of sterile lube to assist movement of tissues, and gentle retropulsion.

Umbilical evagination of the bladder has been reported in a neonatal filly. The bladder prolapsed through the umbilicus such that the mucosa of the bladder was outside (bladder eversion). Correction is surgical.

REFERENCE

1. Kumas C, Maden M. *J Equine Vet Sci*. 2014;34:329.

PATENT URACHUS

Failure of the urachus to close at birth is most common in foals and is very rare in other species. Patent urachus occurs as three syndromes in foals: congenital and present at birth; acquired and secondary to urachal infection or inflammation; or secondary to severe systemic illness, usually sepsis. The urachus is part of the umbilicus during fetal development and drains urine into the allantoic fluid during intrauterine life; after birth, a patent urachus will therefore manifest as urine leaking from the umbilicus. The urine flow varies from a continuous stream during micturition to constant or intermittent dribbling, or a continuous moistening of the umbilical stalk. Healthy foals with congenital patent urachus heal in several days, and no specific treatment is required. Formerly, cauterization with phenol or silver nitrate was practiced, but this treatment has the theoretical potential to induce necrosis and increases susceptibility to infection.

Foals with patent urachus secondary to umbilical disease usually have an enlarged umbilicus, and some have a purulent discharge. Foals that have patent urachus secondary to other umbilical disease might require surgical correction, although most respond to a 7- to 14-day course of antimicrobials. Foals with patent urachus secondary to systemic disease, usually sepsis, should have their other disease treated aggressively and the urachus allowed to close spontaneously, which it usually does. Ultrasonographic examination of the umbilicus of all foals with patent urachus is essential to determine the extent of disease and presence of intraabdominal disease. As with all sick foals, the immune status of foals with patent urachus secondary to umbilical or systemic disease should be determined by measurement of serum IgG concentration, and foals with low serum IgG concentration should receive a blood or plasma transfusion. Cystitis is an occasional sequel to patent urachus, but omphalitis and urachal abscess may also develop as complications. Patent urachus is rarely diagnosed in neonatal ruminants but has been recorded in a lamb.

Urachal abscess is discussed as a subgroup of umbilical abscess in Chapter 19. When the infection is localized in the urachus, there are usually signs of cystitis, especially increased frequency of urination.

RUPTURE OF THE BLADDER (UROPERITONEUM)

Rupture of the bladder is most common in castrated male ruminants as a sequel to obstruction of the urethra by calculi. Rare cases are recorded in cows as a sequel to a difficult parturition, in mares after normal parturition, possibly because of compression of a full bladder during foaling, and in a gelding caused by penile and preputial squamous cell carcinoma.[1] In cattle, abnormal fetal position during prolonged dystocia is suspected to obstruct the urethra and distend the bladder. Subsequent manipulation within the pelvic canal during correction of the dystocia is suspected to lead to rupture of a distended bladder. Occasionally, the urachal remnant can rupture spontaneously in adult cattle, resulting in uroperitoneum. The urachal remnant may be identified using transrectal ultrasonography and a 7.5-MHz transducer.[2] Uroperitoneum in foals is discussed in the next section.

After the bladder ruptures, uroperitoneum results in a series of abnormalities that arise from failure of the excretory process combined with solute and fluid redistribution between the peritoneal fluid and extracellular fluid. The peritoneal membrane serves as a semipermeable membrane through which low molecular weight solutes readily pass. High molecular weight compounds also diffuse across the peritoneal membrane but at a much slower rate. Urine is usually hypertonic, especially in animals whose water intake is decreased by uremia. Osmotic pressure from hypertonic urine promotes movement of extracellular water into the peritoneal cavity. This movement, combined with reduced intake, results in clinical dehydration. Urine usually has a lower concentration of sodium and chloride and higher concentrations of urea, creatinine, potassium, and phosphate than plasma. Diffusion along these concentration gradients across the peritoneal membrane results in a general pattern of azotemia with hyponatremia, hypochloremia, hyperkalemia, and hyperphosphatemia. There are minor differences between species in these general biochemical changes. In particular, the blood concentration of urea rises much more slowly in ruminants than in horses, and hyperkalemia is not as common in ruminants as in horses because excessive potassium can be excreted in the saliva and therefore eliminated in the feces.

Bladder rupture leads to gradual development of ascites from uroperitoneum, ruminal stasis, constipation, and depression. In cattle, uremia may take 1 to 2 weeks to develop to the point in which euthanasia is necessary. The degree of uremia between individual patients can be highly variable. With therapy, the survival rate of steers in one study was 49%. The best predictor of survival among clinical pathology tests was the serum phosphate concentration: all animals with levels greater than 9.0 mg/dL (2.9 mmol/L) died. In mature horses, clinical signs of depression, anorexia, colic, abdominal distension, and uremia develop within 1 to 2 days following rupture.

In cases of ascites or when urinary tract obstruction is evident, it is important in considering treatment and prognosis to determine whether the bladder has ruptured. The urea and creatinine concentrations in plasma or serum can be compared with the values in the peritoneal fluid. The ratio of urea in peritoneal fluid to that in serum is a good guide in the early stages, but after 40 hours the ratio of the peritoneal to serum creatinine greater than 2 : 1 is diagnostic of uroperitoneum. Treatment is surgical with a goal of bladder repair. To avoid the costs of laparotomy in feedlot animals, a urethrostomy is created or an indwelling catheter is placed and the rupture is allowed to repair itself.

REFERENCES

1. May KA, et al. *Equine Vet Educ*. 2008;20:135.
2. Braun U, et al. *Vet Rec*. 2006;159:780.

UROPERITONEUM IN FOALS

ETIOLOGY

Uroperitoneum, the accumulation of urine in the peritoneal cavity, occurs in foals as a result of a variety of situations:

- Congenital (i.e., present at birth) rupture of the bladder
- Bladder rupture associated with sepsis
- Rupture of the urachus, often secondary to sepsis
- Avulsion of the bladder from its urachal attachment, presumably as a result of trauma or strenuous exercise
- Rarely, as embryologic failure of the halves of the bladder to unite (schistocystitis)
- Ureteral defects

The etiology of congenital rupture is unclear, but its association with birth, markedly greater prevalence in colts, and the traumatic nature of the lesion suggest that it occurs during birth as a result of compression of a distended bladder. Intraabdominal pressures of the mare during parturition are large, and these compressive forces are experienced by the foal during phase 2 of parturition. Compression of a distended bladder can cause rupture. The greater prevalence in colts is speculated to be a result of the greater resistance to bladder emptying conferred by the longer urethra of male foals.

Rupture of the bladder occurs as a distinct entity in **septic foals**. The underlying reason for bladder rupture is unclear but is usually related to infection, inflammation, and necrosis of the lower urinary tract. This cause of uroperitoneum in foals is increasingly recognized as the most common, especially among hospitalized foals.

Rupture of the urachus occurs in septic foals. It is probably of similar etiology to rupture of the bladder in septic foals. The urachus of affected foals almost always has infection, inflammation, and necrosis evident on histologic examination.

Avulsion of the bladder from its urachal attachments is presumed to occur as a result of trauma, such as might occur with vigorous exercise. The possibility also exists that there is an underlying defect in affected foals, such as urachitis or omphalitis.

Embryologic failure of the halves of the bladder to unite during organogenesis has been reported anecdotally and in case reports, although adequate documentation of its occurrence is lacking. This defect would be a true congenital anomaly, arising during gestation.

Ureteral defects are an uncommon cause of uroperitoneum in foals. The defects appear to be congenital and more common in fillies. Both ureters can be affected.

The relative frequency of these diseases is that approximately 20% of foals with uroperitoneum do so because of urachal rupture, approximately 30% because of rupture of the dorsal bladder wall, 18% because of rupture of the ventral bladder wall, and the remainder because of multiple defects involving combinations of the urachus and dorsal and ventral bladder. One report of rupture of the urethra and bladder exists in a colt foal.[1]

Uroperitoneum also occurs rarely in **calves** as a consequence of umbilical infection.

EPIDEMIOLOGY

The epidemiology of uroperitoneum is not well documented. The incidence in foals appears to be approximately 0.2%, although this estimate is based on a study conducted 50 years ago. The prevalence in hospitalized foals is 2.5%. Male foals are at greater risk than are females for congenital rupture; more than 80% of foals with this disease are colts. In contrast, there is no sex predilection for development of uroperitoneum in foals with sepsis. The age at diagnosis ranges from 2 to more than 60 days, with most cases recognized within the first 2 weeks of life. The average age at diagnosis is approximately 4 to 5 days, although the age at presentation depends on the underlying cause. Foals with congenital rupture of the bladder or ureteral defects are usually recognized at about 3 to 5 days of age, whereas foals with uroperitoneum secondary to sepsis are usually older (5–9 days of age, but up to 60 days). The prognosis for survival for foals with uroperitoneum depends on the underlying cause and availability of appropriate treatment. Foals with congenital rupture of the bladder that are recognized and treated in a timely fashion have an excellent prognosis (>80%) for survival, whereas those with uroperitoneum secondary to sepsis have a more guarded prognosis (50%–60%) because of the sepsis.

PATHOPHYSIOLOGY

The pathophysiology of uroperitoneum is that of postrenal azotemia. Regardless of the underlying cause of the uroperitoneum, accumulation of urine within the peritoneal cavity results in substantial electrolyte, acid-base, and cardiovascular effects in affected foals. The basic principle is that affected foals are unable to excrete metabolic waste products that are normally excreted in the urine, and are unable to maintain water and electrolyte balance. Young foals derive almost all of their nutritional needs, including water, from mare's milk. Mare's milk has a low sodium concentration (approximately 12 mEq/L) and a higher potassium concentration (25 mEq/L) compared with serum and a dry matter content of 11%. Therefore foals ingest a diet that contains a large quantity of water and potassium but little sodium. Consequently, the urine of foals contains little sodium (7 mEq/L) and has a low osmolality (100 mOsmol/kg). Leakage of urine into the peritoneum, a semipermeable membrane, results in considerable fluid and electrolyte shifts. Partial equilibration of water and electrolytes across the peritoneal membrane results from diffusion of water from the peritoneum with resultant dilution of serum and reductions in serum sodium and chloride concentrations. The low concentration of sodium in uriniferous peritoneal fluid favors diffusion of sodium from the blood into the peritoneal fluid, resulting in a reduction in intravascular sodium content and a consequent reduction in effective circulating volume. Excretion of relatively large quantities of potassium in urine and accumulation of potassium-rich fluid in the peritoneum allows diffusion of potassium into the blood and an increase in plasma potassium concentration.

The peritoneal membrane is permeable to creatinine and urea, as evidenced by the efficacy of peritoneal lavage in the treatment of renal failure in a variety of species, including horses. Consequently, serum creatinine and urea concentrations are higher in foals with uroperitoneum than in unaffected foals. However, equilibration of concentrations of these compounds is not complete and peritoneal fluid concentrations of urea, creatinine, and potassium are higher than those in serum.

Foals with uroperitoneum have compromised circulatory function because of reduced effective circulating plasma (blood) volume, despite having an increase in total body water content. Circulatory function is further impaired by a combination of hyperkalemia, abdominal distension, and accumulation of fluid in the pleural space, resulting in foals with uroperitoneum that have signs of mild to moderate circulatory compromise.

Hyperkalemia and acidosis associated with uroperitoneum predispose affected foals to development of malignant cardiac rhythm disturbances, including ventricular tachycardia and fibrillation. This abnormal cardiac rhythm is a common cause of death of affected foals.

CLINICAL SIGNS

Clinical signs in foals with uroperitoneum depend in part on the underlying disease. Foals with congenital rupture or mild sepsis have progressive signs of lethargy, decreased appetite, mild abdominal discomfort, and abdominal distension. These signs usually first become apparent at 2 to 4 days of age. These foals do not typically have a fever. As the disease progresses and the amount of urine accumulated in the peritoneum increases, foals have progressive distension of the abdomen and make frequent attempts to urinate. Foals that attempt to urinate ventroflex their back (mild lordosis) and have a wide-based stance. This should be contrasted with foals with tenesmus, which characteristically have a narrow-based stance (all four limbs being under the body) and arch their back. Affected foals sometimes produce small quantities of urine, but usually there is lack of urination. Abdominal distension is most apparent when the foal is standing. In moderate to severe cases, there is a readily appreciable fluid wave on ballottement of the abdomen. As abdominal distension increases, the foal's tidal volume is impaired and breathing becomes rapid and shallow. The extremities become cool as cardiovascular function is impaired.

Ventral edema and preputial swelling occur in some foals. Foals with urachal rupture close to or within the abdominal wall or in the subcutaneous tissues will have subcutaneous accumulation of urine (which can be mistaken for ventral edema).

Foals with uroperitoneum secondary to sepsis usually have signs of sepsis as the initial and predominant sign of disease. These signs can range from mild fever and enlargement of the umbilical structures to septic shock and its attendant abnormalities. Initial signs of uroperitoneum in these foals are easily overlooked. As the disease develops, these foals have progressive abdominal distension. Signs of cardiovascular dysfunction can be incorrectly attributed to worsening of sepsis. It is important when treating septic foals to maintain a high index of suspicion and constant vigilance for development of uroperitoneum.

Infusion of contrast agents, such as methylene blue or fluorescein, into the bladder with subsequent detection of these compounds in the peritoneal fluid has been used to diagnose uroperitoneum. However, use of this method of diagnosis is now obsolete except in those instances in which ultrasonographic examination of the foal is not possible.

Imaging

Ultrasonographic examination of the abdomen of foals has simplified detection of uroperitoneum in foals and is the **preferred imaging modality for the detection of excessive peritoneal fluid in foals.** The ultrasound examination is best performed with a 5-MHz sector scan probe, with more detailed examination of the umbilical structures performed using a 7-MHz linear or sector scan probe. However, diagnosis of the presence of excessive peritoneal fluid can be achieved using a 7-MHz linear sector scan probe, such as is routinely used for examination of the mare's reproductive tract. The examination is performed transcutaneously.

Ultrasonography reveals the presence of an excessive quantity of fluid that is minimally echogenic. Intestine, mesentery, and omentum are readily visualized floating in this fluid. The presence of a large quantity of minimally echogenic fluid in the peritoneum of foals is very specific (effectively 100%) for uroperitoneum. The procedure is also sensitive, especially if performed repeatedly to detect changes in the amount of fluid, especially when the initial examination is equivocal. The umbilical structures should be examined closely and the urachus tracked to the bladder. Frequently a defect in the urachus or umbilicus is identified. The thorax of affected foals should also be examined, because foals with large quantities of urine in the peritoneum often have a substantial accumulation of pleural fluid. This can be important when considering anesthesia in these foals.

Radiographic examination of foals with suspected uroperitoneum is rarely performed because of the utility of ultrasonographic examination in this disease. Plain abdominal radiography is of limited usefulness in the detection of uroperitoneum or localizing the source of urine. Positive contrast cystography using a 10% solution of iohexol or similar water-soluble contrast agent administered into the bladder through a Foley catheter can be useful in detection of leaks, especially small leaks that cannot be visualized on ultrasonographic examination. Care should be taken to ensure that the bladder is sufficiently distended to ensure that any leak is visualized. Use of barium contrast medium, or negative-contrast cystography (infusion of air into the bladder), are contraindicated. IV pyelography is of very limited usefulness in the detection of ureteral defects because of the difficulty in localizing the site of the leak.

Electrocardiographic examination can reveal cardiac arrest, atrioventricular block, presumed intraventricular block, ventricular premature complexes, ventricular tachycardia, and ventricular fibrillation. These abnormalities are most likely to occur in foals that are hyperkalemic at the time of induction of anesthesia.

CLINICAL PATHOLOGY

Foals with uncomplicated uroperitoneum have hyponatremia, hypochloremia, hypobicarbonatemia (metabolic acidosis), acidemia, hyperkalemia, and azotemia. Severely affected foals can be profoundly hyponatremic (<110 mEq/L) and hyperkalemic (>7.0 mEq/L). Serum or plasma creatinine and urea nitrogen concentrations are elevated. When interpreting SUN concentrations in foals, it should be kept in mind that the urea concentration in normal foals is much lower than in adults.

Diagnosis based on serum electrolyte abnormalities is confounded in hospitalized foals that are being treated with IV fluids. Administration of fluids prevents the development of hyponatremia and hypochloremia in septic foals that develop uroperitoneum during the course of their disease. However, fluid administration does not prevent the increases in serum creatinine or urea nitrogen concentration.

Hematologic abnormalities reflect any underlying sepsis.

Analysis of **peritoneal fluid** reveals that it has a low specific gravity (<1.010), low total protein concentration (<2.5 g/dL; 25 g/L), and low white cell count (<1000 cells/μL, 1×10^9 cells/L). Peritoneal fluid can have a uriniferous odor, but this is not a reliable diagnostic sign. Peritoneal fluid from foals with uroperitoneum has elevated concentrations of creatinine (usually twice that in a contemporaneous serum sample), urea nitrogen (twice that of serum), and potassium. Microscopic examination of the fluid can reveal calcium carbonate crystals, the presence of which is diagnostic for urine.

NECROPSY FINDINGS

Necropsy examination confirms the presence of uroperitoneum and the structural defect allowing leakage of urine into the abdomen. The defect can have signs of healing, which can make it readily confused with a malformation, because affected foals can survive for days after the rupture occurs, which is sufficient time for partial healing of the defect.

DIFFERENTIAL DIAGNOSIS

Ultrasonographic demonstration of an excessive quantity of poorly echogenic fluid in the abdomen of a foal that is passing little if any urine and that has hyponatremia and hyperkalemia is diagnostic of uroabdomen. Confirmation of the diagnosis can be achieved by measurement of creatinine concentration in the peritoneal fluid. Ultrasonographic examination greatly facilitates the diagnosis.

The principal differential diagnoses for azotemia in foals are uroperitoneum and renal disease. **Primary renal disease** in foals can cause hyponatremia, hyperkalemia, and azotemia, but there is no accumulation of fluid in the peritoneum. Additionally, in primary renal disease there are abnormalities in urine composition (presence of blood, protein, leukocytes, and casts). Hyponatremia and hyperkalemia can occur in foals with **enterocolitis**, but the other clinical signs are diagnostic of this disease. **Addison's disease** (mineralocorticoid deficiency) does occur in foals but is rare, and there is no accumulation of fluid in the abdomen.

TREATMENT

Definitive treatment of uroperitoneum in foals is surgical repair of the defect. However, there is no need for surgery on an emergency basis. Instead, care should be taken to correct life-threatening electrolyte and fluid abnormalities before the foal is subjected to anesthesia. Principles of medical treatment are prevention of potentially lethal cardiac arrhythmia; correction of electrolyte, fluid, and acid-base abnormalities; and relief of abdominal distension.

Potentially life-threatening electrolyte abnormalities, especially hyperkalemia, should be corrected urgently and before any attempted surgical correction of the anatomic defect.

Correction of fluid and electrolyte abnormalities is best achieved by draining the abdomen and ensuring continued voiding of urine while administering isotonic fluids intravenously. Because the foal has normal kidney function, draining urine from the abdomen allows the foal to restore normal serum electrolyte concentrations and fluid balance provided it is allowed to nurse and/or is administered parenteral fluids.

Peritoneal drainage is achieved by placement of a catheter into the abdomen. It should be placed so it remains in place until the electrolyte abnormalities have been corrected and the foal is a suitable candidate for surgical repair of the anatomic defect. An ideal catheter is a Foley balloon-tipped catheter placed into the abdomen through a small (5-mm) incision in the skin and external abdominal wall. The catheter should be placed in the inguinal region and to one side of the linear alba to avoid injury and contamination of a future surgical site and to minimize the chances of the catheter being plugged by omentum. The catheter is inserted under local anesthesia, and the balloon is inflated to secure the catheter in the abdomen. The catheter can be further secured by a suture. Sedation or tranquilization should be avoided in foals at risk of cardiac or respiratory distress because of the electrolyte abnormalities. Urine should be allowed to drain from the catheter into a closed collection system that minimizes the chances of ascending infection of the peritoneum.

Hyperkalemia is usually readily corrected by peritoneal drainage and administration of potassium-free fluid, such as 0.9% sodium chloride. Serum potassium concentration declines quickly when effective peritoneal drainage is obtained, and serum potassium concentrations can normalize in 8 to 12 hours. If emergency management of hyperkalemia is required, administration of 5% dextrose either alone or, if hyponatremia is also present, in 0.9% sodium chloride, is effective in reducing serum potassium concentration. Sodium bicarbonate (1–3 mEq/kg BW, IV) will also decrease serum potassium concentration. Calcium gluconate antagonizes the effect of hyperkalemia on cardiac function and is useful in the treatment of hyperkalemic arrhythmias. The serum potassium concentration should be lower than 5.5 mEq/L before the foal is anesthetized. Mare's milk, which is rich in potassium, should be withheld until the serum potassium concentration is below the required level.

Hyponatremia is resolved by drainage of the peritoneum and administration of 0.9% to 1.8% sodium chloride intravenously. Serum sodium concentration, especially if markedly low, should be corrected slowly to prevent the development of hyponatremic encephalopathy. Serum sodium concentrations should be increased by approximately 1 (mEq/L)/h.

Affected foals should be administered broad-spectrum antibiotics because of the risk of peritonitis and because many foals with uroperitoneum have sepsis. The immune status of young foals should be examined by measurement of serum IgG concentration and, if it is less than 800 mg/dL (8 g/L), the foal should receive 20 to 40 mL/kg of plasma.

Correction of the defect in the bladder, urachus, or urethra is surgical. Nonsurgical management has been described in a foal in which a Foley catheter was inserted in the bladder and left in place for 5 days. The bladder was constantly drained of urine and this allowed the tear to heal. This technique offers an alternative to surgical repair of bladder rupture. However, surgical repair is definitive and is the recommended method of treatment.

Subcutaneous rupture of the urachus can similarly be treated by placement of a Foley catheter through the patent urachus and into the bladder. The defect in the urachus is then allowed to heal and the catheter is removed in 3 to 6 days.

PREVENTION AND CONTROL

There are no recognized means of preventing or controlling this disease. Minimizing the risk of foals developing septic disease is expected to reduce the incidence of uroperitoneum secondary to sepsis.

REFERENCE

1. Castagnetti C, et al. *Equine Vet Educ*. 2010;22:132.

CYSTITIS

Inflammation of the bladder is usually associated with bacterial infection and is characterized clinically by frequent, painful urination (pollakiuria and dysuria) and the presence of blood (hematuria), inflammatory cells, and bacteria in the urine.

ETIOLOGY

Cystitis occurs sporadically as a result of the introduction of infection into the bladder when trauma to the bladder has occurred or when there is stagnation of the urine. In farm animals, the common associations are

- Cystic calculus
- Difficult parturition
- Contaminated catheterization
- Late pregnancy
- As a sequel to paralysis of the bladder; a special case of bladder paralysis occurs in horses grazing sudax or Sudan grass and in horses with equine herpesvirus myoencephalopathy.

In the previous cases, the bacterial population is usually mixed but is predominantly *E. coli*. There is also the accompaniment of specific pyelonephritides in cattle and pigs, associated with *C. renale* and *Eubacterium suis*, respectively. Many sporadic cases also occur in pigs, especially after farrowing. Common isolates from these are *E. coli*, *Streptococcus*, and *Pseudomonas* spp. *C. matruchotii* causes encrusted cystitis in horses.

Enzootic hematuria of cattle resembles cystitis.

PATHOGENESIS

Bacteria frequently gain entrance to the bladder but are usually removed by the flushing action of voided urine before they invade the mucosa. Mucosal injury facilitates invasion, but stagnation of urine is the most important predisposing cause. Bacteria usually enter the bladder by ascending the urethra, but descending infection from embolic nephritis may also occur.

CLINICAL FINDINGS

The urethritis that usually accompanies cystitis causes painful sensations and the desire to urinate. Urination occurs frequently and is accompanied by pain and sometimes grunting; the animal remains in the urination posture for some minutes after the flow has ceased, often manifesting additional expulsive efforts. The volume of urine passed on each occasion is usually small. In very acute cases, there may be moderate abdominal pain, as evidenced by treading with the hindfeet, kicking at the belly and swishing with the tail, and a moderate febrile reaction. Acute retention may develop if the urethra becomes blocked with pus or blood, but this is unusual.

Chronic cases show a similar syndrome, but the signs are less marked. Frequent urination and small volume are the characteristic signs. In chronic cases, the bladder wall may feel thickened on rectal examination and, in horses, a calculus may be present. In acute cases, no palpable abnormality may be detected but pain may be evidenced. Endoscopic examination of the bladder of affected horses reveals widespread inflammation of the cystic mucosa and occasionally the presence of a cystic calculus.

CLINICAL PATHOLOGY

Blood and pus in the urine is typical of acute cases, and the urine may have a strong ammonia odor. In less severe cases, the urine may be only turbid, and in chronic cases there may be no abnormality on gross inspection. Microscopic examination of urine sediment will reveal erythrocytes, leukocytes, and desquamated epithelial cells. Quantitative bacterial culture is necessary to confirm the diagnosis and to guide treatment selection.

NECROPSY FINDINGS

Acute cystitis is manifested by hyperemia, hemorrhage, and edema of the mucosa. The urine is cloudy and contains mucus. In subacute and chronic cases, the wall is grossly thickened and the mucosal surface is rough and coarsely granular. Highly vascular papillary projections may have eroded, causing the urine to be bloodstained or contain large clots of blood. In the cystitis associated with Sudan grass, soft masses of calcium carbonate may accumulate in the bladder, and the vaginal wall may be inflamed and coated with the same material.

TREATMENT

Antimicrobial agents are indicated to control the infection, and determination of the antimicrobial susceptibility of the causative bacteria is essential. Relapses are common unless treatment is continued for a minimum of 7 and preferably 14 days. Repeated bacterial culture of urine at least once during and again within 7 to 10 days after completion of treatment should be used to assess the success of therapy. Recurrence of the infection is usually caused by failure to eliminate foci of infection in the accessory glands and in the bladder wall.

DIFFERENTIAL DIAGNOSIS

The clinical and laboratory findings of cystitis resemble those of pyelonephritis and cystic urolithiasis.

- **Pyelonephritis** is commonly accompanied by bladder involvement and differentiation depends on whether there are lesions in the kidney. This may be determined by rectal examination but in many cases it is not possible to make a firm decision. Provided the causative bacteria can be identified, this is probably not of major importance as the treatment will be the same in either case. However, the prognosis in pyelonephritis is less favorable than in cystitis. Thickening of the bladder wall, which may suggest a diagnosis of cystitis, occurs also in enzootic hematuria and in poisoning by the yellow-wood tree (*Terminalia oblongata*) in cattle and by sorghum in horses.
- **The presence of calculi** in the bladder can usually be detected by rectal examination, by ultrasonographic examination, by endoscopic examination in female ruminants and in both sexes of horses, or by radiographic examination in smaller animals.
- **Urethral obstruction** may also cause frequent attempts at urination, but the urine flow is greatly restricted, usually only drops are voided and the distended bladder can be felt on rectal examination.

The prognosis in chronic cases is poor because of the difficulty of completely eradicating the infection and the common secondary involvement of the kidney. Free access to water should be permitted at all times to ensure a free flow of urine.

UROLITHIASIS IN RUMINANTS

Urolithiasis is common as a subclinical disorder among ruminants raised in management systems where the ration is composed primarily of grain or where animals graze certain types of pasture. In these situations, 40% to 60% of animals may form calculi in their urinary tract. Urolithiasis becomes an important clinical disease of castrated male ruminants when calculi cause urinary tract obstruction and usually obstruction of the urethra. Urethral obstruction is characterized clinically by complete retention of urine, frequent unsuccessful attempts to urinate, and distension of the bladder. Urethral perforation and rupture of the bladder can be sequelae. Mortality is high in cases of urethral obstruction, and treatment is surgical. As a result, prevention is important to limit losses from urolithiasis.

ETIOLOGY

Urinary calculi, or uroliths, form when inorganic and organic urinary solutes are precipitated out of solution. The precipitates occur as crystals or as amorphous "deposits." Calculi form over a long period by a gradual accumulation of precipitate around a nidus. An organic matrix is an integral part of most types of calculus. Several factors affect the rate of urolith formation, including conditions that affect the concentration of specific solutes in urine, the ease with which solutes are precipitated out of solution, the provision of a nidus, and the tendency to concretion of precipitates. These are presented in the following section. Factors that contribute to the clinical syndrome of obstructive urolithiasis are dealt with separately.

EPIDEMIOLOGY

Species Affected

Urolithiasis occurs in all ruminant species but is of greatest economic importance in feeder steers and wethers (castrated lambs) fed heavy concentrate rations and animals on range pasture in particular problem areas. These range areas are associated with the presence of pasture plants containing large quantities of oxalate, estrogens, or silica. When cattle graze pasture containing plants with high levels of silica, uroliths occur in animals of all ages and sexes. The prevalence of uroliths is about the same in cows, heifers, bulls, and steers grazing on the same pasture, and they may even occur in newborn calves. Females and bulls usually pass the calculi, and obstructive urolithiasis is primarily a problem in castrated male animals.

Obstructive urolithiasis is the most common urinary tract disease in breeding rams and goats. There are three main groups of factors that contribute to urolithiasis:

- Those that favor the **development of a nidus** about which precipitation and concretion can occur
- Those that **facilitate precipitation of solutes** on to the nidus
- Those that favor **concretion by cementing precipitated salts** to the developing calculus

Nidus Formation

A nidus favors the deposition of crystals about itself. It may be a group of desquamated epithelial cells or necrotic tissue that may be formed as a result in occasional cases from local infection in the urinary tract. When large numbers of animals are affected, it is probable that some other factor, such as a deficiency of vitamin A or the administration of estrogens, is the cause of excessive epithelial desquamation. When stilbestrol was used as a growth promoter, mortality rates of 20% from obstructive urolithiasis were recorded in wethers receiving stilbestrol implants compared with no mortalities in a control group. Diets low in vitamin A have been suspected as a cause of urolithiasis, but vitamin A deficiency does not appear to be a major causative factor.

Precipitation of Solutes

Urine is a highly saturated solution containing a large number of solutes, many of them in higher concentrations than their individual solubilities permit in a simple solution. Urinary stone formation is currently attributed to supersaturation, crystal growth, and aggregation, with supersaturation and the urinary concentration of promoters and inhibitors playing dominant roles in stone formation.[1] Several factors may explain why solutes remain in solution. Probably the most important factor in preventing precipitation is the presence of **protective colloids** that convert urine into a gel. These colloids are efficient up to a point, but their capacity to maintain the solution may be overcome by abnormalities in one or more of a number of other factors. Even in normal animals, crystals of a number of solutes may be present in the urine intermittently and urine must be considered to be an unstable solution. The physical characteristics of urine, the amount of solute presented to the kidney for excretion, and the balance between water and solute in urine all influence the ease of calculus formation. In most cases, these factors can also be influenced by management practices.

The pH of urine affects the solubility of some solutes, with mixed phosphate and carbonate calculi more readily formed in an alkaline than an acid medium. More important, the urine pH in ruminants is dependent on the urinary strong ion difference, with urine pH increasing with higher urine concentrations of potassium, sodium, magnesium, and calcium (with the effect of potassium predominating). Likewise, urine pH decreases in ruminants with higher urine concentrations of chloride and sulfate.[2] The high urine potassium concentration in herbivores is the main reason that they have an alkaline urine.

Ammonium chloride or phosphoric acid added to the rations of steers increases the acidity of the urine and reduces the incidence of calculi. The mechanism is uncertain but is probably related to the effect of pH on the stability of the urinary colloids or the effect of diuresis. In contrast, variations in pH between 1 and 8 have little influence on the solubility of silicic acid, the form of silica excreted in the urine of ruminants. As a result, dietary supplementation with ammonium chloride does not consistently prevent the formation of siliceous calculi.

The amount of solute presented to the kidney for excretion is influenced by the diet. Some pasture plants can contain up to 6% silica. Although ruminants grazing on these plants absorb only a small portion of the ingested silica, the kidney is the major route of excretion of absorbed silicic acid. The urine of these animals often becomes supersaturated with silicic acid, which promotes the polymerization or precipitation of the silicic acid and calculus formation.

Feeding sodium chloride prevents the formation of silica calculi by reducing the concentration of silicic acid in the urine and maintaining it below the saturation concentration. An excessive intake of minerals may occur from highly mineralized artesian water, or from diets containing high concentrations, particularly of phosphates in heavy-concentrate diets. Sheep with a high dietary intake of phosphorus have an increased concentration of phosphorus in their urine and an increased development of calculi. In cattle, sediment begins to appear in urine when concentrates reach 1.5% of the BW, and urolithiasis formation begins when concentrates have been fed for 2 months at the rate of 2.5% of the animal's BW.

Diets high in magnesium such as some calf milk replacers have been frequently associated with an increasing incidence of obstructive urolithiasis.[3] Supplemental calcium in the diet helps prevent calculus formation when phosphate or magnesium intake is high.

Ingestion of plants with a high oxalic acid content can be a risk factor for formation of calcium carbonate calculi in sheep. Although dietary excesses contribute to certain types of urolithiasis, calculus formation can rarely be recreated experimentally by simple overfeeding. The process of formation of urinary calculi is more complex than a simple dietary excess. However, recognition of associations between diet and some types of urolithiasis has been useful in developing preventive strategies.

Feeding practices can influence the function of the kidney and may contribute to calculus formation. In sheep fed grain in a few large meals, there is a marked reduction in urine volume and a marked increase in urine concentration and calcium excretion at the time of feeding. These short-term changes in urine composition may be factors in the development of uroliths.

The concentration of urine is an important determinant of the concentration of individual solutes in the urine. Although it is difficult to induce urolithiasis by restricting access to water, concentrated urine is a risk factor for calculus formation. Animals can be forced to produce concentrated urine because of lack of easy access to water, a particular problem in pastured animals; lack of familiarity with water delivery systems; and poor quality of available water. Water deprivation can be exacerbated by heavy fluid loss by sweating in hot, arid climates.

Factors Favoring Concretion

Most calculi, and siliceous calculi in particular, are composed of organic matter as well as minerals. This organic component is mucoprotein, particularly its mucopolysaccharide fraction. It acts as a cementing agent and favors the formation of calculi when precipitates are present. The mucoprotein content of urine of feeder steers and lambs is increased by heavy concentrate–low roughage rations, by feeding pelleted rations, even more so by implantation with diethylstilbestrol and, combined with a high dietary intake of phosphate, may be an important cause of urolithiasis in this class of livestock. These high levels of mucoprotein in urine may be the result of a rapid turnover of supporting tissues in animals that are making rapid gains in weight.

Miscellaneous Factors in the Development of Urolithiasis

Stasis of urine favors precipitation of solutes, probably by virtue of the infection that commonly follows, providing cellular material for a nidus. Certain feeds, including cottonseed meal, rice straw, and milo sorghum, are credited with causing more urolithiasis than other feeds. Alfalfa is in an indeterminate position: by some observers it is thought to cause the formation of calculi, by others it is thought to be a valuable aid in preventing their formation. Pelleting appears to increase calculi formation if the ration already has this tendency.

Attempts to produce urolithiasis experimentally by varying any of the previous factors are usually unsuccessful, and natural cases most probably occur as a result of the interaction of several factors. In feedlots a combination of high mineral feeding and a high level of mucoprotein in the urine associated with rapid growth are probably the important factors in most instances. In range animals a high intake of mineralized water, or oxalate or silica in plants, are most commonly associated with a high incidence of urinary calculi, but again other predisposing factors, including deprivation or excessive loss of water, may contribute to the development of the disease. Limited water intake at weaning and in very cold weather may also be a contributory factor.

Composition of Calculi

The chemical composition of urethral calculi varies and appears to depend largely on the dietary intake of individual elements. In semiarid areas such as the great plains of North America and parts of Australia, the dominant pasture grasses have a high content of silica. Cattle and sheep grazing these pastures have a high prevalence of siliceous calculi. Calculi containing calcium carbonate are more common in animals on clover-rich pasture or when oxalate-containing plants abound. Calcium, ammonium, and magnesium carbonate are also common constituents of calculi in cattle and sheep at pasture.

Cattle, sheep, and goats eating a high grain diet in feedlots usually have calculi composed of struvite (magnesium ammonium phosphate, $NH_4MgPO_4.6H_2O$). Cattle, water buffalo, and Boer goats in China fed grain, cottonseed meal, or rice straw as part of their diet may also have crystals present in their urine composed of magnesium potassium phosphate ($KMgPO_4.6H_2O$),[1,3,4] but these crystals do not appear to precipitate to form calculi. High concentrations of magnesium in feedlot rations also cause a high prevalence of struvite calculi in lambs and goats. Experimental feeding of a ration with high magnesium content increases the prevalence of struvite urolithiasis in goats[3] and calcium apatite urolithiasis in calves. Oxalate calculi are extremely rare in ruminants but have been observed in goats and induced experimentally in feedlot cattle. Xanthine calculi in sheep are recorded in some areas in New Zealand where pasture is poor.

Estrogenic subterranean clover can cause urinary tract obstruction in wethers in a number of ways. Soft, moist, yellow calculi containing 2-benzocoumarins, isoflavones and indigotin–indirubin, have been observed. Calculi or unformed sediments of benzocoumarins (urolithins) and 4′-*O*-methylequol, either singly or in various combinations with equol, formononetin, biochanin A, indigotin, and indirubin, also occur. Obstruction is promoted by estrogenic stimulation of squamous metaplasia of the urethral epithelium, accessory sex glandular enlargement, and mucous secretion. Pastures containing these plants are also reputed to cause urinary obstruction by calculi consisting of calcium carbonate. Feedlot lambs receiving a supplement of stilbestrol (1 mg/kg of feed or 2 mg per lamb daily) developed urethral obstruction thought to be caused primarily by plugs of mucoprotein. The accessory sex glands were also enlarged.

Risk Factors for Obstructive Urolithiasis

The risk factors important in the formation of urinary calculi are also important in the development of obstructive urolithiasis.

The size of individual calculi and **the amount of calculus material** are both important in the development of urethral obstruction. Often the obstruction is caused by one stone, although an aggregation of many small struvite calculi often causes obstruction in sheep fed high-concentrate rations.

Once calculi form, the most important factor contributing to the occurrence of obstruction is the diameter of the urethra. Wethers (castrated lambs) and steers (castrated cattle) are most commonly affected because of the relatively small diameter of the urethra in these animals. Castration significantly impacts the diameter of the urethra in steers. When the urethral diameter of late castrates (6 months old) was compared with early castrates (2 months old), it was found to be 8% larger and would be able to expel a calculus that was 13% larger than a calculus passed by early castrates. Bulls can usually pass calculi that are 44% larger than those that could be passed by an early castrated steer.

Occurrence

Urethral obstruction may occur at any site but is most **common at the distal sigmoid flexure** in steers near the insertion of the retractor penis muscle, and in the **vermiform appendage,** distal to the sigmoid flexure, at the distal sigmoid flexure, or subischially in wethers or rams; these are all sites where the urethra narrows.[5] Urolithiasis is as common in females as in males, but obstruction rarely if ever occurs because of the shortness and large diameter of the urethra. Repeated attacks of obstructive urolithiasis are not uncommon in wethers and steers and at necropsy up to 200 calculi may be found in various parts of the tract of one animal. However, generally, a single calculus causes obstruction in cattle, whereas multiple calculi are common in sheep.

In North America, obstructive urolithiasis caused by siliceous calculi is most common in **beef feeder cattle** during the **fall and winter months.** The calves are weaned at 6 to 8 months and moved from pasture to a feedlot in which they are fed roughage and grain. The incidence of obstructive urolithiasis is highest during the early part of the feeding period and during cold weather, when the consumption of water may be decreased.

Although the occurrence of obstructive urolithiasis is usually sporadic, with cases occurring at irregular intervals in a group of animals, outbreaks may occur, affecting a large number of animals in a short time. In outbreaks it is probable that factors are present that favor the development of calculi, as well as the development of obstruction. For example, multiple cases of obstructive urolithiasis can occur in lambs within a few weeks of introducing a concentrated ration. Obstructive urolithiasis increases in occurrence with age but has occurred in lambs as young as 1 month of age.

PATHOGENESIS

Urinary calculi are commonly observed at necropsy in normal animals and in many appear to cause little or no harm. Calculi may be present in the kidneys, ureters, bladder, and urethra. In a few animals, pyelonephritis, cystitis, and urethral obstruction may occur. Obstruction of one ureter may cause unilateral hydronephrosis, with compensation by the contralateral kidney. The major clinical manifestation of urolithiasis is urethral obstruction, particularly in wethers and steers. This difference between urolithiasis and obstructive urolithiasis is an important one. Simple urolithiasis has relatively little importance, but obstructive urolithiasis is a fatal disease unless the obstruction is relieved. Rupture of the urethra or bladder occurs within 2 to 3 days if the obstruction is not relieved and the animal dies of uremia or secondary bacterial infection. Rupture of the bladder is more likely to occur with a spherical, smooth calculus that causes complete obstruction of the urethra. Rupture of the urethra is more common with irregularly shaped stones that cause partial obstruction and pressure necrosis of the urethral wall.

CLINICAL FINDINGS

Calculi in the renal pelvis or ureters are not usually diagnosed antemortem, although obstruction of a ureter may be detectable on rectal examination, especially if it is accompanied by hydronephrosis.[6] Occasionally the exit from the renal pelvis is blocked and the acute distension that results may cause acute pain, accompanied by stiffness of the gait and pain on pressure over the loins. Calculi in the bladder may cause cystitis and are manifested by signs of that disease.

Obstruction of the Urethra by a Calculus

This is a common occurrence in steers and wethers and causes a characteristic syndrome of abdominal pain with kicking at the belly, treading with the hindfeet, and swishing of the tail. Repeated twitching of the penis, sufficient to shake the prepuce, is often observed, and the animal may make strenuous efforts to urinate, accompanied by straining, grunting, and grating of the teeth, but these result in the passage of only a few drops of bloodstained urine. A heavy precipitate of crystals is often visible on the preputial hairs or on the inside of the thighs (Fig. 13-8). Some animals with urethral obstruction will have a dry prepuce because of the absence of urination, although this sign is not specific for urolithiasis.

The passage of a flexible catheter up the urethra, after relaxing the penis by lumbosacral epidural anesthesia, by pudendal nerve block or by administering an ataractic drug, may make it possible to locate the sites of obstructions that are anterior to the sigmoid flexure. However, catheterization of the urethra from the glans penis to the bladder is almost impossible in cattle and ruminants because of the urethral diverticulum and its valve. A precurved coronary catheter has been used to catheterize the bladder of calves and goats but requires fluoroscopic guidance.

Cattle with incomplete obstruction ("dribblers") will pass small amounts of bloodstained urine frequently. Occasionally a small stream of urine will be voided followed by a complete blockage. This confuses the diagnosis. In these animals the calculus is triangular in shape and allows small amounts of urine to move past the obstruction at irregular intervals. However, these instances are rare.

The entire length of the **penis** must be palpated for evidence of a painful swelling from the preputial orifice to the scrotum, above the scrotum to locate the sigmoid flexure, and proximally up the perineum as far as possible.

In **rams**, **bucks**, and **wethers** the **urethral process of the exteriorized penis** must be examined for enlargement and the presence of multiple calculi. Extrusion of the penis is difficult in prepubertal sheep and goats because of the presence of an attachment from the prepuce to the glans penis; loss of this attachment is mediated by testosterone and is usually complete by the onset of puberty, although separation may not occur in castrated animals. Penile extrusion is facilitated by xylazine sedation and positioning the animals with lumbosacral flexion. Abnormal urethral processes should be amputated, and in many animals grit is detected during urethral transection.

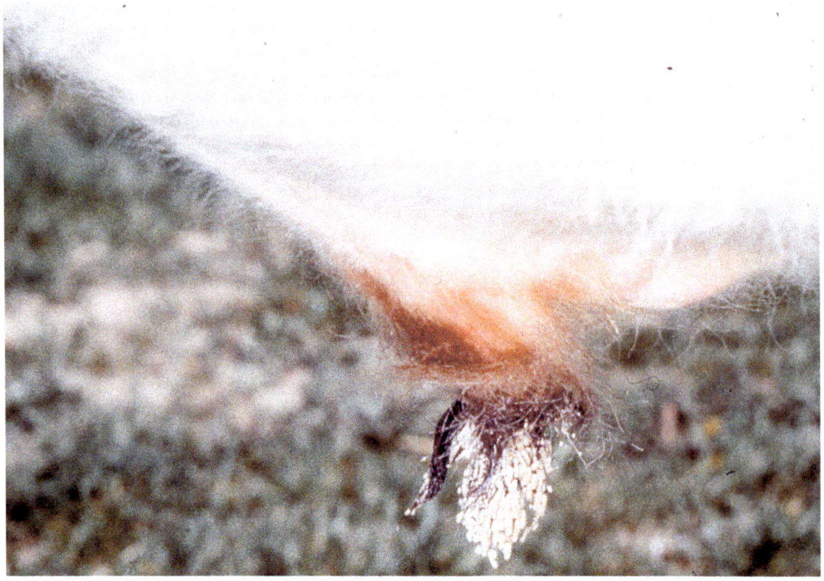

Fig. 13-8 Extensive precipitation of crystals on the preputial hairs of a steer with obstructive urolithiasis.

On rectal examination, when the size of the animal is appropriate, the urethra and bladder are palpably distended and the urethra is painful and pulsates on manipulation.

In rams with obstructive urolithiasis, sudden depression, inappetence, stamping the feet, tail swishing, kicking at the abdomen, bruxism, and anuria or the passage of only a few drops of urine are common. Clinical examination must include inspection of the ventral abdomen for edema, inspection and palpation of the preputial orifice for crystals, palpation of the penis in the area of the sigmoid flexure, and inspection and palpation of the urethral process (vermiform appendage) of the exteriorized penis.

Rupture of Urethra or Bladder

If the obstruction is not relieved, **urethral rupture** or **bladder rupture** usually occurs within 48 hours. With urethral rupture, the urine leaks into the connective tissue of the ventral abdominal wall and prepuce and causes an obvious fluid swelling, which may spread as far as the thorax (Fig. 13-9). This results in a severe cellulitis and toxemia. The skin over the swollen area may slough, permitting drainage, and the course is rather more protracted in these cases. When the bladder ruptures, there is an immediate relief from discomfort but anorexia and depression develop as uremia develops. Two types of bladder rupture have been described: multiple pinpoint perforations in areas of necrosis or discrete tears in the bladder wall. The site of leakage is almost always on the dorsal aspect of the bladder. Complete urethral obstruction therefore results in urethral rupture or bladder rupture and never both in the same animal because pressure is released once rupture occurs.

A fluid wave is detectable on tactile percussion, and the abdomen soon becomes distended. The animal may continue in this state for as long as 2 to 3 days before death occurs. Fibrin deposition around the dorsal surface of the bladder may be palpated per rectum in steers. In rare cases death occurs soon after rupture of the bladder as a result of severe internal hemorrhage.

In rare cases calculi may form in the prepuce of steers. The calculi are top shaped and, by acting as floating valves, cause obstruction of the preputial orifice, distension of the prepuce, and infiltration of the abdominal wall with urine. These cases may be mistaken for cases of urethral perforation.

CLINICAL PATHOLOGY

Urinalysis

Laboratory examinations may be useful in the diagnosis of the disease in its early stages when the calculi are present in the kidney or bladder. The urine usually contains erythrocytes and epithelial cells and a higher than normal number of crystals, which are sometimes accompanied by larger aggregations described as sand or sabulous deposit. Bacteria may also be present if secondary invasion of the traumatic cystitis and pyelonephritis has occurred.

Serum Biochemistry

SUN and creatinine concentrations will be increased before either urethral or bladder rupture occurs and will increase even further afterward. Rupture of the bladder will result in uroabdomen. Because urine has a much lower sodium and chloride concentration and higher osmolality than plasma, equilibration of electrolytes and free water into the abdomen of the ruminant will always result in hyponatremia, hypochloremia, hyperphosphatemia, and hypoosmolality in serum, with the magnitude of the changes reflecting the volume of urine in the abdomen. Hypermagnesemia appears to be a common finding in weaned lambs with urolithiasis,[7] although few studies have reported changes in plasma magnesium concentrations in affected animals. Similar changes in serum biochemistry are present in steers with ruptured urethras, with the magnitude of the changes being smaller than in steers with ruptured bladders. Interestingly, steers with ruptured bladder or urethra typically have serum potassium concentrations within the normal range; this result most probably reflects the combined effects of increased salivary potassium loss in the face of hyponatremia and inappetence. A minority of ruminants with urolithiasis will have hyperkalemia.[8] Prolonged duration of urolithiasis usually results in hypophosphatemia in goats, presumably from increased phosphorus secretion by the salivary glands.[8]

Abdominocentesis and Needle Aspirate of Subcutaneous Tissue

Abdominocentesis is necessary to detect uroperitoneum after rupture of the bladder or needle aspiration from the subcutaneous swelling associated with urethral rupture. However, it is often difficult to identify the fluid obtained from the peritoneal cavity or the subcutaneous tissues as urine other than by appearance and smell or by biochemical examination. Generally, in uroperitoneum, substantial quantities of fluid can be easily obtained by abdominocentesis. Warming the fluid may facilitate detection of the urine odor, although this is a subjective and poorly sensitive diagnostic test.

Ultrasonography

Ultrasonography is an extremely useful aid for the diagnosis of obstructive urolithiasis in rams and bucks, with a 10- to 15-MHz linear probe used to assess the urethra for dilatation proximal to the obstruction or rupture at the site of obstruction and a 5-MHz microconvex or linear probe used to evaluate the bladder and kidneys.[5,9] All parts of the urinary tract must be examined for urinary calculi. The kidneys are examined from the paralumbar fossa and the bladder and urethra transrectally. The kidneys are examined for enlargement, and the renal pelves, medullary pyramids, and urethra examined for dilatation. The size of the bladder should be noted and its contents examined. Distended bladders can reach 20 cm in diameter in adult rams, wethers, and bucks, and ultrasonographically appear as an anechoic (black) area surrounded by a bright white (hyperechoic) line. The bladder diameter should be measured in two dimensions at right angles to each other because the bladder shape changes with

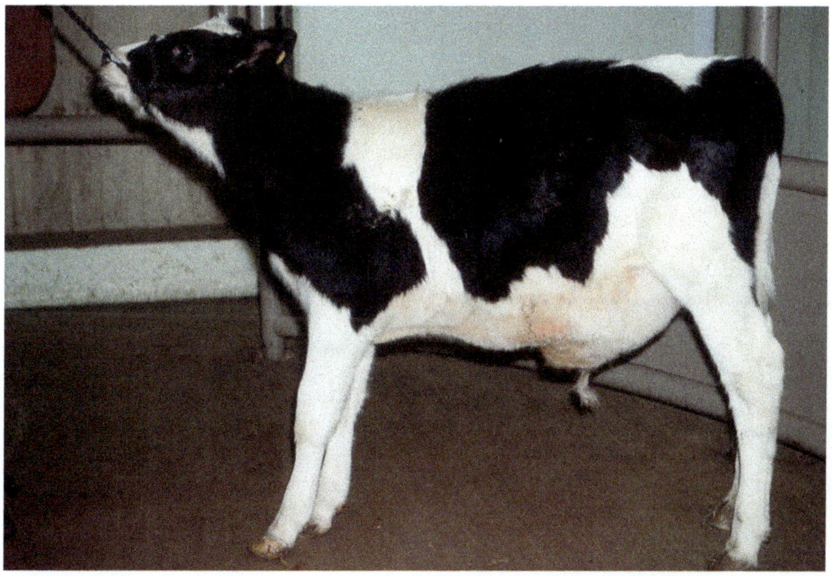

Fig. 13-9 Holstein-Friesian steer with obstructive urolithiasis, urethral rupture, and urine collecting ventrally to the site of rupture. (Photograph graciously provided by Dr. Bruce L. Hull, United States.)

animal movement.[9] A ruptured bladder does not always empty completely. Fibrin tags may be visualized ultrasonographically in animals with uroabdomen or on the dorsal surface of the bladder, which is the usual site for rupture. In rams with obstructive urolithiasis, the urethra and bladder are markedly dilated. Because of severe cystitis, the contents of the bladder appear as multiple, tiny, uniformly distributed echoes. The renal pelves are commonly dilated, and in experimentally induced urethral ligation in male goats, ultrasonographically determined renal dimensions increased after 24 hours of obstruction.[9]

Radiography

Plain radiography is very helpful in small ruminants in which radiopaque calculi (calcium carbonate, calcium oxalate, and silica) are common.[5] Plain radiography helps to identify the best method for surgical correction and confirm resolution of the obstruction, but it is not effective in small ruminants with struvite calculi because the stones are radiolucent and very small in diameter.[5] Contrast radiography using excretory urography, retrograde urethrography, cystourethrography, and normograde cystourethrography via tube cystotomy have also been used because of concerns that the rumen and abdominal viscera (and wool in sheep) obscures the bladder in plain radiographs.

NECROPSY FINDINGS

Calculi may be found in the renal pelvis or bladder of normal animals or of those dying of other diseases. In the renal pelvis they may cause no abnormality, although in occasional cases there is accompanying pyelonephritis. Unilateral ureteral obstruction is usually accompanied by dilatation of the ureter and hydronephrosis. Bilateral obstruction causes fatal uremia. Calculi in the bladder are usually accompanied by varying degrees of chronic cystitis. The urethra or urethral process may be obstructed by one or more stones or may be impacted for a number of centimeters with a fine sabulous deposit.

When rupture of the urethra has occurred, the urethra is eroded at the site of obstruction, and extensive cellulitis and accumulation of urine are present in the ventral abdominal wall. When the bladder has ruptured the peritoneal cavity is distended with urine and there is mild to moderate chemical peritonitis. In areas where urolithiasis is a problem, it is an advantage to determine the chemical composition of the calculi.

DIFFERENTIAL DIAGNOSIS

Obstruction of the urethra in ruminant animals is almost always caused by a calculus and is characterized clinically by anuria or dribbling, swishing of the tail, abdominal pain with kicking at the abdomen or stamping the feet, and a progressively worsening condition.

Nonobstructive urolithiasis may be confused with **pyelonephritis** or **cystitis**, and differentiation may be possible only by rectal examination in the case of vesical calculi or by radiographic examination in smaller animals. Subsequent development of hydronephrosis may enable a diagnosis to be made in cattle. Ultrasonographic examination is extremely useful in sheep and goats.

A rectal examination, if possible, may reveal distension of the bladder and dilatation and pulsation of the urethra if the bladder has not ruptured.

In adults, **rupture of the bladder** is usually the result of obstructive urolithiasis, although other occasional causes of urethral obstruction are observed.

Rupture of the urethra in cattle is characterized by diffuse swelling of the subcutaneous tissues of the ventral body wall, and the skin is usually cooler than normal. It must be differentiated from other causes of swelling of the ventral abdominal wall, including abscesses and herniation of abdominal wall, which can be determined by close physical examination and needle aspiration.

Dilatation of the urethral recess in young cattle is characterized by a midline perineal swelling and may resemble pulsation of the perineal urethra in obstructive urolithiasis. The urethral recess arises from the junction of the pelvic and spongy parts of the urethra at the level of the ischial arch. A fold of urethral mucosa proximal to the recess acts as a valve to prevent the retrograde flow of urine into the pelvic urethra. An abnormally large urethral recess has been described in a calf. When there is dilatation of the urethral recess, during urination the proximal urethra pulses and the swelling may enlarge slightly. There is no urethral obstruction, and urine flows passively from the penis for several minutes after the urethral pulsation ceases. The dilatation can be radiographed using contrast media.

TREATMENT

The treatment of obstructive urolithiasis has traditionally been primarily surgical, including urethral process amputation (rams, wethers, bucks, llamas, and alpacas), prepubic and perineal urethrostomy, laser lithotripsy, tube cystotomy, and bladder marsupialization. Cattle or lambs with obstructive urolithiasis that are near the end of their feedlot feeding period and close to being marketed can be slaughtered for salvage if the result of an antemortem inspection is satisfactory. Animals in the early stages of obstruction before urethral or bladder rupture will usually pass inspection at an abattoir. The presence of uremia warrants failure to pass inspection. Recent studies suggest reasonable treatment response to medical treatment of bucks with urolithiasis.[10]

Rams, bucks, and wethers should all have their glans penis exteriorized and inspected and the urethral process amputated using a scalpel blade. This is best accomplished by having an assistant restrain the animal in a sitting position. The penis is exteriorized by grasping the shaft of the penis within the prepuce and retracting the prepuce to expose the tip of the penis, which is then grasped with a gauze sponge.[10] Exteriorization of the penis can be very difficult in prepubertal rams and bucks because of the presence of a persistent frenulum. Xylazine administration may facilitate exteriorization of the penis but increases urine production and therefore shortens the time to urethral or bladder rupture in animals with a complete obstruction.

It was thought that calculi cannot be dissolved by medical means, but recent studies suggest that administration of specific solutions into the bladder can rapidly dissolve most uroliths, although one report stated that radiopaque calculi (calcium carbonate, calcium oxalate, and silica) do not dissolve readily by urinary acidification by dietary means or infusion of Walpole's solution into the bladder through a tube cystotomy[5] or directly through a long needle.[10] Successful outcomes have occurred following instillation of 30 to 200 mL of an acetic acid solution (Walpole's buffer, pH adjusted to 4.3–4.8; contains 1.16% sodium acetate, 1.09% glacial acetic acid, and 97.75% distilled water) or hemiacidrin solution through a cystotomy catheter or long needle into the bladder after removal of most but not all the urine in the bladder; hemiacidrin is an acidic gluconocitrate solution with magnesium carbonate used for dissolution of magnesium ammonium phosphate and calcium phosphate uroliths in humans. The advantage of hemiacidrin is that it is reportedly less irritating to the urothelium than other acids of similar pH, such as Walpole's solution. The cystotomy tube can be placed surgically or transcutaneously using abdominal ultrasound. The latter technique involves placement of a 12-French sleeved trocar into the lumen of the bladder, followed by removal of the trocar and placement of a 10-French silicone Foley catheter through the sleeve of the trocar into the lumen of the bladder. The balloon on the Foley catheter is then inflated using 0.9% NaCl, the trocar sleeve removed from the abdomen, and the Foley catheter secured to the abdomen. The cystotomy catheter provides an alternative route for urine to leave the bladder and is allowed to drip continuously. The cystotomy catheter is occluded for 30 minutes to 2 hours after infusion of a low pH solution to retain the solution in the bladder and urethra, after this time the solution is drained from the bladder via the cystotomy tube. Checking the pH of the fluid in the bladder using pH strips is thought to be helpful in verifying that the target pH of <5.0 has been reached.[10]

In early stages of the disease or in cases of incomplete obstruction, treatment with smooth muscle relaxants such as phenothiazine derivatives (aminopromazine, 0.7 mg/kg of BW) has been tried to relax the urethral muscle and permit passage of the obstructing calculus; however, treatment efficacy is unknown. Animals treated medically should be observed closely to ensure that urination occurs and that obstruction does not recur. However, field observations indicate that these relaxants are ineffective, and it is difficult to believe that smooth muscle relaxants could be efficacious given that the urethral and periurethral tissue contains very little smooth muscle. Slight sedation induced by acepromazine (0.02 mg/kg IV every 4–6 hours) is of unknown benefit, and if used the sedation should not prevent the animal from standing when approached. A more rational treatment includes parenteral NSAIDs or infiltration of local anesthetic around the origin of the retractor penile muscles or a pudendal nerve block; this theoretically relaxes the retractor penis muscle and straightens the sigmoid flexure, creating a wider and straighter urethral passageway.

Retrograde hydropulsion is only occasionally successful, although it is frequently used as part of the initial treatment. This technique involves catheterization of the urethral orifice with a suitably sized urinary catheter and intermittent injection of 0.9% NaCl containing 2% lidocaine into the urethra in an attempt to flush out the calculi. Frequently, a gritty feeling is detected during this procedure, and one usually is left with the impression that the procedure is creating additional urethral trauma that may contribute to urethral stricture. The addition of lidocaine is thought to decrease urethral spasm but its efficacy and safety are unknown. Retrograde hydropulsion may also pack small crystals more tightly into the urethra. Cystotomy and normograde hydropulsion appear to have a higher success rate than retrograde hydropulsion.

Surgical treatment includes perineal urethrostomy to relieve bladder pressure and for the removal of calculi. This is a salvage procedure, and treated animals can be sent to slaughter for salvage when they have recovered sufficiently to pass antemortem inspection. In a series of 85 cases of surgical treatment of urethral obstruction in cattle, only 35% of animals recovered satisfactorily. In small ruminants, which invariably have multiple calculi, amputation of the urethral process may restore urine flow but usually provides only temporary relief, and the long-term prognosis in sheep and goats is poor because there is a high rate of recurrence of obstruction with stricture formation at the urethrostomy site. A recent surgical modification suggests that urethral stricture formation can be decreased in goats with transection of the penile body attachments from the pelvis and careful apposition of the urethra to the skin.[11] If perineal urethrostomy is unsuccessful, **tube cystotomy** is indicated. Urethroscopy and **laser lithotripsy** have successfully dissolved uroliths in a small number of small ruminants and one steer, but the technique is expensive and not widely available. **Prepubic urethrostomy** has been performed in a small number of small ruminants that have undergone stricture formation following perineal urethrostomy, whereas **urinary bladder marsupialization** by laparotomy or using a laparoscopy-assisted surgical technique[12] offers an alternative surgical method for correction. There is one report of erection failure in a male goat as a sequela to obstructive urolithiasis; erection failure was attributed to vascular occlusion of the corpus cavernosum penis. Surgical correction of urethral dilatation associated with the urethral recess in cattle has been described.

PREVENTION

A number of agents and management procedures have been recommended in the prevention of urolithiasis in feeder lambs and steers. First, and probably most important, the diet should contain an adequate balance of calcium and phosphorus to avoid precipitation of excess phosphorus in the urine. This is the major difficulty in controlling urolithiasis in feedlot ruminants, because their diets are grain rich (and therefore phosphorus rich). The ration should have a Ca : P ratio of 1.2 : 1, but higher calcium inputs (1.5–2.0 : 1) have been recommended, as have formulation of low oxalate and silica diets[5] and low-magnesium diets. Every practical effort must be used to increase and maintain water intake in feeder steers that have just been moved into a feedlot situation. The addition of salt at the level of 4% of the total ration of feeder calves has been shown experimentally to have this effect on both steers and lambs. Under practical conditions, salt is usually fed at a concentration of 3% to 5%, higher concentrations causing lack of appetite. It is thought that supplementary feeding with sodium chloride helps to prevent urolithiasis by decreasing the rate of deposition of magnesium and phosphate around the nidus of a calculus, but it is possible that salt-related diuresis may also play an important role. Feeding of pelleted rations may predispose to the development of phosphate calculi (such as struvite or apatite) by reducing the salivary secretion of phosphorus.

The control of siliceous calculi in cattle fed native range grass hay, which may contain a high level of silica, is dependent primarily on increasing the water intake. The feeding of alfalfa hay is considered to increase urine flow and lower the incidence of urolithiasis but the important reason may be that it contains considerably less silica. As in feedlot animals, water intake can be promoted by supplementing the ration with salt. For yearling (300 kg) steers the daily consumption of 50 g of salt does not prevent the formation of siliceous calculi; at a 200-g daily intake the occurrence of calculi is significantly reduced, and at 300 g daily calculus formation is almost eliminated. For calves on native range, providing supplements ("creep feeds") containing up to 12% salt is effective in eliminating siliceous calculi. This effect is caused by the physical diluting effect of increased water intake promoted by salt supplementation. If the calves consume sufficient quantities of salt to increase the water intake above 200 g/kg BW per day, the formation of siliceous calculi will be completely suppressed. Because siliceous calculi form in the last 60 days before weaning, it is recommended that calves on range be started on creep feed without salt well before weaning and, once calves are established on the supplement, the salt concentration should be gradually increased to 12%. It is usually necessary to increase the salt gradually to this level over a period of several weeks and incorporate it in pellets to facilitate mixing.

An alkaline urine (pH >7.0) favors the formation of phosphate-based stones (struvite and apatite) and calcium carbonate-based stones. Struvite crystallization is reported to occur at urine pH >7.2, and dissolution is reported to occur at urine pH <6.5.[13] Feeding an agent that decreases urine pH to a target range of 6.0 to 6.5 will therefore protect against phosphate and calcium carbonate-based stones. The feeding of ammonium chloride (at 0.5%–2.0% of dry matter intake, approximately 45 g/day to steers, 10 g daily to sheep, and 0.4–0.5 g/kg BW each day to male goats) may prevent urolithiasis caused by struvite or calcium carbonate, but the magnitude of urine acidification achieved varies markedly depending on the acidogenic nature of the diet. The safety of long-term feeding of these diets has not been well documented. A potentially practical method to prevent urolithiasis in goats is to feed a dietary cation anion difference (DCAD) of 0 mEq/kg dry matter, where DCAD = [Na] + [K] − [Cl] − [S] with constituents measured in milliequivalents per kilogram of feed on a dry matter basis.[13] Depending on the aggressiveness of the dosage of ammonium chloride and acidogenicity of the DCAD diet formulation, urine pH decreases over 2 to 5 days before stabilizing.[14] Urine pH should always be closely monitored when adding ammonium chloride to the ration, because clinically relevant acidemia, metabolic acidosis, depression, and inappetence can result from overzealous administration rates, and bone demineralization can theoretically occur with sustained feeding because aciduria promotes hypercalciuria. For range animals, ammonium chloride can be incorporated in a protein supplement and fed at about two-thirds of the earlier dosage. An acidic urine (pH <7.0) favors the formation of silicate stones, so ammonium chloride manipulation of urine pH is not indicated in animals at risk of developing siliceous calculi. However, ammonium chloride may prevent the formation of silica calculi in sheep, which may have been caused by the urine-diluting effects of additional chloride intake.

When urolithiasis is caused by pasture exposure, females can be used to graze the dangerous pastures because they are not as susceptible to developing urinary tract obstruction. In areas where the oxalate content of the pasture is high, wethers and steers should be permitted only limited access to pasture dominated by herbaceous plants. Adequate water supplies should be available, and highly saline waters should be regarded with suspicion. Sheep on lush pasture commonly drink little if any water apparently because they obtain sufficient in the feed. Although the importance of vitamin A in the production of the disease has been decried in recent years an adequate intake should be ensured, especially during drought periods and when animals are fed grain rations in feedlots. Deferment of castration, by permitting greater urethral dilatation, may reduce the incidence of obstructive urolithiasis, but the improvement is unlikely to be significant.

FURTHER READING

Ewoldt JM, et al. Surgery of obstructive urolithiasis in ruminants. *Vet Clin North Am Food Anim Pract.* 2008;24:455.

REFERENCES

1. Sun WD, et al. *Res Vet Sci.* 2010;88:461.
2. Constable PD, et al. *Am J Vet Res.* 2009;70:915.
3. Wang JY, et al. *Res Vet Sci.* 2009;87:79.
4. Sun WD, et al. *Vet J.* 2010;186:70.
5. Kinsley MA, et al. *Vet Surg.* 2013;42:663.
6. Braun U, et al. *Vet Rec.* 2006;159:750.
7. VinodhKumar OR, et al. *Afr J Agric Res.* 2010;5:2045.
8. George JW, et al. *J Am Vet Med Assoc.* 2007;230:101.
9. Ghanem MA, et al. *Alex J Vet Sci.* 2010;31:85.
10. Janke JJ, et al. *J Am Vet Med Assoc.* 2009;234:249.
11. Tobias KM, van Amstel SR. *Vet Surg.* 2013;42:455.
12. Hunter BG, et al. *J Am Vet Med Assoc.* 2012;241:778.
13. Jones ML, et al. *Am J Vet Res.* 2009;70:149.
14. Mavangira V, et al. *J Am Vet Med Assoc.* 2010;237:1299.

UROLITHIASIS IN HORSES

Urolithiasis occurs sporadically in horses. The prevalence is low at about 0.04% to 0.7% of all horse accessions or diagnoses. Animals from about 5 to 15 years of age and older are most often affected, and 76% are males (27% intact and 49% geldings) and 24% are females. The uroliths are most commonly in the bladder (cystic), although they also occur in the renal pelvis, ureters, and urethra. In most cases, there is a single discrete yellowish stone, but a sandy sludge accumulates in cases of paralysis of the bladder. Almost all equine uroliths are composed of calcium carbonate ($CaCO_3$) in the form of calcite, which is the most stable hexagonal crystal form, although other $CaCO_3$ forms such as vaterite (a metastable hexagonal crystal form) and aragonite (an orthorhombic form) have been identified that may be more gray-white in color. The factors that contribute to urolith formation in horses are not understood. Urine from healthy adult horses is characterized by a substantial quantity of mucoprotein, a high concentration of minerals, considerable insoluble sabulous material, and alkalinity. Equine urine is normally supersaturated with calcium carbonate, and it is normal for crystals of calcium carbonate to be present; this is related in some manner with the occurrence of calcium carbonate uroliths in horses. Nephrolithiasis may arise as a sequel to degenerative or inflammatory processes in the kidney in which inflammatory debris serves as a nidus for calculus formation.

The clinical findings of urolithiasis in the horse include:

- Stranguria (straining to urinate)
- Pollakiuria (frequent passage of small amounts of urine), hematuria, and dysuria (difficult urination)
- Incontinence resulting in urine scalding of the perineum in females or of the medial aspect of the hindlimbs in males
- Painful urination with hematuria associated with cystitis
- Weight loss, particularly in horses with nephroliths and chronic renal failure
- Uroabdomen is horses with rupture of the bladder, or less frequently, kidney or ureter
- Bacterial infection of urine is common, usually caused by *E. coli, Staphylococcus* spp., and *Streptococcus* spp.

The bladder wall may be thickened and large calculi in the bladder may be palpable per rectum, just as the hand enters the rectum. Calculi are usually spheroid and have an irregular surface. Large calculi may be observed using transrectal ultrasonography and cystoscopy. Calculi may also be palpated in the ureters, per rectum, or enlarged ureters may be present.

In males, urethral calculi may present with signs of complete or partial obstruction that may be confused with colic of gastrointestinal origin. Horses with urethral obstructions make frequent attempts to urinate but pass only small amounts of blood-tinged urine. Unless rupture has occurred, the bladder is grossly enlarged. The calculus can be located by palpation of the penile urethra and by passage of a lead wire or catheter. If a catheter or lead wire is passed, care should be taken to prevent damage to the urethral mucosa. Bladder rupture leads to uroperitoneum but, if the rupture occurs at the neck of the bladder, urine may accumulate retroperitoneally and produce a large, diffuse, fluid swelling that is palpable per rectum. When rupture occurs, acute signs disappear and are replaced by depression, immobility, and pain on palpation of the abdominal wall. The heart rate rises rapidly, and the temperature falls to below normal.

Urinalysis reveals evidence of erythrocytes, leukocytes, protein, amorphous debris, and calcium carbonate crystals.

Renal calculi are frequently bilateral and affected animals have often progressed to chronic renal failure by the time of diagnosis without having displayed signs of urinary tract obstruction. A history of chronic weight loss and colic in a horse with renal failure indicates the possible presence of renal calculi. Treatment is supportive as for all cases of chronic renal failure.

Treatment for cystic calculi is surgical removal of all calculi and correction of any defect in the bladder. Recurrence of cystic and urethral calculi is common in the horse, which may be related to the failure to remove all calculi. Perineal urethrotomy has been used for removal of cystic calculi in a gelding. Urethral calculi in males are removed through the external urethral orifice or by urethrotomy at the site of obstruction. Some cystic calculi can be removed with the aid of electrohydraulic lithotripsy, laser lithotripsy under endoscopic visualization, or surgery. Extracorporeal shock wave lithotripsy does not appear to have been used in the horse. In large mares with bladder calculi less than 10 cm in diameter, it is possible to remove the calculi manually by passing a very small well-lubricated gloved hand through the urethra into the bladder and retrieving the calculi after administration of epidural analgesia and sedation. Simultaneous palpation per rectum can assist in bringing the calculus to the neck of the bladder. There is one report of laparoscopic removal of a large bladder urolith in a standing gelding.[1] Percutaneous nephrostomy of the right kidney under ultrasonic guidance has been used for short-term diversion of urine in a horse with ureteral calculi.

Control measures typically focus on dietary modifications including decreasing calcium intake, but there appears to be an absence of studies documenting efficacy in control. Water intake should be facilitated and high calcium content feeds, such as alfalfa and clover hay, should be avoided. Ammonium chloride, at 200 mg/kg BW orally twice daily and decreased at biweekly intervals until a dosage of 20 to 60 mg/kg BW is reached, is recommended to maintain the urine pH below 7.0. Urine pH needs to be frequently monitored during supplementation with oral ammonium chloride because of the variability in individual response. Ascorbic acid (1–2 g/kg daily) administered orally is reported to acidify equine urine, but recommended dose rates vary widely and studies documenting treatment efficacy in urolithiasis appear to be lacking.

FURTHER READING

Duesterdick-Zellmer KF. Equine urolithiasis. *Vet Clin North Am Equine Pract.* 2007;23:613-629.
Edwards B, Archer D. Diagnosis and treatment of urolithiasis in horses. *In Pract.* 2011;33:2-10.
Foley A, Brounts SH, Hawkins JF. Urolithiasis. *Comp Contin Ed Pract Vet.* 2009;4:125-133.

REFERENCE

1. Lund CM, et al. *J Am Vet Med Assoc.* 2013;243:1323.

URETHRAL TEARS IN STALLIONS AND GELDINGS

Urethral rents are lesions in the convex surface at the level of the ischial arch in geldings and stallions. The lesions communicate with the corpus spongiosum and cause hemorrhage at the end of urination in geldings or during ejaculation by stallions. Stallions do not have hematuria, despite having a lesion identical to that in geldings, presumably because of the lower pressure in the corpus spongiosum of stallions at the end of urination compared with that in geldings. The disease is apparently caused by contraction of the bulbospongiosus muscle at the end of urination, with a consequent increase in pressure in the corpus spongiosum and expulsion of blood through the rent. The cause of the rent has not been determined. The diagnosis is confirmed by endoscopic examination of the urethra with visualization of the rent in the urethral mucosa. Treatment of the disease is by temporary subischial urethrostomy and sexual rest. Sexual rest alone was successful in one stallion.

URETHRAL DEFECTS

An **anomalous vas deferens** caused a chronic partial urethral obstruction in a 2-year-old Limousin bull, resulting in bilateral hydronephrosis, pyelonephritis of the left kidney, and bilateral ureteral dilatation. There are two reports of a ruptured urinary bladder in neonatal calves apparently caused by a **congenital urethral obstruction** that was corrected by passing a urethral catheter. Congenital urethral obstruction with subsequent hydronephrosis and uroperitoneum is reported in a lamb.

Urethral atresia is recorded rarely in calves and is manifested by failure to pass urine and distension of the patent proximal portion of the urethra.

Imperfect closure of the external male urethra in a series of newborn lambs (**hypospadias**) is recorded with other neonatal defects including atresia ani and diaphragmatic hernia. No genetic influence was suspected, and the cause was unidentified.

Continuous urethral spasm has been reported in a Standardbred mare with a 3-year history of stranguria and pollakiuria.[1] Physical examination, including ultrasonography of the bladder and urethra, was unremarkable. The condition resolved following treatment for 1 month with oral acepromazine (0.04 mg/kg, every 8 hours) and did not recur.

FURTHER READING

Chaney KP. Congenital anomalies of the equine urinary tract. *Vet Clin North Am Equine Pract.* 2007;23:691-696.

REFERENCE

1. Abutarbush SM. *J Equine Vet Sci.* 2014;34:569.

URINARY BLADDER NEOPLASMS

Tumors of the urinary bladder are common only in cattle, and they are associated with bracken poisoning (see the section Bovine Enzootic Hematuria), but they do occur in other circumstances. For example, 18 cows are recorded in one series, with angioma, transitional epithelial carcinoma, and vascular endothelioma as the most common tumors. Abattoir surveys in Canada, the United States, and Australia identified papillomas, lymphomas, adenomas, hemangiomas, and transitional cell tumors of the bladder occurring at low frequencies in slaughter cattle, accounting for 0.01% of all bovine malignancies.[1] Papillomas appear to be associated with the bovine papillomavirus (BPV), and BPV type 1 (BPV-1) and BPV type 2 (BPV-2) are the only viruses known to infect the urothelium of the urinary bladder of healthy cattle. A recent report of a Kaposi-like vascular tumor of the urinary bladder in a cow is available.[2] Most bladder neoplasms develop from focal areas of hyperplasia within the transitional cell layer, and approximately 80% of these can be classified as carcinomas and 17% are papillomas. Because these neoplasms arise from a common site, they can be very similar in gross and histologic appearance and very difficult to differentiate. The immunoenzymatic labeling of intermediate filaments in bovine urinary bladder tumors is an accurate indicator of histogenesis.

Bladder neoplasia caused by squamous cell carcinoma, transitional cell carcinoma, lymphosarcoma, fibromatous polyp, and rhabdomyosarcoma occurs rarely in the horse.[3] Clinical signs included hematuria, weight loss, stranguria, and the secondary development of cystitis. Prognosis is usually poor because of the rapid growth of the neoplasia, likelihood of metastasis, and challenges with obtaining adequate surgical access.

REFERENCES

1. Roperto S, et al. *J Comp Pathol.* 2010;142:95.
2. Pires I, et al. *J Vet Med Sci.* 2009;71:831.
3. Barrell E, Hendrickson DA. *Equine Vet Educ.* 2009;21:267.

BOVINE ENZOOTIC HEMATURIA

SYNOPSIS

Etiology Long-term ingestion of bracken fern, *Pteridium aquilinum,* in cattle with latently infected with bovine papillomavirus type 2.

Epidemiology Enzootic to areas with significant growth of bracken fern; fatal, chronic disease of adult cattle.

Clinical signs Hematuria, anemia, and sometimes palpable lesions in bladder.

Clinical pathology Hematuria.

Necropsy findings Hemangiomas and other neoplastic lesions in bladder mucosa.

Diagnostic confirmation Endoscopic examination of the bladder and biopsy; bladder lesion histopathology.

Treatment None.

Control Eradication of bracken.

ETIOLOGY

Chronic ptaquiloside poisoning caused by the ingestion of *Pteridium aquilinum* (primarily), but also *Pteridium* spp., *Cheilanthes sieberi,* or *Onychium contiguum* is associated with enzootic hematuria in cattle. In the past, the genus was commonly treated as having only one species, *P. aquilinum,* but more recently the genus is being subdivided into approximately 10 species. A high incidence of vesicular carcinomas, similar to the bladder lesions of enzootic hematuria in cattle, has also been recorded in sheep grazing bracken for long periods.

EPIDEMIOLOGY

Enzootic hematuria is an area problem on all continents where bracken grows. Bracken fern is a very common plant worldwide and the only higher order plant known to cause cancer in animals when ingested. There is a strong association between BPV-2 and chronic bracken fern ingestion in cattle with naturally acquired and experimentally induced bladder cancer. The overall prevalence of cancer can reach 10% in endemic areas, such as Sao Miguel Island in the Azores, and the disease may be associated with heavy losses in areas where bracken is a common plant.[1] The disease is usually fatal. Cattle over 3years of age are most often affected, and the disease has also been recorded in sheep and water buffalo exposed to infested pastures for periods exceeding 2 years. The disease occurs mainly on poor, neglected, or recently opened up land and tends to disappear as soil fertility and land management improves. It is not closely associated with a particular soil type, although it is recorded most commonly on lighter soils. The ptaquiloside content of bracken varies considerably between geographic locations, and there is good correlation between its concentration and neoplasia in rats fed bracken from those areas.

PATHOGENESIS

BPV-2 infects the bladder mucosa, producing a latent infection. Chemical carcinogens and immunosuppressants from bracken fern act in a synergistic manner with BPV-2, resulting in neoplastic disease.[2,3] Ptaquiloside from bracken is excreted in the urine and converts to an aglycone dienone intermediate at high urine pH and this substance is the ultimate carcinogen, explaining the location of tumor formation in the bladder. It has been suggested that the dienone reacts with DNA, particularly with adenosine, to initiate carcinogenesis. BPV-2 appears to undergo major changes on cancer development through expression of a viral oncoprotein called E5 and modifying telomerase activity.[4,5]

Hemorrhage from the bladder wall lesions occurs intermittently resulting in ongoing blood loss. Deaths are caused by hemorrhagic anemia.

CLINICAL FINDINGS

Severe cases are manifested by the passage of large quantities of blood, often as clots, in the urine. Hemorrhagic anemia develops and the animal becomes weak and recumbent, and may die after an illness lasting 1 to 2 weeks. Less severe cases are characterized by intermittent, mild clinical hematuria or persistent subclinical hematuria. In these cases, there is a gradual loss of condition over several months and eventually clinical evidence of anemia. On rectal examination, there may be thickening of the bladder wall. Secondary bacterial infection of the bladder may lead to the development of cystitis and pyelonephritis. Cystoscopy reveals the presence of multiple different-sized white to reddish colored nodules protruding into the bladder lumen[2,6] (Fig. 13-10).

CLINICAL PATHOLOGY

Urine dipstick reaction to blood is positively associated with the number and severity of lesions in the bladder.[6] In the absence of gross hematuria, a urine sample should be centrifuged and the deposit examined for erythrocytes. Repeated examinations may be necessary. Nonspecific anemia is detectable by hematologic examination, but clotting time indices (activated partial thromboplastin time, prothrombin time, and D-dimer) are within reference range.[7] Granulocyte and thrombocyte numbers are typically normal. At least one of the viral proteins of BPV-2 (E5 oncoprotein) is expressed in tumors and can be detected using PCR.

NECROPSY FINDINGS

All tissues of the carcass are pale, and the animal is usually emaciated. The urinary bladder contains blood clots or bloodstained urine. The presence of premalignant hemangiomas in the submucosa of the urinary bladder is typical of the disease. A range of other neoplasms may be present, including malignant hemangiosarcoma, hemangioendotheliomas (tumors that are histologically intermediate in appearance between hemangioma and hemangiosarcoma), transitional cell carcinoma, adenoma, fibroma, and papilloma.[2,3,8] The malignant types may have invaded the deeper structures of the bladder and have metastasized to the lumboaortic lymph node (the regional lymph node)[3] or lungs. Tumors expressing p53 mutations appear to be more aggressive.[9] The neoplastic changes in the bladder are accompanied by inflammatory changes of the mucosa and submucosa, including proliferative changes of mucosal epithelium, lymphocytic infiltrates, congestion, edema, and hemorrhage. In some cases, lesions are seen in the ureters and renal pelvis. The severity of the blood loss is not necessarily related to the size or extent of the lesions, and animals may bleed to death when only small localized lesions are present.

DIFFERENTIAL DIAGNOSIS

Diagnosis confirmation is by signs in animals grazing fern-infested pasture and preferably by histopathology of bladder lesions. The differential list includes:
- Cystitis
- Pyelonephritis

Both are usually accompanied by fever, frequent urination, and the presence of pus and debris in the urine. Bacteriologic examination of the urine will reveal the presence of infection.

TREATMENT

Primary

No treatment should be attempted and affected animals should be disposed of at the first opportunity.

Supportive

Blood transfusion may be justified in severe cases and hematinic mixture should be provided in other cases.

CONTROL

A general improvement in nutrition is often followed by a decrease in the number of animals affected. A specific recommendation is to apply gypsum (225–335 kg/hectare) to the pasture as a fertilizer, which is a measure reputed to delay the onset of the disease. Bracken eradication is difficult and should not be undertaken without the advice of the local weed control officer.

FURTHER READING

Dawra RK, Sharma OP. Enzootic bovine haematuria—past, present and future. *Vet Bull.* 2001;71:1R-27R.

Roperto S, Borzacchiello G, Brun R, et al. A review of bovine urothelial tumours and tumour-like lesions of the urinary bladder. *J Comp Pathol.* 2010;142:95.

REFERENCES

1. Resendes AR, et al. *Res Vet Sci.* 2011;90:526.
2. Carvalho T, et al. *J Comp Pathol.* 2006;134:336.
3. Carvalho T, et al. *Vet Pathol.* 2009;46:211.
4. Borzacciello G, et al. *Oncogene.* 2006;25:1251.
5. Yuan Z, et al. *Vet J.* 2007;174:599.
6. Pavelski M, et al. *Semina Ciências Agrárias, Londrina.* 2014;35:1369.
7. Di Loria A, et al. *Res Vet Sci.* 2012;93:331.
8. Roperto S, et al. *J Comp Pathol.* 2010;142:95.
9. Cota JB, et al. *Vet Pathol.* 2014;51:749.

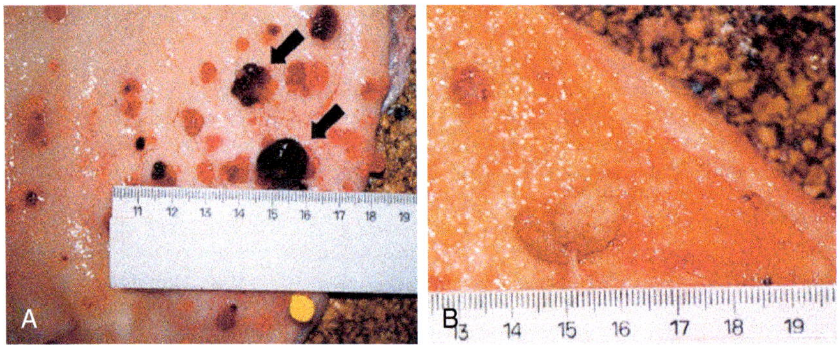

Fig. 13-10 Luminal surface of bladders from cattle with bovine enzootic hematuria. **A,** The bladder contains multiple tumors, with the two tumors (*arrows*) diagnosed as hemangiosarcoma. **B,** The bladder contains a transitional cell carcinoma. (Reproduced with permission from Carvalho T, Pimto C, Peleteiro MC. *J Comp Pathol* 2006; 134:336-346.)

Diseases of the Prepuce and Vulvovaginal Area

ENZOOTIC POSTHITIS (PIZZLE ROT, SHEATH ROT, BALANOPOSTHITIS) AND VULVOVAGINITIS (SCABBY ULCER)

SYNOPSIS

Etiology Multifactorial; organisms that produce urease, usually *Corynebacterium renale*, produce lesions only in certain circumstances of management and urinary composition.

Epidemiology Disease of wether sheep and occasional disease of bulls and goats; may occur as enzootic disease in sheep on high-protein diets and following good rains.

Clinical findings Pustules and scabs at preputial orifice; extension to involve internal prepuce in severe disease with signs of urinary obstruction; ulcers and scabs at the mucocutaneous junction of vulva in ewes; and urine staining of wool predisposes to fly strike. In large mobs of wethers these strikes are often not obvious ("covert strikes"), but are an important means of multiplying *Lucilia cuprina* flies early in the fly season.

Diagnostic confirmation Clinical.

Treatment Dietary restriction, topical disinfectants, and surgical opening of ventral prepuce.

Control Reduction of protein intake; testosterone; hemicastrate or cryptorchid castration.

ETIOLOGY

The etiology of these diseases is **multifactorial**. High urea concentrations in urine, associated with high protein in pasture, result in cytotoxic levels of ammonia when the urea is split by urease-producing organisms present in the prepuce and vagina. Estrogens in pasture, causing swelling and congestion of the prepuce, may predispose to disease. Most often the organism is *C. renale*, but outbreaks of posthitis in sheep associated with other urease-producing organisms (e.g., *R. equi* and *C. hofmannii*) have been described.

Mycoplasma mycoides LC has also been incriminated as a cause of posthitis and vulvovaginitis in sheep.

EPIDEMIOLOGY

The disease is reported primarily from Australia, South Africa, and South America but occurs in all countries with large pastoral sheep industries.

Host Occurrence

Sheep

In Australia, enzootic posthitis occurs most often in Merino sheep, particularly **wethers** over 3 years of age and young rams, but in a severe outbreak young wethers and old rams may also be affected. An ulcerative **vulvitis** often occurs in ewes in the same flocks in which posthitis occurs in wethers and is thought to be a venereal extension of that disease. The disease also occurs in **goats**.

Cattle

Posthitis is uncommon in bulls but is reported to occur at high rates and to be economically important in South America. There appears to be no counterpart to ovine vulvitis in cows.

Source of Infection and Transmission

The causative organism can be recovered from lesions and from the clinically normal prepuce of most sheep. It is also present in the lesions of vulvitis in ewes and posthitis in bulls and Angora goat wethers.

Flies are considered to be probable **mechanical vectors**, and contact with infected soil and herbage is a likely method of spread. Infection at dipping or shearing seems not to be important. Transmission to ewes appears to occur **venereally** from infected rams. Although the natural disease in cattle is usually benign, they may act as reservoirs of infection for sheep on the same farm.

Host and Environmental Risk Factors

Diet and season are the major risk factors. Enzootic posthitis occurs most extensively on lush, **improved pasture** with a high **legume** content and reaches its highest incidence in the autumn in summer rainfall areas and in the spring where the major rainfall is in winter. In these circumstances it can occur in epizootic proportions in wethers. The incidence in affected flocks may be as high as 40%, and in some areas the disease is so common that it is not possible to maintain flocks of wethers.

Factors of lesser importance are continued wetness of the area around the prepuce caused by removal of preputial hairs at shearing; a high-calcium, low-phosphorus diet; and the ingestion of large quantities of alkaline water.

The high incidence in castrates and young rams is probably related to the close adherence of the preputial and penile skins, which separate in mature animals, and to a lesser understood influence of **testosterone**.

Experimental Reproduction

Implantation of the organism on a scarified prepuce in the presence of urine is capable of causing the external ulceration that is characteristic of the disease.

Economic Importance

Many deaths occur because of uremia and secondary bacterial infections and all affected sheep show a severe setback in growth rate and wool production. Young rams that are affected are incapable of mating.

PATHOGENESIS

The organism is capable of hydrolyzing urea with the production of ammonia. It is thought the initial lesion in the wether (the external lesion) is caused by the **cytotoxic effect of ammonia**, produced from urea in the urine by the causative bacteria. This lesion may remain in a static condition for a long period but, when there is a high urea content of the urine associated with a high-protein diet, and continued wetting of the wool around the prepuce, the lesion proceeds to invade the interior of the prepuce, producing the "internal lesion." A similar pathogenesis is postulated for vulvar lesions.

CLINICAL FINDINGS

The primary lesion starts as a pustule, which breaks and forms a soft scab. Small scabs are found on the skin dorsal to the preputial orifice (**external lesion**) and around the external orifice on the nonhaired part of the prepuce. These may persist for long periods without the appearance of any clinical signs. The scab is adherent and tenacious. When extension to the interior of the prepuce occurs (**internal lesion**), there is extensive ulceration and scabbing of the preputial opening, and a hard core can be palpated extending 1 to 2 inches into the prepuce. With pressure, a semisolid core of purulent material can be extruded from the preputial orifice. Affected sheep may show restlessness, kicking at the belly, and dribbling urine as in urethral obstruction. The area is often infested by blowfly maggots. In rams, the development of pus and fibrous tissue adhesions may interfere with urination and protrusion of the penis and cause permanent impairment of function.

Some deaths occur from obstructive uremia, toxemia, and septicemia. During an outbreak many sheep may be affected without showing clinical signs and are detected only when they are subjected to a physical examination. Others recover spontaneously when feed conditions deteriorate.

In ewes the lesions are confined to the lips of the vulva and consist of pustules, ulcers, and scabs. These extend minimally into the vagina. Their presence may distort the vulva, and the ewe may urinate onto the wool with a consequent increased susceptibility to fly strike.

In bulls, lesions are similar to the external lesions, which occur in wethers but rarely there may be invasion of the interior of the prepuce. The external lesions occur at any point around the urethral orifice and may encircle it. Their severity varies from local excoriation to marked ulceration with exudation and edema. There is a tendency for the lesions to persist for several months without treatment and with highly alkaline urine.

CLINICAL PATHOLOGY

Isolation of the causative diphtheroid bacterium may be necessary if there is doubt as to the identity of the disease.

NECROPSY AND DIAGNOSTIC CONFIRMATION

Necropsy is not required, and the diagnosis is clinical.

DIFFERENTIAL DIAGNOSIS

- Ulcerative dermatosis in sheep
- Herpes balanoposthitis in bulls

Obstructive urolithiasis in wethers may superficially resemble posthitis, but there is no preputial lesion.

TREATMENT

The principal measures are restriction of the diet to reduce the urea content of the urine, removal of the wool around the prepuce or vulva to reduce the risk of fly strike, segregation of affected sheep and disinfection of the preputial area, and surgical treatment of severe cases.

Sheep can be removed onto dry pasture and their feed intake restricted to that required for subsistence only. They should be inspected at regular intervals, the wool should be shorn from around the prepuce, and affected animals should be treated individually. Weekly application of a 10% copper sulfate ointment is recommended for external lesions; when the interior of the prepuce is involved, it should be irrigated twice weekly with a 5% solution of copper sulfate, cetrimide (20% in alcohol or water with or without 0.25% acid fuchsin), or 90% alcohol. Penicillin topically, or oxytetracycline or penicillin parenterally, may assist recovery.

In severe cases the only satisfactory treatment is surgical, and surgical treatment is necessary if the prepuce is obstructed. The recommended procedure is to open the ventral sheath by inserting one blade of a pair of scissors into the external preputial orifice and cutting the prepuce back as far as the end of the urethral process; extension beyond this leads to trauma of the penis. Badly affected rams should be disposed of as they are unlikely to be of value for breeding.

TREATMENT AND PROPHYLAXIS

Treatment

Testosterone enanthate (150 mg SC) (R1)

Long-acting Oxytetracycline (20 mg/kg IM) (R2)

Prophylaxis

Testosterone enanthate (75 mg SC) (R1)

IM, intramuscular; SC, subcutaneous.

CONTROL

Subcutaneous implantation with a mix of testosterone esters is highly effective as a preventive, but testosterone propionate is no longer permitted for use in sheep that will be used for human food. Testosterone enanthate is available in some jurisdictions. A single injection of 75 mg is used for prevention and 150 mg for treatment. It is most economical to use preventive treatments coincident with the periods of maximum incidence, the flush of pasture growth in spring and autumn, but timing will vary from district to district.

Alternative control procedures investigated include running male lambs as cryptorchids, called **short scrotum** lambs, in which the testes are pushed into the inguinal canal and a rubber ring is applied to remove the scrotum. Another is to run male lambs as hemicastrates. The prevalence of posthitis is significantly reduced in Merino short scrotum lambs and hemicastrates. There is an increase in live weight, with no increase in fleece weight, but there are obvious masculine characteristics such as horn growth.

FURTHER READING

Radostits O, et al. *Enzooitic Posthitis (Pizzle Rot, Sheath Rot, Balanoposthitis); Vulvovaginitis (Scabby Ulcer). Veterinary Medicine: A Textbook of the Disease of Cattle, Horses, Sheep, Goats and Pigs*. 10th ed. London: W.B. Saunders; 2007: 793-795.

Diseases of the Nervous System

14

Introduction

This chapter focuses on the diagnosis, treatment, and control of large animal diseases primarily affecting the nervous system. In general, the principles of clinical neurology and their application to large animal neurology has not kept pace with the study of neurology in humans and small animals, although remarkable progress has been made in equine neurology over the last 30 years. To a large extent this shortfall is caused by the failure of large-animal clinicians to relate observed clinical signs to a **neuroanatomical location** of the lesion. In many cases this failure has been because of adverse environmental circumstances, or the large size or nature of the animal, all of which adversely impact the quality of the neurologic examination. It may be very difficult to do an adequate neurologic examination on an ataxic belligerent beef cow that is still able to walk and attack the examiner. An aggressive, paretic bull in broad sunlight can be a daunting subject if one wants to examine the pupillary light reflex; ophthalmoscopic examination of the fundus of the eye in a convulsing steer in a feedlot pen can be an exasperating task. Thus at one end of the spectrum is the clinical examination of pigs affected with nervous system disease, which is limited to an elementary clinical examination and necropsy examination. At the other end, neurologic examination of the horse with nervous system disease is very advanced. The global occurrence of bovine spongiform encephalopathy (BSE) has highlighted the importance of accurate clinical diagnosis in adult cattle with neurologic abnormalities.

Discrete lesions of the central nervous system (CNS) resulting in well-defined neurologic signs are not common in agricultural animals. Many diseases are characterized by diffuse neurologic lesions associated with bacteria, viruses, toxins, nutritional disorders, and embryologic defects, and the clinical findings of each disease are similar. Rather than attempting to localize lesions in the nervous system, large-animal practitioners more commonly devote much of their time to attempting to identify whether an animal has diffuse brain edema or increased intracranial pressure, as in polioencephalomalacia (PEM); whether it has clinical signs of asymmetric brainstem dysfunction and depression of the reticular activating system, as in listeriosis; or whether the dysfunction is at the neuromuscular level, as in hypomagnesemic tetany.

Radiographic examination, including myelography, is not used routinely as a diagnostic aid in large-animal practice. The collection of cerebrospinal fluid (CSF) from the different species and ages of large animal without causing damage to the animal or contaminating the sample with blood is a technique that few large-animal veterinarians have mastered. However, the collection of CSF from the lumbosacral cistern is not difficult if the animals are adequately restrained, and the information obtained from analysis of CSF can be very useful in the differential diagnosis of diseases of the brain and spinal cord. Referral veterinary centers are now providing detailed neurologic examinations of horses with nervous system disease, and the clinical and pathologic experience has expanded the knowledge base of large-animal clinical neurology.

In spite of the difficulties, the large-animal practitioner has an obligation to make the best diagnosis possible using the diagnostic aids available. The principles of large-animal neurology are presented in this chapter, and the major objective is to recognize the common diseases of the nervous system by correlating the clinical findings with the location and nature of the lesion. **Accurate neuroanatomical localization of the lesion**(s) remains the fundamental requirement for creating a differential diagnosis list and diagnostic and treatment plan.

A disease such as rabies has major public health implications, and it is important for the veterinarian to be able to recognize the disease as early as possible and to minimize human contact. It is also important to be able to recognize treatable diseases of the nervous system, such as polioencephalomalacia (PEM), listeriosis, and nervous ketosis, and to differentiate these diseases from untreatable and globally important diseases such as Bovine Spongiform Encephalopathy (BSE).

The nontreatable diseases must also be recognized as such, and slaughter for salvage or euthanasia recommended if necessary. There must be a major emphasis on prognosis because it is inhumane and uneconomic to hospitalize or continue to treat an adult cow or horse with incurable neurologic disease for an indefinite period. If they are recumbent, the animals commonly develop secondary complications such as decubitus ulcers and other self-inflicted injuries because of repeated attempts to rise. Very few diseases of the nervous system of farm animals are treatable successfully over an extended period of time. This has become particularly important in recent years with the introduction of legislation prohibiting the slaughter of animals that have been treated with antibiotics until after a certain withdrawal period, which may vary from 5 to 30 days. This creates even greater pressure on the clinician to make a rapid, inexpensive, and accurate diagnosis and prognosis.

Because of limitations in the neurologic examination of large animals, there must be much more emphasis on the history and epidemiologic findings. Many of the diseases have epidemiologic characteristics that give the clinician a clue to the possible causes, thus helping to narrow the number of possibilities. For example, viral encephalomyelitis of horses occurs with a peak incidence during the insect season, lead poisoning is most common in calves after they have been turned out on to pasture, and PEM occurs in grain-fed feedlot cattle and sheep.

The functions of the nervous system are directed at the maintenance of the body's spatial relationship with its environment. These functions are performed by the several divisions of the nervous system including the following:

- Sensorimotor system, responsible for the maintenance of normal posture and gait
- Autonomic nervous system, controlling the activity of smooth muscle and endocrine glands, and thus the internal environment of the body
- Largely sensory system of special senses
- Psychic system, which controls the animal's mental state

The nervous system is essentially a reactive one geared to the reception of internal and external stimuli and their translation into activity and consciousness; it is dependent on the integrity of both the afferent and efferent pathways. This integrative function makes it often difficult to determine in a sick animal whether abnormalities are present in the nervous system; the musculoskeletal system; or acid-base, electrolyte, and energy status. Accordingly, the first step when examining an animal with apparent abnormalities in the nervous system is to determine whether other relevant systems are functioning normally. A decision to implicate the nervous system is often made on the exclusion of other systems.

The nervous system itself is not independent of other organs, and its functional capacity is regulated to a large extent by the function of other systems, particularly the cardiovascular system. Inadequate oxygen delivery caused by cardiovascular disease commonly leads to altered cerebral function because of the dependence of the brain on an adequate oxygen supply.

It is important to distinguish between primary and secondary diseases of the nervous system because both the prognosis and the treatment will differ with the cause.

In primary disease of the nervous system, the lesion is usually an anatomic one with serious, long-range consequences. **In secondary disease,** the lesion, at least in its early stages, is more likely to be functional and therefore more responsive to treatment, provided the defect in the primary organ can be corrected. The clinical findings that should arouse suspicion of neurologic disturbance include abnormalities in the three main functions of the system.

Posture and Gait

An animal's ability to maintain a normal posture and to proceed with a normal gait depends largely on the tone of the skeletal muscle but also on the efficiency of the postural reflexes. Abnormalities of posture and gait are among the best indications of nervous system disease because these functions are governed largely by the coordination of nervous activity. Along with contributing to posture and gait, skeletal muscle tone is characteristic in its own right. However, its assessment in animals is subject to great inaccuracy because of our inability to request complete voluntary relaxation by the patient. In humans it is a very valuable index of nervous system efficiency, but in animals it has serious limitations. The most difficult step whenever there is a defect of gait or posture is to decide whether the defect originates in the skeleton, the muscles, or the nervous system.

Sensory Perceptivity

Tests of sensory perception in animals can only be objective and never subjective, as they can be in humans, and any test used in animals is based heavily on the integrity of the motor system.

Mental State

Depression or enhancement of the psychic state is not difficult to judge, particularly if the animal's owner is observant and accurate. A helpful method for evaluating mental state is to answer the question: Is the animal responding appropriately for its environment? The difficulty usually lies in deciding whether the abnormality is caused by primary or secondary changes in the brain.

Principles of Nervous Dysfunction

Nervous tissue is limited in the ways in which it can respond to noxious influences. Because of its essentially coordinating function, the transmission of impulses along nerve fibers can be enhanced or depressed in varying degrees, with the extreme degree being complete failure of transmission. Because of the structure of the system, in which nerve impulses are passed from neuron to neuron by relays at the nerve cells, there may also be excessive or decreased intrinsic activity of individual cells giving rise to an increase or decrease in nerve impulses discharged by the cells. The end result is the same whether the disturbance is one of conduction or discharge, and these are the only two ways in which disease of the nervous system is manifested. Nervous dysfunction can thus be broadly divided into two forms, **depressed activity** and **exaggerated activity**. These can be further subdivided into four common modes of nervous dysfunction; **excitation (irritation) signs,**

release of inhibition signs, **paresis or paralysis caused by tissue damage**, and **nervous shock**.

MODES OF NERVOUS DYSFUNCTION

Excitation (Irritation) Signs

Increased activity of the reactor organ occurs when there is an increase in the number of nerve impulses received either because of excitation of neurons or because of facilitation of passage of stimuli.

The excitability of nerve cells can be increased by many factors, including stimulant drugs, inflammation, and mild degrees of those influences that in a more severe form may cause depression of excitability. Thus early or mild hypoxia may result in increased excitability, whereas sustained or severe hypoxia will cause depression of function or even death of the nerve cell.

Irritation phenomena may result from many causes, including inflammation of nervous tissue associated with bacteria or viruses, certain nerve poisons, hypoxia, and edema. In those diseases that cause an increase in intracranial pressure, irritation phenomena result from interference with circulation and the development of local anemic hypoxia. The major manifestations of irritation of nervous tissue are tetany, local muscle tremor, and whole-body convulsions in the motor system and hyperesthesia and paresthesia in the sensory system. For the most part the signs produced fluctuate in intensity and may occur periodically as nervous energy is discharged and reaccumulated in the nerve cells.

The area of increased excitability may be local or sufficiently generalized to affect the entire body. Thus a local lesion in the brain may cause signs of excitatory nervous dysfunction in one limb, and a more extensive lesion may cause a complete convulsion.

Release of Inhibition Signs

Exaggeration of normal nervous system activity occurs when lower nervous centers are released from the inhibitory effects of higher centers. The classic example of a release mechanism is experimental decerebrate rigidity caused by transection of the brainstem between the colliculi of the midbrain. This results in an uninhibited extensor tonus of all the antigravity muscles. The head and neck are extended markedly in a posture of opisthotonus, and all four limbs in the quadruped are extended rigidly. The tonic mechanism or myotactic reflex involving the lower motor neuron has been released from the effects of the descending inhibitory upper motor neuron pathways.

Cerebellar ataxia is another example of inhibitory release. In the absence of cerebellar control, combined limb movements are exaggerated in all modes of action including rate, range, force, and direction. In general, release phenomena are present constantly while the causative lesion operates, whereas excitatory phenomena fluctuate with the building up and exhaustion of energy in the nerve cells.

Paresis or Paralysis Caused by Tissue Damage

Depression of activity can result from depression of metabolic activity of nerve cells, and the terminal stage is complete paralysis when nervous tissue is destroyed. Such depression of activity may result from failure of supply of oxygen and other essential nutrients, either directly from their general absence or indirectly because of failure of the local circulation. Infection of the nerve cell itself may cause initial excitation, then depression of function, and finally complete paralysis when the nerve cell dies.

Signs of paralysis are constant and are manifested by muscular paresis or paralysis when the motor system is affected and by hypoesthesia or anesthesia when the sensory system is involved. Deprivation of metabolites and impairment of function by actual invasion of nerve cells or by toxic depression of their activity produce temporary, partial depression of function that is completely lost when the neurons are destroyed.

Nervous Shock

An acute lesion of the nervous system causes damage to nerve cells in the immediate vicinity of the lesion but there may be, in addition, a temporary cessation of function in parts of the nervous system not directly affected. The loss of function in these areas is temporary and usually persists for only a few hours. Stunning is an obvious example. Recovery from the flaccid unconsciousness of nervous shock may reveal the presence of permanent residual signs caused by the destruction of nervous tissue.

Determining the type of lesion is difficult because of the limited range of modes of reaction to injury in the nervous system. Irritation signs may be caused by bacterial or virus infection, by pressure, by vascular disturbance or general hypoxia, by poisons, and by hypoglycemia. It is often impossible to determine whether the disturbance is structural or functional. Degenerative lesions produce mainly signs of paresis or paralysis but unless there are signs of local nervous tissue injury, such as facial nerve paralysis, paraplegia, or local tremor, the disturbance may only be definable as a general disturbance of a part of the nervous system. Encephalopathy is an all-embracing diagnosis, but it is often impossible to go beyond it unless other clinical data, including signalment of the animal, epidemiology, and systemic signs, are assessed or special tests, including radiographic examination and examination of the CSF, are undertaken.

Some information can be derived from a study of the **sign-time relationship** in the development of nervous disease. A lesion that develops suddenly tends to produce maximum disturbance of function, sometimes accompanied by nervous shock. Slowly developing lesions permit a form of compensation in that undamaged pathways and centers may assume some of the functions of the damaged areas. Even in rapidly developing lesions partial recovery may occur in time, but the emphasis is on maximum depression of function at the beginning of the disease. Thus a slowly developing tumor of the spinal cord will have a different pattern of clinical development from that resulting from an acute traumatic lesion of the vertebrae. Another aspect of the rapidity of onset of the lesion is that irritation phenomena are more likely to occur when the onset is rapid and less common when the onset is slow.

Clinical Manifestations of Diseases of the Nervous System

The major clinical signs of nervous system dysfunction include the following:

- **Altered mentation**
- **Involuntary movements**
- **Abnormal posture and gait**
- **Paresis or paralysis**
- **Altered sensation**
- **Blindness**
- **Abnormalities of the autonomic nervous system**

ALTERED MENTATION

Excitation States

Excitation states include **mania**, **frenzy**, and **aggressive behavior**, which are manifestations of general excitation of the cerebral cortex. The areas of the cortex that govern behavior, intellect, and personality traits in humans are the frontal lobes and temporal cortex. The clinical importance of these areas, which are poorly developed in animals, is not great. The frontal lobes, temporal cortex, and limbic system are highly susceptible to influences such as hypoxia and increased intracranial pressure.

Mania

In mania the animal acts in a bizarre way and appears to be unaware of its surroundings. Maniacal actions include licking, chewing of foreign material and sometimes themselves, abnormal voice, constant bellowing, apparent blindness, walking into strange surroundings, drunken gait, and aggressiveness in normally docile animals. A state of delirium cannot be diagnosed in animals, but mental disorientation is an obvious component of mania.

Diseases characterized by mania include the following:

- Encephalitis, e.g., the furious form of rabies, Aujeszky's disease in cattle (pseudorabies, mad itch)

- Degenerative diseases of the brain, e.g., mannosidosis, early PEM, poisoning by *Astragalus* sp.
- Toxic and metabolic diseases of brain, e.g., nervous ketosis, pregnancy toxemia, acute lead poisoning, poisoning with carbon tetrachloride, and severe hepatic insufficiency, especially in horses

Frenzy

Frenzy is characterized by violent activity and with little regard for surroundings. The animal's movements are uncontrolled and dangerous to other animals in the group and to human attendants, and are often accompanied by aggressive physical attacks.

Examples of frenzy in diseases of the nervous system include the following:

- Encephalomyelitides, e.g., Aujeszky's disease.
- Toxic and metabolic brain disease, e.g., hypomagnesemic tetany of cattle and sheep, poisoning with ammoniated roughage in cattle.

Examples of frenzy in diseases of other body systems include the following:

- Acute pain of colic in horses.
- Extreme cutaneous irritation, e.g., photosensitization in cattle. Apparently reasonless panic, especially in individual horses or groups of cattle, is difficult to differentiate from real mania. A horse taking fright at a botfly or a swarm of bees and a herd of cattle stampeding at night are examples.

Aggressive Behavior

Aggression and a willingness to attack other animals, humans, and inert objects is characteristic of the early stages of rabies and Aujeszky's disease in cattle, in sows during postparturient hysteria, in the later stages of chronic hypoxia in any species, and in some mares and cows with granulosa-cell tumors of the ovary. The latter are accompanied by signs of masculinization and erratic or continuous estrus. It is often difficult to differentiate between an animal with a genuine change in personality and one that is in pain or is physically handicapped, e.g., pigs and cattle with atlantoaxial arthroses.

Depressive States

Depressive mental states include somnolence, lassitude, narcolepsy/catalepsy, syncope, and coma. They are all manifestations of depression of cerebral cortical function in various degrees and occur as a result of those influences that depress nervous system function generally, as well as those that specifically affect behavior, probably via the limbic system. It is not possible to classify accurately the types of depressive abnormality and relate them to specific causes, but the common occurrences in farm animals are listed next.

Depression Leading to Coma

In all species this may result from the following:

- Encephalomyelitis and encephalomalacia
- Toxic and metabolic diseases of the brain such as uremia, hypoglycemia, hepatic insufficiency, toxemia, septicemia, and most toxins that damage tissues generally
- Hypoxia of the brain, as in peripheral circulatory failure of periparturient hypocalcemia in dairy cows
- Heat stroke
- Specific poisons that cause somnolence, including bromides, amitraz in horses, methyl alcohol, *Filix mas* (male fern), and kikuyu grass

Syncope

The sudden onset of fainting (syncope) may occur as a result of the following:

- Acute circulatory and heart failure leading to acute cerebral hypoxia
- Spontaneous cerebral hemorrhage, a most unlikely event in adult animals
- Traumatic concussion and contusion
- Lightning strike, electrocution

Narcolepsy (Catalepsy)

Affected animals experience episodes of uncontrollable sleep and literally "fall" asleep. The disease is recorded in Shetland ponies and is thought to be inherited in them, in other horses, and in cattle.

Compulsive Walking or Head Pressing

Head-pressing is a syndrome characterized by the animal pushing its head against fixed objects and into a corner of a pen as well as leaning into a stanchion or between fence posts. Head-pressing should be differentiated from compulsive walking, in which affected animals put their heads down and walk slowly while appearing blind. If they walk into an object, they lean forward and indulge in head-pressing; if confined to a stall they will often walk around the pen continuously or head-press into a corner. The syndrome represents a change in behavior pattern caused by an unsatisfied compulsive drive characteristic of a disorder of the limbic system. Causes include the following:

- Toxic and metabolic brain disease, especially PEM and hepatic encephalopathy
- Diseases manifested by increased intracranial pressure
- Encephalomyelitides

Aimless Wandering

A similar but less severe syndrome to compulsive walking is aimless walking, severe mental depression, and apparent blindness with tongue protrusion and continuous chewing movements, although the animal is unable to ingest feed or drink water. Causes include the following:

- Toxic and metabolic diseases of brain, including poisoning by *Helichrysum* sp. and tansy mustard
- Degenerative brain diseases, e.g., nigropallidal encephalomalacia in horses, ceroid lipofuscinosis in sheep, hydrocephalus in the newborn

INVOLUNTARY MOVEMENTS

Involuntary movements are caused by involuntary muscle contractions, which include gradations from fasciculations, shivering and tremor, to tetany, seizures, or convulsions. Opisthotonus or "backward tone" is a sustained spasm of the neck and limb muscles resulting in dorsal and caudal extension of the head and neck with rigid extension of the limbs.

Tremor

This is a continuous, repetitive twitching of skeletal muscles that is usually visible and palpable. The muscle units involved may be small and cause only local skin movement, in which case the tremor is described as fasciculations; or the muscle units may be extensive and the movement much coarser and sufficient to move the extremities, eyes, or parts of the trunk. The tremor may become intensified when the animal undertakes some positive action. This is usually indicative of cerebellar involvement and is the counterpart of intention tremor in humans. True tremor is often sufficiently severe to cause incoordination and severe disability in gait. Examples of causes of tremor include the following:

- Diffuse diseases of the cerebrum, cerebellum, and spinal cord
- Degenerative nervous system disease, e.g., hypomyelinogenesis of the newborn as in congenital tremor of pigs and calves, poisoning by *Swainsona* sp.
- Toxic nervous system disease caused by a large number of poisons, especially poisonous plants and fungi, *Clostridium botulinum* toxin in shaker foal syndrome; metabolic disease such as hyperkalemic periodic paralysis in the horse; early stages of hypocalcemia in the cow (fasciculations of the eyelids and ears).

Tics

Tics are spasmodic twitching movements made at much longer intervals than in tremor. The intervals are usually at least several seconds in duration and often much longer. The movements are sufficiently widespread to be easily visible and are caused by muscles that are ordinarily under voluntary control. They are rare in large animals but may occur after traumatic injury to a spinal nerve.

Tetany

Tetanus is a sustained contraction of muscles without tremor. The most common cause is *C. tetani* intoxication following localized infection with the organism. The degree of muscular contraction can be exaggerated by stimulation of the affected animal, and the limbs are rigid and cannot be passively flexed easily ("lead pipe" rigidity).

Myoclonus is a brief, intermittent tetanic contraction of the skeletal muscles that results in the entire body being rigid for several seconds, followed by relaxation. Inherited congenital myoclonus (hereditary neuraxial edema) of polled, horned, and crossbred Hereford calves is a typical example. Affected calves are bright and alert and can suck normally, but if they undertake a voluntary movement or are handled their entire body becomes rigid for 10 to 15 seconds.

Convulsions

Convulsions, seizures, fits, or ictus are violent muscular contractions affecting part or all of the body and occurring for relatively short periods as a rule, although in the late stages of encephalitis they may recur with such rapidity they give the impression of being continuous.

Convulsions are the result of abnormal electrical discharges in forebrain neurons that reach the somatic and visceral motor areas and initiate spontaneous, paroxysmal, involuntary movements. These cerebral dysrhythmias tend to begin and end abruptly, and they have a finite duration. A typical convulsion may have a prodromal phase or aura that lasts for minutes to hours, during which the animal is oblivious to its environment and seems restless. The beginning of the convulsion may be manifested as a localized partial convulsion of one part of the body that soon spreads to involve the whole body, when the animal usually falls to the ground thrashing rhythmically. Following the convulsion there may be depression and temporary blindness, which may last for several minutes up to a few hours.

The convulsion may be clonic with typical "paddling" (involuntary movement in which repeated muscle spasms alternate with periods of relaxation). Tetanic or tonic convulsions are less common and are manifested by prolonged muscular spasm without intervening periods of relaxation. True tetanic convulsions occur only rarely, chiefly in strychnine poisoning and in tetanus, and in most cases they are a brief introduction to a clonic convulsion.

Convulsions can originate from disturbances anywhere in the prosencephalon, including cerebrum, thalamus, or even the hypothalamus alone. However, the initiating cause may be in the nervous system outside the cranium or in some other system altogether; convulsions are therefore often subdivided into intracranial and extracranial types. Causes are many and include the following.

Intracranial convulsions are caused by

- Encephalomyelitis, meningitis
- Encephalomalacia
- Acute brain edema
- Brain ischemia, including increased intracranial pressure
- Local lesions caused by trauma (concussion, contusion), abscess, tumor, parasitic injury, hemorrhage
- Inherited idiopathic epilepsy

Extracranial convulsions are caused by brain hypoxia, as in acute circulatory or cardiac failure, and toxic and metabolic diseases of the nervous system, including the following:

- Hepatic encephalopathy
- Hypoglycemia (as in newborn piglets and in hyperinsulinism caused by islet cell adenoma of the pancreas as described in a pony)
- Hypomagnesemia (as in lactation tetany in cows and mares)
- Inorganic poisons, poisonous plants, and fungi; there are too many to give a complete list, but well-known examples are the chlorinated hydrocarbons, pluronics used in bloat control in cattle, *Clostridium* spp.; intoxications, e.g., *C. perfringens* type D and *C. sordellii,* and subacute fluoroacetate poisoning
- Congenital and inherited defects without lesions, e.g., familial convulsions and ataxia in Angus cattle

Involuntary Spastic Paresis

Involuntary, intermittent contractions of large muscle masses may result in spasmodic movements of individual limbs or parts of the body. In most, contractions occur when voluntary movement is attempted. Diseases in this category include the following:

- Stringhalt and Australian stringhalt of horses
- Inherited spastic paresis (Elso heel) of cattle
- Inherited periodic spasticity (stall cramp) of cattle
- Inherited congenital myotonia of cattle
- Inherited myotonia of goats

ABNORMAL POSTURE AND GAIT

Posture

Posture is evaluated with the animal at rest. Abnormal postures may be adopted intermittently by animals in pain, but in diseases of the nervous system the abnormality is usually continuous and repeatable. Deviation of the head and neck from the axial plane or rotation of the head and neck from the horizontal plane (head tilt); drooping of the lips, eyelids, cheeks, and ears; and opisthotonus and orthotonos are examples, although the latter two are often intermittent because they occur as part of a convulsive seizure. Head pressing and assumption of a dog-sitting posture are further examples. Abnormalities of posture and gait are the result of lesions of the brainstem, cerebellum, all levels of the spinal cord, spinal nerve roots, peripheral nerves, neuromuscular junctions, and muscles. The clinical emphasis is on vestibular disease, cerebellar disease, and spinal cord disease. It is important to emphasize that cerebral lesions do not cause abnormalities in posture and gait.

Vestibular Disease

The vestibular system is a special proprioceptive system that assists the animal in maintaining orientation in its environment with respect to gravity. It helps to maintain the position of the eyes, trunk, and limbs in relationship to movements and positioning of the head.

From the vestibular nuclei, the vestibulospinal tracts descend ipsilaterally through the length of the spinal cord. These neurons are facilitatory to ipsilateral motor neurons going to extensor muscles of the limbs, are inhibitory to ipsilateral motor flexor muscles, and are inhibitory to contralateral extensor muscles. The principal effect of unilateral stimulation of this system on the limbs is a relative ipsilateral extensor tonus and contralateral flexor tonus, which promote ipsilateral support of the trunk against gravity. Conversely, a unilateral vestibular lesion usually results in ipsilateral flexor and contralateral extensor tonus, forcing the animal toward the side of the lesion.

The nuclei of cranial nerves (CNs) III, IV, and VI, which control eye movement, are connected with the vestibular system by way of a brainstem tract called the medial longitudinal fasciculus. Through this tract, coordinated eye movements occur with changes in positioning of the head. Through these various pathways, the vestibular system coordinates movements of the eye, trunk, and limbs with head movements and maintains equilibrium of the entire body during motion and rest.

Signs of vestibular disease vary depending on whether there is unilateral or bilateral involvement and whether the disease involves peripheral or central components of the system.

The vestibular influence on balance can be affected

- At the inner ear
- Along the vestibular nerve or
- At the vestibular nucleus in the medulla.

Unilateral excitation or loss of function can be caused by lesions at any of these points.

General signs of vestibular system dysfunction are staggering, leaning, rolling, circling, drifting sideways when walking and a head tilt, and various changes in eye position such as strabismus and nystagmus. The walking in a circle toward the affected side is accompanied by increased tone in the contralateral limbs, which is most easily observed in the contralateral forelimb. Rotation or tilt of the head occurs, and severely affected animals fall to the affected side.

When the lesion affects the inner ear, as in some cases of otitis media, the affected side is turned down, the animal falls to that side, and there may be facial paralysis on the same side if the lesion is extensive and affects CN VII. In the recumbent position, the affected side is held to the ground, and if these animals are rolled over to the opposite side they quickly roll back to the affected side. When the vestibular nuclei are affected, as in listeriosis, the animal falls to the affected side.

Nystagmus and forced circling are common when there is irritation of the vestibular nucleus or the medial longitudinal fasciculus.

Causes of vestibular disease include the following:

- Otitis media interna with involvement of the inner ear
- Focal lesion at the vestibular nucleus, e.g., listeriosis
- Traumatic injury to the vestibular apparatus in the horse caused by fracture of the basisphenoid, basioccipital, and temporal bones; the clinical signs include lack of control of balance, rotation of the head, circling to the affected side, nystagmus, and facial paralysis

In paradoxical vestibular syndrome there is also head tilting, but circling in a direction away from the side of the lesion. Deviation of the head and neck must be distinguished from a head tilt. Asymmetric lesions of the forebrain such as a brain abscess, some cases of PEM, verminous larval migration, or head trauma may cause an animal to hold its head and neck turned to one side, but there is no head tilt and the circle is large in diameter. In fact, the presence of a head tilt (deviation of eyes away from a horizontal plane) accompanied by a tight circle provide clinically useful methods of differentiating a cerebral lesion from a vestibular lesion.

Gait

Gait is assessed when the animal is moving. Neurologic gait abnormalities have two components, **weakness** and **ataxia**. Weakness (paresis) is evident when an animal drags its limbs, has worn hooves, or has a low arc to the swing phase of the stride. When an animal bears weight on a weak limb, the limb often trembles and the animal may even collapse on that limb because of lack of support. While circling, walking on a slope, and walking with the head elevated, an animal frequently will stumble on a weak limb and knuckle over at the fetlock. During manipulation of the limb, the clinician will usually make the subjective observation that the muscle tone is reduced.

Ataxia

Ataxia is an unconscious, general proprioceptive deficit causing incoordination when the animal moves. It is manifested as a swaying from side to side of the pelvis, trunk, and sometimes the whole body (truncal sway). Ataxia may also appear as a weaving of the affected limb during the swing phase of the stride. This often results in abducted or adducted foot placement, crossing of the limbs, or stepping on the opposite foot.

Hypermetria is an increased range of movement and is seen as an overreaching of the limbs with excessive joint movement. Hypermetria without paresis is characteristic of spinocerebellar and cerebellar disease. It is a decreased range of movement that is characterized by a stiff or spastic movement of the limbs with little flexion of the joints, particularly the carpal and tarsal joints.

Dysmetria is a term that includes both hypermetria and hypometria, with goose-stepping being the most common sign. It usually is caused by a lesion in the cerebellum or cerebellar pathway.

In equine degenerative myeloencephalopathy (EDM), there is dysmetria of the hindlimbs and tetraparesis caused by neuraxonal dystrophy originating in the accessory cuneate nuclei. Severely affected horses lift their feet excessively high and stamp them to the ground.

Cerebellar Disease

When cerebellar function is abnormal there is ataxia, which is an incoordination when the animal moves. In general terms, there are defects in the rate, range, and direction of movement. In typical cerebellar diseases, ataxia of the limbs is common and no weakness is evident. In true cerebellar ataxia (e.g., cerebellar hypoplasia), the affected animal stands with the legs wide apart, sways, and has a tendency to fall. Ataxia of the head and neck are characterized by wide, swinging, head excursions; jerky head bobbing; and an intention tremor (nodding) of the head.

The head tremor may be the most obvious sign in mild cases of cerebellar hypoplasia in young foals. The limbs do not move in unison, the movements are grossly exaggerated, muscular strength is usually preserved, and there is a lack of proper placement of the feet (hypermetria and hypometria); falling is common. The fault in placement is the result of poor motor coordination and not related in any way to muscle weakness or proprioceptive deficit. Attempts to proceed to a particular point are usually unsuccessful, and the animal cannot accurately reach its feed or drinking bowl. Examples of cerebellar disease include the following:

- Inherited defects of cerebellar structure or abiotrophy in most breeds of cattle and in Arabian horses[1]
- Congenital cerebellar defects resulting from maternal viral infections such as bovine virus diarrhea (BVD) infection in cattle
- Dysplastic disease of the cerebellum of the horse
- Traumatic injury, e.g., by parasite larvae such as *Hypoderma bovis,* which have caused unilateral cerebellar ataxia in adult cattle
- Tremorgenic mycotoxicoses and ryegrasses
- Cerebellar degeneration in cattle in Uruguay caused by grazing the perennial shrub *Solanum bonariense* ("Naranjillo")[2]
- Encephalomyelitis in which other localizing signs also occur

Spinal Cord Disease

Ataxia caused by cerebellar dysfunction can be difficult to differentiate from the proprioceptive defects and partial motor paralysis (weakness) that occur in animals with spinal cord lesions, and it is most important that this differentiation is made. Spinal cord disease, causing varying degrees of weakness, and ataxia are common in large animals. The weakness is caused by damage to the upper or lower motor neurons and the proprioceptive deficit by damage to the ascending sensory neurons. With a mild or even moderate cervical spinal cord lesion in an adult cow or horse, signs of ataxia and weakness may be evident in the pelvic limbs only, and it can be difficult to determine whether the thoracic limbs are involved.

Close examination of the gait, posture, and postural reactions in the limbs, together with a search for localizing abnormalities, will often be productive in localizing the lesion. Signs of weakness or ataxia may be elicited by gently pushing the hindquarters to one side or pulling the tail to one side as the animal is walked (the sway response). The normal animal resists these movements or steps briskly to the side as it is pushed or pulled. The weak animal can be easily pulled to one side and may stumble or fall and may also tend to buckle or collapse when strong pressure is applied with the hand over the withers and loin regions. The ataxic animal may sway to one side, be slow to protract a limb, cross its hindlegs, or step on its opposite limb.

It is often difficult to distinguish paresis from ataxia, but in most instances it is unimportant because of the close anatomic relationship of the ascending general proprioceptive and descending upper motor neuron tracts in the white matter of the spinal cord. These same abnormal sway responses can be elicited in the standing animal.

The ataxic animal may abduct the outside pelvic limb too far as it is pushed to one side or moved in a small circle. This may appear as a hypermetric movement similar to a stringhalt action and is assumed to be a sign of a general proprioceptive tract lesion. The pushed or circled animal may keep a clinically affected pelvic limb planted in one position on the ground and pivot around it without moving it. The same failure to protract the limb may be seen on backing. It may even force the animal into a "dog-sitting" posture.

Examples of ataxia caused by spinal cord disease include the following:

- Limited trauma to the spinal cord
- The early stages of a developing compression lesion in the vertebral canal

- Degenerative and inflammatory diseases of the nervous system, especially those causing enzootic incoordination in horses and staggers in sheep (both of them dealt with under their respective headings)
- Functional diseases in toxic and metabolic diseases of the nervous system in which lesions have not yet been identified and that are caused mainly by poisons, especially plant materials; typical examples are poisoning by the fungi *Claviceps paspali, Diplodia* spp., *Acremonium lolii,* the grass *Phalaris aquatic,* the ferns *Zamia* and *Xanthorrhea* spp., and herbaceous plants such as *Kallstroemia, Vicia, Baccharis, Solanum, Aesculus,* and *Ficus* spp.
- Heat stress in lambs[3]
- Nutritional deficiency especially of thiamine, occurring naturally in horses poisoned by bracken and horsetail, and experimentally in pigs
- Developmental defects including congenital abnormalities and abiotrophic abnormalities that develop sometime after birth; examples are Brown Swiss weavers and Pietrain creeper pigs.

In many of these diseases, incoordination and paresis are a stage in the development of tetraplegia or paraplegia.

PARESIS AND PARALYSIS

The motor system comprises the following:

- Pyramidal tracts, which originate in the motor cortex
- Extrapyramidal system, which originates in the corpus striatum, red nucleus, vestibular nucleus, and roof of the midbrain
- Peripheral nerves, which originate in the ventral horn cells

The pyramidal tracts are of minor importance in hoofed animals (ungulates), reaching only to the fourth cervical segment. Accordingly, lesions of the motor cortex in farm animals do not produce any deficit of gait. There is also no paresis, although in an acute lesion weakness may be evident for the first day or two. If the lesion is unilateral, the paresis will be on the contralateral side. This is in marked contradistinction to the severe abnormalities of posture and gait that occur with lesions of the pons, medulla, and spinal cord.

The main motor nuclei in these animals are subcortical and comprise the extrapyramidal system, and most combined movements are controlled by nerve stimuli originating in the tectal nuclei, reticular nuclei, vestibular nuclei, and possibly red nuclei. The pyramidal and extrapyramidal tracts comprise the upper motor neurons, which reach to the ventral horn cells of the spinal cord, whose cells, together with their peripheral axons, form the lower motor neurons. Paralysis is a physiologic result in all cases of motor nerve injury, which if severe enough is expressed clinically. The type of paralysis is often indicative of the site of the lesion.

A lesion of the upper motor neuron causes the following:

- **Spasticity with loss of voluntary movement**
- **Increased tone of limb muscles**
- **Increased spinal reflexes**

The spasticity of an upper motor neuron lesion usually occurs with the affected limb in extension. These are all release phenomena resulting from liberation of spinal reflex arcs from higher control.

A lesion of the lower motor neuron causes:

- **Paresis or paralysis with loss of voluntary movement**
- **Decreased tone of the limb muscles**
- **Absence of spinal reflexes**
- **Wasting of the affected muscle (neurogenic atrophy)**

Because injuries to specific peripheral nerves are treated surgically, these are dealt with in surgical textbooks and are not repeated here.

A special form of paralysis is the **Schiff–Sherrington syndrome**, which is common in dogs but recorded rarely in large animals. It is caused by acute, severe compressive injury of the thoracolumbar spinal cord and manifested by extensor rigidity or hypertonia of the forelimbs and hypotonic paralysis of the hindlimbs. Neurons located in the lumbar spinal cord are responsible for the tonic inhibition of extensor muscle alpha motor neurons in the cervical intumescence. The cell bodies of these neurons are located in the ventral gray column from L1-L7, with a maximum population from L2-L4. Their axons ascend to the cervical intumescence. Acute severe lesions cranial to these neurons and caudal to the cervical intumescence will suddenly deprive the cervical intumescence neurons of this source of tonic inhibition, resulting in a release of these latter neurons. This results in extensor hypertonia observed in the thoracic limbs, which can function normally in the gait and postural reactions, except for the hypertonia.

The degree of paresis or paralysis needs to be defined. Paralysis is identified as an inability to make purposeful movements. Thus convulsive, uncontrolled movements as they occur in PEM may still fit a description of paralysis. Paresis, or weakness short of paralysis, can be classified into four categories:

- Animals that cannot rise or support themselves if helped up but can make purposeful movements in attempting to rise
- Animals that cannot rise but can support themselves if helped up
- Animals that can rise but are paretic and can move the limbs well and stumble only slightly on walking
- Animals that move with difficulty and have severe incoordination and stumbling.

Probably the most difficult decision in farm animal neurology is whether a patient's inability to move is because of a nervous or muscular deficit. For example, the horse recumbent because of exertional rhabdomyolysis often resembles a horse with an injured spinal cord. Examples of paresis and paralysis include the following:

- Focal inflammatory, neoplastic, traumatic lesions in the motor pathway. These lesions usually produce an asymmetric nervous deficit.
- Toxic and metabolic diseases of the nervous system in their most severe form, e.g., flaccid paralysis associated with tick bite (*Ixodes holocyclus, Ornithodoros* sp.), poisoning, botulism, and snakebite. Comparable tetanic paralyses include tetanus, lactation tetany of mares, and hypomagnesemic tetany of cows and calves. In contrast to inflammatory, neoplastic, and traumatic lesions in the motor pathway, toxic and metabolic lesions usually produce a symmetric nervous deficit.

Neurogenic Muscular Atrophy

Destruction of the lower motor neurons either within the vertebral canal or peripheral to it causes neurogenic atrophy. Whether or not the atrophy is visible depends on how many neurons and therefore how many muscle fibers are affected.

ALTERED SENSATION

Lesions of the sensory system are rarely diagnosed in animals, except for those affecting sight and the vestibular apparatus, because of the impossibility of measuring subjective responses.

Although animals must experience paresthesia, as in Aujeszky's disease (pseudorabies) in cattle and sheep, the animal's response of licking or scratching does not make it possible to decide whether the diagnosis should be paresthesia or pruritus. Lesions of the peripheral sensory neurons cause hypersensitivity or decreased sensitivity of the area supplied by the nerve. Lesions of the spinal cord may affect only motor or only sensory fiber tracts or both, or may be unilateral.

Although it is often difficult to decide whether failure to respond to a normally painful stimulus is caused by failure to perceive or inability to respond, certain tests may give valuable information. The test usually used is pricking the skin with a needle, or pinching the skin with a pair of forceps, and observing the reaction. In exceptional circumstances, light stroking may elicit an exaggerated response. The **"nibbling"** reaction stimulated by stroking the lumbar back of sheep affected with scrapie is a striking example of hypersensitivity.

In every test of sensitivity, it must be remembered that there is considerable variation between animals and in an individual animal from time to time, and much discretion must be exercised when assessing the response. In any animal, there are also cutaneous areas that are more sensitive than others. The face and the cranial cervical region are highly sensitive, the caudal cervical and shoulder regions less so, with sensitivity increasing over the caudal thorax and lumbar region and to a high degree on the perineum. The proximal parts of the limbs are much less sensitive than the distal parts and sensitivity is highest over the digits, particularly on the medial aspect.

Absence of a response to the application of a painful stimulus to the limbs (**absence of the withdrawal reflex**) indicates interruption of the reflex arc; absence of the reflex with persistence of central perception, as demonstrated by groaning or body movement such as looking at the site of stimulus application, indicates interruption of motor pathways and that central perception of pain persists. In the horse, the response can be much more subtle than in other species, and movements of the ears and eyelids are the best indicators of pain perception. Increased sensitivity is described as **hyperesthesia**, decreased as **hypoesthesia**, and complete absence of sensitivity is described as **anesthesia**. Special cutaneous reflexes include the anal reflex, in which spasmodic contraction of the anus occurs when it is touched, and the corneal reflex, in which there is closure of the eyelids on touching the cornea. The (cutaneous trunci) panniculus reflex is valuable in that the sensory pathways, detected by the prick of a pin, enter the cord at spinal cord segments T1-L3, but the motor pathways leave the cord only at spinal cord segments C8, T1, and T2. The quick twitch of the superficial cutaneous muscle along the whole back, which is the positive response (**panniculus reflex**), is quite unmistakable. Examination of the eye reflexes and hearing are discussed under the section Cranial Nerves (see later).

BLINDNESS

Blindness is manifested as a clinical abnormality by the animal walking into objects that it should avoid. Vision is a cerebral cortical function and is evaluated using the pupillary light reflex, the menace response, and the ability to navigate around a novel obstacle course.

The **pupillary light reflex** is present at birth in large animals but does not need an intact cerebral cortex. This is the reason why ruminants with thiamine-responsive polioencephalomalacia appear blind but have an intact pupillary light reflex; in contrast, ruminants with lead poisoning and a greater extent of cerebral dysfunction appear blind but have a depressed or absent pupillary light reflex. The pupillary light reflex measures the integrity of the retina, optic nerves and chiasm, and oculomotor and pretectal nuclei in the midbrain, and then to a descending motor pathway that includes the oculomotor nerve, ciliary ganglion, and constrictor pupillae muscle.

The **menace or blink response** is used to test the integrity of the entire visual pathway (retina, optic nerves, optic chiasm, optic tract, lateral geniculate nucleus, and internal capsule to the visual area in the cerebrum [occipital lobe]). The visual cortex processes the information and relays signals to the motor cortex. The descending motor pathway receives some input from the cerebellum and proceeds from the ipsilateral pons to the contralateral facial nerve nucleus in the medulla oblongata, and then to the facial nerve, and finally the orbicularis oculi muscle. A threatening gesture of the hand (or even better by the index finger in a pointing manner) toward the eye elicits immediate closure of the eyelids. The finger must come close enough to the eye without touching the tactile hairs of the eyelids or creating a wind that can be felt by the animal. Some stoic, depressed, or even excited animals may not respond to a menace reflex with closure of the eyelids; others may keep the eyelids partially or almost closed. It may be necessary to alert the patient to the risk of injury by touching the eyelids first. The menace response is a learned response that is absent in neonates. Most foals have a menace response by 9 days after birth and most calves by 5 to 7 days after birth. Group housing of neonatal calves appeared to facilitate faster learning of the menace response as a result of more visual threats.[4]

The most definitive test is to make the animal walk an **obstacle course** and place objects in front of it so that it must step over the objects easily. A similar procedure is the only way to test for **night blindness (nyctalopia)**. The area should be dimly lit, but the observer should be able to see the obstructions clearly. A decision that the animal is blind creates a need for examination of the visual pathways.

Central or Peripheral Blindness

Blindness may be central or peripheral. Animals with forebrain lesions are centrally blind, with depressed menace response in one or both eyes, whereas the pupillary light reflexes are usually intact. In peripheral blindness, such as hypovitaminosis A, the menace reflex is absent, and the pupillary light reflexes are also absent.

Blindness can be caused by lesions along the visual pathway, from the eye to the cerebral cortex:

- **Diseases of the orbit** include keratoconjunctivitis, hypopyon, cataract, panophthalmia, mixed ocular defects inherited in white Shorthorn and Jersey cattle, night blindness in Appaloosa horses, and sporadic cases of blindness caused by idiopathic retinal degenerative disease in cattle.
- **Diseases of the retina** include retinal dysplasia of goats, lenticular cataracts caused by poisoning with hygromycin in pigs, and congenital ocular malformations in calves after intrauterine infection with BVD virus (usually accompanied by cerebellar defects).
- **Diseases of the optic nerve and chiasma,** e.g., abscess of pituitary rete mirabile, constriction of optic nerve by diet deficient in vitamin A, tumor of pituitary gland, and injury to the optic nerve, especially in horses after rearing and falling backward. There is a sudden onset of unilateral or bilateral blindness with no ophthalmologic change until 3 to 4 weeks after the injury, when the optic disc becomes paler and less vascular.
- **Metabolic or ischemic lesions of the cerebral cortex** as in PEM, cerebral edema, and hydrocephalus.
- **Localized infectious or parasitic lesions** caused by abscesses or migrating larvae.
- **Functional blindness** in which there is complete, often temporary, apparent blindness in the absence of any physical lesions is seen. Causes are acetonemia, pregnancy toxemia, and acute carbohydrate indigestion (hyper D-lactatemia) of ruminants.
- **Specific poisonings** causing blindness include *F. mas* (male fern), *Cheilanthes* spp. (rock fern), and rape. *Stypandra* spp. cause a specific degeneration of the optic nerves. Lead poisoning in cattle can also cause blindness.

ABNORMALITIES OF THE AUTONOMIC NERVOUS SYSTEM

Lesions affecting the cranial parasympathetic outflow do so by involvement of the oculomotor, facial, vagus, and glossopharyngeal nerves or their nuclei. The effects produced are discussed in the Cranial Nerves section of Special examination of the Nervous System.

In general, the lesions cause abnormality of pupillary constriction, salivation, and involuntary muscular activity in the upper part of the alimentary and respiratory tracts. Lesions of the spinal sympathetic system interfere with normal function of the heart and alimentary tract. For the most part, affections of the autonomic nervous system are of minor importance in farm animals. Central lesions of the hypothalamus can cause abnormalities of heat exchange, manifested as neurogenic hyperthermia or hypothermia and obesity, but they are also of minor importance.

Some manifestations of autonomic disease are important. Autonomic imbalance is usually described as the physiologic basis for spasmodic colic of horses; grass sickness of horses is characterized by degenerative lesions in the sympathetic ganglia; and involvement of the vagus nerve in traumatic reticuloperitonitis of cattle can lead to impaired forestomach and abomasal motility as well as the development of vagus indigestion.

Defects of sphincter control and motility of the bladder and rectum may also be of importance in the diagnosis of defects of sacral parasympathetic outflow and the spinal sympathetic system. The sacral segments of the spinal cord are the critical ones, and loss of their function will cause incontinence of urine and loss of rectal tone. The parasympathetic nerve supply to the bladder stimulates the detrusor muscle and relaxes the sphincter; the sympathetic nerve supply has the reverse function. A spinal cord lesion may cause loss of the parasympathetic control and result in urinary retention. Incontinence, if it occurs, does so from overflow. When the sympathetic control is removed, incontinence occurs but the bladder should empty. Similar disturbances of defecation occur. Both micturition and defecation are controlled by medullary and spinal centers, but some measure of control is regained even when the extrinsic nerve supply to the bladder and rectum is completely removed.

Special Examination of the Nervous System

Veterinarians commonly include several components of a neurologic examination in a complete clinical examination. Most often a diagnosis and differential diagnosis can be made from consideration of the history and the clinical findings. However, if the diagnosis is uncertain it may be necessary to conduct a complete neurologic examination, which may uncover additional clinical findings necessary to make a diagnosis and give a prognosis.

The accuracy of a clinical diagnosis of neurologic diseases in the horse is high. In a study of 210 horses in which a definitive pathologic diagnosis was confirmed, the overall accuracy of clinical diagnosis for all diseases was 0.95; the accuracy ranged from 0.79 to 1.00, the sensitivity varied from 0.73 to 0.95, and the specificity varied from 0.88 to 1.00 for individual disease categories. Some neurologic diseases are therefore underdiagnosed, whereas others are overdiagnosed. The use of careful and thorough clinical examinations and diagnostic techniques, combined with confirmed pathologic diagnoses, will result in more accurate diagnosis and therapy. Retrospective studies of series of ataxic horses, for example, will add to the body of knowledge and improve diagnosis.

NEUROLOGIC EXAMINATION

The primary aim of the neurologic examination is to confirm whether or not a neurologic abnormality exists and to determine the neuroanatomical location of the lesion. A clinicoanatomic diagnosis is necessary before one can develop a list of differential diagnoses and decide whether or not treatment is possible. The format for a precise practical examination procedure that is logical in sequence, easy to remember with practice, and emphasizes the need for an anatomic diagnosis is outlined later. The rationale for the sequence is that the examination starts from a distance to assess posture and mentation and then proceeds to a closer examination that may require placing the animal in stocks or a chute. The examination sequence is therefore suitable for minimally handled beef cattle, dairy cattle, horses, sheep, goats, and New World camelids. The results of the neurologic examination should be documented and not left to memory. There are many standard examination forms available that outline each step in the examination and provide for documentation of the results.

SIGNALMENT AND EPIDEMIOLOGY

The age, breed, sex, use, and value of the animal are all important considerations in the diagnosis and prognosis of neurologic disease. Some diseases occur more frequently under certain conditions, for example, lead poisoning in nursing beef calves turned out to pasture in the spring of the year. *Histophilus somni* meningoencephalitis is most common in feedlot cattle from 6 to 10 months of age, and hypovitaminosis A is most common in beef calves 6 to 8 months of age after grazing dry summer pastures. In the horse, there are several clearly defined diseases that affect the spinal cord including cervical stenotic myelopathy, degenerative myeloencephalopathy, protozoal myelitis, equine rhinopneumonitis myelopathy, rabies polioencephalomyelitis, and equine motor neuron disease. Some of these diseases have distinguishing epidemiologic characteristics that are useful in diagnosis and differential diagnosis. The neurologic examination of the newborn foal is fraught with hazards because of the different responses elicited from those in adults. The differences relate mostly to the temporary dysmetria of gait and exaggerated responses of reflexes.

HISTORY

Special attention should be given to the recording of an accurate history. The questioning of the owner should focus on the primary complaint and when it occurred and how it has changed over time (**the sign-time relationship**). The duration of signs; the mode of onset, particularly whether acute with later subsidence, or chronic with gradual onset; the progression of involvement; and the description of signs that occur only intermittently should be ascertained. When the disease is a herd problem, the morbidity and mortality rates and the method of spread may indicate an intoxication when all affected animals show signs within a very short period. Diseases associated with infectious agents may have an acute or chronic onset. Neoplastic diseases of the nervous system may begin abruptly but are often slowly progressive. For some diseases, such as epilepsy, consideration of the history may be the only way to make a diagnosis. Traumatic injuries have a sudden onset and then often stabilize or improve.

When obtaining a history of convulsive episodes, an estimate should be made of their duration and frequency. The pattern is also important and may be diagnostic, e.g., in salt poisoning in swine. The occurrence of pallor or cyanosis during the convulsion is particularly important in the differentiation of cardiac syncope and a convulsion originating in the nervous system.

HEAD

Behavior

The owner should be questioned about the animal's abnormal behavior, which can include bellowing, yawning, licking, mania, convulsions, aggressiveness, head-pressing, wandering, compulsive walking, and head-shaking. Head-shaking may be photic in origin and can be tested by the application of blindfolds, covering the eyes with a face mask, and observing the horse in total darkness outdoors. In one horse, head-shaking ceased with blindfolding or night darkness outdoors, and became less with the use of gray lenses. Outdoor behavior suggested efforts to avoid light.

Mental Status

Assessment of mental status is based on the animal's level of awareness or consciousness. Coma is a state of complete unresponsiveness to noxious stimuli. Other abnormal mental states include stupor, somnolence, deliriousness, lethargy, and depression. Animals may exhibit opisthotonus, either spontaneously or in response to stimulation (Fig. 14-1). Large animals that are recumbent because of spinal cord disease are usually bright and alert unless affected with complications, which may cause fever and anorexia. Mature beef cattle that are recumbent with a spinal cord lesion and not used to being handled may be quite aggressive and apprehensive.

Head Position and Coordination

Lesions of the vestibular system often result in a head tilt. Lesions of the cerebrum often result in deviation of the head and neck. In cerebellar disease, there may be jerky movements of the head, which are exaggerated by increasing voluntary effort. These fine jerky movements of the head are called intention tremors. Animals with severe neck pain will hold their neck in a fixed position and be reluctant to move the head and neck. Head-shaking in horses has been associated with ear mite infestation, otitis externa, CN dysfunction, cervical injury, ocular disease, guttural pouch mycosis, dental periapical osteitis, and vasomotor rhinitis. However, idiopathic head-shaking in the horse is often associated with evidence of nasal irritation, sneezing and snorting, nasal discharge, coughing, and excessive lacrimation.

Cranial Nerves

Abnormalities of CN function assist in localizing a lesion near or within the brainstem. Some of the information on CN dysfunction is presented in tabular form (Tables 14-1 through 14-6) in addition to the more detailed examination described here.

Olfactory Nerve (Cranial Nerve I)

Tests of smell are unsatisfactory in large animals because of their response to food by sight and sound.

Optic Nerve (Cranial Nerve II)

The only tests of visual acuity applicable in animals are testing the eye preservation (menace) reflex (provoking closure of the eyelids and withdrawal of the head by stabbing the finger at the eye) and by making the animal run a contrived obstacle course. Both tests are often difficult to interpret and must be performed in such a way that other senses are not used to determine the presence of the obstacles or threatened injury. In more intelligent species, a good test is to drop some light object, such as a handkerchief or feather, in front of the animal. It should gaze at the object while it is falling and continue to watch it on the ground. The same method can be applied to young ruminants, which demonstrate normal vision by following the examiner's moving hand at an age so early that they have not yet developed a menace reflex. Ophthalmoscopic examination is an integral part of an examination of the optic nerve.

Oculomotor Nerve (Cranial Nerve III)

This nerve supplies the pupilloconstrictor muscles of the iris and all the extrinsic

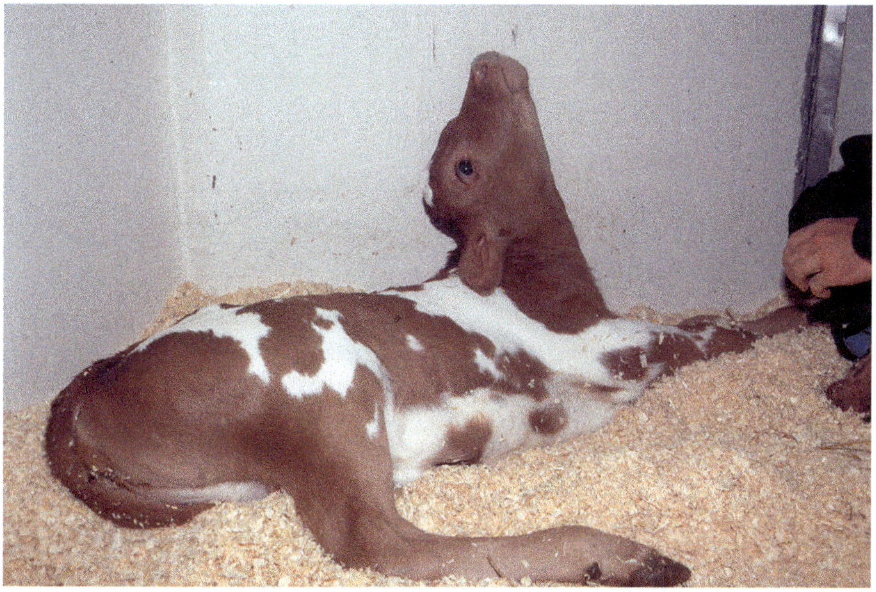

Fig. 14-1 Abnormal mentation in Simmental calf with bacterial meningitis. The calf is exhibiting opisthotonus and is acting inappropriately for its surroundings.

Table 14-1 Correlation between clinical findings and location of lesions in the nervous system of farm animals: abnormalities of mental state (behavior)

Principal sign	Secondary signs	Location of lesion	Example
Mania hysteria/ hyperexcitability	Continuous, leading to paralysis; aggression, convulsions	Cerebrum-limbic system	Peracute lead poisoning, rabies, encephalitis
	Intermittent, acetonuria, signs of hepatic insufficiency	Cerebrum-limbic system	Hypoglycemia, hypoxia
Coma (recumbency with no response to stimuli; dilated pupils)	Gradual development Hypothermia, peripheral vascular collapse. Clinicopathologic tests	Cerebral-brainstem reticular formation (ascending reticular activating system)	Hepatic insufficiency, uremia, toxemia, septicemia
	Sudden onset Normal temperature, pulse/heart rate slow to normal, nosebleed, skin laceration, bruising middle of forehead or poll	Cerebral-brainstem reticular formation (ascending reticular activating system)	Accidental, severe blunt trauma with edema, concussion, contusion of brain
Narcolepsy/catalepsy Uncontrollable sleep	With or without sudden loss of consciousness, intermittent falling caused by loss of voluntary motor function	Brainstem control of cerebral cortex	Inherited in Shetland ponies, American Miniature horses, and Suffolk horses
Compulsive walking and head-pressing, aggressive behavior, grinding of teeth.	Apparent blindness, nystagmus	Cerebral-visual cortex and limbic system	Increased intracranial pressure in polioencephalomalacia
No ataxia	Apparent blindness, no nystagmus, hepatic insufficiency shown on clinical pathology tests	Cerebral-visual cortex and limbic system	Hepatic insufficiency (i.e., ammonia intoxication; in pyrrolizidine poisoning)
Imbecility in neonate; lack of response to normal stimuli; can walk, stand	Blindness	Cerebral cortex absent; hydranencephaly	Intrauterine infection with Akabane or bovine virus diarrhea virus in calves

Table 14-2 Correlation between clinical findings and location of lesion in the nervous system of farm animals: involuntary movements

Principal sign	Secondary signs	Location of lesion	Example
Tremor (continuous repetitive movements of skeletal muscles)	Moderate tetany	No specific focal lesion Generalized disease, e.g., hypomyelinogenesis	Congenital tremor of Herefords Hypomyelinogenesis, shaker pigs, lambs with border disease
	Intention tremor, sensory ataxia	Cerebellum	Cerebellar hypoplasia
	With head rotation	Vestibular apparatus	Otitis media and interna Fracture of petrous temporal bone
Nystagmus	Usually with tetraparesis, impaired consciousness, abnormal pupils, opisthotonus, facial palsy, dysphagia	Cerebellopontine and midbrain areas	Injury, increased intracranial pressure, polioencephalomalacia, listeriosis
	Pendular nystagmus	No lesion	Benign sporadic occurrence in dairy cattle, inherited in Finnish Ayrshire bulls
	Independent episodes	Focus of irritation in cerebral cortex or thalamus, with spread of excitation	Idiopathic or traumatic epilepsy
Convulsions	Continuous, leading to paralysis	Cerebral cortex	Increased intracranial pressure, encephalitis
	Intermittent, related to periods of metabolic stress	Cerebral cortex	Hypomagnesemia (lactation tetany); hypoglycemia (e.g., of baby pigs)
Tenesmus (straining)	Later paralysis of anus, sometimes tail head Sexual precocity in male	Caudal cord segments and cauda equina, stimulation of nerve cells, later paralysis	Rabies, subacute local meningitis
Compulsive rolling	Disturbance of balance, cannot stand, must lie on one side Nystagmus	Vestibular apparatus	Brain abscess, otitis media

Table 14-3 Correlation between clinical findings and location of lesion in the nervous system of farm animals: abnormalities of posture

Principal sign	Secondary signs	Location of lesion	Example
Paresis (difficulty in rising, staggering gait, easily falling)	Persistent recumbency, muscle tone and reflexes variable depending on site of lesion	Loss of function in nervous tissue, e.g., spinal cord, may be upper or motor neuron lesion	Lymphosarcoma affecting spinal cord
	General loss of muscle tone including vascular, alimentary systems	Depression of synaptic or neuromuscular transmission for metabolic reasons or toxic reasons	Periparturient hypocalcemia, botulism, peracute coliform mastitis, tick paralysis
Flaccid paralysis (1) Pelvic limbs only	Thoracic normal Pelvic limbs flaccid, no tone, or reflexes, no anal reflex, urinary incontinence straining initially	Tissue destruction, myelomalacia at lumbosacral cord segments L4 to end osteomyelitis, fracture	Paralytic rabies Spinal cord local meningitis, vertebral body
	Thoracic limbs normal Pelvic limbs normal tone and reflexes, anal reflex normal No withdrawal reflex caudally	Cord damage at thoracolumbar cord segments T3-L3	Spinal cord local meningitis as previously mentioned, damage by vertebral fracture, lymphosarcoma
(2) Thoracic and pelvic limbs	Flaccid paralysis, normal tone and reflexes hindlimbs Absent tone and reflexes in front limbs Atrophy only in front No withdrawal reflex caudally Intact perineal reflex	Cord damage at cervicothoracic segments C6-T2	Fracture of vertebra lymphosarcoma, abscess
	Flaccid paralysis all four legs and neck Unable to lift head off ground Normal tone and reflexes all legs Pain perception persists No withdrawal reflex caudally	Cord damage at upper cervical segments C1-C5	Injury while running or falling, abscess or lymphosarcoma
Spastic paralysis (permanent, no variation, all four limbs in extension, increased tone, exaggerated reflexes, opisthotonus)	Cranial nerve deficits trigeminal to hypoglossal Loss of central perception of pain Depression	Medulla, pons and midbrain	Abscess, listeriosis

Table 14-3 Correlation between clinical findings and location of lesion in the nervous system of farm animals: abnormalities of posture–cont'd

Principal sign	Secondary signs	Location of lesion	Example
Tremor	Tremor (fine or coarse; no convulsions)	Red nucleus and reticular apparatus and midbrain/basal ganglia area tracts	Congenital disease of calves, e.g., hypomyelinogenesis, neuraxial edema
Tetany (all four limbs extended, opisthotonus)	Intense hyperesthesia, prolapse third eyelid	Decreased synaptic resistance generally	Tetanus
Tetanu (variable intensity modifiable by treatment)	Exaggerated response to all external stimuli, i.e., hyperesthesia	Increased neuromuscular transmission	Hypomagnesemia
Paralysis of anus	No anal or perineal reflex May be straining	Damage to spinal cord at segments S1-S3	Injury or local meningitis, early rabies
Paralysis of tail	Flaccid tail with anesthesia	Injury to caudal segments	Injury or local meningitis, early rabies
Opisthotonus	With spastic paralysis, tremor, nystagmus, blindness Part of generalized tetanic state or convulsion	Cerebrum, cerebellum and midbrain Neuromuscular transmission defect, tetanus, hypomagnesemia	Polioencephalomalacia, trauma Tetanus
Falling to one side	Mostly with circling Also with deviation of tail	No detectable lesion in spinal cord	*Xanthorrhea hastile* poisoning

Table 14-4 Correlation between clinical findings and location of lesion in the nervous system of farm animals: abnormalities of gait

Principal sign	Secondary signs	Location of lesion	Example
Circling			
(1) Rotation of the head	Nystagmus, circles, muscle weakness, falls easily, may roll, other cranial nerves affected	Vestibular nucleus	Brain abscess, listeriosis
	Nystagmus, walks in circles, falls occasionally, animal strong Falls easily if blindfolded, sometimes facial paralysis	Inner ear (vestibular canals), cranial nerve VII, facial nerve	Otitis media, otitis interna, fracture petrous temporal bone (horse)
(2) Deviation of the head	Deviation of head and gaze, compulsive walking, depression Can walk straight Balance may be normal	Cerebrum	Brain abscess in calf (infection from dehorning or umbilicus)
	Unable to walk straight Facial paralysis, other cranial nerve deficits, head may be rotated	Medulla	Listeriosis
Cerebellar ataxia	Exaggerated strength and distance of movement, direction wrong Hypermetria Incoordination because of exaggerated movement No paresis	Cerebellum	Inherited cerebellar hypoplasia in all species, especially Arabian horses; *Claviceps paspali* poisoning; Gomen disease a probable plant poisoning; destruction by a virus, especially BVD in cattle; hematoma in the fourth ventricle causes cerebellar displacement Idiopathic cerebellar degeneration in adult cattle
Sensory ataxia	No loss of movement or strength but timing movement wrong, legs get crossed, feet badly placed when pivoting	Damage to sensory tracts in spinal cord	Cervical cord lesion, thoracolumbar if just pelvic limb
Sensorimotor ataxia	Weakness of movement, e.g., scuffing toes, knuckling, incomplete flexion, extension causes wobbly, wandering gait, falls down easily, difficulty in rising	Moderate lesion to spinal cord tracts	Plant poisonings, e.g., sorghum Cervical vertebral compression of spinal cord Degenerative myelopathy

BVD, bovine viral diarrhea.

Table 14-5 Correlation between clinical findings and location of lesion in the nervous system of farm animals: abnormalities of the visual system

Principal sign	Secondary signs	Location of lesion	Example
Blindness (bumps into objects)	Pupillary dilatation No pupillary light reflex No menace reflex	Optic nerve (examine fundus of eye)	Vitamin A deficiency Pituitary rete mirabile abscess Congenital retinal dysplasia of goats
Peripheral blindness or night blindness		Retina	Nutritional deficiency of vitamin A Inherited defect of Appaloosa foals
Central blindness	Pupil normal size Pupillary light reflexes normal	Cerebral cortex	Polioencephalomalacia, lead poisoning
Abnormal dilatation of pupils (mydriasis)	Absence of pupillary light reflex Can see and does not bump into objects	Motor path of oculomotor nerve	Snakebite, atropine poisoning, milk fever
	Absent pupillary light reflex No vision Retinal damage on ophthalmoscopic examination	Retinal lesion	Toxoplasmosis, trauma, ophthalmitis
	Absent pupillary light reflex No vision Retina normal	Optic nerve atrophy and fibrosis	Avitaminosis A in cattle
Abnormal constriction of pupil (miosis)	Diarrhea, dyspnea	Failure to activate acetylcholine	Organophosphate poisoning
	Blindness, coma, semicoma, spastic paralysis	Diffuse lesion	Polioencephalomalacia, acute lead poisoning
Horner's syndrome Drooping upper eyelid, miosis, enophthalmos	Hemilateral sweating and temperature rise side of face and upper neck Unilateral exophthalmus; nasal obstruction	Damage to cranial thoracic and cervical sympathetic trunk	Mediastinal tumor Guttural pouch mycosis Neoplastic space-occupying lesions of the cranium involving the periorbit; perivascular injection around jugular vein or normal intravenous injection of xylazine hydrochloride in normal horses, melanoma at the thoracic inlet in a horse
Nystagmus	See Table 14-2		
Abnormal position of eyeball and eyelids	Dorsomedial deviation of eyeball and eyelid	Trochlear (cranial nerve IV) Facial (cranial nerve VII)	Polioencephalomalacia Listeriosis
	Ventrolateral fixation	Oculomotor (cranial nerve III)	
	Protrusion and medial deviation	Abducent (cranial nerve VI)	Abscess/tumor, e.g., bovine viral leukosis
No palpebral reflex		Deficit sensory branch of cranial nerve V	Trauma
Absence of menace response		Facial nerve (provided vision is present)	Listeriosis
Absence of pupillary light reflex		Oculomotor (provided vision is present)	

Table 14-6 Correlation between clinical findings and location of lesion in the nervous system of farm animals: disturbances of prehension, chewing, or swallowing

Principal sign	Secondary signs	Location of lesion	Example
Inability to prehend or inability to chew	Facial (nasal septal) hypalgesia	Sensory branch of trigeminal (cranial nerve V) dysfunction	Poisoning by *Phalaris aquatica* in cattle Local medullary lesion
	Inappropriate movements of tongue	Hypoglossal (cranial nerve XII) nerve dysfunction	Poisoning by *P. aquatica* in cattle Listeriosis, local medullary lesion
	Inappropriate movements of lips	Facial (cranial nerve VII) nerve dysfunction	Traumatic injury to petrous temporal bone, otitis media and interna, listeriosis, guttural pouch mycosis
	Inadequate chewing movements of jaw	Motor branch of the trigeminal (cranial nerve V) nerve dysfunction	Poisoning by *P. aquatica* in cattle, listeriosis
Inability to swallow (in absence of physical foreign body; in pharyngeal paresis or paralysis)	Regurgitation through nose and mouth, inhalation into lungs causing aspiration pneumonia Inappropriate swallowing movements	Glossopharyngeal (cranial nerve IX) nerve dysfunction. Also vagus (cranial nerve X) Nuclei in medulla globus pallidus and substantia nigra	Abscess or tumor adjacent to nerve Listeriosis, abscess in medulla Poisoning by *Centaurea* sp.

muscles of the eyeball except the dorsal oblique, the lateral rectus, and the retractor muscles. Loss of function of the nerve results in pupillary dilatation and defective pupillary constriction when the light intensity is increased, abnormal position (ventrolateral deviation) or defective movement of the eyeballs, and palpebral ptosis.

The pupillary light reflex is best tested by shining a bright point source of light into the eye, which causes constriction of the iris of that eye (direct pupillary reflex). Constriction of the opposite eye (consensual pupillary light reflex) will also occur. The consensual light reflex may be used to localize lesions of the optic pathways.

Examination of the menace reflex (eye preservation reflex to a menace) and the results of the pupillary light reflex can be used to distinguish between blindness caused by a lesion in the cerebral cortex (central blindness) and that caused by lesions in the optic nerve or other peripheral parts of the optic pathways (peripheral blindness).

As examples, in PEM (central blindness) the menace reflex is absent, but the pupillary light reflex is present. In the ocular form of hypovitaminosis A (peripheral blindness) in cattle, the menace reflex is also absent, the pupils are widely dilated, and the pupillary light reflex is absent. In PEM, the optic nerve, oculomotor nucleus, and oculomotor nerve are usually intact but the visual cortex is not; in hypovitaminosis A, the optic nerve is usually degenerate, which interferes with both the menace and pupillary light reflexes.

Testing of ocular movements can be performed by moving the hand about in front of the face. In paralysis of the oculomotor nerve, there may also be deviation from the normal ocular axes and rotation of the eyeball. There will be an absence of the normal horizontal nystagmus reaction with a medial jerk of the eyeball in response to quick passive movement of the head. Failure to jerk laterally indicates a defect of the abducens nerve.

Trochlear Nerve (Cranial Nerve IV)

This nerve supplies only the dorsal oblique muscle of the eye so that external movements and position of the eyeball are abnormal (dorsolateral fixation) when the nerve is injured. This is common in PEM in cattle, resulting in a dorsomedial fixation of the eyeball. In other words, the medial angle of the pupil is displaced dorsally when the head is held in normal extension.

Trigeminal Nerve (Cranial Nerve V)

The sensory part of the trigeminal nerve supplies sensory fibers to the face and can be examined by testing the palpebral reflex and the sensitivity of the face. The motor part of the nerve supplies the muscles of mastication and observation of the act of chewing may reveal abnormal jaw movements and asymmetry of muscle contractions. There may also be atrophy of the muscles, which is best observed when the lesion is unilateral.

Abducent Nerve (Cranial Nerve VI)

Because the abducent nerve supplies motor fibers to the retractor and lateral rectus muscles of the eyeball, injury to the nerve may result in protrusion and medial deviation of the globe. This is not readily observable clinically. An inherited exophthalmos and strabismus occurs in Jersey cattle.

Facial Nerve (Cranial Nerve VII)

The facial nerve supplies motor fibers for movement of the ears, eyelids, lips, and nostrils, in addition to the motor pathways of the menace, palpebral, and corneal reflexes. The symmetry and posture of the ears, eyelids, and lips are the best criteria for assessing the function of this nerve. Ability to move the muscles in question can be determined by creating a noise or stabbing a finger at the eye. Absence of the eye preservation reflex may be caused by facial nerve paralysis or blindness. Facial paralysis is evidenced by ipsilateral drooping of the ear, ptosis of the upper eyelid, drooping of the lips, and pulling of the philtrum to the unaffected side. There may also be drooling of saliva from the commissures of the lips, and in some cases a small amount of feed may remain in the cheeks of the affected side.

The common causes of damage to the nerve are fracture of the petrous temporal bone, guttural pouch mycosis, and damage to the peripheral nerve at the mandible. A common accompaniment is injury to the vestibular nerve or center. A diagnosis of central, compared with peripheral, nerve involvement can be made by identifying involvement of adjacent structures in the medulla oblongata. Signs such as depression, weakness, and a head tilt would result, and are frequently present in ruminants and New World camelids with listeriosis.

Vestibulocochlear Nerve (Cranial Nerve VIII)

The cochlear part of the vestibulocochlear nerve is not easily tested by simple clinical examination, but failure to respond to sudden sharp sounds, created out of sight and without creating air currents, suggests deafness. The cochlear portion can be tested electronically (the brainstem auditory evoked response, or BAER, test) to diagnose a lesion of the auditory nerve, eliminating the possibility of a central brain lesion. Abnormalities of balance and carriage of the head (rotation around the long axis and not deviation laterally) accompany lesions of the vestibular part of the vestibulocochlear nerve, and nystagmus is usually present.

In severe cases, rotation of the head is extreme, the animal is unable to stand and lies in lateral recumbency; moving to achieve this posture is compulsive and forceful. There is no loss of strength. In some species there is a relatively common occurrence of paralysis of the facial and the vestibular nerves as a result of otitis interna and otitis media. This does occur in the horse but is less common than traumatic injury to the skull as a result of falling.

Pendular nystagmus should not be mistaken as a sign of serious neurologic disease. It is characterized by oscillations of the eyeball that are always the same speed and amplitude and appear in response to a visual stimulus, e.g., a flashing light. Pendular nystagmus is observed most frequently in Holstein Friesian cattle (prevalence of 0.51% in 2932 Holstein Friesian and Jersey cows), is not accompanied by other signs, and there is no detectable histologic lesion. A familial relationship was observed in Ayrshire bulls in Finland.

Glossopharyngeal Nerve (Cranial Nerve IX) and Vagus Nerve (Cranial Nerve X)

The glossopharyngeal nerve is sensory from the pharynx and larynx, and the vagus nerve is motor to these structures. Dysfunction of these nerves is usually accompanied by paralysis of these organs with signs of dysphagia or inability to swallow, regurgitation through the nostrils, abnormality of the voice, and interference with respiration.

Because of the additional role of the vagus nerve in supplying nerve fibers to the upper alimentary tract, loss of vagal nerve function will lead to paralysis of the pharynx and esophagus. Parasympathetic nerve fibers to the stomach are also carried in the vagus, and damage to them could cause hypomotility of that organ. The principal clinical finding in vagus nerve injury is laryngeal and pharyngeal paralysis.

Spinal Accessory Nerve (Cranial Nerve Xi)

Damage to this nerve is extremely rare and the effects are not documented. Based on its anatomic distribution, loss of function of this nerve could be expected to lead to paralysis of the trapezius, brachiocephalic, and sternocephalic muscles and lack of resistance to lifting the head.

Hypoglossal Nerve (Cranial Nerve XII)

As the motor supply to the tongue, the function of this nerve can be best examined by observing the motor activity of the tongue. There may be protrusion and deviation or fibrillation of the organ, which all result in difficulty in prehending food and drinking water. The most obvious abnormality is the ease with which the tongue can be pulled out. The animal also has difficulty in getting it back into its normal position in the mouth, although diffuse cerebral disease can also produce this clinical sign. In lesions of some duration, there may be obvious unilateral atrophy.

POSTURE AND GAIT

The examiner evaluates posture and gait to give a general assessment of brainstem, spinal cord, and peripheral nerve and muscle function. Evaluation of posture and gait consists of determining which limbs are abnormal and looking for evidence of lameness suggesting a musculoskeletal gait abnormality. Weakness and ataxia are the essential components of gait abnormality. Each limb is examined for evidence of these abnormalities. This is done while the animal is standing still, walking, trotting, turning tightly (pivoting), and backing up. To detect subtle asymmetry in the length of the stride, the observer should walk parallel to or behind the animal, step for step. If possible, the gait should also be evaluated while the animal is walking up and down a slope or walking with the head and neck held extended, while blindfolded and while running free in an enclosure.

The best observations are made when the animal is running free, preferably at a fast gait, to avoid abnormalities resulting from being led. Also, slight abnormalities such as a high-stepping gait, slight incoordination of movement, errors of placement of feet, stumbling, and failure to flex joints properly are all better observed in a free animal.

Weakness or paresis is evident when an animal drags its limbs, has worn hooves, or has a low arc to the swing phase of the stride. When an animal bears weight on a weak limb, the limb often trembles and the animal may even collapse on that limb because of lack of support. While circling, walking on a slope, and walking with the head held elevated, an animal frequently will stumble on a weak limb and knuckle over on the fetlock.

The presence of weakness in the limbs of horses or cattle can be determined by pulling the tail while the animal is walking forward. A weak animal is easily pulled to the side and put off stride. While the animal is circling, the examiner can pull on the lead rope and tail simultaneously to assess strength. Ease in pulling the animal to the side occurs because of weakness caused by lesions of the descending upper motor neuron pathway, the ventral horn gray matter level with the limb, or peripheral nerves or muscle. With lower motor neuron lesions, the weakness is often so marked that it is easy to pull an animal to the side while it is standing or walking. In contrast, a weak animal with a lesion of the upper motor neuron pathways will often fix the limb in extension, reflexly, when pulled to one side. It resists the pull and appears strong.

Severe weakness in all four limbs, but with no ataxia and spasticity, suggests neuromuscular disease. Obvious weakness in only one limb is suggestive of a peripheral nerve or muscle lesion in that limb.

Ataxia is an unconscious, general proprioceptive deficit causing poor coordination when moving the limbs and the body. It results in swaying from side to side of the pelvis, trunk, and sometimes the entire body. It may also appear as a weaving of the affected limb during the swing phase. This often results in abducted or abducted foot placement, crossing of the limbs, or stepping on the opposite foot, especially when the animal is circling or turning tightly. Circumduction of the outside limbs when turning and circling is also considered a proprioceptive deficiency. Walking an animal on a slope, with the head held elevated, often exaggerates ataxia, particularly in the pelvic limbs. When a weak and ataxic animal is turned sharply in circles, it leaves the affected limb in one place while pivoting around it. An ataxic gait may be most pronounced when an animal is moving freely, at a trot or canter, especially when attempting to stop. This is when the limbs may be wildly abducted or adducted. Proprioceptive deficits are caused by lesions affecting the general proprioceptive sensory pathways, which relay information on limb and body position to the cerebellum (unconscious proprioception) and to the thalamus and cerebral cortex (conscious proprioception).

Knuckling the flexed foot while the animal stands on the dorsum to determine how long the animal leaves the foot in this state before returning it to a normal position is a test for conscious proprioception in dogs and cats. The test has not been useful in horses and adult cattle but is useful in sheep, goats, New World camelids, and calves. Depressed animals will often allow the foot to rest on the dorsum for prolonged periods. Crossing the limbs and observing how long the animal maintains a cross-legged stance has been used to test conscious proprioception.

Hypermetria is used to describe a lack of direction and increased range of movement, and is seen as an overreaching of the limbs with excessive joint movement. Hypermetria without paresis is characteristic of spinocerebellar and cerebellar disease.

Hypometria is seen as stiff or spastic movement of the limbs with little flexion of the joints, particularly the carpal and tarsal joints. This generally is indicative of increased extensor tone and of a lesion affecting the descending motor or ascending spinocerebellar pathways to that limb. A hypometric gait, particularly in the thoracic limbs, is best seen when the animal is backed up or when it is maneuvered on a slope with the head held elevated. The thoracic limbs may move almost without flexing.

Dysmetria is a term that incorporates both hypermetria and hypometria. Animals with severe cerebellar lesions may have a high-stepping gait but have limited movement of the distal limb joints, especially in thoracic limbs.

The degree of weakness, ataxia, hypometria, and hypermetria should be graded for each limb. The types of gait abnormalities and the degree of weakness reflect various nervous and musculoskeletal lesions. Generally, with focal, particularly compressive, lesions in the cervical spinal cord or brainstem, neurologic signs are one grade more severe in the pelvic limbs than in the thoracic limbs. Thus with a mild, focal, cervical spinal cord lesion, there may be more abnormality in the pelvic limbs with no signs in the thoracic limbs. The anatomic diagnosis in such cases may be a thoracolumbar, cervical, or diffuse spinal cord lesion.

A moderate or severe abnormality in the pelvic limbs, and none in the thoracic limbs, is consistent with a thoracolumbar spinal cord lesion. With a mild and a severe change in the thoracic and the pelvic limb gaits, respectively, one must consider a severe thoracolumbar lesion plus a mild cervical lesion, or a diffuse spinal cord disease.

Lesions involving the brachial intumescence (spinal cord segments C6-T2) with involvement of the gray matter supplying the thoracic limbs, and diffuse spinal cord lesions may both result in severe gait abnormality in the thoracic limbs and the pelvic limbs.

A severely abnormal gait in the thoracic limbs, with normal pelvic limbs, indicates lower motor neuron involvement of the thoracic limbs; a lesion is most likely to be present in the ventral gray columns at spinal cord segments C6-T2 or thoracic limb peripheral nerves of muscle.

Gait abnormalities can occur in all four limbs, with lesions affecting the white matter in the caudal brainstem, when head signs, such as CN deficits, are used to define the site of the lesion. Lesions affecting the cerebrum cause no change in gait or posture.

It is important for clinicians to recognize that a poor level of agreement exists between skilled and experienced observers of gait abnormalities in horses.[5] There is also poor agreement between pathology and clinical signs. The level of agreement is particularly poor when gait abnormalities are subtle. Consequently, there is an important need to develop a set of objective parameters that quantify the severity of ataxia in horses, with appropriate repeatability.

NECK AND FORELIMBS

If a gait abnormality was evident in the thoracic limbs and there was no evidence of brain involvement, then examination of the neck and forelimbs can confirm involvement of the spinal cord, peripheral nerves (spinal cord segments C1-T2), or thoracic limb muscles. The neck and forelimbs are examined for evidence of gross skeletal defects, asymmetry of the neck, and muscle atrophy. The neck should be manipulated from side to side and up and down to detect any evidence of resistance or pain. Localized unilateral sweating of the neck and cranial shoulder is evidence of **Horner's syndrome**, in which there are varying degrees of ptosis; prolapse of the third eyelid; miosis; enophthalmos; and increased temperature of the face, neck, and shoulder. The syndrome is associated with lesions affecting the descending sympathetic fibers in the white matter of the spinal cord or gray matter in the cranial thoracic segments, thoracocervical sympathetic trunk, cervical vagosympathetic trunk, or cranial cervical ganglion and its preganglionic and postganglionic fibers.

Sensory perception from the neck and forelimbs is assessed using a painful stimulus such as a blunt needle or forceps. The local responses as well as the cerebral responses are noted when the skin over the shoulders and down the limbs is pricked.

Gait deficits are evaluated by making the horse or halter-broken ruminant perform a series of movements. Such exercises should include walking and trotting in a straight line, in large circles, in tight circles, backing on a level ground and on a slight slope, walking and trotting over curbs or low obstacles, walking in straight lines and circles, and walking on a slope with the head held elevated. The sway reaction for the thoracic limb is assessed by pushing against the shoulders and forcing the animal first to resist and then to take a step laterally. This can be done while the animal is standing still and walking forward. Pulling the tail and lead rope laterally at the same time will assess the strength on each side of the body. Making the animal turn in a tight circle by pulling the lead rope and tail at the same time will indicate strength; an adult horse should be able to pull the examiner around and should not pivot on a limb or be pulled to the side. Pressing down with the fingers on the withers of a normal animal causes some arching, followed by resistance to the downward pressure. An animal with weakness in the thoracic limbs may not be able to resist this pressure by fixing its vertebral column but will arch its back more than normal and often buckle in the thoracic limbs.

In smaller farm animal species, other postural reactions can be performed. These include wheelbarrowing and the hopping response test. The spinal reflexes are assumed to be intact in animals that are ambulating normally.

If a large mature horse, cow, or pig has a gait abnormality, it is very rare to cast the animal to assess the spinal reflexes. However, spinal reflexes are usually examined in calves, sheep, and goats.

A recumbent animal that can use its thoracic limbs to sit up in the dog-sitting position may have a lesion caudal to spinal cord segment T2. If a recumbent animal cannot attain a dog-sitting position, the lesion may be in the cervical spinal cord. In lambs aged between 4 and 10 weeks with thoracic vertebral body abscesses extending into the epidural space causing spinal cord compression, the thoracic limbs are normal and the lambs frequently adopt a dog-sitting position and move themselves around using the thoracic limbs only. Lambs with a cervical spinal cord lesion are unable to maintain sternal recumbency and have paresis of all four limbs.

However, mature cattle with the downer cow syndrome secondary to hypocalcemia may be unable to use both the thoracic and pelvic limbs. If only the head, but not the neck, can be raised off the ground, there may be a severe cranial cervical lesion. With a severe caudal cervical lesion, the head and neck can usually be raised off the ground but thoracic limb function is decreased and the animal is unable to maintain sternal recumbency.

Assessment of limb function is done by manipulating each limb separately, in its free state, for muscle tone and sensory and motor activity. A limb that has been lain on for some time cannot be properly evaluated because there will be poor tone from the compression. A flaccid limb, with no motor activity, indicates a lower motor lesion to that limb. A severe upper motor neuron lesion to the thoracic limbs causes decreased, or absent, voluntary effort, but there is commonly normal or increased muscle tone in the limbs. This is caused by release of the lower motor neuron, which reflexly maintains normal muscle tone from the calming influence of the descending upper motor neuron pathways.

The tone of skeletal muscle may be examined by passively flexing and extending the limbs and moving the neck from side to side and up and down. Increased muscle tone, spasticity, or tetany may be so great that the limb cannot be flexed without considerable effort. If the spastic-extended limb does begin to flex but the resistance remains, this is known as lead-pipe rigidity, which is seen in tetanus. If after beginning to flex an extended spastic limb the resistance suddenly disappears ("clasp-knife release"), then this suggests an upper motor neuron lesion, which occurs in spastic paresis in cattle.

Flaccidity, or decreased muscle tone, indicates the presence of a lower motor neuron lesion with interruption of the spinal reflex arc.

Localized atrophy of muscles may be myogenic or neurogenic and the difference can be determined only by electromyography (EMG), a technique not well suited to large-animal practice. If the atrophic muscle corresponds to the distribution of a peripheral nerve, then it is usually assumed that the atrophy is neurogenic. In addition, neurogenic atrophy is usually rapid (will be clinically obvious in a few days) and much more marked than either disuse or myogenic atrophy.

Spinal Reflexes of the Thoracic Limbs

Spinal reflexes of the thoracic limbs include the flexor reflex, the biceps reflex, and the triceps reflex. The flexor reflex is tested by stimulation of the skin of the distal limb and observing for flexion of the fetlock, knee, elbow, and shoulder. The reflex arc involves sensory fibers in the median and ulnar nerves, spinal cord segments C6-T2, and motor fibers in the axillary, musculocutaneous, median, and ulnar nerves. Lesions cranial to spinal cord segment C6 may release this reflex from the calming effect of the upper motor neuron pathways and cause an exaggerated reflex with rapid flexion of the limb, and the limb may remain flexed for some time. A spinal reflex may be intact without cerebral perception. Cerebral responses to the flexor reflex include changes in the facial expression, head movement toward the examiner, and vocalization. Conscious perception of the stimulus will be intact only as long as the afferent fibers in the median and ulnar nerves, the dorsal gray columns at spinal cord segments C6-T2, and the ascending sensory pathways in the cervical spinal cord and brainstem are intact.

The laryngeal adductory reflex is of special interest in the examination of ataxic horses. In normal horses, a slap on the saddle region just caudal to the withers causes a flickering adductory movement of the contralateral arytenoid cartilage that is visible by an endoscope. Reflex muscle contraction can be palpated on the dorsolateral surfaces of the larynx. The reflex is absent when there is damage to afferent tracts up the spinal cord, when there is damage to the recurrent laryngeal nerves, and in tense or frightened horses. Elicitation of the reflex is called the **slap test**.

TRUNK AND HINDLIMBS

If examination of the posture, gait, head, neck, or thoracic limbs reveals evidence of a lesion, then an attempt should be made to explain any further signs found during examination of the trunk and hindlimbs that could have been caused by the lesion. If there are only signs in the trunk and hindlimbs, then the lesion(s) must be either between spinal cord segments T2 and S2 or in the trunk and pelvic limb nerves or muscles. It must be remembered that a subtle neurologic gait in the pelvic limbs may be anywhere between the midsacral spinal cord and the rostral brainstem.

The trunk and hindlimbs are observed and palpated for malformations and asymmetry. Diffuse or localized sweating, the result of epinephrine release and sympathetic denervation, is often present in horses affected with a severe spinal cord injury.

Gentle pricking of the skin over the trunk and over the lateral aspects of the body wall on both sides, including on either side of the thoracolumbar vertebral column, will test-stimulate the cutaneous trunci reflex. The sensory stimulus travels to the spinal cord in thoracolumbar spinal nerves at the level of the site of stimulation. These impulses are transmitted up the spinal cord to spinal cord segments C8-T1, where the lateral thoracic nerve is stimulated, causing contraction of the cutaneous trunci muscle, which is seen as a flicking of the skin over the trunk. Lesions anywhere along this pathway will result in suppression or absence of this reflex caudal to the site of the lesion. Degrees of hypalgesia and analgesia have been detected caudal to the sites of thoracolumbar spinal cord lesions, especially if they are severe. In mature cattle with fractured thoracolumbar vertebrae associated with traumatic injury or vertebral body abscesses in calves, the site of the lesion may be able to be localized with this reflex. Sensory perception of pinpricking the trunk and hindlimbs may also be absent caudal to the lesion.

The sway reaction for the pelvic limbs involves pushing against the pelvis and pulling on the tail with the animal standing still and walking forward. An animal that is weak in the pelvic limbs will be easily pulled and pushed laterally, especially while walking. Proprioceptive deficits can be observed as overabduction and crossing of the limbs when a step is taken to the side.

Pinching and pressing down on the thoracolumbar or sacral paravertebral muscles with the fingers causes a normal animal to extend slightly, then fix, the thoracolumbar vertebral column. It also resists the ventral motion and usually does not flex the thoracic or pelvic limbs. A weak animal usually is not able to resist the pressure by fixing the vertebral column; thus it overextends the back and begins to buckle in the pelvic limbs.

In the recumbent animal, examination of the pelvic limbs includes the pelvic limb spinal reflexes, the degree of voluntary effort, and the muscle tone present. Observing the animal attempting to rise on its own or following some coaxing will help to assess the pelvic limbs. The **flexor spinal reflex** is performed by pricking the skin and observing the flexion of the limb; central perception of the painful stimulus is also noted. The afferent and efferent pathways for this reflex are in the sciatic nerve and involve spinal cord segments L5-S3.

The **patellar reflex** is evaluated by placing the animal in lateral recumbency and supporting the limb in a partly flexed position. The intermediate patellar ligament (horses) or patellar ligament (ruminants, pigs, and New World camelids) is then tapped with a heavy metal plexor. This results in extension of the stifle joint. The sensory and motor fibers for this reflex are in the femoral nerve, and the spinal cord segments are L4 and L5. The patellar reflex is hyperactive in newborn farm animals. The gastrocnemius reflex and the cranial tibial reflex are not evaluated because they cannot be reliably induced.

The spinal cord of the calf has more control of basic physical functions than in humans, dogs, and horses. For example, calves are able to retain control of the pelvic limb in spite of experimentally induced lesions that cause hemiplegia in dogs and humans. Also, transection of the spinothalamic tract in the calf cord does not produce an area of hypalgesia or analgesia on the contralateral side as such a lesion would do in a human.

Skin sensation of the pelvic limbs should be assessed independently from reflex activity. The femoral nerve is sensory to the skin of the medial thigh region, the peroneal nerve to the dorsal tarsus and metatarsus, and the tibial nerve to the plantar surface of the metatarsus.

TAIL AND ANUS

Tail tone is evaluated by lifting the tail and noting the resistance to movement. A flaccid tail, with no voluntary movement, is indicative of a lesion of the sacrococcygeal spinal cord segments, nerves, or muscles. Decreased tone in the tail can be detected with severe spinal cord lesions cranial to the coccygeal segment.

The perineal reflex is elicited by lightly pricking the skin of the perineum and observing reflex contraction of the anal sphincter and clamping down of the tail. The sensory fibers are contained within the perineal branches of the pudendal nerve (spinal cord segments S1-S3). Contraction of the anal sphincter is mediated by the caudal rectal branch of the pudendal nerve, and tail flexion is mediated by the sacral and coccygeal segments and nerves (spinal cord segments S1-coccyx). An animal with a flaccid tail and anus, caused by a lower motor neuron lesion, will not have an anal or tail reflex. However, it may still have normal sensation from the anus and tail provided that the sensory nerves and spinal cord and brainstem white matter nociceptive pathways are intact.

Observation of defecation and urination movements and postures contributes to knowledge of the state of the cauda equina. Thus neuritis of the cauda equina is characterized by flaccid paralysis and analgesia of the tail, anus and perineum, rectum, and bladder. There is no paresis or paralysis of the hindlimbs unless lumbosacral segments of the cord are damaged.

PALPATION OF THE BONY ENCASEMENT OF THE CENTRAL NERVOUS SYSTEM

Palpable or visible abnormalities of the cranium or spinal column are not commonly encountered in diseases of the nervous system, but this examination should not be neglected. There may be displacement, abnormal configuration, or pain on deep palpation. These abnormalities are much more readily palpable in the vertebral column and if vertebrae are fractured. Abnormal rigidity or flexibility of the vertebral column, such as occurs in atlantooccipital malformations in Arabian horses and cattle, may also be detectable by manipulation.

COLLECTION AND EXAMINATION OF CEREBROSPINAL FLUID

The collection and laboratory analysis of CSF from farm animals with clinical evidence of nervous system disease can provide useful diagnostic and prognostic information. A case series involving 102 cattle highlighted the clinical utility of CSF analysis in the antemortem diagnoses of nervous diseases.[6]

CSF is formed mostly from the choroid plexuses of the lateral, third, and fourth ventricles by the ultrafiltration of plasma and the active transport of selected substances across the blood-brain barrier; as such CSF should be regarded as a modified ultrafiltrate of plasma. A small amount of CSF is formed from the ependymal lining of the ventricular system, the pia arachnoid and meningeal blood vessels, and the central canal of the spinal cord. The rate of CSF turnover is approximately 1% per minute; accordingly, it takes many minutes for systemic electrolyte or acid-base changes (such as an increase in plasma magnesium concentration in hypomagnesemic beef cattle) to result in detectable and clinically relevant changes in CSF concentrations. CSF in the ventricular system flows caudally and diffuses out of the lateral recess in the fourth ventricle to circulate around the brain and spinal cord. The presence of CSF in the subarachnoid space separates the brain and spinal cord from the bony cranium and vertebral column, which reduces trauma to the underlying delicate nervous tissue. CSF flows within the subarachnoid space of leptomeninges, and it is primarily in this location that CSF equilibrates with the extracellular fluid (ECF) compartment of CNS parenchyma.[6] It also helps regulate intracranial pressure, maintains electrolyte and acid-base homeostasis, serves as an intracerebral transport system for neurotransmitters and hormones, and has excretory functions with the removal of products of cerebral metabolism. CSF analysis therefore provides a clinically valuable insight into diseases of the CNS.

Collection of Cerebrospinal Fluid

CSF can be collected from the **lumbosacral cistern** with sedation (horses) or restraint (ruminants) and the **atlantooccipital cistern (cisterna magna)** using injectable general anesthesia. For collection it is necessary to puncture the subarachnoid space in either the lumbosacral space or cisterna magna. Although there is no substantial difference between the composition of lumbosacral or cisternal CSF samples unless there is a compressive lesion of the spinal cord, the general policy is to sample as close to the lesion as possible, with the exception that atlantooccipital sampling should not be attempted in animals suspected to have increased intracranial pressure. CSF should be collected into a sterile tube and there is no need to add an anticoagulant, even in samples visibly contaminated with blood. Cytology should be performed as soon as possible after collection (ideally within 15 minutes) because the cells rapidly degenerate after collection. The reason for this rapid degeneration appears to be associated with the low oncotic pressure in CSF; the addition of autologous serum to make a 11% serum solution permitted storage of bovine CSF samples for 24 hours at 4°C before cytologic examination was performed with no loss in cell integrity.[7] The addition of serum to CSF in a ratio that provides an approximate final serum solution of approximately 11% should therefore be considered if there is an unavoidable delay before cytologic examination can be performed.[8]

Collection From the Lumbosacral Cistern

The lumbosacral site is preferred because general anesthesia is not required. CSF can be collected from the lumbosacral cistern with relative ease provided that adequate restraint can be achieved and the anatomic landmarks can be identified. It can be collected from the standing or recumbent animal. If recumbent, the animal should be placed in sternal recumbency with hips flexed and the pelvic limbs extended alongside the abdomen. This widens the lumbosacral space to permit correct placement of the spinal needle. Ultrasonographic guidance has been described but is rarely needed.[9]

The site for collection is the midpoint of the lumbosacral space, which can be identified as the midline depression between the last palpable dorsal lumbar spine (L6 in cattle, goats, and horses; L6 or L7 in sheep and pigs; L7 in New World camelids) and the first palpable sacral dorsal spine (usually S2). In well-conditioned animals, these landmarks cannot always be identified; in which case the site is identified as the midpoint of a line connecting the caudal aspect of the tuber coxae. The site is clipped, surgically prepared, and 1 to 2 mL of local anesthetic is administered subcutaneously. Sterile surgical gloves should be worn. Hypodermic spinal needles with stylettes are recommended because ordinary needles commonly plug with tissue. The length and gauge of needle depends on the size of the animal, but at least 15-cm (6-inch) 18-gauge needles are needed for adult horses and cattle. These needles can bend considerably with animal movement, requiring the use of at least an 18-gauge needle; very tall horses may need a 20-cm needle because the depth needed maybe 16 to 18 cm. The following guide is recommended (Table 14-7).

Provided the animal is well restrained and care is exercised in introducing the needle, little difficulty should be encountered. For collection from the lumbosacral space the needle is slowly advanced perpendicular or up to 15 degrees caudal to perpendicular to the plane of the vertebral column. The needle must be introduced in a perfectly vertical position relative to the plane of the animal's vertebral column because of the danger of entering one of the lateral blood vessels in the vertebral canal. Changes in tissue resistance can be felt as the needle point passes sequentially through the subcutaneous tissue and interarcuate ligament; then there is a sudden "'pop" caused by the loss of resistance as the needle point penetrates the ligamentum flavum into the epidural space. Once the needle point has penetrated the dorsal subarachnoid space, CSF will well up in the needle hub within 2 to 3 seconds. Failure to appreciate the changes in resistance as the needle moves down may result in puncture of the conus medullaris, which may elicit an immediate pain response and some discomfort. Movement of the pelvic limbs may dislodge the needle point, with the risk of causing local trauma and hemorrhage in the leptomeninges, which results in blood in the sample. Repeated CSF taps of the lumbosacral space may make it more difficult to obtain an adequate sample volume because of fibrosis of epidural tissue.

Table 14-7 Needle length gauge for lumbosacral cerebrospinal fluid collection

Species and body weight	Length (cm) and gauge of needle
Lambs < 30 kg	2.5 and 20
Ewes 40–80 kg	4.0 and 20
Rams > 80 kg	5.0 and 20
Calves < 100 kg	4.0 and 20
Calves 100–200 kg	5.0 and 18
Cattle > 200 kg	10.0–15.0 and 18

Careful aspiration with a syringe attached to the needle held between the thumb and index finger is usually required to obtain a sample of 2 to 3 mL, which is sufficient for laboratory analysis. This can be facilitated by firmly resting the forearms and wrists on the animal's back. Failure to obtain fluid is usually caused by incorrect direction of the needle, in which the case the bony landmarks of the lumbosacral space (depression) must be rechecked and, with the needle correctly realigned, the procedure repeated. Occasional small rotations of the needle to change the direction of the bevel can be successful in obtaining CSF, particularly in smaller animals.

In animals with a vertebral body abscess and neurologic disease confined to the hindlimbs, CSF may be difficult to obtain from the lumbosacral space because flow is occluded. In these circumstances, if a sample is obtained, the CSF protein may be increased as a result of stagnation of CSF distal to the lesion with exudation or transudation of protein from the lesion (**Froin's syndrome**).

Collection From the Atlantooccipital Cistern (Cisterna Magna)

This site is preferred for intracranial lesions because the fluid is produced in the subarachnoid space and flows caudally down the spinal cord. However, this site is rarely used because of the inherent risk of needle penetration of the brainstem. Xylazine at 0.20 mg/kg body weight (BW) intramuscularly is effective in providing adequate sedation and analgesia for this procedure in cattle. A general anesthetic (such as combined intravenous administration of xylazine and ketamine) is recommended for horses. Ultrasonographic guidance has been described but is rarely needed.

The site is prepared as with the lumbosacral cistern. Ventriflexion of the head and neck of cattle enlarges the space of the cisterna magna and allows easy entry using a styletted spinal needle inserted at a point created by the transection of the transverse line of the cranial rim of the wing of the atlas and the dorsal midline. The needle is advanced carefully and steadily, and the tip is directed rostrally toward the symphysis of the lower jaw. The needle point goes through the skin, ligamentum nuchae, and leptomeninges. In most mature cattle with a BW over 500 kg, a 20-gauge, 10-cm (4-inch) spinal needle will enter the cisterna magna at 5 to 7 cm after going through the ligamentum nuchae, which provides some increased resistance. A 20-gauge 3.8-cm (1.5-inch) needle can be used in sheep, goats, foals, and neonatal calves. The entrance to the cisterna magna is at a depth of approximately 4 to 6 cm in adult horses and 1.5 to 2.5 cm in neonatal foals. Once at the lower range of the anticipated depth to enter the cisterna magna, the spinal needle is advanced 1 to 2 mm at a time. When the needle point punctures the leptomeninges, the animal may move its head slightly. At that point the needle is advanced only 1 to 2 mm and the stylette is then removed. If the end of the needle is in the cisterna magna, CSF will flow out of the needle freely and the manometer can be attached and the pressure measured.

Cerebrospinal Fluid Pressure

CSF pressure can be determined by the use of a manometer attached to the spinal needle. Normal CSF pressures of the cisterna magna in cattle and xylazine/ketamine-anesthetized horses range from 5 to 15 cm H_2O (unknown reference point) and 28 ± 4 cm H_2O (referenced to the right atrium), respectively. When the fluid system is properly connected, occlusion of both jugular veins causes a marked rise in CSF pressure; this is called

Queckenstedt's test. This test involves bilateral jugular vein compression, which results in a sudden increase in intracranial subarachnoid pressure that is transmitted to the cranial subarachnoid space. The resultant CSF pressure wave is transmitted to the lumbar area (when obtaining CSF from the lumbosacral space) in the absence of an obstruction in the spinal subarachnoid space, resulting in an increased flow of CSF.

Variations in CSF pressure are not of much use in clinical diagnosis except in hypovitaminosis A, and measurement of CSF pressure is only indicated in animals with signs of cerebral disease (abnormal mentation) that may have cerebral edema. Care is needed in interpreting results because the pressure is greatly affected by voluntary movement such as tenesmus. CSF pressure is increased in a number of diseases, including PEM, bacterial meningitis, and hypovitaminosis A, reflecting the presence of increased intracranial pressure. Xylazine given intravenously causes a decrease in intracranial pressure in healthy conscious horses. Intracranial pressure is increased in anesthetized horses when their head is placed lower than their heart because of an increase in the hydrostatic pressure gradient.[10] Epidural pressure of cattle changes with change in position from standing to lateral recumbency to dorsal recumbency, and epidural pressure is positive in laterally recumbent animals.

Analysis of Cerebrospinal Fluid

Analysis of CSF has greater diagnostic value than hematology in animals with nervous system disease. CSF can be examined for the presence of protein, cells, and bacteria. The white blood cell count in normal animals is usually less than 5 cells/μL.[11] An increase in the CSF leukocyte count above 5 cells/μL is termed a pleocytosis and is categorized as mild (6 to 49 cells/μL), moderate (50 to 200 cells/μL), or marked (>200 cells/μL). The differential white cell count comprises mostly lymphocytes and monocytes (mononuclear cells predominate); there are no erythrocytes in the CSF of healthy animals with an atraumatic CSF tap. Cytologic examination of CSF is usually done after a Cytospin preparation that carefully concentrates the cells without destroying their architecture. This is needed because the cell count in CSF is usually very low. With bacterial infections of the nervous system, the CSF concentration of protein will be increased and the white blood cell count increased up to 2000 cells/μL with more than 70% neutrophils. A neutrophilic pleocytosis is considered 95% to 100% indicative of an inflammatory process within the CNS. Samples that show visible turbidity usually contain large numbers of cells (>500 cells/μL) and a great deal of protein.

The CSF glucose concentration is usually 60% to 80% of serum glucose concentration; this steady-state value reflects facilitated transport across the blood-brain barrier, absence of binding proteins for glucose in CSF, and nervous tissue metabolism of glucose. However, sudden changes in plasma glucose concentrations are not immediately reflected in CSF glucose concentrations, because CSF turns over at around 1% per minute. Typically, a lag time of up to 3 hours is needed for CSF glucose concentration to be in equilibrium with plasma glucose concentrations. Therefore hyperglycemia from the stress of handling and restraint may not be reflected by an increased CSF glucose concentration.

In cattle, protein concentrations range from 23 to 60 mg/dL, sodium concentrations from 132 to 144 mmol/L, potassium 2.7 to 3.2 mmol/L, magnesium 1.8 to 2.1 mEq/L, and glucose concentrations 37 to 51 mg/dL. In the horse, the reference values for CSF are similar. Neonatal foals under 3 weeks of age have higher CSF protein concentrations than do adult horses. Glucose concentrations peak in the first 48 hours after birth and then decrease to adult values by the second week of life. Concentrations of sodium and potassium are not affected by age and are similar to values reported for adult horses and ponies. In sheep, protein concentrations range from 12 to 60 mg/dL and glucose concentrations from 38 to 63 mg/dL.

Cytokine concentrations in CSF may have prognostic value,[11] and the cytokine gene expression in nucleated cells in CSF may have clinical utility in the diagnosis of specific nervous diseases.[13] The presence of one or more eosinophils in CSF is extremely unusual and should be assumed to indicate the presence of aberrant parasite migration or fungal encephalitis. Theoretically, the CSF glucose concentration will be decreased and CSF lactate concentration will be increased in animals with bacterial meningitis because of bacterial metabolism, but these are unreliable signs and usually do not provide additional information to that provided by determination of CSF leukocyte and protein concentrations. Bacteria may also be cultured from the CSF.

The creatine kinase and lactate dehydrogenase activities in CSF have been examined as an aid in the differentiation of some neurologic diseases. However, creatine kinase activity is considered to be unreliable in the horse; contamination of the sample with epidural fat and dura may increase CSF creatine kinase activity. In contrast, CSF creatine kinase activity >19.5 U/L provided an excellent prognostic test of nonrecovery in sheep with Listeriosis.[12] Insufficient information is available to evaluate the clinical utility of CSF lactate dehydrogenase activity in large animals.

Blood contamination of CSF can make interpretation difficult. A formula has been developed that "corrects" the CSF values for the degree of blood contamination, based on the red blood cell count (RBC) in CSF (RBC_{CSF}) and blood (RBC_{blood}), in which the corrected value for substance X in CSF ($X_{corrected}$, where X is a concentration or activity) is derived from the measured value of X in CSF (X_{CSF}) and blood (X_{blood}) and applying the following formula:

$$X_{corrected} = X_{CSF} - (X_{blood} \times RBC_{CSF} / RBC_{blood}).$$

Calculation of a "corrected" value rarely provides additional insight into the CSF analysis and is not commonly practiced in large animals. Xanthochromia is a slight yellow tinge to CSF that indicates previous erythrocyte lysis or more commonly increased protein concentration. A foamy appearance to the CSF is also suggestive of increased protein concentration.

Protein fractionation of CSF is not routinely performed because it requires sensitive electrophoresis methodology or species-specific radial immunodiffusion assays. Albumin (ALB) concentration in CSF can also be measured using an immunologic technique based on the detection of albumin–antialbumin immune complexes by nephelometry.[7] Calculation of the **albumin quotient** and **IgG index** may be informative in specific neurologic diseases. Theoretically, these calculations can differentiate four blood-brain permeability patterns, normal blood-brain barrier permeability (normal albumin quotient and IgG index), intrathecal IgG production with normal blood-brain barrier permeability (normal albumin quotient and increased IgG index), increased blood-brain barrier permeability without intrathecal IgG production (increased albumin quotient and normal IgG index), and increased blood-brain barrier permeability with intrathecal production of IgG (increased albumin quotient and increased IgG index). The albumin quotient is calculated from the albumin concentration in CSF (ALB_{CSF}) and serum (ALB_{serum}), in which:

$$Albumin\ Quotient = (ALB_{CSF}) \times 100 / (ALB_{serum}).$$

The normal range for albumin quotient in the adult horse is 0.6 to 2.2 for atlantooccipital CSF samples and 0.7 to 2.3 for lumbosacral CSF samples, but the mean is 0.4 to 0.5 in cattle and adult llamas. Because CSF protein is most often derived by disturbance of the blood-brain barrier and inflammation (resulting in an increased CSF albumin concentration), an increased CSF protein concentration is usually accompanied by an increased albumin quotient.

In animals suspected to have increased immunoglobulin production in the CNS (a rare occurrence, and almost always accompanied by disturbance of the blood-brain barrier), the IgG index can be calculated from the IgG concentration in CSF (IgG_{CSF}) and serum (IgG_{serum}), and the albumin concentration in CSF (ALB_{CSF}) and serum (ALB_{serum}), in which:

$$IgG\ Index = (IgG_{CSF}/(IgG_{serum}) \times (ALB_{serum}/ALB_{CSF}/).$$

An IgG index of more than 0.3 is suspected to indicate intrathecal IgG production in the adult horse. This formula corrects the CSF IgG concentration for an increased permeability of the blood-brain barrier; therefore, theoretically it provides a more sensitive method for detecting local production of IgG within the CNS. Calculating the albumin quotient and IgG index is expensive and rarely provides additional information to that provided by CSF protein concentration alone, and for this reason is not commonly performed in large animals.

When antigen-specific titers are measured, two modified CSF indices, the **Goldmann–Witmer coefficient** (***C*-value**) and the **antibody index** (**AI**), can be calculated to distinguish intrathecal versus passively acquired antibodies in the CSF.[14,15] The *C*-value is calculated as

$$C\text{-}value = (IgG_{serum} \times reciprocal\ CSF\ titer)/(IgG_{CSF} \times reciprocal\ serum\ titer).$$

The AI is calculated as the ratio of the specific antibody quotient to the albumin quotient, in which

$$AI = (\{reciprocal\ CSF\ titer\}/\{reciprocal\ serum\ titer\})/(\{CSF\ albumin\ concentration\}/\{serum\ albumin\ concentration\}).$$

The **urine dipstick protein test** provides a useful on-farm assessment of CSF protein concentration and is underutilized in clinical practice. Most dipsticks use the following gradations of trace (<25 mg/dL), 1+ (28–75 mg/dL), 2+ (115–240 mg/dL), and 3+ (470–590 mg/dL), and a study of dog CSF samples indicated that all dogs with a urine dipstick protein of 2+ or greater had increased CSF protein concentration.[16] Similar studies do not appear to have been conducted in large animals.

The **Pandy test** also provides a useful on-farm assessment of CSF protein concentration. The basis for the test is that proteins (globulin and albumin) are precipitated by a saturated solution of phenol in water. The Pandy test uses a 10% solution of carbolic acid crystals dissolved in water (providing a saturated aqueous solution of phenol); the solution is termed Pandy's solution. One milliliter of Pandy's solution is placed in a glass tube and one drop (approximately 0.05 mL) of CSF is carefully layered on top. A turbid appearance at the interface signifies the presence of elevated concentrations of globulin or albumin in the CSF and is regarded as a positive Pandy's reaction (usually a total protein concentration greater than approximately 50 mg/dL). A variant of the test has the sample thoroughly mixed and the degree of turbidity ranked from 1+ (faint turbidity) to 4+ (dense milk-colored precipitate). A negative Pandy's reaction shows no turbidity or precipitate, and this is the expected result in normal CSF samples. A positive control (4+) can be run at the same time by adding a drop of serum or plasma to 1 mL of Pandy's solution. Because Pandy's solution contains phenol, clinicians should wear gloves and protective eyewear when handling the solution, and dispose of used reagents appropriately.

In summary, collection and analysis of CSF from the lumbosacral region provides a practical, safe, and informative diagnostic tool in conscious large animals with neurologic disease. Analysis of CSF in animals with CNS disease has greater diagnostic value than analysis of the leukon or serum biochemical analysis. Routine assessment of CSF should include total protein concentration (including the semiquantitative Pandy test and urine dipstick measurement), erythrocyte count, leukocyte count, and leukocyte differential count. Other analytical procedures on CSF can be performed in specific diseases related to the nervous system.

EXAMINATION OF THE NERVOUS SYSTEM WITH SERUM BIOCHEMICAL ANALYSIS

Arterial Plasma Ammonia Concentration

In animals suspected of having hepatic encephalopathy, measurement of the arterial plasma ammonia concentration provides a clinically useful diagnostic test and a means of monitoring the response to treatment. In monogastrics, ammonia is produced by bacterial degradation of amines, amino acids, and purines in the gastrointestinal tract, by the action of bacterial and intestinal urease on urea in the gastrointestinal tract, and by the catabolism of glutamine by enterocytes. In ruminants, ammonia is derived predominantly from bacterial metabolism in the rumen and catabolism of amino acids in tissue. Absorbed ammonia is normally converted to urea by the liver and to glutamine by the liver, skeletal muscle, and brain. In the presence of hepatic dysfunction, ammonia is inadequately metabolized, resulting in high plasma ammonia concentrations. Ammonia is a direct neurotoxin that alters inhibitory and excitatory neurotransmission in the brain.

Hyperammonemia can be used as a specific indicator of hepatic dysfunction. Normal values for arterial plasma ammonia concentration are less than 29 μmol/L in adult cattle but may reach higher values in the immediate periparturient period. Arterial values are higher than venous values and are preferred for analysis.

Blood gas analysis and serum electrolyte determination should be routinely undertaken in animals with clinical signs of encephalopathy to rule out metabolic causes of cerebral dysfunction.

FURTHER READING

Aleman M. Miscellaneous neurologic or neuromuscular disorders of horses. *Vet Clin North Am Equine Pract*. 2011;27:481-506.

Constable PD. Clinical examination of the ruminant nervous system. *Vet Clin North Am Food Anim Pract*. 2004;20:215-230.

Levine JM, Levine GJ, Hoffman AG, Mez J, Bratton GR. Comparative anatomy of the horse, ox, and dog: the vertebral column and peripheral nerves. *Equine Comp Cont Educ Pract Vet*. 2007;2:279-292.

Schwarz B, Piercy RJ. Cerebrospinal fluid collection and its analysis in equine neurologic disease. *Equine Vet Educ*. 2006;18:243-248.

Scott PR. Cerebrospinal fluid collection and analysis in suspected sheep neurological disease. *Small Rumin Res*. 2010;92:96-103.

REFERENCES

1. Cavalleri JMV, et al. *BMC Vet Res*. 2013;9:105.
2. Verdes JM, et al. *J Vet Diagn Invest*. 2006;18:299.
3. Sprake PM, et al. *J Vet Intern Med*. 2013;27:1242.
4. Raoofi A. *Vet J*. 2009;181:296.
5. Olsen E, et al. *J Vet Intern Med*. 2014;28:630.
6. Stokol T, et al. *Vet Clin Pathol*. 2009;38:103.
7. Goehring LS, et al. *J Vet Diagn Invest*. 2006;18:251.
8. D'Angelo A, et al. *Vet Rec*. 2009;164:491.
9. Aleman M, et al. *J Am Vet Med Assoc*. 2007;230:378.
10. Brosnan RJ, et al. *Am J Vet Res*. 2008;69:737.
11. Ameri M, Mousavian R. *Vet Res Commun*. 2007;31:77.
12. El-Boshy ME, et al. *Small Rumin Res*. 2012;104:179.
13. Pusterla N, et al. *Am J Vet Res*. 2006;67:1433.
14. Furr M, et al. *J Vet Intern Med*. 2011;25:138.
15. Reed SM, et al. *J Vet Intern Med*. 2013;27:1193.
16. Jacobs RM, et al. *Can Vet J*. 1990;31:587.

EXAMINATION OF THE NERVOUS SYSTEM WITH IMAGING TECHNIQUES

Radiography

Examination of the bony skeleton of the head and vertebral column to detect abnormalities that are affecting the nervous system of large animals is commonly used in referral centers. Conventional diagnostic radiography remains the best method for the initial evaluation of trauma to the brain and spinal cord, but usually the trauma needs to have displaced bone for the lesion to be readily visible on a radiograph. Lesions that can be identified on plain radiographs include fractured, luxated, or subluxated vertebra; intervertebral disk prolapse; discospondylitis; osteomyelitis; and neoplasia.[1] The injection of contrast media into the CSF system (**myelography**) is used for the detection of spinal cord compression but is not often performed in large animals because spinal cord depression surgery is rarely undertaken and because sensitivity and specificity estimates are low depending on criteria used for interpretation.[2] In cases of peripheral nerve injury the radiograph of the appropriate limb may reveal the presence of a fracture or space-occupying lesion that has caused dysfunction of the peripheral nerve.

Radiography has been used to diagnose lesions of the tympanic bullae in cattle (otitis interna) characterized by thickening of the bulla wall, increased soft tissue opacity within the bulla, and osteolysis of the bulla wall and trabeculations.[3] Radiography is not as sensitive as computed tomography (CT) for the diagnosis of otitis media, however, because CT provides more detailed information regarding the bony structures of the middle ear[4] and is more sensitive and specific than radiography in the diagnosis of otitis media in calves.[3]

Computed Tomography

CT of the skull has several advantages over radiography because structures are viewed in cross section without superimposition. The use of contrast agents and development of computer software and technology that permit rapid acquisition times and three-dimensional reconstruction allows a large amount of information to be obtained from a CT examination. Numerous diseases of the head of the horse, including those of the brain and cervical spine, can be diagnosed using this technique, but the limiting factors are the weight of the patient (a custom-designed table is required for adult horses and cattle), accessibility for large animals, and the need for general anesthesia.

CT provides an excellent image of skeletal cranial defects and soft tissue defects that differ considerably from surrounding tissue. CT has been used for the antemortem diagnosis of many conditions in foals, horses, and cattle, including cerebral abscess, porencephaly, meningoencephalocele, pituitary adenoma, cervical stenotic myelopathy, spinal cord rupture, and otitis interna/media, and has been used to guide brain biopsy for in vivo diagnosis of an intracranial mass.[4-7] CT provides less contrast resolution than magnetic resonance imaging (MRI), but CT provides better spatial resolution (i.e., is more able to differentiate fine anatomic features such as bone trabeculae), is more widely available, and has a shorter scan acquisition time. In a case series of 57 cases, CT was a useful diagnostic test in horses with abnormal mentation or a history of trauma followed by a period of unconsciousness. In contrast, CT did not provide clinically helpful information in horses with seizures.[8]

Magnetic Resonance Imaging

MRI scanning uses nuclear magnetic resonance to create cross-sectional images based on the magnetic properties of tissues. In general, MRI provides an excellent image of soft tissue defects and is considered superior to CT for intracranial and intraspinal lesions because MRI provides a high contrast between soft tissues and better anatomic detail. MRI can be performed in standing sedated horses; however, these MRI units (typically 0.25 T) produce low-resolution images that may not have sufficient detail to be diagnostic for many nervous diseases. Higher resolution images are produced by more expensive magnets (typically 1.0–3.0 T) that require the patient be immobile. The limiting factors for MRI use are therefore cost (MRI is more expensive than CT), the weight of the patient, accessibility for large animals, and the need for general anesthesia for higher resolution images (usually MRI has a longer imaging time than CT). Other challenges specific to MRI are that the environment provides considerable challenges for the monitoring of anesthesia and the placement of limbs to minimize postanesthetic myopathy/neuropathy syndrome, particularly in horses.[9]

MRI has been used for the antemortem diagnosis of a number of neurologic conditions in foals and horses, including brain abscess, hydrocephalus, nigropallidal encephalomalacia,[10] cerebellar abiotrophy in Arabian horses,[11] cervical stenotic myelopathy,[2] and peripheral nerve sheath tumor (PNST) in the tongue.[12] MRI has also been used to diagnose PEM and cerebellar hypoplasia in calves[13] and PEM, leukoencephalomalacia, and porencephaly and demyelination in sheep and goats.[14] More studies are required documenting the clinical superiority of MRI versus other diagnostic modalities. For instance, MRI can differentiate horses with cervical stenotic myelopathy (CSM) and cervical vertebral stenosis from healthy horses and horses with other causes for ataxia; however, MRI cannot accurately localize the site of cord compression.[2] MRI will be more widely used in the diagnosis of nervous diseases, particularly intracranial and cervical spinal cord disease, as equipment and acquisition costs decrease.

FURTHER READING

Aleman M. Miscellaneous neurologic or neuromuscular disorders of horses. *Vet Clin North Am Equine Pract.* 2011;27:481-506.

Scrivani PV. Advanced imaging of the nervous system in the horse. *Vet Clin North Am Equine Pract.* 2011;27:439-453.

REFERENCES

1. Hughes KJ. *Equine Vet Educ.* 2007;19:460.
2. Mitchell CW, et al. *Vet Radiol Ultrasound.* 2012;53:613.
3. Finnen A, et al. *J Vet Intern Med.* 2011;25:143.
4. Lee K, et al. *Vet Rec.* 2009;165:559.
5. Ohba Y, et al. *J Vet Med Sci.* 2008;70:829.
6. Pease AP, et al. *J Vet Intern Med.* 2011;25:1144.
7. Vanschandevijl K, et al. *J Am Vet Med Assoc.* 2008;233:950.
8. Sogaro-Robinson C, et al. *J Am Vet Med Assoc.* 2009;235:176.
9. Franci P, et al. *Equine Vet J.* 2006;38:497.
10. Jose-Cunilleras E, Piercy RJ. *Equine Vet Educ.* 2007;19:179.
11. Cavalleri JMV, et al. *BMC Vet Res.* 2013;9:105.
12. Schneider A, et al. *Equine Vet Educ.* 2010;22:346.
13. Tsuka T, et al. *Vet Radiol Ultrasound.* 2008;49:149.
14. Schenk HC, et al. *J Vet Intern Med.* 2007;21:865.

Ultrasonography

Ultrasonography of the cricoarytenoideus lateralis muscle has been used as part of the examination of horses with suspected laryngeal hemiplegia and compared with endoscopic findings obtained at rest and during exercise. An 8.4-MHz curvilinear transducer was applied over the larynx and four acoustic windows evaluated. Subjectively assessed increased echogenicity of this muscle had a sensitivity of 94.6% and a specificity of 94.5% for detecting laryngeal hemiplegia.[1] The reported advantages of ultrasonography are that it is widely available, noninvasive, and depicts a real-time view of the tissues.

The supraspinous ligament has been evaluated in horses with and without back pathology using ultrasonography. Linear and sector array transducers (5–10 MHz) were used to obtain longitudinal and cross-sectional views of the supraspinous ligament, and lesions were identified and categorized. All 39 horses studied had at least one site of supraspinous ligament desmitis, and there was no association between desmitis lesions and clinical signs of pain that could be localized to this region.[2]

Ultrasonography has been used to diagnose syringohydromyelia and segmental hypoplasia of the lumbar spinal cord in a 4-day-old Holstein Friesian calf that had been unable to stand since birth. The calf was placed in right lateral recumbency, and lumbosacral flexion was induced to enable widening of ultrasound windows. Diagnostic images of the lumbar spinal cord were obtained in sagittal and transverse orientations at the lumbosacral junction (L6-S1), as well as the proximal lumbar intervertebral junctions up to L2-L3, using a 6- to 10-MHz linear transducer.[3]

An ultrasound imaging technique of the tympanic bullae has been developed for the diagnosis of otitis media in calves.[4] A 7.5-MHz linear probe is applied to the base of the ear without the use of coupling gel and with the calf in a standing position. The probe is applied ventral to the base of the ear and caudal to the mandible. Abnormalities detected included anechoic to hyperechoic content; trabeculae lysis; and thinning, deformation, and rupture of the bulla wall. In calves, ultrasonography has also been used to identify the femoral nerve in calves to assist in the diagnosis of spastic paresis cases that involve the quadriceps muscle (such as in Belgian Blue cattle with a cranially directed hyperextension of the limb) instead of the more common form of spastic paresis that involves the gastrocnemius muscle and a caudally directed hyperextension of the hindlimb.[5,6] Placement of a 5-MHz curved linear array transducer over the dorsal paravertebral space between the fifth and sixth lumbar transverse processes provided the best view of the femoral nerve and permitted selective blocking of the femoral nerve using 4% procaine solution.

ENDOSCOPY (RHINOLARYNGOSCOPY)

Endoscopy (rhinolaryngoscopy) is now a routine technique for the examination of horses with suspected laryngeal hemiplegia, which is a distal axonopathy of the left recurrent laryngeal nerve.

Endoscopic examination of the epidural and subarachnoid space from the atlantooccipital space to the eighth cervical nerve has been performed safely in healthy adult horses.[7] The procedure was performed under general anesthesia. The technique may have clinical utility in the diagnosis of cervical vertebral stenotic myelopathy because physical constraints do not currently permit imaging of the caudal cervical vertebral column by MRI or CT.

Endoscopy has also been used to examine the anatomic structures in the sacrococcygeal area of adult cattle. Cows were restrained and sedated with xylazine (0.03 mg/kg, intravenously). A lidocaine epidural was administered and a flexible endoscope (outside diameter, 2.3 mm) introduced through an introducer set and a small amount of air introduced. The procedure permitted visualization of blood vessels, connective tissue, fat, nerves, and the spinal dura mater.[8]

OPHTHALMOSCOPY

Ophthalmoscopy for the examination of the structures of the eye is important in the diagnosis of diseases affecting the optic nerve such as in vitamin A deficiency and the optic disc edema (papilledema) associated with diffuse cerebral edema.

ELECTROMYOGRAPHY

Electromyographic needle examination is a technique that records the electrical activity generated by single muscle fibers and the summated electrical activity of muscle fibers in individual motor units. The technique involves inserting a recording needle into the muscle of interest and recording the resultant EMG. Typically, animals are unsedated and restrained in stocks or a chute. An abnormal EMG signals include short-duration and low-amplitude motor unit action potentials, which indicate diseased muscle fibers of early or incomplete reinnervation after denervation. Other abnormalities include the presence of fibrillation potentials, positive sharp waves, and complex repetitive discharges that occur when the skeletal cell membrane becomes unstable because of denervation or myopathy.

EMG provides a more practical diagnostic test than electroencephalography (EEG) and provides a sensitive indicator of neurologic dysfunction and assists in the neuroanatomic localization of the lesion.[8] It is especially useful for evaluating peripheral nerve injury and diagnosing hyperkalemic periodic paresis in horses and should be helpful in additional studies on calving-associated paralysis and other peripheral nerve injuries in cattle. EMG can discriminate between lower motor neuron and myogenic disorders, and **nerve conduction studies** can differentiate axonal loss from demyelination. In addition, repetitive stimulation can provide information regarding neuromuscular transmission. Reference values for motor nerve conduction velocity have been developed for calves and, as expected, conduction velocities are related to the nerve fiber diameter.[10]

Somatosensory evoked potentials of the trigeminal complex using the infraorbital nerve have been used in horses to assist in the diagnosis of idiopathic head-shaking. An electrical surface stimulus is applied at a set stimulus rate but variable stimulus currents to a focal area of the buccal mucosa. Recording electrodes placed along the sensory pathway of the trigeminal complex detect the presence or absence of **sensory nerve action potentials** (SNAPs) and nerve conduction velocity.[11] The threshold current required to trigger a SNAP provides clinically useful information about the sensitivity of the anatomic location to stimuli.

EMG has been coupled with transcranial magnetic stimulation to induce magnetic **motor evoked potentials** in the horse. This provides a useful noninvasive evaluation of cervical spinal cord dysfunction in horses with radiologic abnormalities of the cervical vertebrae by detecting the presence of a neuropathy involving the descending motor tracts. However, EMG does not provide information on upper motor neurons; therefore it is not useful in the clinical evaluation of horses suspected to have hindlimb neurologic deficits caused by cervical spinal cord disease.[9]

ELECTROENCEPHALOGRAPHY

EEG has not been used to any significant degree in large animals. It requires sophisticated equipment, a quiet dim environment free from electrical interference, and a quiet patient that has minimal muscular activity. Because of the difficulty in obtaining quality recordings in a conscious large animal, it is preferred that the animal is sedated or anesthetized for the recording, which confounds interpretation of the EEG pattern depending on the anesthetic protocol. Thorough and repeated observations of simultaneously recorded EEG and video may facilitate interpretation of the EEG,[12,13] but the clinical utility of EEG remains uncertain in large animals exhibiting nervous signs consistent with an intracranial lesion. Therefore EEG has been primarily used in large animals as an antemortem or research tool, and its use will probably remain as a complementary test to other neurologic examinations and diagnostic tests at referral institutions.

Recommendations have been made to standardize EEG techniques for animals; these typically involve meticulous preparation of the recording sites on the scalp, and placement of electrodes over the left and right frontal areas, the left and right occipital areas, and the vertex area, and a reference electrode is placed behind the tip of the nose. The addition of other recording sites increases the ability to localize a focal lesion.[12] Neurologic disease is associated with changes in EEG frequency or amplitude, or both, and frequency changes are a more reliable indicator of disease. In general, focal EEG abnormalities indicate a focal lesion in the cortex, whereas diffuse EEG abnormalities indicate diffuse cortical or subcortical lesions or focal subcortical lesions.

EEG has been used to study epilepsy in goats and cattle, congenital hydranencephaly and hydrocephalus in cattle, scrapie in sheep, thiamine-responsive PEM in cattle, and BSE in cattle. When performed under controlled conditions, EEG has been shown to be a useful diagnostic tool for the early diagnosis of equine intracranial diseases, with adequate sensitivity and specificity.

ELECTRORETINOGRAPHY

Flash electroretinography (ERG) is a recording of rod and cone function of the eyes. The animal is sedated (usually with xylazine) and topical 0.5% proparacaine is applied to both eyes to permit the placement of a contact lens electrode on both eyes. Subcutaneous electrodes are then placed at the lateral canthus and midline at the nostrils to provide reference and ground electrodes, respectively. A period of dark adaptation is then implemented, and a standardized flash sequence applied.[10] Decreased B-wave amplitudes during flash ERG have been identified in horses with equine motor neuron disease and attributed to lipofuscin deposits on the retina.

BRAINSTEM AUDITORY EVOKED POTENTIALS

The brainstem auditory evoked potential (BAEP) is a recording of the electrical activity of the brainstem following an acoustic stimulation; as such, BAEP can be used to evaluate the integrity of the auditory pathway. The use of the BAEP permits differentiation of cochlear pathology (including otitis media/interna) from retrocochlear pathology (auditory nerve or brainstem).

BAEP is obtained on a sedated patient (xylazine is frequently used) by recording neuroelectrical activity from generators in the auditory pathway immediately following an acoustic click stimulus, and BAEP waveforms for horses,[14] ponies, foals,[15,16] and calves have been recorded. Such recordings can be useful in evaluating horses suspected to have deafness, vestibular disease, brainstem disease, or temporohyoid osteoarthropathy,[17] as well as calves with otitis media and facial paralysis,[18] and to monitor the response to treatment.[17]

INTRACRANIAL PRESSURE MEASUREMENT

Intracranial pressure has been measured in neonatal foals, although the clinical utility of such measurements in foals has not been demonstrated. Increases in intracranial pressure can cause decreases in cerebral perfusion pressure and irreversible injury to the CNS.

The head-down position in the horse increases the hydrostatic pressure gradient between the heart and brain, increasing mean intracranial pressure in isoflurane-anesthetized horses from 31 to 55 mm Hg when placed in the Trendelenburg position to facilitate abdominal surgery.[19] Similar directional changes in intraocular pressure were measured in adult horses sedated with detomidine.[20] Hydrostatic pressure effects on intracranial pressure have also been observed in isoflurane-anesthetized adult cattle.[21] In other words, large animals suspected to have increased intracranial pressure should be encouraged to keep their heads elevated to prevent cerebral edema formation. In addition, head position must be standardized when intracranial pressure is measured.

KINETIC GAIT ANALYSIS

Lameness is common in large animals and usually results in asymmetric gait abnormalities; lameness caused by selected musculoskeletal abnormalities is discussed in Chapter 15. Ataxia caused by spinal cord disease also causes gait abnormalities that are usually symmetric and particularly evident in the hindlimbs. Diagnostic differentiation of lameness and neurologic causes of gait abnormalities can be challenging, even to experienced practitioners. Consequently, kinetic gait analysis offers an objective quantitative test that may assist in the differentiation of neurologic from musculoskeletal causes for a gait abnormality. Two indices appear to have the greatest clinical utility in identifying the presence of a neurologic gait abnormality: higher lateral force peak and increased variation in vertical force peak in both hindlimbs.[22]

FURTHER READING

Aleman M. Miscellaneous neurologic or neuromuscular disorders of horses. *Vet Clin North Am Equine Pract.* 2011;27:481-506.

Constable PD. Clinical examination of the ruminant nervous system. *Vet Clin North Am Food Anim Pract.* 2004;20:215-230.

MacKay RJ. Brain injury after head trauma: pathophysiology, diagnosis, and treatment. *Vet Clin North Am Equine Pract.* 2004;20:199-216.

Scott PR. Diagnostic techniques and clinicopathologic findings in ruminant neurologic disease. *Vet Clin North Am Food Anim Pract.* 2004;20:215-230.

REFERENCES

1. Chalmers HJ, et al. *Vet Radiol Ultrasound.* 2012;53:660.
2. Henson FMD, et al. *BMC Vet Res.* 2007;3:3.
3. Testoni S, et al. *J Vet Intern Med.* 2012;26:1485.
4. Gosselin VB, et al. *J Vet Intern Med.* 2014;28:1594.
5. De Vlamynck C, et al. *Vet Rec.* 2013;196:451.
6. De Vlamynck CA, et al. *Am J Vet Res.* 2013;74:750.
7. Prange T, et al. *Equine Vet J.* 2011;43:404.
8. Franz S, et al. *Am J Vet Res.* 2008;69:894.
9. Mitchell CW, et al. *Vet Radiol Ultrasound.* 2012;53:613.
10. Schenk HC, et al. *J Vet Intern Med.* 2014;28:646.
11. Aleman M, et al. *J Vet Intern Med.* 2014;28:250.
12. Williams DC, et al. *J Vet Intern Med.* 2008;22:630.
13. Finno CJ, et al. *Vet Ophthalm.* 2012;15(suppl 2):3.
14. Aleman M, et al. *J Vet Intern Med.* 2014;28:1310.
15. Aleman M, et al. *J Vet Intern Med.* 2014;28:1318.
16. Lecoq L, et al. *J Vet Intern Med.* 2015;29:362.
17. Aleman M, et al. *J Vet Intern Med.* 2008;22:1196.
18. Kawasaki Y, et al. *Vet Rec.* 2009;165:212.
19. Brosnan RJ, et al. *Am J Vet Res.* 2008;69:737.
20. Komaromy AM, et al. *Am J Vet Res.* 2006;67:1232.
21. Arai S, et al. *J Vet Med Sci.* 2006;68:337.
22. Ishihara A, et al. *J Am Vet Med Assoc.* 2009;234:644.

Diffuse or Multifocal Diseases of the Brain and Spinal Cord

There are many different causes of diffuse or multifocal nervous system disease in large domestic animals.

- Infectious causes include bacteria, viruses, fungi, and helminth, arthropod, and protozoan parasites.
- Exogenous substances such as lead, salt, selenium, organophosphate insecticides, feed additives such as urea, poisonous plants, and many other chemicals are common causes.
- Endogenous substances such as products of disease in other body systems or of abnormal metabolism such as bacterial toxins, ammonia, and carbon dioxide can cause abnormalities of the nervous system.
- Metabolic and nutritional causes include ischemia secondary to cardiopulmonary disease; hypoglycemia; hypomagnesemia; copper deficiency in pregnant animals; and hyper D-lactatemia in calves, lambs, and kids with neonatal diarrhea and adult ruminants with grain overload.
- Chronic acidemia associated with diarrhea can cause mental depression and ataxia (whereas experimentally induced acute acidemia does not cause mental depression in neonatal calves).
- Idiopathic diseases account for several diseases of the spinal cord of horses.
- Malformation occurs primarily in the developing fetus and results in congenital nervous system disease, which is usually present at birth. Many different teratogens can cause congenital defects. In some cases of inherited disease, the clinical signs do not manifest until sometime after birth.

Responses of Central Nervous System to Injury

The CNS may respond to injury by morphologic changes that include cerebral edema and brain swelling, inflammation, and demyelination. Malformations occur when the CNS is affected during fetal life.

The remainder of this chapter will present the general clinical aspects of the diseases of the nervous system according to anatomic sites and causative agent. The salient features of the etiology, pathogenesis, clinical findings, diagnosis, and treatment of these clinicoanatomic diseases are described. Cerebral hypoxia, hydrocephalus, cerebral edema, meningitis, encephalitis, myelitis, encephalomalacia, and myelomalacia are common to many diffuse or multifocal diseases of the nervous system and are described here.

CEREBRAL HYPOXIA

Cerebral hypoxia occurs when the supply of oxygen to the brain is reduced for any reason. An acute or chronic syndrome develops depending on the acuteness of the deprivation. Initially there are irritation signs followed terminally by signs of loss of function.

ETIOLOGY

All forms of hypoxia, including anemic, anoxic, histotoxic, and stagnant forms cause some degree of cerebral hypoxia, but signs referable to cerebral dysfunction occur only when the hypoxia is severe. Hypoxia of the brain may be secondary to a general systemic hypoxia or be caused by lesions restricted to the cranial cavity.

Cerebral Hypoxia Secondary to General Hypoxia

- Poisoning by hydrocyanic acid or nitrite
- Acute heart failure in severe copper deficiency in cattle
- Anesthetic accidents
- Terminally in pneumonia, congestive heart failure
- During or at birth in foals, hypoxic-ischemic encephalopathy in foals (also known as neonatal encephalopathy, perinatal asphyxia, dummy foal syndrome, or neonatal maladjustment syndrome),[1] or intrapartum hypoxia in calves and lambs caused by prolonged parturition

Cerebral Hypoxia Secondary to Intracranial Lesion

- In increased intracranial pressure
- In brain edema

PATHOGENESIS

The CNS is extremely sensitive to hypoxia, and degeneration occurs if the deprivation is extreme and prolonged for more than a few minutes. The effects of the hypoxia vary with the speed of onset and with the severity. When the onset is sudden, there is usually a transitory period during which excitation phenomena occur, and this is followed by a period of loss of function. If recovery occurs, a second period of excitation usually develops as function returns. In more chronic cases the excitation phase is not observed, and the signs are mainly those of loss of function. These signs include dullness and lethargy when deprivation is moderate and unconsciousness when it is severe. All forms of nervous activity are depressed, but the higher centers are more susceptible than medullary centers and the pattern of development of signs may suggest this.

CLINICAL FINDINGS

Acute and chronic syndromes occur depending on the severity of the hypoxia. Acute cerebral hypoxia is manifested by a sudden onset of signs referable to paralysis of all brain functions, including tetraparesis and unconsciousness. Muscle tremor, beginning about the head and spreading to the trunk and limbs, followed by recumbency, clonic convulsions, and death or recovery after further clonic convulsions is the most common pattern, although affected animals may fall to the ground without premonitory signs. In chronic hypoxia, there is lethargy, dullness, ataxia, weakness, and blindness and in some cases muscle tremor or convulsions. In both acute and chronic hypoxia, the signs of the primary disease will also be evident. Cerebral hypoxia of fetal calves is thought to be a cause of weakness and failure to suck after birth, leading to the eventual death of the calf from starvation. Such hypoxia can occur during the birth process, especially if it is difficult or delayed, or during late pregnancy.

CLINICAL PATHOLOGY AND NECROPSY FINDINGS

There is no distinctive clinical pathology or characteristic necropsy lesion other than those of the primary disease.

DIFFERENTIAL DIAGNOSIS

Clinically there is little to differentiate cerebral hypoxia from hypoglycemia or polioencephalomalacia in which similar signs occur. Irritation and paralytic signs follow one another in many poisonings including lead and arsenic and in most diffuse diseases of the brain including encephalitis and encephalomalacia. The differential diagnosis of cerebral hypoxia depends on the detection of the cause of the hypoxia.

TREATMENT

An increase in oxygen delivery is essential and can usually only be provided by removing the causative agent. A respiratory stimulant (the most effective is doxapram, 2 mg/kg BW, intravenously)[2] may be advantageous in acute cases, and artificial respiration may be necessary and effective.

INCREASED INTRACRANIAL PRESSURE, CEREBRAL EDEMA, AND BRAIN SWELLING

Diffuse cerebral edema and brain swelling usually occur acutely and cause a general increase in intracranial pressure. Cerebral edema is rarely a primary disease, but is commonly an accompaniment of other diseases. Cerebral edema is often a transient phenomenon and may be fatal, but complete recovery or recovery with residual nervous signs also occurs. It is manifested clinically by blindness, opisthotonus, muscle tremor, paralysis, and clonic convulsions.

ETIOLOGY

Diffuse cerebral edema and brain swelling may be **vasogenic**, when there is increased permeability of capillary endothelium, and **cytotoxic** when all the elements of brain tissue, glia, neurons, and endothelial cells undergo swelling. Causes include the following.

Vasogenic Edema

- Brain abscess, neoplasm, hemorrhage, lead encephalopathy, purulent meningitis
- Minor edema after most traumatic injuries, in many encephalitides and many poisonings, including propylene glycol in the horse; probably contributes to the pathogenesis
- Accidental intracarotid injection of promazine in horses
- Leukoencephalomalacia in horses caused by fumonisin consumption
- Septicemia in neonatal foals

Cytotoxic Edema

- Hypoxia
- PEM of ruminants (thiamine deficiency or sulfur toxicosis)
- Salt poisoning of swine

Interstitial Edema

- Hydrocephalus

PATHOGENESIS

Cerebral Edema and Brain Swelling

This disease is potentially life-threatening because of the limited ability for accommodation of increased volume within the confines of the dura and the cranium. CNS parenchyma does not possess a lymphatic system, and the interstitial space between cells, especially in the gray matter, is much narrower than in other tissues. When CNS edema develops, of necessity it largely accumulates within cells, although interstitial fluid will form if cells lyse or if the edema is severe.

Cerebral edema usually occurs to some degree in all pathologic states, whether degenerative or inflammatory or traumatic or neoplastic. Edema around chronic, focal lesions such as abscesses, parasitic cysts, and primary or metastatic tumors in white matter often produce marked swelling. Cerebral hemispheric swelling compresses the underlying brainstem, flattening the rostral colliculi and distorting the aqueduct. As the swollen brain expands and fills the confines of the calvaria, some regions are prone to herniation. If this occurs, the accompanying blood vessels are likely to become occluded, which may result in hemorrhage or infarction. Commonly with brain swelling the caudal lobe of the cerebellar vermis protrudes as a flattened lip over the medulla oblongata toward the foramen magnum.

In vasogenic edema the primary insult is to the wall of cerebral capillaries, allowing the escape of plasma fluid and proteins under the hydrostatic pressure of the circulation. The inciting vascular injury may be brain or spinal cord trauma, vasculitis, a neoplasm, or a cerebrovascular accident. Vasogenic edema affects predominantly the white matter, in which fluid accumulates within the cytoplasm of astrocytes and spreads in the interstitial spaces. Vasogenic edema moves over very long distances and from one hemisphere to the other via the corpus callosum. A chronic epidural abscess involving the frontal lobe can produce sufficient brain swelling from vasogenic edema to induce herniation of the occipital cortex beneath the tentorium cerebelli.

Cytotoxic edema results from an injury to a glial cell that disturbs osmoregulation of that cell by depletion of energy stores and failure of energy-dependent ionic pumps. This leads to cell swelling with fluid and differs from edema in other tissues in which fluid accumulation is interstitial. Cytotoxic edema reflects a specific cellular insult and may result from ischemia or hypoxia, nutritional deficiency, an intoxication, or an inherited metabolic abnormality. Brain swelling from cytotoxic edema is less dramatic than that seen in vasogenic edema. It may affect just the gray matter, just the white matter, or both.

The ECF volume in vasogenic edema is increased by the edema fluid, which is a plasma filtrate containing plasma protein. In cytotoxic edema it is the cellular elements themselves that increase in size. In hypoxia this is because of failure of the adenosine triphosphate (ATP)-dependent sodium pump within the cells. As a result sodium accumulates within the cells and water follows to maintain osmotic equilibrium. In PEM and salt poisoning, the edema of the brain is primary. In salt poisoning in pigs there is an increase in concentration of cations in brain tissue with a sudden passage of water into the brain to maintain osmotic equilibrium. The cause of the edema in PEM of ruminants, associated with a thiamine inadequacy, is unknown. When promazine is injected accidentally into the carotid artery of the horse, it produces a vasogenic edema and infarction generally, but especially in the thalamus and corpora quadrigemina on the injected side. The vasogenic edema surrounding an abscess is localized and is not evident in the white matter.

Cerebral edema and cerebellar herniation have been described in neonatal foals admitted to an intensive care unit for treatment. All foals had septicemia. It was suggested that hypoglycemia, hypoxia, or the alterations in cerebral blood flow associated with septicemia might have initiated injury to cell membranes, resulting in vascular damage and subsequent edema. It is hypothesized that cerebellar herniation occurs in neonatal foals with sepsis because of the inelastic nature of the dural folds and the anatomic rigidity of the neonatal equine skull. This is in contrast to the human infant, in whom cerebral edema occurs in bacterial meningitis but cerebral or cerebellar herniation is not normally a feature. The relatively small brain of the newborn foal is only 1% of total body mass compared with the human infant, which is 12% and in which the brain is enclosed within a large but relatively thin calvarium with sutures that, in the preterm infant at least, can be separated by excess internal pressure.

An increase in intracranial pressure occurs suddenly and, as in hydrocephalus, there is a resulting ischemic anoxia of the brain caused by compression of blood vessels and impairment of blood supply. This may not be the only factor that interferes with cerebral activity in PEM and salt poisoning. The clinical syndrome produced by the rapid rise in intracranial pressure is manifested by involuntary movements such as tremor and convulsions followed by signs of weakness. If the compression of the brain is severe enough and of sufficient duration, ischemic necrosis of the superficial layers of the cortical gray matter may occur, resulting in permanent nervous defects in those animals that recover. Opisthotonus and nystagmus are commonly observed and are probably caused by the partial herniation of the cerebellum into the foramen magnum.

CLINICAL FINDINGS

Although the rise of intracranial pressure in diffuse edema of the brain is usually more acute than in hydrocephalus, the development of clinical signs takes place over a period of 12 to 24 hours and nervous shock does not occur. There is central blindness, and periodic attacks of abnormality occur in which **opisthotonus**, **nystagmus**, **muscle tremor**, and **convulsions** are prominent.

In the intervening periods, the animal is dull, depressed, and blind, and optic disc edema may be present. The involuntary signs of tremor, convulsions, and opisthotonus are usually not extreme, but this varies with the rapidity of onset of the edema. Because of the involvement of the brainstem, in severe cases muscle weakness appears, the animal becomes ataxic, goes down and is unable to rise, and the early signs persist. Clonic convulsions occur terminally, and animals that survive may have residual defects of mentality and vision.

CLINICAL PATHOLOGY

Clinicopathologic observations will depend on the specific disease causing the edema.

NECROPSY FINDINGS

Microscopically the gyri are flattened and the cerebellum is partially herniated into the foramen magnum with consequent distortion of its caudal aspect. The brain has a soft, swollen appearance and tends to sag over the edges of the cranium when the top has been removed. Caudal portions of the occipital lobes herniate ventral to the tentorium cerebelli.

DIFFERENTIAL DIAGNOSIS

Diffuse brain edema causes a syndrome not unlike that of encephalitis, although there are fewer irritation phenomena. Differentiation from encephalomalacia and vitamin A deficiency may be difficult if the history does not give a clue to the cause of the disease. Metabolic diseases, particularly pregnancy toxemia, hypomagnesemic tetany of calves, and lactation tetany, resemble it closely, as do some cases of acute ruminal impaction. In the history of each of these diseases, there are distinguishing features that aid in making a tentative diagnosis. Some of the poisonings, particularly lead, organic mercurial and arsenicals, and enterotoxemia associated with *Clostridium perfringens* type D produce similar nervous signs, and gut edema of swine may be mistaken for diffuse cerebral edema.

TREATMENT

Decompression of the brain is desirable in acute edema. The treatment will depend in part on the cause; the edema associated with PEM will respond to early treatment with thiamine. In general terms, edema of the brain responds to parenteral treatment with hypertonic solutions (mannitol and hypertonic sodium chloride are most often used) and corticosteroids (specifically dexamethasone). Hypertonic solutions are most applicable to cytotoxic edema and corticosteroids to vasogenic edema. This is in addition to treatment for the primary cause of the disease.

Hypertonic solutions open the blood-brain barrier by shrinking endothelial cells and widening the tight junctions.[3] The magnitude of the opening is dependent on the type of hypertonic solution (mannitol and hypertonic saline are used most frequently with mannitol as the first choice treatment) and the achieved plasma concentration. The magnitude of the opening is also dependent on age, with neonates having a "leakier" blood-brain barrier than adults.[3,4] This supports clinical observations that mannitol treatment appears to be more successful in treating neonates suspected to have cerebral edema than adults. The preferred treatment is mannitol given as a 20% solution in a series of bolus intravenous infusions of 0.25 to 1 g/kg BW every 4 to 6 hours. The suggested dose rate has been derived from those recommended for humans and dogs but is very expensive. There are dangers with mannitol: it should not be repeated often, it must not be given to an animal in shock, and it should be given intravenously slowly. A recent meta-analysis suggested that hypertonic saline (1.5–23.5% NaCl at 10–30 mL/kg BW total dose) may be as effective as 20% mannitol in the treatment of cerebral edema, with 7.5% NaCl as the most commonly used osmalality.[5]

Dexamethasone administration (1 mg/kg BW intravenously every 24 hours) is no longer recommended for the treatment of cerebral edema in human infants,[6] and its efficacy in large animals with cerebral edema is uncertain. Dexamethasone is thought to decrease cerebral edema and CSF production and inhibit tumor-induced angiogenesis in patients with intracranial tumors. Hypertonic glucose given intravenously is not recommended because an initial temporary decompression is followed after a 4- to 6-hour interval by a return to pretreatment CSF pressure when the glucose is metabolized.

Diuretics usually produce tissue dehydration too slowly to be of much value in acute cases, but they may be of value as an adjunct to hypertonic solutions or in early or chronic cases. The removal of CSF from the cisterna magna in an attempt to provide relief may cause complications. In some cases the removal of 25 to 75 mL of CSF provides some temporary relief, but the condition becomes worse later because portions of the swollen brain herniate into the foramen magnum. There is no published information available on how much CSF can be safely removed; therefore recommendations cannot be made.

REFERENCES

1. Ringger NC, et al. *J Vet Intern Med*. 2011;25:132.
2. Bleul U, et al. *Theriogenology*. 2010;73:612.
3. Stonestreet BS, et al. *Am J Physiol Regul Integr Comp Physiol*. 2006;291:R1031.
4. Bengtsson J, et al. *Br J Pharmacol*. 2009;157:1085.
5. Mortazarvi MM, et al. *J Neurosurg*. 2012;116:210.
6. Anon. *Pediatr Crit Care Med*. 2012;13:S61.

HYDROCEPHALUS

Obstructive hydrocephalus may be congenital or acquired and is manifested in both cases by a syndrome referable to a general increase in intracranial pressure. Irritation signs of mania, head-pressing, muscle tremor, and convulsions occur when the onset is rapid, and signs of paralysis including dullness, blindness, and muscular weakness are present when the increased pressure develops slowly.

ETIOLOGY

Obstructive hydrocephalus may be congenital or acquired, but in both instances it is caused by defective drainage or absorption of CSF. In the congenital disease, there is an embryologic defect in the drainage canals and foramina between the individual ventricles or between the ventricles and the subarachnoid space, or in the absorptive mechanism, the arachnoid villi.

Congenital Hydrocephalus

Causes include the following:

- Alone, with lateral narrowing of the mesencephalon
- Inherited defects of Hereford, Holstein, Ayrshire, and Jersey cattle
- Inherited combined defects with chondrodysplasia, or in white Shorthorn cattle combined with hydrocephalus, microphthalmia, and retinal dysplasia
- Virus infections of the fetus suggest themselves as possible causes of embryologic defects in the drainage system, but there are no verified examples of this; the cavitation of brain tissue and subsequent accumulation of fluid, hydranencephaly, which occurs after infection with bluetongue virus in lambs, and Akabane virus in calves, is compensatory, not obstructive
- Vitamin A deficiency may contribute
- Other occurrences, sometimes at high levels of prevalence, but without known cause

Acquired Hydrocephalus

Causes include the following:

- Hypovitaminosis A in young growing calves causing impaired absorption of fluid by the arachnoid villi
- Cholesteatoma in choroid plexuses of the lateral ventricles in the horse; these may produce an acute, transient hydrocephalus on a number of occasions before the tumor reaches sufficient size to cause permanent obstruction
- Other tumor or chronic inflammatory lesion obstructing drainage from the lateral ventricles

PATHOGENESIS

Increased intracranial pressure in the fetus and before the syndesmoses of the skull have fused causes hydrocephalus with enlargement of the cranium. After fusion of the suture lines the skull acts as a rigid container, and an increase in the volume of its contents increases intracranial pressure. Although the increase in volume of the contents may be caused by the development of a local lesion such as an abscess, tumor, hematoma or cestode cyst, which interferes with drainage of the CSF, the more common lesion is a congenital defect of CSF drainage.

Clinical and pathologic hydrocephalus has been produced experimentally in animals by creating granulomatous meningitis. The clinical signs included depression, stiffness of gait, recumbency, and opisthotonus with paddling convulsions. The general effects in all cases are the same, the only difference is that local lesions may produce localizing signs as well as signs of increased intracranial pressure. These latter signs are caused by compression atrophy of nervous tissue and ischemic anoxia caused by compression of blood vessels and impairment of blood supply to the brain.

In congenital hydrocephalus the signs observed are usually those of paralysis of function, whereas acquired hydrocephalus, being more acute, is usually manifested first by irritation phenomena followed by signs of paralysis. Edema of the optic papilla is a sign of increased intracranial pressure and may be detected using an ophthalmoscope. Bradycardia occurs inconstantly and cannot be considered to be diagnostic.

CLINICAL FINDINGS

In acquired hydrocephalus there is, in most cases, a gradual onset of general paresis. Initially there is depression, disinclination to move, central blindness, an expressionless stare, and a lack of precision in acquired movements. A stage of somnolence follows and is most marked in horses. The animal stands with half-closed eyes, lowered head, and a vacant expression and often leans against or supports itself on some solid object. Chewing is slow, intermittent, and incomplete, and animals are often observed standing with food hanging from their mouths. The reaction to cutaneous stimulation is reduced, and abnormal postures are frequently adopted. Frequent stumbling, faulty placement of the feet, and incoordination are evidenced when the animal moves, and circling may occur in some cases. Bradycardia and cardiac arrhythmia have been observed.

Although the emphasis is on depression and paresis, signs of brain irritation may occur, particularly in the early stages. These signs often occur in isolated episodes during which a wild expression, charging, head-pressing, circling, tremor, and convulsions appear. These episodes may be separated by quite long intervals, sometimes of several weeks' duration. In vitamin A deficiency in calves, blindness and papilledema are the early signs and an acute convulsive stage occurs terminally.

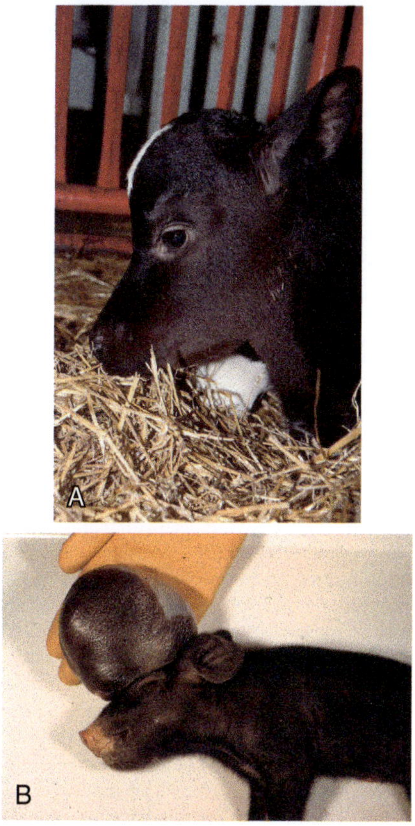

Fig. 14-2 **A,** Holstein Friesian calf with hydrocephalus caused by in utero infection with bovine viral diarrhea virus. The calf was able to suckle but appeared to have diminished responsiveness to its environment. **B,** Piglet with meningocele secondary to in utero hydrocephalus.

Congenitally affected animals are usually alive at birth but are unable to stand and most die within 48 hours. The cranium is sometimes domed, the eyes protrude, and nystagmus is often evident (Fig. 14-2). Meningocele is an infrequent accompaniment.

CLINICAL PATHOLOGY

Examination of the composition and pressure of the CSF will be of value. The fluid is usually normal biochemically and cytologically but the pressure is increased. A marked increase in serum muscle enzyme activity has been observed in calves with congenital hydrocephalus, caused probably to an accompanying muscular dystrophy. Convulsions, if they occur, may contribute to this increase.

NECROPSY FINDINGS

On necropsy the cranium may be enlarged and soft in congenital hydrocephalus. The ventricles are distended with CSF under pressure and the overlying cerebral tissue is thinned if the pressure has been present for some time.

DIFFERENTIAL DIAGNOSIS

Congenital hydrocephalus resembles vitamin A deficiency in newborn pigs, toxoplasmosis, and hydranencephaly if there is no distortion of the cranium.

Acquired hydrocephalus needs to be differentiated from other diffuse diseases of the brain, including encephalitis and encephalomalacia, and from hepatic dystrophies, which resemble it very closely. In these latter diseases, there may be other signs of diagnostic value, including fever in encephalitis and jaundice in hepatic dystrophy. In most cases it is necessary to depend largely on the history and recognition of individual disease entities.

MENINGITIS

Inflammation of the meninges occurs most commonly as a complication of a preexisting disease. Meningitis is usually associated with a bacterial infection and is manifested clinically by fever, cutaneous hyperesthesia, and rigidity of muscles. Although meningitis may affect the spinal cord or brain specifically, it commonly affects both and is dealt with here as a single entity. Meningoencephalitis is common in neonatal farm animals. Primary bacterial meningitis is extremely rare in adult farm animals, with the exception of listeriosis and *H. somni* (formerly *Haemophilus somnus*) infection, although the latter is more a vasculitis than a primary meningitis. The possibility of immunodeficiency should be considered in adult horses with bacterial meningitis. Compared with adults, bacterial meningitis is more common in neonates because their immune system is immature, the blood-brain barrier is incomplete, and umbilical infections are common, providing a nidus of infection.

ETIOLOGY

Most significant meningitides are bacterial, although most viral encephalitides have some meningitic component.

Cattle

- Viral diseases including bovine malignant catarrh, sporadic bovine encephalomyelitis
- Bacterial diseases including listeriosis, *H. somni,* chronic lesions elsewhere in the body possibly associated with meningitis in adult animals; rarely tuberculosis
- Facial paralysis syndrome of calves in the Franklin district of New Zealand[1]

Sheep

- Melioidosis, *S. aureus* (tick pyemia) in newborn lambs
- *Pasteurella multocida* in lambs
- *Mannheimia (Pasteurella) haemolytica* in lambs

Horses

- Strangles, *Pasteurella haemolytica* (also donkeys and mules), *Streptococcus suis, S. equi, Actinomyces* spp., *Klebsiella pneumonia, Staphylococcus aureus,*[2] coagulase-negative staphylococci, *Anaplasma phagocytophilum* (equine granulocytic ehrlichiosis, formerly named *Ehrlichia equi*), *Borrelia burgdorferi,*[3] *Sphingobacterium multivorum,* and *Cryptococcus neoformans.*

Pigs

- Glasser's disease, erysipelas, salmonellosis; *S. suis* type 2 in weaned and feeder pigs

Coliform and streptococcal septicemias are probably the most common causes of meningitis in neonatal farm animals. The infection may originate from omphalophlebitis, bacteremia, or bacterial translocation across the gastrointestinal tract in neonates less than 24 hours of age or with enteritis. Septicemia occurs in all species, especially calves, and may be accompanied by polysynovitis, endocarditis, and hypopyon. The causative bacteria are usually a mixed flora.

Hematogenous infection occurs from other sites also. In neonatal animals, some of the common infections include the following:

- **Calf:** *Escherichia coli*; the disease is most common in calves under several days of age and can occur in less than 24 hours after birth; failure of transfer of colostral immunoglobulins is a common contributing factor
- **Piglet:** *S. zooepidemicus, S. suis* type 1
- **Lamb:** *S. zooepidemicus*

PATHOGENESIS

Inflammation of the meninges causes local swelling and interference with blood supply to the brain and spinal cord but as a rule penetration of the inflammation along blood vessels and into nervous tissue is of minor importance and causes only superficial encephalitis. Failure to treat meningitis associated with pyogenic bacteria often permits the development of a fatal choroiditis, with exudation into CSF, and ependymitis. There is also inflammation around the nerve trunks as they pass across the subarachnoid space. The signs produced by meningitis are thus a combination of those resulting from irritation of both central and peripheral nervous systems. In spinal meningitis, there is muscular spasm with rigidity of the limbs and neck, arching of the back, and hyperesthesia with pain on light touching of the skin. When the cerebral meninges are affected, irritation signs, including muscle tremor and convulsions, are the common manifestations. Because meningitis is usually bacterial in origin, fever and toxemia can be expected if the lesion is sufficiently extensive.

Defects of drainage of CSF occur in both acute and chronic inflammation of the meninges and produce signs of increased intracranial pressure. The signs are general although the accumulation of fluid may be localized to particular sites such as the lateral ventricles.

A newly described mild nonsuppurative meningitis is associated with facial paralysis in calves in a specific geographic location in New Zealand.[1] Affected animals have a fever with unilateral or bilateral dysfunction of the facial nerve (CN VII; buccal and auriculopalpebral branches). The case–fatality rate ranges from 38% to 52%, and affected calves do not have listeriosis or *M. bovis* infection.

CLINICAL FINDINGS

Acute meningitis usually develops suddenly and is accompanied by fever and toxemia in addition to nervous signs. Vomiting is common in the early stages in pigs. There is trismus, opisthotonus, and rigidity of the neck and back. Motor irritation signs include tonic spasms of the muscles of the neck causing retraction of the head, muscle tremor, and paddling movements. Cutaneous hyperesthesia is present in varying degrees, with even light touching of the skin causing severe pain in some cases. There may be disturbance of consciousness manifested by excitement or mania in the early stages, followed by drowsiness and eventual coma.

Blindness is common in cerebral meningitis but not a constant clinical finding. In young animals, ophthalmitis with hypopyon may occur, which supports the diagnosis of meningitis. The pupillary light reflex is usually much slower than normal. Examination of the fundus of the eyes may reveal evidence of optic disc edema, congestion of the retinal vessels, and exudation.

In uncomplicated meningitis the respiration is usually slow and deep, and often phasic in the form of **Cheyne–Stokes breathing** (a breathing pattern characterized by a period of apnea followed by a gradual increase in the depth and rate of respiration) or **Biot's breathing** (an irregular breathing pattern characterized by groups of quick, shallow inspirations followed by periods of apnea). Terminally there is quadriplegia and clonic convulsions.

The major clinical finding of meningoencephalitis in calves under 2 weeks of age was depression, which progressed rapidly to stupor, but the mental state changed to hyperesthesia, opisthotonus, and seizures in unresponsive terminal cases. Meningoencephalitis should be considered in calves that have been treated for the effects of diarrhea with fluid therapy but fail to respond and remain depressed.

In a series of 32 cases of meningitis in neonatal calves, the mean age at admission was 6 days (range, 11 hours to 30 days). The major clinical findings were lethargy (32/32), recumbency (32/32), anorexia and loss of the suck reflex (26/32), and stupor and coma (21/32). The frequencies of other clinical findings were as follows: opisthotonus (9/32), convulsions (7/32), tremors (6/32), and hyperesthesia (6/32). The case–fatality rate was 100%; this case series was accumulated before the widespread availability of third-generation cephalosporins labeled for use in food animals.

Although meningitis in farm animals is usually diffuse, affecting particularly the brainstem and upper cervical cord, it may be quite localized and produce localizing signs, including involvement of the cranial or spinal nerves. Localized muscle tremor, hyperesthesia, and rigidity may result. Muscles in the affected area are firm and board-like on palpation. Anesthesia and paralysis usually develop caudal to the meningitic area. Spread of the inflammation along the cord is usual. Reference should be made to the specific diseases cited under Etiology in this section for a more complete description of their clinical manifestations.

In newborn calves, undifferentiated diarrhea, septic arthritis, omphalophlebitis, and uveitis are frequent concurrent clinical findings. Bacterial meningitis has been reproduced experimentally in calves, resulting in typical clinical signs consisting of convulsions, depression, circling and falling to one side, ataxia, propulsive walking, loss of saliva, tremors, recumbency, lethargy, and nystagmus.

CLINICAL PATHOLOGY

Cerebrospinal Fluid

CSF collected from the lumbosacral space or cisterna magna in meningitis contains elevated protein concentrations, has a high cell count, and usually contains bacteria. The collection of CSF from the lumbosacral space of calves has been described under the section Special Examination of the Nervous System. Culture and determination of antimicrobial susceptibility is strongly recommended because of the low antimicrobial concentrations achieved in the CSF. In a series of meningitis in neonatal calves, the CSF revealed marked pleocytosis (mean 4,000 leukocytes/μL; range, 130–23,270 leukocytes/μL), xanthochromia, turbidity, and a high total protein concentration.

Hematology

Hemogram usually reveals a marked leukocytosis, reflecting the severity of the systemic illness secondary to septicemia.

NECROPSY FINDINGS

Hyperemia, the presence of hemorrhages, and thickening and opacity of the meninges, especially over the base of the brain, are the usual macroscopic findings. The CSF is often turbid and may contain fibrin. A local superficial encephalitis is often present. Additional morbid changes are described under the specific diseases and are often of importance in differential diagnosis. In neonatal calves with meningitis, lesions of septicemia are commonly present at necropsy and *E. coli* is the most common isolated organism.

DIFFERENTIAL DIAGNOSIS

Hyperesthesia, severe depression, muscle rigidity, and blindness are the common clinical findings in cerebral meningitis, but it is often difficult to differentiate meningitis from encephalitis and acute cerebral edema. Examination of the CSF is the only means of confirming the diagnosis before death. Analysis of CSF is very useful in the differential diagnosis of diseases of the nervous system of ruminants. Details are presented in the section Collection and Examination of Cerebral Spinal Fluid. Subacute or chronic meningitis is difficult to recognize clinically. The clinical findings may be restricted to recumbency, apathy, anorexia, slight incoordination if forced to walk, and some impairment of the eyesight. Spinal cord compression is usually more insidious in onset and is seldom accompanied by fever; hyperesthesia is less marked or absent, and there is flaccidity rather than spasticity.

TREATMENT

Most of the viral infections of the nervous system are not susceptible to chemotherapeutics. Some of the larger organisms such as *Chlamydia* spp. are susceptible to broad-spectrum antimicrobial agents such as the tetracyclines and chloramphenicol.

Bacterial infections of the CNS are usually manifestations of a general systemic infection as either bacteremia or septicemia. Treatment of such infections is limited by the existence of the blood-brain and blood-CSF barriers, which prevent penetration of some substances into nervous tissue and into the CSF. Very little useful data exist on the penetration of parenterally administered antibiotics into the CNS of either normal farm animals or those in which there is inflammation of the nervous system.

In humans it is considered that most antimicrobials do not enter the subarachnoid space in therapeutic concentrations unless inflammation is present, and the degree of penetration varies among drugs. Chloramphenicol is an exception; levels of one-third to one-half of the plasma concentration are commonly achieved in healthy individuals; chloramphenicol administration is now much reduced in developed countries because of the idiosyncratic occurrence of aplastic anemia in humans. The relative diffusion of gram-negative antimicrobial agents from blood into CSF in humans is shown in Table 14-8.

The most promising antimicrobial agents for the treatment of bacterial meningitis in farm animals are trimethoprim-sulfonamide combinations, the third-generation cephalosporins, and fluoroquinolones. When treating bacterial meningitis, pharmacodynamic principles suggest that CSF antimicrobial concentrations should have a peak concentration that is at least five times the minimum bactericidal concentration (MBC) of the pathogen, and concentrations above the MBC are required during the entire dosing interval for optimal bactericidal activity.

Table 14-8 Relative diffusion of gram-negative antimicrobials

Excellent with or without inflammation	Good only with inflammation
Sulfonamides	Ampicillin
Third-generation	Carbenicillin
Cephalosporins	Cephalothin
Cefoperazone, cefotaxime	Cephaloridine
Minimal or not good with inflammation	**No passage with inflammation**
Tetracycline	Polymyxin B
Streptomycin	Colistin
Kanamycin	
Gentamicin	

In most instances of bacterial encephalitis or meningitis in farm animals, it is likely that the blood-brain barrier is not intact and that parenterally administered drugs will diffuse into the nervous tissue and CSF to a greater extent than in healthy animals. Certainly, the dramatic beneficial response achieved by the early parenteral treatment of *H. somni* meningoencephalitis in cattle using intravenous oxytetracycline or intramuscular penicillin suggests that the blood-brain barrier may not be a major limiting factor when inflammation is present. Another example of an antibiotic that does not normally pass the blood-brain barrier well but is able to do so when the barrier is damaged is penicillin in the treatment of listeriosis. When cases of bacterial meningoencephalitis fail to respond to antimicrobial agents to which in vitro testing indicates that the organisms are susceptible, other reasons should also be considered. Often the lesion is irreversibly advanced or there is a chronic suppurative process that is unlikely to respond.

Intrathecal injections of antimicrobial agents have been suggested as viable alternatives when parenteral therapy appears to be unsuccessful. However, there is no evidence that such treatment is superior to appropriate parenteral therapy. In addition, intrathecal injections can cause rapid death and therefore are not recommended.

Glucocorticoids may be administered in an attempt to decrease nerve damage resulting from inflammation. Appropriate randomized clinical trials have not been performed in large animals, but steroid administration in adult humans with meningitis was associated with decreased mortality.[4]

FURTHER READING

Fecteau G, George LW. Bacterial meningitis and encephalitis in ruminants. *Vet Clin North Am Food Anim Pract*. 2004;20:363-378.

Johnson AL. Update on infectious diseases affecting the equine nervous system. *Vet Clin North Am Equine Pract*. 2011;27:573-587.

Kessell AE, Finnie JW, Windsor PA. Neurological diseases of ruminant livestock in Australia. III: bacterial and protozoal infections. *Aust Vet J*. 2011;89:289-296.

Scott PR. Diagnostic techniques and clinicopathologic findings in ruminant neurologic disease. *Vet Clin North Am Food Anim Pract*. 2004;20:215-230.

Whitehead CE, Bedenice D. Neurologic diseases in llamas and alpacas. *Vet Clin North Am Food Anim Pract*. 2009;25:385-405.

REFERENCES

1. McFadden AMJ, et al. *New Zeal Vet J*. 2009;57:63.
2. Mitchell E, et al. *Equine Vet Educ*. 2006;18:249.
3. Imai DM, et al. *Vet Pathol*. 2011;48:1151.
4. van de Beek D, et al. *Lancet Infect Dis*. 2004;4:139.

ENCEPHALITIS

Encephalitis is, by definition, inflammation of the brain, but in general usage it includes those diseases in which inflammatory lesions occur in the brain, whether there is inflammation of the nervous tissue or primarily of the vessel walls. Clinically, encephalitis is characterized initially by signs of involuntary movements, followed by signs caused by loss of nervous function. The meninges and spinal cord may be involved in an encephalitis, causing varying degrees of meningoencephalomyelitis.

ETIOLOGY

Many encephalitides of large animals are associated with viruses but other infectious agents are also common. Some causes are as follows.

All Species

- Viral infections including rabies, pseudorabies, Japanese B encephalitis, West Nile virus encephalomyelitis
- Bacterial infections of neonatal farm animals
- Toxoplasmosis, which is not a common cause in any species
- Sarcocystosis
- Verminous encephalomyelitis, which is migration of larvae of parasitic species that normally have a somatic migration route, e.g., *Halicephalobus gingivalis* (previously *H. deletrix* or *Micronema deletrix*) and *Setaria* spp.

Cattle

- BSE
- Viral infections including malignant catarrhal fever, BVD virus, sporadic bovine encephalomyelitis, Akabane virus, and bovine herpesvirus-5 (BHV-5), rarely louping-ill virus,[1] and astrovirus (BoAstV-NeuroS1)[2]
- Bacterial infections including *Listeria monocytogenes, H. somni* (formerly *Haemophilus somnus*), heartwater, and clostridial infections following dehorning of calves
- Migration of *Hypoderma bovis* occasionally to brain and spinal cord
- Newborn calves with in utero protozoal infection of *Neospora caninum*[3]

Sheep

- Scrapie
- Viral infections including louping-ill, visna (associated with maedi-visna virus [MVV]), BVD virus (border disease), and Akabane virus
- Thrombotic meningoencephalitis associated with *H. somni* (formerly *H. ovis*) in lambs
- Bacterial meningoencephalitis in lambs 2 to 4 weeks of age
- Migration of *Oestrus ovis*

Goats

- Scrapie
- Caprine arthritis encephalitis (CAE) virus, Akabane virus

New World Camelids

- Viral infection caused by Eastern equine encephalitis virus[4]
- Bacterial infection caused by *L. monocytogenes*
- Verminous encephalomyelitis caused by *Parelaphostrongylus tenuis* ("meningeal worm" of white-tailed deer)

Horses

- Viral infections including infectious equine encephalomyelitis; Borna disease; equine herpesvirus-1 (EHV-1) myeloencephalopathy; equine infectious anemia; eastern, western, Venezuelan, and West Nile equine encephalomyelitis; Murray Valley encephalitis virus[5,6]; Shuni virus[7]; and rarely louping-ill virus
- Bacterial meningoencephalitis caused by *Anaplasma phagocytophilum* (equine granulocytic ehrlichiosis) and *Borrelia burgdorferi*[8]
- Protozoal myeloencephalitis caused by *Sarcocystis neurona* infection
- Verminous encephalomyelitis caused by *Strongylus vulgaris, P. tenuis* (meningeal worm of white-tailed deer), and *Draschia megastoma*; *Angiostrongylus cantonensis,* which normally migrates through the CNS of the rat, has been found as a cause of verminous encephalomyelitis in foals

Pigs

- Bacterial infections as part of the systemic infections with *Salmonella* and *Erysipelas* spp., rarely *L. monocytogenes*
- Viral infections including hog cholera, African swine fever, encephalomyocarditis, swine vesicular disease, hemagglutinating encephalomyelitis virus, and porcine encephalomyelitis virus

PATHOGENESIS

Compared with other extraneural tissues, the inflammatory response mounted by the nervous system is unique. The CNS is in a sequestered and immunologically dormant state within the body. The capillary endothelial blood-brain barrier restricts free access by blood constituents. The CNS lacks specialized dendritic antigen-presenting cells, and the intrinsic expression by CNS cells of major histocompatibility complex molecules, especially class II, is low. There is no lymphatic system within nervous tissue, but cells and antigens within the CNS drain into the circulation and into the cervical lymph nodes.

The CNS has unique populations of cells consisting of parenchymal cells, which are **neurons** and **neuroglia**. The neuroglia are supporting cells and are subdivided into macroglia and microglia. The macroglia are **astrocytes** and **oligodendrocytes**; the third glial cell type is a **microglial cell**. The brain and spinal cord are enclosed by meninges (**dura**, **arachnoid,** and **pia**), which provide protection, a compartment for CSF circulation (the subarachnoid space), support for blood vessels, and a sheath for the cranial and spinal nerves. Within the brain and spinal cord are the ventricular system and central canal, which are lined by **ependymal cells,** and the **choroid plexuses**, which produce the CSF. Circulation of the CSF moves from the lateral, third, and fourth ventricles into the central canal or through lateral apertures at the cerebellomedullary angle into the subarachnoid space of the brain. CSF in the subarachnoid space drains via specialized **arachnoid granulations** into intracranial venous sinuses, with some draining into venous plexuses associated with cranial and spinal nerves. CSF may also cross the ventricular surface into the adjacent parenchyma.

The histologic characteristics of CNS inflammation include the following:

- Perivascular cuffing
- Gliosis
- Neuronal satellitosis and neuronophagia

A perivascular compartment, actual or potential, exists around all CNS arteries, arterioles, venules, and veins. A characteristic feature of CNS inflammation is perivascular cuffing, which is the accumulation of leukocytes of one or multiple types in the perivascular space. All perivascular cuffing results in vasculitis of some degree. In bacterial diseases, polymorphonuclear cells predominate with a minor component of mononuclear cells. In general, viral diseases are characterized by lymphocyte-rich cells with some plasma cells and monocytes; some arbovirus infections cause a polymorphonuclear cell response. In immune-mediated diseases, there are mixtures of polymorphonuclear and mononuclear cells. In thrombogenic diseases, such as thrombotic meningoencephalitis, vascular occlusion precludes the development of cuffing around injured vessels.

Gliosis is the increased prominence of glial cells, resulting from cytoplasmic swelling and the acquisition of more cell processes, from cell proliferation, or both. Either of the macroglia (oligodendrocytes or astrocytes) or microglia may participate in gliosis.

Neuronal satellitosis occurs when oligodendrocytes react and proliferate in response to degenerating neurons, which may be infected by a virus.

Neuronophagia is the progressive degeneration of the neuron characterized by its piecemeal division and phagocytosis, eventually leaving a dense nodule of glial cells and fragments of the former neuron. Details of the form, functions, and roles of astrocytes in neurologic disease have been reviewed.

Primary demyelination is characteristic of only a small number of inflammatory neurologic diseases and is associated with only a few viruses. The inflammatory neuraxial diseases of large animals include visna in sheep and caprine arthritis encephalitis. The demyelinating process may be initiated directly by the infectious agent alone or by an immunologic response initiated by the agent.

With the exception of the viruses of bovine malignant catarrh and EHV-1, which exert their effects principally on the vasculature, those viruses that cause encephalitis do so by invasion of cellular elements, usually the neurons, and cause initial stimulation and then death of the cells. Those bacteria that cause diffuse encephalitis also exert their effects primarily on vascular endothelium. *L. monocytogenes* does so by the formation of microabscesses. In some diseases, such as meningoencephalitis in cattle associated with *H. somni,* the lesions may be present in the brain and throughout the spinal cord.

Entrance of the viruses into the nervous tissue occurs in several ways. Normally the blood-brain barrier is an effective filtering agent, but when there is damage to the endothelium infection readily occurs. The synergistic relationship between the rickettsias of tick-borne fever and the virus of louping-ill probably has this basis. Entry may also occur by progression of the agent up a peripheral nerve trunk, as occurs with the viruses of rabies and pseudorabies and with *L. monocytogenes.* Entry via the olfactory nerves is also possible.

The clinical signs of encephalitis are usually referable to a general stimulatory or lethal effect on neurons in the brain. This may be in part due to the general effect of inflammatory edema and in part to the direct effects of the agent on nerve cells. In any particular case, one or the other of these factors may predominate, but the tissue damage and therefore the signs are generalized. Clinical signs are often diverse and can be acute or chronic, localized or diffuse, and progressive or reversible. Because of diffuse inflammation in encephalitis, the clinical signs are commonly multifocal and asymmetric. This is not the case in listeriosis, in which damage is usually localized in the pons-medulla. Localizing signs may appear in the early stages of generalized encephalitis and remain as residual defects during the stage of convalescence. In calves with thromboembolic meningoencephalitis caused by *H. somni,* prolonged recumbency may be associated with widespread lesions of the spinal cord. Visna is a demyelinating encephalitis, and caprine leukoencephalomyelitis is both demyelinating and inflammatory and also invades other tissues including joints and lung.

In verminous encephalomyelitis, destruction of nervous tissue may occur in many parts of the brain and in general the severity of the signs depends on the size and mobility of the parasites and the route of entry. One exception to this generalization is the experimental "visceral larva migrans" produced by *Toxocara canis* in pigs when the nervous signs occur at a time when lesions in most other organs are healing. The signs are apparently provoked by a reaction of the host to static larvae rather than trauma caused by migration. Nematodes not resident in nervous tissues may cause nervous signs caused possibly by allergy or by the formation of toxins.

CLINICAL FINDINGS

Because the encephalitides are associated with infectious agents, they are often accompanied by fever, anorexia, depression, and increased heart rate. This is not the case in the very chronic diseases such as scrapie and BSE. In those diseases associated with agents that are not truly neurotropic, there are characteristic signs, which are not described here.

The clinical findings that can occur in encephalitis are combinations of the following:

- **Subtle to marked changes in behavior**
- **Depression**
- **Seizures**
- **Blindness**
- **Compulsive walking**
- **Leaning on walls or fences**
- **Circling**
- **Ataxia**

Bacterial meningoencephalitis in lambs 2 to 4 weeks of age is characterized by lack of suck reflex, weakness, altered gait, and depression extending to stupor, but hyperesthesia to auditory and tactile stimuli. Opisthotonus is common during the terminal stages.

There may be an initial period of **excitement or mania.** The animal is easily startled and responds excessively to normal stimuli. It may exhibit viciousness and uncontrolled activity including blind charging, bellowing, kicking, and pawing. Self-mutilation may occur in diseases such as pseudorabies. Mental depression, including head-pressing, may occur between episodes.

Involuntary movements are variable in their occurrence or may not appear at all. When they do occur, they include convulsions, usually clonic, and may be accompanied by nystagmus, champing of the jaws, excessive frothy salivation, and muscle tremor, especially of the face and limbs. In cattle with malignant catarrhal fever, there is severe depression for a few days followed by the onset of tremors associated with the terminal encephalitis. Unusual irritation phenomena are the paresthesia and hyperesthesia of pseudorabies and scrapie.

Signs caused by loss of nervous function follow and may be the only signs in some instances. Excessive drooling and pharyngeal paralysis are common in rabies. In horses with equine encephalomyelitis, feed may be left hanging from the mouth, although swallowing may not be impaired. The loss of function varies in degree from paresis with knuckling at the lower limb joints, to spasticity of the limbs with resultant ataxia, to weakness and recumbency. Recumbency and inability to rise may be the first clinical finding encountered as in many cases of meningoencephalitis associated with *H. somni.* Hypermetria, a staggering gait and apprehensiveness progressing to belligerency, may occur in a disease such as BSE.

Clinical signs referable to certain anatomic sites and pathways of the brain and spinal cord are manifested by deviation of the head, walking in circles, abnormalities of posture, ataxia, and incoordination but these are more often residual signs after recovery from the acute stages. Progressive ascending spinal cord paralysis, in which the loss of sensation and weakness occur initially in the hindlimbs followed by weakness in the forelimbs, is common in rabies. Residual lesions affecting the CNs do not commonly occur in the encephalitides, except in listeriosis and protozoal encephalitis of horses, both infections predominating in the caudal brainstem.

In the horse with cerebral nematodiasis caused by *S. vulgaris,* the clinical signs are referable to migration of the parasite in the thalamus, brainstem, and cerebellum. There is incoordination, leaning and head-pressing, dysmetria, intermittent clonic convulsions, unilateral or bilateral blindness, and paralysis of some CNs. The onset may be gradual or sudden. The clinical diagnosis is extremely difficult because examination of CSF and hematology are of limited value. A pathologic diagnosis is necessary. In foals with neural angiostrongylosis, tetraparesis was the result of progressive and multifocal neurologic disease.

CLINICAL PATHOLOGY

Clinical pathology may be of considerable assistance in the diagnosis of encephalitis, but the techniques used are for the most part specific to the individual diseases.

Hemogram

In the horse, complete and differential blood counts and serum chemistry profiles are recommended for most neurologic cases.

Serology

Acute and convalescent sera can be submitted when a specific infectious disease is suspected for which a serologic diagnosis is possible.

Cerebrospinal Fluid

Laboratory examination of CSF for cellular content and pathogens may also be indicated. In bacterial meningoencephalitis, analysis of CSF obtained from the lumbosacral space reveals a highly significant increase in protein concentration with marked neutrophilic pleocytosis.

NECROPSY FINDINGS

In some of the common encephalitides there are no gross lesions of the brain apart from those that occur in other body systems and that are typical of the specific disease. In other cases, on transverse section of the brain, extensive areas of hemorrhagic necrosis may be visible, as in meningoencephalitis in cattle caused by *H. somni.* Histologic lesions vary with the type and mode of action of the causative agent. Material for laboratory diagnosis should include the fixed brain and portions of fresh brain material for culture and for transmission experiments.

DIFFERENTIAL DIAGNOSIS

The diagnosis of encephalitis cannot depend entirely on the recognition of the typical syndrome because similar syndromes may be caused by many other brain diseases. Acute cerebral edema and focal space-occupying lesions of the cranial cavity, and a number of poisonings, including salt, lead, arsenic, mercury, rotenone, and chlorinated hydrocarbons, all cause similar syndromes, as do hypovitaminosis A, hypoglycemia, encephalomalacia, and meningitis.

Fever is common in encephalitis but is not usually present in rabies, scrapie, or bovine spongiform encephalopathy; but it may occur in the noninflammatory diseases if convulsions are severe.

In general, the clinical diagnosis rests on the recognition of the specific encephalitides and the elimination of the other possible causes on the basis of the history and clinical pathology, especially in poisonings, and on clinical findings characteristic of the particular disease. In many cases a definite diagnosis can only be made on necropsy. For differentiation of the specific encephalitides, reference should be made to the diseases listed under the previous section Etiology.

Infestation with nematode larvae causes a great variety of signs depending on the number of invading larvae and the amount and location of the damage.

TREATMENT

Specific treatments are dealt with under each disease. Antimicrobials are indicated for bacterial meningoencephalomyelitis. In general, the aim should be to provide supportive treatment by intravenous fluid and electrolyte therapy or stomach tube feeding during the acute phase. Sedation during the excitement stage may prevent the animal from injuring itself, and nervous system stimulants during the period of depression may maintain life through the critical phase. Although there is an increase in intracranial pressure, the removal of CSF is contraindicated because of the deleterious effects of the procedure on other parts of the brain.

FURTHER READING

Johnson AL. Update on infectious diseases affecting the equine nervous system. *Vet Clin North Am Equine Pract.* 2011;27:573-587.

Kessell AE, Finnie JW, Windsor PA. Neurological diseases of ruminant livestock in Australia. III. Bacterial and protozoal infections. *Aust Vet J.* 2011;89:289-296.

Kessell AE, Finnie JW, Windsor PA. Neurological diseases of ruminant livestock in Australia. IV. Viral infections. *Aust Vet J.* 2011;89:331-337.

Whitehead CE, Bedenice D. Neurologic diseases in llamas and alpacas. *Vet Clin North Am Food Anim Pract.* 2009;25:385-405.

REFERENCES

1. Benavides J, et al. *Vet Pathol.* 2011;48:E1.
2. Li L, et al. *Emerg Infect Dis.* 2013;19:1385.
3. Malaguti JMA, et al. *Rev Bras Parasitol Vet Jaboticabal.* 2012;2:48.
4. Nolen-Watson R, et al. *J Vet Intern Med.* 2007;21:846.
5. Gordon AN, et al. *J Vet Diagn Invest.* 2012;24:431.
6. Holmes JM, et al. *Aust Vet J.* 2012;90:252.
7. van Eeden C, et al. *Emerg Infect Dis.* 2012;18:318.
8. Imai DM, et al. *Vet Pathol.* 2011;48:1151.

EPILEPSY

Seizures occur most frequently in conjunction with other signs of brain disease. The syndrome of inherited, recurrent seizures, which continues through life with no underlying morphologic disease process, is true epilepsy, which is extremely rare in farm animals. Familial epilepsy has been recorded in Brown Swiss cattle and Arabian foals.[1]

Residual lesions after encephalitis may cause symptomatic epileptiform seizures, but there are usually other localizing signs. A generalized seizure is manifested by an initial period of alertness, the counterpart of the aura in human seizures, followed by falling in a state of tetany, which gives way after a few seconds to a clonic convulsion with paddling, opisthotonus, and champing of the jaws. The clonic convulsions may last for some minutes and are followed by a period of relaxation. The animal is unconscious throughout the seizure, but appears normal shortly afterward.

Some seizures may be preceded by a local motor phenomenon such as tetany or tremor of one limb or of the face. The convulsion may spread from this initial area to the rest of the body. This form is referred to as jacksonian epilepsy and the local signs may indicate the whereabouts of the local lesion or point of excitation. Such signs are recorded very rarely in dogs and not at all in farm animals. The seizures are recurrent, and the animal is normal in the intervening periods.

EEG has been performed but there are significant challenges in obtaining and interpreting the EEG from a conscious foal. It is not clear whether the EEG recording changed the initial treatment protocol for affected foals, and it should be noted that a diagnosis of epilepsy in humans is made primarily on clinical grounds.[1]

TREATMENT

Treatment is empirical. Seizures in foals can be initially controlled with intravenous diazepam (0.1–0.4 mg/kg; the large dose range suggests that some seizures are of short duration). Long-term seizure control emphasizes oral phenobarbital because of its cost and proven efficacy in humans and dogs. A loading intravenous phenobarbital dose that has been used in foals is 12 to 20 mg/kg diluted in 1 L of 0.9% NaCl and administered over 30 minutes, followed by oral phenobarbital at 6 to 12 mg/kg every 12 hours. The oral dose is adjusted based on clinical response and measured peak and trough serum phenobarbital concentrations. Therapeutic phenobarbital concentrations for horses are unknown, but the therapeutic range in humans is 15 to 40 μg/mL. Once seizure control is established with oral phenobarbital and the foal is seizure free for 6 months, the phenobarbital dose can be decreased by 20% every 2 weeks and the horse closely monitored. If phenobarbital does not provide adequate seizure control, potassium bromide can be tried at a tentative initial oral dose of 25 mg/kg every 24 hours. Clients should wear gloves during administration of potassium bromide.

FURTHER READING

McBride S, Hemmings A. A neurologic perspective of equine stereotypy. *J Equine Vet Sci.* 2009;29:10-16.

REFERENCE

1. Aleman M, et al. *J Vet Intern Med.* 2006;20:1443.

MYELITIS

Inflammation of the spinal cord (myelitis) is usually associated with viral encephalitis. Clinical signs of myelitis are referable to the loss of function, although there may be signs of irritation. For example, hyperesthesia or paresthesia may result if the dorsal root ganglia are involved. This is particularly noticeable in pseudorabies and to a lesser extent in rabies. However, paresis or paralysis is the more usual result of myelitis. There are no specific myelitides in farm animals, with most viral infections producing an encephalomyelitis with variations on the predominance of clinical signs being intracranial or extracranial. Viral myelitis associated with EHV-1 (the equine rhinopneumonitis virus) is now commonplace, and equine infectious anemia and dourine include incoordination and paresis in their syndromes. In goats, CAE is principally a myelitis, involving mostly the white matter.

Equine protozoal myeloencephalitis (EPM) causes multifocal lesions of the CNS mostly on the spinal cord. The most accurate diagnosis is based on histologic findings:

- Necrosis and mild to severe, nonsuppurative myeloencephalitis
- Infiltration of neural tissue by mononuclear cells
- Sometimes giant cells, neutrophils, and eosinophils
- Infiltration of perivascular tissue by mononuclear cells including lymphocytes and plasma cells.

EPM is caused primarily by *S. neurona,* which has the opossum (*Didelphis virginiana*) as the definitive host, raccoons as the most likely intermediate host, and the horse acting as a dead end host. Occasional cases of protozoal myeloencephalitis in horses are associated with *Neospora hughesi.*

Myelitis associated with *N. caninum* infection in newborn calves has been described. Affected calves were recumbent and unable to rise but were bright and alert. Histologically, there was evidence of protozoal myelitis.

ENCEPHALOMALACIA

The degenerative diseases of the brain are grouped together under the name encephalomalacia. By definition encephalomalacia means softening of the brain. It is used here to include all degenerative changes. **Leukoencephalomalacia** and **PEM** refer to softening of the white and gray matter, respectively. **Abiotrophy** is the premature degeneration of neurons caused by an inborn metabolic error of development and excludes exogenous insults of neurons. The underlying cellular defect in most abiotrophies is inherited. The syndrome produced in most degenerative diseases of the nervous system is essentially one of loss of function.

ETIOLOGY

Some indication of the diversity of causes of encephalomalacia and degenerative diseases of the nervous system can be appreciated from the examples that follow, but many sporadic cases occur in which the cause cannot be defined.

All Species

- Hepatic encephalopathy is thought to be caused by high blood levels of ammonia associated with advanced liver disease. This is recorded in experimental pyrrolizidine alkaloid poisoning in sheep, in hepatic arteriovenous anomaly, and thrombosis of the portal vein in the horse. Congenital portacaval shunts are also a cause of hepatic encephalopathy.
- Abiotrophy involves multisystem degenerations in the nervous system as focal or diffuse lesions involving the axons and myelin of neuronal processes. These include a multifocal encephalopathy in the Simmental breed of cattle in New Zealand and Australia and progressive myeloencephalopathy in Brown Swiss cattle, known as "weavers" because of their ataxic gait.
- Poisoning by organic mercurials and, in some instances, lead; possibly also selenium poisoning; a bilateral multifocal cerebrospinal poliomalacia of sheep in Ghana.
- Cerebrovascular disorders corresponding to the main categories in humans are observed in animals, but their occurrence is chiefly in pigs, and their clinical importance is minor.
- Congenital hypomyelinogenesis and dysmyelinogenesis are recorded in lambs (hairy shakers), piglets (myoclonia congenita), and calves (hypomyelinogenesis congenita). All are associated with viral infections in utero. EHV-1 infections in horses cause ischemic infarcts.
- Cerebellar cortical abiotrophy occurs in calves and lambs.

Ruminants

- BSE
- Plant poisons, e.g., *Astragalus* spp., *Oxytropis* spp., *Swainsona* spp., *Vicia* spp., *Kochia scoparia*
- Focal symmetric encephalomalacia of sheep, thought to be a residual lesion after intoxication with *C. perfringens* type D toxin
- PEM caused by thiamine inadequacy in cattle and sheep and sulfur toxicosis in cattle; poliomalacia of sheep caused possibly by an antimetabolite of nicotinic acid
- Progressive spinal myelopathy of Murray Grey cattle in Australia
- Spongiform encephalopathy in newborn polled Hereford calves similar to maple syrup urine disease
- Neuronal dystrophy in Suffolk sheep
- Shakers in horned Hereford calves associated with neuronal cell body chromatolysis
- The abiotrophic lysosomal storage diseases including progressive ataxia of Charolais cattle, mannosidosis, gangliosidosis, and globoid cell leukodystrophy of sheep
- The inherited defect of Brown Swiss cattle known as weavers, and presented elsewhere, is a degenerative myeloencephalopathy
- Swayback and enzootic ataxia caused by nutritional deficiency of copper in lambs
- Prolonged parturition of calves causing cerebral hypoxia and the weak calf syndrome
- Idiopathic brainstem neuronal chromatolysis in cattle
- Bovine bonkers caused by the consumption of ammoniated forages
- Inherited neuronal degeneration in Angora goats

Horses

- Leukoencephalomalacia caused by feeding moldy corn infested with *Fusarium moniliforme,* which produces primarily fumonisin B_1 and, to a lesser extent, fumonisin B_2[1,2]
- Nigropallidal encephalomalacia caused by feeding on yellow star thistle (*Centaurea solstitialis*)[3]
- Poisoning by bracken and horsetail causing a conditioned deficiency of thiamine
- Ischemic encephalopathy of neonatal maladjustment syndrome of foals
- EDM,[4,5] which is associated with vitamin E deficiency

Ruminants and Horses

Neurotoxic Mycotoxins

Swainsonine and slaframine produced by *Rhizoctonia leguminicola* cause mannose accumulation and parasympathomimetic effects. Lolitrems from *A. lolii* and paspalitrems from *C. paspali* are tremorgens found in grasses.

Pigs

- Leukoencephalomalacia in mulberry heart disease
- Subclinical attacks of enterotoxemia similar to edema disease
- Poisoning by organic arsenicals, and salt.

PATHOGENESIS

The pathogenesis of the degenerative diseases can be subdivided into the following:

- **Metabolic and circulatory disorders**
- **Intoxications and toxic-infectious diseases**
- **Nutritional diseases**
- **Hereditary, familial, and idiopathic degenerative diseases**

Metabolic and Circulatory

Hepatic encephalopathy is associated with acquired liver disease, and the resultant hyperammonemia and other toxic factors are considered to be neurotoxic. Disorders of intermediary metabolism result in the accumulation of neurotoxic substances such as in maple syrup urine disease of calves. Lysosomal storage diseases are caused by a lack of lysosomal enzymes, which results in an accumulation of cellular substrates and affecting cell function.

CNS hypoxia and ischemia impair the most sensitive elements in brain tissue, especially neurons. Severe ischemia results in necrosis of neurons and glial elements and areas of infarcts. Gas anesthesia–related neurologic disease occurs in animals that have been deprived of oxygen for more than 5 minutes. The hypoxia is lethal to neurons, and on recovery from anesthesia affected animals are blind and seizures may occur. The typical lesion consists of widespread neuronal damage. Postanesthetic hemorrhagic myelopathy and postanesthetic cerebral necrosis in horses are typical examples.

Hypoglycemia occurs in neonates deprived of milk and in acetonemia and pregnancy toxemia and clinical signs of lethargy, dullness progressing to weakness, seizures, and coma have been attributed to hypoglycemia. However, there are no studies of the CNS in farm animals with hypoglycemia and the effects, if any, on the nervous tissue are unknown.

Intoxications and Toxic-Infectious Diseases

A large number of poisonous substances including poisonous plants, heavy metals (lead, arsenic, and mercury), salt poisoning, farm chemicals, antifreeze, herbicides, and insecticides can directly affect the nervous system when ingested by animals. They result in varying degrees of edema of the brain, degeneration of white and gray matter, and hemorrhage of both the central and peripheral nervous system. Toxic-infectious diseases such as edema disease of swine and focal symmetric encephalomalacia of sheep are examples of endotoxins and exotoxins produced by bacterial infections, which have a direct effect on the nervous system resulting in encephalomalacia.

Nutritional Diseases

Several nutritional deficiencies of farm animals can result in neurologic disease:

- **Vitamin A deficiency** affects bone growth, particularly remodeling of the optic nerve tracts, and CSF absorption. The elevated CSF pressure and constriction of the optic nerve tracts results in edema of the optic disc and wallerian-type degeneration of the optic nerve resulting in blindness.
- **Copper deficiency** in pregnant ewes can result in swayback and enzootic ataxia of the lambs. Copper is an integral element in several enzyme systems such as ceruloplasmin and lysyl oxidase, and copper deficiency affects several organ systems. The principal defect in swayback appears to be one of defective myelination probably caused by interference with phospholipid formation. However, some lesions in the newborn are more extensive and show cavitation with loss of axons and neurons rather than simply demyelination. In the brain, there is a progressive gelatinous transformation of the white matter, ending in cavitation that resembles porencephaly or hydranencephaly. In the spinal cord the lesions are bilateral, and it is suggested that the copper deficiency has a primary axonopathic effect
- **Thiamine deficiency** in ruminants can result in **PEM** or **cerebrocortical necrosis**. Thiamine, mainly as thiamine diphosphate ([TDP]; pyrophosphate), has an important role as a coenzyme in carbohydrate metabolism, especially the pentose pathway. Diffuse encephalopathy may occur characterized by brain edema and swelling, resulting in flattening of the gyri, tentorial herniation, and coning of the cerebellar vermis. Bilateral areas of cerebral cortical laminar necrosis are widespread.

Hereditary, Familial, and Idiopathic Degenerative Diseases

A large number of neurologic diseases of farm animals are characterized by abnormalities of central myelinogenesis. In most instances, the underlying abnormality directly or indirectly affects the oligodendrocyte and is reflected in the production of CNS myelin of diminished quantity or quality or both. Many of these are inherited and manifest from or shortly after birth. They include leukodystrophies, hypomyelinogenesis, spongy degeneration, and related disorders. Neuronal abiotrophy, motor neuron diseases, neuronal dystrophy, and degenerative encephalomyelopathy of horses and cattle are included in this group.

Polioencephalomalacia and Leukoencephalomalacia

PEM appears to be, in some cases at least, a consequence of acute edematous swelling of the brain and cortical ischemia. The pathogenesis of leukoencephalomalacia appears to be related to vasogenic edema as a result of cardiovascular dysfunction and an inability to regulate cerebral blood flow. Whether the lesion is in the gray matter (PEM) or in the white matter (leukoencephalomalacia) the syndrome is largely one of loss of function, although as might be expected irritation signs are more likely to occur when the gray matter is damaged.

CLINICAL FINDINGS

Weakness of all four limbs is accompanied by the following:

- **Dullness or somnolence**
- **Blindness**
- **Ataxia**
- **Head-pressing**
- **Circling**
- **Terminal coma**

In the early stages, particularly in ruminant **PEM**, there are involuntary signs including muscle tremor, opisthotonus, nystagmus, and convulsions.

In equine leukoencephalomalacia, which may occur in outbreaks, initial signs include anorexia and depression. In the neurotoxic form, which is the most common, the anorexia and depression progresses to ataxia, circling, apparent blindness, head-pressing, hyperesthesia, agitation, delirium, recumbency, seizures, and death. An early and consistent sign in affected horses is reduced proprioception of the tongue, which manifests as delayed retraction of the tongue to the buccal cavity after the tongue has been extended. In the hepatotoxicosis form, clinical findings include icterus, swelling of the lips and nose, petechiation, abdominal breathing, and cyanosis. Horses with either syndrome may be found dead without any premonitory signs.

In many of the leukoencephalomalacias, the course may be one of gradual progression of signs, or more commonly a level of abnormality is reached and maintained for a long period, often necessitating euthanasia of the animal. For example, EDM is a diffuse degenerative disease of the equine spinal cords and caudal portion of the brainstem and primarily affects young horses. There is an insidious onset of symmetric spasticity, ataxia, and paresis. Clinical signs may progress slowly to stabilize for long periods. All four limbs are affected, but the pelvic limbs are usually more severely affected than the thoracic limbs. There is no treatment for the disease, no spontaneous recovery and, once affected, horses remain atactic and useless for any athletic function.

CLINICAL PATHOLOGY

There are no clinicopathologic tests specific for encephalomalacia, but various tests may aid in the diagnosis of some of the specific diseases mentioned in this section under Etiology.

NECROPSY FINDINGS

Gross lesions including areas of softening, cavitation, and laminar necrosis of the cortex may be visible. The important lesions are described under each of the specific diseases.

TREATMENT

The prognosis depends on the nature of the lesion. Early cases of thiamine deficiency–induced PEM can recover completely if treated with adequate levels of thiamine. Encephalomalacia caused by sulfur-induced PEM and lead poisoning is more difficult to treat. Young calves with acquired in utero hypomyelinogenesis and horses with myelitis associated with EHV-1 infection can make complete recoveries.

> **DIFFERENTIAL DIAGNOSIS**
>
> The syndromes produced by encephalomalacia resemble very closely those caused by most lesions that elevate intracranial pressure. The onset is quite sudden, and there is depression of consciousness and loss of motor function. One major difference is that the lesions tend to be nonprogressive, and affected animals may continue to survive in an impaired state for long periods.

FURTHER READING

Cebra CK, Cebra ML. Altered mentation caused by polioencephalomalacia, hypernatremia, and lead poisoning. *Vet Clin North Am Food Anim Pract.* 2004;20:287-302.

De Lahunta A. Abiotrophy in domestic animals: a review. *Can J Vet Res.* 1990;54:65-76.

REFERENCES

1. Smith GW, et al. *Am J Vet Res.* 2002;63:538.
2. Foreman JH, et al. *J Vet Intern Med.* 2004;18:223.
3. Chang HT, et al. *Vet Pathol.* 2012;49:398.
4. Finno CJ, et al. *J Vet Intern Med.* 2011;25:1439.
5. Wong DM, et al. *Vet Pathol.* 2012;49:1049.

MYELOMALACIA

Degeneration of the spinal cord (myelomalacia) occurs rarely as an entity separate from encephalomalacia. One recorded occurrence is focal spinal poliomalacia of sheep, and in enzootic ataxia the lesions of degeneration are often restricted to the spinal cord. In both instances there is a gradual development of paralysis without signs of irritation and with no indication of brain involvement. Progressive paresis in young goats may be associated with the virus of CAE and other unidentified, possibly inherited causes of myelomalacia.

Degeneration of spinal cord tracts has also been recorded in **poisoning** by *Phalaris aquatica* in cattle and sheep, by *Tribulus terrestris* in sheep,[1] by sorghum in horses, by 3-nitro-4-hydroxyphenylarsonic acid in pigs, and by selenium in ruminants; the lesion is a symmetric spinal poliomalacia. Poisoning of cattle by plants of *Zamia* spp. produces a syndrome suggestive of injury to the spinal cord but no lesions have been reported. Pantothenic acid (PA) or pyridoxine deficiencies also cause degeneration of the spinal cord tract in swine.

A spinal myelinopathy, possibly of genetic origin, is recorded in Murray Grey calves. Affected animals develop ataxia of the hindlegs, swaying of the hindquarters, and collapse of one hindleg with falling to one side. Clinical signs become worse over an extended period.

Sporadic cases of degeneration of spinal tracts have been observed in pigs. One outbreak is recorded in the litters of sows on lush clover pasture. The piglets were unable to stand, struggled violently on their sides with rigid extension of the limbs and, although able to drink, usually died of starvation. Several other outbreaks in pigs have been attributed to selenium poisoning.

Neuraxonal dystrophy is a progressive degenerative process of CNS axons characterized initially by discontinuous swellings (called spheroids) along the distal section of axons. The spheroids reflect an inability of the neuron to maintain a normal structure and function. Neuraxonal dystrophy has been diagnosed in a number of sheep breeds, including Suffolks in the United States, Coopworth and Romney lambs in New Zealand, and Merino sheep in New Zealand and Australia, where it was previously been called Murrurrundi disease or ovine segmental axonopathy. The disease is consistent with an autosomal recessive disorder.[2]

EDM (neuraxonal dystrophy) affects young horses and has been recorded in the United States, Canada, the UK, and Australia. EDM appears to be inherited with vitamin E intake during growth modifying the clinical expression and is pathologically more advanced form of neuraxonal dystrophy.[3,4] The major clinical signs are referable to bilateral leukomyelopathy involving the cervical spinal cord. There is abnormal positioning and decreased strength and spasticity of the limbs as a result of upper motor neuron and general proprioceptive tract lesions. Hypalgesia, hypotonia, hyporeflexia, muscle atrophy, or vestibular signs are not present, and there is no evidence of CN, cerebral, or cerebellar involvement clinically. Abnormal gait and posture are evident, usually initially in the pelvic limbs but eventually also in the thoracic limbs. There are no gross lesions, but histologically there is degeneration of neuronal processes in the white matter of all spinal cord funiculi, especially the dorsal spinocerebellar and sulcomarginal tracts. The lesion is most severe in the thoracic segments and is progressive.[5]

Motor neuron diseases are a group of nervous disorders characterized by selective degeneration of upper motor neurons and/or lower motor neurons. Common characteristics of motor neuron diseases are muscle weakness or spastic paralysis. Motor neuron diseases have been identified in a number of species and are currently considered incurable.[6] An inherited **motor neuron disease** has been identified in an extended family of Romney lambs. Lower motor neuron signs predominated and affected lambs were euthanized at 4 weeks of age. The disorder was inherited in a simple autosomal recessive manner.[6] **Bovine spinal muscular atrophy** is an inherited motor neuron disease of Brown Swiss cattle characterized by progressive weakness and severe neurogenic muscle atrophy with early postnatal onset and death within the first few months of life.[2]

An inherited lower motor neuron disease has been recorded in pigs. Clinical findings of muscular tremors, paresis, or ataxia developed at 12 to 59 days of age. There is widespread degeneration of myelinated axons in peripheral nerves and in the lateral and ventral columns of lumbar and cervical segments of the spinal cord. Axonal degeneration is present in ventral spinal nerve roots and absent in dorsal spinal nerve roots when sampled at the same lumbar levels.

Equine motor neuron disease is a neurodegenerative condition that affects horses from 15 months to 25 years of age of many different breeds and has been associated with oxidative stress and vitamin E deficiency.[7,8] Progressive weakness, short-striding gait, trembling, long periods of recumbency, and trembling and sweating following exercise are characteristic clinical findings. The weakness is progressive and recumbency is permanent. Appetites remain normal or become excessive. At necropsy, degeneration or loss of somatic motor neurons in the spinal ventral horns, angular atrophy of skeletal muscle fibers, and the presence of lipofuscin deposits in the ventral horns of the spinal cord and retina are characteristic.

Sporadic cases of spinal cord damage in horses include hemorrhagic myelomalacia following general anesthesia and acute spinal cord degeneration following general anesthesia and surgery. Following recovery from the anesthesia, the horse is able to assume sternal recumbency but not able to stand. A hemorrhagic infarct assumed to be caused by cartilage emboli, and a venous malformation causing spinal cord destruction, have also occurred in the horse. The disease must be differentiated from myelitis and spinal cord compression caused by space-occupying lesions of the vertebral canal and cervical, vertebral malformation/malarticulation.

REFERENCES

1. Bourke CA. *Aust Vet J.* 2006;84:53.
2. Krebs S, et al. *Mamm Genome.* 2006;17:67.
3. Finno CJ, et al. *J Vet Intern Med.* 2011;25:1439.
4. Finno CJ, Valberg SJ. *J Vet Intern Med.* 2012;26:1251.
5. Wong DM, et al. *Vet Pathol.* 2012;49:1049.
6. Zhao X, et al. *Heredity.* 2012;109:156.
7. Wijnberg ID. *Equine Vet Educ.* 2006;18:126.
8. Mohammed HO, et al. *Am J Vet Res.* 2012;73:1957.

Focal Diseases of the Brain and Spinal Cord

TRAUMATIC INJURY TO THE BRAIN

The effects of trauma to the brain vary with the site and extent of the injury, but initially nervous shock is likely to occur followed by death, recovery, or the persistence of residual nervous signs. Traumatic lesions of the skull or vertebral column were the most commonly diagnosed nervous diseases of horses at necropsy in a large case series of 4,319 horses with clinical signs of nervous disease, accounting for 34% of all diagnoses.[1]

ETIOLOGY

Traumatic injury to the brain may result from direct trauma applied externally, by violent stretching or flexing of the head and neck, or by migration of parasitic larvae internally. Recorded causes include the following:

- Direct trauma is an uncommon cause because of the force required to damage the cranium. Accidental collisions, rearing forward, falling over backward after rearing are the usual reasons.
- Periorbital skull fractures in horses are caused by direct traumatic injury commonly from colliding with gate posts.
- Cerebral injury and CN injury accounted for a large percentage of neurologic diseases in horses. Young horses under 2 years of age seem most susceptible to injuries of the head.
- Injury by heat in goat kids is achieved with prolonged application of a hot iron used for disbudding
- Pulling back violently when tethered can cause problems at the atlantooccipital junction.
- Animals trapped in bogs, sumps, cellars, and waterholes and dragged out by the head, and recumbent animals pulled onto trailers can suffer dire consequences to the medulla and cervical cord, although the great majority of them come to surprisingly little harm.
- The violent reaction of animals to lightning stroke and electrocution causing damage to central nervous tissue; the traumatic effect of the electrical current itself also causes neuronal destruction.
- Spontaneous hemorrhage into the brain is rare but sometimes occurs in cows at parturition, causing multiple small hemorrhages in the medulla and brainstem.
- Brain injury at parturition, recorded in lambs, calves, and foals, is possibly a significant cause of mortality in the former.

PATHOGENESIS

The initial reaction in severe trauma or hemorrhage is nervous shock. Slowly developing subdural hematoma, a common development in humans, is accompanied by the gradual onset of signs of a space-occupying lesion of the cranial cavity, but this seems to be a rare occurrence in animals. In some cases of trauma to the head, clinical evidence of injury to the brain may be delayed for a few days until sufficient swelling, callus formation, or displacement of the fracture fragments has occurred. Trauma to the cranial vault may be classified, from least to most severe, as **concussion**, **contusion**, **laceration**, and **hemorrhage**.

Concussion

Concussion is usually a brief loss of consciousness that results from an abrupt head injury, which produces an episode of rapid acceleration/deceleration of the brain.

Contusion

With a more violent force, the brain is contused. There is maintenance of structure but loss of vascular integrity, resulting in hemorrhage into the parenchyma and meninges relative to the point of impact. Bony deformation or fracture of the calvaria results in two different kinds of focal lesions:

- Direct (**coup**) contusions immediately below the impact site
- Indirect (**contrecoup**) contusions to the brain at the opposite point of the skull; these hemorrhages result from tearing of leptomeningeal and parenchymal blood vessels.

Laceration

The most severe contusion is laceration in which the CNS tissue is physically torn or disrupted by bony structures lining the cranium or by penetrating objects such as bone fragments. Focal meningeal hemorrhage is a common sequel to severe head injury. Subdural hematomas usually follow disruption of bridging cerebral veins that drain into the dural venous sinuses, but subarachnoid hemorrhages are more common. The importance of these hemorrhages is that they develop into space-occupying masses that indent and compress the underlying brain. Progressive enlargement of the hematoma can result in secondary effects such as severe, widespread brain edema, areas of ischemia, herniations, midline shift, and lethal brainstem compression.

In birth injuries the lesion is principally one of hemorrhage subdurally and under the arachnoid.

Experimental Traumatic Craniocerebral Missile Injury

Traumatic insult of the brains of sheep with a .22 caliber firearm results in a primary hemorrhagic wound track with indriven bone fragments and portions of muscle and skin. There is crushing and laceration of tissues during missile penetration; secondary tracks caused by bone and bullet fragments; widely distributed stretch injuries to blood vessels, nerve fibers, and neurons as a consequence of the radial forces of the temporary cavity that develops as a bullet penetrates tissue; marked subarachnoid and intraventricular hemorrhage; and distortion and displacement of the brain. The lesions are consistently severe and rapidly fatal.

CLINICAL FINDINGS

Clinical signs of neurologic disease usually follows the pattern of greatest severity initially with recovery occurring quickly but incompletely to a point where a residual defect is evident, with this defect persisting unchanged for a long period and often permanently. This failure to improve or worsen after the initial phase is a characteristic of traumatic injury.

With severe injury there is cerebral shock in which the animal falls unconscious with or without a transient clonic convulsion. Consciousness may never be regained, but in animals that recover it returns in from a few minutes up to several hours. During the period of unconsciousness, clinical examination reveals dilatation of the pupils; absence of the eye preservation and pupillary light reflexes; and a slow, irregular respiration, with the irregularity phasic in many cases. There may be evidence of bleeding from the nose and ears, and palpation of the cranium may reveal a site of injury. Residual signs vary a great deal. Blindness is present if the optic cortex is damaged, hemiplegia may be associated with lesions in the midbrain, and traumatic epilepsy may occur with lesions in the motor cortex.

Fracture of the petrous temporal bone is a classic injury in horses caused by rearing and falling over backward. Both the facial and the vestibular nerves are likely to be damaged so that at first the animal may be unable to stand and there may be blood from the ear and nostril of the affected side. When the animal does stand, the head is rotated with the damaged side down. There may be nystagmus, especially early in the course of the disease. The ear, eyelid, and lip on the affected side are also paralyzed and sag. Ataxia with a tendency to fall is common. Some improvement occurs in the subsequent 2 or 3 weeks as the horse compensates for the deficit, but there is rarely permanent recovery. An identical syndrome is recorded in horses in which there has been a stress fracture of the petrous temporal bone resulting from a preexisting inflammation of the bone. The onset of signs is acute but unassociated with trauma.

Fracture of the basisphenoid and/or **basioccipital bones** is also common. These fractures can seriously damage the jugular vein; carotid artery; and glossopharyngeal, hypoglossal, and vagus nerves. The cavernous sinus and the basilar artery may also be damaged and lead to massive hemorrhage within the cranium. Large vessels in the area are easily damaged by fragments of the fractured bones, causing fatal hemorrhage. A midline fracture of the frontal bones can also have this effect.

Other signs of severe trauma to the brain include opisthotonus with blindness and nystagmus and, if the brainstem has been damaged, quadriplegia. There may also be localizing signs, including head rotation, circling, and falling backward. Less common manifestations of resulting hemorrhage include bleeding into the retropharyngeal area, which may cause pressure on guttural pouches and the airways and lead to asphyxia. Bleeding may take place into the guttural pouches themselves.

Newborn lambs affected by birth injury to the brain are mostly dead at birth, or die soon afterward. Surviving lambs drink poorly and are very susceptible to cold stress. In some flocks it may be the principal mechanism causing perinatal mortality.

DIAGNOSIS

Radiography of the skull is important to detect the presence and severity of fractures, which may have lacerated nervous tissue; however, CT is a much more sensitive method for detecting fractures of the calvarium and basilar bone than radiography.[1]

CLINICAL PATHOLOGY

CSF should be sampled from the cerebellomedullary cistern and examined for evidence of RBCs. Extreme care must be taken to ensure that blood vessels are not punctured during the sampling procedure because this would confound the interpretation of the presence of RBCs. The presence of heme pigments in the CSF (xanthochromia) suggests the presence of preexisting hemorrhage; the presence of eosinophils or hypersegmented neutrophils suggests parasitic invasion.

NECROPSY FINDINGS

In most cases a gross hemorrhagic lesion will be evident, but in concussion and nematodiasis the lesions may be detectable only on histologic examination.

DIFFERENTIAL DIAGNOSIS

Unless a history of trauma is available diagnosis may be difficult.

TREATMENT

The principles of treatment of animals exhibiting neurologic abnormalities after a traumatic event are derived from the results of large, controlled, multicenter clinical trials in humans. Similar studies have not been performed in large animals. The general principles are (1) stabilize the patient by ensuring a patent airway, obtaining vascular access and attending to wounds; (2) specific treatment for hyperthermia, because brain defects may result in an inability to regulate core temperature; (3) prevent or treat systemic arterial hypotension; (4) optimize oxygen delivery; (5) ensure adequate ventilation by placing in sternal recumbency whenever possible; (6) decrease pain; (7) monitor plasma glucose concentration and maintain euglycemia; and (8) prevent or treat cerebral edema by having the head elevated or by the intravenous administration of a hyperosmolar agent (20% mannitol as a series of bolus infusions of 0.25–1.0 g/kg BW every 4–6 hours, the latter is an expensive treatment; hypertonic saline, 7.2% NaCl, 2 mL/kg BW every 4 hours for five infusions). Intravenous catheterization should be confined to one jugular vein, and the neck should not be bandaged in an attempt to minimize promotion of cerebral edema by jugular venous hypertension.

Seizures should be treated when they occur by initially administering diazepam at 0.1 mg/kg intravenously. If no improvement is noticed within 10 minutes, then one or two additional doses of diazepam (0.1 mg/kg, intravenously; total dose 0.3 mg/kg, intravenously) should be administered at 10-minute intervals. Midazolam could be substituted for diazepam, but dose rates are not well defined. If this dosage protocol of diazepam does not provide adequate seizure control, then phenobarbitone (20 mg/kg intravenously over 20 minutes) should be administered to effect; the phenobarbitone can be diluted in 0.9% NaCl solution. This should provide seizure control for a number of hours. If seizures return, then oral phenobarbitone (6 mg/kg every 8 hours) can be administered to foals and horses, with a reduction in the oral dose to 3 mg/kg every 8 hours if seizures are controlled. An alternative protocol in horses is a mixture of 12% chloral hydrate and 6% magnesium sulfate to effect at an intravenous administration rate not exceeding 30 mL/min. Euthanasia should be considered to adult ruminants with seizures that are only responsive to intravenous phenobarbitone.

Many anecdotal treatments have been used in large animals, but evidence attesting to their efficacy is lacking. Among the more popular empiric antioxidant treatments are dimethyl sulfoxide (1 g/kg BW IV as a 10% solution in 0.9% NaCl) administered intravenously or by nasogastric tube every 12 hours, vitamin E (α-tocopherol, 50 IU/kg BW administered orally every day), vitamin C (ascorbic acid, 20 mg/kg BW administered orally every day), and allopurinol (5 mg/kg BW administered orally every 12 hours). Corticosteroids have also been advocated; promoted treatments include an antiinflammatory dose of dexamethasone (0.05 mg/kg BW IV every day) or a high dose of methylprednisolone sodium succinate (30 mg/kg BW initial IV bolus, followed by continuous infusion of 5.4 mg/kg BW per hour for 24–48 hours); the latter treatment is prohibitively expensive in large animals and must be given within a few hours of the traumatic event to be effective. Intravenous magnesium sulfate (50 mg/kg BW) in the first 5 to 10 L of intravenous fluids has also been advocated on the basis that it inhibits several aspects of the secondary injury cascade.

The overall short-term survival rate in one case series of 34 cases was 62%.[2] In those animals that recover consciousness within a few hours or earlier, the prognosis is favorable and little or no specific treatment may be necessary other than nursing care. When coma lasts for more than 3 to 6 hours, the prognosis is unfavorable, and slaughter for salvage or euthanasia is recommended. Horses with basilar bone fractures are 7.5 times more likely not to survive as horses without this type of fracture.[2] Treatment for cerebral edema of the brain as previously outlined may be indicated when treatment for valuable animals is requested by the owner. Animals that are still in a coma 6 to 12 hours following treatment are unlikely to improve, and continued treatment is probably not warranted.

FURTHER READING

MacKay RJ. Brain injury after head trauma: pathophysiology, diagnosis, and treatment. *Vet Clin North Am Equine Pract.* 2004;20:199-216.

REFERENCES

1. Laugier C, et al. *J Equine Vet Sci.* 2009;29:561.
2. Feary DJ, et al. *J Am Vet Med Assoc.* 2007;231:259.

BRAIN ABSCESS

Abscesses of the brain are rare, but occur most commonly in young farm animals under 1 year of age and rarely in older animals. They appear to be more common in ruminants than in horses. Brain abscesses were not observed at necropsy in a large case series of 4,319 horses with clinical signs of nervous disease in France.[1] They produce a variety of clinical signs depending on their location and size. Basically the syndrome produced is one of a space-occupying lesion of the cranial cavity with some motor irritation signs. Localized or diffuse meningitis is also common, along with the effects of the abscess.

ETIOLOGY

Abscesses in the brain originate in a number of ways. Hematogenous infections are common, but direct spread from injury to the cranium or via the nasopharynx may also occur.

Hematogenous Spread

The lesions may be single, but are often multiple, and are usually accompanied by meningitis. The infection usually originates elsewhere.

- *Actinobacillus mallei* from glanders lesions in lung
- *Streptococcus zooepidemicus* var. *equi* as a complication of strangles in horses
- *Corynebacterium pseudotuberculosis* in a goat causing an encapsulated abscess in the left cerebellar peduncles
- *Actinomyces bovis* and *Mycobacterium bovis* from visceral lesions in cattle
- *Fusobacterium necrophorum* from lesions in the oropharynx of calves
- *Pseudomonas pseudomallei* in melioidosis in sheep

- *Staphylococcus aureus* in tick pyemia of lambs
- Systemic fungal infections such as cryptococcosis may include granulomatous lesions in brain.

Local Spread

- Via peripheral nerves from the oropharynx, the one specific disease is listeriosis in ruminants and New World camelids.
- Multifocal meningoencephalitis associated with lingual arteritis induced by barley spikelet clusters.
- Space-occupying lesions of facial and vestibulocochlear nerves and geniculate ganglion secondary to otitis media in calves.
- Abscesses of the rete mirabile of the pituitary gland are seen secondary to nasal septal infection after nose-ringing in cattle. *Trueperella* (*Arcanobacterium* or *Actinomyces* or *Corynebacterium*) *pyogenes* is the most common isolate, and several other species of bacteria that cause chronic suppurative lesions have been recovered. Similar abscesses, usually containing *T. pyogenes,* occur in the pituitary gland itself.
- Extensions from local suppurative processes in cranial signs are seen after dehorning from otitis media. The lesions are single and most commonly contain *T. pyogenes* and are accompanied by meningitis.

PATHOGENESIS

Infectious agents can invade the CNS by four routes:

- **Retrograde infection via peripheral nerves**
- **Direct penetrating injuries**
- **Extension of adjacent suppurative lesions**
- **By way of the systemic circulation**

Single abscesses cause local pressure effects on nervous tissue and may produce some signs of irritation, including head-pressing and mania, but the predominant effect is one of loss of function caused by destruction of nerve cells. Multiple abscesses have much the same effect. In single abscesses the signs usually make it possible to define the location of the lesion, whereas multiple lesions present a confusing multiplicity of signs and variation in their severity from day to day, suggesting that damage has occurred at a number of widely distributed points and at different times.

The pituitary abscess syndrome has an uncertain pathogenesis. The pituitary gland is surrounded by a complex mesh of intertwined arteries and capillary beds known as the rete mirabile, which has been identified in cattle, sheep, goats, and pigs but not horses. This extensive capillary network surrounding the pituitary gland makes it susceptible to localization by bacteria that originate from other sources of infection. Nose-ringing of cattle may result in septic rhinitis, which could result in infection of the dural venous sinus system, which communicates with the subcutaneous veins of the head. Bacteria may also reach the rete mirabile by way of lymphatics of the nasal mucosa and cribriform plate. CN deficits occur as a result of the extension of the abscess into the adjacent brainstem.

CLINICAL FINDINGS

General signs include mental depression, clumsiness, head-pressing, and blindness, often preceded or interrupted by transient attacks of motor irritation including excitement, uncontrolled activity, and convulsions. A mild fever is usually present, but the temperature may be normal in some cases.

The degree of blindness varies depending on the location of the abscess and the extent of adjacent edema and meningoencephalitis. The animal may be blind in one eye and have normal eyesight in the other eye or have normal eyesight in both eyes. Unequal pupils and abnormalities in the pupillary light reflex, both direct and consensual, are common. Uveitis, iris bombé, and a collection of fibrin in the anterior chamber of an eye may be present in some cases of multiple meningoencephalitis in cattle. Nystagmus is common when the lesion is near the vestibular nucleus; strabismus may also occur.

Localizing signs depend on the location of lesions and may include cerebellar ataxia, deviation of the head with circling and falling, and hemiplegia or paralysis of individual or groups of CNs often in a unilateral pattern. In the later stages, there may be papilledema. In calves with lesions of the facial and vestibulocochlear nerves and geniculate ganglion, clinical signs may include drooping of the ears and lips, lifting of the nose, slight unilateral tilting of the head, and uncontrolled saliva flow. Inability to swallow may follow and affected calves become dehydrated.

These localizing signs may be intermittent, especially in the early stages, and may develop slowly or acutely.

Pituitary gland abscesses are most common in ruminants, primarily cattle 2 to 5 years of age, but are relatively rare. The most common history includes anorexia, ataxia, depression, and drooling from the mouth with inability to chew and swallow. The most common clinical findings are depression, dysphagia, dropped jaw, blindness, and absence of pupillary light reflexes. Terminally, opisthotonus, nystagmus, ataxia, and recumbency are common. Characteristically, the animal stands with a base-wide stance with its head and neck extended and its mouth not quite closed; there is difficulty in chewing and swallowing, and drooling of saliva. Affected animals are usually nonresponsive to external stimuli. CN deficits are common, and usually asymmetric, multifocal, and progressive. These include reduced tone of the jaw, facial paralysis, strabismus, and a head tilt. There may also be ptosis and prolapse of the tongue. Bradycardia has been recorded in about 50% of cases. Terminally there is opisthotonus, nystagmus, and loss of balance, followed by recumbency.

CLINICAL PATHOLOGY

Cerebrospinal Fluid

Leukocytes, protein, and bacteria may be present in the CSF, but only when the abscess is not contained.

Hematology

In pituitary gland abscessation there may be hematologic evidence of chronic infection including neutrophilia, hyperproteinemia, and increased fibrinogen, although it is unlikely that a pituitary abscess itself is sufficiently large enough to induce these changes.

Imaging

Radiographic examination will not detect brain abscesses unless they are calcified or cause erosion of bone. CT has been used to diagnose a brain abscess in the horse. MRI is the preferred imaging modality to diagnose a cerebral abscess, with mature abscesses having an isointense to hypointense core on T1-weighted images and an isotense to hyperintense core with a hypointense capsule on T2-weighted images.[2]

Electroencephalography

Electroencephalographic assessment of central blindness caused by brain abscess in cattle has been reported.

NECROPSY FINDINGS

The abscess or abscesses may be visible on gross examination and if superficial are usually accompanied by local meningitis. Large abscesses may penetrate to the ventricles and result in a diffuse ependymitis. Microabscesses may be visible only on histologic examination. A general necropsy examination may reveal the primary lesion.

DIFFERENTIAL DIAGNOSIS

Brain abscess is manifested by signs of involuntary movements and loss of function, which can occur in many other diseases of the brain, especially when local lesions develop slowly. This occurs more frequently with tumors and parasitic cysts but it may occur in encephalitis. The characteristic clinical findings are those of a focal or multifocal lesion of the brain, which include the following:

- Localizing signs of hemiparesis and ataxia
- Postural reaction deficit
- Vestibular signs, including head tilt and positional nystagmus
- Cranial nerve deficits

There may be evidence of the existence of a suppurative lesion in another organ, and a high cell count and detectable infection in the CSF to support the diagnosis of abscess. Fever may or may not be present. The only specific disease in which abscess occurs is listeriosis, in which the lesions are largely confined to the medulla oblongata and the characteristic signs include circling and unilateral facial paralysis. Occasional cases may be associated with fungal infections, including cryptococcosis. Toxoplasmosis is an uncommon cause of granulomatous lesions in the brain of most species.

Many cases of brain abscess are similar to otitis media but there is, in the latter, rotation of the head, a commonly associated facial paralysis and an absence of signs of cerebral depression.

The pituitary gland syndrome in cattle must be differentiated from listeriosis, polioencephalomalacia, lead poisoning, other brain abscesses, and thrombomeningoencephalitis. In sheep and goats, *Parelaphostrongylus tenuis* infection and caprine arthritis encephalomyelitis syndrome may resemble the pituitary gland abscess syndrome.

TREATMENT

Parenteral treatment with antimicrobials is indicated but the results are often unsatisfactory because of the inaccessibility of the lesion, with the clear exception being listeriosis. Treatment of pituitary gland abscess is not recommended, and an antemortem diagnosis is rarely obtained. There is one successful report of recovery after surgical excision of the complete abscess in a 1-month-old alpaca.[2]

FURTHER READING

Kessell AE, Finnie JW, Windsor PA. Neurological diseases of ruminant livestock in Australia. III. Bacterial and protozoal infections. *Aust Vet J.* 2011;89:289-296.

Morin DE. Brainstem and cranial nerve abnormalities: listeriosis, otitis media/interna, and pituitary abscess syndrome. *Vet Clin North Am Food Anim Pract.* 2004;20:243-274.

REFERENCES

1. Laugier C. *J Equine Vet Sci.* 2009;29:561.
2. Talbot CE, et al. *J Am Vet Med Assoc.* 2007;231:1558.

TUMORS OF THE CENTRAL NERVOUS SYSTEM

Primary tumors of the CNS are extremely rare in farm animals. They produce a syndrome indicative of a general increase in intracranial pressure and local destruction of nervous tissue. Tumors of the peripheral nervous system are more common.

ETIOLOGY

The reader is referred to the review literature for a summary of available references on the tumors of the CNS of farm animals, which include the following:

- Meningeal tumors in cattle
- Oligodendroglioma in a cow[1]
- Ependymoblastoma in a heifer[2]
- Primitive neuroectodermal tumor with ependymal differentiation in a cow[3]
- Cerebellar medulloblastoma in a calf[4]
- Choroid plexus carcinoma in a goat[5]
- Equine papillary ependymoma
- Lymphoma confined to the CNS in a horse.[6]

PATHOGENESIS

The development of the disease parallels that of any space-occupying lesion, with the concurrent appearance of signs of increased intracranial pressure and local tissue destruction. Many lesions found incidentally at necropsy may not have had any related clinical findings.

CLINICAL FINDINGS

The clinical findings are similar to those caused by a slowly developing abscess and localizing signs depending on the location, size, and speed of development of the tumor. Clinical signs are usually representative of increased intracranial pressure, including opisthotonus, convulsions, nystagmus, dullness, head-pressing, and hyperexcitability. Common localizing signs include circling, deviation of the head, and disturbance of balance.

CLINICAL PATHOLOGY

There are no positive findings in the clinicopathologic examination, which aids in diagnosis.

NECROPSY FINDINGS

The brain should be carefully sectioned after fixation if the tumor is deep-seated.

TREATMENT

There is no treatment.

DIFFERENTIAL DIAGNOSIS

Differentiation is required from the other diseases in which space-occupying lesions of the cranial cavity occur. The rate of development is usually much slower in tumors than with the other lesions.

REFERENCES

1. Kleinschmidt S, et al. *J Comp Pathol.* 2009;140:72.
2. Miyoshi N, et al. *J Vet Med Sci.* 2009;71:1393.
3. Patton KM, et al. *J Am Vet Med Assoc.* 2014;244:287.
4. Bianchi E, et al. *J Vet Intern Med.* 2015;29:1117.
5. Klopfleisch R, et al. *J Comp Pathol.* 2006;135:42.
6. Morrison LR, et al. *J Comp Pathol.* 2008;139:256.

CENTRAL NERVOUS SYSTEM–ASSOCIATED TUMORS

The pituitary gland (hypophysis) consists of the adenohypophysis (pars distalis, intermedia, tuberalis) and the neurohypophysis (pars nervosa). Tumors of the pituitary gland are common in older horses. Cushing's syndrome in horses almost invariably originates from an **adenoma of the pars intermedia** of the pituitary gland. Initially, these animals exhibit only one remarkable sign, namely, hirsutism. Horses with Cushing's disease only do not manifest polyuria and polydipsia. Major sequelae of an adenoma of the pars intermedia of the pituitary gland are type 2 diabetes mellitus and laminitis. Diagnosis of an adenoma of the pars intermedia of the pituitary gland in the horse mainly depends on dynamic endocrinologic function tests. The sensitivity of the adrenocorticotropin test is about 80%.

Pituitary adenomas can arise from other parts of the pituitary gland; there is a report of a nonfunctional chromophobe adenoma located in the pars distalis of an alpaca with depression and compulsive walking.[1]

FURTHER READING

McFarlane D. Equine pituitary pars intermedia dysfunction. *Vet Clin North Am Equine Pract.* 2011;27:93-113.

REFERENCE

1. Gilsenan WF, et al. *J Vet Intern Med.* 2012;26:1073.

METASTATIC TUMORS OF THE CENTRAL NERVOUS SYSTEM

Many primary tumors of nonnervous tissue have the potential for metastasis or localized growth into the CNS.

- **Ocular squamous cell carcinoma** of cattle may invade the cranium through the cribriform plate
- **Lymphomas** of cattle may metastasize to the CNS with either a multicentric distribution or occasionally as the only lesion. Most commonly bovine lymphoma occurs as an epidural mass in the vertebral canal. Intracranial lymphoma usually involves the leptomeninges or the choroid plexus. Clinical signs are related to the progressive compression of the nervous tissue at the site of the mass. Lymphoma in the horse has occurred in the epidural space with spinal cord compression.
- **Thymic lymphosarcoma** rarely metastasizes to the cerebellum and intracranial extradural sites in yearling cattle.[1]
- **Rhabdomyosarcoma** invaded the thoracic spinal cord of a heifer, resulting in posterior paresis.[2]
- **Schwannomas** (also called neuromas) originate from the Schwann cells of cranial or spinal nerve roots except CNs I and II, which are myelinated by oligodendroglia. Local growth of a schwannoma into the thoracic or sacral spinal cord produced clinical signs of spinal cord dysfunction in two adult cattle.[3] Schwannomas occur in adult

horses with no apparent breed or sex predisposition. There is one report of successful treatment of a dermal schwannoma using localized radiation therapy.[4] In domestic animals, schwannomas can be difficult to differentiate from neurofibromas, and consequently, schwannomas and neurofibromas are categorized as PNSTs by the WHO.

- **Malignant melanoma** has been diagnosed in a cow with hindlimb ataxia[3] and in gray horses where they are usually metastases from skin tumors.

CENTRAL NERVOUS SYSTEM–ASSOCIATED MASSES

Cholesterinic granulomas, also known as cholesteatomas, may occur in up to 20% of older horses without any clinical effects. However, they can be associated with significant neurologic disease. Affected horses are usually obese. Cholesterinic granulomas occur in the choroid plexus of the fourth ventricle or in the lateral ventricles and mimic cerebrocortical disease. It has been suggested that cholesterol granulomas result from chronic hemorrhage into the plexus stroma, but the underlying pathogenesis is unknown.

Brownish nodular thickening of the plexuses with glistening white crystals is a common incidental finding in mature and aged horses. Occasionally, deposits in the plexuses of the lateral ventricles are massive and fill the ventricular space and cause secondary hydrocephalus caused by the buildup of CSF behind the mass. CSF may be xanthochromic with an elevated total protein.

Clinical findings include episodes of abnormal behavior such as depression and bolting uncontrollably and running into fences and walls. Some horses exhibit profound depression, somnolence, and reluctance to move. Seizures have also been reported. Other clinical findings reported include decreased performance, aggression, head tilt, incoordination, intermittent convulsions, hindlimb ataxia progressing to recumbency, intermittent circling in one direction, and spontaneous twitching along the back and flank. There are often serious changes in temperament, with previously placid animals becoming violent and aggressive. In others there are outbursts of frenzied activity followed by coma. The horse may be normal between attacks, and these may be precipitated by moving the head rapidly.

These signs are referable to cerebrocortical disease and the differential diagnosis of cholesterol granulomas must include diffuse cerebral encephalopathy caused by abscess, tumor, toxicosis, metabolic disease, encephalomyelitis, trauma, and hydrocephalus. At necropsy, large cholesterol granulomas are present in the choroid plexus.

REFERENCES

1. Tawfeeq MM, et al. *J Vet Med Sci.* 2012;74:1501.
2. Kajiwara A, et al. *J Vet Med Sci.* 2009;71:827.
3. Braun U, Ehrensperger F. *Vet Rec.* 2006;158:696.
4. Saulez MN, et al. *Tydskr S Afr Vet Assoc.* 2009;80:264.

Plant Toxins Affecting the Nervous System

CANNABINOIDS

Cannabinoids are resinoids found in the plant *Cannabis sativa* (marijuana). The toxic principle is the alkaloid tetrahydrocannabinol. Most reports of poisoning are in dogs and humans, but cattle and horses have also been affected. Clinical signs of poisoning in horses include restlessness, hypersensitivity, tremor, sweating, salivation, dyspnea, staggering gait, and death or recovery after a few hours. No significant necropsy lesions are recorded. The toxin is detectable in stomach or rumen contents.

CYNANCHOSIDE

Cynanchoside is found in *Cynanchum* spp. (monkey rope),[1] and a very similar toxin is found in *Marsdenia rostrata* (milk vine), *M. megalantha*,[1] *Sarcostemma brevipedicellatum* (= *S. australe*; caustic vine), and *S. viminale* (caustic bush). It is associated with hypersensitivity; ataxia; muscle tremors; recumbency; tetanic and clonic convulsions; opisthotonus; and death in horses, donkeys, pigs, and ruminants.[1,2] Other less common signs include teeth grinding, dyspnea, salivation, and vomiting.

DITERPENOID (KAURENE) GLYCOSIDES (ATRACTYLOSIDE, CARBOXYATRACTYLOSIDE, PARQUIN, CARBOXYPARQUIN, AND WEDELOSIDE)

Diterpenoid glycoside toxins have been found in the following species:

Atractylis
Atractylodes
Callilepsis
Cestrum
Iphiona
Wedelia
Xanthium

Xanthium strumarium (cockleburr, Noogoora burr) includes the taxa *X. canadense, X. italicum, X. orientale, X. pungens,* and *X. chinense,* and is poisonous to pigs and ruminants. *X. spinosum* (Bathurst burr) is also toxic and assumed to contain diterpenoid glycosides. The two cotyledonary leaves, either within the spiny burrs or just after sprouting, contain the largest amount of toxin and are the usual source of poisoning. The cockleburs occur on most continents. Poisonings are reported from North America, UK, Europe, and Australia. Most deaths occur on flood plains on which the weed is allowed to grow in abundance. After heavy rain the seeds in the burrs sprout and are palatable to all species, especially calves and pigs. Mortalities are also recorded in adult cows and sheep. Burrs may contaminate feed grains and poison livestock fed on the compounded ration.

Cestrum spp. (e.g., *C. parqui, C. laevigatum*), are garden plants originating from South and Central America which, except for *C. diurnum,* also contain a carboxyatractyloside toxin.

Wedelia asperrima (yellow daisy), *W. biflora,* and *W. glauca* contain wedeloside. Severe hepatic necrosis is the principal necropsy finding, and the clinical syndrome and clinical pathology are characteristic of hepatic encephalopathy.

Poisoning by diterpenoid glycoside toxins in pigs and calves is acute, manifested by hyperexcitability, so that the entire herd appears restless, followed by severe depression, rigidity of the limbs and ears, weakness and a stumbling gait, falling easily and recumbency, and clonic convulsions with opisthotonus. Calves may be belligerent. Acute cases die during the first convulsive episode. The course may be as long as 48 hours and terminate in recovery, but death is the usual outcome. The characteristic lesion is hepatic necrosis.

Treatment is not undertaken. Control depends on keeping livestock away from pasture dominated by these weeds, especially when there are large quantities of sprouted *Xanthium* spp. seeds available.

STYPANDROL

Stypandrol (syn. hemerocallin), a binaphthoquinone (binaphthalene tetrol) is found in *Dianella revoluta* (flax lily), *Stypandra glauca* (= *S. imbricata, S. grandiflora*—nodding blue lily), and *Hemerocallis* spp. (day lily). Field cases occur only with *S. glauca* and are characterized by blindness, incoordination, posterior weakness and, eventually, flaccid paralysis and recumbency in grazing ruminants. Dilatation and immobility of the pupil, with retinal vascular congestion, hemorrhage, and papilledema visible ophthalmoscopically, are characteristic. At necropsy there is diffuse status spongiosis in the brain, general neuronal vacuolation, and axonal degeneration of optic nerve fibers and the photoreceptor cells of the retina.[3] Only the young green shoots are poisonous, so that outbreaks occur only in the spring when the plant is flowering.

TROPANE ALKALOIDS

Tropane alkaloids include atropine, hyoscyamine, hyoscine, and scopolamine, found in the following:[4,5]

Atropa belladonna (deadly nightshade)
Datura stramonium (common thorn apple, jimsonweed, gewone stinkblaar)[4]
D. ferox (large thornapple, groot stinkblaar)[4]

Duboisia leichhardtii
D. myoporoides (corkwoods)
Hyoscyamus niger (henbane).

D. stramonium grows universally but cases of poisoning are few, possibly because of its unpalatability, its high toxic dose, and because it produces ruminal atony in cattle. All parts of *Datura* spp. contain belladonna alkaloids with the highest amount in the flowers, followed by the stem, seeds, leaves, and roots.[5] The seeds of the plant are likely to contaminate grain supplies and may be associated with poisoning.[4]

Clinical signs are primarily caused by blockade of peripheral muscarinic receptors innervating smooth muscle, cardiac muscle, and exocrine glands. Ingestion of these plants in sufficient quantity is associated with a syndrome of mydriasis (pupil dilation and blindness), dry mouth, restlessness, tremor, tachycardia, hyperthermia, and frenzied actions.[5] Colic, in particular impaction colic, is reported in horses.[4] Convulsions, recumbency, and death may occur. Cholinesterase inhibitors such as physostigmine may be used to reverse the anticholinergic effects.[4] There are no significant necropsy lesions.

TUTIN

Tutin is a poisonous constituent of the *Coriaria* spp. (tutu trees) in New Zealand. It is associated with a short course of hypersensitivity, restlessness, and convulsions followed by death, with no visible lesions at necropsy.

FURTHER READING

Botha CJ, Naude TW. Plant poisonings and mycotoxicoses of importance in horses in southern Africa. *J S Afr Vet Assoc.* 2002;73:91-97.

Jain MC, Arora N. Ganja (*Cannabis sativa*) refuse as cattle feed. *Indian J Anim Sci.* 1988;58:865-867.

Naudé TW, Gerber R, Smith R, et al. *Datura* contamination of hay as the suspected cause of an extensive outbreak of impaction colic in horses. *J S Afr Vet Assoc.* 2005;76:107-112.

REFERENCES

1. Neto SAG, et al. *Toxicon.* 2013;63:116.
2. Pessoa CRM, et al. *Toxicon.* 2011;58:610.
3. Finnie JW, et al. *J Aust Vet Assoc.* 2011;89:24.
4. Gerber R, et al. *J S Afr Vet Assoc.* 2006;77:86.
5. Krenzelok E. *Clin Toxicol (Phila).* 2010;48:104.

INDOLE ALKALOIDS

A large number of indole alkaloids occur in fungi, especially the *Claviceps* and *Acremonium* spp. In plants there are also some groups of toxins with similar toxic effects, and similar to those of the fungi. The important two are the β-carbolines and the dimethyl tryptamines; followed by the hydroxyl methyl tryptamines, and a miscellaneous group of alstonine and related toxins. Plants included in the latter group that are associated with an incoordination syndrome like phalaris staggers are *Gelsemium sempervirens* (yellow jessamine), *Alstonia constricta* (bitter bark tree), and the mushroom *Psilocybe* spp. (mad or magic mushroom). *Poa hueca* and *Urtica* spp. (stinging nettle) are associated with a more acute syndrome of convulsions and sudden death. *Phalaris* spp. are unusual in that they contain both β-carbolines and methylated tryptamines. Related indole alkaloids of the pyrrolidinoindoline type have poisoned livestock in Australia (idiospermuline in *Idiospermum australiense*) and North America (calycanthine in *Calycanthus* spp.), producing tetanic convulsions.

β-CARBOLINE INDOLEAMINE ALKALOID POISONING

β-Carboline indole alkaloids (harmala alkaloids) in plants include harmaline, tetrahydroharmine, harman, norharman, tetrahydroharman, harmine, harmol, harmalol, peganine, and deoxypeganine.[1] The mechanism of action for these alkaloids is competitive inhibition of monoamine oxidase (primarily MAO-A) resulting in increased serotonin activity.[2] Synthetic forms of these alkaloids are associated with clinical signs similar to those occurring in natural plant poisonings with *Peganum harmala* (African or Turkish rue), *P. mexicana* (Mexican rue), *Phalaris* spp., *T. terrestris* (caltrop, catshead burr), *T. micrococcus* (yellow vine), *Kallstroemia hirsutissima* (hairy caltrop, carpet weed), and *K. parviflora*.[1-3]

The characteristic syndrome, similar to that of an upper motor neuron lesion, includes hypermotility or hypomotility, sometimes sequentially in the same patient, muscle tremor, partly flexed paresis of the thoracic and/or the pelvic limb, hypermetria, a wide-based stance, crossing of the limbs, extension of the neck, swaying of the head, walking backward, sudden jumping movements, sham eating, and terminal convulsions. The net effect, seen in all farm animal species and camels, is one of easy stimulation, by stimulating gait incoordination and stumbling, fetlock knuckling, falling, and recumbency. The signs appear gradually; are similar to, but less severe than, those associated with the methylated tryptamines; and are irreversible. There is axonal degeneration in peripheral nerves. Long-term cases of *T. terrestris* poisoning pivot on their front limbs while their hindlimbs trace a circle. The pivoting is related to the unilateral muscle atrophy of limbs of one side or the other.

FURTHER READING

Allen JRF, Holmstedt BR. The simple β-carboline alkaloids. *Phytochemistry.* 1980;19:1573-1582.

Bourke CA. A novel nigrostriatal dopaminergic disorder in sheep affected by *Tribulus terrestris* staggers. *Res Vet Sci.* 1987;43:347-350.

Moran EA, Couch JF, Clawson AB. *Peganum harmala,* a poisonous plant in the Southwest. *Vet Med.* 1940;35:234-235.

REFERENCES

1. Burrows GE, Tyrl RJ, eds. *Nitrariaceae Lindl. Toxic Plants of North America.* 2nd ed. Hoboken, NJ: Wiley-Blackwell; 2013:833.
2. Herraiz T, et al. *Food Chem Toxicol.* 2010;48:839.
3. Finnie JW, et al. *Aust Vet J.* 2011;89:247.

INDOLIZIDINE ALKALOID TOXICOSIS (LOCOISM, PEASTRUCK)

The two indolizidine alkaloids of plant origin are castanospermine and swainsonine and both of them affect cellular enzyme activity.

CASTANOSPERMINE POISONING

Castanospermine, an indolizidine alkaloid found in the seeds of *Castanospermum australe* (Moreton Bay chestnut tree), is structurally and functionally similar to swainsonine.[1] It inhibits α-glucosidase activity so that affected cattle have been misdiagnosed as heterozygotes for generalized glycogenosis type II (Pompe's disease). The seeds are also associated with hemorrhagic gastroenteritis with myocardial degeneration and nephrosis in cattle and sheep if eaten in large quantities.[1]

SWAINSONINE POISONING

SYNOPSIS

Etiology Poisoning by some plants in the genera of *Astragalus, Oxytropis,* and *Swainsona.* It is associated with induced mannosidosis.

Epidemiology Grazing toxic plants for 2–6 weeks is associated with signs, reversible if pasture is changed.

Clinical pathology Urine content of mannose-containing oligosaccharides is elevated.

Lesions Vacuolation of neurons.

Diagnostic confirmation Swainsonine can be detected in serum, urine, or animal tissues; the endophyte may be detected in the plant.

Treatment No treatment is available.

Control Restrict both the amount of plant and time animals allowed to graze infected pastures.

ETIOLOGY

Swainsonine is an indolizidine alkaloid found in many *Astragalus* spp., *Oxytropis* spp., and *Swainsona* spp. legumes.[2,3] Some *Ipomoea* spp.[4] as well as *Turbina cordata*[5] and *Sida carpinifolia*[6,7] contain swainsonine either alone or in combination with mixtures of other alkaloids. Ingestion of the toxic plants over a long period is associated with an induced lysosomal storage disease in all animal species. Not all plants in a particular species contain swainsonine. In North America there are over 354 different species of *Astragalus* and 22 species of *Oxytropis,* yet only 20 of them are known to contain swainsonine or are associated with locosim.[2] The common plants in which the alkaloid's presence has been identified include the following:

- *Astragalus lentiginosus, A. mollisimus, A. wootonii, A. emoryanus.*[2] Other plants of this genus that are associated with a similar disease, and in which the presence of swainsonine is assumed, are *A. northoxys, A. lentiginosus* var. *waheapensis, A. lusitanicus,* and *A. thurberi.*
- *Oxytropis sericea, O. ochrocephala.*[2] Other plants of this genus that are associated with a similar disease, and in which the presence of swainsonine is assumed, are *O. besseyi, O. condensata, O. lambertii,* and *O. puberula.*
- *Swainsona canescens, S. galegifolia, S. brachycarpa, S. greyana, S. luteola, S. procumbens, S. swainsonioides.*[3]

Undifilum oxytropis (formerly *Embellisa* spp.), a fungal endophyte present in the seeds, has been identified in the genera of *Astragalus* spp. and *Oxytropis* spp. as well as in *S. canescens* and is currently thought to be responsible for the production of swainsonine.[6,8,9] Swainsonine is also synthesized by the fungus *R. leguminicola,* but the disease associated with this fungus is caused by its slaframine content.

EPIDEMIOLOGY

Occurrence

Poisoning is most common in North America (as locoism associated with *Astragalus* spp. and *Oxytropis* spp.) and in Australia as Darling pea or peastruck (*Swainsona* spp.), but it occurs worldwide.[2,3,8] Toxicity from *Oxytropis* spp. has been reported in China, *Ipomea* spp. in goats in Brazil,[4] *T. cordata* in goats in Brazil,[5] *S. carpinifolia* in horses in Brazil,[10] and unknown swainsonine source in a horse in Belgium.[7]

Risk Factors

Animal Risk Factors

All animal species are affected, and experimental administration of the alkaloid to monogastric, farm, and laboratory animals is associated with the typical neuronal *A. lentiginosus* lesions. Horses are highly sensitive to swainsonine and develop clinical signs when fed 0.2 mg swainsonine/kg BW for 60 days followed by cattle and sheep at 0.25 mg/kg BW for 30 to 45 days.[7,11]

Grazing animals must ingest the plants for at least 2 weeks, and more often 6 weeks, before clinical signs appear.[7] The plants are not addicting, but animals appear to have a preference for them over other plants. It may be that the plants are more palatable to them at certain times of the year compared with what other forage is available.[2]

Swainsonine is excreted in the milk and may intoxicate nursing animals.[2]

PATHOGENESIS

Swainsonine is a specific inhibitor of lysosomal α-mannosidase causing accumulation of mannose in lysosomes and thus widespread neurovisceral cytoplasmic vacuolation.[2,3,7] The vacuoles are accumulations of mannose-rich oligosaccharides, including abnormal glycoproteins. Vacuolation reaches its greatest intensity in the CNS, and this is probably related to the predominance of nervous signs in the disease. Vacuolation of the chorionic epithelium may be related to the occurrence of abortion, and a transient infertility is suspected in rams to be the result of a similar lesion in the epithelium of the male reproductive tract. The lesion appears quickly and is reversible if the swainsonine intake ceases. In addition, swainsonine inhibits mannosidase II resulting in an alteration of glycoprotein synthesis, processing, and transport. The net result is a dysfunction of membrane receptors and circulating insulin, as well as impairment of cellular adhesion.[2,7]

CLINICAL FINDINGS

After several weeks of grazing affected pasture adult animals begin to lose condition and young animals cease to grow. The appetite is diminished, and the coat becomes dull and harsh.[2,7,10,11] Several weeks later nervous signs of depression; gait incoordination; muscle tremor; and difficulty in rising, eating, and drinking become apparent. Sheep commonly adopt a "star-gazing" posture, and horses may show nervousness, excitation, rearing over backward when handled, tremors, colic, recumbency, and death.[7,11] Cases may become overexcited if stressed or stimulated. Recovery is likely if the animal is removed from the source of the toxin soon after signs appear. Recovery may be complete or there may be a residual gait incoordination if the animal is excited. Advanced cases may show no improvement, and others become recumbent and die. Calves at high altitudes fed *A. lentiginosus* or *O. sericea* develop a higher incidence of congestive heart failure than calves not fed on the plants.

Pregnant ewes ingesting *Astragalus* spp. plants may abort or produce abnormal offspring with contractures. The defects take the form of small, edematous, or dead fetuses or skeletal deformity.[2,12] There are no such abnormalities recorded with *Swainsona* spp.

CLINICAL PATHOLOGY

Vacuolation in circulating lymphocytes occurs in poisoning caused by *Swainsona* spp., and may have diagnostic significance. Serum levels of α-mannosidase are significantly reduced and swainsonine levels increased. Swainsonine levels reflect the amount being ingested and not the duration of exposure, and quickly return to normal when ingestion of the plants ceases.[7] The urine content of mannose-containing oligosaccharides is greatly increased during the period of intake of swainsonine.

NECROPSY FINDINGS

The characteristic microscopic lesion is fine vacuolation of the cytoplasm in neurons throughout the CNS. Similar vacuolation is present in cells of other organs, especially the kidney, and the fetus in animals poisoned by *Astragalus* spp. High blood and tissue levels of swainsonine are detectable, including in frozen material.

In aborted calves, lambs, and foals there is extensive vacuolation of the chorionic epithelial cells. The skeletal deformities include arthrogryposis and rotation of the limbs about their long axis.

Diagnosis is made by documenting exposure to a swainsonine-containing plant, identifying the clinical signs, and swainsonine serum or tissue concentrations. Recently a quantitative polymerase chain reaction (PCR) method was identified that can measure fungal endophytes in the *Astragalus* spp. and *Oxytropis* spp.[13]

DIFFERENTIAL DIAGNOSIS

Differential diagnosis list

- *Conium* spp. piperidine alkaloids
- Inherited mannosidosis
- *Lupinus* spp. quinolizidine alkaloids
- *Nicotiana* spp. alkaloids

TREATMENT

There is no effective treatment for Swainsonine poisoning. Removal of the affected animals from access to source plants may result in partial or complete recovery, provided the cases are not too advanced.

CONTROL

Pregnant animals should not be exposed to sources of swainsonine, but other stock may be grazed on the plant without ill effect for short, specified periods, namely 4 weeks for sheep and cattle and 2 weeks for horses. The most important factor is the amount of plant material ingested and the amount of time the animal is exposed to the toxin. Animals should not be allowed to graze when toxic plants are palatable and other forage is in short supply. In the western part of the United States, cattle should not be allowed to graze on locoweed-infected pastures until late May or early June, when other grasses have begun to grow. Pastures should not be overstocked because a lack of adequate forage will force animals to graze on locoweed. Animals grazing on locoweed pastures should be monitored closely and moved to a different pasture if they begin to show signs of poisoning. Herbicides may be used to control *Astragalus* spp. and *Oxytropis* spp., but the endophyte is contained in the seeds and they are drought resistant and able overwinter, allowing only for control and not elimination. Attempts to reduce consumption of the toxic plants by creating conditioned reflex aversion, to reduce absorption of ingested swainsonine or by supplementing the diet with bentonite, have not been rewarding.

FURTHER READING

Radostits O, et al. Indolizidine alkaloid poisoning. In: *Veterinary Medicine: A Textbook of the Disease of Cattle, Horses, Sheep, Goats and Pigs*. 10th ed. London: W.B. Saunders; 2007:1870.

Stegelmeier BL, James LF, Panter KE, et al. The pathogenesis and toxicokinetics of locoweed (*Astragalus* and *Oxytropis* spp.) poisoning in livestock. *J Natural Toxins*. 1999;8:35-45.

REFERENCES

1. Stegelmeier BL, et al. *Toxicol Pathol*. 2008;36:651.
2. Cook D, et al. *Rangelands*. 2009;31:16.
3. Finnie JW, et al. *Aust Vet J*. 2011;88:247.
4. Barbosa RC, et al. *Pesq Vet Res*. 2007;27:409.
5. Dantas AFM, et al. *Toxicon*. 2007;49:111.
6. Cook D, et al. *J Agric Food Chem*. 2011;59:1281.
7. Nollet H, et al. *Equine Vet Ed*. 2008;20:62.
8. Grum DS, et al. *J Nat Prod*. 2013;76:1984.
9. Ralphs MH, et al. *J Chem Ecol*. 2008;34:32.
10. Lima EF, Riet-Correa B, Riet-Correa F, et al. Poisonous plants affecting the nervous system of horses in Brazil. In: Riet-Correa F, Pfister J, Schild AL, Wierenga TL, eds. *Poisoning by Plants, Mycotoxins, and Related Toxins*. Oxfordshire, UK: CAB International; 2011:290.
11. Stegelmeier BL, Lee ST, James LF, et al. The comparative pathology of locoweed poisoning in livestock, wildlife, and rodents. In: Pater KE, Ralphs MH, Pfister JA, eds. *Poisonous Plants: Global Research and Solutions*. Oxfordshire, UK: CAB International; 2007:59.
12. Panter KE, Welch KD, Lee ST, et al. Plants teratogenic to livestock in the United States. In: Riet-Correa F, Pfister J, Schild AL, Wierenga TL, eds. *Poisoning by Plants, Mycotoxins, and Other Toxins*. Oxfordshire, UK: CAB International; 2011:236.
13. Cook D, et al. *J Agric Food Chem*. 2009;57:6050.

NEUROGENIC QUINOLIZIDINE ALKALOIDS (*LUPINUS* SPP.)

ETIOLOGY

Alkaloids causing the nervous syndrome include sparteine, lupinine, lupanine, hydroxylupanine, spathulatine, and thermopsine. These vary widely in their toxicity and their concentration in plant species, and within the same species between years, depending largely on the climate. Species of lupin known to contain them are *Lupinus angustifolius* and *L. cosentinii* (synonym *L. digitatus*). Species that are associated with the characteristic nervous syndrome and in which the presence of the alkaloids in the plant is assumed include the following:

L. argenteus
L. caudatus
L. cyaneus
L. greenei
L. laxiflorus
L. leucophyllus
L. leucopsis
L. onustus
L. pusillus

EPIDEMIOLOGY

The alkaloids are present in all parts of the plant but are in their greatest concentration in the seeds and pods; most outbreaks of poisoning occur when livestock graze mature, standing lupins, carrying many pods. Sheep eat the plant more readily and are more commonly affected than cattle or horses. The mortality rate in sheep is high. In cattle, it is usually low but may be as high as 50%.

Other plants in which the alkaloids occur and which are associated with the nervous disease include the following:

Cytisus (synonym *Laburnum*, *Sarothamnus* spp.)
Baptisia spp.
Sophora spp.
Spartium junceum (Spanish broom)
Thermopsis spp.

CLINICAL FINDINGS

In the nervous disease, affected animals may develop dyspnea and depression, followed by coma and death without a struggle. More acute cases have convulsive episodes in which they are dyspneic and staggery, and show frothing at the mouth, clonic convulsions, and grinding of the teeth. A more prolonged disease is reported in cattle poisoned experimentally with *Thermopsis montana*. There is anorexia, depression, edematous swelling of the eyelids, tremor, a stilted gait, arching of the back and a tucked-up abdomen, rough hair coat, and prolonged recumbency.

PATHOLOGY

Severe myopathy results in high aspartate aminotransferase (AST), creatine kinase (CK) and lactic acid dehydrogenase (LDH) activities. The possibility of a myopathy being associated with lupins has been raised because the prevalence of enzootic muscular dystrophy appears to be much higher on lupin than on other pasture. Lupins are low in selenium and vitamin E content, and classical white muscle disease may also occur. Histologic and biochemical examination of affected calves discount myopathy as the primary lesion. In poisoning by *Cytisus* spp., both *C. laburnum* (laburnum) and *C. scoparius* (broom) are associated with fatalities.

FURTHER READING

Panter KE, Maryland HF, Gardner DR, et al. Beef cattle losses after grazing *Lupinus argenteus* (silvery lupine). *Vet Hum Toxicol*. 2001;43:279-282.

NITROCOMPOUND PLANT TOXICOSIS (MILK VETCH)

SYNOPSIS

Etiology Several different toxins; miserotoxin in certain *Astragalus* spp. is the most important.

Epidemiology Limited to geographic distribution of the toxic plants; mostly North America but other countries affected depending on specific plant.

Clinical pathology Nonspecific; methemoglobin values >20%.

Lesions Degenerative lesions in peripheral nerves and spinal cord.

Diagnosis confirmation Associated with isolation of nitrotoxins in tissues and fluids.

Treatment None.

Control Management of pasture to avoid grazing pasture when relevant plants are abundant.

ETIOLOGY

Nitrocompounds (nitrotoxins) poisonous to animals occur in a number of plants, especially in some species of *Astragalus*. They are all glycosides of 3-nitropropionic acid (NPA) or of 3-nitro-ropanol (NPOH). Miserotoxin is the most common and well known toxin; other toxins include cibarian, corollin, coronarian, coronillin, and karakin.[1] The best known occurrences of the nitrocompounds include the following:

- *A. canadensis* (Canadian milk vetch), *A. emoryanus* (Emory's milk vetch), *A. miser* (forest or woody milk vetch), *A. pterocarpus* (winged milk vetch), *A. tetrapterus* (four-wing milk vetch), and others; contain miserotoxin.[1]
- *Corynocarpus laevigatus* (karaka tree); contains karakin.[2]
- *Oxytropis* spp., a plant genus very similar botanically to *Astragalus* spp., is associated with the same diseases as the latter but its toxic agent has not been identified.
- *Securigera varia* (*Coronilla varia*), contains cibarian and others.[1]
- *Indigofera linnaei* (Birdsville indigo), contains karakin and other nitrocompounds.[3]

EPIDEMIOLOGY

Occurrence

The occurrence of these plant poisonings is determined by the presence and ingestion of the specific plants. *Astragalus* and *Oxytropis* spp. are, for the most part, limited in distribution to North America, but poisoning of sheep by *A. lusitanicus* is recorded in Morocco, and of all species by *O. puberula* in Kazakhstan. *Corynocarpus* spp. occur in New Zealand and *Indigofera* spp. are widespread, occurring in North America, Australia, Africa, and Southeast Asia.

Astragalus and *Oxytropis* spp. are herbaceous legumes, most of them are perennial, and they dominate the desert range over large areas of the United States. They provide excellent forage. Only some species contain miserotoxin, but this makes them very destructive and very heavy losses of sheep and cattle may occur.

Risk Factors

Animal Risk Factors

Cattle are the more susceptible. Lactating animals are more susceptible than dry animals. There are reports of the disease in horses in North America and a similar disease in horses in China after grazing *O. kansuensis*

Human Risk Factors

Miserotoxin and its metabolic end products may be excreted in the milk of cows eating these plants.

PATHOGENESIS

In ruminants the glycosides are hydrolyzed in the rumen to NPOH and NPA. Both are absorbed from the rumen and once in the liver, NPOH is further biodegraded to NPA. Nitrous dioxide (NO_2) formed during biodegradation may account for methemoglobinemia.[1] Some nitrite may also be formed resulting in methemoglobinemia in horses and ruminants. The onset of clinical signs is associated with the accumulation of NPA and a resulting neurologic syndrome, characterized principally by nervous signs and the development of degenerative lesions in the CNS. In experimental animals the dose rate and length of exposure to the toxin determine whether the acute or chronic disease occurs. Typically, animals must have consumed nitrotoxin plants for a week or more before showing signs. Morbidity is 10% to 15%; case–fatality rate may be up to 30%.[1]

CLINICAL FINDINGS

Acute Poisoning

Death may occur as soon as 3 hours after the commencement of signs, but the course is usually about 24 hours. Common signs include ataxia or a staggering walk, recumbency, and death from respiratory or cardiac arrest.

Chronic Poisoning

The syndrome in cattle is often referred to as "cracker heels," because of the noise made when rear hooves strike each other.[1] Affected animals lose weight, and develop a poor hair coat, nasal discharge, and poor exercise tolerance. Respiratory distress, with loud stertor (roaring), is more marked in sheep than in cattle and knuckling of the fetlocks and incoordination, followed in some by paraplegia, is more common in cattle. Temporary blindness and drooling of saliva may also be evident. The mortality rate is very high, with the course lasting over several months. Animals that recover have a long convalescence. Death may occur suddenly if affected animals are stressed.

I. linnaei poisoning in horses (synonym Birdsville horse disease) is associated with weight loss, gait incoordination, easy falling, toe dragging, dyspnea, and convulsions.[3] The plant is equally poisonous when dry or green, although most cases occur in the spring when the plant is succulent. Horses need to graze the plant for about 10 days before signs appear. Characteristic signs include segregation and somnolence, with the animal often standing out in the open in the hot sun, apparently asleep when unaffected horses have sought the shade. There is marked incoordination, with the front legs being lifted and extended in an exaggerated manner. The hocks are not flexed, causing the fronts of the hind hooves to be dragged on the ground. The head is held in an unnaturally high position and the tail is held out stiffly. There is difficulty in changing direction, and incoordination increases as the horse moves. The horse commences to sway and at the canter there is complete disorientation of the hindlegs so that the animal moves its limbs frantically but stays in the one spot with the legs becoming gradually abducted until it sits down and rolls over. Terminally there is recumbency with intermittent tetanic convulsions, which may last for up to 15 minutes and during which death usually occurs.

A chronic syndrome may develop in some horses subsequent to an acute attack. Affected animals can move about, but there is incoordination and dragging of the hindfeet with wearing of the toe, and inspiratory dyspnea (roaring) may also occur. No lesions have been described in the nervous system of affected animals. *I. linnaei* contains the toxic amino acid, indospicine, an analog of arginine, and NPA.[3] Poisoned horses may not always develop the liver damage typical of intoxication by indospicine[3]; however, supplementation of the diet with arginine-rich protein feeds prevents development of the disease.[4] Peanut meal (0.5–1 kg/day) and gelatin provide readily available and cheap sources of arginine.

CLINICAL PATHOLOGY

Methemoglobinemia concentrations greater than 20% may occur in cattle and horses. Laboratory procedures for the determination of blood levels of miserotoxin, some other nitrotoxins, and NPOH and NPA are available.

NECROPSY FINDINGS

Brown discoloration of the blood, and extensive petechiation in tissues, are common findings in the acute form of the disease. In the chronic disease, there are degenerative changes in the spinal cord and peripheral nerves, especially the sciatic nerve, as well as areas of necrosis in the thalamus and Purkinje cells in some cerebellar folia, white matter spongiosis in the globus pallidus, and distension of the lateral ventricles.[1] Nonspecific gross lesions include pulmonary emphysema and pneumonia, abomasal ulceration, and pericardial/pleural fluid.

Diagnosis confirmation depends on the identification of the poisonous plants in the environment and the toxins in the plants and animal tissues

> **DIFFERENTIAL DIAGNOSIS**
>
> **Differential diagnosis list (chronic form)**
> - Chronic cyanide poisoning
> - Paspalum staggers
> - Phalaris staggers
> - Ryegrass staggers

TREATMENT

Treatment includes removing animals from the suspected pastures and providing an alternate food source. The use of injectable thiamine has not shown to be of any value. There is no specific treatment for the chronic form of the disease, and some animals may ultimately recover.

CONTROL

Control of the growth of the plants by stimulating growth of competitive grasses, or the widespread use of selective herbicides, is recommended but unlikely to be a practicable procedure in many of the situations in which the plants occur. Experimentally, the use of some herbicides significantly reduces the content of miserotoxin in *A. miser* var. *oblongifolia* in pasture. Variations between species of *Astragalus* spp. in their capacity to produce miserotoxin and store selenocompounds (some of them, e.g., *A. toanus*, do both) provides opportunities to manipulate the grazing of particular fields to best advantage.

FURTHER READING

Anderson RC, Majak W, Rasmussen MA, et al. Toxicity and metabolism of the conjugates of 3-nitropropanol and 3-nitropropionic acid in forages poisonous to livestock. *J Agric Food Chem*. 2005;53:2344-2350.

Benn M, McEwan D, Pass MA, et al. Three nitropropanoyl esters of glucose from *Indigofera linnaei*. *Phytochemistry*. 1992;7:2393-2395.

Majak W, Benn M. Additional esters of 3-nitropropanoic acid and glucose from fruit of the New Zealand karaka tree, *Corynocarpus laevigatus*. *Phytochemistry*. 1994;35:901-903.

Majak W, Stroesser L, Lysyk T, et al. Toxicity and development of tolerance in cattle to timber milkvetch. *J Range Manage*. 2003;56:266-272.

REFERENCES

1. Burrows GE, Tyrl RJ. Nitrotoxicosis (cracker heels). In: *Toxic Plants of North America*. 2nd ed. Hoboken, NJ: Wiley-Blackwell; 2013:515.
2. Noori MA, et al. *Toxicol Environ Chem*. 2007;89: 479.
3. Ossedryver SM, et al. *Aust Vet J*. 2013;91:143.
4. Lima EF, et al. *Toxicon*. 2012;60:324.

PIPERIDINE ALKALOID PLANT TOXICOSIS

ETIOLOGY

The important, identified piperidine alkaloids include coniine, cynapine, nicotine, and lobeline. These alkaloids are primarily neurotoxins; some alkaloids present in *Conium maculatum* and *Nicotiana* spp. are also teratogens and are dealt with separately in Chapter 18.

CONIUM

C. maculatum (poison hemlock) contains five major acetate-based piperidine alkaloids—coniine, *N*-methylconiine, conhydrine, pseudoconhydrine, and γ-coniceine—and a number of other, lesser, alkaloids. γ-Coniceine is likely a precursor of the others and is much more toxic.[1] The concentration of each of the alkaloids in different parts of the plant, in different climates, and at different times of the year is quite variable. For example, the concentration of the γ-coniceine is high in the fruits when they are formed, but there is no significant content in the roots. In the dormant stage, the toxicity of the roots is very high.

EPIDEMIOLOGY

Poison hemlock occurs in most parts of the world. All animal species are affected, with cattle, sheep, goats, horses, and pigs showing the nervous form of the disease. Poisoned cattle, pigs, and sheep also produce deformed offspring, with ewes being much less susceptible than cows and sows. Grazing animals are poisoned by eating the standing plant, the seeds, or roots at the appropriate time of their development. The plant may also be fed in hay or green feed or the seeds may contaminate harvested grain. Milking cows secrete the alkaloids in their milk.

PATHOGENESIS

The alkaloids are associated with two modes of poisoning, paralysis of skeletal muscle by blocking transmission at neuromuscular junctions and by acting as teratogens. All of the major alkaloids are associated with the acute disease. Only coniine and γ-coniceine are known to be teratogenic.

CLINICAL FINDINGS

Clinical signs in the acute, neurologic form of poisoning include tremor, staggering gait, knuckling of fetlocks, belching, vomiting, frequent urination and defecation, drooling of saliva, tachycardia, and pupillary dilation.[2,3] In cows and sows, prolapse of the nictitating membrane occurs, and in affected cows, a characteristic mousy odor of the milk and urine is described. The course in cattle, goats, and horses is only a few hours and terminates in recumbency and death by respiratory paralysis, without convulsions. Sheep are least affected and recovery is common.

CYNAPINE

Cynapine, a piperidine alkaloid found in *Aethusa cynapium* (fool's parsley, lesser hemlock) is associated with dyspnea and gait incoordination in cattle, goats, and pigs.

NICOTIANA

The most common poisonous members of the tobacco family of plants include the following:

Nicotiana tabacum (commercial tobacco)
N. attenuata (wild tobacco)
N. exigua
N. glauca (tree tobacco)
N. megalosiphon
N. trigonophylla (wild tobacco)
N. velutina

The principal toxins include nicotine, anabasine, and anagyrine.[4] Other alkaloids occurring in *Nicotiana* spp., but which are not recorded as having poisoned animals, are nornicotine and anatabine. *Duboisia hopwoodii* (pituri) is another plant with these alkaloids. Several alkaloids may be present in the one plant, but most plant species have a particular alkaloid that predominates. The concentration of the alkaloid varies between parts of the plant and between different stages of growth.

Acute poisoning of livestock ingesting *Nicotiana* spp. or *D. hopwoodii* is associated with muscle tremor, weakness, incoordination, pupil dilation, and recumbency with limb paddling progressing to paralysis. Diarrhea may be present. The alkaloid anabasine is teratogenic.

Tobacco-specific nitrosamines, formed from *Nicotiana* spp. alkaloids, are known to be carcinogenic to laboratory animals, but there is no record of this association in agricultural animals.

LOBELINE

The piperidine alkaloid lobeline is found in the plant *Lobelia berlandieri*. Ingestion of the plant is associated with mouth erosions, salivation, and diarrhea. Necropsy lesions are limited to the lesions of enteritis.

FURTHER READING

Galey FD, Holstege DM, Fisher EG. Toxicosis in dairy cattle exposed to poison hemlock (*Conium maculatum*) in hay: isolation of Conium alkaloids in plants, hay, and urine. *J Vet Diagn Invest.* 1992;4:60-64.

Panter KE, Keeler RF, Baker DC. Toxicoses in livestock from the hemlocks (*Conium* and *Cicuta* spp. *J Anim Sci.* 1988;66:2407-2413.

REFERENCES

1. Odriozola E. Poisoning by plants, mycotoxins, and algae in Argentina livestock. In: Riet-Correa F, Pfister J, Schild AL, Wierenga TL, eds. *Poisoning by Plants, Mycotoxins, and Other Toxins.* Oxford, UK: CAB International; 2011:35.
2. Binev R, et al. *Trakia J Sci.* 2007;5:40.
3. Nicholson SS. *Vet Clin North Am Food Animal Pract.* 2011;27:447.
4. Schep LJ, et al. *Clin Toxicol (Phila).* 2009;47:771.

CORYNETOXINS (TUNICAMINYLURACILS) (ANNUAL RYEGRASS STAGGERS, FLOOD PLAIN STAGGERS, STEWART RANGE SYNDROME)

SYNOPSIS

Etiology Corynetoxins (tunicaminyluracils) present in infected grass (*Lolium rigidum, Lachnagrostis filiformis, Polypogon monspeliensis*) eaten by all species. A similar tunicaminyluracil has been isolated from water-damaged wheat eaten by pigs.

Epidemiology Outbreaks in Australia (summer to early fall) and South Africa when grazing animals ingest infected seedhead galls. Occurs anytime of the year in animals fed infected hay.

Clinical pathology Increased activity of hepatic enzymes in serum; prolonged prothrombin and activated partial thromboplastin time.

Lesions Perivascular edema in meninges and brain; hemorrhages in multiple tissues.

Diagnosis confirmation Tunicaminyluracil in pasture seed heads.

Treatment Magnesium sulfate in horses or small herds. Removal of animals from infected fields or hay; reduce stress.

Control Keep animals off infected pastures; decrease prevalence of infection by various methods (see text); test hay before purchasing.

ETIOLOGY

Nematode larvae infest and are associated with galls in the seedheads of *Lolium rigidum* (Wimmera or annual ryegrass), *Polypogon monspieliensis* (annual beard grass), and *Lachnagrostis filiformis* (formerly *Agrostis avenacea* and commonly referred to as blown or blowaway grass).[1,2] Nematodes in the genus *Anguina* (*A. agrostis, A. funesta, A. paludicola*) transport the corynetoxin producing bacteria *Rathayibacter toxicus* into the cuticle of grass seeds.[1,3,4] Bacteriophages were originally felt to play an integral part, but that may no longer be the case.[2] Corynetoxins (tunicaminyluracils) are glycolipid tunicaminyluracil antibiotics produced in the seedhead gall and sheep, cattle, and horses grazing the pasture are poisoned when they are ingested.[1,3,5] Animals eating corynetoxin-infected hay are poisoned.[1,2]

Other outbreaks have been recorded. In the 1960s, sheep and cattle in the northwestern United States developed a similar neurologic condition when fed fescue infected with *A. agrostis* and *Rathayibacter*-like organisms.[1] Tunicaminyluracil has been isolated from water-damaged wheat, which when fed to pigs is associated with clinical signs and deaths similar to those associated with the tunicaminyluracil on grasses.[1]

EPIDEMIOLOGY

Occurrence

Poisoning that occurs in livestock pastured on *L. rigidum* (termed annual ryegrass toxicity or ARGT) or in those grazing *L. filiformis* (flood plain staggers) has become a very important cause of death losses on farms in western and southern Australia, southern New South Wales, and also in South Africa.[1,3,5] Toxicity associated with ingestion of *P. monspieliensis* (termed Stewart range syndrome) is found in flood-prone portions in southeastern South Australia.[1] Typically, in Australia, infected seed heads are toxic beginning with the dry summer period and continuing until the onset of fall rains.[1,2] Clinical signs do not occur until the stock has been on pasture for several days or up to 12 weeks.[1] Forced exercise and high ambient temperatures precipitate or exacerbate clinical signs.[1,5]

Risk Factors

Animal Risk Factors

The oral dose of tunicamycins in sheep associated with the onset of clinical signs following investigational intraduodenal administration is 150 μg/kg.[6] The subcutaneous lethal dose is much smaller, 30 to 40 μg/kg as a single dose or a set of small sequential doses. The toxins are cumulative if the interval between doses are few days.

Plant Risk Factors

Pasture improvement based on annually alternating crop-pasture rotations seem to predispose to the disease, with the worst outbreaks occurring after the end of a cropping year. This can be avoided by burning the pasture in the autumn. The organism is introduced onto farms by the introduction of infested grass seed or contaminated agricultural implements.[2] *L. rigidum* has become a weed in southern Australia and herbicide-resistant strains have evolved, complicating control measures. Hay made from infested grass remains poisonous for 5 to 6 years. Poisoning associated with *L. filiformis* has occurred in cattle on extensive pasture recently subjected to severe flooding, hence the name flood plain staggers.[1]

PATHOGENESIS

Corynetoxins are similar structurally to tunicamycin antibiotics originally isolated from an actionmycete (*Streptomyces lysosuperificus*).[1] Collectively the group, including corynetoxins, is referred to as tunicaminyluracil antibiotics. They are potent inhibitors of lipid linked *N*-glycosylation of glycoproteins[1] and capable of causing cerebral vascular lesions in experimental animals. Interference with cardiovascular function and vascular integrity leads to interference with oxygenation of tissues, particularly the brain.

CLINICAL FINDINGS

Signs appear when the cattle or sheep are disturbed or stressed, especially by driving. The animals fall in a convulsion with paddling of limbs, nystagmus, opisthotonus, jaw champing and salivation, head nodding, tetanic extension of limbs and, in sheep, posterior extension of the hindlimbs.[1-3] Death may occur during a convulsion or, if left alone, the animal may recover to the point of being able to stand, but there may be gait incoordination caused by hypermetria, stiff gait, a broad-based stance, head swaying, rocking backward and forward, and loss of balance. Intermittent convulsive episodes recur and the animals soon go down again. Death occurs in up to 24 hours. Further cases occur for up to 10 days after affected animals are removed from the pasture.[2] Morbidity and mortality rates may reach as high as 100% in sheep flocks. In surviving ewes, abortion may occur in up to 10% of pregnant sheep.[1]

Poisoning occurs less frequently in horses and stress is often a precipitating factor.[5] Colic with tachycardia, borborygmi, and congested mucous membranes, is often the first sign observed followed by hypermetria, ataxia, muscle tremors, recumbency, convulsions with limb paddling, and death.[5]

CLINICAL PATHOLOGY

Blood levels of liver enzymes, bilirubin, and bile acids are elevated. Prothrombin time and activated partial thromboplastin time are prolonged.[1]

NECROPSY FINDINGS

Necropsy findings are inconsistent and nonspecific. The liver may be enlarged and pale or icteric. There may be hemorrhages in a range of tissues. Histologically, there may be perivascular edema in the brain, particularly in cerebellar meninges. Other lesions may include significant liver damage.

DIFFERENTIAL DIAGNOSIS

Differential diagnosis list:

- Lead poisoning
- Perennial ryegrass staggers
- Phalaris staggers
- Poisoning by any one of a large number of plants in which the toxic agent has not been identified.

TREATMENT

Affected flocks or herds should be removed from a toxic pasture as slowly and as quietly as possible to good-quality feed with shade and water in a place free of disturbance.[1,5] Stress should be kept to a minimum.

No specific antidote or antitoxin is available.[1,5] An antidote was developed by CSIRO in Australia for use early in outbreaks of poisoning, but field trials were disappointing.[7] Pharmacologic measures are impractical in herd situations, although intravenous administration of magnesium sulfate could be used for individual animals. Horses have been treated successfully with an intravenous injection of magnesium sulfate (approximately 100 mg/kg BW; range of 60–200 mg/kg) and supportive measures including flunixin meglumine, dimethyl sulfoxide, and intravenous fluids.[5] Doses of 25 to 150 mg/kg intravenously have been used for hypomagnesemia in horses and may be useful in managing equine cases.[8] It is recommended that magnesium not be administered concurrently with calcium-containing intravenous fluids. Used in combination, calcium is used preferentially at the neuromuscular junction, limiting the effectiveness of magnesium in preventing muscle contractions.[5]

CONTROL

Pasture management in endemic areas should aim to reduce exposure of livestock to mature pastures with seedheads. This may be achieved by a variety of measures such as heavy stocking during winter and spring, harvesting pasture for silage or hay before seeding followed by heavy grazing to remove ryegrass seedlings, burning crop and pasture residues, and herbicide application.[2]

Methods exist for testing hay and are used for hay exported from Australia.[2,9] Recent improvements in testing have shortened the turnaround time considerably.[10] Hay purchased for use within Australia should be tested and accompanied by a declaration stating that testing occurred and the hay is safe for use.[2]

Two cultivars of *L. rigidum* (Guard and Safeguard) resistant to *A. funesta* have been developed that significantly reduce the number of galls per kilogram of hay and the risk of developing ARGT.[2] Pasture application of *Dilophospora alopecuri,* a fungal pathogen of *A funesta,* has been studied, but the results are mixed and may be uneconomical.[11] Immunization against the toxin is promising but difficult as glycolipids are poor immunogens.[1]

FURTHER READING

Bourke CA, Carrigan MJ, Love SCJ. Flood plain staggers, a tunicaminyluracil toxicosis of cattle in north New South Wales. *Aust Vet J.* 1992;69:228-229.

Cockrum PA, Culvenor CCJ, Edgar JA, et al. Toxic tunicaminyluracil antibiotics identified in water-damaged wheat responsible for the death of pigs. *Aust J Agric Res.* 1988;39:245-253.

Riley IT, Gregory AR, Allen JG, et al. Poisoning of livestock in Oregon in the 1940s to 1960s attributed to corynetoxins produced by *Rathayibacter* in nematode galls in Chewings fescue. *Vet Hum Toxicol.* 2003;45:160-162.

REFERENCES

1. Finney JW. *Aust Vet J.* 2006;84:271.
2. Allen JJ. *Microbiology.* 2012;8:18.
3. Finnie JW, et al. *Aust Vet J.* 2011;89:247.
4. Bertozzi T, et al. *Zootaxa.* 2009;2060:33.
5. Grewar JD, et al. *J S Afr Vet Assoc.* 2009;80:220.
6. Haply SL, et al. Dose response of tunicamycins in sheep following intra-duodenal administration. In:

Panter KE, Wierenga TL, Pfister JA, eds. *Poisonous Plants: Global Research and Solutions*. Oxford, UK: CABI; 2007:242.
7. Allen JG, et al. *8th International Symposium on Poisonous Plants (ISOPP8), João Pessoa, Paraiba, Brazil, May 2009*. Oxford UK: CABI; 2011.
8. Plumb DC. Magnesium. In: Plumb DC, ed. *Veterinary Drug Handbook*. 7th ed. Ames, IA: Wiley-Blackwell; 2011:618.
9. Masters AM, et al. *Crop Pasture Sci*. 2006;57:731.
10. Masters AM, et al. *Crop Pasture Sci*. 2011;62:523.
11. Barbetti MJ, et al. *Plant Dis*. 2006;90:229.

MISCELLANEOUS PLANT TOXINS AFFECTING THE NERVOUS SYSTEM (UNIDENTIFIED TOXINS)

Plants with ingestions resulting in signs of gait incoordination, with or without recumbency, convulsions, or lesions of nervous system include the following:

Ageratina altissima
Araujia hortorum (cruel vine)
Berula erecta
Brachychiton populneus (kurrajong tree)
Brachyglottis repanda (rangiora)
Catharanthus spp.
Centella uniflora
Combretum platypetalum
Craspedia chrysantha
Doronicum hungaricum (wild sunflower)
Echinopogon spp. (roughbearded grass)[1]
Ervum spp.
Euphorbia mauritanica
Gomphrena celosioides (soft khaki weed)
Hoya spp. (wax flower)[1]
Idiospermum australiense
Melanthrium hybridum
M. virginicum (bunchflower)
Melica decumbens (dronkgras)
Melochia pyramidata
Modiola caroliniana (creeping mallow)
Pennisetum clandestinum (kikuyu grass)[2,3]
Rhodomyrtus macrocarpa (finger cherry; also is associated with blindness).

E. mauritanica is associated with hypersensitivity, stiffness, tremor, incoordination, recumbency, and convulsions in sheep.[1] *Echinopogon ovatus* poisoning in calves and lambs is characterized by stress-induced episodes of stiff-legged incoordination and easy falling and bellowing followed by spontaneous recovery.

G. celosioides is associated with outbreaks of incoordination in horses in northern Australia. Spontaneous recovery follows removal from the pasture.

P. clandestinum poisoning was originally attributed to rumen acidosis, but the current suggestion is that it is a poisoning associated with the fungi *Fusarium torulosum* growing on the grass, which is an unlikely association in some outbreaks.[2,3] Epidemiologically, the disease occurs concurrently with circumstances conducive to fungal growth, including warmth, moisture, and litter under the grass, often caused by the depredations of heavy infestations of sod webworms (grass caterpillars), African black beetles, leaf hoppers, and armyworm caterpillars (*Pseudoletia separata, Pseudocalymma elegans, Spodoptera exempta*).[2]

Cattle, sheep, and to a lesser extent, goats, show signs of poisoning in late summer and autumn.[2] Clinical signs include depression, hypersalivation, abdominal pain, ruminal tympany and stasis, paralysis of the tongue and pharynx, sham drinking, muscle tremors, incoordination, recumbency, diarrhea, dehydration, and death.[2] In the forestomachs there is distension, mucosal reddening, and extensive microscopically visible necrosis in the rumen and abomasum.

Plant ingestions associated with paralysis in ewes and horses, with lesions of a lysosomal storage disease and prominent neuronal pigmentation in the brain and spinal cord include the following:

Romulea spp. (onion weed)[1]
Solidago chilensis
Stachys arvensis (stagger weed)
Stephania spp.
Trachyandra spp.
T. laxa
T. divaricata.

Romulea bulbocodium is associated with a high incidence of phytobezoars, a level of fertility in ewes as low as 20%, and a severe gait incoordination when stimulated to move.[1] Affected sheep walk with their heads held high, fall easily, struggle momentarily, then relax and get up and walk normally. If they are left on the same pasture for 3 or 4 weeks, they become permanently recumbent.

Plant ingestions resulting in signs of mania (e.g., wild running, hyperexcitability, incoordination, circling, aimless wandering, blindness) include the following:

Burttia prunoides
Pisum sativum

FURTHER READING

Peet RL, Dickson J. Kikuyu poisoning in sheep. *Aust Vet J*. 1990;67:229.

REFERENCES

1. Finnie JW. *Aust Vet J*. 2011;89:247.
2. Bourke CA. *Aust Vet J*. 2007;85:261.
3. Ryley MJ, et al. *Australas Plant Dis Notes*. 2007;2:133.

Fungal Toxins Affecting the Nervous System

Diplodia maydis (synonym *D. zeae, Stenocarpella maydis*) is associated with a serious disease of maize crops called corn cob rot. Infected cobs fed to cattle, sheep, goats, and horses are associated with diplodiosis, a neuromycotoxicosis, reported in Australia, Argentina, Brazil, and most often in South Africa.[1] The toxin has been identified as diplonine; a second toxin, diplodiatoxin, has been identified but may not be related to poisoning.[1] The fungus develops its toxin only after a prolonged (more than 6 weeks) period of growth. This may explain frequent reports that the fungus is not poisonous. The same applies to cultured fungus used to produce the disease experimentally; it must be a culture that is at least 8 weeks old.

Clinical signs in adults include lacrimation, salivation, tremor, ataxia, paresis, and paralysis, but signs disappear when the corn is removed from the diet. If the subjects are females in the second and third trimesters of pregnancy, there may be a very high mortality rate (up to 87%) in stillborn or newborn lambs or calves; many of the dead neonates have widespread degeneration of the CNS. Affected animals recover if feeding of the infected grain is stopped.

At postmortem, a status spongiosus lesion may occur in the brain of affected animals, but in most cases there are no necropsy lesions. Fetuses are much more susceptible, and spongiform lesions in the brain are present in most. Their BWs are less than normal, and the gestation period is also reduced.

FURTHER READING

Odriozola E, Odeon A, Canton G, et al. Diplodia maydis: a cause of death of cattle in Argentina. *New Zeal Vet J* 2005;53:160-161.

REFERENCE

1. Snyman LD, et al. *J Agric Food Chem*. 2011;59: 9039.

TREMORGENIC MYCOTOXINS

Tremorgenic mycotoxins are produced by fungi belonging to the *Penicillium, Aspergillus, Claviceps,* and *Neotyphodium* genera.[1] Over 20 different mycotoxins, all containing a tryptophan indole moiety, affect many different mammals including cattle, sheep, goats, and horses. The fungi grow on a wide variety of foodstuffs including spoiled food, garbage, stored grains, forages (grasses and legumes), malt (beverage) residues, and compost piles.[2,3] Despite the different fungi and mycotoxins, the common neurologic signs of prolonged muscle tremors, ataxia, and stress-exacerbated weakness are similar in most species.[2] Hyperexcitability or depression, tetanic seizures, recumbency, paralysis, and rarely death may occur.[2,4]

Tremorgenic mycotoxins are rapidly absorbed from the gastrointestinal tract, and signs occur anywhere from a few hours to several days, depending on the species and particular mycotoxin. Age is important with younger animals more susceptible than older.[5] They are lipid soluble and easily move across the blood-brain barrier and into the CNS. Excretion is primarily biliary and fecal; little hepatic metabolism occurs.[6]

The mechanism of action is unknown, but generally tremorgenic mycotoxins interfere with inhibitory neurotransmitters (γ-amino butyric acid [GABA] and glycine) and stimulate excitatory neurotransmitters. Treatment is supportive and symptomatic.

Aspergillus-Associated Mycotoxins

Aspergillus clavatus, other Aspergillus spp., and Penicillium spp. produce several tremorgenic mycotoxins associated with outbreaks in cattle and sheep. Verruculogen is the most widely recognized mycotoxin; less recognized mycotoxins produced by these fungi include tryptoquivaline, territrems A and B, and aflatrem. *A. clavatus*–associated mycotoxins have been incriminated in several neurologic outbreaks in sheep and cattle.[2,7,8] Common clinical signs included tremors, posterior paresis, knuckling at the fetlocks, recumbency, and death. The specific mycotoxin may be patulin, although that was not present in all cases.[2]

Bermudagrass Staggers

Cattle in California, Oklahoma, and Texas have developed tremors and neurologic signs after grazing on mature bermudagrass (*Cynodon dactylon*) infected with *C. cynodontis*. Analysis of infected seedheads showed high concentrations of the tremorgens paspalitrems and paspaline-like indole-diterpenes and low concentrations of ergine and ergonovine.[1]

Claviceps-Associated Mycotoxins (*Paspalum* or Dallis Grass Staggers)

Cattle, sheep, and horses may develop "grass staggers" after several days after grazing on mature Bahia grass (*Paspalum notatum*) or Dallis grass (*P. dilatatum*) infected with *C. paspali*.[2,4,8,9] The tremorgenic mycotoxins paspaline and paspalitrems A, B, and C are present in the sclerotia (ergots); paspalitrem B is most commonly associated with the onset of signs in cattle and sheep. Affected animals develop exercise-induced nervousness, odd facial expressions, tremors, ataxia, seizures, and death.

Neotyphodium-Associated Mycotoxins (Perennial Ryegrass Staggers)

Horses, deer, cattle, alpacas, and in particular, sheep grazing on perennial ryegrass (*L. perenne*) in the northwestern United States, Australia, New Zealand, and some parts of Europe have developed neurologic signs similar to other stagger-producing grasses.[2,5,10] Lolitrems A, B, and D and other lolitrem precursors produced by the endophyte *Neotyphodium lolii* are the tremorgenic mycotoxins most involved.[9,10] Lolitrem B (maximum tolerable dose 2 mg/kg BW) is the predominant mycotoxin associated with the onset of signs in sheep and cattle.[2] Signs most often occur in the late summer/early fall when animals are on overgrazed pastures. Tremors begin in the head, progress to the neck and shoulder, and finally include the extremities. Affected animals are uncoordinated and become recumbent or develop seizures when stressed. If removed from infected grasses and not stressed, affected animals recover in 7 days or so.

Penicillium-Associated Mycotoxins

Penitrem A and roquefortines, produced by *Penicillium* spp., are the most common mycotoxins associated with tremors. In general, toxicosis with these mycotoxins are more common in small animals ingesting spoiled food (meats, cheese, nuts, eggs, etc.) and garbage, but cases have occurred in horses, cattle, and sheep. Janthitrem A, B, and C produced by *P. janthinellum* have been associated with outbreaks of staggers in sheep grazing on ryegrass.

FURTHER READING

Cole RJ, et al. Paspalum staggers: isolation and identification of tremorgenic metabolites from sclerotia of *Claviceps paspali*. *J Agric Food Chem*. 1977;25:1197-1201.

Scudamor K, et al. Occurrence and significance of mycotoxins in forage crops and silage: a review. *J Sci Food Agric*. 1998;77:1-17.

REFERENCES

1. Uhlig S, et al. *J Agric Food Chem*. 2009;57:1112.
2. Mostrom MM, et al. *Vet Clin North Am Food Anim Pract*. 2011;27:344.
3. Riet-Correa F, et al. *J Vet Diagn Invest*. 2013;25:692.
4. Moyano MR, et al. *Vet Med (Praha)*. 2010;55:336.
5. Sampaio N, et al. *Anim Prod Sci*. 2008;48:1099.
6. Hooser SB, Talcott PA. Mycotoxins. In: Peterson ME, Talcott PA, eds. *Small Animal Toxicology*. 3rd ed. London, UK: Elsevier; 2013:925.
7. Fink-Gremmels J. *Food Add Contam*. 2008;25:172.
8. Finnie JW, et al. *Aust Vet J*. 2011;89:247.
9. Cawdell-Smith AJ, et al. *Aust Vet J*. 2010;88:393.
10. Di Menna ME, et al. *New Zeal Vet J*. 2012;60:315-328.

MISCELLANEOUS FUNGAL TOXINS AFFECTING THE NERVOUS SYSTEM (UNIDENTIFIED TOXINS)

BLACK SOIL BLINDNESS

This is a mycotoxicosis of grazing cattle, associated with the fungus *Corallocytostroma ornicopreoides* growing on Mitchell grass (*Astrebla* spp.) in pastures on heavy basalt (black soil) soil in tropical northwest Australia. The disease has occurred only once, in a year marked by heavy seasonal rainfall and a longer than usual growing season. Morbidity and mortality were high at the peak of the outbreak. Clinical characteristics include blindness and death within 24 hours. Necropsy lesions include renal tubular nephrosis, rumenoreticulitis, and moderate liver cell damage.

NERVOUS SIGNS

Nervous signs of tremor, gait incoordination, recumbency, and convulsions are the primary toxic effects present after ingestion of *Trichothecium roseum* and *Penicillium cyclopium*.

FURTHER READING

Jubb TF, et al. Black soil blindness: a new mycotoxicosis of cattle grazing Corallocytostroma-infected Mitchell grass (*Astrebla* spp). *Aust Vet J*. 1996;73:49-51.

Other Toxins Affecting the Nervous System

INORGANIC TOXINS AFFECTING THE NERVOUS SYSTEM

LEAD TOXICOSIS (PLUMBISM)

SYNOPSIS

Etiology Accidental ingestion of lead metal or lead-containing substances, ingestion of lead-contaminated feed, or grazing pastures containing excessive lead in the soil.

Epidemiology Occurs in all age groups. One of the most common poisonings of farm livestock, especially in young calves after turn out in spring. In cattle, usually sporadic and caused by ingestion of a single source of lead but outbreaks occur when feed is contaminated. High case–fatality rate if untreated. Sources include discarded lead batteries, lead-based paints, industrial sources of lead, ash residues, pastures near motor vehicle highways, and smelters. Occurs in sheep and horses grazing contaminated pastures.

Clinical pathology Lead levels in blood, feces, liver, kidney; elevated porphyrins in blood.

Lesions Encephalopathy, degeneration of liver and kidney; pale musculature, brain laminar cortical necrosis, intranuclear renal inclusion bodies.

Diagnostic confirmation Toxic levels of lead in blood and tissues.

Treatment Supportive care, removal of large amounts of lead from the gastrointestinal tract, chelation therapy.

Control Identify and prevent access of animals to sources of lead.

ETIOLOGY

Lead poisoning is associated with the accidental ingestion of lead metal or lead-containing compounds; ingestion of feed, usually forage, containing lead; or grazing lead-contaminated pastures.[1,2] The latter two are often associated with environmental pollution. Both organic and inorganic lead are toxic, with organic lead the most bioavailable followed by inorganic lead and then metallic lead.[1,3]

EPIDEMIOLOGY

Where groups of animals have access to the same source of lead, outbreaks occur and the morbidity rate ranges from 10% to 30%. The case–fatality rate may reach 100% but early intensive therapy can be successful and reduce the figure to less than 50%. In one recorded outbreak, in which a discarded 24-V battery was accidentally mixed and ground up into the feed of 80 heifers, 55 of the animals died or were euthanized.

Occurrence

Lead is one of the most common poisonings in farm animals, especially young cattle.[1] Sheep and horses are also affected but not as often.[3,4] Pigs, because of housing conditions, are not often exposed to lead and appear to be more tolerant than other species.

Risk Factors

Animal Risk Factors

Cattle

Data from diagnostic toxicology laboratories illustrate that lead poisoning is one of the most common toxicosis in cattle. In Alberta, Canada, over a period of 22 years, lead poisoning was the most frequently diagnosed toxicoses of cattle, representing 0.68% of all bovine submissions to the provincial diagnostic laboratories. Most cases of poisoning occur during the summer months from May to August, when the cattle have ready access to lead-containing materials such as crankcase oil and batteries that are being changed in agricultural machinery. In many countries the incidence of the disease is highest in cattle in the spring of the year a few days after the animals have been turned out onto pasture.[5] Poisoning is most common in younger cattle, with 52% of the cases reported in animals 6 months of age or less.[6] Younger animals are more susceptible to lead toxicosis presumably because of a higher rate of gastrointestinal tract absorption. In addition, young cattle are especially curious and seem to seek out and find sources of lead. Confined housing of calves with or without overcrowding is often followed by the appearance of pica, which may be associated with boredom and an increase ingestion of lead-containing objects.

Lead poisoning in cattle is usually acute and caused by accidental ingestion of a toxic quantity of lead over a short period of time.[7] The natural curiosity, licking habits, and lack of oral discrimination of cattle makes any available lead-containing material a potential source of poisoning. Cattle will readily drink motor oil; lick older machinery grease, peeling paint, and paint ashes; and chew lead-based batteries. Many countries currently ban leaded gasoline, and in these areas used motor oil may not contain lead as well as motor oil from diesel engines or present-day machinery grease.[8] In ruminants, there is a tendency for metallic lead particles to settle in the reticulum, and poisoning results from the gradual conversion of lead particles to soluble lead acetate. Several epidemics of lead poisoning in domestic animals have been recorded throughout the world in which the source of the metal was contamination of pasture or crops by nearby lead mining or industrial lead operations.[9,10] Animals eating vegetation in these areas may accumulate amounts of lead sufficient to produce clinical signs of lead poisoning.

Buffalo

Lead poisoning in buffalo has been reported and provides interesting comparative data; they may have a higher tolerance to lead than cattle.

Sheep

Sheep are usually affected by eating soil or forage contaminated by environmental sources of lead.

Horses

Horses are much more selective in their eating habits. They usually do not lick old paint cans, lead storage batteries, and peeling paint, and they do seem to find the taste of used motor oil attractive. Lead poisoning in horses is most common when they graze lead-contaminated pastures rather than by the accidental ingestion of a toxic amount of lead.[2,4,10] Young horses are particularly more susceptible than older horses and cattle grazing on the same pasture.

Environmental Risk Factors

Environmental pollution with lead is a common occurrence in cities and surrounding suburbs. For farm animals, significant pollution is more likely to occur near smelters or other industrial enterprises or near major highways where pasture is contaminated by exhaust fumes of automobiles if leaded gasoline is still used in the region. Much of the poisoning is subclinical because of the low level of absorption, but lead-intoxicated animals have served as sentinels for human lead exposure.[11]

Lead is still commonly found in pastures near highways. The lead levels in the whole blood of sheep grazing near main highways in three areas of the Nile delta region of Egypt were 0.062, 0.067, and 0.083 parts per million (ppm). Pasture adjacent to heavily used roads may carry as much as 390 mg/kg of lead, in contrast to 10 mg/kg on lightly used roads.[9,10] The concentration of lead on pasture varies markedly with proximity to the traffic, falling rapidly the greater the distance and with the time of the year. Pastures contaminated by smelters are recorded as carrying 325 mg/kg of lead (equivalent to a daily intake for an animal of 6.4 mg/kg BW).[12] In some locations near lead smelters, lead poisoning is considered to be a predictable occurrence in horses that are allowed to graze on local pastures.[4] As a result horses are either not raised in these areas or hay is imported from other areas. Although ingestion is the principal method of poisoning of animals, inhalation may also be a significant method of entry for cattle grazing close to smelters or highways.

Lead as an environmental contaminant is often combined with cadmium, which has some effects similar to those of lead, thus the effects may be somewhat additive. Experimental poisoning with both elements is associated with reduced weight gain in calves at dose levels up to 18 mg/kg BW of each contaminant, and clinical signs appear at levels above 18 mg/kg BW of each. Lead is also combined with chromate for industrial purposes. The combination is nontoxic when combined with lead at lead intake levels of less than 100 mg/kg BW.

Environmental pollution in the vicinity of lead and zinc-ore processing factories can result in varying degrees of poisoning with lead, zinc, and cadmium.[13] These can be monitored by the analysis of blood, hair, and tissues obtained at necropsy.

Farm or Premise Risk Factors

The relationship between lead concentrations in blood of cattle with lead poisoning and those in the milk is exponential.[14] The lead level in milk is relatively constant up to a blood level of 0.2 to 0.3 mg/L, and increases sharply at higher blood levels. The biological half-life of lead excretion in cattle is between 6 and 14 weeks.[15] Studies in six affected dairy herds reported a variable half-life ranging from 48 to 2507 days.[2] One probable reason for this great variance is the ability of the ruminant to retain variable amounts of metallic lead in the rumen, which acts as a continuing reservoir. Half-life studies do not account for variable intake and retention of a persistent reservoir of toxicant, so the concept of using half-life excretion in dealing with lead-poisoned cattle is not likely accurate. Owners of such cattle should be advised of the potentially long withdrawal period. It may be advisable to test periodically and allow marketing based on actually measured levels or to estimate the costs of such a plan and consider salvage. This recent work casts doubt on the economic utility of holding recovered animals. In acutely sick cows that were emergency slaughtered, the range of lead levels in edible muscle tissue was 0.23 to 0.50 mg/kg. The concentrations in the kidneys ranged from 70 to 330 mg/kg and in the livers 10 to 55 mg/kg.

Human and Public Health Risk Factors

The source of lead intoxication in animals must be identified so humans are not inadvertently poisoned. In one recent study, investigations involving cattle deaths from lead poisoning led to elevated blood levels in a pregnant woman, dog, cat, and remaining cattle.[11]

A major concern with the treatment of lead-poisoned animals, particularly food-producing animals, is the assurance that the edible tissues of recovered animals do not contain toxic levels of lead. The length of time required after successful treatment of cattle with typical clinical lead poisoning before such animals can be sent to slaughter or before the milk can be used safely is not known. It is suggested that treated animals should be appropriately identified[6] and blood lead levels determined once or twice monthly for several months. When the blood lead levels have dropped to background levels for three consecutive samplings at least 2 weeks apart, the animals are assumed to be safe for slaughter. Undocumented field observations suggest that at least 6 months are necessary for background levels to be achieved. Decisions about reaching acceptable residue levels will depend on national or local regulations as well as the economics of maintaining a herd for long periods without sales of milk or meat, and appropriate food safety and public health officials should be consulted in this decision. The lead concentrations in blood and milk from periparturient heifers 7 months after an episode of acute lead poisoning revealed no lead in the milk. Animals that had been severely affected by lead poisoning experienced a transient increase in whole-blood lead concentration at parturition that was not high enough to be considered toxic.

Transmission (Sources of Lead)

Lead poisoning is most common in cattle on pasture, particularly if the pasture is poor and the animals are allowed to forage in unusual places, such as trash dumps.[15,16] Phosphorus deficiency may also be a predisposing factor, because affected animals will chew solid objects as a manifestation of osteophagia. However, cattle on lush pasture may also seek out foreign material to chew. Discarded lead batteries are one of the most common sources of lead poisoning in cattle.[13] In Alberta, Canada, over a period of 22 years, discarded batteries or used crankcase oil accounted for more than 80% of cases for which the source of lead was determined: batteries, 39.5%; used crankcase oil, 31.6%. The batteries are commonly placed in garbage dumps on the farm and, in temperate climate countries, the batteries freeze during the winter months and break open, exposing the plates, which are attractive and palatable for cattle to lick and chew.

The contamination of forage supplies with shotgun lead pellets used in hunting and shooting exercises can serve as a source of lead for cattle grazing the pasture or consuming haylage or silage made from the contaminated field.[1,6] Automobile batteries have been accidentally added to feed mixers in which they are ground by powerful augers and mixed into the feed supply of cattle. Discarded lead-based paint cans are particularly dangerous but fences, boards, the walls of pens, painted canvas, and burlap are also common sources in calves. Painted silos may cause significant contamination of the ensilage. One outbreak of lead poisoning in cattle was associated with silage containing 1200 mg/kg dry matter lead, which had become contaminated by ash and debris left after burning an old lead-containing electrical cable in the silo before it had been filled.

Metallic lead in the form of lead shot, solder, or leaded windows has been associated with mortalities, although, experimentally, sheet lead is not toxic.[1,2,4] Lead sheeting that has been exposed to the weather or subjected to acid corrosion appears to be more damaging, possibly because of the formation of a fine coating of a soluble lead salt. Lead poisoning can be a major hazard in the vicinity of oil fields, and engine sump oil may contain over 500 mg lead per 100 mL. Automotive and other mineral oils are very palatable to young beef calves. As lead use becomes restricted in many countries, grease and lead-contaminated engine oil have become less common sources of lead.[8] Less common but still potent sources of lead are linoleum, roofing felt, putty, automobile oil filters, and aluminum paint. Some of the latter paints contain large quantities of lead, and others none at all. Only lead-free aluminum paint should be used on fixtures to which animals have access.

Lead parasiticide sprays, particularly those containing lead arsenate, were once associated with heavy losses in cattle grazing in recently sprayed orchards or vegetable crops. These are not commonly used now, except in some countries, but cattle may accidentally ingest old stores of the compound.

PATHOGENESIS

The absorption, distribution, and elimination of lead vary depending on the chemical form of lead, amount ingested, age and species of animal, and other physiologic factors. Deficiencies in calcium, iron, and zinc are associated with increased lead absorption and increased toxicity. Lead from salts such as lead sulfate are absorbed more than metallic lead from battery plates.[13] Regardless of the chemical form of the ingested lead, only a small proportion (2%–10%) is absorbed because of the formation in the alimentary tract of insoluble lead complexes, which are excreted in the feces.[1,15] Once absorbed, 60% to 90% of lead is found in erythrocytes and the rest bound to albumin and other proteins.[3] Very little lead is found unbound in the serum. Lead is distributed to first to the soft tissues, especially kidneys and liver, and ultimately to bone, which serves as a storage or "sink" for excess lead. Excretion is slow and primarily through bile and the milk of lactating animals with little excreted in the urine.[1,3,14]

Blood lead concentrations are an excellent marker of exposure in animals. In cows, blood-level concentrations greater than 0.35 ppm have been associated with poisoning[1] and blood lead levels less than 0.1 ppm with normal background exposure. In horses, blood lead levels greater than 0.2 to 0.35 ppm have been associated with poisoning[4] and blood lead levels less than 0.2 ppm with background exposure. Correlation between blood lead levels and milk levels is good; correlation between blood lead levels and the presence or severity of clinical signs is often poor.[14,17]

Lead is transferred across the placental barrier,[17] and high liver levels occur in the lambs of ewes fed more than normal amounts of lead. Calves born from cows experimentally poisoned with lead have elevated levels of lead in bone, kidney, and liver. In a naturally occurring case of lead poisoning in a pregnant heifer, the blood and liver concentrations in the fetus were 0.425 and 4.84 ppm, respectively, which was 72% and 84% of the same tissue lead concentrations of the dam. Hepatic lysosomes of the fetus contained metallic electron densities, which may have been lead.

Several biochemical processes are affected by lead. Lead is a neurotoxicant and at elevated doses it disrupts the blood-brain barrier allowing albumin, water, and electrolytes to enter, resulting in edema. The complete mechanism of action associated with lead's neuropathy is unknown, but its ability to substitute for calcium and/or zinc is involved.[3] Lead mimics or inhibits the action of calcium altering the release of neurotransmitters and activating protein kinases.[3] It also binds to a sulfhydryl group on proteins resulting in inhibition of enzymes, conformational changes in proteins, and alterations in calcium/vitamin D metabolisms.[16] Lead inhibits δ-aminolevulinic acid dehydratase (D-ALAD) and ferrochelatase activity, thus decreasing heme synthesis and hemoglobin production.[2,3,18] This not only plays a role in lead-associated anemia but results in decreased oxygen carrying capacity with the nervous system susceptible to the resulting tissue ischemia.

CLINICAL FINDINGS

Lead is toxic to a number of organ systems including the nervous, gastrointestinal, hematologic, cardiovascular, renal, musculoskeletal, and reproductive systems.[3] The major effects of lead toxicity are often manifested in three main ways[7]:

- Lead encephalopathy
- Gastroenteritis
- Degeneration of peripheral nerves

Clinical signs vary depending on the species, type and amount of lead involved, and duration of exposure. Typically, acute nervous system involvement occurs following the ingestion of large doses in susceptible animals such as calves, alimentary tract irritation following moderate doses, and peripheral nerve lesions following long-term ingestion of small amounts of lead. The nervous signs of encephalopathy and the lesions of peripheral nerve degeneration are caused by the degenerative changes of nervous system tissue. Gastroenteritis is associated with the caustic action of lead salts on the alimentary mucosa.

Cattle

The signs of acute lead poisoning are more common in calves and younger cattle and have a sudden onset and short duration, usually lasting only 12 to 24 hours. Many animals, especially those on pasture, are found dead without any observable signs. Staggering and muscle tremors particularly of the head and neck, with champing of the jaws (chewing gum fits) and frothing at the mouth are obvious. Snapping of the eyelids, rolling of the eyes, and bellowing are common. Blindness and cervical, facial, and auricular twitching are consistent in acute lead poisoning of cattle.[15] The animal eventually falls and intermittent tonic-clonic convulsions occur and may continue until death. Pupillary dilation, opisthotonus, and muscle tremors are marked and persist between the convulsive episodes (Fig. 14-3). There is hyperesthesia to touch and sound, and the heart and respiratory rates are increased. In some cases, particularly in adults, the animal remains standing, is blind, maniacal, charges into fences, attempts to climb or jump over walls, and head-presses strongly against walls or fences. Frenzy is common and some animals appear to attack humans, but the gait is stiff and jerky and progress is impeded. Death usually occurs during a convulsion and is caused by respiratory failure.

The subacute form is more common in adult cattle, and in this form the animal remains alive for 3 to 4 days. Gastrointestinal tract dysfunction is one of the most common abnormalities. Ruminal atony is accompanied by constipation in the early stages. Later a fetid diarrhea occurs in most cases. Grinding of the teeth is common, and hypersalivation may occur. Neurologic signs include dullness, blindness, and some abnormality of gait including incoordination and staggering, and sometimes circling. The circling is intermittent and not always in the same direction and usually occurs when the animal is confined in a small space like a box stall. Muscle tremor and hyperesthesia are common but not as pronounced as in the acute form.

Sheep

Lead poisoning in sheep is usually manifested by a subacute syndrome similar to that seen in adult cattle. There is anorexia and scant feces followed by the passage of dark, foul-smelling feces. Weakness and ataxia follow, often with abdominal pain, but there is no excitement, tetany, or convulsions. Polyuria occurs when the intake of lead is small but with large amounts there is oliguria.

Chronic toxicity is rare, but two syndromes of posterior paresis have been described in young lambs in old lead-mining areas, and tissue levels of lead are abnormally high in both instances. In both syndromes there is gait impairment. Osteoporosis is present in one but in the other there is no suggestion of skeletal changes. In the osteoporotic disease the signs occur only in lambs 3 to 12 weeks of age and never in adults. There is stiffness of gait, lameness, and posterior paralysis. Affected lambs are unthrifty and the bones, including the frontal bones, are very fragile. The paralysis is caused by lesions of the vertebrae, usually affecting one or more of the lumbar bones, resulting in compression of the spinal cord. In the other form, gait abnormalities occur in the same lamb age group and are manifested initially by incomplete flexion of the limb joints so that the feet drag while walking. In a later stage the fetlocks are flexed, the extensor muscles paretic, and the lamb soon becomes recumbent. Recovery is common, although many lambs die of concurrent disease.

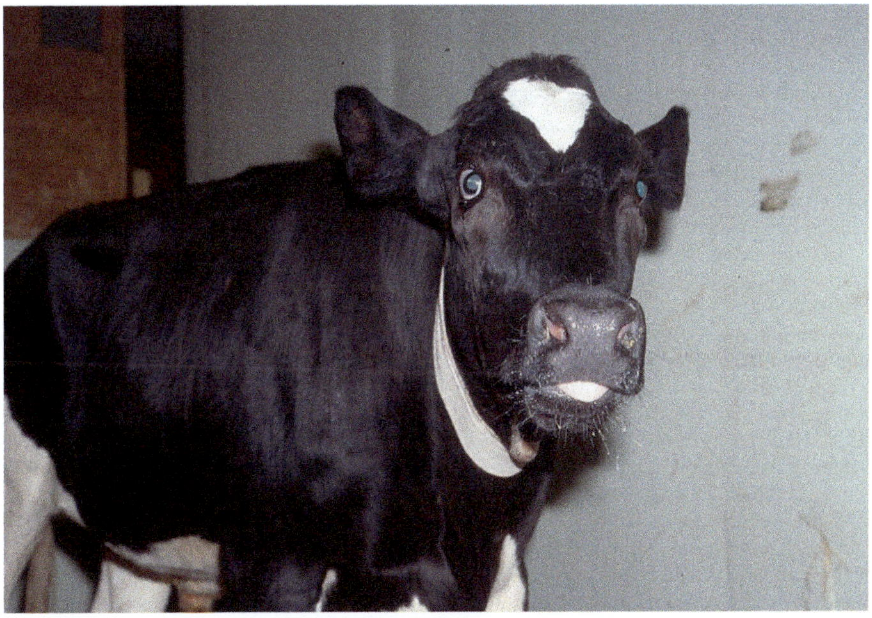

Fig. 14-3 Holstein Friesian steer with acute lead toxicity. Notice the abnormal mentation, contraction of facial muscles, and marked dilatation of the pupils. The bandage around the neck protected an intravenous catheter that was used for daily intravenous Ca-EDTA treatment. The steer recovered following treatment.

Horses

Acute and chronic lead poisoning occurs in horses and ponies, although more rarely than other species. Signs occur most often in horses ingesting contaminated forage or soil found near old lead mines, smelters, and battery recycling depots.[3,4] The clinical findings are extremely variable, but include ataxia, weakness, hypotonia, muscle tremors, rough hair coat, dysphagia, weight loss, dyspnea, roaring or stridor, seizure like movements, colic, and maniacal behavior.[3] A roughened hair coat, pharyngeal dysfunction, and weight loss were the most common clinical findings in 10 case reports involving a total of 68 animals. Some horses died without any previous clinical illness but where clinical signs are apparent they were usually distinct and dramatic rather than subtle. Inspiratory dyspnea associated with paralysis of the recurrent laryngeal nerve is the most common finding. This may be accompanied by pharyngeal paralysis in which recurrent choke and regurgitation of food and water through the nostrils occur. Aspiration pneumonia may result after inhalation of ingesta through the paralyzed larynx. Paralysis of the lips occasionally accompanies the other signs.

Pigs

Early signs include squealing as though in pain, mild diarrhea, grinding of the teeth, and salivation. The disease is usually a prolonged one and listlessness, anorexia, and loss of weight develop followed by muscle tremor, incoordination, partial or complete blindness, enlargement of the carpal joints, and disinclination to stand on the front feet. Convulsive seizures occur in the terminal stages.

CLINICAL PATHOLOGY

Hematology

In chronic lead poisoning, hematologic examination may reveal a normocytic, normochromic anemia in some, and, although basophilic stippling does not occur often enough to be diagnostic, it is recorded in some experimental poisonings.[3] It is recorded as occurring in lead-exposed pigs and a horse. In some, poikilocytosis and anisocytosis were marked. The CSF is approximately normal with slightly elevated leukocyte numbers but no increase in protein or other biochemical components.

Blood Lead

Whole-blood levels are generally the best sample for determining the lead status of the animal. Bovine blood lead reference materials are available and have been certified for many years. Whole-blood levels of lead in normal ruminants are usually below 0.05 to 0.25 ppm; poisoned animals, including horses, usually have levels above 0.35 ppm and deaths begin at 1.0 ppm.[1,3,4] Buffalo may have blood levels above 1.0 ppm and still survive, which suggests that they have a higher tolerance level than cattle. Blood lead concentrations also fluctuate markedly after administration of lead and, consequently, the clinical importance of blood lead concentrations is often questionable and a diagnosis based on this single determinant is equivocal.

Blood lead concentration also has limited value for assessing the effectiveness of therapy for lead poisoning. Blood level concentrations may change rapidly during chelation therapy, often decreasing by 50% or more within 24 hours after initiation of treatment despite certain body tissues still containing high concentrations of lead. Thus the evaluation of biochemical indicators such as **aminolevulinic acid dehydratase (ALA-D)** may be useful. The blood and liver levels of fetuses from pregnant cattle with lead poisoning may be higher than what are considered toxic levels in adults, which suggests concentration in the fetus.

Milk Lead

Only limited information is available on the concentrations of lead that occur in cattle affected with field cases of lead poisoning. Lead levels of 0.13 mg/L of milk have occurred in natural cases with a half-life of 4.6 days. The regulatory limit for lead in bovine milk in the Netherlands is 0.05 mg/L milk. In acute lead poisoning in lactating buffalo pastured near smelters in India, the lead concentrations in milk were 1.13 ppm compared with 0.24 ppm in the milk from buffalo in unpolluted areas. The mean lead concentrations in the forage of poisoned animals were 706 ± 73.0 ppm, compared with the unpolluted area of 78 ± 12 ppm.

Fecal Lead

Fecal levels of lead represent unabsorbed and excreted lead deriving from the bones, and are of limited value unless considered in conjunction with blood levels because ingested lead may have been in an insoluble form and harmless to the animal. When fecal levels are high, it can be assumed that the lead has been ingested in the preceding 2 to 3 weeks, but high blood levels may be maintained for months after ingestion. Thus high blood and low fecal levels indicate that the lead was taken in some weeks previously, but high blood and high fecal levels suggest recent ingestion and significant absorption.

Urinary Lead

Urine lead levels are variable, rarely high (0.2–0.3 mg/L), and although elevated urine levels are usually associated with high blood levels, this relationship does not necessarily hold.

δ-ALA-D

Because of some of the limitations of blood lead, other indirect measurements of lead poisoning, such as the levels of δ-ALA-D in blood, are used to supplement blood lead determinations. For example, the best method of detecting the presence of lead poisoning in its early stages, except in the horse, is the estimation of δ-ALA-D in the blood. The evaluation of δ-ALA-D and blood lead concentrations together can assist in resolving diagnostic situations in which the blood lead concentration is in the questionable range of 0.25 to 0.35 ppm.

δ-ALA-D is important in the synthesis of heme and is probably the most sensitive enzyme in the heme pathway. Inhibition of the enzyme results in a block in the utilization of δ-ALA, a subsequent decline in heme synthesis and a marked increase in the urinary excretion of δ-ALA.[17] In cattle, sheep, and pigs affected with chronic lead poisoning, the plasma levels of δ-ALA-D are decreased, and the urinary levels of δ-ALA are increased before clinical signs are detectable. In sheep, erythrocyte δ-ALA-D is recommended as the most sensitive diagnostic test available.

The disadvantages of the assay for blood δ-ALA-D include age-related variations, particularly in calves[12,18]; the methods used for analysis are not yet uniform and blood must be collected in polystyrene or polyethylene tubes rather than glass tubes and an anticoagulant other than ethylenediaminetetraacetic acid (EDTA) must be used. The levels of δ-ALA-D increase in calves from birth to 10 weeks of age and age-matched controls should be evaluated simultaneously when conducting the test in calves of younger than 6 months of age. In cattle under 1 year of age, δ-ALA-D values of less than 200 mmol of porphobilinogen (PBG)/mL of RBC/h should raise suspicion of their having ingested lead. In this same age range values below 100 mmol would confirm ingestion of lead. In cattle equal to or less than 2 years of age, values of δ-ALA-D of less than 100 mmol of PBG/mL of RBC/h would indicate ingestion of lead.

The dδ-ALA-D is so sensitive to lead that it remains inhibited even after lead exposure has ceased. Following treatment with a chelating agent the blood lead levels will often decline giving a false indication of a positive treatment effect. If the δ-ALA-D levels do not decrease following therapy, it indicates that there is sufficient lead present to continue to suppress the enzyme.

Erythrocyte Protoporphyrin

The levels of free erythrocyte zinc protoporphyrin increase in lead poisoning, and this is indicative of the chronic metabolic effect of lead on the erythroid cells being released from bone marrow into the peripheral circulation. A mean value of 22 μg coproporphyrin per 100 mL of erythrocytes has been determined. It may be of some value along with determinations of blood lead and δ-ALA-D. The use of δ-ALA-D activity and erythrocyte protoporphyrin content as cumulative lead exposure indicators in cows environmentally exposed to lead is recommended.

Plasma δ-Aminolevulinic Acid

In human beings, δ-ALA is suggested as a sensitive marker of trace exposures to lead.[18] Plasma δ-aminolevulinic acid has been evaluated in cattle as a biomarker for acute lead poisoning and the results showed it to be a promising tool.[2,18] Further work is necessary, however, to establish concentrations in unexposed, intermittently exposed, and chronically exposed animals.

NECROPSY FINDINGS

In most acute cases there are no gross lesions at necropsy. In cases of longer standing there may be some degree of abomasitis and enteritis, diffuse congestion of the lungs, and degeneration of the liver and kidney. Epicardial hemorrhages are common. Congestion of meningeal and cerebral vessels may also be observed and hemorrhages may be present in the meninges. An increase in CSF is often recorded but is of minor degree in most cases.

In chronic cases, gross lesions in cattle include cerebrocortical softening, cavitation, and yellow discoloration with the most severe lesions in the occipital lobes. Histologic lesions were most severe at the tips of the gyri. Similar lesions were produced experimentally. Acid-fast inclusion bodies deep in the renal cortex have diagnostic significance. Examination of the contents of the reticulum in ruminants for particulate lead matter is essential. Flakes of paint, lumps of red lead, or sheet lead usually accumulate in this site. Their absence is not remarkable, especially if animals have licked fresh paint, but their presence does give weight to the provisional diagnosis.

Liver and Kidney Lead

The submission of alimentary tract contents and tissues for analysis forms an important part of the diagnosis of lead poisoning, but results must be interpreted with caution.

Cattle

In the kidney cortex 25 mg/kg (ppm) of lead wet weight (WW) is diagnostic and is a more reliable tissue for assay than liver, which may contain 10 to 20 mg/kg WW. The concentrations in the kidney are always much higher than in the liver. A diagnostic laboratory found mean levels in livers of poisoned cattle of 93 μg/g WW, and 438 μg/g WW in kidneys. Tissue lead levels in cattle from industrial areas are significantly higher (liver 0.23 mg/kg WW, kidney 0.42 mg/kg WW) than in cattle from clear air zones (liver and kidney less than 0.1 mg/kg WW).

Horses

Levels of lead at 4 to 7 mg/kg (ppm) WW have been found in the livers of horses dying of chronic lead poisoning but 25 to 250 mg/kg are more likely, and 40 mg/kg WW may occur in the livers of affected pigs.

Samples for Confirmation of Diagnosis

- **Toxicology:** 50 g liver, kidney, and reticulum content (determine lead concentration)
- **Histology:** formalin-fixed cerebral cortex, kidney (light microscopy)

DIFFERENTIAL DIAGNOSIS

In all cases, the possibility of access to lead and the environmental circumstances that may arouse suspicion of other poisonings or errors in management should be considered. Estimation of the lead content of blood and feces should be performed at the earliest opportunity and tissues for necropsy specimens submitted for analysis.

Differential diagnosis list

Cattle (see Table 14-12)

- Arsenic poisoning
- *Claviceps paspali* toxicity
- Diseases resulting in blindness (hypovitaminosis A, ophthalmitis, polioencephalomalacia)
- Hypomagnesemic tetany
- Meningoencephalitis
- Nervous acetonemia

Sheep

- Enzootic ataxia caused by copper deficiency
- Enzootic muscular dystrophy
- Polyarthritis caused by bacterial infection

Horses (see Table 14-11)

- Botulism
- Equine degenerative myeloencephalopathy
- Equine motor neuron disease
- *Equisetum* spp. (horsetail toxicosis)
- Fumonisin toxicosis (equine leukoencephalomalacia)
- Hepatoencephalopathy caused by hepatotoxic plants
- Laryngeal hemiplegia
- Protozoal encephalomyelitis
- Rabies
- Viral encephalomyelitides, including West Nile virus

TREATMENT

Treatment in most animals includes supportive care, preventing further exposure to lead, surgical removal of large amounts of lead from the gastrointestinal tract, and chelation therapy. Supportive care should include the use of tranquilization for those animals with neurologic signs and intravenous fluids to prevent and treat dehydration. Chelation therapy may be used to lower blood level concentrations but may not remove it completely from tissues or affect tissue damage. Large amounts of lead left in the gastrointestinal tract before chelation may result in enhanced or increased absorption of lead. Lead mobilized from tissue sites during chelation may transiently increase blood lead levels and exacerbate clinical signs.

Calcium Versenate

Calcium versenate (calcium disodium EDTA [CaEDTA]) has been used successfully in cases of lead poisoning produced experimentally in calves and in natural cases in cattle and horses.[3,4,14] Cattle may be treated with 73.3 mg/kg/day slow intravenously divided two to three times a day for 3 to 5 days.[19] If necessary, after a rest period of 2 days, an additional 3 to 5 days of treatment may be used. Other doses and dosage regimens are available.[14,19] Horses may be treated with CaEDTA at 75 mg/kg BW divided two to three times a day by slow intravenous infusion for 4 to 5 days.[4,19] If necessary, after a rest period of 2 days, an additional 4 to 5 days of therapy may be used.

The disadvantages of CaEDTA is that it must be given intravenously and there are side effects. Renal and gastrointestinal toxicity may occur with long-term therapy, and essential minerals such as copper and iron may be removed with multiple treatments.[3] Severe neurologic signs and dyspnea occurred in a horse receiving a second round of CaEDTA therapy.[4]

Succimer (Dimercaptosuccinic Acid)

Dimercaptosuccinic acid has been used for many years in human medicine as a specific chelator for arsenic, lead, and mercury. Published doses are available for dogs, cats, and birds but not large animals.[19] Succimer has the advantages of heavy metal specificity, oral administration, and lack of nephrotoxicity.[3]

Thiamine Hydrochloride

When used in combination with CaEDTA, thiamine is a valuable agent for the treatment of lead poisoning. Thiamine hydrochloride reduced the deposition of lead in most tissues, especially liver, kidney, and the central and peripheral nervous system of experimentally poisoned calves. The recommended dose is 2 mg/kg BW intramuscularly, given at the same time as CaEDTA, with a total daily dose not to exceed 8 mg/kg BW.[19]

Magnesium Sulfate

Oral dosing with small amounts of magnesium sulfate has been used on the basis that soluble lead salts will be precipitated as the insoluble sulfate and excreted in the feces.[14] However, the lead is often present in large quantities and in the form of particles, which are only slowly dissolved.

Rumenotomy

Rumenotomy to remove the ingested lead has been used but may be unsatisfactory because of the difficulty in removing particulate material from the recesses of the reticular mucosa. However, it may be appropriate when a valuable animal is affected and it is known that the animal ingested a certain compound of lead, which may be removable from the reticulum and rumen.

TREATMENT AND CONTROL

Cattle

- Calcium versenate (73 mg/kg/day slow IV divided two to three times a day for 3–5 days. Rest × 2 days. Repeat 4–5 days of therapy if need be) (R-2)
- Thiamine HCl (2 mg/kg BW IM, given at the same time as CaEDTA; max 8 mg/kg BW/day) (R-2)

Horses

- Calcium versenate (75 mg/kg BW divided two to three times a day slow IV for 4–5 days. Rest × 2 days. Repeat 4–5 days of therapy if need be) (R-2)
- Thiamine HCl (2 mg/kg BW IM, given at the same time as CaEDTA; max 8 mg/kg BW/day) (R-2)

BW, body weight; CaEDTA, calcium disodium ethylenediaminetetraacetic acid; IM, intramuscular; IV, intravenous.

CONTROL

The following practices are recommended to reduce the incidence of lead poisoning:

- Limit grazing on pastures near lead mines, smelters, or battery recycling depots.
- Use phosphate rock treatment on contaminated pastures (phosphate salts bind to lead yielding low solubility lead phosphates).[4]
- Keep trash out of pastures.
- Do not burn wood or other substances in pastures, and keep animals away from ashes.
- Provide adequate nutrition and consistent feeding practices to minimize pica or abnormal feeding behavior in livestock.
- Consider temporarily adding calcium phosphate to the diet to decrease lead absorption.[4]
- Dispose of or store used lead batteries, motor oil, and leaded petroleum products in areas animals cannot access.

- Use vehicle service and machinery storage areas separate from areas used by livestock.
- Use only lead-free paints on fencing, boards, and buildings.
- Dispose of contaminated carcasses according to Environmental Protection Agency regulations.
- Identify the source of lead intoxication.

FURTHER READING

Radostits O, et al. *Veterinary Medicine: A Textbook of the Disease of Cattle, Horses, Sheep, Goats and Pigs*. 10th ed. London: W.B. Saunders; 2007:1799.

REFERENCES

1. Varga A, et al. *Vet Med Res Rep*. 2012;3:111.
2. Roegner A, et al. *Vet Med Res*. 2013;4:11.
3. Puschner B, et al. *Equine Vet Educ*. 2010;22:526.
4. Allen KJ. *Equine Vet Educ*. 2010;22:182.
5. Mavangira V, et al. *J Am Vet Med Assoc*. 2008;233:955.
6. Sharpe RT, et al. *Vet Rec*. 2006;159:71.
7. Krametter-Froetscher R, et al. *Vet J*. 2007;174:99.
8. Burren BG, et al. *Aust Vet J*. 2010;88:240.
9. Swarup D, et al. *Small Rum Res*. 2006;63:309.
10. Madejón P, et al. *Ecotoxicology*. 2009;18:417.
11. Bischoff K, et al. *J Med Toxicol*. 2010;6:185.
12. Rodríguez-Estival J, et al. *Environ Pollution*. 2012;160:118.
13. Yabe J, et al. *Environ Toxicol Chem*. 2011;30:1892.
14. Aslani MR, et al. *Iran J Vet Sci Technol*. 2012;4:47.
15. Miranda M, et al. *J Vet Med Ser A*. 2006;53:305.
16. Finnie JW, et al. *Austr Vet J*. 2011;89:247.
17. Reis LSLS, et al. *J Med Medical Sci*. 2010;1:560.
18. Kang HG, et al. *J Vet Diagn Invest*. 2010;22:903.
19. Plumb DC. Edetate calcium disodium; thiamine. In: Plumb DC, ed. *Veterinary Drug Handbook*. 7th ed. Ames, IA: Wiley-Blackwell; 2011:366, 970.

MERCURY TOXICOSIS

SYNOPSIS

Etiology Ingestion, inhalation, or dermal exposure to mercury compounds including fungicides, phenylmercury treated grain, contaminated ashes, etc.

Epidemiology Generally organic preparations used in seed grain fed accidentally to livestock.

Clinical pathology High levels of mercury in all tissues; elevated serum urea nitrogen and creatinine concentration; decreased osmolarity, glycosuria, proteinuria, and phosphaturia.

Lesions
- Inorganic salts: acute, gastroenteritis; chronic, nephrosis.
- Organomercurials: neuronal necrosis in brain and spinal nerves.

Diagnostic confirmation High blood, urine, tissue, hair levels of mercury.

Treatment Supportive and symptomatic care; judicious use of chelation in acute cases; treatment of chronic intoxication generally unrewarding.

Control Care in the handling of agricultural and pharmaceutical mercury compounds.

ETIOLOGY

Mercury is a naturally occurring element (heavy metal) that occurs in three different forms.[1] Metallic mercury, an environmental pollutant, comes from sources such as mining, smelting, fossil fuels, volcanoes, and forest fires.[2] It is used in a variety of products including thermometers, button batteries, barometers, and dental fillings. Inorganic mercury (mercury salts) is produced when mercury is combined with a salt such as sulfur or chlorine. Fungicides, disinfectants, antiseptics, and older anthelmintics may contain inorganic mercurial compounds. Organic mercury (organomercurials) is formed when mercury combines carbon to form, among others, methylmercury, ethylmercury, and phenylmercury.

EPIDEMIOLOGY

Occurrence

Stringent state and national standards have made mercury poisoning in animals a rare occurrence. Toxicosis, when it occurs, is most often associated with oral ingestion of an organic mercury compound. In general, this is chronic and caused by accumulation of grain contaminated with mercury in the form of phenylmercury.[3] Acute or chronic poisoning can occur from either inorganic or organic mercury compounds but is generally accidental in nature.[4]

Because of the availability of fungicidal agents other than mercury it is possible to limit the use of mercuric agents by legislation to those excreted rapidly by animals, the phenylmercury compounds, and prohibit those that are most highly retained in animal tissues, the ethyl and methyl compounds.[5] Worldwide use of mercurial fungicides has declined, and poisoning is much less common than in the past. The most common products, when used, are dusts of 5.25% methoxyethylmercury silicate or methylmercury dicyandiamide. These and ethylmercuric chloride are toxic when fed to pigs at the rate of 0.19 to 0.7 6 mg of mercury per kilogram BW per day for 60 to 90 days. Methylmercury dicyandiamide fed to pigs at the rate of 5 to 15 mg/kg is associated with illness, and 20 mg/kg is associated with some deaths with a delay of 3 weeks between dosing and illness.

Treated seed is usually not harmful if it comprises only 10% of the ration and must be fed in large amounts for long periods before clinical illness occurs. A single feeding even of large amounts of grain is thought to be incapable of causing mercury poisoning in ruminants, but horses may be susceptible.

Accidental administration of medicines containing mercury, licking of skin dressings (e.g., mercuric oxide), and absorption from liberally applied skin dressings or combined with dimethyl sulfoxide may be associated with sporadic cases that may occur in horses after application of mercury-containing "blisters." Inorganic mercury salts contaminating lakes or other anaerobic ecologic areas can be reduced and converted to methylmercury and serve as a source of organic mercurial poisoning or food contamination through accumulation in fish or fish meal.

Risk Factors

Animal Risk Factors

The toxicity of mercury compounds depends on their solubility and the susceptibility of the animals. Cattle are highly susceptible, with toxicosis occurring on an average daily intake of mercury, in organic mercury form, of 10 mg/kg BW/day, whereas toxic effects are only obtained in sheep with intakes of 17.4 mg/kg BW/day. In horses, the acute toxic dose inorganic mercury is 5 to 10 g.[5] Chronic ingestion of inorganic mercuric chloride (0.8 g/kg BW/day) for 14 weeks resulted in mercury toxicity.[5]

Human Risk Factors

Meat, liver, and kidneys from animals poisoned by mercury are unsuitable for human consumption. Depending on the form of mercury, milk may not be safe.

PATHOGENESIS

The toxicokinetics of mercury depends on the form and route of exposure. Metallic mercury is primarily absorbed through the respiratory tract with very little by ingestion.[1] It is lipophilic and once distributed to the kidneys it crosses both the blood-brain and placental barriers in which it can remain for extended periods of time. Excretion is via urine and feces and a small amount in milk. Inorganic mercury has limited gastrointestinal absorption (<40%), is not lipophilic, is distributed to several body organs, and accumulates in the kidney.[5] Excretion is via urine and feces with very small amounts in the milk. Organic mercury is almost completely absorbed from the gastrointestinal tract (90%–95%). It is rapidly distributed to the circulatory system, is lipophilic, and crosses both the blood-brain and placental barriers in which it is trapped and accumulates in the brain and fetus, accumulates in RBCs, and undergoes further distribution to body tissues, reaching equilibrium in approximately 4 days. Excretion is very slow and primarily fecal, although some urine and milk excretion occurs.

The mechanism of action relates to the specific form of mercury. Metallic mercury and organic mercury accumulate in the brain and are potent neurotoxicants.[1,5,6] Toxicity from methylmercury is multifactorial. It inhibits protein synthesis in the brain by interfering with aminoacyl tRNA synthetase enzymes, generates excess free radicals, and inhibits antioxidant enzymes resulting in cell death. All forms of mercury accumulate in the kidney, concentrating in the proximal renal tubular cells, producing cell membrane permeability, excess free radical formation, inhibition of antioxidant enzymes, and induction of glutathione and glutathione-dependent enzymes.[1,5] Acute toxicity results in acute tubular necrosis and renal failure; chronic toxicity results in renal interstitial fibrosis and renal failure.[5]

CLINICAL FINDINGS

The toxic effects of mercury depend on the form, route of exposure, dose, and duration of exposure.[1,5] The target organs of both inorganic and organic mercury are the brain and kidney, and this is where the most damage occurs.[1,6,7]

Acute inorganic mercury toxicosis occurs when large amounts of inorganic mercury are ingested. There is an acute gastroenteritis with vomiting of bloodstained material and severe diarrhea.[4] Death occurs within a few hours from shock and dehydration. In less acute cases the patient survives several days. The syndrome includes salivation, a fetid breath, anorexia, oliguria, tachycardia, hyperpnea, and, in some cases, posterior paralysis and terminal convulsions.

Chronic inorganic mercury toxicosis occurs when small amounts of inorganic mercury are ingested over longer periods. Damage to the kidney and nervous system in addition to the gastrointestinal tract is likely to occur.[4] Signs include depression, anorexia, emaciation, a stiff, stilted gait that may progress to paresis, alopecia, scabby lesions around the anus and vulva, pruritus, petechiation and tenderness of the gums and shedding of the teeth, persistent diarrhea, weakness, incoordination, and convulsions.

Chronic organic mercurial poisoning is associated with neurologic syndromes.[4,5] In pigs blindness is accompanied by staggering, gait instabilities, lameness, recumbency, and inability to eat, although the appetite is good. Cattle poisoned in this way show ataxia, neuromuscular incoordination, paresis, recumbency, convulsions, evidence of renal failure, and death. Clinical signs may not develop until 20 days after feeding is commenced. Sheep are similar to cattle, although signs of tetraplegia may occur. Horses show renal disease, neurologic abnormalities, colic, and laminitis.

CLINICAL PATHOLOGY

Mercury can be detected at higher levels than normal in the blood, urine, feces, milk, tissues, and hair of affected animals and in the toxic source material.[1,4,8] Urine is the best source for metallic and inorganic mercury and hair for organic mercury. Generally, blood is useful only for the first 3 to 5 days postexposure as distributed to other tissues occurs.[1] Creatinine and serum urea nitrogen concentrations will be elevated and urinalysis may show reduced osmolarity, glycosuria, proteinuria, and phosphaturia. Less than 0.2% of ingested mercury is excreted in cow's milk.

NECROPSY FINDINGS

In acute cases, there is severe gastroenteritis with edema, hyperemia, and petechiation of the alimentary mucosa. The liver and kidneys are swollen, and the lungs are congested and show multiple hemorrhages. There may be an accompanying catarrhal stomatitis. A crusting focus of dermatitis may be identified if exposure was percutaneous.

Histologically, the renal tubular epithelial cells are swollen and vacuolated, and proteinuria is evident. An ulcerative colitis may also be visible. In chronic toxicity associated with organic mercury compounds there are also degenerative changes in nerve cells in the cortex of the cerebrum, brainstem, and spinal cord. The lesions include neuronal necrosis, neuronophagia, cortical vacuolation, and gliosis. Fibrinoid necrosis of leptomeningeal arterioles may be seen. Other common microscopic changes include degeneration of granular cells of the cerebellar cortex and of Purkinje cells of the myocardium.

Mercury reaches its greatest concentration in the kidney, and this tissue should be submitted for assay. In horses with acute mercury toxicosis, renal tissue with mercury at more than 10 μg/g of mercury is diagnostic.[4] Concentrations of 100 mg/kg may be present in the kidney of animals poisoned with inorganic mercury. With chronic organic mercurial poisoning in swine, levels of mercury up to 2000 mg/kg may be present in the kidney.

Samples for Confirmation of Diagnosis

- **Toxicology:** 50 g kidney, brain is half fresh and half in formalin, 500 g of suspect feed (ASSAY [Hg]); muscle tissue for potential residues in food animal edible tissues
- **Histology:** formalin-fixed kidney, heart, oral and/or skin lesions; half of midsagittally sectioned brain (LM)

DIFFERENTIAL DIAGNOSIS

Differential diagnosis list
- Arsenic toxicosis (especially organic arsenicals in swine)
- Lead toxicosis

TREATMENT

Treatment should be aimed toward removal of the source and providing supportive care. Activated charcoal followed by mineral oil or another laxative should be used in acute cases. Further care includes intravenous fluids to enhance hydration, promote excretion, and correct electrolyte abnormalities, gastrointestinal protectants, and pain medications. Antioxidants, including selenium, have been used in human beings.[9]

There is no true antidote, and the use of chelation agents is controversial. In acute toxicity in horses, intramuscular dimercaprol (BAL) at 3 mg/kg BW every 4 hours × 2 days, followed by 3 mg/kg BW every 6 hours on day 3, and then 3 mg/kg BW twice a day × 10 days has been used.[4] Penicillamine, 3 mg/kg BW orally every 6 hours has also been used effectively.[4] In cattle and swine, intramuscular dimercaprol at 3 mg/kg BW every 6 hours for 4 days, followed by every 12 hours for 10 days has been recommended.[10]

CONTROL

Seed grains dusted with mercury compounds should not be fed to animals.

FURTHER READING

Graeme MD, et al. Heavy metal toxicity, part I: arsenic and mercury. *J Emerg Med.* 1988;16:45-56.
Neathery MW, Miller WJ. Metabolism and toxicity of cadmium, mercury, and lead in animals: a review. *J Dairy Sci.* 1975;58:1767.
Radostits O, et al. Mercury poisoning. In: *Veterinary Medicine: A Textbook of the Disease of Cattle, Horses, Sheep, Goats and Pigs.* 10th ed. London: W.B. Saunders; 2007:1814.

REFERENCES

1. Bernhoft RA. *J Environ Public Health.* 2012;2012:460-508.
2. Krametter-Froetscher R, et al. *Vet J.* 2007;174:99.
3. Bilandzic N, et al. *Food Addit Contam.* 2010;2:172.
4. Schmitz DB. *Vet Clin North Am Equine Pract.* 2007;23:677.
5. Raikwar MK, et al. *Vet World.* 2008;1:28.
6. Chen C, et al. *Sci Total Environ.* 2006;366:627.
7. Chen C, et al. *Environ Health Perspect.* 2006;114:297.
8. Rudy M, et al. *Med Weter.* 2007;63:1303-1306.
9. Shukla SV, et al. *Tox Int.* 2007;14:67.
10. Plumb DC. Dimercaprol. In: Plumb DC, ed. *Veterinary Drug Handbook.* 7th ed. Ames, IA: Wiley-Blackwell; 2011:220.

BORON TOXICOSIS

Boron, an essential element for plant growth, is added to many agricultural fertilizers and presents yet another toxic chemical in the list of farm hazards for animals. Boron compounds such as boric acid or sodium borate are generally of low toxicity and reports of poisoning in cattle rare. In some fertilizers, a solubilized form of boron is used to increase availability thus increasing its toxicity and palatability. Cattle accidentally ingesting a boron-containing fertilizer developed depression, weakness, tremor, and ataxia; other reported signs include short periods of gait spasticity, dorsiflexion of the head, and flutter of the periorbicular muscles, followed by stumbling backward and sternal recumbency, then lateral recumbency, and a quiet death. The case–fatality rate is 100%. There are no gross lesions on necropsy examination.

Experimental dosing with the fertilizer in goats is associated with the previously mentioned syndrome plus head-shaking, ear-flicking, star-gazing (staring), phantom dodging, oral champing, restless weight shifting from foot to foot, sawhorse stance, mild diarrhea, and frequent urination. The goats do not eat or drink but paw food and water as though they are hungry but unable to prehend.

FURTHER READING

Radostits O, et al. *Veterinary Medicine: A Textbook of the Disease of Cattle, Horses, Sheep, Goats and Pigs*. 10th ed. London: W.B. Saunders; 2007:1830.

Sisk DBB, et al. Acute, fatal illness in cattle exposed to boron fertilizer. *J Am Vet Med Assoc*. 1988;193: 943-946.

BROMIDE TOXICOSIS

Bromide salts are available in several forms including sodium bromide, potassium bromide, and methyl bromide.[1-3] Potassium bromide has been added to horse feed and studied in horses for treatment of epilepsy.[1,2] Sodium bromide is commonly used in swimming pools as an alternative to chlorine and in the petroleum industry around oil wells. Methyl bromide is a soil fumigant once commonly used worldwide. Because of its effect on the ozone layer, a planned phase out of methyl bromide will be complete in 2015.[3]

Ingestion of methyl bromide–contaminated oat hay by horses, goats, and cattle and sodium bromide–pelleted feed by cattle has resulted in toxicosis. Clinical signs are neurologic in nature and include ataxia, weakness, and lethargy.

FURTHER READING

Knight HD, Costner GC. Bromide intoxication of horses, goats, and cattle. *J Am Vet Med Assoc*. 1977;171:446.

Knight HD, Reina-Guerra M. Intoxication of cattle with sodium bromide-contaminated feed. *Am J Vet Res*. 1977;38:407.

Lynn G, et al. Grain fumigant residues, occurrence of bromides in the milk of cows fed sodium bromide and grain fumigated with methyl bromide. *J Agric Food Chem*. 1963;11:87-91.

REFERENCES

1. Peacock RE, et al. *Aust Vet J*. 2013;91:320.
2. Raidal SL, et al. *Aust Vet J*. 2008;86:187.
3. Ruzo LO. *Pest Manag Sci*. 2006;62:99.

ORGANIC TOXINS AFFECTING THE NERVOUS SYSTEM

ANTHELMINTIC TOXICOSIS

Anthelmintics are drugs used to treat infections with parasitic worms. This includes both flat worms (e.g., flukes and tapeworms) and round worms (i.e., nematodes). Poisoning associated with most of the newer anthelmintics is rare and usually caused by an accidental overdose in individual animals or a mixing error when added to feed. Older anthelmintics carry the burden of higher toxicity, but fortunately their use has declined dramatically.

COMMONLY USED ANTHELMINTICS

Commonly used anthelmintics include the following groups:

- Amino-acetonitrile derivatives (monepantel)
- Benzimidazoles and probenzimidazoles (albendazole, fenbendazole, etc.)
- Cyclic octadepsipeptides (emodepside)
- Imidazothiazoles (levamisole)
- Macrocyclic lactones ([MLs] ivermectin, moxidectin, doramectin)
- Miscellaneous (Piperazine, clorsulon)
- Praziquantel/epsiprantel
- Salicylanilides/substituted phenols (closantel, rafoxanide, oxyclozanide)
- Tetrahydropyrimidines (pyrantel and morantel)

OLDER ANTHELMINTICS

Older, rarely used anthelmintics include:

- Carbon tetrachloride
- Hexachloroethane
- Hexachlorophene
- Nicotine
- Phenothiazines
- Sumicidin (fenvalerate)
- Tetrachlorethylene

CURRENTLY USED ANTHELMINTICS

Amino-Acetonitrile Derivatives (Monepantel)

Amino-acetonitrile derivatives (ADD) are a group of synthetic compounds with activity against intestinal nematodes. Anthelmintics in this group work by binding to an MPTL-1, nematode-specific acetylcholine receptor.[1] Monepantel, an ADD, was originally marketed in New Zealand as a drench for sheep, but it is now used in Australia, South America, Europe, and other countries.[1,2] Oral administration to sheep at 5× the recommended dose every 3 weeks × 8 treatments did not result in any adverse effects.[1] No adverse effects were noted in ewes when given 3× the recommended dose every 5 days for their entire reproductive cycle.[2]

Benzimidazoles (Albendazole, Fenbendazole, and Thiabendazole) and Probenzimidazoles (Febantel, Netobimin, etc.)

The benzimidazoles are generally not water soluble and thus poorly absorbed from the gastrointestinal tract. Probenzimidazoles must be absorbed and metabolized into their respective active compounds. The mechanism of action of this group is inhibition of parasitic β-tubulin, which generally makes them safe drugs.[3] Many of them, however, are contraindicated in pregnancy because of antimitotic activity with resultant embryo toxicity and teratogenicity.[3,4]

Albendazole, Cambendazole, and Parbendazole

Albendazole at four times the standard dose produces some fetal abnormalities if given early in pregnancy. Cambendazole and parbendazole are teratogens and are specifically contraindicated in pregnant animals, especially during the first third of the pregnancy and at dose rates higher than normal. The safety margin is small, and their use at any dose level is not recommended in these females. Defects produced include rotational and flexing deformities of the limbs, overflexion of the carpal joints, abnormalities of posture and gait, vertebral fusion and asymmetric cranial ossification, cerebral hypoplasia, and hydrocephalus.

Fenbendazole

A dose of fenbendazole and the flukicide bromsalans to cattle either simultaneously or within a few days of each other may be accompanied by deaths. Because fenbendazole and the other tertiary benzimidazoles, oxfendazole and albendazole, are extremely valuable in removing dormant *Ostertagia ostertagi* larvae, it is suggested that Fascol (bromsalans) should not be used when this is an important problem or if 2 weeks should elapse between treatments.

Thiabendazole

At an oral dose rate of 800 mg/kg BW in sheep, transient signs of salivation, anorexia, and depression appear. There are similar signs at larger dose rates, and death is likely at a dose rate of 1200 mg/kg BW. Toxic nephrosis is the cause of death and is reflected in the clinical and pathologic findings of hypokalemia, hypoproteinemia, and uremia.

Cyclic Octadepsipeptides (Emodepside)

Currently emodepside is the only commercially available member of this group, and it is registered in the United States and Europe for use in dogs and cats.[1] It has been used experimentally in sheep and cattle and found to be effective and safe.[1,5] Anthelmintics in the groups have a dual mechanism of action, binding to a SLO-1, calcium-activated potassium channel SLO-1 and binding to am HC110R, latrophilin-like receptor. The result is inhibition of pharyngeal muscle activity in parasites resulting in death.[1,5]

Imidazothiazoles (Levamisole)

All commercial preparations of levamisole consist of the levo isomer. Its mechanism of action is similar to nicotine by causing prolonged depolarization and neuromuscular junction blockade resulting in parasympathetic stimulation and cholinergic type signs.[6,7] The absorption of levamisole is rapid regardless of the route of administration. Elimination is rapid with an elimination half-life of 2.34 hours (intramuscularly) and 5.44 hours (orally) in sheep, 1.44 hours (orally) in goats, and 6.9 hours (intramuscularly) and 9.3 hours (orally) in swine.[8]

There are some human health implications because levamisole may be found in meat, milk, and cheese especially in toxic situations. The withdrawal period of sheep is 13 days, goats 9 days, swine 11 days, and beef and milk from dairy cows 48 hours.[8] A recent study involving six dairy cows receiving levamisole at 5 mg/kg BW and oxyclozanide at 10 mg/kg BW showed levamisole residues greater than 0.83 µg/kg for the first 10 milkings and concentration of levamisole residues in soft, hard, and whey cheeses.[9]

Accidental injection of pigs caused vomiting, salivation, ataxia, recumbency, and a high mortality within a few minutes of injection. In pigs, concurrent treatment with levamisole and pyrantel tartrate resulted in enhanced toxicity of the levamisole.[6]

Sheep accidentally receiving a double dose of levamisole as a drench developed depression, head-shaking, muscle tremors, spastic movements, and diarrhea.[7] Levamisole used during the breeding season has an adverse effect on the semen quality in rams when used as an anthelmintic and on pregnancy in ewes when used as an immunomodulatory agent.[10]

Double doses in goats produce mild depression and ptosis, whereas higher doses produce, in addition, head-shaking, twitching of facial muscles, grinding of teeth, salivation, tail-twitching, increased micturition, and straining.

Following treatment at standard doses, some cattle show signs of lip-licking, increased salivation, head-shaking, skin tremors, and excitability. The excitability is more marked in calves; when released they tend to raise their tails and run around the paddock. Coughing may commence within 15 to 20 minutes, but this is from the death and expulsion of lung worms and stops in 24 hours. With higher doses, the signs are more pronounced, defecation is frequent, and hyperesthesia in the form of a continuous twitching of the skin may be seen.

Macrocyclic Lactones (Ivermectin, Moxidectin, and Doramectin)

Macrocyclic lactones are insecticides, acaricides, and nematicides in a number of species and are covered in a separate chapter.

Miscellaneous (Piperazine and Clorsulon)

Piperazine

Piperazine acts to block neuromuscular transmission in the parasite resulting in flaccid paralysis and rapid expulsion of parasites. Piperazine should not be used in animals with a heavy parasite load, in particular foals, because it may result in an ascarid-impaction colic or intestinal perforation.

Piperazine compounds are relatively nontoxic but poisoning can occur in horses on normal or excessive doses. Signs follow a delay of 12 to 24 hours and include incoordination, pupillary dilation, hyperesthesia, tremor, somnolence, and either swaying while at rest or lateral recumbency. Recovery follows in 48 to 72 hours without treatment.

Clorsulon

Clorsulon is a sulfonamide used primarily in the treatment of liver flukes in cattle and sheep. It has a high margin of safety and few reports of toxicosis. Infected sheep treated with 100 mg/kg showed no adverse effects and neither did uninfected sheep treated with 200 mg/kg and 400 mg/kg. No acute toxic dose is recorded for cattle, although cows treated with 25× the label dose showed no changes in weight gain or feed consumption.[11] Uninfected goats treated with 35 mg/kg every other day for three doses showed no adverse effects.[11] Clorsulon is distributed to muscle and secreted into milk so appropriate precautions need to be taken both with normal use and in overdose situations.

Praziquantel/Epsiprantel

Praziquantel and epsiprantel are effective against cestode parasites in most species of animals and humans.[12] Both products have a wide margin of safety, and reports of toxicity in large animals are scarce.

Salicylanilides/Substituted Phenols (Closantel, Rafoxanide, and Oxyclozanide)

Closantel, rafoxanide, and oxyclozanide are halogenated salicylanilides effective against *Fasciola* spp. in sheep and have approximately the same low level of toxicity if dosed appropriately. They are capable of causing CNS signs including temporary or permanent blindness if overdosed, especially in small rumianants.[13,14] Overdosed sheep and goats developed retinal lesions characterized by necrosis, loss of the photoreceptor layer, and retinal separation.[14] Status spongiosus of the cerebral and cerebellar white matter were consistent findings at postmortem.[14]

All three drugs are highly protein bound and have very long terminal half-lives (closantel, 14.5 days; rafoxanide, 16.6 days; oxyclozanide, 6.4 days) in sheep. Associated with their use are tissue residues and the need for long withholding times.

Tetrahydropyrimidines (Pyrantel and Morantel)

Pyrantel, either as pamoate or tartrate salt, is widely used in horses and pigs and, to a lesser extent, ruminants. Morantel tartrate, the methyl ester, is more widely used in ruminants. There are two mechanisms of action.[15] The first mechanism is inhibition of fumarate reductase, whereas the second mechanism is a direct action on acetylcholine receptors at the neuromuscular junction. It is the second mechanism that is responsible for paralysis and death of the parasite.

All of these drugs have been on the market for over 30 years and are considered safe in most species studied. Pyrantel pamoate is labeled for administration to mares a month before foaling; no adverse reactions were reported when it was administered at the recommended dose to pregnant mares or breeding stallions. No adverse reactions were reported when pyrantel tartrate was administered at the recommended dose to pregnant mares or breeding stallions. Horses dosed with pyrantel tartrate at 100 mg/kg BW developed incoordination, sweating, and an increased respiratory rate. Cattle dosed at 200 mg/kg morantel tartrate (20× the recommended dose) did not exhibit any adverse effects. Morantel tartrate has a 14-day meat withdrawal in cattle, but no milk withholding time.

OLDER ANTHELMINTICS

Carbon Tetrachloride

Carbon tetrachloride is sometimes accidentally administered in excessive quantities but deaths are more common when sheep are given standard doses or cattle are dosed by mouth instead of by injection. Standard doses of 2 mL per sheep to kill adult *Fasciola hepatica* or 1 mL/10 kg BW to obtain efficacy against immature forms, have been widely used but in some circumstances these doses can be highly toxic. Doses as low as 0.5 mL/10 kg BW can be associated with liver damage in calves, and clinical effects are apparent at 1 mL/10 kg BW in goats.

Inhalation of carbon tetrachloride is associated with an immediate and acute depression of the CNS and peripheral and circulatory collapse. Diffuse pulmonary edema occurs and sheep that survive show hepatic and renal damage. Ingestion of toxic doses may result in death within 24 hours because of anesthetic depression and severe pulmonary edema, or may occur 3 to 7 days later resulting from renal and hepatic insufficiency. Deaths are associated with almost complete liver and kidney failure.

In gross overdosing or inhalation there is an immediate onset of staggering, falling, progressive narcosis, collapse, convulsions, and death caused by respiratory failure. Animals that survive this stage or, as in the most common form of carbon tetrachloride poisoning in which animals absorb insufficient dose to produce narcosis, additional signs may be manifested in 3 to 4 days. These include anorexia, depression, muscle weakness, diarrhea, and jaundice. After a further 2 to 3 days affected sheep go down and mild-to-moderate clonic convulsions may occur, but death is always preceded by a period of coma. Survivors are emaciated and weak, and may develop photosensitization or shed their wool. They are very susceptible to environmental stresses, particularly inclement weather, and isolated deaths may occur for several months.

Animals dying after inhalation of the drug show marked pulmonary, hepatic, and renal damage. Those dying of massive oral overdosing may show abomasitis and inflammation of the duodenum. In addition acute hepatic swelling, pallor, and mottling accompanied by centrilobular necrosis and fatty degeneration, and renal lesions of extensive tubular necrosis and degeneration, are observed in animals that die after the ingestion of small doses.

Hexachloroethane

Hexachloroethane is preferred to carbon tetrachloride for the treatment of fascioliasis in cattle, but it is not completely without danger. Deaths are rare (1 in 20,000) cattle treated and in sheep (1 in 40,000), but nonfatal illness is not uncommon. Susceptible groups may show narcosis, muscle tremor, and recumbency after administration of the standard dose (cattle, 15 g per 6 months of age up to a maximum of 60 g; sheep, 0.4 g/kg BW); such animals should be given half this dose on two occasions at 48-hour intervals.

Animals with large overdoses show ataxia, dullness, anorexia, dyspnea, ruminal tympany, and sometimes abdominal pain, diarrhea, and dysentery. Necropsy lesions include acute abomasitis and enteritis, edema of the abomasal mucosa, and hepatic centrilobular necrosis. Treatment with calcium borogluconate as in milk fever elicits a good response.

Hexachlorophene

At high dose rates (25–50 mg/kg BW) hexachlorophene is associated with atrophy of seminiferous epithelium of the testis of young adult rams. Repeated dosing is associated with periportal fatty changes in liver.

Nicotine

Nicotine poisoning seldom occurs in animals except in lambs and calves in which nicotine sulfate is still incorporated in some vermifuges. Doses of 0.2 to 0.3 g nicotine sulfate have been toxic for lambs weighing 14 to 20 kg. Animals in poor condition are more susceptible than well-nourished animals. Animals are affected within a few minutes of dosing and show dyspnea with rapid shallow respirations, muscle tremor and weakness, recumbency, and clonic convulsions. Animals that survive the acute episode may show abdominal pain, salivation, and diarrhea. At necropsy there may be abomasitis and inflammation of the duodenum.

Phenothiazine

Exposure to phenothiazine has occurred in the past from its extensive use as an anthelmintic. Keratitis, a noteworthy sign of poisoning, is most common in calves, rarely in pigs and goats, and usually after a heavy single dose of phenothiazine, but it can occur in a program of daily intake in a dietary premix. Phenothiazine is absorbed from the rumen as the sulfoxide, conjugated in the liver and excreted in the urine as leukophenothiazine and leukothionol. As urine is voided, further oxidation turns the metabolic products to a red-brown dye, phenothiazine and thionol, which may be confused as hematuria or hemoglobinuria.

Cattle are unable to detoxify all the sulfoxide and some escapes into the circulation and can enter the aqueous humor of the eye, causing photosensitization. Other photodynamic agents that cannot enter the eye may also be produced, and they, with the sulfoxide, are associated with photosensitization of light-colored parts of the body. Hyperlacrimation with severe blepharospasm and photophobia commences 12 to 36 hours after treatment and is followed by the development of a white opacity on the lateral or dorsal aspects of the cornea, depending on which is exposed to sunlight. Most animals recover within a few days, particularly if kept inside or in a shaded paddock. If the animals continue to be exposed, a severe conjunctivitis with keratitis may result.

Sumicidin

Sumicidin (fenvalerate) is a synthetic pyrethroid anthelmintic capable of causing nonfatal restlessness, yawning, frothing at the mouth, dyspnea, ear and tail erection, pupillary dilation, ruminal tympany, regurgitation of ruminal contents, staggering, tremor, clonic convulsions, and recumbency after a single oral dose. Single oral doses of >450 mg/kg are lethal. Repeated daily dosing (113 mg/kg BW or 225 mg/kg BW) also causes death after 5 to 15 days.

Tetrachlorethylene

Tetrachlorethylene rarely produces incoordination, which may be evident for 1 or 2 hours after dosing in cattle or sheep. Treatment is not usually necessary.

FURTHER READING

Cornwell RL, Jones RM. Controlled laboratory trials with pyrantel tartrate in cattle. *Br Vet J.* 1970;126:134-141.
Dayan AD. Albendazole, mebendazole and praziquantel. Review of non-clinical toxicity and pharmacokinetics. *Acta Trop.* 2003;86:151-159.
Delatour P, Parish R. *Benzimidazole Anthelmintics and Related Compounds: Toxicity and Evaluation of Residues.* Orlando, FL: Academic Press; 1986.
McKellar QA, Jackson F. Veterinary anthelmintics: old and new. *Trends Parasitol.* 2004;20:456.
McSherry BJ, et al. The hematology of phenothiazine poisoning in horses. *Can Vet J.* 1966;7:3.
Radostits O, et al. Poisoning by anthelmintics. In: *Veterinary Medicine: A Textbook of the Disease of Cattle, Horses, Sheep, Goats and Pigs.* 10th ed. London: W.B. Saunders; 2007:1830.
Van Cauteren H, Vandenberghe J, Hérin V, et al. Toxicological properties of closantel. *Drug Chem Toxicol.* 1985;8(3):101-123.
Von Samson-Himmelstjerna G, et al. Efficacy of two cyclooctadepsipeptides, PF1022A and emodepside, against anthelmintic-resistant nematodes in sheep and cattle. *Parasitology.* 2005;130:343-346.

REFERENCES

1. Epe N, et al. *Trends Parasitol.* 2013;29:129.
2. Malikides N, et al. *New Zeal Vet J.* 2009;57:192.
3. Danaher M, et al. *J Chromatography.* 2007;845:1.
4. Teruel M, et al. *Biocell.* 2011;35:29.
5. Crisford A, et al. *Mol Pharmacol.* 2011;79:1031.
6. Hsu WH, Martin RJ. Antiparasitic agents. In: Hsu WH, ed. *Handbook of Veterinary Pharmacology.* Ames, IA: Wiley-Blackwell; 2013:379.
7. Rahimi S, et al. *Iran J Vet Med.* 2008;6:12.
8. Zanon RB, et al. *J Vet Pharmacol Ther.* 2013;36:298.
9. Whelan M, et al. *J Agric Food Chem.* 2010;58:12204.
10. Pancarci SM, et al. *Bull Vet Inst Pulawy.* 2007;51:253.
11. Lanusse CE, et al. Anticestodal and antitrematodal drugs. In: Rivere JE, Papich MG, eds. *Veterinary Pharmacology and Therapeutics.* 9th ed. Ames, IA: Wiley-Blackwell; 2009:1095.
12. Slocombe J, et al. *Vet Parasitol.* 2007;144:366.
13. Ecco R, et al. *Vet Rec.* 2006;159:564.
14. Van der Lugt JJ, et al. *Comp Pathol.* 2007;136:87.
15. Elsheikha HM, McOrist S. Antiparasitic drugs: Mechanisms of action and resistance. In: Elsheikha HM, Khan NA, eds. *Essentials of Veterinary Parasitology.* Norfolk, UK: Caister Academic Press; 2011:87.

MACROCYCLIC LACTONE (IVERMECTIN, MOXIDECTIN, ETC.) TOXICOSIS

SYNOPSIS

Etiology Exposure to any of the macrocyclic lactone compounds including abamectin, doramectin, eprinomectin, ivermectin, and moxidectin.

Epidemiology Wide application as insecticides, nematicides, and ascaricides. Ivermectin is most popular because of safety and efficacy. Agricultural uses include miticides, ascaricide, and insecticide.

Clinical pathology Nonspecific changes in CBC and elevations in liver enzymes; increases in plasma and milk concentrations of specific compound.

Lesions Nonspecific postmortem lesions.

Diagnostic Confirmation Clinical signs, history of exposure, analysis of tissue or body fluids.

Treatment No antidote, supportive care; intravenous intralipid emulsion in individual cases.

Control Use appropriate dose for size and weight of animal; keep agricultural and crop products stored where animals cannot access them.

CBC, *complete blood count.*

ETIOLOGY

Ivermectin, the most widely recognized of the group, is a semisynthetic ML originally obtained from *Streptomyces avermitilis.*[1] It is approved for oral or injectable use as an endectocide in horses, cattle, sheep, goats, swine, and many other species but not lactating cattle, sheep, and goats.[1,2] Abamectin is a mixture of ivermectin B_{1a} and B_{1b} used primarily as an injectable product in cattle. Other ML endectocides used in livestock include doramectin (injectable and pour-on), eprinomectin (pour-on), and moxidectin (oral, injectable, pour-on).[3-7] They are also agricultural products used on crops and fields as miticides, ascaricides, and insecticides.[8]

EPIDEMIOLOGY

The MLs have a wide margin of safety in most species when used at the recommended doses and according to label directions. Clinical signs of toxicosis in all species involve neurologic dysfunction as well as some gastrointestinal disturbances.[9] Many of the case reports involve younger animals and are caused by an incomplete blood-brain barrier, failure to adequately estimate weight, or massive overdoses.[5,10] There have been case reports of adult horses developing neurologic signs when administered the recommended dose of ivermectin. These may be caused by the presence of a toxic plant, other medications, low body fat, or other physiologic reasons.

Eight-month-old Jersey bull calves receiving 600 µg/kg BW either intravenously or subcutaneously developed neurologic signs including depression, ataxia, and miosis. Calves receiving 8 mg/kg BW developed neurologic signs and became recumbent 24 hours after dosing with ivermectin.[11] Horses receiving 6 to 10 times the recommended dose of ivermectin developed ataxia, depression, and vision impairment within 24 hours of dosing. Three horses displayed classic signs of ivermectin toxicosis after receiving the normal recommended dose and consuming toxic plants in the *Solanum* family.[12]

Occurrence

Poisoning associated with MLs has been reported worldwide in a large number of animal species most often secondary to an inadvertent overdose or misuse of the product. Agricultural use of the product as a miticide, insecticide, or ascaricide opens the door to herd problems should animals be exposed to bulk quantities.

Risk Factors

Animal Risk Factors

Reports of toxicosis are most common in horses and often in foals. In general, a dosing error has occurred and the animal has received several times the recommended dose.[9,10] Signs of toxicosis have been reported with normal doses, but these often occur in conjunction with another compound or substance.[11]

Environmental Risk Factors

MLs are excreted in the feces of treated animals and may contaminate the field or act as a poison to nontarget species either directly through defecation or when manure is spread in a pasture or field.[13,14]

PATHOGENESIS

The pharmacokinetic properties of MLs depend on the dose, specific formulation, and route of administration. In general, MLs are slowly absorbed, widely distributed throughout the body to fat and liver, poorly metabolized, and excreted primarily unchanged in the feces.[1,5] Up to 90% of ivermectin and 77% of moxidectin are excreted via bile into the feces.[1,6] At normal doses they do not cross the blood-brain barrier of healthy, adult large animals, which his due primarily to action of the P-glycoprotein transporter system.[5,6] They are lipophilic, in particular moxidectin, and thus the lack of body fat may play a role in the elimination half-life and toxicity in debilitated animals.[5] In the absence of body fat, MLs concentrate in the serum and may reach levels high enough to overcome the blood-brain barrier.[5]

They exert their toxic effects by binding to GABA and glutamate-gated chloride channels. Binding to glutamate-gated chloride channels results in hyperpolarization and paralysis of the parasite's pharyngeal pump musculature.[1,5,6] Glutamate-gated chloride channels are present only in nematodes and arthropods. In animal species, GABA-gated channels are only found in the CNS and poisoning does not occur unless the P-glycoprotein transporter is overwhelmed or compromised and MLs are allowed to enter.

CLINICAL FINDINGS

Clinical signs in horses are primarily those of neurologic dysfunction.[9,10, 12,15] Intoxicated horses are ataxic and stand base wide with the head down. Muscle tremors, head-pressing, impaired vision, and facial nerve abnormalities including ptosis. have been reported. Mydriasis is commonly reported. Other signs include hyperthermia, colic, seizures, and recumbency. Similar signs have been reported in other species including cattle and pigs.[1]

NECROPSY FINDINGS

Postmortem findings are nonspecific. Tissues and body fluids (serum and milk) may be analyzed for the presence of ML compounds using high-performance lipid chromatography.[16] Gastrointestinal contents, feces, fat, and liver are the best specimens to submit for postmortem analysis.[6]

> **DIFFERENTIAL DIAGNOSIS**
>
> **Differential diagnosis list**
> - Blue-green algae toxicosis
> - Central nervous system trauma
> - Encephalitis
> - Hepatic encephalopathy
> - Organophosphorus compound or carbamate toxicosis

TREATMENT

There is no antidote for ML toxicosis and treatment is symptomatic and supportive. Activated charcoal should be administered in recent overdoses when the animal is stable; multiple doses are recommended because MLs undergo enterohepatic recirculation. Methocarbamol has been recommended for tremors, diazepam or phenobarbital for seizures, and intravenous fluids for rehydration.[9,10,12] Physostigmine is no longer recommended because of the incidence of seizures. Sarmazenil, a benzodiazepine agonist effective at GABA receptor sites, at 0.04 mg/kg BW intravenously every 2 hours × 6 doses has been used with equivocal success.[5,10]

An intravenous intralipid emulsion (ILE) containing 20% soybean oil in water has been used successfully in the treatment of ivermectin and moxidectin overdoses in dogs[17,18] and was successful in treating a large overdose in a miniature Shetland pony.[10] The mechanism of action of ILEs in drug overdoses is not completely understood. When associated with lipophilic drug overdoses, it may act as a vascular "lipid sink," pulling drugs from the CNS back into the systemic circulation in which they can be metabolized and/or excreted.[10] There currently is no specified dose in large animals; the recommended small animal dose is a bolus of 1.5 mL/kg BW slowly over 1 to 3 minutes, followed by an infusion of 0.25 to 0.5 mL/kg BW over 30 to 60 minutes.[19] The dose (0.25 mL/kg BW) may be repeated in 4 to 6 hours if there is no evidence of lipemia in the serum.[10]

> **TREATMENT AND CONTROL**
>
> Sarmazenil (0.04 mg/kg BW IV every 2 hours × 6 doses) (R3)
>
> Intralipid emulsion (20% soybean oil) (1.5 mL/kg BW as IV bolus over 1–3 minutes, followed by an infusion of 0.25–0.5 mL/kg BW over 30–60 minutes) (R2)
>
> *BW, body weight; IV, intravenous.*

CONTROL

Careful attention should be paid to administration as most of the case reports revolve around errors in administration, primarily because of miscalculation of an animal's weight or failure to read and follow directions. As with all anthelmintics and insecticides, MLs should be kept in an area where animals cannot access them.

FURTHER READING

Anderson RR. The use of ivermectin in horses: research and clinical observations. *Comp Cont Edu.* 1994;6:S517-S520.

Toutain PL, Upson DW, Terhune TN, et al. Comparative pharmacokinetics of doramectin and ivermectin in cattle. *Vet Parasitol.* 1997;72:3-8.

REFERENCES

1. Canga AG, et al. *Vet J.* 2009;179:25.
2. Sheridan R, et al. *J Assoc Anal Comm Int.* 2006;89:1088.
3. Durden DA. *J Chromatogr B.* 2007;850:134-146.

4. Gokbulut C, et al. *J Vet Pharmacol Ther.* 2013;36:302.
5. Schumacher J, et al. *Equine Vet Educ.* 2008;20:546.
6. Cobb R, et al. *Parasit Vectors.* 2009;2:1756.
7. Gokbulut C, et al. *Vet Parasitol.* 2010;170:120.
8. Wislocki PG, et al. Environmental aspects of abamectin use in crops. In: Campbell WC, ed. *Ivermectin and Abamectin.* 2nd reissue. Springer-Verlag; 2011:182.
9. Plummer CE, et al. *Vet Ophthalmol.* 2006;9:29.
10. Bruenisholz H, et al. *J Vet Intern Med.* 2012;26:407.
11. Cankas GR, Gordon LR. Toxicology. In: Campbell WC, ed. *Ivermectin and Abamectin.* 2nd reissue. Springer-Verlag; 2011:89.
12. Norman TE, et al. *J Vet Intern Med.* 2012;26:143.
13. Fernandez C, et al. *Soil Sed Contam.* 2009;18:564.
14. Floate KD. *Can J Vet Res.* 2006;70:1.
15. Swor TM, et al. *J Am Vet Med Assoc.* 2009;125:558.
16. Kaoliang P, et al. *Vet Res Commun.* 2006;30:263.
17. Bates N, et al. *Vet Rec.* 2013;172:339.
18. Crandall DE, et al. *J Vet Emerg Crit Care.* 2009;19:181.
19. Plumb DC. Fat emulsion. In: Plumb DC, ed. *Veterinary Drug Handbook.* 7th ed. Ames, IA: Wiley-Blackwell; 2011:409.

ORGANOPHOSPHORUS COMPOUNDS AND CARBAMATE INSECTICIDES

SYNOPSIS

Etiology Poisoning by accidental exposure or overdosing with any one of the very large number of insecticides in these two groups of organic compounds.

Epidemiology Outbreaks occur from overdosing, use of oil-based preparations formulated for use on nonanimal surfaces, dehydrated animals, drift of spray from orchards, field crops to pasture.

Clinical pathology Marked depression of blood cholinesterase levels.

Lesions

Acute disease: no diagnostic lesions.

Delayed neurotoxicity: degenerative lesions in peripheral nerves and spinal cord.

Diagnostic confirmation Depressed cholinesterase levels in blood; organophosphate or carbamate in feed or environment.

Treatment Atropine in large doses to effect or atropine plus 2-PAM; remove residual toxin from hair coat; prevent absorption from gastrointestinal tract with activated charcoal and cathartics.

Control Avoid use in stressed, especially dehydrated, animals. Special constraints with chlorpyrifos.

ETIOLOGY

Organophosphorus (OP) compounds and carbamates act in essentially the same manner therapeutically and toxicologically, but bonding of the compound to the esterase enzyme is irreversible in the OP compounds and spontaneously degradable with the carbamates, rendering the carbamates potentially less dangerous. A large number of compounds are included in the group, and those used for the direct treatment of animals have been selected for their low toxicity. A vast amount of information is available on the relative toxicities of the many compounds but it is not possible to provide details here and the information does not lend itself to summarization.[1]

EPIDEMIOLOGY

Occurrence

All animal species are affected. OP compound and carbamate poisoning in animals may occur less frequently as safer insecticides are developed.[2]

Source of Toxin

- Grazing in recently sprayed areas, particularly orchards in which the most toxic compounds are frequently used
- Spray used on cereal crops and in orchards carried by wind onto pasture fields
- Hay or cubes made from plants sprayed with organophosphate compounds
- Inadvertent access to granular insecticides intended for crops
- Use of old insecticide containers as feeding utensils
- Contamination of water supplies
- Too high a concentration of the insecticide in a spray
- Storage toxicity of some compounds appears to increase with storage
- Application to animals of products containing oily bases designed specifically for spraying on walls or plants

Risk Factors

Animal Risk Factors

Susceptible groups include the following:

- Young animals (but with some compounds adults are more so), stressed, water-deprived, and chilled animals; the increased susceptibility caused by restriction of water intake is noted especially after oral treatment to control warble fly infestations.
- Pregnant females in that congenital defects occur in their offspring.
- Brahman and Brahman-cross cattle appear to be more susceptible to some compounds than other cattle.
- Dorset Down sheep may be especially susceptible.
- Chlorpyrifos is more toxic for male animals with high blood levels of testosterone and is not recommended for use in bulls over 8 months of age.

Environmental Risk Factors

The introduction of these compounds into animal therapeutics as treatments for nematode, botfly, sheep nasal botfly, and warble fly infestations and as insecticidal sprays on plants and soil has increased their importance as possible causes of poisoning and as causes of pollution of milk, meat, and eggs. They also have a role in the poisoning of native birdlife and other nontarget animals.[2]

Transmission

- Formulation used, especially the solvent or vehicle used and droplet size
- Method of application, e.g., the toxicity of pour-ons is delayed by 24 hours compared with sprays

PATHOGENESIS

OP compounds are highly toxic and readily absorbed by ingestion, inhalation, and by percutaneous and perconjunctival absorption. Once absorbed, sulfur-containing OPs (phosphorothioates and phosphorodithioates) are metabolized by mixed function oxidases (MFOs) and sulfur is exchanged for oxygen, thus increasing toxicity. There are two forms of toxicity: cholinesterase inactivation and an OP-induced, delayed neurotoxicity.

Cholinesterase Inactivation

The inactivation of cholinesterase by these OP compounds is associated with an increase in acetylcholine in tissues and increased activity of the parasympathetic nervous system and of the postganglionic cholinergic nerves of the sympathetic nervous system. The toxic effects thus reproduce the muscarinic and nicotinic responses of acetylcholine administration. Differences between the toxicities of compounds depend on the stability of this bonding between esterase and compound, and the toxicity of the substance formed by the bonding.

The muscarinic effects of acetylcholine are the visceral responses of the respiratory system and include marked respiratory distress caused by a decrease in dynamic lung compliance and arterial oxygen tension and an increase in total pulmonary resistance; there is bronchial constriction and increased mucous secretion by bronchiolar glands. In the alimentary tract there is increased peristalsis and salivation. Effects in other systems include hypotension and bradycardia, pupillary constriction, sweating, and abortion.

The nicotinic effects are the skeletal muscle responses of twitching, tremor and tetany, convulsions, opisthotonus, weakness, and flaccid paralysis. There is a difference in the relative muscarinic and nicotinic responses between species, and the visceral effects are more marked in ruminants and the muscular effects more evident in pigs in which posterior paralysis is the common manifestation.

Organophosphorus-Induced Delayed Neurotoxicity

This form of toxicity is manifested by distal axonopathy commencing 1 or 2 weeks after the poisoning incident. There is a dieback of neurons causing regional flaccid paralysis, especially in long neurons. The pathogenesis of this lesion is the toxic end product produced by the interaction between some OP compounds and the esterase, a phosphorylated neurotoxic esterase. The most severe effects are associated with industrial OP compounds. Typical examples include the following:

- Congenital defects in young carried by poisoned pregnant females.
- Bilateral laryngeal hemiplegia in horses.
- Paralytic ileus may possibly be associated with chlorpyrifos toxicosis.

Haloxon, in particular, has this neurotoxic effect because it is associated with only a slight depression in cholinesterase levels, but a neurotoxic response in the form of hindlimb ataxia has been reported in a proportion of treated sheep and pigs. The susceptibility of sheep is determined by each individual's genetic ability to metabolize this class of OP compound.

CLINICAL FINDINGS

Acute Poisoning

In general, signs of acute toxicity in animals may occur within minutes of inhalation or ingestion of solutions of the more toxic compounds and deaths 2 to 5 minutes later. After cutaneous application of dichlorvos to calves clinical signs appear within 30 minutes, peak at about 90 minutes, and disappear in 12 to 18 hours. With less toxic compounds in solid form, signs may not appear for some hours and deaths may be delayed for 12 to 24 hours.

Cattle, Sheep, and Goats

Acute Toxicosis

In acute cholinesterase inactivation the premonitory signs, and the only signs in mild cases, are salivation, lacrimation, restlessness, nasal discharge, cough, dyspnea, diarrhea, frequent urination, and muscle stiffness with staggering. Grunting dyspnea is the most obvious, often audible from some distance because of the number affected. Additional signs include protrusion of the tongue, constriction of the pupils with resulting impairment of vision, muscle tremor commencing in the head and neck and spreading over the body, bloat, collapse, and death with or without convulsions or severe respiratory distress. In sheep and goats, the signs also include abdominal pain. Signs disappear at 12 to 18 hours.

Delayed Neurotoxicity

In these cases, the signs do not appear for at least 8 days and up to 90 days after the poisoning. Signs include posterior incoordination and paralysis. Chlorpyrifos is a specific example of this kind of poisoning. It should not be applied to adult dairy cattle or to mature bulls. The signs include anorexia, depression, recumbency, a distended abdomen, ruminal stasis and diarrhea, and fluid splashing sounds on percussion of the right flank. Severe dehydration develops and may result in death.

Pigs

Acute Toxicosis

In pigs acute cholinesterase inactivation visceral effects (except vomiting) are less pronounced than in ruminants and salivation, muscle tremors, nystagmus, and recumbency are characteristic. In some instances, the syndrome is an indefinite one with muscle weakness and drowsiness the only apparent signs. Respiratory distress and diarrhea do not occur.

Delayed Neurotoxicity

Outbreaks of posterior paralysis occur 3 weeks after dosing with an OP anthelmintic; clinical signs vary in severity from knuckling in the hindlimbs to complete flaccid paralysis. The hindlimbs may be dragged behind while the pigs walk on the front legs. Affected pigs are bright and alert and eat well.

Horses

Acute Toxicosis

Signs include abdominal pain and grossly increased intestinal sounds, a very fluid diarrhea, muscle tremors, ataxia, circling, weakness, and dyspnea. Increased salivation occurs rarely. In foals, fluid diarrhea, which is a transient sign in moderate intoxication, may be expanded to a severe gastroenteritis with heavier dose rates.

Delayed Neurotoxicity Syndrome

Bilateral laryngeal paralysis develops in foals after dosing with an OP anthelmintic.

Miscellaneous Signs of Organophosphorus Poisoning

- Piglets with congenital defects of the nervous system manifested clinically by ataxia and tremors are produced by sows dosed with OP compounds during pregnancy. Teratogenicity may be a characteristic of only some OP compounds, e.g., trichlorfon is teratogenic and dichlorvos is not.
- A significant drop in conception rate when the administration is at the beginning of estrus.
- Most OP compounds are associated with only temporary interference with cholinesterase and are not associated with any permanent effects in recovered animals. With some compounds, especially coumaphos and ronnel, the recovery period may be quite long (up to 3 months in the case of ronnel) because of slow excretion of the compound and the combined compound-esterase complex.
- Absorption of an OP compound may also be associated with significant changes in the patient's cholinesterase status without causing clinical signs.
- Potentiation of the action of succinylcholine chloride can occur for up to 1 month after the administration of the OP compound in horses; the administration of the relaxant to a sensitized horse can be followed by persistent apnea and death. This, and a number of other interactions with drugs that may themselves have toxic effects, means that the manufacturer's instructions for OP compounds must be followed explicitly.

CLINICAL PATHOLOGY

The estimation of cholinesterase in body tissues and fluids is the most satisfactory method of diagnosing this poisoning, but it is essential that proper methods and standards of normality be used. Convincing figures are of the order of 50% to 100% reduction from normal controls. The degree and the duration of the depression of blood cholinesterase levels varies with the dose rate and the toxicity of the compound used. Blood cholinesterase levels are depressed for much longer than clinical signs are apparent, e.g., after dichlorvos poisoning the depression of cholinesterase level in the blood does not reach bottom until 12 hours after application, and the return to normal levels takes 7 to 14 days. Similarly, cholinesterase levels in cattle poisoned with terbufos, an agricultural insecticide, do not commence to rise toward normal until 30 days and are not normal for 150 days after the poisoning incident. Unlike organophosphate insecticides, carbamate insecticide cholinesterase inhibitors may spontaneously reverse binding, and cholinesterase depression may not be detectable in recently poisoned animals.

Suspected food material can be assayed for its content of OP compounds but assays of animal tissues or fluids are virtually valueless and may be misleading.

NECROPSY FINDINGS

There are no gross or histologic lesions at necropsy in acute cholinesterase inactivation cases, but tissue specimens could be collected for toxicologic analysis. Material sent for laboratory analysis for cholinesterase should be refrigerated but not deep frozen.

Distinctive degenerative lesions in peripheral nerves and spinal cord can be seen in delayed neurotoxicity cases, and hypoplasia is visible in the cerebrum, cerebellum, and spinal cord in congenitally affected piglets.

DIFFERENTIAL DIAGNOSIS

Outbreaks of a syndrome of dyspnea, salivation, muscle stiffness, and constriction of the pupils after exposure plus a history of exposure and depressed blood levels of cholinesterase suggest intoxication with these organophosphorus compounds, but diagnostic confirmation requires positive assay results on

Continued

suspected toxic materials. In cattle the morbidity and case–fatality rates are approximately 100%, but in pigs the recovery rate is good and all pigs may recover if intake has been low and access is stopped. With the other poisons listed next, death is much more common in pigs, and residual defects, including blindness and paralysis, occur in a proportion of the survivors.

Differential diagnosis list

Cattle

- Early stages of nicotine poisoning
- Groups of cattle affected by acute bovine pulmonary emphysema and edema (fog fever)
- Sporadic cases of anaphylaxis

Horses

- Lead toxicosis

Pigs

- Arsenic toxicosis
- Avitaminosis A
- Mercury poisoning
- Sodium chloride (salt) poisoning

TREATMENT

Animals that have been dipped or sprayed should be washed with water to which soap or a detergent is added to remove residual OP material. When oral intake has occurred, activated charcoal will adsorb residual toxin in the gut.

Primary treatment is urgent and critical, especially in cattle because of the usually high case–fatality rate. Atropine is the antidote for muscarinic effects, but does not reverse the nicotinic effects of the OP compound, i.e., tremors, spasms, and convulsions. The recommended dose in sheep and goats is 0.5 mg/kg BW with ¼ given intravenously and the remainder intramuscularly or subcutaneously.[3] This should be repeated every 3 to 4 hours for 1 to 2 days with salivation and heart rate guiding therapy. Atropine appears to have low efficacy in sheep. This is not a serious drawback because sheep are much less susceptible than cattle to larger doses of atropine. The recommended dose of atropine in horses is 0.02 to 0.2 mg/kg BW intravenously to effect,[3] but it needs to be given with care because horses are very susceptible to the gastrointestinal effects of atropine.

Oximes, if available and economically feasible, may be useful in the early treatment of poisoning from OP compounds. Their usefulness as antidotes declines rapidly with the passage of time after the poisoning occurs, and they are of doubtful use after 24 hours. The most common oxime is pralidoxime chloride (2-PAM). The recommended dose rate for 2-PAM in ruminants is 25 to 50 mg/kg BW given intravenously as a 20% solution over 6 minutes.[4] In horses 2-PAM at doses of 20 mg/kg BW has given good results.[4] Treatment may need to be repeated for up to 10 days to counteract slower acting compounds such as coumaphos.

TREATMENT AND CONTROL

Ruminants

Atropine sulfate (0.5 mg/kg BW with ¼ given IV and the remainder IM or SC; repeat every 3–4 hours for 1–2 days) (R1)

Pralidoxime chloride (2-PAM) (25–50 mg/kg BW IV as a 20% solution over 6 minutes. Repeat as needed) (R2, depending on economics; not for herd use)

Horses

Atropine sulfate (0.02 to 0.2 mg/kg BW IV to effect; repeat judiciously SC every 1.5–2 hours) (R1, only if needed)

Pralidoxime chloride (2-PAM) (20 mg/kg BW IV; repeat every 4–6 hours as needed) (R2)

BW, body weight; IM, intramuscularly; IV, intravenously; SC, subcutaneously.

CONTROL

Most outbreaks occur after accidental access to compounds. Animals to be treated orally with OP insecticides should be permitted ample fresh drinking water beforehand. Use of chlorpyrifos is restricted to beef cattle and not in calves less than 12 weeks old or in bulls over 8 months of age.

FURTHER READING

Abdelsalam EB. Factors affecting the toxicity of organophosphorus compounds in animals. *Vet Bull.* 1987;57:441-448.

Barrett DS, et al. A review of organophosphorus ester-induced delayed neurotoxicity. *Vet Human Toxicol.* 1985;27:22-37.

Radostits O, et al. Organophosphorus compounds and carbamates. In: *Veterinary Medicine: A Textbook of the Disease of Cattle, Horses, Sheep, Goats and Pigs.* 10th ed. London: W.B. Saunders; 2007:1834.

Savage EP, et al. Chronic neurological sequelae of acute organophosphate pesticide poisoning. *Arch Environ Health.* 1988;43:38.

REFERENCES

1. Karami-Mohajeri S, et al. *Hum Exp Toxicol.* 2011;30:1119.
2. Poppenga RH. *Vet Clin North Am Food Anim Pract.* 2011;27:379.
3. Plumb DC. Atropine. In: Plumb DC, ed. *Veterinary Drug Handbook.* 7th ed. Ames, IA: Wiley-Blackwell; 2011:94.
4. Plumb DC. Pralidoxime chloride (2-PAM chloride). In: Plumb DC, ed. *Veterinary Drug Handbook.* 7th ed. Ames, IA: Wiley-Blackwell; 2011:842.

INDUSTRIAL ORGANOPHOSPHATES

Principal industrial uses of organophosphates are as fire-resistant hydraulic fluids, as lubricants, and as coolants. A number of compounds including tri-*o*-tolyl phosphate, tri-*o*-cresyl phosphate (TOCP), and triaryl phosphates (TAP) have come to veterinary notice as being associated with poisoning in animals. TAPs contain a number of isomers as well as TOCP (e.g., *m*-cresol, *p*-cresol, *o*-cresol), and all of them are more poisonous than TOCP. Poisoning may occur by ingestion or cutaneous absorption.

Clinical signs of delayed neurotoxicity do not occur until several weeks after contact and include irreversible neurologic signs of respiratory stertor, dyspnea, dysuria, knuckling, leg weakness, and posterior paralysis.

Diagnostic confirmation depends on evidence of exposure to the toxicant, signs referable to the nervous system lesions, and a positive assay for the toxicant in the animal's tissues. Necropsy lesions characteristically include neuronal degeneration in the spinal cord and peripheral nerves.

ROTENONE TOXICOSIS

Rotenone has been extensively used in the past to control bovine *Hypoderma* larvae (cattle grubs). It is a neurotoxicant; chronic exposure results in degeneration of neuronal cells, especially dopaminergic neurons.[1] Use as a pesticide and insecticide in the United States is being phased out, in part because of its link to Parkinson's disease in humans.[2]

It has a reputation for low mammalian toxicity but relatively high toxicity to aquatic life. The mammalian oral LD_{50} is 100 to 300 mg/kg, whereas the LD_{50} for fish is less than 100 μg/L of water. Oral absorption in mammals is limited but enhanced by fat in the diet.

Ingesta at necropsy may contain as much as 2000 ppm of rotenone. Signs include salivation, muscle tremor, vomiting, ascending paralysis, incoordination, quadriplegia, respiratory depression, coma, and death. Accidental oral exposure may be treated with activated charcoal, and an osmotic cathartic for decontamination followed by control of seizures is needed. Phenothiazine tranquilizers are contraindicated in rotenone toxicosis.

FURTHER READING

Lapointe N, et al. Rotenone induces non-specific central nervous system and systemic toxicity. *FASEB J.* 2004;18:717-719.

Graham OH, et al. The potential of animal systemic insecticides for eradicating cattle grubs, *Hypoderma* spp. *J Econ Entomol.* 1967;60:1050.

REFERENCES

1. Watabe M, et al. *Mol Pharmacol.* 2008;74:933.
2. Tanner CM, et al. *Environ Health Perspect.* 2011;119:866.

ORGANOCHLORINE INSECTICIDES

SYNOPSIS

Etiology Poisoning by any of the group of insecticides including aldrin, hexachloride, chlordane, DDT, dieldrin, endrin, heptachlor, isodrin, lindane, methoxychlor, or toxaphene.

Epidemiology Accidental or misinformed overdosing. Usage on animals now superceded by other less toxic compounds. Stored or leftover products may accidentally be accessed by animals. It is important because of residues in animal products used in the human food chain.

Clinical pathology Assay of compounds in animal tissues.

Lesions No consistent significant lesions; some animals show pale musculature.

Diagnostic confirmation Chemical assay of liver or brain for acute poisoning; fat or other animal tissue for chronic poisoning.

Treatment. Supportive care only; control hyperthermia and seizures. Removal of residual chemical; activated charcoal for oral detoxification.

Control Do not use these insecticides and store them appropriately.

DDT, *dichlorodiphenyltrichloroethane.*

ETIOLOGY

This group of poisons includes dichlorodiphenyltrichloroethane (DDT), benzene hexachloride (and its pure gamma isomer, lindane), aldrin, dieldrin, chlordane, toxaphene, methoxychlor, dichlorodiphenyldichloroethane, isodrin, endrin, and heptachlor. Methoxychlor is less toxic than DDT, and isodrin and endrin are more toxic than aldrin and dieldrin. Camphor (2-bornanone) is chemically similar to toxaphene and is associated with a similar syndrome when fed accidentally.

EPIDEMIOLOGY

Occurrence

Poisoning with these compounds has been recorded in all animal species. The chlorinated hydrocarbons have come under so much criticism as environmental contaminants that they are rarely used directly on animals, so outbreaks of clinical illness associated with them are much less common than they were.

Risk Factors

Animal Risk Factors

The compounds vary in their ability to pass the skin barrier. Benzene hexachloride, aldrin, dieldrin, and chlordane are readily absorbed. Species susceptibility to skin absorption also varies widely. Very young animals of any species are more susceptible than adults, and lactating and emaciated animals also show increased susceptibility.

Farm or Premise Risk Factors

Many outbreaks are associated with the application to animals of products intended for crops, e.g., endosulfan, and labeled specifically "Not For Animal Use." These insecticides may contaminate soil and persist there for many years. Rooting animals such as pigs are particularly susceptible to this source of poisoning. These compounds are also sometimes fed accidentally and in large amounts in lieu of feed additives, and are associated with acute poisoning. In feedlot animals, signs may continue for as long as a year because of repeated contamination from the environment. Insect baits, e.g., grasshopper baits containing toxaphene and chlordane, used on pasture and for leaf-eating insects on market gardens can be associated with poisoning in livestock, which may eat large quantities of them. These insecticides, especially heptachlor, are incorporated in the soil before the crop of potatoes or maize is sown to control soil pests. Subsequent grazing of the field will cause contamination of the livestock for several years.

Environmental Risk Factors

Organochlorines are closely regulated and banned in many countries primarily because of their persistence in the environment, but some are still widely used in agriculture, principally on growing plants to control insect pests and on stored seed grain to control fungi. If the plants or grain, even milled and by-products, e.g., bran, are fed to animals, they can be associated with problems of tissue residues; if they are fed in sufficient quantities they can be associated with clinical illness.

Human Risk Factors

Because the compounds are soluble in fat and accumulate in body stores they are formidable threats to the meat industry. They are also excreted in significant amounts in milk and enter the human food chain at this point. They are concentrated still further in cream and butter.

Transmission

Ingestion, inhalation, aspiration, and percutaneous absorption are all possible portals of entry so that contamination of feed and application of sprays and dips can all be associated with poisoning.

Method of Application

Dipping of animals is the most hazardous method of application because entry may occur through all portals. Spraying is safer because percutaneous absorption and inhalation are the only portals of entry. The small particle size of the compound and concentration of animals in confined spaces while spraying increase the possibility of poisoning. Oily preparations are not used for animal treatment but are used inadvertently and are readily absorbed through the skin.

Formulation Used

Concentrations of insecticide in formulations used for spraying barns are much higher than those used for animals. Among spray preparations simple solutions are most dangerous followed by emulsions and, least of all, suspensions of wettable powder. Dusting is safest and is preferred to other methods. Preparations for use on plants are often unstable emulsions, which come out of suspension quickly when they reach the plant. If these preparations are used in animal dips, the first few animals through the dip can be heavily contaminated and suffer acute, lethal toxic effects. Although the treatment of pastures to control their insect pests is usually safe to animals grazing, the treated pasture or hay made from it can cause contamination of animal products. This contamination can be avoided by incorporating the insecticide into superphosphate granules ("prills") instead of applying it as sprays or dusts.

PATHOGENESIS

The mechanism of action of organochlorines is to induce repetitive discharge of motor and sensory neurons by interference with axonal transmission of nerve impulses. After absorption, cyclodiene insecticides are activated by the MFO system, and any prior chemical or environmental exposures that increase the MFO system may exacerbate the onset of poisoning. The diphenyl aliphatic (DDT) organochlorines affect sodium channels, prolonging sodium influx and inhibiting potassium efflux at the nerve membrane. The cyclodiene organochlorines competitively inhibit the binding of GABA at receptor sites, resulting in loss of GABA inhibition and resultant stimulation of the neuron. In all organochlorine poisonings recovery may occur, but with smaller animals paralysis follows and finally collapse and death ensue.

Most of the substances accumulate in the fat depots, where they are a potential source of danger in that sudden mobilization of the fat may result in liberation of the compound into the bloodstream and the appearance of signs of poisoning.

CLINICAL FINDINGS

The speed of onset of illness after exposure varies from a few minutes to a few hours, depending on the portal of entry and the compound and its formulation, but it is never very long.

The toxic effects produced by the members of this group include complete anorexia, increased excitability and irritability followed by ataxia, muscle tremor, weakness and paralysis, and terminal convulsions in severe cases. Salivation and teeth grinding occur in large animals and vomiting occurs in pigs. Variations on this clinical syndrome, which is common to all organochlorine intoxications, include the following:

- DDT and methoxychlor chronic poisoning may be associated with moderate liver damage.
- Benzene hexachloride, lindane, chlordane, toxaphene, dieldrin, endrin, aldrin, and heptachlor are associated with an exaggerated syndrome including teeth grinding, champing of jaws, dyspnea, tetany, snapping of the eyelids,

auricular spasms, opisthotonus, frequent micturition, frenzied movements, walking backward, climbing walls, violent somersaults, and aimless jumping. Fever of 5% to 7% above normal may occur, possibly as a result of seizure activity. Seizures may persist for 2 or 3 days if the animal does not die.

CLINICAL PATHOLOGY

Blood, hair, and ingesta can be assayed chemically for specific toxins. The removal of a biopsy from the fat pad near the cow's tail offers a satisfactory means of providing samples for tissue analysis. Organochlorine residues in acutely poisoned animals may reach 4 to 7 ppm in brain or liver.

NECROPSY FINDINGS

At necropsy there are no specific major lesions in the nervous system, but toxic hepatitis and tubular nephritis appear in some cases. Tissue levels need to be high to be good indicators of recent intoxication. If possible, the specimens should be deep frozen, and the suspected compound should be nominated because assay procedures are long and involved.

Samples for Postmortem Confirmation of Diagnosis

- Specimens of hair, if the portal is percutaneous
- Ingesta, if oral intake is probable

DIFFERENTIAL DIAGNOSIS

Differential diagnosis list
- Lead poisoning
- Rabies
- Pseudorabies of cattle
- Polioencephalomalacia
- Thromboembolic meningoencephalitis
- Salt poisoning in pigs

TREATMENT

There is no specific primary treatment. Activated charcoal (2 g/kg) given early by stomach tube will bind pesticide in rumen and reduce further absorption. The use of mineral oil should be avoided because it will increase the absorption of lipid organochlorines. Residual chemical should be removed from the coat with a degreasing soap and copious water rinse. Supportive treatment includes sedation with diazepam or pentobarbital sodium until signs disappear, monitoring and treating hyperthermia, and replacing fluid losses.

Treatment to reduce the contamination of tissues is unsuccessful and in most cases the time required for the contamination to subside varies between compounds but is lengthy, taking 3 to 6 months or longer. For example, cows fed DDT prepartum need an average of 189 days from parturition for the level in the milk fat to decline to 125 ppm. After the source of contamination is removed, drenching of cows with up to 2 kg of activated charcoal followed by daily incorporation in their feed for 2-week intervals has been recommended for this purpose. Neither of these procedures is really practical in the average farm operation. The common procedure for reducing the level of tissue contamination in animals is to put them in a feedlot without any contact with pasture and feed them on energy-intensive rations. Sheep decontaminate much more quickly than cattle, and animals on a high plane of nutrition eliminate the toxins more quickly.

CONTROL

Avoidance of the use of the compounds is recommended.

FURTHER READING

Aslani MR. Endosulfan toxicosis in calves. *Vet Human Toxicol.* 1996;38:364.

Booth NH, McDowell JR. Toxicity of hexachlorobenzene and associated residues in edible animal tissues. *J Am Vet Med Assoc.* 1975;166:591-595.

Marth E. Stunzner D. Toxicokinetics of chlorinated hydrocarbons. *J Hyg Epidemiol Microbiol Immunol.* 1989;33:514-520.

Radostits O, et al. Chlorinated hydrocarbons. In: *Veterinary Medicine: A Textbook of the Disease of Cattle, Horses, Sheep, Goats and Pigs.* 10th ed. London: W.B. Saunders; 2007:1832.

The history of organochlorine pesticides in Australia. (Accessed 10.12.2013, at http://www.apvma.gov.au/products/review/completed/organochlorines_history.php.).

Uzoukwu M, Sleight SD. Effects of dieldrin in pregnant sows. *J Am Vet Med Assoc.* 1972;160:1641-1643.

SODIUM FLUOROACETATE (COMPOUND 1080) TOXICOSIS

ETIOLOGY

Sodium fluoroacetate in the form of compound 1080 is used as a potent rodenticide in agriculture. It is currently used in the United States against coyotes and in Australia and New Zealand against introduced species such as possums.[1,2] It is also formed naturally by fluoride uptake from the soil and water in many plants that are native to Africa, Australia, and Brazil. The toxic dose level for domestic animals including sheep is 0.3 mg/kg BW,[3] and 0.4 mg/kg BW is lethal for cattle. Sublethal doses may be cumulative if given at sufficiently short intervals.

EPIDEMIOLOGY

The use of fluoroacetate in agriculture poses a hazard for grazing farm animals because it is usually spread out across fields combined with cereals, carrots, or bread as bait and is attractive to ruminants.

PATHOGENESIS

Fluoroacetate in the body is converted to fluorocitrate, which inhibits the enzymes aconitase and succinate dehydrogenase in the tricarboxylic acid cycle (Krebs cycle) leading to the accumulation of significant amounts of citrate in tissues and to irreversible cardiac damage. Two actions are manifest: CNS stimulation producing convulsions and myocardial depression with ventricular fibrillation. In sheep the predominant effect with acute poisoning is on the myocardium and the pulmonary system; in pigs and dogs it is the nervous system.

CLINICAL SIGNS

Clinical signs vary widely among species. In herbivores, sudden death in acute cases typically occurs. The animals are found dead without evidence of a struggle, or there are tetanic convulsions and acute heart failure with the animals showing weakness and dyspnea accompanied by cardiac arrhythmia, a weak pulse, and electrocardiographic evidence of ventricular fibrillation.

In sheep with subacute poisoning, the signs are similar but are not apparent when the animal is at rest. When they are disturbed, the nervous signs of tremor and convulsions appear but disappear when the sheep lies down.

Pigs manifest the nervous form of the disease, including hyperexcitability and violent tetanic convulsions. In all cases there is a period of delay of up to 2 hours after ingestion before signs appear.

CLINICAL PATHOLOGY/ NECROPSY FINDINGS

There are no specific lesions, but the tissues contain elevated levels of citrate.

TREATMENT/CONTROL

No specific treatment is available. In cats, calcium gluconate and sodium succinate have been used successfully in the treatment of experimental intoxication.[4] Care in the disposition of baits and highly dependable retrieval of uneaten baits before allowing livestock access to baited fields preempts most mortalities.

FURTHER READING

Radostits O, et al. *Veterinary Medicine: A Textbook of the Disease of Cattle, Horses, Sheep, Goats and Pigs.* 10th ed. London: W.B. Saunders; 2007:1839.

REFERENCES

1. Proudfoot AT, et al. *Tox Rev.* 2006;25:213.
2. Eason C, et al. *New Zeal J Ecol.* 2011;35:1.
3. Gooneratne SR, et al. *Onderstepoort J Vet Res.* 2008;75:127.
4. Collicchio-Zuanaze RC, et al. *Hum Exp Toxicol.* 2006;25:175.

MOLLUSCICIDE TOXICOSIS

Metaldehyde

Metaldehyde is the active ingredient in products used to control slugs and snails (mollusks), mites, and insects.[1-3] It is often used in combination with a carbamate, such as methiocarb, and historically with calcium arsenate.[3] Metaldehyde is often bran based with molasses frequently added to attract snails and slugs. It is a neurotoxicant to all mammals by inhalation, ingestion, and dermal exposure. The mechanism of action is unknown, but it may be related to changes in the concentration of neurotransmitters in the brain. Outbreaks have occurred in cattle, goats, sheep, and horses.[1-3] The acute lethal dose in adult cattle is 0.2 g/kg BW and less in calves[3]; in horses it is 0.1 g/kg BW. The onset of signs varies depending on the concentration and amount ingested, but in cattle it is reported to be 15 minutes to 24 hours postingestion.[3] Prolongation may be caused by delayed rumen absorption.

Ingestion of a toxic amount of metaldehyde causes CNS stimulation with profound muscle tremors and hyperthermia. Other reported signs in ruminants include incoordination, hyperesthesia, hypersalivation, dyspnea, diarrhea, partial blindness, unconsciousness, cyanosis, and death caused by respiratory failure.[2,3] All the signs are exacerbated by excitement or activity. A mortality rate of 3% may be expected. Signs in horses are similar plus heavy perspiration and death in 3 to 5 hours.

There is no antidote, and treatment is largely supportive. Mineral oil and activated charcoal (1–3 doses) may be used to decrease absorption. Muscle tremors and seizures should be controlled with a tranquilizer and/or muscle relaxant. Intravenous fluids should be used to replace and restore fluids and electrolytes. Rumenotomy may be effective if performed before the onset of clinical signs.

Methiocarb

Methiocarb is a carbamate molluscicide used alone or in combination with metaldehyde. It has anticholinesterase and nicotinic and muscarinic activities.[4] The compound is usually in pellet form and dyed blue or yellow so that affected animals can be detected by the blue/yellow staining of their mouths.[3,4]

The signs can vary widely depending on the degree of receptor stimulation. Poisoning of sheep is associated with depression, hypersalivation, diarrhea, dyspnea, aimless wandering, and ataxia. Death is caused by pulmonary edema. Horses show sweating, lacrimation, urine dribbling or polyuria, muscle tremor, hypersalivation, and finally recumbency and death caused by pulmonary edema.[4]

Binding to acetylcholinesterase is reversible so recovery can occur with supportive care. Atropine is an effective antidote but likely will need to be repeated several times, especially if the amount ingested is large. Additional treatment is supportive and aimed toward specific system involvement.

FURTHER READING

Booze TF, Oehme FW. Metaldehyde toxicity: a review. *Vet Human Toxicol.* 1985;27:11-15.

Giles CJ, et al. Methiocarb poisoning in a sheep. *Vet Rec.* 1984;114:642.

REFERENCES

1. Daniel R, et al. *Vet Rec.* 2009;165:575.
2. Guitart R, et al. *Vet J.* 2010;183:249.
3. Valentine BA, et al. *J Vet Diagn Invest.* 2007;19:212.
4. Kaye BM, et al. *Aust Vet J.* 2012;90:221.

STRYCHNINE

Strychnine has been used for years as a rodenticide and avicide. Historically it has been used as an appetite stimulant and laxative and most recently, as a contaminant in LSD and other street drugs. It is an alkaloid derived primarily from seeds and bark of the *Strychnos nux-vomica* tree, although it is found in various amounts in many *Strychnos* spp.

Strychnine poisoning is an uncommon occurrence in large animals and usually associated with accidental overdosing with strychnine preparations or accidental access to strychnine treated bait meant for rodent control. Cattle are particularly susceptible to parenteral administration (30–60 mg of strychnine hydrochloride may be fatal) but less susceptible to oral administration because of destruction of the drug in the rumen. Lethal doses by parenteral injection are 200 to 250 mg in horses, 300 to 400 mg in cattle, and 15 to 50 mg in pigs.

Strychnine is rapidly absorbed from the gastrointestinal tract in monogastric animals and less so by ruminants. Distribution to tissues is rapid as is hepatic metabolism. In most animals, 50% of strychnine is eliminated in 6 hours following a sublethal dose.

It is a potent neurotoxicant and convulsant, exerting its action at the postsynaptic membrane. In the spinal cord, strychnine interferes with the inhibition of motor cell stimulation resulting in simultaneous muscle contraction. In the brain, it interferes with inhibitory responses of the motor neurons resulting in neuronal excitation. The convulsant effects of strychnine are caused by interference with glycine-mediated postsynaptic inhibition. The net effect is that all skeletal muscles become hyperexcited, and tetanic seizures may be provoked by the application of minor external stimuli. In these convulsive episodes there is extension of the limbs, opisthotonus, and protrusion of the eyeballs. The seizures may last for 3 to 4 minutes and are followed by periods of partial relaxation, which become progressively shorter as the disease develops. Hyperthermia may be extreme. Respiratory arrest leads to death.

There is no antidote and treatment is supportive. Animals should be kept in a dark, calm area and not stimulated in any manner. Seizures should be treated with diazepam or a barbiturate. If seizures can be adequately controlled, animals may survive.

FURTHER READING

Boyd RE, et al. Strychnine poisoning. *Am J Med.* 1983;74:507-512.

Ward JC, Garlough FE. Strychnine IV: lethal dose studies on cattle and sheep. *J Am Pharm Assoc.* 1936;125:422-426.

Diseases of the Cerebrum

PSYCHOSES, NEUROSES, AND STEREOTYPY

Psychoses or neuroses are rarely documented in farm animals, whereas **stereotypy** is common, particularly in horses. Stereotypic behavior is repetitive behavior induced by frustration, repeated attempts to cope, or CNS dysfunction. Primary equine stereotypies include crib-biting, weaving, box walking, tongue rolling, and lip movement.

Crib-Biting and Windsucking

Crib-biting or "cribbing" is an oral stereotypic behavior in which the horse grasps an object, usually the feed box or any solid projection, with the incisor teeth, then arches the neck and, by depressing the tongue and elevating the larynx, pulls upward and backward and swallows air, emitting a loud grunt at the same time. This results in erosion of the incisor teeth and intermittent bouts of spasmodic colic and flatulence. Crib-biting must be distinguished from chewing wood from boredom and from pica caused by a mineral deficiency. **Windsucking** (aerophagia) is an oral stereotypic behavior in which the horse flexes and arches the neck and swallows air and grunts, but there is no grasping of objects.

Crib-biting is viewed as a vice and potentially "contagious" problem and affected horses are usually not welcome in stables. Once established, crib-biting is primarily postprandial. Treatments include environmental enrichment (move horse to a stall where they can view more activity; change stall door/walls so that other horses can be seen) and feeding more hay and less concentrate so that feeding takes longer. More aggressive treatments include placement of a crib-strap (a strap placed around the neck of the horse that has two pieces of metal hinges at the ventral area; during arching of the neck the crib-strap tightens around the pharynx) or neurectomy or myectomy. Weaning in a box stall appears to increase the risk of developing crib-biting.

Weaving

Weaving is a locomotor behavior during which the horse moves its head and neck laterally while its weight is moved to the contralateral forelimb, usually while the horse is positioned at the stall door with its head over the stable door into the aisle. There is no specific treatment and closing the top half of the stable door merely moves the activity back into the stall. Feeding hay ad libitum may decrease the time devoted to this activity (anecdotal reports).

Box Walking

The term **box walking** refers to persistent walking around the perimeter of the stall in a circular, repetitive manner. There is no specific treatment, but anecdotal reports suggest that feeding hay ad libitum may decrease the time devoted to this activity. Other stereotypical behavior includes persistent kicking of the stall, in the absence of pruritic lesions of the lower limbs, and cutaneous and subcutaneous mutilation by self-biting.

Farrowing Hysteria in Sows

Hysteria in sows at farrowing is a common occurrence. This syndrome is most common in gilts. Affected animals are hyperactive and restless and they attack and savage their piglets as they approach the head during the initial teat sucking activity after birth. Serious and often fatal injuries result. Cannibalism is not a feature.

When the syndrome occurs, the remaining piglets and freshly born piglets should be removed from the sow and placed in a warm environment until parturition is finished. The sow should then be tested to see if she will accept the piglets. If not, ataractic or neuroleptic drugs should be administered to allow initial sucking, after which the sow will usually continue to accept the piglets.

Azaperone (2 mg/kg BW IM) is usually satisfactory, and pentobarbital sodium administered intravenously until the pedal reflex is lost has been recommended. Promazine derivatives are effective but subsequent incoordination may result in a higher crushing loss of piglets. The piglets' teeth should be clipped.

Affected gilts should be culled subsequently because the syndrome may recur at subsequent farrowing. Where possible, gilts should be placed in their farrowing accommodation 4 to 6 days before parturition and the farrowing environment should be kept quiet at the time of parturition.

Tail-Biting, Ear-Chewing, and Snout-Rubbing in Pigs

The incidence of cannibalism has increased with intensification of pig rearing, and it is now a significant problem in many pig-rearing enterprises. Tail-biting is the most common and occurs in groups of pigs, especially males, from weaning to market age.

Ear-chewing is less common and is generally restricted to pigs in the immediate postweaning and early growing period, although both syndromes may occur concurrently. The incidence of ear-chewing has increased with the practice of docking piglet tails at birth. The lesions are usually bilateral and most commonly involve the ventral part of the ear. Lesions from bite wounds may also occur on the flanks of pigs. There is frequently an association with mange infestation with both of these vices.

A syndrome of snout-rubbing to produce eroded necrotic areas on the flanks of pigs has been described. Affected pigs were invariably colored, although both white and colored pigs acted as agonists.

The causes of these forms of cannibalism in pigs are poorly understood, but they are undoubtedly related to an inadequate total environment. Affected groups are usually more restless and have heightened activity. Factors such as a high population density, both in terms of high pen density and large group size; limited food and competition for food; low protein and inadequate nutrition; boredom; and inadequate environment in terms of temperature, draft, and ventilation have been incriminated in precipitating the onset of these vices.

When a problem is encountered, each of these factors should be examined and corrected or changed if necessary. **Prevention** is through the same measures. Chains or tires are frequently hung for displacement activity but are not particularly effective.

The problem may recur despite all attempts at prevention. Also for economic reasons it is not always possible to implement the radical changes in housing and management that may be necessary to avoid the occurrence of these vices. Because of this, the practice of tipping or docking the piglets' tails at birth has become common as a method of circumventing the major manifestation of cannibalism.

HEAD-SHAKING IN HORSES

Head-shaking by horses is a troubling syndrome associated with hypersensitivity of the trigeminal nerve in most affected horses. The disorder is characterized by repeated, sudden shaking or tossing of the head. It is proposed that a subgroup of horses with defined trigeminal hypersensitivity be classified as having trigeminal-mediated facial dysesthesia.[1]

ETIOLOGY

The etiology is complex and often unclear and conditions associated with head-shaking include the following[2]:

- Ear mites
- Otitis interna/externa
- Ophthalmic disease (uveitis)
- *Trombicula autumnalis* (chiggers) infestation of the muzzle
- Guttural pouch disease (mycosis)
- Stylohyoid arthropathy
- Osteitis of the petrous temporal bone
- Dental disease (wolf teeth, ulceration, periodontal disease, periapical abscess)
- Behavioral abnormalities
- Trigeminal neuralgia
- Optic neuritis
- Photic head-shaking (optic-trigeminal summation)
- Neck pain
- Rhinitis or sinusitis (including fungal sinusitis)[3]
- Ethmoidal disease including hematoma
- Infraorbital neuritis
- Excessive neck flexion by rider
- Equine protozoal myeloencephalitis
- Ill-fitting tack including bit and bridle
- Obstructive airway disease (heaves, laryngeal hemiplegia, epiglottic cysts, etc.)
- Fractures of the nuchal crest[4]
- Surgery of the paranasal sinuses[5]

Most cases of the disease are idiopathic despite intensive investigation of affected horses. Photic head-shaking is a common cause of the disease. Most cases have some seasonal distribution, although the reason for this is undetermined. Trigeminal neuralgia is considered an important cause of the disease. It is not associated with EHV-1 infection of the trigeminal ganglia.[6]

EPIDEMIOLOGY

The epidemiology of the disease is not well defined. The syndrome occurs in horses throughout the world. The syndrome is sporadic, usually affects only one horse on a farm, and does not occur as outbreaks. It has a seasonal occurrence in approximately 60% of horses with the majority first demonstrating head-shaking, or being most affected, during spring and summer. Head-shaking is worst on sunny days, and less severe on cloudy days, in approximately 60% of horses. Sunshine and windy weather worsen the condition in many horses.[7] Seventy-five percent and 80% of affected horses have less severe signs at night or when ridden indoors, respectively.

Affected horses are usually mature adults with onset of head-shaking at 7 to 9 years of age in over half of the cases, although signs can occur in horses as young as 1 year.[2] The disease is reported twice as often in geldings as in mares. There is an apparent predisposition to the disease in Thoroughbreds, but this is not consistently reported. Most affected horses are used for general riding, although this might represent an age effect because the syndrome tends to occur in older horses that are not used for racing. There is no apparent association of temperament and risk of head-shaking.

PATHOGENESIS

The pathogenesis of head-shaking depends on the cause, but it is increasingly persuasive that the majority of cases involve hypersensitivity of the trigeminal nerve.[1,8-10] The trigeminal nerve provides sensory function of the nose and nasal mucosa. Horses affected by head-shaking have low stimulus thresholds for the trigeminal nerve than do healthy horses, although once stimulated nerve conduction is not different between the groups.[9] The lower stimulus threshold likely makes affected horses more sensitive to noxious stimuli. A method is also described for assessment of the trigeminocervical reflex in normal horses.[11] This technique might be useful in head-shaking horses.[10-12]

Head-shaking is related to exposure to bright light in some animals. This is a condition referred to as photic or optic-trigeminal summation because of its similarity to a syndrome in people. Trigeminal neuralgia is thought to cause acute, sharp, and intense pain in the face. Although this cannot be definitively diagnosed in horses, its presence is inferred from the horse's behavior and response to analgesia of the infraorbital or posterior ethmoidal nerves.

CLINICAL FINDINGS

The **clinical signs** of head-shaking are unmistakable. Movements of the head are sudden and apparently spontaneous and involve lateral, dorsal, ventral, or rotatory movement of the nose usually during exercise. Horses rarely have the behavior only at rest, with most affected both at rest and during exercise and about 10% exhibiting signs only during exercise. The action often resembles that of a horse trying to dislodge something from its nose. Approximately 90% of horses have vertical movement of the head (as if flipping the nose). The head-shaking can be so severe it causes lateral, dorsal, or ventral flexion of the neck to the level of the caudal cervical vertebrae, although more commonly only the rostral one-third of the neck is involved, if it is involved at all. Some horses rub their nose on objects, the ground, or their front limbs, sometimes during exercise. Affected horses often snort or sneeze. There can be twitching of the facial muscles and flipping of the upper lip. The movements are sudden and at times appear to catch the horse by surprise. The frequency and/or severity of movements are usually increased during exercise. Severely affected horses can stumble and fall if head-shaking occurs during exercise, rendering the horse unsafe to ride.

A grading system to classify the severity of signs is as follows:

0 No signs of head-shaking
1 Intermittent and mild clinical signs: facial muscle twitching; rideable
2 Moderate clinical signs: definable conditions under which head-shaking occurs; rideable with some difficulty
3 Rideable to unpleasant to do so: difficult to control
4 Unrideable and uncontrollable
5 Dangerous with bizarre behavior patterns

This system might be useful for assessing response to therapy and concisely describing the severity of the signs.

Ancillary testing involves radiography of the skull; endoscopic examination of both nostrils and ethmoidal regions, nasopharynx, larynx, and guttural pouches; otoscopic examination of the external auditory canal and tympanic membrane (difficult to achieve in a conscious horse, a small endoscope is necessary); desensitization of the infraorbital and posterior ethmoidal nerves; biopsy of the nasal mucosa (in horses with suspected rhinitis); radiographic examination of the head and neck; measurement of stimulus threshold for action potentials in the trigeminal nerve,[9] and therapeutic trials including application of contact lenses or masks, or administration of medications (see the following section Treatment).

CLINICAL PATHOLOGY

There are no characteristic hematologic or serum biochemical abnormalities.

NECROPSY FINDINGS

There are no characteristic findings on necropsy, apart from those of any underlying disease. Evidence of lesions in the trigeminal nerve is lacking.

> **DIFFERENTIAL DIAGNOSIS**
>
> The disease must be differentiated from the stereotypic weaving that occurs during stabling and not during exercise.

TREATMENT

The principles of treatment include relief of specific underlying diseases, removal of management or environmental conditions that cause head-shaking, and administration of medications. There is the potential for an important placebo effect, in the owners, for treatment of head-shaking.[13]

If underlying conditions are detected, such as ear mites, dental disease, and other conditions listed in the previous section Etiology, then these conditions should be treated effectively. Effective treatment will alleviate head-shaking, if in fact the condition was the cause of the disease. However, most horses with head-shaking have seasonal or photic disease and treatment is more difficult. A survey of owners of 254 horses with head-shaking revealed that only 129 horses had been treated by a veterinarian and, of those, only 6% had complete resolution of head-shaking, whereas 72% had no response to treatment. Other treatments used were on the advice of lay "back specialists," homeopathy, alternative therapies, or face or head masks. Success rates for these interventions varied between 6% and 27%, with the most success obtained by use of a nose net (27%). Nose nets provided better control of signs than did face or eye masks. These figures on the success of treatment illustrate the refractory, and therefore frustrating, nature of the disease.

Fitting of **nose masks** alleviates or lessens head-shaking in some horses. The design of the nose mask does not appear to be important regarding whether it covers the entire rostral face or just the nostrils. The nose masks were most effective for treatment of up-and-down head-shaking, but not for side-to-side or rubbing behavior.

Blue-tinted **contact lenses** have been suggested for use in horses with photic head-shaking. Others have not found this intervention useful. Administration of sodium cromoglycate eye drops has demonstrated potential in a small number of horses for treatment of seasonal head-shaking, presumably because of the amelioration of the effects of seasonal allergy.[14]

Sclerosis of the infraorbital or posterior ethmoidal nerves is performed in those horses that have reduced or eliminated head-shaking after injection of local anesthetic into the infraorbital foramen or around the posterior ethmoidal nerve. Sclerosis is achieved by injection of 5 mL of 10% phenol in oil. Care must be taken to ensure that the phenol is deposited only around the nerve. The procedure should be done under general anesthesia.

Cyproheptadine (0.3 mg/kg, orally every 12 hours) improved head-shaking in 43 of 61 horses, based on owner-reported efficacy. Responses were usually observed within 1 week of the start of therapy. Others have not replicated this success but found that the combination of **carbamazepine** (4 mg/kg orally every 6 to 8 hours) and cyproheptadine improved clinical signs in seven horses within 3 to 4 days of starting treatment.

Acupuncture and **chiropractic** manipulation appear to be minimally effective.

Prevention of exposure to bright light is an obvious recommendation, but not practical for most horse owners.

Caudal compression of the infraorbital nerve with platinum coils provides a surgical treatment option for horses that do not respond to medical treatment or environmental modification.[15] Of 58 horses treated using caudal compression of the infraorbital nerve a successful outcome was initially achieved in 35 of 57 (63%) horses, but recurrence occurred between 9 and 30 months later in 9 (26%). Surgery was repeated in 10 of 31 (32%) horses. Final success rate, considering only response to the last performed surgery, was 28 of 57 (49%) horses with median follow-up time of 18 months (range 266 months). Nose-rubbing was reported postoperatively in 30 of 48 (63%) horses and resulted in euthanasia of four horses.[16]

Administration of dexamethasone in a pulsed dose schedule (60 mg orally every 24 hours × 4 days, every 3 weeks for 4 months) to 12 horses did not result in improvement of clinical signs in a randomized, placebo-controlled, blinded field trial.[7]

Addition of an unspecified feed supplement to the diet of 44 affected horses in a randomized, blinded placebo controlled study did not detect a beneficial effect of the supplement.[13]

CONTROL

There are no recognized measures for preventing development of the disease.

FURTHER READING

Pickles K, Madigan J, Aleman M. Idiopathic headshaking: is it still idiopathic? *Vet J.* 2014;201:21-30.

REFERENCES

1. Pickles K, et al. *Vet J.* 2014;201:21.
2. Radostits O, et al. Headshaking in horses. In: *Veterinary Medicine: A Textbook of the Disease of Cattle, Horses, Sheep, Goats and Pigs*. London: W.B. Saunders; 2006:2022.
3. Fiske-Jackson AR, et al. *Equine Vet Educ.* 2012;24:126.
4. Voigt A, et al. *J S Afr Vet Assoc.* 2009;80:111.
5. Gilsenan WF, et al. *Vet Surg.* 2014;43:678.
6. Aleman M, et al. *J Vet Intern Med.* 2012;26:192.
7. Tomlinson JE, et al. *J Vet Intern Med.* 2013;27:1551.
8. Roberts V. *Vet J.* 2014;201:7.
9. Aleman M, et al. *J Vet Intern Med.* 2014;28:250.
10. Aleman M, et al. *J Vet Intern Med.* 2013;27:1571.
11. Veres-Nyeki KO, et al. *Vet J.* 2012;191:101.
12. Mayhew J. *Vet J.* 2012;191:15.
13. Talbot WA, et al. *Equine Vet J.* 2013;45:293.
14. Stalin CE, et al. *Vet Rec.* 2008;163:305.
15. Roberts VLH, et al. *Equine Vet J.* 2009;41:165.
16. Roberts VLH, et al. *Equine Vet J.* 2013;45:107.

TAIL-BITING IN SWINE

Tail-biting, which is the chewing or biting or sucking of a tail of a fellow pig, is an example of cannibalism. It is a very complex problem that is widespread and has demanded more attention with time. It is an intractable problem[1,2] that is very unpredictable. It has a high economic impact because of euthanasia, medical costs, other infections, and condemnations. This has increased with intensive farming and is the most serious of the vices of the domestic pig. It is much more important than flank-biting, nosing, or ear-biting. It has been seen in outdoor pigs and on organic units. About 60% of farms in the UK have at one time or another experienced tail-biting in single pigs or as a group problem. It is a serious welfare issue because it often leads to systemic infections from a whole variety of opportunist bacteria, principally *Trueperella pyogenes* and *Streptococcus* spp., which lead to septicemias and particularly spinal abscessation. Both ear-chewing and tail-biting have also increased in recent years.[3] It is assumed that contented pigs do not tail-bite.

Three stages of tail-biting have been recognized[3]:

1. Two-stage initial phase that includes predamage and damage probably related to having no substrates or play items
2. A second stage called sudden or forceful in which there are probably inadequate resources
3. An obsessive phase that includes many of the factors described in stages 1 and 2, principally those associated with genetics, attraction to blood, and protein metabolism upsets

The diagnosis of the condition is very difficult. It occurs under all conditions including outdoors. Possibly 0.5% to 0.7% of docked pigs are bitten and 2% to 4% of undocked pigs. A recent survey in the UK suggested that 90% of farms had pigs that were not bitten, 6% had small problem, and 4% had big problems. Most abattoirs do not record pigs bitten, and many bitten pigs are sent to small abattoirs. There are probably three mild lesions to every one serious lesion and these are probably not recorded.

ETIOLOGY

There are said to be three basic scenarios: (1) gentle chewing that escalates; (2) two-stage biting; and (3) sudden forceful biting, which may be sudden frustration over a lack of a resource.[5,6]

Tail-biting usually begins with one pig doing the biting and one pig being bitten in an environment that for some reason has caused stress. It then spreads rapidly through the whole group as the bitten tail becomes more attractive.

The inadequate total environment for an animal that naturally requires the opportunity to socially interact and demonstrate its natural behavior of inquisitiveness and rooting is often the underlying cause. Abnormal foraging behavior has been suggested as the underlying cause.[6] Abnormalities of ventilation, particularly drafts, appear very unsettling to pigs. The normal pig group is probably under 20 and over that number the individual's place in the hierarchy is probably lost.

EPIDEMIOLOGY

"Belly-nosing" may be one of the behavior patterns that predispose to tail-biting. It is often associated with early weaning and is the persistent rubbing of the snout on the belly of another pig. It may be misdirected suckling behavior.[7] This behavior is not eliminated by providing environmental enrichment, suckling devices, of extra drinkers or nipple feeders. There is a genetic linkage with Landrace pigs[8] and with weight for age.[9]

The condition is found worldwide. It is often more prevalent in males than females and may be part of natural aggressiveness. The real cause is still unknown but is probably a mental reaction on the part of the pig to unsavory living conditions. Under normal circumstances happy pigs root for 18% of the time and probably doze for about 82% of the time. They are really the "couch potatoes" of the domesticated farm animals. If they have nothing to do, they cause trouble. Recent studies have suggested that the "troublesome" pig may be lighter, more active, and possess more "nosing" behavior patterns.[10] Others have suggested that it is the heavier pigs that are bitten.

The causes for tail-biting are multifactorial, but it has to be considered that there may be a bad "psychologically disturbed pig." Once the behavior has started it behaves like an epidemic. Recent studies have suggested that the way the tail is held has a very considerable influence on whether it is bitten or not.

Anal biting may or may not be related to tail-biting. It has certainly been a feature of a few cases of anal irritation in response to oral dosing with Lincocin.

RISK FACTORS

These have been reviewed.[4,5] Traits related to foraging, exploration feeding, motivation to feed, and sociability are heritable.[11,12]

Because of modern genetics, pigs grow faster and are more aggressive. Aggression is also heritable.[13] Some of the breeds may be more heavily bitten, but Hampshires are less frequently bitten. Some pigs may be unable to use food properly because of a metabolic deficiency.

There is a subset of pigs called the fanatical biters who are generally small males with low lightweight gain. These biters have a low growth rate from weaning to finishing. They spend more time chewing than they do rooting. In a poor environment, they will chew other pigs rather than root. Some of these biters have respiratory or alimentary diseases or porcine circovirus type 2 (PCV2) infections. There are other types of pigs that bite.

The tail-biting hypothesis suggests that there may be a big protein demand that is not being met, so there is a protein deficiency as a result of poor intake of food. There may be a dysfunctional autonomic nervous system regulation involving the general sense responses, interrelated illnesses, and suppressed thyroid hormone T_3 production. It may be that there is a lack of tyrosine for serotonin production, which is an important neurotransmitter. Pigs with higher levels of serotonin spend more time rooting, and in the "bit tail blood model" it is found that serotonin-deficient pigs do more biting.

- There may be breed, line, or family predispositions.
- White pigs have more of a problem than colored breeds.
- There is a genetic tendency to be a biter or to bitten.
- Tail-biting is associated with lean tissue growth and backfat thickness

FACTORS INCREASING BITING

- Tails are bitten more frequently when there is a low weight gain (nutrition).
- Males may be more predisposed, but there is less biting in single sex rearing.
- When there are no interests provided and there are no toys with which to play.
- High-density stocking.
- Over stocking.
- Large group sizes.
- Mixing and moving.
- Space postweaning.[14]
- If you move pigs from a straw-based system to a slatted system they will bite much more.
- Insufficient trough space, if feeders are blocked then pigs will bite to get at the feeder.
- Insufficient drinkers.
- Inadequate nutrition.
- Change in ration formulation leading to food sensing.

- Low-protein diets encourage biting and chewing.
- Not enough amino acids (lysine, tryptophan, but true position unknown).
- Low salt.
- Nonsatisfying environments, particularly those with a poor layout, on nonstraw systems are badly affected.
- Boredom (lack of toys).
- Inadequate environment.
- Low temperatures: cold and damp is bad on straw-based systems, and poor-quality straw is a problem.
- High temperatures.
- Fluctuating temperatures.
- Drafts.
- Too high a humidity.

Variable tail docking length is also a factor. The variation in tail anatomy and position is also important.[15]

Concurrent disease, particularly PCV2 infection and skin, disease may predispose to biting.

In a summary, overstocking was thought to be important in 60% of cases, inadequate ventilation in 50%, wrongly positioned ventilation in 50%, and cold drafts in 40%. Sick pigs that are not moved promptly were thought to be important in 60% of outbreaks and boredom in 50%. The other factors were considered to be of lesser importance (below 20%).

CLINICAL FINDINGS

At the start there is no effect on the bitten pig because the end of the tail is relatively insensitive, but as the bitten area extends toward the anus it becomes more painful and the bitten pig shows signs of distress. With continuation the pig may be reluctant to feed, reluctant to move, and eventually become paralyzed as spinal abscessation becomes the reality.

CLINICAL PATHOLOGY

There may be chewed, gnawed, and partially or completely removed tails. In an early study at an abattoir 19.9% of the lesions on the carcasses were related to tail-biting and 61.75 of carcass abscesses were associated with tail-biting.

NECROPSY

At necropsy or in the abattoir it is a bitten tail as well as the abscessation that is most noticeable along the length of the spine as infection tracts along lymphatics and longitudinal spinal veins. In some cases, the carcass is so badly affected that the whole carcass is condemned. In some cases, there will be evidence of flank-biting and ear-biting (sometimes the ear is completely bitten off), which are part of the same disturbed pig syndrome.

TREATMENT

Remove affected pigs to hospital accommodation, pen separately, and treat the wounds by cleaning, disinfection, and topical palliatives and possibly parenteral broad-spectrum antibiotics. Shoot badly affected or paraplegic pigs. Casualty slaughter is not very useful because of the carcass damage.

CONTROL

There is no really successful plan for control that will work all the time. There is a husbandry advisory tool with 100 possible risk factors. The spreadsheet lists 83 factors. Weighted for risk factors the tool shows that a quarter of the farms have no problems and a quarter of the farms have a serious problem. Attend to all the listed factors and even then you will not always remove the problem, but it will certainly be reduced. Nothing is ever completely effective.

First, observe pigs several times a day and remove the biter as soon as it is seen to bite and put it into separate accommodation.

Elevating the salt level to 0.8% often works even though there is already 0.4% in the diet, which is thought to be sufficient. Make sure there is plenty of water available.

The improved environment is one of the most important items, particularly the application of negative pressure systems. Lowering light levels reduces the "glowing effect" of blood-covered surfaces similar to housing broiler birds in infrared lights to reduce "vent pecking."

The provision of an improved environment by providing "playthings" that satisfy the desire of the pig to sniff, inquire, taste, and chew is most important. These items should be malleable, which is why straw or peat, or spent mushroom compost or rubber cords, or even tires[16] are more satisfying than chains. The chains are no good because they slap other pigs and increase the restlessness. Straw provision has the ability to keep pigs occupied for longer than other substrates,[17,18] and it is better if it is provided daily.[19] Housing systems that have had ad libitum feeding systems with multiple feed spaces have had a reduced prevalence of the problem.

This attention to sucking and chewing is the basis of all the saliva tests that have been developed to detect viruses such as porcine reproductive and respiratory syndrome (PRRS) and PCV2 and antibodies to them. Hanging a set of cotton cords in a pen that will soon be sucked by most pigs as part of play will provide a readily accessible sample source for saliva antigens antibodies and many other substances such as acute phase proteins. This does not involve disturbing the pigs or requiring handling and invasive techniques for the individual pig for investigating herd profiles.

The provision of straw is no guarantee that tail-biting will be stopped.[20]

Tail docking is the only technique that does reduce the presence of tail-biting. The conditions attached to use of this practice vary from country to country and often mean that the technique has to be prescribed by a veterinarian only after the presence of a tail-biting problem has been established on that farm. Even tail-docked pigs have evidence of being tail-bitten.[21]

The ideal length of tail docking is not really known. One of the major problems is that tails differ in thickness and length before any consideration of the length to be cut off. Too short a tail, i.e., cut very short, interferes with the nervous control around the anus, may lead to fecal incontinence, and exposes the anus itself to being bitten.

Tail docking produces a neuroma at the site of nerve transection, which results in the formation of many sensitive nerve endings that enable the pig to react more sensitively to any nosing of its tail.

In a recent survey,[18] 62% thought that docking was effective in preventing tail-biting, 47% thought adding straw was helpful, 46% thought that playthings were effective, but only 18% thought reducing stocking density was helpful. The latter may be because of the economic implications of reducing stocking. All in all, reducing stocking density and adding straw together was considered to be the best option.[22]

FURTHER READING

Taylor NR, et al. Tail biting: a new perspective. *Vet J.* 2009;186:137-147.

Taylor NR, et al. The prevalence of risk factors for tail biting. *Vet J.* 2012;194:77-88.

Zonderland JJ Thesis. Talking tails-quantifying the development of tail biting in pigs. 2010; http://edepot.wur.nl/151535.

REFERENCES

1. Edwards SA. *Pig J.* 2011;66:81.
2. Edwards SA. *Vet J.* 2006;171:198.
3. Kritas SK, Morrison RB. *Vet Rec.* 2007;160:149.
4. Taylor NR, et al. *Vet J.* 2012;194:77.
5. Taylor NR, et al. *Vet J.* 2010;186:137.
6. Peeters E, et al. *Appl Anim Behav Sci.* 2006;98:234.
7. Widowski T, et al. *Appl Anim Behav Sci.* 2008;110:109.
8. Bensch CJ, Gonyou HW. *Appl Anim Behav Sci.* 2007;105:26.
9. Torrey S, Widowski TM. *Appl Anim Behav Sci.* 2006;101:288.
10. Zonderland JJ, et al. *Animal.* 2011;5:767.
11. Baumung R. *Archiv Tierzucht.* 2006;49:77.
12. Renadeu D, et al. *Asian Australas J Anim Sci.* 2006;19:593.
13. Turner SP, et al. *Anim Sci.* 2006;82:615.
14. http://www.thepigsite.com/pighealth/article/366/vice-abnormal-behaviour-tail-biting-flank-chewing-ear-biting/ Accessed August 2016.
15. Zonderland JJ, et al. *Appl Anim Behav Sci.* 2009;121:165.
16. Day JEL, et al. *Appl Anim Behav Sci.* 2008;109:249.
17. Scott K, et al. *Appl Anim Behav Sci.* 2006;99:222.
18. Scott K, et al. *Anim Welfare.* 2007;16:53.
19. Scott K, et al. *Appl Anim Behav Sci.* 2007;105:51.
20. Statham P, et al. *Anim Behav Sci.* 2011;134:100.
21. Smulders D, et al. *Anim Welfare.* 2008;17:61.
22. Paul ES, et al. *Vet Rec.* 2007;160:803.

Bacterial Diseases Primarily Affecting the Cerebrum

ENTEROTOXEMIA ASSOCIATED WITH *CLOSTRIDIUM PERFRINGENS* TYPE D (PULPY KIDNEY, OVEREATING DISEASE)

> **SYNOPSIS**
>
> **Etiology** An acute toxemia of ruminants associated with the proliferation of *Clostridium perfringens* type D in the intestines and the liberation of ε-toxin that produces vascular damage and the damage to the nervous system typical of this disease.
>
> **Epidemiology** Lambs 3–10 weeks of age and lambs and calves after weaning. Goats of all ages. Affected animals in good condition and on a rising plane of nutrition.
>
> **Clinical findings** The disease in lambs and calves and young goats has a rapid course with diarrhea, depression, and convulsions. At this age animals are often found dead. Adult goats show more chronic disease with abdominal pain and bloody diarrhea.
>
> **Clinical pathology** Hyperglycemia and glycosuria in sheep.
>
> **Necropsy findings** None specific to all cases. Sheep and some goats may have gross or histologic areas of malacia in internal capsule, lateral thalamus, and cerebellar peduncles.
>
> **Diagnostic confirmation** Epidemiology, clinical and necropsy findings, demonstration of ε-toxin
>
> **Treatment** Anti-ε antitoxin.
>
> **Control** Feed restriction, antitoxin, vaccination.

ETIOLOGY

Enterotoxemia results from the proliferation of *C. perfringens* type D in the small intestine. This organism produces a number of toxins, of which the epsilon toxin is the most important and results in vascular damage and the damage to the nervous system typical of this disease. The presence of *C. perfringens* type D in the intestine does not in itself result in disease unless other factors intercede that promote proliferation and the production of toxin. The natural habitat of the organism is in the intestine and in soil contaminated by feces, although it does not persist in soil for long periods of time.

EPIDEMIOLOGY

Occurrence

Enterotoxemia associated with *C. perfringens* type D is a disease of ruminant animals, primarily of lambs, and is worldwide in its distribution. The common practice of vaccination against this disease has reduced its prevalence, but it is still a common disease.

Although most common in lambs, it is also an important disease of calves and goats. It occurs rarely in adult cattle, deer, domesticated camels, and possibly horses. In pastured sheep, it causes heavy losses, particularly in flocks managed for the production of lamb and mutton. The prevalence in flocks varies a great deal but seldom exceeds 10%. The case–fatality rate approximates 100%. In North America enterotoxemia ranks as one of the main causes of loss among feedlot lambs. In a survey in two feedlots the disease had an annual prevalence of 3.1% and 1.5%; it ranked third in importance as a cause of death despite a policy of vaccination, and the costs of prevention programs were the largest expenditure of all disease prevention programs in the feedlots.

Experimental Reproduction

The disease can be produced experimentally in susceptible sheep, goats, and cattle by the injection into the duodenum of whole culture of *C. perfringens* type D and dextrin or starch. Clinical disease occurs as early as 30 minutes and usually within 6 to 8 hours of the start of duodenal infusion and death 1 to 9 hours following the onset of clinical signs. The disease has also been reproduced by intravenous infusion of epsilon toxin.

Animal and Management Risk Factors

C. perfringens type D normally inhabits the alimentary tract of sheep and other ruminants but only in small numbers. The extent to which it occurs in the alimentary tract varies widely between flocks, although this accounts only in part for the variable prevalence. The organism does not persist for more than 1 year in the soil.

Under certain conditions, the organisms proliferate rapidly in the intestines and produce lethal quantities of epsilon toxin. In most, if not all circumstances, the affected animals are on **highly nutritious diets** and are in very good condition. The husbandry conditions in which the disease occurs include grazing on lush, rapidly growing pasture or young cereal crops, and heavy grain feeding in feedlots. Lambs on well-fed, heavy-milking ewes are particularly susceptible. The occurrence of the disease under these conditions has given rise to the name "overeating disease."

Sheep

The highest incidence of the disease is in suckling lambs between 3 and 10 weeks of age, although lambs as young as 1 to 5 days old can be affected.[1] The risk for disease in this age group is highest when ewes are grazed on lush pastures that result in profuse lactation. The disease can occur following rain in set stocked flocks, and in flocks newly introduced to lush pastures it is often manifested 5 to 14 days after introduction. Larger and more rapidly growing single lambs are more susceptible than twins. Weaned lambs up to 10 months of age are the second most susceptible age group, and again the occurrence of disease is associated with highly nutritious diets. Feeder lambs are most commonly affected soon after they are introduced into feedlots.

Calves

Enterotoxemia in calves is most common between 1 and 4 months of age and the same risk factors pertain as for lambs. Veal calves are particularly at risk. Feeder cattle may develop disease shortly after introduction to the lot. It is a common belief among cattlemen and veterinarians that many unexplained sudden deaths in feeder cattle after the period of acclimatization are caused by this type of enterotoxemia. However, there is no laboratory evidence to support such field observations, and a controlled trial found no protective effect of vaccination.

Goats

Enterotoxemia is a common disease in goats under intensive or extensive grazing systems, occurring in many countries, and is particularly important in countries with a large goat population.[2] The peracute disease in goat kids has the same age occurrence as in lambs, but less acute and chronic forms of enterotoxemia occur in adult goats. Sudden changes in diet appear to be the most common predisposing factor. Disease can occur in vaccinated goats because vaccination is poorly protective against the enteric and chronic form of the disease in this species.[2]

Outbreaks in sheep and goats have followed the administration of phenothiazine and other anthelmintics, and a high incidence has been observed in association with heavy tapeworm infestation.

Horses

Type D enterotoxemia is rare in horses, but it has been suspected in mature horses fed concentrates during a drought. *C. perfringens* type D can be isolated in high numbers from gastric reflux of horses with anterior enteritis.

PATHOGENESIS

In the normal course of events, ingested *C. perfringens* type D are destroyed in large numbers in the rumen and abomasum, although some survive to reach the duodenum, in which multiplication occurs and toxin is produced. Toxemia does not occur because the movement of ingesta keeps the bacterial population and toxin content down to a low level. In certain circumstances, this does not hold and multiplication of the organisms and the production of toxin proceeds to the point in which toxemia occurs.

One of the circumstances has been shown to be the passage of large quantities of starch granules into the duodenum when sheep overeat on grain diets or are changed suddenly from a ration consisting largely of roughage to one consisting mainly of grain. Other factors such as heavy milk feeding may have the same effect. A slowing of alimentary tract movement has also been thought to permit excess toxin accumulation and it may be that any factor that causes intestinal stasis will predispose to the disease. The importance of diet in the production of ruminal stasis has been discussed in diseases of the forestomachs of ruminants.

The epsilon toxin of *C. perfringens* type D is a pore-forming protein that increases the permeability of the intestinal mucosa to this and other toxins, facilitating its own absorption.[3]

A receptor for epsilon toxin has been identified on vascular endothelial cells, and the clinical signs and pathologic findings can be explained by the widespread vascular damage and increase in vascular permeability.

Acute cases are characterized by the development in the brain of degeneration of vascular endothelium; perivascular and intercellular edema; and microscopic foci of necrosis in the basal ganglia, thalamus, internal capsule, substantia nigra, subcortical white matter, and cerebellum. The damage to the vascular endothelium leads to the accumulation of protein-rich fluid effusions observable in heart, brain, and lung. The postmortem autolysis of kidney tissue that occurs so rapidly and is the characteristic of "pulpy kidney" has the same basis.

There is a pronounced hyperglycemia caused by the mobilization of hepatic glycogen; severe hemoconcentration; and elevation of blood concentrations of pyruvate, lactate, and α-ketoglutarate.

In contrast to sheep, goats with enterotoxemia produced by *C. perfringens* type D also have a hemorrhagic enterocolitis that is present in both the natural and the experimental disease. The genesis of this lesion is uncertain, but it is responsible for the major clinical signs that present in goats with this disease.

A degree of natural immunity may be attained by nonlethal exposure to the toxin. Because a proportion of lambs, calves, and kids appear to be exposed to subclinical but antigenic levels of *C. perfringens* toxin, they become immune without having shown signs of illness or without having been vaccinated.[4]

CLINICAL FINDINGS

Lambs

The course of the illness is very short, often less than 2 hours and never more than 12 hours. Many lambs are found dead without previously manifesting signs. In closely observed flocks the first signs may be dullness, depression, yawning, facial movements, and loss of interest in feed. Acute cases may show little more than severe clonic convulsions with frothing at the mouth and rapid death. Cases that survive for a few hours show a green, pasty diarrhea, staggering, recumbency, opisthotonus, and severe clonic convulsions. The temperature is usually normal but may be elevated if convulsions are severe. Death occurs during a convulsion or after a short period of coma.

Adult Sheep

These usually survive for longer periods of up to 24 hours. They lag behind the flock and show staggering and knuckling; champing of the jaws; salivation; and rapid, shallow, irregular respiration. There may be bloat in the terminal stages. Irritation signs, including convulsions, muscle tremor, grinding of the teeth, and salivation, may occur but are less common than in lambs.

Calves

The syndrome is similar to that seen in adult sheep, with nervous signs predominating. Peracute cases are found dead without having shown premonitory signs of illness and with no evidence of struggling. The more common, acute cases show a sudden onset of bellowing, mania, and convulsions, with the convulsions persisting until death occurs 1 to 2 hours later. Subacute cases, many of which recover, do not drink, are quiet and docile, and appear to be blind, although the eye's preservation reflex persists. They may continue in this state for 2 to 3 days and then recover quickly and completely. In an outbreak of the disease in calves all three forms of the disease may be seen. Experimental inoculation of whole or washed cultures of *C. perfringens* type D into the duodenum of 9-month-old calves produced severe clinical signs within 2 to 5 hours of inoculation.[5]

Goats

Diarrhea is a prominent sign in affected goats, especially in those that survive for more than a few days.[2] In the peracute form, which occurs most frequently in young kids, there are convulsions after an initial attack of fever (40.5°C, 105°F) with severe abdominal pain and dysentery; death occurs in 4 to 36 hours. In the acute form, which is more common in adults, there is usually no fever, and abdominal pain and diarrhea are prominent with death or recovery within 2 to 4 days. In chronic cases, the goats may be ill for several weeks and show anorexia, intermittent severe diarrhea and, in some cases, dysentery and the presence of epithelial shreds in the feces. Chronic wasting, anemia, and eventual emaciation also occur with chronic disease in goats.

CLINICAL PATHOLOGY

A high plasma glucose concentration of 8.3 to 11.1 mmol/L (150 to 200 mg/dL) and marked glycosuria are characteristic of the terminal stages of enterotoxemia in sheep, and are supportive for a diagnosis but are not pathognomonic.[6] Hyperglycemia and glycosuria are variably present in goats with the disease and calves with experimentally induced disease.[5]

NECROPSY FINDINGS

The body condition of the animal is usually good, but there is often fecal staining of the perineum and rapid decomposition of the carcass. In peracute cases there may be no gross lesions. More frequently, there is an excess of clear, straw-colored pericardial and thoracic fluid that clots on exposure to air. Many petechiae are present in the epicardium and endocardium, and there is pulmonary edema. Patchy congestion of the abomasal and intestinal mucosae is usual, and the small intestine often contains a moderate amount of thin, creamy ingesta. The content of the large intestine may be watery and dark green.

The characteristic finding of soft, pulpy kidneys is only useful in animals necropsied within a few hours after death because it is nonspecific and merely correlates to a more rapid rate of autolysis. Microscopy of experimentally induced ovine type D enterotoxemia cases confirms that the renal changes represent autolysis and not a true nephrosis.

The liver is dark and congested. The rumen and abomasum of feedlot lambs may be overloaded with concentrates. In goats there is acute fibrinonecrotic and hemorrhagic enterocolitis, although microscopic examination may be needed to detect this change.

In sheep that have not died acutely there may be symmetric areas of hemorrhage, edema, and liquefaction in the brain, especially in the area of the basal nuclei. Again, microscopic evaluation of the tissue is critical.

Gram-stained smears of ingesta from several levels in the small intestine should be examined. In affected animals the short, fat, gram-positive rods dominate the slide to the almost complete exclusion of other bacteria. Bowel filtrates can be tested for toxicity by injection into mice. If the filtrate is toxic, the type of toxin can be determined by protection of the mice with specific antisera. This does not determine the type of clostridia, but detection of β-toxin indicates the presence of types B or C, and ε-toxin indicates the presence of B or D.

The time taken for diagnosis by mouse neutralization tests, as well as humanitarian considerations, has promoted the development of alternative tests. Commercial enzyme-linked immunosorbent assay (ELISA) kits and multiplex PCR assays have become available for toxin detection and require minimal amounts of intestinal content.[6] Nevertheless, it is important to base a diagnosis on epidemiologic, clinical, and pathologic information, not just the detection of toxin at postmortem.

ε-Toxin is stable if frozen, but at average temperatures it is possible to identify the toxin from the intestine of a sheep dead for up to 12 hours. The addition of one drop of chloroform to each 10 mL of ingesta will stabilize the toxin for up to 1 month. Alternatively, intestinal contents can be absorbed on filter paper and shipped at environmental temperatures, with little loss of activity for as long as 74 days as detected by immunoassay. Hyperglycemia and glucosuria may also be detected in necropsy material.

Samples for Confirmation of Diagnosis

- Bacteriology: 20 to 30 mL of intestinal content, frozen in a leak-proof glass or plastic container (ELISA, latex agglutination, bioassay, anaerobic culture, PCR); air-dried smears of ingesta from several levels of gut (cyto-Gram stain)
- Clinical pathology: urine (assay–glucose) (best performed at time of necropsy)
- Histology: fixed colon, ileum, jejunum, entire brain

DIFFERENTIAL DIAGNOSIS

Lambs
- Acute pasteurellosis
- Septicemia associated with *Histophilus somni* (formerly *Haemophilus agni*)
- *Clostridium sordellii*
- Polioencephalomalacia
- Rumen overload

Sheep
- Hypocalcemia
- Hypomagnesemia
- Focal symmetric encephalomalacia (chronic enterotoxemia)
- Rabies
- Pregnancy toxemia
- Louping-ill

Calves
- Lead poisoning
- Polioencephalomalacia
- Hepatoencephalopathy
- *H. somni* (formerly *Haemophilus somni*)

Goats
- Salmonellosis
- Coccidiosis

In lambs, but not in goats, a history of vaccination against the disease is a significant consideration in the ranking of a list of differential diagnoses.

TREATMENT

In general, the clinical course of the disease is too acute for effective treatment. Hyperimmune serum, an efficient short-term prophylactic, is unlikely to be of much value in sick animals because of the acute nature of the disease. In goats the course is longer, and antitoxin in combination with orally administered sulfadimidine may be effective in treatment.[2]

CONTROL

There are three major control measures available: reduction of the food intake, administration of antitoxin, and vaccination. These may be used individually or in combination.

Reduction in Food Intake

Reduction in food intake is the cheapest but least effective in control and is used as a short-term control while waiting for immunity to develop after vaccination. Reduction in food intake will cause a setback in the growth of the lambs and for this reason farmers tend to rely more on vaccination as a control measure. However, exercise of lambs, by mustering or herding around the paddock, may help slow the course of an outbreak.

Antitoxin

Antitoxin can be administered to all sheep as soon as an outbreak commences. The administration of ε-antitoxin 200 IU/kg BW will provide for protective circulating antitoxin levels for 21 to 29 days. Immediate losses are prevented, and in most instances the disease does not recur. Toxoid is cheaper, but to administer it alone at such times may result in further serious losses before active immunity develops.

Vaccination

Immunity in sheep is readily produced by suitable vaccination. A blood level of 0.15 Wellcome unit of ε-antitoxin per milliliter of serum is sufficient to protect sheep. Vaccines available are toxoids, and adjuvants generally improve the antigenicity. Activated alum-precipitated toxoid is the common vaccine in use. A recombinant *C. perfringens* type D toxoid has been shown to induce antibody titers comparable to a traditional toxoid and may offer a more consistent or cost-effective method of vaccine production.[7]

Vaccination of maiden **ewes** twice at an interval of at least 1 month and with the last vaccination approximately 4 weeks before lambing will result in good passive immunity in young lambs, with 97% of lambs having protective antibody levels at 8 weeks of age and a significant proportion at 12 to 16 weeks of age. This is sufficient to protect lambs during their highest risk period. Older ewes that have been vaccinated the previous year receive a single booster vaccination 4 weeks before lambing. Sheep vaccinated for 3 consecutive years can be considered to be permanently immune and to require no further vaccination.

When faced with an outbreak in lambs, the recommended procedure is to administer antiserum and toxoid immediately and repeat the toxoid in a month's time. The simultaneous administration of hyperimmune serum with this vaccine does not interfere with the stimulation of antibody production, nor does the presence of passively derived colostral immunity.

Lambs can be vaccinated with toxoid when 4 to 10 weeks of age and again a month later.

Any vaccination of sheep is not without risk of precipitating blackleg or other clostridial disease, and if these are a severe problem in an area it may be wise to vaccinate a portion of the flock as a pilot test and proceed with vaccination of the remainder only when no complications arise. A multivalent bacterin-toxoid containing antigens to all of the clostridial diseases is commonly used in sheep in these circumstances or where all of these diseases are likely to occur. Vaccination should not be done in sheep with wet fleeces.

Vaccination with toxoid is effective in calves but is not highly effective in goats, having a limited effect in preventing the disease although reducing its incidence and severity.[2] The anti-ε titer in goats following vaccination is variable, sometimes equivalent, but often lower or of shorter duration to that induced in sheep. The reasons for decreased protection following the use of commercial vaccines against type D infections in goats are not fully understood.[2] Thus, goat owners should be advised that vaccination with the current commercial vaccines often provides limited protection against type D infections, even if multiple booster vaccines are given at 3- to 6-month intervals. This occurs especially when a high level of concentrate feeding occurs, such as in dairy production. The use of hyperimmune serum must also be performed with caution in goats, particularly Saanens, which are very prone to anaphylactic reactions. Despite the limitations of protection against the enteric manifestations of the disease, vaccination is protective against the peracute form of the disease and kids should be vaccinated twice, a month apart, commencing at 4 weeks of age with booster vaccinations at 6-month intervals.

Local reactions to vaccination are common in both sheep and goats and may be visible for at least 6 months. In sheep these are generally hidden by the wool, but the vaccination site should be high on the neck and close to the base of the ear to minimize carcass blemish. With goats, especially show goats, the owner should be warned of this occurrence. Goats, especially show goats, should be vaccinated under the loose skin of the axilla, where local reactions will be hidden by the elbow.

FURTHER READING

Allaart JG, van Asten AJAM, Gröne A. Predisposing factors and prevention of *Clostridium perfringens*-associated enteritis. *Comp Immunol Microbiol Infect Dis.* 2013;36:449-464.

Alves GG, et al. Clostridium perfringens epsilon toxin: the third most potent bacterial toxin known. *Anaerobe*. 2014;30:102-107.

Bokori-Brown M, Savva CG, et al. Molecular basis of toxicity of *Clostridium perfringens* epsilon toxin. *FEBS J*. 2011;23:4589-4601.

Morris WE, Dunleavy MV, et al. Effects of *Clostridium perfringens* alpha and epsilon toxins in the bovine gut. *Anaerobe*. 2012;18:143-147.

Radostits O, et al. Enterotoxemia associated with *Clostridium perfringens* type D (pulpy kidney, overeating disease). In: *Veterinary Medicine: A Textbook of the Diseases of Cattle, Horses, Sheep, Goats and Pigs*. 10th ed. London: W.B. Saunders; 2007:841-844.

Uzal FA, Vidal JE, et al. *Clostridium perfringens* toxins involved in mammalian veterinary diseases. *Open Toxicol*. 2010;3:24-42.

Wioland L, Dupont J-L, Bossu J-L, et al. Attack of the nervous system by *Clostridium perfringens* epsilon toxin: from disease to mode of action on neural cells. *Toxicon*. 2013;75:122-135.

REFERENCES

1. Scholes SFE, et al. *Vet Rec*. 2007;160:811.
2. Sumithra TG, et al. *Small Rum Res*. 2013;114:1.
3. Alves GG, et al. *Anaerobe*. 2014;30:102.
4. Veschi JLA, et al. *Vet Immunol Immunopathol*. 2008;125:198.
5. Filho EJF, et al. *Vet Pathol*. 2009;46:1213.
6. Uzal FH, Songer JG. *J Vet Diagn Invest*. 2008;20:253.
7. Lobato FCF, et al. *Vaccine*. 2010;28:6125.

FOCAL SYMMETRIC ENCEPHALOMALACIA

SYNOPSIS

Etiology The disease is a chronic neurologic manifestation of enterotoxemia associated with *Clostridium perfringens* type D ε-toxin, with vascular damage and damage to the nervous system.

Epidemiology Sporadic disease in weaners and mature sheep, usually following a change of pasture, anthelmintic treatment, or supplementary feeding with grain and incomplete vaccination regimens.

Clinical findings Aimless wandering, an inability to eat, and a dummy syndrome are predominant findings

Clinical pathology None reported.

Necropsy findings Gross or histologic areas of malacia in internal capsule, lateral thalamus, and cerebellar peduncles.

Diagnostic confirmation Epidemiology, clinical and necropsy findings.

Treatment Supportive.

Control Complete vaccination.

ETIOLOGY

Lesions of focal symmetric encephalomalacia have been produced in experimental enterotoxemia and by infusion with ε-toxin of *C. perfringens* type D. Similar brain lesions have been described in an experimentally induced case of enterotoxemia in a 9-month-old calf that survived for 8 days.[1]

EPIDEMIOLOGY

Focal symmetric encephalomalacia occurs most often in lambs, weaners, and mature sheep, but lesions consistent with focal symmetric encephalomalacia have also been reported in calves and goats.[2] In grazing sheep. It has the same seasonal occurrence as enterotoxemia but may occur in sheep of poor body condition. In weaners and mature sheep, there is often a history of supplementary feeding of highly fermentable carbohydrate, such as cereal grains, a move to fresh pasture, or of anthelmintic administration 5 to 14 days preceding the occurrence of initial cases. This is often combined with an incomplete history of vaccination, and outbreaks have been associated with the grazing of young green cereal crops. The morbidity is usually low but may approach 15%. The case–fatality rate is high.

CLINICAL FINDINGS

Most often, because of infrequent observation of sheep of this age, the finding of dead sheep is the first indication of the disease. Clinically affected sheep are separate from the group or can be detected by slow movement of the flock. They show no fear of humans or dogs and can be examined without restraint. Blindness, aimless wandering, head-pressing, and incoordination are the predominant findings. More severely affected sheep lie quietly in lateral recumbency with moderate dorsiflexion of the head and show infrequent nystagmus with paddling convulsions. The sheep are unable to eat and most cannot drink, although some affected lambs may still retain a suck reflex. The clinical course varies from 1 to 14 days, with the majority of affected sheep surviving for 5 to 7 days.

NECROPSY FINDINGS

Lesions are confined to the brain, and formalin-fixed samples of this tissue are required for confirmation of the diagnosis. In many cases the characteristic lesions can be detected on macroscopic examination and consist of areas of hemorrhage and softening in the internal capsule, lateral thalamus, and cerebellar peduncles. Malacia, edema, and hemorrhage are visible histologically. Glycosuria is not a feature, and toxin cannot be demonstrated in gut contents.

TREATMENT AND CONTROL

There is no treatment. Less severely affected cases may recover if they are maintained with fluids and nutrients given by stomach tube. Outbreaks cease if the sheep are vaccinated with pulpy kidney vaccine.

FURTHER READING

Finnie JW. Pathogenesis of brain lesions produced in sheep by *Clostridium perfringens* type D epsilon toxin: a review. *Aust Vet J*. 2003;81:219-221.

Wioland L, Dupont J-L, Bossu J-L, et al. Attack of the nervous system by *Clostridium perfringens* epsilon toxin: from disease to mode of action on neural cells. *Toxicon*. 2013;75:122-135.

REFERENCES

1. Filho EJF, et al. *Vet Pathol*. 2009;46:1213.
2. Anon. *Vet Rec*. 2012;171:168.

CEREBROSPINAL ANGIOPATHY

Cerebrospinal angiopathy is a sporadic disease of recently weaned pigs manifested primarily by neurologic signs and wasting. It is probably a form of edema disease. It affects only one or a few pigs within a litter up to 5 weeks after weaning, although a similar condition has been reported in finishing and adult pigs. The disease is characterized by the variety of neurologic signs that it presents. Incoordination and a decreased central awareness are common presenting signs but abnormal head position, aimless wandering, and persistent circling may also be observed. There is usually apparent impairment of vision. Fever is not a feature, and the clinical course may last for several days. Affected animals may die but are often euthanized because of emaciation. Wasting without neurologic disorder may also occur. They are also prone to savaging by unaffected penmates.

Histologically, the disease is characterized by an angiopathy that is not restricted to the CNS. The similarity of the angiopathy to that seen in chronic edema disease has led to postulation that this disease is a sequel to subclinical edema disease. The disease has been reported occurring in pigs 15 to 27 days after experimental *E. coli* infection. The characteristic feature is the presence of perivascular eosinophilic droplets.

The main differential diagnosis is that of spinal or brain abscess and the porcine viral encephalomyelitides. Affected pigs should be housed separately as soon as clinical signs are observed. In view of the nature of the lesion, therapy is unlikely to be of value; however, recovery following treatment with oxytetracycline has been reported.

FURTHER READING

Harding DJD, et al. Cerebrospinal angiopathy in pigs. *Vet Rec*. 1966;79:388.

Viral Diseases Primarily Affecting the Cerebrum

RABIES

SYNOPSIS

Etiology *Lyssavirus* of family Rhabdoviridae

Epidemiology Occurs in all farm animals worldwide except Australia and New

Continued

Zealand. Major zoonoses. Transmitted by bites of infected animal. Different animals are vectors depending on geographic location: foxes in Europe and North America, skunks and raccoons in North America, mongoose in Africa, vampire bats in South America.

Signs Incubation period varies from 2 weeks to several months.

Cattle: *Paralytic form:* bizarre mental behavior (yawning, bellowing), incoordination, decreased sensation of hindquarters, drooling saliva, recumbency, and death in 4–7 days. *Furious form:* hypersensitive, belligerent, then paralysis and death as in paralytic form.

Sheep: Outbreaks common; sexual excitement, wool pulling, attacking, incoordination, and then paralysis.

Horses: Abnormal postures, lameness or weakness, depression, ataxia, pharyngeal paralysis, recumbency, hyperesthesia, biting, loss of anal sphincter tone, death in 4–6 days.

Pigs: Excitement, attack, twitching of nose, clonic convulsions, paralysis.

Clinical pathology No antemortem test.

Lesions Nonsuppurative encephalomyelitis.

Differential diagnosis list

- **Cattle:** Lead poisoning, lactation tetany, hypovitaminosis A, listerial meningoencephalitis, polioencephalomalacia, nervous acetonemia.
- **Sheep:** Enterotoxemia, pregnancy toxemia, louping-ill, scrapie.
- **Horse:** Viral encephalomyelitis, herpes viral paralysis, cerebrospinal nematodiasis, equine degenerative myeloencephalopathy, protozoal encephalomyelitis, neuritis of cauda equina, horsetail poisoning, Borna, Japanese encephalitis, botulism.
- **Pig:** Pseudorabies, Teschen disease, Glasser's disease, and other meningitides (*Escherichia. coli* and *Streptococcus suis*).

Diagnostic confirmation Fluorescent antibody test of brain. Negri bodies histologically.

Treatment None. All rabies cases are fatal.

Control Prevention of exposure. Vaccination of domestic animals and wildlife. Quarantine and biosecurity to prevent entry of virus into country.

ETIOLOGY

Rabies is caused by single-stranded RNA viruses in the genus *Lyssavirus* of the family Rhabdoviridae. The Lyssavirus genome contains about 12 kb, and five separate genes encode for two membrane-associated proteins: matrix (M); glycoprotein (G); and three structural proteins, nucleoprotein (N), phosphoprotein (P), and polymerase (L).[1]

Currently, seven distinct genetic lineages are identified in the genus *Lyssavirus:* classical rabies virus (RABV, genotype 1, which includes a number of variants), Lagos bat virus (LBV, genotype 2), Mokola virus (MOKV, genotype 3), Duvenhage virus (DUUV, genotype 4), European bat lyssavirus (EBLV, subdivided into genotype 5 and genotype 6), and the Australian bat lyssavirus (ABLV, genotype 7). It was recognized long ago that the strain of virus known as the "street" rabies virus differed in some way from "fixed" strains that had been cultivated for vaccine production (grown in cell culture or passaged through serial generations of laboratory animals). A large number of rabies virus strains are adapted to particular host species but remain infective for any mammal.

EPIDEMIOLOGY

Occurrence

Rabies occurs in all warm-blooded animals. The disease occurs in cattle, sheep, horses, and pigs, in most countries, except the insular countries that exclude it by rigid quarantine measures or prohibition of the entry of dogs. However, the genus *Lyssavirus* can still cause surprises. In 1996 and 1998, two women died in Queensland, Australia, from infections with a newly discovered rabies-related virus (Australian bat lyssavirus). In 2002 a man died in Scotland after contracting European bat lyssavirus rabies indicating that after a century of apparent freedom from rabies, the disease is now enzootic in the UK.

Europe

In Europe, sylvatic rabies is a major problem for which the **red fox** is the principal vector. The disease is still spreading from a focal point that developed in Poland in the mid-1930s. It is endemic in Yugoslavia and Turkey, and has spread westward to Germany, Denmark, Belgium, Czechoslovakia, Austria, Switzerland, and France. Spread continues at the rate of about 30 to 60 km (18–37 miles) per year, and the threat to the UK increases each year.[2] Finland had been free of rabies since 1959, but in 1988 sylvatic rabies occurred with the raccoon dog as the vector.

United States

Information on rabies surveillance in the United States is published annually by the Centers for Disease Control and Prevention (CDC). In 2013, 92% of cases occurred in wild animals, 4.2% in cats, 1.5% in cattle, and 1.5% in dogs. The disease occurred in raccoons, bats, skunks, foxes, sheep and goats, horses and mules, mongoose, rodents and lagomorphs, and humans.

The most frequently reported rabid wildlife cases occurred in raccoons, skunks, bats, and foxes. The relative contributions of those species continue to change in recent decades because of fluctuations in enzootics of rabies among animals infected with several distinct variants of the rabies virus. Endemic raccoon rabies occurs in the Appalachian mountain range and the entire eastern seaboard of the United States. Endemic skunk rabies occurs mainly in three geographic regions: the north central United States and the Canadian provinces of Manitoba, Saskatchewan, and Alberta; south central United States; and California. Within these broad areas, the disease persists in enzootic foci and erupts every 6 to 8 years. Experimental studies suggest that the species specificity of endemic rabies is caused by differences in the pathogenicity of variants of rabies virus. Skunk rabies peaks in the spring and early winter, which is probably a reflection of certain life history events within the skunk population.

The prevalence of rabies in bats in the United States is about 7%, and transmission to humans is rare even though sensational journalism has caused many people to consider bats as a serious threat to health. Trends in national surveillance for rabies among bats in the United States from 1993 to 2013 have consistently found a diffuse geographic pattern of rabies in bats throughout the continental United States. Although spillover infection of bat variants of rabies among terrestrial animals such as dogs and cats are rare, these variants of rabies virus have been associated with 92% of the indigenously acquired human rabies infections in the United States since 1990.

Canada

The arctic fox variant of rabies invaded most of Canada south of 60°N and east of the Rocky Mountains in the early 1950s largely by the migration of **arctic foxes** into the populated areas. It died out in most of that range, but persisted for over 40 years in southern Ontario with sporadic incursions into narrow adjacent strips in western Quebec and northern New York. The principal vectors were red foxes (*Vulpes vulpes*) and, to a lesser extent, striped skunks (*Mephitis mephitis*). From 1957 to 1989, Ontario experienced more animal rabies cases than almost every North American jurisdiction almost every year, and over 95% of those cases were limited to the southernmost 10% of the province's land area.

A second major outbreak, involving striped **skunks**, progressed from North Dakota into the Prairie Provinces during the late 1950s and 1960s. In the 1990s, the endemic areas in Canada are southern Ontario, which accounts for 85% of the Canadian diagnoses, and the Prairie Provinces where rabies is endemic in skunks. In western Canada, the main reservoirs of the rabies virus are skunks, bats, and foxes.

Africa

Rabies occurs in most countries in the African continent, but the reported incidence is surprisingly low for an area with such a high population of wild carnivores. The incidence of rabies, and the range of species involved, is increasing in Africa, and a number of wildlife hosts has been identified, including wild dogs, jackals, and mongoose.

In South Africa over a 4-year period, of all the domestic animal rabies cases reported, cattle accounted for half of the rabies cases in domestic animals. The **mongoose** accounted for 70% of the wild animal cases reported. Widespread distribution of the rabies virus occurs when the young mongooses are evicted from their parents' territory during the winter months, forcing them to scatter over a wide area. This increases the probability of domestic animals coming in contact with rabid animals.

South America, Latin America, and the Caribbean

Rabies in cattle is a major economic and public health problem in South America, where vampire bat–transmitted rabies results in cyclic outbreaks. Bovine paralytic rabies is endemic in the tropical regions extending from northern Mexico, to northern Argentina, and on the island of Trinidad.

Distribution of Virus Variants

The *Lyssavirus* genus belongs to the Rhabdoviridae family of the Mononegavirales order and includes unsegmented RNA viruses causing rabies encephalomyelitis. They are well fitted to vectors belonging to the orders Carnivora (flesh-eating mammals including skunks) and Chiroptera (the order which comprises all of the 178 genera in 16 families of bats). Seven genotypes have been delineated within the genus. These genotypes are divided into two immunopathologically and genetically distinct phylogroups. Phylogroup I includes two African genotypes: *Mokola virus*, which has been isolated from shrews and cats, although its reservoir remains unknown, and *Lagos bat virus*, which has been found mainly in frugivorous bats but also in an insectivorous bat. Phylogroup II has five genotypes: *DUUV* (Africa), EBLV-1 (Europe), EBLV-2 (Europe), *Australian bat lyssavirus* (Australia), and the classical RABV (worldwide). Members of the genotypes *Duvenhage virus*, EBLV-1, and EBLV-2 are exclusively found in insectivorous bats, members of the genotype *Australian bat lyssavirus* are found in both insectivorous and frugivorous bats, and members of the genotype RABV are found in carnivorous and American bats (insectivorous, frugivorous, and hematophagous). The fact that lyssaviruses are well established in two ecologically distinct mammal orders may very likely be the consequence of successful host switching.

Analysis of 36 carnivoran and 17 chiropteran lyssaviruses representing the main genotypes and variants strongly supports the hypothesis that host switching occurred in the history of the lyssaviruses. In fact, lyssaviruses evolved in chiroptera long before the emergence of carnivoran rabies, very likely following spillover from bats. Using dated isolates, the emergence of carnivoran rabies from chiropteran lyssaviruses is estimated to have occurred 888 to 1459 years ago. In Europe, bat rabies is associated with two specific virus strains: European bat lyssavirus type 1 and European bat lyssavirus type 2. European bat lyssavirus type 1 isolates have been found in serotine bats in France. European bat lyssavirus type 2 has now been found in Daubenton's bats in England and Scotland.

In North America, variants of rabies virus are maintained in the wild by several terrestrial carnivore species, including raccoons, skunks, and a number of bat species. Each antigenically and genetically distinct variant of the virus in mammalian species occurs in geographically discrete areas and is strongly associated with its reservoir species. Within each area, a spillover of rabies into other species occurs, especially during epidemics. Temporal and spatial analysis of skunk and raccoon rabies in the eastern United States indicated that epidemics in raccoons and skunks moved in a similar direction from 1990 to 2000. However, there is no evidence that the raccoon rabies virus variant is cycling independently in the skunk population of the eastern United States or that the variant has undergone any genetic adaptations among skunks.

Within broad geographic regions, rabies infections in terrestrial mammals can be linked to distinct virus variants, identified by panels of monoclonal antibodies or by genetic analysis. These analyses have demonstrated substantial differences between isolates from various parts of the world and conventional vaccines do not fully protect against some of the naturally occurring antigenic variants that exist in nature. Most outbreaks of rabies tend to be host species specific. Each variant is maintained primarily by **intraspecific transmission** within a dominant reservoir, although spillover infection of other species may occur within the region. Geographic boundaries of the currently recognized reservoirs for rabies in terrestrial mammals have been established. Reservoirs for rabies virus are found worldwide. The virus is maintained at endemic and epidemic levels in a wide variety of Carnivora and Microchiroptera (bats) species.

The geographic boundaries of the currently recognized reservoirs for rabies in terrestrial species in North America are as follows:

- Raccoons in the southeastern United States
- Red and arctic foxes in Alaska, resulting in spread across Canada as far east as Ontario, Quebec, and the New England states
- Striped skunks in California, the north central states, and the south central states
- Gray foxes in small reservoirs in Arizona
- Coyotes in south Texas as a result of spread from domestic dogs in a long-standing reservoir at the Texas–Mexico border

In Ontario, wildlife rabies persists in two predominant species: the red fox and the striped skunk. Molecular epidemiology studies indicate that there is no host specificity, but there are very clear and consistent differences in the virus from distinct geographic regions. In Canadian studies, two major antigenic groups can be distinguished among the rabies virus isolates examined. One group is found in Ontario, Quebec, and the Northwest Territories and is represented in the wild by endemic red fox and striped skunk rabies that originated in northern Canada. The second group is found in Manitoba where striped skunk rabies is endemic.

Overlying the disease in terrestrial mammals are multiple, independent reservoirs for rabies in several species of insectivorous bats. Distinct viral variants can be identified for different bat species, but geographic boundaries cannot be defined for rabies outbreaks in the highly mobile bat species.

Methods of Transmission

The source of infection is always an infected animal, and the method of spread is almost always by the **bite** of an infected animal, although contamination of skin wounds by fresh saliva may result in infection. Not all bites from rabid animals result in infection because the virus is not always present in the saliva; the virus may not gain entrance to the wound if the saliva is wiped from the teeth by clothing. The virus may appear in the milk of affected animals, but spread by this means is unlikely as infection. The rabies virus is relatively fragile, susceptible to most standard disinfectants, and dies in dried saliva in a few hours.

One of the most important parameters in rabies models is the transmission rate, or the number of susceptible animals infected by a diseased animal per unit of time. In a population of 19 raccoons feeding at a concentrated, common food source available during the summer in rural eastern Ontario, raccoons bite and are bitten an average of 1.0 to 1.3 times per hour, respectively.

Because of the natural occurrence of rabies in animals in caves inhabited by infected insectivorous bats, inhalation as a route of infection came under suspicion. It is now accepted that interbat spread, and spread from bats to other species is principally by bites, but that infection by inhalation also occurs. That infection can occur by ingestion has been put to use in devising systems of vaccinating wildlife by baiting them with virus-laden baits.

Animal Vectors

Traditionally, the dog, and to a minor extent the cat, have been the main source animals.

However, native fauna, including foxes, skunks, wolves, coyotes, vampire, insectivorous and fruit-eating bats, raccoons, mongoose, and squirrels provide the major source of infection in countries where domestic Carnivora are well controlled. In general, foxes are less dangerous than dogs, because foxes tend to bite only one or two animals in a group, whereas dogs will often bite a large proportion of a herd or flock. Raccoons and skunks are major reservoirs of rabies in North America.

Bats are the most important species in which subclinical carriers occur. Multiplication of the virus without invasion of the nervous system is known to occur in fatty tissues in bats and may be the basis of the "reservoiring" mechanism in this species. Violent behavior is rare in rabid animals of this species, but it has been observed. Bats represent a serious threat of spread of rabies because of their migratory habits. Most spread is within the species, but the threat to humans and animal species by bats cannot be completely disregarded. Although rodents can be infected with the rabies virus they are not thought to play any part in the epidemiology of rabies, either as multipliers or simply as physical carriers of the virus. Many of the viruses they carry are rabies-like rather than classical rabies.

Rabies has occurred in swine herds where the skunk population is high, where farms were settled from rough terrain resulting in considerable interface between wildlife and domestic animals, and in which the management system allows the pigs to run free on the premises. The disease has occurred in pigs reared in a closed feeder barn where access by wildlife was very unlikely.

There is a difference in the role between vectors. For example, in Europe it is thought that foxes carry the infection into a new area, but other species disseminate it within an area. Foxes are the principal vectors and, as in Canada, cattle are the principal receptors. In western Canada, the main reservoirs of infection are skunks, bats, and foxes. This would have important consequences for control programs based on wildlife surveillance.

Domestic livestock like cattle are rarely a source of infection, although chance transmission to humans may occur if the mouth of a rabid animal is manipulated during treatment or examination. The virus may be present in the saliva for periods up to 5 days before signs are evident.

Seasonal Spread

Spread of the disease is often seasonal, with the highest incidence in the late summer and autumn because of large-scale movements of wild animals at mating time and in pursuit of food. In Canada, the frequency of rabies infection in livestock populations increases in the fall when adolescent foxes mature, begin mating behavior, and travel over large areas.

Latent Infection

Because of rapid developments in virologic techniques, especially serologic screening of animal populations to obtain presumptive diagnoses of the presence of a virus in the population, the question of latent infection and inapparent carriers of rabies has assumed some importance. The presence of rabies antibodies in animals in a supposed rabies-free area is likely to arouse concern. Inapparent carriers do occur in bats and there is some evidence that latent infections can occur in other species.

Zoonotic Implications

The disease in unvaccinated and untreated humans has always been considered **fatal**. The prime importance of rabies is its transmissibility to humans, with veterinarians being at special risk. European data indicate that by far the greatest proportion of humans requiring pretreatment for rabies have been exposed to a rabid domestic animal, and not a wild one. Human rabies is extremely rare in countries where canine rabies is controlled by regular vaccination.

Economic Importance

Rabies is not of major economic importance in farm animals, although individual herds and flocks may suffer many fatalities. The economic costs of rabies in a country are associated with pet animal vaccinations, animal bite investigations, confinement and quarantine of domestic animals that bite humans or that are suspected of exposure to rabid animals, salaries of animal control officers, laboratory diagnosis, the costs of preexposure and postexposure prophylaxis and treatment and consultation, public education, staff training, and clerical costs.

PATHOGENESIS

Following the deep introduction of rabies virus by the bite of a rabid animal, initial virus multiplication occurs in striated muscle cells at the site. The neuromuscular spindles then provide an important site of virus entry into the nervous system, which may also occur at motor end plates. In the olfactory end organ in the nares, neuroepithelial cells are in direct contact with the body surface, and these cells extend without interruption into the olfactory bulb of the brain. Following entry of the virus into nerve findings, there is invasion of the brain by passive movement of the virus within axons, first into the spinal cord, and then into the brain. The immune response during this phase of the infection is minimal and explains why neutralizing antibody and inflammatory infiltration are usually absent at the time of onset of encephalitic signs. Antibody titers reach substantial levels only in the terminal stages of the disease. Following entry of rabies virus to the CNS, usually in the spinal cord, an ascending wave of neuronal infection and neuronal dysfunction occurs.

The primary lesions produced are in the CNS, and spread from the site of infection occurs only by way of the peripheral nerves. This method of spread accounts for the extremely variable incubation period, which varies to a large extent with the site of the bite. Bites on the head usually result in a shorter incubation period than bites on the extremities. The severity and the site of the lesions will govern to a large extent whether the clinical picture is primarily one of irritative or paralytic phenomena. The two extremes of the paralytic or dumb form and the furious form are accompanied by many cases that lie somewhere between the two. Gradually ascending paralysis of the hindquarters may be followed by severe signs of mania, which persist almost until death. Destruction of spinal neurons results in paralysis, but when the virus invades the brain, irritation of higher centers produces manias, excitement, and convulsions. Death is usually caused by respiratory paralysis. The clinical signs of salivation, indigestion and pica, paralysis of bladder and anus, and increased libido all suggest involvement of the autonomic nervous system, including endocrine glands. At death, there are viral inclusions and particles in almost all neurons in the brain, spinal cord, and ganglia, but none in the supportive cells of the CNS. Electron microscopic examination also shows the presence of the virus in the cornea, which it reaches centrifugally along the peripheral nerves.

Virus reaches the salivary glands and many other organs in the same way, but the highly infective nature of saliva arises from passage of the virus along the olfactory nerve to taste buds and other sensory end organs in the oropharynx, rather than from the salivary glands. Experimentally, infection of nonnervous tissues in skunks and foxes has been reproduced in the adrenal medulla, cornea, and nasal glands. The virus may be found in milk, in some organs and in fetuses, but the virus cannot be demonstrated in the blood at any time.

Variations in the major manifestations as mania or paralysis may depend on the source of the virus. Virus from vampire bats almost always causes the paralytic form. "Fixed" virus that has been modified by serial intracerebral passage causes ascending paralysis in contrast to "street" virus, which more commonly causes the furious form. The site of infection and the size of the inoculum may also influence the clinical course. There is also a geographic difference in the proportion of animals affected by the furious or paralytic form of the disease. In the Americas most cases are paralytic. In Africa and India most cases in farm animals are the furious form.

The disease is always fatal, but infrequently an experimentally infected animal shows clinical signs of the disease but recovers. There are two recent records of spontaneous recovery in man, and the occurrence of nonfatal rabies in all species has been reviewed. There appears to be no field occurrence in domestic animals of the finding in experimentally infected mice that some strains of virus invade only peripheral nerves and spinal ganglia leaving a number of survivors with permanent nervous disability. The pathogenesis of recovery from rabies is important relative to vaccination and serologic testing to determine the incidence and prevalence of the disease.

CLINICAL FINDINGS

Among farm animals, cattle are most commonly affected. The incubation period in naturally occurring cases is about 3 weeks, but varies from 2 weeks to several months in most species, although incubation periods of 5 and 6 months have been observed in cattle and dogs.

Cattle

Experimentally, in cattle the average incubation period was 15 days and the average course of the disease was 4 days. Unvaccinated cattle had shorter incubation and clinical duration of disease than vaccinated cattle. Major clinical findings included excessive salivation (100%), behavioral change (100%), muzzle tremors (80%), vocalization (bellowing 70%), aggression, hyperesthesia and/or hyperexcitability (70%), and pharyngeal paralysis (60%). The furious form occurred in 70%.

In the **paralytic form**, knuckling of the hind fetlocks, sagging and swaying of the hindquarters while walking, and often deviation or flaccidity of the tail to one side, are common early signs. Decreased sensation usually accompanies this weakness and is one of the best diagnostic criteria in the detection of rabies. It is most evident over the hindquarters. Tenesmus, with paralysis of the anus, resulting in the sucking in and blowing out of air, usually occurs late in the incoordination stages just before the animal becomes recumbent. This is a characteristic finding but it may be transient or absent. Drooling of saliva is one of the most constant findings. The **yawning movements** are more accurately described as voiceless attempts to bellow, and voiceless bellowing is considered a helpful clinical sign for distinguishing rabid cows from nonrabid cows, and when sound is generated in rabid cattle, the bellowing is of a higher pitch than normal.[3] When paralysis occurs, the animal becomes recumbent and unable to rise. Bulls in this stage often have paralysis of the penis. Death usually occurs 48 hours after recumbency develops and after a total course of 6 to 7 days.

In **furious rabies,** the animal has a tense, alert appearance, is hypersensitive to sounds and movement, and is attracted to noise so that it may look intently or approach as though about to attack. In some cases, it will violently attack other animals or inanimate objects. These attacks are often badly directed and are impeded by the incoordination of gait. Frequently, loud bellowing is usual at this stage. The sound is characteristically hoarse and the actions are exaggerated. Sexual excitement is also common, with bulls often attempting to mount inanimate objects. Multiple collections of semen for artificial insemination have been made during very short periods from bulls that later proved to be rabid. With this violent form of the disease, the termination is characteristically sudden. Severe signs may be evident for 24 to 48 hours and the animal then collapses suddenly in a paralyzed state, dying usually within a few hours.

There is no consistent pattern in either the development or the range of signs. Body temperatures are usually normal but may be elevated to 39.5°C to 40.5°C (103°F-105°F) in the early stages by muscular activity. Appetite varies also. Some animals do not eat or drink, although they may take food into the mouth. There is apparent an inability to swallow. Others eat normally until the terminal stages. The course may vary from 1 to 6 days. So wide is the variation in clinical findings that any animal known to be exposed and showing signs of spinal cord or brain involvement should be considered rabid until proved otherwise.

Sheep and Goats

In sheep experimentally infected, the average incubation period was 10 days, and the average course of the disease was 3 days. Major clinical findings included muzzle and head tremors (80%); aggressiveness, hyperexcitability, and hyperesthesia (80%); trismus (60%); salivation (60%); vocalization (60%); and recumbency (40%). The furious form occurred in 80% of sheep. In one large-scale outbreak in sheep, deaths occurred 17 to 111 days after exposure.

Rabies often occurs in a number of animals at one time because of the ease with which a number of sheep can be bitten by a dog or fox. Clinically, the picture is similar to that seen in cattle. The minority of animals show sexual excitement, attacking humans or each other, and vigorous wool pulling; sudden falling after violent exertion, muscle tremor, and salivation are characteristic. Excessive bleating does not occur. Most sheep are quiet and anorectic. Goats are commonly aggressive, and continuous bleating is common.

Horses

Most recorded cases in horses are lacking in distinctive nervous signs initially, but incline to the paralytic form of the disease. Experimentally, the average incubation period was 12 days and the average duration of disease was 6 days. Unvaccinated animals had shorter incubation periods and duration of clinical disease. Muzzle tremors were the most frequently observed and most common initial signs. Other clinical findings included pharyngeal paresis (71%), ataxia or paresis (71%), and lethargy or somnolence (71%). The furious form occurred in 43% of cases, some of which began as the dumb form. The paralytic form was not observed.

In naturally occurring cases, the initial clinical findings may include abnormal postures, frequent whinnying, unexplained aggressiveness and kicking, biting, colic, sudden onset of lameness in one limb followed by recumbency the next day, high-stepping gait, ataxia, apparent blindness, and violent head-tossing. Lameness or weakness in one leg may be the first sign observed, but the usual pattern of development starts with lassitude, then passes to sternal recumbency and lateral recumbency, followed by paddling convulsions and terminal paralysis.

In a series of 21 confirmed cases in horses, the clinical findings at the time of initial examination included ataxia and paresis of the hindquarters (43%), lameness (24%), recumbency (14%), pharyngeal paralysis (10%), and colic (10%). The major clinical findings observed over the course of hospitalization included recumbency (100%), hyperesthesia (81%), loss of tail and anal sphincter tone (57%), fever ~38.5°C (52%), and ataxia and paresis of the hindquarters (52%). Mean survival time after the onset of clinical signs was 4 days (range, 1–7 days). Clinical findings of the furious form of rabies, such as aggressiveness (biting), compulsive circling, and abnormal vocalization, were evident in only two horses. Supportive therapy, given to nine horses, had no effect on survival time and did not correlate with the detection of Negri bodies at necropsy. Horses developing the furious form show excitement, become vicious, and bite and kick. Their uncontrolled actions are often violent and dangerous and include blind changes, sudden falling, and rolling and chewing of foreign material or their own skin. Hyperesthesia and muscular twitching of the hindlimbs followed by crouching and weakness are also recorded in the horse.

Pigs

Pigs manifest excitement and a tendency to attack, or dullness and incoordination. Affected sows show twitching of the nose, rapid chewing movements, excessive salivation, and clonic convulsions. They may walk backward. Terminally, there is paralysis and death occurs 12 to 48 hours after the onset of signs. The clinical findings in pigs are extremely variable, and individual cases may present in a variety of ways and only one or two of the classical findings may occur.

CLINICAL PATHOLOGY

No antemortem laboratory examination is of diagnostic value, but tests for lead on blood, urine, and feces may help to eliminate lead poisoning as a possible diagnosis. Virus neutralization tests are available, but the presence of antibodies is not diagnostic. Other available tests are passive hemagglutination, complement fixation, radioimmunoassay, and indirect fluorescent antibody staining. These are used to determine immune status rather than as a diagnostic aid. An ELISA is available for measurement of rabies-specific antibody in the sera of major domestic and wildlife reservoirs in North America.

NECROPSY FINDINGS

Confirmation of a diagnosis of rabies depends on careful laboratory examination of fresh brain. The recommended laboratory procedure includes the following tests and it is recommended that at least two of them be used on all specimens.

- The most widely used test is the fluorescent antibody test (**FAT**) on impression smears from the brain. Current recommendations include sampling of the hippocampus, **medulla oblongata**, cerebellum, or gasserian ganglion.[4] However, a recent publication stipulates that the hippocampus and cerebellum are less desirable samples than the thalamus, pons, or medulla for the detection of viral antigen, and that the current sampling recommendations stem from the visibility of Negri bodies, rather than the true distribution of viral antigen. An FAT can be completed in approximately 2 hours and is accurate when done routinely by experienced personnel because it detects all genotypes if a potent conjugate is used.[5] The reliability of FAT confirmed by the mouse inoculation test is over 99%. Those specimens that are negative on FAT, and have contact with humans, are inoculated into experimental mice. The incubation period in mice before clinical signs are seen averages 11 to 12 days (range of 4–18 days), and death occurs in 7 to 21 days. The mouse brain is harvested as soon as signs appear and is submitted to the same tests described earlier. Thus a positive result can be obtained as soon as 4 to 7 days after inoculation. Some mice must be left for the full 21 days because only a negative result at that time can give a complete negative to the test. A tissue culture infection test is now available, which allows demonstration of the virus in stained tissue culture cells within 4 days. This may replace the mouse inoculation test.
- A dot **ELISA** is available for the detection of rabies antigen in animals. It is rapid, simple, economical and, in comparison with the FAT, the agreement is 95%.
- A **histologic search** for Negri bodies in tissue sections has results available in 48 hours. Because of false-positive diagnoses the technique is in some disrepute.
- An **immunohistochemical (IHC)** test for rabies can be used on formalin-fixed, paraffin-embedded brain tissues of domestic animals and wild animals when fresh tissues are not available. In some cases, the brain tissue may be negative for the rabies virus using standard diagnostic techniques, but IHC tests may detect the presence of antigen.
- A **reverse transcriptase** (RT-)**PCR** test has been found of value in detecting rabies infection in decomposed brain samples that were negative by the direct FAT.

The histopathologic changes of rabies infection include a nonsuppurative encephalomyelitis and ganglioneuritis, with neuronal necrosis and the formation of glial nodules. Negri bodies are most commonly found in the Purkinje cells of the cerebellum in ruminants. Spongiform change has also been reported in the brain of a heifer infected with rabies virus.

Samples for Confirmation of Diagnosis

- **Histology:** half of midsagittally sectioned brain, cervical spinal cord (including root ganglia), gasserian ganglion, parotid salivary gland (LM, IHC)
- **Virology:** half of midsagittally sectioned brain, cervical spinal cord (FAT, BIOASSAY).

Note the zoonotic potential of this organism when handling carcass and submitting specimens.

DIFFERENTIAL DIAGNOSIS

The diagnosis of rabies is one of the most difficult and important duties that a veterinarian is called on to perform. Because in most cases there is a probability of human exposure, failure to recognize the disease may place human life in jeopardy. It is not even sufficient to say that if rabies occurs in the area one will classify every animal showing nervous signs as rabid, because nervous signs may not be evident for some days after the illness commences. In addition, many animals suffering from other diseases will be left untreated. The best policy is to handle all suspect animals with extreme care but continue to treat them for other diseases if such treatment appears to be indicated. If the animal is rabid, it will die and the diagnosis can then be confirmed by laboratory examination.

Several diseases are characterized by signs of abnormal mental state or paralysis, or a combination of both (see Table 14-9 for the horse; Table 14-10 for cattle). Rabies must be differentiated from the following common diseases affecting the nervous system, according to species.

Cattle and sheep

- Lead poisoning. In acute and subacute lead poisoning in cattle the clinical findings are similar to those of furious and dumb rabies. In acute lead poisoning, the common clinical findings are blindness, convulsions, champing of the jaws with the production of frothy saliva, and twitching of the eyelids and ears. In subacute lead poisoning in cattle there is blindness, stupor, head-pressing, grinding of the teeth, and almost no response to treatment. Rabid cattle are usually not blind, and signs of motor irritation such as convulsions and twitching of the facial muscles usually do not occur. However, there are signs of bizarre mental behavior, such as wild gazing, bellowing, yawning, attacking, and compulsive walking.
- Lactation tetany occurs in lactating cattle on lush pasture in the spring during cold wet and windy weather, and is characterized by hyperesthesia, tremors, convulsions, recumbency, and rapid death.
- Vitamin A deficiency occurs in groups of young cattle from 6 months to 18 months of age not receiving adequate carotene intake or vitamin A supplementation and is characterized by blindness in the ocular form and episodes of tremors and convulsions.
- Polioencephalomalacia in cattle and sheep is characterized by blindness, nystagmus, opisthotonus, and convulsions; bellowing, loss of sensation, and tenesmus do not occur.
- Listeriosis in cattle and sheep is manifested by localizing signs of circling and facial nerve paralysis.
- Enterotoxemia in sheep is usually confined to lambs on heavy carbohydrate diets.
- Pregnancy toxemia is a disease of pregnant ewes and is readily differentiated by the presence of ketonuria.
- Louping-ill in sheep is transmitted by insects, has a seasonal occurrence, and a localized geographic distribution.

Horses

In horses, rabies must be differentiated from several diseases of the nervous system (summarized in Table 14-11).

The most common include diseases include viral encephalomyelitis, herpes virus myeloencephalopathy, cerebrospinal nematodiasis, equine degenerative myeloencephalopathy, equine protozoal myeloencephalitis, neuritis of the cauda equina, horsetail poisoning, Borna, Japanese encephalitis, and botulism.

Pigs

In pigs, rabies must be differentiated from pseudorabies, Teschen disease, and involvement of the brain in several other diseases of the pigs, such as hog and African swine fever, meningitis associated with *Streptococcus suis* type II, *Haemophilus* spp., Glasser's disease, *Escherichia coli,* septicemia, and erysipelas.

Text continued on p. 1237

Table 14-9 Diseases of horses characterized by signs of intracranial or disseminated lesions of the central nervous system

Disease	Etiology and epidemiology	Clinical and laboratory findings	Treatment and control
Infection causes			
Viral encephalomyelitis (WEE, EEE, VEE)	Summer season Insect vector, usually mosquitoes Young nonvaccinated horses at greatest risk, outbreaks may occur	Stage of slight hyperexcitability and mild fever initially, impaired eyesight, circling and walking Stage of mental depression, somnolence, leaning, feed hanging from mouth, unsteady Stage of paralysis, unable to swallow, weakness, recumbency; dies 2–4 days after onset Serology for diagnosis	Supportive therapy, thick bedding Recovery rate 60%–75% Vaccinate foals at 6 months of age and other horses for the first time, twice 2 weeks apart and once or twice annually thereafter
Rabies	All age groups, knowledge of disease in area, wildlife Usually single animal affected Not common	Ascending paralysis, hypersalivation, will bite Ataxia and paresis of hindlimbs, lameness, recumbency, pharyngeal paralysis, colic, loss of tail and sphincter tone, fever Dies in 1 week Immunofluorescent antibody testing on brain for positive diagnosis	No treatment All die Vaccinate horses if anticipate outbreak
Herpesvirus myeloencephalopathy (EHV-1)	Can occur as outbreaks Neurologic disease usually preceded by fever Mature horses	Symmetric ataxia and paresis, bladder paralysis, recumbency may occur, spontaneous recovery possible, CSF (hemorrhage or xanthochromia) Vasculitis with subsequent focal malacia in gray and white matter of brain and spinal cord	No specific therapy Antiinflammatory drugs may be useful Use of corticosteroids is controversial Recovery may occur spontaneously
WNE	West Nile virus Late summer in temperate regions Can occur as epizootics Now enzootic in most of North America	Fever, muscle fasciculations, weakness, ataxia, depression, cranial nerve disease, recumbency Prominent signs of spinal cord precede sign of intracranial disease in most cases	Supportive Antiserum Interferon Antiinflammatory. drugs including corticosteroids Prevention by vaccination
Borna	Virus Direct transmission Germany and other European countries Disease is recorded in Japan Low morbidity, high case–fatality rate	Pharyngeal paralysis, muscle tremor, flaccid paralysis, course 1–3 weeks Viral encephalomyelitis with inclusion bodies	No treatment
Japanese encephalitis	Japanese encephalitis virus Sporadic Asia including Japan and China, parts of Oceania including New Guinea and Torres Strait Pig is mammalian amplifying host Vector mosquitoes, birds infected	Fever, lethargy, jaundice, dysphagia, incoordination, staggering, recovery in 1 week Serology	Spontaneous recovery Vaccination in endemic areas
Protozoal myeloencephalitis	*Sarcocystis neurona* Single animal affected Infectious but not contagious	Any central nervous system disorder. Usually causes ataxia but can cause cerebral and cranial nerve disease	Antiprotozoal medications (pyrimethamine + sulphonamide, ponazuril, or nitazoxanide) Vaccine available in the United States, but not recommended
Cerebrospinal nematodiasis (verminous encephalitis)	Migration of larval stages of *Strongylus vulgaris, Habronema* sp., and *Filaroides* *Micronema deletrix* (*Helicephalobolus*) *deletrix* Not common	Clinical signs referable to gray matter lesions are common Hypalgesia, hyporeflexia, hypotonia, muscle atrophy and cerebral, cerebellar and cranial nerve involvement Progressive encephalitis, incoordination, sensory deficits, blindness in one or both eyes, course of several days Pleocytosis of CSF Hemorrhage and malacia of thalamus, brainstem, cerebellum	Ivermectin or moxidectin at usual doses High dose benzimidazole Antiinflammatory drugs Parasite control
Brain abscess	Sporadic Often a complication of strangles	Obtunded mentation, variable signs of intracranial disease Leukocytosis Variable pleocytosis and increased protein concentration in CSF CT scan	Antimicrobials Surgical drainage Prognosis is poor

Continued

Table 14-9 Diseases of horses characterized by signs of intracranial or disseminated lesions of the central nervous system—cont'd

Disease	Etiology and epidemiology	Clinical and laboratory findings	Treatment and control
Physical			
Traumatic injury to the brain	History of traumatic injury (falling, rearing-up and falling backward)	Coma, depression, hemorrhage from nose and ears, blindness, cranial nerve deficits Often rupture of longus capitus muscle	Antiinflammatory drugs, mannitol Fair to poor prognosis
Facial nerve paralysis	Associated with prolonged surgical recumbency and compression of facial nerve	Facial nerve paralysis lasting several days Paralysis of ear, eyelid, lip, nostril on one side No alteration in sensation or vestibular function	Supportive
Lightning strike	Observed lightning strike or history of recent thunderstorm activity	Death is most common Horses that survive strike often have prominent signs of vestibular disease	Supportive Recovery is possible
Fracture or arthritis of the temporal-stylohyoid articulation, otitis media	Sporadic in older horses	Acute onset circling, head tilt, nystagmus, unilateral facial paralysis, dysphagia	Antibiotics, antiinflammatory drugs, supportive care
Intoxications			
Horsetail poisoning (*Equisetum arvense*)	Ingestion of plants mixed with hay Not common	Incoordination, swaying from side to side, muscle tremor recumbency, bradycardia, cardiac arrhythmia	Thiamine parenterally. Good response
Equine leukoencephalomalacia (fumonisin toxicosis)	Horses eating moldy corn grain contaminated with *Fusarium moniliforme* fungus	Muscle tremor, weakness, staggering gait, dysphagia, depression	None
Hepatoencephalopathy associated with hepatotoxic plants (*Crotalaria, Senecio* and *Amsinckia*)	Horses on inadequate pasture forced to eat poisonous plants More than one animal may be affected Geographic distribution	Develops slowly, commonly ill for 2–3 weeks previously, depression, pushing, ataxia, hypertonic face and lips, yawning, compulsive walking, loss of weight, icterus, photosensitization occasionally Serum liver enzymes elevated and liver function tests abnormal Hyperammonemia Gross and histopathologic liver lesions	No treatment Prevent access to poisonous plants
Lead poisoning	Grazing on pastures contaminated by atmospheric lead from nearby factories, not common now	Usually a chronic disease Inspiratory dyspnea caused by paralysis of recurrent laryngeal nerve Pharyngeal paralysis, dysphagia, aspiration pneumonia, paralysis of lips, weakness and recumbency Ingestion of large amounts causes subacute form similar to that seen in cattle	Calcium versenate
Yellow-star thistle poisoning (*Centaurea* sp., anigropallidal encephalomalacia of horses)	Ingestion of yellow-star thistle in California and Australia Summer months on weedy pasture	Difficult prehension, fixed facial expression with mouth held half open, hypertonic face and lips, persistent chewing movements and rhythmic protrusion of tongue, yawning and somnolence but easily aroused, aimless walking, slight stiffness of gait, high mortality Malacia of globus plants pallidus and substantia nigra	No treatment Prevent access to poisonous plants
Botulism	Ingestion of preformed toxin of *Cl. botulinum* in decaying grass or spoiled silage, hay or grain. Sporadic in horses. Endemic in foals in some areas of North America	Flaccid paralysis of skeletal muscles leading to weakness, stumbling and recumbency. Mentation normal. Skin sensation normal. Paralysis of tongue and thoracic muscles. Die in 2–4 days. Some recover. Filtrates of intestinal tract into laboratory animals	Supportive therapy, antitoxins. Vaccination in enzootic areas. Prevent contamination of feed by animal carcasses
Tetanus	Wounds infected with *Clostridium tetani* Sporadic	Generalized tetany of all skeletal muscles Fever, hyperesthesia, protrusion of third eyelid, trismus, recumbency followed by tetanic convulsions, die in 5–10 days	Prognosis unfavorable Dark stall, penicillin, muscle relaxants, supportive therapy and antitoxin parenterally or into subarachnoid space Toxoid vaccination
Metabolic and idiopathic			
Lactation tetany	Lactating mares, suckling foals Hypocalcemia	Acute onset of generalized stiffness, trismus, no hyperesthesia, no prolapse of third eyelid, diaphragmatic flutter, soft heart sounds Serum hypocalcemia	Rapid response to calcium borogluconate intravenously

Table 14-9 Diseases of horses characterized by signs of intracranial or disseminated lesions of the central nervous system—cont'd

Disease	Etiology and epidemiology	Clinical and laboratory findings	Treatment and control
Idiopathic epilepsy of Arabians	Single horse First noticed from shortly after birth up to 6 months of age Etiology unknown	Recurrent episodes of typical clonic-tonic convulsions lasting 10–15 minutes, loss of consciousness, sweating, tachycardia, spontaneous defecation No lesions	Control seizures with phenobarbital or potassium bromide Spontaneous recovery as foals mature
Idiopathic epilepsy of adult horses	Sporadic disease Unknown cause Can be associated with brain lesions detectable on EEG or CT	Tonic-clonic convulsions Variable periodicity and intensity	Control seizures acutely with diazepam and in the long term with phenobarbital and/or potassium bromide Spontaneous recovery unlikely
Cerebellar hypoplasia of Arabian and Swedish Gotland foals	Inherited Signs noticeable from 2–6 months of age	Defective eye blinks, ataxia, head-nodding, slight tremor of head and neck, intention tremor of the head, high-stepping gait, difficulty in rising, legs wide apart, difficulty in jumping over obstacles, fall backward if dorsiflex head and neck Cerebellar hypoplasia grossly or histologically	Eliminate carrier animals
Lower motor neuron disease	Associated with stabling and no access to pasture Sporadic North America and Europe Low serum vitamin E concentrations	Weight loss, weakness, muscle fasciculations, maintained appetite Normal mentation Low serum vitamin E concentration Diagnosis by muscle biopsy	No definitive cure Some cases stabilized with administration of oral vitamin E Poor prognosis for return to function

Note: Other less common diseases affecting the nervous system of horses include space-occupying lesions (cholesteatomas of old horses, tumors), intracranial myiasis caused by migration of Hypoderma bovis, *hydrocephalus in young horses, the accidental injection of an ataractic drug into the carotid artery, and bacterial meningitis in young horses as a sequel to streptococcal infection.*
CSF, cerebrospinal fluid; CT, computed tomography; EEE, eastern equine encephalitis; EEG, electroencephalogram; EHV-1, equine herpesvirus-1; VEE, Venezuelan equine encephalitis; WEE, western equine encephalitis; WNE, West Nile encephalomyelitis.

Table 14-10 Differential diagnosis of diseases of cattle with clinical findings referable to brain dysfunction

Disease	Epidemiology	Clinical findings	Clinical pathology and pathology	Response to treatment
Lead poisoning	All ages of calves and cows on pasture with access to dumps Discarded lead batteries, used crankcase oil, lead-based paint common sources Case–fatality rate high	Acute in calves Blindness and "chewing gum" champing of jaws, convulsions, charging, rapid death Subacute in adults: blindness, stupor, head-pressing, grinding teeth, rumen static, protozoa dead	Blood and tissue for lead Encephalomalacia	Will respond favorably to treatment in early stages if not too severe but most cases do not return to normal Calcium versenate and thiamine hydrochloride Must be concerned about disposition of meat and milk of treated animals
Polioencephalomalacia	Grain-fed rapidly growing feedlot cattle May occur on pasture containing plants and water high in sulfates Outbreaks occur	Sudden onset, blindness, tremors and shaking of head, twitching of ears, head-pressing, opisthotonus, nystagmus, strabismus, rumen contractions normal, CSF pressure increased	Blood biochemistry (see text) Brain for histopathology	Responds to thiamine in early stages Cases caused by sulfate toxicity may not respond
Hypovitaminosis A	Calves 6–8 months of age most commonly but mature cows too off dry summer pasture (CSF form) Young rapidly growing cattle fed deficient ration for several months (ocular form)	CSF form: sudden onset; syncope and convulsions followed by recovery, eyesight and pupils normal Nyctalopia CSF pressure increased Ocular form: blindness in daylight, pupils dilated and fixed, optic disc edema Syncope and convulsions may also occur Usually preceded by nyctalopia but missed by owner	Plasma and liver vitamin A Optic nerve constriction Squamous cell metaplasia of parotid ducts	CSF form: recover in 48 hours following treatment with vitamin A injections Ocular form: will not recover because of optic nerve degeneration

Continued

Table 14-10 Differential diagnosis of diseases of cattle with clinical findings referable to brain dysfunction—cont'd

Disease	Epidemiology	Clinical findings	Clinical pathology and pathology	Response to treatment
Haemophilus meningoencephalitis (thromboembolic meningoencephalitis)	Feedlot cattle (8–12 months), outbreaks, preceded by respiratory disease in group High case fatality if not treated early	Found down, fever common, ataxic, not usually blind, fundic lesions, irritation signs uncommon, weakness and paresis common, synovitis, laryngitis, pleuritis May die in 8–10 hours Myocardial abscesses may also occur	Neutrophilia CSF contains neutrophils Typical gross lesions in brain Pleuritis, pneumonia, synovitis, myocardial abscesses	Respond favorably to antimicrobials if treated early Later, high case–fatality rate
Listeria meningoencephalitis	Sporadic Fed silage Yearlings and adults	Unilateral facial paralysis, deviation of head and neck, mild fever, endophthalmitis, may be recumbent	CSF for cells Brain for histopathology	Recovery may occur. Antimicrobials Residual signs in survivors common
Nervous signs with coccidiosis (see text)	In 20% of young cattle affected with dysentery caused by coccidiosis Case fatality may exceed 50%	Tonic-clonic convulsions, normal eyesight, hyperesthesia, normal temperature, dysentery, may live 2–4 days	Oocysts in feces	Unfavorable response to treatment Must control coccidiosis
Rabies	Cattle exposed to wildlife, one or more affected, all ages, incubation 3 weeks to few months	Quiet and dull (dumb form) or excitable and easily annoyed (furious form) Bellowing, yawning, drooling, saliva, eyesight normal, tenesmus, ascending paralysis beginning with anesthesia over tail head, progressive course, dies in 4–6 days, usually no gross muscular tremors or convulsions, mild fever early	Hemogram normal Brain for laboratory diagnosis	None
Bovine spongiform encephalopathy (BSE)	Mostly in dairy cattle; epizootic began in Britain in 1986; long incubation period; caused by scrapie-like agent in protein concentrate made from sheep carcasses following change in processing procedures	Insidious onset, clinical course several weeks, change in behavior, hyperesthesia, ataxia, loss of body weight, stare, agnostic behavior, kick during milking, knuckling, falling, progressive weakness leading to recumbency	None	None
Pseudorabies	Disease of pigs transmitted to cattle by bites	Intense, local pruritus at site of bite, excitement, bellowing, convulsions, paralysis, death 2–3 days	Tissues for injection into rabbit Histopathology of brain	None
Hypomagnesemic tetany (lactation tetany)	Lactating dairy cows on lush pasture, late pregnant beef cows, cold, windy weather in spring May be precipitated by long transportation or deprivation of feed and water Outbreaks occur Seen in yearlings too Case mortality can be high	Acute: sudden onset of irritability, hyperesthesia; convulsions, recumbency, loud heart sounds, tachycardia, polypnea. Subacute: gradual onset (2–4 days), hyperirritable, difficult to handle, stilted gait, falling, stumbling, sudden movement may precipitate convulsion	Serum magnesium level slow	Responds to magnesium sulfate early
Nervous acetonemia	2–6 weeks postpartum High-producing cow Single animal	Sudden onset, bizarre mental behavior, chewing, licking, bellowing, hyperesthesia, sweating	Ketonuria, hypoglycemia	Responds to glucose parenterally and/or propylene glycol orally
Bovine bonkers (bovine hysteria)	Mature cattle and calves consuming ammoniated feeds (lucerne hay, bromegrass hay, fescue hay, wheat hay, maize stalks or silage) May also occur when animals have access to molasses-urea-protein blocks Toxic agent may be substituted imidazole formed by combination of soluble carbohydrates and ammonia Usually occurs when high-quality forage treated with ammonia concentrate of more than 3% dry matter by weight Can occur in nursing cows fed ammoniated feedstuffs	Periodic episodes of hyperexcitability, bellowing, running, charging, circling, convulsions, weaving, episodes last 30 seconds and may recur every 5–10 minutes Some die Most recover following removal of feed	Information not available	Recover spontaneously following removal of feed source

Table 14-10 Differential diagnosis of diseases of cattle with clinical findings referable to brain dysfunction—cont'd

Disease	Epidemiology	Clinical findings	Clinical pathology and pathology	Response to treatment
Hepatic encephalopathy (i.e., ragwort poisoning)	Cattle with access to plants containing pyrrolizidine alkaloids Many cattle may be affected	Loss of body weight, gradual onset of aggressive behavior, ataxia, muscular tremors, recumbency, convulsions, tenesmus and bellowing	Hyperbilirubinemia, decreased excretion of bromsulphthalein (BSP) Liver lesions	No treatment
Brain abscess	Sporadic, young cattle (6 months to 2 years of age) may have history of previous infections	Localizing signs, rotation or deviation of head and neck, loss of equilibrium, circling, mild fever, may be blind in one eye, nystagmus one eye	Neutrophilia, neutrophils in CSF	Unfavorable response to therapy
Enterotoxemia caused by *Clostridium perfringens* type D	Calves 2–4 months of age sucking high producing cows grazing on lush pastures Outbreaks occur Uncommon	Peracute: found dead. Acute: bellowing, mania, convulsions, blindness, death in 1–2 hours Subacute: dull, depressed, blind	Hyperglycemia (150–200 mg/dL), glycosuria marked Smear intestinal contents Recover toxin (mouse protection tests)	Hyperimmune serum Most die Vaccination effective
Whole-milk hypomagnesemic tetany of calves	Calves 2–4 months of age on whole milk Also in calves on milk replacers, concentrates and hay and occasionally in nursing calves on pasture	Sudden alertness, hyperesthesia, head-shaking, opisthotonus, muscular tremors, frothing at mouth, convulsions, heart rate 200–250 beats/min	Serum magnesium levels usually below 0.8 mg/dL	Magnesium sulfate intravenously gives good response, must follow up daily because of previous depletion of bone reserves

TREATMENT

No treatment should be attempted after clinical signs are evident. If the bite is seen, immediately after exposure, irrigation of the wound with 20% soft soap solution or a solution of benzalkonium chloride for at least 5 minutes may prevent the establishment of the infection. The area exposed to potential infection should be doused with iodine solution or a 40% to 50% alcohol solution if iodine is unavailable.[2] Immediate and thorough washing of all bite wounds and scratches with soap and water is perhaps the most effective measure for preventing rabies in veterinarians bitten by rabid animals. In experimental animals, simple local wound cleansing has been shown to markedly reduce the likelihood of rabies. Postexposure vaccination is unlikely to be of value in animals, because death usually occurs before appreciable immunity has had time to develop. Euthanasia of suspect animals must be avoided, particularly if human exposure has occurred, because the development of the disease in the animals is necessary to establish a diagnosis. Antirabies serum may become available for animal treatment at some future date. **In some countries, cases of rabies in farm animals are notifiable to the animal health and disease regulatory bodies.**

CONTROL

The major goal of rabies control in domestic and wild animals is the reduction or elimination of human rabies. The most rational approach to reducing human rabies is to reduce the prevalence and incidence of disease in animals. In developed countries, this has been accomplished by vaccination of dogs and cats, leaving much rabies in wildlife to be controlled. In countries without wildlife reservoirs, such as the Philippines, it would be economically advantageous to eliminate dog rabies. In Africa, where the incidence of rabies as well as the range of species involved is increasing, there is a need to develop new and economical methods of vaccinating domestic animals.

Dogs remain the major vector for transmission to humans in developing countries and are responsible for an estimated 59,000 human deaths worldwide annually.[6,7] Preexposure immunization for individuals, like veterinarians, who are at high risk to rabies, has been recommended by the World Health Organization (WHO), because it reduces risk and provides a more rapid anamnestic response, eliminating the need for human globulin should exposure occur. Rabies preexposure vaccination is now mandatory in many veterinary colleges. Despite some mild adverse reactions, immunization against rabies is an important prophylaxis measure well accepted by veterinary students.

For farm animals, there are two useful control techniques: the **prevention of exposure** and **preexposure vaccination**.

Prevention of Exposure to the Virus

This can be achieved by controlling access of wildlife species that are likely to come into contact with the farm livestock in particular areas or through vaccination of the wildlife. Foxes accounted for a very large proportion (85% in Europe) of wildlife rabies, and a control program aimed at reducing their population using poison or traps was attempted until the 1970s. This method of population reduction failed to control outbreaks or reduce enzootic rabies.

Point infection control has been shown to be highly successful in controlling raccoon rabies. This involves the use of three tactics: population reduction, trap-vaccinate-release, and oral vaccination with baits to control the spread of raccoon rabies.

Preexposure Vaccination of Humans

The most successful form of rabies prevention is preexposure vaccination. In human medicine, there are no reported cases of rabies deaths in anyone who has had preexposure vaccination followed by a booster vaccination if exposed. The CDC has published the recommendations of the Advisory Committee on Immunization Practices (ACIP) for human rabies prevention, which indicate that rabies preexposure vaccination should be offered to persons more likely to be exposed to rabies virus than the population of the United States at large. The recommendations of the ACIP for preexposure prophylaxis and maintenance of a detectable antibody titer differ depending on the estimated degree of risk of exposure to the virus. Four risk categories have established: continuous, frequent, infrequent, and rare. The classification depends on factors such as the occupation of the individual and geography.

With directed continuing education, common sense, first aid, and the availability of modern biologic agents, human rabies is nearly always preventable. Rabies preexposure vaccination is recommended for anyone at increased risk of exposure to rabies, including veterinarians, veterinary students who work in university veterinary teaching hospitals, laboratory staff working with rabies, vaccine producers, animal and wildlife control personnel, and zoologists. The standard preexposure regimen is three doses of vaccine intramuscularly or intradermally on days 0, 7, and 28 (or 21). A booster dose after 1 year increases and prolongs the antibody response. This preexposure vaccination permits postexposure vaccination to consist of two doses of vaccine on days 0 and 3 instead of five doses on days 0, 3, 7, 14, and 28 and avoids the need for postexposure of administration of human rabies immunoglobulin.

Postexposure Vaccination of Humans

Modern postexposure treatment is highly successful if done adequately. Wound care with infiltration of the wound with human rabies immunoglobulin and active rabies immunization is essential, especially after severe exposure. Postexposure treatment is assumed to neutralize or inactivate virus while it is still in the wounds, before it gains access to the nervous system where it is protected from the immune system. Therefore treatment after exposure to rabies virus is very urgent, even if the patient was bitten months before.

Postexposure Vaccination of Domestic Animals

An effective postexposure protocol for unvaccinated domestic animals exposed to rabies includes immediate vaccination against rabies, a strict isolation period of 90 days, and administration of booster vaccinations during the third and eighth weeks of the isolation period. The protocol has been effective in dogs, cats, cattle, and horses.

Vaccination of Domestic Animals

A *Compendium of Animal Rabies Control* is published annually by the National Association of State Public Health Veterinarians in the United States and Canada. It provides recommendations for immunization procedures in domestic animals and the vaccines licensed and marketed in the United States. Detailed information is provided on preexposure vaccination, management of dogs and cats and livestock, postexposure management, and control methods in wild animals. Such publications should be consulted when necessary. In general, for cattle, sheep, and horses, the primary vaccination is given at 3 months of age and boosters given annually. Farm livestock in endemic areas where clinical cases of rabies occur are common should be vaccinated.

In countries where vampire bats are a major vector for rabies in farm livestock, vaccination of livestock is necessary, but in countries such as Argentina vaccination does not support a cost-benefit analysis.

Vaccines

Almost all rabies vaccines for domestic animals are inactivated. Inactivated tissue culture cell vaccines given to cattle result in neutralizing antibodies in 1 month after the primary vaccination. A booster given 1 year later increases the titers, which are detectable 1 year after the booster. A vaccine inactivated with binary ethylenimine, and containing aluminum hydroxide adjuvant, provides excellent protection for up to 3 years and is very useful for the control of rabies in cattle in Latin America where the vampire bat is the main vector.

Vaccinal antibodies are present in the colostrum of vaccinated cows and it is recommended that, where cattle are vaccinated annually, calves be vaccinated at 4 months of age and again when 10 months of age, but vaccination should be delayed 6 months for calves born to and receiving colostrum from previously vaccinated dams.[8] However, in areas with endemic and epizootic rabies, calves can be vaccinated as early as 2 months of age and be protected in the presence of passive immunity from colostral antibodies provided they are revaccinated 4 months later.[9] Calves from unvaccinated dams can be protected by vaccinating them at 17 days of age. Postvaccinal paralysis does not occur after its use. Coadministration of levamisole (6 mg/kg, subcutaneously) with vaccination does not increase the vaccine titer; however, the effect on cell-mediated immunity was not specifically evaluated in that study.[10]

Vaccination of Wildlife

Mass oral vaccination of terrestrial wild animals is a rabies control method that is feasible, effective, and internationally accepted. It is based on the concept of applied herd immunity. The vaccines are efficacious when fed as vaccine baits. The factors affecting acceptance of baits for delivery of oral rabies vaccine to raccoons have been examined.

The oral immunization of foxes has resulted in a substantial decrease in the number of rabies cases in Europe. As a result of oral vaccination of the red fox (*V. vulpes*) against rabies, using hand and aerial distribution of vaccine-laden baits, the rabies virus has almost been completely eradicated from Western and Central Europe. The same dramatic decrease occurred in southern Ontario, Canada. In most countries, vaccine baits were distributed twice yearly during the spring (March to May) and autumn (September to October). Several European countries have become rabies free: Belgium, Luxembourg, France, Italy, Switzerland, Finland, and the Netherlands.

Progress has been made in applying oral rabies vaccination to contain and eliminate some strains of terrestrial rabies in North America. Raboral V-RG is the only rabies vaccine licensed for use in the United States. It has not produced sufficient levels of population immunity in skunks in the wild at the current dose, and it may be less effective in skunks than in other species. Skunks are a major contributor to rabies in North America and this has raised concerns about an independent maintenance cycle for raccoon rabies in skunks. The national rabies management goals of virus containment and elimination will likely remain elusive until an oral vaccine is licensed that is immunogenic in all terrestrial rabies reservoir species. Vaccination will succeed in reducing or eradicating rabies only if a sufficient proportion of the target population can be immunized. Mathematical modeling techniques are now being tested to examine the population biology of rabies in wildlife species such as raccoons and skunks.

It is notable that no practical vaccination methods have been developed for bats. Phylogenetic analyses of viruses from bats and carnivores suggest a historical basis for still existing viral origins caused by interactions between these taxa. Thus the possibility for pathogen emergence resulting from transmission by rabid bats with subsequent perpetuation among other animals cannot be discounted easily on any continent.

Quarantine and Biosecurity

The most effective method of preventing the entry of rabies into a country free of the disease is the imposition of a quarantine period of 4 to 6 months on all imported dogs. This system has successfully prevented the entry of the disease into island countries, but has obvious limitation in countries that have land borders. The occurrence of the disease in two dogs in the United Kingdom in 1969 to 1970 in which the incubation period appeared to last 7 to 9 months suggests that the more usual period of 6 months may give incomplete protection. Therefore vaccination on two occasions with an inactivated vaccine while the animal is still in quarantine for 6 months is the current recommendation. To require a longer period of quarantine would encourage evasion of the law by smuggling. The situation in the UK, and in any country where the disease does not occur, is a vexed one. It is possible to rely chiefly on quarantine and act swiftly to stamp the disease out if it occurs. The shock eradication program would include quarantine of, and vaccination in, a risk area, ring vaccination around it, and destruction of all wildlife. This procedure is likely to be adopted in countries where the risk is small, such as Australia. Where the risk is great, consideration must be given to mass vaccination of wildlife by baits, because wildlife are the cracks in the defense armor. The use of combined vaccines containing rabies vaccine in other vaccines used in dogs would be an effective and panic-free way of increasing the immune status of the pet population.

FURTHER READING

Bellotto A, et al. Overview of rabies in the Americas. *Virus Res.* 2005;111:5-12.

Dyer JL, Yager P, Orciari L, et al. Rabies surveillance in the United States during 2013. *J Am Vet Med Assoc.* 2014;245:1111-1123.

REFERENCES

1. Papaneri AB, et al. *Virus Res.* 2015;197:54.
2. Banyard AC, et al. *Virus Res.* 2010;152:79.
3. Den K, et al. *Am J Trop Med Hyg.* 2012;86:528.
4. Chandrashekhara N, et al. *Indian J Field Vet.* 2013;8:49.
5. Shankar BP. *Veterinary World.* 2009;2:74.
6. Reddy RVC, et al. *Infect Genet Evol.* 2014;27:163.
7. Hampson K, et al. *PLoS Negl Trop Dis.* 2015;9:e0003709.
8. Yakobson B, et al. *Prev Vet Med.* 2015;121:170.
9. Filho OA, et al. *Res Vet Sci.* 2012;92:396.
10. Cazella LN, et al. *Vet Rec.* 2009;165:722.

PSEUDORABIES (AUJESZKY'S DISEASE)

The disease was first described in cattle and was known then as pseudorabies because of the similarity to rabies and thereafter Aujeszky's disease after the Hungarian physician who first isolated the virus.

SYNOPSIS

Etiology Aujeszky's disease virus (suid herpesvirus 1) (SuHV-1).

Epidemiology Found in pigs worldwide and major economic importance in swine-raising areas. High prevalence of infection; lower incidence of disease. Infected pig source of infection; latent infection is characteristic; spread occurs within herds, between herds, and from infected carriers; long-distance aerosol transmission occurs from area to area; immunity follows infection or vaccination.

Signs Fever, incoordination, recumbency, convulsion, and death in piglets. Coughing, nasal discharge, sneezing, and dyspnea in older growing pigs. In cattle and sheep, intense pruritus at site of bite, excitement, circling, convulsions, fever, recumbency, paralysis, and death in 48 hours or less.

Clinical pathology Serology for virus-neutralizing antibodies. Detection of virus in tissues.

Lesions Viral encephalitis.

Diagnostic confirmation Detection of virus in tissues; serology; inclusion bodies in nervous tissue and respiratory tract.

Differential diagnosis

Swine
- Viral encephalomyelitis (Teschen disease)
- Rabies
- Streptococcal meningitis
- Hog cholera
- African swine fever
- Glasser's disease
- Septicemias (*Escherichia coli*, erysipelas, salmonella)
- Bowel edema
- Salt poisoning
- Reproductive insufficiency (parvovirus).

Cattle and sheep
- Nervous form acetonemia
- Rabies C
- Acute lead poisoning.

Treatment None.

Control Depopulation and repopulation, test and removal, segregation of progeny, and vaccination with subunit vaccines that distinguish between infected and vaccinated pigs.

ETIOLOGY

Pseudorabies is caused by porcine herpesvirus-1 (SuHV-1), Aujeszky's disease virus, or pseudorabies virus (PRV), of the genus *Varicellovirus*, a member of the family of Herpesviridae,[1] subfamily Alphaherpesvirinae. It exists as a single serotype. Many cell lines are used for PRV culture. There are four major genome types; Type 1 is found in the United States and Europe; Type 2 is found in central Europe, Type 3 is found in Eastern Europe, and Type 4 is found only in Asia.

EPIDEMIOLOGY

Occurrence

PRV primarily affects pigs and occurs incidentally in other species. It has a worldwide distribution except for Norway, Australia, and most of the islands of Southeast Asia. Control programs have eliminated the condition in many countries,[2] leaving isolated pockets in Northern Ireland and in France. It is still endemic in eastern and southeastern Europe, Latin America, Africa, and Asia. For example, in Poland from 2005 to 2009 around 0.4% of the population was infected.[3] In countries where the disease has been eradicated vaccination is not allowed.

The disease persists in feral pigs, wild boar, and hybrids[4,5] at quite high levels in many European countries and also in the United States[2] and these permanently threaten the domestic pig population.

The reservoir of Aujeszky's disease has shifted from domestic pigs to wild and feral pig populations and circulates unchecked in many countries.[6] Thus the identification of reservoirs and the epidemiologic surveillance is becoming more difficult.

PRV is primarily a disease of pigs, and naturally occurring cases in cattle, sheep, dogs, cats, rats, and horses are rare and usually fatal. Many other species have also been affected, but only pigs survive the infection. Infection in other species often occurs when pigs cohabit with other species.

Morbidity and Case Fatality

Typically, the disease spreads rapidly in infected herds over a period of 1 to 2 weeks, and the acute stage of the outbreak lasts 1 to 2 months. In sucking pigs, the morbidity and mortality rates approach 100%, but in mature swine there may be no clinical signs, and affected animals usually recover. The highest morbidity occurs initially in unweaned piglets, but as the outbreak continues and piglets become passively immunized through the sow's colostrum, the major incidence may occur in weanlings.

In recent years, there has also been an increase in the morbidity and case–fatality rates in older pigs associated with the intensification of pig rearing and the dominance of more virulent strains.

Risk Factors

Animal Risk Factors

The seroprevalence of infection varies widely between herds, and between breeding and finishing pigs within herds. The most important animal risk factors of virus persistence are herd size and the population density of the sows in the herd. Endemic infection is more likely in herds of breeding sows with more than 66 sows. In breeding herds, spread of infection is positively associated with increasing size of the herd, having the gilts in the same barn as the sows (gestation barn), and serologic evidence of infection in the finishing pigs. The seroprevalence of infection is low in quarantined breeding herds, which makes them prime candidates for elimination of the disease by test and removal.

In the early period of a compulsory vaccination program with gI-deleted vaccines, in an area endemically infected with the disease, the seroprevalence of infected breeding females is higher in farrow–finish than farrow–feeder herds. Mandatory vaccination is beneficial in both herds but the pattern is linear in farrow–feeder herds and curvilinear in farrow–finish herds, and is more rapid in the early period of the program. In the farrow–finish herds, the odds of infected breeding females were associated positively with seropositivity in the finishing pigs of the herd and with the density of the pigs in the county in which the herd is located. In Belgium the presence of finishing pigs in the same herd increased the chances of being infected. The spread and transmission of the virus between herds can be reduced by a reduction in the contact rate between the herds and their size and by a reduction of the transmission within the herd.

The factors associated with circulation of the virus within herds include confinement of finishing pigs, concurrent infection with *Actinobacillus pleuropneumoniae*, the length of time since the herd has been under quarantine, and the presence of clinical disease.

In general, PRV does not increase the susceptibility of animals to infection with other pathogens.

The primary risk factors associated with seroprevalence of the virus in 500 swine herds in Illinois included total confinement and density of infected herds in the geographic area. It was calculated in Belgium that if there were over 455 pigs per squared kilometer, then there was a 10-fold increase in the risk of PRV. Total confinement is associated with higher seroprevalence, presumably because of increased density of population and increased risk of transmission. Seroprevalence is higher in vaccinated herds, increases over the course of the eradication program, and decreases with an increased time between quarantine and the development of a herd plan. In the Netherlands, the risk factors contributing to seroprevalence of infection in breeding herds included the presence of finishing pigs, production type (producers of finishing pigs had a higher prevalence than producers of breeding stock), vaccination of sows during nursing (compared with vaccinating all sows simultaneously at 5-month intervals, or vaccination during the second half of gestation), pig density in the municipality in which the herd was located (seroprevalence increased with higher pig density), herd size of fewer than 100 sows, average within-herd parity (seroprevalence increased with higher within-herd parity), replacement pigs raised on the premises, and vaccine strain administered to the sows.

Environmental Risk Factors

The virus is resistant to environmental conditions depending on pH, humidity, and temperature. The virus may survive for 2 to 7 weeks in an infected environment and for up to 5 weeks in meat. The infectivity of the virus in an aerosol decreases by 50% in 1 hour. Environments at 4°C supported the survival of the virus in aerosol better than at 22°C. The virus is lipophilic and sensitive to several commonly used disinfectants. Sodium hypochlorite (5.25%) is the most desirable and practical disinfectant. Suspensions of the virus in saline G solution and on the solid fomites, whole corn, and steel remained infectious for at least 7 days. Loam soil, straw, and concrete supported survival of the virus at 25°C for up to 1 week. During shipment of pigs, bedding material and surfaces in contact with pigs may become contaminated. Rinsing a needle between sampling may reduce the probability of mechanically transmitting the disease.

Pathogen Factors

Field strains of the virus differ in virulence. Numerous genomically different strains of the virus exist, and restriction endonuclease (RE) analysis can distinguish between virus isolates, which is useful for identifying new isolates of the virus as they appear in pig populations. In Denmark, restriction fragment analyses of older clinical isolates, and of isolates from all the virologically confirmed outbreaks since 1985, indicated the introduction of foreign strains. Strain variation in virulence has been observed in field isolates and produced by laboratory attenuation. Virulence also affects the tropism of the virus. Many of the highly virulent strains are neuroinvasive; many of the moderately virulent or mild strains are not neuroinvasive but affect the respiratory tract. The highly adapted or vaccinal strains often acquire a tropism for the reproductive systems. Inactivation of several genes that are not essential for viral replication can reduce the virulence of the virus.

Some field strains of the virus from Poland and Hungary have been identified by restriction fragment pattern analysis as derivatives of conventionally attenuated vaccine strains. This is considered a rare event but must be considered in relationship to trade in semen from vaccinated boars or trade in live animals between disease-free areas and areas in which vaccination with live attenuated strains is practiced.

Methods of Transmission

Pseudorabies is not very contagious and large quantities of the virus are required to infect pigs except very young piglets. Larger doses of virus are needed for oral infection than nasal infection. In feral pig and wild boar populations it appears to be venereal transmission that is more important.[7] It can be transmitted transplacentally, especially in the last third of gestation. It can also be passed through the colostrum. In milk excretion of virus takes place for 2 to 3 days following infection. Virus can be transmitted for up to 12 days in semen following infection. Venereal transmission of latent infection in sows and boars has been suspected, but there is no direct evidence. The virus cannot usually be isolated from urine.

In a study of PRV in wild swine in the United States it was found that the virus was found in the oral cavity of feral pigs and was widely distributed in the tonsils, salivary glands, taste buds, and even mucosa in the region of the tusks.[8]

Infected swine shed virus in large quantities from all body excretions, secretions, and aerosols. Virus shedding starts 1 to 2 days after infection, reaches a peak at 2 to 5 days, and may last up to 17 days. Virus can be isolated from the oropharynx for 18 to 25 days.

Pigs, and possibly rodents, appear to be the primary host for the virus. The virus is present in the nasal discharge and in the mouth of affected pigs on the first day of illness and for up to 17 days after infection. This suggests that short-length aerosol transmission is a common occurrence within buildings or units but long distance transmission is still doubted. After infection and recovery pigs may be regarded as carriers.

Within Herds

Transmission within herds occurs by direct oral–nasal contact between infected and susceptible pigs and aerosols from projection of discharges during sneezing, but it may also occur via contaminated drinking water and feed. Transmission within herds is independent of the size of the population.

The transmission of virus decreases rapidly following the start of a vaccination program, but extensive spread can still occur even among finishing pigs vaccinated twice. Vaccinated pigs may shed more virulent virus but there are no significant differences in magnitude of transmission. Mixing of chronically infected pigs with seronegative pigs may not result in seroconversion in the seronegative pigs until a clinical outbreak of disease occurs.

Between Herds

Transmission between herds is caused by the introduction of infected animals, and the virus may still be introduced into vaccinated breeding herds. Other methods of transmission have been suggested, including farm laborers, vehicles, feedstuffs, rodents, and wild or domestic animals, the carcasses of dead infected animals, and infected food and water.

Within an Area

Transmission within an area is a major problem and not well understood. Some evidence indicates that area spread may be associated with markets and the frequency of delivery of pigs to market per year. In France, it has been suggested that the presence of an infected herd within 1 km is an important factor in the spread of PRV. The concurrent occurrence of an outbreak of disease on many farms in the same area in Denmark suggested long-distance airborne transmission of the virus.

Infection is spread by airborne transmission. Sneezing probably generates the airborne virus. In a series of outbreaks in Britain between 1981 and1982, 7 of 11 were found likely to have been transmitted by aerosol on meteorologic grounds. Airborne spread occurred between herds 2 to 9 km apart. An epidemic in Denmark in 1987 to 1988, associated with foreign strains of the virus, suggests that airborne transmission occurred across the German–Danish border, especially as a southerly wind was blowing during the period of transmission.

Computer modeling based on the mean dose of virus received by an animal at a farm downwind can be used to predict the airborne spread of the virus.

The virus is inactivated in meat after 35 days of storage at −18°C (0.5°F). Meat from infected pigs may cause infection when fed to dogs.

Latency

Pigs that recover from infection are latent carriers of the virus for life. Reactivation, followed by shedding and spreading the virus, may occur following stress such as transport or farrowing, or by the administration of corticosteroids. Serologic testing of latent carriers detects the antibody response to the whole virus or to a PRV virus glycoprotein. During natural infection, the virus replicates at the site of infection, usually in the oronasal areas. The virus gains entry into the nerve endings and ascends by retrograde axonal transport to the cell body in the trigeminal ganglion. Viral components can be found in both the trigeminal ganglion and the tonsils. The tonsil is a primary site of virus replication and serves as an area for monitoring virus shedding during acute infection and reactivation. The virus can be isolated from tissue fragments of pigs clinically recovered from disease for up to 13 months and followed by a challenge with the live virus, which may be shed by sows for up to 19 months after initial infection. Virus gene products can be found in the trigeminal ganglia and tonsils for many weeks following acute infection. Latent infection can also occur in vaccinated pigs.

Other Species

The rarity of spread to other species is caused by scanty nasal discharge and the improbability of the discharge coming into contact with abraded skin or nasal mucosa of animals other than pigs. The disease has occurred in sheep and cattle following the use of a multidose syringe previously used in infected swine. It may spread from normal or clinically affected pigs to animals of other species, but does not usually spread between animals of the other species. For example, sheep and calves can be infected experimentally, but there is no evidence that they excrete the virus. The disease may occur in pigs, sheep, and cattle on the same farm. Brown rats may be a minor source of infection but are unlikely to be an important reservoir; they are capable of spreading the disease to dogs. The wild Norway rat is thought to have only a minor role in the transmission of the disease to farm animals. The virus causes fatal disease in dogs, which are usually infected from close association with infected pigs. The raccoon can be infected experimentally, but is not considered to be a long-term subclinical carrier of the virus. The possible role of wild animals in transmission of PRV in swine has been examined with inconclusive results. It has been seen in Kodiak, polar, and Himalayan bears fed on a diet of raw pig's heads. Five viral isolates were recovered from latently infected wild boar originating from two regions of East Germany, but in the Netherlands the wild boar were said to be rarely affected. The PRV infections in the wild boar in Germany are said to exist in the country as an endemic infection and persist completely separately from the domestic population and also do not appear to affect it. The sacral ganglia and trigeminal ganglia of wild pigs were said to be a source of infection. The latency was shown in 9/16 sacral ganglia, 7/16 trigeminal ganglia, and 5/13 tonsils from feral swine in the United States, but even so most of the transmission in feral swine is expected to be venereal. The experimental infection of wild boars and domestic pigs with different strains has been performed and the clinical signs depended on the strain but the wild boar could infect the domestic strains and vice versa. The low virulence strains were highly adapted to the wild boar.

Immune Mechanisms

When infected with a virulent strain of the virus, pigs develop an immune response that can completely, or almost completely, prevent the virus from replicating after the pig becomes reinfected. Following natural infection, sows acquire immunity, which is transferred to their piglets in the colostrum and persists in the piglets until 5 to 7 weeks of age. Following intranasal challenge, piglets with colostral immunity from naturally infected sows are protected from clinical disease, but not against subclinical infection.

Vaccination of pigs with attenuated PRV virus prevents clinical disease and death that may otherwise follow exposure to the virulent virus. Vaccination does not, however, prevent either acute or latent infection with virulent virus. Consequently, vaccinated pigs, as well as nonvaccinated pigs that survive infection with the virulent virus, can become virus carriers and a source of the virus following reactivation of a latent infection. This is of vital importance in eradication programs in which it is necessary to identify infected pigs regardless of their vaccination status. Maternal immunity interferes with inactivated virus vaccination much more than with live virus vaccination.

Vaccination of pregnant sows induces a maternal immunity, which protects piglets from experimental disease. However, latent infection of young pigs with highly virulent virus can develop in the absence of clinical signs. The virus can reach the uterine and fetal tissues, via infected mononuclear cells, which is the presence of circulating antibodies induced on vaccination. Vaccination of piglets before challenge exposure has little or no effect on the rate of establishment of virus latency, but vaccination does reduce shedding after subsequent experimental reactivation of the virus with dexamethasone. Attenuated tyrosine kinase-negative vaccine strains of the virus can also establish a reactivatable, latent infection.

In growing and finishing pigs in quarantined herds, the serologic status is unpredictable because the infection may continue to spread, may cease temporarily, or may cease altogether. Evaluation of the serologic status of the boars in a breeding herd does not accurately reflect the serostatus of the herd.

It has been suggested that the T cells are more important than the B cells in the clearance of PRV from the host, and it has been shown that strong T-cell–mediated responses after challenge produce the best protection.

Economic Importance

The economic losses associated with pseudorabies in swine are caused by clinical disease and the costs of serologic analysis and vaccination programs. Economic loss estimates must include the measurement of losses during and immediately after clinical outbreaks of disease and the indirect losses incurred until after eradication of the disease. Losses have been estimated at $25 to $50 per sow per year; these include only losses during the period of the outbreak and the direct losses attributable to death and abortions. When expanding the observations of economic losses to 3 months after the termination of the outbreak, estimated losses may be as high as $145 per sow per year. Economic analyses of the losses in a commercial farrow–finish herd of 240 breeding-age sows in the United States revealed that the major part of the loss was caused by death of suckling pigs at 76% of total loss, nursery pig mortality accounted for 12.6% of total net loss, sow culling and deaths accounted for 9.4% of net loss, and market pig deaths accounted for 1.2% of net losses.

The costs of eradicating PRV vary depending on the methods used. Depopulation–repopulation is the most expensive method because it requires culling of animals, clean-up costs, and downtime, which represents the largest proportion of expense. In addition, the probability of reinfection following repopulation is a risk.

Test and removal is the most inexpensive, and segregation of offspring is an intermediate cost. The cost of eradicating the virus from a swine herd can be in excess of $220 per inventoried sow; some estimates are much higher. In large breeding herds or finishing herds with the continual influx of susceptible pigs, the disease may become endemic. PRV may also be a significant cause of reproductive inefficiency in pig herds, and infection within the herd may be initially manifested by abortions in the sow herd, followed later by the more typical occurrence of neurologic disease in suckling and growing pigs. The economic losses from the disease can be very high because of mortality in young pigs, decreased reproductive performance, and the necessity to depopulate to eradicate the disease from a herd. An economic assessment of an epidemic of PRV in a 150-sow farrow–finish operation on selected production and economic variables has been made. The mean litter size remained the same throughout the period of observation, but there was a twofold increase in suckling pig mortality and 3.5-fold increase in stillbirths during the months of the epidemic compared with the period before the epidemic. Following the epidemic, suckling pig mortality was 14% greater and stillbirth rate was 71% greater than during the months preceding the outbreak. The major economic losses (88% of the total loss) were related to breeding herd removal/depopulation and production downtime.

PATHOGENESIS

The portal of entry is through abraded skin, oral mucosa, or via the intact nasal mucosa. Strain differences in the effect of historical PRV strains in porcine respiratory nasal mucosa explants shows that there were differences in the strains.[8] The virus is pantropic and affects tissues derived from all embryonic layers. Receptor and receptor-binding virion proteins that can mediate the virus entry into the cell and cell-to-cell spread have been described. The various glycoproteins of the virus are required for various stages of virion morphogenesis. For example, deletion of glycoproteins gE, gI, and gM inhibits the virion maturation. Pseudorabies glycoprotein gK is a virion structural component involved in virus release from the cell but not viral entry, and its presence is important to prevent immediate reinfection. Viremia occurs with localization of the virus in many viscera, but with multiplication occurring primarily in the upper respiratory tract. Viral and cell interactions have been described in detail.[9] Spread to the brain occurs by way of the olfactory, glossopharyngeal, or trigeminal nerves, i.e., via the autonomic nerves. It can pass across synapses and infect higher level neurons.[10] Cells with the common leukocyte antigen CD45+ populate the CNS-infected areas from the local capillaries, and the number of cells is increased in proportion to the number of infected neurons. Virus disappears from the brain by the eighth day, coinciding with the appearance of neutralizing antibody in the blood. When the virus gains entry through a skin abrasion, it quickly invades the local peripheral nerves, passing along them centripetally and causing damage to nerve cells. It is this form of progression that causes local pruritus in the early stages of the disease, and encephalomyelitis at a later stage when the virus has invaded the CNS. In pigs, pruritus does not develop after intramuscular injection, but a local paralysis indicative of damage to low motor neurons occurs before invasion of the CNS in some pigs. In cattle, pruritus of the head and neck is usually associated with respiratory tract infection, whereas perianal pruritus is usually caused by vaginal infection.

The inoculation of PRV into the nasal cavities or brain results in signs of encephalitis instead of local pruritus. With oral inoculation, there is an initial stage of viral proliferation in the tonsillar mucosa, followed by systemic invasion, localization, and invasion of the CNS along peripheral and autonomic nerve trunks and fibers. Lesions of Auerbach's myenteric plexus and the skin may also occur. The peripheral blood mononuclear cells, tonsils, lymph nodes, and bone marrow are a poor source of virus after experimental infection. The trigeminal ganglia and olfactory bulb are good sources of virus. The virus may be present in the trigeminal ganglion of a naturally infected sow without any history of clinical disease. Experimental inoculation of the virus into young pigs can result in a mild pneumonia, which may progress to a severe suppurative bronchopneumonia.

The virus can invade the uterus and infect preimplantation embryos, which can lead to degeneration of the embryo and reproductive failure. Virulent PRV virus can cause lesions in the uterine endothelium and ovarian corpora lutea of pigs in early pregnancy, and gene-deleted mutant virus vaccine given intravenously during estrus can cause ovarian lesions, which may affect fertility. Through the use of embryo transfer procedures, infected embryos may disseminate the virus from donors to recipients.

In other species the virus tends to be restricted to the nervous system.

CLINICAL FINDINGS

Pigs

The incubation period in natural outbreaks is about 1 day but may be from 1 to 8 days. The major signs are referable to infection of the respiratory, nervous, and reproductive systems. There is considerable variation in the clinical manifestation, depending on the virulence and tropism of the infecting strain. Nervous system disease is the major manifestation, but with some strains, respiratory disease may be the initial and prime presenting feature. There is also strain variation in the pattern of age susceptibility.

Young pigs a few days to a month old are most susceptible. Very young sucklings develop an indistinct syndrome, but prominent nervous signs occur in older piglets. A febrile reaction, with temperatures up to 41.5°C (107°F), occurs before the onset of nervous signs. Incoordination of the hindlimbs causing sideways progression is followed by recumbency, fine and coarse muscle tremors, and paddling movements. Lateral deviation of the head, frothing at the mouth, nystagmus, slight ocular discharge, and convulsive episodes appear in a few animals. A snoring respiration with marked abdominal movement occurs in many, and vomiting and diarrhea in some affected pigs. Deaths occur about 12 hours after the first signs appear. In California, a consistent sign has been blindness caused by extensive retinal degeneration.

In growing and adult pigs, the disease is much less severe but there is considerable variation depending on the virulence of the infecting strain. In growing pigs, mortality falls with increasing age and is generally less than 5% in pigs at 4 to 6 months of age. With some strains, fever is a prominent sign, whereas depression, vomiting, and sometimes marked respiratory signs, including sneezing, nasal discharge, coughing, and severe dyspnea are common. Trembling, incoordination, and paralysis and convulsions follow, and precede death. With others, the disease may be manifested at this age by mild signs of posterior incoordination and leg weakness. In adults, fever may not be present, and the infection may cause only a mild syndrome of anorexia, dullness, agalactia, and constipation. However, virulent strains may produce acute disease in adults, characterized by fever, sneezing, nasal pruritus, vomiting, incoordination and convulsions, and death. Infection in early pregnancy may result in embryonic death, or abortion, and early return to estrus. An abundant vaginal discharge may occur. Infection in late pregnancy may result in abortion, or in the subsequent birth of mummified fetuses, which may involve all or only part of the litter. Abortion may result from the effects of fever or from viral infection of the fetus.

Concurrent infection has been described with PCV2, and PRRS and swine influenza virus, and in these cases the resultant disease is more likely to be a severe proliferative and necrotizing pneumonia.[11]

Cattle, Sheep, and Goats

There may be sudden death without obvious signs of illness. More commonly, there is intense, local pruritus with violent licking, chewing, and rubbing of a particular body part. Itching may be localized to any part of the body surface, but is most common about the head, the flanks, or the feet, which are the sites most likely to be contaminated by virus. There is intense excitement during this stage, and convulsions and constant bellowing may occur. Maniacal behavior, circling, spasm of the diaphragm, and opisthotonus are often evident. A stage of paralysis follows in which salivation, respiratory distress, and ataxia occur. The temperature is usually increased, sometimes to as high as 41°C to 41°C (106°F-107°F). Final paralysis is followed by death in 6 to 48 hours after the first appearance of illness. A case of nonfatal PRV in a cow is recorded. There is also a report of PRV occurring in feedlot cattle in which there were nervous signs, bloat, and acute death, but no pruritus. In young calves, it is characterized clinically by encephalitis, no pruritus, erosion in the oral cavity and esophagus, and a high case-fatality rate. An outbreak in sheep was associated with skin abrasions acquired at shearing. Affected ewes were dull, inappetent, and had a fever of 41.1°C. About 23 of 29 affected sheep developed the "mad itch," with nibbling of their fleece and frenzied attempts to bite one area of the skin and rub it against the wall and bars of their pen. Terminally, recumbency, tremors, and opisthotonus were common, and death occurred within 12 to 24 hours after onset. Five farm cats also became ill and died; the virus was isolated from the brain of one cat. In goats, rapid deaths, unrest, lying down and rising frequently, crying plaintively, profuse sweating, and spasms and paralysis terminally are characteristic. There may be no pruritus.

The clinical findings in dogs and cats are similar to those in cattle, with death occurring in about 24 hours. In France, cases in dogs have been linked to strains of virus from wild boars.

CLINICAL PATHOLOGY

Serology

The commonly used serologic tests for PRV-specific antibodies are the serum neutralization (SN) and ELISA tests.

Serum Neutralization Test

The SN test using the Shoppe strain has been the gold standard against which other serologic tests are compared and has been most widely used because of its sensitivity and specificity. Specific virus-neutralizing (VN) antibodies are detectable in the serum of recovered pigs, and this test is in routine use for herd diagnosis and survey purposes. Antibody is detectable on the seventh day after infection, reaches a peak about the 35th day, and persists for many months. Paired serum samples taken as early as possible, and about 3 weeks later, show a marked antibody rise. However, the SN test lacks the sensitivity necessary for detection of pigs with low levels of humoral titers of specific SN antibodies, which can be enhanced by using the Bartha gIII strain.

Some herds may have no serologic evidence of previous infection or current spread of the virus but have single reactors in the herd that may be infected with the virus. Such singleton reactors may be found in herds being monitored serologically for presence of infection. These singleton reactors may be infected with strains of the virus that are relatively avirulent.

Enzyme-Linked Immunosorbent Assay

The ELISA test is more sensitive than the SN test, especially early in the immune response to PRV antigens. However, because of its high sensitivity, screening ELISAs yield some false positives, which must be confirmed by another test, such as another ELISA, SN test, or latex agglutination test. False positives are unlikely to be caused by infection with other herpesviruses. ELISA has also been used as a meat juice test with high sensitivity (93%) and specificity (98%).

The indirect ELISA is a more rapid and convenient procedure, offering many advantages over the SN test for routine serodiagnostic work. An indirect ELISA, using whole blood collected onto paper disks, is a rapid and convenient test and eliminates the costs of using vacutainer tubes and separating the blood. An indirect ELISA based on recombinant and affinity-purified glycoprotein E of PRV to differentiate vaccinated from naturally infected animals has been developed. An indirect ELISA has been developed in the Czech Republic that can be used because of its high sensitivity and specificity for blood serum on frozen pork samples. It has allowed the demonstration of PRV in meat juice with only marginal titers in the blood.

Commercial ELISA kits are available and some are more specific than others. A highly sensitive and specific competitive ELISA based on baculovirus-expressed PRV glycoprotein gE and gI complex has been described. This allows detection as early as 2 weeks postinfection and can handle large numbers of tests without the need to handle live virus.

In countries where vaccination is regularly used for control of the disease, an assay to serologically distinguish infected from vaccinated pigs is critical. Although a vaccination program will reduce the circulation of virus in the field, it will not eliminate the virus from the pig population. To eradicate the virus, the ability to differentiate infected from vaccinated pigs is crucial. Several commercial ELISA kits can differentiate between vaccinated and naturally infected pigs. Differentiation is possible when vaccine virus strains have either a natural, or a genetically engineered, deletion that encodes for either gI, gIII, or gX genes. Commercial ELISA kits that specifically detect antibody responses to gI of the virus offer considerable advantages as diagnostic tests for the virus, with a sensitivity of 99.2% and specificity of 100%. The gI ELISA is able to distinguish infected pigs from those vaccinated with gI-negative vaccines. The field strains of the virus produce antibodies to gI when inoculated into pigs. Unvaccinated pigs, or pigs vaccinated with gI-negative vaccines, that become subclinically infected with field strains of the virus may be detected with the gI–ELISA for a long time after infection. Thus pigs that are seropositive in the gI–ELISA have either been infected with PRV or have been vaccinated with gI-positive vaccines; gI-seronegative pigs can be considered to be uninfected. Eradication of the virus from swine herds is possible by gI–ELISA testing, and culling gI-seropositive pigs in herds using gI-negative vaccines.

Detection of pigs in the latent phase of infection can be done serologically. Pigs of any age that survive the acute infection phase become latent carriers for life, and serologic testing consistently detects animals in the latent phase of infection if the test detects the antibody response to the whole virus or to a reliable PRV glycoprotein. Of several serologic tests examined, the gI and gIII marker systems, which performed with similar sensitivity as the screening tests, were superior to the gX marker system in detecting antibodies in infected pigs.

Detection of Virus

In infected pigs the virus is usually present in nasal secretions for up to 10 days. A common method for the diagnosis of PRV in sows is to take swabs from the nasal mucosa and vagina. Polyester and wire swabs shipped in 199 tissue culture medium supplemented with 2% fetal bovine serum (FBS) buffered with 0.1% sodium bicarbonate and HEPES will yield optimum recovery of the virus. Wooden applicator sticks with cotton wool have antiviral activity and recovery of the virus may not be possible after 2 days, which is of practical importance if the samples are shipped by mail. The virus can be demonstrated in nasal cells by immunofluorescence and immunoperoxidase techniques. It can be detected by direct filter hybridization of nasal and tonsillar specimens from live pigs. The virus survives on tonsil swabs taken with Dacron-tipped applicators for up to 72 hours in cell culture medium under transport.

New PCR techniques have been used and they can differentiate between true and false serologic positives when single reactor pigs have been found. A molecular beacon RT-PCR for the detection of PRV, African swine fever (ASF), PCV2, and Porcine Parvovirus has been described[12] and for the detection of PRV, ASF, and PRRS.[13] A multiplex PCR for PRV, porcine respiratory coronavirus, and PCV2 has been described.[14]

Loop-mediated isothermal amplification (LAMP) for rapid detection and differentiation of wild-type PRV and gene-deleted virus vaccines was described.[15]

NECROPSY FINDINGS

There are no gross lesions typical and constant for the disease, and in some cases lesions are absent or minimal and diagnosis must rely on laboratory examination. When pruritus has occurred, there is considerable damage to local areas of skin and extensive subcutaneous edema.

Gross lesions in the upper respiratory tract are the most obvious and these include necrotic rhinitis, conjunctivitis, laryngitis, and tracheitis. The lungs show congestion, edema, and some hemorrhages. Hemorrhages may be present under the endocardium and excess fluid is often present in the pericardial sac. In pigs, there are additional lesions of visceral involvement. Slight splenomegaly, meningitis, and excess pericardial fluid are observed, and there may be small necrotic foci in the spleen and liver. In sows, there may be a necrotizing placentitis and endometritis. Foci of hepatic, splenic, or pulmonary necrosis may be seen in aborted fetuses.

Histologically, in all species, there is severe and extensive neuronal damage in the spinal cord, paravertebral ganglia, and brain. Perivascular cuffing and focal necrosis are present in the gray matter, particularly in the cerebellar cortex. Intranuclear inclusion bodies occur infrequently in the degenerating neurons and astroglial cells, particularly in cerebral cortex in the pig. These inclusions are of considerable importance in differential diagnosis. Necrotizing lesions with inclusion-body formation in the upper respiratory tract and lungs is strongly suggestive of porcine pseudorabies. Ultrastructural observations have been made that included syncytia, cellular debris and macrophages, and lymphocytes with vacuoles in their cytoplasm. Virus may be detected by direct fluorescent antibody examination or by growth in tissue culture. The tissues of the head and neck regions of nonimmune pigs yield virus most consistently and in the highest concentration after challenge. The immunoperoxidase test can be used to study the distribution of the virus in different tissues. Latent virus can be detected using a DNA hybridization dot blot assay. Whenever possible, whole carcasses and fetuses should be submitted for laboratory examination. The location of the optimal neural samples, including the paravertebral ganglia, has been described for sheep. The placental lesions in pregnant sows that have aborted from natural infection with pseudorabies consist of necrotizing placentitis and the presence of intranuclear inclusions. In an experimental infection of loops of intestine it was shown that there was necrosis of the follicles in the Peyer's patches and degeneration of the epithelial cells in the crypts and villi and degeneration of the cells in the myenteric plexuses. Intranuclear inclusion bodies were found 2 to 4 days after inoculation. The primary target of the wild PRV was the macrophages of the subepithelial area of the dome of the Peyer's patch.

Samples for Confirmation of Diagnosis

- Histology: half of midsagittally sectioned brain, spinal cord with paravertebral ganglia, gasserian ganglion, placenta, liver, lung, spleen, tonsil, and retropharyngeal lymph node (LM) should be collected. IHC has been used to confirm cases in countries where the disease is rare and other corroborating evidence is lacking. In situ hybridization has also been used Can also collect muscle samples for meat juice ELISAs.
- Virology: brain, spinal cord, liver, spleen, tonsil, retropharyngeal lymph node (FAT, ISO). CSF is not good for virus isolation. The best source is the trigeminal ganglion in the domestic pig and the sacral ganglia in feral pigs. Viral isolation takes about 2 to 5 days. There are several PCRs available[5] and also nested PCRs and RT-PCRs.[16,17]

DIFFERENTIAL DIAGNOSIS

The different clinical forms of pseudorabies in pigs and ruminants resemble several diseases.

Teschen disease occurs in similar forms in certain areas; the diagnosis is dependent on serology and pathology.

Rabies is rare in pigs and is usually accompanied by pruritus at the site of the bite.

Streptococcal meningitis is restricted to sucking pigs of 2–6 weeks of age, the lesions are usually obvious at necropsy, and the causative organism is readily cultured from the meninges. The response to treatment with penicillin is good and is of value as a diagnostic test.

Encephalopathy associated with hog cholera, African swine fever, salmonellosis, Glasser's disease, *Escherichia coli* septicemia and erysipelas are considerations, and are usually obvious at necropsy.

Bowel edema causes typical edema of the head and eyelids in weaner pigs as well as a rapid death.

Salt poisoning causes typical intermittent nervous signs, with a typical history of water deprivation.

Respiratory form of pseudorabies should be considered in any outbreak of respiratory disease that is poorly responsive to usually effective therapeutic measures.

Reproductive inefficiency associated with enterovirus (SMEDI) and parvovirus infections closely resembles that associated with pseudorabies and requires laboratory differentiation by virus isolation and serologic testing.

In cattle the local pruritus is distinctive, but the disease may be confused with the nervous form of acetonemia in which paresthesia may lead to excitement. The rapid recovery that ordinarily occurs in this form of acetonemia is an important diagnostic point. The furious form of rabies and acute lead poisoning cause signs of mania, but pruritus does not occur.

SMEDI, *stillbirth, mummification, embryonic death, and infertility.*

TREATMENT

There is no treatment.

CONTROL

The control of pseudorabies is difficult and currently unreliable because normal healthy pigs may be infected and shed the virus for up to several months. One of the most important future concerns is the infection in wild boar[18] and their illegal transportation across countries.[19]

An important principle in control and eradication of the disease is the reproduction ratio, R_0, which is defined as the average number of new infections caused by one typical infectious animal. When $R_0 > 1$, the infection can spread; when $R_0 < 1$, the infection will disappear. In eradication programs it is essential that R be less than 1 and the infection will die out in the herd.

Strategies Available

The methods of control or eradication include depopulation and repopulation, test and removal, segregation of progeny, and vaccination. The selection of a strategy for the control or elimination of the disease depends on the following: (1) source of the herd infection; (2) method of transmission of the virus; (3) survival of the virus in the environment; (4) sensitivity and specificity of the diagnostic test; (5) risk factors in the herd, which include type of operation, degree of herd isolation, prevalence of infection, value of the genetic material, level of management expertise, and availability of suitable virus-free replacement swine if depopulation and repopulation is chosen as a strategy.

The eradication of the disease from small herds was described in Hungary. In this country the shared use of boars, the pig density, and the infection in the surrounding area were the most significant influences on the spread and control of the disease.

Breeding stock producers favor eradication, farrow–finish producers that do not sell breeding stock or feeder pigs are generally more concerned with the reduction of losses from clinical PRV infection than with eradication. In the United States offsite all in/all out finishing was more frequent among the successful farms than the unsuccessful ones. The unsuccessful farms also had other infected herds within 3.2 km (2 miles) and often no cleaning or disinfection.

Economics of Control and Eradication

Depopulation–repopulation is the most expensive form of eradication, the segregation of progeny method the is next expensive, and the test and removal method is the most inexpensive per sow. A computerized decision-tree analysis and simulation modeling can evaluate the economics of control and eradication strategies. The optimal alternative is to test and remove seropositive animals if the initial prevalence is ~57%; otherwise vaccination of sows only is preferred. Vaccination may be recommended at lower prevalence rates as a conservative approach. Eradication by test and removal combined with the use of gene-deleted vaccines is advantageous at any prevalence rate of infection. Depopulation and repopulation is not the best option under any circumstances. Once formulated, a decision-tree analysis can be adapted to the prevailing economic or epidemiologic conditions.

Determination of Prevalence of Infection

In large herds, the virus must be eliminated from the growing–finishing pigs and the breeding herd. Large herds that are virus positive are infected in both groups; smaller herds are frequently infected in only the breeding herd. An initial step in eradication is to determine the prevalence of infection. Representative samples of finishing pigs older than 4 months, and of breeding sows, gilts, and boars are tested. On the basis of the test results and the risk factors in the herd, a cost-effective plan can be devised for the individual herd.

Depopulation and Repopulation

When the prevalence of infection in the herd is over 50%, eradication can be achieved by depopulation and repopulation with virus-free breeding stock. However, depopulation is the most expensive method and is not compatible with the retention of valuable pedigree stock. The entire herd is depopulated over a period of months as the animals reach market weight. After removal of the animals the entire premises are cleaned and disinfected. Repopulation should be delayed at least 30 days after the final disinfection, and swine should originate from a pseudorabies-free qualified herd and be isolated on the premises and retested 30 days after introduction. All herd additions should be isolated and tested 30 days after introduction.

Test and Removal

The test and removal program is recommended when the prevalence of infection in the herd is below 50%. This method requires testing of the entire breeding herd and immediate removal of all seropositive animals; 30 days after removal of seropositive animals, the herd is retested, and if necessary at 30-day intervals, until the entire herd tests are negative. Following a second negative test, the testing regimen may be changed to test only 25% of the herd every 4 months. Seropositive animals are identified and culled. The test and removal method is superior to the vaccination system as a method of control. Valuable genetic material from breeding stock that is seropositive may be salvaged using embryo transfer techniques. Embryos may be transferred safely to susceptible recipient gilts from sows that have recovered from infection, but not from sows that are in the active stages of infection. The virus does not penetrate the outer covering of the embryo, but it can become attached to it so that it may physically transfer to the uterus of the recipient. This transfer of infection may occur if the donor sow is in the active phase of infection.

Offspring Segregation

The objective of this strategy is to raise a PRV-negative breeding herd to replace the infected herd. Once the herd is diagnosed as PRV infected, a regular schedule of vaccination is instituted. Gilts are vaccinated at first breeding, and both sows and gilts are vaccinated 2 to 4 weeks before farrowing to provide a high level of colostral immunity to their piglets. Offspring are removed at weaning and raised apart from the infected herd. At 4 months of age, and then again before breeding, the segregated replacements are tested for antibody. Because colostral immunity is no longer detectable by 4 months of age, any animals over 4 months of age that are seropositive are considered pseudorabies infected. As the gilts reach reproductive maturity, the old sow herd is replaced. Segregation between the infected sow herd and the clean gilt herd is maintained until all positive sows have been removed and the facilities disinfected. Groups of seronegative pigs are identified and combined into larger groups to establish a new herd. The original herd is gradually depopulated and the premises cleaned and disinfected. The new herd is then monitored on a regular basis.

Control Programs in Effect

PRV was first diagnosed in the North Island of New Zealand in 1976, an eradication program was started in 1989, and the virus was cleared from the North Island in 1997.

A pseudorabies control program was introduced in England in 1983 when the infection was spreading rapidly. New legislation imposed restrictions on the movement of pigs where clinical signs of the disease were present in the herd. The first part of the eradication scheme involved testing all of those herds previously known to have PRV. Within several months after the beginning of the eradication campaign, 417 herds had been slaughtered, involving 342,275 pigs, of which 72.5% were salvaged. Only 121 herds had been known to be previously infected, while the remaining 296 herds had been identified through trace backs and reports of new cases. By 1985 it was concluded that the disease was well controlled in England with only 10 to 14 infected herds remaining. Farmers were compensated for all animals slaughtered and also for consequential loss associated with the loss of stock. The cost of the eradication program was financed by a levy on all pigs normally marketed for slaughter in England. In 1995 England was free of Aujeszky's disease. Following the successful use of the gene-deletion vaccination and an eradication program the Netherlands and Germany are free of the disease. In Sweden the herds were declared free from 12 to 53 months after the start of the program. Now, in Northern Ireland, PRV is more widespread than it ever was in Britain before the eradication program. Because the infection rate is over 50%, an eradication program based on slaughter of infected herds would destroy the swine industry. Thus the control program in Northern Ireland is based on the use of vaccination, the culling of seropositive animals, and the gradual introduction of seronegative animals.

In the United States the national pseudorabies eradication program was implemented in 1989 as a joint State-Federal-Industry–sponsored program. Pilot projects were conducted in Iowa, Illinois, Pennsylvania, Wisconsin, and North Carolina from 1984 to 1987. In the pilot projects, 97.5% of 116 herds that were initially PRV positive were successfully cleared of infection. This indicated that eradication of PRV virus from herds of swine can be efficiently achieved and is most effective applied on an area basis. The introduction of the gene-deleted PRV vaccines in the program was the technical breakthrough needed to be able to offer the national eradication program, since it was now possible to distinguish between naturally infected and vaccinated animals. The program consisted of the following: stage I, preparation; stage II, control; stage III, mandatory herd clean-up; stage IV, surveillance; and stage V, free. As of 2004, commercial swine operations in all 50 states of the US were considered free of PRV; however, endemic infection exists in feral pigs in a number of states. Endemic PRV infection remains a concern for commercial herds.

When an outbreak of the disease occurs in a susceptible herd the mortality may be very high, and the first consideration is to prevent spread to uninfected sows and litters and pregnant sows from infected pigs. They should be attended by separate personnel, or adequate barriers to mechanical transmission of infection should be arranged. On affected premises, cattle should be separated from pigs, and dogs and cats should be kept from the area. The affected herd should be quarantined, and all pigs sold off the farm should be for slaughter only.

Vaccines and Vaccination

Vaccination is used to reduce clinical disease when outbreaks occur or when the disease is endemic in the herd. An effective immunity develops after natural infection or vaccination, and piglets from immune sows are protected from clinical disease during the nursing period by colostral immunity. However, the presence of circulating antibody does not prevent infection, the development of latency, and subsequent activation and excretion of the virus. However, vaccination reduces viral shedding after natural infection. On farms in which the disease is endemic or outbreaks have occurred, vaccination of the sows, and management procedures to reduce the spread of infection, have markedly reduced preweaning mortality and reproductive failures. Field studies in large numbers of herds in which the sows were vaccinated three times annually show that the reproduction ratio was below 0.66, which is significantly below,[1] and massive spread of the virus does not occur.

It is often virtually impossible to prevent the spread of infection in a susceptible herd and vaccination of all pigs at risk, especially pregnant sows, is recommended. The vaccine reduces losses in infected herds, limits the spread of infection, and decreases the incidence in endemic areas. With a properly controlled and monitored vaccination and culling program in a breeding herd, it is possible to control clinical disease and reduce the infection pressure. All breeding stock present during an outbreak are subsequently vaccinated regularly until they are all culled, which removes the major sources of virulent virus. Following this phase, newly introduced gilts and boars are tested, and monitored regularly. This is considered to be less costly than the test and slaughter policy.

However, in vaccinated herds, the virus continues to circulate and an accurate epidemiologic analysis is not possible because titers caused by vaccination cannot be distinguished from those caused by natural infections.

Control of the diseases in many countries has always been based on compulsory intensive vaccination of the entire population.

Vaccines

Conventional modified live virus and inactivated virus vaccines have been available. Both vaccines will reduce the incidence rate and severity of clinical disease in an infected herd. They also reduce the field virus shedding and latency in the trigeminal ganglion after exposure to field virus. The vaccine efficiency is, however, markedly influenced by the modified live virus vaccine strain and the route of administration. The vaccine genotype plays a very important role in the effectiveness of the vaccine program. Recently needle-free transdermal vaccination using a modified live PRV vaccine has been described, preventing the loss of any needles in the carcass. Cell-mediated immunity in the form of cytotoxic T cells may play an important part in the effectiveness of the vaccine. The deficiencies of inactivated vaccines in producing virus-specific interferon-γ (IFN-γ) can be enhanced by the use of simultaneous administration of interleukin-12, which appears to upregulate Th1/Th2 expression.

Pregnant Sows

Vaccination of pregnant sows induces SN antibodies, which are transferred to the newborn piglets and provide protection against infection. Vaccination during pregnancy produces more protection against PRV for piglets than sow vaccination before mating. A better protection was observed in sows vaccinated with an attenuated virus than in sows vaccinated with inactivated virus. Piglets rely on colostral and milk antibodies for protection, and the vaccination of piglets born from vaccinated sows does not produce a significant serologic response until the piglets are about 12 weeks of age. Maternally derived antibodies may disturb or even block the development of active humoral responses.[20] Earlier vaccination of piglets from infected or vaccinated sows is ineffective because high levels of maternal antibodies interfere with a serologic response stimulated by the vaccine. Maternal immunity interferes with the development of active immunity from vaccination until at least 15 weeks of age, even when the colostral titers are low. Thus in a situation in which the majority of sows have been infected or vaccinated, vaccination of weaned pigs may not yield desirable results. Both inactivated virus and attenuated live virus vaccines provide similar results when piglets born from vaccinated sows are vaccinated before colostral immunity has waned.

Growing and Finishing Pigs

The optimal vaccination strategy for growing and finishing pigs in an eradication program is controversial. In eight persistently infected herds' vaccinations, both intranasally and intramuscularly, were made at 4 and 10 weeks of age. Only one vaccination is given to finishing pigs in endemic areas in Europe. However, this does not reduce the prevalence of infection in finishing pigs in herds with a high prevalence. Double vaccination of finishing pigs will reduce the spread of the virus, but extensive spread can still occur. The presence of maternal antibodies may interfere with the induction of antibodies, and double vaccination 4 weeks later may boost immunity. Mean daily weight gain was also improved by a second vaccination with a direct economic benefit.

Marker or Subunit Vaccines

A major development in vaccination against pseudorabies has been the introduction of genetically engineered live vaccine strains used to make marker or subunit vaccines. Vaccination with modified live gene-deleted vaccines is now an integral part of pseudorabies eradication programs worldwide. The most common gene deletions are for glycoproteins E (gE) or gI and G (gG) or gX, and gIII. A gD/gE-negative vaccine was described. In Europe, use of gE vaccines has become the standard. These vaccines, in conjunction with a companion diagnostic test, can distinguish between naturally infected and vaccinated animals. Colostrum can also be used to monitor antibodies against gI protein of the virus.

A study comparing intranasal and intramuscular vaccination showed that pigs given both vaccines (intranasally and intramuscularly) had a significantly better clinical and virologic protection after challenge than the single intranasal vaccination. The recombinant vaccines are able to circumvent the inhibition of active immunity that occurs when maternally derived antibody is still present. Animals vaccinated with a deleted vaccine are not able to mount an immune response against the protein whose gene has been deleted in the vaccine virus genome. In contrast, wild-type virus-infected animals produce antibodies against all the viral glycoproteins. Differentiating ELISAs, specific for the deleted marker protein, then allow discrimination between infected animals, which can be culled from the herd, and vaccinated animals. These vaccines reduce the severity of clinical disease and viral shedding. However, the presence of colostral antibodies in growing pigs may interfere with an immune response, which may result in increased virus excretion on challenge exposure. Repeated vaccination is needed to provide some protective immunity against challenge exposure to virulent virus.

These mutants have also been rendered thymidine kinase-deficient (TK−) mutants, and are avirulent and immunogenic. Pigs inoculated with these mutants are resistant to experimental challenge with the virulent virus, and the virulent virus cannot be recovered from the ganglia, which suggests that vaccination reduced colonization of the ganglia. The ideal vaccine strain should prevent clinical disease and mortality, should not be transmitted to nonimmunized animals, and should prevent colonization of the ganglia by a potential superinfecting virulent virus reducing the natural reservoir of the virus. The TK− mutant virus possesses these desirable characteristics. The high efficacy of recently constructed gI-negative deletion mutant vaccines of PRV virus provide a sound basis for implementing the "gI" approach to the future control of the disease.

Piglets born from sows vaccinated with deleted (gIII, TK) strains at 3 days and 9 and 11 weeks of age developed detectable antibodies that lasted up to 100 days of age when vaccinated. Maternal antibodies in piglets from sows vaccinated with gIII-deleted vaccine decay to undetectable levels at 7 weeks of age. The vaccination of piglets at 3 days of age with the same vaccine results in a priming effect, which protects the piglets against virulent virus challenge at 7 weeks of age. Thus effective protection could be provided by active immunization from birth through weaning, in the nursery, and into the growing and finishing stages of production. Piglet vaccination at 10 and 14 weeks was considered to be the optimal time for vaccination.[21]

Although genetically engineered live virus vaccines have been shown to be efficacious and safe, there is a possibility of spread between vaccinated and unvaccinated animals, of persistence in the field and of recombination between different vaccine strains, which can lead to enhanced virulence. New viral mutants lacking glycoproteins gD, gE, gG, and gI may form the basis for the development of new vaccines that do not recombine. A gB deletion vaccine has been described for intranasal use and has been shown to produce both local and serum antibodies. Recently a DNA vaccine was shown to give as good a response as gD plasmid vaccine, but the DNA vaccine had to be given intradermally. It can overcome maternally derived antibody, and the vaccine described in this case still gave protection against infectious PRV challenge at the end of the finishing period.

Even more radical is a vaccine with a granulocyte-macrophage colony stimulating factor.

Experimentally, immunized pigs can be latently infected with the wild-type virus without being detected by the gE-specific ELISA routinely used to discriminate between infected and vaccinated pigs. Thus gE seronegative pigs may still be infected and be a source of infection.

Remarkable progress has been made with the use of gI-deleted vaccines. Intensive regional vaccination of finishing pigs with a gI-deleted vaccine, along with companion diagnostic tests, reduced the seroprevalence in infected finishing herds from 81% to 19% in 2 years. Vaccination increases the virus dose needed for establishment of infection and decreases the level and duration of virus excretion after infection. In the control group, with routine disease control, no significant change in seroprevalence occurred. The consistent application of intensive vaccination of all breeding herds in a region, including those herds participating in a production chain, can also decrease the prevalence of infection in heavily infected areas. The intensive regional vaccination did not completely eliminate virus infections within these herds; the source of infection was not determined. It is suggested that the virus either circulated at a low level within herds, or its introduction or reactivation did not lead to an extensive spread of the virus. A voluntary vaccination program on individual farms was unsuccessful in reducing the prevalence of virus-infected breeding pigs. The importation of breeding stock from outside the area is associated with a higher prevalence of virus-infected pigs because of lack of vaccination. The introduction of infections can be reduced by purchasing virus-free animals and by increasing farm biosecurity procedures.

Vaccination of breeding herds three times annually to ensure a high level of immunization can lead to elimination of the disease when the reproduction ratio is less than one.

The method used for vaccination may influence the effect of the vaccine. Using glycoprotein vaccines, intramuscular vaccination in the neck, and six-point intradermal vaccination in the back provided the best protection; six-point intradermal injections resulted in a better vaccination than two-point injections. BW changes and viral excretion after challenge were compared with VN titers, antigen-specific IgG and IgA responses in serum, and virus-specific lymphoproliferative responses in peripheral blood during the immunization period.

An intensive eradication program in farrow–finish herds using a gI-deleted vaccine in breeding and growing–finishing pigs, and decreases of movement and mixing of growing–finishing pigs was successful in 3 years. The initial goal was to decrease viral spread in the growing–finishing pigs, which enabled production of seronegative replacement gilts. Increases in the number of sows culled, combined with an increase in the number of seronegative replacement gilts, resulted in a decrease in seroprevalence of sows. Bimonthly serologic monitoring indicated minimal spread of the virus in the growing–finishing pigs after 1 year. Eighteen months after the initiation of the program, the test and removal of seropositive sows commenced in all herds. All herds were released from quarantine within 3 years, indicating that eradication can be achieved by vaccination and management changes designed to minimize the spread of virus combined with test-and-removal procedures.

An attenuated gI-deleted–TK-deleted vaccine was used to eradicate the virus from a large farrow–finish herd in Sweden. At the start of the program, 86% of the breeding animals were seropositive. The breeding stock was vaccinated every 4 months and monitored serologically. Seropositive sows and boars were culled at an economic rate. The herd was declared gI negative 39 months after the start of the program. Monitoring the herd for another 4 years, until all vaccinated animals had been culled, revealed the herd free of the virus.

In New Zealand, progress toward eradication using a subunit vaccine is reported. Those farms that combined vaccination with good management techniques, intensive testing, and culling eradicated the wild virus infection within 2 years; those that made little or no progress has less than satisfactory standards of hygiene and did not practice an intensive testing and culling program.

Vaccination of both breeding stock and growing pigs is recommended. A combined vaccination–eradication program for the disease would generally comprise four phases:

1. A systematic and intensive vaccination campaign
2. Screening of pigs for gI antibodies
3. Economic culling of infected breeding pigs
4. Final ending of vaccination.

Piglets at 3 days of age can be vaccinated with one of these genetically engineered vaccines and be protected from experimental challenge at 5 weeks of age.

A recent study has shown that infection with PRRS virus does not inhibit the development of a vaccine-induced protection against PRV.

Vaccination of wild boar with an attenuated live vaccine has been shown to protect against infection.[22]

Vaccination of cattle with an inactivated vaccine is recommended where they are in close contact with swine and where a low level of exposure is likely.

REFERENCES

1. Davison AJ. *Vet Microbiol.* 2010;143:52.
2. Hahn EC, et al. *Vet Microbiol.* 2010;143:45.
3. Lipowski A, et al. *Medycyna Wet.* 2009;85:771.
4. Muller T, et al. *Epidemiol Infect.* 2010;12:1.
5. Muller T, et al. *Arch Virol.* 2011;156:1691.
6. Toma B. *Epidemiol Sante Anim.* 2013;63:141.
7. Smith G. *PrevVet Med.* 2012;103:145.
8. Glorieux S, et al. *Vet Microbiol.* 2009;136:141.
9. Nauwynck H, et al. *Vet Res.* 2007;38:229.
10. Pomeranz L, et al. *Microbiol Mol Biol Rev.* 2006;69:462.
11. Morandi F, et al. *J Comp Pathol.* 2010;142:74.
12. McKillen J, et al. *J Virol Methods.* 2007;140:155.
13. Sami L, et al. *Acta Vet Hung.* 2007;55:267.
14. Lee C-S, et al. *J Virol Methods.* 2007;139:39.
15. Zhang C-F, et al. *J Virol Methods.* 2010;169:239.
16. Tombacz D, et al. *BMC Genomics.* 2009;10:491.
17. Ma WJ, et al. *J Vet Diagn Invest.* 2008;20:440.
18. Boadella M, et al. *BMC Vet Res.* 2012;8:7.
19. Wilson S, et al. *J Wildl Dis.* 2009;45:874.
20. Pomorska-Mol M, et al. *Vet Microbiol.* 2010;144:450.
21. Markowska-Daniel I, et al. *Bull Vet Inst Pulawy.* 2009;53:169.
22. Maresch C, et al. *Vet Microbiol.* 2013;161:20.

SPORADIC BOVINE ENCEPHALOMYELITIS (BUSS DISEASE AND TRANSMISSIBLE SEROSITIS)

Sporadic bovine encephalomyelitis (SBE) is associated with a chlamydia, and characterized by inflammation of vascular endothelium and mesenchymal tissue. There is secondary involvement of the nervous system, with nervous signs, in some cases.

ETIOLOGY

The disease is associated with specific strains of *Chlamydophila* (*Chlamydia*) *pecorum.*[1,2] It resists freezing but is highly susceptible to sodium hydroxide, cresol, and quaternary ammonium compounds in standard concentrations. The chlamydia can be passaged in guinea pigs and hamsters and adapted to grow in the yolk sac of developing chick embryos.

EPIDEMIOLOGY

Occurrence

The disease has been reported only from the United States, Europe, Japan, Israel, and Australia,[1] but a provisional diagnosis has been made in Canada and South Africa. In the United States it was most common in the midwestern and western States, but there have been no reports of its occurrence for the last 30 years.

Sporadic cases or outbreaks occur in individual herds. Although the disease has not reached serious economic proportions in the endemic infection, there is some serologic evidence that widespread subclinical infections occur.

Only cattle and buffalo are affected, and calves less than 6 months of age are most susceptible. Other domestic and experimental species appear to be resistant. There is no seasonal incidence and cases appear at any time of the year. A strong and apparently persistent immunity develops after an attack of the disease.

Prevalence of Infection

Morbidity and Case–Fatality Rates

The occurrence is sporadic, but outbreaks have occurred resulting in severe loss from both deaths of animals and loss of condition. Morbidity rates average 12.5% (5–50%) and are highest in calves (25%) and lowest in animals over a year old (5%). Mortality rates average about 31% and are higher in adults than in calves. In affected herds a stage of herd immunity is reached when only introduced animals and newborn calves are susceptible.

Method of Transmission

The method of spread is not known but is suspected to be fecal–oral.[1] Spread from farm to farm does not occur readily. On some farms only sporadic cases may occur, but on others one or two cases occur every year. In still other herds the disease occurs in outbreak form, with a number of animals becoming affected within a period of about 4 weeks. The epidemiology of SBE resembles in many ways that of malignant catarrhal fever in cattle. The organism can be isolated from many organs, including liver, spleen, and CNS, and from the blood, feces, urine, nasal discharges, and milk in the early stages of the disease. There is some evidence that the organism is eliminated in the feces for several weeks after infection.

PATHOGENESIS

The causative agent is not specifically neurotropic and attacks principally the mesenchymal tissues and the endothelial lining of the vascular system, with particular involvement of the serous membranes. Encephalomyelitis occurs secondarily to the vascular damage. Neurologic signs may be caused by infection with specific strains; *C. pecorum* genotype ST 23 has been associated with SBE cases from Australia, England, and the United States,[1] whereas other strains have been isolated from cattle with pneumonia and polyarthritis[2] and calves with poor weight gain.[3]

CLINICAL FINDINGS

Affected calves are depressed and inactive, but the appetite may be unaffected for several days. Nasal discharge and salivation with drooling are frequently observed. A **fever is common** (40.5°C-41.5°C, 105°F-107°F), and remains high for the course of the disease. Dyspnea, coughing, a mild catarrhal nasal discharge, and diarrhea may occur. During the ensuing 2 weeks, difficulty in walking and lack of desire to stand may appear. Stiffness with knuckling at the fetlocks is evident at first, followed by staggering, circling, and falling. Opisthotonus may occur but there is no excitement or head-pressing. The course of the disease varies between 3 days and 3 weeks. Animals that recover show marked loss of condition and are slow to regain the lost weight.

CLINICAL PATHOLOGY

Hematology

In experimental cases, leukopenia occurs in the acute clinical stage. There is a relative lymphocytosis and depression of polymorphonuclear cells.

Detection of Agent

The causative agent can be isolated from the blood in the early clinical phase, and can be used for transmission experiments in calves and guinea pigs, and for culture in eggs. Elementary bodies are present in the guinea pig tissues and yolk-sac preparations.

Serology

Serologic methods, including a complement fixation test for the detection of circulating antibody, are available although there is difficulty in differentiating antibodies to the chlamydia from those to the typical psittacosis virus.

NECROPSY FINDINGS

A fibrinous peritonitis, pleurisy, and pericarditis, accompanied by congestion and petechiation, are characteristic. In the early stages, thin serous fluid is present in the cavities, but in the later stages this has progressed to a thin fibrinous net covering the affected organs, or even to flattened plaques or irregularly shaped masses of fibrin lying free in the cavity. Histologically, there is fibrinous serositis involving the serosa of the peritoneal, pleural, and pericardial cavities. A diffuse encephalomyelitis involving particularly the medulla and cerebellum, and a meningitis in the same area, are also present. Minute elementary bodies are present in infected tissues and in very small numbers in exudate. The necropsy findings are diagnostic for SBE, and confirmation can be obtained by the complement fixation test or SN tests.

DIFFERENTIAL DIAGNOSIS

Clinically, the disease resembles other encephalitides of cattle. The epidemiology and pathogenesis resembles malignant catarrhal fever in cattle, but the mortality rate is much lower, there are no ocular or mucosal lesions, and the serositis of SBE does not occur in bovine malignant catarrh. A viral encephalomyelitis of calves (Kunjin virus) has been identified, but has not been associated with clinical signs of disease of the nervous system. An encephalomyocarditis virus, a primary infection of rodents that also occurs in primates and causes myocarditis in pigs, has been transmitted experimentally to calves but without causing significant signs of disease.

Listeriosis is usually sporadic and is accompanied by more localizing signs, especially facial paralysis and circling.

Rabies may present a very similar clinical picture, but the initial febrile reaction and the characteristic necropsy findings as well as the epizootiologic history of SBE should enable a diagnosis to be made.

Lead poisoning can be differentiated by the absence of fever, the more severe signs of motor irritation, and the shorter course of the disease. Because of the respiratory tract involvement, SBE may be easily confused with pneumonic pasteurellosis, especially if outbreaks occur, but in the latter disease nervous signs are unusual and the response to treatment is good.

SBE, *sporadic bovine encephalomyelitis.*

TREATMENT

Broad-spectrum antimicrobials control the agent in vitro. However, clinical results with chlortetracycline and oxytetracycline have been irregular, but may be effective if used in the early stages of the disease.

CONTROL

Control measures are difficult to prescribe because of lack of knowledge of the method of transmission. It is advisable to isolate affected animals. No vaccine is available.

REFERENCES

1. Jelocnik M, et al. *BMC Vet Res.* 2014;10:121.
2. Kaltenboeck B, et al. *Vet Microbiol.* 2009;135:175.
3. Poudel A, et al. *PLoS ONE.* 2012;7:e44961.

BORDER DISEASE (HAIRY SHAKER DISEASE OF LAMBS, HAIRY SHAKERS, HYPOMYELINOGENESIS CONGENITA)

SYNOPSIS

Etiology Pestivirus strains in the border disease and bovine virus diarrhea genotypes.

Epidemiology Congenital disease transmitted by persistently infected sheep, rarely cattle.

Clinical findings Abortions, stillbirths, barren ewes, and the birth of small weak lambs, some of which have an abnormally hairy birth coat, gross tremor of skeletal muscles, inferior growth, and a variable degree of skeletal deformity.

Clinical pathology None specific.

Lesions Hypomyelination in brain and spinal cord of lamb.

Diagnostic confirmation Detection of virus and/or demonstration of serologic response.

Treatment Supportive.

Control Avoid infection of pregnant sheep. Identify and cull persistently infected animals.

ETIOLOGY

The causal agent, border disease virus (BDV), is a pestivirus within the family Flaviviridae. Four members of the pestivirus genus have been identified; bovine virus diarrhea virus

(BVDV) types 1 and 2, classical swine fever virus, and BDV. Isolates from border disease predominantly fall within the BDV genotype, but sheep and goat isolates also fall in the BVDV genotypes. Pestiviruses consist of a single strand of RNA and were originally named after the host from which they were isolated. However, their interspecies transmissibility means an increasing reliance on phylogenetic studies based on sequences generated from relatively well conserved regions of the viral genome, such as the 5′ untranscribed region. On this basis BDV can be phylogenetically segregated into at least seven clusters, subtypes BDV-1 to BDV-7.[1]

Strains of BDV have differing pathogenicity, and variations in pathogenicity also result from interactions between the virus and different host genotypes, specifically between different breeds of sheep. Persistent infections in sheep are associated with noncytopathic strains of virus. An isolate of BDV, now designated as BDV-5, caused a leukopenic enterocolitis in sheep and growing lambs in the Aveyron region of France (Aveyron disease).[2] The disease caused high mortality in sheep in this region in 1984 but has not occurred since then.

EPIDEMIOLOGY

Occurrence

Border disease was originally described in the border country between England and Wales. It has subsequently been reported from most of the major sheep-producing countries and probably occurs in all of them. The disease occurs primarily in sheep, and less often in goats and free-living ruminants, such as chamois.[3] The prevalence of infection is much higher than the incidence of clinical disease because the latter only occurs when there is infection during pregnancy. BDV-1 has been detected in sheep from Australia, New Zealand, UK, and United States; BDV-2 from ruminants in Germany; BDV-3 in Switzerland and Austria; BDV-4 in Spain; BDV-5 and BDV-6 in France; and BDV-7 in Turkey.[1]

Studies on seroprevalence suggest that pestivirus infections in sheep and goats are less common than in cattle, but there are considerable differences in seroprevalence between different geographic areas and flocks. Flock seroprevalence in different regions or countries generally falls within the range of 5% to 50%. The prevalence of seropositive females within positive flocks is influenced by age, with a lower seroprevalence in sheep 4 to 8 months of age than in older sheep. Seroprevalence is higher in flocks with persistently infected sheep, but there can still be a significant proportion of seronegative sheep present in a flock containing persistently infected sheep.

Source of Infection

Infection can be introduced into a flock with the purchase of persistently infected replacement sheep. Persistently infected sheep excrete virus in nasal secretions, saliva, urine, and feces, and provide the major source of infection. A proportion of persistently infected sheep may survive to adulthood and may breed successfully to produce further persistently infected sheep. However, the breeding efficiency of persistently infected sheep is poor, and the probability of establishing lines of persistently infected sheep appears less than with the equivalent infection in cattle.

Virus is also present in the placenta and fetal fluids at the birth of persistently infected lambs and in the products of abortion resulting from infection with the virus in early pregnancy. In flocks where there is a long lambing period it is possible that this could provide a source for clinical disease in late-lambing ewes. Field observations suggest that transmission during the lambing period is limited.

Calves persistently infected with BVDV can infect sheep, and in countries where pregnant sheep and cattle are housed in close proximity during the winter this can be an important source of infection for outbreaks of border disease. In some countries this appears to be the major source, and studies in both Northern Ireland and the Republic of Ireland suggest that cattle are the primary source of infection for sheep in those countries. There is also evidence that bovine strains are important in goat infections. In contrast BDV is the predominant ovine pestivirus in Great Britain and New Zealand.

Free-living deer are also a potential source of infection. Outbreaks of disease have also occurred after vaccinating pregnant goats with an Orf vaccine contaminated with a pestivirus.

Transmission

Natural transmission is by sheep-to-sheep contact, but successful experimental transmission has followed both oral and conjunctival challenge.

The spread of infection within a susceptible flock is facilitated by factors such as close contact at mating time or mustering and aggregating sheep for any purpose. There is an increased risk for explosive outbreaks of border disease where animals are housed in early pregnancy.

Host Risk Factors

Border disease may occur as an outbreak or as a sporadic disease. When infection is introduced into a susceptible flock in early pregnancy, an outbreak with infertility, abortion, and congenital disease in lambs from all ages of ewes is likely. Subsequently, older sheep in the flock will have acquired immunity and disease occurs only in introduced sheep and maiden ewes. Persistently infected ewes have reduced fertility but will give birth to congenitally affected lambs throughout their breeding life. The disproportional occurrence of outbreaks of clinical disease in certain breeds suggests that they may have higher rates of persistently infected individuals.

Experimental Reproduction

Border disease is readily reproduced by the experimental oral, conjunctival, and parenteral infection of pregnant ewes before 80 days' gestation. Experimental disease can be produced with both BDV and BVDV strains.

The following have been produced experimentally, although there are strain differences in clinical and pathologic manifestations:

- Placentitis
- Abortions
- Mummified fetuses
- Congenital malformations, including hydrocephalus, porencephaly, cerebellar hypoplasia and dysplasia, and arthrogryposis
- Fetal growth retardation
- Hypomyelinogenesis
- Birth of weak lambs with nervous disorders
- A hairy birth coat

Experimental infections of pregnant cows with BDV results in similar defects with placentitis, mummification, and abortion of fetuses; intrauterine growth retardation with abnormal osteogenesis; and hypomyelinogenesis.

The disease has also been produced experimentally in goat kids by inoculation of pregnant goats but there are no abnormalities of hair coat, and embryonic mortality and abortion are more common than in the experimental disease in ewes.

Economic Importance

The effect of infection varies with the immune status of the flock and whether infection occurs during pregnancy. In fully susceptible flocks, abortion and neonatal lamb loss resulting from infection can be 25% to 75% of the expected lamb crop depending on the strain of the virus. An assessment of the economic losses caused by infertility, abortion, neonatal losses, and low carcass weight indicate that an outbreak of border disease can result in a potential reduction of income in excess of 20%.

Where sheep and cattle are comingled, the presence of BDV in sheep could also jeopardize efforts to control and eradicate pestivirus (BVDV) from cattle herds. Persistently infected sheep readily transmit BDV to seronegative calves; thus the antigenic similarity between the two viruses will complicate attempts to demonstrate freedom from BVD in cattle by serology.[4]

PATHOGENESIS

Nonpregnant Sheep

In adolescent and adult nonpregnant sheep, infection and viremia are subclinical. The intramuscular inoculation of immunocompetent lambs with BDV results in a mild transient disease and a subsequent reduction in growth rate, but no gross or microscopic lesions.

Pregnant Sheep

When BDV infects susceptible pregnant ewes the virus infects the placenta to produce an acute necrotizing placentitis and it subsequently invades the fetus. This may result in early embryonic death, abortion and stillbirth, the birth of lambs with malformations and/or neurologic abnormalities, the birth of small weak lambs that are immunosuppressed, or the birth of lambs with no clinical abnormality. The ultimate outcome of the infection depends on the age of the fetus, the properties of the strain of the virus, the dose of the virus, the genotype of the host, and the ability of the fetus to respond to the virus. Immune competence to the virus in the fetus develops between approximately 61 and 80 days' gestation; thus fetal age at the time of infection determines the outcome of infection.

Infection in Early Pregnancy

Fetal death occurs when there is infection of the fetus with virulent strains before the development of immune competence and uncontrolled viral replication. Prenatal death is more likely to follow infections in early pregnancy, but is recorded with infections from 45 to 72 days' gestation.

Persistent infections occur in lambs that survive infection in early pregnancy before the development of immune competence and result from maternal infections between 21 and 72 days' gestation but never later. The virus is present in all organs, and lambs born persistently infected will remain so for their lifetime, with few exceptions; persistent infections have been recorded to at least 5 years of age.

Most persistently infected sheep are unable to produce a specific antibody to BDV, but some show intermittent seropositivity with low antibody levels or occasionally undergo frank seroconversion. The humoral response to other pathogens and antigens is normal. However, cell-mediated immunity is compromised, with change in T-cell populations and a deficiency in lymphocyte function. Persistently infected lambs are more susceptible to intercurrent disease and commonly die before reaching maturity.

Hypomyelinogenesis occurs in persistently infected lambs and resolves spontaneously in lambs that survive to the age of 6 months. Most of these lambs exhibit neurologic dysfunction at birth, varying from a continuous light tremor to tonic-clonic contraction of the skeletal muscles involving the whole body and head (shakers).

A deficiency of the thyroid T_3 and T_4 hormones has been detected in lambs affected with border disease and may be the basic cause of the lack of myelination. The enzyme 2,3-cyclic nucleotide-3-phosphodiesterase is associated with normal myelination and depends on normal amounts of thyroid hormone. The deficiency in thyroid hormones may also result in the reduced rate of weight gain that occurs in infected lambs. Other studies suggest a direct infection of oligodendroglia with the virus as the cause of the defective myelination.

Fleece abnormality also occurs in persistently infected lambs and results from an enlargement of the primary hair follicles and a concurrent reduction in the number of secondary follicles. The resulting hairiness is caused by the presence of large medullated primary fibers. BDV appears to have no effect on the skin and birth coat of coarse-fleeced breeds of sheep or on goats.

Intrauterine growth retardation is a common feature of infection with BDV and is initiated shortly after infection. Deformities of the skeleton include abnormally shortened long bones and a reduction in crown–rump length and the long axis of the skull, which results in lambs appearing more compact and short-legged than normal (goat lambs). In the long bones there is evidence of growth arrest lines and disturbed osteogenesis and ossification.

Some persistently infected lambs do not have nervous signs or abnormalities of the fleece and are phenotypically normal. This limits the value of identification of infected lambs based on the presence of clinical abnormality at birth.

In Midpregnancy

When fetal infection occurs during the period of development of the ability to mount an immune response (between approximately 61 and 80 days' gestation), the effect is variable. Some fetuses infected at this stage respond with a severe inflammatory process in the CNS with nodular periarteritis, necrosis, and inflammation of the germinal layers of the brain. Resultant lesions are hydranencephaly, cerebellar dysplasia, and multifocal retinal atrophy; such lambs exhibit behavioral abnormalities and more severe neurologic disease than shaker lambs.

Infection in Late Pregnancy

Infection of the fetus after 80 days' gestation is likely to be controlled or eliminated by a fetal immune response. These lambs are born without clinical disease, and are virus negative, but have precolostral circulating antibody.

Goats

In goats, fetal death is the major outcome of infection of the pregnant doe with both BDV and BVDV, and infections before 60 days' gestation almost invariably result in reproductive failure. Persistently infected shaker kids and clinically normal kids are born with infections around 60 days' gestation but are a less common manifestation of the disease than occurs in sheep. The caprine fetus develops immune competence against pestiviruses between 80 and 100 days' gestation.

Enteric Disease

Experimental inoculation of a homologous strain of the BDV into persistently infected but clinically recovered lambs results in a severe clinical syndrome. This is characterized by persistent diarrhea and respiratory distress associated with an inflammatory lymphoproliferative response in the CNS, intestines, lungs, heart, and kidney. A similar syndrome is seen in some persistently infected sheep that survive early life and reach weaning. This syndrome resembles certain aspects of mucosal disease in cattle, in which it is postulated that superinfection of persistently viremic immunotolerant cattle with a homologous strain of BVDV results in fatal mucosal disease. In such animals a specific and dynamic equilibrium exists between an attenuated form of the virus and the immunotolerant host. Disturbance of this equilibrium either by injection of the homologous strain of BDV, or some other factor, results in fatal disease.

CLINICAL FINDINGS

The most obvious and characteristic features of border disease are evident at birth and relate to conformation and growth, fleece type, and neurologic dysfunction. An increased proportion of barren ewes will also be apparent in severe outbreaks.

Conformation

Affected lambs may have a lower birth weight than uninfected lambs, a decreased crown–rump length, and a shorter tibia/radius length so that they have a boxy appearance. The head has a shortened longitudinal axis and the cranium may be slightly domed (goat, lambs).

Fleece

The fleece, when dry, appears hairy and rough because of long hairs rising above the fleece to form a halo, especially over the nape, back, flanks, and rump. This feature is most evident in medium-wool and fine-wool breeds and is not observed in the coarse kempy-fleeced breeds, such as the Scottish Blackface. The halo kemp fibers are shed with time and are most evident in the first 3 weeks of life. Some lambs have abnormal pigmentation occurring as patches of pigmented fleece or hair, or a totally pigmented fleece. This can occur in white-faced sheep.

Neurologic Dysfunction

Neurologic dysfunction is manifest, with rhythmic tremors of the muscles of the pelvis and upper parts of the hindlimbs, or of the whole body, resulting in a characteristic jerking movement, and of the head and neck with rhythmic bobbing of the head (shaker lambs). In some less severe cases, only fine tremors of the ears and tail are evident. Tremors are most apparent during movement, and are absent while the lamb is sleeping. The tremors usually decline in severity as the lamb matures and may seem to disappear unless the animal is stressed. More severely affected lambs have difficulty in rising, and if able to stand with assistance exhibit an erratic gait especially of the hindquarters. Paralysis does not occur. Affected lambs are often unable to nurse the ewe because they cannot hold onto the teat. They appear languid and lie around listlessly. They do not suck as they should and bloat continuously, and the ewes' udders become engorged with milk.

Behavioral and visual defects with circling, head-pressing, nystagmus, and gross incoordination are seen in lambs with the type of infection producing hydranencephaly and cerebellar dysplasia. These lambs are of lighter birth weight but have normal birth coats.

Growth Rate

Growth rate is reduced, affected lambs are unthrifty, and the majority will die before or at weaning time from parasitism, pneumonia, a mucosal disease-like syndrome, or nephritis. With good nursing care, they can be reared, but deaths may occur at any age. Puberty may be delayed and, in males, the testes are flabby and may not develop normally. A study of lambs in a Spanish feedlot found that BDV-positive lambs (by RT-PCR or ELISA) were 12% (3.3 kg) lighter after 41 days of lot feeding because of significantly lower average daily gain, 260 g per head per day compared with 320 g per head per day in BDV-negative lambs.[5] BDV-positive lambs also had double the chance of having diarrhea or respiratory signs.

Reproductive Performance

Impaired reproductive performance of the flock occurs from low fertility, abortion, and poor viability of lambs. Abortions usually are not noticed until lambing when it is evidenced by an unexpected increase in barren ewes. In goats, where there is often closer observation, the aborted fetuses may be reasonably well developed, small and underdeveloped, or autolyzed and unrecognizable as a fetus in expelled fetal fluid.

CLINICAL PATHOLOGY

There are no consistent changes in hematology or blood chemistry. Persistently infected lambs have changes in lymphocyte subpopulations, with a reduction in T lymphocytes and an altered CD8:CD4 ratio.

Virus can be detected in blood and tissues by virus isolation, antigen ELISAs, and RT-PCR techniques (both conventional and real time). These are specialist techniques, but an RT-PCR ELISA may be a cost-effective and sensitive alternative for nonspecialist laboratories.[6] Antibody can be detected by antibody ELISAs or SN tests, and a combination of serology and virus isolation is usually used in the diagnosis of border disease.

Detection of Persistently Infected Sheep

For diagnosis of border disease in newborn lambs, precolostral blood samples should be taken from both clinically normal and affected lambs. Persistently infected sheep are seronegative and BDV can be isolated from leukocytes in the blood buffy coat. Lambs infected late in gestation will be seropositive but virus negative. Persistently infected lambs that have received colostrum from their dam will be seropositive until they lose maternal passive immunity.

Persistently infected adolescent and adult sheep in a flock can be identified by the detection of virus in blood; however, this is expensive in large flocks and an alternative is to test all sheep for antibody and then culture the buffy coat of seronegative sheep. Antigenic differences between laboratory strains and field virus can result in false-negative serology, and serologic studies are best done with the homologous virus.

Abortion

Serologic tests are of limited value as an aid to the diagnosis of abortion associated with BDV infection. The infection of the ewe that results in abortion occurs several weeks before clinical disease is apparent, and unless prospective samples can be taken there is little chance of a rise in antibody titers in paired samples. Seropositivity in ewes indicates that the flock has been exposed to pestivirus but does not incriminate it in a disease process. Seronegativity indicates that BDV is not the cause of the abortion, with the exception that aborting ewes, who themselves are persistently infected, will have no antibody titer.

NECROPSY FINDINGS

Gross findings may be normal, or may include an abnormal wool coat and a reduction in the size of the brain and spinal cord. Arthrogryposis, hydranencephaly, porencephaly, and cerebellar dysplasia may also be present. Histologically, there is a deficiency of stainable central myelin, with neurochemical and histochemical evidence of demyelination or myelin dysmorphogenesis. In most sheep the myelin defect resolves substantially during the first few months of life. The brain, which has been very small, returns to normal weight, and chemical composition and degree of myelination. The histologic lesions of the skin consist of primary follicle enlargement, increased primary fiber size, and an increased number of medullated primary fibers.

Virus can be demonstrated by immunofluorescent staining of cryostat sections of tissues from affected lambs or by IHC staining of formalin-fixed material. Preferred tissues for such tests include brain, thyroid gland, and skin. Virus titers reach high levels in the placentomes, so caruncles or cotyledons should be cultured for virus. Isolates are noncytopathic and the presence of viral antigens must be demonstrated by direct or indirect immunofluorescence or immune peroxidase techniques.

Because of the closely related character of this pestivirus and BVDV, diagnostic tests to confirm infection parallel those for BVDV. Fetal serology can be useful for confirming exposure in abortions and stillbirths. PCR and ELISA techniques may be substituted for virus isolation if available.

In the brain of naturally infected cases, viral antigens and RNA are found in the neuropil, glial, and neuronal cells, especially in periventricular areas, cerebellum, and brainstem.[7] Cell death occurs in both BDV-infected and adjacent cells by the activation of pathways that cause apoptosis, which are associated with the increased expression of nitric oxide synthases.[8,9]

Samples for Confirmation of Diagnosis

- **Histology:** formalin-fixed skin, spinal cord, half of midsagittally sectioned brain, skin, thyroid, distal ileum, colon, cecum, thymus, spleen, liver, heart, kidney (LM, IHC)
- **Serology:** heart blood serum/thoracic fluid (virus neutralization)
- **Virology:** placenta/caruncle, thymus, lymph node, spleen, thyroid, brain, ileum (ISO, FAT, ELISA, PCR).

DIFFERENTIAL DIAGNOSIS

Congenital disease
- Swayback (copper deficiency)
- Caprine encephalomyelitis

Abortion
- Enzootic abortion
- Listeriosis
- Toxoplasmosis
- Leptospirosis
- Rift Valley fever
- Akabane disease

TREATMENT

There is no specific treatment for border disease. With care and nursing, many affected lambs will survive the immediate neonatal period, but they grow poorly, are very susceptible to intercurrent disease during the growing period, and it is generally not economic to attempt to raise these lambs.

CONTROL

The principles are to attempt to engender flock immunity and to avoid exposing sheep to infection in early pregnancy. Persistently infected sheep are a continuous source of infection and those that survive to breeding age can perpetuate the disease. They should be identified and culled.

The problem is with their identification, because some persistently infected lambs show no clinical or phenotypic abnormality. Lambs that are clinically affected at birth should be permanently identified because the tremor and fleece abnormality disappear at 1 to 2 months of age and the lambs may no longer be recognizable as infected. Persistently infected animals can be identified by serologic screening of the ewe lambs intended for replacement stock at 6 months of age (after maternal passive immunity has waned), followed by virus isolation in seronegative animals, but this is expensive and only practical in small flocks. An alternative is to keep no replacement ewes from an affected lamb crop.

Persistently infected sheep can be run with the flock when it is not pregnant, particularly with the replacement ewes, in an attempt to produce infection and immunity before pregnancy. They should be removed before breeding. Although this can result in "natural vaccination," the rates of infection and seroconversion in replacement females can be low. In theory, cattle BVDV vaccines could be used to produce immunity but their efficacy would depend on a significant relatedness to the BDV under consideration.

In most flocks a serious outbreak of the disease is followed by minor disease in subsequent years, with the flock developing immunity in the initial outbreak.

In flocks that are free of infection, replacement ewes and rams should be screened for infection before purchase or quarantined after arrival on the farm. Newly introduced sheep should be kept separate from the main flock until after lambing. Ideally, cattle should not be pastured or housed with pregnant sheep.

FURTHER READING

Radostits O, et al. Border disease (hairy shaker disease of lambs, hairy shakers, hypomyelinogenesis congenita). In: *Veterinary Medicine: A Textbook of the Diseases of Cattle, Horses, Sheep, Goats and Pigs*. 10th ed. London: W.B. Saunders; 2007:1414-1418.

REFERENCES

1. Strong R, et al. *Vet Microbiol*. 2010;141:208.
2. Dubois E, et al. *Vet Microbiol*. 2008;130:69.
3. Marco I, et al. *Res Vet Sci*. 2009;87:149.
4. Braun U, et al. *Vet Microbiol*. 2015;168:98.
5. González JM, et al. *Vet Rec*. 2014;174:69.
6. Dubey P, et al. *J Virol Methods*. 2015;213:50.
7. Toplu N, et al. *Vet Pathol*. 2011;48:576.
8. Dincel GC, Kul O. *PLoS ONE*. 2015;10:e0120005.
9. Dincel GC, Kul O. *Histol Histopathol*. 2015;30:1233.

VISNA

SYNOPSIS

Etiology Neurovirulent strains of maedi-visna virus, a lentivirus.

Epidemiology Occurs in association with maedi but endemic visna only recorded in Iceland.

Clinical findings Afebrile disease with insidious onset. Progressive ataxia and wasting, long clinical course.

Clinical pathology Pleocytosis and elevated protein, virus, virus proteins, and antivirus antibody in cerebrospinal fluid.

Lesions Chronic demyelinating encephalomyelitis.

Diagnostic confirmation Histology, demonstration of virus, PCR.

Treatment None.

Control As for ovine progressive pneumonia.

ETIOLOGY

Visna is the neurologic manifestation of maedi-visna disease caused by infection with Maedi-Visna Virus (MVV). This virus is a single-stranded RNA, nononcogenic lentivirus within the retrovirus family. There are neurovirulent and nonneurovirulent strains of MVV, and neurovirulence is enhanced by intracerebral passage of virus. There is a high degree of relatedness between MVV, the ovine lentivirus associated with ovine progressive pneumonia (OPP), and the Caprine Arthritis Encephalitis (CAE) virus. These ovine and caprine lentiviruses share nucleotide homology and serologic properties and are now regarded as a viral continuum and referred to as small ruminant lentiviruses (SRLV).[1]

Visna usually occurs in conjunction with maedi lesions in the lungs, with up to 18% of sheep affected by maedi having histologic lesions of visna in the brain.

EPIDEMIOLOGY

Occurrence

Visna is a disease of sheep and rarely of goats. It was originally a significant cause of death in the epizootic of maedi-visna that occurred in Iceland from 1933 to 1965. It always occurred in association with maedi, but was sporadic and generally less important than the pulmonary manifestation of the infection. The exception was in some flocks in which it was the major manifestation of the maedi-visna disease complex, but visna not been seen in Iceland since 1951 and maedi-visna has since been eradicated from that country.

Despite the widespread occurrence of maedi-visna or OPP in many countries, visna is now an uncommon disease, and a high prevalence of neurologic disease has seldom been recorded in countries other than Iceland. The reason for this is not known but might be from an increased susceptibility of the Icelandic breed of sheep to the neurologic form of the disease, or to differences in the neurovirulence of different strains of the virus. In Britain, MVV was first detected in the late 1970s, and the initial clinical expression was largely maedi (dyspnea), but occasionally with coexistent visna.

Experimental Transmission

Sheep experimentally infected by intracerebral inoculation spread MVV to commingled sheep. The incubation period and the course of the disease are both protracted, with clinical signs not appearing until 2 years after experimental inoculation.

PATHOGENESIS

The virus infects cells of the monocyte–macrophage lineage and replicates its RNA genome via a DNA intermediate provirus, which is integrated into the chromosomal DNA of the host cell. Replication is limited and does not proceed beyond the synthesis of provirus in most cells. Persistent production of viral antigen results in lymphocytic hyperplasia.

There are two basic lesions, an inflammatory lesion that is not related to the occurrence of nervous signs, and a focal demyelination in the brain and spinal cord, the occurrence of which is related to the appearance of paresis. Experimental immunosuppression reduces the severity of lesions by suppressing the cellular proliferative response without suppressing the growth of the virus, whereas postinfection immunization enhances the severity of experimental visna. Viral nucleic acid and proteins are present in oligodendrocytes, and demyelination is thought to be a direct effect of the virus on these cells as well as a sequel to the inflammatory response they provoke.

CLINICAL FINDINGS

The disease has an insidious onset, and the early clinical signs include lagging behind the flock because of ataxia and body wasting. The body wasting and the hindlimb ataxia are progressive. Affected animals show hypermetria and may stumble or fall as they traverse uneven ground or when making sudden turns. There is no fever, and a normal appetite and consciousness are retained. Additional signs include severe tremor of the facial muscles and knuckling of the distal limbs so that the animal stands on the flexed tarsi. Some animals may show a head tilt, aimless wandering, circling, and blindness.[2]

The clinical picture is not unlike that of scrapie without the pruritus. During the course of the disease, periods of relative normality may occur. Affected animals may show clinical signs for several months before final paralysis necessitates slaughter. The disease is always fatal, and the clinical syndrome in goats is the same as for sheep.

CLINICAL PATHOLOGY

There are an increased number of mononuclear cells in the CSF, an elevated protein, and positive Pandy test. The pleocytosis is variable during the course of the disease. Virus, virus antigen, and antibody are also demonstrable in CSF. Serologic tests are detailed under the section on ovine progressive pneumonia in chapter 12.

NECROPSY FINDINGS

Muscle wasting and an interstitial pneumonia may be visible but there are no gross changes in the CNS. The characteristic histologic lesion is patchy, demyelinating encephalomyelitis. The inflammatory infiltrate is predominantly composed of lymphocytes and macrophages. Demyelination occurs in the white matter of the cerebrum and cerebellum, and in the spinal cord. The histologic character of the lung is typical of ovine lentivirus-associated pneumonia. Isolation of the virus is difficult. Typical neural lesions and a positive serologic titer usually suffice for confirmation of the diagnosis. IHC tests and PCR-based assays have been successfully used to confirm this lentiviral infection in lung, mammary gland, and even third eyelid, but the use of these tests to confirm of the infection in CNS tissues is not well documented.

Samples for Confirmation of Diagnosis

- **Histology:** fixed spinal cord, half of midsagittally sectioned brain, lung, mammary gland, joint synovium (IHC, LM)
- **Serology:** serum (Agar gel immunodiffusion test, ELISA)
- **Virology:** chilled brain, spinal cord, lung, mammary gland (PCR, ISO).

DIFFERENTIAL DIAGNOSIS

Visna is a sporadic disease of mature sheep with an insidious onset of muscle wasting, progressive ataxia, and a long clinical course. These characteristics differentiate it from other diseases of sheep manifest with ataxia.

Differentials include

- Scrapie
- Delayed organophosphate toxicity
- Cerebrospinal nematodiasis
- Segmental axonopathy (Murrurrundi disease)

TREATMENT AND CONTROL

There is no treatment for visna. It usually occurs in conjunction with signs of maedi and is a comparatively rare disease by itself. Control procedures are as for those suggested for OPP/maedi. It is possible to greatly reduce the prevalence, and even eradicate the disease, by either (1) testing all sheep with an ELISA and removing seropositive sheep from the flock, or (2) by removal of lambs at birth and rearing them in isolation from other sheep. Testing all sheep at shorter intervals (3–6 months) with a combination of serology and PCR tests can reduce the prevalence more rapidly but is more costly.

Many jurisdictions have developed accreditation programs for flocks to establish that they have a low risk of infection with MVV. Once flocks are seronegative they are subjected to testing at various intervals, typically 1 to 3 years depending on an assessment of the biosecurity risk and the presence of untested sheep on the same farm holding.

There is currently no effective vaccine against MVV, and in some cases candidate vaccines have enhanced viremia and/or the immune-mediated pathology of the disease.[3] The difficulty in developing effective vaccines is common among the lentiviruses, with various approaches including attenuated vaccines, vector vaccines, and proviral DNA vaccines having little success.

Marker-assisted genetic selection, to identify those sheep less susceptible to infection with MVV, has the potential to supplement existing control measures. For example, in a trial involving 187 lambs, the probability of infection following natural exposure to OPP virus (a related virus that is part of the SRLV continuum) was 3.6 times greater in crossbred lambs with susceptible or heterozygous diplotype to ovine transmembrane protein gene 154 (TEM154 diplotype "1 3" or "3 3") compared with lambs with diplotype "1 1."[4] This is an active research area and it is expected that additional markers will be identified with future investigations.

FURTHER READING

Blacklaws B. Small ruminant lentiviruses: immunopathogenesis of visna-maedi and caprine arthritis and encephalitis virus. *Comp Immunol Infect Dis.* 2012;35:259-269.

Radostits O, et al. Visna. In: *Veterinary Medicine: A Textbook of the Diseases of Cattle, Horses, Sheep, Goats and Pigs.* 10th ed. London: W.B. Saunders; 2007:1413-1414.

REFERENCES

1. Le Roux C, et al. *Curr HIV Res.* 2010;8:94.
2. Christodouloplous G. *Small Rumin Res.* 2006;62:47.
3. Blacklaws B. *Comp Immunol Microbiol Infect Dis.* 2012;35:259.
4. Leymaster KA, et al. *J Anim Sci.* 2013;91:5114.

CAPRINE ARTHRITIS ENCEPHALITIS

SYNOPSIS

Etiology Retrovirus (a small ruminant lentivirus).

Epidemiology Persistent infection with perinatal and horizontal spread. Management of herd influences extent of seropositivity.

Clinical findings This disease of goats is characterized by arthritis, especially of the carpal joints (big knee), in mature goats, and acute leukoencephalomyelitis in young goats. Indurative mastitis, and less commonly chronic pneumonia and chronic encephalomyelitis, occur in older goats.

Clinical pathology Increased mononuclear cell count in cerebrospinal fluid. Lower or inverted CD4:CD8 ratio in peripheral blood.

Lesions Chronic polysynovitis, degenerative joint disease in adults. Nonsuppurative demyelinating encephalomyelitis. Interstitial pneumonia.

Diagnostic confirmation Microscopic lesions and agar gel immunodiffusion test.

Treatment None.

Control Segregation of the newborn from seropositive animals, and feeding of virus-free colostrum and milk. Prevention of horizontal transmission. Regular testing with segregation or culling.

ETIOLOGY

Caprine arthritis encephalitis (CAE), maedi-visna, and Ovine Progressive Pneumonia (OPP) viruses are single-stranded RNA, nononcogenic lentiviruses within the retrovirus family. They have a tropism for monocytes, macrophages, and dendritic cells, but not T lymphocytes. This is an important determinant of their pathogenesis because they induce a persistent infection that can cause lymphoproliferative changes in the lung, mammary tissues, brain, and joints. There is a high degree of relatedness between these lentiviruses, with shared nucleotide homology and serologic properties. Consequently, CAE, maedi-visna, and OPP viruses are now regarded as a viral continuum known as SRLV.[1]

There are genetically distinct isolates of CAE virus and they may differ in virulence. Because of the nature of the virus, recombination during replication, hence antigenic drift, is common and may facilitate persistence of the virus in the host and the development of disease. Based on analysis of *gag* and *pol* genomic regions, SRLVs have been placed into five clusters (A to E), with A and B further divided into at least 13 and 3 subtypes, respectively. Some of these are geographically restricted, such as cluster C in Norway, whereas others appear more dispersed, probably reflecting the active trading of animals. In Canada, molecular analysis of goat and sheep isolates of SRLV from herds or flocks with only sheep or goats reveals a relatively simple arrangement, with goats infected with B1 subtype and sheep with A2 subtype, respectively. However, on farms with both goats and sheep, there is evidence of crossover between sheep and goats, and vice versa, and mixed infections in both species.[2] Consequently, mixed flocks of goats and sheep may represent an active source for the evolution of these viruses, with a CAE-like virus responsible for severe outbreaks of arthritis in sheep in Spain and mixed infections confirmed in many European countries and North America.[2-4]

EPIDEMIOLOGY

Geographic Occurrence

There is serologic evidence of infection in most areas of the world, including Europe, the UK, North America, Africa, Arabia, Australia, New Zealand, and South America. Although there is sampling bias, one study found marked differences in prevalence between countries, with a lower prevalence in developing countries that did not import dairy-type goats from North America or Europe. This may also reflect the absence of management factors that have a high risk of propagating infection in some countries, such as the pooling of colostrum. Other countries, such as New Zealand, have a low prevalence with the occurrence of CAE mainly in exotic importations.

There may also be variation in seroprevalence within countries. For example, in the United States, the prevalence of infection in goats in the western and middle parts of the country is approximately 50% of all goats tested, which is about twice that in the eastern and Rocky Mountain areas. Herd seroprevalence is greater than 60% in all regions. The seroprevalence within herds shows clustering, with most herds falling into either high or low seroprevalence groups. There are area differences in age prevalence of seropositivity, with some surveys showing no difference and others showing an increasing prevalence with increasing age.

Clinical disease is much less common than infection, and the annual incidence of disease in heavily infected flocks is usually low and approximates 10%.

Host Risk Factors

Breeds

All breeds are susceptible to infection but several studies have recorded apparent differences in breed susceptibility, which may reflect differences in management practices such as feeding practices of colostrum and milk, or genetic differences in susceptibility. There is often a higher prevalence of seropositive goats in family-owned farms compared with institutional herds, which might reflect a greater movement of goats or comingling with other herds among the former.

Housed Rocky Mountain goats (*Oreamnos americanus*) have developed clinical disease attributed to infection with CAE virus, including interstitial pneumonia and synovial changes. Three of four affected goats had been fed raw goat milk from a source later found to have CAE virus.[5]

Age

There is no age difference in susceptibility to experimental infection. Some herds show similar seroprevalence across age groups, whereas others show an increasing seroprevalence with increasing age. These differences probably reflect differences in management between herds and differences in the relative importance of the mechanisms of transmission between herds. Increasing prevalence with age reflects management systems that increase the risk of acquiring infection from horizontal transmission. Leukoencephalomyelitis occurs predominantly in young kids and arthritis in older goats.

Method of Transmission

More than 75% of kids born to infected dams may acquire infection, which can be potentially transmitted to them by several routes. Infection can also occur in older goats.

Colostrum and Milk

Observation of the natural disease and experimental studies indicate that the primary mode of transmission is through the colostrum and milk. The presence of antibody in colostrum does not prevent infection. The virus can be isolated both from the cells in the milk and from cell-free milk from infected dams. Kids born of noninfected dams, but fed colostrum and/or milk from infected dams, can become infected. A single feeding of infected milk can be sufficient to infect a kid. Conversely, the risk of infection is much lower in kids that are removed from the doe immediately after birth and reared on pasteurized milk, and many can be reared free from infection.

Other Perinatal Transmission

Intrauterine infection can occur, but appears to be infrequent and not of major significance in the control of the disease. The disease can be transmitted by contact both during and following the perinatal period, and perinatal transmission is most important in the epidemiology of the disease. Perinatal transmission can result from contact with vaginal secretions, blood, saliva, or respiratory secretions, with the relative importance of these not clearly known.

Contact Transmission

Horizontal transmission occurs at all ages, and older goats can be infected by oral challenge with virus. Contact transmission will result in the spread of the disease when an infected animal is introduced into an infection-free herd and has been one cause of spread in countries in which the infection has been introduced with imported animals.

Prolonged comingling of uninfected with infected animals is likely to promote horizontal transmission.

Other Routes

Milk contains virus-free and virus-infected cells and shared milking facilities increase the risk of cross-infection. This possibly results from the transfer of infected cells in milk during the milking process. Both iatrogenic and venereal transmissions are possible but are probably of limited significance.

Experimental Reproduction

Arthritis and mastitis have been reproduced by oral, intravenous, and intraarticular challenge with CAE virus, although pneumonia is often not a feature of the experimental disease. Leukoencephalomyelitis in young lambs can be reproduced by intracerebral challenge, but this form of the disease has not been reproduced by more natural challenge routes. Strains of the virus can be neuroadapted by passage and show increased neurovirulence but not neuroinvasiveness, suggesting that these are separate characteristics.

The relatedness between caprine and the ovine lentiviruses was first evident with experimental infections, with the CAE-type virus transferred to lambs by feeding them infected colostrum. This experimental infection was followed by viremia and seroconversion, but some strains of the virus produced no clinical or histopathologic evidence of disease. Goat kids have been similarly infected with the maedi virus. The arthritic form of the disease has been produced experimentally in cesarean-derived kids injected with virus isolated from the joints of infected goats.

Economic Importance

There is a high prevalence of infection in many countries, and several have opted for national or breed-associated control programs. There is a higher cull rate in infected herds, with as many as 5% to 10% of goats culled each year for arthritis, and affected animals cannot be entered for show. Seropositive herds have a higher incidence of disease.

There are conflicting reports on the effect of infection on productivity in goat herds, but seropositive goats can have significantly lower milk production (around 10%), a reduced length of lactation, lower 300-day yields of milk, and impaired reproductive performance compared with seronegative goats.

PATHOGENESIS

Animals infected at birth remain persistently infected for life, although only a proportion, typically from 10% to 30%, will develop clinical disease. The virus persistently infects some cells of the monocyte–macrophage type, and the expression and shedding of virus occurs as infected monocytes mature to macrophages.[1] Disease is associated with the host's immune response to the expressed virus. The development of neutralizing antibody does not arrest viral replication because of ongoing expression of antigenic variants of the virus with differing type-specific neutralization epitopes. However, the immune complexes are thought to be the basis for the chronic inflammatory changes in tissues. Goats vaccinated with CAE virus develop more severe clinical disease following challenge compared with nonvaccinated controls. The lesions are lymphoproliferative and followed by a multisystem disease syndrome. This primarily involves synovial-lined connective tissue, causing chronic arthritis, in the udder, causing swelling and hardening of the glands (with or without mastitis), and in the lungs causing a chronic interstitial pneumonia.

A retrovirus infection, detected by electron microscopy and the presence of RT activity, is suspected as the cause of an immunodeficiency syndrome in llamas characterized by failure to thrive, anemia, leukopenia, and recurrent infection, but this has not been reported since 1992.

CLINICAL FINDINGS

Joints

Arthritis occurs predominantly in adult goats and is a chronic hyperplastic synovitis, which is usually noticeable only in the carpal joints. This gives rise to the lay term of big knee, although tarsal joints may also be affected. The onset may be insidious or sudden, and unilateral or bilateral. Goats may be lame in the affected leg, but this is usually not severe. Affected goats may live a normal life span but some gradually lose weight, develop poor hair coats, and eventually remain recumbent most of the time and develop decubitus ulcers. Dilatation of the atlantal and supraspinous bursae occurs in some cases. The course of the disease may last several months. The arthritis may be accompanied by enlargement and hardening of the udder and by interstitial pneumonia, although this may be clinically inapparent. There can be herd and area differences in the clinical expression of the disease. For example, in some outbreaks in Australia pneumonia, rather than arthritis, has been the predominant clinical sign.

Radiographically, there are soft tissue swellings in the early stages and calcification of periarticular tissues and osteophyte production in the later stages. Quantitative joint scintigraphy provides an accurate noninvasive method for assessing the severity of the arthritis in a live animal.

Brain

Leukoencephalitis occurs primarily in 1- to 5-month-old kids. The syndrome is characterized by unilateral or bilateral posterior paresis and ataxia. In the early stages, the gait is short and choppy, followed by weakness and eventually recumbency. In animals that can still stand, there may be a marked lack of proprioception in the hindlimbs (Fig. 14-4). Brain involvement is manifested by head tilt, torticollis, and circling. Affected kids are bright and alert and drink normally. Kids with unilateral posterior paresis usually progress to bilateral posterior paresis in 5 to 10 days. The paresis usually extends to involve the forelimbs, so that tetraparesis follows, and most kids are euthanized. The interstitial pneumonia that often accompanies the nervous form of the disease is usually not severe and not clinically obvious.

Udder

Indurative mastitis, or hard bag, is often initially detected a few days after kidding. The udder is firm and hard but no milk can be expressed. There is no systemic illness and no bacterial mastitis. Recovery is never complete but there may be some gradual improvement.

CLINICAL PATHOLOGY

The synovial fluid from affected joints is usually brown to red-tinged, and the cell count is increased up to 20,000 μL with 90% mononuclear cells. The CSF may contain an increased mononuclear cell count. There is a reduction in monocytes in peripheral blood, a decrease in the number of CD4+ lymphocytes, and a lower or inverted CD4:CD8 ratio.

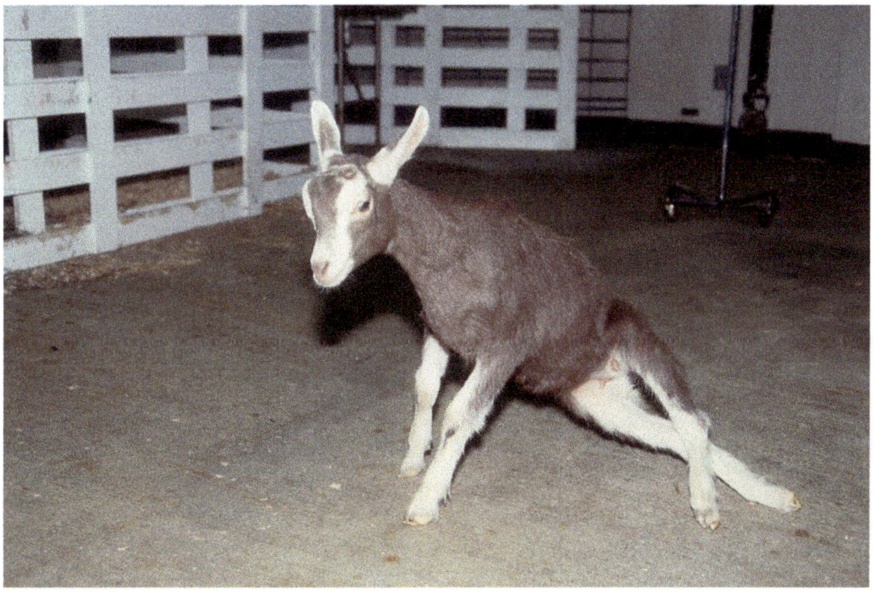

Fig. 14-4 A 3-month-old Toggenburg kid with advanced progressive neurologic signs caused by infection with caprine arthritis encephalitis virus. The goat has normal mentation but is exhibits asymmetric weakness (hindlimbs worse than forelimbs) and proprioceptive abnormalities.

Serologic Testing

For the live animal, there are a number of test systems available whose sensitivity and specificity varies. The agar gel immunodiffusion test (AGID) and a variety of commercial ELISA tests are the most widely used, and the latter usually has a higher sensitivity and specificity. Differences in the performance of the ELISA tests may be related to the peptides they use and the types of SRLV present.[6] Maternal antibody is lost by approximately 3 months of age, hence a seropositive test in a goat older than 6 months is considered evidence of infection. Most animals have a persistent antibody response and remain seropositive for life, although some infected goats may become seronegative over time.

A negative test does not rule out the possibility of infection because there may be a considerable delay between infection and the production of detectable antibody. It is possible that in some infected goats there is insufficient virus expression to lead to an antibody response.

A competitive-inhibition ELISA, which detects antibody to the surface envelop of the virus, has very high sensitivity and specificity and may be more useful in determining the status of individual animals, such as before the movement of goats. Other tests with potentially greater sensitivity and/or specificity are described, but are not generally available. For example, serum adenosine deaminase activity is used as a biochemical marker of HIV infection in humans, and is elevated in goats infected with CAE, but is not a routinely available veterinary test.[7]

Other Tests

A more cost-effective way of monitoring CAE in dairy goats may be testing the bulk tank milk. In Norwegian dairy flocks, an ELISA for testing bulk tank milk detected a within-herd prevalence of CAE of at least 2%, with a sensitivity of 73% and specificity of 87%.[8] Identification of the presence of CAE is usually provided by isolation of the virus from tissue explants into tissue culture. PCR can be used to detect the presence of viral antigen or proviral DNA. Most primers for diagnostic purposes are selected to detect the broadest possible range of SRLV strains, whereas those selected for research purposes may take a type-specific approach.[2] A rapid detection assay based on LAMP has been developed for detecting CAEV proviral DNA in whole blood and whole-blood samples and separated mononuclear cells.[9] This assay can be performed in less well-equipped laboratories as well as in the field.

NECROPSY FINDINGS

In the arthritic form of CAE, there is emaciation and chronic polysynovitis, with degenerative joint disease affecting most of the joints of animals submitted for necropsy. Periarticular tissues are thickened and firm and there is hyperplasia of the synovium. The local lymph nodes are grossly enlarged and a diffuse interstitial pneumonia is usually present. Mammary glands are frequently involved, although gross changes are restricted to induration and increased texture. Microscopically, lymphoplasmacytic infiltrates of the interstitial tissues of mammary gland, lung, and synovium are characteristic. In the neural form the diagnostic lesions are in the nervous system and involve the white matter, especially of the cervical spinal cord and sometimes the cerebellum and the brainstem. The lesion is a bilateral, nonsuppurative demyelinating encephalomyelitis. The infiltrating mononuclear leukocytes tend to be more numerous in the periventricular and subpial areas. There is usually also a mild, diffuse, interstitial pneumonia in this form of the disease. In some cases, a severe lymphoplasmacytic interstitial pneumonia with extensive hyperplasia of type II pneumocytes can occur in the absence of neurologic disease.

Culture of the virus is difficult but can be attempted. A variety of nucleic acid recognition tests, including in situ hybridization, PCR, and IHC, have been developed. For most cases, confirmation of the diagnosis is based on the characteristic microscopic lesions, preferably supported by antemortem serology.

Samples for Confirmation of Diagnosis

- **Histology:** formalin-fixed lung, bronchial lymph node, mammary gland, synovial membranes, half of midsagittally sectioned brain, spinal cord (LM, IHC)
- **Serology:** blood (ELISA, AGID, PCR)
- **Virology:** lung, synovial membrane, mammary gland, hindbrain (PCR, virus isolation).

DIFFERENTIAL DIAGNOSIS

The differential diagnosis of the arthritic form of the disease includes the other infectious arthritides, such as those associated with mycoplasma and chlamydia.

Leukoencephalitis must be differentiated from:

- Swayback caused by copper deficiency
- Spinal abscess
- Cerebrospinal nematodiasis
- Listeriosis
- Polioencephalomalacia

TREATMENT

There is no treatment likely to be of value for any form of CAE.

CONTROL

A measure of control can be achieved by testing the herd every 6 months, and segregating or culling of seropositive animals. More complete control is dependent on preventing/minimizing perinatal transmission of infection to the kid, particularly colostrum and milk transmission, coupled with identifying infected animals and maintaining them physically separated from the noninfected animals or culling them from the herd.

Because of the evidence of transmission of SRLV between sheep and goats, the presence of each species needs to be considered when developing control programs for CAE of goats or OPP of sheep.

Prevention of Perinatal Transmission

Early recommendations for control concentrated on reducing transmission via milk and colostrum, but it is now recognized that this must be coupled with segregation. Newborn kids should be removed from the dam immediately at birth. There should be no contact with the dam, and fetal fluids and debris should be rinsed off the coat. Heat-treated goat colostrum or cow colostrum should be fed, followed by pasteurized milk or a commercial milk replacer. The kid should be segregated from the doe and other infected animals. In herds that feed pasteurized colostrum and milk there is a significant difference in subsequent seroconversions between those that segregate the kids at birth and for rearing and those that do not.

Test and Segregate/Cull

Animals over 3 months of age should be tested by ELISA or AGID every 6 months, and seropositive animals segregated or (preferably) culled from the herd. The interval between infection and seroconversion varies between goats, and the optimal interval for testing has not been determined. More frequent testing may be needed for large herds with a high seroprevalence. Segregation of seropositive and seronegative goats is essential because horizontal spread in adult goats is important in maintaining and increasing infection rates in some herds, and even a brief contact time can allow transmission. Where culling is not practiced, seropositive goats should be milked after seronegative ones, and the use of common equipment, such as for ear-tagging, tattooing, and vaccinating, should be avoided.

Several countries have programs for herd accreditation of freedom from infection. The stringency of these schemes varies, and they may be governmental or breed society accreditation programs. Typically, they require that all adults in the herd test negative on two herd tests at a 6-month interval. There are also restrictions on the movement and purchase of animals, and periodic serologic surveillance. For example, a scheme in Norway has been quite successful, with only 5 of 406 flocks (1.2%) being reinfected over a 10-year period.[8]

Vaccination and Genetic Selection

There is currently no effective vaccine against the SRLVs, including CAE, maedi-visna, or OPP viruses, and in some cases candidate vaccines have enhanced viremia and/or the immune-mediated pathology of the disease.[1] The difficulty in developing effective vaccines is common among the lentiviruses, with various approaches, including attenuated vaccines, vector vaccines, and proviral DNA vaccines having little success. The reasons are obscure, but probably relate to the underlying dysfunction in T-cell–mediated immune responses.

However, marker-assisted genetic selection, to identify animals less susceptible to infection, has the potential to supplement existing control measures. For example, in a trial investigating the control of OPP in lambs, the probability of infection following natural exposure to OPP virus was 3.6 times greater in crossbred lambs with susceptible or heterozygous diplotype to ovine transmembrane protein gene 154 (TEM154 diplotype 1 3 or 3 3) compared with lambs with diplotype 1 1.[10] Similar studies have not yet been undertaken in goats, but this is an active research area and it is expected that additional markers for conditions caused by SRLV will be identified in future.

FURTHER READING

Blacklaws B. Small ruminant lentiviruses: immunopathogenesis of visna-maedi and caprine arthritis and encephalitis virus. *Comp Immunol Infect Dis.* 2012;35:259-269.

Hermann-Hoesing LM, et al. Diagnostic assays used to control small ruminant lentiviruses. *J Vet Diagnost Invest.* 2010;22:843-855.

Radostits O, et al. Caprine arthritis encephalitis (CAE). In: *Veterinary Medicine: A Textbook of the Diseases of Cattle, Horses, Sheep, Goats and Pigs.* 10th ed. London: W.B. Saunders; 2007:1410-1413.

REFERENCES

1. Blacklaws B. *Comp Immunol Microbiol Infect Dis.* 2012;35:259.
2. Fras M, et al. *Infect Genet Evol.* 2013;19:97.
3. Glaria I, et al. *Vet Microbiol.* 2009;138:156.
4. Gjerset B, et al. *Virus Res.* 2007;125:153.
5. Patton KM, et al. *Vet Diagn Invest.* 2012;24:392.
6. de Andrés X, et al. *Vet Immunol Immunopathol.* 2013;152:277.
7. Rodrigues LF, et al. *Small Rumin Res.* 2012;108:120.
8. Nagel-Alne GE, et al. *Vet Rec.* 2015;176:173.
9. Huang J, et al. *Arch Virol.* 2012;157:1463.
10. Leymaster KA, et al. *J Anim Sci.* 2013;91:5114.

OVINE ENCEPHALOMYELITIS (LOUPING-ILL)

SYNOPSIS

Etiology Louping-ill virus, flavivirus.

Epidemiology Disease of sheep (and red grouse), and occasionally other domestic animals and man, transmitted by *Ixodes ricinus.* Occurs predominantly in lambs and yearling sheep in Great Britain and Europe in the spring, associated with tick rise.

Clinical findings Fever, neurologic dysfunction, muscle tremor, incoordination, bounding gait. Recovery or convulsions and death.

Lesions Nonsuppurative encephalitis.

Diagnostic confirmation Serology, demonstration of virus.

Control Vaccination, tick control.

ETIOLOGY

Louping-ill virus belongs to the genus *Flavivirus,* which is divided into eight groups, one of which is the tick-borne encephalitis group. Louping-ill is antigenically related to the tick-borne encephalitis viruses. The latter circulate in Europe and Asia and are a serious zoonotic disease for humans, but do not infect sheep.[1] Louping-ill virus occurs in Great Britain, Ireland and Norway, but similar disease occurs elsewhere and there is antigenic diversity between isolates from different geographic areas. Viruses that are closely related to louping-ill virus, and that cause very similar disease but in different regions of the world, include Russian spring-summer encephalitis, Turkish sheep encephalitis, Spanish sheep encephalitis, Spanish goat encephalitis,[2] and Greek goat encephalitis viruses. In sheep, concurrent infection with the agent of tick-borne fever *Ehrlichia* (*Cytoecetes*) *phagocytophila* enhances the pathogenicity of the virus.

EPIDEMIOLOGY

Occurrence

Geographic Occurrence

Louping-ill was originally considered to be restricted to the border counties of Scotland and England but is now recognized as also occurring in upland grazing areas of Scotland, in Ireland, southwest England, and in Norway; related viruses and diseases occur in Spain, Bulgaria, Greece, and Turkey. The distribution of the disease is regulated by the occurrence of the vector tick *Ixodes ricinus,* which requires suitable hosts and a ground layer microclimate of high humidity throughout the year. In these areas, louping-ill can be a common infection and may be a significant cause of loss.

Host Occurrence

Louping-ill virus can infect and produce disease in a wide variety of vertebrates including man, but predominantly sheep are affected because of their susceptibility and the fact that they are the main domestic animal species that graze the tick-infested areas. Nonruminant species, such as alpaca and horses, and wild ungulates such as chamois,[3] have also been infected.

Although sheep (and red grouse) are the only animals that commonly develop clinical disease, *I. ricinus* feeds on a number of different hosts and the adult tick requires a large mammalian host. As a consequence, seropositivity and occasional clinical disease occur in all other domestic species, especially goat kids, but also cattle, horses, alpaca,[4] pigs, and humans.

Traditionally, pigs have not been free-ranged on upland tick-infested areas, but they are susceptible to experimental infection by all routes.

Red deer (*Cervus elaphus*) and roe deer (*Capreolus capreolus*) are hosts for the tick in Scotland, and the elk (*Alces alces*) may be in Sweden. Infection in these species is usually subclinical; however, when these animals are subjected to the stress of captivity, clinical illness is more likely to occur. This may be important to commercial deer farmers.

Transmission

Tick Transmission

The reservoir for the disease and the major vector is the three host tick *I. ricinus,* which requires a single blood meal at each stage of development. Changes in the distribution of the tick are probably introducing this and other tick-borne disease into previously unaffected areas. The tick feeds for approximately 3 weeks every year and completes its life cycle in 3 years. The larval and nymphal stages will feed on any vertebrate, but the adult female will engorge and mate only on larger mammals. The tick becomes infected by feeding on a viremic host and the virus translocates to the salivary gland of the subsequent stage to provide a source of infection at feeding in the following year. Transstadial transmission of the virus occurs, but transovarial transmission does not; thus only the nymph and adult ticks are capable of transmitting the disease. The tick is seasonally active at temperatures between 7°C and 18°C. Most ticks feed in the spring, with peak activity dependent on the latitude and elevation of the pasture, but generally occurring in April and May. In some areas there is a second period of activity of a separate population of *I. ricinus* in the autumn during August and September. Although infected ticks can transmit the infection to a large number of vertebrate hosts, only sheep, red grouse (*Lagopus scoticus*), and possibly horses, attain a viremia sufficient to infect other ticks and act as maintenance hosts. Grouse amplify the virus, deer amplify the vector, and hares (*Lepus timidus*) amplify both. Infection in red grouse is accompanied by a high mortality, and the louping-ill virus is essentially maintained in an area by a sheep–tick cycle and hare tick cycle.

Nontick Transmission

Although the major method of spread is by the bites of infected ticks, spread by droplet infection is of importance in man, and the infection can be transmitted in animals by hypodermic needle contamination and other methods. The virus is not very resistant to environmental influences and is readily destroyed by disinfectants. Pigs fed the carcasses of sheep that had died of louping-ill become infected with the louping-ill virus. The virus is excreted in the milk of experimentally infected female goats, and infects sucking kids to produce an acute disease. Virus is also excreted in the milk of ewes during the acute stages of infection but, paradoxically, does not result in the transmission of the infection to lambs. Grouse can be infected by eating infected ticks, and this is considered a major mechanism of infection for grouse.

Host and Environmental Risk Factors

The epidemiology of disease is dictated by the biology of the tick and so disease is seasonal, occurring during spring when the ticks are active. The prevalence of infection, as measured by seropositivity, is high in areas where the disease is enzootic. In these areas, the annual incidence of disease varies but there are cases every year and they occur predominantly in yearlings and in lambs. In enzootic areas, the majority of adult sheep have been infected and are immune. Colostral immunity from these ewes will protect their lambs for approximately 3 months, and these lambs are resistant to infection during the spring rise of the ticks. Ewe lambs that are retained in the flock are susceptible to infection at the second exposure the following spring. In the UK there are concerns that the density and range of ticks is increasing because of changes in climate and land management; thus the distribution of tick-borne disease is also changing.[5]

The proportion of infected animals that develop clinical disease in any year is estimated to vary from 5% to 60% and is influenced by the intensity of the tick vector; the immune status of the flock; the age at infection; nutritional status; and factors such as cold stress, herding, and transport, and the occurrence of intercurrent disease. Naive animals introduced to an enzootic area are at high risk for infection and clinical disease.

Intercurrent infection with *E.* (*Cytoecetes*) *phagocytophila* and *Toxoplasma gondii* have been shown to increase the severity of experimental tick-borne fever in young lambs, but the relevance of this association to naturally occurring disease is uncertain. It would appear that concurrent infection with louping-ill and tick-borne fever is unlikely to occur in the field in young lambs because colostral immunity will protect against infection with the louping-ill virus, whereas colostral immunity is not protective against tick-borne fever. Similarly, the superinfection of *Rhizomucor pusillus* on this concurrent infection has been observed in experimental conditions, but is not a commonly recorded observation in natural disease.

Zoonotic Implications

Louping-ill is a zoonosis. The major risk for veterinarians is with the postmortem examination and handling of tissues from infected animals. Laboratory workers, and shepherds and abattoir persons who handle infected sheep, are also at risk. The occurrence of virus in the milk of goats and sheep is a risk for human disease where raw milk is consumed.

PATHOGENESIS

After tick-borne infection, the virus proliferates in the regional lymph node to produce a viremia that peaks at 2 to 4 days and declines with the development of circulating antibody before the development of clinical disease. Invasion of the CNS occurs in the early viremic stage in most if not all infected animals, but in most the resultant lesions are small and isolated and there is no clinical neurologic disease. The occurrence of clinical disease is associated with the replication of the virus in the brain, severe inflammation throughout the CNS, and necrosis of brainstem and ventral horn neurons. The reason for more severe disease in some animals appears to be related to the rapidity and extent of the immune response. Animals that survive exposure to louping-ill virus have an earlier immune response to the infection and have high concentrations of antibody in the CSF.

In experimental studies, there is a more severe and prolonged viremia and a higher mortality from louping-ill when there is concurrent infection with tick-borne fever. Sheep with tick-borne fever have severe neutropenia, lymphocytopenia, defective cellular and humoral immunologic responses, and high mortality associated with concurrent infection with this agent is thought to be from enhanced viral replication of the louping-ill virus. The dual infection in experimental sheep also facilitates fungal invasion and a systemic mycotic infection with *R. pusillus.*

CLINICAL FINDINGS

In most sheep, infection is inapparent. There is an incubation period of 2 to 4 days followed by a sudden onset of high fever (up to 41.5°C, 107°F) for 2 to 3 days followed by a return to normal. In animals that develop neurologic disease, there is a second febrile phase during which nervous signs appear. Affected animals stand apart, often with the head held high and with twitching of the lips and nostrils. There is marked tremor of muscle groups and rigidity of the musculature, particularly in the neck and limbs. This is manifested by jerky, stiff movements and a bounding gait, which gives rise to the name louping-ill. Incoordination is most marked in the hindlimbs. The sheep walks into objects and may stand with the head pressed against them. Hypersensitivity to noise and touch may be apparent. Some animals will recover over the following days, although there may be residual torticollis and posterior paresis. In others, the increased muscle tone is succeeded by recumbency, convulsions, and paralysis, and death occurs as early as 1 to 2 days later. Young lambs may die suddenly with no specific nervous signs.

The clinical picture in cattle is very similar to that observed in sheep, with hyperesthesia, blinking of the eyelids, and rolling of the eyes, although convulsions are more likely to occur in cattle, and in the occasional animals that recover from the encephalitis there is usually persistent signs of impairment of the CNS.

Horses also show a similar clinical picture to sheep, with some showing a rapidly progressing nervous disease with a course of approximately 2 days and others a transient disorder of locomotion with recovery in 10 to 12 days.

The infection is usually subclinical in adult goats but the virus is excreted in the milk and kids may develop severe acute infections. In humans an influenza-like disease followed by meningoencephalitis occurs after an incubation period of 6 to 18 days. Although recovery is common, the disease can be fatal and residual nervous deficiencies can occur.

CLINICAL PATHOLOGY

The initial viremia that occurs with infection declines with the emergence of serum antibody and virus is no longer present in the blood at the onset of clinical signs. Hemagglutination inhibition (HI), complement-fixing, and neutralizing antibodies can be detected in the serum of recovered animals. HI and complement-fixing antibodies are relatively transient, but neutralizing antibodies persist. HI IgM antibody develops early in the disease and can be used as an aid to diagnosis in animals with clinical disease. Analysis of CSF is usually not considered because of the zoonotic risk.

Molecular tests, including conventional and real-time RT-PCR, can target specific viruses in this tick-borne encephalitis virus group, and a pan-flavirvirus test has been developed.[6]

NECROPSY FINDINGS

No gross changes are observed. Histologically, there are perivascular accumulations of cells in the meninges, brain, and spinal cord, with neuronal damage most evident in cerebellar Purkinje cells and, to a lesser extent, in the cerebral cortex. Louping-ill virus can be demonstrated in formalin-fixed tissues by the avidin-biotin–complex immunoperoxidase technique.

Samples for Confirmation of Diagnosis

- **Virology:** chilled brain, halved midsagitally (VI, RT-PCR)
- **Histology:** fixed brain, other half (LM, IHC)
- **Molecular:** CNS tissue, blood, ticks (conventional and real-time RT-PCR)

DIFFERENTIAL DIAGNOSIS

The disease is restricted to areas in which the vector tick occurs.

- In lambs, the disease has clinical similarities with delayed swayback, spinal abscess, and some cases of tick pyemia. Spinal abscess occurs shortly following a management procedure such as docking or castration or with tick pyemia; it has a longer clinical course, is commonly present at C7-T2, and can be established by radiographic examination. Tick pyemia can also occur in flocks that have louping-ill, and the determination of the contribution of each disease to flock mortality relies on clinical, epidemiologic, and postmortem examination.
- In yearlings, the disease has similarities to spinal ataxia caused by trauma, to gid (*Coenurus cerebralis*), and to the early stages of polioencephalomalacia.
- In adults, the disease in sheep resembles some stages of acute neurologic diseases, including scrapie, tetanus, hypocalcemia, hypomagnesemia, pregnancy toxemia, and listeriosis.

TREATMENT

An antiserum has been used and is protective if given within 48 hours of exposure, but is of no value once the febrile reaction has begun. However, it is not commercially available. Animals with clinical disease should be sedated if necessary during the acute course of the disease and kept in a secluded and dark area with general supportive care.

CONTROL

The prevention of louping-ill requires either the prevention of exposure of sheep to tick-infested pastures or the immunization of animals before exposure. Immunization has been the traditional approach.

Historically, a formalinized tissue vaccine derived from brain, spinal cord, and spleen was used and provided excellent immunity in enzootic areas. The vaccine was not without risk for persons manufacturing it and at one stage led to an outbreak of scrapie where the vaccine was prepared from sheep incubating the disease. Currently, vaccination is with a formalin-killed tissue culture–derived vaccine administered in an oil adjuvant. A single dose of this vaccine will give protection for at least 1 year and possibly up to 2 years. The vaccine is used in the autumn, or in the early spring 1 month before the anticipated tick rise, in all ewe lambs that will be held for flock replacements. Vaccination of pregnant ewes twice in late pregnancy is recommended to ensure adequate passive immunity to the lambs via the colostrum. A recombinant vaccine has also been shown to offer protection against infection.

The limited geographic occurrence of this disease and commercial economics has, and may, restrict the availability of vaccines. Consequently tick control, or the elimination of infection from pastures, may be required in the future. The intensity of tick infestation of pastures can be reduced by influencing the microclimate that they require for survival. In some areas this can be achieved by ditching and drainage of the pastures. The control of the causative tick using acaricides provides some protection against disease.

Epidemiologic, modeling, and experimental studies indicate that sheep, red grouse, and hares are the only maintenance hosts for the virus and this, coupled with the fact that there is no transovarial transmission of the virus in the tick, offers a potential method for eradication of the infection from an area. However, this approach (the elimination of wildlife hosts) is increasingly unacceptable in relationship to game and wildlife conservation, may have unintended consequences and is probably of dubious benefit-cost in relationship to alternate methods of control.[7]

FURTHER READING

Estradapena A, Farkas R, Jaenson TGT, et al. *Ticks and Tick-Borne Diseases: Geographical Distribution and Control Strategies in the Euro-Asia Region.* Wallingford, UK: CABI Publishing; 2003.

Radostits O, et al. Ovine encephalomyelitis (louping-ill). In: *Veterinary Medicine: A Textbook of the Diseases of Cattle, Horses, Sheep, Goats and Pigs.* 10th ed. London: W.B. Saunders; 2007:1414-1418.

REFERENCES

1. Jeffries CL, et al. *J Gen Virol.* 2014;95:1005.
2. Mansfield KL, et al. *J Gen Virol.* 2015;96:1676.
3. Ruiz-Fons F, et al. *Eur J Wildl Dis.* 2014;60:691.
4. Cranwell MP, et al. *Vet Rec.* 2008;162:28.
5. Sarginson N, et al. *In Pract.* 2009;31:58.
6. Johnson N, et al. *Vector Borne Zoonotic Dis.* 2010;10:665.
7. Harrison A, et al. *J Appl Ecol.* 2010;47:926.

WEST NILE, KUNJIN, AND MURRAY VALLEY ENCEPHALITIS

SYNOPSIS

Etiology Flavivirus including West Nile virus (lineages 1 and 2) including Kunjin virus, and Murray Valley encephalitis virus. Closely related to Japanese encephalitis virus.

Epidemiology Maintained in a bird–mosquito cycle. Mammals are incidentally infected. Enzootic in Africa, North America, Pakistan, southern Europe, and Australia. Epizootics. Affects a wide variety of species with a major impact on humans and horses.

Clinical signs Weakness, incoordination, altered mentation, muscle fasciculations, recumbency.

Clinical pathology MAC-ELISA for diagnosis.

Lesions Polioencephalomyelitis.

Diagnostic confirmation MAC-ELISA, PCR, clinical signs, lesions.

Treatment None specific. Supportive care.

Control Vaccination. Mosquito control.

MAC-ELISA, *M antibody-capture enzyme-linked immunosorbent assay.*

ETIOLOGY

Encephalitis in horses, humans, and other species is associated with West Nile virus, an arthropod-borne flavivirus in the Japanese encephalitis virus group. Other viruses in the group include Japanese encephalitis virus (Japan and Southeast Asia), St. Louis encephalitis virus (United States), Kunjin virus (now considered a subtype of West Nile virus, Australia),[1,2] Murray Valley encephalitis virus (Australia),[3-5] and Rocio virus (Brazil). Murray Valley virus causing encephalomyelitis in horses in southeastern Australia is endemic to northern Australia.[4] Viruses causing, or suspected of causing encephalomyelitis in equids, are listed in Table 14-11.[6]

The virus was first isolated in 1937 from a human with fever in Uganda. There are at least two lineages of the virus, with one lineage (Lineage 1) isolated from animals in central and North Africa, Europe, Israel, and

Table 14-11 Viruses causing encephalomyelitis in horses. reproduced with permission.[6]

Virus species	Geographic location	Reservoir species	Equine syndrome
Alphavirus			
Eastern equine encephalitis virus	North/South/Central America, Caribbean	Birds, rodents, snakes	Encephalomyelitis
Western equine encephalitis virus	North/South America	Birds, rodents, snakes	Encephalomyelitis
Venezuelan equine encephalitis virus	Central/South America, Caribbean	Cotton rat	Encephalomyelitis
Ross River virus	Australia, Papua New Guinea	Marsupial and placental mammals	Systemic: hemolymphatic Neurologic ataxia
Semliki Forest virus	East and West Africa	Unknown	Encephalomyelitis
Flavivirus			
Japanese encephalitis	Asia, India, Russia, Western Pacific	Birds, swine	Encephalomyelitis
Murray Valley	Australia, Papua New Guinea	Birds, horses, cattle, marsupials, and foxes	Encephalomyelitis
Kunkin virus	Australia	Water birds: herons and ibis	Encephalomyelitis
St. Louis encephalitis	North, Central and South America	Birds	Serologic only recorded
Usutu	Europe, Africa	Birds	Serologic only recorded
West Nile	Africa, Middle East, Europe, North, Central and South America, Australia	Passerine birds (crows, sparrows, robins)	Encephalomyelitis
Louping-ill	Iberian Peninsula, UK	Sheep, grouse	Encephalomyelitis
Powassan	North American, Russia	Lagomorphs, rodents, mice, skunks, dogs, birds	Encephalomyelitis
Tick-borne encephalitis	Asia, Europe, Finland, Russia	Small rodents	Encephalomyelitis
Bunyavirus			
California serogroup: California encephalitis, Jamestown Canyon, La Crosse, Snowshoe hare	North America (United States and Canada), parts of eastern Asia	Rodents and lagomorphs	Encephalomyelitis

North America, whereas the other (Lineage 2) is enzootic in central and southern Africa with outbreaks of disease in humans in central Europe, Greece, and Russia.[6-10] The recent outbreak in North America was associated with a Lineage 1 (Clade a) virus of African origin almost identical to that isolated from diseased geese in Israel, and which subsequently acquired a mutation that enhanced its capacity to reproduce in mosquitos and its virulence in corvid birds and other species.[11] Viruses of both lineages can circulate at the same time in the same geographic region. Virus of either lineage can cause disease, although that of Lineage 1 appears to be associated with more severe disease in horses and other species. Kunjin virus, a West Nile virus (Lineage 1, Clade b), causes encephalomyelitis in horses in Australia.[12,13] An outbreak in Australia in 2011 was associated with unusually wet weather (see later) and emergence of a strain of West Nile virus (WNVNSW2011) that had at least two amino acid changes associated with increased virulence of WNVNY99 (the strain associated with the epidemic in North America in 1999).[12] The WNV(KUN) NSW2011 strain also had adaptations that increased the amount of virus in material (saliva) regurgitated by mosquitos, which could have increased the rate of vector transmission of the virus.[14] The WNVNSW2011 strain did not have all the virulence attributes of the WNVNY99 strain.[15]

Murray Valley encephalitis virus causes encephalomyelitis in horses in Australia.[3]

The West Nile virus causes disease in humans, horses, birds (including geese, raptors, and corvids), sheep, alpaca, and dogs. Experimental inoculation of little ravens (*Corvus mellori*) with WNVKUN resulted in infection and viremia but not clinical disease.[13]

EPIDEMIOLOGY

Distribution

West Nile encephalitis virus is enzootic to Africa and sporadic outbreaks of the disease occurred in the 1960s in Africa, the Middle East, and southern Europe. Recently outbreaks affecting horses and other animals have occurred in southern France, Tuscany, Israel, and other parts of southern Europe. There is serologic evidence of common and widespread infection of equids with West Nile virus in Pakistan and Tunisia.[16,17]

The virus was introduced into New York City in North America in 1999 and subsequently spread widely across the continent, including Canada, Mexico, and the Caribbean, reaching the west coast by 2004. The virus caused widespread deaths of wild birds and disease and death in humans, horses, and other species in North America during this period.

Introduction of the infection to North America was associated with an epizootic of disease that over several years moved across the continent. During the initial years of the epizootic there were large numbers of cases in horses (15,000) and humans (4,000) and death of at least 16,500 birds. As the front of the epizootic moved across the country, the infection became enzootic and the number of cases in horses in these regions decreased markedly over those in the first year.

Infection by Kunjin virus (a strain of West Nile virus) rarely causes disease of horses in areas in which it is endemic (northern Australia) but was associated with an outbreak of neurologic disease in horses in southeastern Australia after a decade-long drought broke with record rains resulting in sixfold increases in vector density.[1,12] The outbreak did not extend into the subsequent year.[12] There is serologic evidence of infection by flaviviruses (including Kunjin and/or Murray Valley encephalitis virus in 15%–18% of horses in southeast Queensland, where infection is presumed to be endemic and clinical disease is rare.[18]

Viral Ecology

The virus is maintained by a cycling between amplifying hosts, usually birds, and insect vectors. Large mammals, including horses and humans, are incidentally infected and are not important in propagation of the virus. Amplifying hosts are those in which the viremia is of a sufficient magnitude and duration (1–5 days) to provide the opportunity to infect feeding mosquitoes. Mammals, and in particular horses, are generally not amplifying hosts because of the low level of viremia.

The virus is spread by the feeding of ornithophilic mosquitoes, usually of the genus *Culex* with mosquitos of the *C. pipiens* group being effective vectors.[19,20] The principal vectors for West Nile virus include Africa, *C. univittatus*; Europe, *C. pipiens, C. modestus,* and *Coquillettidia richiardii*; Asia, *C. quinquefasciatus, C. tritaeniorhynchus,* and *C. vishnui*; United States, *C. pipiens* complex including *C. pipiens* and *C. restuans* in the northeastern and north central United States, *C. tarsalis* in the Great Plains and western United States; and *C. nigripalpus* and *C. quinquefasciatus* in southeastern United States.[21] *C. annulirostris* and a variety of other native and introduced species of mosquitos are actual or potential vectors of West Nile virus in Australia.[21]

Infected mosquitoes carry the virus in salivary glands and infect avian hosts during feeding. The virus then multiplies in the avian host causing a viremia that may last for up to 5 days. Mosquitoes feeding on the avian host during the viremic phase are then infected by the virus. This pattern of infection of amplifying hosts and mosquitoes is repeated such that the infection cycles in these populations. Increases in mosquito number, such as occur at the end of the summer, and enhanced viral replication in mosquitoes at higher ambient temperatures, increase the likelihood that avian hosts, or incidental hosts, will become infected. This results in an increase in the incidence of disease in late summer and early autumn.

The principal avian host and vector species vary markedly between geographic regions. In North America the house sparrow (*Passer domesticus*) is the principal amplifying host and *C. pipiens* is the principal vector. *C. pipiens,* and other mosquito vectors, feed almost exclusively on passerine and columbiform birds early in the season, but later in the summer in temperate regions switch to feeding on mammalian hosts. This change in feeding behavior is associated with increased frequency of infection and disease in mammals, including horses and humans, in the late summer.

The virus cycles between the avian host and insect vectors year round in tropical regions. However, in temperate regions in which mosquitoes do not survive during the winter the mechanism by which the virus survives over winter is unknown.

The primary vector involved in Murray Valley encephalitis virus transmission is the mosquito *C. annulirostris.*[1,3] Wading birds, particularly the rufous night heron (*Nycticorax caledonicus*) appear to be the principal natural reservoirs of Murray Valley encephalitis virus and West Nile virus in Australia.[1]

Transmission

Transmission is only by the bite of infected insect vectors. There is no evidence of horizontal spread of infection among horses. The disease can be spread in humans by transfusion of blood or transplantation of organs obtained from an infected person.

Animal Risk Factors

The disease occurs in parts of the world as epidemics, apparently associated with sporadic introduction of the virus into nonendemic regions, such as the Mediterranean littoral and parts of central Europe.[22] Introduction of the virus to these regions occurs infrequently enough that horses have no active immunity and are susceptible to infection and disease. Horses immune through either natural infection or vaccination are resistant to the disease. The effect of immunity was evidenced in North America by the marked decrease in morbidity and mortality among horses after the epizootic waned and the disease became enzootic. The decrease in morbidity was attributed to both natural and vaccinal immunity. Interestingly, although the number of cases in horses decreased rapidly, there was not a similar decrease in the number of human cases, perhaps because of the lack of a vaccine for use in humans.

Horses of all ages appear to be equally susceptible to infection. Disease is reported in horses aged from 5 months to >20 years. There does not appear to be any predilection based on breed or sex. Polymorphism in horse genome is associated with susceptibility to disease, including a haplotype associated with the promoter region of the OAS1 gene.[23]

Morbidity and Case Fatality

The incidence of the disease during an epizootic can be as high as 74 cases per 1000 horses at risk. The case–fatality rate for West Nile virus encephalomyelitis in horses in North America treated in the field is 22% to 44%, whereas it is 30% to 43% of horses in referral centers.[24] The case–fatality rate for West Nile virus (Kunjin) and Murray Valley encephalitis virus infected horses in Australia with signs of disease is 5% to 20%.[1]

Zoonotic Implications

Infection of humans by West Nile virus or Murray Valley encephalitis virus can result in fatal encephalitis, although less severe disease or inapparent infection is more common.[7,12,25] The virus has zoonotic potential and tissues from potentially infected animals and virus cultures should be handled in containment level 3 facilities, particularly material from potentially infected birds.

PATHOGENESIS

Horses are infected by the bite of infected mosquitoes. Feeding by as few as seven infected mosquitoes is sufficient to cause infection in seronegative horses. Viremia, which persists for less than 2 days, occurs 2 to 5 days after feeding by infected mosquitoes. West Nile encephalitis occurs in only a small proportion of infected horses. The virus localizes in cells in the CNS where it induces a severe polioencephalomyelitis with the most severe lesions being in the spinal cord. Lesions are often evident in the ventral horn of the spinal cord, which is consistent with clinical signs of weakness.

CLINICAL FINDINGS

The incubation period of Wes Nile virus after natural infection is estimated to be 8 to 15 days. Fever occurs early in the disease but is uncommon at the time that signs of neurologic disease become evident. Affected horses are often somnolent, listless, or depressed, although hyperexcitability has been reported. The signs of neurologic disease, including muscle fasciculation, weakness, and incoordination, develop within a period of hours and can progress over several days. Muscle fasciculations are common in the head and neck, but can occur in any muscle group. Weakness is most pronounced in limb and neck muscles and severely affected horses are recumbent with flaccid paralysis. Signs of neurologic disease are usually, but not reliably, bilaterally symmetric. Altered mentation, blindness, and cranial nerve abnormalities, if they occur, usually become evident after signs of spinal cord disease are apparent.

Weakness with or without ataxia is present in almost all affected horses, whereas altered mentation is detected in approximately 66% of horses. Cranial nerve abnormalities are evident in approximately 40% of horses, whereas apparent blindness or lack of menace reflex occurs in 3% to 7% of horses.

Median recovery time for horses treated in the field is 7 days, with a range of 1 to 21 days.

The prognosis depends on the severity of clinical signs. Horses that become recumbent and unable to rise are approximately 50 times more likely to die than are horses that remain able to stand while affected by the disease. Most horses that survive the initial disease do not have signs of neurologic dysfunction 6 months later.

Murray Valley encephalitis in horses causes signs consistent with encephalitis including fever, depressed mentation, abnormalities in cranial nerves including paralysis of the facial muscles, ataxia, and recumbency.[3,5] The clinical course can be prolonged.

Other Species

Disease associated with West Nile virus is documented in small numbers of other species, including squirrels, chipmunks, bats, dogs, cats, reindeer, sheep, alpaca, alligators, and a harbor seal during intense periods of local viral activity. West Nile virus infection in dogs is usually subclinical.[26] The disease in camelids is characterized by acute recumbency and altered mentation.

CLINICAL PATHOLOGY

Affected horses are often mildly lymphopenic, and hyperbilirubinemic (likely from anorexia), and occasionally azotemic. These changes are not diagnostic of West Nile or Murray Valley encephalitis.

CSF is abnormal in approximately 70% of horses with signs of neurologic disease. Abnormalities include mononuclear pleocytosis and elevated total protein concentration.[6]

Serologic Tests

Antibody can be identified in equine serum by IgM capture ELISA (IgM capture ELISA, M antibody-capture ELISA [MAC-ELISA]), HI, IgG ELISA, or plaque reduction neutralization (PRN).[27,28] Equine West Nile-specific IgM antibodies are usually first detectable 7–10 days after infection and persist for 1 to 2 months. Because the incubation period of the disease after infection by bite of infected mosquitoes is at least 8 days, West Nile-specific IgM is usually present at the time of development of clinical signs of the disease. MAC-ELISA is therefore a useful test in the diagnosis of the disease.

West Nile virus neutralizing antibodies are detectable in equine serum by 2 weeks postinfection and can persist for more than 1 year. In some serologic assays, antibody cross-reactions with related flaviviruses (St. Louis encephalitis virus or Japanese encephalitis virus), can be encountered. The PRN test is the most specific among West Nile serologic tests and all affected horses have titers ≥1:100 4 to 6 weeks after recovering from the disease, and 90% of horses maintain this titer 5 to 7 months after recovery.

Detection by MAC-ELISA of West Nile-specific IgM in serum at dilutions greater than 1:400, in the presence of appropriate clinical signs, is considered diagnostic of West Nile virus. Similarly, a fourfold increase in PRN titer in serum collected during the acute and convalescent stages of the disease, in the absence of vaccination and in the presence of appropriate clinical signs, is considered diagnostic.

Identification of West Nile Virus

The virus can be grown in cell culture, and viral nucleic acid can be demonstrated in tissues of infected animals by RT-PCR.[29,30] Note that infected horses have much lower concentrations of virus than do infected birds, and failure to demonstrate viral antigen in infected horses is not uncommon, especially if less sensitive techniques, such as IHC, are used.

NECROPSY FINDINGS

Gross lesions are infrequently seen. When present they consist of multifocal areas of congestion and hemorrhage within the medulla oblongata, midbrain, and spinal cord. Histopathologic changes include a nonsuppurative poliomeningoencephalomyelitis with multifocal glial nodules and neuronophagia. The inflammatory changes and viral distribution are concentrated in the rhombencephalon and spinal cord, with comparatively little damage to the cerebrum. One IHC study of naturally infected horses concluded that examination of the spinal cord is required to accurately identify West Nile virus infection. Another report, in which RT-PCR was used, concluded that high-quality samples of medulla were sufficient to detect the presence of the virus. Postmortem confirmation of the diagnosis through virus isolation is possible, but the sensitivity is generally inferior to molecular biology-based techniques. RT-PCR is generally superior to IHC. The processing of tissue from multiple CNS sites is recommended to increase the chances of finding a virus-rich focus. High concentrations of West Nile virus are not found in non-CNS tissues of infected equids, in contrast to the distribution of the virus in many other species.

Samples for Confirmation of Diagnosis

- **Virology:** minimum sample is half of sagittally sectioned hindbrain (must include medulla). Ideally a segment of thoracolumbar spinal cord as well. Submit samples chilled (VI, RT-PCR)
- **Histology:** same samples, fixed in formalin (LM, IHC, RT-PCR).

Note the zoonotic potential of this disease when collecting and submitting specimens. Some authorities recommend using containment level 3 precautions when handling potentially infected tissues, such as that from birds.

DIFFERENTIAL DIAGNOSIS

Differential diagnoses for West Nile encephalitis include (Table 14-11) the following:

- Eastern and Western encephalitis
- Venezuelan equine encephalitis
- Equine herpesvirus-1 myeloencephalopathy
- Hendra virus infection
- Rabies
- Botulism
- Hepatic encephalopathy
- Borna disease
- Equine protozoal myeloencephalitis
- Leukoencephalomalacia
- Lower motor neuron disease

TREATMENT

There is no specific treatment for West Nile encephalitis, although administration of IFN or hyperimmune globulin has been advocated. Affected horses are often administered nonsteroidal antiinflammatory drugs such as flunixin meglumine, dimethyl sulfoxide, or corticosteroids in an attempt to reduce inflammation in neural tissue. Administration of corticosteroids minimally but statistically significantly increases the likelihood of survival, but this practice is controversial. Treatment is based on supportive care and prevention of complications of neurologic disease and includes assistance to stand, including use of a sling support, administration of antimicrobials, and maintenance of hydration and nutrition.

CONTROL

Control of disease associated with West Nile virus and other flaviviruses is achieved by vaccination and minimization of exposure. It is important to recognize that factors affecting vector density, as happened in Australia in 2011, introduction of new vectors, or emergence of virus strains with higher virulence can affect incidence of the disease and require revision of existing control measures.[12,25,31] Elimination of the virus is not practical given that it cycles through avian and insect vectors and that the horse is incidentally infected.

Vaccination is effective in preventing development of disease, and reduces the likelihood of death in horses with West Nile encephalitis by approximately two to three times.[32-34] Vaccination is an important aspect of controlling the disease. There is no evidence that administration of the inactivated virus vaccine increases the risk of fetal loss in mares. Vaccination prevents viremia in most horses following exposure to West Nile virus-infected mosquitoes. Vaccination induces an IgG, but not an IgM, response in horses providing a means of identifying recently naturally infected horses from those with vaccine-induced serologic results.[32]

Both inactivated virus vaccine and a live canarypox-vectored recombinant vaccine are available in North America.[6] The inactivated virus vaccine should be administered in two doses at an interval of 3 to 6 weeks in early summer in the first instance, and then again once to twice yearly before the season of peak disease incidence. Foals from unvaccinated mares should be administered the vaccine beginning at 2 to 3 months of age, and foals of vaccinated mares should be administered the vaccine beginning at 7 to 8 months of age. Vaccination of foals that acquired passive immunity from the dam can be effective at inducing active immunity when the first dose of vaccine is administered at 3 months of age.[35]

Administration of the recommended two doses of inactivated virus vaccine fails to induce an adequate plaque reduction titer in approximately 14% of horses 4 to 6 weeks after vaccination and in 30% of horses 5 to 7 months after vaccination. This effect was especially evident in horses >10 years of age. These results indicate that some horses will not develop protective immunity against West Nile virus despite administration of vaccine in the recommended dose and interval.

Minimization of exposure of horses to the virus includes reducing the population density of mosquitoes and protecting horses from being bitten. Reducing the population of mosquitoes includes widespread spraying with insecticides and elimination of mosquito breeding sites. Widespread spraying in cities is used when the disease is a risk for humans but is not practical for controlling mosquitoes in rural areas. Environmental concerns make this approach to control unacceptable in many regions.

Removal of larval habitat by draining standing water is recommended for control of West Nile virus, although the efficacy of this approach has not been demonstrated. Standing water includes not just dams and ponds but also poorly maintained outdoor swimming pools, bird baths, discarded vehicle tires, and other receptacles that could hold water. Use of larvicidal compounds in standing water is recommended by some authorities.

Minimizing the frequency with which horses are bitten by mosquitoes has the potential to reduce the risk of contracting the disease. However, specific recommendations are not available. Housing during periods of peak mosquito activity, especially at dawn and dusk, might reduce the risk of disease.

FURTHER READING

Long MT. West Nile virus and equine encephalitis viruses new perspectives. *Vet Clin North Am Equine Pract*. 2014;30:523-540.

McVey DS, et al. West Nile Virus. *Rev - Off Int Epizoot*. 2015;2:431-439.

REFERENCES

1. Roche SE, et al. *Aust Vet J*. 2013;91:5.
2. Frost MJ, et al. *Emerg Infect Dis*. 2012;18:792.
3. Barton AJ, et al. *Aust Vet J*. 2015;93:53.
4. Mann RA, et al. *J Vet Diagn Invest*. 2013;25:35.
5. Gordon AN, et al. *J Vet Diagn Invest*. 2012;24:431.
6. Long MT. *Vet Clin North Am Equine Pract*. 2014;30:523.
7. McVey DS, et al. *Rev Sci Tec*. 2015;34:431.
8. Chaintoutis SC, et al. *Emerg Infect Dis*. 2013;19:827.
9. Ciccozzi M, et al. *Infect Genet Evol*. 2013;17:46.
10. McMullen AR, et al. *J Gen Virol*. 2013;94:318.
11. Añez G, et al. *PLoS Negl Trop Dis*. 2013;7:e2245.
12. Prow NA. *Int J Environ Res Public Health*. 2013;10:6255.
13. Tee SY, et al. *Aust Vet J*. 2012;90:321.
14. van den Hurk AF, et al. *Parasit Vectors*. 2014;7.
15. Setoh YX, et al. *J Gen Virol*. 2015;96:1297.
16. Bargaoui R, et al. *Transbound Emerg Dis*. 2015;62:55.
17. Zohaib A, et al. *Epidemiol Infect*. 2015;143:1931.
18. Prow NA, et al. *Int J Environ Res Public Health*. 2013;10:4432.
19. Amraoui F, et al. *PLoS ONE*. 2012;7.
20. Andreadis TG. *J Am Mosq Control Assoc*. 2012;28:137.
21. Jansen CC, et al. *Int J Environ Res Public Health*. 2013;10:3735.
22. Sedlak K, et al. *Epid Mik Imun*. 2014;63:307.
23. Rios JJ, et al. *PLoS ONE*. 2010;5:e10537.
24. Epp T, et al. *Can Vet J*. 2007;48:1137.
25. Selvey LA, et al. *PLoS Negl Trop Dis*. 2014;8:2656.
26. Bowen RA, et al. *Am J Trop Med Hyg*. 2006;74:670.
27. Long MT, et al. *J Vet Intern Med*. 2006;20:608.
28. Wagner B, et al. *Vet Immunol Immunopathol*. 2008;122:46.
29. Brault AC, et al. *J Med Entomol*. 2015;52:491.
30. Toplu N, et al. *Vet Pathol*. 2015;52:1073.
31. Kock RA. *Rev - Off Int Epizoot*. 2015;34:151.
32. Khatibzadeh SM, et al. *Am J Vet Res*. 2015;76:92.
33. Long MT, et al. *Equine Vet J*. 2007;39:491.
34. Minke JM, et al. *Vaccine*. 2011;29:4608.
35. Davis EG, et al. *Equine Vet J*. 2015;47:667.

JAPANESE ENCEPHALITIS

Japanese encephalitis is a neurologic disease of humans, horses, and cattle caused by Japanese encephalitis virus. The disease is an important zoonosis in Asia, arising as a result of virus infection of amplifying hosts (pigs) transmitted by mosquitos from the avian wildlife reservoir. Horses, cattle, and humans are not important in the propagation of the disease because of the low levels of viremia in these species. There is an effective vaccine.

ETIOLOGY

Japanese encephalitis flavivirus (JEV), a member of the Flaviviridae family (which also includes Murray Valley encephalitis virus, Kunjin virus, and West Nile virus), all of which cause disease in humans, horses, and other mammals, and Usutu virus, which causes disease only in birds.[1-3] JEV, an enveloped virus of about 50 nm in diameter, has a nonsegmented, single-stranded, positive-sense RNA genome of about 11 kb in length.[3] The genome has one long open reading frame (ORF) that encodes a single polyprotein is cleaved cotranslationally and posttranslationally into three structural proteins and seven nonstructural proteins. The three structural proteins are the capsid (C), precursor to membrane (prM), and envelope (E) proteins.[3] Based on the nucleotide sequence of genomic RNA, JEV is classified into five major genotypes.[4-9] Genotype 1 occurs in the People's Republic of China, Vietnam, South Korea, Northern Thailand, Cambodia, Japan, Australia, India, and Chinese Taipei; Genotype 2 occurs in Southern Thailand, Malaysia, Indonesia, Northern Australia, and Papua New Guinea; Genotype 3 is present in Indonesia, Malaysia, Nepal, Sri Lanka, India, Indochinese Peninsula, Philippines, Chinese Taipei, South Korea, People's Republic of China, Vietnam, and Japan; Genotype 4 was isolated only during 1980 and 1981 in Indonesia; and Genotype 5 occurs Malaysia, Tibet (China), and South Korea (Fig. 14-5).[2,4,5,9] JEV RNA has been detected in dead birds and a *C. pipiens* mosquitos in Italy.[10]

The virus cycles between avian and mammalian amplifying hosts and the mosquitoes (Fig. 14-6).[2] The natural maintenance reservoir for JEV are birds of the family Ardeidae (herons and egrets), which do not demonstrate clinical disease but do have high levels of viremias. The pig is the principal mammalian amplifying host among domestic animals. Horses, cattle, sheep, goats, dogs, cats, and humans become infected but likely play only a minor role in the spread of the virus because of the low level of viremia in these species. There are a number of species of mosquito important in the biology of the virus:[11,12] *C. tritaeniorhynchus* is the primary vector, whereas *C. gelidus*, *C. fuscocephala*, and *C. annulirostris* are considered as secondary/regional vectors. The virus has been detected in *Anopheles peditaeniatus Leicester*, *A. barbirostris* (*van der Walp*), and *A. subpictus* in India.

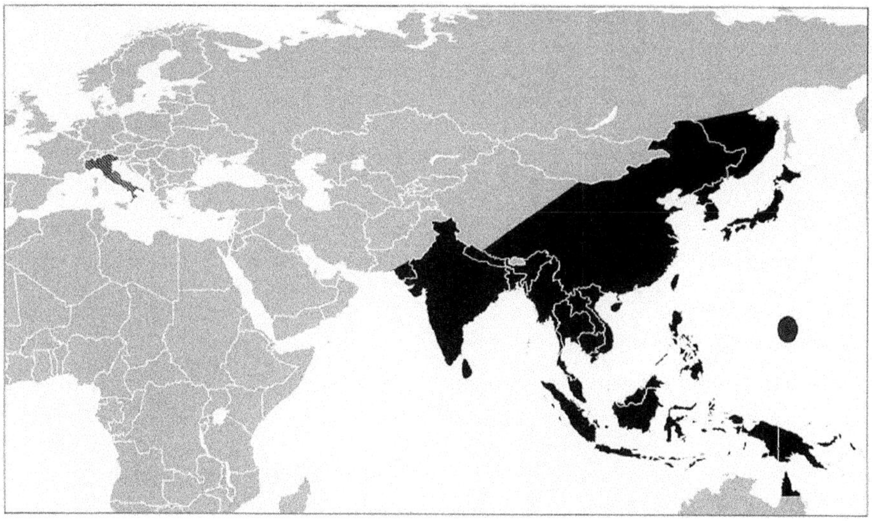

Fig. 14-5 Distribution of Japanese Encephalitis Virus as of 2015. Viral genome has been detected in dead birds and mosquitos in Italy, but the virus has not been isolated nor disease consistent with Japanese encephalitis detected in that country. (reproduced with the permission of the World Organisation for Animal Health (OIE, www.oie.int). Fig. 2 of Morita K., et al., Japanese encephalitis. *In* New developments in major vector-borne diseases. Part II: Important diseases for veterinarians (S. Zientara, D. Verwoerd & P.-P. Pastoret..., eds). *Rev. Sci. Tech. Off. Int. Epiz.*, 34 (2), page 443. doi: 10.20506/rst.34.2.2370.)

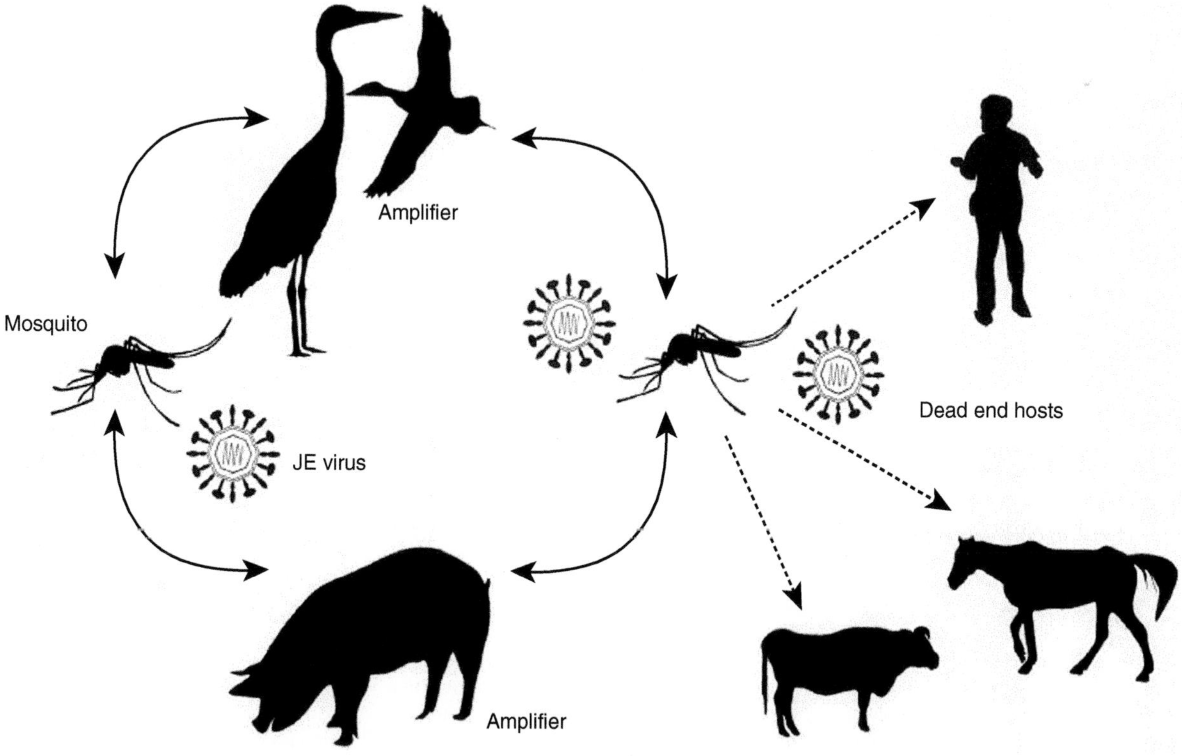

Fig. 14-6 Transmission cycle of Japanese encephalitis virus between amplifiers (pigs and wild birds) and mosquito vectors (especially *Culex tritaeniorhynchus*), including the infection of dead-end hosts (humans, horses, cattle). (reproduced with the permission of the World Organisation for Animal Health (OIE, www.oie.int). Fig. 3 of Morita K., et al., Japanese encephalitis. *In* New developments in major vector-borne diseases. Part II: Important diseases for veterinarians (S. Zientara, D. Verwoerd & P.-P. Pastoret..., eds). *Rev. Sci. Tech. Off. Int. Epiz.*, 34 (2), page 444. doi: 10.20506/rst.34.2.2370.)

Aedes koreicus, a potential vector of JEV, is reported for the first time in northern Italy/Switzerland (it has been reported in Belgium and parts of central Europe), continuing a pattern of climate change-induced incursions of insect vectors of important viral diseases into Europe.[13] *Ochlerotatus detritus* (syn. *Aedes detritus*), a temperate zone (British) mosquito can be infected by JEV in laboratory settings and might be a competent vector in the field, although this remains to be established.[11]

The virus is destroyed by heating for 30 minutes above 56°C and the thermal inactivation point (TIP) is 40°C. It is inactivated in acid environment of pH 1 to 3 but stable in alkaline environment of pH 7 to 9. The virus is very labile, is sensitive to ultraviolet light and gamma irradiation, and does not survive well in the environment.

EPIDEMIOLOGY

The disease in humans, horses, pigs, or cattle occurs **throughout the Orient and Southeast Asia** and has extended into Papua New Guinea, the Torres Strait, and northern Australia. Outbreaks of disease occurred in the Torres Strait in 1995, and disease in humans has occurred rarely in northern Australia. Outbreaks of disease have not occurred in Australia, despite large populations of wild pigs, wading birds, and mosquitoes probably because the mosquitoes prefer to feed on marsupials, which are poor hosts for JEV.

Sporadic clinical cases of JEV in horses have been reported in various countries including Japan, Hong Kong, Taiwan, and India.[4,14,15] Horse deaths are now uncommon in Japan with few to none reported in several decades,[2,15] because of vaccination of most horses, but 15% to 70% of race horses have antibodies to JEV that are not induced by vaccination. Antibodies against JEV were detected in 67 of 637 (10.5%) horses in India screened between 2006 and 2010.[14] Seroepidemiologic surveys of cattle in Japan reveal that about 68% of animals are positive. Disease in horses and humans occurs in China. The prevalence of the disease is related to the population of pigs, the main amplifying host; the mosquito vector; and susceptible human and equine hosts. Japanese encephalitis virus HI seroprevalence was 74.7% (95% CI = 71.5%–77.9%), JEV IgM seroprevalence was 2.3% (95% CI = 1.2%–3.2%) in pigs at slaughter in Laos, with greater prevalence during the monsoonal season.[16] Factors affecting the number of mosquitoes include availability of suitable habitat, such as a rice field in which survival of mosquito larvae is enhanced by application of nitrogenous fertilizers and the presence of phytoplankton, which provide food and shelter for the larvae.

CLINICAL SIGNS

The **clinical manifestations** of the disease in horses vary widely in severity.[15] Mild cases show fever up to 39.5°C (103°F), anorexia, sluggish movements, and sometimes jaundice for 2 to 3 days only. A more severe form of the disease includes lethargy with variable febrile periods (as high as 41°C), with a pronounced stupor, bruxism and chewing motions, difficulty in swallowing, petechiation of mucosa, incoordination, neck rigidity, apparent impaired vision, paresis, and paralysis. Recovery usually occurs within about a week. More severe cases show pronounced lethargy, mild fever, and somnolence. Jaundice and petechiation of the nasal mucosa are usual. There is dysphagia, incoordination, staggering, and falling. There is also a hyperexcitable form of the disease characterized by high fevers (41°C or higher), profuse sweating and muscle tremors, aimless wandering, behavioral changes manifested by aggression, loss of vision, collapse, coma, and death. This severe type of the disease is uncommon, representing only about 5% of the total cases, but is more likely to terminate fatally. In most cases complete recovery follows an illness lasting from 4 to 9 days. The disease occurs in foals and can manifest as encephalitis.[14]

Infection of **cattle, sheep, and goats** is usually clinically inapparent and of little overall significance, although rare cases of clinical disease occur in these species.[2,17,18] Widespread losses, however, have been reported in **swine**, particularly in Japan. The disease occurs as a nonsuppurative encephalitis in pigs under 6 months of age. Sows abort or produce dead pigs at term, and the disease has economic importance because of these losses.

CLINICAL PATHOLOGY

A variety of tests are available to detect antibodies to JEV or viral RNA. A latex agglutination test provides accurate detection of antibodies in the field. However, definitive diagnosis of Japanese viral encephalitis should not be based exclusively on serology because infection with antigenically related viruses including Murray Valley encephalitis virus, Kunjin virus, and West Nile virus can cause false-positive (from the perspective of JEV) results. Isolation of this flavivirus is difficult, and bioassay techniques are comparatively slow. As a result, detection via PCR is likely to be increasingly utilized. Tests to detect viral RNA in mammalian tissues or mosquitos are available.[19-23]

NECROPSY FINDINGS

There are no characteristic gross changes. As is typical of most viral encephalitides, microscopic changes include a nonsuppurative encephalomyelitis, focal gliosis, neuronal necrosis, and neuronophagia. Lesions in piglets following experimental infection are glial cell aggregates and perivascular cuffing throughout the olfactory tract and pyriform cortex. JEV antigens were detected in the cytoplasm and neuronal processes of small nerve cells in the granule cell layer of the olfactory bulb, in the neuronal processes of the olfactory tract, and in the cytoplasm of neurons in the pyriform cortex.[24]

IHC can be used to demonstrate this virus in formalin-fixed, paraffin-embedded sections.

ZOONOSIS[25,26]

Japanese encephalitis virus is endemic in 24 countries in the WHO Southeast Asia and Western Pacific regions with more than 3 billion people at risk of infection. Japanese encephalitis is the main cause of viral encephalitis in people in many countries of Asia occurring in almost 68,000 clinical cases yearly. Children are at greatest risk, with adults in endemic areas having protective immunity as a consequence of childhood infection. Most JEV infections are mild (fever and headache) or without apparent symptoms, but approximately 1 in 250 infections results in severe disease characterized by rapid onset of high fever, headache, neck stiffness, disorientation, coma, seizures, spastic paralysis, and death.[25] Although symptomatic JEV is rare, the case–fatality rate among those with encephalitis can be as high as 30%. Permanent neurologic or psychiatric sequelae occur in 30% to 50% of people with clinical encephalitis. There is no effective, specific treatment and care of affected people includes symptomatic treatment. Safe and effective vaccines are available to prevent JEV in people and consequently the WHO recommends JEV vaccination in all regions in which the disease is a recognized public health problem.[25]

Samples for Confirmation of Diagnosis

- **Virology:** 5 mL chilled CSF fluid, chilled brain (split along midline) (ISO, BIOASSAY, PCR)
- **Histology:** fixed samples of the other half of brain, lung, spleen, liver, heart (LM, IHC)

Note the zoonotic potential of this organism when handling carcass and submitting specimens.

DIFFERENTIAL DIAGNOSIS

Differential diagnosis in horses include[27] other equine viral encephalitides (Eastern, Western, Venezuelan, Murray Valley, West Nile), African horse sickness, Borna disease, EHV infection, equine infectious anemia, acute babesiosis, hepatic encephalopathy, rabies, tetanus, botulism, cerebral nematodiasis or protozoodiasis, or leukoencephalomalacia (*F. moniliforme*).

Differential diagnoses for pigs include[27] Menangle virus infection, porcine parvovirus infection, classical swine fever, porcine reproductive and respiratory syndrome, Aujeszky's disease (pseudorabies), La Piedad Michoacan paramyxovirus (blue eye paramyxovirus), hemagglutinating encephalomyelitis, encephalomyocarditis virus, porcine brucellosis, Teschen/Talfan, water deprivation/excess salt, and any other causative agent of stillbirth, mummification, embryonic death, and infertility (SMEDI) or encephalitis in newborns.

TREATMENT AND CONTROL

There is no specific treatment for the disease.

Control is by vaccination. Formalinized **vaccines** afford excellent protection in pigs and horses. A delta inulin-adjuvanted, inactivated cell culture-derived JEV vaccine was safe and well tolerated and induced a strong JEV-neutralizing antibody response in all foals and pregnant mares. The neutralizing activity was passively transferred to their foals via colostrum. Foals that acquired passive immunity to JEV via maternal antibodies had evidence of maternal antibody interference to subsequent vaccination at ~35 days, but not at 1 year of age.[28]

The virus is inactivated by organic and lipid solvents, common detergents, iodine, phenol iodophors of 70% ethanol, 2% glutaraldehyde, 3% to 8% formaldehyde, and 1% sodium hypochlorite.[27]

REFERENCES

1. Ziegler U, et al. *Vector Borne Zoonotic Dis.* 2015;15:481.
2. Morita K, et al. *Rev - Off Int Epizoot.* 2015;34:441.
3. Unni SK, et al. *Microbes Infect.* 2011;13:312.
4. Cherian SS, et al. *Arch Virol.* 2015;160:3097.
5. Li M-H, et al. *PLoS Negl Trop Dis.* 2011;5:1231.
6. Nabeshima T, et al. *Future Virol.* 2010;5:343.
7. Schuh AJ, et al. *J Gen Virol.* 2010;91:95.
8. Su C-L, et al. *PLoS Negl Trop Dis.* 2014;8:e3122.
9. Takhampunya R, et al. *Virol J.* 2011;8.
10. Ravanini P, et al. *Eurosurveillance.* 2012;17:2.
11. Mackenzie-Impoinvil L, et al. *Med Vet Entomol.* 2015;29:1.
12. van den Hurk AF, et al. *Annu Rev Entomol.* 2009;54:17.
13. Suter T, et al. *Parasit Vectors.* 2015;8:402.
14. Gulati BR, et al. *J Vet Sci.* 2012;13:111.
15. Yamanaka T, et al. *J Vet Med Sci.* 2006;68:293.
16. Conlan JV, et al. *Am J Trop Med Hyg.* 2012;86:1077.
17. Kako N, et al. *BMC Vet Res.* 2014;10.
18. Katayama T, et al. *J Clin Microbiol.* 2013;51:3448.
19. Cha G-W, et al. *PLoS ONE.* 2015;10:e0127313.
20. Chen YY, et al. *Transbound Emerg Dis.* 2014;61:37.
21. Deng J, et al. *J Virol Methods.* 2015;213:98.
22. Dhanze H, et al. *Arch Virol.* 2015;160:1259.
23. Glushakova LG, et al. *J Virol Methods.* 2015;214:60.
24. Yamada M, et al. *J Comp Pathol.* 2009;141:156.
25. Japanese encephalitis fact sheet 386. World Health Organisation, 2014. (Accessed 06.12.2015, at http://www.who.int/mediacentre/factsheets/fs386/en/.).
26. Ghosh D, et al. *PLoS Negl Trop Dis.* 2009;3:e437.
27. Japanese encephalitis. 2013. (Accessed August, 2016, at www.oie.int/fileadmin/Home/eng/Animal_Health_in_the_World/docs/pdf/Disease_cards/JAPANESE_ENCEPHALITIS.pdf.).
28. Bielefeldt-Ohmann H, et al. *Vet Res.* 2014;45.

EASTERN AND WESTERN EQUINE ENCEPHALOMYELITIS

SYNOPSIS

Etiology Eastern encephalitis and Western encephalitis viruses.

Epidemiology Disease limited to the Americas. Arthropod, usually mosquito-borne virus. Mammals, including horses, are accidental hosts. Horse is dead-end host for EEE and WEE. Case–fatality rate 5%–70%. WEE and EEE occur as sporadic cases and as outbreaks. Both diseases affect humans.

Clinical signs Fever, muscle fasciculation, severe depression, head-pressing, incoordination, recumbency, opisthotonus and paddling, and death.

Clinical pathology Leukopenia.

Lesions Nonsuppurative encephalomyelitis.

Diagnostic confirmation Virus isolation and identification. Identification of viral antigen by indirect immunofluorescence. Serologic confirmation of exposure, preferably demonstrating an increase in hemagglutination inhibition, virus neutralization, or complement fixation titer.

Treatment No specific treatment. Supportive care.

Control Vaccination with formalin-inactivated vaccines (EEE, WEE). Insect control.

EEE, *eastern equine encephalitis;* WEE, *western equine encephalitis.*

ETIOLOGY

Equine encephalomyelitis is associated with one of the two immunologically distinct arthropod-borne alphaviruses (family Togaviridae): **eastern equine encephalomyelitis** virus (EEE) and **western equine encephalomyelitis** virus (WEE).

- There is one EEE virus strain, but two antigenic variants: North American and South American.[1]
- WEE likely arose as a recombinant of EEE and Sindbis virus. There are strains of WEE from Argentina, Brazil, and South Dakota that differ antigenically, and there are four major lineages of WEE in California whose geographic distributions overlap.

All the viruses are extremely fragile and disappear from infected tissues within a few hours of death. Both EEE and WEE cause disease in humans.[2] **WEE** is the least virulent of these viruses in horses and humans and incidence of disease in humans appears to be declining.[3,4] Transmission cycles are depicted in Fig. 14-7.

EPIDEMIOLOGY

These encephalitis viruses cause disease in horses, humans, pigs, and various birds including ratites[5,6] and domestic pheasants.

Distribution

Equine eastern and western encephalomyelitis viruses are restricted to the Americas. The two viruses have distinct geographic ranges that may overlap: **EEE** is restricted to South America and North America typically east of the Mississippi River, whereas **WEE** is found west of the Mississippi River and predominantly in the western United States and Canada, although it also occurs in Florida and South America. There is recent evidence of extension of the range of EEE into northern Maine and Vermont and the emergence of the disease in Tennessee.[6-11]

Viral Ecology

Humans, horses, cattle, pigs, dogs, and ratites are accidental hosts of the virus. The EEE and WEE viruses are normally maintained in a host–vector relationship by cycling between mosquitoes, and some other hematophagous insects, and the definitive host. However, there are some important differences in the ecology of the different viruses.

Western Equine Encephalomyelitis

The definitive hosts of endemic WEE are wild birds, which are not clinically affected, and the vectors are the mosquitoes *C. tarsalis* (in the western United States) and *Culiseta melanura* (in the eastern and southern United States). Infected mosquitoes bite susceptible birds, usually nestlings or fledglings that then develop viremia. Mosquitoes are infected by feeding on viremic birds or by vertical transmission. Vertical transmission is likely an important overwintering mechanism in WEE, and possibly EEE.

Epidemics of WEE are uncommon, but sporadic individual cases are not. Epidemics of WEE are associated with factors that increase the number of infected mosquitoes or their feeding on susceptible (unvaccinated) horses. The disease in horses occurs in midsummer and fall, and is associated with a change in the feeding habits of *C. tarsalis.* Horses, and humans, are dead-end hosts because the viremia in these species is not sufficiently severe to allow infection of feeding **mosquitoes.**

Eastern Equine Encephalomyelitis

The primary **maintenance cycle of EEE virus** is transmission between passerine birds by the mosquito *C. melanura,* an inhabitant of drainage ditches and swamps. However, other mosquitoes, including *Aedes sollicitans* and *A. vexans,* can propagate the virus through infection of large shore birds. The Carolina chickadee and yellow-crowned night heron are the most common avian hosts in the southeastern United States. Virus is detected in *C. melanura* and *Anopheles quadrimaculatus* mosquitos in Florida in February, both of which feed on the black-crowned night heron (*Nycticorax nycticorax*), The yellow-crowned night heron (*Nyctanassa violacea*), anhinga (*Anhinga anhinga*), and great blue heron (*Ardea herodias*), suggesting a means for the virus cycle to overwinter.[12] There is increasing evidence that snakes could be a reservoir for the virus, with high seroprevalence rates for antibody to EEE.[13,14] The reservoir of the virus during winter might involve the vertical

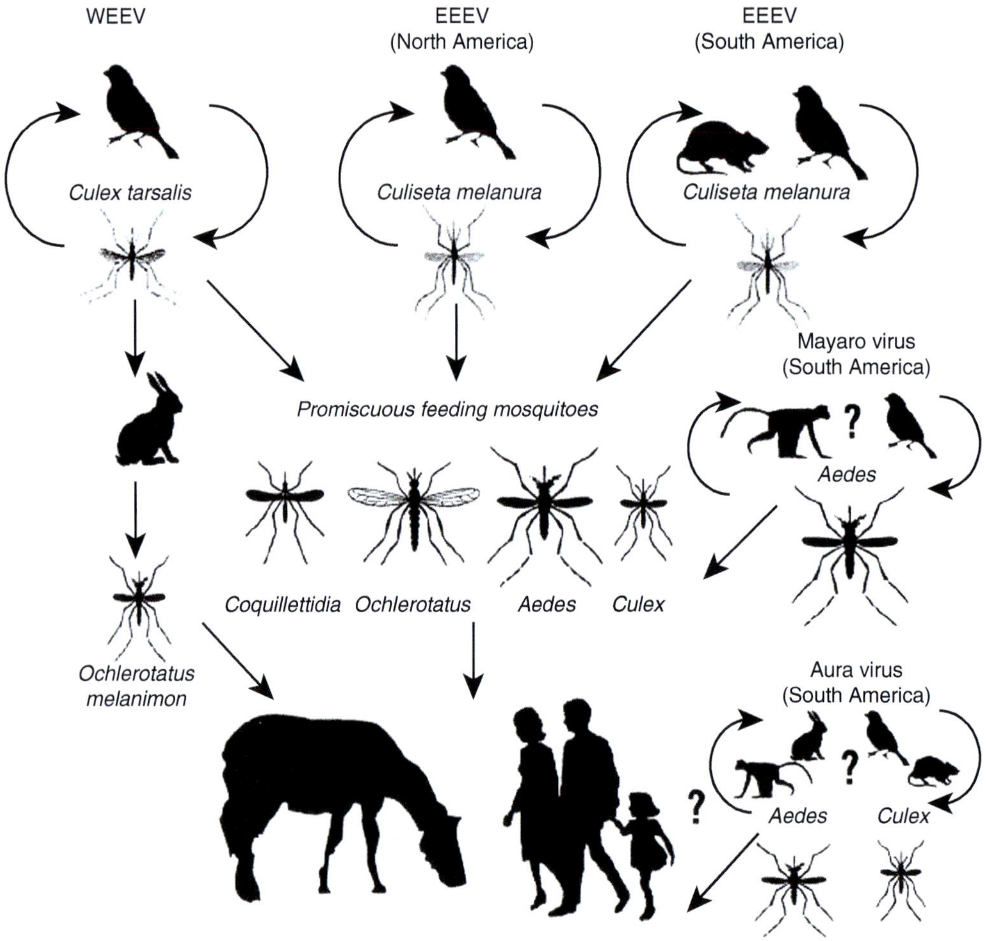

Fig. 14-7 Transmission cycles for infection with Western Equine Encephalitis Virus and Eastern Equine Encephalitis Virus in the Americas. (reproduced with the permission of the World Organisation for Animal Health (OIE, www.oie.int). Adapted from Fig. 1 of Arechiga-Ceballos N. & A. Aguilar-Setién, Alphaviral equine encephalomyelitis (Eastern, Western and Venezuelan). *In* New developments in major vector-borne diseases. Part II: Important diseases for veterinarians (S. Zientara, D. Verwoerd & P.-P. Pastoret..., eds). *Rev. Sci. Tech. Off. Int. Epiz.,* 34 (2), page 492. doi: 10.20506/rst.34.2.2374.)

transmission of infection to larvae that survive the winter.

The vertebrate host in South America has not been identified, but cotton rats and house sparrows both have the potential to be vectors.[15] The virus in North America likely has Florida as its overwintering site with subsequent seasonal spread into other states of the United States and into Eastern Canada.[1,12]

Horses are usually dead-end hosts, although viremia can be sufficiently severe in some horses to permit infection of mosquitoes.

Epidemics of EEE have occurred in the provinces of Ontario and Quebec; in virtually all the states of the United States east of the Mississippi River; in Arkansas, Minnesota, South Dakota, and Texas; in many of the Caribbean Islands; in Guatemala, Mexico, and Panama; and in Argentina, Brazil,[2,16] Columbia, Ecuador, Guyana, Peru, Suriname, and Venezuela. EEE continues to cause significant death losses annually in horses in Florida, primarily in unvaccinated horses. It is suggested that the incidence of clinical disease caused by EEE in Florida is much higher than reported, and there is a need to increase public awareness about the importance of vaccination, particularly in foals. **Unexpected epizootics** occur in inland states of the United States, and frequently the source of the infection is undetermined, although **meteorologic factors** that allow rapid movement of infected mosquitoes may be important.[5] For instance, in 1972, outbreaks of EEE occurred in Quebec, Canada, and in Connecticut, which originated with mosquitoes carried on surface winds from Connecticut to Quebec, a distance of 400 km, in 14 to 16 hours at a speed of 25 to 30 km/h and a temperature of 15°C. There may be a continual cycle of EEE virus in mosquitoes and birds in the southeastern United States, from where the virus could be distributed by infected mosquitoes on the wind along the Gulf and Atlantic Coasts and up the Mississippi Valley.

There is an increased likelihood of detecting the virus in mosquitos near wooded areas in Florida, an observation that is consistent with the patchy occurrence of the disease in that state.[17] An outbreak of EEE in equids, a llama, and pheasants in Maine was associated with unusually high numbers of *C. melanura* that year.[8]

Animal Risk Factors

Recovered horses are resistant to infection for at least 2 years, and vaccination confers immunity of variable duration (see under the section Control). **Unvaccinated horses** are at increased risk of disease; the risk of a vaccinated horse contracting EEE is only 0.14 that of an unvaccinated horse. The disease is more severe, and case fatality is higher, in unvaccinated horses than in vaccinated horses. The case fatality in young foals from nonimmune mares, which are infected with WEE, is always high, often as high as 100%.

Housing and **exposure to mosquitoes** are important risk factors for EEE, and presumably WEE. During an outbreak in 1831, only horses kept at pasture were affected. The use of **insect repellants** reduces the odds of a horse being infected with EEE to 0.04 that of an unprotected horse. Similarly, keeping horses at pasture near woods increases the risk of disease by almost four times, and the presence of **swamp land** increases the risk by over two times. Horses kept in areas with **high precipitation** have an increased risk of the disease, presumably because of the density of mosquitoes in these areas.

Morbidity and Case Fatality

Morbidity varies widely depending on seasonal conditions and the prevalence of insect vectors; cases may occur sporadically or in the form of severe outbreaks affecting 20% or more of a group. The prevalence of infections, as judged by serologic examination, is much higher than the clinical morbidity with ~9% of horses in Quebec serologically positive for EEE but with a much lower rate of occurrence of clinical disease.[18] The **case–fatality rate** differs with the strain of the virus; in infection with the WEE virus it is usually 20% to 30% and with the EEE it is usually between 40% and 80% and may be as high as 90%.

Zoonotic Implications

The **susceptibility of humans** to the causative virus gives the disease great public health importance. Humans can become infected with the EEE and the WEE virus.[2]

PATHOGENESIS

Inapparent infection is the mildest form of the disease and may be characterized by only a transient fever. A more severe form of the disease is manifested by tachycardia, depression, anorexia, occasional diarrhea, and fever.

A transitory **viremia** occurs at the height of the fever. Penetration of the virus into the **brain** does not occur in all cases, and the infection does not produce signs, other than fever, unless involvement of the CNS occurs. The lesions produced in nervous tissue are typical of a viral infection and are localized particularly in the **gray matter of the cerebral cortex, thalamus, and hypothalamus**, with minor involvement of the medulla and spinal cord. It is this distribution of lesions that is responsible for the characteristic signs of mental derangement, followed at a later stage by paralysis. The early apparent blindness and failure to eat or drink appear to be cortical in origin. True blindness and pharyngeal paralysis occur only in the late stages.

CLINICAL FINDINGS

The diseases associated with EEE and WEE viruses are **clinically indistinguishable**. The **incubation period** for EEE is 1 to 3 days and is 2 to 9 days for WEE. Uncomplicated disease usually lasts about 1 week. In the initial viremic stage there is fever, which may be accompanied by anorexia and depression, but the reaction is usually so mild that it goes unobserved. In the experimental disease, the temperature may reach 41°C (106°F) persisting for only 24 to 48 hours, with signs of neurologic dysfunction appearing at the peak of the fever. Animals that have signs of neurologic disease for more than 24 hours are often not pyrexic.

Initial signs of neurologic disease include hypersensitivity to sound and touch, and in some cases transient periods of excitement and restlessness, with apparent blindness. Horses can have a period of anorexia and colic before onset of signs of neurologic disease. Affected horses may walk blindly into objects or walk in circles and in severe cases can mimic signs of horses with catastrophic intestinal disease. Involuntary muscle movements occur, especially tremor of shoulder and facial muscles and erection of the penis. A stage of severely depressed mentation follows. Affected horses stand with the head hung low; they appear to be asleep and may have a half-chewed mouthful of feed hanging from the lips. At this stage the horse may eat and drink if food is placed in its mouth. The pupillary light reflex is still present. The animal can be aroused, but soon relapses into a state of somnolence.

A stage of **paralysis** follows. There is inability to hold up the head, and it is often rested on a solid support. The lower lip is pendulous and the tongue protrudes from the mouth. Unnatural postures are adopted, with the horse often standing with the weight balanced on the forelegs or with the legs crossed. Head-pressing or leaning back on a halter are often seen. On walking, there is obvious incoordination, particularly in the hindlegs, and circling is common. Defecation and urination are suppressed, and the horse is unable to swallow. Complete paralysis is the terminal stage. The horse goes down, is unable to rise, and usually dies within 2 to 4 days from the first signs of illness. A proportion of affected horses do not develop paralysis and survive, but have persistent neurologic deficits.

Pigs

EEE causes an encephalitis and myocarditis of piglets less than 2 weeks of age. The disease is characterized by incoordination, seizures, vomition, weight loss, and paddling. Recovered piglets can have retarded growth.

Ratites and Pheasants

The disease in emus is characterized by vomiting, bloody diarrhea, and depression with absent to minimal signs of neurologic disease.[5] Pheasants display signs of neurologic disease and aberrant behavior such as excessive aggressive pecking and mortality rates of 30%.[8] Wild turkeys are rarely clinically infected, although they can become infected.[8]

CLINICAL PATHOLOGY

There are no characteristic hematologic or biochemical abnormalities. The absence of biochemical indication of liver disease (hyperbilirubinemia, increased activity in serum of liver-specific enzymes such as sorbitol dehydrogenase or γ-glutamyl transferase, absence of hyperammonemia) rules out hepatic encephalopathy.

Diagnostic confirmation is achieved by one or more of the following:

- Isolation of virus from an affected animal
- Detection of viral antigen or nucleic acid in an animal with appropriate clinical signs
- Seroconversion or an increase in serum titer of sick or recovered animal

Virus isolation provides definitive proof of infection. However, viremia may have resolved by the time nervous signs have developed, and it can be advantageous to sample febrile animals instead of animals showing more advanced signs of the disease. Virus can be cultured in intracranially inoculated suckling mice, weanling mice, guinea pigs, cell culture, newly hatched chicks, or embryonated eggs. Viral genome can be detected, and isolates can be identified, by quantitative RT-PCR,[19-21] or by complement fixation, HI, virus neutralization, immunofluorescent assay (IFA), and antigen capture ELISA.

Acute and convalescent sera taken 10 to 14 days apart for the presence of neutralizing, hemagglutination-inhibiting, or complement-fixing antibodies in the serum of affected or in-contact horses, is of value in detecting the presence of the virus in the group or in the area. A fourfold increase in complement-fixing antibodies is considered positive.

Demonstration of viral nucleic acid in tissue, blood, or insects by PCR test may be a useful indicator of the presence of the virus. There may be sufficient viral antigen to be detected by ELISA in clinical material, and this may provide a useful test in the early stages of an epidemic.

The presence of a high HI, complement fixation and neutralizing antibody in a **single serum sample** obtained from a horse during the acute phase of illness associated with the WEE virus can be used as presumptive evidence of infection with this virus. However, antibodies against the WEE virus can persist for years, are produced after vaccination with WEE or WEE/EEE bivalent vaccines, and in foals might be caused by colostral immunity. Therefore a single serum sample cannot be used to make a confirmed diagnosis of WEE using the HI, complement fixation or neutralization tests. Horses infected experimentally or naturally with either the WEE or the EEE virus do not produce detectable HI or neutralizing antibody for 5 to 10 days after infection.

Circulating antibody appears on or near the day of onset of clinical illness. Infection with the WEE virus results in the production of serum IgM specific to WEE, and the ELISA test is a rapid, sensitive, and specific test for IgM against WEE and EEE viruses. Additionally, the ratio of titers of EEE and WEE can be useful in detecting infection by EEE; ratios of >8:1 are highly suggestive of EEE infection.

NECROPSY FINDINGS

The brain meninges may appear congested, but there are generally no gross changes. Histologic examination of the brain reveals perivascular accumulations of leukocytes and damage to neurons. The gray matter of the forebrain and midbrain are the most severely affected areas. Lesions associated with EEE antigen are also present in myocardium, stomach, intestine, urinary bladder, and spleen.

Cell culture and transmission experiments using brain tissue as an inoculum are the traditional means of confirming a diagnosis and require that the brain be removed within an hour of death. Transmission is by intracerebral inoculation of brain tissue into sucking mice or duck embryo tissue culture. Fluorescent antibody tests have been developed to detect EEE virus in brain tissue. A PCR-based diagnostic test is available for EEE virus. Lesions similar to those seen in horses have also been described in a beef cow infected with EEE. **The disease in piglets** is characterized by disseminated perivascular cuffing, gliosis, focal necrosis of the cerebral cortex, and multifocal myocardial necrosis.

Samples for Postmortem Confirmation of Diagnosis

- Half of midsagittally sectioned brain and liver and spleen should be submitted for fluorescent antibody and PCR testing, virus isolation and bioassay.
- Half of midsagittally sectioned brain, fixed in formalin, should be submitted for light microscopic examination.

Note the zoonotic potential of these organisms when handling the carcass and submitting specimens.

DIFFERENTIAL DIAGNOSIS

Clinically, the disease has very great similarity to the other viral encephalomyelitides, from which it can often be discriminated by the geographic location of the horse, and to the hepatic encephalopathies and a number of other diseases (see later and in Table 14-12).

West Nile encephalitis is predominantly a myelitis with later development of signs of neurologic disease, whereas EEE and WEE have predominant signs of encephalopathy.

- Rabies.
- Borna disease (occurs in Europe).
- Japanese encephalitis (occurs in Asia).
- Various other viral infections that are geographically restricted.
- Hepatic encephalopathy, such as that associated with poisoning by *Crotalaria*, *Senecio*, and *Amsinckia* spp.; acute serum hepatitis or hepatopathy.
- Botulism causes weakness evident as muscle fasciculation, recumbency, and dysphagia, but does not cause cerebral signs (irritation, behavioral abnormalities).
- Yellow star thistle poisoning (*Centaurea solstitialis*, and poisoning by fumonisins (*Fusarium moniliforme*) can produce similar clinical signs to that of the encephalitides, with the exception of fever.

TREATMENT

There is no definitive or specific treatment. Supportive treatment may be given with the intention to prevent self-inflicted injury and maintain hydration and nutritional status.

CONTROL

Control of viral encephalomyelitis of horses is based on the following:

- Accurate clinical and laboratory diagnosis of the disease in horses
- Use of sentinel animals to monitor the presence of the virus in the region
- Quarantine of infected horses to stop movement of virus donors
- Insect abatement when deemed necessary
- Vaccination of all horses.

Vaccination

Vaccination of horses is important for the control of EEE and VEE.[3,22] Formalin-inactivated EEE and WEE virus vaccines are available (see Table 14-14 in Venezuelan Equine Encephalitis) and are effective, although over 50% of horses with EEE had been vaccinated within the previous year. This apparent poor protection can be explained by many horses not developing a detectable change in antibody titer after vaccination with a bivalent vaccine and rapid decreases in antibody titer from a peak value achieved 2 to 4 weeks after vaccination. Vaccines are available as univalent or bivalent preparations and in combination with other antigens (for instance, tetanus toxoid). Horses should be vaccinated well in advance of the anticipated encephalomyelitis season in a given area. Vaccination against both strains of the virus is advisable in areas where the strain has not been identified or where both strains exist. The currently recommended vaccination schedule consists of two doses of the vaccine initially, 10 days apart, followed by annual revaccination using two or three doses.[22] **Annual revaccination** is currently recommended because the duration of effective immunity beyond 1 year is not known. It is probable that the initial two-dose vaccination lasts for up to 3 to 4 years. The emphasis in a vaccination program should be on the young horses.

Colostral antibody can be detected in the blood of foals from vaccinated dams for up to 6 to 7 months, after which time it declines rapidly. Foals from vaccinated dams should be vaccinated at 6 to 8 months of age and revaccinated at 1 year of age. Foals from unvaccinated dams may be vaccinated at 2 to 3 months of age and again at 1 year of age. Colostral antibodies in the foal will prevent the development of autogenous antibodies, and foals vaccinated when less than 6 months should be revaccinated when they are 1 year old or, in high-risk areas. Foals from vaccinated mares should be vaccinated at 3, 4, and 6 months of age.

Experimental DNA vaccines hold promise for the prevention of WEE.

Protection From Insects

Housing of horses indoors at night, especially in fly-proofed stables, and the use of insect repellents may restrain the spread of the virus. Use of insect repellents decreases the risk of EEE in horses to 0.04 that of unprotected horses.

Widespread spraying of insecticides to reduce the population of the vector insects has been used in the control of VEE; however, such measures are not practical for preventing sporadic cases of EEE or WEE, and the environmental impact of widespread insecticide use should be considered.

Complete eradication of the virus appears to be impossible because of the enzootic nature of the ecology of the virus. The horse is an accidental host for EEE and WEE virus making elimination of the virus impossible with methods currently available.

Zoonotic Aspects of Control

Control of the disease in humans in areas where the disease may occur is dependent on insect control, and a monitoring and surveillance early warning system is necessary to decide whether or not to take control measures. In areas where WEE occurs, clinical cases of the disease in unvaccinated horses usually precede the occurrence of the disease in humans. The establishment of a reporting system in which practicing veterinarians report all clinical cases of the disease in horses will also assist in predicting potential epidemics of WEE virus infection in the human population. Serologic surveys of wildlife may also serve as good indicators of the geographic distribution and seasonality of circulation of these viruses and provide an early warning system before the detection of human cases.

FURTHER READING

Arechiga-Ceballos N, et al. Alphaviral equine encephalomyelitis (Eastern, Western and Venezuelan). *Rev - Off Int Epizoot*. 2015;34:491-510.

Long MT. West Nile virus and equine encephalitis viruses new perspectives. *Vet Clin North Am Equine Practice*. 2014;30:523-533.

REFERENCES

1. White GS, et al. *Am J Trop Med Hyg*. 2011;84:709.
2. Carrera J-P, et al. *N Engl J Med*. 2013;369:732.
3. Arechiga-Ceballos N, et al. *Rev - Off Int Epizoot*. 2015;34:491.

4. Zacks MA, et al. *Vet Microbiol.* 2010;140:281.
5. Chenier S, et al. *Can Vet J.* 2010;51:1011.
6. Saxton-Shaw KD, et al. *PLoS ONE.* 2015;10:e0128712.
7. Mukherjee S, et al. *J Med Entomol.* 2012;49:731.
8. Lubelczyk C, et al. *Am J Trop Med Hyg.* 2013;88:95.
9. Lubelczyk C, et al. *Vector Borne Zoonotic Dis.* 2014;14:77.
10. Molaei G, et al. *Parasit Vectors.* 2015;8:516.
11. Mutebi J-P, et al. *Vector Borne Zoonotic Dis.* 2015;15:210.
12. Bingham AM, et al. *Am J Trop Med Hyg.* 2014;91:685.
13. White G, et al. *Am J Trop Med Hyg.* 2011;85:421.
14. Graham SP, et al. *Am J Trop Med Hyg.* 2012;86:540.
15. Arrigo NC, et al. *Emerg Infect Dis.* 2010;16:1373.
16. de Novaes Oliveira R, et al. *Arch Virol.* 2014;159:2615.
17. Vander Kelen PT, et al. *Int J Health Geogr.* 2012;11:47.
18. Rocheleau J-P, et al. *Vector Borne Zoonotic Dis.* 2013;13:712.
19. Armstrong PM, et al. *Vector Borne Zoonotic Dis.* 2012;12:872.
20. Brault AC, et al. *J Med Entomol.* 2015;52:491.
21. Zink SD, et al. *Diag Microbiol Infect Dis.* 2013;77:129.
22. Long MT. *Vet Clin North Am Equine Pract.* 2014;30:523.

VENEZUELAN EQUINE ENCEPHALOMYELITIS

SYNOPSIS

Etiology Venezuelan encephalitis virus (types IAB, IC, and, to a lesser extent, IE), an alphavirus.

Epidemiology Disease limited to the Americas. Arthropod-borne, usually mosquito-borne, virus. VEE occurs as epidemics associated with mutation of virus and associated movement from enzootic to epizootic cycles. Virus cycles between sylvatic rodents (and probably not birds) and mosquitos in enzootic areas. Equids and humans are amplifying hosts important in propagation of VEE in epizootics. Care–fatality rate 5%–70% for equids.

Clinical findings Fever, muscle fasciculation, severe depression, head-pressing, incoordination, recumbency, opisthotonus and paddling, and death.

Clinical pathology Leukopenia.

Lesions Nonsuppurative encephalomyelitis.

Diagnostic confirmation Virus isolation and identification. RT-PCR provides more rapid identification of virus. Identification of viral antigen by indirect immunofluorescence. Serologic confirmation of exposure, preferably demonstrating an increase in hemagglutination inhibition, virus neutralization, or complement fixation titer.

Treatment No specific treatment. Supportive care.

Control Vaccination with formalin-inactivated or modified live virus is effective. Vaccines being developed with newer technologies. Insect control.

RT-PCR, *reverse transcriptase-polymerase chain reaction.*

ETIOLOGY

Venezuelan equine encephalomyelitis (VEE) is associated with an arthropod-borne alphavirus (family Togaviridae) VEE. The VEE complex has one virus, VEE, with six antigenically related subtypes: I, VEE; II, Everglades; III, Mucambo; IV, Pixuna; V, Cabassou; and VI, AG80-663. Within subtype I are at least five variants (IAB, IC, ID, IE, and IF). Epidemic (pathogenic) VEE in horses is associated with variants IAB (originally identified as distinct variants, A and B are now considered the same variant) IC, and IE; all other subtypes of I (D-F), and other variants of VEE virus (II-VI), are usually nonpathogenic for horses and are found in sylvatic or enzootic, nonequine cycles, although they can cause disease in humans.[1] The pathogenic variant, IAB, has been detected in cryptic circulation up to 8 years after an epizootic.[2] The infection cycles between rodents and mosquitos as an enzootic cycle not associated with disease in equids or humans (Fig. 14-8). Birds might be involved in this enzootic cycling. Disease occurs when pathogenic variants of the virus become established and cycle between humans or horses, both of which have high levels of viremia, and mosquitos.[1,3]

Outbreaks of disease in horses and humans occur infrequently, but can affect large numbers of equids and humans when they do occur. Outbreaks were documented in Mexico in 1993 and 1996, and in Venezuela and Columbia in the autumn of 1995. The Columbian outbreak affected 90,000 people and killed an estimated 4000 horses. The strain involved in the Columbian outbreak was IC, whereas that involved in the Mexican outbreaks was a variant of the usually nonpathogenic IE. The outbreak in Mexico was associated with a variant of VEE that did not cause viremia in horses, although it was capable of causing neurologic disease in this species, and it might have been this attribute that abbreviated the course of the epidemic. There is evidence of continuing enzootic circulation of VEE IE in southern Mexico.[4,5]

The virus is extremely fragile and disappears from infected tissues within a few hours of death.

EPIDEMIOLOGY

Venezuelan equine encephalitis virus infects a range of species including rodents, humans, equids, cattle and dogs.[5] It causes disease in humans and equids.

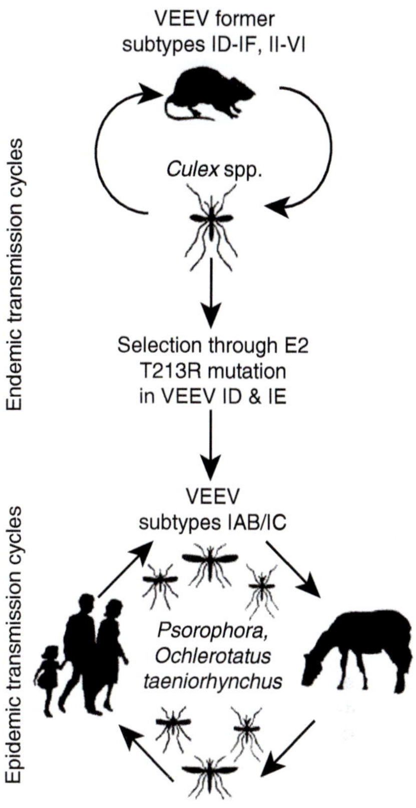

Fig. 14-8 Epidemiology of Venezuelan Equine Encephalitis virus in enzootic (endemic) and epizootic (epidemic) cycles. Note the need for mutation of the virus for development and establishment of epizootics. (reproduced with the permission of the World Organisation for Animal Health (OIE, www.oie.int). Adapted from Fig. 1 of Arechiga-Ceballos N. & A. Aguilar-Setién, Alphaviral equine encephalomyelitis (Eastern, Western and Venezuelan). *In* New developments in major vector-borne diseases. Part II: Important diseases for veterinarians (S. Zientara, D. Verwoerd & P.-P. Pastoret..., eds). *Rev. Sci. Tech. Off. Int. Epiz.*, 34 (2), page 492. doi: 10.20506/rst.34.2.2374.)

Distribution

Pathogenic or epizootic VEE is found in northern South America, Central America, Mexico and, rarely, in the southern United States. The epizootic variants are currently exotic to the United States. Enzootic VEE strains have been identified in the Florida Everglades (subtype II), Mexico (variant IE), Central American countries (variant IE), Panama (variants ID and IE), Venezuela (variant ID), Colombia (variant ID), Peru (variants ID, IIIC, and IIID), French Guiana (variant IIIB and subtype V), Ecuador (variant ID), Suriname (variant IIIA), Trinidad (variant IIIA), Brazil (variants IF and IIIA and subtype IV), and Argentina (subtype VI). In an atypical ecologic niche, variant IIIB has been isolated in the United States (Colorado and South Dakota) in an unusual association with birds.[3]

Viral Ecology

VEE exists as both nonpathogenic and pathogenic strains. **Nonpathogenic VEE viruses** persist in sylvatic cycles in northern South America, Central America, and parts of the southern United States, and are important because they are the source of the epizootic strains of the virus that emerge at infrequent intervals. The enzootic strains also confound the diagnosis of VEE because of the extensive serologic cross-reactivity among endemic and epidemic VEE viruses. However, recent advances in diagnostic techniques may have solved this diagnostic problem. The nonpathogenic viruses are maintained in rodents associated with swamps, and transmitted by mosquitoes of the genus *Culex,* and perhaps other hematophagous insects. Humans, horses, cattle, pigs, dogs, and ratites are accidental hosts of the virus. **Epidemics of VEE** occur irregularly, the latest being in northern Columbia in 1995, and Mexico in 1993 and 1996. The source of virus during outbreaks is infected horses. **Horses** develop a profound viremia and are **amplifying hosts** that aid in the spread of the epizootic; other domestic species, including cattle, pigs, and goats, are not considered to be amplifiers of the virus. During epizootics, all species of mosquitoes that feed on horses, including *Aedes, Psorophora,* and *Deinocerites* species, are thought to be capable of spreading the infection, although *O. taeniorhynchus* is thought to be the principal vector responsible for transmission of VEE virus during outbreaks, whereas *Culex* (*Melanoconion*) species mosquitoes transmit enzootic strains of VEE virus.[6] Epizootics end as the population of susceptible horses decreases below a critical level, either by death or vaccination. The **reservoir of the virus between outbreaks**, which may be up to 19 years, was unknown until it was demonstrated that epidemic VEE type IAB virus arises by **mutation of endemic strains** (types ID-F and II-VI), or that type IE (enzootic) mutates into an epizootic form serologically very similar to IE. This mutation of the endemic virus into the epidemic form has occurred on at least three occasions associated with epidemics of VEE. It is likely that pathogenic strains of VEE will continue to emerge in areas where the nonpathogenic strains of the virus are endemic.

Animal Risk Factors

Recovered horses are resistant to infection for at least 2 years, and vaccination confers immunity of variable duration (see under the section Control). **Housing** and **exposure to mosquitoes** are important risk factors for EEE, and presumably VEE.

Morbidity varies widely depending on seasonal conditions and the prevalence of insect vectors; cases may occur sporadically or in the form of severe outbreaks affecting 20% or more of a group. The prevalence of infections, as judged by serologic examination, is much higher than the clinical morbidity; for example, up to 72% of horses examined in the Gulf region of Mexico had antibodies to VEE virus (variant IE).[5] Only 0.8% of horses in Trinidad have serologic evidence of infection.[7]

The **case-fatality rate** is usually 40% to 80% and may be as high as 90% with VEE.

Zoonotic Implications

The **susceptibility of humans** to the causative virus gives the disease great public health importance. Humans can become infected with sylvatic and epizootic VEE subtypes. A recent outbreak of VEE in Columbia caused 75,000 human cases, 300 fatalities, and killed approximately 4000 horses. **Human infections** generally follow equine infections by approximately 2 weeks. The infection in humans is usually a mild, influenza-like illness in which recovery occurs spontaneously. When clinical encephalitis does occur, it is usually in very young or older people. Occurrence of the disease in humans can be limited by the use of a vaccine in horses, thus limiting the occurrence of the disease in horses in the area. There is a strong relationship between the **mosquito population** and the incidence of the disease in horses and in humans. The occurrence of the disease in humans may be predicted by an unusually high activity of virus in mosquitoes. There are usually, but not always, widespread mortalities in horses before the disease occurs in humans. VEE infections, and disease, of epizootic or enzootic virus have occurred among **laboratory workers** as a result of aerosol infections from laboratory accidents, from handling of infected laboratory animals, or inhalation of cage debris of infected laboratory animals.[3] Human VEE virus infections have originated by aerosol transmission from the cage debris of infected laboratory rodents and from laboratory accidents. Those who handle infectious VEE viruses or their antigens prepared from infected tissues or cell cultures should be vaccinated and shown to have demonstrable immunity in the form of a VEE virus-specific neutralizing antibody.

All procedures producing aerosols from VEE virus materials should be conducted in biosafety cabinets at containment level 3.[3]

VEEV viruses are highly infectious via the aerosol route for humans and has been developed as a biologic weapon in the United States and in the former Soviet Union.[6]

The TC83 live attenuated VEE virus vaccine may be **teratogenic** in humans.

PATHOGENESIS

Inapparent infection is the mildest form of the disease and may be characterized by only a transient fever. A more severe form of the disease is manifested by tachycardia, depression, anorexia, occasional diarrhea, and fever.

Viremia persists throughout the course of the disease in VEE, and the blood provides a source of infection for biting insects. Transplacental transmission of the VEE virus can occur in pregnant mares infected near term. The virus is present in saliva and nasal discharge, and this material can be used to transmit the disease experimentally by intranasal instillation.

Penetration of the virus into the **brain** does not occur in all cases and the infection does not produce signs, other than fever, unless involvement of the CNS occurs. The lesions produced in nervous tissue are typical of a viral infection and are localized particularly in the **gray matter of the cerebral cortex, thalamus, and hypothalamus**, with minor involvement of the medulla and spinal cord. It is this distribution of lesions that is responsible for the characteristic signs of mental derangement, followed at a later stage by paralysis. The early apparent blindness and failure to eat or drink appear to be cortical in origin. True blindness and pharyngeal paralysis occur only in the late stages.

CLINICAL FINDINGS

The diseases associated with the different viruses are **clinically indistinguishable**. The **incubation period** for VEE is 1 to 6 days. Uncomplicated disease usually lasts about 1 week. In the initial viremic stage there is fever, which may be accompanied by anorexia and depression, but the reaction is usually so mild that it goes unobserved. In the experimental disease, the temperature may reach 41°C (106°F) persisting for only 24 to 48 hours, with nervous signs appearing at the peak of the fever. Animals that have shown nervous signs for more than 24 hours may then have a temperature within the normal range.

Early nervous signs include hypersensitivity to sound and touch, and in some cases transient periods of excitement and restlessness, with apparent blindness. Affected horses may walk blindly into objects or walk in circles. **Involuntary muscle movements** occur, especially tremor of shoulder and facial muscles and erection of the penis. A stage of **severe mental depression** follows. Affected horses stand with the head hung low; they appear to be asleep and may have a half-chewed mouthful of feed hanging from the lips. At this stage the horse may eat and drink if food is placed in its mouth. The pupillary light reflex is still present. The animal can be aroused, but soon relapses into a state of somnolence.

A stage of **paralysis** follows. There is inability to hold up the head, and it is often rested on a solid support. The lower lip is pendulous and the tongue may hang out. Unnatural postures are adopted, with the horse often standing with the weight balanced on the forelegs or with the legs crossed. **Head-pressing** or leaning back on a halter are often seen. On walking, there is obvious incoordination, particularly in the hindlegs, and circling is common. Defecation and urination are suppressed, and the horse is unable to swallow. Complete paralysis is the terminal stage. The horse goes down, is unable to rise, and usually dies within 2 to 4 days from the first signs of illness. A proportion of affected horses do not develop paralysis and survive but have persistent neurologic deficits.

In the experimental infection of horses with the endemic strain of the **VEE virus**, a fever and mild leukopenia occurs. Following infection with the epidemic strain of the virus, a high fever and severe leukopenia are common, and a high level of neutralizing antibodies develop about 5 to 6 days after infection. Clinical findings include profound depression, accompanied by flaccidity of lips, partially closed eyelids, and drooped ears; some horses chew continuously and froth at the mouth. In the terminal stages, there is recumbency and nystagmus.

CLINICAL PATHOLOGY

There are no characteristic **hematologic or biochemical abnormalities**. The **absence of biochemical indication of liver disease** (hyperbilirubinemia, increased activity in serum of liver-specific enzymes such as sorbitol dehydrogenase and γ-glutamyl transferase, absence of hyperammonemia) rules out hepatic encephalopathy.

Diagnostic confirmation is achieved by one or more of the following:

- Isolation of virus from an affected animal
- Detection of viral antigen or nucleic acid in an animal with appropriate clinical signs
- Seroconversion or an increase in serum titer of sick or recovered animal.

Virus isolation provides definitive proof of infection. However, viremia may have resolved by the time nervous signs have developed, and it may be advantageous to sample febrile animals instead of animals showing more advanced signs of the disease. Virus can be cultured in intracranially inoculated suckling mice, weanling mice, guinea pigs, cell culture, newly hatched chicks, or embryonated eggs. Virus isolates can be identified by complement fixation, HI, virus neutralization, PCR, IFA, and antigen capture ELISA. A recently developed indirect fluorescent test using monoclonal antibodies enables the differentiation of endemic from epidemic strains of VEE. Interpretation of the results of serologic tests of horses in an area where endemic, nonpathogenic VEE virus exists is difficult because of the cross-reaction between endemic and epidemic strains of the virus. Therefore in areas where there is endemic, nonpathogenic VEE, demonstration of the presence of antibodies should not be considered persuasive evidence of the presence of the disease.

Acute and convalescent sera taken 10 to 14 days apart for the presence of neutralizing, hemagglutination-inhibiting, or complement-fixing antibodies in the serum of affected or in-contact horses, is of value in detecting the presence of the virus in the group or in the area. A fourfold increase in complement-fixing antibodies is considered positive.

Demonstration of viral nucleic acid in tissue, blood, or insects by PCR test is a useful indicator of the presence of the virus.[8] Use of modern bioinformatic techniques can enable viral genotyping, facilitating diagnosis and forensic and epidemiologic investigations.[9] There can be sufficient viral antigen to be detected by ELISA in clinical material, and this may provide a useful test in the early stages of an epidemic.

NECROPSY FINDINGS

The brain meninges may appear congested, but there are generally no gross changes. Histologic examination of the brain reveals perivascular accumulations of leukocytes and damage to neurons. The gray matter of the forebrain and midbrain are the most severely affected areas. In some cases of VEE, liquefactive necrosis and hemorrhage are visible in the cerebral cortex. Cell culture and transmission experiments using brain tissue as an inoculum are the traditional means of confirming a diagnosis and require that the brain be removed within an hour of death. Transmission is by intracerebral inoculation of brain tissue into sucking mice or duck embryo tissue culture. Fluorescent antibody tests have been developed to detect VEE virus and EEE virus in brain tissue.

Samples for Postmortem Confirmation of Diagnosis

- Half of midsagittally sectioned brain and liver and spleen should be submitted for fluorescent antibody and PCR testing, virus isolation and bioassay.
- Half of midsagittally sectioned brain, fixed in formalin, should be submitted for light microscopic examination.

Note the zoonotic potential of these organisms when handling the carcass and submitting specimens.

DIFFERENTIAL DIAGNOSIS

Clinically, the disease has very great similarity to the other viral encephalomyelitides, from which it can often be discriminated by the geographic location of the horse, and to the hepatic encephalopathies and a number of other diseases (see next).

- Rabies.
- West Nile virus encephalomyelitis.
- Hendra disease (occurs in Australia).
- Borna disease (occurs in Europe).
- Japanese encephalitis (occurs in Asia).
- Various other viral infections that are geographically restricted.
- Hepatic encephalopathy, such as that associated with poisoning by *Crotalaria, Senecio,* and *Amsinckia* spp.; acute serum hepatitis or hepatopathy.
- Botulism causes weakness that is evident as muscle fasciculation, recumbency, and dysphagia, but does not cause cerebral signs (irritation, behavioral abnormalities).
- Yellow star thistle poisoning (*Centaurea solstitialis*) and poisoning by fumonisins can produce similar clinical signs to that of the encephalitides, with the exception of fever.

TREATMENT

There is no definitive or specific treatment. Supportive treatment may be given with the intention to prevent self-inflicted injury and maintain hydration and nutritional status.

CONTROL

Control of VEE of horses is based on the following:

- Accurate clinical and laboratory diagnosis of the disease in horses
- Use of sentinel animals to monitor the presence of the virus in the region
- Quarantine of infected horses to stop movement of virus donors
- Insect abatement when deemed necessary
- Vaccination of all horses

Vaccination

Vaccination of horses is important not only because it minimizes the risk of disease in vaccinated horses but also because it prevents viremia, subsequent infection of feeding mosquitoes, and propagation spread of VEE. There are a number of commercial vaccines available (Table 14-12).

One of the most important aspects of the control of VEE is the vaccination of the horse population to minimize the number of horses that are viremic and serve as amplifying hosts. A **tissue culture-attenuated virus vaccine, TC83**, is available for immunization of horses against VEE. The vaccine is considered to be safe and efficacious. Concerns about reversion to virulence and safety have prompted the development of DNA and chimeric vaccines, of which a number of experimental vaccines are reported.[10-15] The World Organization for Animal Health specifies vaccination by the TC83 attenuated virus vaccine or a formalin-killed virus vaccine.[3]

A **highly effective immunity** is produced within a few days following vaccination, and serum-neutralizing antibodies persist for 20 to 30 months. The vaccine causes a mild fever, leukopenia, and a viremia and, because of conflicting reports about its capacity to cause abortion, should not be used in pregnant mares. Antibodies to the heterologous alphaviruses, WEE and EEE, existing at the time of TC83 vaccination, may suppress the VEE antibody response to the vaccine.

Table 14-12 Commercial vaccines against alphaviral equine encephalomyelitis available for equines

Name*	Uses	Administration**
Equiloid Innovator: Encephalomyelitis vaccine-tetanus toxoid	For the vaccination of healthy horses as an aid in the prevention of equine encephalomyelitis caused by Eastern and Western viruses, and tetanus	Inject one 1-mL dose intramuscularly using aseptic technique Administer a second 1-mL dose 3–4 weeks after the first dose
Fluvac Innovator 4 Encephalomyelitis-influenza vaccine-tetanus toxoid	For vaccination of healthy horses as an aid in the prevention of equine encephalomyelitis caused by Eastern and Western viruses, equine influenza from type A2 viruses, and tetanus	Inject one 1-mL dose intramuscularly using aseptic technique Administer a second 1-mL dose 3–4 weeks after the first dose
Fluvac Innovator 5 Encephalomyelitis-rhinopneumonitis-influenza vaccine-tetanus toxoid	For vaccination of healthy horses as an aid in the prevention of equine encephalomyelitis caused by Eastern and Western viruses, equine rhinopneumonitis caused by type 1 and 4 herpesviruses, equine influenza caused by type A2 viruses, and tetanus	Inject one 1-mL dose intramuscularly using aseptic technique Administer a second 1-mL dose 3–4 weeks after the first dose
Fluvac Innovator 6 Encephalomyelitis-rhinopneumonitis-influenza vaccine-tetanus toxoid	For vaccination of healthy horses as an aid in the prevention of equine encephalomyelitis caused by Eastern, Western, and Venezuelan viruses, equine rhinopneumonitis caused by type 1 and 4 herpesviruses, equine influenza caused by type A2 viruses, and tetanus	Inject one 1-mL dose intramuscularly using aseptic technique Administer a second 1-mL dose 3–4 weeks after the first dose
Fluvac Innovator Triple-E FT Encephalomyelitis-influenza vaccine-tetanus toxoid	For vaccination of healthy horses as an aid in the prevention of equine encephalomyelitis caused by Eastern, Western, and Venezuelan viruses, equine influenza caused by type A2 viruses, and tetanus	Inject one 1 mL dose intramuscularly using aseptic technique Administer a second 1-mL dose 3–4 weeks after the first dose
Triple-E T Innovator Encephalomyelitis vaccine-tetanus toxoid	For intramuscular vaccination of healthy horses as an aid in the prevention of equine encephalomyelitis caused by Eastern, Western, and Venezuelan viruses, and tetanus	Inject one 1-mL dose intramuscularly using aseptic technique Administer a second 1-mL dose 3–4 weeks after the first dose
WEST Nile Innovator + EW Encephalomyelitis-West Nile virus vaccine	For vaccination of healthy horses as an aid in the prevention of viremia caused by West Nile virus, and as an aid in the prevention of equine encephalomyelitis caused by Eastern and Western viruses	Inject one 1-mL dose intramuscularly using aseptic technique Administer a second 1-mL dose 3–4 weeks after the first dose
West Nile Innovator + EWT Encephalomyelitis-West Nile virus-tetanus toxoid	For vaccination of healthy horses as an aid in the prevention of viremia caused by West Nile virus, and as an aid in the prevention of equine encephalomyelitis caused by Eastern and Western viruses and tetanus	Inject one 1-mL dose intramuscularly using aseptic technique Administer a second 1-mL dose 3–4 weeks after the first dose
West Nile-Innovator + VEWT Encephalomyelitis-West Nile virus-tetanus toxoid	For vaccination of healthy horses as an aid in the prevention of viremia caused by West Nile virus, and as an aid in the prevention of equine encephalomyelitis caused by Eastern, Western, and Venezuelan viruses and tetanus	Inject one 1-mL dose intramuscularly using aseptic technique Administer a second 1-mL dose 3–4 weeks after the first dose

**Commercial name and vaccine components*
***Recommended vaccination protocol*

However, the response to the vaccine is adequate to provide protection against VEE, and the interference is not considered significant. There is inconclusive evidence that WEE and EEE antibodies protect horses against infection with virulent VEE virus, or conversely that VEE antibodies protect against infection with WEE and EEE viruses. Simultaneous vaccination using formalin-inactivated EEE, WEE, and VEE (the TC83 strain of VEE) is effective and recommended in areas where all three viruses may be present.

Protection From Insects

Housing of horses indoors at night, especially in fly-proofed stables, and the use of **insect repellents** might restrain the spread of the virus.

Widespread spraying of insecticides to reduce the population of the vector insects has been used in the control of VEE in humans, along with vaccination of horses. **Complete eradication** of the virus appears to be impossible because of the enzootic nature of the ecology of the virus: epidemic VEE arising by chance mutation of endemic strains of VEE, makes elimination of the virus impossible with methods currently available.

REFERENCES

1. Arechiga-Ceballos N, et al. *Rev - Off Int Epizoot.* 2015;34:491.
2. Medina G, et al. *Am J Trop Med Hyg.* 2015;93:7.
3. Venezuelan equine encephalitis. OIE, 2008. (Accessed August, 2016, at www.oie.int/fileadmin/Home/eng/Animal_Health_in_the_World/docs/pdf/Disease_cards/VEE.pdf.).
4. Deardorff ER, et al. *Am J Trop Med Hyg.* 2010;82:1047.
5. Adams AP, et al. *PLoS Negl Trop Dis.* 2012;6:31875.
6. Zacks MA, et al. *Vet Microbiol.* 2010;140:281.
7. Thompson NN, et al. *Vector Borne Zoonotic Dis.* 2012;12:969.
8. Belen Pisano M, et al. *J Virol Methods.* 2012;186:203.
9. Gardner SN, et al. *J Virol Methods.* 2013;193:112.
10. Paessler S, et al. *Vaccine.* 2009;27:D80.
11. Fine DL, et al. *J Virol Methods.* 2010;163:424.
12. Dupuy LC, et al. *Clin Vaccine Immunol.* 2011;18:707.
13. Tretyakova I, et al. *Vaccine.* 2013;31:1019.
14. Carossino M, et al. *Vaccine.* 2014;32:311.
15. Rossi SL, et al. *PLoS Negl Trop Dis.* 2015;9:e0003797.

EQUID HERPESVIRUS-1 MYELOENCEPHALOPATHY, ABORTION, AND NEONATAL SEPTICEMIA

SYNOPSIS

Etiology EHV-1 causes respiratory disease of adults, abortion, neonatal septicemia, and myeloencephalopathy. Infection by specific variants of the virus increases the likelihood of the clinically important manifestations of infection—myeloencephalopathy and/or abortion.

Epidemiology Transmission between horses and by mediate contagion. Lifelong latency of infection with periodic reactivation of virus shedding. Respiratory disease, abortion, and myeloencephalopathy occur prominently as outbreaks, but can affect sole animals.

Clinical signs Upper respiratory disease, abortion, neonatal septicemia, and neurologic disease with incontinence, ataxia, and recumbency.

Clinical pathology No pathogenic changes in hemogram or serum biochemistry profile. Detection of viral DNA and variant genotyping by RT-PCR in nasal swabs or white blood cells, seroconversion or increase in titer using an ELISA able to differentiate between EHV-1 and EHV-4.

Diagnostic confirmation Virus isolation from, or polymerase chain reaction test on, blood, nasopharyngeal swabs or tissue. Seroconversion or increase in titer.

Treatment There is no specific treatment, although acyclovir, an antiviral agent, has been administered. Symptomatic treatment of neurologic signs in horses with myeloencephalopathy.

Control Infection is ubiquitous. Management including quarantine, maintaining mares in small bands, and education of staff about importance of control measures to prevent outbreaks of abortion or myeloencephalopathy. Vaccination for prevention of abortion. Quarantine. Hygiene.

EHV-1, *equid herphesvirus-1;* RT-PCR, *reverse transcriptase-polymerase chain reaction.*

Herpesviruses infecting equids (such as horses, donkeys, mules, and zebra) are all viruses with a linear, double-stranded DNA genome in the order Herpesvirales, family Herpesviridae.[1] Equid herpesviruses (EHV)-1, 3, 4, 8 (syn. asinine herpesvirus-3), and 9 (a virus infecting gazelle) are Alphaherpesvirinae (alphaherpesviruses) in the genus *Varicellovirus*. EHV-6 (syn. asinine herpesvirus-1) is tentatively assigned to this genus. EHV-2, 5, and 7 (syn. asinine herpesvirus-2) are Gammaherpesvirinae (gammaherpesviruses).[1] There is also a zebra gammaherpesvirus, which appears to be associated with disease in nonequids housed in proximity to zebras (see later).[2,3]

Five herpesviruses have been associated with various diseases of horses and foals (EHV-1 to 5). Common names are "equine abortion virus" for EHV-1, "cytomegalovirus" for EHV-2, "equine coital exanthema virus" for EHV-3, and "rhinopneumonitis virus" for EHV-4 (although this term is sometimes used, confusingly, for EHV-1). Related herpesviruses (asinine herpesvirus-1 to 6, some of which have been recently classified or identified as EHVs[1]) infect, and some cause disease in, donkeys, mules, or horses.[4-7] Some asinine herpesviruses cause a fatal interstitial pneumonia or neurologic disease in donkeys.[8]

Infection by EHV-1, EHV-4, or both is common, if not ubiquitous, in equids worldwide with most animals infected while juveniles and latent virus in trigeminal ganglia[9] and other tissues maintaining that infection. EHV-4 causes respiratory disease and, rarely, abortion. EHV-1 causes respiratory disease but also causes individual cases or outbreaks of myeloencephalopathy, abortion, and neonatal septicemia. Certain variants of EHV-1, detectable by examination of viral genome, are associated with increased risk of myeloencephalopathy, abortion, or both.

A partial list of disease syndromes attributed to EHV and asinine herpesvirus infection and the viruses associated with them include the following:

- **Upper respiratory tract disease** of adult horses, weanlings, and older foals is caused principally by EHV-4, although disease attributable to EHV-1 occurs. EHV-2 causes respiratory disease, including pneumonia, of foals, and rarely upper respiratory disease of adults.
- **Abortion** in horses is almost always associated with EHV-1, although rare sporadic cases are associated with EHV-4. EHV-7 (syn. asinine herpesvirus-2, a gammaherpesvirus) was associated with abortion in a donkey.[4]
- **Perinatal disease** of foals, including birth of sick and weak foals and development of viral septicemia within 48 hours of birth, is associated with EHV-1.
- **EHV-1 myeloencephalopathy** (EHM) is associated with EHV-1 and rarely, if ever, with EHV-4. In donkeys it has been associated with an asinine gammaherpesvirus.[8]
- **Coital exanthema** is associated with EHV-3, and genital disease is an unusual manifestation of EHV-1 infection.
- **Equine multinodular pulmonary fibrosis** in horses is associated with infection by EHV-5.[10,11]
- **Lymphoma** in horses is tentatively associated with infection by EHV-5.[12,13]
- **Chorioretinitis** is associated with EHV-1 infection.[14]
- **Dermatitis** (erythema multiforme) is associated with EHV-5 infection in horses.[15]
- **Neurologic disease or abortion** in gazelle, onagers, and polar bears is caused by EHV-9 or EHV-1 originating from zebra.[2,3,16,17]

The following discussion focuses on myeloencephalopathy, abortion, and neonatal septicemia in equids associated with infection by EHV-1. Respiratory disease caused by EHV-4 and EHV-1 is discussed elsewhere in this text as are other manifestations of EHV infection.

ETIOLOGY

EHV-1 is an alphaherpesvirus, a DNA virus with 76 ORFs. EHV-1 and EHV-4 are closely related and have extensive antigenic cross-reactivity but are genetically and biologically distinct viruses with different disease profiles.[18,19] Phylogenetic mapping ("trees") and genetic fingerprinting for EHV-1 are not available, as they are for many other viruses (see the section on Equine Influenza in Chapter 12 as an example), and are needed to investigate links between outbreaks and associations with virulence.

Although EHV-1 virus is genetically stable, with limited genetic divergence and differences in strains of less than 0.1%, genetic variants of EHV-1 exist and some have differing biologic characteristics.[20] Analysis of ORF 68 reveals at least 19 distinct DNA sequences allowing identification of 6 major strain groups of EHV-1.[20] Importantly, a single nucleotide polymorphism (SNP) (A-G) at position 2254 in the DNA polymerase gene (DNA_{pol}, ORF 30) that results in substitution of asparagine (N) by aspartic acid (D) at position 752 in the DNA polymerase protein is not limited to any one strain. Variants of the virus are therefore classified as N752 or D752, irrespective of the particular strain.[20] This suggests that the D752/N752 mutation has occurred multiple times.[21] The original isolation of EHV-1 in 1941 was of the D752 phenotype.[21]

The D752 variant is isolated more frequently than is N752 from horses with myeloencephalopathy and, increasingly, abortion.[22-27] Infection with the D752 variant increases the risk of myeloencephalopathy by 160× compared with that of infection with N752.[28] These data are based on retrospectively collected data that were not randomly collected, and this relative risk estimate could change markedly, although the association between increased risk of EHM and infection by D752 is well accepted.[18,19,21,23,24,29] However, horses can develop EHM when infected by the N752 variant in approximately 25% of cases (noting the uncertainty around this estimate).[28]

The N752 variant is the one most commonly reported as infecting asymptomatic horses.[28,30] Although estimates are potentially biased by the sampling method used in various epidemiologic studies, the D752 variant was identified in 3%, 10.8%–19.4%, 7.4%, 24%, and 10.6% of horses positive for EHV-1 sampled in Japan, the United States, Argentina, France, and Germany, respectively.[31] Horses can be infected by both variants of the disease simultaneously, and each variant can cause disease (D752 variant causing neurologic disease in the dam and N752 causing abortion).[32] Both D752 and N752 variants were both isolated from trigeminal ganglia of 12 of 153 horses examined postmortem for reasons other than EHV-associated disease, indicating that symptomatic dual infection is common. One or the other variant, but not both, were isolated from a further 9/153 horses.[9] Similarly, of 70 Thoroughbred racehorses examined postmortem because of death secondary to catastrophic musculoskeletal injuries, 2 carried only a latent neurotropic strain of EHV-1, 6 carried a nonneurotropic genotype of EHV-1, and 10 were dually infected with neurotropic and nonneurotropic EHV-1.[33] Among 132 mares from central Kentucky sampled postmortem, latent EHV-1 DNA was detected in the submandibular lymph node tissues of 71 (54%). Thirteen (18%) of the 71 latently infected horses were infected with the D752 variant, of which 11 were also infected with the N752 variant.[30] The remainder were infected with only the N752 variant.

The D752 variant of EHV-1 differs from the N_{752} variant in that it causes higher levels of white blood cell–associated viremia (up to 10-fold), infects CD4+ and CD8+ cells to a greater extent but CD14 + and B cells to a lesser extent, and is less sensitive to aphidicolin, a drug targeting the viral polymerase.[34] The D752 variant is also more virulent in experimentally infected horses, with those infected with the D752 variant having higher rectal temperatures, a longer period of pyrexia after infection (3 days versus 1 day), and greater severity of nasal discharge, but no difference in nasal shedding of virus. Horses experimentally infected with D752 variant developed EHM, whereas those infected with the N752 variant did not, although uniform development of EHM in horses or ponies experimentally infected with D752 variant is not present in other studies of the disease.[34] The D752 variant infects submucosal immune cells in respiratory explants to a greater extent than does the N752 variant.[35] CSF from horses infected by D752 was abnormal, whereas that from horses infected with N752 was not abnormal.[34]

It is unclear whether viral load is associated with the outcome of clinical disease, although one study of a small number of horses (seven) treated at a referral institution, identified viral loads in nasal fluid and blood that were 1000× and 100× greater in nonsurviving horses with EHM. These findings require confirmation because of the small number of horses examined and in surviving (five) and nonsurviving groups (two).[36]

Both N752 and D752 variants can cause disease. Virulence is associated with presence of a functional gp2 protein, which is apparently responsible for viral egress from infected cells, and glycoprotein D and cell-surface glycosaminoglycans that are needed for efficient entry of EHV-1 into cells.

The most important clinical syndromes associated with EHV-1 infection are abortion, neonatal septicemia, and myeloencephalopathy. Genital disease is an unusual manifestation of EHV-1 infection. Infection with EHV-1 causes retinitis and fatal disease in camelids. It also causes disease in wild equids including zebras and neurologic disease in black bears (*Ursus americanus*), Thomson's gazelles (*Eudorcas thomsonii*), guinea pigs (*Cavia porcellus f. dom.*) Indian rhinoceros (*Rhinoceros unicornis*), and polar bears in zoologic parks in which these animals are in proximity to equids (such as zebra).[37-39] It is associated with abortions and stillbirths in guinea pigs.[37]

EPIDEMIOLOGY

Occurrence

Infection with EHV-1 is endemic in horse populations worldwide, and many adult horses have serologic evidence of infection. Serologic surveys, which provide an index of the extent of infection in the sampled population, performed before 1995 were hindered by the lack of an assay able to differentiate immune responses to EHV-1 from those to EHV-4. Furthermore, the advent of vaccines eliciting serum antibodies against EHV-1/4, and the inability of diagnostic tests to differentiate between antibodies induced by vaccination or natural infection, complicates assessment of the prevalence of serum antibodies to EHV-1/4. Seroprevalence of EHV-1–specific antibodies is 9% to 28% in adult Thoroughbred horses, 26% of Thoroughbred broodmares, 11% of Thoroughbred foals, and 46% to 68% of 1- and 2-year-old Thoroughbred race horses in Australia. Sixty-one percent of 82 normal horses and horses with upper respiratory tract disease had antibodies to EHV-1 in New Zealand. Of 70 Thoroughbred race horses examined postmortem, 18 (26%) and 58 (83%) horses were PCR positive for the gB gene of EHV-1 and EHV-4, respectively, in at least one of trigeminal ganglia, bronchial, or submandibular lymph nodes sampled. Twelve horses were dually infected with EHV-1 and EHV-4.[33]

The EHV-1 D752 variant has been detected in equids in North America, Europe (the Netherlands, France, Belgium, and Germany), Australia, New Zealand, and South America.[18,27,30-32,40-43] It likely occurs worldwide given that it is not a recent mutation, having been detected in samples collected in the 1940s.[21] EHM is rarely reported in the Southern Hemisphere with the first case described in New Zealand in 2013.[18]

Upper respiratory tract disease associated with EHV-1 infection has been suggested to occur as outbreaks, although this is not well documented. Signs of infectious upper respiratory disease affected 20% of Thoroughbred race horses at one race track in Canada over a 3-year period, and seroconversion to EHV-1 occurred in 5% to 18% of these horses, whereas the vast majority of horses seroconverted to influenza. However, all horses that seroconverted to EHV-1 also either seroconverted to influenza virus or had been recently vaccinated with a vaccine containing EHV-1. These results suggest that the stress of influenza disease may have triggered reactivation of latent EHV-1 infection in some horses, suggesting that EHV-1 did not have a primary role in the outbreak of respiratory disease. Similarly, in England, EHV-1 was not associated with clinical respiratory disease in Thoroughbred racehorses. EHV-1 was isolated from foals with purulent nasal discharge and respiratory disease concurrent with neurologic disease among the dams in Australia.

Abortion caused by EHV-1 occurs as both sporadic cases and as epizootics (abortion storms).[27,40,44] Approximately 3% of abortions in mares are attributable to EHV-1 infection, although the actual incidence probably varies widely among years and geographic regions. Outbreaks of EHV-1 abortion and birth of nonviable foals occurs sporadically on farms with sometimes catastrophic losses. Loss of foals through abortion or birth of nonviable foals can be as high as ~60% of pregnant mares on the farm.[27,40,44] Initial cases can, in the absence of appropriate control measures, rapidly spread the infection and prompt diagnosis, and implementation of control measures is important to limit the spread of infection.[27,29] Vaccination with killed EHV-1 vaccine during late gestation does not reliably prevent the disease, although conventional wisdom is to ensure that mares are well vaccinated (see the section Control).[27] EHV-4 rarely causes abortion in mares. Disease of neonates associated with EHV-1 occurs both sporadically and as outbreaks in which up to 25% of foals may be affected. Foals infected in utero usually die soon after birth, whereas those infected in the period after birth may have milder disease and a lower mortality rate (6%). One-third of viremic foals may not seroconvert, based on the complement fixation test.

Myeloencephalopathy occurs as sporadic cases but more often presents as an epizootic within a stable or barn or within a localized area. Morbidity rates in exposed horses range from 1% to 90%, mortality rates of 0.5% to 40%, and case–fatality rates of ~15%–75%.[25,32,41,43,45,46] The attack rate (number of horses with disease/number of horses infected) in outbreaks of the D752 variant is 22% to 50%.[20] Pregnant or nursing mares are suggested to be at greater risk of this disease, but outbreaks occur on premises, such as riding schools or race tracks, where there are no foals or pregnant mares.

Method of Transmission

EHV-1 is highly infectious, as evidenced by transmission of infection despite stringent biosecurity measures in referral hospitals, riding schools, and so on.[32,46,47] Transmission occurs by the inhalation of infected droplets or by the ingestion of material contaminated by nasal discharges or aborted fetuses/placenta/fetal fluids. Viral loads in nasal fluids in horses with EHM or aborted fetuses and associated tissues and fluids can be very high.[36,48] Other routes of infection are not recognized, although EHV-1 binds in vitro to embryos, and binding persists after 10 cycles of washing, suggesting that embryo transfer has the potential to transmit infection.[49] This route of infection has not been demonstrated as being important, or indeed possible, in the spread of spontaneous disease. EHV-1 DNA, but not EHV-4, was detected in semen samples of 51 of 390 stallions, illustrating the potential for spread of the virus during mating or artificial insemination.[50]

The virus is efficiently transmitted to in-contact animals, and rapid spread of infection results from close contact of an infected animal with susceptible horses. Infection can be spread over short distances in the absence of physical contact or fomite transmission. This likely occurs by airborne spread of virus in droplets of aerosolized nasal secretions.

Infections always arise from other horses, either by direct contact or via fomites. Mediate infection from virus on fomites such as tack, veterinary equipment, vehicles, and housing occurs because the virus survives for 14 to 45 days outside the animal. The source of the virus is always one of the following:

- A horse or foal with active infection
- A fetus, fetal membranes, or reproductive tract secretions of a mare immediately after abortion or birth of a weak foal
- Virus shed by horses in which latent infection has reactivated.

Horses and foals are infectious during the active stage of disease and, because horses become **latently infected**, during subsequent periods of viral reactivation and shedding. Latent infection occurs by inclusion of virus in immune cells (CD8+ T cells) in trigeminal ganglia, submandibular lymph nodes, and likely other immunologically active tissues.[9,30,51] Latent infection by EHV-1 virus can be reactivated by administration of corticosteroids or other immunosuppressants but, at least in experimental situations, the resulting level of viremia is very low and in-contact susceptible horses were not infected.[51]

Virus is detectable in nasal fluids of approximately 70% of horses when they first exhibit clinical signs of EHM and for up to 9 days after development of it.[32,47] The duration of nasal shedding is not related to age, duration of fever, or severity of clinical signs.[32]

There is good circumstantial evidence, such as the occurrence of abortion, neonatal disease, or myeloencephalopathy in closed herds, to support a role for latency and reactivation in the genesis of the disease, although the importance of reversion from latency has been questioned. The duration of latency is unknown but is assumed to be lifelong. Latent EHV-1 virus is detectable in the trigeminal ganglion and CD5/CD8 lymphocytes. Reactivation of the virus might not result in clinical signs in the host animal, but there is shedding of virus in nasal secretions. Consequently, clinically normal animals harbor latent virus that can infect susceptible animals during periods of reactivation. This feature of the disease has obvious importance in the prevention, control, and management of outbreaks of disease.

Abortion storms are usually attributable to an index case with the following:

- A latently infected mare that sheds virus from the respiratory tract, but does not abort
- A mare that aborts an infected conceptus
- A mare that sheds virus from the respiratory tract, and then aborts

Mares usually, but not always, abort from EHV-1 infection only once in their lifetime. A likely scenario in abortion storms is the reactivation of latent virus in a resident horse with subsequent shedding of virus in nasal secretions or, if the mare aborts, fetal tissues and uterine fluids. Contamination of the environment or horse-to-horse contact spreads infection to susceptible cohorts (primary transmission). The infected cohorts then further spread the virus to other horses in that band of mares (secondary transmission), which then spread infection among other bands of mares and foals, paddocks or fields of horses, or farms (tertiary transmission).

Outbreaks of **myeloencephalopathy** likely occur through similar mechanisms. Most outbreaks are associated with an index case or introduction of a horse with signs of infectious respiratory disease, with subsequent development of new cases in horses that have either direct or indirect (aerosol or fomite) contact with the index case.[25,43,46,47] Horses with clinical signs of myeloencephalopathy excrete the virus in nasal fluids, often in high concentrations,[36] and for periods of time up to 14 days (nasal shedding of the virus has been demonstrated up to 9 days after the onset of clinical signs of EHM)[32] and can spread the disease, contrary to previous supposition. This has important implications for handling and care of affected horses, especially those severely affected horses that may be referred for intensive or specialized care. Extreme care should be exercised when accepting horses with EHM, or suspected EHM, to referral facilities or hospitals because these animals can cause nosocomial spread of infection and disease among hospitalized equids.[46,47] Furthermore, equids infected nosocomially can spread the infection when they return home.

Cycling of Infection

Studies on Thoroughbred stud farms in Australia have demonstrated the temporal sequence of events that contribute to spread of EHV-1 infection in that region and these studies likely have relevance to other regions of the globe. There is a cyclical pattern in which horses are infected at a young age and the source of infection is, depending on the age of the foal, either its dam or other foals. Foals are infected by EHV-1 and shedding virus in nasal secretions as young as 11 days of age, often without development of clinical signs but usually associated with mucopurulent nasal discharge. Peak incidences of cases of respiratory disease associated with EHV-1 are late during the foaling season before weaning, and again after weaning when foals from several groups are housed together. The source of infection in foals before weaning is mares and, as the number of foals in the herd increases over the course of the foaling season, other foals. Weanlings spread the disease among their herd during the period shortly after weaning when foals from more than one group are mixed. The incidence density of new cases among weanlings can be as high as 13 new cases per 1000 foal weeks. The disease associated with these outbreaks is mild and without long-term consequences to the foal or weanling. However, the presence of foals excreting large quantities of EHV-1 has the potential to increase the risk of viral abortion in late-term mares in contact with these foals. Furthermore, the presence of respiratory disease associated with EHV-1 and shedding of virus by foals is associated with development of myeloencephalopathy in mares.

Risk Factors

Risk factors for EHM include the following[21]:

- Presence of susceptible equids: based largely on age (>5 years) and immune status (there are no reports of horses affected twice by the disease, suggesting long-lasting immunity).
- Introduction of EHV-1: almost always associated with a horse shedding the virus, either as a result of new infection or recrudescence of latent infection.
- Presence of the D752 variant: although disease can occur associated with infection by N752.
- Season: there appears to be higher incidences of the disease in the Northern Hemisphere in autumn, winter, and spring.
- Pyrexia: horses that are pyrexic during an outbreak are more likely to develop EHM.
- Movement of new horses onto the property, or use of horses in riding schools.[32]
- Possible associations with sex (increased risk if female) or breed (pony), although these associations are not consistent in all or most studies and are of limited usefulness in controlling or managing the disease.[43,46,47]

Immunity

Immunity to EHV-1 is mediated by cytotoxic T cells, which explains the limited efficacy of inactivated virus vaccines that have minimal effect in stimulating cytotoxic T cells despite being capable of inducing a humoral immune response.[52] The presence of EHV-1 cytotoxic T-cell precursors correlates well with protection from experimental infection, and some of the EHV-1 antigens responsible for this resistance have been identified.[53-55] Mares usually only abort from EHV-1 infection once in their lifetime, and there are no reports of horses developing myeloencephalopathy more than once.

Lack of antibodies to EHV-1 was identified as a risk factor in an outbreak of EHM in a herd of mares with foals at foot. Mares with strong antibody responses to EHV-1 did not develop disease.

Economic Importance

Disease associated with EHV-1 is of considerable economic importance because of the loss of training time and opportunities to perform during convalescence and quarantine, the loss of pregnancies during abortion storms, and deaths caused by myeloencephalopathy and infection of neonates.

PATHOGENESIS

The three organ systems involved in clinical disease associated with EHV-1 infection are the respiratory tract, uterus and placenta, and CNS. The common final pathway for injury in each of these body systems is damage to vascular endothelium with subsequent necrosis, thrombosis, and ischemia.

Following EHV-1 exposure to the upper respiratory tract, virus can be detected in the soft palate and mainstem bronchus within 12 hours, and at all levels of the respiratory tract by 24 hours. The virus gains access to the body after binding to respiratory mucosal epithelium where it forms plaques that do not extend into submucosal tissues.[35] In the respiratory tract there is an initial phase after infection of nasal epithelium[56] in which there is rapid proliferation of the virus in the nasal, pharyngeal, and tonsillar mucosae, with subsequent penetration and infection of local blood vessels. This is followed by a systemic, viremic phase in which the virus is closely associated with blood lymphocytes (especially CD172a(+)),[56] from which it can be isolated. Infection induces increased production of IFN-γ by T lymphocytes.[54] Absence of viral antigens on the surface of EHV-1–infected peripheral blood mononuclear cells explains their ability to avoid complement-mediated lysis. This activity, combined with the immunosuppression that accompanies EHV-1 infection,[55,57-59] allows dissemination of the infection to the reproductive tract and CNS. Immunosuppression is mediated by production in EHV-1–infected cells of an "early protein" that interferes with peptide translocation by the transporter associated with antigen processing. Immunosuppression is evident as reduced in vitro proliferation of peripheral blood monocytes and downregulation of expression of major histocompatibility complex class I molecules on the surface of infected cells. It is from this point that the invasion of lungs, placenta, fetus, and nervous tissue occur. Movement of infected mononuclear cells into target tissues is associated with expression of adhesion molecules by endothelium in the gravid uterus and in leukocytes.

Viral infection of endothelium results in death of endothelial cells, inflammation, activation of clotting factors and platelets, increases in markers of fibrin degradation, and formation of blood clots in small vessels.[60-62] This thrombotic disease causes ischemia of neighboring tissues with subsequent necrosis and loss of function. Another theory is that deposition of antigen–antibody complexes in small vessels results in an Arthus reaction with subsequent ischemia, necrosis, and loss of function. However, recent demonstration that mares with no antibody titer to EHV-1 were at increased risk of developing myeloencephalopathy does not support a role for type III hypersensitivity in this disease. Regardless of the underlying mechanism, clinical signs are a result of vasculitis and necrosis of tissue in the CNS and reproductive tract. This is in contrast to neurologic disease associated with herpesvirus in other species, in which the nervous system disease is a direct result of infection of neural tissues.

Abortion is caused by damage to the placenta, endometrium, or fetus. Placental lesions include vasculitis, focal thrombosis, and infarction of the microcotyledons of the pregnant uterus. The fetus is infected and there are diagnostic lesions present in many aborted foals, including massive destruction of lymphocytes in the spleen and the thymus. In those abortions in which there is no lesion or evidence of virus infection in the foal, there may be extensive damage to the endometrium caused by an endothelial lesion and its attendant vasculitis, thrombosis, and secondary ischemia.

Foals that are infected in utero but survive to full term may be stillborn or weak and die soon after birth with pulmonary, hepatic, and cardiac lesions. EHV-1 infection in foals not infected before or at birth is usually a self-limiting, mild infection of the upper respiratory tract with an accompanying leukopenia and a transitory immune suppression, although uveitis and occasionally death occur in a small number of foals. Virus can be isolated from the nasal mucus and the buffy coat of the blood for some time after clinical signs have disappeared.

The pathogenesis of **myeloencephalopathy** in horses contrasts with herpesvirus encephalitis of other species in which there is viral infection of neuronal tissue. The myeloencephalopathy in horses is, as discussed earlier, the result of vasculitis, thrombosis, and subsequent ischemia of neural tissue. Impairment of blood flow results in hypoxia and dysfunction or death of adjacent neural tissue.

CLINICAL FINDINGS

EHV-1 infection manifests as several forms of disease on a farm such that nervous system involvement can occur in an outbreak in which abortion and respiratory disease also feature, although more commonly one form of the disease (myeloencephalopathy or abortion) occurs alone or with mild respiratory disease. Foals, stallions, and mares can be affected with one or the other form of the disease, although it is most commonly seen in adult horses. Onset of neurologic signs is usually, but not invariably, preceded by cases of respiratory disease, fever, limb edema, or abortion.

Myeloencephalopathy

Myeloencephalopathy initially occurs in an index case, which might or might not have had signs of infectious respiratory disease alone or with signs of neurologic disease. Signs of neurologic disease develop in other horses approximately 6 to 14 days after disease in the index case. Disease then develops in a number of horses over a short period of time (3–10 days). Outbreaks in a stable can evolve rapidly.[25,43,46,47]

Fever, without signs of respiratory disease, often precedes signs of neurologic disease by 24 to 72 hours. The onset of neurologic signs is usually rapid, with the signs stabilizing within 1 to 2 days. Fever is more common (odds ratio 20×, 95% CI 3.4–390) in horses that go on to develop EHM, but the presence of limb edema or severity of nasal discharge are not associated with the likelihood of developing EHM during an outbreak of the disease.[32,46] Thirteen percent of 61 horses with fever recorded during an outbreak of abortion and EHM developed signs of EHM.[25] Six of seven pregnant mares aborted.

Signs are variable but usually referable to spinal white matter involvement. Affected horses have variable degrees of ataxia and paresis manifest as stumbling, toe dragging, pivoting, and circumduction that is most severe in the hindlimbs. Signs are usually symmetric. There is often hypotonia of the tail and anus.

Fecal and urinary incontinence are common and affected horses often dribble urine, have urine scalding of the skin of the perineum and legs, and require manual evacuation of the rectum. The severity of signs can progress to hemiplegia or paraplegia manifesting as recumbency and the inability to rise. Less commonly, CN deficits, such as lingual or pharyngeal paresis, head tilt, nystagmus, or strabismus, are present. Affected horses are usually alert and maintain their appetite.

Severity of neurologic disease varies among horses within an outbreak, and the prognosis is related to the severity of disease. In general, horses that become recumbent have a poor prognosis for both short-term and long-term survival despite intensive nursing care.[43,46,47] However, less severely affected horses have a good prognosis for survival, with case–fatality rates as low as 2% to 3% in some outbreaks. Horses with mild signs of neurologic disease often recover completely and return to their previous level of performance, although some have persistent neurologic deficits after 1 year.

Abortion

Outbreaks of abortion might not be preceded by clinically apparent respiratory disease. The incidence of abortion is highest in the last third of pregnancy, particularly in the 8- to 10-month period but can occur as early as the fifth month. Abortion occurs without premonitory signs, and the placenta is usually not retained. Frequently there is no mammary development. Affected mares sometimes have prolapse of the uterus. Some foals are stillborn, whereas others are weak and die soon after birth.

Abortion storms are often long-lasting, with a period of 17 to 22 days separating the index case from cases caused by secondary transmission of the virus, suggesting an incubation period of 2 to 3 weeks. Experimental infections induce abortion 15 to 65 days after intranasal inoculation of the virus. Although most abortions then occur within 1 month of the first secondary cases, abortions on a farm can continue for many months.[27]

Neonatal Viremia and Septicemia

In utero EHV-1 infection causes abortion or the birth of infected foals, some of which are normal at birth, but become weak and die within 3 to 7 days of birth with signs of respiratory distress and septicemia. A less severe form of the disease, characterized by pyrexia, nasal discharge, and chorioretinitis, occurs in slightly older foals that are apparently infected after birth. Affected foals that survive sometimes do not have serum antibodies to EHV-1. Death may be associated with secondary bacterial infection with *E. coli* or *Actinobacillus equuli,* although EHV-1 infection alone is sufficient to cause death.

Respiratory Disease

The classical respiratory tract form of the disease (rhinopneumonitis) is virtually indistinguishable on the basis of clinical signs from the other upper respiratory tract diseases of horses and is identical to that associated with EHV-4.

CLINICAL PATHOLOGY

Results of hematologic and serum biochemical examinations are neither specific nor diagnostic. EHV-1 infection of adult horses results in leukopenia that is attributable to both neutropenia and T-cell lymphopenia, with B-cell lymphocytosis occurring during the recovery period. EHV-1 septicemia of foals is characterized by profound leukopenia, neutropenia with a left shift, and lymphopenia. An approach to achieving prompt antemortem diagnosis of EHM is suggested in Fig. 14-9.[63]

CSF of horses with EHV-1 encephalomyelopathy is characteristically xanthochromic and has an increased total protein concentration (>1 g/L) with a normal white cell count.[32,64] The interpretation of EHV-1 antibody in CSF is uncertain, although normal horses are not expected to have detectable antibodies to EHV-1 in the CSF.

Serologic tests are of critical importance in diagnosis and control of EHV infections. Many horses have serum antibodies to EHV-1 and EHV-4 as a result of previous infection or vaccination. Thus the demonstration of antibodies is not in itself sufficient to confirm a diagnosis of the disease. Complement-fixing antibody appears on the 10th to 12th day after experimental infection but persists for only a limited period. Demonstration of a threefold to fourfold increase in the serum concentration of specific complement-fixing antibodies in acute and convalescent serum samples provides persuasive evidence of recent infection. Complement-fixing antibodies persist for only a short time (several months) while VN

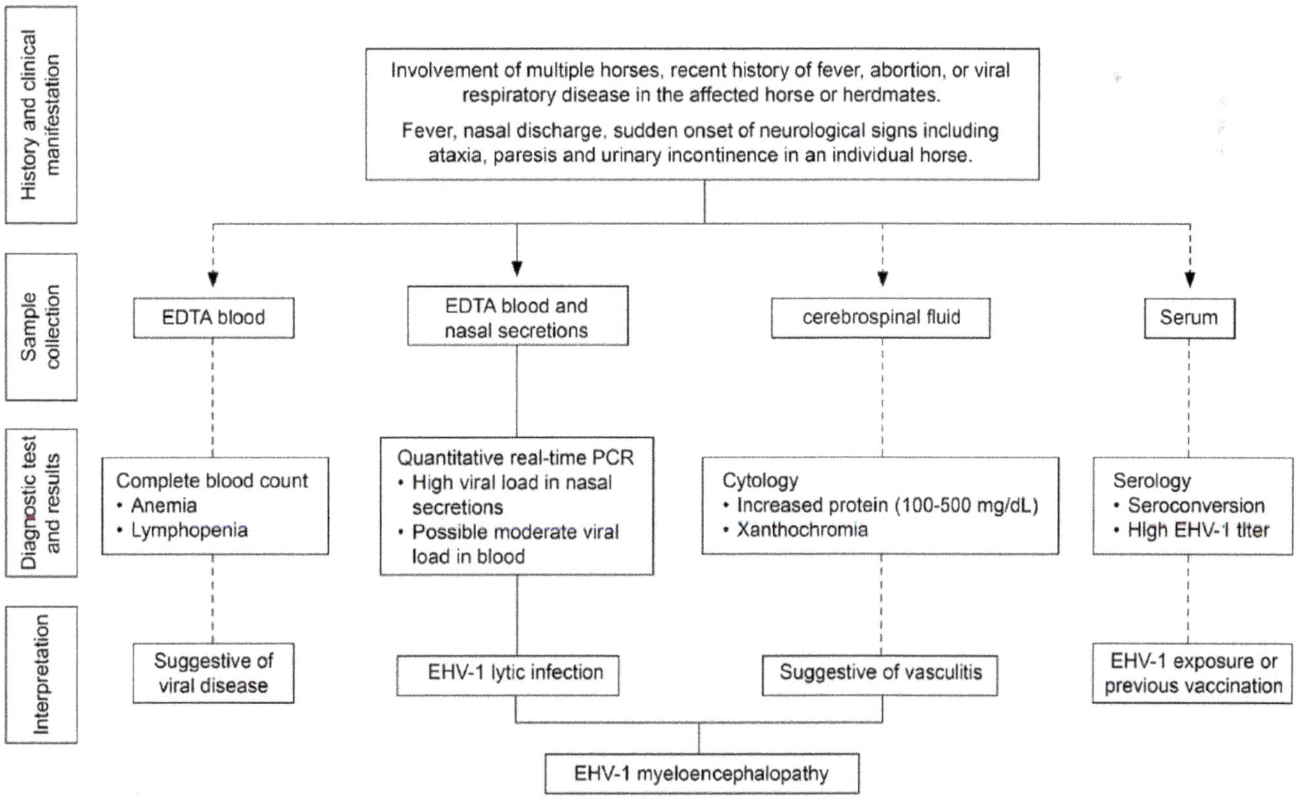

Fig. 14-9 Methodology for rapid antemortem diagnosis of equine herpesvirus-1 (EHV-1) myeloencephalopathy in horses with signs of nervous system disease. Solid lines represent a diagnostic pathway. *EDTA,* ethylenediaminetetraacetic acid. (Reproduced, with permission, from Pusterla N, Wilson WD, Madigan JE, Ferraro GL. Equine herpesvirus-1 myeloencephalopathy: a review of recent developments. *Vet J* 2009;180:279-289.)

antibodies persist for over a year, and testing for them is therefore a more reliable means of determining that previous infection with the virus has occurred. Until recently, serologic differentiation of antibodies to EHV-1 and EHV-4 was not possible. However, highly specific **ELISA** tests based on differences between EHV-1 and EHV-2 in the variable region of the C terminus of glycoprotein G, at least one of which is commercially available, have been developed that can differentiate between antibodies to EHV-1 and EHV-4 in horse serum. The ELISA is reported to be more sensitive, easier to perform, more rapid, and more reproducible than the virus neutralization test. Importantly, the ELISA test is able to differentiate between infections associated with EHV-1 and EHV-4.[65,66]

Identification of the virus in nasal swabs, or blood buffy coat, or tissue by culture or a PCR test provides confirmation of infection.[67-71] The use of seminested or multiplex PCR or qPCR, which avoids the risk of carryover contamination, provides rapid identification of EHV-1 viral genome in nasopharyngeal swabs, blood, and other tissues. The test is at least as sensitive as viral isolation in identifying presence of virus. Rapid identification of virus shedding using qPCR can facilitate monitoring and interventions to prevent spread of infection and additional examination or prophylactic treatment of infected horses.

Appropriate PCR testing can determine whether the EHV-1 is the D752 or N752 variant. This information can be important in epidemiologic investigations and might have implications for administration of antiviral therapy, although this is unclear, but generally does not influence management of a disease outbreak.[21,72]

The virus can be isolated in tissue culture, chick embryos and hamsters, from either nasal washings or aborted fetuses, and has growth characteristics that differentiate it from EHV-4.[73]

Samples of nasopharyngeal exudate for virus isolation are best obtained from horses during the very early, febrile stages of disease, and are collected via the nares by swabbing the nasopharyngeal area with a 5 × 5-cm gauze sponge attached to the end of a 50-cm length of flexible, stainless steel wire encased in latex rubber tubing. A guarded uterine swab devise can also be used. After collection, the swab should be removed from the wire and transported promptly to the virology laboratory in 3 mL of cold (not frozen) fluid transport medium (serum-free minimal essential medium with antibiotics). Virus infectivity can be prolonged by the addition of bovine serum albumin or gelatin to 0.1% (w/v).

NECROPSY FINDINGS

Macroscopic findings in **aborted fetuses** include petechial and ecchymotic hemorrhages, especially beneath the respiratory mucosae. The most consistent finding is an excess of clear yellow fluid in the pleural and peritoneal cavities. Focal hepatic necrosis and slight icterus may also be present. In some aborted fetuses the cut surface of the spleen reveals unusually prominent lymphoid follicles, which are swollen from necrosis and edema. Acidophilic intranuclear inclusion bodies may be evident histologically in a variety of cell types, including the bronchiolar and alveolar epithelium, hepatocytes, and dendritic cells of the lymphoid tissues. Although the microscopic pathology is unimpressive, examination of the placenta via IHC techniques can be a useful aid in the diagnosis of EHV-1–induced and EHV-4–induced abortions. In foals that are alive at birth but die soon afterward there is usually massive pulmonary congestion and edema, with collapse of the lung and hyaline membrane development in those that survive longer.

In the **nervous or paralytic form** of the disease there is an acute disseminated myeloencephalopathy. Hemorrhages may be visible grossly but often there are no macroscopic changes. Disseminated vasculitis occurs in the experimental disease, and the malacic lesions present in the nervous tissue are the result of leakage from these damaged vessels. The virus can be isolated from the brain, and the isolation is facilitated by use of an indirect peroxidase stain to establish the location of the virus. The virus infects endothelial cells within the CNS but has also been demonstrated within neurons and astrocytes and has been linked to chorioretinitis in a foal. In rare cases the virus may cause lesions in other tissues, such as the intestinal mucosa and spleen or pharynx.

The laboratory examination of aborted fetuses should include a search for virus by tissue culture and IHC or PCR techniques, as well as a histologic examination of the lung and liver for the presence of inclusion bodies. A direct FAT has also been used. A serologic examination of the foal may provide useful information in those cases in which attempts at isolation are negative but seroconversion has occurred. However, a recent study found that fetal serology was an unreliable means of diagnosing EHV-1 abortion, and that IHC was slightly more sensitive than virus isolation.

Samples for Confirmation of Diagnosis

- **Virology:** chilled lung, liver, spleen, thymus, and thoracic fluid of aborted fetuses or neonates. Spinal cord or brain of horses with nervous disease (VI, PCR, FAT, serology).
- **Histology:** fixed lung, liver, spleen, thymus, and trachea from fetuses or neonates.
- Fixed brain and spinal cord from several sites, as well as Bouin's fixed eye should be examined in adults with nervous disease (LM, IHC).

DIFFERENTIAL DIAGNOSIS

Respiratory disease in horses is associated with a variety of agents (Table 12-14).

Abortion can be associated with leptospirosis, *Salmonella abortusequi,* placentitis associated with *Streptococcus zooepidemicus* or *Escherichia coli,* associated with mare reproductive loss syndrome, or congenital abnormalities, among other causes. When other pregnant mares are at risk, abortion in a late-term mare should always be considered to be caused by EHV-1 until proved otherwise.

Neurologic diseases with clinical presentations similar to that associated with EHV-1 include rabies, equine protozoal myeloencephalitis, neuritis of the cauda equina (equine polyneuritis), trauma, acute spinal cord compression (cervical stenotic myelopathy), and equine degenerative myelopathy. Fever is rare in other neurologic diseases of horses, and any horse with neurologic disease and fever or a history of fever within the previous week should be considered to have EHV-1 myeloencephalopathy. Outbreaks of posterior paresis or ataxia, especially in horses without fever, should prompt consideration of ingestion of intoxicants such as *Astragalus* spp., *Swainsona* spp., or sorghum. Ryegrass staggers can produce similar signs of ataxia.

Neonatal septicemia can be associated with *E. coli, Streptococci* spp., and other bacteria, especially in foals with failure of transfer of maternal immunoglobulins.

EHV-1, equid herphesvirus-1.

TREATMENT

Because of the highly contagious nature of EHV-1 infections, horses with respiratory disease, abortion, or neurologic disease, especially if these occur as an outbreak, should be isolated until the cause of the disease is identified.

There is **no specific treatment** for the diseases associated with EHV infection, although acyclovir and other antiviral drugs are used on occasion to treat horses in outbreaks of myeloencephalopathy.[46]

Horses with EHM require intense supportive care. Nursing care to prevent urine scalding, pressure sores, and pneumonia is important in horses with myeloencephalopathy. Recumbent or severely ataxic horses should be supported to stand if at all possible. Although a rope tied to the tail and slung over an overhead beam may be used to assist the horse to stand, a sling may be necessary to support more severely affected horses. Nursing care is important to prevent development of pressure sores in recumbent horses or those supported by slings. The perineum of incontinent horses should be cleaned frequently, and salves or ointments to protect the skin applied. Some horses require catheterization of the bladder to relieve distension. Enemas, accompanied by careful manual evacuation of the rectum, might be needed to promote passage of feces.

Administration of corticosteroids to these horses is controversial, but many clinicians administer dexamethasone sodium phosphate (0.05–0.25 mg/kg intramuscularly every 12–24 hours) or prednisolone (1–2 mg/kg orally or parenterally every 24 hours) for 2 to 3 days. Administration of corticosteroids may be contraindicated because of the presence of replicating virus in affected horses. The use of antiplatelet drugs or antithrombotic compounds has received anecdotal support, but there is no evidence that they do not harm affected horses and similarly no evidence of efficacy.

Administration of drugs to inhibit viral replication has merit and is attempted during outbreaks of disease. The challenges of this approach are that the infection is well advanced by the time clinical signs of neurologic disease are detected, especially in cases early in the disease outbreak before purposeful monitoring is in place, pharmacokinetics and pharmacodynamics of the available drugs are unknown or imperfectly known, and the drugs are expensive. Antiviral drugs considered for use in horses with EHM include acyclovir, valacyclovir, penciclovir (after oral administration of its prodrug famciclovir), ganciclovir, and valganciclovir.[74-78] Acyclovir is effective against EHV-1 in vitro, and pharmacokinetic studies suggest that administration of 10 mg/kg orally every 4 to 6 hours (five times daily) or 10 mg/kg intravenously every 8 hours results in acceptable concentrations of drug in the blood. However, further investigation reveals that there is a large variation between individual horses in the absorption of acyclovir with consequent failure to obtain therapeutic concentrations in many horses.[79] The in vitro activity of acyclovir, ganciclovir, cidofovir, adefovir, 9-(2-phosphonylmethoxyethyl)-2,6-diaminopurine (PMEDAP) and foscarnet against three abortigenic isolates and three neuropathogenic isolates of EHV-1 revealed variable activity of cidofovir and limited to no activity of foscarnet.[80]

Current recommendations for the prophylaxis and treatment of horses with EHM include administration of acyclovir (10–20 mg/kg every 5–8 hours, orally for 7 days) or ganciclovir IV at 2.5 mg/kg every 8 h for 24 h followed by maintenance dosing of 2.5 mg/kg every 12 h, or orally at 30–40 mg/kg every 8–12 h for 7 days.[72] The efficacy of these compounds has not been demonstrated in appropriate clinical trials, and earlier comments about the variability in oral bioavailability of acyclovir should be noted.

Neonatal foals with septicemia should be treated aggressively with **antibiotics** and **supportive care**, including enteral or parenteral nutrition and fluid administration (see the section Clinical Assessment and Care of Critically Ill Newborns in Chapter 19). Treatment with acyclovir has been reported. Failure of transfer of passive immunity should be rectified with oral or intravenous administration of colostrum or plasma, respectively.

CONTROL

Recommendations for programs to prevent introduction of infection and to control EHM and abortion outbreaks are available from several sources and might vary between countries.[18,21,29,81]

Prevention of Infection

The general principles include the following:

- Enhanced immunity, currently attempted by vaccination
- Subdivision and maintenance of the farm population in groups of horses to minimize spread of the infection
- Minimize risk of introduction of infection by new horses
- Minimize risk of reactivation of latent infection in resident horses
- Develop plans for implementation of these routine control measures, and for actions in the event of an abortion
- Educate management and staff as to the importance of strict adherence to these procedures

The relative importance of each of these measures has not been determined, but implementation of control measures, including allocation of mares to small bands based on anticipated foaling date, quarantine of new introductions, and vaccination of pregnant mares, has reduced the incidence of EHV-1 abortion in central Kentucky. The most striking association has been an apparent reduction in the incidence of abortion storms. It must be emphasized that vaccination does not replace any of the other management procedures in control of this disease and that abortions have occurred among vaccinated mares on farms on which the other management procedures have been ignored.

Vaccination

Vaccination against respiratory disease and abortion associated with EHV-1 is widely practiced despite lack of clear-cut evidence that vaccination reduces the incidence or severity of either of these diseases. Information regarding field efficacy of EHV vaccines is lacking, and that derived from experimental challenge models is often contradictory or incomplete. Give these caveats, the following recommendations are made based on generally accepted practices.

None of the currently available vaccines, of which there are approximately 14 worldwide, consistently prevent infection of vaccinated horses or provide complete protection against disease associated with EHV-1.[21,52,72] The principal objective of vaccination has been to protect mares against abortion associated with EHV-1, although vaccines intended to prevent rhinopneumonitis and containing both EHV-1 and EHV-4 are available. Additionally, vaccination of mares is intended to reduce transmission of EHV-1 to foals in an attempt to interrupt the cyclical nature of infection on stud farms. Vaccines consisting of a modified live EHV-1, inactivated EHV-1, or a mixture of inactivated EHV-1 and EHV-4 are available for intramuscular or intranasal administration to horses. Both inactivated and modified live EHV-1 vaccines elicit virus-neutralization and complement fixation antibody responses in horses, although high antibody titers are not necessarily related to resistance to infection.

Resistance to infection might be more closely related to cytotoxic T-cell responses. Widespread use of a combined EHV-1 and EHV-4 killed virus vaccine in Australia has not reduced serologic evidence of infection in foals on farms where mares are vaccinated, although the vaccine was effective in preventing disease induced by experimental infection. Complicating assessment of vaccine efficacy is the variable response to vaccination by some mares and foals, with certain animals having minimal responses to vaccination, which in other horses elicits a strong immune response. Efforts are underway to develop modified live vaccines that can be administered intranasally. Intranasal administration of one such EHV-1 vaccine induced protection against experimentally induced EHV-1 (and EHV-4) respiratory disease and abortion in mares, and prevented infection of foals even when administered in the presence of maternally derived antibodies. An alternative approach is the development of subunit vaccines using the envelope glycoprotein D, which has been shown to elicit protective immunity in laboratory animal models of EHV-1 disease and administration of which induces VN antibody and glycoprotein D–specific ELISA antibodies in horses. Current modified live vaccines appear to induce a more restricted IgG isotype than does natural infection, which could partly account for their limited efficacy.[53]

Despite the incomplete protection afforded by vaccines, vaccination against EHV-1 is an important part of most equine herd health programs in the vaccination of pregnant and nonpregnant mares, foals, and adult horses. The intent of vaccination of mares is to prevent abortion associated with EHV-1. One inactivated virus vaccine is reported to decrease the incidence of abortion by 65%, although others have not been able to replicate this success and there are reports of abortion storms on farms of well-vaccinated mares. An inactivated virus vaccine containing EHV-1 and EHV-4 prevented abortion in five of six mares exposed experimentally to EHV-1, whereas all six nonvaccinated mares aborted. Mares are vaccinated with the inactivated vaccine during the fifth, seventh, and ninth months of gestation. Additional vaccinations at breeding and 1 month before foaling are recommended by some authorities.

No vaccines are currently licensed with the claim of preventing EHM, and the disease occurs in well-vaccinated horses. Concerns that the disease might represent a "second hit" as a result of vaccination and subsequent infection have not received widespread support and do not have empirical evidence that is in any way supportive.[21]

Foals are an important source of infection and control of infection in foals is considered critical to control of infection on a farm. Consequently, attention has been paid to the responses of foals to vaccination at various ages, given the risk of passive immunity interfering with vaccination and the early age at which foals are infected by EHV-1. Current recommendations vary with some authorities recommending vaccination of foals after 5 months of age, to avoid the interfering effect of passive immunity on response to vaccination. However, vaccination of foals at this age likely misses the period of time when foals are first infected by EHV-1 from their dam or other mares in the band. One recommendation is that foals should be vaccinated in their third month, with revaccination 1 month and 6 months later. Modified live virus vaccine is given to foals at 3 to 4 months of age, and nonpregnant mares and other horses are given two doses administered 3 months apart followed by revaccination every 9 months. Because of the short duration of immunity following vaccination, frequent vaccination, perhaps at intervals as short as 3 months, of horses at high risk is recommended. However, the efficacy of such a program is uncertain.

Subdivision of Horses on a Farm

Maintenance of small groups of horses of similar age and reproductive status is recommended to minimize the chances of spread of infection. Pregnant mares, after weaning of foals, should be maintained in a herd that does not have access to foals, weanlings, nonpregnant mares, or other equids (donkeys). Similarly, weaned foals should be separated from horses of other ages in recognition of the high rate of infection and viral shedding in weanlings. Failure to adhere to these procedures can result in rapid spread of infection and abortions among at-risk mares. Pregnant mares should be combined into small groups (~10) early in pregnancy based on their anticipated foaling dates. Multiparous mares should not be mixed with mares that are pregnant for the first time.

Management practices should be introduced that minimize the opportunities for viral spread. Ideally, pregnant mares are handled using facilities separate from those used to handle mares with foals or weanlings. If common facilities must be used, pregnant mares should be handled first, after thorough cleaning of the facility, followed by mares with foals and finally weanlings and other horses.

Minimize Risk of Introduction of Infection

The only sources of virus are recrudescence of latent infection and introduction by newly arrived horses shedding virus. All horses must be considered as potentially shedding EHV-1 on arrival at a farm and should be isolated from resident horses. Introduction of new horses to the small groups of pregnant mares should be avoided if at all possible, or if absolutely necessary preceded by a 21-day isolation period. If at all possible, avoid mingling resident and nonresident mares even after quarantine of nonresident animals.

Prevention of Reactivation of Latent Infection

The factors inciting reactivation of latent infection and viral shedding are unknown. However, stressful events, such as transportation or other disease, have the potential to cause reactivation of latent infection. For this reason pregnant mares should not be shipped within 8 weeks of expected foaling and all efforts, including vaccination, should be made to prevent other infectious diseases.

Control of Outbreaks

The principles underlying control of abortions or EHM caused by EHV-1 include the following:

- Early and rapid diagnosis
- Prevention of spread of infection
- Treatment of individual cases

These aims are approached through six stages:

1. **Preliminary recognition of the problem (outbreak):** typically by owners or trainers recognizing the presence of sick horses.
2. **Preliminary veterinary investigation:** conducted by a veterinarian on, usually, their first response to the owner's concerns and leading to a presumptive clinical diagnosis.
3. **Establishing the diagnosis:** use of appropriate laboratory and other testing to confirm or rule out specific diagnoses.
4. **Understanding and managing the outbreak:** this is complex because it involves an understanding of the biology and epidemiology of the disease, the financial and social context of the outbreak, and assessment of the feasibility, and cost-effectiveness, of potential interventions.
5. **Establishing freedom of infection:** documenting the end of the outbreak and confirming freedom from infection by the offending agent.
6. **Return the premise to normal function and activity.**

Control of Outbreaks of Myeloencephalopathy

Diagnostic criteria for EHM are set out in the six stages list earlier. Adult horses with rapid onset of signs of nervous system disease, with or without fever, should be considered to have EHM until proven otherwise.

Outbreaks of EHV-1–induced neurologic disease often occur in riding schools and similar situations where there is constant movement of horses on and off the property. As such it is exceedingly difficult to institute control measures that prevent introduction of the disease and that are compatible with the use of the horses. Having said that, the principles outlined earlier for preventing introduction of infection onto breeding farms also apply for prevention of myeloencephalopathy at riding stables.

Reports of outbreaks of EHM in stables and veterinary hospitals have underscored the highly infectious nature of the disease.[25,46,47] EHV-1 is spread from infected horses, which can have virus in nasal fluid before onset of clinical signs, by aerosol, and on fomites. It is critical to prevent spread by diligent attention to biosecurity, including spread by personnel and aerosol. Infected horses should be isolated in a separate air space to uninfected or at risk horses.

Detailed instructions for handling outbreaks of neurologic disease attributable to EHV-1 are available and provide advice on quarantine, disinfection, and sample collection. There is no "one size fits all," and the recommendations should be modified or adopted with a full understanding of the financial, social, and psychologic context of managing the outbreak. Guidelines for managing an outbreak of EHM include the following[21,29,72,82]:

- Affected horses should be isolated because they are infectious.
- The diagnosis should be confirmed by virus isolation, PCR, or histologic examination of tissues from affected horses that die or are euthanized.
- Potentially affected horses should be tested to determine whether they are excreting the virus (nasal swabs).
- There should be no movement of horses on or off the premises for at least 21 days after the last case has occurred.
- Movement among bands of horses on the farm should be avoided.
- Animals should leave or move between bands only when there is no evidence of continued active infection in their group.
- Vaccination in the face of an outbreak of EHM is not recommended. Clinically affected horses should not be vaccinated.
- Prophylactic use of acyclovir has been reported, although the efficacy of this practice is unknown.

Table 14-13 Three-tiered approach to managing an outbreak of equine herpesvirus myeloencephalopathy.

	Three tiers of approach		
Action	*Gold tier*	*Silver tier*	*Bronze tier*
Segregate the population into small discrete groups that can be managed discretely to avoid infection transferring between them	**Yes** The smaller the groups the better to minimize the impact of ongoing disease and possibly reduce later laboratory test costs	**Yes** The smaller the groups the better to minimize the impact of ongoing disease and possibly reduce later laboratory test costs	**Yes** The smaller the groups the better to minimize the impact of ongoing disease and possibly reduce later laboratory test costs
Collect samples	**Collect full set from all animals** NP swab in VTM, serum (5–10 mL) and heparinized whole blood (30 ml)	**Collect partial set from all animals** NP swab in VTM and serum (5–10 mL)	**Collect partial set from all animals** NP swab in VTM and serum (5–10 mL)
Test samples	**Test full set from all animals** NP swab by qPCR, serum by CFT and heparinized blood by virus isolation	**Test partial set from all animals** NP swab by qPCR and serum by CFT	**Do not test, but freeze** the partial set from all animals for possible testing later
Observe for clinical disease (neurologic disease and/or abortion noting that pregnant mares should only be considered clear once they have a foaled successfully and have a healthy foal at foot)	**Observe all groups for 3–4 weeks**: If no clinical disease is observed in a group: collect NP swabs and sera (pair with already tested sample in CFT) and test, consider EHV-1 free if all results are negative If clinical disease is observed in a group: immediately collect and test a full set of samples from all horses in the affected group Remove positives to an isolation area Repeat after 2–3 weeks and only consider EHV-1 free when all results are negative	**Observe all groups for 3–4 weeks**: If no clinical disease is observed in a group: collect NP swabs and sera (pair with already tested sample in CFT) and test, consider EHV-1 free if all results are negative If clinical disease is observed in a group: immediately collect and test a full set of samples from all horses in the affected group Remove positives to an isolation area Repeat after 2–3 weeks and only consider EHV-1 free when all results are negative	**Observe all groups for 3–4 weeks**: If no clinical disease is observed in a group: collect NP swabs and sera (pair with frozen samples in CFT) and test, consider EHV-1 free if all results are negative If clinical disease is observed in a group: immediately collect a full set of samples from all the affected group and test all, including frozen, samples Remove positives to an isolation area Repeat after 2–3 weeks and only consider EHV-1 free when all results are negative

CFT, complement fixation test; NP, nasopharyngeal; qPCR, quantitative polymerase chain reaction; VTM, virus transport medium.
Reproduced from Gonzalez-Medina S et al: Equine Vet J *2015; 47:142.*

A suggested, three-tiered approach to managing an outbreak of EHM is depicted in Table 14-13.

Abortion

Rapid Diagnosis

Every abortion in a late-term mare should be considered to be associated with EHV-1 until proven otherwise. Therefore rapid and early diagnosis of the abortion or of EHM is important to instituting control measures. In regions with large numbers of breeding mares, **all** abortions in mares should be investigated by detailed postmortem examination of the fetus and serologic examination of the mare.

Prevention of Spread

Diligent and concerted efforts must be made to prevent dissemination of infection from the initial focus in cases of abortion. Delay in doing so increases the incidence of abortion and prolongs the outbreak.[27] Infected fetal tissues and fluids, and contaminated materials such as bedding, should be placed in impervious containers and either transported to a laboratory for examination or destroyed by incineration. Samples for laboratory examination should be handled to prevent spread of infection. Facilities and equipment that might have been contaminated should be disinfected by thorough cleaning followed by application of a phenolic or iodophor disinfectant.

The mare should be isolated until results of laboratory examination are negative for EHV-1 or until the second estrus, at which time it is unlikely that there is shedding of virus from the reproductive tract. Other mares in the same band as the mare that aborted should be considered exposed and at risk of abortion. These mares should be held in strict isolation until the results of laboratory examination are negative for EHV-1, or until they foal or abort. Other recommendations for horse movement include the following:

- When an abortion occurs on the stud, no mares should be allowed to enter or leave it until the possibility of EHV-1 infection is excluded. However, maiden and barren mares, i.e., mares that have foaled normally at home but that are not in foal, coming from home studs where no signs of the disease are occurring, may be admitted because they are considered not to be infected.
- If EHV-1 infection is identified on the stud, all pregnant mares ready to foal that season (i.e., late-pregnant mares) should remain at the stud until they have foaled. The incubation period for EHV-1 abortion ranges between 9 and 121 days.
- All nonpregnant animals and mares that have foaled should remain at the stud for 30 days after the last abortion.

The main problem that arises in this program is in deciding what to do with mares that come into contact with the respiratory disease but not the abortion disease. This may occur very early in pregnancy and prolonged isolation would be onerous. The decision usually depends on the owner's risk aversion and the availability of facilities to maintain long-term isolation.

FURTHER READING

Gonzalez-Medina S, Newton JR. Equine herpesvirus-1:dealing pragmatically but effectively with an ever present threat. *Equine Vet J.* 2015;47:142-144.

Lunn DP, et al. Equine herpesvirus-1 consensus statement. *J Vet Intern Med.* 2009;23:450-461.

Pusterla N, Hussey GS. Equine herpesvirus 1 myeloencephalopathy. *Vet Clin North Am Equine Pract.* 2014;30:489-506.

REFERENCES

1. Davison AJ, et al. *Arch Virol.* 2009;154:171.
2. Schrenzel MD, et al. *Emerg Infect Dis.* 2008;14:1616.
3. Rebelo AR, et al. *Can J Vet Res.* 2015;79:155.

4. LeCuyer TE, et al. *J Vet Diagn Invest*. 2015;27:749.
5. De Witte FG, et al. *J Vet Intern Med*. 2012;26:1064.
6. Bell SA, et al. *Vet Microbiol*. 2008;130:176.
7. Rushton JO, et al. *Vet J*. 2014;200:200.
8. Vengust M, et al. *J Vet Diagn Invest*. 2008;20:820.
9. Pusterla N, et al. *Vet Rec*. 2010;167:376.
10. Wong D, et al. *JAVMA*. 2008;232:898.
11. Williams KJ, et al. *PLoS ONE*. 2013;8:e63535.
12. Vander Werf KA, et al. *J Equine Vet Sci*. 2014;34:738.
13. Vander Werf K, et al. *J Vet Intern Med*. 2013;27:387.
14. Hussey GS, et al. *Vet Res*. 2013;44:118.
15. Herder V, et al. *Vet Microbiol*. 2012;155:420.
16. Abdelgawad A, et al. *PLoS ONE*. 2015;10:e0138370.
17. Ibrahim ESM, et al. *Arch Virol*. 2007;152:245.
18. Dunowska M. *New Zeal Vet J*. 2014;62:171.
19. Ma G, et al. *Vet Microbiol*. 2013;167:123.
20. Nugent J, et al. *J Virol*. 2006;80:4047.
21. Lunn DP, et al. *J Vet Intern Med*. 2009;23:450.
22. Allen GP. *Am J Vet Res*. 2008;69:1595.
23. Pronost S, et al. *Equine Vet J*. 2010;42:672.
24. Pronost S, et al. *Vet Microbiol*. 2010;145:329.
25. Walter J, et al. *Acta Vet Scand*. 2013;55.
26. Stasiak K, et al. *BMC Vet Res*. 2015;11.
27. Schulman ML, et al. *Equine Vet J*. 2015;47:155.
28. Perkins GA, et al. *Vet Microbiol*. 2009;139:375.
29. Gonzalez-Medina S, et al. *Equine Vet J*. 2015;47:142.
30. Allen GP, et al. *Equine Vet J*. 2008;40:105.
31. Tsujimura K, et al. *J Vet Med Sci*. 2011;73:1663.
32. Burgess BA, et al. *J Vet Intern Med*. 2012;26:384.
33. Pusterla N, et al. *Vet J*. 2012;193:579.
34. Goodman LB, et al. *PLoS Pathog*. 2007;3:e160.
35. Vandekerckhove AP, et al. *J Gen Virol*. 2010;91:2019.
36. Estell KE, et al. *Equine Vet J*. 2015;47:689.
37. Wohlsein P, et al. *Vet Microbiol*. 2011;149:456.
38. Abdelgawad A, et al. *Vet Microbiol*. 2014;169:102.
39. Guo X, et al. *J Vet Med Sci*. 2014;76:1309.
40. Damiani AM, et al. *Vet Microbiol*. 2014;172:555.
41. Gryspeerdt A, et al. *Vlaams Diergeneeskundig Tijdschr*. 2011;80:147.
42. Mori E, et al. *Rev - Off Int Epizoot*. 2011;30:949.
43. van Galen G, et al. *Vet Microbiol*. 2015;179:304.
44. Bazanow BA, et al. *Polish J Vet Sci*. 2014;17:607.
45. Pronost S, et al. *Transbound Emerg Dis*. 2012;59:256.
46. Henninger RW, et al. *J Vet Intern Med*. 2007;21:157.
47. Goehring LS, et al. *J Vet Intern Med*. 2010;24:1176.
48. Gardiner DW, et al. *Vaccine*. 2012;30:6564.
49. Hebia I, et al. *Theriogenology*. 2007;67:1485.
50. Hebia-Fellah I, et al. *Theriogenology*. 2009;71:1381.
51. Pusterla N, et al. *J Vet Intern Med*. 2010;24:1153.
52. Paillot R, et al. *Open Vet Sci J*. 2008;2:68.
53. Goodman LB, et al. *Clin Vaccine Immunol*. 2012;19:235.
54. Paillot R, et al. *Dev Comp Immunol*. 2007;31:202.
55. Wimer CL, et al. *Vet Immunol Immunopathol*. 2011;140:266.
56. Gryspeerdt AC, et al. *Vet Microbiol*. 2010;142:242.
57. Luce R, et al. *Equine Vet J*. 2007;39:202.
58. Ma G, et al. *J Virol*. 2012;86:3554.
59. Sarkar S, et al. *Vet Immunol Immunopathol*. 2015;167:122.
60. Andoh K, et al. *Virus Res*. 2015;195:172.
61. Goehring LS, et al. *J Vet Intern Med*. 2013;27:1535.
62. Stokol T, et al. *PLoS ONE*. 2015;10:e0122640.
63. Pusterla N, et al. *Vet J*. 2009;180:279.
64. Goehring LS, et al. *Vet J*. 2010;186:180.
65. Amer HM, et al. *Afr J Microbiol Res*. 2011;5:4805.
66. Yildirim Y, et al. *Iranian J Vet Res*. 2015;16:341.
67. Hu Z, et al. *Appl Microbiol Biotech*. 2014;98:4179.
68. Pusterla N, et al. *J Vet Diagn Invest*. 2009;21:836.
69. Pusterla N, et al. *Vet J*. 2009;179:230.
70. Smith KL, et al. *J Clin Microbiol*. 2012;50:1981.
71. Stasiak K, et al. *Polish J Vet Sci*. 2015;18:833.
72. Pusterla N, et al. *Vet Clin North Am Equine Pract*. 2014;30:489.
73. Equine rhinopneumonitis (equine herpesvirus 1 and 4). OIE, 2015. (Accessed 07.02.2016, at http://www.oie.int/fileadmin/Home/eng/Health_standards/tahm/2.05.09_EQUINE_RHINO.pdf.).
74. Carmichael RJ, et al. *J Vet Intern Med*. 2010;24:712.
75. Carmichael RJ, et al. *J Vet Pharmacol Ther*. 2013;36:441.
76. Garre B, et al. *Vet Microbiol*. 2009;135:214.
77. Maxwell LK, et al. *J Vet Pharmacol Ther*. 2008;31:312.
78. Tsujimura K, et al. *J Vet Med Sci*. 2010;72:357.
79. Wong DM, et al. *Equine Vet Educ*. 2010;22:244.
80. Garre B, et al. *Vet Microbiol*. 2007;122:43.
81. Dunowska M. *New Zeal Vet J*. 2014;62:179.
82. Equine herpesvirus 1 and 4 related diseases. American Association of Equine Practitioners, 2013. (Accessed 07.02.2016, at http://www.aaep.org/custdocs/EquineHerpesvirusFinal030513.pdf.).

PERUVIAN HORSE SICKNESS VIRUS

Peruvian horse sickness virus is an Orbivirus associated with causing neurologic disease in horses in Peru with a mortality rate of approximately 1.25% and a case–fatality rate of 78%.[1] A genetically identical virus has been isolated from horses dying of neurologic disease in northern Australia.[2] Serologic surveillance in that area demonstrates antibody to Peruvian horse sickness virus in 11% of horses. The disease is described as causing motor incoordination, sagging jaw, tooth grinding, and stiff neck with death in 8 to 11 days.

REFERENCES

1. Attoui H, et al. *Virology*. 2009;394:298.
2. Mendez-Lopez MR, et al. *J Vector Ecol*. 2015;40:355.

POWASSAN VIRUS

The **Powassan virus**, a flavivirus that is spread by the bite of infected ticks,[1] occurs in Ontario and the eastern United States, and produces a nonsuppurative, focal necrotizing meningoencephalitis in horses. Approximately 13% of horses sampled in Ontario in 1983 were serologically positive to the virus. Experimental intracerebral inoculation of the Powassan virus into horses resulted in a neurologic syndrome within 8 days. Clinical findings include a "tucked-up" abdomen, tremors of the head and neck, slobbering and chewing movements resulting in foamy saliva, stiff gait, staggering, and recumbency. There is a nonsuppurative encephalomyelitis, neuronal necrosis, and focal parenchymal necrosis. The virus has not been isolated from the brain.

REFERENCE

1. Dupuis AP II, et al. *Parasit Vectors*. 2013;6:185.

NIGERIAN EQUINE ENCEPHALITIS

Nigerian equine encephalitis, a disease with low morbidity but high mortality, is characterized by fever, generalized muscle spasms, ataxia, and lateral recumbency of 3 to 5 days' duration. The virus has not been identified, but the only report describes the lesions as consistent with an alphavirus, although Lagos bat virus, a pathogenic lyssavirus, is highly endemic in this area.

MAIN DRAIN VIRUS ENCEPHALITIS

The **main drain virus** has been isolated from a horse with severe encephalitis in California.[1] Clinical findings included incoordination, ataxia, stiffness of the neck, head-pressing, inability to swallow, fever, and tachycardia. The virus is transmitted by rabbits and rodents and by its natural vector, *Culicoides variipennis*.

REFERENCE

1. Wilson WC, et al. *Rev - Off Int Epizoot*. 2015;34:419.

BORNA DISEASE

Borna disease is an **infectious encephalomyelitis** of horses and sheep first recorded in Germany. It is associated with a negative sense, single-stranded RNA virus classified as *Bornavirus* within the order Mononegavirales. There is a recently recognized avian variant of Borna disease virus, which causes disease in birds.[1]

The disease and the virus in horses are indistinguishable from EEE. Borna disease is now recognized as a subacute meningoencephalitis in horses, cattle, sheep, rabbits, and cats in Germany, Sweden, and Switzerland.[2] There are reports of encephalitis with Borna disease virus genome detected in lesions by PCR in a horse and a cow in Japan. The disease apparently occurs in New World camelids.[3] Encephalitis associated with Borna disease virus was detected in young ostriches in Israel. The disease does not appear to be a common cause of nonsuppurative encephalitis in pigs.[4] Serologic evidence of infection by Borna disease virus is widespread both geographically and in the range of species.[5,6]

Borna disease virus is suspected of causing disease in humans, including lymphocytic meningoencephalitis, but infection is not associated with an increased prevalence of psychiatric disorders. Others suggest that the presence of circulating Borna disease virus immune complexes (Borna disease virus antigen and specific antibodies) is associated with severe mood disorders in humans. The role, if any, of Borna disease virus in human neurologic or psychiatric disease has not been established with any certainty and is the subject of considerable debate.[1]

Detection of Borna disease virus **genome** by PCR analysis suggests that, although the spontaneous disease in horses and sheep occurs predominantly if not exclusively in Europe, clinically unapparent Borna disease virus infection is widespread in a number of species including horses, cattle, sheep, cats, and foxes. However, concern has been raised that some of these reports might be based on flawed laboratory results as a consequence of contamination of PCR assays. **Antibodies** to Borna disease virus in serum or CSF have been detected in horses in the eastern United States, Japan, Iran, Turkey, France, and China, and in healthy sheep and dairy cattle in Japan. In areas in which the disease is not endemic, between 3% (United States) and 42% (Iran) of horses have either antibodies or Borna disease virus nucleic acid, detected by PCR, in blood or serum. Similarly, approximately 12% to 20% of horses have serologic evidence of exposure to Borna disease virus in areas of Europe in which the disease is endemic. Antibodies to Borna disease virus and nucleic acid have been detected in humans in North America, Europe, and Japan. Closed flocks of sheep and herds of horses have evidence of persistent infection of some animals, based on serologic testing. It is worth noting that animals infected with the virus and those who are clinically ill may have undetectable to very low antibody titers.

The method of transmission of infection between animals is unknown, but it is thought to be horizontal by inhalation or ingestion. Seropositive, clinically normal horses and sheep can excrete virus in conjunctival fluid, nasal secretions, and saliva, suggesting that they might be important in the transmission of infection. Removal of all seropositive and Borna disease virus RNA-positive sheep from a closed flock did not prevent seroconversion of other animals in the flock the following year. The possibility of vertical transmission is raised by the finding of Borna disease virus RNA in the brain of a fetal foal of a mare that died of Borna disease.

There is a seasonal distribution to the prevalence of the disease, with most cases in horses occurring in spring and early summer. The virus has not been isolated from arthropods, including hematophagous insects.

The **morbidity** in Borna disease is not high, approximately 0.006% to 0.23% of horses affected per year in endemic areas of Germany, but most affected animals die.

The **pathogenesis** of the disease involves infection of cells of the CNS. It is assumed that the virus gains entry to the CNS through trigeminal and olfactory nerves, with subsequent dissemination of infection throughout the brain. Viral transcription and replication occurs within the cell nucleus. Viral replication does not appear to result in damage to the infected neuron. However, infected cells express viral antigens on their surface, which then initiate a cell-mediated immune response by the host that then destroys infected cells (immunosuppression prevents development of the disease). The inflammatory response is largely composed of CD3 lymphocytes. The disease is subacute; infection and the development of lesions may take weeks to months. Clinically inapparent infection appears to be common in a number of species, including horses.

In **field outbreaks** the incubation period is about 4 weeks and possibly up to 6 months.

Clinical signs of the disease in horses include the following:

- Moderate fever
- Pharyngeal paralysis
- Lack of food intake
- Muscle tremor
- Defects in proprioception
- Hyperesthesia
- Blindness or visual defects[7]

Lethargy, somnolence, and flaccid paralysis are seen in the terminal stages, and death occurs 1 to 3 weeks after the first appearance of clinical signs. Infection without detectable clinical signs is thought to be common on infected premises. The frequency with which Borna disease virus is detected in horses with gait deficits is greater than in clinically normal horses, suggesting a role for the virus in inducing subtle disease.

The presentation of the disease in cattle is similar to that in horses, with affected animals having reduced appetite, ataxia, paresis, and compulsive circling. The disease ends in the death of the animal after a 1- to 6-week course.

Hematology and routine serum biochemistry are typically normal, with the exception of fasting-induced hyperbilirubinemia in anorexic horses. Clinicopathologic identification of exposed animals is achieved with complement fixation, ELISA, Western blot, or indirect immunofluorescent tests.

At **necropsy** there are no gross findings, but histologically there is a lymphocytic and plasmacytic meningoencephalitis, affecting chiefly the brainstem, and a lesser degree of myelitis. The highest concentration of virus is in the hippocampus and thalamus. The diagnostic microscopic finding is the presence of intranuclear inclusion bodies within neurons, especially in the hippocampus and olfactory bulbs. The virus can be grown on tissue culture and demonstrated within tissues by immunofluorescence and immunoperoxidase techniques. Borna disease virus can also be detected in formalin-fixed, paraffin-embedded brain tissues using a nested PCR.

Specific **control measures** cannot be recommended because of the lack of knowledge of means of transmission of the virus. The role of inapparently infected horses in transmission of the disease is unknown, and there is no widespread program for testing for such horses. An attenuated virus vaccine was produced by continued passage of the virus through rabbits and used in the former East Germany until 1992. However, its use was discontinued because of questionable efficacy.

FURTHER READING

Lipkin WI, et al. Borna disease virus—Fact and fantasy. *Virus Res.* 2011;162:162-172.

REFERENCES

1. Lipkin WI, et al. *Virus Res.* 2011;162:162.
2. Lutz H, et al. *J Feline Med Surg.* 2015;17:614.
3. Jacobsen B, et al. *J Comp Pathol.* 2010;143:203.
4. Bukovsky C, et al. *Vet Rec.* 2007;161:552.
5. Bjornsdottir S, et al. *Acta Vet Scand.* 2013;55:77.
6. Kinnunen PM, et al. *J Clin Virol.* 2007;38:64.
7. Dietzel J, et al. *Vet Pathol.* 2007;44:57.

TESCHOVIRUS INFECTIONS

Important enteric viruses of the pig belong to the Picornaviridae particularly enteroviruses, teschoviruses and sapeloviruses (formerly porcine enterovirus A or porcine enterovirus).

SEROTYPES

The most important disease of this group is Teschen itself, which was restricted to a particular region around the town of Teschen in Czechoslovakia and the surrounding parts of Eastern Europe.[1,2] The mild forms of the disease have occurred elsewhere and are referred to as Talfan or in the past poliomyelitis suum or benign enzootic paresis, and these are probably present worldwide.

SYNOPSIS

Etiology Porcine enteroviruses capable of causing encephalomyelitis. Teschen virus, Talfan virus, and others.

Epidemiology Certain European countries, Scandinavia, and North America. Morbidity 50%; case fatality 70%–90%. Teschen in Europe. Talfan in UK. Viral encephalomyelitis in North America. Transmitted by direct contact.

Signs Acute Teschen: fever, stiffness, unable to stand, tremors, convulsions, and death in few days

Subacute Talfan: milder than acute form. Most common in pigs under 2 weeks of age. Morbidity and case–fatality rate 100%. Outbreaks. Hyperesthesia, tremors, knuckling of fetlocks, dog-sitting, convulsions, blindness, and death in a few days. Milder in older growing pigs and adults.

Clinical pathology Virus-neutralization tests.

Lesions Nonsuppurative encephalomyelitis.

Diagnostic confirmation Demonstrate lesion and identify virus.

Differential diagnosis list

- Pseudorabies
- Hemagglutinating encephalomyelitis virus

Treatment None.

Control Outbreaks will cease and herd immunity develops.

ETIOLOGY

Originally, there were at least 13 enterovirus members, and these are now reclassified. The viruses are resistant to environmental effects (in one study of disinfectants only sodium hypochlorite was effective), are stable, and easily cultivated. The only known host is the pig, and the viruses are not zoonotic.

Important enteric viruses belong to the Picornaviridae and the genera *Enterovirus*, *Teschovirus*, and *Sapelovirus* (these were formerly known as porcine enterovirus A or porcine enterovirus serotype B.[1] In a survey of 206 viral isolates 97 (47%) were identified as teschoviruses, 18% as sapeloviruses, and 3% as adenoviruses.[3]

Porcine enteric picornaviruses produce asymptomatic infections as well as reproductive disorders, diarrhea, pneumonia, and dermal lesions. These viruses were previously classified as enteroviruses. They are now reclassified into three groups on the basis of genomic sequences: (1) porcine teschoviruses (PTVs) with 11 different serogroups; (2) porcine enterovirus B, which corresponds to the former enterovirus serotypes 9 and 10; and (3) porcine sapelovirus (PSV), which corresponds to former enterovirus type 8 and has a single serotype that is divided into antigenic variants (PEV 8a, 8b, and 9c). It is associated with reproductive disease, diarrhea, and pneumonia.

It appears that PTV-1, the most virulent type, is only found in Central Europe (there have been a number of independent isolates, such as the Konratice and Reporyje strains) and Africa. Talfan virus, isolated from England, and other unnamed isolates appear less virulent. Teschen and Talfan virus occur in subgroup 1, which is now called porcine enterovirus group 1 (PEV-1), but isolates from encephalomyelitis are also associated with other subgroups. The other PTVs and PSV are ubiquitous. Porcine enterovirus B (PEV-9 and PEV-10) is found in Italy, UK, and Japan.[4]

A PTV caused respiratory distress and acute diarrhea in China in 50-to 70-day-old pigs.[5] PTV-8 (a sapelovirus in the new classification) caused a SMEDI-like syndrome in China,[6,7] in which approximately 80 gilts aborted and many piglets were stillborn or died soon after birth; samples from most were PTV positive.

Within subgroups, strains may be further differentiated using a complement fixation test and monospecific sera. There is variation in virulence between strains, and with many strains, clinical encephalitis following infection appears to be the exception rather than the rule. Most of the infections are subclinical.

Polioencephalomyelitis is associated with PTV-1, 2, 3, and 5; reproductive disease is associated with PTV-1, 3, and 6; diarrhea is associated with PTV-1, 2, 3, and 5; pneumonia is associated with PTV-1, 2, and 3; pericarditis and myocarditis have been associated with PTV-2 and 3; and cutaneous lesions are associated with PTV-9 and 10.

EPIDEMIOLOGY

Occurrence and Prevalence of Infection

There is serologic evidence that the disease occurs throughout the world. The most severe form of the disease, Teschen disease, appears to be limited to Europe and Madagascar, but the milder forms occur extensively in Europe (Hungary, 2012), Scandinavia, and North America (2002–2007) and recently in Japan (2012). The recent outbreak in the United States (Indiana) was ascribed to porcine enterovirus Serogroup 5 or 6 with the only characteristic feature being the histologic lesions of polioencephalomyelitis. Losses caused by the disease result primarily from deaths.

Serologic surveys in areas where the disease occurs indicate that a high proportion of the pig population is infected without any clinical evidence of the disease. In the majority of field occurrences, porcine encephalomyelitis is a sporadic disease affecting either one or a few litters, or a small number of weaned pigs.

Morbidity and Case Fatality

The morbidity rate is usually about 50% and the case–fatality rate 70% to 90% in Teschen. Talfan is much milder, and the morbidity rate below 6%.

Methods of Transmission

Infection is transmitted by the fecal–oral route and therefore by ingestion and possibly by aerosol. The virus replicates primarily in the intestinal tract, particularly the lower intestine and the ileum but also in the respiratory tract. Replication is thought to be in the reticuloendothelial cells of the lamina propria. There may be a viremia in the Teschen type of disease but not in the mild forms. Piglets may pick up the infection after weaning when the maternal antibody disappears. Many strains can infect the pig. They can be infected at any age with a strain that they have not been exposed to before. When infection first gains access to a herd, the spread is rapid and all ages of pigs may excrete virus in their feces.

Risk Factors

Animal Risk Factors

Depending on the virulence of the infecting strain, clinical disease primarily affects young pigs but may occur in older pigs at the same stage. As infection becomes endemic and herd immunity develops, excretion of the virus is largely restricted to weaned and early grower pigs. Adults generally have high levels of serum antibody, and suckling piglets are generally protected from infection by colostral and milk antibody. Sporadic disease in suckling pigs may occur in these circumstances in the litters of nonimmune or low-antibody sows, and may also occur in weaned pigs as they become susceptible to infection. In the recent outbreak in the United States, the major factor was the rapid decline of the maternal antibody in the piglets (<21 days). Seroconversion then coincided with the increased mortality in the herd.

Pathogen Risk Factors

The causative viruses will infect only pigs and are not related to any of the viruses that cause encephalomyelitis in other species. They are resistant to environmental conditions, including drying, and are present principally in the CNS and intestine of affected pigs.

PATHOGENESIS

The virus multiplies in the intestinal and respiratory tracts and Teschen produces a viremia. Invasion of the CNS may follow, depending on the virulence of the strains and the age of the pig at the time of infection. There is some strain difference in the areas of the CNS primarily affected, which accounts for variations in the clinical syndrome. Histopathologic evidence of encephalitis may be the only evidence of disease.

CLINICAL FINDINGS

Acute Viral Encephalomyelitis (Teschen Disease)

An incubation period of 10 to 12 days is followed by several days of fever (40°C-41°C, 104°F-106°F). Signs of encephalitis follow, although these are more extensive and acute after intracerebral inoculation. They include stiffness of the extremities, and inability to stand, with falling to one side followed by tremor, nystagmus, and violent clonic convulsions. Anorexia is usually complete, and vomiting has been observed. There may be partial or complete loss of voice caused by laryngeal paralysis. Facial paralysis may also occur. Stiffness and opisthotonus are often persistent between convulsions, which are easily stimulated by noise and often accompanied by loud squealing. The convulsive period lasts for 24 to 36 hours. A sharp temperature fall may be followed by coma and death on the third to fourth day, but in cases of longer duration the convulsive stage may be followed by flaccid paralysis affecting particularly the hindlimbs. In milder cases, early stiffness and weakness are followed by flaccid paralysis without the irritation phenomena of convulsions and tremor. In a recent case in the UK, the pigs were off-color, showed anterior limb paralysis, and were reluctant to rise and were therefore euthanized. Pigs were bright and keen to eat and drink.

Subacute Viral Encephalomyelitis (Talfan Disease)

The subacute disease is milder than the acute form, and the morbidity and mortality rates are lower. The disease is most common and severe in pigs less than 2 weeks of age. Older sucking pigs are affected too, but less severely and many recover completely. Sows suckling affected litters may be mildly and transiently ill. The morbidity rate in very young litters is often 100% and nearly all the affected piglets die. In litters over 3 weeks old there may be only a small proportion of the pigs affected. The disease often strikes suddenly—all litters in a piggery being affected within a few days—but disappears quickly, with subsequent litters being unaffected. Clinically, the syndrome includes anorexia, rapid loss of condition, constipation, frequent vomiting of minor degree, and a normal or slightly elevated temperature. In some outbreaks, diarrhea may precede the onset of nervous signs, which appear several days after the illness commences. Piglets up to 2 weeks of age show hyperesthesia, muscle tremor, knuckling of the fetlocks, ataxia, walking backward, a dog-sitting posture and terminally lateral recumbency, with paddling convulsions, nystagmus, blindness, and dyspnea.

The Dresden type of teschovirus caused an ataxia and recumbency in a large group of pigs about 5 days after removal of the sows and housing in the production unit. Older pigs (4 to 6 weeks of age) showed transient anorexia and posterior paresis, manifested by a swaying drunken gait, and usually recovered completely and quickly. In the Japanese outbreak, the pigs had at 40 days of age a flaccid paralysis of the hindlimbs and became recumbent, although they could move using their forelegs. After the initial group of affected piglets the disease disappeared.

Individual instances or small outbreaks of "leg weakness" with posterior paresis and paralysis in gilts and sows may also occur with this disease.

CLINICAL PATHOLOGY

Serology

Virus-neutralization and complement fixation are useful serologic tests. Antibodies are detectable in the early stages and persist for a considerable time after recovery. Because nearly all pigs are positive, it is only meaningful when paired serum samples are examined. There is a good ELISA for the detection of teschovirus serology.

Detection of Virus

It is absolutely necessary to collect tissues from acutely ill animals. If they have been ill for several days, the viruses have probably disappeared.

The virus is present in the blood of affected pigs in the early stages of the disease and in the feces in very small amounts during the incubation period before the signs of illness appear. Isolated viruses can be identified by virus neutralization, complement fixation, and immunofluorescence. Brain tissue is usually used as a source of virus in transmission experiments. A nested PCR has recently been described in which all 13 serotypes and field isolates were detected using three sets of primer pairs. It is more rapid and less time-consuming as a test than tissue culture and serotyping. Now RT-PCR can be used to detect viral RNA. New nested RT-PCRs have been developed to differentiate the viruses from each other.

NECROPSY FINDINGS

There are no gross lesions except muscle wastage in chronic cases. The lesions are only found by the microscope and are most severe in cases of Teschen. Microscopically, there is a diffuse nonsuppurative encephalomyelitis and ganglioneuritis with involvement of gray matter predominating. This takes the form of perivascular cuffing with mononuclear cells, focal gliosis, neuronal necrosis, and neuronophagia. The brainstem and spinal cord show the most extensive lesions, often with the most severe lesions in the cord. These take the form of degenerated or necrotic nerve cells in the ventral horns, glial nodules, occasional hemorrhage, and a diffuse infiltration of mononuclear cells. In the white matter the changes were not so severe. Infiltration of mononuclear cells was also seen in the dorsal root ganglia (together with degenerated ganglion cells and neuronophagia) spinal nerves, and sciatic nerves. Swollen myelin sheaths and axonal spheroids were seen in the peripheral nerves. Meningitis, particularly over the cerebellum, is an early manifestation of the disease. No inclusion bodies are visible in neurons, in contrast to many cases of pseudorabies. Virus can be isolated from the brain and spinal cord early in the disease course, and from the blood during the incubation period. Recovery of the virus from the gastrointestinal tract does not confirm the diagnosis because asymptomatic enteric infection is common. Isolation attempts may prove unrewarding, necessitating the correlation of clinical, serologic, and necropsy findings to confirm the diagnosis. Recently an experimental infection with PEV-3 produced tremors and paralysis 3 to 7 days postinfection with all the animals having pericarditis and myocarditis.

Samples for Confirmation of Diagnosis

- Histology: half of midsagittally sectioned brain, spinal cord including spinal ganglia, gasserian ganglion (LM)
- Virology: half of midsagittally sectioned brain, spinal cord (ISO, FAT)

In the recent German cases the virus was isolated from all the tissues examined but not from the blood. A technique using monoclonal antibodies has been described that can be used either as an immunofluorescent agent or for immunoelectron microscopy. In the recent Japanese description cytopathogenic agents were recovered from the tonsil, brainstem, and cerebellar homogenates. The PCR products from these were then sequenced and the isolate confirmed as PTV. Isolation of virus is not easy and needs to be from the brain and spinal cord. There are no firm indications of when to take material and a good consistent site in the brain for isolation.

> **DIFFERENTIAL DIAGNOSIS**
>
> The diagnosis of diseases causing signs of acute cerebral disease in pigs is difficult because of the difficulty in neurologic examination of pigs, and the diagnosis usually depends on extensive diagnostic laboratory work particularly in histopathology.
>
> Pseudorabies and hemagglutinating encephalomyelitis virus disease are similar clinical syndromes. In general, viral diseases, bacterial diseases, and intoxications must be considered as possible groups of causes; careful selection of material for laboratory examination is essential. The differentiation of the possible causes of diseases resembling viral encephalomyelitis is described in the section Pseudorabies.

IMMUNITY

Pigs mount a classical humoral response with IgM and IgG and it may be that IgA is important to prevent entry beyond the intestinal epithelium.

TREATMENT

There is no treatment.

CONTROL

The sporadic occurrence of the disease in a herd is usually an indication that infection is endemic. When outbreaks occur, the possibility that introduction of a new strain has occurred should be considered. However, by the time clinical disease is evident, it is likely that infection will be widespread and isolation of affected animals may be of little value. A closed-herd policy will markedly reduce the risk of introduction of new strains into a herd, but there is evidence that they can gain access by indirect means. The sporadic nature of the occurrence of most incidents of porcine encephalomyelitis does not warrant a specific control program.

Teschen disease is a different problem. Vaccines prepared by formalin inactivation of infective spinal cord and adsorption onto aluminium hydroxide have been used extensively in Europe. Two or three injections are given at 10- to 14-day intervals and immunity persists for about 6 months. A modified live virus vaccine is also available.

In the event of its appearance in a previously free country, eradication of the disease by slaughter and quarantine should be attempted if practicable. Austria reported eradication of the disease, which had been present in that country for many years. A slaughter policy was supplemented by ring vaccination around infected premises.

FURTHER READING

Kouba V. Teschen disease, eradication in Czechoslovakia: a historical report. *Vet Med (Praha)*. 2007;54:550-560.

REFERENCES

1. Tseng CH, Tsai HJ. *Virus Res*. 2007;129:104.
2. Kouba V. *Vet Med (Praha)*. 2007;54:550.
3. Tseng CH, Tsai HJ. *Virus Res*. 2007;129:104.
4. Buitrago D, et al. *J Vet Diagn Invest*. 2007;22:763.
5. Sozzi E, et al. *Transbound Emerg Dis*. 2010;57:434.
6. Zhang CF, et al. *J Virol Methods*. 2010;167:208.
7. Lin W, et al. *Arch Virol*. 2012;157:1387.

Prion Diseases Primarily Affecting the Cerebrum

INTRODUCTION

The transmissible spongiform encephalopathies (TSEs) are a group of progressive neurologic disorders that are transmissible and affect a number of animal species and humans (Table 14-14). They are nonfebrile with long incubation periods and a long course of disease.

There is a debate about the nature of the infective agent causing TSEs. An abnormal folded isoform, designated PrP^{Sc}, of a host-encoded cell-surface glycoprotein (prion protein, PrP^{c}) accumulates during disease and is associated closely with infectivity. The function of PrP^{C} is not known and the mechanism by which PrP^{C} is converted to PrP^{Sc} is uncertain. PrP^{Sc} is rich in β-sheets and can be isolated as insoluble aggregates. A theory is that the transmissible agent is the abnormal isoform of the prion protein and that, in the infected host, this can recruit further alternatively folded prion protein by acting as a template for protein folding. With this theory the long incubation period of prion diseases reflects the rise in level and deposition of PrP^{Sc} in a variety of tissues, including brain, eventually resulting in fatal spongiform encephalopathy.

Scrapie affects sheep and goats and is the prototypic disease for the group in domestic and wild animals.

Although scrapie in sheep has been recognized for over 200 years, the recent epidemic of Bovine Spongiform Encephalopathy (BSE) has focused public attention and scientific research on the TSEs. With scrapie, and other TSEs, transmission can be effected by crude or purified extracts of brain or other tissues from affected animals, and the infective agent is very resistant to ionizing and ultraviolet irradiation and to reagents that damage or modify nucleic acids. This, along with other experimental findings, has led to proposals that the infectious agent in scrapie, and other TSEs, is the PrP^{Sc} itself, and not a small, unconventional virus or virino as previously proposed. The structure of the infecting PrP^{Sc} is thought to imprint on the normal cellular precursor PrP^{c}, resulting in a change to the abnormal isoform, which is protease resistant and accumulates in cells.

Naturally occurring TSEs, such as sporadic Creutzfeldt–Jakob (vCJD) in humans or transmissible mink encephalopathy in mink, are associated with individual species or with closely related species as with scrapie in sheep, goats, and mouflon (*Ovis orientalis musimon*) and chronic wasting disease (CWD) in mule deer (*Odocoileus hemionus*), white-tailed deer (*O. virginianus*), and elk (*Cervus elaphus nelsoni*).

The results of attempts at interspecies transmission of these diseases are variable. Although, by definition, each TSE is transmissible, the species to which they will transmit varies between the TSE, and can be influenced by the route of challenge; the tissues that contain infection also vary according to the particular TSE. Frequently they do not transmit. Successful primary transmission between different mammalian species typically requires a larger dose to affect disease than would be required for transmission to the same species. Also, usually, parenteral or intracerebral routes are required and success is greater with young animal recipients. This is the so-called "species barrier," which may be absolute or partial because it will affect only a proportion of animals on first passage, or may result in an extended incubation period on first passage.

When using transmission studies to detect the presence of one of these agents, optimal sensitivity is with a recipient host of the same species. Transgenic mice may eliminate this barrier.

The gold-standard technique for the diagnosis of TSE agents is the passage of tissue in panels of inbred mice, which is a technique known as "strain typing." Until recently this was the only way to differentiate scrapie and BSE. BSE presents with a characteristic incubation period, pattern of distribution, and relative severity of the changes in the brain of the different mouse strains (the lesion profile), which is distinct from all scrapie strains tested.

When examining TSEs as a group, one cannot extrapolate the transmission particulars of one TSE to another and one cannot extrapolate risk factors or epidemiology from one to another, and certainly generalizations from an experimental model to a natural disease across a species barrier is scientifically inappropriate.

The literature on this subject is large. This section will discuss scrapie in sheep and goats, and BSE, which are the two TSEs of agricultural animals. It will also discuss the risk for BSE in sheep. CWD in deer is briefly described but has not shown any evidence for transmission to agricultural animals other than deer.

Table 14-14 Transmissible spongiform encephalopathies in animals and humans

Disease	Acronym	Species	Etiology	First described
Creutzfeldt–Jakob disease	CJD	Man	Sporadic familial iatrogenic	1920
Gerstmann-Straussler-Scheinker	GSS	Man	Familial	1936
Kuru		Man	Acquired	1957
Fatal familial insomnia	FFI	Man	Familial	1992
Variant Creutzfeldt–Jakob disease	vCJD	Man	Acquired	1996
Scrapie		Sheep, goats, mouflon	Natural	1738
Transmissible mink encephalopathy	TME	Mink	Acquired	1964
Chronic wasting disease	CWD	Deer, elk	Natural	1980
Bovine spongiform encephalopathy	BSE	Cattle	Acquired	1986
Zoo ungulate transmissible spongiform encephalopathy	Zoo ungulate TSE	Nyala, kudu, gemsbok, oryx	Acquired	1986
Feline spongiform encephalopathy	FSE	Zoo cats (puma, cheetah and domestic cats)	Acquired	1990

BOVINE SPONGIFORM ENCEPHALOPATHY (MAD COW DISEASE)

Classical BSE is an afebrile, slowly progressive neurologic disorder affecting adult cattle. It is a subacute TSE that is uniformly fatal once cattle show signs of nervous disease. TSEs are caused by accumulation of β-sheets of prion proteins in nervous tissue, leading to slowly progressive neurodegeneration and death. Current knowledge suggests that classical BSE originated from a sporadic spongiform encephalopathy preexistent in the cattle population, and that the causative prion was fed to genetically susceptible cattle in contaminated animal protein feeds.

SYNOPSIS

Etiology Epizootic disease was most likely caused by a bovine prion called the classical bovine spongiform encephalopathy strain that was fed back to genetically susceptible cattle in contaminated meat-and-bone meal. Major concern for zoonotic potential. Some countries have documented the presence of atypical bovine prion strains (H-type, L-type) at an extremely low prevalence.

Epidemiology Has occurred as an epidemic in Great Britain associated with the feeding of infected meat-and-bone meal. Sporadic in other countries.

Clinical findings Nonfebrile disease of adult cattle, with long clinical course. Disturbance in behavior, sensitivity, and locomotion.

Clinical pathology None specific.

Diagnostic confirmation Histology, demonstration of prion protein.

Treatment None.

Control Slaughter eradication. Avoidance of feeding ruminant-derived protein to ruminants.

The disease is of considerable importance mainly because it has zoonotic potential and has spread to many countries. The cost of control is very high.

ETIOLOGY

Classical BSE is a prion-associated TSE that causes disease primarily in cattle and also in a number of other species, including humans.

The stability of the lesion profile in cattle and experimental infection studies strongly suggests that the bovine epidemic in the UK, and the subsequent extended epizootic in other countries, was caused by transmission of a single stable bovine prion.[1]

A number of alternative hypotheses were originally offered for the epidemic in the UK. The most popular initial theory was that BSE was caused by transmission of a strain of scrapie that was modified to infect cattle. However, BSE has many characteristics that distinguishes it from conventional scrapie strains, and there is no evidence that cattle develop infection or neurologic disease after 8 or 10 years of oral administration of the scrapie agent.[1,2] Another hypothesis was that the agent could have entered into meat-and-bone meal (MBM) from the carcass of an animal that died in a zoo or a safari park in the UK. This hypothesis was based on the method of carcass disposal for these animals (many were rendered and not incinerated) and because of the high susceptibility of certain African ungulates and zoo carnivores to BSE infection. An additional hypothesis proposed that MBM from the Indian subcontinent was the source. The UK government has conducted several inquiries into the source of the BSE agent and the cause of the outbreak including the Phillips report in 2000 and the Horn report in 2001, but these reports were not conclusive.

The mass exposure of cattle in the UK to this agent, and the subsequent development of a disease epizootic in cattle in the latter half of the 1980s and the early 1990s, is currently thought to have been the consequence of a change in the method of processing of MBM prepared from slaughtered cattle latently infected with the classical BSE strain. This change in processing permitted the prion to persist in the feed, which was fed back to cattle to create a positive feedback loop. Subsequent recycling of the agent in MBM prepared from latently infected slaughter cattle amplified its occurrence until an epidemic of neurologic disease in adult cattle was identified. In hindsight, it was not a wise decision to turn an evolutionary herbivore into a carnivore by feeding contaminated MBM to cattle.

There appear to be at least three different strains of prions identified from cattle with BSE. Discriminatory testing of 370 BSE cases in the EU between 2001 and 2011 indicated that 83% were classical BSE, which transmits to humans as vCJD, 7% were atypical high-type (H-type) BSE first diagnosed in the United States in 2004, and 10% were atypical low-type (L-type) BSE.[1] The L-type has been identified in cattle from Belgium, Canada, Germany, Italy, and Japan, whereas the H-type has been identified in cattle from France, Germany, Japan, the Netherlands, Poland, Sweden, Switzerland, the UK, and the United States. It is likely that atypical forms of BSE (H-type, L-type) represent a rare, sporadic, spontaneous disease in cattle related to old age, with some similarities to sporadic CJD in humans or the Nor98 variant of scrapie in sheep and goats.[3] Only 42 cases of atypical BSE had been reported by 2010, and all were in cattle at least 8 years of age with the exception of a possible case in a 23-month-old heifer.[4]

EPIDEMIOLOGY

Occurrence

Geographic Occurrence

Classical BSE was first described in Great Britain in 1987, but the BSE inquiries considered it likely that there had been several undetected cycles of BSE in the southwest England in the 1970s and early 1980s. Following its description in 1987, the disease developed to an epizootic with over 183,000 cases, of which more than 95% were detected before 2000. The epidemic in the UK peaked at an annual total of more than 37,000 clinical cases in 1992. The disease was recognized in Northern Ireland in 1998 and in the Republic of Ireland in 1999. The disease was subsequently recognized in Switzerland, Portugal, and France in the early 1990s and then became widespread to involve 27 countries by 2015.

Cases have occurred in imported British cattle in Oman and the Falkland and Channel Islands. Countries that have had cases of BSE in native-born cattle are Austria, Belgium, Canada, Czech Republic, Denmark, Finland, Germany, Greece, Ireland, Israel, Italy, Japan, Luxembourg, the Netherlands, Poland, Portugal, Slovakia, Slovenia, Spain, Switzerland, UK, and the United States.

Occurrence in Cattle

Great Britain

In Great Britain, the first known clinical case of classical BSE probably occurred in 1985. The annual incidence subsequently increased and the disease became a major epizootic in the late 1980s. The disease was declared notifiable, and a statutory ban on the feeding of ruminant-derived protein to ruminants was introduced in 1988. A more extensive ban on feeding any animal protein to any agricultural animal was later implemented to avoid feed cross-contamination. The annual incidence peaked in 1992 and has fallen every year since to produce a bell-shaped epidemic curve at approximately the year 2000, with some cases every year since (Fig. 14-10). The reduction from the peak in 1992 is attributed to the 1988 ruminant-feed ban with the delay in response an effect of the incubation period of this disease. Britain has had the greatest number of affected cattle and, consequently, provides the majority of information on the disease.

Herd Type

A great proportion of cases have occurred in **dairy and dairy crossbred herds**, and by 2002 62% of dairy herds in Great Britain had experienced one or more cases. In contrast, 17% of **beef** herds had cases in the same time period. There has been no apparent breed predisposition. In both herd types, the risk for cases increased significantly with increasing herd size. A significant proportion of the cases in beef cattle herds have occurred in animals purchased into the herds from dairy herds. The reason for this difference in herd type is thought to be the greater use of concentrates in dairy cattle.

The disease has occurred in all regions of the country but was most prevalent in southwest England. Although the disease

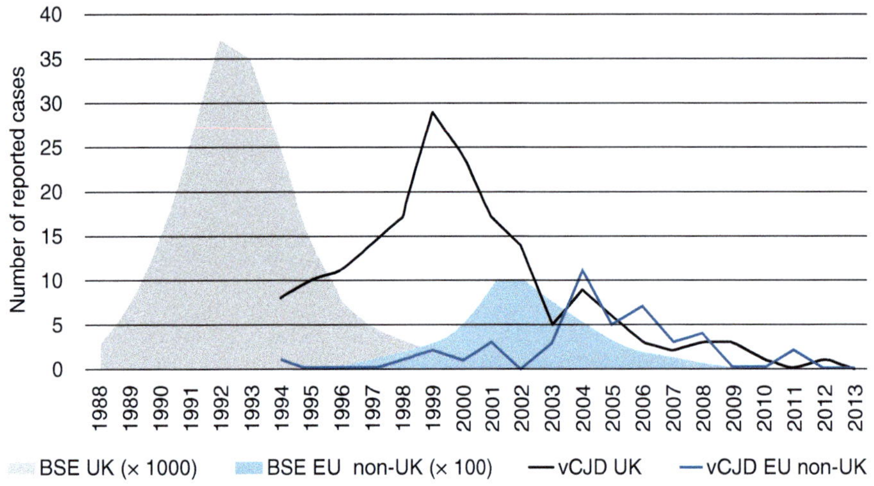

Fig. 14-10 The number of reported bovine spongiform encephalopathy (BSE) cases in cattle and variant Creutzfeldt–Jakob (vCJD) cases in humans by date of onset in the UK and in the European Union (EU) excluding the UK from 1988 to 2013. Note the different multiplier for BSE and vCJD cases in the UK and EU non-UK. (Published with permission from the European Centre for Disease Prevention and Control. http://ecdc.europa.eu/en/healthtopics/Variant_Creutzfeldt-Jakob_disease(vCJD)/Pages/factsheet_health_professionals.aspx.)

developed to an epizootic within the country, the disease does not occur as an epizootic within affected herds and most experience either single cases or a limited number of cases. The average **within-herd incidence** has remained below 2% since the disease was first described.

Northern Ireland and Republic of Ireland

In Northern Ireland classical BSE was recognized in 1998 and in the Republic of Ireland in 1999, but epizootic disease occurred Great Britain and Northern Ireland. The epidemiologic features in both countries were similar to that in Great Britain, but the incidence has been lower. In Northern Ireland the incidence was approximately one-tenth of that in Great Britain. The yearly incidence of the disease peaked in 1994 in Northern Ireland but jumped unexpectedly in the Republic of Ireland in 1996 to 1998 and has remained high since. The source of infection in both countries is thought to have been MBM imported from Great Britain. In the Republic of Ireland there has been geographic clustering with a higher incidence in two counties possibly associated with the location of feed suppliers.

European Continent and Iberian Peninsula

On the European continent classical BSE was recognized in Switzerland in 1999 and shortly after on the Iberian peninsula in Portugal. Both countries showed a case incidence with evidence of an epidemic curve. However this was not mirrored in EU member states in the continent, in which only sporadic cases were reported in the 1990s, and it appears that the disease in this region was unrecognized, underreported, and was more widespread than recorded. Apparently cattle with typical clinical manifestations and fallen stock with clinical signs that should have led to a suspicion of BSE were misdiagnosed or not reported.

Switzerland established a surveillance system in 1999 testing fallen cattle, emergency slaughter, and normal cattle using Prionics Western blot rapid testing methods. This surveillance method was rapidly adopted by EU member countries so that all but two had recorded cases by the end of 2001. In France, between the first notified case in 1991 and the establishment of mandatory testing in 2000, there were 103 cases detected by passive surveillance, but it is estimated that 301,200 cattle were infected with BSE during this period. The first report of L-type BSE was from Italy in 2004.

North America

Canada experienced a case of classical BSE in a cow imported from Great Britain in 1993, but the first case in an indigenous Canadian cow occurred in 2003 in Alberta. Trace back on 40 herds and slaughter of over 2000 suspects were all negative. The molecular profile of the BSE agent from this case was very similar to the UK BSE strains and had no relationship to the agent associated with **CWD** in deer and elk. In 2003 a Canadian cow that had been exported to the United States as a young calf developed complications at parturition, was shipped as a nonambulatory cow, and was discovered as a classical BSE case under a routine monitoring program of downer cows. Canada had two more cases of classical BSE in 2005. By 2009, Canada had reported 14 cases of classical BSE, with 1 H-type and 1 L-type.

The United States had a case of atypical H-type BSE in a native-born cow in 2004. The affected cow had a new prion coding gene (E211K) that suggested the possible existence of a genetic susceptibility to developing clinical signs.[5] A second case of atypical H-type BSE has been reported in the United States. Genetic studies have indicated that susceptibility to classical BSE does not appear to be related to genetic differences in the prion coding gene.[6]

Japan

Japan had reported 33 cases of BSE (32 classical and 1 atypical in a 16-year-old Japanese black cow) by 2007. Cases were attributed to imported infected cattle and imported fat that was used in a milk replacer formulation fed to calves.[7]

Age Incidence

TSEs as a group have long and variable incubation periods, with genetic susceptibility to clinical disease playing a major role in the age of onset of clinical signs. BSE, like scrapie, has a **long incubation period**, 2.5 to at least 8 years and possibly for the life span of cattle and is a disease that affects mature animals. Epidemiologic studies suggest that most affected cattle have been infected as calves, with the mean incubation period decreasing with increasing dose. Risk is greatest in the first 6 months of life and between 6 and 24 months of age risk is related to feeding patterns of proprietary concentrates. Adult cattle are at low risk for infection.

The **modal age at onset** of clinical signs is between 4 and 5 years, but there is a skewed distribution with the youngest age at onset recorded at 22 months and the oldest at 15 years. During the course of the outbreak in the UK there has been a change in the age distribution of cases in both Britain and Northern Ireland, consistent with a sudden decrease in exposure as a result of the bans on ruminant protein feeding. The clinical course is variable, but the case fatality is 100%. There is a variation in risk associated with the calendar month of birth-related to seasonal differences in calf management and exposure to ruminant protein in calf feeds.

The majority of the occasional cases of BSE currently being diagnosed in the UK are attributed to residual contamination of raw feed, but may also reflect a very low level prevalence of atypical BSE cases.[1,8]

Other Species

Spongiform encephalopathies have been identified in seven species of **ungulates** in zoos or wildlife parks in Great Britain since the occurrence of the disease in cattle. These animals had been fed MBM, but the apparently shorter incubation period suggests that they might be more susceptible to infection than cattle and there is evidence for horizontal transmission.

Feline spongiform encephalopathy (FSE) also has been recorded in **domestic cats** in Great Britain since 1990 and in zoo felids. The **zoo felids** had been fed cattle carcasses unfit for human consumption, or the zoo had a history of BSE in exotic ruminants and fed culled carcasses to other zoo animals. Transmission studies in mice with the agents associated with these encephalopathies in zoo ungulates and felids suggest that they are the same strain that causes BSE. The initial concern that there would be an outbreak of FSE in domestic cats did not occur, and only 89 cases were confirmed to the end on 2003.

Method of Natural Transmission

Ingestion of Meat-and-Bone Meal

The initial epidemiologic studies suggested that the disease in the UK was an extended common-source epidemic, and the only common source identified in these initial studies was the feeding of proprietary concentrate feedstuffs. Epidemiologic studies also suggested that the presence of MBM in proprietary concentrates was the proxy for affected cattle to have been exposed to a scrapie-like agent, and this conclusion is supported by case–control studies examining feeding practices to calves that subsequently developed the disease. This hypothesis explains **breed differences** in incidence because concentrates are not commonly fed to beef calves in the UK; it also can account for geographic differences in incidence. The oral route of challenge is known to be an inefficient route for the transmission of the agents associated with spongiform encephalopathies, and this is thought to be the reason for the low within-herd incidence of the disease in the face of a common exposure.

MBM is manufactured by the rendering industry from tissues discarded in slaughterhouses and from down and dead livestock. The outbreak of BSE in Great Britain was temporarily preceded by a change in the method of processing of MBM to a continuous process with a cessation of the use of hydrocarbon fat solvents. It is postulated that this change permitted the cycling of unrecognized but extremely low-incidence cases of classical BSE. The initial exposure probably occurred from 1981 to 1982 and, subsequently, the agent recycled from infected cattle carcasses and offal used in the preparation of MBM. Rendering procedures have subsequently been devised to minimize survival of the agent.

The marked fall in disease incidence following the introduction of the feed ban in 1987 in the UK substantiated the importance of ingestion of MBM as the major method of infection. Bans in Europe were largely introduced in 1990.

Born-After-the-Ban

In the UK and in other countries a number of cattle that were born-after-the-ban (BAB; French acronym NAIF) have developed the disease. Most of these were born in the years immediately following the ban and their numbers have decreased in subsequent years but still continue at low levels. A case–control study found that vertical or horizontal transmission was not an important cause of these cases. It is thought that MBM that was already in the food chain at the time, in mills and on the farm, was fed until it was depleted.

In several countries the occurrence of BAB cases has been geographically clustered, and also associated with certain birth cohorts. In the UK the clustering was related to areas with high concentrations of pigs and poultry, and it is thought that there was cross-contamination of feedstuffs in feedmills. This is certainly possible with an infective dose of 1 g or less for cattle.

More recently, there has been concern about cattle in the UK that have developed BSE but that were born after the implementation of the reinforced feed ban in 1996 (BARBs). Up to 2005, there have been approximately 100 cases. Again there is no evidence of maternal or lateral transmission and the inadvertent use of illegal feed material residual on farms is suspected.[9]

Non–Feed-Borne Transmission

There is no epidemiologic evidence for significant horizontal or vertical transmission of the disease in cattle, although the studies suggest that minor horizontal transmission may occur to birth cohorts of calves that subsequently develop BSE. This type of transmission is of minor importance to the perpetuation of the disease in a country, but it may be of significance to human health, and birth cohorts are included in trace backs of infection in the United States and Canada.

Vertical Transmission

In the absence of other mechanisms of transmission, vertical transmission is not considered significant for the perpetuation of the disease in an epidemic form. There is an **enhanced risk** for the disease in calves born to infected cows, and this is higher in calves born after the onset of clinical disease in the cow. This may be the result of exposure, at birth, to high infectivity in birth products because there is no evidence for infection and transmission in embryo transplants. However, no detectable infectivity has been found in placentas from cows with the disease.

A very elegant experiment that examined the risk for transmission of BSE via embryo transfer that used recipient cattle sourced from New Zealand and donor cows clinically affected with BSE, bred to bulls that did and did not have clinical BSE, concluded, after a 7-year observation period on the progeny, that embryos were unlikely to carry BSE.

Modeling the BSE epidemic in the UK indicated a constant and relatively high basic reproduction number (R_0) that is defined as the expected number of secondary infections produced in a susceptible population by a typical infected host. If $R_0 > 1$, then the agent can persist indefinitely; initial estimates for R_0 before the first feed ban in 1988 ranged from 10 to 12. This degree of infectivity was consistent with the potential that a maximally infectious animal could infect up to 400 other cattle. Since the feed ban, the value for R_0 is thought to have decreased to 0 to 0.25, indicating that the disease will soon disappear.

Risk for Occurrence of Disease in Countries

Changes in the method of processing MBM have occurred in countries other than the UK, and scrapie occurs in sheep in other countries. However, the major risk for the occurrence of the disease in other countries is the importation of latently infected cattle and/or the importation of infected MBM. This risk can be substantially avoided by prohibiting the feeding of MBM to cattle.

An assessment in 1996 of risk for the occurrence of BSE in the United States concluded that the potential risk of an epizootic was small and that there are substantial differences in the strength of the risk factors between the United States and the UK. These result from differences in proportional numbers of sheep and cattle, differences in the nature of the beef and dairy industries, the type of animal used for beef production and the age at slaughter, and differences in the practice of feeding ruminant-derived protein in calf rations, which is uncommon in the United States. Thus the risk of an outbreak similar to that in the UK was considered negligible. However, a case in a native-born cow in the United States occurred in 2005. This, and contemporary cases in Canada suggested that infected MBM was imported to the North American continent at some time, or that in the United States, the case reflected the very low incidence of spontaneous atypical BSE in cattle. The cases in both countries occurred in cattle that were born before the ban on feeding MBM imposed in both countries in 1997.

Countries with largely pastoral cattle are at low risk.

The International Animal health code of the OIE describes five BSE risk categories for countries based on the importation of cattle from at-risk countries, the importation of potentially infected MBM, the consumption of MBM by cattle and other animals, animal feeding practices, livestock population structure, rendering practices, and the potential for recycling of BSE. In order of increasing incidence of BSE these categories are BSE free, BSE provisionally free, minimal BSE risk, moderate BSE risk, and high BSE risk.

Experimental Reproduction

Although studies on the transmissibility and experimental reproduction of BSE were established before the occurrence of human cases of BSE (vCJD), they have been **critical in determining the risk** of cattle products for human disease and the risk for disease in other species.

In cattle, disease has been experimentally reproduced by oral and intracerebral inoculation with infected cattle brain homogenates.

Oral, intravenous, and intracerebral inoculation of sheep with infected cattle brain homogenates also results in disease. Disease has also been reproduced in goats and mink by parenteral challenge. In pigs, disease has been produced by intracerebral challenge with infected brain homogenates but not oral challenge. It has not been produced by any route of challenge in poultry and is not produced by oral challenge in farmed deer.

Infectivity of Tissues

Brain, spinal cord, and retina are tissues that are infective to cattle or laboratory animals from natural cases of BSE. The tissues that are infective to cattle or laboratory animals from experimentally infected cattle are brain, spinal cord, retina, distal ileum, bone marrow, trigeminal nerve, and lingual lymph tissue. The infective dose of brain material from a cow with classical BSE appears to be <1 mg of brain tissue.[10]

Parenteral injection of BSE brain:
- Transmits from cattle to cattle, mice, goats, sheep, pigs, mink, guinea pig

Orally fed BSE brain:
- Transmits from cattle to cattle, mice, mink, sheep and goats
- Not to pigs or farmed deer

Other tissues including the major visceral organs, striated muscle, and tissue common for human consumption were negative by mouse bioassay, indicating that no infectivity could be detected. These tissues are currently being reexamined for infectivity using the most sensitive assay known, intracerebral infection into the host species, which in this case the host is cattle. These studies are ongoing but, at last report have only confirmed the results of the negative mouse bioassays. There is no evidence of infectivity in milk based on the fact that calves suckling cows with clinical BSE do not themselves develop BSE when mature and also on the lack of infectivity with intracerebral injection of mice.

Strongest evidence of absence of infection in milk is the study that examined and found no increase in incidence of BSE in calves born to dams with BSE that suckled these cows during clinical disease compared with calves that suckled clinically normal dams. There is species susceptibility (no barrier) strength in this study.

BSE, *bovine spongiform encephalopathy.*

Economic Importance

BSE is not of major economic significance to individual herds in countries in which it is endemic because of the low within-herd incidence. In most countries, compensation will cover cases detected by passive surveillance and, with active surveillance, most of the costs if there is selective culling in affected and trace back herds. However, it is arguable that this disease is the **most economically devastating** agricultural animal disease in the developed world.

The disease has been of major economic importance in the UK and is estimated to have cost £600 billion. This has been from the national cost associated with detection and control procedures, the cost of compensation, and the cost of disposal of affected animals. These costs, along with the cost of loss of export markets, are very high.

Worldwide, the public has developed an extreme concern for the public health risk associated with BSE infection in cattle and, consequently, all countries have been mandated or encouraged to develop active surveillance programs. Not to do so runs the risk of loss of overseas markets and loss of home consumption of beef in favor of other meats. Further, the detection of a single case of BSE by these active surveillance programs results in the loss of export markets for the country and a severe fall in cattle prices for countries that rely on exports in their cattle industries.

BSE is also arguably the disease that has been used most to influence trade in live cattle and cattle products with no science-base or attention to the internationally adopted OIE Terrestrial Animal Health Code. This is largely because of the success of local political influence of ranches and farmers.

It is further arguable that the money spent, for reasons of public health, on this relatively minor zoonotic disease, by far outweighs its relative importance as a cause of human disease.

Zoonotic Implications

Concerns that this disease could transmit to man were raised a very short time after its initial diagnosis. These unfortunately proved true in 1996 when a new form of CJD was reported. Although, with the initial cases, there was reservation as to causality, studies showed the agent associated with this disease is similar to that associated with BSE and the FSEs; there is now no doubt that this is a form of BSE in man. It differs from CJD in that it affects young people with a mean age onset in the third decade of life. In humans there is evidence for genetic susceptibility, and all cases have been homozygous for methionine at codon 129. The disease has been termed **variant CJD** (vCJD).

The disease occurred in the UK despite the progressive bans on human consumption of beef products that contained infectivity that were implemented in 1998 and subsequently tightened further as new information on potential infectivity became available. It is possible that exposure of affected humans occurred in the early and mid-1980s, before the recognition of the disease. There was initially extreme concern that there would be a very large outbreak in humans. However, this has not occurred. The total number of deaths form vCJD in the UK has reached 150. The peak number of deaths occurred in the year 2000, and the outbreak appears to have reached a plateau and is possibly in decline, although the nature of the outbreak will be dependent on the range of incubation periods in humans. More than 200 individuals had succumbed to this infection worldwide by 2015.

Although there is no evidence of direct transmission to humans, veterinarians and animal handlers should take appropriate precautions when handling nervous system tissues of infected animals. Cow's milk appears to provide a negligible risk of contracting vCJD disease.[11]

PATHOGENESIS

Information on the pathogenesis and development of BSE in cattle was initially derived from studies published from Great Britain in the 1990s that studied the spatial and temporal development of infectivity and pathologic change in cattle after oral challenge with a 100-g dose of BSE-affected brain homogenate sourced from naturally clinically affected cattle. The experimental cattle were killed sequentially following challenge, and infectivity in tissues was subsequently determined initially by infectivity assays by intracerebral and intraperitoneal injection into panels of inbred mice and subsequently by infectivity studies by intracerebral challenge of cattle to exclude any species barrier effects.

- Long incubation period (5 years)
- Oral infection
- Infection of Peyer's patches, to brainstem via vagus nerve
- Accumulation of abnormal prions destroys brain slowly

BSE prions spread by two antegrade pathways from the gastrointestinal tract to the CNS: (1) via the splanchnic nerves, mesenteric and celiac ganglion complex, and lumbar/caudal thoracic spinal cord and (2) via the vagus nerve.[12] Following oral challenge of calves, infectivity was initially detectable in the distal ileum, in the Peyer's patches, but no infection is demonstrable in other lymphoreticular organs. Infectivity was identified at 4 months postinfection and was unchanged in magnitude at 24 months postinfection, revealing no decline or clearance of the agent from ileal Peyer's patches.[13] Infectivity was demonstrable in the cervical and thoracic dorsal root ganglia at 32 to 40 months after infection and in the trigeminal ganglion at 36 to 38 months. Traces of infectivity were shown in sternal bone marrow in cattle killed 38 months postexposure. The earliest presence of abnormal PrP and infectivity in the CNS occurred 32 months postexposure, before any typical diagnostic histopathologic changes in the brain. The onset of clinical signs and pathologic change in the brain occur at approximately the same time. Infectivity of peripheral nerves such as the sciatic nerve appears to be a secondary event after infection of the CNS.[12,13]

More recent reports of the oral experimental dosing studies have indicated that the 50% infective dose for classical BSE was 0.15 g of brain homogenate, with higher oral doses increasing the likelihood of developing BSE.[14] In addition, the incubation period decreased as the infective dose increased. In other words, an increase in the incidence of classical BSE disease indicates an increase in exposure, and a decrease in the age of clinical signs indicates a larger infective dose.

CLINICAL FINDINGS

The disease is insidious in onset and the clinical course progresses over several weeks, varying from 1 to 6 months in duration. There is a **constellation of clinical signs** with alterations in behavior, temperament, posture, sensorium, and movement, but the clinical signs are variable from day to day, although they are progressive over time Cattle that show behavioral, sensory, and locomotor abnormality together are highly suspect for BSE. The predominant **neurologic signs** are apprehensive behavior, hyperesthesia, and ataxia, and a high proportion of cases lose body condition and have a diminishing milk yield during the clinical course of the disease. Cattle with BSE do not always show neurologic signs in the initial stages of the disease, and animals with BSE may be sent to slaughter for poor production before the onset of clinical nervous signs. Cattle with vacuolar changes in the brainstem usually have more severe clinical abnormalities; this observation is consistent with vacuolar change reflecting a more advanced histologic lesion.[15]

Clinical signs in BSE

- Change in temperament and behavior
  - Apprehension, excitable, unusual kicking, head-tossing when haltered, separation from group
- Change in posture and movement
  - Abnormal posture and ataxia
- Fall in milk production
- **No antemortem test available**

Behavioral changes are gradual in onset and include changes, such as a reluctance to pass through the milking shed or to leave a vehicle or a pen, a change in milking order, and a reluctance to pass through passageways. Affected cattle are disoriented and may stare, presumably at imaginary objects, for long periods. There is hyperesthesia to sound and touch, with twitching of the ears or more general muscle fasciculation and tremors. Many throw their head sideways and show head-shaking when the head or neck is touched.

Other changes in **temperament** include the avoidance of other cows in loose housing but antagonistic behavior to herdmates and humans when in confined situations. Affected animals may kick during milking and show resistance to handling. Some cows show excessive grooming and licking and may show the equivalent of the scrapie scratch reflex.

Bradycardia, associated with increased vagal tone and not occurring because of decreased food intake, is reported and may persist despite the cow's nervousness during clinical examination.

Relatively early in the course of the disease there is **hindlimb ataxia** with a shortened stride, swaying gait, and difficulty in negotiating turns. This should be especially examined as animals exit transport vehicles or are trotted through an area. Knuckling, stumbling, and falling, with subsequent difficulty in rising, is common in the later stages of the disease. Cows show **progressive weakness**, with ataxia and weight loss, and before the common recognition of the disease, they were sent to slaughter because of locomotor disabilities or changes in temperament.

It has been recommended that the reaction of the animal to sudden noise, sudden light, sudden movement, and sudden touch be used as a test. Sudden noise is tested by clanging two metal objects together out of sight of the animal (the **bang test**), sudden light is tested with a camera flash (the **flash test),** sudden movement is tested by waving a clipboard toward the cow from a short distance (the **clipboard test),** and sudden touch is tested by touching the animal on the hindlimbs with a soft stick (**stick test**). Abnormal reactions to these tests include being startled, head-tossing, salivation, snorting, running away, or panicky circling and kicking out on touch. These tests have been found positive in BSE suspects that had a history of behavioral change but did not show abnormalities of gait.

Cattle infected with atypical BSE (H-type, L-type) appear more dull and to have a greater degree of difficulty in rising than cattle with classical BSE; otherwise they have similar clinical findings.[16] Abnormal BAEPs have been reported at the onset of neurologic signs in classical BSE-infected cattle and manifest as prolonged peak latency of waves III and V and prolonged I-V latency.[17] Prion accumulation in the auditory brainstem nuclei of BSE-infected cattle[18] may contribute to their hyperresponsiveness to the bang test.

Electroencephalographic and evoked potential diagnostic methods have been proposed as antemortem diagnostic test methods but require further evaluation and would seem impractical for routine use. Antemortem assessment of retinal function and morphology identified changes 11 and 5 months before the onset of unequivocal clinical signs in cattle experimentally infected by intracranial inoculation with classical BSE and H-type BSE.[19] Strain-specific differences in retinal function, the amount of prion accumulated in the retina, and the retinal glial response to disease were also identified.

Clinical Signs and Passive Surveillance

There is no reliable preclinical test for BSE, and clinical recognition of BSE is the major component of passive surveillance.

At the peak of the outbreak in Great Britain, BSE was confirmed in 85% of suspects picked by passive surveillance. This percentage fell to 56% later in the outbreak. Farmers were fully compensated at notification and well informed and so were probably motivated to contact their veterinarian. Veterinarians were also very aware of the clinical presentation of BSE and observant at livestock markets and while testing for tuberculosis and at abattoirs. Relatively high success rates were also found in Switzerland in which approximately 59% of animals notified with BSE were confirmed. However, in other countries, passive surveillance was an utter failure.

Although an aid to surveillance of a disease, passive surveillance of BSE based on clinical signs is an insensitive method of disease detection; targeting surveillance of emergency slaughtered cattle and fallen stock is 40 times more likely to detect cases of BSE than notification on the basis of clinical signs. One study found that the odds of finding a BSE case was 49 times higher in the fallen stock and 58 times higher in emergency slaughtered cattle greater than 24 months of age compared with passive surveillance of clinical disease.

CLINICAL PATHOLOGY

There is no specific test for the antemortem diagnosis of this disease. Apolipoprotein E and two unidentified proteins are present in the CSF from clinical cases but not normal cattle, and the presence of a 30-kDa, 14-3-3 protein in CSF in affected cows is reported, but there is no information of specificity.

NECROPSY FINDINGS

There are no abnormalities in gross pathology, and diagnosis is dependent on histologic findings or testing of brainstem samples using validated tests based on in situ IHC or Western immunoblots, with the obex and rostral brainstem being the subsampled region of choice.[12] The preferred method for determining prevalence is immunology-based rapid tests, which are validated to detect classical BSE disease-associated prions. These tests typically apply proteinase K to destroy the cellular isoform of the prion protein (PrP^{c}) while maintaining a proteinase K–resistant disease-associated isoform (PrP^{sc}). This approach has identified three types of BSE: classical type (C-type), H-type, and L-type, with the H and L designation referring to the apparent molecular weights of the proteins.[20]

Major histologic changes are in the brainstem, and the pathognomonic lesion is a bilaterally symmetric intracytoplasmic vacuolation of neurons and gray matter neuropil. The occurrence of vacuolation in the solitary tract and the spinal tract of the trigeminal nerve in the medulla oblongata is the basis of the statutory diagnosis of the disease in Great Britain. In Great Britain, statutory diagnosis is achieved by an examination of a single brainstem section obtained via the foramen magnum and obviating the need of extracting the brain with the associated risk of aerosol production. This sampling location has the potential to miss some cattle infected with atypical BSE.[21]

Scrapie-associated fibrils can be visualized by electron microscopy. Government regulatory agencies are usually responsible for the confirmation of this diagnosis and typically distribute specific protocols regarding the collection of samples and disposal of carcasses from suspect animals.

Samples for Confirmation of Diagnosis

- Immunology-based rapid tests: fresh brainstem
- Histology: formalin-fixed brain, including midbrain and entire medulla oblongata (LM).

Note the zoonotic potential of this disease when handling carcass and submitting specimens.

DIFFERENTIAL DIAGNOSIS

The disease should be considered in the differential diagnosis of any progressive neurologic disease in cattle. Primary differentials on clinical signs include the following:

- Hypomagnesemia
- Nervous acetonemia
- Rabies
- Lead poisoning
- Listeriosis
- Polioencephalomalacia
- Tremorgenic toxins

TREATMENT AND CONTROL

There is no treatment for the disease.

Detection of BSE in Surveillance and Control Programs

Passive surveillance has been used in many countries. Suspect disease is notifiable with compulsory slaughter and compensation and disposal of the carcass by incineration. The limitations of passive surveillance were described earlier and, in most countries, passive surveillance has been replaced with some form of active surveillance.

Active surveillance was initially directed at a targeted proportion of culled animals, animals manifesting neurologic disease, rabies suspects negative for rabies, fallen (down) cattle, and emergency slaughter categories, and a proportion of cattle, or all cattle, over 24 to 30 months (depending on country) that were presented for slaughter for human consumption. In slaughter cattle, **the sampling frame was set to detect BSE at a prevalence rate of one mature animal in a million mature animals**. The ability to conduct active surveillance, particularly on slaughter cattle, has been allowed by the development of rapid tests that can be conducted and read while the carcass is being held so that positive test cattle are not released for human consumption. Positive rapid tests need to be confirmed by histology and IHC. More recently, because the average age of BSE cases has been over 11 years, meaning that they were born before the date of the reinforced feed ban, the majority of EU countries have now raised the age limit for testing to 72 months for healthy slaughtered cattle (or even stopped testing) and to 48 months for fallen stock and emergency slaughter categories.[1]

In the United States, following the case of BSE in an imported cow, the United States Department of Agriculture (USDA) implemented an intensive national testing program for BSE that concentrated on a targeted high-risk population. The purpose is to help discover if BSE is in the United States and, if so, at what level. The intention is to sample as many cattle over a 12- to 18-month period as possible with the goal of examining 268,500 cattle. This would allow a detection rate of 1 in 10 million with a 99% confidence level. The cattle will be over 30 months of age and include nonambulatory cattle, cattle that are too weak to walk, cattle that are moribund, cattle with neurologic signs, rabies suspects that are negative, and dead cattle.

Control of BSE in Cattle

Control programs use the following assumptions:

- Infection and disease in cattle is introduced through feeding contaminated feed containing infected MBM or greaves.
- The source of infection to cattle can be eliminated by effective prohibition on feeding infected feed.
- There is no significant horizontal or vertical transmission.

Based on this, most countries have established a ban on the feeding of ruminant protein to ruminants. This was done in 1987 in the UK, the mid-1990s in most European countries, and in 1997 in Canada, the United States and Mexico. There is, however, a strong argument for banning all mammalian protein for feeding to all livestock. The experience of several countries with animals that were born after the ban shows that cross-contamination in feed mills can occur. Although the removal of **specified risk materials** (SRMs), (brain, spinal cord, eyes, tonsil, thymus, spleen, and intestines) from cattle carcasses should reduce the risk of the BSE agent being in the subsequent rendered carcass, it obviously does not eliminate it. More detail of the regulations and of control procedures is available.

These control procedures, initiated in the UK, were effective in changing the course of their epidemic, which is now on the wane.

Measures to Protect Human Health

High-risk animals, such as **downer cows**, should be kept out of the human food chain and not rendered for MBM. Infection is present in the tissues listed as **SRMs** (brain, spinal cord, eyes, tonsil, thymus, spleen, and intestines), which are removed from the carcass at slaughter. The removal of SRMs also protects against the risk posed by cattle that may be incubating the disease yet do not show any clinical signs. Together with a ban on products such as mechanically recovered meat that could be contaminated with SRMs, excluding SRMs from the human food chain is the most important food safety measure to protect public health.

However, this may not be sufficient. The method of slaughter with captive bolt guns can result in the widespread dissemination of brain within the carcass with dissemination by blood into the pulmonary tissues and elsewhere. Also, the method of splitting the carcass and spinal cord can result in significant carcass contamination and contamination of the slaughterhouse environment. Methods to decrease the risk of contamination of the carcass at slaughter have been suggested.

Based on transmission and infectivity experiments cattle under 30 months of age are considered to have very low risk of being infected, but there can be a risk in endemic countries with cattle over this age. Some countries with a high incidence of BSE have banned cattle over 30 months of age for human consumption.

FURTHER READING

Al-Zoughool M, Cottrell D, Elsaadany S, et al. Mathematical models for estimating the risks of bovine spongiform encephalopathy (BSE). *J Toxicol Environ Health B Crit Rev*. 2015;18:71-104.

Hamir AN, Kehrli ME, Kunkle RA, et al. Experimental interspecies transmission studies of the transmissible spongiform encephalopathies to cattle: comparison to bovine spongiform encephalopathy in cattle. *J Vet Diagn Invest*. 2011;23(3):407.

Harmon JL, Silva CJ. Bovine spongiform encephalopathy. *J Am Vet Med Assoc*. 2009;234:59-72.

REFERENCES

1. Acin C. *Vet Rec*. 2013;173:114.
2. Konold T, et al. *Vet Rec*. 2013;173:118.
3. Gavier-Widén D, et al. *J Vet Diagn Invest*. 2008;20:2.
4. Dobly A, et al. *BMC Vet Res*. 2010;6:26.
5. Richt JA, Hall SM. *PLoS Pathog*. 2008;4:e1000156.
6. Goldmann W. *Vet Res*. 2008;39:30.
7. Yoshikawa Y. *J Vet Med Sci*. 2008;70:325.
8. Ortiz-Pelaez A, et al. *Vet Rec*. 2012;170:389.
9. Wilesmith JW, et al. *Vet Rec*. 2010;167:279.
10. Wells GA, et al. *J Gen Virol*. 2007;88:1363.
11. Tyshenko MG. *Vet Rec*. 2007;160:215.
12. Hoffman C, et al. *J Gen Virol*. 2007;88:1048.
13. Masujin K, et al. *J Gen Virol*. 2007;88:1850.
14. Fast C, et al. *Vet Res*. 2013;44:123.
15. Konold T, et al. *BMC Vet Res*. 2010;6:53.
16. Konold T, et al. *BMC Res Notes*. 2012;8:22.
17. Arai S, et al. *Res Vet Sci*. 2009;87:111.
18. Greenlee MHW, et al. *PLoS ONE*. 2015;10:e0119431.
19. Fukada S, et al. *J Comp Pathol*. 2011;145:302.
20. Polak MP, Zmudzinski JF. *Vet J*. 2012;191:128.
21. Konold T, et al. *BMC Res Notes*. 2012;5:674.

BOVINE SPONGIFORM ENCEPHALOPATHY AND SHEEP

There is considerable speculation and concern that the agent of BSE could have become established in small ruminants. BSE can be readily experimentally transmitted to sheep and goats and produces clinical signs and lesions similar to scrapie. There is further concern following a recent report of the transmission of the agent from challenged ewes to their lambs. Further, the risk to human health from the ingestion of meat from sheep may be even greater than that from cattle because of the widespread distribution of the BSE agent in the lymphoid tissue of infected sheep.

In the UK and Europe concentrates are commonly fed to meat-producing breeds of sheep in late pregnancy and early lactation and less commonly to their lambs. They are also fed to milk-producing sheep breeds and to lactating goats. Concentrates fed during the 1980s and 1990s could have contained infected MBM, and this risk would have lasted until the total ban on feeding MBM to all farm animals in 1996 in the UK and 2001 in Europe.

The inclusion of MBM in concentrate rations for small ruminants was less than that for cattle, and the proportion of concentrate ration fed was also lower. This, coupled with the fact that prion diseases require a larger infective dose to produce disease in a cross-species to that required to produce the disease in the same species (the **species barrier** effect) may have resulted in an infective dose to sheep that was too low to establish infection.

The possibility that BSE did establish in sheep during the BSE epidemic in Britain is not supported by a study that examined the incidence and new infection rates of scrapie flocks in Britain covering the period from 1962 to 1998. This study found no evidence of a change in scrapie occurrence before, during, or following the BSE epidemic and no temporal or spatial correlations of scrapie occurrence with the BSE epidemic. There have been other studies that have examined the risk factors for transmission of BSE to sheep and the possibility that it could be perpetuated by sheep-to-sheep transmission. Most have concluded that the risk that BSE has established in sheep is low but, with current knowledge, cannot rule out the possibility.

There are no reports of naturally occurring cases of BSE detected in sheep. However, there is one report of a TSE in a goat in France that was found to have IHC and immunoblotting characteristics compatible with BSE, and, following injection into mice, incubation times compatible with those recorded for experimental ovine BSE.[1]

Experimental Transmission

BSE can be experimentally transmitted to sheep and goats by intracerebral, oral, and intravenous routes using BSE-infected cow brain. The PrP genotype affects the incubation period in both Cheviot and Romney sheep. PrP genotypes ARQ/ARQ and AHQ/AHQ are associated with short incubation periods (approximately 18–36 months) following challenge and also with disease susceptibility. One study further suggests that AHQ/ARQ sheep have a similar susceptibility to infection, and that sheep homozygous for alanine (A) at codon 131 and glutamine (Q) at codon 171 are more susceptible to BSE than any other genotype. In contrast, the PrP genotype ARR/ARR is associated with a long incubation period in sheep challenged intracerebrally, and ARR/ARR sheep are resistant to BSE challenged orally and do not have infectivity in their tissues. The ARR allele appears dominant in this respect because sheep carrying at least one ARR allele in combination with any other allele have a longer incubation period. PrP genotype VRQ/VRQ appears to have an intermediate incubation period.

Texel and Lacaune sheep with PrP ARQ/ARQ genotypes are susceptible. However, in these studies the survival of some sheep with susceptible genotypes suggests that factors other than the PrP genotype has influence on survival. Challenge dose in all of these studies has been high.

In a recent study, 30 ewe lambs were dosed orally, at 6 months of age, with 5 g of infected cattle brain and subsequently mated. Twenty-four developed clinical disease between 655 and 1065 days postinoculation and two lambs, born before their dams had clinical disease, also subsequently developed clinical disease. This study indicated that the agent of BSE can transmit either in utero or perinatally in sheep. There is no information on other routes of transmission and if they exist.

PATHOGENESIS

Following challenge of sheep with BSE, infectivity has been found in intestinal Peyer's patches as early as 5 months postinfection and in enteric nerves and spinal cord after 10 months with widespread dissemination throughout the lymphoreticular system and peripheral nervous system by 21 months.[1]

CLINICAL SIGNS

The clinical signs reported in affected experimental animals are not well described in many of the experimental challenge studies but have varied in different studies. In one study, sheep and goats showed sudden onset of ataxia, which progressed rapidly to recumbency. There was little evidence of pruritus and the clinical course was very short, lasting between 1 and 5 days in the majority of animals with one goat showing progressive weight loss over 3 weeks before it was culled. Genotype had no influence on the duration of the clinical course. In another study in sheep only, the clinical course was approximately 3 months and affected sheep showed pruritus with fleece loss and ataxia and behavioral change. Ataxia, weight loss, and pruritus were considered constant in another.

In an experiment designed to test specifically if clinical signs could be used for differentiation between scrapie and BSE, two different groups of sheep were inoculated with each agent. The duration of clinical signs varied quite markedly within both groups with a mean of approximately 9 days for each group but a variation in both from 1 to over 80 days. As with natural scrapie, there was considerable variation in the nature of the clinical signs, but there was no marked difference in the frequencies of clinical signs between the two groups, except that ataxia was the first sign noticed in a significantly greater proportion of the BSE-challenged group, whereas pruritus was the first noticed sign in a significantly greater proportion of the scrapie-challenged group.

DISPOSITION OF DISEASE-ASSOCIATED PRP

Genotype and route of inoculation influence the disposition of disease-associated PrP in lymphoreticular system tissues (tonsil, spleen, and mesenteric lymph node). The most conspicuous effect is the absence of disease-associated PrP in peripheral lymph tissue in ARR/ARR genotype sheep and lack of infectivity, and there appears to be an inverse relationship between this disposition and the incubation period. Route of inoculation influences the relative intensity of disposition in tonsil, spleen, and mesenteric lymph node.

Following experimental infection of sheep with BSE, disease-associated PrP can be detected in tonsil biopsies 11 to 20 months after challenge but, in contrast to scrapie, disease-associated PrP is not detected in biopsies of lymphoid tissue from the third eyelid.

DIAGNOSIS

The diagnosis of BSE in clinically affected cattle can be achieved with several techniques, including the analysis of symptoms, histopathology, and the detection of the disease-associated form of the prion protein, by immunocytochemistry, Western blot, or ELISA. The profiling of vacuoles in the affected host had shown a remarkable uniformity over the year and from different geographic regions. However, this is not true with scrapie and the variation in the host brain with scrapie would not allow differentiation from BSE on histologic findings. The diagnosis of BSE in sheep presents problems, and the similarity of the clinical signs and pathology between scrapie and BSE could easily result in naturally occurring cases of BSE in sheep being misdiagnosed as scrapie.

Strain Tying

The gold-standard technique for the diagnosis of TSE agents is the passage of tissue in panels of inbred mice, a technique known as strain typing. Until recently this was the only way to differentiate the two diseases. BSE presents with a characteristic range of incubation periods and a pattern of distribution and relative severity of changes in the brain of the different mouse strains (the lesion profile), which is distinct from all scrapie strains tested. However, this method of diagnosis is both expensive and time-consuming.

There has been a wide search for a differential test system in including prion protein profiling, studies in glycosylation and glycoform ratios, and other molecular and biochemical studies that are detailed elsewhere. A recent promising set of studies suggests that the site of truncation of disease-associated PrP during partial digestion by proteases located in lysozymes appears different for sheep scrapie and experimental BSE. After digestion by exogenous enzymes, the BSE PrP molecule is shorter than that of scrapie stains giving rise to different IHC patterns, and this is supported by Western blot studies. Unlike scrapie, the intracellular truncation site of ovine BSE PrP is influenced by the cell type in which it accumulates, giving distinct patterns of immunolabeling with different PrP antibodies. Epitope labeling shows that the shortest fragment of disease-associated PrP occurs in tangible body macrophages followed by glial cells and neurons. It appears that this difference in truncation of PrP in experimentally infected BSE sheep is not influenced by route of inoculation or by genotype or by sheep bred, and it is proposed that truncation patterns, as detected by immunoblotting and IHC, can be used in surveys for BSE in sheep.

CONTROL

If BSE is or does establish in small ruminants in a country, there is significant concern for human health. The distribution of BSE infection in the carcasses of cattle is limited and can be removed by the ban of the use of SRMs (largely brain, spinal cord, and offal). In contrast, the distribution of the BSE agent in infected sheep is widespread, and it would be virtually impossible to remove this by trimming or selective organ removal from a carcass for human consumption. Also, lymphocytes in milk could be infected.

Active surveillance for TSEs in sheep and goats has been increased in the EU, and several rapid tests for use in sheep and goats are now available.[2] In the UK, a worst-case scenario, published in 2001 in a contingency plan to address BSE in sheep, threatened the national herd with slaughter, largely on the grounds that an epidemic of BSE in sheep could be harder to contain than was the case for BSE in cattle and that lamb could present a greater risk to consumers than beef. A more recent UK contingency plan would allow PrP genotype ARR homozygous sheep and ARR heterozygous sheep for human consumption. This plan is the same as the EU, except that there are differences in the maximum age allowed at slaughter between the UK and the EU recommendations.

The risk for BSE in sheep was a major incentive for the development of national breeding programs for the control of scrapie, and possible BSE, including the National Scrapie Plan in the UK, launched in 2001, and the National Scrapie Eradication Program in the United States. The purpose in these breeding programs is to select against highly susceptible genotypes and select for the highly resistant genotype.

REFERENCES

1. Harmon JL, Silva CJ. *J Am Vet Med Assoc.* 2009;234:59.
2. van Keulen LJM, et al. *Arch Virol.* 2008;153:445.

SCRAPIE

SYNOPSIS

Etiology A transmissible agent (prion, a proteinaceous infectious particle) that is highly resistant to chemical and physical agents, and appears not to contain DNA. Susceptibility of sheep to developing clinical disease after infection is determined by genetics.

Epidemiology Transmitted primarily by contact with infected sheep and from environmental contamination; very long incubation period.

Clinical findings Nonfebrile disease of adult sheep, goats, and mouflons with insidious onset and long clinical course. Clinical disease is rare in goats and mouflons. Affected animals show behavioral change, tremor, pruritus and locomotor disorder, and wasting.

Clinical pathology Demonstration of scrapie prion protein by immunostaining of the obex in brain and selected lymphoid tissue elsewhere.

Lesions Vacuolation of gray matter neuropil and neuronal perikarya, neuronal degeneration, gliosis.

Diagnostic confirmation Demonstration of scrapie prion protein.

Treatment None.

Control Slaughter eradication. Genetic testing and selection/culling.

Scrapie is a nonfebrile, fatal, chronic disease of adult sheep, goats, and mouflons (one of two ancestors of all modern sheep breeds) characterized clinically by pruritus and abnormalities of gait, and by a very long incubation period. It is the prototypic disease for a group of diseases known as **TSEs**. This group also includes **CWD** of deer and elk; **transmissible mink encephalopathy;** and FSE, CJD, and other spongiform encephalopathies of humans, and the relatively new disease, **BSE**, which is described separately under that heading. In Iceland scrapie is known as ***rida***, in France as ***la tremblante***, and in Germany as ***traberkrankheit***.

ETIOLOGY

There has been a significant historical debate over the etiology of this disease. The current consensus view is that scrapie is associated with an infectious agent, but that the incubation period for clinical manifestation of the disease and the susceptibility of the host to developing clinical disease after infection is determined by genetics. In other words, to develop clinical disease caused classical scrapie, an animal must be exposed to the infectious agent and have a susceptible genotype.

Scrapie can be transmitted experimentally to other sheep and to certain laboratory animals, and infection induces the production in the brain, and some other tissues, of amyloid fibrils called scrapie-associated fibrils or prion rods. The main constituent of these is a disease-specific, protease-resistant neuronal membrane glycoprotein termed the **prion protein**, or PrP^{Sc}. PrP^{Sc} is an abnormal isoform of a host-coded membrane glycoprotein, PrP^{C}, and the TSEs are characterized by the accumulation of PrP^{Sc} in neuronal and other tissue.

Transmission can be effected by crude or purified extracts of brain or other tissues from affected sheep, and the infective agent is very resistant to ionizing and ultraviolet irradiation and to reagents that damage or modify nucleic acids. This, along with other experimental findings, has led to the accepted view that the infectious agent in scrapie is PrP^{Sc} itself, and not a small, unconventional virus or virino as previously proposed. The structure of the infecting PrP^{Sc} is thought to imprint on the normal cellular precursor PrP^{C}, with the template resulting in a change to the abnormal isoform which is protease-resistant and accumulates in cells.

More than 20 different **strains** of scrapie have been identified based on the following:

- Strain typing by differences in incubation time of the experimental disease in inbred strains of mice of different genotype
- The type, pattern, severity, and distribution of lesions in the brain of the different strains of experimental animals (lesion profiles)
- Resistance to thermal inactivation
- The type of disease produced in sheep and experimental animals (e.g., drowsy versus pruritic manifestations in goats)
- The ability of a strain to produce disease in different species of experimental animals

It is proposed that strain differences reflect differences in replicating information carried within the conformational state of the PrP^{Sc}. The more important strains identified are called **classical scrapie strains**, comprising strain A and strain C (thought to be the most prevalent strain in the United States), and **atypical (or discordant or nonclassical) scrapie strains**, comprising the Nor98 strain and other discordant strains. Coinfection of strains can occur with scrapie.

Nor98 was first reported in 1998 in five unrelated Norwegian sheep that had PrP^{Sc} in a different location (cerebellum) than usually reported with scrapie. Nor98 has now been identified in sheep in a number of countries. Atypical scrapie is thought to arise spontaneously and not be associated with an infective source.[1] Interestingly, atypical scrapie is usually not clinically apparent, but there are reports of sheep infected with atypical scrapie strains exhibiting some of the typical clinical signs of classical scrapie, particularly rear limb ataxia.[1,2] Atypical scrapie caused by Nor98 has been diagnosed in sheep in Australia and New Zealand; these are two countries that do not have classical scrapie.[3] Atypical scrapie is not considered rare compared with classical scrapie and appears to occur at a constant prevalence in different countries.[4]

EPIDEMIOLOGY

Occurrence

Geographic Occurrence and Incidence

Scrapie in sheep occurs enzootically in the UK, Europe, and North America. Outbreaks have been reported in Australia, New Zealand, India, the Middle East, Japan, and Scandinavia, principally in sheep imported from enzootic areas. Australia and New Zealand used vigorous importation, quarantine, and culling policies to prevent subsequent entry of the disease and are considered free of disease.

The true prevalence of the disease both within and between countries is not known because there has been no test to detect the presence of infection in individual sheep or in flocks at all stages of infection. This is further confounded by secrecy about the existence of scrapie in many flocks and breeds. This secrecy results from a fear of economic penalties that could result from the admission of infection.

In Great Britain, where the disease is enzootic and has been recognized for over 250 years, the true incidence is unknown, although a questionnaire survey in 1988 suggests that one-third of sheep flocks are infected. In infected flocks the annual incidence ranges from 0.4 to 10 cases per 100 sheep per year, with a mean of 1.1 cases per 100 sheep per year. However, the annual incidence can approach 20% of the adult flock, on occasions up to 40%, and in flocks where there is no selection against the disease the annual incidence and mortality can reach a level that results in disbandment of the flock or its nonsurvival.

Farmer consultation with a veterinarian about a case of scrapie and farmer reporting of cases of scrapie are notoriously low. Historically, this is because factors such as the stigma associated with having scrapie diagnosed in a purebred flock and concerns for future sales or, in the case of commercial flocks, a lack of incentive to consult and a lack of concern because nothing can be done to cure the present case or prevent future cases. In England, it has been estimated that only 13% of farmers who had a suspected case of scrapie in the past 12 months reported it. Possibly, the chance of improvement through genetic selection will alter this farmer trait.

In the United States the disease is thought to have been introduced in 1947, and by 1992 was found in 657 flocks in 39 states. In 2007 the prevalence of infection in the United States was estimated at 0.1% to 0.3%.

Host Occurrence

Age

Scrapie is a disease of **mature sheep,** although most are exposed as young sheep, and the incidence decreases with age at exposure. The age-specific incidence in **sheep** is highest between 2.5 and 4.5 years of age and cases rarely occur under 18 months of age. Natural disease in **goats** is rare. The age at death is similar to that in sheep, with a range from 2 to 7 years. The **case–fatality rate**, with time, is 100%. The death loss is added to by the slaughter of infected and in-contact animals in countries where control and eradication is a practice.

Breed

Scrapie occurs in both sexes and in the majority of breeds, although the incidence is higher in some breeds than others. Breed differences in prevalence occur in several countries; an example would be the high prevalence in the Suffolk breed in the United States relative to white-faced breeds and in some Hill breeds in the UK. These probably reflect breed and flock differences in genetic susceptibility to the development of clinical disease. Similarly, the occurrence of outbreaks of scrapie may result from the introduction of infection to a genetically susceptible flock or to a change in the genetic structure of flocks that are infected.

Methods of Transmission

Knowledge of transmission of scrapie is based primarily on the experimental disease and observations of the natural disease in experimental flocks.

Sources and Routes of Infection

The usual method of introduction into unaffected flocks is by the purchase of preclinically infected sheep. Infectivity can be demonstrated in the placenta, fetal fluids, saliva, colostrum, and milk of naturally occurring cases,[5-7] and in the oral cavity of sheep with preclinical scrapie,[8] but has not been demonstrated in the urine or feces of natural cases, even though it can be demonstrated in the intestine. Ingestion of infected material appears the most likely route of infection, but scarification of the skin and conjunctival inoculation will also allow infection. Hay mites have been found to harbor the agent on scrapie-infected properties and have been proposed as a reservoir for infection.

Horizontal Transmission

This is the usual method of spread, and the placenta is considered the major source of infection for the mother to her lamb, and to other lambs in close contact. Under natural conditions the disease in flocks often runs in families, and whether or not a lamb contracts scrapie appears to depend primarily on the current or future scrapie status of its dam. It is common for all the VQR/VQR lambs from dams dying of classical scrapie to develop scrapie.

Scrapie can also transmit between sheep in close contact, and this can occur from sheep in the preclinical phase of the disease. Scrapie can be transmitted by blood transfusion. The importance of this route of infection in field infections appears low because successful transmission appears to require at least 400 mL of blood.

Under natural conditions, scrapie occurs in sheep and occasionally spontaneously in goats. Under experimental conditions, scrapie has been observed to spread from sheep to goats by contact, and the little evidence available on the natural disease in goats is consistent with the view that the scrapie can be maintained by contagion in a herd of goats living apart from infected sheep.

Vertical Transmission

There is a greater risk for scrapie in lambs born to infected dams, but this most probably reflects horizontal transmission at birth from placentas. There are conflicting results between studies that have examined transmission by embryo transfer, and the importance of vertical transmission to the epidemiology of the natural disease remains to be determined. However, epidemiologic studies suggest that it is of rare occurrence, and there is significant evidence against the occurrence of in utero transmission. The agent has not been demonstrated in the testes or semen of rams.

Environment

An infected environment can also be the source, and scrapie-free sheep can develop disease after grazing pasture previously grazed by scrapie-infected sheep, with infection by ingestion or possibly via abrasive lesions. Environmental infection can occur from the products of parturition and, although the scrapie agent has not been demonstrated in feces, it is suspected as being so in infected animals. The duration of infectivity on inanimate materials such as pasture has not been defined, but field and experimental observations indicate that it is a long time, probably in excess of 16 years under some conditions.[9,10]

Iatrogenic Transmission

An outbreak of scrapie occurred in the 1930s following the use of a vaccine against louping-ill prepared from the brains of sheep. More recently, the use of a vaccine against contagious agalactia has been epidemiologically linked to an outbreak of scrapie in sheep and goats in Italy where there was a high attack rate and high mortality affecting several birth cohorts.

Genetics

Scrapie is recorded in most breeds of sheep, but there are breed, family, and individual differences in susceptibility. There is substantial genetic control of the incidence of disease, and in both the natural and experimental disease, genetics is a major determinant of susceptibility with the susceptibility of sheep strongly linked to certain polymorphisms in the sheep PrP gene.

In earlier studies, experimental challenge and breeding showed that sheep could exhibit a long or short incubation period following challenge, and that this difference in incubation period or susceptibility was determined by a single gene called **scrapie incubation period** (*Sip*). There is a similar gene in mice (*Sinc*) that determines incubation period and susceptibility following experimental challenge. The *Sip* gene has two alleles, *sA* and *pA*, which, respectively, shorten or prolong the experimental incubation period for most strains of the scrapie agent. The subsequent recognition of prion protein (PrP) and its association with scrapie led to the recognition of the gene that encodes PrP, which was found congruent to *Sip* in sheep, and *Sip* genetics have been entirely superseded by PrP genetics.

Sheep have one pair of genes that influence susceptibility to scrapie known as the prion protein genes. These code for a normal prion protein in the cell (PrP^C), which has 254 amino acids with each codon in the gene encoding for a specific amino acid at a particular location on PrP^C. PrP^C can be converted to a scrapie prion protein molecule (PrP^{Sc}) in infected sheep which, when it accumulates in the CNS, causes disease. The susceptibility of sheep to this conversion, and thus to scrapie, is **strongly associated with certain polymorphisms at codons 136, 154, and 171**. It is thought that there are at least two groups of scrapie TSE strains, one of which is influenced primarily by the amino acid at codon 136 and the other group by the amino acid at codon 171. Within these there may be subtypes because resistance to some 136-type TSEs can be affected by the amino acid at codon 154.

- At codon 136 valine (V) is linked to scrapie susceptibility and alanine (A) is linked with resistance
- At codon 154 histidine (H) is linked to susceptibility and arginine (R) to resistance
- At codon 171 glutamine (Q) and histidine (H) are linked to susceptibility and arginine (R) to resistance.

- The notations used for descriptions of the prion protein (PrR) genotype vary in different countries.
- The susceptibility of sheep to scrapie is strongly associated with polymorphisms at codons 136, 154, and 171 in the prion protein gene.
- The amino acids associated with these polymorphisms are alanine, valine, histidine, arginine, and glutamine.
- In the description of the PrP genotype these are given the letters A, V, H, R, and Q, respectively.
- The PrP genotype is listed in the order of codon 136 followed by 154 and then 171.
- The amino acid at each codon is listed according to the letter designation for each of the two alleles separated by a backslash. Examples are ARR/ARR or ARR/VQR. These could also be expressed as $AA_{136}RR_{154}RR_{171}$ and $AV_{136}RQ_{154}RR_{171}$.
- In sheep in the United States the polymorphisms at codon 171 are the major determinant of scrapie susceptibility. Polymorphisms at codon 154 play a minor role and are usually not listed as part of the PrP genotype.
- Genotypes in the United States are usually referred to using the letters of the amino acids in numerical order codon 136 followed by codon 171.
- The previous examples would be AA RR and AV RR.
- They can also be referred to using the codon number followed by the corresponding amino acid 136AA, 171RR and 136AV, 171RR or the amino acid followed by the codon.
- Often only the amino acids at codon 171 are listed.

Of the possible alleles from these polymorphisms, only five, ARR, ARQ, VRQ, AHQ, ARH, are commonly seen. The relationship between PrP genotype and susceptibility to scrapie is shown in Table 14-15 using the groupings of the British National Scrapie Plan.

It can be seen from Table 14-15 that in the Britain, the VQR allele confers the greatest degree of susceptibility and that ARR is associated with resistance. Estimates that quantify risk in the British national flock based on genotypes of the sheep, and those of scrapie-affected sheep, are available but they are not strongly concordant. There is also an effect of PrP genotype on the incubation period, with the most susceptible genotypes (VQR) having the shortest incubation period and dying of scrapie at a younger age.

The frequency and distribution of the various PrP genotypes varies considerably between flocks and between breeds of sheep. There are also some marked between-breed differences in susceptibility with the same PrP genotype.

Susceptibility in the Suffolk and other black-faced breeds in the United States appears less complex than in other breeds and is strongly associated with sheep that are homozygous for glutamine at the 171 codon (171QQ) of the PrP gene, but is rare in sheep heterologous for glutamine and arginine (171QR) or homozygous for arginine (171RR) at codon 171. Suffolks are the predominant breed affected with scrapie in the United States. They lack the VRQ allele, and the ARQ/ARQ genotype is the genotype that confers the greatest susceptibility. The association between genotype and susceptibility, as defined in the scrapie eradication plan of the USDA, in the United Sates is shown in Table 14-16.

Factors other than the PrP genotype influence susceptibility to scrapie because not all sheep with a susceptible genotype challenged with scrapie subsequently develop the disease. Also, there are some breed differences in the level of resistance or susceptibility conferred by a given genotype. For example, ARQ/ARQ Suffolk sheep are highly susceptible to scrapie, whereas ARQ/ARQ Cheviots are relatively resistant. Breed differences in PrP genotype scrapie disease linkage and disease pattern differences with atypical strains of scrapie may be associated with polymorphisms in the PrP gene promoter. Atypical scrapie caused by to Nor98 strain is most common in sheep in Europe carrying phenylalanine (F) at position 141 or the PrP genotypes ARR/ARR, ARR/ARQ, and AHQ/ARQ.[11-13]

Table 14-15 PrP genotype and susceptibility to scrapie in national scrapie program in Great Britain

NSP Type	Main characteristic	Genotypes	Comments
1	ARR homozygous	ARR/ARR	Genetically most resistant
2	ARR heterozygous non-VQR	ARR/AHQ ARR/ARQ ARR/ARH	Sheep that are genetically resistant to scrapie, but will need careful selection when used for further breeding
3	**Non-ARR and non-VQR**	AHQ/AHQ ARQ/AHQ AHQ/ARH ARH/ARH ARQ/ARH ARQ/ARQ	Sheep that genetically have little resistance to scrapie and will need careful selection when used for further breeding Group 3 risk varies and can depend on breed, e.g., ARQ/ARQ Suffolk are highly susceptible ARQ/ARQ Cheviots are relatively resistant
4	**ARR/VQR heterozygous**	ARR/VRQ	Sheep that are genetically susceptible to scrapie and should not be used for breeding unless in the context of a controlled breeding
5	**VQR and non-ARR**	AHQ/VRQ ARQ/VRQ ARH/VRQ VRQ/VRQ	Sheep that are highly susceptible to scrapie and should not be used for breeding

NSP, *National Scrapie Program.*

Table 14-16 Scrapie susceptibility and genotype as defined by the U.S. Scrapie Eradication Plan

Genotype	Susceptibility
1. AA RR	Sheep that are resistant
2. AA QR	Sheep that are rarely susceptible
3. AV QR	Sheep that are susceptible to some scrapie strains that are thought to occur with low frequency in the United States
4. AA QQ	Sheep that are highly susceptible
5. AV QQ	Sheep that are highly susceptible
6. VV QQ	Sheep that are highly susceptible

There is less information on the genetics of scrapie in **goats**. There is high variability in the goat PrP gene that possibly can be exploited to select for goat-specific scrapie-resistant PrP genotypes. An initial report indicated that the H_{154}, Q_{211}, and K_{222} single nucleotide polymorphisms were associated with a high resistance to classical scrapie.[14]

Risk Factors

Exposure Factors

There is a dose–response relationship in naturally occurring scrapie. The high incidence in some Icelandic flocks is attributed to a high level of exposure, resulting from a long winter housing period with a higher risk for disease in lambs born in the winter housing period.

Factors that influence exposure risk will vary with the management systems, which can vary markedly between countries. With that caveat, risk factors that have been identified in case–control studies include the following:

- A higher risk for scrapie in larger flocks and in pedigree flocks
- A greater risk in flocks that lamb communally in group pens compared with those that lamb in individual pens or outside on pasture
- A greater risk in flocks that disposed of the placenta in the compost and spread sheep compost on the land
- A lower risk in flocks in which cow compost is spread on the land
- A greater risk in flocks that purchased replacement sheep through the market
- A greater risk where different flocks share pastures or rams

Age at Exposure

Lambs exposed at birth have a shorter incubation period and higher risk for scrapie than lambs exposed at 6 to 9 months of age. Similarly, lambs or goats removed from infected dams at birth to a scrapie-free environment have a lower incidence of scrapie than those removed at later times.

Infection Status of Parents

Lambs born to affected ewes are at increased risk for scrapie, and the offspring from an infected ewe and an infected ram are at greater risk than those born from an infected ewe and an uninfected ram. However, even in high-incidence herds a considerable proportion of disease cannot be attributed to parental scrapie status and results from horizontal transmission. Also, the number of genetically susceptible sheep in an affected flock can increase the infection pressure.

Goats

Scrapie in goats is rare, and most cases arise in goats that are in close contact with infected sheep. Scrapie can spread from goat to goat with no sheep contact.

Experimental Reproduction

The agent is present in the brain, spinal cord, lymph nodes, intestinal tract tissue, and spleen of infected sheep, and has been extracted from sheep and goat brain. Experimentally, the disease can be transmitted to sheep, goats, mice and other laboratory animals using these tissues, and by a variety of routes of inoculation. The experimental disease has a long incubation period that varies with the strain of the agent and the genetics of the recipient. Transmission of the disease to sheep has also been effected by the oral or intracerebral administration with fetal membrane material from known infected ewes. Accidental transmission is recorded following vaccination against louping-ill, with vaccine contaminated by the agent of scrapie, and resulted in widespread dissemination of the disease.

Pathogen Risk Factors

The scrapie agent can be maintained in tissue culture, and infectivity is retained with passage. It can also be perpetuated in experimental animals. Infectivity also survives for remarkable periods in dead and formalinized tissues; infected brain homogenates buried in soil for 3 years retain their infectivity. It is highly resistant to physical and chemical influences and can survive decontamination processes that are effective against conventional viruses. It is capable of withstanding the usual virucidal procedures and is not destroyed by boiling, by rapid freezing and thawing, or by exposure to ether or 20% formalin. Conventional heat treatments may reduce infectivity, but the agent is remarkable resistant to heat and steam sterilization at 27 psig (132°C) is required to totally destroy it. Chemical inactivation can be achieved with sodium hypochlorite providing 2% (20,000 ppm) of available chlorine acting for 1 hour, and by 4% sodium hydroxide.

Economic Importance

Scrapie is of major concern to pedigree flocks and, if present and public, will curtail the sale of sheep and effectively result in the dissolution of the flock. Some countries have, or have had, eradication schemes. The disease is also of major international importance because of the embargos maintained by several countries against sheep from enzootic areas.

Zoonotic Implications

There is no evidence for transmission of scrapie to humans or for a risk to public health.

PATHOGENESIS

In both sheep and mice, the agent shows a predilection for tissues of the lymphoreticular system in which it replicates during the incubation period before invading the nervous system. In naturally infected sheep, replication begins in the tonsil, retropharyngeal lymph node and Peyer's patches, and gut-associated lymphoid tissue, which probably reflects the oral route of infection. PrP^{Sc} subsequently becomes disseminated to other lymph nodes and the spleen. There may be a considerable period, ranging from 14 months to 7 years, before there is infection of the brain, and during this infection in the lymphoreticular system probably provides the reservoir for maternal and horizontal transmission. The action of the PrP genotype may be to delay neural invasion, in which case it is possible that a nonclinical carrier state may exist for scrapie.

How the scrapie agent reaches the CNS is not certain, but it is probably through transportation across intestinal villous enterocytes[15] and subsequent infection of the autonomic nervous system. Gut-associated lymphoid nodules in the Peyer's patches have a substantial network of nerve fibers and are probably the site for neuroinvasion. The scrapie agent has been detected in lymphoid nodules of the Peyer's patches of the gut as early as 5 months after oral infection.

Infection in the brain of sheep is initially in the diencephalon and medulla oblongata, with subsequent spread and replication in other areas of the brain. Characteristically, there is a noninflammatory, vacuolar degeneration of gray matter and the presence of PrP^{Sc} in scrapie-associated fibrils. Infection results in the posttranslational modification of this protein so that it becomes resistant to proteinases and to normal clearance and, consequently, accumulates in the cell.

PrP^{Sc} is also present in the placenta and in the trophoblast cells of the placentomes but not in the endometrium, myometrium, associated nerve plexuses, or in the fetus. The presence of PrP^{Sc} in the placenta is determined by the fetal PrP gene, and PrP^{Sc} is not present in the placenta of fetuses carrying one or two ARR alleles.

CLINICAL FINDINGS

Incubation

The incubation period varies from several months to several years. Scrapie is a nonfebrile disease and the onset is insidious, but as the disease progresses clinical signs become more obvious and severe. The **clinical course** is protracted, varying from 2 to 12 months, but lasting in most cases for about 6 months. Affected animals usually show **behavioral change, tremor, pruritus, and locomotor disorder.** A clinical examination protocol to detect classical and atypical scrapie in sheep has been developed.[16,17]

Early Signs

The earliest signs are transient, nervous phenomena occurring at intervals of several weeks or under conditions of stress. These episodes include sudden collapse and sudden changes of behavior, with sheep charging at dogs or closed gates.

Rubbing and biting at the fleece then begins but are often unobserved because of their infrequent occurrence. The apparent **pruritus** is manifested chiefly over the rump, thighs, and tail base. The poll and dorsum of the neck may also be involved and, less commonly, the neck in front of the shoulder and the ribs behind the elbow. The affected areas have approximate bilateral symmetry. In this early stage a stilted gait is often observed. A general loss of condition may also be observed as an early sign, although the appetite may not be severely affected.

Advanced Cases

More advanced cases show intense pruritus, muscle tremor and marked abnormalities of gait, and severe emaciation. **Persistent rubbing** causes loss of wool over the areas mentioned previously. Scratching with the hindfeet and biting at the extremities also occurs. Hematoma of the ears and swelling of the face may result from rubbing. Light or deep pressure, pinpricking, and application of heat or cold may elicit the characteristic "nibbling or scrapie scratch" reaction, during which the animal elevates the head and makes nibbling movements of the lips and licking movements with the tongue (Fig. 14-11). The sheep's expression suggests that the sensations evoked are pleasant ones. The reaction may not be observed consistently, often disappearing when the sheep is excited or in new surroundings.

Simultaneously with the development of pruritus there is serious **impairment of locomotion**. Hindlimb abnormalities appear first. There is incomplete flexion of the hock, shortening of the step, weakness, and lack of balance. The sense of spatial relationship appears to be lost, and the sheep is slow to correct abnormal postures. Adduction occurs during extension, and abduction occurs during flexion. When the animal is attempting to evade capture, gross incoordination of head and leg movements is likely and the animal often falls. Convulsions, usually transient but occasionally fatal, may occur at this time.

General hyperexcitability is evident. In the animal at rest an intermittent nodding and jerking of the head and fine tremor of superficial muscles may also be observed. In some cases, nystagmus can be produced by rotating the head sideways. Other clinical signs include inability to swallow, although prehension is unaffected; vomiting; loss of bleat; and blindness. A change of voice to a trembling note is often most noticeable.

Anorexia is not evident in most cases until the last 4 to 5 weeks and results in rapid loss of BW. Abomasal distension and impaction occurs in a small number of cases. Pregnancy toxemia may occur as a complication in pregnant ewes during this stage of scrapie. Finally, the sheep reaches a stage of extreme emaciation and inability to move without becoming readily fatigued. Sternal recumbency follows and lateral recumbency with hyperextension of the limbs is the final stage. Pyrexia is not evident at any time.

In a detailed study in 129 sheep with scrapie the proportional occurrence of signs was hindlimb ataxia 71%, head tremor 61%, altered mental status 57%, positive nibble reflex 51%, crouching position 51%, teeth grinding 44%, low head carriage 38%, body condition score of less than 1.5, 38%, and conscious proprioceptive deficits of limbs 36%. The occurrence of clinical signs was examined in relationship to the PrP genotype. The nibble reflex was strongly associated with PrP genotypes ARQ/ARQ and ARQ/ARH.

In goats, the clinical course in naturally occurring cases lasts from 2 to 24 weeks. Clinical signs are similar to those in sheep, and hyperesthesia, ataxia, and pruritus are common, but loss of weight is less common. In lactating goats the first sign may be a reluctance to permit milking. Dribbling and regurgitation of ruminal contents are also recorded in one-third of cases.

In most countries the disease is reportable to government authorities.

CLINICAL PATHOLOGY

There are no changes in hematologic or serum biochemistry parameters. The **IHC test on the obex** and other parts of the brain is the confirmatory test at some laboratories of the OIE and is considered the gold standard test in the United States. At least four ELISA tests are approved for scrapie surveillance at slaughter in the EU. Western blots on retropharyngeal lymph nodes obtained at slaughter have a sensitivity approaching that of IHC.[18] Atypical scrapie is best diagnosed using cerebellum as the tissue for analysis.

Until recently there has been no **antemortem** test for scrapie; however, PrP^{Sc} can be detected in cells by IHC methods and is present in the lymphoid tissue of some sheep with scrapie in the preclinical phase of the disease. **Palatine tonsillar biopsy** has detected PrP^{Sc} in lambs of susceptible genotypes as young as 5 months of age and in the tonsils of nonchallenged susceptible lambs at 9 to 10 months of age that were born and maintained in a scrapie environment. However, tonsil biopsy requires general anesthesia and is not a practical on-farm technique.

Biopsy of **lymphoid follicles in the third eyelid** or **rectum** is more practical, requires only restraint, sedation using xylazine, and local analgesia, and the techniques are being investigated for the preclinical diagnosis of scrapie in surveillance programs. In scrapie-positive sheep, PrP^{Sc} can be detected in third

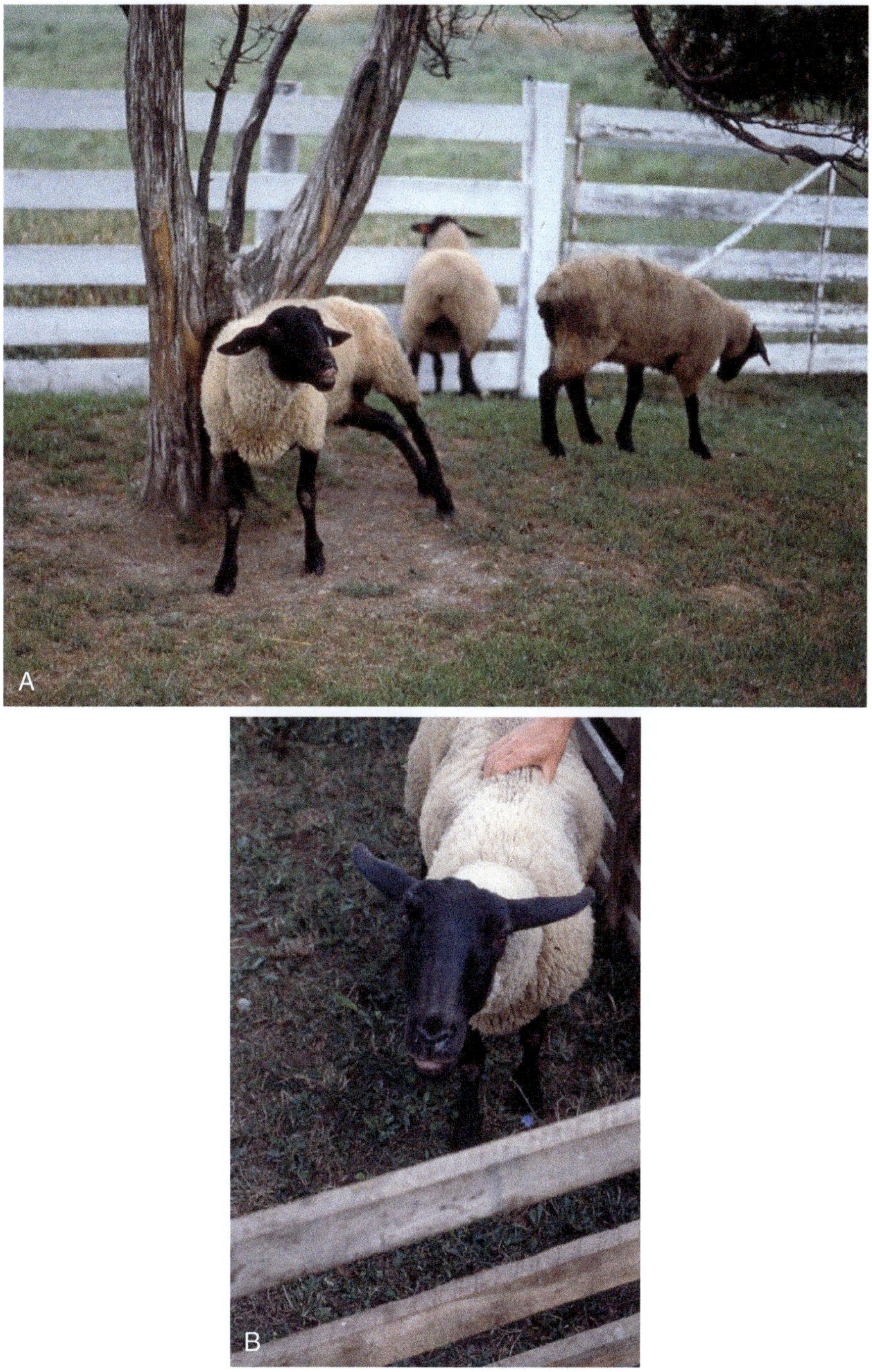

Fig. 14-11 **A,** Clinical signs of scrapie in Suffolk ewes located in the midwest region of the United States. The ewe on the left is pruritic, which is manifested as rubbing against the tree. The same ewe is also showing a positive nibble reflex (scrapie scratch reaction) with an upper lip curl and protruded tongue. The ewe on the right is losing weight and has an abnormally low head carriage. **B,** A positive result to the scrapie scratch reaction test. Rubbing/scratching the back over the thoracic vertebrae results in a slight elevation of the head, an upper lip curl, licking of the lips, and a pleasing look in the eyes of sheep with scrapie.

eyelid biopsies by 14 months of age, obtained from the palpebral side of the third eyelid. Histamine-containing eye drops improve the success of collecting a sample with adequate lymphoid follicles for examination. However, lymphoid follicles may not be present in sufficient numbers in third eyelid biopsies for evaluation in up to 60% of adult sheep sampled, and the sensitivity of third eyelid biopsy and rectal mucosa biopsy in detecting scrapie-infected sheep is 40% and 36%.[19] It is unlikely that lymphoid tissue will ever achieve an adequately high test sensitivity because a large number of infected animals have minimal or no PrP^{Sc} in lymphoid tissue.

Research is ongoing about developing an accurate test that can detect serum biomarkers of early and late phase scrapie or PrP^{Sc} in blood.[20] It has been suggested that the disease could be diagnosed antemortem by EEG, but this has been disputed.

NECROPSY FINDINGS

Significant gross findings are restricted to traumatic lesions caused by rubbing, and to emaciation and loss of wool; gross distension of the abomasum has been recorded in some natural cases.

The essential histopathologic lesion in scrapie is the **vacuolation of gray matter neuropil** in the spinal cord, medulla, pons, and midbrain, and the consequential wallerian degeneration in dorsal, ventral and ventrolateral columns of the spinal cord, and in nerve fibers in the cerebellar peduncles and the optic nerve. In addition, there is degeneration of the cerebellar and hypothalamoneurohypophyseal systems. There are different strains of the scrapie agent that can result in differing clinical signs and pathology. Scrapie-associated fibrils are present in infected brain. Histologic findings are diagnostic in many cases but can be supplemented with the immunodetection of PrP^{Sc} in brain tissue by in situ IHC and Western immunoblots. The breed of the sheep affects the magnitude of neuropil vacuolation, and variation also is associated with the PRP genotype within breeds.

Atypical strains of scrapie (Nor98) are recognized that differ from the usual strains in their vacuolation patterns and their disease-specific, protease-resistant PrP^{Sc} disposition patterns. These strains can also produce disease in PrP genotypes not normally affected, including Prp genotype ARR/ARR.

DIFFERENTIAL DIAGNOSIS

The characteristic signs of behavioral change, tremor, pruritus, and locomotor disorder occurring during a period of prolonged illness should suggest the possibility of this disease. The long incubation period, slow spread, and high case–fatality rate should also be considered when making a diagnosis. Diseases that may require differentiation include the following:

Diseases with signs of nervous dysfunction
- Louping-ill
- Pregnancy toxemia
- Rabies
- Pseudorabies
- Visna.

Skin diseases
- External parasites
- Wool loss

Treatment No treatment has proved capable of changing the course of the disease.

CONTROL

Individual Flocks

The maintenance of a closed ewe flock is critical to the control of this disease. If ewes need to be purchased from outside flocks, they should be from certified flocks or, better still, selected by PrP genotype testing for 171RR or 171QR genotype. The rams should be 171RR or 171QR genotypes. Ewes should be isolated at lambing and lambed individually with disposal of placenta by burning.

National Eradication

In countries that do not have the disease, and where it is inadvertently introduced with imported sheep, the approach is slaughter eradication of the infected flock and all in-contact animals. The aim is to eliminate the disease from the country, and the approach is usually successful because it has the full support of the sheep industry and the government.

Flock Eradication

The eradication of scrapie in countries where it is enzootic has less chance of success. Eradication programs vary and may involve the whole flock or just the family lines of the infected sheep. Programs in the United States since 1952 have varied from compulsory slaughter eradication of the affected flock and source flocks, to bloodline eradication, and finally from discontinuation to a voluntary certification scheme.

During this period there was no antemortem diagnostic test for scrapie and the identification of infected farms and flocks relied on owners submitting suspect or clinical cases for postmortem and histologic diagnosis. Owners are unlikely to put their flocks at risk if there is inadequate compensation for the results of their action, if they perceive that other flock owners are not cooperating with the control program, or if they question the validity of the eradication policy, which is attested to by the experience in the United States.

Iceland is currently attempting an eradication program that involves depopulation of infected farms and areas. The farms are left without sheep for a 2-year period during which there is extensive cleaning and disinfection of the farm area before repopulation with scrapie-free sheep. The program is a national thrust but very expensive. This approach has also been apparently successful in virtually eliminating, if not eradicating, the disease in Iceland. Norway is also attempting eradication in a similar manner. In both countries the disease was geographically clustered.

Genetic Control and National Programs

The occurrence of scrapie and the concern for BSE in sheep has led many countries to develop national breeding programs for the control of scrapie and potential BSE. Examples are the National Scrapie Plan in the UK and the National Scrapie Eradication Program in the U.S. National Scrapie Plan. The overall aim is to identify sheep genetically resistant to scrapie on the basis of their genotype (ARR) and to and breed them to create a national flock with scrapie resistance. Genetic testing will allow the selection of resistant sheep for breeding and the culling of susceptible sheep, particularly in breeds such as the Suffolk in which the genetics of susceptibility appear relatively simple.

The **UK** has a Voluntary **National Scrapie Flocks Scheme** and a National Scrapie Plan which, under EU regulations, become compulsory for flocks that have had a case of scrapie after July 2004. Under the Compulsory Scrapie Flocks Scheme farmers with confirmed scrapie cases on their farms will either have their sheep flocks genotype tested so that those animals more susceptible to disease can be identified and removed or the whole flock slaughtered and disposed of. All goats on affected holdings also will be slaughtered and disposed of. Testing of breeding rams will also become compulsory for all purebred flocks and any other flocks producing and selling homebred rams for breeding. All rams carrying VRQ PrP genotypes will be slaughtered or castrated. Allied to this will be a voluntary ewe-testing scheme.

A mathematical model of the program has examined the time that it would take to eliminate scrapie from the national flock. The results suggest eradication is feasible but the process could take decades and would be expensive. Surprisingly whole-flock culling was more efficient in terms of time to eradication than genetic typing and selective culling. Not surprising was the finding that the **most important factor** influencing the efficacy of control at the national level was the ability to identify affected flocks. It was suggested that investing money in obtaining better notifications and in conducting trace backs and active surveillance of animals slaughtered for human consumption and animals found dead on farms would be a good investment.

In the **United States**, all breeding sheep must be individually identified with a unique flock and individual number. The **Scrapie Flock Certification** program monitors flocks over time and assigns certified status to flocks with no evidence of scrapie. Although this program has strict requirements of identification and reporting, it is not based on genetic testing.

The **United States** also has a **USDA Genetics-Based Flock Cleanup and Monitoring Plan.** This program targets scrapie-infected and source flocks. The sheep in these flocks are genotyped, sheep with susceptible genotypes are removed (as are all goats), and the flock is placed under surveillance for 5 years. Flocks that are exposed to scrapie are placed on a monitoring program, and if scrapie is detected the genetics-based cleanup program would begin.

There is concern that breeding for the selection for certain PrP genotypes and reduction or elimination of other PrP genotypes could affect other **desirable genetic characteristics** and reduce the overall "genetic pool." This will need to be determined for individual breeds, but preliminary analyses that have involved several breeds suggest that reproductive traits, muscle mass, wool quality, live weight gain, and carcass characteristics are not affected, at least in some breeds.

There has also been concern that **rare breeds** could be threatened in the face of an occurrence of scrapie and subsequent disposition of the flock based on the PrP genotype. Interestingly, there is a good representation of ARR and some breeds have very high frequencies.

FURTHER READING

Bulgin MS, Melson SS. What veterinary practitioners should know about scrapie. *J Am Vet Med Assoc.* 2007;230:1158-1164.

Fast C, Groschup MH. Classical and atypical scrapie in sheep and goats. In: *Prions and Diseases.* Vol. 2. New York: Springer; 2013.

Hunter N. Scrapie—uncertainties, biology and molecular approaches. *Biochim Biophys Acta.* 2007;1772:619-628.

Prusiner SB. Molecular biology of prion diseases. *Science.* 1991;252:1515-1522.

REFERENCES

1. Simmons HA, et al. *BMC Vet Res.* 2009;5:8.
2. Benestad SL, et al. *Vet Res.* 2008;39:19.
3. Kittelberger R, et al. *J Vet Diagn Invest.* 2010;22:863.
4. Fediaevsky A, et al. *BMC Vet Res.* 2008;4:19.
5. Vascellari M, et al. *J Virol.* 2007;81:4872.
6. Konold T, et al. *BMC Vet Res.* 2008;4:14.
7. Konold T, et al. *BMC Vet Res.* 2013;9:99.
8. Maddison BC, et al. *J Infect Dis.* 2010;201:1672.
9. Georgsson G, et al. *J Gen Virol.* 2006;87:3737.
10. Seidel B, et al. *PLoS ONE.* 2007;2:e435.
11. Lühken G, et al. *Vet Res.* 2007;38:65.
12. Andréoletti O, et al. *PLoS Pathog.* 2011;7:e1001285.
13. Saunders GC, et al. *J Gen Virol.* 2006;87:3141.
14. Corbiére F, et al. *J Gen Virol.* 2013;94:241.
15. Jeffrey M, et al. *J Pathol.* 2006;209:4.
16. Konold T, Phelan L. *J Vis Exp.* 2014;83:e51101.
17. Konold T, Phelan L. *Vet Rec.* 2014;174:257.
18. Langeveld JPM, et al. *BMC Vet Res.* 2006;2:19.
19. Monleón E, et al. *Vet Microbiol.* 2011;147:237.
20. Batxelli-Molina I, et al. *BMC Vet Res.* 2010;6:49.

CHRONIC WASTING DISEASE

CWD has recently emerged, or been recognized, in the United States as a TSE of captive and free-ranging cervids. The ability of this infection to transmit laterally between cervids, coupled with the longevity of the agent in the environment and the common grazing land of infected cervids and cattle and sheep, has resulted in concern that CWD in cervids might be a risk to livestock, and subsequently to humans, similar to BSE. There has also been concern that it might be transmitted directly from infected cervids to hunters dressing carcasses or consuming deer meat. There is no evidence for either of these risks.

The known natural hosts for CWD are mule deer (*O. hemionus*), white-tailed deer (*O. virginianus*), Rocky Mountain elk (*C. elaphus nelsoni*), and less frequently Shiras moose (*Alces alces shirasi*). CWD was originally recorded in the late 1960s as a chronic wasting syndrome of unknown etiology in captive mule deer in research facilities in Colorado and Wyoming. It was subsequently established that the disease was a TSE, and CWD has subsequently been found affecting cervids in captivity in several states in the United States and also in the provinces of Saskatchewan and Alberta, Canada. The occurrence in captive and farmed cervids in these different geographic areas is likely the result of transfer of animals between them, and the disease has recently been reported in Korea in cervids imported from North America. The disease continues to expand in prevalence and range in North America.

CWD has a focus and may have originated in free-ranging deer and elk in north central Colorado and southeastern Wyoming; however, in recent years it has been detected in free-ranging cervids east of the Mississippi and in a much broader area of North America. It is not certain whether this is caused by spread or because of improved surveillance. Based on comparisons of the CNS lesions and the glycoform patterns, the CWD agent is the same in captive and free-ranging deer.

There is strong evidence from outbreaks in captive deer that lateral transmission is of major importance in the transmission of CWD. The agent accumulates in gut-associated lymphoid tissues early in the infection, and saliva and feces are the likely source of horizontal infection with contamination of the environment.

The disease can be transmitted experimentally between cervids, and there is evidence for genetic susceptibility. The prion associated with CWD is not the same as that associated with BSE. In a recent study, it was shown that infection, with amplification of prion protein in brain tissue, can be transmitted to cattle by intracerebral inoculation of CWD-infected deer brain. Six years following challenge less than 50% of the challenged cattle showed amplification of the infection and none had histologic evidence of spongiform encephalopathy. It was concluded that if infection via the oral route did occur in cattle it would be unlikely that it would result in amplification of the abnormal prion within the life span of cattle.

Clinically the disease in cervids is manifested initially by changes in behavior not commonly observed in free-ranging cervids, and the major manifestation is a marked fall in body condition. In the terminal stages, there may be ataxia and excitability. The clinical course varies from a few days to a year but averages 4 months. Diagnosis is by histologic examination of the brain or more commonly by the demonstration of PrP^{CWD} in brain tissue by IHC. Antemortem biopsy of lymphatic tissue in tonsils and retropharyngeal lymph nodes as well as rectal biopsy have all been proven to be useful in diagnosing preclinical and subclinically infected animals, with diagnostic performance approaching testing brain tissue. Because prions in cervids with CWD are heavily shed in saliva and ocular secretions, diagnostic tests are currently under development using these fluids.

Control of CWD appears to be unsuccessful because of its horizontal transmission, as well as occurrence in wildlife that migrate over large distances and that are naturally shy. Eradication appears very unlikely.

FURTHER READING

Gilch S, Chitoor N, Taguchi Y, et al. Chronic wasting disease. *Top Curr Chem*. 2011;305:51-78.

Sigurdson CJ. A prion disease of cervids: chronic wasting disease. *Vet Res*. 2008;39:41.

Parasitic Disease Primarily Affecting the Cerebrum

COENUROSIS (GID, STURDY)

Coenurosis is the disease caused by invasion of the brain and spinal cord by the intermediate stage of *Taenia multiceps*. The syndrome produced is one of localized, space-occupying lesions of the CNS. In most countries the disease is much less common than it used to be and relatively few losses occur.

ETIOLOGY

The disease is associated with *Coenurus cerebralis*, the intermediate stage of the tapeworm *T. multiceps*, which inhabits the intestine of dogs and wild Canidae. The embryos, which hatch from eggs ingested in feed contaminated by the feces of infested dogs, hatch in the intestine and pass into the bloodstream. Only those embryos that lodge in the brain or spinal cord survive and continue to grow to the coenurid stage. *C. cerebralis* can mature in the brain and spinal cords of sheep, goats, cattle, horses, and wild ruminants, and occasionally humans, but clinical coenurosis is primarily a disease of sheep and occasionally goats[1] and cattle.[2] Infection in newborn calves, acquired prenatally, has occasionally been observed.

PATHOGENESIS

The early stages of migration through nervous tissue usually passes unnoticed, but in heavy infections an encephalitis may be produced. Most signs are caused by the mature coenurus, which may take 6 to 8 months to develop to its full size of about 5 cm. The cystlike coenurus develops gradually and causes pressure on nervous tissue, resulting in its irritation and eventual destruction. It may cause sufficient pressure to rarefy and soften cranial bones, leading to a larger volume of calvarium, compared with uninfected controls.[3]

CLINICAL FINDINGS

In acute outbreaks caused by migration of larval stages, sheep show varying degrees of blindness, ataxia, muscle tremors, nystagmus, excitability, and collapse. Sheep affected with the mature *Coenurus* show an acute onset of irritation phenomena including a wild expression, salivation, frenzied running, and convulsions. Deviation of the eyes and head may also occur. Some animals may die in this stage, but a large number proceed to the second stage of loss of function phenomena, the only stage in most affected animals. The most obvious sign is slowly developing partial or complete blindness in one eye. Dullness, clumsiness, head-pressing, ataxia, incomplete mastication, and periodic epileptiform convulsions are the usual signs. Papilledema may be present. Localizing signs comprise chiefly deviation of the head and circling; there is rotation of the head with the blind eye down, and deviation of the head with circling in the direction of the blind eye.

In young animals local softening of the cranium may occur over a superficial cyst and rupture of the cyst to the exterior may follow, with final recovery. When the spinal cord is involved, there is a gradual development of paresis and eventually inability to rise. Death usually occurs after a long course of several months.

CLINICAL PATHOLOGY

Clinicopathologic examinations are not generally used in diagnosis in animals, and serologic tests are not sufficiently specific to be of value. Radiologic examinations are helpful in defining the location of the cyst, especially if there is a prospect of surgical intervention. MRI provides more detailed information regarding cyst size and location.[3]

NECROPSY FINDINGS

Thin-walled cysts may be present anywhere in the brain but are most commonly found on the external surface of the cerebral hemispheres. In the spinal cord the lesions are most common in the lumbar region but can be present in the cervical area. Local pressure atrophy of nervous tissue is apparent, and softening of the overlying bone may occur.

DIFFERENTIAL DIAGNOSIS

The condition needs to be differentiated from other local space-occupying lesions of the

Continued

cranial cavity and spinal cord, including abscess, tumor, and hemorrhage. In the early stages the disease may be confused with encephalitis because of the signs of brain irritation. Clinically there is little difference between them and, while clinical signs and local knowledge may lead to a presumptive diagnosis, demonstration of the metacestode is essential.

TREATMENT AND CONTROL

Surgical drainage of the cyst may make it possible to fatten the animal for slaughter, and surgical removal with complete recovery is possible in a majority of cases. The life cycle can be broken most satisfactorily by control of mature tapeworm infestation in dogs. Periodic treatment of all farm dogs with a tenicide is essential for control of this and other more pathogenic tapeworms. Carcasses of livestock infested with the intermediate stages should not be available to dogs.

Anthelmintic agents appear to have efficacy in treating coenurosis in naturally infected sheep, as demonstrated by degeneration of the cysts in treated animals.[4] Best results were obtained with oral albendazole (25 mg/kg), or combined oral fenbendazole (500 mg) and oral praziquantel (500 mg) The clinical effect of such treatment is undetermined.

REFERENCES

1. Nourani H, Kheirabadi KP. *Comp Clin Pathol.* 2009;18:85.
2. Giadinis ND, et al. *Vet Rec.* 2009;164:505.
3. Manunta ML, et al. *Am J Vet Res.* 2012;73:1913.
4. Ghazaei C. *Small Rumin Res.* 2007;71:48.

HALICEPHALOBUS

H. gingivalis (*H. deletrix; Micronema deletrix*) is a small nematode that has been found in horses on rare occasions. Like *Pelodera*, it is a free-living saprophytic organism that has the ability to become an opportunistic parasite. *H. gingivalis,* however, invades the deeper tissues where it reproduces. Enormous numbers may be seen in granulomatous lesions that grow to several centimeters in diameter. Lesions may be found near the eye, in the prepuce, nares, or the maxilla. The latter may be sufficiently large to cause the hard palate to bulge, displacing the molars and causing difficulty in mastication.[1] Putative hematogenous spread gives rise to similar lesions in the kidney,[2] which may be misdiagnosed as renal neoplasia. The worm also invades the brain,[3-5] spinal cord, and heart,[6] but here the lesions are usually microscopic and consist of discrete granulomata with a vascular orientation. In the brain lesions are predominantly in the cerebrum with numerous intralesional worms.[5] Affected horses may show a wide variety of clinical signs including lethargy, ataxia, and incoordination leading to recumbency and death.[1,6] Diagnosis of superficial lesions is by demonstration of worms and larvae in biopsy samples, but more often *H. gingivalis* infection is identified retrospectively in histologic sections following necropsy.[7] The worms are 250 to 430 μm long, have a characteristic bilobed pharynx, and often contain a single large egg. PCR and sequencing have been used to identify *H. gingivalis* definitively.[3] This infection must be considered in the differential diagnosis of equine cerebrospinal nematodosis.[3,4] Treatment with ivermectin at the maximum safe dose has been attempted, although the susceptibility of the worm to this compound is uncertain.[1] Experimental tests have indicated that *H. gingivalis* adult worms and larvae have remarkable tolerance to ivermectin.[8]

REFERENCES

1. Henneke C, et al. *Acta Vet Scand.* 2014;2:22.
2. Henneke C, et al. *Dansk Vettisskr.* 2014;56:56.
3. Akagami M, et al. *J Vet Med Sci.* 2007;69:1187.
4. Hermosilla C, et al. *Equine Vet J.* 2011;43:759.
5. Jung JY, et al. *Vet Med Sci.* 2014;76:281.
6. Adedeji AO, et al. *Vet Clin Pathol.* 2015;44:171.
7. Sant'Ana FJF, et al. *Bra J Vet Res Anim Sci.* 2012;5:12.
8. Fonderie P, et al. *Parasitology.* 2012;139:1301.

Metabolic Diseases Primarily Affecting the Cerebrum

POLIOENCEPHALOMALACIA (CEREBROCORTICAL NECROSIS) OF RUMINANTS

SYNOPSIS

Etiology Several different causes including thiamine inadequacy, sulfate toxicity.

Epidemiology Sporadic disease in young well-nourished ruminants on high-level grain diets and not synthesizing sufficient thiamine. Ingestion of preformed thiaminase in certain plants or production by ruminal microbes may also cause destruction of thiamine. May also occur in cattle and sheep of all ages ingesting excess amounts of sulfates in feed and water.

Signs Sudden blindness, ataxia, staggering, head-pressing, tremors of head and neck, ear-twitching, champing fits, clonic-tonic convulsions, recumbency, opisthotonus, rumen contractions normal initially, pupils usually normal and responsive, nystagmus, death may occur in 24–48 hours. Hydrogen sulfide odor of ruminal gas in sulfate toxicity.

Clinical pathology Erythrocyte transketolase activity decreased and thiamine pyrophosphate effect increased but both measurements difficult to interpret; blood thiamine concentrations decreased but are not reliable in thiamine inadequacy form. Increased hydrogen sulfide content in rumen gas and increased thiosulfate concentration in urine in sulfur-induced form.

Lesions Diffuse cerebral edema, flattened dorsal gyri, coning of cerebellum, multifocal to linear areas of fluorescence in gray and white matter borders of cortical gyri and sulci.

Diagnostic confirmation Fluorescence of gray and white matter of cortical gyri and sulci of brain.

Differential diagnosis list

Cattle
- Lead poisoning
- Hypovitaminosis A
- Sodium chloride toxicity
- *Histophilus somni* meningoencephalitis

Sheep
- Pregnancy toxemia
- *Clostridium perfringens* type D enterotoxemia
- Focal symmetric encephalomalacia
- Lead poisoning.

Goats
- Pregnancy toxemia
- *C. perfringens* type D enterotoxemia
- Closantel overdosage[1]
- Lead poisoning

Treatment Thiamine hydrochloride parenterally.

Control Thiamine supplementation of diet. Avoid excess feeding or access to sulfate in feed and water supplies.

ETIOLOGY

Historically, PEM was considered to be caused by a thiamine inadequacy. It is important to realize that PEM is a histologic description of a cerebral injury affecting predominantly the gray matter, and that there are several different causes of PEM in ruminants. The current preference is to discuss PEM in relationship to a suspected etiology.

Thiamine Inadequacy

Thiamine (vitamin B_1) is synthesized only in bacteria, fungi, and plants but is an essential nutrient for animals. Consequently, animals must obtain thiamine from their diet. The evidence that a thiamine inadequacy can be associated with the disease includes the following:

- Affected animals respond to the parenteral administration of thiamine if given within a few hours after the onset of clinical signs
- Affected animals have biochemical findings consistent with thiamine pyrophosphate ([TPP], also known as TDP) inadequacy (TPP is the biologically active form of thiamine)
- The clinical signs and pathologic lesions can be reproduced in sheep and cattle by the administration of large daily

doses of pyrimidine containing structural analogs of thiamine, principally amprolium, given orally or intraperitoneally.

Excess Dietary Sulfur

Elemental sulfur in the rumen is metabolized by two pathways: (1) reduction of sulfate (SO_4^{2-}) to sulfide (S^{2-}), which is then incorporated into sulfur-containing compounds such as cysteine and methionine that are used by rumen bacteria and (2) reduction of sulfate to sulfide, which is converted to hydrosulfide (HS^-) at normal rumen pH (pKa of $S^{2-} + H^+ \leftrightarrow HS^-$ is 11.96). Hydrosulfide is in equilibrium with hydrogen sulfide in the rumen because the pKa for the equilibrium reaction: $HS^- + H^+ \leftrightarrow H_2S$ is 7.04).[2] The practical significance of these equilibrium reactions is that sulfate metabolism results in higher levels of H_2S in rumen gas (and H_2S is assumed to be the toxic agent) at lower rumen values for pH. These equilibria reactions help to explain the association between high sulfate intakes, high-grain diets, and increased risk of sulfur-associated PEM. The ingestion of excessive quantities of sulfur from the diet and water supply can cause the disease in cattle and sheep without any change in the thiamine status of the tissues. An increased dietary sulfur intake may increase the metabolic demand for thiamine, possibly to offset the damaging effect of hydrogen sulfide on brain tissue.[3]

EPIDEMIOLOGY

Occurrence

PEM occurs sporadically in young cattle, sheep, goats, and other ruminants. In North America, UK, Australia, and New Zealand, the disease is most common in cattle and sheep that are being fed concentrate rations under intensified conditions such as in feedlots. An inadequate amount of roughage can result in a net decrease in the synthesis of thiamine. The disease is most common in well-nourished thrifty cattle 6 to 18 months of age (peak incidence 9–12 months of age) that have been in the feedlot for several weeks. Feedlot lambs may also be affected only after being on feed for several weeks. The disease also occurs in goats and in antelope and whitetail deer. It may affect goats from 2 months to 3 years of age and is commonly associated with milk-replacer diets in kids or concentrate feeding in older goats. The disease occurs only rarely in adult cattle, which may be a reflection of the greater quantities of roughage they usually consume. However, there are recent reports of the disease occurring in adult cows on pasture with access to drinking water containing excessive concentrations of sulfates.

Morbidity and Case Fatality

Accurate morbidity and case–fatality data are not available, but outbreaks can occur suddenly in which up to 25% of groups of feeder cattle may be affected, with case-fatality rates from 25% to 50%. Case–fatality rates are higher in young cattle (6–9 months) than in the older age group (12–18 months), and mortality increases if treatment with thiamine is delayed for more than a few hours after the onset of signs. In feedlot lambs, it has been suggested that approximately 19% of all deaths are caused by PEM.

Risk Factors

When PEM was first described in 1956, and for about 30 years, it was considered to be a thiamine deficiency conditioned by dietary factors such as high-level grain feeding and inadequate roughage. PEM was most common in well-nourished young cattle from 6 to 12 months of age that were being fed high-level grain rations. The scientific investigations centered on the effects of dietary factors, such as grain diets, and the presence of thiaminases in certain diets on thiamine metabolism in the rumen. In recent years, it has become clear that the disease is not etiologically specific because many different dietary factors have been associated with the occurrence of the disease, and in some instances the thiamine status of the affected animals is within the normal range. Notable examples are the recent observations linking dietary sulfate with the occurrence of the disease.

Dietary Risk Factors

Although there has been general agreement that thiamine inadequacy is associated with the cause of PEM, the possible mechanisms by which this occurs are uncertain. Thiamine inadequacy in ruminants could, theoretically, occur in any of the following situations in which inadequate net microbial synthesis of thiamine in the rumen may occur:

- Concentrate-fed animals receiving inadequate roughage
- Impaired absorption and/or phosphorylation of thiamine
- Presence of a thiamine inhibitor in the tissues of the host
- Lack of sufficient or appropriate apoenzyme or coenzyme-apoenzyme binding for thiamine-dependent systems
- Increased metabolic demands for thiamine in the absence of increased supply
- Increased rate of excretion of thiamine resulting in its net loss from the body

Thiamine can be destroyed by thiaminases of which significant amounts can be found in the rumen contents and feces of cattle and sheep affected with naturally occurring PEM.

Thiamine Inadequacy

In cattle under farm conditions, using erythrocyte transketolase activity as a measurement of thiamine status, up to 23% of cattle under 2 years of age and 5% over 2 years may be in a thiamine-low state. Newly weaned beef calves on a hay diet are not subject to a thiamine deficiency, but a low and variable proportion of young cattle on barley-based feedlot diets (1.7%) may have some evidence of thiamine deficiency based on a TPP activity effect in excess of 15%. The supplementation of the diet of feedlot steers on an all-concentrate barley-based diet with thiamine at 1.9 mg/kg dry matter resulted in an increase in average daily gain and final carcass weights. Thus some animals may be marginally deficient in thiamine, which may be associated with decreased performance in cattle fed all-concentrate diets. However, thiamine supplementation of cattle on all-concentrate diets does not consistently result in improved animal performance. The experimental disease can be produced in young lambs fed a thiamine-free milk diet, and it may be unnecessary to postulate that thiamine analogs produced in the rumen are essential components of the etiology.

Thiaminases

A major factor contributing to PEM in cattle and sheep is a progressive state of thiamine deficiency caused by the destruction of thiamine by bacterial thiaminases in the rumen and intestines. Certain species of thiaminase-producing bacteria have been found in the rumen and intestines of animals with PEM. *Bacillus thiaminolyticus* and *Clostridium sporogenes* produce thiaminase type I and *B. aneurinolyticus* produces thiaminase type II. Although there is good circumstantial evidence that the thiaminases from these bacteria are the real source of thiaminases associated with the disease, it is not entirely certain. The experimental oral inoculation of large numbers of thiaminase type I producing *C. sporogenes* in lambs did not result in the disease.

Certain species of fungi from moldy feed are also thiaminase producers, but the evidence that they destroy thiamine and are associated with PEM is contradictory and uncertain.

The factors that promote the colonization and growth of thiaminase-producing bacteria in the rumen are unknown. Attempts to establish the organism in the rumen of healthy calves or lambs have been unsuccessful. Thiaminases have also been found in the rumen contents and feces of normal animals, which may suggest the existence of a subclinical state of thiamine deficiency. Poor growth of unweaned and weaned lambs can be associated with a thiaminase-induced subclinical thiamine deficiency. Weekly testing of young lambs over a period of 10 weeks revealed that 90% of unthrifty lambs were excreting high levels of thiaminase in their feces; low levels of thiaminase activity were present in 20% of clinically normal animals, and there were significant differences in the mean erythrocyte transketolase activity of the unthrifty animals excreting thiaminase compared with the thiaminase-free normal animals.

Field and laboratory investigations have supported an association between inferior growth rate of weaner sheep in Australia and a thiaminase-induced thiamine deficiency. Thiaminase activity has been detected in the feces of lambs at 2 to 5 days of age, with the levels increasing for 10 days and then declining over the next 3 to 4 weeks. Decreased erythrocyte transketolase activity indicated a thiamine insufficiency in lambs with high thiaminase activity, and mean growth rates were 17% less than lambs with low thiaminase activity. The oral supplementation with thiamine at 2 to 3 weeks of age was the most appropriate prevention and treatment for subclinical thiamine deficiency.

The parenteral or oral administration of thiamine to normal calves raised under farm conditions resulted in a marked reduction in the percentage TPP effect, which is an indirect measurement of thiamine inadequacy. Goats with PEM were found to have elevated ruminal and fecal thiaminase activities, low erythrocyte transketolase activity, elevated TPP effect, low liver and brain thiamine levels, and elevated plasma glucose levels compared with goats not affected with the disease. With the increased interest in goat farming, some breeders attempted to improve body condition of breeding stock for sale or show by feeding grain or concentrate, which creates a situation similar to feedlot rearing of sheep and cattle that is conducive to the establishment of thiaminases in the rumen and the occurrence of PEM.

High levels of thiaminase type I are present in the rhizomes of bracken fern (*Pteridium aquilinum*) and horsetail (*Equisetum arvense*). The feeding of the bracken fern rhizomes (*P. esculentum*) to sheep will cause acute thiamine deficiency and lesions similar to those of PEM, but neither of these plants is normally involved in the natural disease. The disease has occurred in sheep grazing the Nardoo fern (*Marsilea drummondii*) in flood-prone or low-lying wet areas in Australia. The fern contains a high level of thiaminase type I activity.

Amaranthus blitoides (prostrate pigweed) may contain high levels of thiaminase and be associated with PEM in sheep.

Sulfur-Induced Polioencephalomalacia

PEM has been associated with diets high in sulfur, particularly in the form of sulfate. A high concentrate of sulfates in the diet of cattle has been associated with episodes of the disease in 6- to 18-month-old cattle. Inorganic sulfate salts in the form of gypsum (calcium sulfate) added to feedlot rations to control the total daily intake of the diet may cause PEM. Seasonal outbreaks have occurred in feedlot beef cattle between 15 and 30 days after introduction to a **high-sulfur diet,** and the risk may increase when water is an important source of dietary sulfur, and during hot weather, when the ambient temperatures exceeded 32°C.

Initial outbreaks may follow the use of a **new well of water containing more sulfate** than water used previously from another well, increasing from a monthly incidence of 0.07% to 0.88%. Growing cattle consume 2.4 times more water when the temperature is 32°C than at 4°C; consequently total ingestion of sulfur by consumption of high-sulfate water increases during hot weather. The feed contained 2.4 g of SO_4/kg dry matter with a total sulfur content of 0.20%. Samples of drinking water contained between 2.2 and 2.8 g of SO_4/L. During hot weather daily sulfur ingestion from feed and water combined was estimated to be 64 g per animal corresponding to total dietary sulfur of approximately 0.67% of dry matter. Daily SO_4 ingestion was approximately 160 g per animal. The ruminal sulfide levels were much higher 3 weeks after entering the feedlot, when the incidence of the disease was greatest, than 2 months after entering the feedlot when the risk of the disease was low.

In western Canada, there is an association between PEM and high levels of sodium sulfate in water, and range cows are usually affected when certain waters become concentrated with this salt during the summer months. Water containing high levels of magnesium sulfate, often called ***gyp water*** (for gypsum water) is common in the western plains and intermountain areas of the United States and Canada. Ideally, water for livestock consumption should contain less than 500 ppm sulfate, and 1000 ppm is considered the maximum safe level in water for cattle exposed to moderate dietary sulfur levels or high environmental temperatures. A level of 2000 ppm of sulfate in drinking water is the taste discrimination threshold for cattle. Performance of feedlot cattle is reduced when offered water with sulfate levels of 2000 ppm or higher. The National Research Council states that the requirement of sulfur in feed to be 1500 to 2000 ppm for both growing and adult beef cattle; 4000 ppm is considered the maximum tolerated dose. Ruminant diets normally contain between 1500 to 2000 ppm (0.15%–0.20% sulfur).

Based on National Research Council guidelines, 30 g of sulfur is the calculated maximum tolerated dose of sulfur for a 650-lb (294-kg) steer consuming 16.25 lb (7.39 kg; 2.5% BW) of feed daily. If the ambient temperature reaches 32°C, a 650-lb steer can drink 14.5 gallons (53.9 L) of water daily, Consumption of 14.5 gallons of water containing 3000 ppm sulfate results in a daily intake of 55 g of sulfur. A feed intake of 2.5% BW would also consume 22.2 g of sulfur from feed containing 3000 ppm sulfur for a total daily intake of 77.2 g of sulfur from both feed and water, which is 2.5 times the maximum tolerated dose.

In some surveys, water supplies in western Canada contained 8447 ppm of total dissolved solids and 5203 ppm of sulfate. A survey of the sulfate concentrations in water on farms found that high levels of sulfate can have a detrimental effect on the thiamine status of the cattle on those farms. Cattle exposed to sulfate concentrations >1000 ppm had blood thiamine levels lower than those drinking water with low levels <200 ppm. This raises the possibility that a subpopulation of cattle under such circumstances could be marginally deficient in thiamine.

The total dietary intake of sulfur by cattle must be considered when investigating sulfur as a cause of PEM. In a study of one farm, water from a 6.1-m well containing 3875 mg/L of total dissolved solids with 3285 mg/L of sodium sulfate was associated with PEM in heifers 6 months of age. However, the water contributed about 20% of the total sulfur content in the diet of the heifers, and 60% of the dietary sulfur intake was supplied by the hay and 20% by the grain supplement. The hay contained 0.4% total sulfur, which is at the maximum tolerable level for cattle and at the upper limit for hay. The hay consisted of variable amounts of kochia (*Kochia scorpia*) and Canada thistle (*Cirsium arvense*). *K. scorpia* (summer cypress or Mexican fireweed) is high in sulfur content and has been associated with the disease in range cattle.

The levels of sulfate in water that have affected feed intake in cattle have varied from 2800 to 3340 mg sulfate/L, whereas other studies found no reduction in feed intake with levels up to 7000 mg/L. It appears that the different effects of sulfur toxicity for similar sulfur contents in saline water are attributed to the total sulfur intake. Outbreaks of the disease may occur in adult cattle on pasture drinking water containing 7200 ppm of sodium sulfate. Thus established guidelines for saline drinking water are not applicable when cattle are fed feeds grown in saline areas.

A combination of excessive intake of sulfur and a low dietary intake of trace minerals, especially copper, may affect the thiamine status of a cattle herd and contribute to PEM. Sulfur adversely affects both thiamine and copper status in sheep. A nutritionally related PEM has also been reproduced in calves fed a semipurified, low-roughage diet of variable copper and molybdenum concentrations and it was not related to copper deficiency. The disease has occurred in cattle in New Zealand fed chou moellier (*Brassica oleracea*), which contained sulfur concentrations of 8500 mg/kg dry matter. The morbidity was 25% and mortality 46% despite rapid conventional therapy. Sulfur-associated PEM has also occurred in Australia when cattle grazed extensive stands of *Sisymbrium irio* (London rocket), *Capsella bursapastoris* (shepherd's purse), and *Raphanus raphanistrum* (wild radish), which all contain high sulfur content and are in the Brassicaceae (Cruciferae) family.[4]

Ammonium sulfate used as a urinary acidifier in the rations of cattle and sheep has been associated with outbreaks of PEM. Morbidity rates ranged from 16% to 48% and mortality rates from 0% to 8%. Affected animals did not respond to treatment with thiamine.

Outbreaks have occurred in sheep exposed to an alfalfa field previously sprayed with 35% **suspension of elemental sulfur**. The disease can be induced experimentally in lambs by the administration of sodium hydrosulfide into the esophagus and has occurred in lambs 3 to 4 weeks after being fed a concentrate ration containing 0.43% sulfur. Feeding experimental diets containing inorganic sulfur to young lambs was associated with PEM, and supplementation of those diets with thiamine decreased the severity of the lesions. Rumen microbes are able to reduce sulfate to sulfides, which may be directly toxic to the nervous system. Feeding calves (115–180 kg) a semipurified diet high in readily fermentable carbohydrate, without long fiber, and with added sodium sulfate for a total sulfur content of 0.36% resulted in PEM within 21 days of the introduction of the experimental diet. An odor of hydrogen sulfide was frequently detected on passage of a stomach tube into the rumen of all calves during the experiment. The total thiamine concentrations in affected and control calves remained within normal limits.

The dietary content of copper, zinc, iron, and molybdenum may also have important modifying influences on sulfur toxicosis. Molybdenum and copper can combine with sulfur to form insoluble copper thiomolybdate. Copper, zinc, and iron form insoluble salts with sulfide, and their expected effect would be to decrease the bioavailability of sulfide in the rumen. Conversely, low, but not necessarily deficient, dietary contents of these divalent metals could be prerequisites for excess absorption of sulfide to occur. PEM is not associated with copper deficiency, but copper and sulfur metabolism are interdependent. An excess of dietary sulfur may result in depression of serum copper, or alternatively, low serum copper may potentiate the actions of toxic levels of sulfur. Chronic copper poisoning in a lamb has been associated with PEM. It is suggested that the copper toxicity may have caused decreased hepatic function resulting in increased plasma concentration of sulfur containing amino acids which, may have predisposed to sulfur toxicity encephalomalacia.

Major dietary sulfur sources are inorganic salts that are fed in acidogenic diets to control periparturient hypocalcemia in dairy cattle, the by-products of grain processing, such as distillers grains, corn gluten meal, and brewers grain, and molasses, beet pulp, and alfalfa hay. Prolonged feeding of barley malt sprouts to cattle in Turkey has resulted in PEM caused by the high sulfur content of barley sprouts.[5] Similarly, molasses toxicity occurred in Cuba in cattle fed on a liquid molasses-urea feeding system with limited forage. The clinical and necropsy findings were identical to PEM; however, molasses toxicity is not thiamine responsive and can be reversed by feeding forage.

Other Dietary Circumstances

Deprivation of Feed and Water. In some outbreaks there is a history of deprivation of feed and water for 24 to 28 hours, because of either a managerial error or frozen water supplies. In other cases, a rapid change in diet appears to precipitate an outbreak. Some outbreaks are associated with a temporary deprivation of water for 24 to 36 hours, followed by sudden access to water and an excessive supply of salt, a situation analogous to salt poisoning in pigs, but these require more documentation to ensure that they indeed are not salt poisoning.

In sheep flocks, a drastic change in management, such as occurs at shearing time, will precipitate outbreaks in which only the yearlings are affected. Changing the diet of sheep from hay to corn silage resulted in a decrease in thiamine concentrations in ruminal fluid to about 25% of control values on hay. The cause of the drop in thiamine concentrations is unknown.

***Phalaris Aquatica* "PEM-Like" Sudden Death in Sheep and Cattle.** The Mediterranean perennial grass *P. aquatica* (formerly *P. tuberosa*) can cause sudden death in sheep and cattle throughout southern Australia. The nervous form of the disease is similar clinically to PEM but atypical because of the very rapid onset and the absence of either neuronal necrosis or malacia in cerebral cortical sections from affected animals. The available evidence suggests that this form of phalaris sudden death is more likely to involve a peracute form of ammonia toxicity than a peracute form of PEM.

PATHOGENESIS

Thiamine Inadequacy Polioencephalomalacia

High levels of thiaminases are formed in the rumen, which destroy thiamine that is naturally synthesized. The circumstances in the diet or in the rumen that allow for the development of high levels of thiaminases are unknown but may be related to the nature of the ruminal microflora in young cattle and sheep fed concentrate rations, which results in the development of ruminal acidosis. These rations may also allow for the development and growth of thiaminase-producing bacteria which, combined with a smaller net synthesis of thiamine in the rumens of concentrate-fed ruminants, could explain the higher incidence in feedlot animals. Experimentally PEM has been produced in lambs by continuous intraruminal infusion of a highly fermentable diet. Animals changed very rapidly to high-concentrate rations develop increased ruminal thiaminase levels.

The possibility that intraruminal thiaminases may also create thiamine analogs capable of acting as thiamine antimetabolites and accentuating the disease has been studied, but the results are inconclusive. The presence of naturally occurring second substrates (cosubstrates) in the rumen could produce, by the thiaminase type I reaction, a potent thiamine antimetabolite capable of accentuating the condition. In vitro studies have shown that thiaminase only caused rapid destruction of thiamine when a second substrate was added, and a large number of drugs commonly used as anthelmintics or tranquilizers may be active as second substrates. Many compounds found in the rumen of cattle are potential cosubstrates.

Amprolium has been used extensively to produce the lesions in the brains of cattle and sheep that are indistinguishable from the naturally occurring disease. However, because amprolium has been found in the brain tissue, the experimental disease should perhaps be known as "amprolium poisoning encephalopathy." The administration of other antagonists such as oxythiamine and pyrithiamine does not produce the disease. This suggests that PEM is a particular form of thiamine deficiency in which the supply of thiamine is reduced by the action of intraruminal thiaminase. Thus the thiamine status of the animal will be dependent on dietary thiamine intake, thiamine synthesis, the presence of thiaminase in the rumen, and the effects of possible antimetabolites. Subclinical states of thiamine deficiency probably exist in apparently normal cattle and sheep being fed diets that are conducive to the disease. This suggests that in outbreaks of the disease the unaffected animals of the group should be considered as potential new cases and perhaps treated prophylactically.

Thiamine is an essential component of several enzymes involved in intermediary metabolism and a state of deficiency results in increased blood concentration of pyruvate, a reduction in the lactate to pyruvate ratio and depression of erythrocyte transketolase. These abnormalities affect carbohydrate metabolism in general, but in view of the specific requirements of the cerebral cortex for oxidative metabolism of glucose, it is possible that a thiamine inadequacy could have a direct metabolic effect on neurons. The brain of the calf has a greater dependence on the pentose pathway for glucose metabolism, in which pathway the transketolase enzyme is a rate-limiting enzyme. Ultrastructural examination of the brain of sheep with the natural disease reveals that the first change that occurs is an edema of the intracellular compartment, principally involving the astrocytes and satellite cells. This is followed by neuronal degeneration, which is considered secondary. It has been suggested that the edema may be caused by a reduction in ATP production following a defect of carbohydrate metabolism in the astrocyte. There are three basic lesions that are not uniform: compact necrosis, edema necrosis, and edema alone. This may suggest that a uniform etiology such as thiamine deficiency cannot be fully supported.

In the cerebral cortex of affected animals, autofluorescent spots are observed under ultraviolet 365-nm illumination and are a useful diagnostic aid. The distribution of autofluorescence corresponds to that of mitochondria in cerebrocortical neurocytes in affected calves, suggesting that metabolic impairment occurs and the autofluorescent substance is produced in the mitochondria. Mitochondrial swelling and disorganization of cristae are also observable in brain tissue, but are not specific to PEM.

Sulfate-Induced Polioencephalomalacia

Diets high in sulfur result in hydrogen sulfide production in the rumen and anaerobic bacteria from rumen samples of cattle fed high-carbohydrate, short-fiber diets with added sulfate will generate hydrogen sulfide in rumen fluid broth medium. Rumen microflora adapt to higher dietary sulfate content over a period of 10 to 12 days before they are capable of generating potentially toxic concentrations of sulfide. In experimental sulfate diets, which induce PEM, the rumen pH decreases during the transition to the experimental diet and acidic conditions in the rumen favor increased rumen gas cap concentrations of hydrogen sulfide. With a change of pH from 6.8 to 5.2, the percentage of hydrogen sulfide in the rumen gas cap increased from 47% to 97%.

Hydrogen sulfide gas concentration gradually increases in the rumen of sheep during the first 4 weeks on ingesting a medium-concentrate corn and alfalfa-based diet that contained substantial amounts of distillers grains.[6] Hydrogen sulfide is thought to be detoxified by the liver via oxidation to sulfate. Hydrogen sulfide absorbed across the ruminal wall into the portal circulation is not considered a likely mechanism of toxicity because absorbed hydrogen sulfide will be detoxified. However, a portion of the eructated hydrogen sulfide can be absorbed across the alveolar membrane directly into pulmonary capillaries, effectively bypassing hepatic detoxification before reaching the brain. If ruminants inhale 60% of eructated gases, inhalation of hydrogen sulfide could be a route of systemic sulfide absorption, in addition to gastrointestinal absorption. Sulfide inhibits cellular respiration leading to hypoxia, which may be sufficient to create neuronal necrosis in PEM. The nervous system lesions of sulfur toxicosis are indistinguishable from lesions in the naturally occurring disease.

Acute Cerebral Edema and Laminar Necrosis

Acute cerebral edema and laminar necrosis occur and the clinical signs are usually referable to increased intracranial pressure from the edema and the widespread focal necrosis. Recovery can occur with early treatment, which suggests that the lesions are reversible up to a certain point. EEGs of buffalo calves with amprolium-induced PEM found decreased frequency patterns, occasional spindles, and decreased voltage patterns during the onset of clinical signs. In the comatose stage, there was little evidence of electrical activity. EEGs of animals treated with thiamine hydrochloride found normal awake patterns.

CLINICAL FINDINGS

Cattle

Animals may be found dead without premonitory signs, especially beef cattle on pasture. The clinical findings are variable but characteristically, there is a sudden onset of **blindness; walking aimlessly; ataxia; muscle tremors**, particularly of the head with ear-twitching; **champing of the jaws** and frothy salivation; and **head-pressing** (which is really compulsive forward walking stopped by a wall), and the animal is difficult to handle or move (Fig. 14-12). Dysphagia may be present when one attempts to force feed hay by hand. Grinding of the teeth is common. Initially, the involuntary movements may occur in episodes, and convulsions may occur, but within several hours they become continuous. The animal usually then becomes recumbent, and there is marked opisthotonus; nystagmus; clonic-tonic convulsions, particularly when the animal is handled or moved; and tetany of the forelimbs is common. The temperature is usually normal but elevated if there has been excessive muscular activity. The heart rate may be normal, subnormal, or increased and is probably not a reliable diagnostic aid.

Rumen movements remain normal for a few days, which is an important distinguishing feature from lead poisoning in which the rumen is static.

The **menace reflex is always absent** in the acute stage, and its slow return to normal following treatment is a good prognostic sign. The **palpebral eye-preservation reflex is usually normal**. The pupils are usually of normal size and responsive to light. In severe cases the pupils may be constricted. Dorsal strabismus caused by stretching of the trochlear nerve is common. Nystagmus is common and may be vertical or horizontal. Optic disc edema is present in some cases but is not a constant finding.

Calves 6 to 9 months of age may die in 24 to 48 hours, whereas older cattle up to 18 months of age may survive for several days. Recovery is more common in the older age group.

In less severe cases, affected animals are blind, head-press into walls and fences, and remain standing for several hours or a few days. In outbreaks, some cattle will be sternally recumbent; others remain standing with obvious blindness, whereas others are anorexic, mildly depressed, and have only partial impairment of eyesight. Those with

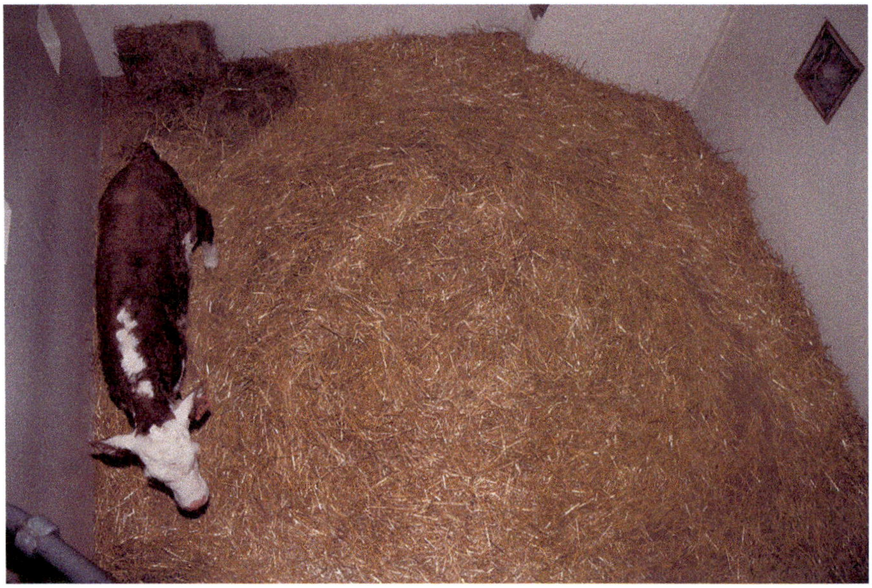

Fig. 14-12 Weaned Polled Hereford calf with polioencephalomalacia. The calf has been walking in the same direction in the stall for many hours (as indicated by the straw). The diameter of the circle is determined by the width of the stall. The calf was blind and depressed, but was neurologically normal 48 hours later after aggressive treatment with intramuscular thiamine.

some eyesight will commonly return to almost normal. Some survivors are permanently blind to varying degrees but may begin to eat and drink if assisted. Some cases will recover following treatment and may grow and develop normally.

Evidence of recovery within a few hours following treatment with thiamine indicates that the disease is associated with thiamine inadequacy. A failure of response indicates the possibility of sulfur toxicity PEM.

Sheep

Sheep usually begin to wander aimlessly, sometimes in circles, or stand motionless and are blind, but within a few hours they become recumbent with opisthotonus, extension of the limbs, hyperesthesia, nystagmus, and periodic tonic-clonic convulsions (Fig. 14-13). Hoggets affected at shearing time may show blindness and head-pressing but, if fed and watered, usually recover within a few days. Occasional animals show unilateral localizing signs, including circling and spasmodic deviation of the head. In goats, early signs may include excitability and elevation of the head. Blindness, extreme opisthotonus, and severe extensor rigidity and nystagmus are common.

In sulfur-induced PEM in sheep introduced to a diet containing 0.43% sulfur, clinical signs occurred 15 to 32 days later and consisted of depression, central blindness, and head-pressing, but no hyperesthesia, nystagmus, or opisthotonus were observed. In sulfur toxicity in lambs with PEM, the rumen contents may have a strong odor of hydrogen sulfide (rotten egg smell).

There are some reports from Australia of unthriftiness in unweaned and weaned lambs associated with thiamine deficiency caused by the presence of thiaminases in the alimentary tract. In affected flocks the incidence of ill-thrift in lambs is much higher than the usual incidence and other causes of unthriftiness were ruled out. Affected lambs lose weight, may have chronic diarrhea, and become emaciated and die of starvation. In some flocks, clinical signs of PEM may occur in a small percentage of animals. The disease is most common in early July, which is the coldest part of the year in Australia for lambs that are born in May and June. In affected lambs the fecal thiaminase levels are high and the blood transketolase level activity is increased above normal. Treatment of affected lambs with thiamine resulted in an increase in growth rate.

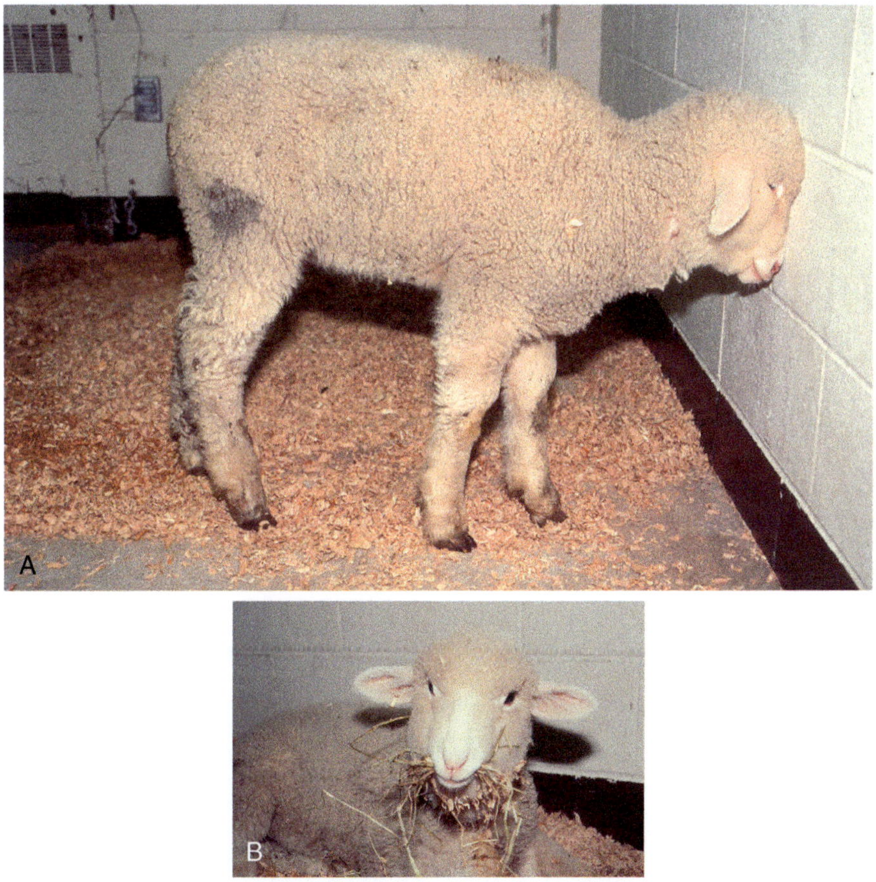

Fig. 14-13 A, Weanling sheep with acute polioencephalomalacia demonstrating slow progressive walking that is interrupted by a wall. This is mistakenly called head-pressing. B, The same weanling sheep 24 hours later after repeated intravenous thiamine injections. The sheep has stopped progressive walking and the appetite has partially returned; however, the sheep is not fully aware and could not identify that it was still eating. It made a full recovery.

CLINICAL PATHOLOGY

Thiamine Inadequacy Polioencephalomalacia. The biochemical changes occurring in cattle and sheep with the thiamine-deficiency PEM have not been well defined diagnostically based on thoroughly investigated naturally occurring clinical cases. However, some estimates are available including the changes that occur in the experimental disease. Interpretation of the values may also be unreliable if the animals have been treated before death. Because of challenges with the availability and cost of laboratory tests, the most practical method to confirm a diagnosis of PEM caused by thiamine inadequacy is the clinical response to treatment with thiamine.

In animals, thiamine is present as free thiamine, thiamine monophosphate (TMP), TDP (more commonly known as TPP, which is the biologically active form), and thiamine triphosphate (TTP). The role of TMP and TTP is not well known at this time. The critical forms to measure are therefore free thiamine and TPP.[3] The **thiamine concentrations** of blood of animals with PEM have varied widely and may be difficult to interpret because of the possibility of thiamine analogs inducing deficiency even when blood thiamine levels are normal. However, this would not apply when blood thiamine concentrations are below normal. A normal reference range of 75 to 185 nmol/L is suggested for both cattle and sheep, and levels below 50 nmol/L are considered indicative of deficiency. In normal goats, the mean thiamine content of blood was 108 nmol/L, with a range of 72 to 178 nmol/L. In goats with PEM, blood thiamine levels were less than 66 nmol/L with a mean of 29 nmol/L. Levels as low as 1.8 to 3.6 μg/dL (6–12 nmol/L) have been found in suspected cases of PEM. The thiamine concentrations of liver, heart, and brain of cattle and sheep with PEM are decreased. The levels of blood pyruvate and lactate are also increased and thiamine pyrophosphate–dependent enzymes such as pyruvate kinase are decreased. The thiaminase activity of the feces is increased. Laboratory reference ranges should be used to evaluate blood thiamine concentrations because of analytical differences related to whether the measurement relates to free thiamine, total thiamine, or TPP.

The **erythrocyte transketolase activity** is decreased in confirmed cases of thiamine-inadequacy PEM. Transketolase is an important enzyme in the pentose pathway and requires TPP. Measurement of transketolase activity in erythrocytes is attractive because a blood sample is readily obtained and this is a biologic assay. Unfortunately, the assay must be run soon after blood collection and is not widely available. Erythrocyte transketolase activities in normal sheep range from 40 to 60 IU/mL RBCs. A variant of the transketolase test involves the addition of a standard amount of TPP, with the percentage increase in erythrocyte transketolase activity being recorded; this is called the TPP effect. A TPP effect of 30% to 50% is commonly found in normal healthy cattle and sheep, and an increase to above 70% to 80% occurs in animals with PEM.

It is important to note that decreased erythrocyte transketolase activities, an increased TPP effect, and decreased blood thiamine concentrations would be expected in animals that have been inappetent for a number of days because thiamine is a water-soluble vitamin within minimal body stores. For example, cattle with pneumonia or simple indigestion had lower plasma thiamine concentrations (1.00 and 0.50 μg/mL, respectively) than healthy cattle (1.70 μg/mL).[7] Sheep with acute ruminal lactic acidosis had a mean TPP effect on erythrocyte transketolase activity of 109% compared with 22% in a health control group.[8] Measurements of erythrocyte transketolase activity, increased TPP effect, and blood TPP concentration should therefore be obtained from healthy animals in the same pen as the affected animal to adjust for the effect of feed intake on the measured values.

The **hemogram** is usually normal; the total and differential leukocyte counts may indicate a mild stress reaction, a finding that may be useful in differentiation from encephalopathies caused by bacterial infections.

CSF pressure taken at the cisterna magna is increased from a normal range of 12 to 16 cm H_2O to levels of 20 to 35 cm H_2O. The level of protein in the CSF may be normal to slightly or extremely elevated. A range from 15 to 540 mg/dL with a mean value of 90 mg/dL in affected cattle is recorded. There may also be a slight to severe pleocytosis in the CSF in which monocytes or phagocytes predominate.

Brain Imaging Function. MRI of a 2-month-old Holstein Friesian calf with thiamine-inadequacy PEM indicated a laminar hyperintense T2-weighted image of the cerebral cortex from the parietal to occipital lobes that predominantly affected the gray matter.[9] The visual evoked potentials are abnormal in ruminants with thiamine-responsive PEM.

Sulfate-Induced Polioencephalomalacia

Sulfur-induced PEM is most commonly differentiated from other causes of PEM in ruminants by the lack of responsiveness to thiamine injections and calculation of total sulfur intake from feed and water. Measurement of ruminal hydrogen sulfide content or urinary thiosulfate concentration offers promise as useful diagnostic tests.

Ruminal Hydrogen Sulfide Measurement. Changes in rumen gas cap H_2S concentrations are larger than changes in rumen fluid H_2S concentrations, and estimation of rumen gas H_2S concentration may be a practical method of detecting pathologic increases in ruminal hydrogen sulfide gas. A simple and rapid method has been developed for measuring the H_2S concentration of ruminal gas under field conditions, and an excellent description of the procedure is available.[2,6] In brief, the left paralumbar fossa is clipped and aseptically prepared. A sterile 7.6- to 10.2-cm 12- to 18-gauge needle with stylet is introduced into the gas cap of the rumen by way of the left paralumbar fossa. The needle is then connected to a calibrated H_2S detector tube. In cattle with sulfate-induced PEM increases in ruminal gas H_2S may be as high as 100 times more than control animals; however, ruminal pH has a marked effect on the measured value for H_2S,[2] suggesting that test interpretation needs to be adjusted for rumen pH to improve diagnostic accuracy. The hydrogen sulfide test is more accurate when applied to healthy animals in the same pen as an animal showing clinical signs of sulfate-induced PEM, because affected animals have a markedly reduced appetite and therefore lower sulfate intake and higher ruminal pH.

Urine thiosulfate concentrations appear to provide a useful diagnostic tool for sulfate-induced PEM in ruminants. Thiosulfate ($S_2O_3^{2-}$) is produced by incomplete oxidation of sulfide and by partial reduction of sulfate and therefore an increase in urine or plasma thiosulfate concentration reflects an increase in dietary sulfate intake or ruminal sulfide concentration. Thiosulfate concentrations in urine are stable for 8 hours at room temperature and 24 hours when stored at 4°C, and marked increases in urine thiosulfate concentrations occur when cattle are fed a high-sulfate diet, with the greatest increase occurring after feeding.[2] The urine thiosulfate concentration does not need to be normalized to urine creatinine concentration.

Brain Function. The effects of high dietary sulfur on brain function have been examined using evoked potentials techniques. Altered nerve conduction pathways occur in sheep fed high-sulfur diets without supplemental thiamine compared with animals that have received thiamine.

NECROPSY FINDINGS

Diffuse cerebral edema with compression and yellow discoloration of the dorsal cortical gyri is evident, and the cerebellum is pushed back into the foramen magnum with distortion of its posterior aspect.

In recovered animals, there is macroscopic decortication about the motor area and over the occipital lobes. The lesion can be identified grossly using ultraviolet illumination, which results in a fluorescence that indicates necrosis of brain and engulfment of necrotic tissue by lipophages. In general, there is a good correlation between the presence of characteristic fluorescence and the biochemical changes in cases of PEM. A small percentage of false negatives may occur.

Histologically, the lesions are widespread but most common in the cerebral cortex. There is bilateral laminar necrosis and necrosis of deeper cerebral areas. The necrosis is most prominent in the dorsal occipital and parietal cortex, but bilateral areas of necrosis are also seen less frequently in the thalamus, lateral geniculate bodies, basal ganglia, and mesencephalic nuclei. Lesions of the cerebellum are also present. The severity and distribution of the lesions probably depend on the interrelationships between clinical severity, age of affected animal, and length of illness before death.

Subnormal levels of thiamine are detectable in the liver and brain of calves with the natural disease, and low levels are also found in the experimental disease. In the molasses-induced disease in Cuba, the tissue thiamine levels were within the normal range.

In some cases of sulfur-associated PEM, the rumen contents have a strong odor of hydrogen sulfide (the rotten egg smell).

DIFFERENTIAL DIAGNOSIS

The biochemical tests described under the section Clinical Pathology are not practical. The diagnosis must be made on the basis of clinical findings and the readily available simple tests that rule out other diseases that resemble polioencephalomalacia. A careful consideration of the epidemiologic history often assists in the diagnosis.

Cattle

The differential clinical diagnosis for cattle is summarized in Table 14-12. Polioencephalomalacia in cattle occurs primarily in young growing animals 6–9 months of age on concentrate rations and is characterized clinically by a sudden onset of blindness, muscular tremors of the head and neck, head-pressing, nystagmus, and opisthotonus. The disease also occurs in mature beef cattle on pasture containing a high level of sulfate in their water and feed.

In cattle the disease must be differentiated from the following:

- **Acute lead poisoning,** which is most common in calves after spring turnout but occurs in adult cattle too and is characterized by central blindness, tremors, convulsions, uncontrollable activity with bellowing, champing fits, hyperexcitability, rumen stasis, and death in several hours. Early treatment may be successful.
- **Subacute lead poisoning** characterized by blindness, stupor, head-pressing, rumen stasis, weak palpebral reflexes, and no response to therapy.
- **Hypovitaminosis A** is characterized by a history of a vitamin A–deficient diet and nyctalopia, peripheral blindness, dilated and fixed pupils, optic disc edema, and transient convulsions followed by recovery.

- ***Histophilus somni* meningoencephalitis** characterized by sudden onset of ataxia, recumbency, fever, depression with eyes closed, lesions of the fundus, marked changes in hemogram, enlarged joints, and death in several hours if not treated early.

Sheep

In sheep polioencephalomalacia must be differentiated from the following:

- **Enterotoxemia (pulpy kidney disease) caused by *Clostridium perfringens* type D** in unvaccinated sheep, especially feedlot lambs, in which the clinical findings are almost identical; it occurs under the same management conditions as polioencephalomalacia. Enterotoxemia in lambs usually develops within several days after being placed on a grain ration, whereas polioencephalomalacia occurs after several weeks of grain feeding. Glycosuria in pulpy kidney disease may assist the diagnosis, but a necropsy is usually more informative
- **Focal symmetric encephalomalacia** also resembles polioencephalomalacia but is sporadic, usually involves only a few animals, and will not respond to treatment.

Goats

In goats the disease must be differentiated from enterotoxemia, pregnancy toxemia, lead poisoning, and meningoencephalitis.

TREATMENT

Thiamine Hydrochloride

The treatment of choice for thiamine-inadequacy PEM is thiamine hydrochloride at 10 mg/kg BW by slow intravenous injection initially and followed by similar doses every 3 hours for a total of five treatments. Bolus intravenous thiamine injections have been associated with collapse but are not usually fatal. Intramuscular injections of thiamine can be given instead of intravenous injections in animals that are difficult to handle with no discernable effect on treatment efficacy. When treatment is given within a few hours of the onset of signs, a beneficial response within 1 to 6 hours is common, and complete clinical recovery can occur in 24 hours. Goats and sheep will commonly respond within 1 to 2 hours. For those that take longer to recover, the eyesight and mental awareness will gradually improve in a few days and the animal will usually begin to eat and drink by the third day after treatment. Transfaunation of rumen fluid from roughage-fed cattle may improve appetite and rumen function in those responding slowly. In sheep, following treatment with thiamine, the blood transketolase activity begins to return to normal in 2 to 4 hours and is considered normal 24 hours after treatment.

Some cattle improve to a subnormal level within a few days and fail to continue to improve. These are usually affected with diffuse cortical and subcortical necrosis and will usually not improve further in spite of continued treatment. Those that return to a clinically normal state will usually do so by 48 hours or sooner after initial treatment. Those that are still clinically subnormal and anorexic by the end of the third day will usually remain at that level and should be slaughtered for salvage.

General treatment of cerebral edema (such as intravenous infusions of 20% mannitol at 0.25–1 g/kg BW or 7.2%–7.5% NaCl solution at 4–5 mL/kg BW, and parenteral dexamethasone (1 mg/kg BW, intravenous, see the section Increased Intracranial Pressure, Cerebral Edema, and Brain Swelling, earlier in this chapter) is theoretically indicated as part of the initial treatment of severely affected animals; however, clinical trials have not been conducted as to whether general treatment for cerebral edema provides a beneficial response above that provided by thiamine administration alone for ruminants with PEM caused by thiamine inadequacy. Both mannitol and dexamethasone are very expensive when administered to adult cattle, sheep, and goats.

Treatment is ineffective in advanced cases, but unless an accurate history is available on the length of the illness, it is usually difficult to predict the outcome until 6 to 12 hours following treatment. Thus it is usual practice to treat most cases with thiamine at least twice and monitor the response. If there is no beneficial response in 6 to 8 hours, emergency slaughter for salvage should be considered.

The oral administration of thiamine or thiamine derivatives is indicated when thiaminases are thought to be in the alimentary tract. Thiamine hydrochloride, at a rate of 1 g for lambs and kids and 5 g for calves in a drench, is recommended. However, because the action of thiaminase type I on thiamine may result in the production of thiamine analogs, which may act as inhibitors of thiamine metabolism, thiamine derivatives, which are resistant to thiaminases, lipid soluble and absorbed from the intestine, are being explored as therapeutic and prophylactic agents. Thiamine propyl disulfide can depress the thiaminase activities in the ruminal fluid of sheep with PEM within 2 hours after oral administration. The blood pyruvate levels and transketolase activities are also restored to normal and treated animals recovered clinically.

Outbreak Management

In outbreaks, the in-contact unaffected animals on the same diet as the affected animals may be on the brink of clinical disease. The diet should be changed to one containing at least 50% roughage or 1.5 kg of roughage per 100 kg BW. Thiamine may be added to the ration at the rate of 50 mg/kg of feed for 2 to 3 weeks as a preventive against clinical disease, followed by a level of 20 to 30 mg/kg of feed (cattle and sheep) if the animals remain on a diet that may predispose them to the disease.

Sulfur-Induced Polioencephalomalacia

There is no specific treatment for PEM caused by sulfate toxicity. The use of thiamine hydrochloride in doses given earlier is recommended, and may be successful in some cases, particularly when administered early in the disease course.

TREATMENT AND CONTROL

Treatment

Thiamine inadequacy form

Thiamine HCl (10 mg/kg BW by slow IV or IM every 3 hours for at least five treatments) (R-1)
- In severe acute cerebral edema
  - 20% mannitol IV (0.25–1.0 g/kg) or
    - 7.2%–7.5% NaCl IV (4–5 mL/kg) (R-2)
  - Dexamethasone (1 mg/kg, IV, once) (R-2)
- Rumen transfaunation if prolonged off feed (R-2)
- Oral drench with thiamine (1 g to lambs/kids, 5 g to calves) if thiaminases are suspected (R-2)

Sulfur-induced form

Thiamine HCl (10 mg/kg BW by slow IV or IM every 3 hours for at least five treatments) (R-2)

Treat suspected cerebral edema (R-2)

Control

Thiamine inadequacy form

Alter intraluminal environment by increasing roughage or changing source of roughage (R-2)

Supplement ration with thiamine at 3 mg/kg dry matter of feed (R-2)

Remove amprolium from diet (R-2)

Sulfur-induced form

Decrease overall sulfur intake in ration and water (R-1)

Restrict access to pastures with Brassicaceae family plants that have high sulfur content (R-1)

BW, body weight; IM, intramuscularly; IV, intravenously.

CONTROL

Thiamine Supplementation

A rational approach to the control of PEM associated with thiamine inadequacy is to supplement the rations of concentrate-fed cattle and sheep with thiamine on a continuous basis. The daily requirements for protection have not been determined using controlled feeding trials, but a rate of 3 mg/kg dry matter of feed for cattle and sheep has been recommended. This level may not be protective in all situations, and response trials may be necessary to determine protective levels for different situations. Levels up to 20 to 30 mg/kg of feed may be necessary for protection. Most natural feedstuffs for ruminants contain thiamine at about

2 mg/kg dry matter, which when combined with the thiamine synthesized in the rumen will meet the requirements. However, the presence of thiaminases in the rumen will necessitate dietary supplementation with thiamine, but the optimal amount that will provide protection under practical conditions is uncertain.

The intramuscular injection of 500 mg thiamine three times weekly into 6-month-old calves raised under practical farm conditions will steadily reduce the percentage TPP effect to zero in about 6 weeks. The daily oral administration of 100 mg thiamine to young calves fed initially on milk substitutes and then on concentrates and hay results in a decrease in percentage pyrophosphate effect.

For animals fed diets associated with thiamine inadequacy, it is recommended that thiamine be added to the diet at the rate of 5 to 10 mg/kg dry matter. Cattle and sheep on concentrate-fed rations must also receive supplements containing all necessary vitamins and minerals, especially cobalt, a deficiency of which may be associated with some outbreaks of the disease.

Feeding Roughage

The minimum amount of roughage, which should be fed to feedlot cattle and sheep to prevent the disease and still maintain them on high levels of concentrates is unknown. A level of 1.5 kg of roughage per 100 kg BW has been recommended, but this may not be economical for the feedlot whose profits are dependent on rapid growth in grain-fed cattle. Supplementation of the diet with thiamine appears to be the only alternative.

The prevention of the disease in sheep that are being moved long distances or gathered together for shearing and other management practices will depend on ensuring an ample supply of roughage and water and avoiding drastic changes in management.

Sulfate Toxicity PEM

The prevention of the disease associated with a high sulfur intake in the feed and water supplies will depend on analysis of the feed and water for sulfate and making appropriate adjustments in the sources of feed and water to decrease the intake of sulfur to safe levels.

FURTHER READING

Apley MD. Consideration of evidence for therapeutic interventions in bovine polioencephalomalacia. *Vet Clin North Am Food Anim Pract*. 2015;31:151-161.

Burgess BA. Polioencephalomalacia. *Large Animal Veterinary Rounds*. 2008;8:3.

Niles GA, Morgan SE, Edwards WC. The relationship between sulfur, thiamine and polioencephalomalacia—a review. *Bovine Pract*. 2002;36:93-99.

REFERENCES

1. Sakhaee E, Derakhshanfar A. *J S Afr Vet Assoc*. 2010;81:116.
2. Drewnoski ME, et al. *J Vet Diagn Invest*. 2012;24:702.
3. Amat S, et al. *Res Vet Sci*. 2013;95:1081.
4. McKenzie RA, et al. *Aust Vet J*. 2009;87:27.
5. Kul O, et al. *J Vet Med A Physiol Pathol Clin Med*. 2006;53:123.
6. Neville BW, et al. *J Anim Sci*. 2010;88:2444.
7. Irmak K, et al. *Kafkus Univ Vet Fak Derg*. 1998;4:63.
8. Karapinar T, et al. *J Vet Intern Med*. 2008;22:662.
9. Tsuka T, et al. *Vet Radiol Ultrasound*. 2008;49:149.

THIAMINE DEFICIENCY (HYPOTHIAMINOSIS)

The disease caused by deficiency of thiamine in tissues is characterized chiefly by signs of neurologic disease. PEM of ruminants is discussed in the previous section.

ETIOLOGY

Thiamine deficiency can be primary; caused by deficiency of the vitamin in the diet; or secondary, because of destruction of the vitamin in the diet by thiaminase. A primary deficiency is unlikely under natural conditions because most plants, especially seeds, yeast, and milk contain adequate amounts.

Thiamine is normally synthesized in adequate quantities in the rumen of cattle and sheep on a well-balanced roughage diet. The degree of synthesis is governed to some extent by the composition of the ration, a sufficiency of readily fermentable carbohydrate causing an increase of synthesis of most vitamins of the B complex, and a high intake in the diet reducing synthesis. The etiology of PEM has been discussed in detail previously. Microbial synthesis of thiamine also occurs in the alimentary tract of monogastric animals and in young calves and lambs, but not in sufficient quantities to avoid the necessity for a dietary supply, so that deficiency states can be readily induced in these animals with experimental diets. Thiamine is relatively unstable and easily destroyed by cooking.

The coccidiostat, amprolium, is a thiamine antagonist and others are produced by certain plants, bacteria, fungi, and fish.

EPIDEMIOLOGY

One of the best examples of secondary thiamine deficiency is inclusion of excess raw fish in the diet of carnivores, resulting in destruction of thiamine because of the high content of thiaminase in the fish.

Two major occurrences of secondary thiamine deficiency are recorded. In horses, the ingestion of excessive quantities of **bracken fern** (*P. aquilinum*) and **horsetail** (*E. arvense*) causes nervous signs because of the high concentration of thiaminase in these plants. The disease has been induced in a pig fed bracken rhizomes, and the possibility exists of it occurring under natural conditions. It also occurs in horses fed large quantities of turnips (*Beta vulgaris*) without adequate grain. The second important occurrence of thiamine deficiency is in the etiology of PEM and is discussed under that heading.

A thiaminase-induced subclinical thiamine deficiency causing suboptimal growth rate of weaner lambs has been described. Higher levels of thiaminase activity were present in the feces and rumen contents of lambs with poor growth rate compared with normal lambs. *B. thiaminolyticus* was isolated from the feces and ruminal fluids of affected lambs and supplementation of thiaminase-excreting lambs with intramuscular injections of thiamine hydrochloride was associated with significantly improved growth rate.

Thiamine deficiency occurs in sheep being subjected to live export from Australia to the Middle East. Sheep that died or were clinically ill and euthanized had significantly lower hepatic and ruminal thiaminase concentrations than clinically healthy control sheep. A high proportion had thiamine concentrations comparable with those found in sheep that die with PEM. The evidence indicates that the thiamine deficiency is a primary one associated with deprivation of feed during transportation to the preembarkation feedlots. The low feed intake and failure of the ruminal microbes to adapt, thrive, and synthesize a net surplus of thiamine during alterations in the ruminal environment are considered to be major contributing factors.

PATHOGENESIS

The only known function of thiamine is its activity as a cocarboxylase in the metabolism of fats, carbohydrates, and proteins and a deficiency of the vitamin leads to the accumulation of endogenous pyruvates. Although the brain is known to depend largely on carbohydrates as a source of energy, there is no obvious relationship between a deficiency of thiamine and the development of the nervous signs that characterize it. PEM has been produced experimentally in preruminant lambs on a thiamine-free diet. There are other prodromal indications of deficiency disease. For example, there is a decrease in erythrocyte precursors and in erythrocyte transketolase. Additional clinical signs are also in the circulatory and alimentary systems, but their pathogenesis cannot be clearly related to the known functions of thiamine. Subclinical thiamine deficiency caused by thiaminases in the alimentary tract is associated with low erythrocyte transketolase activities and elevated TPP effects, which may explain the poor growth rate.

CLINICAL FINDINGS

Bracken Fern (*P. aquilinum*) and Horsetail (*E. arvense*) Poisoning in the Horse

Incoordination and falling and bradycardia caused by cardiac irregularity are the cardinal clinical signs of bracken fern poisoning in the horse. These signs disappear after the parenteral administration of thiamine. Similar clinical effects occur with horsetail.

Swaying from side to side occurs first, followed by pronounced incoordination, including crossing of the forelegs and wide action in the hindlegs. When standing, the legs are placed well apart and crouching and arching of the back are evident. Muscle tremor develops and eventually the horse is unable to rise. Clonic convulsions and opisthotonus are the terminal stage. Appetite is good until late in the disease when somnolence prevents eating. Temperatures are normal and the heart rate slow until the terminal period, when both rise to above normal levels. Some evidence has also been presented relating the occurrence of hemiplegia of the vocal cords in horses with a below normal thiamine status. Neither plant is palatable to horses and poisoning rarely occurs at pasture. The greatest danger is when the immature plants are cut and preserved in meadow hay.

Experimental Syndromes

These syndromes have not been observed to occur naturally but are produced readily on experimental rations.

In **pigs**, inappetence; emaciation; leg weakness; and a fall in body temperature, respiratory rate, and heart rate occur. The ECG is abnormal and congestive heart failure follows. Death occurs in 5 weeks on a severely deficient diet. In calves, weakness, incoordination, convulsions, and retraction of the head occur, and in some cases there is anorexia, severe scouring, and dehydration.

Lambs 1 to 3 days old placed on a thiamine-deficient diet show signs after 3 weeks. Somnolence, anorexia, and loss of condition occur first, followed by tetanic convulsions.

Horses fed amprolium (400–800 mg/kg BW daily) developed clinical signs of thiamine deficiency after 37 to 58 days. Bradycardia with dropped heartbeats, ataxia, muscle fasciculation and periodic hypothermia of hooves, ears, and muzzle were the common signs, with blindness, diarrhea, and loss of BW occurring inconstantly.

CLINICAL PATHOLOGY

Blood pyruvic acid levels in horses are raised from normal levels of 2 to 3 μg/dL to 6 to 8 μg/dL. Blood thiamine levels are reduced from normal levels of 8 to 10 μg/dL to 2.5 to 3.0 μg/dL. ECGs show evidence of myocardial insufficiency. In pigs, blood pyruvate levels are elevated and there is a fall in blood transketolase activity. These changes occur very early in the disease. In sheep subjected to export, liver and rumen thiamine concentrations and erythrocyte transketolase activities were all below levels found in clinically normal sheep.

NECROPSY FINDINGS

No macroscopic lesions occur in thiamine deficiency other than nonspecific congestive heart failure in horses. The myocardial lesions are those of interstitial edema, and lesions are also present in the liver and intestine.

In the experimental syndrome in pigs, there are no degenerative lesions in the nervous system, but there is multiple focal necrosis of the atrial myocardium accompanied by macroscopic flabbiness and dilatation without hypertrophy of the heart.

DIFFERENTIAL DIAGNOSIS

Diagnosis of secondary thiamine deficiency in horses must be based on the signs of paralysis and known access to bracken fern or horsetail. A similar syndrome may occur with poisoning by the following:

- *Crotalaria* spp.
- Perennial ryegrass
- *Indigofera enneaphylla*
- Ragwort (*Senecio jacobaea*)

It is accompanied by hepatic necrosis and fibrosis. The encephalomyelitides are usually accompanied by signs of cerebral involvement, by fever, and by failure to respond to thiamine therapy.

TREATMENT

In clinical cases the injection of a solution of the vitamin produces dramatic results (5 mg/kg BW given every 3 hours). The initial dose is usually given intravenously followed by intramuscular injections for 2 to 4 days. An oral source of thiamine should be given daily for 10 days and any dietary abnormalities corrected.

CONTROL

The daily requirement of thiamine for monogastric animals is generally 30 to 60 μg/kg BW. The addition of yeast, cereals, grains, liver, and meat meal to the ration usually provides adequate thiamine.

THIAMINASE TOXICOSIS

SYNOPSIS

Etiology Thiaminases occur naturally in *Marsilea* spp., *Cheilanthes* spp., *Pteridium* spp., and *Equisetum* spp. ferns or fernlike plants.

Epidemiology Horses fed hay containing bracken; pigs eating bracken, especially rhizomes.

Clinical pathology Low blood concentrations of thiamine; high blood concentrations of pyruvate.

Lesions Similar to vitamin B_1 (thiamine) deficiency in horses; cardiac lesions in pigs.

Diagnostic confirmation. Low blood and urine levels of thiamine.

Treatment Injectable thiamine gives excellent results, provided thiamine source is withdrawn.

Control Limit access to plants.

ETIOLOGY

The identified thiaminases that are important to animals occur in ferns or fernlike plants and catalyze the decomposition of thiamine. Thiaminases are of two types, methyltransferase and hydrolase. The hydrolases are not found in plants but only in the rumen, presumably as metabolites produced by ruminal bacteria from specific precursors in the plants. The thiaminase content of the ferns varies widely, being highest at a period of rapid growth and after being grazed severely. Thiaminase activity occurs in the fronds of the ferns *M. drummondii, Cheilanthes sieberi,* and *P. aquilinum* in descending order of magnitude. Plants containing thiaminases are usually deficient in thiamine.

The ferns that are sources of thiaminase and the animal species affected are as follows:

- Horses: *Pteridium* spp. (bracken fern), *E. arvense* (horsetail), *E. fluviatile, E. hyemale, E. palustre, E. ramosissimum, E. sylvaticum, M. drummondii* (Nardoo)[1]
- Sheep: *M. drummondii, C. sieberi* (mulga or rock fern)[1]
- Cattle: *C. sieberi, Dryopteris borreri, D. filix-mas*

EPIDEMIOLOGY

Occurrence

Thiaminase poisoning associated with *Pteridium* spp. and *Equisetum* spp. occurs most often in horses fed hay contaminated by the ferns and is most toxic if the hay is cut when the fronds are very young. The standing plants are unpalatable and rarely eaten by these animals unless no other feed is available. In grazing horses ingesting 20% to 25% of their diet as thiaminase-containing plants, signs occur in 3 to 4 weeks; horses grazing on a pasture with thiaminase-containing plants providing close to 100% of their diet may show signs in as little as 10 days.[2,3] Stabled horses fed heavily contaminated hay may show signs in a short period of time, depending on how much thiaminase is present in the hay.

Thiaminase deficiency is less common in pigs and the clinical signs not as obvious.[3] Grazing pigs may root out and eat *Pteridium* rhizomes, which contain a much higher concentration of the thiaminase than the fronds. Sheep grazed on pastures dominated by *M. drummondii* on floodplains in inland Australia or forced to graze *C. sieberi* are poisoned.[1]

Grazing cattle may be forced to eat the ferns because of lack of other feed and when the fern is at a toxic, rapidly growing stage, but they are not affected by thiamine deficiency. They succumb to a hemorrhagic disease.[4]

PATHOGENESIS

A state of thiamine deficiency is created by the destruction of thiamine in the alimentary tract. The activities of enzymes that require thiamine, are impaired and there is an accumulation in tissues of pyruvate and lactate.[3] The relationship between the intake of the thiaminase and the nervous signs is not adequately explained. That a relationship exists is suggested by the development of brain lesions of PEM in sheep poisoned by *M. drummondii* and in those fed experimentally on the rhizomes of *P. aquilinum.*[3]

CLINICAL FINDINGS

Affected horses sway from side to side, show gait incoordination, including crossing the forelimbs and a wide action in the hindlimbs. Abnormal postures include a wide stance, arching of the back, and crouching. Muscle tremor, cardiac irregularity, and bradycardia are evident. Terminally, the animal falls easily, becomes recumbent and hyposensitive to external stimuli, and makes convulsive movements. The heart rate and the temperature become elevated. Additional signs seen in horses poisoned by *M. drummondii* include carrying the head close to the ground, whinnying, partial blindness, nodding of the head, twitching of the ears, and frequent yawning.

Pigs fed bracken fern rhizomes (33% of diet) developed anorexia and nonspecific signs. At 8 weeks they deteriorated rapidly and death occurred at 10 weeks.[3] Postmortem lesions were cardiac in nature. In another report, 4 of 22 piglets died when a pregnant sow was poisoned with bracken fern.[3]

Sheep poisoned by *M. drummondii* may be affected by an acute or a chronic syndrome. The acute form of the disease is characterized by the sudden onset of dyspnea, depression, and recumbency and death in 6 to 8 hours. The chronic syndrome is indistinguishable from PEM. Sheep affected by *Cheilanthes* spp. poisoning are hyposensitive to external stimuli, including being blind, and walk slowly and with an uncoordinated gait.

Cattle poisoned by *Dryopteris* spp. are also blind and hyposensitive. Many recover but remain blind.

CLINICAL PATHOLOGY

The characteristic findings attributable to a nutritional deficiency of thiamine are present. These include depression of blood levels of thiamine and transketolase and elevation of levels of blood pyruvate.

NECROPSY FINDINGS

In naturally occurring cases in horses, there are no lesions recorded other than the nonspecific ones of acute or congestive heart failure. PEM has been seen in sheep and, in pigs, an enlarged mottled heart and congestion of the lungs and liver indicate the presence of congestive heart failure.

Diagnostic confirmation is based on low blood thiamine levels.

DIFFERENTIAL DIAGNOSIS

Differential diagnosis list

- Hepatic encephalopathy
- Infectious encephalitides
- *Crotalaria* spp., *Senecio jacobea* toxicosis
- Staggers syndromes, e.g., ryegrass staggers, paspalum staggers, phalaris staggers

TREATMENT

In the early stages, the administration of thiamine and removal of the dietary source of thiaminase are the critical procedures and recovery is to be expected. In horses, an intravenous injection of 0.5 to 1 g of thiamine followed by intramuscular administration for 3 to 5 days is recommended.[2,5] The response to treatment is usually excellent.

CONTROL

Large-scale control is attempted by a combination of pasture management, application of herbicide, and mowing in early spring, but it is expensive and subject to error; thus professional agrochemical advice is desirable. Draining water from marshy areas and improving drainage will encourage grasses and legumes to compete with and outgrow these plants.

FURTHER READING

Radostits O, et al. Thiaminase poisoning. In: *Veterinary Medicine: A Textbook of the Disease of Cattle, Horses, Sheep, Goats and Pigs*. 10th ed. London: W.B. Saunders; 2007:1882.

REFERENCES

1. Finnie JW, et al. *Aust Vet J*. 2011;89:247.
2. Martinson K, et al. Horsetail and brackenfern. In: Martinson K, Hovda LR, Murphy M, eds. *Plants Poisonous or Harmful to Horses in North Central United States*. Minneapolis, MN: University of Minnesota Press; 2007:17.
3. Vetter J. *Acta Vet Hung*. 2009;18:183.
4. Plessers E, et al. *Vlaams Diergeneeskundig Tijdschr*. 2013;82:31.
5. Plumb DC. Thiamine HCl (Vitamin B1). In: Plumb DC, ed. *Veterinary Drug Handbook*. 7th ed. New York: Wiley and Sons; 2011:970.

SALT TOXICITY (SODIUM CHLORIDE TOXICOSIS)

SYNOPSIS

Etiology Ingestion of excessive amounts of sodium chloride or normal intake of sodium but limited water intake.

Epidemiology Multiple sources of excess salt in the diet and limitations of drinking water.

Clinical pathology High serum levels of sodium and chloride; increased plasma osmolarity; eosinopenia in pigs. High salt content in water or feed.

Lesions
Acute: gastroenteritis plus neurologic abnormalities.

Chronic: eosinophilic meningitis in pigs; polioencephalomalacia in pigs and cattle. High rumen, brain, and CSF levels of sodium.

Diagnostic confirmation Elevated sodium content of rumen and brain. CSF sodium exceeds serum sodium. Elevated sodium in aqueous or vitreous humor.

Treatment
Peracute with no signs: remove source of salt and allow free choice water; monitor closely.

Acute and chronic with signs: remove source of salt, restrict water intake, IV fluid replacement.

Control Limit intake of salt-rich water, whey, concentrate mixes; ensure adequate drinking water supply at all times.

CSF, *cerebrospinal fluid;* IV, *intravenous.*

ETIOLOGY

Sodium and chloride are the main ions responsible for maintaining osmotic balance in the ECF. Any alteration in serum concentrations, either through increased salt intake or decreased water consumption is likely to result in salt toxicity.[1,2]

Feed and water containing excessive quantities of salt are unpalatable to animals but excessive quantities of salt are sometimes ingested, especially in saline drinking waters. Specific details about the degree of salinity of drinking water compatible with health in animals are difficult to provide, because of the variation in the kinds of salts that occur in natural saline waters. Hypernatremia may also occur secondary to limited water intake such as occurs in cold environments when there is no access or water has frozen.

EPIDEMIOLOGY

Occurrence

Salt poisoning will occur wherever bore water is used for livestock drinking. It is reported principally from Australia, North America, and South Africa. Other sources of excessive salt include the following:

- Saline drinking water, especially after a change from fresh water, and especially if the animals are thirsty.[3]
- Water accumulating in salt troughs during drought periods.
- Grazing on salt marshes or drinking water obtained from salt marshes.[3]
- Swill fed to pigs containing excessive amounts of salt from bakery dough residues, butcher shop brine, cheese factory salt whey, or salted fish waste.
- Excessive sodium sulfate given to pigs as treatment for gut edema if the water intake is restricted.
- Oil field brine.[2]

Salt poisoning associated with water deprivation may occur from:

- Temporary restriction of the water supply to pigs of 8 to 12 weeks of age and lambs and calves fed prepared feeds containing the standard recommendation of 2% salt; poisoning occurs when the animals are again allowed access to unlimited water.
- Pigs brought into new pens where drinking water is supplied in automatic drinking cups that are not be accustomed to their use and fail to drink for several days until they learn to operate the cups.
- Feeder lambs and calves may also be deprived of water when their water troughs are frozen over.

Risk Factors

Animal Risk Factors

Swine are the most susceptible animals and have generated the most clinical reports of toxicity.[4] Sheep, beef cattle, and dry dairy cattle appear to be less susceptible than milking dairy cows, which are in turn less susceptible than horses. Heavy milking cows, especially those in the early stages of lactation, are highly susceptible to salt poisoning because of their unstable fluid and electrolyte status.

Many animals may be clinically affected and the mortality rate may be high when animals are kept under range conditions and have to depend on saline water supplies for drinking purposes. In animals kept under intensive conditions salt poisoning occurs only sporadically, but most affected animals die and heavy losses may occur in groups of pigs.

High salt intakes may be used in sheep to restrict food intake during drought periods and in the control of urolithiasis in feeder wethers, but salt poisoning does not occur if there is free access to water. Rations containing up to 13% of sodium chloride have been fed to ewes for long periods without apparent ill-effects, although diets containing 10% to 20% and water containing 1.5% to 2% sodium chloride do reduce food consumption. This may be of value when attempting to reduce feed intake but can be a disadvantage when sheep are watered on saline artesian water.

Toxic doses for acute sodium chloride poisoning in pigs, horses, and cattle are 2.2 g/kg BW and in sheep 6 g/kg. The toxicity of salt is significantly influenced by the age and BW of the subject. For example, dose rates that kill pigs of 6.5 to 10 kg BW have little effect on pigs of 16% to 20 kg BW. Water concentrations of 1000 mg Na/L water are associated with chronic problems in dairy cattle, including decreased production.[2]

Farm Risk Factors

Saline waters often contain a mixture of salts and those containing high levels of magnesium or fluorine may be quite toxic. Water containing 0.2% to 0.5% magnesium chloride may be associated with reduced appetite and occasional diarrhea in sheep, especially if the sodium chloride content is also high, but water containing similar quantities of sodium sulfate does not have any harmful effect. Variation between bore waters includes differences in the relative proportions of the acid radicals, particularly sulfates, carbonates, and chlorides.

Environmental Risk Factors

Environmental temperatures have an effect on toxicity, with signs occurring in the summer on water containing levels of salt that appear to be nontoxic in the winter. Australian recommendations are that the maximum concentration for sodium chloride or total salts in drinking water should not exceed 1.3% for sheep, 1% for cattle, and 0.9% for horses. South African and Canadian recommended levels are much lower, but there does not appear to be any proof that such low levels of total and individual salts are necessary.

PATHOGENESIS

Acute Poisoning

When excessive amounts of salt are ingested, gastroenteritis occurs because of the irritating effects from the high concentrations of salt. Dehydration and diarrhea result and are exacerbated by the increased osmotic pressure of the alimentary tract contents. Salt is absorbed from the gastrointestinal tract and may be associated with the involvement of the CNS.

Chronic Poisoning

Where the defect is one of decreased water but normal salt intake, there is an accumulation of sodium ions in tissues, including the brain, over a period of several days. An initial high sodium accumulation may inhibit anaerobic glycolysis, preventing active transport of sodium out of the cerebrospinal compartment. When water is made available in unlimited quantities, it migrates to the tissues to restore normal salt–water equilibrium. This is associated with acute cerebral edema and the appearance of signs referable to a sudden rise in intracranial pressure. The response is the same in all species, but in pigs there is also an accumulation of eosinophils in nervous tissue and the meninges. The sodium ion is the one that accumulates in the tissues, and identical syndromes are produced by the feeding of sodium propionate or sodium sulfate. It has also been observed that the feeding of soluble substances such as urea, which are excreted unchanged by the kidney, may be associated with anhydremia and an increase in the sodium ion concentration in brain tissue and the development of encephalomalacia.

This form of salt poisoning is chronic only in the sense that the sodium ion accumulates gradually. The clinical syndrome is acute in much the same way as the syndrome is acute in chronic copper poisoning. There is an apparent relationship between this form of salt poisoning and PEM in all species.[5,6] Many outbreaks of the latter disease occur in circumstances that suggest chronic salt poisoning. Sheep adapt to a continuous high salt intake (up to 1.3% sodium chloride in the drinking water) by significant changes in numbers of microflora in the rumen, but this is not usually accompanied by any change in total metabolic activity. The same level of intake in sheep is associated with some mortality; chronic diarrhea; and reduction in fertility, weight gain, and wool growth.

CLINICAL FINDINGS

Subclinical Salt Poisoning

Lower levels of intake can suppress food intake and growth without overt clinical signs. This occurs in heifers drinking water containing 1.75% sodium chloride; the animals only maintain weight at a salt level of 1.5% and show suboptimal weight gains when the water contains 1.25% sodium chloride. Drinking water containing 0.25% salt significantly reduces the milk yield of high-producing dairy cows.

Acute Salt Poisoning

With large doses, vomiting, diarrhea with mucus in the feces, abdominal pain, and anorexia occur. The more common syndrome, occurring 1 to 2 days after ingestion, includes opisthotonus, nystagmus, tremor, blindness, paresis, and knuckling at the fetlocks.[7] There may be a nasal discharge and polyuria. A period of recumbency with convulsions follows and affected animals die within 24 hours of first becoming ill. Sheep show similar signs. In swine the signs include weakness and prostration, muscle tremor, clonic convulsions, coma, and death after a course of about 48 hours.

Subacute Poisoning

This syndrome in cattle and sheep on saline drinking water includes depression of appetite; thirst; constant bawling, especially in calves; loss of BW; dehydration; hypothermia; weakness; and occasional diarrhea. Incoordination, collapse, and tetanic convulsions with frothing from the mouth and nose may occur if the animals are forced to exercise. Acetonemia may be a complication in lactating cows.

Chronic Salt Poisoning

Chronic toxicity occurs most often in pigs. Lack of appetite, constipation, thirst, restlessness, and pruritus occur 2 to 4 days after exposure. A characteristic nervous syndrome follows within 12 to 24 hours. Initially there is apparent blindness and deafness, with the pig remaining oblivious to normal stimuli and wandering about aimlessly, bumping into objects, and pressing with the head. There may be circling or pivoting on one front leg. Recovery may occur at this stage or epileptiform convulsions begin, recurring at remarkably constant time intervals, usually 7 minutes, accompanied by tremor of the snout and neck. Clonic contractions of the neck muscles may be associated with jerky opisthotonus until the head is almost vertical causing the pig to walk backward and assume a dog-sitting posture. This may be followed by a clonic convulsion in lateral recumbency, with jaw champing, salivation, and dyspnea. Death may occur from respiratory failure or the pig relaxes into a state of coma for a few moments, revives, and wanders about aimlessly until the next episode occurs. The pulse and temperature are normal except in convulsive pigs when both may be elevated.

CLINICAL PATHOLOGY

Serum sodium concentrations are elevated appreciably above normal levels (135–145 mmol/L) to about 160/170 to 210 mmol/L.[1,8] An eosinopenia is also evident during this stage and a return to normal levels usually indicates recovery. In cattle the same changes occur but there is no eosinopenia. CSF sodium concentration exceeds serum sodium concentration.

NECROPSY FINDINGS

In acute salt poisoning of cattle, there is marked congestion of the mucosa of the omasum and abomasum. The feces are fluid and dark. Animals that have survived for several days show hydropericardium and edema of the skeletal muscles. Gastroenteritis may be evident in some pigs poisoned with large doses of salt, but in chronic poisoning there are no gross lesions. Histologically, the neurologic lesions of acute poisoning are restricted to expansion of perivascular spaces in the brain. In contrast, the microscopic changes in chronic salt poisoning in pigs are quite diagnostic. The expansion of perivascular spaces typical of acute cerebral edema is accompanied by meningitis featuring large numbers of eosinophils, which extend along Virchow–Robin spaces into the brain tissue. In pigs that survive there may be residual PEM, especially of the cerebral cortex. Chemical estimation of the amount of sodium and chloride in tissues, especially brain, may be of diagnostic value. Brain sodium levels exceeding 1,800 ppm are considered diagnostic in cattle and swine.[2]

Samples for Confirmation of Diagnosis

- **Toxicology:** 50 g liver, skeletal muscle, brain, serum, CSF, aqueous, or vitreous humor, feed, water (assay for sodium concentration)
- **Histology:** formalin-fixed half of sagittally sectioned brain (LM)

DIFFERENTIAL DIAGNOSIS

Differential diagnosis list
Bacterial meningoencephalitis
Gut edema occurs in rapidly growing pigs
Mulberry heart disease in older pigs
Polioencephalomalacia
Pseudorabies
Viral encephalomyelitis

TREATMENT

Treatment of both acute and chronic salt poisoning is the immediate removal of the toxic feed or water.[8] Further treatment involves correcting hypernatremia and serum hyperosmolality.

Acute Toxicity

If the animals have not yet shown clinical signs, allow access to water and monitor closely for several days. In those animals showing an acute onset of clinical signs (less than 12–24 hours), serum sodium concentration may be lowered by 1 mmol/L/h.[8] Intravenous fluids of choice include 5% dextrose in water or 0.45% sodium chloride in well-hydrated animals and 0.9% sodium chloride or an isotonic crystalloid in hypovolemic animals.[1,8]

Chronic Toxicity

Initially, access to fresh water should be restricted to small amounts at frequent intervals; unlimited access may be associated with a sudden increase in the number of animals affected. In advanced cases animals may be unable to drink and water may have to be administered by stomach tube. Serum sodium levels in those animals with toxicity of several days' duration or those with an unknown duration of hypernatremia should be decreased by no more than 0.5 mmol/L/h.[8] Fluid choices again depend on whether the animal is volume depleted or well hydrated.

If possible, serum sodium concentration should be measured and the following formula used to calculate the free-water deficit:

$$\textit{Free-water deficit } (L) = 0.6 \times BW\ (kg) \times ([\textit{current serum sodium concentration}/\textit{reference range serum sodium concentration}] - 1)$$

No more than 50% of the free-water deficit should be replaced in the first 24 hours, with the remainder replaced over the subsequent 24 to 48 hours.

Supportive treatment includes gastrointestinal protectants, diuretics for pulmonary edema, and mannitol or hypertonic saline to decrease brain edema should it occur.

CONTROL

Both salt and water should be freely available at all times. Drinking water for all classes of livestock should not contain more than 0.5% sodium chloride or total salts. Water containing a high concentration of fluoride or magnesium is particularly dangerous to livestock and should be avoided. In cold weather, access to water should be monitored on a daily basis. Diets fed to pigs should not contain more than 1% salt. The manner in which whey is fed to pigs (with minimum water intake) makes prevention difficult unless the whey can be kept salt free at the cheese factory.

FURTHER READING

Radostits O, et al. Sodium chloride poisoning. In: *Veterinary Medicine: A Textbook of the Disease of Cattle, Horses, Sheep, Goats and Pigs*. 10th ed. London: W.B. Saunders; 2007:1824.

Senturk S, Huseyin C. Salt poisoning in beef cattle. *Vet Hum Toxicol*. 2004;46:26-27.

Weeth HJ, Haverland LH. Tolerance of growing cattle for drinking water containing sodium chloride. *J Anim Sci*. 1961;20:518-521.

REFERENCES

1. Goldkamp C, et al. *Comp Contin Educ Vet*. 2007;29:140.
2. Morgan SE. *Vet Clin North Am Food Animal Pract*. 2011;27:286.
3. Ollivett TL, et al. *J Vet Intern Med*. 2013;27:592.
4. Heydarpour F, et al. *Toxicol Environ Chem*. 2008;90:1115.
5. de Sant'Ana FJF, et al. *Braz J Vet Pathol*. 2010;3:70.
6. Macri SM, et al. *Vet Pathol Online*. 2013;0300985813498782.
7. Heydarpour F, et al. *Toxicol Environ Chem*. 2008;90:1035.
8. Abutarbus SM, et al. *Can Vet J*. 2007;48:184.

VITAMIN A DEFICIENCY (HYPOVITAMINOSIS A)

A deficiency of vitamin A may be caused by an insufficient supply of the vitamin in the ration or its defective absorption from the alimentary canal. In young animals, the manifestations of the deficiency are mainly those of compression of the brain and spinal cord. In adult animals, the syndrome is characterized by night blindness, corneal keratinization, pityriasis, defects in the hooves, loss of weight, and infertility. Congenital defects are common in the offspring of deficient dams. Vitamin A may also provide a protective effect against various infectious diseases and enhance many facets of the immune system.

SYNOPSIS

Etiology Dietary deficiency of vitamin A or its precursors.

Epidemiology Primary vitamin A deficiency in animals fed diet deficient in vitamin A or its precursors. Common in cattle grazing dry pastures for long periods. Occurs when diet of hand-fed animals is not supplemented with vitamin A.

Signs

Cattle: Night blindness. Loss of body weight. Convulsions followed by recovery. Episodes of syncope. Permanent blindness with dilated pupils and optic disc edema.

Pigs: Convulsions, hindleg paralysis, congenital defects.

Clinical pathology Low levels plasma vitamin A.

Necropsy findings Squamous metaplasia of interlobular ducts of parotid gland. Compression of optic nerve tracts and spinal nerve roots. Degeneration of testes.

Diagnostic confirmation Low levels of plasma vitamin A and squamous metaplasia of interlobular ducts of parotid glands.

Differential diagnosis list

Cattle

- Polioencephalomalacia
- Hypomagnesemic tetany
- Lead poisoning
- Rabies
- Meningoencephalitis
- Peripheral blindness caused by bilateral ophthalmitis.

Pigs

- Salt poisoning
- Pseudorabies
- Viral encephalomyelitis
- Spinal cord compression caused by vertebral body abscess

Treatment Vitamin A injections.

Control Feed diets with adequate carotene. Supplement diet with vitamin A. Parenteral injections of vitamin A at strategic times.

ETIOLOGY

Vitamin A deficiency may be primary disease, caused by an absolute deficiency of vitamin A or its precursor carotene in the diet, or a secondary disease, in which the dietary supply of the vitamin or its precursor is adequate, but their digestion, absorption, or metabolism is interfered with to produce a deficiency at the tissue level.

EPIDEMIOLOGY

Primary Vitamin A Deficiency

Primary vitamin A deficiency is of major economic importance in groups of young growing animals on pasture or fed diets deficient in the vitamin or its precursors. In the UK, primary vitamin A deficiency occurs in housed cattle fed a ration containing little or no green forage. Animals at pasture receive adequate supplies of the vitamin, except during prolonged droughts, but animals confined indoors and fed prepared diets may be deficient if not adequately supplemented. For example, a diet of dried sugar beet pulp, concentrates, and poor-quality hay can result in hypovitaminosis A in confined beef cattle.

Ruminants on Pasture

Primary vitamin A deficiency occurs in beef cattle and sheep on dry range pasture during periods of drought. Clinical vitamin A deficiency does not always occur under these conditions because hepatic storage is usually good and the period of deprivation not sufficiently long for these stores to reach a critically low level. Young sheep grazing natural, drought-stricken pasture can suffer serious depletion of reserves of the vitamin in 5 to 8 months, but normal growth is maintained for 1 year at which time clinical signs develop. Adult sheep may be on a deficient diet for 18 months before hepatic stores are depleted and the disease becomes evident. Cattle may subsist on naturally deficient diets for 5 to 18 months before clinical signs appear. However, during the annual dry season (October to June), herds of cattle, sheep, and goats in the Sahelian region of West Africa are managed on dry grasses and shrubby ligneous plants, which fail to provide maintenance levels of crude protein and vitamin A. These substandard conditions result in vitamin A deficiency characterized by night blindness, xerophthalmia, retarded growth rates, reproductive failures, and increased mortality. The pastoral herders associate the cure of night blindness with the consumption of green vegetation and will purposefully herd livestock into green vegetation areas when available. Certain ethnic groups of pastoral herders depend on ruminant milk as their principal source of vitamin A, and night blindness in lactating and pregnant women as well as in young children appears after the onset of night blindness in their cattle and sheep during the latter half of the dry season. Therefore increasing vitamin A levels in the milk of cows may alleviate the clinical signs of vitamin A deficiency in herder families.

Primary vitamin A deficiency is still relatively common in beef cattle that depend on pasture and roughage for the major portion of their diet. Beef calves coming off dry summer pastures at 6 to 8 months of age are commonly marginally deficient.

Maternal Deficiency

A maternal deficiency of vitamin A can result in herd outbreaks of congenital hypovitaminosis A in calves. In one such occurrence, out of 240 heifers fed a vitamin A–deficient ration, 89 calves were born dead and 47 were born alive but blind and weak and died within 1 to 3 days after birth. Blindness with dilated pupils, nystagmus, weakness, and incoordination were characteristic. In another occurrence in the UK, 25% of the calves born from maternally vitamin A–deficient heifer dams had ocular abnormalities.

The status of the dam is reflected in the status of the fetus only in certain circumstances because carotene, as it occurs in green feed, does not pass the placental barrier, and a high intake of green pasture before parturition does not increase the hepatic stores of vitamin A in newborn calves, lambs, or kids and only to a limited extent in pigs. However, vitamin A in the ester form, as it occurs in fish oils, will pass the placental barrier in cows. Feeding of these oils, or the parenteral administration of a vitamin A injectable preparation before parturition, will cause an increase in stores of the vitamin in fetal livers. Antepartum feeding of carotene and the alcohol form of the vitamin does, however, cause an increase in the vitamin A content of the colostrum. Young animals depend on the dam's colostrum for their early requirements of the vitamin, which is always highest in colostrum and returns to normal levels within a few days of parturition. Pigs weaned very early at 2 to 4 weeks may require special supplementation. Pregnant beef cows wintered on poor-quality roughage commonly need supplementation with vitamin A throughout the winter months to ensure normal development of the fetus and an adequate supply of the vitamin in the colostrum at parturition.

Adequacy of Supplements

The addition of vitamin A supplements to diets may not always be sufficient to prevent deficiency. Carotene and vitamin A are readily oxidized, particularly in the presence of unsaturated fatty acids. Oily preparations are thus less satisfactory than dry or aqueous preparations, particularly if the feed is to be stored for any length of time. Pelleting of feed may also cause a serious loss up to 32% of the vitamin A in the original feedstuff.

Heat, light, and mineral mixes are known to increase the rate of destruction of vitamin A supplements in commercial rations. In one study, 47% to 92% of the vitamin A in several mineral supplements was destroyed after 1 week of exposure to the trace minerals, high relative humidity, sunlight, and warm temperatures.

Feedlot Cattle

The disease still occurs in feedlot cattle in some parts of North America when feedlot cattle are fed rations low in carotene or vitamin A over a period of several months. The onset of clinical signs in growing feedlot cattle is typically seen 6 to 12 months after feeding a diet deficient in carotene or vitamin A. Small farm feedlots may feed their cattle a cereal grain such as barley and barley straw with no vitamin supplementation or inadequate supplementation. Grains, with the exception of yellow corn, contain negligible amounts of carotene, and cereal hay is often a poor source. Any hay cut late, leached by rain, bleached by sun, or stored for long periods loses much of its carotene content. The carotene content of yellow corn also deteriorates markedly with long storage. Moreover, under conditions not yet completely understood, the conversion by ruminants of carotene present in feeds such as silage may be much less complete than was formerly thought.

In feedlot cattle, the disease is most common in steers fed the same ration as heifers that may remain clinically normal. It is suggested that sexual dimorphism may be caused by the production of vitamin A by the corpus luteum of heifers.

Pigs

Young pigs on a deficient diet may show signs after several months, but as in other animals, the length of time required before signs appear is governed to a large extent by the status before depletion commences. As a general rule it can be anticipated that signs will appear in pigs fed deficient rations for 4 to 5 months; variations from these periods are probably caused by variations in the vitamin A status of the animal when the deficient diet is introduced. Congenital defects occur in litters from deficient sows, but the incidence is higher in gilts with the first litter than in older sows. It is presumed that the hepatic stores of vitamin A in older sows are not depleted as readily as in young pigs. Feeding white maize bran without supplementation can result in congenital defects in litters and paralysis in adult pigs.

Horses

Adult horses may remain clinically normal for as long as 3 years on a deficient diet.

Secondary Vitamin A Deficiency

Secondary vitamin A deficiency may occur in cases of chronic disease of the liver or intestines because much of the conversion of carotene to vitamin A occurs in the intestinal epithelium and the liver is the main site of storage of the vitamin. Highly chlorinated naphthalenes interfere with the conversion of carotene to vitamin A, and animals poisoned with these substances have a very low vitamin A status. The intake of inorganic phosphorus also affects vitamin A storage, low phosphate diets facilitating storage of the vitamin. This may have a sparing effect on vitamin A requirements during drought periods when phosphorus intake is low and an exacerbating effect in stall-fed cattle on a good grain diet. However, phosphorus deficiency may lower the efficiency of carotene conversion. Vitamins C and E help to prevent loss of vitamin A in feedstuffs and during digestion. Additional factors, which may increase the requirement of vitamin A, include high environmental temperatures and a high nitrate content of the feed, which reduces the conversion of carotene to vitamin A and rapid rate of gain. Both a low vitamin A status of the animal and high levels of carotene intake may decrease the biopotency of ingested carotene.

The continued ingestion of mineral oil, which may occur when the oil is used as a preventive against bloat in cattle, may cause a depression of plasma carotene and vitamin A esters and the carotene levels in buffer fat. Deleterious effects on the cattle are unlikely under the conditions in which it is ordinarily used because of the short period for which the oil is administered and the high intake of vitamin A and carotene.

PATHOGENESIS

Vitamin A is essential for the regeneration of the visual purple necessary for dim-light vision, for normal bone growth, and for maintenance of normal epithelial tissues. Deprivation of the vitamin produces effects largely attributable to disturbance of these functions. The same tissues are affected in all species. However, there is a difference in tissue and organ response in the different species and particular clinical signs may occur at different stages of development of the disease. The major pathophysiologic effects of vitamin A deficiency are as follows.

Night Vision and Ocular Abnormalities

Ability to see in dim light is reduced because of interference with regeneration of visual purple. Ocular abnormalities occur because of disruption to ocular, retinal, and optic nerve development from midpregnancy onward.[1]

Cerebrospinal Fluid Pressure

An increase in CSF pressure is one of the first abnormalities to occur in hypovitaminosis A in calves. It is a more sensitive indicator than ocular changes and, in the calf, it occurs when the vitamin A intake is about twice that needed to prevent night blindness. The increase in CSF pressure is caused by impaired absorption of the CSF from reduced tissue permeability of the arachnoid villi and thickening of the connective tissue matrix of the cerebral dura mater. The increased CSF pressure is responsible for the syncope and convulsions, which occur in calves in the early stages of vitamin A deficiency. The syncope and convulsions may occur spontaneously or be precipitated by excitement and exercise. It is suggested that the CSF pressure is increased in calves with subclinical deficiency and that exercise further increases the CSF pressure to convulsive levels.

Bone Growth

Vitamin A is necessary to maintain normal position and activity of osteoblasts and osteoclasts. When deficiency occurs, there is no retardation of endochondral bone growth, but there is incoordination of bone growth in that shaping, especially the finer molding of bones, does not proceed normally. In most locations this has little effect but may cause serious damage to the nervous system. Overcrowding of the cranial cavity occurs with resulting distortion and herniations of the brain and an increase in CSF pressure up to four to six times normal. The characteristic nervous signs of vitamin A deficiency, including papilledema, incoordination, and syncope, follow. Compression, twisting, and lengthening of the cranial nerves and herniations of the cerebellum into the foramen magnum, causing weakness and ataxia, and of the spinal cord into intervertebral foramina results in damage to nerve roots and localizing signs referable to individual peripheral nerves. Facial paralysis and blindness caused by constriction of the optic nerve are typical examples of this latter phenomenon. The effect of excess vitamin A on bone development by its interference with vitamin D has been discussed elsewhere. Dwarfism in a group of pigs in a swine herd was suspected to be caused by vitamin toxicosis.

Epithelial Tissues

Vitamin A deficiency leads to atrophy of all epithelial cells, but the important effects are limited to those types of epithelial tissue with a secretory as well as a covering function. The secretory cells are without power to divide and develop from undifferentiated basal epithelium. In vitamin A deficiency these secretory cells are gradually replaced by the stratified, keratinizing epithelial cells common to nonsecretory epithelial tissues. This replacement of secretory epithelium by keratinized epithelium occurs chiefly in the salivary glands, the urogenital tract (including placenta but not ovaries or renal tubules), and the periocular glands and teeth (disappearance of odontoblasts from the enamel organ). The secretion of thyroxine is markedly reduced. The mucosa of the stomach is not markedly affected. These changes in epithelium lead to the clinical signs of placental degeneration, xerophthalmia, and corneal changes.

Experimental vitamin A deficiency in lambs results in changes in the epithelium of the small intestine characterized by vesicular microvillar degeneration and disruption of the capillary endothelium. Diarrhea did not occur.

Embryologic Development

Vitamin A is essential for organ formation during growth of the fetus. Multiple congenital defects occur in pigs and rats and congenital hydrocephalus in rabbits on maternal diets deficient in vitamin A. In pigs, administration of the vitamin to depleted sows before the 17th day of gestation prevented the development of eye lesions but administration on the 18th day failed to do so. A maternal deficiency of vitamin A in cattle can result in congenital hypovitaminosis A in the calves, characterized by blindness with dilated pupils, nystagmus, weakness, and incoordination. Constriction of the optic canal with thickening of the dura mater results in ischemic necrosis of the optic nerve and optic disc edema resulting in blindness. Retinal dysplasia also occurs. Thickening of the occipital and sphenoid bones and doming of the frontal and parietal bones with compression of the brain also occur. Dilated lateral ventricles may be present and associated with increased CSF pressure.

Immune Mechanisms

The effects of vitamin A and β-carotene on host defense mechanisms have been uncertain and controversial for many years. Some workers claim that the incidence and severity of bacterial, viral, rickettsial, and parasitic infections are higher in vitamin A–deficient animals. It is possible that vitamin A and β-carotene afford protection against infections by influencing both specific and nonspecific host defense mechanisms. The protective effect of vitamin A may be mediated by enhanced polymorphonuclear neutrophil function, but this effect is also influenced by the physiologic status of the animal such as lactation status in dairy cattle. Experimentally, a severe vitamin A deficiency in lambs is associated with alterations in immune function, but the exact mechanism is unknown.

CLINICAL FINDINGS

Similar syndromes occur in all species, but because of species differences in tissue and organ response, some variations are observed. The major clinical findings are set out in the following sections.

Night Blindness

Inability to see in dim light (twilight or moonlit night) is the earliest sign in all species, except in the pig, in which it is not evident until plasma vitamin A levels are very low. This is an important diagnostic sign.

Xerophthalmia

True xerophthalmia, with thickening and clouding of the cornea, occurs only in the calf. In other species, a thin, serous mucoid discharge from the eyes occurs, followed by corneal keratinization, clouding and sometimes ulceration, and photophobia.

Ocular Abnormalities

A range of ocular deformities, including cataract formation, lens luxation, microphthalmia, and reduction in the size of the optic nerve head, occurred in calves with low serum vitamin A and E concentrations (Fig. 14-14).[1] Mean vitamin A concentration was 0.47 µmol/L (reference range 0.87 to 1.75 µmol/L) and the mean vitamin E concentrations was 2.28 µmol/L (reference range 3.0 to 18 µmol/L).

Changes in the Skin

A rough, dry coat with a shaggy appearance and splitting of the bristle tips in pigs is characteristic, but excessive keratinization, such as occurs in cattle poisoned with chlorinated naphthalenes, does not occur under natural conditions of vitamin A deficiency. Heavy deposits of branlike scales on the skin are seen in affected cattle. Skin disease occurs in Angus calves (~8 months of age) with vitamin A deficiency and is characterized by alopecia, severe epidermal and follicular orthokeratosis, and acanthosis. Affected animals responded to vitamin A supplementation.[2]

Dry, scaly hooves with multiple, vertical cracks are another manifestation of skin changes and are particularly noticeable in horses.

A seborrheic dermatitis can be observed in deficient pigs but is not specific to vitamin A deficiency.

Body Weight

Under natural conditions, a simple deficiency of vitamin A is unlikely to occur and the emaciation commonly attributed to vitamin A deficiency may be largely caused by multiple deficiencies of protein and energy. Although inappetence, weakness, stunted growth, and emaciation occur under experimental conditions of severe deficiency, in field outbreaks severe clinical signs of vitamin A deficiency are often seen in animals in good condition. Experimentally, sheep maintain their BW under extreme deficiency conditions and with very low plasma vitamin A levels.

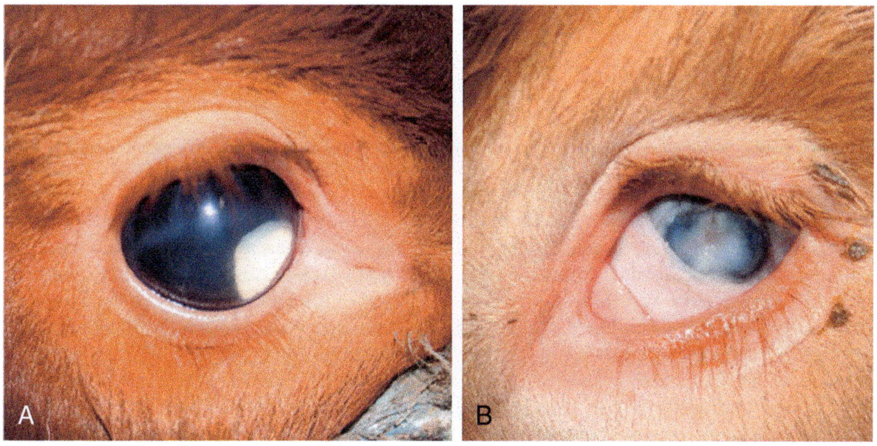

Fig. 14-14 Lens dislocation **(A)** and ocular rupture **(B)** in Simmental calves with hypovitaminosis A. (Reproduced with permission from Anon. *Vet Rec* 2014;174:244.)

Reproductive Efficiency

Loss of reproductive function is one of the major causes of loss in vitamin A deficiency. Both the male and female are affected. In the male, libido is retained but degeneration of the germinative epithelium of the seminiferous tubules causes reduction in the number of motile, normal spermatozoa produced. In young rams, the testicles may be visibly smaller than normal. In the female, conception is usually not interfered with, but placental degeneration leads to abortion and the birth of dead or weak young. Placental retention is common.

Dairy ewes on a diet low in vitamin A have increased somatic cell counts, possibly indicating a predisposition to mastitis in animals with hypovitaminosis A.[3]

Nervous System

Signs related to damage of the nervous system include the following:

- **Paralysis** of skeletal muscles caused by damage of peripheral nerve roots
- **Encephalopathy** caused by increased intracranial pressure
- **Blindness** caused by constriction of the optic nerve canal

These defects occur at any age but are most common in young, growing animals; they have been observed in all species except horses.

Paralysis

The paralytic form is manifested by abnormalities of gait caused by weakness and incoordination. The hindlegs are usually affected first and the forelimbs later. In pigs, there may be stiffness of the legs, initially with a stilted gait or flaccidity, knuckling of the fetlocks and sagging of the hindquarters. Complete limb paralysis occurs terminally.

Convulsions

Encephalopathy, associated with an increase in CSF pressure, is manifested by convulsions, which are common in beef calves at 6 to 8 months, usually following removal from a dry summer pasture at weaning time. Spontaneously, or following exercise or handling, affected calves will collapse (syncope) and during lateral recumbency a clonic-tonic convulsion will occur, lasting for 10 to 30 seconds. Death may occur during the convulsion or the animal will survive the convulsion and lie quietly for several minutes, as if paralyzed, before another convulsion may occur. Affected calves are usually not blind and the menace reflex may be slightly impaired or hyperactive. Some calves are hyperesthetic to touch and sound. During the convulsion there is usually ventroflexion of the head and neck, sometimes opisthotonus and, commonly, tetanic closure of the eyelids and retraction of the eyeballs. Outbreaks of this form of hypovitaminosis A in calves have occurred and the case–fatality rate may reach 25%. The prognosis is usually excellent; treatment will effect a cure in 48 hours, but convulsions may continue for up to 48 hours following treatment.

Seizures and acute death attributable to hypovitaminosis A and D have occurred in feeder pigs fed ground red wheat and whole milk and housed in a barn with no exposure to sunlight. Lethargy, inappetence, diarrhea, and vomiting and progression to convulsions were characteristic.

Blindness

The ocular form of hypovitaminosis A occurs usually in yearling cattle (12–18 months old) and up to 2 to 3 years of age. These animals have usually been on marginally deficient rations for several months. Night blindness may or may not have been noticed by the owner. The cattle have usually been fed and housed for long periods in familiar surroundings and the clinical signs of night blindness may have been subtle and not noticeable. A computer-based algorithm for using pupillary light reflex responses to detect cattle with incipient visual loss or mild impairment of vision caused by hypovitaminosis A was not effective in detecting affected cattle.[4] The first sign of the ocular form of the disease is blindness in both eyes during daylight. Both **pupils** are **widely dilated and fixed** and will not respond to light. Optic disc edema may be prominent and there may be some loss of the usual brilliant color of the tapetum. Varying degrees of peripapillary retinal detachment, papillary and peripapillary retinal hemorrhages, and disruption of the retinal pigment epithelium may also be present. The **menace reflex** is usually totally absent, but the **palpebral and corneal reflexes** are present. The animal is aware of its surroundings and usually eats and drinks, unless placed in unfamiliar surroundings. The CSF pressure is increased in these animals, but not as high as in the calves described earlier. Convulsions may occur in these cattle if forced to walk or if loaded onto a vehicle for transportation. The prognosis for the ocular form with blindness is unfavorable and treatment is ineffective because of the degeneration of the optic nerves. Exophthalmos and excessive lacrimation are present in some cases.

Congenital Defects

Congenital defects have been observed in piglets and calves. In piglets, complete absence of the eyes (**anophthalmos**) or small eyes (**microphthalmos**), incomplete closure of the fetal optic fissure, degenerative changes in the lens and retina, and an abnormal proliferation of mesenchymal tissue in front of and behind the lens are some of the defects encountered.

Ocular abnormalities in newborn calves from maternally vitamin A–deficient heifers included corneal dermoid, microphthalmos, aphakia (absence of lens) and in some cases, both eyes covered by haired skin.[5] Cardiac defects, including ventricular septal defect and overriding aorta, are reported in a limited number of cases of calves with hypovitaminosis A, but the relationship is unclear.[5]

Other congenital defects attributed to vitamin A deficiency in pigs include cleft palate and harelip, accessory ears, malformed hindlegs, subcutaneous cysts, abnormally situated kidneys, cardiac defects, diaphragmatic hernia, aplasia of the genitalia, internal hydrocephalus, herniations of the spinal cord, and generalized edema. Affected pigs may be stillborn, or weak and unable to stand, or may be quite active. Weak pigs lie on their sides, make slow paddling movements with their legs, and squawk plaintively.

Other Diseases

Increased susceptibility to infection is often stated to result from vitamin A deficiency. The efficacy of colostrum as a preventive against diarrhea in calves was originally attributed to its vitamin A content, but the high antibody content of colostrum is most important.

Anasarca. Edema of the limbs and brisket has been associated with vitamin A deficiency in feedlot cattle, especially steers. The pathogenesis is not understood. The edema can be extensive, include all four limbs, ventral body wall, and extend to the scrotum. Heifers were unaffected.

CLINICAL PATHOLOGY

Plasma Vitamin A

Vitamin A levels in the plasma are used extensively in diagnostic and experimental work. Plasma levels of 20 μg/dL are the minimal concentration for vitamin A adequacy. Papilledema is an early sign of vitamin A deficiency, which develops before nyctalopia and at plasma levels below 18 μg/dL. Normal serum vitamin A concentrations in cattle range from 25 to 60 μg/dL. In pigs, levels of 11.0 μg/dL have been recorded in clinical cases, with normal levels being 23 to 29 μg/dL. In experimental vitamin A deficiency in lambs, serum levels declined to 6.8 μg/dL (normal lambs at 45.1 μg/dL).

The clinical signs may correlate with the serum concentrations of vitamin A. In one outbreak, feedlot cattle with serum concentrations between 8.89 and 18.05 μg/dL had only lost BW, those between 4.87 and 8.88 μg/dL had varying degrees of ataxia and blindness, and those below 4.88 μg/dL had convulsions and optic nerve constriction. Clinical signs can be expected when the levels fall to 5 μg/dL. For complete safety, optimum levels should be 25 μg/dL or above.

Plasma Retinol

Some information on the plasma retinol values in stabled Thoroughbred horses is available. The mean plasma level of retinol in 71 horses 2 to 3 years of age was 16.5 μg/dL. The serum retinol levels in racing Trotters in Finland are lower than during the summer months, which is a reflection of the quality of the diets.

Plasma Carotene

Plasma carotene levels vary largely with the diet. In cattle, levels of 150 μg/dL are optimum and, in the absence of supplementary vitamin A in the ration, clinical signs appear when the levels fall to 9 μg/dL. In sheep, carotene is present in the blood in only very small amounts even when animals are on green pasture.

Hepatic Vitamin A

A direct relationship between plasma and hepatic levels of vitamin A need not exist because plasma levels do not commence to fall until the hepatic stores are depleted. A temporary precipitate fall occurs at parturition and in acute infections in most animals. The secretion of large amounts of carotene and vitamin A in the colostrum of cows during the last 3 weeks of pregnancy may greatly reduce the level of vitamin A in the plasma.

Hepatic levels of vitamin A and carotene can be estimated in the living animal from a biopsy specimen. Biopsy techniques have been shown to be safe and relatively easy, provided a proper instrument is used. Hepatic levels of vitamin A and carotene should be of the order of 60 and 4.0 μg/g of liver, respectively. These levels are commonly as high as 200 to 800 μg/g. Critical levels at which signs are likely to appear are 2 and 0.5 μg/g for vitamin A and carotene, respectively.

Cerebrospinal Fluid

CSF pressure is also used as a sensitive indicator of low vitamin A status. In calves, normal pressures of less than 100 mm of saline rise after depletion to more than 200 mm. In pigs, normal pressures of 80 to 145 mm rise to above 200 mm in vitamin A deficiency. An increase in pressure is observed at a blood level of about 7 μg vitamin A per deciliter of plasma in this species. In sheep, normal pressures of 55 to 65 mm rise to 70 to 150 mm when depletion occurs. In the experimentally induced disease in cattle, there is a marked increase in the number of cornified epithelial cells in a conjunctival smear and distinctive bleaching of the tapetum lucidum as viewed by an ophthalmoscope. These features may have value as diagnostic aids in naturally occurring cases.

NECROPSY FINDINGS

Gross changes are rarely observed at necropsy. Careful dissection may reveal a decrease in the size of the cranial vault and of the vertebrae. Compression and injury of the cranial and spinal nerve roots, especially the optic nerve, may be visible. In outbreaks in which night blindness is the primary clinical sign, atrophy of the photoreceptor layer of the retina is evident histologically, but there are no gross lesions.

Congenital ocular abnormalities in newborn calves from vitamin A–deficient heifer dams included aphakia, absence of a uveal tract and aqueous humor, microphthalmos, bony outgrowths of the occipital bone, compression of the cerebellum, and cardiac abnormalities similar to the tetralogy of Fallot.

Squamous metaplasia of the interlobular ducts of the parotid salivary gland is strongly suggestive of vitamin A deficiency in pigs, calves, and lambs, but the change is transient and may have disappeared 2 to 4 weeks after the intake of vitamin A is increased. This microscopic change is most marked and occurs first, at the oral end of the main parotid duct. Abnormal epithelial cell differentiation may also be observed histologically in a variety of other sites such as the tracheal, esophageal, and ruminal mucosae; preputial lining; pancreatic ducts; and urinary epithelium. Hypovitaminosis A has also been associated with an increased incidence of pituitary cysts in cattle. Secondary bacterial infections, including pneumonia and otitis media, are also common, due at least in part to the decreased barrier function of the lining epithelia.

The abnormalities that occur in congenitally affected pigs have already been described.

Samples for Confirmation of Diagnosis

- **Toxicology:** 50 g liver, 500 g feed ASSAY (Vit A)
- **Histology:** formalin-fixed parotid salivary gland (including duct), rumen, pituitary, pancreas, brain (including optic nerves), cervical spinal cord (including nerve roots); Bouin's fixed eye (LM).

DIFFERENTIAL DIAGNOSIS

When the characteristic clinical findings of vitamin A deficiency are observed, a deficiency of the vitamin should be suspected if green feed or vitamin A supplements are not being provided. The detection of papilledema and testing for night blindness are the easiest methods of diagnosing early vitamin A deficiency in ruminants. Incoordination, paralysis, and convulsions are the early signs in pigs. Increase in CSF pressure is the earliest measurable change in both pigs and calves. Laboratory confirmation depends on estimations of vitamin A in plasma and liver, with the latter being most satisfactory. Unless the disease has been in existence for a considerable time, response to treatment is rapid. For confirmation at necropsy, histologic examination of parotid salivary gland and assay of vitamin A in the liver are suggested.

The salient features of the differential diagnosis of diseases of the nervous system of cattle are summarized in Table 14-12.

Cattle

Convulsive form of vitamin A deficiency in cattle must be differentiated from the following:

- **Polioencephalomalacia**: characterized by sudden onset of blindness, head-pressing, and tonic-clonic convulsions, usually in grain-fed animals but also in pastured animals ingesting an excess of sulfate in water and grass
- **Hypomagnesemic tetany**: primarily in lactating dairy cattle on pasture during cool windy weather; characterized by hyperesthesia, champing tonic-clonic convulsions, normal eyesight and tachycardia, and loud heart sounds
- **Lead poisoning**: in all age groups, but most commonly in pastured calves in the spring; characterized by blindness, tonic-clonic convulsions, champing of the jaw, head-pressing, and rapid death
- **Rabies**: in all age groups; characterized by bizarre mental behavior, gradually progressive ascending paralysis with ataxia leading to recumbency, drooling saliva, inability to swallow, normal eyesight, and death in 4–7 days.

Ocular form of vitamin A deficiency in cattle must be differentiated from those diseases of cattle characterized by central or peripheral blindness:

- Central blindness:
  Polioencephalomalacia
  Lead poisoning
  Meningoencephalitis
- Peripheral blindness:
  Bilateral ophthalmitis caused by ocular disease

Loss of body condition in cattle, failure to grow, and poor reproductive efficiency are general clinical findings not limited to vitamin A deficiency.

Pigs

Convulsive form of vitamin A deficiency in pigs must be differentiated from the following:

- Salt poisoning
- Pseudorabies
- Viral encephalomyelitis
- Organic arsenic poisoning.

Paralytic form of vitamin A deficiency in pigs must be differentiated from the following:

- Spinal cord compression caused by vertebral body abscess.

Congenital defects similar to those caused by vitamin A deficiency may be caused by deficiencies of other essential nutrients, by inheritance or by viral infections in early pregnancy in all species. Maternal vitamin A deficiency is the most common cause of congenital defects in piglets. Final diagnosis depends on the necropsy findings, analysis of feed and serum vitamin A of the dams.

TREATMENT

Vitamin A

Animals with curable vitamin A deficiency should be treated immediately with vitamin A at a dose rate equivalent to 10 to 20 times the daily maintenance requirement. As a rule, 440 IU/kg BW is the dose used. Parenteral injection of an aqueous rather than an oily solution is preferred. The response to treatment in severe cases is often rapid and complete, but the disease may be irreversible in chronic cases. Calves with the convulsive form caused by increased CSF pressure will usually return to normal in 48 hours following treatment. Cattle with the ocular form of the deficiency and that are blind will not respond to treatment and should be slaughtered for salvage.

Hypervitaminosis A

Daily heavy dosing (about 100 times normal) of calves causes reduced growth rate, lameness, ataxia, paresis, exostoses on the planter aspect of the third phalanx of the fourth digit of all feet, and disappearance of the epiphyseal cartilage. Persistent heavy dosing in calves causes lameness, retarded horn growth, and depressed CSF pressure. At necropsy, exostoses are present on the proximal metacarpal bones and the frontal bones are thin. Very high levels fed to young pigs may cause sudden death through massive internal hemorrhage and excessive doses during early pregnancy are reputed to result in fetal anomalies. However, feeding vitamin A for prolonged periods at exceptionally high levels is unlikely to produce severe embryotoxic or teratogenic effects in pigs.

CONTROL

Dietary Requirement

The minimum daily requirement in all species is 40 IU of vitamin A per kilogram BW, which is a guideline for maintenance requirements. In the formulation of practical diets for all species, the daily allowances of vitamin A are commonly increased by 50% to 100% of the daily minimum requirements. During pregnancy, lactation, or rapid growth the allowances are usually increased by 50% to 75% of the requirements. The supplementation of diets to groups of animals is governed also by their previous intake of the vitamin and its probable level in the diet being fed. The rate of supplementation can vary from 0 to 110 IU/kg BW per day (1 IU of vitamin A is equivalent in activity to 0.3 μg of retinol; 5 to 8 μg β-carotene has the same activity as 1 μg of retinol).

Nutrient studies have indicated that preruminant Holstein calves being fed milk replacer should receive 11,000 IU of vitamin A per kilogram dry matter for optimum growth and to maintain adequate liver vitamin A stores.

The amounts of the vitamin to be added to the ration of each species to meet the requirements for all purposes should be

Table 14-17 Daily dietary allowances of vitamin A

Animal	Vitamin A (IU/kg BW daily)
Cattle	
Growing calves	40
Weaned beef calves at 6–8 months	40
Calves 6 months to yearlings	40
Maintenance and pregnancy	70–80
Maintenance and lactation	80
Feedlot cattle on high energy ration	80
Sheep	
Growth and early pregnancy and fattening lambs	30–40
Late pregnancy and lactation	70–80
Horses	
Working horse	20–30
Growing horse	40
Pregnant mare	50
Lactating mare	50
Pigs	
Growing pigs	40–50
Pregnant gilts and sows	40–50
Lactating gilts and sows	70–80

obtained from published recommended nutrient requirements of domestic animals. Some examples of daily allowances of vitamin A for farm animals are set out in Table 14-17.

Supplementation Method

The method of supplementation will vary depending on the class of livestock and the ease with which the vitamin can be given. In **pigs**, the vitamin is incorporated directly into the complete ration, usually through the protein supplement. In **feedlot and dairy cattle** receiving complete feeds, the addition of vitamin A to the diet is simple. In **beef cattle**, which may be fed primarily on carotene-deficient roughage during pregnancy, it may not be possible to supplement the diet on a daily basis. However, it may be possible to provide a concentrated dietary source of vitamin A on a regular basis by feeding a protein supplement once weekly. The protein supplement will contain 10 to 15 times the daily allowance, which permits hepatic storage of the vitamin.

Parenteral Injection

An alternative method to dietary supplementation is the intramuscular injection of vitamin A at intervals of 50 to 60 days at the rate of 3,000 to 6,000 IU/kg BW. Under most conditions, hepatic storage is good and optimum plasma and hepatic levels of vitamin A are maintained for up to 50 to 60 days. In pregnant beef cattle the last injection should not be more than 40 to 50 days before parturition to ensure adequate levels of vitamin A in the colostrum. Ideally, the last injection should be given 30 days before parturition, but this may not be practical under some management conditions. Administration of vitamin A palmitate by intramuscular injection (3500 IU/kg BW) increased plasma vitamin A concentrations by 24 hours and these elevated concentrations persisted for at least 8 days.[6] The effect of a single administration of vitamin A on liver vitamin A concentrations, the biologic reservoir for the vitamin, was not determined.

The most economical method of supplementing vitamin A is, in most cases, through the feed and when possible should be used.

The use of injectable mixtures of vitamins A, D, and E is not always justifiable. The injection of a mixture of vitamins A, D, and E of feeder cattle in northern Australia before transport did not, contrary to anecdotal evidence, reduce weight loss associated with transportation. Cattle in Queensland and northwestern Australia have very high concentrations of hepatic vitamin A and in fact, drought-stricken cattle in the terminal stages of malnutrition have also had high liver concentration. The indiscriminate use of vitamin A preparations in cattle is a public health concern because some bovine livers may contain high levels of vitamin A, which are potentially teratogenic for pregnant women.

Oral Vitamin A

The oral administration of a single bolus of vitamin A at a dose of 2.8 mg/kg BW to debilitated Sahelian cattle during the dry season was effective in raising the milk levels of vitamin A and was as effective as adding 10 g of the powder to the drinking water. Both the powder and bolus products provided high levels of vitamin A in milk within 3 days of treatment and according to herder testimonials, night-blind people consuming milk from cattle previously treated with either oral vitamin A preparation were no longer affected with night blindness.

REFERENCES

1. Anon. *Vet Rec*. 2014;174:244.
2. Baldwin TJ, et al. *J Vet Diagn Invest*. 2012;24:763.
3. Koutsoumpas AT, et al. *Small Rumin Res*. 2013;110:120.
4. Han S, et al. *Comput Electron Agric*. 2014;108:80.
5. Millemann Y, et al. *Vet Rec*. 2007;160:441.
6. Koutsoumpas AT, et al. *Small Rumin Res*. 2013;109:28.

NICOTINIC ACID DEFICIENCY (HYPONIACINOSIS)

Nicotinic acid or niacin is essential for normal carbohydrate metabolism. Because of the high content in most natural animal feeds, deficiency states are rare in ordinary circumstances, except in pigs fed rations high in corn. Corn has both a low niacin content and a low content of tryptophan, which is a niacin precursor. A low-protein intake exacerbates the effects of the deficiency, but a high-protein intake is not fully protective.

In ruminants, synthesis within the animal provides an adequate source. Even in young calves, signs of deficiency do not occur, and because rumen microfloral activity is not yet of any magnitude, extraruminal synthesis appears probable. There are preliminary indications that dietary supplementation with niacin alters muscle fiber composition (increased type 1 (oxidative) versus type 2) in pigs and sheep.[1,2]

The oral supplementation of niacin in the diet of periparturient dairy cows may result in an increase in serum inorganic phosphorus and a decrease in serum potassium, calcium, and sodium concentrations. Niacin has been used to study the effects of artificially induced ketonemia and hypoglycemia in cattle through inducing changes in nonesterified fatty acid concentrations.[3]

The daily requirements of niacin for mature pigs are 0.1 to 0.4 mg/kg BW, but growing pigs appear to require more (0.6–1 mg/kg BW) for optimum growth.

Experimentally induced nicotinic acid deficiency in pigs is characterized by inappetence, severe diarrhea, a dirty yellow skin, with a severe scabby dermatitis and alopecia. Posterior paralysis also occurs. At necropsy, hemorrhages in the gastric and duodenal walls, congestion and swelling of the small intestinal mucosa, and ulcers in the large intestine are characteristic and closely resemble those of necrotic enteritis caused by infection with *Salmonella* spp.

Histologically, there is severe mucoid degeneration followed by local necrosis in the wall of the cecum and colon. Experimental production of the disease in pigs by the administration of an antimetabolite to nicotinamide causes ataxia or quadriplegia, accompanied by distinctive lesions in the gray matter of the cervical and lumbar enlargements of the ventral horn of the spinal cord. The lesions are malacic and occur in the intermediate zone of the gray matter. The identical lesions and clinical picture have been observed in naturally occurring disease.

The oral therapeutic dose rate of nicotinic acid in pigs is 100 to 200 mg; 10 to 20 g/tonne of feed supplies have sufficient nicotinic acid for pigs of all ages. Niacin is low in price and should always be added to pig rations based on corn.

REFERENCES

1. Khan M, et al. *Acta Vet Scand.* 2013;55:85.
2. Khan M, et al. *BMC Vet Res.* 2013;9:177.
3. Pires JAA, et al. *J Dairy Sci.* 2007;90:3725.

PYRIDOXINE (VITAMIN B_6) DEFICIENCY (HYPOPYRIDOXINOSIS)

A deficiency of pyridoxine in the diet is not known to occur under natural conditions. Experimental deficiency in pigs is characterized by periodic epileptiform convulsions and at necropsy by generalized hemosiderosis with a microcytic anemia, hyperplasia of the bone marrow, and fatty infiltration of the liver. Less severe deficiency impairs weight gain and alters biochemical markers of sulfur-containing amino acid metabolism.[1] The daily requirement of pyridoxine in the pig is of the order of 100 µg/kg BW or 1 mg/kg of solid food, although higher levels have been recommended on occasion. Certain strains of chickens have a high requirement for pyridoxine and the same may be true of pigs.

Experimentally induced deficiency in calves is characterized by anorexia, poor growth, apathy, dull coat, and alopecia. Severe, fatal epileptiform seizures occur in some animals. Anemia with poikilocytosis is characteristic of this deficiency in cows and calves.

REFERENCE

1. Zhang Z, et al. *Animal.* 2009;3:826.

PANTOTHENIC ACID DEFICIENCY (HYPOPANTOTHENOSIS)

PA is essential in metabolism because of its incorporation into coenzyme A and acyl carrier protein, both of which are central to energy metabolism. PA is ubiquitous in fodder, in addition to which microorganisms in the rumen synthesize the compound.[1] However, it is not clear if synthesis meets the requirements of dairy cows. The role of PA in ruminant nutrition is reviewed.[1]

Deficiency under natural conditions has been recorded mainly in pigs on rations based on corn.

In pigs, a decrease in weight gain caused by anorexia and inefficient food utilization occurs first. Dermatitis develops with a dark brown exudate collecting about the eyes and there is a patchy alopecia. Diarrhea and incoordination with a spastic, goose-stepping gait are characteristic. At necropsy, a severe, sometimes ulcerative, colitis is observed constantly, together with degeneration of myelin.

Calcium pantothenate (500 µg/kg BW/day) is effective in treatment and prevention. As a feed additive, 10 to 12 g/tonne of calcium pantothenate is adequate.

Experimentally induced PA deficiency in calves is manifested by rough hair coat, dermatitis under the lower jaw, excessive nasal mucus, anorexia and reduced growth rate, and is eventually fatal. At necropsy, there is usually a secondary pneumonia, demyelination in the spinal cord and peripheral nerves, and softening and congestion of the cerebrum.

REFERENCE

1. Ragaller V, et al. *J Anim Physiol Nutr.* 2011;95:6.

Metabolic and Toxic Encephalomyelopathies

A number of metabolic defects and a very large number of poisons, especially poisonous plants and farm chemicals, cause abnormalities of function of the nervous system. Those plants that cause degenerative nervous system disease are listed under the section Encephalomalacia; those that cause no detectable degenerative change in tissue are listed here. More detailed information on toxins that are primary neurotoxins are addressed in this chapter based on the predominant neuroanatomic location affected. This section includes those toxins that do not have a predilection for a specific neuroanatomic location.

An incomplete list of metabolic abnormalities and toxins that can cause nervous system dysfunction are as follows.

Abnormalities of Consciousness and Behavior

- Hypoglycemia and ketonemia of pregnancy toxemia (with degenerative lesions in some) and acetonemia
- Depression caused by hyponatremia and strong ion (metabolic) acidosis associated with diarrhea and dehydration, particularly in neonatal animals
- Hypomagnesemia of lactation tetany
- Hyper-D-lactatemia in neonatal calves, lambs, and kids and adult ruminants with grain overload
- Primary hyperammonemia and hepatic encephalopathy[1,2]
- Unspecified toxic substances in uremic animals
- Exogenous toxins, including carbon tetrachloride, hexachloroethane, and trichloroethylene
- Plants causing anemic and histotoxic hypoxia, especially plants causing cyanide or nitrite poisoning
- Poison plants, including *Helichrysum* spp., tansy mustard, male fern, kikuyu grass (or a fungus, *Myrothecium* sp. on the grass)

Abnormality Characterized by Tremor and Ataxia

- Weeds, including *Conium* spp. (hemlock), *Eupatorium* spp. (snakeroot), *Sarcostemma* spp., *Euphorbia* spp. and *Karwinskia* spp.
- Ivermectin toxicosis in horses[3]
- Bacterial toxins in shaker foal syndrome (probably)
- Fungal toxins, e.g., *Neotyphodium (Acremonium) lolii,* the endophyte fungus of ryegrass staggers

Convulsions

- Metabolic deficits, including hypoglycemia (piglets, ewes with pregnancy toxemia), hypomagnesemia (of whole milk tetany of calves, lactation tetany, cows and mares), hypernatremia
- Nutritional deficiencies of vitamin A (brain compression in calves and pigs), pyridoxine (experimentally in calves)
- Inorganic poisons, including lead (calves),[4] mercury (calves), farm chemicals such as organic arsenicals (pigs), organophosphates, chlorinated hydrocarbons, strychnine, urea, metaldehyde
- Bacterial toxins, including *C. tetani, C. perfringens* type D
- Fungal toxins, e.g., *C. purpurea*
- Grasses, including Wimmera ryegrass (*Lolium rigidum*) or the nematode on it, *Echinopogon ovatus*
- Pasture legumes: lupines
- Weeds: *Oenanthe* spp. (hemlock water dropwort), *Indigofera* spp. (in horses), *Cicuta* spp. (water hemlock), *Albizia tanganyicensis, Sarcostemma* spp., *Euphorbia* spp.
- Trees: laburnum, oleander, supplejack (*Ventilago* spp.)

Ataxia Apparently Caused by Proprioceptive Defect

- Grasses: *Phalaris tuberosa* (aquatica) (and other *Phalaris* spp.), *Lolium rigidum, E. ovatus*
- Weeds: *Romulea bulbocodium,* sneezeweed (*Helenium* spp.), *Indigofera* spp., Iceland poppy (*Papaver nudicaule*), *Gomphrena* spp., *Malva* spp., *Stachys* spp., *Ipomoea* spp., *Solanum esuriale*
- Trees: *Kalmia* spp., *Erythrophloeum* spp., *Eupatorium rugosum*
- Ferns: *Xanthorrhoea* spp., *Zamia* spp.; induced thiamine deficiency caused by bracken and horsetail poisoning

Involuntary Spastic Contraction of Large Muscle Masses

This includes, for example, acquired (Australian) equine reflex hypertonia (formerly known as Australian stringhalt) associated with ingestion of the Australian dandelion *Hypochaeris radicata*, European dandelion *Taraxacum officinale*, or mallow *Malva parviflora*).

Tremor, Incoordination, and Convulsions

There is an additional long list of plants that cause diarrhea and nervous signs, especially ataxia, together, but whether the latter are caused by the former or caused by neurotoxins is not identified.

The nervous signs include tremor, incoordination, and convulsions.

Paresis or Paralysis

Many of the toxic substances and metabolic defects listed previously cause paresis when their influence is mild and paralysis when it is severe. Some of the items appear in both lists. Because an agent appears in one list and not the other list is not meant to suggest that the agent does not cause the other effect. It is more likely that it occurs in circumstances that are almost always conducive to the development of a mild syndrome (or a severe one, as the case may be).

- **Disturbance of function** at neuromuscular junctions, e.g., hypocalcemia, hypomagnesemia, hypokalemia (as in downer cows), tetanus, botulism and hypoglycemia of pregnancy toxemia in cows and ewes, and tick paralysis. Hypophosphatemia has not been demonstrated to be a definitive cause of weakness in cattle.
- **Nutritional deficiency**, but including only experimentally induced deficiency of nicotinic and PAs: biotin and choline, cause posterior paresis and paralysis in pigs and calves.
- **Toxic diseases** of the nervous system, including disease associated with many chemicals used in agriculture, e.g., piperazine, rotenone, 2,4-D and 2,4,5-T, organophosphates, carbamates, chlorinated hydrocarbons, propylene glycol, metaldehyde, levamisole, toluene, carbon tetrachloride, strychnine, and nicotine sulfate.

FURTHER READING

Dawson DR. Toxins and adverse drug reactions affecting the equine nervous system. *Vet Clin North Am Equine Pract.* 2011;27:507-526.

Divers TJ. Metabolic causes of encephalopathy in horses. *Vet Clin North Am Equine Pract.* 2011;27:589-596.

Finnie JW, Windsor PA, Kessell AE. Neurological diseases of ruminant livestock in Australia. II: toxic disorders and nutritional deficiencies. *Aust Vet J.* 2011;89:247-253.

REFERENCES

1. Hughes KJ, et al. *Vet Rec.* 2009;164:142.
2. Pillitteri CA, Craig LE. *Vet Pathol.* 2012;50:177.
3. Swor TM, et al. *J Am Vet Med Assoc.* 2009;235:558.
4. Krametter-Froetscher R, et al. *Vet J.* 2007;174:99.

Inherited Diseases Primarily Affecting the Cerebrum

INHERITED CONGENITAL HYRDOCEPHALUS

Hydrocephalus is the distention of the ventricular system of the brain, caused by increased production of CSF by the choroid plexus, obstruction of normal CSF flow, or decreased absorption of CSF at the arachnoid villi in the venous sinuses.[1]

Cattle

Congenital hydrocephalus without abnormality of the frontal bones occurs sporadically but is also known to be an inherited defect in Holstein and Hereford and possibly in Ayrshire and Charolais cattle. Two specific inherited entities have been described. In one there is obstruction of drainage of the CSF from the lateral ventricles, which become distended with fluid and may cause bulging of the forehead, often sufficient to cause fetal dystocia. Hereford calves with this defect have partial occlusion of the supraorbital foramen, a domed skull, and poorly developed teeth; at necropsy the cerebellum is found to be small and there may be microphthalmia and skeletal muscle myopathy. They are usually born a few days prematurely, are small in size, and are unable to stand or suck. In some cows the amniotic fluid is increased in volume.

Another form of inherited hydrocephalus caused by malformation of the cranium and with no enlargement of the cranium has also been observed in Hereford cattle. The ventricular dilatation is not marked, and microphthalmia and cerebellar hypoplasia are not features. Affected calves may be alive at birth but are blind and unable to stand. Some bawl continuously and some are dumb. They do not usually survive for more than a few days. At necropsy there is internal hydrocephalus of the lateral ventricles with marked thinning of the overlying cerebrum. Other lesions include constriction of the optic nerve, detachment of the retina, cataract, coagulation of the vitreous humor, and a progressive muscular dystrophy. The condition is inherited as a recessive character.

Internal hydrocephalus inherited in combination with multiple eye defects in White Shorthorns is dealt with elsewhere, as are noninherited forms of the disease.

Sheep

A defect comparable to the Dandy–Walker syndrome in humans and characterized by internal hydrocephalus caused by obstruction of the foramina of Magendie and Lushka occurs in several breeds of sheep, especially Suffolk, and in cattle. Affected lambs are stillborn or die within a few hours of birth; because of the grossly enlarged cranium many cause dystocia, which can only be relieved by a fetotomy.

Horses

A Standardbred stallion sired a number of hydrocephalic foals in a pattern that suggested the inheritance of a dominant mutation in the germline and in the form of a single locus defect. Affected foals caused dystocia and were all stillborn. There is one report of an unsuccessful outcome following placement of ventriculoperitoneal shunt in an attempt to manage hydrocephalus in a Quarter Horse colt.[2]

Hydrocephalus has been observed more commonly in Friesian horses than other breeds. Affected foals have a malformed petrosal bone, which causes a narrowing of the jugular foramen.[1] Hydrocephalus in Friesian foals is thought to be caused by diminished absorption of CSF into the systemic circulation at the venous sinus because of the abnormally small jugular foramen. This type of hydrocephalus has been genetically linked in humans and dogs to chondrodysplasia.[1]

Pigs

Congenital hydrocephalus in Yorkshire and European pigs has been recorded. The abnormality varies from a small protrusion of dura (meningocele) to an extensive brain hernia in which the cerebral hemispheres protrude through the frontal suture, apparently forced there by increased fluid pressure in the lateral and third ventricles. The condition is thought to be inherited in a recessive manner, but exacerbated in its manifestation by a coexisting hypovitaminosis A. An outbreak of congenital meningoencephalocele in Landrace pigs is recorded in circumstances suggesting that it was inherited.

REFERENCES

1. Sipma KD, et al. *Vet Pathol.* 2013;50:1037.
2. Bentz BG, Moll HD. *J Vet Emerg Crit Care.* 2008;18:170.

INHERITED HYDRANENCEPHALY AND ARTHROGRYPOSIS

The defect is recorded in Corriedale sheep, and breeding trials indicate that it is inherited as an autosomal recessive character. Most affected lambs are found dead but facial deformity, including shortening of the mandible and distortion of the facial bones will be evident. At necropsy the predominant finding is the fixation and deformity of the joints of the limbs and vertebral column, and the almost complete absence of a cerebral cortex.

INHERITED PROSENCEPHALY

Recorded in Border Leicester sheep, this defect takes the form of fusion of the cerebral hemispheres and a single lateral ventricle. It is widespread in the breed in Australia and is inherited as an autosomal recessive character. Most affected lambs are stillborn. Live ones have dyspnea caused by gross shortening of the nasomaxillary region creating a severely overshot mandible and interference with sucking. Blindness, nystagmus, and recumbency are constant signs. The cerebrum and the cranial cavity are much smaller than normal.

INHERITED MULTIFOCAL SYMMETRIC ENCEPHALOPATHY

Two forms of the disease are recorded, in **Simmental** and in **Limousin** and Limousin-cross cattle. The Limousin calves are normal at birth but from about 1 month of age develop a progressive forelimb hypermetria, hyperesthesia, blindness, nystagmus, weight loss, and behavioral abnormalities, especially aggression. The signs gradually worsen for up to 4 months when euthanasia is necessary. Necropsy lesions include brain swelling; optic chiasma necrosis; and multifocal, symmetric areas of pallor, up to 0.5 cm diameter in the brain. These lesions show partial cavitation and multiple, pathologic abnormalities, especially myelin lysis and vacuolation and demyelination. The distribution of cases suggests an inherited defect.

The disease in Simmental and Simmental-cross cattle recorded in Australia and New Zealand also has a distribution suggesting an inherited defect. The disease is clinically similar to that in Limousin cattle except that affected animals are not blind and it develops later at 5 to 8 months. Calves may survive longer, up to 12 months and, although the characteristic abnormality of gait is hypermetria, the hindlimbs are affected, not the forelimbs. Other signs observed are dullness, a swaying gait and, terminally, gradually developing opisthotonus and forelimb hypertonia in extension. Necropsy lesions are also similar to those in the Limousins, but the distribution is in the midbrain and the entire brainstem.

A multifocal symmetric necrotizing encephalomyelopathy in Angus calves has been described. Clinically affected calves exhibited ataxia, nystagmus, strabismus, muscular tremors, opisthotonus, bruxism, hyperesthesia, tetanic spasms, and episodic convulsions at 2 to 6 weeks of age. Death occurred 4 to 7 days after the onset of clinical signs. Lesions consisted of symmetric degenerative foci affecting the dorsal vagal motor, lateral cuneate, and olivary nuclei in the medulla oblongata, and occasionally in the spinal cord, substantia nigra, and cerebellar peduncles. Although an inherited basis for the disease is suspected, the etiology is unknown.

MAPLE SYRUP URINE DISEASE (BRANCHED-CHAIN KETO ACID DEHYDROGENASE DEFICIENCY)

Calves affected by this disease may be stillborn. Live calves are normal at birth and develop signs only at 1 to 3 days of age. It is inherited as an autosomal recessive and occurs principally in Poll Hereford, Hereford, and Poll Shorthorn cattle but probably also occurs in other breeds. There is molecular heterogeneity between the breeds, and tests based on detection of the mutation could be prone to error. Hair roots are good sources of target DNA for genotyping cattle for the mutation in one of the genes coding for the branched-chain α-keto acid dehydrogenase enzyme. This avoids the errors created by hemopoietic chimerism when blood is used for the test.

The disease is caused by an accumulation of branched-chain amino acids, including valine, leucine, and isoleucine. The mutation responsible for maple syrup urine disease in Poll Shorthorns and genotyping Poll Shorthorns and Poll Herefords for the maple syrup urine disease alleles has been determined. The mutations responsible for maple syrup urine disease and inherited congenital myoclonus are present in the Australian Poll Hereford population.

Clinical signs include dullness, recumbency, tremor, tetanic spasms and opisthotonus, a scruffy coat, blindness, and severe hyperthermia. When held in a standing position, some calves have tetanic paralysis and others have flaccid paralysis. Terminal coma is followed by death after a course of 48 to 72 hours. The urine smells of burnt sugar (because of the presence of branched-chain amino acids), and this smell is the source of the name.[1]

At necropsy there is a characteristic severe spongiform encephalopathy similar to that found in comparable hereditary aminoacidurias in humans.[1] Final identification can be made based on the elevated ratios of branched : straight chain amino acids in nervous tissue.

REFERENCE

1. O'Toole D, et al. *J Vet Diagn Invest*. 2005;17:546.

INHERITED CITRULLINEMIA

This autosomal recessive disease is inherited in Australian Holstein Friesians, American Holstein Friesians, and Red Holstein Friesians in Europe.

Affected calves are normal at birth but develop signs in the first week of life and die 6 to 12 hours after the onset of illness. The signs are depression, compulsive walking, blindness, head-pressing, tremor, hyperthermia, recumbency, opisthotonus, and convulsions. Argininosuccinate synthetase deficiency is the likely cause. Blood citrulline levels are of the order of 40 to 1200 times normal, and the assay can be used to detect heterozygotes. The alternative method of detecting heterozygotes is to use a PCR test, which RE test designed to identify the mutation that causes the disease. Prenatal diagnosis has been achieved by examination of cell cultures derived from amniotic fluid.

INHERITED NEONATAL SPASTICITY

The defect is recorded in Jersey and Hereford cattle. Affected calves are normal at birth but develop signs 2 to 5 days later. The signs commence with incoordination and bulging of the eyes and a tendency to deviation of the neck causing the head to be held on one side. Subsequently, the calves are unable to stand and on stimulation develop a tetanic convulsion in which the neck, trunk, and limbs are rigidly extended and show marked tremor. Each convulsion is of several minutes' duration. Affected calves may survive for as long as a month if nursed carefully. There are no gross or histologic lesions at necropsy. Inheritance of the defect is conditioned by a single, recessive character.

DODDLER CALVES

This is an inherited congenital defect in Hereford cattle produced by intensive breeding of half-siblings, and it is no longer recorded. It was characterized by continuous clonic convulsions, nystagmus, and pupillary dilatation. Stimulation by touch or sound exacerbated the convulsions.

INHERITED IDIOPATHIC EPILEPSY OF CATTLE

Idiopathic epilepsy has been reported as an inherited condition in Brown Swiss cattle and appears to be inherited as a dominant character. Typical epileptiform convulsions occur, especially when the animals become excited or are exercised. Attacks do not usually commence until the calves are several months old and disappear entirely between the ages of 1 and 2 years.

FAMILIAL NARCOLEPSY

Affected horses, including Lipizzaners,[1] Shetlands, Miniature Horses, Icelandic foals, and Suffolk foals, suffer recurrent episodes of several minutes' duration during which they fall and lie motionless, without voluntary or involuntary movements except respiratory and eye movements. Between episodes there is no clinical abnormality. Handling or the excitement of feeding may precipitate an attack, and a sharp blow may terminate one.

A genetic cause is suspected in horses based on the occurrence of the disease in three fillies born to the same sire.[1] A physostigmine provocation test (0.06 mg/kg BW intravenously) has been used, and a positive result is a cataplectic attack or clinical worsening of the sleepiness over the following hour. The genetic basis has not been confirmed in horses but is suspected to be an autosomal dominant trait with incomplete penetrance.[1]

FURTHER READING

Mignot EJM, Dement WC. Narcolepsy in animals and man. *Equine J.* 1993;25:476.

REFERENCE

1. Ludvikova E, et al. *Vet Q.* 2012;32:99.

Congenital and Inherited Encephalomyelopathies

INHERITED LYSOSOMAL STORAGE DISEASES

These are diseases in which there is a genetically determined deficiency of a specific lysosomal hydrolase enzyme causing a defective degradation of carbohydrates, proteins, and lipids within lysosomes. These diseases are currently grouped into glycoproteinoses, mucopolysaccharidoses, sphingolipidoses, and mucopolysaccharidoses. Enzyme deficiencies associated with lysosomal storage diseases in agricultural animals include α-mannosidase, β-mannosidase, GM_1 gangliosidosis, GM_2 gangliosidosis,[1,2] β-glucocerebrosidase (Gaucher disease),[3] α-*N*-acetylglucosaminidase (NAGLU),[4] acid-sphingomyelinase (Niemann–Pick disease),[5] and an incompletely characterized form.[6,7] The lysosomes themselves are concerned with hydrolyzing polymeric material, which enters the vacuolar system, and converting it to monomeric units, such as monosaccharides, amino acids, and nucleotides, which can be dealt with by the better known metabolic processes. As a result of the deficiency, upstream metabolic substrates accumulate in the lysosomes and downstream metabolites are markedly reduced.

Lysosomal storage diseases can also be caused by poisonings, and these are addressed elsewhere in this chapter. The best known ones are caused by poisoning with *Swainsona,*[8] *Astragalus, Oxytropis,* and *Ipomoea* spp.[9-12], *Side* spp.[13], and *Phalaris* spp. (the chronic form of that disease).

The diseases included in this section are not strictly diseases of the nervous system because the lysosomes in both **neuronal** and **visceral** sites are affected, but the effects of the disease are most obvious in terms of nervous system function.

MANNOSIDOSIS

Mannosidosis is the best known group of the inherited lysosomal storage diseases in agricultural animals.

α-Mannosidosis

This is a lysosomal storage disease in which a deficiency of the enzyme α-mannosidase results in the accumulation of a metabolite rich in mannose and glucosamine in secondary lysosomes in neurons, macrophages, and reticuloendothelial cells of lymph nodes, causing apparent vacuolations in these cells. Similar vacuoles are found in exocrine cells in pancreas, abomasum, and lacrimal and salivary glands. Storage appears to be cumulative in the fetus, but after birth stored material is lost from the kidney into the urine via desquamated tubular epithelium. On the other hand, postnatal storage continues in the brain, pancreas, and lymph nodes. The disease occurs in Angus, Murray Grey, and Galloway cattle, is inherited as a simple recessive, and is recorded as occurring in the United States, Australia, and New Zealand.

Clinically it is characterized by ataxia, fine lateral head tremor, slow vertical nodding of the head, intention tremor, an aggressive tendency, failure to thrive, and death or the necessity of euthanasia at about 6 months of age. These signs appear almost immediately after birth up to several months later and worsen over a period of up to 3 to 4 months. The signs are bad enough to require euthanasia during the first week of life in many cases. The first sign observed is a swaying of the hindquarters, especially after exercise or with excitement. The stance becomes wide based and the gait jerky, stilted and high stepping, with slight overflexion of the hindquarters so that the animal appears to be squatting as it moves.

The nervous signs are exacerbated by excitement, diarrhea is common, and the calves are usually stunted and unthrifty. They are also aggressive and attempt to charge but are usually impeded by their incoordination. Many calves die after having shown general ill-thrift and with minimal nervous signs. Death may occur from paralysis and starvation, or to misadventure, and some calves appear to die during a "fit" following a period of excitement. Many others are euthanized because of persistent recumbency. The nervous syndrome of mannosidosis is well known; affected calves will die. An α-mannosidosis is recorded in Galloway cattle and is manifested by stillbirth, moderate hydrocephalus, enlargement of the liver and kidneys, and arthrogryposis.

Normal heterozygotes carrying genes for mannosidosis are identifiable because of their reduced tissue or plasma levels of α-mannosidase. The mannosidase test for α-mannosidase in goats is specific and does not cross-react with α-mannosidase.

Advances in molecular biology have now led to the development of a more accurate test based on DNA technology. DNA tests based on the PCR have been developed for the detection of two breed-specific mutations responsible α-mannosidosis. One of the mutations is responsible for α-mannosidosis in Galloway cattle. The other mutation is uniquely associated with α-mannosidosis in Angus, Murray Grey, and Brangus cattle from Australia. The latter mutation was also detected in Red Angus cattle exported from Canada to Australia as embryos. The two breed-specific mutations may have arisen in Scotland and by the export of animals and germplasm disseminated to North America, New Zealand, and Australia.

A control program can be based on the identification of heterozygotes using PCR-based assays for detection of breed-specific mutations. A program of screening cattle in herds that produce bulls for sale to commercial herds should stop the spread of the disease very quickly, because the number of heterozygous females in the population will be irrelevant to the continuation of the disease in the absence of affected sires.

The α-mannosidosis gene prevalence is now insignificant and disease incidence has been reduced from an estimated 3000 cases/year to negligible levels.

β-Mannosidosis

β-Mannosidosis occurs in Salers cattle and Anglo-Nubian goats and has been recorded in a sheep. In cattle, some affected calves are stillborn. The remainder of calves are euthanized forthwith because of the severity of the congenital defects.

Calves are affected at birth with craniofacial deformity and inability to stand. The cranium is domed and there is mild prognathism; narrow palpebral fissures; and a tough, hidebound skin. When in sternal recumbency, the head is moved in a combined motion of circling and bobbing, eventually converting the calf to lateral recumbency, in which it remains until passively returned to the sternal position, where nystagmus and tremor become evident. There is no suck reflex at any time. In lateral recumbency there is opisthotonus and paddling convulsions.

In the goats the condition is present at birth and characterized clinically by tetraplegia, tremor, deafness, and nystagmus, and an inexorably fatal termination. Additional signs include bilateral Horner's syndrome, carpal contractures, pastern joint hyperextension, thickened skin, and a dome-shaped skull. Although retinal ganglion cells are badly affected, there appears to be no defect of vision. It is an autosomal recessive defect that is very similar to α-mannosidosis.

The diagnosis is confirmed by a reduced level of β-mannosidase in the blood.

Necropsy findings include a deficiency of cerebral cortical and cerebellar substance, distended lateral ventricles, and bilateral renomegaly. The biochemical defect is one of acidic β-mannosidase, and is conditioned by an autosomal recessive character. The carrier rate of the causative gene is very high in the Salers breed.

REFERENCES

1. Porter BF, et al. *Vet Pathol.* 2011;48:807.
2. Torres PA, et al. *Mol Genet Metab.* 2010;101:357.
3. Karageorgos L, et al. *J Inherit Metab Dis.* 2011;34:209.
4. Karageorgos L, et al. *J Inherit Metab Dis.* 2007;30:358.
5. Saunders GK, Wenger DA. *Vet Pathol.* 2008;45:201.
6. Mikami O, et al. *J Vet Med A Physiol Pathol Clin Med.* 2006;53:77.
7. Masoudi AA, et al. *Anim Sci J.* 2009;80:611.
8. Dantas AFM, et al. *Toxicon.* 2007;49:111.
9. Barbosa RC, et al. *Toxicon.* 2006;47:371.
10. Armien AG, et al. *Vet Pathol.* 2007;44:170.
11. Mendonca D, et al. *Acta Vet Brno.* 2011;80:235.
12. Armien AG, et al. *J Vet Diagn Invest.* 2011;23:221.
13. Furlan FH, et al. *Vet Pathol.* 2009;46:343.

GANGLIOSIDOSIS

At least five types of gangliosidosis are known to occur in humans and animals. Two (GM_1 and GM_2 gangliosidosis) have thus far been identified in agricultural animals.

GM_1 Gangliosidosis

GM_1 gangliosidosis occurs in cattle and sheep. In Friesian cattle it is inherited as a lysosomal storage disease in which the activity of an enzyme, β-galactosidase, in nervous tissue is greatly reduced. As a result, there is an accumulation of the ganglioside (GM_1) in the tissue. Clinical signs of progressive neuromotor dysfunction and a reduction in growth rate appear at about 3 months of age. The growth rate is reduced, and the animal is in poor condition, blind, and has a staring coat. The neuromotor signs include lack of response to external stimuli, sluggish mastication and swallowing, hindquarter sway while walking, a wide stance, a tendency to fall, reluctance to move, stiff high-stepping gait, aimless walking, head-pressing, and convulsions. Abnormal electrocardiogram (ECG) tracings are common. The blindness results from lesions in the retina and the optic nerve. Ophthalmoscopic examination of the retina is recommended as an aid to diagnosis. A positive diagnosis is made on the grounds of intraneuronal lipid storage plus reduced β-galactosidase activity plus identification of the stored lipid. The stored ganglioside is visible under the electron microscope as stacks and concentric whorls of lamellae. In the live animal enzyme assays are performed on leukocytes. The enzymatic defect is also detectable in liver, skin, and leukocytes.

GM_1 gangliosidosis is also present in Suffolk and Suffolk-cross sheep. Visceral and neuronal lysosomal storage are both evident but the neuronal lesion is more severe. Deficiencies of β-galactosidase and α-neuraminidase are evident. Affected sheep become ataxic at 4 to 6 months old and worsen to recumbency and death in up to 2 months.

GM_1 gangliosidosis has been reported from England in "Coopworth Romney" lambs closely related to a ram imported from New Zealand.

GM_2 Gangliosidosis

GM_2 gangliosidosis (Tay–Sachs disease) occurs in sheep and pigs and is an autosomal recessive lysosomal storage disease caused by defects in the genes that code for hexosaminidase. In Jacob sheep, progressive accumulation of GM_2 ganglioside results in in cortical blindness, proprioceptive deficits, and ataxia in all four limbs within 6 to 8 months of birth.[1,2]

GM_2 gangliosidosis has also been identified in Yorkshire pigs and also causes decreased growth rate, incoordination appearing after 3 months of age, gray-white spots in the retina and dark blue granules in neutrophils, and azurophilic granules in lymphocytes. A serum enzyme assay is a suitable method of detecting "carrier" heterozygous pigs. The test is based on the amount of *N*-acetyl-β-D-hexosaminidase in tissues.

REFERENCES

1. Porter BF, et al. *Vet Pathol.* 2011;48:807.
2. Torres PA, et al. *Mol Genet Metab.* 2010;101:357.

GAUCHER DISEASE TYPE 2

Gaucher disease is an autosomal recessive lysosomal storage disease caused by mutations in the β-glucocerebrosidase gene. Gaucher disease is the most common lysosomal storage disorder in humans and is divided into three subtypes based on the level of neurologic involvement and clinical signs: (1) type 1, nonneuronopathic; (2) type 2, acute neuronopathic; and (3) type 3 (subacute neuronopathic).[1]

Type 2 Gaucher disease has been reported in Southdown sheep in Victoria, Australia.[1] Affected lambs were unable to stand and exhibited continued shaking and shivering. Lambs could be bottle-fed but their neurologic status did not improve. Affected lambs also had a thickened leathery skin in the abdominal and cervical regions. Glucocerebrosidase activity was markedly reduced in leukocytes and cultured skin fibroblasts and glucocerebrosidase content was increased in the brain, liver, and blood.

REFERENCE

1. Karageorgos L, et al. *J Inherit Metab Dis.* 2011;34:209.

BOVINE MUCOPOLYSACCHARIDOSIS TYPE IIIB

Mucopolysaccharidosis IIIB is an autosomal recessive lysosomal storage disease caused by mutations in the NAGLU gene. NAGLU is intimately involved with the degradation of heparin sulfate in lysosomes; gene mutations therefore result in intralysosomal storage of heparin sulfate.

Mucopolysaccharidosis IIIB has been reported in cattle in Queensland, Australia.[1] Animals were normal at weaning at 6 to 8 months of age; clinical signs developed progressively from 12 months onward and included loss of herding instinct, aimless wandering, tendency to stand alone, becoming very placid and sedate in nature, and development of excessively hairy ears. Animals survived to 3 to 5 years of age, and terminally developed progressive ataxia, a stumbling gait, and excessive weight loss.

REFERENCE

1. Karageorgos L, et al. *J Inherit Metab Dis.* 2007;30:358.

SPHINGOMYELINASE DEFICIENCY (NIEMANN–PICK DISEASE TYPE A) IN CATTLE

Sphingomyelinase deficiency (Niemann–Pick disease) is a lysosomal storage disease caused by mutations in the sphingomyelinase gene and is described as three forms in humans: type A (early onset of neurologic disease in infancy), B, and C. Sphingomyelinase is involved with catalyzing the conversion of sphingomyelin to ceramide and phosphorylcholine.

Sphingomyelinase deficiency (type A) has been diagnosed in a 5-month-old Hereford calf in Virginia.[1] The calf had a 4-week history of abnormal and progressive neurologic signs, including hypermetria, wide-based stance, ataxia, and positional strabismus.

REFERENCE

1. Saunders GK, Wenger DA. *Vet Pathol.* 2008;45:201.

GLOBOID CELL LEUKODYSTROPHY (GALACTOCEREBROSIDOSIS)

Globoid cell leukodystrophy has been identified in Poll Dorset sheep in Australia. Incoordination in the hindlimbs progresses until the animals are tetraplegic. Only histologic changes are evident at necropsy. These include myelin destruction and the accumulation of characteristic globoid cells in nervous tissue. There is greatly decreased galactocerebrosidase activity in affected tissue.

INHERITED NERVOUS SYSTEM ABIOTROPHIES

These diseases are characterized by **premature, progressive loss of functionally related and discrete populations of neurons.** As a result, most affected animals are born normal but develop signs of a progressive neurologic disease that is either fatal or leads to such a serious neurologic deficit that euthanasia is the only reasonable solution. In a few rare diseases the patient is abnormal at birth but worsens, and usually dies, during the neonatal period. Again there are exceptions, and in rare cases complete recovery has been reported. The genetic nature of some of the cases included may not be certain; they are included here if the evidence that they are inherited can be reasonably presumed. An important distinction is that **abiotrophy implies premature aging,** which is different from degeneration, which is a term that implies an extrinsic etiology. From a clinical perspective nervous system degeneration can appear identical to nervous system abiotrophy, and a firm diagnosis of abiotrophy usually requires histologic examination unless the species, breed, or availability of specific diagnostic tests permits antemortem diagnosis of abiotrophy. At the moment the abiotrophic diseases cannot be treated. The lysosomal storage diseases, listed in the preceding section, represent a specific group of abiotrophic diseases.

FURTHER READING

Siso S, Hanzlicek D, Fluehmann G, et al. Neurodegenerative diseases in domestic animals: a comparative review. *Vet J.* 2006;171:20-38.

NEURONAL CEROID LIPOFUSCINOSIS

The neuronal ceroid lipofuscinoses are a group of inherited neurodegenerative lysosomal storage diseases of humans and other animals, inherited as autosomal recessive traits. They are grouped together because of common clinical and pathologic phenomena related to brain and retinal atrophy, premature death, and accumulation of a fluorescent lipopigment in neurons and many other cell types within the body. Molecular genetic studies have identified mutations in eight different genes (*CLN1, CLN2, CLN3, CLN5, CLN6, CLN6, CLN8,* and *CTSD*) that can result in neuronal ceroid lipofuscinoses.[1-4]

The disease is recorded in Devon cattle,[1] South Hampshire sheep,[2,3,4] Rambouillet sheep, Borderdale sheep,[5] Merino sheep, Nubian goats, and Vietnamese pot-bellied pigs.[6] It resembles neuronal ceroid lipofuscinosis of humans and is not strictly a primary lysosomal disorder; it is classified as a proteolipid proteinosis, and provides a good animal model for discussing the similar disease (Batten disease) of humans. Secondary lysosomes in animals with neuronal ceroid lipofuscinoses fill with subunit c of mitochondrial ATP synthase because of excessive peroxidation of polyunsaturated fatty acids. The mechanism of the accumulation is that protein is formed, which is normal for mitochondria, but is misdirected so that it accumulates in the lysosome. The disease in Devon cattle is caused by a single base duplication in the bovine *CLN5* gene.[1] The disease in Merino sheep is a subunit c–storing abnormality, clinically and pathologically similar to ceroid lipofuscinosis in South Hampshire sheep, which is caused by a missense mutation in the ovine *CLN6* gene.[2,3] The disease in Borderdale sheep is caused by a nucleotide substitution in the ovine *CLN5* gene.[5]

The occurrence of neuronal ceroid lipofuscinosis in South Hampshire and Borderdale sheep in New Zealand have been well described. The severity of neurodegeneration and minor differences in the ultrastructure of storage material suggests this is a different disease from other forms of ovine ceroid lipofuscinosis, which accumulate the subunit c of mitochondrial ATP synthase. An autosomal recessive mode of inheritance is considered probable.

Clinical findings include slowly progressive ataxia of the hindlimbs, commencing usually at about 4 months but possibly as late as 18 months of age, and lasting for 6 months leading to euthanasia at up to 4 years. Inability to keep up with the flock is noticed first, followed by a sawhorse stance, obvious ataxia, severe depression, and an increasing failure of the menace and pupillary light reflexes. Terminal blindness is a constant sign. Positional nystagmus, circling, and head-pressing occur in some. Eating, drinking, and defecation are normal, but there is slight weight loss. A blood test has been developed to detect the genetic mutation in South Hampshire sheep.[2] CSF is altered in sheep with advanced diseased, characterized by increased lactate, acetate, and tyrosine concentrations and decreased myo-inositol and scyllo-inositol and citrate concentrations.[3]

The lesion in lambs and calves is atrophy of the cerebrum, especially the optic cortex, with eosinophilic granulation of neurons and macrophages in the CNS followed by progressive retinal atrophy. There is a progressive storage of lipopigment in nervous tissue, especially retinal photoreceptors; its presence can be demonstrated by quantitative autofluorescence using a modified slit lamp microscope. Other clinicopathologic aids include lysosomal enzyme assay, organ biopsy, and CT, which reveals the enlargement of the lateral ventricles of the brain resulting from cerebral atrophy.

Neuronal ceroid lipofuscinosis has been described in three horses. Clinically, there was developmental retardation, slow movements, and loss of appetite at 6 months of age. Torticollis, ataxia, head tilt, and loss of eyesight were present at 1 year of age. There were abnormalities in posture and movements, decreased spinal reflexes, and some CN dysfunction, dorsal strabismus, and absence of the menace reflex. At necropsy, there was flattening of the gyri and discoloration of the brain. Histologically, eosinophilic, autofluorescent material in the perikarya of neurons was present throughout the brain, spinal cord, neurons of the retina, submucosa, and myenteric ganglia and in glial cells.

Neuronal ceroid lipofuscinosis has been described in a 2-year-old Vietnamese pot-bellied pig.[6] Ataxia had progressed to tetraparesis over a 3-month period, with terminal development of a head tilt and intermittent nystagmus. The pig did not appear to be blind.

REFERENCES

1. Houweling PJ, et al. *Biochimi Biophys Acta.* 2006;1762:890.
2. Tammen I, et al. *Biochim Biophys Acta.* 2006;1762:898.
3. Pears MR, et al. *J Neurosci Res.* 2007;85:3494.
4. Kay GW, et al. *Neurobiol Dis.* 2011;41:614.
5. Frugier T, et al. *Neurobiol Dis.* 2008;29:306.
6. Cesta MF, et al. *Vet Pathol.* 2006;43:556.

CONGENITAL NECROTIZING ENCEPHALOPATHY IN LAMBS

This condition, defined by its pathology, was a common diagnosis of neurologic disease in lambs under 7 days of age by the Veterinary Laboratories Agency in the north of England.[1] Affected flocks had single or multiple cases, with up to 10% morbidity of lambs in a flock. All cases came from ewes carrying multiple fetuses, but there is variation in the clinical signs of sibling lambs. The most severely affected may be stillborn, with less severely affected lambs born weak, small, and unable to rise with ataxia and head tremor. Some lambs survive but may have residual signs of cerebellar dysfunction. The common lesion is superficial cerebrocortical neuronal necrosis. A significant proportion also has necrosis of the Purkinje cells in the cerebellum and leukoencephalopathy of the thalamus and brainstem. It is possible that this syndrome reflects hypoglycemia consequent to negative energy balance in late pregnancy.

REFERENCE

1. Scholes SFE, et al. *Vet Rec.* 2007;160:775.

LAVENDER FOAL SYNDROME

Lavender foal syndrome is a congenital, inherited, autosomal recessive disease of Egyptian Arab foals characterized by signs of neurologic disease evident at birth and unusual dilute coat color.[1] The disease is caused by a mutation in the MYO5A gene that is a single-base deletion in a conserved region of the tail domain.[2] The deletion produces a truncated protein product through the insertion of a premature stop codon (p.Arg1487AlafsX13). There is a prevalence of carriers in Egyptian Arabian horses of 10.3% (heterozygotes),[3] and within Arabs the allele frequency is estimated at 0.0162, with no alleles detected in Thoroughbred, Standardbred, Morgan, Quarter Horse, or Percheron horses.[4] The carrier prevalence of LFS in Arabian foals in South Africa for the 2009/2010 season was 11.7% (95% confidence interval [CI] 7.6–17.0%).[5]

There is a dilute (lavender) coat color and signs of central neurologic disease including inability to stand, paddling, opisthotonus, and torticollis with apparently normal peripheral reflexes (blink to bright light, triceps, patellar, and cutaneous truncal).[1] There are no characteristic hematologic and serum biochemical abnormalities. There is no effective treatment.

Gross necropsy examination does not reveal any consistent or diagnostic abnormalities apart from the dilute hair coat. An assay for the genetic mutation is available and provides confirmation of diagnosis. Testing of Egyptian Arabians enables avoidance of carrier-to-carrier matings, and thus the disease.[3]

REFERENCES

1. Page P, et al. *J Vet Intern Med.* 2006;20:1491.
2. Bierman A, et al. *Anim Gen.* 2010;41:199.
3. Brooks SA, et al. *PLoS Genet.* 2010;6:e000909.
4. Gabreski NA, et al. *Anim Gen.* 2012;43:650.
5. Tarr CJ, et al. *Equine Vet J.* 2014;46:512.

INHERITED HYPOMYELINOGENESIS (CONGENITAL TREMOR SYNDROMES OF PIGLETS)

Congenital tremor of pigs has a multiple etiology and some of the causes are not yet identified. The disease is also known as *myoclonia congenita* or trembling pig syndrome or jumpy pig disease. Gilts are particularly affected. The types are shown in Table 14-18 and the features in Table 14-19. They can only be differentiated by pathology and particularly neurochemistry. The essential lesion is the same in all cases and is a hypomyelination of the brain and spinal cord. The infectious forms are discussed elsewhere.

There are two inherited forms. One is congenital tremor Type A-III, which is found in Landrace pigs and Landrace crosses. It is sometimes known as Landrace trembles. Type A-III is a sex-linked recessive gene carried by the sow. It is associated with females, high growth rates, lean carcasses, and pale colored meat characterized by the presence of poorly myelinated axons in all parts of the CNS. It is also known as congenital cerebrospinal hypomyelinogenesis. The sows produce piglets that have reduced numbers of oligodendrocytes and therefore cannot myelinate nerve fibers. The tremor disappears when the piglets are asleep.

The other inherited form is Type A-IV of British Saddleback pigs. It is not common. The specific defect in A-IV is one of fatty acid metabolism, which results in hypomyelination and demyelination. (A similar disorder but a monogenic autosomal recessive tremor has also been described in Saddleback /Large White crosses).

The structural abnormalities in the type A-III disease have been identified; splayleg is a common accompaniment.

Both diseases are characterized by muscle tremor, incoordination, difficulty in standing, and some squealing. The A-III disease occurs only in males. Both are inherited as recessive characteristics.

Table 14-18 Diagnostic taxonomy of congenital tremor in pigs

Cause	AI	AII	AIII	AIV	AV	B
Field observations	**Virus hog cholera**	**Virus unknown**	**Genetic S-L recessive**	**Genetic autosomal recessive**	**Chemical trichlorfon**	**Unknown**
Proportion of litters affected	High	High	Low	Low	High	Variable
Proportion of pigs affected within litter (approximately)	>40%	>80%	25%	25%	>90%	Variable
Mortality among affected pigs	Medium to high	Low	High	High	High	Variable
Sex of affected pigs	Both	Both	Male	Both	Both	Any
Breed of dam (pure or crossbred)	Any	Any	Landrace	Saddleback	Any	Any
Recurrence in successive litters of same parents	No	No	Yes	Yes	Yes	?
Duration of outbreak	<4 months	<4 months	Indefinite	Indefinite	<1 month	?

Table 14-19 Key features of the six types of congenital tremor described in pigs

Type	Cause	Key features
A1	Hog Cholera	Dysgenesis Cerebellar hypoplasia Small cord Demyelination Swollen oligodendrocytes
AII	Congenital tremor virus PCV2	Swollen oligodendrocytes
AIII	Inherited autosomal recessive sex linked in landrace	Reduced oligodendrocytes Reduced myelination Hypoplasia of cord
AIV	As previously noted in Saddleback Also Landrace/Saddleback cross syndrome	Demyelination Cerebral, cerebellar and cord hypoplasia
AV	Trichlorfon toxicity	Cerebellar hypoplasia affected 45–79 days' gestation, particularly 75–79
B	Unknown	No special features

FURTHER READING

Harding DJD, et al. Congenital tremor AIII in pigs, an hereditary sex-linked cerebrospinal myelinogenesis. *Vet Rec.* 1973;92:527.

Kidd ARM, et al. A-IV A new genetically-determined congenital nervous disorder in pigs. *Br Vet J.* 1986;142:275.

Diseases Primarily Affecting the Cerebellum

INHERITED CEREBELLAR DEFECTS

Several inherited cerebellar defects occur congenitally in calves, lambs, and foals. Lesions of the cerebellum may or may not be grossly or clinically obvious. They all need to be differentiated from similar defects known to be caused by intrauterine viral infections such as swine fever, bovine mucosal disease, and bluetongue.

Cerebellar Hypoplasia

This occurs in Herefords, Guernseys, Holsteins, Shorthorns, and Ayrshires and appears to be conditioned by a factor inherited in a recessive manner. Most calves are obviously affected at birth. While lying down, there is no marked abnormality, although a moderate lateral tremor of the neck occurs, causing a gentle side-to-side swaying of the head. Severely affected calves are blind; they have widely dilated pupils and their pupils do not react to light. Such calves are unable to stand, even when assisted, because of flaccidity of limb muscles. When less severely affected animals attempt to rise, the head is thrown back excessively, the limb movements are exaggerated in force and range and are grossly incoordinated, and many calves are unable to rise without assistance. If they are placed on their feet, the calves adopt a straddle-legged stance with the feet wide apart and the legs and neck extended excessively. On attempting to move, limb movements are incoordinated and the calf falls, sometimes backward because of overextension of the forelimbs. Affected animals drink well but have great difficulty in getting to the teat or pail, with attempts usually wide of the mark. There are no defects of consciousness and no convulsions. Tremor may be evident while standing and there may be postrotational nystagmus after rapid lateral head movements. Sight and hearing are unimpaired and, although complete recovery does not occur, the calf may be able to compensate sufficiently to enable it to be reared to a vealing weight. Diagnosis can be confirmed by MRI.

At necropsy the most severe defect comprises complete absence of the cerebellum; hypoplasia of the olivary nuclei, the pons, and optic nerves; and partial or complete absence of the occipital cortex. Less severe defects include a reduction in size of the cerebellum and absence of some neuronal elements in a cerebellum of normal size.

Although the disease is dealt with generally as an inherited one. There is no firm evidence to substantiate this view, and there are sporadic, noninherited cases in other breeds.

Cerebellar Atrophy of Lambs (Daft Lamb Disease 1)

This has been recorded in many sheep breeds in Britain, Corriedales in Canada and New Zealand, and in Drysdales. Affected lambs are normal at birth but are weak and unable to rise without assistance. At 3 days of age it is obvious that there is severe incoordination of limb movement, opisthotonus, tremor, and a straddle-legged stance. At necropsy the cerebellum may be of normal size but on histologic examination there is gross atrophy of cerebellar neurons. The disease appears to be conditioned by a recessive gene but not as a simple homozygous recessive. A clinically similar disease has been observed in Border Leicester lambs. There is no histopathologic lesion in the cerebellum, but there are significant lesions in the cervical muscles and the nerve supply to them. The disease is inherited, most likely as an autosomal recessive trait.

Star-Gazing Lambs (Daft Lamb Disease 2)

A hereditary disease clinically similar to cerebral cortical atrophy has been described in newborn Leicester lambs in the UK but without histologic evidence of Purkinje cell loss, which is considered the hallmark of "cerebellar abiotrophy." Affected lambs exhibit "dorsal arching of the neck with the head being pressed backward," which is also described as star-gazing. Histologic lesions are present in neck muscles and nerves, but it is uncertain if these are primary or secondary.

Hereditary Lissencephaly and Cerebellar Hypoplasia in Churra Lambs

Lissencephaly is a very rare developmental intracranial disorder of animals that results from defects in neuronal migration. The gross result is a very simplified folding of the cerebrum and cerebellum with the presence of only a few broad gyri.

Lissencephaly and cerebellar hypoplasia have been identified in Churra lambs in Spain. Affected lambs were abnormal at birth, exhibiting weakness, inability to stand, and muscular rigidity. The cerebral cortex was disorganized histologically and the cerebellum was reduced in size. Pedigree analysis indicated a monogenic autosomal pattern of inheritance.[1] The genetic defect was a 31 base pair deletion in the coding area for the RELN gene, which plays an important role in neuronal migration and layer formation.[2] The deletion results in formation of a premature termination codon, resulting in the absence of protein expression.

REFERENCES

1. Perez V, et al. *BMC Vet Res.* 2013;9:156.
2. Suarez-Vega A, et al. *PLoS ONE.* 2013;8:e81072.

Inherited Ataxia of Calves

This is a true cerebellar ataxia inherited as a recessive character in Jerseys, Shorthorns, and Holsteins. Clinically the condition resembles cerebellar hypoplasia except that signs may not occur until the calves are a few days to several weeks old. At necropsy the cerebellum is normal in size but histologically aplasia of neurons is evident in the cerebellum and also in the thalamus and cerebral cortex. An inherited condition, manifested by cerebellar ataxia that does not develop until calves are 6 weeks to 5 months old, has also been recorded but the cerebellum is small and macroscopically abnormal. Conspicuous degeneration of cerebellar Purkinje cells is evident on histologic examination.

Familial Convulsions and Ataxia in Cattle

A neurologic disease is recorded as being inherited in Aberdeen Angus cattle and their crossbreeds and Charolais. In young calves there are intermittent attacks of convulsions, and in older animals these are replaced by a residual ataxia. The first signs appear within a few hours of birth; up to several months later there are single or multiple tetanic convulsions lasting for 3 to 12 hours. As these episodes disappear a spastic goose-stepping gait becomes apparent in the forelimbs and there is difficulty placing the hindlimbs. The characteristic necropsy lesion is a very selective cerebellar cortical degeneration. A proportion of cases make a complete recovery. The epidemiology of the disease is consistent with the operation of an autosomal dominant gene with incomplete penetrance.

Inherited Congenital Spasms of Cattle

This condition has been recorded only in Jersey cattle and appears to be conditioned by a factor inherited in a recessive manner. Affected calves show intermittent, vertical tremor of the head and neck, and there is a similar tremor of all four limbs that prevents walking and interferes with standing. Although the calves are normal in all other respects, they usually die within the first few weeks of life. No histologic examinations have been reported, but a cerebellar lesion seems probable.

Cerebellar Abiotrophy

This disease occurs in Holstein and Poll Hereford cross calves, Aberdeen Angus cattle and their crossbreds and Charolais cattle, Merino sheep, alpaca,[1] Arabian horses,[2-6] and pigs. The pathologic feature of cerebellar abiotrophy is disorganization of the Purkinje cells in the granular layer of the cerebellum, with subsequent disorganization of the molecular and granular layers. The etiology is thought to be abnormal migration of the Purkinje cells through the cerebellum during development, resulting in premature neuronal degeneration of Purkinje cells.[4]

Cattle

In the calves, ataxia appears for the first time when they are 3 to 8 months old. The calves are not blind but they often fail to exhibit a menace reflex. The onset of clinical signs is sudden but progression is slow or inapparent. Some become recumbent. Those that remain standing have a spastic, dysmetric ataxia and a broad-based stance and they fall easily and have a fine head tremor. All are strong and have good appetites. Abiotrophy, or premature aging, is evident only microscopically and consists of axonal swellings and segmental degeneration and loss of cerebellar Purkinje cells. The disease appears to be inherited, but recovery of some late cases is recorded.

Familial convulsions and ataxia is characterized as being inherited in Aberdeen Angus cattle and their crossbreds and Charolais. In young calves there are intermittent attacks of convulsions, and in older animals these are replaced by a residual ataxia. The first signs appear within a few hours of birth; up to several months later there are single or multiple tetanic convulsions lasting for 3 to 12 hours. As these episodes disappear a spastic goose-stepping gait becomes apparent in the forelimbs and there is difficulty placing the hindlimbs. The characteristic necropsy lesion is a very selective degeneration of the cerebellar cortex. A proportion of cases make a complete recovery. The epidemiology of the disease is consistent with the operation of an autosomal dominant gene with incomplete penetrance.

Sheep

The disease in sheep does not appear until about 3 years of age. There is incoordination and dysmetria so that the gait is awkward and disorganized and there is frequent falling. There are also a reduced menace response, an apprehensive manner, and a wide-based stance in the hindlimbs. At necropsy there is diffuse cerebellar degeneration and severe loss of Purkinje cells.

Alpaca

Neurologic abnormalities were first detected at 18 months of age, at which time intention tremors, hypermetria, and a wide-based stance were evident.[1] CSF analysis was within normal limits and the cerebellum appeared smaller than expected on CT.

Horses

The disease is recorded principally in Arabian horses but occurs also in the Australian pony, which was developed from the Arab, and in the Gotland breed from Sweden. A similar clinical syndrome occurs in the Oldenberg breed, but the pathologic picture is quite different.

The disease may be present at birth but is often not observed until the foal is 2 to 6 months old with the latest recognition being between 9 and 24 months of age. The characteristic signs are vertical head-nodding (some cases show horizontal head tremors), especially when excited, and ataxia, which is most noticeable at a fast gait. It may not be evident while the foal is walking. Very badly affected foals are unable to stand or suckle at birth, less severe ones are normal until about 4 months of age when head-nodding becomes obvious. The degree of ataxia varies from slight incoordination to inability to stand. A goose-stepping gait, which slams the front feet into the ground, occurs in some. All foals can see but there is an absence of the menace reflex in many. Nystagmus is not recorded as occurring in this disease. The first antemortem confirmatory test to be developed was **computer-assisted MRI brain morphometry,** which is used to determine the presence of a relatively smaller cerebellum and relatively larger cerebellar CSF space compared with size-matched horses.[3] Diagnosis has historically been made on the basis of breed and age of the animal, clinical signs, slow progression of disease, and elimination of other differential diagnoses.[2] The recent development of a DNA test on hair roots that detects the presence of the putative cerebellar abiotrophy gene mutation[4-6] should make antemortem diagnosis much more straightforward in Arabian horses.

Necropsy findings are limited to histopathologic lesions in the cerebellum. These include widespread loss of Purkinje cells and the presence of a gliosis. There are no degenerative lesions in the spinal cord. In the similar disease in Oldenberg horses the cerebellum is often reduced in size. The disease is an abiotrophy—a premature aging of tissues.

The disease is inherited as an autosomal recessive trait in Arabian horses.[4] An SNP has been identified in affected Arabian horses and may induce the disease by decreasing MUTYH expression, which is a DNA glycosylase that removes adenine residues.[5] The frequency of the allele is estimated at approximately 10.5% in the U.S. Arabian population, which is high.[6] The gene mutation has been identified at a low level in three breeds with Arabian ancestry (Trakehner; Bashkir Curly Horses, also known as North American Curly horses; and Welsh ponies).[6]

Pigs

A congenital progressive cerebellar abiotrophy is also reported in piglets of the offspring of Saddleback sows and an unrelated Large White boar. The disorder behaves epidemiologically like an inherited disease conditioned by a simple autosomal recessive trait. Clinical signs include dysmetria, ataxia, and tremor at standing but not at rest. There is gradual adjustment so that the piglets can walk and stand at 5 weeks of age, but by 15 weeks they are no longer able to do so. Affected pigs also have a coarse matted hair coat caused by a disproportionate number of coarse hairs to fine hairs. Histopathologic lesions are confined to the cerebellum in which there is a significant loss of Purkinje cells.

REFERENCES

1. Mouser P, et al. *Vet Pathol.* 2009;46:1133.
2. Foley A, et al. *Equine Vet Educ.* 2011;23:130.
3. Cavalleri JMV, et al. *BMC Vet Res.* 2013;9:105.
4. Brault LS, et al. *Am J Vet Res.* 2011;72:940.
5. Brault LS, et al. *Genomics.* 2011;97:121.
6. Brault LS, Penedo MCT. *Equine Vet J.* 2011;43:727.

Diseases Primarily Affecting the Brainstem and Vestibular System

OTITIS MEDIA/INTERNA

Infection of the middle ear (**otitis media**) occurs in young animals of all species but especially dairy calves and pigs, to a lesser extent feedlot cattle and lambs, and rarely foals. The infection may gain entrance from the external ear (e.g., caused by ear mite infestation) or hematogenously, but the spread is chiefly an ascending infection of the eustachian tubes in a young animal from a respiratory tract infection. Extension of infection into the inner ear leads to **otitis interna.**

Pigs

Otitis media was present in 68% of 237 pigs that were slaughtered because of illness. It is suggested that otitis media in pigs develops first as an acute inflammation in the auditory tube and then extends to other parts of the ear and brain. When abscesses form at the ventrum of the brainstem, the vestibulocochlear nerve is usually involved in the lesion. Infection in the ear may extend into the brain by following the auditory nerve. Perilymph filling the scala vestibuli and scala tympani is also a possible tract for the extension of the infection because there is a communication between the perilymph-filled spaces of the bony labyrinth and the subarachnoid space.

Calves and Lambs

The highest prevalence is in suckling dairy calves and weaned cattle and sheep in feedlots where the disease is probably secondary to respiratory tract infection. Outbreaks of otitis media/interna have occurred in beef calves from 6 to 10 weeks of age on pasture with their dams; mixed cultures of *E. coli, Pseudomonas* spp., and *Acinetobacter* spp. were isolated. Otitis media/interna in suckling dairy calves can also occur in outbreaks, and *M. bovis* is frequently isolated from the middle and inner ears of affected calves.

The onset of clinical signs commonly includes dullness, fever, inappetence, tachypnea, and a purulent discharge from the affected ear accompanied by rotation of the head (in otitis interna) and drooping of the ear a few days later because of involvement of the facial nerve in the inflammation. Deep palpation at the base of the ears may elicit a pain response.

Rotation of the head, with the affected side down, and facial paralysis may occur on the same side, and walking in circles with a tendency to fall to the affected side is common. In most cases the animals are normal in other respects, although depression and inappetence can occur in advanced cases (Fig. 14-15).

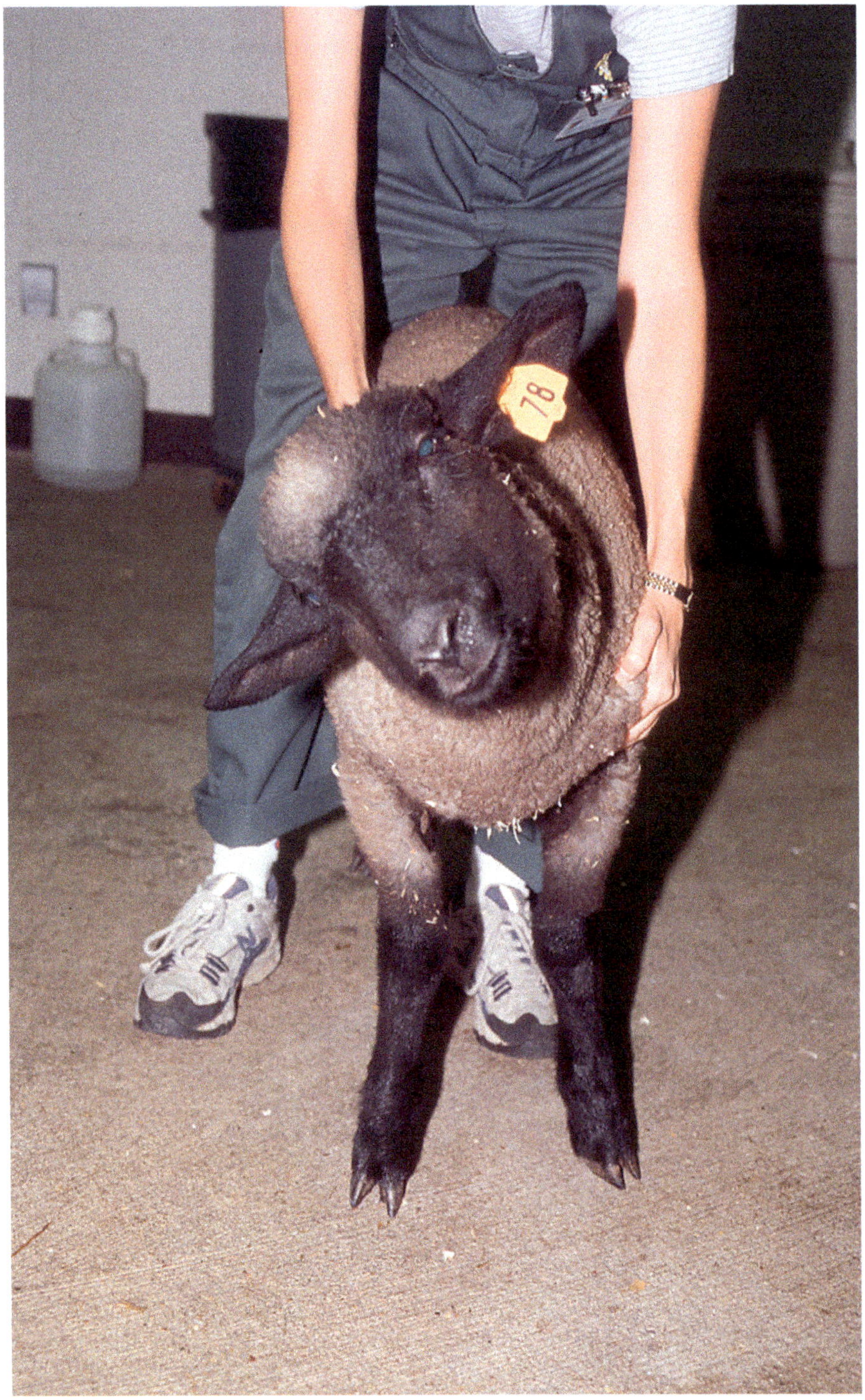

Fig. 14-15 Otitis media/interna on the right side of a recently weaned Suffolk sheep. Notice the marked deviation of the line between the two eyes from horizontal.

Horses

Otitis media/interna occurs in horses, and two clinical syndromes have been described. **The first syndrome** is primary otitis media characterized by abnormal behavior, including head-tossing, head-shaking, and ear-rubbing. Violent, uncontrollable behavior includes throwing themselves on the ground, rolling, and thrashing. This may progress to involve the bony structures of the temporal and proximal stylohyoid bones, resulting in a degenerative arthritis and eventual fusion of the temporohyoid bone.

The second syndrome is characterized by an acute onset of neurologic deficits. Commonly, there is vestibulocochlear nerve and often facial nerve dysfunction characterized by head tilt to the side of the lesion, nystagmus with the slow component to the affected side, and weakness of the extensor muscles on the affected side resulting in an ataxia or reluctance or refusal to stand. Horses that can stand often will lean on walls for support of the affected side.

Definitive diagnosis is dependent on either a positive tympanocentesis or, in the majority of cases, bony proliferation of the temporal bone and proximal part of the stylohyoid bone, or lysis of the tympanic bulla, as determined by radiography or CT. Otoscopic examination should be performed to determine whether there is purulent material in the auditory canal and whether the tympanic membrane is ruptured or bulging outward.

Radiography has been used to diagnose lesions of the tympanic bullae in cattle (otitis interna), characterized by thickening of the bulla wall, increased soft tissue opacity within the bulla, and osteolysis of the bulla wall and trabeculations.[1] Radiography is not as sensitive as CT for the diagnosis of otitis media; however, because CT provides more detailed information regarding the bony structures of the middle ear[2,3] and is more sensitive and specific than radiography in the diagnosis of otitis media in calves.[1] CT was used to provide an excellent anatomic description of the external acoustic meatus, tympanic cavity, and tympanic bulla of the llama.[4] Ultrasonography has also been used to diagnose otitis media in calves.[5] A 7.5-mHz linear probe is applied to the base of the ear without the use of coupling gel and the calf in a standing position. The probe is applied ventral to the base of the ear and caudal to the mandible. Abnormalities detected included anechoic to hyperechoic content; trabeculae lysis; and thinning, deformation, and rupture of the bulla wall. The lesions can be subtle in early cases and, consequently, test sensitivity is low in animals with acute or subacute clinical presentations.

Tympanocentesis is done under general anesthesia in horses or sedation in ruminants by directing a 15-cm needle through the tympanic membrane visualized with the aid of an otoscope. The technique is somewhat difficult because of the long and angled external auditory canal. Sterile 0.9% NaCl (0.5–1 mL) is injected into the tympanic cavity and then, after a few seconds, withdrawn. A positive tap consists of withdrawal of a cloudy or yellow fluid, which on analysis may contain evidence of pus and can be sampled for culture and antimicrobial susceptibility. An alternative method uses a 15-cm sterile polypropylene catheter that has the appropriate stiffness for puncturing the tympanic membrane but sufficient flexibility to advance along the external acoustic meatus.[3]

DIFFERENTIAL DIAGNOSIS

The disease needs to be differentiated from otitis externa, in which the head may be carried in a rotated position, but usually intermittently, and this is accompanied by head-shaking and the presence of exudate and an offensive smell in the ear canal, and from cerebral injury or abscess, and similar lesions of the upper cervical cord. All of these are characterized by deviation of the head, not rotation. At necropsy the tympanic bulla contains pus, and a variety of organisms, such as staphylococci, streptococci, *Pasteurella haemolytica,* and *Neisseria catarrhalis,* may be isolated.

TREATMENT

Treatment consists of broad-spectrum antimicrobials daily for 4 weeks and antiinflammatory agents. The prognosis with treatment with fluoroquinolones is very good in calves, although a 50% mortality rate has been reported in calves that were not treated with other antimicrobial agents. The use of lincomycin at 6.5 mg/kg BW combined with spectinomycin at 10 mg/kg BW intravenously twice daily for 5 days has been reported to be successful for the treatment of otitis media in beef calves. Anecdotal reports exist of the use of a knitting needle to rupture the tympanic membrane in cattle, with rapid resolution of the head tilt because of the decreased pressure in the middle ear. Bilateral tympanic bulla osteotomy has been performed in an affected calf, resulting in a rapid resolution of the head tilt.

FURTHER READING

Duarte ER, Hamdan JS. Otitis in cattle, an etiological review. *J Vet Med B.* 2004;51:1-7.

Morin DE. Brainstem and cranial nerve abnormalities: listeriosis, otitis media/interna, and pituitary abscess syndrome. *Vet Clin North Am Food Anim Pract.* 2004;20:243-273.

REFERENCES

1. Finnen A, et al. *J Vet Intern Med.* 2011;25:143.
2. Lee K, et al. *Vet Rec.* 2009;165:559.
3. Kawasaki Y, et al. *Vet Rec.* 2009;165:212.
4. Concha-Albornoz I, et al. *Am J Vet Res.* 2012;73:42.
5. Gosselin V, et al. *J Vet Intern Med.* 2014;28:1594.

LISTERIOSIS

SYNOPSIS

Etiology *Listeria monocytogenes.* Ubiquitous in farm environment.

Epidemiology Ruminants, particularly sheep. Prime occurrence is seasonal associated with feeding silage with high listerial growth. Also following management-induced stress. Commonly manifest with multiple cases in a group.

Clinical findings Most commonly encephalitis with brainstem and cranial nerve dysfunction or abortion in last third of pregnancy. Less commonly septicemia in periparturient and neonatal sheep and goats, enteritis in weaned sheep, spinal myelitis, uveitis, and occasionally mastitis.

Clinical pathology Culture, PCR. Pleocytosis and elevated protein in cerebrospinal fluid with encephalitis.

Lesions Microabscesses in brainstem in listerial encephalitis, spinal cord in spinal myelitis, abomasum, intestine, liver, and mesenteric lymph nodes in enteritis. Visceral lesions in septicemia.

Diagnostic confirmation Culture and histopathology.

Treatment Penicillin or oxytetracycline. Must be given early in clinical disease.

Control Control of listerial growth in feeds. Vaccination.

ETIOLOGY

There are currently six species classified within the genus *Listeria,* but only *L. monocytogenes* and *L. ivanovii* (previously classified as *L. monocytogenes* serotype 5) are pathogenic for domestic animals. *L. ivanovii* is only mildly pathogenic and is an occasional cause of abortion in sheep and cattle. Aborted fetuses have suppurative bronchopneumonia and lack the multifocal hepatocellular necrosis commonly seen in abortions associated with *L. monocytogenes. L. innocua* is occasionally associated with encephalitis in ruminants that is clinically and pathologically similar to that associated with *L. monocytogenes.* Most, but not all, reports of both infections record that the animals were being fed silage.

L. monocytogenes is widespread in nature and has characteristics that allow its survival and growth in a wide variety of environments. There is a highly diverse range of strains, some of which have the capability of causing disease in animals and humans.

Optimal growth temperatures are between 30°C and 37°C but the organism can grow and reproduce at temperatures between 1°C and 45°C. It can grow between pH 4.5 and 9.6 although growth at low pH is minimal at low temperatures. The organism is susceptible to common disinfectants.

L. monocytogenes can be divided into 16 serovars on the basis of somatic and flagellar antigens, and there is considerable genetic diversity between serovars. Serovars 4b, 1/2a and 1/2b, and 3 are most commonly isolated from diseased animals but there are geographic differences. Virulent strains can multiply in macrophages and monocytes and produce a hemolysin, listeriolysin O, which is thought to be a major virulence factor.

EPIDEMIOLOGY

Occurrence

Geographic

Although the organism is widespread in nature, clinical disease in animals occurs mainly in the northern and southern latitudes and is much less common in tropical and subtropical than in temperate climates. The disease is important in North America, Europe, the UK, New Zealand, and Australia.

Seasonal

In the northern hemispheres listeriosis has a distinct seasonal occurrence, probably associated with seasonal feeding of silage, with the highest prevalence in the months of December through May, but seasonal occurrence is not a feature in Australia.

Host

Listeriosis is primarily a disease of ruminants, particularly sheep, and the major diseases associated with *L. monocytogenes* are encephalitis and abortion. In ruminants it also produces syndromes of septicemia, spinal myelitis, uveitis, gastroenteritis, and mastitis. Occasional septicemic disease occurs in horses and pigs.

- **Encephalitis/meningitis** usually occurs sporadically, affecting a single animal in a herd or flock or a few individuals over several weeks. The mean attack rate in 50 affected flocks in Britain was 2.5% with a range of 0.1% to 13.3%. More serious outbreaks can occur with attack rates as high as 35% and cases occurring over a 2-month period. The disease occurs in sheep older than 6 weeks but may be more prevalent in lambs between 6 and 12 weeks of age and ewes over 2 years of age. The case–fatality is high, especially in sheep, because the short clinical course often precludes treatment.
- **Abortion** may also occur sporadically, which is usually true in cattle, but in sheep and goats it is more common as an outbreak with an attack rate that frequently approaches 10%.
- **Spinal myelitis** is an uncommon manifestation but is recorded as occurring in 0.8% to 2.5% of sheep in affected flocks and in all ages of sheep 4 weeks following spray dipping. Spinal myelitis also occurs sporadically in cattle 12 to 18 months of age.

- **Septicemic disease** is also a less common manifestation of infection with *L. monocytogenes* but can occur as an outbreak with a high case fatality in newborn lambs and kids and also in periparturient ewes and does.
- **Keratoconjunctivitis/uveitis** occurs in both sheep and cattle and has been associated with silage feeding from big bales or ring feeders. This condition presents a distinct entity that is not associated with systemic infection with *Listeria.*
- **Gastroenteritis** has been reported primarily by veterinary diagnostic labs in Great Britain and New Zealand as a sporadic disease affecting sheep after weaning. It occurs during the winter months most commonly in sheep fed baleage or silage. Cases occur 2 days or more after the onset of feeding. Less commonly, cases occur in sheep on root crops or on pasture where the quality of the pasture is poor and they are at high stocking densities.
- **Mastitis** is uncommon but can occur in cattle, sheep, and goats. It results in contamination of milk with *L. monocytogenes.* The more common source of *L. monocytogenes* in raw milk is fecal contamination. In a Danish study of quarter milk samples from over a million cows in 36,199 herds, 0.4% of cows had listerial mastitis and 1.2% of herds had infected cows.

Source of Infection

The organism is common in the environment and infection is not limited to agricultural animals. *L. monocytogenes* has been isolated from 42 species of mammals and 22 species of birds as well as fish, crustaceans, and insects. It is truly **ubiquitous in the environment** and can be commonly isolated from animal feces, human feces, farm slurry, sewerage sludge, soil, farm water troughs, surface water, plants, animal feeds, and the walls, floors, drains, and so forth of farms and other environments. The ability to form biofilms may assist in its survival in the environment and may assist in perpetuating its presence in water troughs on infected farms.

Most feed hays, grains, and formulated feeds have the potential to contain *L. monocytogenes* but, with most, low levels of available water restrict its multiplication.

In ruminants *L. monocytogenes* can be isolated from the feces and nasal secretions of healthy animals and has been isolated from the feces of cattle in 46% of 249 herds examined and from 82% of samples of feedstuffs. In a French survey 5% of small ruminant fecal samples were found positive for *L. monocytogenes.* Fecal material from wild birds in agricultural regions may also contain large amounts of *L. monocytogenes* that can contribute to the contamination of feed, water, bedding material, and soils.[1] Exposed sheep may become latent carriers, shedding the pathogen in feces and milk.[1]

In temperate climates the prevalence of *L. monocytogenes* in the feces of ruminants appears to vary with the season, being higher in the winter period. It is also increased during periods of environmental stress and in association with the stress of lambing and transport. The presence in feces and secretions can also be influenced by the number of the organism in feeds fed to the animals. In herds where there is a high proportion of cattle excreting in feces, the organism can be isolated from dried fecal dust on walls and most farm surfaces.

L. monocytogenes is not isolated from the feces or environment in all farms and its presence in isolable numbers is largely a reflection of its presence in feed, or the presence of animals with intestinal carriage. It is apparent that in some healthy herds and flocks there may be a multitude of different strains in the silage and feed, water troughs, feces, and environment in a single herd.

The presence of *L. monocytogenes* in bulk tank milk or milk filters is used as a measure of farm infection prevalence. Obviously this measure is influenced by the management and environmental conditions on farms that might result in fecal contamination of the teats. Although bulk tank and milk filter infection rates provide information of possible value to measures of environmental contamination and risk for human exposure, there is no evidence that this measure has any relationship to risk for animal disease on the farm being studied.

Silage

L. monocytogenes is commonly present in silage, but it does not multiply to any significant extent in effectively preserved silage, which is characterized by anaerobic storage, high density, a high concentration of organic acids, and a pH below 4.5. *Listeria* can multiply in silage above pH 5.0 to 5.5, the critical pH depending on the dry matter content. *L. monocytogenes* may be present in silage that is **poorly fermented,** but it can also occur in pockets of **aerobic deterioration** in otherwise good silage and this is most common. These areas are often indicated by mold growth and occur at the edges of the clamp and in the top few inches of the surface in plastic-covered clamps where air has circulated under the plastic. Thus the growth of *L. monocytogenes* is a surface problem in silage, except those that are poorly fermented, and occurs in small areas sporadically over the surface of a silage.

The risk for contamination of silage with *Listeria* is higher when it contains **soil**, which may be incorporated from molehills present in the field and in the front of the clamp during final packing. An **ash content** of greater than 70 mg/kg dry matter indicates soil contamination.

Big bale silage may have a higher risk for listerial infection than conventional silage because of its lower density, poor fermentation, greater surface area relative to clamp silage, and greater risk for mechanical damage to the plastic covering.

Moist preserved feeds other than grass silage are at risk for listerial growth; listeriosis is recorded, for example, in association with the feeding of moist brewers grains, wet spoiled hay bales, and silage made from commodity by-products such as orange and artichoke waste. A relatively rapid method for the quantitative assessment of the occurrence and distribution of *Listeria* in suspect silage is available.

Infective material also derives from infected animals in the feces, urine, aborted fetuses and uterine discharge, and in the milk. Although immediate spread among animals in a group has been demonstrated, field observations suggest that mediated contagion by means of inanimate objects also occurs. **Woody browse** may be a risk factor for goats.

Transmission

With septicemic disease and abortion, the organism is transmitted by ingestion of contaminated material. Lambs that develop septicemic disease may acquire infection from contamination on the ewe's teat, from the ingestion of milk containing the organism from ewes or does with subclinical bacteremia, through the navel from the environment, and also as a congenital infection. The encephalitic form of the disease results from infection of the terminals of the trigeminal nerve consequent to abrasions of the buccal mucosa from feed or browse or from infection of tooth cavities. Spinal myelitis is thought to result from growth up spinal nerves subsequent to body area infections.

Outbreaks of encephalitis that occur in sheep after introduction to silage usually commence about 3 to 4 weeks later, although there is wide variation, and one study of a large number of outbreaks found the median time of this period to be 44 days. This delay reflects the time for ascending infection.

Commonly, the serotype isolated from the brain of an affected animal is also present in the silage being fed. However, the recent development of methods for genetic analyses of *L. monocytogenes* has demonstrated that serotyping is a relatively crude tool for epidemiologic studies and in many instances, although the isolate from brain may be the same serotype as that from silage, there is no relationship on genetic analysis. Possibly this reflects differences in strains at different sites in silage and the difference between the time of sampling of the silage and the time when the affected cow ate it.

Septicemic disease in sheep and goats usually occurs within 2 days of introduction to silage and abortions 6 to 13 days later.

Risk Factors

Despite the ubiquity of *L. monocytogenes*, only a small proportion of animals develop clinical disease. A number of predisposing factors have been observed, or proposed, as risk factors for disease. These include factors that cause a lowering of the host animal's resistance and factors that increase the infection pressure of the organism. In farm animals the latter appear the most important.

Host Management Risk Factors

Observed risk factors include the following:

- Poor nutritional state
- Sudden changes of weather to very cold and wet
- Stress of late pregnancy and parturition
- Transport
- Long periods of flooding with resulting poor access to pasture

Differences in susceptibility between species are apparent with sheep being considerably more likely to develop clinical disease than cattle. Area outbreaks affecting several flocks can occur in sheep on poorly drained and muddy pastures following floods, but outbreaks are also described in droughts. Overcrowding and unsanitary conditions with poor access to feed supplies may predispose housed sheep.

Breed difference in susceptibility (Angora goats and Rambouillet sheep) has been observed in some studies but not in others.

Pathogen Risk Factors

Factors that increase the infection pressure largely involve a massive multiplication of *L. monocytogenes* in the feed or environment. The feeding of grass or corn silage as a major risk factor for the occurrence of listeriosis has been recognized for many decades. The increase in use of silage for feed in ruminants may be the reason for the apparent increase in the prevalence of the disease in recent years. Silage may also exert its effect by increasing the susceptibility of the host to listerial infection, although this has been disputed.

The organism persists for as long as 3 months in sheep feces and has been shown to survive for up to 11.5 months in damp soil, up to 16.5 months in cattle feces, up to 207 days on dry straw, and for more than 2 years in dry soil and feces. It is resistant to temperatures of −20°C (−6°F) for 2 years and is still viable after repeated freezing and thawing.

Experimental Reproduction

Oral or parenteral challenge of nonpregnant sheep and goats will produce a bacteremia with minor clinical signs of pyrexia and depression in animals with no preexisting antibody. Clinical disease is more severe in young animals and the infection clears with the development of an immune response. The challenge of animals with preexisting antibody is not associated with clinical disease, although there may be a bacteremia. Lactating animals secrete the organism in milk during the bacteremic period. Prior challenge of goats with *L. ivanovii* or *L. innocua* does not protect against subsequent challenge with *L. monocytogenes*.

Several studies have shown that oral, conjunctival, and parenteral challenge of **pregnant animals** results in more severe signs of septicemia and can be followed by **abortion**, although this is not an invariable sequel. Encephalitis has not been reproduced experimentally by intravenous challenge, although meningoencephalitis may occur following this route of challenge in young lambs. **Encephalitis** has been reproduced experimentally by the injection of organisms into the buccal mucosa or the tooth pulp cavity, with the organism traveling centripetally via the trigeminal nerve to reach the brainstem.

Zoonotic Implications

In humans, listeriosis is considered a foodborne infection of sporadic occurrence producing septicemia, meningoencephalitis, abortion, and infection in other organs as well as neonatal infection. Although outbreaks of listeriosis associated with contaminated food receive the most public attention, **sporadic listeriosis** is the more common presentation. Although all age groups are susceptible the disease incidence is the highest among people 65 years and older followed by young children (0–4 years) and immunocompromised patients.[2] In the EU a disease incidence of 0.3 and in the United States of 0.8 per 100,000 population have been reported.[1-4] The case fatality is high, and overall approximately 25% of reported cases die. Although the incidence increased at the beginning of the millennium, incidence rates have been stable over the last years.[4]

Although there is a potential for zoonotic transmission, the majority of human exposures to the organism, and the risk for disease, result from contamination of foods during processing and from the particular ability of the organism to grow at refrigerator temperature and in organic material with high salt content.

High disease prevalence and numbers of *L. monocytogenes* have been linked to certain foods such as soft cheese, smoked fish, pate, deli meats, unpasteurized milk, fermented raw meat sausages, hot dogs, and deli salads.[2,3]

Milk products have been incriminated in some outbreaks of the disease. Numerous studies have shown that *L. monocytogenes* is commonly present in low numbers (usually less than 1 organism per milliliter) in raw milk from some herds. In the vast majority of herds this is the result of fecal contamination during the milking process or other environmental contamination. Rarely, its presence in raw milk is from an animal with subclinical mastitis and in this case its numbers in bulk tank milk are much higher (2,000–5,000 organisms per milliliter), even when there is a single cow or goat with *L. monocytogenes* mastitis. In goats and sheep the presence in raw milk may also be the result of a subclinical bacteremia.

There have been concerns that the organism might survive pasteurization, especially if present in phagocytes. D-values for *Listeria* in milk have been determined to be in the range of 0.9 seconds at 71.1°C. The legal limit for high-temperature/short-time pasteurization in the United States is 71.7°C for 15 seconds, and this temperature is sufficient to inactivate numbers far beyond those present in raw milk. There is no evidence that the organism will survive correct pasteurization procedures.

Bulk tank infection rates are higher in winter and spring and cross-sectional and case–control studies have shown that the risk for detecting *L. monocytogenes* in bulk milk is higher in those herds that used a bucket milking system rather than a pipeline system. It is also higher in herds fed component feeds, fed leftover feed, fed from plastic feed bunks, and from feed bunks with a low frequency of cleaning, It is lower in herds that practice premilking teat disinfection.

Farmers or others who consume **raw milk** need to be aware of the risk of infection, especially if they fall within at-risk categories. There may be a particular risk with milk from goats and sheep fed silage. People associated with agriculture are also more liable to direct zoonotic transmission of listerial disease. **Dermatitis** with a papular and pustular rash occurs on the arms of **veterinarians** following the handling of infected dystocia cases and aborted fetuses. **Conjunctivitis** is also recorded in agricultural workers handling infected livestock.

Although *L. monocytogenes* rarely causes disease in **pigs,** it is present in the tonsils and feces of some pigs at slaughter and this presence is a potential source of contamination of the carcass and the slaughterhouse environment. There is a significantly higher prevalence in the tonsils of fattening pigs than in those of sows. The organism can be isolated from the floors, walls, and feed in pig units. Wet feeding, poor hygiene, and a short spelling period between batches of pigs in the finishing house have been found to be risk factors for infection in pigs. Paradoxically, disinfecting the pipeline used for wet feeding was associated with a higher risk of fecal contamination than no disinfection at all.

A further concern for indirect zoonotic risk of *L. monocytogenes* is the presence of the organism in the feces on infected farms and the potential for fecal or windborne dust spread to adjacent fields that may contain crops for human consumption.

PATHOGENESIS

In most animals, ingestion of the organism, with penetration of the mucosa of the intestine, leads to an inapparent infection with prolonged fecal excretion of the organism and to a subclinical bacteremia, which clears with the development of immunity. The bacteremic infection is frequently subclinical and may be accompanied by excretion of the organism in milk. Septicemic listeriosis, with or without meningitis, is most common in neonatal ruminants and in adult sheep and goats, particularly if they are pregnant and when the infection challenge is large.

The organism is a facultative intracellular pathogen that can infect cells, including intestinal cells, by directed endocytosis. It can survive and grow in macrophages and monocytes. Bacterial superoxide dismutase protects against the bactericidal activity of the respiratory burst of the phagocyte and listeriolysin O disrupts lysosomal membranes, allowing the organism to grow in the cytoplasm. The experimental mouse model indicates that cell-mediated immunity is important in protection against listerial infection, but studies in goats suggest that the clearance of bacteremic infection and resistance to infection are also strongly associated with humoral antibody.

In **pregnant animals,** invasion of the placenta and fetus may occur within 24 hours of the onset of bacteremia. Edema and necrosis of the placenta lead to **abortion,** usually 5 to 10 days postinfection. Infection late in pregnancy results in **stillbirths** or the delivery of young that rapidly develop a fatal septicemia. Maternal **metritis** is constant and if the fetus is retained a fatal listerial septicemia may follow. Infection of the uterus causing abortion and intrauterine infection occurs in all mammals.

Encephalitis/Meningitis

Encephalitis/meningitis in ruminants occurs as an acute inflammation of the brainstem or the meningeal membranes and is usually focal. Invasion of the CNS can occur by at least three different mechanisms.[5] These include the following:

- Retrograde (centripetal) migration into the brain within the axon of CNs
- Transport across the blood-brain barrier within parasitized leukocytes
- Direct invasion of endothelial cells by blood-borne bacteria

In cases without systemic infection centripetal translocation of the pathogen along the trigeminal or other CNs following penetration of the traumatized buccal mucosa, the shedding of deciduous or permanent teeth, and following periodontitis may result in encephalitis. Meningitis is thought to be associated with hematogenous translocation of the pathogen through parasitized endothelial cells or leukocytes.

The incubation period after experimental inoculation of the tooth pulp was at least 3 weeks even though lesions were detectable in the brainstem within 6 days of inoculation.[5] Clinical signs are characterized most strongly by an **asymmetric** disorder of CN function, in particular the trigeminal, facial, vestibular, and glossopharyngeal nerves, but there is some variation in the involvement of individual CNs depending on the distribution of lesions in the brainstem. Lesions in the sensory portion of the trigeminal nucleus and the facial nucleus are common and lead to ipsilateral facial hypalgesia and paralysis; involvement of the vestibular nucleus is also common and leads to ataxia with circling and a head tilt to the affected side. The additional signs of dullness, head-pressing, and delirium are referable to the more general effects of inflammation of the brain developing in the agonal stages. Spread of the infection along the optic nerve may result in endophthalmitis in sheep and cattle.

Spinal Myelitis

Spinal myelitis possibly results from ascending infection in the sensory nerves of the skin following dermatitis from prolonged wetting of the fleece.

Mastitis

L. monocytogenes is rarely found to be a cause of **clinical mastitis** in cattle, despite the fact that it can be common in the dairy environment, suggesting that this pathogen is not a particularly invasive or perpetuating organism for the udder. Infection of the mammary gland appears to primarily occur hematogenously.[1]

Enteritis

An acute diarrheal condition in sheep with clinical signs and morphologic changes resembling salmonellosis from which *L. monocytogenes* can be recovered has been recognized since the early 1990s.[6] Cases are frequently linked to feeding poor-quality silage and may occur within 2 days of feeding silage heavily contaminated with *L. monocytogenes.* The mechanisms through which *Listeria* invade the gastrointestinal mucosa are not yet understood, but infection seems to depend more on the ingested dose and the age of the animal than on predisposing conditions or immune status of the animal.[7] Lesions occur in the abomasum, small intestine, large intestine, mesenteric lymph nodes, and liver.[6]

CLINICAL FINDINGS

When disease occurs it is usual to have an outbreak of either encephalitis or abortion. Encephalitis is the most prevalent manifestation in sheep. Septicemia in lambs may occur in conjunction with abortion but it is rare to have all three syndromes on the same farm, at least in the same temporal period. There are always exceptions to such generalities, and the occurrence of septicemia, abortion, and encephalitis in a flock of sheep is possible.

Listerial Encephalitis/Meningitis

Sheep

In sheep, early signs are separation from the flock and depression with a hunched stance. Sheep approached during this early stage show a frenetic desire to escape but are uncoordinated because they run and fall easily. The syndrome progresses rapidly with more severe depression to the point of somnolence and the development of signs of CN dysfunction. Fever, usually 40°C (104°F) but occasionally as high as 42°C (107°F), is common in the early stages of the disease but the temperature is usually normal when overt clinical signs are present.

Signs vary between individual sheep but incoordination, head deviation sometimes with head tilt, walking in circles, unilateral facial hypalgesia, and facial paralysis are usually present. Facial hypalgesia can be detected with pressure from a hemostat, and the facial paralysis is manifested with drooping of the ear, paralysis of the lips, and ptosis on the same side of the face as the hypalgesia. This may be accompanied by exposure keratitis, often severe enough to cause corneal ulceration. Strabismus and nystagmus occur in some. Panophthalmitis, with pus evident in the anterior chamber of one or both eyes, is not uncommon in cattle that have been affected for a number of days. Also there is paresis of the muscles of the jaw, with poor tone or a dropped jaw, in which case prehension and mastication are slow and the animal may stand for long periods drooling saliva and with food hanging from its mouth.

The position of the head varies. In many cases there is deviation of the head to one side with the poll–nose relationship undisturbed (i.e., there is no rotation) but in others there is also head tilt. The head may be retroflexed or ventroflexed depending on the localization of the lesions and in some cases may be in a normal position. The deviation of the head cannot be corrected actively by the animal, and if it is corrected passively the head returns to its previous position as soon as it is released. Progression is usually in a small-diameter circle in the direction of the deviation. There is ataxia, often with consistent falling to one side, and an affected sheep may lean against the examiner or a fence. The affected animal becomes recumbent and is unable to rise, although often still able to move its legs. Death is caused by respiratory failure.

Cattle

In cattle, the clinical signs are essentially the same but the clinical course is longer (Fig. 14-16). In adult cattle the course of the disease is usually 1 to 2 weeks, but in sheep and calves the disease is more acute, with death occurring in 2 to 4 days.

Goats

In goats the disease is similar to that in the other species, but in the young goat the onset is very sudden and the course short, with death occurring in 2 to 3 days (Fig. 14-17).

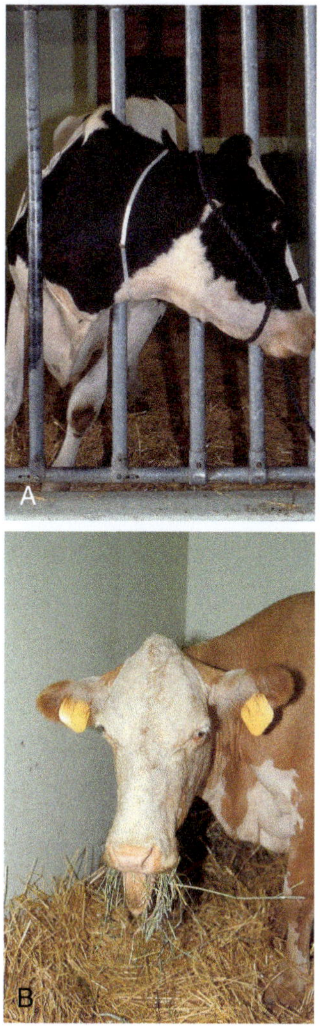

Fig. 14-16 **A,** Two-year-old Holstein Friesian heifer with listeriosis. The heifer is exhibiting clinical signs of a left brainstem lesion in the vicinity of the vestibulocochlear nerve nucleus (cranial nerve VIII) manifested as extensor thrust from the right side and tight circles to the left (circling is impeded by placement in the headgate). **B,** Three-year-old Simmental cow with listeriosis. The cow is exhibiting depression, weakness of the tongue and jaw muscles, and lack of sensation that she has hay in her mouth. Some of these clinical signs are also seen in cattle with rabies or esophageal obstruction (choke). Both animals responded well to intravenous oxytetracycline treatment.

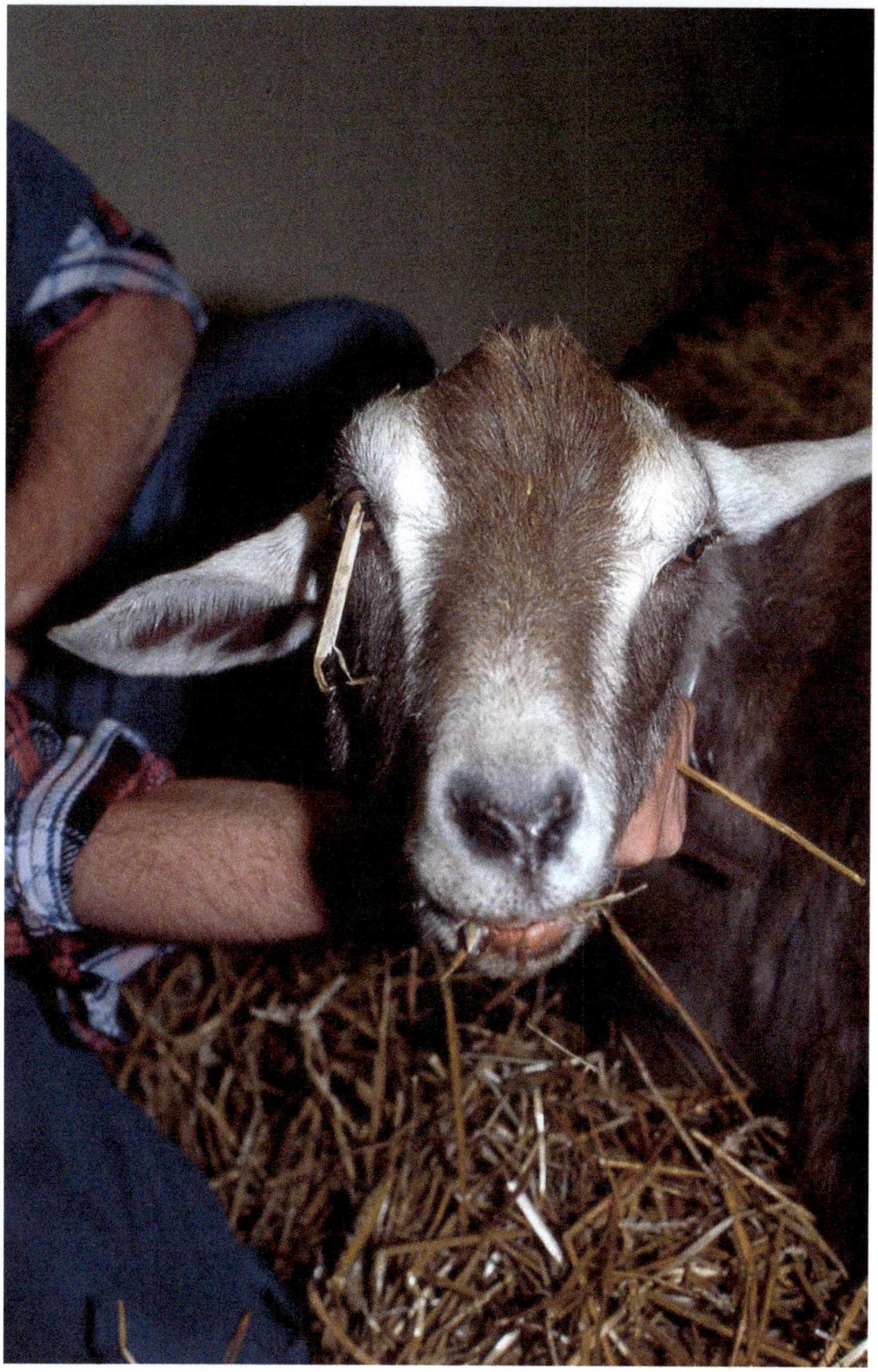

Fig. 14-17 Two-year-old goat with listeriosis. The goat has depression of the right corneal branch of the trigeminal nerve (cranial nerve V) because it does not detect the straw on its right eye, and the right facial nerve (cranial nerve VII) because it has a right ear droop, deviation of the philtrum to the left, and flaccid right upper lip. The goat was unable to stand and appeared depressed.

Listerial Abortion

Outbreaks of abortion are recorded in cattle but are more common in sheep and in goats. Abortion caused by this organism is rare in pigs.

Cattle

In cattle, abortion or stillbirth occurs sporadically and usually in the last third of pregnancy; retention of the afterbirth is common, in which case there is clinical illness and fever of up to 40.5°C (105°F). Abortion has been observed soon after the commencement of silage feeding but does not always have this association.

Sheep and Goats

In sheep and goats abortions occur from the 12th week of pregnancy onward, the afterbirth is usually retained, and there is a blood-stained vaginal discharge for several days. There may be some deaths of ewes from septicemia if the fetus is retained. In both species the rates of abortion in a group are low but may reach as high as 15%. On some farms, abortions recur each year.

Abortion Caused by *Listeria Ivanovii*

This occurs as a sporadic disease in cattle and has no distinguishing clinical features from that associated with *L. monocytogenes*. Outbreaks in sheep are manifested with abortion and stillbirth but particularly with the birth of live infected lambs, which seldom survive long enough to walk or suck.

Septicemic Listeriosis

Acute septicemia caused by *L. monocytogenes* is not common in adult ruminants but does occur in monogastric animals and in newborn lambs and calves. There are no signs suggestive of nervous system involvement, the syndrome being a general one comprising depression, weakness, emaciation, pyrexia, and diarrhea in some cases, with hepatic necrosis and gastroenteritis at necropsy. The same syndrome is also seen in ewes and goats after abortion if the fetus is retained. A better defined but less common syndrome has been described in calves 3 to 7 days old. Corneal opacity is accompanied by dyspnea, nystagmus, and mild opisthotonus. Death follows in about 12 hours. At necropsy there is ophthalmitis and serofibrinous meningitis. Septicemic listeriosis is recorded in a foal.

Mastitis

Infection in the udder may involve a single quarter or both quarters; it is chronic and poorly responsive to treatment. There is a high somatic cell count in milk from the affected quarter, but the milk appears normal.

Spinal Myelitis

There is fever, ataxia with initial knuckling of the hindlimbs progressing to hindlimb weakness, and paralysis. In some cases, both in sheep and cattle, there is also paresis and paralysis of the front limbs. There is no evidence of CN involvement, and affected animals are initially mentally alert, bright, and continue to eat. However, there is rapid deterioration and affected animals are commonly humanely destroyed.

Keratoconjunctivitis, Uveitis

There is swelling of the iris and constriction of the pupil; white focal lesions are evident on the internal surface of the cornea with floccular material in the anterior chamber. Advanced cases have pannus and corneal opacity.

Enteritis in Sheep

Reported clinical signs include lethargy, anorexia, and diarrhea or sudden death. Pregnant ewes may abort.

CLINICAL PATHOLOGY

The CSF in cases of encephalitis has a moderately to markedly increased protein concentration and leukocyte count. Neutrophils are the predominant cell type with lymphocytes contributing not more than 20% of cells.[8] *L. monocytogenes* is not detectable by culture or PCR.

The organism can be cultivated from vaginal secretions for up to 2 weeks after abortion, and a proportion of aborting animals also have *L. monocytogenes* in the milk and feces.

Serologic tests (agglutination and complement fixation tests) have been used but lack the predictive value required for diagnostic use. Ruminants commonly have antibody to *Listeria* and high titers are often encountered in normal animals in flocks and herds where there have been clinical cases. Nucleic acid–based techniques can be used to determine the source of a strain of *L. monocytogenes* in an outbreak.

NECROPSY FINDINGS

Typically, there are no distinctive gross changes associated with listerial **encephalitis**. Histologic examination of CNS tissue is necessary to demonstrate the microabscesses that are characteristic of the disease. These are present in the brainstem in listerial encephalitis and in the cervical and/or lumbar spinal cord in outbreaks of spinal myelitis. Sampling of the forebrain will typically result in a false-negative diagnosis. Cold enrichment techniques are advisable when attempting to isolate the organism. Gram staining of paraffin-embedded tissue may permit confirmation of the diagnosis in cases for which suitable culture material is unavailable. Alternative test methods such as fluorescent antibody or immunoperoxidase tests are available in some laboratories. In one retrospective study comparing diagnostic methods, immunoperoxidase staining was superior to bacterial culture when correlated with histopathologic changes.

Visceral lesions occur as multiple foci of necrosis in the liver, spleen, and myocardium in the **septicemic form** and in **aborted fetuses**. Aborted fetuses are usually edematous and autolyzed, with very large numbers of bacteria visible microscopically in a variety of tissues. In aborting dams, there is placentitis and endometritis in addition to the lesions in the fetus.

Sheep with **enteritis** show ulcerative and hemorrhagic abomasitis and reddening of the small intestinal mucosa.[6] In a small number of cases typhlocolitis is diagnosed at necropsy; histologically, there are microabscesses throughout the intestine and a characteristic infiltration of degenerating neutrophils in the mucosa lamina muscularis of the abomasum.[6]

Samples for Confirmation of Diagnosis

Central Nervous System Listeriosis

- **Bacteriology:** half of midsagittally sectioned brain, **including brainstem**, chilled or frozen (CULT, FAT)
- **Histology**: formalin-fixed half of midsagittally sectioned brain, **including brainstem**; appropriate segment of spinal cord if spinal myelitis suspected (LM, IHC)

Septicemia and Abortion

- **Bacteriology:** chilled liver, spleen, lung, placenta, fetal stomach content (CULT, FAT)
- **Histology:** formalin-fixed liver, spleen, lung, brain, placenta, fetal intestine (LM, IHC).

Enteritis

- **Bacteriology:** abomasum, small intestine, large intestine, mesenterial lymph nodes (CULT)
- **Histology:** formalin-fixed abomasum, small intestine, large intestine, mesenterial lymph nodes (LM, IHC).

DIFFERENTIAL DIAGNOSIS

Encephalitis
- Pregnancy toxemia in sheep
- Nervous ketosis in cattle
- Rabies
- Gid
- Polioencephalomalacia
- Middle ear disease
- Scrapie

Abortion
- Sheep
- Cattle

Gastroenteritis
- Salmonellosis

Keratoconjunctivitis/Uveitis
- Contagious ophthalmia
- Infectious bovine keratoconjunctivitis

TREATMENT

Penicillin is considered the drug of choice for treatment of listeriosis but it only has a bacteriostatic effect on *L. monocytogenes*.[2] Cephalosporins are ineffective because of minimal or nonexistent affinity of listerial penicillin-binding protein 3 and 5.[2,5]

A recent study exploring the prevalence of in vitro resistance of *L. monocytogenes* strains isolated from dairy farms found all strains to be resistant to cephalosporins, streptomycin, and trimethoprim. Over 90% of isolated strains were resistant to ampicillin and 66% were resistant to florfenicol. Resistance to penicillin G was determined for 40% of isolated strains.[9]

Penicillin administered at a dose of 44 000 IU/kg BW every 12 hours or every 24 hours given intramuscularly for 10 to 14 days is among the most commonly used treatments for listerial encephalitis/meningitis. Initiating the therapy with a loading dose of penicillin of 200,000 IU/kg as a water-soluble formulation given intravenously has been proposed.[10] The intravenous treatment of oxytetracycline (10 mg/kg BW every 12 hours or 20 mg /kg BW every 24 hours for 10 days) has been reported as being reasonably effective in meningoencephalitis of cattle but less so in sheep.

The use of nonsteroidal antiinflammatory drugs (NSAIDs) to address pain resulting from meningitis may be indicated but warrants close monitoring of the patient's hydration status to prevent renal damage. The use of glucocorticoids has been proposed with the objective to prevent abscess formation in the CNS.[1] Concerns have been raised since increased listerial shedding through milk was reported in cattle infected with *L. monocytogenes* treated with dexamethasone.[11]

The recovery rate depends largely on the time that treatment is started after the onset of clinical signs. If severe clinical signs are already evident, death usually follows in spite of treatment. Usually the course of events in an outbreak is that the first case dies but subsequent cases are detected sufficiently early for treatment. Dehydration, acid-base imbalances, and electrolyte disturbances must also be corrected. Cases of spinal myelitis are poorly responsive to treatment.

Treatment of listerial iritis is with systemic antibiotics in the early stages coupled with subpalpebral corticosteroid and atropine to dilate the pupil.

Supportive treatment with thiamine, to compensate for decreased thiamine production during the disease, and glucocorticoids to prevent formation of microabscesses in the CNS have been proposed. Correction of metabolic acidosis, resulting from excessive bicarbonate loss with drooling saliva, may be indicated.

TREATMENT AND CONTROL

Treatment

Encephalitis

Procaine penicillin G (200,000 IU/kg IV as initial loading dose) (R-2)

Procaine penicillin G (22,000 IU/kg every 12 hours or 44,000 IU/kg every 24 hours IM, for 10–14 days (R-2)

Oxytetracycline (10 mg/kg IV every 12 hours or 20 mg/kg IV every 24 hours for 10–14 days) (R-2)

Cephalosporins (R-4)

Thiamine (10 mg/kg slow IV every 24 hours) (R-2)

Flunixin meglumine (1 mg/kg every 24 hours IV) (R-2)

Dexamethasone (1 mg/kg IV single treatment) (R-3)

Control

Ensure pH of silage is < 5.0 (R-2)

Don't feed strongly spoiled sections of silage (R-2)

IM, intramuscularly; IV, intravenously.

CONTROL

Control is difficult because of the ubiquitous occurrence of the organism, the lack of a simple method of determining when it is present in high numbers in the environment, and a poor understanding of the risk factors other than silage. Where the risk factor is silage, there may be some merit in the recommendation that a change of diet to include heavy feeding of silage should be made slowly, particularly if the silage is spoiled or if listeriosis has occurred on the premises previously. Tetracyclines can be fed in the ration of animals at risk in a feedlot. When possible, the obviously spoiled areas of silage should be separated and not fed.

Other recommendations on the feeding of silage include avoid making silage from fields in which molehills may have contaminated the grass; avoid soil contamination when filling the clamp; avoid using additives to improve fermentation; and avoid silage that is obviously decayed, or with a pH of greater than 5 or an ash content of more than 70 mg/kg of dry matter.

Silage removed from the clamp should be fed as soon as possible.

Where uveitis is a problem, feeding systems that avoid eye contact with silage should be used.

A live attenuated **vaccine** has been shown to induce protection against intravenous challenge, and a live attenuated vaccine in use in Norway for several years is reported to reduce the annual incidence of the disease in sheep from 4% to 1.5%. An economic model is available for determining whether vaccination should be practiced. Commercial killed vaccines are available for the control of the disease in some countries, and some companies will also produce autogenous vaccines on request. The efficacy of vaccination still requires further determination; however, when economics or food availability on the farm dictate that contaminated silage must be fed, consideration might be given to vaccination as a means of providing some protection.

FURTHER READING

Anon. *Listeria monocytogenes*. Recommendations by the national advisory committee on microbiological criteria for foods. *Int J Food Microbiol*. 1991;14:185-246.

Drevets DA, Bronze MS. Listeria monocytogenes: epidemiology human disease, and mechanisms of brain invasion. *Immunol Med Microbiol*. 2008;53:151-165.

Farber JM, Peterkin PI. *Listeria monocytogenes*, a food-borne pathogen. *Microbiol Rev*. 1991;55:476-511.

Fenlon DR. Listeria monocytogenes in the natural environment. In: Ryser ET, Martin EH, eds. *Listeria, Listeriosis and Food Safety*. 2nd ed. New York: Marcel Dekker; 1998.

Gitter M. Veterinary aspects of listeriosis. *PHLS Microb Dig*. 1989;6(2):38-42.

Gray ML, Killinger AH. *Listeria monocytogenes* and listeric infections. *Bacteriol Rev*. 1966;30:309.

Low JC, Donachie W. A review of *Listeria monocytogenes* and listeriosis. *Vet J*. 1997;153:9-29.

Scarratt WK. Ovine listeric encephalitis. *Compend Contin Educ Pract Vet*. 1987;9:F28-F32.

REFERENCES

1. Brugere-Picoux J. *Small Rum Res*. 2008;76:12.
2. Allerberger F, Wagner M. *Clin Microbiol Infect*. 2010;16:16.
3. Kramarenko T, et al. *Food Control*. 2013;30:24.
4. European centre for disease prevention and disease control. Annual epidemiological report 2012. (Accessed 29.09.2013, at http://www.ecdc.europa.eu/en/publications/Publications/Annual-Epidemiological-Report-2012.pdf.).
5. Drevets DA, Bronze MS. *Immunol Med Microbiol*. 2008;53:151.
6. Fairley RA, et al. *J Comp Pathol*. 2012;146:308.
7. Zundel E, Bernard S. *J Med Microbiol*. 2006;55:1717.
8. Scott PR. *Small Rum Res*. 2010;92:96.
9. Srinivasan V, et al. *Foodborne Pathog Dis*. 2005;2:201.
10. Scott PR. *Small Rum Res*. 2013;110:138.
11. Welsley IV, et al. *Am J Vet Res*. 1989;50:2009.

Diseases Primarily Affecting the Spinal Cord

TRAUMATIC INJURY

Sudden severe trauma to the spinal cord causes a syndrome of immediate, complete, flaccid paralysis caudal to the injury because of spinal shock. This is so brief in animals it is hardly recognizable clinically. Spinal shock is soon followed by flaccid paralysis in the area supplied by the injured segment and spastic paralysis caudal to it.

ETIOLOGY

Trauma is the most common cause of monoplegia in large animals. There are varying degrees of loss of sensation, paresis, paralysis, and atrophy of muscle.

Physical Trauma

- Animals falling off vehicles, through barn floors
- Osteoporotic or osteodystrophic animals, especially aged broodmares and sows, spontaneously while jumping or leaning on fences
- Spondylosis and fracture of thoracolumbar vertebrae in old bulls in insemination centers
- Cervical vertebral fractures account for a large percentage of spinal cord injuries in horses
- Trauma caused by excessive mobility of upper cervical vertebrae may contribute to the spinal cord lesion in wobbles in horses
- Dislocations of the atlantooccipital joint are being reported increasingly
- Stenosis of the cervical vertebral canal at C2-C4 in young rams, probably as a result of head-butting
- Fracture of T1 vertebra in calves turning violently in an alleyway wide enough to admit cows
- Vertebral fractures in 7- to 10-month-old calves escaping under the headgate of a chute and forcefully hitting their

backs (just cranial to the tuber coxae) on the bottom rail of the gate
- Vertebral fractures in neonatal calves associated with forced extraction during dystocia
- Lightning strike may cause tissue destruction within the vertebral canal.

Parasitic Invasion

- Cerebrospinal nematodiasis, e.g., *P. tenuis, Setaria* spp. in goats and sheep, *Stephanurus dentatus* in pigs, *P. tenuis* in moose, causing moose sickness
- *Toxocara canis* experimentally in pigs
- *S. vulgaris* in horses and donkeys
- *Hypoderma bovis* larvae in cattle

Local Ischemia of the Spinal Cord

- Obstruction to blood flow to the cord by embolism, or of drainage by compression of the caudal vena cava, e.g., in horses during prolonged dorsal recumbency under general anesthesia; in pigs caused by fibrocartilaginous emboli, probably originating in injury to the nucleus pulposus of an intervertebral disk

PATHOGENESIS

The lesion may consist of disruption of nervous tissue or its compression by displaced bone or hematoma. Minor degrees of damage may result in local edema or hyperemia or, in the absence of macroscopic lesions, transitory injury to nerve cells, classified as concussion. The initial response is that of spinal shock, which affects a variable number of segments on both sides of the injured segment and is manifested by complete flaccid paralysis. The lesion must affect at least the ventral third of the cord before spinal shock occurs. When the shock wears off, the effects of the residual lesion remain. These may be temporary in themselves and completely normal function may return as the edema or the hemorrhage is resorbed. In sheep, extensive experimental damage to the cord may be followed by recovery to the point of being able to walk, but not sufficiently to be of any practical significance.

Traumatic lesions usually affect the whole cross-section of the cord and produce a syndrome typical of complete transection. Partial transection signs are more common in slowly developing lesions. Most of the motor and sensory functions can be maintained in 3-month-old calves with experimental left hemisection of the spinal cord.

In a retrospective study of dystocia-related vertebral fractures in neonatal calves, all the fractures were located between T11 and L4, with 77% occurring at the thoracolumbar junction. All but one case was associated with a forced extraction using unspecified (53%), mechanical (28%), or manual (17%) methods of extraction. Traction is most commonly applied after the fetus has entered the pelvic canal. Manual traction varies from 75 kg of pressure applied by one man to 260 kg of pressure applied by three or more men. The forces applied in mechanical traction vary from 400 kg for a calf puller to over 500 kg for a tractor. The transfer of these forces to the vertebrae and to the physeal plates at the thoracolumbar junction could readily cause severe tissue damage. In a prospective study of vertebral fractures in newborn calves, all fractures were located at the thoracolumbar area, especially the posterior epiphysis of T13.

CLINICAL FINDINGS

Spinal shock develops immediately after severe injury and is manifested by flaccid paralysis (reflex loss) caudal to a severe spinal cord lesion. There is a concurrent fall in local blood pressure caused by vasodilatation and there may be local sweating. Stretch and flexor reflexes and cutaneous sensitivity disappear but reappear within a half to several hours, although hypotonia may remain. The extremities are affected in most cases and the animal is unable to rise and may be in sternal or lateral recumbency. The muscles of respiration may also be affected, resulting in interference with respiration. The body area supplied by the affected segments will eventually show flaccid paralysis and disappearance of reflexes and muscle wasting, all representative of a lower motor neuron lesion.

When the injury is caused by invasion by parasitic larvae, there is no stage of spinal shock but the onset is acute, although there may be subsequent increments of paralysis as the larva moves to a new site.

Neonatal calves with dystocia-related vertebral fractures are weak immediately after birth or remain recumbent and make no effort to rise.

Sensation may be reduced at and caudal to the lesion, and hyperesthesia may be observed in a girdle-like zone at the cranial edge of the lesion as a result of irritation of sensory fibers by local inflammation and edema. Because of interference with the sacral autonomic nerve outflow there may be paralysis of the bladder and rectum, although this is not usually apparent in large animals. The vertebral column should be examined carefully for signs of injury. Excessive mobility, pain on pressure, and malalignment of spinous processes may indicate bone displacements or fractures. Rectal examination may also reveal damage or displacement, particularly in fractures of vertebral bodies and in old bulls with spondylosis.

Residual signs may remain when the shock passes off. This usually consists of paralysis, which varies in extent and severity with the lesion. The paralysis is apparent caudal to and at the site of the lesion. The reflexes return except at the site of the lesion. There is usually no systemic disturbance but pain may be sufficiently severe to cause an increase in heart rate and prevent eating.

Recovery may occur in 1 to 3 weeks if nervous tissue is not destroyed, but when extensive damage has been done to a significantly large section of the cord there is no recovery and disposal is advisable. In rare cases animals that suffer a severe injury continue to be ambulatory for up to 12 hours before paralysis occurs. In such instances it may be that a fracture occurs but displacement follows at a later stage during more active movement. Recovered animals may be left with residual nervous deficits or with postural changes such as torticollis.

Fracture of the Cervical Vertebrae in Horses

In horses fracture/dislocation of cranial cervical vertebrae is fairly common. Affected animals are recumbent and unable to lift the head from the ground. However, they may be fully conscious and able to eat and drink.[1] It may be possible to palpate the lesion, but a radiograph is usually necessary. Lesions of the caudal cervical vertebrae may permit lifting of the head but the limbs are not moved voluntarily. In all cases the tendon and withdrawal reflexes in the limbs are normal to supernormal.

Spondylosis in Bulls

Old bulls in artificial insemination centers develop calcification of the ventral vertebral ligaments and subsequent spondylosis or rigidity of the lumbar area of the vertebral column. When the bull ejaculates vigorously, the calcified ligaments may fracture, and this discontinuity may extend upward through the vertebral body. The ossification is extensive, usually from about T2-L3, but the fractures are restricted to the midlumbar region. There is partial displacement of the vertebral canal and compression of the cord. The bull is usually recumbent immediately after the fracture occurs but may rise and walk stiffly several days later. Arching of the back, slow movement, trunk rigidity, and sometimes unilateral lameness are characteristic signs. Less severe degrees of spondylosis have been recorded in a high proportion of much younger (2- to 3-year-old) bulls, but the lesions do not appear to cause clinical signs.

CLINICAL PATHOLOGY

Radiologic examination may reveal the site and extent of the injury, depending on the amount of surrounding muscle mass. CSF obtained from the lumbosacral space may reveal the presence of xanthochromia or intact RBCs, suggesting preexisting hemorrhage.

NECROPSY FINDINGS

The abnormality is always visible on macroscopic examination. In neonatal calves with dystocia-related vertebral fractures, hemorrhage around the kidneys, around the adrenal glands, and in the perivertebral muscles is a common finding and a useful indicator that a thoracolumbar fracture is present. In addition to the vertebral fracture, subdural and epidural hemorrhage, myelomalacia, spinal cord compression, severed spinal cord, and fractured ribs are common findings.

DIFFERENTIAL DIAGNOSIS

Differentiation from other spinal cord diseases is not usually difficult because of the speed of onset and the history of trauma, although spinal myelitis and meningitis may also develop rapidly. Other causes of recumbency may be confused with trauma, especially if the animal is not observed in the immediate preclinical period. In most diseases characterized by recumbency, such as azoturia, acute rumen impaction, and acute coliform mastitis, there are other signs to indicate the existence of a lesion other than spinal cord trauma. White muscle disease in foals is characterized by weakness, and the serum creatine kinase activity will be increased.

TREATMENT

Treatment is expectant only, and surgical treatment is rarely attempted. Large doses of corticosteroids or nonsteroidal antiinflammatory agents are recommended to minimize the edema associated with the spinal cord injury. Careful nursing on deep bedding with turning at 3-hour intervals (ideally, but at least 3 times a day in animals that are not "creepers"), massage of bony prominences, and periodic slinging may help to carry an animal with concussion or other minor lesion through a long period of recumbency. In well-muscled cattle especially, recumbency beyond a period of about 48 hours is likely to result in widespread necrosis of the caudal muscles of the thigh and recovery in such cases is improbable. A definitive diagnosis of a vertebral fracture with paralysis usually warrants a recommendation for euthanasia.

FURTHER READING

Divers TJ. Acquired spinal cord and peripheral nerve disease. *Vet Clin North Am Food Anim Pract.* 2004;20:231-242.

Dyson SJ. Lesions of the equine neck resulting in lameness of poor performance. *Vet Clin North Am Equine Pract.* 2011;27:417-437.

REFERENCE

1. Muno J, et al. *Equine Vet Educ.* 2009;21:527.

SPINAL CORD COMPRESSION

The gradual development of a space-occupying lesion in the vertebral canal produces a syndrome of progressive weakness and paralysis. A preexisting inflammatory or neoplastic lesion of the vertebral body may result in spontaneous fracture of the vertebral body and compression of the spinal cord.

ETIOLOGY

Compression of the spinal cord occurs from space-occupying lesions in the vertebral canal; the common ones are as follows.

Tumors

The most commonly occurring tumor in animals is lymphomatosis in which the nerve trunks and invades the vertebral canal, usually in the lumbosacral region and less commonly in the brachial and cervical areas. This tumor is particularly common in adult cattle with multicentric lymphosarcoma caused by bovine leukosis virus infection (Fig. 14-18).

Rare tumors include fibrosarcomas, metastases, plasma cell myeloma, angioma, melanoma in a horse, hemangiosarcoma in a horse, neurofibroma, and lymphosarcoma, e.g., in horses, vascular hamartoma in a goat.

Vertebral Body or Epidural Abscess

Vertebral body abscesses (osteomyelitis) are most common in neonatal farm animals and are generally in association with a chronic suppurative lesion elsewhere in the body.

- Docking wounds in lambs, bite wounds in pigs, and chronic suppurative pneumonia in calves are common occurrences for vertebral body abscesses. Polyarthritis and endocarditis may also be present. The original site of infection may have resolved when the clinical signs referable to the spinal cord abscess appear.
- Compression of the spinal cord is caused by enlargement of the vertebral body abscess into the vertebral canal and there may or may not be deviation of the vertebral canal and its contents.[1] Epidural abscesses causing compression

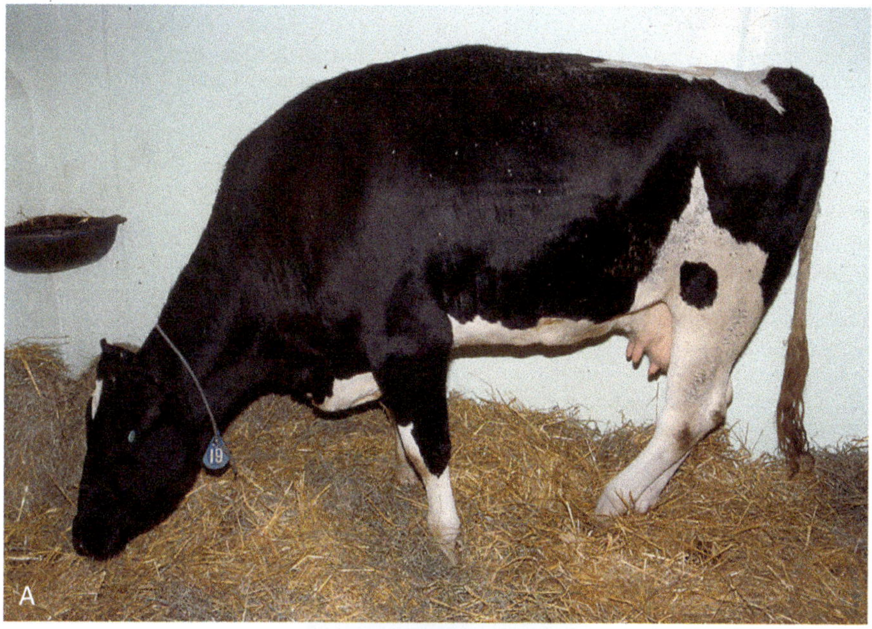

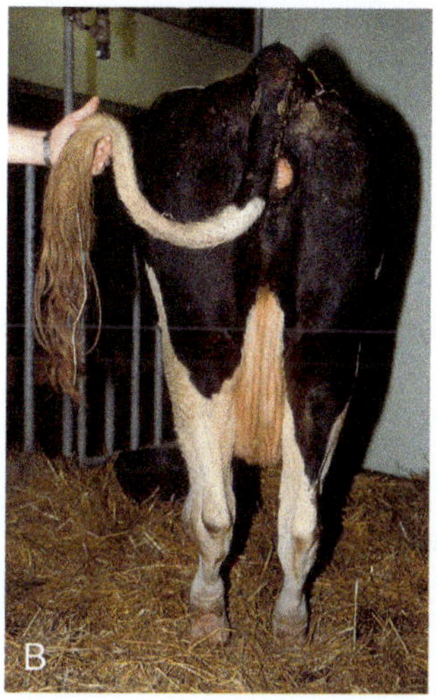

Fig. 14-18 **A,** Bilateral posterior paresis in a 5-year-old Holstein Friesian cow with spinal lymphosarcoma caused by infection with enzootic bovine leukosis virus. **B,** Caudal view of the same cow, demonstrating marked paresis of the tail and hindlegs and poor milk production.

of the spinal cord, and not associated with vertebral bodies, occur in lambs.
- Hematogenous spread may also occur from *Trueperella* (*Arcanobacterium* or *Actinomyces* or *Corynebacterium*) *pyogenes* in cattle, *A. bovis* in cattle with lumpy jaw, and *Corynebacterium pseudotuberculosis* in sheep.
- Multiple cases of compressive myelopathy have been reported in cattle following intramuscular injection of an oil containing vaccine in the lumbar area.[2]
- Cervical myelomalacia in a lamb and an alpaca developed after attempted intramuscular injections in the neck[3]
- A pyogranulomatous lesion in the sacral region of horse extended into the sacral vertebral canal, resulting in reduced anal and tail tone and urinary overflow incontinence.[4]

Bony Lesions of Vertebra

- Exostoses over fractures with no displacement of vertebral bodies.
- Similar exostoses on vertebral bodies of lambs grazing around old lead mines.
- Hypovitaminosis A in young growing pigs causing compression of the nerve roots passing through the vertebral foramina.
- Congenital deformity or fusion of the atlantooccipital axial joints in calves, foals, and goats.
- Congenital spinal stenosis of calves.
- Protrusion of an intervertebral disk is identifiable by myelogram or at necropsy,[5] although rare in large animals. The degenerative lesions in disks in the neck of the horse resemble the Hansen type 2 disk prolapses in dogs.
- Progressive paresis and ataxia also occur rarely in diskospondylitis in horses, an inflammatory condition focused on a single intervertebral joint that often results from a septic process.[6,7] Diskospondylitis has been diagnosed in a 4-month-old calf with a stiff gait and umbilical abscess,[8] an adult goat with paraplegia,[9] and an alpaca with paraparesis.[10]
- Spondylosis occurs, which is a degenerative condition characterized by extensive osteophytes on the vertebral body axis. *Spondylus* is an old Greek name meaning vertebra. Spondylosis usually affects the ventral or lateral aspects of multiple adjacent vertebrae. It is a progressive disease affecting contiguous vertebrae because of biomechanical stresses.[6] Ankylosing spondylosis typically cause lameness rather than compression of cord and paresis/paralysis.

Adult sows and boars may have degeneration of intervertebral disks and surrounding vertebral osteophytes. Less commonly are ankylosing spondylosis, arthrosis of articular facets, defects in annulus fibrosus and vertebral end plates, and vertebral osteomyelitis or fracture. These lesions of ankylosing spondylosis cause lameness in boars and sows rather than compression of cord and paresis/paralysis. These are not to be confused with the many extravertebral causes of posterior lameness or paralysis in adult pigs, which are discussed in Chapter 15.

Vertebral Subluxation or Compressive Myelopathy

- Cervicothoracic vertebral subluxation in Merino sheep in Australia and Columbia lambs in the United States
- Compressive cervical myelopathy in yearling Texel and Beltex sheep caused by fatty nodules encroaching into the dorsal vertebral canal at C6-C7[11]

Ataxia in Horses

This is a major problem and has numerous potential causes:
- Nonfatal fractures of the skull (basisphenoid, basioccipital, and petrous temporal bones)
- Nonfatal cervical fractures
- Atlantooccipital instability
- Cervical vertebral malformation (equine cervical vertebral stenotic myelopathy) caused by stenosis of the cranial vertebral orifice of C3-C7[12]; this may be effective as a compression mechanism only if the vertebrae adopt exaggerated positions
- Abnormal growth of interarticular surfaces
- Dorsal enlargement of caudal vertebral epiphyses and bulging of intervertebral disks
- Formation and protrusion of false joint capsules and extrasynovial bursae
- Spinal myelitis caused by parasitic invasion or EHV-1 virus, even louping-ill virus and probably others
- Spinal abscess usually in a vertebral body
- *Onchocerca* sp.–induced spinal cord compression and axonopathy[13]
- Spinal hematomas[14] causing ataxia, paresis, and neck pain
- Cerebellar hypoplasia (most commonly the inherited version in Arabian foals)
- Degenerative myelomalacia/myelopathy (cause unknown)
- Fusion of occipital bone with the atlas, which is fused with the axis
- Hypoxic–ischemic neuromyopathy in aortoiliac thrombosis
- Tumors of the meninges

PATHOGENESIS

The development of any of the lesions listed previously results in the gradual appearance of motor paralysis or hypoesthesia, depending on whether the lesion is ventrally or dorsally situated. In most cases there is involvement of all motor and sensory tracts, but care is necessary in examination if the more bizarre lesions are to be accurately diagnosed. There may be hemiparesis or hemiplegia if the lesion is laterally situated. Paraparesis or paraplegia is caused by a bilateral lesion in the thoracic or lumbar cord and monoplegia by a unilateral lesion in the same area. Bilateral lesions in the cervical region cause tetraparesis to tetraplegia (quadriplegia).

Vertebral osteomyelitis in young calves is most common in the thoracolumbar vertebrae and less commonly in the cervical vertebrae. The abscess of the vertebral body gradually enlarges and causes gradual compression of the spinal cord, which causes varying degrees of paresis of the pelvic limbs and ataxia. The abscess may extend into adjacent intervertebral spaces and result in vertebral arthritis with lysis of the articular facets. The onset of paresis and paralysis may be sudden in cases of abscessation or osteomyelitis of the vertebrae, which may fracture and cause displacement of bony fragments into the vertebral canal with compression and traumatic injury of the spinal cord. Vertebral body abscesses between T2 and the lumbar plexus will result in weakness of the pelvic limbs and normal flexor withdrawal reflexes of the pelvic limbs. Lesions at the site of the lumbar plexus will result in flaccid paralysis of the pelvic limbs.

In horses with cervical vertebral malformation, compression of the spinal cord results in necrosis of white matter and some focal loss of neurons. With time, secondary wallerian-like neuron fiber degeneration in ascending white matter tracts cranial to the focal lesion and in descending white matter tracts caudal to the lesion occurs. Astrocytic gliosis is a prominent and persistent alteration of the spinal cord of horses with chronic cervical compressive myelopathy and is associated with nerve fiber degeneration at the level of the compression and in well-delineated areas of ascending and descending nerve fiber tracts. It is possible that the persistent astrocytic gliosis may prevent, or slow, recovery of neurologic function in affected horses.

CLINICAL FINDINGS

Varying degrees of progressive weakness of the thoracic limbs or pelvic limbs may be the initial clinical findings. With most lesions causing gradual spinal cord compression, difficulty in rising is the first sign, then unsteadiness during walking caused by weakness, which may be more marked in one of a pair of limbs. The toes are dragged along the ground while walking and the animal knuckles over on the fetlocks when standing. Finally, the animal can rise only with assistance and then becomes permanently recumbent. These stages may be passed through in a period of 4 to 5 days.

The paralysis will be flaccid or spastic depending on the site of the lesion and reflexes will be absent or exaggerated in the respective states. The dog-sitting position in large animals is compatible with a spinal lesion caudal to the second thoracic vertebral segment. Calves with vertebral osteomyelitis caudal to T2 are usually able to sit up in the dog-sitting position; they are bright and alert and will suck the cow if held up to the teat. In some cases, extensor rigidity of the thoracic limbs resembles the Schiff–Sherrington syndrome and indicates a lesion of the thoracic vertebrae.

Lesions involving the lumbar plexus will result in flaccid paralysis of the pelvic limbs and an absence of the flexor withdrawal reflexes. Lesions involving the sacrococcygeal vertebrae will cause a decrease in tail tone, decreased or absent perineal reflex, and urinary bladder distension.

Pain and hyperesthesia may be evident before motor paralysis appears. The pain may be constant or occur only with movement. In vertebral body osteomyelitis in the horse, vertebral column pain and a fever may be the earliest clinical abnormalities. With neoplasms of the epidural space, the weakness and motor paralysis gradually worsen as the tumor enlarges.

Considerable variation in signs occurs depending on the site of the lesion. There may be local hyperesthesia around the site of the lesion and straining to defecate may be pronounced. Retention of the urine and feces may occur. There is usually no detectable abnormality of the vertebrae on physical examination.

Calves with congenital spinal stenosis are usually unable to stand or can do so only if assisted. There are varying degrees of weakness and ataxia of the pelvic limbs. They are bright and alert and will suck the cow if assisted. Those that survive for several weeks will sometimes assume the dog-sitting position.

In the wobbler horse, circumduction of the limbs with ataxia is typical. The ataxia is usually pronounced in the pelvic limbs, and weakness is evident by toe dragging and the ease with which the horse can be pulled to one side while walking. Ataxia with hypometria is often evident in the thoracic limbs, especially while walking the horse on a slope and with the head elevated.

CLINICAL PATHOLOGY

Radiographic examination of the vertebral column should be performed if the animal is of a suitable size. Myelography is necessary to demonstrate impingement on the spinal cord by a stenotic vertebral canal. The **CSF** may show a cellular reaction if there is some invasion of the spinal canal.

NECROPSY FINDINGS

Gross abnormalities of the vertebrae and the bony spinal canal are usually obvious. Those diseases of the spinal cord characterized by degeneration without gross changes require histologic techniques for a diagnosis.

DIFFERENTIAL DIAGNOSIS

Differentiation between abscess, tumor, and exostosis in the vertebral canal is usually not practicable without radiographic examination. Vertebral osteomyelitis is difficult to detect radiographically, particularly in large animals, because of the overlying tissue. In bovine lymphosarcoma there are frequently signs caused by lesions in other organs. A history of previous trauma may suggest exostosis. The history usually serves to differentiate the lesion from acute trauma.

- Spinal myelitis, myelomalacia, and meningitis may resemble cord compression but are much less common. They are usually associated with encephalitis, encephalomalacia, and cerebral meningitis, respectively.
- Meningitis is characterized by much more severe hyperesthesia and muscle rigidity.
- Rabies in the dumb form may be characterized by a similar syndrome but ascends the cord and is fatal within a 6-day period.

In the newborn there are many congenital defects in which there is defective development of the spinal cord. Most of them are not characterized by compression of the cord, because the diminished function is caused in most cases by an absence of tissue. **Spina bifida**, **syringomyelia**, and **dysraphism** are characterized by hindquarter paralysis or, if the animal is able to stand, by a wide-based stance and overextension of the legs when walking. Some animals are clinically normal.

A generalized degeneration of peripheral nerves such as that described in pigs and cattle causes a similar clinical syndrome and so does **polyradiculoneuritis**. A nonsuppurative **ependymitis**, **meningitis**, and **encephalomyelitis**, such as occurs in equine infectious anemia, may also cause an ataxia syndrome in horses.

Paresis or paralysis of one limb (monoplegia) is caused by lesions in the ventral gray matter, nerve roots, brachial and lumbosacral plexus, and peripheral nerves and muscles of the limbs.

TREATMENT

Successful treatment of partially collapsed lumbar vertebra by dorsal laminectomy has been performed in calves.[1] Surgical treatment of cervical vertebral malformation (fusion of affected cervical vertebrae) is performed in horses, but in farm animals treatment is usually not possible and in most cases slaughter for salvage is recommended. Spinal hematomas of the cervical cord in horses can recover spontaneously but surgical decompression may be helpful in chronic cases.[14]

FURTHER READING

Divers TJ. Acquired spinal cord and peripheral nerve disease. *Vet Clin North Am Food Anim Pract.* 2004;20:231-242.

REFERENCES

1. Zani DD, et al. *Vet Surg.* 2008;37:801.
2. Ubiali DG, et al. *Pesq Vet Bras.* 2011;31:997.
3. Johnson AL, et al. *J Vet Intern Med.* 2012;26:1481.
4. Cudomre LA, et al. *Aust Vet J.* 2012;90:392.
5. Fews D, et al. *Vet Comp Orthop Traumatol.* 2006;19:187.
6. Denoix JM. *Equine Vet Educ.* 2007;19:72.
7. Wong DM, et al. *J Am Vet Med Assoc.* 2015;247:55.
8. Hammond G, et al. *Vet Rec.* 2006;158:600.
9. Levine GJ, et al. *Vet Radiol Ultrasound.* 2006;47:585.
10. Zanolari P, et al. *J Vet Intern Med.* 2006;20:1256.
11. Penny C, et al. *J Vet Intern Med.* 2007;21:322.
12. Hoffman CJ, Clark CK. *J Vet Intern Med.* 2013;27:317.
13. Hestvik G, et al. *J Vet Diagn Invest.* 2006;18:307.
14. Gold JR, et al. *J Vet Intern Med.* 2008;22:481.

BACK PAIN IN HORSES

The subject of back pain, and its relationship to lameness, is a very important one in horses. There is often a lesion in the vertebral canal and by pressing on the cord or peripheral nerves it causes gait abnormalities that suggest the presence of pain, or they actually cause pain. Spondylosis, injury to dorsal spinous processes, and sprain of back muscles are common causes of the same pattern of signs. Because these problems are largely orthopedic ones, and therefore surgical, their discussion is left to other authorities.

It is necessary in horses to differentiate spinal cord lesions from acute nutritional myodystrophy and subacute tying-up syndrome. Those diseases are characterized by high serum creatine kinase and AST activities.

Parasitic Diseases Primarily Affecting the Spinal Cord

EQUINE PROTOZOAL MYELOENCEPHALITIS

SYNOPSIS

Etiology *Sarcocystis neurona,* a protozoon. *Neospora hughesi* is an uncommon cause.

Epidemiology Sporadic disease occasionally occurring as localized epidemics. Endemic throughout most of the Americas. Disease is infectious but not contagious. The definitive host in North America is the opossum (*Didelphis* spp.), and other opossum species in South America.

Clinical signs Variable, but commonly asymmetric spinal ataxia, focal, neurogenic muscle atrophy, with or without cranial nerve dysfunction.

Clinical pathology No characteristic changes in blood or cerebrospinal fluid. Demonstration of intrathecal production of

Continued

antibodies to specific surface proteins (especially SnSAG2, 4/3) by measurement of antibodies in paired serum and CSF samples (ELISA).

Diagnostic confirmation Histologic demonstration of *S. neurona* or *N. hughesi* in nervous tissue.

Lesions Nonsuppurative myeloencephalitis with schizonts and merozoites in neurons, glial cells, and leukocytes.

Treatment Antiprotozoal agents, including ponazuril, diclazuril, or a combination of a sulfonamide and pyrimethamine.

Control Prevent exposure to *S. neurona* by minimizing fecal contamination by opossums of feed. No vaccine available.

ETIOLOGY

The cause is *S. neurona,* an apicomplexan protozoan that causes myeloencephalitis in equids, sea otters, cats, raccoons, red pandas, dogs, and a small number of other mammalian species.[1-3] Fatal encephalitis in Southern sea otters and EPM in horses is strongly linked to *S. neurona* sporocysts shed by opossums.[4,5] Isolates of *S. neurona* can vary in their antigenic composition because some immunodominant surface proteins (SnSAG 1, 2, 3, and 4) vary in either or both of their presence or antigenicity among strains of *S. neurona.* For instance, some strains of *S. neurona* (e.g., SN4), including some that are virulent in horses, lack the major surface antigen SnSAG-1.[6] This heterogeneity in the surface antigen composition of different *S. neurona* isolates could be an important consideration for development of serologic tests and prospective vaccines for EPM.[6]

Neospora spp., including *N. hughesi,* cause myeloencephalitis in horses less frequently than does *S. neurona.*[7-9]

The subsequent discussion refers to EPM caused by *S. neurona,* with specific points made in respect to *N. hughesi.*

EPIDEMIOLOGY

EPM occurs in horses and ponies in Canada, the United States, Central America, and Brazil. Reports of neurologic disease in horses with antibodies to *S. neurona* in France have yet to be confirmed but might represent cases of EPM in native horses outside of the Americas. The disease is reported in other countries in only horses imported from the Americas, and seroprevalence to *S. neurona*-specific antigens in Europe is rare in horses not imported from the Americas.[10] Distribution of the disease appears to correlate with the range of the definitive host, *Didelphis virginiana* in North America, or the related species *D. marsupialis* and *D. albiventris* in South America. The disease has not been reported in donkeys and mules. Neurologic disease associated with *S. neurona* has been reported in armadillos, sea otters, harbor seals, skunks, raccoons, zebra, lynxes, dogs, porpoises, and cats.[2,3,11,12]

The disease usually occurs sporadically in endemic areas, although epidemics on individual farms are reported. The incidence of EPM is estimated to be 14 new cases per 10,000 horses per year. The **case–fatality rate** is approximately 7%, although up to 14% of horses are sold or given away because they are affected by EPM. Approximately 40% of horses recover completely and another 37% improve but do not recover from the disease. Another study reports that only 55% of horses with EPM examined at a referral hospital were alive a minimum of 3 years after diagnosis and treatment.

Seroepidemiologic studies, based on detection by Western immunoblot test of multiple antibodies to *S. neurona* in serum, indicate that 45% to 60% of horses in the United States are exposed to the agent but do not develop disease.[13] Antibodies to *S. neurona* are present in ~49% of 495 horse sera tested with the rSnSAG2/4/3 trivalent ELISA in the Durango state of Mexico, and antibodies to *N. hughesi* are present in 3.0% of horse sera tested (rNhSAG1 ELISA and confirmed by Western blot of *N. hughesi* tachyzoite antigen) in the same region.[14] Approximately 26% of horses in Argentina have antibodies to *S. neurona,* and 39% of horses with neurologic disease are positive versus 22% of clinically normal horses.[15] Four percent of horses in southern Brazil have serum antibodies to *N. hughesi.*[16] Among horses in Israel, 12% of healthy horses are seropositive for antibodies to *N. hughesi*, and 21% of horses with neurologic disease and 38% of mares that aborted are seropositive.[17]

Rates of seropositivity to *S. neurona, N. hughesi,* or both in North America are reported, and differences in proportion of submitted samples are positive for either or both species identified based on month of submission and various animal-related factors. However, the sample was not random and results could have been heavily affected by sampling bias.[18]

Vaccination with a product containing killed *S. neurona* induces a detectable antibody response in both serum and, in approximately 50% of horses, in the CSF.

Risk Factors

Risk factors for development of EPM include season of the year, with the highest incidence of new cases in the summer and fall; age; use; protection of feed; and presence of opossums on the farm.[19] The disease occurs in horses from 2 months to 19 years of age. Horses <1 year of age are at lower risk of developing disease than are horse 1 to 4 years of age. Older horses are less likely to develop the disease. Protection of feed from contamination by opossum feces is associated with a decreased risk of disease, whereas the presence of opossums on the premises was associated with an increased risk of disease. Horses used primarily for racing and showing are at increased risk for developing EPM with an annual incidence of 38 new cases per 10,000 horses for horses used for racing compared with an incidence of 6 cases per 10,000 horses for horses used for pleasure or farm work. Horses used for showing or competition have the highest annual incidence of 51 cases per 10,000 horses per year. The presence of previous illness is a risk factor for development of EPM. Transportation for 55 hours increases the susceptibility to EPM of horses experimentally infected with *S. neurona.* Relative to neurologic (non-EPM) control horses, horses with EPM are more likely to be ≥2 years old and to have a history of cats residing on the premises. Relative to nonneurologic control horses, horses with EPM are more likely to be used for racing or Western performance.[20]

Transmission

S. neurona has the two-host life cycle (predator–prey) typical of other *Sarcocystis* and *Toxoplasma* spp.[21,22] The definitive host is the opossum, *D. virginiana,* and intermediate hosts include raccoons,[23] cats, skunks, sea otters, armadillos, and cowbirds (*Molothrus ater*).[24] The domestic cat, nine-banded armadillo, raccoon, cowbird, and skunk can be infected by ingestion of sporocysts and develop sarcocysts in muscle, which when fed to opossums, induces shedding of sporocysts, confirming the potential for these species to serve as intermediate hosts. Cats living on farms at which EPM has been diagnosed in horses have a higher rate of seroprevalence (40%) than do cats living in a city (10%), providing evidence for a role of cats in the epidemiology of the disease. However, others have detected a lower prevalence of seropositivity (5%) to *S. neurona* among cats in Texas and conclude that cats are not likely to play an important role in the epidemiology of EPM. At least in those areas where raccoons are present they are probably the most important intermediate host.

The definitive host is infected by ingestion of sarcocysts of *S. neurona* encysted in muscle of the intermediate host. The intermediate host is infected by ingestion of sporocysts derived from rupture oocysts passed in the feces of the definitive host. Sporocysts can remain infective in the environment for months, but are probably, based on behavior of other *Sarcocystis* spp. oocysts, killed by drying, high humidity, or freezing and thawing. Birds and insects also serve as transport hosts. Sporocysts ingested by the intermediate host undergo schizogony and ultimately form infective sarcocysts in muscle. *S. neurona* sarcocysts have been detected in the muscle of a 4-month-old filly, suggesting that horses might serve as intermediate hosts of the organism. This finding needs to be confirmed because the conventional wisdom is that in horses *S. neurona* does not complete schizogony and remains as uninfective merozoites in neural tissue. *S. neurona* sarcocysts do not occur in the muscle of horses; therefore horses are not infective to other animals.

There is no evidence of transplacental infection of foals.

The definitive and intermediate hosts of *N. hughesi* have not been determined. Dogs are the definitive host of the closely related *N. caninum*. *N. hughesi* can be transmitted transplacentally from mares to foals, and it is suggested that infection with this organism can persist in a band of horses by vertical transmision.[25,26]

PATHOGENESIS

Details of the pathogenesis of EPM are unknown. It is assumed that after infection, probably by ingestion, sporocysts excyst and release sporozoites, which penetrate the gastrointestinal tract and enter endothelial cells. Subsequently, meronts (schizonts) develop and on maturation rupture and release merozoites. Schizonts are present in cells of the CNS, including neurons, glial cells, and intrathecal macrophages. Schizonts multiply in the infected cells, as evidenced by the presence of merozoites. Infection induces a nonsuppurative inflammation, characterized by accumulations of lymphocytes, neutrophils, eosinophils, and gitter cells. Infection of neurons, and the associated inflammatory reaction, disrupt normal nervous function and contribute to the clinical signs of weakness, muscle atrophy, and deficits in proprioception.

Mechanisms permitting infection and proliferation of the organism have not been well defined. Horses with EPM have lesser cell-mediated immunity than do asymptomatic horses, and the decrease in cell-mediated immunity appears to be caused by *S. neurona* suppressing immune responses to parasite-derived antigens. However, foals with severe combined immunodeficiency administered *S. neurona* do not develop neurologic disease, despite prolonged parasitemia and infection of visceral organs by the organism, whereas immunocompetent horses do not have prolonged parasitemia but do develop neurologic disease.

CLINICAL FINDINGS

The incubation period after experimental infection of young horses ranges between 28 and 42 days, but is not known for the spontaneous disease.

The clinical findings of EPM in horses are protean, and in endemic areas EPM should be considered as a diagnosis in any horse with clinical signs referable to the nervous system. *S. neurona* can infect any area of the brain and spinal cord, and may affect more than one site in an individual horse, resulting in the wide range of neurologic abnormalities associated with this disease.

Clinical signs of EPM range from barely perceptible changes in gait or behavior to recumbency, muscle atrophy, or seizures. The onset of **signs** can be insidious and gradual, or acute and rapidly progressive. Affected horses do not have increased temperature or heart rate, unless complications of the nervous disease occur.

Spinal ataxia, evident as weakness, hypometria, or hypermetria, and defects in proprioception are common manifestations of EPM. Multifocal spinal or cervical disease causes all four limbs to be affected, whereas lesions caudal to the cervical intumescence cause signs in the rear limbs only. Signs of spinal ataxia range from subtle changes in gait, which are difficult to differentiate from obscure lameness caused by musculoskeletal disease, through obvious spinal ataxia evident as truncal sway, toe dragging, and circumduction of feet, to spontaneous falling and recumbency. **Asymmetry** of clinical signs, in which one limb is affected more than the contralateral limb, is highly suggestive of EPM because CSM and equine degenerative myelopathy usually cause symmetric ataxia.

Lesions in the sacral cord cause signs of **cauda equina syndrome**, including tail paresis and urinary and fecal incontinence.

Lesions affecting spinal cord gray matter cause focal, **asymmetric muscle atrophy**, absent reflexes, or focal areas of **sweating**. Muscles frequently affected include the quadriceps, biceps femoris, epaxial muscles, and the supraspinatus/infraspinatus group. EPM can present as a brachial plexus injury evident as radial nerve paralysis.

CN disease is a common manifestation of EPM. Common syndromes include the following:

- **Vestibular disease** (CN VIII), evident as circling, nystagmus, head tilt, and falling toward the affected side
- **Unilateral facial nerve paralysis** (CN VII), evident as ear droop, lack of palpebral or corneal reflex and menace on the affected side, and displacement of the upper lip and nares away from the side of the lesion
- **Dysphagia** (CNs IX, X, XII) and persistent dorsal displacement of the soft palate
- **Tongue paralysis** (CN XII)
- **Masseter atrophy** and weakness (CN V)
- **Hypalgesia** (lack of sensation) of the nostrils and skin of the face (CN V)

EPM might also manifest as changes in personality and behavior, head-shaking, and seizures.

Clinical disease caused by infection by *N. hughesi* is clinically indistinguishable from that associated with *S. neurona*.[8,9]

CLINICAL PATHOLOGY

There are no characteristic changes in the hemogram or serum biochemical variables. **Diagnosis** has focused on the demonstration of antibodies to *S. neurona* in serum or CSF by Western blot, indirect fluorescence testing, or ELISA. The important concept is use of paired serum and CSF samples to demonstrate intrathecal production of antibodies to differentiate infection associated with neurologic disease from clinically inapparent infection.[13,27-29]

The sensitivity and specificity of Western blot (Sn 80%–89%, Sp 38%–87% on serum, and Sn ~88% and Sp 44%–89% in CSF); indirect FAT (IFAT) (Sn 59%–94%, Sp 71%–100% in serum, and Sn 65%–100%, Sp 90%–99% in CSF); SAG1 ELISA (Sn 13%–68%, Sp 71%–97% in serum); and SAG2,4/3 ELISA (Sn 30%–86%, Sp 37%–88% in serum, Sn 77%–96% and Sp 58%–96% in CSF) for detection of EPM have been recently reviewed.[13,28,29] The combination of serum and CSF testing using tests to detect antibodies to SAG2, 4/3 surface proteins were the most sensitive and specific for diagnosis of horses with clinical signs of neurologic disease.[28,29]

Interpretation of the results of **Western blot** analysis of **CSF** for IgG antibodies to *S. neurona* is problematic because of the potential for blood contamination of the sample during collection, and the high sensitivity but low specificity of the test. Blood contamination of the sample is problematic in horses that are seropositive for antibodies to *S. neurona* and in which it is desired to know if antibodies are present in CSF. Contamination of CSF with blood can introduce antibodies from serum into the otherwise antibody-free CSF, causing a "false"-positive test. Contamination of CSF with small quantities of blood with high concentrations of antibodies to *S. neurona* might not be detectable using RBCs, albumin quotient, or immunoglobulin index, but could yield a positive result on Western blot testing.

Foals of seropositive mares acquire antibodies, but not infection, by ingestion of colostrum from the dam. These antibodies can be detected in both serum and CSF of foals. The mean time for foals to become seronegative for antibodies to *S. neurona* is 4.2 months. Detection of antibodies to *S. neurona* in serum or CSF of foals less than 4 to 6 months of age, even those with neurologic disease, should be interpreted with caution as the antibodies are likely derived from the dam.

An **IFAT** reliably detects antibodies to *S. neurona* in serum and CSF of infected horses.[28] This test has the advantages of providing quantitative results, is cheaper to perform, and is more accurate than immunoblots in the detection of antibodies.

Examination of other variables in CSF is of limited use in the diagnosis of EPM, and measurement of creatine kinase activity in CSF has no diagnostic usefulness. The use of the **albumin quotient** or **IgG index** to detect blood contamination of CSF, or the intrathecal production of IgG, is unreliable and not useful in the diagnosis of EPM.

NECROPSY

Lesions are limited to the spinal cord and brain, with the exception of neurogenic muscle atrophy. Gross lesions of hemorrhage and malacia may be visible in the CNS tissue. The lesions are asymmetric, but may be more frequently encountered in the cervical and lumbar intumescences of the spinal cord. Histologic examination reveals multifocal necrosis of the nervous tissue with an accompanying infiltration of macrophages, lymphocytes, neutrophils, and occasional eosinophils. This reaction is predomnantly nonsuppurative and usually includes a degree of perivascular cuffing. Schizonts or free merozoites may be evident in tissues but are difficult to locate without IHC stains. The sensitivity of screening for the parasite in hematoxylin and eosin–stained sections of nervous tissue from cases with histologic changes suggestive of EPM was only 20%. The sensitivity improved to 51% when IHC staining of the tissue was used. The same interpretative problems encountered when testing antemortem CSF samples apply when the fluid is collected at postmortem. Isolation in cell culture systems is possible but rarely attempted in diagnostic laboratories. PCR tests for these apicomplexan parasites can yield false negatives because of the random distribution of the parasite within CNS tissue.

Samples for Confirmation of Diagnosis

- **Histology:** fixed spinal cord (several levels, including cervical and lumbar intumescences) and half of brain, including the entire brainstem, CN VII in some cases (LM, IHC, PCR).

DIFFERENTIAL DIAGNOSIS

The clinical diagnosis of EPM should be based on the detection of unequivocal neurologic abnormalities consistent with EPM, ruling out of other causes of neurologic disease (listed next) and the detection of antibodies to *S. neurona* or N. hughesi in uncontaminated samples of cerebrospinal fluid and serum to confirm intrathecal production of specific antibodies.[13] A favorable response to treatment specific for EPM increases the likelihood that the horse has EPM. A definitive diagnosis can only be achieved by necropsy.

- Spinal ataxia.
- Cauda equina syndrome: EPM should be differentiated from polyneuritis equi, equine herpesvirus-1 myelopathy, and injection of long-acting anesthetics or alcohol around sacral nerve roots.
- Peripheral nerve lesions: other causes of focal muscle atrophy, such as brachial plexus injury, damage to the supraspinatus nerve, or disuse atrophy can be differentiated from EPM on history and clinical signs.
- Cranial nerve disease: signs of vestibular disease, facial or trigeminal nerve dysfunction, and dysphagia associated with EPM should be differentiated from the following:
  - Middle ear infection
  - Guttural pouch mycosis
  - Arthritis and fracture of the temporohyoid articulation
  - Head trauma

TREATMENT

Specific treatment of EPM involves the administration of **antiprotozoal drugs** including ponazuril, diclazuril, nitazoxanide, or the combination of pyrimethamine and sulfadiazine.

Administration of the combination of sulfadiazine (or similar drug, 20 mg/kg, orally) and pyrimethamine (1–2 mg/kg, orally) every 24 hours given 1 hour before feeding is effective in approximately 60% to 70% of cases.[13] This treatment is continued for at least 90 days if complete resolution of clinical abnormalities occurs, or longer if the signs of EPM do not resolve. **Adverse effects** of the administration of a combination of a sulfonamide and pyrimethamine include enterocolitis, anemia, and abortion. Folic acid is often added to the diet of horses being treated for EPM, but this cannot be recommended because of its lack of efficacy in preventing anemia in treated horses and its ability to cause severe congenital abnormalities in foals born to treated mares and anemia and leukopenia in adult horses. Orally administered synthetic folates interfere with normal folate metabolism in horses being administered antifolate drugs resulting, paradoxically, in folate deficiency. Adequate intake of folates in antiprotozoal-treated horses can be assured by feeding a diet containing good quality green foliage.

Ponazuril, an active metabolite of toltrazuril, is usually administered at a dosage of 5 mg/kg BW orally once daily for 28 days. At this dosage, and at 10 mg/kg orally once daily for 28 days, administration of the drug results in resolution of clinical signs in approximately 60% of horses with EPM. The initial dosage is 5 mg/kg every 24 hours, which is continued for 28 days if signs of improvement are evident after 14 days. If signs of improvement are not seen after 14 days, the dosage is increased to 10 mg/kg orally every 24 for 14 days. Few adverse effects are noted, even at 30 mg/kg orally once daily for 28 days. **Diclazuril,** which is available in the United States as a pelleted product for oral administration to horses, is similarly effective and free of serious adverse effects.[13,30-32]

Nitazoxanide administration was associated with adverse effects including fever, anorexia, diarrhea, and worsening of clinical signs of neurologic disease. It is no longer recommended for treatment of EPM.

The decision to **stop treatment** in horses that do not completely recover is difficult. Some authorities recommend resampling CSF and continuing treatment until antibodies to *S. neurona* are no longer detectable. However, given that normal horses often have antibodies in their CSF, and that some treated horses never lose their positive Western blot test, the decision to stop treatment should not be based entirely on this variable.

Some horses have a transient worsening of clinical signs in the first week of treatment. This is presumed to be from the effect of the antiprotozoal agent causing death of protozoa with subsequent inflammation and further impairment of neurologic function. Relapse of the disease occurs in some horses when administration of antiprotozoal medication is stopped.

Supportive treatment of affected horses includes antiinflammatory drugs (flunixin meglumine, 1 mg/kg intravenously, every 8–12 hours; dimethyl sulfoxide, 1 g/kg as a 10% solution in isotonic saline intravenously, every 24 hours for 3 days) and nutritional support for horses that cannot eat. Flunixin meglumine is often administered twice daily for the first 3 to 5 days of treatment with ponazuril or nitazoxanide, purportedly to reduce the inflammatory effects of death of protozoa in the CNS.

Treatment of EPM associated with infection by *N. hughesi* is based on the same principles and medications as treatment of disease associated with *S. neurona*.[8]

CONTROL

Preventing contamination of feed and water with opossum feces is essential for preventing EPM in animals. Sporocysts of *S. neurona* are resistant to the usual concentrations of many of the conventional disinfectants including sodium hypochlorite (bleach), 2% chlorhexidine, 1% betadine, 5% benzyl chlorophenol, 13% phenol, 6% benzyl ammonium chloride, and 10% formalin. The organism is killed by heating to 55°C for 15 minutes or 60°C (140°F) for 1 minute. Although survival of sporocysts in different environmental conditions outdoors has not been tested, sporocysts remained viable at 4°C (131°F) for months.[22]

Because protection of feed from contamination by opossums has been demonstrated to reduce the risk of horses developing EPM, it is prudent to use measures to reduce the exposure of animals and feed to opossum feces, and possibly feces of birds that might act as transport hosts.

There is interest in pharmacologic means of preventing infection of horses by *S. neurona*. Pyrantel pamoate has some efficacy against *S. neurona* in vitro but daily administration (2.6 mg/kg BW in feed) does not prevent *S. neurona* infection of horses. Daily administration of low doses of **diclazuril** to foals in endemic areas significantly reduces the rate of seroconversion.[30-32]

There is no vaccine available for prevention of EPM associated with either *S. neurona* or *N. hughesi*.[22]

FURTHER READING

Dubey JP, et al. An update on Sarcocystis neurona infections in animals and equine protozoal myeloencephalitis (EPM). *Vet Parasitol.* 2015;209:1-42.

Reed SM, et al. Equine protozoal myeloencephalitis: an updated consensus statement with a focus on parasite biology, diagnosis, treatment and prevention. *J Vet Intern Med.* 2016;30.

REFERENCES

1. Dubey JP, et al. *Vet Parasitol.* 2014;202:194.
2. Dubey JP, et al. *Vet Parasitol.* 2011;183:156.
3. Cooley AJ, et al. *Vet Pathol.* 2007;44:956.
4. Sundar N, et al. *Vet Parasitol.* 2008;152:8.
5. Rejmanek D, et al. *Vet Parasitol.* 2010;170:20.
6. Howe DK, et al. *Int J Parasit.* 2008;38:623.
7. Wobeser BK, et al. *Can Vet J.* 2009;50:851.
8. Finno CJ, et al. *J Vet Intern Med.* 2007;21:1405.
9. Finno CJ, et al. *Vet Ophthalmol.* 2010;13:259.
10. Arias M, et al. *Vet Parasitol.* 2012;185:301.
11. Ellison S, et al. *Intern J Appl Res Vet Med.* 2012;10:243.
12. Hsu V, et al. *J Parasitol.* 2010;96:800.
13. Reed S, et al. *J Vet Intern Med.* 2016;30:491.
14. Yeargan MR, et al. *Parasite.* 2013;20:29.
15. More G, et al. *J Equine Vet Sci.* 2014;34:1051.
16. de Moura AB, et al. *Rev Bras Parasitologia Vet.* 2013;22:597.
17. Kligler EB, et al. *Vet Parasitol.* 2007;148:109.
18. Pusterla N, et al. *Vet J.* 2014;200:332.
19. Morley PS, et al. *J Vet Intern Med.* 2008;22:616.
20. Cohen ND, et al. *JAVMA.* 2007;231:1857.
21. Howe DK, et al. *Vet Clin North Am Equine Pract.* 2014;30:659.
22. Dubey JP, et al. *Vet Parasitol.* 2015;209:1.
23. Dryburgh EL, et al. *J Parasitol.* 2015;101:462.
24. Mansfield LS, et al. *Vet Parasitol.* 2008;153:24.
25. Pusterla N, et al. *J Parasitol.* 2011;97:281.
26. Antonello AM, et al. *Vet Parasitol.* 2012;187:367.
27. Johnson AL, et al. *J Vet Intern Med.* 2010;24:1184.
28. Johnson AL, et al. *J Vet Intern Med.* 2013;27:596.
29. Reed SM, et al. *J Vet Intern Med.* 2013;27:1193.
30. Hunyadi L, et al. *J Vet Pharmacol Ther.* 2015;38:243.
31. MacKay RJ, et al. *Am J Vet Res.* 2008;69:396.
32. Pusterla N, et al. *Vet J.* 2015;206:236.

CEREBROSPINAL NEMATODIASIS (ELAPHOSTRONGYLOSIS)

Cerebrospinal nematodiasis, cerebrospinal elaphostrongylosis (CSE) or neurofilariosis are disease of sheep, goats, and camelids caused by infestation of the brain and spinal cord with the nematode *Elaphostrongylus* and related genera. This genus is closely related to the lungworms of small ruminants but is found in the cranial subarachnoid space, cranial venous sinuses, and occasionally in the spinal subarachnoid space. *Parelaphostrongylus tenuis* occurs in white-tailed deer[1] and moose[2] in eastern North America and parts of western Canada, *E. cervi* in deer, sheep, and goat in Europe[3-5] and New Zealand, and *E. rangiferi* in reindeer in Scandinavia. *P. odocoilei* has been found to infect bighorn sheep in North America.[6] Eggs or larvae are carried to the lungs, undergo a tracheal migration, and the first-stage larvae are passed in the feces. The larvae are quite resistant to adverse environmental conditions and enter slugs or snails to develop into infective larvae. The lifecycle is complete when infected molluscs are ingested by deer and the larvae penetrate the abomasum and migrate, possibly along spinal nerves, to the spinal cord where they develop into adults and migrate into the subarachnoid space.

Clinical signs are not seen in infected deer, but in sheep, goats and New World Camelids the worm continually moves through nervous system tissue causing limping and incoordination followed by almost complete paralysis of the hindlimbs or of the neck, body, and all four legs.[3,7-9] There are usually no signs of cerebral involvement, and affected animals remain bright and continue to eat. If given supportive treatment, they may survive for at least 1 month. *P. tenuis* also transmits to moose and is responsible for the nervous signs in "moose sickness," including the following[4]:

- Weakness
- Incoordination
- Circling
- Impaired vision
- Blindness
- Abnormal carriage of the head
- Paralysis
- Lack of fear of man
- Aggressiveness

Histopathologic lesions include axonal degeneration and swelling, perivascular cuffing, presence of hemosiderin-laden macrophages, and increased numbers of eosinophils.[9,10]

Clinical signs of spinal cord disease attributed to Parelaphostrongylus tenuis appear to diminish after treatment with high doses of oral fenbendazole (50 mg/kg, daily for five days), although randomized clinical trials have not been completed to confirm this impression.

No reliable treatment is available for CSE. Ivermectin has no effect on the adult worms, possibly because the large molecules of this compound cannot pass the blood-brain barrier.[5] One clinical report describes the treatment of 17 light to moderately affected goats with an NSAID (flunixin meglumine) together with ivermectin and fenbendazole for 5 days.[6] Complete recovery occurred in three, partial recovery in eight, but euthanasia was necessary for the remainder.

REFERENCES

1. Jacques CN, et al. *J Wildl Dis.* 2015;51:670.
2. Maskey JJ Jr, et al. *J Wildl Dis.* 2015;51:670.
3. Alberti EG, et al. *J Helminthol.* 2011;85:313.
4. Morandi F, et al. *J Wildl Dis.* 2006;42:870.
5. Sironi G, et al. *Parasitologia.* 2006;48:437.
6. Huby-Chilton F, et al. *J Wildl Dis.* 2006;42:877.
7. Tschuor AC, et al. *Schweiz Arch Tierheiikd.* 2006;148:609.
8. Dobey CL, et al. *J Vet Diagn Invest.* 2014;26:748.
9. Whitehead CE, Bedenice D. *Vet Clin North Am Food Anim Pract.* 2009;25:385.
10. McIntosh T, et al. *Can Vet J.* 2007;48:1146.

SETARIA

Setaria spp. are long (5- to 10-cm) thread-like filarial nematodes commonly found in the peritoneal cavity of most domestic animals. *S. labiato-papillosa* is a cosmopolitan parasite of cattle, whereas *S. digitata* and the closely related, and perhaps synonymous, species *S. marshalli* occur only in Asia.[1] *S. equina* is found worldwide in horses. *S. tundra* infects and causes significant economic losses in reindeer in Finland.[2,3] Adult females produce motile embryos (microfilariae) that circulate in the peripheral blood of the infected animal and are taken up by mosquitoes. Infective larvae develop in the intermediate host and are released when the mosquito subsequently feeds. *S. labiato-papillosa* reaches maturity in cattle in 8 to 10 months. Despite their size, the presence of these worms in the abdominal cavity causes no significant clinical effect.

Serious disease may result if *S. labiato-papillosa* or *S. digitata* infect animals other than their own natural host, especially horses, sheep, goats, and humans. In these hosts, they migrate in an abnormal manner causing epizootic cerebrospinal nematodosis (with local names including lumbar paralysis and kumri) when they invade the brain and spinal cord. Juvenile *S. digitata* may also invade the eye. Although *Setaria* is found in cattle in many countries, cerebrospinal nematodosis is largely restricted to Israel, Japan, China, Korea, India, and Sri Lanka. The incidence is increasing in Taiwan, and a single case has been reported from the United States. Ocular filariasis is seen most commonly in Japan. These diseases occur during summer and autumn when the vectors are most prevalent. The cerebrospinal form sometimes occurs in epidemic proportions, causing the death of horses, sheep, and goats.

Cerebrospinal nematodiosis may be rapid in onset with affected animals dying within a few days or it may occur gradually over a few days. There may be acute or subacute paresis with weakness and incoordination or paralysis involving the hindlegs most commonly, but sometimes all four legs are involved. Recovery is only partial in many animals but others show only a mild neurologic disorder, which gradually becomes indiscernible. There are no systemic signs and the animals may continue to eat. Other diseases causing similar clinical signs include enzootic equine ataxia in horses and paralytic rabies in sheep and goats as lesions as well as traumatic injury, spinal cord abscess, warble fly larvae, *S. vulgaris*, or *H. gingivalis*.

At necropsy, there are no macroscopic changes and sections need to be taken from many levels of the spinal cord to find histologic lesions. Focal areas of malacia or microcavitation are seen and in adjacent sites there may be loss of myelin, axonal swelling, degeneration, and gitter cell formation. Migratory pathways are indicated by necrotic tracts. Where nervous signs have been present for only a few days, a worm or worm fragments may occasionally be found. Molecular techniques have been developed for identifying the responsible species.

S. tundra causes peritonitis, perihepatitis, and significant decrease in body condition score in reindeer calves.[2,3] Treatment of infected reindeer with ivermectin (0.2 mg/kg, subcutaneously) has up to 95% efficacy of worm elimination.[2] Application of biting insect repellant (deltamethrin) significantly decreases *S. tundra* infections in reindeer.[2]

Anthelmintics will not resolve existing lesions but may prevent further damage. Little has been published on treatment or control. Ivermectin gave moderate efficacy (80%–88%) against adult *S. equina* in ponies. In a field study, none of 221 goats and sheep injected twice with ivermectin at a dose of 0.2 mg/kg developed setariasis, whereas 17 of 303 noninjected animals suffered from the disease.

FURTHER READING

Taylor MA, Coop RL, Wall RL. *Veterinary Parasitology*. Oxford, UK: Wiley-Blackwell; 2007.

REFERENCES

1. Laaksonen S, et al. *Acta Vet Scand*. 2008;50:49.
2. Laaksonen S, et al. *Vet Rec*. 2007;160:835.
3. Nakano H, et al. *J Vet Med Sci*. 2007;69:413.

Toxic Diseases Primarily Affecting the Spinal Cord

STRINGHALT

Stringhalt is an involuntary, exaggerated flexion of the hock during walking. It can affect one or both hindlimbs. Classic stringhalt occurs sporadically, is usually unilateral, and is usually irreversible without surgical intervention. Stringhalt can also occur secondarily to injury to the dorsal metatarsus.

A clinically identical disease, Australian stringhalt, occurs in outbreaks in Australia, New Zealand, California, Japan, Europe, the UK, Brazil, and Chile.[1-5] The outbreaks tend to occur in late summer or autumn and are related to drought conditions or overgrazing of pasture with consequent ingestion of plants that would otherwise not be eaten. Outbreaks in Australia, California, and Virginia are related to the ingestion of ***Hypochaeris radicata*** (flatweed, cats ear).[4] Other plants suspected to play a role in the etiology include *Taraxacum officinale* (dandelion), *Arctotheca calendula* (capeweed), or *Malva parviflora* (mallow) but good evidence of the role of any of these latter plants is lacking.

The **pathogenesis** of the disorder is likely related to the presence of toxins in *H. radicata*, especially after it is stressed.[6] The toxin or toxins have not been identified but are unlikely to be mycotoxins.[4] The disease has been **experimentally induced** by feeding a colt 9.8 kg per day for 19 days of *H. radicata* harvested fresh from a pasture on which horses had developed disease.[5] The disease resolved when the colt was fed *H radicata* from a pasture with unaffected horses. Signs in the colt resolved within 15 days of last feeding the toxic plant.[5]

Clinical signs are distinctive. The abnormal movement is only elicited when the horse begins to move forward. The characteristic movement occurs in mildly affected horses when they are backed or turned. Most cases are manifested by a flexion of the hock that can be violent enough for the horse to kick itself in the abdomen. The hoof is held in this position for a moment and then stamped hard on the ground. If both hindlegs are affected, progress is very slow and difficult and the horses often use a bunny-hopping gait. In the most severe cases the horse is unable to rise without assistance. The horse's general health is unaffected, although it may be difficult for it to graze. Some cases have other signs of neurologic disease such as stiffness of the forelimbs or respiratory distress caused by laryngeal paralysis. Many affected horses have unilateral (usually left) laryngeal hemiplegia evident on endoscopic examination of the larynx.

EMG examination reveals markedly abnormal activity including prolonged insertion activity, fibrillation potentials, and positive waves at rest and enhanced EMG activity in the right lateral digital extensor muscle on muscle contraction consistent with denervation. The changes are most severe in the long digital extensor muscle. Most horses recover without treatment, although complete recovery might not occur for over 1 year.

Biopsy of the superficial peroneal nerve and the long digital extensor muscle can be useful in providing an antemortem diagnosis. The superficial peroneal nerve of an affected horse had loss of large myelinated fibers, axonal degeneration, and myelin splitting.[7]

There are no characteristic abnormalities in a complete blood count or serum biochemical profile. Pathologic findings are restricted to a peripheral neuropathy in the tibial, superficial peroneal, and medial plantar nerves and in the left and right recurrent laryngeal nerves. Lesions in affected muscles are consistent with denervation atrophy and fiber type grouping.

The signs of the disease are characteristic. Differential diagnosis of the disease involving one leg is ossifying myopathy of the semimembranosus and semitendinosus muscles. Lead toxicosis can induce similar signs in horses.

Recovery is spontaneous in most cases (50% over an 8-month period in one large case series).[2]

Treatment with phenytoin (15 mg/kg orally daily for 14 days) effects some improvement but the signs recur within 1 or 2 days after treatment is discontinued.[2] Myotenectomy of the lateral digital extensor muscle and tendon is reported to provide immediate relief in affected horses, even in those horses with severe bilateral disease.

Control involves the prevention of overgrazing of pastures, particularly during droughts, and restricting or eliminating access to *H. radicata*.

REFERENCES

1. de Pennington N, et al. *Vet Rec*. 2011;169:476.
2. Domange C, et al. *J Anim Physiol Nutr*. 2010;94:712.
3. Schultze C, et al. *Pferdeheilkunde*. 2009;25:115.
4. El Hage C. *Investigation Into the Cause of Australian Stringhalt*. Canberra: Rural Industries Research and Development Corporation; 2011:1.
5. Araujo JAS, et al. *Toxicon*. 2008;52:190.
6. MacKay RJ, et al. *Toxicon*. 2013;70:194.
7. Armengou L, et al. *J Vet Intern Med*. 2010;24:220.

Inherited Diseases Primarily Affecting the Spinal Cord

SPASTIC PARESIS OF CATTLE (ELSO HEEL)

This disease occurs in the Holstein, Aberdeen Angus, Red Danish, Ayrshire, Beef Shorthorn, Poll Hereford, Murray Grey, and many other breeds of cattle. It has been observed in crossbred Brahman cattle and in an Ayrshire × Beef Shorthorn crossbred steer. The disease occurs principally in calves, with signs appearing from several weeks to 6 months or more after birth. Occasional cases are reported as developing in adult European cattle, and there is one report of the occurrence of the disease in adult Indian cattle. The disease was first termed Elso heel based on its first description in 1922 as a heritable disease from an East Friesian bull named Elso II. The preferred name spastic paresis was first used in 1932 to emphasize the primary defect.[1]

It has been held for a long time that the disease is inherited, and the principal argument has centered on the mode of inheritance. Attempts to determine this have shown that the rate of occurrence in planned test matings is so low that, if inheritance is involved, it can only be the inheritance of a susceptibility to the disease. It is suggested that different time appearances represent a single disease entity with varying expressivity, with the late forms affected by cumulative environmental factors. A proposed hypothesis is of a gene with increased penetrance in the homozygote, with weak penetrance in the heterozygote, acting on a polygenic basis

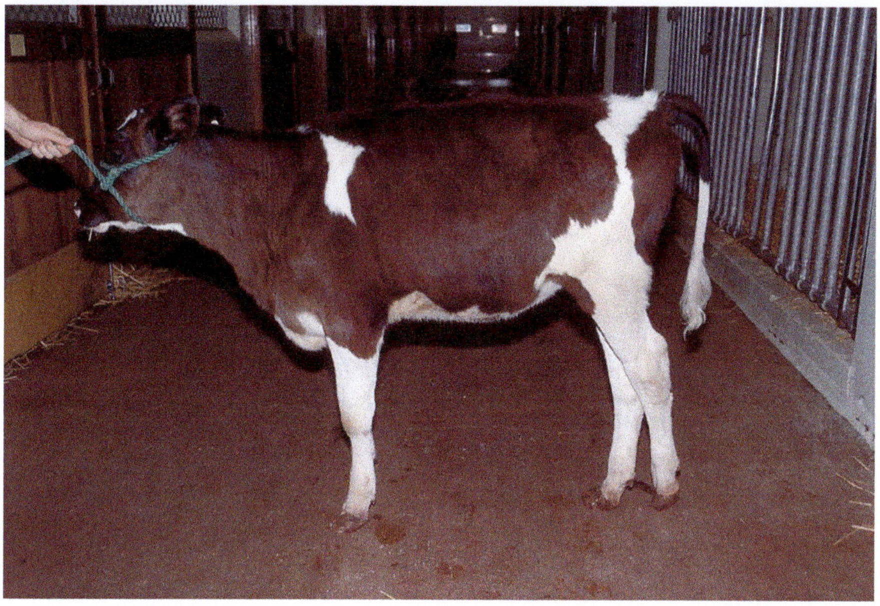

Fig. 14-19 Spastic paresis in an 8-month-old Holstein Friesian heifer. Both hindlegs are excessively straight, the left hindleg is held caudally and above the ground, and the tail is characteristically held away from the body.

dependent on external factors. Males appear to be affected more often than females, but a clear sex predilection has not been identified. The prevalence of disease appears to be <1% in all breeds.[1] Infectious agents causing transmissible subacute spongiform encephalopathies interacting with trace elements such as lithium have been suggested as etiologic agents, but there is no evidence to support this hypothesis.

In all forms of the disease in most cattle breeds (exceptions being the Belgian Blue and Romagnola in which the excessive tone occurs in the quadriceps femoris muscle; the lesion is usually bilateral) there is excessive tone of the gastrocnemius muscle and straightness of the hock, usually more marked in one hindleg. If only one leg is affected, it may be thrust out behind while the calf is walking and advanced with a restricted, swinging motion often without touching the ground. There is no resistance to passive flexion of the limb and the animal appears normal while sitting. Clinical signs are most exaggerated after immediately encouraging a sitting animal to stand. The gastrocnemius and perforatus muscles are rigid and in a state of spastic contraction. There is a characteristic elevation of the tail (Fig. 14-19). The lameness becomes progressively worse and affected animals spend much time lying down. Much BW is lost and the animal is usually destroyed between 1 and 2 years of age.

Minor lesions described as regressive changes in the neurons of the red nucleus, in the reticular substance, and in the lateral vestibular nucleus are of doubtful significance, as are the observed reduction in inorganic phosphate and ascorbic acid levels in the blood and CSF of affected calves. A lower than normal CSF concentration of a central neurotransmitter, dopamine, could also be an effect rather than a cause.

There are demonstrable lesions on radiologic examination of the tarsus with remodeling of the calcaneus bone and development of an enlarged and irregular epiphysis of the calcaneus caused by chronic and repetitive strain that straightens the hindlimb. Extensive examinations of muscles and tendons have failed to reveal histologic abnormalities. The absence of any structural lesion and the variation in intensity of the abnormality suggests that it is a functional one. An **overactive stretch reflex** is thought to be responsible for the clinical signs, possibly caused by defective glycinergic synaptic transmission and alteration of calcium signaling proteins (Fig. 14-20).[1,2]

The diagnosis of spastic paresis is based on history, signalment, clinical signs, and progressive nature of the disease. A genetic test is currently unavailable because the underlying gene defect(s) have yet to be identified. An epidural injection of 0.38% procaine solution diminishes the clinical signs of spastic contracture within 10 to 15 minute and has provided a useful supporting diagnostic test when the gastrocnemius is the principal muscle of contracture; it is less helpful in cases of spastic contraction of the quadriceps. In the latter case ultrasound-guided infiltration around the femoral nerve with local anesthetic solution may be attempted.[1,3]

In Europe, affected animals are kept for breeding purposes, especially if they are double-muscled. They are kept because of the efficacy of the curative surgical operation (partial tibial neurectomy) and for the high incidence of double-muscling in such calves. In the Holstein breed, and several German breeds, bulls that sire affected calves have been observed to have very straight hocks and to suffer from various forms of stifle and hock lameness early in life.

The only effective treatment is surgical. Several surgical techniques including tenectomy, partial tibial neurectomy, and triple tenectomy have been described. The most effective technique appears to be partial tibial neurectomy performed under caudal epidural anesthesia with electrical stimulation used to identify the tibial nerve.[4] In a large case series on 113 Belgian Blue calves with spastic paresis, a telephone follow-up of the owners 3 months later revealed good results in 83%, a considerable improvement in 4%, severe hyperflexion of the hock necessitating early culling for slaughter in 5%, and in 8% there was little or no improvement.

FURTHER READING

De Vlamynck C. Bovine spastic paresis: current knowledge and scientific voids. *Vet J.* 2014;202:229-235.

REFERENCES

1. De Vlamynck C. *Vet J.* 2014;202:229.
2. Pariset L, et al. *BMC Vet Res.* 2013;9:122.
3. De Vlamynck CA, et al. *Am J Vet Res.* 2013;74:750.
4. Milne MH. *UK Vet.* 2007;12:1.

INHERITED CONGENITAL MYOCLONUS (HEREDITARY NEURAXIAL EDEMA)

This congenital defect of the nervous system has been reported only in Poll Hereford cattle or their crossbreds and appears to be transmitted by inheritance in an autosomal recessive pattern. A similar disease has been tentatively recorded in Peruvian Paso horses. At birth affected calves are unable to sit up or rise and are very sensitive to external stimuli, manifested by extreme extensor spasm, including fixation of thoracic muscles and apnea, especially if lifted and held upright. The response is one of hyperesthesia with myoclonic jerks of skeletal muscles in response to external stimuli or spontaneously. The intellect of the calves seems unaffected, vision is normal, they drink well, and can be reared but at a great cost in time. Intercurrent disease is common and calves usually die of pneumonia or enteritis before they are 1 month old.

All affected calves have subluxations of the hip joints or epiphyseal fractures of the femoral head caused by muscle spasms in the fetus. Their gestation length is shorter than that of normal calves by 9 days.

There are no microscopic lesions in the CNS, but there is a biochemical defect—severe alterations in spinal cord glycine-mediated neurotransmission. The specific and marked defect in glycine receptors and the increase in neuronal uptake of glycine are

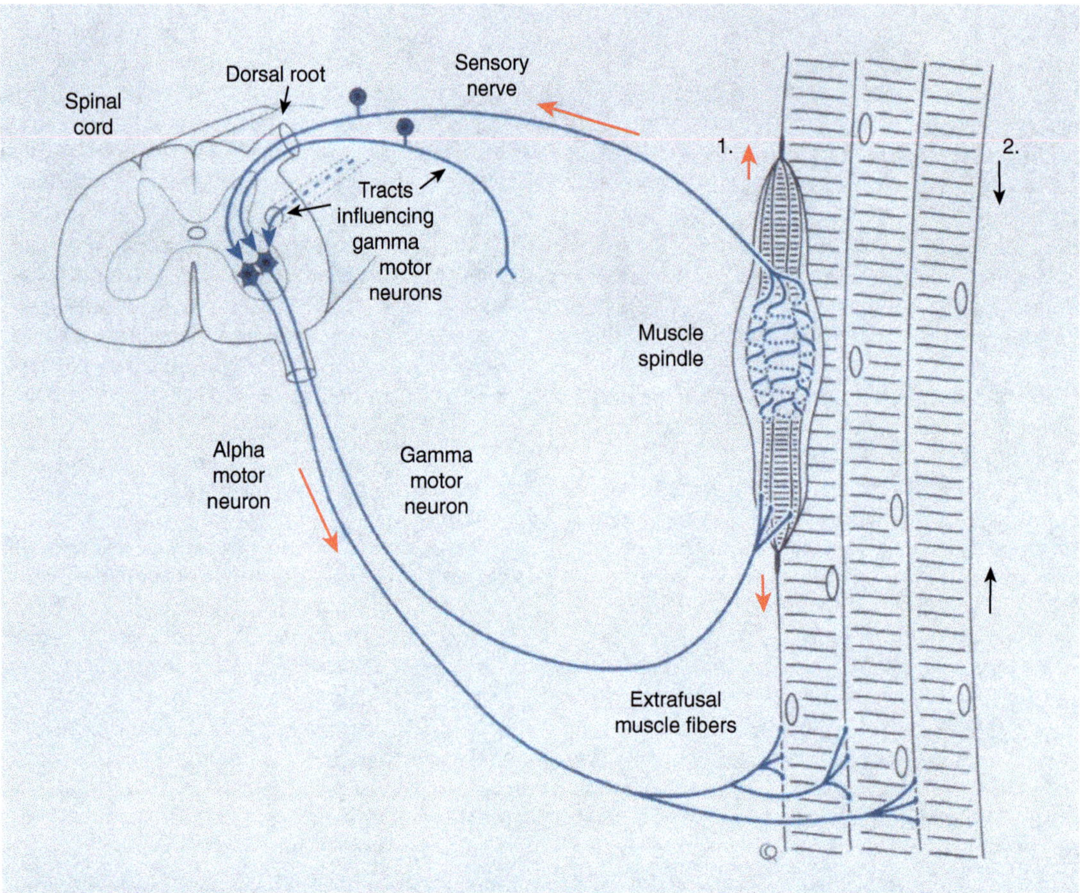

Fig. 14-20 Simplified drawing of the γ-motor neuron system. In cattle with spastic paresis, spinal cord neurons are thought to provide defective control to the γ-motor neuron system, most likely by overstimulation or sufficient inhibition. During the normal stretch reflex the extrafusal skeletal muscle fibers are lengthened, stretching the muscle spindle. This stretch is detected and a signal sent via the afferent axon to the dorsal root. The signal is then sent directly to the α-motor neurons, resulting in muscle contraction. γ-Motor neurons in the ventral spinal cord that are controlled by the central nervous system appear to inappropriately modulate the sensitivity of the stretch reflex system, resulting in sustained and excessive contraction. (Reproduced with permission from De Vlamynck C. *Vet J* 2014; 202:229-235.)

accompanied by a change in the major inhibitory system in the cerebral cortex. It has also been shown that there is a specific and marked deficit of [^{3}H] strychnine-binding sites in the spinal cord. The disease needs to be differentiated from two other congenital, presumed hereditary, diseases of newborn Herefords—maple syrup urine disease and "congenital brain edema"—in which spongy degeneration of the CNS is accompanied by severe edema of the gray and white matter. These two diseases are assumed to represent those cases of congenital disease, originally bracketed with inherited congenital myoclonus, in which there was vacuolation of nervous tissue in the CNS.

INHERITED SPINAL DYSMYELINATION

Bovine spinal dysmyelination is a congenital neurologic disease occurring in several national cattle breeds upgraded with American Brown Swiss cattle. The disease was first described in the Red Danish Dairy breed. In Denmark, all cases are genetically related to the ABS bull White Cloud Jason's Elegant. It is inherited as an autosomal recessive trait. Genetic mapping of the gene in crossbred American Brown Swiss cattle to the bovine chromosome II has been done.

Clinically, in calves there is lateral recumbency, opisthotonus, limb extension, normal to increased reflexes, and mental alertness. Dysmyelination is present, including axonal degeneration and astrogliosis, in spinal tracts, especially the ascending gracile funiculus and dorsolateral spinocerebellar tracts and the descending sulcomarginal tract. This is probably the same defect as spinal muscular atrophy.

INHERITED NEURODEGENERATION (SHAKER CALF SYNDROME)

This is an inherited, degenerative disorder of horned **Hereford** calves. Newborn calves show severe tremor, difficulty in rising, spastic gait, and aphonia. Terminally there is spastic paraplegia. Histologically, there are accumulations of neurofilaments within neurons. A similar disease in **Holstein Friesians** occurs only in males. There are severe degenerative changes in the spinal cord with spongiform lesions and some cavitation. It has the epidemiologic distribution of a sex-linked recessive mutation.

INHERITED SPINAL DYSRAPHISM

This is found as a congenital defect in Charolais calves and is associated with arthrogryposis and cleft palate. Spinal cord anomalies can be associated with a large number of vertebral abnormalities because of the close association of spinal cord and vertebral column during embryology. Other developmental defects that lead to congenital abnormalities include spinal cord hypoplasia and syringomyelia (tubular cystic cavitation containing CSF that extends over several spinal cord segments) in calves[1,2]; however, many of these developmental abnormalities are accidents of embryology and do not necessarily imply the presence of an inherited condition.

REFERENCES

1. Binanti B, et al. *Anat Histol Embryol.* 2012;42:316.
2. Burnside WM, et al. *J Am Vet Med Assoc.* 2014;244:661.

INHERITED CONGENITAL POSTERIOR PARALYSIS

Two inherited forms of congenital posterior paralysis are recorded in cattle. In Norwegian Red Poll cattle posterior paralysis is apparent in affected calves at birth. Opisthotonus and muscle tremor are also present. No histologic lesions have been found. The disease is conditioned by an inherited recessive factor. In Red Danish and Bulgarian Red cattle a similar condition occurs but there is spastic extension of the limbs, particularly the hindlimbs, and tendon reflexes are exaggerated. Histologic examination has revealed degenerative changes in midbrain motor nuclei. Both defects are lethal because of prolonged recumbency.

An inherited posterior paralysis has been recorded in several breeds of swine in Europe. Affected pigs are able to move their hindlimbs but are unable to stand on them. They are normal in other respects. Degeneration of neurons is evident in cerebral cortex, midbrain, cerebellum, medulla, and spinal cord. The disease is conditioned by the inheritance of a recessive character. An inherited progressive ataxia is also recorded in Yorkshire pigs.

INHERITED BOVINE DEGENERATIVE AXONOPATHY

Reported in Holstein Friesian calves in Australia, most affected calves are affected at birth by recumbency; hyperesthesia or depression; rigidity of limbs; tremor, especially of the head; nystagmus, apparent blindness, and the development of opisthotonus and tetanic spasms when stimulated. At necropsy the consistent lesion is a severe, diffuse, axonal swelling and loss in the spinal cord and brainstem. The cause is unknown but the indicators point to an inherited cause.

DEGENERATIVE AXONOPATHY OF TYROLEAN GREY CATTLE

A new neurologic disease was identified in Tyrolean Grey cattle in Switzerland in 2003 and was initially named Demetz syndrome.[1] The clinical presentation is similar to that seen in weaver syndrome of Brown Swiss cattle but clinical signs are first evident at 4 to 6 weeks of age. Calves exhibit mild ambulatory paraparesis with moderate to severe ataxia being more severely affected in the hindlimbs. The disease is progressive and affected calves are usually slaughtered by 10 months of age.

A mutation in the mitofusin 2 gene (a mitochondrial membrane protein) was identified that truncates the last 22 amino acids. Pedigree analysis indicated that the gene mutation occurred before 1972, and gene testing indicated a current carrier frequency of approximately 10%. Marker assisted selection is currently being used to eliminate degenerative axonopathy from this breed.

REFERENCE

1. Drogemuller C, et al. *PLoS ONE.* 2011;6:e18931.

CENTRAL AND PERIPHERAL AXONOPATHY OF MAINE ANJOU (ROUGE-DES-PRÉS) CATTLE

A new neurologic disease was identified in Maine Anjou cattle in France in 2008. Affected calves were 1 to 4 months of age and exhibited mild to severe truncal ataxia with mild to moderate paraparesis. The pelvic limbs were much more severely affected than the thoracic limbs. Clinical signs were rapidly progressive and calves became recumbent within 1 to 3 weeks of being examined, at which time they were euthanized. Mentation remained normal for the calves.

Histopathologic examination revealed marked degeneration of axons and myelin and the dorsolateral and ventromedial funiculi of the distal spinal cord (important tracts for transmitting proprioceptive information from the hindlimbs), lateral vestibular nuclei, caudal cerebellar peduncles, and thoracic nuclei.

INHERITED PROGRESSIVE DEGENERATIVE MYELOENCEPHALOPATHY (WEAVER SYNDROME) OF BROWN SWISS CATTLE

The defect is inherited in Brown Swiss cattle. It appears first in calves when they are 6 months to 2 years old, with a small number more than 2 years, and is manifested by progressive bilateral hindlimb weakness and proprioceptive deficits causing difficulty in rising and a weaving, hypermetric gait, goose-stepping with the forelimbs, and dragging the hindlimbs. The limb reflexes are normal. The calves are bright and alert throughout. There is a broad-based stance and finally recumbency and, after a course of 12 to 18 months, inevitable euthanasia. Necropsy lesions include axonal degeneration, including spheroid formation, and vacuolation of white matter in the cerebellum and at all levels of the spinal cord but especially in the thoracic segment. There is some neurogenic atrophy of muscles but there is no muscular dystrophy. The defect can be identified by examination of chromosomes. It appears to be linked chromosomally with high milk yield traits.

INHERITED PROGRESSIVE ATAXIA

This well-recognized disease occurs in Charolais cattle. The first onset of signs is at about 12 months of age when the gait is seen to be stiff and stumbling, especially in the hindlimbs, and the hindtoes are dragged. The ataxia may be asymmetric, and the animal cannot back up. The ataxia progresses over a period of 1 to 2 years. Affected animals tend to be down a lot and have difficulty in rising and posturing for urination. Urination is abnormal; it is a squirting but continuous flow that soils the tail. Some affected animals nod their heads from side to side when excited. Both males and females are affected. It has been described occurring in 2-year-old Charolais steer in New Zealand. Characteristic necropsy lesions are confined to the CNS and are histopathologic. The white matter of the cerebellum and internal capsule contains multiple foci of oligodendroglial dysplasia. The somatic lymph nodes contain nodules of hyperplastic lymphoid follicles, some catarrh of the medullae of the nodes, and an accumulation of eosinophils.

INHERITED SPINAL MYELINOPATHY

There is a progressive spinal myelinopathy of Murray Grey cattle, similar to that seen in Charolais cattle. It is possibly genetic in origin. Some calves are affected at birth; others do not become affected until 1 year old. The syndrome is one of a progressing paresis, without significant ataxia leading to paresis and permanent recumbency. There are degenerative lesions in spinal cord, midbrain, and cerebellum. The disease is conditioned by an autosomal recessive gene.

INHERITED PERIODIC SPASTICITY OF CATTLE

Inherited periodic spasticity has been observed in Holstein and Guernsey cattle and usually does not appear until the animals are adults. A recent report described it in a Canadian Hereford bull with an early onset between 1 and 2 years of age. It is a particular problem in mature bulls maintained in artificial insemination centers. In the early stages the signs are apparent only on rising; the hindlimbs are stretched out behind and the back depressed (Fig. 14-21). Marked tremor of the hindquarters may be noted. Initially the attacks persist only for a few seconds but are of longer duration as the disease progresses and may eventually last for up to 30 minutes. Movement is usually impossible during the attacks. The tetanic episodes fluctuate in their severity from time to time but there is never any abnormality of consciousness. Lesions of the vertebrae have been recorded but no lesions have been found in the nervous system. Idiopathic muscle

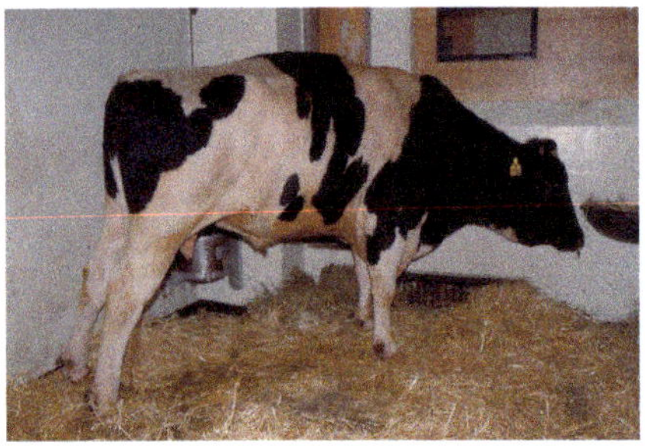

Fig. 14-21 Inherited periodic spasticity in a Holstein Friesian bull. The signs are apparent only on rising; the hindlimbs are stretched out behind and the back depressed.

cramps have been suggested as a cause. The disease is familial and the mode of inheritance appears to be by inheritance of a single recessive factor with incomplete penetrance.

Administration of the spinal cord depressant, mephenesin (3–4 g/100 kg BW given orally in three divided doses and repeated for 2–3 days) controls the more severe signs. A single course of treatment may be effective for some weeks.

NEURAXONAL DYSTROPHY

Neuraxonal dystrophy represents a heterogeneous group of degenerative diseases of genetic or acquired etiology that is characterized by spheroidal swellings of axons called spheroid bodies, which is the result of accumulation of axoplasmic organelles including neurofilaments. The change may be physiologic (caused by normal aging) or pathologic and are categorized as primary (familial) or secondary (acquired).[1] EDM is considered a more severe variant of neuraxonal dystrophy and is discussed separately.

NEURAXONAL DYSTROPHY OF SHEEP (SEGMENTED AXONOPATHY)

This is reported in Suffolk, Merino, Romney, Perendale, Coopworth, and crossbred sheep.[1] An inherited defect (autosomal recessive) is suspected in all cases. Abnormalities appear related to abnormal axonal transport and the inability to maintain integrity of the axon and their associated myelin sheaths.[2]

In **Coopworth sheep** the lambs are affected at birth but have a progressive syndrome in which cerebellar and proprioceptive signs predominate. Most die by 6 weeks of age. Large axonal spheroids are present in the spinal cord and midbrain, and there is a severe depletion of Purkinje cells in the cerebellum.

In **Suffolk** sheep the disease does not appear until 1 to 6 months; signs are a gradual onset of ataxia, followed by recumbency, leading to death or euthanasia. Spheroids in CNS axons are characteristic, mostly in the spinal cord and cerebellum, and contain large amounts of amyloid precursor protein.[1]

The disease in **Merinos** is in fine-wool sheep, is probably the same disease as that previously called **Murrurrundi disease**, and does not appear until 4 to 6 years of age. Most cases require euthanasia after about 2 months but some mild cases survive for up to 3 years. The clinical signs include a wide-based stance, dysmetria of all limb movements with a pronounced hypermetria of the forelimbs resulting in frequent falling, a fine intention tremor of the head, and a diminished menace reflex. A similar disease of medium-wool Merinos, characterized by progressive posterior ataxia and degeneration of sensory tracts in thoracic segments of spinal cord, commencing after 5 months of age and terminating fatally before 2 years of age, is also recorded in Australia. It is probably also an inherited defect

NEURAXONAL DYSTROPHY OF HORSES

In horses, neuraxonal dystrophy has been reported in **Quarter Horses, Haflingers, Morgans, Appaloosas, Paso Finos, and Standardbreds** with a familial occurrence present in a number of breeds.[3,4] The onset of clinical signs can be as early as a few months of age. Common neurologic abnormalities include ataxia, proprioceptive positioning deficits, dysmetria, a wide-based stance, obtundation, and an inconsistent menace response with no detectable visual impairment.[3] Clinical progression can be very slow over a few months to years, and in some cases stabilization of clinical signs may occur.[3] It can be difficult to clinically differentiate neuraxonal dystrophy from **EDM**; however, the latter is considered a more severe clinical variant of neuraxonal dystrophy.[5] Clinical signs of ocular disease are not detectable and the results of ERG and EEG are within the normal range.[6] Lesions at necropsy are only apparent microscopically and include specific tracts and nuclei in the caudal medulla and spinal cord, with occasional involvement of the cerebellum.

REFERENCES

1. Finnie JW, et al. *Aust Vet J.* 2014;92:389.
2. Jolly RD, et al. *New Zeal Vet J.* 2006;54:210.
3. Aleman M, et al. *J Am Vet Med Assoc.* 2011;239:823.
4. Brosnahan MM, et al. *J Vet Intern Med.* 2009;23:1303.
5. Finno CJ, et al. *J Vet Intern Med.* 2013;27:177.
6. Finno CJ, et al. *Vet Ophthalmol.* 2012;15(suppl 2):3.

CAPRINE PROGRESSIVE SPASTICITY

A possibly inherited progressive paresis of Angora goats is recorded in Australia. Signs first appear at about 2 months of age, commencing with lethargy, followed by ataxia, then paresis progressing to sternal recumbency and eventual euthanasia. Tendon reflexes are normal but the kids have difficulty getting to their feet, especially in the hindlimbs. The gait is ataxic with frequent stumbles, and the kids are unwilling to run. At necropsy there are many large, clear vacuoles in many neurons of the spinal cord, posterior brainstem and midbrain, and degeneration of nerve fibers in the same areas and peripheral nerves.

INHERITED SPONTANEOUS LOWER MOTOR NEURON DISEASES

Motor neuron diseases involve selective degeneration of upper and/or motor neurons. Upper motor neurons originate in the cranial vault, where they stimulate contraction of muscles. In comparison, lower motor neurons connect the brainstem and spinal cord to the muscle fibers.[1] Effective treatments for motor neuron diseases have yet to be identified.

A lower motor neuron disease in newborn Romney lambs has been described.[1] Lambs are normal at birth but within 1 week they developed weakness and ataxia, which progressed until they were unable to stand. The principal histologic lesions were degeneration and loss of neurons in the ventral horns of the spinal cord and brainstem, wallerian degeneration of ventral rootlets and motor nerves, and associated denervation atrophy of skeletal muscle fibers. Large fibrillar spheroids were found in white and gray matter including nuclei in the brainstem. One missense mutation on the sheep called the ATP/GTP-binding protein 1 gene was identified in all affected animals, exhibiting recessive pattern of inheritance.[1] This binding protein plays a role in protein turnover by cleaving peptides into amino acids. A similar, though not identical, disease of newborn lambs has been recorded in a Dorset Down flock affecting about 20% of lambs. They lay with hindlimbs tucked under the body and forelimbs splayed sideways.

This progressive disease of Yorkshire piglets 5 to 10 weeks of age is presumed to be inherited. Clinical signs include hindlimb tremor, weakness, and ataxia appearing at 2 to 5 weeks of age. The gait includes fetlock knuckling, short choppy steps, and a tendency to collapse after a few steps. Segmental and postural reflexes are normal. By 10 weeks there is complete hindlimb paralysis, the pig is in sternal recumbency, and front limb paralysis has begun. The appetite is good and the pig is bright and alert. On necropsy there is symmetric degeneration and loss of motor neurons in the spinal cord in some ventral spinal nerve roots.

REFERENCE

1. Zhao X, et al. *Heredity.* 2012;109:156.

INHERITED SPINAL MUSCULAR ATROPHY

A progressive ataxia, weakness, muscle atrophy, and recumbency develops in young calves, mostly during the first 2 weeks of life.

Sensory functions are unimpaired. Some are already affected at birth and some may be stillborn. No new cases occur after 3 months of age. Conditioned by an autosomal recessive gene the defect occurs in Red Danish cattle, which originated from Brown Swiss, German Braunvieh, and American Brown Swiss. The primary lesion is degeneration of ventral horn cells of the spinal cord, without involvement of the brainstem or cerebellum. The visible lesion is the secondary atrophy of the denervated muscles.

INHERITED HYPOMYELINOGENESIS (CONGENITAL TREMOR OF PIGS)

Congenital tremor of pigs has a multiple etiology and some of the causes are not yet identified. The two inherited diseases are noted here: congenital tremor type A-IV of British Saddleback pigs and congenital tremor type A-III, a sex-linked inherited form of cerebrospinal hypomyelinogenesis of Landrace pigs. The A-IV disease is characterized by the presence of poorly myelinated axons in all parts of the CNS. The specific defect in A-IV is one of fatty acid metabolism. The structural abnormalities in the A-III disease have been identified; splayleg is a common accompaniment.

Both diseases are characterized by muscle tremor, incoordination, difficulty in standing, and some squealing. The A-III disease occurs only in males. Both are inherited as recessive characters.

PORCINE CONGENITAL PROGRESSIVE ATAXIA AND SPASTIC PARESIS

This is an autosomal recessive disorder of pigs in Switzerland with a yet to be identified gene defect. Clinical signs of a spastic gait with progressive ataxia become evident within 3 days of birth, and the condition is lethal. Male and female pigs are equally affected. Pedigree analysis has identified a boar born in 1978 that was used widely for artificial insemination as the originator of the genetic defect.

REFERENCE

1. Genini S, et al. *J Anim Breed Genet.* 2007;124:269.

EQUINE DEGENERATIVE MYELOENCEPHALOPATHY (EQUINE NEURAXONAL DYSTROPHY)

EDM is characterized by **symmetric, slowly progressive spasticity and ataxia** in foals and horses less than 2 years of age. The disease occurs in most breeds in North America and Europe and is reported in captive zebra and Mongolian Wild Horses in North America. Neuronal dystrophy of the cuneate and gracilis nuclei is considered a form of EDM and is likely the underlying pathophysiologic process of EDM.[1]

The prevalence of the disease varies widely, with up to 40% of susceptible animals on a farm being affected, although the disease is usually sporadic. There is a familial predisposition to the disease apparently involving an increased requirement for vitamin E, although other factors, including housing, are contributory. Foals from dams that had an EDM-affected foal were at a significantly higher risk (relative risk = 25) of developing EDM than foals from other dams. The occurrence of clusters of cases involving related horses is supportive of a genetic component with inheritance as in an autosomal dominant with variable expression or polygenic manner, although this has not been confirmed in all breeds.[2-4] The disease in Quarter Horses is highly heritable and appears to be polygenic.[2,4]

EDM occurs in Standardbreds, Paso Finos, Quarter Horses, Mongolian horses, Appaloosas, Haflingers, Arabians, Morgans, Lusitanos, Thoroughbreds, Paint horses, Tennessee Walking Horses, Norwegian Fjord Horses, Welsh Pony, and various mixed breeds.[1] There is no sex predilection.

The pathogenesis of the disease is unknown. Abnormal expression of integral synaptic vesicle, synaptic vesicle-associated presynaptic plasma membrane, and cytosolic proteins was observed in two Arabian horses with equine degenerative myeloencephalopathy; however, abnormal α-tocopherol transfer protein does not appear to contribute to the disease.[4] These proteins have a role in trafficking, docking, and fusion of neuronal synaptic vesicles, and this finding suggests that there is disruption of axonal transport in equine degenerative myeloencephalopathy. A role for oxidative stress and damage to neurons is supported by documentation of markers of oxidative stress in nervous tissue and low serum and/or CSF vitamin E concentrations in two horses with EDM and not in healthy control horses.[5] Low vitamin E concentrations in serum are often associated with the disease, but in one small study only foals with a genetic predisposition to the disease, and having a low serum vitamin E concentration, developed the disease. Foals with low serum vitamin E concentrations that did not have the genetic predisposition to the disease did not develop EDM.[6] Loss of axons leads to defects in neurologic function and consequent gait abnormalities.

The clinical signs are those of a slowing progressive spinal ataxia that stabilizes when the animal is 2 to 3 years of age. Age of onset ranges from birth to 36 months, although most cases have clinical signs by 6 to 12 months of age. Affected foals and yearlings have symmetric signs that are most severe in the hindlimbs, of ataxia characterized by pivoting, circumduction, truncal sway, and difficulty performing complex movements such as backing or walking with the head elevated. At rest, severely affected horses may have an abnormal posture. The cutaneous trunci reflex may be absent. Spontaneous recovery does not occur, but progression to death is unusual. Radiography and myelography of the cervical spine does not reveal evidence of compression of the spinal cord. The disease is not associated with abnormalities detected on ocular examination, ERG or EEG.[7]

Serum vitamin E concentrations can be normal or low in affected horses, and this is not a reliable test for diagnosis of the disease.[1-3] The hemogram, serum biochemical profile, and CSF analysis are normal. There are no gross lesions on necropsy. Histologic lesions include neuronal atrophy, accumulation of lipofuscin-like pigment, and glial cell proliferation.

Differential diagnoses are listed in Table 14-20 later in the chapter, under the Equine Cervical Vertebral Compressive Myelopathy section. Diagnosis is achieved by exclusion of other causes, of abnormal gait without fever or disease in other body systems in horses, such as compressive myelopathy and equine protozoal myeloencephalopathy.

No treatment is curative, but vitamin E (6000 IU orally once daily) may prevent progression of signs. Supplementation of at-risk foals and yearlings with vitamin E can prevent the disease, although results are not equivocal.[1,6]

REFERENCES

1. Finno CJ, et al. *J Vet Intern Med.* 2012;26:1251.
2. Aleman M, et al. *JAVMA.* 2011;239:823.
3. Finno CJ, et al. *J Vet Intern Med.* 2011;25:1439.
4. Finno CJ, et al. *J Vet Intern Med.* 2013;27:177.
5. Wong DM, et al. *Vet Pathol.* 2012;49:1049.
6. Finno CJ, et al. *J Vet Intern Med.* 2015;29:1667.
7. Finno CJ, et al. *Vet Ophthalmol.* 2012;15:3.

EQUINE CERVICAL VERTEBRAL COMPRESSIVE MYELOPATHY (WOBBLER, "WOBBLES," FOAL ATAXIA, EQUINE SENSORY ATAXIA, CERVICAL VERTEBRAL INSTABILITY)

SYNOPSIS

Etiology Unknown. The clinical signs are the result of cervical spinal cord compression as a result of abnormalities in the cervical spine.

Epidemiology Two predominant manifestations. Sporadic or endemic disease of young horses with young, rapidly growing male horses most commonly affected. Separate presentation in middle-aged and older horses in which it is sporadic.

Clinical signs Spinal ataxia evident as truncal sway, ataxia, and paresis usually more

Continued

severe in the hindlimbs. Radiographic evidence of narrow spinal canal.

Clinical pathology None.

Lesions Malacia and wallerian degeneration in the cervical spinal cord.

Differential diagnosis Equine degenerative myelopathy, equine protozoal myeloencephalitis, trauma, equine infectious anemia, cerebrospinal nematodiasis, West Nile encephalomyelitis, equine herpesvirus-1 myelopathy, osteomyelitis, cervical vertebral epidural hematoma, aortoiliac thrombosis, congenital vertebral malformation, diskospondylitis, and ryegrass staggers.

Diagnostic confirmation Radiography. Positive contrast myelography. Necropsy.

Treatment Antiinflammatory drugs. Surgical fusion of vertebrae.

Control None.

ETIOLOGY

The cause of neurologic disease is extradural compression of the cervical spinal cord, hence the term **compressive myelopathy.** The compression may be **static**, that is, the compression is present constantly with the neck in a neutral position, or **dynamic** and only present intermittently when the neck is either flexed or extended. The second situation is often referred to as cervical vertebral instability.

The etiology of CSM in most cases is not known. The disease in young horses is caused by malformation and malarticulation of the cervical vertebrae and could represent part of the osteochondritis dissecans spectrum of diseases.[1,2] There can be combinations of articular process osteophytosis, interarcuate ligament hypertrophy, dorsal laminal thickening, vertebral body end plate flaring, and synovial cysts. Importantly, changes in soft tissue associated with the bony lesions can contribute to the compressive myelopathy. Dynamic instability is associated with vertebral instability and subluxation and is most common in the cranial vertebrae (C3-C5).

Copper deficiency has been mooted as one cause of the bony lesions, as have high calorie rations and diets high in soluble carbohydrate.[2]

The disease in older horses is secondary to osteoarthritis of the articular processes. An inciting cause has not been identified.

Several basic syndromes of compressive myelopathy, based on age of occurrence, are recognized:

- CSM in immature horses (<3 years of age, depending on breed) that is often associated with developmental joint disease in the axial and appendicular skeleton. A fundamental underlying predisposing defect appears to be a narrow diameter of the cervical vertebral canal. Compression is a result of the lesions described earlier.
- Cervical vertebral instability is a disease of horses less than 1 year of age that is often associated with malformations of one or more of the cervical vertebrae.[3]
- Compressive myelopathy in mature horses, >4 years (usually >7 years) of age, associated with osteoarthritis of the articular facets of the caudal cervical vertebrae, with subsequent impingement of the vertebral canal by bony and soft tissue proliferative lesions.
- Miscellaneous causes of cervical cord compression by neoplasia (melanoma, sarcoma, lymphoma), trauma (cervical vertebral fractures), arachnoid or synovial cysts, epidural hematoma[4] or, rarely, discospondylitis.[5]

An alternative categorization is based on the nature of the bony lesion and not on the cause of compression of the spinal cord. **Type 1 cervical vertebral malformation** occur in horses <2 years of age that have vertebral changes that likely began in the first few months of life, including malformations causing stenosis of the vertebral canal, malformations at the articulations of the vertebrae including osteochondrosis, and enlarged physeal growth regions. **Type II cervical vertebral malformations** tend to occur in older horses with severe osteoarthritic lesions of the vertebral articulations.

EPIDEMIOLOGY

Occurrence

The disease in mature horses occurs sporadically throughout the world.

The disease in young horses is sometimes endemic on farms or studs and in particular lines of horses. There is a suggestion of a familial tendency for the disease, although this has not been well documented.

The **morbidity rate** can be as high as 25% of each foal crop on individual Thoroughbred farms, although the overall frequency of the disease in the general horse population is much lower. Among Thoroughbreds born on four stud farms in Europe and North America, the disease has an annual prevalence of diagnosis of 1.3% (range of 0.7%–2.1% over the study period) and annual prevalence on farms varying from 0% to 5.8%.[6]

Compressive myelopathy was detected in 83 of 4318 horses subject to necropsy examination in Normandy, France.[7] Fifteen percent of horses with a diagnosis of neurologic disease had cervical compressive myelopathy. There were more males affected than females.[7]

Risk Factors

Animal Risk Factors

Risk factors for CSM identified in a study of 1618 horses at 22 veterinary teaching hospitals in North America are summarized in Table 14-20.

The **disease in young horses** is commonly recognized in Thoroughbred, Standardbred, Warmblood, and Quarter horses, with Arabians and other breeds less likely to be diagnosed with the disease.[8] Ponies are rarely, if ever, affected. Horses less than 4 years of age are at greater risk of the disease, with most cases occurring in 1- to 3-year-old horses. Males, either intact or gelded, are more likely to be affected than are females.[8]

Table 14-20 Association of horse factors associated with a diagnosis of cervical stenotic myelopathy in 811 horses with cervical stenotic myelopathy and 805 control horses

Variable	Or (95% CI)	*P* value
Sex		
Gelding	2.0 (1.5–2.6)	<0.001
Sexually intact male	2.4 (1.8–3.2)	<0.001
Female	1 (Referent)	NA
Breed		
Arabian	0.6 (0.3–0.9)	0.035
Standardbred	0.5 (0.3–0.7)	<0.001
Thoroughbred	1.7 (1.3–2.3)	<0.001
Tennessee Walking Horse	2.3 (1.1–4.7)	0.019
Warmblood	1.9 (1.1–3.1)	0.020
Other breeds	0.6 (0.4–0.8)	0.006
Quarter Horse	1 (Referent)	NA
Age		
<6 mo	2.4 (1.4–3.9)	<0.001
6–11 mo	6.6 (3.8–11.5)	<0.001
12 to 23 mo	16.4 (10.5–25.8)	<0.001
2 to <4 y	7.2 (4.9–10.5)	<0.001
4 to <7 y	3.1 (2.1–4.6)	<0.001
7–10 y	1.1 (0.7–1.8)	0.65
≥10 y	1 (Referent)	NA

OR, odds ratio; NA, not applicable.
From Levine JM, et al. JAVMA 2008;233:1453

The **disease in older horses** is characterized by a slight predominance of male horses with overrepresentation of Warmbloods, which could represent a breed or use predisposition, and median age at diagnosis of 8 years.[1]

Horses with CSM have a narrower spinal canal than do unaffected animals and this condition, with degenerative joint disease of the articular facets and thickening of the ligamentum flavum, contributes to the greater likelihood that the horse will have spinal cord compression.

It is suspected that predisposition to the disease is heritable, but this has not been demonstrated by appropriate studies.

The disease in mature horses tends to be in horses used for athletic endeavors and is uncommon in broodmares or retired animals.

PATHOGENESIS

The disease is attributable to injury to the spinal cord as a result of compression by either soft tissue (joint capsule, intervertebral ligaments, or, rarely, intervertebral disk material) or cartilage and bone.

Constant or intermittent pressure on the spinal cord causes dysfunction or necrosis of white matter and neurons at the site of compression, degeneration of fibers of ascending tracts cranial to the site of compression, and of descending tracts caudal to the compression. The ascending tracts are those associated with general proprioception, whereas the descending tracts are upper motor neurons. These tracts are located superficially in the dorsolateral aspect of the cervical spinal cord and damage to them results in signs of ataxia and weakness. Tracts from the caudal limbs are more superficial, and therefore more easily injured, than tracts associated with the cranial limbs. Consequently, clinical signs are usually more severe in the hindlimbs. The spinal cord lesions are usually, but not always, bilaterally symmetric, as are the clinical signs. Proprioceptive pathways are disrupted, causing the signs of ataxia (incoordination) typical of the disease. Clinical signs vary depending on the site of the lesion (see later).

CLINICAL FINDINGS

The onset of clinical signs is sometimes acute in young horses with CSM and there can be a history of trauma, such as falling. However, the onset of clinical signs of CSM in both young and mature horses is usually gradual and insidious, and in mildly affected horses the nervous disease can be mistaken for lameness of musculoskeletal origin. Affected horses are bright and alert and have a normal appetite. There can be evidence of pain on manipulation of the neck or on firm pressure over the lateral facets, especially in mature horses with osteoarthritis of the caudal cervical vertebral facets.[1] There can be focal muscle atrophy adjacent to affected cervical vertebrae in older horses.

The severity of clinical signs varies from barely detectable to recumbency. There are no defects of al nerves, with the occasional exception of the cervicofacial reflex. The severity of signs of CSM are often graded according to the following:

Grade 0: no gait deficits at the walk
Grade 1: no gait deficits identified at the walk and deficits only identified during further testing (head elevation, backing, walking on a slope, stepping over obstacles, circling, tail pull at rest and while walking)
Grade 2: deficits noted at the walk
Grade 3: marked deficits noted at the walk
Grade 4: severe deficits noted at the walk and might fall or nearly fall at normal gaits
Grade 5: recumbent and unable rise without assistance

The **two primary defects in gait** in affected horses are related to defects in upper motor neuron function and general proprioception. These two primary deficiencies in neurologic function contribute to clinical signs characterized as ataxia, paresis, dysmetria, and spasticity. **Ataxia** is the incoordinated movement of limbs and is evident as interference of one limb with another (such as one foot stepping on another when the horse is tightly circled), knuckling of the fetlock joint (which can also be a sign of weakness), unusual placement of feet (excessively wide-based or narrow-based stance, incomplete or delayed return of the foot to its normal position after it is relocated to an abnormal position, excessive circumduction of the outside foot during tight circling), stumbling, and/or swaying of the trunk during walking in a straight line. **Paresis** is weakness and is evident in its most extreme form as inability of the horse to rise. In less extreme manifestations it is evident as knuckling of the fetlock joint, stumbling when walking downhill or over obstacles, and ease of pulling the horse to one side by the tail when it is walking. **Dysmetria** refers to uneven gait typified by undershoot or overshoot of the limb such that the hoof is in an incorrect position. **Spasticity** is a result of loss of inhibition of lower spinal reflexes by the upper motor neurons and results in a stilted or stiff gait.

Mildly affected horses may have deficits that are difficult to detect and only apparent under saddle or at high speed. The owner might complain of poor performance of a racehorse or dressage animal, of an animal that frequently changes leads, or that is poorly gaited. Careful examination can reveal excessive circumduction of the hindfeet, stumbling, and pacing when the head is elevated.

Moderately affected animals have truncal sway (the body of the horse and hindquarters swaying laterally when the horse is walked in a straight line) and excessive circumduction of the hindfeet. There can be a floating gait of the hindlimbs and scuffing of the toe. Having the horse move in a very tight circle about the examiner often causes the circumduction to become worse in the outside hindleg and the horse to place one foot on top of the other. Affected horses will sometimes pace when walked in a straight line with the head elevated. Blindfolding the horse does not exacerbate the signs. Affected horses will stumble when walked over low objects, such as a curb, and will knuckle at the fetlocks and stumble when walked down a steep hill.

Severely affected horses often fall easily when moved or are unable to stand. The horses are bright and alert, but anxious, and display marked truncal sway and ataxia. When standing, they will often have their legs in markedly abnormal positions.

Horses with lesions in the cervical spinal cord cranial to C6-C7 have signs in both forelimbs and hindlimbs. The hindlimbs are more severely affected and the signs are usually, but not always, bilaterally symmetric.[9] Approximately 43% of affected horses have asymmetric gait abnormalities.[9] Lesions of the cervical intumescence (C6 to T2) may cause signs that are more severe in the forelimbs than in the hindlimbs. Lesions at this site may also cause signs typical of brachial plexus injury. Focal muscle atrophy is not characteristic of CSM or cervical vertebral instability and there are never signs of CNC, cerebral, or cerebellar disease.

After initial progression the clinical signs usually stabilize or partially resolve. However, complete spontaneous recovery is very unusual. Death is unusual unless it is by misadventure, although many affected animals are killed for humane or economic reasons.[8]

Neurologic Examination

A tentative diagnosis of cervical compressive myelopathy is often made based on the clinical examination. Although this assessment is relatively straightforward for severely affected horses, the detection of neurologic abnormalities on physical examination is more challenging for horses with milder forms of the disease. This becomes important as additional diagnostic investigations might not be warranted in all cases of horses with clear-cut signs of cervical compressive myelopathy, but might be indicated in horses with less severe signs of the disease.

The reliability of the neurologic examination of horses has been investigated very little. The agreement between expert or trained observers for overall grade of neurologic abnormality was good (intraclass correlation coefficient of 0.74) when horses of all grades were considered (grades 0–4), but very poor for horses ≤ Grade 1 (intraclass coefficient (ICC) = 0.08) and only moderate (0.43) for horses ≥ Grade 2.[10] The higher ICC for the overall assessment was because observers could easily agree on differences

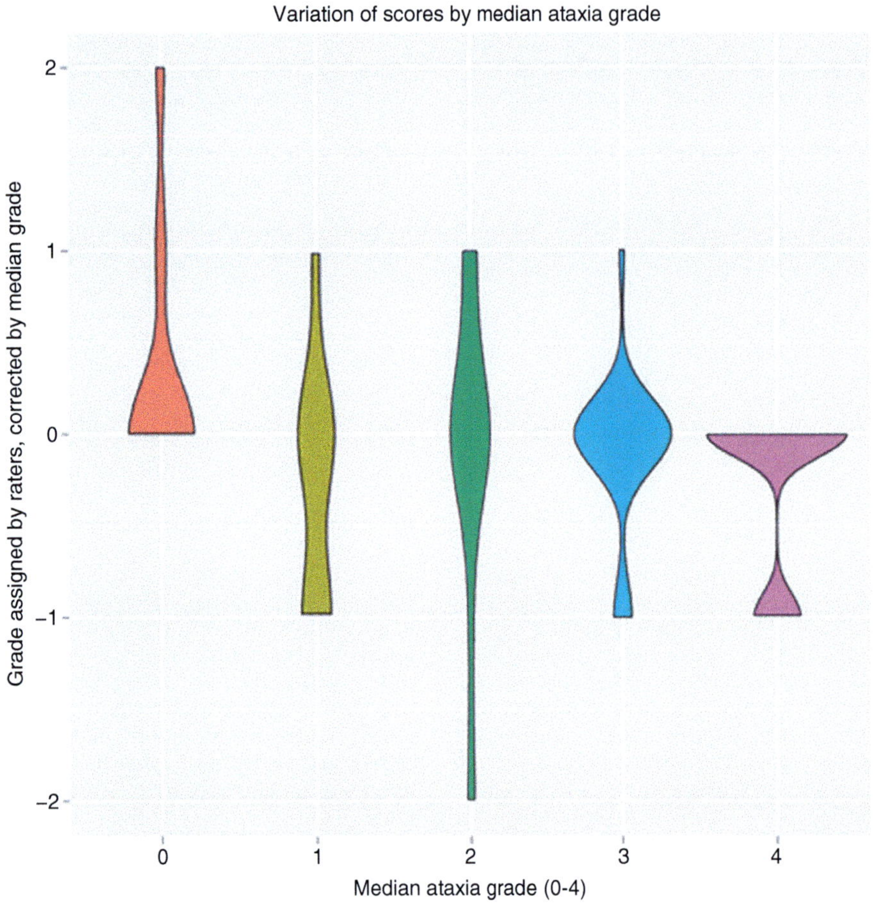

Fig. 14-22 Violin plot of the variation in individual ratings grouped by the median rating for each horse during live scoring only. To align the ratings around 0, each score was subtracted from the median score of the horse. A violin plot is similar to a boxplot, with the addition of the density of data points illustrated by an increase in width. This figure reveals that most grades have a fluctuation of 1 degree more or less than the median; however, grades 0 and 3 are condensed around the median illustrating better agreement, whereas grade 2 stretches from −2 to + 1 grades from the median. (From Olsen E, Dunkel B, Barker WHJ, et al. Rater Agreement on Gait Assessment During Neurologic Examination of Horses. *J Vet Int Med* 2014;28:630.)

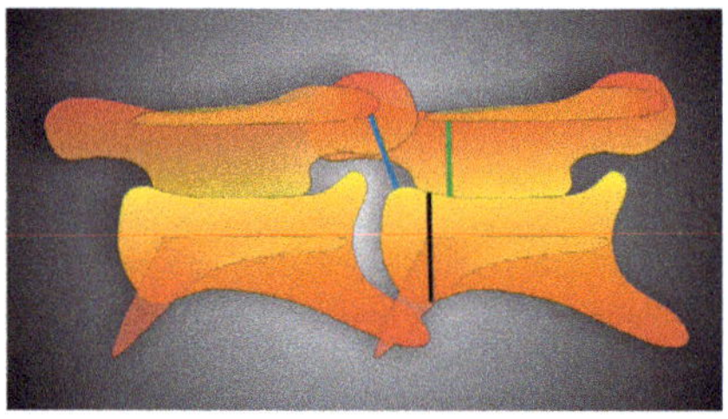

Fig. 14-23 Schematic drawing of the cervical vertebrae illustrating the sagittal ratios: the intravertebral sagittal ratio is calculated as the ratio of the minimum sagittal diameter of the spinal canal (green line) to the maximum sagittal diameter of the vertebral body, taken at the cranial aspect of the vertebra and perpendicular to the spinal canal (black line). The intervertebral sagittal ratio is the ratio of the minimal distance taken from the most cranial aspect of the vertebral body to the most caudal aspect of the vertebral arch of the more cranial vertebra (blue line) and the maximal sagittal diameter of the vertebral body (black line). (Reproduced with permission from Van Biervliet J. An evidence-based approach to clinical questions in the practice of equine neurology. *Vet Clin Nth Am Equine Pract* 2007;23(2):317-328.)

between severely affected and unaffected horses. Greatest lack of agreement was for horses that had Grade 2 neurologic signs (Fig. 14-22).[10]

It is recommended in human medicine that an ICC must be >0.9 for it to be useful for decision making in individual patients,[11] and on this basis the current methods for neurologic examination for horses are not acceptable for clinical use.[10] It is the authors' opinion that the current neurologic grading system for examination of horses continue to be used because it provides a structured way of completing the examination. The results of the examination should be considered in light of its poor reliability, especially for horses with severity of median Grade 2, and interpreted with caution.

Ancillary Diagnostic Tests

The "slap test," in which the response of the arytenoid cartilages to a slap on the thorax is examined through an endoscope, has poorer sensitivity and specificity for detecting spinal cord disease than does a routine neurologic examination.

Acupuncture has no proven value in the diagnosis of cervical compressive myelopathy and should not be used for this purpose.

Radiographic Examination

Radiographic examination of the cervical vertebral column of potentially affected horses is often undertaken because there are frequently lesions of the bone associated with cervical compressive myelopathy. Radiographic examination includes plain radiographs taken from the lateral aspect with the horse standing or myelography using injection of radiopaque dye to allow visualization of the subarachnoid space and detection of extradural compression of this space.

Examination of both plain and contrast radiographs is potentially enhanced by use of one or more of a number of measures and ratios intended to detect and quantify extradural compression of the cord.

Radiographic signs detectable on plain radiographs of the cervical spine in horses with compressive myelopathy include the following:

- Encroachment of the caudal vertebral physis dorsally into the spinal canal ("ski jump lesion") caused by physeal enlargement
- Extension of the arch of the vertebra over the cranial physis of the next vertebra
- Sclerosis of the spinal canal
- Kyphosis, or subluxation, between adjacent vertebra
- Degenerative joint disease of the articular facets evident as osteoarthritis and bony proliferation

However, these signs are also common in normal horses and have poor predictive value. The overall agreement, relative sensitivity, and relative specificity, respectively, for identification of radiographic abnormalities (compared with the gold standard of necropsy examination) in affected horses is 66% (76/116 horses); 63% and 67% for identification of articular process osteophytosis; 61% (71/116), 42%, and 83% for vertebral canal stenosis; and 78% (91/116), 56%, and 85% for vertebral column subluxation.[9] Radiography appears to have useful specificity but limited sensitivity in the diagnosis of bony lesions associated with cervical compressive myelopathy. Use of additional views, such as oblique views of the caudal cervical vertebrae. can enhance the diagnostic value of radiography.[12]

Intervertebral and **intravertebral** ratios have been calculated to assist with diagnosis of CSM (Fig. 14-23). The ratios in and of themselves have variable intraobserver and interobserver reliability with ratios varying by 5% to 10% within and between observers.[13,14] Interobserver agreement in measurements is poor and intraobserver agreement is good across the six most cranial sites but poor for caudal sites.[14] Intraobserver and interobserver variability is sufficient to affect clinical interpretation of radiographs and should be considered when interpreting radiographic examinations with suspected spinal cord disease.

An intravertebral sagittal ratio of the spinal canal to vertebral body diameter of less than 50% for C4-C6 is associated with a 26- to 41-fold increase in the probability of a compressive myelopathy for horse >320 kg; in a separate study all horses with a value of this ratio of less than 0.485 had at least one compressive lesion.[15] An intervertebral ratio can also be calculated and it has diagnostic utility that might be slightly greater than that of the intravertebral ratio.[2,15] The results of these tests are not definitive and a healthy horse can have ratios below this cutoff and affected horses can have normal ratios.[16,17] It is important to recognize that the utility of **intravertebral** (and other) ratios is dependent on the pretest likelihood that the horse has cervical compressive myelopathy. The ratios should therefore be considered in light of other clinical findings. Importantly, neither the intravertebral nor intervertebral ratios predict the site of compression, which can only be detected by myelographic examination.[2]

Myelography has been considered to provide the definitive antemortem confirmation of spinal cord compression, but recent studies demonstrate that it is not a perfect diagnostic test and that results should be interpreted cautiously.[2] The sensitivity of this technique, using a 50% reduction in the width of the dorsal dye column as a cutoff for diagnosis of the disease, is 53% (95% CI 34%–72%, $n = 22$) and the specificity is 89% (95% CI of 84%–93%, $n = 228$) (Fig. 14-24).[2] Others have found similar values for sensitivity and specificity with values of 47% and 78%, respectively, for older horses with compressive myelopathy at caudal cervical sites.[1] These values indicate a test with a relatively high false-negative rate but low false-positive rate for neutral views and indicate that a positive finding on myelography is highly suggestive of the disease, but that a negative finding does not eliminate the possibility of the disease. The **false-positive rate** is increased to 12% to 27% for compression at midcervical sites during neck flexion. Myelography is superior in diagnosing compressive lesions at C6-C7 than at more proximal sites. Occasionally the compression is lateral rather than dorsoventral and is not readily apparent on routine myelography.

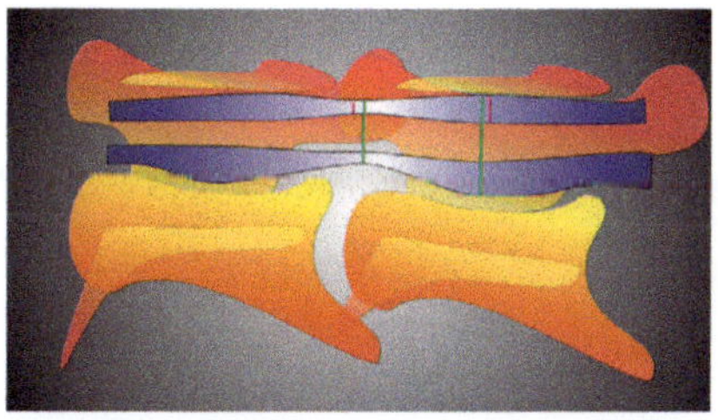

Fig. 14-24 Schematic drawing of cervical myelogram illustrating the dural diameter reduction (green lines) and the dorsal myelographic column reduction (pink lines). (Reproduced with permission from Van Biervliet J. An evidence-based approach to clinical questions in the practice of equine neurology. *Vet Clin Nth Am Equine Pract* 2007;23(2):317-328.)

Myelography has been described in standing, conscious horses, but this technique is not sufficiently well described to allow its recommendation at this time.[18]

Ex situ (postmortem) MRI examination of cervical vertebrae and spinal cord of normal and CSM-affected horses is more accurate than is interpretation of standing lateral radiographs.[17] However, both **CT and MRI** of horses with CSM are limited by the restricted views of the neck of adult horses. This prevents comprehensive examination of the cervical spine.[19,20]

Endoscopy of the epidural and subarachnoid spaces is reported in a horse with confirmed cervical compressive myelopathy.[21,22] The diagnostic or therapeutic value of this procedure is yet to be established.

The **prognosis** for horses with CSM is guarded. Sixty-four percent of affected horses were euthanized, presumably for economic or humane reasons.[9] However, the prognosis depends on the severity of clinical signs and the intended use of the horse. The criteria for euthanasia depend on the danger of the horse to itself (for instance, falling and injuring itself) or its attendants. Horses that are at high risk of self-injury or of injuring their attendants might qualify for humane euthanasia. However, horses with milder signs of disease compatible with their intended use, such as stallions or females with low-grade signs of the disease and reproductive potential, can be treated conservatively and live long lives.

It is imperative to consider the risk to riders or handlers associated with care or competing the horse when deciding on the fate of an affected horse.

The prognosis for horses intended for **athletic use** is less clear. Twenty-one of 70 Thoroughbred racehorses with cervical compressive myelopathy went on to race.[23] The likelihood of a horse racing was inversely related to the severity of its clinical signs.[23]

CLINICAL PATHOLOGY

Hematologic and serum biochemical values are usually within reference ranges in affected horses. CSF from affected horses can have increased protein concentration, but this finding is neither characteristic nor specific for compressive myelopathy. However, other causes of spinal ataxia can cause characteristic changes in the CSF and examination of the fluid might assist in ruling out these diseases.

Measurement of creatine kinase activity in CSF has no diagnostic value in horses.

NECROPSY FINDINGS

Gross examination reveals degeneration of the articular facets in many affected horses.

Impingement of soft tissues, especially the ligamentum flavum and joint structures, or cartilage and osteophytes into the spinal canal may be apparent. The spinal canal may be narrow. It may be indented and soft at the site or sites of compression. Histologically, there is nerve fiber swelling, widespread degeneration of myelin, and astrocytic gliosis. Cranial to the compressive lesion, wallerian degeneration is evident in the dorsal and lateral funiculi, although caudal to the compression these changes are most evident in the ventral and central lateral funiculi. Slight atrophy of cervical muscles is sometimes evident. There is histologic evidence of stretching and tearing of the ligamentum flavum and joint capsule at affected joints, especially C6 or C7.

DIFFERENTIAL DIAGNOSIS

Equine degenerative myelopathy, equine protozoal myeloencephalitis, trauma, equine infectious anemia, cerebrospinal nematodiasis (*Hypoderma* spp., *Setaria* sp., *Halicephalobus deletrix*), equine herpesvirus-1 myelopathy, aortoiliac thrombosis, West Nile encephalomyelitis, congenital vertebral malformation (especially in Arabian foals), discospondylitis, tumors involving the spinal canal (melanoma, lymphoreticular neoplasia, hemangiosarcoma),[5,24] extradural hematoma,[25] vertebral osteomyelitis, fibrocartilaginous embolic, postanesthetic myelopathy,[26] and ryegrass staggers (see Table 14-21).

TREATMENT

Medical treatment of the acute disease consists of rest and administration of antiinflammatory drugs (dexamethasone 0.05–0.25 mg/kg intravenously or intramuscularly every 24 hours; flunixin meglumine 1 mg/kg intravenously every 8–12 hours; phenylbutazone 2.2–4.4 mg/kg orally every 12–24 hours; and/or dimethyl sulfoxide, 1 g/kg as a 10% solution in isotonic saline intravenously every 24 hours for three treatments).

Treatment of arthritis of the facets of mature horses can be achieved by injection of the articular facet joints with corticosteroids (40 mg of methylprednisolone acetate).[27] Injection of the joint is facilitated by ultrasonographic guidance. Injection of the joints with antiinflammatory drugs is assumed to result in reduction in inflammation and soft

Table 14-21 Differential diagnosis of disease causing spinal ataxia in adult horses

Disease	Etiology and epidemiology	Clinical signs and lesions	Treatment and prognosis
Cervical compressive myelopathy (cervical stenotic myelopathy, cervical vertebral instability)	Sporadic; young, rapidly growing males; more common in Thoroughbreds, Standardbreds, and Warmblood horses; syndrome in mature horses caused by arthritis or articular facets.	Symmetric ataxia often of sudden onset; may be associated with trauma; hindlimbs most severely affected; compression of cervical spinal cord demonstrated by myelography; CSF normal	Medical treatment of rest and antiinflammatory drugs; poor prognosis; surgical correction by ventral stabilization
Equine degenerative myelopathy	Young horses (<3 years); familial incidence of increased requirement for vitamin E	Gradual onset symmetric ataxia that stabilizes at about 3 years of age; no radiographic abnormalities in cervical spinal cord; CSF normal	Guarded prognosis; vitamin E 5–20 IU/kg per day in feed may prevent progression; no cure; death uncommon
Equine protozoal myeloencephalitis	*Sarcocystis neurona* or *Neospora hughesi* in spinal cord or brain; Americas only; infectious but not contagious	Any sign of central nervous system dysfunction; usually gradual onset of asymmetric spinal ataxia, focal muscle atrophy or weakness; CSF contains antibody to *S. neurona,* but also found in normal horses	Ponazuril 5–10 mg/kg orally daily for 28 days; older, but effective, treatment is pyrimethamine, 1 mg/kg orally and sulfadiazine, 20 mg/kg orally every 24 hours for 90–120 days; Nitazoxanide 25 mg/kg orally once daily for 2 days followed by 50 mg/kg orally for 26 days; Vaccination not recommended
Equine herpesvirus-1 myeloencephalopathy	EHV-1; infectious and contagious. Sporadic; outbreaks occur often preceded by fever or upper respiratory tract disease	Ascending paralysis with fecal and urinary incontinence, recumbency, normal mentation; CSF xanthochromic and increased protein concentration; lesion is vasculitis and malacia	Valacyclovir for prophylactic therapy at a dose of 30 mg/kg orally every 8 hours for 2 days, then 20 mg/kg every 12 hours for 1–2 weeks Corticosteroids controversial Nursing care; poor prognosis Vaccination potentially effective
West Nile encephalitis	West Nile virus; transmitted by bite of infected mosquito; horse is dead-end host and does not develop sustained viremia; enzootic to Mediterranean littoral and North America; Increased recognition in other areas (Australia, Kunjin); peak disease risk is late summer	Weakness, muscle fasciculations, altered mentation; recumbency	No specific treatment; nursing care; corticosteroids controversial; hyperimmune serum available in some areas; interferon has been used but efficacy uncertain
Trauma	Sudden onset; more common in young horses	Spinal ataxia, varying degrees of weakness and proprioceptive deficits; recumbency Radiographic lesions present occasionally CSF may contain red blood cells	Antiinflammatory drugs; rest
Ryegrass staggers	Intoxication by lolitrems produced by *Acremonium lolii* growing on perennial ryegrass; outbreaks of disease in horses on affected pasture	Ataxia, stiff gait, tremor, hypersensitivity, recumbency; no histologic lesions	Remove source of toxin; rapid recovery without other treatment
Parasite migration	Sporadic. *Strongylus* sp., *Hypoderma* sp., and filaroids (*Setaria* sp.).	Wide variety of clinical signs; progressive ataxia; CSF may contain eosinophils	Ivermectin 0.2 mg/kg orally Antiinflammatory drugs
Congenital anomalies	Sporadic; cause spinal cord compression or lack of neural tissue, e.g., spina bifida	Recumbency, ataxia present at birth	No treatment
Neoplasia	Melanoma, lymphosarcoma, hemangiosarcoma, metastatic neoplasia, multiple myeloma	Variable depending on site; usually extradural tumor although can be secondary to vertebral body involvement and pathologic fracture	No practicable treatment

tissue swelling with consequent reduced compression of the cervical spinal cord. There is no objective prospective assessment of the efficacy of this treatment

A "paced growth" program of slowed growth achieved by nutritional restriction of young horses (foals and weanlings) has been suggested as conservative treatment for immature horses with compressive myelopathy or at high risk of developing the disease.

Surgical fusion of cervical vertebrae is useful in the treatment of mild to moderately affected horses, although because of issues of safety of future riders there are concerns by some authorities about the advisability of this treatment.

CONTROL

Control measures are not usually used, although ensuring an appropriate diet and growth rate of at-risk animals would be prudent.

FURTHER READING

Nout YS, Reed SM. Cervical stenotic myelopathy. *Equine Vet Educ.* 2003;15:212.

REFERENCES

1. Levine JM, et al. *J Vet Intern Med.* 2007;21:812.
2. Van Bierviiet J. *Vet Clin North Am Equine Pract.* 2007;23:317.
3. Unt VE, et al. *Equine Vet Educ.* 2009;21:212.
4. Gold JR, et al. *J Vet Intern Med.* 2008;22:481.
5. Nout YS. *Equine Vet Educ.* 2009;21:569.
6. Oswald J, et al. *Vet Rec.* 2010;166:82.
7. Laugier C, et al. *J Equine Vet Sci.* 2009;29:561.
8. Levine JM, et al. *JAVMA.* 2008;233:1453.
9. Levine JM, et al. *JAVMA.* 2010;237:812.
10. Olsen E, et al. *J Vet Intern Med.* 2014;28:630.
11. Kottner J, et al. *J Clin Epidemiol.* 2011;64:96.
12. Withers JM, et al. *Equine Vet J.* 2009;41:895.
13. Scrivani PV, et al. *Equine Vet J.* 2011;43:399.
14. Hughes KJ, et al. *J Vet Intern Med.* 2014;28:1860.
15. Hahn CN, et al. *Vet Radiol Ultrasound.* 2008;49:1.
16. Hudson NPH, et al. *Equine Vet Educ.* 2005;17:34.
17. Janes JG, et al. *Equine Vet J.* 2014;46:681.
18. Rose PL, et al. *Vet Radiol Ultrasound.* 2007;48:535.
19. Mitchell CW, et al. *Vet Radiol Ultrasound.* 2012;53:613.
20. Sleutjens J, et al. *Vet Q.* 2014;34:74.
21. Prange T, et al. *Equine Vet J.* 2012;44:116.
22. Prange T, et al. *Equine Vet J.* 2011;43:317.
23. Hoffman CJ, et al. *J Vet Intern Med.* 2013;27:317.
24. Raes EV, et al. *Equine Vet Educ.* 2014;26:548.
25. Santos FCCD, et al. *Equine Vet Educ.* 2014;26:306.
26. Ragle C, et al. *Equine Vet Educ.* 2011;23:630.
27. Birmingham SSW, et al. *Equine Vet Educ.* 2010;22:77.

EQUINE MOTOR NEURON DISEASE

Equine motor neuron disease is a **neurodegenerative disease** of horses in the United States, Canada, Europe, UK, and South America.[1-3] The disease is associated with low intake, and abnormally low serum concentrations, of vitamin E, possibly exacerbated by excessive intake of copper or iron.[4-6] The disease can be induced by feeding horses a diet with a low concentration of vitamin E, with development of clinical signs of the disease taking at least 18 months and up to 38 months.[5,7]

The disease affects horses of all breeds, with Quarter Horses most commonly affected, and the incidence of the disease increases with age (horses older than 2 years). The disease is associated with stabling and lack of access to pasture, and the risk of the disease increases with decreasing serum vitamin E concentration.

The pathogenesis of the disease is unknown but is suspected to be caused by oxidative injury to neurons subsequent to vitamin E deficiency. However, not all horses that develop the disease have a clear oxidant stress or decrease in antioxidant capacity.[8] The clinical signs are attributable to degeneration of motor neurons in the ventral horns of the spinal cord, with subsequent peripheral nerve degeneration and widespread neurogenic muscle atrophy.

The onset of **clinical signs** is usually gradual, but in a small proportion of affected horses the first sign is an acute onset of profound muscle weakness. Chronically affected horses have weight loss in spite of a normal or increased appetite, pronounced trembling and fasciculation of antigravity muscles, increased recumbency, and a short-strided gait. They often assume a posture with all feet under the body and a low head carriage, and frequently shift weight, which are all signs attributable to muscle weakness. The tail head is elevated in a large proportion of severely affected horses, which is likely a result of atrophy of the sacrocaudalis dorsalis medialis muscle. Profound flaccidity (weakness) of the tongue with lesions in the hypoglossal nuclei is reported and must be differentiated from botulism.[9] Retinal examination often reveals accumulation of lipofuscin-like pigment in the tapetal fundus.

EMG, under either general or regional anesthesia, is a useful diagnostic aid.[8] Characteristic findings include spontaneous fibrillation potentials and trains of positive sharp waves.

Lesions of redistribution of mitochondrial enzyme stain and anguloid atrophy of myofibers in sacrocaudalis dorsalis medialis muscle of adult horses with vitamin E–responsive muscle atrophy might represent a variant, or early stage, of equine motor neuron disease.[10]

The prognosis is poor for horses with advanced disease and most of these horses do not return to normal function and are destroyed, although the disease stabilizes in some cases that can then live for a number of years after diagnosis. Approximately 40% of cases will have stable clinical signs (no improvement) and 20% will continue to deteriorate after diagnosis and initiation of treatment. Early recognition and correction of diet with or without supplementation with vitamin E can result in recovery.

There is often a mild increase in serum creatine kinase activity. Horses with equine motor neuron disease have abnormal oral and intravenous glucose tolerance tests characterized by peak glucose concentrations that are lower than expected. The lower peak plasma glucose concentration is attributable to a 3× greater rate of glucose metabolism (removal from blood) in affected horses compared with normal horses. There is also evidence that horses with equine motor neuron disease are more sensitive to insulin than are normal horses.

Affected horses often have **serum vitamin E concentrations** that are below the reference range (<1.0–2.0 μg/dL, <1.0–2.0 μmol/L). Horses with equine motor neuron disease have higher spinal cord copper concentrations than do normal horses, but the diagnostic or clinical significance of this observation is unclear.

Examination of CSF is not useful in arriving at a diagnosis.

Examination of muscle from horses with equine motor neuron disease reveals a coordinated shift from characteristics of slow muscle to those of fast twitch muscle including contractile and metabolic functions of muscle. There is a lower percentage of myosin heavy chain type 1 fibers, higher percentages of hybrid IIAX and IIX fibers, atrophy of all fibers, and reduced oxidative capacity, increased glycolytic capacity, and diminished intramuscular glycogen concentrations, among other changes, in affected horses compared with normal horses.

The disease must be differentiated from botulism and other causes of weakness in adult horses. **Diagnostic confirmation** can be achieved by examination of a biopsy of the sacrocaudalis dorsalis medialis muscle or the spinal accessory nerve. The sacrocaudalis dorsalis medialis muscle is preferred because that muscle is predominantly composed of type 1 fibers and is severely affected by the disease. Examination of biopsy of this muscle has a sensitivity of approximately 90%.

Necropsy examination reveals moderate to severe diffuse muscle atrophy. Predominant histologic findings at necropsy examination include degeneration of neurons in ventral horns at all levels of the spinal cord. Muscle atrophy is evident because angular fibers, with predominantly type 1 fibers, or a combination of type 1 and type 2 fibers, are affected. There is accumulation of lipofuscin in the fundus and in capillary endothelium of the nervous tissue.

Treatment consists of administration of vitamin E. There are eight isoforms of vitamin E, and RRR-α-tocopherol, the naturally occurring form, is the most potent antioxidant. Synthetic vitamin E contains all isomers, whereas "natural" vitamin contains only one, the RRR isomer. Administration of lyophilized, water-soluble D-α-tocopherol (RRR-α-tocopherol) is apparently superior to administration of the DL-α-tocopherol acetate in increasing concentrations of vitamin E in blood of horses.[4] The usual dose is 4 IU of D-α-tocopherol (RRR-α-tocopherol) per kilogram BW orally once daily or 5000 to 7000 IU of α-tocopherol per 450-kg horse per day.[4] Supplementation results in improvement in 40% of affected horses within 6 weeks, with some appearing normal at 12 weeks.[4]

Control measures should ensure that horses have adequate access to pasture or are supplemented with good quality forage and/or vitamin E. Horses without access to green pasture should be supplemented with 1 U of vitamin E per kilogram BW per day.[4]

FURTHER READING

Finno CJ, Valberg SJ. A comparative review of vitamin E and associated equine disorders. *J Vet Intern Med.* 2012;26:1251-1266.

Wijnberg ID. Equine motor neurone disease. *Equine Vet Educ.* 2006;18:126-129.

REFERENCES

1. McGowan CM, et al. *Vet J.* 2009;180:330.
2. Delguste C, et al. *Can Vet J.* 2007;48:1165.
3. McGorum BC, et al. *Equine Vet J.* 2006;38:47.
4. Finno CJ, et al. *J Vet Intern Med.* 2012;26:1251.
5. Divers TJ, et al. *Am J Vet Res.* 2006;67:120.
6. Syrja P, et al. *Equine Vet Educ.* 2006;18:122.
7. Mohammed HO, et al. *Acta Vet Scand.* 2007;49:17.
8. Wijnberg ID. *Equine Vet Educ.* 2006;18:126.
9. Robin M, et al. *Equine Vet Educ.* 2016;28:434.
10. Bedford HE, et al. *JAVMA.* 2013;242:1127.

Diseases Primarily Affecting the Peripheral Nervous System

The **peripheral nervous system** consists of **cranial** and **spinal nerve** components. As such, the peripheral nervous system includes the dorsal and ventral nerve roots, spinal ganglia, spinal and specific peripheral nerves, CNs and their sensory ganglia, and the peripheral components of the autonomic nervous system.

ETIOLOGY

There are several different causes of peripheral nervous system disease.

Inflammatory

Polyneuritis equi, also known as **neuritis of the cauda equina** or **cauda equina syndrome**, is a rare and slowly progressive demyelinating granulomatous disease affecting peripheral nerves in the horse. Polyneuritis equi is characterized by signs of lower motor neuron lesions, primarily involving the perineal region but also affecting other peripheral nerves, especially CNs V and VI. CNs VIII, IX, X, and XII also may be involved. Clinical signs of perineal region paresis/paralysis predominate and manifest as varying degrees of hypotonia; hypalgesia; and hyporeflexia of the tail, anus, and perineal region. Degrees of urinary bladder paresis and rectal dilatation are also present. Differential diagnoses include sacral or coccygeal trauma, equine herpes myeloencephalopathy, equine protozoal myeloencephalitis, rabies, and equine motor neuron disease.

Cranial neuritis with guttural pouch mycosis and empyema in the horse may cause abnormalities of swallowing, laryngeal hemiplegia, and Horner's syndrome if the glossopharyngeal and vagal nerves are involved in the inflammatory process of the guttural pouch.

Acquired **myasthenia gravis** has been diagnosed in a 7-month-old Hereford heifer with a 5-day history of recumbency caused by symmetric generalized neuromuscular weakness.[1] The heifer stood with no assistance within 1 minute of edrophonium chloride (0.1 mg/kg intravenously) and was able to stand for 24 hours. Three additional episodes of prolonged recumbency responded to edrophonium, with an increasing period between episodes. Additional treatment was dexamethasone intramuscularly for 5 days. Acquired myasthenia gravis was diagnosed and attributed to an autoimmune disease directed against acetylcholine receptors at the neuromuscular junction. Congenital myasthenia gravis, caused by a homozygous mutation in the acetylcholine receptor gene, has been diagnosed in Braham calves in South Africa.[2]

Degenerative

Equine laryngeal hemiplegia, often called roaring, is a common disease of the horse in which there is paralysis of the left cricoarytenoid dorsalis muscle resulting in an inability to abduct the arytenoid cartilage and vocal fold, which causes an obstruction in the airway during inspiration. Endoscopic examination reveals asymmetry of the glottis. On exercise, inspiratory stridor develops as the airflow vibrates a slack and adducted vocal fold. The abnormality is caused by idiopathic distal degeneration of axons in the left recurrent laryngeal nerve, with the disease characterized as a bilateral mononeuropathy.[3] The left recurrent laryngeal nerve is more severely affected than the right because it is longer and is the longest nerve in the horse (see Chapter 12 for more details).

Diaphragmatic paralysis has been identified in 11 alpacas aged 2 to 12 months. Respiratory dysfunction was present, manifested as tachypnea, pronounced inspiratory effort, and arterial hypercapnia and hypoxemia.[4] The paralysis appeared bilateral in all seven alpacas imaged using fluoroscopy. Histologic examination revealed phrenic nerve degeneration in all six alpacas necropsied, with long nerves also demonstrating degeneration in two alpacas. The etiology was not identified.[4]

Traumatic

Injection injuries to peripheral nerves may result from needle puncture, the drug deposited, pressure from an abscess or hematoma, or fibrous tissue around the nerve. The sciatic nerve has been most commonly affected in cattle because historically most intramuscular injections were given deep in the hamstring muscles. Young calves were particularly susceptible because of their small muscle masses. Current recommendations in cattle are that intramuscular injections should be administered cranial to the shoulder.

Femoral nerve paralysis in calves occurs in large calves born to heifers with dystocia. The injury occurs when calves in anterior presentation fail to enter the birth canal because their stifle joints become engaged at the brim of the pelvis. Traction used to deliver these calves causes hyperextension of the femur and stretching of the quadriceps muscle and its neural and vascular supplies. In most cases the right femoral nerve is affected. Such calves are unable to bear weight on the affected leg within days after birth, the quadriceps muscle is atrophied, and the patella can be luxated easily. The patellar reflex is absent or markedly reduced in the affected limb because this reflex requires an intact femoral nerve and functional quadriceps muscle. Varying degrees of rear limb paresis result, accompanied by varying degrees of hindlimb gait abnormality. Skin analgesia maybe present over the proximal lateral to cranial to medial aspect of the tibia. At rest, the affected leg is slightly flexed and the hip on the affected side is held slightly lower. During walking, the animal has difficulty in advancing the limb normally because the limb collapses when weight bearing. In severe cases of muscle atrophy, the patella is easily luxated both medially and laterally. Injury to the femoral nerve is relatively easy to clinically identify, and there is usually no need to perform EMG studies of atrophied quadriceps muscle to document denervation.

Calving paralysis is common in heifers that have experienced a difficult calving. Affected animals are unable to stand without assistance; if they do stand, the hindlimbs are weak and there is marked abduction and inability to adduct. It has always been erroneously thought that traumatic injury of the obturator nerves during passage of the calf in the pelvic cavity was the cause of the paresis; however, detailed pathologic and experimental studies have demonstrated that most calving paresis/paralysis is caused by damage to the sciatic nerve. Experimental transection of the obturator nerves does not result in paresis. The term **obturator nerve paralysis** should only be used for postparturient cattle with an inability to adduct one or both hindlimbs, and calving paralysis in the preferred descriptive term for hindlimb paresis/paralysis occurring in the immediate postparturient period.

Damage to the sciatic nerve results in rear limb weakness and knuckling of the fetlocks; the latter clinical sign is an important means for differentiating sciatic nerve damage from obturator nerve damage (Fig. 14-25). The patellar reflex in ruminants with sciatic nerve damage is normal or increased, because the reflex contraction of the quadriceps muscle group by the femoral nerve is unopposed by the muscles of the hindlimb innervated by the sciatic nerve.

The peroneal nerve is most frequently damaged by local trauma to the lateral stifle where the peroneal nerve runs in a superficial location lateral to the head of the fibular bone. Damage to the peroneal nerve leads to knuckling over of the fetlock joint from damage to the extensor muscles of the distal limb, resulting in the dorsal aspect of the hoof resting on the ground when the animal is standing. Full weight can be borne on the

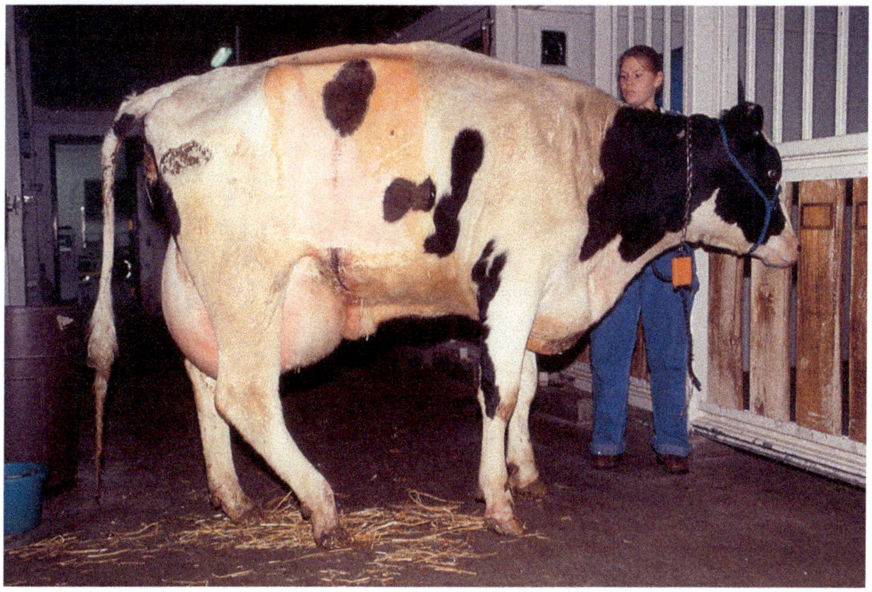

Fig. 14-25 Three-year-old Holstein Friesian cow with mild paresis of the right sciatic nerve. The hock is dropped relative to the normal unaffected left leg, and the fetlock has the characteristic knuckling. The cow has had a left displaced abomasum surgically corrected by a right flank incision and is being treated for concurrent mastitis.

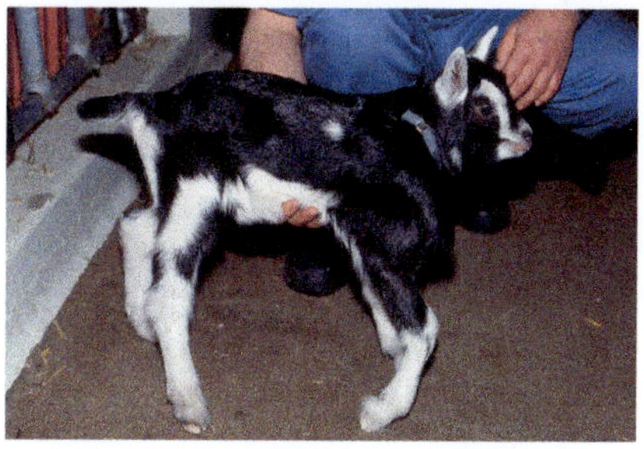

Fig. 14-27 One-week-old kid with brachial plexus avulsion of the right forelimb. The right limb "appears" longer than the unaffected left limb and the right elbow appears dropped. The right front leg cannot support weight and is not advanced in a normal manner during walking. The right leg received excessive traction during correction of a dystocia.

affected limb when the digit is placed in its normal position, but immediately on walking the digit is dragged. There is a loss of skin sensation on the anterior aspect of the metatarsus and digit.

Damage to the tibial nerve causes mild hyperflexion of the hock and a forward knuckling of the fetlock joint. Tibial nerve damage is very rare, and most cases described as tibial nerve damage are actually sciatic nerve damage.

The radial nerve is most susceptible to traumatic damage because it courses distally and laterally over the later condyle of the humerus. Radial nerve paresis is most common when heavy adult cattle are placed in lateral recumbency, such as corrective foot trimming in bulls. Care must be taken in these animals to pad the area around the elbow and to ensure that the time spent in lateral recumbency is minimized. Clinical signs of radial nerve paresis include inability to advance the front limb with the ability to bear weight when the limb is placed directly under the animal in the normal position (Fig. 14-26). In advanced cases, the cranial aspect of the fetlock is dragged along the ground and the area needs to be protected from severe abrasion injury using a splint or cast.

Brachial plexus injury, including avulsion, is rare in large animals, because the muscle mass is usually sufficient to prevent overextension of the front limb. It is a rare outcome of correction of dystocia in goats, particularly when relatively excessive traction is applied to one front limb during delivery. Clinical signs of brachial plexus avulsion include a complete inability to bear weight on the limb and a dropped elbow relative to the unaffected limb (Fig. 14-27).

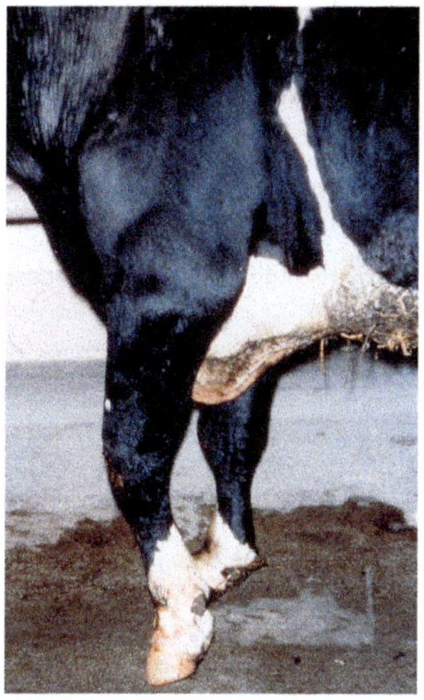

Fig. 14-26 Mild radial nerve paresis in a Holstein Friesian bull. Swelling is present over the lateral aspect of the elbow. Paresis was present immediately after taking the animal off a foot table for corrective foot trimming.

Metabolic and Nutritional

PA deficiency may occur in pigs fed diets based solely on corn (maize). Affected animals develop a goose-stepping gait caused by degenerative changes in the primary sensory neurons of the peripheral nerves.

Toxic

Heavy metal poisoning including **lead and mercury poisoning in horses** has been associated with clinical signs of degeneration of peripheral CNs, but these are not well documented.

Tumors

A multicentric schwannoma causing chronic ruminal tympany and forelimb paresis has been recorded in an aged cow. Neoplastic masses were present throughout the body, and both right and left brachial plexuses were involved. The peripheral nerves of each brachial plexus were enlarged. Large tumor masses were present on the serosal surfaces of the esophagus, pericardial sac and epicardium, and within the myocardium, endocardium, and the ventral branches of the first four thoracic spinal nerves. A large mass was present in the anterior mediastinum near the thoracic inlet.

Autonomic Nervous System

Equine grass sickness (equine dysautonomia, grass sickness, mal Seco) in the horse is a polyneuropathy involving both the peripheral nervous system (autonomic and enteric nervous systems) as well as the CNS.[5-7] Equine grass sickness occurs primarily in Scotland, although cases have been reported elsewhere in Europe, and in Patagonia and the Falkland Islands.[8] The disorder is characterized by a peracute to chronic alimentary tract disease of horses on pasture (hence the name). Gastrointestinal stasis is partial or complete. Peracute cases are in shock and in a state of collapse with gastric refluxing. Acute, subacute, and chronic cases also occur. Degenerative changes occur in the autonomic ganglia (especially the celiac–mesenteric, and stellate), thoracic sympathetic chain, ciliary, cranial and caudal cervical, the craniospinal sensory ganglia, and selected nuclei in the CNS. EMG reveals the presence of a neuropathy of skeletal muscles.[8] The etiology is unknown but neurotoxin involvement is suspected, possibly *Clostridium botulinum* type C/D.

FURTHER READING

Constable PD. Clinical examination of the ruminant nervous system. *Vet Clin North Am Food Anim Pract.* 2004;20:185-214.

Divers TJ. Acquired spinal cord and peripheral nerve disease. *Vet Clin North Am Food Anim Pract.* 2004;20:231-242.

REFERENCES

1. Wise LN, et al. *J Vet Intern Med.* 2008;22:231.
2. Thompson PN, et al. *J Anim Sci.* 2007;85:604.
3. Dupuis MC, et al. *Mamm Genome.* 2011;22:613.
4. Byers S, et al. *J Vet Intern Med.* 2011;25:380.
5. Shotton HR, et al. *J Comp Pathol.* 2011;145:35.
6. Wales AD, Whitwell KE. *Vet Rec.* 2006;158:372.
7. Lyle C, Pirie RS. *In Pract.* 2009;31:26.
8. Wijnberg ID, et al. *Equine Vet J.* 2006;38:230.

TETANUS

ETIOLOGY

Tetanus is caused by *C. tetani,* a gram-positive, spore-forming obligate anaerobe bacillus. It is a ubiquitous organism and a commensal of the gastrointestinal tract of domestic animals and humans. The organism forms highly resistant spores that can persist in soil for many years. The spores survive many standard disinfection procedures, including steam heat at 100°C (212°F) for 20 minutes but can be destroyed by heating at 115°C (239°F) for 20 minutes. After a period of anaerobic incubation spores germinate to their vegetative form, which starts replicating and producing a complex of exotoxins causing the clinic signs characteristic for this condition. The toxins produced are **tetanolysin, tetanospasmin,** and **neurotoxin** or nonspasmolytic toxin.

SYNOPSIS

Etiology Muscle spasm from action of the exotoxin tetanospasmin produced by the vegetative stage of *Clostridium tetani.*

Epidemiology Marked difference in species susceptibility with horses being most and cattle being least susceptible. Usually a history of a wound or other tissue trauma. Occurs as isolated cases but also as outbreaks in young ruminants following castration and docking.

Clinical findings Generalized muscular rigidity and spasms, hyperesthesia, prolapse of third eyelid, trismus, ears pulled caudally, bloat in ruminants, convulsions, respiratory arrest, and death. High case fatality.

Necropsy findings None. May demonstrate the organism in necrotic tissue in some cases.

Diagnostic confirmation Diagnosis is based on characteristic clinical signs and wound history. No definitive antemortem test or pathognomonic postmortem lesion. A bioassay consisting of injecting mice with infectious material to induce characteristic clinical signs is used.

Treatment Objectives are to prevent further production of exotoxin, neutralize residual toxin, control muscle spasms until the toxin is eliminated or destroyed, maintain hydration and nutrition, provide supportive treatment.

Control Regular prophylactic vaccination with tetanus toxoid of susceptible animals, vaccination and administration of tetanus antitoxin to unvaccinated animals with fresh wounds, antibiotic therapy in animals with wounds that are contaminated or at risk to be contaminated.

EPIDEMIOLOGY

Occurrence

Tetanus occurs in all parts of the world and is most common in closely settled areas under intensive cultivation. It occurs in all farm animals, mainly as individual, sporadic cases, although outbreaks are occasionally observed in young cattle, young pigs, and lambs following wound management procedures.[1]

Case–Fatality Rate

In young ruminants the case–fatality rate is over 80%, but the recovery rate is high in adult cattle. In horses it varies widely between areas. In some areas almost all animals die acutely, and in others the mortality rate is consistently about 50%.[2,3]

Source of Infection

C. tetani organisms are commonly present in the feces of animals, especially horses, and in the soil contaminated by these feces. Surveys in different areas of the world show it is present in 30% to 42% of soil samples. The survival period of the organism in soil varies widely from soil to soil.

Transmission

The **portal of entry** is usually through deep puncture wounds, but the spores may lie dormant in the tissues for some time and produce clinical illness only when tissue conditions favor their proliferation. For this reason, the portal of entry is often difficult to identify. Puncture wounds of the hooves are common sites of entry in horses. Introduction to the genital tract at the time of parturition is the usual portal of entry in cattle. A high incidence of tetanus may occur in young pigs following castration and in lambs following castration, shearing, docking, vaccinations, or injections of pharmaceuticals, especially anthelmintics. Docking by the use of elastic band ligatures is reputed to be especially hazardous. **Neonatal tetanus** occurs when there is infection in the umbilical cord associated with unsanitary conditions at parturition. Cases of tetanus in ruminants after thermic dehorning and ear-tagging have been reported.[1]

Outbreaks of **"idiopathic tetanus"** occur occasionally in young cattle without a wound being apparent, usually in association with the grazing of rough, fibrous feed, and it is probable that toxin is produced in wounds in the mouth or gastrointestinal tract or is ingested preformed in the feed. Proliferation in the rumen may also result in toxin production.

Animal Risk Factors

The neurotoxin of *C. tetani* is exceedingly potent, but there is considerable variation in susceptibility between animal species, and horses are the most susceptible and cattle the least susceptible. The variation in prevalence of the disease in the different species is partly caused by this variation in susceptibility but is also because exposure and wound management practices are more likely to occur in some species than in others.

Importance

Tetanus is important because of its high case fatality and the very long convalescence in the survivors. In regions of the world where horses, donkeys, and mules still play an important role in the rural economy and where vaccination is uncommon, the economic impact of tetanus can be considerable.[2]

PATHOGENESIS

The tetanus spores remain **localized** at their site of introduction and do not invade surrounding tissues. Spores germinate to their vegetative form to proliferate and produce **tetanolysin, tetanospasmin,** and **neurotoxin** only if certain environmental conditions are attained, particularly a lowering of the local tissue oxygen tension. Toxin production may occur immediately after introduction if the accompanying trauma has been sufficiently severe, or if foreign material has also been introduced to the wound, or may be delayed for several months until subsequent trauma to the site causes tissue damage. The original injury may be inapparent by then. Of the three mentioned exotoxins, **tetanospasmin is the most relevant** for the pathophysiology of the condition. Although **tetanolysin** was found to promote local tissue necrosis, its role in the pathogenesis of tetanus remains doubtful. The role of the more recently identified neurotoxin, or nonspasmogenic toxin, which is a peripherally active for the pathophysiology of tetanus, is currently unknown.

Tetanospasmin diffuses to the systemic circulation, is bound to motor end plates, and travels up peripheral nerve trunks via retrograde intraaxonal transport to the CNS. The exact mechanisms by which the toxin exerts its effects on nervous tissue are not known, but it blocks the release of neurotransmitters such as GABA and glycine, which are essential for the synaptic inhibition of gamma motor neurons in the spinal cord. There it leads to an unmodulated spread of neural impulses produced by normally innocuous stimuli, causing exaggerated responses and a state of constant muscular spasticity. No structural lesions are produced. Death occurs by asphyxiation caused by fixation of the muscles of respiration.

CLINICAL FINDINGS

The **incubation period** varies between 3 days and 4 weeks, with occasional cases occurring as long as several months after the infection is introduced. In sheep and lambs cases appear 3 to 10 days after shearing, docking, or castration.

Clinical findings are similar in all animal species. Initially, there is an increase in **muscle stiffness**, accompanied by muscle tremor. There is **trismus** with restriction of jaw movements; **prolapse of the third eyelid;** stiffness of the hindlimbs causing an unsteady, straddling gait; and the tail is held out stiffly, especially when backing or turning. Retraction of the eye and prolapse of the third eyelid (a rapid movement of the third eyelid across the cornea followed by a slow retraction) is one of the earliest and consistent signs (with the exception of sheep) and can be exaggerated by sharp lifting of the muzzle or tapping the face below the eye. Additional signs include an anxious and alert expression contributed to by an erect carriage of the ears, retraction of the eyelids and dilation of the nostrils, and hyperesthesia with exaggerated responses to normal stimuli (Fig. 14-28).

The animal may continue to eat and drink in the early stages but mastication is soon prevented by tetany of the masseter muscles and saliva may drool from the mouth. If food or water is taken, attempts at swallowing are followed by regurgitation from the nose. Constipation is usual and the urine is retained, partly as a result of the inability to assume the normal position for urination. The rectal temperature and pulse rate are within the normal range in the early stages but may rise later when muscular tone and activity are further increased. In cattle, particularly young animals, bloat is an early sign but is not usually severe and is accompanied by strong, frequent rumen contractions.

As the disease progresses, muscular tetany increases and the animal adopts a **sawhorse posture** (Figs. 14-29 and 14-30). Uneven muscular contractions may cause the development of a curve in the spine and deviation of the tail to one side. There is great difficulty in walking and the animal is inclined to fall, especially when startled. Falling occurs with the limbs still in a state of **tetany** and the animal can cause itself severe injury. Once down it is almost impossible to get a large animal to its feet again. Tetanic convulsions begin in which the tetany is still further exaggerated. Opisthotonus is marked, the hindlimbs are stuck out stiffly behind and the forelegs forward. Sweating may be profuse and the temperature rises, often to 42°C (107°F). The convulsions are at first only stimulated by sound or touch but soon occur spontaneously. In fatal cases there is often a transient period of improvement for several hours before a final, severe tetanic spasm during which respiration is arrested.

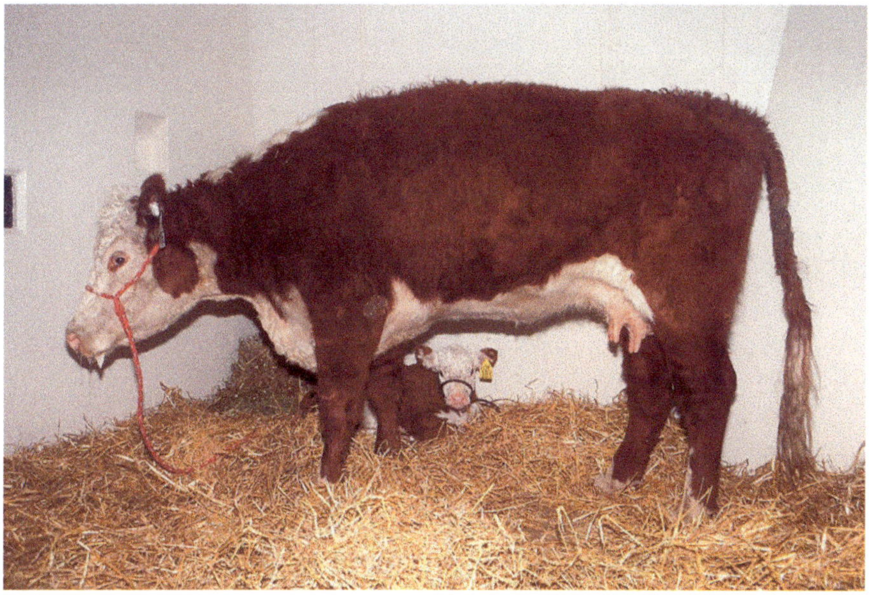

Fig. 14-28 Polled Hereford cow exhibiting early signs of tetanus with healthy calf. The tail is held slightly away from the perineum, the ears are back, the eyes have a surprised expressed with slight prolapse of the nictitating membrane, and saliva is drooling from the mouth. The cow calved 7 days previously and had a retained placenta and metritis.

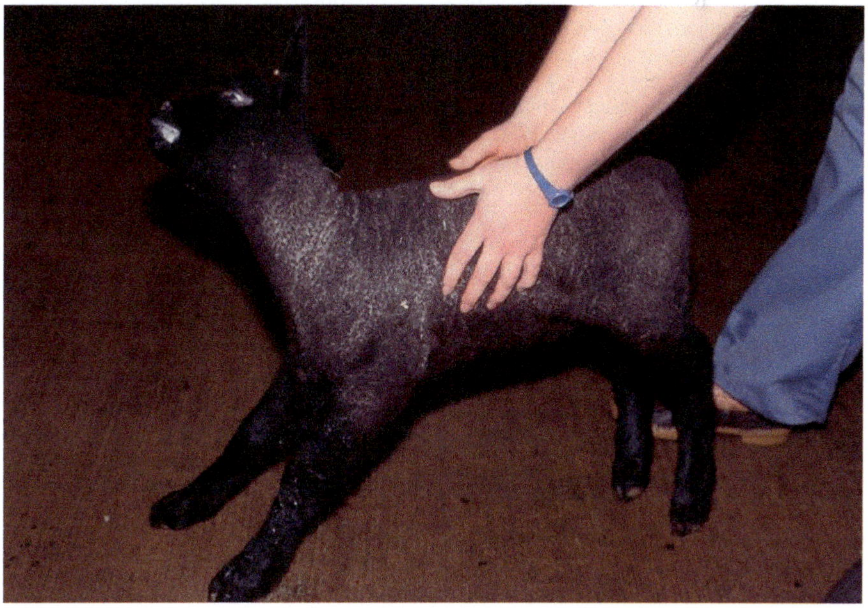

Fig. 14-29 Suffolk lamb with tetanus after castration using a band. The lamb is exhibiting a sawhorse stance caused by generalized muscle rigidity and drooling of saliva.

The **course of the disease** and the **prognosis** vary both between and within species. The **duration** of a fatal illness in horses and cattle is usually 5 to 10 days, but sheep usually die on about the third or fourth day. A long incubation period is usually associated with a mild syndrome, a long course, and a favorable prognosis. **Mild cases** that recover usually do so slowly, with the stiffness disappearing gradually over a period of weeks or even months. The prognosis is poor when signs rapidly progress. Animals vaccinated in the past year have a better prognosis, as do horses that have received parenteral penicillin and tetanus antitoxin and in which the wound was aggressively cleaned when fresh.

CLINICAL PATHOLOGY

There are no specific abnormalities in blood or CSF and no antemortem test confirming

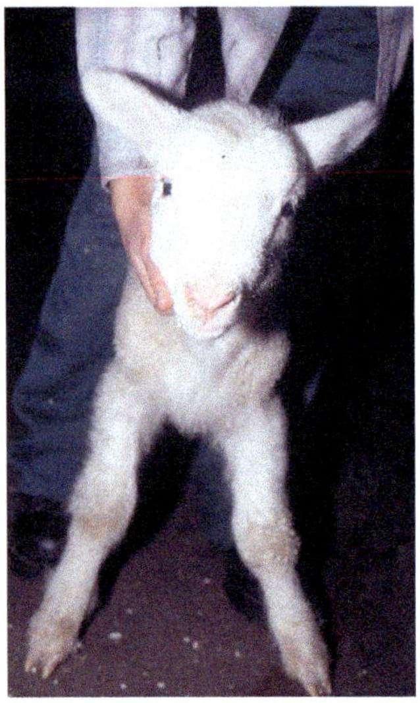

Fig. 14-30 Corriedale lamb with tetanus after tail docking. Note the ear and eyelid retraction and generalized stiffness.

the diagnosis. Blood levels of tetanus toxin are usually too low to be detected. Gram-stain of wound aspirates is considered of limited value because sporulated as well as vegetative forms of *C. tetani* resemble other anaerobic bacteria. Culturing the pathogen is difficult because of the low number of organisms normally present and the strict anaerobic conditions required for culture. Culture in combination with PCR has been used for identification of *C. tetani.*[1] A bioassay consisting of injecting infectious material into the tail base of mice and observing for onset of characteristic clinical signs is possible.[2]

NECROPSY FINDINGS

There are no gross or histologic findings by which a diagnosis can be confirmed, although a search should be made for the site of infection. Culture of the organism is difficult but should be attempted. If minimal autolysis has occurred by the time of necropsy, the identification of large gram-positive rods with terminal spores ("tennis-racket morphology") in smears prepared from the wound site or spleen is supportive of a diagnosis of tetanus.

Samples for Confirmation of Diagnosis

- Bacteriology: air-dried impression smears from spleen, wound site (cyto, Gram stain), culture swab from wound site in anaerobic transport media; spleen in sterile, leak-proof container (anaerobic CULT, bioassay).

DIFFERENTIAL DIAGNOSIS

Fully developed tetanus is so distinctive clinically that it is seldom confused with other diseases. The muscular spasms, the prolapse of the third eyelid, and a recent history of accidental injury or surgery are characteristic findings. However, in its early stages or mild forms, tetanus may be confused with other diseases.

All species
- Strychnine poisoning
- Meningitis

Horses
- Hypocalcemic tetany (eclampsia)
- Acute laminitis
- Hyperkalemic periodic paralysis
- Myositis, particularly after injection in the cervical region.

Ruminants
- Hypomagnesemia (cows, sheep and calves)
- White muscle disease
- Polioencephalomalacia
- Enterotoxemia.

TREATMENT

These are the main principles in the treatment of tetanus:
- Eliminate the causative bacteria
- Neutralize residual toxin
- Control muscle spasms until the toxin is eliminated or destroyed
- Maintain hydration and nutrition
- Provide supportive treatment

There are no structural changes in the nervous system, and the management of cases of tetanus depends largely on keeping the animal alive through the critical stages.

Elimination of the organism is usually attempted by the parenteral administration of penicillin in large doses (44,000 IU/kg), preferably by intravenous administration. Other antimicrobials that have been proposed include oxytetracycline (15 mg/kg), macrolides, and metronidazole. If the infection site is found, the wound should be aggressively cleaned and debrided but only after antitoxin has been administered, because debridement, irrigation with hydrogen peroxide, and the local application of penicillin may facilitate the absorption of the toxin.

The objective of administering **tetanus antitoxin** is to neutralize circulating toxin outside the CNS. The use of tetanus antitoxin is most appropriate in wounded animals that are susceptible to but unvaccinated against tetanus or with uncertain vaccination history. Because binding of tetanospasmin to neural cells is irreversible and because the tetanus antitoxin is unable to penetrate the blood-brain barrier, administration of antitoxin is of little value once signs have appeared. After the experimental administration of toxin, antitoxin is of limited value at 10 hours and ineffective by 48 hours. The recommended doses vary widely and range from 10,000 to over 300,000 IU per treatment, given intravenously, intramuscularly, or subcutaneously once or repeatedly, but reported treatment outcomes are inconsistent. Local injection of some of the antitoxin around the wound has also been proposed. There have been a number of attempts to justify the treatment of early cases of equine tetanus by intrathecal injection of antitoxin, but there is limited evidence of therapeutic value and the procedure carries risk.

The use of **tetanus toxoid** has also been recommended for patients with tetanus, but an antibody response may take 2 to 4 weeks and a booster vaccination is required in previously unvaccinated animals. The effectiveness of this treatment in previously unvaccinated animals is therefore doubtful. When combining tetanus toxoid and antitoxin, both compounds should be administered on different sites using different syringes.

Relaxation of the muscle tetany can be attempted with various drugs. Chlorpromazine (0.4–0.8 mg/kg BW intravenously, or 1.0 mg/kg BW intramuscularly, three or four times daily) and acepromazine (0.05 mg/kg BW three to four times daily) administered until severe signs subside, are widely used in horses. A combination of diazepam (0.1–0.4 mg/kg) and xylazine (0.5–1.0 mg/kg intravenously or intramuscularly) may be effective in horses refractory to phenothiazine tranquilizers.

Hydration can be maintained by intravenous or stomach-tube feeding during the critical stages when the animal cannot eat or drink. The use of an indwelling tube should be considered because of the disturbance caused each time the stomach tube is passed. Feed and water containers should be elevated, and the feed should be soft and moist.

Additional supportive treatment includes slinging of horses during the recovery period, when hyperesthesia is diminishing. Affected animals should be kept as quiet as possible and provided with dark, well-bedded quarters with nonslip flooring and plenty of room to avoid injury if convulsions occur. Administration of enemas and catheterization may relieve the animal's discomfort. This level of nursing, plus penicillin, ataractic drugs, and antitoxin for an average of 14 days, can deliver something like a 50% recovery by an average of 27 days, but the cost is high. A rumenostomy may be required in ruminant patients with recurrent bloat.

Horses that fall frequently sustain bone fractures and may need to be destroyed.

TREATMENT AND CONTROL

Treatment

Penicillin G (30,000 IU/kg IM or IV every 12–24 hours) (R-1)

Procaine penicillin (44,000 IU/kg IM every 12–24 hours) (R-1)

Oxytetracycline (15 mg/kg IV every 24 hours) (R-2)

Tetanus antitoxin (10,000–50, 000 IU per dose IM or IV once or repeatedly) (R-2)

Tetanus antitoxin (30,000–50,000 IU per dose intrathecal) (R-3)

Sedation horses

Chlorpromazine (0.4–0.8 mg/kg IV or IM every 6–8 hours) (R-1)

Acepromazine (0.05–0.1 mg/kg IV or IM every 6–8 hours) (R-1)

Diazepam (0.01–0.4 mg/kg IV or IM) (R-1)

Xylazine (0.5–1 mg/kg IV or IM) (R-1)

Sedation cattle

Diazepam (0.5–1.5 mg/kg IV or IM)

Xylazine (0.05–0.15 mg/kg IV or 0.1–0.3 mg/kg IM)

Sedation sheep

Acepromazine (0.05–0.1 mg/kg IV or IM every 6–8 hours) (R-1)

Diazepam (0.2–0.5 mg/kg IV or IM (every 6–8 hours) (R-1)

Control

Regular vaccination if tetanus toxoid (R-1)

Tetanus antitoxin (1500 IU per dose IM in unvaccinated animals with fresh wounds) (R-1)

IM, intramuscularly, IV, intravenously.

CONTROL

Many cases of tetanus could be avoided by proper skin and instrument disinfection at castrating, docking, and shearing time. These operations should be performed in clean surroundings; in the case of lambs docked in the field, temporary pens are preferred over permanent yards for catching and penning.

Passive Immunity

Short-term prophylaxis can be achieved by the injection of 1500 IU of tetanus antitoxin. The immunity is transient, persisting for only 10 to 14 days.

Tetanus Antitoxin

Tetanus antitoxin should be given to any horse with a penetrating wound or deep laceration, and the wound should also be cleaned aggressively. Tetanus toxoid can be administered at the same time as tetanus antitoxin, provided they are injected at different sites and using different syringes. Animals that suffer injury are usually given an injection of antitoxin and one of toxoid to ensure complete protection.

Tetanus antitoxin is often routinely given to **mares** following foaling and to newborn foals. In some areas the risk for tetanus in young foals is high and repeated doses of antitoxin at weekly intervals may be required for protection.

On farms where the incidence of tetanus in **lambs** is high, antitoxin is usually given at the time of docking or castration; 200 IU has been shown to be effective. The risk for tetanus in calves is lower than in lambs and tetanus antitoxin is not commonly given at the time of castration.

There is a risk for **serum hepatitis** in horses that have been given tetanus antitoxin and, while this risk is small, a policy of routine active immunization of the mare to provide the mare with active immunity and the foal with passive colostral immunity is preferred to one that relies on antitoxin. Provided foals get an adequate supply of colostrum they are protected during the first 10 weeks of life by active vaccination of the mare during the last weeks of pregnancy. Prevention of tetanus in newborn lambs is also best effected by vaccination of the ewe in late pregnancy.

Active Immunity

Available vaccines are formalin-inactivated adjuvanted toxoids; they induce long-lasting immunity. Primary vaccination requires two doses 3 to 6 weeks apart. Protective titers are obtained within 14 days of the second injection and last for at least a year and up to 5 years.

Traditionally **foals** have received primary vaccination at 3 to 4 months of age; however, there is evidence that maternal antibodies acquired by foals born to mares vaccinated shortly before parturition significantly inhibit the antibody response of the foal to primary vaccination until it is 6 months of age and that primary vaccination should be delayed until that age.

Although immunity lasts longer than 1 year, it is common to revaccinate horses yearly with a single booster injection. Pregnant mares should receive a booster injection 4 to 6 weeks before foaling to provide adequate colostral immunity to the foal.

Ewes are immunized with a similar schedule except that the primary doses are usually given at a managementally convenient time when the flock is yarded. A prelambing booster vaccination is given yearly. Commonly, commercial vaccines for sheep also contain antigens for other clostridial diseases for which sheep are at high risk.

Vaccination of **cattle** is usually not considered unless an outbreak of the disease has occurred in the immediate past and further cases may be anticipated.

REFERENCES

1. Valgaeren B, et al. *Vlaams Tiergeneesk Tijdschr.* 2011;80:351.
2. Kay G, Knottenbelt DC. *Equine Vet Educ.* 2007;19:107.
3. Reichmann P, et al. *J Equine Vet Sci.* 2008;28:518.

BOTULISM

SYNOPSIS

Etiology Neurotoxin produced by *Clostridium botulinum* during vegetative growth. *C. botulinum* types B, C, and D and, on rare instances, type A are associated with disease in animals but the type prevalence varies geographically.

Epidemiology Ingestion of preformed toxin in which feed preparation or storage allows multiplication of the organism in the feed with toxin production. Contamination of feed with carrion containing toxin. Consumption of carrion on pasture by phosphorus-deficient animals. Risk factors often result in multiple cases. Toxicoinfections with toxin production from organisms in the intestine or wounds are more uncommon.

Clinical findings Early muscle tremor, progressive symmetric weakness, and motor paralysis leading to recumbency. Mydriasis, ptosis, weak tongue retraction; sensation and consciousness retained until death.

Necropsy findings None specific.

Diagnostic confirmation Demonstration of toxin in intestinal contents, serum, or feed. Demonstration of organisms in feed, intestinal contents, or wounds.

Treatment Type-specific antiserum and supportive treatment.

Control Avoidance of exposure by feed management. Vaccination.

ETIOLOGY

The causative organism *C. botulinum,* a spore-forming obligate anaerobe, produces neurotoxins during vegetative growth. Spores can survive in the environment for over 30 years. Under favorable conditions of warmth and moisture the spores germinate and vegetative cells multiply rapidly, elaborating a stable and highly lethal neurotoxin (BoTN) which, when ingested, or absorbed from tissues, causes the disease. The toxin is also capable of surviving for long periods, particularly in bones. Seven antigenically distinct **toxin types** (A-G), some with subtypes, have been identified. Farm animal disease is produced primarily by types B, C, D, and occasionally type A. Type A, B, E, and F toxins are generally related to human botulism.[1] Botulinum neurotoxin forming *C. botulinum* species are divided into groups I to IV depending on their physiologic properties.[1]

- **Group I**: proteolytic *C. botulinum* type A, B and F. These types degrade protein such as milk, serum, meat, and chicken protein
- **Group II**: nonproteolytic *C. botulinum,* includes nonprotelytic type B and F and all type E
- **Group III:** *C. botulinum* type C and D
- **Group IV:** *C. botulinum* type G.

The **geographic distribution** of these types varies considerably. In a study in the United States, type A was found in neutral or alkaline soils in the west, whereas types B and E were in damp or wet soil all over, except that B was not found in the south. Type C was found in acid soils in the Gulf coast, and type D in alkaline soils in the west. Microorganisms capable of inhibiting *C. botulinum* were present, with or without the clostridia, in many soils. Type B is also common in soils in the UK and in Europe. Types C and D are more common in warm climates.

The organism is present in the **alimentary tract** of animals that have recently ingested contaminated material and may be introduced into new areas in this way, or by birds and blowflies. In healthy animals with normal intestinal fauna and motility *C. botulinum* does not multiply in the gastrointestinal tract

EPIDEMIOLOGY

Occurrence

Botulism has **no geographic limitations**, with isolated cases and sporadic outbreaks occurring in most countries. The source of exposure to toxin and the risk for disease differ between regions because of differences in food storage, feeding, and management practices. **Outbreaks** associated with ingestion of toxin in conserved feeds are more common in the northern states of the United States and in Europe, whereas outbreaks in animals on pasture are reported primarily from South Africa, Australia, and the Gulf coast area of the United States. The disease usually occurs in a number of animals at one time and has a high case–fatality rate.

Source of Infection

Most incidents of botulism are associated with the ingestion of preformed toxin (**forage botulism**). Toxin in feeds may result from the primary growth of *C. botulinum* in the feed or from the contamination of the feed with toxin-containing carrion (**carrion-associated botulism**). Less common sources are growth with toxin production in wounds (**wound botulism**) or growth and toxin production in the alimentary tract (**toxicoinfectious botulism**).

Forage Botulism

Forage botulism occurs when pH, moisture, and anaerobic conditions in the feedstuff allow the vegetative growth of *C. botulinum* and the production of toxin. This can occur in a number of spoiled stored forages. Cereal silages carry a risk in the United States. Silage and hay may spoil to a stage suitable for the growth of *C. botulinum*. This is most likely if the forage is very succulent or is wet by rain when it is made.

Big bale silage is a particular risk. The type of forage ensiled in big bales often has insufficient water-soluble carbohydrate for adequate lactic acid fermentation to achieve a stable low pH, and the higher dry matter content can also lead to a higher pH. Clostridial multiplication is inhibited below pH 4.5. Most non–carrion-associated botulism is caused by type B strains, and horses appear to be especially susceptible.

Proliferation of the organism can occur in **decaying vegetable material**. The disease has also occurred in horses fed on spoiled vegetables and potatoes contaminated by *C. botulinum* and on alfalfa haylage packed in airtight aluminum foil envelopes. Grass clippings allowed to accumulate and decay in a pile have poisoned horses, as has round bale hay that spoiled after rain. Decaying grass at the base of old tussocks and in trampled stubble are known to be suitable sites for growth of *C. botulinum*. Cases have occurred with brewers grains, and high-moisture grain has the potential for toxicity.

Carrion-Associated Botulism

This is almost always the cause of botulism in animals on pasture, and carrion is also a common cause of botulism in animals on conserved feeds. Carrion includes domestic and wild animals and birds. In endemic botulism areas, the carcasses of dead animals are invaded by *C. botulinum*, and high concentrations of toxin are produced such that very small amounts of flesh or bone have lethal concentrations. Most outbreaks of carrion-associated botulism are associated with **type C and D strains**; these strains produce much higher concentrations of toxin in carrion than type A and B strains. Toxin can persist in carrion for at least 1 year. Where the carcasses of rodents, cats, and birds contaminate hay or silage, toxin can leach out and contaminate surrounding hay or other feeds to cause multiple cases of botulism. In one instance a single mouse carcass is thought to have contaminated 200,000 tons of alfalfa cubes. A common source in Australia is hay made at the time of a mouse plague. At such times even good, fresh hay can contain a great deal of carrion. In another recorded incident 427 of 444 dairy cattle died after ingesting feed contaminated with BoTN type C from a cat carcass.

Poultry manure and ensiled **poultry litter** have caused outbreaks of botulism when used as fertilizers, as has poultry litter used for bedding cattle.[2] Outbreaks of botulism have occurred in cattle and sheep grazing pastures that have been fertilized with poultry manure or poultry litter. Cattle and sheep may eat poultry litter piled on a pasture before disposal. It is probable that the source of toxin in poultry litter is from poultry carcasses. Disease is usually caused by *C. botulinum* type D and occasionally type C.[2]

Direct carrion ingestion can occur where **cattle** subsist on a **chronically phosphorus-deficient diet** and manifest osteophagia, with subsequent ingestion of carrion. The disease is likely to occur in outbreak form. In **sheep**, pica is more usually associated with a dietary **deficiency of protein** or net energy. Occasional outbreaks occur that are caused by drinking of **water** contaminated by carcasses of dead animals. A not uncommon occurrence is livestock drinking lake water contaminated by the carcasses of ducks and other waterfowl that have died of botulism. Wetlands where outbreaks of avian botulism have occurred are likely to have repeated occurrences because of soil contamination.

Wound Botulism

Wound botulism is a **toxicoinfectious form of botulism** where the toxin is produced in wounds infected by *C. botulinum*.[3] Wound botulism is rare but is recorded in horses following castration, with omphalophlebitis, umbilical hernias treated with clamps, with an infected wound and in association with an injection abscess.

Toxicoinfectious Botulism

This results when toxin is produced by *C. botulinum* present in the intestine. Two conditions in horses, **equine grass sickness** (see Equine grass sickness in Chapter 7) and the **shaker foal syndrome,** are potential forms of toxicoinfectious botulism. The **shaker foal syndrome** is a disease of young foals up to 8 months of age with the highest prevalence in foals 3 to 8 weeks of age.

The disease occurs sporadically in the United States, Australia, and the UK but may occur repeatedly on some farms. *C. botulinum* type B has been isolated from the feces of naturally occurring cases of the disease, and the condition has been produced experimentally by the intravenous injection of *C. botulinum* toxin.

In cattle a toxicoinfection with *C. botulinum* is suspected to be the cause of a CWD reported to occur with increased incidence in northern and eastern Germany.[4,5] The condition was coined as **chronic or "visceral" botulism** and is thought to be caused by an enteral dysbiosis, allowing *C. botulinum* to grow in the ruminant intestinal tract and to expose the organism to subclinical doses of BoTN over a long time.[4,5] Symptoms associated with this condition are very unspecific including indigestion, lameness and ataxia, weight loss and drop in milk production, tucked-up abdomen, labored breathing, edema in brisket and legs, recumbency, and even death in advanced stages.[4] Although in many reported cases of herd outbreaks the diagnosis was solely based on clinical presentation and by ruling out other differential diagnosis, in several cases feces and intestinal content of affected or death animals were positively tested for *C. botulinum*.[4] The causative relationship is nonetheless under contentious debate because *C. botulinum* spores can routinely be isolated from feces of clinically healthy cattle.[6]

Experimental Reproduction

Cows challenged with type C botulinum toxin intravenously showed initial signs of constipation and straining at defecation 48 hours after injection and weakness, decreased tail tone, decreased tongue tone, and muscle fasciculation of large-muscle groups between 76 and 92 hours. Weakness progressed to total posterior paresis between 80 and 140 hours in these cattle. On a weight-for-weight basis, cattle were considered to be 13 times more sensitive than mice to type C botulinum toxin.

Risk Factors

Animal Risk Factors

Botulism is most common in birds, particularly the domestic chicken and wild waterfowl. Cattle, sheep, and horses are susceptible but pigs, dogs, and cats appear to be resistant. The horse appears to be particularly susceptible to type B toxin. Cattle and sheep are usually affected by types C and D.

Environment Risk Factors

Botulism in range animals has a seasonal distribution. Outbreaks are most likely to occur during drought periods when feed is sparse, phosphorus intake is low, and carrion is plentiful. Silage-associated botulism is also seasonal with the feeding of silage. A key epidemiologic factor identified during recent botulism outbreaks in Europe and Great Britain was the proximity to broiler chicken litter.[2] The variation that occurs in the geographic distribution of the various types, and in carrion versus non–carrion-associated botulism is an important factor when considering prophylactic vaccination programs.

Importance

Severe outbreaks with high case–fatality rates can occur when contaminated feed is fed to large numbers of animals. Under extensive grazing conditions massive outbreaks of carrion-associated botulism also occur unless the animals are vaccinated.

Zoonotic Implications

BoTN is identified as a possible agent for bioterrorism. Furthermore an increasing number of large botulism outbreaks in cattle herds in the past decades have raised public health concerns associated with the consumption of meat or milk originating from affected herds.[1,7,8] In Germany, anecdotal reports of farmers having developed clinical signs resembling symptoms observed in their livestock suspected to suffer of a chronic form of botulism have contributed to these concerns.[9] Notwithstanding there is no evidence to support the assumption that there could be transmission between humans and animals.[1,7] Even the cases in which farm personnel and cattle were affected by a condition thought to be associated with *C. botulinum* different types of *C. botulinum* were isolated from people and cattle.[4,9]

The available evidence for the occurrence of human cases associated with meat and milk consumption has been reviewed.[7] No human cases of clinical botulism that were associated with the consumption of meat or milk derived from animals with botulism or healthy animals from herds affected by botulism were identified.[7] No cases of calves contracting clinical botulism from the consumption of raw milk in herds affected by botulism or cases of other species (dogs) contracting botulism from the consumption of fresh meat were available.[7]

Only one report of a cow affected by clinical botulism has been published in which BoTN was found in one mastitic quarter. The interpretation of this result is complicated by the fact that the BoTN affecting this animal was BoTN type C, whereas the BoNT type E was isolated in milk.[1] Furthermore the toxin was retrieved in a mastitic quarter but not the remaining three clinically healthy quarters. It has therefore been suggested that the BoNT retrieved in this quarter was either produced locally or is the result of contamination.[1] Cows are relatively sensitive to BoTN, whereas the toxin is rarely detectable in the blood of clinical cases. The excretion of BoTN in relevant amounts through the mammary gland is therefore considered to be unlikely. Nonetheless because of the mentioned uncertainties the meat and milk from cattle that have botulism should not be used for human consumption.

PATHOGENESIS

The toxins of *C. botulinum* are neurotoxins and produce functional paralysis without the development of histologic lesions. Botulinum toxins are absorbed from the intestinal tract or the wound and carried via the bloodstream to peripheral cholinergic nerve terminals including neuromuscular junctions, postganglionic parasympathetic nerve endings, and peripheral ganglia. The heavy chain of the toxin is responsible for binding to the receptors and translocation into the cell and the light chain of the toxin for resultant blockade of the release of acetylcholine at the neuromuscular junction. Flaccid paralysis develops and the animal may die of respiratory paralysis.

CLINICAL FINDINGS

Cattle and Horses

Signs usually appear 3 to 17 days after the animals gain access to the toxic material, but occasionally as soon as day 1, the incubation period is shorter as the amount of toxin available is increased. **Peracute cases** die without prior signs of illness, although a few fail to take water or food for a day beforehand. The disease is not accompanied by fever, and the characteristic clinical picture is one of progressive symmetric muscular paralysis affecting particularly the limb muscles and the muscles of the jaw, tongue, and throat. Muscle weakness and paralysis commence in the hindquarters and progress to the forequarters, head, and neck. The onset is marked by very obvious muscle tremor and fasciculation, often sufficient to make the whole limb tremble. Colic may be an initial sign in horses.

In most cases the disease is **subacute**. Restlessness, incoordination, stumbling, knuckling, and ataxia are followed by inability to rise or to lift the head. Mydriasis and ptosis occur early in the clinical course; mydriasis can be prominent in type C botulism in the horse. Skin sensation is retained. Affected animals lie in sternal recumbency with the head on the ground or turned into the flank, not unlike the posture of a cow with parturient paresis. Tongue tone is reduced, as is the strength of tongue retraction. In some cases the tongue becomes paralyzed and hangs from the mouth, the animal is unable to chew or swallow, and it drools saliva. In others there is no impairment of swallowing or mastication and the animal continues to eat until the end. This variation in signs is often a characteristic of an outbreak; either all the cases have tongue paralysis or all of them do not have it. Ruminal movements are depressed. Defecation and urination are usually unaffected, although cattle may be constipated. Paralysis of the chest muscles results in a terminal abdominal-type respiration. Sensation and consciousness are retained until the end, which usually occurs quietly, and with the animal in lateral recumbency, 1 to 4 days after the commencement of illness.

Occasional field cases and some experimental cases in cattle show **mild signs** and recover after an illness of 3 to 4 weeks. These chronic cases show restlessness and respiratory distress followed by knuckling, stumbling, and disinclination to rise. Anorexia and adipsia are important early signs but are often not observed in pastured animals. In some there is a pronounced roaring sound with each respiration. The roaring persists for up to 3 months. During the major part of the illness the animals spend most of their time in sternal recumbency. In some animals there is difficulty in prehending hay but concentrate and ensilage may be taken. This disability may persist for 3 weeks.

A syndrome ascribed to toxicosis with BoTN type B and manifested with anorexia, decline in milk production, dysphagia, a fetid diarrhea, regurgitation, and profuse salivation without myesthesia, paresis, and recumbency is reported in cattle in the Netherlands and Israel. In these cases death occurred as a result of aspiration pneumonia.

With **toxicoinfectious botulism** in foals, muscle tremor is often a prominent early sign. If the foal can walk, the gait is stiff and stilted and the toes are dragged. If the foal sucks, milk drools from the mouth; if it attempts to eat hay some of the material is regurgitated through the nostrils. Constipation occurs consistently. There is a rapid progression to severe muscular weakness and prostration, with the foal going down and being unable to rise. If it is held up, there is a gross muscle tremor, which is not evident when the foal is lying down. Prostrate foals are bright and alert, have normal mentation and pain perception, and have dilatation of the pupils with a sluggish pupillary light reflex. During the latter period of the illness there is a complete cessation of peristalsis. The temperature varies from being slightly elevated to slightly depressed. Death occurs about 72 hours after the onset of signs and is caused by respiratory failure.

Sheep

Sheep do not show the typical flaccid paralysis of other species until the final stages of the disease. There is stiffness while walking and incoordination and some excitability in the early stages. The head may be held on one side or bobbed up and down while walking (**limber neck**). Lateral switching of the tail, salivation, and serous nasal discharge are also common. In the terminal stages there is abdominal respiration, limb paralysis, and rapid death.

Goats

Because of different feeding habits of sheep and goats the risk of exposure to BoTN of goats is considerably lower compared with sheep or cattle. Although goats look for bushes and shrubs on which to browse, cattle and sheep graze along the ground and are therefore more likely to ingest BoTN from contaminated waste spread over pasture.[8]

Pigs

Authentic reports in this species are rare. Clinical signs include staggering followed by recumbency, vomiting, and pupillary dilatation. The muscular paralysis is flaccid and affected animals do not eat or drink.

CLINICAL PATHOLOGY

There are no changes in hematologic values or serum biochemistry that are specific to botulism. In many cases under field conditions the diagnosis is solely based on clinical presentation and by ruling out potential differential diagnoses.

Laboratory diagnosis of botulism in the live or dead animal is difficult because of the lack of sensitive confirmatory laboratory tests. Laboratory confirmation is attempted by the following:

- Detection of preformed toxin in serum, intestinal tract contents, or feed
- Demonstration of spores of *C. botulinum* in the feed or gastrointestinal contents
- Detection of antibody in recovering or clinically normal at-risk animals.

Detection of toxin using bioassay in mice where mice are inoculated intraperitoneally coupled with toxin neutralization with polyvalent antitoxin is considered the most sensitive test currently available. Nonetheless the rate of positivity in clinical cases particularly when testing serum is low, which has been explained by the much higher sensitivity to BoNT of cattle and horse compared with mice and the rapid binding of BoNT in the neuromuscular junctions, leaving low to no amounts of free BoNT in blood. Currently gastrointestinal content or fecal material is preferred over fecal material for the detection of BoNT.[5,7]

In outbreaks of botulism it is not uncommon to have only a proportion of clinically affected animals, or none, test positive. Protection with monovalent antitoxin allows type identification. Toxin detection by an ELISA test appears less sensitive than mouse bioassay. Toxin production or carrion contamination can potentially occur in a number of feeds; however, the majority of outbreaks are associated with contamination in hay or silage and suspect feeds should be tested in mice for toxin. To get around the problem of lack of sensitivity with the mouse test, suspect feed has been fed to experimental cattle. Alternatively, one can make an infusion of the feed sample and use this as the sole drinking water supply for experimental animals. The problem with all feeding experiments is that the BoTN is likely to be very patchy in its distribution in the feed.

Failure to produce the disease in animals vaccinated against botulism, when deaths are occurring in the unvaccinated controls, has also been used as a diagnostic procedure.

Demonstration of spores of *C. botulinum* in the feed being fed or the feces of affected animals supports a diagnosis of botulism because botulism spores are rarely detected in the feces of normal foals and adult horses. Although the testing of gastrointestinal contents from clinically suspect cases in cattle is frequently used as diagnostic tool particularly when toxicoinfectious botulism is suspected, this approach is considered to lack specificity because the postmortem growth of environmental *C. botulinum* spores would result in false-positive results.[2,4,9] Furthermore *C. botulinum* can be isolated from the majority of fecal samples of healthy slaughter cows.

The detection of antibody in chronically affected animals and at-risk herdmates or as retrospective diagnosis by an ELISA test has been used to support a diagnosis in outbreaks of type C and type D botulism. Increased antibody prevalence over time or increased antibody prevalence in an affected group compared with a similar group nearby was reported by some authors.[10]

NECROPSY FINDINGS

There are no specific changes detectable at necropsy, although the presence of suspicious feedstuffs in the forestomachs or stomach may be suggestive. There may be nonspecific subendocardial and subepicardial hemorrhages and congestion of the intestines. Microscopic changes in the brain are also nonspecific, consisting mainly of perivascular hemorrhages in the corpus striatum, cerebellum, and cerebrum. Nonetheless, unless classic flaccid paralysis was observed clinically, the brain should be examined histologically to eliminate other causes of neurologic disease. The presence of *C. botulinum* in the alimentary tract is a further test. The presence of toxin in the gut contents is confirmatory if found but is often misleading, because the toxin may have already been absorbed. The presence of the toxin in the liver at postmortem examination is taken as evidence that the disease has occurred. In addition to traditional bioassays, such as the mouse protection test, newer methods for toxin detection include ELISA techniques, and a recently described immuno-PCR assay.

Samples for Confirmation of Diagnosis

- Bacteriology: suspected contaminated feed material, feces, rumen and intestinal contents, plus serum from clinically affected herdmates (bioassay, anaerobic CULT, ELISA)
- Histology: formalin-fixed brain.

DIFFERENTIAL DIAGNOSIS

A presumptive diagnosis is made on the clinical signs and history, occurrence in unvaccinated animals, and the ruling out of other diseases with a similar clinical presentation. The symmetric motor paralysis of botulism with muscle paralysis that progresses to recumbency in 1–4 days is a major differential for botulism from other causes of neurologic dysfunction in large animals.

Ruminants

- Periparturient hypocalcemia, characterized by low serum calcium concentrations and responsiveness to parenteral calcium administration
- Hypokalemia, characterized by marked hypokalemia
- Tick paralysis
- Paralytic rabies
- Poisoning by *Phalaris aquatica*
- Organophosphate/carbamate poisoning
- Louping-ill in sheep

Horses

- Equine encephalomyelitis
- Equine herpesvirus-1 myeloencephalopathy
- Atypical myopathy of unknown etiology; the condition that presents frequently fatal myopathy can be differentiated by the characteristic increase in serum creatine kinase activity and the presence of hemoglobinuria
- Equine motor neuron disease
- Hyperkalemic periodic paralysis
- Hepatic encephalopathy
- Paralytic rabies
- Ionophore toxicity
- Myasthenia gravis

TREATMENT

Recent studies report a survival rate in foals of 96% which was achieved by the early administration of antitoxin (before complete recumbency) coupled with a high quality of intensive care fluid therapy, enteral or parenteral feeding, nasal insufflation with oxygen, and mechanical ventilation if required. Duration of hospitalization was approximately 2 weeks. Antitoxin was considered essential to the high success rate in this report and this would limit the success of treatment geographically because antitoxin to the various BoTN types is not available universally. Specific or **polyvalent antiserum** is available in some countries and, if administered early in the course at a dose of 30,000 IU for a foal and 70,000 IU for adult horses, can improve the likelihood of survival. A single dose is sufficient, but it is expensive.

Animals should be confined to a stall with **supportive fluid therapy** and enteral feeding. Muzzling may be required to prevent aspiration pneumonia and frequent turning to prevent muscle necrosis and decubital ulcers. Bladder catheterization may be required in horses that do not urinate, and mechanical ventilation may be necessary for recumbent horses. Mineral oil is used to prevent constipation, and antimicrobial drugs are used to treat secondary complications such as aspiration pneumonia. Therapy should avoid the use of drugs that deplete the neuromuscular junction of acetylcholine, such as neostigmine, and those, such as procaine penicillin, tetracyclines, and aminoglycosides, that potentiate neuromuscular weakness.

A rapid progression of signs suggests a poor prognosis, and treatment should only be undertaken in subacute cases in which signs develop slowly and there is some chance of recovery. The prognosis in recumbent horses is grave.

Where groups of animals have had the same exposure factor, the remainder of the animals in the group should be vaccinated immediately.

Vaccination with either type-specific or combined BoNT toxoid in clinically affected animals is ineffective because binding of BoNT to neuromuscular junctions is irreversible.

TREATMENT AND CONTROL

Treatment

Polyvalent antiserum (30,000 IU for a foal and 70,000 IU for an adult horse, single dose) (R-2)

Control

Vaccinate with multivalent BoTN toxoid IM (R-2)

BoTN, botulin toxin, IM, intramuscularly.

CONTROL

In range animals, **correction of dietary deficiencies** by supplementation with phosphorus or protein should be implemented if conditions permit. Hygienic **disposal of carcasses** is advisable to prevent further pasture contamination but may not be practicable under range conditions. **Vaccination** with type-specific or combined (bivalent C and D) toxoid is practiced in enzootic areas in Australia and southern Africa. Type B and C vaccines would be more appropriate for prevention of disease in North America and Europe. The immunity engendered by vaccination is type specific. The number and interval of vaccinations required varies with the vaccine, and the manufacturer's directions should be followed. In horses, the disease is usually sporadic and caused by accidental contamination of feed or water; vaccination is seldom practiced in this species. Some local reactions are encountered after vaccination in horses but they are seldom serious. Vaccination of the mare may not prevent the occurrence of botulism in foals.

A common problem that arises when the disease appears to have resulted from feeding contaminated silage, hay, or other feed is what to do with the residue of the feed. In these circumstances the stock should be vigorously vaccinated with a toxoid on three occasions at 2-week intervals and then feeding of the same material can be recommenced.

FURTHER READING

Jones T. Botulism. *In Pract.* 1996;18:312-313.

Lindström M, Myllykoski J, Sivelä S, et al. *Clostridium botulinum* in cattle and dairy products. *Crit Rev Food Sci Nutr.* 2010;50:281-304.

Smith LDS, Sugiyama H. *Botulism, the Organisms, Its Toxins, the Disease.* Springfield, IL: Charles C Thomas; 1988.

Whitlock RH. Botulism, type C: experimental and field cases in horses. *Equine Pract.* 1996;18(10):11-17.

Whitlock RH, Buckley C. Botulism. *Vet Clin North Am Equine Pract.* 1997;13:107-128.

REFERENCES

1. Lindström M, et al. *Crit Rev Food Sci Nutr.* 2010;50:281.
2. Kennedy S, Ball H. *Vet Rec.* 2011;168:638.
3. Whitlock RH, McAdams S. *Clin Tech Equine Pract.* 2006;5:37.
4. Krüger M, et al. *Anaerobe.* 2012;18:221.
5. Böhnel H, Gessler F. *Vet Rec.* 2013;172:397.
6. Brooks CE, et al. *Vet Microbiol.* 2010;144:226.
7. ACMSF (Advisory committee on the microbiological safety of food) 2006. (Accessed August, 2016, at http://acmsf.food.gov.uk/sites/default/files/mnt/drupal_data/sources/files/multimedia/pdfs/botulismincattlereport1206.pdf.).
8. ACMSF (Advisory committee on the microbiological safety of food) 2009. (Accessed August 2016, at http://acmsf.food.gov.uk/sites/default/files/mnt/drupal_data/sources/files/multimedia/pdfs/botulisminsheepgoats.pdf.).
9. Rodloff AC, Krüger M. *Anaerobe.* 2012;18:226-228.
10. Mawhinney I, et al. *Vet J.* 2012;192:382-384.

TICK PARALYSIS

Infestations with a several species of ticks are associated with paralysis of animals. Dogs are most commonly affected but losses can occur in cattle, sheep, goats, llamas, horses, and a variety of wild animals. At least 31 species in seven genera of ixodid ticks and seven species in three genera of argasid ticks have been implicated in tick paralysis. The most important tick species for livestock are given in Table 14-22. *D. andersoni* is the most common cause of tick paralysis in livestock in North America; *D. occidentalis* is associated with paralysis in cattle, horses, and deer.[1] In Australia, *I. holocyclus* is the predominant tick associated with paralysis, whereas *I. rubicundus* and *Rhipecephalus evertsi* are common in Africa.[1] Animals in Europe and Asia have developed tick paralysis from *I. ricinus* and *Hyalomma punctata.*[1]

The toxin of *D. andersoni* interferes with liberation or synthesis of acetylcholine at the muscle fiber motor end plates.[2] The disturbance is functional and paralysis of the peripheral neurons is the basis for clinical

Table 14-22 Ticks reported to cause paralysis in livestock

Animal	Tick	Country
Sheep, calves, goats	*Dermacentor andersoni* *D. occidentalis*	United States, Canada United States
Calves, lambs, foals, goats	*Ixodes holocyclus*	Australia
Sheep, goats, calves	*I. pilosus*	South Africa
Sheep, goats, calves, antelopes	*I. rubicundus*	South Africa
Sheep, goats	*I. ricinus*	Crete, Israel
Lambs	*Rhipicephalus evertsi*	South Africa
Calves, sheep, goats	*Hyalomma punctata*	South Africa, Europe, Japan
Sheep	*H. aegyptium*	Yugoslavia
Sheep	*Ornithodorus lahorensis*	Central Asia
Cattle, sheep, goats	*Amblyomma cajannense*	Central, South America
Cattle	*R. evertsi*	Africa

signs. Continuous secretion of toxin by a large number (35–150) of partly engorged female ticks that have been attached for 5 to 8 days is necessary to produce paralysis, with complete recovery occurring within 24 hours when the ticks are removed. The disease is generally confined to calves and yearlings. Clinically, there is an ascending, flaccid paralysis commencing with incoordination of the hindlimbs, followed by paralysis of the forelimbs and chest muscles, causing lateral recumbency.[1] Respiration is grossly abnormal; there is a double expiratory effort and the rate is slow (12–15 breaths per minute) but deep. Death, caused by respiratory failure, may occur in 1 to 2 days, but the course is usually 4 to 5 days. The mortality rate may be as high as 50% in dogs, but is usually much lower in farm animals.

I. holocyclus have been shown to paralyze calves of 25 to 50 kg BW. Between 4 and 10 adult female ticks are required to produce this effect and paralysis occurs 6 to 13 days after infestation occurs. The ticks under natural conditions parasitize wild fauna, and infestations of other species occur accidentally. The disease is limited in its distribution by the ecology of the ticks and the natural host fauna. The paralysis characteristic of the disease is associated with a toxin secreted by the salivary glands of female ticks, which is present in much greater concentration in the glands of adults than in other stages. The severity of the paralysis is independent of the number of ticks involved; susceptible animals may be seriously affected by a few ticks.[1]

Hyperimmune serum is used in the treatment of dogs, but in farm animals removal of the ticks in the early stages is usually followed by rapid recovery. Control necessitates eradication of the ticks or host fauna. The general principles of tick control are outlined in Chapter 11. The use of appropriate insecticides is an effective preventive.

FURTHER READING

Sonenshine DE, Lane RS, Nicholson WL. Ticks (*Ixodia*). In: Mullen G, Durden L, eds. *Medical and Veterinary Entomology*. New York: Academic Press; 2002:517-558.

REFERENCES

1. Gwaltney-Brant SM, Dunayer E, Youssef H. Terrestrial zootoxins. In: Gupta RC, ed. *Veterinary Toxicology*. Amsterdam: Elsevier; 2012:969.
2. Lysyk TJ. *J Med Entomol*. 2009;46:358.

OVINE "KANGAROO GAIT" AND FENUGREEK STAGGERS

SYNOPSIS

Etiology Not known.

Epidemiology Seasonal occurrence involving only adult female sheep that are lactating, or in some cases, pregnant. Spontaneous recovery following cessation of lactation in most cases, but sometimes only 50%, but not always all affected sheep.

Clinical findings Bilateral forelimb locomotor disorder.

Lesions Edema of brain and spinal cord in early cases; axonal degeneration of the radial nerve followed by regeneration in more chronic cases (those greater than 6 weeks' duration).

Treatment Supportive.

Control None recognized.

ETIOLOGY

This is a neuropathy with no known cause. In Australia similar clinical and pathologic signs are associated with grazing mature plants or the stubble of fenugreek (*Trigonella foenum-graecum*), which is an annual winter-spring legume from which the seed is harvested as a condiment for human food.[1]

EPIDEMIOLOGY

Occurrence

This condition is recorded in Australia, New Zealand, and the UK. It is manifested by incoordination, including an acute onset of a high-stepping forelimb gait and bounding hindlimb gait.

Risk Factors

It occurs only in adult ewes with an onset in late pregnancy or early lactation. Spontaneous recovery occurs following cessation of lactation, and occasionally while ewes are still nursing lambs, although in Australia often only 50% of ewes recover completely.[1] The cumulative annual incidence varies between flocks but is usually less than 1%.

In the areas of northern England and southern Scotland the condition is significantly more common in upland and lowland flocks than in those hill grazing. Stocking density is higher in affected flocks than that in nonaffected flocks. Onset occurs while on pasture between March and June with a separate smaller peak in October. This seasonal occurrence could be a reflection of the parturition status of flocks or an effect of seasonal influences.

In Australia cases have been recorded in lactating ewes grazing improved pastures from June (winter) to February (summer) and the grazing of fenugreek crop or stubble in summer.

PATHOGENESIS

Clinical signs can be attributed to the generalized neuropathy affecting principally the radial nerves. Subsequent to the axonal degeneration a remyelination of the radial nerve occurs, explaining the clinical recovery. For cases not associated with ingestion of fenugreek, bilateral compression of the radial nerves is suggested as a cause, but there is no knowledge of how such an injury can occur. Despite the differences in diet, the similar clinical and pathologic presentation of kangaroo gait and fenugreek staggers has prompted the suggestion that these may be related entities.[1] Nevertheless there are some key differences; the initial acute stage of fenugreek staggers in Merino sheep is sometimes lethal and is later associated with weight loss, whereas kangaroo gait is not and seems to be restricted to larger meat breeds.

CLINICAL FINDINGS

These include incoordination, a high-stepping forelimb and bounding hindlimb gait, arched back, and proprioceptive deficits (knuckling of fore and occasionally hind fetlocks). There is bilateral forelimb paresis and palpable loss of muscle bulk in the forelimbs. The forelimbs and hindlimbs of affected sheep are positioned centrally under the body and so when they are pressed affected sheep move with a characteristic hopping or kangaroo gait. Affected ewes lie down more frequently and may graze on their knees but continue to eat and effectively suckle their lambs.

CLINICAL PATHOLOGY

There are no consistent abnormalities in hematology, blood biochemistry, or trace element analysis of affected sheep.

NECROPSY FINDINGS

In early cases there are signs of acute edema in the brain and spinal cord (wallerian degeneration of ventral motor tracts, spongy changes in the neuropil, and swollen astrocytes). This progresses to a peripheral neuropathy, with axonal degeneration of the myelinated fibers of the radial nerve fibers in longer standing cases (6 weeks or more), and then regeneration in recovering cases.

DIFFERENTIAL DIAGNOSIS

Romulosis, a condition associated with grazing fungus-infected onion grass (*Romulea rosea*), can cause incoordination and a similar hopping gait (bunny-hopping).

Foot rot or foot abscess involving the front feet can induce the same grazing behavior, but there is no problem in differentiation when the limbs and feet are examined.

Hypocalcemia in sheep occurs in late pregnancy or during lactation, and in the developing stages there is incoordination and muscle weakness. However, there is rapid progression to complete muscular paresis and a dramatic response to treatment.

Spinal abscess or fracture.

TREATMENT

Without the knowledge of etiology there is no specific treatment. Easy access to food and water should be provided.

FURTHER READING

Radostits O, et al. Ovine "kangaroo gait." In: *Veterinary Medicine: A Textbook of the Disease of Cattle,*

Horses, Sheep, Goats and Pigs. 10th ed. London: W.B. Saunders; 2007:2019.

REFERENCE

1. Bourke C. *Aust Vet J*. 2009;87:99.

POLYNEURITIS EQUI (CAUDA EQUINA SYNDROME)

Polyneuritis equi (formerly cauda equina neuritis) is a demyelinating, inflammatory disease of peripheral nerves of adult horses. The **etiology** of the disease is unknown although infectious (adenovirus, EHV-1), immune (autoimmune disease), and toxic etiologies have been suggested, without conclusive substantiation. Adenovirus was isolated from two of three horses with the disease, but this observation has not been repeated, and it appears unlikely at this time that adenovirus is the cause of polyneuritis equi. EHV-1 is not consistently isolated from affected horses.

The disease occurs in adult horses in Europe and North America but has not been reported from the Southern Hemisphere. The prevalence in a group of 4319 horses subject to postmortem examination in Normandy was 0.2% (one case).[1] The disease is usually sporadic with single animals on a farm or in a stable affected. However, outbreaks of the disease can affect multiple horses from the same farm over a number of years.

The **pathogenesis** of the disease involves nonsuppurative inflammation of the extradural nerves and demyelination of peripheral nerves. Initial inflammation of the nerves causes hyperesthesia, which is followed by loss of sensation as nerves are demyelinated. Both motor and sensory nerves are affected, with subsequent weakness, paresis, muscle atrophy, urinary and fecal retention and incontinence, and gait abnormalities.

The inflammatory response is characterized by an abundance of **T lymphocytes**, in addition to B lymphocytes, macrophages, giant cells, eosinophils, and neutrophils in the perineurium and endomeurium.[2] The T cells are CD8+ cytotoxic T lymphocytes with rare CD4+ helper T lymphocytes.[3] This, with electron microscopic imaging, evidence of "myelin stripping" by macrophages and the presence of antibodies to the myelin P2 protein has been interpreted as indicative of immune-mediated activity against myelin.[2,4] This immune response might be toward the myelin as a primary target or could be the result of bystander activity in which other agents, potentially viruses, induce an immune response that is directed against myelin.

The **acute disease** is evident as abrupt onset of hyperesthesia of the perineum and tail head, and perhaps the face, evident as avoidance of touching, and chewing or rubbing of the tail. The hyperesthesia progresses to hypalgesia or anesthesia of the affected regions.

The disease usually has a more **insidious onset** with loss of sensation and function occurring over days to weeks. The most common presentation is that of cauda equina syndrome with bilaterally symmetric signs of posterior weakness, tail paralysis, fecal and urinary incontinence and retention, and atrophy of the gluteal muscles. Tail tone is decreased or absent and the tail is easily raised by the examiner. The anus is usually atonic and dilated. There are signs of urinary incontinence with urine scalding of the escutcheon and hindlegs. Rectal examination reveals fecal retention and a distended bladder that is readily expressed. Male horses can have prolapse of the penis with maintained sensation in the prepuce, which is a finding consistent with the separate innervation of these anatomic regions. Affected horses can also have ataxia of the hindlimbs, but this is always combined with signs of cauda equina disease.

Signs of **CN dysfunction** occur as part of the disease, but not in all cases. CN dysfunction can be symmetric, but is usually asymmetric. Nerves prominently involved in the genesis of clinical signs are the trigeminal (CN V), facial (CN VII), and hypoglossal nerve (CN XII), although all CNs can be affected to some extent. Involvement of the CNs is evident as facial paralysis (CN VII), weakness of the tongue (CN XII), and loss of sensation in the skin of the face (CN V). There can be loss of movement of the pinnae (CN VII) and head tilt (CN VIII). Laryngeal paralysis can be present (CN X). The buccal branches of CN VII can be enlarged and palpable over the masseter muscles ventral to the facial crest.

Not all clinical signs occur in all horses and, depending on the stage and severity of the disease, some animals can have loss of sensation as the only abnormality, especially during the early stages of the disease.

EMG is consistent with denervation with prolonged insertion potentials, positive sharp waves, and fibrillation. Per rectal **ultrasound examination** of the extradural sacral nerve routes as they exit the ventral sacral foramina reveals enlargement and a diffusely mottled, hypoechoic appearance.[3]

Biopsy of the sacrocaudalis dorsalis lateralis muscle can provide antemortem diagnosis of the disease. Affected horses have intense lymphocytic and histiocytic infiltration around the terminal nerves within the muscle, often obliterating architecture of the nerves but sparing the myofibers.[3] There is neurogenic atrophy of the muscle fibers.

The disease is inexorably progressive, the prognosis for life is hopeless, and the course of the disease is usually less than 3 months.

Clinical pathologic abnormalities are not diagnostic. There is sometimes a mild neutrophilic leukocytosis and hypergammaglobulinemia. Serum vitamin E concentrations are usually normal. Analysis of CSF demonstrates mild mononuclear pleocytosis and increased protein concentrations, but these changes are not diagnostic of the disease. Horses with polyneuritis equi have antibodies to P2 myelin protein in serum, but the diagnostic value of this test has not been determined.

Necropsy findings are definitive for the disease. Gross findings include thickening of the epidural nerve roots that is most severe in the cauda equina. The bladder and rectum can be distended. There can be evidence of fecal and urine scalding and self-trauma of the perineum. There can be thickening of the facial nerves. Microscopic changes are characterized by a granulomatous inflammation of the extradural nerves, although radiculoganglioneuritis and myelitis can also occur. There is loss of axons with demyelination and signs of remyelination. There is profound infiltration of nerves by macrophages, moderate to marked infiltration of cytotoxic T lymphocytes, and lesser infiltration of B lymphocytes.[3] Inflammatory cells are initially lymphocytes, plasma cells, and macrophages. As the inflammation becomes more severe or chronic there is extensive proliferation of fibroblasts and fibrocytes in addition to infiltration of lymphocytes and macrophages. There is axonal degeneration with proliferation of the perineurium. The chronic inflammatory changes result in loss of peripheral neural architecture. Lesions are present in many regions of the spinal cord, but are most severe in the sacral division and cauda equina. Lysosomal accumulations are present in the semilunar, geniculate, and sympathetic chains and granulomatous lesions in the celiac-mesenteric ganglion. Lesions of the CNs similarly involve infiltration with lymphocytes and histiocytes, and the inflammation can extend to the terminal branches of the nerves.

The **diagnosis** of polyneuritis equi is based on the presence of clinical signs of the disease, ruling out other diseases causing similar clinical signs, and necropsy examination. Diseases with manifestations similar to polyneuritis equi include the following:

- EHV-1 myeloencephalopathy
- Migrating parasites (Table 14-21, **differential diagnosis of disease causing spinal ataxia in horses**)
- Sorghum-Sudan grass neuropathy
- Equine protozoal myeloencephalitis
- Ryegrass staggers (*A. lolii*)
- Dourine
- Trauma to the sacral vertebral column
- Abscess or neoplasia involving the sacral or caudal lumbar vertebral column
- Meningitis
- Intentional alcohol sclerosis of tail head nerves in Quarter Horses.

There is no definitive **treatment** for polyneuritis equi. Administration of antiinflammatory agents, including corticosteroids, appears to be without sustained benefit.

Supportive care includes evacuation of the rectum and bladder and maintenance of hydration and provision of adequate nutrition. Feeding a diet that softens feces, or administration of fecal softeners or lubricants, can be beneficial. Bethanecol (0.05–0.1 mg/kg every 8–12 hours, orally) might increase bladder tone. Topical administration of petroleum jelly or similar products can protect the skin of the perineum and escutcheon from fecal and urine scalding.

REFERENCES

1. Laugier C, et al. *J Equine Vet Sci.* 2009;29:561.
2. van Galen G, et al. *Equine Vet J.* 2008;40:185.
3. Aleman M, et al. *J Vet Intern Med.* 2009;23:665.
4. Hahn CN. *Equine Vet J.* 2008;40:100.

SCANDINAVIAN KNUCKLING SYNDROME (ACQUIRED EQUINE POLYNEUROPATHY)

This is a recently recognized syndrome of metatarsophalangeal joint extensor paresis in horses in Scandinavia.[1-3] The disease appears to be widespread in Sweden, Norway, and Finland occurring as clusters of disease outbreaks on farms.[1] The etiology is uncertain, although preserved feed is considered the source of an unidentified toxin.

A report described the risk factors and outcome of 42 cases distributed over 13 farms in Scandinavia from 2007 to 2009. Cases occurred between December and May with an overall prevalence of 27% and on-farm prevalence of 11% to 71% (for farms with >6 horses) although the number of cases, and affected farms, varies markedly from year to year.[2,4] The case–fatality rate was 29% in the epidemiology study[1] and 53% (40 of 75) in a case series.[2] The disease was less prevalent in horses >12 years of age, and younger horses had a greater chance of surviving the disease.

Clinical signs were typified by bilateral knuckling of the hindlimbs, which was most apparent on circling. Mild to moderate pelvic limb weakness was detected in 16 of 42 horses.[1] A small proportion of cases (3/42) had mild forelimb signs of weakness and knuckling. There was focal muscle atrophy of hindlimb musculature in seven cases. Mentation and vital signs (temperature, pulse, and respiratory rate) were within normal limits. The disease usually has a slow onset, but some affected horses developed severe signs with hours.[2] The median duration of clinical signs in affected horses that recover is 4.4 months (range 1–17 months) and survivors can recover completely.

Routine hematology and serum biochemical analysis do not reveal consistent abnormalities, apart from increased creatine kinase and AST activity in recumbent horses.[2]

Lesions are restricted to the peripheral nervous system and are evident in sciatic, peroneal, radial, and plantar digital nerves.[2,3] Lesions include areas of thick, swollen axons with subperineural accumulation of mucoid material. There is lymphohistiocytic infiltration of nerves and mild to moderate loss of myelinated nerve fibers.[3] Swollen axons and large vacuoles were present in sections of the lumbar tumescence. There are no lesions detected in the brain.[2]

Treatment consists of supportive and nursing care. Control measures are not reported.

REFERENCES

1. Grondahl G, et al. *Equine Vet J.* 2012;44:36.
2. Hanche-Olsen S, et al. *J Vet Intern Med.* 2008;22:178.
3. Hahn CN, et al. *Equine Vet J.* 2008;40:231.
4. Wolff C, et al. *BMC Vet Res.* 2014;10:265.

PERIPHERAL NERVE SHEATH TUMORS

PNSTs are most commonly benign tumors of the peripheral nervous system with a rare occurrence in veterinary medicine.[1] Most commonly affected species are dogs and cattle.[1] Tumors are composed of components of the peripheral nerve, including Schwann cells, perineural cells, fibroblasts and collagen. While in human medicine PNSTs are subdivided into **neurofibromas** and **schwannomas**, dependent on the predominant cell type and other histologic characteristics, this distinction is less clearly defined in veterinary medicine.[2,3] The existence of true neurofibromas as described in humans has been questioned.[1,2] PNSTs that can occur on any location of the peripheral nervous system most commonly originate from autonomic nerves such as cardiac and intercostal nerves or the brachial plexus.

CLINICAL FINDINGS

In cattle, PNSTs are generally asymptomatic and found incidentally during physical examination or slaughter. Clinical signs are uncommon but can include limb paresis or paralysis, recurrent bloat and vagal indigestion, cardiac insufficiency, and chronic wasting.[1,3,4] The cutaneous presentation is rare but can present as single or multiple indolent cutaneous masses between 1 and over 15 cm in diameter that are well demarcated. In some instances PMSTs may infiltrate surrounding tissue, immobilizing the mass and complicating surgical excision.

CLINICAL PATHOLOGY

Diagnosis must be confirmed histologically. Important features included the concurrent presence of highly and poorly cellular areas of Schwann cells. Nerve fibers are absent in schwannomas but may be found in neurofibromas. Immunohistostaining is used to confirm the presence of Schwann cells and to differentiate between schwannomas and neurofibromas.[1,2]

TREATMENT

Treatment of accessible masses (cutaneous form) is rarely required but may be indicated either for cosmetic reasons as an excisional biopsy or to remove the mass integrally. Although the prognosis in most cases is excellent, tumors with infiltrative growth may recur because of incomplete excision of abnormal c ells.

REFERENCES

1. Schöniger S, Summer BA. *Vet Pathol.* 2009;46:904.
2. Nielsen AB, et al. *J Comp Pathol.* 2007;137:224.
3. Pavarini SP, et al. *Acta Vet Scand.* 2013;55:7.
4. Beytut E. *J Comp Pathol.* 2006;134:260.

Diseases of the Musculoskeletal System

15

Diseases of the organs of support, including muscles, bones, and joints, have much in common in that the major clinical manifestations of diseases that affect them are lameness, failure of support (weakness), insufficiency of movement, and deformity. Insufficiency of movement affects all voluntary muscles, including those responsible for respiratory movement and mastication, but lameness and failure of support are manifestations of involvement of the limbs.

Various classifications of the diseases of the musculoskeletal system, based on clinical, pathologic, and etiologic differences, are in use, but the simplest is that which divides the diseases into **degenerative** and **inflammatory** types. This classification system is used in this chapter.

- The degenerative diseases of muscles, bones and joints are distinguished as myopathy, osteodystrophy, and arthropathy, respectively.
- The inflammatory diseases are myositis, osteitis and osteomyelitis, and arthritis, respectively.

Principal Manifestations of Musculoskeletal Disease

LAMENESS

Lameness is an abnormal gait or locomotion characterized by limping or not bearing full weight on a leg, usually associated with localized pain in the musculoskeletal system. Lameness must be distinguished from **ataxia**, which is an abnormal gait characterized by lack of coordination of muscular action, usually because of a lesion of the central or peripheral nervous system.

Weakness (paresis) is the inability to maintain a normal posture and gait, usually because of a lesion of muscle or generalized weakness as a result of an abnormal systemic state (e.g., shock), a metabolic abnormality (e.g., hypocalcemia or hypokalemia), or starvation. Weakness can also be caused by a lesion in the spinal cord or peripheral nerves.

The incidence and severity of lameness in livestock populations varies tremendously because of differences in management systems (grazing versus confinement, concrete versus slatted floors, free stall design and use by dairy cattle, frequency of foot trimming, etc.), nutrition, genetics, age, body weight, and many other factors. For example, certain breeds may be more susceptible to diseases of the feet and legs than others. Osteoarthritis occurs most commonly in old animals. Diseases of the legs of dairy cattle occur most commonly at the time of parturition and during the first 50 days of lactation. Diseases of the feet of dairy cattle occur most commonly in days 50 to 150 of the lactation period. Often the etiology is complex, and a definitive etiologic diagnosis cannot be made. This makes clinical management difficult and often unrewarding. The direct monetary costs for the treatment of lame animals are not high, but the actual treatment of either individual animals or groups of animals is time-consuming and laborious. The condemnation of animals to slaughter because of lesions of the musculoskeletal system also contributes to the total economic loss.

When lameness is a herd problem, not only are the economic losses increased, but clinical management becomes very difficult. The epidemiologic factors that contribute to lameness include the following:

- Injuries as a result of floor surfaces
- Persistently wet, unhygienic ground conditions
- Overcrowding and trampling during transportation and handling
- Nutritional inadequacies
- Undesirable skeletal conformation
- Failure to provide regular foot trimming

Because of the difficulty inherent in the differentiation of diseases causing lameness, and other abnormalities of gait and posture, a summary is presented in Table 15-1. It does not include lameness in racing horses, which is described in textbooks on lameness in horses, or diseases of the nervous system that interfere with normal movement and posture. These are discussed in Chapter 14.

ABNORMAL POSTURE AND MOVEMENT

As a group, diseases of the musculoskeletal system are characterized by reduced activity in standing up and moving and by the adoption of unusual postures.[1] Abnormal movements include weakness (limpness) or stiffness and lack of flexion. Abnormal postures include persistent recumbency, including lateral recumbency. There may be signs of pain on standing, moving, or palpation. There is an absence of signs specifically referable to the nervous system. Differentiation from diseases of the nervous system and from each other may be aided by specific biochemical, radiologic, or hematologic findings that indicate the system involved. Specific epidemiologic findings may indicate the location of the lesion (which may be secondary) in muscle, bones, or joints, as set out in Table 15-1.

DEFORMITY

Atypical disposition, shape, or size of a part of the musculoskeletal system constitutes a deformity. This may occur in a number of ways, and be caused by the following defects.

Muscle and Tendon Defects

- Congenital hypermobility of joints, inherited and sporadic
- Congenital flexed or stretched tendons of limbs causing contracture of joints or hyperextension
- Inherited congenital splayleg of pigs
- Muscle hypertrophy (doppelender, culard) of cattle
- Acquired asymmetric hindquarters of pigs

Defects of the Skeleton

- Dwarfism—inherited miniature calves, achondroplastic dwarves; short legs of inherited congenital osteopetrosis; nutritional deficiency of manganese; acorn calves
- Giant stature—inherited prolonged gestation, not really giantism, only large at birth
- Asymmetry—normal wither height, low pelvis height of hyena disease of cattle
- Limbs—complete or partial absence, inherited or sporadic amputates; curvature of limbs in rickets; bowie or bentleg of sheep poisoned by *Trachymene* spp.
- Head—inherited and sporadic cyclopean deformity; inherited probatocephaly (sheep's head) of calves; inherited moles,

Table 15-1 Differential diagnosis of diseases of the musculoskeletal system

Disease and clinical findings	Epidemiologic findings	Clinical pathology	Necropsy findings	Examples
Myasthenia				
Paresis, paralysis, and incoordination	Ischemia or reduced supply of energy or electrolytes.	Hypoglycemia, hypocalcemia, hypokalemia, hypomagnesemia	Reversible malfunction	Iliac thrombosis, toxemia, milk fever, lactic acidosis, some poisonous plants
Myopathy				
Either stiff gait, disinclination to move, board-like muscles *or* weakness, pseudoparesis or paralysis, difficulty rising, staggery gait, flabby muscles. Always bilateral, mostly hindlimbs.	Often precipitated by sudden increase in muscular work. Usually diet-dependent and related to: (1) high carbohydrate intake (2) deficiency in selenium/vitamin E intake (3) Ingestion of myopathic agents (e.g., in poisonous plants, cod liver oil)	Marked elevations in serum activity of CPK and AST. Myoglobinemia and possibly myoglobinuria.	White, waxy, swollen, "fish flesh" muscle.	*Horses:* Azoturia (equine paralytic myoglobinuria, tying up, equine rhabdomyolysis, equine atypical myopathy); postanesthetic myositis. *Pigs:* Porcine stress syndrome, selenium deficiency, inherited splaylegs. *Cattle:* Selenium/vitamin E deficiency (enzootic muscular dystrophy), poisoning by *Cassia occidentalis, Karwinskia humboldtiana,* ischemic necrosis of recumbency. *Sheep:* Approximately the same; exertional rhabdomyolysis.
Myositis				
Acute inflammation, swelling, pain; may be associated with systemic signs if infectious. Chronic manifested by atrophy, contracture of joint, incomplete extension.	Related to trauma or specific infectious disease. Atrophy, pallor in chronic.	As for myopathy, plus hematologic response when infection present.	Bruising, edema, and hemorrhage in acute.	Blackleg, false blackleg (malignant edema). Eosinophilic myositis in beef cattle. Traumatic injury by strain of muscle or forceful impact.
Osteodystrophy				
Stiff gait, moderate lameness often shifting from leg to leg, arched back, crackling sounds in joints while walking. Disinclination to move; horses affected early race very poorly.	Absolute deficiency and/or relative imbalance of dietary calcium, phosphorus, and vitamin D. Most apparent in rapidly growing, working, and heavy milk-producing animals.	Radiographic evidence of osteoporosis, deformed epiphyseal lines, broadness of epiphyses. Subperiosteal unossified osteoid.	Osteoporosis, subepiphyseal collapse of bone at pressure points. Fracture of soft bones. Bone ash determinations of Ca, P, and Mg content of bones.	*Cattle:* Phosphorus deficiency, Marie's disease. Hypovitaminosis D. Calcium deficiency. Poisoning by *Trachymene glaucifolia* (bowie or bentleg).
Severely affected animals disinclined to stand, recumbent much of time. Fractures common. Bones soft (e.g., frontal bones) to digital pressure. Deformities of bones (e.g., bowing, pelvic collapse). Ready detachment of tendons and ligaments.				*Horses:* Osteodystrophia fibrosa as a result of low calcium diet, or to poisonous plants containing large amounts of oxalate (see under oxalate poisoning). *Pigs:* Osteodystrophia fibrosa attributable to low Ca and high P in diet.
Osteomyelitis				
Pain, swelling (little), toxemia, fever; may be discharge through sinus.	Only of specific disease.	Radiographic evidence of rarefaction, new bone growth.	Osteomyelitis.	Actinomycosis, brucellosis in pigs and cattle. Necrotic and atrophic rhinitis disease in pigs.
Arthropathy (osteoarthritis)				
Lameness with pain on walking, standing, palpation. Some enlargement but not gross.	(1) Inherited predisposition in cattle (2) Dietary excess of phosphorus, relative deficiency of calcium	Excessive sterile brownish fluid with floccules. Radiologic evidence of joint erosion, epiphyseal deformity, new bone growth peripherally.	Erosion of cartilage and bone, ligament rupture, new bone growth (epiphytes) around edge of joint.	*Cattle:* Degenerative joint disease (of young beef bulls), inherited osteoarthritis. *Horses:* As early part of osteodystrophy syndrome.

Continued

Table 15-1 Differential diagnosis of diseases of the musculoskeletal system—cont'd

Disease and clinical findings	Epidemiologic findings	Clinical pathology	Necropsy findings	Examples
Slackness in joints, may be ligament rupture, crepitus.	(3) Very rapid increase in body weight in young (4) Heavy milk production during many lactations		Excess brownish sterile clear fluid containing floccules.	*Pigs:* Epiphysiolysis of femurs of young breeding boars. Osteochondrosis.
Arthritis				
Acute: Sudden onset, severe pain, very lame, sore to touch, swelling and heat in joint.	Most commonly in young via navel infection and bacteremia, or residual from septicemia of neonate.	Aspiration of fluid under very sterile conditions shows leukocytes and somatic cells in large numbers. Culture may be positive but often negative.	*Acute:* Inflammation or suppuration, increased fluid content. *Chronic:* Thickened synovial membrane.	*Cattle: Mycoplasma* spp., *Erysipelothrix rhusiopathiae Streptococcus* and *Staphylococcus* spp., *Escherichia coli,*
Chronic: Continuous pain, recumbency, may be toxemia if infectious. Joint may be visibly swollen but may be normal in appearance. Pain may be evident only when animal stands on joint.		Joint fluid may appear normal in chronic case	Increased amount of clear fluid. Erosion of articular cartilage	*Salmonella* spp. in newborn. *Brucella abortus,* *Mycoplasma* spp. and *Chlamydophila* spp. *Pigs: E. Erysipelothria rhusiopathiae, Mycoplasma* spp. *Sheep: Corynebacterium pseudotuberculosis,* *E. rhusiopathiae, Histophilus somni, Mannheimia haemolytica, Actinobacillus seminis,* *Chlamydophila* spp., *Mycoplasma* spp. *Horses:* Foal septicemias.
Tenosynovitis, cellulitis, lymphangitis, bursitis				
Inflammation of other supporting tissues. Visible, painful enlargements.	Sporadic as a result of trauma or localization of systemic infection.	Culture of aspirate from local lesion.	Inflammation of affected part. Acute hemorrhagic or chronic, suppurative.	*Horses and cattle:* Bursitis—*B. abortus.* Tenosynovitis—*Histophilus somni,* cattle, *Streptococcus equi* horse, *Histophilus somni,* sheep.
Interdigital dermatitis (footrot)				
Severe foot lameness. Visible local lesion at skin–horn junction, necrotic smell, horn underrun. Allied similar conditions have less severe lesions.	Severe epidemics in wet, warm weather in sheep. Infection soil-borne. Some farms have disease persistently.	Culture of infectious agent, swab from depth of lesion.	Necrosis of soft tissue.	*Sheep:* Footrot—*Bacteroides nodosus;* foot scald—avirulent *B. nodosus;* foot abscess—*F. necrophorus;* *Trueperella pyogenes;* interdigital dermatitis—*F. necrophorum.* *Cattle:* Footrot—*F. necrophorum, B. nodosus.*
Laminitis				
Severe foot pain, separation of horn from sensitive laminae, rotation of the pedal bone. Metabolic, traumatic, or infectious types.	Sporadic except infectious type in sheep related to dipping. Possibly inherited susceptibility to metabolic laminitis in cattle.	Very high blood pressure. Radiologic demonstration of P_3 rotation.	Infection or hemorrhage/ edema, sensitive laminae.	*Sheep: Erysipelothrix rhusiopathiae*—postdipping laminitis. *Horses*—traumatic as a result of continuous pawing. *All species:* Metabolic associated with heavy grain feeding—in mares with retained placenta and metritis.
Damage to horn of hoof				
Severe foot pain if sensitive laminae affected. Horn damage obvious.	Related to hard, abrasive surfaces—pigs and dairy cattle; soft underfoot—cows indoors on wet bedding.	None.	Foot-horn lesion only.	*Cattle:* Stable footrot on soft footing; sole wear on rough concrete. *Pigs:* Sole wear on rough concrete, predisposed by biotin deficiency in diet. *Horses:* Thrush and canker on soft wet underfoot.

Table 15-1 Differential diagnosis of diseases of the musculoskeletal system—cont'd

Disease and clinical findings	Epidemiologic findings	Clinical pathology	Necropsy findings	Examples
Traumatic injuries of feet of newborn piglets				
Severe lameness in piglets 1–8 days of age. Bruising of sole, congestion, and swelling followed by peeling, erosion, and cracking of horn of sole; both claws and accessory digits injured more often on medial aspect, and incidence in hindfeet twice that of forefeet; abrasions of skin of carpal joints common; accessory digits involved too. Ascending secondary bacterial infection resulting in tenosynovitis and septic arthritis. Most piglets recover following antibacterial therapy.	Newborn piglets raised on concrete or slatted floors. Distribution of lesions related to sucking behavior of piglets, the backward, outward, and downward thrusting movements of the hindlegs while sucking.	None.	Erosion, necrosis, congestion, fissures, and hemorrhage of horn of sole and sensitive laminae of digit. Secondary tenosynovitis and arthritis.	*Piglets:* Newborn piglets raised on concrete, expanded metal, or plastic slatted floors.
Coronitis dermatitis at coronet				
Lesions vary from granuloma through vesicles, erosions. Lameness in all, but severity varies with type of lesion. Essential to examine oral mucosa.	Acute outbreaks of lameness as a result of coronitis in any species raises specter of food-and-mouth disease.	Microbiology of material from local lesion.	Local lesions only.	*Sheep:* Bluetongue, foot-and-mouth disease, vesicular stomatitis, ecthyma, strawberry footrot, ulcerative dermatosis, heel dermatitis (*B. nodosus*), strongyloidosis. *Cattle:* Foot-and-mouth disease, vesicular stomatitis, bovine virus diarrhea, bovine malignant catarrh, epitheliogenesis imperfecta. *Pigs:* Foot-and-mouth disease, vesicular exanthema of swine, swine vesicular disease, vesicular stomatitis. *Horses:* Vesicular stomatitis, greasy heel, chorioptic mange.

AST, aspartate aminotransferase; CPK, creatine phosphokinase.

bulldog calves; acquired atrophic rhinitis of pigs

Joint Defects

- Inherited congenital ankylosis of cattle causing fixation of flexion
- Joint enlargement of rickets and chronic arthritis

SPONTANEOUS FRACTURES

Spontaneous fractures occur uncommonly in farm animals, with the exception of physeal fractures of the metacarpus and metatarsus in young ruminants, and preexisting diseases are usually present in fractures not associated with a traumatic incident, such as the following:

- Nutritional excess of phosphorus causing osteodystrophia in horses
- Nutritional deficiency of calcium causing osteodystrophia in pigs
- Nutritional deficiency of phosphorus or vitamin D in ruminants causing rickets and/or osteomalacia; hypervitaminosis A may contribute
- Nutritional deficiency of copper
- Chronic fluorine intoxication

PAINFUL ASPECTS OF LAMENESS

Musculoskeletal pain can be caused by lacerations and hematomas of muscle, myositis, and space-occupying lesions of muscle. Osteomyelitis, fractures, arthritis, joint dislocations, and sprains of ligaments and tendons are also obvious causes of severe pain. Among the most painful of injuries are swollen, inflammatory lesions of the limbs caused by deep penetrating injury or in cattle by extension from footrot. Amputation of a claw, laminitis, and septic arthritis are in the same category. Ischemia of muscle and generalized muscle tetany, as occurs in electroimmobilization, also appear to cause pain.

Research on the pathophysiology and pharmacology of pain associated with lameness in animals indicates that the thresholds to painful stimuli change in response to pain (wind-up), and this change is seen as an indication of an alteration in nerve function or in nociceptive processing at higher levels. In flocks of sheep with severe lameness as a result of footrot, affected sheep had a lower threshold to a mechanical nociceptive stimulus than matched controls, and their thresholds remained low when tested 3 months later, after the apparent resolution of the foot lesions. Thus hyperalgesia persisted in severely lame sheep for at least 3 months. It is suggested that *N*-methyl-D-aspartate receptors are involved in the development of this long-term hypersensitivity. Similar findings have been reported in dairy heifers affected with claw lesions during the peripartum period.

Relief of Musculoskeletal Pain

Several aspects of relieving pain in agricultural animals are important. Cost has always been a deterrent to the use of local anesthetics and analgesics, but with changing attitudes, the need to control pain is more apparent. Treatment of the causative lesion is a major priority, but the lesion may be painful for varying lengths of time.[2] Relief and the control of pain should be a major consideration. Details on the use of analgesics are presented in Chapter 4.

REFERENCES

1. Shearer JK, et al. *Vet Clin North Am Food A.* 2012;28:535.
2. Shearer JK, et al. *Vet Clin North Am Food A.* 2013;29:135.

EXAMINATION OF THE MUSCULOSKELETAL SYSTEM

The clinical examination of the musculoskeletal system and the feet of farm animals includes the following special examinations.

Analysis of Gait and Conformation

Inspection of the gait of the animal is necessary to localize the site of lameness. Evaluation of its conformation may provide clues about factors that may contribute to lameness. Information related to gait and abnormalities of the nervous system is presented in Chapter 15. Details on the examination of farm animals for lameness are available in textbooks on lameness in horses and cattle. Computer-assisted analysis of gait (kinematics) and hoof loading (via force plates) are commonly used in equine practice and are increasingly being used in research studies related to lameness in cattle and pigs.[1]

Close Physical Examination

A close detailed physical examination of the affected area is necessary to localize the lesion. This includes passive movements of limbs to identify fractures, dislocations, and pain on movement. Muscles can be palpated for evidence of enlargement, pain, or atrophy.

Radiography

Radiography remains an extremely useful diagnostic method for diseases of bones and joints and soft tissue swelling of limbs, which cannot be easily defined by physical examination. Detailed radiographic information about the joint capsule, joint cavity, or articular cartilage can be obtained using negative (air), positive, or double-contrast arthrography.

The widespread availability of digital imaging systems (direct radiography [DR]) now permits radiographs to be immediately examined on-site, rather than following development in the clinic. This ensures that good-quality images are obtained in all views, and the information is used in real time to direct treatment.[2] The price of digital radiography systems continues to decrease but is still significant relative to ultrasonography.

Ultrasonography

Most large animal veterinary practices have an ultrasound machine that is used for transrectal pregnancy diagnosis in cattle and horses and transabdominal pregnancy diagnosis in sheep and goats. Use of these machines with a 5.0- or 7.5-MHz linear transducer provides a rapid on-farm method for evaluating musculoskeletal, tendon, and joint diseases. Ultrasonography is cheaper and provides different information than that provided by radiography; it is also less invasive than joint fluid aspiration and analysis. Detailed information about the use of ultrasonography to diagnose bovine musculoskeletal disorders is available.[3,4] Recent advances in ultrasound technology, including harmonic imaging, compound imaging, three-dimensional (3D) imaging, elastography, and fusion imaging will increase the clinical utility of ultrasonography in ambulatory practice.[5,6]

Ultrasonographic examination of the stifle region in cattle has successfully imaged homogeneously echogenic patellar and collateral ligaments, the combined tendon of the long digital extensor and peroneus tertius muscles, the popliteal tendon, the anechoic articular cartilage of femoral trochlea, the echogenic menisci, and the hyperechoic bone surfaces were imaged successfully. The boundaries of the joint pouches became partially identifiable only when small amounts of anechoic fluid were present in the medial and lateral femorotibial joint pouches. The main indication for ultrasonography of the bovine stifle is evaluation of acute septic and traumatic disorders of the region, when specific radiographic signs are often nonspecific or absent. The cruciate ligaments could not be imaged in live cattle. The cruciate ligaments are identifiable using ultrasonography in the horse, in which flexion of the hindlimb is a routine procedure necessary for identification of these structures.

The main indication for ultrasonographic examination of the carpal region in cattle is the evaluation of septic and traumatic disorders of the carpal joints and tendon sheaths. Each tendon and tendon sheath in the carpal region must be scanned separately. The use of a stand-off pad is recommended because it permits adaptation of the rigid transducer to the contours of the carpus. The carpal joint pouches and tendon sheath lumina are not clearly defined in healthy cattle. Thus the ability to image these structures indicates the presence of synovial effusion. Ultrasonographic imaging can be used to differentiate the pathologic changes in the soft tissue structures of digital flexor tendon sheaths of cattle.

Ultrasonography is a valuable diagnostic aid for septic arthritis. Joint effusion, which is one of the earliest signs of septic arthritis; the accurate location of soft tissue swelling; the extent and character of joint effusion; and involvement of concurrent periarticular synovial cavities or other soft tissue structures can be imaged by ultrasonography. The ultrasonogram can image the presence of small hyperechogenic fragments within the joint, which appear very heterogeneous. Normal synovial fluid is anechoic and appears black on the sonogram. A cloudy appearance is usually associated with the presence of pus.

Ultrasonography has been used to evaluate the anatomy of the elbow, carpal, fetlock, and stifle joints of clinically normal sheep using a 7.5-MHz linear transducer with a stand-off pad. The anatomic structures that could be consistently identified in normal ovine joints included bone, articular cartilage, ligaments, and tendons. In sheep with chronic arthritis/synovitis, the gross thickening of the joint capsule is visible as a hyperechoic band up to 20 mm thick.

Arthrocentesis and Synovial Fluid Interpretation

Joint fluid is collected by needle puncture of the joint cavity (arthrocentesis) and examined for the presence of cells, biochemical changes in the joint fluid, and the presence of infectious agents.

Analysis of synovial fluid is a fundamental requirement for differentiating septic arthritis from degenerative arthritis, and fluid parameters are summarized in Table 15-3 later in this chapter. A number of inflammatory biomarkers in synovial fluid have been evaluated in research studies, but the leukocyte count and differential, erythrocyte count, total protein concentration, and an index of viscosity usually provide sufficient information for clinical use.

Arthrocentesis can result in joint contamination with hair when a 20-g needle is inserted. Angled needle insertion reduces joint contamination relative to perpendicular insertion.[6] Insertion of a spinal needle with the stylet in place also reduces joint contamination with hair, relative to insertion without the stylet. A larger-diameter needle (19 g) had a higher risk of hair contamination after arthrocentesis than a 20-g needle.[7]

Arthroscopy

Special endoscopes are available for inspection of the joint cavity and articular surfaces (arthroscopy). Diagnostic and surgical arthroscopy are now commonplace in specialized equine practice. Surgical arthroscopy is rapidly replacing conventional arthrotomy for the correction of several common surgical conditions of the musculoskeletal system of the horse. Accurate quantification of equine carpal lesions is possible when the procedure is performed by an experienced arthroscopist. Convalescent time following surgery is decreased and the cosmetic appearance improved compared with arthrotomy. A synovial membrane biopsy can be examined histologically and for infectious agents and may yield useful diagnostic information. Surgical arthroscopy is being increasingly used in referral cattle practice.[8]

Serum Biochemistry and Enzymology

When disease of bone or muscle is suspected, the serum concentration of calcium and phosphorus, the serum alkaline phosphatase activity, and the serum activity of two muscle-derived enzymes, creatinine kinase (CK) and aspartate aminotransferase (AST), also known as serum glutamic oxaloacetic transaminase (SGOT), may be useful. Both CK and AST are sensitive indicators of muscle cell damage, with CK also being specific. Equations have been developed that relate the change in serum CK activity to grams of skeletal muscle tissue damaged; this methodology should be widely applied in the clinical management of livestock with musculoskeletal injury because it is sufficiently sensitive to pick up skeletal muscle damage as a result of an intramuscular (IM) antibiotic injection.[9]

Other serum biochemical indicators of muscle damage that have been used in experimental studies include myoglobin, a low-molecular-weight protein that is an early marker of muscle damage, and two indices of muscle damage: myosin, a high-molecular-weight protein, and 3-methylhistidine, a posttranslationally modified amino acid released after myosin or actin degradation.[9] In normally hydrated animals with normal renal function, it is important to understand that serum creatinine concentration provides a useful index of skeletal muscle mass. This is covered in more detail in Chapter 13.

The serum concentrations of calcium and phosphorus and the serum alkaline phosphatase activity are much less sensitive indicators of osteodystrophy.

Muscle Biopsy

A muscle biopsy may be useful for microscopic and histochemical evaluations.

Infrared Thermography

Infrared thermography has been increasingly applied to the diagnosis of inflammatory conditions of muscles and tendons, in that acute inflammation is associated with localized heat that can be detected by using a camera capable of imaging the infrared spectrum.[10,11,12]

Nuclear Scintigraphy

Technetium-labeled bone scanning has been available for decades at major referral institutions, but the use of nuclear scintigraphy has declined with the increased availability and resolution of ultrasonographic and magnetic resonance imaging (MRI) units. Nevertheless, scintigraphy is still a valuable diagnostic method for bone diseases such as osteomyelitis of the vertebral column in adult horses and cattle when the lesion is surrounded by a large mass of superimposing muscle.[13]

Magnetic Resonance Imaging

MRI is increasingly being used for the diagnosis of musculoskeletal disease and related research studies.[14,15] As a cross-sectional imaging modality, it provides outstanding tissue contrast and multiple views of the region of interest. Because of the high cost of purchasing and maintaining MRI equipment, this modality is only available at large referral centers, and even then, specially constructed tables have to be made to permit imaging of adult horses and cattle under general anesthesia. High-quality images can usually be obtained from the carpus and hock to the hoof or foot. It is anticipated that rapid advances will be made in the clinical application of MRI to the diagnosis of specific musculoskeletal injuries, such as evaluating cartilage damage and navicular disease in horses.[14,15]

Computed Tomography

Computed tomography (CT) has not been used much for the clinical analysis of musculoskeletal tissue. It is anticipated that continued advances in MRI technology will continue to make this the preferred anatomic technology, despite the development of CT units in Europe that can accommodate the standing horse.[16]

Nutritional History

Because the most important osteodystrophies and myopathies are nutritional in origin, a complete nutritional history must be obtained. This should include an analysis of the feed and determination of the total amount of intake of each nutrient, including the ratio of one nutrient to another in the diet.

Environment and Housing

When outbreaks of lameness occur in housed cattle, sheep, goats, and pigs, the quality of the floor must be examined to evaluate the possibility of floor-related injuries.

REFERENCES

1. Stavrakakis S, et al. *Livestock Sci.* 2014;165:104.
2. Nelson NC, Zekas LJ. *Vet Clin Equine.* 2012;28:483.
3. Kofler J. *Vet Clin North Am Food A.* 2009;25:687.
4. Kofler J, et al. *Vet Clin North Am Food A.* 2014;30:11.
5. Neelis DA, Roberts GD. *Vet Clin Equine.* 2012;28:497.
6. Wahl K, et al. *Vet Surg.* 2012;41:391.
7. Waxman SJ, et al. *Vet Surg.* 2015;44:373.
8. Lardé H, Nichols S. *Vet Clin North Am Food A.* 2014;30:225.
9. Lefebvre HP, et al. *Vet Res.* 1996;27:343.
10. Stokes JE, et al. *Vet J.* 2012;193:674.
11. Alsaaod M, et al. *Vet J.* 2014;199:281.
12. Alsaaod M, et al. *Sensors (Basel).* 2015;15:14513.
13. Selberg K, Ross M. *Vet Clin Equine.* 2012;28:527.
14. Winter MD. *Vet Clin Equine.* 2012;28:599.
15. Pease A. *Vet Clin Equine.* 2012;28:637.
16. van Weeren PR, Firth EC. *Vet Clin Equine.* 2008;24:153.

Diseases of Muscles

MYASTHENIA (SKELETAL MUSCLE ASTHENIA)

The differential diagnosis of paresis, paralysis, and incoordination should include a consideration of skeletal muscle weakness unrelated to primary neurogenic hypotonia or to permanent muscle injury, including myopathy and myositis. Most of the syndromes that fall into this group of myasthenia have been described in detail elsewhere in this book and are referred to briefly here only to complete the list of abnormalities of skeletal muscle that affect gait and posture. Unlike myopathy and myositis, they are reversible states.

The common causes of myasthenia in farm animals are as follows:

- **Ischemia** in iliac thrombosis in the horse and neonatal calf and after recumbency in cows with parturient paresis. The end stage is myonecrosis and is not reversible.
- **Metabolic effect on muscle fibers**—causes include hypokalemia, hypocalcemia, and possibly hypophosphatemia (in parturient paresis of dairy cows), hypomagnesemia (in lactation tetany), hypoglycemia of newborn pigs, and lactic acidemia after engorgement on grain.
- **Toxins**—general toxemia is a cause. Also, many plant toxins exert an effect on skeletal muscle activity. Although in most cases the mode of the action of the toxin is unknown (hypoglycin A is a notable exception), the toxins have been listed as neurotoxins.

MYOPATHY

The term *myopathy* describes the noninflammatory degeneration of skeletal muscle that is characterized clinically by muscle weakness and pathologically by hyaline degeneration of the muscle fibers. The serum activities of some muscle enzymes are elevated, and myoglobinuria is a common accompaniment.

ETIOLOGY AND EPIDEMIOLOGY

The most important myopathies in farm animals are a result of nutritional deficiencies of vitamin E and selenium and the effects of unaccustomed exercise. In humans, in contrast, the muscular dystrophies occur as inherited defects of muscle or degenerative lesions caused by interruption of their nerve supply. The skeletal myopathies can be classified into primary and secondary myopathies.

A retrospective analysis of the case records in a veterinary teaching hospital over a 9-year period revealed that the most common myopathy in horses was exercise-associated muscle disorder (69%). The remainder consisted of postexhaustion syndrome (9%), infectious myopathies (11%), immunologic myopathy (6%), nutritional myopathy (5%), and hyperkalemic periodic paralysis (2%).

The major causes of myopathy in farm animals and their epidemiologic determinants are as follows.

Enzootic Nutritional Muscular Dystrophy

A nutritional deficiency of vitamin E and/or selenium is a common cause of enzootic nutritional muscular dystrophy in young calves, lambs, foals, and piglets. Factors enhancing or precipitating onset include rapid growth, highly unsaturated fatty acids in the diet, and unaccustomed exercise. The disease also occurs in adult horses.

Exertional or Postexercise Rhabdomyolysis

Exertional or postexercise rhabdomyolysis is not known to be conditioned by vitamin E (selenium) deficiency and occurs as equine paralytic myoglobinuria (tying-up syndrome, azoturia) in horses after unaccustomed exercise or insufficient training. It also occurs in sheep chased by dogs, in cattle after running wildly for several minutes, and as capture myopathy during capture of wildlife.

Equine Atypical Myopathy (Seasonal Pasture Myopathy)

Equine atypical myopathy was originally referred to as *atypical myoglobinuria*, but was renamed to *atypical myopathy* to reflect the underlying pathologic process rather than a possible clinical sign. The first reports were in the United Kingdom, and following a large outbreak in northern Germany in fall 1995, the disease has now been recognized in most of Europe. A similar disease has been reported in the United States and named *seasonal pasture myopathy*. Cases have also been reported from Australia and New Zealand.

Affected horses at pasture have a sudden onset of clinical signs consistent with an acute, non-exercised-related myopathic process. The causative toxin appears to be **hypoglycin A,** which is found in the seeds of maple trees.

Equine Polysaccharide Storage Myopathy

Equine polysaccharide storage myopathy is a metabolic disease being recognized with increasing frequency in many breeds of horse. It occurs in Quarter horses, Appaloosa, and Paint-related breeds. The disease represents a group of diseases with similar clinical signs and pathology but different etiology. Some horses have a mutation in the glycogen synthase 1 (*GYS1*) gene that affects carbohydrate metabolism, including Percheron and Belgian draught horses.

Metabolic

Hyperkalemic periodic paralysis occurs in certain pedigree lines of North American show Quarter horses.

Degenerative Myopathy

Degenerative myopathy occurs in newborn calves, sheep, and goats infected by Akabane virus in utero.

Inherited Myopathies

Porcine stress syndrome, which is discussed under that heading, now includes pale, soft, exudative pork encountered at slaughter and malignant hyperthermia following halothane anesthesia. Certain blood types in pigs have been used as predictors of stress susceptibility, and malignant hyperthermia in Pietrain pigs is genetically predetermined. Most of these myopathies of pigs thus have an inherited basis, and the stress of transportation, overcrowding, and handling at slaughter precipitates the lesion and rapid death.

Congenital myopathy of Braunvieh–Brown Swiss calves is thought to be inherited. Affected calves become progressively weak and recumbent within 2 weeks of birth.

Doubling-muscling in cattle and **splaylegs of newborn pigs** are also considered to be inherited. A **dystrophy-like myopathy** in a foal has been described and is similar to human muscular dystrophy. **Dystrophy of the diaphragmatic muscles** in adult Meuse–Rhine–Yessel cattle is thought to be inherited. **Xanthosis** occurs in the skeletal and cardiac muscles of cattle and is characterized grossly by a green iridescence.

Toxic Agents

Certain myopathies are caused by poisonous plants, including *Cassia occidentalis, Karwinskia humboldtiana, Ixioloena* spp., *Geigeria* spp., and lupins. A special case is enzootic calcinosis of all tissues, especially muscle, and the principal signs are muscular. It is caused by poisoning by *Solanum malacoxylon, Tricetum* spp., and *Cestrum* spp. Another special case is equine atypical myopathy.

Ischemia

Ischemic myonecrosis occurs in the thigh muscles of cattle recumbent for approximately 48 hours or more and is discussed in detail under the heading "Downer Cow Syndrome." Iliac thrombosis in horses is an important cause of ischemic myopathy and has been reported in neonatal calves.

Neurogenic

Neurogenic muscular atrophy occurs sporadically as a result of traumatic injury and subsequent degeneration or complete severance of the nerve supply to skeletal muscle. The myopathy in arthrogryposis associated with the Akabane virus is thought to be a result of lesions of the lower motor neurons supplying the affected muscles. It has been suggested that cattle with muscular hypertrophy may be more susceptible to the effects of exercise and the occurrence of acute muscular dystrophy. Suprascapular nerve paralysis in the horse (sweeney) is a traumatic neuropathy resulting from compression of the nerve against the cranial edge of the scapula.

Neoplasms

Neoplasms of striated muscle are uncommon in animals. Rhabdomyosarcomas are reported in the horse, affecting the diaphragm and causing loss of body weight, anorexia, and respiratory distress.

PATHOGENESIS

Primary Myopathy

The characteristic change in most cases of primary myopathy varies from hyaline degeneration to coagulative necrosis, affecting particularly the heavy thigh muscles and the muscles of the diaphragm. Myocardial lesions are also commonly associated with the degeneration of skeletal muscle and when severe will cause rapid death within a few hours or days. The visible effects of the lesions are varying degrees of muscle weakness, muscle pain, recumbency, stiff gait, inability to move the limbs, and the development of respiratory and circulatory insufficiency.

In primary nutritional muscular dystrophy associated with a deficiency of vitamin E and/or selenium there is lipoperoxidation of the cellular membranes of muscle fibers, resulting in degeneration and necrosis. The lesion is present only in muscle fibers, and the histologic and biochemical changes that occur in the muscle are remarkably similar irrespective of the cause. Variations in the histologic lesion occur but indicate variation in the severity and rapidity of onset of the change rather than different causes.

Myoglobinuria

Because of the necrosis of muscle, myoglobin is excreted in the urine, and **myoglobinuric nephrosis** is an important complication, particularly of acute primary myopathy. The degree of myoglobinuria depends on the severity of the lesion, with acute cases resulting in marked myoglobinuria, and on the age and species of animal affected. Adult horses with myopathy may liberate large quantities of myoglobin, resulting in dark-brown urine. Yearling cattle with myopathy release moderate amounts, and the urine may or may not be colored; calves with severe enzootic nutritional muscular dystrophy may have grossly normal urine. In all species the renal threshold of myoglobin is so low that discoloration of the serum does not occur.

Muscle Enzymes

An important biochemical manifestation of myopathy is the increased release of muscle cell enzymes that occurs during muscle cell destruction. Creatine kinase (CK) and serum glutamic oxaloacetate transaminase are both elevated in myopathy; CK, particularly, is a more specific and reliable indication of acute muscle damage. Increased amounts of creatinine are also released into the urine following myopathy.

Exertional Rhabdomyolysis

In exertional rhabdomyolysis in horses there is enhanced glycolysis with depletion of muscle glycogen, the accumulation of large amounts of lactate in muscle and blood, and the development of hyaline degeneration of myofibers. Affected muscle fibers are richer in glycogen in the acute stage of "tying-up" than in the late stages, suggesting increased glycogen storage in the early phase of the disease compared with normal healthy horses. During enforced exercise there is local muscle hypoxia and anaerobic oxidation, resulting in the accumulation of lactate and myofibrillar degeneration. The pathogenesis of postanesthetic myositis in horses is uncertain. A significant postischemic hyperemia occurs in horses that develop postanesthetic myopathy. Postanesthetic recumbency can occur in the horse with polysaccharide storage myopathy.

Types of Muscle Fiber Affected

In most animals, skeletal muscle is composed of a mixture of fibers with different contractile and metabolic characteristics. Fibers with slow contraction times have been called slow-twitch or type I fibers, and those with fast contraction time are fast-twitch or type II fibers. Histochemically, type I and II fibers can be differentiated by staining for myofibrillar ATPase. Type II fibers can be subgrouped into type IIA and IIB on the basis of acid preincubations. Several different characteristics of these muscle fibers have been studied in the horse. There are variations in the percentage of each type of fiber present and in composition of muscle fibers dependent on genetic background, age, and stage of training. There are also variations in the muscle fibers within one muscle and between different muscles. The histochemical characteristics of equine muscle fibers have been examined:

- Type I fibers are characterized by strong aerobic capacity, compared with type IIA.
- Type IIA fibers are more glycolytic and have strong aerobic and moderate to strong anaerobic capacities.
- Type IIB fibers are characterized by a relatively low aerobic and a relatively high anaerobic capacity and are glycolytic.

The histochemical staining characteristics of normal equine skeletal muscle have been examined and serve as a standard for comparison with data obtained from skeletal muscles with lesions.

Secondary Myopathy Resulting From Ischemia

In secondary myopathy resulting from ischemia there may be multiple focal areas of necrosis, which causes muscle weakness and results in an increase of muscle enzymes in the serum. The degree of regeneration with myofibers depends on the severity of the lesion. Some regeneration occurs, but there is considerable tissue replacement. In aortic and iliac thrombosis in calves under 6 months of age the thrombosis results in acute to chronic segmental necrosis of some skeletal muscles and coagulation necrosis in others.

Neurogenic Atrophy of Muscle

In neurogenic atrophy there is flaccid paralysis, a marked decrease in total muscle mass, and degeneration of myofibers, with failure to regenerate unless the nerve supply is at least partially restored.

CLINICAL FINDINGS

The nutritional myopathies associated with a deficiency of vitamin E and/or selenium occur most commonly in young, rapidly growing animals and may occur in outbreak form, particularly in calves and lambs. The details are presented under the heading "Vitamin E and Selenium Deficiency."

Primary Myopathy

In general terms, in acute primary myopathy there is a sudden onset of weakness and pseudoparalysis of the affected muscles, causing paresis and recumbency and, in many cases, accompanying respiratory and circulatory insufficiency. The affected animals will usually remain bright and alert but may appear to be in pain. The temperature is usually normal but may be slightly elevated in severe cases of primary myopathy. Cardiac irregularity and tachycardia may be evident, and myoglobinuria occurs in adult horses and yearling cattle. The affected skeletal muscles in acute cases may feel swollen, hard, and rubbery, but in most cases it is difficult to detect significant abnormality by palpation. Animals with acute cases of primary myopathy may die within 24 hours after the onset of signs.

Acute Nutritional Myopathy

Although acute nutritional myopathy in horses occurs most commonly in foals from birth to 7 months of age, acute dystrophic myodegeneration also occurs in adult horses. There is muscle stiffness and pain, myoglobinuria, edema of the head and neck, recumbency, and death in a few days. A special occurrence of myopathy has been recorded in suckling Thoroughbred foals up to 5 months of age. The disease occurs in the spring and summer in foals running at pasture with their dams and is unassociated with excessive exercise. In peracute cases there is a sudden onset of dejection, stiffness, disinclination to move, and prostration, with death occurring 3 to 7 days later. Lethargy and stiffness of gait are characteristic of less acute cases. There is also a pronounced swelling and firmness of the subcutaneous tissue at the base of the mane and over the gluteal muscles. There may be excessive salivation, desquamation of lingual epithelium, and board-like firmness of the masseter muscles. The foals are unable to suck because of inability to bend their necks. Spontaneous recovery occurs in mild cases, but most severely affected foals die.

Severe nutritional myopathy of the masseter muscles in a 6-year-old Quarter horse stallion has been reported. The masseter muscles were swollen and painful, and there was exophthalmos and severe chemosis with protrusion of the third eyelids. The mouth could be opened only slightly, and masticatory efforts were weak. Serum enzymology supported a diagnosis of nutritional muscular dystrophy, and the concentrations of vitamin E and selenium in the blood and feed were lower than normal.

Tying-Up

In tying-up in horses there is a very sudden onset of muscle soreness 10 to 20 minutes following exercise. There is profuse sweating and the degree of soreness varies from mild, in which the horse moves with a short, shuffling gait, to acute, in which there is a great disinclination to move at all. In severe cases, horses are unable to move their hindlegs, and swelling and rigidity of the croup muscles develops. Myoglobinuria is common.

Postanesthetic Myositis

Horses with postanesthetic myositis experience considerable difficulty during recovery from anesthesia. Recovery is prolonged, and when initial attempts are made to stand, there is lumbar rigidity, pain, and reluctance to bear weight. Some affected horses will be able to stand within several hours if supported in a sling. The limbs may be rigid and the muscles firm on palpation. In severe cases the temperature begins to rise—reminiscent of malignant hyperthermia. Other clinical findings include anxiety, tachycardia, profuse sweating, myoglobinuria, and tachypnea. Death may occur in 6 to 12 hours. Euthanasia is the only course for some horses. In the milder form of the syndrome, affected horses are able to stand but are stiff and in severe pain for a few days.

Exertional Rhabdomyolysis

In horses, the clinical findings are **variable** and range from poor performance to recumbency and death. Signs may be mild and resolve spontaneously within 24 hours or severe and progressive.

The **usual presentation** is a young (2- to 5-year-old) female racehorse with recurrent episodes of stiff gait after exercise. The horse does not perform to expectation and displays a **short-stepping gait** that may be mistaken for lower leg lameness. The horse may be reluctant to move when placed in its stall, be apprehensive and anorexic, and frequently shift its weight. More severely affected horses may be unable to continue to exercise, have **hard and painful muscles** (usually gluteal muscles), sweat excessively, be apprehensive, refuse to walk, and be tachycardic and tachypneic. Affected horses may be hyperthermic. Signs consistent with abdominal pain are present in many severely affected horses. Deep-red urine (myoglobinuria) occurs but is not a consistent finding. Severely affected horses may be recumbent and unable to rise.

Many different manifestations of equine polysaccharide storage myopathy occur. All manifestations are related to dysfunction, which results in pain, weakness, segmental fiber necrosis, stiffness, spasm, atrophy, or any combination of these. The muscles most severely affected are the powerful rump, thigh, and back muscles, including the gluteals, semimembranosus, semitendinosus, and longissimus.

In exertional rhabdomyolysis in sheep chased by dogs, affected animals are recumbent, cannot stand, and appear exhausted, and myoglobinuria is common. Death usually follows. A similar clinical picture occurs in cattle that have run wildly for several minutes.

Hyperkalemic Periodic Paralysis

Initially there is a brief period of myotonia with prolapse of the third eyelid. In severe cases, the horse becomes recumbent and the myotonia is replaced by flaccidity. Sweating occurs, and generalized muscle fasciculations are apparent, with large groups of muscle fibers contracting simultaneously at random. The animal remains bright and alert and responds to noise and painful stimuli. In milder cases, affected horses remain standing, and generalized muscle fasciculations are prominent over the neck, shoulder, and flank. There is a tendency to stand base-wide. When the horse is asked to move, the limbs may buckle, and the animal appears weak. The horse is unable to lift its head, usually will not eat, and may yawn repeatedly early in the course of an episode. The serum potassium levels are elevated above normal during the episodes.

Secondary Myopathy Resulting From Ischemia

In secondary myopathy resulting from ischemia (e.g., downer cow syndrome), the affected animal is unable to rise, and the affected hindlegs are commonly directed behind the cow in the frogleg attitude. The appetite and mental attitude are usually normal. No abnormality of the muscles can be palpated. With supportive therapy, good bedding, and the prevention of further ischemia by frequent rolling of the animal, most cows will recover in a few days.

In calves with aortic and iliac artery thrombosis there is an acute onset of paresis or flaccid paralysis of one or both pelvic limbs. Affected limbs are hypothermic and have diminished spinal reflexes and arterial pulse pressures. The diagnosis can be defined using angiography. Affected calves die or are euthanized because treatment is not undertaken.

Neurogenic Atrophy

With neurogenic atrophy there is marked loss of total mass of muscle, flaccid paralysis, loss of tendon reflexes, and failure of regeneration. When large muscle masses are affected (e.g., quadriceps femoris in femoral nerve paralysis in calves at birth), the animal is unable to bear normal weight on the affected leg.

Dystrophy of the Diaphragmatic Muscles

In dystrophy of the diaphragmatic muscles in adult Meuse–Rhine–Yessel cattle there is loss of appetite, decreased rumination, decreased eructation, and recurrent bloat. The respiratory rate is increased, with forced abdominal respirations, forced movement of the nostrils, and death from asphyxia in a few weeks.

Severe diaphragmatic necrosis in a horse with degenerative myopathy as a result of polysaccharide storage myopathy has been described. Affected horses may have severe respiratory distress and respiratory acidosis, and they do not respond to supportive therapy.

DIAGNOSIS

Muscle-Derived Serum Enzymes

The serum activity of the muscle enzymes is characteristically elevated following myopathy as a result of release of the enzymes from altered muscle cell membranes. CK is a highly specific indicator of both myocardial and skeletal muscle degeneration. Plasma CK activity is related to three factors: the amount and rate of CK released from an injured muscle into plasma, its volume of distribution, and its rate of elimination. CK has a half-life of about 4 to 6 hours; following an initial episode of acute myopathy, serum activity of the enzyme may return to normal within 3 to 4 days if no further muscle degeneration has occurred. Levels of AST are also increased following myopathy; however, because the enzyme is present in other tissues, such as the liver, it is not a reliable indicator of primary muscle tissue degeneration.

Because AST has a longer half-life than CK, the levels of AST may remain elevated for several days following acute myopathy. The daily monitoring of both CK and AST levels should provide an indication of whether active muscle degeneration is occurring. A marked drop in serum CK activity and a slow decline in serum AST activity suggest that no further degeneration is occurring, whereas a constant elevation of CK suggests active degeneration.

In acute nutritional muscular dystrophy in calves, lambs, and foals the serum CK activity will increase from normal values of below 100 IU/L to levels ranging from 1,000 to 5,000 IU/L and even higher. The levels of CK in calves will increase from a normal of 50 IU/L to approximately 5,000 IU/L within a few days after being placed outdoors followed by unconditioned exercise. The amount of skeletal muscle damaged can be estimated based on the change in the amount of CK activity over time (specifically, the area under the serum CK activity–time relationship) and species-specific pharmacokinetic values related to CK clearance.[1]

The measurement of serum activity of glutathione peroxidase is a useful aid in the diagnosis of myopathy as a result of selenium deficiency.

In downer cows with ischemic necrosis of the thigh muscles, the serum CK and AST activities will be markedly elevated and will remain elevated if muscle necrosis is progressive in cows that are not well bedded and rolled from side to side several times daily to minimize the degree and extent of ischemic necrosis.

High serum activities of CK (1000 IU/L and greater) usually indicate acute primary myopathy. Levels from 500 to 1000 IU/L may be difficult to interpret in animals recumbent for reasons other than primary myopathy. This will necessitate a careful reassessment of the clinical findings, history, and epidemiology.

In horses with acute exertional rhabdomyolysis (paralytic myoglobinuria) the serum CK activity will range from 5000 to 10,000 IU/L. Following vigorous exercise in unconditioned horses, the serum CK and AST activity will rise as a result of increased cell membrane permeability associated with the hypoxia of muscles subjected to excessive exercise. Lactate dehydrogenase (LDH) activity has also been used as a biochemical measurement of the degree of physical work done by horses in training. With progressive training in previously unconditioned horses there is no significant change between rest and exercise in the serum CK, AST, and LDH activities. In horses with postanesthetic myositis the serum CK activity may exceed 100,000 IU/L, the serum calcium is decreased, and the serum inorganic phosphorus is increased. In naturally occurring cases of exertional rhabdomyolysis in horses the most consistent acid–base abnormality may be hypochloremia rather than metabolic acidosis as has been assumed.

Muscle Biopsy

Investigation of the structural and biochemical alterations of muscle tissue in myopathy include biopsy techniques. Needle biopsies require specialized Bergstrom muscle biopsy needles, which are expensive, and most practitioners do not have them on hand. Open biopsy is recommended to obtain a strip of muscle. Biopsy of either the semimembranosus or semitendinosus muscles, at a site between the base of the tail and the tuber ischium, provides an adequate sample. Muscle biopsy samples can be processed for either frozen section or routine formalin-fixed, paraffin-embedded sections. The frozen section is considered the gold standard.

Inclusions of periodic acid–Schiff (PAS)-positive, amylase-resistant complex polysaccharide are abnormal and characteristic findings in muscle of equine polysaccharide storage myopathy.

Histochemical techniques can be used on muscle biopsies of horses with muscular disease and animals with congenital and inherited myopathies.

Myoglobinuria

Myoglobinuria is a common finding in adult horses with acute paralytic myoglobinuria but is not a common finding in acute nutritional muscular dystrophy in young farm animals, except perhaps in yearling cattle with acute muscular dystrophy. The myoglobinuria may be clinically detectable as a red-brown or chocolate-brown discoloration of the urine. This discoloration can be differentiated from that caused by hemoglobin by spectrographic examination or with the use of orthotoluidine paper strips. Urine becomes dark when myoglobin levels exceed 40 mg/dL of urine. Discoloration of the plasma suggests hemoglobinuria. Both myoglobin and hemoglobin give positive results for the presence of protein in urine. Porphyria causes a similar discoloration, although this may not be evident until the urine has been exposed to light for some minutes. The coloration is lighter, pink to red rather than brown, and the urine is negative to the guaiac test and fluoresces with ultraviolet light. Creatinuria accompanies acute myopathy but has not been used routinely as a diagnostic aid.

Electromyography is a special technique for the evaluation of the degree of neurogenic atrophy.

NECROPSY FINDINGS

Affected areas of skeletal muscle have a white, waxy, swollen appearance like fish flesh. Commonly only linear strips of large muscle masses are affected, and the distribution of lesions is characteristically bilaterally symmetric. Histologically, the lesion varies from a hyaline degeneration to a severe myonecrosis, with subsequently the disappearance of large groups of muscle fibers and replacement by connective tissue. Calcification of the affected tissue may be present to a mild degree in these cases.

The lesions in exertional rhabdomyolysis in the horse are of a focal distribution and consist of hyaline degeneration with insignificant inflammatory reaction and slight calcification. The degenerative changes affect primarily the fast-twitch fibers, which have a low oxidative capacity and are used when the horse runs at very close to its maximum speed.

DIFFERENTIAL DIAGNOSIS

Most myopathies in farm animals occur in rapidly growing, young animals and are characterized clinically by a sudden onset of acute muscular weakness and pain, often precipitated by unaccustomed exercise. There may be evidence of a dietary deficiency of vitamin and selenium in the case of nutritional muscular dystrophy. A sudden onset of recumbency or stiffness in young farm animals that are bright and alert should arouse suspicion of acute muscular dystrophy. Primary myopathies are not common in adult cattle, sheep, or pigs, but myopathy secondary to recumbency for other reasons does occur.

Secondary myopathy as a result of aortic and iliac thrombosis in calves must be differentiated from other common causes of hindlimb paresis, including traumatic injury to the spinal cord, spinal cord compression as a result of vertebral body abscess, nutritional muscular dystrophy, myositis and nerve damage as a result of trauma of intramuscular injections, and clostridial myositis.

The exertional myopathies in the horse in training are usually readily obvious. Creatine kinase (CK) is a valuable aid to diagnosis. In special circumstances, such as neurogenic myopathy, muscle biopsy and electromyography may be useful additional diagnostic aids. The histologic and histochemical staining characteristics of equine muscle have been described and serve as a standard for comparison with abnormal muscle.

Myositis may present a similar syndrome but is usually present as a secondary lesion in a clinically distinguishable primary disease or is accompanied by obvious trauma or toxemia.

TREATMENT

Vitamin E and selenium are indicated for the treatment of nutritional muscular dystrophy, and the details are provided under that heading. The treatment of exertional rhabdomyolysis in horses has not been well defined because of the uncertain etiology, but enforced rest and the relief of pain, if necessary, seem logical. Supportive therapy for any case of myopathy, particularly severe cases in which there is persistent recumbency, consists of the following:

- Liberal quantities of thick bedding, such as at least 6″ (15 cm) of straw hay
- Removal from solid floors to softer ground
- Frequent turning from side to side to minimize secondary myopathy
- Provision of fluid therapy to prevent myoglobinuric nephrosis
- A palatable, nutritious diet

With the exception of the sporadically occurring congenital and inherited myopathies of farm animals, all the nutritional and exertional myopathies are amenable to treatment if it is begun early and if adequate supportive therapy is provided.

In myopathies associated with systemic acidosis, the use of a solution of sodium bicarbonate may be indicated. Dietary sodium bicarbonate at the rate of 2% of total dry matter intake has been used for the treatment of exertional rhabdomyolysis in a horse. Horses with postanesthetic myositis must be considered as critical care patients for 18 to 24 hours. Maintenance of adequate renal perfusion is vital. Large quantities of intravenous polyionic balanced electrolyte fluids (50 to 100 L) must be given over a 24-hour period. Dantrolene sodium at 4 mg/kg body weight (BW) given orally immediately upon recognition of clinical signs is efficacious.

CONTROL

The nutritional myopathies in farm animals can be satisfactorily prevented by the provision of adequate quantities of dietary vitamin E and selenium in the maternal diet during pregnancy or at the strategic times in postnatal life. The prevention of exertional myopathy in the horse depends on a progressive training program and avoidance of sudden unaccustomed exercise in animals that are in good body condition and have been inactive. Similarly, in general terms, the prevention of porcine stress syndrome will depend on careful handling and transportation techniques combined with genetic selection of resistant pigs.

FURTHER READING

Naylor RJ. Polysaccharide storage myopathy—the story so far. *Equine Vet Educ*. 2015;27:414-419.

Valberg SJ, McCue ME, Mickelson JR. The interplay of genetics, exercise, and nutrition in polysaccharide storage myopathy. *J Equine Vet Sci*. 2011;31:205-210.

Votion DM. The story of equine atypical myopathy: a review from the beginning to a possible end. *ISRN Vet Sci*. 2012;article ID 281018.

REFERENCE

1. Lefebvre HP, et al. *Vet Res*. 1996;27:343.

MYOPATHY OF HORSES

Diseases of the muscles of horses include conditions that induce rhabdomyolysis (literally, dissolution or liquefaction of muscle) and, less commonly, conditions in which function of the muscle is impaired but there is not rhabdomyolysis. Rhabdomyolysis is characterized biochemically by marked increases in the activity in serum of muscle-derived enzymes, such as creatine kinase (CK) and aspartate aminotransferase (AST). The diagnosis of rhabdomyolysis presents no great challenge, but determining the underlying disease condition usually requires a more sophisticated approach than just measuring CK and AST activity in serum.

ETIOLOGY

Horses are affected by a number of diseases of muscle (Table 15-2), and diagnosis of the particular disease based solely on clinical signs might not be possible because of the limited range of manifestations of muscle disease. A useful differentiator is whether development of clinical signs is associated only with exercise or also occurs at rest. Classical exercise-induced rhabdomyolysis presents as signs of muscle disease during or soon after the completion of exercise, whereas signs of some inherited defects or intoxications are evident without the stimulus of exercise. Other muscle diseases can be apparent at rest and are exacerbated by exercise.

Myopathies of equids can be grouped according to their etiopathogenesis:

- **Genetic anomalies**—polysaccharide storage myopathy (type I), malignant hyperthermia, glycogen branching enzyme deficiency, hyperkalemic periodic paralysis, recurrent exertional rhabdomyolysis of Thoroughbreds (suspect), mitochondrial myopathy (specific genetic anomaly not identified), and myotonia in foals. More will be discovered with advent of access to the equine genome and ready access to advanced molecular technologies
- **Environmental or management**—unaccustomed exercise, heat stress or stroke, inconsistent exercise
- **Nutritional**—vitamin E/selenium deficiency (white-muscle disease, masseter myonecrosis), diet high in nonstructural (soluble) carbohydrates
- **Intoxications**—ingestion of hypoglycin A in *Acer negundo* or *Acer pseudoplantanus* seeds, inophores (monensin, salinomycin), tremetone (white snake root, rayless goldenrod [*Isocoma pluriflor*]), or *Cassia occidentalis,* or snake bite (*Notechis scutatus* and likely other elapid and crotalid snakes)
- **Infectious**—localized infections (clostridial myositis), *Streptococcus equi* myositis, *Salmonella* spp. myositis, associated with *Anaplasma phagocytophila* infection
- **Inflammatory or infarctive**—as part of purpura hemorrhagica (infarctive) or immune myositis (inflammatory)
- **Metabolic**—sarcopenia with pituitary pars intermedia dysfunction
- **Unknown**—sporadic exercise-induced rhabdomyolysis, recurrent exercise-induced rhabdomyolysis, polysaccharide storage myopathy type II

PATHOGENESIS

Exercise-induced rhabdomyolysis occurs because of abnormal responses of the muscle to contractions during exercise. Although the exact pathogenesis of exercise-induced muscle damage has not been demonstrated in horses, it likely involves accumulation of normal metabolites to excessive levels in all or part of the cell, formation of abnormal metabolites, or inadequate provision of energy to maintain homeostasis of myocytes during sustained or repetitive contractions. The critical common event is likely accumulation of calcium in the cytosol as a consequence of damage to the sarcolemma and sarcoplasmic reticulum and impaired function of calcium channels and pumps. Reduction of the cytosolic calcium concentration is achieved by the sarcoplasmic reticulum calcium-ATPase pump and calcium transport across the sarcolemma by the Na^+/K^+ pump and the Ca^+/Na^+ exchanger. Abnormal cytosolic calcium concentrations result in activation of intracellular proteases and other enzymes, leading to damage to cell constituents, including the cell membrane, with subsequent leakage of cell contents into interstitial fluid and blood. This is evident clinically as increases in activity in blood (serum, plasma) of muscle-derived enzymes (CK, AST, lactate dehydrogenase [LDH]) and concentration of myoglobin in blood and urine.

DIAGNOSIS

Diagnosis of muscle diseases of horses is made using combinations of history and clinical signs, hematologic or biochemical examination of blood or urine, electromyography, exercise challenge tests, muscle biopsy, and genetic testing.

Clinical signs common to most muscle disease are varying degrees of exercise intolerance, gait abnormalities characterized by short strides or a stilted gait, pain on palpation of affected muscles, muscle fasciculation, myoglobinuria, and muscle atrophy. Not all signs are present in every disease of muscle, and horses can be clinically normal between episodes. Clinical signs of particular diseases are discussed under those topics elsewhere in this text.

There are no changes in routine hematology that are characteristic of all diseases of muscle or are discriminatory among muscle diseases. Most muscle diseases are associated with elevations in serum activity of **muscle-derived enzymes** (CK, AST, LDH). The most commonly measured enzymes are CK and AST. Serum concentrations of CK increase within minutes to hours of injury to the muscle and decline to baseline concentrations within 1 to 2 days of muscle cell membranes regaining their integrity. CK has an elimination half-life of approximately 2 hours in the plasma of horses, which accounts for the rapid reduction in activity in serum. Conversely, AST has a longer elimination half-life, and activity both increases and declines more slowly than that of CK. Horses with injury to muscle that resolved several days previously can therefore have normal activity of CK and elevated activity of AST in serum.

Plasma concentrations of **vitamin E and selenium**, or red cell glutathione peroxidase activity, are usually within the reference interval for healthy animals, with the exception of foals with white-muscle disease and adults with masseter myonecrosis.

Urinalysis of samples collected during the active phase of the disease can contain myoglobin. **Myoglobinuria** should be distinguished from hematuria (by centrifugation of the sample) or hemoglobinuria (by measurement of hemoglobin or myoglobin concentrations). Myoglobinuria kidney injury can cause the presence of granular casts in urine sediment. Urine and serum collected when the horse does not have clinical signs of muscle disease have been proposed to be useful in detecting abnormalities in body content of sodium, potassium, chloride, calcium, and phosphate. Calculation of **fractional excretion of electrolytes** have limited, if any, utility in the diagnosis of causes of exertional rhabdomyolysis.

Muscle biopsy is useful in providing a histologic diagnosis and is diagnostic in a number of diseases of muscle of horses. For muscle biopsy to be useful, the disease being considered must affect the muscle biopsied, the sample should be collected and transported to the laboratory in way that ensures that it is diagnostic, and the sample should be processed and examined in a laboratory accustomed to handling muscle biopsies. Open biopsies, as opposed to collection using a Bergstrom needle, are preferred for clinical samples.

Genetic testing is available for several diseases, and more tests will become available with advances in the field. Demonstration of mutations documented to cause muscle disease in a horse with compatible clinical signs can be considered diagnostic of the disease.

Additional testing can include imaging (ultrasonographic examination, scintigraphy), exercise testing, electromyography, analysis of targeted compounds in body fluids (e.g., methylenecyclopropyl acetic acid in horses with suspect hypoglycin A intoxication), and necropsy.

A rational diagnostic approach combining clinical signs, historical information, genetic testing, and muscle biopsy has been described (Fig. 15-1).[1]

TREATMENT

Treatment should be directed at the underlying disease, and specifics are provided under each disease topic.

Table 15-2 Common or well-characterized myopathies of equids*

Disease	Etiology	Risk factors	Clinical signs	Diagnosis	Treatment	Control
Exertional myopathy						
Sporadic exertional rhabdomyolysis	Unknown.	Unaccustomed exercise, heat stress or stroke, electrolyte imbalances.	Signs of acute rhabdomyolysis (see text).	Elevated serum activity of muscle-derived enzymes.	Supportive. Pain relief. Ensure adequate hydration.	Avoid known risk factors.
Recurrent exertional rhabdomyolysis (RER)	Idiopathic, presumed inherited in Thoroughbreds and Standardbreds.	Breed and diet in some instances.	Recurrent episodes of acute rhabdomyolysis.	Elevated serum activity of muscle-derived enzymes. Genetic testing. Muscle biopsy.	Supportive during acute episodes.	High-fat diet—for RER in Thoroughbreds and other light horse breeds. Dietary modification for PSSM (see following entry). Regular and consistent exercise. Turn out to pasture. Dantrolene (1–3 mg/kg PO q24h).
Polysaccharide storage myopathy type I (PSSM1)	Mutation in glycogen synthase gene (GYS1) leading to higher activity of glycogen synthase in muscle.	Quarter horse and related breeds, draft breeds (Belgians and Percherons), particularly in Europe, and Warmbloods. Many breeds affected. Intermittent exercise.	Exertional rhabdomyolysis (clinical or subclinical). Stiff gait, myalgia, and exercise intolerance. Some horses with histologic lesions are clinically normal. Homozygotes more severely affected than heterozygotes.	Genetic testing. Muscle biopsy.	Supportive.	Dietary control. High-fat, high-fiber diet with low content of soluble nonstructural carbohydrates. Regular, consistent exercise.
Polysaccharide storage myopathy type II (PSSM2)	No demonstrated abnormality in GSY1 gene or glycogen synthase activity. Unknown cause.	Disease documented in many breeds.	Exertional rhabdomyolysis (clinical or subclinical). Stiff gait, myalgia and exercise intolerance. Some horses with histologic lesions are clinically normal.	Examination of muscle biopsy. Rule out PSSM1 by genetic testing.	Supportive.	Dietary control. High fat, high fiber diet with low content of soluble nonstructural carbohydrates. Regular, consistent exercise.
Muscle sprains	Associated with exercise.	Exercise.	Localized muscle pain, stiff gait, ultrasonographic or scintigraphic abnormalities.	Clinical signs, response to treatment, results of imaging. Muscle-derived enzymes minimally elevated.	Rest. Nonsteroidal antiinflammatory drugs.	Prudent exercise and training schedules.
Mitochondrial myopathy	Deficiency of Complex I enzymes in respiratory chain of mitochondria. Other causes likely to be identified.	Exercise. Arabian breed.	*No rhabdomyolysis.* Severe exercise intolerance with signs of discomfort (sweating, short-strided gait).	Muscle-derived enzymes in serum not elevated. Accumulation of lactate out of proportion to exercise intensity or duration. Electron microscopy of muscle tissue.	Rest.	None. Consider wisdom of breeding affected horses.
Nonexertional myopathy						
Glycogen-branching enzyme deficiency	Fatal autosomal recessive mutation of glycogen branching enzyme (GBE1).	Foals of Quarter horse and related breeds.	Abortion and stillbirth. Neonates are hypoglycemic, weak, recumbent; die soon after birth.	Hypoglycemia. Minimal elevations in muscle derived enzymes. Accumulation of abnormal polysaccharide in muscle.	None.	Breeding programs.

Continued

Table 15-2 Common or well-characterized myopathies of equids*—cont'd

Disease	Etiology	Risk factors	Clinical signs	Diagnosis	Treatment	Control
Malignant hyperthermia	Heterozygous, nonsynonymous polymorphism attributable to mutation in RyR1 gene (ryanodine receptor 1).	Quarter horse breed. Anesthesia.	Clinically normal until anesthetized, then hyperthermia, tachycardia, arrhythmias, rhabdomyolysis, and death.	Clinical signs. Elevated serum creatine kinase activity (but not in peracute cases). Detection of mutation by genetic analysis.	Supportive.	Detection of genetic abnormality before anesthesia.
Hyperkalemic periodic paralysis	Autosomal-dominant trait attributable to missense mutation in sodium channel gene (SCN4A).	Quarter horse or related breed. Familial and congenital.	Asymptomatic through episodic disease with occasional death. Muscle fasciculation and tremor. Episodic collapse with myotonia, prolapse of third eyelid, sweating, recumbency.	Measurement of serum potassium concentration (elevated) during episode. Genetic analysis.	Measure to reduce serum potassium concentration (dextrose, fluids, insulin).	Acetazolamide. Low-potassium diet. Prudent breeding program.
Myotonia	Hereditary. Genetic basis has not been identified.	Quarter horse, Thoroughbred, Anglo-Arabian foals.	Disease evident in foals. Generalized muscle stiffness. Dimpling of muscle on pressure (percussion). Weakness.	Classic electromyography of myotonic discharges (dive bomber).	None.	Prudent breeding programs.
Purpura hemorrhagica myopathy	Purpura hemorrhagica. Infarction of muscles.	As for purpura hemorrhagica.	Usually 2–4 weeks after respiratory infection. Acute-onset muscle pain, swelling, abnormal gait, plus signs of purpura hemorrhagica. High case-fatality rate.	Clinical signs. Increased serum activity of muscle-derived enzymes. Muscle biopsy.	Treatment of purpura hemorrhagica. Supportive. Pain relief.	Prevention of respiratory disease.
Immune myositis	Idiopathic.	More common in Quarter horses, but can affect any breed.	Severe muscle atrophy. No rhabdomyolysis at time of detection of atrophy.	Muscle biopsy—histiocytic lymphocytic myositis.	Administration of corticosteroids. Expect full recovery with or without treatment.	None.
Streptococcal myositis	Infection by *Streptococcus equi.*	Risk factors for infection by *S. equi.*	Acute- to peracute-onset myalgia, stiff gait, swelling and pitting edema of epaxial muscles.	Demonstration of muscle disease and rhabdomyolysis with *S. equi* infection.	Aggressive support care, antibiotic administration, NSAIDs.	Prevention of infection by *S. equi.*
Clostridia myositis	Infection by *Clostridium septicum* or other clostridia.	Trauma, intramuscular injections.	Acute-onset fever, tachycardia, localized pain over previous injection site or site of trauma.	Demonstration of clostridia in wound fluids.	Aggressive supportive care, administration of antimicrobials that block protein synthesis (tetracycline).	First aid of wounds, use of hygienic injection technique.
Masseter myonecrosis	Likely selenium deficiency. Role for vitamin E unclear.	Horses on selenium-deficient diet.	Swelling and pain of masseter muscles, trismus; some horses have stilted gait and evidence of myocardial disease.	Clinical signs. Ultrasonographic examination of muscle and heart. Measurement of serum selenium concentration or red cell glutathione peroxidase activity.	Support. Administration of selenium with or without vitamin E	Ensure diet contains adequate selenium.

Table 15-2 Common or well-characterized myopathies of equids*—cont'd

Disease	Etiology	Risk factors	Clinical signs	Diagnosis	Treatment	Control
White-muscle disease	Selenium deficiency.	Foals in regions with low selenium in fodder.	Acute-onset weakness, stiff gait, recumbency, myoglobinuria.	Measurement of serum selenium concentration or red cell glutathione peroxidase activity. Increase serum activity of muscle-derived enzymes.	Supportive. Administration of selenium with or without vitamin E.	Ensure adequate selenium status of mares and foals.
Atypical, pasture-associated myopathy	Ingestion of hypoglycin A in seeds of maple trees, *Acer negundo* (USA) or *Acer pseudoplantanus* (Europe).	Access to seeds of *A. negundo* or *A. pseudoplantanus,* usually by horses at pasture.	Acute onset of weakness, muscle fasciculations, myoglobinuria, recumbency, and death.	Increased concentrations of methylenecyclopropyl acetic acid in serum of affected horses.	Supportive.	Avoid exposure to seeds of *A. negundo* or *A. pseudoplantanu.*
Tremetone toxicosis	Rayless goldenrod (*Isocoma pluriflora*), white snakeroot.	Ingestion of plant.	Weakness, muscle fasciculation, tachycardia, arrhythmia, death over 5–7 days.	Increased serum CK and AST activity and troponin-I concentration. Necropsy with degeneration of myocardium and skeletal muscle.	Supportive.	Prevent access to the plants.
Envenomation by snakes	Documented as a consequence of envenomation by Australian tiger snake (*Notechis scutatus*).	Exposure to habitat of snakes.	Acute-onset anxiety, weakness, muscle fasciculations, myoglobinuria, death.	Demonstration of toxin in blood, body tissue, fluids, or urine. Elevated serum activity of muscle-derived enzymes.	Antivenom. Supportive care.	Avoid exposure to snakes.
Ionophore intoxication	Ingestion of ionophores such as salinomycin, monensin, lasalocid, maduramicin, or narasin.	None.	Anorexia, weakness, stiff gait, colic, recumbency, tachycardia, sudden death, myoglobinuria.	Historical exposure. Necropsy. Detection of ionophore in stomach contents.	Supportive. No specific antidote.	Ensure that horses do not have access to feed containing ionophores.
Fibrotic myopathy	Injury to hamstring muscles (semimembranosus and others).	Exercise. Congenital forms exist.	Foot-slapping gait. Firmness on palpation of hamstring region. Not painful. No response of gait to analgesics.	Differentiate from stringhalt. Palpation of affected muscles. Ultrasound examination.	Surgery.	None.

**Not all myopathies are associated with rhabdomyolysis, and some are evident at rest. Details of each disease can be found under that topic.*
AST, aspartate aminotransferase; CK, creatine kinase; NSAIDs, nonsteroidal antiinflammatory drugs.

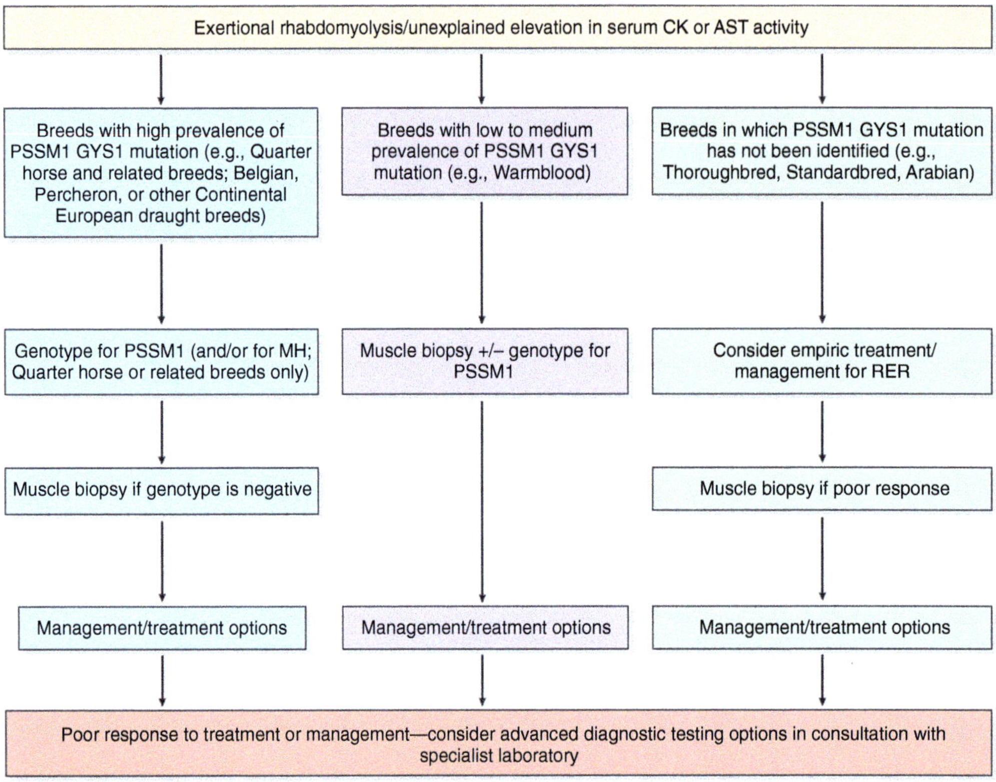

Fig. 15-1 Diagnostic approach to horses with exertional myopathy or persistent increases in serum activity of creatine kinase and aspartate aminotransferase. The approach differs depending on the breed of horse (and hence pretest probability of disease and documented genetic abnormalities). MH, malignant hyperthermia; RER, recurrent exertional rhabdomyolysis (Reproduced with permission from Piercy RJ and Rivero J. Muscle disorders of equine athletes. In Hinchcliff KW, Kaneps AJ, and Geor RJ (eds): Equine Sports Medicine and Surgery: Basic and clinical sciences of the equine athlete, 2nd edition. W.B. Saunders. London. 2014:109.)

There are some general principles and treatments for management of acute rhabdomyolysis regardless of its underlying cause. The treatment chosen depends on the severity of the disease. The **general principles** are rest; correction of dehydration and electrolyte abnormalities; prevention of complications, including nephrosis and laminitis; and provision of analgesia.

Mildly affected horses (heart rate < 60 bpm, normal rectal temperature and respiratory rate, no dehydration) can be treated with rest and phenylbutazone (2.2 mg/kg, orally or intravenously [IV] every 12 hours for 2 to 4 days). Horses should be given mild exercise with incremental increases in workload as soon as they no longer have signs of muscle pain. Access to water should be unrestricted.

Severely affected horses (heart rate > 60 bpm, rectal temperature > 39° C [102° F], 8% to 10% dehydrated, reluctant or unable to walk) should not be exercised, including walking back to their stable, unless it is unavoidable. Isotonic, polyionic **fluids**, such as lactated Ringer's solution, should be administered IV to severely affected horses to correct any hypovolemia and to ensure a mild diuresis to prevent myoglobinuric nephropathy. Less severely affected horses can be treated by administration of fluids by nasogastric intubation (4 to 6 L every 2 to 3 hours). Although it has been recommended that urine should be alkalinized by administration of mannitol and sodium bicarbonate (1.3% solution IV, or 50 to 100 g of sodium bicarbonate orally every 12 hours) to minimize the nephrotoxicity of myoglobin, this therapy is not effective in humans at risk of myoglobinuric nephrosis. Affected horses should not be given diuretics (e.g., furosemide) unless they are anuric or oliguric after restoration of normal hydration.

Phenylbutazone (2.2 to 4.4 mg/kg, IV or orally, every 12 to 24 hours), **flunixin meglumine** (1 mg/kg IV every 8 hours), or **ketoprofen** (2.2 mg/kg IV every 12 hours) should be given to provide **analgesia. Mild sedation** (acepromazine 0.02 to 0.04 mg/kg IM, or xylazine 0.1 mg/kg IM, both with butorphanol, 0.01 to 0.02 mg/kg) can decrease muscle pain and anxiety. Tranquilizers with vasodilatory activity, such as acepromazine, should only be given to horses that are well hydrated. **Muscle relaxants,** such as methocarbamol, are often used but have no demonstrated efficacy. Dantrolene is used for prevention and does not have demonstrated efficacy in treatment of acute disease.

Recumbent horses should be deeply bedded and repositioned by rolling every 2 to 4 hours. Severely affected horses should not be forced to stand.

CONTROL

Control measures should be specific for the particular disease wherever possible (see discussion of the specific diseases elsewhere in this text).

Prevention of the sporadic, idiopathic disease centers on ensuring that horses are fed a balanced ration with adequate levels of vitamin E, selenium, and electrolytes and have a regular and consistent program of exercise. Despite lack of clear evidence for a widespread role for **vitamin E or selenium deficiency** in exertional rhabdomyolysis, horses are often supplemented with 1 IU/kg vitamin E and 2.5 µg/kg selenium daily in the feed. Care should be taken not to induce selenium toxicosis.

Sodium bicarbonate (up to 0.5 to 1.0 g/kg body weight [BW] daily in the ration) and other electrolytes are often added to the feed of affected horses, but their efficacy is not documented. **Phenytoin** has proven useful in the treatment of recurrent rhabdomyolysis. It is administered at a dose rate of 6 to 8 mg/kg, orally, every 12 hours, and the dose is adjusted depending on the degree of sedation produced (a reduced dose should be used if the horse becomes sedated) or lack of effect on serum CK or AST activity. Phenytoin can be administered to horses for months. **Dimethylglycine, altrenogest, and progesterone** are all used on occasion in horses with recurrent rhabdomyolysis, but again without demonstrated efficacy. **Dantrolene** might be effective in treatment of recurrent exertional rhabdomyolysis in Thoroughbred horses (see section on Recurrent Exertional Rhabdomyolysis later in this chapter).

The feeding of high-fat, low-soluble-carbohydrate diets is useful in the prevention of recurrent exertional rhabdomyolysis in Thoroughbred horses and polysaccharide storage myopathy in Quarter horses. The usefulness of this practice in preventing sporadic, idiopathic exertional rhabdomyolysis has not been demonstrated.

FURTHER READING

Piercy RJ, Rivero J. Muscle disorders of equine athletes. In: *Equine Sports Medicine and Surgery: Basic and Clinical Sciences of the Equine Athlete.* 2nd ed. London: W.B. Saunders; 2014:109.

REFERENCE

1. Piercy RJ, Rivero J. Muscle disorders of equine athletes. In: *Equine Sports Medicine and Surgery: Basic and Clinical Sciences of the Equine Athlete.* 2nd ed. London: W.B. Saunders; 2014:109.

MYOSITIS

Myositis may arise from direct or indirect trauma to muscle and occurs as part of a syndrome in a number of specific diseases, including blackleg, foot-and-mouth disease, bluetongue, ephemeral fever, swine influenza, sarcosporidiosis, and trichinosis, although clinical signs of myositis are not usually evident in the latter. Sporadic cases of a localized infectious myositis of skeletal muscles, associated with *Escherichia coli,* may occur in calves. An asymptomatic eosinophilic myositis is not uncommon in beef cattle and may cause economic loss through carcass condemnation. The cause has not been determined.

Acute Myositis of Limb Muscles

Acute myositis is accompanied by severe lameness, swelling, heat, and pain on palpation (Fig. 15-2). There may be accompanying toxemia and fever. In chronic myositis there is much wasting of the affected muscles, and this is difficult to differentiate clinically from atrophy as a result of other causes. Biopsy of the muscles may be necessary to confirm the diagnosis.

Injury to the gracilis muscle can cause acute, severe lameness in performance Quarter horses. Horses competing in barrel racing may be susceptible to gracilis muscle injury because the muscle functions to adduct the hindlimb. The prognosis is good for returning to athletic use after an adequate period of muscle healing and mild exercise. However, fibrotic myopathy or muscle atrophy can be a complication of the injury resulting in persistent gait deficits.

In horses, traumatic myositis of the posterior thigh muscles may be followed by the formation of fibrous adhesions between the muscles (fibrotic myopathy) and by subsequent calcification of the adhesions (ossifying myopathy). External trauma can result in fibrotic myopathy, but it may also be associated with excessive exercise or secondary to intramuscular injections. Occasionally similar lesions may be seen in the foreleg. The lesions cause a characteristic abnormality of the gait in that the stride is short in extension and the foot is suddenly withdrawn as it is about to reach the ground. The affected area is abnormal on palpation.

Generalized myositis ossificans, an inherited disease of pigs, is also characterized by deposition of bone in soft tissues. In traumatic injuries caused by penetration of foreign bodies into muscle masses, ultrasonography may be used to detect fistulous tracts and the foreign bodies.

Extensive damage to or loss of muscle occurs in screwworm and sometimes blowfly infestation, although the latter is more of a cutaneous lesion, and by the injection of necrotizing agents. For example, massive cavities can be induced in the cervical muscles of horses by the intramuscular injection of escharotic iron preparations intended only for slow IV injection. Similarly, necrotic lesions can result from the IM injection of infected or irritant substances. Horses are particularly sensitive to tissue injury, or are at least most commonly affected. Some common causes are chloral hydrate, antimicrobials suspended in propylene glycol, and even antimicrobials alone in some horses.

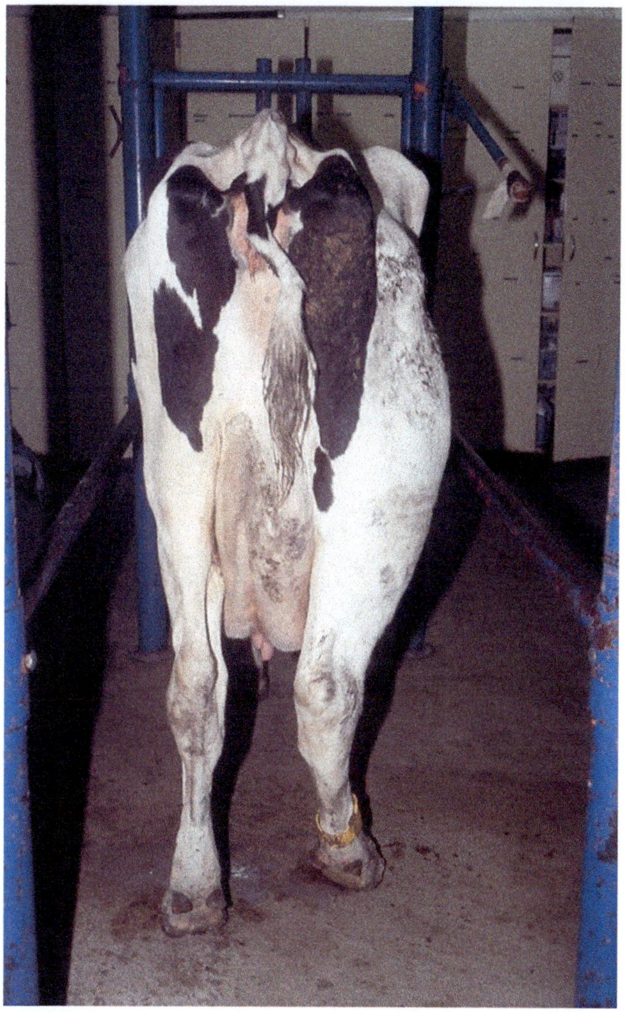

Fig. 15-2 **Myositis centered in the right lateral distal femur region of a lactating dairy cow as a result of a penetrating wound. The cow also has a fractured and shortened tail as a result of a traumatic injury when a calf.**

Injection-Site Lesions in Cattle

Muscle lesions associated with injection sites in the cattle industry are a source of major economic loss because of the amount of trim required at slaughter. The presence of injection-site lesions in whole muscle cuts, such as the top sirloin and outside round, limits their use and value. The occurrence of injection-site lesions in muscle remains among the top five quality challenges for both beef and dairy market cows and bulls. Because injection-site lesions are concealed in muscles and/or are under subcutaneous fat, they are seldom found during fabrication at the packing plant and appear instead during wholesale/retail fabrication or at the consumer level.

Historically, most IM injections were given in the gluteals and the biceps femoris muscles, which are prime cuts of beef. Surveys of injection sites in beef cattle in North America have found lesions in a significant percentage of prime cuts of beef. Lesions consisting of clear scars and woody calluses are mature and probably originated in calfhood; scars with nodules or cysts are less mature, occurring later in the feeding period. It is now recommended that all **IM injections be given in the cervical muscles** (in front of the shoulder). Reducing the incidence of injection-site lesions requires that manufacturers of biological and antibiotic preparations develop less irritating formulations. Products should be formulated for subcutaneous use whenever possible and administered in the neck muscles, which are not prime cuts of beef.

The outcome of an IM injection depends on the nature of the lesion produced. Myodegeneration following IM injections of antibiotics in sheep results in full muscle regeneration within less than 3 weeks. Necrosis following the injection results in scar formation with encapsulated debris, which persists for more than a month and leaves persistent scar tissue.

An outbreak of myositis, lameness, and recumbency occurred following the injection of water-in adjuvanted vaccines into the muscles of the left and right hips of near-term pregnant beef cattle. Within 24 hours, some cattle were recumbent, some had non-weight-bearing lameness, and, within 10 days, 50% of the herd developed firm swellings up to 24 cm in vaccination sites. Histologically, granulomatous myositis with intralesional oil was present. The swellings resolved over a period of 6 months. The acute transient lameness was attributed to the use of two irritating biological vaccines in the hip muscles of cows near parturition.

Injection-Site Clostridial Infections in Horses

Clostridial myositis, myonecrosis, cellulitis, and malignant edema are terms used to describe a syndrome of severe necrotizing soft tissue infection associated with *Clostridium* spp. Affected horses typically develop peracute emphysematous soft tissue swelling in the region of an injection or wound within hours of the inciting cause.

Myositis can occur following the IM or inadvertent perivascular administration of a wide variety of commonly administered drugs. In a series of 37 cases, the lesion occurred in most cases within 6 to 72 hours of a soft tissue injection, and most lesions were in the neck musculature.

Aggressive treatment of clostridial myositis can be associated with a survival rate of up to 81% for cases resulting from *Clostridium perfringens* alone; survival rates for other *Clostridium* spp. are lower. A combination of a high dose of IV antibiotic therapy, surgical fenestration and aggressive debridement, antiinflammatory and analgesic therapy, and general supportive care is recommended.[1]

REFERENCE

1. Adam EN, et al. *Vet Clin Equine*. 2006;22:335.

Diseases of Bones

OSTEODYSTROPHY

Osteodystrophy is a general term used to describe those diseases of bones in which there is a failure of normal bone development or abnormal metabolism of bone that is already mature. The major clinical manifestations include distortion and enlargement of the bones, susceptibility to fractures, and interference with gait and posture.

ETIOLOGY

The common causes of osteodystrophy in farm animals include the following.

Nutritional Causes

Calcium, Phosphorus, and Vitamin D

Absolute deficiencies or imbalances in calcium–phosphorus ratios in diets cause the following conditions:

- Rickets in young animals (e.g., growing lambs fed a diet rich in wheat bran)
- Absolute deficiencies of calcium in beef calves on intensive rations with inadequate supplementation
- Osteomalacia in adult ruminants

Osteodystrophia fibrosa in the horse occurs most commonly in animals receiving a diet low in calcium and high in phosphorus.

Osteodystrophia fibrosa in pigs occurs as a sequela to rickets and osteomalacia, which may occur together in young, rapidly growing pigs that are placed on rations deficient in calcium, phosphorus, and vitamin D following weaning.

Copper Deficiency

- Osteoporosis in lambs
- Epiphysitis in young cattle

Other Nutritional Causes

- Inadequate dietary protein and general undernutrition of cattle and sheep can result in severe osteoporosis and a great increase in ease of fracture.
- Chronic parasitism can lead to osteodystrophy in young, rapidly growing ruminants.
- Hypovitaminosis A and hypervitaminosis A can cause osteodystrophic changes in cattle and pigs.
- Prolonged feeding of a diet high in calcium to bulls (such as high-quality alfalfa) can cause nutritional hypercalcitoninism, replacement of trabecular bone in the vertebrae and long bones with compact bone, and neoplasms of the ultimobranchial gland.
- Multiple vitamin and mineral deficiencies are recorded as causing osteodystrophy in cattle. The mineral demands of lactation in cattle can result in a decrease in bone mineral content during lactation with a subsequent increase during the dry period.

Chemical Agents

- Chronic lead poisoning is reputed to cause osteoporosis in lambs and foals.
- Chronic fluorine poisoning causes the characteristic lesions of osteofluorosis, including osteoporosis and exostoses.
- Grazing the poisonous plants *Setaria sphaceleta, Cenchrus ciliaris,* and *Panicum maximum* var. *trichoglume* causes osteodystrophia in horses.
- Enzootic calcinosis of muscles and other tissues is caused by the ingestion of *Solanum malacoxylon, Solanum torvum, Trisetum flavescens* (yellow oatgrass), and *Cestrum diurnum,* which exert a vitamin D–like activity.
- Bowie or bentleg, a disease caused by poisoning with *Trachymene glaucifolia,* is characterized by extreme outward bowing of the bones of the front limbs.

Inherited and Congenital Causes

There are many inherited and congenital defects of bones of newborn farm animals, which are described and discussed later in this chapter. In summary, these include:

- Achondroplasia and chondrodystrophy in dwarf calves and some cases of prolonged gestation
- Osteogenesis imperfecta in lambs and Charolais cattle. There is marked bone fragility and characteristic changes on radiologic examination.
- Osteopetrosis in Hereford and Angus calves
- Congenital chondrodystrophy of unknown origin ("acorn" calves)
- Inherited exostoses in horses; inherited thicklegs and inherited rickets of pigs, which are well-established entities

Angular deformities of joints of long bones as a result of asymmetric growth-plate activity are common in foals and are commonly repaired surgically. The distal radius and distal metacarpus are most often affected, the distal tibia and metatarsal less commonly. Physiologically immature foals subjected to exercise may develop compression-type fractures of the central or third tarsal bones. Some of these foals are born prematurely or are from a twin pregnancy. Retained cartilage in the distal radial physis of foals 3 to 70 days of age presents without apparent clinical signs.

Physitis is dysplasia of the growth plate, characterized by an irregular border between the cartilage and the metaphyseal zone of ossification, an increase in the lateromedial diameter of the physis, and distoproximally oriented fissures at the medial aspect of the metaphysis, which originate at the physis. In some cases, these may result in bilateral tibial metaphyseal stress fractures in foals.

Abnormal modeling of trabecular bone has been recognized in prenatal and neonatal calves. Abnormalities included growth retardation lines and lattices, focal retention of primary spongiosa, and the persistence of secondary spongiosa. Intrauterine infection with viruses such as bovine virus diarrhea (BVD) may be a causative factor.

Physical and Environmental Causes

Moderate osteodystrophy and arthropathy may occur in rapidly growing pigs and cattle raised indoors and fed diets that contain adequate amounts of calcium, phosphorus, and vitamin D. Those animals raised on slatted floors or concrete floors are most commonly affected, and it is thought that traumatic injury of the epiphyses and condyles of long bones may be predisposing factors in osteochondrosis and arthrosis in the pig (leg weakness) and epiphysitis in cattle. Experimentally raising young calves on metal slatted floors may result in more severe and more numerous lesions of the epiphysis than occurs in calves raised on clay floors. Total confinement rearing of lambs can result in the development of epiphysiolysis and limb deformities. However, the importance of weight-bearing injury as a cause of osteodystrophy in farm animals is still uncertain. In most reports of such osteodystrophy, all other known causes have not been eliminated.

Chronic osteodystrophy and arthropathy have been associated with undesirable conformation in the horse.

Vertebral exostoses are not uncommon in old bulls and usually affect the thoracic vertebrae (T2 and T12) and the lumbar vertebrae (L2 to L3), which are subjected to increased pressure during the bending of the vertebral columns while copulating. The exostoses occur mainly on the ventral aspects of the vertebrae, fusing them to cause immobility of the region. Fracture of the ossification may occur, resulting in partial displacement of the vertebral column and spinal cord compression. The disease is commonly referred to as spondylitis or vertebral osteochondrosis and also occurs less commonly in adult cows and in pigs. It is suggested that the annulus fibrosus degenerates and that the resulting malfunctioning of the disk allows excessive mobility of the vertebral bodies, resulting in stimulation of new bone formation. A similar lesion occurs commonly in horses and may affect performance, particularly in hurdle races and cross-country events. The initial lesion may be a degeneration of the intervertebral disk.

Some types of growth-plate defects occur in young, rapidly growing foals, and these are considered to be traumatic in origin. Failure of chondrogenesis of the growth plate may be the result of crush injuries in heavy, rapidly growing foals with interruption of the vascular supply to the germinal cells of the growth plate. Asymmetric pressures as a result of abnormal muscle pull or joint laxity may slow growth on the affected side and result in limb angulation.

Femoral fractures occur in newborn calves during the process of assisted traction during birth. Laboratory compression of isolated femurs from calves revealed that the fracture configurations and locations are similar to those found in clinical cases associated with forced extraction. The breaking strength of all femurs fell within the magnitude of forces calculated to be created when mechanical devices are used to assist delivery during dystocia. It is suggested that the wedging of the femur in the maternal pelvis and resulting compression during forced extraction accounts for the occurrence of supracondylar fractures of the femur of calves delivered in anterior presentation using mechanical devices in a manner commonly used by veterinarians and farmers.

Tumors

Osteosarcomas are highly malignant tumors of skeletoblastic mesenchyme in which the tumor cells produce osteoid or bone. Osteosarcomas are the most common type of primary bone tumor in animals such as dogs and cats but are rare in horses and cattle. Most tumors of bone in large animals occur in the skull. A periosteal sarcoma on the scapula has been recorded in the horse and an osteosarcoma of the mandible in a cow.

PATHOGENESIS

Osteodystrophy is a general term used to describe those diseases of bones in which there is a failure of normal bone development or abnormal metabolism of bone that is already mature. There are some species differences in the osteodystrophies that occur with dietary deficiencies of calcium, phosphorus, and vitamin D. Rickets and osteomalacia have a similar pathogenesis, with the end result being decreased or defective bone mineralization. In broad terms, rickets is the failure of endochondral ossification in growing bone, whereas osteomalacia is disrupted remodeling in mature bone. Rickets and osteomalacia occur primarily in ruminants fed a deficient diet, osteodystrophia fibrosa occurs in horses, and all three may occur in pigs.[1]

Rickets

Rickets is a disease of young, rapidly growing animals in which there is a **failure of provisional calcification of the osteoid** plus a **failure of mineralization of the cartilaginous matrix of developing bone**. There is also failure of degeneration of growing cartilage and formation of osteoid on persistent cartilage, with irregularity of osteochondral junctions and overgrowth of fibrous tissue in the osteochondral zone. Rickets is most commonly caused in ruminants by a deficiency of vitamin D or phosphorus.[2] Genetic causes of rickets exist, one of which is a simple autosomal-recessive inheritance in Corriedale sheep in New Zealand.[3,4]

Failure of provisional calcification of cartilage results in an increased depth and width of the epiphyseal plates, particularly of the long bones (humerus, radius, ulna and tibia) and the costal cartilages of the ribs. The uncalcified, and therefore soft, tissues of the metaphyses and epiphyses become distorted under the pressure of weight-bearing, which also causes medial or lateral deviation of the shafts of long bones. There is a decreased rate of longitudinal growth of long bones and enlargement of the ends of long bones as a result of the effects of weight, causing flaring of the diaphysis adjacent to the epiphyseal plate. Within the thickened and widened epiphyseal plate, there may be hemorrhages and minute fractures of adjacent trabecular bone of the metaphysis, and in chronic cases the hemorrhagic zone may be largely replaced by fibrous tissue. These changes can be seen radiographically as "epiphysitis" and clinically as enlargements of the ends of long bones and costochondral junctions of the ribs. These changes at the epiphyses may result in separation of the epiphysis, which commonly affects the femoral head. The articular cartilages may remain normal, or there may be subarticular collapse resulting in grooving and folding of the articular cartilage and ultimately degenerative arthropathy and osteochondrosis. Eruption of the teeth in rickets is irregular, and dental attrition is rapid. Growth of the mandibles is retarded and is combined with abnormal dentition. There may be marked malocclusion of the teeth.

Osteomalacia

Osteomalacia is a **softening of mature bone as a result of extensive resorption of mineral deposits** in bone and failure of mineralization of newly formed matrix. There is no enlargement of the ends of long bones or distortions of long bones, but spontaneous fractures of any bone subjected to weight-bearing are common.

Osteodystrophia Fibrosa

Osteodystrophia fibrosa may be superimposed on rickets or osteomalacia and occurs in secondary hyperparathyroidism. Diets low in calcium or that contain a relative excess of phosphorus cause secondary hyperparathyroidism. There is extensive resorption of bone and replacement by connective tissue. The disease is best known in the horse and results in swelling of the mandibles, maxillae, and frontal bones (the "**bighead**" syndrome). Spontaneous fracture of long bones and ribs occurs commonly.

Radiographically there is extreme porosity of the entire skeleton.

Osteoporosis

Osteoporosis is defined as a systemic skeletal disease characterized by low bone mass and microarchitectural deterioration of bone tissue, with a consequent increase in bone fragility and increased susceptibility to fractures.[5] In osteoporosis, the bone becomes porous, light, and fragile, and it fractures easily. Osteoporosis is uncommon in farm animals and is usually associated with general undernutrition and intestinal parasitism rather than specifically a deficiency of calcium, phosphorus, or vitamin D.[6] Copper deficiency in lambs may result in osteoporosis as a result of impaired osteoblastic activity. Chronic lead poisoning in lambs also results in osteoporosis as a result of deficient production of osteoid. In a series of 19 lactating or recently weaned sows with a history of lameness, weakness, or paralysis, 10 had osteoporosis and pathologic fractures, and six had lumbar vertebral osteomyelitis. Bone ash, specific gravity of bone, and the ratio of cortical to total bone were significantly reduced in sows with osteoporosis and pathologic fractures.

Ovariectomized sheep that are fed an acidogenic (calcium-wasting) diet and administered corticosteroids develop osteoporosis, which is being used as a model to study the disease in humans.[6,7]

Osteodystrophy of Chronic Fluorosis

Osteodystrophy of chronic fluorosis is characterized by the development of exostoses on the shafts of long bones as a result of periosteal hyperostosis. The articular surfaces remain essentially normal, but there is severe lameness because of the involvement of the periosteum and encroachment of the osteophytes on the tendons and ligaments.

Congenital Defects of Bone

Congenital defects of bone include complete (**achondroplasia**) and partial (**chondrodystrophy**) failure of normal development of cartilage. Growth of the cartilage is restricted and disorganized, and mineralization is reduced. The affected bones fail to grow, leading to gross deformity, particularly of the bones of the head.

CLINICAL FINDINGS

In general terms there is weakening of the bones as a result of defective mineralization and osteoporosis, which results in the **bending of bones**, which probably causes pain and shifting lameness—one of the earliest clinical signs of acquired osteodystrophy. The normal weight and tension stresses cause distortion of the normal axial relationships of the bones, which results in the bowing of long bones. The distortions occur most commonly in young, growing animals. The distal ends of the long bones are commonly enlarged at the level of the epiphyseal plate, and circumscribed swellings of the soft tissue around the epiphyses may be prominent and painful on palpation.

The effects of osteodystrophy on appetite and body weight will depend on the severity of the lesions and their distribution. In the early stages of rickets in calves and pigs the appetite and growth rate may not be grossly affected until the disease is advanced and causes considerable pain. Persistent recumbency as a result of pain will indirectly affect feed intake unless animals are hand-fed.

Spontaneous fractures occur commonly and usually in mature animals. Common sites for fractures include the long bones of the limbs, pelvic girdle, femoral head, vertebrae, ribs, and transverse processes of the vertebrae. Ordinary hand pressure or moderate restraint of animals with osteomalacia and osteodystrophia fibrosa is often sufficient to cause a fracture. The rib cage tends to become flattened, and in the late stages affected animals have a slab-sided appearance of the thorax and abdomen. Separations of tendons from their bony insertions also occur more frequently and cause severe lameness. The osteoporotic state of the bone makes such separations easy. Any muscle group may be affected, but in young cattle in feedlots, separations of the gastrocnemius are the most common. Thickening of the bones may be detectable clinically if the deposition of osteoid or fibrous tissue is excessive or if exostoses develop, as in fluorosis. Compression of the spinal cord or spinal nerves may lead to paresthesia, paresis, or paralysis, which may be localized in distribution. Details of the clinical findings in the osteodystrophies caused by nutritional deficiencies are provided later in this chapter.

Calcinosis of cattle is characterized clinically by chronic wasting; lameness; ectopic calcifications of the cardiovascular system, lungs, and kidneys; ulceration of joint cartilage; and extensive calcification of bones.

DIAGNOSIS

The **laboratory analyses** that are indicated include the following:

- Serum calcium and phosphorus concentration
- Serum alkaline phosphatase activity
- Feed analysis for calcium, phosphorus, vitamin D, and other minerals when indicated (such as copper, molybdenum, and fluorine)
- Bone ash chemical analysis
- Histopathology of bone biopsy
- Radiographic examination of the skeleton
- Single-photon absorptiometry, a safe and noninvasive method for the measurement of bone mineral content, is now available.

Radiographic examination of the affected bones and comparative radiographs of normal bones are indicated when osteodystrophy is suspected. Radiographic examination of slab sections of bone is a sensitive method for detecting abnormalities of trabecular bone in aborted and young calves.

Serum calcium and **phosphorus** concentrations in nutritional osteodystrophies may remain within the normal range for long periods, and not until the lesions are well advanced will abnormal levels be found. Several successive samplings may be necessary to identify an abnormal trend.

Serum alkaline phosphatase activity may be increased in the presence of increased bone resorption, but this is not a reliable indicator of osteodystrophy. Increased serum levels of alkaline phosphatase may originate from osseous tissues, intestine, or the liver, but osseous tissue appears to be the major source of activity.

Nutritional history and **feed analysis** results will often provide the best circumstantial evidence of osteodystrophy. In vitamin D–dependent rickets, serum 25(OH) D_3 concentrations will be decreased. In phosphorus-dependent rickets, serum 25(OH)D_3 will be normal or increased with normal to decreased parathyroid (PTH) concentrations. Urine calcium-to-phosphorus ratios below 0.05 suggest a calcium or vitamin D deficiency, whereas ratios above 1 reflect phosphorus deficiency.[1]

The definitive diagnosis is best made by a combination of chemical analysis of bone, histopathologic examination of bone, and radiography. The details for each of the common osteodystrophies are discussed under the appropriate headings.

NECROPSY FINDINGS

The pathologic findings vary with the cause, and the details are described under each of the osteodystrophies elsewhere in the book. In general terms, the nutritional osteodystrophies are characterized by bone deformities, bones that may be cut easily with a knife and that bend or break easily with hand pressure, and in prolonged cases the presence of degenerative joint disease. In young growing animals the ends of long bones may be enlarged, and the epiphyses may be prominent and circumscribed by periosteal and fibrous tissue thickening. On longitudinal cut sections the cortices may appear thinner than normal, and the trabecular bone might have been resorbed, leaving an enlarged marrow cavity. The epiphyseal plate may be increased in depth and width and appear grossly irregular, and small fractures involving the epiphyseal plate and adjacent metaphysis may be present. Separation of epiphyses is common, particularly of the femoral head. The calluses of healed fractures of long bones, ribs, vertebrae, and the pelvic girdle are common in pigs with osteodystrophy. On histologic examination there are varying degrees of severity of rickets in young, rapidly growing animals and osteomalacia in adult animals, and osteodystrophia fibrosa is possible in both young and adult animals.

DIFFERENTIAL DIAGNOSIS

In both congenital and acquired osteodystrophy the clinical findings are usually suggestive. There are varying degrees of lameness, stiff gait, long periods of recumbency and failure to perform physical work normally, and progressive loss of body weight in some cases, and there may be obvious contortions of long bones, ribs, head, and vertebral column. The most common cause of osteodystrophy in young, rapidly growing animals is a dietary deficiency or imbalance of calcium, phosphorus, and vitamin D. If the details of the nutritional history are available and if a representative sample of the feed given is analyzed, a clinical diagnosis can be made on the basis of clinical findings, nutritional history, and response to treatment. In some cases, osteodystrophy may be attributable to overfeeding, such as might occur in rapidly growing, large foals.

However, often the nutritional history may indicate that the animals have been receiving adequate quantities of calcium, phosphorus, and vitamin D, which necessitates that other, less common causes of osteodystrophy be considered. Often the first clue is an unfavorable response to treatment with calcium, phosphorus, and vitamin D. Examples include copper deficiency in cattle, leg weakness in swine of uncertain etiology—but perhaps there is weight-bearing trauma and a relative lack of exercise because of confinement—or chemical poisoning such as enzootic calcinosis or fluorosis. These will require laboratory evaluation of serum biochemistry, radiography of affected bones, and pathologic examination. The presence of bony deformities at birth suggests congenital chondrodystrophy, some cases of which appear to be inherited, whereas some are attributable to environmental influences.

TREATMENT

The common nutritional osteodystrophies attributable to a dietary deficiency or imbalance of calcium, phosphorus, and vitamin D will usually respond favorably following the oral administration of a suitable source of calcium and phosphorus combined with parenteral injections of vitamin D. The oral administration of dicalcium phosphate, at the rate of 3 to 4 times the daily requirement, daily for 6 days, followed by a reduction to the daily requirement by the 10th day, combined with one injection of vitamin D at the rate of 10,000 IU/kg BW, is recommended. Affected animals are placed on a diet that contains the required levels and ratios of calcium, phosphorus, and vitamin D. The oral administration of the calcium and phosphorus will result in increased absorption of the minerals, which will restore depleted skeletal reserves. Calcium absorption is increased in adult animals following a period of calcium deficiency; young animals with high growth requirements absorb and retain calcium in direct relation to intake. General supportive measures include adequate bedding for animals that are recumbent.

The treatment of the osteodystrophies resulting from causes other than calcium and phosphorus deficiencies depends on the cause. Copper deficiency will respond gradually to copper supplementation. There is no specific treatment for the osteodystrophy associated with leg weakness in pigs, and slaughter for salvage is often necessary. Overnutrition in young, rapidly growing foals may require a marked reduction in the total amount of feed made available daily.

Oxytetracycline has been used for the treatment of flexural deformities of the distal interphalangeal joints of young foals. It is postulated that oxytetracycline chelates calcium, rendering it unavailable for use for striated muscle contraction. It is considered effective for obtaining a short-term moderate decrease in metacarpophalangeal joint angle in newborn foals.

Hemicircumferential periosteal transection and elevation has gained wide acceptance for correction of angular limb deformities in young foals.

REFERENCES

1. Madson DM, et al. *J Vet Diagn Invest.* 2012;24:1137.
2. Mearns R, et al. *Vet Rec.* 2008;162:98.
3. Dittmer KE, et al. *J Comp Path.* 2009;141:147.
4. Dittmer KE, et al. *Vet J.* 2011;187:369.
5. Klopfenstein Bregger MD, et al. *Vet Comp Orthop Traumatol.* 2007;20:18.
6. Braun U, et al. *Vet Rec.* 2009;164:211-217.
7. Kielbowicz Z, et al. *Pol J Vet Sci.* 2015;18:645.

HYPERTROPHIC OSTEOPATHY (MARIE'S DISEASE)

Although hypertrophic osteopathy is more common in dogs than in the other domestic animals it has been observed in horses,[1-4] cattle,[5] sheep, New World camelids, and captive cervids.[6] The term *hypertrophic osteoarthropathy* is used in humans where there is joint involvement, but the term *hypertrophic osteopathy* is preferred in large animals because the joints are never affected.

Hypertrophic osteopathy is characterized by proliferation of the periosteum, leading to the formation of periosteal bone, and bilateral symmetric enlargement of bones, usually the long bones of limbs and in advanced cases in the horse, the ventral mandible.[1,4] The enlargement is quite obvious and in the early stages is usually painful and often accompanied by local edema. On radiographic examination there is a shaggy periostitis and evidence of periosteal exostosis. The pathogenesis is obscure, but the lesion appears to be neurogenic in origin associated with an increased blood flow to the limbs, with unilateral vagotomy causing regression of the bony changes. Stiffness of gait and reluctance to move are usually present, and there may be clinical evidence of the pulmonary lesion with which the disease is frequently, but not always, associated (the condition was called *hypertrophic pulmonary osteopathy* for many years). Such pulmonary lesions are usually chronic, neoplastic, or suppurative processes such as tuberculosis. Cases of hypertrophic osteopathy have been diagnosed in horses without evidence of intrathoracic disease.[1] In one mare with a large granulosa thecal cell tumor, clinical signs of hypertrophic osteopathy decreased after surgical excision of the tumor.[2]

The majority of reports in large animals are in horses, where the lesions are found more commonly around but not involving the joints of distal limbs.[1] Radiographs of the distal limbs reveal periosteal new bone involving the metaphysis or diaphysis or both. The new bone appears smooth and speculated or has a palisade-like appearance perpendicular to the cortex, with chronic cases having other and less active bony changes.[1]

The disease is considered to be incurable, unless the thoracic lesion can be removed, but there are occasional reports of clinical improvement following prolonged administration of antiinflammatory agents[1] or antibiotics.[3] Affected animals are usually euthanized. At necropsy the periostitis and exostosis are evident, and most, but not all, have gross evidence of chronic intrathoracic disease.[1,2] There is no involvement of the joints.

REFERENCES

1. Enright K, et al. *Equine Vet Educ.* 2011;23:224.
2. Packer M, McKane S. *Equine Vet Educ.* 2012;24:351.
3. Lewis NL, et al. *Equine Vet Educ.* 2011;23:217.
4. Bayless R, et al. *Israel J Vet Med.* 2014;69:151.
5. Guyot H, et al. *Can Vet J.* 2011;52:1308.
6. Ferguson NM, et al. *J Vet Diagn Invest.* 2008;20:849.

OSTEOMYELITIS

ETIOLOGY AND PATHOGENESIS

Inflammation of bone (**osteitis**) or bone and bone marrow (**osteomyelitis**) is uncommon in large animals except when infection is introduced by traumatic injury or by the hematogenous route. **Bacteria can reach bone by any of three routes:**

- Hematogenously
- By extension from an adjacent focus of infection
- By direct inoculation through trauma or surgery

Focal metaphyseal osteomyelitis can occur following open fractures in the horse. Specific diseases that may be accompanied by osteomyelitis include actinomycosis of cattle and brucellosis, atrophic rhinitis, and necrotic rhinitis of pigs. Nonspecific, hematogenous infection with other bacteria occurs sporadically and is often associated with omphalitis, abscesses from tail-biting in pigs, or infection of castration or docking wounds in lambs.

Foals and calves under 1 month of age and growing cattle 6 to 12 months of age may be affected by osteomyelitis in one or more bones. The majority of foals with suppurative polyarthritis have a polyosteomyelitis of the bones adjacent to the affected joints. In a series of cases of tarsal osteomyelitis in foals there was usually evidence of infectious arthritis. Osteomyelitis of the pubic symphysis associated with *Rhodococcus equi* in a 2-year-old horse has been described. The lameness was localized to the pelvis and was associated with a fever and an inflammatory leukogram.

The infections occur commonly in the metaphysis, physis, and epiphysis, which are sites of bony growth and thus susceptible to blood-borne infections. The metaphyseal blood vessels loop toward the physis and ramify into sinusoids that spread throughout the metaphyseal region. Blood flow through the sinusoids is sluggish and presents an ideal environment for propagation of bacteria. Lesions occur on both sides of the physis in both the metaphysis and the epiphysis. Multiple lesions are common and support the explanation that septic emboli are released from a central focus.

In a series of 445 cattle with bone infection of the appendicular skeleton, a distinction was made between hematogenous and posttraumatic origin (wound/fracture). Bone infection was classified into four types according to the site of infection: Type 1 is metaphyseal and/or epiphyseal osteomyelitis close to the growth plate; type 2 is primary subchondral osteomyelitis, mostly accompanied by septic arthritis; type 3 is infectious osteoarthritis with subchondral osteomyelitis, implying that infection in the subchondral bone originates from the infection. Type 4 includes bone infections that cannot be categorized in the other groups. Hematogenous osteomyelitis was 3.2 times more frequent than posttraumatic osteomyelitis. *Trueperella* (*Arcanobacterium* or *Corynebacterium*) *pyogenes* was the most common etiologic agent. Approximately 55% of the affected animals with osseous sequestration had physical evidence of lacerations, contusions, abrasions, or puncture wounds from a previous traumatic event.

Hematogenous osteomyelitis in cattle can be of two types:

- Physeal type, in which an infection generally of metaphyseal bone originates at or near the growth plate, usually affecting the distal metacarpus, metatarsus, radius, or tibia
- Epiphyseal type, in which an infection originates near the junction of the subchondral bone and the immature epiphyseal joint cartilage, most often affecting the distal femoral condyle epiphysis, the patellar, and the distal radius

Epiphyseal osteomyelitis is usually a result of infection with *Salmonella* spp. and is most common in calves under 12 weeks of age. The physeal infections are usually caused by *T. pyogenes* and occur most commonly in cattle over 6 months of age.

Osseous Sequestration in Cattle

Osseous sequestration is a common orthopedic abnormality in cattle and horses. In most cases, the lesions develop in the bones of the distal portion of the limbs (Figs. 15-3 and 15-4). Sequestration is associated with trauma that results in localized cortical ischemia and bacterial invasion secondary to loss of adjacent periosteal and soft tissue integrity and viability. The soft tissues covering the bones that comprise the distal portions of the limbs fail to provide adequate protection and collateral blood supply to the bone.

Osteomyelitis Secondary to Trauma

In horses, osteomyelitis is a frequent sequela to wounds of the metacarpal and metatarsal bones and the calcaneus. These bones have limited soft tissue covering, which may predispose them to osteomyelitis following traumatic injury. Similarly, a portion of the lateral aspect of the proximal end of the radius has limited soft tissue covering. Penetrating and nonpenetrating wounds in this region therefore may result in serious consequences even though they may initially appear to be minor. Because lesions may be an extension of septic arthritis, a thorough examination of the wound area is necessary.

Inflammation of Bone Marrow

Acute inflammation of the bone marrow commonly accompanies bacterial sepsis, resulting in either multifocal microabscesses or perivascular infiltrates of neutrophils, fibrin, edema, and hemorrhage. The most common abnormality associated with fibrinous inflammation is disseminated intravascular coagulopathy. Discrete granulomas may occur in the marrow of animals with systemic mycotic disease, idiopathic granulomatous disease, and serous atrophy of fat.

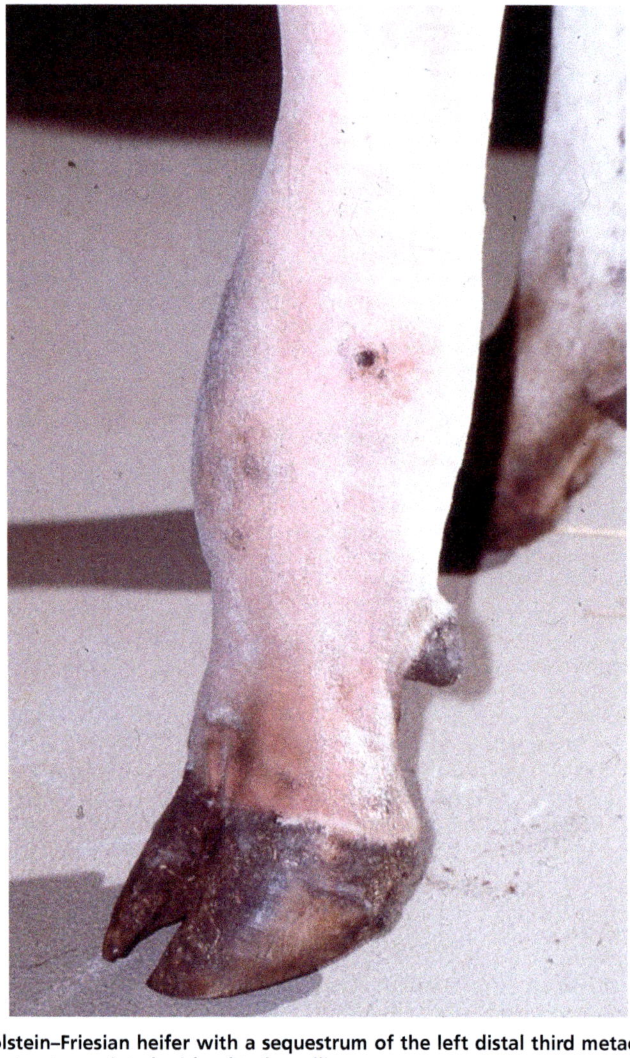

Fig. 15-3 **Holstein–Friesian heifer with a sequestrum of the left distal third metacarpal bone with draining tract associated with a hard swelling.**

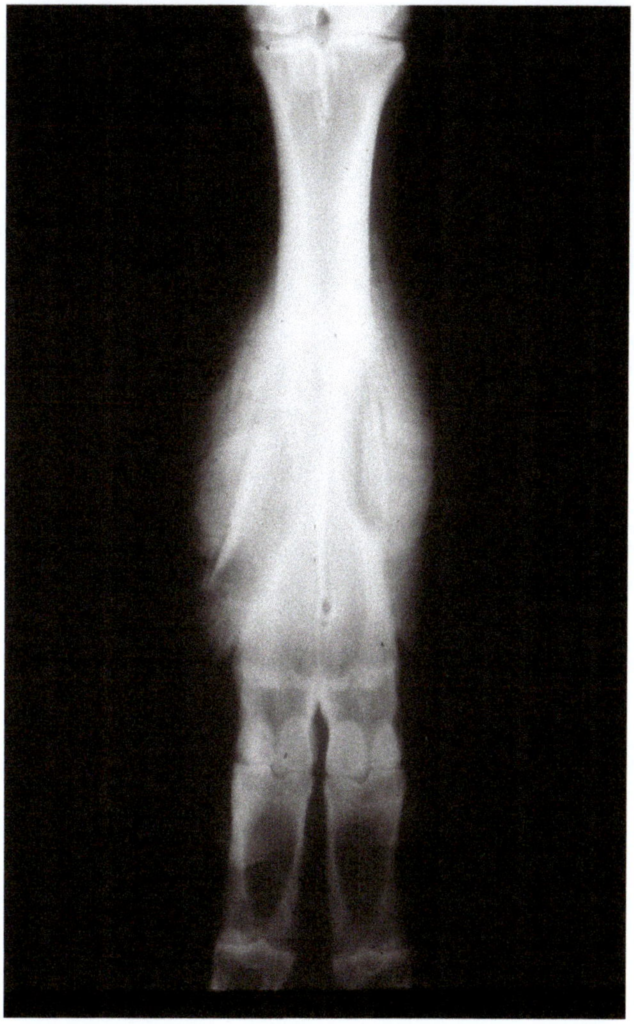

Fig. 15-4 **Palmar-dorsal radiograph of the limb of the heifer in Figure 15-3 showing involucrum laterally and medially (thick sheath of periosteal new bone surrounding a sequestrum) and marked bone proliferation on the cortical surface.**

CLINICAL FINDINGS

The common clinical findings of osteomyelitis include the following:

- Lameness
- Generalized soft tissue swelling and inflammation
- Pain on palpation of the affected area
- Chronic persistent drainage
- Secondary muscle atrophy of the affected limb

Erosion of bone occurs, and pus discharges into surrounding tissues, causing cellulitis or phlegmon, and to the exterior through sinuses, which persist for long periods. The affected bone is often swollen and may fracture easily because of weakening of its structure. When the bones of the jaw are involved, the teeth are often shed, and this, together with pain and the distortion of the jaw, interferes with prehension and mastication. Involvement of vertebral bodies may lead to the secondary involvement of the meninges and the development of paralysis. Lameness and local swelling are the major manifestations of involvement of the limb bones.

Most osseous sequestra in cattle are associated with the bones of the extremities, most commonly the third metacarpal or metatarsal bone. Cattle 6 months to 2 years of age are most likely to have a sequestrum compared with animals less than 6 months of age.

The lesions are typically destructive of bone and cause severe pain and lameness. Those associated with *Salmonella* spp. are characteristic radiographically in foals and calves. *T. pyogenes, Corynebacterium* spp., and *E. coli* may also be causative agents. Affected animals are very lame, and the origin of the lameness may not be obvious. A painful, discrete soft tissue swelling over the ends of the long bones is often the first indication. The lameness characteristically persists in spite of medical therapy, and the animal may become lame in two or more limbs and spend long periods recumbent.

Osteomyelitis affecting the cervical vertebrae, usually the fourth to sixth vertebra, causes a typical syndrome of abnormal posture and difficulty with ambulation. Initially there is a stumbling gait, which then becomes stiff and restricted and with a reluctance to bend the neck. Soon the animal has difficulty eating off the ground and must kneel to graze pasture. At this stage there is obvious atrophy of the cervical muscles, and pain can be elicited by deep, forceful compression of the vertebrae with the fists. There is no response to treatment, and at necropsy there is irreparable osteomyelitis of the vertebral body and compression of the cervical spinal cord. Radiologic examination is usually confirmatory.

Cervicothoracic vertebral osteomyelitis in calves between 2 and 9 weeks of age is characterized by difficulty in rising with a tendency to knuckle or kneel on the forelimbs, which are hypotonic and hyporeflexic. Pain can be elicited on manipulation of the neck. The lesion usually involves one or more of the vertebrae from C6 to T1. *Salmonella dublin* is commonly isolated from the vertebral lesion.

DIAGNOSIS

Radiographs are an essential part of the diagnosis. **Radiographic changes** include the following:

- Necrotic sequestrum initially
- New bone formation
- Loss of bone density

Radiographic lesions are characteristically centered at the growth and extend into both metaphysis and epiphysis.

Nuclear scintigraphy, which is only available at large referral centers, can be useful in identifying osteomyelitis in areas of bone surrounded by a large amount of muscle, which minimizes the ability to detect subtle radiographic lesions.

Culture of the inflammatory exudate and necrotic sequestra removed surgically is necessary to determine the species of bacteria and their antimicrobial susceptibility. Samples of bone obtained at surgery provide the most accurate culture results compared with specimens obtained from the draining sinuses, which may yield a mixed flora. Specimens should consist of sequestra and soft tissues immediately adjacent to bone thought to be infected. Special transport media are desirable for optimum culture results. Anaerobic bacteria are frequently associated with osteomyelitis and should be considered when submitting samples for culture.

NECROPSY FINDINGS

At necropsy the osteomyelitis may not be obvious unless the bones are opened longitudinally and the cut surfaces of the metaphysis and epiphysis are examined.

DIFFERENTIAL DIAGNOSIS

A differential diagnosis for a destructive lesion in the end of a long bone of a foal or calf would include the following: a healing fracture, traumatic periostitis or osteitis, bone tumor, nutritional osteodystrophy and infection of the bone as a result of external trauma, fracture, extension from adjacent infection or hematogenous spread. The absence of equal pathologic involvement in the comparable parts of long bones and the young age of the animal will usually suggest infection of bone. The pathologic features of multiple-bone infection in foals are described.

TREATMENT

Despite advances in antimicrobial therapy and refined diagnostic techniques, the clinical management of osteomyelitis is difficult. Medical therapy alone is rarely completely successful because of the poor vascularity of the affected solid bone, the inaccessibility of the infection, and the potential for development of a biofilm slime layer by bacteria. In cases of long-term infection or those with extensive bone necrosis, surgery is generally recommended to remove sequestra, devitalized tissue, and sinus tracts that are harboring large numbers of bacteria. Good results are obtained when the affected bone is removed and standard wound management practices are implemented.[1] A retrospective case series of 108 thoroughbred foals with septic osteomyelitis secondary to bacteremia indicated that 81% were discharged from the hospital, and 48% successfully raced.[2]

In septic physitis, the implantation of homologous cancellous bone grafts following debridement of necrotic bone, the application of a walking cast for 4 to 5 weeks, and antimicrobial therapy for 2 weeks is usually a successful approach. Absolute asepsis is a fundamental requirement for successful application of a bone graft; after debridement of the necrotic bone, the cavity is flushed with saline and aqueous ampicillin or a combination of penicillin G potassium and ceftiofur.

Antimicrobials are an integral part of the treatment, and selection of the most appropriate drug should be based on identification and susceptibility testing of the organism. Initial treatment may be based on the most common isolates, and a combination of penicillin G and gentamicin or amikacin provides an excellent initial treatment in horses until culture and susceptibility results are available. Aminoglycosides such as gentamicin or amikacin do not provide an ideal initial treatment option in food-producing animals because of the extensive slaughter withdrawals associated with their use. Ideally, parenteral antimicrobial therapy should be continued for a minimum of 10 days and ideally 4 to 6 weeks following surgical curettage. However, in a series of osteomyelitis of the calcaneus of adult horses, there was no difference in the survival rate of animals between those treated surgically and those treated medically. Likewise, a retrospective study of 108 Thoroughbred foals with osteomyelitis secondary to septicemia did not demonstrate an improved success rate with surgical debridement.[2]

Most anaerobic bacteria associated with osteomyelitis are sensitive to penicillin and the cephalosporins, but some species of *Bacteroides fragilis* and *Bacteroides asaccharolyticus* and other species of *Bacteroides* are known to produce beta-lactamases, which can inactivate penicillin and cephalosporin. Metronidazole and clindamycin will penetrate bone and can be considered for use in the horse, but metronidazole is not permitted to be used in food-producing animals in some countries.

Regional perfusion of the distal limb may be helpful as part of the initial treatment by providing higher antimicrobial concentrations at the site of infection. A tourniquet made of latex tubing is placed at a suitable location on the limb proximal to the site of infection. In regional intravenous perfusion, a large superficial vein is identified, and the overlying skin is disinfected. A butterfly catheter is inserted into the vein and a water-soluble antimicrobial agent that is minimally cytotoxic, such as penicillin G potassium or ceftiofur, is infused intravenously and the tourniquet left in place for 30 minutes to facilitate diffusion into infected tissues.

In regional osseous perfusion, an intraosseous infusion screw is inserted using aseptic technique into the medullary cavity, and appropriate water-soluble antimicrobial agents are periodically infused without the use of a tourniquet. The intraosseous screw is left in place under a sterile wrap in between infusions.

FURTHER READING

Goodrich LR. Osteomyelitis in horses. *Vet Clin Equine.* 2006;22:389-417.

Hardy J. Etiology, diagnosis, and treatment of septic arthritis, osteitis, and osteomyelitis in foals. *Clin Tech Equine Pract.* 2006;5:309-317.

REFERENCES

1. Neil KM, et al. *Aust Vet J.* 2010;88:4.
2. Lischer CJ. *Equine Vet Educ.* 2009;21:76.

TAIL-TIP NECROSIS IN BEEF CATTLE

Tail-tip necrosis occurs in cattle housed in confinement on slatted floors. The disease has occurred in steers, heifers, and bulls being fed for beef production, and less frequently in dairy cattle.

The lesion is most commonly caused by a traumatic injury of the tail caused by tramping of the tail by other animals.[1] The tail tip of a lying bull usually is away from the animal's body and therefore accessible for tramping by herdmates. Focal damage is more severe when the tail tip is tramped on slatted floors. Tail-tip necrosis is rare in dairy cattle confined in free stalls because most cows lie down in free stalls and their tails are thereby relatively protected from being tramped. Less frequently, the lesion starts as a ball of manure on the tail switch of animals with loose feces; the manure accumulates until a large dry fecal mass (up to 15 cm in diameter) is present on the tip of the tail. The presence of the hard fecal mass increases the likelihood of damage to the tail tip, particularly when animals are confined.

The lesion begins at the tip of tail followed by varying degrees of extension proximally. Initially, the tip of the tail is swollen, followed by inflammation and infection with *Trueperella pyogenes.* Histopathologic changes are compatible with cutaneous ischemia as a pathogenic mechanism. Extension of the infection can result in metastases to other parts of the body, resulting in abscesses and osteomyelitis. Affected cattle do not grow normally, and deaths from pyemia may occur. The morbidity is about 5%. Approximately 10% of affected animals may be condemned for osteomyelitis and abscessation.

Risk Factors

Risk factors include slatted concrete floors, close confinement, warm seasons, and a body weight above 200 kg. The risk increases as the space allotment, expressed as kg animal per m^2 pen, increases from approximately 165 kg/m^2. Tail tramping is more frequent in slatted-floor pens with lower space allotment (1.5 m^2 per head) than in similar pens with higher space allotment (2.4 m^2 per pen head). In an Ontario study, no case of tail-tip necrosis was diagnosed in solid-floor barns, whereas 1.36% of cattle in slatted-floor barns were either treated or slaughtered for tail-tip necrosis. In a mail survey of feedlots in Ontario, 96% of 71 feedlots with slatted floors, but only 5% of 184 feedlots with solid floors, reported a problem with tail-tip necrosis from 1982 to 1986. Of 441 tails inspected at slaughter plants, 35% were affected, with 3% involving skin lacerations and infection, and 4% were amputated before slaughter. Most cases occur from May to September when the temperature is above 18° C (64 F). This may be associated with increased contamination as a result of increased humidity and temperature under confinement conditions.

In slatted-floor barns, abnormal locomotor patterns occur in 20% to 25% of the times when animals get up and lie down. When animals get up abnormally, they first rise from the front, then consequently assume a dog-like sitting posture. To obtain momentum to rise in the rear, they then start to sway back and forth. The tail may become pinched between the hock of the rocking animal and the floor, resulting in blunt trauma to the tip of the tail.

TREATMENT

Treatment consists of early amputation combined with intensive antimicrobial therapy. Early detection is important. During warm months, cattle confined on slatted floors and weighing more than 200 kg should be closely inspected at least 2 or 3 times weekly. This includes palpation of all tail tips because early lesions are difficult to see.

CONTROL

Control is dependent on providing sufficient space for housed cattle on slatted floors.

REFERENCE

1. Ural K, et al. *Kafkas Univ Vet Fak Derg.* 2007;13:203.

LAMINITIS OF HORSES

SYNOPSIS

Etiology Degeneration of the sensitive lamellae of the hoof. Syndromes of endocrinopathic, sepsis-associated, supporting limb and concussive laminitis are recognized. Pasture-associated laminitis is considered a form of endocrinopathic laminitis.

Epidemiology Disease involving single animals. As a sequela to severe systemic disease induced by colic, enterocolitis, metritis, and grain engorgement. Horses worked on hard surfaces. Horses or ponies at pasture, and especially obese horses and ponies and those with hyperinsulinemia as a result of insulin resistance or equine metabolic syndrome. Horses with pituitary pars intermedia dysfunction. Horses with unilateral lameness often develop laminitis in the contralateral, supporting limb.

Clinical signs Lameness, ranging from mild to sufficiently severe to cause the horse to be recumbent, involving both front feet, and occasionally all four feet.

Clinical pathology None characteristic of the disease.

Diagnostic confirmation Physical examination. Radiography.

Treatment There is no single effective treatment. Control of pain by administration of nonsteroidal antiinflammatory drugs is important. Administration of vasodilatory agents, anticoagulants, frog and sole support, and corrective hoof trimming and shoeing are all used with variable success. Chilling of the limb (cryotherapy) in horses at high risk (e.g., diarrhea, metritis) during the prodromal or acute phase is promising but unproven as yet in prospective clinical trials.

Control Prophylaxis for acute, severe diseases. Aggressive treatment of systemic disease associated with metritis, colic, and enterocolitis, including digital cryotherapy. Prevent unrestricted access to feeds rich in soluble carbohydrates. Maintain optimal body condition. Treat existing equine metabolic syndrome (insulin resistance) or pituitary pars intermedia dysfunction.

Laminitis refers to a spectrum of processes and clinical signs related to breakdown of the connection between of the basement membrane of the secondary dermal lamellae and the basal cells of the secondary epidermal lamellae, with subsequent disruption of the anatomic relationship between the hoof and the distal phalanx. Understanding of the condition is dependent on a specialized vocabulary and jargon, including the following:[1,2]

- **Hoof**—the layers of integument of the foot from the secondary epidermal lamella distally (outward, toward the hoof surface). The keratinized portion of the hoof is the hoof capsule.
- **Distal phalanx**—the most distal of the bones in the limb of the horse (synonyms of pedal bone, P3, or third phalanx)
- **Lamellae** (colloquially, "laminae")—primary and secondary lamellae originate from the inside of the hoof and from the surface of the distal phalanx. Primary lamellae give rise to secondary lamellae. The basal cells of the primary and secondary epidermal lamellae attach the hoof to the basement membrane of the primary and secondary lamellae of the distal phalanx through numerous anchoring points, the hemidesmosomes (Fig. 15-5).[3] Hemidesmosomes are composed of multiple anchoring filaments that connect to laminin-5, a unique glycoprotein that attaches to type IV collagen in the lamina densa of the basement membrane. Type VII collagen connects the lamina densa to the distal phalanx. laminin-5 in the basement membrane is connected through the hemidesmosomes by integrin (which crosses the cell wall) and plectin to the cytoskeleton of the basal cell. Protein BP-180 is associated with the hemidesmosomes and might be involved in anchoring. Basal cells are connected to one another by desmosomes (containing cadherins, a group of compounds responsible for cell–cell adhesion).[3]
- **Parietal integument** (incorrectly, "lamellar integument")—that part of the space between the hoof capsule and distal phalanx occupied by the lamellae, parts of the dermis, and all subcutaneous tissue.

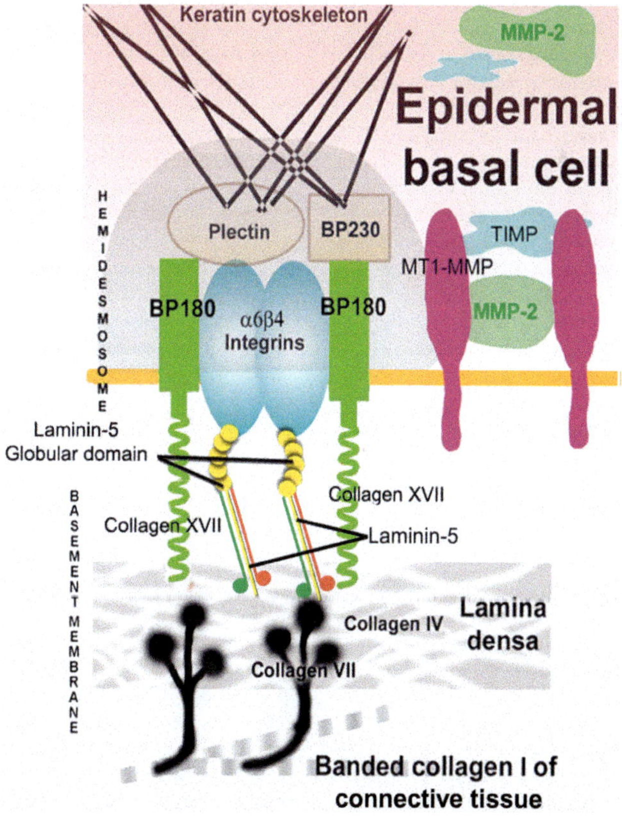

Fig. 15-5 Depiction of the structure of a hemidesmosome and lamina densa, which provide the connection between the basal cell and basement membrane. Note the variety of proteins, including glycoproteins and collagen, that provide tight attachment of the distal phalanx to the hoof. (Reproduced with permission from Pollit C. The anatomy and physiology of the suspensory apparatus of the distal phalanx. *Vet Clin North Am Equine* 2010; 26:29–49.)

- **Laminitis**—the conventional definition is that of a clinical syndrome of foot pain, usually in an acute setting, in horses resulting from separation of the dermal and epidermal lamellae. Laminitis implies an inflammatory component or etiopathogenesis, which does not appear to always be present in all phases of the disease.
- **Prodromal laminitis** (developmental laminitis)—that phase between initiation of the disease process in the foot and appearance of clinical signs.
- **Acute laminitis**—that phase between first development of signs of foot pain and displacement of the distal phalanx (often 72 hours but variable and displacement does not occur in all cases).
- **Chronic laminitis**—phase of the disease after displacement has occurred. It can be further divided into early chronic laminitis, chronic active laminitis, and chronic stable laminitis.
- **Acute founder**—clinical signs of laminitis (strong digital pulses, toe relieving stance, and frequent weight shifting) plus signs of disruption of the normal gross anatomy of the foot evident as supracoronary depressions or radiographic evidence of rotation or distal displacement of the distal phalanx within the hoof ("sinking").
- **Chronic founder**—clinical signs of concave dorsal hoof wall, abnormally wide dorsal white lines, and divergent growth rings in the hoof wall. Sometimes referred to as "chronic laminitis," this syndrome is not characterized by continued disruption of the lamellae but rather represents the sequelae to laminitis or acute founder. If there is ongoing disruption of the epidermal-dermal connection, then this would be laminitis or acute founder.
- **Prolapse of the sole**—a consequence of distal displacement of the distal phalanx resulting in loss of concavity of the sole.
- **Penetration of the sole**—progression of prolapse of the sole to the point where the dermis or pedal bone protrudes through the sole.

ETIOLOGY

The proximate cause of laminitis is acute degeneration of the connections between the basal cells of the primary and secondary epidermal lamellae and the basement membrane of the primary and secondary dermal lamellae. Loss of these connections can lead to microscopic and macroscopic disruption of the normal architecture of the foot and development of clinical signs of foot pain. The factors inciting or leading to breakdown of the epidermal-dermal connections within the hoof are uncertain and the subject of much active investigation.

Laminitis is recognized in a number of settings, which could have differing inciting causes:

- **Endocrinopathic** laminitis—laminitis associated with hormonal influences favoring hyperinsulinemia and often associated with insulin resistance as part of equine metabolic syndrome (EMS) or pasture associated laminitis.[4] Hyperinsulinemia is an experimental model for inducing laminitis.[5,6] Endocrinopathic laminitis, associated with either EMS or pituitary pars intermedia dysfunction, is responsible for most cases of laminitis, with estimates ranging from 71% to 89% of cases.[4,7]
- **Sepsis-related** laminitis—horses with septic illness characterized by signs of a systemic inflammatory response (fever, tachycardia, depression), such as horses with enterocolitis, pneumonia and/or pleuritis, and postpartum septic metritis, or after ingestion of large quantities of soluble carbohydrate, are at increased risk of laminitis.
- **Weight-bearing** laminitis—horses that chronically bear more weight on one limb, such as animals with severe persistent unilateral lameness, often develop laminitis in the weight-bearing limb.
- **Concussive** laminitis—associated with prolonged or unaccustomed exercise on a hard surface.
- **Toxic** laminitis—exposure to shavings of black walnut (*Juglans nigra*) causes laminitis. The mechanism involves a severe systemic inflammatory response, and this category of laminitis could share basic mechanisms with that caused by sepsis. Black walnut has been used as an experimental model of laminitis but is now considered less clinically relevant.[8]
- Sustained (lasting 48 hours) digital hyperthermia does not cause laminitis.[9]

EPIDEMIOLOGY

For such a common and important disease, the epidemiology of laminitis is poorly documented.[10] Quantitative analysis and identification of putative risk factors is available from few studies, and in many instances such studies do not have clear case definitions or rely on lay reporting of the diagnosis and presence of potential risk factors, with the result that conclusions are unreliable and conflicting. There is a pressing need for well-designed, comprehensive studies that address the prevalence, risk factors, and outcome of spontaneously occurring laminitis in non-hospital settings.

A recent systematic review of the scientific literature reporting on risk factors for laminitis concluded that there is limited evidence to support a role for many of the putative risk factors for laminitis.[10] Based on the reporting in the 6 highest-quality reports of 17 reviewed, the following conclusions were made:[10]

- Age—good evidence that increasing age is a risk factor for laminitis, although some studies did not find this association for acute laminitis
- Sex (gender)—inconsistent evidence; most studies did not find an association
- Breed—inconsistent evidence; most studies did not find an association
- Height—no evidence of an association
- Bodyweight—inconsistent evidence
- General obesity—no evidence
- Cresty neck—weak evidence
- Health variables—no evidence
- Exercise—weak evidence that reduced exercise level is a risk factor
- Endotoxemia—weak evidence, noting that experimental endotoxemia does not cause laminitis
- Pituitary pars intermedia dysfunction—no evidence
- Seasonality—inconsistent evidence
- Weather—weak evidence

Some of these results are surprising and likely will be revised as additional studies are conducted. As noted in the following discussion, there is consensus on several risk factors for development of laminitis that are not reflected in the results of the systematic review cited previously. In the absence of multiple high-quality epidemiologic studies, the results of the systematic review should be considered in light of other knowledge.

Occurrence

Single sporadic cases are the rule for **horses,** in which the disease is usually related to individual risk factors such as obesity, systemic illness, or lameness. An estimated 13% of horse operations in the United States have a horse with laminitis at any one time, and laminitis accounts for 7.5% to 15.7% of all lameness in horses.[11] A study of 1000 horses on a single farm in East Anglia (UK) found annual that annual incidence rates for laminitis varied from 7.9% to 17.1%, that 33% of animals diagnosed once with laminitis has a repeat episode of the disease, and that 24% of animals with laminitis had a repeat episode in the same year.[12] Laminitis accounts for up to 40% of hoof problems in horses, depending on the use of the horse. Approximately 5% of horses with laminitis die or are euthanized. Among cases occurring in the field (as opposed to veterinary hospitals), approximately 74% recover and become sound, with 8% improving but continuing to be lame.[11] However, approximately 10% of horses that developed laminitis had a permanent change in their primary use as a result of having developed laminitis.

Within the United Kingdom, 30% of all cases of laminitis are speculated to be caused by grazing lush pasture, 21% as a result of pituitary pars intermedia dysfunction, 13% by obesity, and 9% attributable to equine metabolic syndrome (cited in[4]). Laminitis accounts for approximately 4.4% of reported diseases in equids in the United Kingdom.[13]

Risk Factors

Animal Risk Factors

There are few studies that provide quantitative estimates of risk factors for equids developing laminitis.

Phenotype

There is a consensus that ponies and horses at increased risk of developing pasture-associated laminitis have a particular phenotype characterized by regional and generalized obesity.[14] Although not borne out by the systematic review, there appears to be considerable diverse evidence that ponies, and especially obese ponies, are at high risk of developing pasture-associated laminitis.[14,15] This risk also applies to obese horses and especially those of "easy keeper" or "thrifty" breeds such as Andalusians, Quarter horses, Morgan, and Arabians. The risk of laminitis is associated with insulin resistance, and not all obese horses or ponies are insulin resistant. Ponies at increased risk might be identified by a variety of means, including measurement of plasma or serum insulin concentration 2 hours after ingestion of glucose (1 g/kg orally).[16] Ponies with exaggerated insulin response are at increased risk of developing laminitis.

Hyperinsulinemia

Available evidence clearly indicates a propensity for ponies and horses at risk of insulin resistance (obesity, equine metabolic syndrome) to have a higher incidence of laminitis, especially if they are kept on pasture. These equids are considered to develop endocrinopathic laminitis.[15-20] A unifying feature of these horses and ponies is the presence, or presumed presence, of hyperinsulinemia.[14] Reports indicate that between 10% to 22% of obese horses and 28% of ponies in Australia have hyperinsulinemia. Insulin concentrations are higher (138 vs. 315 pmol/L) in ponies with a history of laminitis than in younger ponies of similar body condition that have never had laminitis,[15,21] and are higher in previously laminitic ponies that have a higher body-condition score than unaffected ponies.[14] The affected ponies are also insulin resistant based on a higher insulin : glucose ratio or the reciprocal of the square root of plasma insulin concentration (RISQI).[15,21] Similarly, hyperinsulinemia is common in horses presenting to veterinary hospitals with a complaint of laminitis—from 21 of 36 (58%) to 13 of 30 (43%).[7,22]

Horses or ponies with documented hyperinsulinemia or pituitary pars intermedia dysfunction (PPID) are at increased risk of having laminitis.[7] Horses of 15 years of age or older in Queensland with PPID diagnosed by seasonally adjusted plasma adrenocorticotropic hormone (ACTH) concentrations were 4.7 times as likely to have laminitis compared with similarly aged horses without PPID.[23] Aged horses with hyperinsulinemia (>20 μU/mL) were 10 times more likely to have laminitis than were horses without documented hyperinsulinemia.[23] Laminitis in horses with PPID is associated with hyperinsulinemia but not at a greater rate than for horses that do not have PPID,[23] suggesting that the hyperinsulinemia present in some horses with PPID might be coincidental in the horse has both EMS and PPID and that it is the EMS that predisposes to hyperinsulinemia and laminitis. Although not supported by the systematic review, clinical evidence clearly supports a link between insulin resistance (hyperinsulinemia) or PPID and risk of laminitis.

The disease is more common in the United States during spring and summer (1.3% in spring and 0.4% in winter in the central United States) and during May in the United Kingdom.[12] Increasing number of hours of sunlight has been linked to the risk of laminitis in horses at pasture—a reflection of the effect of sunlight to increase the content of nonstructural carbohydrate in pasture and not of a biological effect of sunlight on the horses.[12]

The disease is very uncommon in foals and horses less than 8 months of age, then increases in frequency with increasing age such that horses greater than 20 years of age have an incidence of the disease roughly 3 times that of horses between 5 and 20 years of age. This apparent age distribution could represent, among other factors, an increase in prevalence of PPID as horses and ponies age.

Trauma and other physical factors such as excessive work on hard surfaces, increased weight-bearing on one limb, and persistent pawing can contribute to the development of the disease in horses. Standing for periods of days during transport can predispose to laminitis.

Laminitis is associated with many **systemic illnesses** of horses. Horses with illness attributable to colic, diarrhea, pleuropneumonia, and metritis are prone to develop laminitis. **Potomac horse fever** (equine neorickettsiosis) is frequently a cause of laminitis in horses, and laminitis is the major cause of death from this disease. Approximately 28% of horses with **anterior enteritis** (duodenitis/proximal jejunitis) develop laminitis, usually within 2 days of developing enteritis. There are anecdotal reports that suggest that administration of **corticosteroids** (dexamethasone, triamcinolone) causes or exacerbates laminitis, but this association has not been proved.[24-26] Laminitis is common in horses that engorge on grain or similar feeds containing a high concentration of soluble carbohydrates. Ingestion of large quantities of lush pasture has been anecdotally associated with increased risk of laminitis, especially among ponies. It is thought that the presence of a high concentration of soluble carbohydrates in the grass is responsible for the increased risk of laminitis.

Supporting Limb Laminitis

Development of laminitis in a limb bearing a disproportionate amount of the horse's weight for prolonged periods of time is a frequent occurrence among horses treated for severe chronic unilateral lameness or subject to fracture repair requiring casting of the limb. Of 113 horses that received half-limb or full-limb casts, 14 (12%) developed confirmed supporting limb laminitis.[27] Risk factors significantly associated with development of laminitis included body weight of the horse and duration of casting in weeks, with horses requiring full-limb casts or transfixion pin casts more likely to develop this complication than horses requiring half-limb casts. Supporting hindlimbs (for the contralateral hindlimb) were as likely to be affected as supporting forelimbs.

Horses hospitalized for treatment of laminitis, or those that develop laminitis during hospitalization for other diseases, have risk factors that differ from those of horses with pasture-associated laminitis. Endotoxemia (defined clinically, not by measurement of blood endotoxin concentration, and therefore more appropriately referred to as toxemia) was the only factor associated with development of laminitis.[28] This study provides evidence that severe systemic inflammation increases the risk of laminitis, but it provides no evidence of the effect of endotoxemia.

Importance

Death is unusual in horses with laminitis that do not have other severe systemic illness, but the severe lameness can cause a great deal of inconvenience, and affected horses can develop permanent deformities of the feet. Some have to be euthanized on humane grounds.

Of 107 horses with pasture-associated laminitis, 77 had a "good" outcome as assessed by a panel of veterinarians, and 47 of 79 animals used for riding before developing laminitis were being ridden 8 weeks later. Five of the initial 107 animals were euthanized by 8 weeks after development of the disease, and those that were more severely affected (based on Obel grade of lameness) were more likely to have been euthanized.[29]

Among 247 hospitalized horses that died or were euthanized because of laminitis and 344 horses that developed laminitis but did not die, factors increasing the risk of death because of laminitis were being Thoroughbred (odds ratio [OR] = 1.57) or a racehorse (OR = 1.76), treatment with flunixin meglumine (OR = 1.76), distal displacement of the third phalanx (OR = 2.68), pneumonia (OR

= 2.87), and lameness of Obel grade II (OR = 2.99), grade III (OR = 9.63), or grade IV (OR = 20.48) compared with Obel grade I.[30]

PATHOGENESIS

The pathogenesis of laminitis is complex and in most cases involves systemic disease that is at least partially expressed in the foot. Evidence for laminitis being part of a systemic disease and not only a localized disease of the foot includes observations that analysis of a panel of tissue samples from horses with experimentally induced laminitis revealed that degradation of laminin-332 and collagen type IV, both proteins found in the basement membrane of the hoof, occurs in the skin and stomach in addition to the hoof lamellae.[31] Additionally, systemic inflammatory responses, including infiltration of neutrophils, are noted in lung, skin, liver, and gastrointestinal tract of horses with black walnut–induced laminitis.[32-34] These findings suggest that systemic inflammation and degradation of proteins common to a wide range of tissues, and including the basement membrane, are common to many epithelial tissues during equine laminitis, suggesting a systemic pathogenesis for at least some forms of this disease.

The local pathogenic process common to all forms of laminitis is disruption of the connective tissue (involving laminin-5 and collagen types IV and VII) providing connections between the lamellar basal cells and the basement membrane of the third phalanx.[35] Carbohydrate overload is associated with up-regulation of genes expressing MMP-13 (matrix metalloproteinase 13) and localized loss of collagen I, fibronectin, chondroitin, and keratin sulfate glycosaminoglycans in secondary lamellae.[36]

It is possible, indeed likely, that a more than one type of insult to basal cells or basement membrane can result in loss of adhesion between the basal cell and the basement membrane—sometimes referred to as dyshesion—or degeneration of the basement membrane. As a consequence of the loss of these connections, the weight of the horse is no longer transmitted through the numerous lamellae to the hoof wall but is instead transmitted toward the sole of the foot.

Loss of the connection between the third phalanx and hoof allows the third phalanx to **rotate** within the hoof capsule, likely in response to the torque applied by the deep digital flexor tendon, and/or to displace ventrally (**sink**) within the hoof as a result of weight transmitted through the third phalanx; or there can be a combination of these changes. Rotation of the third phalanx causes the sole to be pushed downward or "dropped," and the point of the toe of the third phalanx may actually penetrate the sole. Serum accumulates in the space created by degeneration of the laminae and displacement of the third phalanx, and there is breakdown of the white line.

Exactly what the mechanism is that links the risk factors listed previously to the laminar degeneration, the basis of the separation, is unknown. There are differences in the microscopic lesions induced by either **hyperinsulinemia or models of sepsis-induced laminitis** (carbohydrate overload, oligofructose [OF] administration), suggesting that the inciting mechanisms in each from of laminitis could differ,[37] with subsequent common events resulting in the clinical signs of laminitis.[38] Calprotectin, a marker of the presence or activation of neutrophils, expression in lamellae was absent in control horses, moderate in hyperinsulinemic horses, and marked in OF-treated horses, indicating that hyperinsulinemia induces less leukocyte emigration than carbohydrate overload at 48 hours after initiation of the inciting cause.[37] Laminitis induced by administration of black walnut is characterized by early (1.5 hours) marked infiltration of neutrophils and expression of neutrophil adhesion molecules in lamellar endothelial cells and cytokines favoring extravasation of neutrophils into lamellae.[39-42] There are similar changes during carbohydrate overload laminitis but with a somewhat delayed time frame with some extravasation of leukocytes, which are predominantly monocytes and macrophages (compare with neutrophils in black walnut laminitis), during the prodromal phase but maximal accumulation in lamellar tissues at the onset of clinical signs.[43-46] Similarly, there is increased mRNA concentrations for IL-1 beta, IL-6, IL-12p35, COX-2, E-selectin, and ICAM-1 in laminae from horses with Obel grade I lameness but not during the prodromal phase in horses with carbohydrate-induced laminitis.[43]

The majority of laminar inflammatory events appear to occur at or near the onset of lameness in the carbohydrate-overload (CHO) model, whereas many of these events peak earlier in the prodromal (developmental) stages in the black walnut extract–model. This suggests that, in addition to circulating inflammatory molecules, there may be a local phenomenon in the CHO model resulting in the simultaneous onset of multiple laminar events, including endothelial activation, leukocyte emigration, and proinflammatory cytokine expression.[43] CHO laminitis is associated with increases in mRNA of various CXC and CC chemokines during either the prodromal or clinical phase, or both, and in the increase in expression of a wide range of proinflammatory genes.[45,47] CHO-induced laminitis is associated with marked changes in fecal microbiota, including overgrowth of gram-negative bacteria.[48] Inflammatory signaling is a consistent entity in the pathophysiology of laminitis, although there is evidence that leukocyte appearance in lamellar tissues is not the first event in the pathogenesis of laminitis but has a key early role in the development of lesions and progression of the disease.

Hyperinsulinemia (with euglycemia) induced by prolonged (up to 72 hours) infusion of insulin and glucose results in development of clinical and histologic signs of laminitis in insulin-sensitive horses and in ponies.[5,49-51] The concentrations of insulin required to induce laminitis in insulin-sensitive horses are very high (>1000 µU/mL), although lesions, but not clinical signs, have been detected in horses in which insulin concentrations approximated 200 µU/mL as a result of infusion of glucose.[6] Microscopic lesions induced by infusion of insulin during the prodromal (development) phase of laminitis have been well characterized and contrasted with those of carbohydrate overload.[51-53] There is no detectable calprotectin present before 48 hours (about the time of onset of clinical signs of laminitis), whereas secondary epidermal lamellar width decreases, and there is histomorphological evidence of epidermal basal (and suprabasal) cell death after 6 hours of hyperinsulinemia.[50,53] Increased cellular proliferation in the secondary epidermal lamellae, infiltration of the dermis with small numbers of leukocytes, and basement membrane (BM) damage occurred later at 24 and 48 hours. Narrowing of the secondary epidermal lamellae was progressive over the 6- to 48-hour period.[50] There were signs of apoptosis of basal cells. Cellular lesions preceded leukocyte infiltration and BM lesions, indicating that the latter changes may be secondary or downstream events in hyperinsulinemic laminitis to initial insults to basal cells.[50]

A role for insulin-like growth factor (IGF) has been proposed, with insulin acting as an agonist for the IGF receptor. Cell proliferation occurs in the lamellae during insulin-induced laminitis, and in other species high concentrations of insulin can activate receptors for the powerful cell mitogen IGF-1.[54] It is speculated that stimulation of the IGF-1 receptor by insulin could lead to inappropriate lamellar epidermal cell proliferation and lamellar weakening, a potential mechanism for hyperinsulinemic laminitis.[54]

Hyperinsulinemia causes increases in plasma concentrations of pentosidine, an advanced glycoxidation end product indicative of inflammation, which could indicate a role for glucose toxicity in the genesis of endocrinopathic laminitis.[21] However, the failure to detect advance glycoxidation products in the lamellae of horses during the prodromal phase of laminitis induced by hyperinsulinemic–hyperglycemic clamp, although these products were detected when clinical signs of laminitis had developed, and the lack of evidence of oxidative stress do not lend support to oxidative stress and protein glycosylation playing a central role in the pathogenesis of acute, insulin-induced laminitis.[55] The insulin-independent glucose transporter GLUT-1 was increased in lamellar tissue in the developmental stages of insulin-induced laminitis compared with control horses, although the importance of this observation is unclear.[55] There does not appear to be a role for toll-like receptor 4 (TLR4) in the development of hyperinsulinemic laminitis in otherwise healthy horses.[56]

Hyperinsulinemia in isolated (ex vivo) hooves of healthy horses increases vascular resistance and lamellar endothelin-1 expression and perfusion of isolated lamellar veins with cortisol and insulin.[57] Exposure of isolated lamellar veins to cortisol increases maximum contractility to the vasoconstrictors (noradrenaline and 5-hydroxytryptamine) and decreases the maximal contraction to endothelin-1, whereas exposure to insulin decreases contractility of vessels to phenylephrine and endothelin-1 (ET-1).[58] It is possible that short-term cortisol excess could enhance venoconstrictor responses to 5-hydroxytryptamine and noradrenalin in laminar veins in vivo, thereby predisposing to laminitis.[58] The authors conclude that a reduction in the ability of insulin to counteract alpha-adrenoreceptor and ET-1-mediated contraction, likely to occur in subjects with insulin resistance, could further exacerbate venoconstriction in animals prone to laminitis. These mechanisms could also predispose horses with PPID or EMS to laminitis.[58] Others have demonstrated that insulin resistance, which is associated with hyperinsulinemia, increases vascular reactivity and response to various vasoconstrictors and has, in the absence of direct experimental evidence in horses or ponies, been speculated to contribute to excessive vasoconstriction in the dermis of susceptible horses.[20] Short-term hyperinsulinemia increases vascular resistance in the equine digit and increases expression of ET-1 in the laminar tissue, providing a possible explanation for a role for insulin in perfusion of the digit.[57] Furthermore, laminitis induced by IV infusion of insulin is associated with warmth of the hoof, which is considered evidence of vasodilatation in the foot. It is plausible that there is a combination of these mechanisms, beginning with digital venoconstriction and ending in arteriovenous shunting, that could lead to hypoxemia of lamella and loss of integrity of the basal cells or basement membrane.

Other theories for the etiopathogenesis of laminitis include the following:

- Ischemia of the laminae with subsequent dysfunction or death of basal cells or degeneration of the basement membrane—proposed causes of ischemia include vasoconstriction, development of arteriovenous shunts, interstitial edema, and presence of microthrombi in digital vessels. Ischemia as a result of microthrombus formation is no longer considered a potential cause of laminitis. However, there is evidence from experimental laminitis, both black walnut and carbohydrate models, that there are changes to the microvasculature of the dermis, possibly secondary to changes in circulating concentrations of vasoactive amines or contractile activity of vessels in the hoof.[57,59-63] Alternatively, increases in capillary filtration pressure, resulting from venoconstriction, might cause edema and increased interstitial pressure with subsequent ischemia of the laminae.[11]
- Enzymatic digestion of connective tissues of the lamella by matrix metalloproteins (MMPs) induced by circulating factors including products of *Streptococcus bovis* infection has been proposed as a cause of the loss of integrity of the basal cell–basement membrane junction. Recent evidence indicates that MMP-9 is not involved in this process because it remains in the inactive proenzyme form during the prodromal (developmental) phase of oligofructose-induced laminitis, although MMP-13 might be.[36,64,65] However, other proteinases, such as ADAMT-4, and metalloproteinases might be involved in affecting basal cell or basement membrane function. Interesting, ADAMT-4 is located primarily in the basal cells and not in the matrix, calling into question its role in basement membrane integrity or disruption of adhesion between basal cells and the basement membrane.[66,67] Alternatively, elevated ADAMT-4 expression and versican depletion could be associated with abnormal basal cell function and disruption of adhesion.[68]
- Infusion of endotoxin does not induce laminitis in healthy horses or ponies, nor does the systemic inflammatory response induced by administration of endotoxin manifest as expression of genes of proinflammatory cytokines in the lamellae.[69] Many of the inciting causes of laminitis are diseases that are associated with **endotoxemia** or, more generally, toxemia, and in experimental models endotoxin was detectable in the blood of horses that developed laminitis, suggesting that endotoxin could contribute to the development of the disease. However, infusions of endotoxin do not cause laminitis, although endotoxin does impair endothelium-dependent relaxation and augments adrenergic contraction of palmar digital arteries.
- Theories for development of laminitis in a supporting limb include loss of intermittent weight-bearing with a reduction in vascular perfusion of the hoof and ischemia of the lamellae.[70]
- There is no evidence that laminitis is an autoimmune disease.[71]

The disease occurs in three distinct phases: (1) a developmental stage in which lesions are detectable in the sensitive laminae but during which there are no clinical signs, (2) the acute phase from the development of the first clinical signs through to rapid resolution or to rotation or ventral displacement of the third phalanx, and (3) the chronic stage evidenced by rotation of the third phalanx with or without ventral displacement and characterized by variable but persistent pain.

CLINICAL FINDINGS

The disease presents as both an acute disease and as a chronic disease. The severity of the acute disease varies considerably from very mild with rapid (5 to 7 days) recovery, to severe with progression to the chronic, refractory stage.

Severity of lameness attributable to laminitis can be graded according to a scale proposed by Obel in 1948:

Grade 0—normal

Grade 1—horse alternately and intermittently lifts its feet; lameness is not evident at a walk but the gait is short and stilted at a trot.

Grade 2—there is a stilted gait at the walk, but the horse moves willingly; a foot may be lifted by a handler without the horse resisting.

Grade 3—the horse moves reluctantly and resists attempts by a handler to lift a foot.

Grade 4—the horse refuses to move and does so only if forced.

The reliability of this system has been assessed, and it has reasonable intraobserver reliability (weighted kappa statistic of 0.54) when using all four (five) grades, which increases to 0.69 when reduced to three categories (sound, grades I and II combined, and grades III and IV combined).[72] Interobserver agreement (58 veterinarians in primary opinion equine practice) was 0.43 (moderate agreement) for the unweighted kappa statistic and 0.65 (substantial agreement) for the weighted kappa statistic when all four (five) grades were used. When grades were lumped into the three categories, the interobserver agreement increased to 0.52 and 054 for unweighted and weighted kappa statistics, respectively. Importantly, there was 83% agreement on detection of severely affected animals (of the three lumped grades).[72] These results are similar to those of a study comparing use of a visual analog scale, Obel grade, and clinical grading system. All methods of assessing severity of laminitis had acceptable intra- and interobserver agreement, with more experienced observers having greater reliability.[73] These studies demonstrate that the Obel grading system is useful for clinical description of laminitis and therefore assessment of the response to therapy.

The **acute disease** develops rapidly; apparently normal horses can founder within hours. Signs of the disease are entirely attributable to pain in the feet. All hooves can be affected, but more commonly the forefeet are affected and the hindfeet are spared. The disease is rarely unilateral except in cases in which the disease develops because of severe lameness in the contralateral limb or repeated pawing. Mild, or early, disease is apparent as a resistance to movement and repetitive and frequent shifting of weight from one foot to the other. There is a characteristic shuffling gait.

More severe disease is apparent as refusal to move or to lift a hoof. At this stage the horse has an anxious expression that can be accompanied by muscle fasciculation, sweating, a marked increase in heart rate to as high as 75/min, and rapid and shallow respiration. There is a characteristic posture with all four feet being placed forward of their normal position, the head held low, and the back arched. There is usually a great deal of difficulty in getting the animal to move, and when it does so the gait is shuffling and stumbling, and the animal evidences great pain when the foot is put to the ground. The act of lying down is accomplished only with difficulty, often after a number of preliminary attempts. There is also difficulty in getting the animals to rise, and some horses may be recumbent for long periods. It is not unusual for horses to lie flat on their sides. In occasional cases, the separation of the wall from the laminae is acute, and the hoof is shed. There may be exudation of serum at the coronet, and this is considered a sign of impending sloughing of the hoof and a poor prognosis.

Clinical signs in laminitis include pain on palpation around the coronet and a marked withdrawal response when hoof testers are applied to the hoof. The intensity of the pulse in the palmar digital artery, palpable over the abaxial aspects of the proximal sesamoid, of affected feet is markedly increased over normal. In horses in which the third phalanx is displaced distally (sinks), a concavity can be palpable at the coronary band. Infiltration of the palmar digital nerves at the level of the proximal sesamoid with local anesthetic agents provides marked, but not complete, relief.

In the **chronic stages** of the disease, there is separation of the wall from the sensitive laminae and a consequent dropping of the sole. The hoof wall spreads and develops marked horizontal ridges, and the slope of the anterior surface of the wall becomes accentuated and concave. Horses with chronic or refractory laminitis may continue to feel much pain, lose weight, and develop decubitus ulcers over pressure points because of prolonged recumbency. Loss of integrity of the sole and disruption of the white line can allow infection to develop in the degenerate lamellae. The infection can spread to involve the pedal bone, causing a septic pedal osteitis. The lameness might abate, but the animal becomes lame easily with exercise and can suffer repeated, mild attacks of laminitis.

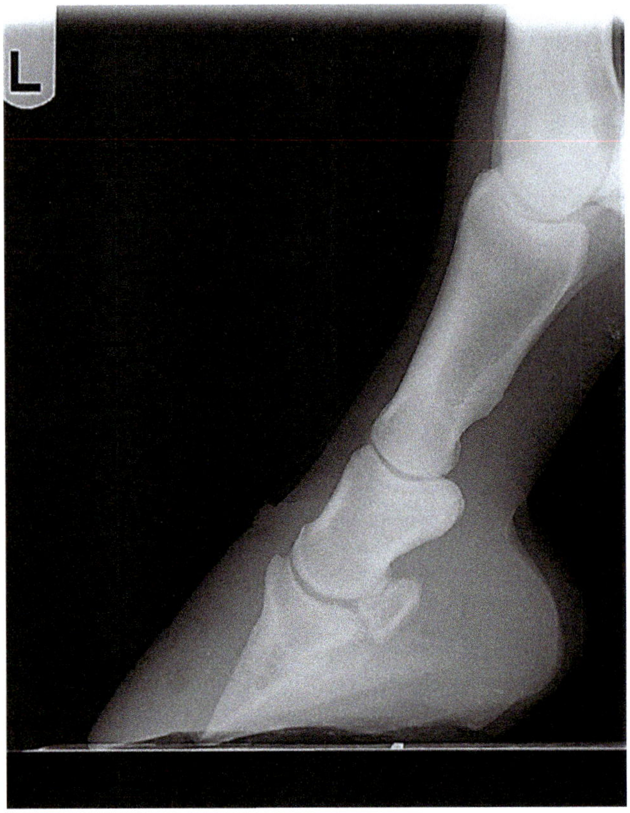

Fig. 15-6 **Radiograph of a horse demonstrating rotation of the distal phalanx with likely penetration of the sole. The coronary band is indented, and there is no evidence of sinking. There is not osteolysis of the distal phalanx.** (Reproduced with permission.[75])

Radiographic examination of the feet is an essential component in evaluation of horses with laminitis. The standard radiographic views that should be obtained to aid assessment of horses with laminitis are the lateromedial, horizontal dorsopalmar, and dorsal 45 degrees proximal palmarodistal oblique views.[74] A variety of objective measures have been developed to aid in the interpretation of radiographic examinations of the feet of laminitic horses (Figs. 15-6 and 15-7), and these are discussed in detail elsewhere.[74]

Initially and in mild cases, changes in the position of the distal phalanx are not evident. Radiographs of more severe or advanced cases will demonstrate rotation of the distal phalanx within the hoof, evident as a tilting of the most distal aspect of the third phalanx toward the sole. The space created by rotation of the pedal bone can fill with gas or serum and be evident as a radiolucent line between the pedal bone and the dorsal hoof wall. Displacement of the pedal bone toward the sole will be evident in approximately 25% of cases as a thickening of the dorsal hoof wall and reduction of the distance between the sole and solar aspect of the distal phalanx. Chronic or refractory cases can have osteopenia of the pedal bone with proliferation of bone at the toe.

Prognosis

The radiographic examination provides information of prognostic value, although because of differing radiographic techniques and interpretations the value of combining separate research studies to develop firm guidelines is difficult.[74] Horses that return to their previous level of athletic function after a bout of laminitis have pedal bone rotation of less than 5.5 degrees, whereas horses that can no longer perform as athletes usually have more than 11.5 degrees of rotation, although there are exceptions to this rule and the prognosis should be developed through a holistic assessment of the horse (level of pain, number of feet involved, sole penetration).[74] Therefore, these values should only be used as rough guidelines. The general rule is that the greater the degree of rotation or extent of displacement of the distal phalanx, the worse the prognosis for return to function and pain-free living.

Objective radiographic variables include the distance between the proximal aspect of the hoof wall (marked on the radiographic image by a piece of wire or strip of metal stuck to the dorsal hoof wall) and the

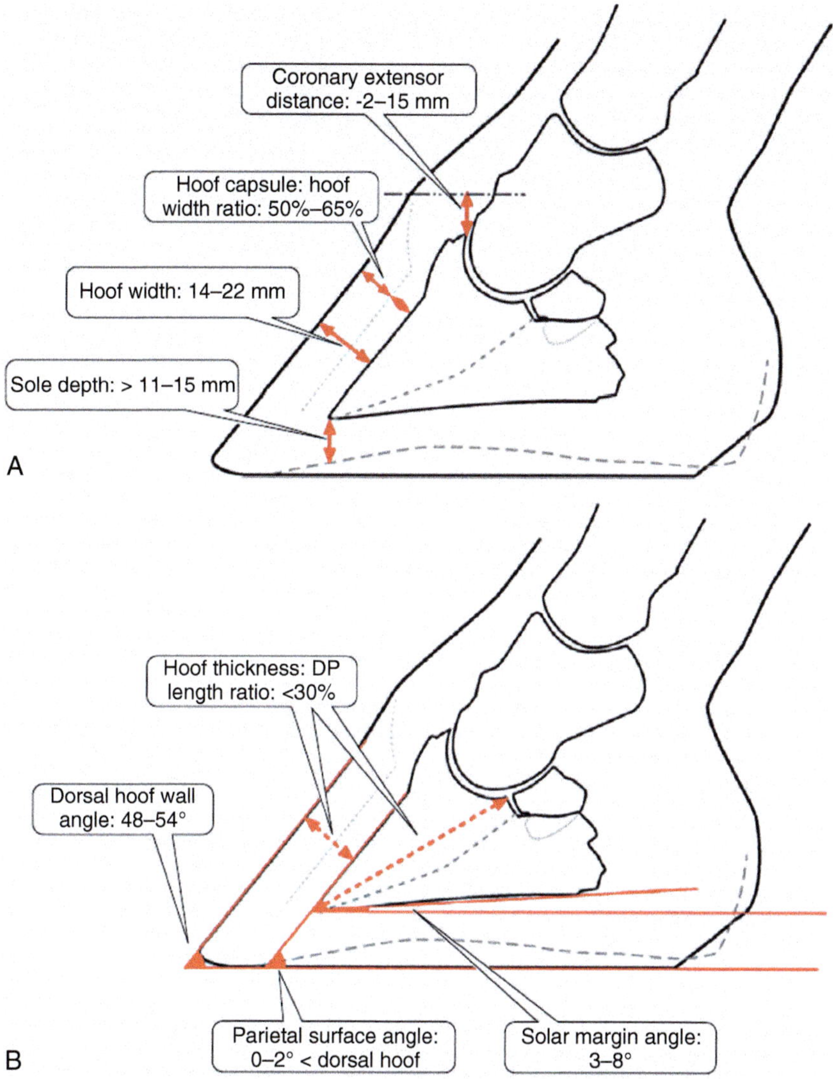

Fig. 15-7 Diagrams showing the normal radiologic distances and proportions in the front feet of sound horses. Care must be taken in interpretation of these values because there is marked individual (breed and size) variability, and many can also be altered by farriery; the measurements in these diagrams do not represent the absolute minimum and maximum of normal values; rather. they are representative of the center of the range. (Reproduced with permission.[74])

proximal limit of the extensor process of the distal phalanx (the "founder" distance), and the distance between the dorsal hoof wall and the dorsal cortex of the distal phalanx. Although values for these measures vary among breeds and with the size of the horse, most normal horses will have a "founder" distance of 4.1 ± 2.2 (standard deviation) mm and a wall thickness of 16.3 ± 2.4 mm. Intensively managed horses with signs of sinking (medial, lateral, or vertical) had an overall success rate of 18% (17/95), whereas nonsinkers (horses with or without apparent rotation) with laminitis had a 71% (107/150) success rate.[75]

CLINICAL PATHOLOGY

There are no changes that are characteristic of the disease.

NECROPSY FINDINGS

The disease is not usually fatal, but severely affected animals are often euthanized. In acute cases, there may be evidence of colitis, grain overload, or retained placenta and metritis in mares. No reliable gross findings are visible on the feet, but a midsagittal section of the hoof may reveal congestion, hemorrhage, and slight separation of the dorsal surface of P3 from the epidermal laminae of the inner surface of the horny hoof wall in severe cases. The separation of P3 becomes more obvious in subacute and chronic cases, leading to a ventral rotation of the phalanx. In some cases the degree of rotation of P3 results in perforation of the sole.

Histologic examination is required only in acute cases, and confirmation of the diagnosis in such instances demands that the foot be cut into slab sections and fixed shortly after the death of the animal, before even moderate autolysis can ensue. Microscopically, the lesions are degeneration and necrosis of epithelial cells of the laminae, separation of epithelial cells from the basement membrane, and loss of the basement membrane.

> **DIFFERENTIAL DIAGNOSIS**
>
> **Horses**
> Rhabdomyolysis, tetanus, colic, and spinal ataxia may all mimic the immobility and pain of laminitis, but there is no pain in the feet in these diseases, and other distinguishing characteristics are apparent on careful clinical examination.

TREATMENT

The adage "where facts are few experts are many" (Donald R. Gannon) applies well to the treatment of laminitis. There are few well-designed studies of the treatment of naturally occurring laminitis, and thus the choice of treatment is based on personal experience, extrapolation from our imperfect understanding of the pathogenesis of the disease, the availability of certain drugs, and current fashion. Indeed, the treatment of laminitis might one day be chronicled to demonstrate the power of "expert" opinion to determine treatments, many of which are now recognized as useless. A fascinating example is that of the application of nitroglycerin patches to the pasterns of horses with laminitis or at increased risk of laminitis. A multitude of horses were treated in this way, some to the extent that they were rendered hypotensive, at considerable direct cost and opportunity cost, and all for naught. Although not intended to discount the opinion of experts in the treatment of laminitis, it is a salutary tale demonstrating the strength of fashion and fad in promoting ineffective treatments of this important disease.

In general, the treatments can be grouped into several classes, based on the intended intervention. These are as follows:

- Removal of the causative agent or treatment of the inciting disease
- Pain relief and minimization of inflammation
- Prevention of further damage to lamellae and rotation or distal displacement of the pedal bone
- Promotion of keratinization and hoof growth

The efficacy of administration of analgesic, antiinflammatory, anticoagulant, and vasodilatory drugs and mechanical support of the hoof has never been demonstrated in appropriate clinical trials. There is evidence that local cryotherapy (cooling of the distal limb) is effective in reducing the clinical signs and severity of lesions of oligofructose-induced experimental laminitis,[76] with limited although supportive clinical evidence.[77]

Acute laminitis is an emergency, and treatment should be started without delay because early and aggressive therapy might enhance the chances of recovery.

Treatment of Inciting Process or Disease

The inciting disease should be treated aggressively and every attempt made to remove any causative agent.

Horses with systemic inflammatory disease (colitis, metritis, etc.) should be treated aggressively to reduce the likelihood that they will develop laminitis. Treatment of colitis, metritis, pleuropneumonia, colic, and other diseases is dealt with under those topics.

Horses with laminitis should be rested and housed in stalls that are well bedded with sand or soft shavings. Horses suspected of having PPID, insulin resistance, or EMS[17] should have the diagnosis confirmed and appropriate therapy instituted.

Cryotherapy or Digital Cooling

There is experimental, and some clinical, evidence that chilling of the feet is effective in preventing development of laminitis and in attenuating the effects of established (acute) laminitis induced experimentally.[77,78]

Progression of experimental laminitis (CHO model) can be prevented by cooling (chilling) of the feet of horses during the prodromal and acute phases of the disease.[76,78] Cooling of the distal limbs of horses administered 10 g/kg body weight of oligofructose markedly reduced the clinical signs of laminitis and development of histologic lesions in the feet of treated horses. Cooling in the experimental model began at the time of administration of oligofructose and continued for 72 hours. Horses treated by immersion of the limbs in cold water (0.5 to 2.0° C; 33–36 F) had only mild signs of lameness (grade I or less) at all times up until euthanasia at 72 hours.[76] Furthermore, chilling of the limbs significantly reduced expression of a range of genes of proinflammatory proteins and increased expression of an antiinflammatory protein during both the prodromal and clinical phases of disease.[79]

Chilling of limbs after the onset of laminitis induced by oligofructose prevents lamellar structural failure and reduces the severity of damage to lamellae.[80] Chilling (cryotherapy) of feet was initiated as soon as Obel grade II lameness was detected (horses were examined every 4 hours) and continued until euthanasia 36 hours after onset of lameness. Horses were also administered phenylbutazone (8 mg/kg IV—a high dose) and had continuous peripheral nerve block to alleviate foot pain. The frequency of weight shifting was significantly reduced in chilled feet, as assessed by pedometer, which was inferred as indicating less pain in chilled feet. It is important to consider that model was one of experimental laminitis, chilling was initiated less than 4 hours after onset of lameness, and chilling was maintained continuously for the duration of the study (36 hours). Whether the treatment would be as effective for other forms of laminitis or if initiated later in the development of lameness, and the optimal duration of chilling, are not known.

A **retrospective case-control study** identified that horses at risk of developing laminitis secondary to colitis were 0.14 (95% confidence interval [CI] 0.04 to 0.51) times less likely to develop laminitis if treated with digital cryotherapy.[77]

It has been practice for some time by both laypeople and veterinarians to cool the feet of acutely laminitic horses. With evidence that chilling reduces clinical and biochemical/genetic signs of inflammation in the feet of horses with induced laminitis, there is justification for clinical trials to determine the usefulness of this treatment in horses with acute or ongoing (chronic, active) laminitis. Prophylactic chilling of the feet of horses at high risk of developing laminitis, such as those with colitis, pleuropneumonia, metritis, and grain engorgement, could be considered, recognizing that there is a history of proposed treatments for laminitis that have not lived up to their promise. Protocols for chilling of limbs in a clinical setting have not been developed or demonstrated to be effective and without important adverse effects. It is important that any such protocols address issues such as the optimal time for starting cooling of limbs in horses with acute laminitis, duration of treatment, how to rewarm the limb, whether all limbs or only the forelimbs should be cooled, efficacy in differing forms of laminitis (endocrinopathic, sepsis-associated, supporting limb, concussive), and long-term outcome. Techniques have been developed to assist in monitoring the distal limb temperatures of horses during limb chilling.[81]

Analgesics and Antiinflammatory Drugs

A mainstay of the treatment of both acute and chronic laminitis is the use of nonsteroidal antiinflammatory drugs (NSAIDs). These are administered to provide pain relief, and there is no evidence that they delay progression of the disease.

Phenylbutazone, at doses of 2.2 to 4.4 mg/kg IV or orally every 12 to 24 hours, is an effective analgesic in cases of mild to moderate laminitis. Higher doses (6.6 mg/kg every 12 to 24 hours) can be required in severe cases. However, the potential for phenylbutazone toxicosis, evident as colic, gastrointestinal ulceration, nephrosis, hypoproteinemia, leukopenia, and hyponatremia, is dose related, and high doses of phenylbutazone should only be used for at most several days and only in horses experiencing severe pain. **Flunixin meglumine** (1.1 mg/kg, IM or IV every 8 to 12 hours) or **ketoprofen** (2.2 mg/kg, IM every 12 to 24 hours) are also effective analgesics. Their concurrent use with phenylbutazone can enhance pain relief but also increases the risk of NSAID toxicosis. A number of other NSAIDs are available for use in horses (meloxicam, firocoxib) and might be useful for management of pain in some horses. The use of aspirin is dealt with under "Anticoagulants."

Narcotic analgesics such as butorphanol, morphine, and meperidine (pethidine) provide effective pain relief; α-2 agonists such as **xylazine and detomidine** provide only brief respite from the pain.

Horses with severe lameness (Obel grade III or IV) might benefit from administration of drug cocktails including tramadol and subanesthetic doses of ketamine (0.6 mg/kg per hour IV)[82] or constant-rate infusions of a mixture of an α-2 agonist, a narcotic, and ketamine.[83] The use of objective assessment tools to assess the severity of pain and response to administration of analgesics is preferred over unstructured assessment of pain.[83]

Local analgesia of the foot with agents such as lidocaine or bupivacaine provides marked pain relief. However, analgesia is usually only brief, depending on the agent used, and has the disadvantage of causing the horse to bear more weight on the affected limbs. Local analgesia can be useful in facilitating relocation of the horse, hoof trimming, corrective shoeing, or application of sole and frog support, but not as a routine treatment.

Lidocaine, administered intravenously as a constant-rate infusion, has been advocated as an antiinflammatory drug for the treatment of laminitis. However, evidence from the black-walnut model of laminitis does not indicate efficacy in reducing markers of inflammation.[84]

Because of suspicion that **corticosteroids** induce or exacerbate laminitis, at this time their use is contraindicated in the treatment of laminitis.[24-26,85,86]

Vasodilatory Drugs

Vasodilatory drugs are used on the premise that vasoconstriction is an important mechanism underlying the development or progression of acute laminitis. Several classes of drugs have been used, including α-adrenergic antagonists such as phenoxybenzamine and phentolamine, drugs with multiple mechanisms of action such as acepromazine and isoxsuprine, and nitric oxide donors such as glyceryl trinitrate (nitroglycerine) and L-arginine. None of the vasodilatory drugs should be used in horses with compromised cardiovascular function or dehydration.

Phenoxybenzamine and phentolamine are not readily available and have limited use. Phenoxybenzamine causes sedation. **Acepromazine** is a potent vasodilator, principally because of its α-adrenergic antagonist activity, that is currently used occasionally in the treatment of acute laminitis.[12] Acepromazine increases blood flow to the digit, but its effect on nutritive flow to the lamellae is unknown, as is the case for all the vasodilators. The effect of Acepromazine persists for approximately 90 minutes after IV administration. Acepromazine can be administered at dose rates ranging from 0.01 to 0.05 mg/kg, IM, every 6 to 12 hours. Sedation may be considerable at the higher doses and/or with more frequent administration and might be a desired effect in reducing movement (and hence potential for further damage to lamellae) and anxiety. **Isoxsuprine** is a combined α-antagonist and β-agonist that increases blood flow to the leg but not to the foot in normal horses. It has been used at doses of 1 to 1.5 mg/kg orally every 12 hours. Pentoxifylline (4.4 mg/kg orally q8h), which increases red blood cell deformability, does not increase digital blood flow in normal horses.

Application of **nitroglycerine** a nitric oxide donor, to the palmar digital arteries of affected horses has been reported to increase or not affect blood flow to the dorsal hoof wall. However, the effect of these substances on the course of the disease is unknown. In spontaneous cases of acute laminitis, nitroglycerine has been applied to the skin over both palmar digital arteries of affected feet at a dose of 15 to 30 mg per artery, once daily. However, because of lack of evidence of efficacy and the potential for systemic hypotension secondary to systemic absorption of the drug, its use is no longer recommended.

Anticoagulants

Anticoagulant drugs are administered to prevent the development of microthrombi within the hoof. Current evidence does not support an important role for microthrombi in the development of laminitis. However, activated platelets do accumulate in lamellar vessels and release vasoactive compounds.[59] Aspirin is a very poor analgesic in horses but is used because it reduces platelet aggregation in normal horses by blocking formation of thromboxane A_2. However, thromboxane may not be an important cause of platelet aggregation in horses. Aspirin is administered at a dose of 10 mg/kg orally every 48 hours. The efficacy of aspirin in the treatment of laminitis has not been determined.

Heparin in sufficient doses prolongs blood clotting, provided that there is adequate antithrombin III in the patient's blood. Heparin has been reported to prevent or to have no effect on the development of laminitis in horses with anterior enteritis or colic, respectively. Heparin can be administered at 40 to 80 IU/kg IV or subcutaneously (SC) every 8 to 12 hours for 3 to 5 days. Anemia can develop during heparin administration but resolves rapidly when administration of the drug is stopped.

Administration of low-molecular-weight heparin is proposed as prophylaxis for laminitis in horses at high risk of the disease. A study of horses admitted for colic surgery included 304 horses treated with low-molecular-weight heparin between 1995 and 2007 and 56 horses, admitted before 1995, that were not treated with the compound found that the prevalence of horses developing laminitis in the treatment group (3.3%; 95% CI, 1.7% to 6.2%) was significantly lower than in the control group (10.7%; 95% CI, 4.4% to 22.6%).[87] However, horses in the control group were a historical control, and there might well be other factors that contributed to the reduction in incidence of laminitis, such as improved preoperative, intraoperative, and postoperative care. This one study cannot be considered to provide proof of efficacy.

Mechanical Support

Mechanical support to provide pain relief, minimize further damage to lamellae, and in an attempt to prevent rotation or distal displacement of the pedal bone is an important part of the care of horses with acute laminitis.

Support of the frog and/or sole can be achieved using packing material such as dental acrylic or firm plastic or silicone that is molded to conform to the shape of the sole. Some clinicians prefer to use **wedge pads** to elevate the heel and reduce tension in the deep digital flexor tendon, with the aim of preventing rotation of the distal phalanx by reducing "break-over" forces. Trimming of the toe could achieve the same effect.

Housing the horse on sand or other soft bedding is frequently recommended.

Corrective shoeing of horses with chronic laminitis is widely practiced, and there are proponents of a wide variety of shoe types (fullered egg-bar, heart-bar, glue-on shoes). Appropriate hoof care, which might include shoeing, is important in managing horses with chronic laminitis. Interestingly, there was not a difference among shoe types in efficacy for pain relief in horses with chronic laminitis.

Promotion of Healing

Methionine has been given to both acute and chronic laminitis cases on the known requirement for methionine in the chondroitin complex of collagen. There is some rationale for the treatment, but it seems more appropriate as a supportive than as a principal treatment. The oral dose rate is 10 g/day for 3 days followed by 5 g/day for 10 days.

Antibiotics might be indicated to treat secondary infection of the degenerate lamellae.

Rest is important in the convalescent phase. Horses with no rotation or sinking of the pedal bone should be rested after resolution of the clinical signs. Return to work should be gradual. Horses that develop rotation or sinking of the pedal bone should be monitored both by physical examination and radiographic examination. It will be many months before horses with even mild rotation can be returned to work. Horses with severe rotation or sinking will likely never resume active work, although they may become pasture sound.

TREATMENT

Summary of treatment of acute laminitis

Depending on the cause, treatment of acute laminitis should include:

- Chilling of the limb (cryotherapy) (R-1)
- Administration of nonsteroidal antiinflammatory drugs (R-1)
- Administration of vasodilators (acepromazine) (R-2)
- Support of the frog and/or sole (R-1)
- Application of nitroglycerin (R-4)
- Aggressive treatment of the inciting disease (R-1)
- Trimming the hoof, distal phalanx realignment, and corrective shoeing (R-1)

Chronic Laminitis

The **prognosis** for return to normal of horses with chronic or refractory laminitis (laminitis of more than 1 week's duration) is poor (see previous discussion for the use of radiography to determine prognosis).

Treatment includes NSAIDs for pain relief, corrective shoeing (egg-bar or heart-bar shoes), trimming of the hoof (shortening the toe or complete removal of the dorsal hoof wall), and realignment of the distal phalanx.[88] Rehabilitating rotational displacement usually involves shoeing changes that move the center of pressure of the foot caudally from its normal position under the toes, decrease tension on the deep digital flexor tendon to reduce rotational forces on the distal phalanx that act to increase the distance between the distal phalanx and dorsal hoof wall, provide axial support of load structures within the perimeter of the wall (sole, frog, bars), and ease break-over in all directions (medial, lateral, and dorsally) in an effort to reduce distraction forces on the lamellae during movement.[75] Methods to move the center of pressure caudally and decrease tension on the deep digital flexor tendon using bar shoes and a heel elevation are recommended.[75] Use of a wedge to counteract rotational forces might be beneficial.[75]

Tenotomy of the deep digital flexor can provide relief, but the efficacy of this procedure in affecting long-term outcome has not been well demonstrated.[11,75]

CONTROL

The disease is not readily subject to control because of its sporadic nature, with the exception of management of diseases that increase risk of laminitis, such as PPID, insulin resistance, and EMS. Details of the management of these conditions is provided elsewhere.

Moderate exercise by nonobese ponies previously affected with laminitis reduced serum amyloid A concentrations and haptoglobin concentrations and led to reductions in exercise-induced increases in postexercise serum insulin concentrations.[89] These results suggest a beneficial role for relatively low-intensity exercise (10 minutes enforced walking followed by 5 minutes of trotting) on inflammation in ponies at risk of laminitis.

FURTHER READING

Katz LM, Bailey SR. A review of recent advances and hypotheses on the pathogenesis of acute laminitis. *Equine Vet J*. 2012;44:752-761.

Pollitt C. Advances in laminitis. Parts 1 and 2. *Vet Clin North Am-Equine*. 2010;26(1-2):1-466.

REFERENCES

1. Eustace RA. *Vet J*. 2010;183:245.
2. Parks AH, et al. *Equine Vet Educ*. 2009;21:102.
3. Pollitt CC. *Vet Clin Equine*. 2010;26:29.
4. Wylie CE. *Vet J*. 2013;196:139.
5. Asplin KE, et al. *Vet J*. 2007;174:530.
6. de Laat MA, et al. *Vet J*. 2012;191:317.
7. Karikoski NP, et al. *Dom Anim Endocrin*. 2011;41:111.
8. Belknap J, et al. *Equine Vet J*. 2012;44:749.
9. de Laat MA, et al. *Vet J*. 2012;192:435.
10. Wylie CE, et al. *Vet J*. 2012;193:58.
11. Radostits O, et al. Laminitis of horses. In: *Veterinary Medicine: A Textbook of the Diseases of Cattle, Horses, Sheep, Goats and Pigs*. 10th ed. London: Saunders; 2007:2030.
12. Menzies-Gow NJ, et al. *Vet Rec*. 2010;167:690.
13. Slater J. *Vet Rec*. 2014;175:271.
14. Treiber KH, et al. *JAVMA*. 2006;228:1538.
15. Carter RA, et al. *Equine Vet J*. 2009;41:171.
16. Borer KE, et al. *J Anim Sci*. 2012;90:3003.
17. Frank N, et al. *J Vet Int Med*. 2010;24:467.
18. Geor RJ. *Vet Clin Equine*. 2009;25:39.
19. McGowan C. *J Equine Vet Sci*. 2008;28:603.
20. Tadros EM, et al. *Equine Vet Educ*. 2013;25:152.
21. Valle E, et al. *Vet J*. 2013;196:445.
22. Knowles EJ, et al. *Equine Vet J*. 2012;44:226.
23. McGowan TW, et al. *Equine Vet J*. 2013;45:74.
24. Bailey SR. *Vet Clin Equine*. 2010;26:277.
25. Bailey SR, et al. *Equine Vet J*. 2007;39:7.
26. Bathe AP. *Equine Vet J*. 2007;39:12.
27. Virgin JE, et al. *Equine Vet J*. 2011;43:7.
28. Parsons CS, et al. *JAVMA*. 2007;230:885.
29. Menzies-Gow NJ, et al. *Vet Rec*. 2010;167:364.
30. Orsini JA, et al. *Can Vet J*. 2010;51:623.
31. Visser MB, et al. *J Comp Pathol*. 2011;145:80.
32. Chiavaccini L, et al. *Vet Immunol Immunopath*. 2011;144:366.
33. de la Rebiere de Pouyade G, et al. *Vet Immunol Immunopath*. 2010;135:181.
34. Stewart AJ, et al. *Vet Immunol Immunopath*. 2009;129:254.
35. Pollitt CC. *Equine Laminitis: Current Concepts*. Canberra, Australia: Rural Industries Research and Development Corporation; 2008.
36. Wang L, et al. *J Vet Int Med*. 2014;28:215.
37. de Laat MA, et al. *J Comp Pathol*. 2011;145:399.
38. Katz LM, et al. *Equine Vet J*. 2012;44:752.
39. Belknap JK, et al. *Equine Vet J*. 2007;39:42.
40. Black SJ. *Vet Immunol Immunopath*. 2009;129:161.
41. Loftus JP, et al. *Am J Vet Res*. 2007;68:1205.
42. Faleiros RR, et al. *J Vet Int Med*. 2009;23:174.
43. Leise BS, et al. *Equine Vet J*. 2011;43:54.
44. Faleiros RR, et al. *J Vet Int Med*. 2011;25:107.
45. Faleiros RR, et al. *Vet Immunol Immunopath*. 2011;144:45.
46. Visser MB, et al. *Vet Immunol Immunopath*. 2011;144:120.
47. Budak MT, et al. *Vet Immunol Immunopath*. 2009;131:86.
48. Moreau MM, et al. *Vet Microbiol*. 2014;168:436.
49. Asplin KE, et al. *Equine Vet J*. 2010;42:700.
50. de Laat MA, et al. *Vet J*. 2013;195:305.
51. Nourian AR, et al. *Equine Vet J*. 2009;41:671.
52. Nourian AR, et al. *Equine Vet J*. 2007;39:360.
53. Karikoski NP, et al. *Am J Vet Res*. 2014;75:161.
54. de Laat MA, et al. *Vet J*. 2013;197:302.
55. de Laat MA, et al. *Vet Immunol Immunopath*. 2012;145:395.
56. de Laat MA, et al. *Vet Immunol Immunopath*. 2014;157:78.
57. Gauff F, et al. *Equine Vet J*. 2013;45:613.
58. Keen JA, et al. *J Vet Pharmacol Ther*. 2013;36:382.
59. Bailey SR, et al. *Vet Immunol Immunopath*. 2009;129:167.
60. Eades SC, et al. *Am J Vet Res*. 2007;68:87.
61. Eades SC, et al. *Am J Vet Res*. 2006;67:1204.
62. Peroni JF, et al. *Equine Vet J*. 2005;37:546.
63. Peroni JF, et al. *J Appl Phys*. 2006;100:759.
64. de Laat MA, et al. *Vet Immunol Immunopath*. 2011;140:275.
65. Loftus JP, et al. *Vet Immunol Immunopath*. 2009;129:221.
66. Pawlak E, et al. *Am J Vet Res*. 2012;73:1035.
67. Wang L, et al. *Am J Vet Res*. 2012;73:1047.
68. Belknap JK, et al. *Equine Vet J*. 2012;44:738.
69. Kwon S, et al. *Vet Immunol Immunopath*. 2013;155:1.
70. Orsini JA. *Equine Vet J*. 2012;44:741.
71. Steelman SM, et al. *Vet Immunol Immunopath*. 2013;153:217.
72. Menzies-Gow NJ, et al. *Vet Rec*. 2010;167:52.
73. Vinuela-Fernandez I, et al. *Vet J*. 2011;188:171.
74. Sherlock C, et al. *Equine Vet Educ*. 2013;25:524.
75. Morrison S. *J Equine Vet Sci*. 2011;31:89.
76. van Eps AW, et al. *Equine Vet J*. 2009;41:741.
77. Kullmann A, et al. *Equine Vet J*. 2014;46:554.
78. van Eps AW, et al. *Equine Vet J*. 2014;46:625.
79. van Eps AW, et al. *Equine Vet J*. 2012;44:230.
80. van Eps A, et al. *Equine Vet J*. 2014;46:625-630.
81. Reesink HL, et al. *Am J Vet Res*. 2012;73:860.
82. Guedes AGP, et al. *Am J Vet Res*. 2012;73:610.
83. Dutton DW, et al. *Equine Vet Educ*. 2009;21:37.
84. Williams JM, et al. *Equine Vet J*. 2010;42:261.
85. Cornelisse CJ, et al. *Equine Vet Educ*. 2013;25:39.
86. Dutton H. *Equine Vet J*. 2007;39:5.
87. de la Rebiere de Pouyade G, et al. *J Vet Emerg Crit Care*. 2009;19:113.
88. O'Grady SE. *Equine Vet Educ*. 2006;18:214.
89. Menzies-Gow NJ, et al. *Equine Vet J*. 2013;46:317-321.

LAMINITIS IN RUMINANTS AND SWINE

SYNOPSIS

Etiology Degeneration of the sensitive laminellae of the hoof.

Epidemiology
Cattle: An endemic disease of some herds of high-producing dairy cattle, and in feedlots. Associated with ruminal acidosis, either clinical or subclinical.

Clinical signs
Cattle: Inapparent to severe lameness, most common in the hindfeet. Predisposition to other infectious or traumatic diseases of the foot.

Clinical pathology None characteristic of the disease.

Diagnostic confirmation Physical examination. Radiography.

Treatment
Cattle: Nonsteroidal antiinflammatory drugs. Corrective hoof care.

Control
Cattle: Dietary control to prevent ruminal acidosis. Correction of housing and flooring problems.

ETIOLOGY

Laminitis is caused by acute degeneration of the sensitive primary and secondary lamellae of the hoof. The cause of this degeneration is unknown, although the disease can be induced by administration of oligofructose (17 g/kg, orally) to dairy heifers.[1,2] The disease is less well characterized than that of horses, and several conditions are often classified as laminitis. Laminitis in dairy cattle occurs as part of a spectrum of foot diseases.[3,4] There is a detailed description of the radiographic (CT) anatomy of the digit of cattle.[5]

EPIDEMIOLOGY

Occurrence

In **cattle** the disease can occur as clusters in herds and on farms where a predisposition appears to be inherited or where access to large quantities of soluble carbohydrate are available, such as for high-producing dairy cows or feedlot cattle. On farms of high-producing dairy cattle the prevalence may be as high as 78%. The prevalence of laminitis-related hoof lesions in Norwegian dairy cattle is 18%,[6] although the prevalence is lower in Switzerland.[7] Among Swiss cattle, 5.4% had signs of subclinical laminitis, and 3.3% had signs of chronic laminitis.[7] A recent study of 1352 dairy cows in Israel detected lameness in 387 (28.6%).[8] Of these lame cows, 320 (82.7%) had 591 lesions that could be associated with subclinical laminitis.[8]

Risk Factors

Cattle and Sheep

Subclinical laminitis that predisposes to the development of other diseases of the hoof occurs in calves and first-calf heifers and is common in intensively fed feedlot cattle. Laminitis, conditioned by the inheritance of an autosomal-recessive gene, is recorded in Jersey heifers.[9] There may be an association between the disease in feedlot ruminants and **ruminal acidosis**. Administration of oligofructose to dairy heifers induced ruminal acidosis, with clinical signs of laminitis (hoof pain and abnormal gait) occurring by 30 hours after administration and being most severe at 3 to 5 days.[1]

Beef cattle being prepared for shows are often grossly overfed on high-grain rations and become affected with a chronic form of the disease that markedly affects their gait and may cause permanent foot deformity. The disease occurs in dairy cattle fed improper rations, especially first-calf heifers and cattle of herds attempting to increase milk production, and it is not uncommon for the disease to present as a herd problem.

Among **dairy cattle,** the heifers are usually the most affected, and the disease usually develops soon after calving, with more than 50% of cases occurring in the period 30 days before and 30 days after calving. There may be a relationship between being introduced to the herd, with the frequent harassment by dominant cows, when heavily pregnant, and when the surface of the yards is rough. Housing can be important, including standing in slurry or having to twist and turn in narrow passageways and races, and there is an association between the prevalence of the disease and rough concrete floors.

Diet is an important risk factor for development of laminitis in heifers. Diets of wet, fermented grass silage are associated with a greater risk of laminitis than are diets rich in dry unfermented straw and a concentrate. Furthermore, transition from a low-net-energy diet to a high-net-energy diet immediately after calving increases the risk of subclinical mastitis in Holstein dairy cows.

The disease is also reported to occur after metritis, retained placenta, mastitis, and mammary edema, but the incidence is not usually very high.

Pigs

Laminitis has been recorded in pigs, but the disease is difficult to diagnose in this species, and many cases secondary to other diseases (e.g., postparturient fever) can be missed. The disease is also recorded when pigs are fed very heavy concentrate diets.

Importance

Subclinical laminitis of dairy cattle predisposes to other hoof disease that decrease milk production.[10]

PATHOGENESIS

The pathogenesis of laminitis in cattle, sheep, and pigs is unclear but likely has some similarity to that in horses (see "Laminitis in Horses"), with increased expression of genes coding inflammatory or proinflammatory products in corium of cattle with induced laminitis.[11] The links between nutrition and lameness in cattle have been reviewed.[12] Chronic laminitis leads to a low resistance of claw horn to mechanical insults in the dorsal wall, abaxial wall, and sole,[13] which could explain why laminitis predisposes cattle to other foot lesions.

CLINICAL FINDINGS

Cattle and Sheep

In cattle and sheep the clinical picture is similar to but less marked than that observed in the horse.

In **calves 4 to 6 months** of age, and in heifers, an acute syndrome similar to that seen in the horse has been described. Affected animals lie down much of the time and are reluctant to rise. When they attempt to rise, they remain kneeling for long periods. Their standing posture is with all four feet bunched together with the back arched; they shift their weight from foot to foot frequently and walk with a shuffling, painful gait. The feet are painful when squeezed and later become flattened and enlarged and look as though slippers are being worn. There is severe ventral rotation of the third phalanx.

In **adult cows** some cases have acute signs, whereas others show only local lesions. These include sole ulcers and patchy changes in the horn, including softening, waxy yellow discoloration, and red–brown patches suggestive of previous hemorrhage. The cow is chronically lame.

Young bulls are very susceptible to laminitis and may develop abnormalities of gait and posture, such as a stilted gait and frequent knuckling of the fetlocks, which may mislead the diagnostician.

Chronic laminitis in adult cows is characterized by a smaller anterior hoof wall-sole angle, down from 55 degrees to 35 degrees, a concave anterior wall, and the appearance of horizontal grooves (growth arrest lines) around the entire claw. The sole is usually dropped a little, and bruising and sole ulcers may be present. Overgrowth of the sole of the lateral claw may reach the point of creating a false or double sole. The white line is greatly widened and disrupted, and stones and other debris may be impacted in it.

Chronic, traumatic laminitis is most common in heifers when they are first introduced into the milking or dry herds. Housing them on concrete and exposing them to frequent confrontations with bossy cows lead to the development of sole hemorrhages and inflammation of the laminae.

Radiographic signs in cattle include rarefaction of the pedal bone, particularly the toe, and the development of osteophytes at the heel and on the pyramidal process.

Pigs

In sows the clinical signs are similar and include arching of the back, bunching of the feet, awkwardness of movement, increased pulsation in the digital arteries, and pain when pressure is applied to the feet.

CLINICAL PATHOLOGY

There are no changes that are characteristic of the disease.

NECROPSY FINDINGS

Histologic examination of claws from heifers killed 72 hours after overload showed changes consistent with acute laminitis, including stretched lamellae, wider basal cells with low chromatin density, and a thick, wavy, and blurry appearance of the basement membrane.[2,14]

DIFFERENTIAL DIAGNOSIS

Cattle

- White-muscle disease, epiphysitis, other primary diseases of the foot

TREATMENT

Although similar principles to those used to determine treatment of laminitis in horses are likely to apply to cattle, treatment in cattle is usually limited to administration of NSAIDs (aspirin 20 mg/kg, orally every 12 hours, phenylbutazone 4.4 mg/kg orally every 48 hours, or flunixin meglumine 1.0 mg/kg IV every 12 hours). The inciting cause (metritis, ruminal acidosis) should be treated aggressively.

CONTROL

Cattle and lambs that are brought into feedlots should be gradually introduced to grain feeds and a higher forage:grain ratio provided in the feed. Calves should not be fed intensively on grain until they are 14 months old because of the high frequency of internal hoof lesions at the earlier ages. Some protection against laminitis in dairy cattle in intensive units is gained by careful planning of housing cubicles to make them more comfortable and less damaging to the feet and by providing more straw in the cubicles. Exercise should be provided around calving time. Vaccination with a gram-negative bacterin-endotoxoid combination vaccine has provided some protection against laminitis induced by grain overload. Dietary supplementation of biotin (20 mg per head per day) improves hoof health of primiparous dairy cows and may be beneficial in reducing the incidence or severity of lameness in a herd. This treatment might not improve objective indicators of hoof health, but it does improve production.

Selection of traits for foot and leg conformation in Norwegian Red cattle is not associated with a reduced risk of disease of the claws.[15]

REFERENCES

1. Danscher AM, et al. *J Dairy Sci.* 2009;92:607.
2. Danscher AM, et al. *J Dairy Sci.* 2010;93:53.
3. Capion N, et al. *Vet Rec.* 2008;163:80.
4. Capion N, et al. *Vet J.* 2009;182:50.
5. Tsuka T, et al. *J Dairy Sci.* 2014;97:6271.
6. Fjeldaas T, et al. *Acta Vet Scand.* 2007;49.
7. Becker J, et al. *Schweiz Arch Tierheilkd.* 2014;156:71.
8. Sagliyan A, et al. *Israel J Vet Med.* 2010;65:27.
9. Radostits O, et al. Laminitis in ruminants and pigs. In: *Veterinary Medicine: A Textbook of the Diseases*

of Cattle, Horses, Sheep, Goats and Pigs. London: Saunders; 2006:2034.
10. Vatandoost M, et al. *J Anim Vet Adv*. 2009;8:880.
11. Osorio JS, et al. *J Dairy Sci*. 2012;95:6388.
12. Lean IJ, et al. *Livestock Sci*. 2013;156:71.
13. Hinterhofer C, et al. *Vet J*. 2007;174:605.
14. Mendes HMF, et al. *Pesquisa Veterinaria Brasileira*. 2013;33:613.
15. Odegard C, et al. *J Dairy Sci*. 2014;97:4522.

Diseases of Joints

DEGENERATIVE JOINT DISEASE (OSTEOARTHROPATHY) AND OSTEOCHONDROSIS

There are two common noninfectious conditions of the joint, degenerative joint disease and osteochondrosis. The terms *degenerative joint disease* and *osteoarthropathy* are used here to describe noninfectious lesions of the articular surfaces of joints characterized by the following:

- Degeneration and erosion of articular cartilage
- Eburnation of subchondral bones
- Hypertrophy of bone surrounding the articular cartilage, resulting in lipping and spur formation at the joint margins

In contrast, a separate condition is **osteochondrosis** (dyschondroplasia), which is a degeneration of both the deep layers of the articular cartilage and the epiphyseal plate—**a defect in endochondral ossification**—that occurs most commonly in pigs and horses but also occurs in cattle. Osteochondrosis in horses is one of a number of conditions included in **developmental orthopedic disease**, which is a catch phrase that includes a number of skeletal conditions of the rapidly growing horse.[1]

ETIOLOGY AND EPIDEMIOLOGY

The etiology of degenerative joint disease and osteochondrosis is not clear in some cases. In most of the commonly occurring cases, the lesions are considered to have a genetic basis and to be multifactorial and perhaps secondary to conformational defects resulting in excessive joint laxity, acute traumatic injury of a joint, the normal aging process, and nutritional deficiencies. The etiologic information is primarily circumstantial, and some of the epidemiologic observations that have been associated with degenerative joint disease and osteochondrosis of farm animals are outlined here.

Nutritional Causes

- Secondary to, or associated with, rickets, osteomalacia, bowie, and osteodystrophia fibrosa
- Coxofemoral arthropathy in dairy cattle associated with aphosphorosis
- Experimental diets deficient in manganese or magnesium, causing arthropathy and joint deformity in some calves—magnesium supplementation of foals decreased the prevalence of osteochondrosis.[2]
- Copper deficiency is thought to be related to osteochondrosis and enlargement of limb joints in foals on pasture and pigs fed experimental copper-deficient diets, and deficiency appears to impair the repair of damaged bone.[1]
- Experimental riboflavin deficiency in pigs

Toxic Causes

- As part of the enzootic calcinosis syndrome caused by poisoning with *Solanum malacoxylon* and others
- Fluorosis in cattle
- Chronic zinc poisoning in pigs and foals

Steroid Induced

The intraarticular injection or prolonged parenteral administration of corticosteroids in horses may lead to degenerative joint disease.

Biomechanical Trauma

- **Acute traumatic injury**—injury to, for example, joint surfaces, menisci, and ligaments, especially the cruciate ligaments of the stifle joints of breeding bulls, may lead to chronic progressive osteoarthritis. Injuries to the femorotibial ligaments of horses can predispose to osteoarthropathy of the stifle joint.
- **Repeated subacute trauma** to joint surfaces can lead to degenerative arthropathy. This is common in young racehorses in training, which may have their joint surfaces and surrounding tissues made susceptible to injury because of conformational defects and subtle deficiencies of calcium and phosphorus. Hard running surfaces may also contribute to the onset of degenerative joint disease.
- **Trauma caused by movement** is suspected of contributing to the erosive lesions on the articular surfaces of some horses affected by enzootic incoordination, the intervertebral joints of caudal thoracic and cranial lumbar vertebrae of old bulls with spondylitis, and the condition of bulls with inherited spasticity. Coxofemoral osteoarthritis may occur in aged horses with joint instability and in calves with hip dysplasia.

Degenerative coxofemoral arthropathy occurs in **young beef bulls** as early as 9 months of age. A congenital shallow acetabulum may predispose bulls to this condition. It may be secondary to hip dysplasia, but in some cases there is no evidence of this. The large, weight-bearing joints subjected to the greatest movement and concussion appear to be most susceptible. Rapidly growing bull calves appear to be most susceptible, and some of them have an inherited susceptibility.

Aging Process

Degenerative arthropathy in aged dairy cows and bulls may be a manifestation of the normal aging process. Degenerative joint disease and vertebral osteophysis occur in middle-aged bulls.

Osteoarthrosis of the distal tarsal joints (hock), commonly known as **bone spavin**, is common in Icelandic horses and strongly related to age. In Icelandic horses aged 6 to 12 years and used for riding, the prevalence of radiographic signs of osteoarthrosis in the distal tarsus increased from 18% in horses 6 years of age up to 54% in 12-year-old horses. The age of onset of radiographic signs reflect a predisposition to bone spavin and indicates a trait with medium to high heritability. There is a high prevalence of chondronecrosis in young Icelandic horses, indicating an early onset and slow progression of disease. The disease is the most common cause of culling as a result of disease in riding horses in the age group of 7 to 17 years.

Osteoarthrosis of the antebrachial joint of riding horses has been described. Affected animals were aged mares that developed osteoarthrosis and ankylosis. The cause is unknown.

Osteochondrosis

Osteochondrosis occurs in rapidly growing **cattle** raised in confinement on hard, usually concrete, floors and with minimal exercise. Osteochondrosis has been reported in rapidly growing bull beef calves fed a diet lacking adequate calcium, sodium, copper, and vitamins A, D, and E and grazing on improved native pasture, in which a common ancestral sire and gender (all males) might have been contributing factors. Severe osteochondrosis of multiple joints but with remarkable changes in the humeral head and glenoid of both shoulder joints in 10-month-old beef calves has been described.

Osteochondrosis in feedlot cattle may be associated with a high-calorie diet and rapid growth rate. It is thought that weight-bearing trauma in these rapidly growing animals is sufficient to cause degenerative lesions of certain joints, especially in animals with a skeletal conformation that results in abnormal stress on certain weight-bearing condyles of long bones. In a series of 42 cases of stifle lameness in cattle, 18 had evidence of subchondral bone cyst and ranged in age from 6 to 18 months. Subchondral bone cyst is considered as a common clinical manifestation of osteochondrosis.

Osteochondrosis similar to that seen in pigs has been recorded in purebred **Suffolk lambs** raised in a system designed to produce rapidly growing, high-value **rams**. The disease has been recorded in a single pedigree Suffolk ram.

Osteochondrosis is an important cause of lameness in **horses**. It is usually seen in young rapidly growing animals, and it affects males more commonly than females. Mares that are fed concentrates during pregnancy are more likely to produce foals that will develop clinical signs associated with osteochondrosis. Moreover, foals kept entirely on pasture for their first year of life are less affected with osteochondrosis than foals housed in box stalls.[3,4] The predilection sites of osteochondrosis in the horse and their general order of incidence are hock, stifle, scapula-humeral joint, fetlock, and cervical spine. The stifle, hock, and scapula-humeral joints are more commonly affected, but many other joints may also be affected, including the metatarsal and metacarpal bones and, rarely, the acetabula of young foals. There is a nutritional component to osteochondrosis, with magnesium supplementation of foals decreasing the prevalence[2] and copper deficiency appearing to interfere with normal bone-repair processes.[1] There is also a genetic component to osteochondrosis, but the mechanism has not been identified.

The epidemiology, heritability, and body measurements and clinical findings of osteochondrosis of hock and fetlock joints in Standardbred trotters have been examined. The incidence of the disease is high in the Swedish Standardbred population and well developed by the age of 18 months. The incidence of osteochondrosis is higher in horses born later in the foaling season than earlier, and the incidence was related to body size: affected horses were taller at the withers and had a greater circumference of the carpus. This suggests that differences in body size at birth and the first few months of the foal's life are of major importance in the development of osteochondrosis. The heritability estimates of osteochondrosis in the hock and fetlock joints of 753 Standardbred trotters 6 to 21 months of age were 0.52 and 0.21, respectively.

Osteochondrosis and arthrosis are considered to be major causes of "leg weakness" in rapidly growing **pigs**. Restricting the energy intake appears to decrease the prevalence and severity of osteochondrosis when gilts are examined at 100 kg, and osteochondrosis is more common in pigs with faster growth rates from weaning to 3 months of age.[5] The prevalence and severity of osteochondrosis in growing pigs are probably not related to floor type. Recent work has shown a significant relationship between body conformation and the presence of joint lesions. Pigs with a narrow lumbar region, broad hams, and a large relative width between the stifle joints are highly susceptible to poor locomotor ability as a result of lesions in the elbow and stifle joints, the lumbar intervertebral joints, and the hip joint.

PATHOGENESIS

A brief review of the structure and biochemistry of the normal articular joint will serve as background for understanding the pathogenesis of osteoarthropathy.

Articular cartilage is a tissue consisting of chondrocytes scattered in a matrix of collagen fibers and an amorphous intercellular substance containing proteoglycans. Articular cartilage contains no nerves, is avascular, and has a high matrix-to-cell ratio. The chondrocytes are the only living matter in cartilage, produce the fine strands of collagen, and are engaged in protein and proteoglycan synthesis. The matrix of the cartilage consists of water-soluble proteoglycans interspersed with collagen fibers, which are arranged in parallel rows superficially and crisscross rows closer to the calcified layer. This enables the cartilage to withstand shearing stresses superficially and compression more deeply.

The proteoglycans are glycosaminoglycan–protein complexes, bound by a link glycoprotein to a linear hyaluronic acid molecule. The glycosaminoglycans in articular cartilage are chondroitin 4-sulfate, chondroitin 6-sulfate, and keratan sulfate. About 75% of the proteoglycans exist on aggregates that protect them from degradation, and because of their high water content, they form large polyanionic complexes that have considerable elastic resistance to compression.

Nutrition of the articular cartilage is provided via the synovial fluid and is dependent on the capillary flow to the synovial membrane. Nutrients flow through the synovial fluid and diffuse through the cartilage to the chondrocytes. Proteoglycans are synthesized by the chondrocytes and secreted to the cell exterior. Proteoglycans are also degraded intracellularly by lysosomes. The normal equilibrium between anabolism and catabolism is maintained by several different low-molecular-weight proteins. When the equilibrium is disturbed and shifts toward catabolism, degeneration occurs.

Primary Osteoarthropathy

Primary osteoarthropathy is a result of normal aging processes and ordinary joint usage. The initial lesions occur in the superficial layers of the articular cartilages where, with increasing age, there is loss of the normal resilience of the cartilage, a lowering of the chondroitin sulfate content, and reduction in the permeability of the cartilaginous matrix, which results in progressive degeneration of the articular cartilage. There is grooving of the articular cartilage, eburnation of subchondral bone, and secondary hypertrophy of marginal cartilage and bone, with the formation of pearl-like osteophytes. In experimentally induced arthritis in the horse, the major changes include synovitis, increased synovial effusion, and superficial fibrillation with chondrocyte necrosis in the articular cartilage. These are comparable to the early changes in naturally occurring degenerative joint disease.

Secondary Osteoarthropathy

Secondary osteoarthropathy appears to be initiated by injuries or congenital conformational defects that create greater shearing stresses on particular points, in contrast to the intermittent compressive stresses typical of ordinary weight-bearing. These irregular stresses result in cartilaginous erosion, increased density of subchondral bone at points of physical stress, and proliferation of bone and cartilage at the articular margins.

Following acute trauma, the initial changes are often characterized by acute synovitis and capsulitis. As a result of the inflammatory response, leukocytes, prostaglandins, lysosomal enzymes, and hyaluronidase enter the synovial fluid, which becomes less viscous, affecting the nutrition of the cartilage. There is some evidence of immune complexes associated with collagen-type-specific antibodies in horses with secondary osteoarthritis. Cytokines can be detected in the synovial fluid after racing in horses with degenerative joint disease. The cartilage matrix undergoes a variety of changes, possibly because of chondrocyte damage with lysosomal enzyme release or as result of collagen fiber injury. There is an increase in water content and loss of orientation of the collagen fibers. Proteoglycans are lost, and although increased chondrocyte activity synthesizes proteoglycans, they are of lower molecular weight and altered glycosaminoglycan composition. This leads to loss of elasticity and surface integrity of the cartilage, resulting in increased friction, blistering, and ulceration. There is additional lysosomal enzyme release from the chondrocytes, resulting in matrix destruction and further proteoglycan destruction. The degrading enzymes enter the altered matrix and cause further degradation.

The first stage of matrix degradation involves discoloration, softening, and blistering of the tangential layer of the cartilage surface, a process known as early fibrillation. As the fissuring extends to the radial layer, microfractures occur, with loss of cartilage fragments (detritus) into the synovial fluid. As the cartilage is destroyed, the underlying bone is exposed and becomes sclerotic. Bony proliferation occurs in the floor of the cartilage lesions, whereas osteophyte formation occurs at the joint margins. The pathogenesis of degenerative joint disease indicates that the ideal treatment would be the use of a substance that would promote synthesis of matrix components and retard catabolic processes.

The major proteoglycan in cartilage is a high-molecular-weight aggrecan that contains chondroitin sulfate and keratin sulfate chains located on specific regions of the core protein. These macromolecules are continuously released into the synovial fluid during normal cartilage matrix metabolism. Cartilage proteoglycans are degraded early in the course of joint disease and released from the cartilage into the synovial fluid, where they can be identified.

In horses with degenerative joint disease, proteoglycan fragments—glycosaminoglycans—have been determined in equine synovial fluid as indicators of cartilage metabolism in various types of arthritides. The intraarticular injection of corticosteroids depresses chondrocyte metabolism, alters the biochemical composition, and causes morphologic changes in the articular cartilage, which remains biochemically and metabolically impaired for several or more weeks.

In **femoral-tibial osteoarthrosis of bulls**, the secondary degenerative joint lesions are a result of rupture of the attachments of the lateral meniscus resulting in mechanical instability in the joint, with unusual mechanical stresses on the articular cartilage leading to degeneration. The cranial cruciate ligament becomes progressively worn and eventually ruptures, resulting in loss of all joint stability and the development of gross arthrosis. In cattle with severe degenerative joint disease of the coxofemoral joints, an acetabular osseous bulla may develop at the cranial margin of the obturator foramen.

Osteochondrosis

Osteochondrosis (dyschondroplasia) is characterized by a focal disturbance of the normal differentiation of the cells in the growing cartilage as a result of failure of the blood supply. The failure is associated with the process of incorporating blood vessels into the ossification front during growth,[6] but, experimentally, bacteremia can also result in vascular occlusion. The end result is a focal ischemic chondronecrosis, which can lead to formation of pseudocysts and true cysts in the subchondral bone.[7] **Osteochondrosis should therefore be considered as a disease that occurs multifocally at predilection sites.** Both the metaphyseal growth plate (the growth zone of the diaphysis) and immature joint cartilage (the growth zone of the epiphysis) are affected. The loss of normal differentiation of the cartilage cells results in failure of provisional calcification of the matrix and endochondral ossification ceases. Degeneration and necrosis of blood vessels in cartilage canals results in ischemia of an area of growing cartilage, followed by chondrocyte degeneration and death. The initial lesion occurs in growing cartilage, and *dyschondroplasia* is a more appropriate term. The primary lesion of osteochondrosis directly affects the differentiation and maturation of the cartilage cells and the surrounding matrix that are destined to become replaced by bone. This can occur at the two sites of endochondral ossification in long bones—the articular/epiphyseal cartilage complex and the metaphyseal growth plate. In osteochondrosis, the capillary buds fail to penetrate the distal region of the hypertrophic zone, which leads to a failure of the final stages of cartilage maturation and modification of the surrounding matrix. These changes lead to retention and thickening of cartilage with subsequent weakening of the articular/epiphyseal cartilage complex.

Typical lesions in the horse involve extensive cartilaginous and subchondral bone degeneration with flap formation and, ultimately, loose pieces in the joint. This is usually referred to as osteochondritis dissecans and is associated with synovial effusion and varying degrees of synovitis. Osteochondral fracture associated with severe pathologic changes to the subchondral bone occurs most commonly on the trochlear ridges and the lateral or medial malleoli of the hock. It is likely that osteochondrosis lesions develop in foals within the first few months of extrauterine life, which is much earlier than originally thought.

In **rapidly growing pigs** raised in confinement with minimal exercise, **osteochondrosis and arthrosis** are seen as degeneration of the deep layer of the articular cartilage and adjacent subchondral bone with degenerative lesions of the epiphyseal plate. Lesions in the epiphyseal plate may result in epiphysiolysis, which occurs most commonly in the femoral head. The typical lesions are usually symmetric and commonly involve the elbow, tarsocrural, stifle, and hip joints and the distal epiphyseal plate of the ulna.[5] Lesions also occur in the intervertebral articulations. The lesions are common in pigs when they are examined at slaughter (90 to 100 kg BW), and there might have been no evidence of clinical abnormality, or a proportion of the pigs with severe lesions might have been affected with leg-weakness syndrome. Osteochondrosis and *Erysipelothrix rhusiopathiae* are the most common causes of nonsuppurative joint disease of pigs examined at the abattoir. Thus not all lesions are clinical.

CLINICAL FINDINGS

The major clinical characteristic is a chronic lameness that becomes progressively worse over a long period of time and does not usually respond to treatment. The disease is insidious and generally not clinically apparent in the early stages. A common clinical history is that the affected animal becomes progressively more lame over a period of weeks and months and prefers long periods of recumbency. The lesion may develop slowly over a period of weeks and months during the convalescent stages of an acute traumatic injury to the joint when recovery is expected but the animal continues to be lame.

There is usually difficulty in flexing affected joints normally, which results in a stiff and stilted gait. In cattle confined to stanchions, one of the earliest and persistent signs is shifting of weight from limb to limb. In dairy cattle, as the lesions become more painful, there is a decline in appetite and milk production, prolonged recumbency, and considerable difficulty in rising from the recumbent state. In the early stages, there may be an apparent remission of the lameness, but relapses are common. The bony prominences of the joint eventually appear more prominent than normal, which is a result of disuse muscle atrophy of the affected limbs. Acute and marked distension of the joint capsule is not as common as it is in an infectious or suppurative arthritis, but joints can slowly distend over weeks to months (Fig. 15-8). The joint capsule of palpable joints is usually not painful on palpation. Passive flexion of affected joints may be painful, and it may be possible to elicit crepitus as a result of detached pieces of cartilage and bone and osteophytes surrounding the articular cartilage. However, crepitus is most common in the large movable joints, such as the stifle, and commonly in osteoarthropathy secondary to acute traumatic injury of the meniscus and cranial cruciate ligament of the joint.

Osteochondrosis in cattle is characterized by chronic long-standing lameness, either with or without joint effusion. Joint fluid analysis is usually normal or indicates nonseptic inflammation. The stifle joint is most commonly affected, followed by the hock joint. In osteochondrosis in young, rapidly growing bulls there is reluctance to move, stiffness, enlargement of the ends of long bones, and a straightened joint. Although there may be clinical evidence of lameness in less than 40% of affected cattle, radiographically, 88% of the lesions are bilateral. Young breeding bulls in the early stages of coxofemoral arthropathy may be reluctant to perform the breeding act and yet appear to have sufficient libido.

Osteochondrosis in the horse is characterized by a wide range of clinical signs, and in some cases lesions are not accompanied by clinical signs. The most common sign of osteochondrosis is a nonpainful distension of an affected joint. In foals under 6 months of age, a tendency to spend more time lying down is common. This is accompanied by joint swelling, stiffness, and difficulty keeping up with the other animals in the group. An upright conformation of the limbs may also be present. In yearlings or older animals the common clinical signs are stiffness of joints, flexion responses, and varying degrees of lameness.

In the horse with osteochondrosis of the shoulder joint there is intermittent lameness, characterized by a swinging leg and shoulder lameness with pain elicited by extension, flexion, or abduction of the limb. Secondary joint disease is also a common finding. In a retrospective study of osteochondrosis dissecans in 21 horses, affected animals were 8 months to 5 years of age. The usual age of onset of clinical abnormalities was 18 to 24 months. The common presenting complaints included joint effusion and lameness of

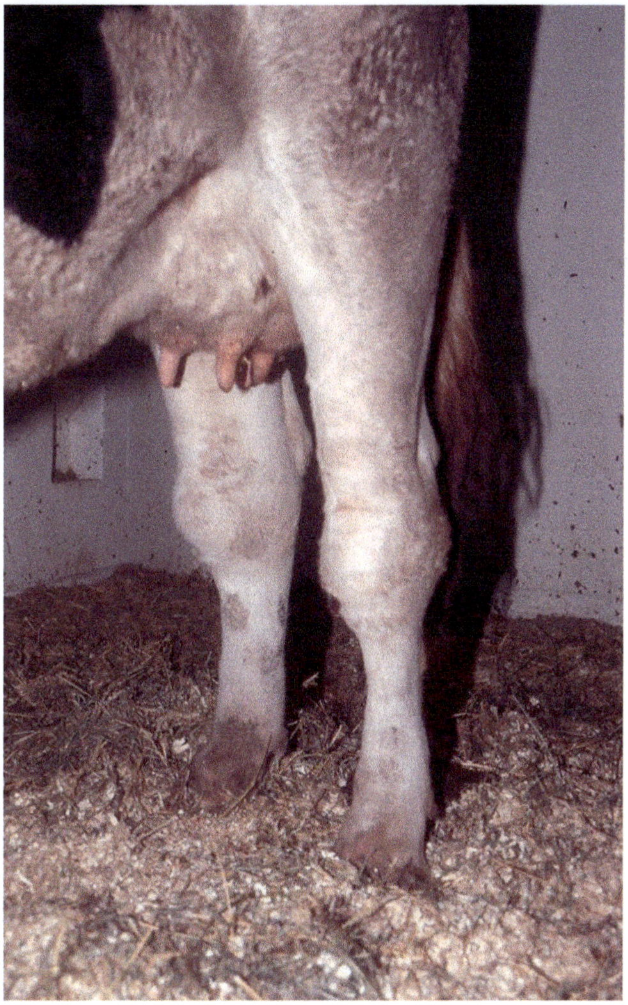

Fig. 15-8 **Bilateral tarsitis in a lactating Holstein–Friesian cow. Note the marked joint effusion centered on both tarsal joints and the excessively straight hindlimbs.**

Table 15-3 Laboratory evaluation of synovial fluid in diseases of the joints

Synovial fluid analysis	Normal joint	Degenerative arthropathy	Infectious arthritis
Gross appearance	Colorless, clear	Pale yellow, may contain flocculent debris	Turbid, yellow
Total volume	—	Normal or slight increase	Usually marked increase
Clot formation	No clot	No clot	May clot within minutes after collection
Erythrocytes (μL)	<4,000	6,000–12,000	4,000–8,000
Leukocytes (μL)	<250	250–1,000	50,000–150,000
Neutrophils (%)	7	10–15	80–90
Lymphocytes (%)	35–40	45–50	4–8
Monocytes (%)	45–50	35–40	1–3
Microbiology	—	—	May be able to culture bacteria, mycoplasma, or virus, but not always
Total protein (g/dL)	1.2–1.8	1.6–1.8	3.2–4.5
Relative viscosity	—	Slightly reduced	Decreased
pH	—	—	Decreased

Other laboratory analyses of synovial fluid include the following: sugar content, alkaline phosphatase activity, lactic dehydrogenase activity, aldolase activity, glutamic oxaloacetic transaminase activity, glutamic pyruvic transaminase activity, mucinous precipitate quality.

either gradual or sudden onset. The prevalence was higher in males than in females.

Common clinical findings in **pigs with osteochondrosis** are hyperflexion of the carpus, limb bowing, adduction of both forelegs at the level of the carpus, hyperextension of the fore and hind phalanges, and anterior curvature of the tarsus. One of the first clinical abnormalities of osteochondrosis and epiphysiolysis in young breeding boars may be inability to mount the sow—impotentia coeundi. Locomotory dysfunction involves primarily the hindlegs. There is pronounced swaying of the hindquarters and crossing of the hindlegs with each step, which makes the pig appear uncoordinated. Epiphysiolysis of the head of the femur occurs in young pigs from 5 months to 1 year of age. There is usually a history of slight to moderate lameness, sudden in onset and affecting one or both hindlimbs. The onset of lameness may coincide with some physical activity such as breeding, farrowing, or transportation. The lameness is progressive, and in about 7 to 10 days the animal is unable to use its hindlegs. Crepitus may be audible on circumduction of the affected limb, and radiography may reveal the separation.

DIAGNOSIS

Joint Fluid

The changes in the synovial fluid of joints affected with degenerative arthropathy are usually unremarkable and can be readily distinguished from the changes in infectious arthritis. A summary of the laboratory evaluation of synovial fluid in diseases of the joints is set out in Table 15-3. The isolation of an infectious agent from the synovial fluid of a diseased joint suggests the presence of septic arthritis, but failure to isolate an organism must not be interpreted as the presence of a noninfectious arthritis. In well-advanced cases of septic arthritis the number of organisms may be small, or they might have been phagocytosed by neutrophils in the joint fluid.

Total protein concentration and viscosity of synovial fluid of horses can be determined. Normal values are available, and the concentration and molecular weight distribution of hyaluronate in synovial fluid from clinically normal horses and horses with diseased joints have been compared. Synovial fluid viscosity is reduced in horses with infectious and chronic arthritides and with radiographic evidence of cartilage degeneration. The synovial fluid hyaluronate concentration can be used as a diagnostic marker for chronic traumatic arthritis. However, high-molecular-weight proteoglycans or other markers in the synovial fluid cannot be used for diagnosing or monitoring degenerative joint disease.

Infrared spectroscopy measures the infrared absorption patters of molecules in synovial fluid when exposed to infrared light. Infrared spectroscopy of synovial fluid indicated that the infrared patterns from equine joints with traumatic arthritis differed from the pattern for corresponding healthy joints.[8] It remains to be determined whether this technology provides additional clinical information to that obtained by the routine analysis of synovial fluid. **Hematology and serum biochemistry** should be combined with appropriate hematology and serum biochemistry where indicated, although the results rarely change treatment protocols or prognosis. The concentration of hyaluronic acid in synovial fluid can be determined using an assay technique. The determination of serum calcium and phosphorus may reveal the existence of a dietary deficiency or imbalance of minerals.

Radiography

Radiography of the hock joints in a craniomedial–caudolateral oblique view and of the fetlock joints in lateromedial view are standard techniques for the diagnosis of osteochondrosis in the horse. Those joints with abnormal radiographs may be radiographed from additional perspectives. Horses with bony fragments or defects at the cranial edge of the intermediate ridge of the distal aspect of the tibia or defects at the lateral trochlea of the talus can be classified as having osteochondrosis. The radiographic progression of femoropatellar osteochondrosis in horses under 1 year of age at the onset of clinical signs has been examined. The full extent of the radiographic lesions may take several weeks to develop.

Arthroscopy

Arthroscopic examination and surgery of affected joints of horses with osteochondrosis can provide considerably more information than is possible from clinical and radiographic examination alone.

NECROPSY FINDINGS

In **degenerative joint disease** the joint cartilage is thin or patchily absent, and polished subchondral bone is evident. The articular surfaces are irregular and sometimes folded. Exposed bone may be extensively eroded, and osteophytes (small bony excrescences, appearing like pearls) may be present on the nonarticular parts of the joint on the circumference of the articular cartilage. The synovial fluid is usually only slightly increased in volume and appears amber-colored. Menisci and intraarticular cartilages and ligaments may be entirely absent, and there may be areas of calcification in the joint capsule and cartilages free in the synovium. When the stifle is affected, fractures of the head of the tibia occur commonly, usually a chip of the lateral condyle having become separated. In such cases, fractures of the lateral condyle of the distal end of the femur may follow. With either of these fractures, lameness is extreme, and the animal may often refuse to rise. When the hip joint of bulls is affected, the head of the femur becomes smaller and more flattened than normal, the acetabulum is shallower, and the round ligament is usually ruptured.

In **osteochondrosis** there is splitting and invagination of articular cartilage, loss of articular cartilage, chip fractures of condyles, exposed and collapsed subchondral bone, osteophyte formation around the circumference of the articular cartilage, and loose pieces of cartilage in the joint. In **equine osteochondrosis (dyschondroplasia)**, the histologic lesions can be divided into two groups. In one group, there are accumulations of small rounded chondrocytes, areas of necrosis, and chondrocyte clusters. In the second group, there are alterations in the appearance of the mineralized matrix, areas of necrosis, chondrocyte clusters, and an alteration in type VI collagen immunoreactivity within the chondrocyte clusters.

In the epiphyseal plates (e.g., the distal ulna in pigs with osteochondrosis), the cartilage is uneven and thickened, with hemorrhage, fibrous tissue, collapse of bone tissue in the metaphysis, and epiphyseal separation. Complete separation of the epiphysis occurs most commonly at the head of the femur. The ultrastructural appearance of normal epiphyseal cartilage of the articular–epiphyseal cartilage complex in growing swine has been examined and serves as a standard for comparison with the lesions in affected pigs. The lesions may be present in pigs at an early age as part of the usual growth pattern of cartilages.

DIFFERENTIAL DIAGNOSIS

Osteoarthropathy is characterized clinically by a chronic lameness that becomes progressively worse and usually does not respond to treatment. The gait is stiff, there is disuse muscle atrophy, the bony prominences of the joint are more apparent, but usually there is no marked distension and pain of the joint capsule, as in infectious arthritis. Examination of synovial fluid may aid in differentiation from septic arthritis.

Radiographically, there is erosion of articular cartilage, sclerosis of subchondral bone, and periarticular accumulations of osteophytes. In the early stages of the disease in large animals, radiographic changes may not be visible, and repeated examinations may be necessary.

The radiographic changes of osteochondrosis in the shoulder joint of the horse consist of the following:

- Alteration in the contour of the humeral head and glenoid cavity
- Periarticular osteophyte formation
- Sclerosis of the subchondral bone
- Bone cyst formation

TREATMENT

The treatment of arthropathy depends largely upon correction of the cause, but in most cases the lesions are progressive and irreparable, and food-producing animals should be slaughtered for salvage. Tarsal degenerative joint disease in cattle has been treated with intraarticular injections of corticosteroids and has provided temporary relief from pain and discomfort. However, the corticosteroids do not promote healing of the joint, and their use in arthropathy may actually accelerate erosion of articular cartilage, loss of joint sensation, and the development of "steroid arthropathy."

In the horse, there are many choices available for controlling inflammation in osteoarthritis. Treatment is symptomatic and largely nonspecific, but the long-term administration of antiinflammatory agents remains a central part of the treatment of equine joint disease.[9]

Nonsteroidal Antiinflammatory Agents and Opioids

Several nonsteroidal antiinflammatory drugs (NSAIDs), such as **phenylbutazone**, **flunixin meglumine**, **ketoprofen**, **naproxen**, and **carprofen**, are available treatment options. Each has associated toxicities. They are now the most commonly used drugs because of their analgesic, antipyretic, and antiinflammatory properties. They inhibit some component of the enzyme system that converts arachidonic acid into prostaglandins and thromboxanes. All cells, including chondrocytes and synoviocytes, possess arachidonic acid as a fatty acid constituent of phospholipids. Once released, arachidonic acid is oxidized by either cyclooxygenase (COX) or 5-lipooxygenase. COX oxidation leads to prostaglandin production, whereas lipoxygenase oxidation leads to leukotriene formation. The effect of NSAIDs is primarily from inhibiting COX, which blocks arachidonic acid conversion to prostaglandin.

Phenylbutazone is the most commonly used NSAID around the world to treat arthritis in horses, but oral administration at 2 mg/kg every 12 hours did not appear to have a clinically relevant effect on joint tissue metabolism.[10] This suggests that the major clinical effect of phenylbutazone in horses with osteoarthritis is analgesia. Some countries, such as the United States, do not permit the use of phenylbutazone in food-producing animals. The oral administration of **meloxicam** (0.6 mg/kg BW once daily) altered joint tissue metabolism, as demonstrated by decreased synovial fluid concentrations of PGE_2, substance P, bradykinin, and matrix metalloproteinase activity in horses with experimentally induced synovitis.[9] This suggests that meloxicam may have beneficial effects in limiting cartilage catabolism during acute synovitis.

Intraarticular morphine administration (0.05 mg/kg BW or 120 mg) is associated with substantial analgesic effects and beneficial antiinflammatory effects, resulting in less joint swelling and lower synovial fluid total protein concentration; leukocyte count;

and PGE2, bradykinin, and substance P concentrations in horses with experimentally induced acute synovitis.[11,12] The mechanism for the antiinflammatory effect of morphine is unknown.

Intraarticular Steroids

Various steroidal formulations for intraarticular administration are available, and correct dosage, frequency of administration, indications, and toxicity are factors to consider for each drug. They include methylprednisolone acetate, betamethasone, and triamcinolone acetonide.

Chondroprotective Agents

Various **chondroprotective** drugs, such as intraarticular **hyaluronic acid** and **polysulfated glycosaminoglycan**, and the oral neutraceutic agents **glucosamine-chondroitin sulfate** are also used to control inflammation and provide viscosupplementation. The allotransplantation of synovial fluid into the joints of horses with arthropathies has been examined.

There is a notable lack of treatment information based on randomized, blinded, placebo-controlled clinical trials in the horse to identify the efficacy of therapeutic agents for both symptomatic and disease-modifying activity in degenerative joint disease. Until there are validated outcome measures that can be used practically in clinical trials, there will always be uncertainty about whether these therapeutic agents have any real disease-modifying action.

Hyaluronic Acid

The beneficial effects of hyaluronic acid are claimed to be improved viscosity of the synovial fluid and thereby improved rheologic properties, lubrication of unloaded joints, and provision of an antiinflammatory and analgesic effect. The changes in the synovia following the intraarticular injection of **sodium hyaluronate** into normal equine joints and after arthrotomy and experimental cartilage damage have been examined, but in general the results are inconclusive.

Polysulfated Glycosaminoglycan

Polysulfated glycosaminoglycan has been reported to induce articular cartilage matrix synthesis and to decrease matrix degradation. Experimentally, intraarticular injection of **polysulfated glycosaminoglycan** provides some protection against chemically induced articular cartilage damage but not against physical defects of articular cartilage in the horse. The polysulfated glycosaminoglycans inhibit lysosomal enzymes and neutral proteases. A survey of the use of polysulfated glycosaminoglycans by equine practitioners for the treatment of lameness in horses found that the drug is moderately effective overall and is considered most beneficial in the treatment of subacute degenerative joint disease. Its efficacy for incipient and chronic forms of degenerative joint disease is considered comparable to that of sodium hyaluronate.

The prevention of further trauma should be ensured, and possible nutritional causes should be corrected. The treatment of active disease, particularly in soft tissues, that is contributing to articular degeneration includes rest, immobilization, physical therapy, intraarticular injections of corticosteroids, NSAIDs, joint lavage, and intraarticular injection of sodium hyaluronate, all of which have been used with variable success.

Other Treatments

Surgical therapy includes curettage of articular cartilage, removal of osteophytes, and surgical arthrodesis. In a retrospective study of stifle lameness in 42 cattle admitted to two veterinary teaching hospitals over a period of 6 years, 18 had radiographic evidence of subchondral bone cyst without radiographic evidence of degenerative joint disease. The prognosis in those with a subchondral bone cyst was favorable, with 75% returning to their intended function, whereas in cases of, septic arthritis only 22% returned to normal.

Chemical arthrodesis using the intraarticular injections of monoiodoacetate (MIA) has been described as an alternative to surgical arthrodesis for the treatment of degenerative joint disease of the distal tarsal joints. MIA causes an increase in intracellular concentration of adenosine triphosphate, resulting in inhibition of glycolysis and cell death. It causes dose-dependent cartilage degeneration characterized by cartilage fibrillations, chondrocyte death, and glycosaminoglycan and proteoglycan depletion. MIA produces reliable radiographic and histologic ankylosis of the distal tarsal joints. Resolution of the lameness required 12 months and occasionally longer. Soundness was achieved in 82% and 85% of horses at 12 and 24 months, respectively. Complications of the injections were uncommon and were probably related to periarticular injection or leakage of MIA, or to use of higher concentrations or volumes. Postinjection pain was marked in a small number of horses but was transient and managed effectively with analgesic drugs. The procedure is controversial. Some clinicians argue that arthrodesis should only be used where lameness is localized to the tarsometatarsal and centrodistal joints with objective means such as local analgesic techniques and when other more conservative treatments have failed.

CONTROL AND PREVENTION

Prevention of osteoarthropathy will depend on recognition and elimination of the predisposing causes: provision of an adequate diet and the avoidance of overnutrition during the first 3 months of extrauterine life, regular exercise for confined animals, the provision of suitable flooring to minimize persistent concussion, and the use of breeding stock that have a body conformation that does not predispose to joint lesions.

FURTHER READING

Laverty S, Girard C. Pathogenesis of epiphyseal osteochondrosis. *Vet J*. 2013;197:3-12.

Lewczuk D, Korwin-Kossakowska A. Genetic background of osteochondrosis in the horse—a review. *Anim Sci Papers Rep*. 2012;30:205-218.

Olstad K, Ekman S, Carlson CS. An update on the pathogenesis of osteochondrosis. *Vet Pathol*. 2015;52:785-802.

Richardson DW, Loinaz R. An evidence-based approach to selected joint therapies in horses. *Vet Clin Equine*. 2007;23:443-460.

Ytrehus B, Carlson CS, Ekman S. Etiology and pathogenesis of osteochondrosis. *Vet Pathol*. 2007;44:429-448.

REFERENCES

1. van Weeren PR, Jeffcott LB. *Vet J*. 2013;197:96.
2. Counotte G, et al. *J Equine Vet Sci*. 2014;34:668.
3. Robert C. *Vet Rec*. 2013;doi:10.1136/vr.f310.
4. Vander Heyden J, et al. *Vet Rec*. 2012;doi:10.1136/vr.101034.
5. van Grevenhof EM, et al. *Livestock Sci*. 2012;143:85.
6. Lecocq M, et al. *Equine Vet J*. 2008;40:442.
7. Olstad K, et al. *Vet Pathol*. 2015;52:862.
8. Vijarnsorn M, et al. *Am J Vet Res*. 2006;67:1286.
9. de Grauw JC, et al. *Equine Vet J*. 2009;41:693.
10. de Grauw JC, et al. *Vet J*. 2014;201:51.
11. Lindegaard C, et al. *Am J Vet Res*. 2010;71:69.
12. van Loon JPAM, et al. *Equine Vet J*. 2010;42:412.

SEPTIC ARTHRITIS SYNOVITIS

Inflammation of the synovial membrane and articular surfaces as a result of infection occurs commonly in farm animals. It is characterized by varying degrees of lameness and a warm, swollen, and painful joint. The synovial fluid is usually abnormal, containing an increased leukocyte count and the pathogens causing the arthritis. The arthritis may be severe enough to cause systemic illness, and in some cases a draining sinus tract may occur.

ETIOLOGY AND EPIDEMIOLOGY

Specific bacterial infections of the joints are most common in newborn farm animals, in which localization of infection occurs in joints following bacteremia or septicemia. Surveys of Thoroughbred studs have shown that the incidence of infectious arthritis is higher in foals with other perinatal abnormalities and in which the ingestion of colostrum was delayed for more than 4 hours after birth. Calves with hypogammaglobulinemia are particularly susceptible to bacteremia and meningitis, ophthalmitis, and arthritis. Some of the important infectious causes of arthritis are as follows.

Calves

- Nonspecific joint-ill from omphalophlebitis associated with *Trueperella pyogenes, Fusobacterium necrophorum, Staphylococcus* spp.
- *Erysipelothrix rhusiopathiae* sporadically in older calves

- *Salmonella dublin, Salmonella typhimurium,* and *Mycoplasma bovis*

Lambs
- *E. rhusiopathiae* in newborn and recently tail-docked lambs
- Sporadic cases associated with *F. necrophorum, Staphylococcus* spp., *Corynebacterium pseudotuberculosis, Histophilus somni, Mannheimia haemolytica*
- *Chlamydophila* spp. causes polyarthritis extensively in feedlot lambs
- Tick pyemia is associated with *Staphylococcus aureus.*

Foals
- Part of neonatal septicemia, with gram-negative bacteria predominating[1]
- *Actinobacillus equuli, Rhodococcus equi, Salmonella abortivoequina* in the newborn
- *Chlamydophila* spp. has caused polyarthritis in foals.

Piglets
- Streptococci, Lancefield groups C, E, and L
- *Streptococcus suis*
- *E. rhusiopathiae* in pigs of any age—up to 65% of joints of pigs at slaughter are affected, and up to 80% of the farms from which the pigs come do not vaccinate for erysipelas. Mortality in preweaning groups of pigs may affect 18% of litters and 3.3% of the piglets, with a herd mortality of 1.5%
- In a 4-year period in a swine research station, 9411 piglets were born alive, and 9.8% were treated for lameness. About 75% of the cases were observed in piglets under 3 weeks of age. The incidence of lameness was much higher in piglets born from sows of parity 3 (11.4%) compared with piglets born to sows of parity 4 to 7 (8%).

Cattle
- *Histophilus somni* is a cause of synovitis.
- *Mycoplasma agalactia* var. *bovis* is a common cause of synovitis, arthritis, and pneumonia in young feedlot cattle.
- *Mycoplasma bovigenitalium* may cause mastitis in cows, with some animals developing arthritis.
- *Mycoplasma mycoides* may cause arthritis in calves vaccinated with the organism against contagious bovine pleuropneumonia. Calves already sensitive to the organism develop an immediate-type allergic reaction of the synovial membrane.
- *Brucella abortus*—occasional cows with brucellosis develop arthrodial synovitis.
- Some cases of ephemeral fever have sterile arthritis.
- BVD virus in young bulls, rarely
- Idiopathic septic arthritis in dairy heifers—the etiology is unknown.
- Septic arthritis of the proximal interphalangeal (pastern) joint in cattle as a result of perforating wounds—*T. pyogenes* is the most common cause in cattle.

Sheep and Goats
- As part of melioidosis
- *Mycoplasma* spp. of serositis—arthritis
- *Streptococcus dysgalactiae* in lambs and kids[2,3]

Horses
- Septic arthritis after penetrating wounds, intraarticular injection of corticosteroids, and surgery; young foals under 6 months of age usually associated with septicemia; adult horses without a known etiology.
- In a series of 34 cases of monoarticular infectious arthritis in adult horses admitted to a veterinary teaching hospital over a period of 10 years, 16 had a penetrating wound over the joint, 4 had a puncture wound of the sole, and in 5 the infection was iatrogenic (3 had received intraarticular corticosteroids, 1 had received intraarticular anesthesia, and 1 had sepsis after a purulent thrombophlebitis); in 9 cases, no cause could be determined.
- Spread to the joints from generalized strangles.
- Rare cases of nonerosive polysynovitis in a horse, possibly immunologic and immune-mediated polysynovitis in foals.
- *Acedosporium prolificans,* a newly recognized opportunistic fungus, has been associated with an incurable arthritis and osteomyelitis in a mature horse.

Pigs
- Glasser's disease
- *Mycoplasma* spp. in synovitis and arthritis of growing pigs, especially in housed pigs
- *Brucella suis* commonly infects bones, especially vertebrae, and joints.

All Species
Sporadic cases are a result of the following:
- Traumatic perforation of the joint capsule
- Spread from surrounding tissues (e.g., footrot to interphalangeal joints in cattle and pigs, interdigital abscess in sheep)
- Hematogenous spread from suppurative lesions, commonly in udder, uterus, diaphragmatic abscess, infected navel or tail, castration wound

PATHOGENESIS
In infectious arthritis that is hematogenous in origin there is usually a synovitis initially, followed by changes in the articular cartilages and sometimes bone. With almost any systemic infection, there may be localization of the infectious agent in the synovial membrane and joint cavity. The synovial membrane is inflamed and edematous, and there are varying degrees of villous hypertrophy and deposition of fibrin. Bacteria colonize synovial membranes, which makes treatment difficult. The synovitis causes distension of the joint capsule with fluid, and the joint is painful and warm. Successful treatment and elimination of infection at this early stage of synovitis will minimize changes in articular cartilage and bone, and healing will result. A progressive infectious synovitis commonly results in pannus formation between articular surfaces, with erosion of articular cartilage, infection of subchondral bone, and osteomyelitis. In the chronic stages, there is extensive granulation tissue formation, chronic synovitis, and degenerative joint disease with osteophyte formation, and ankylosis is possible. Depending on the organism, the arthritis may be suppurative or serofibrinous. Suppurative arthritis is particularly destructive of cartilage and bone, and commonly there is rupture of the joint capsule. In foals with septic arthritis, there may be a concurrent polyosteomyelitis, usually in either the epiphysis and/or the metaphysis of the long bones.

Calves With Experimentally Induced Infectious Arthritis
Septic arthritis induced by *E. coli* is a reliable and reproducible model of infectious arthritis in laboratory animals, including horses and calves. The inoculation of *E. coli* into the tarsal joint of newborn colostrum-fed calves resulted in septic arthritis in all calves. Clinic signs of septic arthritis appeared on day 2 after infection and persisted until day 9 for all calves. *E. coli* was cultured from synovial fluid on day 2 for one calf and until day 4 for five other calves. Polymerase chain reaction (PCR) for *E. coli* was positive in the synovial fluid of all calves. Synovial fluid neutrophil and white blood cell counts were increased on days 2 to 4. All bacterial cultures were negative on day 8, although clinicopathologic signs of inflammation persisted until day 20. Rapid recovery occurred within 1 week when an appropriate treatment was begun early in the course of the disease.

Lambs With *Streptococcus dysgalactiae* Polyarthritis
Streptococcus dysgalactiae is the most common cause of septic arthritis in lambs under 4 weeks of age in the United Kingdom.[3] It appears that a small proportion of ewes carry *S. dysgalactiae* in vaginal secretions, milk, and other secretions, and *S. dysgalactiae* can survive on straw or hay for up to 5 to 6 weeks.[2] The route of entry of *S. dysgalactiae* into lambs is uncertain but appears to be either via the umbilicus or following ingestion.[4]

Foals With Septicemia

Septicemic foals may develop infectious arthritis and a concurrent polyosteomyelitis because of the patency of transphyseal vessels in the newborn foal; this allows spread of infection across the physes with the development of lesions in the metaphysis, epiphysis, and adjacent to the articular cartilage. The syndrome is classified into four types according to the location of the lesions:

- A foal with **S-type** septic arthritis has synovitis without macroscopic evidence of osteomyelitis. This is most commonly seen in the first 2 weeks of life.
- Foals with **E-type** septic arthritis also have osteomyelitis of the epiphysis at the cartilage–subchondral bone junction. This is most commonly seen at 3 to 4 weeks of life.
- Those with **P-type** infections have osteomyelitis directly adjacent to the physis and do not have septic arthritis, although there may be a nonseptic effusion of the closest joint.
- Foals with **T-type** have an initial infection of the small cuboidal bones of the carpus and tarsus that spreads into the carpal or tarsal joints.

Horses

Septic arthritis has been reproduced experimentally in horses and the sequential synovial fluid changes monitored. Following intraarticular inoculation of *S. aureus,* clinical signs are evident as early as 8 hours after infection. A high and persistent neutrophilia is one of the earliest and most accurate diagnostic abnormalities. The total white blood cell count rises within 12 to 24 hours to a mean value of 100×10^9/L. Total protein also increases. Synovial fluid acidosis also occurs in infectious arthritis, which may interfere with the antibacterial activity of some antimicrobials. In experimental arthritis, the synovial pH declined from a mean value of 7.43 to 7.12. Bacteria could be detected in 40% of the smears of infected synovial fluid samples, and primary cultures of the fluid were positive in 70%. The intraarticular inoculation of *E. coli* into horses induces a reliable, reproducible, and controlled model of infectious arthritis consistent with the naturally occurring disease and has been used to evaluate the efficacy of gentamicin for treatment. The injection of *E. coli* lipopolysaccharide into various joints of horses can cause clinical signs of endotoxemia, and the synovial fluid total nucleated cell count and total protein are linearly responsive in increases in endotoxin.

Endothelin (ET)-1, a 21-amino-acid polypeptide, is locally synthesized in the joints of horses with various forms types of joint disease. It induces a potent and sustained vasoconstriction. Synovial fluid concentrations of ET-1 varies among horses with joint disease, with higher concentrations in animals with joint sepsis suggesting a pathogenic role in septic arthritis.

Synovial fluid in infectious arthritis in the horse may contain the proteolytic enzymes collagenase and caseinase, which may derive from both synovial cells and neutrophils. These enzymes are involved in the degradation of connective tissue and loss of cartilage matrix. Lavage of affective joints is intended to remove these enzymes.

Infectious arthritis may occur following traumatic injury to a joint, but the pathogenesis is obscure. Traumatic injury of the joint capsule resulting in edema and inflammation may allow latent organisms to localize, proliferate, and initiate a septic arthritis.

Septic arthritis occurs rarely in adult horses following injection of an intraarticular medication or elective equine arthroscopy without antimicrobial prophylaxis. In a retrospective and prospective case series involving 16,624 injected joints, the risk of septic arthritis was 1 case per 1,279 injections, with veterinarian and type of corticosteroid (triamcinolone and dexamethasone) being risk factors for infection.[5] The significant effect of the veterinarian suggests the presence of variable attention to strict aseptic technique. In 444 consecutive equine arthroscopies performed without prophylactic antimicrobial therapy, the incidence of septic arthritis in horses after surgery was 0.7%, which was similar to the infection rate (0.9%) in other studies where horses received antimicrobial prophylaxis.[6]

CLINICAL FINDINGS

Inflammation of the synovial membrane causes pain and lameness in the affected limb, sometimes to the point that the animal will not put it to the ground. Pain and heat are usually detectable on palpation, and passive movement of the joint is resented. The joint may be swollen, but the degree will depend on the type of infection. Pyogenic bacteria cause the greatest degree of swelling and may result in rupture of the joint capsule. Some enlargement of the epiphysis is usual, and this may be the only enlargement in nonpyogenic infections, particularly those associated with *E. insidiosa.*

Fever, inappetence to anorexia, endotoxemia, loss of body weight, and discomfort may occur in animals with only one severely affected joint or when several joints are less severely affected. In many of the neonatal infections, there will also be an accompanying omphalophlebitis (Fig. 15-9) and evidence of lesions in other organs and tissues, particularly the liver, endocardium, and meninges. Arthritis in older animals may also be accompanied by signs of inflammation of the serous membranes and endocardium when the infection is the result of hematogenous localization.

The joints most commonly involved are the hock, stifle, and knee, but infection of the fetlock, interphalangeal, and intervertebral joints is not uncommon. In chronic cases, there may by physical impairment of joint movement because of fibrous thickening of the joint capsule, periarticular ossification, and, rarely, ankylosis of the joints. Crepitus may be detectable in joints where much erosion has occurred.

In newborn and young animals, involvement of several joints is common. The joints may become inflamed simultaneously or serially. Lameness is often so severe that affected foals lie down in lateral recumbency most of the time and may have to be assisted to rise. Decubitus ulcerations as a result of

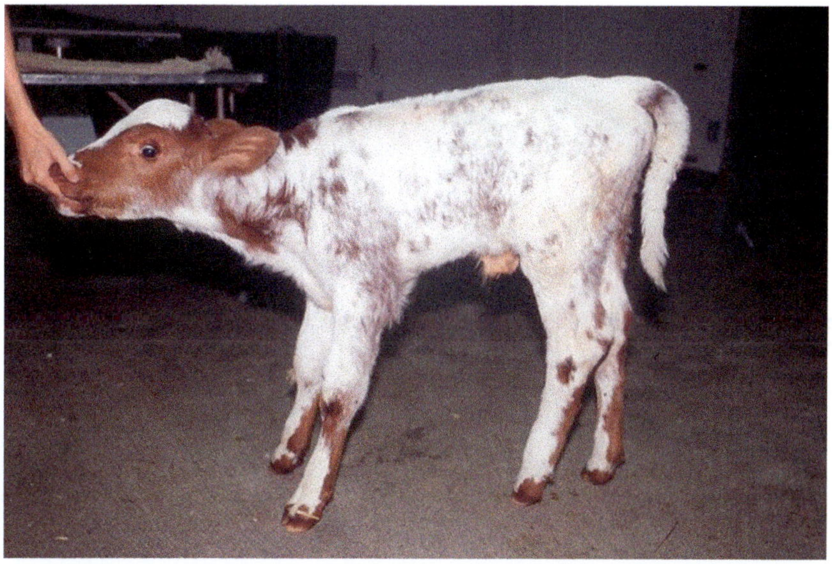

Fig. 15-9 Very early signs of septic arthritis of the left hock joint in a 7-day-old Shorthorn calf. The calf did not suckle colostrum and had a slightly enlarged and painful umbilicus of 2 days in duration. Decreased weight-bearing on the left leg with palpable joint distention of the left hock has just become evident.

prolonged recumbency are common. The gait may be so impaired as to suggest ataxia of central origin.

The **prognosis** in cases of advanced septic arthritis is poor. Neglected animals may die or have to be destroyed because of open joints or pressure sores. The subsequent development of chronic arthritis and ankylosis may greatly impede locomotion and interfere with the usefulness of the animal.

DIAGNOSIS

The diagnosis of septic arthritis requires aseptic arthrocentesis of infected joint(s) and synovial fluid analysis, including bacterial culture of the fluid. An important therapeutic question to be answered is whether infection is confined to the synovial structure of the joint or whether infection includes cartilage and subchondral bone (osteomyelitis). Imaging modalities are designed to identify extension of infection deeper to the synovial structures, of which radiography has been extensively used and is very helpful in chronic cases.

Arthrocentesis

Aspiration of joint fluid for culture and analysis is necessary for a definitive diagnosis. Careful disinfection of the skin and the use of sterile equipment is essential to avoid the introduction of further infection. Intravenous diazepam (0.1 mg/kg BW) is helpful is sedating foals for arthrocentesis. Joint fluid should be collected using an 18-g or 16-g needle to facilitate removal of viscous or purulent fluid.

Analysis of Joint Fluid

Total and differential cell count, total protein concentration, and specific gravity are determined. The classical changes in synovial fluid in large animals with septic arthritis are increased leukocyte count (particularly neutrophils), an increased protein concentration, and decreased fluid viscosity.

In infectious arthritis, the volume of joint fluid is increased, and the total leukocyte count is increased, with a high percentage (80% to 90%) of neutrophils. The severity of infectious arthritis may be manifested systemically by a leukocytosis with a marked regenerative left shift. In degenerative joint disease, the volume may be normal or only slightly increased, and the total and differential leukocyte count may be manifested within the normal range. In traumatic arthritis, there may be a marked increase in the number of erythrocytes. Special biochemical examinations of joint fluid are available that measure for viscosity, strength of the mucin clot, and concentrations of certain enzymes. The laboratory findings in examination of the joint fluid are summarized in Table 15-3.

Culture of Joint Fluid

Joint fluid must be cultured for aerobic and anaerobic bacteria and on specific media when *Mycoplasma* spp. infection is suspected. It is often difficult to isolate bacteria from purulent synovial fluid. The rates of recovery of organisms vary from 40% to 75%. In one study of suspected infectious arthritis in 64 horses admitted to a veterinary teaching hospital over a period of 8.5 years, positive cultures were obtained from 55% of the joints sampled. The most common organisms were *S. aureus, E. coli,* and *Pseudomonas aeruginosa,* accounting for more than half the isolates obtained.

There is no single test that is reliable for the diagnosis of septic arthritis. Failure to isolate organisms on culture does not exclude a bacterial cause, and organisms are often not observed in synovial fluid smears. Poor collection, storage, and laboratory techniques; prior administration of antibiotics; or partial success of the immune system in containing the infection may explain the failure to detect organisms. Arthrocentesis should be done before antibiotics are given, and a blood culture bottle should be inoculated immediately, a Gram stain made, and culture for anaerobes included. Positive cultures from synovial fluid can be expected in only about 65% of cases.

A biopsy sample of synovial membrane may be more reliable than synovial fluid for culture, but there is little evidence based on comparative evaluations to support such a claim. PCR has been examined in in vitro studies to detect selected bacterial species in joint fluid compared with microbial culture. The benefits would include rapid and accurate diagnosis infectious arthritis, ability to detect bacteria in synovial fluid in the presence of antimicrobial drugs, and diagnosis of infectious arthritis when culture results are inconclusive. However, initial studies found no difference between microbial culture and PCR analyses.

Serology of Joint Fluid

Serologic tests may be of value in determining the presence of specific infections with *Mycobacterium mycoides, Salmonella* spp., *Brucella* spp., and *E. insidiosa.* Radiographic examination may aid in the detection of joint lesions and can be used to differentiate between inflammatory and degenerative changes. In foals with arthritis and suspected osteomyelitis there may be radiographic evidence of osteolysis of the metaphysis or epiphysis.

Radiography

Radiography of the affected joint will often reveal the nature and severity of the lesions. Typical radiographic findings of septic arthritis include osteolytic lesions of the articular cartilage, increased width of intraarticular joint space, and soft tissue swelling. Osteomyelitic changes are seen in some cases. Because radiographic changes usually appear after 2 to 3 weeks when destruction of subchondral bone has become extensive, it may be necessary to take a series of radiographs several days apart before lesions are detectable.

Ultrasonography

Arthrosonography is an effective, fast, and noninvasive complement to traditional diagnostic techniques (arthrocentesis and radiography) for comprehensive evaluation of the pathology of joints and associated tendons of cattle and horses.[7] Ultrasonography should be performed before arthrocentesis because joint distention facilitates imaging, and the introduction of air into the joint can interfere with interpretation of ultrasonographic images. Ultrasonography is particularly valuable in septic arthritis cases that are the result of trauma and to assist in the identification of foreign bodies.

Ultrasonographic changes are variable and primarily depend on the duration of infection.[7] Distension of the joint cavities can be imaged; assessment of the echogenicity, acoustic enhancement, and ultrasonographic character of the exudate correlates well with findings by arthrocentesis, arthrotomy, or at necropsy. Joint effusion, which is the earliest indication of septic arthritis, can usually be detected with ultrasound by an experienced operator in the early stages. The synovial membrane, synovial fluid, ligaments, tendons, and periarticular soft tissue, only inadequately imaged by radiography, can be imaged with ultrasonography. In advanced septic arthritis, ultrasonography provides accurate information on the location of the soft tissue swelling, the extent and character of the joint effusion, and the involvement of concurrent periarticular synovial cavities.

Arthroscopy

Endoscopy is now used widely to define joint abnormalities more clearly and to gain access to the joint cavity as an aid in the treatment of septic arthritis.

Nuclear Scintigraphy

Nuclear scintigraphy is considered much more sensitive than radiography for detecting the presence of subchondral (cortical) bone involvement and can be performed in the standing sedated horse. Scintigraphy is only found at large referral hospitals and usually cannot be scheduled on the same day as admission because the diagnostic agents need to be ordered and delivered. Consequently, the use of nuclear scintigraphy for identifying the extent of infection in acute cases of septic arthritis has declined. Scintigraphy remains a valuable diagnostic technique in adult horses with chronic septic arthritis, particularly of the proximal limbs and vertebral column.

Magnetic Resonance Imaging and Computed Tomography

These imaging modalities are only found at large referral hospitals and require general anesthesia to prevent movement during image acquisition. In general, the duration of anesthesia for imaging is shorter with magnetic resonance imaging (MRI) than computed tomography (CT). MRI and CT provide excellent anatomic information on articular structures, but imaging is usually confined to the distal limbs, including the carpus and hock, of adult horses and cattle because units are designed for human use.

MRI is regarded as the gold standard method for diagnosing subchondral osteomyelitis associated with septic arthritis in human medicine and is therefore likely to provide the best imaging modality for identifying the anatomic location of early cases of septic arthritis in large animals.[8] Magnetic resonance findings in adult horses with septic arthritis include diffuse hyperintensity within bone and extracapsular tissue on fat suppressed images, bone sclerosis, and cartilage and subchondral bone damage.[9] Intravenous gadolinium administration usually identifies synovial enhancement.[9] CT has the advantage of speed, permitting the evaluation of multiple joints, which is particularly advantageous in foals with septic arthritis.

NECROPSY FINDINGS

The nature of the lesions varies with the causative organism. The synovial membrane is thickened and roughened, and there is inflammation and erosion of the articular cartilage. There is usually an increase in the amount of synovial fluid present, varying from a thin, clear, serous, brownish fluid through a thicker, serofibrinous fluid to pus. There may be some inflammation of the periarticular tissues in acute cases and proliferation of the synovial membrane in chronic cases. In the latter, plaques of inspissated necrotic material and fibrin may be floating free in the synovial fluid. Infectious arthritis caused by *T. pyogenes* is characterized by extensive erosion and destruction of articular cartilage and extensive suppuration. There may be a primary omphalophlebitis in newborn animals, and metastatic abscesses may be present in other organs.

DIFFERENTIAL DIAGNOSIS

Infectious arthritis is characterized clinically by swollen joints that are painful and warm to touch, along with lameness of varying degrees of severity. The volume of joint fluid is usually markedly increased, and the leukocyte count is increased, with a high percentage of neutrophils. In the early stages of synovitis and in chronic nonsuppurative arthritis, the joint may not be visibly enlarged, and careful examination by palpation may be necessary to reveal abnormalities of the joint capsule. Lameness is common, however, even though only slight in some cases, and should arouse suspicion of the possibility of arthritis.

The diseases of the musculoskeletal system that cause lameness and stiffness of gait include the following:

- Degenerative joint disease
- Osteodystrophy and epiphysitis
- Osteomyelitis
- Degenerative myopathy
- Myositis
- Traumatic injuries of tendons and ligaments

Diseases of the nervous system, especially the peripheral nerves and spinal cord, may be confused with arthritis unless the joints are examined carefully.

Some severe cases of polyarthritis may cause recumbency that may be erroneously attributed to the nervous system.

Degenerative joint disease is characterized by an insidious onset of moderate lameness and stiffness of gait that becomes progressively worse over several weeks. The joint capsule is usually not grossly enlarged and not painful, and there is usually no systemic reaction. The total leukocyte count in the joint fluid is only slightly increased, and the differential count may be normal. Chronic arthritis is often difficult to differentiate clinically from degenerative joint disease. Chronic arthritis is more common in young animals than in older animals such as rapidly growing yearling bulls, adult bulls, and aged dairy cows and horses, in which degenerative arthropathy is most common. A sudden onset of acute lameness and marked swelling of a joint with severe pain suggests an infectious arthritis or traumatic injury to the joint. Marked swelling of several joints suggests infectious polyarthritis.

Osteodystrophy is characterized by the following:

- Lameness and stiffness of gait
- Usually, an absence of joint-capsule abnormalities
- Enlargements and deformities of the long bones in growing animals
- A number of animals being affected at about the same time

Radiography may reveal the abnormal bones, and the nutritional history may explain the cause.

Degenerative myopathy causes acute lameness and a stiff and trembling gait, often leading to recumbency and absence of joint or bone involvement.

Traumatic sprains of tendons or ligaments and fractures of the epiphyses may cause lameness and local pain; when they involve periarticular tissues, they may be difficult to differentiate from arthritis.

Arthritis is never present at birth and apparent fixation of the joints should arouse suspicion of a congenital anomaly. The differentiation between arthritis and diseases of the peripheral nerves or spinal cord, both of which can cause lameness or recumbency, may be difficult if the arthritis is not clinically obvious. Diseases of the peripheral nerves cause lameness as a result of flaccid paralysis and neurogenic atrophy. Lesions of the spinal cord usually result in weakness of the hindlimbs, weak or absent withdrawal reflexes, and loss of skin sensation.

TREATMENT

Parenteral Antimicrobials

Treatment should focus on **early diagnosis**; **removal of infected fluids and tissue** via joint lavage (tidal or though and through), arthroscopy, arthrotomy, or possibly closed suction drainage; **effective antimicrobial therapy**; and **controlling inflammation**. Acute septic arthritis should be treated as an emergency to avoid irreversible changes in the joint. The conservative approach is the use of antimicrobials given parenterally daily for several days and up to a few weeks in some cases, but this provides a lower success rate than when antimicrobial treatment is accompanied by removal of infected fluids and tissue. Antimicrobials that perfuse into septic joints in therapeutic concentrations when administered parenterally include the natural and synthetic penicillins, cephalosporins, tetracycline, trimethoprim-potentiated sulfonamides, neomycin, gentamicin, kanamycin, and amikacin, with species preferences regarding preferred antimicrobial protocols.

The relative efficacy of antimicrobials administered parenterally versus by intraarticular injections is uncertain. Trimethoprim–sulfadiazine, given to calves parenterally, results in therapeutic concentrations of the drug in the synovial fluid of calves, and penetrability was not enhanced or restricted by experimental joint inflammation. Oxytetracycline and penicillin given parenterally readily penetrate the synovial membrane of both normal neonatal calves and those with experimental arthritis. Because peak synovial joint fluid levels of oxytetracycline and penicillin exceeded the minimum inhibitory concentrations for organisms such as *T. pyogenes*, the use of parenteral antimicrobials for the treatment of infectious arthritis in calves is appropriate. Ceftiofur at 1 mg/kg BW intravenously every 12 hours for 20 days, along with joint lavage, was successful in treating experimental septic arthritis associated with *E. coli*. The duration of antibiotic therapy is empirical; 3 weeks is recommended. Cephapirin administered parenterally to normal calves or those with arthritis resulted in synovial fluid levels approximately 30% of serum levels. The use of ampicillin trihydrate in calves with suppurative arthritis, at a dose of 10 mg/kg BW intramuscularly, resulted in a peak serum concentration of 2.5 µg/mL, 2 hours after injection; the highest concentration in normal synovial fluid was 3.5 µg/mL at 4 hours, and the highest concentration in suppurative synovial fluid was 2.7 µg/mL at 2 hours. Marbofloxacin at 4 mg/kg BW intramuscularly daily for 10 days was effective for the treatment of infectious arthritis in calves.

In **foals** and **horses** with septic arthritis, the selection of the antimicrobial of choice will depend on the suspected cause of the arthritis. The antimicrobial susceptibilities of bacterial isolates from horses with septic arthritis/synovitis or osteomyelitis after fracture repair vary widely. A combination of a cephalosporin and amikacin is recommended before culture and susceptibility results are available. Commonly used dosage protocols include penicillin G potassium (22,000 IU/kg BW IV every 6 hours) with aminoglycoside gentamicin (11 mg/kg BW IV every 24 hours) or amikacin (20 mg/kg BW IV every 24 hours) or the third-generation cephalosporin ceftiofur (2.2 mg/kg BW IM every 12 hours). In azotemic foals, care needs to be taken while administering aminoglycosides, and monitoring should be in place to detect nephrotoxicity. Amoxicillin at 40 mg/kg BW IV is effective for the treatment of infectious joint disease in horses. The administration of trimethoprim-sulfadiazine at 30 mg/kg BW orally once daily to horses with experimentally induced *S. aureus* arthritis was ineffective in maintaining adequate levels of both drugs in infected synovial fluid. In contrast, the use of the same drug at 30 mg/kg BW orally given every 12 hours was effective in maintaining therapeutic concentrations of both drugs in the serum and in the joint fluid. Amphotericin B given intravenously daily for up to 30 days combined with joint drainage has been used for the treatment of *Candida* sp. arthritis in the horse.

In **piglets at 2 weeks of age, streptococcal arthritis** is most likely, and it will respond quickly to penicillin given parenterally. Likewise, acute arthritis associated with erysipelas in pigs will respond beneficially if treated early before there is pannus formation.

Synovitis caused by *Histophilus somni* infection responds quickly to systemic treatment. However, in other specific types of infectious arthritis the response is poor, and recovery, if it does occur, requires several days or a week. Mycoplasmal arthritis in cattle is relatively nonresponsive to treatment, and affected cattle may be lame for up to several weeks before improvement occurs; complete recovery may not occur. Chronic arthritis as a result of infection of pigs with *E. insidiosa* will commonly develop into a rheumatoid-like arthritis and be refractory to treatment.

Failure to respond to conservative therapy has been attributed to the following:

- Inadequate concentrations of antimicrobials achieved in the joint cavity
- Presence of excessive amounts of exudate and fibrin in the joint, making the infectious agent inaccessible to the antimicrobial
- Antimicrobial-resistant infections

It is often not possible to determine which situation is responsible.

If conservative treatment is not providing sufficient improvement and the value of the animal warrants extended therapy, a joint sample should be obtained for culture and susceptibility testing. The most suitable antimicrobial may then be given parenterally and/or by intraarticular injection. Strict asepsis is necessary to avoid introduction of further infection.

Intraarticular Antimicrobials

Antimicrobials infused into the joint should not be cytotoxic, and gentamicin (500 mg), amikacin (125 mg), soluble ceftiofur, and cefazolin (500 mg) are commonly used with minimal to no apparent effects on developing cartilage. The combined intraarticular and intravenous administration of gentamicin to normal horses can result in concentrations 10 to 100 times greater than after intravenous administration alone. In addition, gentamicin concentration in synovial fluid remained above the minimum inhibitory concentration for many common equine bacterial pathogens for at least 24 hours after treatment. The intraarticular administration of gentamicin is advantageous for the treatment of infectious arthritis in animals in which the systemic administration of the drug may be contraindicated, especially in the presence of impaired renal function or endotoxemia. Continuous infusion of gentamicin into the tarsocrural joint of horses for 5 days is an acceptable method of treating septic arthritis.

Antimicrobial-impregnated polymethylmethacrylate beads and gentamicin-impregnated collagen sponges have been used for the treatment of orthopedic infections involving bone, synovial structures, and other soft tissues. The antimicrobials diffuse from the nonbiodegradable beads in a bimodal fashion. There is a rapid ("burst") release of 5% to 45% of the total amount of antimicrobial within the first 24 hours after implantation and then a sustained elution that persists for weeks to months, depending on the antimicrobial used. For effective diffusion, the antimicrobials must be water soluble, heat stable, and available in powder form. Aminoglycosides (gentamicin, amikacin) and third-generation cephalosporins (e.g., ceftiofur) have been incorporated most commonly into the beads, but to be successful the drug must retain its antimicrobial effect after heating. The major disadvantage with polymethylmethacrylate beads is that they must be removed because they act as a foreign body and also provide unknown slaughter withdrawal times in food-producing animals. Long-term placement of intraarticular catheters has also been used in horses with septic arthritis, but aseptic methods must be maintained at the catheter site and during continuous or intermittent antimicrobial infusion, which can be challenging in a mobile animal. Moreover, a catheter should always be considered a two-way street and a potential vehicle for bacterial contamination of the joint. Whether placement of intraarticular catheters, polymethylmethacrylate beads, or gentamicin-impregnated collagen sponges have any substantive clinical advantages over intraarticular injections at approximately 3-day intervals has not been determined. Intraarticular ceftiofur injection every 3 days accompanied by wound management has become favored by some in the treatment of septic arthritis of the distal interphalangeal joint in cattle.

Regional limb perfusion with antimicrobials has been used for the treatment of experimentally induced septic arthritis. The antimicrobial is infused under pressure to a selected region of the limbs through the venous system. The concentration of the antimicrobial in the septic synovial fluid will usually exceed those obtained by intravenous administration. However, there are insufficient data available to evaluate the procedure in naturally occurring cases of septic arthritis. Therapeutic concentrations of cefazolin are achieved in the synovial fluid of clinically normal cows when injected intravenously distal to a tourniquet, and the technique could be used as an alternative to systemic administration of antimicrobials to provide adequate concentrations in a joint cavity. Regional limb perfusion appears better suited to treatment of more extensive infections such as septic arthritis secondary to penetrating wounds or accompanied by infected tendons or osteomyelitis.

Lavage of Joint

Drainage of the affected joint and through-and-through lavage of the joint is also desirable along with the systemic administration of antimicrobials. Aspiration and distension–irrigation of the joint cavity using polyionic electrolyte solutions buffered to a pH of 7.4 is recommended (Fig. 15-10). The irrigation removes exudates and lysozymes that destroy articular cartilage. A through-and-through lavage system may also be used with drainage tubes. General or local anesthesia should be provided. The distended joint is identified by palpation, the hair is clipped short, and the skin is prepared with appropriate surgical disinfection. A 2-cm 16-g needle is inserted into the joint cavity, avoiding direct contact with the bones of the joint. A second needle is inserted into the joint as far as possible from the first needle to cause any fluid perfused into the joint to pass through as much of the joint cavity as possible. Next, 0.5 to 1 L of a balanced crystalloid solution such as lactated Ringer's solution warmed to 37° C (99 F) is flushed through the joint using a hand-pumped pressure bag to keep a steady fluid flow into the joint. The only antimicrobial solution documented to be safe to be added to joint lavage solutions is 0.1% povidone-iodine solution, which produces minimal synovitis and no articular cartilage damage or joint irritation.

Arthroscopy

Arthroscopy provides excellent visualization of most parts of an affected joint and can be

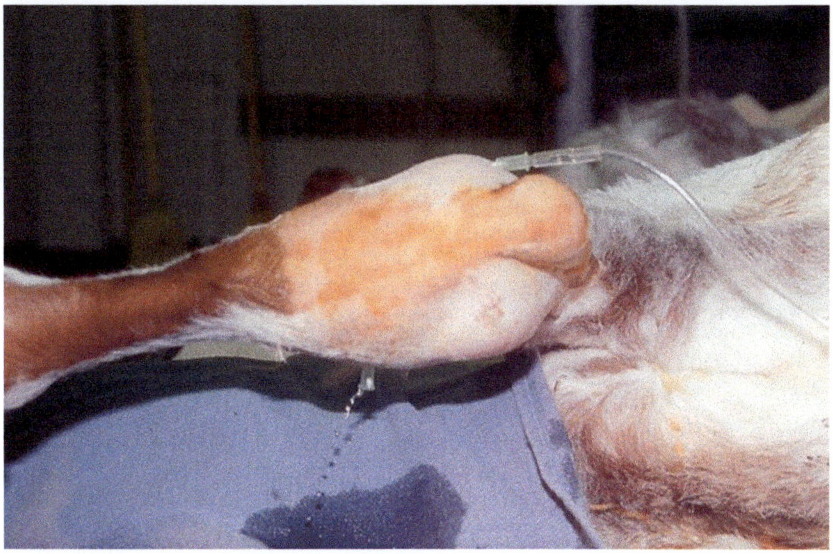

Fig. 15-10 Through-and-through needle lavage of the left hock joint of the Shorthorn calf in Figure 15-9. Warmed lactated Ringer's solution is lavaged through the joint with periodic joint distention (present) to facilitate lavage of the entire joint. The calf made a complete recovery.

used to access the joint for the treatment of septic arthritis. The endoscope can be used to explore and debride the affected joint during the same intervention. Purulent exudate can be removed, and necrotic areas within the synovial membrane can be debrided.

Surgical Drainage and Arthrotomy

Failure to respond to parenteral and intraarticular medication may require surgical opening of the joint capsule, careful debridement, and excision of synovium and infected cartilage and bone. This may be followed by daily irrigation of the joint cavity with antimicrobials and saline. A lavage system can be established and the joint cavity infused with an antimicrobial and saline daily for several days. Arthrotomy with lavage was more effective in eliminating joint infections by providing better drainage than arthroscopy, synovectomy, and lavage. However, with arthrotomy the risk of ascending bacterial contamination is greater, and the major difficulty is to eliminate the infection from the joint and incision site. Infected sequestra and osteomyelitis of subchondral bone will prevent proper healing. Curettage of septic physeal lesions in foals may be necessary.

Open drainage and intraarticular and parenteral antimicrobials have been used to treat persistent or severe septic arthritis/tenosynovitis. Although joint lavage through needles is still effective in many horses with acute infectious arthritis or tenosynovitis, in those with chronic or recurring septic arthritis, open drainage is indicated to remove the inflammatory exudate from the synovial space. Infected synovial structures are drained through a small (3-cm) arthrotomy incision left open and protected by a sterile bandage. Joint lavage using antimicrobials is done daily, and parenteral antimicrobials are given intensively.

Septic pedal arthritis in cattle may be treated successfully by the creation of a drainage tract to promote adequate drainage. In cattle with septic arthritis of the digit, placement of a wooden block under the unaffected digit decreases weight-bearing on the affected digit and provides for earlier, less painful ambulation.

Arthrodesis or Artificial Ankylosis

Surgical arthrodesis can be used for the treatment of chronic septic arthritis in horses and calves. Septic arthritis of the distal interphalangeal joint is a common complication of diseases of the feet of cattle. Facilitated ankylosis of the joint is a satisfactory alternative to amputation of the affected digit in valuable breeding animals. In a series of 12 cases of septic arthritis of the distal interphalangeal joint treated by use of facilitated ankylosis, the success rate was 100%.

Physical Therapy

The local application of heat, by hot fomentations or other physical means, is laborious, but if practiced frequently and vigorously, it will reduce the pain and local swelling. Analgesics are recommended if there is prolonged recumbency. Persistent recumbency is one of the problems in the treatment of arthritis, particularly in foals. The animal spends little time feeding or sucking and loses much condition. Compression necrosis over bony prominences is a common complication and requires vigorous preventive measures.

Stall rest for at least 3 to 4 weeks is recommended to minimize excessive exercise because the joint cartilage appears to be more vulnerable to injury after an acute inflammatory episode.

Antiinflammatory Agents and Adjunctive Therapy

NSAIDs are used routinely parenterally to decrease the inflammatory response and to provide analgesia. A common dose rate in foals with septic arthritis is 1.1 mg/kg BW IV every 24 hours for flunixin meglumine. In experimental synovitis in the horse, similar to septic arthritis, phenylbutazone was more effective than ketoprofen in reducing lameness, joint temperature, synovial fluid volume, and synovial fluid prostaglandin. Topical application of a fentanyl transdermal "patch" to the thorax or groin may provide additive analgesia, but scheduled drug requirements and reporting may make such treatment impractical.

Hyaluronic acid is protective for joint health because it is an important constitutive component of articular cartilage and synovial fluid. Horses with septic arthritis have depleted hyaluronic acid content, and consequently foals with septic arthritis benefit from the intraarticular administration of hyaluronic acid (10 mg) because this results in glycosaminoglycan loss from articular cartilage and has antiinflammatory properties.

Prognosis for Survival and Athletic Use in Horses With Septic Arthritis

The factors affecting the prognosis for survival and athletic use in 93 foals treated for septic arthritis have been examined. The femoropatellar and tarsocrural joints were most commonly affected. Osteomyelitis or degenerative joint disease were detected in 59% of the foals. Failure of transfer of passive immunity, pneumonia, and enteritis were common. Treatment consisted of lavage, lavage and arthroscopic debridement with or without partial synovectomy, or lavage and arthrotomy to debride infected bone and parenteral antibiotics. Seventy-five foals survived and were discharged from hospital, and approximately one-third raced. Isolation of *Salmonella* from synovial fluid was associated with an unfavorable prognosis for survival, and multisystemic disease was associated with an unfavorable prognosis for survival and ability to race. The key to successful outcome for septic arthritis is rapid diagnosis and initiation of treatment. The presence infection in multiple joints is associated with a poor outcome.[1]

In a series of 507 horses treated for joint disease at one equine hospital during a period of 7 years, the risk factors affecting discharge from the hospital were examined; 58% of foals, 78% of yearlings, and 94% of racing adults were discharged. Foals with a less severe lameness, duration of less than 1 day, and infectious arthritis had increased odds of discharge.

Factors associated with the short-term survival rate of 81 foals with septic arthritis were evaluated. Seventy-seven percent of the foals were discharged from the referral hospital, with nonsurvival being associated with multiple joint involvement; detection of gram-negative, mixed bacterial intraarticular infection; and the presence of degenerate neutrophils in the joint fluid.[10] Initiation of treatment within 24 hours of first evidence of clinical abnormalities and the use of multiple treatment modalities were positively associated with survival.[10] In general, little information is available about athletic performance in horses following septic arthritis.

CONTROL

The control of infectious arthritis is of major importance in newborn farm animals. The early ingestion of adequate quantities of good-quality colostrum and a clean environment for the neonate are necessary. The prophylactic use of antimicrobials may be considered to reduce incidence. Some of the infectious arthritides associated with specific diseases can be controlled through immunization programs. For example, vaccination of piglets at 6 to 8 weeks of age will provide protection against both the septicemic and arthritic forms of erysipelas.

FURTHER READING

Annear MJ, Furr MO, White NA 2nd. Septic arthritis in foals. *Equine Vet Educ.* 2011;23:422-431.

Desrochers A, Francoz D. Clinical management of septic arthritis in cattle. *Vet Clin North Am Food A.* 2014;30:177-203.

Haerdi-Landerer MC, Habermacher J, Wenger B, Suter MM, Steiner A. Slow release antibiotics for treatment of septic arthritis in large animals. *Vet J.* 2010;184:14-20.

Hardy J. Etiology, diagnosis, and treatment of septic arthritis, osteitis, and osteomyelitis in foals. *Clin Tech Equine Pract.* 2006;5:309-317.

Paradis MR. Septic arthritis in the foal: what is the best imaging modality? *Equine Vet Educ.* 2010;22:334-335.

REFERENCES

1. Hepworth-Warren KL, et al. *J Am Vet Med Assoc.* 2015;246:785.
2. Rutherford SJ, et al. *Vet Rec.* 2014;10.1136/vr101753.
3. Rutherford SJ, et al. *Vet Rec.* 2015;10.1136/vr.102781.
4. Lacasta D, et al. *Small Ruminant Res.* 2008;78:202.
5. Steel CM, et al. *Aust Vet J.* 2013;91:268.
6. Borg H, et al. *Vet Surg.* 2013;42:262.
7. Beccati F, et al. *Vet Radiol Ultrasound.* 2015;56:68.
8. Gaschen L, et al. *Vet Radiol Ultrasound.* 2011;52:627.
9. Easley JT, et al. *Vet Radiol Ultrasound.* 2011;52:402.
10. Vos NJ, Ducharme NG. *Irish Vet J.* 2008;61:102.

LAMENESS IN PIGS AND DEGENERATIVE JOINT DISEASE (OSTEOCHONDROSIS, OSTEOARTHROSIS, EPIPHYSIOLYSIS AND APOPHYSIOLYSIS, LEG WEAKNESS IN PIGS)

LEG DISORDERS

Leg disorders are divided into three major groups[1]: (1) infectious arthritis, (2) physical injuries, and (3) osteochondrosis.

Leg weakness is a locomotory disability of pigs that is not associated with infectious disease. It is a combination of noninfectious arthropathy and osteopathy and is a significant cause of culling in pig herds. The causes are defects of conformation, osteochondrosis (including epiphysiolysis), arthrosis, lumbar intervertebral disk degeneration, and spondylosis. The clinical syndrome varies from lameness to difficulty in rising to recumbency. The characteristic signs are carrying a hindleg, sitting on the haunches for long periods of time, and a shuffling gait. All of the conditions affecting the limbs are related to the growth patterns in the respective limb bones. Rickets is seen from 8 weeks to physeal closure, osteomalacia from 8 weeks onward, osteochondrosis (OCD) from 0 to 30 weeks, epiphyseal separation from 15 weeks to physeal closure, and spondylosis in older sows or boars.

LAMENESS

Lameness is deviation from normal gait. Joint kinetics have been described,[2] and lameness is closely associated with floor conditions.[3] One of the key decisions in examining pigs that are not showing signs of normal locomotion is to ascertain whether the pigs have abnormalities in the nervous, skeletal, muscular, or joint systems. In most cases lameness will involve the joints for a variety of reasons because these are the most stressed structures in the locomotory system. Patience in examination is essential, and noting the progression of signs is also very important. What the clinician will see and what the pathologist and laboratory diagnostician sees are usually two different things.

Lameness in pigs is associated with several etiologic disease groups: (1) trauma and bone fractures; (2) infections, such as arthritis, abscesses, tendonitis, and osteomyelitis; (3) overgrown feet, heels/claws, and wear conformation; and (4) osteochondrosis/osteoarthropathy, which is probably the most important group. The most common combination is trauma/infection/weak conformation.

AGE-RELATED CHANGES IN PIGS

Young Pigs

Examination of young pigs for lameness is not easy. They are quick on their feet, bunch often, and need to be marked individually for further identification. You need to identify and mark those that are not walking or behaving normally or, if very young, not suckling properly. In young pigs purulent arthritis is common (usually *S. suis*, but may be others, including streptococci, *S. aureus*, *E. coli*).[4-6] In a Swedish study, 75% of lame piglets had polyarthritis (more than one joint affected).[5]

The risk factors[7] include the following:

- Poor mothering, poor milk supply, poor colostral antibody protection, and agalactia
- Skin lesions, particularly at the carpal joints as piglets struggle to suckle
- Foot lesions associated with very poor flooring—rough edges, jagged metal (always worse than plastic), old plastic, poor concrete finish, and so forth—which causes damage to the tender feet of neonates, leading to bruised heels, erosion of heels, coronary band lesions, and subsequently septic arthritis
- Arthritis is ubiquitous, principally as a result of bad hygiene in the farrowing house; the importation of nonimmune gilts; poor management; no all-in/all-out system; improper cleaning, disinfection, and drying; lack of bedding; fully slatted floors; and lack of creep heating and feeding.

Most of the factors in the first two categories have disappeared by weaning because the piglet skin hardens and underfloor conditions generally improve.

The situation can be improved by proper management of sows and gilts; batch farrowing followed by cleaning, disinfection, and drying; proper building maintenance; bird and rodent control; treatment of sows for agalactia; use of cross-fostering if there are large litters; and use of vaccines if appropriate. It was shown that repairing floors and doubling the straw decreased the amount of abrasions,[5] and the level of lameness decreased from week 1 to week 3.

Osteodystrophy has been associated with hypervitaminosis A in growing pigs.

Growers and Finishers

In growers and finishers all of the groupings of disease type are important. See how they react to walking. Usually lame pigs have an arched back, sit for longer periods, are reluctant to stand or move, are easily bullied, and tend to sit or lie down as soon as possible. If they are not lame they get up quickly and move quickly. In these animals the infectious causes involve *M. hyosynoviae*, *M. hyorhinis*, *S. aureus*, *Erysipelothrix* spp., and *H. parasuis*. In addition, OCD is important. In a survey of 1000 pigs,[8] 14% had OCD, and every pig with OCD gained 100 g/day less than the unaffected pigs.

The risk factors include low herd immunity (need to increase by exposure or vaccination); the importation of carriers onto the farm (e.g., *S. suis*, *Erysipelas* spp., *M. hyosynoviae*, and *H. parasuis* in particular); mixing of different ages of pigs (need all-in/all-out system by age); and stress as a result of excessive mixing, moving, and handling (reduce if possible).

A hereditary form of rickets has been described in which there is no enzyme to convert D2 to D3 in the kidney. Normally, rickets derived from dietary causes is normally seen in pigs of 2 to 6 months, and they have swollen joints, particularly the carpal, humeral, elbow, and stifle joints. Cases of rickets from dietary causes are very uncommon and should not happen in this day and age, but cases do occur, particularly in the pigs of "back garden" and enthusiastic amateurs. The clinical signs include a stunted and unthrifty appearance, lameness, fractured long bones, and paresis. In young, weaned, growing pigs, there is a failure of mineralization of the osteoid and cartilage matrix, especially in the growth plates. At necropsy, the bones are pale and soft, particularly the ribs, which bend rather than snap under pressure and are radiolucent. Because the bones bend and don't fracture, there is often evidence of recent or healing fractures.

Rickets develop as a result of the following:

- Inadequate concentrations of calcium, phosphorus, and/or vitamin D in the ration
- Improperly balanced calcium and phosphorus in the ration, resulting in a ratio greatly different from 1 to 2:1
- Inadequate concentrations of the active vitamin D
- No vitamin D synthesis in a dark environment
- No proper ration analysis
- Excess iron in the diet

Kyphosis/lordosis ("kinky back" or lordosis/kyphosis) can be seen as a congenital abnormality, but it has also been seen in association with precocious behavior causing relaxation of the spinal ligaments and also by breeding for extra vertebrae in the spinal column, resulting in too much muscle weight for the skeleton.

Older Animals

In older animals the disease is mainly of the infectious disease group, particularly polyarthritis and spondylitis. The risk factors are low herd immunity, the importation of carriers, mixing of pigs with different immunities, and episodes of stress. In these animals prevention is by isolation and quarantine of new imports, thorough mixing of pigs to ensure equal susceptibility and resistance, vaccination where possible (use the right strain, store vaccines correctly, and use them properly), and, importantly, reduction of adverse nutrition (look after P, Ca, and ratios, and make sure they are mixed at the right proportions).

A case-control study of factors associated with arthritis detected at slaughter in pigs from 49 farms in Finland showed that 93% to 96% of pigs had osteochondritic lesions in joints, both in the control group and the group with high incidence of arthritis at slaughter, and infection was found only rarely.[9] Bursitis is a common feature in this age group,[10] as are other foot lesions.[11,12] Osteomyelitis is an uncommon problem but may result in lameness or pathologic fractures of vertebrae with compression of the spinal cord. It may follow septicemia or a local progression, as in tail-biting abscessation.

Adults

In a survey of cull sow bone and joint integrity in the Moorepark Research Farm herd in Ireland, it was found that there was no relationship between lameness and joint pathology in sows. Osteochondritic lesions were found in all the sows and were most common in the medial condyle of the humerus and the anconeal process of the ulna.[13,14] A study of lameness and fertility in sows and gilts in loose-housed herds in Finland[15] showed that 8.8% of the animals (646 in 21 herds) were lame. The most common clinical diagnoses were osteochondrosis, infected skin lesions, and claw lesions. Sows on slatted floors had twice the chance of being lame than those on solid floors. Yorkshire pigs were more likely to be lame than Landrace or crossbred pigs. Lameness was not a risk factor for nonpregnancy. With sows, fighting in loose-housing systems is an important factor, especially if there are limited numbers of feeders. Slipping on concrete-based flooring systems with badly drained, water-soaked floors is also a hazard. In these cases rubber mats may help. In sows there is commonly medial claw atrophy (hypoplasia) and an overgrown lateral claw. Quite often it is the younger animals that are affected, especially in loose-housed animals. Lesions at the coronary band are also not uncommon. Claw lesions may be primary, with secondary conditions to follow. In two commercial sow herds,[16] less than 4% of sows had lameness, with heel erosions being the most common cause and overgrowth of dewclaws second.

One of the most common lesions in this age group is cracked feet, either of the sole or wall or heels; affected animals are lame, but if treated, a proportion will always get better. OCD in sows will often cause an intermittent lameness, whereas animals with arthritis are persistently lame. In a survey of sows at casualty slaughter in 2005, 22% had fractures, 12% arthroses, and 15% osteomyelitis in the spine and other arthritides. All of the four groups are a problem in sows. Lameness is always on the list of culling for sows.[17]

Prevention is attention to all the items previously listed: inspect, trim, and treat feet regularly; check for wet floors, sharp edges, and newly laid concrete (treat with sodium carbonate); correct width of slats for age of animal; remove steps and steep slopes; check drainage angles; improve hygiene; perform regular cleaning, disinfection, and drying; reduce fighting; provide manipulable materials, particularly straw; have stable subgroups and provide good feeding and ad lib water; improve horn quality, possibly by increasing biotin and vitamin E in the diet; and, most important, improve genetic selection techniques.

Piglets often have fractures if laid on by sows, especially if they are hypoglycaemic or weak. Older piglets may fracture bones when they are stuck in fences or equipment. Finishing pigs may fracture bones during transport. Fractures found in several animals at the same time may be a result of electrocution or sometimes outdoor lightning strike. Vertebrae, particularly in the thoracic area of the spine, humerus, neck of the scapula, pelvis, and neck of the femur are the usual sites. Sometimes the fractures are in the lumbosacral junction, resulting in separation of spinal cord and nerves. In these cases decomposition occurs quickly. Fractures have been described as part of lactational osteoporosis (downer sows) that occurred in first-litter sows when they were moved from the farrowing quarters and involved the pelvis, spine, femur, and other bones. It was caused by early mating, rapid growth rates, high milking yield of the sows, large litters, and insufficient nutrients in the diet to provide for both milk and sow growth, and thus calcium and phosphorus were drawn from the skeleton. Lactational osteoporosis is a result of an imbalance between bone formation (osteoblast activity) and bone resorption (osteoclast activity). There is often calcium deficiency. Sows bones decalcify to mobilize calcium for milk production. The specific gravity of bone in these animals will be 1.018, whereas the normal is 1.022. The ratio of cortex to total area is 0.2 or less compared with 0.3 in the normal cross section of the sixth rib. The bones are structurally normal but of lower mass. Complicating factors include long periods of restricted exercise (sow stalls, farrowing crates), and it is particularly a problem during the first litter when gilts are still growing and there is an even higher demand for calcium and phosphorus. At necropsy the most frequent sites for lesions are the proximal one-third of the humerus and the proximal one-third of the femur. Comminuted spiral fractures extend from the metaphysis down into the diaphysis.

Osteomalacia has been described as a result of deficiencies or imbalances of calcium, phosphorus, and vitamin D but may also be a result of the inability to consume sufficient food. Large quantities of unmineralized osteoids develop, thereby weakening the bones. This is attributable to a higher secretion of parathyroid hormone in the lactating sow.

Proliferative osteitis of the femoral greater trochanter and medial epicondyle of the humerus has been described, usually in gilts after the first weaning. Affected animals are seen dog-sitting, and they rise with pain and discomfort; the pathology is a hemolytic mass in the muscle.

Ankylosing spondylitis has been identified in culled sows and boars at abattoirs, but it is thought that the condition starts as early as the first year of life. Pigs have a painful lumbar region, may develop kyphosis, and waddle when walking or drag the hindfeet. The cause is probably multiple—wear and tear, spinal trauma, poor nutrition, genetics, arthritis of spinal joints, and so on.

Vertebrae may eventually fuse when alleviation occurs. Spondylosis results in bridging of the vertebrae, with possible trapping of the vertebrae.

Arthrosis is sometimes referred to as arthropathy, osteoarthrosis, or osteoarthritis and is a nonspecific degenerating condition of cartilage that develops in chronic joint disease. The incidence increases with age (animals less than 18 months had 7% incidence, but those over 18 months had 82%). It is the result of instability resulting from osteochondrosis and the surface lesions in the joint that have filled with osseous repair tissue. Pathologically, the lesions include fibrillation of joint cartilage, ulceration of the articular surface, osteophyte production, and thickened synovial membranes and joint capsule.

Tumors are not common but include an osteosarcoma of the maxilla occluding the nasal cavity, secondary tumors from a malignant melanoma, congenital melanomas, and multiple myeloma[18] and a glioblastoma in the ventral cerebral cortex of a 6-month-old Yorkshire gilt.

OSTEOCHONDROSIS

Leg weakness in pigs is a very loose term that includes a wide variety of conditions and is best discarded. Degenerative joint disease would be a much better general term to describe the lameness of young rapidly growing pigs affected with noninfectious joint diseases, which include osteochondrosis (OC), epiphysiolysis, and degenerative osteoarthrosis (OA). Degenerative joint disease is characterized by varying degrees of intermittent but progressive lameness in rapidly growing pigs from 4 to 8 months of age, and pathologically it is characterized by the presence of OA and OC. The disease is of major economic importance because of the high culling rate of breeding-age swine.

Degenerative joint disease is, in fact, a dyschondroplasia that affects growth cartilage, both physeal and epiphyseal, in most breeds of rapidly growing pigs, which results in cartilage and bone lesions.

The term *dyschondroplasia* should be used to describe the majority of lesions affecting growth plates, especially physeal growth cartilage or physes and lesions involving the articular epiphyseal cartilage complex (AECC). Dyschondroplasic foci may undergo calcification and ossification; alternatively, the chondrocytes may die, and the necrotic chondrocytes and the denatured matrix are removed by fibrous connective tissue that ossifies. Occasionally, features develop at the chondro-osseous interface with the metaphysis or within the calcified portion of the zone of hypertrophying chondrocytes; cysts or clefts that contain blood persist and appear to stop the ossification front. Osteochondrosis is defined as a focal disturbance of endochondral ossification and is regarded as having a multifactorial etiology, with no single factor accounting for all aspects of the disease. The most commonly cited factors are genetics, rapid growth, anatomic conformation, trauma, and dietary imbalances. Only heredity and anatomic conformation are confirmed by the scientific data. The term *osteochondrosis* should be used to describe a group of syndromes that cause limb deformities or degenerative joint disease in young, fast-growing pigs of either sex. Currently the consensus is that it is the effect of rapid growth (early excess weight) and lack of exercise on the developing cartilage that is at fault. The lesions appear to develop when pigs are less than 1 month old, when there is little muscle mass, indicating that heavy musculature is not the prime cause but helps in the exacerbation of the disorder. It has been observed in pigs as young as 1 day old. However, in these young pigs the AEEC and growth plates are proportionately thicker and possibly susceptible to stress. This results in a thickening of part of the growth plate that causes interference with metaphyseal growth. This in turn results in deformation of bones, joints, and ultimately limbs. It is this distortion that may lead to incongruity of joints, with subsequent development of osteoarthritis and other degenerative joint diseases.

In the past, many of the lesions affecting the AEEC were examined at a stage when degenerative joint disease (DJD) had already become established. In these cases, the articular surface was advanced, and subchondral bone was often exposed. However, examination of early lesions shows that the lesions are initiated as microscopic foci of chondrolysis at or near the interface of the articular cartilage and epiphyseal growth cartilage. The lesions may progress at this site, and lysed cartilage persists in the deeper layers of the AEEC, at the chondro-osseous interface, and within the bone of the epiphysis. The recently replicated cells die, and there is either failure of matrix production or disruption of the formed matrix. Clusters of chondrocytes often develop at the periphery of the lesion in an attempt to repair the lesion. The soft denatured cartilage is probably subject to further damage during joint movement, so that flaps, fissures, and craters develop. When the AEEC is breached and subchondral bone is in contact with the joint space, the joint becomes painful, and lameness develops.

There is a consensus view that vascular injury within cartilage canals is part of the pathogenesis, although there are opponents of this view. With no normal vascularization, there is no subsequent ossification. The position with regard to OCD has recently been summarized[19] and describes it as being a premature regression of the blood supply to the epiphyseal growth cartilage, leading to ischemic necrosis of the cartilage canals. Research suggests that there are three different manifestations of OCD: (1) *osteochondrosis latens* (OCL), where there are foci areas of cartilage necrosis at the epiphyseal growth cartilage that are not visible grossly but are visible on microscopic examination; (2) *osteochondrosis manifesta* (OCM), where endochondral ossification becomes visible on microscopic and radiographic examination as thickened or uneven cartilage; and (3) *osteochondritis dissecans* (OCD), characterized by lesions of fissured articular cartilage protruding into the underlying bone.

There is still much confusion as to whether there is an association between OCD and lameness. Our considered opinion is that it is referable to the individual animal and depends entirely on the extent and severity of the lesion, the joints affected, the "meatiness" of the animal, and the age at which the animal is affected. In many cases, the situation is complicated by secondary processes such as osteomyelitis, fractures, and damage to greater trochanter and tubercle.

Epiphysiolysis and apophysiolysis are now considered to be part of the abnormalities of the AEEC, with fractures occurring at the weakened epiphyseal sites in the femur and tuber ischiadicum, respectively.

Diagnosis of these conditions is achieved by ruling out other causes of lameness and then by confirming with a postmortem examination of cull sows.

SYNOPSIS

Etiology The specific cause is unknown but is probably a failure of vascularization of cartilage.

Epidemiology Occurs in majority of breeds of rapidly growing pigs and young breeding females and males. Lesions are commonly present at slaughter. May be related to nutrition and rapid growth rate, genetic predisposition, and type of flooring, but there are no reliable correlations.

Signs There may be no clinical findings or possibly lameness and inability to breed.

Clinical pathology Radiographic evidence of osteochondrosis.

Lesions Osteochondritic lesions of varying degrees of development, severity, and healing.

Diagnostic confirmation Lesions at necropsy.

Differential diagnosis list As listed for the various ages.

Other causes of lameness include the following:

- Polyarthritis attributable to infectious causes
- Laminitis
- Nutritional osteodystrophy attributable to calcium, phosphorus, and vitamin D imbalance
- Hypovitaminosis A causing hindlimb paresis

Treatment None.

Control Uncertain. Select breeding stock with sound legs and gait.

ETIOLOGY

The cause of the articular abnormalities is not known. The etiology and factors underlying these syndromes are poorly defined, partly because of the difficulty of definitive clinical examination of affected pigs and the frequent lack of apparent significant pathologic changes in necropsy examination of mild cases. There are no specific associations between degenerative joint disease and infectious diseases.

The growth plates that close last are the ones that are most susceptible (medial condyles of humerus and femur, ulna, costochondral junctions, and the 6th to 8th lumbar vertebrae). Many terms have been used to describe the condition, including osteochondritis, osteoarthritis, degenerative joint disease, arthropathy, arthritis, polyarthritis, and metaphyseal dysplasia, to name but a few. Most of these titles are inaccurate because the condition has its origin in the growth cartilage, and bones are affected secondarily.

EPIDEMIOLOGY

Occurrence

Recently, a study of 9,411 newborn piglets showed that 9.8% were treated for lameness. For parity 3 sows, the level had risen to 11.4%, but by parities 4 to 7, only 8% were treated. The treatments were in pigs of less than 3 weeks of age in 73% of the cases. Litters with 12 or more pigs had the highest incidences of lameness. Osteoarthritic changes are strongly associated with osteochondrotic changes in the humeral and femoral condyles. Osteochondrosis has been recorded as early as 1 day of age, so the lesions may be congenital. There may be some degree of change in up to 85% of pigs.

The osteochondrosis complex (OCD) is the most common cause of lameness in breeding pigs.[20]

However, a recent study[14] has shown no relationship between lameness and OCD, but all the sows studied had evidence of OCD (particularly in the medial condyle of the humerus and anconeal process of ulna).

We can say, in summary, that nearly all sows have some evidence of leg weakness, and in many circumstances leg weakness is a cause of culling. The reason for this is quite simple: the legs are the components of locomotion that are most influenced by genetics, nutrition, management, environment, and microorganisms and infection. Overfeeding is the cause that results in too much weight and not enough bone to support the weight.

There is a correlation between body conformation and the presence of joint lesions. Pigs with a narrow lumbar region, broad hams, and a large relative width between the stifle joints were highly susceptible to poor locomotory ability as a result of lesions in the elbow and stifle joints, the lumbar intervertebral joints, and the hip joint. It is postulated that inherited weakness of muscle, ligaments, cartilage, and joint conformation results in local overloading of the joint and the development of OC and OA. Some breeds, such as the Duroc, have more problems of structure and movement in the front legs than the rear, but OC is not responsible for the leg weakness. OC has been recorded in wild boar–Swedish Yorkshire crossbred pigs, in which the growth rate was low. It is probably not related to floor type. It is not associated with adventitious bursitis.

The intensification of the swine industry has required that pigs grow rapidly and with high feed efficiency. Under such intensified conditions, rapidly growing pigs develop lesions of the bones and joints, especially the femur. Most pigs near market weight have varying degrees of OC. Except for severe lesions, which usually occur in a relatively small proportion of the total population examined, the lesions seen at slaughter often have no detrimental effect on the growth rate of pigs up to market weight. An advanced degree of OC, however, can result in severe degenerative joint disease and lameness in breeding stock. The disease occurs in both male and female pigs, and the incidence of lame pigs can be as high as 20% to 30%. It is a particular problem in gilt and boar testing stations, where it may necessitate slaughter of affected animals before the testing period is complete. The lesions develop most commonly in growing pigs, particularly boars from 20 to 30 weeks of age, raised in confinement. The onset occurs when pigs are between 4 and 8 months of age, which coincides with a period of maximal growth rate. The peak period of clinical manifestation is from the late grower stage until 18 months of age, although the effect of OA may carry through to the adult period. Extensive multicentric degenerative joint disease in adult sows and boars can cause severe lameness, which often warrants euthanasia. However, sows ranging in age from 1.5 to 3.0 years and culled for impaired reproductive performance, with no history of lameness, may have lesions of the femoral condylar surface.

Risk Factors

Numerous risk factors contribute to the disease, including nutrition and rate of growth, genetic and breed predisposition, sex, type and quality of flooring, and exercise and confinement conditions. The pig carries 53% to 51% of its weight on the forelimbs and 47% to 49% on the hindlegs when young, but the weight supported on the hindlimbs is greater at 90-kg and 105-kg body weights. In a study of gilts and sows in Denmark, approximately 12% of gilts showed stiff locomotion, but 53% of gilts had at some time showed the same sign. Buck-kneed forelegs, upright pasterns, legs turned out wide, standing under position, and swinging hindquarters were associated with stiff locomotion or lameness. Weak pasterns on the hindfeet were associated with stiff locomotion and lameness. Weak pasterns on hindlegs and splayed digits on forelegs were associated with brisk movement (freedom from locomotor problems). The following leg weakness signs at the gilt stage were found to have a significant effect on the longevity of the sows: buck-kneed forelegs, swinging hindquarters, and standing under position on the hindlegs.

Nutrition and Rate of Growth

The disease is associated with rapid early growth, but it does not appear to be related to protein, vitamins A and D, or calcium and phosphorus imbalance in the ration. Maximal mineralization of bones is not necessary to prevent leg weakness. Only almost complete absence of calcium and phosphorus causes lameness. Disturbances of the Ca:P ratio below 0.5 or over 3.0 are necessary to produce lameness. Recently it has been suggested that long-term acidosis may be associated with the condition because bone is not formed as phosphorus is removed from the bone. In this context the acidification of pig diets has been suggested as a contributory cause. It has also been shown that the presence of deformed forelimbs is not associated with low levels of vitamin C in plasma. Rapid growth, especially during the early period, was thought to have a significant influence on the occurrence, and there is also some breed variation in susceptibility. However, in some feeding trials of pigs from weaning to slaughter weight, there was no direct effect of rapid growth rate on the incidence and severity of OC. In other feeding trials, average daily gain of gilts was an important factor in the severity of lesions of OC. Decreasing the rate of gain by restricting energy intake appeared to decrease the prevalence and severity of OC when gilts were slaughtered at 110 kg. However, it was shown that when pigs were fed waste food and grew more slowly, they had an increased prevalence and score for OC compared with pigs fed a commercial feed concentrate. Decreasing the concentration of protein in the diet of gilts from 16% to 12% resulted in less longitudinal bone growth but did not decrease the incidence of OC. A simple association between growth rate and the incidence or severity of joint lesions has not been consistently demonstrated, and a reduction in the growth rate of pigs does not control the disease.

A significant favorable association between leg action and daily gain has been noted. There has also been speculation that growth hormone could influence the development of lesions of OC by exerting a direct effect on differentiation and colonization of epiphyseal chondrocytes. There is no consistent relationship between the incidence of osteochondrosis and selection of pigs for lean tissue growth rate. It may be simply that more feed means more growth, which makes the stress on developing cartilage greater and therefore predisposes to OC.

Genetic and Breed Predisposition

It has been proposed for many years that selection of pigs for increased growth rate resulted in a concomitant increase in the incidence and severity of musculoskeletal disease. Genetic studies indicate that the heritabilities of leg weakness are low to moderate (0.1 to 0.3). A more recent study suggested from 0.01 to 0.42 for leg weakness and OC and that both are associated with production traits (lean percentage and back-fat thickness). Genetic analysis of the incidence of OC and leg weakness in the Swedish pig progeny testing scheme revealed a low to moderate heritability. Genetic control of leg weakness has been achieved by various researchers, and thus inheritance is probably an important risk factor for this disease complex. The genetics of leg weakness have been described in Finnish Large White and Landrace populations. Meaty breeds are the most severely affected, including the Duroc and the Dutch and Swedish Landrace.

Inheritance may not be polygenic; it may be just one gene that controls OC, the MEP gene.

Osteochondrosis also occurs in crossbred Wild Boar–Yorkshire pigs with a genetically decreased growth rate, raised under the same conditions as finishing pigs. The distribution and extent of OC was similar to that of purebred Swedish Yorkshire pigs. This suggests that it is not limited to rapidly growing pigs. There are significant breed differences in the periarticular and meniscal ossifications seen on x-ray. Recently the quantitative trait loci for locomotion and osteochondrosis-related traits have been identified in Large White–Meishan crossbred pigs. Correlations between breeding values for longevity and for OC were low but significant, in a favorable direction. Higher OC scores were associated with a higher risk of being culled.

It has been seen in wild boar in Slovenia.

Type of Flooring

Insecure footing because of unfavorable floor surfaces and the presence of foot lesions may change the posture of the animal and cause local overloading of certain joints. The effect of the quality of floor has been examined, and there is no clear evidence that the hardness of floor contributes to an increased incidence of leg weakness associated with joint disease. However, the incidence and severity of joint lesions may be related to the duration of confinement in pigs confined individually. Exercise will prevent abnormalities such as bow legs, flexion of the carpus, and sickle-legs from impairing the mobility of boars, but it does not influence the severity of joint lesions. The milder syndromes of poor movement and lameness associated with defects in leg conformation in the grower stage are not necessarily associated with bone or joint lesions and may regress spontaneously or improve if affected pigs are placed on pasture. However, severe lameness at this age, and occurring in replacement stock and young adults, is frequently associated with severe bone and joint lesions, which may be irreversible. A recent study has looked at type of floor (solid floor plus straw, solid floor no straw, and fully slatted). The slatted floors were worst for leg weakness and the floors with straw best. The different types of floor affected leg weakness and claw disorders differently.

Trauma probably exacerbates the late lesions by damaging further the blood supply to the blood vessels of the cartilage.

Exercise and Confinement

There is some limited evidence that a high lean growth rate may predispose toward leg weakness under confinement rearing. It may be that the growth rate at different ages is more important. Trauma during handling, penning, and transportation may be associated with a relatively high frequency of OC, but the evidence is very limited. A high stocking density had an adverse effect on four of the signs of leg weakness (knock knees, turned-out forelimbs or hindlimbs, standing with the legs under the body). A recent study of housing and treadmill training did not show any adverse effects on leg weakness. It has even been seen in pigs on grass and on deep litter and in wild boar.

Economic Importance

In Scandinavia, breeding pigs culled because of lameness had a 100% frequency of OC or OA, and up to 40% of boars in a performance test station had osteochondrosis or osteoarthrosis. A conservative estimate suggests that 3% of sows and 10% of boars are culled for unsoundness associated with OC and OA. The hidden costs include a reduced pool for selection of high-performance boars and gilts, the maintenance of pigs that cannot be used for breeding, increased mortality among piglets crushed by lame sows, reduced feed intake and growth rate in lame pigs, and transportation costs of replacement stock.

PATHOGENESIS

The initial stage of pathogenesis is thought to consist of the formation of fragile cartilage, failure of chondrocyte differentiation, subchondral bone necrosis, and failure of blood supply to the growth cartilage. Some of the literature supports the idea that the failure of blood supply is the crucial lesion, either from the epiphyseal or metaphyseal side. In a summary, the primary lesion could be described as a focal ischemic necrosis of growth cartilage initiated by necrosis of cartilage canal blood vessels. The necrotic cartilage does not undergo mineralization or vascular penetration, and then focal failure of endochondral ossification occurs when the ossification front approaches the lesion.

The condition has been seen as early as 1 day of age, and the lesions develop with age. The essential lesion is the necrosis of cartilage canals and surrounding cartilage. Lesions may be seen to be developing and healing at the same time. In growing animals, the superficial layer of joint cartilage is articular cartilage, and the deeper layer is epiphyseal cartilage that undergoes endochondral ossification as the animal matures. The articular cartilage persists in the mature animal, whereas the epiphyseal cartilage becomes a layer of calcified cartilage and underlying subchondral bone. The cartilage of the physis is known as the growth plate and is involved in metaphyseal growth. The normal growth plate cartilage has a well-ordered structure, with the chondrocytes of the proliferative and hypertrophic regions arranged into columns.

Osteochondrosis is a generalized disease in which there are focal areas of failure of endochondral ossification in the physeal (metaphyseal growth) and epiphyseal growth cartilage. The underlying defect may be an abnormality of the chondrocytes, which do not undergo normal hypertrophic ossification. They accumulate rough endoplasmic reticulum, lipid droplets, and mitochondria. The surrounding matrix contains deposits of electron-dense material that may prevent normal vascularization and therefore ossification. The hypertrophic region is disorganized and greatly extended compared with normal tissue. The matrix surrounding the clustered chondrocytes is altered compared with that in normal cartilage. The primary abnormality is an increased thickness of the joint cartilage combined with degenerative changes that result in infoldings and erosion of the articular cartilage. Defects of the growth plates (physes) result in short, deformed bones.

Pathologically, severe clinical cases are characterized by osteochondrosis and secondary degenerative joint disease, especially involving the medial aspects of the larger joints; epiphysiolysis; and lumbar intervertebral disc degeneration and spondylosis. Osteochondrosis has been used to encompass lesions involving the physes and the articular epiphyseal complexes. However, because of morphologic changes that have been observed in growing pigs, dyschondroplasia is now the preferred term to be used generically and then qualified by the location and nature of the morphologic description because the causes may be different.

Osteochondrosis occurs commonly in growing pigs at predilection sites of the medical condyle of the humerus and femur, the epiphyseal plates of the distal ulna, and the femoral head and the intervertebral joints. The 6th to 8th costochondral junctions may also be affected. It may heal spontaneously or it may progress to osteochondritis dissecans and OA. Its progression in either direction is influenced by local loading and by joint stability, which depends on joint shape and muscle and ligamentous support. The age-related changes and OC in the articular and epiphyseal cartilage have been described. The cartilage increases with age up to 5 weeks and then begins to decrease in thickness. Deleterious influences such as defects in conformation; heavy musculature with skeletal immaturity; muscular weakness resulting from myofibrillar hypoplasia, myopathies, or lack of exercise; inadequate flooring; or even simple trauma may adversely affect this progression and lead to severe skeletal change.

Porcine synovial fluid contains both hyaluronic acid and chondroitin sulfate, and ratio of chondroitin sulfate to hyaluronic acid is not influenced by relatively advanced stages of osteochondrosis. Treatment of lame boars with glycosaminoglycan polysulfate improves leg soundness score and results in an increase in the hyaluronic acid concentration of the cubitus joint synovial fluid and in the proportion of aggregated proteoglycans in the articular cartilage of the medial femoral condyle. It is suggested that the hyaluronic acid accounts for most of the viscosity of synovial fluid and for efficient lubrication of the joint.

Well-established lesions typical of OC associated with the physes can be found in young pigs between 25 and 30 days of age. The earliest change associated with a dyschondroplasia of the physis is a focus of persistent hypertrophied chondrocytes that do progress but heal. Lesions associated with physes and articular epiphyseal complexes develop continuously and regress as pigs grow older. Changes in cartilage canal vessels appear to be important in the pathogenesis. There is no evidence that vascular damage is a factor in the pathogenesis of the lesions.

Because foci of dyschondroplasic lesions are associated with physes of pigs between birth and the stage of rapid growth, they could be regarded as part of the usual growth patterns in contemporary commercial swine. However, clinical signs of dyschondroplasias, or degenerative joint disease secondary to dyschondroplasias, usually do not appear until pigs are almost 6 months of age.

Radiologic Monitoring of Lesions

Osteochondrosis can be diagnosed radiologically. Radiologically, the lesions were similar in Yorkshire pigs and Landrace but more severe in the Landrace and similar to the Danish Landrace.

The development of epiphyseal osteochondrosis in pigs from 42 to 147 days of age has been followed radiologically. Osteochondritic lesions were seen radiologically in the articular–epiphyseal (A-E) complexes of the humeral condyles of 42-day-old pigs and in the femoral condyles at 63 days of age, in contrast to earlier reports indicating that lesions were not visible radiologically until 100 days of age. The osteochondrosis lesions of the A-E complexes develop, become progressive, and subsequently become either stable, regressive, or even more progressive as the pigs grow. This supports the observations that the lesions develop and become progressive and regress as the pigs grow. The humeral medial condyles have more pronounced lesions and are more frequent than the lateral ones.

Radiologic monitoring of the development and sequelae of physeal osteochondrosis lesions of the growth plate cartilage and A-E complexes of the forelimbs and hindlimbs in young breeding swine found that the majority of distal ulnar lesions healed by 18 to 20 months, and some started fusing at 18 to 21 months. The distal ulna healed without complications in most animals, and the most severe lesions healed faster than the mild or moderate ones. In a recent study, periarticular ossifications at the elbow joint were found in the radiographs at a prevalence of 0.9%. Meniscal ossifications were seen as single or multiple foci at the cranial aspect of the joint at a prevalence of 2.6% and had a bilateral occurrence of 20%. Meniscal ossifications were associated with turned-out hindlegs and stiff locomotion in the hindlegs and negatively associated with growth rate.

CLINICAL FINDINGS

Palpation is an important method of examination of lame pigs. Lame pigs are usually stiff on either front or back legs or both. The key is to send affected animals for slaughter quickly on diagnosis, provided they are fit to travel and inspected at the abattoir or rapidly placed in a quarantine area to prevent further injury and to supervise the effects of treatment.

OC and OA produce leg weakness that varies in severity from locomotor abnormality resulting from conformation and leg defects such as narrow lumbar area and broad hips, hyperflexion of the carpus, bowing of the forelimbs and "knock knees," hyperextension of the phalanges, and lateral angulation of the foot and sickle hocks, to more severe lameness and, in the extreme, inability to rise and paresis. Nine signs of leg weakness are described: buck-kneed forelegs, steep hock joints, turned-out forelimbs and hindlimbs, upright pasterns on the hindlegs, stiff locomotion, standing under on the hindlimbs, swaying hindquarters, goose-stepping hindlegs, and lameness and tendency to slip. The four most common signs are buck knees, small inner claws on forefeet, small inner claws on hindfeet, and upright pasterns on the hindlegs.

The clinical syndrome is a locomotor disorder usually involving the hindlimbs. Often the most rapidly growing pigs are lame. The lameness may be acute, intermittent, chronic, progressive, or a combination of these. An insidious onset is common, and pigs are unwilling to move, the stride is shortened, and the limbs are held in partial flexion. The carpal joints may be underextended while the metacarpophalangeal joints are overextended, giving the limb an abnormal S-shaped profile. The pelvic limbs are commonly held straight, and the back is slightly arched. In some cases, affected animals will assume a kneeling position with flexed carpal joints and walk on those joints.

Mild cases show stiffness, especially immediately after a period of lying down, and lameness. Slowness to rise and a tendency to walk with short steps on tiptoes, frequently in association with a marked inward curve of hindlimb motion during forward progression and side-to-side motion of the buttocks, are frequently seen. More severely affected pigs sit on their hindquarters and are reluctant to stand. They carry one or both hindlimbs more forward under the body and walk with a short, goose-stepping gait. Wasting is not a feature except in severely affected animals, and the locomotor disorder may be minor unless exacerbated by physical exertion.

The syndrome is of particular importance in breeding animals because it may interfere with successful mating. Boars may show initial interest in mounting but subsequently slide off the sow or dummy before mating is complete, presumably as a result of the pain of the limb lesions.

There may be no meaningful association between visual scores for physical soundness in the live animal and the degree of joint damage. Some pigs with severe lesions are not lame; conversely, other pigs are severely lame with minor lesions.

Epiphysiolysis

Separation of the epiphyses probably occurs when the process of endochondral ossification reaches or approaches the cartilage defect. The resulting fracture may extend in a jagged crack through primary and secondary spongiosa. It may be that the traumatic forces applied to the epiphyseal cartilage at the site of empty spaces near atrophic blood vessels or at eosinophilic streaks cause further separation and epiphyseal lysis.

The defect involves the proximal femoral epiphysis. There is separation along the proximal femoral epiphysis and the metaphyseal bone. It is a traumatic occurrence at a site of a growth defect in the cartilage with a combination of excess tension in the hip joint across a weakened physeal region in the femur, which then separates. It occurs from 5 months to 3 years of age (epiphyses fuse at 3 to 7.5 years of age). It may develop from an extended eosinophilic streak (area of matrix degeneration) or from areas of necrosis in the growth of cartilage rather than from areas of metaphyseal dysplasia.

Usually, it is a severe and sudden-onset lameness, occasionally insidious. Animals lie down, are unable to rise unless assisted, and usually eat and drink. It may be unilateral or bilateral, and manipulation reveals crepitation. It can be confused with fractures of the femur, spinal canal abscesses, or lumbosacral fractures. It may become a center of necrosis if secondary bacterial infection occurs.

Epiphysiolysis contributes to the leg-weakness complex. In this case, repeated trauma and consequent microfractures significantly contribute to the retention of a thick and irregular epiphyseal cartilage and to fibrous tissue formation. Epiphysiolysis of the femoral head produces severe unilateral lameness, and if bilateral, it is usually manifest by marked reluctance to rise and severe locomotor disability. Initial signs are frequently deceptively mild and follow physical exertion, such as in mating, transport, farrowing, or fighting, but they progress to severe lameness over a 7- to 10-day period.

Apophysiolysis

Epiphysiolysis of the tuber ischii is known as apophysiolysis. It may also occur following physical exertion but is more common in second- or third-parity sows and is manifest by "paralysis," with the hindlimbs in forward extension under the body of the sow. These animals dog-sit and are unable to rise. In many instances, the injury occurs when the animals arrive on the farm or are first mated. In pigs the anconeal process does not arise from a separate ossification center, so apophysiolysis of the anconeal process is a better description than epiphysiolysis of the anconeal process.

Bilateral separation of the ischiatic tuberosities along their physes has been recognized in young sows. Most affected animals are heavily pregnant, most dog-sit with the hindlimbs forward, and palpation elicits crepitus. It is associated with slippery floors excessively pulling the biceps femoris tendons from the tuber ischiadicum. Unilateral lesions cause a moderate to severe lameness, but bilateral separation may prevent the sow from rising or walking. The pain and muscle contraction frequently make it difficult to determine the site and severity of the lesion by simple clinical examination, and palpation following general anesthesia or radiography may be required for proper clinical assessment. Physical examination should include complete palpation of all limbs for heat, swelling, and pain. The palpable parts of the pelvis should be examined, with particular emphasis on the ischial tuberosities. Passive flexion, extension, and rotation of each limb along with auscultation over the joint may reveal evidence of crepitus or a pain response.

Although the lesions of the physes and articular epiphyseal complexes are detectable in pigs under 14 days of age, they are not detectable radiographically in live animals until the pigs are over 100 days of age. Only 21% of the lesions associated with the physes and 22% of the lesions associated with the articular epiphyseal complexes were detectable in radiographs of bones of live pigs.

Meniscal ossifications were observed as simple or multiple small, smooth, firm, and irregular swellings in the cranial horn of the lateral meniscus. The periarticular osseous foci were seen as focal firm swellings at the craniomedial aspect of the elbow joint.

CLINICAL PATHOLOGY

The carpal, elbow, tarsal, and stifle joints can be radiographed for evidence of joint lesions, with the lesions then scored according to a system. It is also possible to use ultrasonics for diagnosis.

NECROPSY FINDINGS

At necropsy, the cartilage is not normal, and cracks, fissures, and necrosis are seen below the cartilage. The pathology has been reviewed for osteochondrosis.[19]

The scapulohumeral, humeroradioulnar, carpal, coxofemoral, femorotibial, and tarsal joints should be examined. Typically, in osteochondrosis, the changes are feathery hypertrophy of villi, focal full-thickness cartilage buckles, ulcers or flaps of cartilage, and no changes in the draining lymph nodes. Joint mice and synovitis may also be seen. Deformation, or even fractures, may occur in the long bones.

Histologically, osseous trabeculae may be seen with clusters of chondrocytes; between the trabeculae, lined by flat osteoblasts, there are adipocytes. The osseous center is formed of mineralized cartilage that has blended into more or less fibrous cartilage, but toward the joint cavity the meniscal ossifications are covered by hyaline cartilage.

DIFFERENTIAL DIAGNOSIS

The syndrome must be differentiated from other diseases that cause lameness and paralysis in growing and young adult pigs, including the following: infectious polyarthritis; laminitis; traumatic foot lesions; foot lesions produced by biotin deficiency and footrot; osteodystrophy resulting from calcium, phosphorus, and vitamin D imbalance in rations; vitamin A deficiency; and viral encephalomyelitis.

TREATMENT

There is no effective treatment. Early cases may recover spontaneously after being placed outside on pasture or housed individually, inside, on deep straw litter. Recently it has been suggested that meloxicam at a dosage of 0.4 mg/kg is efficacious and safe for the treatment of noninfectious locomotor disorders in pigs. Treatment with 2.5-D vitamin D had no effect on the incidence and severity of OC/OA lesions. Animals that are affected with clinical signs should be removed from the herd quickly for casualty slaughter and, if necessary, should be humanely destroyed as soon as possible.

CONTROL

Because the etiology is unknown, it is not possible to provide specific control measures. The hereditary nature of the disease suggests that the selection of breeding stock with sound legs and a low incidence of lesions would be an effective long-term control measure. Genetic control of leg weakness has been documented by various researchers. Selection of boars for leg soundness has dramatic effects on the structural soundness of their crossbred progeny, and therefore selection of structurally sound replacements must be maintained if leg weakness in market or breeding pigs is to be avoided. Divergent selection for leg soundness in Duroc pigs has been dramatic. Progeny of leg-soundness sires had significantly better measures for all leg traits at 104 kg than did progeny of leg-weakness sires. Differences between the two progeny groups indicated that the realized heritability for front-leg soundness exceeded 0.50.

Selection of breeding stock will require careful genetic selection, examination of all pigs that are to be retained for breeding, and necropsy of siblings of affected pigs of the same gender, to identify genetic lines of pigs that have a low incidence of lesions. A recent study showed that the increase in wild boar alleles in crosses with Large White pigs reduced the prevalence of OC. It has been suggested that the selection of pigs based on the joint lesion score could lead to a better leg and joint condition both visually and pathologically. Reduction of growth rate and exercise may help, but they are not a real methods of control. Improvement of nutrition and housing may help to remove the traumatic component of cartilage damage. Increasing the calcium and phosphorus in the diet also does not help.

REFERENCES

1. Jensen TB, Toft N. *Pig News Info.* 2009;30:1.
2. Thorup VM, et al. *J Anim Sci.* 2008;86:992.
3. Kilbride AL, et al. *Animal Welfare.* 2009;18:215.
4. Zoric M, et al. *Acta Vet Scand.* 2009;51:23.
5. Zoric M, et al. *Acta Vet Scand.* 2008;50:37.
6. Zoric M. *Pig J.* 2010;63:1.
7. Holmgren N, et al. *Swedish, Vet J.* 2008;60:11.
8. Busch ME, Wachmann H. *Vet J.* 2010;188:197.
9. Heinonen M, et al. *Vet Rec.* 2007;160:573.
10. Gillman CE, et al. *Prev Vet Med.* 2009;doi:10.1016/j.prevet-med.2009.05.023.
11. Gillman CE, et al. *Prev Vet Med.* 2008;83:308.
12. Kilbride AL, et al. *Prev Vet Med.* 2008;83:272.
13. Kirk RK, et al. *Acta Vet Scand.* 2008;50:5.
14. Ryan WF, et al. *Vet Rec.* 2010;166:268.
15. Heinonen M, et al. *Vet Rec.* 2006;159:383.
16. Sonderman J, et al. *Proc Am Assoc Swine Vet.* 2009;40:283.
17. Engblom L, et al. *Livestock Sci.* 2009;106:76.
18. Rintisch V, et al. *Berl Munch Tierarztl Wschr.* 2010;123:70.
19. Ytrehus B, et al. *Vet Pathol.* 2007;44:429.
20. Busch ME, et al. *Dansk Vet.* 2007;2:24.

Infectious Diseases of the Musculoskeletal System

BORRELIOSIS (LYME BORRE LIOSIS, LYME DISEASE)

SYNOPSIS

Etiology Spirochete *Borrelia burgdorferi sensu lato* complex with different genospecies. In North America, genospecies *B. burgdorferi sensu stricto;* in Europe, *B. burgdorferi sensu stricto, B. afzelii,* and *B. barinii.* Other genospecies possibly associated with clinical disease are *B. spielmanii, B bisentii, B. lusitaniae,* and *B. valaisiana*

Epidemiology Occurs in North and South America, Europe, Asia, and Australia in cattle, sheep, horses, dogs, and humans. Transmitted by *Ixodes* spp. ticks from small wild animals, which are host reservoirs to domestic animals and humans. Larval ticks feed on small mammals; nymphal ticks feed on a broader range of hosts, including rodents, birds, sheep, and cattle; adult ticks feed on deer, horses, cattle, and dogs. All stages feed on humans.

Signs In horses: chronic weight loss, sporadic lameness, persistent fever, swollen joints, muscle stiffness, depression, anterior uveitis, neurologic signs, abortion, and weak foals. In cattle and sheep: polyarthritis, chronic weight loss, fever.

Clinical pathology Serology (indirect immunofluorescent antibody test [IFAT], enzyme-linked immunosorbent assay [ELISA]), culture, polymerase chain reaction (PCR), immunohistochemistry (IHC).

Lesions Polysynovitis, lymphadenopathy, interstitial myocarditis, nephritis, meningoencephalitis.

Treatment Tetracyclines and penicillin.

Control No specific control measures available; tick control.

ETIOLOGY

Borrelia burgdorferi, a gram-negative aerobic, microaerophilic, motile, spiral-shaped bacterium belonging to the family Spirochaetaceae, is the causative agent of Lyme borreliosis (Lyme disease). The *Borrelia burgdorferi sensu lato* complex comprises at least 12 genospecies, of which only a few have been associated with clinical disease. Of these different species, *B. burgdorferi sensu stricto, B. afzelii,* and *B. garinii* have been recognized as pathogens associated with clinical disease in mammals. The more recently identified species *B. spielmanii, B. bisentiii, B. lusitaniae,* and *B. valaisiana* have also been incriminated as potentially pathogenic species in humans and mammals.[1]

EPIDEMIOLOGY

Occurrence and Prevalence of Infection

A disease complex consistent with Lyme borreliosis in humans with characteristic skin lesions was first described at the end of the nineteenth century, but the etiology of the condition remained unknown until 1982, when W. Burgdorfer identified the causative agent.[2] Currently, Lyme borreliosis is recognized as the most common vector-borne disease in the northern hemisphere.[3] The disease predominantly occurs in North America and Europe but has also been reported in parts of Asia and in Latin American countries, including Brazil, Mexico, and Colombia.[1]

In the United States the infection is primarily prevalent in three regions: the Northeast (from Massachusetts to Maryland), the Midwest (Wisconsin and Minnesota), and the Pacific region (California and Oregon). The disease occurs most commonly in areas with an appropriate density of the insect vector, intermediate hosts, and the environmental conditions favoring transmission.

The different genospecies of *B. burgdorferi sensu lato* differ in their geographic occurrence. Whereas **in North America** Lyme disease is most commonly associated with ***B. burgdorferi sensu stricto,*** in **Europe,** ***B. afzelii*** is most prevalent in the north, ***B. burgdorferi sensu stricto*** in the western part of the continent, and ***B. lusitaniae*** in the Mediterranean basin. *B. spielmanii* has been isolated in Germany, France, the Netherlands, Hungary and Slovenia, the Ukraine, and other countries. *B. valaisiano* was found to occur in central Europe, the United Kingdom, and Russia.[1]

The prevalence of vector ticks infected with *B. burgdorferi sensu lato* has been studied in different countries and occurs at rates of 22% to 35% in Germany, 10% to 35% in the Netherlands, 40% in Bulgaria, 38% in Slovakia, 5.4% in Poland, and 12.9% in Ontario, Canada.[4-9] The prevalence of infection with *B. burgdorferi* for different animal species has been studied for different geographic regions. These data must be interpreted cautiously because they reflect the degree of exposure of an animal population (seroprevalence) but are not associated with the prevalence of clinical disease (disease prevalence).

Cattle

Seroprevalence studies of cattle in the United Kingdom indicate that the seropositivity rate increased from 44% to 67% after the cattle were turned out to a pasture heavily infested with ticks. The seropositivity rate was found to be higher in cattle with digital dermatitis ("Morbus Mortellaro"; 71%) than in cattle without the lesions (7.3%). This observation nonetheless should be interpreted cautiously because there was a significant age difference between cows with digital dermatitis (adult cows) and unaffected cows (1- to 3-year-old heifers), and an effect of age on the seroprevalence rate is well established in other animal species.[4]

In a study conducted during the grazing period of 2002 in Bavaria, Germany, including nearly 300 cattle, a seroprevalence of 45.6% was determined. Within-herd prevalence rates ranged from 20% to 100%. The antibody titer was associated with the number of ticks found on the animal but not with its age.[10]

In Japan, the seroprevalence of infection varied from 8% to 15% and was higher during the summer months; cows with arthritis had higher titers to the organism than healthy cows. Similar observations have been made in dairy cows in Minnesota and Wisconsin in areas with endemic *B. burgdorferi* infections. In Wisconsin, the peak seasonal incidence of clinical disease in horses and cattle occurs in May, June, and October, which correlates with emergence of *I. dammini* in the spring, usually March and April, and again in September.

Sheep

Seroprevalence studies in sheep infested with *Ixodes ricinus* in Scotland indicate an infection rate in lambs of 2.7%, with 24% to 40% in young sheep and 0% to 6% in ewes. There is also evidence for transmission of Lyme disease to sheep in Cumbria in the United Kingdom in grassland and heath communities where wild fauna are uncommon and sheep are thought to be the main host for all feeding stages of the tick. However, there was no evidence of clinical disease associated with the infection. Serologic surveys of infection in sheep in Norway indicate that 10% of animals tested are seropositive with the enzyme-linked immunosorbent assay (ELISA) test, with a range of 0% to 20% between counties. The geographic distribution of seropositive animals correlated with the known distribution of *I. Ricinus,* with the highest proportion of seropositive animals found in the southern coastal areas of Norway. The majority of animals appear to become infected during the first 2 years of life; the animals were all healthy at the time of sampling.

Horses

Geographic surveillance of horses in Europe and North America suggests that exposure of horses to *B. burgdorferi* is widespread. Seroprevalence rates for horses have been reported from several European countries, including France (31% to 48%),[11] Germany (16.1%), Sweden (16.8%), Denmark (29%), Italy (15.3% to 24.3%),[12,13] Poland (25.6%),[14] and Slovakia (47.8%).[13]

Serologic surveys of horse populations in the United States revealed that in the New Jersey–Pennsylvania area, approximately 10% of horses have significant serum antibody titers to the organism. Infection appears to be uncommon in horses in Texas. In Cape Cod horses, the seroprevalence was 35%, which was found to be age-specific and considered to be a reflection of exposure because of the relative absence of disease. It was found that 7% to 13% of horses admitted to a veterinary teaching hospital were seropositive to the organism and the frequency of antibody response varied according to the geographic origin of the horses. A retrospective study on seroprevalence of infection with *B. burgdorferi* in Minnesota based on 1260 serum samples submitted to a diagnostic laboratory between 2001 and 2010 revealed an average seroprevalence of 58.7%.[15] Because of the selection bias in this study, which was based on blood samples obtained from horses with health issues, this value likely overestimates the overall prevalence in the equine population in the region.

Lyme disease in the horse is rare but it is clinically important in the United Kingdom. In areas where the disease occurs in humans, the seroprevalence of infection in horses was 49% compared with 3% to 4% in horses from other areas. Horses with unexplained lameness associated with fever and tick infestation had high levels of antibody to the organism. Within endemic areas, up to 60% of mares and yearlings on one farm were serologically positive. On such farms, there may be a clustering of clinical cases in foals after weaning. However, there is no evidence that abortion in mares is associated with infection.

Wildlife

In Ontario, epidemiologic studies indicate a widespread but low level or scattered distribution of infection in wildlife reservoirs in the south, with occasional spillover into human and canine populations. Serologically, the organism was found to be circulating in populations of white-footed mice, field mice, and white-tailed deer.

A serologic survey including over 600 wild boars in the Czech Republic found seroprevalence rates between 8.9% and 25.0% depending on the region of the country, with the highest prevalence rates in the rural and forested regions. Seroprevalence rates increased in the spring months of March and April, with peak values in May.[16]

Zoonotic Implications

Lyme borreliosis was first recognized when a cluster of suspected juvenile rheumatoid arthritis cases occurred among residents of Lyme, Connecticut. An arthropod-transmitted disease was suspected as the etiologic agent because, in addition to recurrent, short-lived joint pain, patients had an expanding, red, annular rash resembling erythema chronicum migrans similar to a lesion identified in Europe in the late nineteenth century associated with tick bites, and the rash was responsive to penicillin. An infectious cause was confirmed when spirochetal bacteria isolated from *Ixodes* ticks and from blood, cerebrospinal fluid (CSF), and other tissues of patients were shown to be identical. Subsequently, *B. burgdorferi* was identified in ticks in numerous regions of the United States, and infection was associated with clinical disease in other animals, including dogs and horses.

The disease has been recognized in most areas of the United States and in at least 20 countries spanning every continent. In the United States, the northeastern states of Connecticut, Massachusetts, and New York; the midwestern states of Wisconsin, Minnesota, Michigan, Illinois, and Indiana; and the western states of California and Nevada are considered as the most endemic areas, especially in wooded and grassy parts of these regions.

Lyme borreliosis is the most common tick-transmitted disease of humans in the northern hemisphere. In the United States, roughly 20,000 clinical cases are reported to the Centers for Disease Control and Prevention every year. Depending on the region, this is equivalent to incidence rates of up to 10 per 100,000 population.[1] Incidence rates reported from European countries vary widely and range from 0.6 per 100,000 population in Ireland and the United Kingdom to 130 per 100,000 in Austria to 155 per 100,000 in Slovenia.[17]

The geographic prevalence of borreliosis in humans and animals is related to the distribution of the various *Ixodes* spp. and the location of herds of deer, which are preferred hosts for the ticks. Geographic areas with dense vegetation and high humidity promote the development of the tick. Risk of infection is correlated with the opportunity of being bitten by an infected tick and dependent on the density of vector ticks in an endemic area, the proportion of ticks infected, and the duration and extent of the susceptible host's activities in that area.

Methods of Transmission

B. burgdorferi cycles between reservoir hosts and tick vectors. Reservoir hosts are defined as those animal species that can infect a significant number of ticks feeding on them but do not normally develop clinical disease. Reservoir hosts are critical for maintaining the agent in a geographic region. At present, 16 species of birds, 7 medium-sized mammals, and 9 small mammal species are considered to be able to transmit *B. burgdorferi* to vector ticks.[4] The white-footed mouse (*Peromyscus leucopus*) is considered to be the main reservoir for *B. burgdorferi* in the eastern United States. Rodents incriminated as reservoir hosts in the western part of the United States include the white-footed mouse, the brush mouse (*Peromyscus boylii*), the western gray squirrel (*Sciurus griseus*), the duskyfooted wood rat (*Neotoma fuscipes*), and the California kangaroo rat (*Dipodomys californicus*).[1] It is suggested that migrating birds acting as carriers may account for the widespread nature of the infection. Pheasants and some passerine birds, including European blackbirds and song thrushes, are considered to be maintenance hosts.

Ungulates, including deer, sheep, cattle, and goats, feed large numbers of ticks, and seroprevalence rates in these species in tick-infested regions can be high. Nonetheless, an increasing body of evidence suggests that ungulates do not infect a high proportion of ticks—most of which are adult-stage ticks—that feed on them.[17]

The spirochete is **transmitted by *Ixodes* ticks,** including *I. scapularis,* the deer tick, in the northeastern and midwestern United States; *I. pacificus,* the black-legged tick, in the western United States; *I. ricinus,* the sheep tick, in Europe; and *I. persulcatus* in Asia. The life cycle of an ixodid tick is 2 to 3 years and includes the stages of egg, larvae, nymph, and adult. Ticks transmit spirochetes during feeding with their saliva. Spirochetes migrate from the midgut, where they are found in unfed ticks, to the tick's salivary glands, a migration that is thought to be activated by ingestion of blood. Because ixodid ticks only feed once at each developmental stage, infection is usually acquired by one stage and transmitted by the next (transstadial transmission). Ticks in the larval stage feed on small mammals and are not infected before their meal, suggesting that transovarial transmission does not occur. Both immature stages of the tick (larvae and nymphs) feed on the white-footed mouse, which makes the life cycle of the organism dependent on horizontal transmission from infected nymphs to mice in the early summer and from infected mice to the larvae in late summer. White-footed mice are susceptible to oral infection and transmit the infection to one another by direct contact. Infection with the spirochete does not cause clinical or pathologic changes or alter the biological features of the mouse. These combined factors indicate a long-standing relationship between the mouse and the spirochete. Nymphal ticks feed on a broader range of animal species, such as rodents, squirrels, birds, dogs, sheep, and cattle. Infected nymphs can transmit *B. burgdorferi* to their second host, and uninfected nymphs can contract infection from an infected host. The adult tick feeds primarily on larger animals such as deer, horses, cattle, sheep, and dogs. All three stages of the tick will feed on humans.

The white-tailed deer is the preferred host for the adult stage of the tick and often harbors large numbers of adult ticks. Adult ticks are likely to be responsible for transmission of infection to horses and cattle.

Transmission of Lyme disease requires prolonged attachment of the tick to its host of at least 18 hours.[4] This lag time between attachment of the tick and infection of the host has been proposed to be caused by the delay between activation of *B. burgdorferi* in the tick's midgut at the onset of a blood meal and the appearance of the bacterium in the tick's salivary glands.[17]

The ticks *Dermacentor variabilis* and *Amblyomma americanum*, tabanid flies, and mosquitoes have also been shown to carry the organism.

The organism can be found in the urine of infected animals, and it is possible that transmission may occur through close contact without the bite of a tick. Infected cattle purchased from an endemic area could shed the organisms in the urine and transmit them to animals in a different herd.

Transplacental transmission of the organism from infected dams to their fetuses also occurs through in utero infection and can be a cause of mortality in foals and calves.

PATHOGENESIS

Borrelia are highly motile and invasive, and they localize in selected tissues, thereby evading the host's immune response.[4] They spread through tissues and can directly transcytose endothelial layers. *B. burgdorferi* predominantly migrates within connective tissue, which may protect it from humoral antibodies. Following infection there is multisystemic inflammation, resulting in polyarthritis, generalized lymphadenitis, pleuritis, peritonitis, interstitial pneumonia, encephalitis, and in utero infection causing in fetal infection. In humans, the progression of Lyme borreliosis is divided into early localized, early disseminated, and late stages. In humans, the skin is the most frequently affected tissue. Erythema migrans, borrelial lymphocytoma, acrodermatitis chronica atrophicans, neuroborreliosis, myocarditis, arthritis, and ocular disease are possible outcomes of infection.

Borreliosis has been reproduced in ponies by exposure to *Ixodes* ticks infected with *B. burgdorferi*. Infection with *B. burgdorferi* was detected in skin biopsies and various tissues at necropsy by culture and PCR. Clinical signs were limited to skin lesions, all ponies seroconverted, and there were no significant other lesions.

Immune Mechanisms

B. burgdorferi is able to persist in the mammalian host because of active immune suppression, induction of immune tolerance, phase and antigenic variation, intracellular seclusion, and incursion into immune privileged sites, all of which are survival strategies. Vaccination with outer surface protein A (OspA) from the organism prevented *B. burgdorferi* infection in animal and human studies. Vaccination of 1-year-old ponies with recombinant OspA (*osp. A* gene derived from *B. burgdorferi* B31) with adjuvant (aluminum hydroxide) followed by challenge with *B. burgdorferi*–infected adult ticks provided protection against skin infection compared with unvaccinated controls.

CLINICAL FINDINGS

The symptoms of Lyme borreliosis in animals are poorly defined, and a broad spectrum of clinical manifestations have been attributed to *B. burgdorferi* infection. High seroprevalence rates in different animal species in endemic regions with low disease prevalence suggest that the large majority of infected animals remain asymptomatic.[18] On the other hand, the diagnosis of Lyme borreliosis is often based on clinical signs consistent with the disease (e.g., lameness or arthritis) in combination with positive serology, which can be considered as presumptive diagnosis at best. To complicate matters, many of the symptoms associated with Lyme disease have not been reproducible under experimental conditions.[18]

Horses

Infection with *B. burgdorferi* in horses in the majority of cases does not cause clinical disease, as is suggested by the large number of seroconverted animals without history of disease. Clinical signs attributed to *B. burgdorferi* infection in horses include chronic weight loss, persistent mild fever, intermittent or shifting lameness, laminitis, swollen joints, muscle stiffness, and anterior uveitis. Neurologic signs such as depression, behavioral changes, dysphagia, head tilting, and encephalitis have also been reported. Polyarthritis and swelling of tendon sheaths in horses of all ages are commonly reported. Infection of pregnant mares has been associated with abortion and the birth of weak foals that die soon after birth. An unexplained increase in early embryonic loss or failure of conception in mares has been associated with Lyme disease antibodies but not confirmed.

Cattle

In cattle, signs and symptoms attributed to infection with *B. burgdorferi* include persistent mild fever, chronic weight loss, decreased milk production, lameness, and polyarthritis.[1] Erythema of the udder or the skin between the digits and edematous lesions on the hairless skin of the udder have been described in cows with *B. burgdorferi* infection.

Sheep

In sheep, lameness, swollen joints, unthriftiness, and a persistent fever are commonly reported clinical signs.

CLINICAL PATHOLOGY

Detection of Organism

B. burgdorferi is difficult to isolate because it is present in low numbers in blood or tissues. The microorganism is fastidious, is microaerophilic, and requires enriched bacteriologic media, making culture slow, difficult, and expensive; special stains are required to visualize it. Aseptically collected blood, cerebrospinal fluid, urine, and colostrum can be examined under dark-field microscopy or in a culture.

Amplification of plasmid or chromosomal DNA of the microorganism by **polymerase chain reaction (PCR)** can be attempted, but because of the low number of microorganisms, lack of detection does not rule out infection.[1] On the other hand, positive PCR confirms the presence of bacterial DNA but does not prove the pathogen was alive, and it could be the result of leftover fragments from a previous infection.[18] **Immunohistochemistry** has been used to detect bacterial antigen in tissue.[1]

Serology

Serologic testing is the most practical method of making at least a presumptive diagnosis of *B. burgdorferi* infection. Serum and synovial fluid samples may contain antibodies to the organism in horses. The indirect immunofluorescent antibody (IFA) test has been used with reliable results in horses and cattle. The ELISA is ideal for high-volume testing; the results are quantitative, and the test can detect total immunoglobulin or class-specific IgM and IgG antibodies to the organism. An ELISA and immunoblots using certain antigens of the spirochete are more specific for the diagnosis of Lyme borreliosis in horses. Western blotting techniques and the ELISA have been used for serologic surveys and for examination of synovial fluids of horses in the United Kingdom, where the incidence of infection is common in some areas. The positive results in horses are not as a result of cross-reactions with *Leptospira*, which has been suspected.

Subclinical infections are common in domestic animals, and the interpretation of serologic results must be done in conjunction with the clinical findings. Antibody titers higher than 1/64 or 1/100 are considered as positive. Positive antibody results are an aid to diagnosis but are not conclusive evidence of current infection or clinical disease. False-positive results may be a result of infection with other *Borrelia* species.

NECROPSY FINDINGS

Polysynovitis, lymphadenopathy, and emaciation are present. Multifocal interstitial myocarditis, glomerulonephritis, interstitial pneumonitis, and polysynovitis have been described in cattle. In the horse, polysynovitis and meningoencephalitis have been reported. Using PCR amplification of DNA, necropsy tissues may be positive for *B. burgdorferi* DNA.

Samples for Confirmation of Diagnosis

- **Bacteriology**—kidney, joint synovium, lung, choroid plexus (PCR)

- **Histology**—formalin-fixed kidney, joint synovium, heart, brain, lung, lymph node (LM, IHC)

DIFFERENTIAL DIAGNOSIS

Diagnosis is dependent on recognition of clinical signs, a history of possible exposure to infection by the bites of ticks, and identification of the spirochete in the affected animal. Because clinically normal animals have antibodies to the organism, a positive antibody result is not conclusive of current infection or clinical disease. Other diseases causing muscle stiffness, lameness, polyarthritis, lymphadenopathy, and fever must be considered in the differential diagnosis.

TREATMENT

Procaine penicillin, oxytetracycline, doxycycline (10 mg/kg PO q12h for 3 weeks) and ceftiofur (2.2 mg/kg IM q12h) have been used for treatment of Lyme disease in horses. Experimentally infected horses treated with oxytetracycline for 3 weeks were negative on culture and PCR following treatment.[4] Penicillin or oxytetracycline daily for 3 weeks has also been recommended for use in cattle.

Treatment recommendations are largely based on empirical evidence, and the efficacy of these treatments is difficult to assess. In many cases where the treatment was found to be effective, the diagnosis was presumptive; an unapparent coinfection with another pathogen cannot be ruled out. For example, horses with presumed Lyme disease that responded to oxytetracycline may actually have been infected with *Anaplasma phagocytophilum,* which is transmitted by the same vector, causes similar clinical signs, and is highly susceptible to tetracycline.[4]

TREATMENT

- Procaine penicillin G (44,000 IU/kg q24 IM, for 3 weeks) (R-2)
- Oxytetracycline (6 to 12 mg/kg IV q24h for 3 weeks) (R-2)

CONTROL

Prevention of Lyme borreliosis in domestic animals and humans is dependent on reduction of the risk of tick bites at the environmental or individual animal level. Knowledge of the ecologic requirements for the tick-borne diseases that are present in an area is necessary for selection and implementation of the most effective integrated prevention strategies. Protective measures may include the avoidance of tick-infested areas; the use of protective clothing, repellents, and acaricides; tick checks; and modifications of landscapes in or near residential areas. After a tick bite has occurred in humans, the body of the tick should be grasped with medium-tipped tweezers as close to the skin as possible and removed by gently pulling the tick straight out, without twisting motions.

A commercial adjuvanted vaccine is available for use in dogs. An experimental vaccine composed of recombinant OspA protected ponies against *B. burgdorferi* infection, and further studies are necessary to determine duration of protection after vaccination, safety, and cross-protection against the possible heterogeneous OspA structures that may be present among new *B. burgdorferi* strains isolated in the United States.

A human vaccine was available in the United States but was withdrawn by the manufacturer in 2002. Problems included poor demand, high costs, the need for a series of three vaccinations and boosters to maintain adequate titers, failure to obtain adequate titers in a small subset of vaccines, and theoretical concerns with vaccine-induced autoimmune arthritis.[1]

FURTHER READING

Butler CM, Houwers DJ, Jongejan F, van der Kolk JH. *Borrelia burgdorferi* infections with special reference to horses: a review. *Vet Quart.* 2005;27:146-156.

Divers TJ, Chang YF, Jacobson RH, McDonough SP. Lyme disease in horses. *Comp Cont Educ Pract Vet.* 2001;23:375-381.

Embers ME, Ramamoorthy R, Phillip MT. Survival strategies of *Borrelia burgdorferi,* the etiologic agent of Lyme disease. *Microbes Infect.* 2004;6:312-318.

Fritz CL, Kjemtrup AM. Lyme borreliosis. *J Am Vet Med Assoc.* 2003;223:1261-1270.

Littman MP, Goldstein RE, Labato MA, Lappin MR, Moore GE. ACVIM small animal consensus statement on lyme disease in dogs: diagnosis, treatment, and prevention. *J Vet Intern Med.* 2006;20:422-434.

Stanek G, Strle F. Lyme borreliosis. *Lancet.* 2003;362:1639-1647.

REFERENCES

1. The Center for Food Security and Public Health. At <http://www.cfsph.iastate.edu/Factsheets/pdfs/lyme_disease.pdf>; 2011 Accessed 09.02.14.
2. Gern L, Falco RC. *Rev Sci Tech Off Int Epiz.* 2000;19:121-135.
3. Higgins R. *Rev Sci Tech Off Int Epiz.* 2004;23:569-581.
4. Butler CM, et al. *Vet Quart.* 2005;27:146-156.
5. Runge M, et al. *J Verbr Lebensm.* 2010;5:317-375.
6. Strube C, et al. *Berl Münch Tierärztl Wschr.* 2011;124:512-517.
7. Morshed MG, et al. *J Med Entomol.* 2006;43:762-773.
8. Cisak E, et al. *Ann Agric Environ Med.* 2006;13:301-306.
9. Gassner F, et al. *Appl Environ Microbiol.* 2008;74:7136-7144.
10. Lengauer H, et al. *Berlin Münch Tierärztl Wschr.* 2006;119:335-341.
11. Maurizi L, et al. *Vector-Borne Zoonot.* 2010;10:535-537.
12. Ebani VV, et al. *Ann Agric Environ Med.* 2012;19:237-240.
13. Veronesi F, et al. *Vet Microbiol.* 2012;160:535-538.
14. Stefancikova A, et al. *Ann Agric Environ Med.* 2008;15:37-43.
15. Durrani AZ, et al. *J Equine Vet Sci.* 2011;31:427-429.
16. Juricova Z, Hubalek Z. *Vector-Borne Zoonot.* 2009;9:479-482.
17. EUCALB. At <http://www.eucalb.com>; 2009 Accessed 10.02.14.
18. Littman MP, et al. *J Vet Intern Med.* 2006;20:422-434.

MALIGNANT EDEMA, CLOSTRIDIAL MYONECROSIS (GAS GANGRENE)

SYNOPSIS

Etiology Acute wound infection associated with organisms of the genus *Clostridium.*

Epidemiology All ages and species of animals are susceptible. Sporadic disease affecting individual animals following injections; outbreaks following contamination of wounds produced by management procedures.

Clinical findings Acute onset with fever and toxemia. Inflammation and swelling at site of a wound, with heat, edema, pain on palpation, and usually subcutaneous emphysema.

Clinical pathology No diagnostic change in hematology or serum biochemistry. Fluorescent antibody staining.

Necropsy findings Gangrene of the skin with edema of the subcutaneous and intermuscular connective tissue around the site of infection.

Diagnostic confirmation Demonstration of the causal organisms by fluorescent antibody staining.

Treatment Antibiotics, surgical debridement.

Control Vaccination. Prophylactic antibiotics.

ETIOLOGY

Clostridium septicum, C. chauvoei, C. perfringens, C. sordellii, and *C. novyi* have all been isolated from lesions typical of malignant edema of animals. In some cases there can be mixed infections. The occurrence of malignant edema caused by *C. chauvoei* is discussed in the section on blackleg.

C. sordellii has been associated chiefly with malignant edema of cattle, but it has been found to be a cause of malignant edema and swelled head in sheep. However, swelled head of rams, in which the lesions of malignant edema are restricted to the head, is most commonly associated with *C. novyi* infection.

In a retrospective study of 37 horses with clostridial myonecrosis, *C. perfringens* was isolated from 68%, *C. septicum* from 16%, and the remainder were mixed infections with these two species. *C chauvoei, C. novyi,* and *C. fallax* have been isolated incidentally.

EPIDEMIOLOGY

All ages and species of animals are affected. The clostridia bacteria that cause malignant edema are **common inhabitants** of the animal **environment** and intestinal tract, and although some of the causative species have a restricted distribution, the disease has a worldwide occurrence. The disease occurs sporadically, affecting individual animals, except in circumstances where a management procedure in a group of animals results in an outbreak.

Source of Infection

The infection is usually **soil-borne**, and the resistance of spores of the causative clostridia to environmental influence leads to **persistence** of the infection for long periods in a local area. A dirty environment that permits contamination of wounds with soil is the common predisposing cause.

Transmission

In most cases a wound is the **portal of entry**. Deep puncture wounds accompanied by trauma provide the most favorable conditions for anaerobial growth, and malignant edema occurs most frequently under such conditions. Infection may occur through surgical or accidental wounds following vaccination, intramuscular injection of drugs, venipuncture, or through the umbilical cord in the newborn. Dormant spores of *C. perfringens* and other clostridial species can be found in the normal muscle of horses, and it is possible in some cases that these may be activated by anaerobic conditions produced by the injected material.

Animal and Management Risk Factors

In horses, intramuscular injection of drugs, commonly in association with the treatment of colic, is the common precipitating factor.[1] Certain drugs may have a greater propensity to initiate muscle necrosis and disease, but these drugs are also commonly used in the treatment of colic. Perivascular leaking of drugs is also a precipitating cause in horses. In all species there is risk with the intramuscular injection of drugs such as anthelmintics and nutritional supplements, some of which can cause significant tissue damage at the site, particularly if proper asepsis is not practiced.

Outbreaks can occur in sheep after management practices such as shearing and docking, or following lambing. Outbreaks have also been observed in cattle following **parturition**, sometimes associated with lacerations of the vulva. An unusual method of infection occurs when crows that have eaten infected carrion carry the infection to live, weak sheep and to lambs when they attack their eyes. Castration wounds in pigs and cattle may also become infected. Unless treatment is instituted in the early stages the death rate is extremely high.

The practice of **dipping** sheep immediately after they are shorn may cause a high incidence of malignant edema if the dip is heavily contaminated. The disease **"swelled head,"** a form of malignant edema, occurs in young rams 6 months to 2 years old when they are run in bands and fight among themselves.

Importance

Outbreaks of malignant edema are probably less common as a result of education of farmers and the availability of vaccines. In the wrong circumstances and with improper hygiene, severe disease can still occur.

PATHOGENESIS

Potent necrotoxins are produced in the local lesion and cause death when absorbed into the bloodstream. Locally the exotoxins cause extensive edema and necrosis followed by gangrene.

CLINICAL FINDINGS

Clinical signs appear within 6 to 48 hours of infection. There is always a local lesion at the **site of infection** consisting of a soft, doughy swelling with marked local erythema accompanied by severe pain on palpation. At a later stage the swelling becomes tense and the skin dark and taut. Emphysema may or may not be present, depending on the type of infection, and may be so marked as to cause extensive frothy exudation from the wound. With *C. novyi* infections, there is no emphysema. A high fever (41 to 42° C; 106 to 107° F) is always present; affected animals are depressed, are weak, and show muscle tremor and usually stiffness or lameness. The mucosae are dry and congested and have very poor capillary refill. The illness is of short duration, and affected animals die within 24 to 48 hours of the first appearance of signs. New cases continue to appear for 3 to 4 days after shearing or other precipitating cause.

When infection occurs at **parturition**, swelling of the vulva accompanied by the discharge of a reddish-brown fluid occurs within 2 to 3 days. The swelling extends to involve the pelvic tissues and perineal region. The local lesions are accompanied by a profound toxemia, and death occurs within 1 to 2 days.

In **"swelled head"** of rams, the edema is restricted initially to the head. It occurs first under the eyes and spreads to the subcutaneous tissues of the head and down the neck.

In **pigs**, the lesions are usually restricted to the axilla, limbs, and throat and are edematous, with very little evidence of emphysema. Local skin lesions consisting of raised, dull red plaques distended with clear serous fluid containing *C. septicum* and causing no systemic illness may be encountered in pigs at abattoirs.

In horses, emphysema, detected by palpation or ultrasound, is an early sign.[1]

CLINICAL PATHOLOGY

Antemortem laboratory examination of affected farm animals is not usually undertaken, usually because there are carcasses for postmortem examination.

Examination of a Gram-stained smear of aspirated fluid from edematous swellings or swabs from wounds will give an early diagnosis, allowing therapy early in the course of the disease. A PCR has been developed to allow the rapid identification and differentiation of the clostridia associated with malignant edema in livestock.

Hematologic examination in horses may reveal abnormal white blood cell counts, either leukocytosis or leukopenia with toxic degeneration of granulocytes and a regenerative left shift. Elevated activity of muscle enzymes such as CPK, AST, and LDH match the degree of muscle tissue involvement. Blood-gas analysis conducted in affected horses revealed severe acidemia and metabolic acidosis.[1]

NECROPSY FINDINGS

Tissue changes occur rapidly after death, particularly in warm weather, and this must be kept in mind when evaluating postmortem findings. There is usually gangrene of the skin with edema of the subcutaneous and intermuscular connective tissue around the site of infection. There may be some involvement of underlying muscle, but this is not marked. The edema fluid varies from thin serum to a gelatinous deposit. It is usually bloodstained and contains bubbles of gas, except in *C. novyi* infections when the deposit is gelatinous, clear, and contains no gas. A foul, putrid odor is often present in infections with *C. perfringens* and *C. sordellii.*

Subserous hemorrhages and accumulations of serosanguineous fluid in body cavities are usual. In "swelled head" of rams, the edema of the head and neck may extend into the pleural cavity and also involve the lungs.

The **histologic** picture of malignant edema consists of abundant edema fluid, emphysema, and neutrophils within the connective tissues. Muscle is not spared, but the damage is focused along fascial planes.

Samples for Confirmation of Diagnosis

- Bacteriology—fascial tissue, placed in an airtight container; four air-dried smears of fluid from lesion (anaerobic CULT, FAT)
- Histology—fixed sample of lesion

DIFFERENTIAL DIAGNOSIS

The association of profound toxemia and local inflammation and emphysema at the site of a wound is characteristic.

- **Blackleg**—the disease is differentiated from blackleg by the absence of typical muscle involvement and the presence of wounds
- **Anthrax** in pigs and horses
- **Photosensitivity** in white-faced sheep with swelled head

TREATMENT

Affected animals should be treated as emergency cases because of the acute nature of the disease. Specific treatment requires the administration of penicillin (high doses of crystalline penicillin intravenously, repeated at 4- to 6-hour intervals) or a broad-spectrum antibiotic. Antitoxin aids in controlling the toxemia but is expensive and must be given very early in the course of the disease. An NSAID and supportive therapy are recommended. Local treatment consists of surgical incision to provide drainage, along with irrigation with hydrogen peroxide. In horses, early and aggressive treatment with myotomy and fasciotomy, repeated if indicated, coupled with IV potassium penicillin is reported to allow recovery rates approaching 70%. The success rate in treating horses with infections with *C. perfringens* was higher than that with *C. septicum.*

TREATMENT AND CONTROL

Treatment

Penicillin G sodium/potassium (40,000 IU/kg IV q6–8h) (R-2)

Surgical incisions to drain and flush with dilute H_2O_2

Flunixin meglumine (2.2 mg/kg IV q24h) (R-2)

Ketoprofen (3 mg/kg IM q24h) (R-2)

Carprofen (1.4 mg/kg IM as single dose) (R-2)

Meloxicam (0.5 mg/kg SC/IV as single dose) (R-2)

Diclofenac (2.5 mg/kg IM as single dose) (R-2)

Control

Penicillin (44,000 IU/kg IM q24 for 3 days for animals at risk) (R-2)

CONTROL

Hygiene at lambing, shearing, castration, and docking is essential to the control of the infection in sheep. Vaccination with a specific or multivalent clostridial bacterin-toxoid will prevent the occurrence of the disease in enzootic areas. Penicillin can be given prophylactically to animals at risk for the disease.

FURTHER READING

Hatheway CL. Toxigenic clostridia. *Clin Microbiol Rev.* 1990;3:66-98.

Lewis C. Aspects of clostridial disease in sheep. *In Pract.* 1998;20:494-500.

Songer JG. Clostridial diseases of animals. In: Rood JI, McClane BA, Songer JG, Titball RW, eds. *The Clostridia: Molecular Biology and Pathogenesis.* London: Academic Press; 1997:153-182.

Songer JG. Clostridial diseases of small ruminants. *Vet Res.* 1998;29:219-232.

REFERENCE

1. Recknagel S, et al. *Tierarztl Prax Grosstiere.* 2009;37:255-262.

BLACKLEG

SYNOPSIS

Etiology Infectious necrotizing myositis associated with *Clostridium chauvoei.* Common in cattle but occurs occasionally in other species.

Epidemiology Cattle 6 months to 2 years of age that are rapidly growing and on a high plane of nutrition. Seasonal occurrence in warm, wet months. There are often multiple cases in at-risk animals. Sheep of all ages—occurs as outbreaks predisposed by wounds from shearing, docking, castration, dystocia.

Clinical findings Lameness and pronounced swelling of upper limb. Myonecrosis of skeletal or cardiac muscles, severe toxemia, and a high case-fatality rate. May be found dead.

Clinical pathology Culture from needle biopsy. No diagnostic change in hematology or serum biochemistry.

Necropsy findings Myositis; dark, rancid odor, metallic sheen on the cut surface.

Diagnostic confirmation Fluorescent antibody identification of *C. chauvoei* in lesion.

Treatment High doses of penicillin in early stages. Surgical debridement.

Control Vaccination.

ETIOLOGY

Blackleg, or clostridial myositis of skeletal and/or heart muscle tissue, is associated with *Clostridium chauvoei (feseri)*, a gram-positive, spore-forming, rod-shaped bacterium. The spores are normally found in soil and are highly resistant to environmental changes and disinfectants and persist in soil for many years.

EPIDEMIOLOGY

Occurrence

Blackleg is an acute febrile disease primarily affecting cattle and sheep, with worldwide occurrence. The condition is characterized by severe necrotizing myositis of striated and occasionally cardiac muscle tissue and severe toxemia with high mortality. Although black leg is widely considered a disease of ruminants, available reports suggest that swine, mink, freshwater fish, wales, frogs, and ostriches are also susceptible to infection. In recent years at least two cases of fatal disease associated with *C. chauvoei* in humans have been reported.[1,2] Although sheep of any age can be affected, cattle between 6 months and 2 years of age most commonly develop clinical disease. The disease incidence shows a seasonal pattern, with peak incidences observed during the warmer period of the year. In general, several animals of a herd or flock are affected within a short period of time. The disease is enzootic in particular areas, especially when they are subject to flooding. The **case-fatality rate** in blackleg approaches 100%.

Source of Infection

Blackleg is a **soil-borne** infection. In sheep, infection with *C. chauvoei* is assumed to predominantly occur through penetrating lesions of the skin or mucosa, but the primary portal of entry for the organism in cattle is still in dispute. It is presumed that infection primarily occurs through the mucosa of the digestive tract after ingestion of contaminated feed or may be associated with erupting teeth. Spores of *C. chauvoei* have been found in the spleen, liver, and alimentary tract of healthy animals, and contamination of the soil and pasture may occur from infected feces or decomposition of carcasses of animals that died of the disease. Clinical disease develops when spores are caused to proliferate by yet undetermined mechanisms. Tissue trauma and anoxia have been incriminated as potential triggers.

Transmission

Whereas in cattle the disease usually occurs without a history of trauma, in sheep, skin wounds from **shearing**, **docking,** and **vulvar or vaginal lacerations from parturition** or the fresh **navel** at birth are the most common routes through which *C. chauvoei* penetrates and infects muscle tissue to cause clinical disease. Infections of the vulva and vagina of the ewe at **lambing** may cause serious outbreaks, and the disease has occurred in groups of young ewes and rams up to a year old, usually as a result of infection of skin wounds caused by **fighting**. Occasional outbreaks have occurred in sheep **after vaccination** against enterotoxemia. Presumably the formalinized vaccine causes sufficient tissue damage to permit latent spores of the organism to proliferate.

A special occurrence is in **fetal lambs**. Ewes exposed to infection at shearing develop typical lesions, but ewes treated with penicillin are unaffected, except that the pregnant ewes in the latter group show distended abdomens, weakness, and recumbency as a result of edema and gas formation in the fetus, from which *C. chauvoei* can be isolated.

Risk Factors

Environment Risk Factors

Blackleg of cattle has a **seasonal incidence**, with most cases occurring in the warm months of the year. The highest incidence may vary from spring to autumn, likely depending on when calves reach the susceptible age group. There appears to be an increased disease incidence in years of high rainfall, which has been explained by increased anaerobiosis in water-saturated soils in combination with enhanced pasture growth stimulating feed intake of pastured cattle.[3] Outbreaks of blackleg in cattle have occurred following excavation of soil, which suggests that disturbance of the soil may expose and activate latent spores.

An outbreak of blackleg has also been reported in housed cattle in a nonendemic blackleg area in Norway.[4]

Animal Risk Factors

Blackleg is usually a disease of cattle and to a lesser degree of sheep, but outbreaks of the disease have been recorded in deer and horses. In cattle, the disease is most commonly seen in young stock between the ages of 6 months and 2 years, although disease occurs occasionally in younger animals and cattle up to 3 years. In the field, **risk factors** include rapidly growing cattle and a high plane of nutrition. Elevation of the nutritional status of sheep by increased protein feeding increases their susceptibility to blackleg. In sheep, there is no restriction to age group. In calves and sheep, atypical outbreaks of sudden death occur in which the lethal lesion is a clostridial cardiac myositis.

In pigs, blackleg is not common, although a gas gangrene type of lesion may be associated with *C. chauvoei* or *C. septicum* infection.

Economic Importance

Blackleg is a cause of severe financial loss to cattle raisers in many parts of the world. For the most part, major outbreaks are prevented by vaccination, although outbreaks still occur occasionally in vaccinated herds or cattle incompletely vaccinated.

PATHOGENESIS

With spores of *Cl. chauvoei* normally found in soils, ingestion of such spores through contaminated pasture or silage is unavoidable. Spores of *C. chauvoei* have been found not only in the digestive tract but also the spleen and liver healthy animals. Because *C. chauvoei* appears to be present in tissue in a dormant state before disease occurs blackleg—at least in cattle—has also be termed as "endogenous" clostridial infection, in contrast to malignant edema that is considered an exogenous infection, because the pathogen gains access to the tissue through mucosal or skin breaks and directly causes clinical disease.[5]

Whereas in sheep the clinical disease in most cases has been related to tissue laceration and trauma, the stimulus that results in growth of the latent bacterial spores in cattle is unknown. There is usually no history of trauma. Once returned to its vegetative state, *C. chauvoei* produces a number of toxins, such as oxygen-stable and oxygen-labile hemolysins, DNase, hyaluronidase, and neuramidase, which cause severe **necrotizing myositis** locally in skeletal muscles and a **systemic toxemia** that is usually fatal.

CLINICAL FINDINGS

Cattle

If the animal is observed before death there is severe lameness, usually with pronounced swelling of the upper part of the affected leg. On closer examination the animal will be found to be very depressed, have complete anorexia and ruminal stasis, and have a high temperature (41° C; 106° F) and pulse rate (100 to 120/min). Pyrexia is not present in all cases. In the early stages, the swelling is hot and painful to the touch but soon becomes cold and painless, and edema and emphysema can be felt. The skin is discolored and soon becomes dry and cracked.

Although the lesions are usually confined to the upper part of one limb, occasional cases are seen where the lesions are present in other locations, such as the base of the tongue, the heart muscle, the diaphragm and psoas muscles, the brisket, and the udder. Lesions are sometimes present in more than one of these locations in one animal. The condition develops rapidly, and the animal dies quietly 12 to 36 hours after the appearance of signs. Many animals die without signs having been observed.

Sheep

When blackleg lesions occur in the limb musculature in sheep, there is a stiff gait, and the sheep is disinclined to move because of severe lameness in one limb or, more commonly, in several limbs. The lameness may be severe enough to prevent walking in some animals but be only moderate in others. Subcutaneous edema is not common and gaseous crepitation cannot be felt before death. Discoloration of the skin may be evident, but skin necrosis and gangrene do not occur.

In those cases where infection occurs through **wounds** of the skin, vulva, or vagina, there is an extensive local lesion. Lesions of the head may be accompanied by severe local swelling as a result of edema, and there may be bleeding from the nose. In all instances, there is high fever, anorexia, and depression, and death occurs very quickly. Sheep and cattle with cardiac myositis associated with *C. chauvoei* are usually found dead.

Horses

The clinical syndrome in horses is not well defined. Pectoral edema, stiff gait, and incoordination are recorded.

CLINICAL PATHOLOGY

The disease is usually so acute that necropsy material is readily available but, failing this, it may be possible to obtain material suitable for cultural examination by needle puncture or swabs from wounds. There are no constant changes in hematologic parameters or serum biochemistry.

NECROPSY FINDINGS

Cattle found dead of blackleg are often in a characteristic position: lying on the side with the affected hindlimb stuck out stiffly. Bloating and putrefaction occur quickly, and bloodstained froth exudes from the nostrils and anus. Clotting of the blood occurs rapidly. Incision of the affected muscle mass reveals dark-red to black, swollen tissue with a rancid odor and thin, sanguineous fluid containing bubbles of gas. Freshly cut surfaces are often dry and may have a metallic sheen. The heart and all skeletal muscles, including those of the tongue, diaphragm, and lumbar region, must be checked because the lesion may be small and escape cursory examination. The thoracic cavity and the pericardial sac may contain excess bloodstained fluid with variable amounts of fibrin. This serositis is often overlooked or is misinterpreted as a component of pleuropneumonia. The lungs are usually congested and may be atelectatic as a result of abdominal tympany.

In **sheep**, the muscle lesions are more localized and deeper, and the **subcutaneous edema is not so marked, except around the head**. Gas is present in the affected muscles but not in such large amounts as in cattle. When the disease has resulted from infection of skin wounds, the lesions are more obvious superficially, with subcutaneous edema and swelling and involvement of the underlying musculature. When invasion of the genital tract occurs, typical lesions are found in the perineal tissues and in the walls of the vagina and occasionally the uterus. In the special case of pregnant ewes, typical lesions may involve the entire fetus and cause abdominal distension in the ewe.

Histologically, blackleg cases feature myonecrosis, edema, emphysema, and an unimpressive neutrophilic cellulitis. Organisms may be few in number but can usually be seen in tissue sections. Smears from the affected tissue should be made and material collected for bacteriologic examination. The isolation and identification of *C. chauvoei* and *C. novyi* is difficult because of the fastidiousness of these species in culture and rapid postmortem contamination of the tissues by clostridial species from the gastrointestinal tract. Thus it is essential that tissues be examined as soon after death as possible. Most laboratories use fluorescent antibody tests performed on tissue smears to complement (or substitute) anaerobic culture.

"False blackleg" may be associated with *C. septicum* and *C. novyi*, but this disease is more accurately classified as malignant edema. Mixed infections with *C. chauvoei* and *C. septicum* are not uncommon, but the significance of *C. septicum* as a cause of the disease is debated. However, in a study of 176 cases of clostridial myositis in cattle, *C. chauvoei* either alone or with *C. septicum* was demonstrated in 56%. In 36%, *C. novyi* was found alone or with *C. septicum*. This indicates that maximum protection to cattle can be provided only by a multivalent vaccine that contains the antigens of *C. chauvoei*, *C. novyi*, and *C. septicum*. A multiplex PCR based on the flagellin gene sequence has been used to identify pathogenic clostridia in clinical specimens.

Samples for Confirmation of Diagnosis

- Bacteriology—muscle, placed in air-tight container; four air-dried impression smears of surface of freshly cut lesion (anaerobic CULT, FAT, PCR)
- Histology—fixed samples of suspected muscle lesion

DIFFERENTIAL DIAGNOSIS

In establishing a diagnosis when a number of animals are found dead in a group not kept under close observation and postmortem decomposition is so advanced that little information can be obtained, one must depend on one's knowledge of local disease incidence, season of the year, age group affected, and pasture conditions, and on a close inspection of the environment in which the animals have been maintained. More frequent observation should be established so that sick animals or fresh cadavers will be available for examination.

- **Malignant edema**—in typical cases of blackleg in cattle a definite diagnosis can be made on the clinical signs and the necropsy findings. Definitive identification of *Clostridium chauvoei* is by fluorescent antibody staining. Diagnosis on gross postmortem findings from other causes of clostridial myositides is hazardous and may result in improper recommendations for control
- **Anthrax**
- **Lightning strike**
- **Bacillary hemoglobinuria**
- Other causes of sudden unexpected death

TREATMENT

Treatment of affected animals with **penicillin and surgical debridement** of the lesion, including fasciotomy, is indicated if the animal is not moribund. Recovery rates are low because of the extensive nature of the lesions. Large doses (44,000 IU/kg BW) should be administered, commencing with crystalline penicillin intravenously and followed by longer-acting preparations. Blackleg **antiserum** is unlikely to be of much value in treatment unless very large doses are given.

TREATMENT AND CONTROL

Treatment

Penicillin G sodium/potassium (44,000 IU/kg IV q6–8h) (R-2)

Clostridium chauvoei antitoxin (only in early stages, but doubtful efficacy)

Control

Multivalent clostridial vaccine including at least *C. chauvoei*, *C. septicum*, and *C. novyi* (R-2)

Penicillin (44,000 IU/kg IM q24 for 3 days for animals at risk) (R-2)

CONTROL

Cattle

On farms where the disease is enzootic, annual vaccination of all cattle between 3 and 6 months with two vaccinations given 4 weeks apart followed by an annual booster vaccination is generally recommended. This should be done just before the anticipated danger period, usually spring and summer. Maternal immunity persists for at least 3 months and will interfere with active immunity in calves vaccinated before this age.

In an **outbreak**, all unaffected cattle should be vaccinated immediately and injected with penicillin intramuscularly. Movement of the cattle from the affected pasture is advisable. If antibiotics are not given, new cases of blackleg may occur for up to 14 days until immunity develops, and constant surveillance and the early treatment of cases will be necessary.

Sheep

With sheep in areas where the disease is enzootic, the **maiden ewes** should be vaccinated twice, with the last vaccination given about 1 month before lambing and a subsequent yearly booster given at the same time before lambing. This will prevent infection of the ewes at lambing and will also protect lambs against umbilical infection at birth and infection of the tail wound at docking, provided the tail is docked at a young age. If an **outbreak** commences in a flock of ewes at lambing time, prophylactic injections of penicillin and antiserum to ewes requiring assistance are recommended.

A single vaccination of **wethers** can also be carried out 2 to 3 weeks before **shearing** if infection is anticipated. Because of the common occurrences of the disease in young sheep, vaccination before they go on to pasture and are exposed to infection of skin wounds from fighting is recommended in danger areas. The duration of the immunity in these young vaccinated animals is relatively short, and ewes in particular must be revaccinated before they lamb for the first time. Clostridial vaccines have **poorer antigenicity** in sheep and goats than in cattle.

In both sheep and cattle, it is advisable to use a **combined vaccine** containing at least *C. chauvoei*, *C. septicum*, and *C. novyi*, where these organisms occur in the area and cause clostridial myositis.

There is limited information on which to base the previous recommendations because there is limited information on the **efficacy** of available individual manufacturers' vaccines.[6] There is variability in the immune response and its duration with different vaccines. **Vaccine failure** has been associated with an inadequate spectrum of the antigens in the vaccine, and in these circumstances a bacterin prepared from a local strain of *C. chauvoei* is preferred. Vaccines combined with anthelmintics or with trace elements are used in some areas to minimize the number of injections required when processing sheep.

It is important that **carcasses** of animals dying of blackleg are destroyed by burning or deep burial to limit soil contamination.

FURTHER READING

Hatheway CL. Toxigenic clostridia. *Clin Microbiol Rev.* 1990;3:66-98.

Songer JG. Clostridial diseases of animals. In: Rood JI, McClane BA, Songer JG, Titball RW, eds. *The Clostridia: Molecular Biology and Pathogenesis.* London: Academic Press; 1997:153-182.

Songer JG. Clostridial diseases of small ruminants. *Vet Res.* 1998;29:219-232.

Useh NM, Nok AJ, Esievo KAN. Pathogenesis and pathology of blackleg in ruminants; the role of toxins and neuraminidase. A short review. *Vet Q.* 2003;25:155-158.

REFERENCES

1. Nagano N, et al. *J Clin Microbiol.* 2008;46:1545-1547.
2. Wearherhead JE, Tweardy DJ. *J Infect.* 2012;64:225-227.
3. Useh NM, et al. *Vet Rec.* 2006;158:100-101.
4. Groseth PK, et al. *Vet Rec.* 2011;169:339.
5. Odani JSJ. *Vet Diagn Invest.* 2009;21:920-924.
6. Uzal F. *Vet Clin North Am Food A Pract.* 2012;28:71-77.

BOVINE FOOTROT (INFECTIOUS BOVINE PODODERMATITIS, INTERDIGITAL PHLEGMON, INTERDIGITAL NECROBACILLOSIS, FOUL IN THE FOOT)

SYNOPSIS

Etiology Biotypes A and AB of *Fusobacterium necrophorum*. Other organisms can facilitate infection.

Epidemiology All ages susceptible. Infected feet are source of infection. Transmission highest where conditions are wet underfoot and in wet, humid seasons.

Clinical findings Sudden onset of lameness and fever, drop in milk production with typical fissuring, necrotic lesion in the skin at the top of the interdigital cleft.

Clinical pathology Not routinely done.

Diagnostic confirmation Clinical findings. Culture may be done.

Treatment Antimicrobials.

Control Avoidance of abrasive underfoot conditions. Footbaths, antimicrobials, vaccination.

ETIOLOGY

Footrot is usually described as a contagious disease as a result of localized infection by *F. necrophorum*, a gram-negative non–spore-forming anaerobe.[1,2] Other bacteria, primarily *Porphyromonas levii* (originally classified as *Prevotella melaninogenica* or *Bacteroides melaninogenicus*),[3] are present at variable rates in clinically infected cattle and may play a role in the development of clinical disease. Experimentally, the subcutaneous inoculation of only *F. necrophorum* into the interdigital skin of cattle will result in typical lesions of interdigital phlegmon.

F. necrophorum has traditionally been categorized into four biotypes: A (called *F. necrophorum* subsp. *necrophorum*), B (called *F. necrophorum* subsp. *funduliforme*), AB (taxonomic status is unresolved), and C (which is nonpathogenic). The majority of isolates of *F. necrophorum* obtained from the feet of cattle and sheep belong to biotypes A and AB; they produce a soluble exotoxin, a **leukotoxin**, that is produced by *F. necrophorum* strains carrying the *lktA* gene. Leukotoxin appears to play an important role in the pathogenesis of clinical disease. The isolates obtained from lesions that are not classified as interdigital necrobacillosis and from clinically normal feet are predominantly biotype B and cause few experimental lesions and produce little or no leukotoxin.

Strains of *Bacteroides nodosus* that are associated with the nonprogressive form of ovine footrot are occasionally isolated from the feet of cattle with footrot[1,2] and cause mild interdigital dermatitis. It is possible they may predispose to the much more severe dermatitis that characterizes bovine interdigital phlegmon.

EPIDEMIOLOGY

Occurrence

The disease is common in most countries and accounts for 5% to 15% of cases of lameness in dairy cattle.

Usually the disease is sporadic, but under favorable conditions, as many as 25% of a group may be affected at one time. An epidemiologic study of footrot in pastured cattle in Denmark over a 12-year period revealed that annual incidence ranged from 0.1% to 4.8%, but in most years it was below 1%. The incidence was higher in some breeds than others, higher in some geographic areas than others (usually where the fields were smaller and soil higher in pH), and higher 4 to 8 weeks after periods of high rainfall.

Transmission

Discharges from the feet of **infected animals** are the probable source of infection. Duration of the infectivity of pasture or bedding is unknown. Infection gains entrance through **abrasions** or damage to the skin in the interdigital cleft. Introduction of the infection to a farm by transient cattle is often observed, but again the disease may not develop on some farms in spite of the introduction of the infection. Contaminated footbaths can be a source of infection.

Environmental Risk Factors

In many but not all regions, the incidence is much higher during **wet, humid weather** or when conditions are **wet underfoot**. Stony ground, lanes filled with sharp gravel and pasturing on coarse stubble also predispose to the condition. A high incidence can occur, with beef cattle at high stocking densities on irrigated pastures. The observation that the disease is common on some farms and does not occur at all on others suggests that there may be factors that limit the persistence of infectivity in certain soils or environments.

Abrasions to the skin of the feet are more likely to occur when the skin is swollen and soft as a result of continual wetting. The increased incidence in wet summer and autumn months may be so explained in part, although wet conditions may also favor persistence of the infection in pasture. In housed cattle, the incidence is higher in **loose-housed** cattle than tied cattle. Unhygienic cubicle passageways and poorly maintained straw beds may predispose to infection.

Host Risk Factors

Cattle of all ages, including young calves, may be affected, but the disease is much more common in adults. The highest incidence occurs in cows in the **first month of lactation**. A field observation is that *Bos indicus* cattle are much more resistant to infectious footrot than *Bos taurus* breeds, and variations in prevalence have been observed among dairy breeds.

Economic Importance

Footrot is of greatest economic importance in dairy cattle, in which it reaches the highest level of incidence because of the intensive conditions under which they are kept. A 2010 study estimated that each case of footrot costs dairy producers US$121.[4] In beef cattle at range the incidence is usually low, but many cases may occur in purebred herds and in feedlot cattle. Lame cows will lie down for longer and eat less, have difficulty rising, and are at greater risk for teat trampling and mastitis. Loss of production occurs, and an occasional animal may suffer a serious involvement of the joint and other deep structures of the foot necessitating amputation of a digit. The disease is not fatal, but some cases may have to be slaughtered because of joint involvement.

PATHOGENESIS

The pathogenesis is not completely understood, but with the experimental SC inoculation of the virulent biotype of *F. necrophorum* into the interdigital skin of cattle, the typical lesion of footrot develops in approximately 5 days. This suggests that any injury or constant wetting of the skin of the cleft that interferes with its integrity will allow the organism to invade the tissues. There is acute swelling and necrosis of the skin and SC tissues, which may spread to adjacent tendon sheaths, joint capsules, and bone if treatment is delayed or ineffective.

CLINICAL FINDINGS

Severe foot **lameness** appears suddenly, usually in one limb only, and may be accompanied by a moderate systemic reaction with a **fever** of 39 to 40° C (103 to 104° F). There is temporary depression of milk yield in cows, and affected bulls may show temporary infertility. The animal puts little weight on the leg, although the limb is carried only when severe joint involvement occurs. Swelling of the coronet and **spreading of the claws** are obvious.

The typical lesion occurs in the skin at the top of the **interdigital cleft** and takes the form of a **fissure** with swollen, protruding edges that may extend along the length of the cleft or be confined to the anterior part or that part between the heel bulbs. Pus is never present in large amounts, but the edges of the fissure are covered with **necrotic material,** and the lesion has a **characteristic odor**. Occasionally in early cases no external lesion may be visible, but there is lameness and swelling of the coronet. Such cases are usually designated "blind fouls" and respond well to parenteral treatment. A hand-held infrared thermographic unit may be helpful in identifying cattle with footrot, particularly when the difference in temperature between the plantar aspect is compared with the other hindfoot or front foot.[5]

A more severe form of the disease that is peracute in onset and refractory to conventional therapy has been termed "super foul" or "super footrot," although there does not seem to be a persuasive reason to develop a descriptive term from separate footrot. With this type there is sudden onset of acute lameness, severe interdigital swelling, and rapid progression to necrosis and deep erosion of the interdigital space with swelling of soft tissue above the coronary band. The hindfeet or all four feet may be affected.

Spontaneous recovery is not uncommon, but if the disease is left untreated, the lameness usually persists for several weeks, with adverse effects on milk production and condition. The incidence of **complications** is also higher if treatment is delayed, and some animals may have to be destroyed because of local **involvement of joints and tendon sheaths.** In such cases the lameness is severe, the leg is usually carried, and the animal strongly resents handling of the foot. Swelling is usually more obvious and extends up the back of the leg. There is poor response to medical treatment, and surgical measures are necessary to permit drainage. **Radiologic examination** may be of value in determining the exact degree of involvement of bony tissue.

Long continued irritation may result in the development of a wart-like mass of fibrous tissue, the **interdigital fibroma**, in the anterior part of the cleft and chronic mild lameness. Interdigital fibroma occurs commonly without the intervention of footrot, the important cause being inherited defects in foot conformation in heavy animals.

CLINICAL PATHOLOGY

Bacteriologic examination is not usually necessary for diagnosis, but direct smears of the lesion will usually reveal large numbers of a mixture of *Fusobacterium* and *Bacteroides* spp. Routine differentiation between virulent and nonvirulent bovine isolates of *F. necrophorum* can be done by assessment of the cultural characteristics of the colonies grown on blood agar. Proteomic analysis of plasma from cattle with footrot identified increased concentrations of innate immune recognition molecules, acute-phase proteins, and cell-adhesion and cytoskeletal proteins.[6]

> **DIFFERENTIAL DIAGNOSIS**
>
> The characteristic site, nature, and smell of the lesion; the pattern of the disease in the group; and the season and climate are usually sufficient to indicate the presence of true footrot.

NECROPSY FINDINGS

Necropsy examinations are rarely carried out in cases of footrot. Dermatitis is followed by necrosis of the skin and subcutaneous tissues. In complicated cases there may be suppuration in joints and tendon sheaths.

Interdigital Dermatitis/Stable Footrot

Interdigital dermatitis occurs commonly in cattle that are housed for long periods. Although the condition occurs most commonly when the cattle are kept under unsanitary conditions, it is also seen in well-managed herds. The causative agent has not been established, but *Bacteroides nodosus* can be isolated.

The initial lesion is an outpouring of sebaceous exudate at the skin–horn junction, particularly at the bulbs of the heel. There is a penetrating foul odor, the lesion is painful to touch, and there is little swelling and no systemic reaction. More than one foot is commonly affected. In long-standing cases there is separation of the horn at the heel bulb, and this is followed by secondary bacterial infection of the sensitive structures of the foot. Often there is a purulent dermatitis of the interdigital space. Stable footrot does not respond satisfactorily to the standard parenteral treatments used in footrot, but local treatments as set out as follows are effective.

Verrucose Dermatitis

Verrucose dermatitis is a proliferative inflammatory lesion of the **skin of the plantar surface** of the foot extending from the bulb of the heels to the fetlock joint. The condition is seen particularly in feedlot cattle that are overcrowded in wet muddy conditions and may occur in outbreaks. **All four feet** may be affected, there is considerable pain and lameness, and, on smear of the lesion, *F. necrophorum* is present in large numbers. The treatment of verrucose dermatitis consists of washing the affected skin with a disinfectant soap, followed by daily applications of 5% copper sulfate solution. When many animals are affected, a daily walk-through and soaking in a foot bath containing the copper sulfate solution is very effective.

Traumatic Injury

Traumatic injury to bones and joints, puncture by foreign bodies, bruising of the heels, and gross overgrowth of the hoof can usually be distinguished by careful examination of the foot. **Laminitis** is the major cause of lameness in most herds, but with this condition there are no skin lesions present.

TREATMENT

Parenteral administration of antibiotics or sulfonamides and local treatment of the foot lesion are necessary for best results. **Immediate treatment** as soon as possible after the onset of swelling and lameness will give excellent recovery in 2 to 4 days. In the experimental disease, when treatment was delayed for a few days after the onset of signs, severe lesions developed and recovery was extended. Under field conditions, the disease may be present in cattle at pasture for several days before being recognized, making it necessary to confine them for daily treatment until recovery is apparent.

Antimicrobials

Long-acting antimicrobial formulations are preferred to decrease labor associated with daily treatment and hospital pen space requirements.[7] Oxytetracycline, 10 mg/kg BW IV daily, or long-acting tetracycline, 20 mg/kg BW IM, is preferred because of cost and excellent efficacy, but some prefer ceftiofur because of injection-site swelling and longer withdrawal period with oxytetracycline. Tulathromycin (2.5 mg/kg SC) and Florfenicol (40 mg/kg SC) are also effective as one-time treatments. Ceftiofur, 1 to 1.1 mg/kg BW IM, or procaine penicillin G, 22,000 IU/kg BW IM twice daily, or once daily for 3 consecutive days, are effective but need multiple treatments. Sodium sulfadimidine (150 to 200 mg/kg BW) solution given by IV injection is highly effective. Sulfabromomethazine at the rate of 30 g/kg grain was given for two consecutive days to calves weighing 150 kg, and results were excellent. Sulfonamides are not approved for use in lactating dairy cattle in many countries.

Local Treatment

Local treatment necessitates restraint of the affected leg, and this procedure is greatly facilitated by a restraint table or the administration of a very small dose of xylazine. The foot is scrubbed, all necrotic tissue is curetted away, and a local dressing is applied under a pad or bandage. Any **antibacterial**, and preferably **astringent**, dressing appears to be satisfactory. A wet pack of 5% copper sulfate solution is cheap and effective. Any suitable antibacterial ointment preparation may be applied and secured with a bandage, which may be left on for several days. The main advantage of local treatment is that the foot is cleaned and kept clean. If conditions underfoot are wet, the animal should be kept stabled in a dry stall.

In cattle running at pasture, or in the case of large numbers of feedlot cattle, examination of the foot and local treatment are often omitted because of the time and inconvenience involved. However, identification of the animal with a marker is considered necessary in outbreaks to avoid unnecessary confusion in the days following, and examination of the foot is deemed necessary to ensure that foreign bodies are not involved. Local treatment may not be necessary in the early stages of the disease if the animal can be prevented from gaining access to wet, muddy areas.

Surgical Drainage

Surgical drainage may be necessary in refractory cases or when complications with spread to deeper tissues have occurred.

CONTROL

Prevention of foot injuries by filling in muddy and stony patches in barnyards and lanes will reduce the incidence of the disease. Lanes and bedding should be kept clean and dry. The incorporation of biotin in the diet, although reducing the incidence of lameness caused by white-line lesions, has no effect on the incidence of interdigital phlegmon.

Footbaths

Provision of a footbath containing a 5% to 10% solution of formaldehyde or copper sulfate, in a doorway so that cattle have to walk through it twice daily, will practically eliminate the disease on dairy farms. A mixture of 10% copper sulfate in slaked lime is often used in the same manner. Similar measures can be adopted for small groups of beef animals; however, it is thought that providing dry footing and removing abrasive objects provides more effective control than footbaths.

Antibacterials

Feeding chlortetracycline to feedlot cattle 500 mg/head per day for 28 days, followed by 75 mg/d throughout the finishing period, has been recommended, but controlled comparative trials have not been carried out. The feeding of organic iodides (200 to 400 mg) of ethylene diamine dihydroiodide (EDDI) in the feed daily has been used for many years as a preventive against the disease in feedlot cattle. Feeding EDDI in an ad libitum salt mixture at a level of 0.156% EDDI (0.125% iodine) is also effective in reducing the incidence of footrot. Dosing cattle daily with zinc sulfate by including it in the feed has no prophylactic effect.

Vaccination

Commercial vaccines against bovine interdigital phlegmon are available, but their efficacy has not been established in controlled comparative trials. A mineral-oil adjuvant vaccine containing whole cells or fractions of *F. necrophorum* provided about 60% protection from experimentally induced interdigital phlegmon. A similar vaccine containing *Bacteroides nodosus* appeared to reduce the severity of lesions but not the incidence compared with nonvaccinates.

TREATMENT AND CONTROL

Treatment

- Oxytetracycline (20 mg/kg IM/SC of long-acting formulation) (R-1)
- Ceftiofur crystalline suspension (long-acting formulation, 6.6 mg/kg, once) (R-1)
- Tulathromycin (2.5 mg/kg SC, once) (R-1)
- Florfenicol (40 mg/kg SC, once) (R-1)
- Procaine penicillin 22,000 IU/kg IM daily for at least 3 days) (R-2)
- Oxytetracycline (6.6 mg/kg IM daily for 3 days) (R-2)
- Ceftiofur sodium (1.1 or 2.2 mg/kg IM BW daily for 3 days) (R-2)
- Florfenicol (20 mg/kg IM, repeated at 48 hours) (R-2)

Control

- Decrease moisture on the ground by scraping and improving drainage (R-1)
- Minimize exposure to items that traumatize the interdigital cleft (R-1)
- Vaccination using a bacterin against *Fusobacterium necrophorum* and leukotoxin (R-3)

FURTHER READING

Apley MD. Clinical evidence for individual animal therapy for papillomatous digital dermatitis (hairy heel wart) and infectious bovine pododermatitis (footrot). *Vet Clin North Am Food A*. 2015;31:81-95.

Nagaraja TG, Narayanan SK, Stewart GC, Chengappa MM. *Fusobacterium necrophorum* infections in animals: pathogenesis and pathogenic mechanisms. *Anaerobe*. 2005;11:239-246.

REFERENCES

1. Bennett G, et al. *Res Vet Sci*. 2009;87(3):413.
2. Sun DB, et al. *African J Microbiol Res*. 2011;5:667.
3. Sweeney M, et al. *Vet Ther*. 2009;10:E1.
4. Cha E, et al. *Prev Vet Med*. 2010;97:1.
5. Main DCJ, et al. *Vet Rec*. 2012;doi:10.1136/vr100533.
6. Sun D, et al. *PLoS ONE*. 2013;8:e55973.
7. van Donkersgoed J, et al. *Vet Ther Res Applied Vet Med*. 2008;9:157.

BOVINE DIGITAL DERMATITIS, PAPILLOMATOUS DIGITAL DERMATITIS OF CATTLE (MORTELLARO'S DISEASE), FOOT WARTS, HAIRY FOOT WARTS, "HEEL WARTS"

SYNOPSIS

Etiology Causative agent(s): primary causative agents are thought to be anaerobic spirochetes *Treponema medium/Treponema vincentii*–like, *Treponema phagdenis*–like, and *Treponema denticola/Treponema putidum*–like, and other foot-adapted *Treponema* strains. Other bacterial may play a role in establishing clinical disease.

Epidemiology Worldwide disease after first report in 1974; more common in dairy cattle housed in wet, unhygienic conditions.

Clinical findings Lesions located most commonly on caudal aspect of hindfeet; early lesions have a red, granular (strawberry-like) appearance and are very painful; mature lesions are less painful and more proliferative and may have long wart-like projections.

Diagnostic confirmation Clinical signs are sufficiently diagnostic; no additional diagnostic tests required.

Treatment Sustained topical treatment with topical bandage over gauze with 10 mL oxytetracycline in oil (100 mg/mL) is considered the gold standard treatment.

Control Footbaths—5% copper sulfate (not in European Union), 5% formaldehyde—new proprietary formulations are under active development; vaccination ineffective.

Digital dermatitis (DD) is a painful, erosive, papillomatous-like lesion of the skin of the feet of cattle. The region proximal and adjacent to the interdigital skin midway between the heel bulbs of the plantar surface of the foot is most frequently affected. Early lesions are circumscribed, with a red, granular appearance and variable degrees of proliferation of filiform papillae. Mature lesions tend to be more proliferative and may have long papillary fronds. Lameness is severe, particularly when evaluated against the size and location of the lesion, and economic losses result from decreased milk production and reproductive performance.

ETIOLOGY

The etiology is uncertain, but it is very likely that anaerobic spirochetes in the genus *Treponema* play a primary role in infection. A mixed population of gram-negative bacteria, including anaerobes, microaerophilic organisms, and spirochetes, has been demonstrated in or isolated from DD lesions, but spirochetes are consistently observed in superficial lesions and deeper layers of the epidermis in cattle with DD. At least 17 different spirochetal phylotypes within the genus *Treponema* have been identified in lesions,[1] and the most common isolates are *Treponema medium/Treponema vincentii*–like; *Treponema phagdenis*–like; and *Treponema denticola/Treponema putidum*–like, with the latter being recognized as a new species, *Treponema pedis*.[2,3,4] Other bacterial may play a role in establishing clinical disease. PCR measurement of a small subunit of ribosomal RNA or its gene (16S rDNA) has been used for phylogenetic analysis, with *T. phagedenis*–like or *T. denticola/T. putidum*–like in 51% of DD cases and *T. medium/T. vincentii*–like in 38% of DD cases.[2,5] The phylogenetic cluster distribution appears to vary from country to country, leading to the suggestion that the total amount of treponemes is an important determinant of disease outcome, with the presence of specific phylotypes being of lesser importance.[6] Quantitative 16s rRNA clonal analysis indicates that all DD isolates are more than 99% identical to *T. phagedenis*–like, which is an inhabitant of the human genital tract.[7] *Treponema* spp. have been isolated from the gingival tissue of 14% of dairy cattle, but only in the housing season and only in cattle with visible DD lesions, and from the rectal tissue of 15% of dairy cattle.[8] This finding suggests colonization of sites other that the foot in dairy cattle. Cow feces and environmental manure slurry have been shown to be potential reservoirs of treponemes that cause DS.[9]

A spirochete isolated from cases of severe virulent ovine footrot in Australia and the United Kingdom and Ireland is closely related to a treponeme isolated from human periodontitis and bovine digital dermatitis. This suggests the possibility of cross-species transmission, and that a number of spirochetes could be involved in the pathogenesis of either DD or severe virulent ovine footrot.

EPIDEMIOLOGY

Occurrence and Prevalence of Infection

The disease was first described in Italy in 1974 as **Mortellaro's disease**. It occurs primarily in dairy cattle and has been reported as a cause of lameness in dairy cattle worldwide, although beef cattle can also be affected. Surveys of dairy farms in California in the United States found that 25% to 75% of farms have had the disease, and about 10% of cows have been affected, with a range from 1% to 99% of cows in affected herds.

Factors associated with high herd incidence of DD (>5%) include geographic location, herd size, type of land lactating cows accessed on a daily basis, flooring type where lactating cows walked, percent of cows born off the farm, use of a primary hoof trimmer who trimmed cows' hooves on other farms, and lack of washing of hoof-trimming equipment between cows. It is likely that undisinfected hoof-trimming equipment plays a role in transmission of infection from farm to farm.[10] Seasonal differences occur and may be a result of a combination of weather, housing, and management. The incidence may be higher during the winter months, when the weather is cold and wet and cows are kept in confined housing, than during the summer months when cows are on pasture.

Risk Factors

Host Risk Factors

First-parity cows have the highest odds of DD, and the odds decrease, in a dose–effect manner, as parity increases. The odds of DD increase with increasing days in lactation.

Other risk factors include loose housing, slatted floors, housing under wet and unhygienic conditions, and the introduction of subclinically infected cows into susceptible populations. The plantar and palmar regions of the foot may be more conducive to the development of DD because these anatomic sites are exposed to more moisture. Exposure to slurry increases the permeability of the skin and therefore the susceptibility to DD.[11] Epidemiologic observations indicate that the risk of DD is associated with environmental conditions that cause moist feet in commercial dairy herds. Interdigital dermatitis and heel horn erosion predispose the foot to DD, and all three diseases appear to have similar causative mechanisms that focus on increased exposure of the foot to moisture.[6] Moreover, feet affected with clinical DD lesions have an increase prevalence in heel horn erosion, further supporting a common etiology for these foot conditions.[12] Nonhealing white-line disease and sole ulcers appear to be more common in herds endemically affected with DD,[13] and *T. medium*/*T. vincentii*–like is consistently isolated from these lesions.[14]

The greater incidence of the lesions in the hindfeet is considered to be associated with more exposure to deeper slurry during feeding times than the forelimbs. The plantar and palmar regions of the interdigital cleft are therefore more susceptible to being continually moist compared with the more open dorsal locations. The bovine gut and feces appear to be an important reservoir of infection,[15] but direct skin-to-skin contact could also be an important transmission route for DD treponemes.[16] The anatomic location of DD lesions also has an effect on the efficacy of topical treatment with antibiotics.

Immune Mechanisms

T. phagedenis–like spirochetes isolated from active DD lesions in dairy cattle are associated with serum IgG_2 antibodies, and most react with lipopolysaccharide. Both the antibody and blastogenic responses were reduced in convalescent dairy cattle, suggesting the immune response to the spirochetes has short duration. The presence of IgG_2 spirochete antibodies detected by ELISA does not necessarily describe an active immune protective response by affected cows but reflects prior infection and repeated exposures to treponemes.

Cattle and sheep with DD and severe virulent ovine footrot, respectively, and that may be infected by the same group of treponemes, have increased seropositivity rates to both treponeme isolates, with different patterns of reactivity between farms.

Environmental and Management Risk Factors

Case-control studies in dairy farms indicate that the odds of having a higher proportion (>5%) of affected cows were about 20 times more likely in dairy farms with muddier corrals than in farms with drier ground surfaces in corrals. The disease appears to be more common in free-stall confined herds where feet are constantly exposed to moisture and manure conditions. The feet often become coated with a layer of dried feces, which may provide the anaerobic conditions necessary for bacterial growth.

Buying replacement heifers was associated with a 4.7-fold increase in the odds of a higher occurrence of disease than in herds that did not purchase heifers. There also may be a positive relationship between risk and the number of heifers purchased. Herd size was positively associated with the presence of the disease. Cows in dairy herds that used a footbath were less likely to have DD than those herds not using one. Animals housed in a straw yard were 3.2 times less likely to be affected compared with cattle on slatted floors. Feeding with a larger variety of dietary components (hay, milk, concentrates plus silage) was a protective measure.

Pathogen Risk Factors

Molecular typing of DD-associated *Treponema* isolates has found some genetic relatedness to those of the related human-associated *Treponema* spp. associated with human periodontal disease. These *Treponema* strains have adhesion properties and produce high levels of chymotrypsin-like protease and high levels of proline iminopeptidase, which are major virulence factors.

Economic Importance

The economic losses associated with the lameness accompanying DD in lactating cows include loss in milk production, the effects on reproductive performance, and the costs of treatment, including the time required to recognize the lesions, the costs of individual medication of affected cows if necessary, and the costs of construction and maintenance of a footbath. Lameness has an important effect on milk yield, with the total mean estimated reduction in milk yield per 305-day lactation being 360 kg. Lameness has an important effect on reproductive performance. Dairy cows with claw lesions have a higher calving-to-conception interval and a greater number of services per conception.

PATHOGENESIS

DD is an acute or chronic ulcerative lesion of the skin of the bulbs of the heel or interdigital cleft. In the early stages of the lesion, there is loss of superficial keratin, with a concurrent thickening of the epithelium by both hyperplasia and hypertrophy of epithelial cells. Superficial layers are eosinophilic and undergo necrotic change with the appearance of small holes. Large numbers of spirochetes are present around the holes. Loss of superficial layers of keratin stimulates epidermal proliferation and hyperplasia. In advanced cases, large numbers of spirochetes infiltrate the eroded dermis and may destroy the epidermis. DD is characterized by erosion of the superficial layers of the epidermis, epithelial hyperplasia and hypertrophy, pain, and mild swelling. Lesions usually occur on the hindfeet and are prone to bleeding. Early lesions are circumscribed with a red, granular (strawberry-like) appearance and variable degrees of proliferation of filiform papillae. Mature lesions are more proliferative and may have long wart-like projections, thus the term "hairy wart" disease.

CLINICAL FINDINGS

DD typically occurs in dairy cattle as lameness episodes of variable severity. Affected cattle can be lame and reluctant to move. The affected limb is often held trembling in partial flexion as if the animal is in pain. Less severely affected limbs are rested on the toes and animals may walk on their toes, which become markedly worn and may even expose the sensitive laminae. Affected cattle lose weight and may not eat normally if they have to walk some distance to obtain feed. Milk production may decline if the lesions are severe enough.

Clinical inspection of the foot has been the most effective diagnostic procedure. Lesions are confined to the digits and do not occur above the dewclaws. The feet of the hindlimbs are most commonly affected. The plantar surface of the feet is most commonly affected, but the palmar aspects may also be involved. The majority of lesions are medium to large, measure 2 to 4 cm across at their largest dimension, and are **located on the skin at its junction with the soft perioplic horn of the heel and midway between the two claws**. Most lesions are situated proximal and adjacent to the plantar/palmar interdigital space and rarely involve the interdigital skin. The surface of the lesion is moist, prone to bleeding, and intensely painful to the touch. The lesions are circular to oval in shape, raised, and variable in color and in degree of papillary proliferation. The washed surfaces are typically red and granular or a composite of white–yellow, gray, brown, or black papillary areas mixed with red granular areas (strawberry-like) (Fig. 15-11). Filiform papillae commonly protrude from the surface of the lesions. Most lesions are circumscribed or delineated by a discrete line of raised hyperkeratotic skin with long wart-like projections. The lesions are restricted to the skin and do not extend into the deeper soft tissues. If untreated, DD can persist for months associated with persistent lameness, reduced milk production, impaired reproductive performance, and premature culling.

More advanced lesions may lead to progressive separation of horn from the sensitive laminae, resulting in a typical underrun sole that may extend forward from the heel to reach halfway to the toe. Outbreaks of the disease may occur in dairy herds, in which up to 75% of all cows may be affected over a period of several months.

The presence and nature of any DD lesions on the plantar aspect of the foot are categorized using a scoring system.[17] The scoring system utilizes the size of the lesion, pain reaction, and clinical appearance and consists of five categories:

- M0, normal skin, no signs of disease
- M1, small (0.5 to 2 cm in diameter) DD lesion that is usually not painful
- M2, erosive hyperemic DD lesion greater than 2 cm in diameter that is usually painful on palpation (Fig. 15-11)
- M3, healing stage of M2 manifest as the presence of a scab with minimal pain
- M4, hyperkeratotic cutaneous DD lesion that is usually not painful on palpation (Fig. 15-11)

The consensus view is that lesion progression proceeds as follows: M0 → M1 → M2 → M3 → M4, although definitive experimental evidence is lacking. The duration of M3 appears to be very short. Lesion area (as measured by digital photography) appears to provide the most sensitive measure of treatment efficacy but has not been frequently applied.

A screening method for the detection of lesions of dairy cattle has been described. At the milking parlor and once the cows are in place for milking, a water hose is used to wash the cows' feet. Then, using a powerful flashlight, the digits are carefully inspected for DD lesions. A DD case is defined as a cow with a circular or oval-shaped, well-demarcated, alopecic, moist, erosive foot lesion, surrounded by a white hyperkeratotic ridge or hypertrophic hairs. Lesions bleed easily and are very painful. When struck by a concentrated jet of water from a hose, the animal frequently reacts by pulling the foot away and sometimes shaking it. The screening method has a sensitivity of 0.72 and a specificity of 0.99. This method can be approximated by turning a parlor hose fully on and using the following scoring system: (0) no movement of the foot after application of the water stream; (1) cow picks up foot and returns it to the floor within 2 seconds of application of the water stream; (2) cow picks up the foot and holds the foot up above the floor for more than 2 seconds. Use of a borescope (an extended rigid tube that provides a focused visual image of the foot at the end of the scope) in the milking parlor does not provide any additional diagnostic information to that provided by application of a water hose to wash the cows' feet.[18]

Infrared thermography does not appear to be of clinical value in detecting DD lesions and is of marginal clinical value in detecting other skin and claw lesions.[18] Improvement in clinical utility can be obtained by examining clean feet and comparing hindfeet to front feet,[19] but these requirements make the test impractical.

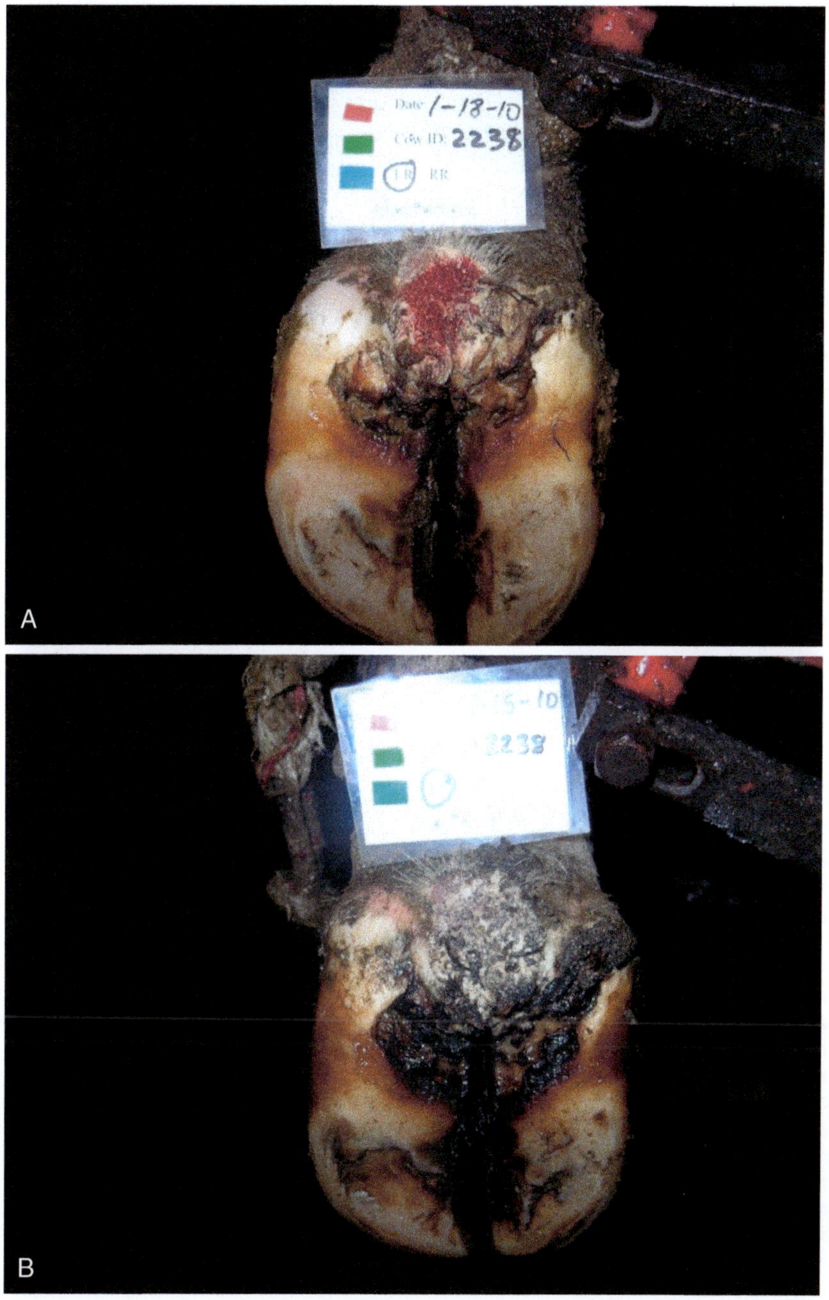

Fig. 15-11 Progression of a painful M2 lesion (A) to a mature M4 lesion accompanied by heel horn erosion (B) 4 weeks later on the same foot of a 3-year-old Holstein–Friesian cow. Pictures generously provided by Dr. Tessa Marshall, United States.

CLINICAL PATHOLOGY

Detection of Organism

Smears of the exudate and scrapings of the surface of the lesions are submitted for culture and for staining for spirochetes. Culture is extremely difficult, which has resulted in the increased application of PCR to identify the presence of spirochetes.

Dark-field microscopy of the scrapings may reveal profuse motile spirochetes with vigorous rotational and flexing movements. Biopsy specimens of the lesions can be submitted for histologic examination and special silver staining to identify the spirochetes.

Serology

Using an ELISA, in cattle with DD, there is a significant humoral response to certain strains of spirochetes isolated from lesions.[20] Animals without DD lesions show little or no response.

PATHOLOGY

The majority of lesions are 2 to 4 cm across their largest dimension, circular to oval, raised, and variable in color. Washed surfaces are typically either extensively red and granular or a composite of white–yellow, gray, brown, and/or black papillary areas interspersed with red granular areas. The surface of the lesions is covered by filiform papillae, 0.5 to 1 mm in caliber and 1 to 3 mm in length. Most lesions are characteristically circumscribed or delineated by a discrete line of raised hyperkeratotic skin, often bearing erect hairs 2 to 3 times longer than normal. The surfaces are also partially to completely alopecic, moist, prone to bleed, and intensely painful to touch. Histologically active lesions are characterized by zones of acute degeneration, necrosis, and inflammatory cell infiltration within the stratum corneum, usually associated with focal thinning. Using immunocytochemical staining and PCR of lesion biopsies, *Treponema* spp. has consistently been identified.

DIFFERENTIAL DIAGNOSIS

Digital dermatitis must be differentiated from the following:

Interdigital dermatitis—moist, gray thickening of the skin, with focal areas of shallow ulceration and hyperkeratosis. It is less painful and rarely has a granular, tufted, or papillomatous surface.

Heel horn erosion (slurry heel)—occurs commonly in dairy cows standing for long periods in slurry. The intact smooth horn of the heel develops deep, black fissures, which may become totally eroded. There is no liquefaction necrosis of keratin characteristic of digital dermatitis.

Interdigital necrobacillosis (footrot)—a necrotizing infection of the interdigital skin. There is marked painful, deep swelling of the tissues of the interdigital cleft; cracking of the skin may occur, with release of a foul-smelling discharge. Response to treatment with antimicrobials is good unless the lesion is advanced.

Verrucose dermatitis—occurs in cattle kept in deep muddy yards and is characterized by marked painful proliferative dermatitis of the plantar surface of pastern from the bulbs of the heels to the fetlocks. *Fusobacterium necrophorum* is usually present in the lesions. Affected cattle are lame and respond to topical treatment and use of a footbath with a suitable antimicrobial.

Interdigital fibroma (corn)—develops from the fold of skin adjacent to the axial wall of the hoof in the interdigital space. The lesion consists of firm fibrous tissue and may extend the entire length of the interdigital cleft. Lameness is caused by the presence of the corn in the interdigital cleft; advanced corns must be removed surgically.

TREATMENT

Treatment and control of DD have used two main approaches: (1) individual treatment of lesions by application of a topical antibiotic or disinfectant at the lesion site or, less frequently, parenteral antibiotic treatment, or (2) herd treatment using footbaths.[21,22] Evaluation of treatment efficacy is challenging because the M2 lesion appears to have a much higher level of infectivity than other lesion categories. Mathematically derived models of transition rates indicate that the speed in identifying acute M2 lesions and the efficacy of treatment of M2 lesions play important roles in determining whether lesions become more severe or heal.[17] The challenge is that accurate diagnosis requires clinical inspection of the foot, which is labor intensive.[20] Consequently, efficacy studies are frequently confounded by case definitions. Many treatments have not undergone rigorous evaluation and are likely to be ineffective. As an example, a survey of 65 French dairy farmers identified 30 different products that were used for individual treatment of DD and 31 products that were used for herd treatment of cows with DD.[23] The large number of treatments emphasizes the need for more randomized clinical trials related to treatment and control of DD.

Topical Antimicrobials

The consensus view is that the gold standard treatment is topical antimicrobial application with 10 mL of long-acting oxytetracycline (200 mg/mL in an oil base) in cotton ball or gauze, covered by a bandage, resulting in 2 g of tetracycline applied per treatment. The oil formulation is thought to help retain the antimicrobial in the gauze, resulting in sustained topical antimicrobial exposure. This treatment protocol does not result in detectable milk residues, and field efficacy is supported by in vitro susceptibility results; however, this treatment is not practical when large numbers of animals are affected. Moreover, there is one report that this treatment protocol resulted in a low healing rate in cows with a large lesion size in an endemic herd that had long-term application of tetracycline for treating DD.[24] An alternative equivalent treatment that does not require a bandage is application of a tetracycline paste consisting of 175 mL of propylene glycol, 175 mL of vinegar, and 150 g of tetracycline hydrochloride applied directly to the lesion with a paintbrush, resulting in 2 to 5 g of tetracycline applied per treatment.[25] This treatment protocol exposes more tetracycline to the environment than treatment involving application of a foot bandage. In general, application of a bandage over the lesion after application of a treatment should result in longer topical application times, and consequently it should be expected that a topical treatment followed by bandaging should be more effective than topical spray without bandaging.[26]

In vitro studies have identified the following minimum bactericidal concentrations for 90% of *Treponema* spp. isolated from DD lesions:[2,7,16] penicillin G (<0.06 to 0.19 μg/mL), erythromycin (<0.06 to 0.19 μg/mL), ampicillin (<0.06 to 4 μg/mL), oxytetracycline (0.5 to 6 μg/mL), ceftiofur (6 to 8 μg/mL), spectinomycin (48 μg/mL), lincomycin (8 to 48 μg/mL), enrofloxacin (8 to 192 μg/mL), rifampin (>128 μg/mL). These results support the routine use of topical oxytetracycline and suggest that topical lincomycin will be ineffective and that topical macrolides might provide an effective treatment.

Topical antimicrobial sprays or ointments are used on individual animals after the lesions have been cleaned. Direct spraying of the lesions with oxytetracycline at 25 mg/mL in 20% glycerine in deionized water once daily for 5 days using a garden-type spray applicator was effective. Only affected cows and individual lesions should be treated. The anatomic location of DD lesions has an effect on the efficacy of topical treatments. The use of oxytetracycline solution (25 mg/mL in distilled water) as a topical spray on cows with DD lesions was most effective on lesions located on the heels or dewclaws compared with those in the interdigital cleft; this result confirms the obvious conclusion that topical treatments need to be applied directly on the lesion and not near the lesion to be effective.

Oxytetracycline solution (100 mg/mL), acidified ionized copper solution, acidified sodium chlorite, or placebo given as a topical spray three times daily, after washing the lesions, for 3 weeks was effective in decreasing the lameness associated with the disease. In a Swedish dairy herd, topical oxytetracycline was more effective for the treatment of DD in cattle with heel-horn erosion than hoof trimming alone and more effective than glutaraldehyde. The use of an oxytetracycline solution topically at doses of 15 mL of a solution containing 100 mg oxytetracycline/mL sprayed twice daily for 7 days, or a one-time application of a bandage of cotton soaked with 20 mL of a solution containing 100 mg oxytetracycline/mL, has a low risk of causing volatile antibiotic residues in milk. Topical treatment with chlortetracycline cured painful digital dermatitis lesions at 79% per week (M2 to other categories).[27]

Lincomycin at a dose of 25 mL of a solution containing 0.6 mg lincomycin/mL or valnemulin at a dose of 25 mL of a solution containing 100 mg/mL valnemulin, given as an individual topical spray for two treatments 48 hours apart, resulted in significant improvement within 14 days after the first treatment.

Nonantibiotic Topical Formulations

The efficacy of oxytetracycline has been compared with nonantibiotic solutions, a commercial preparation of soluble copper, peroxide compound and a cationic agent, 5% copper sulfate, acidified ionized copper solution, hydrogen peroxide–peroxyacetic acid solution, and tap water for the treatment of DD. The commercial formulation of soluble copper, peroxide compound, and a cationic agent appeared to be as effective as oxytetracycline. A nonantimicrobial cream containing soluble copper with peroxide and a cationic agent was compared with topical lincomycin. The efficacy of the treatments was not different for decreasing pain or lesion activity, but lincomycin was more effective in decreasing lesion size and preventing recurrence. Cows with 3 or more lactations were more likely to have a healed lesion at 29 days compared with first- and second-lactation cows.

The efficacy of a number of disinfectants, including proprietary formulations, has been evaluated in vitro. A 5% copper sulfate solution was extremely effective in killing *Treponema* spp., but its effectiveness was markedly affected by the presence of manure.[28] Organic chemicals such as glutaraldehyde and formaldehyde (formalin) were effective in vitro and have the benefit of being degraded in manure, but they are not as effective as 5% copper sulfate. Salicylic acid applied under a bandage is effective.[26] A nonantibiotic proprietary formulation based on a reduced soluble copper solution, peroxide compound, and a cationic agent was most effective for the treatment of DD, once daily for 5 days, compared with other similar formulations and oxytetracycline.

A nonantibiotic paste, Protexin Hoof-Care, containing formic acid (6.8%), acetic acid (3.74%), copper (3.29%), and zinc sulfate (0.40%), and essential oils (peppermint/eucalyptus, 0.16%) with a pH of 3.5 has been compared under controlled conditions with topical oxytetracycline and is considered an effective alternative to the antibiotic for the treatment of DD. Only one topical application is required after cleaning the lesion. Advantages include the following: no prescription is required, no withdrawal time is required, and it does not result in any concerns about antibiotic residue in meat or milk.

Cleaning the Surface of the Lesion

It is very important to wash and clean the surface of the lesion with a disinfectant soap before the topical administration of any medication. Topical treatment failures are commonly associated with failure to adequately wash and clean the surface of the lesion.

Bandaging the Lesion

Whether or not the lesion should be bandaged after cleaning and medicating is controversial. Bandaging requires additional restraint to handle the leg and foot, is labor intensive, and is an additional cost. However, field observations indicate topical treatment under a bandage is particularly effective, with most cows showing remarkable improvement in 24 to 48 hours. Furthermore, when properly applied, the bandage and the topical medication have the potential of reaching lesions in the interdigital cleft.

Antimicrobials Parenterally and Topically

Antimicrobial therapy is indicated and effective, and various methods of administration have been used, including parenteral and topical application in individual animals and footbaths for medication of large numbers of animals.

Parenteral Antimicrobials

Although parenteral antibiotic treatment can be effective (depending on the antimicrobial class), milk withdrawal and cost are major concerns regarding this being a routine recommendation. Procaine penicillin, at 18,000 U/kg BW IM twice daily for 3 days, or intramuscular ceftiofur sodium at 2 mg/kg daily for 3 days, was highly successful for the treatment of DD in dairy cattle in California. IV regional administration of tetracycline hydrochloride into the lower lateral digital or median vein after application of a tourniquet proximally on the limb provides has been used[29] but appears to provide a much more complicated treatment protocol that topical tetracycline and bandage. However, the use of parenteral antimicrobials on an individual basis is labor intensive, costly, and not feasible when large numbers of animals are involved. In addition, drug residues in the milk are more likely when animals are treated parenterally. Recurrence after treatment may also occur. In one report, the lesions recurred in 18% of cows treated with antibiotics parenterally.

Footbaths

Some veterinarians prefer to focus treatment protocols on footbaths. The benefits of footbaths include mass treatment and a potential decrease in the transmission of infection from carrier cows to noninfected animals. Footbaths containing antimicrobials and germicides have been used for treatment of groups of animals and for control of the disease. The most important benefit of using footbaths is that all animals are treated for DD at the same time. Types of footbaths include walk-through and stand-in (stationary). The walk-through footbath, commonly located in milking-parlor exit lanes, is most popular in loose housing systems. Portable walk-through footbaths constructed of rubber, fiberglass, or hard plastic are also available and can be relocated as needed. The portable footbath is also the most convenient type for individual treatment situations that may involve bathing two, or possibly all four, feet for prolonged periods. Unfortunately, only a small number of randomized clinical trials have been published that document the efficacy of footbath solutions or topical antiseptic solutions in treating and preventing DD in lactating dairy cows. Copper sulfate is the most commonly used antiseptic footbath solution to treat and control DD because of its widespread availability, low cost, and ease of use. Repeated topical application of 8% copper sulfate solution has been shown to be effective in healing DD lesions, but is not as effective as daily application of a topical chlortetracycline spray to the lesion.[30] Copper sulfate footbaths have been shown to have some efficacy at reducing DD lesions, whereas other studies have shown little to no response. A 2015 systematic review[31] identified only one study that clearly demonstrated the efficacy of copper sulfate footbaths in decreasing the number of cattle with DD lesions; however, that one study provided unequivocal evidence of efficacy.[32] This study demonstrated that a 5% copper sulfate footbath solution applied at 4 consecutive milkings each week was effective in healing DD lesions but did not alter the new infection rate of cows with DD.[32] Copper sulfate footbaths also help to harden the horn on the foot,[33] but it is unclear what role this might play in preventing or treating DD. An acidified ionized copper sulfate footbath solution has been shown to be superior to a 4% formaldehyde (formalin) footbath in preventing new cases of DD.[34] Negative aspects of formaldehyde use include irritation to mucous membranes and carcinogenic effects in humans.[33]

After 150 to 300 cows pass through, the copper sulfate solution in the footbath is thought to become ineffective and is disposed of by land application. Government agencies have expressed concern that the frequent application of $CuSO_4$ solutions in footbaths will result in unacceptably high concentrations of copper in the soil; for example, the use of $CuSO_4$ solutions in footbaths has been restricted to low concentrations (0.5% $CuSO_4$) in the Netherlands,[27] and 5% $CuSO_4$ footbath solutions are not permitted in the European Union. There is therefore widespread interest in developing alternative antiseptic solutions for the treatment and control of DD in dairy cattle. A well-controlled study in Denmark failed to document efficacy of commercially available hoof-care products containing glutaraldehyde, quaternary ammonium compounds, or organic acids (acetic acid, peracetic acid, and hydrogen peroxide) in treating and preventing DD in dairy cattle.[35]

Optimal footbath dimensions are 3.0 to 3.7 m long, 0.5 to 0.6 m wide, and a 28-cm step-in height.[36] Proper construction includes systems for efficient drainage, cleaning, and refilling. Footbaths should be filled to a depth of at least 10 cm (4 in.) to ensure coverage of the typical lesion site for DD. The capacity of a rectangular footbath varies according to its dimensions, which can be calculated using the formula: width × length × depth × 7.46 = capacity in gallons. (Multiplying the number of gallons by 3.8 will provide capacity in liters.) The size of the footbath needed will depend on the number of feet that will be treated with the system. Footbaths must be carefully monitored for excessive contamination with dirt and feces.

Not only is the optimal footbath formulation unknown, but the optimal footbath frequency is also unknown. It has been suggested to use hygiene scoring to determine the frequency of foot bathing, whereby 20% of cows in the free-stall barn are scored; if more than 50% of the cows receive a score of "poor," then the footbath frequency should be 5 days a week. The maximum number of cows that can be treated with a footbath varies according to the cleanliness of the cows, size of the bath, type and concentration of the medication used, housing system, weather conditions, and cow flow patterns. One recommendation suggests one footbath is sufficient for 150 to 200 cows and that DD may be controlled with a single monthly passage through a footbath containing 5 to 10 g/L of oxytetracycline or 1 to 3 g/L of lincomycin in 200 L of water or erythromycin at a rate of 50 g/150 L of water. A common recommendation is that a foot bath can treat 150 to 200 cows per change of solution, used three times per week in outbreaks, once every week or two for maintenance. Other observations, however, suggest that as few as 30 to 50 cows through a footbath may cause major shifts in pH and solids loading, and the largest increment of change in pH occurred with the passage of the first 32 cows through the bath.

Some footbaths are set up with a "prerinse" water bath to reduce contamination of the active ingredients by gross fecal matter on the feet of the cows. It is unclear whether this prerinse footbath provides any advantages. In summary, footbaths make biological sense for the treatment and control of DD. However, most of the recommendations regarding their use, footbath formulation, frequency of use, and optimum number of cows are based on uncontrolled field observations.

Antibiotics in Footbaths

Antibiotics are commonly used in footbaths for the treatment and control of DD, but their use should be discouraged. Use of footbath solutions containing antimicrobials, such as tetracycline, chlortetracycline, lincomycin, or erythromycin, has decreased in popularity because of concerns over antimicrobial residues in the environment and the potential for increased antimicrobial resistance in bacteria. Most of the antibiotics require a veterinary prescription and must be used according to specific recommendations and compliance with withdrawal periods as necessary. Antibiotics in footbaths are rapidly neutralized in the presence of excessive contamination from mud and manure. This is a significant limitation in large herds or in housing situations in which muddy conditions are present.

Tetracycline in 6 to 8 g/L of water has been used in a footbath for treatment of DD. Tetracycline powder (324 g/lb) at 20 to 40 g per gallon (U.S.) to deliver 0.5% to 1% has been used. Lincomycin mix at 0.5 to 4 g/gallon (U.S.) is also used. A mixture of lincomycin and spectinomycin in 150 g/200 L of water for treatment and 125 g/200 L of water for control was also effective. Walking cows through a footbath containing erythromycin, at a concentration of 35 mg erythromycin/L, after two consecutive milkings is effective. Four days after treatment, four of the measured signs (exudation, reddening, creaminess, and pain) were all significantly improved.

Treatment Failure

The possible causes of treatment failure include inconsistent application of treatments or the failure to periodically retreat all feet of all cows in the herd every 2 to 3 months with a topical spray, improper formulation of the medication, the neutralization of the antibiotics by manure, and the inaccessibility of the medication when the lesion is in the interdigital cleft. In addition, ideally lesions should be washed and cleaned thoroughly before applying the medication.

CONTROL

Because the risk factors that predispose to the lesions are uncertain, specific environmental control strategies have not been examined using controlled field trials. Recurrence rates of DD vary from 40% to 52% after 7 to 12 months. Thus it makes biological sense to have an infectious disease control system in place in the herd to provide optimum control.

- **Housing, environment, and management.** The high incidence of the disease in dairy cattle in drylot and free-stall housing suggests that a high infection rate may be associated with high population density and contamination of bedding and the environment. Providing environmental conditions that promote clean and dry ground surfaces and bedding appears to be a logical strategy. Improving cow comfort by providing clean stalls, corrals, and alleys and dry and comfortable bedding, reducing the stocking rate, and improving ventilation to allow drying of stalls and alleys may decrease the incidence and severity of clinical cases. Hoof trimming, mobile tilt tables, and livestock trailers should be thoroughly cleaned and disinfected to prevent potential transmission of the agent of DD. The optimal disinfectant has not been identified.
- **Biosecurity.** For herds that are free of DD, the most important control consideration is the purchase of herd replacements. According to the 1996 NAHMS survey in the United States, the odds of DD infection were 8 times greater in herds that purchased replacements from outside sources compared with those that did not. Herd replacements should be purchased from herds known to be free of DD. Quarantine procedures may be applicable but often impractical.
- **Footbath.** Successful control is possible by single passage of cattle through a footbath containing 5 to 6 g/L oxytetracycline or 150 g lincomycin/spectinomycin in 200 L water; however, use of antimicrobials in footbaths should be discouraged. For optimum results the heels of affected cows should be spray washed before entering the footbath. Repeating the footbath treatment in 4 to 6 weeks is recommended. Regular footbaths with 5% copper sulfate solution and formalin 3% to 5% solution once weekly, according to the incidence of the disease, may be necessary in certain circumstances. Regular inspection of the feet of cattle is recommended to monitor the occurrence of the lesions.
- **Vaccination.** There is no evidence that a vaccine is effective for the control of DD. An effective vaccine will be challenging to develop. Koch's postulates have not been fulfilled for DD, and natural immunity does not appear to be long lasting. Humoral immunity is elicited in cows with DD, and clinical disease is less common in older cows.

TREATMENT AND CONTROL

Treatment

Topical antimicrobial application with 10 ml of long-acting oxytetracycline (200 mg/ml) in cotton ball or gauze, covered by a foot bandage (R-1)

Application of a tetracycline paste consisting of 175 mL of propylene glycol, 175 mL of vinegar, and 150 g of tetracycline hydrochloride applied directly to the lesion with a paintbrush (R-2)

Direct spraying of lesions with oxytetracycline at 25 mg/mL in 20% glycerine in deionized water once daily for 5 days (R-2)

Control

Optimal footbath formulation and frequency of application is unknown; some evidence supporting use of weekly (or more frequent) footbaths with 5% copper sulfate solution (not permitted in the European Union) or formaldehyde 3% to 5% solution (R-2)

Footbath containing an antimicrobial (R-3)

Vaccination with *Treponema* bacterin (R-3)

FURTHER READING

Apley MD. Clinical evidence for individual animal therapy for papillomatous digital dermatitis (hairy heel wart) and infectious bovine pododermatitis (footrot). *Vet Clin North Am Food A.* 2015;31:81-95.

Refaai W, Van Aert M, Abd El-Aal AM, Behery AE, Opsomer G. Infectious diseases causing lameness in cattle with a main emphasis on digital dermatitis (Mortellaro disease). *Livestock Sci.* 2013;156:53-63.

REFERENCES

1. Rasmussen M, et al. *Vet Microbiol.* 2012;160:151.
2. Evans NJ, et al. *J Clin Microbiol.* 2009;47:689.
3. Sullivan LE, et al. *Vet Microbiol.* 2015;178:77-87.
4. Klitgaard K, et al. *J Clin Microbiol.* 2013;51:2212.
5. Evans NJ, et al. *Vet Microbiol.* 2008;130:141.
6. Knappe-Poindecker M, et al. *J Dairy Sci.* 2013;96:7617.
7. Yano T, et al. *J Clin Microbiol.* 2009;47:727.
8. Evans NJ, et al. *Vet Microbiol.* 2012;156:102.
9. Klitgaard K, et al. *Appl Environ Microbiol.* 2014;80:4427.
10. Sullivan LE, et al. *Vet Rec.* 2014;doi:10.1136/vr.102269.
11. Palmer MA, et al. *Animal.* 2013;7(10):1731.
12. Gomez A, et al. *J Dairy Sci.* 2014;98:927.
13. Kofler J, et al. *Vet J.* 2015;204:229.
14. Sykora S, et al. *Vet J.* 2015;205:417.
15. Zinicola M, et al. *PLoS ONE.* 2015;10(3):doi:10.1371/journal.pone.0120504.
16. Evans NJ, et al. *Vet Microbiol.* 2012;156:102.
17. Döpfer D, et al. *Vet J.* 2012;193:648.
18. Stokes JE, et al. *Vet J.* 2012;193:679.
19. Alsaaod M, et al. *Vet J.* 2014;199:281.
20. Gomez A, et al. *J Dairy Sci.* 2014;97:4864.
21. Laven RA, Logue DV. *Vet J.* 2006;171:79.
22. Nuss K. *Vet J.* 2006;171:11.
23. Relun A, et al. *Animal.* 2013;7(9):1542.
24. Nishikawa A, Taguchi K. *Vet Rec.* 2008;163:574.
25. Cutler JHH, et al. *J Dairy Sci.* 2013;96:7550.
26. Scultz N, Capion N. *Vet J.* 2013;198:518.
27. Holzhauer M, et al. *Vet Rec.* 2008;162:41.
28. Hartshorn RE, et al. *J Dairy Sci.* 2013;96:3034.
29. Rodrigues CA, et al. *J Vet Pharmacol Ther.* 2010;33:363.
30. Stevancevic M. *Acta Vet.* 2009;59:437.
31. Thomsen PT. *J Dairy Sci.* 2015;98:2539.
32. Speijers MHM, et al. *J Dairy Sci.* 2010;93:5782.
33. Fjeldaas T, et al. *J Dairy Sci.* 2013;97:2835.
34. Holzhauer M, et al. *Vet J.* 2012;193:659.
35. Thomsen PT, et al. *J Dairy Sci.* 2008;91:1361.
36. Cook NB, et al. *Vet J.* 2012;193:669.

INFECTIOUS FOOTROT IN SHEEP

SYNOPSIS

Etiology *Dichelobacter nodosus.* Strains vary in virulence to produce benign and virulent footrot.

Epidemiology Main source of infection is lesion discharge from other infected sheep. *D. nodosus* typically survives in the environment for only a few days. Highly contagious disease with high attack rate in warm, wet conditions. Lesions are present on both claws of the foot and commonly in more than one foot. Significant effect on productivity.

Clinical findings Inflammation of the skin at the skin–horn junction in the interdigital area with underrunning of the soft horn in benign (nonprogressive) footrot. Progresses to underrunning of the hard horn and inflammation of the sensitive laminae in virulent (progressive) footrot and severe lameness.

Clinical pathology Gram-stained smears and culture to confirm the presence of the organism; protease and polymerase chain reaction (PCR) tests for strain virulence.

Diagnostic confirmation Clinical.

Treatment and control Topical treatment with bactericides in footbaths at time of transmission to minimize new infections, parenteral antibiotics for treating virulent footrot, vaccination, culling. Goats and cattle can carry *D. nododus* and so must be included in control programs.

ETIOLOGY

Dichelobacter (*Bacteroides*) *nodosus* is the essential causal pathogen. It is a highly specialized organism in the small taxonomic group, the Cardiobacteriaciae. *F. necrophorum* aids *D. nodosus* in the invasion of the foot and contributes in the inflammatory reaction. Two other bacteria, a treponeme originally known as *Spirochaeta* (*Treponema*) *penortha* and a motile fusiform bacillus, are commonly present in affected feet but are thought to have no primary etiologic importance.

The type IV fimbriae of *D. nodosus* are recognized as a major virulence factor, are highly immunogenic, and provide the basis for the classification of *D. nodosus* strains into two major classes based on the genetic organization of the fimbrial gene region, with class I containing strains of serogroups A, B, C, E, F, G, I, and M and class II consisting of serogroups D and H. The serologic diversity observed in the fimbriae is as a result of sequence variation in the fimbrial subunit protein and the fimbriae are the major immunoprotective antigens, although protection is serogroup-specific.

Within this typing scheme there are strains that have major and minor prevalence in the disease. For example, footrot introduced into Norwegian flocks around 2008 was predominantly serogroup A, with 96% of virulent isolates belonging to this serogroup.[1]

EPIDEMIOLOGY

Geographic Occurrence

Footrot of sheep is common in all countries where there are large numbers of sheep, except that it does not occur in arid and semiarid areas unless the sheep have access to wet areas such as subirrigated swales.

Host Occurrence

Sheep are the species principally affected, but goats are also susceptible. Infection has been identified in farmed red deer and in cattle and is considered the cause of overgrown and deformed claws in wild mouflon in Europe. With environmental conditions of moisture and warmth, the disease in sheep has a high attack rate, and a large proportion of a group of sheep can be affected within 1 to 2 weeks. Both claws of a foot and more than one foot (usually all) on the sheep will be affected. The disease is common, and in high-risk areas the prevalence of infected flocks is high.

Source of Infection

The source of infection of *D. nodosus* is discharge from the active or chronic infection in the feet of affected animals. The major reservoir of infection for virulent strains of sheep is other sheep because the isolates from cattle and deer generally produce the benign form of footrot in sheep. Culture has demonstrated that the organism does not usually survive in the environment for more than a few days, 2 weeks at the most, although PCR techniques suggest that maximum environmental survival could be up to 24 days.[2] It can survive virtually indefinitely in lesions on chronically infected feet.

Two classifications of footrot have made based on the site of survival and perpetuation of the organism in a flock and the importance of this to control strategies:

1. **Virulent footrot (progressive footrot) and intermediate footrot**—strains survive between footrot transmission periods in pockets of infection in previously underrun ovine hoof
2. **Benign footrot (nonprogressive footrot)**—strains survive in the interdigital skin, and the organism can be demonstrated in the interdigital skin of a high proportion of asymptomatic sheep and cattle.

Methods of Transmission

Infection is usually introduced into a flock by the introduction of carrier sheep, although sheep can become infected from the environment when footrot-free sheep use yards, roads, or trucks that have been used by footrot-infected sheep in the immediate past. For example, transmission occurred when sheep were held for 1 hour in a yard that 4 hours previously had contained a flock of sheep in which less than 1% had footrot. Spread within a flock is facilitated by the flocking nature of sheep and heavy environmental contamination around communal drinking and feeding areas. Spread from ewe to lamb in intensive systems can be rapid, within 5 to 13 hours.[3,4]

Host Risk Factors

Age and Sex

Footrot occurs in sheep of all ages, with rams or ram lambs often more severely affected than ewes.[4] In a flock outbreak, the age-specific incidence and severity of lesions in ewes tends to increase with age, and older lambs have more severe lesions than younger lambs. Prior natural infection does not provide immunity at a subsequent challenge for sheep that have had the disease. However, sheep do vary in their resistance or susceptibility to footrot infection. This appears to be, in part, immunologically mediated, with the ability of some sheep to mount a strong T-cell response and to produce agglutinating antibodies to *D. nodosus* fimbriae being an important factor in conferring resistance to severe infection.

Breed

Merino sheep are the most susceptible to footrot. British breeds, particularly Romney Marsh, are less susceptible and suffer from a milder form of the disease; they respond better to vaccination by suffering fewer subsequent attacks of footrot but have worse reactions to a multivalent vaccine than Merinos. In the natural disease, some animals never become infected, a few become infected but recover, and most become infected and persist as chronic cases. There is evidence that this variation is genetically determined, and selection for resistance, based on exposure to the disease and rigorous culling of affected individuals, has been demonstrated in Merino, Corriedale, Romney, Perrendale, and Targhee breeds.[4] Substantial genetic variation in resistance to footrot has been demonstrated, both within flocks and between the progeny of different sires, among both Merino and Sottish Blackface breeds.[5,6]

Environmental Risk Factors

Climate and Season

Moistness of the pasture and environmental temperature are major determinants for the transmission of footrot. Wetness and warmth favors persistence of the bacteria in pasture and increases the susceptibility of feet to injury and dermatitis, thus facilitating spread of the disease from carrier sheep. There must be continued moisture on the ground for transmission to occur. Thus in drier temperate climates, such as Australia, transmission tends to occur predominantly in the spring and, to a lesser degree, autumn. In cooler, wetter temperate climates, such as New Zealand and the United Kingdom, the transmission period can be much longer. The daily mean temperature must also be above 10° C (50° F) for transmission to occur, and so in colder climates transmission is reduced or does not occur during the winter. There is a linear relationship between the prevalence of farms with footrot and yearly rainfall.

Transmission and outbreaks of footrot occur in winter in housed sheep when conditions underfoot are wet and in summer with sheep on irrigated pastures.

Management

Any practice that concentrates sheep in small areas will favor spread of the disease when environmental conditions favor transmission. Routine foot trimming may increase risk of infection and clinical disease.

Failure to isolate introduced sheep until their footrot status has been determined, straying sheep, and the presence of at least one footrot-infected farm within a 1-km radius with severe footrot are confirmed risk factors for the introduction of footrot into a flock.[7,8]

Pasture Type

Footrot is commonly associated with lush or improved, irrigated, and clover-dominant pastures. Long mature grass may result in interdigital abrasions as it is dragged through the interdigital space and facilitates infection, as may penetration of interdigital skin by barley grass seeds (*Hordeum murinum*). Skin penetration by larvae of the nematode *Strongyloides* spp. may also predispose to infection.

Pathogen Factors

The major *D. nodosus*–encoded virulence factors that have been implicated in the disease are type IV fimbriae and extracellular proteases, and the fimbrial subunit gene, *fimA,* is essential for virulence.

There is considerable variation in the virulence of strains of *D. nodosus.* Some produce benign footrot, whereas others produce deep lesions that facilitate their survival and confound eradication programs. As a result, they have traditionally been subdivided into benign, intermediate, and virulent strains to conform with the types of clinical footrot they are associated with in the field. The virulence of each strain depends on its keratinolytic capacity; virulent strains produce more extracellular protease, and an earlier production of elastase, than benign strains. The separation of the hard horn of the claw from the germinal layer, which is a characteristic of virulent footrot, has been associated with infection with strains that produce a heat-stable protease with a single isoenzyme pattern, whereas benign strains have thermolabile protease. Infection associated with more than one strain is reported, and up to five serogroups including up to eight strains have been reported from a single foot.

The genome of *D. nodosus* has been fully sequenced,[9] and this has allowed further investigation of the factors that determine its virulence. Acidic protease V2 (AprV2) is the main thermostable protease responsible for most elastase activity and differs from its benign counterpart, AprB2, by only a single amino acid.[10] It is one of three thermostable proteases that act synergistically, the others being AprV5 and a basic protease, BprV. AprV5 is needed to activate all three proteases, whereas BprV degrades hoof horn matrix more efficiently than its counterpart from benign strains, BprB.[11]

A molecular genetic analysis of *D. nodosus* isolates from four European countries, Switzerland, France, Germany, and Norway, found a perfect correlation between the clinical presentation of footrot and the presence of either AprV2 or AprB2.[12]

Economic Importance

Benign footrot is generally considered to cause little if any economic effect, and its occurrence is confined to the warm, wet seasons. However, even benign footrot infections can depress body weight, wool growth, and wool quality in some countries, especially in Merinos.

In contrast, virulent footrot causes a severe loss of body condition, and this, combined with a moderate mortality rate, a reduction in wool production, the disruption of the general routine of the farm, and the expense of labor and materials to treat the disease adequately, makes footrot one of the most costly of sheep diseases. Estimates of the total annual cost to industry in Australia are estimated at $32.3 m and $12.1 m for virulent and benign footrot, respectively, and £24 m in Britain.[13,14] In addition, there are welfare concerns, societal pressures encountered by owners of footrot-infected flocks, and, in control areas, the community costs of statutory footrot control programs.

In controlled studies, virulent footrot causes an 11% depression in body weight and an 8% reduction in clean fleece weight of affected sheep. The magnitude of the loss can be related to the virulence of the infecting organism and the severity of disease.

The effects on body weight are most severe during the active transmission period of the organism and development of clinical disease, but there may be compensatory growth during the recovery period. Both greasy and clean fleece weight are significantly depressed by footrot, with a linear association between the extent of the depression and the severity of the disease. Wool fiber diameter is also decreased, which can partially compensate for decreased fleece weight in the final price for wool. Some sheep with severe disease may develop a break in the wool, which can then incur price discounts of up to 50%.

Feet of sheep affected with footrot are attractive to blowfly strike. Necrotic exudate with accompanying maggots from affected feet can be deposited on the fleece to result in a focus of body strike.

PATHOGENESIS

Maceration of the interdigital skin from prolonged wet conditions underfoot allow for infection with *F. necrophorum*. This initial local dermatitis associated with infection with *F. necrophorum* at the skin and the skin–horn junction may progress no further, but the hyperkeratosis induced by this infection facilitates infection by *D. nodosus* if it is present. The preliminary dermatitis has been named "ovine interdigital dermatitis" and is also called "foot scald."

OVINE INTERDIGITAL DERMATITIS, FOOT SCALD

This disease is seasonal and occurs when moist conditions underfoot, or trauma from pastures or frost, produce maceration of the interdigital skin, allowing invasion by *Fusobacterium necrophorum,* a ubiquitous organism in feces and soil.

Lesions are in the interdigital space, where there is hyperemia, or swelling and blanching, and wetness of the interdigital skin. There is no, or only minimal, separation at the skin–horn junction ("underrun"). Lambs are more commonly affected, particularly in spring, but the disease can involve all ages of sheep. Most or all feet on a sheep are affected, and it is present in a large proportion of the age cohort of the flock.

In Australia and New Zealand, the disease is not usually associated with severe or chronic lameness and is often found incidentally when examining sheep for other reasons.

In Britain it is reported as a common cause of lameness, but this might reflect a lack of cultural differentiation from the less virulent forms of infectious footrot that can present with identical clinical findings. Examining Gram-stained air-dried smears of lesion material will reveal the absence of *Dichelobacter nodosus.*

Control is by avoiding grazing lambs on long grass or in muddy conditions. The disease will regress spontaneously when the pasture dries up or sheep are moved to drier paddocks, but it can be treated with topically applied oxytetracycline or by walking animals through a footbath containing 10% zinc sulfate (preferably standing in the solution for 1 to 3 minutes, then allowing the feet to dry on grating or in a woolshed) or 3% formalin.

Ovine interdigital dermatitis can predispose to infectious footrot or to foot abscess.

Benign and Virulent Footrot

It is assumed that the pili of *D. nodosus* facilitate attachment of the organism to the epithelium of the foot. When the feet of sheep with interdigital dermatitis are colonized with a strain of *D. nodosus* that has little keratinolytic ability, there is underrunning of the soft horn but no further progression, and this infection has been given the name of benign or nonprogressive footrot. Benign footrot cannot be easily distinguished on clinical examination from ovine interdigital dermatitis. Colonization with keratinolytic and virulent strains leads to the clinical disease of virulent footrot. The underrunning lesion is the result of keratolytic activity, and the associated inflammation is a consequence of a combined activity of *D. nodosus* and *F. necrophorum*. A designation of intermediate footrot is used to provide a midclassification of severity between benign and virulent footrot, with the classification of infected sheep into these categories based on a foot lesion scoring system (see following discussion). There is much difficulty in specifying exactly the characteristics of these clinical forms in natural outbreaks, partly because more than one strain is commonly involved, but also because the severity of the lesions is modulated by breed, previous treatments, and varying geographic and climatic conditions.

CLINICAL FINDINGS

Sheep

Virulent Footrot

In a flock, a sudden onset of lameness of several sheep is the usual presenting sign of footrot because the disease is not detected before this occurs. The pain associated with infection is severe, and affected sheep will limp or carry the affected leg. Usually more than one foot is affected, and affected sheep may graze on their knees.

On close examination the earliest sign of virulent footrot is swelling and moistness of the skin of the interdigital cleft and a parboiled and pitted appearance at the skin–horn junction in the cleft. This inflammation is accompanied by slight lameness, which increases as necrosis underruns the horn in the cleft. The underrunning starts as a separation of the skin–horn junction at the axial surface just anterior to the bulb of the heel and proceeds down the axial surface and forward and backward. There is destruction of the epidermal matrix beneath the hard horn, which is subsequently separated from the underlying tissues. In severe cases both the axial and the abaxial wall and the sole are underrun, and deep necrosis of tissue may lead to the shedding of the horn case. The separation may not be obvious on superficial visual examination but can be detected by trimming the feet with a knife or secateurs. There is a small amount of distinctive, gray, foul-smelling exudate, but abscessation does not occur.

Both claws of the one foot will be involved, and commonly more than one foot is involved. When extensive underrunning has occurred, lameness is severe. A systemic reaction, manifest by anorexia and fever, may occur in severe cases. Recumbent animals become emaciated and may die of starvation. Secondary bacterial invasion and/or fly strike may result in the spread of inflammation up the legs.

Benign Footrot

Benign footrot is manifest with interdigital lesions, a break at the skin–horn junction, and separation of the soft horn, but the disease does not progress beyond this stage to severe underrunning of the hard horn of the foot. The interdigital skin becomes inflamed and covered by a thin film of moist necrotic material; the horn is pitted and blanched.

It is difficult to distinguish between an established infection with benign footrot and the early stages of virulent footrot. With virulent footrot, it is common to find all stages and severity levels of the disease in the same flock. A large number of sheep (e.g., 100 in large flocks or mobs) should be examined to differentiate benign from virulent footrot, and it may be necessary to reexamine the flock after a period of time to determine whether the disease has progressed to the virulent type.

Scoring Systems

Several scoring systems, based on severity and persistence, have been devised to aid in epidemiologic and control programs and can be used to categorize the severity of disease, hence the virulence of associated strains of *D. nodosus,* within a flock. In the Australian system, a score of 0 (normal foot) to 4 (severe underrun) is allocated to each foot of each sheep, then the score is used to classify the severity of disease in that flock or a cohort.[4] Feet scored 0 have no evidence of necrosis or inflammation or cleavage of horn. Scores of 1 and 2 are confined to sheep with interdigital lesions, whereas a gradation of scores from 3 to 4 reflects progressive underrunning and separation of horn from the underlying laminar, with 3 representing underrunning of the soft horn. In this score system, most benign footrot cases score 1 or 2, with some allowance for scores of 3. Intermediate footrot in a cohort is defined when 1% to 10% of the cohort have a score of 4. Virulent footrot is defined by greater than 10% of the cohort with a score of 4. It has been suggested that the scoring system may not always be reliable because the severity of disease can be influenced by climate. However, a large field study in Australia found that a cohort of sheep with scores defining intermediate footrot maintained that clinical classification when moved to a climate that would have promoted the development of more severe disease. Evaluation of the repeatability of scoring systems has found that scoring is usually consistent within the same observer, but that differences can arise between observers through observer bias and different observer thresholds.[15,16]

Symptomless Carriers

Symptomless carriers may be affected for periods of up to 3 years. Most such animals have a misshapen foot, and a pocket of infection beneath underrun horn can be found if the foot is pared. A less common form of the chronic disease is an area of moist skin between the claws without obvious involvement of the claw.

Goats

Footrot is associated with *D. nodosus* and is manifested by severe interdigital dermatitis. There may be some separation of the skin-horn junction at the axial surface, but the disease is less invasive, and there is much less underrunning of the horn of the sole or the abaxial surface of the foot compared with sheep.

Cattle

Infection with *D. nodosus* is also associated primarily with a severe interdigital dermatitis, and there may be lameness. There is fissuring and hyperkeratosis of the interdigital skin, with pitting and erosion at the skin-horn junction in the cleft. There is also fissuring, pitting, and erosion on the horny bulbs of the heel. There may be underrunning at the heel, but it is usually minimal.

CONTAGIOUS OVINE DIGITAL DERMATITIS (CODD)

CODD is a relatively new disease described in the United Kingdom and is still poorly understood.[17,18]

It is manifest with severe, rapidly spreading lameness and is more common in adults than lambs. Commonly there is a history of poor response to conventional methods of footrot control. The initial lesion is a proliferative or ulcerative lesion at the coronet, with subsequent extensive underrunning of the hoof horn and, in some cases, complete separation of the hoof. Interdigital lesions are absent. It may affect only one claw on one foot. Spirochetes similar to the *Treponema* isolates from bovine digital dermatitis are associated with CODD lesions, but these are also recovered from heathy feet.[19]

Fusobacterium necrophorum and *Dichelobacter nodosus* may also be present in some flocks. Their contribution to CODD is unclear, although vaccination against *D. nodosus* had a mild protective effect against new CODD infections (32% compared with 62% against footrot).[18]

Response to formalin and zinc sulfate footbaths is poor, but the disease responds to long-acting parenteral amoxicillin.[17,18] Topical application of lincomycin and spectinomycin solutions has also been used.

CLINICAL PATHOLOGY AND NECROPSY FINDINGS

In countries that do not have a large sheep industry, identification of *D. nodosus* in most laboratories is made by examining an air-dried smear of exudate, taken from underneath some underrun horn at the advancing edge. Smears can be stained with Gram stain or a fluorescein-stained antibody.

In countries with lager sheep industries and where footrot is more common, culture of *D. nodosus,* examination of protease type, and the use of highly sensitive PCR tests are undertaken. PCR tests can be used to detect gene sequences and identify particular strains and are useful where eradication from flocks or areas is the aim.[20,21] Gene probes and nucleotide sequencing, to differentiate virulent from benign strains, are also used in regions with eradication programs and in epidemiologic studies.

The two most commonly used protease tests are the gelatin gel and elastase protease thermostability tests. A comparison of tests, using more than 2800 isolates collected from 12 flocks in southeastern Australia, found that 91%, 64%, and 41% were classed as virulent by the gelatin gel, elastase, and *intA* PCR tests, respectively.[19] The latter tests for an inserted genetic element that is unrelated to protease, and it was developed as a further test for cases where a gelatin gel test indicated a virulent *D. nodosus* isolate but this was inconsistent with a field assessment of benign footrot.[22]

Serum antibody develops as early as 2 weeks after natural infection, and the level obtained is proportional to the severity of the early clinical disease. The antibody response is not long lasting, falling to pre-infection levels within a few months after resolution of the foot lesions. An ELISA for serologic detection of infected sheep has some value for diagnosis of flock infection, but it lacks specificity and is inaccurate in older sheep and so is not routinely used.

Necropsy of sheep for diagnosis of footrot is not needed.

DIFFERENTIAL DIAGNOSIS

Diagnosis of virulent footrot is clinical, is based on a whole-flock approach, and postmortem examination is not necessary.

Because of the rigorous control measures required sometimes by law to control or eradicate infectious footrot of sheep, it is imperative that the diagnosis be made with great care. The greatest problem is in the identification of carrier sheep in the nontransmitting periods. A number of conditions may be confused with footrot, especially when they occur under the same environmental conditions (Table 15-4).

- **Foot abscess**—a major differential and can be present in several sheep in a flock at the same time. It usually affects only one foot, is not contagious, and is characterized by extensive suppuration. The abscess occurs in a single claw on the foot, and there is obvious local heat and pain on palpation.
- **Contagious ovine digital dermatitis**
- **Shelly toe**—the name given to a condition where there is separation of the wall of the foot in Merino sheep and occasionally in other breeds on improved pasture. The abaxial wall of the hoof separates from the sole near the toe, and the crevice formed becomes packed with mud, gravel, and manure. The hoof in the region is dry and crumbly. The cause is not known but it is probably a form of laminitis.
- **Suppurative cellulitis**—associated with *Fusobacterium necrophorum,* commences as an ulcerative dermatitis of the pastern above the bulb of the heel and extends up the leg to the knee or the hock and more deeply into subcutaneous tissues.

Other diseases with foot lameness include:

- Contagious ecthyma
- Bluetongue
- Foot-and-mouth disease
- Ulcerative dermatosis
- Strawberry footrot
- Laminitis
- Lameness associated with *Erysipelothrix insidiosa,* and occurring after dipping

TREATMENT AND CONTROL

The time-honored method of treatment of footrot has been the application of topical bactericidal agents to the foot. These agents are most effective early in the transmission period, before any extensive underrunning of the horn. When there is underrunning of the horn, the underrun horn must be removed so as to expose the infection to the topical agent. This approach has been used successfully for treatment, control, and eradication purposes. However, it requires extensive paring of affected feet, which is labor intensive, time consuming, and distressing to both the operator and the sheep. Consequently, paring is now recommended mainly for diagnosis, and treatments usually minimize the need for extensive paring of the feet. These include the use of topical zinc sulfate, the use of parenteral antibiotics, and the recognition of vaccination as an adjunct to treatment and a strategy for control.

Where eradication of virulent or intermediate footrot from a flock is the aim, control measures are usually applied during the periods favorable for transmission. This reduces the number of infected sheep that have to be treated more intensively once transmission is reduced or negligible.

Topical Treatment

In general, parenteral treatment with antibiotics, without paring of the feet, has replaced topical antimicrobial treatment of individual or small numbers of sheep. To be reasonably effective most topical treatments require that all underrun horn be carefully removed so that the antibacterial agent can come into contact with infective material. This necessitates painstaking and careful examination and paring of all feet because as incomplete paring will leave pockets of infection. With severely underrun feet, it is impossible to expose all of the underrun areas without

Table 15-4 Differential diagnosis of lameness accompanied by foot lesions in sheep

Disease	Epidemiology	Foot lesions	Other lesions	Other clinical signs	Response to treatment	Diagnostic microbiology
Infectious footrot	Serious outbreaks in wet, warm weather. High morbidity. Few chronic lame sheep in dry seasons.	Interdigital dermatitis, underrunning of horn medial aspect of claw. Strong smell of necrotic horn.	—	Very severe lameness. Walk on knees.	To penicillin and streptomycin, erythromycin excellent.	*Dichelobacter nodosus* on smear, or fluorescent antibody test
Benign footrot (scald)	High morbidity in wet, warm weather. Disappears with dry weather.	Interdigital dermatitis, no smell, almost no underrunning of horn.	—	Mild lameness.	Not treated.	*D. nodosus* avirulent strains not distinguishable microbiologically
Infectious bulbar necrosis	Adult sheep, usually less than 10% affected. Serious in wet seasons.	Toe abscess usually in front feet. Heel abscess in hindfeet. Swelling, pain, discharge of pus.	—	Very severe lameness.	Good to sulfonamides or penicillin-streptomycin.	*F. necrophonum* and *Actinomyces (Corynebacterium pyogenes)*
Contagious ecthyma	Lambs mostly or nonimmune adults. Dry summer.	Raised proliferative lesions with tenacious scabs on coronet skin.	Lesions around mouth almost always.	Rarely lambs have septicemia. Lameness mild only.	—	—
Ulcerative dermatitis	Spread by physical contact at mating. Morbidity usually 20%.	Raw granulating ulcers in interdigital space and on cornet. No pus.	Around mouth and genitalia usually.	Moderate lameness.	—	—
Bluetongue	Insect-borne disease. Variable morbidity.	Coronitis, separation of horn. Are late in syndrome.	Severe erosions around mouth and nasal cavities.	High fever, salivation. Severe lameness and recumbency.	—	Virus isolation
Strawberry footrot	In summer, high morbidity; carrier sheep infect.	Proliferative dermatitis, piled up scabs. Heal in 5–6 weeks. Coronet to knee or hock.	—	No itching or lameness.	—	*Dermatophilus congolensis*
Foot-and-mouth disease	May present like outbreak of contagious footroot.	Vesicles at coronary band and skin of interdigital cleft.	Vesicles in mouth.	All ages.	—	Virus demonstration
Infestation with *Strongyloides* or trombiculid mites	Wet summer conditions. Local distribution only.	Nonspecific dermatitis of skin of lower legs.	—	—	Organophosphates for trombiculids.	Parasites in scrapings

causing hemorrhage because it may be necessary to remove all of the sole and the wall of the claw. Very sharp instruments, including a knife and hoof secateurs, are needed to do the job properly, and they should be disinfected after each use. The parings should be collected and buried or burned. Sheep restraint cradles make the task of paring safer, more accurate, and less arduous for the operator.

With small numbers of sheep, topical treatment may be applied by brush, spray, or aerosol. Topical treatments are likely to be washed off the feet, and thus their efficacy under wet conditions is inevitably reduced. Local applications include chloramphenicol (10% tincture in methylated spirits or propylene glycol), oxytetracycline (5% tincture in methylated spirits), cetyltrimethyl ammonium bromide or cetrimide (20% alcoholic tincture), zinc sulfate (10% solution), copper sulfate (10% solution), and Dichlorophen as a 10% solution in either diacetone alcohol or ethyl alcohol.

Chloramphenicol is prohibited for use in food animals in many countries. It is also expensive, but it is reasonably effective under both wet and dry conditions. Oxytetracycline must be used as a 5% tincture for optimum results and is not as efficient as chloramphenicol under wet conditions, but it gives reasonable results when the weather is dry. Cetrimide is a relatively cheap product and appears to be as effective as chloramphenicol under all conditions. It is likely that in different countries, with different climates and environmental conditions, the efficiency of particular treatments will vary. When only a few sheep are affected, bandaging may help maintain local concentrations of the topical preparation.

Footbathing for Treatment and Control

Footbathing is a more practical approach to topical treatment and is used for control during transmission periods when dealing with large numbers of sheep. All sheep should be footbathed, but it is good practice to divide the flock into affected and unaffected mobs or groups by examination before the initial footbathing, then graze them separately following footbathing to minimize subsequent infection of uninfected sheep.

After several footbaths and inspections the majority of the flock should be free of infection, and the residual infected sheep are culled.

Preparations suitable for footbathing include 10% zinc sulfate, with or without a surfactant to aid wetting, 5% formalin, or 5% copper sulfate. Regardless of the agent used, it is recommended that the sheep be kept standing on concrete, wooden slats, or dry ground for 1 to 2 hours after treatment, although this may be logistically difficult with large flocks.

The relative merits and disadvantages of the various preparations used are as follows.

Zinc Sulfate Solution (10% to 20%)

Zinc sulfate solution is as effective as formalin, is more pleasant to use, and is generally the preferred topical chemical for the treatment of footrot. Its ability to penetrate the hoof horn is enhanced by the addition of the surfactant sodium lauryl sulfate to the footbath solution. Significant cure rates can be achieved without prior paring, which removes a significant labor cost from the treatment and control of the disease.

Cure rates, without paring, are higher in sheep that have moderate rather than severe lesions in their feet. Some paring of chronically affected, overgrown feet may be required to allow the treatment access to pockets of infection in the anterior aspects of the sole and also of feet that have underrunning that has progressed to the abaxial area of the digit. Sheep are stood for 1 hour in a footbath containing a 10% to 20% zinc sulfate solution with 2% sodium lauryl sulfate with sufficient depth to cover the coronet. The treatment is repeated in 5 days, then after a further 21 days the sheep are individually examined to determine their status and retreated or culled, depending on the strategy of treatment and control in the flock. Zinc sulfate footbathing can provide protection to the foot against reinfection for periods of at least 2 weeks and can be used effectively during periods of active spread of the disease. Repeated daily footbathing (10 min each day for 5 days) in a zinc sulfate solution with surfactant has eradicated (as opposed to controlled) virulent footrot in sheep associated with some strains but was ineffective against a strain that produced severe underrunning.

Thirsty sheep that drink from the footbath may die of acute zinc poisoning, and contamination with zinc can defoliate pasture at the exit of the footbath.

Formalin Solution (5%)

Formalin solution does not deteriorate with pollution but causes extreme discomfort to sheep that have heavily pared feet. Consequently, its use for sheep with severe lesions is discouraged on humane grounds. The feet of the sheep must be pared and all infected areas exposed before treatment. Formalin is unpleasant to work with in enclosed areas and has toxicity for humans, and its use may be banned in some countries for this reason. Sheep should be passed through the footbath every 1 to 4 weeks during periods of high risk for transmission.

The use of solutions containing more than 5% formalin, footbathing at intervals of less than 1 week, or prolonged footbathing may cause irritation of the skin. Farmers can be neglectful in maintaining proper concentrations of formalin in footbaths, and frequent use of the bath combined with hot weather can result in a concentration of 30% formalin. Such concentrations cause extensive cellulitis around the coronets, and a high proportion of animals may be so badly affected that they need to be destroyed. The hoof horn also becomes hardened and deformed. The safest precaution is to empty the footbath and prepare a new mixture.

Copper Sulfate Solution (5%)

Copper sulfate solution colors the wool, deteriorates with pollution, corrodes metal, and may cause excessive contamination of the environment with copper. The feet of the sheep must be pared and all infected areas exposed before treatment. Copper sulfate footbathing appears to harden the horn, which can be an advantage but also a disadvantage if further paring is required at a later date. A patented copper salt preparation (not copper sulfate) has reasonable efficacy without the disadvantages of copper sulfate.

Antibiotic Treatment

Footrot can be treated with antibiotics without the necessity of paring of the feet. Treatment is considerably more effective if done during dry periods and when the sheep are kept on dry floors for 24 hours after treatment, because in wet conditions the concentration of antibiotic at the tissue level is much reduced. In conditions are unfavorable for eradication, such as in the United Kingdom, prompt treatment of lame sheep with parental antibiotics is associated with a significantly lower prevalence of lameness compared with farmers who treated by foot-paring and applying topical treatment (<2% compared with 9%).[23,24]

D. nodosus is susceptible in vitro to penicillin, cefamandole, clindamycin, tetracycline, chloramphenicol, erythromycin, sodium cefoxitin, tylosin tartrate, nitrofurazone, and tinidazole and has the least susceptibility to sulfonamides and the aminoglycosides. However, in vitro tests may have little relevance to field application because of differences in the penetrance of antibiotics to the affected part of the foot.

Antibiotics and their dosage shown to be effective against virulent footrot are presented in the accompanying box. Many of these treatments are "off label," and some are not approved for use on sheep in some countries. Choice of antibiotic will be influenced by the withholding period required before sheep culled because they are not cured can be sent to market. Use of lincomycin/spectinomycin in sheep has precipitated severe outbreaks of salmonellosis in some flocks.

TREATMENT AND CONTROL

Treatment:

- Penicillin/streptomycin (single IM dose of 70,000 U/kg procaine penicillin and 70 mg/kg dihydrostreptomycin) (R-1)
- Erythromycin (single IM dose of 10 mg/kg) (R-1)
- Long-acting oxytetracycline (single IM dose of 20 mg/kg) (R-1)
- Lincomycin/spectinomycin (single SC dose of 5 mg/kg lincomycin and 10 mg/kg spectinomycin) (R-2)
- Gamithromycin (single SC dose of 6 mg/kg) (R-2)[25]
- Long-acting amoxicillin (single IM dose of 15 mg/kg) (R-2)[18]

Control:

- Multivalent or autogenous mono- or bivalent vaccination (R-1)

Australian studies with large numbers of sheep have demonstrated cure rates of approximately 90% using oxytetracycline, erythromycin, and lincomycin/spectinomycin, and slightly less for penicillin/streptomycin. Following treatment, sheep are kept in a dry environment for 24 hours, such as a wool shed, then moved to a "clean" dry pasture and inspected 3 to 4 weeks later. At this time sheep that are still clinically affected (i.e., not cured) are culled.

Reinfection will occur in footrot spread periods; thus, in general, the use of antibiotics for control of footrot should be confined to the summer period when there is reduced or no spread. Cure can occur even in severely affected sheep, and extensive paring before treatment does not improve cure rates. Cure rates fall to 60% if sheep are in a wet environment following treatment, although cure rates are improved slightly if sheep are footbathed at the time of antibiotic administration.

In naturally infected sheep on 10 farms in southern Germany, significantly higher cure rates were recorded 3 weeks after treatment with gamithromycin (94%) compared with oxytetracycline (79%), although this study involved only 20 sheep per farm.[25] Antimicrobial resistance has been reported in anaerobic bacteria isolated from ovine footrot,[26] and all farms had used oxytetracycline in topical applications for at least 3 years. Consequently, a decreased susceptibility to oxytetracycline may have contributed to this result.

Antibiotics are particularly valuable for the treatment of late-pregnant sheep that develop footrot, where more prolonged yarding for footbathing, paring, and topical treatment could lead to problems such as pregnancy toxemia. Antibiotics have no role in the prevention of footrot, but a combination of vaccination and antibiotic treatment can increase cure rates, especially in areas that have extended transmission periods and so are not well suited to eradication programs.[18]

Vaccination

Vaccination against footrot can significantly increase short-term resistance to infection and is an important component of control strategies, especially in circumstances where climate and management practices make other control strategies difficult to apply. Vaccination also shortens the clinical course in infected sheep and can be used as a treatment strategy. In neither case is vaccination 100% effective.

Pilus antigens are the major host-protective immunogens and confer protection against challenge with homologous strains. Immunity is associated with circulating antibody, but high levels of pilus-specific circulating antibody are required for adequate diffusion into the epidermis and protection against the disease. There is a positive correlation between antibody titer and footrot resistance in the first few months following vaccination. Immunity can be passively transferred with gammaglobulins from immunized sheep to naive recipients and from vaccinated ewes to their lambs via colostrum to provide protection for the first 8 weeks of life.

Vaccines must contain adjuvants for an adequate antibody response, and vaccination with oil-adjuvant vaccines is accompanied by significant local reaction, including local swelling at the injection site and abscessation in a proportion of animals. This reaction is more severe in British breeds than in Merinos. In milk goats and sheep, vaccination can result in a significant drop in milk production. The potential gains from vaccination need to be weighed against this effect in a decision to use vaccination as a method of control rather than other control procedures.

Multivalent Vaccines

Commercial multivalent vaccines have contained up to 10 strains of *D. nodosus* representative of the most common serogroups associated with footrot. The extent to which these vaccines will give protection or promote earlier cure depends on the relationship of the vaccine pilus types to those associated with the footrot problem. Vaccine failure is generally attributable to the occurrence of footrot associated with strains of the organism not present in the vaccine or for which there is no cross-protection, and to individual animal variation in response. It is now recognized that there is a limitation to the number of strains that can be incorporated in current vaccines because of antigenic competition. Mixing different *D. nodosus* fimbriae in vaccines may lead to inadequate host responses to individual antigens, and an alternative approach is to identify *D. nodosus* strains present in a given geographic region, enabling the development of optimized and localized strain-specific vaccines.[5,27-30]

Field trials have shown a wide variation in the therapeutic effect of multivalent vaccination, with a reduction in footrot incidence varying from 27% to 54% in sheep in which there was no routine foot care to 69% to 91% in flocks in which vaccination was coupled with routine foot care such as trimming and footbathing. The effect is to reduce the incidence, severity, and duration of the infection. The improvement seems to be as a result of accelerated healing of the lesions with some protection against reinfection. For optimum effect, two vaccinations are required, and the duration of this effect depends on the adjuvant and the breed of sheep. Even so, the duration of the protection is limited to 4 to 12 weeks in most studies. It can be very effective in control when coupled with a culling policy of sheep that remain clinically infected.

Whereas vaccination is of value for control of an existing flock infection, it may not be economic to use vaccination as a strategy to prevent infection of a footrot-free flock. The use of footrot vaccines may be prohibited in areas where there are footrot eradication programs.

Mono- and Bivalent Vaccines

The use of vaccines targeting only the strains of *D. nodosus* present was first tested in 40 flocks in Nepal with a recombinant fimbrial vaccine against two virulent serogroups. These were vaccinated annually for 4 years, with no virulent footrot detected after the first year of vaccination.[5] Subsequently, a monovalent whole-cell vaccine was used for 2 years in a chronically infected flock in Bhutan, and footrot was not detected after the first year of vaccination.[27] Further trials were conducted in two Australian flocks.[28] In the first, the prevalence of infection was reduced from 44% to 0.5% within 4 months of a monovalent vaccination, and no cases were detected 16 months later. In the second, a bivalent vaccine reduced the prevalence from 8.5% to 0.3% after 6 months, with no cases detected 18 months after vaccination. In both cases a few sheep that were not fully cured within 6 to 12 weeks of the second dose of vaccine ("nonresponders") had to be culled from each flock.

Where multiple virulent serotypes are present, sequential vaccination with specific mono- or bivalent vaccines has been demonstrated to be an effective strategy.[29] This was undertaken after antigenic competition was demonstrated when bivalent vaccines were administered concurrently, but not when given 3 or more months apart.[29] Virulent footrot was eradicated from 5 of 12 commercial flocks that had 3 or less serogroups at the start of the study.[5,29] Where one or two serogroups were present, there was a rapid reduction in prevalence. However, where multiple serogroups were present, additional rounds of vaccination with different bivalent vaccines were given at 1-year intervals.[29] This controlled but did not eliminate all strains of virulent footrot in the remaining trial flocks, and so shortening the intervaccination interval was proposed as a means of accelerating this program.[5,29,30]

Summary of Control Procedures in Infected Flocks

The objective of control programs in a footrot-infected flock is to maintain the lowest possible prevalence of disease by reducing the incidence of new infections and preventing the development of advanced lesions. This is achieved most cost-effectively through strategies that are based on whole-flock control, with minimal need for handling of individual animals. This less-labor-intensive approach is most likely to be adopted by sheep owners and includes routine footbathing, with or without vaccination, during transmission periods. Sheep that are affected with virulent footrot can also be treated with parenterally administered antibiotics or culled, depending on the relative proportion affected. The exact timing of these operations will vary by country and the prevailing climatic conditions.

Genetic Selection

Whereas there are breed effects on susceptibility and an apparent high heritability for resistance, genetic selection for resistance has not been used in control programs on farms. Resistance can be determined by direct challenge of a candidate ram, which is undesirable in ram-breeding flocks, but antibody response to vaccination cannot be used as a surrogate.

ERADICATION

Eradication of virulent footrot is a desirable but not always feasible objective. The simplest form of eradication is destocking (culling) the whole flock or just those mobs affected with virulent footrot. This assumes that it will be possible to restock with sheep that have a high degree of assurance of not being infected with virulent footrot, but this is not always the case. Eradication can also be achieved through treatment and control programs, especially in climates where the transmission periods are shorter. Conversely, eradication is more difficult where rainfall is heavy and pastures remain moist for most of the year.

Area eradication of virulent footrot is more challenging, task but has proceeded satisfactorily in several regions in Australia and in Norway.[31,32] In the Australian state of New South Wales, choice of eradication strategy was influenced by flock size, with destocking more often chosen for smaller flocks (those less than 500 sheep). Time spent in quarantine was considerably shorter when specialist contractors were used to inspect and treat sheep and longest when footbathing was the main eradication option chosen.[31] In Norway, virulent footrot has been eradicated from about 70% of the flocks in which this was attempted.[32]

Currently the eradication of benign footrot is not justified economically, nor is it possible with existing knowledge because benign footrot strains can be carried in the interdigital skin of asymptomatic sheep.

The principles for successful eradication from a flock have been described as follows:[5]

1. Correct diagnosis of the form of footrot present in the flock
2. Knowledge of seasonal trends and patterns of transmission in that environment
3. Ability of the operator (or contractor) to recognize footrot in its different forms
4. Acceptance that eradication is a costly and time-consuming investment
5. Understanding that in flocks with a high initial prevalence, it may take 2 or more years to eradicate the disease
6. Acceptance that eradication should only be attempted if the flock can protect itself from reinfection, either from neighboring flocks or introduced sheep

Further, eradication programs are based on the following facts:

1. *D. nodosus* persists in the flock in infected feet.
2. Infection in the foot can be detected and the infected sheep cured or culled.
3. The organism does not persist in pasture for long periods and does not transmit in dry periods.

Paddocks kept free of sheep for 14 days can be considered free of infection. If all infected animals are culled or cured and infection removed from the pasture, eradication is achieved. Eradication of the disease should be undertaken during a dry summer season, but active measures must be taken to reduce the incidence of infection and spread during the transmission period in the preceding spring. Regular footbathing, at intervals of 1 to 4 weeks, and possible vaccination are usually parts of this strategy.

In the eradication phase during the nontransmission period, all feet of sheep are examined, and affected or suspicious sheep are segregated. When examinations are carried out during dry weather, the feet are likely to be hard and the disease at a quiescent stage. In such circumstances minor lesions may be missed, necessitating careful "diagnostic" trimming and examination of all feet. Clean sheep are run through a footbath (10% zinc sulfate or 5% formalin) and put into fresh fields, whereas the affected sheep are isolated and treated with antibiotics and/or footbathing. Sheep that do not respond may be treated intensively, for example, with an additional antibiotic treatment or two footbathings for 1 hour in 10% zinc sulfate, but preferably should be culled. The apparently clean mob should be reinspected at least twice more during the nontransmission period to ensure these sheep are in fact not infected. Eradication programs often fail because too much effort is invested in trying to cure the infected sheep rather than reinspecting the clean ones.

In areas where flocks are small and there are insufficient fields to carry out this program completely, it has been found to be sufficient to treat all affected sheep weekly but to put all affected sheep back in the flock and the flock back onto the infective pasture, provided conditions are dry.

Culling is an important strategy in footrot eradication, and if the number of infected sheep is small, immediate culling may be the most economic strategy. The use of autogenous mono-and bivalent vaccines can successfully eradicate virulent footrot, with a dramatic decrease in cases within 3 to 6 months of vaccinating.[27-30] Culling of persistent cases that do not respond to the vaccine is an important part of this strategy.

Introduced Sheep

Most breakdowns in eradication occur because of inefficient examination and treatment or the introduction of affected sheep without first checking that they are free from the disease. Introduced sheep should be run as a separate group from the main flock until they have been proven to be footrot-free following a transmission period. Similar isolation of introduced sheep should also be practiced in flocks free of the disease. This is also an important management practice in flocks that have disease to minimize the risk of introduction of different strains of the organism.

FURTHER READING

Abbot KA, Lewis J. Current approaches to the management of ovine footrot. *Vet J.* 2005;169:28-41.

Allworth B. Challenges in ovine footrot control. *Small Rum Res.* 2014;118:110.

Bennett GN, Hickford JG. Ovine footrot: new approaches to an old disease. *Vet Microbiol.* 2011;148:1-7.

Radostits O, et al. Infectious footrot in sheep. In: *Veterinary Medicine: A Textbook of the Diseases of Cattle, Horses, Sheep, Goats and Pigs.* 10th ed. London: W.B. Saunders; 2007:1070-1077.

REFERENCES

1. Cederlöf SE, et al. *Acta Vet Scand.* 2013;55:4.
2. Gilhuus M, et al. *Vet Microbiol.* 2013;163:142.
3. Raadsma HW, Egerton JR. *Livestock Prod Sci.* 2013;156:106.
4. Muzafar M, et al. *Vet Microbiol.* 2015;179:53.
5. Raadsma HW, Dhungyel OP. *Livestock Prod Sci.* 2013;156:115.
6. Nieuwhof GJ, et al. *Animal.* 2008;2:1427.
7. Kaler J, Green LE. *Prev Vet Med.* 2009;92:52.
8. Grøneng GM, et al. *Prev Vet Med.* 2014;113:241.
9. Myers GS, et al. *Nat Biotechnol.* 2007;25:569.
10. Kennan RM, et al. *PLoS Pathog.* 2010;6:e1001210.
11. Wong W, et al. *J Biol Chem.* 2011;286:42180.
12. Strauble A, et al. *Vet Microbiol.* 2014;168:177.
13. Lane J, et al. MLA Report BAHE.0010, March 2015.
14. Nieuwhof GJ, Bishop SC. *Anim Sci.* 2005;81:57.
15. Conington J, et al. *Vet Res Commun.* 2008;32:583.
16. Foddai A, et al. *BMC Vet Res.* 2012;8:65.
17. Duncan JS, et al. *Vet Rec.* 2011;169:606.
18. Duncan JS, et al. *Vet J.* 2014;201:295.
19. Sayers G, et al. *J Clin Microbiol.* 2009;47:1199.
20. Dhungyel O, et al. *Vet Microbiol.* 2013;162:756.
21. Frosth S, et al. *Acta Vet Scand.* 2012;54:6.
22. Cheetham BF, et al. *Vet Microbiol.* 2006;116:166.
23. Wassink GJ, et al. *Prev Vet Med.* 2010;96:93.
24. Kaler J, et al. *J Vet Intern Med.* 2010;24:420.
25. Strobel H, et al. *Vet Rec.* 2014;174:46.
26. Lorenzo M, et al. *Vet Microbiol.* 2012;157:112.
27. Gurung RB, et al. *Vet J.* 2006;172:356.
28. Dhungyel OP, et al. *Vet Microbiol.* 2008;132:364.
29. Dhungyel OP, et al. *Vacc.* 2013;31:1701.
30. Dhungyel OP, Whittington RJ. *Vacc.* 2010;28:470.
31. Mills K, et al. *Aust Vet J.* 2012;90:14.
32. Vatn S, et al. *Small Rumin Res.* 2012;106:11.

FOOT ABSCESS IN SHEEP

Foot abscess includes two diseases: heel abscess and toe abscess.

HEEL ABSCESS/INFECTIOUS BULBAR NECROSIS

Heel abscess follows damage to the interdigital skin. This may be physical damage from sharp stones or stubble, or from friction produced by overgrown feet, but most commonly results as an extension from ovine interdigital dermatitis into the soft tissues of the heel associated with *Fusiformis necrophorum* and *Arcanobacterium (Actinomyces; Corynebacterium) pyogenes.* In interdigital dermatitis, the organisms can invade deep into the interdigital skin. The joint capsule of the distal interphalangeal joint is extremely vulnerable to invasion on the axial interdigital area, and this leads to abscessation.

Most flocks experience cases of heel abscess, but the yearly incidence is usually less than 1%. Heel abscess occurs mainly during very wet seasons, as does footrot, but the former is limited largely to adult sheep, especially ewes heavy in lamb, and rams. Interdigital dermatitis and heel abscess are frequently present in the flock at the same time. An increased prevalence in a flock of young rams may be a result of close flocking and increased muddying of pasture because of this high concentration of livestock. Usually only one foot and one claw will be involved, although in severe outbreaks all four feet may become affected. Most commonly, the medial claw of the hindfoot is affected.

In the initial stages the affected digit is hot and painful. There is an acute lameness—the affected sheep holds the foot off the ground while walking. There is swelling and inflammation of the interdigital skin and pain on pressure across the heel. Pressure in this area may result in the discharge of pus from sinuses in the interdigital space. When the phalangeal joints are involved, there is severe swelling at the back of the claw, and the infection may extend to break out at one or more points above the coronet, with a profuse discharge of pus.

Treatment of Heel Abscess

The treatment of foot abscess is by surgical drainage, parenteral treatment with sulfonamides or a combination of penicillin and streptomycin, and the application of a local bandage. Therapy should be continued for several days. Recovery is not rapid. Because of the frequent involvement of the distal interphalangeal joints with heel abscess, treatment with antibiotics without surgical intervention is unlikely to be successful, but some cases heal spontaneously in 6 to 8 weeks.

TOE ABSCESS

Toe abscess is a lamellar suppuration with purulent underrunning of the horn at the toe. It results from damage to the sole, white line, or wall of the foot and is a common sequela to overgrown feet. Most commonly, it involves a digit on the **front** feet. The affected digit is hot, and there is pain on pressure across the sole and toe. There is severe lameness, swelling of the coronet with pain and heat apparent, and usually rupture and purulent discharge at the coronet between the toes. Penetration to deeper structures may also occur.

Treatment of Toe Abscess

The only treatment of toe abscess is by surgical drainage, and the response is rapid. Toe granuloma can be a sequela, but more commonly toe granuloma is a response to overzealous foot paring.

FURTHER READING

Radostits O, et al. Foot abscess in sheep. In: *Veterinary Medicine: A Textbook of the Diseases of Cattle, Horses, Sheep, Goats and Pigs*. 10th ed. London: W.B. Saunders; 2007:1077-1079.

LAMB ARTHRITIS

In the United Kingdom, *Streptococcus dysgalactiae* is a significant cause of outbreaks of arthritis in lambs, especially during the first 3 weeks of life. It occurs more commonly in lambs that are lambed indoors. Affected lambs are lame in one or more legs and are often found recumbent. There is minimal joint swelling in the initial stage of the disease, and for this reason differential diagnoses include nutritional myopathy, swayback, and spinal abscess. Infection is present in any joint but most common in the tarsal and atlanto-occipital joints. Some die with systemic disease and myocarditis. Survivors may be chronically lame.

CHLAMYDIAL POLYARTHRITIS

Virulent chlamydia, including *Chlamydia* (formerly *Chlamydophila*) *pecorum*, can be isolated from the joints and eyes of lambs with polyarthritis.[1,2] Intestinal infection with *C. pecorum* is also common in pastured lambs between 3 and 9 months of age, but it is not associated with clinical disease.

Chlamydial polyarthritis is a common disease of sheep in feedlots in the United States, but the mortality rate is low. The strain associated with arthritis is not common in the United Kingdom, and polyarthritis in the United Kingdom has been associated with a chlamydial strain distinct from *C. pecorum*. Outbreaks of polyarthritis caused by *C. pecorum* have also been reported with increased frequency in 3- to 6-month-old lambs Australia.[2] In sheep grazing pasture the morbidity may be as high as 80%, but deaths are usually less than 1%. PCR testing has demonstrated that mixed infections of *Chlamydophila* are often present in the conjunctivae of sheep, but there is no consistent association with the onset of disease.[2]

In calves, the disease is uncommon but often fatal, and response to treatment is poor; affected calves are often destroyed. The experimental disease in calves begins as chlamydemia, followed by localization in the joints.

The clinical signs in calves and lambs include gross swelling of most limb joints but especially the larger joints, lameness, stiffness, unwillingness to move, recumbency, depression, conjunctivitis, and fever of 39° to 42° C (102° to 108° F). The navel is unaffected, but there may be signs caused by localization of the infection in other organs (e.g., pneumonia, encephalomyelitis, and renal abscess). Clinically, the disease is indistinguishable from polyarthritis caused by other infections such as *Mycoplasma* and *Haemophilus* spp.

Response to treatment with oxytetracycline is variable, and residual effects of infection, such as poor growth and ill-thrift, commonly occur.

FURTHER READING

Jelocnik M, Frentiu FD, et al. Multilocus sequence analysis provides insights into molecular epidemiology of Chlamydia pecorum infections in Australian sheep, cattle and koalas. *J Vet Micro*. 2010;140:405-417.

Nietfeld JC. Chlamydial infections in small ruminants. *Vet Clin N Am Food A*. 2001;17:301.

REFERENCES

1. Jelocnik M, et al. *J Vet Microbiol*. 2010;140:405.
2. Polkinghorne A, et al. *Vet Microbiol*. 2009;135:142.

CHRONIC PECTORAL AND VENTRAL MIDLINE ABSCESS IN HORSES (PIGEON FEVER)

C. pseudotuberculosis biovar equi has been associated with a high regional prevalence of chronic abscessation in horses in California, Texas, and Colorado and can cause disease in horses in other states.[1] Six phenotypes are recognized on culture, but there is no association between phenotype and clinical form of the disease.[2]

The incidence of the disease is 9.2 per 10,000 horses and appears to be increasing, and this change might be related to climatic changes.[1,3] The disease is most prevalent in Texas (35 cases per 10,000 horses), Colorado (18 per 10,000), and Oregon (12 cases per 10,000), with California reporting 6 cases per 10,000 horses.[1] Within Texas, prevalence of the disease increased from 0.9 in 2005 to 10 cases per 100,000 horses at risk in 2011.[4] There is no apparent breed or sex predisposition and cases occur in horses of all ages, but the majority are adult horses and there are few cases under 1 year of age.[1] Usually, only a single horse on a farm is affected. A small proportion of farms have endemic infection, with a prevalence of disease of 5% to 10% and recurrent infections each year. In some years spread to naive horses results in epidemic disease.

Cases can occur in all months of the year but are most common in dry months in autumn, with a peak prevalence in November, December, and January; internal abscesses are more common in late autumn and January, with a smaller peak in June and July, and ulcerative lymphangitis is more common in March, April, and May.[1,4] There is a variation in the prevalence from year to year, and[1,4] in both Texas and California, years with high prevalence of the disease have been preceded by seasons with higher-than-normal rainfall and conditions that promote high insect populations. Insects, such as horn flies (*Habronema irritans*), that produce a ventral midline dermatitis during feeding may predispose to infection, and the organism has been detected by PCR populations of *H. irritans, Stomoxys calcitrans,* and *Musca domestica*. Feeding of infected house flies (*Musca domestica*) on experimentally induced wounds on the pectoral region caused disease in ponies, demonstrating that house flies are mechanical vectors of infection and can spread the disease to equids.[5] Flies are not the host of the organism, being mechanical vectors only, and the source appears to be soil. *C. pseudotuberculosis* persists and multiplies in a variety of soil types and under a range of environmental conditions.[6] Addition of feces to the soil enhances growth of the organism.[6]

Patterns of spatial and temporal clustering indicate that disease is transmitted directly or indirectly from horse to horse with an incubation period of 3 to 4 weeks.

The disease occurs in a region where caseous lymphadenitis is also common in sheep, although the disease in sheep is usually caused by *C. pseudotuberculosis biovar ovis*. Stable hygiene, insect control, and isolation of infected horses might aid in control.

Disease caused by *C. pseudotuberculosis* occurs in captive elk, although the biovar involved is not reported.[7]

External Abscesses

The most common form of the disease is an external abscess (97% of reported cases), with internal abscess formation (2%) and ulcerative lymphangitis (1%) being much less common manifestations of infection.[1] However, the most common clinical manifestation of infection varies geographically, with California reporting 49% of cases as being internal abscesses and ulcerative lymphangitis being most common in Texas (96%).[1] These occur in a variety of areas on the body, but in the majority of cases they are in the pectoral, axillary, inguinal, or ventral midline regions.[8] Affected horses are usually markedly lame. The abscesses can reach a diameter of 10 to 20 cm, with a surrounding area of edema, before they rupture 1 to 4 weeks later. Clinical signs include local swelling, lameness, pain on palpation, ventral edema, reluctance to move, midline dermatitis, fever, and depression in the early stage, followed eventually by rupture of the abscesses.

Treatment of external abscesses is by hot packs to encourage opening and by surgical drainage and lavage. Ultrasound can aid in the detection of deeper abscesses. NSAIDs can be used to control swelling and pain. Recovery rates are excellent and are not improved by antimicrobial therapy.

Internal Abscesses

Internal abscesses occur at a variety of sites but predominantly in the liver and can occur in horses with no external abscessation. The diagnosis should be suspected in horses, in the region and the season, with a clinical history of external abscess, fever, anemia, and colic and laboratory evidence of leukocytosis with neutrophilia, anemia, hyperglobulinemia, hyperfibrinogenemia, and elevated activity of hepatic-associated enzymes.[8] Abdominocentesis in most cases shows an elevated protein and nucleated cell count, and the organism can be cultured.

Treatment is with antimicrobial therapy, but the case-fatality rate is high if the abscess cannot be drained. *C. pseudotuberculosis* is sensitive to concentrations of most common antibiotics achieved in vivo with MIC90 values for chloramphenicol less than or equal to 4 µg/mL, enrofloxacin less than or equal to 0.5 µg/mL, gentamicin less than or equal to 0.25 µg/mL, penicillin at 0.25 µg/mL, rifampin less than or equal to µg/mL, tetracycline less than or equal to 2 µg/mL, trimethoprim-sulfamethoxazole (TMS) less than or equal to 0.5 µg/mL, ceftiofur at 2 µg/mL, and doxycycline less than or equal to 2 µg/mL.[9]

The value of a **synergistic hemolysis inhibition serologic** test in diagnosis has been examined. The test was useful for detecting internal infection in horses that did not have external abscesses (likelihood ratio of 2.98 [95% CI 2.2 to 4.1] with a titer ≥ 512), but it was not useful when horses had external abscesses.[10]

An autogenous vaccine has given protection against experimental challenge, but in field trials, there has been no difference in the incidence of infection between vaccinated and control horses.

Otitis media interna, meningitis, and unilateral orchitis are documented forms of the disease.[11,12] *C. pseudotuberculosis* is also recorded as a cause of pericarditis and pleuritis in a horse and in association with suppurative facial dermatitis following trauma.

REFERENCES

1. Kilcoyne I, et al. *JAVMA*. 2014;245:309.
2. Britz E, et al. *Vet J*. 2014;200:282.
3. Spier SJ. *Equine Vet Educ*. 2008;20:37.
4. Szonyi B, et al. *J Equine Vet Sci*. 2014;34:281.
5. Barba M, et al. *J Vet Int Med*. 2015;29:636.
6. Spier SJ, et al. *Vet Rec*. 2012;170.
7. Kelly EJ, et al. *J Wildlife Dis*. 2012;48:803.
8. Nogradi N, et al. *JAVMA*. 2012;241:771.
9. Rhodes DM, et al. *J Vet Int Med*. 2015;29:327.
10. Jeske JM, et al. *JAVMA*. 2013;242:86.
11. Gonzalez M, et al. *Equine Vet Educ*. 2008;20:30.
12. Rand CL, et al. *Equine Vet Educ*. 2012;24:271.

INFECTIOUS POLYARTHRITIS (GLÄSSER'S DISEASE, PORCINE POLYSEROSITIS, AND ARTHRITIS)

SYNOPSIS

Etiology *Haemophilus parasuis* (HPS) rarely a primary pathogen in respiratory disease.

Epidemiology Common in pigs postweaning to 4 months of age. Sporadic outbreaks. Environmental stressors are risk factors. There may be significant losses.

Signs Sudden onset of anorexia, dyspnea, lameness, swollen joints, fever, nervous signs, and death. Three types: hyperacute (death), acute, and endemic. Glässer's disease not yet seen in wild boar.

Clinical pathology Culture organisms from serous membranes.

Lesions Peritonitis, pleuritis, synovitis, meningitis.

Diagnostic confirmation Culture organism and a variety of new techniques.

Differential diagnosis Erysipelas, mycoplasmal and streptococcal arthritis, other serositis; also *Actinobacillus pleuropneumoniae* infection, vitamin E deficiency, *Escherichia coli*, and *Actinobacillus suis*.

Treatment Antimicrobials.

Control Minimize stressors at weaning and in nursery barns. Limited commercial vaccines.

Glässer's disease is a contagious disease of young pigs characterized by arthritis, pericarditis, pleurisy, peritonitis, and meningitis. In a study in the United Kingdom, it was found to be common in herds with a history of chronic respiratory disease.

ETIOLOGY

Initially, the agent was thought to be *Haemophilus influenzae* suis, but it is now known to be *Haemophilus parasuis* (HPS). Now recognized as one species, it is, however, extremely pleomorphic. It is a gram-negative bacterium that requires V factor for its growth. A modified classification of 15 major serotypes has been achieved, although many are still untypeable. The current serotyping is based on reactions between antisera and surface antigens, which leads to a classification based on 15 serotypes. Serotyping originally used a GID test, but this has been replaced by indirect hemagglutination assay (IHA), which has increased the proportion of typeable strains from 60% to 80%. The study of these polysaccharides is under way.[1-3]

Most studies have shown that serotypes 4 and 5 are the most common strains involved in Glässer's disease. In many instances, the serotype is not an indicator of virulence because different strains within one serotype may have a different virulence. HPS, as with other *Haemophilus* spp., has an affinity for the mucosa of the oropharyngeal and upper respiratory tract. HPS can be isolated from the nasal cavity, tonsillar area, and trachea. Several strains may be found in the same nose, and there may be several types in the same herd.[4] HPS isolates are genetically heterogeneous within the same serovar and between serovars. The gene content and diversity of the loci encoding the biosynthesis of the capsular polysaccharides of the 15 serovars have recently been described.[5]

EPIDEMIOLOGY

The colonization of the respiratory tract is rapid, with 50% of pig noses colonized by 7 days and 100% by 60 days,[4] and there is a turnover of the strains.

Most countries have different distributions of serotypes. In the United Kingdom, 5 is the most common, followed by 4 and 7 in equal numbers, and the rest are largely nontypeable. In Denmark, 5 is followed by 13 and 4 and then the nontypeable.

It may be a true commensal organism in the upper respiratory tract. It is responsible for severe polyserositis in young pigs, and it may also occasionally cause arthritis in older pigs and the individual sow. The organism, like the others with a similar name, *Actinobacillus suis* and *Streptococcus suis*, has been called one of the "suis-cides" of pigs, which are responsible for considerable economic loss in high-health herds and herds that practice very early weaning. HPS is also commonly isolated from lungs with lesions of enzootic pneumonia.

Pigs infected with virulent isolates of HPS can remain healthy and serve as reservoirs for transmission to naïve pigs, and heterologous protection is possible.[6]

Although the disease occurs worldwide, reports used to be rare and mainly from Europe. However, since the onset of separate-site production and the occurrence of porcine reproductive and respiratory syndrome, virulent forms of swine influenza, and diseases associated with porcine circo virus type 2 (PCV-2), HPS has become one of the most common of the so-called secondary infections. It is a significant contributor to the porcine respiratory disease complex (PRDC). When it first appears in naive or specific-pathogen-free herds, it may be a common cause of sudden death; such cases may be numerous, and these situations it also affects younger animals. When the disease becomes endemic, it may affect older animals, with fewer sudden deaths but more chronic polyserositis. The disease has also been observed in Australia, the United States, Canada, and the United Kingdom. The disease accounted for less than 1% of total mortalities of pigs submitted to veterinary diagnostic laboratories over an 11-year period in Ontario. However, the disease was the second most common cause of mortality in test station boars. In a survey of 19 excellent specific-pathogen-free pig herds, 16 were positive, and the average number of culture-positive pigs per herd was 6/10 for positive herds.

It is probably spread by aerosol and certainly by nose-to-nose contact. The disease occurs as sporadic outbreaks—usually in weanling to 4-month-old pigs that have been recently chilled, transported, weaned, or moved to different pens. The onset is sudden, with several pigs in the group affected, and occurs within 2 to 7 days of the initiating stress. Occasionally, it causes arthritis in older animals, or even sow herds. The case-fatality rate is high in untreated pigs. Acute myositis in primary specific-pathogen-free sows has been associated with HPS.

Little is known of the method of transmission of the disease. The causative organisms are facultative pathogens and can be frequently isolated from pig lungs diseased from other causes, even though they are generally not present in normal lungs. It is probable that a respiratory carrier state does exist and that invasion with subsequent septicemia and polyserositis is initiated by stress situations in young pigs that have lost maternal immunity but have not yet gained active immunity. Piglets probably acquire the infection soon after birth, but maternal antibody protects them from clinical disease until they are 2 to 4 weeks of age. Animals that are weaned early are likely to have this infection, so the supposition is that most pigs acquire the infection at or immediately after birth. *H. parasuis* has been found in the tonsil using IHC and EM.

There are several pathogenic serovars of HPS. Serotypes 3, 6, 7, 8, 9, and 11 are considered to be avirulent; 15 more pathogenic; and 1, 4, 5, 10, 12, 13, and 14 virulent. However, this pattern cannot be considered permanent because genes can be shared, and in any case up to 50% of isolations are considered nontypeable. In the United States and Canada, 15.2% were classified as nontypeable, 26.2% in Germany, 29.3% in Spain, and 41.9% in Australia. In a particular pig herd, many strains can be isolated, but in most cases, one or two strains predominate. In many herds the nontypeable outnumber the typeable. Of seven reference strains examined, only serotypes 1 and 5 were pathogenic, and the seven strains have common antigenic determinants. Within specific-pathogen-free herds, many herds have common strains; no strains are common to both conventional and specific-pathogen-free herds, which is a reflection of little or no movement of pigs between these types of herd. Specific-pathogen-free pigs are often free of this organism and are highly susceptible to the infection, even at several months of age, if they are mixed with conventionally raised pigs that may be infected. Outbreaks with rapid spread and high mortality have been reported in specific-pathogen-free pigs. It has been suggested that the causative bacteria are common in most herds and that the disease arises only when pigs from uninfected herds are introduced to a contaminated environment, especially if they have been exposed to environmental stress during transport. When infection is introduced into a previously noninfected herd, the disease may act as a contagious disease until herd immunity is developed or the infection eliminated. Recently it has been suggested that the nasal cavity strains may be nonpathogenic and form a completely different population to the pathogenic strains. Serotypes from nasal and tracheal cultures were shown to be similar in one study. They found that there was a lower level of colonization in the litters of the young sows. The genetic diversity of the strains is not well understood. Several serotypes may be isolated from the same herd or even from the same pig. High-pathogenicity porcine respiratory and reproductive syndrome virus (PRRSV) has been shown to accelerate the colonization and load of HPS in conventional pigs.[7]

The organism probably does not survive outside the host, and therefore transmission is direct, with most of the transmission occurring during birth.

PATHOGENESIS

One of the key factors may be that maternal antibody does not last a long time and may be gone by 2 to 4 weeks of age but will last until 6 to 8 weeks if sow antibody titers are high. It is the animals that become infected after their maternal protection has waned that have resulting clinical disease. Serovar 5 is highly virulent when inoculated into specific-pathogen-free piglets at 6 to 8 weeks of age. Bordetella bronchiseptica increases HPS colonization of the nasal cavity. However, it is also said that previous infection with PRRSV has no effect on the occurrence. The severity of the disease increases with the increase in the dose of the organisms.

The nonpathogenic isolates probably only colonize the upper respiratory tract. The pathogens colonize the upper respiratory tract and then descend to the lower respiratory tract by evading phagocytosis[8,9] and by using adhesion factors.[10] The pathogens escape from the respiratory tract,[11] enter the bloodstream, and attach to the endothelial cells;[11,12] they survive because the capsule prevents the killing of the organism.[4] Entrance to the bloodstream is more likely when the animal is stressed or immunity is suspect. The organism then establishes the pathology at the serosal surfaces using hemolysins, proteases, and neuraminidases. The outcome is determined by the innate and adaptive immunity (colostrum, previous exposure, concurrent infections, etc.). The blood cellular immune responses have been described, which suggests that there is an increased trafficking of inflammatory cells.[13] There is a response to iron restriction.[14] The pathogen enters the endothelial cells and induces apoptosis and produces IL-6 and IL-815.[16] The virulent strains survive against the phagocytes and complement system, and the nonvirulent are phagocytosed. HPS acquires iron for growth through the surface receptors.[17]

The precise relationship between protein patterns, serovars, and virulence potential remains to be defined. The major virulence factors and the protective antigens are still largely unknown. Only a small number of organisms in the region of 104 to 106 are sufficient to produce disease. The pathogenesis has recently been described.[15] A new technique called differential display reverse transcription PCR (RT-PCR) has been used to search for virulence factors. The pathogenic HPS may have an outer membrane protein, fimbriae, and lipopolysaccharides; a cytotoxin has yet to be described, but it may be a membrane neuraminidase. The outer membrane protein may be important, and it is iron regulated.[18] Fibrinous meningitis, polyserositis, and polyarthritis are typical. Fatal septicemia can occur spontaneously or following the intraperitoneal inoculation of pigs with HPS. The intranasal inoculation of HPS into cesarean-derived colostrum-deprived pigs results in a suppurative rhinitis, which may represent an initial event in the pathogenesis of the systemic infection in pigs. After infection with HPS, there was a highly significant rise in radical formation, and monocyte proliferation was reduced. Neutrophils reacted inconsistently. In this experimental study, the CD25+ marker cells were markedly reduced. Experimental infections showed that not all field isolates are pathogenic, and it may be that route of infection and dosage are most important in determining the outcome of infections. In a new study, polyacramide gel electrophoresis (PAGE) typing of HPS and virulence potential based on site were looked at together. PAGE group I had 83.4% of the isolates from the upper respiratory tract (these were mostly of serotype 3 or nontypeable), but of the PAGE group II isolates, 90.7% of all the isolates were from the systemic sites (these are mostly serotypes 1, 2, 4, 5, 12, and 14). It may be that there is also a tropism for some sites because some strains are only found in the brain and others in the pericardium. This means that the systemic sites are the best sites for the identification of pathogenic HPS. Most practitioners have the opinion that the problem is more apparent when there is predisposing viral infection, particularly porcine respiratory and reproductive syndrome (PRRS), swine influenza, or porcine circo virus type 2 (PCV-2). Although most practitioners would say that the prevalence of PRRS-associated HPS infections has increased the natural occurrence of HPS, experimental confirmation is lacking. Only PRRS consistently increased the isolation of HPS from the lung.

On the other hand, both PRRS and *B. bronchiseptica* increase the colonization of the upper respiratory tract by HPS. There is no additive effect here. There is no doubt that the occurrence of the vasculitis plays a part in the pathogenesis.

CLINICAL FINDINGS

The incubation period depends on the strain.[11] Clinical disease occurs because of a mismatch between immunity and colonization by virulent strains. This may be a result of early decline of colostral immunity, later or slow HPS colonization, mixed pig flows, and the purchase of breeding stock that are carriers.

In the naive herd and where specific-pathogen-free animals have entered commercial herds, sudden death may be the only feature. Some people are of the opinion that there may be polyserositic, arthritic, and meningitic forms. A virulent type 10 outbreak has been described.[19] A wide variety of signs may be seen, including fever, depression, and reluctance to move, progressing to prostration, convulsions, and sudden death. The depression is a marked feature. The mortality rate may be high, and many pigs that survive become "poor doers."

The onset is sudden, with a fever, an unusual rapid and shallow dyspnea with noisy lung fields, an anxious expression, extension of the head, and mouth-breathing. There may be a serous nasal discharge, and coughing may occur. Depression and anorexia are observed. The animals are very lame, stand on their toes, and move with a short, shuffling gait. All the joints are swollen and painful on palpation, and fluid swelling of the tendon sheaths may also be clinically evident. In many animals there may be just a single joint affected, which is often the hock. A red to blue discoloration of the skin appears near death. Most cases die 2 to 5 days after the onset of illness. Animals that survive the acute stage of the disease may develop chronic arthritis, and some cases of intestinal obstruction caused by peritoneal adhesions occur. Meningitis occurs in some pigs, particularly when these are naive or where there is an acute onset, and is manifested by muscle tremor, paralysis, and convulsions. Although Glässer's disease can occur in pigs of any age, weanling pigs are most commonly and most seriously affected. In chronic cases, pigs may lose part of an ear as a result of ischemic necrosis. There may be also wasting piglets, which fade and die. In some instances in which there is a severe peritonitis, there may be scrotal swelling as the fluid drains down the tunica vaginalis.

Another type of syndrome of necrosis of the masseter muscles was described in which sows had swollen, cyanotic heads, with HPS isolated from the affected muscles. Purulent rhinitis has also been described.

CLINICAL PATHOLOGY

The disease is essentially a polyserositis and arthritis, and as a result the organism is recoverable from joint fluid and pleural exudate. Material aspirated from joints may be serous, fibrinous, or purulent. It may just be a few fibrin tags that have organized from an initial fibrinous exudate. The disease can be diagnosed serologically on the presence of precipitins in the serum of recovered pigs, and complement-fixing antibody can be detected following infection. But these are not reliable methods. In an experiment in which 183 specific-pathogen-free pigs were given infections, the hemoglobin concentrations and hematocrit fell. Leukopenia developed 1 to 2 days after infection, with leukocytosis later. Any changes in the cerebrospinal fluid were not related to the clinical signs. One of the common findings in HPS infections is vitamin E deficiency, and this is most likely to be as a result of the toxic oxygen radical damage.

NECROPSY FINDINGS

Glässer's disease generally is associated with three main lesions: fibrinous polyserositis and arthritis, signs of septicemia, and toxemia.

In some cases there are no gross lesions, and all that is seen is a small amount of peritoneal fluid or a very thin fibrin strand (tag).

Serofibrinous or fibrinous pleuritis, pericarditis, and peritonitis are usually present, but the exudate is scanty in some cases. Pneumonia may also be apparent. There is inflammation and edema of the periarticular tissues, and the joint cavities contain turbid fluid and discoid deposits of yellowish-green fibrin. A suppurative rhinitis is also possible. A fibrinopurulent meningitis is common. In specific-pathogen-free pigs, the lesions may be minimal, and only successful isolation of the organism permits the differentiation of Glässer's disease from other causes of sudden death. The distinction may be a difficult one because of the fastidious culture requirements of HPS. Eventually, all surfaces are covered with a thick mat of fibrin, and the individual organs may be difficult to recognize. This eventually becomes fibrotic. The spleen and liver may be enlarged.

Histologically, acutely affected serosal surfaces are thickened by neutrophils entrapped in a matrix of fibrin. As these lesions age, fibrous adhesions may develop and lead to chronic pleuritis, arthritis, and pericarditis. Such cases are often culture-negative, even when selective media are used. Most isolates are made from the lungs. Petechial hemorrhages may also be found on the kidney (the so-called "turkey egg," which is not pathognomonic for anything except septicemia in its widest sense, with over 30 agents known to cause it).

Samples for Confirmation of Diagnosis

Bacteriology

The collection of samples from animals that have been dead for several hours is not worth considering even at the best of times and certainly not when HPS is suspected. An acutely affected live pig, freshly autopsied, will give much better results, especially if there is no overheating of the carcass postmortem or subsequent cooling because the organism is temperature-sensitive. Transport media to the laboratory will also be beneficial in recovery rates. It is said that culture of the nasal swabs will be as rewarding as collecting tracheal swabs, but it is likely that the larynx and below are normally sterile. What you isolate from the nasal cavity may then be a commensal population of largely nontypeable species, whereas the trachea harbors the pathogenic forms. Other authors say that they are the same serotypes. These authors have also found that a lower level of colonization was found in the litters of young sows, and a low level of colonization at weaning probably predisposed pigs to clinical disease in the nursery, assuming the presence of a virulent serotype.

Culture swabs from serosal surfaces, including joints and meninges. It is essential to collect samples from areas that are not enclosed in fibrin. Nasal swabs are more easily collected than tracheal but may indicate a different population of HPS. It is usually said that it is difficult to isolate from fluids but is easier from the lesions. It is necessary to have a fresh pig with no antibiotic therapy. It may also be necessary to use Amies transport medium to preserve HPS on the way to the laboratory.

H. parasuis is a gram-negative rod existing as a coccobacillus to long filamentous chains. There is usually a capsule, but the expression of this is influenced by culture. NAD or V factor is required for growth (chocolate agar or staph streak, and then there is satellite growth). The availability of NAD may determine growth capabilities. After 24 to 48 hours the colonies are small, translucent, and nonhemolytic on chocolate agar.

Histology

Histology includes formalin-fixed brain, synovial membranes, liver, lung (LM). Immunohistochemistry can be used to show the organisms in the cytoplasm of neutrophils and macrophages in the lungs and in the mononuclear cells in the subscapular and medullary sinuses of the lymph nodes. Immunofluorescence was observed on the bronchiolar epithelium in the alveoli and in the lung parenchyma.

Modern techniques have been applied. The results are better if you use both the Angen[20] and Olvera[8] PCR techniques, with few false positives.

Serology

Recently, an indirect hemagglutination test has been described for the serotyping of field isolates. A new indirect hemagglutination technique has just been described, and it is rapid and effective. It is also much more sensitive than the immunodiffusion test.

DIAGNOSIS

The best cases to examine are those that have received no antibiotics and are acute cases. The organism is very likely to die out if subjected to too much heat or cold.

There is a need to have the samples taken from the lesions as quickly as possible, transported to the laboratory quickly in transport media (Amies medium), preferably chilled if overnight transport, and plated as quickly as possible. It requires to be cultured on chocolate agar or blood agar with a staph streak.

Once cultured, strain typing can be achieved. There are 15 strains and many that are untypeable. The relative strain virulence is shown in Table 15-5.

Table 15-5 Virulence of strains

HPS serotype	Virulence	Effects
1, 5, 10, 12, 13, 14	High	Death within 96 hours
2, 4, 15	Moderate	Severe polyarthritis
8	Low	Mild lesions
3, 6, 7, 9, 11	Nonpathogenic	No signs or lesions

Novel genotyping was first described in 2008, and an improved species specific PCR has been described since.[15] The complete genome of HPS was described.[2,10] Demonstration of HPS requires culture and PCR identification. There is a correlation between clinicopathologic outcome and the typing of HPS field strains.[21]

A detailed analysis of diagnostic analyses and the occurrence of strains in the Netherlands is available,[22] in which strains 3 and 10 were not identified. In this study ERIC-PCR and *hsp60* gene typing were also employed because 145 of the strains could not be serotyped.

A multiplex nested PCR has been described[23] that works for *S. suis* and *M. hyorhinis* and HPS. It is extremely useful when samples are negative after isolation and can be used on formalin-fixed and paraffin-embedded tissues as well.

Usually, HPS can be identified by either of two conventional PCR20 tests or by an RT-PCR,[24] but sometimes *A. indolicus* gives a false positive. A RT-PCR for HPS has been validated.[25] However, a recent paper has suggested that it may fail to recognize an HPS strain, so false negatives may be found.[26]

Researchers in China have described loop-mediated isothermal amplification for rapid detection of HPS and found it more sensitive than nested PCR. It appears to be best used for internal organs and tissues because there are many nonpathogenic types of HPS in the respiratory tract.

The first improvement in the diagnosis of HPS occurred with the development of an oligonucleotide-specific plate hybridization assay that could be used on the nasal swabs. The assay detects fewer than 100 cfu/mL in a pure culture and gives a positive result when HPS is present in the ratio of 1 : 103 to 1 : 104 in a mixed culture. The assay is more sensitive than culture for detection of HPS in nasal swabs.

In-situ hybridization will demonstrate a patchy to multifocal distribution of HPS in the lung. A repetitive-element-based PCR (rep-PCR) has been developed, which is a technique that compares very favorably with traditional microbiology. The rep-PCR uses repetitive sequences within the bacterial genome to produce strain-specific fingerprints, allowing comparison and differentiation between *H. parasuis* strains. This enables comparison of these strains and allows the source of virulent strains to be identified.

Another new technique is ERIC-PCR, and this is very successful compared with conventional microbiological techniques. Identification and differentiation of *H. parasuis* using a species-specific PCR with subsequent DNA fingerprinting using the digestion of PCR products using Hind III endonuclease has been described. This restriction fragment length polymorphism (PCR-RFLP) enabled eight patterns to be determined for the nontypeable strains.

Recently, a technique for the computer-based analysis of HPS protein fingerprints has been described that is a considerable improvement on serotyping. It was shown that there is a high genetic diversity within the serovars. At least 12 different strains within the type 4 serovar, and genetic diversity in the other serotypes as well, were described. Nontypeable isolates were divided into 18 genotypes. The major advantage of this technique is that there is no need for isolation, culture, and biochemical identification of the isolates. In addition, all strains can be identified, not just those of certain serotypes. At the moment, there is no direct demonstration of a linkage between PCR-RFLP, OMP patterns, and serotyping and rep-PCR. In a recent study, 32 strains were grouped into six serovars and 11 genotypes. This led to the hypothesis that HPS strains with a similar distribution of repetitive sequences can express different antigens. A lot of work is still required to relate genome classification to the real virulence of the strain.

DIFFERENTIAL DIAGNOSIS

The clinical signs and pathology are not pathognomic because similar pictures can be seen with Escherichia coli, Mycoplasma hyosynoviae, Mycoplasma hyorhinis, Erysipelothrix rhusiopathiae, and Streptococcus suis.

The unusual combination of arthritis, fibrinous serositis, and meningitis is sufficient to make a diagnosis of Glässer's disease, but differentiation from the many similar disease entities apparently caused by other agents can only be confirmed by bacteriologic examination.

The disease may be confused with erysipelas, mycoplasma arthritis, and streptococcal arthritis on clinical examination. Mycoplasmosis is a much milder disease and is manifested principally by the presence of a few unthrifty or lame pigs in the litter just before weaning, rather than an acute outbreak with a high mortality. Differentiation between cases of Glässer's disease with meningitis and the other diseases of the nervous system in young pigs, especially streptococcal meningitis and Teschen disease, may not be possible without necropsy examination.

TREATMENT

Pigs are usually ill with this disease, and thus parenteral treatment is required first. A high

Table 15-6 Antimicrobial resistance in Spain and the UK.[27]

	Spain	UK
Florfenicol	0	0
Penicillin	60	0
Erythromycin	40	0
Tilmicosin	40	0
Enrofloxacin	20	0
Ceftiofur	7	0
Tiamulin	40	3
Ampicillin	57	7
Oxytetracycline	40	7
Trimet/sulpha	53	10
Spectinomycin	23	10
Gentamycin	27	10
Neomycin	33	20

proportion of HPS strains are resistant or multiresistant.[27] In China, over 70% of the strains were resistant to enrofloxacin.[28] Resistance has been reported for penicillin, and certain strains are resistant to tetracyclines, erythromycin, and other aminoglycosides (Table 15-6). This requires attention to the sensitivity patterns of the organism in different countries. If pigs are sick with HPS, then parenteral treatment is a must as the first step. This can be followed by water medication for at least 5 days. It has long been known that ill animals will not eat, but it is currently appreciated that sick pigs do not drink as much as when they are healthy, and therefore there is the tendency to underdose until they are well enough to drink their normal amounts.

Treatment with penicillin, trimethoprim–sulfadoxine, or oxytetracycline is effective in the early stages of the disease.

Tilmicosin can be used for effective treatment because it is concentrated in the macrophages and neutrophils. These can migrate to the site of infection, and therefore there may be higher levels of antibody in the tissue. Long-acting medication can also be useful (tulathromycin, ceftiofur).

CONTROL

It is essential to protect high-herd-health units by not importing new stock into a unit also thought to be free, and vice versa, because both groups can be exposed. Never bring high-herd-health stock into a low-health unit. Multisourcing pigs into a grow-out unit is especially suicidal.

Control of PRRS and PCV-2 is important because HPS is associated with both of these.[29,30] Control is only possible if there is (1) diagnosis of infection, (2) identification of prevalent strains, (3) use of autogenous vaccines, and (4) management of new strains.

There are three main approaches:

1. Prophylactic medication
2. Optimization of pig immunity
3. Management techniques to maximize immunity

IgG antibodies kill HPS via the classical complement pathway.[31,32] It is therefore best to vaccinate piglets before weaning, or the sows to boost maternal antibody, but if you do, then delay vaccinating the piglets until maternal antibody has waned. Always vaccinate the replacement breeding stock.

Avoidance of undue exposure to adverse environmental conditions at weaning is recommended. Avoidance of undue fluctuations of temperature is absolutely essential. Prophylactic dosing at the time of shipping or medication of feed or drinking water on arrival with the previously mentioned drugs may be of value in preventing outbreaks. Feeding a mixture of 3% sulfamonomethoxine and 1% trimethoprim at 160 and 240 ppm for 5 days and challenging with *H. parasuis* at 3 days prevented clinical disease, and bacteria were not recovered. There are resistance genes for tetracyclines and beta-lactam antibiotics.[33] Maternal antibody does not interfere with vaccination of pigs at 1 to 3 weeks of age. Maternal immunity lasts about 20 days, but if the sows are vaccinated, then it may last 60 days.[4]

Humoral immunity is protective against experimental Glässer's disease.[34] A formalin-killed bacterin administered before weaning with two injections at 5 and 7 weeks of age has proved highly effective in preventing the disease. A formalin-killed whole-cell culture bacterin developed in Ontario is effective in protecting 4-week-old pigs against experimental challenge with the organism. A recent trial showed that vaccinating sows at 80 and 95 days of pregnancy with a commercial bacterin containing HPS 2, 3, and 5 was useful in reducing pneumonic lesions and arthritic joint changes in subsequently challenged piglets. Vaccination of piglets seemed to have no effect, and vaccination of the sows seemed to have no effect on the colonization of the nasal mucosa by HPS or on the timing of colonization.

Autogenous vaccines against homologous strains have been shown to work, but vaccination failures do occur. There may be little cross-protection between strains. A new serotype 5 vaccination was described, and the subsequent challenge with serotypes 1, 12, 13, and 14 produced different responses in control pigs.

The vaccines against this bacterium are whole-cell bacterins that are protective only against serotypes 1, 4, 5, and 6.[35] Vaccination has three important components. First, there is the decision of commercial or autogenous vaccination, and this depends on the strains in the field and whether they are in the commercial vaccine. Second, the timing of vaccination should take into account the length of persistence of maternal antibody and the peak of piglet mortality. If this peak is at 2 to 3 weeks, then the sows should be vaccinated. The piglets should then be vaccinated at weaning and 2 weeks later. Third, because sow and piglet vaccination together is not recommended because the sow's vaccination can produce maternal antibody that interferes with the piglet's active immunity, you should make a choice of one or the other. A new departure is the production of a genetically inactivated vaccine, the ghost vaccine.[36]

Recently, the technique of introducing known populations of live HPS to the young piglet shortly after birth, thus allowing a slow rate of acquisition of organisms, has been advocated. All-in/all-out by age is absolutely essential to prevent carry-over of infection, and it is likely that nose-to-nose transmission is important, so solid partitions between different litters may help.

When it comes to disinfection, it has been suggested that chloramine may be useful[37] in deactivating HPS.

FURTHER READING

Kielstein P, Rapp-Gabriel V. Designation of the 15 serovars of H. parasuis on the basis of immunodiffusion using heat-stable antigen extracts. *J Clin Microbiol.* 1992;30:862-865.

Olvera A, Segales J, Aragon V. Update on the diagnosis of HPS infections in pigs and novel genotyping methods. *Vet J.* 2007;174:523-529.

REFERENCES

1. Perry MB, et al. *Carb Res.* 2013;doi:10.1016/J.carres.04.023.
2. Xu C, et al. *Vet J.* 2013;195:200.
3. Martinez-Moliner V, et al. *Microbiol.* 2012;158:2117.
4. Cerdd-Cuellar M, et al. *Vet Microbiol.* 2010;145:315.
5. Howell KJ, et al. *J Bacteriol.* 2013;195:e 4264.
6. Brockmeier SL, et al. *Clin Vacc Immunol.* 2013;20:1466.
7. Yu J, et al. *Vet Microbiol.* 2012;158:316.
8. Olvera AM, et al. *Vet Microbiol.* 2007;123:230.
9. Costa-Hurlado M, et al. *Vet Res.* 2012;43:57.
10. Olvera AM, et al. *Vet J.* 2007;174:522.
11. Aragon V, et al. *Vet Microbiol.* 2010;142:387.
12. Frandoloso R, et al. *Vet Microbiol.* 2012;154:347.
13. de la Fuente AJM, et al. *Res Vet Sci.* 2009;86:230.
14. Metcalf DS, MacInnes JL. *Can J Vet Res.* 2007;71:181.
15. Bouchet B, et al. *Microbial Pathogen.* 2009;46:108.
16. Vanier G, et al. *Microbiol.* 2006;152:135.
17. del Rio M, et al. *Vet Res.* 2006;37:49.
18. Mullins MA, et al. *J Bacteriol.* 2009;191:5988.
19. Strugnell BW, Woolfenden NJ. *Pig J.* 2011;65:43.
20. Angen V, et al. *Vet Microbiol.* 2007;119:266.
21. Yue M, et al. *J Bacteriol.* 2009;191:1359.
22. Dijkman R, et al. *Res Vet Sci.* 2012;93:585.
23. Kang I, et al. *Can J Vet Res.* 2012;76:195.
24. Turni C, et al. *Vet Microbiol.* 2009;108:1123.
25. Turni C, et al. *J Appl Microbiol.* 2010;108:1323.
26. Turni C, Blackall PJ. *J Vet Diag Invest.* 2011;23:355.
27. de la Fuente AJM, Tucker AW. *Vet Microbiol.* 2007;120:184.
28. Zhou M, et al. *Vaccine.* 2009;27:5271.
29. Li JK, et al. *Prev Vet Med.* 2009;91:274.
30. Palzer A, et al. *Vet Rec.* 2008;162:267.
31. Zhou SM, et al. *FEMS Microbiol Lett.* 2012;326:109.
32. Zhou SM, et al. *Vet J.* 2013;196:111.
33. De la Fuente AJM, et al. *J Com Path.* 2009;140:169.
34. san Millan A, et al. *Antomicrob Agents Chemother.* 2007;51:2260.
35. Dijkman R, et al. *Res Vet Sci.* 2012;93:589.
36. Hu M, et al. *Clin Vacc Immunol.* 2013;20:795.
37. Rodriguez-Ferri EF, et al. *Res Vet Sci.* 2010;88:385.

ARTHRITIS RESULTING FROM ERYSIPELAS

ERYSIPELAS IN SHEEP

Erysipelas in sheep is caused by infection with the soil-borne organism *Erysipelas rhusiopathiae* (formerly *Erysipelas insidiosa*). Pigs are the most important reservoir of infection, with up to 50% of healthy pigs carrying the bacterium in lymphoid tissues. The disease in sheep is manifested as arthritis in lambs, postdipping lameness, and rarely endocarditis. Sheep other than newly born lambs deprived of colostrum are generally quite resistant to infection with this organism.

Arthritis in Lambs

Acute and chronic forms of arthritis are seen.[1] Acute nonsuppurative arthritis occurs most commonly after tail docking, especially when a cold knife is used, but can also follow umbilical infections at or soon after birth. The organism persists in the soil and gains entry via the umbilicus or tail-docking and/or mulesing wounds. The latter practice is used to make merino lambs less susceptible to flystrike, mainly in Australia, but is gradually being phased out. Up to 50% of lambs marked may be affected, especially if tail docking is performed in muddy or unhygienic conditions. The mortality rate is low, but some affected lambs lose weight and have permanently swollen joints, leading to trimming of meat or rejection of the whole carcass at abattoirs.

Clinical signs appear about 14 days after birth or tail docking. There is a sudden onset of lameness with some swelling of the affected joints, typically the carpus, tarsus, hock, or stifle. Recovery is slow, and a high proportion of affected lambs have chronic lameness and swollen joints.

Chronic fibrinous polyarthritis also occurs in 2- to 6-month-old lambs, affecting several joints, and lambs may be lame on all four legs.[1] Up to 20% of lambs may be affected, although severe outbreaks with a higher prevalence are associated with spreading pig slurry or running free-range pigs on areas grazed by sheep. Arthritis in mature ewes can also occur in these circumstances.[2]

At necropsy the joint capsule is thickened, and there may be erosions of articular cartilage and slightly increased amount of synovial fluid that has a turbid appearance. There is no obvious suppuration as occurs with septic arthritis caused by streptococcal infection. In chronic cases the organism is usually only isolated from joints, but PCR testing indicates that it is also a multisystemic disease.[1]

Improved hygiene at tail docking will usually reduce the prevalence of *Erysipelas* arthritis, but a formalin-killed bacterin is available in many countries and may be indicated where there is a persistently high prevalence of infection.

Postdipping Lameness

The use of plunge dips to control ectoparasites in sheep can be followed by a high incidence of laminitis if the insecticide solution does not contain a suitable disinfectant. Dips that become grossly contaminated with organic matter are most likely to cause *Erysipelas* infection. The organism gains entry through skin abrasions and causes cellulitis, with extension to the laminae of the feet but without involving the joints. Up to 90% of a flock may be affected, although the incidence is usually about 25%. Similar outbreaks of lameness caused by *Erysipelas rhusiopathiae* have occurred without dipping, usually when sheep have to walk through wet, muddy areas likely to be contaminated with the organism.

Severe lameness begins 2 to 4 days after dipping, usually in one leg. The affected legs are hot and swollen from the coronet to halfway up the metacarpus or metatarsus, and the hair over the affected area usually falls out. Sheep rapidly lose body condition, but deaths are rare except in recently weaned lambs, in which septicemia may develop. Affected lambs show fever, malaise, and anorexia.

At necropsy there is subcutaneous edema of the area, sometimes with hemorrhage and inflammation extending to the coronet of the feet. Most cases recover spontaneously in 10 to 14 days, but long-acting penicillin will assist recovery. Wet dipping is now less common, but where dipping is still routinely practiced the use of fresh dipping solution each day and inclusion of a bacteriostatic agent into the solution will help prevent this condition.

Postdipping lameness can be differentiated from footrot by the history of recent dipping and lack of underrunning of the hoof tissue, from foot abscess by the lack of abscessation, and from strawberry footrot by the lack of any proliferative dermatitis.

REFERENCES

1. Ersdal C, et al. *Vet Path*. 2015;52:635.
2. Scott P. *Livestock Health*. 2013;18:80.

MYCOPLASMA HYOSYNOVIAE IN PIGS

Mycoplasmal arthritis caused by *M. hyosynoviae* occurs in growing and finishing pigs from 35 kg upward and is characterized clinically by lameness, frequently in newly purchased stock.

ETIOLOGY

M. hyosynoviae causes arthritis in growing pigs. *M. hyoarthrinosa* has been associated with a syndrome similar to that produced by *M. hyosynoviae*, but they may be the same species. Other mycoplasmas, including *M. flocculare* and *Acholeplasma* spp., have been isolated from pigs but appear to have no propensity to produce arthritis.

EPIDEMIOLOGY

M. hyosynoviae is a causative organism with a very wide heterogeneity and is resident on the pharyngeal mucosa and tonsil. Shedding is less frequent than with *M. hyorhinis*, and the organism cannot usually be isolated from the pharynx of piglets before 7 weeks of age and is regarded as rare before 12 weeks. This is true even when most of the sows in a herd are tonsillar carriers. There is a very varied pattern of carriage. It appears that transference is fairly rare but can be the source of infection for the other littermates. There is some variation in virulence between strains. With virulent strains, bacteremia with subsequent arthritis follows within a few days of minor stress, such as vaccination, movement, regrouping, or a change in weather. The overall prevalence of clinical disease appears to be low, but it achieves significance in certain herds that experience a persistent problem. The reasons for this are still unclear. Infection profiles between herds vary considerably. In some herds in the United Kingdom, the incidence may be higher, with 21% of sows culled because of lameness primarily associated with *M. hyosynoviae*. It appears that there is a latent period between the tonsillar infection and the development of generalized infection and arthritis, which may be accounted for by the long persistence of maternal antibodies of 8 to 16 weeks. The active serologic response possibly indicating immunity only seems to occur when there is the onset of arthritis. It is more prevalent in heavily muscled pigs with straight-legged conformation, and there is variation in breed susceptibility. Morbidity in problem herds is generally 5% to 15% but may reach 50%. Mortality is rare, but 2% to 15% may become chronically affected.

Abattoir studies have suggested that 5% to 10% of pigs may be affected. Transmission of infection is by direct contact or possibly by aerosol infection.

M. hyosynoviae can survive drying for up to 4 weeks and may be capable of survival in the environment for longer periods than most mycoplasmas. A further consideration of the importance of these diseases must be given to their possible contribution to the occurrence of carcass condemnation from arthritis.

PATHOGENESIS

The most important thing to remember about pathogenesis is that pigs can carry the infection in their tonsils and their synovial fluid without clinical signs of lameness and may therefore not be diagnosed as carriers and can act as a potential source of infection to others.

Systemic infection by mycoplasma may occur following stress. Clinical disease is manifest if localization occurs, but this is probably the exception rather than the rule. In the experimental disease, the incubation period varies from 4 to 10 days. After experimental intranasal infection with *M. hyosynoviae*, septicemia usually takes about 2 to 4 days to manifest. *M. hyosynoviae* produces synovitis with some arthritis, especially in the larger joints of the hindlimbs.

CLINICAL FINDINGS

Diagnosis is often difficult to make clinically. Often there is no fever and perhaps only a change in the gait of the pig. In these herds the sows are nearly always culled for lameness before the fourth parity, which constitutes a huge economic loss. Failure to treat leads to chronic lameness. Clinical disease occurs primarily in pigs over 3 months of age and in replacement stock brought into these problem herds.

With *M. hyosynoviae* infection, there is a sudden onset of acute lameness in one or more limbs, usually without fever. Lameness may be referable to one or more joints, and the stifle, hock, and elbow joints are most commonly affected. In many cases the pigs may lie in sternal recumbency. The lameness is severe, although clinical swelling of the affected joint may be minimal. In the majority of affected pigs, clinical recovery occurs after 3 to 10 days, but some may become permanently recumbent. In the United Kingdom, the condition is often associated with delivery of high-herd-health gilts to more conventional farms, with the condition occurring 2 days to 4 weeks after the delivery or with a change of housing. Other outbreaks have followed the introduction of pigs to straw yards, whereas contemporary animals kept in fully slatted accommodation have been unaffected. *M. hyosynoviae*-infected pigs may require humane slaughter.

CLINICAL PATHOLOGY

Blood cell counts remain within the normal range, but there is an increase in leukocytes and protein in synovial fluid. The organisms may be detected by immunofluorescent techniques, and complement-fixing antibody develops following infection.

PATHOLOGY

Synovial hypertrophy with an increased amount of serosanguinous synovial fluid occurs in affected joints with hyosynoviae. Sometimes the amount of fluid is considerable. Chronic cases show thickening of the joint capsule with a varying degree of articular erosion and pannus formation. Joint lesions are most likely to be found in the carpus, shoulder, stifle, and tarsus. Quite often with *M. hyosynoviae* infections, one joint—usually the hock—is affected.

Microscopically, there is usually edema, hyperemia, hyperplasia of synovial cells, and an increased density of subsynovial cells. Lymphocytes and plasma cells are present in the affected serosal and synovial membranes of subacute to chronic cases. There is often a significant villus hypertrophy of the synovial membrane. In the chronic phase, there may be some fibrosis. A full description of the phases of infection has recently been described. The organism is more easily demonstrated during the acute stage of the disease.

DIAGNOSIS

Clinical signs may help. Joint fluid may be helpful in that it is often clear or yellowish-brown and may contain flakes of fibrin. In streptococcal arthritis, the fluid is often hemorrhagic and turbid.

Samples for Confirmation of Diagnosis

- Histology—synovial membrane, liver, lung, heart. Sometimes the mycoplasmas can be seen between the synoviocytes on the tips of the villi of the synovial membrane.
- Mycoplasmology—culture swabs from serosal surfaces, joints. Selective media is usually required to suppress *M. hyorhinis.*
- *M. hyosynoviae* is best grown in anaerobic conditions, where it outgrows *M. hyorhinis.*
- Synovial fluid has been taken from the hock joint under general anesthesia and cultured. Isolation from the joints of lame pigs was twice as high as from littermates that were not lame. Approximately 8% to 9% of synovial fluid samples from nonpatent arthritis samples from Danish slaughterhouse pigs were positive. The same authors also showed that blood culture was also effective.
- Antigen detection. An in situ hybridization technique for the differentiation of *M. hyosynoviae, M. hyorhinis,* and *M. hyopneumoniae* has been described for use with formalin-fixed tissues.
- PCR can be used to amplify a p36 or p46 gene to differentiate *M. hyorhinis* and *M. hyosynoviae* infections for use in cultures and in blood samples.
- Serology—it has been shown that herds with *M. hyosynoviae* arthritis had higher serologic responses and more carriers among growers of 16-week-old pigs than did the unaffected herds, but by the end of the finishing period, the serologic response and carrier prevalence were as high in herds with arthritis as without.
- An indirect ELISA has been developed using membrane lipoprotein antigens and appears to be specific.

The differential diagnosis of mycoplasma infections must include *S. suis* and *H. parasuis.*

TREATMENT

When gilts and sows are treated, they do not appear to have a reduced overall survival time, indicating that treatment is cost-effective.

Treatment with tylosin at 1 to 2 mg up to 15 mg/kg BW IM or Lincomycin at 2.5 mg/kg BW IM for 3 consecutive days has been recommended. Lincomycin was effective in one outbreak, but the outbreak flared up again as soon as it was removed. Oxytetracycline also can be used. Early treatment of *M. hyosynoviae* arthritis with 8 mg of betamethasone IM has been found to reduce the occurrence of chronic lameness. Tiamulin at both 10 and 15 mg/kg BW IM daily for 3 days is effective for treatment of pigs affected with arthritis associated with *M. hyosynoviae* and is as effective as Lincomycin. Recently, enrofloxacin has been used at 2.1 mg/kg IM or SC for 3 days. It is essential to treat the in-contacts and to isolate the treated animals until the clinical signs have disappeared. Valnemulin was highly active against *M. hyosynoviae,* whereas tiamulin and enrofloxacin were much less active.

CONTROL

The control of mycoplasmal joint disease rests largely in the avoidance of stress situations. The administration of tylosin or tetracyclines in the drinking water or feed during unavoidable stress such as weaning can reduce the incidence. The use of tiamulin as a single injection before moving pigs from one house to another was sufficient to prevent 50% of the cases of the disease. Early weaning at 3 to 5 weeks of age has been recommended as a method of preventing infection of pigs with *M. hyosynoviae* and thus of reducing the occurrence of the disease in growing pigs. However, in one study *M. hyosynoviae* was not eliminated in herds where the piglets were commingled after 4 weeks and reared in herds using all-in/all-out management. In fact, the herd had widespread infection when the herd was 4 months old. The authors concluded that elimination of *M. hyosynoviae* requires that the pigs are moved immediately from weaning at an age of no more than 4 weeks. If newly arrived gilts are under threat, usually 14 to 21 days after arrival, then a course of treatment such as Lincomycin in the water for 2 to 3 days may prevent the infection.

FURTHER READING

Hagedorn-Olsen T Mycoplasma hyosynoviae arthritis in pigs. PhD thesis, Royal Veterinary and Agricultural University, Copenhagen, Denmark; 1997.

FOOTROT IN PIGS (BUSH FOOT)

Footrot in pigs is similar clinically to footrot in other species. It is a term describing septic conditions of the claws of the foot, which burst at the coronet.

ETIOLOGY

The majority of cases result from secondary infection of traumatic lesions. These are erosions of the sole and wall of the claw that occur in pigs reared on rough, abrasive flooring. These lesions do not usually produce lameness, unless they are extensive, but when pigs are also reared in dirty conditions, infection and subsequent lameness may occur.

Foot lesions are common in pigs of all ages, and bruising of the sole–heel junction, one of the earliest lesions observed, can be seen in piglets less than 24 hours old. If the bruising is severe and further trauma is not prevented, necrosis will follow quickly. The cause may be a combination of factors, including trauma, contact dermatitis, and subsequent infection. Wet conditions underfoot may cause maceration of the horn and exacerbate the abrasive effect of the flooring. Foot abscess in neonatal pigs is associated with being reared on woven-wire floors. Dietary deficiency, especially biotin deficiency, may also result in foot lesions that predispose to secondary infection.[1,2]

Fusiformis necrophorum, Trueperella pyogenes, Staphylococci and an unidentified spirochete have been isolated from affected feet. In an outbreak of the disease on a semiextensive pig farm, *Dichelobacter nodosus* and other anaerobic bacteria, including *Prevotella, Peptostreptococcus, Fusobacterium, Porphyromomonas, Bacteroides,* and *Eubacterium,* have also been isolated from affected feet.

EPIDEMIOLOGY

The disease is probably universal. A study of the prevalence and distribution of foot lesions in finishing pigs in England found that 94% of pigs had at least one foot lesion. The prevalence of the different lesions was as follows: toe erosion (33%), sole erosion (62%), heel erosion (13%), heel flaps (14%), white-line lesions (55%), false sand cracks (24%), and wall separation (11%). The hindfeet are more commonly affected than the front feet, and on each foot the lateral digits were significantly more frequently affected than the medial digits. Sole erosions, heel flaps, wall separation, and false sand cracks were observed more frequently on the lateral than the medial digit.

Erosive lesions on the foot are common and have been reported at an incidence as high as 65%. They have been reproduced experimentally, and the nature of the flooring has a marked influence on claw wear in pigs. Recently poured alkaline concrete and poorly laid concrete with constituents leading to a rough abrasive surface lead to a high incidence. A slope inadequate to allow proper drainage may also be an important predisposing factor. All ages of pigs are susceptible, but clinical lameness is uncommon. In individual herds where the unfavorable predisposing factors prevail, a high incidence of infection and clinical lameness can occur. The disease may cause reproductive inefficiency as a result of reluctance to stand or mount for mating.

PATHOGENESIS

Perforation of the horn leads to infection of the sensitive laminae. The infection may track up the sensitive laminae to the coronary band and discharge to the exterior. Elastolytic activity is a virulence factor involved in the pathogenesis of footrot in pigs associated with *Dichelobacter nodosus* and *Prevotella melaninogenica.*

CLINICAL FINDINGS

Where the disease is caused by abrasion of the horn by rough concrete surfaces, a number of characteristic lesions occur, including the following:

1. Erosion of the sole at either the toe or the heel
2. Bruising of the sole with hemorrhagic streaks in the horn
3. Separation of the hard horny wall from the heel or sole to produce a fissure at the white line
4. A false sand crack in the posterior third of the lateral wall of the claw

In the majority of cases these do not produce lameness, and they do not have any apparent effect on productivity. However, when they are extensive, where infection has occurred, and when more than one foot is affected, severe lameness is apparent. In most cases only the lateral digit of one foot is affected. Heat and obvious pain when moderate pressure is applied to the affected claw are constant findings. Necrosis extends up between the sole and sensitive laminae and may discharge at the coronet, causing the development of a granulomatous lesion, or it may extend to deeper structures of the foot with multiple sinuses discharging to the exterior. A minimal amount of purulent material is present. Productivity is affected with this type of lesion. With deeply infected feet, the recovery rate is only fair with treatment. A permanently deformed foot may result, and destruction of the pig may be necessary in severe cases. Secondary abscessation in other parts of the body is an occasional sequela and may result in partial carcass condemnation.

Foot abscesses in neonatal pigs are characterized by necrotic pododermatitis, severe osteomyelitis, arthritis, and tenosynovitis. The primary sites of injury are located at either the point of the toe at the white line, the bulb of the heel, or the haired skin around the coronet, including the interdigital area. The least severe lesions are superficial abrasions or ulcerations of the hoof wall, heel bulb, or interphalangeal skin, with only minimal inflammatory changes in deeper tissues. The most severely affected digits have focal superficial abscesses, or deep, diffuse, purulent inflammation and fibrosis around tendons, joints, and bones. The hindlimbs are more commonly affected than the forelimbs, and in the hindlimbs the medial claws are most likely to have lesions, whereas in the forelimbs the lateral claws are more likely to be affected. Approximately 6% of piglets develop foot abscess before weaning. About one-third of litters may be affected, and most litters have only one or two affected pigs. Discharge of pus from the coronary band is common, and the horny claw may slough, leaving sensitive laminae of one or more claws or accessory digits exposed. Skin necrosis may be present over the carpi, fetlocks, hocks, coronary bands, and elbows in about 75% of pigs during the first week of life.

CLINICAL PATHOLOGY

Bacteriologic examination of discharges from the lesions may aid in deciding the treatment to be used. In foot abscesses of neonatal pigs, bacteria isolated include the following:

- *Trueperella pyogenes*
- *Staphylococcus* spp.
- Beta-hemolytic *Streptococcus* spp.
- *Actinobacillus* spp.
- *Escherichia coli*

NECROPSY FINDINGS

Necrosis of the laminar tissue with indications of progression from an infected sole are the usual findings. There may be progression to tenosynovitis.[3]

DIFFERENTIAL DIAGNOSIS

Most other causes of lameness in pigs are not manifested by foot lesions. Bursitis, adventitious bursitis, and laminitis may occasionally be found. In young pigs they are not uncommon as a result of bad flooring (sharp metal and plastic and coarse concrete). These are seen as early as 24 hours, peak at 4 to 8 days, and are usually gone by 14 days. In adult pigs housed indoors, an overgrowth of the hoof may occur and be followed by underrunning of the sole, necrosis, and the protrusion of granulation tissue, causing severe lameness and often persistent recumbency. The general appearance of these feet is not unlike that of canker in horses. Swelling of the hoof is caused by an extensive fibrous tissue reaction. Vesicular exanthema and foot-and-mouth disease are characterized by the presence of vesicular lesions on the coronets and snout.

TREATMENT

There are few published reports of treatment of footrot in pigs. Rubber mats in the farrowing house may prevent some of the worst effects for piglets. Use of a broad-spectrum antimicrobial or penicillin given parenterally seems rational, and the use of Nuflor was said to be a successful treatment.

CONTROL

Prevention of excessive wear of the feet by the use of adequate bedding and less abrasive flooring in pig pens is suggested as a reasonable control measure. Slats should be round edged and have a minimum width of at least 100 mm. Any existing dietary deficiency should be corrected. Of particular interest is the response to biotin supplementation of the diet of pigs in the prevention of foot lesions of various kinds. Regular foot care and paring of excessive growth is important. Formalin foot baths (5% to 10%, 2 to 3 times a week) may also reduce bacterial infection.

REFERENCES

1. Fitzgerald RF, et al. *Livestock Sci.* 2012;145:230.
2. Knauer M, et al. *Prev Vet Med.* 2007;82:198.
3. Kilkbride AL, et al. *BMC Vet Res.* 2009;5:31.

ROSS RIVER VIRUS

ETIOLOGY

Ross River virus is an alphavirus within the Semliki Forest complex of togaviruses. These are small enveloped viruses with a single-stranded, positive sense RNA genome. There is considerable sequence homology between Getah and Ross River virus genomes.[1] Ross River virus causes disease in both humans and horses.

EPIDEMIOLOGY

Ross River virus is found in most areas of continental Australia, Tasmania, West Papua and Papua New Guinea, New Caledonia, Fiji, Samoa, and the Cook Islands.[2] There is geographic genetic variability among isolates of Ross River virus. There is serologic evidence of lack of infection of cattle by RRV in the Coromandel region of New Zealand.[3]

The virus is arthropod borne, and infection is through the bite of an infected mosquito. The virus is maintained in the mosquito–vertebrate–mosquito host cycle typical of arboviruses. The vertebrate hosts of Ross River virus include a large number of eutherian, marsupial, and monotreme mammals and birds.[2] Macropod species, including kangaroos and wallabies, are assumed to be the most important amplifying hosts, although this is debated. There is a high prevalence of serologically positive Western Grey kangaroos (48%).[4]

There is a high incidence of Ross River virus infection of horses in endemic regions of Australia, and the prevalence was shown to be increased with year-round mosquito activity. The proportion of seropositive horses in Queensland, an area in with year-round mosquito activity, was approximately 80%, whereas that of horses around the Gippsland lakes in southern Australia, a region with seasonal mosquito activity, was 50%. Outbreaks of clinical disease attributed to Ross River virus infection of horses occurred in southeastern Australia in late 2010 and early 2011 and were also associated with serologic and virological evidence of infection by Murray Valley encephalitis virus and Kunjin virus (a lineage of West Nile virus).[5] During the outbreak, which was associated with unusually wet summer conditions in an area characterized by hot, dry summers, 392 horses on 271 premises were suspected or confirmed to have been infected by one or more of these arboviruses.

Zoonotic Implications

Disease associated with Ross River virus infection is common in humans in Australia, with an estimated 4800 cases per year, and much larger numbers during epidemics of the disease.[2] The horse is thought to be an amplifying host of the virus because experimentally infected horses can infect mosquitoes. Direct transmission from the horse, however, would be primarily occupational. The disease in humans is characterized by mild pyrexia and constitutional signs initially, with subsequent development of a rash on the skin and oral lesions. Arthritis or arthralgia is common and affects primarily the wrists, knees, ankles, and small joints of the extremities. These signs and symptoms can persist for 2 to 3 months, and the disease can relapse.

CLINICAL SIGNS

The disease associated with Ross River virus infection of horses is typified by pyrexia; petechial hemorrhages; submandibular lymphadenopathy; lameness, including "stiffness"; swollen joints or distal limbs; inappetence; reluctance to move; and mild colic.[5,6] Horses are often described as being ataxic, although the neurologic basis of this sign is unclear. Any previous skepticism regarding the pathogenicity of Ross River virus in horses was addressed by the outbreak of disease caused by Ross River virus during 2010 and 2011 in southeastern Australia. Disease associated with confirmed Ross River virus infection was characterized by ataxia, stiff gait, depression, edema, listlessness, pyrexia, and reluctance to walk. Horses infected experimentally with Ross River virus have minimal clinical signs of disease. The duration of disease caused by Ross River virus in horses is uncertain, and some veterinarians consider that the disease can persist for weeks to months, and it can recur in horses.

There are insufficient reports of disease to determine whether characteristic or diagnostic abnormalities in serum biochemistry or hematology occur in affected horses. An elevated concentration of fibrinogen in plasma was reported in all of three horses with the presumptive disease that were tested.

DIAGNOSIS

Diagnosis of infection by Ross River virus is confirmed by virus isolation from serum or heparinized blood samples collected during the acute phase of the disease or detection in serum of antibodies to the virus. Detection of IgM antibodies to Ross River virus is indicative of recent infection, whereas detection of IgG or neutralizing antibodies is indicative of more distant infection. Seroconversion confirms exposure, and presumably infection, by the virus. Isolation of Ross River virus has been achieved from horses with IgM antibody to the virus but not with IgG antibody, likely because of the temporal pattern of antibody appearance in the blood of infected horses.[6] In addition to culture of the virus in mice or tissue culture, Ross River virus can be detected in blood and synovial fluid using an RT-PCR. It is important to remember that subclinical infection of horses in endemic regions is very common and that this high rate of subclinical infection increases the risk of incorrect diagnosis of infection by the virus. It is possible that clinical abnormalities in a horse with Ross River viremia or serum antibodies to the virus are actually not attributable to infection by Ross River virus. This is extremely significant in that there are no reports of postmortem examination of horses with disease confirmed to be caused by Ross River Virus. Thus case definition in terms of postmortem confirmatory diagnostics has not been established.

TREATMENT

Treatment of affected horse is supportive. Affected horses might benefit from administration of analgesics and antipyretics such as phenylbutazone. Administration of antimicrobials is not indicated in uncomplicated cases.

CONTROL

Control measures have not been evaluated, but minimizing the exposure of horses to infected mosquitoes is prudent, although the efficacy of this technique in preventing infection is unknown. There is no vaccine to prevent infection or disease of horses by Ross River Virus. There is an experimental vaccine for humans.[7]

REFERENCES

1. Zhai Y-g, et al. *J Gen Virol.* 2008;89:1446.
2. Jacups SP, et al. *Vector-Borne Zoonot.* 2008;8:283.
3. McFadden AMJ, et al. *NZ Vet J.* 2009;57:116.
4. Potter A, et al. *Vector-Borne Zoonot.* 2014;14:740.
5. Roche SE, et al. *Aust Vet J.* 2013;91:5.
6. El-Hage CM, et al. *Aust Vet J.* 2008;86:367.
7. Wressnigg N, et al. *Clin Vac Immunol.* 2015;22:267.

Nutritional Diseases Affecting the Musculoskeletal System

SELENIUM AND/OR VITAMIN E DEFICIENCIES

Several diseases of farm animals are associated with a deficiency of either selenium (Se) or vitamin E (VE) alone or in combination, usually in association with predisposing factors such as dietary polyunsaturated fatty acids, unaccustomed exercise, and rapid growth in young animals. All of these diseases are described under one heading because both Se and VE are important in the etiology, treatment, and control of the major diseases caused by their deficiencies.

There are also **selenium–vitamin E–responsive diseases** because, with some exceptions, they can be prevented by adequate supplementation of the diet with both nutrients. In some regions of the world, particularly New Zealand and in parts of Australia and North America, diseases such as ill-thrift in sheep and cattle and poor reproductive performance respond beneficially to Se. Although these cases usually occur in Se-deficient regions, they may not be attributable solely to Se deficiency. Thus there are some reasonably well-defined **selenium-deficiency diseases** and some ill-defined **"selenium-responsive" diseases**.

There is more concern with these diseases now because it is becoming increasingly important to make sure that milk and meat are not deficient in Se and VE from the human nutrition point of view. Deficient meat makes for deficient humans.

More and more oxidants, antioxidants, and oxidative stress disorders are featuring in human and animal diseases. At least theoretically, oxidative stress should be easily prevented with antioxidants, but such therapy is controversial.[1]

In addition, there is an increasing recognition of the importance of toxic oxygen radicals (free-oxygen radicals) produced in the body that are neutralized by antioxidants and that may or not be effective resulting in an oxidative stress.[2,3] This focus is particularly important in ruminant medicine[4] with respect to sepsis, mastitis, pneumonia, and retained placenta.

ETIOLOGY

The Se- and VE-responsive or deficiency diseases of farm animals are caused by diets deficient in Se and/or VE, with or without the presence of conditioning factors such as an excessive quantity of polyunsaturated fatty acids in the diet. Almost all of the diseases that occur naturally have been reproduced experimentally using diets deficient in Se and/or VE. Conversely, the lesions can usually be prevented with Se and VE supplementation. In certain instances, such as, for example, in hand-fed dairy calves, the incorporation of excessive quantities of polyunsaturated fatty acids was a major factor in the experimental disease. The presence of polyunsaturated fatty acids in the diet may cause a conditioned VE deficiency because the vitamin acts as an antioxidant. In the case of naturally occurring muscular dystrophy in calves, lambs, and foals on pasture, the myopathic agent, if any, is unknown, and selenium is protective. However, Se is not protective against the muscular dystrophy associated with the feeding of cod liver oil to calves.

SYNOPSIS

Etiology Dietary deficiencies of selenium and vitamin E and conditioning factors such as dietary polyunsaturated fatty acids.

Epidemiology

- **Enzootic muscular dystrophy** occurs in young, rapidly growing calves, lambs, goat kids, and foals born to dams in selenium-deficient areas with unsupplemented diets. Occurs worldwide and common in Australasia, United Kingdom, and Great Plains of North America where soils are deficient in selenium. Vitamin E deficiency in animals fed poor-quality forage and diets high in polyunsaturated fatty acids. Outbreaks of muscular dystrophy precipitated by exercise.
- **Mulberry heart disease** in finishing pigs.
- **Selenium-responsive diseases** occur in Australasia and are not obvious clinically but respond to selenium supplementation. Selenium and vitamin E deficiency may be involved in reproductive performance, retained placenta in cattle, and resistance to infectious disease such as bovine mastitis. Controversial.

Signs Muscular dystrophy characterized by groups of animals with stiffness, weakness, and recumbency; severe in myocardial form. Mulberry heart disease characterized by outbreaks of sudden death in finishing pigs.

Clinical pathology Increased plasma levels of creatine kinase. Low serum levels of selenium and vitamin E. Glutathione peroxidase activity.

Necropsy findings Bilaterally symmetric pale skeletal muscle; pale streaks in myocardial muscle. Hyaline degeneration of affected muscle.

Diagnostic confirmation Low selenium and vitamin E in diet and tissues; increased creatine kinase and muscle degeneration.

Differential diagnosis list

Acute muscular dystrophy in calves and yearlings

- *Haemophilus somnus* septicemia
- Pneumonia

Subacute enzootic muscular dystrophy:

- **Musculoskeletal diseases**—polyarthritis, traumatic or infectious myopathies (blackleg), osteodystrophy, and fractures of long bones
- **Diseases of the nervous system**—spinal cord compression, *Haemophilus somnus* meningoencephalitis and myelitis, organophosphatic insecticide poisoning
- **Diseases of the digestive tract**—carbohydrate engorgement resulting in lactic acidosis, shock, dehydration, and weakness
- Muscular dystrophy in lambs and kids—enzootic ataxia and swayback
- Muscular dystrophy in foals—traumatic injury to the musculoskeletal system and polyarthritis; meningitis; traumatic injury to the spinal cord

Treatment Vitamin E selenium parenterally.

Control Selenium and vitamin E supplementation of diet; strategic oral and/or parenteral vitamin E and selenium to pregnant dams or young animals on pasture.

Se is an essential nutrient for animals, and diseases caused by Se inadequacy in livestock are of worldwide distribution.

Biological Functions of Selenium and Vitamin E (VE)

Selenium

Selenium is the component of over 30 selenoproteins[5] that protect cells from damage by free radicals, the cause of many chronic diseases.[6] The Se is present as selenocysteine in the selenoproteins. It is the 21st amino acid. The selenoproteins also participate in the metabolism of thyroid hormones, control reproductive functions, and exert neuroprotective effects. In addition to its antiproliferative and antiinflammatory effects, SE also stimulates the immune system via the macrophages, neutrophils, and lymphocytes. Se stimulates the T-helper cells, cytotoxic T cells, and natural killer (NK) cells. It is aided by VE and sulfur-containing amino acids. Se-containing proteins may have a role in muscle formation and repair.[7] Deficiencies can result in nutritional muscular dystrophy (white-muscle disease) in lambs, kids, calves, and poultry; exudative diatheses in poultry; and necrotic liver degeneration and mulberry heart disease in pigs. In cattle, it is also associated with parturition problems, placental retention, and metritis. Se deficiency also contributes to the formation of ovarian cysts and increased early embryonic mortality. VE and Se also facilitate leukocyte migration into the mammary glands and enhance neutrophil phagocytosis, which helps in the fight against mastitis.

One of these proteins is selenoprotein W, first identified in sheep suffering from Se deficiency; the majority of its functions are unknown, but it serves as an antioxidant, responds to stress, and is involved in cell immunity.[8] In sheep given sodium selenite and selenium nanoparticles, it was shown that expression of transferrin and its receptor genes was considerably increased during supplementation by both Se components for 10 to 20 days and then decreased significantly.[9] It is close to sulfur in terms of properties.[10] It is largely absorbed through the duodenum and the cecum by active transport through a sodium pump.

Long-term supplementation (0.3%) with organic Se modulates the gene-expression profiles in leukocytes of adult pigs; 28 genes were up-regulated and 24 down-regulated by the Se supplementation, leading to improved expression of genes that are related to enhanced immunity of pigs.[11]

Glutathione Peroxidases and Tissue Peroxidation

Se is a biochemical component of the enzyme glutathione peroxidase (GSH-PX).[12] The activity of the enzyme in erythrocytes is positively related to the blood concentration of Se in cattle, sheep, horses, and pigs and is a useful aid for the diagnosis of Se deficiency and to determine the Se status of the tissues of these animals. The enzyme from the erythrocytes of both cattle and sheep contains 4 g atoms of selenium per 1 mol of enzyme. Se is also a component of thyroid gland hormones and is very important in converting T4 to T3 (i.e., inactive to active).[13]

Plasma GSH-PX protects cellular membranes and lipid-containing organelles from peroxidative damage by inhibition and destruction of endogenous peroxides, acting in conjunction with VE to maintain the integrity of these membranes. Hydrogen peroxide and lipid peroxides are capable of causing irreversible denaturation of essential cellular proteins, which leads to degeneration and necrosis. GSH-PX catalyzes the breakdown of hydrogen peroxide and certain organic hydroperoxides produced by glutathione during the process of redox cycling. This dependence of GSH-PX activity on the presence of Se offers an explanation for the interrelationship of Se, VE, and sulfur-containing amino acids in animals. The sulfur-containing amino acids may be precursors of glutathione, which in turn acts as a substrate for GSH-PX and maintains sulfhydryl groups in the cell. Se is also a component of several other proteins, such as the selenoprotein of muscle (selenoflagellin), Se-transport proteins, and the bacterial enzymes formate dehydrogenase and glycine reductase. Se also facilitates significant changes in the metabolism of many drugs and xenobiotics. For example, Se functions to counteract the toxicity of several metals, such as arsenic, cadmium, mercury, copper, silver, and lead.

Vitamin

VE is important in the general immune response because it affects the blood cell populations and, in particular, the persistence of the immune response. Together with vitamins A and D and Se, it increases reproductive performance.[14]

The term "vitamin E" is a generic description encompassing two families of lipid-soluble compounds, the tocopherols and the tocotrienols, of which alpha-tocopherol is the most active.[15] VE is an antioxidant that prevents oxidative damage to sensitive membrane lipids by decreasing hydroperoxide formation. The vitamin has a central role in protection of cellular membranes from lipoperoxidation, especially membranes rich in unsaturated lipids, such as mitochondria, endoplasmic reticulum, and plasma membranes.

Cows discriminate against the 2S isomers of the synthetic form, which contains all eight isomers (4 of 2R and 4 of 2S). This means that 1 g of all-rac is actually 0.5 g of the RRR form.[15]

It has been observed that low serum alpha-tocopherol levels are possibly indicative of a disposition to left-sided displaced abomasum in early-lactating dairy cows.[16] Organic farms have more VE than conventional ones, and grass clover silage is the best source of VE compared with hay, maize, or grain. Silage is a better source of tocopherols than hay as a result of high storage losses in the latter, and ensiled grasses and legumes have more VE than maize silage.[17]

Interrelationships Between Selenium and Vitamin E

An important interrelationship exists between Se, VE, and the sulfur-containing amino acids in preventing some of the nutritional diseases caused by their deficiency. If VE prevents fatty acid hydroperoxide formation, and the sulfur amino acids (as precursors of GSH-PX) and Se are involved in peroxide destruction, these nutrients would produce a similar biochemical result, that is, lowering of the concentration of peroxides or peroxide-induced products in the tissues. Protection against oxidative damage to susceptible nonmembrane proteins by dietary Se, but not by VE, might explain why some nutritional diseases respond to Se but not to VE. On the other hand, certain tissues or subcellular components may not be adequately protected from oxidant damage because they are inherently low in GSH-PX even with adequate dietary Se. Damage to such tissues would be expected to be aggravated by diets high in unsaturated fatty acids and to respond adequately to VE but not to Se. The variations in GSH-PX activity between certain tissues, such as liver, heart, skeletal, and myocardial muscles, would explain the variations in the severity of lesions between species.

There are both selenium-dependent GSH-PX and nonselenium-dependent GSH-PX activities in the tissues and blood. The nonselenium-dependent enzyme does not contain Se and does not react with hydrogen peroxide but shows activity toward organic hydroperoxide substrates. The spleen, cardiac muscle, erythrocytes, brain, thymus, adipose tissue, and striated muscles of calves contain only the selenium-dependent enzyme. The liver, lungs, adrenal glands, testes, and kidney contain both enzymes. Hepatic tissue contains the highest level of nonselenium-dependent enzyme.

VE can prevent a toxic reaction to oral iron (ferrous sulfate) or iron dextran IM. When 0.1 ppm of Se and 50 IU VE/kg are added during the gestation of sows, glutathione peroxidase activity increased in 2-day-old pigs, especially if the iron injection is given before colostrum ingestion.

EPIDEMIOLOGY

Enzootic Nutritional Muscular Dystrophy

Enzootic nutritional muscular dystrophy (NMD) was the first disorder linked with Se and was associated with a high mortality, especially in ruminants, and impaired production in growing and adult animals.

Occurrence

This type of muscular dystrophy occurs in all farm animal species, but most commonly in young, rapidly growing calves, lambs, goat kids, and foals born from dams that have been fed for long periods, usually during the winter months, on diets low in Se and VE. It is an important cause of mortality in goat kids from birth to about 3 months of age. Goat kids may require more Se than lambs or calves, which may explain the higher incidence of the disease in kids. The disease in kids may also be associated with low α-tocopherol levels and normal Se status.

NMD in horses occurs most commonly in foals to about 7 months of age. In reported cases, the concentration of Se in the blood of the mares was subnormal, the concentrations of Se and VE in the feedstuffs were subnormal, the level of unsaturated fatty acids in the feed was high, and VE and Se supplementation prevented the disease. The disease is not well recognized in adult horses, but sporadic cases of dystrophic myodegeneration are recorded in horses from 5 to 10 years of age. The disease also occurs in grain-fed yearling cattle. Stressors such as being turned outdoors after winter housing, walking long distances, the jostling and movement associated with vaccination, and dehorning procedures and similar management practices are often precipitating factors. The disease has occurred in steers and bulls 12 to 18 months of age under feedlot conditions. There may even be laboratory evidence of subclinical myopathy in normal animals in a group from which an index case occurred. Outbreaks of severe and fatal NMD have occurred in heifers, at the time of parturition, that were previously on a diet deficient in both Se and VE. The disease may also occur sporadically in adult horses that are deficient in Se. Muscular dystrophy has occurred in Bohemian Red Poll mature dairy cows in the Czech Republic moved from a stanchion barn into loose box housing that resulted in increased locomotor activity and stress associated with the change in housing conditions.

Myopathy and hepatic lipidosis in weaned lambs deficient in VE without concurrent Se deficiency has been described.

There are two major syndromes of myopathy:

- An acute form—myocardial dystrophy, which occurs most commonly in young calves and lambs and occasionally foals
- A subacute form—skeletal muscular dystrophy, which occurs in older calves and yearling cattle.

The two forms are not mutually exclusive.

Geographic Distribution

NMD occurs in most countries of the world but is common in the United Kingdom, the United States, Scandinavia, Europe, Canada, Australia, and New Zealand. In North America, it is common in the Northeast and Northwest and uncommon on the relatively high-Se soils of the Great Plains, where Se toxicity has occurred. It is one of most common deficiency diseases of farm livestock in the United States. In the Czech Republic, the incidence of Se deficiency in cattle is high and most frequently diagnosed in heifers, feeder bulls, grazed beef cattle, and dairy cows in the dry period. Surveys of live cattle in the Czech Republic and in cattle tissues obtained at slaughter have found significant deficiency of Se. Poor-Se status, as assessed from blood, muscle, and liver Se concentrations, was found in 80%, 70%, and 73% of the tested animals, respectively. White-muscle disease has occurred in lambs in Turkey, where the levels of Se in the hay and soil are deficient. The mean values of Se in the soil and hay were 0.03 ppm and 0.07 ppm, respectively.

NMD is endemic in grazing goats on the Mexican plateau because of Se deficiency in the soil and forages. In two different locations of the plateau, the concentration of Se in the soil was 0.047 and 0.051 ppm; in the forages, 0.052 and 0.075 ppm; and in the serum of goats, 0.02 and 0.21 ppm, respectively. The pH of the soil was 6.1 and 5.9, respectively. The mean concentration of Se in the serum of kids with clinical signs of NMD was 36% lower compared with kids from the same farm that were normal.

Based on bulk-tank milk Se concentrations compared with serum Se concentrations in dairy herds in Prince Edward Island, Canada, 59% of the herds were at some point marginal or deficient in Se, which places them at risk of disease and suboptimal production. The periods of greatest risk were in the fall and winter, when 5% and 4%, respectively, of herds fell in the range of true deficiency. Herds in which Se supplementation was provided from a commercial dairy concentrate were over 4 times more likely to be selenium adequate than herds not using this method, and adjusted average daily milk yield was 7.6% greater in herds determined to be selenium adequate compared with selenium-marginal herds. In Chile, bulk-tank milk samples may show low levels of Se as a result of low-Se soil.[18]

Soils, and therefore the pastures they carry, vary widely in their Se content, depending largely on their geological origin. In general, soils derived from rocks of recent origin (e.g., the granitic and pumice sands of New Zealand) are notably deficient in Se. Soils derived from igneous rocks are likely to be low in Se. Sedimentary rocks, which are the principal parent material of agricultural soils, are richer in Se. Forage crops, cereal grains, and corn grown in these areas are usually low in Se content (below 0.1 mg/kg dry matter [DM]) compared with the concentration in crops (above 0.1 mg/kg DM) grown in areas where the available soil Se is much higher and usually adequate. The disease occurs in pigs, usually in association with other more serious diseases, such as mulberry heart disease and hepatosis dietetica.

Selenium in Soil, Plants, and Animals

Selenium in Soils

Soils containing less than 0.5 mg/kg of Se are likely to support crops and pastures with potentially inadequate Se concentrations (<0.05 mg/kg DM).

Selenium in Plants

Plants vary in their uptake of Se, but it is not a requirement for plant growth. The Se content of different pasture species on the same soil type does vary widely, but slow-growing and more deeply rooting species contain slightly higher concentrations. In New Zealand, the most deficient soils consist of rhyolitic pumice in the central volcanic plateau of the North Island. Peat soils in the Waikaito River Valley are also deficient. North Island coastal sands and stony soils in several locations are considered to be selenium responsive, whereas most of the South Island is at least marginally deficient.

Se deficiency occurs in most soils in the Balkan region; for example, the Se in wheat is so low that the daily requirement would not be met.[19] In the United States, the states of the Pacific Northwest and of the northeastern and southeastern seaboard are generally low in Se. In Canada, western prairie grains generally contain relatively high levels of Se, whereas in the eastern provinces, soils and feedstuffs usually have low Se concentrations. Most soils in the Atlantic provinces of Canada are acidic, and consequently, the forages are deficient in Se. Most forage samples contain less than 0.10 mg/kg DM of Se, and enzootic nutritional muscular dystrophy is common throughout the region.

Surveys in the United Kingdom found that the Se status may be low in sheep and cattle fed locally produced feedstuffs without any mineral supplementation. In some surveys, up to 50% of farms were low in Se, which places a large number of animals at risk. There are also differences in the Se concentrations of different feeds grown in the same area. For example, in some areas 75% of cattle fed primarily corn silage, or 50% of the cattle fed sedge hay, might be receiving diets inadequate in Se.

Factors Influencing the Availability of Soil Selenium to Plants. The Se concentration in soil varies with type, texture, and organic matter of the soil and with rainfall. In a study of various diets, it was found that the availability of Se increased when a 70% grain diet was fed, as a result of the high content of nonstructural carbohydrates.[20] Other influencing factors include the following:

- **Soil pH**—alkalinity encourages Se absorption by plants, and the presence of a high level of sulfur, which competes for absorption sites with Se in both plants and animals, with both factors reducing availability.
- The assimilation by plants is influenced by the physicochemical properties of the soil (redox status, pH, and microbial activity).
- Variation between plants in their ability to absorb selenium—**"selector" and "converter" plants** are listed under the heading of "Selenium Poisoning"; legumes take up much less Se than do grasses.
- **Seasonal conditions also influence the selenium content of pasture**, with the content being lowest in the spring and when rainfall is heavy. Blood Se levels in dairy cows in the United States were lower during the summer and fall than during the winter and spring. In this way, a marginally deficient soil may produce a grossly deficient pasture if it is heavily fertilized with superphosphate, thus increasing its sulfate content, if the rainfall is heavy and the sward is lush and dominated by clover as it is likely to be in the spring months.

Environmental sulfur from various anthropogenic activities has been suspected to be a significant factor in contributing to several health problems in livestock. Livestock producers near natural sour gas desulfurization plants have reported that sulfur emissions are responsible for an increased occurrence of nutritional muscular dystrophy, weak calves, and retarded growth. Experimentally, a moderate increase in dietary sulfur does not impair Se and copper status or cause related disease in cattle.

Selenium in Animals

There may be wide variations in the serum Se concentrations and glutathione peroxidase activities in cattle grazing forages of various Se concentrations within the same geographic area. The Se status of beef cows can vary between geographic areas within a region of a country, which is likely attributable to variations in Se concentration of the soil and plants in these areas. Beef herds from areas with adequate soil levels of Se, herds provided with supplemental feed on pasture, and herds in which pregnancy diagnosis was done had higher average herd blood Se values than other herds. In growing cattle the recommended dose is 100 mu g/kg

DM, and for pregnant and lactating females it is 200 mu per g/kg. In a study of Belgian Blue cattle, it was found that they have a higher requirement for Se as a result of the hypermusculature of the breed[21] and that yeast selenite provided the best response in the dams.

Some species have a greater ability to concentrate Se than other species. For example, Norwegian reindeer meat has more Se than beef, lamb, mutton, pork, or chicken.[22]

Vitamin E

There may be an antioxidant interaction with proinflammatory cascades involving important signal transduction elements. There may be an antiinflammatory property of compounds that could shift the TH1–TH2 type of immune balance toward a TH2-type immunity.[23]

Cows supplemented with VE had a lower rate of culling and mastitis and a reduced level of retained fetal membranes, from 6.5% to 3.0%, compared with nonsupplemented diets. There was no effect on milk yield, reproductive performance, or uterine infections.[24] The relationship between plasma VE and milk VE is too poor for milk VE to be used as a primary test for VE deficiency.[25]

VE deficiency occurs most commonly when animals are fed inferior-quality hay or straw or root crops. Cereal grains, green pasture, and well-cured fresh hay contain adequate amounts of the vitamin.

Alpha-tocopherol levels are high in green grasses and clovers, but there are wide variations in the concentrations from one area to another. The serum α-tocopherol levels are higher in calves born from cows fed grass silage than in those born from cows fed the same grass as hay. Many factors influence the α-tocopherol content of pasture and hence the animals' intake. The level of α-tocopherol in pasture declines by up to 90% as it matures. Levels as low as 0.7 mg/kg DM have been reported in dry summer pastures grazed by sheep. The α-tocopherol content of ryegrass and clover pasture ranges from 22 to 350 mg/kg DM and 90 to 210 mg/kg DM, respectively. After harvesting and storage, the α-tocopherol content of pasture and other crops may fall further, sometimes to 0. Preservation of grain with propionic acid does not prevent the decline. Thus the dietary intake of α-tocopherol by cattle and sheep may be expected to vary widely and lead to wide variations in tissue levels. The plasma VE status of horses is highest from May to August in Canada when fresh grass is being grazed and lowest when the horses are being fed harvested or stored feed during the same period. Plasma VE levels in dairy cows in the United States were higher during the summer and fall than during the winter and spring.

Outbreaks of NMD may occur in yearling cattle fed on high-moisture grain treated with propionic acid as a method of inexpensive storage and protection from fungal growth. There is a marked drop in the VE content of acid-treated grain and an increase in the levels of peroxides of fat, which is consistent with a loss of naturally occurring antioxidants such as the tocopherols (secondary VE deficiency). In these situations, the levels of Se in the feed were below 0.05 mg/kg DM, which is inadequate and emphasizes the interdependence of Se and VE. The α-tocopherol content of moist grain (barley and maize) stored for 6 months, with or without propionic acid, falls to extremely low levels compared with conventionally stored grain, in which the α-tocopherol levels usually persist over the same length of time. Selenium-deficient barley treated with sodium hydroxide to deplete it of vitamin E can be used to induce NMD when fed to yearling cattle. The disease may occur in sucking lambs with low plasma α-tocopherol levels and an adequate Se status, which indicates that the sparing effect of each nutrient may not occur over the broad spectrum of clinical deficiencies.

Polyunsaturated Fatty Acids in Diet

Diets rich in polyunsaturated fatty acids (PUFAs), such as cod liver oil, other fish oils, fishmeal used as a protein concentrate, lard, linseed oil, soybean, and corn oils, have been implicated in the production of NMD, particularly in calves fed milk replacers containing these ingredients. The disease can be reproduced experimentally in young ruminant cattle, 6 to 9 months of age, by feeding a diet low in VE and Se and adding linolenic acid. There are widespread lesions of myodegeneration of skeletal and myocardial muscles. Fresh spring grass containing a sufficient concentration of linolenic acid to equal the amount necessary to produce NMD in calves may explain the occurrence of the naturally occurring disease in the spring months. The oxidation during rancidification of the oils causes destruction of the vitamin, thus increasing the dietary requirements (a conditioned vitamin E deficiency), and the presence of myopathic agents in the oils may also contribute to the occurrence of the disease. The lack of specificity of VE in the prevention of muscular dystrophy in some circumstances is indicated by its failure and by the efficiency of Se as a preventive agent in lambs on lush legume pasture.

Supplementation with fish oil and barium selenite and its effects on carcass characteristics and muscle fatty acid of late-season lambs finished on grass or concentrate has been studied.[26] It was found that fish oil is of some help in concentrate diets but not in grass-based diets. Barium sulfate helps if there is no concentrate in the diet but is of little use if the lambs are fed on concentrate- or fish-oil-enriched diets.

Other Myopathic Agents in Diet

Not all of the myopathic agents that may be important in the development of NMD in farm animals have been identified. Unsaturated fatty acids in fish and vegetable oils may be myopathic agents in some outbreaks of NMD of calves and lambs. Lupinosis-associated myopathy in sheep is a substantial skeletal muscle myopathy encountered in weaner sheep grazing lupin stubbles infected with the fungus *Phomopsis* spp. Affected sheep have a stiff gait, walk reluctantly, stand with their back humped and their feet under the body, and have difficulty getting to their feet.

Unaccustomed Exercise

Historically, NMD occurred most commonly in rapidly growing, well-nourished beef calves 2 to 4 months of age, shortly following unaccustomed exercise. This was commonplace in countries where calves were born and raised indoors until about 6 to 8 weeks of age, when they were turned out onto new pasture in the spring of the year. This has been a standard practice in small beef herds in the United Kingdom, Europe, and North America. A similar situation applies for ewes that lambed indoors and the lambs were let out to pasture from 1 to 3 weeks of age. Thus unaccustomed activity in calves and lambs, such as running and frolicking following their turn-out onto pasture, is an important risk factor but is not necessarily a prerequisite for the disease. In lambs, the vigorous exertion associated with running and sucking may account for the peracute form of myocardial dystrophy in young lambs on deficient pastures and from deficient ewes. In older lambs up to 3 months of age, outbreaks of acute NMD and stiff-lamb disease may be associated with the driving of flocks long distances. A similar situation applies for calves that are moved long distances from calving grounds and early-spring pastures to lush summer pastures. The wandering and bellowing that occur in beef calves weaned at 6 to 8 months of age may precipitate outbreaks of subacute NMD. Degenerative myopathy of yearling cattle (feedlot cattle, housed yearling bulls, and heifer replacements) is now being recognized with increased frequency. The disease resembles subacute NMD of calves and in the United Kingdom is often seen when yearlings are turned outdoors in the spring of the year after being housed during the winter and fed poor-quality hay or straw or propionic-acid-treated grain. Unaccustomed exercise is a common precipitating factor. However, the disease has occurred in housed yearling bulls with no history of stress or unaccustomed exercise but whose diet was deficient in Se and VE.

In horses subjected to exercise, there is an increase in erythrocyte malondialdehyde, a product of peroxidation, but Se supplementation has no beneficial effect. There is inconclusive evidence that a selenium–vitamin E deficiency causes NMD in adult horses. There is no evidence that paralytic myoglobinuria and "tying-up" syndrome are a result of a deficiency of selenium and vitamin E.

Congenital Nutritional Muscular Dystrophy

Congenital NMD is rare in farm animals. Isolated cases have been reported.

Similarly, NMD can occur in calves and lambs only a few days of age, but rarely. Se readily crosses the bovine placenta, and fetal Se is always higher than the maternal status. There is no evidence that weak-calf syndrome is associated with Se deficiency. Long-term parenteral supplementation with either Se alone or in combination with VE had no effect on the incidence of weak-calf syndrome.

An investigation of aborted bovine fetuses with lesions of heart failure, specifically cardiac dilatation or hypertrophy, along with a nodular liver and ascites compared with aborted fetuses without such lesions and nonaborted fetuses from the abattoir found myocardial necrosis and mean selenium levels of 5.5 μmol/kg in the fetuses with heart lesions, 6.5 μmol/kg in the fetuses without heart lesions, and 7.5 μmol/kg selenium in the fetuses from the abattoir. This suggests that Se deficiency in bovine fetuses may cause myocardial necrosis and heart failure. Normal levels of selenium in the liver and kidney tissue of bovine fetuses derived from the abattoir were 7.5 ± 5.2 μmol/kg and 4.4 ± 1.1 μmol/kg, respectively.

In pigs, NMD has been produced experimentally on VE- and Se-deficient rations but is usually only a part of the more serious complex of mulberry heart disease and hepatosis dietetica.

Vitamin E–Selenium Deficiency Syndrome

The combination of mulberry heart disease, hepatosis dietetica, exudative diathesis, and nutritional myopathy, also known as vitamin E–selenium deficiency (VESD) syndrome, occurs in pigs, usually as a serious disease. Nutritional muscular dystrophy may also occur in pigs. The occurrence of edema in various tissues has also been suggested as a possible result of Se or VE deficiency. Impaired spermatogenesis and increased susceptibility to the effects of swine dysentery have also been suggested as responses to reduced levels of these two substances. There is a suspicion that the problems become more common as the pig grows more quickly and the requirements and demands for antioxidants are increased at the same time that the provision of fat-soluble vitamins is increasingly difficult. In addition, there is a very small difference between the therapeutic and toxic levels of Se, and Se toxicosis has occurred in an attempt to prevent Se deficiency. A more recent complication is the realization that we have been using inorganic Se to provide Se in the diet, whereas in the plant, most of the Se is organic in the form of L-selenomethionine, an Se analog of the amino acid methionine. In the pig, as in other species, Se is thought to serve as an antagonist to toxic free radicals and act in concert with other substances such as vitamin C. Little is known about Se metabolism in the pig. In the pig, there is very little transfer of fat-soluble products across the placenta, so there is very little reserve of VE in the new born pig. Immediately after birth, the young pig gets its VE from the colostrum and milk of the sow. If the sow has low body stores or is fed a ration low in VE, then the piglet will be very low in VE when it is weaned. SE and VE can substitute for each other in a limited way in the pig. In the pig, the diet has the most influence. Diets rich in polyunsaturated fatty acids, copper, vitamin A, or mycotoxins may reduce the availability of VE. As dietary vitamin A levels increase, serum and liver α-tocopherol concentrations decline, suggesting a reduced absorption and retention of α-tocopherol when weaned pigs were fed high dietary vitamin A levels. Se antagonists or crops from inherently low-soil-Se fields may also make the situation worse. In pigs, NMD has been produced experimentally on VE- and Se-deficient rations but is usually only a part of the more serious complex of mulberry heart disease and hepatosis dietetica. Microangiopathy is most common in weaned pigs and may be particularly related to VE deficiency.

There is conflicting evidence on the effect of the antioxidative vitamins C and E on the reproductive performance of sows. In some studies, increasing dietary VE in the diet during gestation may have increased the litter size and reduced the preweaning piglet mortality. A similar response has been seen following intramuscular injection of sows with VE and Se, but the injection of vitamin C has produced no improvement. A recent study has confirmed that there was no effect on the reproductive performance of sows and the growth performance of piglets when supplemented by both vitamin E and C. Vitamin E and Se given to immature gilts for flushing purposes led to the formation of fewer but larger corpora lutea after ovulation, probably as a result of the progression of a smaller number of follicles to the ovulatory stage. Vitamin E and Se increased the development of the uterus but did not influence the number of piglets at farrowing.

VESD occurs naturally in rapidly growing pigs, usually during the postweaning period (3 weeks to 4 months), particularly during the early finishing period. The lowest concentration of VE in piglets was at day 45 after farrowing, but it may be that the Se status of the newborn piglets may be more important for their health than their VE status. The first 3 to 4 weeks following the move to the finishing house is the most dangerous period for a low VE level, and it is important to remember that there is considerable individual variation. Serum VE declines after weaning, and even with VE supplementation it takes 2 to 3 days for levels to rise. There appears to be a temporary decreased absorption of the vitamin in the immediate postweaning period, and this in turn leads to the reduction of the stored vitamin E reserves. It is usually associated with diets deficient in both Se and vitamin E and those that may contain a high concentration of unsaturated fatty acids. Such diets include those containing mixtures of soybean, high-moisture corn, and cereal grains grown on soils with low levels of Se. The feeding of a basal ration of cull peas, low in Se and VE, to growing pigs can cause the typical syndrome, and low tissue levels of Se are present in pigs with spontaneously occurring hepatosis dietetica. It has been shown that feeding diets containing linseed oil reduced the VE levels in the diet but increased the skatole levels. However, there are reports of naturally occurring mulberry heart disease of pigs in Scandinavia in which the tissue levels of Se and VE are within normal ranges compared with normal pigs. In Ireland, in spite of supplementation of pig rations with VE and Se at levels higher than that necessary to prevent experimental disease, spontaneous mulberry heart disease may still occur. Affected pigs have lower tissue vitamin E levels than control pigs, which suggests an alteration in α-tocopherol metabolism unrelated to dietary Se and PUFA contents.

Natural occurrence of the disease complex in pigs is not uncommonly associated with diets containing 50% coconut meal, fish-liver-oil emulsion, fish scraps with a high content of unsaturated fatty acids, or flaxseed, which produces yellow and brown discoloration of fat preventable by the incorporation of adequate amounts of α-tocopherol or a suitable antioxidant. The quality of the dietary fat does not necessarily influence blood VE levels, but the presence of oxidized fat reduces the resistance of the red blood cells against peroxidation. The higher requirement for VE by pigs fed oxidized fat may be a result of the low VE content in such fat. It has recently been shown that the inclusion of 0.3 ppm Se to the diet of postweaning piglets resulted in better performance than non-Se-supplemented diets, irrespective of the level of VE in the ration (up to 200 ppm).

Mulberry Heart Disease

Mulberry heart disease (MHD) is the most common form of Se and VE deficiency of pigs. It occurs most commonly in rapidly growing feeder pigs (60 to 90 kg) in excellent condition being fed on a high-energy diet low in VE and Se. The true causal mechanism is not known, but it can be prevented by supplementation with VE. It can also occur when it would appear that the level in the diet and in the serum or tissues appear to be satisfactory. The diets most commonly incriminated are soybean, corn, and barley. Mean liver concentrations of VE were lower in pigs with MHD than in pigs that died of causes other than MHD. The α-tocopherol content of corn is usually low, and it is virtually absent from solvent-extracted soybean meal. Both are low in Se. The use of high-moisture corn may further exacerbate the tocopherol deficiency. The level of PUFAs in the diet was thought to be an important etiologic factor, but this is now not considered to be a necessary prerequisite. Outbreaks of the disease may occur in which 25% of susceptible pigs are affected, and the case-mortality rate is about 90%. The disease has occurred in young piglets and in adult sows.

Hepatosis Dietetica

Hepatosis dietetica appears to be less common than mulberry heart disease, but the epidemiologic characteristics are similar. It appears to be less common because the Se levels in supplements were raised to 0.3 ppm. It affects young, rapidly growing pigs up to 3 to 4 months of age. NMD in pigs usually occurs in cases of mulberry heart disease and hepatosis dietetica, but it has occurred alone in gilts.

Selenium-Responsive Disorders

A variety of diseases have been known as selenium-responsive disorders because they respond beneficially to the strategic administration of Se. These include the following: **ill-thrift** in lambs and calves on pasture; **lowered milk production** in cows; **white-muscle disease** in lambs, calves, and kids; **lowered fertility** and **embryonic death** in sheep and cattle; **retained fetal membranes**, **metritis**, **poor uterine involution**, and **cystic ovaries** in cows; subclinical **mastitis** and **impaired immune function** in cattle; and **prematurity**, **perinatal death**, and **abortion** in cattle. Of these, only ill-thrift, lowered fertility, lowered milk production, and white-muscle disease have been reported in New Zealand.

The pathogenesis of these selenium-responsive diseases is not well understood, but it would appear that the Se deficiency is only marginal. Most investigations into selenium-responsive diseases have occurred in selenium-deficient areas in which diseases such as NMD of calves and lambs occur. The evidence that Se deficiency in breeding ewes can result in a decline in reproductive performance has not been substantiated experimentally. Reproductive performance was not affected in ewes on a selenium-depleted diet.

Selenium-responsive unthriftiness in sheep has received considerable attention in New Zealand, where the response to Se administration has been most dramatic, compared with Australia, where the syndrome has also been recognized but where the response is much smaller. The oral administration of Se to lambs in these areas results in greater body-weight gains from weaning to 1 year of age compared with lambs not receiving Se supplementation. The mean fleece weight of selenium-treated lambs is also greater.

The diagnosis of selenium-responsive unthriftiness depends on analyses of the soil, pasture, and animal tissues for Se and response to trials of Se supplementation. A deficiency state might be encountered when the Se content of the soil is below 0.45 mg/kg, the pasture content is below 0.02 mg/kg DM, the liver content is below 21 μg/kg (0.27 μmol/kg wet weight [WW]), and wool concentrations are below 50 to 60 μg/kg (0.63 to 0.76 μmol/kg). For the blood in selenium-responsive unthriftiness of sheep, the following criteria are suggested for mean blood selenium status (μg/dL):

- Deficient = 1.0
- Doubtful = 1.1 to 1.9
- Normal = ~2.0

The GSH-PX activity is a good index of the Se status of sheep with a selenium-responsive disease. If measured on a regular basis, it can provide an indication of the Se status of grazing sheep in individual flocks. Single measurements of GSH-PX activity may fail to detect recent changes in grazing area, differences in pasture species and pasture composition, and alterations in the physiologic state of the animals.

Subclinical Selenium Insufficiency

Subclinical insufficiencies of Se in grazing ruminants are widespread over large areas of southern Australia. The plasma concentrations of affected sheep flocks are low, there are no obvious clinical signs of insufficiency in the ewes, and there are significant responses in wool production and fiber diameter to Se supplementation. The incidence of estrus and fertility is not affected by Se supplementation. Live weights at birth, in midlactation, and at weaning were increased in lambs born to selenium-supplemented and crossbred ewes and in lambs born as singletons. Clean fleece weight at 10 months of age was increased by 9.5% and fiber diameter by 0.3 μm in lambs born to ewes that had received supplementary Se. Differences in fleece weight and live weight were not detected at 22 months, suggesting that subclinical Se insufficiency in early life did not permanently impair productivity if Se status subsequently increased.

Temporal variations in glutathione peroxidase activity in sheep can be used to identify seasons of the year with the highest risk of Se deficiency. In the Mediterranean area, lambs born in the spring/summer are at higher risk of selenium-deficiency related diseases. Lambs born in autumn/winter are from ewes gestating during the summer, when supplementation with cereal grains is provided.

Se is a component of type I iodothyronine deiodinase, which catalyzes the extrathyroidal conversion of thyroxine (T4) to the more active tri-iodothyronine (T3). Sheep grazing pastures low in Se frequently have higher circulating T4 and lower circulating T3 concentrations than sheep receiving Se supplementations.

When ewes grazing pastures low in Se were supplemented with thiocyanate (to cause iodine insufficiency), iodide, and Se, there was no evidence of clinical deficiencies. Growth rates of lambs were not affected by the thiocyanate of their dams during mid-pregnancy, but plasma T3 and T4 concentrations were depressed in ewes receiving thiocyanate. The iodide supplementation increased thyroid hormone concentrations in ewes but depressed plasma T3 concentrations in lambs. Supplementation of sheep grazing pastures low in Se with both Se and thyroid hormones improved wool characteristics, live-weight gain, and blood Se, but there was no evidence of an interaction between the Se and the hormones. Thus it seems unlikely that the decline in the quantity of T3 produced, or of T4 utilized for T3 production, in selenium-deficient sheep is responsible for the observed differences in the productivity of selenium-deficient and supplemented sheep. The thyroids have a major role in regulating thermogenesis, and lambs born to ewes supplemented with iodide tend to have higher rectal temperatures during cold stress. The thermoregulatory ability of the perinatal lamb is not adversely affected by subclinical Se deficiency.

In a survey of the status of VE and Se of the livers of cull ewes and market lambs raised in Ontario, Se was present at marginal levels in 3.3% of cull ewe samples and in 43% of market lamb samples. VE was low to deficient in 10% of cull ewe samples and in 90% of market lamb samples. In cull ewes, there was a strong relationship between Se and VE. A large percentage of samples with marginal Se values had adequate VE, which may indicate that the sheep had access to high levels of VE but received inadequate levels of supplement containing Se.

An evaluation of the trace mineral status of beef cows in Ontario found that 96% of cull cows were deficient in blood Se. Based on analysis of serum samples from cattle in Iowa and Wisconsin, subclinical Se deficiency is common in the cattle population. The serum levels may be adequate for reproductive performance but marginal for optimal resistance to mastitis or for adequate transfer of selenium to the calf.

In moose in northwestern Minnesota, declining numbers of moose have been associated with low trace elements, particularly copper and selenium.[27]

Reproductive Performance

The roles of reactive oxygen species in female reproduction have been reviewed,[28] and nutritional management is important.[29] The published information on the effects of VE and Se deficiency or of dietary supplementation with one or the other or both on reproductive performance in farm animals is conflicting and controversial. Reproductive performance is complex and dependent on the interaction of many factors. Reproductive inefficiency is likewise complex, and it is difficult to isolate one factor, such as a deficiency of VE or Se, as a cause of reproductive inefficiency. Conversely, it is difficult to prove that supplementation with these nutrients will ensure optimum reproductive performance. The roles of cellular reactive oxygen species, oxidative stress, and antioxidants in the outcome of pregnancy have been reviewed.[30] Many vitamins and trace elements have a dual role in mammals in that they (a) control or are involved in the metabolic processes and/or gene expression and (b) spend most of their time in trapping radical oxygen species. Any deficiencies will produce high rates of radical oxygen species production.[31]

Pigs

Selenium and vitamin E improve the in vitro maturation, fertilization, and growth to blastocysts of porcine oocytes.[32]

Sheep

The evidence about the effect of Se and VE deficiency on reproductive performance in sheep is conflicting. Observations in the 1960s concluded that Se deficiency caused embryonic deaths 20 to 30 days after fertilization in ewes. But Se supplementation of ewes that were low or marginal in Se status did not improve reproductive performance. Experimental studies using selenium-deficient diets in ewes have been unable to find any adverse effects of Se depletion on ewe conception rates, embryonic mortality, or numbers of lambs born. The parenteral administration of Se to pregnant ewes between 15 and 35 days after mating resulted in a reduced embryonic survival rate and is not recommended during the first month of pregnancy.

Cattle

VE supplementation can have significant effects on the health and some aspects of fertility in lactating dairy cows. VE supplementation of dairy cows has its most beneficial effect of reducing the incidence of mastitis when used at rates of at least 1000 IU per day during the dry period and early lactation. The primary effect of VE supplementation is on the immune system. The importance of Se and VE for the maintenance of optimum reproductive performance is not clear. The IM injection of dairy cattle at 3 weeks prepartum did not have any effect on average days to first estrus or first service, average days to conception, services per conception, or number of uterine infusions required. The prepartum IM injection of VE and Se at 3 weeks prepartum increased the percentage of cows pregnant to first service, reduced the number of services per conception, decreased the incidence of retained placenta, and reduced the interval from calving to conception. In a randomized field trial in a large dairy herd in the United States, oral supplementation of pregnant first-calf dairy heifers with Se using a commercially available sustained-release intraruminal selenium bolus increased blood Se concentrations in treated animals at 30 days after treatment until after calving. However, based on data analyzed at midlactation and late lactation, there were no differences between treated and control groups in somatic cell count, days not pregnant, total milk production, or times bred. The use of an intraruminal pellet of Se at two different levels in dairy herds in New Zealand was evaluated in yearling heifers. The recommended dose was effective in elevating whole-blood GSH-PX activity and Se concentrations to over 10 times those of control animals. Milk production was increased, and there was a trend toward decreased somatic cell counts. There were no differences in calving-first-service or calving-conception intervals, or in the percentage of animals pregnant to first or all services. In other observations, there was an improvement in first-service conception rate and significantly higher blood levels of GSH-PX following the treatment of dairy cows with oral Se pellets. The inconsistent results obtained following the use of Se and VE in pregnant cows may be related to the Se status of the animals; in some herds the blood levels are marginal, and in others the levels are within the normal range.

Winter-fed lactating Norwegian dairy cows were found to have an adequate plasma levels of VE and marginal to adequate levels of blood Se. Silage was the most important source of VE, and selenium-supplemented commercial concentrates were the most important source of selenium. No significant differences in VE or Se status were found between cows with or without recorded treatments of mastitis, parturient paresis, or reproductive abnormalities.

Retained Fetal Placenta

A high incidence (more than 10%) of retained fetal membranes has been associated with marginal levels of plasma Se compared with herds without a problem. In some cases, the incidence could be reduced to below 10% by the injection of pregnant cattle with Se and VE at approximately 3 weeks prepartum, whereas in other studies similar prepartum injections neither reduced the incidence nor improved reproductive performance. A single injection of Se 3 weeks prepartum can reduce the number of days postpartum required for the uterus to reach minimum size and reduce the incidence of metritis and cystic ovaries during the early postpartum period. The parenteral administration of a single injection of 3000 mg VE prepartum to dairy cows of all ages decreased the incidence of retained placenta and metritis to 6.4% and 3.9%, respectively, in the treated group, compared with 12.5% and 8.8% in the control group. The injection, 20 days prepartum, of 50 mg of Se and 680 IU of VE reduced the incidence of retained fetal membranes in one series, but it did not have this effect in another series. The plasma Se concentration at parturition ranged from 0.02 to 0.05 ppm in control cows, in which there was an incidence of 51% retained membranes, and from 0.08 to 0.1 ppm in treated cows, in which the incidence was reduced to 9%. A dietary level of 0.1 mg/kg DM Se is recommended to minimize the incidence of the problem. The complex nature of the etiology of retained fetal membranes also requires a well-designed experimental trial to account for all of the possible factors involved. In a study in Croatia, where the soils are generally deficient, it was found that there is a high level of retained fetal membranes in cattle associated with low levels of Se and VE.[33] VE supplementation during the dry period has reduced the risk of retained fetal membranes, and it is said that the synthetic forms of VE are more effective in this regard.[34]

Mammary Gland Function

One of the techniques for protection against mastitis is to increase the immunity of the bovine mammary gland. Se affects the innate and adaptive immune mechanisms of the mammary gland.[35] VE also reduces the incidence of mastitis.[36] VE supplementation was shown to have an adverse effect on the occurrence of clinical and subclinical mastitis in high doses. The level at dry-off of 14.5 mu mol/L was a risk factor for clinical mastitis. It is therefore necessary to assess the exact level at which VE affects udder health.

In buffaloes, Se helps to combat mastitis because it increases neutrophil phagocytosis and antioxidant levels during acute mastitis in riverine buffaloes.[37]

Transport Stress

VE, Se, and vitamins A and D have been shown to prevent lipid peroxidation and oxidative stress associated with long-term transportation stress in cattle.[38]

Resistance to Infectious Disease

Several trace elements, particularly copper, Se, and zinc, affect immune function, but the effects of supplementation are equivocal. However, adding VE may reduce bovine respiratory disease morbidity but have some effect on performance.[39]

Many studies have examined the role of Se and VE resistance to infectious disease. Most of the evidence is based on in vitro studies of the effects of deficiencies of Se or VE or supplementation with the nutrients on leukocyte responses to mitogens, or on the antibody responses of animals to a variety of pathogens. The status of Se and VE in an animal can alter antibody response, phagocytic function, lymphocyte response, and resistance to infectious disease. The deficiency of VE or Se reduces neutrophil function during the periparturient period. Se and iodine administration in prepartum cows may enhance the calf immune system.[40] The administration of VE and Se during the dry period can influence mammary gland health and milk cell counts in dairy ewes. In general, a deficiency of Se results in immunosuppression, and supplementation with low doses of Se augments immunologic functions.

A deficiency of Se has been shown to inhibit the following:

- Resistance to microbial and viral infections
- Neutrophil function
- Antibody production
- Proliferation of T and B lymphocytes in response to mitogens
- Cytodestruction of T lymphocytes and natural killer lymphocytes

VE and Se have interactive effects on lymphocyte responses to experimental antigens.

VE supplementation of transport-stressed feedlot cattle is associated with reduced serum acute-phase protein concentrations compared with control animals. Supplementation of the diet of cattle arriving in the feedlot with VE had beneficial effects on humoral immune response and recovery from respiratory disease.

The parenteral administration of Se and VE during pregnancy in dairy cows has a positive effect on the increase of Se and VE concentrations in blood, increase of Se and immunoglobulin concentrations in colostrum, and increase of T3 concentration in blood on the day of parturition. In addition, there was a trend toward a decreased incidence of clinical mastitis.

Neutrophil Function

Se deficiency can affect the function of polymorphonuclear neutrophils (PMNs), which are associated with physiologic changes in GSH-PX levels. In calves on an experimental selenium-deficient diet, the oxygen consumption and the activities of GSH-PX were lower than normal in neutrophils. The feeding of 80 to 120 mg of Se/kg of mineral mixture provided ad libitum was shown to be an effective method of increasing blood Se in a group of cattle and to optimize the humoral antibody response experimentally. It is suggested that blood Se levels over 100 µg/L are necessary to maintain optimum immunocompetence in growing beef cattle. In selenium-deficient goats, the production of leukotriene B_4, a product of neutrophil arachidonic acid lipoxygenation and a potent chemotactic and chemokinetic stimulus for neutrophils, is decreased, resulting in dysfunction of the neutrophils. A deficiency of Se in pregnant sows impairs neutrophil function, and VE deficiency impairs function of both neutrophils and lymphocytes, which may result in increased susceptibility of their piglets to infectious diseases. It is suggested that selenium supplementation be maintained at 0.3 mg/kg of the diet.

Neutrophils from postparturient dairy cows with higher levels of Se have greater potential to kill microbes, and cattle with greater superoxide production may have higher milk production. VE is a fat-soluble membrane antioxidant that enhances the functional efficiency of neutrophils by protecting them from oxidative damage following intracellular killing of ingested bacteria. Peripartum immunosuppression in dairy cows is multifactorial but is associated with endocrine changes and decreased intake of critical nutrients. Decreased phagocytosis and intracellular killing by neutrophils occurs in parallel with decreased dry matter intake and decreased circulating VE. Because neutrophils are the primary mechanism of uterine defense and mammary health, the role of VE on the health of dairy cows during the transition period has been examined. Compared with control cows given a placebo, the parenteral administration of VE 1 week prepartum had no effect on the incidence of retained placenta, clinical mastitis, metritis, endometritis, ketosis, displaced abomasum, or lameness. However, there was a decreased incidence of retained placenta in cows with marginal pretreatment VE status. An increase in α-tocopherol of 1 µg/mL in the last week prepartum reduced the risk of retained placenta by 20%. In addition, serum nonesterified fatty acid concentration greater than or equal to 0.5 mEq/L tended to increase the risk of retained placenta by 80%, and in the last week prepartum, a 100 ng/mL increase in serum retinol was associated with a 60% decrease in the risk of early-lactation clinical mastitis.

Immune Response

The effects of Se deficiency and supplementation on the immune response of cattle to experimental infection with the infectious bovine rhinotracheitis virus and sheep to parainfluenza-3 virus indicate that a deficiency can affect the humoral response and that supplementation enhances the response. The administration of Se either alone or in combination with VE can improve the production of antibodies against *E. coli* in dairy cows. Pigs fed a deficient diet develop an impaired cell-mediated immunity as measured by lymphocyte response to mitogenic stimulations. Supplementation of the diets of young pigs with Se levels above those required for normal growth have increased the humoral response, but not in sows. The wide variations in antibody responses that occur in these experiments indicate that there is a complex relationship between the Se status of the host, humoral immune responses, and protective immunity. The concept of using selenium supplementation to enhance antibody responses in sheep to vaccines is probably unfounded. However, the administration of sodium selenite to sheep vaccinated against enzootic abortion (*Chlamydophila abortus*) increased the antibody response, but not when given with vitamin E. The Se sources provided to mares may influence the immune function of foals at 1 month of age.[41] In sheep with footrot, an improved immune response is found after a higher blood serum Se response is found.[42]

Experimentally, VE can stimulate the immune defense mechanisms in laboratory animals and cattle. In most cases, the immunostimulatory effects of additional VE are associated with supplementation in excess of levels required for normal growth. The parenteral administration to calves of 1400 mg of VE weekly increases their serum VE concentrations and lymphocyte stimulation indices. Similarly, in growing pigs, a serum VE concentration above 3 mg/L is necessary to achieve a significant response of the lymphocytes to stimulation with mitogens.

The administration of a daily 2500 IU RRR-alpha-tocopherol to pregnant mares stimulated maternal IgG and IgM production in colostrum and enhanced VE and IgM status in foals.[43]

General Resistance

These changes may render selenium-deficient animals more susceptible to infectious disease, but there is no available evidence to indicate that naturally occurring deficiencies are associated with an increase in the incidence or severity of infectious diseases. Neutrophils from selenium-deficient animals lose some ability to phagocytose certain organisms, but how relevant this observation is in naturally occurring infections is unclear. Field studies of the incidence and occurrence of pneumonia in housed calves found that Se status was not a risk factor.

Transfer of Selenium and Vitamin E to the Fetus, Colostrum, and Milk

Selenium

In sheep, Se is transferred across the placenta to the fetus, and maternal Se status during gestation is positively associated with fetal and newborn lamb Se status. Supplementation of gestating ewes with Se will improve the Se status of the lambs at birth. Supplementing ewes with VE and Se during pregnancy increased the weight of lambs at weaning by about 2 kg above those on a marginal level of Se., and organic Se produced better lamb viability.[44] However, after birth, the Se of the lamb is depleted quickly, by about 18 days after birth. Thus continued intake of Se by the lamb is necessary to maintain normal Se status during the postnatal period. The colostrum of ewes contains higher levels of Se than ewe milk. The Se content of ewe's milk decreases rapidly after parturition, reaching a stable level by 1 week postpartum. Supplementation of ewes during lactation results in higher milk Se concentration and higher blood Se in lambs. Supplementation of ewes has been shown to prevent nutritional myodegeneration in nursing lambs in selenium-deficient flocks.

There is a highly significant relationship between blood Se of cattle and milk Se concentration. As in sheep, in cattle, Se is transferred across the placenta to the fetus and across the mammary barrier into the colostrum and milk.

Pigs

The maternal intake of Se affects fetal liver Se, and newborn piglets have lower liver Se concentrations compared with their dams, regardless of Se intake of sows during gestation. Thus compared with cattle and sheep, the relatively high concentration of Se needed in the diets of young rapidly growing piglets may be partially a function of limited placental transport or hepatic deposition of Se and may explain why the piglet is more susceptible to Se deficiency than the sow.

Vitamin E

The transfer of VE across the placenta to the fetus in sheep and cattle is limited. Plasma levels of VE in the fetus and in newborn lambs (before ingestion of colostrum) are lower than in the ewe. VE supplementation of the ewe in late gestation results in insignificant increases of the serum VE in the lamb. However, supplementation of the ewe in the last month of pregnancy increases the VE content of colostrum and milk. Colostrum of the ewe is a rich source of VE for the neonatal lamb, containing 5 to 11 times more VE than milk at 1 week postpartum. The parenteral administration of sodium selenite to ewes at lambing increases the VE content of milk of ewes over the first 5 weeks of lactation, indicating a potential positive effect of Se repletion on VE transfer to milk.

Neonatal Morbidity and Mortality

Based on some preliminary observations of the Se content of hair samples of young calves, higher Se levels in newborn calves may have some protective effect against morbidity as a result of neonatal disease. Similarly, neonatal piglets with high blood levels of GSH-PX activity may be more resistant to infectious diseases or other causes of neonatal mortality. Administration of VE and Se to dairy cows in late pregnancy resulted in the production of increased quantities of colostrum, and the calves had increased quantities of GSH-PX at birth and 28 days of age, but the improved Se status did not provide any improvement in passive immunity or growth.

Supplementing Se to beef cows grazing selenium-deficient pastures with a salt mineral mix containing 120 mg selenium/kg of mix increased the Se status of the cows and increased the serum IgG concentration, or enhanced transfer of IgG from serum to colostrum, and increased the Se status of the calves. The parenteral administration of 0.1 mg Se and 1 mg of vitamin E/kg BW at midgestation did not affect the production of systemic or colostral antibodies. Supplementation of dairy cows at dry-off with Se at 3 mg/d as selenite via an intraruminal bolus resulted in sufficient transfer of Se to meet a target concentration of more than 2.2 μg of selenium/g of liver DM in newborn calves. Milk Se is a useful indicator of animal and herd Se status.[45]

Mastitis

There is some evidence that a dietary deficiency of VE may be associated with an increased incidence of mastitis in dairy cattle. An increased incidence of mastitis during the early stages of lactation coincides with the lowest plasma concentration of VE. Supplementation of the diet of dairy cows beginning 4 weeks before and continuing for up to 8 weeks after parturition with vitamin E at 3000 IU/cow per day, combined with an injection of 5000 IU 1 week before parturition, prevented the suppression of blood neutrophil and macrophage function during the early postpartum period compared with controls. The VE prevented the suppression of blood neutrophils during the postpartum period. Cows in both the treated and control groups were fed diets containing Se at 0.3 ppm of total dry matter. When Se status in dairy cows is marginal, plasma concentrations of α-tocopherol should be at least 3 μg/mL. Cows receiving a dietary supplement of about 1000 IU/d of VE had 30% less clinical mastitis than did cows receiving a supplement of 100 IU/d of VE. The reduction was 88% when cows were fed 4000 IU/d of VE during the last 14 days of the dry period.

The Se status of dairy cows may also have an effect on the prevalence of mastitis and mammary gland health. Dairy herds with low somatic cell counts had significantly higher mean blood GSH-PX and higher whole-blood concentrations of Se than in herds with high somatic cell counts. The prevalence of infection caused by *Streptococcus agalactiae* and *Staphylococcus aureus* was higher in herds with the high somatic cell counts compared with those with the low somatic cell counts. This suggests that phagocytic function in the mammary gland may be decreased by a marginal Se deficiency. In a survey of cattle in herds in Switzerland, those with chronic mastitis had lower serum levels of Se than healthy control herds. Experimental coliform mastitis in cattle is much more severe in selenium-deficient animals than selenium-adequate animals. The severity was in part a result of the increased concentrations of eicosanoids.

Milk neutrophils from cows fed a selenium-deficient diet have significantly reduced capacity to kill ingested *E. coli* and *S. aureus*, compared with cells from cows fed a selenium-supplemented diet. However, other experimental results are not as convincing.

In pasture-based heifers injected with barium sulfate before calving and fed diets with 1.3 or 2.5 mg of Se/d precalving and during lactation, respectively, there was no clinical mastitis observed in the first month of lactation.[46] Se deficiency may predispose to mastitis in sheep, and examination of the Se status may indicate which ewes may develop ovine mastitis.[47]

Lambs supplemented with Se were also able to deal with oxidative stress generated from *H. contortus* infections by the provision of higher GSH-Px levels.[48]

Blood Abnormalities

In young cattle from areas where NMD is endemic, and particularly at the end of winter housing, the erythrocytes have an increased susceptibility to hemolysis following exposure to hypotonic saline. During clinical and subclinical white-muscle disease in calves, there is a significant increase in both the osmotic and the peroxidative hemolysis of the erythrocytes. This defect is thought to be the result of alterations in the integrity of cell membranes, of which tocopherols are an essential component. Abnormalities of the bone marrow associated with VE deficiency in sheep have been described, and abnormal hematologic responses have been described in young, rapidly growing pigs on an experimental SE- and VE-deficient diet. VE deficiency in sheep results in increased hemolytic susceptibility of erythrocytes, which may provide a basis for a single functional test for VE deficiency in sheep.

Anemia characterized by a decreased packed cell volume, decreased hemoglobin concentration, and Heinz-body formation has been observed in cattle grazing on grass grown on peaty muck soils in the Florida everglades. Se supplementation corrected the anemia, prevented Heinz-body formation, increased the body weight of cows and calves, and elevated blood Se. In a study of supplementation,[49] it was found that the Se levels stabilized in the liver and plasma by 56 to 112 days, whereas the whole-blood and red blood cell (RBC) concentrations were still increasing through 224 days of supplementation, regardless of the form of supplemental Se.

In lambs with WMD, there was a significant increase in serum total sialic acid (TSA) and lipid-bound sialic acid (LBSA), together with a significant decrease in serum Se and VE concentrations. Within 1 month of treatment, the changes were reversed.[50]

Equine Nutritional Myopathy

In areas of severely Se-deficient soil, such as the Pacific Northwest of the United States, there is the possibility of Se deficiency myopathy; this can occur in horses of any age, but more usually it occurs in foals, most commonly up to 2 weeks of age. VE deficiency occurs in horses that eat marginal- or poor-quality grass hay with no access to pasture and no VE supplementation. Affected foals are born to deficient mares. They are weak at birth or shortly after. They may become recumbent but are generally bright and alert. The weakness of the tongue and pharyngeal muscles makes it difficult to suckle. The affected horses are usually stabled, and the condition occurs mostly in late winter or early spring; in the very deficient Northwest, it can occur at any time of the year. The temporal or masseter muscles are often predisposed, with swelling and stiffness of these muscles and impaired mastication. There may be dysphagia and impaired prehension of food. There is often general weakness and a stiff, short-strided gait. The muscles may be pale, and the most severely affected muscles are those that do the most work. Often this means the neck muscles during attempts to suckle. The gross appearance depends on the duration of the condition and may involve the heart. In animals that die, there are often areas of severe necrosis. In the more subacute cases there are areas of repair and regeneration together with new areas of necrosis. In these animals diagnosis is based on the geographic area, history, clinical signs, increased levels of CK and AST, and gross and histologic lesions.

Fatal myocardial degeneration in an adult Quarter horse with Vitamin E deficiency but normal Se has been described.[51] There were pale and firm foci in the heart.

Congenital white-muscle disease also occurs in deer calves.[52]

Equine Degenerative Myeloencephalopathy

Equine degenerative myeloencephalopathy, also sometimes called neuronal dystrophy, is seen pure and mixed breeds of horses. It has also been seen in zebras and in Morgan and Haflinger horses. Clinically, it is a symmetric spasticity with ataxia and paresis of the limbs.

Equine degenerative myeloencephalopathy, which may have an inherited basis, has been associated with VE deficiency. The VE status is low in some affected horses, and supplementation with the vitamin was associated with a marked reduction in the incidence of the disease. In some premises affected with the condition, the administration of VE reduced the incidence. On the other hand, however, serum VE and blood GSH-PX activities determined in horses with histologically confirmed diagnosis of the disease compared with age-matched controls failed to reveal any differences, and the findings did not support a possible role for VE deficiency as a cause. Foals sired by a stallion with degenerative myeloencephalopathy and with neurologic deficits consistent with the disease during their first year of life had lower plasma levels of α-tocopherol when the levels were determined serially beginning at 6 weeks to 10 months of age than did age-matched controls. Absorption tests with VE revealed that the lower α-tocopherol levels were not attributable to an absorption defect. The lesions are usually microscopic and are found as axonal degeneration in the spinal cord, with the dorsal spinocerebellar tracts in the lateral funiculi and some areas of the ventral funiculi severely affected. Myelin loss is secondary to axonal loss. In the brain, there are eosinophilic spheroids in the brainstem nuclei.

Equine Motor Neuron Disease

Equine motor neuron disease is a neurodegenerative disease of the somatic lower motor neurons resulting in a syndrome of diffuse neuromuscular disease in the adult horse. Case-control studies found the mean plasma VE concentrations in affected horses were lower than that of control horses. Adult horses are affected with the risk peaking at 16 years of age. In addition to the role of VE depletion, other individual and farm-level factors contribute to the risk of developing the disease.

Generalized Steatitis

Steatitis in farm animals and other species may be associated with VE and/or Se deficiency. Most cases in horses have involved nursing or recently weaned foals. Generalized steatitis in the foal has been described as either generalized cachexia as a result of steatitis alone or as a primary myopathy or myositis, with steatitis of secondary importance. The terms used have included steatitis, generalized steatitis, fat necrosis, yellow-fat disease, polymyositis, and muscular dystrophy. The relationships between steatitis and VE and Se deficiency in the horse are not clear, and there may not be any. Many more clinical cases must be examined in detail before a cause–effect relationship can be considered.

PATHOGENESIS

Dietary Se, sulfur-containing amino acids, and VE act synergistically to protect tissues from oxidative damage. GSH-PX, which is selenium dependent, functions by detoxifying lipid peroxides and reducing them to nontoxic hydroxy fatty acids. Vitamin E prevents fatty acid hydroperoxide formation. High levels of PUFAs in the diet increase the requirements for VE, and with an inadequate level of Se in the diet, tissue oxidation occurs, resulting in degeneration and necrosis of cells. VE protects cellular membranes from lipoperoxidation, especially membranes rich in unsaturated lipids, such as mitochondric, endoplasmic reticulum, and plasma membranes. Thus dietary PUFAs are not a prerequisite for the disease. Diets low in Se and/or VE do not provide sufficient protection against the "physiological" lipoperoxidation that occurs normally at the cellular level.

The relative importance of Se, VE, and sulfur-containing amino acids in providing protection in each of the known diseases caused by their deficiency is not clearly understood. Se has a sparing effect on VE and is an efficient prophylactic against muscular dystrophy of calves and lambs at pasture, but it does not prevent muscular dystrophy in calves fed on a diet containing cod liver oil. The current understanding of the biochemical function of Se and its relation to VE and the mechanisms of action of Se and VE in protection of biological membranes have been reviewed.

Nutritional Muscular Dystrophy

A simplified integrated concept of the pathogenesis of the NMD would be as follows. Diets deficient in Se and/VE permit widespread tissue lipoperoxidation, leading to hyaline degeneration and calcification of muscle fibers. One of the earliest changes in experimental Se deficiency in lambs is the abnormal retention of calcium in muscle fibers undergoing dystrophy, and Se supplementation prevents the retention of calcium. Unaccustomed exercise can accelerate the oxidative process and precipitate clinical disease. Muscle degeneration allows the release of enzymes, such as lactate dehydrogenase, aldolase, and creatine phosphokinase, the last of which is of paramount importance in diagnosis. Degeneration of skeletal muscle is rapidly and successively followed by invasion of phagocytes and regeneration. In myocardial muscle, replacement fibrosis is the rule.

In calves, lambs, and foals, the major muscles involved are skeletal, myocardial, and diaphragmatic. The myocardial and diaphragmatic forms of the disease occur most commonly in young calves, lambs, and foals, resulting in acute heart failure, respiratory distress, and rapid death, often in spite of treatment. The skeletal form of the disease occurs more commonly in older calves, yearling cattle, and older foals and results in weakness and recumbency; it is usually less severe and responds to treatment. The biceps femoris muscle is particularly susceptible in calves, and muscle biopsy is a reliable diagnostic aid.

In foals with NMD, there is a higher proportion of type IIC fibers and a lower proportion of type I and IIA fibers than in healthy foals. The type IIC fibers are found in fetal muscle and are undifferentiated and still under development. During the recovery period, fibers of types I, IIA, and IIB increase and the proportion of type IIC fibers decreases. A normal fiber type composition is present in most surviving foals 1 to 2 months after the onset of the disease.

Acute NMD results in the liberation of myoglobin into the blood, which results in myoglobinuria. This is more common in horses, older calves, and yearling cattle than in young calves, whose muscles have a lower concentration of myoglobin. Hence, the tendency to myoglobinuria will vary depending on the species and age of animal involved.

Subclinical Selenium Insufficiency

Se deficiency affects thyroid hormone metabolism and may explain the cause of ill-thrift. The conversion of the iodine-containing hormone thyroxine (T4) to the more potent triiodothyronine (T3) is impaired in animals with low Se status, and iodothyronine deiodinase is a selenoprotein that mediates this conversion.

VESD Syndrome and Others

The pathogenesis of mulberry heart disease, hepatosis dietetica, exudative diathesis, and muscular dystrophy of pigs is not yet clear. VE and Se are necessary to prevent widespread degeneration and necrosis of tissues, especially the liver, the heart, skeletal muscle, and blood vessels. Se and VE deficiency in pigs results in massive hepatic necrosis (hepatosis dietetica), degenerative myopathy of cardiac and skeletal muscles, edema, microangiopathy, and yellowish discoloration of adipose tissue. Myocardial and hepatic calcium concentrations are increased in pigs with mulberry heart disease. In addition, there may be esophagogastric ulceration, but it is uncertain whether or not this lesion is caused by a Se and/or VE deficiency. Anemia has also occurred and has been attributed to a block in bone-marrow maturation, resulting in inadequate erythropoiesis, hemolysis, or both. However, there is no firm evidence that anemia is a feature of Se and VE deficiency in pigs. The entire spectrum of lesions has been reproduced experimentally in pigs with natural or purified diets deficient in Se and VE or in which an antagonist was added to inactivate VE or Se. However, in some studies, the Se content of tissues of pigs that died from mulberry heart disease was similar to that of control pigs without the disease.

The extensive tissue destruction in pigs may account for the sudden-death nature of the complex (mulberry heart disease and hepatosis dietetica) and the muscle stiffness that occurs in some feeder pigs and sows of farrowing time with muscular dystrophy. The tissue degeneration is associated with marked increases in serum enzymes related to the tissue involved. An indirect correlation between VE intake and peroxide hemolysis in pigs on a deficient diet suggests that lipoperoxidation is the ultimate biochemical defect in pigs and that VE and Se are protective.

It is thought now that the disease is associated with the lack of balance between free-radical generation and scavenging of these radicals that is called oxidative stress. Scavengers include superoxide dismutase, glutathione peroxidase, vitamin C, and vitamin E. Se is included because it is a component of glutathione peroxidase. Deficiency of these scavengers can lead to cellular injury and death.

In these pigs, there are other complicating factors that may make the condition multifactorial. These include stress, increased iron tissue concentrations, increased calcium and decreased magnesium concentrations, and diets containing corn oil, PUFAs, aflatoxins, excess vitamin A, or dried distiller grains. Individual animals may also have a genetic predisposition.

CLINICAL FINDINGS

Nutritional muscular dystrophy is frequently diagnosed in cattle in Europe, but diagnosis based on samples is the only way to confirm the diagnosis because the clinical signs are rarely pathognomonic.[53]

Acute Enzootic Muscular Dystrophy

Affected animals may collapse and die suddenly after exercise without any other premonitory signs. The excitement associated with the hand-feeding of dairy calves may precipitate peracute death. In calves under close observation, a sudden onset of dullness and severe respiratory distress, accompanied by a frothy or blood-stained nasal discharge, may be observed in some cases. Affected calves, lambs, and foals are usually in lateral recumbency and may be unable to assume sternal recumbency even when assisted. When picked up and assisted to stand, they feel and appear limp. However, their neurologic reflexes are normal. Their eyesight and mental attitude are normal, and they are usually thirsty and can swallow unless the tongue is affected. The heart rate is usually increased up to 150 to 200/min and often with arrhythmia, the respiratory rate is increased up to 60 to 72/min, and loud breath sounds are audible over the entire lung fields. The temperature is usually normal or slightly elevated. Affected animals commonly die 6 to 12 hours after the onset of signs, in spite of therapy. Outbreaks of the disease occur in calves and lambs in which up to 15% of susceptible animals may develop the acute form and the case-fatality approaches 100%.

Subacute Enzootic Muscular Dystrophy

Subacute enzootic muscular dystrophy is the most common form in rapidly growing calves, often referred to as "white-muscle disease" and, in young lambs, "stiff-lamb disease." Affected animals may be found in sternal recumbency and be unable to stand, but some make an attempt to stand (Fig. 15-12). If they are standing, the obvious signs are stiffness, trembling of the limbs, weakness, and, in most cases, an inability to stand for more than a few minutes. The gait in calves is accompanied by rotating movements of the hocks and in lambs by a stiff, goose-stepping gait. Muscle tremor is evident if the animal is forced to stand for more than a few minutes. On palpation the dorsolumbar, gluteal, and shoulder muscle masses may be symmetrically enlarged and firmer than normal (although this may be difficult to detect). Most affected animals retain their appetite and will suck if held up to the dam or eat if hand-fed. Major involvement of the diaphragm and intercostal muscles causes dyspnea with labored and abdominal-type respiration. The temperature is usually in the normal range, but there may be a transient fever (41° C; 105° F) as a result of the effects of myoglobinemia and pain. The heart rate may be elevated, but there are usually no rhythmic irregularities. Following treatment, affected animals usually respond in a few days, and within 3 to 5 days they are able to stand and walk unassisted. In sheep with stiff-lamb disease, there were heart arrhythmias resulting from myocardial degeneration. In these lambs with low VE and Se, there were seven different arrhythmias detected.[54]

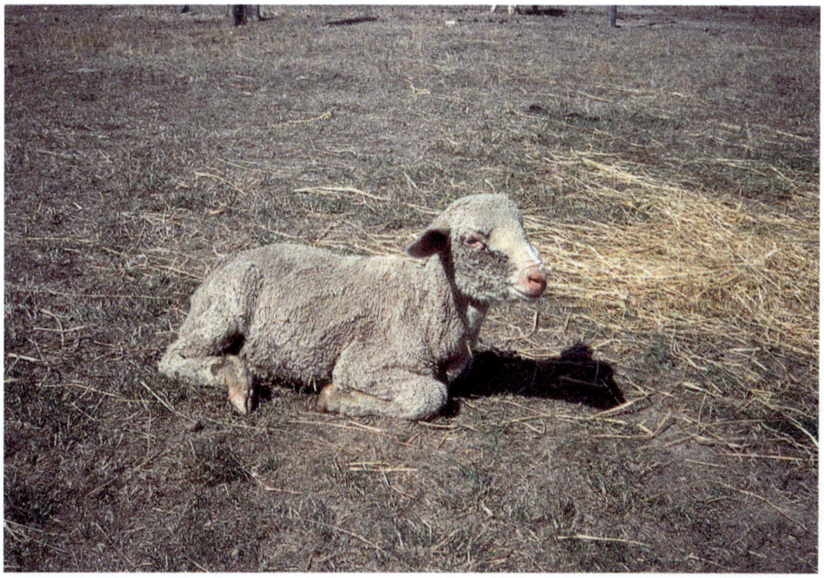

Fig. 15-12 Subacute enzootic muscular dystrophy in a recently weaned Merino lamb. The weanling is bright, alert, and responsive, with a good appetite, but it is unable to stand for more than a few seconds.

In alpacas grazing the same pastures as sheep, it was found that the sheep had higher blood Se levels but the alpacas had higher plasma Se levels.[55]

In some cases, the upper borders of the scapulae protrude above the vertebral column and are widely separated from the thorax. This has been called the "flying scapula" and has occurred in outbreaks in heifers from 18 to 24 months of age within a few days to 3 weeks after being turned out in the spring following loose-housing conditions throughout the winter.[56] The abnormality is a result of bilateral rupture of the serratus ventralis muscles and has also been reported in a red deer. Occasionally, the toes are spread, and there is relaxation of carpal and metacarpal joints or knuckling at the fetlocks and standing on tip-toe, inability to raise the head, difficulty in swallowing, inability to use the tongue, and relaxation of abdominal muscles. Choking may occur when the animals attempt to drink. In "paralytic myoglobinuria" of yearling cattle, there is usually a history of recent turning out on pasture following winter housing. Clinical signs occur within 1 week and consist of stiffness, recumbency, myoglobinuria, hyperpnea, and dyspnea. Severe cases may die within a few days, and some are found dead without premonitory signs. In rare cases, lethargy, anorexia, diarrhea, and weakness are the first clinical abnormalities recognized, followed by recumbency and myoglobinuria.

Congenital muscular dystrophy has been described in a newborn calf. The calf was still recumbent 13 hours after birth and had increased serum creatine kinase and decreased serum VE and Se levels. Recovery occurred following supportive therapy and VE and Se administration.

Subcapsular liver rupture in lambs has been associated with VE deficiency in lambs, usually those under 4 weeks of age. Affected lambs collapse suddenly, become limp, and die within a few minutes or several hours after the onset of weakness.

In **foals, muscular dystrophy** occurs most commonly during the first few months of life and is common in the first week. The usual clinical findings are failure to suck, recumbency, difficulty in rising, and unsteadiness and trembling when forced to stand. The temperature is usually normal, but commonly there is polypnea and tachycardia. The disease in foals may be characterized by an acute, fulminant syndrome, which is rapidly fatal, or a subacute syndrome characterized by profound muscular weakness. Failure of passive transfer, aspiration pneumonia, and stunting are frequent complications. In the subacute form, mortality rates may range from 30% to 45%.

In **adult horses with muscular dystrophy**, a stiff gait, myoglobinuria, depression, inability to eat, holding the head down low, and edema of the head and neck are common. The horse may be presented initially with clinical signs of colic.

In **pigs, muscular dystrophy** is not commonly recognized clinically because it is part of the more serious disease complex of mulberry heart disease and hepatosis dietetica. However, in outbreaks of this complex, sucking piglets, feeder pigs, and sows after farrowing may exhibit an uncoordinated, staggering gait suggestive of muscular dystrophy.

Subclinical nutritional muscular dystrophy occurs in apparently normal animals in herds at the time clinical cases are present. The serum activity of creatine kinase may be elevated in susceptible animals for several days before the onset of clinical signs; following treatment with VE and Se the serum enzyme activity returns to normal. Grossly abnormal electrocardiograms occur in some animals and may be detectable before clinical signs are evident.

Juvenile mortality in captive lesser kudu was reported at Basle Zoo as a result primarily of WMD caused by a diet deficient in both VE and Se.[57]

Vitamin E/Selenium Deficiency in Pigs

In pigs the total antioxidant pool is the important feature because Se and ascorbic acid are sparing for vitamin C and alpha-tocopherol.[58] Usually, they occur separately, but rarely MHD and HD occur together; even more rarely, you may find that there is NMD as well. There is a suspicion that the occurrence of two or more together has recently become more common, but this in fact may be a result of the greater awareness of both conditions. Two or more conditions require supplementation with both VE and Se.

Mulberry Heart Disease

MHD is usually seen in pigs from a few weeks to 4 months of age. The incidence of the disease is generally low. These pigs are nearly always the best of the group, and it may be that this rate of growth increases the demand for VE and Se. Nearly always the animals are found dead, so clinical signs are not often seen. Death usually results from arrhythmias associated with the myocardial necrosis.

More than one pig may be found dead. When seen alive, animals show severe dyspnea, cyanosis, and recumbency, and forced walking can cause immediate death. In some outbreaks, about 25% of pigs will show a slight inappetence and inactivity; these are probably in the subclinical stages of the disease. The stress of movement, inclement weather, or transportation will precipitate further acute deaths. The temperature is usually normal, the heart rate is rapid, and irregularities may be detectable. The feces are usually normal.

Hepatosis Dietetica

In hepatosis dietetica, most pigs are found dead. Very few cases show other signs. In occasional cases, before death there will be dyspnea, severe depression, vomiting, staggering, diarrhea, and a state of collapse. Some pigs are icteric. Outbreaks also occur similar to the pattern in mulberry heart disease. Muscular dystrophy is an almost consistent necropsy finding in both mulberry heart disease and hepatosis dietetica but is usually not recognized clinically because of the seriousness of the two latter diseases. Clinical muscular dystrophy has been described in gilts at 11 months of age. About 48 hours after farrowing, there was muscular weakness, muscular tremors, and shaking. This was followed by collapse, dyspnea, and cyanosis. There were no liver or heart lesions. In experimental Se and VE deficiency in young, rapidly growing pigs, a subtle stiffness occurred along with a significant increase in the creatinine phosphatase (CPK) and serum glutamic-oxaloacetic transaminase (SGOT) values.

CLINICAL PATHOLOGY

Myopathy

Plasma Creatine Kinase

Plasma creatine kinase (CK) is the most commonly used laboratory aid in the diagnosis of NMD. The enzyme is highly specific for cardiac and skeletal muscle and is released into the blood following unaccustomed exercise and myodegeneration. In cattle and sheep, its half-life is 2 to 4 hours, and plasma levels characteristically decline quickly unless there is continued myodegeneration but remain a good guide to the previous occurrence of muscle damage for a period of about 3 days. The normal plasma levels of CK (IU/L) are as follows: sheep, 52 ± 10; cattle, 26 ± 5; horses, 58 ± 6; and pigs, 226 ± 43. In cattle and sheep with NMD, the CK levels will be increased, usually above 1000 IU/L and commonly to 5000 to 10,000 IU/L, and not uncommonly even higher. Following turn-out of housed cattle onto pasture, the CK levels will increase up to 5000 IU/L within a few days. The CK levels will usually return to normal levels within a few days following successful treatment. Persistent high levels suggest that muscle degeneration is still progressive or has occurred within the last 2 days. Measurement of plasma CK activity could be used to monitor recovery of animals treated for nutritional myopathy.

Aspartate Aminotransferase

Aspartate aminotransferase (AST) activity is also an indicator of muscle damage, but it is not as reliable as the CK because increased AST levels may also indicate liver damage. The AST activity remains elevated for 3 to 10 days because of a much longer half-life than CK. In acute cases, levels of 300 to 900 IU/L in calves and 2000 to 3000 IU/L in lambs have been observed. In normal animals of these species, serum levels are usually less than 100 IU/L.

The magnitude of the increase in AST and CK is directly proportional to the extent of muscle damage. Both are elevated initially; an elevated AST and declining CK would suggest that muscle degeneration is no longer active. The levels of both enzymes will be increased slightly in animals that have just been turned out and subjected to unaccustomed exercise, horses in training, and in animals with ischemic necrosis of muscle as a result of recumbency caused by diseases other than muscular dystrophy. However, in acute muscular dystrophy, the levels are usually markedly elevated.

Selenium Status

Although information on the critical levels of Se in soil and plants is accumulating gradually, the estimations are difficult and expensive. Most field diagnoses are made on the basis of clinicopathologic findings, the response to treatment, and control procedures using selenium. The existence of NMD is accepted as presumptive evidence of Se deficiency, which can now be confirmed by analyses of GHS-PX and the concentrations of Se in soil, feed samples, and animal tissues. Tentative critical levels of the element are as follows:

- **Forages and grains**: A content of 0.1 mg/kg DM is considered adequate.
- **Soil**: Soils containing less than 0.5 mg/kg are likely to yield crops inadequate in selenium concentration.
- **Animal tissues, blood, and milk**: The concentrations of Se in various tissues are reliable indicators of the Se status of the animal. There is a positive correlation between the Se content of feed and the Se content of the tissues and blood of animals ingesting that feed, and the values fluctuate with the dietary intake of the element.

Three tests can be used to assess Se status in cattle and sheep: serum and whole-blood Se and glutathione peroxidase activity. Serum Se responds more rapidly to the administration of Se than whole-blood Se. There is a similar delay in glutathione peroxidase activity to Se supplementation. Blood or serum Se status is most consistently measured at the herd level. Interlaboratory differences in thresholds for deficiency exist, and results should be considered based on laboratory-specific guidelines.

The recommended blood Se reference ranges for New Zealand livestock have been used in several publications.

Reference ranges for Se and VE in serum, blood, and liver of sheep and goats in the United States are available.

Selenium Status in Horses

In New Zealand, the reference ranges for blood used for Se status in horses are as follows: adequate, greater than 1,600 nmol/L (128 ng/mL); marginal, 450 to 1,600 nmol/L (36 to 128 ng/mL); and deficient, less than 450 nmol/L (36 ng/mL).

Kidney Cortex and Liver

Normal liver Se concentrations range from 1.2 to 2.0 μg/g DM, regardless of species or age. Levels of 3.5 to 5.3 μg/g (44 to 67 nmol/g) DM in the kidney cortex and 0.90 to 1.75 μg/g (11 to 22 nmol/g) DM in the liver of cattle are indicative of adequate Se. Levels of 0.6 to 1.4 μg/g (8 to 18 nmol/g) in the kidney cortex and 0.07 to 0.60 μg/g (0.9 to 8 nmol/g) in the liver represent a deficient state.

The Se content of bovine fetal liver samples collected at an abattoir contained 0.77 μg/mL WW and 0.13 μg/mL WW, from dairy breeds and beef breeds of cattle, respectively. Mean liver Se levels from aborted bovine fetuses with myocardial lesions were 5.5 μmol/kg, 6.5 μmol/kg in fetuses without myocardial lesions, and 7.5 μmol/kg in fetuses from the abattoir, which suggests that Se deficiency may be the cause of abortion.

Blood and Milk

Blood and milk levels of Se are used as indicators of Se status in cattle and the effect of dietary supplementation. Serum Se values increase gradually with age from starting ranges for neonates of 50 to 80 ng/mL for calves and sheep and 70 to 90 for foals and pigs. Expected or normal values for adults are in the ranges of 70 to 100 for cattle, 120 to 150 for sheep, 130 to 160 for horses, and 180 to 220 for pigs.

Dams of affected calves have levels of 1.7 ng/mL (22 nmol/L) in blood and 4.9 ng/mL (62 nmol/L) in milk; their calves have blood levels of 5 to 8 ng/mL (63 to 102 nmol/L). Normal selenium-supplemented cows have 19 to 48 ng/mL (241 to 609 nmol/L) in blood and 10 to 20 ng/mL (127 to 253 nmol/L) in milk, and their calves have blood levels of 33 to 61 ng/mL (419 to 774 nmol/L). Mean Se concentrations in the blood of normal mares are 26 to 27 ng/mL (329 to 342 nmol/L). In Thoroughbred horses, Se concentrations in serum range from 39.5 to 118.5 mg/mL (40 to 160 ng/mL; 0.5 to 2.0 μmol/L), and there are significant differences between various stables of horses.

Bulk-Tank Milk

The bulk-tank milk Se levels are closely related to the mean herd blood and milk levels and have the potential to be a low-cost, noninvasive means of evaluating herd Se levels to determine Se deficiency in the dairy herd. Bulk-tank Se concentrations are an accurate reflection of the herd Se status over the range of Se intakes typical of dairy herds in an area.

Glutathione Peroxidase

There is a direct relationship between the GSH-PX activity of the blood and the Se levels of the blood and tissues of cattle, sheep, horses, and pigs. The normal Se status of cattle is represented by whole-blood Se concentration of 100 ng/mL (1270 nmol/L) and blood GSH-PX activity of approximately 30 mU/mg hemoglobin.

There is a high positive relationship ($r = 0.87$ to 0.958) between blood GSH-PX activity and blood Se concentrations in cattle. Blood Se levels less than 50 ng/mL are considered as selenium-deficient, levels between 50 and 100 ng/mL (126.6 nmol/L) are marginal, and those greater than 100 ng/mL are adequate. Comparable whole-blood levels of GSH-PX are deficient if less than 30 mU/mg hemoglobin, marginal if 30 to 60 mU/mg, and adequate if greater than 60 mU/mg hemoglobin. There is some evidence of variation in GSH-PX activities between breeds of sheep; levels may also decrease with increasing age. Low levels in some breeds of sheep may also be a reflection of adaptation to low Se intake because of low levels of Se in the soil and forages.

The GSH-PX activity is a sensitive indicator of the level of dietary Se intake and the response to the oral or parenteral administration of Se. Because Se is incorporated into erythrocyte GSH-PX only during erythropoiesis, an increase in enzyme activity of the blood will not occur for 4 to 6 weeks following administration of Se. Plasma GSH-PX will rise more quickly and will continue to increase curvilinearly with increasing dietary Se levels because it is not dependent on incorporation of the Se into the erythrocytes. The liver and Se concentration and serum GSH-PX activity may respond to changes in dietary Se more rapidly than either whole-blood Se or erythrocyte GSH-PX activity. The response in GSH-PX activity may depend on the Se status of the animals at the time when Se administered. Larger increases in the enzyme activity occur in selenium-deficient animals. The GSH-PX activity in foals reflects the amount of Se given to the mare during pregnancy.

The sandwich ELISA is a simplified method for the estimation of GSH-PX activity and Se concentration in bovine blood and can be used for rapid screening of the Se status of a large number of cattle. The GSH-PX activity of whole-blood samples has been used to assess the Se status of cattle in the Czech Republic.

The GSH-PX activity can be determined rapidly using a spot test, which is semiquantitative and can place a group of samples from the same herd or flock into one of three blood Se categories: deficient, low marginal, and marginal adequate. A commercial testing kit known as the Ransel Kit is now available. Because of the instability of GSH-PX plasma, GSH-PX activity in sheep, cattle, and pigs should be measured in fresh plasma or stored at −20° C (−4° F). For absolute measurements, it is suggested that pig plasma GSH-PX activity be measured immediately after separation from the blood cells or be assayed within 24 hours under specified laboratory conditions.

Vitamin E Status

VE occurs in nature as a mixture of tocopherols in varying proportions. They vary widely in their biological activity so that chemical determination of total tocopherols is of much less value than biological assay. Tocopherol levels in blood and liver provide good information on the VE status of the animal. However, because of the difficulty of the laboratory assays of tocopherols, they are not commonly done, and insufficient reliable data are available. Analysis of liver from clinically normal animals on pasture reveals a mean α-tocopherol level of 20 mg/kg WW for cattle and 6 mg/kg WW for sheep. The corresponding ranges were 6.0 to 53 mg/kg WW for cattle and 1.8 to 17 mg/kg WW in sheep. The critical level below which signs of deficiency may be expected are 5 mg/kg WW for cattle and 2 mg/kg WW for sheep. Tocopherol levels in the serum of less than 2 mg/L in cattle and sheep are considered to be critical levels below which deficiency diseases may occur. However, if the diet contains adequate quantities of Se, but not an excessive quantity of PUFAs, animals may thrive on low levels of serum tocopherols. In growing pigs, the serum VE levels are between 2 and 3 mg/L. In summary, there are insufficient reliable data available on the VE status on animals with NMD to be of diagnostic value.

The mean plasma VE level in clinically normal horses of various ages and breeds was 2.8 μg/mL. The optimal method for storing equine blood before α-tocopherol analysis is in an upright position in the refrigerator for up to 72 hours. If a longer period is needed, the serum or plasma should be separated, blanketed with nitrogen gas, and frozen in the smallest possible vial; the α-tocopherol in these samples will be stable at −16° C (3° F) for at least 3 months.

A summary of the GSH-PX activity, tocopherol levels, and Se levels in blood and body tissues of animals deficient in Se appears in Table 15-7. Normal values are also tabulated for comparison. Both the abnormal and normal values should be considered as guidelines for diagnosis because of the wide variations in levels between groups of animals. The level of dietary Se may fluctuate considerably, which may account for variations in GSH-PX. Se reference ranges to determine Se status of sheep and cattle in New Zealand are shown in Table 15-8.

In the early stages of the subclinical form of NMD in lambs, there may be a decrease in serum Se and glutathione peroxidase activity and an increase in the activity of aspartate aminotransferase (AST), creatine kinase (CK), and lactate dehydrogenase (LDH) compared with healthy lambs. The LDH-isoenzyme activity is useful for detection of subclinical forms of NMD because of significant increases in the activity of the LDH_5-muscle fraction.

Table 15-7 Glutathione peroxidase (GSH-PX) activity and selenium concentration in blood and body tissues of animals deficient in selenium

Species	Clinical state or degree of deficiency	Erythrocyte GSH-PX activity μmol/min at 37° C/g hemoglobin	Serum selenium (μg/mL)	Liver selenium (μg/g DM)
Cattle	Normal or adequate	19.0–36.0	0.08–0.30	0.90–1.75
	Marginal	10.0–19.0	0.03–0.077	0.45–0.90
	Deficient	0.2–10.0	0.002–0.025	0.07–0.60
Sheep	Normal or adequate	60–180	0.08–0.50	0.90–3.50
	Marginal	8–30	0.03–0.05	0.52–0.90
	Deficient	2–7	0.006–0.03	0.02–0.35
Horse	Adequate	30–150	0.14–0.25	1.05–3.50
	Deficient	8–30	0.008–0.55	0.14–0.70
Pigs	Adequate	100–200	0.12–0.30	1.40–2.80
	Deficient	<50	0.005–0.60	0.10–0.35

Table 15-8 Selenium reference range to determine selenium status of sheep and cattle in New Zealand

	Deficient	Marginal	Adequate
Sheep			
Blood selenium (nmol/L)	<130	130–250	>250
Liver selenium (nmol/kg fresh tissue)	<250	250–450	>450
Cattle			
Blood selenium (nmol/L)	<130	130–250	>250
Liver selenium (nmol/kg fresh tissue)	<600	600–850	>850
Serum selenium (nmol/L)	<85	85–140	>250
Blood glutathione peroxidase (Ku/L −25°C)	<0.5	0.5–2.0	>2.0

Farmed Red Deer

Reference range data for liver and blood selenium in red deer are limited. White-muscle disease has occurred in young deer with blood and liver Se concentrations of 84 to 140 nmol/L and 240 to 500 nmol/kg fresh tissue, respectively. No growth-rate response to Se supplementation occurred in 1-year-old deer when blood Se concentrations were less than 130 nmol/L, the range in which a growth rate response would be expected in sheep.

Pigs

An increase in the activity of several plasma enzymes occurs in Se and VE deficiencies of pigs. The measurement of AST, CPK, LDH, and isocitrate dehydrogenase can be used to detect the onset of degeneration of skeletal and myocardial muscles and liver. However, these are not commonly used for diagnostic purposes because of the acuteness of the illness. The determination of the levels of Se in feed supplies, tissues, and blood of affected pigs is much more useful as an aid to diagnosis and for guidelines for supplementation of the diet.

In Se–VE deficiency in pigs, serum Se values of less than 2.5 ng/mL (3.2 nmol/L), hepatic Se of less than 0.10 mg/kg (1.3 μmol/kg), plasma α-tocopherol values of less than 0.40 μg/mL, and hepatic α-tocopherol concentrations of less than 0.75 μg/g of tissue are common. In a recent study, the VE level was less than 2 ppm in 25% of pigs with gross and microscopic lesions of MHD. In a recent study, results suggested that supplementation with a surfeit level of VE reduced the response to endotoxin (i.e., a reduced response to the peak levels of IL-6).

The diagnostic criteria for the VESD complex in pigs in New Zealand indicate that liver VE concentrations greater than 10 μmol/kg are adequate, with less than 2.5 μmol/kg associated with deficiency. Corresponding estimates for serum VE are greater than 2.5 μmol/L and less than 0.8 μmol/L, respectively. Liver Se concentrations of greater than 2200 nmol/kg are adequate, with 1100 to 2200 nmol/kg being in the marginal range and less than 1100 nmol/kg being deficient. Deficiency levels for blood are in the range of 400 to 1500 nmol/L. These values must be interpreted along with the concentration of PUFAs in the diet.

There is a close relationship between blood VE and resistance of erythrocytes against lipid peroxidation. The supplementation of the diet of pigs with VE will increase both the serum levels of VE and the resistance of the erythrocytes to lipid peroxidation.

NECROPSY FINDINGS

The gross appearance of the muscle lesions is quite constant, but the distribution of affected muscles varies widely in different animals. Affected groups of skeletal muscle are bilaterally symmetric and contain localized white or gray areas of degeneration and necrosis. These areas may be in streaks, involving a large group of muscle fibers that run through the center of the apparently normal muscle or as a peripheral boundary around a core of normal muscle. In the diaphragm, the distribution of damaged bundles gives the tissue a radially striated appearance. The affected muscle is friable and edematous and may be mineralized. Secondary pneumonia often occurs in cases where the muscles of the throat and chest are affected. In cases with myocardial involvement, white areas of degeneration are visible, particularly under the endocardium of the left ventricle in calves and of both ventricles in lambs. The lesions may extend to involve the interventricular septum and papillary muscles and have a gritty character consistent with mineralization. Pulmonary congestion and edema is common.

Histologically, the muscle lesions in all species are **noninflammatory**. Hyaline degeneration is followed by coagulation necrosis and variable degrees of mineralization.

Other than a variable degree of muscular atrophy, gross lesions are not seen in horses with **equine motor neuron disease**. Confirmation of the diagnosis relies on histologic identification of characteristic degeneration and loss of motor neurons of the spinal cord ventral horns. However, a very strong presumptive diagnosis can be achieved by microscopic confirmation of neurogenic atrophy in the sacrocaudalis dorsalis muscle or axonal degeneration in the spinal accessory nerve.

A generalized **steatitis** has been described in newborn foals less than 2 months of age. The microscopic appearance of this yellow-brown fat consists of necrotic fat infiltrated by neutrophils, macrophages, and giant cells. Steatitis and nodular panniculitis have also been reported in a 3-year-old VE–Se-deficient mare.

In **mulberry heart disease**, the carcass is in good condition. All body cavities contain excessive amounts of fluid and shreds of fibrin. In the peritoneal cavity, the fibrin is often in the form of a lacy net covering all the viscera. The liver is enlarged, appears mottled, and has a characteristic nutmeg appearance on the cut surface. The lungs are edematous, and excessive fluid in the pleural cavities is accompanied by collapse of the ventral lung field. The pericardial sac is filled with gelatinous fluid interlaced with bands of fibrin. Beneath the epicardium and endocardium are multiple hemorrhages of various sizes. Usually, this hemorrhage is more severe on the right side of the heart. This gives the heart the typical mottled appearance, which is caused by areas of necrosis and areas of hemorrhage.

Histologically, the characteristic lesion is widespread myocardial congestion, hemorrhage, and myofiber degeneration. Multiple fibrinous microthrombi are within the myocardial capillaries, and occasionally degenerative changes are visible in the walls of small arterioles in many organs, including the heart. Malacia of cerebral white matter or, more rarely, the molecular layer of the cerebellum may occur and is attributable to microvascular damage. Microscopic lesions consistent with dietary microangiopathy may also be found in arterioles and capillaries of the heart, kidneys, liver, stomach, intestine, mesentery, skeletal muscle, and skin. It should be stressed that in some cases, the disease course is so rapid that morphologic changes are not discernible in the myocardial cells. Because it can be extremely difficult to distinguish mulberry heart disease from *S. suis* septicemia histologically, it is prudent to also attempt bacteriologic culture when attempting to confirm the diagnosis.

In **hepatosis dietetica,** the liver is swollen and turgid and has a mottled to mosaic-like appearance throughout its lobes. Many of the lobules are distended and reddish in color. There is in fact an irregular distribution of hepatic necrosis and hemorrhage. The gall bladder may be edematous, and there may also be myocardial necrosis and pulmonary edema. Typically, the disease course is so rapid that jaundice does not develop. Histologically, there is a distinct lobular distribution of hemorrhage, degeneration, and necrosis.

In **NMD** of pigs, the lesions are often only visible at the microscopic level and consist of areas of bilaterally distributed areas of muscular degeneration. The changes include hyalinization, loss of striations, and fragmentation of myofibers. The sections are difficult to cut because of the presence of calcium in the myocytes. A mild degree of NMD may accompany some cases of hepatosis dietetica.

Samples for Confirmation of Diagnosis

- **Toxicology**—50 g liver (ASSAY [Se] [VE])
- **Histology**—formalin-fixed skeletal muscle (multiple sites), heart (both left and right ventricular walls), and brain (including cerebral hemisphere) (LM). It may require special stains to show the presence of calcium in the sections. In biopsies from medial gluteal muscles using a Bergstrom needle, there were ragged red fibers of type I and IIA. Muscle fiber atrophy and subsarcolemmal aggregates in type I and IIA fibers were also found. More severely affected horses had inflammatory infiltrate, collagen proliferation, phagocytosis, necrosis, and calcification.[59]
- **Bacteriology** (for mulberry heart disease only)—heart, liver, swab from pericardial sac (CULT)

DIFFERENTIAL DIAGNOSIS

Nutritional muscular dystrophy (NMD)
NMD is most common in young rapidly growing animals fed a ration deficient in selenium and vitamin E or whose dams were on a deficient, unsupplemented ration throughout the winter months. Characteristically, the disease is sudden in onset, and several animals are affected initially or within a few days, particularly following unaccustomed exercise. In the acute form, generalized weakness and a state of collapse are common. In the subacute form, the major clinical findings are stiffness in walking, long periods of recumbency or total recumbency, inability to stand, a normal mental attitude and appetite, and no abnormal neurologic findings to account for the recumbency. The creatine phosphokinase (CPK) levels are markedly elevated.

Calves and yearlings
Acute enzootic muscular dystrophy in calves with myocardial involvement must be differentiated from other diseases causing generalized weakness, toxemia, and shock.

These include the following:

- **Septicemias**: *Haemophilus* septicemia resulting in weakness, recumbency, and fever
- **Pneumonia**: Pneumonic pasteurellosis causing dyspnea, toxemia, fever, and weakness

Subacute enzootic muscular dystrophy, in which skeletal muscle lesions predominate, must be differentiated from other diseases of young calves and yearlings characterized clinically by paresis and paralysis. The subacute form is more common in yearlings and young cattle and is characterized by recumbency, with other body systems being within relatively normal ranges. The other diseases include the following:

- **Musculoskeletal diseases**—polyarthritis, traumatic or infectious myopathies (blackleg), osteodystrophy and fractures of long bones
- **Diseases of the nervous system**—spinal cord compression, *Hemophilus* meningoencephalitis and myelitis, organophosphatic insecticide poisoning
- **Diseases of the digestive tract**—carbohydrate engorgement resulting in lactic acidosis, shock, dehydration, and weakness

Lambs and kids
In lambs with "stiff-lamb" disease, there is stiffness and a stilted gait, affected animals

Continued

prefer recumbency, and they are bright and alert and will suck the ewe if assisted. The serum levels of CPK and serum glutamic-oxaloacetic transaminase (SGOT) are also markedly elevated. Differentiation may be necessary from enzootic ataxia and swayback, but in these two diseases, stiffness is not characteristic, but rather, weakness and paresis.

Foals

In foals, NMD must be differentiated from acute diseases of the musculoskeletal and nervous system causing abnormal gait, weakness, and recumbency. They include the following:

- Polyarthritis
- Meningitis
- Traumatic injury to the spinal cord

Mulberry heart disease

Mulberry heart disease must be differentiated from other common causes of sudden death in pigs in which the diagnosis is made at necropsy:

- Acute septicemias attributable to salmonellosis, erysipelas, pasteurellosis, and anthrax
- Porcine stress syndrome
- Gut edema
- Intestinal volvulus, heat exhaustion, suffocation during transportation

TREATMENT

Because of the overlapping functions of Se and VE and because it is not always possible to know the relative etiologic importance of one nutrient or the other in causing some of the acute conditions already described, it is recommended that a combined mixture of selenium and α-tocopherol be used in treatment. α-Tocopherol is the most potent form of the tocopherols and is available in a number of pharmaceutical forms, which also vary in their biological activity. It has become necessary to express the unitage of VE in terms of international units of biological activity (1 IU:1 mg synthetic racemic α-tocopherol acetate; natural D-α-tocopherol acetate 1 mg: 1 IU and natural D-α-tocopherol 1 mg: 0.92 IU). It is also obvious that we need to know how to use organic Se (Se-enriched yeast) because this is likely to be much more valuable as a supplement than sodium selenite as a component of the 30+ selenoproteins.

In cattle, a blend of ammonium chloride, VE, and Se is recommended for the treatment of retained fetal membranes.[60]

Organic selenium (Se-enriched yeast) is a strategy to increase the benefits of the replacement of sodium selenite.[61] Se-enriched yeast increases milk selenium at parturition and weaning.[62]

Nutritional Muscular Dystrophy

For treatment of NMD in calves, lambs, and foals, a mixture containing 3 mg Se (as sodium or potassium selenite) and 150 IU/mL of DL-α-tocopherol acetate, given IM at 2 mL/45 kg BW, is recommended. One treatment is usually sufficient. Animals with severe myocardial involvement will usually not respond to treatment, and the case-mortality rate is about 90%. However, all in-contact animals in the herd (calves, lambs, and foals) should be treated prophylactically with the same dose of Se and VE. They should be handled carefully during treatment to avoid precipitating acute muscular dystrophy. Animals with subacute skeletal muscular dystrophy will usually begin to improve by 3 days following treatment and may be able to stand and walk unassisted within 1 week.

Animals sometimes do not respond to either VE or Se or treatment with both.

Supplementation of lambs with Se had no significant effect on performance and blood hematology, but it increased blood G-Th-P and serum T3 but decreased serum T4 compared with nonsupplemented lambs. Se-enriched yeast significantly improved the disgestibility.[63] In outbreaks of mulberry heart disease, hepatosis dietetica, and related Se- and VE-deficiency diseases in pigs, all clinically affected pigs and all pigs at risk should be treated individually with a combination of Se/VE parenterally, at first to prevent any further sudden deaths. It can then be followed by oral administration.

CONTROL

It is necessary to adapt production systems to take into account changes in climatic systems, which can alter the feeding constituents and increase vitamin and mineral requirements and alter the balance between gestation and sources of stress.[31]

Se status is now associated with improved immune function, arthropathy, and cardiomyopathy. Most important, it protects against oxidative stress and aids in regulation of thyroid hormone metabolism.[64]

The control and prevention of the major diseases caused by Se and VE deficiencies can generally be accomplished by the provision of both nutrients to susceptible animals fed on deficient rations.

Provide Selenium and Vitamin E

Over the years, both the VE levels and Se levels in the diets have increased but particularly the former. This is in response to the more rapid growth rates of pigs but also the realization that pigs are coping with many more oxidative disease states. Outdoor pigs usually have sufficient levels of both unless the soil is Se deficient. A recent study from China has suggested that dietary zinc at 85 mg/kg, Se at 0.40 mg/kg, and vitamin E at 45 IU/kg is appropriate for crossbred sows.

Although Se alone is protective against a greater spectrum of diseases than is VE, there are situations in which VE is more protective. Both Se and VE should be provided when the diets are deficient in both nutrients, but this may not apply in every situation. Most of the emphasis has been on Se supplementation at the expense of VE, which is more expensive and less stable. Most injectable VE and Se preparations are adequate in Se but insufficient in VE.

There have been several attempts to supplement weaner pigs with a VE preparation. Besides individual injections, it is possible to supplement weaner pigs with water supplementation. Pigs will usually drink even if they are not eating. A recent study showed that the supplementation of drinking water with high doses of VE (150 mg of DL-α-tocopherol acetate) was effective in maintaining serum VE levels over the weaning period. This was even true when the intake of food over the weaning period was very low (it can be as low as 0.2 to 0.3 kg) and there was a temporary malabsorption in the intestine. It takes about 100 IU/L of water to provide a good VE blood serum value.

Maternal Transfer to Newborn

Treatment with organic and inorganic Se improves the growth rate, humoral immune response, and antioxidant status of the lambs.[65] Se supplementation in cattle and ewes is associated with increased embryo production, higher fetal mass, and reduced levels of retained placenta. There is a complex relationship between supplementation (source of Se, time, length of time, presence of interfering elements, and the diet feeding regime). A 79-mg Se pill to dairy cows 3 weeks before expected calving date significantly elevated blood Se levels in cows after calving.[66] Nearly always, calf VE levels are lower than cow VE levels.[67]

Diseases caused by Se deficiency are preventable by the administration of Se to the dam during pregnancy or directly to the young, rapidly growing animal. Se is transported across the placenta and provides protection for the neonate. Oral supplementation with Se in beef cattle will provide enough to maintain blood levels in the dam and for adequate transfer to the fetus, which can sequester Se when the levels are low in the dam. The colostrum of selenium-supplemented cattle also contains an adequate amount of Se to prevent severe selenium-deficiency diseases. However, by 7 days after parturition, the levels in milk may be inadequate to maintain adequate serum levels in calves. The strategic administration of Se and VE before the expected occurrence of the disease is also a reliable method of preventing the disease.

Selenium Is Potentially Toxic

Selenium toxicosis is seen as a chronic problem (alkali disease) or as an acute selenosis (blind staggers). In a study of Se toxicity in lambs, it was found that sodium selenite administration led to decreased VE levels in the liver, but selenomethionine (organic Se) did not.[68] This study suggests that the chemical form of the ingested Se must be known to interpret tissue, blood, and serum concentrations. It can be associated with severe depression, dyspnea, congested mucous membranes, watery diarrhea, and colic spasms,[69] and high levels of Se can be found in heart muscle, liver, and kidney. Chronic selenosis has also been described in camels.[70]

Because Se is toxic, any treatment and control program using it must be carefully monitored. Se injected into or fed to animals concentrates in liver, skeletal muscle, kidney, and other tissues, and withdrawal periods before slaughter must be allowed. There is some concern that Se may be a carcinogen for humans. The only tissues that appear likely to consistently accumulate more than 3 to 4 mg/kg of Se are the kidney and liver, and these are very unlikely to constitute more than a very small part of the human diet. There have been no reports of untoward effects of Se on human health when it has been used at nutritional levels in food-producing animals. The incorporation of Se into commercially prepared feeds for some classes of cattle and pigs has been approved in some countries. A recent case in Norway showed the hazards of Se contamination in the case of an iron supplement. Se toxicosis has been fairly regularly reported. Se toxicosis in pigs seen as progressive apathy, paralysis, and sudden death has been described.[71]

Pigs that are deficient may be more susceptible to other diseases. Pigs with NMD often have the appearance of pneumonic pigs because the diaphragm is weak and the pigs are dyspneic.

Deficient and small pigs may be more susceptible to the effects of iron, and when this is given by injection there may be large numbers of dead piglets as a result of iron toxicity. In these cases, the heart lesions resemble those of MHD.

In a recent case of Se toxicosis in sheep associated with excessive sodium selenite in commercial supplement,[72] there were hemorrhages throughout the lung lobes and edema. Toxicity is greater than 250 umol/kg DM, and in these sheep the levels were 325 to 400 umol/kg DM. Se-accumulating plants are thought not to occur in the United Kingdom, and these sheep were thought to have been given free-access minerals from bags with 7628 to 8771 ppm of selenium.

Selenium in Milk Supplies

The use of Se in the diet of lactating dairy cows has caused concern about possible adulteration of milk supplies. However, the addition of Se to the diets of lactating dairy cows at levels that are protective against the deficiency diseases does not result in levels in the milk that are hazardous for human consumption. The feeding of excessive quantities of Se to dairy cattle would cause toxicity before levels became toxic for humans. Se supplementation to colostrum increased the IgG amounts and Se concentration in blood plasma in newborn calves.[73]

Dietary Requirement of Selenium

The dietary requirement of Se for both ruminants and nonruminants is 0.1 mg/kg DM of the element in the diet. There may be Nutritionally important differences in the Se status between the same feeds grown in different regions and between different feeds within a region. Even within a region featuring high Se concentrations, some feeds may contain levels of Se below the 0.1 mg/kg minimum requirement for livestock. Thus an Se analysis of feeds appears necessary to supplement livestock appropriately. Some geographic areas are known to be deficient in Se, and the feeds grown in these areas must be supplemented with Se and VE on a continuous basis. Some reports indicate that surveys have found that dairy producers are providing insufficient supplementary Se in the ration to meet the recommended Se intake for lactating dairy cows. Long-term administration of organic Se in the form of Se yeast provides higher blood and tissue concentrations than repeated parenteral administration of recommended therapeutic doses of inorganic Se.

Grass-based diets elevate precursors of VE and vitamin A. Argentinian beef contains more α -tocopherols, beta carotene, ascorbic acid, and glutathione than feedlot beef.[74]

There is an improvement in the preventative antioxidant systems of cows fed Se-enriched yeast.[75]

Avoidance of high-sulfate diets is desirable, but provision of adequate Se overcomes the sulfate effect.

Glutathione Peroxidase Activity

Whole-blood GSH-PX activity is a way of monitoring Se status but is not as reliable in pigs as in sheep and cattle. Levels of the enzyme increased significantly over a 12-week period when beef cattle were receiving organic or inorganic Se. Levels were higher in the group receiving organic Se. It was shown that combinations of Se injections and supplementation could help maintain Se and GSH-Px blood status in beef cattle heifers.[76]

Pigs

In growing pigs, both Se and vitamin E at 30 IU/kg DM of feed are necessary for the prevention of the diseases caused by diets deficient in vitamin E and Se. Supplementation of the diet of the sow will result in an adequate transfer to the piglets. Satisfactory protection of the diseases of pigs caused by VE/Se deficiency depends on the correct balance between Se, α-tocopherol, and PUFAs in the diet and the presence of a suitable antioxidant to conserve the α-tocopherol.

Different Methods of Supplementation

The prevention of the major diseases caused by Se and VE deficiencies can be achieved by different methods, including the following:

- Dietary supplementation in the feed or water supplies
- Individual parenteral injections
- Oral administration
- Pasture top dressing

The method used will depend on the circumstances of the farm, the ease of administration, the cost, the labor available, the severity of the deficiency that exists, and whether or not the animals are being dosed regularly for other diseases, such as parasitism. The subcutaneous injection of barium selenate, the administration of an intraruminal pellet, and the addition of Se to the water supply were compared in cattle; each method was effective for periods ranging from 4 to 12 months.

Dietary Supplementation

The inclusion of Se and VE in the feed supplies or salt and mineral mixes has been generally successful in preventing the major diseases caused by deficiencies of these two nutrients. The currently available data do not support the use of supplemental injections of VE for beef cattle because the benefits are greater when VE is fed.[77]

Selenium Dose

Individual Injections

Injections of Se and VE have been used successfully for prevention, particularly in circumstances where the diet cannot be easily supplemented. Following the IM injections of sodium selenite into calves, lambs, and piglets, the Se concentration of the tissues, particularly the liver, increases and then declines to reach preinjection levels in 23 days in calves and 14 days in lambs and piglets. Adequate sources of vitamin E also must be provided. Injectable preparations of Se and VE are usually adequate in Se and deficient in VE, and it may not be possible to correct a marginal deficiency of VE in pregnant beef cattle, for example, by IM injection of a Se and VE preparation that contains an inadequate concentration of VE. The current label dose of injectable Se, 0.055 mg Se/kg BW, which is therapeutically adequate for NMD, is not sufficient for long-term Se supplementation of cattle on a Se-deficient diet. Copper and Se supplementation by parenteral administration can be combined when both deficiencies are present.

Subcutaneous Injections

Cattle and Sheep. A slow-release preparation of barium selenate for SC injection is now available for use in cattle and sheep. An SC injection of 1 mg selenium/kg BW to ewes 3 weeks before breeding elevated the Se level in milk during lactation and increased the Se concentration and GSH-PX activity in the blood of the lambs during the period when they are at greatest risk from selenium-deficiency diseases. At a dose of 1 mg selenium/kg BW to pregnant ewes, the GSH-PX activity is increased and maintained at adequate levels for up to 5 months. There is adequate transfer of Se to the lambs, providing protection for up to 12 weeks of age, which covers the period when lambs are at greatest risk. A dose of 1.2 mg selenium/kg BW provided adequate Se status for as long as two consecutive lambing seasons. Barium selenate at 1 mg selenium/kg BW SC provides protection in young sheep for at least 3 months and is not associated with risk of Se toxicity or unacceptable residues of Se in tissues other than the site of injection. A dose of 1 mg selenium/kg BW (barium selenate) to cattle SC increased the GSH-PX activity within 4 weeks and was maintained at high levels for up to 5 months.

Pigs. The SC injection of barium selenate of pregnant sows at 0.5 to 1.0 mg selenium/kg BW resulted in a significant difference in GSH-PX activity in the piglets from treated sows compared with untreated controls. The SC injection of barium selenate at 2.5 mg selenium/kg BW into pigs weighing 20 kg also maintained blood levels of selenium and GSH-PX activity during the most rapid growing period. The relative safety of barium selenate is a result of its slow rate of release from the site of injection. By comparison, when Se is administered as a soluble salt, such as sodium selenite, acute toxicity may occur at doses of 0.45 mg selenium/kg BW. Treatment with barium selenate increases the concentration of Se in blood, liver, and muscle and persists for at least 4 months. One disadvantage of barium selenate is that a large residue persists at the site of injection for long periods. The use of sodium selenite also increases tissue and blood concentrations of Se, but they begin to decline by 23 days. The bovine liver rapidly removes approximately 40% of injected Se salts (soluble) from the systemic plasma, binds it to a plasma component, and releases it back into circulation within 1 hour of injection.

Farmed Red Deer. A long-acting barium selenate given subcutaneously to red deer on pasture, at 0.5, 1.0, or 2.0 mg Se/kg BW, elevated blood Se concentrations from 105 nmol/L preinjection for at least 377 days, with peak levels of 1894, 1395, and 818 nmol/L for high, medium, and low doses, respectively. Pastures contained 10 to 30 mg Se/kg DM. There was no significant difference in growth rate between treated and control deer. The preparation produced fewer and less severe SC tissue reactions than previous preparations. Young, rapidly growing deer seem less sensitive to Se deficiency, as measured by weight gain, than sheep and cattle, suggesting that reference ranges for those species are not appropriate for deer.

Oral Selenium and Anthelmintics

Oral dosing using sodium selenite is sometimes combined with the administration of anthelmintics and vaccinations. The dose should approximate 0.044 mg/kg BW. A routine program in a severely deficient area comprises three doses of 5 mg of selenium (11 mg sodium selenite) each to ewes, one before mating, one at midpregnancy, and one 3 weeks before lambing, along with four doses to the lambs. The first dose to lambs (of 1 mg) is given at docking and the others (2 mg each) at weaning and then at 3-month intervals. A 100-day controlled release anthelmintic capsule containing 13.9 mg of selenium will protect lambs from Se deficiency for at least 180 days.

Both Se and cobalt can be incorporated into an anthelmintic program. The levels of GSH-PX activity may be monitored on a regular basis following the drenching with Se and provide a good indication of Se availability and the Se status of grazing sheep.

Pasture Top Dressing

The application of sodium selenate as a top dressing to pasture is now practiced and permitted in some countries. Top dressing at the approved rate of 10 g selenium/ha is effective for 12 months and has a toxicity margin of safety of about 20 times. Sodium selenate is now used in preference to sodium selenite because only about one-fifth is required to raise the pasture level of Se to the same concentrations provided by sodium selenite. Top dressing of severely deficient pumice soils in New Zealand prevented deficiency for at least 12 months, sheep were protected against white-muscle disease in sheep, and reproduction performance and weight gains were improved. It is recommended that sodium selenate be applied annually to all selenium-deficient soils at the rate of 10 g selenium/ha added to the superphosphate fertilizer or as prills of sodium selenate alone. Top dressing is an economical alternative to individual animal dosing, particularly in severely deficient areas with a high stocking rate. At the approved rate, no adverse effects are anticipated for human or animal health or for the environment. Se-enriched fertilizer increases the Se level of hay to a level that is recommended for horses (0.1 mg/kg DM).[78]

Muscular Dystrophy

Under most conditions, NMD of calves and lambs can be prevented by providing Se and VE in the diets of the cow or ewe during pregnancy at 0.1 mg/kg DM of actual Se and α-tocopherol at 1 g/d per cow and 75 mg/d per ewe. If possible, the supplementation should be continued during lactation to provide a continuous source of Se to the calves and lambs. Under some conditions the level of 0.1 mg/kg DM may be inadequate. In some circumstances, the optimal Se concentration in the feed is considerably higher than 0.1 mg/kg DM, and levels up to 1.0 mg/kg DM in the feed result in increases in GSH-PX activity, which may be beneficial; however, the cost-effectiveness has not been determined. Pregnant ewes being fed on alfalfa hay may require selenium at a level of up to 0.2 mg/kg DM to prevent white-muscle disease in their lambs. Young, rapidly growing cattle, particularly beef cattle, likely to receive hay and straw deficient in Se and those that are fed high-moisture grain should receive a supplement of Se at the rate of 0.1 mg/kg DM and α-tocopherol at 150 mg/d per head. If selenium-supplemented concentrates are used as part of a feeding program for dairy cows, it is not necessary to provide additional Se by parenteral injection.

Lambs are born with a low serum level of VE, but the concentration increases rapidly after the ingestion of colostrum. Supplementation of pregnant ewes with α-tocopherol, either as a single IM dose (500 mg 2 weeks before lambing) or orally (150 mg daily during 3 to 4 weeks before lambing) results in a marked increase in the levels of the vitamin in the serum and colostrum. The VE concentration in colostrum was 5 to 11 times higher than in milk 1 week after lambing.

VE supplementation of the feed of weaner sheep by oral drench or feed additive is effective in increasing plasma α-tocopherol concentrations. This is the most practical method for housed sheep and prevents subclinical myopathy. The IM oily injection was slow to increase plasma levels of tocopherols and did not prevent myopathy in grazing experiments. VE supplements have no beneficial effects on wool quality or quantity in grazing sheep, and unless certain flocks are susceptible to VE deficiency myopathy, it is not recommended.

Beef Cattle and Sheep

Salt–Mineral Mixture

NMD can be prevented in unweaned beef calves and lambs by the inclusion of Se (14.8 mg/kg) and VE (2700 IU/kg) in the mineral supplement provided ad libitum to the pregnant cows and ewes on a selenium-deficient ration during the latter two-thirds of gestation and for the first month of lactation. Under most conditions this will provide Se at 0.1 mg/kg DM in the diet.

The provision of **sodium selenite in a salt–mineral mixture** to provide 90 mg of selenium/kg salt–mineral mixture on a year-round basis, even under range conditions, increased GSH-PX activity levels into normal ranges in beef cows for 3 months when fed to extremely deficient animals. Calves of these cows had increased weaning weights and decreased incidence of infectious diseases, but the trial was uncontrolled. The provision of 30 mg selenium/kg salt–mineral mixture was insufficient to raise the GSH-PX activity levels to normal ranges. Peak blood selenium levels were achieved in weaned beef calves supplemented with 80 and 160 mg selenium/kg in free-choice salt–mineral mixtures for a period of 108 days. In some jurisdictions, it may be necessary for the veterinarian to prescribe a supplement containing higher levels than those permitted by legislation. A level of 25 mg/kg selenium of a salt–mineral mixture provided ad libitum for sheep will result in sufficient levels of Se in the dam's blood and milk to prevent Se deficiency diseases. Each ewe must consume from 8 to 12 g of the salt–mineral mixture per day.

Se deficiency in grazing and forage-fed cattle is widespread in the United States and other countries. Calves may be severely depleted of Se and selenium-dependent glutathione peroxidase but exhibit no clinical signs of deficiency unless they are subjected to an oxidant or other types of stress. Nursing beef calves may be at risk of Se deficiency if their dams are not supplemented with Se. Even when sodium selenite is used in a free-choice mineral supplement designed to deliver 2 mg of Se daily, calves are still at risk for Se deficiency for up to 90 days. Se supplementation of pregnant beef cows with seleno-yeast in a free-choice mineral mixture increased the whole-blood Se and GSH-PX activity of both cows and calves and was much superior to sodium selenite.

In some parts of the world, it is recommended that animals be allowed to graze saltbrush, which produces a higher quality of sheep and goat meat with less fat, more lean meat, and higher VE levels.[79]

The supplementation of beef cattle in late gestation with oral VE, 1000 IU/head per day, influenced the VE status of cows that calved in late winter to a greater extent than that of cows calving in late summer because of the high VE content in the pasture-based summer diet. Calves from supplemented cows had higher serum VE levels than calves from unsupplemented cows. Winter-born calves from supplemented Hereford cows had heavier 205-day adjusted weaning weights than did winter-born calves from unsupplemented cows. Supplementation did not affect vitamin E or IgG concentrations in cows that calved in late summer, and it did not affect calf growth.

Dairy Cattle

Selenium

The legal commercial Se supplementation of complete rations for dairy cattle in the United States has been increased from 0.1 to 0.3 mg/kg DM of complete feed. At this rate, a lactating cow consuming 20 kg of DM/d would consume about 6 mg supplemental selenium in addition to that naturally present in the feedstuffs. Current recommendations indicate that Se intake for lactating and gestating dairy cattle should range from 5 to 7 mg/d for adequate concentrations in serum or plasma that would range from 70 to 100 ng of selenium/mL serum. Such supplementation should result in improved Se status of the newborn, improved concentration of Se in colostrum, and improved health of the calves. The effects of Se supplementation in dairy cattle on reproductive performance is equivocal. Some studies over a period of two lactations revealed no effect on reproductive performance, whereas others report an improvement in dairy cattle in a district considered to be marginally deficient in selenium. Intakes of inorganic Se as sodium selenite in amounts of 50 mg/d for 90 days or 100 mg/d for 28 days by adult dairy cows (10 to 30 times the nutritional requirement) did not cause any health problems. The toxic dose for cattle ranges from 0.25 to 0.5 mg/kg BW.

Milk replacers for dairy calves should contain a suitable antioxidant and be supplemented with 300 IU/kg DM of α-tocopherol acetate at the rate of 0.1 mg/kg DM of the milk replacer.

Vitamin E

Dietary or parenteral supplementation of VE to dairy cows during the peripartum period has consistently improved the function of neutrophils and macrophages. However, the effects of supplementation of dry dairy cows with VE in the feed or parenteral administration of VE before parturition on the incidence of disease have been variable. The amount of supplemental VE fed per day during the prepartum period has ranged from 1000 to 3000 IU/day. Feeding 1000 IU/day of supplemental VE to dry cows when adequate Se was supplemented reduced the incidence of retained placenta. The prepartum subcutaneous injection of dairy cows with 3000 IU of VE, 1 week before expected calving, had no significant effect on the incidence of retained placenta, clinical mastitis, metritis, endometritis, ketosis, displaced abomasum, or lameness. VE administered to cows with marginal pretreatment VE status had a reduced risk of retained placenta. In cows with adequate serum VE, there was no reduction in the incidence of any disease.

Based on health and immune function in cows, plasma concentrations of α-tocopherol in peripartum cows should be approximately 3 μg/mL. To maintain these blood values, dry cows and heifers fed stored forages during the last 60 days of gestation require approximately 1.6 IU of supplemental vitamin E/kg BW (approximately 80 IU/kg DMI). Increased intake of VE of cows and heifers during the prepartum period also increases the VE in colostrum. Milk is not a major source of VE, but colostrum contains high concentrations of α-tocopherol (3 to 6 μg/mL). To reduce the incidence of mastitis in lactating cows being fed stored forages, the recommendation for VE is 0.8 IU/kg BW (approximately 20 IU/kg DMI). When fresh forage is fed, there is less need for supplemental VE. The intake of polyunsaturated fatty acids increases the VE requirement, and additional VE may be required when protected unsaturated fats are fed. VE supplementation increases the response to vaccination,[80] and supplementation to pregnant and lactating ewes blunts the immune suppression that make take place over the parturition period. High levels of copper given to sheep during the final 3 weeks of pregnancy has a negative effect on the serum VE concentrations at 72 hours postpartum.[81] High levels of iodine in late pregnancy also seem to preprogram ewes to low VE levels from colostrum,[82] and therefore the presence of NMD in the neonate should be checked.

Although Se alone is protective against a greater spectrum of diseases than is VE, there are situations in which VE is more protective. Both Se and VE should be provided when the diets are deficient in both nutrients, but this may not apply in every situation. NMD can occur in ruminants with VE deficiency and an adequate Se status. Most of the emphasis has been on Se supplementation at the expense of VE, which is more costly and less stable. Most injectable VE and Se preparations are adequate in Se but insufficient in VE.

Selenium-Responsive Reproductive Performance and Growth

Sheep

In situations of Se deficiency, reproductive performance of ewes may be improved by Se or Se/Ve supplementation. Survival of lambs and live weights at birth and at weaning may be increased by Se supplementation. Single injections of Se before mating and lambing had no significant effects on estrus, fertility, prolificacy, and the number of lambs born and reared to 28 days in 2-year-old ewes. Two consecutive injections of Se (before mating and lambing) significantly increased the incidence of estrus, fertility, and lamb body weight at 28 days and daily weight gains for 28 days in 3-year-old ewes compared with controls. The injection of Se/VE did not significantly improve reproductive performance in 2- or 3-year-old ewes in the flock not considered Se deficient. Injected VE and Se can improve semen characteristics and reproductive performance of rams during the hot season.[83]

Weak-Calf Syndrome

The parenteral injection of Se and iodine to pregnant cattle in Ireland did not significantly reduce the incidence of the weak-calf syndrome, which is often attributed to a Se deficiency.

Pigs

The injection of Se (0.06 mg/kg BW) into piglets under 1 week of age, repeated at weaning time and into the sow 3 weeks before farrowing, will be effective. The minimum lethal dose of Se for piglets is 0.9 mg/kg BW, which provides a reasonably wide range of safety. A high concentration of Se in the diet of pregnant sows in the last half of gestation has been associated with hemorrhagic lesions on the claws of newborn piglets.

Horses

Little information is available on the need of horses for Se, but the optimum intake is 6 mg/week or 2.4 µg/kg BW daily. The oral supplementation of 1 mg selenium/d increases blood Se concentrations above levels associated with myodegeneration in horses and foals. In New Zealand, for horses on pasture, the injection of barium selenate, at a dose of 0.5 mg Se/kg BW, aseptically at a deep intramuscular site was efficacious in correcting the Se status of mares grazing pasture with a Se content of 0.01 to 0.07 mg/kg DM. Some local swelling will occur.

To ensure nutritional adequacy and to have an adequate safety margin, adult Standardbred horses should receive 600 to 1800 mg DL-α-tocopherol daily in their feed. The parenteral administration of VE and Se to mares in late pregnancy and to their foals beginning at birth will increase blood Se to adequate levels. In selenium-deficient areas or when mares are fed selenium-deficient hay, prepartum injections of Se/VE are indicated, followed by intermittent injection of the foals or supplementation of the diet with Se at 0.1 mg/kg DM.

Intraruminal Selenium Pellets

Sheep

Intraruminal Se pellets, similar to those used in cobalt deficiency, have produced satisfactory blood levels of Se for up to 4 years in ewes at pasture. A satisfactory pellet is composed of 0.5 g elemental Se and finely divided metallic iron. The technique is efficient, but not completely, because of wide variations between animals in the absorption rate of the Se. The average delivery of Se is 1 mg/d, and there is no danger of toxicity. In sheep grazing selenium-deficient pastures, the ruminal pellets increase the Se status and weight gains compared with controls. About 15% of treated sheep reject the pellets within 12 months, and in varying degrees the pellets acquire deposits of calcium phosphate. Sheep fed pellets recovered from sheep have low selenium levels, which suggests a low release of Se from pellets that have been in the rumen of other sheep for several months. The peak levels of Se occur 3 months after administration; there is a rapid decline in activity between 5 and 13 months. Sustained-released boluses containing sodium selenite, cobalt sulfate, potassium iodide, manganese sulfate, zinc oxide, sulfate, and vitamins A, D, and E have also been formulated to provide long-term maintenance of Se levels.

A soluble glass bolus containing zinc, cobalt, and Se administered to ram lambs increased the Se status of the animals and increased sperm motility, percentage of live sperm, and sperm responding to hypo-osmotic swelling test (an assay to determine plasma membrane permeability).

High-density compressed pellets containing both sodium selenite and cobalt carbonate have been developed for cattle and sheep. The sheep pellet weighs 6 g and contains 276 mg Se and 765 mg Co. A 6-g bolus given to ewes before mating resulted in improved lambing performance, an increase in the percentage of twin lambs.

Cattle

A Se pellet containing 10% selenium and 90% iron grit is available for cattle and will maintain plasma Se and GSH-PX activity above the critical level for up to 2 years. When given to beef cows in the last 3 months of pregnancy, the Se levels in milk were found to be higher than in controls, and the Se status of the calves was sufficient to prevent NMD. The use of these pellets at 2, 3, and 4 times the recommended dose in growing cattle weighing 300 to 350 kg did not cause toxicosis, and the Se levels in the tissues at slaughter were not a risk for humans.

Use of the intraruminal Se pellets in dairy cattle in New Zealand resulted in improved growth and milk production in herds where the Se status was below the adequate range, but there was no effect on udder health and reproductive performance.

High-density compressed pellets containing both sodium selenite and cobalt carbonate have been developed for cattle and sheep. For cattle, the pellets weigh 18 g and contain 4.6% selenium and 12.75% cobalt (828 mg Se and 2295 mg Co). In both beef cows and growing cattle, the boluses increased blood glutathione peroxidase activity for at least 1 year.

A sustained-release intrareticular bolus is an osmotic pump designed to release 3 mg selenium into the reticulo-rumen. It is intended to provide Se supplementation for 120 days in grown heifers and pregnant beef cattle.

A soluble glass bolus containing zinc, copper, and Se resulted in an increased antibody response.[84]

Selenium Toxicity and Residues

Selenium intoxication can occur following the administration of toxic amounts of an Se salt. The use of selenium selenite instead of sodium selenate and giving a dose of 5 times the intended dose resulted in a high mortality within several hours after administration. Animals deficient in Se are more susceptible to Se toxicosis than those that are selenium-adequate. The pharmacokinetics of Se toxicity in sheep given selenium selenite parenterally has been examined. When oral preparations of Se and monensin are given concurrently as part of a routine dietary management practice, there is greater risk of Se intoxication than if the Se is given alone. Administration of monensin sodium at a constant, safe dosage enhanced the toxicity of Se, as demonstrated by increased severity of the signs of intoxication, fatalities, and tissue Se concentrations and intensified gross, histopathologic, and biochemical changes. There is some concern about Se supplementation of beef cattle being a potential source of contamination for nearby aquatic systems, but there is no evidence that this has occurred.

Selenium Responsiveness

The response to Se supplementation is proportional to the degree of deficiency, and supplementation of animals that have adequate Se intakes is unlikely to significantly improve growth rate. In New Zealand, for selenium-deficient lambs, the potential for a growth response to Se supplementation is strongly related to blood Se concentration. Economically significant live-weight gains of greater than 10 g/d can occur when initial blood Se concentrations are less than 130 nmol/L. This is the basis for the development of reference curves using blood Se concentration to diagnose Se deficiency and predict growth responses to lambs.

Although many methods of supplementation of Se are efficacious, they can differ widely in their cost and convenience of administration. The objective of any micronutrient supplementation program should be to optimize the return on investment. The least-cost option that provides adequate supplementation for the required period should be recommended initially.

Veterinarians are the professionals in the best position to offer advice on cost-effectiveness supplementation. To retain this position, they must provide sound recommendations based on micronutrient analysis of animal tissue and defensible reference ranges that are supported by production response data. Monitoring micronutrient status in animal tissue should be encouraged to ensure that regulatory requirements are met and that deficiency and excessive use are avoided. Circumvention of veterinary involvement in the diagnosis and treatment of micronutrient supplementation can lead to greater use of supplements when not indicated, higher costs to farmers, and low cost-to-benefit ratios for the industry

Depot and bolus preparations have revolutionized the treatment of deficiencies of cattle and sheep that are grazed extensively where there is little opportunity for frequent administration. The relatively short duration of a single drench or injection of Se salts such as sodium selenite should be noted. The use of fertilizer applications is gaining widespread acceptance on farms with high stocking rates.

FURTHER READING

Baldi A, et al. Influence of antioxidants on ruminant health. *Feed Comp.* 2006;26:19-25.

Faye B, Seboussi R. Selenium in camels—a review. *Nutrients*. 2009;1:30.
Guyot H, Rollin F. Diagnosis of selenium and iodine deficiencies in bovines. *Ann Med Vet*. 2007;151:166.
Lykkesfeldt J, Svendsen O. Oxidants and antioxidants in disease: oxidative stress in farm animals. *Vet J*. 2007;173:502.
Lyons MP, et al. Selenium in food chain and animal nutrition: lessons from nature–review. *Asian-Australasian J Anim Sci*. 2007;20:1136.
Mehdi Y, et al. Selenium in the environment, metabolism and involvement in body functions. *Molecules*. 2013;18:3292.
Willshire JA, Payne JH. Selenium and vitamin E in dairy cows—a review. *Cattle Practice*. 2011;19:22.
Zarczynska K, et al. Effects of selenium on animal health. *J Elem*. 2013;18:329.

REFERENCES

1. Lykkesfeldt J, Svendsen O. *Vet J*. 2007;173:502.
2. Spears JW, Weiss WP. *Vet J*. 2008;176:70.
3. Sordillo LM, Aitken SL. *Vet Immunol Immunopathol*. 2009;128:104.
4. Celi P, et al. *Immunopathol Immunotoxicol*. 2011;33:233.
5. Lyons MP, et al. *J Anim Sci*. 2007;16:435.
6. Zarczynska KP, et al. *J Elem*. 2013;18:329.
7. Rederstorff M, et al. *Cellular Molec Life Sci*. 2006;63:52.
8. Whanger PD, et al. *Biochim Biophys Acta-General*. 2009;1790:1448.
9. Kojouri GA, et al. *Res Vet Sci*. 2012;93:275.
10. Mehdi Y, et al. *Molecules*. 2013;18:3292.
11. Song K-D, et al. *Anim Sci J*. 2013;84:238.
12. Elijah MRH, et al. *Jap J, Vet Res*. 2007;54:163.
13. El Ghany Hefnawy A, Tortora-Perez JL. *Small Rumin Res*. 2010;89:185.
14. Ahmed WM, et al. *Global Vet*. 2012;8:172.
15. Politis I, et al. *Animal*. 2012;6:1427.
16. Qu Y, et al. *J Dairy Sci*. 2007;96:3012.
17. Kalac P. *Fd Chem*. 2011;125:307.
18. Ceballos A, et al. *Archiv Med Vet*. 2013;45:33.
19. Manojlovic M, Singh BR. *Acta Agric Scand B*. 2012;62:673.
20. Del Razo-Rodriguez OE, et al. *Czech, J Anim Sci*. 2013;58:253.
21. Guyot H, et al. *Livestock Sci*. 2007;111:259.
22. Hassan AA, et al. *Nutrients*. 2012;4:724.
23. Zaknun D, et al. *Int Arch Allergy Immunol*. 2012;157:1130.
24. Bourne N, et al. *Vet J*. 2008;177:381.
25. Bourne N, et al. *Livestock Sci*. 2007;106:57.
26. Annett RW, et al. *Animal*. 2011;5:1923.
27. Murray DL, et al. *Wildl Monog*. 2006;166:1.
28. Rizzo A, et al. *Reprod Dom Anim*. 2012;47:344.
29. Roche JF. *Anim Reprod Sci*. 2006;96:282.
30. Al-Gubory KHY, et al. *Int J Biochem Cell Biol*. 2010;42:1634.
31. Aurorusseau B, et al. *Reprod Nutr Develop*. 2006;46:601.
32. Tareq KMA, et al. *J Reprod Develop*. 2012;58:621.
33. Asic K, et al. *Acta Agric Sloven*. 2008;92(Supp2):155.
34. Bourne N, et al. *Theriogenol*. 2007;67:494.
35. Salman S, et al. *Anim Hlth Res Rev/Conf Res Work Anim Dis*. 2009;10.
36. Heinrichs AJ, et al. *Vet Microbiol*. 2009;134:172.
37. Muicheljee R. *Vet Res Commun*. 2008;32:305.
38. Aktas MS, et al. *Livestock Sci*. 2011;141:76.
39. Duff CC, et al. *J Anim Sci*. 2007;85:823.
40. Giles A, et al. *Rev Med Vet*. 2009;160:10.
41. Montgomery JB, et al. *J Eq Vet Sci*. 2012;32:352.
42. Hall JA, et al. *Vet Res*. 2011;42:99.
43. Bondo T, Jensen SK. *J Anim Physiol Anim Nutrit*. 2011;95:214.
44. Munoz C, et al. *Animal*. 2008;2:64.
45. Bertoni G, et al. *Italian J Anim Sci*. 2009;8:491.
46. Ceballos-Marquez A, et al. *J Dairy Sci*. 2010;93:4602.
47. Giadinis ND, et al. *Small Rum Res*. 2011;95:193.
48. do Reo Leal ML, et al. *Vet Res Commun*. 2010;34:549.
49. Brennan KM, et al. *Biol Trace Element Res*. 2011;144:504.
50. Deger Y, et al. *Biol Trace Element Res*. 2008;121:39.
51. Bargiye R, et al. *J Eq Vet Sci*. 2007;27:405.
52. Pourliotis K, et al. *NZ Vet J*. 2009;57:44.
53. Guyot H, Rollin F. *Ann Med Vet*. 2007;151:166.
54. Kojouri GA, et al. *Small Rum Res*. 2009;84:65.
55. Judson GJ, et al. *Anim Product Sci*. 2011;51:873.
56. Jobse KW, et al. *Tijd Diergeneesk*. 2008;133:704.
57. Besselmann D, et al. *J Zoo Wildl Med*. 2008;39:86.
58. Bertinato J, et al. *Nutrition J*. 2007;6:7.
59. Amorim RM, et al. *Pesq Vet Brasil*. 2011;31:579.
60. Brozos CN, et al. *Livestock Sci*. 2009;124:210.
61. Cozzi G. *Animal*. 2011;5:1531.
62. Davis PA, et al. *Prof Anim Scient*. 2008;24:52.
63. Alimohamady R, et al. *Biol Trace Elem Res*. 2013;154:45.
64. Palmieri C, Szarek J. *J Elementology*. 2011;16:143.
65. Kumar N. *Anim Fd Sci Technol*. 2009;153:77.
66. Geishauser T, et al. *Pract Tierarzt*. 2012;93:938.
67. Maas J, et al. *J Vet Diag Invest*. 2008;20:86.
68. Tiwary AK, et al. *J Vet Diag Invest*. 2006;18:61.
69. Schiavon E, et al. *Large Anim Rev*. 2007;13:3.
70. Seboussi R, et al. *J Camel Pract Res*. 2009;16:25.
71. Nathues H, et al. *Can Vet J*. 2010;51:515.
72. Strugnell BW, et al. *Vet Rec*. 2010;167:707.
73. Kamada H, et al. *J Dairy Sci*. 2007;90:5665.
74. Descalzo AM, Sancho AM. *Meat Sci*. 2008;79:423.
75. Calamari L, et al. *Livestock Sci*. 2011;142:128.
76. Chorfi Y, et al. *Can Vet J*. 2011;52:1089.
77. Cusack P, et al. *Prev Vet Med*. 2009;88:229.
78. Montgomery JB, et al. *Anim Fd Sci Tech*. 2011;170:63.
79. Pearce KL, et al. *Small Rum Res*. 2010;91:29.
80. Anugu S, et al. *Small Rum Res*. 2013;111:83.
81. Boland TM, et al. *Animal*. 2008;2:197.
82. Boland TM, et al. *Anim Sci*. 2008;82:310.
83. Ali ABT, et al. *Italian J Anim Sci*. 2009;8:743.
84. Kendall NR, et al. *Livestock Sci*. 2012;148:81.

MASSETER MYONECROSIS

Degeneration of the masseter muscles causes dysphagia and trismus in adult horses and Miniature horses.[1] The disease is associated with abnormally low serum or blood concentrations of vitamin E or selenium in some affected horses, and ingestion of tetrachlorvinphos, an organophosphate, was associated with the disease in Miniature horses.[1,2] Muscles of locomotion and cardiac muscle can be affected in addition to disease of the masseter muscle. Clinical signs include acute onset of dysphagia, trismus, salivation, and swelling of the masseter muscles. These can progress to weight loss, gait abnormalities, atrophy of the masseter muscle, teeth grinding or quidding of feed, and unexpected death. Ultrasonography of the masseter muscles reveals hyperechoic lesions with patchy blurring of the fascia, indicative of inflammation and edema.[3] There is electrocardiographic and echocardiographic evidence of myocardial disease in some horses. These signs include tachycardia (after resolution of hypovolemia and pain) with supraventricular and ventricular extrasystole and diminished left ventricular systolic (decreased ejection fraction and fractional shortening) and diastolic function (increased isovolumic relaxation time).[3]

Horses with extensive involvement of other muscles can have myoglobinuria. Signs of dysphagia and trismus are related to dysfunction of the masseter muscle.[4] Gait abnormalities are related to disease in muscles of locomotion, and unexpected death is probably a result of the cardiac lesions. Serum activity of creatine kinase and aspartate aminotransferase is elevated in acute cases. Serum concentrations of troponin are elevated in horses with involvement of the myocardium.[3] Necropsy examination reveals diffuse swelling, muscle pallor, and white streaking of masseter muscle in acutely affected animals. Lesions are also detected in muscles of locomotion and myocardium in some horses. Chronic cases have atrophy of affected muscle. Histologic changes include swelling, fragmentation and loss of striations of myocytes in acute cases, and degenerating fibers replaced by fibrosis in chronic cases. Treatment is symptomatic, and affected horses can require enteral or parenteral delivery of nutrients. Vitamin E and selenium status should be determined and supplements administered if indicated. Prevention should focus on ensuring that horses in geographic regions in which vitamin E or selenium are deficient in feeds are supplemented with these micronutrients.

REFERENCES

1. Myers CJ, et al. *Equine Vet J*. 2006;38:272.
2. Radostits O, et al. Masseter myonecrosis. In: *Veterinary Medicine: A Textbook of the Diseases of Cattle, Horses, Sheep, Goats and Pigs*. 10th ed. London: W.B. Saunders; 2006:1686.
3. Schefer KD, et al. *J Vet Int Med*. 2011;25:1171.
4. Aharonson-Raz K, et al. *Vet Rec*. 2009;164:597.

SPORADIC EXERTIONAL RHABDOMYOLYSIS IN HORSES (AZOTURIA, TYING-UP)

The disease discussed here is that of sporadic acute exertional rhabdomyolysis that occurs as a single event in a horse and does not have a tendency to recur. The recurrent disease is discussed toward the end of this chapter under "Congenital/Inherited Musculoskeletal Disease."

ETIOLOGY

The etiology of most cases of *sporadic* acute exertional rhabdomyolysis is unknown, although suggested causes include hypothyroidism, sodium or potassium deficiency, viral infection, high-carbohydrate diets, and abnormalities in metabolic function. The most common cause is performing exercise of unaccustomed intensity or duration, which can result in metabolic exhaustion and hyperthermia. However, the disease is not always associated with severe exertion or hyperthermia, and it can occur with as little exercise as slow draft work or turn-out to pasture after stabling. An important contributing factor is a prolonged period (days to weeks) of rest in a horse previously accustomed to regular exercise. The disease occurs in young horses as a result of vitamin E/selenium deficiency, although this is an uncommon cause in adult horses.

Rhabdomyolysis not associated with exercise occurs during general anesthesia maintained by inhalation of halothane in horses of a specific genotype or in horses at pasture in Europe. Rhabdomyolysis also occurs in horses with *S. equi* infection (strangles).

Recurrent exertional rhabdomyolysis is a recognized syndrome in Thoroughbred horses and is dealt with separately.

It is likely that most cases of sporadic exertional rhabdomyolysis are a result of a combination of predisposing factors, with the disease precipitated by a bout of exercise. The difficulty in detecting the presence of predisposing factors contributes to the sporadic nature of the disease.

EPIDEMIOLOGY

The sporadic disease is almost always associated with exercise that is either enforced, as with horses in training or competition, or spontaneous, as with young horses turned out to pasture after a prolonged period of stabling.[1] Clinical signs occur in horses within minutes to hours of the cessation of exercise, although signs can be apparent in horses during prolonged exercise. The epidemiology of the sporadic disease has not been well defined, in contrast to that of recurrent exertional rhabdomyolysis, and the subsequent discussion includes some of the epidemiology of each because it is not always possible to determine whether one episode of exertional rhabdomyolysis is the only occurrence in that animal or will reoccur.

Interpretation of reports of prevalence and risk factors for exertional rhabdomyolysis is difficult because studies to date have mostly not differentiated between the recurrent exertional rhabdomyolysis of Thoroughbreds, polysaccharide storage myopathy of Quarter horses and related breeds, and the sporadic disease in other breeds. The **incidence** or 1-year period prevalence of exertional rhabdomyolysis is as follows: 1.5% in ponies in Australia; 4.9% in Thoroughbred racehorses in the United States, Australia, and Great Britain; 6.1% in National Hunt Thoroughbreds in Great Britain; 4% to 5% in 2- to 3-year-old Thoroughbreds in the United Kingdom;[2] and up to 13.5% in polo ponies in the United States and Great Britain. Polo, racing, rodeo, Western, and show jumping are all associated with a high period prevalence (>5% per annum) of exertional rhabdomyolysis.

Risk factors for exertional rhabdomyolysis include exercise, breed and use, and sex. Overall, horses that exercise are approximately 10 times more likely to develop the disease than are sedentary horses, and among breed/use groups, polo horses are approximately 3 times more likely to develop the disease than are horses used for racing. Horses used for racing are more likely to have episodes of the disease than are horses used for pleasure riding or "other" uses, although racing and breed (Thoroughbred or Standardbred) are confounding factors. Female racehorses are three times more likely to have episodes of exertional rhabdomyolysis than are male (intact or castrated) racehorses, and young female Thoroughbreds are at greatest risk. Among National Hunt horses in Great Britain, females are 24 times as likely to have an episode of the disease as are males. Female polo ponies are not more likely to develop the disease. Thoroughbred racehorses and polo ponies, but not National Hunt horses, with a nervous or "flighty" temperament are more likely to experience episodes of the disease. Other apparent risk factors include a rest day before hard exercise, feeding greater than 4.5 kg of grain per day, lameness, playing polo at a level for which the horse is not fit, and playing early in the season.

The disease occurs repeatedly in 74% of affected Thoroughbred racehorses in Great Britain and in 20% of affected polo ponies.

The disease is of considerable **economic impact** because of its frequent occurrence in athletic horses, recurrent nature, and need to rest affected horses. On average, affected Thoroughbred racehorses cannot train for 6 days after an episode, and approximately two-thirds of affected horses are unable to race because of the disease. Polo ponies lose an average of 7 days of training after an episode of exertional rhabdomyolysis. The effect of the loss of training days for each episode is magnified because of the recurrent nature of the disease in a large proportion of affected horses. Approximately 6% of the wastage of Thoroughbred racehorses in Australia is attributable to exertional rhabdomyolysis.

PATHOGENESIS

The disease is a result of dysfunction and death of myocytes with subsequent release of cellular constituents, including the enzymes creatine kinase, aspartate aminotransferase and carbonic anhydrase, and myoglobin. The proximate cause of myocyte death is uncertain, but it is not related to accumulation of lactic acid, as previously supposed. Proposed mechanisms include oxidant injury to cells as a result of increased oxidant formation during exercise or inadequate antioxidant activity. Apart from horses deficient in vitamin E and/or selenium, which are rare, there is no indication that oxidant injury is a common cause of rhabdomyolysis in horses.

Cell death is likely linked to abnormal accumulation of calcium in intracellular fluids secondary to deranged energy and/or membrane function. Necrosis of myocytes causes pain and inflammation in the muscle, with infiltration of inflammatory cells. Healing and regeneration of myocytes occurs over a period of weeks in the absence of further episodes of myonecrosis.

Release of cellular constituents results in electrolyte abnormalities, primarily hypochloremic metabolic alkalosis, a systemic inflammatory response, and pigmenturia. Severely affected horses can have metabolic acidosis. Myoglobin and possibly other cell constituents are nephrotoxic, and acute renal failure can develop as a result of myoglobinuric nephrosis. Pain and loss of muscle function cause a stilted, short-stepping gait.

CLINICAL FINDINGS

The clinical findings are variable and range from poor performance to recumbency and death. Signs can be mild and resolve spontaneously within 24 hours or be severe and progressive.

Clinical findings are very similar to those observed in horses with sporadic acute exertional rhabdomyolysis that occurs as a single event in a horse (see earlier section in this chapter), except that clinical signs recur. The most common presentation of recurrent exertional rhabdomyolysis is a horse that does not perform to expectation and displays a stiff or short-stepping gait that can be mistaken for lower leg lameness. The horse might be reluctant to move when placed in its stall, be apprehensive and anorexic, paw, and frequently shift its weight. More severely affected horses can be unable to continue to exercise, have **hard and painful muscles** (usually gluteal muscles), sweat excessively, tremble or have widespread muscle fasciculations, be apprehensive, refuse to walk, and have elevated heart and respiratory rates. Affected horses can be hyperthermic, especially soon after exercise. Signs consistent with abdominal pain are present in many severely affected horses. Deep-red urine (myoglobinuria) occurs but is not a consistent finding. Severely affected horses are often recumbent.

CLINICAL PATHOLOGY

Mildly affected or apparently nonaffected horses have moderate increases in **serum creatine kinase** (CK) (20,000 to 50,000 IU/L), **aspartate aminotransferase** (AST), and **lactate dehydrogenase** (LDH) activity. Severely affected horses have large increases in CK (>100,000 IU/L) and other muscle-derived enzymes. Serum CK and AST activities peak approximately 5 to 6 and 24 hours after exercise, respectively, and in the absence of further muscle damage, serum AST might not return to normal levels for 7 to 10 days. The half-life of CK activity in serum is approximately 12 hours, and serum CK declines rapidly in the absence of continuing muscle damage. The persistence of increased AST activity, compared with CK, is useful in identifying affected horses days or weeks after the episode.

Serum myoglobin concentrations increase markedly during exercise in affected horses and decline within 24 to 48 hours. Serum carbonic anhydrase III activity is increased in horses with exertional rhabdomyolysis.

Severely affected horses are often **hyponatremic** (<130 mEq/L), **hyperkalemic** (>5.5 mEq/L), **hypochloremic** (<90 mEq/L), azotemic (increased serum urea nitrogen and creatinine concentrations), and **acidotic** or **alkalotic**. Hemoconcentration (hematocrit > 50%, 0.5 L/L) and increased serum total protein concentration (>80 g/L) indicative of dehydration are common. Serum bicarbonate concentration can be falsely markedly elevated in animals with severe rhabdomyolysis because of cellular constituents released from damaged muscle that interfere with the analytical method when automated clinical chemistry analyzers are used. **Myoglobinuria** is detectable either grossly or on chemical analysis and should be differentiated from hemoglobinuria or hematuria. Measurement of **urinary excretion of electrolytes**, although popular in the past, is of no use in diagnosing, treating, or preventing exertional rhabdomyolysis.

Muscle biopsy during the acute or convalescent stages reveals myonecrosis of type II (fast-twitch, oxidative) fibers, mild myositis, and fibrosis.

NECROPSY FINDINGS

Horses dying of exertional rhabdomyolysis have widespread degeneration of striated muscle, principally the muscles of exertion, but often involving the diaphragm and heart. Affected muscles tend to be dark and swollen but may have a pale, streaked appearance. The kidneys are swollen and have dark-brown medullary streaks. Dark-brown urine is present in the bladder. Histologic examination reveals widespread necrosis and hyaline degeneration of predominantly type II (fast-twitch, oxidative) fibers. In horses with recurrent disease, there may be evidence of myofiber regeneration. Myoglobinuric nephrosis is present in severely affected horses.

Samples for Postmortem Confirmation of Diagnosis

- Formalin-fixed kidney and affected muscle for light microscopic examination

DIAGNOSTIC CONFIRMATION

Biochemical confirmation of muscle damage by demonstration of increased serum CK or AST activity, in conjunction with appropriate clinical signs, provides the diagnosis.

DIFFERENTIAL DIAGNOSIS

- Muscle cramping induced by ear tick (*Otobius megnini*)
- Polysaccharide storage myopathy of Quarter horses and related breeds
- Emerging or newly recognized myopathies, such a vacuolar myopathy in Warmbloods[3]
- Ionophore intoxication (monensin, lasalocid, salinomycin, narasin, maduramicin)
- Infection by *Anaplasma phagocytophilum*[4]
- Equine lower motor neurone disease (acute form)
- White snake root (*Eupatorium rugosum*) or rayless goldenrod (*Isocoma pluriflora*)
- Hyperkalemic periodic paralysis
- Laminitis
- Colic
- Pleuritis
- Aorto-iliac thrombosis

TREATMENT

The treatment chosen depends on the severity of the disease. The **general principles** are rest; correction of dehydration and electrolyte abnormalities; prevention of complications, including nephrosis and laminitis; and provision of analgesia.

Mildly affected horses (heart rate < 60 bpm, normal rectal temperature and respiratory rate, no dehydration) may be treated with rest and phenylbutazone (2.2 mg/kg, orally or IV every 12 hours for 2 to 4 days). Horses should be given mild exercise with incremental increases in workload as soon as they no longer have signs of muscle pain. Access to water should be unrestricted.

Severely affected horses (heart rate > 60 bpm, rectal temperature > 39° C [102° F], 8% to 10% dehydrated, reluctant or unable to walk) should not be exercised, including walking back to the stable, unless it is unavoidable. Isotonic, polyionic **fluids**, such as lactated Ringer's solution, should be administered IV to severely affected horses to correct any hypovolemia and to ensure a mild diuresis to prevent myoglobinuric nephropathy. Less severely affected horses can be treated by administration of fluids by nasogastric intubation (4 to 6 L every 2 to 3 hours). Although it has been recommended that urine should be alkalinized by administration of mannitol and sodium bicarbonate (1.3% solution IV, or 50 to 100 g of sodium bicarbonate orally every 12 hours) to minimize the nephrotoxicity of myoglobin, this therapy is not effective in humans at risk of myoglobinuric nephrosis. Affected horses should not be given diuretics (e.g., furosemide) except if they are anuric or oliguric after correction of hypovolemia.

Phenylbutazone (2.2 to 4.4 mg/kg, IV or orally, every 12 to 24 hours), **flunixin meglumine** (1 mg/kg IV every 8 hours), or **ketoprofen** (2.2 mg/kg IV every 12 hours) should be given to provide **analgesia. Mild sedation** (acepromazine 0.02 to 0.04 mg/kg IM, or xylazine, 0.1 mg/kg IM, both with butorphanol, 0.01 to 0.02 mg/kg) may decrease muscle pain and anxiety. Tranquilizers with vasodilatory activity, such as acepromazine, should only be given to horses that are well hydrated. **Muscle relaxants**, such as methocarbamol, are often used but have no demonstrated efficacy.

Recumbent horses should be deeply bedded and repositioned by rolling every 2 to 4 hours. Severely affected horses should not be forced to stand.

CONTROL

Prevention of the sporadic, idiopathic disease centers on ensuring that horses are fed a balanced ration with adequate levels of vitamin E, selenium, and electrolytes and have a regular and consistent program of exercise. Despite lack of clear evidence for a widespread role for **vitamin E or selenium deficiency** in exertional rhabdomyolysis, horses are often supplemented with 1 IU/kg vitamin E and 2.5 μg/kg selenium daily in the feed. Care should be taken not to induce selenium toxicosis.

Sodium bicarbonate (up to 0.5 to 1.0 g/kg BW daily in the ration) and other electrolytes are often added to the feed of affected horses, but their efficacy is not documented. **Phenytoin** has proven useful in the treatment of recurrent rhabdomyolysis. It is administered at a dose rate of 6 to 8 mg/kg, orally, every 12 hours, and the dose is adjusted depending on the degree of sedation produced (a reduced dose should be used if the horse becomes sedated) or lack of effect on serum CK or AST activity. Phenytoin can be administered to horses for months. **Dimethylglycine, altrenogest, and progesterone** are all used on occasion in horses with recurrent rhabdomyolysis, but again, without demonstrated efficacy.

The feeding of high-fat, low-soluble-carbohydrate diets is useful in the prevention of recurrent exertional rhabdomyolysis in Thoroughbred horses and polysaccharide storage myopathy in Quarter horses. The usefulness of this practice in preventing sporadic, idiopathic exertional rhabdomyolysis has not been demonstrated.

FURTHER READING

Piercy RJ, Rivero J. Muscle disorders of equine athletes. In: *Equine Sports Medicine and Surgery: Basic and Clinical Sciences of the Equine Athlete.* 2nd ed. London: W.B. Saunders; 2014:109.

REFERENCES

1. Radostits O, et al. Sporadic exertional rhabdomyolysis of horses. In: *Veterinary Medicine: A Textbook of the Disease of Cattle, Horses, Sheep, Goats and Pigs.* 10th ed. London: W.B. Saunders; 2007:1683.
2. Wilsher S, et al. *Equine Vet J.* 2006;38:113.
3. Massey CA, et al. *Neuromusc Dis.* 2013;23:473.
4. Hilton H, et al. *J Vet Int Med.* 2008;22:1061.

DIETARY DEFICIENCY OF PHOSPHORUS, CALCIUM, AND VITAMIN D AND IMBALANCE OF THE CALCIUM: PHOSPHORUS RATIO

A dietary deficiency or disturbance in the metabolism of calcium, phosphorus, or vitamin D, including imbalance of the calcium : phosphorus ratio, is the principal cause of the **osteodystrophies,** which can occur in a number of forms:

- **Osteomalacia**—a reduction in the strength of bones secondary to defective bone mineralization typically caused by inadequate or imbalanced levels of available phosphate and calcium, vitamin D deficiency, or because of excessive resorption of calcium from the bone, such as is caused by hyperparathyroidism. There is a reduction in the mineral : matrix ratio in bone in that there is less mineral than expected for the bone mass. The disease is histologically evident as increased osteoid (unmineralized matrix).
- **Osteoporosis**—a reduction in bone mass, with associated increased risk of fracture, in which there is a proportionate reduction in both the mineral and the matrix (protein, osteoid) content of bone. The remaining bone is essentially normal but is insufficient in quantity. The disease is typically evident as thin bone cortices on sectioning or radiographic examination.
- **Rickets**—a disease caused by vitamin D deficiency, resulting in aberrant calcium and phosphorus metabolism, that affects young animals and is characterized osteomalacia. Affected animals are described as "rachitic."

Osteodystrophia fibrosa—also referred to osteitis fibrosa (incorrectly, because this is not an inflammatory condition) or fibrous osteodystrophy. A form of osteomalacia in which mineralized bone is replaced by unmineralized fibrotic tissue under the influence of prolonged hyperparathyroidism, secondary to a high phosphorus : low calcium ratio in feed in horses, calcium deficiency in pigs, or chronic renal disease in some species.

The etiology and pathogenesis of these disorders is discussed in more detail in the sections of this text dealing with those diseases. It is important to note that the interrelations of calcium, phosphorus, and vitamin D metabolism are complex, and the importance of these and related factors (age, overall nutritional status, other mineral deficiencies or excesses) in clinical disease is often very difficult to define.

In an attempt to simplify this situation, the diseases in this section are covered in the following order:

Calcium deficiency (hypocalcicosis)
- Primary: an absolute deficiency in the diet
- Secondary: when the deficiency is conditioned by some other factor, principally an excess intake of phosphorus

Phosphorus deficiency (hypophosphatosis)
- Primary: an absolute deficiency in the diet
- Secondary: when the deficiency is conditioned by some other factor; although in general terms an excessive intake of calcium could be such a factor, specific instances of this situation are lacking

Vitamin D deficiency (hypovitaminosis-D)
- Primary: an absolute deficiency intake of the vitamin
- Secondary: when the deficiency is conditioned by other factors of which excess carotene intake is the best known.

In different countries with varying climates, soil types, and methods of husbandry, these individual deficiencies are of varying importance. For instance, in South Africa, northern Australia, and North America, the most common of the deficiencies just listed is that of phosphorus deficiency; vitamin D deficiency is uncommon. In Great Britain, Europe, and parts of North America, a deficiency of vitamin D can also be of major importance.[1,2] Animals are housed indoors for much of the year, they are exposed to little ultraviolet irradiation, and their forage may contain little vitamin D. Under such conditions, the absolute and relative amounts of calcium and phosphorus in the diet need to be greater than in other areas if vitamin D deficiency is to be avoided. In New Zealand, where much lush pasture and cereal grazing are used for feed, the vitamin D status is reduced not only by poor solar irradiation of the animal and plant sterols, but in addition, an antivitamin D factor is present in the diet, possibly in the form of carotene.

Now that the gross errors of management with respect to calcium and phosphorus and vitamin D are largely avoided, more interest is devoted to the marginal errors; in these, diagnosis is not nearly so easy, and the deficiency can be evident only at particular times of the year. The conduct of a response trial in which part of the herd is treated is difficult unless they are hand-fed daily; there are no suitable reticular retention pellets or long-term injections of calcium or phosphorus because the daily requirement is so high. Two methods suggest themselves:

1. Analysis of ash content of samples of spongy bone from the tuber coxae
2. The metabolic profile method

The latter program may have some value as a monitoring and diagnostic weapon in the fields of metabolic disease, nutritional deficiency, and nutritional excesses.

Absorption and Metabolism of Calcium and Phosphorus

In ruminants, dietary calcium is absorbed by the small intestine according to body needs, whereas in equids there is greater obligatory absorption of calcium, and it is less dependent on vitamin D (and its metabolites) than in ruminants.[3,4] Whereas young animals with high growth requirements absorb and retain calcium in direct relation to intake over a wide range of intakes, adult male ruminants, irrespective of intake, absorb only enough calcium to replace that lost by excretion into urine and intestine, retaining none of it. Calcium absorption is increased in adult animals during periods of high demand, such as pregnancy and lactation, or after a period of calcium deficiency, but a substantial loss of body stores of calcium appears to be necessary before this increase occurs. The dietary factors influencing the efficiency of absorption of calcium include the nature of the diet, the absolute and relative amounts of calcium and phosphorus present in the diet, and the presence of interfering substances. The calcium in milk is virtually all available for absorption, but the calcium in forage-containing diets has an availability of only about 50%. The addition of grain to an all-forage diet markedly improves the availability of the calcium.

Phosphorus is absorbed by young animals from both milk and forage-containing diets with a high availability (80% to 100%), but the availability is much lower (50% to 60%) in adult animals. Horses fed diets containing adequate amounts of calcium and phosphorus absorb 50% to 65% of the calcium and slightly less than 50% of the phosphorus present in a variety of feedstuffs. In grains, 50% to 65% of the phosphorus is in the phytate form, which is utilizable by ruminants, but not as efficiently by nonruminants such as the horse and pig. An average availability of 70% has been assumed for phosphorus in early-weaning diets for young pigs, and a value of 50% is assumed for practical cereal-based feeds as supplied to growing pigs, sows, and boars.

The metabolism of calcium and phosphorus is influenced by the parathyroid hormone, calcitonin, and vitamin D (Fig. 15-13), although there are important differences in calcium homeostasis between ruminants and equids.[5-8] For instance, equids have much lower serum vitamin D concentrations, greater absorption of calcium by the small intestine (duodenum), and greater renal excretion of calcium than do ruminants.[4,8,9] In all mammalian species, parathyroid hormone is secreted in response to hypocalcemia and stimulates the conversion of 25-dihydroxycholecalciferol to 1,25-dihydroxycholecalciferol (1,25-DHCC). Parathyroid hormone and 1,25-DHCC together stimulate bone resorption, and 1,25-DHCC alone stimulates active intestinal absorption of calcium.[10] Calcium enters the blood from bone and intestine, and when the

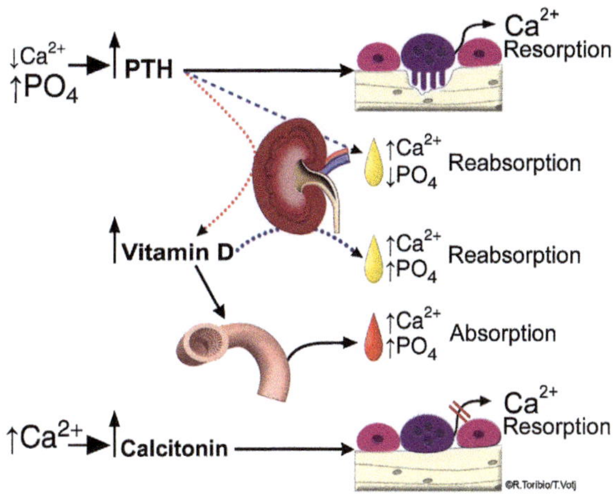

Fig. 15-13 Calcium and phosphate homeostasis. A decrease in extracellular Ca^{2+} concentrations or an increase in phosphate (PO_4) concentrations leads to a parathyroid hormone (PTH) release from the parathyroid gland, which in turn increases renal reabsorption of Ca^{2+}, renal activation of vitamin D, urinary PO_4 excretion, and bone resorption. In turn, vitamin D increases intestinal absorption and renal reabsorption of Ca^{2+} and PO_4. An increase in Ca^{2+} concentration stimulates the thyroid gland to secrete calcitonin to inhibit osteoclastic bone resorption. (Courtesy of Ramiro E. Toribio, DVM, MS, PhD, and Tim Vojt, Columbus, OH; Reproduced with permission.[8])

serum calcium level increases above normal, parathyroid hormone is inhibited and calcitonin secretion stimulated. The increased calcitonin concentration blocks bone resorption, and the decreased parathyroid hormone concentration depresses calcium absorption. Most calcium absorption occurs in the small intestine, with equids absorbing a greater proportion of dietary calcium than ruminants.[5] Detailed descriptions of the physiology of calcium metabolism are available in the section "Milk Fever (Hypocalcemia)" and in reviews.[6]

REFERENCES

1. Hymoller L, et al. *J Dairy Sci.* 2010;93:2025.
2. Hymoller L, et al. *Brit J Nutr.* 2012;108:666.
3. Breidenbach A, et al. *Vet Res.* 1998;29:173.
4. Rourke KM, et al. *Gen Comp Endocrin.* 2010;167:6.
5. Cehak A, et al. *Comp Biochem Physiol.* 2012;161:259.
6. Goff JP. *Vet Clin North Am Food A.* 2014;30:359.
7. Hymoller L, et al. *J Equine Vet Sci.* 2015;35:785.
8. Toribio RE. *Vet Clin Equine.* 2011;27:129.
9. Pozza ME, et al. *Vet J.* 2014;199:451.
10. Christakos S. *Arch Biochem Biophys.* 2012;523:73.

CALCIUM DEFICIENCY

Calcium deficiency can be primary or secondary, but in both cases, the end result is a type of osteodystrophy, with the specific disease depending largely on the species and age of the animals affected.

SYNOPSIS

Etiology Primary dietary deficiency of calcium is uncommon. Secondary calcium deficiency can be induced by marginal calcium intake and high phosphorus intake.

Epidemiology Sporadic. Not common if diets adequate.

Signs Poor growth and dentition. Tetany can occur in lactating ewes. Inappetence, stiffness, fracture of long bones. Specific diseases include rickets, osteomalacia, and osteodystrophia fibrosa.

Clinical pathology Serum calcium and phosphorus. Radiography.

Necropsy findings Osteoporosis; low ash content of bone.

Diagnostic confirmation Histology of bone and bone ash analyses.

Differential diagnosis list See differential diagnosis of each specific disease.

Treatment Calcium salts parenterally (for tetany) and orally (for prolonged correction of deficiency).

Control Adequate calcium and phosphorus levels in diet.

ETIOLOGY

A primary deficiency attributable to a lack of calcium in the diet is uncommon, although a secondary deficiency attributable to a marginal calcium intake aggravated by a high phosphorus intake is not uncommon. In ponies, such a diet depresses intestinal absorption and retention of calcium in the body, and the resorption of calcium from bones is increased as a result of hyperparathyroidism (secondary nutritional hyperparathyroidism—see discussion of osteodystrophia fibrosa later in this section). Hypoparathyroidism, either primary or secondary to renal disease, reduces intestinal and renal reabsorption of calcium and causes seizures and muscle fasciculation.[1-3]

EPIDEMIOLOGY

Calcium deficiency is a sporadic disease occurring in particular groups of animals rather than in geographically limited areas. Although death does not usually occur, there can be considerable loss of function and disabling lesions of bones or joints.

Horses in training, cattle being fitted for shows, and valuable stud sheep are often fed artificial diets containing cereal or grass hays that contain little calcium and grains that have a high content of phosphorus. The secondary calcium deficiency that occurs in these circumstances is often accompanied by a vitamin D deficiency because of the tendency to keep animals confined indoors. Pigs are often fed heavy concentrate rations with insufficient calcium supplement. Dairy cattle can occasionally be fed similarly imbalanced diets, the effects of which are exaggerated by high milk production.

There are no well-established records of calcium deficiency in grazing cattle, but there are records of low calcium intake in feedlots accompanied by clinical osteodystrophy. There is also a well-recognized field occurrence of calcium deficiency in young sheep in southeast Australia. Outbreaks can affect many sheep and are usually seen in winter and spring, following exercise or temporary starvation. In most outbreaks, the characteristic osteoporosis results from a long-term deprivation of food as a result of poor pasture growth. Occasional outbreaks occur on green oats used for grazing. The calcium intake in some cases is as low as 3 to 5 g/week in contrast to the requirement of 3 to 5 g/d. Sheep in the Kalahari Desert develop osteoporosis as a result of low calcium intake and low-grade fluorosis.[4] Goats deficient in calcium, phosphorus, and vitamin D develop osteoporosis.[5] Copper deficiency is associated with osteoporosis in young sheep.

High protein intake and rapid growth have been suggested as contributory factors in the development of skeletal problems in young horses (developmental orthopedic disease [DOD]). The cause of DOD in young horses is multifactorial and related to mineral imbalances in the diet, genetic predisposition,[6] trauma, and maternal[7] and foal nutritional status. For instance, wither height at 30 days of age, age of the mare, breed, regularity of exercise, Ca/P level in the mare and foal rations, group size in pasture, and the type and frequency of handling were identified as risk factors for DOD in foals in France.[8] Although excessive energy intake is sometimes blamed, a concentration of dietary protein of 20%, which is significantly above the National Research Council (NRC) recommended level of 14%, is neither helpful nor harmful to growing horses. The high protein intake did not affect the rate of growth, height, and circumference of cannon bones compared with horses receiving the lower 14% diet. The high-protein diet did not result in hypercalciuria and did not affect calcium absorption or calcium retention.

In females there is likely to be a cycle of changes in calcium balance, with a negative balance occurring in late pregnancy and early lactation and a positive balance in late lactation and early pregnancy and when lactation has ceased. The negative balance in late pregnancy is in spite of a naturally occurring increased absorption of calcium from the intestine at that time, at least in ewes.

PATHOGENESIS

The main physiologic functions of calcium are the formation of bone and milk, participation in the clotting of blood, and the maintenance of neuromuscular excitability. In the development of osteodystrophies, dental defects, and tetany, the role of calcium is well understood; however, the relation between deficiency of the element and lack of appetite, poor growth, loss of condition, infertility, and reduced milk flow is not readily apparent. The disinclination of the animals to move about and graze and poor dental development may contribute to these effects.

Experimentally, feeding young lambs a diet low in calcium and phosphorus for 12 weeks results in soft and pliable ribs with thickening of the costochondral junctions, reduction in feed intake by about 34%, significant changes in plasma calcium and phosphorus concentrations, and changes in dry matter digestibility. Feeding repletion diets results in complete remineralization of rib bones but only partial remineralization of the metatarsal bones.

Nutritional factors other than calcium, phosphorus, and vitamin D can be important in the production of osteodystrophies, which also occur in copper deficiency, fluorosis,[4] and chronic lead poisoning. Vitamin A is also essential for the development of bones, particularly those of the cranium.

CLINICAL FINDINGS

The clinical findings, apart from the specific syndromes described later, are less marked in adults than in young animals, in which there is decreased rate or cessation of growth and dental maldevelopment. The latter is characterized by deformity of the gums, poor development of the incisors, failure of permanent teeth to erupt for periods of up to 27 months, and abnormal wear of the permanent teeth as a result of defective development of dentine and enamel, occurring principally in sheep.

A calcium deficiency can occur in lactating ewes and sucking lambs, whose metabolic requirements for calcium are higher than in dry and pregnant sheep. There is a profound fall in serum calcium. Tetany and hyperirritability do not usually accompany hypocalcemia in these circumstances, probably because it develops slowly. However, exercise and fasting often precipitate tetanic seizures and parturient paresis in such sheep. This is typical of the disease as it occurs in young sheep in southeast Australia. Attention is drawn to the presence of the disease by the occurrence of tetany, convulsions, and paresis, but the important signs are ill-thrift and failure to respond to anthelmintics. Serum calcium levels will be as low as 5.6 mg/dL (1.4 mmol/L). There is lameness, but fractures are not common even though the bones are soft. A simple method for assessing this softness is compression of the frontal bones of the skull with the thumbs. In affected sheep, the bones can be felt to fluctuate.

Pigs fed on heavy concentrate rations may develop a hypocalcemic tetany, which responds to treatment with calcium salts. Tetany may also occur in young, rapidly growing cattle in the same circumstances.

Inappetence, stiffness, tendency of bones to fracture, disinclination to stand, difficult parturition, reduced milk flow, loss of condition, and reduced fertility are all nonspecific signs recorded in adults.

SPECIFIC SYNDROMES

Primary Calcium Deficiency

No specific syndromes are recorded, although the complex relationship between overall nutrition, including concentration or amount of calcium in the diet, and bone development should be noted.

Secondary Calcium Deficiency

Rickets, osteomalacia, osteoporosis, osteodystrophia fibrosa of the horse, goat, and pig and degenerative arthropathy of cattle are the common syndromes in which secondary calcium deficiency is one of the specific causative factors.[5] In sheep, rickets is seldom recognized, but there are marked dental abnormalities. Rickets has been produced experimentally in lambs by feeding a diet low in calcium. There is an inherited form of rickets in Corriedale sheep.[9-11]

CLINICAL PATHOLOGY

Because of the effect of the other factors listed previously on body constituents, examination of specimens from living animals may give little indication of the primary cause of the disturbance. For example, hypocalcemia need not indicate a low dietary intake of calcium. Data on serum calcium and phosphorus concentrations and plasma alkaline phosphatase activity, radiographical examination of bones, and balance studies of calcium and phosphorus retention are all of value in determining the presence of osteodystrophic disease, but determination of the initial causative factor will still depend on analysis of feedstuffs and comparison with known standard requirements. Serum calcium concentration can be within the normal range in most cases, although calcium deficiency is followed, at least in sheep, by a marked fall in serum calcium levels to as low as 3.5 mg/dL (0.87 mmol/L). In an uncomplicated nutritional deficiency of calcium in sheep, there is only a slight reduction in the radiopacity of bone, in contrast to sheep with a low phosphorus and vitamin D status, which show marked osteoporosis. The response to dietary supplementation with calcium is also of diagnostic value.

NECROPSY FINDINGS

True primary calcium deficiency is extremely rare, but when it does occur, severe osteoporosis and parathyroid gland hypertrophy are the significant findings. The cortical bone is thinned, and the metaphyseal trabeculae appear reduced in size and number. The ash content of the bone is low because the bone is resorbed before it is properly mineralized.

Calcium deficiency secondary to other nutritional factors is common and typically induces the form of osteodystrophy known as osteodystrophia fibrosa (see subsequent description). In most instances, the confirmation of a diagnosis of hypocalcinosis at necropsy includes an analysis of the diet for calcium, phosphorus, and vitamin D content.

Samples for Confirmation of Diagnosis

- **Toxicology**—long bone (ASSAY [ash]); feed (ASSAY [Ca] [P] [Vit D])
- **Histology**—formalin-fixed section of long bone (including metaphysis), parathyroid (LM)

DIFFERENTIAL DIAGNOSIS

A diagnosis of calcium deficiency depends on proof that the diet is, either absolutely or relatively, insufficient in calcium, that the lesions and signs observed are characteristic, and that the provision of calcium in the diet alleviates the condition. The diseases that may be confused with calcium deficiency are described under the diagnosis of each of the specific disease entities.

The close similarity between the dental defects in severe calcium deficiency of sheep and those occurring in chronic fluorosis may necessitate quantitative estimates of fluorine in the teeth or bone to determine the cause.

TREATMENT

The response to treatment is rapid, and the preparations and doses recommended here are effective as treatment. Parenteral injections of calcium salts are advisable when tetany is present. When animals have been exposed to dietary depletion of calcium and phosphorus over a period of time, it is necessary to supplement the diet with calcium and phosphorus during dietary mineral repletion.

CONTROL

The provision of adequate calcium in the diet, the reduction of phosphorus intake where it is excessive, and the provision of adequate vitamin D are the essentials of both treatment and prevention. Some examples of estimated minimum daily requirements for calcium, phosphorus, and vitamin D are set out in Table 15-9. These are estimated minimum requirements and may need to be increased by a safety factor of 10% to allow for variation in individual animal requirements, the biological availability of nutrients in the feedstuffs, and the effect which total amount of feed intake has on absolute intake of minerals. For example, the use of a complete pig ration on a restricted basis may require that the concentration of both calcium and phosphorus be increased for that ration to deliver the actual total quantity of calcium and phosphorus necessary to meet a particular requirement for growth, pregnancy, or lactation. The information in Table 15-9 is presented as a guideline. When investigating a nutritional problem of formulating rations, it is recommended that the most recently available publications on the nutrient requirements of domestic animals be consulted.

Ground limestone is most commonly used to supplement the calcium in the ration, but it should be prepared from calcite and not from dolomite. Variations in availability of the calcium in this product occur with variations in particle size, with a finely ground preparation being superior in this respect. Bone meal and dicalcium phosphate are more expensive, and the additional phosphorus may be a disadvantage if the calcium : phosphorus ratio is very wide. Alfalfa, clover, and molasses are also good sources of calcium but vary in their content. The optimum calcium : phosphorus ratio is within the range of 2 : 1 to 1 : 1. In cattle, absorption of both elements is better at the 2 : 1 ratio. For optimum protection against the development of urolithiasis in sheep, a ratio of 2 to 2.5 calcium to 1 phosphorus is recommended.

The dustiness of powdered limestone can be overcome by dampening the feed or adding the powder mixed in molasses. Addition to salt or a mineral mixture is subject to the usual disadvantage that not all animals partake of it readily when it is provided in a free-choice manner, but this method of supplementation is often necessary in pastured animals. High-producing dairy cows should receive the mineral mixture in their ration and have access to it in boxes or in blocks.

REFERENCES

1. Durie I, et al. *J Vet Int Med.* 2010;24:439.
2. Schwarz B, et al. *Equine Vet Educ.* 2012;24:225.
3. Toribio RE. *Vet Clin Equine.* 2011;27:129.
4. Simon MJK, et al. *Osteoporosis Int.* 2014;25:1891.
5. Braun U, et al. *Vet Rec.* 2009;164:211.
6. Corbin LJ, et al. *Mamm Genome.* 2012;23:294.
7. Vander Heyden L, et al. *Vet Rec.* 2013;172:68.
8. Lepeule J, et al. *Prev Vet Med.* 2011;101:96.
9. Thompson KG, et al. *NZ Vet J.* 2007;55:137.
10. Dittmer KE, et al. *J Comp Pathol.* 2009;141:147.
11. Zhao X, et al. *PLoS ONE.* 2011;6.

PHOSPHORUS DEFICIENCY

SYNOPSIS

Etiology Usually a primary deficiency in the diet; may be conditioned by vitamin D deficiency.

Epidemiology Primary phosphorus (P) deficiency occurs in arid regions with low phosphorus content in soil. Most commonly chronic, but transient and acute P deficiency thought to occur in lactating dairy cattle in early lactation. Occurs under range conditions in beef cattle and sheep. Occurs in pigs not supplemented with sufficient phosphorus.

Signs Feed intake depression and anorexia are most commonly encountered sign with chronic P deficiency. Young animals grow slowly and develop rickets. Adults develop osteomalacia, unthriftiness, weight loss, reduced feed consumption, reluctance to move, leggy appearance, and fractures. Impaired milk production, growth rate, and fertility, presumably from energy and nutrient deficiency as a result of feed-intake depression. Recumbency and acute intravascular hemolysis (postparturient hemoglobinuria) in high-producing cows in early lactation have empirically been associated with hypophosphatemia and P depletion.

Clinical pathology Serum inorganic phosphorus. Phosphorus content of diet.

Necropsy findings Rickets and osteomalacia; lack of mineralization of bones.

Diagnostic confirmation Radiography of long bones, histology of bone lesions; bone ash analyses.

Differential diagnosis Those diseases resembling rickets and osteomalacia. Milk fever and downer cow syndrome in periparturient recumbent cattle. Other disorders associated with intravascular hemolysis in cases of periparturient hemoglobinuria.

Treatment Phosphate salts orally or intravenously, vitamin D.

Control Supplement diets with adequate phosphorus, calcium, and vitamin D.

ETIOLOGY

Phosphorus (P) deficiency occurs predominantly in arid regions of the world with low P content in soil. Phosphorus deficiency is encountered whenever the daily dietary P intake is insufficient to cover the requirements for maintenance and production and the organism has to recur to the mobilization of bone P. Under most circumstances P deficiency is chronic, and signs and symptoms associated with it occur after dietary P deprivation over months to years.

In dairy cattle, a rather acute and transient period of P deficiency is thought to occur in the first days to weeks of lactation and has been associated with recumbency and acute intravascular hemolysis in early-lactating cows. Rations with marginal P content in combination with low feed intake around calving are thought to result in inadequate P intake to cover for the suddenly increasing P requirements for milk production at the onset of lactation. The assumption that the commonly observed periparturient hypophosphatemia is an indicator for P depletion is, however, under contentious debate, and the clinical relevance of subnormal plasma inorganic phosphorus (Pi) levels in affected cows is uncertain.[1] Pronounced hypophosphatemia is also seen around parturition in mastectomized cattle, which don't produce any milk. Furthermore, even severe hypophosphatemia is often seen in healthy fresh cows not showing any clinical signs or symptoms.[1]

EPIDEMIOLOGY

Geographic Occurrence

Chronic P deficiency has a distinct geographic distribution depending largely upon the P content of the parent rock from which the soils of the area are derived, but also upon the influence of other factors, such as excessive calcium, aluminum, or iron, which reduce the availability of P to plants. Large areas of grazing land in many countries are of little value for livestock production without P supplementation. In New Zealand, for example, where fertilization of pasture with superphosphate has been practiced for many years, P deficiency may still occur in dairy herds because of inadequate maintenance of application over several years. Animals in affected areas mature slowly and are inefficient breeders, and additional losses as a result of botulism and defects and injuries of bones may occur. Apart from areas in which frank P deficiency is seen, it is probable that in many other areas a mild degree of deficiency is a limiting factor in the production of meat, milk, and wool.

Heavy leaching by rain and constant removal by cropping contribute to P deficiency in the soil, and the low P levels of the plant cover may be further diminished by drought conditions. Pastures deficient in P are classically also deficient in protein.

Cattle

The earliest report of naturally occurring P deficiency in grazing cattle was at Armoedsvlakte in the Northern Cape of South Africa. The disease was called **aphosphorosis,** and animals with the disease demonstrated a depraved appetite characterized by the desire to eat wood, bones, rocks, and other such materials, a behavior known as **pica**. In severely affected regions, cattle often died from botulism from eating bones from old carcasses contaminated with *Clostridium botulinum* toxin. In advanced states of aphosphorosis, animals developed bone malformations that were associated with stiffness in

Table 15-9 Examples of estimated daily requirements of calcium, phosphorus, and vitamin D

Species, kg body weight, and function	Calcium	Phosphorus	Vitamin D
	(G/ANIMAL)		
Dairy cattle			
Growing heifers (large breeds)			300 IU/kg dry matter (DM) intake
159	15	12	
300	24	18	
400	26	20	
Growing heifers (small breeds)			
100	9	7	
200	15	11	
300	19	14	
Growing bulls (large breeds)			
300	27	20	
400	30	23	
500	30	23	
Maintenance of mature lactating cows			
400	17	13	
500	20	15	
600	22	17	
Maintenance and pregnancy			
400	23	18	
500	29	22	
600	34	26	
Milk production	Add 2–3 g calcium and 1.7–2.4 g phosphorus to the maintenance requirements for each kg of milk produced.		
	(% OF RATION)		
Beef cattle			
Dry mature pregnant cows	0.16	0.16	300 IU/kg DM intake
Cows nursing calves	0.30	0.25	
Bulls, growth and maintenance	0.26	0.20	
Growing heifers (200-kg live weight gaining 0.8 kg/d)	0.33	0.26	
Growing steers (200-kg live weight gaining 0.8 kg/d)	0.36	0.28	
Sheep			
Ewes			
Maintenance	0.30	0.28	250–300 IU/kg DM intake
Pregnant (early)	0.27	0.25	
Pregnant (late)	0.24	0.23	
Lactating	0.52	0.37	200 IU/kg DM intake
Rams			
(40- to 120-kg live weight)	0.35	0.19	200 IU/kg DM intake
Lambs			
Early weaned (10- to 30-kg live weight)	0.40	0.27	150 IU/kg DM intake
Finishing (30- to 55-kg live weight)	0.30	0.20	
Horses			
Mature horses (400- to 600-kg live weight)	0.30	0.20	6–8 IU/kg body weight
Mares (400- to 600-kg live weight)			
Last 90 days of pregnancy	0.38	0.30	
Peak of lactation	0.50	0.40	
Growing horses (400-kg mature weight)			
3 months old	0.68	0.43	
6 months old	0.68	0.48	
12 months old	0.45	0.30	
Growing horses (500-kg mature weight)			
3 months old	0.69	0.44	
6 months old	0.82	0.51	
12 months old	0.43	0.28	
Pig			
Growing pigs (10- to 100-kg live weight)	0.65	0.50	200 IU/kg ration
Breeding pigs (gilts, sows, boars)	0.75	0.50	275 IU/kg ration

the forelegs, with a characteristic lameness referred to as "styfsiekte" in South Africa, "creeps" in Texas, and "pegleg" in Australia.

A survey of the mineral status of bones of cattle at abattoirs in western New South Wales, Australia, found evidence of osteodystrophy based on ash density. They represented cattle attempting to grow in a poor season, often female, in poor body-fat condition, light in body weight, and mostly from red soils known to be deficient in P.

Cattle constantly grazing pasture in the southern hemisphere appear to require somewhat less P in the diet (0.20% is probably adequate) than do higher-producing, partly housed livestock. The dietary requirements of P recommended by the NRC for beef cows weighing 450 kg may exceed the basic requirements. Over a period of several gestations, a daily allowance of 12 g of P per day per animal was deemed to be adequate for beef cows. Cattle given a P-deficient diet did not develop detectable signs of P deficiency until after 6 months of deprivation of this mineral.[2]

Hypophosphatemia in periparturient dairy cows is widespread, affecting at least 10% of fresh dairy cows, and it is often interpreted as a sign of dietary P deficiency in the periparturient period.[1,3,4] Hypophosphatemia in early lactation has been associated with syndromes such as postparturient hemoglobinuria, a form of intravascular hemolysis that is thought to be caused by increased fragility of red blood cell in P-deficient states and postparturient recumbency that is not responsive to intravenous treatment with calcium salts.[1,5]

Sheep and Horses

Sheep and horses at pasture are much less susceptible to the osteodystrophy of P deficiency than are cattle, and their failure to thrive on P-deficient pasture is probably attributable in part to the low protein content of the pasture. In fact, there has been no clear demonstration of a naturally occurring P deficiency in sheep.

There is some limited evidence that the plasma inorganic phosphorus (Pi) levels in Thoroughbred racehorses may be related to certain feeding regimens and to racing performance. Horses fed cubed or pelleted dietary supplement have plasma Pi concentrations consistently below an accepted mean of 1.03 mmol/L (3.2 mg/dL). It is suggested that a rapid rate of passage of the ingesta may affect P absorption. Other observations indicate that some of the best track performers had significantly lower plasma Pi concentrations compared with some of the worst performers.

Pigs

A primary deficiency can occur in pigs kept in confinement and not provided with sufficient dietary P. Lactating sows are more commonly affected than growing pigs. In some situations, in the cereal grains, the phytate levels are so high and phytase levels so low that rickets and osteomalacia are common in the pig population.

Secondary Phosphorus Deficiency

Secondary P deficiency is the result of hyperparathyroidism or vitamin D deficiency. This is of minor importance compared with the primary P deficiency. A deficiency of vitamin D is not necessary for the development of osteodystrophy, although with suboptimal P intakes deficiency of this vitamin becomes critical. Excessive intake of calcium does not necessarily result in secondary P deficiency, although it may cause a reduction in weight gains, probably as a result of interference with digestion, and may contribute to the development of P deficiency when the intake is marginal. The presence of phytic acid in plant tissues, which renders phytate-P unavailable to nonruminant species, is a major consideration in pigs but of only minor importance in ruminants, except that increasing intakes of calcium may reduce the availability of phytate-P even for ruminants. Rock phosphates containing large amounts of iron and aluminum have been shown to be of no value to sheep as a source of P. A high intake of magnesium, such as that likely to occur when magnesite is fed to prevent lactation tetany, may cause hypophosphatemia if the P intake of dairy cows is already low.

PATHOGENESIS

Of the body P, 80% to 85% is located in the skeleton, where it is deposited in a metabolically inert form together with calcium as hydroxyapatite. Hydroxyapatite is the compound that provides bone with its characteristic structural rigidity and stability. Bone P also functions as an important P reservoir that can be mobilized when body requirements temporarily exceed dietary intake. The remainder of the body P is available as dissolved P that is either encountered as inorganic phosphate (Pi) or forming part of organic molecules such as phospholipids, phosphocreatine, different adenosine molecules, or various carbohydrate metabolites. Phosphorus is a predominantly intracellular mineral, of which only small amounts are located in the extracellular space. Phosphorus bound in phospholipid molecules is essential for the structural stability of cell membranes that are composed of these phospholipids. The availability of soluble Pi in the intracellular space is essential for a plethora of biochemical reactions, especially those concerned with energy metabolism and transfer. Phosphorus furthermore functions as a buffer in rumen fluid, urine, and the intracellular space. Rumen microbes that are of critical importance for ruminant nutrition are inherently dependent of adequate P supply, which is not only provided by feed but also by the salivary glands, which produce large amounts of saliva rich in P.

Inadequate dietary P supply will result in the mobilization of hydroxyapatite, from which will release P together with calcium. Prolonged P deficiency is therefore associated with abnormal development of bone tissue, known as osteodystrophy.

Experimentally, female beef cattle fed diets containing less than 6 g of P/day developed an insidious complex syndrome characterized by weight loss, rough hair coat, abnormal stance, and lameness. Spontaneous fractures occurred in the vertebrae, pelvis, and ribs. Some affected bones were severely demineralized, and the cortical surfaces were porous, chalky white, soft, and fragile. The osteoid tissue was not properly mineralized.

Experimental dietary P depletion in cattle results in a rapid and marked decline in serum Pi. When markedly P deficient diets are fed over months, affected animals develop an avid appetite for old bones. The long-term signs include decreased weight gain in growing animals or loss of body condition in adult animals, feed-intake depression, reduced bone density as determined by radiography, and reduced bone weight, which are consistent with osteodystrophy. Serum Pi concentrations tend to increase despite of ongoing dietary P deprivation with activation of counterregulatory mechanisms that are reflected in increased plasma 1,25-dihydroxyvitamin D, reduced plasma concentrations of parathyroid hormone, and increased renal calcium excretion.

Muscle weakness to the point of recumbency is thought to be another symptom of P depletion, particularly in early-lactating dairy cows. The proposed underlying mechanism is a deficiency of Pi that may result in decreased concentration of phosphorylated molecules such as phosphocreatine and adenosine triphosphate (ATP) that are essential for energy storage on a cellular level. It has been proposed that it is through a depletion of these energy-storing molecules that P deficiency may result in muscle weakness and recumbency in periparturient cattle.[6] Nevertheless, it should be noted that disturbed muscle function has only been associated with hypophosphatemia in fresh cows but is not a common feature of chronic P deprivation in cattle. Doubts about the causative association between P deficiency and recumbency in cattle have furthermore been raised because of the impossibility of experimentally inducing recumbency through dietary P depletion in cattle and because of the variable response to treatment with P salts in recumbent hypophosphatemic cows.[1]

A decline of the intracellular ATP concentration, this time of red blood cells, is the presumed mechanism behind intravascular hemolysis observed in fresh cows with postparturient hemoglobinuria (see also the discussion of postparturient hemoglobinuria). Red blood cells (RBCs) require ATP to maintain their osmotic stability. A decrease of the ATP concentration in P depleted human RBCs to 15% of normal values resulted in increased osmotic fragility of erythrocytes that was associated with intravascular hemolysis. In cattle, hypophosphatemia has been reported in many but not all cases of postparturient hemoglobinuria, and response to treatment with phosphate salts is variable.[5,7] In a recently published study in which dairy cows were fed a ration over 40% deficient for several weeks, the plasma Pi concentration dropped by over 60% within days, whereas the Pi concentration of RBCs and their osmotic resistance remained unchanged.[7] The authors concluded that dietary P depletion causing pronounced hypophosphatemia is not generally associated with intracellular P depletion of RBCs or increased osmotic fragility, and that the plasma Pi concentration is an unsuitable indicator for the intracellular P content of RBCs.[7]

Decreased fertility was historically one of the predominant symptoms associated with P deficiency in cattle. Because there is no known mechanism through which P deficiency would directly affect fertility and because P depletion is commonly associated with feed-intake depression, weight loss, and decreased milk production along with reproductive failure, it is more likely that poor fertility is a result of a negative energy and nutrient balance rather than a specific effect of P on a (yet undetermined) reproductive function.

The pathophysiologic effects of low dietary P in pigs have been examined. Determination of the serum concentrations of parathyroid hormone, 1,25-$(OH)_2$ D, and osteocalcin were monitored in Romanian Landrace pigs originating from herds with dietary P deficiency. Serum Pi concentrations were negatively correlated with those of 1,25-$(OH)_2$ D. In lactating animals and sucklings, the linear relationships were not present. Serum Pi concentrations positively correlated with those of PTH, and 1,25-$(OH)_2$ D concentrations were negatively correlated. The serum concentrations of 1,25-$(OH)_2$ D and osteocalcin were positively correlated. Milk P concentrations ranging from 3.1 to 7.5 mmol/L were correlated positively with urinary Pi concentrations ranging from 0.3 to 11.4 mmol/L. In conclusion, similar to other species, P homeostasis is achieved in pigs by feedback mechanisms between P, PTH, and 1,25-$(OH)_2$ D, and osteocalcin production is induced by 1,25-$(OH)_2$ D.

CLINICAL FINDINGS

A plethora of clinical signs and conditions, such as unthriftiness, anorexia, pica, impaired growth and fertility, muscle weakness, lameness, recumbency, intravascular hemolysis, osteomalacia, and many more, have been associated with P deficiency in ruminants and other species.

Primary P deficiency is common only in cattle and is associated with chronic dietary P deprivation. In the experimental production of P deficiency in beef or dairy cattle, several months to years on a P-deficient diet are necessary before clinical signs develop.

Young animals grow slowly and develop rickets. In adults there is an initial subclinical stage followed by osteomalacia. In ruminants of all ages, a reduction in voluntary feed intake is a first sign of P deficiency and is the basis of most of the general systemic symptoms to follow, which are retarded growth, weight loss, low milk yield, and reduced fertility. For example, in severe P deficiency in range beef cattle, the calving percentage has been known to drop from 70% to 20%. The development and wear of teeth are not greatly affected, in contrast with the severe dental abnormalities that occur in a nutritional deficiency of calcium. However, malocclusion may result from poor mineralization and resulting weakness of the mandible. More advanced stages of P deficiency occurring in severely P-deficient regions are associated with reluctance to move, abnormal stance, and increased incidence of bone fractures. The animals have a leggy appearance with a narrow chest and small girth, the pelvis is small, and the bones are fine and break easily. The chest is slab-sided as a result of weakness of the ribs, and the hair coat is rough and lacking in pigment. In areas of severe deficiency, the mortality rate may be high as a result of starvation, especially during periods of drought when deficiencies of P, protein, and vitamin A are severe. Osteophagia is common and may be accompanied by a high incidence of botulism.

Cows in late pregnancy often become recumbent, and although they continue to eat, they are unable to rise. Such animals present a real problem in drought seasons because many animals in the area may be affected at the same time. Parenteral injections of P salts are ineffective, and the only treatment that may be of benefit is to terminate the pregnancy by the administration of corticosteroids or by cesarean section.

A more acute form of P deficiency is thought to occur in the first days to weeks of lactation in mature, high-yielding dairy cows. Hypophosphatemia in these animals has been associated with periparturient recumbency that is unresponsive to IV treatment with calcium salts. Affected animals are recumbent but mentally alert, with normal or only slightly decreased feed intake. They continue making attempts to stand and tend to creep around.

Another condition associated with P depletion and hypophosphatemia in dairy cattle in early lactation is postparturient hemoglobinuria. The disorder affects individual mature animals in the first days to weeks of lactation and is characterized by massive intravascular hemolysis, resulting in the excretion of large amounts of hemoglobin in urine (see also the discussion of postparturient hemoglobinuria).[7]

Although sheep and horses in P-deficient areas do not develop clinically apparent osteodystrophy, they are often of poor stature and unthrifty and may develop perverted appetites. An association between low serum or plasma Pi and infertility in mares has been suggested, but the evidence is not conclusive. The principal sign in affected sows is posterior paralysis.

CLINICAL PATHOLOGY

Serum Phosphorus

The concentration of serum or plasma Pi is the most commonly used parameter to assess the P status of an individual animal independent of the species. Although the serum Pi concentration reflects the short-term dietary P supply and the body's P pool size reasonably well, it is less suited to diagnose chronic P deficiency because compensatory mobilization of P reserves from bone tend to increase the Pi concentration in serum or plasma, thereby masking P depletion at least partially. Marked individual and diurnal fluctuations of the serum Pi concentration further complicate the interpretation of this parameter on an individual animal basis.[1]

Serum Pi levels are affected by such factors as age, milk yield, stage of pregnancy, breed, dietary P content, time of sample collection relative to feeding, and the blood vessel from which the blood sample is collected. Rapid and pronounced changes of the serum Pi level in the range of 10% to 30% can occur as a result of sudden shifts of P from the extracellular to the intracellular space, for instance, after strenuous physical exercise or oral or parenteral administration of carbohydrates.[1] Hypophosphatemia diagnosed in one single sample collected from one animal is therefore an unreliable indicator for the P status of that individual or a group of animals. The diagnostic value of the serum P concentration is complicated by the fact that clinical signs are not consistently observed with a certain degree of hypophosphatemia. For instance, serum Pi levels below 0.6 mmol/L (1.9 mg/dL) in cattle have been associated with intravascular hemolysis and recumbency, whereas even lower concentrations are often measured in healthy dairy cows.[1] To obtain comparable results it is advisable to collect blood from the same blood vessel at standardized times relative to feeding.

Reference ranges for cattle given in the literature are 1.4 to 2.6 mmol/L (4.0 to 8.0 mg/dL) and 1.9 to 2.6 mmol/L (6.0 to 8.0 mg/dL) for adult and growing animals, respectively. The reference ranges for sheep and goats are 1.6 to 2.4 mmol/L (5.0 to 7.3 mg/dL) and 1.3 to 3.0 mmol/L (4.2 to 9.1 mg/dL), respectively. Juvenile and growing individuals have higher serum Pi because of enhanced intestinal Pi uptake, presumably to provide sufficient Pi for adequate bone mineralization. The reference ranges for serum Pi for horses and swine are 1.0 to 1.8 mmol/L (3.1 to 5.6 mg/dL) and 2.1 to 3.3 mmol/L (6.5 to 10.2 mg/dL) respectively.

Dietary Phosphorus Content

Estimating the dietary P content is among the most reliable methods to estimate the P status of one or several animals, provided the feed intake can also be quantified. For pastured cattle, estimation of the dietary P content based on the P content in soil has been proposed. A P content in soil above 8 ppm was not associated with any signs of P deficiency, whereas negative effects on feed intake, growth, and fertility became apparent in cattle pastured for prolonged periods on soils with a P content between 7 and 8 ppm. Signs became more prominent in animals kept on soils with a P content between 4 and 6 ppm and were most severe on soils with a P content below 4 ppm.

The association between dietary P intake and the concentrations of P in feces has been explored in several studies. Although the effect of the dietary P content on the intestinal absorption rate of P is well established, neither rumen fluid samples nor fecal grab samples were found to reliably identify P depleted animals. Specifically, when P-depleted animals show feed-intake depression, a clinical sign often associated with P deficiency, fecal output decreases. This can translate into unchanged or even increased fecal P, although the total fecal P output is decreased.[1]

Bone Ash Concentrations

Determination of total bone ash concentrations and bone calcium and P concentrations from a sample of rib can provide useful diagnostic information and comparison to normal values. Nonetheless the bone P content is slow to respond to changes in dietary P supply, which means that the nutritional history has a strong impact on the mineral content of fresh bone. The P content in fresh bone is considered an excellent indicator for the body P reserves, but not for the current dietary P supply or the P pool size. Because obtaining bone biopsies is impractical under field conditions, determination of bone P content is largely restricted to postmortem examination or research.[1]

NECROPSY FINDINGS

The necropsy findings are those of the specific diseases, rickets, and osteomalacia.

DIFFERENTIAL DIAGNOSIS

A diagnosis of phosphorus (P) deficiency depends on evidence that the diet is lacking in P and that the lesions and signs are typical of those caused by P deficiency and can be arrested or reverted by the administration of P. Differentiation from those diseases that may resemble rickets and osteomalacia is dealt with under those headings.

Milk fever and downer cow syndrome in periparturient recumbent cattle.

Other disorders associated with intravascular hemolysis in cases of periparturient hemoglobinuria.

TREATMENT

For P supplementation in ruminants, either oral or parenteral treatment has been proposed. For metabolism and cell function, the organism requires P as inorganic phosphate (PO_4). Accordingly, P must be supplemented in a form that either contains phosphate or as a compound that can be hydrolysed to phosphate. Most pharmaceutical products containing P and labeled for parenteral administration in animals contain phosphite (Po_2), hypophosphite (PO_3), or organic P compounds such as toldimfos (dimethylamino-methylphenyl-phosphinate) or butafosfan (butylamino-methylethyl-phosphoric acid), which the body does not appear to convert to phosphate. These compounds must thus be considered to be unsuitable for P supplementation.

The preparation of a custom-made solution either with 300 mL of distilled water containing 30 g of NaH_2PO_4 or 500 mL of deionized water containing 90 g of $Na_2HPO_4 \times 12H_2O$, which are to be administered intravenously as a single dose to an adult cow, have been proposed in the literature (both equivalent to approximately 8 g of P) but are extra-label treatments. Both solutions are only suitable for IV administration, and their effect on the plasma Pi concentration is short lived, lasting for less than 2 hours when administered as an IV bolus.

Because of the rapid and sustained effect of orally administered P salts, this treatment route is preferred over the parenteral treatment. Oral administration of monosodiumdihydrogen phosphate (300 g) or monopotassium dihydrogen phosphate (250 g), both providing approximately 60 g of P, were found to increase the plasma Pi concentration in hypophosphatemic dairy cows within 3 to 4 hours of treatment and for at least 12 hours.[8] Monocalcium phosphate (250 g, also equivalent to approximately 60 g P) was less effective than monosodium phosphate and monopotassium phosphate, but more effective than dicalcium phosphate.[8,9]

TREATMENT AND CONTROL

Treatment

Cattle:

Monosodium dihydrogen phosphate (36 g NaH_2PO_4 dihydrate in 300 mL distilled water IV as single dose) (R-2)

Disodium monohydrogen phosphate (90 g $Na_2HPO_4 \times 12\ H_20$ in 500 distilled water IV as single dose) (R-2)

Monosodium dihydrogen phosphate (300 g NaH_2PO_4 PO q12h for 1 to 3 days) (R-1)

Monopotassium dihydrogen phosphate (250 g KH_2PO_4 PO q12h for 1 to 3 days) (R-2)

Monocalcium dihydrogen phosphate (250 g Ca $[HPO_4]_2$ PO q12h for 1 to 3 days) (R-2)

Dicalcium monohydrogen phosphate (300 g $CaHPO_4 \times 2H_20$ PO q12h for 1 to 3 days) (R-3)

Monosodium dihydrogen phosphate IM or SC (R-3)

Disodium monohydrogen phosphate IM or SC (R-3)

Butafosfan (butylamino-methylethyl-phosphoric acid) (R-3)

Toldimfos (dimethylamino-methylphenyl-phosphinate) (R-3)

Control

Bone meal, calcium-phosphate salts, sodium-phosphate salts, and sodium-pyrophosphate may be provided in supplementary feed or by allowing free access to their mixtures with salt.

Fertilization of P-deficient pastures with phosphate.

CONTROL

Phosphorus deficiencies in grazing livestock can be prevented by direct treatment of the animal through supplementing the diet or the water supply, or indirectly by approximate fertilizer treatment of the soils. Hand-fed animals are supplemented with P in their diets.

Phosphorus Requirements

Cattle

The P requirements for cattle in various stages of the production cycle have varied widely worldwide. Estimates of daily P requirements for cattle have been adjusted over the past decades based on evidence indicating that the digestibility of dietary P has been underestimated in the past, particularly in ruminants.[10] Apparent P requirements can vary for a variety of reasons: differences among breeds of cattle, P availability in the feed, whether animals are pen fed or free grazing, possible interactions between nutrients, and the effects of disease and parasitism.

Dairy Cattle

There is widespread belief among producers and consultants that reproductive performance in dairy cows can be improved by feeding P above recommended levels. The current NRC recommendations for early-lactation (90 days in milk) diets are 0.36% P (DM basis) for cows milking 45 kg/d and 0.35% P for cows milking 35 kg/d. The NRC recommends up to 0.42% dietary P for the highest-producing cows during the first few weeks of lactation.[10]

Several studies indicate that dietary P at 0.38 to 0.40% is sufficient for high producing dairy cows. Depending on feed ingredients, this concentration of P can be obtained with no or minimum supplementation with P of a standard North American or European dairy cow ration. Negative effects on milk yield and feed intake were observed in dairy cows fed ration with a dietary P content below 0.31% of feed dry matter over several months.[1] Cows conserve P when fed diets low in P by reducing P excretion in feces.

The transition period from late gestation to lactation presents a particular challenge for the mechanisms regulating the P homeostasis. In the last weeks of gestation, the dietary P content is often limited to reduce the risk of periparturient paresis.[10] With the onset of lactation, daily P requirements increase suddenly while daily feed intake is at a nadir. This situation may indeed result in a transiently negative P balance during the first days of lactation, which is likely to contribute to the commonly encountered hypophosphatemia in fresh cows. However, the mechanisms driving this periparturient hypophosphatemia are not well understood, and the degree of P depletion in affected cows has never been examined in detail, but has rather just been extrapolated from the observed declines in plasma Pi levels.[1] Hypophosphatemia shortly after calving is an unreliable indicator for P depletion because this decline in plasma Pi levels has not only been attributed to P losses through the mammary gland but also to hormone-induced compartmental shifts of P from the extracellular to the intracellular space.[1]

It is deemed unlikely that increasing the amount of dietary P in late pregnancy and early lactation will be able to prevent periparturient hypophosphatemia because this imbalance seems to occur secondary to hypocalcemia.[10]

Environmental Implications of Phosphorus Feeding of Livestock

In the European Union and the United States, environmental pollution with P from cattle manure has received increased attention over the past decades, and incentives with the objective to reduce the P content in ruminant fecal material have been implemented in many countries.

Ideally, P is recycled into the soil/plant/animal system, from which only the P incorporated into the animal system escapes. In a sustainable dairy farming system, the amount of P expelled in the form of manure must be limited to the amount that crops need for maximum growth. However, because of high livestock intensities and excessive amounts of P in feed, overapplication of P from manure occurs, leading to P accumulation in the soil and finally leaching, thus causing eutrophication of surface waters. Reducing the dietary P intake of cattle has been identified as an effective way to reduce the amount of P in manure and thereby contain environmental pollution with P.

The current recommendations for dairy cattle from the NRC are to provide phosphorus at 0.32% to 0.42% of dry matter intake.[10] These are lower than the previous recommendation of 0.5% of dry matter intake. Based on calculation of P losses and the true absorption coefficient using data on saliva production, saliva P content, and the efficiency of P absorption, the P requirement recommended for dairy cows in the Netherlands are as follows: P requirement (g/d per 600-kg cow) = 19 + 1.43 × 1 kg milk. This recommendation is up to 22% lower than the current recommendation for high-yielding dairy cows used in the United Kingdom.

Surveys in the United States revealed that dairy diets contain approximately 0.45% to 0.50% P (DM basis), an amount that is about 20% in excess of estimated requirements. A reduction of the dietary P content by 20% was estimated to result in a 25% to 30% reduction in the P content of manure and a similar reduction in the amount of land required to accommodate the manure. Phosphorus is the most expensive nutrient in typical mineral–vitamin formulations for dairy cattle. Feeding a diet containing 0.45% P versus one containing 0.55% would save about $0.05/cow daily; for a 100 cows over 1 year, this would save about $1825.00.

Simulation models of the long-term effects of changes in feeding, cropping, and other production strategies on P loading and the economics of 100-cow and 800-cow dairy farms in southeastern New York found that the most easily implemented change was to reduce the supplemented mineral P fed to that required to meet the current NRC recommended amounts, which would provide an annual increase in farm profit of about $22.00 per cow.

The overfeeding of P has important environmental implications. Phosphorus excretion increases linearly as P intake is increased above the requirement. Once P requirements are met, all of the excess dietary P is excreted in the feces. This excess P accumulates in the environment, primarily by the recycling of manure to land as fertilizer for crop production. The surface runoff of this excess P promotes the eutrophication of surface waters (eutrophication is the accidental or deliberate promotion of excessive growth of one kind of organism to the disadvantage of other organisms in the ecosystem). Therefore, close monitoring of P inputs in the livestock industry is important to reduce the risk of eutrophication of lakes and streams. Reducing dietary intake closer to the requirement will require frequent and accurate feed analysis, quantification of dry matter intake, and ration management to ensure that formulated diets are mixed and delivered to the cows properly. Phosphorus reduction will be achieved by precision of feeding of dairy cattle. Portable and rapid tests are now available to determine the level of P in dairy cattle manure. These hand-held tools can yield real-time measurements of dissolved P and total P in manure.

The effects of feeding low amounts of P to high-yielding dairy cows have been examined extensively in numerous studies.[10] Lactating dairy cows were fed diets containing 67%, 80%, and 100%, respectively, of the P requirements recommended by the Dutch Committee on Mineral Nutrition for a period of 21 months. Nearly 5 months after the beginning of the feeding trial, the milk yield and milk lactose content of the 67% group decreased significantly. It was concluded that rations for high-yielding dairy cows should not have a P content lower than 3.0 g/kg (or 0.3%) DM. The P supply with the 80% ration was considered to be just sufficient.

The supplementation of dietary P above levels recommended by the NRC (0.38% considered adequate or 0.48% excessive) did not improve duration or intensity of estrus in dairy cows. Large lactation studies have shown that feeding P in excess of 0.37% of diet DM, which corresponds closely to the NRC P requirements, did not affect milk production, milk composition, or animal health. Digestion studies and P retention data also support the NRC recommendations.[10]

Beef Cattle

There has been a notable lack of research into the P requirements of grazing beef cattle of various age groups and under varying soil and forage conditions, which has created considerable confusion and disagreement about the P requirements. The effects of P fertilizer on forage P levels and seasonal changes in P concentration are well understood, but the availability of P in different forage species, at different stages of maturity, and grown under different management schemes and environmental conditions is not well understood.

The details of the phosphorus requirements for beef cattle of various age groups are available in the NRC publication *Nutrient Requirements of Beef Cattle*, which was updated in 2000.[2]

Feedlot Cattle

The P requirement of finishing feedlot calves is less than 0.16% of diet DM or 14.2 g/d. Typical grain-based feedlot cattle diets do not require supplementation of inorganic mineral P to meet P requirements. Plasma P, performance, and bone characteristics indicate that P requirements are less than the predicted requirements and should be modified. Supplementation of mineral P in finishing diets is an unnecessary economic and environmental cost for beef feedlot producers and should be discontinued.

Pigs

The estimated dietary P requirements for maximum growth and feed efficiency of pigs at 3 to 5, 5 to 10, 10 to 20, 20 to 50, 50 to 80, and 80 to 120 kg, as a percentage of diet (90% DM) are 0.70%, 0.65%, 0.60%, 0.50%, 0.45%, and 0.40%, respectively. The form in which P exists in natural feedstuffs influences the efficiency of its utilization. In cereal grains, grain byproducts, and oilseed meals, about 60% to 75% of the P is organically bound in the form of phytate, which is poorly available to nonruminant species. The biological availability of P in cereal grains is variable, ranging from less than 15% in corn to approximately 50% in wheat, which has naturally occurring phytase enzyme. The P in inorganic phosphorus supplements also varies in bioavailability. The P in ammonia, calcium, and sodium phosphates is highly available.

Phosphorus Supplementation

Bone meal, calcium-phosphate salts, sodium-phosphate salts, and sodium-pyrophosphate may be provided in supplementary feed or by allowing free access to their mixtures with salt or more complicated mineral mixtures. The availability of the phosphorus in feed supplements varies, and this needs to be taken into consideration when compounding rations. For cattle, mineral sources with the highest absorption coefficients for P are monosodium dihydrogen phosphate (absorption coefficient 0.9), ammonium phosphates and monocalcium phosphate (absorption coefficient 0.80), followed by dicalcium phosphate (absorption coefficient 0.75).[10] The relative biological values for young pigs in terms of phosphorus are as follows: dicalcium phosphate or rock phosphate, 83%; steamed bone meal, 56%; and colloidal clay or soft phosphate, 34%. It is suggested that in deficient areas adult dry cattle and calves up to 150 kg BW should receive 225 g bone meal/week, growing stock over 150 kg BW 350 g/week, and lactating cows 1 kg weekly, but experience in particular areas may indicate the need for varying these amounts. The top dressing of pasture with superphosphate is an adequate method of correcting the deficiency and has the advantage of increasing the bulk and protein yield of the pasture, but it is often impractical under the conditions in which the disease occurs.

The addition of phosphate to drinking water is a much more satisfactory method, provided the chemical can be added by an automatic dispenser to water piped into troughs. Adding chemicals to fixed tanks introduces errors in concentration, excessive stimulation of algal growth, and precipitation in hard waters. Monosodium dihydrogen phosphate (monosodium orthophosphate) is the favorite additive and is usually added at the rate of 10 to 20 g/20 L of water. Superphosphate may be used instead but is not suitable for dispensers, must be added in larger quantities (50 g/20 L), and may contain excess fluorine. A reasonably effective and practical method favored by Australian dairy farmers is the provision of a supplement referred to as "super juice." Plain superphosphate at a rate of 2.5 kg in 40 L of water is mixed and stirred vigorously in a barrel. When it has settled for a day, the "super juice" is ready for use and is administered by skimming off the supernatant and sprinkling 100 to 200 mL on the feed of each cow.

FURTHER READING

Grünberg W. Treatment of phosphorus balance disorders. *Vet Clin North Am Food A.* 2014;30:383-408.

Karn JF. Phosphorus nutrition of grazing cattle: a review. *Anim Feed Sci Technol.* 2001;89:133-153.

National Research Council. Minerals. In: *Nutrient Requirements of Beef Cattle.* 7th rev. ed., updated 2000. Washington, DC: National Academy of Sciences; 2000 [Ch. 5].

National Research Council. Minerals. In: *Nutrient Requirements of Dairy Cattle.* 7th rev. ed. Washington, DC: National Academy of Sciences; 2001 [Ch. 7].

National Research Council. Minerals. In: *Nutrient Requirements of Swine.* 10th rev. ed. Washington, DC: National Academy of Sciences; 1998 [Ch. 4].

Valk H, Beyen AC. Proposal for the assessment of phosphorus requirements of dairy cows. *Livestock Prod Sci.* 2003;79:267-272.

REFERENCES

1. Grünberg W. *Vet Clin North Am Food A.* 2014;30:383-408.
2. National Research Council. Minerals. In: *Nutrient Requirements of Beef Cattle.* 7th rev. ed., updated 2000. Washington, DC: National Academy of Sciences; 2000 [Ch. 5].
3. Macrae AI, et al. *Cattle Practice.* 2012;20:120-127.
4. Macrae AI, et al. *Vet Rec.* 2006;159:655-661.
5. Stockdale C, et al. *Aust Vet J.* 2005;83:362-366.
6. Goff JP. *Vet Clin North Am Food A.* 2014;30:359-381.
7. Grünberg W, et al. *J Vet Intern Med.* 2014;doi:10.1111/jvim.12497.
8. Idink MJ, Grünberg W. *Vet Rec.* 2015.
9. Grünberg W, et al. *Br J Nutr.* 2013;110:1012-1023.
10. National Research Council. Minerals. In: *Nutrient Requirements of Dairy Cattle.* 7th rev. ed. Washington, DC: National Academy of Sciences; 2001 [Ch. 7]

VITAMIN D DEFICIENCY

SYNOPSIS

Etiology Deficiency of preformed vitamin D and, less commonly, insufficient exposure to ultraviolet solar irradiation.

Epidemiology Uncommon because diets are supplemented. Occurs in animals in countries with relative lack of UV irradiation, especially in winter months; animals raised indoors for long periods. Can occur in young grazing animals in winter months. The is marked species variation in susceptibility to effects of vitamin D deficiency.

Signs Reduced productivity; poor weight gain; reduced reproductive performance. Rickets in young animals (see that topic); osteomalacia in adults.

Clinical pathology Serum calcium and phosphorus. Plasma vitamin D.

Necropsy findings Lack of mineralization of bone.

Diagnostic confirmation Histology of bone lesions.

Differential diagnosis list See rickets and osteomalacia.

Treatment Administer vitamin D parenterally and oral calcium and phosphates.

Control Supplement diets with vitamin D. Injections of vitamin D when oral supplementation not possible.

Vitamin D deficiency is usually caused by insufficient solar irradiation of animals or their feed, or inadequate concentrations of vitamin D in rations of housed animals, and is manifested by poor appetite and growth and in advanced cases by osteodystrophy (rickets or osteomalacia).

ETIOLOGY

A lack of ultraviolet solar irradiation of the skin, coupled with a deficiency of preformed vitamin D complex in the diet, leads to a deficiency of vitamin D in tissues.

EPIDEMIOLOGY

Although the effects of clinically apparent vitamin D deficiency have been largely eliminated by improved nutrition, the subclinical effects have received little attention. For example, retarded growth in young sheep in New Zealand and southern Australia during winter months is corrected or prevented by vitamin D administration.

However, general realization of the importance of this subclinical vitamin D deficiency in limiting productivity of livestock has come only in recent years. This is partly a result of the complexity of the relations between calcium, phosphorus, and vitamin D and their common association with protein and other deficiencies in the diet. Much work remains to be done before these individual dietary essentials can be assessed in their correct economic perspective.

Vitamin D is available to animals from either or both of isomerization of 7-dehydrocholesterol (7-DHC) in the skin to vitamin D_3 during exposure to ultraviolet light or ingestion of vitamin D_2 or D_3 in the diet.[1]

Ultraviolet Irradiation

The intensity of ultraviolet light that reaches the skin of the animal depends on latitude and altitude. The lack of ultraviolet irradiation becomes important as distance from the equator increases and the sun's rays are filtered and refracted by an increasing depth of the earth's atmosphere. Cloudy, overcast skies, smoke-laden atmospheres, and winter months exacerbate the lack of irradiation. When the incidence angle of sun striking the skin is less than 35 degrees, as occurs during winter at latitudes of 31 degrees or higher, there is insufficient penetration of ultraviolet light to convert 7-DHC to previtamin D_3.[1] Reduced grazing time of cattle during summer at higher latitudes (56 degrees) is linearly associated with serum vitamin D concentrations.[2] The production of vitamin D_3 by dairy cows is directly correlated with the amount of skin exposed to ultraviolet radiation, and blanketing cows reduces vitamin D_3 production.[3]

The effects of poor irradiation are felt first by animals with dark skin (particularly pigs and some breeds of cattle) or heavy coats (particularly sheep), by rapidly growing animals, and by those that are housed indoors for long periods. The concentration of plasma vitamin D_3 recorded in grazing sheep varies widely throughout the year. During the winter months in the United Kingdom, the levels in sheep fall below what is considered optimal, whereas in the summer months, the levels are more than adequate. There is a marked difference in vitamin D status between sheep with a long fleece and those that have been recently shorn, especially in periods of maximum sunlight. The higher blood levels of vitamin D in the latter group are probably a result of their greater exposure to sunlight. Pigs reared under intensive farming conditions and animals being prepared for shows are susceptible especially if the diet is marginal or deficient in vitamin D.[4]

Dietary Vitamin D

The importance of dietary sources of preformed vitamin D must not be underestimated. Irradiated plant sterols with antirachitic potency occur in the dead leaves of growing plants. Variation in the vitamin D content of hay can occur with different methods of curing. Exposure to irradiation by sunlight for long periods causes a marked increase in antirachitic potency of the cut fodder, whereas modern hay-making technique with its emphasis on rapid curing tends to keep vitamin D levels at a minimum. Grass ensilage also contains very little vitamin D.

Based on a survey of the concentrations of vitamin D in the serum of horses in the United Kingdom, the levels may be low. In the absence of a dietary supplement containing vitamin D, the concentrations of 25-OH D_2 and 25-OH D_3 are, respectively, a reflection of the absorption of vitamin D_2 from the diet and of biosynthesis of vitamin D_3.

Information on the vitamin D requirements of housed dairy cattle is incomplete and contradictory. It appears, however, that in some instances natural feedstuffs provide less-than-adequate amounts of the vitamin for optimum reproductive performance in high-producing cows.

Grazing Animals

The grazing of animals, especially in winter and on lush green feed including cereal crops, leads to a high incidence of rickets in the young. An antivitamin D factor is suspected because calcium, phosphorus, and vitamin D intakes are usually normal, but the condition can be prevented by the administration of calciferol. Carotene, which is present in large quantities in this type of feed, has been shown to have antivitamin D potency, but the existence of a further rachitogenic substance seems probable. The rachitogenic potency of this green feed varies widely according to the stage of growth and virtually disappears when flowering commences. Experimental overdosing with vitamin A causes a marked retardation of bone growth in calves. Such overdosing can occur when diets are supplemented with the vitamin and may produce clinical effects.

Exposure of animals to solar radiation is important in metabolism of vitamin D, with previtamin D_3 formed in the skin. Skin pigmentation—specifically, melanin—influences the amount of ultraviolet exposure needed to produce vitamin D_3. A longer time in sunlight is required for maximum previtamin D_3 formation in dark-skinned animals.[1]

The importance of vitamin D to animals is now well recognized, and supplementation of the diet where necessary is usually performed by the livestock owner. Occasional outbreaks of vitamin D deficiency are experienced in intensive systems where animals are housed and in areas where specific local problems are encountered (e.g., rickets in sheep on green cereal pasture in New Zealand).

Animal Risk Factors

Most herbivores efficiently produce vitamin D_3 in the skin, and shorn sheep have higher concentrations of vitamin D_3 than do unshorn sheep.[1] However, New World camelids are particularly susceptible to vitamin D deficiency, likely as a result of their heavy fleece and evolution in the Andes and attendant exposure to high levels of solar radiation. Movement to lower altitudes, higher latitudes, or housing denies them access to the required amount of sunlight.[1,5-7] Inherited rickets in Corriedale sheep is caused by excessive vitamin D catabolism as a result of overexpression of the gene for 25-hydroxyvitamin D3-24-hydroxylase, the enzyme responsible for catabolism of vitamin D.[8,9] The disease occurs in housed fattening pigs, likely as a result of errors in feed formulation resulting in vitamin D deficiency.[4]

Foals have lower serum vitamin D concentrations than do adult horses.[10]

PATHOGENESIS

Vitamin D is a complex of substances with antirachitogenic activity. Increasingly in human medicine, vitamin D is recognized as also having important roles in immune function and resistance to neoplasia and cardiovascular disease.[11,12] The important components are as follows:

- Vitamin D_3 (cholecalciferol) is produced from its precursor 7-dehydrocholesterol in mammalian skin by natural irradiation with ultraviolet light (270 to 315 nm) over the course of 3 days.[1]
- Vitamin D_2 is present in certain plants, such as sun-cured hay, as a result of conversion of ergosterol to vitamin D_2 by ultraviolet light. Vitamin D_2 is present in and is produced by ultraviolet irradiation of plant sterols.
- Vitamin D_4 and D_5 occur naturally in the oils of some fish.

Vitamin D produced in the skin or ingested with the diet and absorbed by the small intestine is transported to the liver. In the liver, 25-hydroxycholecalciferol is produced, which is then transported to the kidney, where at least two additional derivatives are formed by 1-α-hydroxylase. One is 1,25-dihydroxycholecalciferol (DHCC), and the other is 24,25-DHCC. Under conditions of calcium need or calcium deprivation, the form predominantly produced by the kidney is 1,25-DHCC. At present, it seems likely that 1,25-DHCC is the metabolic form of vitamin D most active in eliciting intestinal calcium transport and absorption and is at least the closest known metabolite to the form of vitamin D functioning in bone mineralization. The metabolite also functions in regulating the absorption and metabolism of the phosphate ion and especially its loss from the kidney. A deficiency of the metabolite may occur in animals with renal disease, resulting in decreased absorption of calcium and phosphorus, decreased mineralization of bone, and excessive losses of the minerals through the kidney. A deficiency of vitamin D per se is governed in its importance by the calcium and phosphorus status of the animal.

Because of the necessity for the conversion of vitamin D to the active metabolites, there is a lag period of 2 to 4 days following the administration of the vitamin parenterally before a significant effect on calcium and phosphorus absorption can occur. The use of synthetic analogs of the active metabolites such as 1-α-hydroxycholecalciferol (an analog of 1,25-DHCC) can increase the plasma concentration of calcium and phosphorus within 12 hours following administration and has been recommended for the control of parturient paresis in cattle.

Maternal Status

Maternal vitamin D status is important in determining neonatal plasma calcium concentration. There is a significant correlation between maternal and neonatal calf plasma concentrations of 25-OH D_2, 25-OH D_3, 24,25-$(OH)_2$ D_2, 24,25-$(OH)_2$ D_3, and 25,26-$(OH)_2$ D_3. This indicates that the vitamin D metabolite status of the neonate is primarily dependent on the 25-OH D status of the dam. The maternal serum concentrations of calcium, phosphorus, and magnesium do not determine concentrations of these minerals found in the newborn calf. The ability of the placenta to maintain elevated plasma calcium or phosphorus in the fetus is partially dependent on maternal 1,25-$(OH)_2$ D status. Parenteral cholecalciferol treatment of sows before parturition is an effective method of supplementing neonatal piglets with cholecalciferol via the sow's milk and its metabolite via placenta transport.

Calcium : Phosphorus Ratio

When the calcium : phosphorus ratio is wider than the optimum (1 : 1 to 2 : 1), vitamin D requirements for good calcium and phosphorus retention and bone mineralization are increased. A minor degree of vitamin D deficiency in an environment supplying an imbalance of calcium and phosphorus might well lead to disease, whereas the same degree of vitamin deficiency with a normal calcium and phosphorus intake could go unsuspected. For example, in growing pigs, vitamin D supplementation is not essential provided calcium and phosphorus intakes are rigidly controlled, but under practical circumstances, this may not be possible.

The minor functions of the vitamin include maintenance of efficiency of food utilization and a calorigenic action, with the metabolic rate being depressed when the vitamin is deficient. These actions are probably the basis for the reduced growth rate and productivity in vitamin D deficiency. Some evidence suggests that vitamin D may have a role in the immune system. Local production of 1,25-$(OH)_2$ D by monocytes may be important in immune function, particularly in the parturient dairy cow.

Other Roles for Vitamin D

Vitamin D is now recognized in humans to have important roles in immune function, cancer, and cardiovascular disease as a result of a diverse range of biological actions, including induction of cell differentiation, inhibition of cell growth, immunomodulation, and control of hormonal systems. In addition, 1,25-dihydroxyvitamin D (calcitriol), through the vitamin D receptor, has an immunoregulatory role in both the innate and adaptive immune systems and exerts pleiotropic effects on numerous tissues.[12]

CLINICAL FINDINGS

The most important effect of lack of vitamin D in farm animals is reduced productivity. A decrease in appetite and efficiency of food utilization cause poor weight gains in growing stock and poor productivity in adults. Reproductive efficiency is also reduced, and the overall effect on the animal economy can be severe. The underlying mechanisms are unclear but could be related to the recently recognized pleiotropic effects of vitamin D (calcitriol).

In the late stages, lameness, which is most noticeable in the forelegs, is accompanied in young animals by bending of the long bones and enlargement of the joints. This latter stage of clinical rickets may occur simultaneously with cases of osteomalacia in adults. An adequate intake of vitamin D appears to be necessary for the maintenance of fertility in cattle, particularly if the phosphorus intake is low. In one study in dairy cattle, the first ovulation after parturition was advanced significantly in vitamin D-supplemented cows.

CLINICAL PATHOLOGY

Serum Calcium and Phosphorus

A pronounced hypophosphatemia occurs in the early stages and is followed some months later by a fall in serum calcium. Plasma alkaline phosphatase levels are usually elevated. The blood picture quickly returns to normal with treatment, often several months before the animal is clinically normal. Typical figures for beef cattle kept indoors are serum calcium 8.7 mg/dL (10.8 normal), 2.2 mmol/L (2.7 normal); serum inorganic phosphate 4.3 mg/dL (6.3 normal), 1.1 mmol/L (1.6 normal); and alkaline phosphatase 5.7 units (2.75 normal).

Plasma Vitamin D

The normal ranges of plasma concentrations of vitamin D and its metabolites in the farm animal species are now available and can be used to monitor the response of the administration of vitamin D parenterally or orally in sheep. The serum concentrations of vitamin D in the horse have been determined.[10]

NECROPSY FINDINGS

The pathologic changes in young animals are those of rickets, whereas in older animals there is osteomalacia. In all ages, a variable amount of osteodystrophia fibrosa may develop, and distinction of the origin of these osteodystrophies based on only gross and microscopic examination is impractical. A review of management factors and a nutritional analysis of the feed are essential. The samples for confirmation of the diagnosis at necropsy are as per calcium deficiency.

> **DIFFERENTIAL DIAGNOSIS**
>
> A diagnosis of vitamin D deficiency depends on evidence of the probable occurrence of the deficiency and response of the animal when vitamin D is provided. Differentiation from clinically similar syndromes is discussed under the specific osteodystrophies.

TREATMENT

It is usual to administer vitamin D in the dose rates set out under "Control." Affected animals should also receive adequate calcium and phosphorus in the diet.

CONTROL

Supplementation

The administration of supplementary vitamin D to animals by adding it to the diet or by injection is necessary only when exposure to sunlight or the provision of a natural ration containing adequate amounts of vitamin D is impractical.

A total daily intake of 7 to 12 IU/kg BW is optimal. Sun-dried hay is a good source, but green fodders are generally deficient in vitamin D. Fish liver oils are high in vitamin D, but they are subject to deterioration on storage, particularly with regard to vitamin A. They have the added disadvantages of losing their vitamin A and D content in premixed feed, of destroying vitamin E in these feeds when they become rancid, and of seriously reducing the butterfat content of milk. Stable water-soluble vitamin A and D preparations do not suffer from these disadvantages. Irradiated dry yeast is probably a simpler and cheaper method of supplying vitamin D in mixed grain feeds.

Stable water-soluble preparations of vitamin D are now available and are commonly added to the rations of animals being fed concentrate rations. The classes of livestock that usually need dietary supplementation include the following:

- Calves raised indoors on milk replacers
- Pigs raised indoors on grain rations
- Beef cattle receiving poor-quality roughage during the winter months
- Cattle raised indoors for prolonged periods and not receiving sun-cured forage containing adequate levels of vitamin D—these include calves raised as herd replacements, yearling cattle fed concentrate rations, bulls in artificial insemination centers, and purebred bulls maintained indoors on farms.
- Feedlot lambs fed grain rations during the winter months or under totally covered confinement
- Young, rapidly growing horses raised indoors or outdoors on rations that may not contain adequate concentrations of calcium and phosphorus—this may be a problem in rapidly growing, well-muscled horses receiving a high level of grain.

Because there is limited storage of vitamin D in the body, compared with the storage of vitamin A, it is recommended that daily dietary supplementation be provided when possible for optimum effect.

Injection

In situations where dietary supplementation is not possible, the use of single IM injections of vitamin D_2 (calciferol) in oil will protect ruminants for 3 to 6 months. A dose of 11,000 units/kg BW is recommended and should maintain an adequate vitamin D status for 3 to 6 months.

In mature nonpregnant sheep weighing about 50 kg, a single IM injection of 6000 IU/kg body weight produced concentrations of 25-hydroxyvitamin D_3 at adequate levels for 3 months. The parenteral administration of vitamin D_3 results in both higher tissue and plasma levels of vitamin D_3 than does oral administration, and IV administration produces higher plasma levels than does IM injection. The timing of the injection should be selected so that the vitamin D status of the ewe is adequate at the time of lambing. The vitamin D_3 status of lambs can be increased by the parenteral administration of the vitamin to the pregnant ewe. Dosing pregnant ewes with 300,000 IU of vitamin D_3 in a rapidly available form, approximately 2 months before lambing, provides a safe means of increasing the vitamin D status of the ewe and the newborn lambs by preventing seasonally low concentrations of 25-hydroxyvitamin D_3. In adult sheep, there is a wide margin of safety between the recommended requirement and the toxic oral dose, which provides ample scope for safe supplementation if such is desirable. In adult sheep given 20 times the recommended requirements for 16 weeks, there was no evidence of pathologic calcification. Oral dosing with 30 to 45 units/kg BW is adequate, provided treatment can be given daily. Massive oral doses can also be used to give long-term effects (e.g., a single dose of 2 million units is an effective preventive for 2 months in lambs). Excessive doses may cause toxicity, with signs of drowsiness, muscle weakness, fragility of bones, and calcification in the walls of blood vessels. The latter finding has been recorded in cattle receiving 10 million units/d and in unthrifty lambs receiving a single dose of 1 million units, although larger doses are tolerated by healthy lambs.

FURTHER READING

Dittmer KE, Thompson KG. Vitamin D metabolism and rickets in domestic animals: a review. *Vet Pathol.* 2011;48:389-407.

O'Brien MA, et al. Vitamin D and the immune system: beyond rickets. *Vet J.* 2012;194:27.

REFERENCES

1. Dittmer KE, et al. *Vet Pathol.* 2011;48:389.
2. Hymoller L, et al. *Brit J Nutr.* 2012;108:666.
3. Hymoller L, et al. *J Dairy Sci.* 2010;93:2025.
4. Madson DM, et al. *J Vet Diagn Invest.* 2012;24:1137.
5. Stieger-Vanegas SM, et al. *Aust Vet J.* 2013;91:437.
6. Van Saun RJ. *Small Rumin Res.* 2006;61:153.
7. Van Saun RJ. *Vet Clin North Am Food A.* 2009;25:797.
8. Dittmer KE, et al. *Res Vet Sci.* 2011;91:362.
9. Zhao X, et al. *PLoS ONE.* 2011;6.
10. Pozza ME, et al. *Vet J.* 2014;199:451.
11. Dittmer K. *Vet J.* 2012;194:5.
12. O'Brien MA, et al. *Vet J.* 2012;194:27.

VITAMIN D INTOXICATION

Vitamin D intoxication has occurred in cattle, horses, alpacas and llamas, and pigs after the parenteral or oral administration of excessive quantities of the vitamin. It also occurs in horses, cattle, and sheep after ingestion of hay or silage containing large amounts of *Trisetum flavescens* (yellow oat grass).[1,2]

In cattle, large parenteral doses of vitamin D_3 (15 to 17 million IU) result in prolonged hypercalcemia, hyperphosphatemia, and large increases in plasma concentrations of vitamin D_3 and its metabolites. Clinical signs of toxicosis occur within 2 to 3 weeks and include marked anorexia, loss of body weight, dyspnea, tachycardia, loud heart sounds, weakness, recumbency, torticollis, fever, and a high case-fatality rate. Pregnant cows 1 month before parturition are more susceptible than nonpregnant cows.

Hypercalcemia and hypervitaminosis D occurred in 17-day-old lambs being fed a milk replacer. The vitamin D content of the milk replacer was not excessive; there was no explanation for the abnormalities in the lamb, which recovered when the milk replacer was changed. Serum concentrations of calcium were high at 23.61 mg/dL and 23.09, respectively, in the two lambs.

Accidental vitamin D_3 toxicosis has occurred in horses fed a grain diet that supplied 12,000 to 13,000 IU/kg BW of vitamin D_3 daily for 30 days, equivalent to about 1 million IU vitamin D_3/kg of feed. Clinical findings included anorexia, stiffness, loss of body weight, polyuria, and polydipsia. There was also evidence of hyposthenuria, aciduria, soft tissue mineralization, and fractures of the ribs. Calcification of the endocardium and the walls of large blood vessels are characteristic.

Vitamin D intoxication occurs in pigs, usually as a result of errors in mixing of rations, and can result in polydipsia, polyuria, and weight loss.[3] Severe toxicosis in pigs occurs at a daily oral dose of 50,000 to 70,000 IU/kg BW. Signs include a sudden onset of anorexia, vomiting, diarrhea, dyspnea, apathy, aphonia, emaciation, and death. Clinical signs are commonly observed within 2 days after consumption of the feed containing excessive vitamin D. At necropsy, hemorrhagic gastritis and mild interstitial pneumonia are commonly present. Arteriosclerosis with calcification of the heart base vessels may also be visible macroscopically in poisoned cattle. Osteoporosis with multiple fractures has been observed in subacute to chronic hypervitaminosis D in pigs. Histologically, there is widespread soft tissue mineralization, with a predilection for the lung and gastric mucosa, and elastin-rich tissue, such as blood vessels. Changes in bone vary with the duration of exposure to toxic levels of the vitamin.

Research notes development of vitamin D intoxication in New World camelid cria supplemented with vitamin supplements that provided doses of 4000 to 13,000 IU/kg per day over several days.[4] The recommended dose of vitamin D to crias is a single parenteral dose of 1000 to 2000 IU/kg BW every 7 to 11 weeks.[4] Clinical signs of intoxication in the supplemented crias included weakness and inappetence. There was azotemia, hypercalcemia, and hyperphosphatemia.[4] Treatment was for acute renal failure.

Assay of the various metabolites of vitamin D in tissues is difficult. The diagnosis is therefore usually confirmed by correlating microscopic changes with a history of exposure to toxic levels of vitamin D.

Samples for Confirmation of Diagnosis

- **Toxicology**—500 g of suspect feed (ASSAY [Vit D])
- **Histology**—formalin-fixed lung, stomach/abomasum, proximal aorta, lung, bone (LM)

REFERENCES

1. Bockisch F, et al. *Tieraerztliche Praxis Ausgabe Grosstiere Nutztiere.* 2015;43:296.
2. Franz S, et al. *Vet Rec.* 2007;161:751.
3. Anon. *Vet Rec.* 2014;175:452.
4. Gerspach C, et al. *J Vet Intern Med.* 2010;24:443.

RICKETS

SYNOPSIS

Etiology Deficiencies of any or combination of phosphorus and vitamin D, and less commonly calcium. Inherited forms are recognized in sheep and pigs.

Epidemiology Young, rapidly growing animals. No longer common. In calves on phosphorus-deficient diets (range or housed). In grazing lambs as a result of lack of solar irradiation. Rare in foals and pigs.

Signs Stiff gait and lameness, enlargement of ends of long bones, curvature of long bones, prolonged periods of recumbency. Delayed dentition.

Clinical pathology Elevated alkaline phosphatase; low serum calcium and phosphorus. Lack of density of bone radiographically.

Necropsy findings Abnormal bones and teeth. Bone shafts are soft, epiphyses enlarged. Ratio of bone ash to organic matter is decreased.

Diagnostic confirmation Histology of bone, especially epiphyses.

Differential diagnosis list
- Epiphysitis
- Congenital and acquired abnormalities
- Infectious synovitis

Treatment Vitamin D injections; calcium and phosphate orally.

Control Supplement deficient diets with calcium, phosphorus, and vitamin D.

Rickets is a disease of young growing animals caused by impaired mineralization of physeal and epiphyseal cartilage during endochondral ossification and of newly formed osteoid.[1] Osteomalacia is the failure of calcification of osteoid in adult animals (i.e., after closure of the growth plate). The essential lesion is a failure of provisional calcification with persistence of hypertrophic cartilage and enlargement of the epiphyses of long bones and the costochondral junctions (so-called "rachitic rosary" of humans). The poorly mineralized bones are susceptible to fracture, compression, or both.

ETIOLOGY

Rickets is caused by an absolute or relative deficiency of any or a combination of calcium, phosphorus, or vitamin D in young growing animals. The effects of the deficiency are also exacerbated by a rapid growth rate.

An inherited form of rickets has been described in pigs. It is indistinguishable from rickets caused by nutritional inadequacy. The inherited form of the disease in Corriedale sheep is associated with increased expression of the gene for 25-hydroxyvitamin D3-24-hydroxylase, the enzyme responsible for catabolism of vitamin D.[2,3]

EPIDEMIOLOGY

Clinical rickets is not as important economically as the subclinical stages of the various dietary deficiencies that produce it. The provision of diets adequate and properly balanced with respect to calcium and phosphorus and sufficient exposure to sunlight are mandatory in good livestock production. Rickets is no longer a common disease because these requirements are widely recognized, but the incidence can be high in extreme environments, including purely exploitative range grazing, intensive feeding in fattening units, and heavy dependence on lush grazing, especially in winter months.

Rickets is a disease of young, rapidly growing animals and occurs naturally under the following conditions.

Calves

Primary phosphorus deficiency in phosphorus-deficient range areas and vitamin D deficiency in calves housed for long periods are the common circumstances. Vitamin D deficiency is the most common form of rickets in cattle raised indoors for prolonged periods in Europe and North America. Grazing animals may also develop vitamin D deficiency rickets at latitudes where solar irradiation during winter is insufficient to promote adequate dermal photobiosynthesis of vitamin D_3 from 7-dihydrocholesterol. Rickets has occurred in yearling steers in New Zealand wintered on swede (*Brassica napus*) crop deficient in phosphorus.

In young, rapidly growing cattle raised intensively indoors, a combined deficiency of calcium, phosphorus, and vitamin D can result in leg weakness characterized by stiffness, reluctance to move, and retarded growth. In some cases, rupture of the Achilles tendon and spontaneous fracture can occur. The Achilles tendon may rupture at the insertion of, or proximal to, the calcaneus.

Lambs

Lambs are less susceptible to primary phosphorus deficiency than cattle, but rickets does occur under the same conditions. Green cereal grazing and, to a lesser extent, pasturing on lush ryegrass during winter months may cause a high incidence of rickets in lambs; this is considered to be a secondary vitamin D deficiency. An outbreak of vitamin D–deficiency rickets involving 50% of lambs aged 6 to 12 months grazing new grass and rape occurred during the early winter months in Scotland. In the South Island of New Zealand, where winter levels of solar irradiation are low, rickets occurs in hoggets grazing green oats, or other green crops, which have been shown to contain high levels of rachitogenic carotenes. The disease occurs in sheep flocks in northern England, likely for similar reasons to the disease occurring in New Zealand.[4] A vitamin D–responsive rickets has occurred in twin lambs at 3 to 4 weeks of age.

Pigs

Rickets in young pigs occurs in intensive fattening units.[5] The cause is assumed to imbalances or mixing errors resulting in feed that contains excessive phosphate (high-cereal diets), or vitamin D and calcium deficiencies.

Foals

Rickets is uncommon in foals under natural conditions, although it has been produced experimentally.

New World Camelids

Llamas and alpacas are particularly susceptible to rickets secondary to vitamin D deficiency,[6-9] a consequence of them evolving at high altitudes with consequent high exposure to solar radiation. Movement to lower altitudes, where the increased atmospheric depth reduces solar radiation, or indoor housing, reduces the opportunity for dermal production of vitamin D.

PATHOGENESIS

Dietary deficiencies of calcium, phosphorus, and vitamin D result in defective mineralization of the osteoid and cartilaginous matrix of developing bone. There is persistence and continued growth of hypertrophic epiphyseal cartilage, increasing the width of the epiphyseal plate. Poorly calcified spicules of diaphyseal bone and epiphyseal cartilage yield to normal stresses, resulting in bowing of long bones and broadening of the epiphyses, with apparent enlargement of the joints. Rapidly growing animals on an otherwise good diet will be first affected because of their higher requirement of the specific nutrients.

CLINICAL FINDINGS

The subclinical effects of the particular deficiency disease will be apparent in the group of animals affected and have been described in the earlier general section. Clinical rickets is characterized by the following:

- Stiffness in the gait
- Enlargement of the limb joints, especially in the forelegs
- Enlargement of the costochondral junctions
- Long bones showing abnormal curvature, usually forward and outward at the carpus, in sheep and cattle
- Lameness and a tendency to lie down for long periods

Outbreaks affecting 50% of a group of lambs have been described. Arching of the back and contraction, often to the point of virtual collapse, of the pelvis occur, and there is an increased tendency for bones to fracture.

Eruption of the teeth is delayed and irregular, and the teeth are poorly calcified, with pitting, grooving, and pigmentation. They are often badly aligned and wear rapidly and unevenly. These dental abnormalities, together with thickening and softness of the jaw bones, may make it impossible for severely affected calves and lambs to close their mouths. As a consequence, the tongue protrudes, and there is drooling of saliva and difficulty in feeding. In less severely affected animals, dental malocclusion may be a significant occurrence. Severe deformity of the chest may result in dyspnea and chronic ruminal tympany. In the final stages, the animal shows hypersensitivity, tetany, and recumbency and eventually dies of inanition.

CLINICAL PATHOLOGY

The plasma alkaline phosphatase activity is commonly elevated, but serum calcium and phosphorus levels depend on the causative factor. If phosphorus or vitamin D deficiencies are the cause, the serum phosphorus level will usually be below the normal lower limit of 3 mg/dL. The serum concentrations of 25-hydroxyvitamin D_3 and 25-hydroxyvitamin D_2 are markedly decreased in vitamin D–deficient rickets compared with the normal values of greater than 5 ng/mL. Serum vitamin D concentrations as low as 0.4 ng/mL have been reported in lambs with vitamin D–responsive rickets. Serum calcium levels will be low only in the final stages. In leg weakness of young, rapidly growing cattle, the serum concentration of 25-hydroxyvitamin D may be nondetectable, and the serum levels of calcium and inorganic phosphorus may be low.

Radiographic examination of bones and joints is one of the most valuable aids in the detection of rickets. Rachitic bones have a characteristic lack of density compared with normal bones. The ends of long bones have a "woolly" or "moth-eaten" appearance and have a concave or flat, instead of the normal convex, contour. Surgical removal of a small piece of costochondral junction for histologic examination has been used extensively in experimental work and should be applicable in field diagnosis.

NECROPSY FINDINGS

Apart from general poorness of condition, the necropsy findings are restricted to abnormal bones and teeth. The bone shafts are softer and larger in diameter, in part because of the subperiosteal deposition of osteoid tissue. The joints are enlarged, and on cutting, the epiphyseal cartilage can be seen to be thicker than usual. Histologic examination of the epiphysis is desirable for final diagnosis. In sheep, the best results are obtained from an examination of the distal cartilages of the metacarpal and metatarsal bones.

A valuable diagnostic aid is the ratio of ash to organic matter in the bones. Normally the ratio is 3 parts of ash to 2 of organic matter, but in rachitic bone this may be depressed to 1:2, or to 1:3 in extreme cases. A reduction below 45% of the bone weight as ash also suggests osteodystrophy. Because of the difficulty encountered in repeating the results of bone ash determinations, a standardized method has been devised in which the ash content of green bone is determined, using either the metacarpus or metatarsus and the ash content related to the age of the animal, as expressed by the length of the bone. Although normal standards are available only for pigs, the method suggests itself as being highly suitable for all species.

Samples for Confirmation of Diagnosis

- **Toxicology**—long bone (ASSAY [ash]); 500 g feed (ASSAY [Ca] [P] [Vit D])
- **Histology**—formalin-fixed long bone (including growth plate) (LM)

DIFFERENTIAL DIAGNOSIS

Rickets occurs in young, rapidly growing animals and is characterized by stiffness of the gait and enlargement of the distal physes of the long bones, particularly noticeable on the metacarpus and metatarsus as circumscribed painful swellings. A history of a dietary deficiency of any of calcium, phosphorus, or vitamin D will support the clinical diagnosis. Radiographic evidence of widened and irregular physes suggests rickets. Copper deficiency in young cattle under 1 year of age can also result in clinical, radiographic, and pathologic findings similar to rickets. Clinically, there is an arched back, severe stiffness of gait, reluctance to move, and loss of weight. There are marked swellings of the distal aspects of metacarpus and metatarsus, and radiographically there is a widened zone of cartilage and lipping of the medial and lateral areas of the physeal plate. Copper concentration in plasma and liver are low, and there is usually dietary evidence of copper deficiency.

Epiphysitis occurs in rapidly growing yearling cattle raised and fed intensively under confinement. There is severe lameness, swelling of the distal physes, and radiographic and pathologic evidence of a necrotizing epiphysitis. The etiology is uncertain but thought to be related to the type of housing.

Congenital and acquired abnormalities of the bony skeletal system are frequent in newborn and rapidly growing foals. Rickets occurs, but only occasionally. "Epiphysitis" in young foals resembles rickets and is characterized by enlargements and abnormalities of the distal physes of the radius, tibia, third metacarpal, and metatarsal bones and the proximal extremity of the proximal phalanx. There may or may not be deviation of the limbs caused by uneven growth rates in various growth plates. The suggested causes include improper nutrition, faulty conformation and hoof growth, muscle imbalance, overweight, and compression of the growth plate. Recovery may occur spontaneously or require surgical correction.

Rickets in pigs is uncommon and the diagnosis can be difficult. The disease is usually suspected in young, rapidly growing pigs in which there is stiffness in the gait, walking on tip-toes, enlargements of the distal ends of long bones, and dietary evidence of a marginal deficiency of calcium or phosphorus. The radiographic and pathologic findings may suggest a rickets-like lesion.

Mycoplasmal synovitis and arthritis clinically resemble rickets of pigs. There is a sudden onset of stiffness of gait, habitual recumbency, a decrease in feed consumption, and enlargements of the distal aspects of the long bones, which may or may not be painful; spontaneous recovery usually occurs in 10 to 14 days. The locomotor problems in young, growing pigs raised in confinement and with limited exercise must be considered in the differential diagnosis. In performance testing stations, up to 20% of boars may be affected with leg weakness.

Rickets in lambs must be differentiated from chlamydial and erysipelas arthritis, which are readily diagnosed at necropsy.

TREATMENT AND CONTROL

Recommendations for the treatment of the individual dietary deficiencies (calcium, phosphorus, and vitamin D) are presented under their respective headings. Lesser deformities recover with suitable treatment, but gross deformities usually persist. A general improvement in appetite and condition occurs quickly and is accompanied by a return to normal blood levels of phosphorus and alkaline phosphatase. The treatment of rickets in lambs with a vitamin A, vitamin D_3, calcium borogluconate solution containing magnesium and phosphorus parenterally and supplementation of the diet with bone meal and protein resulted in a dramatic response. Recumbent animals were walking within a few days.

FURTHER READING

Dittmer KE, Thompson KG. Vitamin d metabolism and rickets in domestic animals: a review. *Vet Pathol.* 2011;48:389-407.

REFERENCES

1. Dittmer KE, et al. *Vet Pathol.* 2011;48:389.
2. Dittmer KE, et al. *Res Vet Sci.* 2011;91:362.
3. Zhao X, et al. *PLoS ONE.* 2011;6.
4. Mearns R, et al. *Vet Rec.* 2008;162:98.
5. Madson DM, et al. *J Vet Diagn Invest.* 2012;24:1137.
6. Schroeder C, et al. *Tieraerztliche Praxis Ausgabe Grosstiere Nutztiere.* 2008;36:343.
7. Stieger-Vanegas SM, et al. *Aust Vet J.* 2013;91:437.
8. Van Saun RJ. *Small Rumin Res.* 2006;61:153.
9. Van Saun RJ. *Vet Clin North Am Food A.* 2009;25: 797.

OSTEOMALACIA

SYNOPSIS

Etiology Absolute or relative deficiency of any one or combination of calcium, phosphorus, and vitamin D in adult animals.

Epidemiology Primarily in cattle and sheep on phosphorus-deficient diets. In feedlot animals as a result of excessive phosphorus without complementary calcium and vitamin D.

Signs Reduced productivity, licking and chewing inanimate objects, stiff gait, moderate nonspecific lameness, shifting from leg to leg, crackling sounds while walking, arched back, lying down for long periods. "Milk lameness" in high-producing dairy cows on deficient diet.

Clinical pathology Increased alkaline phosphatase, decreased serum phosphorus levels. Decreased density of long bones radiographically.

Necropsy findings Decreased density of bones; erosions of articular cartilages.

Diagnostic confirmation Histology of bones.

Differential diagnosis list

- Chronic fluorosis
- Polysynovitis and arthritis
- Spinal cord compression

Treatment As for calcium, phosphorus, and vitamin D deficiency.

Control Adequate supplementation of diet.

Osteomalacia is a disease of mature animals affecting bones in which endochondral ossification has been completed. The characteristic lesion is osteoporosis and the formation of excessive uncalcified matrix (osteoid). Lameness and pathologic fractures are the common clinical findings.

ETIOLOGY

In general, the etiology and occurrence of osteomalacia are the same as for rickets, except that the predisposing cause is not the increased requirement of growth but the drain of lactation, pregnancy, or both.

EPIDEMIOLOGY

Osteomalacia occurs in mature animals under the same conditions and in the same areas as rickets in young animals, but it is recorded less commonly. Its main occurrence is in cattle in areas seriously deficient in phosphorus. It occurs in goats.[1] It is also recorded in sheep, again in association with hypophosphatemia. In pastured animals, osteomalacia is most common in cattle, and sheep raised in the same area are less severely affected. In feedlot animals, excessive phosphorus intake without complementary calcium and vitamin D is likely as a cause, especially if the animals are kept indoors. It also occurs in sows that have recently weaned their pigs after a long lactation period (6 to 8 weeks) while on a diet deficient in calcium. A marginal deficiency of both phosphorus and vitamin D will exaggerate the condition. Intensively fed yearling cattle with inadequate mineral supplementation may be affected with spontaneous fractures of the vertebral bodies, pelvic bones, and long bones, leading to recumbency.[1] Simply handling the animals through a chute for routine activities such as tuberculin testing may precipitate the fractures.

PATHOGENESIS

Increased resorption of bone mineral to supply the needs of pregnancy, lactation, and endogenous metabolism leads to osteoporosis and weakness and deformity of the bones. Large amounts of uncalcified osteoid are deposited around the diaphyses. Pathologic fractures are commonly precipitated by sudden exercise or handling of the animal during transportation. There is evolving understanding of the role of fibroblast growth factor 23 in this disease and other diseases (rickets) associated with abnormalities in calcium, phosphorus, or vitamin D metabolism.[2]

CLINICAL FINDINGS

Ruminants

In the early stages, the signs are those of phosphorus deficiency, including lowered productivity and fertility and loss of condition. Licking and chewing of inanimate objects begins at this stage and may bring their attendant ills of oral, pharyngeal, and esophageal obstruction; traumatic reticuloperitonitis; lead poisoning; and botulism.

The signs specific to osteomalacia are those of a painful condition of the bones and joints and include a stiff gait; moderate lameness. often shifting from leg to leg; crackling sounds while walking; and an arched back. The hindlegs are most severely affected, and the hocks may be rotated inward. The animals are disinclined to move, lie down for long periods, and are unwilling to get up. The colloquial names "pegle," "creeps," "stiffs," "cripples," and "bog lame" describe the syndrome aptly. The names "milkleg" and "milk lameness" are commonly applied to the condition when it occurs in heavily milking cows. Fractures of bones and separation of tendon attachments occur frequently, often without apparent precipitating stress. In extreme cases, deformities of bones occur; when the pelvis is affected, dystocia may result. Finally, weakness leads to permanent recumbency and death from starvation.

Pigs

Affected sows are usually found recumbent and unable to rise from lateral recumbency or from the dog-sitting position. The shaft of one femur or the neck of the femur is commonly fractured. The fracture usually occurs within a few days following weaning of the pigs. The placing of the sow with other adult pigs usually results in some fighting and increased exercise, which commonly precipitates the pathologic fractures.

CLINICAL PATHOLOGY

In general, the findings are the same as those for rickets, including increased serum alkaline phosphatase and decreased serum phosphorus levels. Radiographic examination of long bones shows decreased density of bone shadow.

NECROPSY FINDINGS

It can be difficult to discern any gross changes as the epiphyses are seldom enlarged, and the altered character of cancellous bone may not be macroscopically visible. Cortical bone may be somewhat thinned, and erosions of the articular cartilages have been recorded in cattle suffering from primary phosphorus deficiency. The parathyroid glands may be enlarged. Histologically, abnormal osteoid covers trabeculae, and a degree of fibrous tissue proliferation is often evident. Analysis reveals the bones to be lighter than normal with a low ratio of ash to organic matter.

Samples for Confirmation of Diagnosis

- **Toxicology**—long bone (ASSAY [ash]); 500 g feed (ASSAY [Ca] [P] [Vit D])
- **Histology**—formalin-fixed bone, parathyroid (LM)

> **DIFFERENTIAL DIAGNOSIS**
>
> The occurrence of nonspecific lameness with pathologic fractures in mature animals should arouse suspicion of osteomalacia. There may be additional evidence of subnormal productivity and reproductive performance and dietary evidence of a recent deficiency of calcium, phosphorus, or vitamin D.
>
> A similar osteoporotic disease of cattle in Japan has been ascribed to a dietary deficiency of magnesium. The cattle are on high-concentrate, low-roughage diets and have high serum calcium and alkaline phosphatase levels but a low serum magnesium level. The osteoporosis is observable at slaughter, and clinical signs observed are those of intercurrent disease, especially ketosis, milk fever, and hypomagnesemia. Reproductive and renal disorders occur concurrently.
>
> In **cattle** it must be differentiated from **chronic fluorosis** in mature animals, but the typical mottling and pitting of the teeth and the enlargements on the shafts of the long bones are characteristic. In some areas (e.g., northern Australia) where the water supply is obtained from deep subartesian wells, the two diseases may occur concurrently. Analysis of water supplies and foodstuffs for fluorine may be necessary in doubtful cases.
>
> In sows, **osteomalacia** with or without pathologic fractures must be differentiated from **spinal cord compression** as a result of a vertebral body abscess and chronic arthritis resulting from erysipelas.

TREATMENT AND CONTROL

Recommendations for the treatment and control of the specific nutritional deficiencies have been described under their respective headings. Some weeks will elapse before improvement occurs, and deformities of the bones are likely to be permanent.

REFERENCES

1. Braun U, et al. *Vet Rec*. 2009;164:211.
2. Hardcastle MR, et al. *Vet Pathol*. 2015;52:770.

OSTEODYSTROPHIA FIBROSA

Osteodystrophia fibrosa is similar in its pathogenesis to osteomalacia, but it differs in that soft, cellular, fibrous tissue is laid down as a result of the weakness of the bones instead of the specialized uncalcified osteoid tissue of osteomalacia.[1] It occurs in horses, goats, and pigs.[2-4] The disease occurs in large animals, principally equids, as a result of secondary nutritional hyperparathyroidism.[4] Renal hyperparathyroidism, as is widely recognized in dogs, is rare to nonexistent in equids.[1]

ETIOLOGY

A secondary calcium deficiency resulting from excessive phosphorus feeding is the

common cause in horses and probably also in pigs. The disease also occurs in horses grazing tropical or subtropical pastures containing buffel, pangola, setaria, kikuyu, green panic, guinea, signal, and purple pigeon grasses. These tropical grasses contain oxalate, which interferes with mineral utilization by horses by forming calcium oxalate, which renders the calcium unavailable for intestinal absorption.[4] Grasses with more than 0.5% oxalate or calcium : oxalate ratios of less than 0.5 result in a negative calcium balance and are capable of inducing hypocalcemia in horses.[4] The disease can be readily produced in horses on diets with a ratio of calcium : phosphorus of 1 : 2.9 or greater, irrespective of the total calcium intake. Calcium : phosphorus ratios of 1 : 0.9 to 1 : 1.4 have been shown to be preventive and curative. With a very low calcium intake of 2 to 3 g/d and a calcium : phosphorus ratio of 1 : 13, the disease may occur within 5 months. With a normal calcium intake of 26 g/d and a calcium : phosphorus ratio of 1 : 5, obvious signs appear in about 1 year, but shifting lameness may appear as early as 3 months.

The disease is reproducible in pigs on similar diets to those just described and also on diets low in both calcium and phosphorus. The optimum calcium : phosphorus ratio is 1.2 : 1, and the intake for pigs should be within the range of 0.6% to 1.2% of the diet.

EPIDEMIOLOGY

Osteodystrophia fibrosa is principally a disease of horses and other Equidae and to a lesser extent of pigs. It occurs in goats. Previously, among horses, those engaged in heavy city work and in racing were more likely to be affected because of the tendency to maintain these animals on unbalanced diets. Widespread adoption of use of commercial diets and recognition of the importance of correct mineral nutrition has likely decreased the importance of this disease in these animals. The disease in developed countries is now restricted to equids fed inadequate or imbalanced diets. The major occurrence is in horses fed a diet high in phosphorus and low in calcium. Such diets include cereal hays combined with heavy grain or bran feeding. Legume hays, because of their high calcium content, are preventive.

The disease may reach endemic proportions in army horses moved into new territories, whereas local horses, more used to the diet, suffer little. Although horses may be affected at any age after weaning, it is the 2-to-7-year age group that suffers most, probably because they are the group most likely to be exposed to the rations that predispose to the disease.

A novel occurrence has been recorded of an endemic form of the disease affecting large numbers of horses at pasture.[4] The dietary intake of calcium and phosphorus and their proportions were normal. The occurrence was thought to be caused by the continuous ingestion of oxalate in specific grasses: *Cenchrus ciliaris, Panicum maximum* var. *trichoglume, Setaria anceps, Brachiaria mutica,* and *Pennisetum clandestinum.*

PATHOGENESIS

Defective mineralization of bones follows the imbalance of calcium and phosphorus in the diet, and a fibrous dysplasia occurs. This may be in response to the weakness of the bones, or it may be more precisely a response to hyperparathyroidism stimulated by the excessive intake of phosphorus. The weakness of the bones predisposes to fractures and separation of muscular and tendinous attachments. Articular erosions occur commonly, and displacement of the bone marrow may cause the development of anemia.

CLINICAL FINDINGS

Horse

As in most osteodystrophies, the major losses are probably in the early stages before clinical signs appear or on diets where the aberration is marginal. In horses, a shifting lameness is characteristic of this stage of the disease, and arching of the back may sometimes occur. The horse is lame, but only mildly so, and in many cases, no physical deformity can be found by which the seat of lameness can be localized. These signs probably result from relaxation of tendon and ligaments and appear in different limbs at different times. Articular erosions may contribute to the lameness. In more advanced cases, severe injuries, including fracture and visible sprains of tendons, may occur, but these are not specific to osteodystrophia fibrosa, although their incidence is higher in affected than in normal horses. Fracture of the lumbar vertebrae while racing has been known to occur in affected horses.

The more classical picture of the disease has largely disappeared because cases are seldom permitted to progress to this advanced stage. Local swelling of the lower and alveolar margins of the mandible is followed by soft, symmetric enlargement of the facial bones, which may become swollen so that they interfere with respiration. Initially these bony swellings are firm and pyramidal and commence just above and anterior to the facial crests. The lesions are bilaterally symmetric and prevent full occlusion of the incisors. Flattening of the ribs may be apparent, and fractures and rupture or avulsion of ligaments might occur if the horse is worked. There may be obvious swelling of joints and curvature of long bones. Severe emaciation and anemia occur in the final stages.

Pigs

In pigs, the lesions and signs are similar to those in the horse, and in severe cases, pigs may be unable to rise and walk and show gross distortion of limbs and enlargement of joints and the face. In less severe cases, there is lameness, reluctance to rise, pain on standing, and bending of the limb bones, but normal facial bones and joints. With suitable treatment, the lameness disappears, but affected pigs may never attain their full size. The relationship of this disease to atrophic rhinitis is discussed under the latter heading.

Goats

An outbreak of the disease has been recorded in goats receiving a diet of wheat straw (60%) and 40% barley for 89 months. The ratio of calcium to phosphorus in the diet was 1 : 1.8. Affected goats were 9 to 10 months of age, with a history of stunted growth, lameness, diarrhea, and tongue protrusion. Clinically, there was symmetric enlargement of the face and jaws, tongue protrusion, prominent eyeballs, and tremor. The enlarged bones were firm and painful on palpation. The hindlimbs were bent outward symmetrically from the tarsal joints.

CLINICAL PATHOLOGY

There are no significant changes in blood chemistry in horses affected with severe osteodystrophia fibrosa. However, the serum calcium level will tend to be lower than normal, the serum inorganic phosphorus higher than normal, and the alkaline phosphatase activity higher than normal. The levels of diagnostic alkaline phosphatase have not been determined. Affected horses may be unable to return their serum calcium levels to normal following the infusion of a calcium salt. Radiographic examination reveals increased translucency of bones, especially of the mandibles.

NECROPSY FINDINGS

The entire skeleton is abnormal in this severe form of metabolic bone disease, but the change is most notable in the mandibular, maxillary, and nasal bones, which may appear thickened and distorted. The fleshy tissue that replaces normal cancellous bone in these sites is also present in the metaphyses of the long bones. Microscopically, there is proliferation of fibrous tissue and markedly increased osteoclast activity along thinned and abnormally oriented bony trabeculae. The parathyroid glands are enlarged. It must be remembered that osteodystrophia fibrosa is a lesion, not a disease. The pathway to this lesion usually involves a dietary imbalance in calcium and phosphorus, but the kidneys should also be examined to rule out the possibility of renal secondary hyperparathyroidism.

Samples for Confirmation of Diagnosis

- **Toxicology**—bone (ASSAY [ash]); 500 g feed (ASSAY [Ca] [P] [Vit D])
- **Histology**—formalin-fixed bone, parathyroid gland, kidney (LM)

DIFFERENTIAL DIAGNOSIS

In the early stages, the diagnosis may be difficult because of the common occurrence of traumatic injuries to horses' legs. A high incidence of lameness in a group of horses warrants examination of the ration and determination of their calcium and phosphorus status. An identical clinical picture has been described in a mare with an adenoma of the parathyroid gland. Inherited multiple exostosis has been described in the horse.

In pigs, osteodystrophia can be the result of hypovitaminosis A and experimentally as a result of manganese deficiency.

TREATMENT AND CONTROL

A ration adequately balanced with regard to calcium and phosphorus (calcium : phosphorus should be in the vicinity of 1 : 1 and not wider than 1 : 1.4) is preventive in horses, and affected animals can only be treated by correcting the existing imbalance. Even severe lesions may disappear in time with proper treatment. Cereal hay may be supplemented with alfalfa or clover hay, or finely ground limestone (30 g daily) should be fed. Dicalcium phosphate and bone meal are not as efficient because of their additional content of phosphorus.

FURTHER READING

Stewart J, et al. Bighead in horses—not an ancient disease. *Aust Equine Vet.* 2010;29:55-62.

REFERENCES

1. Toribio RE. *Vet Clin Equine.* 2011;27:129.
2. Braun U, et al. *Vet Rec.* 2009;164:211.
3. John E, et al. *Intas Polivet.* 2007;8:458.
4. Stewart J, et al. *Aust Equine Vet.* 2010;29:55.

"BOWIE" OR "BENTLEG" IN LAMBS

Bowie is a disease of lambs of unknown etiology characterized by carpus valgus, and less commonly carpus varus, resulting in a lateral displacement of the carpus and medial displacement of the hooves. The lesions differ from those of rickets. It has been observed only on unimproved range pasture in New Zealand and in South Africa. The cause is unknown, although phosphorus deficiency has been suggested. A similar syndrome has been produced by the feeding of wild parsnip (*Trachemene glaucifolia*) and, experimentally, by the feeding of a diet low in both calcium and phosphorus. There is no clear genetic component to the disease in South Africa.

Improvement of the pasture by top dressing with superphosphate and sowing-improved grasses is usually followed by disappearance of the disease. Only sucking lambs are affected, and cases occur only in the spring at a time when rickets does not occur. Up to 40% of a group of lambs can be affected without breed differences in incidence. Signs of the disease can be evident at 3 to 4 weeks of age.

The disease has also been reported from South Africa, where it occurs primarily in ram lambs and develops from as early as 3 months up to 1 year of age. There is gradual bending of the forelimbs, with the hooves turned inward and the carpal joints turned outward. Animals of the South African Mutton Merino breed had significantly higher plasma phosphorus concentrations than those of the Merino and Dohne Merino breeds. The plasma calcium : phosphorus ratio was lower in affected lambs and their ewes, and this converse ratio is thought to result in an induced plasma ionized calcium deficiency leading to improper calcification of bone.

Some tenderness of the feet and lateral curvature at the knees can be seen as early as 2 to 3 weeks of age, and marked deformity is present at 6 to 8 weeks, with maximum severity at weaning. The forelimbs are more commonly affected than the hindlimbs. Carpus varus occurs in rare cases. The sides of the feet become badly worn, and the lateral aspects of the lower parts of the limbs can be injured and be accompanied by lameness. The lambs grow well at first, but by the time of weaning, affected lambs are in poor condition because of their inability to move about and feed properly. A rather similar syndrome has been observed in young Saanen bucks, but the condition showed a tendency to recover spontaneously.

At necropsy lesions are restricted to the radius and metacarpus with medial collapse of the distal radial epiphysis and consequent carpus valgus. There is often excessive synovial fluid in the carpal joints; in the later stages, there are articular erosions. Increased deposition of osteoid is not observed.

Supplementation of the diet with phosphorus or improvement of the pasture seems to reduce the incidence of the disease. Dosing with vitamin D or providing mineral mixtures containing all trace elements is ineffective.

DEGENERATIVE JOINT DISEASE AND OSTEOARTHRITIS

Degenerative joint disease in food animals describes severe, progressive, nonseptic arthropathy in growing animals that is the result of one or more processes that lead to damage to articular cartilage and consequent osteoarthritis. The insult can be to cartilage or underlying bone as a result of metabolic, nutritional, congenital, or traumatic causes but can be difficult to identify because the insult to tissues causing the disease usually occurs weeks to months before clinical signs of disease. Degenerative joint disease can affect almost any diarthrodial joint. The most severe disease occurs when affected joints are loaded with weight.[1] The disease is well documented and researched in racehorses in which it is the end result of damage to articular cartilage.[2,3]

According to some studies, greater than 90% of steers are affected by osteoarthritis, and it is an important cause of infertility in beef bulls.[4] The disease is most often seen in the stifle joint, where the predilection sites are the medial and lateral condyles and the patellar groove. Most lesions are bilateral.[1,4,5]

Degenerative arthropathy occurs in cattle of all breeds but reaches its highest incidence as a sporadic disease of young beef bulls. The disease has been identified as hip dysplasia because of the preexisting shallow contour of the acetabulum. It is considered to be inherited as a recessive characteristic and exacerbated by rapid weight gain in young animals. The occurrence of the condition in these animals is usually associated with rearing on nurse cows, housing for long periods, provision of a ration high in cereal grains and byproducts (i.e., a high phosphorus : calcium ratio), and possibly with an inherited straight conformation of the hindlegs. Although the disease occurs in all beef breeds, there is a strong familial tendency that appears to be directly related to the rate of body-weight gain and the straightness of the hindleg. If the potential for rapid weight gain is being realized in animals being force fed, the rate of occurrence appears to be dependent on their breeding, and animals in the same herd that are allowed to run at pasture under natural conditions are either not affected or are affected at a much later age. Thus animals in a susceptible herd can show signs as early as 6 months of age if they are heavily hand-fed and raised on dairy cow foster mothers. In the same herd, signs do not appear until 1 to 2 years of age if supplementary feeding is not introduced until weaning and not until 4 years if there is no significant additional feeding.

Clinically there is a gradual onset of lameness in one or both hindlegs. The disease progresses, with the lameness becoming more severe over a period of 6 to 12 months. In some animals, there is a marked sudden change for the worse, usually related to violent muscular movements, as in breeding or fighting. In severely affected animals, the affected limb is virtually useless; on movement, distinct crepitus can often be felt and heard over the affected joints. This can be accomplished by rocking the animal from side to side or having it walk while holding the hands over the hip joints.

An additional method of examination is to place the hand in the rectum close to the hip joint while the animal is moved. Passive movement of the limb may also elicit crepitus or louder clinking or clicking sounds. The hip joints are always most severely affected, but in advanced cases, there may be moderate involvement of the stifles and minimal lesions in other joints. Affected animals lie down most of the time and are reluctant to rise and to walk. The joints are not swollen, but in advanced cases, local atrophy of muscles may be so marked that the joints appear to be enlarged. There is a recorded occurrence in which the lesions were confined mainly to the front fetlocks.

Radiographic examination can provide confirmatory or diagnostic evidence but is restricted to facilities with equipment suited to these examinations.

At **necropsy,** the most obvious finding is extensive erosion of the articular surfaces, often penetrating to the cancellous bone, and disappearance of the normal contours of the head of the femur or the epiphyses in the stifle joint. The synovial cavity is distended, with an increased volume of brownish, turbid fluid; the joint capsule is much thickened and often contains calcified plaques. Multiple small exostoses are present on the periarticular surfaces. When the stifle is involved, the cartilaginous menisci, particularly the medial one, are very much reduced in size and may be completely absent. In cattle with severe degenerative changes in the coxofemoral joint, an acetabular osseous bulla may be present at the cranial margin of the obturator foramen.[1]

Adequate calcium, phosphorus, and vitamin D intake and a correct calcium : phosphorus ratio in the ration should be ensured. Supplementation of the ration with copper at the rate of 15 mg/kg has also been recommended for the control of a similar disease.

Degenerative joint disease of cattle is recorded on an enzootic scale in Chile and is thought to be attributable to gross nutritional deficiency. The hip and tarsal joints are the only ones affected, and clinical signs appear when animals are 8 to 12 months old. There is gross lameness and progressive emaciation. An inherited osteoarthritis is described under that heading. Sporadic cases of degenerative arthropathy, with similar signs and lesions, occur in heavy-producing, aged dairy cows and are thought to be caused by long-continued negative calcium balance. Rare cases also occur in aged beef cows but are thought to be associated with an inherited predisposition. In both instances the lesions are commonly restricted to the stifle joints.

Degenerative arthropathy of the distal interphalangeal joints and sesamoid bones occurs in calves (Fig. 15-14). Affected animals have moderate to severe lameness of one or both forelimbs but no discernible distension of the joint. Treatment is palliative, involving administration of NSAIDs (meloxicam or phenylbutazone, where permitted by regulatory authorities) or surgery.[6]

Osteoarthritis occurs in the stifle joint of dairy breed bulls. Seventy-two percent (39/54) of stifle joints and 85% (23/27) of dairy bulls 31 to 60 months of age had at least one gross lesion, and 94% of the lesions were localized to the distal end of the femur, with the patellar groove and the lateral trochlear ridge being predilection sites.

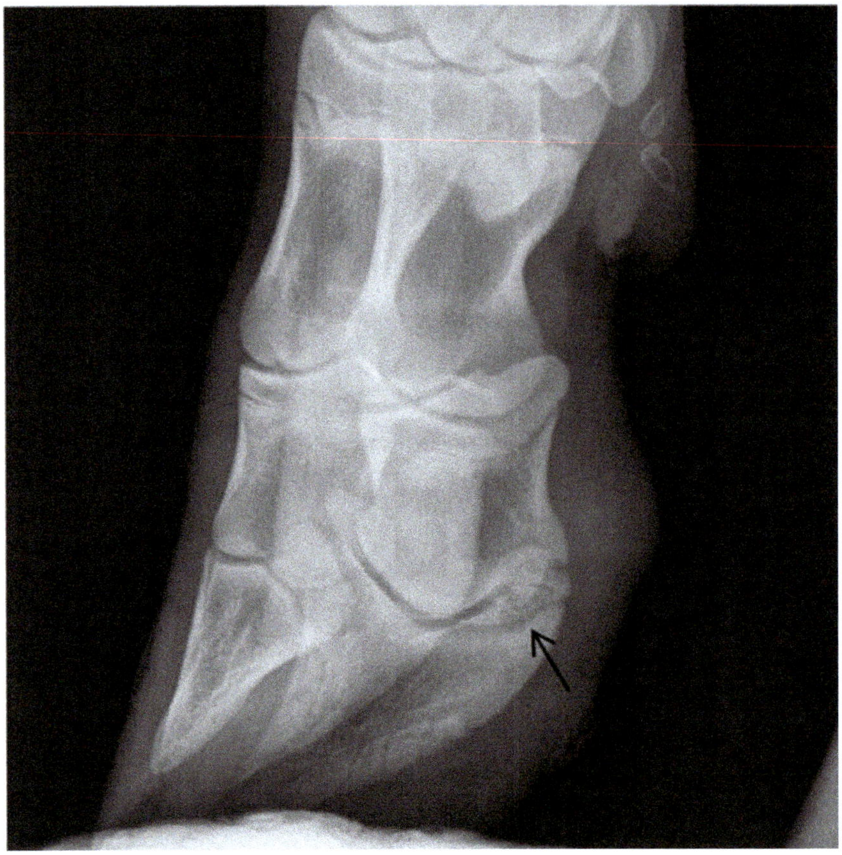

Fig. 15-14 Degenerative joint disease (arrow) affecting P2 to P3 of a calf. (Reproduced with permission.[6])

Osteoarthritis of one or both temporomandibular joints occurs in ~1.3% of Soay sheep on the island of St. Kilda, being more common in older ewes.[7] Osteoarthritis also occurs in the elbows of sheep.[8] It can be bilateral, in which case the sheep have a characteristic stance with both hindfeet placed more cranially, under the abdomen, apparently in an effort to reduce weight-bearing by the forelegs. There is no definitive treatment.[8]

FURTHER READING

Nichols S, Larde H. Noninfectious joint disease in cattle. *Vet Clin North Am Food A.* 2014;30:205-220.

REFERENCES

1. Heinola T, et al. *J Comp Pathol.* 2013;148:335.
2. McCoy AM. *Vet Pathol.* 2015;52:803.
3. Nichols S, et al. *Vet Clin North Am Food A.* 2014;30:205.
4. Persson Y, et al. *Acta Vet Scand.* 2007;49.
5. Heinola T, et al. *Vet J.* 2014;200:88.
6. Mulon P-Y, et al. *JAVMA.* 2009;234:794.
7. Arthur C, et al. *Vet J.* 2015;203:120.
8. Scott PR. *Vet Rec.* 2001;149:652.

MANGANESE DEFICIENCY

A dietary deficiency of manganese (Mn) can cause skeletal deformities, both congenitally and after birth, and infertility.

ETIOLOGY

A primary deficiency occurs endemically in some areas because of a geological deficiency of manganese in the local rock formations. Apart from a primary dietary deficiency of manganese, the existence of factors depressing the availability of ingested manganese is suspected. An excess of calcium and/or phosphorus in the diet increases the requirements of manganese in the diet of calves and is considered to reduce the availability of dietary manganese to cattle generally.

Congenital chondrodystrophy in calves has been associated with a manganese deficiency, and there are outbreaks of congenital skeletal defects in calves suspected to be attributable to manganese deficiency.[1-3]

EPIDEMIOLOGY

Soils containing less than 3 mg/kg of manganese are unlikely to be able to support normal fertility in cattle. In areas where manganese-responsive infertility occurs, soils on farms with infertility problems have contained less than 3 mg/kg of manganese, whereas soils on neighboring farms with no infertility problems have had levels of more than 9 mg/kg. A secondary soil deficiency is thought to occur, and one of the factors suspected of reducing the availability of manganese in the soil to plants is high alkalinity. Thus heavy liming is associated with manganese-responsive infertility. There are three main soil types on which the disease occurs:

- Soils low in manganese, which have low output even when pH is less than 5.5
- Sandy soils, where availability starts to fall
- Heavy soils, where availability starts to fall at a pH of 7.0

Many other factors are suggested as reducing the availability of soil manganese, but the evidence is not conclusive. For example, heavy liming of soils to neutralize sulfur dioxide emissions from a neighboring smelter is thought to have reduced the manganese intake of grazing animals.

Herbage on low-manganese soils, or on marginal soils where availability is decreased (possibly even soils with normal manganese content), is low in manganese. A number of figures are given for critical levels. It is suggested that pasture containing less than 80 mg/kg of manganese is incapable of supporting normal bovine fertility, and that herbage containing less than 50 mg/kg is often associated with infertility and anestrus. The Agricultural Research Council believes that although definite figures are not available, levels of 40 mg/kg DM in the diet should be adequate. Other authors state that rations containing less than 20 mg/kg DM may cause anestrus and reduction in conception rates in cows and the production of poor-quality semen by bulls. Most pasture contains 50 to 100 mg/kg DM. Skeletal deformities in calves occur when the deficiency is much greater that just noted; for example, a diet containing more than 200 mg/kg DM is considered to be sufficient to prevent them.

Rations fed to pigs usually contain more than 20 mg/kg DM of manganese, and deficiency is unlikely unless there is interference with manganese metabolism by other substances.

There are important variations in the manganese content of seeds, an important matter in poultry nutrition. Maize and barley have the lowest content. Wheat or oats have 3 to 5 times as much, and bran and pollard are the richest natural sources, with 10 to 20 times the content of maize or wheat. Cows' milk is exceptionally low in manganese.

Diets high in iron reduce duodenal activity of manganese transporters in calves, although the clinical importance of this finding is unclear.[4]

PATHOGENESIS

Manganese plays an active role in bone-matrix formation and in the synthesis of chondroitin sulfate, which is responsible for maintaining the rigidity of connective tissue. In manganese deficiency, these are affected deleteriously, and skeletal abnormalities result. Only 1% of manganese is absorbed from the diet, and the liver removes most of it, leaving very low blood levels of the element.

CLINICAL FINDINGS

In cattle, the common syndromes in confirmed or suspected manganese deficiency are infertility, stillbirth, perinatal loss, calves with congenital limb deformities, and calves that manifest poor growth, dry coat, and loss of coat color.[2,3] The deformities include knuckling over at the fetlocks, enlarged joints, and, possibly, twisting of the legs. The bones of affected lambs are shorter and weaker than normal, and there are signs of joint pain, hopping gait, and reluctance to move.

Heifers fed a low-manganese diet (16 mg Mn per kg DM of diet) during pregnancy had impaired fetal growth and development evident as lower birth weight than calves from heifers fed 50 mg of Mn per kg DM, superior brachygnathism, unsteadiness, disproportionate dwarfism, and swollen joints.[5] A severe congenital chondrodystrophy in Charolais calves occurred on one farm. The limbs were shortened and the joints enlarged. The pregnant cows were fed on apple pulp and corn silage, both of which were low in manganese.

An outbreak of congenital skeletal malformations in Holstein calves was characterized clinically by small birth weights (average 15 kg). Abnormalities included joint laxity, doming of the foreheads, superior brachygnathia, and a dwarflike appearance as a result of the short length of the long bones. The features of the head were similar to those of the wildebeest. The majority of affected calves were dyspneic at birth, and snorting and grunting respiratory sounds were common. Affected calves failed to thrive, and most were culled because of poor performance.

A manganese-responsive infertility has been described in ewes and is well known in cattle. In cattle, it is manifested by slowness to exhibit estrus and failure to conceive, often accompanied by subnormal size of one or both ovaries. Subestrus and weak estrus have also been observed.

Functional infertility was once thought to occur in cattle on diets with calcium-to-phosphorus ratios outside the range of 1:2 to 2:1. This was not upheld on investigation but might have been correct if high calcium-to-phosphorus intakes directly reduced manganese (or copper or iodine) availability in diets marginally deficient in one or other of these elements.

In pigs, experimental diets low in manganese cause reduction in skeletal growth; muscle weakness; obesity; irregular, diminished, or absent estrus; agalactia; and resorption of fetuses or the birth of stillborn pigs. Leg weakness, bowing of the front legs, and shortening of bones also occur.

CLINICAL PATHOLOGY

The blood of normal cattle contains 18 to 19 μg/dL (3.3 to 3.5 μmol/L) of Mn, although considerably lower levels are sometimes quoted. The livers of normal cattle contain 12 mg/kg (0.21 mmol/kg) of Mn and down to 8 mg/kg (0.15 mmol/kg) in newborn calves, which also have a lower content in hair. The Mn content of hair varies with intake. The normal level is about 12 mg/kg (0.21 mmol/kg), and infertility is observed in association with levels of less than 8 mg/kg (0.15 mmol/kg). In normal cows, the Mn content of hair falls during pregnancy from normal levels of 12 mg/kg (0.21 mmol/kg) in the first month of pregnancy to 4.5 mg/kg (0.08 mmol/kg) at calving. All of these figures require much more critical evaluation than they have received before they can be used as diagnostic tests.

Although tissue manganese levels in normal animals have been described as being between 2 and 4 mg/kg (0.04 and 0.07 mmol/kg), in most tissue there appears to be more variation between tissues than this. However, tissue levels of manganese do not appear to be depressed in deficient animals, except for in the ovaries, in which levels of 0.6 mg/kg (0.01 mmol/kg) and 0.85 mg/kg (0.02 mmol/kg) are recorded in contrast to a normal level of 2 mg/kg (0.04 mmol/kg).

Thus, there is no simple, single diagnostic test permitting detection of manganese deficiency in animals. Reproductive functions, male and female, are most sensitive to manganese deficiency and are affected before possible biochemical criteria (e.g., blood and bone alkaline phosphatase, and liver arginase levels) are significantly changed. The only certain way of detecting moderate deficiency states is by measuring response to supplementation. Clinical findings in response to treatment that may provide contributory evidence of manganese deficiency are set out in the following discussion.

NECROPSY FINDINGS

In congenital chondrodystrophy in calves, the limbs are shortened, and all the joints are enlarged. Histologically, there is poor cartilage maturation with excessive amounts of rarefied cartilage matrix. The major histologic abnormality in the physes is disorderly development of the zones of cartilage hypertrophy, with reduced number and irregular arrangement of hypertrophic chondrocytes; similar but less severe changes are present in the zones of cartilage proliferation.[3] There are degenerative changes in the chondrocytes and severe reduction in the mucopolysaccharide content of all body hyaline cartilage.

TREATMENT AND CONTROL

The NRC estimated the maintenance requirement (0.002 of available Mn/kg BW) of dairy cows from dietary concentrations of Mn reported to cause Mn deficiency in cattle. Based on NRC of 2001 equations, the maintenance requirement for Mn represents 82% of the total Mn requirement for a nonlactating, late-gestation cow and 53% for a cow producing 40 kg/d of milk. Fecal loss of endogenous Mn is assumed to comprise the entire maintenance requirement. Assuming typical dry matter intake (DMI), a diet with approximately 14 mg Mn/kg DM will meet the requirement for a 700-kg nonlactating cow during the last month of lactation. Recent research has determined that Mn intake had to equal 580 mg/d to meet the metabolic fecal Mn requirement. The corresponding dietary concentrations, assuming DMIs of 21 and 12 kg/d for lactating and dry cows, respectively, were 28 and 49 mg/kg DM. These concentrations are approximately 1.6 and 2.7 times higher than those needed to meet the Mn requirements for lactating and dry cows, respectively, as calculated using the 2001 NRC dairy nutrient requirements model. Supplementation of 50 mg of Mn/kg of DM to the control diet of heifers was sufficient to overcome any signs of Mn deficiency in calves; the control diet contained ~17 mg Mn per kg DM.[5]

For pigs, the recommended dietary intakes are 24 to 57 mg manganese per 45 kg BW. Expressed as a proportion of food intake, the recommended dietary level is 40 mg/kg DM in feed. The manganese requirements for gestation and lactation are 20 ppm of the diet.

Supplementation with high levels of manganese to cattle fed a copper-deficient diet can further impair copper absorption, with consequent reductions in the growth and health of cattle.[6]

REFERENCES

1. Anon. *Vet Rec.* 2013;172:389.
2. Cave JG, et al. *Aust Vet J.* 2008;86:130.
3. McLaren PJ, et al. *Vet Pathol.* 2007;44:342.
4. Hansen SL, et al. *J Dairy Sci.* 2010;93:656.
5. Hansen SL, et al. *J Dairy Sci.* 2006;89:4305.
6. Hansen SL, et al. *Brit J Nutr.* 2009;101:1068.

BIOTIN (VITAMIN H) DEFICIENCY (HYPOBIOTINOSIS)

Biotin, or vitamin H, has several important biochemical functions. It is a cofactor in several enzyme systems involved in carboxylation and transcarboxylation reactions and consequently has a significant effect on carbohydrate metabolism, fatty acid synthesis, amino acid deamination, purine synthesis, and nucleic acid metabolism. Biotin is found in almost all plant and animal materials and, being required in very small quantities, is unlikely to be deficient in diets under natural conditions, especially because microbial synthesis occurs in the alimentary tract.

Cattle

Biotin is now considered a significant factor in lameness of cattle.[1-5] Biotin is important for the differentiation of epidermal cells, which are required for normal production of keratin and hoof horn tissue. Biotin also acts as a cofactor in carboxylase enzymes and is an important factor in both gluconeogenesis and fatty acid synthesis. Significant differences in the fatty acid profile of horn tissue of cattle with claw lesions have been observed. Biotin supplementation reduces clinical white-line disease, reduces horn lesions, and improves horn quality by strengthening the intercellular cementing material between keratinocytes. Improved hoof integrity in intensively managed dairy cows has occurred following biotin supplementation. However, a long period of supplementation is required before the effect of the vitamin on hoof health care is expressed. In addition, there can be improved milk production, milk composition, and cow fertility with biotin supplementation, although this finding is not consistent across studies.[6]

Biotin is synthesized in the rumen, and absolute biotin deficiency has not been recognized. However, ruminal synthesis of biotin may be compromised by acidic conditions in the rumen, which may increase the need for supplementation of biotin in the diet of high-producing dairy cows. In the dairy cow in the periparturient period and early lactation, the levels of biotin may decrease. A decrease in plasma biotin levels of dairy cows at 25 days in milk (DIM) has been noted, returning to constant levels from 100 DIM until the end of lactation. Feeding supplemental biotin at 20 g/d during the last 16 days postpartum and at 30 g/d from calving through to 70 days postpartum elevated concentrations of plasma and milk compared with cows unsupplemented with biotin. Supplemental biotin also elevated plasma glucose and lowered nonesterified fatty acids, which indicates that supplemental biotin is involved in hepatic gluconeogenesis. The triacylglycerol concentration in liver tended to decrease at a faster rate within 2 days after parturition.

Supplementation of young, extensively managed cattle with 12.5 mg of diluted powdered biotin, or a control treatment, for 40 consecutive days revealed an effect of biotin to increase average hoof growth of 11.3 +/− 0.72 mm in supplemented cattle versus 7.2 +/− 0.78 mm over the 40 days.[2] There was a positive effect of biotin supplementation on the growth of the angle and length of the dorsal hoof wall and the hoof sole length, and on resistance to wearing, in young, extensively managed cattle.[2] The supplementation of Holstein cows in the Atherton Tablelands in Australia with biotin at 20 mg/head per day resulted in improved locomotion scores compared with unsupplemented cows. In the wet summer period, the number of lame cows observed by the farmer was significantly fewer during the rainy period for the biotin-supplemented herds, and animals in the herd required fewer antibiotic treatments than unsupplemented herds. Most hoof lesions were most commonly observed in the outer claws of the hindlimb.

In a randomized control field trial on five commercial dairy farms in Gloucestershire, southwest United Kingdom, the effect of parity and duration of supplementation with oral biotin at 20 mg/d on white-line disease was studied over a period of 18 months. The incidence of white-line disease increased with increasing parity independent of biotin supplementation from 2 cases per 100 cow-years in primiparous cows to 15.5 cases per 100 cow-years in all multiparous cows, but up to 47.7 cases per 100 cow-years for cows in parities = 5. Supplementation with biotin reduced white-line disease lameness by 45% in multiparous cows down to 8.5 cases per 100 cow-years, whereas the effect of biotin supplementation in primiparous cows was not significant. A supplementation of length of at least 6 months was required to reduce the risk of white-line lameness in multiparous cows. The overall incidence rate of lameness (per 100 cows per year) was 68.9, with a range of 31.6 to 111.5 per farm. The incidence rates of the four most frequently reported causes of lameness were sole ulcer, 13.8; white-line separation, 12.7; digital dermatitis, 12.0; and interdigital necrobacillosis, 7.1 per 100 cows per year. The incidence of lameness was highly variable between farms. However, when the data from all farms were pooled, the risk of lameness caused by white-line separation in cattle supplemented with biotin was approximately 50%. Approximately 130 days of biotin supplementation is required before a significant difference in white-line lesion lameness occurs.

A controlled 14-month field trial evaluated the effect of biotin supplementation on hoof lesions, milk production, and reproductive performance of dairy cows housed in the same free-stall facility with the same environment, base diet, and management. Supplemented cows received 20 mg/d by computer feeder. The feet of a select number of cows were trimmed three times at 6-month intervals, and hoof health was evaluated. At the final hoof trimming, the incidence of sole hemorrhages was significantly higher in the control group (50%) compared with the supplemented group (24%). No cases of lameness occurred. Milk production and fat yield increased in all parities, and fertility was improved in first-calf heifers.

It is possible that biotin improves the quality of claw horn, which encourages the replacement of defective horn, improves healing, and makes it less likely for sole lesions to develop from laminitis in its early stages. The administration of biotin at 40 mg per day for 50 days to dairy cows with uncomplicated sole ulcers resulted in significant improvement in histologic horn quality of the newly formed epidermis covering the sole ulcer. Biotin supplementation at 20 mg/d did not affect the tensile strength of the white line.

Vertical fissures, or sand cracks, are vertical cracks of the hoof that may extend across the coronary band and continue to the bearing surface of the dorsal wall of the claw. Sand cracks are common in beef cattle in western Canada. One survey, 37.5% of beef cows were affected with one or more cracks. Supplementary dietary biotin at 10 mg/head per day significantly increased serum levels of biotin and increased claw hardness compared with unsupplemented cows. After 18 months, 15% of the biotin-supplemented cows had vertical fissures compared with 35% in the unsupplemented cows.

Sheep

There is evidence from a small number of studies that biotin supplementation of the diets of sheep improves hoof health.[7]

Pigs

The principal source of biotin for the pig is the feed it receives, and feeds vary greatly in their biotin content and in the biological availability of that biotin. Diets based on cereals with a low available biotin content may provide insufficient dietary biotin for the maintenance of hoof horn integrity in pigs. The biotin content in basal diets fed to pigs has varied from 29 to 15 μg/kg available biotin, and supplementation of these diets has resulted in improvements in litter size. Continuous feeding of sulfonamides or antibiotics may induce a deficiency. An antivitamin to biotin (avidin) occurs in egg white, and biotin deficiency can be produced experimentally by feeding large quantities of uncooked egg white.

In pigs, experimental biotin deficiency is manifested by alopecia, dermatitis, and painful cracking of the soles and the walls of the hooves.

Naturally occurring outbreaks of lameness in gilts and sows associated with lesions of the soles and the walls of the hooves, which responded to biotin supplementation, have now been well described. The severe lameness and long course of convalescence have been responsible for a high rate of culling in breeding animals. In gilts fed a basal diet with a low level of biotin (32 μg available biotin/kg) from 25 kg live weight to 170 days of age, there were no significant differences in the number of lesions and claws affected compared with gilts fed a biotin-supplemented diet (350 μg available biotin/kg). However, between 170 days of age and the first weaning, the incidence of hoof lesions increased markedly. Over the next four litters, the incidence of lesions increased with the age of the sow. The predominant lesions in the foot were cracks, which occurred mainly in two associated regions: the heel/toe junction and the heel and the sidewall and adjacent white-line region of the toe. Supplementation of the diet of breeding sows with biotin at an early stage of development makes a significant contribution to the maintenance of horn integrity.[8]

Affected animals become progressively lame after being on a biotin-deficient ration for several months. Arching of the back and a haunched stance with the hindlegs positioned forward occurs initially. This posture has been described as a "kangaroo-sitting" posture. The foot pads become softer and the hoof horn less resilient. The feet are painful, and some sows will not stand for breeding. Deep fissures at the wall–sole junction may extend upward beneath the wall horn, and gaping cracks may separate the toe and heel volar surfaces. The foot pads initially show excessive wear; later, longitudinal painful cracks develop. In well-developed cases, the foot pads appear enlarged, and the cracks are obvious and covered by necrotic debris. The foot pads of the hindfeet are usually more severely affected than those of the forefeet, and the lateral digit is more frequently affected. The dewclaws also are affected by cracks and the accumulation of necrotic tissue.

Skin lesions also develop in affected gilts and sows. There is gradual alopecia, particularly over the back, the base of the tail, and the hindquarters. The hairs are more bristly than normal and break easily. The alopecia is accompanied by a dryness of the skin.

As the lesions of the feet and skin develop there is a marked drop in the serum biotin concentrations, which is considered as a sensitive index of biotin deficiency. Adequate biotin status may be indicated by serum biotin levels (ng/L) greater than 700; marginal, 600 to 700; inadequate, 400 to 600; and deficient, below 400. Compression and hardness tests made on external hoof have also been used as an indirect measure of biotin adequacy in pigs. The tests indicate that significant improvements in the strength and hardness of pig hoof horn are produced by biotin. Supplementation of the diet with biotin does not affect either horn growth or wear rates. Biotin supplementation does affect the structure of the coronary epidermis; there is an increase in the density of the horn tubules in the stratum medium, the horny squames in the stratum medium are more tightly packed, and the tubules are more clearly defined.

Reproductive performance of sows is also influenced by their biotin status. Supplementation of the diet with biotin may increase litter size, increase the number of pigs weaned, decrease the mean interval in days from weaning to service, and improve conception rate. Over a period of four parities, piglet production increased by 1.42 pigs/sow year.

Biotin Requirements

Pigs

The daily requirements of biotin for pigs have not been well defined, but certain amounts have been associated with an absence of lameness and improved reproductive performance. Basic diets for gilts contain 35 to 50 μg/kg, and the addition of 350 to 500 μg/kg is recommended. This provides a daily intake of 4.0 to 5.0 mg/sow per day. The response to dietary supplementation may take several months; therefore, supplementation should begin at weaning. The details of biotin studies in pigs, including experimental deficiency, the absorption and synthesis of biotin, biotin availability in feedstuffs, and the biotin requirements of the growing pig, are available.

Supplementation of a basal diet, calculated to contain 56 μg/kg available biotin with daily allowances of biotin at 1160 μg/sow per day in pregnancy and 2320 μg/sow per day in lactation, produced significant improvements in litter size in second- and fourth-parity sows. It is suggested that the requirement is in excess of 175 μg available biotin per 1 kg of diet. In a swine herd with a lameness problem, the supplementation of the sow's ration during pregnancy and lactation with daily intakes of biotin of 400 and 800 μg/sow per day, respectively, and the rations of the weaners and growers to 150 and 250 was effective.

Horses

The dietary supplementation of horses with 10 to 30 mg biotin/d for 6 to 9 months is considered to be effective as an aid in the treatment of weak horn hoof in horses. The hoof horn quality of more than two-thirds of the Lippizaner horses had moderate to severe changes: microcracks visible in the transition from the middle to the inner zone of the coronary horn; separation of the sole from the coronary horn in the region within the white zone. Biotin supplementation for 19 months improved horn quality. Continuous dietary supplementation with biotin at a daily dose of 20 mg is necessary to improve and maintain hoof horn quality in horses with less-than-optimum-quality hooves.

REFERENCES

1. Barker ZE, et al. *Animal Welfare*. 2012;21:563.
2. Franco da Silva LA, et al. *Can Vet J*. 2010;51:607.
3. Lean IJ, et al. *Livestock Sci*. 2013;156:71.
4. Osorio JS, et al. *J Dairy Sci*. 2012;95:6388.
5. Randhawa SS, et al. *Vet Res Comm*. 2008;32:599.
6. Ferreira G, et al. *J Dairy Sci*. 2007;90:1452.
7. Bampidis VA, et al. *Anim Feed Sci Tech*. 2007;134:162.
8. van Riet MMJ, et al. *Livestock Sci*. 2013;156:24.

Toxic Agents Affecting the Musculoskeletal System

HYENA DISEASE OF CATTLE

Hyena disease of cattle occurs worldwide and is characterized clinically by a lateral body appearance similar to the hyena. The cause is unknown for some cases, but sustained excessive intake of vitamin A and vitamin D_3 in young calves appears to be the most likely cause of hyena disease by suppressing differentiation and proliferation in chondrocytes and osteoblasts. This effect is clinically detectable because of **premature closure of the physis of long bones**. A small number of cases may be a result of systemic viral disease of young calves.

In some naturally occurring cases in yearlings from one large dairy herd, approximately 1% of calves were affected annually. Affected calves had received vitamins A and D_3 immediately after birth, and from birth to weaning they received the same vitamins from fresh milk, whole corn, a customized feed mix, and a milk supplement. The mean daily intake of vitamin A from birth to 6 weeks of age was approximately 80,000 IU and 6,300 IU of vitamin D_3, and progressively less vitamin A and D_3 was fed from 6 weeks until weaning at 3 months. The NRC recommendations for daily vitamin intake are 2100 IU of vitamin A at birth, increasing to 6360 IU at 2 months, and 330 IU of D_3, increasing to 990 IU over the same period. Experimentally, the IM injection of vitamins A and D (2,000,000 IU and 300,000 IU, respectively) on the first day after birth followed by 30,000 IU/kg BW added to the milk replacer daily resulted in gross lesions in the proximal tibial growth plates in 3 weeks. Excessive amounts of vitamin D_3 appear to promote the primary effect of vitamin A on premature closure of the physis. For example, daily administration of vitamin A (30,000 IU/kg BW) in milk replacer fed to lambs resulted in premature closure of the distal growth plate in the femur and proximal growth plate in the tibia, but clinical signs of hyena disease were not detected.[1]

The premature closure of the growth plates of the long bones results in a marked dissimilarity in growth and development between the forequarters and the hindquarters, the latter being comparatively underdeveloped. This gives the animal the classic contours of the hyena, and this resemblance is heightened by a crest of thick, stiff bristles along the back in the midline. An aggressive attitude also develops. Affected calves are normal at birth and only develop the abnormality at 5 to 6 months of age. The femur and tibia are shorter in affected than in normal animals. There are accompanying difficulties of locomotion, with a tendency to fall sideways, and to frequently adopt a position of lateral recumbency. The gait is described as "bunny-hopping."

German Simmental, Charolais, Black Pied, German Holstein–Friesian, and German Red Pied cattle have been involved. Genetic analysis appears to indicate that the disease is inherited as a simple recessive trait with incomplete penetrance, but this is obviously not so in some herds.

The lesion is a chondrodystrophy affecting particularly the long bones and the lumbar vertebrae. Gross examination and radiography of the longitudinal slabs of the humeri, tibias, and femurs reveal focal to almost complete closure of the physes, with physes subjected to compression being more severely affected more than those subjected to tension.

FURTHER READING

Espinasse J, Parodi AL, Constantin A, Viso M, Laval A. Hyena disease in cattle: a review. *Vet Rec.* 1986;118:328-330.

Rothenberg AB, Berdon WE, Woodard JC, Cowles RA. Hypervitaminosis A-induced premature closure of the epiphyses (physeal obliteration) in humans and calves (hyena disease): a historical review of the human and veterinary literature. *Pediatr Radiol.* 2007;37:1264.

REFERENCE

1. Azimpour S, Mortazavi P. *Comp Clin Pathol.* 2013;22:941.

CALCINOGENIC GLYCOSIDE POISONING (ENZOOTIC CALCINOSIS)

SYNOPSIS

Etiology Ingestion of calcinogenic glycosides in a few specific poisonous plants.

Epidemiology Enzootic disease in all species in regions where toxic plants occur.

Clinical pathology Elevated blood calcium and phosphorus concentration; tissue calcification visible on x-ray.

Lesions Calcification of all tissues; degenerative arthritis in all limb joints.

Diagnostic confirmation Identification of specific plant.

Treatment None.

Control Remove and keep animals away from toxic plants.

ETIOLOGY

Calcinogenic glycosides occur in very small quantities in plant leaves. The aglycone (nonsugar) radical is a vitamin D_3 sterol, a 1,25-$(OH)_2D_3$-like compound. Hydrolysis of the glycoside releases the vitamin D_3 analog, causing the development of calcification of soft tissues, similar to hypervitaminosis D. The plants in which these glycosides have been identified are *Solanum malacoxylon* (i.e., *S. glaucophyllum, S. glaucum, S. glaucescens, S. glaucumfrutescens*), *Nierembergia veitchii*, and *Cestrum diurnum* (wild jessamine).[1]

Other plants in which the presence of calcinogenic glycosides is suspected are *Stenotaphrum secundatum* (crab grass) in Jamaica, *S. linnaeanum* (= *S. hermannii, S. sodomaeum*; apple of Sodom), *S. torvum* (devil's fig), and *Trisetum flavescens* (yellow or golden oat grass) in Europe.[1,2]

The plants are weeds of pasture and are readily eaten by livestock, especially in drought years when other forage is scarce.[2] The glycosides are very stable and resist drying and storage for periods of longer than a year. Heating reduces the toxicity of *Solanum malacoxylon* significantly but has little effect on that of *Trisetum flavescens.*

EPIDEMIOLOGY

Occurrence

Enzootic calcinosis and its causative plants occur in most countries. The disease associated with *Solanum* spp. occurs in tropical and subtropical regions, including Africa, Argentina, Brazil, Cuba, Papua New Guinea, the West Indies, and Hawaii. *Cestrum diurnum* poisoning occurs in the far southern United States, especially Florida, Texas, and California. Tentative diagnoses have been made in India and Israel. In Jamaica the disease is known as "Manchester wasting disease," in Hawaii as "naalehu," and in South America as "espichamento" or "enteque seco."

In Austria and Germany, *T. flavescens* is a common component of alpine pasture and is associated with the onset of signs about 18 months after cattle are put onto the infested pasture. Resident cattle show clinical signs at about 3 years of age. The grass is most toxic when it is young, and the clinical signs are worse when the cattle are at pasture.

Risk Factors

Animal Risk Factors

Both sexes and all ages of all animal species are affected—ruminants most commonly, horses less so. Pigs and sucking lambs are least susceptible.

PATHOGENESIS

The glycoside ingested in the plant is hydrolyzed by rumen microbes, intestinal mucosal enzymes, and bone cells to form the vitamin D_3 analog.[2] Absorption of the active substance results in a dramatic increase in the uptake of calcium from the diet. Blood levels of calcium are markedly increased, and this is followed by deposition of calcium in soft tissues. The mode of action of the glycoside is similar to that of 1,25-dihydroxycholecalciferol.

CLINICAL FINDINGS

The disease is chronic and may persist for several years. It is characterized by wasting, reluctance to walk, a stiff gait, constant shifting of the weight from foot to foot, and a disinclination to get up or to lie down.[1,2] Forced exercise is associated with severe distress; some animals may become aggressive. Affected animals stand for long periods with the back arched and the legs stiffly extended. Calcification of blood vessels may be palpable, for example, during rectal examination. Cardiac murmurs are audible. Clinical signs subside if the animals are removed from the causative feed, but resorption of calcium deposits in tissues is minimal even years after removal from the affected pastures. Animals left on the toxic pasture eventually become recumbent and die. Fetuses may be affected.

CLINICAL PATHOLOGY

Serum concentrations of calcium and phosphorus increase by 20% to 25%, with increases of up to 3.4 mmol/L of calcium and 4 mmol/L of phosphorus.[2] Tissue calcification should be detectable radiologically. Anemia is common in animals poisoned by *Solanum malacoxylon.*

NECROPSY FINDINGS

Nonspecific emaciation, anasarca, and ascites are common. Calcification of all blood vessels, including the aorta and coronary arteries, and of the endocardium, is the most readily visible, characteristic lesion. Calcification is also present in the pleura; the lung parenchyma, which is usually emphysematous; in most other viscera; and in tendons and ligaments.[3] Degenerative arthritis occurs in the limb joints.

> **DIFFERENTIAL DIAGNOSIS**
>
> The history, clinical findings, and discovery of specific toxic plants will provide diagnostic confirmation. Repeated overdosing with vitamin D, by injection or administration in compounded feeds, replicates the clinical and necropsy findings.

TREATMENT AND CONTROL

No practicable treatment is available. Careful management of affected pasture in Europe has been shown to significantly reduce the losses as a result of the disease.

FURTHER READING

Haussler MR, Wasserman RH, McCain TA, et al. 1, 25-dihydroxyvitamin D3-glycoside: identification of a calcinogenic principle of *Solanium malocoxylon. Life Sci.* 1976;15:1049-1056.

Hughes MR, McCain TA, Chang SY, et al. Presence of 1, 25-dihydroxyvitamin D3-glycoside in the calcinogenic plant *Cestrum diurnum. Nature.* 1977;268:347-349.

Mello JRB. Calcinosis—calcinogenic plants. *Toxicon.* 2003;41(1):1-12.

REFERENCES

1. Y Santos C, Capelli A, Sosa S, et al. Enzootic calcinosis of sheep in Uruguay. In: Riet-Correa, Pfister J, Schild AL, Wierenga TL, eds. *Poisoning by Plants, Mycotoxins, and Other Toxins.* Oxfordshire: CAB International; 2011:448.
2. Santos C, et al. *J Vet Diag Invest.* 2012;24:423.
3. Barros SS, et al. *Vet Path.* 2006;43:494.

HYPOGLYCIN A INTOXICATION OF HORSES (ATYPICAL MYOPATHY [MYOGLOBINURIA] IN GRAZING HORSES)

Hypoglycin A intoxication of horses is a syndrome of acute myoglobinuria occurring in horses at pasture in Great Britain, Ireland, Europe, North America, and, possibly, Australia and New Zealand.[1-6] The disease is caused by ingestion of seeds of the maple trees *Acer negundo* (box elder) in the United States and *Acer pseudoplantanus* in Europe.[6-8] The toxic compound is hypoglycin A (L-a-amino-methylenecyclopropylpropionic acid), which is metabolized to methylenecyclopropylacetic acid (MCPA). MCPA can be detected in the blood of affected horses[9] and is a potent inhibitor of multiple acyl-CoA dehydrogenases causing a specific abnormal pattern of accumulation of blood acylcarnitines and urine organic acids.[7] This pattern was recognized in affected horses before the causative agent was identified.[5]

The potential of other maple trees (*Acer palmatum* [Japanese maple], *A. saccharum* [sugar maple], *A. spicatum* [mountain maple], and possibly others) to cause this disease is unknown, although these species contain, or likely contain, hypoglycin A.[10]

The disease has a strong seasonal distribution, with most, but not all, cases occurring in autumn.[1,4,11,12] Occurrence of the disease is sporadic but usually affects more than one animal in a band of equids. Horses, ponies, and zebras have been affected.[11] Localized outbreaks involving large numbers of horses are reported.[11] Risk of the disease in Europe increases with increasing time at pasture, presence of wood or dead leaves in the pasture, lack of supplemental feeding, and presence of trees.[11,12] Wind speed and speed of wind gusts is greater immediately preceding outbreaks of the disease than at other times.[7]

There does not appear to be a breed or sex predilection to development of the disease. Younger horses might be at greater risk of the disease, but this could simply reflect the age distribution of horses at pasture in areas in which the disease occurs. Atypical myopathy occurs almost exclusively in horses at pasture and is not associated with enforced exercise.

The case-fatality rate is usually 60% to 70% but can be much higher.[11] Prognosis is directly related to the severity of clinical signs, such as tachycardia, tachypnea, recumbency, sweating, anorexia, and dyspnea.[13]

Clinical signs are those characteristic of acute rhabdomyolysis and include an abrupt onset of stiffness and reluctance to move. Affected horses might be noticed to be depressed or have reduced activity for 1 to 2 days before onset of clinical signs.[11] Horses can be affected up to 4 days after being removed from pasture.[11] Progression to lateral recumbency is rapid, occurring within hours of the initial onset of signs. Recumbency is often the first indication of this disease observed in horses at pasture. Horses forced to stand have tremors and difficulty walking. Lumbar and gluteal muscles can be firm. Affected horses are tachycardic and tachypneic. Respiratory distress, presumably secondary to degeneration of intercostal muscle and the diaphragm, is common in recumbent horses in the terminal stages of the disease. There is discolored urine (pigmenturia). There are abnormal ventricular arrhythmias and impaired myocardial function, which can persist for at least 10 weeks in affected horses.[14] Affected horses usually die or are euthanized within 24 to 72 hours of onset of clinical signs.[11]

Serum biochemical abnormalities include massively increased serum activities of creatine kinase, lactate dehydrogenase, and aspartate aminotransferase. Serum concentrations of troponin T, a marker of myocardial damage, are above normal in most affected horses. Serum concentrations of vitamin E and/or selenium and red cell activity of glutathione peroxidase are not consistently abnormally low. Serum concentrations of acylcarnitines are abnormal, with elevations of concentrations of short-, medium-, and long-chain compounds.[6,7] Urine concentrations of ethylmalonic acid, methylsuccinic acid, lactic acid, adipic acid, butyrlglycine, isovalerylglycine, and hexanoglycine are increased in affected horses.[7]

The acid–base status of affected horses is a mixture of respiratory alkalosis, lactic acidosis, and strong iron difference (SIDm) alkalosis.[15] Abnormalities in serum sodium, potassium, and chloride concentrations are usually small.[15]

Necropsy examination does not reliably reveal gross evidence of muscle disease, although there can be swelling, edema, and localized hemorrhage into muscles. There are hemorrhagic or pale areas in the ventricular myocardium of some horses. Histologic examination reveals the presence of widespread degeneration of myocytes, without inflammation, in muscles of locomotion and respiration. Within a muscle group, some fibers are severely affected, whereas other neighboring fibers are apparently normal. The ventricular myocardium has lesions of muscle degeneration in some horses. Myoglobinuric nephrosis is a consistent finding in horses that die spontaneously or are euthanized in the terminal stages of the disease.

Definitive diagnosis is based on the presence of clinical signs of muscle disease, large elevations in serum activity of muscle-derived enzymes, and necropsy examination.

Treatment is supportive because there is no definitive antidote for hypoglycin A.[16,17] Affected and at-risk horses should be removed from the pasture and prevented from eating more seeds of *A. negundo* or *A. pseudoplantanus.* Consideration should be given to administering activated charcoal to reduce absorption of further toxin from the gastrointestinal tract (500 g per 500-kg horse, orally). Some affected horses are in pain and should be administered analgesics. Hydration and electrolyte and acid: base balance should be maintained.

Administration of antioxidants and muscle relaxants is recommended but is without objective evidence of efficacy.[16,17]

Control centers around preventing horses and ponies from eating the seeds (samaras) of *Acer negundo* or *A. pseudoplantanus*. The seeds can be blown into pastures from trees bordering the pasture—consistent with wind speeds being higher immediately preceding outbreaks than at times when the disease did not occur.[7]

REFERENCES

1. Hollyer J, et al. *Irish Vet J*. 2010;63:612.
2. McKenzie RK, et al. *NZ Vet J*. 2013;61:367.
3. Quist EM, et al. *Vet Pathol*. 2011;48:E52.
4. Sponseller BT, et al. *J Vet Int Med*. 2012;26:1012.
5. van der Kolk JH, et al. *Mol Gen Metab*. 2010;101:289.
6. Votion DM, et al. *Equine Vet J*. 2013;n/a.
7. Valberg SJ, et al. *Equine Vet J*. 2013;45:419.
8. Unger L, et al. *J Vet Int Med*. 2014;28:1289.
9. Votion DM, et al. *Equine Vet J*. 2014;46:146.
10. Gillman JH, et al. *Equine Vet J*. 2014;46:135.
11. van Galen G, et al. *Equine Vet J*. 2012;44:614.
12. van Galen G, et al. *J Vet Emerg Crit Care*. 2010;20:528.
13. van Galen G, et al. *Equine Vet J*. 2012;44:621.
14. Verheyen T, et al. *J Vet Int Med*. 2012;26:1019.
15. van Galen G, et al. *J Vet Int Med*. 2013;27:186.
16. van Galen G, et al. *Equine Vet Educ*. 2013;25:264.
17. van Galen G, et al. *Equine Vet Educ*. 2013;25:308.

PLANT POISONINGS WITH KNOWN TOXINS

AMINOPROPIONITRILE

3-Aminopropionitrile is a poisonous substance found in *Lathyrus* spp. (wild peas), for example, *Lathyrus hirsutus* (wild winter pea), sometimes sown with grasses to provide early-spring grazing. Signs of toxicity in cattle grazing mature plants bearing seed pods consist of salivation, sawhorse stance, head held low, continuous head and ear movements, trance-like gaze, diminished responsiveness, reluctance to move, pain in the feet causing lameness, sitting with the feet under the body, and a marked disinclination to rise. Other signs include lameness, stumbling gait, recumbency, and paddling convulsions. The signs are exacerbated by driving or other stimulation. Necropsy findings are limited to nonspecific lesions such as pulmonary congestion.

PLANT POISONINGS WITH SUSPECTED OR UNIDENTIFIED TOXINS

JUGLONE

Juglone, a poisonous resinoid found in the shavings of *Juglans nigra* (black walnut tree), has been suspected as being associated with lameness and edema of the lower limbs in horses bedded on the shavings, but juglone is present in the bark and leaves, not the heartwood from which the shavings are made. The lesions are produced by an increase in local capillary blood pressure.

A similar syndrome is associated with *Berteroa incana* (hoary alyssum). Swelling of the distal limbs and fever are consistent signs associated with ingestion of this plant. Signs appear 18 to 36 hours after ingestion of the plant and disappear 2 to 4 days after the plant is removed. Abortions have been reported but may be secondary to the high fever. An alternative syndrome of severe gastroenteritis plus intravascular hemolysis is also recorded in horses fed hay contaminated by *Berteroa incana*.

MYOPATHY—WITH GAIT INCOORDINATION, RECUMBENCY, ELEVATED CPK

- *Karwinskia humboldtiana*—coyotillo
- Small amounts of *Senna* (= *Cassia*) spp. ingested over a long period are associated with skeletal muscle myopathy and/or paralysis. In *Senna occidentalis* poisoning in horses and goats, the early signs are anorexia and diarrhea followed by hyperpnea, tachycardia, ataxia, staggering, and recumbency. At autopsy there is a fatal cardiomyopathy. The muscle lesion is accompanied by marked elevations of SGOT and CPK levels. Similarly, in pigs, early diarrhea may be followed by lateral recumbency and skeletal muscle myopathy.

FURTHER READING

Radostits O, et al. *Veterinary Medicine: A Textbook of the Disease of Cattle, Horses, Sheep, Goats and Pigs*. 10th ed. London: W.B. Saunders; 2007:1883.

ALUMINUM TOXICOSIS

Aluminum is one of the potentially toxic elements introduced into the diets of animals by the deposition of soluble salts in acid rain, powder particles in factory effluent, accidental dosing, or absorption by plants.

Case reports in large animals are rare, and most of the toxicologic information comes from human data or investigational studies using rats, mice, and rabbits. Frank et al. reported polioencephalomalacia associated with elevated aluminum levels in Simmental calves,[1] and Easterwood et al. reported phosphine gas generation in horses accidentally receiving aluminum phosphide in their feed.[2] It should be pointed out that the toxin associated with aluminum phosphide intoxication is the toxic gas phosphine and not aluminum.

Absorption of aluminum is poor following oral, dermal, and inhalation exposure. Following absorption, it is distributed to other tissues, with the highest concentration in the bone.[3] Chronic exposure to aluminum results in sequestration in the bone, from which it is slowly released. Aluminum readily crosses the blood–brain barrier and placental barrier, resulting in neurotoxicity and developmental toxicity.[4,5] Excretion is through the urine, with very little bile and fecal excretion.[3]

Clinical signs depend on specific organs, but deposition in the bone is associated with osteoarthritis and anemia. Other organs affected include the heart (myocardial infarction), brain (cognitive dysfunction and other neurotoxic effects), liver, and kidney.

There is no treatment, and diagnosis depends on finding aluminum in the liver and kidney. Aluminum levels of 6 to 11 ppm in the liver and 4 to 5 ppm in the kidney of sheep and cattle are considered toxic amounts.

FURTHER READING

Allen VG, Robinson DL, Hembry FG. Aluminum in the etiology of grass tetany in cattle. *J Anim Sci*. 1980;50:44.

Allen VG. Influence of dietary aluminum on nutrient utilization in ruminants. *J Anim Sci*. 1984;59:836-844.

Frank AA, Hedstrom OR, Braselton WE, et al. Multifocal polioencephalomyelomalacia in Simmental calves with elevated tissue aluminum and decreased tissue copper and manganese. *J Vet Diagn Invest*. 1992;4:353-355.

REFERENCES

1. Frank AA, et al. *J Vet Diagn Invest*. 1992;4:353-355.
2. Easterwood L. *J Am Vet Med Assoc*. 2010;236:446.
3. Krewski D, et al. *J Toxicol Environ Health B*. 2007;10:1.
4. Domingo JL, Aluminum, Gupta RC, eds. *Reproductive and Developmental Toxicology*. Elsevier; 2011:407.
5. Kumar V, Gill KD. *Arch Toxicol*. 2009;83:965.

FLUORIDE TOXICOSIS

SYNOPSIS

Etiology Toxic amounts of fluoride are found in water (naturally or contaminated), soil, and plants contaminated by industry pollution, mineral mixes with excessive fluoride, and older insecticides, anthelmintics, and rodenticides containing sodium fluoride, sodium fluorosilicate, and sodium fluoroacetate. Fluoroacetate may also be found in several plant species, such as *Dichapentalum* spp., *Gastrolobium* spp. *Oxylobium* spp., and others.

Epidemiology Most often associated with continuous ingestion of small but toxic amounts of fluoride in the diet or drinking water.

Clinical pathology Elevated serum and urine levels of fluoride; elevated serum levels of Ca, BUN, and ALP in some cases.

Lesions

Live animals: Dental fluorosis—mottling and erosion of permanent teeth. Osteofluorosis with lameness and unthriftiness.

Postmortem: Osteoporosis; widespread exostoses. Dental enamel and dentin hypoplasia.

Diagnostic confirmation Fluoride assay of forage, soil, or water; blood and urine of affected animals; bones and teeth at necropsy.

Treatment Primarily supportive; activated charcoal is not recommended; oral calcium, magnesium, or aluminum to bind fluoride in gastrointestinal tract.

Control Good nutritional plane; keep young animals off and rotate stock if water or forage contaminated; keep fluoride in feed less than 2%; use of aluminum salts in feed of questionable efficacy.

ETIOLOGY

Fluoride is present in some concentration in almost all animal feed and water sources, so exposure not only occurs but continues throughout the lifetime. Both acute and chronic poisoning occur. Acute toxicosis in large animals is very rare and generally occurs after exposure to an older commercial product, such as sodium fluoride, sodium fluorosilicate, or sodium fluoroacetate, or to volcanic ash.[1,2] Chronic toxicosis is associated with the ingestion of high-fluoride-containing rock salt phosphate supplements, fluoride-contaminated forage or soil, and water either naturally containing excess fluoride or that has been contaminated with fluoride.[3-6] The severity of the poisoning depends on the amount ingested, the solubility of the fluoride compound, the species, diet, and the animal's age.[1,7] Death losses are rare and restricted largely to acute poisoning, with the major losses taking the form of unthriftiness associated with chronic fluorosis.

EPIDEMIOLOGY

Occurrence

Fluoride intoxication has been observed in most countries, usually in association with specific natural or industrial hazards. In Europe and Great Britain, losses are greatest on summer grazing of pastures contaminated by industrial fumes, including dust from factories converting rock phosphate to superphosphate and effluent from aluminum smelters. Iceland and parts of the southern Andes Mountains are extensively affected by contamination from volcanic ash. Drinking water from deep wells, industrial contamination of pasture, and the feeding of fluoride-bearing phosphatic supplements are the common associations in North America. Deep wells also are an important source in Australia and South America. In Africa the important association is the feeding of phosphatic rock supplements.

In experimentally induced fluorosis in cattle, mottling of the tooth enamel occurs at intakes of 27 mg/kg in the diet, but there is no pitting until levels of 49 mg/kg are fed. Bony lesions are slight at intakes of 27 mg/kg, moderate at 49 mg/kg, and marked at 93 mg/kg, and milk production in dairy cows is thought not to be affected by intakes of 50 mg/kg of fluoride in the diet until about the fourth lactation. A more recent view is that the existing tolerance level for dairy cows of 40 mg/kg is too high and will lead to serious loss of production and some dental fluorosis in high-producing cows.[1]

Risk Factors

Animal Risk Factors

Host factors are age and species. Daily intakes of 0.5 to 1.7 mg/kg BW of fluoride as sodium fluoride produce dental lesions in growing animals without affecting general well-being. Intakes equal to twice these amounts are consumed by adult animals without ill effect. In heifers a continuous intake of 1.5 mg/kg BW per day is sufficient to be associated with severe dental fluorosis without affecting growth rate or reproductive function. However, extensive osteofluorosis and periods of severe lameness will occur. The fluoride content of the bones of newborn calves depends on the dam's intake of fluoride in the last 3 to 4 months of pregnancy and not on her own bone composition.

Most recorded occurrences of fluorosis are in cattle. Sheep are less susceptible than cattle, and it is rarely reported in horses. A continuous intake of 1 mg/kg BW is the maximum safe limit for ruminants; an intake of 2 mg/kg BW produces clinical signs. In pigs an intake of 1 mg/kg BW added fluoride for long periods has no deleterious effect.

Fetal effects are small. The current view is that placental passage is infinitesimal in amount, but historically, cases of neonatal dental fluorosis have been identified in cattle.[3] Fluoride does not occur in significant quantities in the milk or colostrum of poisoned cows.[1]

Environmental Risk Factors

Fluoride occurs naturally in rocks, particularly in association with phosphate, and these rocks, the soils derived from them, and the surface water leaching through the soils may contain toxic quantities of fluoride. In such areas the soil content of fluoride may be as high as 2000 to 4000 mg/kg, even up to 12,000 mg/kg, and the levels in water up to 8.7 mg/kg; soil fluoride varies in its solubility from 10% to 20%. Levels of fluoride likely to be toxic to animals are not usually encountered in natural circumstances; interference by humans is necessary in most instances to increase fluoride ingestion above the critical level.

Contamination from industrial factories by smoke, vapor, or dust may produce pasture containing 20 to 50 mg/kg of fluoride. Factories producing aluminum by the electrolytic process, iron and steel with fluoride-containing fluxes, superphosphate, glazed bricks, copper, glass, and enamels are likely to be potent sources and may be associated with toxic levels of contamination as far as 14 km downwind from the factory. Dust from factories manufacturing superphosphate from rock phosphate may contain as much as 3.3% fluoride. Industrial plants engaged in the calcining of ironstone have also been incriminated as sources of fluoride.

Contamination by effluent is a complex problem because of variation in the form of the contaminating compound. Grass can absorb and retain gaseous fluoride from the ambient air, but physical deposit of liquids and dust is the critical form of contamination.[5,6] Two of the common effluent substances are hydrofluoric acid and silicon tetrafluoride, both of which are as toxic as sodium fluoride, and dental lesions occur in 100% of young ruminants on an intake of 14 to 16 mg/kg DM of these substances. Severe cases occur on pasture or hay containing more than 25 mg/kg DM, and similar lesions develop much more rapidly on pasture containing 98 mg/kg DMr. Fluoracetamide is also known to be a toxic factory effluent.

Dust and gases from volcanic eruptions may also be associated with acute fatal fluoride intoxication in the period immediately after the eruption, and contamination of pasture may be sufficient to be associated with subsequent chronic intoxication in animals eating the herbage, although the fluoride content of the contaminated materials decreases very rapidly if rain falls. Iceland is particularly afflicted with fluoride intoxication deriving from this source.

Top dressing of pasture with phosphatic limestone is commonly associated with fluorosis. Most phosphatic limestones, particularly those from North Africa, are rich in fluoride (0.9% to 1.4%). Nonphosphatic limestones contain insignificant amounts.

Supplementary Feeding of Phosphates

The common occurrence of phosphorus deficiency in animals has led to the search for cheap phosphatic materials suitable for animal feeding. Rock phosphates are commonly used, and many deposits contain dangerous amounts of fluoride (3% to 4%).[8] The fluoride content of the mineral can be reduced, but the cost encourages the use of marginally safe material.

The major occurrence of water-borne fluoride intoxication is from water obtained from deep wells or artesian bores. The available data suggest that although minor tooth lesions occur at 5 mg/kg of fluoride, it is not until levels of 10 mg/kg are exceeded that excessive tooth wear occurs and the nutrition of the animal is impaired. More serious systemic effects do not occur until the water contains 30 mg/kg.

Miscellaneous sources of fluoride include the ingestion of superphosphate itself, but a supernatant liquid of a suspension of the fertilizer will contain no fluoride. Some wood preservatives may contain large quantities of fluoride, which may be associated with acute poisoning in some circumstances.

Farm Risk Factors

Animals that are housed in the winter and grazed only during the summer and fall on pasture contaminated by factory effluent may show considerable clinical improvement in clinical signs during the winter and an annual recrudescence of signs when the animals are outside.[9]

Human Risk Factors

Although it is possible for animal tissues to contain amounts of fluoride in excess of permissible amounts, this is not usually so in chronic fluorosis. The fluoride content of milk in these circumstances is below that permitted in fluoridated drinking water (1 mg/L).

PATHOGENESIS

Absorption from the gastrointestinal (GI) tract depends on the form ingested, with soluble forms such as sodium fluoride being more bioavailable than fluoride found in contaminated feed, soil, or water. Once absorbed, fluoride is distributed throughout the body, primarily to bone and teeth. Excretion is renal.[10]

Acute intoxication, as a result of the ingestion of large amounts of soluble fluorides (e.g., sodium fluoride), occurs rapidly, with signs appearing 30 to 60 minutes after ingestion. The mechanism of action is unknown but may be attributable to the development of hydrofluoric acid in the GI tract, onset of systemic hypocalcemia, decreased Na/K ATPase activity, or the inhibition of glycolysis.[10]

Chronic ingestion results in the deposition of fluoride in the bones and/or teeth of affected animals.[7] Deposition in bone occurs throughout life but in teeth only in the formative stages.[1,7] In bones, fluorides alter mineralization, crystal structure, and remodeling of bone by replacing hydroxyl groups in the hydroxyapatite of the bone crystalline structure. The degree of deposition varies, being greatest on the periosteal surface of the long bones where exostoses commonly develop. These bony changes are often referred to as skeletal fluorosis or osteofluorosis.

During tooth formation, fluorides inhibit the action of ameloblasts and odontoblasts, resulting in failure of the developing tooth to accept minerals. Thus tooth lesions occur only if the intake is high before the teeth have erupted, but bone lesions occur at any stage.

When the tissue levels of fluoride are moderate, characteristic lesions as a result of hypoplasia of enamel appear in the teeth. During this time the fluoride levels in bone can increase slowly without appreciable bone changes. The facility of storage in bone explains the long latent period that occurs in animals subjected to chronic intoxication. Lesions generally begin on the medial side of the proximal metatarsal bones and expand to include the mandibles, metacarpal bones, and ribs. Abnormalities, once they occur, result in lameness and are generally symmetric and bilateral.[1] At very high levels the storage capacity of bone and teeth is exceeded, and blood and urine levels rise. The bone lesions of osteomalacia and osteoporosis, with accompanying pathologic fractures, are associated with excessive mobilization of calcium and phosphorus to compensate for their increased urinary excretion in conjunction with fluoride.

The kidney is the primary tissue affected, but other tissues in which degenerative changes may occur are the bone marrow, adrenal glands, heart muscle, and central nervous system.[2,10,11] A severe anemia may rarely occur as a result of toxic depression of bone-marrow activity, although this is not a constant or expected sign.

CLINICAL FINDINGS

Acute Intoxication

The syndrome includes dyspnea, complete anorexia, vomiting, and diarrhea in pigs and ruminal stasis with constipation or diarrhea in ruminants.[1,2] Vomiting acts as a protective mechanism, and toxic doses in pigs may be eliminated in this way without the development of other signs. Nervous signs are characteristic and include ataxia, muscle tremors and weakness, a startled expression, pupillary dilatation, hyperesthesia, and constant chewing. Tetany, convulsions, and collapse and death follow within a few hours.

Chronic Intoxication

Because of the distinct clinical separation between animals with dental lesions and those that have, in addition, signs of lameness and general ill-health, it is customary to refer to two forms of the disease: dental fluorosis and osteofluorosis. Lesions of the teeth and bones are characteristic, and the signs are largely referable to these lesions. Tooth changes are the earliest and most diagnostic sign but may not produce clinical effects until other signs have developed.[12] Consequently, they are often missed until other clinical findings suggest that the teeth be examined.

Dental Fluorosis

The permanent teeth exposed to intoxication before eruption will be affected and perhaps those of animals exposed in utero. The earliest and mildest sign is mottling with the appearance of pigmented (very light yellow, green, brown, or black) spots or bands arranged horizontally across the teeth. Occasional vertical bands may be seen where pigment is deposited along enamel fissures. Mottling and staining occur on incisors and cheek teeth and are not evident when the affected tooth erupts, and in fact they may not appear until some months later. The cheek teeth are usually more dramatically affected than the incisors but are very difficult to examine clinically. If the period of exposure to intoxication has been limited only some of the teeth may be affected, but the defects will always be bilateral.

Mottling may not progress any further, but if the intoxication has been sufficiently severe, defective calcification of the enamel leads to accelerated attrition or erosion of the teeth, usually in the same teeth as the mottling. The mottled areas become pits, and the teeth are brittle and break and wear easily and unevenly. Patterns of accelerated attrition are dependent on the chronologic occurrence of the intoxication and the eruption time of the teeth. Uneven and rapid wear of the cheek teeth makes proper mastication impossible. Infection of the dental alveoli and shedding of teeth commonly follow. The painful condition of the teeth and inability to prehend and masticate seriously reduce the food intake and are associated with poor growth in the young and unthriftiness and acetonemia in adults. Affected cattle may lap cold drinking water to avoid the discomfort occasioned by normal drinking. Eruption of the teeth may be abnormal, resulting in irregular alignment.

A standard for the classification of fluorosis has been proposed based on the degree of mottling, pitting, and rate of wear of the teeth. The effects of dental mottling, pitting, and excessive wear of incisors can be used to estimate the exposure periods of cattle during odontogenesis. The additional clinically apparent abnormalities include delayed eruption of permanent incisor teeth, necrosis of alveolar bone resulting in recession of bone and gingiva, oblique eruption of permanent teeth, hypoplasia of teeth, wide spaces between teeth, and rapid development of any dental lesions.

Osteofluorosis

Lameness most marked in the loins, hip joints, and hindlimbs and unthriftiness in animals of any age are the signs usually observed first.[11,12] The occurrence of hip lameness or fractures of the third phalanx on a herd scale in cattle is thought to be diagnostic of fluorosis. Pain is evinced on pressure over limb bones and particularly over the bulbs of the heels. The bones may be palpably and visibly enlarged. This is most readily observed in the mandible, sternum, metacarpal, and metatarsal bones and the phalanges. This overall thickness may be subsequently replaced by well-defined exostoses. The bones are subject to easy fracture. These well-defined lesions occur only in advanced cases and are often accompanied by extensive tooth lesions in young animals. In addition to the cases affected by generalized lameness, there are cases that show a sudden onset of very severe lameness, usually in a forelimb, associated with transverse fracture of the third phalanx.

Other Effects

Reproduction, milk yield, and wool growth are not usually considered to be adversely affected except indirectly by the reduced food intake. Severely lame animals may have lowered reproductive performance indirectly as a result of physical dysfunction that interferes with mating.

Additional signs, including diarrhea and anestrus and other forms of infertility in cattle, diarrhea in sheep, and polydipsia and polyuria in pigs, are recorded in the naturally occurring disease but cannot be considered as constant or pathognomonic. Horses with chronic fluorosis have lameness; dental lesions, including excessive molar abrasion; and hyperostotic lesions of the metatarsus, metacarpus, mandible, and ribs.

CLINICAL PATHOLOGY

Normal cattle have blood levels of up to 0.2 mg fluoride per mg/dL of blood and 2 to 6 mg/kg in urine. Cattle on fluoride intakes sufficient to cause intoxication may have blood levels of 0.6 mg/dL and urine levels of 16 to 68 mg/kg, although blood levels are often normal. Such high levels may not be an indication of high intakes immediately preceding the examination because heavy deposits in bones may be associated with abnormally high blood and urine fluoride levels for some months after the intake has been reduced to normal. Urine levels should be corrected to a specific gravity of 1.040. Serum calcium may be low or normal, phosphorus levels are usually normal, and there is a significant correlation between the amount of fluoride fed and the concentration of alkaline phosphatase in the serum.[2,12] The increase in phosphatase activity is probably related to the abnormal formation of bone and may be 3 to 7 times the normal level.

Radiographic changes of bones containing more than 4000 mg/kg of fluoride include increased density or abnormal porosity, periosteal feathering and thickening, increased trabeculation, thickening of the compact bone, and narrowing of the marrow cavity. Spontaneous rib fractures show incomplete union. Good data are available for fluoride concentrations in rib bones, and estimations of fluoride content in biopsy samples of ribs have been used in the clinicopathologic study of the disease. Samples of tail bone and the spongiosa of the tuber coxae have also been used for these purposes.

NECROPSY FINDINGS

Severe gastroenteritis is present in acute poisoning, and there may be degenerative changes in the renal tubular epithelium. In chronic fluorosis the bones have a chalky, white appearance; are brittle; and have either local or disseminated exostoses, particularly along the diaphyses. Intraarticular structures are not primarily affected, although there may be some spurring and bridging of the joints. Histologically, there is defective and irregular calcification of newly formed trabecular bone and active periosteal bone formation. Hypoplasia of the enamel and dentin are consistent physical and histologic defects in the teeth of affected young animals. Young animals may also develop thickened growth plates and widened metaphyses that are grossly similar to rachitic changes. Degenerative changes in kidney, liver, heart muscle, adrenal glands, and central nervous system have been reported in severe cases. Degeneration of the bone marrow and consequent aplastic anemia also occur.

Chemical examination of necropsy specimens is valuable in the diagnosis because the fluoride content of bones from poisoned animals is greatly increased. Levels of up to 1200 mg/kg of bone on a dry, fat-free basis are observed in normal animals but may be increased up to 3000 mg/kg in animals exposed to fluoride and showing only mottling of the teeth. Animals showing severe clinical signs have levels greater than 4000 mg/kg of bone on a dry, fat-free basis; after prolonged heavy feeding, levels may be as high as 1.04%. Care must be taken in selecting the bone samples because of the great variation in the concentration of fluoride that occurs between different bones. Good data are available for comparison between metacarpal, metatarsal, rib, pelvic, and mandibular bones and antlers of deer. Mandibles usually show the greatest concentrations; in the long bones, the distal and proximal quarters are more sensitive indicators than the center half.

Diagnostic confirmation depends on fluoride assay of forage, soil, or water; blood and urine of affected animals; and bones and teeth at necropsy.

Samples for Confirmation of Diagnosis

- **Toxicology**—mandible/metacarpal/metatarsal, rib, vertebrae for evidence of osteofluorosis; urine from affected animals for evidence of recent exposure (ASSAY [F])
- **Histology**—formalin-fixed metacarpal/metatarsal/mandible (LM)

DIFFERENTIAL DIAGNOSIS

ACUTE:
- Heavy metal toxicosis
- Nephrotoxic mycotoxicosis
- Oak (*Quercus* spp.) toxicosis
- Plant toxins (*Amaranthus* spp., *Isotropis* spp., *Lantana* spp.)

Chronic:
- Chronic selenium toxicosis
- Degenerative joint disease/osteoarthritis
- Enzootic calcinosis
- Ephemeral fever in cattle
- Nutritional deficiency of phosphorus
- Nutritional deficiency of vitamin D
- Osteodystrophia fibrosa in horses
- White-muscle disease

TREATMENT

Treatment, apart from removing the animals from the source of fluoride, is largely impractical and supportive in nature. In acute ingestions, most animals die before there is time for treatment. With chronic ingestions, no improvement in dental or osseous lesions can be anticipated, but there may be amelioration of the other clinical signs. Activated charcoal is not recommended because fluoride does not bind well to it. Calcium, magnesium, or aluminum may be used to bind hydrofluoric acid produced in the stomach, and because of their insolubility they are safe even in large quantities.[13,14] Intravenous calcium should be used if hypocalcemia or tetany are present.

CONTROL

- Where fluoride levels are marginal, careful husbandry, including the watering of young growing stock on fluoride-free supplies, permitting only adults to be watered on the dangerous supplies, and rotating the animals between safe and dangerous waters at 3-month intervals, may make it possible to utilize land areas otherwise unsuitable for stock raising. In some areas, dairy herds may have to be maintained by the purchase of replacements rather than by the rearing of young stock. In areas where long-term ingestion of fluoride is likely to occur, the aim should be to provide a diet of less than 50 mg/kg of the total diet of dairy cows. Adequate calcium and defluorinated phosphorus intakes should be ensured because these reduce bone storage of fluoride.
- Phosphate feed supplements should contain no more than 0.2% fluoride for milking or breeding cattle or 0.3% for slaughter cattle, and they should not comprise more than 2% of the grain ration if the fluoride content is of this order. Some deposits of rock phosphate have much higher contents of fluoride than others, and commercial defluorination makes these toxic deposits safe for animal feeding.
- Bone meal in some areas may contain excessive quantities of fluoride and should be checked for its fluoride content.
- Water from deep wells and artesian bores should be assayed for fluoride content before use. The fluoride content of drinking water can be reduced (from 10 to 0.95 mg/kg) by adding freshly

slaked lime to the water; 500 to 1000 mg/kg should be added, and the water must be allowed to settle for 6 days. The method requires the use of large storage tanks.
- Aluminum salts are the principal substances used to detoxicate food and water. They are unpalatable and relatively ineffective, reducing the accumulation of fluoride in bone by only 20% to 30%, and are thus referred to as "alleviators." Extensive field trials of aluminum as an alleviator have not justified its use as a practicable control measure in average circumstances.

FURTHER READING

Clark RG, Hunter AC, Steward DJ. Deaths in cattle suggestive of subacute fluoride poisoning following ingestion of superphosphate. *NZ Vet J.* 1976;24:193.

Radostits O, et al. Fluorine poisoning. In: *Veterinary Medicine: A Textbook of the Disease of Cattle, Horses, Sheep, Goats and Pigs.* 10th ed. London: W.B. Saunders; 2007:1816.

Wheeler SM, Fell LR. Fluorides in cattle nutrition. *Nutr Abst Rev.* 1983;53:741-766.

REFERENCES

1. Poppenga RH. *Vet Clin North Am Food A.* 2011;27:373.
2. DeBey BM, et al. *J Vet Diagn Invest.* 2007;19:305.
3. Begum A, et al. *Rasayan J Chem.* 2008;4:774.
4. Bombik E, et al. *Bull Vet Inst Pulawy.* 2010;54:63.
5. Skinner G, et al. *Bios.* 2008;79:61.
6. McGrath D, et al. *J Plant Nutr Soil Sci.* 2010;173:548.
7. Mishra PC, et al. *Bioscan.* 2007;2:31.
8. Zanetti MC, et al. Fluoride availability from rock phosphate in sheep. In: Schlegel P, Durosy A, Jongbloed A, eds. *Trace Elements in Animal Production Systems.* Netherlands: Wageningen Academic Pub; 2008:303.
9. Grace ND, et al. *NZ Vet J.* 2007;55:77.
10. Barbier O, et al. *Chem Biol Interact.* 2010;188:319.
11. Ulemale AH, et al. *Vet World.* 2010;3:526.
12. Ranjan RD, et al. *Indian J Anim Sci.* 2009;79:546.
13. Lohakare J, et al. *Revista Brasileira de Zootecnia.* 2013;42:751.
14. Whitford AM. *Monogr Oral Sci.* 2011;22:66.

Congenital Defects of Muscles, Bones, and Joints

Defects of the musculoskeletal system are among the most common congenital abnormalities in farm animals. In cattle, 476 such defects are listed. Many of them are lethal, and most of the remainder are life-threatening because of interference with grazing or the prehension of food. Many of them occur in combinations, and thus single defects are uncommon. For example, most axial skeletal defects and cleft palates occur in calves that already have arthrogryposis.

Because of the very large volume of literature involved it is not possible to deal with all the recorded defects here, and the text is limited to those defects that are thought to be of general importance. Whether or not they are inherited or have an environmental cause is often not known, and thus an etiologic classification is not very effective—nor is an anatomic or pathologic classification, so we are reduced to a classification based on abnormal function.

WEAKNESS OF SKELETAL MUSCLES

A number of sporadic myopathies are recorded in cattle and sheep. Causes have not been determined in most of them. Splayleg in pigs has been well described and occurs in most countries.

CONGENITAL HYPERPLASIA OF MYOFIBER

There is only one identified state of congenital hyperplasia; it is the inherited form of doppelender, double muscling, or culard of cattle, described under "Myofiber hyperplasia." The principal cause of the bulging muscles is an increase in the number of myofibers in the muscle.

OBVIOUS ABSENCE OR DEFORMITY OF SPECIFIC PARTS OF THE MUSCULOSKELETAL SYSTEM

Some of these defects are inherited and include the following:
- Achondroplastic dwarfism, inherited miniature calves, bulldog calves
- Umbilical or scrotal hernia, cryptorchidism
- Tail deformity (kinking), taillessness
- Reduced phalanges, including hemimelia (individual bones missing), amputates (entire limbs missing), vestigial limbs (all parts present but limbs miniaturized)—amputates in outbreak form are recorded in cattle and produced experimentally by irradiation injury of sows, cows, and ewes during early pregnancy
- Inherited arachnomyelia (spidery limbs) of calves
- Congenital thickleg of pigs, osteopetrosis of calves, muscular hypertrophy of calves
- Cyclopean deformity—the inherited form is associated with prolonged gestation. The toxic form associated with ingestion of *Veratrum californicum.*
- Displaced molar teeth, mandibular prognathism—agnathia in lambs takes a variety of forms, including complete absence of the lower jaw and tongue.

FIXATION OF JOINTS

Because arthrogryposis, which has been used to convey the description of joint fixation, strictly means fixation in flexion, the term **congenital articular rigidity** has been introduced. The immobilization of the joint may be attributable to lack of extensibility of muscles, tendons, ligaments, or other tissues around the joint; to deformity of articular surfaces; or, theoretically, to fusion between the bones at the articular surface. Muscle contracture, which is the principal cause of joint fixation, has been produced experimentally and occurs naturally as a result of primary muscle atrophy or of atrophy resulting from denervation. Articular surface deformity is usually associated with gross deformity of the limb bones and is usually identifiable, but the principal problem in the diagnosis of congenital articular rigidity is to determine what the pathogenesis might have been and, beyond that, what was the specific cause.

Congenital fixation of joints can be caused by some well-known entities, as follows.

Cattle

- Hereditary congenital articular rigidity (HCAR) with cleft palate in Charolais
- HCAR with normal palates in Friesians, Danish Reds, Swedish, Shorthorns
- Inherited arthrogryposis
- Inherited multiple-tendon contracture
- Sporadic cases of congenital joint deformity as described for foals
- Inherited multiple ankylosis of Holstein–Friesian cattle
- Environmentally induced congenital articular rigidity caused by the following:
  - Intrauterine infection with Akabane virus
  - Ingestion of lupins
  - Ingestion of *Astragalus* and *Oxytropis* spp. (locoweeds)
  - Sorghum, Johnson grass, Sudan grass
  - Dietary deficiency of manganese

Sheep and Goats

- Inherited congenital articular rigidity in Merino sheep
- Infection with Akabane virus
- Infection with Schmallenberg virus
- Poisonous plants as for cattle
- Poisoning with parbendazole and cambendazole.

Foals

- **"Contracted" foals** having congenital axial and appendicular contractures of joints have been report in the United States; the cause unknown, but it is not thought to be inherited. Deformities include torticollis, scoliosis, and thinning of ventral abdominal wall, sometimes accompanied by eventration, asymmetry of the skull, and flexion contracture in distal limb joints.
- **Congenital articular rigidity** also occurs in foals from mares fed on hybrid Sudan grass pastures.

- **Sporadic cases of congenital joint deformity** occur in foals and calves. They are manifested usually by excessive flexion of the metacarpophalangeal joints, causing affected animals to "knuckle" at the fetlocks and sometimes walk on the anterior aspect of the pastern. A similar defect occurs in the hindlegs. Many mild cases recover spontaneously, but surgical treatment may be required in badly affected animals. The cause in these sporadic cases in unknown, and necropsy examination fails to reveal lesions other than excessive flexion of the joints caused by shortening of the flexor tendons. Rarely such fixations are associated with spina bifida or absence of ventral horn cells of the spinal cord.

Piglets

- Inherited congenital articular rigidity
- Nutritional deficiency of vitamin A
- Poisonous plants, hemlock (*Conium maculatum*), *Prunus serotina,* Jimson weed (*Datura stramonium*), tobacco wastes

CONGENITAL ARTHROGRYPOSIS AND HYDRANENCEPHALY, AKABANE DISEASE, CACHE VALLEY VIRUS DISEASE, SCHMALLENBERG VIRUS

SYNOPSIS

Etiology Akabane virus in the Simbu serogroup of *Orthobunyavirus,* Cache Valley virus in the Bunyamwera serogroup of *Orthobunyavirus,* Schmallenberg virus in the Simbu serogroup of *Orthobunyavirus.*

Epidemiology Transmission by hematophagous insects. Outbreaks occur when cattle or sheep are infected in early pregnancy.

Clinical findings Teratogenic pathogen that results in abortions, stillbirths, and birth of calves (Akabane virus, Schmallenberg virus) and lambs or kids (Cache Valley virus, Schmallenberg virus) with skeletal deformities and neurologic disorders (arthrogryposis-hydranencephaly syndrome).

Necropsy findings Necrotizing nonsuppurative encephalomyelitis and polymyositis. Arthrogryposis and hydranencephaly.

Control Vaccination or exposure of breeding females to natural infection before pregnancy.

ETIOLOGY

Akabane virus and Cache Valley viruses are both members of the genus *Orthobunyavirus* in the family Bunyaviridae, with Akabane virus and Schmallenberg virus being members of the Simbu serogroup of the genus *Orthobunyavirus* and Cache Valley virus being a member of the Bunyamwera serogroup of the genus *Orthobunyavirus.* There are a large number of members of the *Orthobunyavirus* genus, and several can produce clinically inapparent infections in ruminants, but Akabane virus and Cache Valley virus produce fetal disease when they infect the dam in early pregnancy. There are subtypes of these viruses.

Other *Bunyavirus* that have been associated with natural or experimentally produced fetal disease in ruminants include the following:

- Simbu serogroup—Aino and Peaton viruses
- Bunyamwera serogroup—Main Drain viruses
- California serogroup—LaCrosse and San Angelo viruses

Antibodies to the related, but as far as is known nonpathogenic, Australian Douglas virus and Tinaroo virus have been detected in cattle, sheep, goat, buffalo and deer.

EPIDEMIOLOGY

Occurrence

Akabane

Serologic studies suggest that infection occurs in cattle, sheep, goats, horses, donkeys, camels, pigs, and buffaloes, but disease occurs only in calves, lambs, and goat kids.

The disease is most common in calves and has been recorded as the cause of epizootics of abortion, stillbirths, and congenital malformation in calves, with high attack rates in affected herds in two north–south geographic bands. The first band extends from Japan/Korea through Taiwan to Australia.[1,2] The second band extends from the Middle East to South Africa. Congenital disease in lambs is less common but is recorded in Israel and Australia. The virus has also been isolated from insect vectors in Africa and is the probable cause of the "rigid lamb syndrome" in Zimbabwe.

Serologic surveys suggest widespread distribution of the virus in the Middle East, Asia and South East Asia, and in parts of Africa. Whereas infection in adult cattle is common in endemic areas, reports of clinical disease are rare, but neurologic disease associated with infection in cattle 2 to 7 years of age has been observed. Akabane viruses have been divided genetically into four groups (I to IV), with group I being further divided into two subgroups (Ia, Ib).[1,3,4] Genogroup Ia strains are found primarily in Japan and Taiwan and appear to have a stronger neurovirulence than genogroup II strains that have been isolated from Japan and Korea. Genogroup Ib strains have been isolated in Japan and Israel. Genogroup III strains have been isolated from Queensland in Australia, whereas a strain isolated in Kenya represents genogroup IV.[1,3,4]

Cache Valley

There is serologic evidence that infection occurs in sheep, goats, horses, cattle, pigs, and several wildlife species but clinical disease is recorded only in sheep. The disease in sheep is recorded as an occasional epizootic in flocks in North America. Cache Valley virus is one of the more common *Orthobunyaviruses* in North America and has been isolated from mosquito pools collected in 22 states and several provinces in Canada and Mexico and also in Central and South America. Cache Valley is an agricultural valley in northern Utah and southeast Idaho in the United States.

Schmallenberg

A new disease in dairy cattle was identified in autumn 2011 in northwest Germany and the Netherlands. Viral genome sequences were identified in pooled blood from three affected sick dairy cows from a farm near Schmallenberg in northwest Germany, hence the name Schmallenberg virus (SBV). Serologic studies indicate that SBV was not present in domestic ruminants in northern Europe before 2011, and that the epizootics constituted introduction of the new virus into a susceptible population. Genomic studies indicate that SBV belongs to the species Sathuperi and may represent the ancestor of the reassortant Shamonda virus.

Antibodies against SBV have been identified in roe deer, red deer, European fallow deer, mouflons, bison, New World camelids, and wild boar in northern and west-central Europe.[5]

Aino and Shamonda

Aino virus is present and thought to be a cause of disease in Australia, Japan, and Israel. Serologic studies in Australia show a similar distribution in cattle to Akabane but at a lower prevalence, and clinical disease is much less common than with Akabane virus. Aino virus and Shamonda virus can induce congenital malformations in sheep and goats.

Source of Infection

The viruses are maintained through a cycle involving vectors, in which there is probably transovarial transmission, and a susceptible vertebrate population. Replication occurs in both vertebrate and insect populations.

Akabane

Viremia in cattle is short-lived, lasting 1 to 9 days, and long-term carriers are not thought to occur. Herbivores appear essential to the vector–virus–host cycle, and there is serologic evidence of infection in cattle, sheep, goats, camels, horses, and buffaloes. In endemic areas, breeding females are infected before their first pregnancy, and therefore clinical signs are not observed in their offspring. Clinical signs occur at the north and south end of the two bands, where weather effects determine expansion of vectors out of the endemic region. This accounts for intermittent "outbreaks" of congenitally affected calves in southern Australia, Japan, and Korea.

In Australia, transmission is by the bites of midges *Culicoides brevitarsis* and *C. nebeculosus.* The virus has been isolated from *C. brevitarsis,* and this is probably the major vector; serologic data in Australia show that most identified infections are within the known habitat of *C. brevitarsis.* Vertical infection occurs, but introduction of the virus into the bovine uterus in semen causes no developmental defects. Ruminants do not become persistently infected.

The vectors for Akabane disease in Japan and Korea are *C. brevitarsis, Culicoides oxystoma, Aedes vexans,* and *Culex tritaeniorhynchus.*

Cache Valley

The Cache Valley virus has been isolated predominantly from mosquitoes. The primary amplifying vertebrate hosts are unknown, but white-tailed deer are suspected to play a role as a disease reservoir.[6]

Schmallenberg

Biting midges, including *C. dewulfi, C. chiopterus,* and *C. obsoletus* complex are thought to be important vectors for SBV transmission in Belgium and Denmark and presumably contiguous countries.

Aino

Aino virus has been isolated from mosquitoes and midges, including *C. brevitarsis.* Serologic studies show antibody in cattle, sheep, goats, and buffalo but not camels, dogs, or horses.

Host and Environmental Risk Factors

The seasonal and geographic pattern of epizootics of abortions and premature births are determined by the distribution of vectors and the availability of susceptible ruminant populations in early pregnancy. Global warming is thought to be contributing to extension of vectors into geographic regions north and south of the typical infection belts and therefore disease epidemics.[1,3,7]

Akabane

In the north of Australia, *C. brevitarsis* is active throughout the year, cattle are infected with Akabane virus before their first pregnancy, and disease does not occur. Epizootics occur in southern Australia when *C. brevitarsis* extends its range of distribution, probably by wind-borne spread from the north, to infect immunologically naive herds. Abortions and premature births commence in the autumn, with clinical cases of arthrogryposis and hydranencephaly occurring in midwinter.

Wind-borne introduction of *Culicoides* spp. is also postulated as the means of introduction of infection in Israel. The movement of immunologically naive pregnant cattle into an enzootic area can be the result in severe outbreaks in those herds.

The disease is likely to disappear for intervals of 5 to 10 years, until there is combination of a susceptible population and a heavy vector population. Occurrences of the disease are also dependent on the presence of susceptible early-pregnant females at the time that the vectors are plentiful. These conditions are provided by a series of years of drought in an enzootic area, so that there are no insect vectors, no infection, and no immunization activity of prepubescent females, followed by a wet season when the vectors are plentiful.

Cache Valley

Outbreaks occur after a long period of drought and winter frosts reducing the population of mosquito vectors and resulting in populations of seronegative ewes. Mating in the summer appears to be a major risk factor, allowing sheep to be in the susceptible stage of pregnancy during the vector season. Many outbreaks are in areas that interface between suburban and rural environments.

Schmallenberg

Retrospective analysis of stored serum samples indicates that SBV was introduced into Europe in spring or early summer of 2011, probably first along the border of the Netherlands with northwest Germany. It is interesting to note that SBV emerged in the same region of Europe in 2011 as did bluetongue strain 8 in 2006.

Experimental Reproduction

Disease has been reproduced by inoculation into early-pregnant cattle, sheep, and goats.

Zoonotic Implications

Bunyavirus infections occur in humans from bites from infected insect vectors.

PATHOGENESIS

Akabane

Viremia occurs in the dam for 2 to 4 days, with an antibody peak 4 to 5 days after the viremia and a subsequent secondary rise. The dam is unaffected, but there is a focal viral persistence in cotyledons and subsequent viremia in the fetus.

Inflammatory and degenerative lesions occur in the central nervous system, but tissue tropism and damage are determined by the age of the fetus and its ability to mount an immune response. Three forms, or principal manifestations, of the disease in an affected herd are described. The first is arthrogryposis occurring in calves infected at an older age than others (fetus infected at 105 to 174 days of pregnancy). The second is arthrogryposis accompanied by hydranencephaly. The third is hydranencephaly only (infected between days 76 and 104 of pregnancy).

With arthrogryposis, there is almost complete absence of ventral horn cells in the spinal cord and an accompanying neurotropic failure of muscle development. Contracture of the joints results. The hydranencephaly is manifested by a partial or complete failure of development of the cerebral cortex. The brainstem and cerebellum are usually normal.

Several other manifestations have been described. They include prearthrogryposis groups of calves with incoordination and a mild to moderate nonsuppurative encephalitis, along with other calves with flaccid paralysis and active secondary demyelination in motor areas of the spinal cord. Some calves are unable to stand and have thickened dorsal cranial bones, hydranencephaly involving anterior and midbrainstem, and a diminutive cerebellum. The infection with Akabane virus is also credited with causing abortion, stillbirth, and premature birth. There are reports from Japan and South Korea where encephalomyelitis as a result of Akabane virus is thought to have been acquired after birth,[2,8] and experimental inoculation of young calves with the Iriki variant of Akabane virus has induced encephalitis.

Lesions produced in **lambs** by experimental inoculation of the ewes during early pregnancy (days 32 to 36) include skeletal muscle atrophy and degeneration, and inflammatory and degenerative lesions in the cerebrum; the lesions in the central nervous system vary from porencephaly to hydranencephaly. There are also brachygnathism, scoliosis, hypoplasia of the lungs, agenesis or hypoplasia of the spinal cord, and arthrogryposis. Lesions are also present in fetuses of ewes inoculated between 29 and 45 days of gestation.

Cache Valley

Ovine fetuses are susceptible to the teratogenic effects between 28 and 48 days of gestation.[9] Destructive lesions occur in the central nervous system, but infection of fetal membranes with a reduction in the volume of amniotic fluid and constriction by membranes around the fetus are thought to contribute to the occurrence of arthrogryposis.

Schmallenberg

The acute phase of infection in adult ruminants produces a viremia of 5 to 6 days in duration.[10] In utero infection of the lamb appears to be determined by the absence or presence of a functional blood–brain barrier, explaining the window for experiment infection of 28 to 50 days (placentomes are initially present on day 28; the blood–brain barrier becomes functional on day 50 of gestation).

Arthrogryposis is secondary to transplacental infection resulting in abnormal development of motor neurons of the ventral horn of the fetal spinal cord. This results in hypoplasia of the limb musculature, neurogenic muscle atrophy, and subsequent fixation (ankyloses) of the joints.

CLINICAL FINDINGS

Akabane

Infection in adult cattle is most commonly clinically inapparent, unless there is dystocia, but neurologic disease manifests with hypersensitivity, tremor, and ataxia has been recorded. In calves, the two syndromes, arthrogryposis and hydranencephaly, occur separately—arthrogryposis in the early stages of the outbreak and hydranencephaly at the end. Cases of calves with both defects occur in the middle of the outbreak. In some outbreaks, only one of the manifestations of the disease is seen.

Calves with arthrogryposis almost always are the subjects of difficult birth requiring physical assistance. They are small and significantly underweight, but they are fully mature in terms of teeth eruption and hair coat and hoof development. They are unable to rise, stand, or walk. One or more limbs is fixed at the joints; there is a congenital articular rigidity. The limb is usually fixed in flexion, but it may be in extension. The joint becomes freely movable if the tendons around it are severed; that is, there is no abnormality of the articular surface. The muscles of affected limbs are severely wasted. Kyphosis or scoliosis are common.

Calves with hydranencephaly have no difficulty rising and walking. The major defects are a lack of intelligence and blindness. They will suck if put onto the teat, but if this is not done, they stand and vocalize and have no apparent dam-seeking reflex. A few calves have microencephaly and are more severely affected. They are dummies, very uncoordinated in gait, and unable to stand properly, and they move erratically when stimulated. These cases appear at the very end of the outbreak.

In addition to the skeletal and neurologic diseases, cases of abortion, stillbirth, and premature birth are also regarded as being associated with Akabane virus infection in cows. They are usually recorded at the beginning of the outbreak before the neurologic defects occur.

Cache Valley

Affected flocks have a higher rate of stillbirth and mummified fetuses. Congenital malformations in liveborn lambs include arthrogryposis of one or more limbs, scoliosis, and torticollis, and neurologic signs are similar to those seen in calves with Akabane disease.

Schmallenberg

Adult cattle exhibit clinical signs of decreased milk production and fever, and some have diarrhea, with the duration of illness ranging from 1 to 6 days. Clinical disease has not been reported in sheep or goats.

Embryonic deaths, abortions, stillbirths, and arthrogryposis–hydranencephalopathy syndrome in newborn lambs and kids are the most common clinical abnormalities observed following infection of pregnant ewes and does. These abnormalities in lambs and kids are almost identical to those produced by Akabane virus in calves. Teratogenic effects were also observed in cattle, but at a much lower rate than in sheep and goats. A presumptive diagnosis of SBV teratogenicity is made in lambs, kids, and calves in Europe if stillbirth, premature or mummified fetuses, or abnormal neonates present with two or more of the following abnormalities: arthrogryposis, hydranencephaly, torticollis, scoliosis, kyphosis, brachygnathia inferior, muscle atrophy, joint malformations, ataxia, paresis, behavioral abnormalities, or blindness.

CLINICAL PATHOLOGY

The presence of specific antibody in fetal sera or the precolostral sera of neonates is diagnostic, but its absence does not exclude the diagnosis if infection precedes the development of immunologic competence. Precolostral sera from several animals should be tested, and most cases are positive at high titer. A rising titer with paired samples from the dam, or a high titer in the serum of surviving neonates, is suggestive of recent infection but not confirmatory for disease. Serologic tests include microneutralization, hemagglutination inhibition, agar gel immunodiffusion (AGID), and an ELISA test.

Virus can be detected using real-time RT-PCR and culture in specific cell lines. RT-qPCR testing of blood is of reduced value because the period of viremia is short, but brainstem material provides the best tissue for testing teratogenic fetuses.[11] A humoral immune response mounted by the fetus can clear SBV from the fetus during gestation; consequently, SBV antibody testing of fetal heart blood or dam blood should be combined with RT-PCR testing of brainstem tissue for confirmation of SBV infection.[11,12]

NECROPSY FINDINGS

The primary lesions with Akabane, Cache Valley, and Schmallenberg infections in the fetus are a **necrotizing nonsuppurative encephalomyelitis and polymyositis**.

In calves and lambs with arthrogryposis, there is severe muscle atrophy, fixation of joints by tendon contracture, and normal articular surfaces. The joints are easily released by cutting the surrounding tendons. Histologically, there may be almost complete absence of ventral horn cells in the spinal cord. This lesion may be localized to one segment of the cord, and viral antigen may be demonstrated via immunohistochemistry.

In calves and lambs with hydranencephaly, the cerebral hemispheres are completely absent, and the vacant space is filled with fluid enclosed by the normal meninges. In a few cases the lesions will be limited to porencephaly. In most, the brainstem and cerebellum lack cavitations, but diminution of their size may be recorded.

Samples for Confirmation of Diagnosis

- **Virology**—2 mL fetal heart blood and maternal serum for serology performed using ELISA[13]
- **Histology**—brain, spinal cord, muscle (LM, IHC)

DIFFERENTIAL DIAGNOSIS

Akabane virus disease in calves, Cache Valley virus disease in lambs and kids, and Schmallenberg virus disease in calves, lambs, and kids, because they are manifest epidemiologically and are well-defined and easily recognizable entities. Differentials include the following:

- Lupine-induced arthrogryposis in calves
- Manganese deficiency in calves
- Heritable forms of arthrogryposis and/or micrencephaly
- Fetal infection with bluetongue virus, Rift Valley fever virus, or pestivirus

Cattle in Japan may also produce hydranencephalic calves, which are recumbent, opisthotonic, and unable to suckle at birth, when infected during pregnancy by the Chuzan virus. The virus, a member of the Polyam subgroup of orbiviruses, is transmitted by *Culicoides oxystoma*.

In Africa, infection with flaviviruses, including West Nile, Banzi, and AR5189, also causes abortion, stillbirth, and congenital brain malformations.

TREATMENT AND CONTROL

No treatment is contemplated because affected calves, lambs, and kids are not viable and cannot be humanely kept alive.

Vector control is not possible with current knowledge, and vaccination provides the most effective method of control.

Killed vaccines for Akabane virus have proved very effective against natural exposure and are available in Japan and Australia. Japanese data suggest vaccines should include genogroup Ia strains because these strains have a stronger neurovirulence,[14] and vaccine failures has been attributed to antigenic variation among Akabane virus strains.[15] Vaccination requires two inoculations before pregnancy and an annual booster. Maternally derived antibodies against Akabane virus appear to last 4 to 5 months in colostrum-fed calves, and they last slightly longer in beef calves than dairy calves,[16] possibly as a result of a higher colostral titer in beef calf colostrum as a result of smaller colostral volumes. The economics of annual vaccination against Akabane virus is dictated by the risk of disease in regions subject to periodic outbreaks of disease.

Vaccines are not commercially available for Cache Valley virus.

Killed vaccines are commercially available for Schmallenberg virus in the United Kingdom and France, but they have not been widely used. Vaccination of calves with a commercially available Japanese vaccine against Akabane virus, Aino virus, and Chuzan virus did not provide cross-protection against SBV.[17] Preliminary data on a small number of vaccinated sheep suggest that protection against detectable viremia is provided after one injection of a SBV vaccine.[18] Early lambing flocks and pedigree flocks have been more likely to employ vaccination in the United Kingdom.[19] The seroprevalence in ranges widely from herd to herd, and determination of seroprevalence within a herd could be used to guide the decision regarding the need to vaccinate. Individual blood testing is not practical in this regard, and for cattle, determining the titer of a bulk-tank milk sample does not provide a sufficiently accurate test of herd seroprevalence.[20] Maternally derived antibodies against SBV last at least 2 years in adult cattle after natural infection and 5 months in their colostrum-fed calves;[21] on this basis, an initial vaccination series could start at 6 months of age if indicated.

Spread of SBV infection from farm to farm appears to be primarily a result of vector movements on the wind, and thus application of animal movement restrictions, including a total animal movement ban, is likely to have little impact on farm-to-farm transmission of infection.[22] In the Schmallenberg virus outbreak in Europe, cattle that had access to pasture for grazing in 2011 were 2.6 times more likely to deliver ered malformed calves than cattle that were housed inside.[23] Specific control measures may not be economically indicated in cattle because the decrease in milk production is mild and transient, non-SBV-associated mortality in adult cattle has been reported, and the incidence of fetal abnormalities is low.[24] Housing sheep to minimize contact with midges has been shown to decrease seroprevalence within a flock. The seroprevalence in the endemic area is lower in goat herds than sheep flocks; this has been attributed to differences in housing, with goats being more likely to be kept indoors with decreased exposure to midges. The use of insecticides or repellants on pregnant ewes and does is not likely to be efficacious, but experimental data are lacking. Changing the timing of lambing and kidding so that the second month of gestation occurs during cold ambient temperatures when midges are not active will theoretically decrease the incidence of teratogenic effects resulting from SBV. This recommendation has been supported by epidemiologically studies indicating lower odds of SBV-induced fetal malformations in sheep flocks that started breeding in October versus August.[25]

A number of European countries, including Germany, France, and the Netherlands, made it mandatory to report the birth of malformed lambs, kids, and calves on farms seropositive for SBV. The numbers of abnormal lambs, kids, and calves born decreased in 2013 and 2014, most likely because of the development of herd immunity and high seroprevalence. Reemergence and spread of SBV within Europe is considered likely.

FURTHER READING

Beer M, Conraths FJ, van der Poel WHM. Schmallenberg virus—a novel orthobunyavirus emerging in Europe. *Epidemiol Infect.* 2013;141:1-8.

Ganter M, Eibach R, Helmer C. Update on Schmallenberg virus infections in small ruminants. *Small Rumin Res.* 2014;118:63-68.

Lievaart-Peterson K, Luttikholt SJM, van den Brom R, Velleme P. Schmallenberg virus infection in small ruminants—first review of the situation and prospects in northern Europe. *Small Ruminant Res.* 2012;106:71-76.

Tarlinton R, Daly J, Dunham S, Kydd J. The challenge of Schmallenberg virus emergence in Europe. *Vet J.* 2012;194:10-18.

REFERENCES

1. Oem JK, et al. *Vet Microbiol.* 2012;158:250.
2. Kamata H, et al. *J Comp Path.* 2009;140:187.
3. Kobayashi T, et al. *Virus Res.* 2007;130:162.
4. An DJ, et al. *Vet Microbiol.* 2010;140:49.
5. Mouchantat S, et al. *Vet Res.* 2015;46:99.
6. Andreadis TG, et al. *Vector-Borne Zoonot.* 2014;14:763.
7. Oem JK, et al. *J Comp Path.* 2012;147:101.
8. Lee JK, et al. *Vet Rec.* 2007;161:236.
9. Hoffmann AR, et al. *J Virol.* 2012;86:4793.
10. Wernike K, et al. *Vet Microbiol.* 2013;166:461.
11. de Regge N, et al. *Vet Microbiol.* 2013;162:595.
12. Bouwstra RJ, et al. *Vet Microbiol.* 2013;165:102.
13. Oem JK, et al. *Trop Anim Health Prod.* 2014;46:261.
14. Kono R, et al. *BMC Vet Res.* 2008;4:20.
15. Bangphoomi N, et al. *J Vet Med Sci.* 2014;76:1471.
16. Tsutsui T, et al. *J Vet Med Sci.* 2009;71:913.
17. Hechinger S, et al. *Vet Res.* 2013;44:114.
18. Hechinger S, et al. *Vet Res.* 2014;45:79.
19. Roger P. *In Pract.* 2015;37:33.
20. Daly JM, et al. *BMC Vet Res.* 2015;11:56.
21. Elbers ARW, et al. *BMC Vet Res.* 2014;10:103.
22. Gubbins S, et al. *Prev Vet Med.* 2014;116:380.
23. Veldhuis AMB, et al. *Prev Vet Med.* 2014;116:412.
24. Veldhuis AMB, et al. *Vet Microbiol.* 2014a;168:281.
25. Luttikholt S, et al. *PLoS ONE.* 2014;9(6):e100135.

HYPERMOBILITY OF JOINTS

- This is recorded as an inherited defect in Jersey cattle. Affected animals are unable to rise or stand because of the lack of fixation of limb joints. The joints and limbs are usually all affected simultaneously and are so flexible that the limbs can be tied in knots. Causes include the following:
  - Inherited joint hypermobility in Jersey cattle
  - Heredity in Holstein–Friesian cattle, which also have pink teeth as a result of absence of enamel
  - In inherited congenital defects of collagen formation, including dermatosparaxis, hyperelastosis cutis, and Ehlers–Danlos syndrome in cattle
  - Sporadically in newborn animals

Inherited Diseases of Muscles

GLYCOGEN STORAGE DISEASES

A number of glycogen storage diseases have been detected in large animal species. The glycogen storage diseases discussed here are those that result in accumulation of abnormal concentrations of glycogen in muscle, either within lysosomes or within myocytes. These diseases include polysaccharide storage myopathy (glycogen storage disease type I) in various breeds of horses and as a result of a mutation in the gene encoding the enzyme glycogen synthase (addressed in detail later in the discussion of other inherited myopathies of the horse), glucosidase deficiency (glycogen storage disease type II) in sheep and cattle, and glycogen phosphorylase deficiency (glycogen storage disease type V) in sheep and cattle. Glycogen storage disease types II and V are discussed in the following sections.

GENERALIZED GLYCOGENOSIS (GLYCOGEN STORAGE DISEASE TYPE II)

Generalized glycogenosis is a glycogen storage disease. Glycogen storage disease type II (GSD II; generalized glycogenosis), which resembles Pompe's disease in humans, occurs in Corriedale sheep, Shorthorn, and Brahman beef cattle, and it is caused by mutant alleles of the glucosidase alpha acid (GAA), creating a loss of function. Glucosidase is a lysosomal enzyme catabolizing glycogen to glucose. The heredity is autosomal recessive. In Brahman cattle, the glycogenosis is caused by two mutations; the mutation in exon 7 is a dinucleotide deletion (c.1057_1058delTA) causing frameshift, and the mutation in exon 13 is the cytosine-to-thymine transition (c.1783C>T) coding for stop codons in exons 8 and 13, respectively.[1] The mutation in exon 9 (c.1351C>T) reduces glucosidase activity, and MspI polymorphism is a silent mutation in exon 16 (c.2223G>A). In Shorthorn cattle, glycogenosis type II is caused by a single mutation that is a deletion (c.2454_2455delCA). The genetic abnormality was not detected in a survey of Charolais, Czech Spotted (Czech Simmental), Belgian Blue, Limousine, Blonde d'Aquitaine, Aberdeen Angus, and Beef Simmental sires reared in the Czech Republic, although the number of animals tested was small for some breeds (Czech Simmental, 62; Charolais, 34; Belgian Blue, 6; Limousine, 4; Blonde d'Aquitaine, 4; Beef Simmental, 2; and Aberdeen Angus, 1).[1]

In Brahman cattle, there is a common mutation affecting many Australian Brahmans and a less common one affecting descendants of one imported bull. In addition, a third mutation is associated with significantly reduced α-glucosidase activity, but not sufficient to cause clinical disease in the homozygous state.

Clinical signs include poor growth, muscle weakness, incoordination of gait, and difficulty in rising. The animals become permanently recumbent. The disease is identified as a lysosomal storage disease, with lesions present in skeletal and cardiac muscle and central nervous tissue. During the course of the disease there is progressive muscular damage and acute degeneration of muscle fibers in the terminal stage. Affected Brahman calves die at 8 to 9 months of age and British breed cattle at over 1 year. Only histopathologic lesions are evident and include extensive vacuolation and accumulations of granular material in affected tissues. Among the biochemical lesions are greatly diminished α-glucosidase activity in liver and muscle and a correspondingly high level of glycogen. Animals in affected herds are divisible into normal heterozygotes and homozygotes on the basis of α-1,4-glucosidase activity in lymphocytes or in muscle, especially the semitendinosus muscle.

Genotyping methods using hair root and blood samples to test Shorthorn cattle for generalized glycogenosis are available, and PCR assays have been developed to genotype Brahman cattle for loss-of-function alleles within the acidic α-glucosidase gene.

FURTHER READING

Jolly RD, Blair HT, Johnstone AC. Genetic disorders in sheep in New Zealand: a review and perspective. *NZ Vet J.* 2004;52:52-64.

REFERENCE

1. Citek J, et al. *J Vet Med A.* 2007;54:257.

GLYCOGEN STORAGE DISEASE TYPE V (MUSCLE GLYCOGEN PHOSPHORYLASE DEFICIENCY)

Glycogen storage disease Type V (akin to McArdle's disease in humans) has been recorded in Charolais cattle in North America and Merino sheep in Australia.[1] Type V is inherited as an autosomal-recessive trait, and the mutation in sheep has been identified as an adenine-for-guanine substitution at the intron 19 3′ splice site, with subsequent lack of myophosphorylase activity.[2] There is mildly elevated muscle glycogen concentration and elevated serum creatine and aspartate aminotransferase activity. Severely affected animals can develop rhabdomyolysis, which may be accompanied by myoglobinuria.

In Charolais cattle, glycogen storage disease type V is usually seen in calves at several weeks or months of age and is associated with exercise intolerance or reduced capacity for exercise. Calves lag behind their dam or herd and may become temporarily recumbent for several minutes; with continuous exercise there are further periods of collapse and recumbency, which can become prolonged. Not all homozygous animals are clinically affected if they are allowed to "pace their exercise," and some animals have been known to breed despite muscle weakness.

The disease in Merino sheep is associated with exercise intolerance and increased concentrations of glycogen in muscle.[1,2]

A PCR restriction fragment length polymorphism test has been used to identify heterozygous individuals in a Charolais herd in New Zealand that were otherwise normal. Using a similar test, a Blonde d'Aquitaine crossbred calf with a double-muscled phenotype and suspected of having myophosphorylase deficiency based on clinical findings of brown-colored transparent urine after exercise, pain, and elevated creatine kinase was considered negative. The gene maps to chromosome 29.[3]

REFERENCES

1. Howell JM, et al. *Neuromusc Dis.* 2014;24:167.
2. Tan P, et al. *Neuromusc Dis.* 1997;7:336.
3. Citek J, et al. *J Vet Med A.* 2007;54:257.

INHERITED DIAPHRAGMATIC MUSCLE DYSTROPHY

Inherited diaphragmatic muscle dystrophy is an inherited defect in diaphragmatic muscle of Meuse–Rhine–Yssel and Holstein–Friesian cattle appearing in adults and characterized by anorexia, decreased rumination, and eructation leading to recurrent bloat, dyspnea, abdominal respiration, nostril dilatation, and death from asphyxia after a course of several weeks. The disease is a result of a mutation involving one of the genes for heat shock protein 70 (HSP70), resulting in markedly reduced HSP70 concentrations in muscle of affected animals.[1] Loss of HSP70 function causes accumulation of glycogen phosphorylase enzyme protein in muscle. Necropsy lesions comprise degenerative changes in diaphragmatic and thoracic muscles.

REFERENCE

1. Sugimoto M, et al. *Anim Genet.* 2003;34:191.

CONGENITAL MYASTHENIA GRAVIS

Congenital myasthenic syndrome occurs in Brahman cattle in South Africa and is reported in a Hereford heifer in the United States. Affected Brahman calves develop progressive muscular weakness, beginning at birth and up to 3 to 4 weeks of age. Within 1 week they are unable to stand without assistance. Some calves are able to stand and walk for 30 to 45 minutes before collapsing, but they are still able to suck their dams. The calves remain alert and continue sucking but may collapse after 20 to 60 seconds. The weakness becomes progressively worse, and affected calves are usually euthanized. Hematology and serum biochemistry are normal, and muscle biopsies do not reveal any abnormalities.

The disease was traced to two founder animals as the most likely original carriers. Pedigree analysis revealed no ancestors common to all known carriers, but rather that the mutation had been introduced at least twice into the South African Brahman population, probably via animals imported from the United States.[1]

The underlying defect is a homozygous 20-base-pair (bp) deletion in the gene, muscular acetylcholine receptor (bov*CHRNE*), coding for the subunit of the nAChR at the neuromuscular junction. A PCR-based DNA test, using blood or semen, has been developed and validated. The test makes it possible to differentiate rapidly and accurately between homozygous wild-type, heterozygous, and homozygous affected animals. Overall prevalence of carriers among 1453 animals tested in South Africa was 0.97% (0.50% to 1.68%, 95% confidence interval). Heterozygosity for the CHRNE 470del20 mutation is associated with a 13.3-kg increase in adjusted 600-day body weight, providing evidence of a selective advantage for carrier animals and an explanation of the relatively high prevalence of the disease.[1]

The disease in a Hereford heifer was characterized as recurrent recumbency and upper eyelid ptosis. Both recumbency and ptosis resolved within 1 minute of IV administration of edrophonium (0.1 mg/kg) and persisted for up to 48 hours.[2] The heifer was first examined at 7 months of age and was slaughtered at 11 months of age.

REFERENCES

1. Thompson PN, et al. *J Anim Sci.* 2007;85:604.
2. Wise LN, et al. *J Vet Int Med.* 2008;22:231.

BOVINE FAMILIAL DEGENERATIVE NEUROMUSCULAR DISEASE

Bovine familial degenerative neuromuscular disease has been reported as occurring in Gelbveih cattle in several separate beef herds in the United States. Affected animals are 4 to 20 months of age, and the case-fatality rate is 100%. Clinical findings include ataxia, weakness, and terminal recumbency. Gross and histologic muscle lesions were indicative of nutritional muscular dystrophy with no myocardial lesions. Acute to chronic lesions in most large skeletal muscle groups consist of degeneration, necrosis, regeneration, fibrosis, and atrophy. Fibrinoid necrosis of arterioles is a common feature in multiple tissues. Lesions in the spinal cord white matter and peripheral nerves consisted of degeneration of the dorsal columns and axons, respectively. Chronic interstitial nephritis with fibrosis, hyaline droplet change, and tubular epithelial vacuolar change were most severe in older calves. Vitamin E levels were abnormally low in most affected calves. Pedigree analysis found a common ancestry for all but one of the affected calves. It is hypothesized that a hereditary metabolic defect, possibly involving antioxidant metabolism, may be the causative factor.

INHERITED UMBILICAL HERNIA

Umbilical hernias in cattle have been considered to be inherited defects for many years, but the evidence is uncertain.

Umbilical hernias are commonly identified in dairy heifers. In 18 commercial dairy herds in New York, 15% of heifer calves had umbilical hernias during the first 3 months of age. The economic costs of umbilical hernias include the cost of medical and surgical treatment and the loss in value for breeding animals.

It has been generally accepted that umbilical hernias may be inherited in a dominant or recessive mode. Some studies have found the risk of hernias was higher in some breeds, with the incidence being much higher in Holstein cattle than other breeds such as Angus, Ayrshire, Brown Swiss, Charolais, Guernsey, Hereford, Jersey, and Shorthorn. However, aspects other than genetic factors may be important. For example, many veterinarians have observed that umbilical infections commonly lead to umbilical hernia by slowing closure of the umbilicus. It is unlikely that the responsible genes are sex-linked, in spite of the apparent greater incidence in females. Umbilical hernias in Holstein–Friesian cattle can also be conditioned by a dominant character with incomplete penetrance or be caused by environmental factors. In a case-control study to determine risk factors associated with identification of an umbilical hernia during the first 2 months after birth in Holstein heifers, the sire and umbilical infection were associated with risk of a hernia. Heifers born to sires with = 3 progeny with an umbilical hernia were 2.31 times as likely to develop a hernia as were heifers born to sires with = 2 progeny with an umbilical hernia. Heifers with umbilical infection were 5.65 times as likely to develop a hernia as were heifers without umbilical infection. Attributable proportion analysis found that the frequency of umbilical hernias in Holstein heifers with umbilical infection would have been reduced by 82% if umbilical infection had been prevented.

The risk factors for congenital umbilical hernias in German Fleckvieh calves offered for sale at livestock markets were examined. An umbilical hernia was defined as a palpable opening in the abdominal wall of the umbilical region greater than 1.5 cm, even if no hernia had developed. Inflammation, abscesses, or fistulae were excluded. Data from 53,105 calves were collected from 77 livestock markets over a 2-year period. The overall incidence of congenital hernia was 1.8%. The analyses found significant effects for sex of calf, birth type, age of calf at examination, market place and date, sire line, sire, and frequency of affected herdmate calves in male calves. The incidence was 2.2% in males and 1.5% in females. The calves varied from 3 to 8 weeks of age. The diameter of hernial openings was between 1.5 and 9 cm, with 47% of affected calves with a hernia measuring greater than 3 cm. A significantly higher incidence occurred in twin or triplet calves. Shorter gestation periods increased the risk of hernias linearly by a factor of 1.3% for 10 days. There were differences in the incidence of hernias according to sire lines, but the heritability estimates were low, varying from $h = 0.04$ (>100 progeny) or $h = 0.05$ (>25 or 50 progeny). However, analysis of the data found no evidence for a monogenic autosomal-recessive inheritance. The analyses indicated that the incidence of congenital umbilical hernia observed could not be explained by one autosomal-recessive gene locus; it seems much more likely that more than one gene locus is involved, or a mixed multifactorial monogenic mode of inheritance may be the underlying genetic mechanism. It is suggested that the incidence of congenital umbilical hernias could be reduced if all breeding bulls are examined as calves and a veterinary certificate confirms a closed umbilical ring.

Breeders should be aware of the implications of congenital hernias, and, thus, congenital hernia should get more attention in the selection process of young sires.

Breeding studies and genotyping using the Canadian Holstein bull Glenhapton Enhancer have provided evidence that Enhancer is the carrier of a major dominant or codominant gene with partial penetrance for umbilical hernia. Five sons of Enhancer produced progeny with greater than 10% frequency of umbilical hernia, whereas the progeny of three sons had less than 3% frequency umbilical hernia. Genotyping of grand-progeny found significant differences in paternal allele frequencies between the affected and unaffected progeny groups for a marker BMS1591 on bovine chromosome 8(BTA8). The umbilical hernia–associated paternal allele originated from Enhancer.

MYOFIBER HYPERPLASIA (DOUBLE MUSCLING, DOPPELENDER, CULARD)

EPIDEMIOLOGY

Myofiber hyperplasia is an inherited condition characterized by an increased bulk of skeletal muscles as a result of the presence of a greater-than-normal number of muscle fibers that occurs in Charolais, Belgian Blue (Fig. 15-15), Piedmont, and South Devon breeds. The condition is recorded only rarely in sheep (Texel breed).[1] Pietrain pigs (see following discussion) exhibit many of the characteristics of double-muscled cattle, including large muscle mass and susceptibility to stress.

The condition in Belgian Blue cattle is attributable to a mutation in the MSTN gene that regulates myostatin production.[1-3] Inhibition of myostatin, through a loss-of-function mutation, results in increases in muscle fiber number and muscle mass. The disease in Belgian Blue cattle, and presumably in other breeds of cattle and sheep,

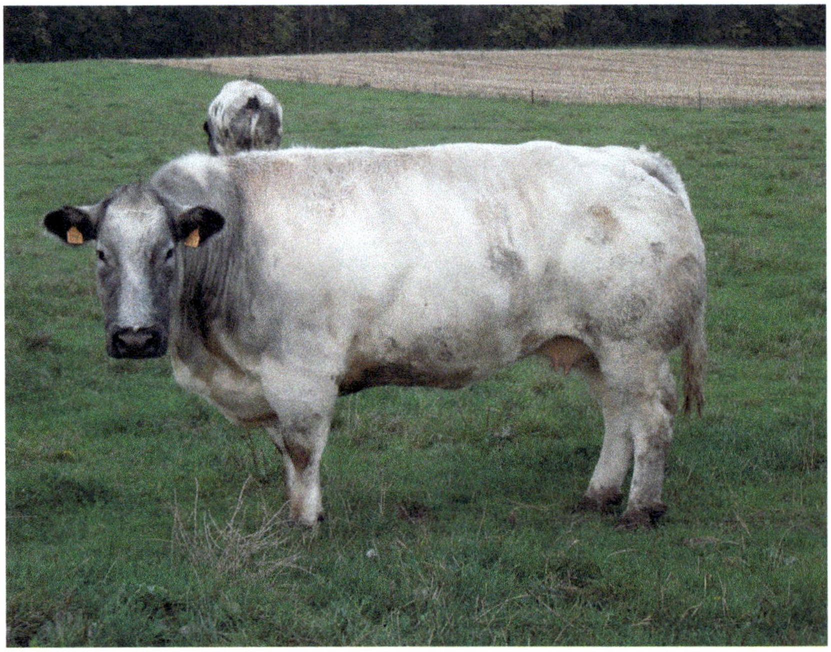

Fig. 15-15 Myofiber hyperplasia in a Belgian Blue cow.

is transmitted as an autosomal-recessive characteristic. A similar mutation in Thoroughbred horses is associated with superior sprint (<1600 m) racing performance.[4,5] The mutation has been induced experimentally in Meishan pigs.[6]

The mutation of MSTN was "fixed" in the Belgian Blue breed in the 1990s as a result of strong selection pressure for the double-muscle phenotype.[2] Subsequent continued selection pressure has resulted in increases in frequency of other haplotypes favoring increased lean muscle mass, resulting in a polygenic basis for the current phenotype. Selection of the phenotype is currently limited because of the occurrence of crooked-tail syndrome (see section on Inherited Taillessness and Tail Deformity later in this chapter) in animals homozygous for the MRC2 gene, which encodes protein Endo180. Animals heterozygous for the MRC2 mutation do not have crooked-tail syndrome and have enhanced muscularity.[7]

CLINICAL FINDINGS

Severely affected cattle show a marked increase in muscle mass most readily observed in the hindquarters, loin, and shoulder; an increase in the muscle: bone ratio; and a decrease in body fat.[8] Affected calves demonstrate above-average weight gains during the first year of life if well fed and managed, although mature size is somewhat reduced. Well-marked grooves along the intramuscular septa in the hindquarters are a distinguishing feature, as is an apparent forward positioning of the tail head. Macroglossia, prognathism, and a tendency toward muscular dystrophy and rickets have been observed in affected calves. Electrocardiographic abnormalities have been reported. The condition often gives rise to dystocia and the need for frequent caesarian section to deliver viable calves.[9] There is also a very high incidence of Elso heel in affected cattle, and this interferes greatly with their economic value. Other associated defects are brachygnathia, deviation of the incisor arch, and, in Belgian Blue and White cattle, greater susceptibility than normal to laryngitis and bronchopneumonia.

CLINICAL PATHOLOGY

Blood lactate is increased, as is susceptibility to stress. These findings are interpreted as being indicators of cell-membrane fragility, which is also manifested by fragility of the erythrocytes.

NECROPSY FINDINGS

The skin is thinner than normal, and the muscle mass is characterized by a disproportionate number of glycolytic anaerobic fibers.

REFERENCES

1. Clop A, et al. *Nat Genet.* 2006;38:813.
2. Druet T, et al. *BMC Genet.* 2014;15.
3. Grobet L, et al. *Nat Genet.* 1997;17:71.
4. McGivney BA, et al. *Anim Genet.* 2012;43:810.
5. Petersen JL, et al. *Anim Genet.* 2014;45:827.
6. Qian L, et al. *Sci Rep.* 2015;5.
7. Sartelet A, et al. *Anim Genet.* 2012;43:604.
8. Kolkman I, et al. *Animal.* 2010;4:661.
9. Kolkman I, et al. *Reprod Dom Anim.* 2012;47:365.

INHERITED SPLAYED DIGITS

Recorded only in Jersey cattle, this defect appears to be conditioned by an inherited gene, most likely a monogenic autosomal-recessive gene. Lameness becomes apparent at 2 to 4 months of age, with the toes becoming increasingly widely spread and the toes themselves misshapen. Walking and standing are painful, especially on the front feet, so that some animals graze and walk on their knees. Affected animals either lie down increasingly or stay standing for very long periods. The apparent abnormality is a defect of the muscles and ligaments holding the phalanges together.

INHERITED PROGRESSIVE MUSCULAR DYSTROPHY

Inherited progressive muscular dystrophy is a primary skeletal muscle disease of sheep with a strong probability of having a genetic mode of transmission. It is recorded in Merino flocks in Australia and is characterized by a gradually progressive failure to flex the joints of the hindlimbs commencing at 3 to 4 weeks of age. Eventually the limbs are rigid at all times, and running becomes impossible. The forelimbs and the head and neck are normal. Affected sheep are easily detected when they are 1 year old and will have mobility problems by the time they are 2 to 3 years old. At necropsy there are pale areas in skeletal muscle and sometimes the muscles of the diaphragm in those sheep that have a tendency to bloat. The histopathology and histochemistry of the muscle lesions are comparable with those of inherited muscle atrophies in humans.

PSEUDOMYOTONIA OF CATTLE, CONGENITAL MUSCULAR DYSTONIA-1

SYNOPSIS

Etiology Pseudomyotonia (PMT) and congenital muscular dystonia-1 (CMD1) are caused by dysfunctional sarcoplasmic reticulum Ca^{2+}-ATPase (SERCA1) that is caused by a mutation in the ATP2A1 gene that encodes SERCA1.

Epidemiology PMT is predominantly observed in Italian beef cattle breeds; CMD1 has only been reported in Belgian Blue cattle.

Clinical findings Increased resting muscle tone; exercise-induced, transient muscle stiffness that resolves within seconds to minutes and may result in adaptation of a sawhorse-type posture or flipping over. Congenital, nonprogressive. Animals with PMT can reach adult age; calves with CMD1 die in the first weeks of life.

Diagnostic confirmation Genome analysis to identify gene mutation.

Treatment None available.

Control Check parents of confirmed cases for presence of gene defect and exclude from future breeding. In population with high prevalence of gene defect, test breeding bulls for gene defect.

ETIOLOGY

Pseudomyotonia (PMT) of cattle is a congenital muscular condition similar to Brody's disease in humans that is clinically indistinguishable from myotonia.[1,2] Congenital muscular dystonia-1 (CMD1) is a condition thus far only reported in Belgian Blue calves that is clinically distinct from PMT.[3] The underlying cause for both conditions was determined to be a malfunction of the **sarcoplasmic reticulum Ca^{2+}-ATPase isoform 1 (SERCA1)** as a result of a **missense mutation in the ATP2A1 gene** that encodes SERCA1.[1,2] It is inherited in an autosomal-recessive manner.[4]

EPIDEMIOLOGY

Bovine congenital pseudomyotonia has been described in Italian Chianina and Romagnola cattle and as a single case in a Dutch Improved Red and White crossbreed calf.[1,5] Congenital muscular dystonia in contrast has only been described in Belgian Blue cattle.[3] Two distinct point mutations in the ATP2A1 gene have been identified, with one consistently occurring in Italian cattle breeds and one identified in Belgian Blue and in one Dutch Improved Red and White crossbreed calf.[4] Although the mutation described in Italian breeds has only be associated with PMT, the mutation observed in Belgian Blue calves, and thus generally associated with CMD1, was also found in the single animal, where it presented clinically as PMT.[1,5]

The incidence of CMD in Belgian Blue calves, which comprises CMD1 but also the clinically similar but etiologically different condition CMD2, has been given as 0.1% to 0.2%.[3] The prevalence of the PMT gene defect in the Italian Chianina sire population used for artificial insemination was 13.6% for the period between 2007 and 2011, and the prevalence in the male progeny selected for a performance testing program was 13.4%.[6]

PATHOGENESIS

PMT and CMD1 are both caused by a malfunction of the **sarcoplasmic reticulum Ca^{2+}-ATPase isoform 1 (SERCA1)**.[1,5] In normal skeletal muscle fibers, contraction and relaxation are determined by Ca^{2+} interaction with contractile proteins. Ca^{2+} is normally stored in the lumen of the sarcoplasmic reticulum, and its release into the cellular cytoplasm induces muscle contraction. At the end of a contraction cycle, SERCA1 proteins pump excessive Ca^{2+} ions back from the cytoplasm into the sarcoplasmic reticulum to initiate relaxation. Impaired function of SERCA1 delays the removal of Ca^{2+} from the cytosol of muscle fibers, thereby prolonging the contractile phase.[5]

CLINICAL FINDINGS

Although PMT and CMD1 are caused by the same gene defect, the clinical presentation of both conditions differs markedly.

Congenital Muscular Dystonia Type 1 (CMD1)

CMD1 is a fatal congenital and nonprogressive condition of Belgian Blue calves.[3] The disease is characterized by exercise-induced pronounced episodes of generalized muscle contractures. During such episodes the affected calf has stiffened limbs and is unable to move or may even flip over with the extremities extended. Impaired swallowing has also been reported, and affected calves usually die in the first weeks of life as a result of respiratory complications.[3]

Pseudomyotonia (PMT)

PMT in cattle is a congenital and nonprogressive disease characterized by a generally increased muscle tone and exercise induced episodes of generalized muscle stiffness. Affected animals are reported to have a stiff or clumsy gait from birth on, and forcing them to move faster than at their own pace will trigger an episode of transient muscle contracture lasting from 20 seconds to over 1 minute. During this episode the animal is unable to move as a result of rigidity of the limbs. It either adopts a saw-horse type posture or may even flip over with all of the limbs extended. After a variable time period lasting from a few seconds to over a minute, the muscle contracture resolves progressively and the animal returns to its normal behavior. Although affected animals are often thought to have a neurologic affliction, the condition is purely a muscular disorder and is not associated with any neurologic deficiencies. In contrast to CMD1, animals with PMT can reach adult age.[5]

CLINICAL PATHOLOGY

Clinically, the condition is indistinguishable from myotonia, a chloride channel disorder, occurring incidentally in cattle as consequence of a spontaneous mutation in the ClCN1 gene (see also "Myotonia of Goats"). Percussing large muscle bellies either with the fingers or a percussion hammer will fail to produce local muscle fasciculation (**percussion myotonia**) in calves with PMT or CMD1, which would be characteristic for myotonia. **Electromyographic examination** is unremarkable, which also allows for differentiation of the condition from myotonia.[1,5]

Genome analysis to confirm the presence of a mutation in the **ATP2A1 gene** is required to make the definitive diagnosis. DNA analysis is also required to rule out congenital myotonia type 2 (CMD2) in Belgian Blue cattle, which is caused by a nonsense mutation in the gene encoding the inhibitory glycine receptor.[3]

TREATMENT

There is currently no specific treatment available.

NECROPSY FINDINGS

Necropsy examination has been not reported to yield remarkable findings.

CONTROL

With the condition being inherited in an autosomal-recessive manner, it has been recommended to test parents of a calf confirmed with PMT or CMD1 for the presence of the gene defect. Parent animals recessively carrying the gene defect are clinically healthy but should not be used for breeding. For populations with high prevalence of the gene defect, it is advisable to systematically check breeding bulls for the presence of the mutations before using their semen for breeding.[6]

REFERENCES

1. Testoni S, Boni P, Gentile A. *Vet Rec.* 2008;163:252.
2. Drögemüller C, et al. *Genomics.* 2008;92:474-477.
3. Charlier C, et al. *Nat Genet.* 2008;40:449-454.
4. Murgiano L, et al. *BMC Vet Res.* 2012;8:186.
5. Grunberg W, et al. *Neuromuscular Disord.* 2010;20:467-470.
6. Murgiano L, et al. *Vet J.* 2013;195:238-240.

OVINE HUMPYBACK

Ovine humpyback is probably a form of heat stroke that affects Merino wethers in western Queensland (Australia). It is characterized by a stiff, short gait when sheep are forced to walk for about a kilometer. The sheep stops walking and adopts an arched-back posture, and the body temperature is significantly elevated. Blood samples reveal a low number of lymphocytes. The condition occurs predominantly in summer, when sheep are in full wool, and the hyperthermia and ataxia disappear when sheep are shorn. Environmental temperatures at the time of the greatest prevalence of the disease are commonly 40° C (104 F).

FURTHER READING

Radostits O, et al. Focal symmetrical encephalomalacia. In: *Veterinary Medicine: A Textbook of the Diseases of Cattle, Horses, Sheep, Goats and Pigs.* 10th ed. London: W.B. Saunders; 2007:2015.

MYOTONIA OF GOATS (FAINTING GOATS)

SYNOPSIS

Etiology Chloride channel disorder caused by a gene mutation affecting the ClCN-1 gene.

Epidemiology Myotonia of goats is the characteristic trait of an uncommon American goat breed, the fainting goat.

Clinical findings Increased resting muscle tone; transient muscle stiffness after startling the animal that resolves within seconds to minutes and may result in adaptation of a sawhorse-type position or flipping over. Congenital, nonprogressive.

Diagnostic confirmation Muscle percussion, electromyography, genetic analysis to identify gene mutation.

Treatment Not treated.

Control Not applicable.

ETIOLOGY

Myotonia of goats describes an inherited condition that is characterized by an abnormal delay in muscle relaxation following voluntary forceful muscle contraction.[1] The underlying cause is a structural and functional defect of the **skeletal muscle chloride channel 1 (ClC1)** that is essential to restore and maintain the membrane potential of muscle cells at the resting level. A missense mutation of the ClCN1 gene encoding the skeletal muscle ClC1 in so-called fainting goats has been identified and has been associated with decreased muscle chloride conductance resulting from a decreased number of functional chloride channels on muscle cell membranes.[2]

Anecdotal evidence suggests that the myotonic goat phenotype is transmitted as an autosomal-dominant trait, although many herds have been inbred, resulting in clinical presentation reminiscent of human recessive generalized myotonia (or Becker myotonia) with recessive inheritance.[1]

Historically the fainting goats played an important role in the process of unraveling the etiology and pathophysiology of congenital myotonia, a condition also affecting humans and other species.[2]

EPIDEMIOLOGY

Occurrence

Myotonia in goats was first reported in the 1880s in Tennessee, United States, where several does and one buck with signs of nervousness and stiffness appear to have been introduced by a transient farm worker.[3] Since then, the progeny of these animals have become established in the area. These goats, which are now a recognized breed, **the fainting goat,** became popular in the region as shepherds used them to protect their flocks from predators. During a predator attack, the fainting goat would become startled and develop a characteristic episode of muscle stiffness, making it an easy prey, while the rest of the flock would be able to make an escape.

Currently there are two strains of this breed, which is indigenous to the United States. The original strain in Tennessee and the eastern part of the United States consists of smaller animals, whereas fainting goats found in and around Texas have been selectively bred for the meat market and are larger and heavy rumped, with a deep chest. The Livestock Breed Conservancy has this goat breed listed as a conservation priority livestock breed, with an estimated world population below 10,000 head.[4]

Economic Importance

Myotonic goats are considered a rare breed. Although historically their main purpose appears to have been to serve as prey animals to protect flocks from predators, this use has fallen out of practice. Today the main purposes are meat production and amusement. Myotonia is generally accompanied by muscle fiber hypertrophy, yielding greater muscle mass, less body fat, and higher bone-to-meat ratio than other breeds. Frequently this breed is kept as pet for its fainting spells for the owners' amusement, which has led to ethical concerns about breeding animals with this gene defect.

PATHOGENESIS

The missense mutation in the ClCN1 gene results in the transcription into a faulty chloride channel 1 protein that reduces the sarcolemmal chloride conductance. With normal chloride conductance across muscular cell membranes, chloride moves in and out of the cell until the intracellular concentration is adjusted to set the chloride equilibrium potential equal to the resting potential. The function of chloride is to rapidly return the membrane potential of the contracted and thus depolarized cell to the resting membrane potential, thereby allowing muscle relaxation. A reduced number of functional chloride channels on the sarcolemmal membrane reduces the velocity with which the membrane potential can be returned to the resting level, which has two important consequences: (1) a lower electrical stimulus is required to trigger an action potential, resulting in increased excitability the muscle cell; and (2) after initial depolarization, the membrane potential very slowly returns to a normal resting membrane potential. Until the resting membrane potential is reached, the actual membrane potential is closer to the threshold voltage needed to trigger a new action potential, which can result in spontaneous action potentials that are not triggered by neuromuscular transmission. Such autonomous action potentials will cause persistent muscle contraction and delayed muscle relaxation after an initial voluntary muscle activity, which are characteristic for myotonia.[1,5]

CLINICAL FINDINGS

The congenital condition that is characterized by a delay in muscle relaxation following an initial voluntary contraction is present from birth and is nonprogressive. Although affected goats are referred to as fainting goats, the condition is a purely muscular disorder and not associated with any neurologic deficits. The severity can vary from very mild to severe, and it appears that goats are able to adjust to the condition with age. Myotonia is not associated with pain.

A typical presentation is a slightly to moderately increased resting muscle tone that may result in a clumsy or stiff gait in animals with severe myotonia. Myotonic episodes and muscular stiffness can be triggered by startling the animal and thereby inducing a forceful initial movement. Because of delayed muscle relaxation, initially contracted muscles remain tensed for a period of between 10 seconds and 1 minute or longer and relax progressively thereafter. During this prolonged phase of muscle contraction, animals may either remain in a sawhorse-type position or may flip over with extended, stiffened limbs. Once muscle contraction resolves, the animal returns to normal attitude and behavior.

CLINICAL PATHOLOGY

The presentation is characteristic, with animals being affected from birth by inducible myotonic episodes. Clinically the diagnosis can be supported by percussing large muscle bellies either with the fingers or a percussion hammer. In myotonic animals, muscle percussion triggers local muscle fasciculation (**percussion myotonia**) that lingers for several seconds. **Electromyographic examination** reveals increased insertional activity when inserting myography needles into muscle tissue and continued high-frequency discharges that outlast normal motor unit responses by several seconds.

To confirm the diagnosis, DNA analysis to confirm the presence of mutation in the ClCN1 gene is required.[6]

NECROPSY FINDINGS

Necropsy examination is not usually undertaken for diagnostic purposes.

FURTHER READING

Lossin C, George AL. Myotonia congénita. *Adv Genet.* 2008;63:25-55.

Tang CY, Chen TY. Physiology and pathophysiology of ClC-1: mechanisms of a chloride channel disease, myotonia. *J Biomed Biotech.* 2011;article ID 685328,

REFERENCES

1. Lossin C, George AL. *Adv Genet.* 2008;63:25-55.
2. Beck CL, et al. *Proc Nat Acad Sci.* 1996;93:11248-11252.
3. Clark SL, et al. *J Nerv Ment Dis.* 1939;90:297-309.
4. American Livestock Conservancy. At <http://albc-usa.etapwss.com/images/uploads/docs/PriorityLivestock2013.pdf>; 2013 Accessed 10.01.13.
5. Tang CY, Chen TY. *J Biomed Biotech.* 2011;article ID 685328.
6. Wijngber ID, et al. *Neuromuscular Dis.* 2012;22:361-367.

MYOTONIA CONGENITA AND MYOTONIC DYSTROPHY

Myotonia is the prolonged contraction of muscle as a result of delayed relaxation. It can be present soon after birth or develop as a progressive disease.

The **congenital** form in horses (New Forest ponies),[1] goats, and Murrah buffalo is an inherited disorder of muscle membrane hyperexcitability caused by mutations in the voltage-gated chloride channel gene CLCN1. The mutation reduces sarcolemmal chloride conductance and delays relaxation of the muscle.[1,2] It is transmitted as an autosomal-recessive trait in ponies.[1] The disease is evident as generalised myotonia evident soon after birth. The disease is not progressive, but there is not treatment. Control is based on breeding programs.

The disease in horses **myotonia dystrophia** is evident as increased muscle tone, increased muscle bulk or muscle atrophy, stilted gait, and weakness.[3] Electromyographic examination reveals the classic myotonic discharges. Affected horses can have testicular atrophy and cataracts. The disease is progressive. There are no characteristic changes in blood or serum. Muscle biopsy demonstrates dystrophic changes, with variations in fiber size and fiber-type grouping. There is no effective treatment, and control is through avoidance of breeding of affected animals.

REFERENCES

1. Wijnberg ID, et al. *Neuromusc Dis.* 2012;22:361.
2. Borges AS, et al. *Neuromusc Dis.* 2013;23:206.
3. Ludvikova E, et al. *Vet Quart.* 2012;32:187.

RECURRENT EXERTIONAL RHABDOMYOLYSIS IN THOROUGHBRED AND STANDARDBRED HORSES

ETIOLOGY

Recurrent exertional rhabdomyolysis is a recognized syndrome in Thoroughbred, Standardbred, and Arabian racehorses. A genetic basis is considered likely, with heritability of 0.42,[1] but has not been demonstrated. Genome-wide scans and linkage analyses map candidate genes to the genomic region between UCDEQ41 and TKY499 on ECA12 (*Equus caballus* chromosome 12) or regions on ECA16 or ECA 20.[1,2] The differences between the two studies, with one mapping to ECA16[2] and the other to ECA12 and ECA20,[1] might be attributable to the study of different populations of horses (North America vs. Japan), phenotyping (disease classification), or laboratory techniques. The RYR1, CACNA1S, and ATP2A1 genes are not linked to recurrent exertional rhabdomyolysis in Thoroughbreds,[3] nor do affected Standardbred horses have the GSY1 mutation identified as a cause of polysaccharide storage myopathy in Quarter horses, draft horses, and other breeds.[4] Mutations in genes expressing monocarboxylate transporter 1 and CD147 are not associated with the disease.[5]

Recurrent exertional rhabdomyolysis in Thoroughbreds is likely to be a complex genetic disease resulting from one or more genes having a major effect, with expression affected by modifying genes, environment, or sex.[2,6]

EPIDEMIOLOGY

Interpretation of reports of prevalence and risk factors for exertional rhabdomyolysis are imprecise because of difficulties in distinguishing the disease from other causes of rhabdomyolysis, including the sporadic disease. The **incidence** or 1-year period prevalence of exertional rhabdomyolysis is as follows: 4.9% in Thoroughbred racehorses in the United States, Australia, and Great Britain; 6.1% in National Hunt Thoroughbreds in Great Britain; and 4% to 5% in 2- to 3-year-old Thoroughbreds in the United Kingdom.[7] The annual incidence in Standardbred racehorses in Sweden is 6.4 (95% CI 4.6% to 8.2%) per 100 horses.[4] Annual incidence in 22 Standardbred training yards in Sweden ranged from 1.7 to 20 cases per 100 horses.[4]

Risk factors for recurrent exertional rhabdomyolysis include exercise and sex. Female racehorses are 3 times more likely to have episodes of exertional rhabdomyolysis than are male (intact or castrated) racehorses, and young female Thoroughbreds are at greatest risk. Among 2- to 4-year-old Thoroughbreds in the United Kingdom, 76% to 78% of occurrences of "tying-up" are in females, and female Standardbreds in Sweden are 7 times more likely (95% CI 2.1 to 23.4) to be affected by the disease than are males.[4] Among National Hunt horses in Great Britain, females are 24 times as likely to have an episode of the disease as are males. Thoroughbred racehorses and Standardbred horses (odds ration [OR] 7.9, 95% CI 2.3 to 27)[4], but not National Hunt horses, with a nervous or "flighty" temperament are more likely to experience episodes of the disease.[8]

The disease occurs repeatedly in 74% of affected Thoroughbred racehorses in Great Britain and in 20% of affected polo ponies.

The disease is of considerable **economic impact** because of its frequent occurrence in athletic horses, its recurrent nature, and the need to rest affected horses.[8] On average, affected Thoroughbred racehorses cannot train for 6 days, and Standardbreds for 7 days, after an episode,[4,8] and approximately two-thirds of affected horses are unable to race because of the disease. The effect of the loss of training days for each episode is magnified because of the recurrent nature of the disease in a large proportion of affected horses. Approximately 6% of the wastage of Thoroughbred racehorses in Australia is attributable to exertional rhabdomyolysis.

Interestingly, Standardbred horses in the United Kingdom with recurrent exertional rhabdomyolysis have enhanced performance.[4]

PATHOGENESIS

The cellular defect has not been identified and fully explicated. Muscle from affected horses has abnormal contraction and relaxation kinetics and is hypersensitive to exposure to caffeine in vitro, but connection with development of the disease is unclear. Affected French Trotters have a characteristic micro-RNA profile in muscle, although this might represent a response to muscle damage rather than the mi-RNA's involvement in development of the disease.[9]

The disease is attributable to dysfunction and death of myocytes with subsequent release of cellular constituents, including the enzymes creatine kinase, aspartate aminotransferase, and carbonic anhydrase, and myoglobin. The proximate cause of myocyte death is uncertain, but it is not related to accumulation of lactic acid.

Cell death is likely linked to abnormal accumulation of calcium in intracellular fluids secondary to deranged energy and/or membrane function. Necrosis of myocytes causes pain and inflammation in the muscle, with infiltration of inflammatory cells. Healing and regeneration of myocytes occurs over a period of weeks in the absence of further episodes of myonecrosis.

Release of cellular constituents results in electrolyte abnormalities, primarily a hypochloremic metabolic alkalosis, a systemic inflammatory response, and pigmenturia. Severely affected horses can have a metabolic acidosis. Myoglobin, and possibly other cell constituents, is nephrotoxic, and acute renal failure can develop as a result of myoglobinuric nephrosis. Pain and loss of muscle function cause a stilted, short-stepping gait.

CLINICAL FINDINGS

The clinical findings are variable and range from poor performance through classic signs of muscle pain, stiffness, and reluctance to move, to recumbency and death, although the latter are rare with recurrent exertional rhabdomyolysis. Most affected horses have more than one episode of the disease each year while in training, and some can have numerous episnodes (up to 20).[4,8]

The most common presentation is of a horse that does not perform to expectation and displays a stiff or **short-stepping gait** that can be mistaken for lower leg lameness. The horse might be reluctant to move when placed in its stall, be apprehensive and anorexic, paw, and frequently shift its weight. More severely affected horses can be unable to continue to exercise, have **hard and painful muscles** (usually gluteal muscles), sweat excessively, tremble or have widespread muscle fasciculations, be apprehensive, refuse to walk, and have elevated heart and respiratory rates. Affected horses can be hyperthermic, especially soon after exercise. Signs consistent with abdominal pain are present in many severely affected horses. Deep-red urine (myoglobinuria) occurs but is not a consistent finding. Severely affected horses are often recumbent.

Among affected Standardbred horses, clinical signs are evident in 98% of horses within 1 hour of exercise. Clinical signs include stiffness in all cases (44), sweating (86%), pain or evident distress (43%), swollen or firm gluteal muscles (23%), and recumbency (2%).[4]

CLINICAL PATHOLOGY

Mildly affected or apparently nonaffected horses have moderate increases in **serum creatine kinase** (CK) (20,000 to 50,000 IU/L), **aspartate aminotransferase** (AST), and **lactate dehydrogenase** (LDH) activity. Severely affected horses have large increases in CK (>100,000 IU/L) and other muscle-derived enzymes. Serum CK and AST activities peak approximately 5 to 6 and 24 hours after exercise, respectively, and in the absence of further muscle damage, serum AST might not return to normal levels for 7 to 10 days. The half-life of CK activity in serum is approximately 2 hours, and in the absence of continuing muscle damage, serum CK declines rapidly. The persistence of increased AST activity, compared with CK, is useful in identifying affected horses days or weeks after the episode.[8]

Serum myoglobin concentrations increase markedly during exercise in affected horses and decline within 24 to 48 hours. Serum carbonic anhydrase III activity is increased in horses with exertional rhabdomyolysis.[8]

Severely affected horses are often **hyponatremic** (<130 mEq/L), **hyperkalemic** (>5.5 mEq/L), **hypochloremic** (<90 mEq/L), azotemic (increased serum urea nitrogen and creatinine concentrations), and **acidotic** or **alkalotic**. Hemoconcentration (hematocrit > 50%, 0.5 L/L) and increased serum total protein concentration (>80 g/L) indicative of dehydration are common. Serum bicarbonate concentration can be falsely markedly elevated in animals with severe rhabdomyolysis because of cellular constituents released from damaged muscle that interfere with the analytical method when automated clinical chemistry analyzers are used. **Myoglobinuria** is detectable either grossly or on chemical analysis and should be differentiated from hemoglobinuria or hematuria.

Measurement of **urinary excretion of electrolytes**, although popular in the past, is of no use in diagnosing, treating, or preventing exertional rhabdomyolysis.

Muscle biopsy during the acute or convalescent stages reveals myonecrosis of type II (fast-twitch, oxidative) fibers, mild myositis, and fibrosis.

NECROPSY FINDINGS

Horses dying of exertional rhabdomyolysis have widespread degeneration of striated muscle, principally the muscles of exertion, but often involving the diaphragm and heart. Affected muscles tend to be dark and swollen but may have a pale, streaked appearance. The kidneys are swollen and have dark-brown medullary streaks. Dark-brown urine is present in the bladder. Histologic examination reveals widespread necrosis and hyaline degeneration of predominantly type II (fast-twitch, oxidative) fibers. In horses with recurrent disease, there may be evidence of myofiber regeneration. Myoglobinuric nephrosis is present in severely affected horses.

Samples for Postmortem Confirmation of Diagnosis

- Formalin-fixed kidney and affected muscle for light microscopic examination (LM)

DIAGNOSTIC CONFIRMATION

Biochemical confirmation of muscle damage by demonstration of increased serum CK or AST activity, in conjunction with appropriate clinical signs, provides the diagnosis.

DIFFERENTIAL DIAGNOSIS (See Table 15-2)

- Muscle cramping induced by ear tick (*Otobius megnini*)
- Ionophore intoxication (monensin, lasalocid, salinomycin, narasin, maduramicin)
- Infection by *Anaplasma phagocytophilum*[10]
- White snake root (*Eupatorium rugosum*) or rayless goldenrod (*Isocoma Pluriflora*),
- Laminitis
- Colic
- Pleuritis
- Aorto-iliac thrombosis

TREATMENT AND CONTROL

TREATMENT OF RECURRENT EXERTIONAL RHABDOMYOLYSIS IN THOROUGHBRED AND STANDARDBRED HORSES

Treatment of Acute disease

- Nonsteroidal antiinflammatory drugs—phenylbutazone (2.2 to 4.4 mg/kg IV or PO q12–24h) or **ketoprofen** (2.2 mg/kg IV every 12 h) (R-1)
- Rest (R-1)
- Fluid therapy—as needed (R-1)
- Acepromazine or similar sedatives (R-2)
- Furosemide (R-3)

Control

- Consistent exercise schedule (R-1)
- Dietary modifications (R-1)
- Dantrolene sodium (R-2)
- Phenytoin (R-3)

The treatment chosen depends on the severity of the disease. The **general principles** are rest; correction of dehydration and electrolyte abnormalities; prevention of complications, including nephrosis and laminitis; and provision of analgesia, and are the same as for all acute myopathies with rhabdomyolysis.

Mildly affected horses (heart rate < 60 bpm, normal rectal temperature and respiratory rate, no dehydration) may be treated with rest and phenylbutazone (2.2 mg/kg, orally or IV every 12 hours for 2 to 4 days). Horses should be given mild exercise with incremental increases in workload as soon as they no longer have signs of muscle pain. Access to water should be unrestricted.

Severely affected horses (heart rate > 60 bpm, rectal temperature > 39° C [102° F], 8% to 10% dehydrated, reluctant or unable to walk) should not be exercised, including walking back to the stable, unless it is unavoidable. Isotonic, polyionic **fluids**, such as lactated Ringer's solution, should be administered IV to severely affected horses to correct any hypovolemia and to ensure a mild diuresis to prevent myoglobinuric nephropathy. Less severely affected horses can be treated by administration of fluids by nasogastric intubation (4 to 6 L every 2 to 3 hours). Although it has been recommended that urine should be alkalinized by administration of mannitol and sodium bicarbonate (1.3% solution IV, or 50 to 100 g of sodium bicarbonate orally every 12 hours) to minimize the nephrotoxicity of myoglobin, this therapy is not effective in humans at risk of myoglobinuric nephrosis. Affected horses should not be given diuretics (e.g., furosemide) except if they are anuric or oliguric after correction of hypovolemia.

Phenylbutazone (2.2 to 4.4 mg/kg, IV or orally, every 12 to 24 hours), **flunixin meglumine** (1 mg/kg IV every 8 hours), or **ketoprofen** (2.2 mg/kg IV every 12 hours) should be given to provide **analgesia**. **Mild sedation** (acepromazine 0.02 to 0.04 mg/kg IM, or xylazine, 0.1 mg/kg IM, both with butorphanol, 0.01 to 0.02 mg/kg) might decrease muscle pain and anxiety. Tranquilizers with vasodilatory activity, such as acetylpromazine (acepromazine), should only be given to horses that are well hydrated. **Muscle relaxants**, such as methocarbamol, are often used but have no demonstrated efficacy.

Recumbent horses should be deeply bedded and repositioned by rolling every 2 to 4 hours. Severely affected horses should not be forced to stand.

CONTROL

Although the cause has not been identified, a number of preventive measures are used, including the following: ensuring consistency of exercise (i.e., every day); dietary interventions to provide a high-fat, low-soluble-carbohydrate diet, with reduction of the amount of soluble carbohydrate in the diet on days when the horse will not exercise; and administration of dantrolene sodium.

Despite lack of clear evidence for a role for **vitamin E or selenium** deficiency in recurrent exertional rhabdomyolysis, horses are often supplemented with 1 IU/kg vitamin E and 2.5 μg/kg selenium daily in the feed. Care should be taken not to induce selenium toxicosis.

Sodium bicarbonate (up to 0.5 to 1.0 g/kg BW daily in the ration) and other electrolytes are often added to the feed of affected horses, but their efficacy is not documented. **Phenytoin** is administered at a dose rate of 6 to 8 mg/kg, orally, every 12 hours, and the dose is adjusted depending on the degree of sedation produced (a reduced dose should be used if the horse becomes sedated) or lack of effect on serum CK or AST activity. Phenytoin can be administered to horses for months, although its efficacy has not been demonstrated. **Dimethylglycine, altrenogest, and progesterone** are all used on occasion in horses with recurrent rhabdomyolysis, but again without demonstrated efficacy.

The feeding of high-fat, low-soluble-carbohydrate diets is useful in the prevention of recurrent exertional rhabdomyolysis in Thoroughbred horses,[4] and dietary modifications that reduce feeding of grain (oats) are common in Standardbred horses in Sweden (and likely elsewhere).[4]

Administration of **dantrolene sodium** (1 to 3 mg/kg, PO q24 h) has been advocated for prevention or amelioration of recurrent exertional rhabdomyolysis, and the pharmacokinetics of dantrolene in horses have been determined.[11,12] Dantrolene reduces calcium efflux from the sarcoplasmic reticulum and is a muscle relaxant. Plasma concentrations are greatest when it is administered with feeding, and feed restriction for more than 4 hours before oral administration decreases gastrointestinal absorption of dantrolene.[11] There is only relatively weak laboratory or field trial evidence of the efficacy of dantrolene in prevention of the disease.[13]

FURTHER READING

Piercy RJ, Rivero J. Muscle disorders of equine athletes. In: *Equine Sports Medicine and Surgery: Basic and Clinical Sciences of the Equine Athlete.* 2nd ed. London: W.B. Saunders; 2014:109.

REFERENCES

1. Tozaki T, et al. *Anim Genet.* 2010;41:80.
2. Fritz KL, et al. *Anim Genet.* 2012;43:730.
3. Dranchak PK, et al. *Am J Vet Res.* 2006;67:1395.
4. Isgren CM, et al. *PLoS ONE.* 2010;5.

5. Mykkanen AK, et al. *Res Vet Sci*. 2011;91:473.
6. Barrey E, et al. *Anim Genet*. 2012;43:271.
7. Wilsher S, et al. *Equine Vet J*. 2006;38:113.
8. Radostits O, et al. Sporadic acute exertional rhabdomyolysis in horses. In: *Veterinary Medicine: A Textbook of the Diseases of Cattle, Horses, Sheep, Goats and Pigs*. 10th ed. London: W.B. Saunders; 2007:1683.
9. Barrey E, et al. *Equine Vet J*. 2010;(suppl):303.
10. Hilton H, et al. *J Vet Int Med*. 2008;22:1061.
11. McKenzie EC, et al. *Equine Vet J*. 2010;42:613.
12. Knych HKD, et al. *J Vet Pharmacol Ther*. 2011;34:238.
13. Holmes MA. *Equine Vet Educ*. 2007;19:97.

POLYSACCHARIDE STORAGE MYOPATHY OF HORSES

Polysaccharide storage myopathy, a myopathy of principally Quarter horses and related breeds, but also occurring with high frequency in draft breeds, is characterized by excessive accumulations of amylase-resistant glycogen (evident as amylase-resistant polysaccharide on periodic acid–Schiff [PAS] staining) in muscle and signs of exertional rhabdomyolysis. One form of the disease is associated with a specific mutation in the GYS1 gene (polysaccharide storage myopathy 1 [PSSM1]) and another with an identical phenotype but without the same genetic abnormality (PSSM2).[1]

ETIOLOGY

PSSM1 is the result of a single missense G-to-A gain-of-function mutation in the skeletal muscle glycogen synthase (GYS1) gene that results in a histidine (H) substitution for arginine (R) in the enzyme.[1,2] The mutation is dominant, with both homozygotic (AA, both H alleles) and heterozygotic (GA, one H allele, one R allele) animals affected. Homozygotes for the H allele are more severely affected than are heterozygotes, as indicated by accumulation of amylase-resistant polysaccharide in muscle and elevated resting serum CK and AST activities.[3] The mutation is conserved in the haplotype of many affected horse breeds, has been present in horses for over 1200 years, and is widely distributed among breeds of horses, with the mutation identified in over 30 breeds.[2] The gene is well characterized in equids.[4]

The etiology of PSSM2 is not known, but it is not associated with the same mutation as PSSM1.

EPIDEMIOLOGY

A polysaccharide storage myopathy characterized by accumulation of polysaccharide in muscle was described in Quarter horses and other breeds and subsequently recognized as being either of amylase-resistant polysaccharide or amylase-sensitive polysaccharide. Approximately 48% of 831 muscle samples from horses with PSSM tested positive for the GYS1 mutation, with 16% of horses with amylase-sensitive polysaccharide accumulation having the H allele and 70% of horses with amylase-resistant having the allele. Of the 831 horses, 31 (3.7%) were homozygous for the H allele (gene AA), 379 (45.6%) were heterozygous (HR for enzyme, GA for gene), and 430 were homozygous normal (RR for enzyme, GG for gene). The presence of the mutated gene (heterozygous form) increases the risk of clinical exertional rhabdomyolysis by 7 times in Warmblood horses.[5]

The disease and mutation are recognized in many breeds, with the greatest frequency in Quarter horses and related breeds and draft breeds worldwide.[1,6-14] Allele frequencies are available for PSSM in horses in the United States (Percheron, 0.346; Belgian, 0.242; Paint, 0.041; Quarter horse, 0.034; Appaloosa, 0.030; Morgan, 0.005; Shire, 0.003; Thoroughbred, 0.000) and Europe (South German Coldblood, 0.117; Saxon-Thuringian Coldblood, 0.068; Shire, 0.000; Hanoverian, 0.000).[14] The GYS1 mutation was detected in 11 breeds, with a prevalence of genetic susceptibility to type 1 PSSM from 0.5% to 62.4%. The GYS1 mutation was not found in the sampled Thoroughbreds, Akhal-Tekes, Connemaras, Clydesdales, Norwegian Fjords, Welsh Ponies, Icelandics, Schleswig Coldbloods, or Hanoverians, but failure to detect the mutation does not guarantee its absence from the breed, although it does imply a low prevalence.[14]

PSSM, based on examination of muscle biopsy from a convenience sample of 164 Quarter horses, occurs in 6% to 12% of overtly healthy Quarter horses in the United States.[6] Allele frequencies for type 1 PSSM among Quarter horses in the United States range from 0.055 to 0.155, depending on the population sampled.[15]

The mutation, and disease, are common in Percheron and Belgian draft horses in Europe, and the disease is reported in Normandy Cob draft horses.[11,16] Of a nonrandom selection of continental European draught horses belonging to 13 breeds, 62% (250 of 403) tested were found to carry the mutant allele.[9] The highest percentages of GYS1-positive horses were found in the Belgian trekpaard (92%, 35 of 38 horses tested), Comtois (80%, 70 of 88), Netherlands trekpaard (74%, 17 of 23), Rheinisch-Deutsches kaltblut (68%, 30 of 44), and Breton (64%, 32 of 51).[9] There is genetic evidence of historical selection pressure in favor of the mutated genotype in Belgium draft horses, but not in American Quarter horses.[17]

The mutation has not been detected in purebred Thoroughbred, Standardbred, and Arabian horses.[1,18]

It appears that the GYS1 mutation arose in heavy (draft) breeds of horses in Europe over 1200 years ago, as indicated by its high frequency in European draft breeds, but not English draft breeds, and the lower prevalence of the mutation in lighter breeds.[9] Light breeds with closely kept stud books that have prevented ingress of genes over centuries, such as Thoroughbreds and Standardbreds, do not carry the mutant gene.

Animal risk factors for exertional rhabdomyolysis include breed (as discussed previously) but not sex or age.[6,19] Quarter horses that carry a mutation of the RYR1 (ryanodine) gene and the mutated GYS1 gene have more severe expression of the disease.[20]

Prolonged periods of rest or irregular exercise schedules are risk factors for development of exertional rhabdomyolysis associated with the disease.

PATHOGENESIS

Mutation of the GYS1 gene causes increased activity in muscle glycogen synthase activity without an increase in activity of glycogen branching enzyme.[2] There is subsequent accumulation of amylase (diastase)-resistant polysaccharide (polyglucosan)—proglycogen and macroglycogen with fewer branching points and more straight chains—in skeletal muscle.[2,21] The reason that accumulation of polysaccharide causes myopathy and exertional rhabdomyolysis is unclear. It does not appear to be related to availability of energy within the cell, although this is uncertain, and it could be related to physical damage caused by accumulation of polysaccharide in vacuoles within predominantly type 2A fibers of homozygous horses.[3]

CLINICAL FINDINGS

The clinical findings are variable and range from sporadic to episodic exertional rhabdomyolysis of varying severity. Notably, 6% to 12% of overtly healthy (asymptomatic) Quarter horses in the United States have histologic evidence of the disease.[6] The acute clinical syndrome does not vary importantly from that of other exertional rhabdomyolysis syndromes. Horses with PSSM1 do not have important cardiac abnormalities as part of their disease syndrome.[22]

Muscle biopsy reveals accumulation of amylase (diastase)-resistant polysaccharide (PAS-positive) inclusions in vacuoles in predominantly, but not exclusively, type 2A and type 2X fibers.[3] Examination of muscle biopsies from candidate horses should be done with consideration of the risk of false-positive findings, especially if the amylase-resistant nature of the polysaccharide is not determined. Horses with PSSM2 will have excess accumulation of amylase-resistant polysaccharide but will not have the mutation in the GYS1 gene. PSSM is most accurately diagnosed in muscle biopsy specimens on the basis of appearance of amylase-resistant, abnormal polysaccharide, not amylase-sensitive glycogen, regardless of fixation technique.[23]

CLINICAL PATHOLOGY

Most Quarter horses and related breeds, but not draft breeds, with the GYS1 mutation have elevations in serum CK and AST at rest.[3] Mildly affected or apparently nonaffected horses have moderate increases in serum CK, AST, and LDH activity after moderate exercise. Severely affected horses have large increases in CK and other muscle-derived enzymes. Serum CK and AST activities peak approximately 5 to 6 and 24 hours after exercise, respectively, and in the absence of further muscle damage, serum AST might not return to normal levels for 7 to 10 days.

NECROPSY FINDINGS

Gross lesions may vary depending on whether or not the horse died from severe rhabdomyolysis or was euthanized after being recumbent. Affected muscles may be pale pink or diffusely red-tinged, which can be mistaken for autolysis. Any of the large power muscle groups and the diaphragm can be affected. The kidneys may be swollen and dark red as a result of myoglobinuria. In chronic cases with repeated episodes, muscle atrophy may be marked, or the muscles may be of normal size but contain pale streaks where myofibers have been replaced by fat.

Microscopically, the presence of amylase-resistant, abnormal polysaccharide inclusions in the cytoplasm of type 2 myocytes is the most sensitive and specific diagnostic indicator for polysaccharide storage myopathy.[23] Other lesions, such as fiber atrophy, internal nuclei, and fatty infiltration, may be present. Muscles most often affected include the semimembranosus, semitendinosus, gluteal, longissimus, and pectoral muscles and the diaphragm.[24]

Samples for Postmortem Confirmation of Diagnosis

Samples of semimembranosus, semitendinosus, gluteal, and diaphragmatic muscles for H & E and PAS stains are used for confirmation of the diagnosis. Frozen sections of biopsies are better suited for studying myopathies because many histopathologic features of skeletal muscle are obscured by formalin fixation.[23]

DIAGNOSTIC CONFIRMATION

Biochemical confirmation of muscle damage is achieved by demonstration of increased serum CK or AST activity in horses with compatible clinical signs. In breeds with known or strongly suspected genetic basis for PSSM1, gene testing for the GYS1 mutation provides evidence of the PSSM1. Confirmation is achieved by examination of a muscle biopsy (see Diagnostic Algorithm in Fig. 15-1). If the muscle biopsy demonstrates the presence of amylase-resistant polysaccharide and the horse is negative for the AA or AG mutation in the GYS1 gene, then the horse has PSSM2.

DIFFERENTIAL DIAGNOSIS (See Table 15-2)

- Muscle cramping induced by ear (*Otobius megnini*)
- Laminitis
- Colic
- Pleuritis
- Aorto-iliac thrombosis
- Other myopathies

TREATMENT

The treatment chosen depends on the severity of the disease. The **general principles** are rest; correction of dehydration and electrolyte abnormalities; prevention of complications, including nephrosis and laminitis; and provision of analgesia, and are the same as for all acute myopathies with rhabdomyolysis (see "Myopathies of Horses").

CONTROL

The feeding of high-fat, low-soluble-carbohydrate diets is useful in the prevention of clinical signs in affected horses with either PSSM1 or PSSM2 and is reported to be useful in controlling the disease.[19] Horses should have a regular exercise program, preferably with frequent turn-out to pasture, and be fed a diet rich in long-chain fatty acids with low starch content (<10%) and high in fat (10% of digestible energy).[25-27]

FURTHER READING

Piercy RJ, Rivero J. Muscle disorders of equine athletes. In: *Equine Sports Medicine and Surgery: Basic and Clinical Sciences of the Equine Athlete.* 2nd ed. London: W.B. Saunders; 2014:109.

REFERENCES

1. McCue ME, et al. *J Vet Int Med.* 2008;22:1228.
2. McCue ME, et al. *Genomics.* 2008;91:458.
3. Naylor RJ, et al. *PLoS ONE.* 2012;7.
4. Echigoya Y, et al. *Molecular Bio Rep.* 2011;38:461.
5. Johlig L, et al. *Equine Vet J.* 2011;43:240.
6. McCue ME, et al. *JAVMA.* 2007;231:746.
7. McGowan CM, et al. *Vet J.* 2009;180:330.
8. Stanley RL, et al. *Equine Vet J.* 2009;41:597.
9. Baird JD, et al. *Vet Rec.* 2010;167:781.
10. Schwarz B, et al. *Vet Rec.* 2011;169:583.
11. Herszberg B, et al. *Anim Genet.* 2009;40:94.
12. Colgan S, et al. *Aust Vet J.* 2006;84:436.
13. Stanley R, et al. *Equine Vet Educ.* 2007;19:143.
14. McCue ME, et al. *Anim Genet.* 2010;41:145.
15. Tryon RC, et al. *JAVMA.* 2009;234:120.
16. Larcher T, et al. *Vet Pathol.* 2008;45:154.
17. McCoy AM, et al. *J Heredity.* 2014;105:163.
18. Isgren CM, et al. *PLoS ONE.* 2010;5.
19. Hunt LM, et al. *Equine Vet J.* 2008;40:171.
20. McCue ME, et al. *Neuromusc Dis.* 2009;19:37.
21. Brojer JT, et al. *Am J Vet Res.* 2006;67:1589.
22. Naylor RJ, et al. *J Vet Int Med.* 2012;26:1464.
23. Firshman AM, et al. *Vet Pathol.* 2006;43:257.
24. van Vleet J, et al. Maxie M, ed. *Jubb, Kennedy and Palmers' Pathology of Domestic Animals.* 5th ed. Edinburgh: W.B. Saunders; 2007:185.
25. Aleman M. *Neuromusc Dis.* 2008;18:277.
26. Borgia LA, et al. *Am J Vet Res.* 2010;71:326.
27. Finno CJ, et al. *Equine Vet J.* 2010;42:323.

EQUINE HYPERKALEMIC PERIODIC PARALYSIS

SYNOPSIS

Etiology Defect in sodium channel of skeletal muscle.

Epidemiology Disease of Quarter horses and crossbreds. Inherited as an autosomal-dominant trait with variable penetrance.

Clinical signs Episodes of muscle fasciculation, stridor, muscle weakness, and flaccid paralysis.

Clinical pathology Hyperkalemia during episodes. Gene probe to detect mutated gene.

Lesions None.

Treatment Palliative. Potassium-free intravenous fluids. Acetazolamide.

Control Selective breeding. Low-potassium diet.

ETIOLOGY

Hyperkalemic periodic paralysis (HYPP) is caused by a heritable defect in the sodium channel of skeletal muscle. The mutation, of which only one form has been identified, results in substitution of a cytosine for guanine, with consequent replacement of phenylalanine by leucine in a transmembrane protein regulating sodium flux across the cell membrane and T-tubule.[1] The disease is transmitted as an autosomal-codominant trait, with the result that homozygotes are more severely affected than heterozygotes, and phenotypic expression (disease severity) differs among heterozygotes.

EPIDEMIOLOGY

The disease is familial and affects Quarter horse and crossbred descendants of a single Quarter horse sire, Impressive. More than 50,000 registered Quarter horses are related to known carriers of the disease. Quarter horses with the disease are presumably selected because they outperform unaffected animals in the Halter classes in which they compete at horse shows, although recent rule changes have changed this practice. The disease occurs in breeds derived from or crossed with Quarter horses, including Appaloosas, American Paint horses, and crossbreds. Of 651 elite performance American Quarter horses, 200 control American Quarter horses, and 180 control American Paint horses (APHs), allele frequency for HYPP in all animals was 0.008, APHs had high prevalence of HYPP of 0.025, and Halter horses had significantly greater allele frequency for HYPP of 0.299,[2] consistent with the alleles associated with the desired phenotype. Approximately 14% of 51 Quarter horses in Mexico have the N/H genotype, with 2% having the H/H genotype. Allele frequencies were 0.157 N and 0.843 normal.[3]

The disease is inherited in an **autosomal-codominant** manner. Therefore 50% of the offspring of the breeding of a heterozygote and a normal animal will carry the trait, as will 75% of the offspring of the breeding of two heterozygotes. Of the breeding of two heterozygotes, 50% of progeny will be heterozygotes, 25% homozygotes for the mutated gene, and 25% homozygotes for the normal gene. Animals homozygous for the abnormal gene are uncommon, representing only 0.9% of animals tested for the disease. The low prevalence of the homozygote genotype is likely a reflection of severity of disease and the reduced likelihood that homozygotic animals will reach sexual maturity.

The risk of a **heterozygous** animal being affected with periodic paralysis is variable. Most heterozygous horses appear normal and never experience an attack, whereas others have severe episodes starting at a young age. **Homozygous** horses are much more likely to have severe manifestations of the disease at a young age.

PATHOGENESIS

The abnormality in the sodium channel coded for by the mutated gene predisposes the horse to episodes of complete depolarization of the muscle membrane and flaccid paralysis. The mutation in the sodium channel increases the probability that any one channel is open, with the result that the resting membrane potential in affected horses is higher (less negative and closer to the depolarization threshold) than that of normal horses. This results in frequent depolarizations of individual muscle fibers, causing muscle fasciculations. The weakness associated with severe episodes of the disease results from failure of sodium channels to close after depolarizations. Opening of potassium channels when the muscle is depolarized results in movement of potassium out of the muscle cell and the development of hyperkalemia.

CLINICAL SIGNS

The disease in **heterozygous** animals is characterized by periods of muscle fasciculation and tremor that progress to weakness, paralysis, and recumbency. Such episodes may last minutes to hours, and most resolve spontaneously. Horses often sweat, have prolapse of the third eyelid, and have contractions of facial and locomotor muscles during episodes. Episodes may be mistaken for colic. Inspiratory stertor commonly noted during episodes is probably attributable to laryngeal and pharyngeal dysfunction.

Episodes are more frequent and severe in **homozygous** animals, and signs of **laryngeal and pharyngeal dysfunction**, such as stridor and dysphagia, occur in almost all of these animals. Endoscopic examination of homozygotes reveals pharyngeal collapse, laryngopalatal dislocation, and laryngeal paralysis. The disease can manifest in foals as young as 7 days of age. The severity of signs in some homozygotes diminishes with age.

Electromyographic demonstration of myotonic discharges, prolonged insertional activity, and doublets and triplets is a sensitive and specific indicator of the disease.

Horses with HYPP have reduced exercise tolerance compared with normal horses. Homozygotic horses have laryngospasm, airway obstruction, hypoxia, hypercapnia, and ventricular depolarizations during intense exercise, which is not recommended for these horses.

CLINICAL PATHOLOGY

Hyperkalemia (>5.5 mEq/L) during or immediately after episodes is characteristic of the disease, although the existence of a normokalemic variant has been suggested.

Diagnostic confirmation has in the past been achieved by provocative testing by administering potassium chloride (88 to 166 mg/kg, orally) to suspect horses. However, the development of genotyping has rendered provocative testing obsolete and, for humane reasons and because of the risk of death, its use is not recommended. The **test of choice** for demonstrating the presence of the mutated gene is a specific **gene probe**. The probe can be applied to various tissues, but blood or hair, with attached root (a plucked hair), are preferred for diagnostic testing of live animals. This test classifies horses as normal, heterozygous, or homozygous but does not indicate the propensity of heterozygotes to exhibit the disease. Samples can be analyzed in the United States at the Veterinary Genetics Laboratory of the University of California (www.vgl.ucdavis.edu).

DIFFERENTIAL DIAGNOSIS

- Colic
- Laminitis
- Hypocalcemia
- Botulism
- Exertional rhabdomyolysis
- Upper airway obstruction

NECROPSY FINDINGS

There are no characteristic findings on necropsy examination.

TREATMENT

Acute Episodes

Most acute episodes resolve spontaneously or with only minor treatment. The aim in treating more severe or prolonged episodes is to **reduce the plasma potassium concentration** by intravenous infusion of isotonic potassium-free fluids such as sodium chloride, sodium bicarbonate, or dextrose.[4] Some authors recommend infusion of calcium gluconate, but others caution against its use. A practical approach is the slow IV administration of 0.25 to 0.5 mL of 23% calcium gluconate per 1 kg of body weight (125 to 250 mL for a 500-kg horse) diluted in isotonic sodium chloride or, preferably, 5% dextrose. Administration of $NaHCO_3$ at 1 mL/kg IV has been suggested.

Prevention of Episodes

Maintaining affected horses on a **low-potassium diet** reduces the frequency with which episodes occur. Alfalfa (lucerne); some oils, including soyabean; molasses; lite salt (a mixture of KCl and NaCl); and many sweet feeds are potassium rich and should be avoided. Grass hay (timothy) and straw and oats, corn, and barley are low in potassium. There are commercial feeds that have a guaranteed low concentration of potassium. Alternatively, diets can be formulated using feed of known potassium concentration, as determined by feed analysis. Care should be taken that diets are nutritious and contain appropriate concentrations and ratios of calcium and phosphorus.

Acetazolamide (2 to 4 mg/kg, every 12 hours) reduces the severity and frequency of episodes and is widely used to control the disease. The drug is poorly absorbed in horses, but the concentration required in plasma of horses to achieve a pharmacodynamic effect is lower than that of humans.

CONTROL

The disease is heritable, and carriers are readily identified; thus, a breeding program to eliminate the disease is feasible.

REFERENCES

1. Radostits O, et al. Equine hyperkalemic periodic paralysis. In: *Veterinary Medicine: A Textbook of the Diseases of Cattle, Horses, Sheep, Goats and Pigs*. 10th ed. London: W. B. Saunders; 2007:1965.
2. Tryon RC, et al. *JAVMA*. 2009;234:120.
3. Riojas-Valdes V, et al. *African J Biotech*. 2014;13:1323.
4. Pang DSJ, et al. *Vet Anaesth Analg*. 2011;38:113.

MALIGNANT HYPERTHERMIA IN HORSES

Malignant hyperthermia is a disease of Quarter horses and other breeds induced by exposure to halothane, succinylcholine, or similar depolarizing agents and various other stressors. It also occurs in pigs, dogs, and humans.[1] The disease in Quarter horses is caused by a mutation in the RyR1 gene, with subsequent dysfunction of calcium handling within the cell.[2] There is excessive release of calcium from the sarcoplasmic reticulum on exposure to halothane, with development of hyperthermia, hypercapnia, and lactic acidosis, and often death.[2] There is no apparent breed, age, or sex predilection for the sporadic disease. Breed is clearly a predilection for affected Quarter horses. The mutation in Quarter horses can be detected by analysis of the genome.[3]

The clinical signs are rapid onset of hyperthermia, sweating, muscle fasciculation, tachycardia, tachypnea, and muscle rigidity in anesthetised horses. There is acidosis, hypercapnea, and, in acute cases, increases in serum activity of CK. Elevations in CK might not be evident in horses that die peracutely. Treatment is supportive and includes prompt removal of the inciting agent (halothane), cooling, correction of acid : base and electrolyte abnormalities, and prevention of myoglobinuric nephrosis.

REFERENCES

1. Aleman M. *Neuromusc Dis.* 2008;18:277.
2. Aleman M, et al. *J Vet Int Med.* 2009;23:329.
3. Nieto JE, et al. *J Vet Int Med.* 2009;23:!619.

PORCINE STRESS SYNDROME (MALIGNANT HYPERTHERMIA)

SYNOPSIS

Etiology Inherited defect caused by an autosomal-recessive gene at a single locus with incomplete penetrance. Also known as the halothane-sensitivity gene, or porcine stress syndrome (PSS) mutation, which is a single-point mutation of nucleotide 1843 in the skeletal muscle gene for the calcium-release channel of the sarcoplasmic reticulum.

Epidemiology Worldwide in major breeds of swine: Landrace, Yorkshire, Duroc, Pietrain, and Poland China. Market-weight pigs and adult sows and boars. Prevalence of defective gene varies between breeds and countries. Syndromes precipitated by stress of transportation, high environmental temperatures and humidity, exhaustive exercise, and halothane anesthesia. Major economic importance because of deaths and poor-quality pork.

Signs

- Porcine stress syndrome: death during transportation
- Malignant hyperthermia: induced by halothane anesthesia; results in muscular rigidity and death
- Pale, soft, exudative pork: rapid rigor mortis after slaughter followed by excessive dripping of carcass and pale, watery pork; dark, firm, and dry pork is a variation
- Back-muscle necrosis: reluctance to move, acute swelling and pain over back; some may die; subacute form also possible

Clinical pathology Halothane test. Blood creatine kinase test. Blood typing. DNA-based test for PSS mutation gene.

Lesions Pale skeletal muscles in PSS deaths. Pale muscles in back-muscle necrosis.

Diagnostic confirmation—necropsy findings. Identification of homozygous animals with tests.

Differential diagnosis list

- Mulberry heart disease
- Acute septicemias attributable to salmonellosis, erysipelas, pasteurellosis, and anthrax
- Intestinal volvulus
- Heat exhaustion
- Suffocation during transportation.

Treatment None.

Control Genetic selection. Reduction of environmental and management stressors.

ETIOLOGY

Considerable attention from breeders has greatly reduced the occurrence of this condition in recent years.

Three closely related stress syndromes occur in pigs. Porcine stress syndrome (PSS) is characterized by acute death induced by stressors such as transport, high ambient temperature, exercise, and fighting, which results in progressive dyspnea, hyperthermia, disseminated vasoconstriction, and the rapid onset of rigor mortis. Pale, soft, and exudative pork (PSE) occurs postmortem in some pigs slaughtered by conventional methods. Malignant hyperthermia (MH) is a drug-induced stress syndrome characterized by muscle rigidity and hyperthermia occurring in susceptible pigs following the use of halothane or the muscle relaxant suxamethonium. Back-muscle necrosis of pigs is a special manifestation of PSS.

Malignant hyperthermia also occurs in humans. PSS is caused by an inherited defect as a result of an autosomal-recessive gene at a single locus with incomplete penetrance. It is also known as the halothane sensitivity gene, or PSS mutation, which is single-point mutation of nucleotide 1843 in the skeletal muscle gene for the calcium-release channel of the sarcoplasmic reticulum. The PSS defect renders muscle hypersensitive to stimulation by various stressors. In stress-susceptible pigs there is a rapid onset of anaerobic glycolysis and loss of control of skeletal muscle metabolism in response to stress and anoxia.

The gene is commonly known as the halothane-sensitivity gene (HAL gene) because pigs with the homozygous genotype can be identified with the halothane test, which results in malignant hyperthermia. The halothane gene is located within a group of blood-type genes on the same chromosome, allowing identification of affected pigs by blood typing. A single-point mutation in the porcine gene for the skeletal muscle ryanodine receptor channel is associated with malignant hyperthermia in five major breeds of heavily muscled swine. There is then massive muscle contraction and release of heat. Comparison of the sequences of the HAL genes of PSS and normal pigs revealed a single mutation at nucleotide 1843 in the cDNA derived from the HAL gene.

EPIDEMIOLOGY

Prevalence and Occurrence

This subject needs to be kept in perspective. It has recently been suggested that only 4% of inferior-quality meat is a result of genetics (halothane positive), with the remainder being caused by preslaughter and post-slaughter treatment.

PSS occurs worldwide, but there is considerable breed and area variation in its prevalence. In some European countries the prevalence is a major problem in pig production because of the inadvertent selection for this trait in genetic improvement programs. This underlies the problems of selection based purely on performance and production characteristics.

The prevalence of PSS in the swine population can be determined by the use of screening tests applied on the farm or when pigs enter swine performance test stations. The halothane test and the CK test are useful for this purpose. A DNA-based test with 99% accuracy is also available. In European breeds, the prevalence varies from 0% to 88%, with up to 100% in the Pietrain breed. The prevalence of halothane susceptibility is low in the Danish Landrace breed in Denmark. Based on the halothane test, 1.5% of young boars entering a Record of Performance Test Station in Canada were positive reactors. The reactors originated from 7.5% of 107 herds. The halothane succinylcholine test was a more sensitive test because 18% of the same pigs were identified as reactors.

Using a DNA-based test, in a survey of 10,245 breeding swine of various breeds from 129 farms in the United States, Canada, and England, approximately 1 of 5 pigs was a heterozygous carrier of the PSS mutation, and 1% were homozygous. The prevalence of the PSS mutation was 97% for 58 Pietrain, 35% for 1962 Landrace, 15% for 718 Duroc, 19% for 720 Large White, 14% for 496 Hampshire, 19% for 1727 Yorkshire, and 16% for 3446 crossbred swine. The PSS gene frequencies for these breeds were 0.72, 0.19, 0.08, 0.10, 0.07, 0.10, and 0.09, respectively. The PSS mutation has also been identified in Poland China and Berkshire breeds. These gene frequencies were 30% to 75% lower in Canadian swine than in U.S. swine, with the exception of Yorkshires, for which the gene frequency is threefold in Canadian swine.

Risk Factors

Animal Risk Factors

Susceptibility to the PSS is inherited, and the biochemical events leading to PSE, transport death, or malignant hyperthermia are triggered by several external influences or stressors in the living animal. PSS probably occurs in all breeds of pigs, but the incidence is highest in pigs selected for heavy muscling, and stress-susceptible pigs are leaner and more meaty. These include the Pietrain and Poland China breeds and also some European strains of Landrace, where a score for muscling and growth rate, feed conversion, and back fat has been included in the selection index. A recent study has shown that there are considerable breed differences, in that halothane-stress-susceptible pigs and Hampshires suffer more severely from heat stress than Yorkshires, Danish Landrace, and Duroc boars.

There is a correlation between halothane susceptibility and carcass traits. Halothane status is the most important factor influencing pork quality, although preslaughter handling and stunning method also influence the carcass quality.

Halothane-positive animals usually score higher for visual conformation of the loin and ham than halothane-negative pigs. The progeny of reactor boars are also more susceptible than the progeny of nonreactors. Until recently it was thought that the major limitation of the halothane test was that it identified only those pigs that are stress-susceptible to the syndrome. It is now known that the halothane-sensitivity gene is expressed in heterozygous pigs, where it is likely to cause poor carcass quality.

Landrace pigs can be divided into those that are sensitive to halothane and develop PSE pork postmortem, those that are resistant to halothane but develop PSE pork, and those resistant to halothane and PSE pork (the normal pig). Muscle from pigs susceptible to malignant hyperthermia and PSE pork has significantly higher glucose-6-phosphate levels and lower phosphocreatine under thiopentone anesthesia than muscle from pigs susceptible to PSE and normal pigs. Altered muscle fiber type is not the primary basis of the disease complex.

Environmental and Management Risk Factors

The most important precipitating factors are transportation at high environmental temperatures and humidity, exhaustive exercise, and, under experimental conditions, the more specific reaction toward the anesthetic halothane. Response of pigs to transport is dependent on genotype, particularly at high temperatures such as 36° C (97 F). Experimentally, psychological mechanisms can precipitate the PSS. The effects of mixing, transportation, and duration of lairage can have profound effects on the carcass characteristics of susceptible pigs. Death during transportation and PSE are associated with fear, defensive or aggressive reactions in unfamiliar social environments, and conflict with other unfamiliar pigs or people. Other activities that may trigger malignant hyperthermia include restraint, mating, farrowing, fighting, and vigorous exercising.

Economic Importance

The economic losses associated with PSS are attributable to mortality from transport death and inferior meat quality as a result of PSE pork. As a result of the excessive rates of production of lactic acid and heat, sarcoplasmic proteins denature, thereby causing a deterioration of the water-binding capacity of muscle. The increased osmotic activity resulting from end products of hypermetabolism causes an influx of water from the extracellular space, resulting in hemoconcentration and increased intramyofiber water content. The muscle becomes pale, soft, and exudative, sour-smelling, and loose textured. The shrinkage resulting from water loss during storage, transport, and processing of the carcass is the major cause of wholesale losses at pork-packing plants. PSE carcasses yield less bacon, and the drip loss from fresh PSE meat is more than doubled compared with normal carcasses. Another cause of lost revenue with MH-susceptible swine is their decreased average daily weight gains, conception rates, litter sizes, and boar breeding performance.

PATHOGENESIS

The molecular basis for susceptibility to the PSS is a hypersensitive triggering mechanism of the calcium-release channel of skeletal muscle sarcoplasmic reticulum. The calcium channel, also known as the ryanodine receptor, plays a critical role in the initiation of muscle contraction. The PSS defect renders muscle hypersensitive to stimulation by various stressors. Stress-susceptible pigs cannot tolerate stress and lose control of skeletal muscle metabolism. The stress may be from external influences such as transportation, fear and excitement, or halothane anesthesia. There is excessive catecholamine release and the sudden onset of anaerobic glycolysis of skeletal muscle, excessive production of lactate, and excessive heat production, which, in conjunction with peripheral vasoconstriction, leads to hyperthermia. Following exertional or thermal stress, susceptible pigs undergo more extensive physiologic change than do resistant pigs. Halothane-sensitive pigs are more susceptible to becoming nonambulatory when subjected to multiple stressors and may be more prone to producing inferior pork products. The blood glucose concentrations are dependent on the MH genotype, with the homozygous-positive animals having the highest levels and the homozygous-negative animals having the lowest. The changes in carbohydrate metabolism at rest in MH-positive animals are caused by latent increases of intracellular Ca^{2+} concentrations. Under physical load conditions there is higher lipolysis, which may be the result of an indirect activation of the lipolytic system via catecholamine-induced cAMP turnover.

Depending on the nature, severity, and duration of the stress, the syndrome may manifest in different ways:

- The porcine stress syndrome causes rapid death following severe stress.
- The PSE pork and dark, firm, dry (DFD) pork are seen after slaughter, which might have been preceded by mild stressors during lairage.
- The malignant hyperthermia is drug-induced.

PSE pork is attributed to increased glycolysis after slaughter. In muscles that develop DFD pork, the muscle glycogen is already depleted before slaughter. When PSE develops in a muscle, pH drops to values lower than 5.8 at 45 minutes after death. In normal muscles, the pH decreases from approximately 7 in living muscles to 5.3 to 5.8 at 24 hours after death. The lower pH in PSE muscles, combined with a high carcass temperature within the first hour after death, causes the proteins in the muscles to denature. This contributes to the pale color of PSE meat and to its reduced water-holding capacity. Development of muscles with PSE characteristics seems to be initiated by a combination of lower muscle pH already at exsanguination and a faster pH decrease.

Malignant hyperthermia is the drug-induced and often fatal stress syndrome occurring in susceptible pigs within 3 minutes following the inhalation of a mixture of halothane and oxygen. Susceptible pigs develop limb rigidity and a hyperthermia, which are not easily reversed and may result in death. There is an increased rate of intracellular ATP hydrolysis leading to a progressive failure of ATP-dependent Ca^{2+} accumulation by the sarcoplasmic reticulum and/or the mitochondria, with a rise in myoplasmic concentration of Ca^{2+} and consequent contraction of muscle. The same molecular defect occurs in lymphocytes from affected susceptible pigs. There is no histomorphometric evidence of cardiac abnormalities in MH-susceptible pigs. The mitochondria from predominantly red muscle fibers have a greater calcium-binding capacity than those from predominantly white-muscle-fiber areas. There is extreme rigidity of skeletal muscles, hyperthermia, tachycardia, cardiac arrhythmia, an increase in oxygen consumption, lactate formation and high-energy phosphate hydrolysis in muscle, respiratory and metabolic acidosis, and a rise in the CK activity and concentrations of potassium, lactate, glucose, free fatty acids, and catecholamines in blood. There is a large release of glucose and potassium from the liver, which contributes to the hyperglycemia and hyperkalemia. There is a marked α-adrenergic stimulation, which is responsible for the heat production in MH-susceptible pigs. However, the β-adrenergic response in stress-sensitive and stress-resistant pigs is inconsistent. The lactic acidemia is severe because of the overproduction of lactate peripherally and failure of normal lactate uptake.

Malignant hyperthermia can also be induced using methoxyflurane, isoflurane and enflurane, and succinylcholine.

Exposing stress-susceptible pigs to halothane or exercise induces glycolysis, but the mechanisms are different. There are no histochemical differences between muscles of susceptible and normal swine. There is some indication that halothane causes a transient but significant vasoconstrictive action, which could be a contributing factor in initiating the severe reactions in malignant hyperthermia. Electron microscopy of platelets from stress-susceptible pigs reveals a defect characterized by dilatation of the open canalicular system.

CLINICAL FINDINGS

Porcine Stress Syndrome (Transport Death)

Death during or following transport to market may be significant and is more prevalent when overcrowding occurs and during the hot summer period. If seen alive, affected pigs initially show a rapid tremor of the tail, general stiffness associated with increased muscular rigidity, and dyspnea to the extent of mouth-breathing. The body temperature is elevated, often beyond the limits of the clinical thermometer, and there are irregularly shaped areas of skin blanching and erythema. At this stage the affected pig is frequently attacked by other pigs within the group. The pig collapses and dies shortly afterward, and the total time course of the syndrome is generally of the order of 4 to 6 minutes.

Malignant Hyperthermia

Malignant hyperthermia is also a manifestation of the PSS. It may be induced in stress-susceptible pigs by stress and injectable (succinyl choline, acepromazine, ketamine) or inhalation anesthesia with potent volatile anesthetics such as halothane or isoflurane. It is characterized by the development during anesthesia of increased muscle metabolism with muscular rigidity, lactic acidosis, a marked increase in basal metabolic rate, increased oxygen consumption and carbon dioxide production, severe hyperthermia and tachycardia, tachyarrhythmia, and death. Death is a result of the peripheral circulatory changes that are produced by severe acidosis, vasoconstriction, hyperkalemia, reduced cardiac output, and hypotension. Once fully developed, the syndrome is irreversible. The syndrome poses a hazard in swine anesthesia, which can be averted by prior medication with dantrolene and has received considerable study as a model for an analogous syndrome in humans. It has also been used as a method for determining stress susceptibility for genetic selection programs.

Pale, Soft, and Exudative Pork

In stress-susceptible pigs, after slaughter, the inferior quality of the meat, with its pale, soft, exudative (PSE) characteristics, is obvious. This is caused by excessive postmortem glycolysis with lactic acid production and a rapid fall in muscle pH, with depigmentation and reduced water binding as a consequence. In affected muscle, rigor mortis occurs rapidly after slaughter but then decreases, so that affected carcasses have been "set" and postmortem drip is excessive. Affected pork has a pH of less than 6 and generally a temperature of 41° C (106° F) or greater 45 minutes after slaughter, compared with the normal pork with a pH above 6 and a temperature less than 40° C (104° F). This causes denaturation of muscle proteins, leading to affected meat that has inferior taste, cooking, and processing qualities and does not accept curing as readily. The occurrence of this syndrome is considerably influenced by the stress of transport and handling before and during slaughter, and this aspect of the syndrome is of major economic importance. Rapid chilling helps prevent PSE, but chill type has no effect.

Dark, Firm, and Dry Pork

Dark, firm, and dry (DFD) pork has darker color and higher ultimate pH than normal meat. In muscles that develop DFD, the muscle glycogen is already depleted before slaughter, which may be related to prolonged transport with fasting.

Back-Muscle Necrosis

Acute necrosis of the longissimus dorsi occurs in German Landrace pigs and other breeds. The acute syndrome lasts approximately 2 weeks and is characterized by swelling and pain over the back muscles, with arching or lateral flexion of the spine and reluctance to move. The swelling and pain then subside, but there is atrophy of the affected muscle and development of a prominent spinal ridge. Some regeneration may occur after several months. Acute cases may die. The syndrome occurs in young adults weighing from 75 to 100 kg. The mild form may be undetectable except for pigs lying down near the feed trough. In the severe form, affected pigs may assume the dog-sitting position with a hunched-up back.

CLINICAL PATHOLOGY

Several testing methods are available for predicting susceptibility.

Halothane Test

The halothane test is highly reliable for the identification of pigs that are homozygous for the single recessive gene responsible for susceptibility to PSS. However, the test is not 100% accurate because of the incomplete penetrance of the halothane sensitivity trait (not all homozygous MH-susceptible pigs react by developing limb rigidity). Penetrance of the halothane sensitivity trait is estimated to vary from 50% to 100% depending on the breed, herd, and investigators. The test detects the worst clinical outcomes, and it will not identify all the pigs that will develop PSE. There is now evidence that it will detect the heterozygote. Stress-susceptible pigs are sensitive to halothane at 8 weeks of age, and if the anesthetic challenge is removed immediately after obvious signs of limb rigidity develop and before the development of fulminant hyperthermia, the mortality from the procedure is negligible. Pigs that remain unreactive for a challenge period of 5 minutes are considered normal.

A halothane-sensitive muscle defect can be present in certain individuals that do not develop rigid malignant hyperthermic episodes on brief exposure to halothane. A longer halothane exposure combined with succinylcholine is required if these false negatives are to be identified. The halothane test has good predictive value for the occurrence of PSE. However, there may be breed variations, as mentioned previously.

A decrease in the amplitude of the phosphocreatine (PCr) signal in the in vivo 31 P nuclear magnetic resonance spectrum of skeletal pigs is an early and 100% predictive measurement for the detection of malignant hyperthermia in anesthetized piglets. Nuclear magnetic resonance techniques such as magnetic resonance imaging and magnetic resonance spectroscopy are sensitive diagnostic aids for detecting the onset of PSS in young animals and for following the metabolic changes in muscle tissue during the syndrome.

Halothane concentration markedly affects the outcome of halothane testing, and either higher halothane concentrations or longer exposure might be required to identify positive reactors in a heterogeneous population. The ionophore A23187, a lipophilic carboxylic antibiotic that binds and transports divalent cations across both natural and artificial membrane bilayers, allows clear differentiation between the muscles of normal and pathologic animals and may be a useful adjunct to the halothane test.

Blood Creatine Kinase Levels

The blood creatine kinase (CK) levels are higher in stress-susceptible pigs. Pigs are subjected to a standard exertion test, and blood samples are taken 8 to 24 hours later and analyzed for CK. The original research indicated a good correlation between CK levels and the halothane test. There is also an increase in CK levels in pigs as they are transported from the farm to the abattoir. However, not all pigs that develop PSE have increased serum levels of CK. Increased CK activity is highest in stress-susceptible pigs of a certain phenotype Phi-B, and their total plasma CK levels are higher than those of nonreactors. The initial test was modified so that blood could be collected as drops on a filter paper and sent to a laboratory for identification by a bioluminescent technique. A recent evaluation of a commercial CK screening test using the method of bioluminescence compared with the halothane challenge test on young boars entering a Record of Performance Test Station revealed that it was an inadequate indicator of susceptibility to PSS or MH. In a different study the CK levels of piglets 8 to 10 weeks of age predicted halothane-induced stress syndrome with an accuracy of 87% to 91%.

Plasma pyruvate kinase activity has been compared with CK activity as an indicator of PSS. Both enzymes are increased significantly in homozygous halothane-reacting pigs compared with nonreacting pigs. Pyruvate kinase activity was less variable within groups than CK activity, which may allow more effective discrimination between the two different genotypes. However, age-related effects and the failure to identify heterozygotes may restrict the use of plasma pyruvate activity as a diagnostic test.

Blood Typing

Blood typing is also used as a method for the identification of susceptible pigs. On one of the chromosomes of the pig, a region with four known loci has been identified. These loci contain the genes responsible for variants of the enzymes 6-phosphogluconate dehydrogenase and phosphoferose isomerase (PHI). The H-blood group system is determined by one of the loci, and halothane sensitivity is also determined by genes at a locus in this region. This region is of special interest because a close connection has been found between this and important carcass traits such as the PSE condition. Thus blood grouping may be used to detect halothane-sensitive pigs and heterozygote carriers.

A DNA-based blood test can now be used to detect the HAL gene status. It can be adapted for rapid batch analysis of many samples simultaneously, is less invasive, and can be applied to as little as 50 µL of blood. The test is more than 99% accurate, is cost-effective, and can be used to determine the prevalence of the PSS mutation in various breeds of swine in various countries. A recent study showed that 23% of pigs classified as Hal-1843–free based on a DNA test responded abnormally to halothane anesthesia.

Pale, Soft, and Exudative Pork

Pale, soft, and exudative pork (PSE) is evaluated by a meat quality index that combines meat color, pH at 24 hours postmortem, and water-binding capacity. Susceptible lines can be identified by carcass inspection and the results applied to sibling or progeny selection. A recent approach is the measurement of mitochondrial calcium efflux. Mitochondria isolated from Mm longissimus dorsi muscle exhibit a rate of Ca^{2+} efflux twice that of normal pigs. Most of the tests readily predict the worst examples of the syndrome but are not sufficiently precise to be able to identify tendencies toward it, which restricts their value in breeding programs.

Erythrocyte Osmotic Fragility

Erythrocyte osmotic fragility may be correlated with malignant hyperthermia and is being examined as a possible aid in the determination of susceptibility.

Other Tests

Any reliable test that can identify stress-susceptible pigs without using halothane testing is attractive. Increased peroxidation of the erythrocytes may be an improved diagnostic test for PSS. Differences in the levels of cortisol, creatinine, aspartate aminotransferase, and lactate dehydrogenase are highly significant between halothane-sensitive and halothane-negative lines of pigs.

An allele-specific PCR (AS-PCR) technique has been developed. A PCR followed by reduction endonuclease assay has been developed and used on plucked hair as a source of genomic DNA. In a test with this method, 9 of 12 Pietrains tested were homozygous or heterozygous. A one-step procedure has been developed called mutagenically separated PCR (MS-PCR).

NECROPSY FINDINGS

In PSS, rigor mortis is present immediately following death, and carcass putrefaction occurs more rapidly than normal. The viscera are congested, and there is usually an increased quantity of pericardial fluid and pulmonary congestion and edema. The muscles—especially the gluteus medius, biceps femoris, and longissimus dorsi—are pale, wet, and soft. In back-muscle necrosis, these changes appear grossly to be confined to the epaxial musculature. Histologically, the lesions in skeletal muscle may be minimal and are easily obscured by autolysis. In some instances only interstitial edema is visible, whereas in animals that have survived repeated episodes there is obvious phagocytosis of degenerate myofibers, with ongoing regeneration and fibrosis. The most typical microscopic finding is hypercontraction of myofibers, characterized by division of the cell into irregularly sized segments by transverse and sometimes branching bands. Degenerate sarcoplasm of a floccular or sometimes hyaline character may be present. Degenerative changes may also be detected in myocardial cells.

Samples for Confirmation of Diagnosis

- Genetic analysis—50 g frozen muscle (DNA ANALYSIS) and hair for PCR tests
- Histology—formalin-fixed skeletal muscle (several sections, including longissimus dorsi), heart (LM)
- Biochemistry—it has been reported that pigs with PSS develop metabolic acidosis in association with respiratory acidosis, which is manifested as lower values of acid–base excess and HCO_3—with higher H^+ concentrations and P_{CO_2} compared with resistant pigs.

DIFFERENTIAL DIAGNOSIS

The acute nature of porcine stress syndrome (PSS) and its relation to stress serve to differentiate it from most other syndromes causing sudden death in market- and adult-sized pigs. The sudden death syndrome must be differentiated from:

- Mulberry heart disease
- Acute septicemias attributable to salmonellosis, erysipelas, pasteurellosis, and anthrax
- Other causes of sudden death, including intestinal volvulus, heat exhaustion, and suffocation during transportation
- Hypocalcemic tetany resulting from severe vitamin D deficiency, which can produce a similar clinical syndrome
- Porcine viral encephalomyelitis, which can also result in a similar clinical syndrome in post-weaned pigs; pathologic and biochemical examinations differentiate these from the PSS

TREATMENT

Early recognition enables successful treatment. Any drug administration should cease. Aggressive cooling using icepacks and alcohol baths should be instituted. The acute syndromes are usually not treated. Several drugs are available for the protection of pigs against drug-induced malignant hyperthermia. A combination of acepromazine and droperidol will delay the onset or prevent the occurrence of halothane-induced malignant hyperthermia. Dantrolene is also effective for treatment and prevention. The therapeutic dose is 1 to 3 mg/kg BW IV and 5 mg/kg orally as a preventative. Carazolol is effective for the prevention of transport death when given 3 to 8 hours before transportation and improves meat quality compared with untreated susceptible animals. Acute back necrosis has been treated successfully with isopyrin and phenylbutazone. Experimentally, the supplementation of the diets of stress-susceptible pigs with vitamin E and C will provide some protective effect on cell-membrane integrity.

CONTROL

The control of this syndrome depends on genetic selection and possible eradication of the PSS mutation and reduction of the severity of stress imposed on pigs.

Genetic Selection

The best strategy for control of this complex is not clear. Several factors must be considered. Swine homozygous for the PSS mutation are at very high risk for developing PSS and severe PSE to make them useful for market pigs. They are used primarily as a source of the PSS mutation for breeding programs and research purposes. Using swine that are heterozygous for the PSS mutation as market pigs may be advantageous. They benefit from the positive effects of the mutation, have minimal risk of developing PSS, and may have acceptable prevalence and severity of PSE, if the environmental and management risk factors that precipitate PSE are minimized during marketing and slaughter. The mutation is not a prerequisite for leanness and muscularity, and it is possible for breeders to eradicate the gene from their breeding stock. The negative effects of the halothane gene on fresh pork quality are well known. However, such a policy may result in the loss of an easily accessible and cost-effective selection criterion for favorable carcass characteristics. The PSS mutation has been used successfully in most swine breeds for increasing leanness and muscling. With the development of the DNA-based test for the PSS mutation, the mutation can be selected for with high precision and accuracy, and its expression can be finely controlled in a breeding program.

The various testing methods described under "Clinical Pathology" are used to identify pigs with the halothane gene. The tests can be applied to breeding stock entering swine performance test stations or on a herd basis. A reliable diagnostic test such as a DNA-based blood test to identify the gene will provide the basis for elimination of the gene or its controlled inclusion in swine breeding programs.

Management of Stressors

Control through reduction of stress is not easily applied because frequently the syndrome is induced by routine minor procedures within the piggery. The incidence of transport deaths or the necessity for immediate slaughter salvage of severely stressed pigs on arrival at the abattoir and the occurrence of PSE meat characteristics are a significant economic problem in some countries. The necessity to climb an upper deck in the transport poses a significant stress, and the use of single-deck transports or mechanical lifts for multiple-deck transports, and the shipment of pigs in containers, has resulted in a decreased incidence. The provision of spacious, well-ventilated transport vehicles and spray-cooling of pigs on arrival at the holding pens is also beneficial. Pigs should not be slaughtered directly after arrival at the abattoir and should be rested for at least 1 to 2 hours if they have been stressed only by transportation. In cases of severe physical exertion, even more time should be allowed for recovery. Where possible transport distance should be kept to a minimum, and transport should be avoided on excessively hot days.

PIETRAIN CREEPER PIGS

A progressive muscular weakness is found in stress-susceptible Pietrain pigs. A similar condition might have been seen in Landrace. It was originally described in one to three herds in the United Kingdom. It is probably an autosomal-recessive gene and is a progressive familial myopathy. In each litter one-quarter to one-third of piglets may be affected. The syndrome commences with muscle tremor at 2 to 4 weeks of age, in the hindlimbs progressing to the forelimbs, followed by reluctance to stand, limbs being flexed, and standing on tip-toe, with walking on flexed carpal joints leading to complete recumbency by 12 weeks of age. At this stage the pigs move with a creeping gait with the limbs flexed. The pigs remain alert and feed and grow normally. There are no neuropathologic lesions, but there are myopathic changes, especially in the forelimbs. In these muscles there are very variable muscle cells with internal nuclei.

FURTHER READING

Wells GAH, et al. A progressive familial atrophy of the Pietrain pig: the clinical syndrome. *Vet Rec.* 1980;106:556.

ASYMMETRIC HINDQUARTER SYNDROME OF PIGS

Asymmetric hindquarter syndrome of pigs was first reported in Germany and Belgium and was recognized in the United Kingdom in 1968. In these cases perineurial fibrosis was a feature, and it was thought that the condition resulted from either a neurogenic atrophy or a periarticular fibrosis extending to the peripheral nerves.

In this syndrome variable asymmetry of the hindquarters is evident during early growth of the animal and obvious by 80 kg live weight. An asymmetric distribution of subcutaneous fat is also noted, and possibly skin dimpling. The muscle most frequently affected is the semimembranosus, followed by the semitendinosus, biceps femoris, adductor femoris, and gracilis. The muscles show changes that can be described as myofibril degeneration, interstitial fibrosis, and dystrophic changes.

Several breeds, including Landrace, Large White, and Hampshire, have been found affected, but the problem is generally restricted to certain herds and to certain families within these herds, suggesting that a genetic liability exists for this condition. The mechanism of inheritance studied from test matings is not simple. Whatever the cause, there is a marked reduction in the number of muscle fibers. Both sexes may be involved, and the condition may involve either hindlimb.

Despite a marked reduction in muscle mass, there is no detectable abnormality in gait. The cause is unknown, although it appears to result from suboptimal muscle growth rather than degenerative loss. In the only cases recorded from outside Europe, a group of seven Australian pigs were examined in detail; in one of these pigs the affected semitendinosus weighed only 41% of the normal, unaffected one. Perineural fibrosis and myopathy have been observed in some cases.

FURTHER READING

Done JT, et al. Asymmetric hindquarter syndrome (AHQS) in the pig. *Vet Rec.* 1975;96:482.

PORCINE CONGENITAL SPLAYLEG (SPLAYLEG SYNDROME IN NEWBORN PIGS)

Porcine congenital splayleg (PCS) is also called spraddle leg, but more usually myofibrillar hypoplasia. This may be an erroneous term because this hypoplasia occurs in many normal pigs and may be a normal feature of postnatal muscle growth. This clinical condition of splayleg occurs in newborn piglets in most countries and is characterized by a temporary inability to stand with the hindlimbs.

ETIOLOGY

The etiology is unknown, but based on epidemiologic evidence, it is multifactorial. The current hypothesis is that the disease is caused by an interaction of genetic and non-genetic factors, a polygenic mode, or expression of many genes without dominance.

Splayleg is not characterized by general muscular atrophy in the affected hindlimbs.[1]

The studies of Czech workers have suggested that the patho-morphology of the condition resembles that of glucocorticoid-induced myopathy in humans and animals. Dexamethasone given to minisows from the first to the last days of pregnancy produced a disorder characterized by splayleg syndrome with retardation of both muscle growth and myofibrillogenesis in their newborn piglets. It has also been experimentally produced following the administration of pyrimethamine.

There may be pathways indicated in gene expression for the further investigation of congenital splayleg.[2] It may be that the combined differential expression of MAFbx (a major atrophy marker) and P311 (a novel protein down regulated in all PCS muscles) is of potential in the diagnosis of subclinical PCS.[3]

EPIDEMIOLOGY

The prevalence of the disease in the United Kingdom is 0% to 4%, and the morbidity in affected herds varies from 2% to 27%. The case-fatality rate is approximately 50% and is attributable to crushing, chilling, and starvation because affected piglets are not able to move around normally. The disease is more common in the Pietrain, Welsh, Landrace, and Large White breeds of swine; Landrace pigs may be especially susceptible. This suggests a genetic basis, but test-matings, with the exception of a few, have not been successful in reproducing the disease. On most farms the disease affects both male and female piglets. In a recent retrospective analysis of the incidence of the disease in a swine herd over a period of 5 years, the overall frequency was 1.74 times greater in males than females, and the birth weight of splayleg piglets tended to be subnormal. The environmental factors that have been associated with some outbreaks include slippery floors, a dietary choline deficiency, and the ingestion of **Fusarium toxin** by pregnant sows. Choline deficiency is unlikely to be a factor, and no other factors have been substantiated as etiologic factors or epidemiologic determinants.

PATHOGENESIS

The pathogenesis of the disease is unclear. In affected pigs there is myofibrillar hypoplasia, but this is also a feature of many muscles in normal pigs. There are simply too few maturing type I fibrils in the muscles, particularly of the foreleg, lumbar epaxial group, and the hindlimb, to carry weight. The semitendinosus appears to be the most significantly affected muscle. However, because myofibrillar hypoplasia may also be present in normal unaffected littermates, it has been difficult to explain the pathogenesis of the muscular weakness. The use of morphometrics has enabled the detailed determination of the myofibrillar hypoplasia. In addition to myofibrillar hypoplasia, in splayleg pigs there is a higher content of sarcoplasmic RNA, reflected ultrastructurally by the presence of numerous ribosomes. The extramyofibrillar space was also filled with glycogen in splayleg pigs. In myofibrillar hypoplasia induced with glucocorticoids given to the pregnant sow, none of the pigs had splaylegs, but the extramyofibrillar space contained little glycogen. There were also many glycogen-filled phagosomes and residual bodies, indicating a difference in the metabolism of glycogen in the first 2 or 3 days after birth. In a study of natural cases there was hypoplasia, but there was an increased accumulation of glycogen, especially within the large extramyofibrillar spaces, in comparison with the normal pigs. These authors also found an anomalous distribution of glucose-6-phosphatase in splayleg-affected muscles, in that the activity was concentrated at the periphery of the extremely dilated cisternae of the sarcoplasmic reticulum. In the normal muscles this enzyme activity was normal. This distribution could account for the slower utilization of glycogen in affected muscles and therefore would account for the build-up. Quantitative image analysis of skeletal muscle revealed that the arrangement of the myofibrils within the fascicles of affected and unaffected pigs was different.

Some studies have found both quantitative (hypoplastic type) and qualitative (dystrophic type) insufficiencies in affected pigs that represent a temporary perinatal developmental disturbance. This could explain the muscular weakness and the recovery that occurs.

CLINICAL FINDINGS

There is a temporarily impaired functionality of the hindleg muscles immediately after birth. Essentially, the adductors are not as powerful as the abductors.

Larger litters may be more affected, possibly because these tend to be born earlier. The clinical signs are usually obvious in 2 to 3 hours after birth when the litter should be standing and walking around the creep area. Affected piglets are unable to stand, their hindlimbs are splayed sideways or forward, and the animals rest in sternal recumbency. Sometimes the forelimbs are also splayed. Most severely affected piglets are unable to move; less severely affected animals are able to move slightly. Many pigs have soiled hindlimbs and perineum as a result of being unable to stand. As a result, the piglets are likely to be crushed or have difficulty gaining access to their source of nourishment. Affected piglets are normal in other respects, have a normal appetite, and will suck the sow if placed near a teat. In the experimental induction there was hypoplasia but no clinical signs, which is further evidence for suggestions that the condition has a threshold for clinical signs and has strong maternal influences.

TREATMENT

Treatment can be successful. If the pigs are able to suck or if they are fed artificially for 2 to 4 days, recovery will occur within 1 week in about 50% of cases. The ambulatory capacity of affected pigs can be improved, and mortality reduced, by taping or loosely tying together the hindlimbs for a period of up to 1 week. The method of loose tying of the hindlimbs consists of a figure-of-eight bandage (2.5-cm-wide adhesive tape) being fixed around the metatarsal bones, leaving a space between the legs of up to 7 cm depending on the size of the piglet. The legs should be tied together within a few hours after the syndrome is obvious; a delay of several hours will decrease the prognosis. The provision of a nonslip floor surface such as a carpet or sack may also be helpful. Many farmers will tell you that repeated massaging of the limbs will also improve the survival rate.

CONTROL

Whether or not to cull the boar depends on the pedigree value of the animal, the incidence of the disease, and the probability that the boar is responsible. There is no evidence that the disease is monogenic. However, the incidence is highest in the Landrace breed, which suggests a hereditary predisposition. In deciding whether to use a suspected carrier animal, there is a need to distinguish between different situations. The consequences of disease are felt differently at the different levels of organization of the pig industry. A boar of high merit for performance traits may be more economical to retain as breeding stock even though some progeny are affected with the disease than a less superior boar whose progeny are unaffected. If stress of the pregnant sow is a factor, control of the disease may be dependent on the selection of stress-resistant boars and sows.

Concurrent disease should be controlled; producers report a higher percentage of splayleg piglets after a period of porcine respiratory and reproductive syndrome (PRRS) infection. There are also suggestions that induced early farrowing and zearalenone poisoning may also be complicating factors to prevent.

FURTHER READING

Papatsiros VG, et al. The splay leg syndrome in piglets: a review. *Am J Anim Vet Sci.* 2012;7:80-83.

REFERENCES

1. Boettcher D, et al. *Dev Biol.* 2008;132:301.
2. Maack S, et al. *Int J Biol Sci.* 2009;5:331.
3. Ooi P, et al. *BMC Vet Res.* 2006;2:23.

Inherited Diseases of Bones

Congenital skeletal abnormalities are relatively common in large animals and can be genetic, teratogenic, or nutritional in origin.[1-3] Exposure of developing fetuses to a wide variety of toxic compounds, maternal mineral deficiencies or imbalances, or exposure to one of a number of infectious agents at certain stages of gestation can create skeletal lesions indistinguishable from those caused by a genetic abnormality. In some cases, teratogenic or nutritional causes of skeletal abnormalities can appear very similar to genetic causes, and distinguishing among them can be challenging.[3] For example, chondrodysplasia associated with intrauterine zinc or manganese deficiency have similar clinical features and histologic lesions to mild forms of hereditary chondrodysplasia.[3] Therefore, historical data are essential in any attempt to distinguish genetic and acquired causes of skeletal lesions; as many animals as possible should be examined, and samples should be collected for future analysis, such as genetic testing.

ETIOLOGY

Over 350 defects in cartilage and bone development are identified in humans.[4] Although substantially fewer are identified in large animals, this large number in humans underscores the many potential diseases in animals. The situation in many production animal industries is compounded by the "founder effect" and widespread use of elite sires by means of artificial insemination that leads to the frequent emergence of recessive genetic defects, which cause important economic and animal welfare concerns.[2,5] Table 15-10, modified from Dittmer and Thompson,

Table 15-10 Inherited skeletal diseases of livestock with known mutations and proposed mechanisms.

Disease	Breed/mutation/OMIA no.	Proposed mechanism
Bulldog chondrodysplasia	Dexter cattle, other miniature cattle breeds Mutated gene, Aggrecan (*ACAN*), OMIA: 001271-9913	ACAN is the main proteoglycan expressed by chondrocytes during cartilage. formation in the primordial limb bud.
Angus dolichocephalic long-nosed dwarfism	Angus cattle Mutated gene; cGMP-dependent type II protein kinase (*PRKG2*); OMIA: 001485-9913	PRKG2 is required for growth-plate development because it regulates SOX9, a critical transcription factor involved in endochondral ossification and the control of growth-plate collagens type II and X.
Ellis van Creveld syndrome 2	Japanese Brown cattle, Gray Alpine cattle	Part of the primary cilia, thought to have a role in regulating sonic hedgehog, a key regulator of skeletal development.
Arachnomelia	Italian Brown, Simmental, German Fleckvieh, and Brown Swiss cattle Mutated gene; molybdenum cofactor synthesis step 1 (*MOCS1*), sulfite oxidase (*SUOX*); OMIA: 001541-9913, 000059-9913	Increased sulfite levels result in atypical bone development.
Osteopetrosis with gingival hamartomas	Belgian Blue cattle Mutated gene; chloride/proton exchanger, lysosomal anion transporter (*CLCN7*); OMIA: 001887-9913	CLCN7 and associated subunit osteopetrosis associated transmembrane protein (Ostm1) are on lysosome membranes and the ruffled border of osteoclasts. Mutations in CLCN7 and Ostm1 impair acidification of resorption lacunae.
Osteopetrosis	Red Angus cattle Mutated gene; anion exchange transporter (*SLC4A2*); OMIA: 000755-9913	The SLC4A2 transporter exchanges bicarbonate ions for chloride ions. As a result of proton secretion during acidification of resorption lacunae, mutations in this transporter result in accumulation of bicarbonate ions, leading to toxic osteoclast alkalinization.
Marfan syndrome	Japanese Black cattle Mutated gene; fibrillin 1 (*FBN1*); OMIA: 000628-9913	Fibrillin is a component of the extracellular microfibrils present in connective tissues. Fibrillins regulate TGF-b and BMP availability, and the decreased bone mineral density and decreased mechanical strength seen in Marfan syndrome are thought to be attributable to increased activation of TGF-b signaling.
Autosomal-recessive hypophosphatemic rickets, type I	Corriedale sheep Mutated gene; dentin matrix protein 1 (*DMP1*); OMIA: 001542-9940	Dentin matrix protein 1 (DMP1) is a noncollagenous bone protein involved in bone mineralization. In addition, decreased DMP1 results in increased FGF23 and subsequent phosphaturia.
Spider lamb syndrome	Suffolk sheep, Hampshire sheep Mutated gene; fibroblast growth factor receptor 3; OMIA: 001703-9940	Mutation removes FGFR3 inhibition of chondrocytes entering the hypertrophic chondrocyte phase, resulting in increased length of long bones.
Texel chondrodysplasia	Texel sheep Mutated gene; sodium-sulfate transporter (*SLC13A1*); OMIA: 001400-9940	In addition to changes in the cartilage matrix, undersulfation of cartilage proteoglycans leads to altered Indian hedgehog signaling, resulting in decreased chondrocyte proliferation.[2,5]
Schmid metaphyseal chondrodysplasia	Yorkshire pig Mutated gene; collagen, type X, alpha 1 chain (*COL10A1*); OMIA: 001718-9825	Type X collagen is expressed by hypertrophic chondrocytes, and this mutation prevents trimerization of the collagen X chains.
Vitamin D–dependent rickets type I	Hannover pig Mutated gene, 25-hydroxyvitamin D 1-α-hydroxylase (*CYP27B1*); OMIA: 000837-9825	CYP27B1 is required for the formation of active vitamin D (1,25-dihydroxyvitamin D). Decreased active vitamin D leads to hypocalcemia and hypophosphatemia, impaired cartilage and bone mineralization, and decreased chondrocyte apoptosis.

Modified from Dittmer and Thompson.[3]

provides a listing of currently recognized inherited skeletal diseases of livestock, the associated mutations, and mechanisms underlying the disease.[3]

PATHOGENESIS

Bone development and remodeling is a complex process involving timely expression and control of numerous genes and epigenetics factors, and there is increasing understanding of the role of these factors in creation of bone and cartilage.[4,6] The large number of genes involved in osteogenesis and cartilage formation and development, and the crucial and nonredundant role of many of these genes, means that a wide range of skeletal defects occur in humans and domestic animals. A variety of transcription and growth factors are identified as being involved in the pathogenesis of skeletal defects. This allows etiologic, rather than morphologic, classification of diseases and abnormalities. **Osteochondrodysplasia** (or skeletal dysplasia) includes generalized abnormalities in chondro-osseous tissues, whereas *dysostosis* refers to a localized malformation of an individual bone or group of bones.[2] Osteochondrodysplasias are now mostly classified according to the underlying defect, rather than the morphologic presentation.[7] Most of the skeleton develops through processes involving endochondral ossification, and abnormalities in cartilage formation or structure can have widespread effects on the skeleton. Defects in cartilage formation that result in skeletal abnormalities are called **chondrodysplasia. Achondroplasia**, referring to an absence of cartilage, should be reserved for diseases characterized by a lack of cartilage, rather than abnormalities in its composition or structure.[2]

CLINICAL FINDINGS

Animals with acquired defects often have substantial variation in clinical signs and lesions and can improve over time, whereas animals with disease caused by genetic defects usually have a consistent clinical presentation and pathology. Clinical signs of the various diseases are described under those headings.

Diagnosis

If a disease is determined to be of genetic origin, a number of approaches can be used to detect mutations, include sequencing candidate genes, single-nucleotide polymorphism array with genome-wide association studies, and exome or whole-genome sequencing.[3] Use of genome-wide, high-density single-nucleotide polymorphism (SNP) panels, or next-generation genomic analysis, combined with an understanding of livestock populations, allows for rapid positional identification of genes and mutations that cause inherited defects.[5] However, a thorough understanding of the history of the animal's disease, its clinical presentation, and its lesions is essential for establishing a reliable diagnosis.

Differential diagnoses for inherited skeletal diseases of animals are shown in Table 15-11 (modified from Dittmer and Thompson).[3]

TREATMENT AND CONTROL

There is no effective treatment for genetic diseases, and affected animals are usually euthanized. Control is based on an understanding of the mode of inheritance, identification of carrier animals (for diseases with recessive inheritance), and selective breeding or testing and removal of heterozygotes from the breeding pool.

FURTHER READING

Thompson KG, et al. Inherited disorders of skeletal development in sheep. *Vet J*. 2008;177:324-333.

Online Mendelian Inheritance of Animals. University of Sydney. (Accessed June 30, 2016 at <http://omia.angis.org.au/home/>.)

REFERENCES

1. Thompson KG. *Small Rumin Res*. 2008;76:112.
2. Thompson KG, et al. *Vet J*. 2008;177:324.
3. Dittmer KE, et al. *Vet Pathol*. 2015;52:851.
4. Krakow D, et al. *Genet Med*. 2010;12:327.
5. Charlier C, et al. *Nat Genet*. 2008;40:449.
6. Pitsillides AA, et al. *Nat Rev Rheum*. 2011;7:654.
7. Rimoin DL, et al. *Am J Med Genet*. 1998;79:376.

INHERITED OSTEOGENESIS IMPERFECTA

The term *osteogenesis imperfecta* covers a heterogeneous group of connective tissue diseases caused by quantitative or qualitative defects in type I collagen.

The disease is recorded as being inherited in Holstein–Friesian cattle and New Zealand Romney sheep.

Cattle

It is transmitted as an autosomal-dominant trait. Calves are clinically abnormal at birth, with the main presenting signs being bright-pink teeth and slackness of the flexor tendons on all four feet so that the animals are unable to stand. The calves become progressively worse, to the point where they cannot walk. The full list of abnormalities in this syndrome includes smaller-than-normal body size at birth, a dome-shaped cranial vault, and fragility of bones, manifested by multiple fractures occurring during birth. The defect is one of connective tissue cells in which there is a faulty production of collagen and intercellular cement. Radiologic examination demonstrates growth-arrest lines and multiple fractures in the long bones and thin dentine and enamel layers on the teeth, which are pink because of the exposed condition of the enlarged pulp. The excessive mobility of the joints results from the small bulk of the ligaments and tendons.

A syndrome of simple bone fragility occurs in Charolais cattle and is called osteogenesis imperfecta.

Sheep

The disease in New Zealand Romney sheep[1] is similar to that in Holstein–Friesian cattle with additional lesions of thickness of the diaphyses and reduction in size of the medullary cavity, moderate brachygnathia inferior, subcutaneous edema, skin fragility, and a dark blue color of the sclera. It is inherited as an autosomal dominant trait, and was thought to have developed as a new mutation in the testicular cell line of the parent ram.

REFERENCE

1. Thompson KG, et al. *Vet J*. 2008;177:324.

INHERITED DWARFISM

Most inherited food animal dwarfs are chondrodysplastic, and the disease occurs in cattle and sheep.

Sheep

Brazilian hair sheep of the Cabugi breed, which are typically shorter and more compact than other breeds, have a form of skeletal dysplasia characterized by lambs born with craniofacial abnormalities and dwarfism that die at 2 to 6 months of age.[1] Dwarf lambs are much smaller than normal, with short legs, a domed head with superior brachygnathism, sternal deformities, and exophthalmic eyes situated more laterally in the head than normal. There is disproportionate shortening of the appendicular bones. The disease is inherited as an incomplete dominant trait, with the shortened face, a feature of the Cabugi breed, representing the heterozygous state and the more severe, often lethal, dwarfism occurring in homozygotes.

A syndrome of **dwarfism, brachygnathia, cardiomegaly, and renal hypoplasia syndrome** occurs in Poll Merino/Merino sheep in Australia.[2] The disease is a lethal genetic disorder associated with homozygosity in genetic material located toward the distal end of chromosome OAR2, from 220,932,050 to 221,939,408, which includes approximately 25 genes.[3] Segregation analysis suggests the disorder is transmitted as an autosomal trait with a recessive mode of inheritance. Affected lambs are dwarfs with multiple defects in the skeleton, heart, liver, and kidneys.

Cattle

Snorter Dwarfs

Snorter dwarfs are no longer important because of successful efforts in eliminating carriers of the gene. These calves are short-legged with short, wide heads and protruding lower jaws. The mandibular teeth may protrude 2 to 4 cm beyond the dental pad, preventing effective grazing and necessitating hand-feeding if the animal is to survive. There is protrusion of the forehead and distortion of the maxillae, and obstruction of the respiratory passages results in stertorous respiration and dyspnea. The tip of the tongue usually protrudes from the mouth, and the eyes bulge. There is some variation between affected animals in their appearance at birth. In most cases the defects are as just described, but they become more exaggerated as the calf grows. In addition, abdominal enlargement and persistent bloat develop. The head is disproportionately large. The calves fail to grow normally and are about half the weight of normal calves of the same age.

The predominant form of the condition appears to be inherited as a simple recessive character, although the relationship of the "compress" types to the total syndrome is more complex. Heterozygotes vary widely in conformation, but some of them show minor defects that may be attractive to cattle breeders who were seeking a chunkier, short-legged type of animal. For this reason, indiscriminate selection toward the heterozygote undoubtedly occurred, resulting in widespread dissemination of the character. Herefords and Aberdeen Angus are the breeds most commonly affected, but similar dwarfs occur also in Holstein and Shorthorn cattle, and typical dwarf animals have been produced by mating heterozygous Aberdeen Angus and Herefords. Besides the shortness of limbs, there is also a looseness of attachment of limbs and abnormal mobility of joints. The disorder of dolichocephalic long-nosed dwarfism in American Angus cattle is attributable to a nonsense mutation in exon 15 of cGMP-dependent type II protein kinase (PRKG2).[4]

Ellis van Creveld syndrome (bovine chondrodysplastic dwarfism) occurs Grey Alpine cattle, Japanese Brown cattle, and

Table 15-11 Differential diagnoses for inherited skeletal diseases of animals

Disease	Clinical signs and lesions
Abnormal head shape	
Genetic	Usually has recessive inheritance, so only small numbers of animals affected. Breeds: Angus, Dexter, Japanese Brown, Tyrolean Grey, and Holstein–Friesian cattle; Texel, Merino, and Cabugi sheep; Danish Landrace pigs. Clinical signs have a consistent presentation, typically with minimal variation. Normal liver zinc and manganese concentrations. Shortened long bones (mild to severe depending on the gene affected), epiphyses potentially mushroomed, domed head, + brachygnathia inferior. Decreased thickness of physes, particularly hypertrophic zone; histologic lesions present in severe forms but mild or nonexistent in other forms.
Chondroplasia—nutritional	Prevalence generally higher than expected for inherited forms of chondrodysplasia. History of drought or adverse weather events during pregnancy and exposure of pregnant animals to unusual supplementary feeding or toxic plants. Variation in severity of dwarfism and twisted limbs; animals with mild cases improve after birth. Shortened long bones, epiphyses can be mushroomed. Decreased thickness of physes, particularly hypertrophic zone; histologically, lesions may be mild or nonexistent. Low liver zinc or manganese concentrations; if deficiency occurred for a finite period during gestation, zinc or manganese concentrations can return to normal.
Plant toxins	*Veratrum californicum* toxicity in sheep: shortening metacarpal/metatarsal + other bones, fusion of metacarpal bones, arthrogryposis, hypermobility of hock joints. Wild lupins (*Lupinus* spp.): cattle; shortening and rotation of limb bones, flexion contracture, arthrogryposis.
Vitamin A intoxication	Pigs: shortening of long bones, abnormally shaped long bones and carpal/tarsal bones, osteoporosis. Calves: possibly associated with "'hyena disease"; premature closure of hindlimb growth plates, segmental narrowing of physes.
Vertebral abnormalities	
Brachyspina	Cattle; smaller-than-normal size, shortened vertebral column as a result of fusion of vertebrae, and long thin limbs. Irregular areas of ossification separated by cartilage, fusion of epiphyses, and diaphysis of adjacent vertebrae.
Complex vertebral malformation	Cattle; smaller-than-normal size, consistent arthrogryposis of forelimbs + hindlimbs, shortening of cervical and thoracic vertebral column, hemivertebrae, fused vertebrae, scoliosis. Cardiac abnormalities in ~50% of cases.
Shortened spine	*Veratrum californicum:* cattle; decreased coccygeal vertebrae, arthrogryposis. Parbendazole toxicosis: compression/fusion vertebrae, absence of various limb bones, curvature of long bones.
Scoliosis, kyphosis, torticollis	Wild lupins: see also craniofacial defects and shortened limbs. Conium maculatum: cattle, sheep, pigs; + arthrogryposis, carpal flexure, cleft palate *Nicotiana tabacum, N. glauca:* cattle/pigs; + arthrogryposis, brachygnathia. Locoweed (*Astragalus* spp., *Oxytropis* spp.): cattle/sheep; also brachygnathia. *Lathyru* spp., *Vicia* spp.: cattle/sheep; + arthrogryposis, rotation of forelimbs.
Manganese deficiency	Cattle; congenital spinal stenosis and premature closure of growth plates associated with Mn deficiency but not proven.
Limb abnormalities	
Syndactyly	Autosomal recessive with incomplete penetrance and variable expression in Holstein–Friesian, Angus, Chianina, Hereford, Simmental, German Red Pied, Indian Hariana, and Japanese native cattle. Right forelimb most commonly involved, but all limbs may be affected. *Veratrum californicum* toxicosis in cattle.
Angular limb deformity	*Trachymene* spp.: sheep; outward bowing, particularly of forelimbs. Locoweed (*Astragalus* spp., *Oxytropis* spp.): cattle/sheep; also limb contractures, osteoporosis.
Congenital hyperostosis	Severe edema: soft tissues of limbs (particularly antebrachium). Radiating trabeculae of new periosteal bone.
Tibial hemimelia	Bilateral tibial hemimelia, cryptorchidism, ventral abdominal hernia, + meningocele.
Abnormalities in multiple axial and appendicular bones	
Spider lamb syndrome	Excessively long limbs and neck leading to angular limb deformities, scoliosis/kyphosis, sternal deformities, Roman nose, degenerative joint disease. Multiple irregular islands of ossification in epiphyseal cartilage.
Schmallenberg virus, Akabane virus, bunyaviruses	Arthrogryposis (Schmallenberg, Akabane); torticollis, kyphosis, scoliosis, lordosis (Schmallenberg); brachygnathia inferior (Schmallenberg); and central nervous system abnormalities (Schmallenberg, Akabane, bluetongue virus).
Plant toxins	Wild lupins, *Conium maculatum, Nicotiana* spp.

Modified from Dittmer KE, Thompson KG. Approach to investigating congenital skeletal abnormalities in livestock. Veterinary pathology. 2015; 52:851.

Tyrolean Grey cattle, in which it is an autosomal-recessive defect with the phenotype of short limbs, joint abnormality, and ateliosis.[5,6] Long bones of affected animals have insufficient endochondral ossification with irregularly arranged chondrocyte, abnormal formation of cartilaginous matrix, and partial disappearance of the epiphyseal growth plates. The mutated gene is Ellis van Creveld syndrome 2 gene (EVC2),[5,6] also known as LIMBIN; OMIA: 000187-9913, causing a defect in the primary cilia, which is thought to have a role in regulating sonic hedgehog, a key regulator of skeletal development.

These disorders should not be mistaken for chondrodysplasia caused by nutritional deficiencies, which characteristically occur with a much higher incidence in affected herds after periods of drought or nutritional stress.[7-9]

Inherited Congenital Achondroplasia With Hydrocephalus

First recorded as **bulldog calves** in Dexter cattle, this inherited defect has since been observed in a variety of forms in other breeds, including Jerseys, Guernseys, Holsteins, and Japanese Brown cattle. Chondrodysplasia in the Holstein–Friesian breed sharing morphologic features with the Dexter bulldog calves have been reported from the United States, the Netherlands, Great Britain, and recently in Denmark. Dexter bulldog–type calves have occurred in French and Danish Holstein calves in a familial pattern related to the sire Igale Masc, and it is likely that the genetic disorder is present in the Holstein breed worldwide.

Characteristic features of lethal chondrodysplasia (Dexter bulldog) calves in Australian Dexter cattle include abortion, disproportionate dwarfism, a short vertebral column, marked micromelia, a relatively large head with retruded muzzle, cleft palate and protruding tongue, and a large abdominal hernia.[5] Histologic changes in limb bones are consistent with failure of endochondral ossification. Dexter chondrodysplasia is considered to be inherited in an incompletely dominant manner, with the homozygous form producing the congenital lethal condition. Based on analysis of the contribution of three obligate heterozygotes whose semen has been widely used in artificial insemination in Australia, it is estimated that the heterozygote frequency is 19% within the registered Australian Dexter herd.

Affected calves are often aborted, but some reach full term and cause fetal dystocia because of the extreme hydrocephalus. The forehead bulges over a foreshortened face with a depressed, short nose. The tongue protrudes, the palate is cleft or absent, the neck is short and thick, and the limbs are shortened. Accompanying defects are fetal anasarca and hydrops amnii in the dam.

The defect is primarily chondrodystrophy rather than achondroplasia; the nasal bones and maxillae do not grow. Hydrocephalus develops because of the deformed cranium. In most breeds the condition is inherited as a simple recessive character, but a dominant form has occurred in Jerseys. The heterozygous form in Dexters is easily recognized by the shortness of the limbs. The heterozygote in other breeds is normal in appearance.

Miscellaneous Dwarfs

Other types of dwarfs have been described and include **"compress"** and **"compact"** cattle in Herefords and Shorthorns and various other forms of **proportional dwarfs**. For example, in Charolais, miniature calves have been recorded that are exact replicas of normal calves but weigh only 5 to 16 kg at birth and are born 2 or more weeks prematurely. Most are dead at birth or die soon after so that the condition is effectively lethal. Proportional dwarfs occur also in Simmentals.

Other forms of chondrodystrophy, including "bulldog calves" and a form that causes fatal nasal obstruction in the German Black Spotted breed of cattle, have also been recorded. In the latter there are multiple deformities of limb bones, and the condition appears to be inherited as a result of the influence of a single recessive gene.

REFERENCES

1. Dantas FPM, et al. *J Comp Pathol.* 2014;150:245.
2. Shariflou MR, et al. *Aust Vet J.* 2011;89:254.
3. Shariflou MR, et al. *Anim Genet.* 2013;44:231.
4. Koltes JE, et al. *Proc Nat Acad Sci.* 2009;106:19250.
5. Murgiano L, et al. *PLoS ONE.* 2014;9.
6. Muscatello LV, et al. *Vet Pathol.* 2015;52:957.
7. Dittmer KE, et al. *NZ Vet J.* 2015;63:174.
8. White PJ, et al. *Prev Vet Med.* 2010;94:178.
9. White PJ, et al. *Vet J.* 2012;193:336.

CONGENITAL OSTEOPETROSIS

Osteopetrosis is a skeletal disorder of humans and animals characterized by the formation of overly dense bones. The disease is reported in Angus, Red Angus, Hereford, Simmental, and Holstein cattle.[1] The inherited defect is recorded in Aberdeen Angus calves, which are stillborn and undersized. The major manifestations are shortening of the mandible with protrusion of the tongue, impaction of the lower molars, a patent fontanelle, and the characteristic lesion of shortness of the long bones and absence of a marrow cavity in them. The absence of the marrow cavity, caused by defective remodeling of the bone, gives it a homogeneous shaft, leading to the colloquial name of "marble bone." Genetically affected calves are typically aborted late in gestation, display skull deformities, and exhibit a marked reduction of osteoclasts. The disease is caused by a deletion mutation within bovine SLC4A2,[1] encoding an anion exchanger protein, causing loss of SLC4A2 function that induces premature cell death and likely results in cytoplasmic alkalinization of osteoclasts, which, in turn, may disrupt acidification of resorption lacunae.

REFERENCE

1. Meyers SN, et al. *BMC Genet.* 2010;11.

INHERITED PROBATOCEPHALY (SHEEPSHEAD)

This defect is inherited in Limousin cattle. The cranial bones are deformed so that the head resembles that of a sheep. The accompanying defects in the heart, buccal cavity, tongue, and abomasum increase the chances of an early death.

INHERITED ATLANTO-OCCIPITAL DEFORMITY

(See "Congenital Defects of the Nervous System.")

INHERITED AGNATHIA

Partial or complete absence of the mandibles with ventral displacement of the ears occurs in sheep and is categorized as a lethal recessive because the sheep are unable to graze properly.

INHERITED DISPLACED MOLAR TEETH

Inherited as a simple recessive character, the defect of displaced molar teeth usually results in the death of affected calves within the first week of life. The six premolars of the lower jaw are impacted or erupted in abnormal positions, often at grotesque angles. The mandible is shorter and narrower than normal. There is no abnormality of the incisors or upper jaw.

INHERITED JAW MALAPPOSITION

Defective apposition of upper and lower incisors, or lower incisors and dental pad, in ruminants may result in inefficient grazing and malnutrition. Abnormal protrusion of the mandible (mandibular **prognathism**) is of most importance in ruminants, and there is good evidence that abnormal length of the mandible is inherited. Among British breeds of **cattle** the defect is more common in beef than in dairy breeds. In Herefords and Angus the inheritance is thought to be conditioned by a single recessive gene.

Brachygnathia, underdevelopment of the mandible, has also been recorded in Dairy Shorthorn, Jersey, Holstein, Ayrshire, and Simmental cattle, with the defect so severe in some cases that the animals are unable to suck. In Angus cattle, brachygnathia can occur linked to a generalized degenerative joint disease, in which all joint surfaces are involved. Affected animals, detected at a few days to 4 months of age, are not viable. Inheritance of the defect is probably conditioned by a recessive gene.

A less severe degree of **brachygnathia** has been recorded in Merino and Rambouillet **sheep**. The mode of inheritance is suggested to be by the interaction of several pairs of genes. Brachygnathia occurs in Poll Merinos in Australia as part of the lethal brachygnathia, cardiomegaly, and renal hypoplasia syndrome.[1] The disorder is also caused by intrauterine infection by the Schmallenburg virus.[2]

Mandibular prognathism occurs as a part of other, more general defects, including achondroplastic dwarfism and inherited displaced molar teeth. It is associated with mutations in the MATN1 gene in donkeys.[3]

Brachygnathia is also seen in **horses** but is not recognized as inherited. Maxillary prognathism is associated with two SNPs within a region on the distal end of chromosome ECA 13 in horses.[4]

REFERENCES

1. Shariflou MR, et al. *Anim Genet.* 2013;44:231.
2. Wagner H, et al. *Berliner Munchener Tierarztliche Wochenschrift.* 2014;127:115.
3. Rodrigues JB, et al. *Gene.* 2013;522:70.
4. Signer-Hasler H, et al. *PLoS ONE.* 2014;9.

INHERITED CRANIOSCHISIS (CRANIUM BIFIDUM)

The disease occurs in a number of pig breeds, but has been shown to be inherited only in Poland China pigs and their crossbreds. There is a deficit in the cranial bones, and meningoceles or encephaloceles may result. The pigs are not viable. Genetic experiments have shown the inheritance to be of a recessive character with varying penetrance.

Many single cases of cranial and spinal deformity in farm animals have been likened to the human Arnold–Chiari malformation, but a specific syndrome of protrusion of the medulla oblongata and the cerebellum through the foramen magnum into the spinal canal has not been identified in a hereditary context in these species. Cases of cranium bifidum are reported on lambs and calves, but the inherited basis, if any, is unclear.[1-3]

REFERENCES

1. Lopez MJ, et al. *Large Anim Pract.* 2000;21:16.
2. Mirshahi A, et al. *Iran J, Vet Surg.* 2012;7:85.
3. Yadegari M, et al. *Res Op Anim Vet Sci.* 2013;3:387.

INHERITED CRANIOFACIAL DEFORMITY

The defect is incompatible with life. One form in Border Leicester lambs is characterized by a variable degree of nasomaxillary hypoplasia, often associated with incomplete cerebral development with less pronounced sulci and gyri than normal. It appears to be inherited in a simple autosomal-recessive mode. A similar lethal defect is recorded in Angus cattle (as brachygnathia superior) in association with generalized degenerative joint disease.

Cyclopia (cyclops anomaly) is commonly associated with ingestion of plants, such as *Veratrum californicum,* containing cyclopamine, which is an inhibitor of the sonic hedgehog pathway.[1-3] Cyclopia of other cause, or unknown cause, occurs sporadically.[4]

REFERENCES

1. Lee ST, et al. *J Agric Food Chem.* 2014;62:7355.
2. Welch KD, et al. *J Appl Toxicol.* 2009;29:414.
3. Welch KD, et al. *Int J Poison Plant Res.* 2012;2:54.
4. Zeiss CJ, et al. *Vet Ophthalmol.* 2008;11:30.

INHERITED ARACHNOMELIA (INHERITED CHONDRODYSPLASIA)

Cattle

Arachnomelia, a suspected inherited disease of Simmental, Brown Swiss, Italian Brown calves, Fleckvieh,[1] and other European breeds of cattle, is manifested by excessively long, thin distal extremities, which give the calves a spidery look—hence the term *arachnomelia.* The bones are fragile, and there is curvature of the spine, foreshortening of the mandible, and associated cardiac and vascular defects. In Swiss Braunvieh cattle it is combined with arthrogryposis. The mutation is a 2-bp deletion mutation c.1224_1225delCA in exon 11 of the molybdenum cofactor biosynthesis protein 1 (MOCS1) gene in Simmental and Fleckvieh cattle[1,2] and a 1-bp insertion c.363-364insG in the sulfite oxidase (SUOX) gene of Brown Swiss cattle.[3] It is inherited as a simple recessive trait.

Sheep

Spider Lamb Syndrome

A hereditary chondrodysplasia is recorded in Suffolk and Hampshire lambs in which the limbs are thin and disproportionately long and have abnormal positions of the bones near the joints, causing abnormalities of posture. The disease is caused by a nonsynonymous T > A transversion in the highly conserved tyrosine kinase II domain of a positional candidate gene, fibroblast growth factor receptor 3 (FGFR3).[4] The mutant FGFR3 allele has an additive effect on long-bone length, suggesting that the disease is not inherited as a strict monogenic, mendelian recessive trait but is determined primarily by the presence of the mutant FGFR3 allele and influenced by an animal's genetic background. In contrast to FGFR3 mutations causing dwarfism in humans, this single-base change results in a skeletal overgrowth. There is also less muscle than normal. In severe cases the deformities are obvious at birth and may be lethal. In less severe cases the deformities do not become apparent until the lambs are several weeks old. The defects are readily visible in x-rays before clinical signs develop, and affected lambs can be detected in this way. The diagnostic lesion is multiple irregular islands of ossification in the upper limb joints. Spinal deformities, especially kyphoscoliosis, and cranial deformities, including a roman nose, deviation of the nose poll axis, and shortening of the mandible, are observed in some lambs (Fig. 15-16).

Inheritance by an autosomal-recessive gene with complete penetrance and variable expressivity has been established as the cause in Suffolks. The defect is thought to be one of deficiency of an insulin-like growth factor (IGF) and IGF-binding proteins. Differentiation from arthrogryposis-hydranencephaly is important because of the superficial similarity of the two diseases.

Inherited Chondrodysplasia in Texel Sheep

A chondrodysplasia resulting in a dwarfing phenotype has occurred in a Texel sheep flock as a newly recognized recessively inherited genetic disease of the Texel breed. The disorder in this breed is attributable to a 1-bp deletion of T (g.25513delT) at the 107bp position of exon 3 in the SLC13A1 gene (solute carrier family 13 [sodium/sulfate symporters], member 1). The mutation g.25513delT shifts the open reading frame of SLC13A1 to introduce a stop codon and truncate C-terminal amino acids.[5] Heterozygotes appear clinically normal. Affected lambs appear normal at birth but show evidence of dwarfism, wide-based stance, and exercise intolerance as early as 1 week of age. Death usually occurs within 3 months, often after developing bilateral varus deformity of the forelimbs. Some severely affected lambs die with respiratory distress, probably as a result of tracheal collapse. Gross and microscopic lesions of variable severity were present in the tracheal, articular, epiphyseal, and physeal cartilage. In severe cases, articular cartilage in major joints was eroded from weight-bearing surfaces. The trachea was flaccid, was abnormally kinked, and had thickened cartilaginous rings and a narrow lumen. Affected sheep that survived to breeding age commonly developed severe degenerative joint disease. Histologically, chondrocytes were disorganized and surrounded by concentric rings of abnormal fibrillar material, and the matrix often contained focal to coalescing areas of chondrolysis. The disease has considerable potential as a suitable model for studying various forms of therapy for human chondrodysplasia.

REFERENCES

1. Seichter D, et al. *Anim Genet.* 2011;42:544.
2. Jiao S, et al. *PLoS ONE.* 2013;8.
3. Chu Q, et al. *Yichuan.* 2013;35:623.

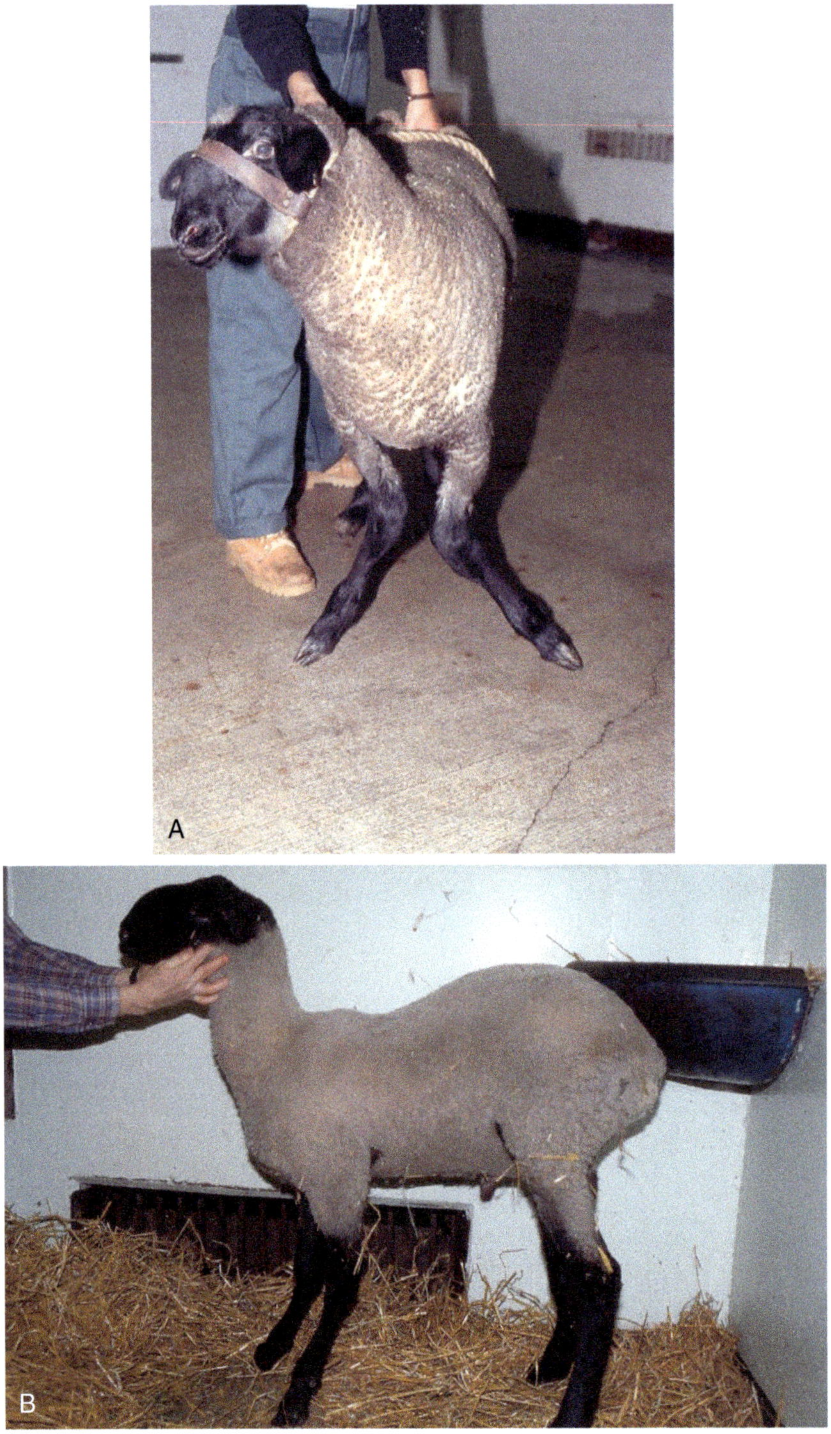

Fig. 15-16 Spider lamb syndrome in two yearling Suffolk lambs. A, A wether with marked angular limb abnormalities and disproportionately long, thin legs. B, A wether with a roman nose, shortening of the mandible, and kyphoscoliosis.

4. Beever JE, et al. *Anim Genet*. 2006;37:66.
5. Zhao X, et al. *Anim Genet*. 2012;43:9.

COMPLEX VERTEBRAL MALFORMATION IN HOLSTEIN CALVES

A lethal congenital defect of the axial skeleton of purebred Holstein calves has been reported in Denmark, the United States, and the United Kingdom. It is caused by a mutation in the gene *SLC35A3* coding a uridine-diphosphate-*N*-acetylglucosamine transporter.[1] A single-base transversion of guanine to thymine has been located in the abnormal allele at position 559. It is present in both copies of the allele, and the mutation is lethal. It is a simple recessive genetic defect that requires that both the sire and the dam of an affected calf are carriers.

Most affected calves are born between day 250 and 285 of gestation. Approximately 80% of homozygous affected fetuses are aborted before gestation day 260. Birth weights are reduced. Most affected calves are stillborn, but affected calves occasionally are born alive. Euthanasia must be performed for humanitarian reasons.

In premature, stillborn, and neonatal affected calves, the defect is characterized by congenital growth retardation, malformed vertebrae, and tetramelic arthrogryposis. There is shortening of the cervical and thoracic parts of the vertebral column as a result of multiple hemivertebrae, fused and misshaped vertebrae, and scoliosis. Growth retardation and vertebral malformation are typical lesions. Malformation of the head, primarily in the form of dysplasia or palatoschisis, also occurs.

Symmetric flexures of the carpal and joints and the metacarpophalangeal joint in combination with a slight lateral rotation of the phalanges are also present. Similar low-grade arthrogryposis is present in the pelvic limbs. Heart defects were present in 50% of affected calves (interventricular septal defects, dextroposition of the aorta, and eccentric hypertrophy of the right ventricle).

Retrospective genotyping of affected calves according to the mutation in the *SLC35A3* gene determined that there were homozygous affected, heterozygote, and homozygous normal genotypes. The morphologic expression of the malformation is wide, but certain aspects such as growth retardation, vertebral malformation, and symmetric arthrogryposis are nearly constant findings. A presumptive diagnosis of the malformation can be made in most cases based on necropsy findings combined with pedigree analysis and genotyping. Breeding studies were carried out in Denmark using selected cows that were progeny of sires with a heterozygous genotype for the malformation and were pregnant after insemination with semen from another sire with heterozygous malformation genotype. The number of calves born with the malformation was less than expected, suggesting increased intrauterine mortality. Fertility traits in Holsteins are severely affected by the malformation phenotype of the fetus. If the fetus is homozygous for the malformation, 29% of the cows will abort before gestation day 100, increasing to 45% at day 150 and 77% at day 260. Rates of nonreturn to service, frequency of calvings after the first insemination, and interval from insemination to next calving were significantly reduced by a fetal malformation phenotype.

Pedigree analysis and DNA analyses of semen from sires used for insemination have found a widely branched familial occurrence of the malformation in the Holstein breed.

The mutation in the *SCL35A3* gene has been traced to the U.S. sire Penstate Ivanhoe Star, born in 1963, and his widely used son Carlin-M Invanhoe Bell, born in 1974. Descendants of this bull in China have a heterozygote carrier frequency of 9.54% and 16.7% in Poland.[2,3] The frequency of carriers in Girolando dairy cattle in Brazil is less than 2%.[4] The malformation mutation is not restricted to descendants of the American Holstein–Friesian bull Carlin-M Ivanhoe Bell. Through these sires and elite sires genetically related to them, the defect has been disseminated in the Holstein breed worldwide. PCR testing is available to detect heterozygotes.[2] Testing is available on registered or registerable Holstein animals only through the Holstein Association (Holstein USA), through one of the National Association of Animal Breeders' member AI organizations, or at the Van Haeringen Laboratorium, Wageningen, the Netherlands.

REFERENCES

1. Thomsen B, et al. *Genome Res.* 2006;16:97.
2. Zhang Y, et al. *J Anim Sci, Biotech.* 2012;3.
3. Rusc A, et al. *Pol J Vet Sci.* 2013;16:579.
4. Paiva DS, et al. *Gen Mol Res.* 2013;12:3186.

INHERITED REDUCED PHALANGES (AMPUTATES, ACROTERIASIS, ECTROMELIA)

The defect of inherited reduced phalanges has been recorded in cattle and appears to be inherited as a single recessive character.[1,2] The limbs are normal down to the metacarpal and metatarsal bones, which are shorter than usual, but the first two phalanges are missing, and the normal hooves and third phalanges are connected to the rest of the limb by soft tissues only. The calves are unable to stand but can crawl about on their knees and hocks.

Hereditary Hemimelia

The bilateral absence of the distal half of the limb (e.g., the patella) and shortening or absence of the tibia, often accompanied by hydrocephalus, meningoceles, ventral abdominal hernia, and cryptorchidism, comprise the syndrome known as tibial hemimelia. It is inherited in the Galloway breed of cattle. An autosomal-recessive mode of inheritance is assumed. A concerted program of eradicating the defect has been undertaken, based on test matings and examination for defects of 90-day fetuses obtained by terminating pregnancy with prostaglandin. Hemimelia and amelia also occur in sheep.[3]

Hereditary Peromelia of Mohair Goats

The syndrome of hereditary peromelia of mohair goats includes agenesis of the phalanges and parts of the metacarpus and metatarsus affecting one or more limbs; it follows an autosomal-recessive mode of inheritance.

Amputates

An even more serious defect, in which the mandible and all the bones below the humerus and stifle are vestigial or absent, has been reported in British, French, and German Friesians. It appears to be conditioned by the inheritance of a single recessive gene. Similar "amputates" have been shown not to be inherited. The disease occurs in Italian buffalo, in which it is associated with chromosomal instability.[4,5]

REFERENCES

1. Droegemueller C, et al. *BMC Genet.* 2007;8.
2. Duchesne A, et al. *Genomics.* 2006;88:610.
3. Scholes SFE, et al. *Vet Rec.* 2008;163:96.
4. Albarella S, et al. *Mutagenesis.* 2009;24:471.
5. Szczerbal I, et al. *Vet Pathol.* 2006;43:789.

INHERITED CLAW DEFORMITY

Extra claws (**polydactylism**) and fusion of the claws (**syndactylism**) are known hereditary defects of cattle, the former in the Normandy breed and the latter in Holsteins, Angus, Hereford, and Chianina.[1,2] Polydactyly in pigs appears to be inherited, in some forms, as an autosomal-recessive trait with incomplete penetrance, although the genetic abnormality is unclear.[3]

Dactylomegaly (enlarged dewclaws), often associated with syndactyly or deviation of the adjacent major digit and creating a clubfooted appearance, may be inherited in Shorthorn cattle. In most cases they cause no more than inconvenience but an association of syndactyly with susceptibility to hyperthermia is recorded, and some of these animals die of hyperthermia when subjected to high environmental temperatures.

Adactyly is a recorded but less-well-defined defect in cattle and sheep in which the hooves are absent at birth.

There is good field evidence that **corkscrew claw** or **curled toe** is an inherited defect in cattle, especially in beef breeds, but also in Holstein–Friesians. It is almost always the lateral claw that is affected. In some breeds it is more common in the hindfeet; in others it is more common in the front feet. In the affected digit the third phalanx is much smaller than normal and is narrower and longer. The soft tissue and the horn are correspondingly deformed so that the horn grows much longer and narrower and tends to curl over the sole so that the cow walks on the wall of the hoof. The claw also curls over the front of the other digit of the limb. There are often cracks in the front of the claw, originating at the coronet and causing serious lameness. All affected animals suffer gait abnormalities as they get older and heavier. Much of this is attributable to distortion and wear of the articular surfaces in the companion claw, which has to carry much more weight than is usual. Marked changes in the affected digit are detectable by anteroposterior radiography.

REFERENCES

1. Droegemueller C, et al. *BMC Genet.* 2007;8.
2. Duchesne A, et al. *Genomics.* 2006;88:610.
3. Gorbach D, et al. *J Hered.* 2010;101:469.

INHERITED MULTIPLE EXOSTOSIS

Multiple exostosis affecting both cortical and medullary bone of the limbs and ribs has been described in Quarter horses and Thoroughbreds in the United States. The lesions are visible externally but cause little apparent inconvenience. It is inherited as a single autosomal-dominant gene. Restriction nuclease analysis is used to diagnose the disease.

INHERITED CONGENITAL HYPEROSTOSIS (THICK FORELIMBS OF PIGS)

This defect is thought to be caused by the inheritance of a simple recessive character. Affected piglets show obvious lesions at birth, and although many of them die or are destroyed immediately, a proportion of them may survive. The forelimbs are markedly enlarged below the elbows, and the skin is tense and may be discolored. There is difficulty in standing and moving about, and starvation and crushing contribute to the mortality rate. There is extensive edema of the subcutaneous tissues, thickening of the bones, and roughness of the periosteum. It is thought that the primary lesion is a separation of the periosteum from the bone.

INHERITED RICKETS

An inherited form of rickets occurs in purebred Corriedale sheep in New Zealand, with an incidence of up to 20 lambs out of 1600 over a 2-year period. Affected sheep have decreased growth rate, thoracic lordosis, and angular limb deformities, with low serum calcium and phosphate concentrations and normal 25 hydroxyvitamin D and 1,25 dihydroxyvitamin D_3 concentrations.[1-3] The disease is inherited as a simple autosomal-recessive disorder caused by a nonsense 250C/T mutation on exon 6 in the dentin matrix protein 1 gene (DMP1).[4] This mutation introduces a stop codon (R145X) and could truncate C-terminal amino acids. Affected sheep are "T T" genotypes, carriers are "C T," phenotypically normal related sheep are either "C T" or "C C," and unrelated normal sheep from other breeds are "C C." A simple diagnostic test can identify carriers with the defective "T" allele. Necropsy examination reveals segmental thickening of physes, growth-arrest lines, collapse of subchondral bone of the humeral head, thickened cortices, and enthesophytes around distal limb joints.[5] other features include hypertrophic chondrocytes at sites of endochondral ossification; inappropriate and excessive osteoclastic resorption; microfractures; and wide, unmineralized osteoid seams lining trabeculae and filling secondary osteons.[5]

The disease of pigs is indistinguishable from rickets as a result of nutritional inadequacy.[6] The pigs are healthy at birth. Subsequently there is hypocalcemia, hyperphosphatemia, and increased serum alkaline phosphatase activity. The defect is a failure of active transport of calcium through the wall of the small intestine.

REFERENCES

1. Dittmer KE, et al. *Vet J.* 2011;187:369.
2. Dittmer KE, et al. *Res Vet Sci.* 2011;91:362.
3. Thompson KG, et al. *NZ Vet J.* 2007;55:137.
4. Zhao X, et al. *PLoS ONE.* 2011;6.
5. Dittmer KE, et al. *J Comp Pathol.* 2009;141:147.
6. Dittmer KE, et al. *Vet Pathol.* 2011;48:389.

INHERITED TAILLESSNESS AND TAIL DEFORMITY

Complete absence of the tail or deformity of the appendage occur relatively commonly as a congenital defect. The disease "crooked-tail syndrome" in Belgian Blue cattle is attributable to a loss-of-function mutation of the bovine MRC2 gene that impairs production of Endo18 protein. Affected cattle have signs of impaired endochondral ossification and skeletal and muscular malformations. The mutation is also associated with muscular attributes in heterozygotes, including double muscling (as a result of a defect in the myostatin gene), that are desirable traits and result in 25% of Belgian Blue cattle being carriers for the condition.[1]

A syndrome of **vertebral and spinal dysplasia** occurs in Holstein cattle. There are tail malformations and neurologic dysfunction, with gait abnormalities of the hindlimbs. The deformities and neurologic dysfunctions vary from subtle or mild (limited to tail deformities) to paraparesis. The syndrome is inherited in a dominant mode with incomplete penetrance.[2]

REFERENCES

1. Fasquelle C, et al. *PLoS Genet.* 2009;5.
2. Kromik A, et al. *Vet J.* 2015;204:287.

CONGENITAL CHONDRODYSTROPHY OF UNKNOWN ORIGIN (CCUO, "ACORN" CALVES, CONGENITAL JOINT LAXITY AND DWARFISM, CONGENITAL SPINAL STENOSIS)

A noninherited condition has been described in the United States, Europe, Africa, Australia, and New Zealand that resembles inherited dwarfism.[1] The disease occurs in poor-range areas and is thought to be attributable to a maternal nutritional deficiency during the middle trimester of pregnancy.[2] The specific dietary factors involved have not been determined.

Cases are characterized by damage to physeal growth plates with subsequent failure of growth of long bones. Abnormal osseous development of the head causes superior brachygnathia. Shortening of the shafts of the long bones of the limbs is accompanied by rotated limbs and bending at the joints, and calves nurse and stand with difficulty. Deformities of the nasal turbinates and trachea are often present and frequently lead to breathing difficulties. Incoordination, arching of the back, and a tendency to bloat, which may cause death, also occur. The dentition is normal. Muscle spasticity, wry neck, circling, falling backward, and goose-stepping occur rarely. Serologic results for Akabane virus, Aino virus, bovine virus diarrhea virus, and Bluetongue are typically negative.[3]

Most of the calves are born alive; in badly affected herds, as many as 15% of calves may be affected. The original name for the condition (Acorn calves) was derived from the common occurrence of acorns in the diet of affected herds, although the acorns are not thought to have any etiologic significance. Currently, an unknown nutritional deficiency or deficiencies, possibly including manganese,[3] during the second trimester is thought to be the cause.

REFERENCES

1. White PJ, et al. *Prev Vet Med.* 2010;94:178.
2. White PJ, et al. *Prev Vet Med.* 2010;96:36.
3. Cave JG, et al. *Aust Vet J.* 2008;86:130.

Inherited Diseases of Joints

INHERITED ARTHROGRYPOSIS (INHERITED MULTIPLE TENDON CONTRACTURE)

Inherited fixation of limb joints present at birth is recorded in many breeds of cattle, especially in Belgian Blue, Shorthorn, Charolais, Piedmont, and Swedish Dole. It is inherited as a single recessive mutation in the *PIGH* gene in Belgian Blue cattle.[1] The disease occurs in Swiss Large White pigs as part of the **arthrogryposis multiplex congenita** complex of clinical abnormalities that includes inferior brachygnathism and spinal curvature.[2]

There are many environmental causes of the disease, the most well recognized of which are Schmallenberg and Akabane virus infection of early pregnancy (discussed under that heading).[3]

Simple Arthrogryposis

The limbs of affected calves are fixed in flexion or extension and cause dystocia as a result of abnormal positioning and lack of flexibility. There is no involvement of joint surfaces, and the joints can be freed by cutting the surrounding tendons or muscles. There is atrophy of limb muscles, and those calves that are born alive are unable to stand and usually die or are destroyed within a few days.

Arthrogryposis With Dental Dysplasia

Arthrogryposis with dental dysplasia in cattle appears to be inherited in a dominant manner. The teeth are soft, fleshy, and easy to bend. There is no defect of bones or joints other than marked softness and the presence of excess cartilage at the epiphyses. There is abnormal ossification of the cartilage. The calves are of normal size, do not cause dystocia, and, although they are unable to stand because of the excessive flexibility of the limbs, they can suck. Hypostatic pneumonia usually develops and causes death of the calf.

Arthrogryposis With Palatoschisis

Arthrogryposis with palatoschisis (SAP) is inherited as a simple recessive trait with low penetrance in pure French Charolais in France and high penetrance in 7/8 Charolais cattle in Canada, where the gene frequency is high in purebred and crossbred Charolais. Among crossbred Charolais cattle the homozygous condition is almost always markedly expressed and lethal, but a high percentage of purebred homozygous cattle show slight to no visible effect of the gene and survive. Because of the low rate of prevalence in France, attempted eradication does not appear to be economical.

In this syndrome all limbs are usually affected but the front limbs more than the hindlimbs, and the more distal joints are more rigidly fixed than proximal ones. The muscles of affected limbs are atrophic and pale in color. Histologic changes in the spinal cord suggest that the muscle atrophy is neurogenic. In affected calves the gestation period may be longer than normal by an average of 2 weeks.

Arthrogryposis With Multiple Defects

In Simmentals a combined set of defects includes arthrogryposis, often with the limbs in a wraparound position around the body, underdevelopment of the mandible, curvature of the spine, and defects of the heart and main vessels.

Arthrogryposis in Species Other Than Cattle

Inherited arthrogryposis has also been recorded in Merino and Corriedale **sheep** and in Norwegian Landrace **pigs,** in which it is thought to be inherited as a simple recessive trait. The Corriedale defect is associated with other lesions, including brachygnathia inferior, hydranencephaly, and thoracic scoliosis. Inherited arthrogryposis in pedigree Suffolk lambs has been described.[1] Breeding studies using superovulation and embryo transfer were used to increase the numbers of offspring from females that were carrying the gene or genes responsible for the defect, which is inherited as an autosomal-recessive trait.

Ovine heritable arthrogryposis multiplex congenita is a congenital syndrome in lambs characterized by curvature, hunching, and twisting of the thoracic spine, with associated abnormalities of the ribs and sternum, distal arthrogryposis of the carpal and tarsal joints, and cleft hard and soft palate or palatoschisis (a median fissure of the palate) and is an autosomal-recessive inherited disease.[4] Affected lambs are born full term but die shortly after birth. Affected lambs have slightly reduced body weight (as a result of low muscle mass) compared with normal newborn lambs of the same flock. The syndrome is similar to **bovine heritable arthrogryposis multiplex congenita** in Angus cattle and **porcine heritable arthrogryposis multiplex congenita.**[2]

An inherited arthrogryposis also occurs in Norwegian Fjord **horses.** The arthrogryposis affects the hindlimbs, and there are accompanying defects of polydactyly, palatoschisis, and brachygnathia in some. Most foals are unable to stand, and the defect must be considered to be a lethal one.

INHERITED MULTIPLE ANKYLOSES

Multiple ankylosis affecting all limb joints has been recorded as an inherited congenital defect of Holstein calves. The abdomen of the dam shows marked enlargement at month 6 to 7 of pregnancy, and this may occasion some respiratory distress. Excessive fetal fluids are present, and insertion of the hand per rectum is impeded by the distended uterus. Abortion during the last month of pregnancy is a common occurrence. Affected fetuses have a very short neck, ankylosed intervertebral joints, and varying degrees of ankylosis of all limb joints. The limbs are fixed in flexion, and there is some curvature of the spine. Fetal dystocia always occurs, and embryotomy or cesarean section is necessary to deliver the calf.

Ankylosis of limb joints combined with **cleft palate** occurs occasionally in Charolais cattle and is suspected of being inherited. **Ankylosis of the coffin joint**, developing at several weeks of age, has been reported in Simmental calves. The etiology of the condition is not clear.

REFERENCES

1. Sartelet A, et al. *BMC Genet.* 2015;16:316.
2. Haubitz M, et al. *Mol Cell Prob.* 2012;26:248.
3. Agerholm JS, et al. *Acta Vet Scand.* 2015;57.
4. Tejedor MT, et al. *J Comp Pathol.* 2010;143:14.

INHERITED PATELLAR SUBLUXATION

Unilateral or bilateral subluxation occurs as an inherited defect in *Bos indicus* cattle and in water buffalo (*Bubalus bubalis*). Shetland ponies also have a predisposition, and a monogenic autosomal-recessive transmission is suspected. There is periodic lameness, with the affected limb held in rigid extension; the patella is displaced medially.[1]

REFERENCE

1. Busschers E. *Equine Vet Educ.* 2009;21:464.

INHERITED HYPERMOBILITY (LAXITY) OF JOINTS

Inherited hypermobility of joints is recorded only in Jersey cattle. It has assumed great importance because of the great popularity of a sire that carried the gene. There is abnormal flexure and extension of all joints but especially the hock, stifle, hip, knee, elbow, and shoulder joints. The muscles are much atrophied, and the joints look very enlarged as a result. It is impossible for the calves to stand, but they are bright, alert, and eat well. The limbs are so flexible that they can be bent into extraordinary positions and almost tied in knots. A drawer sign, a displacement of the articular surfaces laterally, produced by manual pressure, can be elicited easily and with a displacement of up to 2 cm. There are no detectable lesions in the nervous or musculoskeletal systems. Although the disease is known to be inherited as a simple autosomal-recessive trait, it has also been seen in circumstances that preclude inheritance being the cause.

INHERITED HIP DYSPLASIA

An inherited defective development of the acetabulum occurs in Dole horses. There is no clinical evidence of the disease at birth, but osteoarthritis of the joint and disruption of the round ligament develop subsequently. Hip dysplasia occurs in Belgian Blue cattle.[1]

REFERENCE

1. Van Vlierbergen B, et al. *Vet Rec.* 2007;160:910.

16 Diseases of the Skin, Eye, Conjunctiva, and External Ear

Introduction

The major functions of the skin are:

- To maintain a normal body temperature
- To maintain a normal fluid and electrolyte balance within the animal
- To create a mechanical barrier to protect the body from noxious agents and organisms
- To act as a sensory organ perceiving those features of the environment that are important to the subject's survival

In general, these functions are not greatly impeded by most diseases of the skin of large animals, with the exceptions of failure of the sweating mechanism, which does seriously interfere with body temperature regulation, and severe burns or other skin trauma, which may cause fatal fluid and electrolyte loss.

The major effects of skin diseases in large animals are esthetic and economic but can also present a considerable animal welfare concern. Discomfort and scratching interfere with normal rest and feeding, and when the lips are affected, there may be interference with prehension. The unsightly appearance of the animal distresses the owner. There is loss of the economic coat, and the sales value and acceptability of animals for transport and appearance in exhibitions is greatly reduced.

Primary/Secondary Lesions

Diseases of the skin may be primary or secondary in origin. In primary skin disease the lesions are restricted initially to the skin, although they may subsequently spread from the skin to involve other organs. Conversely, cutaneous lesions may be secondary to disease originating in other organs. Differentiation between primary and secondary skin diseases should be attempted by seeking evidence that organs other than the skin are affected. If there is no such evidence produced during a thorough clinical examination of the patient, it is reasonable to assume that the disease is primary. Even if involvement of other organs is diagnosed, it is still necessary to determine whether the involvement constitutes the primary state or whether it has developed secondarily to the skin disease. This decision can be based on the chronology of the signs, elicited by careful history taking, and a detailed knowledge of the individual diseases likely to be encountered.

Taking an accurate anamnesis and doing a complete clinical examination must precede the careful examination of the skin itself, using the proper technique of examination. The veterinarian may need to employ advanced diagnostic procedures such as histopathological examination of a biopsy specimen to define the type of lesion present.

The purpose of this chapter is to describe the basic skin lesions so that the differential diagnosis, up to the point of defining the type and nature of the lesion, the pathoanatomical diagnosis, can be accomplished. A definitive etiologic diagnosis requires further examination and is included in the discussion of the specific diseases.

Clinical Signs and Special Examination

A general clinical examination is followed by a special examination of the skin and must include inspection and, in most cases, palpation. Additional information can be obtained by taking swabs for bacteriologic examinations, scrapings for examination for dermatophytes and metazoan parasites, and biopsy for histopathological examination.

Biopsy material should include abnormal, marginal, and normal skin. Artifacts are common in biopsy specimens, including nonrepresentative sampling, crushing the specimen by forceps or hemostat, and inadequate fixation.

A Wood's lamp finds a special use in the examination of the skin for dermatophytes.

Descriptions of lesions should include size, depth to which they penetrate topographic distribution on the body, and size of the area affected. Abnormalities of sebaceous and sweat secretion, changes in the hair or wool coat, and alterations in color and temperature of the skin should be noted, as should the presence or absence of pain or pruritus.

Lesions

An accurate definition of the lesions, summarized in Table 16-1, is an essential part of a dermatologic patient's clinical record. The table makes a primary differentiation into discrete and diffuse lesions, and these categories need to be further categorized in terms

Table 16-1 Terms used to identify skin lesions

Name of lesion	Nature of lesion	Relation to skin surface	Skin surface
Scales	Dry, flaky exfoliations	On surface only, no penetration of skin	Unbroken
Excoriations	Traumatic abrasions and scratches	Penetration below surface	Variable skin surface damage—depends on severity
Fissures	Deep cracks	Penetrate into subcutis	Disrupted
Dry gangrene	Dry, horny, black, avascular, shield-like	Above skin, usually all layers affected	Removed
Early, moist gangrene	Blue-black, cold, oozing serum	In plane of skin or below	Complete depth of subcutis
Keratosis	Overgrowth of dry, horny, keratinized epithelium	Above skin	Undamaged stratum corneum is retained
Acanthosis	Like keratosis but moist, soft	Above skin	Prickle cell layer swollen; is really part of skin
Hyperkeratosis	Excessive overgrowth of keratinized, epithelium-like scab	Above skin	Skin surface unbroken
Parakeratosis	Adherent to skin	Above skin	Cells of stratum corneum nucleated and retained; really part of skin
Eczema	Erythematous, itching dermatitis	Superficial layer of epidermis affected	Weeping, scabby disruption of surface
Hypermelanosis	Increased deposits of melanin (e.g., melanosis, meloderma)	In epidermis or dermis	Unbroken
Hypomelanosis	Decreased deposits of melanin	In epidermis or dermis	Unbroken
Discrete lesions			
Vesicle, bleb, bulla, blister	Fluid (serum or lymph)-filled blister 1–2 cm diameter	Above skin surface, superficial	Unbroken but will slough
Pustule	Pus-filled blister, 1–5 mm	Above, superficial	Will rupture
Wheal	Edematous, erythematous, swellings, transitory	Above, all layers affected	Undamaged
Papules (pimples)	Elevated, inflamed, necrotic center, up to 1 cm diameter	Above surface, all layers affected	Points and ruptures
Nodules, nodes	Elevated, solid, up to 1 cm diameter Acute or chronic inflammation. No necrotic center	Above surface, all layers	Surface unbroken
Plaque	Larger nodule, up to 3–4 cm diameter	All layers affected; raised above surface	Surface unbroken
Acne	Used synonymously with *pimple* but strict meaning is infection of sebaceous gland	Above surface of skin; all layers affected	May point and rupture
Comedo	Plugged (sebum, keratin) hair follicle	Raised above skin	May rupture
Impetigo	Flaccid vesicle, then pustule, then scab, up to 1 cm diameter	Raised above skin; very superficial	Upper layers destroyed
Scab (or crust)	Crust of coagulated, blood, pus, and skin debris	Raised above skin	Disrupted, depth varying with original lesion
Macule (patch)	Small area of color change; patch is larger	Within superficial layers	Unbroken

of size (e.g., they may be limited diffuse lesions or extensive localized ones).

Abnormal Coloration

The parameter of abnormal coloration includes jaundice, pallor, and erythema. In animals these conditions are rarely visible in light-colored skins. Red–purple discoloration of the skin of septicemic, white pigs may be dramatic, but no diagnostic significance can be attached to its degree. Early erythema is a common finding where more definite skin lesions are to develop, as in early photosensitization. The blue coloration of early gangrene (e.g., of the udder and teat skin in the early stages of peracute bovine mastitis associated with *Staphylococcus aureus*) is characterized by coldness and loss of elasticity.

Hypopigmentation of the skin may be general, as in albino, pseudoalbino, and lethal white animals. Local patches of hypopigmentation are characteristic of vitiligo and leukoderma.

Pruritus

- **Pruritus or itching** is the sensation that gives rise to scratching.
- **Hyperesthesia** is increased sensitivity to normal stimuli.
- **Paresthesia** is perverted sensation, a subjective sensation, and not diagnosed in animals.

All sensations that give rise to rubbing or scratching are therefore included with pruritus, more properly defined as scratching. Pruritus can arise from peripheral or central stimulation. When it is peripheral in origin, it is a primary cutaneous sensation, similar to heat, cold, pain, and touch; it differs from pain because it is purely epidermal, whereas pain can still be felt in areas of skin denuded of epidermis. Thus itching does not occur in the center of deep ulcerations or in very superficial lesions, such as those of ringworm, where only the hair fibers and keratinized epithelium are involved. Itching can be elicited over the entire skin surface but is most severe at the mucocutaneous junctions. Common causes include the following.

Cattle

- Sarcoptic and chorioptic mange
- Lice infestation
- Nervous acetonemia
- Aujeszky's disease

Sheep

- Lice, mange, ked, blow-fly, and itch-mite infestations
- Scrapie

Horses

- Chorioptic mange on the legs
- Queensland (sweet) itch along the dorsum of the body
- Lice infestation
- Perianal pruritus from *Oxyuris equi* infestation

Pigs

- Sarcoptic and chorioptic mange
- Lice infestation

All Species

- Early stages of photosensitive dermatitis
- Urticarial wheals in an allergic reaction
- **"Licking syndromes,"** such as those that occur in cattle on copper-deficient diets, are accompanied by pica and the licking of others as well as themselves. They are examples of depraved appetites developed in response to nutritional deficiency and are not a response to pruritus.
- **Itching of central origin** derives mainly from the scratch center below the acoustic nucleus in the medulla. It may have a structural basis, as in scrapie and pseudorabies, or it may be functional in origin, as in the nervous form of acetonemia. The only lesions observed are those of a traumatic dermatitis with removal of the superficial layers to a variable depth, breakage or removal of the hairs, and a distribution of lesions in places where the animal can bite or rub easily.

Secretion Abnormalities of Skin Glands

The activity of the **sweat glands** is controlled by the sympathetic nervous system and is for the most part a reflection of body temperature. Excitement and pain may cause sweating as a result of cerebral cortical activity. A generalized form of hyperhidrosis, apparently inherited, has been recorded in Shorthorn calves. Local areas of increased or decreased sweating may arise from peripheral nerve lesions or obstruction of sweat gland ducts. A generalized anhidrosis is recorded in horses and occasionally in cattle.

Excess secretion of sebum by **sebaceous glands** causes oiliness of the skin or seborrhea, but its pathogenesis is poorly understood.

Abnormalities of Wool and Hair Fibers

Deficiency of hair or wool in comparison to the normal pilosity of the skin area is **alopecia** or **hypotrichosis**.

Hirsutism, abnormal hairiness, manifested by a long, shaggy, and usually curly coat, is most common in aged ponies with adenomas of the pars intermedia of the pituitary gland.

The character of the fiber may also vary with variations in the internal environment. For example, in copper deficiency the crimp of fine wool fibers is lost, and the wool becomes straight and "steely." Alternation in coat color, achromotrichia, may be generalized or segmental along the fiber.

FURTHER READING

Knotterbelt DC. The approach to the equine dermatology case in practice. *Vet Clin Equine.* 2012;25:131-153.

Metz M, et al. Pruritus: an overview of current concepts. *Vet Dermatol.* 2011;22:121-131.

Outerbridge CA. Cutaneous manifestations of internal diseases. *Vet Clin North Am Small.* 2013;43:135-152.

Paterson S, Ball C. A practical approach to equine dermatology. *In Pract.* 2013;35:190-196.

Principles of Treatment of Diseases of the Skin

PRIMARY TREATMENT

For a specific treatment, accurate diagnosis of the condition and the identification of underlying cause must precede the selection of any topical or systemic treatment. Hair coat and debris on and around the affected area must be removed to enable topical applications to come into direct contact with the affected skin. In bacterial diseases susceptibility tests on cultures of the organism are advisable. Bacterial resistance to antimicrobials used in veterinary dermatologic practice is a concern. The uncritical use of antimicrobials either locally or systemically should be avoided to contain the development of bacterial resistance to microbials. Specific skin diseases caused by bacteria, fungi, and metazoan parasites are reasonably amenable to treatment with the appropriate specific remedy. Identification of the fungal or parasitic organism presumably causing the disease allows for selection of a pharmacologic substance and route of administration with documented efficacy against the agent in question and can prevent frustrating treatment failures.

Removal of the causative agent in allergic diseases and photosensitization may be impossible, and symptomatic treatment may be the only practicable solution. Symptomatic treatment may also be indicated for welfare reasons in cases where the underlying cause of the disorder could not (yet) be identified. The veterinarian must be aware that in these cases antiinflammatory treatment, although indicated, may complicate further diagnostic workup. In some instances the primary disease may be confounded by the presence of a secondary agent, which can lead to confusion in diagnosis.

SUPPORTIVE TREATMENT

Supportive treatment may include prevention of secondary infection by the use of bacteriostatic ointments or dressings and the prevention of further damage from scratching.

- Effective treatment of pruritus depends on the reduction of central perception of itch sensations by the use of ataractic, sedative, or narcotic drugs administered systemically or on successful restraint of the mediator between the lesion and the sensory end organ. In the absence of accurate knowledge of the pathogenesis of pain, it is usual to resort to local anesthetic agents, which are short-lived in their activity, and corticosteroids, which are longer-acting and effective, provided that vascular engorgement is part of the pruritus-stimulating mechanism.
- When large areas of skin are involved, it is important to prevent the absorption of toxic products by continuous irrigation or the application of absorptive dressings. Losses of fluid and electrolytes should be compensated by oral or parenteral administration of fluids containing the necessary electrolytes.
- Ensure an adequate dietary intake of protein, particularly sulfur-containing amino acids, to facilitate the repair of skin tissues.
- Boredom contributes significantly to an animal's response to itch stimuli, and close confinement of affected animals is best avoided.

FURTHER READING

Matousek JL, Campbell KL. A comparative review of cutaneous pH. *Vet Dermatol.* 2002;13:293-300.

Schwarz S, Noble WC. Aspects of bacterial resistance to antimicrobials used in veterinary dermatological practice. *Vet Dermatol.* 1999;10:163-176.

Scott DW. *Large Animal Dermatology.* Philadelphia: WB Saunders; 1988.

Diseases of the Epidermis and Dermis

PITYRIASIS

Primary pityriasis is characterized by excessive bran-like scales on the skin and is caused by overproduction of keratinized epithelial cells. The etiology is uncertain. The diagnosis is based on clinical presentation and can be supported by further diagnostic testing ruling out other differential diagnoses. Proposed causative or predisposing factors are as follows:

- Hypovitaminosis A
- Nutritional deficiency of B vitamins, especially of riboflavin and nicotinic acid, in pigs, or linolenic acid, and probably other essential unsaturated fatty acids
- Poisoning by iodine

Secondary pityriasis is characterized by excessive desquamation of epithelial cells and usually associated with the following:

- Scratching in flea, louse, and mange infestations
- Keratolytic infection (e.g., with ringworm fungus)

Pityriasis scales are accumulations of keratinized epithelial cells, sometimes softened and made greasy by the exudation of serum or sebum. Overproduction, when it occurs, begins around the orifices of the hair follicles and spreads to the surrounding stratum corneum.

Primary pityriasis scales are superficial, accumulate where the coat is long, and are usually associated with a dry, lusterless coat. Itching or other skin lesions are not features. Secondary pityriasis is usually accompanied by the lesions of the primary disease.

Pityriasis rosea or pustular psoriaform dermatitis is a skin condition of piglets that is clinically and histopathologically distinct from human pityriasis rosea (see also **"Pityriasis rosea"**).

Pityriasis is identified by the absence of parasites and fungi in skin scrapings.

DIFFERENTIAL DIAGNOSIS

- Hyperkeratosis (see following discussion)
- Parakeratosis (see following discussion)
- Swine erysipelas (for pityriasis rosea in pigs)
- Porcine dermatitis and nephropathy syndrome (for pityriasis rosea in pigs)
- Ringworm (for pityriasis rosea in pigs)

TREATMENT

Primary treatment requires correction of the primary cause.

Supportive treatment commences with a thorough washing, followed by alternating applications of a bland emollient ointment and an alcoholic lotion. Salicylic acid is frequently incorporated into a lotion or ointment with a lanolin base.

HYPERKERATOSIS

Epithelial cells accumulate on the skin as a result of excessive keratinization of epithelial cells and intercellular bridges, interference with normal cell division in the granular layer of the epidermis, and hypertrophy of the stratum corneum.

Local hyperkeratosis may be caused by the following:

- Mechanical stress on pressure points (e.g., elbows, hocks, or brisket) when animals lie habitually on hard surfaces
- Mechanical and/or chemical stress (e.g., **teat-end keratosis** of dairy cows that can be caused by improper milking machine settings, overmilking, improper use of teat sanitizers or cold weather)
- Parasitism (e.g., hyperkeratotic form of sarcoptes mange of pigs and small ruminants)

Generalized hyperkeratosis may be caused by the following:

- Poisoning with highly chlorinated naphthalene compounds
- Chronic arsenic poisoning
- Inherited congenital ichthyosis
- Inherited dyserythropoiesis–dyskeratosis
- Infection with *Scopulariopsis brevicaulis*, a fungus, was recently associated with generalized hyperkeratosis in a calf and a goat kid.[1,2]

The skin is dry, scaly, thicker than normal, usually corrugated, hairless, and fissured in a gridlike pattern. Secondary infection of deep fissures may occur if the area is continually wet. However, the lesion is usually dry, and the plugs of hyperkeratotic material can be removed, leaving the underlying skin intact.

Confirmation of the diagnosis is by the demonstration of the characteristically thickened stratum corneum in a biopsy section, which also serves to differentiate the condition from parakeratosis (see also "Parakeratosis") and inherited ichthyosis (see also "Congenital and Inherited Skin Defects").

Primary treatment depends on correction of the cause. Supportive treatment is by the application of a keratolytic agent (e.g., salicylic acid ointment).

REFERENCES

1. Ogawa S, et al. *J Comp Pathol.* 2008;138:145-150.
2. Ozturk D, et al. *Bull Vet Pullawy.* 2009;53:361-363.

PARAKERATOSIS

Parakeratosis, a skin condition characterized by incomplete keratinization of epithelial cells, can have various causes:

- Caused by nonspecific chronic inflammation of cellular epidermis
- Associated with dietary deficiency of zinc
- Part of an inherited disease (described later in the chapter)

The initial lesion comprises edema of the prickle cell layer, dilatation of the intercellular lymphatics, and leukocyte infiltration. Imperfect keratinization of epithelial cells at the granular layer of the epidermis follows, and the horn cells produced are sticky and soft, retain their nuclei, and stick together to form large masses, which stay fixed to the underlying tissues or are shed as thick scales.

The lesions may be extensive and diffuse but are often confined to the flexor aspects of joints (referred to historically in horses as **mallenders** and **sallenders**). Initially the skin is reddened, followed by thickening and gray discoloration. Large, soft scales accumulate, are often held in place by hairs, and usually crack and fissure; their removal leaves a raw, red surface. Hyperkeratosis scales are thin and dry and accompany an intact, normal skin.

Parakeratosis in pigs is most commonly seen in swine 2 to 4 months of age and responds to dietary supplementation of zinc. Zinc deficiency in affected animals can be absolute or relative. The latter can be caused by excessive dietary calcium or phytic acid content or by a deficiency in essential fatty acids, which all interfere with the intestinal absorption of zinc.

The diagnosis is made based on the clinical presentation and can be confirmed by the identification of imperfect keratinization in a histopathological examination of a biopsy or a skin section at necropsy.

DIFFERENTIAL DIAGNOSIS

- Hyperkeratosis
- Pachyderma
- Ringworm
- Sarcoptic mange
- Greasy pig disease (*Staphylococcus hyicus* infection)
- Inherited ichthyosis
- Inherited parakeratosis of calves
- Inherited dermatosis vegetans in pigs
- Inherited epidermal dysplasia

TREATMENT

Primary treatment requires correction of any nutritional deficiency (specifically, correcting zinc and preventing excessive dietary calcium content).

Supportive treatment includes removal of the crusts by the use of keratolytic agent (e.g., salicylic acid ointment) or by vigorous scrubbing with soapy water, followed by application of an astringent (e.g., white lotion paste), which must be applied frequently and for some time after the lesions have disappeared.

PACHYDERMA

Pachyderma, including scleroderma, is thickening of the skin affecting all layers, often including subcutaneous tissue, and usually localized but often extensive, as in lymphangitis and greasy heel in horses. There are no specific causes, with most cases being a result of a nonspecific chronic or recurrent inflammation.

In affected areas the hair coat is thin or absent, and the skin is thicker and tougher than usual. It appears tight and, because of its thickness and reduced volume of subcutaneous tissue, cannot be picked into folds or moved easily over underlying tissue. The skin surface is unbroken, and there are no lesions and no crusts or scabs as in parakeratosis and hyperkeratosis.

Confirmation of the diagnosis depends on histopathological examination of a biopsy. The cells in all layers are usually normal, but the individual layers are increased in thickness. There is hypertrophy of the prickle cell layer of the epidermis and enlargement of the interpapillary processes.

DIFFERENTIAL DIAGNOSIS

Parakeratosis
Cutaneous neoplasia
Papillomatosis

TREATMENT

Primary treatment requires removal of the causal irritation, but in well-established cases little improvement can be anticipated, and surgical removal may be a practical solution when the area is small. In early cases local or systemic corticosteroids may effect a recovery.

IMPETIGO

Impetigo is a superficial eruption of thin-walled, small vesicles, surrounded by a zone of erythema, that develop into pustules, then rupture to form scabs.

In humans, impetigo is specifically a streptococcal infection, but lesions are often invaded secondarily by *staphylococci*. In animals the main organism found is usually a staphylococcus. The causative organism appears to gain entry through minor abrasions, with spread resulting from rupture of lesions causing contamination of surrounding skin and the development of secondary lesions. Spread from animal to animal occurs readily.

Two specific examples of impetigo in large animals are as follows:

- **Udder impetigo** (udder acne) of cows
- **Contagious impetigo,** also known as **exudative epidermitis** (see also "Udder Impetigo") or "**greasy pig disease,**" caused by *Staphylococcus hyicus* (see also "Exudative Epidermitis/Greasy Pig Disease")

Confirmation of the diagnosis is by isolation of *staphylococci* from vesicular fluid.

DIFFERENTIAL DIAGNOSIS

Cowpox/buffalopox, in which the lesions occur almost exclusively on the teats and pass through the characteristic stages of pox
Pseudocowpox, in which lesions are characteristic and also restricted in occurrence to the teats
Pityriasis rosea (for greasy pig disease)
Sarcoptic mange (for greasy pig disease)
Ringworm

TREATMENT

Primary treatment with antibiotic topically is usually all that is required because individual lesions heal so rapidly (see also under "Greasy Pig Disease").

Supportive treatment is aimed at preventing the occurrence of secondary lesions and spread of the disease to other animals. Twice-daily bathing with an efficient germicidal skin wash is usually adequate.

URTICARIA

Urticaria (hives) is a skin condition characterized by development of topical dermal edema becoming apparent as cutaneous wheals. Horses are the most commonly affected species. In acute cases hives appear suddenly and regress within hours. Longer-lasting or even chronic cases are characterized by the continuous recurrence of new wheals on the skin for days or even months. Urticaria can occur as localized allergic reaction only affecting parts of the skin or as part of a more severe systemic allergic reaction.

ETIOLOGY

Although urticaria in many cases is of allergic origin, nonallergic causes such as physical stress on the skin (e.g., through squeezing [pressure urticaria or dermatographism] or exposure to low ambient temperature [cold urticaria]) can result in the development of urticaria.

In horses chronic urticaria is most commonly associated with feed allergies. Specifically, in some of the chronic and recurrent cases a causative allergen cannot be found and the underlying etiology remains obscure. In humans the presence of serum immunoglobulin G (IgG) autoantibodies targeting immunoglobulin E (IgE) or the IgE receptor has been documented in a subset of patients with chronic urticaria of unknown etiology. An autoimmune basis for chronic urticaria has therefore been proposed.[1,2]

Primary urticaria can be caused by the following:

- Insect stings
- Contact with stinging plants
- Ingestion of unusual food, with the allergen, usually a protein
- Occasionally an unusual feed item (e.g., garlic to a horse)
- Administration of a particular drug (e.g., penicillin, streptomycin, possibly guaifenesin or other anesthetic agent)
- Allergic reaction in cattle following vaccination for foot-and-mouth disease
- Death of warble fly larvae in tissue
- Milk allergy when Jersey cows are dried off
- Transfusion reaction
- Cutaneous vasculitis (purpurea hemorrhagica)
- Local skin trauma (dermatographism)
- Temperature induced (heat, cold, sunlight)
- Infection—parasitic, bacterial, fungal, viral

Secondary urticaria occurs as part of a syndrome, such as the following:

- Respiratory tract infections in horses, including strangles and the upper respiratory tract viral infections
- Erysipelas in pigs

PATHOGENESIS

Degranulation of mast cells liberating chemical mediators of inflammation that result in the subsequent development of dermal edema is the presumed cause for the development of urticaria. A primary dilatation of capillaries causes cutaneous erythema. Exudation from the damaged capillary walls causes local edema in the dermis, and a wheal develops. Only the dermis, and sometimes the epidermis, is involved. In extreme cases the wheals may expand to become seromas, when they may ulcerate and discharge. The lesions of urticaria usually resolve in 12 to 24 hours, but in recurrent urticaria an affected horse may have persistent and chronic eruption of lesions over a period of days or months.

CLINICAL FINDINGS

Wheals, mostly circular, well-delineated, steep-sided, easily visible elevations in the skin, appear very rapidly and often in large numbers, commencing usually on the neck but being most numerous on the body. They vary from 0.5 to 5 cm in diameter, with a flat top, and are tense to the touch. There is often no itching, except with plant or insect stings, and no discontinuity of the epithelial surface, exudation, or weeping. Pallor of the skin in wheals can be observed only in unpigmented skin. Other allergic phenomena, including diarrhea and slight fever, may accompany the eruption. The onset of the lesions is acute to peracute, with the wheals developing within minutes to hours after exposure to the triggering agent. When associated with severe adverse systemic responses, including apnea, respiratory arrest, atrial fibrillation, cardiac arrest, or sudden death, the case qualifies as one of anaphylaxis.

Subsidence of the wheals within 24 to 48 hours is usual, but they may persist for 3 to 4 days because of the appearance of fresh lesions. In some very sensitive horses, dermatographism, the production of a continuous wheal following the pattern of a blunt-pointed instrument drawn across the skin, can be demonstrated about 30 minutes later.

Urticaria lasting 8 weeks or longer is classified as chronic or recurrent urticaria, which may require testing for atopic disease using intradermal skin testing and serum testing for antigen-specific IgE.

Adverse reactions in dairy cattle following annual vaccination for foot-and-mouth disease are characterized by wheals (3 to 20 mm in diameter) covering most of the body, followed by exudative and necrotic dermatitis. The affected areas become hairless, and the wheals exude serum and become scabbed over. Edema of the legs is common, and vesicles occur on the teats. The lesions appear 8 to 12 weeks postvaccination and may persist for 3 to 5 weeks. Loss of body weight and lymphadenopathy also occur. Pruritus, depression, and a drop in milk yield are common. Adverse effects of parenteral administration of penicillin streptomycin in the form of a type I hypersensitivity reaction that was associated with rapid development of urticaria have been reported.[3]

CLINICAL PATHOLOGY

The diagnosis in most cases is based on the clinical presentation, possibly in combination with a history of local or systemic exposure to a potential allergen. Biopsies show that tissue histamine levels are increased, and there is a local accumulation of eosinophils. Blood histamine levels and eosinophil counts may also show transient elevation.

Opinions over the usefulness of intradermal skin tests in horses are strongly divided. Although intradermal testing may be of use in some cases, results are often difficult to interpret, and the panel of available allergens may not be the most appropriate for horses.[4] Intradermal tests in horses without atopy and horses with atopic dermatitis or recurrent urticaria using environmental allergens indicate a greater number of positive reactions for intradermal tests in horses with atopic dermatitis or recurrent urticaria compared with horses without atopy. This provides evidence of type I IgE-mediated hypersensitivity for these diseases.

DIFFERENTIAL DIAGNOSIS

Urticaria is manifested by a sudden appearance of a crop of cutaneous weals, sometimes accompanied by restlessness, mostly in horses, occasionally in cattle. Identification of the etiology is also helpful in diagnosis but is often difficult, depending on a carefully taken history and examination of the environment.

The **differential diagnosis list** is limited to angioedema, but in urticaria the lesions can be palpated in the skin itself. Angioedema involves the subcutaneous tissue rather than the skin, and the lesions are much larger and more diffuse. The two conditions may appear in the same animal at the same time.

TREATMENT

Primary Treatment

Spontaneous recovery is common in acute cases with incidental exposure to an allergen. In chronic or recurrent cases identification and removal of the allergen must be a priority. A change of diet and environment, especially exposure to the presumably causal insects or plants, is standard practice.

Supportive Treatment

Corticosteroids, antihistamines, or epinephrine by parenteral injection provides the best and most rational treatment, especially in the relief of the pruritus. One treatment is usually sufficient, but lesions may recur. The local application of cooling astringent lotions such as calamine or white lotion or a dilute solution of sodium bicarbonate is favored. In large animal practice parenteral injections of calcium salts are used, with apparently good results.

Long-term medical management of persistent/chronic urticaria involves the administration of corticosteroids and/or antihistamines. Oral administration or prednisone or prednisolone at the lowest possible dose on alternate days is the method of choice. The antihistamine of choice is oral hydroxyzine hydrochloride, initially at 1 to 2 mg/kg administered twice daily or three times daily, followed by gradual reduction to a minimum maintenance dose required to keep the horse free of lesions.

TREATMENT

Acute anaphylaxis with urticaria in horses:
- Epinephrine: 3 to 5 mL/450 kg of a 1:1000 solution IM or SC (can be combined with steroids) (R-1)

Acute urticaria in horses:
- Dexamethasone soluble 0.01 to 0.1 mg/kg IV or IM q24 h for 3 to 7 days (R-1)

Chronic or recurrent urticaria:
- Prednisolone 0.25 to 1.0 mg/kg IV or PO q24 h. Reduce to 0.2 to 0.5 mg/kg q48 h (R-1)
- Dexamethasone 0.01 to 0.02 mg/kg PO q48-72 h (R-1). Further reduce dose until the lowest dose keeping the animal free of signs is determined.
- Hydroxyzine hydrochloride 0.5 to 1.0 mg/kg IM or PO q8 h (R-2)
- Diphenhydramine hydrochloride 0.7 to 1 mg/kg q12 h (R-2)
- Chlorpheniramine 0.25 to 0.5 mg/kg q12 h (R-2)

FURTHER READING

Evans AG. Urticaria in horses. *Compend Contin Educ Pract Vet.* 1997;15:626-632.

Knottenbelt DC. The approach to the equine dermatology case. *Vet Clin Equine.* 2012;28:131-153.

Stannard AA. Immunologic diseases. *Vet Dermatol.* 2000;11:163-178.

REFERENCES

1. Caplan AP, Greaves M. *Clin Exp Allerg.* 2009;39:777-787.
2. Vonakis BM, Saini SS. *Curr Opin Immunol.* 2008;20:709-716.
3. Omidi A. *Can Vet J.* 2009;50:741-744.
4. Knottenbelt DC. *Vet Clin Equine.* 2012;28:131-153.

DERMATITIS AND DERMATOSIS

SYNOPSIS

Etiology Any disease of skin, including those characterized by inflammation. All pathogens, infectious, chemical, physical, allergic, autoimmune.

Epidemiology Sporadic or outbreak; acute or chronic course; cosmetic to lethal; of most importance because of constraints on movement, sale, or exhibition; may affect animal welfare.

Clinical signs Primarily localized to skin, including lesions varying from parakeratosis and pachyderma to weeping, through necrosis, vesicles, and edema. Secondarily signs of shock, toxemia, anaphylaxis.

Clinical pathology Positive findings in the area of skin swabs or scrapings.

Necropsy lesions Inflammatory, degenerative, or vascular lesions in skin biopsy.

Diagnostic confirmation Positive finding in skin biopsy.

Treatment Primary treatment is removal of the (presumed) causative agent; supportive treatment includes treatment for pruritus, secondary infection, shock, toxemia, or fluid and electrolyte loss.

ETIOLOGY

Some of the identifiable occurrences of dermatitis in food animals and horses are as follows.

All Species

- Mycotic dermatitis as a result of *Dermatophilus congolensis*, in horses, cattle, and sheep
- *S. aureus*, a common finding in cases in all species, either as a sole pathogen or combined with other agents
- Ringworm
- Photosensitive dermatitis
- Chemical irritation (contact dermatitis) topically
- Arsenic—systemic poisoning
- Mange mite infestation—sarcoptic, psoroptic, chorioptic, demodectic mange

- Trombidiiform mite infestation (tyroglyphosis)
- Biting flies, especially *Culicoides* spp.; observed most commonly in horses, but also in other species
- *Stephanofilaria* spp. dermatitis
- *Strongyloides (Pelodera)* spp. dermatitis
- Besnoitiosis (*Besnoitia* spp.)

Cattle

- Udder impetigo (udder acne)—*Staphylococcus* spp.
- Udder cleft dermatitis of cattle
- Dermatitis interdigitalis (see following discussion)
- Ulcerative mammillitis—udder and teats only
- Cutaneous botryomycosis of the udder caused by a combination of trauma and infection by *Pseudomonas aeruginosa*
- Cowpox/buffalopox
- Flexural seborrhea
- Lumpy skin disease of cattle—painful nodules (2 to 5 cm) develop over the entire body, caused by pox virus, serotype *lumpy skin disease virus* (LSDV)
- Foot-and-mouth disease—vesicles around natural orifices; vesicular stomatitis with lesions on teats and coronet
- Bovine virus diarrhea, bovine malignant catarrh, bluetongue—erosive lesions around natural orifices, eyes, coronets
- Potato dermatitis in cattle, horses, and swine associated with prolonged feeding of potato distillery wastes; erythematous skin disease of distal limbs suspected to be of allergic origin
- Dermatitis as a result of the ingestion of *Vicia villosa* and *Vicia dasycarpa*
- Bovine exfoliative dermatitis

Sheep and Goats

- Strawberry footrot—proliferative pustular dermatosis linked to spirochete-like organisms and *Dermatophilus* and *Rhizobium*
- Dermatophilosis (lumpy wool disease, rain scald)—*Dermatophilus congolensis*
- Fleece rot—constant wetting and associated with *Pseudomonas aeruginosa*
- Staphylococcal dermatitis—exudative dermatitis around eyes, ears, and base of horns in sheep; vesicles possibly present on teats and udder in goats
- Sheeppox
- Contagious ecthyma—*Parapoxvirus* (*Orf*)
- Ulcerative dermatosis—caused by similar but antigenically distinct virus to Orf
- Rinderpest, peste de petits ruminants, bluetongue—as for cattle
- Foot-and-mouth disease and vesicular stomatitis
- Itch-mite (*Psorergates ovis*) infestation
- Blow-fly infestation (cutaneous myiasis)
- Elaeophoriasis (*Elaeophora* spp. infestation)
- Caprine idiopathic dermatitis
- Postdipping necrotic dermatitis (see following discussion).

Horses

- Staphylococcal pyoderma caused by *S. aureus/Staphylococcus intermedius*
- *Staphylococcus hyicus* in a syndrome reminiscent of greasy heel
- Dermatophytes, including ringworm, follicular dermatitis, hyphomycosis (pythiosis), tinea versicolor dermatitis
- Summer eczema (also Queensland or sweet itch)—sensitivity to *Culicoides* spp. sandflies
- Dermatophilosis/rain scald—*D. congolensis*
- *Actinomyces viscosum* causing skin pustules and nodules
- Horsepox
- Canadian horsepox
- Viral papular dermatitis (see following discussion)
- Vesicular stomatitis—vesicles around natural orifices
- Vesicular dermatitis around nasal area, eyes, and ears in horses stabled on shavings of a tree of the *Quassia* spp.
- Spongiotic vesicular dermatitis of unknown etiology
- Sporotrichosis
- Atopic dermatitis (IgE-mediated hypersensitivity)
- Chronic eosinophilic dermatitis (see following discussion)
- Pemphigus, lupus erythematosus, erythema multiforme, eosinophilic dermatitis and stomatitis (described separately in following discussion)
- Molluscum contagiosum (see following discussion)
- Linear hyperkeratosis (see following discussion)
- Nodular necrobiosis
- Equine aural plaque (see following discussion)
- Uasin Gishu disease
- Cutaneous habronemiasis
- Equine tropical lichen (see following discussion)
- Midline ventral dermatitis as a result of infestation with *Hydrotaea irritans* (horn fly and buffalo fly)
- Trombidiiform mites, e.g., *Pyemotes tritici* and *Acarus (Tyroglyphus) farinae*
- Ulcerative dermatitis, thrombocytopenia and neutropenia in neonatal foals (see Alloimmune hemolytic anemia of the newborn (neonatal isoerythrolysis, isoimmune hemolytic anemia of the newborn).

Pigs

- Ulcerative granuloma—*Borrelia suilla*
- Contagious epidermitis—*Staphylococcus hyicus* ("greasy pig disease")
- Pig pox
- Swine vesicular disease, vesicular exanthema of swine, foot-and-mouth disease—vesicles around natural orifices
- Contact with fresh parsnip tops, celery
- Sunburn
- Porcine necrotic ear syndrome (see following discussion)
- Nonspecific nutritional dermatitis—experimental nutritional deficiency of nicotinic acid, riboflavin, pantothenic acid, biotin
- Pityriasis rosea
- Idiopathic chronic recurrent dermatoses

Special Local Dermatitides

Special local dermatitides include dermatitis of the teats and udder, the bovine muzzle and coronet, and flexural seborrhea, and are dealt with under their respective headings.

PATHOGENESIS

Dermatitis is an inflammation of the deeper layers of the skin involving the blood vessels and lymphatics. The purely cellular layers of the epidermis are involved only secondarily. The noxious agent causes cellular damage, often to the point of necrosis, and, depending on the type of agent responsible, the resulting dermatitis varies in its manifestations. It may be acute or chronic, suppurative, weeping, seborrheic, ulcerative, or gangrenous. In all cases there is increased thickness and increased temperature of the part. Pain or pruritus is present, and erythema is evident in unpigmented skin. Histologically there is vasodilatation and infiltration with leukocytes and cellular necrosis. These changes are much less marked in chronic dermatitis.

CLINICAL FINDINGS

Affected skin areas first show erythema and increased warmth. The subsequent stages vary according to the type and severity of the causative agent. There may be development of discrete vesicular lesions or diffuse weeping. Edema of the skin and subcutaneous tissues may occur in severe cases. The next stage may be the healing stage of scab formation; if the injury is more severe, there may be necrosis or even gangrene of the affected skin area. Spread of infection to subcutaneous tissues may result in a diffuse cellulitis or phlegmonous lesion. A distinctive suppurative lesion is usually classified as pyoderma. Deep lesions that cause damage to dermal collagen may cause focal scarring and idiopathic fibrosing dermatitis (see following discussion).

A systemic reaction is likely to occur when the affected skin area is extensive. Shock, with peripheral circulatory failure, may be present in the early stages. Toxemia as a result of absorption of tissue breakdown products, or septicemia as a result of invasion via unprotected tissues, may occur in the later stages.

Individual dermatitides are as follows:

- **Interdigital dermatitis** is a low-grade exudative inflammation of the interdigital skin of cattle housed indoors and standing continuously in slurry. This condition has been linked to *Dichelobacter nodosus*.
- **Ovine postdipping necrotic dermatitis** is associated with *P. aeruginosa* and related to dipping in solutions containing no bacteriostatic agent. Necrotic lesions (1 to 3 cm in diameter), with cellulitis down to the underlying muscle, occur only along the backline and may be related to trauma during dipping. It may be accompanied by an outbreak of fatal otitis media with *P. aeruginosa* present in the lesion.
- **Ovine atopic dermatitis**: Only the wool-less parts of the skin are affected by symmetric erythema, alopecia, lichenification, and excoriation. Only occasional sheep in the flock are affected, and these are affected each summer, with remission during the winter months.
- **Caprine idiopathic dermatitis**: Alopecic, exudative dermatitis of all ages and both sexes of pygmy goats is characterized by hair loss and scaling and crusting around the eyes, lips and chin, ears, poll, perineum, and ventral abdomen. Histologically the lesions have a psoriasis-like form.
- **Chronic equine eosinophilic dermatitis** is characterized by marked acanthosis and hyperkeratosis, and eosinophilic granulomas in the pancreas, salivary glands, and other epithelial organs. The systemic involvement is accompanied by severe weight loss. The disease is chronic, and the cause unknown.
- **Spongiotic vesicular dermatitis** has been described in horses. Lesions are characterized by a multifocal, exudative, oozing dermatitis characterized histologically by epidermal spongiotic vesicles and perivascular eosinophilic, neutrophilic, and mixed mononuclear inflammation. Some horses are pruritic.
- **Equine nodular necrobiosis (eosinophilic granuloma)**: Firm, small (up to 1 cm in diameter) nodules, usually a number of them, occur on the sides of the trunk and neck. A hypersensitivity reaction to insect bites has been proposed as the underlying cause. The lesions consist largely of an accumulation of eosinophils.
- **Molluscum contagiosum** is a chronic, progressive dermatitis characterized by raised, hairless lesions 0.5 to 2 cm in diameter, covered by soft keratin, that bleed profusely when the horse is groomed. The lesions are on the face, shoulders, trunk, lateral aspects of limbs, fetlocks, and pasterns. Histologic examination identifies the disease because of the presence of characteristic inclusions in cells. These are thought to be poxvirus virions, but the virus cannot be cultivated from the lesions. There is no specific treatment
- **Systemic lupus erythematosus** (SLE) is an extensive dermatitis, manifested as a scaly, crusty dermatitis of the face, neck, and trunk, with loss of hair over the lesions, edema of the limbs, and mild to moderate lymph node enlargement. Multiple ulcers 11 cm in diameter are present on the oral mucosa, especially the mucocutaneous junctions of the lips and nares, and on the tongue. There is a severe systemic reaction, including a marked loss of body weight, a temperature up to 39.5°C (103.1 F), heart rate of 80/min, respiratory rate up to 60/min, painful swollen joints containing sterile serous fluid, stiff gait, reluctance to move, and persistent lateral recumbency. SLE is an immune-mediated disease with a characteristic histopathology including a necrotizing lymphocytic dermatitis and focal accumulations of lymphocytes in the liver, membranous glomerulonephritis, and synoviocyte hyperplasia. An antinuclear antibody test is diagnostic. No treatment is effective, and the disease runs a chronic progressive course marked by remissions and exacerbations.
- **Discoid lupus erythematosus** is an uncommon, benign variant of the systemic disease, with cutaneous lesions similar to those in the major disease but with no involvement of other tissues.
- **Erythema multiforme** is a self-limiting skin disease of horses and cattle characterized by macular, papular, urticarial, or bullous skin lesions but without any abnormality of the epidermis or loss of hair, and with no apparent itching or pain. The lesions occur symmetrically on most parts of the body, persist for long periods, and increase in size up to 5 cm to form annular or crescent-shaped wheals. Spontaneous disappearance of the lesions after about 3 months is usual. Symptomatic treatment may be effective but is not usually necessary.
- **Equine aural plaque**: Multiple white plaques, resembling papilloma and about 1 cm in diameter, develop on the inner surface of the ear pinna of horses. This condition has been associated with the papillomavirus that is thought to be transmitted by biting insects.
- **Equine tropical lichen** is an intensely irritating, papular eruption in the skin on the side of the neck, under the mane, on the shoulders, and at the tailhead, occurring in summer and recurring annually. The disease closely resembles the cutaneous sensitivity to *Culicoides* spp. but responds dramatically to treatment with ivermectin. Microfilariae, thought to be *Onchocerca* spp., can be found in histologic sections.
- **Linear hyperkeratosis** is most common in horses, especially Quarter horses. One case has been recorded in cattle. Lesions appear spontaneously in horses 1 to 5 years old and persist, usually for life. They appear first as isolated scaly lumps, which then coalesce to form a ridge, usually vertical, 3 to 4 cm wide and up to 70 cm long, of hyperkeratotic, hairless skin. There may be one or more lesions, commonly on the sides of the neck and chest. Symptomatic treatment appears to have no effect on the lesions.
- **Idiopathic fibrosing dermatitis**: As the end stage of several severe dermatoses, this causes damage to dermal collagen. Manifested by multiple fibrous plaques in the skin caused by sclerosis of the skin or subcutis, it resembles human morphea and the skin granulomas of animals.
- **Porcine dermatitis–nephropathy syndrome**, an idiopathic low-morbidity but highly fatal disease of feeder pigs, is characterized by papular vascular dermatopathy, systemic necrotizing vasculitis, and exudative and proliferative glomerulonephritis. Skin lesions are full-depth necrosis appearing as multiple flat red–blue papules up to 2 cm in diameter (which may coalesce to form large plaques) on any part of the body. Some pigs die of glomerulonephritis without skin lesions having been apparent. Many cases that show only skin lesions recover spontaneously in several weeks. The disease may disappear if the commercial grain ration used is ground more coarsely.
- **Porcine necrotic ear syndrome** is an extensive necrosis of the edges of the ears. The cause is unknown, but the possibility that a combination of *S. hyicus* infection and trauma by biting by pen mates is the cause seems high.
- **Porcine idiopathic chronic, recurrent dermatitis** has been recorded in sows in specific farrowing houses. Boars and piglets were not affected, and lesions disappeared as soon as the sows left the houses. Annular macules 11 cm in diameter and patches of erythema 11 cm in diameter occur only on white skin. There are no systemic signs.
- **Equine staphylococcal pyoderma** is a serious disease because the lesions are intractable to treatment and are so painful to touch that the horse is hard to handle, and the presence of the lesions under the harness, where they

commonly are, prevents the horse from working kindly. Harness horses are at a particular disadvantage. Individual lesions are raised nodules, 3 to 5 mm in diameter, covered by a small, easily removed scab. When these lift, they take a tuft of hair with them, and a small crater is left. A little pus exudes, and only a red serous fluid can be expressed. Individual lesions last a long time, at least several weeks, and fresh crops occur, causing the disease to spread slowly on the animal.

Pemphigus

Pemphigus is an autoimmune disease of the skin occurring in mature horses, usually 5 years of age or older, as well as in foals. Vesicles and pustules are usually very difficult to find because they progress rapidly to crusts, exfoliation, alopecia, and scaling.[1] There are a number of manifestations, of which pemphigus foliaceus is the most common. Pemphigus vulgaris and bullous pemphigoid, in contrast, are rare. Pemphigus is a chronic autoimmune disease often accompanied by severe weight loss.

Pemphigus foliaceus is not only the predominant form of pemphigus but also the most common autoimmune disease of the horse. The classic, but rarely seen, primary lesion is a vesicle or pustule. Usually, the earliest lesions visible are crusted papules best seen in lightly or nonhaired skin adjacent to mucocutaneous junctions—the nostrils, eyelids, or lips. Lesions rapidly coalesce to form multifocal or diffuse areas of crusting. Pemphigus foliaceus occurs as a generalized scabby, weeping dermatitis, but it may be localized as circumscribed, circular lesions in the mouth and vulva and on the skin at mucocutaneous junctions. The lesions are subepidermal bullae, from which the top layer can be pulled away, and are sore to the touch. In some cases the lesions are around the coronary bands on all limbs. Edema, urticaria, pruritus, and pain of the extremities, especially the hindlimbs, and the ventral abdominal region may result in pronounced lameness.

The differential diagnoses include all skin diseases caused by scaling and crusting. These include dermatophytosis, dermatophilosis, staphylococcal dermatitis and folliculitis, systemic granulomatous disease, and primary or idiopathic abnormalities of keratinization.

The diagnosis is based on history, clinical presentation, skin cytology, and histopathology. Immunohistochemical staining and direct immunofluorescence examination, consisting of a fluorescein–antihorse IgG applied to the lesion, can confirm the diagnosis. Corticosteroid or gold (aurothioglucose) therapy has been reported to result in improvement, but an inexorable deterioration is usual. Pemphigus foliaceus is recorded in goats as a widespread disease characterized by the presence of scales, sometimes in heavy crusts, and involvement of the coronets.

CLINICAL PATHOLOGY

Examination of skin scrapings or swabs for parasitic, bacterial, or other agents is essential. Culture and sensitivity tests for bacteria are advisable to enable the best treatment to be selected. Skin biopsy may be of value in confirming the diagnosis and determining the causal agent. In allergic or parasitic states there is usually an accumulation of eosinophils in the inflamed area. In mycotic dermatitis organisms are usually detectable in the deep skin layers, although they may not be cultivable from superficial specimens.

DIAGNOSIS

The clinical features of dermatitis are apparent. The characteristic features of the etiologic types of dermatitis are described under each specific disease. **Diagnostic confirmation** is by histopathological demonstration in a biopsy specimen.

> **DIFFERENTIAL DIAGNOSIS**
>
> **Hyperhidrosis** and **anhidrosis** are dysfunctions of sweating and have no cutaneous lesion.
>
> **Cutaneous neoplasm** is differentiable on histopathological examination.
>
> **Epitheliogenesis imperfecta** is a congenital absence of all layers of skin.
>
> **Vascular nevus** is a congenital lesion commonly referred to as a "birthmark."

TREATMENT

Primary treatment must be to remove the noxious physical or chemical agent from the environment or to supplement the diet to repair a nutritional deficiency. The choice of a suitable treatment for infectious skin disease will depend on the accurate identification of the etiologic agent.

Supportive treatment includes both local and systemic therapy. Local applications may need to be astringent, either as powders or lotions in the weeping stage or as greasy salves in the scabby stage. The inclusion of corticosteroids or antihistamine preparation is recommended in allergic states, and it is desirable to prescribe sedative or anesthetic agents when pain or pruritus is severe.

If shock is present, parenteral fluids should be administered. If the lesions are extensive or secondary bacterial invasion is likely to occur, parenterally administered antibiotics or antifungal agents may be preferred to topical applications. To facilitate skin repair, a high-protein diet or the administration of protein hydrolysates or amino acid combinations may find a place in the treatment of valuable animals. Nonspecific remedies such as gold-containing remedies (e.g., aurothioglucose) are commonly used in autoimmune diseases such as pemphigus.

The use of vaccines as prophylaxis in viral and bacterial dermatitides must not be neglected. Autogenous vaccines may be most satisfactory in bacterial infections. An autogenous vaccine is particularly recommended in the treatment of staphylococcal dermatitis in horses and bovine udder impetigo, in which long and repeated courses of treatment with penicillin produce only temporary remission. An autogenous vaccine produces a cure in many cases.

REFERENCE

1. Yu A. *Proc Am Assoc Eq Pract*. 2006;52:492-497.

PHOTOSENSITIZATION

> **SYNOPSIS**
>
> **Etiology** Caused by the accumulation of photosensitizing substances (PSs) in the skin, resulting in the local irritation of unprotected, unpigmented skin after exposure to sunlight. Four types of photosensitization are differentiated based on the underlying etiology.
>
> Type I, or primary, caused by intake of primary PS.
>
> Type II, as a result of inherited defects of porphyrin metabolism.
>
> Type III, or hepatogenous, as a result of liver damage and ensuing faulty excretion of phylloerythrin.
>
> Type IV, or idiopathic, as a result of undetermined etiology.
>
> **Epidemiology** Exposure to PSs and sunlight of specific wavelength. Similar incidence of sporadic cases and outbreaks. Always life-threatening condition unless exposure to sunlight can be avoided.
>
> **Clinical signs** Primary cases have cutaneous signs only (erythema, edema, necrosis, gangrene of light-colored skin or mucosae exposed to sunlight). Secondary cases have also signs of hepatic dysfunction (jaundice, prostration, short course, death) or porphyrin metabolism.
>
> **Clinical pathology** Nil for evidence of photosensitivity. In secondary cases there is evidence of the primary disease.
>
> **Necropsy lesions** Only skin lesions in primary cases. Secondary cases show liver lesions or evidence of porphyrin accumulation.
>
> **Differential diagnosis** Clinical evidence of restriction of damage to white, wool-less skin on body dorsum and lateral aspects of limbs, teats, corneas, and tongue and lips.
>
> **Treatment** Primary: remove from exposure to sunlight and PS. Supportive: treat for infection, shock, toxemia.

ETIOLOGY AND EPIDEMIOLOGY

Photosensitization is caused by exposure of tissue containing certain photoactive substances to light of specific wavelength. Substances with the potential to accumulate in skin and get activated by solar irradiation are termed **photosensitizing substances (PSs)**. Skin containing an excess of PSs that is exposed to sunlight while unprotected by hair, wool, or pigmentation is most affected. PSs release unstable high-energy molecules when exposed to a wavelength of light above 320 nm that reacts with substrate molecules in the skin. The result is the formation of free radicals causing cell damage in outer cells and becoming clinically apparent as inflammation, edema, ulceration, and even necrosis of the skin.

Photosensitization differs from sunburn in that it requires the presence of a photosensitizing agent, it is triggered by exposure to a wavelength of light between 320 and 400 nm (in contrast to sunburn, which in most cases is the result of exposure to light with lower wavelength), its onset is rapid (in contrast to the more delayed onset with sunburn), and skin lesions are considerably more severe than with sunburn.

Based on the origin of the photosensitizing agent, photosensitization has been classified into four classes, as follows:

- **Type I,** primary photosensitization caused by PSs of exogenous origin (no underlying primary pathology of the organism)
- **Type II,** photosensitization caused by aberrant pigment metabolism
- **Type III,** hepatogenous photosensitization caused by disturbed liver function
- **Type IV,** idiopathic photosensitization that is of undetermined etiology

Another form of photosensitization that is of little importance in livestock is the **photoallergic photosensitization** related to an immunologic response involving T-cell-mediated delayed hypersensitivity.

Type I, Primary Photosensitization

Exogenous PSs can enter the organism through oral ingestion (e.g., PSs contained in feed), parenteral administration (e.g., certain drugs), or direct absorption through skin. In livestock oral ingestion is the most common route of exposure, with PSs being either contained in the diet or, less commonly, an orally administered drug. Photosensitization as a result of the ingestion of exogenous photodynamic agents usually occurs when the plant is in the lush green stage and is growing rapidly. Livestock are affected within 4 to 5 days of going to pasture, and new cases cease soon after the animals are removed. In most cases the plant responsible must be eaten in large amounts and will therefore usually be found to be a dominant inhabitant of the pasture. All species of animals are affected by photodynamic agents, although susceptibility may vary between species and between animals of the same species. PSs that occur naturally in plants include the following:

- Dianthrone derivatives—hypericin in *Hypericum perforatum* (St. John's wort) and other *Hypericum* spp. and fagopyrin in seeds and dried plants of *Fagopyrum esculentum* (buckwheat)
- Furocoumarins in *Cymopterus* spp. (wild carrot), *Ammi majus*, and *Thamnosma texana*
- Perloline from perennial ryegrass (*Lolium perenne*)
- Cocoa shells in feedlot rations causing photosensitization in feedlot calves
- Gluten metabolites in dairy cattle concentrates being fed to horses
- *Erodium moschatum*, an exotic weed in South Africa, causing photosensitization in sheep
- Unidentified photodynamic agents in *Medicago denticulata* (burr trefoil) and the aphids that infest it, and in *Brassica* spp., *Erodium* spp., and *Trifolium* spp.

Drug-related photosensitization has been reported after oral treatment with phenothiazine, an antiparasitic drug, and anecdotally after treatment of cows with corticosteroids to induce parturition (photosensitive dermatitis of the teats, escutcheon, and udder).

Type II, Photosensitization as a Result of Aberrant Pigment Metabolism

The PSs associated with type II photosensitization are porphyrins that may accumulate in an organism with disturbed heme synthesis. The only known examples in domestic animals are the two rare inherited conditions of **congenital porphyria erythropoietica** (pink tooth) and **congenital protoporphyria erythropoietica** described in Limousin cattle.

Type III, Hepatogenous Photosensitization

Hepatogenous photosensitization is the most common form of the disorder in livestock. The PS is invariably **phylloerythrin**, a normal end product of chlorophyll metabolism excreted in the bile. When biliary secretion is obstructed by hepatitis or biliary duct obstruction, phylloerythrin accumulates in the body and may reach levels in the skin that make it sensitive to light. Although hepatogenous photosensitization is more common in animals grazing green pasture, it can occur in animals fed entirely on hay or other stored feeds and in animals exposed to hepatotoxic chemicals (e.g., carbon tetrachloride). There appears to be sufficient chlorophyll, or breakdown products of it, in stored feed to produce critical tissue levels of phylloerythrin in affected animals. The following list includes those substances or plants that are common causes of hepatogenous photosensitization. The individual plants are discussed in more detail in the section on poisonous plants.

Plants Containing Hepatotoxins

- *Pithomyces chartarum* fungus on perennial ryegrass, causing **facial eczema of sheep**
- *Periconia* spp. fungus on Bermuda grass
- Cyanobacteria associated with blue-green algae (water bloom) on drinking water in ponds, dams, and dugouts—*Microcystis flosaquae*
- Lupins—*Lupinus angustifolius* plus the accompanying fungus, *Phomopsis leptostromiformis*
- Signal grass (*Brachiaria decumbens* and *Brachiaria brizantha*), a common component of established pastures in Brazil
- Alligator weed (*Alternanthera philoxeroides*), a South American aquatic plant causing photosensitization in dairy cattle in Australia and New Zealand
- Weeds, including lantana (*Lantana camara*), *Lippia rehmanni*, sacahuiste (*Nolina texana*), coal oil bush (*Tetradymia* spp.), alecrim (*Holocalyx glaziovii*), ngaio (*Myoporum laetum*), *Crotalaria retusa*, ragwort (*Senecio jacobea*), *Sphenosciadium* spp.

Plants Containing Steroidal Saponins

The following plants containing steroidal saponins cause crystal-related cholangiohepatopathy:

- *Agave lecheguilla*, *Narthecium ossifragum*, *Panicum* spp. (panic and millet grasses), and *Tribulus terrestris* (caltrop, geeldikkop), plants that are grazed particularly by sheep
- *Narthecium ossifragum* (bog asphodel)—Sheep (lambs) grazing on pastures containing *N. ossifragum* on the west coast of Norway and in Scotland, northern England, Ireland, and the Faroe Islands have been affected by alveld, a hepatogenous photosensitivity disease. The disease is known as alveld (literally, "elf fire") in Norway; plochteach, saut, or yellowses in the British Isles; and ormajuka ("worm disease") in the Faroe Islands. Pastures containing *N. ossifragum* in these countries are commonly used for grazing sheep. Photosensitization of sheep grazing this plant usually occurs in 2- to 6-month-old lambs and is rarely seen in adult sheep. It produces similar clinical signs to those resulting from facial eczema, a disease most commonly seen in New Zealand and associated with the fungal toxin sporidesmin.

Congenitally Defective Hepatic Function

Inherited congenital photosensitivity in Corriedale and Southdown lambs is an inherited defect in the excretion of bile pigment.

Type IV, Photosensitization of Uncertain Etiology

In the following diseases it has not been possible to ascertain whether the photosensitization is primary or as a result of hepatic insufficiency:

- Feeding on rape or canola (*Brassica rapa*), kale, lucerne or alfalfa (*Medicago sativa*), burr medic or burr trefoil (*Medicago denticulata*), *Medicago minima*, *Trifolium hybridum* (alsike or Swedish clover), and *Erodium cicutarium* and *Erodium moschatum* (lamb's tongue, plantain)
- Cattle feeding on water-damaged or moldy alfalfa hay or alfalfa silage; extensive outbreaks usually with no signs suggestive of hepatic disease
- Cattle, sheep, and horses grazing lush pasture; many clinical cases occur sporadically
- Corticosteroids used systemically to terminate parturition in cows
- Phenanthridium used in the treatment of trypanosomiases

PATHOGENESIS

Penetration of light rays to sensitized tissues causes local cell death and tissue edema. Irritation is intense because of the edema of the lower skin level, and loss of skin by necrosis or gangrene and sloughing is common in the terminal stages. Nervous signs may occur and are caused either by the photodynamic agent, as in buckwheat poisoning, or by liver dysfunction.

Hepatogenous photosensitization involves production of a toxin, by a higher plant, fungus, or cyanobacterium (algae), that causes liver damage or dysfunction, resulting in the retention of the photosensitizing agent phylloerythrin.

CLINICAL FINDINGS

General Signs

Skin lesions are limited to lightly or unpigmented skin directly exposed to light; pigmented parts of the integument remain unaffected. Early signs include erythema and swelling of the muzzle, nasal and ocular discharge, and photophobia. Local edema is often severe and may cause drooping of the ears; closure of the eyelids and nostrils, causing dyspnea; and dysphagia as a result of swelling of the lips. As the disease progresses, fissuring followed by sloughing of the thick skin is observed. Keratitis may be present and become severe enough to cause blindness. Behavioral changes are a result of intense irritation and include restlessness and scratching and rubbing of affected skin parts. When the teats are affected, the cow may kick at them and walk into ponds to immerse the teats in water, sometimes rocking backward and forward as if to cool the affected parts. In nursing ewes there may be resentment toward the lambs sucking, and heavy lamb mortalities as a result of starvation may result. General depression, anorexia, and even recumbency may occur but are related to liver injury and disturbed liver function.

Skin Lesions

Skin lesions are initially erythema, followed by edema and subsequent weeping with matting and then shedding of clumps of hair, and finally gangrene. The lesions have a characteristic distribution, restricted to the unpigmented areas of the skin and to those parts that are exposed to solar rays. They are most pronounced on the dorsum of the body, diminishing in degree down the sides, and are absent from the ventral surface. The demarcation between lesions and normal skin is very clear-cut, particularly in animals with broken-colored coats.

Predilection sites for lesions are the ears; conjunctiva, causing opacity of the lateral aspect of the cornea; eyelids; muzzle; face; lateral aspects of the teats; and, to a lesser extent, the vulva and perineum. In solid black cattle dermatitis will be seen at the lips of the vulva, on the edges of the eyelids, and on the cornea. Linear erosions often occur on the tip and sides of the tongue in animals with unpigmented oral mucosa. In severe cases the exudation and matting of the hair and local edema cause closure of the eyelids and nostrils. In the late stages necrosis or dry gangrene of affected areas leads to sloughing of large areas of skin.

Systemic Signs

Systemic signs include shock in the early stages, as a result of extensive tissue damage. There is an increase in the pulse rate, with ataxia and weakness. Subsequently a considerable elevation of temperature (41° to 42° C, 106° to 107° F) may occur.

Nervous Signs

Nervous signs, including ataxia, posterior paralysis and blindness, and depression or excitement, are often observed. A peculiar sensitivity to water is sometimes seen in sheep with facial eczema: when driven through water, they may lie down in it and have a convulsion.

CLINICAL PATHOLOGY

In most cases a presumptive diagnosis can be made based on clinical presentation in combination with the history of the patient (recently pastured, access to certain plants, etc.). There are no specific diagnostic tests to confirm photosensitization.

Hepatogenous photosensitization can be diagnosed by analysis of plasma phylloerythrin concentration using a spectroscopic method. Plasma or serum fluorescence can be used to measure the elevation of phylloerythrin above normal levels before hepatogenous photosensitization. The levels of phylloerythrin in plasma of lambs grazing *N. ossifragum* are increased from a normal of less than 0.05 μg/mL to more than 0.3 μg/mL when clinical signs of photosensitization are observed. Levels in skin are also increased.

In lambs in which facial eczema was experimentally induced by dosing with the mycotoxin sporidesmin, the plasma concentrations of phylloerythrin were increased from a normal of less than 0.1 μmol/L to 0.3 μmol/L when clinical signs were evident. The concentration of phylloerythrin in the skin began increasing 2 to 3 days later than that in the blood.

Determining the presence of liver damage or disturbed liver function is indicated. Icterus is highly suggestive of hepatogenous hypersensitization but should be confirmed by measuring the serum activity of specific liver enzymes and the serum bilirubin concentration.

NECROPSY FINDINGS

In primary photosensitization, lesions are restricted to white-haired or pale-skinned areas of skin or mucosa that have been exposed to sunlight, and they vary from necrosis to gangrene. Lesions characteristic of hepatic injury or metabolic defects of porphyrin metabolism are described elsewhere.

Diffuse hepatocellular hydropic degeneration and hyperplasia of the smooth endoplasmic reticulum associated with marked multifocal cholangitis in the portal triads with bile duct proliferation are characteristic of the hepatic lesions of sheep grazing *Brachiaria decumbens*. Foam cells are present in the liver and mesenteric and hepatic lymph nodes of cattle grazing *Brachiaria* spp. Hepatocellular degeneration is the primary event in alveld photosensitization in sheep. High concentrations of conjugated episapogenins are present in both the liver and bile in alveld-affected lambs.

DIFFERENTIAL DIAGNOSIS

The diagnosis of photosensitivity depends almost entirely on the distribution of the lesions. It can be readily confused with other dermatitides if this restriction to unpigmented and hairless parts is not kept in mind.

Mycotic dermatitis is often mistaken for photosensitization because of its tendency to commence along the back line and over the rump, but it occurs on colored and white parts alike.

Frequent wetting, as in periods of heavy rainfall, along the back in horses or cattle with a dense hair coat.

Bighead of rams associated with *Clostridium novyi* infection may also be confused with photosensitization, but the local swelling is an acute inflammatory edema, and many clostridia are present in the lesion.

Keratitis sometimes seen in photosensitization can been confused with those of pinkeye, but that disease is not accompanied by extensive dermatitis.

Continued

Sunburn is a very rare differential that has been reported in white swine, closely shorn sheep, and white-faced horses only.

Treatment

Primary treatment includes immediate removal from direct sunlight, prevention of ingestion of further toxic material, and the administration of laxatives to eliminate toxic materials already eaten. In areas where the disease is enzootic the use of dark-skinned breeds may make it possible to utilize pastures that would otherwise be too dangerous.

Local treatment is governed by the stage of the lesions. Nonsteroidal antiinflammatory drugs (NSAIDs), corticosteroids, or antihistamines can be administered parenterally and adequate doses maintained. To avoid septicemia, the prophylactic administration of antibiotics may be worthwhile in some instances.

FURTHER READING

House JK, et al. Primary photosensitization in cattle ingesting silage. *J Am Vet Med Assoc*. 1996;209:1604.
Plumlee KH. Photosensitization in ruminants. *Vet Med*. 1995;90:605-612.

Diseases of the Hair, Wool, Follicles, and Skin Glands

ALOPECIA AND HYPOTRICHOSIS

ETIOLOGY

Alopecia and hypotrichosis are defined as lack of hair in any quantity on a normally haired body surface.[1] In contrast to alopecia, which describes hair loss of a skin surface with previously normal hair growth, hypotrichosis refers to a condition where there was no hair growth or abnormally low hair growth in the first place. Some texts define alopecia simply as hair loss and subdivide alopecia into a congenital and an acquired form, the former also being referred to as hypotrichosis. Acquired alopecias are further subdivided into cicatrical and noncicatricial alopecia.

Both may be caused by the following conditions.

Failure of Follicles to Develop

- Congenital hypotrichosis
- Hypotrichosis in piglets without dental dysplasia

Loss of Follicles

- Cicatricial alopecia as a result of scarring after deep skin wounds that destroy follicles—Cicatricial alopecia occurs following permanent destruction of the hair follicles, and regrowth of hair will not occur. Examples include physical, chemical, or thermal injury; severe furunculosis; neoplasia; and certain infections, such as cutaneous onchocerciasis.

Failure of the Follicle to Produce a Fiber

Congenital

- Inherited symmetric alopecia
- Congenital hypotrichosis/hypotrichosis and anodontia defect (alopecia of variable degree associated with incomplete dentation, mainly occurring in male calves)
- Hypotrichosis in Polled Hereford calves
- Lethal hypotrichosis in Holstein–Friesian calves (generalized alopecia, with sparse hair on muzzle, eyelids, and ears—affected calves die within hours of life)
- Viable hypotrichosis in different cattle breeds (Guernsey, Jersey, Holstein–Friesian: generalized alopecia with sparse hair growth on legs, tail, eyelids, and ear pinnae)
- Hair-coat-color-linked follicle dysplasia
- Inherited dyserythropoiesis and dyskeratosis
- In baldy calves combined with adenohypophyseal hypoplasia
- Congenital hypothyroidism (goiter) as a result of iodine deficiency in the dam

Acquired

- Neurogenic alopecia as a result of peripheral nerve damage
- Infection in the follicle
- Epidermolysis bullosa in calves[2]
- Alopecia areata of horses and, less commonly, cows characterized by one or more round lesions of nonpruritic, nonscarring alopecia over the face, neck, shoulders, and brisket[3]
- Bovine besnoitiosis[4]

Loss of Preformed Fibers

- Dermatomycoses—ringworm
- Mycotic dermatitis in all species as a result of *D. congolensis*
- Metabolic alopecia subsequent to a period of malnutrition or severe illness (e.g., calves having suffered severe diarrhea or calves with incomplete function of the reticular groove reflex [rumen drinker calves])[5]
- Alopecia of calves fed milk replacer containing fats of nonanimal origin (whale, palm, or soya oil); fibers grown during the period of nutritional or metabolic stress have a zone of weakness and are easily broken
- Traumatic alopecia as a result of excessive scratching or rubbing associated with louse, tick, or itch-mite infestations; rubbing against narrow doors, feed troughs, or tethers in confined housing; rubbing against harness in working animals
- Poisoning by thallium, selenium, arsenic, mercury, or the tree *Leucaena leucocephala*
- Idiopathic hair loss from the tail-switch of well-fed beef bulls
- Sterile eosinophilic folliculitis of cattle
- Wool slip
- In many primary skin diseases (e.g., parakeratosis, hyperkeratosis, dermatitis, cutaneous neoplasia, sarcoid, pythiosis), hair loss at the site of local lesions

PATHOGENESIS

In inherited hair defects the underlying cause can be disturbed hair follicle formation resulting in a reduced hair follicle quantity or disturbed functionality of hair follicles that are present in adequate numbers. Noncicatricial alopecia is caused by reversible trauma to previously functional hair follicles by inflammation or mechanical trauma, which results in disturbed or interrupted synthesis in the hair bulb and ensuing shedding or fracture of hairs. Cicatricial alopecia is characterized by an irreversible destruction of hair follicles most commonly caused by physical, chemical, or thermal injury or severe inflammation.

Chemical depilation produced by cytotoxic agents, such as cyclophosphamide, occurs as a result of induced cytoplasmic degeneration in some of the germinative cells of the bulb of the wool follicle. The alteration in cell function is temporary, so that regrowth of the fiber should follow.

The pathogenesis of alopecia areata, primarily occurring in horses but also in cattle, has been associated with damage to growing hair mediated by T lymphocytes presumably specific for antigens of the hair matrix (autoimmune disease).[3] A genetic predisposition for alopecia areata has been discussed for humans.

CLINICAL FINDINGS

When alopecia is a result of breakage of the fiber, the stumps of old fibers or developing new ones may be seen. When fibers fail to grow, the skin is shiny and in most cases is thinner than normal. In cases of congenital follicular aplasia, the ordinary covering hairs are absent, but the coarser tactile hairs around the eyes, lips, and extremities are often present. Absence of the hair coat makes the animal more susceptible to the effects of sudden changes of environmental temperature. There may be manifestations of a primary disease and evidence of scratching or rubbing.

Alopecia areata in horses primarily affects the mane, head, and tail, whereas in cattle extensive alopecia affecting large parts of the body has been reported.[3,6] Cases reported in the literature are primarily from animals showing first signs at adult age.[3,6] In cattle a predisposition of black-haired breeds (Black

Angus, Aberdeen Angus, Eringer) has been proposed.[3]

Congenital hypotrichosis results in alopecia that is apparent at birth or develops within the neonatal period.

CLINICAL PATHOLOGY

If the cause of the alopecia is not apparent after the examination of skin scrapings or swabs, a skin biopsy will reveal the status of the follicular epithelium. Alopecia areata is characterized by bulbar and peribulbar lymphocyte infiltration, primary targeting anagen hair follicles.[3] In early stages several biopsies may be required to identify this pattern of infiltration. More advanced stages show dysplastic follicles with mild to moderate concentric fibrosis surrounding rudiments of hair bulbs.[5]

DIFFERENTIAL DIAGNOSIS

Diagnostic confirmation of alopecia is by visual recognition, the diagnostic problem being to determine the primary cause of the hair or fiber loss.

TREATMENT

Primary treatment consists of removing the causes of trauma or other damage to fibers. In cases of faulty follicle or fiber development treatment is not usually attempted.

FURTHER READING

Anonymous. Alopecia in the horse—an overview. *Vet Dermatol.* 2000;11:191-203.

Mecklenburg L. An overview on congenital alopecia in domestic animals. *Vet Dermatol.* 2006;17:393-410.

Pascoe RR. Alopecia, diagnosis and treatment. *Equine Pract.* 1993;15:8-16.

REFERENCES

1. Mecklenburg L. *Vet Dermatol.* 2006;17:393-410.
2. Foster AP, et al. *J Comp Pathol.* 2010;142:336-340.
3. Valentine B, et al. *J Vet Diagn Invest.* 2012;24:405-407.
4. Rostaher A, et al. *Vet Dermatol.* 2010;21:329-334.
5. Lorenz I, et al. *Dtsch Tierarztl Wochenschr.* 2007;114:231-235.
6. Hoolahan DE, et al. *Vet Dermatol.* 2013;24:282-285.

ACHROMOTRICHIA

Achromotrichia is a deficient pigmentation in hair or wool fiber, which may manifest as follows:

- Bands of depigmentation in an otherwise black wool fleece are the result of a transitory deficiency of copper in the diet.
- Cattle on diets containing excess molybdenum and deficient copper show a peculiar speckling of the coat caused by an absence of pigment in a proportion of hair fibers. The speckling is often most marked around the eyes, giving the animal the appearance of wearing spectacles.
- General loss of density of pigmentation in all coat colors (e.g., Hereford cattle shade off from their normal deep red to a washed-out orange)

LEUKODERMA AND LEUKOTRICHIA

Several skin diseases of the horse are characterized by an acquired loss of melanin pigment in the epidermis or hair. Melanocytes in the epidermis and those in the hair bulbs are frequently affected independently. Leukotrichia occurs when the melanocytes in the hair bulbs lose their normal amount of melanin pigment. When the melanocytes in the epidermis are affected and the skin loses normal pigmentation, the abnormality is leukoderma. Whereas leukotrichia can be observed as a single entity, leukoderma is most commonly associated with leukotrichia.

ETIOLOGY

The etiology and pathogenesis of leukoderma are unknown, but trauma, inflammation, autoimmune reactions against melanocytes, local injections with epinephrine-containing local anesthetics, and defects of the autonomous nervous system have been discussed. Specific forms of leukoderma have been linked to hereditary gene defects (see following discussion).

PATHOPHYSIOLOGY

The unknown underlying cause appears to result in acquired loss of functional melanocytes.

CLINICAL FINDINGS

The forms of leukotrichia/leukoderma have been reported in horses:

- **Reticulated leukotrichia**: Alopecia and ensuing leukotrichia in a characteristic cross-hatched or reticulated pattern. Yearlings and occasionally older animals are affected, and Quarters horses appear to be predisposed.
- **Spotted leukotrichia**: Multiple, sharply demarcated area of leukotrichia of 1 to 3 cm in diameter.
- **Juvenile Arabian leukoderma**: Most common form of leukoderma in horses, reported in young Arabian and occasionally in Quarter horses. One- to 2-year-old animals develop leukoderma on eyelids, periocular skin, muzzle, nares, genitalia, anus perineum, and inguinal region.
- **Hyperesthetic leukotrichia**: Condition of unknown etiology that is characterized by the development of single or multiple very painful crusts on the dorsal midline from withers to tail. Crusts disappear and pain resolves after 2 to 3 months, while leukotrichia persists.
- **Albinism and lethal white foal syndrome:** Albinism refers to a congenital lack of melatonin pigment in skin, hair, and other normally pigmented tissues. Albinism can occur as partial or complete albinism, the latter being inherited as autosomal-dominant trait that is only viable in the heterozygous state. The homozygous state results in a nonviable embryo that is resorbed in early gestation. A different form of lethal white foal syndrome results in homozygous expression of the associated trait and affects a subset of American Paint horses with the so-called frame overo color pattern.

CLINICAL PATHOLOGY

A reduced number of melanocytes within epidermis and follicular epithelium in combination with complete loss of melanin pigment from the epidermis are typical findings.

TREATMENT

No specific treatment is currently available

FURTHER READING

Pigmentary disorders. *Vet Dermatol.* 2000;11:205-210.

VITILIGO

Vitiligo is a presumably acquired autoimmune disorder characterized by patchy depigmentation of the skin described in horses, cattle, and other species.

ETIOLOGY

Although the etiology of vitiligo is still unknown, evidence corroborating the hypothesis that vitiligo is an acquired autoimmune disease associated with the production of antimelanocyte antibodies has accumulated over the last decades.[1] Other etiologies discussed in the literature are an increased susceptibility of melanocytes to certain melatonin precursor molecules or local nerve injuries. A genetic etiology is suspected in Arabian horses and Holstein–Friesian cattle.

PATHOPHYSIOLOGY

The underlying cause results in a complete, although sometimes reversible, loss of functional melanocytes in a small area of the dermis.

CLINICAL FINDINGS

Vitiligo has been reported in different breeds, without apparent gender predisposition. Although the condition can develop at any age, it most commonly is observed in young animals. Typical presentation is a patchy depigmentation of the skin of the muzzle, eyelids, and occasionally anus and other body regions. The degree of depigmentation can vary over time, and the condition may even completely resolve, making the interpretation of anecdotal treatment successes difficult. The defect is esthetic only.

CLINICAL PATHOLOGY

Histopathological examination reveals a complete absence of melanocytes from affected areas. Increased numbers of Langerhans cells and epidermal vacuolization have been reported in some cases.[1]

TREATMENT

No specific treatment with confirmed efficacy is currently available. Anecdotal reports of improvement after supplementation of vitamins and minerals (vitamin A and copper) are available.[1] Because of the possible genetic predisposition, the use of affected animals for breeding has been discouraged.

FURTHER READING

Montes LF, et al. Value of histopathology in vitiligo. *J Dermatol.* 2003;42:57-61.
Sandoval-Cruz M, et al. Immunopathogenesis of vitiligo. *Autoimmun Rev.* 2011;10:762-765.

REFERENCE

1. Montes LF, et al. *J Eq Vet Sci.* 2008;28:171-175.

SEBORRHEA

ETIOLOGY

The etiology of seborrhea is still not understood. Historically seborrhea was considered to be the result of excessive secretion of sebum onto the skin surface. More recently seborrhea was classified as disease of abnormal cornification and keratinization of the skin rather than of excessive sebum production because there is little evidence for abnormal function of the sebaceous glands. In large animals it is always secondary to dermatitis or other skin irritations that result in excessive crusting, scaling, or oiliness, such as the following:

- Exudative epidermitis of pigs associated with *S. hyicus*
- Greasy heel of horses, including infection with *S. hyicus*
- Greasy heel of cattle
- Flexural seborrhea of cattle
- Besnoitiosis of cattle associated with *Besnoitia besnoiti*

CLINICAL FINDINGS

In primary seborrhea there are no lesions, only excessive greasiness of the skin. The sebum may be spread over the body surface like a film of oil or be dried into crusts, which can be removed easily. Sebaceous glands may be hypertrophied.

Flexural Seborrhea

Flexural seborrhea is most common in young periparturient dairy cows. Severe inflammation and a profuse outpouring of sebum appear in the groin between the udder and the medial surface of the thigh or in the median fissure between the two halves of the udder. Extensive skin necrosis follows, causing a pronounced odor of decay, which may be the first sign observed by the owner (see also under "Udder Cleft Dermatitis"). Irritation may cause lameness, and the cow may attempt to lick the part. Shedding of the oily, malodorous skin leaves a raw surface beneath; healing follows in 3 to 4 weeks.

Greasy Heel of Cows

Cows grazing constantly irrigated, wet pastures or in very muddy conditions in tropical areas may develop local swelling, with deep fissuring of the skin and an outpouring of vile-smelling exudate on the back of the pastern of all four feet but most severely in the hindlimbs. Affected animals are badly lame, and their milk yield declines sharply. Moving the cows to dry land and treating systemically with a broad-spectrum antibiotic effects a rapid recovery.

Greasy Heel of Horses (Scratches)

Greasy heel occurs mostly on the hind pasterns of horses that stand continuously in wet, unsanitary stables. Some cases do occur in well-managed stables. It has been suggested that secondary infections associated with either *S. aureus* and *D. congolensis* may be causative factors. Dermatophytosis, chorioptic mange, and photosensitization are also possible causative factors.

Lameness and soreness to touch are a result of excoriations called scratches on the back of the pastern that extend down to the coronary band. The skin is thick and greasy; if neglected, the condition spreads around to the front and up the back of the leg. This involvement can be severe enough to interfere with normal movement of the limb.

CLINICAL PATHOLOGY

The diagnosis is based on the clinical presentation and on ruling out other skin conditions resulting in abnormal cornification and keratinization. The primary cause of the seborrhea may be diagnosed by a suitable examination for the presence of parasitic or bacterial pathogens. Histopathology may be supportive to rule out other causes.

DIFFERENTIAL DIAGNOSIS

The lesion is characteristic, and diagnostic confirmation is by histopathological examination of a biopsy specimen; the principal difficulty is to determine the primary cause. All the types listed may be mistaken for:

Injury, commonly wire cuts or rope burn

Flexural seborrhea for injury, usually a result of straddling a gate or wire fence

Greasy heel of horses for chorioptic mange

TREATMENT

With secondary seborrhea the primary objective of treatment must be to resolve the underlying cause. Topical and symptomatic treatment of the affected skin is indicated for relief and to assist in control of the disease. Seborrheic shampoos and lotions can either be keratolytic or keratoplastic. Keratolytic products may initially worsen the scale production by chemically debriding the stratum corneum but will eventually result in reduced scale formation. Particularly during the initial phase, frequent washing of the affected skin to remove debrided cells is important. Keratoplastic ointments slow the mitotic rate of the epidermis, thereby reducing scale formation. Emollients are useful after washing the skin to rehydrate, lubricate, and soften the skin. In severe cases associated with pyoderma or even skin necrosis, the use of local and systemic broad-spectrum antibiotics may be indicated.

FOLLICULITIS

ETIOLOGY

Etiology includes inflammation and possibly infection of hair follicles that can be caused by suppurative organisms (often *staphylococci*), secondary to follicular trauma, obstruction of sebaceous gland ducts, or more rarely as result of an autoimmune reaction. Identifiable forms of folliculitis as individual diseases include the following:

- Staphylococcal dermatitis of horses
- Contagious acne of horses
- Benign facial folliculitis of sucking lambs
- Staphylococcal folliculitis of goats
- Bovine sterile eosinophilic folliculitis

PATHOGENESIS

Depending on the underlying etiology, inflammatory cells infiltrate the walls and lumen of hair follicles. With more extensive inflammation, neutrophils may also infiltrate perifollicular tissue, resulting in formation of larger abscesses (**furunculosis**). Increased pressure and tissue lysis will result in a rupture of the hair follicle with an ensuing granulomatous dermal reaction.

CLINICAL FINDINGS

Folliculitis may present with skin lesions in almost any location of the skin. Early stages present as papules or pustules with hairs emerging through the lesions. Involvement of the hair follicle allows one to differentiate this condition from impetigo, where the hair follicle is not involved.[1] Later focal crusting and alopecia and pruritus may develop. Pustule rupture leads to contamination of the surrounding skin and development of further lesions, such as ulcerations and draining tracts. Severe cases can be associated with pain, pyrexia, and feed-intake depression. Chronic folliculitis can affect skin pigmentation and cause permanent destruction of hair follicles, which results in cicatricial alopecia.

In **bovine sterile eosinophilic folliculitis**, the multiple lesions are crusted, alopecic,

3- to 5-cm-diameter nodules on all parts of the body except the limbs. They are composed largely of eosinophilic cells and are negative on culture.

Staphylococcal folliculitis in goats can be generalized, with pustules developing in the periocular and periauricular area, ventral abdomen, medial thighs, and distal limbs.[1] Involvement of the udder skin can occasionally occur.

Benign folliculitis of suckling lambs can develop from the first week of life and consists of small pustules and crusts on the lips, nostrils, ventral tail, and perineum. The condition resolves spontaneously over several weeks.

CLINICAL PATHOLOGY

Swabs should be taken for bacteriologic and parasitologic examination. Histopathological findings include microabscesses associated with hair follicles, along with abscessation and necrosis of the epidermis, dermis, and subcutaneous tissue. Cellular infiltration with mononuclear cells and granulocytes is another common finding.

DIFFERENTIAL DIAGNOSIS

Diagnostic confirmation is by demonstration of infection of hair follicles in a biopsy specimen.

Udder impetigo of cattle; lesions do not involve hair follicles in the first place.

Dermatophytosis

Dermatophilosis

Besnoitiosis of cattle

Viral infections caused by BHV (types 1, 2, and 4), BVD, bovine *parapox virus*, cowpox, buffalopox, bluetongue virus, vesicular stomatitis, foot-and-mouth disease

Exudative epidermitis of pigs (greasy pig disease) as a result of *S. hyicus*, with extensive seborrheic dermatitis

Ulcerative dermatitis of face in adult sheep

Ecthyma (orf)

Facial eczema of sheep; caused by hepatogenous photosensitization

Leg dermatitis down to coronet of sheep

Chronic pectoral and ventral midline abscesses in horses as a result of *Corynebacterium pseudotuberculosis;* not a skin lesion but it resembles furunculosis.

TREATMENT

Primary treatment consists of identifying and eliminating possible primary causes. Topical treatment commences with clipping and cleaning the skin by washing followed by a disinfectant rinse, for instance, with chlorhexidine-based products. Affected areas should be treated with antibacterial ointments or lotions. If the lesions are extensive, the parenteral administration of antibiotics is recommended. The course of treatment should last 1 week; in chronic cases this may need to be at least 1 month; a broad-spectrum preparation is recommended.

For **supportive treatment**, infected animals should be isolated and grooming tools and blankets disinfected.

REFERENCE

1. Foster AP. *Vet Dermatol.* 2012;23:e42-e63.

Diseases of the Subcutis

SUBCUTANEOUS EDEMA (ANASARCA)

ETIOLOGY

Extensive accumulation of edema fluid in the subcutaneous tissue is part of general edema and is caused by the same diseases, as follows.

Increased Hydrostatic Pressure

- Congestive heart failure
- Vascular compression by a mass (e.g., anterior mediastinal lymphosarcoma, large hematoma)
- Vascular obstruction of blood vessels or lymphatic vessels (e.g., thrombophlebitis or thrombosis)

Hypoproteinemic (Hypooncotic) Edema

- Reduced albumin production in the liver associated with chronic inflammation or liver insufficiency (e.g., fascioliasis or liver cirrhosis)
- Nephrotic syndrome with protein loss into urine (e.g., renal amyloidosis in cattle)
- Protein-losing enteropathy (e.g., intestinal nematodiasis or paratuberculosis in cattle)

Increased Blood Vessel Permeability

- Inflammation (e.g., **dourine** of horses or equine infectious anemia, bacterial infections by *Clostridium* spp. or *Anthrax*)
- Allergic reaction (e.g., purpura hemorrhagica of horses, insect stings)

Fetal Anasarca

- Some pigs with congenital goiter also have myxedema, especially of the neck.
- Sporadic cases resulting from unknown causes are sometimes associated with deformities (e.g., in Awassi sheep).
- Congenital absence of lymph nodes and some lymph channels causes edema to be present at birth.

DIFFERENTIAL DIAGNOSIS

Diagnostic confirmation is by clinical detection of serous fluid in a subcutaneous site.

In male ruminants, **extravasation of urine** as a result of urethral obstruction and rupture.

Subcutaneous hemorrhage, hematoma or seroma, which is not necessarily dependent, nor bilaterally symmetric.

Ventral hernia, usually unilateral and does not pit on pressure.

Cellulitis, usually asymmetric, hot, often painful, does not pit on pressure and can be sampled by needle puncture.

PATHOGENESIS

Alteration in the balance between the hydrostatic pressure of intravascular fluids, the blood and lymph, and the osmotic pressure of those fluids or changes in the integrity of the filtering mechanism of the capillary endothelium (leaky vessels) leads to a positive advantage by the hydrostatic pressure of the system and causes a flow of fluid out of the vessels into the tissues.

CLINICAL FINDINGS

There is visible swelling, either local or diffuse. The skin is puffy and pits on pressure; there is no pain unless inflammation is also present. In large animals the edema is usually confined to the ventral aspects of the head, neck, and trunk and is seldom seen on the limbs.

CLINICAL PATHOLOGY

Anasarca is a clinical diagnosis, but many estimates (e.g., arterial blood pressure, serum and urine protein levels) provide contributory evidence. Normal total protein concentrations in serum or plasma allow one to rule out hypooncotic edema. Differentiation between obstructive and inflammatory edema can be made by cytologic and bacteriologic examination of the fluid.

TREATMENT

Primary treatment requires correction of the primary causal abnormality. Supportive treatment will also depend on the underlying cause but can consist of transfusing plasma or whole blood in cases of hypooncotic edema, or antiinflammatory or diuretic therapy in cases of inflammatory or allergic edema.

ANGIOEDEMA (ANGIONEUROTIC EDEMA)

ETIOLOGY

Transient, localized subcutaneous edema as a result of an allergic reaction and caused by endogenous and exogenous allergens provokes either local or diffuse lesions. Angioedema occurs most frequently in cattle and horses on pasture, especially during the period when the pasture is in flower. This suggests that the allergen is a plant protein. Fish meal may also provoke an attack.

Recurrence in individual animals is common. Angioedema can also occur as adverse reaction to parenteral administration of certain antibiotics, vaccines, blood, plasma, or other IV fluids.

PATHOGENESIS

The precise type of hypersensitivity reaction has not yet been determined, but most cases appear to be associated with a type I or type III hypersensitivity reaction. After an initial erythema, local vascular dilatation is followed by leakage of plasma through damaged vessels.

CLINICAL FINDINGS

Local lesions most commonly affect the head, with diffuse edema of the muzzle, eyelids, conjunctiva, and cheeks. Occasionally only the conjunctiva is affected, so that the eyelids are puffy, the nictitating membrane is swollen and protruding, and lacrimation is profuse. Affected parts are not painful to touch, but shaking the head and rubbing against objects suggest irritation. Salivation and nasal discharge may be accompanying signs.

Perineal involvement includes vulvar swelling, often asymmetric, and the perianal skin, and sometimes the skin of the udder, is swollen and edematous. When the **udder** is affected, the teats and base of the udder are edematous and cows may paddle with the hind limbs, suggesting irritation in the teats. Edema of the lower limbs, usually from the knees or hocks down to the coronets, is a rare sign.

Systemic signs are absent, except in those rare cases where angioedema is part of a wider allergic response, when bloat, diarrhea, and dyspnea may occur, often with sufficient severity to require urgent treatment.

CLINICAL PATHOLOGY

The blood eosinophil count is often within the normal range, but may be elevated from a normal level of 4% to 5% up to 12% to 15%.

DIFFERENTIAL DIAGNOSIS

Diagnostic confirmation is found with sudden onset and disappearance of edema at the typical sites.

Subcutaneous edema as a result of vascular pressure occurs mostly in dependent parts and is not irritating.

In horses, and rarely in cattle, angioedema may be simulated by **purpura hemorrhagica**, but hemorrhages are usually visible in the mucosae in purpura.

TREATMENT

Primary treatment to remove the specific cause is usually impossible, but affected animals should be removed from the suspected source of allergens. Cattle running at pasture should be confined and fed on dry feed for at least a week.

Supportive treatment to relieve the vascular lesion is always administered even though spontaneous recovery is the rule. In acute cases with suspected anaphylaxis, epinephrine should be administered parenterally. For subacute cases, corticosteroids or other antiinflammatories are preferred over antihistamines or epinephrine; usually only one injection is required.

TREATMENT

Acute anaphylaxis with angioedema:
- Epinephrine: 3 to 5 mL/ 450 kg of a 1 : 1000 solution IM or SC (can be combined with steroids) (R-1)

Acute angioedema in horses:
- Dexamethasone soluble 0.01 to 0.1 mg/kg IV or IM q24 h for 3 to 7 days (R-1)
- Hydroxyzine hydrochloride 0.5 to 1.0 mg/kg IM or PO q8 h (R-2)
- Diphenhydramine hydrochloride 0.7 to 1 mg/kg q12 h (R-2)
- Chlorpheniramine 0.25 to 0.5 mg/kg q12 h (R-2)

SUBCUTANEOUS EMPHYSEMA

ETIOLOGY

Emphysema, free gas in the subcutaneous tissue, occurs when air or gas accumulates in the subcutaneous tissue as a result of the following:

- Air entering through a cutaneous wound made surgically or accidentally, particularly in the axilla or inguinal region
- Extension from pulmonary emphysema
- Air entering tissues through a discontinuity in the respiratory tract lining (e.g., in fracture of nasal bones; trauma to pharyngeal, laryngeal, and tracheal mucosa caused by external or internal trauma, as in lung puncture by a fractured rib; trauma to the trachea during an attempt to pass a nasoesophageal tube; following a tracheal wash procedure to assist in the diagnosis of respiratory disease where the trachea does not seal quickly to air movement after removal of the trocar)
- Extension from vaginal lacerations in cattle, particularly in cattle with vaginal prolapse and following dystocia, or cattle with puerperal metritis and gas accumulation in the uterus
- Gases migrating from abdominal surgery because the abdominal cavity is usually at a negative pressure relative to atmospheric pressure
- Gas gangrene infection

PATHOGENESIS

Air moves very quickly in a dorsal manner through fascial planes, especially when there is local muscular movement. For example, when a lung is punctured, or in cases of severe interstitial pulmonary edema, air escapes under the visceral pleura and passes to the hilus of the lung, and hence to beneath the parietal pleura, between the muscles, and into the subcutis, particularly between the dorsal aspects of the scapulae.

CLINICAL FINDINGS

Visible subcutaneous swellings are soft, painless, fluctuating, and grossly crepitant to the touch, but there is no external skin lesion. In gas gangrene, discoloration, coldness, and oozing of serum may be evident. Affected areas of skin are moderately painful to touch. Emphysema may be sufficiently severe and widespread to cause stiffness of the gait and interference with feeding and respiration. The source of the subcutaneous emphysema is usually directly ventral to the most severely affected area, which is usually along the back.

CLINICAL PATHOLOGY

Clinical pathology is not necessary except in cases of gas gangrene, when a bacteriologic examination of fluid from the swelling should be carried out to identify the organism present.

DIFFERENTIAL DIAGNOSIS

Diagnostic confirmation is based on the observation of crepitus and the extreme mobility of the swelling; these distinguish emphysema from other superficial swellings.

Anasarca, dependent and pits on pressure (see previous discussion).

Hematoma, seroma at injury sites, confirmed by needle puncture (see following discussion).

Cellulitis is accompanied by toxemia, confirmed by needle puncture.

TREATMENT

Primary treatment is to address the source of the air, but this may be impossible to locate or to close. **Supportive treatment** is only necessary in the extremely rare case where emphysema is extensive and incapacitating, in which case multiple skin incisions may be necessary. Gas gangrene requires immediate and drastic treatment with antibiotics.

LYMPHANGITIS

Lymphangitis is characterized by inflammation and enlargement of the lymph vessels and is usually associated with lymphadenitis.

ETIOLOGY

Lymphangitis in most cases is a result of local skin infection with subsequent spread to the lymphatic system. Common causes are as follows.

Cattle

- Bovine farcy caused by *Mycobacterium farcinogenes* and *Mycobacterium senegalense*
- Cutaneous tuberculosis associated with atypical mycobacteria, rarely *Mycobacterium bovis*

Horse

- Epizootic lymphangitis (equine histoplasmosis) as a result of *Histoplasma capsulatum var. farciminosum*
- Ulcerative lymphangitis as a result of *Corynebacterium pseudotuberculosis*
- Glanders (farcy) caused by *Burkolderia mallei*
- Sporotrichosis
- Sporadic lymphangitis
- Strangles in cases where bizarre location sites occur
- In foals, ulcerative lymphangitis associated with *Streptococcus zooepidemicus*

PATHOGENESIS

Spread of infection along the lymphatic vessels causes chronic inflammation and thickening of the vessel walls. Abscesses often develop, with discharge to the skin surface through sinuses.

CLINICAL FINDINGS

An indolent ulcer usually exists at the original site of infection. The lymph vessels leaving this ulcer are enlarged, thickened, and tortuous and often have secondary ulcers or sinuses along their course. Local edema may result from lymphatic obstruction. In chronic cases much fibrous tissue may be laid down in the subcutis, and chronic thickening of the skin may follow. The medial surface of the hindlimb is the most frequent site, particularly in horses.

CLINICAL PATHOLOGY

Bacteriologic examination of discharge for the presence of the specific bacteria or fungi is common practice.

TREATMENT

Primary treatment requires vigorous, early surgical excision or specific antibiotic therapy.

Supportive treatment is directed toward removal of fluid and inflammatory exudate and relief of pain.

PANNICULITIS

Panniculitis is diffuse inflammation of subcutaneous fat that has been associated with a number of causes, such as trauma, infection, postinjection site inflammation, insect bite, neoplasia, drug eruption, and dietary factors (excessive intake of polyunsaturated fatty acids or vitamin E deficiency). Deep-seated, firm, and painful nodules or plaques that can reach a diameter of 15 cm or more, often in large numbers, anywhere over the body but especially on the neck and sides, most commonly occur in young horses and rarely in cattle. The lesions may fluctuate greatly in size and number, or even disappear spontaneously. In a few cases there is transient fever, reduced feed intake, and weight loss. Lameness may be evident in horses with extensive lesions.

Diagnosis is by histologic examination of a biopsy specimen. At necropsy examination there are no other lesions. The lesions reduce in size and number after the administration of dexamethasone but recur when treatment stops.

HEMATOMA

Hematoma refers to extravasation of whole blood into the subcutaneous tissues.

ETIOLOGY

Accumulation of blood in the subcutaneous tissues beyond the limit of that normally caused by trauma may be a result of defects in the coagulation mechanism or a result of increased permeability of the vessel wall.

Common causes include the following:

- Traumatic rupture of large blood vessel
- Dicoumarol poisoning from moldy sweet clover hay
- Purpura hemorrhagica in horses
- Bracken poisoning in cattle; other granulocytopenic diseases manifested principally by petechiation, with lesions observed only in mucosae
- Systemic disease associated with disseminated intravascular coagulopathy (DIC)
- Hemangiosarcoma in subcutaneous sites
- Neonatal bovine pancytopenia
- Inherited hemophilia

PATHOGENESIS

Leakage of blood from the vascular system can cause local swellings, which interfere with normal bodily functions but are rarely sufficiently extensive to cause signs of anemia.

CLINICAL FINDINGS

Subcutaneous swellings resulting from hemorrhage are diffuse and soft, with no visible effect on the skin surface. There may be no evidence of trauma. Specific locations of subcutaneous hemorrhages in horses include the frontal aspect of the chest—as a result of fracture of the first rib in collisions at full gallop, and often fatal through internal hemorrhage—and perivaginal at foaling, causing massive swelling of the perineum and medial aspect of the thigh.

CLINICAL PATHOLOGY

Visual examination of a needle aspirate confirms the existence of subcutaneous hemorrhage. Diagnosis of the primary cause is greatly assisted by platelet counts and prothrombin, clotting, and bleeding times.

TREATMENT

Primary Treatment

Primary treatment targets removal or correction of the cause.

Supportive Treatment

The hematoma should not be opened until clotting is completed, except in the case of a massive hemorrhage that is interfering with respiration, defecation, or urination. If blood loss is severe, blood transfusions may be required. Parenteral injection of coagulants can be justified if the hemorrhages are recent and severe.

DIFFERENTIAL DIAGNOSIS

Hematomas as a result of coagulopathies are usually associated with hemorrhages into other tissues, both manifestations being a result of defects in clotting or capillary wall continuity. Single hematomas (e.g., from trauma) must be differentiated from abscesses, seromas, and neoplasias.

Diagnostic confirmation is by needle puncture of the swelling, avoiding excessive blood loss (that would decrease pressure on the leaking vessel) and contamination of a possibly sterile fluid pocket.

NECROSIS AND GANGRENE

Necrosis is tissue death; gangrene is sloughing of dead tissue. When either change occurs in the skin, it involves the dermis, epidermis, and subcutaneous tissue.

Different types of gangrene are recognized:

- **Dry gangrene** is primarily caused by arterial occlusion resulting in tissue ischemia. Affected tissue appears dry and shrunken, with dark discoloration and a clear demarcation line from healthy tissue. There is no bacterial infection or putrefaction because bacteria fail to survive in the desiccated tissue.
- **Wet gangrene** is most common after sudden blockage of venous blood flow resulting in ischemia while the affected tissue is saturated with stagnant blood. Tissue trauma (e.g., from mechanical trauma or burns) and ischemia result in release of tissue water and give the affected area a moist and swollen appearance. Because the moist and protein-rich tissue facilitates bacterial growth, infection with saprogenic microorganisms is common. This infection results in the putrid and rotten aspect and odor of the tissue and may cause septicemia.
- **Gas gangrene** is caused by *C. perfringens* (see also "Malignant Edema").

ETIOLOGY

Severe **damage to the skin** in the following categories causes gangrene:

- Severe or continued trauma (e.g., pressure sores, saddle and harness galls, carpal or tarsal necrosis in recumbent animals)
- Strong caustic chemicals (e.g., creosote)
- Severe cold or heat, with bushfires and stable fires being the worst offenders. Frostbite is an unusual occurrence in animals unless the patient has a circulatory deficit (e.g., in the neonate, in severe shock or toxemia).
- Beta-irradiation
- **Infections**, especially:
  - Erysipelas and salmonellosis in pigs
  - Clostridial infections in cattle, affecting subcutis and muscle
  - Staphylococcal mastitis in cattle; pasteurella mastitis in sheep
  - Bovine ulcerative mammillitis of the udder and teats
- **Local vascular obstruction**—obstruction by thrombi or arterial spasm causes skin gangrene but includes deeper structures, also from poisoning by:
  - *Claviceps purpurea*
  - *Festuca arundinacea* (probably as a result of an accompanying fungus)
  - *Aspergillus terreus*
  - Mushrooms
- Intradermal injection of local anesthetics containing epinephrine have been associated with dry gangrene of injected skin in cattle.

Similar cutaneous and deeper-structure involvement occurs in systemic infections in which bacterial emboli block local vessels (e.g., in salmonellosis in calves, and after tail vaccination of calves with *Mycoplasma mycoides*).

Other Causes

- Final stages of photosensitive dermatitis and flexural seborrhea
- Screw-worm infestation

PATHOGENESIS

The basic cause of gangrene is interference with local blood supply by external pressure; by severe swelling of the skin, as in photosensitization; or by arteriolar spasm or damage to vessels by bacterial toxins.

CLINICAL FINDINGS

With **dry gangrene** the lesion is dry from the beginning, and the area is cold and sunken, with red-brown discoloration and without offensive odor, resembling mummified tissue. Bacterial infection is commonly not present. Sloughing of dry tissue may take a long time, and the underlying surface usually consists of granulation tissue.

With **wet gangrene** the initial lesion is moist and oozing, and the affected area is swollen, raised, discolored, and cold. Separation occurs at the margin, and the affected skin may slough before it dries; the underlying surface is raw and weeping. Because wet gangrene is in most cases accompanied by infection with saprophytic pathogens, affected tissue often has a putrid and rotten aspect and odor. Systemic disease may result from absorption of toxic products from tissue breakdown and bacteria, resulting in septicemia.

The presentation of **gas gangrene** is discussed under "Malignant Edema."

> **DIFFERENTIAL DIAGNOSIS**
>
> Confirmation of the diagnosis is by visual recognition.
>
> Gangrenous mastitis in cows or ewes.
>
> Photosensitive dermatitis.
>
> *Claviceps purpurea* poisoning.

TREATMENT

Primary treatment requires removal of the etiologic insult.

Supportive treatment comprising the application of astringent and antibacterial ointments may be required in cases of wet gangrene to facilitate separation of the gangrenous tissue and to prevent bacterial infection. Aggressive tissue debridement of necrotic tissue and in severe cases amputation of affected body parts may be required. Systemic antibiotics do not reach gangrenous tissue but are indicated whenever septicemia is suspected.

SUBCUTANEOUS ABSCESS

Most subcutaneous abscesses are matters of purely local and esthetic concern, but if they are sufficiently extensive and present with active **localized infection**, they may cause mild toxemia. Their origins include the following.

Trauma

Most subcutaneous abscesses are the result of traumatic skin penetration with resulting infection. For example, **facial subcutaneous abscesses** are common in cattle eating roughage containing foxtail grass (*Hordeum jubatum*). Several animals in a herd may be affected at one time. The awns of these plants migrate into the cheek mucosa, causing subcutaneous abscesses containing *Trueperella* (formerly *Arcanobacterium*) *pyogenes* and *Actinobacillus* spp. The abscesses contain purulent material, are well encapsulated, and must be surgically drained and treated as an open wound. Medical therapy with parenteral antimicrobials and iodine is ineffective.

Hematogenous

Rarely the infection reaches the site via the bloodstream (e.g., chronic pectoral abscesses of horses, infections in foals with *R. equi*, infections in all species with *Corynebacterium pseudotuberculosis*, infections in lambs with *Histophilus somni* or *Pseudomonas pseudomallei*).

Extension

Abscesses may originate by **extension** from lesions of furunculosis, pyoderma, or impetigo or by **contiguous spread** by contact from an internal organ (e.g., from traumatic reticuloperitonitis).

CUTANEOUS CYSTS

Cysts contained by an epithelial wall enclosing amorphous contents or living tissue may be congenital, inherited defects or acquired as a result of inappropriate healing of accidental wounds. They are smooth, painless, about 1.5 to 2.5 cm in diameter, round, and usually fluctuating, although inspissated contents may make them feel quite hard. The skin and hair coat over them are usually normal, although some may leak mucoid contents onto the skin. Epidermoid cysts are lined with skin; dermoid cysts usually contain differentiated tissue such as sebaceous glands and hair follicles; dentigerous cysts contain teeth or parts of them. Acquired cysts include apocrine, sebaceous, and keratin varieties.

Developmental cysts, which are present from birth, are usually located at specific anatomic sites, and include the following:

- **Branchial cysts** in the neck, formed from an incompletely closed branchial cleft
- **False nostril cysts** in horses
- **Wattle cysts** in goats

Cysts may occur anywhere on the body, but most commonly they are found near the dorsal midline. In horses a common site is the base of the ear.

Other diseases that cause cutaneous nodules in horses include collagenolytic granuloma, mastocytosis, amyloidosis, lymphoma, sarcoidosis, and infestation with *Hypoderma* spp.

Surgical excision for cosmetic reasons is common practice.

GRANULOMATOUS LESIONS OF THE SKIN

Granulomatous lesions are chronic inflammatory nodules, plaques, and ulcers; they are cold, hard, and progress slowly, often accompanied by lymphangitis and lymphadenitis. In many cases there is no cutaneous discontinuity or alopecia. Some of the common causes in animals are as follows.

Cattle

- Bovine farcy caused by *M. farcinogenes* and *M. senegalense*
- Actinobacillosis (botryomycosis) caused by *Actinobacillus lignieresi*

- Infestation with *Onchocerca* spp.
- Infestation with larvae of *Hypoderma* spp.
- Infection with *Mucor* spp. fungi in thick-walled nodules in the skin on the posteroventral aspect of the udder
- Lechiguana associated with the sequential infection with *Dermatobia hominis* and *Mannheimia granulomatosis*. The condition has been reported in Brazilian cattle, which develop very large granulomata consisting of fibrous tissue that develop in subcutaneous sites in any part of the body.[1]

Sheep

- Strawberry footrot—*D. congolensis*
- Ecthyma
- Ulcerative lesions of lower jaw and dewlap associated with *A. lignieresi*

Horses

- Tumorous calcinosis, which causes hard, painless, spherical granulomata, up to 12 cm in diameter, near joints and tendon sheaths, especially the stifle joint
- Cutaneous amyloidosis
- Collagenolytic granuloma (nodular necrobiosis)—the most common nodular skin disease of the horse. The etiology is unknown. There are multiple firm nodules located in the dermis, ranging in size from 0.5 to 5 cm in diameter. The overlying skin surface and hair are usually normal. Biopsy reveals collagenolysis. Treatment consists of surgical removal and possibly the administration of corticosteroids.
- Botryomycosis, or bacterial pseudomycosis, results from bacterial infection at many sites, often accompanied by a foreign body. Lesions on the limbs, brisket, ventral abdomen, and scrotum vary in size from nodules to enormous fungating growths composed of firm inflammatory tissue riddled by necrotic tracts, leading to discharging sinuses, often containing small yellow-white granules or "grains." Surgical excision is the only practicable solution.
- Equine eosinophilic granuloma—nonalopecic, painless, nonpruritic, firm nodules, 2 to 10 cm in diameter and covered by normal skin, develop on the neck, withers, and back of horses, especially in the summer. The cause is unknown, and palliative treatment, surgical excision, or corticosteroid administration is usually provided.
- Systemic granulomatous disease (equine sarcoidosis)—a rare disease of horses characterized by skin lesions and widespread involvement of the lungs, lymph nodes, liver, gastrointestinal tract, spleen, kidney, bones, and central nervous system
- *Burkolderia mallei*—cutaneous farcy or glanders
- *Actinomadura* spp. and *Nocardia brasiliensis*—painless mycetomas
- *Histoplasma farciminosum*—epizootic lymphangitis
- *Corynebacterium pseudotuberculosis*—ulcerative lymphangitis
- *Habronema megastoma* and *Hyphomyces destruens* as causes of swamp cancer, bursattee, Florida horse leech, and blackgrain mycetoma
- Infestation with *Onchocerca* spp.
- Chronic urticaria

Pigs

- *Actinomyces* spp. and *B. suilla* cause lesions on the udder.

REFERENCE

1. Andrade GB, et al. *Vet Res Comm.* 2008;32:65-74.

Non-Infectious Diseases of the Skin

INSECT BITE HYPERSENSITIVITY IN HORSES (EQUINE SEASONAL ALLERGIC DERMATITIS)

Insect bite hypersensitivity (IBH) is an intensely pruritic dermatitis of horses caused by hypersensitivity to insect bites, especially *Culicoides* spp. and, less frequently, *Simulium* spp.

ETIOLOGY

The disease is caused by type I (immediate) hypersensitivity to salivary antigens introduced into the skin by the bites of sandflies and other insects. There may be a lesser role for type IV (cell-mediated) hypersensitivity in the disease. *Culicoides brevitarsus* is the cause in Australia, *Culicoides pulicaris* in the United Kingdom and Europe, and *Culicoides obsoletus* in Canada. *Stomoxys calcitrans*, the stable fly, and *Simulium* spp. cause the disease. The distribution of the skin lesions and seasonal nature of the disease are related to the feeding habits of the inciting insect. For instance, *C. pulicaris* has a predilection for landing at the mane and tail, and this is where the lesion is most commonly seen.

EPIDEMIOLOGY

The prevalence of the disease varies depending on environmental factors, and possibly characteristics of the local horse population. Up to 60% of horses are reported to be affected in areas of Queensland, Australia; 22% in Israel; and 18% of Icelandic horses in Norway. The prevalence in Switzerland is very low in regions above 1000 m and 1.6% in lower areas. The prevalence of the disease in Dutch Shetland Ponies (>7000) assessed over 3 years was 8.8%.[1]

The disease is quite common worldwide in areas where **hot and humid summer weather** favors the causative insects: Sweden, the United Kingdom, Japan, Israel, Hong Kong, North America, Australia, the Philippines, India, and France. Most cases occur during **summer,** and lesions disappear during cooler weather. Lesions disappear when the horses have been stabled in insect-proof barns for several weeks or are moved outside the geographic range of the inciting insect.

The disease is characteristically sporadic and affects only a few of a group of horses. However, because the predilection to the disease is inherited, there may be multiple cases among related animals on a farm. The prevalence of the disease increases with age; 3.4% of Icelandic horses 1 to 7 years of age compared with 32% of horses older than 14 years were affected.

The disease has a demonstrated genetic basis in some breeds, including heritability of 0.08 (standard error [SE] = 0.02) on the observed binary scale and 0.24 (SE = 0.06) on the underlying continuous scale in Dutch Shetland ponies.[1] Variants in the major histocompatibility complex (MHC) class II region are associated with disease susceptibility, with the same allele (COR112:274) associated with the disease in Icelandic ponies and Exmor ponies. In addition, homozygosity across the entire MHC class II region is associated with a higher risk of developing the disease ($p = 0.0013$).[2] Genes not encoding MHC and associated with IBH in Old Kaldruby horses include interferon gamma (IFNG), transforming growth factor beta 1 (TGEB1), Janus kinase 2 (JAK2), thymic stromal lymphopoietin (TSLP), and involucrin (IVL).[3] Expression of genes associated with allergy and immunity in the skin of affected horses indicates a role for these pathways in the disease.

PATHOGENESIS

Reaginic antibodies (IgE) produced in response to exposure to proteins in insect saliva bind to mast cells in the skin; when exposed to the antigen, they are associated with degranulation of the mast cell. Horses with IBH have IgE antibodies that react with constituents of the salivary gland of *Culicoides* spp., whereas horses that do not have the disease have IgG, but not IgE, antibodies against *Culicoides* spp. salivary gland antigens. Horses that have not been exposed to *Culicoides* spp. do not have either antibody to the insect salivary gland antigen. IgE antibodies against *Culicoides* spp. are present on a seasonal basis in horses that do not have evidence of the disease, indicating that the presence of these antibodies, although necessary for development of the diseases, is not sufficient and that other factors are involved.[4]

The antigen in saliva of *Culicoides* sp. and *Simulium* spp. has identical IgE epitopes, demonstrating that the disease in some horses is caused by IgE-mediated cross-reactivity to homologous allergens in the saliva of both species.[5] A specific antigen in midge (*Culicoides sonorensis*) saliva associated with IgE reaginic antibodies and causing both in vivo and in vitro activity mimicking IBH is a 66 kDa protein referred to as Cul s 1.[6]

Degranulating mast cells and intradermal or subcutaneous lymphocytes release various vasoactive substances and cytokines that cause inflammation and accumulation of eosinophils in the skin of affected areas and eosinophilia. The distribution of the lesions on patients reflects the insects' preferred feeding sites. Ponies with seasonal allergic dermatitis have greater numbers of circulating CD5+ and CD4+ T lymphocytes than do normal animals. Increased numbers of CD3+ T lymphocytes, most of which are CD4+, and eosinophils are present in the skin of affected ponies after injection of *Culicoides* antigen. Furthermore, in eotaxin and monocyte chemoattractant protein (MCP) 1, but not MCP-2 or MCP-4, mRNA expression is upregulated in skin biopsies of sweet itch lesions, demonstrating a mechanism for accumulation of eosinophils and T-2 lymphocytes in the lesions.

CLINICAL FINDINGS

Lesions are usually confined to the base of the tail, rump, along the back, withers, crest, poll, ears, and, less commonly, ventral midline. In severe cases the lesions may extend down the sides of the body and neck and onto the face and legs.

Pruritus is intense, especially at night, and the horse scratches against any fixed object for hours at a time. In the early stages, slight, discrete papules, with the hair standing erect, are observed. Constant scratching may cause self-mutilation, severe inflammatory lesions, and loss of hair. Scaliness and loss of hair on the ears and tail base may be the only lesions in mildly affected horses.

CLINICAL PATHOLOGY

Affected animals have **eosinophilia** and thrombocytosis.

Diagnosis is facilitated by skin biopsy, fungal culture, parasitologic examination of skin scrapings, and intradermal sensitivity testing. **Skin biopsy** of early lesions, before trauma masks the true picture, reveals edema, capillary engorgement, and eosinophilic and mononuclear perivascular infiltration. Fungal culture and parasitologic examination of **skin scrapings** are useful only in that they rule out dermatophytosis, onchocerciasis, and strongyloidosis. **Intradermal skin testing** demonstrates immediate and delayed sensitivity reactions to extracts of *Culicoides* spp. and *Stomoxys* spp. Recommended concentrations of insect antigen in the testing solution are 60 to 250 PNU per mL,[7] or 1 : 1000 w/v concentration of *Culicoides* spp. extracts relevant to the locality, providing useful support for a clinical diagnosis of equine insect hypersensitivity.[8]

Testing of serum for specific IgE antibodies holds potential for enhancing diagnostic strategies, but because of the detection of IgE antibodies against *Culicoides* spp. and *Simulium* spp. antigens in healthy horses,[4] the poor concordance between results of skin hypersensitivity testing and serum IgE concentration,[9] and the poor performance of serologic testing with enzyme-linked immunosorbent assay (ELISA) that uses the high-affinity IgE receptor (Fc epsilon R1 alpha),[10] serologic testing is currently not recommended.

> **DIFFERENTIAL DIAGNOSIS**
>
> Infection with larvae of *Onchocerca* spp., *Strongyloides* spp., or *Dermatophilus congolensis* can produce similar lesions. Alopecia of the tailhead may be caused by *Oxyuris equi*.

TREATMENT

The principles of treatment are removal of the inciting cause and suppression of the hypersensitivity reaction.

Removal of the inciting cause is achieved by preventing horses from being exposed to the inciting insects. This can be achieved by relocating the horse to a geographic region where the insects do not occur, stabling of the horse in an insect-proof stable during the periods of the day (early evening) when the insects are most active, or applying agents that kill the insects or otherwise prevent them from alighting on and biting the horse.

Suppression of the immediate hypersensitivity reaction or its sequelae can be achieved by administration of corticosteroids (prednisolone, 1 mg/kg orally every 24 hours initially, then reducing to as low of a maintenance dose as possible).

Hyposensitization (allergen-specific immunotherapy) has received attention for its potential efficacy in desensitizing affected horses. Two controlled clinical trials did not demonstrate a beneficial effect (although the placebo effect on the owners was impressive) in a representative sample of horses. These trials were blinded and used objective measures of efficacy.[11] A retrospective study using owner-reported responses (reduction in antipruritic therapy) found a response in 57% of horses.[12] There is insufficient high-quality evidence to support use of allergen-specific immunotherapy as routine treatment for IBH.

CONTROL

Reduce Exposure to Biting Midges

Horses should be housed in insect-proof buildings or, at a minimum, buildings that limit exposure of horses to midges by closure of doors and covering of windows with gauze. Impregnation of gauze with an insecticide further reduces biting rates. Stables should be situated in areas that have minimal midge populations, such as on hilltops or well-drained sites. Midge numbers on individual farms should be reduced by habitat alteration, so that areas of damp, organically enriched soils are eliminated.[13] Widespread use of insecticides is unlikely to be environmentally acceptable.

The feeding pattern of midges is such that housing of horses during the crepuscular periods and at night will significantly reduce biting rates and likelihood of infection. Horses kept at pasture should have insect repellents applied regularly and especially to provide protection during periods of high insect-biting activity. Diethyltoluamide, or DEET (*N,N*-diethyl-*meta*-toluamide), is the only commercially available repellent with documented activity against *Culicoides* spp. Application of deltamethrin (10 mL of 1% solution) to the skin of horses did not reduce the frequency of midge feeding in an experimental trial in the United Kingdom.[14] Installation of alphacypermethrin-impregnated mesh in jet stalls reduced the attach rate of *Culicoides* spp. by 6- to 14-fold and markedly reduced the number of *Culicoides* spp. insects collected from horses housed in the stalls compared with sentinel horses, suggesting that this might be a useful means of reducing exposure of housed horses to midges.[15]

REFERENCES

1. Schurink A, et al. *J Anim Sci*. 2009;87:484.
2. Andersson LS, et al. *Immunogenetics*. 2012;64:201.
3. Vychodilova L, et al. *Vet Immunol Immunopath*. 2013;152:260.
4. Wilkolek PM, et al. *Polish J Vet Sci*. 2014;17:331.
5. Schaffartzik A, et al. *Vet Immunol Immunopath*. 2010;137:76.
6. Langner KFA, et al. *Int J Parasit*. 2009;39:243.
7. Baxter CG, et al. *Vet Dermatol*. 2008;19:305.
8. van Oldruitenborgh-Oosterbaan MMS, et al. *Vet Dermatol*. 2009;20:607.
9. Morgan EE, et al. *Vet Immunol Immunopath*. 2007;120:160.
10. Frey R, et al. *Vet Immunol Immunopath*. 2008;126:102.
11. Ginel PJ, et al. *Vet Dermatol*. 2014;25:29.
12. Stepnik CT, et al. *Vet Dermatol*. 2012;23:29.
13. Carpenter S, et al. *Med Vet Ent*. 2008;22:175.
14. Robin M, et al. *Vet Rec*. 2015;176.
15. Page PC, et al. *Vet Parasitol*. 2015;210:84.

SEASONAL ALLERGIC DERMATITIS OF SHEEP

A disease similar to seasonal dermatitis (insect bite hypersensitivity) of horses (see "Equine Seasonal Allergic Dermatitis," in this chapter) occurs in sheep in the United Kingdom, Brazil, Israel, and likely elsewhere.[1-3] The disease is also reported in goats in Brazil and suspected in New World camelids (alpacas) in New York State.[4,5] Up to one-third of a sheep flock can be affected, with the disease remitting and affected sheep appearing to fully or almost fully recover during the dry season in Brazil, or during winter in higher latitudes.[1] Because of the seasonal appearance of the disease during periods

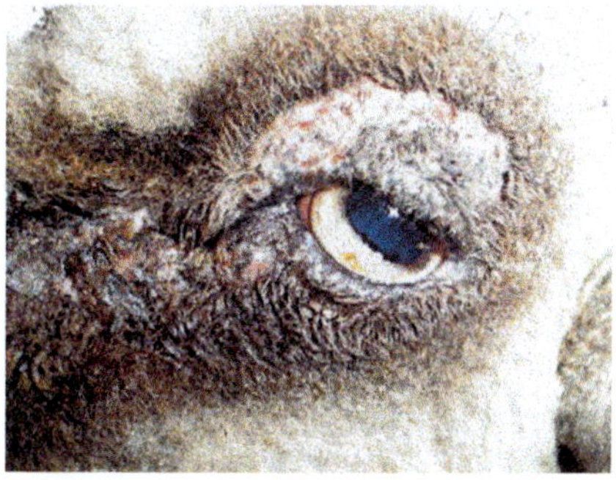

Fig. 16-1 Lesions of seasonal allergic dermatitis in a Hampshire Down sheep. (Reproduced with permission from Correa TG et al. *Vet Parasitol* 2007; 145:181.[6])

when midges are present or most active, a cutaneous sensitivity to *Culicoides* spp., especially *C. obsoletus* in the United Kingdom or *Culicoides insignis* in Brazil, is suspected.[6] Cutaneous sensitivity to ground-up *Culicoides* spp. is present in affected sheep, and observed bites by *C. insignis* in sheep in Brazil caused pruritus.[6] Allergic dermatitis occurs in sheep infested with fleas (*Ctenocephalides* spp.), although rarely are sheep infested by fleas.[7] Similar skin lesions can occur in sheep infested with lice (*Bovicola ovis*) or scabies (*Psoroptes ovis*).[8] The equivalent disease in horses has a genetic basis, and this should be considered in sheep.[2,9]

The lesions are similar to those in horses and are located principally on the teats, udder, and ventral midline, but also on the tips of the ears, around the eyes, and on the nose and the lips (Fig. 16-1). Initially there is erythema and small red papules followed by development of alopecia and crust formation. The skin of the affected sheep is whitish and irregularly thickened, with alopecia, crusts, and intense pruritus. Histologically the lesions represent the changes characteristic of immediate (type I) hypersensitivity, evident as perivascular eosinophilic dermatitis.[6] Histologic lesions of the epidermis are hyperkeratosis, acanthosis, hypergranulosis, and moderate spongiosis with infiltration of the dermis by eosinophils, macrophages, and plasma cells. There are no diagnostic changes in the differential blood count. Treatment, if provided, should include topical or systemic administration of antihistamines or corticosteroids, although both might be restricted for use in food animals, and there is no formal evidence of efficacy. Affected animals recover when they are not exposed to midges.[1] Control is based on preventing or minimizing exposure to midges.

A very similar disease occurs in cattle in Japan. It is thought to be a result of an allergy to the bite of an external parasite.

REFERENCES

1. Portela RA, et al. *Pes Vet Brasil.* 2012;32:471.
2. Shrestha M, et al. *J Heredity.* 2015;106:366.
3. Yeruham I, et al. *Vet Rec.* 2000;147:360.
4. Macedo JTSA, et al. *Pes Vet Brasil.* 2008;28:633.
5. Scott DW, et al. *Vet Dermatol.* 2011;22:2.
6. Correa TG, et al. *Vet Parasitol.* 2007;145:181.
7. Yeruham I, et al. *Vet Dermatol.* 2004;15:377.
8. Shu D, et al. *Vet Immunol Immunopath.* 2009;129:82.
9. Schurink A, et al. *J Anim Sci.* 2009;87:484.

ANHIDROSIS (NONSWEATING SYNDROME, PUFF DISEASE, DRY COAT)

Anhidrosis refers to the reduced or absent capacity to produce sweat. It affects horses and cattle. Reduced ability to sweat affects horses in hot and humid climates. Affected horses are unable to maintain their body temperature within safe limits, especially during or after exercise, and suffer heat stress and a reduction in athletic performance. The only effective treatment is to move the horses to a cooler environment.

ETIOLOGY

The etiology of anhidrosis is unknown, but it involves a reduction in the sensitivity of the sweat gland to β-2 adrenergic stimulation, the normal stimulus for sweating in the horse. Hypothyroidism does not contribute to anhidrosis, although anhidrotic horses have an exaggerated thyroid-stimulating-hormone response to administration of thyroid-releasing hormone.[1] The etiologic or pathogenic importance of this observation is unclear.

EPIDEMIOLOGY

The disease occurs in horses, and rarely in cattle, in countries with hot, humid climates, including tropical and semitropical regions.

The overall prevalence in horses is approximately 2% to 6% in Florida, with the highest prevalence in southern Florida (4.3%) and lowest in northern Florida (0.08%).[2] The prevalence of affected farms is 11%. There is no reported sex or color predilection. Thoroughbred horses and Warmblood horses in Florida are 4.4 (95% confidence interval [CI] 1.2 to 15.5) times and 13.9 (2.5 to 77.5) times as likely to have the disease as are Quarter horses.[2] None of 190 Arabian horses were affected.[2] Horses with a family history of the disease are approximately 6 times more likely to be affected.[2]

Both native and imported horses are affected, although horses born in the western and midwestern United States are at 2.5 times the risk of developing the disease as are native-born horses.[2] Among native horses, the age of onset of the condition ranges from 1 year to 10 years. Foals, especially of draft breeds, can be affected. Horses imported to endemic areas usually do not develop the disease within 1 year. The incidence and severity of the disease are highest in the hotter season, with most affected horses first exhibiting signs of the disease in the summer.[2]

The disease is rarely fatal unless severely affected horses are exercised in the heat, in which case death from heat stroke can occur. The major importance of the disease is the inability of affected horses to exercise and compete in athletic events.

PATHOGENESIS

Sweat is produced in horses by apocrine sweat glands that have a single type of secretory cell. The sweat glands are epitrichial (associated with a hair follicle) and have a density of about 800 per square centimeter, with a greater volume density of sweat glands in the summer compared with winter, in skin of healthy Thoroughbreds.[3] Evaporation of sweating is responsible for elimination of approximately 70% of the heat load of exercising horses (with a further ~20% attributable to evaporation from the respiratory tract).[4] Evaporation is essential for heat transfer because the latent energy of evaporation of 1 mL of water is 2.2 kJ (2260 kJ/kg of water). High heat transfer from the horse to the environment is possible because of the **high sweating rate** of strenuously exercising horses of up to 3300 g per meter square of skin surface area per hour or 10 to 12 liters per horse per hour.[4] The sweat of horses during exercise is alkaline (pH 8.0 to 8.9), is slightly hyperosmolar compared with plasma (290 to 340 mm Osmol), and has sodium concentrations that approximate those of plasma, potassium concentrations approximately 10 times those of plasma, and chloride concentrations double those of plasma.

The sweat glands are well innervated, and sweating is controlled by a combination of hormonal (β-2 adrenergic) and neural factors.[4] The apocrine sweat glands respond in vitro to both purinergic stimuli, including adenosine triphosphate (ATP), adenosine diphosphate (ADP), and uridine triphosphate (UTP), and application of isoprenaline, a β-agonist.[5,6] Both β-adrenoreceptor and purinergic receptors are present on the basolateral aspects of the sweat glands, but not the apical aspect.[6] Responses to isoprenaline or purinergic stimulants by sweat glands of anhidrotic horses are much reduced compared with those of sweat glands from unaffected horses.[6] The defect in sweating of anhidrotic horses is a consequence of failure of the gland to respond to either of the agonists for sweat production. This breakdown of cellular secretory function is thought to be the prime cause of lack of sweating, as opposed to earlier suggestions of obstruction of the sweat gland duct.[6]

Sweat production increases with increasing concentrations of epinephrine in blood up to a peak value, after which sweating rates decline. Anhidrotic horses have lower initial and peak rates of sweat production and lower overall sweat production than do normal horses during intravenous (IV) infusion of epinephrine.[7] Suggested, but unproved, mechanisms for decreased sweat production by anhidrotic horses includes diminished glandular sensitivity to epinephrine, failure of secretory function, blocking of sweat gland ducts, fatigue of the gland, and gland atrophy.

Sweating is the predominant means by which horses dissipate heat. Reduction in the capacity to produce sweat results in an inability to effectively control body temperature during exercise and when temperature and humidity are high. The elevation in body temperature results in tachypnea in an attempt to dissipate heat through the respiratory tract. Hyperthermia impairs performance and, if severe, can result in heat shock, a systemic inflammatory response syndrome, and death.

CLINICAL FINDINGS

The most apparent clinical sign is lack of sweating in response to an appropriate stimulus, such as exercise. In severely affected horses, sweating is limited to the perineum, brisket, and areas under the mane and saddle. Less severely affected horses have a diminished sweat response and do not lather during exercise. The skin becomes dry and scurfy and loses its elasticity, and there may be alopecia, especially of the face.

Affected animals become extremely tachypneic when heat stressed, leading to the colloquial term for the disease, "dry puffer."[1] Affected horses have abnormally high respiratory rates after exercise that persist for at least 30 minutes after 30 minutes of lunging exercise. Affected horses have a respiratory rate twice that of healthy horses after exercise (60 bpm vs. 120 bpm).[1] The animal's appetite declines, and it loses weight. Athletic performance is severely compromised. Affected horses have higher body temperatures during exercise than unaffected horses, and this difference can persist for at least 30 minutes.[1]

Diagnostic confirmation is achieved by demonstrating reduced sweating in response to intradermal injection of epinephrine or the β-2 adrenergic agonists terbutaline and salbutamol. A crude test involves the intradermal injection of 0.1 mL of a 1 : 1000 dilution of epinephrine. If the horse sweats, then it is not considered to be completely anhidrotic. A semiquantitative test using epinephrine, terbutaline, or salbutamol may be useful in identifying partially anhidrotic horses. Normal horses sweat when 0.1 mL of 1 : 1,000,000 epinephrine is injected, whereas partially anhidrotic horses sweat only with higher concentrations (1 : 10,000 or 1 : 1000). Injections are usually made using small-gauge needles (25 g) into the skin over the lateral aspects of the neck. Terbutaline (0.1 mg/mL) injected intradermally induces sweating in approximately 4 minutes (+/− 1.7 min) in healthy horses and 10.5 minutes (+/− 7 min) in anhidrotic horses.[1]

A further refinement is the **quantitative intradermal terbutaline** sweat test in which 0.1 mL of solutions of terbutaline of 0.001, 0.01, 0.1, 1, 10, 100, and 1000 mg/mL are injected into the skin of the horse.[8] Preweighed absorbent pads are then taped over each site, removed after 30 minutes, and weighed. The amount of sweat produced is quantified as the change in weight of the pad. This technique, although not described in anhidrotic horses, provides a means of quantifying the sweat test.

The **prognosis** is poor for athletic function for affected animals that remain in hot and humid environments, but the condition may resolve if the horse is moved to a cool climate.

CLINICAL PATHOLOGY

Plasma epinephrine concentrations are reported to be higher in affected horses than in unaffected horses, but this has not been a consistent finding among studies.

NECROPSY FINDINGS

There are no characteristic gross lesions at necropsy. Histologic examination of the skin of affected horses reveals abnormalities in sweat gland morphology, including flattening of cells, loss of luminal microvilli, and a reduction in the number of secretory vesicles.[7] These findings are thought to be a consequence, rather than a cause, of the disease.

TREATMENT AND CONTROL

There is **no specific treatment** that restores the horse's ability to sweat, other than movement to a cooler climate. Affected horses for which translocation to a cooler environment is not feasible benefit from housing in air-conditioned stables so that exposure to high ambient temperatures is minimized. Exercise of affected horses during the coolest periods of the day is sensible. Affected horses are frequently administered **electrolyte supplements**, but these are without demonstrated benefit. However, as with all working horses, an adequate intake of sodium, potassium, and chloride should be ensured.

Administration of **thyroid hormone supplements** is not warranted and might be dangerous because they cause an increase the metabolic rate, and therefore heat production, of affected horses. **Vitamin E** administration has no demonstrated efficacy.

Removal of affected animals to cooler climates is often necessary, although air-conditioning of stables and maintenance of horses in higher country where they can be returned after a day's racing may enable susceptible horses to be kept locally.

FURTHER READING

Jenkinson DM, Elder HY, Bovell DL. Equine sweating and anhidrosis part 1: equine sweating. *Vet Derm.* 2006;17:361-392.

Jenkinson DM, Elder HY, Bovell DL. Equine sweating and anhidrosis part 2: anhidrosis. *Vet Derm.* 2007;18:2-11.

REFERENCES

1. Breuhaus BA. *J Vet Int Med.* 2009;23:168.
2. Johnson EB, et al. *J Am Vet Med Assoc.* 2010;236:1091.
3. Sneddon JC, et al. *Vet Dermatol.* 2008;19:163.
4. Jenkinson DM, et al. *Vet Dermatol.* 2006;17:361.
5. Bovell DL, et al. *Vet Dermatol.* 2013;24:398.
6. Wilson DCS, et al. *Vet Dermatol.* 2007;18:152.
7. Jenkinson DM, et al. *Vet Dermatol.* 2007;18:2.
8. MacKay RJ. *Equine Vet J.* 2008;40:518.

WETNESS (MACERATION)

Frequent exposure to wetting, sufficient to keep the skin permanently wet for long periods, results in maceration with loss of dermal integrity and predisposes to fleece rot in sheep and mycotic or bacterial dermatitis in all species. In horses it leads to a superficial dermatitis along the dorsum, especially over the croup, and is known as scald. Frequent immersion of the lower limbs of cattle on irrigated pasture causes dermatitis on the backs of the pasterns, leading to mycotic dermatitis. Digital dermatitis of cattle can be induced by prolonged wetness of the skin, resulting in maceration, and inoculation with *Treponema* spp.[1] Wetting also predisposes to hypothermia in the young.

Standing in cold water for a period of more than 3 days causes the immersed parts to become edematous and congested and slough their skin in the form of a cuff around the limb. Recovery is slow and incomplete.

REFERENCE

1. Gomez A, et al. *J Dairy Sci.* 2012;95:1821.

COCKLE

Cockle is a superficial nodular dermatitis of sheep recorded only in New Zealand that results in nodules in the skin that are of economic importance to the leather industry. The presence of cockle downgrades the value of the pelt, which is rendered unsuitable for suede and clothing.

Cockle is not usually diagnosed clinically, but examination by close inspection of the skin over the upper shoulder region after close shearing has high specificity for detection. The lesions are the result of an immune response in some sheep to infestation with the biting louse *B. ovis*. The occurrence of cockle and its severity are positively correlated with the severity of the louse infestation, and sheep that develop lesions have *B. ovis*-specific homocytotropic antibody. Serum histamine concentrations are significantly higher in louse-infested lambs than louse-naïve lambs.

Lesions commence on the neck and shoulders and may extend over the entire pelt. Widely distributed lesions, termed scatter cockle, are attributed to infestation with *B. ovis*, and this is the most common cause, but rib cockle may be a hypersensitivity to infestation with the sheep ked *Melophagus ovinus*. Pelt lesions in the dorsal midline region are usually a result of infection with *D. congolensis*.

CONTROL

Control rests with the control of *B. ovis*. For cockle control, sheep should be treated off-shears with pour-on or spray-on insecticide and, as soon as practical after shearing, treated by saturation dipping. Saturation dipping is required to significantly reduce louse populations. Prelambing dipping is also recommended to reduce the risk of lambs acquiring louse infestations.

FURTHER READING

Radostits O, et al. Cockle. In: *Veterinary Medicine: A Textbook of the Disease of Cattle, Horses, Sheep, Goats and Pigs*. 10th ed. London: W.B. Saunders; 2007:2041.

WOOL SLIP, WOOL LOSS

Wool slip is a condition in which housed ewes, shorn in winter, lose part of their fleece and develop bald patches over a large area of the rear half of the back. This commonly starts at the base of the tail and progresses to the rump and back and less commonly the neck. There is no systemic disease; the skin is normal. Histologic examination of skin biopsies shows that in affected sheep the wool follicles are in the active anogen stage rather than the inactive telogen phase of unaffected cohort sheep, and the wool regrows immediately following loss. The loss of wool starts 2 to 3 weeks after shearing. All breeds are equally susceptible, and there is no effect of age or whether the sheep are carrying single or twin lambs; up to 40% of a flock may be affected. The wool loss occurs because of a premature and synchronized shedding of wool fibers and not because of a pathologic process that damages the wool fiber. Wool shedding can be induced experimentally by prolonged treatments with corticosteroids, and the current explanation for the wool shedding that occurs with the wool-slip syndrome is that blood corticosteroid levels rise after the stress of shearing and are maintained for a long period because of the trauma of being housed and shorn and kept in the cold. Blood zinc concentrations in sheep affected with wool slip are within the normal range, and there is no epidermal change as occurs in zinc deficiency.

The prevention of the condition is aimed at reducing the severity and length of the stress period by shearing the sheep at the time of entry to winter housing and ensuring a good nutritional plane in the postshearing period. This hypothesis as to cause may not be correct because the syndrome has also been seen in the summer in Wiltshire shorn sheep that had little history of stress in the period immediately preceding the wool slip.

Wool slip should not be confused with the normal shedding of wool that occurs in breeds such as the Wiltshire or Shetland in the spring period. Loss of wool along the backline also occurs in older longwool sheep and may be exacerbated by lambs playing or sleeping on the ewe.

Impairment of wool growth and a thinning of fiber diameter can occur during the course of any severe disease, such as bluetongue, pregnancy toxemia, or footrot, temporarily affecting the growth of the fleece. This results in a segment of the wool fiber that has decreased tensile strength, and the condition has the name *tender wool*. Following recovery from the inciting disease the wool growth is normal, but there is a line of wool with poor tensile strength in the staple. This can be observed in the intact fleece as a line of decreased fiber diameter, often with a change in crimp character and discoloration as a result of entrapment of dust. The wool may break if the staple on either side of this break is sharply snapped between the fingers. The fleece may subsequently be shed in part or in whole at the level of the defect, a condition known as wool break. Tender wool downgrades the value of a fleece and has economic significance in wool-producing sheep.

Zinc deficiency can reduce keratinization, reduce wool growth, and occasionally result in fleece loss in sheep. Wool loss associated with pruritus occurs in association with external parasite infestations and with scrapie and pseudorabies in ruminants.

Pelodera dermatitis, characterized by thickening of the skin and complete wool loss in affected skin areas, has been recorded in winter-housed sheep where there was poor bedding management. The condition affected the majority of the ewes at risk. The parasite *Pelodera (Rhabditis) strongyloides* is a free-living nematode commonly present in decaying organic material but can invade hair follicles to produce an inflammatory response. Histologic examination of the skin showed the presence of the parasite in wool follicles and infiltration of eosinophils and mast cells in connective tissue. Affected skin areas were those that had contact with the bedding when the sheep were lying down, and large numbers of the nematode were found in the bedding. Clinical signs regressed with the more frequent provision of new bedding and disinfection of the stable.

WOOL EATING

Wool eating can occur as a result pica associated with micronutrient deficiency. A condition called *shimao zheng*, occurring in a region of the Gansu province of China, has wool eating as its primary manifestation. The disease has a seasonal occurrence, with the peak incidence in January through April. Both goats and sheep are affected, but the incidence and severity are much higher in goats, where 90% may show signs. Affected animals bite the wool or hair off their own or other animals' bodies, particularly in the hip, belly, and shoulder areas. Histology on biopsies shows heavily keratinized epithelial cells, a decreased number of hair follicles, and aggregated foci of lymphocytes in the dermis. Controlled trials have shown that the condition can be corrected by supplementation with sulfur, copper, and iron. Wool eating is also recorded in Israel, possibly associated with trace-element copper and zinc deficiency, and in housed superfine Merino sheep in Australia fed grain-based supplements, where it is corrected by the provision of roughage in the form of hay. Wool and hair loss in individual sheep and cattle in association with excessive licking have been recorded and are postulated as psychogenic dermatoses.

FURTHER READING

Radostits O, et al. Wool slip, wool loss. In: *Veterinary Medicine: A Textbook of the Disease of Cattle, Horses, Sheep, Goats and Pigs*. 10th ed. London: W.B. Saunders; 2007:2041-2042.

IDIOPATHIC NASAL/PERIORAL HYPERKERATOTIC DERMATOSIS OF CAMELIDS (MOUTH MUNGE)

Idiopathic nasal/perioral hyperkeratotic dermatosis is a common skin condition of llamas and has anecdotally been reported in alpacas. The ailment is characterized by a thickening of the stratum corneum of the epidermis resulting in hyperkeratotic plaques and crusts in the perinasal and perioral region. Similar skin lesions may occur on the perineum, ventral abdomen, medial hind- and forelegs, axillae, and inguinal region, in which case the condition is more globally referred to as idiopathic hyperkeratosis.[1] The etiology of this condition is poorly understood but has been categorized as zinc-responsive dermatosis because cases responsive to high oral doses of zinc have been reported.

CLINICAL FINDINGS

Individual animals of either sex between 6 and 24 months of age are commonly affected. Animals present with thick papular crusts and plaques covering the periocular and perioral area, occasionally obstructing the nostrils. Secondary dermatitis that waxes and wanes is common, but pruritus is usually mild or absent.[2]

CLINICAL PATHOLOGY

The diagnosis is based on clinical presentation and by ruling out other differentials. Histologic examination of skin biopsies shows epidermal and follicular orthokeratotic hyperkeratosis that can be associated with dermal infiltration with lymphocytes, macrophages, and occasionally eosinophiles.[1] The degree of infiltration is dependent on the extent of secondary inflammation.[3] The treatment outcome of diagnostic therapy consisting of oral zinc supplementation will contribute to confirming or refuting the diagnosis.[3]

The usefulness of measuring the serum zinc concentration in affected animals is doubtful because the condition could not be linked to subnormal plasma zinc concentrations in affected animals.[4]

DIFFERENTIAL DIAGNOSIS
Chorioptic mange
Dermatophilosis
Dermatophytosis
Viral contagious pustular dermatitis
Bacterial dermatitis

TREATMENT

Supplementing the diet with zinc, either by offering zinc-enriched feed or by supplementing organic or anorganic zinc, for a minimum of 2 months has been suggested. Current recommendations are to supplement either zinc sulfate (2 g/d and animal) or zinc methionine (4 g/d and animal) for a period of 2 to 3 months before reassessing the patient to determine the treatment effect.

Treatments targeting at resolving secondary dermatitis consist of local and/or systemic administration of antibiotics. The topical use of a 7% iodine tincture to control secondary dermatitis and of chlorhexidine-based shampoos to loosen hyperkeratic crusts has been recommended. The use of topical or systemic glucocorticoids has been proposed in cases not responsive to antibiotic therapy.

TREATMENT

Oral treatment:
- Zinc sulfate (2 g/d and animal q24 PO for 2 to 3 months) (Q2)
- Zinc methionine (4 g/d and animal q24 PO for 2 to 3 months) (Q2)

Topical treatment:
- Chlorhexidine-based shampoo (3%, once to twice a week locally) (Q1)
- Topical treatment for secondary dermatitis:
- Iodine tincture (7%, once to twice a week locally) (Q2)
- Topical antibiotic skin ointments (based on culture and sensitivity testing to control secondary dermatitis) (Q2)
- Topical skin ointments containing glucocorticoids in cases unresponsive to antibiotics (Q2)

Systemic treatment:
- Systemic antibiotics (based on culture and sensitivity testing to control secondary dermatitis) (Q2)
- Systemic glucocorticoids in cases unresponsive to oral zinc supplementation and antibiotic therapy (Cave: pregnant animals) (Q2)

REFERENCES

1. Foster A, et al. *In Pract.* 2007;29:216-223.
2. Scott DW, et al. *Vet Dermatol.* 2010;22:2-16.
3. Zanolari P, et al. *Tierarztl Prax.* 2008;36:421-427.
4. Clauss M, et al. *Vet J.* 2004;167:302-305.

Bacterial Diseases of the Skin

METHICILLIN-RESISTANT *STAPHYLOCOCCUS AUREUS*

Staphylococcal skin disease in animals[1] is not uncommon and includes udder dermatitis in cattle; secondary infections to chorioptic mange or orf in goats (may also be *S. chromogenes* and occasionally *S. hyicus*); dermatitis of the head in sheep; and in pigs, usually *S. hyicus* but also possibly *S. sciuri*, *S. rostri*, *S. pasteuri*, *S. hominis*, *S. warneri*, *S. hemolyticus*, *S. epidermidis* (may be methicillin resistant), and *S. chromogenes*.[2]

INTRODUCTION

Methicillin (formerly meticillin in the United Kingdom) was introduced into human medicine in the 1950s to treat penicillinase-resistant *S. aureus* (SA).

Methicillin-resistant *S. aureus* (MRSA) strains have an altered protein-penicillin binding protein (PBP2a) that has a low affinity for all beta-lactam antibiotics (i.e., penicillins and cephalosporins). The protein is encoded by the *mecA* gene.

The MRSA strains may also have or not have a penicillinase enzyme (a beta-lactamase). *Spa*-typing is a method of typing *S. aureus* based on repeats located on several housekeeping genes.

Multilocus sequence typing (MLST) is a method of typing based on the sequence of several housekeeping genes. Similar sequence types may be grouped together in clonal complexes (CCs).

This protein is encoded by the gene *mecA*, which resides on a mobile genetic element called a staphylococcal chromosomal cassette (SCC*mec*). The detection of this gene is the best detection for MRSA.[3]

Methicillin is no longer used in human medicine, but oxacillin, nafcillin, and cloxacillin, which are very similar, are still used, although the resistance to these is usually lower than it is to methicillin.

The serious problem is that MRSA organisms are also often resistant to other antimicrobials, in particular aminoglycosides, macrolides, tetracyclines, and fluoroquinolones.[4]

Human Public Health

MRSA organisms cause infections, can be carried both persistently or intermittently, can colonize, and can also cause contamination. The infection can be mild or severe and sometimes fatal. There is a wide range of human prevalence in many countries. In some countries, a certain lineage may be most common.

Over the years, the types found in humans will change as new clones arise and they introduce new toxins.[5] The type CC398 is the most common animal type isolated from humans and is associated with increased mortality and morbidity. It also carries endotoxin genes but has only once been associated with food poisoning.

These bacteria have been an important cause of nosocomial infections for over 40 years.[6]

Type CC398 is a poor persistent colonizer of humans.[7] It is also less transmissible than non-ST398 in humans and in Dutch animals.[8]

Very rarely are these large animal-associated MRSA organisms responsible for serious infections in humans, although they have been found in deep-seated infections in skin and soft tissue and in pneumonia and septicemia. However, in most cases these infections with hospital-acquired MRSA (HA-MRSA) are inapparent, except when there is stress, such as in surgical situations or in immunocompromised patients.

A new strain has arisen in the Netherlands with no link to existing established Dutch risk factors for acquisition. In one study, a quarter of the 5545 MRSA isolates were from defined risk groups; 26% were CC398, and 74% were non-CC398.[9] Increases in CC398 have occurred in patients with or without contact with livestock and have led to an increase in carriers and infections.[10] Over the period from 2002 to 2008, there was a 925% increase in the number of cases in the laboratory database. Most cases involved CC398, with *spa* type *t*567 particularly overrepresented in sepsis and post-trauma osteomyelitis. CC398 was also more likely to be multiresistant than other types of MRSA. Simply put, the increase in CC398 has led to more carriers and infections.

MRSA accounts for approximately 20% of all bloodstream infections in U.S. hospitals and approximately 65% of the *S. aureus* infections in intensive care units, and it killed approximately 18,000 Americans in 2005.

Veterinarians

The carriage of MRSA by veterinarians in Australia attending a conference in 2009 has been investigated.[11] Industry and government veterinarians had the lowest levels of MRSA carriage at 0.9% prevalence. Those with horses as a major workload had 11.8% prevalence, and those on horse work only had 21.4% prevalence. Veterinarians with a dog and cat practice had 4.9% prevalence. The conclusion was that MRSA was an occupational hazard for those working in clinical practice in Australia.

A study of veterinarians showed that MRSA and livestock-associated MRSA (LA-MRSA) infection levels were 9.5% and 7.5%, respectively, in Belgium and Denmark (all Danish MRSA are LA-MRSA). A strong association was found with live pigs.[12] At the 2008 meeting of the American College of Veterinary Surgeons, a survey sampled 341 people; 17% of the veterinarians and 18% of the technicians were positive for MRSA. Contact with small ruminants in the previous 30 days, living with a person with MRSA diagnosed in the previous year, and working where there is a person specifically in charge of an infection control program were associated with colonization.[13]

Veterinary students conducting diagnostic investigations were also sampled.[14] Thirty students visited 40 pork farms and found MRSA on 30% of the farms; 22% of the students picked up the infection following exposure, but all were clear within 24 hours of the visit.

Pig Farmers

Thirty-five persons were screened for MRSA and sent on holiday; 27 of the farmers (77%) carried MRSA at least transiently. For 59% of the farmers, the infection was not cleared after the holiday away from pigs.[15]

Butchers

Colonization of butchers with LA-MRSA has been documented in markets in Hong Kong;[16] 300 pork butchers were sampled, and 17 were positive. Although five strains were health-care associated, the high incidence of *t*899 (CC9) suggests that cross-contamination from pork products occurs quite frequently.

Animal MRSA

Animal MRSA strains are found in farm animals, and it is likely that people in contact with these animals and their families, such as veterinarians, farmers, farm workers, and abattoir workers, may acquire these organisms. In the European Union, there are many animal MRSA types, but the most common type in farm animals is CC398. It is found commonly in pigs, veal calves, and broiler chickens. This type does not appear to be a risk to abattoir workers. There is also no evidence, as yet, that this strain can cause infection or generate carriers in humans when found in food. Where workers work full time, the incidence of MRSA is higher, and less if part time.

In general, the presence of multiple virulence profiles within a MRSA genotype in an animal species suggests possible reverse zoonosis and the potential for new MRSA clones by gaining or losing additional genes.[16]

If the *staphylococci* are resistant, then treatment with antibiotics to which the *staphylococci* are resistant can increase the proportion of infected pigs and increase the numbers of bacteria present. Generally, MRSA organisms are poor responders to treatment, and infected patients have a high death rate.

For years, the problem was restricted to hospitals (HA-MRSA). These strains were the main group for over 40 years, and they are resistant to many antibiotics. Since then, the incidence of HA-MRSA has decreased and now only accounts for about 20% of all infections, particularly those occurring in intensive care units.

Community-associated MRSA (CA-MRSA) developed in the 1960s, and strains were found outside of hospitals. In particular, these strains were isolated from cats, dogs, and horses and consisted of *S. intermedius* and *S. pseudointermedius*. It is now estimated that CA-MRSA may account for about 13,000 infections annually that require hospitalization, with a resultant 1400 deaths.

In 2003, large-animal-associated MRSA (LA-MRSA) strains were discovered. These were largely CC398, as determined by MLST. In different countries various types are found. For example, in Germany CC5, CC9, and CC97 are often found. In a German study of 14,036 MRSA samples, there were 578 *spa* types.[17] Where there are large numbers of these, such as in pigs, the possibility of colonization and infection rises.[18] LA-MRSA strains share some virulence factors with human strains, but they also have distinct virulence factors.[19] Exchange of these genes encoding virulence factors may extend the host range and thereby threaten public health.

ETIOLOGY

Three types of MRSA are currently recognized, as described in the previous sections: HA-MRSA, CA-MRSA, and LA-MRSA. Originally, the HA-MRSA strains were most common, then the CA-MRSA strains became problematic as the incidence of HA-MRSA decreased, and currently LA-MRSA strains are receiving increased attention.[20]

The CC398 (ST 398) type is 12 times more likely to be carried by pig farmers than nonfarmers, and cattle farmers are more than 20 times more likely to be carriers. LA-MRSA strains, which do not spread rapidly in the human population, emerged in the 1960s following poor response to treatment. It is now thought that half of the swine herds in Iowa carry LA-MRSA CC398. Pig farmers in Switzerland were found to be carriers of CC398.[21]

LA-MRSA strains were first described in a pig in 2003 and in other species in 2005 and 2007,[22,23] and since then cases have occurred in several countries.[24-28] LA-MRSA strains are an important source of infection in humans. It is thought that people spending a lot of time with pigs are at a higher risk of testing positive.[29] LA-MRSA strains were first noticed as spreading to humans in 2008 after cases reached hospitals in the Netherlands[30] and Denmark. Pig exposure has been cited as an important factor in LA-MRSA colonization in humans.[31,32] There is apparent transmission between pigs, pig farmers, and their families.[33] Pig farmers are 760 times more likely to be colonized by LA-MRSA than the general population.[22] LA-MRSA strains are not typable by pulsed field gel electrophoresis (PFGE) because of the presence of a novel DNA methylation enzyme. For this reason, *spa* types have been isolated from pigs and their human contacts; however, the majority are classified as sequence type (ST) 398 by MLST, suggesting that ST398 strains are adept at colonizing pigs and can be transmitted between pigs and their human contacts.

MRSA infections spreading from dogs and horses to humans are not usually important causes of infection; they tend to be sporadic and involve human skin infection.

In one study, 4 out of 13 workers at a teaching and research farm had MRSA, but a variety of animals (dairy cattle, beef cattle, sheep, horses, pigs, and goats) did not.[34] A unique sequence was found in pigs in Europe, and it was found that the new MRSA clone ST398 belonged mainly to random *spa* types *t*034, *t*011, and *t*108. ST398 is considered the main reservoir of LA-MRSA infection, and it is the main type that subclinically affects pigs. The transmission of ST398 to humans is dependent on the intensity of the animal contact,[35] but spread to the local community is not very frequent.[36]

CC398 is the predominant clone in animals.[37] Genes confirming metal resistance are commonly found in CC398, and only a few non-CC398 types carry these genes. This suggests that the use of metal-containing compounds in pig production may aid in the selection for LA-CC398.

EPIDEMIOLOGY

Distribution

MRSA can be found in nearly any location. It has been found in Korea[38] in a variety of forms in pigs (ST398, ST541, and HA-ST72). It has been found in Italy in a slaughterhouse study, suggesting a high risk from pork products. It was found in Sweden in cattle.[39] In the United States, United Kingdom, and Denmark, it has been found in pigs and pig workers.[40] At the equine hospital in Turkey,[41] 48% of the horses, 92.3% of the clinical staff, and 71.4% of the environmental samples were positive for MRSA. In France, three MRSA strains belonging to *t*034 *spa* were identified.[42] *S. aureus* was identified in 59/60 necropsies where *staphylococci* were implicated, and the organism was associated with 1.7% of the total equine deaths. The other case was associated with *S. pseudointermedius*.

In a study of veterinary hospital environments, MRSA was found in 12% of the environments. In the small-animal hospital, it was 16%; equine hospital, 4%; and large-animal hospital, 0%. The strain was usually type *spa* 100, which is commonly found in the United States.[43] MRSA was found in fattening pigs in Germany (152/290), all of which were ST398 cases. In Belgium, pigs were found to be already colonized in the farrowing house.[44] Various strains were found in Japan, including ST398 and ST9, but also ST5, ST97, and ST705.[45] In Belgium, 94% of the open farms and 56% of the closed farms were found to be infected,[46] and management and age-related trends were found to be important. There is a low level of MRSA incidence in Switzerland.[21] In Ireland, MRSA has been found in horses and dogs, but not cats,[47] and in three distinct clones (CC5, CC8, and CC22).[47]

Colonization

Colonization commences at birth, and piglets born to positive sows rapidly become infected; thus, by weaning, all the offspring are positive.

Subclinical nasal infection is common in pigs.[25,48] In other studies, the prevalence was found to increase rapidly after weaning but then fall during the finishing period,[44] and the strains were found to circulate from the nursery unit to the finishing unit. Where there is a doubling of veal calf, cattle, and pig populations in a municipality, there appears to be an increase of MRSA over the other types of *S. aureus* in the population.[18]

Pigs in slaughterhouses were found to be colonized by MRSA in different EU countries.[24,29,40,49]

Transmission

Air inlets and outlets have been found to be contaminated, contributing to MRSA transmission. Regular airborne transmission of LA-MRSA and deposition, strongly influenced by wind direction and season, up to 300 m was found in MRSA-positive pig farms.[50,51] LA-MRSA is regularly found downwind of pig and poultry barns (73% and 44%, respectively) but at low concentrations, suggesting that colonization is unlikely.

In a study in Denmark, MRSA was found in the dust and in five different age groups of pigs.[52,53] Inside pig and poultry barns, the levels were much higher. MRSA has also been found in the exhaust air from piggeries. In one study, 85% of all barns had MRSA in the air, and boot swabs and feces were also positive.[51]

In one study, nine fomites were investigated, and all transmitted MRSA to pig skin, except soap.[54] The nonporous fomites were able to transmit to the pig skin many weeks after contamination. In one study it was found that use of mobile phones by healthy workers in the health-care industry raised the possibility of transferring infection to workers, patients, and people outside the hospital.[55]

MRSA can be considered a contaminant of the environment[51] and has been detected on field surfaces.[56] There is a highly significant positive association between nasal carriage of MRSA in animals and the ability to isolate MRSA from dry surfaces.[57]

Pig workers have a significant risk of transmission.[58] Transmission to humans is associated with contact time, which is why workers are more likely to be carriers than the other members of the family. People who visit farms regularly to buy eggs or milk, or even for private farm visits, are more likely to be colonized.

Shower units on conventional swine farms have been shown to be infected.[59] MRSA can be isolated at postmortem examinations.[60] In a recent study, it was found that pharyngeal tissues had a high level of MRSA and thus may be more important in transmission than was previously thought because nose-to-nose contact with infected pharyngeal tissues is possible.[61]

In an experimentally induced infection with two sequence types (ST398 and ST9) and four commonly found *spa* types (*t*011, *t*08, *t*034, and *t*899), it was found to be difficult to produce carriage after nasal/gastrointestinal infection of piglets. Vaginal inoculation of the sow resulted in persistent carriage of *t*011-ST398 and *t*899-ST9 in all newborn piglets.[62] A low-dose inoculation was shown to be capable of horizontal transmission between pigs.[63] The major risk of transmission of ST398 is probably through trading of piglets.[64]

In a U.S. study in Ohio, 3% of the pigs were found to be positive for MRSA before slaughter, 11% in the lairage, and 2% in the carcasses, along with 4% of the retail pork.[65] The most common type was ST5, followed by ST398.

RISK FACTORS

Management is an important factor, although direct transmission is probably the most important. Animal carriers and human carriers present a hazard.

Risk factors also include herd size. The larger the herd, the more likely it is that MRSA is present.

Low incidence at birth is common, which slowly increases and stays positive for weeks, and then the prevalence slowly declines. In one study, 33% of sows were infected before farrowing, but the level had risen to 77% before weaning. Transmission rates were higher in preweaning pigs than in postweaning pigs[66] and spread rapidly in weaned piglets.[67]

There are usually up to three *spa* types per herd. The sow herd determines the production-chain levels of infection. The level of infection in piglets depends on the sow's colonization.

In all systems, the prevalence decreases with age.[68,69] If a pig herd is positive, people can be positive. If the pigs are positive, then farm dust certainly will be. Environmental contamination is therefore a risk. In one study, MRSA was found in dust, boots, socks, feces, air, and the shower units.[59]

In dairy herds the use of antibiotics is a risk factor, as are dairy hygiene and the age of the cow population. In pigs, LA-MRSA may persist without the use of antibiotics.[70]

If there are no positive pigs, then usually there are no positive people.[71] Farm visits are associated with the acquisition of MRSA, but most of these cases are only temporary.[27] At the 2006 International Pig Veterinary Society (IPVS) conference, 276 pig vets from a large number of countries were sampled, and 12.5% tested positive for MRSA.

On Swiss pig farms, it was shown that SA (including MRSA), endotoxin, and fungi levels were higher in the winter, so there may be a seasonal effect.[72] The incidence of MRSA is higher in zinc-treated and antibiotic-treated pigs.[73]

Pigs

It is generally acknowledged that the pig is the main reservoir for MRSA in large animals. *S. hyicus* is usually present in pigs but differs from *S. aureus* in that it does not have the *mecA* gene. Other species in pigs may include *S. chromogenes*, *S. epidermidis*, *S. sciuri*, *S. warneri, and S. xylosus*. A new species (*S. rostri*) has been found in the nasal cavity of pigs in Switzerland.[74]

There is known transfer between pigs and humans,[23,33,75,76] but it rarely spreads to the community.[77] Under some circumstances, MRSA strains can also produce enterotoxin. MRSA strains have been implicated in swollen ears, umbilical abscesses, vegetative endocarditis, subcutaneous abscesses, foot lesions, arthritis, osteomyelitis, mastitis, metritis, and enteritis.

There is a low incidence of MRSA in the United States compared with Europe. MRSA has been found in pigs in France, the Netherlands, Denmark, and Singapore.[24,40,78] In one study of Irish pigs, no cases of MRSA were found, and only two workers tested positive.[79] In finishing units in Italy, 11 different *spa* types were found, and this report identified ST9 for the first time in Europe and ST1 and ST97 for the first time in pigs.[80] In Spain, slaughter pigs are commonly affected with CC398 and CC97.[81] Free-range pigs in Spain are also infected (CC398 and *t*1011).[82] In Belgium, 94% of pigs on open farms were infected, compared with 56% of pigs on closed farms.[67] Thus far, in pigs in Europe, ST398 does not seem to be highly resistant to most antibiotics, with the exception of tetracyclines and perhaps macrolides.

The existence of lineages in species has been shown; for example, cattle often have CC133 and CC151, CC5 is common in poultry, and CC8 is common in horses. In pigs, the most common clonal complex is CC398,[83] which is different from the HA-MRSA and CA-MRSA in strains in humans,[48,84] but CC30, CC9, and CC49 have all been found. There are differences in colonization patterns of the different MRSA types in pigs.[85] CC9 is most common in Asia; ST8 has been found on a Norwegian pig farm, and the low occurrence suggests that this strain may be less able to colonize and persist on pig holdings.[86] There is considerable heterogeneity of the resistance genes in the complex, so CC398 may acquire multiple antimicrobial antiresistance genes.[87] It easily acquires genetic material, and therefore strains with increased resistance will develop.

ST398 seems to prefer pigs but has no host specificity.[88] The same authors suggested that ST398 has an apparent lack of virulence genes in a unique genetic background. It does not, for example, usually produce Panton-Valentin E leukocidin.

In a study in the Netherlands, it was found that the MRSA strains were usually resistant to at least three but sometimes five out of six antibacterials.[89]

There may be a link with cephalosporin usage in pigs.[90]

In Switzerland, there is a low level of MRSA in pigs, although transfer to humans may happen frequently. This low level is a result of the very low level of antibiotic use for pigs in Switzerland.[21] MRSA ST49 was found in Switzerland, and it has been suggested that it has been selected in the Swiss pig husbandry because a nearly threefold increase was noted over a 3-year period.[91]

MRSA is commonly present in pigs in Denmark as a reservoir, but not in other species.[92] In pigs, it has been shown that 74% of the CC398 strains from Denmark had a reduced susceptibility to zinc chloride,[93] which is important as a reflection of the use of zinc oxide to prevent *Escherichia coli* scours.

In a study of slaughterhouse pigs in Switzerland, it was found that 89% of farms screened[54] were positive for SA. Although no MRSA strains were found, there was widespread antimicrobial resistance, particularly to penicillin (62.5%) and tetracycline (33.3%). The *S. aureus* isolates belonged to Ridon *spa* types *t*034, *t*208, and *t*899.[94]

In a large study of herds in the Netherlands (202 pig farms), MRSA was present in 67% of the breeding herds and 71% of the finishing herds. MRSA was found in 40% of small herds and 80% of the larger herds.

A study in pigs and people in Canada in 2008 showed that 45% of the farms were affected, but only 24.9% of the pigs[29] and 20% of the farmers. The most common type was the same as that found in Europe, CC398 of *spa* type 539 (Ridon *t*034). The same strains were found in the pigs and personnel on the five farms where human colonization was present.

A pig can be colonized with several strains at any one time.

Cattle

MRSA has been associated with mastitis in cattle.[95,96] In a Belgian study, the presence of *mecA* was investigated in 118 MRSA strains from 118 different farms with *S. aureus* mastitis, and MRSA was found in 11 samples; all were CC398 (*t*011 or *t*567).[97] Non *S. aureus* MRSA strains have also been studied in veal calves, dairy cows, and beef cattle, and most of the organisms were *S. sciuri*, *S. lentus*, *S. fleurette*, and occasionally *S. epidermidis*.[98] In a long-term study of MRSA ST1, *t*127 mastitis in a dairy cow was reported.[99]

The first isolations from bulk-tank milk in the United Kingdom were described in 2012,[100] and in these strains a *mecC* homologue was described. In a subsequent study of UK cattle veterinarians, only 8/307 delegates were positive for MRSA, and none had the *mecC* homologue.[101,102]

MRSA has been found in milk from the udder in Switzerland and at high levels in milk in Africa. It was found to be present at quite high levels in Iran (28%), but at low levels in India and Japan. It can invariably be found on the skin of the udder and the inside of the thigh. Generally, in Europe, the United States, and Canada, the level of MRSA in cattle is quite low. In a study of U.S. bulk-tank milk samples, only 4% had MRSA (6/150).[103]

The most common MRSA strain is generally CC398, but there may be more than one strain of different types on the same farm, which suggests that subtypes may have been imported onto the farms or that a strain of CC398 has undergone diversification.[104]

In one study, 88% of dairy farms had MRSA (90/102), 458/2151 (28%) of the cattle were positive, 32% of the farmers were positive, and only 8% of the family members were positive; the prevalence in the humans decreased in the vacation periods.

A novel *mecA* homologue has been found in humans and cattle in Denmark. In a study in Denmark, a new *mecC* gene was discovered. In a study of 411 cows, it was found that 3.9% had MRSA, and all were positive for *mecA*, negative for *mecC*, and negative for Panton–Valentine-leukocidin (PVL).[105] The MRSA-positive level was much lower than in Dutch pigs and veal calves.

In a study of 36 German dairy herds, CC398 strains were found in all 36; no PVL genes were detected, but a hemolysin gene was found.[106] In another German study, it was found that where dairy cattle were kept in an area with a large number of pigs, the MRSA level was approximately 2%; where there were no pigs, the level was less than 1%.[107]

In the Netherlands, in a study during 2008 to 2009, over 50,000 milk samples were examined from 14 different dairy herds, and only 14 MRSA strains were found. All were CC398 and the usual *spa* types (*t*011, *t*108, and *t*889) commonly found in pigs. Not all of the strains possessed PVL genes, and all were resistant to two or more antibiotics.

In the United Kingdom, a study of *S. aureus* in milk samples showed that 31/940 were resistant to cefoxitin and/or oxacillin, and 3/24 tested positive for the novel *mecA* variant. This variant is 70% homologous to the *mecA* gene, and it is located on a newly recognized SCC *mecA* element designated SCC *mecXI*. Most isolates were MLST 1245, CC130, and *spa* type *t*843.[100]

A study showed the correlation between MRSA in humans and the percentage of positive cows in a herd; 36% of human nasal swabs and 61% of bovine nasal swabs were positive. In addition, 44% of bulk milk tests were also positive.

A new type showing resistance to cefoxitin and/or oxacillin has been detected in bulk milk and mastitis cases in England and Wales and also in humans from England and Denmark. The isolates are negative for the *mecA* gene and in latex agglutination tests for PBP2, encoded by *mecA* in standard tests. This new variant *mecA* gene was found in 13/940 samples examined. Most of these isolates were MLST 1245, CC130, and *spa* type *t*843.

In a study of beef cattle in the United States, MRSA was not isolated from 491 nasal swabs and 488 fecal samples.[108]

Veal Calves

In a study in veal calf farms, it was found that 38% of farmers had MRSA, and 16% of family members also had MRSA. Carriage was related to contact, and a family member was more likely to be positive when the farmer was positive. Only a small percentage consisted of persistent carriers, and only 7.5% were not CC398.[109]

In a study of rose and white veal calves, it was found that rose veal calves had less MRSA than white veal calves, and the conclusion was that care had to be gene taken in the use of antibiotics.[110] Conversely, it has been suggested that MRSA increased in calves with the length of the production cycle but was not related to antibiotic use.[109]

A high carriage rate of LA-MRSA was found in Belgian veal calves compared with other farm types, and they were significantly more resistant to antibiotics than the pig strains. Most were CC398 in the multispecies survey, but MRSA CC130 and CC599 carrying the *mecC* gene were detected in the beef and dairy cattle.[111]

Sheep and Goats

S. aureus is widely carried in sheep and goats and shows considerable diversity.[112,113] It has been isolated from goats with mastitis.[114] In a study of 179 sheep, 41% were positive; in a small sample of goats, 11/17 were positive. Twelve ST types were found and 26 *spa* types. Most commonly these were ST133. Only three MRSA strains were found in all of the positive strains, and two were ST130 and 1 ST398.[115]

Small Animals

MRSA was first recognized in dogs and cats in the United States. In pets, the MRSA strains can include a number of species, including *S. epidermidis*, *S.*

pseudoepidermidis, *S. hemolyticus*, *S. hominis*, *S. capitis*, *S. cohnii*, and *S. warneri*.[116,117] It usually passes from humans to pets and then back again. Usually, the strains in pets are the same as those found in the local hospitals.

A strain harboring the *mecA* gene has been isolated from humans, dogs, cats, and a guinea pig in Germany.[118]

In a study in the United States of dogs, cats, horses, pigs, and other species, 24 isolates were resolved into four PFGE clones (USA100, USA300, USA500, and USA800) and into sequence types (ST5, ST8, ST105, ST830, and ST956; or two clonal complexes, CC5 and CC8).[119]

A study of companion animals in the London area found that 26/1692 samples were positive for MRSA. Animals presented for treatment were more likely to be positive than healthy animals. MRSA carriage was rare, and it is likely that companion animals were contaminated vectors rather than true reservoirs.[120,121] A case-control study in the United Kingdom showed that significant risk factors for MRSA were the number of antimicrobial courses, the number of days admitted to veterinary clinics, and the presence of surgical implants. A risk study in the United States and Canada in dogs showed that both MRSA and methicillin-sensitive *S. aureus* (MSSA) were common on the ears of pets and that the risk factors were antibiotic treatments (beta-lactams and fluoroquinolones) and intravenous catheterization. MRSA did not transmit readily from apparently healthy dog to healthy dog in a study carried out in a rescue center.[122]

Horses

Humans who work with horses are sometimes affected by MRSA. MRSA can cause serious skin disease and soft tissue infections in horses. It is most easily cultured from the nostril, with carriage from 55 to 771 days.[123] The most vulnerable horse appears to be the long-term hospitalized horse.[124] Exposure to veterinary care may predispose both healthy horses and horse handlers to MRSA.[125]

MRSA was first recognized in horses in 1996 and since then has become a problem in horse clinics in Europe and North America. Originally, the strain was CC8 (*t*8 and *t*254), but this strain has been replaced by CC398, and recent evidence suggests that human strains may appear in horses. The horse is likely a low-level contributor to LA-MRSA in Belgium, where CA-MRSA is at a low level.[126]

MRSA was recognized in horses in the United States in 2005. In one study in the United States, it was not found on a pleasure horse farm but was found on a racehorse farm, where 61% of nasal samples and 71% of environmental samples tested positive.[127]

In the United States, the most common strain is CC500, whereas in Europe it is CC398, which is highly prevalent in horses and veterinary personnel at equine clinics.

In the Netherlands, there were no cases of MRSA in 2002, but by 2008 MRSA was found to be present in 375 of the SA samples. The CC398 strain currently predominates (*t*1011, *t*2123, and *t*064).

During an outbreak in a teaching hospital, some of the personnel tested positive, in addition to 57% of the environmental samples, including samples from the students' and staff members' rooms. In another study, 81 swabs from 42 horses on four farms were examined, and 11 species of *staphylococci* were found; 17/42 were untypable.[128]

MRSA was reported in Sweden in 2012, where 8/10 horses were infected in a veterinary hospital and two other infected horses were found close by. In another hospital study, 12/84 horses and 16/139 staff at a veterinary teaching hospital had MRSA. ST5 was the culprit. The risk was greater in the veterinarians and in the full-time rather than the part-time staff.[129]

The first strain of MRSA isolated in horses in the United Kingdom was ST398 from two horses and reported in 2009.[130]

A survey of horses admitted to the Berne University Clinic showed that 2.2% of the horses had MRSA.[131]

It has been found in Lusitano horses at the Lisbon teaching hospital.[132]

In a large study of 209 racehorses, 13 veterinarians, and 14 environmental surfaces, it was found that 48.3% of the equines, 92.3% of the vets, and 71% of the environmental samples were positive for a variety of staphylococcal species.[41]

In another study of nasal swabs from horses, 42 strains of MRSA were found,[133] again from a variety of staphylococcal species (*S. sciuri*, *S. xylosus*, *S. lentus*, *S. aureus*, and *S. capitis*). All the species contained the *mecA* gene.

Other Species

Poultry

People working with broilers have higher levels of MRSA than the general population (5.5% compared with < 0.1%) in the Netherlands. However, the level is lower than in those working with pigs and veal calves.[134] In another Dutch study of broiler flocks, slaughterhouses, and personnel, it was found that the risk was greater when dealing with live animals. Over 36% of the flocks were positive and 6% of the broilers. During the production day the level of MRSA infection increased from 8% to 35%. Most strains were ST398, but there were also large numbers of ST9.

In a study of mixed pig and poultry farms,[135] MRSA was most frequently isolated from the cloaca, nose, pharynx, and skin under the wings. There was a low prevalence in the broilers (0% to 28%) on the farm, but 82% to 92% of the pigs had MRSA. The broilers may be less sensitive to the ST398 strain than pigs. The farmer may have been part of the cause of the spread of the MRSA from the pigs to the poultry on the same mixed farm.

Turkeys

A study showed that 18/120 turkey farms had MRSA, as did 22/59 people on the farms. Those with frequent access were most likely to test positive.[136]

Donkeys

In a study of donkeys in Sicily, 40/46 donkeys were found to be positive for *staphylococci*. Of the 80 isolates examined, 52/80 were *S. aureus*. Nine genera were found; most of these were MSSA, and only 14 were MRSA. The *mecA* gene was found in 6/52 SA cases.

Donkeys could be a reservoir for the CC133 lineage.

Wild Boar

So far no important MRSA cases have been found in wild boar.[137]

Backyard Pigs

A study in the United States of backyard pigs suggested that there were no major differences from domestic commercial pigs,[138] and that in all probability there was no greater risk for human infection from these pigs.

In a study of farms in Connecticut (considered noncommercial) and their pig handlers (263 pigs and 9 humans on 35 farms), it was found that 51% of farms, 30% of pigs, and 22% of the handlers were positive for MRSA. The swine had HA-MRSA, CA-MRSA, and LA-MRSA, but the humans only had HA -strains of MRSA. The PVL gene was found in 7/8 of MRSA isolates, and this was the first time this gene had been found in pigs in the United States.[139]

Camels

MRSA has been described in an alpaca, which was infected with a human epidemic clone.[140]

Fish

MRSA have been isolated from Tilapia. In one study, 559 isolates of *staphylococci* were obtained; 198 (35%) were *S. aureus*, and 98 (50%) of these were MRSA.[141]

Zoo Animals

There are few reports of MRSA in zoo animals (skin in an elephant, rumen in a Moufflon, digit of a rhinoceros).[142]

Other Sources

Holding Areas

The abattoir holding area may act as a reservoir for MRSA, but this area does not appear to disseminate MRSA into the processing lines.[143]

Working in a lairage area or in a dehairing area was the major risk factor for MRSA carriage in pig slaughterhouse workers. The overall prevalence is low and decreases along the slaughterhouse line.[144]

The high prevalence of nasal carriage in slaughterhouse workers is largely associated with working with pigs.[144,145]

State Fairs

A study at two state fairs in the United States showed that only 25/157 pigs (15.9%) were positive for *S. aureus*, and only two MRSA cases were found.[146]

Food

There is no doubt that MRSA acquired on the farm can be transferred through to processing, but there is no significant evidence of cross-contamination between carcasses.[147]

In a German study the contamination rate was highest in nasal swabs at stunning (64.7%) and was low in carcasses (6%), meat at processing (4.2%), and final products (2.8%). MRSA can be identified at all points in the food chain.[148,149]

Food may be contaminated by MRSA, but there is no evidence that this leads to increased carriage rates in humans, either in food handlers or the public. It has been found in meat,[150, 151] and its incidence in meat was not uncommon.[152] MRSA can enter the slaughterhouse on or in animals and therefore does occur in raw meat emanating from the abattoir. ST398 has been found in up to 11.9% of retail meat samples in several studies in different parts of the world.[153]

In a study of retail meat samples (raw pork, chicken, beef, and turkey) from stores in Iowa, there was an overall presence of 16% positivity for MRSA, but only two isolates from pork were positive, although one had the PVL gene. The study suggested that MRSA rates in retail meat supplies, especially pork, were low.[154]

In Denmark, imported broiler meat had the highest levels of MRSA (18%), followed by imported pork (7.5%) and Danish pork (4.6%). In the same study, CC398 was found in Danish beef (1.4%). In addition to ST398, CC30 was also found for the first time.[155]

The transfer of MRSA from retail pork products to food-contact surfaces and the potential for consumer exposure has been described.[156] Pork loins, bacon, and fresh pork sausage were inoculated with mixed MRSA, vacuum packed, and stored for 2 weeks at 5 degrees C (41 F); the products were then placed on knives, cutting boards, and a human skin model for 5 minutes. Transfer to the cutting board occurred in 39% to 49%, to the knives in 17% to 42%, and to the human skin model in 26% to 36%. The transfer ranged from 2.2% to 5.2% across all products and contact surfaces.

PATHOGENESIS

S. aureus can produce many virulence factors, including protein A, technoic acid, coagulase, staphylokinase, deoxyribonuclease (DNase), lipase, hyaluronic acid, leucocidin, enterotoxins, and exfoliative toxins.

PATHOLOGY

MRSA has been detected in less than 1% of all pig postmortems. It is found both as a primary pathogen and as mixed infections, mainly in suckling and weaned pigs. Joints are more often affected than tissues. MRSA organisms live in clusters between the cilia or as singletons on the cilia in the respiratory tract. There are no morphologic changes when pig tracheal explants are experimentally infected. In an experimental infection,[157] there was colonization of lymph nodes (ileocecocolic).

DIAGNOSIS

MRSA organisms can be identified by phenotypic methods or genotyping. Samples are taken directly from lesions, biopsies, or blood culture onto selective and nonselective media. Contamination can be detected by swabbing noses (individuals), sampling dust (in herds and flocks), and food sampling. Increased sensitivity is obtained when using selective liquid enrichment media. *Spa* typing is available for lineage studies.[158]

Diagnosis of MRSA is based on culture, colony morphology, MLST on the protein A gene sequencing (*spa* typing), coagulase testing, antimicrobial sensitivity testing, and confirmation with Ceftiofur resistance and polymerase chain reaction (PCR) for the *mecA* gene.

CONTROL

Control should focus on the careful use of antimicrobials and consistent application of hygiene measures to reduce the spread of infection.[159] The reduction of access and exposure to pigs is most important. This means that movement restrictions and farm-level hygiene measures are the only possibilities.

There should be methods for harmonizing the sampling, detecting, and quantifying of MRSA in humans and animals and for detecting MRSA as a contaminant in food and the environment. Professionals connected with animals should also be tested on entry to the hospital. Transfer from animals to humans is difficult to control. Hand washing before and after contact is essential, as is avoiding direct contact with nasal secretions, saliva, and wounds. MRSA organisms can be killed with photodynamics.[160]

There is a clear difference between colonization and infection with MRSA.[161] Disinfection programs may temporarily reduce MRSA strains for the sow and piglets, but they do not result in a complete removal.[162] These programs are more effective in farrowing units than in finishing units.[163] Control programs in abattoirs should involve reduction in carcass contamination.[164]

FURTHER READING

Fitzgerald JR. Livestock associated *Staphylococcus aureus*; origin, evolution, and public health threat. *Trends Microbiol.* 2012;20:192-198.

Heller J, Hughes K. MRSA in horses. *In Pract.* 2013;35(1):30-35.

Voss A, et al. MRSA in pig farming. *Emerg Infect Dis.* 2005;11:1965-1966.

REFERENCES

1. Foster AP. *Vet Derm.* 2012;23:342.
2. Vanderhaeghen W, et al. *Vet Microbiol.* 2012;158:123.
3. Vanni M, et al. *Veterinaria.* 2012;26:19.
4. Deurenberger RH, et al. *Clin Microbiol Infect.* 2007;13:222.
5. Graveland H, et al. *Prev Vet Med.* 2012;107:180.
6. de Lencastre H, et al. *Curr Opin Microbiol.* 2007;10:428.
7. Graveland H, et al. *Int J Med Microbiol.* 2011;301:630.
8. Bootsma MCJ, et al. *J Roy Soc Interface.* 2011;8:578.
9. Lekkerkerk WSH, et al. *Clin Microbiol Infect.* 2012;18:656.
10. Wulf MWH, et al. *Europ J Clin Microbiol Inf Dis.* 2012;31:61.
11. Jordan D, et al. *Aust Vet J.* 2011;89:152.
12. Garcia-Graelis C, et al. *Epid Infect.* 2012;140:388.
13. Burstiner L, et al. *Vet Surg.* 2010;39:150.
14. Frana TS, et al. *PLoS ONE.* 2013;8:1.
15. Koeck R, et al. *J Hosp Infect.* 2011;79:292.
16. Lin Y, et al. *Clin Med Res.* 2011;9:7.
17. Koeck R, et al. *PLoS ONE.* 2013;8:2.
18. Feingold BJ, et al. *Emerg Infect Dis.* 2012;18:1841.
19. Fluit AC, et al. *Clin Microbiol Infect.* 2012;18:735.
20. Koeck R, et al. *Deutsch Arz Int.* 2011;108:761.
21. Oppliger A, et al. *Appl Env Micrbiol.* 2012;78:8010.
22. Voss A, et al. *Emerg Infect Dis.* 2005;11:1965.
23. Van Loo I, et al. *Emerg Infect Dis.* 2007;13:1834.
24. de Neeling AJ, et al. *Vet Microbiol.* 2007;122:366.
25. Smith TC, et al. *PLoS ONE.* 2009;4:e4258.
26. Huber H, et al. *Euro Surveill.* 2010;15:19542.
27. van Cleef BA, et al. *Epidemiol Infect.* 2010;138:756.
28. Horgan M, et al. *Vet J.* 2011;190:255.
29. Khanna T, et al. *Vet Microbiol.* 2008;128:298.
30. Van Rijen MM, et al. *Clin Infect Dis.* 2008;46:261.
31. Vandenbroucke-Grauls CMJE, Beaujen DJMA. *Ned Tijds Gen.* 2006;150:1710.
32. Rijen MV, et al. *Clin Microbiol Infect.* 2007;13:S446.
33. Huijsdens XW, et al. *Ann Clin Microbiol Antimicrob.* 2006;5:26.
34. Aquino GDV, et al. *Zoonoses Public Health.* 2012;59:1.
35. Graveland H, et al. *PLoS ONE.* 2011;6:e16830.
36. Cuny C, et al. *PLoS ONE.* 2009;2:e6800.
37. Otter JA, French GL. *Lancet Infect Dis.* 2010;10:227.
38. Lim S-K, et al. *Vet Microbiol.* 2012;155:88.
39. Unnerstad HE, et al. *Svensk Vet.* 2012;64:35.
40. Guardabassi L, et al. *Vet Microbiol.* 2007;122:384.
41. Asiantas O, et al. *J Vet Med Sci.* 2012;74:1583.
42. Haenni M, et al. *J Vet Diagn Invest.* 2010;22:953.
43. Hoet AE, et al. *Vector Zoo Dis.* 2011;11:609.
44. Dewaele I, et al. *Vet Sci Dev.* 2011;1:e1.
45. Asai T, et al. *Jpn J Infect Dis.* 2012;65:551.
46. Crombe F, et al. *Microb Drug Resist.* 2012;18:125.
47. Abbott Y, et al. *Epidem Infect.* 2010;138:764.
48. Smith TC, Pearson N. *Vector Zoo Dis.* 2009;11:327.
49. Schwarz S, et al. *J Antimicrob Chemother.* 2008;61:282.
50. Schulz J, et al. *Appl Environ Microbiol.* 2012;78:5666.
51. Friese A, et al. *Vet Microbiol.* 2012;158:129.
52. Espinosa-Gongora C, et al. *Vet Rec.* 2012;170:564.
53. Espinosa-Gongora C, et al. *Epidem Infect.* 2012;140:1794.
54. Desai R, et al. *Am J Infect Control.* 2011;39:219.
55. Ustun C, Cihanigiroglu M. *J Occup Environ Hyg.* 2012;9:538.

56. Friese A, et al. *Berl Munch Tierarztl Wschr.* 2013;126:175.
57. Peterson AE, et al. *Vet Microbiol.* 2012;160:539.
58. Comland O, Hoffmann L. *Ann Agric Env Med.* 2012;19:637.
59. Larson KRL, et al. *J Ag Safety Health.* 2012;18:5.
60. Wolf PJ, et al. *Vet Microbiol.* 2012;158:136.
61. Gibbons JF, et al. *Vet Microbiol.* 2013;162:771.
62. Moodley W, et al. *Epidem Infect.* 2011;139:1594.
63. Jovy E, et al. *Lett Appl Microbiol.* 2012;54:518.
64. Espinosa-Gongora C, et al. *Vet Rec.* 2012;doi:10.1136/vr.100704.
65. Molla B, et al. *J Clin Microbiol.* 2012;50:3687.
66. Broens EM, et al. *Vet Microbiol.* 2012;155:381.
67. Crombe F, et al. *Appl Env Microbiol.* 2012;78:1631.
68. Verhegghe M, et al. *Vet Microbiol.* 2013;162:679.
69. Weese JS, et al. *Zoonoses Public Health.* 2011;58:238.
70. Broens EM, et al. *BMC Vet Res.* 2012;8:58.
71. Overesch G, et al. *Schweiz Arch Tierheilk.* 2013;155:339.
72. Masclaux FG, et al. *Annls Occup Hyg.* 2013;57:550.
73. Moodley A, et al. *Vet Microbiol.* 2011;152:420.
74. Stegman R, Perreten V. *Vet Microbiol.* 2010;145:165.
75. Denis O, et al. *Emerg Infect Dis.* 2009;15:98.
76. Graveland H, et al. *PLoS ONE.* 2011;6:e16830.
77. Cuny C, et al. *PLoS ONE.* 2009;4:e6800.
78. Sergio DMB, et al. *J Med Microbiol.* 2007;56:1107.
79. Horgan M, et al. *Vet J.* 2012;190:255.
80. Battisti A, et al. *Vet Microbiol.* 2010;142:361.
81. Gomez-Sanz E, et al. *Food Pathog Dis.* 2010;7:1269.
82. Porrero MC, et al. *Vet Microbiol.* 2012;156:157.
83. Vanderhaeghen W, et al. *Vet Microbiol.* 2012;158:123.
84. Smith TC, Pearson N. *Vector Zoo Dis.* 2010;11:327.
85. Szabo I, et al. *Appl Environ Microbiol.* 2012;78:541.
86. Sunde M, et al. *J Vet Diagn Invest.* 2011;23:348.
87. Argudin MA, et al. *Appl Env Microbiol.* 2011;77:3052.
88. Jamrozy DM, et al. *PLoS ONE.* 2012;7:e40458.
89. Van Der Wolf PJ, et al. *Vet Microbiol.* 2012;158:136.
90. Burch DGH. *Pig Progress.* 2010;26:14.
91. Overesch G, et al. *BMC Vet Res.* 2011;7:30.
92. Hasman H, et al. *Vet Microbiol.* 2012;141:326.
93. Aarestrup FM, et al. *Vet Microbiol.* 2010;142:455.
94. Riesen A, Perreten V. *Schweiz Arch Tierheilk.* 2009;151:425.
95. Frey Y, et al. *J Dairy Sci.* 2013;96:2247.
96. Pilla RVV, et al. *Vet Rec.* 2012;170:312.
97. Vanderhaeghen W, et al. *Vet Microbiol.* 2010;144:166.
98. Vanderhaeghen W, et al. *J Anim Chemother.* 2013;68:300.
99. Pilla R, et al. *Vet Rec Case Rep.* 2013;doi:10.1136/vetreccr.100510rep.
100. Paterson GK, et al. *Eurosurveillance.* 2012;17:20327.
101. Paterson GK, et al. *J Anitmicrob Chemother.* 2012;67:2809.
102. Paterson GK, et al. *PLoS ONE.* 2013;8:e68463.
103. Haran KP, et al. *J Clin Microbiol.* 2012;50:688.
104. Fessler AT, et al. *Vet Microbiol.* 2012;160:77.
105. Van Duijkeren E, et al. *Vet Microbiol.* 2010;141:96.
106. Kreauskon K, et al. *J Dairy Sci.* 2012;95:4382.
107. Friedrich A, et al. *Ther Umsch.* 2012;66:195.
108. Weese JS, et al. *Zoonoses Public Health.* 2012;59:144.
109. Graveland H, et al. *PLoS ONE.* 2012;6:2.
110. Bos MEH, et al. *Prev Vet Med.* 2012;105:155.
111. Vandendriessche S, et al. *J Anim Chemother.* 2013;68:1510.
112. Porrero MC, et al. *Lett Appl Microbiol.* 2012;54:280.
113. Gharsa H, et al. *Vet Microbiol.* 2012;156:367.
114. Aras Z, et al. *Small Rum Res.* 2012;102:68.
115. Eriksson J, et al. *Vet Microbiol.* 2013;163:110.
116. Cooper KS. *Vet Med.* 2012;107:516.
117. Kern A, Perrenden VD. *J Ant Chemother.* 2013;68:1266.
118. Walther B, et al. *Emerg Inf Dis.* 2012;18:2017.
119. Lin Y, et al. *Clin Med Res.* 2011;9:17.
120. Loeffler A, Lloyd DH. *Epidem Infect.* 2010;138:595.
121. Loeffler A, et al. *Epidem Infect.* 2011;139:1019.
122. Loeffler A, et al. *Vet Microbiol.* 2010;141:178.
123. Bergstrom K, et al. *Vet Microbiol.* 2013;163:388.
124. Van den Eede A, et al. *Vet J.* 2012;193:408.
125. Van den Eede A, et al. *Vet Micrbiol.* 2013;163:313.
126. Maddox TW, et al. *Eq Vet J.* 2012;44:289.
127. Peterson AE, et al. *Vet Microbiol.* 2012;160:539.
128. Van Meurs MLJGM, et al. *Infection.* 2013;41:339.
129. Schwabe MJ, et al. *Vet Microbiol.* 2013;162:907.
130. Loeffler A, et al. *J Hosp Infect.* 2009;72:1.
131. Panchaud Y, et al. *Schweiz Arch Tierheilk.* 2010;152:176.
132. Couto N, et al. *J Equine Vet Sci.* 2012;32:300.
133. Mallardo K, et al. *Irpologia.* 2010;21:23.
134. Geenen P, et al. *Epidem Infect.* 2013;141:1099.
135. Pletinckx LJ, et al. *Inf Gen Evol.* 2011;11:2133.
136. Richter A, et al. *Epidem Infect.* 2012;140:2223.
137. Meemken D, et al. *Appl Environ Microbiol.* 2013;79:1739.
138. Gordoncillo MJ, et al. *Zoonoses Public Health.* 2012;59:212.
139. Osadebe LU, et al. *Zoonoses Public Health.* 2013;60:234.
140. Still JW, et al. *Canad Vet J.* 2012;53:670.
141. Atyaih MAS, et al. *Vet Microbiol.* 2010;144:502.
142. Vercammen F, et al. *J Zoo Wildl Med.* 2012;43:159.
143. Hawken P, et al. *Food Control.* 2013;31:473.
144. Gilbert MJ, et al. *Occup Environ Med.* 2012;69:472.
145. Van Cleef BAGL, et al. *Epidem Infect.* 2012;138:706.
146. Driessler AE, et al. *Vet Rec.* 2012;170:495.
147. Hawken P, et al. *J Food Protect.* 2013;76:624.
148. Beneke B, et al. *J Food Prot.* 2011;74:126.
149. Tenhagen B-A, et al. *Vet Rec.* 2009;165:589.
150. Lozano C, et al. *J Antimicrob Chemother.* 2009;64:1325.
151. de Jonge R, et al. *Eurosurveillance.* 2010;15:19712.
152. Weese JS, et al. *Lett Appl Microbiol.* 2010;51:338.
153. Kluytermans JA. *Clin Microbiol Infect.* 2010;16:11.
154. Hanson BM, et al. *J Infect Public Health.* 2011;4:169.
155. Agerso Y, et al. *Vet Microbiol.* 2012;157:246.
156. Snyder HL, et al. *J Food Protect.* 2013;76:2087.
157. Szabo I, et al. *Appl Envir Microbiol.* 2012;78:541.
158. Graveland HJ, et al. *Vet Microbiol.* 2009;139:121.
159. Nes A, Wolf MWH. *Wien Tierartzl Mschr.* 2012;99:315.
160. Eichner A, et al. *Photochem Photoderm Sources.* 2013;12:135.
161. Brasse K, et al. *Tier Umschau.* 2012;67:260.
162. Pletinckx LJ, et al. *J Appl Microbiol.* 2013;114:1634.
163. Merialdi G, et al. *Res Vet Sci.* 2013;94:425.
164. Lassok B, Tenhagen BA. *J Food Protect.* 2013;76:1095.

DERMATOPHILOSIS (MYCOTIC DERMATITIS CUTANEOUS STREPTOTRICHOSIS, SENKOBO DISEASE OF CATTLE, LUMPY WOOL OF SHEEP)

The disease is commonly called mycotic dermatitis in sheep and cutaneous streptotrichosis in cattle, although other local names exist including Senkobo skin disease in central Africa, Kirchi in Nigeria, and Saria in Malawi. Dermatophilosis is a name common to the disease in all species.

SYNOPSIS

Etiology *Dermatophilus congolensis*

Epidemiology Organism present in minor carriage lesions on face and feet. Serious disease occurs when body skin is broken by shearing or insect bites, or macerated by prolonged wetting, coupled with management practices that promote transmission. The disease has significant importance in cattle in tropical areas, whereas in high-rainfall temperate climates it occurs mainly in sheep and horses. In tropical areas ticks promote severe infection in cattle by suppression of immune function.

Clinical findings Sheep: hard crusts distributed over backline palpable in fleece. Cattle and horses: nonpruritic crusting dermatitis, initially with paintbrush tufts of hair. In cattle in tropical areas, extensive skin lesions.

Clinical pathology Branching filaments containing cocci in pairs.

Diagnostic confirmation Clinical. Organisms in scrapings or biopsy sections, culture, polymerase chain reaction (PCR).

Treatment Antibiotics. Topical antibacterial in horses.

Control Avoidance of skin trauma and of management practices that promote transmission. Use of topical bactericides to prevent infection of shear cuts, and of skin in risk periods. Acaricides in cattle.

ETIOLOGY

D. congolensis is the infective agent but requires damage to the skin from other causes to establish infection. The organism is dimorphic and grows as branched filamentous mycelia containing dormant zoospores that are transformed by moisture to the infective stage of motile isolated cocci. There is considerable genetic diversity between isolates. Isolates from the same geographic region are not necessarily closely genetically related, although genotypic variation between isolates is correlated with the host species.

EPIDEMIOLOGY

Occurrence

Geographic Occurrence

The disease occurs in all areas of the world but can be epizootic in tropical and subtropical areas of the world, where it can result in considerable economic loss. Surveys of large numbers of cattle in Africa report prevalence rates approaching 15%, with a 100% infection rate in some herds at the time of peak seasonal prevalence. In temperate climates the disease is usually sporadic but can still be of considerable economic importance where predisposing factors pertain. For example, an incidence ranging from 10% to 66% was recorded in nine dairy herds, where shower cooling was the predisposing factor to disease.

High prevalence in sheep flocks occurs in the high- and medium-rainfall areas of Australia. Significant clinical disease has been reported as far north as Canada, the northern United States, and Scotland, and as far south as New Zealand.

Host Occurrence

Disease occurs in cattle, sheep, goats, horses, and donkeys, and occasionally in deer, pigs, camels, and wildlife species. Animals of all ages are susceptible, including sucklings a few weeks old.

Source of Infection

The major source of infection for outbreaks of clinical disease exists with minor active lesions on the face and feet in otherwise healthy carrier animals, and with infection in scabs still carried in the hair and wool from healed lesions.

D. congolensis is not highly invasive and does not normally breach the barriers of healthy skin. These barriers include the stratum corneum, the superficial wax layer produced by the sebaceous glands, and, on the body of sheep, the physical barrier of the wool. On the feet and face, these barriers are easily and commonly broken by abrasive terrain or thorny and spiny forage and feedstuffs.

Dermatophilus may infect these lesions and may be transmitted mechanically by feeding flies to result in minor infection on the face and feet. This subclinical carriage form of the disease is common in most herds and flocks, and the minor lesions are most evident at the junction of the haired and nonhaired areas of the nares and of the claws and dewclaws. Minor lesions may also be present in the haired areas of the face and feet and on the scrotum and, in lambs, on the skin along the dorsal midline of the back. They are of no clinical significance to the animal except that they provide a source of more serious infection when other areas of the skin surface are predisposed to infection.

Transmission

Transmission occurs from the carriage lesions by contact from the face of one animal to the fleece or skin of another, and from the feet to the skin during mounting. Infection can be transmitted mechanically by flies and ticks and mediate infection by contaminated dips.

Environmental and Management Risk Factors

Sheep

Prolonged wetting of the fleece is the major risk factor and leads to emulsification of the wax barrier and maceration of the skin surface with disruption of the stratum corneum. A prolonged and heavy rain is sufficient to do this, especially if followed by warm and humid weather that retards drying of the fleece. Increased environmental humidity and temperature, as distinct from wetting of the skin, does not appear to promote the development of lesions. Moisture releases infective zoospores from carriage lesions, and these may be carried mechanically by flies that are attracted to the wet wool. The motile zoospores are aided in their movement to the skin surface by the moisture of the fleece and their positive chemotactic response to carbon dioxide at the skin surface.

A protracted wetting period of the fleece can also occur following dipping, jetting, or spraying of sheep for external parasites when these procedures are conducted at periods greater than 1 to 2 months after shearing; the incidence of mycotic dermatitis in sheep has been shown to increase with the time period between shearing and dipping. The infection onto the fleece comes primarily from the lesions on the face and feet and is promoted by tightly yarding sheep following these procedures.

Shearing cuts also destroy the barriers of the skin, and cuts may become infected mechanically by flies, physically by tight yarding after shearing, and by mediate infection in **dips** when sheep are dipped immediately following shearing. The resultant lesions do not spread over the body but provide a significant source of infection for other sheep in the flock when management or climatic circumstances lead to a high degree of flock skin susceptibility. Skin infection can also occur following infection with contagious ecthyma.

Cattle

Temperate Zones

Outbreaks in herds and severe disease in individuals are uncommon but can occur associated with high rainfall, with attack rates of 50%. There is a particular tendency for lesions to occur on the rump and back in females and males, probably as a result of the introduction of infection through minor skin abrasions caused by mounting. Lesions down the flanks of cattle may also result from abrasions and direct infection from the dewclaws during mounting. Other penetrating lesions caused by eartags or biting flies can also result in minor lesions.

The use of periodic showers or continual misting to cool cattle during hot periods is a risk factor for infection in dairy herds. Intercurrent disease and stress are also risk factors, and in infected dairy herds a higher incidence has been observed during the first weeks of parturition in first-calf heifers that also had endometritis or mastitis.

Tropical Zones

Climate is the most important risk factor and in tropical and subtropical regions; the disease has its highest incidence and severity during the humid, high-rainfall season. Animals in which the disease regresses are usually reinfected repeatedly in successive wet seasons. As in sheep, the disease in cattle requires disruption of natural skin barriers. However, prolonged wetting of the skin of cattle does not appear to be a major predisposing factor by itself, and the seasonal occurrence is associated with a concomitant increase in tick and insect infestation.[1] For example, a study in Ethiopia found that although prevalence was higher in cattle in the wet season, in both seasons, infestation with *Ambylomma variegatum* significantly affected the occurrence of disease, with infested cattle having a risk 7 times higher.

Tick infestation, particularly with *A. variegatum*, *Hyalomma asticum*, and *Boophilus microplus*, is strongly associated with the occurrence of extensive lesions of dermatophilosis, which can be minimized by the use of acaricides.

The lesions of dermatophilosis on the body do not occur at the predilection sites for ticks, and it is thought that the importance of tick infestation relates to a tick-produced immune suppression in the host rather than mechanical or biological transmission.

Lesions do occur at predilection sites for biting insects, mainly *Stomoxys* spp., *Lyperosia* spp., *Glossinia* spp., *Calliphoria* spp., and mosquitoes. In Africa the disease is often combined with demodicosis to produce Senkobo disease, a more severe and often fatal combination.

Trauma to the skin produced by thorny bushes and the ox-pecker bird (*Buphagus africanus africanus*) can also initiate lesions.

Horses

Biting flies (*Stomoxys calcitrans*) are thought to act as mechanical vectors of the infection, and the housefly (*Musca domestica*) can carry infection. Skin damage from trauma or from ectoparasites can predispose for disease, as does wetting from rainfall or from **frequent washing**.

HOST RISK FACTORS

There are breed differences in susceptibility in cattle and sheep. In Africa, the N'dama and Muturu cattle breeds and native sheep are resistant, whereas Zebu, White Fulani, Renitleo,[2] and European breeds are susceptible. Within-breed differences in susceptibility are also apparent, and genetic markers have been identified in Zebu cattle and Merino sheep. Susceptibility in cattle can be influenced by genetic selection. For example, selection against susceptibility to dermatophilosis, based on a BoLA-*DRB3/DQB* class II haplotype, reduced the prevalence of disease in

Brahman cattle in Martinique from 76% to 2% over 5 years.

In the Merino, sheep of the strong- or medium-wool strains are more susceptible. Open-fleeced sheep and sheep with a low-wax and high-suint content in their fleece are more prone to infection.

PATHOGEN RISK FACTORS

D. congolensis does not live well off the body and in the normal environment, and it is susceptible to the external influences of pH and moisture fluctuations. In the laboratory it can survive for 4 years in otherwise sterile broth culture and for at least 13 years in dry scab material kept at room temperature.

EXPERIMENTAL DISEASE

Local lesions, but not with spread to extensive disease, can be readily reproduced in sheep and cattle by removal of the skin wax followed by local challenge. Genetic differences modulate the severity of the lesion that occurs.

ECONOMIC IMPORTANCE

Sheep

Damage to the fleece causes severe losses, up to 30% loss of value of wool and 40% loss of skin value, and may be so extensive in lambs that spring lambing has to be abandoned. Other losses in sheep are caused by interference with shearing and a very great increase in susceptibility to blow-fly infestation.

Cattle

In Africa the disease in cattle causes great losses and many deaths, and the it ranks as one of the four major bacteriologic diseases with equivalent importance to contagious bovine pleuropneumonia and brucellosis. Goats in the same area also suffer a high incidence. Losses are from direct animal loss, decreased work ability of affected oxen, reproductive failure from vulval infection or infection on the limbs of males preventing mounting, death from starvation of calves of dams with udder infection, loss of animal meat and milk production, and downgrading of hides. In temperate climates deaths are uncommon, but cows that fail to respond to treatment and have to be culled are not infrequent. In a study in nine herds in Israel, death or culling rates from this disease ranged from 2% to 17%, and there was an average 23% fall in milk production in affected cattle. Reproductive inefficiency is a common accompaniment in severe cases.

Zoonotic Implications

Human infection is reported, such as on the hand of a veterinarian working with infected sheep, but contagion from livestock is rare in spite of ample opportunity.

PATHOGENESIS

The natural skin and wool waxes act as effective barriers to infection. Minor trauma, or maceration by prolonged wetting, allows establishment of infection and multiplication of the organism in the epidermis. The formation of the typical pyramid-shaped crusts is caused by repeated cycles of invasion into the epidermis by hyphae, bacterial multiplication in the epidermis, rapid infiltration of neutrophils, and regeneration of the epidermis. The organism in the scab is the source for the repeated and expanding invasion, which occurs until immunity develops and the lesion heals. The scab then separates from the healed lesion but is still held loosely in place by hair or wool fibers. In sheep, the extensive maceration of skin that can occur with prolonged fleece wetting can result in extensive skin lesions under the fleece. In cattle, tick infestation suppresses immune function and promotes the spread of the lesion. Secondary bacterial invasion may occur and gives rise to extensive suppuration and severe toxemia.

CLINICAL FINDINGS

Sheep

Lesions are commonly not visible in sheep because they are obscured by the fleece, but the crusts can be palpated as hard masses at the surface of the skin (**lumpy wool disease**) and typically are distributed irregularly over the dorsal midline, with "ribs" spreading laterally and ventrally. The crusts are roughly circular, thick, up to 3cm, often distinctly **pyramidal** with a concave base, and often pigmented, and the underlying skin is moist and reddened. The muzzle, face, and ears, and the scrotum of rams, may also be involved. The health of the animal is unaffected unless the lesions are widespread.

Heavy mortalities can occur in very young **lambs,** where there can be extensive lesions over the body. Many develop cutaneous blow-fly myiasis, and in occasional cases a secondary pneumonia resulting from the organism may cause the death of the animal.

Cattle

The early lesion is a pustule, and the hair over the infected site is erect and matted in tufts (paintbrush lesions) with greasy exudate forming crumbly crusts that are hard to remove. These develop into scabs that are greasy and fissures at flexion points, and finally to scabs that are hard, horny, and confluent. The scabs vary in color from cream to brown, are 2 to 5 cm in diameter, and are often in such close apposition that they give the appearance of a mosaic. In the early stages the crusts are very tenacious, and attempts to lift them cause pain. Beneath the crusts there is granulation tissue and some pus. In the later stages, the dermatitis heals and the crusts separate from the skin and are held in place by penetrating hairs, but they are easily removed.

Lesions occur on the neck, body, and back of the udder and may extend over the sides and down the legs and the ventral surface of the body. Commonly they commence along the back from the withers to the rump and extend halfway down the ribcage. In some animals the only site affected is the flexor aspect of the limb joints, the inguinal area, or between the forelimbs.

In young calves, infection commences on the muzzle, probably from contact with the infected udder or because of scalding by milk in bucket-fed calves, and may spread over the head and neck.

Horses

Lesions in horses are similar to those in cattle. The hairs are matted together over the lesion, and an exudative dermatitis produces a firm mat of hairs and debris just above the skin surface. If this hair is plucked, the entire structure may lift off, leaving a characteristic ovoid, slightly bleeding skin area. No pruritus or irritation is apparent, although the sores are tender to the touch.

Infection can appear on the head, beginning at the muzzle and spreading up the face to the eyes, and if sufficiently extensive may be accompanied by lacrimation and a profuse, mucopurulent nasal discharge. In some horses the lesions are confined to the lower limbs, with a few on the belly. In very bad environmental conditions the lesions may be widespread and cover virtually the whole of the back and sides. The lesions on lower limbs are most common behind the pastern, around the coronet, and on the anterior aspect of the hind cannon bones. If the underlying skin cracks, the horse can become very lame. This variable distribution of lesions may depend on the inciting skin trauma.

Goats

Lesions appear first on the lips and muzzle and then spread, possibly by biting, to the feet and scrotum. They may extend to all parts of the body, especially the dorsal midline and inside the thighs. In some cases lesions commence on the external ear. Heavy crust formations may block the ear canal and the external nares.

CLINICAL PATHOLOGY

The causative organism may be isolated from scrapings or a biopsy section and is much easier to isolate from an acute case than a chronic one. Polymyxin B sulfate can be used to suppress contaminants. Typical branching organisms with double rows of zoospores can be seen in a stained impression smear made directly from the ventral surface of a thick scab pressed firmly onto a slide. The organism can also be demonstrated by fluorescent antibody. ELISA and counterimmunoelectrophoresis have been used to detect serologic evidence of infection, and a real-time PCR test for rapid detection of *D. congolensis* has been developed in Spain.[3]

NECROPSY FINDINGS

In animals that die, there is extensive dermatitis, sometimes a secondary pneumonia, and often evidence of intercurrent disease.

Samples for Confirmation of Diagnosis

- **Bacteriology**—affected skin and draining lymph node (CYTO FUNGAL CULT)
- **Histology**—formalin-fixed samples of these tissues (LM)

DIFFERENTIAL DIAGNOSIS
Ringworm
Staphylococcal dermatitis/folliculitis
Scabies
Pediculosis
Fleece rot—sheep
Other causes of dermatitis are listed in Tables 16.3 and 16.4.

TREATMENT

Sheep

Bactericidal dips are used but have limited efficacy because topical treatments do not penetrate the scab to the active lesion; they are more appropriate for control.

Antibiotic treatment at high dose for a single treatment is effective in reducing the proportion of active lesions in an affected flock. Antibiotics that are effective include procaine penicillin combined with streptomycin at a dose of 70,000 units/kg and 70 mg/kg, respectively; erythromycin at 10 mg/kg; long-acting tetracycline at 20 mg/kg; and combination of lincomycin and spectinomycin at a dose of 5 mg/kg and 10 mg/kg, respectively; all treatments are given intramuscularly. Treatments appear effective in wet weather. The usual strategy is to treat 8 weeks before shearing so that there is time for the lesions to heal and shearing to occur without interference from active lesions. Sheep may be dipped in a bactericidal dip after shearing, as detailed under "Control." An alternate approach is to cull affected sheep.

Cattle

With the disease that occurs in temperate areas, tetracycline (5 mg/kg body weight [BW]) repeated weekly as required is recommended, and long-acting tetracycline (20 mg/kg BW) in one injection is reported to give excellent results in cattle. Parenteral procaine penicillin G (22,000 IU/kg IM) daily for 3 days is also reported as efficacious.

With the disease that occurs in tropical areas and associated with tick infestation, there is no completely satisfactory treatment in herds with extensive involvement or those being constantly reinfected or exposed to predisposing causes. In general terms, better results are obtained during dry weather and in dry climates. In tropical Africa, treatments that are reasonably effective elsewhere are of little or no value.

Parenteral treatment with antibiotics, as described previously, can be used and should be used in conjunction with acaricides when ticks are present.

Horses

Topical therapy is most commonly used in horses, coupled with removal from whatever is causing prolonged wetness of the skin. Although horses generally respond well, in bad weather even they can be recalcitrant to treatment. Scabs can be removed by grooming under sedation and the lesions treated topically daily with povidone–iodine or chlorhexidine until the lesions heal. Benzoyl peroxide has keratolytic, antibacterial, and follicular flushing properties and is reported to be effective in therapy when applied topically at a concentration of 2.5%.

Severe cases can be treated daily for 3 days with procaine penicillin G at 20,000 units/kg intramuscularly alone or in combination with streptomycin at 10 mg/kg IM.

CONTROL

The principal approach, where possible, is the avoidance of predisposing factors. The disease usually disappears in dry weather. Isolation of infected animals and avoidance of contact by clean animals with infected materials such as grooming tools is desirable. Affected sheep should be shorn and/or dipped last.

Close yarding of sheep or factors that promote face-to-skin contact immediately after shearing or after dipping should be avoided. Insecticidal dips should contain a bactericide. Where dipping immediately after shearing is a risk factor, the severity of infection can be reduced by delaying dipping, for example, from the 1st to the 10th day after shearing, or by dipping in zinc sulfate immediately following shearing with later dipping in an insecticide. Alternatively, pour-on insecticides can be used.

Bactericidal dips will give some protection to sheep. Spraying or dipping of sheep in a 0.5% to 1.0% solution of zinc sulfate immediately after shearing is used to prevent infection of shear cuts. Spraying or dipping sheep in a 1% solution of alum (potassium aluminum sulfate) provides protection against infection for up to 70 days, with alum rendering the organism nonmotile, and can be used to provide protection during the rainy season in woolled sheep. Alum strips from the dip, and the dip requires frequent replenishment, with the amount depending on wool length. An alternate treatment is to dust alum along the back of the sheep.

With cattle in tropical areas, **tick control** (see Tick Infestations in this chapter) is most important in control of dermatophilosis. Attempts at prophylaxis by vaccination in both sheep and cattle have been unsuccessful; immunity appears to be isolate-specific.

FURTHER READING

Norris BJ, Colditz IG, Dixon TJ. Fleece rot and dermatophilosis in sheep. *Vet Microbiol.* 2008;128:217-230.

Radostits O, et al. Dermatophilosis (mycotic dermatitis, cutaneous streptotrichosis, Senkobo disease of cattle, lumpy wool of sheep). In: *Veterinary Medicine: A Textbook of the Diseases of Cattle, Horses, Sheep, Goats and Pigs.* 10th ed. London: W.B. Saunders; 2007:1048-1051.

REFERENCES

1. Chatikobo P, et al. *Trop Anim Health Prod.* 2009;41:1289.
2. Razafindraibe H, et al. *Annal NY Acad Sci.* 2006;1081:489.
3. Garcia A, et al. *J Vet Sci.* 2013;14:491.

SKIN TUBERCULOSIS

Chronic indurative lesions of the skin in cattle, occurring usually on the lower limbs, are called "skin tuberculosis" because they frequently sensitize affected animals to tuberculin.

ETIOLOGY

Acid-fast organisms can often be found in the lesions in small numbers. They have not been identified and are probably not true pathogens. Iatrogenic lesions may be caused by aluminum adsorbed vaccines that produce subcutaneous granulomas, which are colonized by acid-fast bacteria.

EPIDEMIOLOGY

The disease occurs in most countries of the world, particularly where animals are housed and incur minor abrasions and pressure sores. The frequent occurrence of lesions on the lower extremities suggests **cutaneous abrasions** as the probable portal of entry of the causative organism.

The lesions cause little inconvenience but are unsightly, and affected animals may give a suspicious or positive reaction to the tuberculin test when they are in fact free of tuberculosis. This becomes important when herds and areas are undergoing eradication and attention is focused on any condition that complicates the tuberculin test.

PATHOGENESIS

Tuberculoid granulomas occur at the site of infection, with spread along local lymphatic vessels but without involvement of lymph nodes.

CLINICAL FINDINGS

Small lumps 1 to 2 cm in diameter appear under the skin. The **lower limbs** are the most common site, particularly the forelimbs, and spread to the thighs and forearms, and even to the shoulder and abdomen, may occur. The lesions may be single or multiple and often occur in **chains** connected by thin cords of tissue. The nodules are attached to the skin; they may rupture and discharge thick cream-to-yellow pus. Ulcers do not persist. Individual lesions may disappear, but complete recovery to the point of disappearance of all lesions is unlikely if the lesions are large and multiple.

CLINICAL PATHOLOGY

Affected animals may react to the tuberculin test. Bacteriologic examination of smears of pus may reveal the presence of acid-fast bacteria.

NECROPSY FINDINGS

The lesions comprise much fibrous tissue, usually containing foci of pasty or inspissated pus, and are sometimes calcified.

> **DIFFERENTIAL DIAGNOSIS**
>
> In herds with tuberculosis, reactors that have lesions of skin tuberculosis are disposed of in the usual way. In herds free of tuberculosis, a positive reaction to the tuberculin test in animals with skin tuberculosis is usually taken to be nonspecific; the affected animal is retained, provided it is negative on retest.
>
> **Bovine farcy** (see also "Bovine Farcy")
>
> **Ulcerative lymphangitis** (see also "Ulcerative Lymphangitis").

TREATMENT AND CONTROL

Treatment and control measures are not usually instituted, although surgical removal may be undertaken for cosmetic reasons.

MYCOBACTERIUM ULCERANS INFECTION (BURULI OR BAIRNSDALE ULCER)

Mycobacterium ulcerans causes progressive ulcers in the skin of humans, dogs, cats, alpacas, horses and wildlife.[1-5] Pigs can be infected experimentally.[6] The disease in humans occurs in at least 30 countries,[5] often as geographic clusters associated with water bodies. Wildlife, such as the common brushtailed possum (*Trichosurus vulpecula*) and ring-tailed possum (*Pseudocheirus peregrinus*) in southeastern Australia, are proposed as important components of the disease infection cycle, with *M. ulcerans* detected in the feces of 41% of possums in areas in which the disease is endemic and less than 1% in nonendemic areas.[5] Clusters of the disease in people are spatially associated with the presence of possums.[7] A relationship between wildlife and domestic animal disease has not been investigated or reported. The organism can be detected in a number of species of mosquitoes, although the importance of these species in spread of the infection and causation of disease is unclear.[7]

Infection by the organism causes extensive and progressive necrosis of the skin and underlying soft tissue, usually of the limbs or extremities. The disease is reported in the thigh of one horse and the withers and fetlock of another,[1] and the distal limb and face, respectively, of two alpacas.[4] Infection causes both ulcerating and nonulcerating granulomatous lesions in dogs and cats.[2] One of two horses affected died as a result of the disease, as did both alpacas.[1,4]

Diagnosis is by the demonstration of the organisms by Ziehl–Neilson staining of biopsies of lesions with confirmation by culture or, more conveniently and presumably with greater sensitivity, by PCR detection of *M. ulcerans* genome.[1,2,4]

Treatment is by surgical excision of the lesion. Therapy with antimycobacterial drugs such as rifampin, clarithromycin, or fluoroquinolones can be considered but is limited because of drug-induced toxicoses, including diarrhea, difficulty in long-term administration, and expense.

There are no accepted control measures. The disease has zoonotic potential, and affected animals and samples should be handled accordingly.

REFERENCES

1. van Zyl A, et al. *Aust Vet J.* 2010;88:101.
2. O'Brien CR, et al. *Aust Vet J.* 2011;89:506.
3. Malik R, et al. *Vet Dermatol.* 2013;24:146.
4. O'Brien C, et al. *Aust Vet J.* 2013;91:296.
5. Fyfe JAM, et al. *PLoS Neglect Trop Dis.* 2010;4.
6. Bolz M, et al. *PLoS Neglect Trop Dis.* 2014;8.
7. Carson C, et al. *PLoS Neglect Trop Dis.* 2014;8.

FLEECE ROT IN SHEEP

> **SYNOPSIS**
>
> **Etiology** Dermatitis associated with growth of chromogenic *Pseudomonas aeruginosa* following prolonged wetting of the skin of sheep.
>
> **Epidemiology** Occurs with high incidence in sheep with susceptible fleece characters in wet seasons. Major risk factor for body flystrike.
>
> **Clinical findings** Dermatitis with fleece coloration over the backline.
>
> **Diagnostic confirmation** Clinical.
>
> **Control** Selection of sheep with resistant fleece characters.

ETIOLOGY

Fleece rot develops as an exudative dermatitis following wetting of the fleece by rain. The growth of toxigenic strains of *Pseudomonas aeruginosa* is thought to be the major cause of the dermatitis, and the fleece coloration that usually accompanies it, but other *Pseudomonas* spp., including *P. maltophilia*, have been incriminated in the genesis of the condition. The enzyme phospholipase C in *P. aeruginosa* is a virulence determinant for this disease.

EPIDEMIOLOGY

Occurrence

The disease is common in most parts of Australia and occurs in South Africa and also in areas of New Zealand. Its occurrence is associated with wet years, and in these circumstances the incidence in affected flocks varies from 40% to 100%.[1,2]

Environmental and Host Risk Factors

Fleece rot occurs in sheep only in wet seasons and when the fleece is predisposed to wetting by its physical characters.

Prolonged rainfall, sufficient to wet sheep to the skin for a week, is required for this condition to occur. Young sheep (those < 10 months) are more susceptible than old, and heritable differences in fleece characters affect the susceptibility of individual sheep. These characters are probably related to the ease with which the skin can be wetted.

Fleece Characteristics

The degree of "grip" and body skin wrinkling are unimportant as factors affecting susceptibility, but fleece weight, fiber diameter and variability, staple density, and neck wrinkle are positively correlated with susceptibility. These characteristics produce visible differences between fleeces. Resistant sheep have closely packed elliptical wool staples with blocky tips and even crimp. Susceptible fleeces have thin staples of unevenly crimped wool and with a fringe-tipped appearance as a result of the protrusion of thicker wool fibers above the top of the staple. This fringed appearance is visible along the back and sides. Susceptible flocks are characterized by fleeces with longer, heavier, thicker staples with lower crimp frequency and higher fiber diameter and variability.

Fleeces with a high wax content are less susceptible, probably because of the waterproofing effect of the wax. This view is supported by the observation that disruption of the sebaceous layer on the skin increases its susceptibility to wetting.

Greasy fleece color has been found to be a good predictor of susceptibility to fleece rot in some studies but not others. Wool with a high suint content is highly susceptible.

Experimental Production

The disease can be reproduced experimentally by inoculating *P. aeruginosa* epicutaneously and wetting the fleece.

Economic Importance

Fleece rot causes considerable financial loss because of the depreciation in the value of the damaged fleeces and the increased need for chemical applications to treat or prevent body flystrike, for which it is a major risk factor.

PATHOGENESIS

With prolonged wetting, conditions of high humidity in the fleece microenvironment and the availability of rich nutrients from serous exudates and indigenous suint allow the proliferation of opportunistic skin and fleece bacteria, including *P. aeruginosa*, and result in dermatitis. The predominant bacterium is usually *P. aeruginosa*, which inhibits the growth of other bacteria, and its pyocyanin produces a green color. Its rapid growth is accompanied by the production of the dermonecrotic toxin phospholipase C, which exacerbates the dermatitis and initiates the inflammatory cascade that draws neutrophils and lymphocytes into the skin.

In the experimental disease there is outpouring of serous exudate and infiltration of leukocytes into dermis, but *P. aeruginosa* is localized as aggregates at the leading front of the seropurulent exudate and never penetrates the dermis.

Other discolorations may occur depending on the predominance of a particular chromogenic bacterium, many of which belong to *Pseudomonas* spp. *P. maltophilia* can result in yellow–brown coloration, and *P. indigofera* results in blue coloration.

The odor produced by the bacteria and the serum protein on the skin surface is very attractive to blow flies, and most body strikes are a result of preexisting fleece-rot lesions. To add a further complication, *P. aeruginosa* also proliferates in the presence of organophosphorous insecticides and facilitates its biodegradation.

Sequencing of 16SrRNA genes to identify bacteria present before and after the onset of disease in an experimental flock at Trangie in Australia identified several new bacteria associated with fleece rot, and the bacterial populations differed between susceptible and resistant sheep.[3] It was concluded that although *P. aeruginosa* may be associated with severe fleece-rot lesions, there may be other bacteria associated with susceptibility or resistance to this condition. Subsequently, investigation of single-nucleotide polymorphisms between susceptible and resistant sheep identified 155 genes that were differentially expressed.[4] Fibulin (FBLN1) and fatty acid binding protein 4 (FAB4) were identified as key factors in resistance to fleece rot. If validated in larger populations, these could enable marker-assisted selection to increase the resistance of Merino sheep to fleece rot.[4]

CLINICAL FINDINGS

Lesions occur most commonly over the withers and along the back. In active cases, the wool over the affected part is always saturated, and the tip is more open than over unaffected areas. The wool is leached and dingy and in severe cases can be plucked easily. The skin is inflamed, and serous exudate produces bands of matted and colored fibers across the staple. The coloration of the fibers is commonly green, but may be yellow, yellow–brown, or red–brown and occurs in fibers at skin level or extending the full length of the staple.

The general health of the sheep is unaffected in typical fleece rot, but severe ulcerative dermatitis with mortality associated with *P. aeruginosa* can occur. For example, chronic ulcerative and necrotic dermatitis associated with *P. aeruginosa*, occurring on the tail, udder, and legs of sheep and accompanied by green coloration of the surrounding fleece, was recorded following excessive rain in the Mediterranean climate zone of Israel.

CLINICAL PATHOLOGY AND NECROPSY FINDINGS

Autopsy examinations are not carried out, and laboratory examination of the living animal is not usually necessary.

There are differences in the inflammatory response and in peripheral blood lymphocyte subsets between fleece-rot-resistant and susceptible sheep, with several different mechanisms likely to occur in resistant sheep.[2]

DIAGNOSIS

Fleece rot resembles mycotic dermatitis in body distribution and predisposing factors, but the typical scab is not present in fleece rot.

CONTROL

Treatment is unlikely to be of value, but some degree of control may be effected by selection of fleece-rot-resistant sheep for use in susceptible localities. In these same localities, shearing before the wet season should facilitate drying of the fleece and lessen susceptibility, although the variable and unpredictable timing of rainfall means that no shearing time will reliably prevent fleece rot. The heritability of resistance to fleece rot has been estimated to be between 0.35 and 0.4; thus, selective breeding programs have been advocated, with genetically selected lines showing increased resistance in high-risk environments.[2]

Considerable effort was invested into the investigation of vaccines against fleece rot in the 1980s and 1990s.[2] These reduced the severity of fleece rot in pen experiments, often by up to 60%, but when the infecting serotype of *P. aeruginosa* differed from the vaccine strain there was little cross protection.

REFERENCES

1. Radostits O, et al. Fleece rot in sheep. In: *Veterinary Medicine: A Textbook of the Diseases of Cattle, Horses, Sheep, Goats and Pigs*. 10th ed. London: W.B. Saunders; 2007:1081-1082.
2. Norris BJ, et al. *Vet Microbiol*. 2008;128:217.
3. Dixon TJ, et al. *Aust J Agric Res*. 2007;58:739.
4. Smith WJM, et al. *BMC Vet Res*. 2010;6:27.

BOLO DISEASE

This disease of the fleece of predominantly merino and Döhne merino sheep appears confined to the Eastern Cape province of South Africa and gets its name from the region where it was first described. An unclassified *Corynebacterium* spp. closely resembling *Corynebacterium pseudodiphtheriticum* and *Corynebacterium urealyticum* can be isolated from the skin of affected sheep. This organism is rarely isolated from the skin of sheep with normal fleeces. The disease can be experimentally reproduced by the topical application of the organism onto the intact skin of newly shorn sheep and sheep in 5-month wool, and the organism persists in the produced lesions for at least 169 days.

Bolo disease is a disease of medium- and medium–strong-wool Merino sheep having dense fleeces with a high yolk content. It occurs in sheep on natural grazing. There is no sex predilection, but older and poor-conditioned sheep are more severely affected. It can occur in semiarid climates, and there is no apparent seasonal or climatic influence or influence of external parasites. The attack rate in a flock can be as high as 90%, and the disease has considerable economic impact because as the wool is of inferior quality and low economic value.

Lesions occur most commonly on the sides of neck and the shoulders and are more easily seen in unshorn sheep as well-defined, dark gray to black patches and bands that vary in number and in size (20 mm to 30 cm in diameter) and are sunk below the surface of the tips of the surrounding staple. The underlying skin is red–purple in color, is tender to the touch, and breaks easily. There is a yellow sticky exudate on the surface of the skin and in between the wool fibers, resulting in a spiky staple. On freshly shorn sheep, the affected areas are chalky white.

Histologically there is acanthosis, superficial and follicular hyperkeratosis and hyperpigmentation, and sebaceous gland hypertrophy.

Treatment regimens are not defined, but high-dose parenteral penicillin as used in mycotic dermatitis might be effective.

Bolo disease can be differentiated from fleece rot and mycotic dermatitis by its clinical presentation and the epidemiologic circumstances in which it occurs.

FURTHER READING

Radostits O, et al. Bolo disease. In: *Veterinary Medicine: A Textbook of the Disease of Cattle, Horses, Sheep, Goats and Pigs*. 10th ed. London: W.B. Saunders; 2007:798.

STRAWBERRY FOOTROT OF SHEEP (PROLIFERATIVE DERMATITIS)

Strawberry footrot of sheep is a proliferative dermatitis of the lower limbs of sheep.

ETIOLOGY

The causative agent is thought to be *D. congolensis* (*Dermatophilus pedis*).[1]

EPIDEMIOLOGY

The disease is recorded in the United Kingdom and occurs extensively in some parts of Scotland and in Australia. It is not fatal, but severely affected animals do not make normal weight gains. Up to 100% of animals in affected flocks may show the clinical disease.

All ages and breeds appear susceptible, but under natural conditions lambs are more commonly affected. Most outbreaks occur during the summer months, and lesions tend to disappear in cold weather. Although the disease is recorded naturally only in sheep, it can be transmitted experimentally to man, goats, guinea pigs, and rabbits. Complete immunity does not develop after an attack, although sheep recently recovered from contagious ecthyma may show a transient resistance.

The natural method of transmission is unknown, but the frequency of occurrence of lesions at the knee and coronet suggests infection from the ground through cutaneous injuries. Dried crusts containing the causative agent are infective for long periods, and ground contamination by infected animals, or infection from carrier animals, is the probable source of infection.

PATHOGENESIS

Histologically, the lesions are those of a superficial epidermitis similar to that of contagious ecthyma.

CLINICAL FINDINGS

Most cases appear 2 to 4 weeks after sheep have been moved onto affected, pasture but incubation periods of 3 to 4 months have been observed. Small heaped-up scabs appear on the leg from the coronet to the knee or hock. These enlarge to 3 to 5 cm in diameter and become thick and wart-like. The hair is lost, and the lesions may coalesce. Removal of the scabs reveals a bleeding, fleshy mass resembling a fresh strawberry, surrounded by a shallow ulcer. In later stages the **ulcer** is deep and pus is present. There is no pruritus or lameness unless lesions occur in the interdigital space. Most lesions heal in 5 to 6 weeks, but chronic cases may persist for 6 months.

CLINICAL PATHOLOGY

Swabs and scrapings should be examined for the causative organism.

> **DIFFERENTIAL DIAGNOSIS**
>
> Lesions of strawberry footrot closely resemble those of contagious ecthyma but are restricted in their distribution to the lower limbs, whereas lesions of contagious ecthyma occur mostly on the face and less often on the legs. On careful examination, often both leg and face lesions are present. The absence of a systemic reaction and the proliferative character of the lesions differentiate it from sheeppox.

TREATMENT

There is little information on treatment. Antibiotics as used in dermatophilosis should be effective. In an unusual outbreak of lameness affecting 40% of a flock, with lesions resembling strawberry footrot but from which no organisms were isolated, the response to topical antibiotic and preparations was poor, although lesions did become less painful after bathing affected areas in a solution of lincomycin/spectinomycin.[2] Systemic treatment with tilmicosin and long-acting amoxicillin did assist healing.[2]

CONTROL

In the light of present knowledge, isolation of infected sheep and the resting of infected fields are the only measures that can be recommended.

REFERENCES

1. Radostits O, et al. Strawberry footrot. In: *Veterinary Medicine: A Textbook of the Disease of Cattle, Horses, Sheep, Goats and Pigs*. 10th ed. London: W.B. Saunders; 2007:1051.
2. van Burgt GM, et al. *Vet Rec*. 2011;168:569.

CONTAGIOUS ACNE OF HORSES (CANADIAN HORSEPOX, CONTAGIOUS PUSTULAR DERMATITIS)

Contagious acne of horses is characterized by the development of pustules, particularly where the skin comes in contact with the harness.

ETIOLOGY

Corynebacterium pseudotuberculosis is the specific cause of this disease.

EPIDEMIOLOGY

The disease is spread from animal to animal by means of contaminated grooming utensils or harnesses. An existing seborrhea or folliculitis as a result of blockage of sebaceous gland ducts by pressure from the harness probably predisposes to infection. Inefficient grooming may also be a contributing cause.

Contagious acne is of limited occurrence and causes temporary inconvenience when affected horses are unable to work.

PATHOGENESIS

Infection of the hair follicle leads to local suppuration and the formation of pustules, which rupture and contaminate surrounding skin areas. Occasional lesions penetrate deeply and develop into indolent ulcers.

CLINICAL FINDINGS

The skin lesions usually develop in groups in areas that come into contact with the harness. The lesions take the form of papules that develop into pustules varying in diameter from 1 to 2.5 cm. There is no pruritus, but the lesions may be painful to touch. Rupture of the pustules leads to crust formation over an accumulation of greenish-tinged pus. Healing of lesions occurs in about 1 week, but the disease may persist for 4 or more weeks if successive crops of lesions develop.

CLINICAL PATHOLOGY

Swabs of the lesions can be taken to determine the presence of *C. pseudotuberculosis*.

> **DIFFERENTIAL DIAGNOSIS**
>
> Ringworm
> Staphylococcal pyoderma
> Nodular necrobiosis
>
> **Diagnostic confirmation**
>
> Isolation of *C. pseudotuberculosis* from lesions

TREATMENT

Affected animals should be rested until all lesions are healed. Frequent washing with a mild skin disinfectant solution followed by the application of antibacterial ointments to the lesions should facilitate healing and prevent the development of further lesions. Parenteral administration of antibiotics may be advisable in severe cases.

CONTROL

Infected horses should be rigidly isolated, and all grooming equipment, harnesses, and blankets must be disinfected. Grooming tools must be disinfected before each use. Vaccination is not likely to be effective because of the poor antigenicity of the organism.

EXUDATIVE EPIDERMITIS (GREASY PIG DISEASE)

ETIOLOGY

The condition of exudative dermatitis (marmite disease) is similar to staphylococcal scalded skin syndrome in humans associated with *S. aureus*. It is a skin condition of pigs of all ages. One human case of *S. hyicus* septicemia has been recorded.

S. hyicus is the cause of exudative epidermitis (EE) in suckling and weaned piglets. It also causes several other diseases sporadically in different animal species, bacteriuria in pigs, polyarthritis in pigs, abortion in pigs, flank biting and necrotic ear lesions, and pneumonia. It is a normal inhabitant of the skin of adults. Virulence is associated with toxins.[1,2]

In other species it has been associated with skin infections in horses, donkeys, and cattle; subclinical mastitis in cows; and osteomyelitis in heifers.

A second species, *Staphylococcus chromogenes*, is part of the normal skin flora of pigs, cattle, and poultry. It had been considered nonpathogenic until EE was associated with it in 2005. These strains produced exfoliative toxin type B (ExLB), which was identified by PCR. A third species, *Staphylococcus sciuri*, has also caused EE.[3]

> **SYNOPSIS**
>
> **Etiology** *Staphylococcus hyicus* of at least six serotypes and many phage types.
>
> **Epidemiology** Affects suckling and weanling piglets under 6 weeks of age; peak incidence under 1 week of age. Morbidity 20% to 100%; case fatality 50% to 75%. Organism carried by sow. Introduced by carriers.
>
> **Signs** Marked cutaneous erythema and pain, dehydration, extensive greasy exudate; peracute cases die; less severe cases may survive. May cause ear necrosis syndrome.
>
> **Clinical pathology** Bacterial culture of skin.
>
> **Necropsy findings** Exudative epidermitis; degenerative changes in kidney.
>
> **Diagnostic confirmation** Culture of organism.
>
> **Differential diagnosis** See Table 16-2.
>
> **Treatment** Penicillin parenterally.
>
> **Control** Sanitation and hygiene of pens. In outbreaks, isolate affected piglets and sows.

EPIDEMIOLOGY

Occurrence

The disease occurs in all pig-producing countries. Most cases of exudative epidermitis occur in suckling and weaned piglets under 6 weeks of age, with a peak incidence in piglets under 1 week. Occasionally groups of pigs up to 3 months of age may be affected. Within litters the incidence is high; often all piglets are affected. The morbidity will vary from 20% to 100% and the case fatality rate from 50% to 75%. The organism has been isolated from the joint fluid of lame pigs affected with arthritis.[3] In 28% and 26% of studies of cases of exudative epidermitis, no cases of toxigenic *S. hyicus* could be detected. In a recent study of 314 cases in Denmark, it was shown that 20% had exfoliatum toxin A, 33% had B, 18% had C, and 22% had D in 60% of cases of EE investigated.

Method of Transmission

The source of the organism is unknown, but the gilt or sow is probably an inapparent carrier. It can be isolated from the skin of healthy in-contact piglets and healthy sows. It can be frequently isolated from the vagina of prepubertal gilts, and the majority of the litters from the same gilts may be colonized by the organism within 24 hours after farrowing. The maternal strains of *S. hyicus* persisted on the skin of the offspring piglets for the first 3 weeks of the piglets' lives—the critical period for outbreaks of exudative epidermitis. The organism has also been isolated from the atmosphere of buildings housing affected pigs. Bacteriophage typing of *S. hyicus* subspp. hyicus isolated from pigs with or without exudative epidermitis revealed two or more phage patterns in the isolates from each pig with the disease and a single-phage pattern in isolates from healthy pigs. It may also spread by aerosol.

Risk Factors

Animal Risk Factors

Field evidence suggests that environmental stress of various kinds, including agalactia in the sow and intercurrent infection, predisposes to the disease. Lesions commonly develop first over the head, apparently in association with bite wounds, which occur when the needle teeth have not been cut or have been cut badly. Other factors include fighting following mixing of litters, excessive humidity over 70%, and following sarcoptic mange. The presence of the disease in a swine herd can account for a 35% reduction in the margin of output over feed and veterinary costs over a 2-month period. It may also occur as a result of floor injuries.

Pathogen Risk Factors

Strains of *S. hyicus* can be divided into virulent and avirulent strains with regard to ability to produce exudative epidermitis in experimental piglets; both types of strain can be isolated simultaneously from diseased piglets. It has been shown that different types of *S. hyicus* expressing different types of toxin may be present in the same diseased pig.

S. hyicus produces an exfoliative toxin that can be used to reproduce the disease. There are several toxins, including ExLA, ExLB, ExLC, ExLD, SHETa, and SHETb.[4] Toxigenic *S. hyicus* is isolated more freely from diseases than healthy pigs.[5] Strains of the organism isolated from a large number of Danish pig herds indicated different electrophoretic motility and plasma-mediated antibiotic resistance patterns. The antibiotic and plasmid profiles of strains isolated from pig herds may be a reflection of the use of antibiotics in those herds. Different types of toxin are produced.

Recently the genes encoding for the exfoliative toxins SHETb, ExLA, ExLB, ExLC, and ExLD have been identified and sequenced.

The condition has been seen more frequently in cases of PRRS and PCV-2 infections. It is very resistant to drying and can persist in the environment.

The organism has been found as a frequent inhabitant of the skin of cattle and has been isolated from cattle with skin lesions. Naturally occurring lesions of dermatitis of the lower limbs of horses and similar lesions over the neck and back of donkeys have been recorded. Experimentally, the organism can cause lesions in horses similar to those of exudative epidermitis. A concurrent infection with *D. congolensis* has also been reported.

PATHOGENESIS

S. hyicus has cytotoxic activity for porcine keratinocyte cells in culture, particularly the cells of the stratum granulosum. At least six toxins have been found. There is also a virulence factor that helps resist phagocytosis by binding IgG.[6] The organism also produces a coagulase, streptokinase lipase, and has a fibronectin-like substance that aids attachment to skin cells.

The exfoliative toxins are actually epidermolysins that are active against desmoglein-1, which is a desmosomal cadherin-like molecule involved in cell-to-cell adhesion. The ExLs can cause blister formation in the porcine skin by digesting porcine desmoglein-1 in a similar way to exfoliative toxins of *S. aureus*.

The earliest lesion is a subcorneal pustular dermatitis involving the interfollicular epidermis. Exfoliation follows with sebaceous exudation and formation of a crust. In the well-developed case there is a thick surface crust composed of orthokeratotic and parakeratotic hyperkeratosis and neutrophilic microabscesses with numerous colonies of gram-positive cocci.

Although the principal lesion is an inflammatory–exudative reaction in the corium and upper layers of the epidermis, the disease is probably a systemic rather than a local one. Experimental infection of gnotobiotic pigs leads to dermatitis of the snout and ears, then the medial aspect of the thighs, the abdominal wall, and the coronets. The lesions can be produced experimentally by using crude extracellular products and a partially purified exfoliative toxin.

CLINICAL FINDINGS

The morbidity varies from 10% to 100% and the mortality from 5% to 90%, with an average of 25%. It is usually self-limiting, and as immunity rises, it may well disappear.

In the peracute form, which occurs most commonly in piglets only a few days of age, there is a sudden onset of marked cutaneous erythema, with severe pain on palpation, evidenced by squealing. Anorexia, severe dehydration, and weakness are present, and death occurs in 24 to 48 hours. The entire skin coat appears wrinkled and reddened and is covered with a greasy, gray-brown exudate that accumulates in thick clumps around the eyes, behind the ears, and over the abdominal wall. In the less acute form, seen in older pigs 3 to 10 weeks of age, the greasy exudate becomes thickened and brown and peels off in scabs, leaving a deep-pink-colored to normal skin surface. There is no irritation or pruritus. In the subacute form, the exudate dries into brown scales that are most prominent on the face, around the eyes, and behind the ears. In a small percentage of pigs, the chronic form occurs and the course is much

Table 16-2 Differential diagnosis of diseases of swine with skin lesions

Disease	Epidemiology	Clinical and laboratory findings	Response to treatment
Swinepox	Mainly suckling piglets. High morbidity but low mortality except in very young piglets. Usually associated with swine louse infestation.	Papules, vesicles, and circular red-brown scabs on ventral belly wall and over the sides and back. Pox characteristics.	None required except for insect and louse control. Spontaneous recovery in 3 weeks.
Skin necrosis	Suckling piglets. High morbidity with abrasive flooring.	Abrasion and necrosis starting shortly after birth and reaching maximum severity at about 1 week. Anterior aspect of carpus more common site but also fetlock, hock, elbow, and coronet. Bilateral. Necrosis and erosion of anterior two or three pairs of teats.	Usually none required. Recovery in 3–5 weeks. Protect area with tape if severe, plus topical antiseptics. Teat necrosis will render animal unsuitable for selection and breeding. Correction of flooring.
Exudative epidermitis (greasy pig disease)	Entire litters of sucklings pigs, most severe under 1 week of age, occurs up to 10 weeks, high case fatality in younger pigs.	Marked cutaneous erythema with seborrhea, severe dehydration, and death in piglets under 10 days. Older piglets covered with greasy exudate and recover. *S. hyicus* on culture.	Piglets under 10 days of age die in spite of therapy. Older pigs may survive with penicillin treatment topically and parenterally.
Dermatosis vegetans	Inherited and congenital, high morbidity. High case fatality by 8 weeks.	Erythema and edema of coronets, uneven brittle hooves, dry brown crusts on belly wall, giant-cell pneumonia. Club foot.	None indicated. Genetic control.
Pityriasis rosea	One or more piglets in litter after weaning. High morbidity, nil mortality.	Lesions begin as small, red, flat plaques that enlarge from 1–2 cm diameter with a prominent ring of erythematous skin covered in center by thin, dry, brown, loose scales. Lesions usually coalesce, forming a mosaic pattern, especially on belly. Scraping negative. No growth depression.	None required. Emollient to soothe the lesion. Recovery occurs in 4–8 weeks.
Parakeratosis (zinc deficiency)	Weaners and feeder pigs on diet low in zinc and high in calcium. Herd problem, high morbidity, no mortality.	Erythematous areas on ventral abdomen and symmetrically over back and legs develop into thick crusts and fissures. No pruritus. Skin scrapings negative. Growth rate depression.	Add zinc to diet 100 ppm. Adjust calcium. Recovery in 2–6 weeks.
Ringworm	Feeder and mature pigs. Usually several pigs within pen or shed. High morbidity with *M. nanum* in sows.	Centrifugally progressing ring of inflammation surrounding an area with scabs, crusts, and brown or black exudate. May reach large size. Bristles usually intact. No pruritus. Positive skin scrapings and hair. No ground depression.	Fungicides. In growers, spontaneous recovery in 8–10 weeks if well nourished. *M. nanum* in sows is persistent and responds poorly.
Facial dermatitis	Suckling piglets. High incidence in litters associated with fighting. Low mortality.	Lesions on cheeks—usually bilateral abrasions which become infected. Scabs hard and brown and difficult to remove. Overlie a raw shallow bleeding ulcer. Occasional extension to other areas.	Usually none indicated. Topical antibacterials. Clip teeth at birth.
Ulcerative granuloma	Young pigs but all ages. Sporadic Infection following abrasion. Poor hygiene.	Large swollen tumorous mass with several discharging sinuses. Central slough and ulcer.	Fair, depending on site. Surgical removal and/or sulfadimidine and streptomycin.
Sarcoptic mange	All ages of pigs. Herd problem. Reservoir of infection in sows. High morbidity. Nil mortality.	Intense pruritus. Mites on scraping. Erythematous spots with scale and minor brown exudation. Especially evident in thin skin areas. Secondary trauma to skin and bristles from rubbing. If severe, intense erythema. Chronic infections, thickening and wrinkling of skin. Depression or weight gain.	Good response to vigorous therapy with ascaricides. Treat on herd basis.
Allergic dermatoses to *Tyroglyphus* spp. (harvest mites)	Weaner and feeder pigs few weeks after eating dry ground feed from autonomic feeders.	Pinpoint erythematous spots and fragile scales. Intense pruritus. Skin scraping positive for mites.	Spontaneous recovery common. Insecticide effective.
Erysipelas	Feeder and adult pigs, occasionally weaners. Variable morbidity. Low mortality if treated early.	Small red spots developing to characteristic rhomboidal lesion, raised and red in color. Lesions may become joined and lose their characteristic shape. Progress to necrosis and desquamation. Fever and other signs of septicemia.	Penicillin.

longer; there is thickening with wrinkling of the skin and thick scabs that crack along flexion lines, forming deep fissures. Most peracute cases die, whereas piglets with the less severe forms will survive if treated. Some pigs are affected with ulcerative glossitis and stomatitis.

In older pigs lesions may be very limited. Sometimes just the ears are affected. Abortion in a sow has been attributed to the organism. In some cases pigs are dehydrated and emaciated. Surface lymph nodes may be enlarged or edematous. The condition is much more common when there are the immunosuppressive disorders (Porcine reproductive and respiratory syndrome virus, Porcine circovirus 2, Swine Influenza Virus).

CLINICAL PATHOLOGY

Bacterial examination of skin swabs may reveal the presence of S. hyicus. A phage typing system can be used to determine the presence of virulent strains and to distinguish them from less virulent strains.

NECROPSY FINDINGS

Necropsy of these dehydrated, unthrifty piglets often reveals a white precipitate in the renal papillae and pelvis. Occasionally this cellular debris causes ureteral blockage. Some piglets also have a mild ulcerative glossitis and stomatitis. Microscopically, there is separation of the cells of the epidermis in the upper stratum spinosum, exfoliation of the skin, erythema, and serous exudation. The crusting dermatitis features a superficial folliculitis and a hyperkeratotic perivascular dermatitis with intracorneal pustules and prominent bacterial colonies. Degenerative changes are visible in the renal tubular epithelium.

DIAGNOSIS

Diagnosis is usually made on the basis of clinical signs and lesions.

Samples for confirmation of diagnosis include the following:

- Bacteriology—samples of acute skin lesions for culture are best if the skin underneath the crusts is sampled or the local lymph nodes. The organism forms 3- to 4-mm white, nonhemolytic colonies on blood agar. It is catalase- and mannitol-negative but hyaluronidase-positive. Selective media can be used (potassium thiocyanate),
- Histology—formalin-fixed skin (multiple sites), kidney (LM)
- A PCR is available but requires a pure culture and large numbers of organisms to be successful. An ELISA has been developed for the toxins.[7]

DIFFERENTIAL DIAGNOSIS

Exudative epidermitis may resemble several skin diseases of pigs of all age groups (Table 16-2). However, in exudative epidermitis there is no pruritus or fever. In mange there is pruritus, and the lesions can be scraped. Ringworm can be cultured or skin scrapings made for microscopy. Pityriasis rosea is erythematous and self-limiting. Zinc deficiency in 2- to 4-month-old pigs is particularly found in Landrace, and the lesions are dry. Swinepox is usually local and rarely fatal. Careful gross examination of the lesions, particularly their distribution, the state of the hair shaft, the character of the exudate, and the presence or absence of pruritus, must be considered, along with skin scrapings and biopsies.

TREATMENT

In severely affected animals, injection is best followed by water and feed medication. Experimentally infected piglets respond favorably to a topical application of cloxacillin 10,000 IU/g of lanolin base and 1% hydrocortisone combined with parenteral cloxacillin. Treatment must be administered as soon as the lesions are visible. Procaine penicillin G at a dose of 20,000 IU/kg BW intramuscularly daily for 3 days is also recommended. The antimicrobial sensitivities determined in one field investigation revealed that all isolates were sensitive to novobiocin, neomycin, and cloxacillin. Novobiocin may be the antimicrobial of choice because *staphylococci* are universally sensitive to this antibiotic. However, there is no available information on the efficacy of antimicrobials for naturally occurring cases of exudative epidermitis. A study has suggested that lincomycin, amoxicillin, and cetaloxin (off-label use) seem to work well in the United Kingdom. Erythromycin, sulfathiazole, and trimethoprim may be the most useful drugs, whereas penicillin and tetracyclines may not be very useful. Resistance to penicillin, erythromycin, streptomycin, sulphonamides, and tetracycline is fairly common. There is, however, no correlation between genes and resistance patterns.[2] Naturally occurring cases in piglets under 10 days of age respond poorly, whereas older pigs recover with a skin wash using a suitable disinfectant soap. The most successful treatment is antibiotics and skin washing for a period of at least 5 to 7 days. It is also essential to make sure that there is sufficient dietary provision of zinc, biotin, fat, selenium, and vitamin E in the diet. Because there is dehydration, electrolyte therapy may help.

CONTROL

Improved hygiene, lower humidity, and dimmed lighting all help, as will control of concurrent infectious disease. Teeth clipping also reduces skin damage. Soft bedding also reduces skin damage (e.g., chopped straw is better than straw).

The infected accommodation should be cleaned, disinfected, and left vacant before another farrowing sow is placed in the pen. Strict isolation of the affected piglets and their dam is necessary to prevent spread throughout the herd. Dead piglets should be removed promptly from the premises, and in-contact sows should be washed with a suitable disinfectant soap. Maternal antibodies will protect piglets in the first few weeks of life. Prophylactic medication in feed or water has also helped.

Autogenous vaccines have been used, with varying degrees of success. It is important to use a strain that produces the exfoliative toxin, so the recent development of PCRs that identify the genes for toxin development will ensure that the right isolate is used for the autogenous vaccine. It will also facilitate the development of a commercial vaccine.

A novel approach to the control is bacterial interference. Experimentally, the precolonization of the skin of gnotobiotic piglets with an avirulent strain of *S. hyicus* will prevent the experimental reproduction of the disease with the virulent strain of the organism.

REFERENCES

1. Futagawa-Saito F, et al. *Vet Microbiol.* 2007;124:370.
2. Futagawa-Saito F, et al. *J Vet Med Sci.* 2009;71:681.
3. Chen S, et al. *PLoS ONE.* 2007;2:e147.
4. Nishifuji K, et al. *J Derm Sci.* 2008;49:21.
5. Kanbar T, et al. *J Vet Sci.* 2008;9:327.
6. Rosander A, et al. *Vet Microbiol.* 2011;149:273.
7. Voytenko AV, et al. *Vet Microbiol.* 2006;116:211.

ULCERATIVE DERMATITIS (GRANULOMATOUS DERMATITIS) OF PIGS

Ulcerative granuloma is an infectious disease of pigs originally associated with the spirochete *Borrelia suilla* (formerly *B. suis*) and more recently *T. pedis*.[1] In some cases it has become more common where there is PCV2 infection. It is characterized by the development of chronic ulcers of the skin and subcutaneous tissues. It can be confused with necrotic ear syndrome and, more importantly, with swine vesicular disease when there are granulating lesions at the coronary groove.

For sows, it occurs most commonly under conditions of poor hygiene. Lesions occur on the central abdomen of sows and on the mammary glands. The lesions expand, often to 20 to 30 cm in diameter, on the belly of the sow. They are usually single or in small numbers. In adult animals there is considerable inconvenience if the lesions are permitted to develop. Necrotic ulcers on the udders of sows may continue to develop and extend deeper into areas with fistulae, and sloughing may result.

The faces of sucking piglets are affected, suggesting infection of cutaneous or mucosal abrasions as the portal of entry. In some instances, these outbreaks have followed episodes of severe fighting. Initially the lesions are small, hard, fibrous swellings that ulcerate in 2 to 3 weeks to form a persistent ulcer with raised edges and a center of excessive granulation tissue covered with sticky, gray pus. All you may see is a grayish, crusty, weeping lesion that may spread. There is often coinfection with *S. hyicus* or beta-hemolytic streptococci, and the lesions may be contaminated by *Trueperella* (*Arcanobacterium*) *pyogenes*. The lesions commence about the lips and erode the cheeks, and sometimes the jawbone, and often cause shedding of the teeth.

In young pigs, usually at 5 to 7 weeks of age, the whole litter may be affected. Here the lower margin of both ears close to the junction with the neck, with extensive tissue destruction and sloughing, is affected. The major diagnostic problem is that the initial spirochetal lesions may be secondarily infected with environmental organisms such as *Fusobacterium* spp. or *T. pyogenes*, and the underlying spirochetes may be missed unless smears are viewed. The pathology usually involves edema, erythema, necrosis, ulceration, and purulent lesions. In young pigs there may be heavy losses as a result of severe damage to the face.

Differential diagnosis may include abscesses, foreign bodies, granulomas, and pressure necrosis. In growing pigs, the lesions need to be differentiated from necrotic lesions resulting from snout rubbing and ear biting, and those resulting from excessive self-trauma with mange infestation. It may be mistaken for lesions of *Actinomycosis* and *Nocardia* in sows, and swabs should be taken from the ulcers for bacteriologic examination. A fresh smear of the exudates usually shows the spirochetes, and if necessary they can be stained by silver stains or viewed in histologic sections. A course of potassium iodide given orally (1 g/35 kg up to 3 g) or a 5-day period of injections of penicillin are the methods of treatment. Topical tetracycline spray has been used effectively with early lesions followed by tetracycline injection in the deeper-seated and more chronic cases. Dusting with sulphanilamide, arsenic trioxide, or tartar emetic has also been recommended. Removal of large granulomas surgically has also been tried. Fly repellents should be used to prevent flystrike.

The injection of 0.2 mL of a 5% solution of sodium arsenite into the substance of the lesion is reported to give good results. Improvement in hygiene, particularly at the times of routine treatments, and disinfection of skin wounds should reduce the incidence in affected piggeries.

REFERENCE

1. Pringle M, Fellstrom C. *Vet Microbiol*. 2010;142:461.

Viral Diseases of the Skin

PAPILLOMAVIRUS INFECTION (PAPILLOMATOSIS, WARTS)

SYNOPSIS

Etiology Papillomaviruses (PVs), including bovine papillomaviruses 1 through 13, equine papillomaviruses 1 through 7, and various other host-specific papillomaviruses.

Epidemiology Occur in all countries in all species but most common in young cattle and horses. Transmission is by direct contact and fomites. Risk factors for PV-associated diseases include ingestion of bracken fern (enzootic hematuria, alimentary squamous-cell carcinoma in cattle) and increasing age (penile squamous-cell carcinoma in equids).

Clinical findings Solid outgrowths of epidermis, may be sessile or pedunculated. Most common type in cattle occurs on head and neck and has cauliflower-like appearance, but lesion site and appearance vary with papilloma type. Alimentary (squamous epithelium) warts and squamous-cell carcinoma in cattle. Enzootic hematuria (bladder carcinoma) in cattle. In the horse, lesions are on the face and lips. Penile and prepucial papillomatosis and squamous-cell carcinoma in horses. Aural plaques in horses. Sarcoids in horses.

Clinical pathology None specific.

Lesions Papilloma or fibropapilloma.

Diagnostic confirmation Histology and DNA identification by polymerase chain reaction (PCR) in biopsy or tissue scraping.

Treatment Removal by surgery or cryosurgery. Vaccination with autogenous vaccine. Application of imiquimod 5% cream to aural plaques.

Papillomaviruses appear to infect all groups of amniotes, having been isolated from 54 species, including mammals, birds, and reptiles.[1] Study of this group of viruses is historically important in the context of demonstration of the possibility of a viral etiology for some neoplastic diseases.[2] Diseases associated with infection by papillomaviruses range from nonneoplastic lesions on epithelial surfaces (skin, urogenital tract, gastrointestinal tract) through to neoplasms, including in humans (human papillomavirus and cervical cancer).[3] Cutaneous warts in cattle, horses, sheep, and goats are benign tumors induced by host-specific papillomaviruses. These infect epithelial cells, causing hyperproliferative lesions that are benign and self-limiting and that, in most cases, spontaneously regress. The virus is also associated with neoplastic diseases, including bladder cancer in cattle ingesting bracken fern, carcinoma of the upper alimentary tract of cattle (usually associated with ingestion of bracken fern), and squamous-cell carcinoma of the penis and prepuce in horses. Papillomaviruses are usually quite host specific, with the exception of some bovine papillomaviruses, and require close contact for spread of infection.

ETIOLOGY

Papillomaviruses (PVs) are members of the Papillomaviridae family, which have a characteristic circular double-stranded DNA genome of around eight kilobase pairs (kbp) that usually contains at least six relatively conserved open reading frames (ORFs) in an early (E1, E2, E6, E7) and a late (L1, L2) region.[4] Papillomaviruses are characterized genetically by the L1 ORF.[4] To date, at least 112 nonhuman papillomaviruses have been identified, and there is the anticipation that more will be detected.[1] It appears that each species carries a suite of papillomaviruses—for example, 13 bovine papillomavirus (BPV) types have been identified in cattle (BPV-1 through BVP-13), 15 canine papillomavirus (CPV) types in dogs (CPV-1 through CPV-15), and 7 equine caballus papillomavirus (EcPV) types in horses (EcPV-1 through EcPV-7). The feline sarcoid-associated virus has been proposed as BPV-14; it can infect cattle but has not been demonstrated in horses.[5]

Unusually, horses are also infected by BPV-1 and/or BPV-2, and possibly BPV-13,[6] which are associated with development of sarcoids (see "Sarcoids" for further discussion).[7] Papillomaviruses have been isolated from camels, goats, deer, sheep, and pigs, usually from papillomas or similar epithelial lesions.[1] BPV-1 and BPV-2 are associated with papillomas in yaks and sarcoids in zebra, giraffes, and sable antelope.[8-10] New papillomaviruses continue to be identified.[11]

Cattle types show some site predilection or site specificity, as exemplified by the following partial listing:

- **BPV-1**—frond fibropapillomas of teat and skin and penile fibropapilloma
- **BPV-1 and BPV-2**—fibropapilloma of the skin of the anteroventral part of the body, including the forehead, neck, and back;[12] the common cutaneous wart
- **BPV-2**—cauliflower-like fibropapillomas of the anogenital and ventral abdominal skin
- **BPV-2**—associated with bladder cancer in cattle in association with the ingestion of bracken fern (*Pteridium* spp.) (see "Enzootic Hematuria")[13]
- **BPV-3**—cutaneous papilloma
- **BPV-4**—papilloma of the esophagus, esophageal groove, forestomaches, and small intestine; capable of becoming malignant, particularly in animals fed bracken fern; has site specificity to the upper alimentary tract

- **BPV-5,** and to a lesser extent BPV-1 and BVP-2, in fibropapilloma/papilloma of the mouth, esophagus, rumen, and reticulum of cattle and water buffalo[14]
- **BPV-5**—rice grain fibropapilloma on the udder; has also been demonstrated in cutaneous skin warts
- **BPV-6**—frond epithelial papillomas of the bovine udder and teats
- **BPV-7, BPV-9, and BPV-10**—lesions of the teats and udder[15,16]
- **BPV-10**—lingual papilloma[17]
- **BPV-12**—associated with papillomas[18]

Although a single BPV type is detected in an individual papilloma, a single animal can have papillomas at different sites associated with different BPV types.

Other papilloma of cattle that have regional distribution and may have separate antigenic identity are as follows:

- Oral papillomas, mostly in adult cattle and apparently reaching a high incidence, up to 16% in some areas; these are probably BPV-4
- Papilloma of the larynx in steers
- Papillomavirus has been observed in squamous-cell carcinoma of bovine eyes, although its etiologic role is unclear.

Other skin lesions in which papillomavirus plays an etiologic role are:

- Equine sarcoid, which is associated with BPV-1 and BPV-2, and possibly BPV-13 (see "Sarcoid," in this chapter)
- Squamous-cell carcinoma of sheep (likely OaPV-3, although this can be isolated from the skin of healthy sheep)[19]
- Epithelial tumors in goats (although the causal relationship is not clear)[20]
- Cauliflower-like tumor of the external nares in a chamois[21]

Equids

Papillomas, aural plaques, and squamous-cell carcinoma in horses are associated with infection by one of the seven equine papillomaviruses.[1] Cutaneous papilloma, including of the penis, and aural or genital plaques are associated with infection by EcPV-1 through EcPV-6.[1] EcPV-7 was isolated from a penile mass that was not histologically classified.[4] Penile papillomas are associated with infection by EcPV-2.[22] EcPV-2 DNA was detected in abnormal tissue in 15 of 16 cases of penile squamous-cell carcinoma, 8 of 8 cases of penile intraepithelial neoplasia, 4 of 4 cases of penile papilloma, and 1 of 2 lymph nodes containing metastatic tumor cells. EcPV-2 DNA was detected in 4 of 39 of penile swabs of healthy horses and in 0 of 20 vulvovaginal swabs.[23] Coinfection by more than one EcPV appears to be common.[4] Infection by equine papillomavirus EcPV-2, as demonstrated by detection of EcPV-2 DNA in lesions,[24] is associated with squamous-cell carcinoma of the genitalia of horses,[25] being transcriptionally active in tumor but not semen or swabs of healthy horses,[26] and detected in 91 of 103 tissue samples of horses with penile or preputial carcinoma and in 1 of 12 samples from horses free of the disease.[27] There is no evidence to date that EcPV-3 is associated with carcinoma of the penis or prepuce. Papillomavirus DNA is not detected in periocular squamous-cell carcinoma of horses.[28]

Sarcoids in equids are discussed under that topic.

Pigs

Papillomavirus specific to pigs has been isolated from skin of healthy pigs, but has not been associated with disease.[29]

EPIDEMIOLOGY

Occurrence

Papillomatosis has an international occurrence in all animal species, and sarcoids and urogenital tumors occur in almost all populations of horses. There are few studies of the seroprevalence of papillomaviruses in healthy animals. Five of 50 horses without evidence of skin disease or urogenital tumors in Switzerland had EcPV-2-specific DNA amplified but not EcPV-2-specific antibodies detected, 14 of 50 horses had antibodies against EcPV2 but no DNA detected, and both antibodies and viral DNA were detected in 4 of 50 horses. Neither specific antibodies nor viral DNA were found in 27 of 50 horses (54%).[30]

BPV-1 or BPV-2 infection is common in horses and cattle, being detectable by PCR and/or reverse transcription PCR (RT-PCR) in 14 of 70 blood samples (20%) and in 11 of 31 semen samples (35%) from healthy horses,[31] and in 8/12 blood samples of healthy cattle and in 8/9 samples from cattle with papillomatosis. Six of 8 papilloma-free cattle that were positive for BPV also had evidence of expression of BPV in blood.[32]

Papillomaviruses were detected in 28/45 of samples of horses with aural plaques, of which 4/45 were solely EcPV-3 and 17/45 were solely EcPV-4, with 7/45 being coinfected. Viral DNA was not detected in 17/45 of samples. Neither EcPV-3 nor EcPV-4 was detected in samples from 10 horses that did not have aural skin lesions.[33] Similar results demonstrating presence of papillomavirus antigen or EcPV DNA in papillomas, aural plaques, and sarcoids supports the etiologic associated between the virus and these diseases.[34]

Origin of Infection and Transmission

The method of spread is by **direct contact** with infected animals, with infection gaining entry through **cutaneous abrasions**. Viruses can also persist on inanimate objects in livestock buildings and infect animals rubbing against them. BPV-1 DNA is present in flies (*Musca domestica*, *Fannia carnicularis*, and *Stomoxys calcitrans*) trapped in stables of donkeys with sarcoids, suggesting the possibility that flies, and especially biting flies (*S. calcitrans*), are potential vectors.[35] The presence of BPV-1 and BPV-2 in blood of both horses and cattle raises the possibility of spread by biting flies independent of them feeding on actual lesions.

The means of transmission of the virus causing penile and preputial papillomas and squamous-cell carcinoma is unclear. Venereal transmission is possible, but lesions occur in animals that are not and have not been sexually active (e.g., geldings).

Crops of warts sometimes occur around eartags, at branding sites, or along scratches made by barbed wire, and they can be spread by tattooing implements, by dehorning shears, and by procedures such as tuberculin testing.

An extensive outbreak of perianal warts is recorded in beef heifers, the infection having been spread by rectal examination for pregnancy. A high prevalence of papillomas on the larynx of feedlot steers is ascribed to implantation of the virus in contact ulcers, which are also entry sites for *Fusobacterium nodosus* (a cause of calf diphtheria), so that the two diseases may occur in the one animal. An outbreak of periorbital papillomatosis in cattle is recorded in association with a heavy periorbital infestation with *Haematopinus quadripertusus.*

Animal Risk Factors

All species may be affected by papillomas or fibropapilloma, but it is most commonly reported in cattle and horses. With cattle, usually several animals in an age group are affected. Alimentary papillomas occur in up to 20% of cattle ingesting bracken fern, but in less than 4% of other cattle.[3]

Outbreaks have been recorded in sheep and goats, but the disease is uncommon in sheep. It is also uncommon in pigs, usually affecting the genitalia.

Papillomavirus infection is widespread in nondomestic species, including birds and reptiles, and is associated with disease in many of these species (see previous discussion).[1]

Age

Cutaneous papillomas of the head and neck occur predominantly in young animals, the lack of susceptibility of adults to natural infection being ascribed to immunity acquired by apparent or inapparent infection when young. The occurrence of cutaneous warts and their severity can be influenced by factors that induce immunosuppression, and latent infection has converted to clinical disease with the administration of immunosuppressive agents. Congenital infection is recorded in the foal and calf, but it is rare.

Alimentary papillomas in cattle, teat papillomas in cattle, and papillomas on the mammary glands of goats occur, or persist, at all production ages.

Squamous-cell carcinoma of the penis or prepuce occurs mostly in older horses (mean age 20 y) and without apparent breed predilection.[36]

Experimental Production

The supernatant from a suspension of wart tissue, injected intradermally (ID) or applied to skin scarifications, is an effective means of experimental production of the disease. Lesions are restricted to the site of inoculation. Cutaneous and oral papillomas have been transmitted in cattle, and cutaneous papillomas have been transmitted in sheep and horses. The incubation period after experimental inoculation in cattle is 3 to 8 weeks but is usually somewhat longer after natural exposure.

Economic Importance

Cutaneous warts are quite common in young cattle, especially when they are housed, but ordinarily they cause little harm and regress spontaneously. In purebred animals they may interfere with sales and shows because of their unsightly appearance. Animals with extensive lesions may lose condition, and secondary bacterial invasion of traumatized warts can occur. Warts on the teats of dairy cows often cause interference with milking. In horses, the lesions are usually small and cause little inconvenience, but they are esthetically unattractive.

Urogenital lesions in equids, predominantly penile and preputial papillomas, can progress to squamous-cell carcinoma, which carries a poor prognosis unless treated early in the disease.[36]

PATHOGENESIS

The virus infects the basal keratinocytes, replicating its genome in the differentiating spinous and granular layers and causing the excessive growth that is characteristic of wart formation.[2] Expression of the late structural proteins of the virus is limited to the differentiated cells of the squamous layer where the new virus particles are encapsulated and shed into the environment as the cells die. The tumor contains epithelial and connective tissues and can be a papilloma or a fibropapilloma, depending on the relative proportions of epithelial and connective tissue present; papillomas contain little connective tissue, and fibropapillomas are mostly fibrous tissue, with very little epithelial tissue. Papillomas are the result of basal-cell hyperplasia without viral antigen production. Fibropapillomas are uncommon in horses but are the common lesion in cattle, sheep, and wild ruminants. Latent infection in the skin and lymphocytes has been demonstrated in cattle.

CLINICAL FINDINGS

Warts are solid outgrowths of epidermis that are sessile or pedunculated. Other papillomavirus-associated diseases include penile or prepucial lesions in horses, alimentary lesions in ruminants, enzootic hematuria in cattle ingesting bracken fern, and squamous-cell carcinoma of the urogenital or alimentary tracts.

Cattle

In cattle, warts occur on almost any part of the body, but when numerous animals in a group are affected it is common to find them all affected in the same part of the body. The most common papillomas occur in the skin of cattle under 2 years of age, most commonly on the head (Fig. 16-2), especially around the eyes, and on the neck and shoulders (Fig. 16-3), but they may spread to other parts of the body. They vary in size from 1 cm upward, and a dry, horny, cauliflower-like appearance is characteristic. In most animals they regress spontaneously, but the warts may persist for 5 to 6 months, and in some cases for as long as 36 months, with serious loss of body condition.

Warts on the **teats** manifest with different forms depending on the papillomavirus type and may show an increasing frequency with age. The **frond forms** have filiform projections on them and appear to have been drawn out into an elongated shape of about 1 cm in length by milking machine action. If sharp traction is used, they can often be pulled out by the roots.

The second form is the flat, round type, which is usually multiple, always sessile, and up to 2 cm in diameter. The third form has an elongated structure appearing like a **rice grain**. Teat warts may regress during the dry period and recur with the next lactation.

Perianal warts are esthetically unattractive, but they do not appear to reduce activity or productivity. **Genital warts** on the vulva and penis make mating impracticable because the lesions are of large size, are friable, and bleed easily. They commonly become infected and flyblown. They occur on the shaft or on the glans of the penis in young bulls, may be single or multiple, are pedunculated, and frequently regress spontaneously.

Alimentary tract papillomas can occur anywhere from the mouth to the rumen. They often appear as lines of warts, suggesting a predisposing effect of trauma as a result of ingestion of roughage. Papillomas occur on the lateral and dorsal aspects of the tongue, soft palate, oropharynx, esophagus, esophageal groove, and rumen. Papillomas occurring in the esophageal groove and in the reticulum are a cause of chronic ruminal tympany. Papillomas also can progress to squamous-cell carcinoma in cattle, with an inevitable fatal outcome.[3]

Less common manifestations of papillomatosis in cattle include lesions in the **urinary bladder**, which cause no clinical signs but may predispose to enzootic hematuria. BPV-4 papillomas in the upper alimentary tract of cattle being fed bracken fern are the focus for transformation to squamous-cell carcinomas. Cattle fed bracken fern are immunosuppressed, which promotes the persistence and spread of the papillomavirus, and mutagens in bracken fern cause neoplastic transformation of papilloma cells.

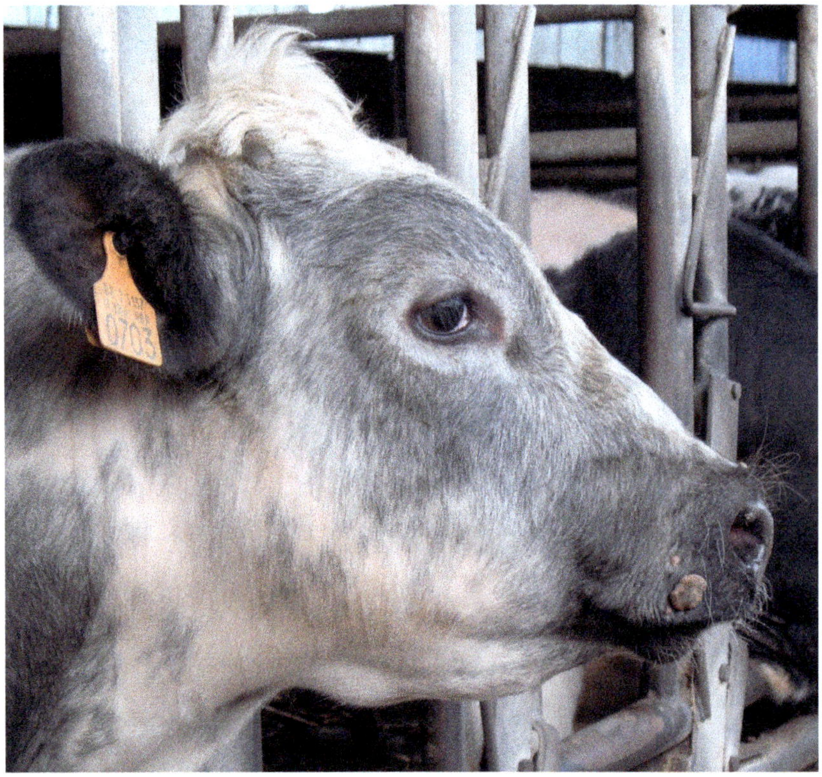

Fig. 16-2 Warts on the face of a yearling Belgian Blue bull.

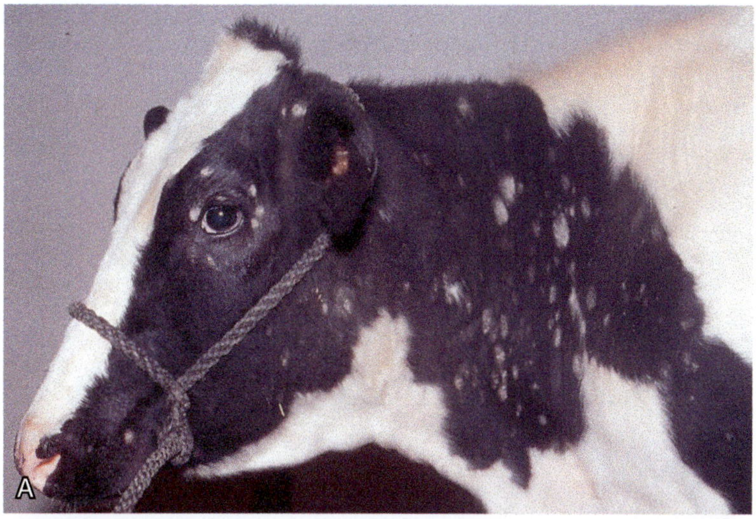

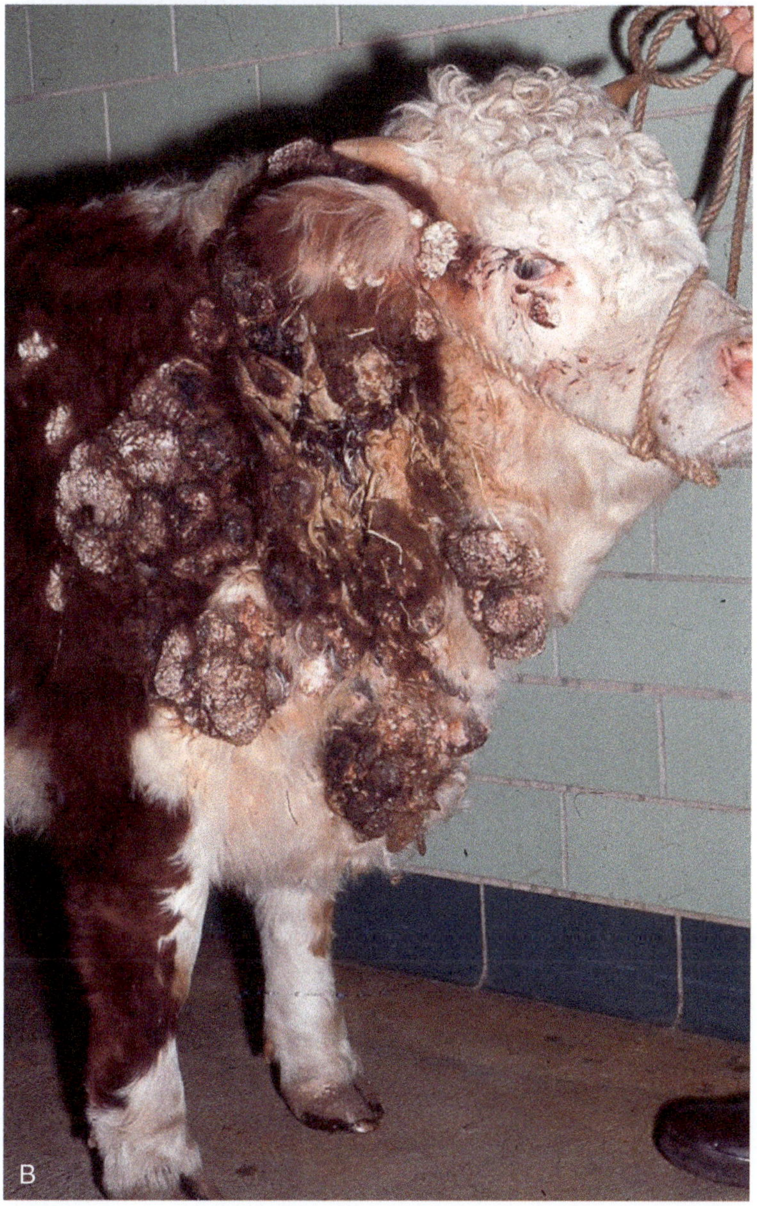

Fig. 16-3 **A, Warts (papillomas) on the neck and shoulders of a Holstein–Friesian heifer. B, Extensive warts (papillomas) on the face, neck, and shoulder of a yearling Hereford bull.**

Goats

Papillomas most commonly occur on the face and ears but may occur on the skin generally, especially on unpigmented skin. Most completely regress, others regress and recur, and occasional lesions progress to carcinomas. Papillomas that occur on the teats are persistent and may spread through the herd.

Horses

Warts are confined to the lower face, the muzzle, nose, and lips, and are usually sessile and quite small, rarely exceeding 1 cm in diameter. Papillomas also occur on the penis and prepuce of both geldings and stallions,[36] and much less commonly on the vulva. All ages can be affected. Spontaneous recovery of papillomas on the head is usual, but the warts may persist for 5 to 6 months.

Aural plaques in horses are well-delineated lesions that affect the concave aspect of the pinna with a flat surface of whitish keratinous crust covering a shiny and erythematous skin surface. Lesions are single or multiple and coalescing and, in some cases, can cover almost the entire surface of one or both pinnae (Fig. 16-4).[37] The lesions are usually not pruritic, but some horses with aural plaques resist bridling or handling of the ears. A common concern is cosmetic in show horses.

Squamous-cell carcinoma of the penis and prepuce is usually evident as ulcerations or mass lesions and can be complicated

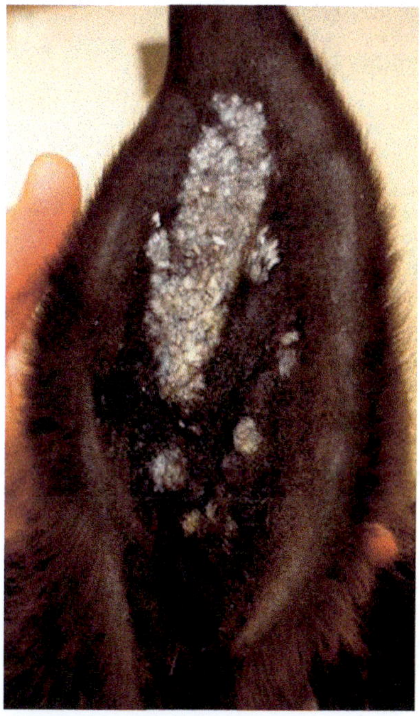

Fig. 16-4 **Coalescing plaques covered with a keratinous crust occupying most of the concave aspect of the horse's left ear, as viewed from the front.** (Reproduced from Torres SMF et al. *Vet Dermatol* 2010; 21:503.)

by secondary bacterial infection.[36] Approximately 40% of affected horses have purulent or blood-stained preputial discharge. Preputial edema or the inability to prolapse the penis occurs in approximately 10% of horses.[36] Lesions are most commonly (~80%) located on the glans of the penis and can have papillomas neighboring the neoplastic tumor. Metastasis to inguinal lymph nodes is common as the disease progresses and is more likely in horses with poorly differentiated tumor.[27] Intrathoracic (lung) metastases are rare. Survival is related to the degree of differentiation of the tumor (log rank $P < 0.001$), with a greater proportion of horses with less differentiated tumors dying of the disease (papilloma, 8.3%; G1, 26.1%; G2, 26.3%; G3, 63.3%; where G1 = well differentiated, G2 = moderately differentiated, and G3 = poorly differentiated) (Fig. 16-5).[27]

CLINICAL PATHOLOGY

There are no specific changes in the hemogram or blood chemistry of affected cattle. As noted previously, papillomavirus can be detected in blood and semen of healthy and affected animals, varying with the species of animal and papillomavirus.

Biopsy of a lesion can be used to differentiate papillomas from squamous-cell carcinoma. Biopsy of classic "warts" is unnecessary. However, it may be advisable when large growths are found on horses to determine whether the lesion is a verrucose form of sarcoid. Microscopically, true papillomas consist of a hyperplastic epidermis with scant dermal tissue, whereas in fibropapillomas the dermal component tends to predominate. The need to identify the specific virus in a crop of warts creates a requirement for serologic and histologic examinations.

Detection of viral DNA is achieved by RT-PCR or PCR, and serologic tests are available to determine exposure to some papillomaviruses.[16,18,27,38-40] As with all PCR assays, care must be taken to ensure that the appropriate primers are used.[40]

> **DIFFERENTIAL DIAGNOSIS**
>
> Clinically, there is little difficulty in making a diagnosis of dermal papillomatosis, with the possible exception of atypical papillomas of cattle, probably associated with an unidentified type of the papillomavirus. These lesions are characterized by an absence of dermal fibroplasia and are true papillomas rather than fibropapillomas. All ages of animals can be affected, and the lesions persist for long periods. They are characteristically discrete, low, flat, and circular, and they often coalesce to form large masses. They do not protrude like regular warts, and the external fronds are much finer and more delicate.
>
> **Horses:**
>
> Sarcoid
>
> Melanoma

TREATMENT

Warts can be removed by surgery or cryosurgery. Crushing of a proportion of small warts, or the surgical removal of a few warts, has been advocated as a method of hastening regression, but the tendency for spontaneous recovery makes assessment of the results of these treatments very difficult. Partial resection of a wart(s) in a horse does not always promote resolution of the residue. Surgical removal can be followed by vaccination with an autogenous vaccine, although the efficacy of this approach is unclear. There is anecdotal concern that surgical intervention, and even vaccination, in the early stages of wart development may increase the size of residual warts and prolong the course of the disease.

Aural plaques in horses can be treated by application of imiquimod, an immunomodulator, and antiviral agents, as 5% cream applied three times a week, every other week, for 6 weeks to 8 months. Crusts were removed before each application of the cream and required sedation in most horses. Complete resolution of lesions was noted in all horses at the cessation of treatment, and the long-term resolution rate was 88%.[37] Imiquimod is used for treatment of penile papillomas and squamous-cell carcinoma in humans, but its use in horses for this purpose is not reported. Imiquimod is used for treatment of sarcoids in horses.[41]

Vaccination

For cattle, autogenous vaccines prepared from wart tissues of the affected animal are effective in many cases. Commercially available vaccines are available for cattle but may be less efficacious; an autogenous vaccine prepared for a specific problem has the advantage of including the local virus types. The vaccine is prepared from homogenized wart tissue that is filtered and inactivated with formalin. Because of the different BPV types, care is required in the selection of the tissues. In general terms they can be selected based on tumor type, location, and histologic composition. The alternative is to use many types of tissue in the vaccine. Animal-to-animal variation in regression following vaccination of a group of calves with a vaccine prepared from a single calf in the group has been attributed to more than one BPV type producing disease in the group. The stage of development is also important, and the virus is present in much greater concentration in the epithelial tissue of older warts than young ones. The vaccine can be administered subcutaneously, but better results are claimed for ID injection. Dosing regimens vary, but 2 to 4 injections 1 to 2 weeks apart are commonly recommended. Recovery in 3 to 6 weeks is recorded in 80% to 85% of cases where the warts are on the body surface or penis of cattle, but in only 33% when the warts are on the teats. The response of low, flat, sessile warts to vaccination is poor. Development of DNA vaccines for prophylaxis or therapy (which will likely use different genes) is active but experimental at this time.[42]

Other treatments no longer commonly used include the injection into the wart of

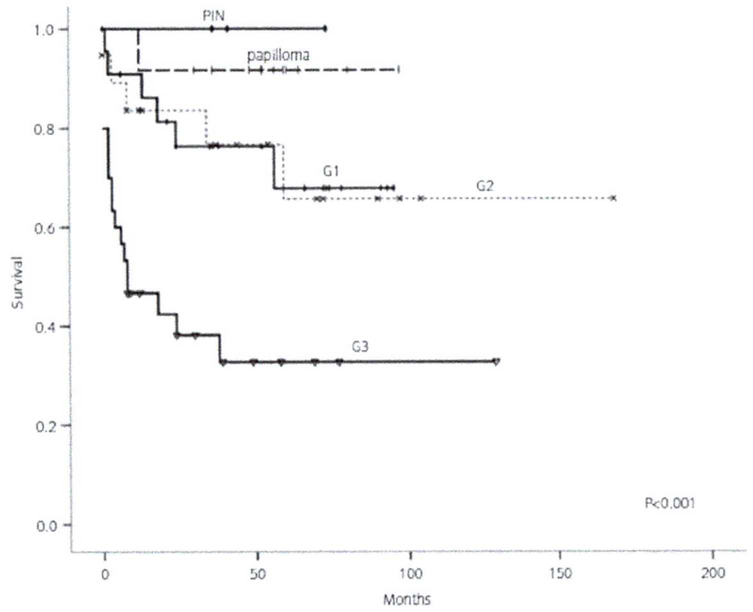

Fig. 16-5 Survival of horses with penile or preputial papilloma, or squamous-cell carcinoma (G1, well differentiated; G2, moderately differentiated; and G3, poorly differentiated. PIN, penile intraepithelial neoplasia). (Reproduced from van den Top JGB et al. *Equine Vet J* 2015; 47:188.)

proprietary preparations containing antimony and bismuth or the intralesional injection of bacille Calmette–Guérin (BCG).

CONTROL

Specific control procedures are usually not instituted or warranted because of the unpredictable nature of the disease and its minor economic importance.

Vaccination has been shown experimentally to be an effective prevention method and gives complete protection in cattle against stiff experimental challenge. The vaccine must contain all serotypes of the papillomavirus because they are very type-specific.

Avoidance of close contact between infected and uninfected animals should be encouraged, and the use of communal equipment between affected and unaffected animals should be avoided.

FURTHER READING

Munday JS. Bovine and human papillomaviruses: a comparative review. *Vet Pathol*. 2014;51:1063-1075.

Rector A, van Ranst M. Animal papillomaviruses. *Virology*. 2013;445:213-223.

REFERENCES

1. Rector A, et al. *Virol*. 2013;445:213.
2. Cheville NF. *Vet Pathol*. 2014;51:1049.
3. Munday JS. *Vet Pathol*. 2014;51:1063.
4. Lange CE, et al. *J Gen Virol*. 2013;94:1365.
5. Munday JS, et al. *Vet Microbiol*. 2015;177:289.
6. Lunardi M, et al. *J Clin Micro*. 2013;51:2167.
7. Nasir L, et al. *Vet Microbiol*. 2013;167:159.
8. Bam J, et al. *Transbound Emerg Dis*. 2013;60:475.
9. van Dyk E, et al. *J S Afr Vet Assoc*. 2011;82:80.
10. Williams JH, et al. *J S Afr Vet Assoc*. 2011;82:97.
11. Melo TC, et al. *Gen Mol Res*. 2014;13:2458.
12. Pangty K, et al. *Transbound Emerg Dis*. 2010;57:185.
13. Cota JB, et al. *Vet Microbiol*. 2015;178:138.
14. Kumar P, et al. *Transbound Emerg Dis*. 2015;62:264.
15. Hatama S, et al. *Vet Microbiol*. 2009;136:347.
16. Tozato CC, et al. *Brazil J Micro*. 2013;44:905.
17. Zhu W, et al. *Vet J*. 2014;199:303.
18. Araldi RP, et al. *Gen Mol Res*. 2014;13:5644.
19. Alberti A, et al. *Virol*. 2010;407:352.
20. Simeone P, et al. *Open Vet J*. 2008;2:33.
21. Mengual-Chulia B, et al. *Vet Microbiol*. 2014;172:108.
22. Knight CG, et al. *Vet Dermatol*. 2011;22:570.
23. Bogaert L, et al. *Vet Microbiol*. 2012;158:33.
24. Lange CE, et al. *Vet Pathol*. 2013;50:686.
25. Scase T, et al. *Equine Vet J*. 2010;42:738.
26. Sykora S, et al. *Vet Microbiol*. 2012;158:194.
27. van den Top JGB, et al. *Equine Vet J*. 2015;47:188.
28. Newkirk KM, et al. *J Vet Diagn Invest*. 2014;26:131.
29. Stevens H, et al. *J Gen Virol*. 2008;89:2475.
30. Fischer NM, et al. *Vet Dermatol*. 2014;25:210.
31. Silva MAR, et al. *Transbound Emerg Dis*. 2014;61:329.
32. Silva MAR, et al. *Gen Mol Res*. 2013;12:3150.
33. Gorino AC, et al. *Vet J*. 2013;197:903.
34. Postey RC, et al. *Canad J Vet Res*. 2007;71:28.
35. Finlay M, et al. *Virus Res*. 2009;144:315.
36. van den Top JGB, et al. *Equine Vet J*. 2008;40:528.
37. Torres SMF, et al. *Vet Dermatol*. 2010;21:503.
38. Bogaert L, et al. *BMC Biotechnol*. 2006;6.
39. Kawauchi K, et al. *J Virol Meth*. 2015;218:23.
40. Silva MAR, et al. *J Virol Meth*. 2013;192:55.
41. Nogueira SAF, et al. *Vet Dermatol*. 2006;17:259.
42. Lima EG, et al. *Gen Mol Res*. 2014;13:1121.

SARCOID

SYNOPSIS

Etiology Locally aggressive benign fibroblastic tumors of the skin associated with bovine papillomavirus (BVP) types 1 and 2 (BVP-1 and BVP-2).

Epidemiology Common tumor of equids, including horses, donkeys, mules, and zebras. Breed differences in prevalence. Transmission by close contact and infection of wounds.

Clinical findings Single or multiple lesions in the skin of limbs, lips, eyelids, eye, penile sheath, and base of the ears. Can present as warty growth or have the appearance of granulation tissue or as nodules beneath the skin. Spontaneous regression is rare.

Diagnostic confirmation Histopathology.

Treatment No single treatment modality has an advantage. Surgical excision, cryosurgery, immunotherapy, radiation, and local chemicals (intralesional cisplatin, acyclovir) are used.

Control None recognized.

ETIOLOGY

The cause of sarcoid in horses, mules, and donkeys is associated with infection by bovine papillomavirus (BPV) types 1 or 2, and possibly BPV-13.[1-6] Infection of young horses with BPV-1 virions induces nodular skin lesions 11 to 32 days after inoculation.[7] DNA of both types can be demonstrated in sarcoid tumors by PCR, as can the major transforming gene of BPV, E5, although papillomavirus has not been isolated from these tumors, nor have papillomavirus particles been demonstrated.[8] Variants of BPV-1 associated with sarcoids in horses have greater activity in equine cells than in bovine cells, indicating some adaptation or predilection of this variant for equine tissues.[9] The causative virus (BPV-1 or BPV-2) appears to vary geographically, with ~80% of cases in western Canada associated with BPV-2, as opposed to reports from other countries in which BPV-1 predominates.[10]

Genomic studies reveal that BPV-1 associated with sarcoids in horses likely diverged on multiple occasions from that in cattle at least 50,000 years before the present, and possibly much earlier, and well before domestication of either horses or cattle.[11]

It is speculated that this is a nonproductive infection in which viral DNA exists episomally, and a "hit-and-run" mechanism for pathogenesis has been proposed, in which infection by the virus, which resolves, induces changes that then lead to neoplastic transformation of tissue.[6]

However, given the demonstration of genetic susceptibility to sarcoid,[12] the cause is almost certainly multifactorial, with virus infection being an inciting event in susceptible animals. There does not appear to be a role for mutation in the tumor suppressor gene, *p53*, in the development of sarcoid in horses.

EPIDEMIOLOGY

Occurrence and Prevalence

Horses, donkeys, mules and zebras are affected, as are giraffes and sable antelope.[13-16] Skin lesions histologically similar to those in equids also occur in felids.[17] Equine sarcoid is the **commonest neoplasm** in horses, representing about 20% of all equine tumors diagnosed at necropsy, ~46% of all neoplastic skin lesions in horses at two sites in North America, and lesions in 21 of 68 horses examined in a first-opinion practice in the United Kingsom.[18,19] Sarcoids were the histologic diagnosis in 42% of skin samples submitted to veterinary diagnostic laboratories in Canada.[10]

Sarcoid tumors occur in 0.7% to ~11% of 3-year-old Swiss warmbloods[20] and 0.4% of Freiberger horses in Switzerland. Sarcoids made up 53% of all tumors located on the head and body.[18] Sarcoids occurred as solitary tumors in more than 99% of horses.[18]

Methods of Transmission

Transmission can be by infection of wounds, and castration is thought to be a risk factor, with flies as possible vectors. Close contact may facilitate transmission. BPV DNA has been detected in flies (*M. autumnalis*, *M. domestica*) and biting stable flies (*S. calcitrans*) associated with horses and donkeys with sarcoids.[21]

Experimental Reproduction

The disease has been transmitted with sarcoid tissue and cell free supernatant from minced sarcoid tumors. The disease has also been reproduced with bovine papillomavirus, although the experimentally produced tumors subsequently regressed, which seldom occurs with natural sarcoid.[6]

Animal Risk Factors

Horses with sarcoids had a mean age of 7 years (95% CI, 7.9 to 8.5 years). Horses with fibroblastic sarcoids are younger (median age of 5 years, range 0.6 to 25 years) than those with nodular (median 7, range 1.0 to 23), occult (median 7, range 1.1 to 21), verrucose (median 6, range 0.5 to 19), or mixed (median 6, range 0.5 to 31) sarcoids.[10] This wide age range highlights that sarcoids occur in young horses in addition to more aged animals. Risk of sarcoids was not associated with age or breed in two studies,[10,18] but other studies report that Appaloosa, Arabian, and Quarter horses are at greater risk than are Standardbreds or Thoroughbreds. Donkeys were overrepresented in one study,[10] and prevalence of disease was greater in populations of inbred zebra populations than in outbred populations (53% vs. 2%).[13]

There is a **genetically based susceptibility** to the disease, and the predisposition of horses to sarcoid is associated with the type of **major histocompatibility complex,** although this association is not universally accepted.[12] There are quantitative trait loci on equine chromosome (ECA) 20, 23, and 25 associated with genes that regulate virus replication and host immune responses.[22] Approximately 40% of the susceptibility to the disease in Swedish Halfbred horses is attributable to an autosomal-dominant equine leukocyte antigen (ELA)-linked gene. However, Swiss Warmbloods are no more likely to have the disease if their parent is diagnosed with sarcoids than if the sire is free of the disease.[20]

Environmental Risk Factors

Lesions commonly occur on traumatized areas.

PATHOGENESIS

The virus infects fibroblasts, and the infection is nonproductive. Viral DNA can be detected in lesional tissue, although viral load varies only slightly with clinical type of sarcoid.[2,23] However, intralesional viral load is directly associated with the severity of the disease.[24] It is thought that virus capsids of BVP are not found in equine sarcoids because papillomaviruses are usually host specific and the expression of virus capsids of the bovine papillomavirus requires the cellular environment of keratinocytes of the host species. Fibroblasts isolated from sarcoids are highly invasive, an attribute related to the high level of viral gene expression,[2,24] matrix metalloproteinase upregulation,[25] and production of viral oncoproteins.[26-28] Protein products of E5 and E6 enhance cell proliferation and, in vitro, increased invasion in EqS02a cells, and E7 enhances independence of cell anchorage independence, all attributes of neoplastic cells.[29] Elevated expression of phosphorylated p38 occurs in fibroblasts infected with BPV-1 as a result of the expression of BPV-1 E5 and E6 with enhancement of phosphorylation of the MK2 kinase, a substrate of *p38*, suggesting cellular mechanisms for the neoplastic transformation of infected cells.[30] Expression levels of FOXP3, interleukin-10, and interferon gamma mRNA (markers of regulatory T cells) and BPV-1 E5 copy numbers are significantly increased in lesional compared with tumor-distant skin samples from horses with sarcoids, suggesting local, regulatory, T-cell-induced immune suppression.[27]

Sarcoids do not regress, in contrast to the majority of papillomavirus infections, probably because expression of BPV in equine cells elicits immune evasion mechanisms.

CLINICAL FINDINGS

Sarcoids are localized proliferations of epidermal and dermal tissue that may remain small and dormant for many years and then undergo a stage of rapid, cancer-like growth. The lesions show moderate malignancy but do not metastasize to other sites, although there are sometimes (~2% of horses or 20% 30% of horses with sarcoids) multiple lesions.[10,20] Sarcoids occur as single or, more commonly, multiple lesions or clusters in the skin. The lesions occur anywhere on the body, but are more common on the head. Tumors on the head are 2.3 (95% CI, 2.0 to 2.7) times as likely to be sarcoids, compared with any other tumor type. Of 746 horses with sarcoids, 41% were on the head, 20% on the limbs, 16% on the neck or shoulder, 11% on the abdomen, 8% on the axilla or chest, and 5% in paragenital regions.[10]

Several forms of sarcoid are described:

- Verrucous (warty) sarcoid is a dry, horny, cauliflower-like surface that is usually partially or completely hairless. It may be broad based (sessile) or pedunculated. Verrucous sarcoids occur most commonly on the face, body, groin, and sheath area.
- Fibroblastic sarcoid has a similar appearance to that of proud flesh or excessive granulation tissue. It is often a firm, fibrous nodule in the dermis, although the surface may be ulcerated. It is found most commonly at sites of previous wounds and also the eyelid and limbs.
- A combination of both of the forms just described ("mixed")
- Occult sarcoid is typically an area of slightly thickened skin that has a roughened surface. It is usually partially hairless. Interference with these slow-growing sarcoids, including attempts at treatment, should be avoided; such interference can cause the tumor to proliferate. They occur most commonly around the mouth and eyes and on the neck.

CLINICAL PATHOLOGY

Confirmation of the diagnosis requires a **biopsy specimen** for histologic examination. Because sarcoids are usually associated with excessive granulation tissue and pyogranulomatous debris, the preferred specimen is a **transverse section of the excised tumor.** If punch biopsies are to be collected, then care should be taken that they include a representative section of the tumor, not just peripheral granulation tissue and edematous nontumor material. Examination by a pathologist accustomed to examining equine skin sections is important because the tumor has some features in common with papillomas and sarcomas and can be easily misdiagnosed.

PCR has been used to detect and quantitate BPV DNA.[31,32]

DIFFERENTIAL DIAGNOSIS

Cutaneous habronemiasis
Phycomycosis
Fibromas
Granulation tissue
Squamous-cell carcinoma, especially of the penis and eyelid
Other skin tumors, including melanoma, by examination of a biopsy of the lesion
Papillomatosis

TREATMENT

Surgical excision results in the return of the tumor in a significant proportion of animals within 6 months, often with overproliferation. BPV DNA can be detected in normal skin immediately surrounding sarcoids, and the recurrence has been speculated to reflect activation of latent BPV in normal tissue surrounding the tumor, although this interpretation is not supported by objective measurement of viral load in skin margins of the excised lesions.[33]

Intralesional administration of **cisplatin**, an oncolytic agent with in vitro activity against sarcoids cells,[34] by injection into the sarcoids or by electrochemotherapy, results in cure rates of 96% and 98%, respectively.[35,36] The protocol for intralesional injection of cisplatin in sesame seed oil is as follows:[36]

1. Crystalline lyophilized cisplatin powder is reconstituted with sterile water at a concentration of 10 mg/mL and mixed with medical-grade sesame seed oil (60%) and sorbitan monooleate (7%) by use of the pumping method just before administration (3.3 mg of cisplatin/mL of mixture).
2. Dosing objective is to deliver 1 mg of cisplatin per cubic centimeter of tumor. Tumor volume is calculated from the formula $V = \pi \times D1 \times D2 \times D3/6$, where D1 through D3 are tumor diameters measured with Vernier calipers.
3. Four intratumoral administrations of cisplatin are given at 2-week intervals of a series of intratumoral and peritumoral injections in 1 or 2 parallel planes, depending on the tumor size. The cisplatin emulsion is injected through narrow-bore needles (22 or 25 gauge). The spacing between injection rows is uniform, with a separation of 6 to 8 mm. The spacing between planes of injection is approximately 1 cm.

The largest dose of cisplatin to an adult horse should be not greater than 85 mg. Adverse reactions include moderate skin irritation. The treatment can be combined with surgical debulking of the lesion, with cisplatin administration begun when the surgical site has healed.[36]

Administration of **imiquimod** 5% cream to sarcoids three times weekly resulted in a cure rate of 60% in a study involving 15 horses.[37] Topical application of acyclovir (5%

cream) daily for 2 months to 47 sarcoids in 22 horses resulted in cure of 68%, with regression of tumor size in the remaining horses.[38]

Cryotherapy is associated with a much lower recurrence rate, but its use is limited by the anatomic location of the tumor. For instance, cryotherapy is not recommended for periocular lesions because of the risk of damaging nearby ocular tissues. The efficacy of cryotherapy may be enhanced by the use of thermocouples to monitor the temperature of the lesion to ensure adequate freezing. At least two or three freeze–thaw cycles are necessary.

Radiation therapy using radon-222, gold-198, radium-226, cobolt-60, or iridium-192 has been used and is indicated for recurrent or surgically inaccessible sarcoids such as periocular sarcoid. Radiation therapy is also useful for treating sarcoids of the body and legs. Local hyperthermia induced by a radiofrequency current of 2 MHz is also reported to be effective.

Immunotherapy, by injection of live organisms, killed bacilli, or cell-wall extract of the bacillus of Calmette and Guerin (BCG) have been successful on occasion, but their efficacy depends on the size of the lesion, its anatomic location, and possibly its type. Immunotherapy may work by inducing tumor-specific immunity. Adverse effects include local reactions characterized by edema and systemic anaphylactoid reactions after the second or third injections if commercial, whole-cell vaccines are used. Vaccines composed of cell-wall fractions in oil are free of such reactions and have given good results in periocular lesions, but sarcoids of the axilla did not react favorably. Large sarcoids or cases with multiple lesions may also respond poorly. Immunotherapy using mycobacterial cell-wall skeleton combined with trehalose dimycolate has resulted in total tumor regression.

Autogenous vaccines might result in the regression of existing sarcoids but have the risk of inducing new tumors and are not recommended for routine therapy. Use of acupuncture to treat sarcoids is reported, but there is little scientific justification for using this procedure.[39]

As yet, no single treatment modality is universally successful in the treatment of sarcoid. In a study in 92 horses comparing outcome, a successful outcome was obtained in 79% of horses treated with cryosurgery, 67% of those treated with BCG vaccination, 82% of those treated with conventional excision, and 71% of those treated using carbon dioxide laser. Greater success rates are reported for intralesional administration of cisplatin, and possibly for imiquimod and acyclovir.[35-38]

FURTHER READING

Taylor S, Haldorson G. A review of equine sarcoid. *Equine Vet Educ.* 2013;25:210-216.

REFERENCES

1. Lunardi M, et al. *J Clin Micro.* 2013;51:2167.
2. Bogaert L, et al. *J Gen Virol.* 2007;88:2155.
3. Nasir L, et al. *Vet Microbiol.* 2013;167:159.
4. Rector A, et al. *Virol.* 2013;445:213.
5. Torres SMF, et al. *Vet Clin Equine.* 2013;29:643.
6. Munday JS. *Vet Pathol.* 2014;51:1063.
7. Hartl B, et al. *J Gen Virol.* 2011;92:2437.
8. Wilson AD, et al. *Vet Microbiol.* 2013;162:369.
9. Nasir L, et al. *Virol.* 2007;364:355.
10. Wobeser BK, et al. *Can Vet J.* 2010;51:1103.
11. Trewby H, et al. *J Gen Virol.* 2014;95:2748.
12. Christen G, et al. *Vet J.* 2014;199:68.
13. Marais HJ, et al. *J S Afr Vet Assoc.* 2007;78:145.
14. Marais HJ, et al. *J Wildl Dis.* 2011;47:917.
15. van Dyk E, et al. *J S Afr Vet Assoc.* 2011;82:80.
16. Semieka MA, et al. *J Adv Vet Res.* 2012;2:276.
17. Orbell GMB, et al. *Vet Pathol.* 2011;48:1176.
18. Schaffer PA, et al. *J Am Vet Med Assoc.* 2013;242:99.
19. van der Zaag EJ, et al. *Pferdeheilkunde.* 2012;28:697.
20. Studer S, et al. *Schweiz Arch Tierheilkd.* 2007;149:161.
21. Finlay M, et al. *Virus Res.* 2009;144:315.
22. Jandova V, et al. *Schweiz Arch Tierheilkd.* 2012;154:19.
23. Bogaert L, et al. *Vet Microbiol.* 2010;146:269.
24. Haralambus R, et al. *Equine Vet J.* 2010;42:327.
25. Yuan Z, et al. *Virol.* 2010;396:143.
26. Corteggio A, et al. *J Gen Virol.* 2011;92:378.
27. Maehlmann K, et al. *Vet J.* 2014;202:516.
28. Mosseri S, et al. *Vet J.* 2014;202:279.
29. Yuan Z, et al. *J Gen Virol.* 2011;92:773.
30. Yuan Z, et al. *J Gen Virol.* 2011;92:1778.
31. Bogaert L, et al. *Vet Pathol.* 2011;48:737.
32. Wobeser BK, et al. *J Vet Diagn Invest.* 2012;24:32.
33. Taylor SD, et al. *J Equine Vet Sci.* 2014;34:722.
34. Finlay M, et al. *Vet Res.* 2012;43.
35. Tamzali Y, et al. *Equine Vet J.* 2012;44:214.
36. Theon AP, et al. *J Am Vet Med Assoc.* 2007;230:1506.
37. Nogueira SAF, et al. *Vet Dermatol.* 2006;17:259.
38. Stadler S, et al. *Vet Rec.* 2011;168:187.
39. Thoresen AS. *Am J Trad Chin Vet Med.* 2011;6:29.

COWPOX AND BUFFALOPOX

SYNOPSIS

Etiology Cowpox and buffalopox virus are members of the genus *Orthopoxvirus* in the family Poxviridae. Buffalopox is a close variant of vaccinia virus.

Epidemiology Cowpox is endemic in the population of certain rodents in Europe and East Asia. Cattle are a rare and incidental host. Buffalopox is a (re) emergent disease occurring in buffaloes, cattle, and humans in India and neighboring countries. The natural host of buffalopox virus has not yet been identified. Spread of both viruses is by contact.

Clinical findings Typical pox lesions on the teats and udder. Erythema, papules with a zone of hyperemia around the base, vesiculation, pustular stage, and scab.

Clinical pathology Electron microscopy, polymerase chain reaction (PCR).

Diagnostic confirmation Electron microscopy, PCR, and virus isolation.

Treatment Palliative.

Control Sanitation to prevent spread between cows.

ETIOLOGY

Cowpox virus (CPXV) and buffalopox virus (BPXV) are members of the genus *Orthopoxvirus* in the family Poxviridae. Other orthopoxviruses infecting agricultural animals include horsepox, Uasin Gishu, and camelpox. All orthopoxviruses are antigenically extremely similar, but they can be identified by a combination of phenotypic and genetic tests.

CPXV received its name as a result of the association of this agent with skin lesions on the teat and udder skin of dairy cattle. Notwithstanding, it is probably a misnomer because infection of cattle is rare, whereas infection is widespread among rodents in Europe and western Asia.

EPIDEMIOLOGY

Occurrence

Infection with CPXV is **endemic in wild rodents** such as voles (*Microtus* spp.) in **Great Britain, Europe, and western Asia**, with infection in different rodent species acting as the reservoir host in different geographic areas. Domestic cats are commonly infected from hunting rodents, but CPXV infection can occur in a number of different mammalian species, one of which is cattle. The clinical syndrome of cowpox in cattle is now extremely rare, but it occurs sporadically in Europe. In recent decades, reemergence of CPXV infections in cats, zoo animals, and humans has been reported.[1]

BPXV was first isolated in India in the early 1930s, and disease outbreaks affecting buffaloes, cattle, and humans have been reported in India, Nepal, Pakistan, Egypt, and Indonesia since then.[2] BPXV is considered an important emerging or reemerging zoonotic viral infection in regions with a large buffalo population.[3] A similar but **distinct vaccinia-like virus** has been associated with disease outbreaks among cattle and humans in **Brazil.**[2]

Origin of Infection and Transmission

The origin of CPXV infection is most probably from infected farm cats or humans. **Transmission** from cow to cow within a herd is effected by milkers' hands or teat cups. Spread from herd to herd is probably effected by the introduction of infected animals, by carriage on milkers' hands, and in the absence of either of these methods, transport by biting insects is possible. In a herd in which the disease is enzootic, only heifers and new introductions develop lesions. Milkers recently vaccinated against smallpox may serve as a source of infection for cattle, although the **vaccinia virus**, the smallpox vaccine virus, is a different virus.

BPXV is most commonly isolated from buffaloes, cattle, and people having direct and frequent contact with these animals. Although a primary host species functioning as virus reservoir has not yet been identified for BPXV, peridomestic rodents have been incriminated as potential vectors.[4] Because disease outbreaks in buffalo herds are often associated with high disease occurrence among animal handlers and caretakers, transmission from animal to animal by means of people as vectors is considered to play an important role.[3]

It is generally assumed that the virus gains access to tissues through injuries to teat skin, and extensive outbreaks are likely to occur when the environment is conducive to teat injuries. Spread is rapid within a herd and immunity is solid, so that the disease tends to occur in sharp outbreaks of several months in duration, with subsequent immunity protecting the cattle for at least several years.

Economic Importance

Losses are a result of inconvenience at milking time because of the soreness of the teats and from occasional cases of mastitis, which develop when lesions involve teat sphincters and decreased milk production.

Zoonotic Implications

Human cowpox is not common, although the disease incidence has increased over the past decades, an observation that has been explained by increasing susceptibility of the human population to poxvirus infection following discontinuation of smallpox vaccination in most parts of the world.[5] Clinical cases in humans usually consist of one or a few lesions on the hand and face with minimal systemic reaction and are most commonly traced back to infected cats or occasionally rats rather than cattle.[1]

An increasing incidence of clinical cases of BPXV and Brazilian vaccinia-like virus infection has been reported in humans, particularly among animal caretakers and animal handlers in India but also in Brazil, and has become a serious public health concern in some countries.[2,3] Consumption of unpasteurized milk of affected animals has been incriminated as potential route of virus transmission from animal to human.

PATHOGENESIS

Five stages of a **typical pox eruption** can be observed. After an incubation period of 3 to 6 days, a roseolar erythema is followed by firm, raised papules light in color but with a zone of hyperemia around the base. Vesiculation, a yellow blister with a pitted center, follows. The subsequent pustular stage is followed by the development of a thick, red, tenacious scab.

In experimentally produced **vaccinia virus** mammillitis (produced by inoculation of smallpox vaccine), the lesions have three zones: a central brown crusty area of necrosis, surrounded by a gray–white zone of microvesicle formation, again surrounded by a red border as a result of congestion. The lesions are essentially hyperplastic.

CLINICAL FINDINGS

Typical **lesions** are similar for CPXV and BPXV infection and may be seen at any stage of development, but they are mostly observed during the scab stage, with the vesicle commonly having been ruptured during milking. True cowpox scabs are 1 to 2 cm in diameter and are thick, tenacious, and yellow–brown to red in color. In cows being milked, scab formation is uncommon, with the scab being replaced by a deep ulceration.

Distribution of the lesions is usually confined to the teats and lower part of the udder. Soreness of the teats develops, and milk letdown may be interfered with; the cow usually resents being milked. Secondary mastitis occurs in a few cases. Individual lesions heal within 2 weeks, but in some animals fresh crops of lesions may cause the disease to persist for a month or more. In severe cases, lesions may spread to the insides of the thighs, and rarely to the perineum, vulva, and mouth. Sucking calves may develop lesions around the mouth. In bulls, lesions usually appear on the scrotum.

Ulcerative skin lesions with raised edges frequently affected by secondary bacterial or fungal infection are commonly observed on the ears of nonlactating cattle and buffaloes infected with BPXV.[3]

CLINICAL PATHOLOGY

The virus can be propagated in tissue culture, and differentiation is possible by electron microscopy. The presence of virus-related DNA sequences can be identified by means of PCR.

DIFFERENTIAL DIAGNOSIS

- A number of skin diseases may be accompanied by lesions on the udder and can easily be confused with cowpox if the lesions are advanced in age. Most outbreaks of teat skin disease that clinically resemble classical cowpox are associated with vaccinia virus from contact with a recently vaccinated person.
- Pseudocowpox
- Bovine ulcerative mammillitis associated with bovine herpesvirus-2 and bovine herpesvirus-4
- Vesicular stomatitis and foot-and-mouth disease
- Udder impetigo
- Teat chaps and frostbite
- Black spot

CONTROL

Prevention of spread is difficult because the virus responsible for the disease is readily transmitted by direct or indirect contact. Udder cloths, milking machines, and hands should be disinfected after contact with infected animals. Dipping of the teats in an alcoholic tincture of a suitable disinfectant, such as quaternary ammonium compounds, is usually satisfactory in preventing immediate spread. Although the prevalence and significance of CPXV infection in cattle is too low to warrant the development of vaccines, the emergence of buffalopox in buffalo and cattle herds and the ensuing zoonotic risk in some parts of the world may warrant considering the development of vaccines against BPXV for certain regions of the world.[3]

REFERENCES

1. Kurth A, Nitsche A. The challenge of highly pathogenic microorganisms. In: Schafferman A, et al., eds. *Berlin: Springer Science+Business Media BV*. 2010:157-164.
2. Singh RK, et al. *Indian J Virol*. 2012;23:1-11.
3. Venkatesan G, et al. *Vet Ital*. 2010;46:439-448.
4. Abrahao JS, et al. *PLoS ONE*. 2009;10:e7428.
5. Bray M. *Am J Trop Med Hyg*. 2009;80:499-500.

PSEUDOCOWPOX (MILKERS' NODULE)

SYNOPSIS

Etiology Parapoxvirus.

Epidemiology Primarily affects cows in early lactation. Low, but progressive, morbidity in herd. Spread during milking.

Clinical findings Vesicles, pustules, formation of a thick scab elevated by granulating tissue. Key distinguishing feature is horseshoe-shaped ring of small scabs surrounding granulating tissue on the teat.

Clinical pathology Vesicle fluid for electron microscopy.

Diagnostic confirmation Electron microscopy.

Treatment Antiseptics and emollient ointment.

Control Milking hygiene.

ETIOLOGY

Pseudocowpox virus is a member of the genus *Parapoxvirus*, with close similarity to the viruses of infectious papular stomatitis of cattle and contagious ecthyma of sheep and goats. It is possible that pseudocowpox virus (PCPV) might be identical to bovine papular stomatitis virus (BPSV).[1,2] The pseudocowpox virus was previously known as parapoxvirus bovis 2.

EPIDEMIOLOGY

Occurrence

Pseudocowpox is reported in **most countries**. In an affected herd the rate of spread is relatively slow and may result in the disease being present in the herd for up to a year. The **morbidity** rate approximates 100%, but at any given time it varies between 5% and 10%, and occasionally up to 50%.

Origin of Infection and Transmission

The source of infection is **infected cattle**. The method of **transmission** includes physical transport by means of contaminated milkers' hands, washcloths, and teat cups. The virus cannot penetrate mucosa, and a preexisting discontinuity of it is necessary for the virus to gain entry. Transmission by biting insects seems likely. The virus can be isolated from the mouths of calves sucking affected calves, and from the semen of bulls.

Animal Risk Factors

Freshly calved and **recently introduced** cattle are most susceptible, but **all adult cattle** in a herd, including dry cows, are likely to be affected. The disease does not appear to occur in animals less than 2 years of age unless they have calved. There is no seasonal variation in incidence. Little immunity develops, and the disease is likely to recur in the herd within a short time.

Economic Importance

Pseudocowpox is relatively benign, with most losses occurring as a result of difficulty in milking and an increase in the incidence of mastitis.

Zoonotic Implications

The disease is transmissible to humans, with infection usually resulting in the development of milkers' nodule on the hand.

PATHOGENESIS

Transmission most commonly occurs at milking time and is mechanical, with the potential for transmission from cow to calf by suckling. The disease can be reproduced by the introduction of the virus onto scarified areas of skin. The lesions are characterized by hyperplasia of squamous epithelium.

CLINICAL FINDINGS

Acute and chronic lesions occur, and there may be up to 10 lesions on one teat (the udder is very rarely infected). **Acute lesions** commence as erythema followed by the development of a vesicle or pustule, which ruptures after about 48 hours, resulting in the formation of a thick scab. Pain is moderate and present only in the prescab stage. The scab, varying in size from 0.5 to 25 mm in diameter, becomes markedly elevated by developing granulating tissue beneath it; the scabs drop off 7 to 10 days after lesions appear, leaving a **horseshoe-shaped ring** of small scabs surrounding a small, wart-like granuloma, which may persist for months. The disease tends to disappear from a herd after 18 to 21 days but may recur cyclically about 1 month later. There are reports of lesions occurring occasionally in cows' mouths.

Chronic lesions also commence as erythema, but progress to a stage in which yellow–gray, soft, scurfy scabs develop. The scabs are readily rubbed off at milking, leaving the skin corrugated and prone to chapping. There is no pain, and the lesions may persist for months.

Milkers' nodules are clinically indistinguishable from human lesions associated with ecthyma virus. The lesions vary from multiple vesicles to a single, indurated nodule.

An outbreak of pseudocowpox infection occurred in Brazil, characterized by the presence of severe vesicular, papulopustular, and proliferative scabby lesions on the muzzle of 14 crossbred calves that did not have contact with dairy cattle.[2] The lesions started as macules and papules on the muzzle that progressed to vesicles, pustules, and scabs with a clinical course of 10 to 15 days, at which time the lesions spontaneously resolved. Nucleotide sequencing of the virus isolated from the lesions revealed 97% homology with pseudocowpox virus and only 84% homology with bovine popular stomatitis virus.[2]

CLINICAL PATHOLOGY AND NECROPSY FINDINGS

Material for examination by tissue culture or electron microscopic examination, the latter being highly recommended as a diagnostic procedure, should include fluid from a vesicle.

> **DIFFERENTIAL DIAGNOSIS**
>
> Differentiation of those diseases in which lesions of the teat are prominent is dealt with in the preceding section on cowpox.

TREATMENT

Locally applied ointments of various kinds appear to have little effect on the lesions. The recommended treatment includes the removal of the scabs, which should be burned to avoid contaminating the environment, application of an astringent preparation, such as triple dye, after milking and an emollient ointment just before.

CONTROL

Recommended measures, such as treatment and isolation of affected cows or milking them last, the use of disposable paper towels for udder washing, and disinfection of teat cups, appear to have little effect on the spread of the disease. An iodophor teat dip is recommended as the most effective control measure because it appears to exert some antiviral effect. An effort should be made to reduce teat trauma because infection is facilitated by discontinuity of the skin.

REFERENCES

1. Yaegashi G, et al. *J Vet Med Sci*. 2013;75:1399.
2. Cargnelutti JF, et al. *J Vet Diagn Invest*. 2012;24:437.

LUMPY SKIN DISEASE (KNOPVELSIEKTE)

> **SYNOPSIS**
>
> **Etiology** Lumpy skin disease virus, of the genus *Capripoxvirus* (closely related to sheep and goatpox viruses).
>
> **Epidemiology** Previously enzootic in sub-Saharan Africa, but expanded into most of Africa in the 1970s. The disease is now actively spreading in the Middle East, with outbreaks in Israel, Lebanon, Turkey, Syria, Iran, Azerbaijan, and North Cyprus. Epizootics interspersed with periods of sporadic occurrence. Transmission by contact and a range of sucking/biting arthropod vectors.
>
> **Clinical findings** Fever, nodular lesions on the skin and mucous membranes and lymphadenopathy. A proportion of cattle develop generalized infection, with high mortality. Losses accrue from damage to hides, decreased milk yield and growth, abortion, deaths, and disruption of international trade. Necrotic plugs of tissue highly susceptible to secondary infection and flystrike.
>
> **Clinical pathology** Intracellular, eosinophilic inclusion bodies in biopsy material. Virus isolation. Fluorescent antibody, serum neutralization, and polymerase chain reaction (PCR) tests.
>
> **Necropsy findings** Nodules in skin, upper alimentary tract, respiratory tract.
>
> **Diagnostic confirmation** Biopsy and histology. Virus isolation to differentiate from pseudo lumpy skin disease caused by bovine herpesvirus-2.
>
> **Treatment** Supportive.
>
> **Control** Vaccination, control of movement of cattle from affected areas.

ETIOLOGY

Lumpy skin disease (LSD) is a severe systemic disease of cattle associated with the Neethling poxvirus, a *Capripoxvirus*. It has close antigenic relationship to sheeppox and goatpox viruses, which are in the same genus. There appears to be a difference in virulence between strains.

EPIDEMIOLOGY

Occurrence

The disease used to be confined to sub-Saharan Africa, but spread to many other African countries in the 1970s, then Egypt (outbreaks occurred in 1988 and 2006; the disease is now enzootic) and Israel (outbreaks in 1989, 2006-2007, and 2012). In Israel it was initially eradicated by slaughter of infected and in-contact animals, but vaccination using Sheeppox, and more recently Neethling strain vaccine, has since been used. The virus is actively spreading within and from the Middle East, with cases confirmed in Kuwait (1991), Lebanon (1993), the United Arab Emirates (2000), Bahrain (2003), Oman (2010), Turkey and Syria (2013), Jordan (2013), Iran and Iraq (2013), Azerbaijan and North Cyprus.[1-3] There is a risk it could be introduced into European countries, mainly through the illegal movement of animals but also within vectors.[2,3]

Some outbreaks are associated with severe and generalized infections and a high mortality rate, whereas others have few obviously affected animals and no deaths. In general, outbreaks are more severe following introduction of the infection into a region and then abate, probably associated with the development of widespread immunity. Morbidity rates can reach 80% during epizootics, but typically range from 10% to 30% in enzootic areas. In Kenya, the disease is milder, with a lower morbidity rate and an average case fatality of 2%. Outbreaks in Israel produced no direct mortality from the disease. A resurgence of the disease in South Africa was associated with higher rainfall and a decrease in the use of vaccination.

Origin of Infection and Transmission

The virus is present in the nasal and lacrimal secretions, semen, and milk of infected animals. However, direct contact is not thought to be the major source of transmission, with most cases associated with transmission by an arthropod vector. LSD virus has been isolated from *S. calcitrans* and *M. confiscata* and transmitted experimentally using *S. calcitrans* and *Ablyomma* and *Rhipicephalus* ticks, with evidence that the virus may be transmitted vertically and overwinter in these tick species.[4,5] Other vectors are suspected, including *Biomyia*, *Culicoides*, *Glossina*, and *Musca* spp. However, although the virus was detected in mosquitoes (*Anopheles stephensi*, *Culex quinquefascuatus*), stable flies, and biting midges (*Culicoides nebeculosis*) after feeding on cattle with lumpy skin disease, infection did not transmit to susceptible cattle when these arthropods were subsequently allowed to feed on them.

Transmission via infected semen used in artificial breeding has been demonstrated experimentally.[6]

Risk Factors

Animal Risk Factors

All ages and types of cattle are susceptible, although very young calves and lactating and malnourished cattle develop more severe clinical disease. Recently recovered animals are immune for about 3 months.

British breeds, particularly Channel Island breeds, are much more susceptible than zebu types, both in numbers affected and the severity of the disease. Wildlife species are not affected in natural outbreaks, although there is concern that they might be reservoir hosts in interepidemic periods, such as African buffalo (*Syncerus caffer*) in the Kruger National Park in South Africa.[7] Typical skin lesions, without systemic disease, have been produced experimentally with Neethling virus in sheep, goats, giraffes, impalas, and Grant's gazelles, but wildebeests were resistant. Natural cases of lumpy skin disease were recorded in water buffalo (*Bubalis bubalis*) during an outbreak in Egypt in 1988, but morbidity was much lower than for cattle (1.6% vs. 30.8%).

Environmental Risk Factors

Outbreaks tend to follow waterways. Extensive epizootics are associated with high rainfall and high levels of insect activity, with peaks in the late summer and early autumn. Introduction of new animals and communal grazing have been identified as risk factors for LSD infection in Ethiopia.[8]

Pathogen Risk Factors

Capripoxviruses are resistant to drying and able to survive freezing and thawing, but most are inactivated by temperatures above 60° C (140 F).

Experimental Transmission

Experimental transmission can be achieved with ground-up nodular tissue, blood, or virus grown in tissue culture given by intranasal, ID, or IV routes. Although lumpy skin disease is characterized by generalized nodular skin lesions, less than 50% of natural or experimental infections develop generalized skin nodules. The length of viremia is not correlated with the severity of clinical disease.

Economic Importance

The mortality rate is usually low (although it can be 10% or more), but economic losses are high. There is reduced feed intake, a reduction in milk production, and occurrence of secondary mastitis associated with lesions on the teats. Losses also accrue from hide damage, reduced body condition, decreased fertility in bulls, and abortion in cows. There has always been a high risk of LSD spreading out of Africa, and it is now actively spreading in the Middle East. It is also a potential agent for agricultural bioterrorism.

PATHOGENESIS

In the generalized disease there is viremia and fever, followed by localization in the skin and development of inflammatory nodules. Following ID inoculation, local lesions develop at the challenge site but without viremia and systemic infection.

CLINICAL FINDINGS

The incubation period is typically 2 to 4 weeks in field outbreaks and 7 to 14 days following experimental challenge. In severe cases there is an initial rise of temperature, which lasts for over a week, occasionally accompanied by lacrimation, nasal discharge, salivation, and lameness. Multiple intradermal nodules appear suddenly about a week later, often initially on the perineum. They are round and firm, 1 to 4 cm in diameter, and flattened, and the hair on them stands on end. They vary from a few to hundreds and, in most cases, are confined to the skin. However, lesions can occur elsewhere, such as in the nostrils and on the turbinates, causing mucopurulent nasal discharge, respiratory obstruction, and snoring; in the mouth, as plaques and then ulcers, causing salivation; on the conjunctiva, causing severe lacrimation; and on the prepuce or vulva, spreading to nearby mucosal surfaces. In most cases the nodules disappear rapidly, but they may persist as hard lumps or become moist and necrotic, then slough.

Lymph nodes draining the affected area become enlarged, and local edema can occur, particularly of the limbs. When the yellow center of nodules slough, this can expose underlying tissues, including testicles or tendons. Lesions where skin is lost may remain visible for long periods. When lesions coalesce, large areas of raw tissue can be exposed, and these are susceptible to invasion with screwworm fly larvae. Lesions in the respiratory tract are often followed by pneumonia.

Convalescence usually takes 4 to 12 weeks, and pregnant cows may abort.

CLINICAL PATHOLOGY

The virus can be cultivated from lesions, and the viral antigen can be detected by a variety of PCR tests. Viral DNA can be detected in the skin up to 90 days after infection using PCR, which is much longer than the virus can be isolated. An antigen ELISA has also been used with samples collected early in the course of the disease, before the development of neutralizing antibodies. Electron microscopy will identify capripox virions in skin biopsies or scabs. This must be used in combination with the history of generalized nodular skin disease; capripox can be distinguished from parapoxvirus (the agent of bovine papular stomatitis) and pseudocowpox, but it is morphologically similar to cowpox and vaccinia viruses. Histopathology of lesions reveals a granulomatous reaction in the dermis and hypodermis, with intracellular, eosinophilic inclusion bodies in early lesions.

Virus neutralization is the most specific serologic test, but immunity is predominantly cell mediated, and thus it may fail to detect low concentrations of antibodies in many exposed cattle. The agar gel immunodiffusion (AGID) and indirect fluorescent antibody tests are less specific, producing false positives as a result of cross-reaction with bovine papular stomatitis and pseudocowpox viruses.

NECROPSY FINDINGS

The skin lesions are described under "Clinical Findings." Similar lesions are present in the mouth, pharynx, trachea, skeletal muscle, bronchi, and stomachs, and there may be accompanying pneumonia. The superficial lymph nodes are usually enlarged. Respiratory distress and death are often the result of respiratory obstruction by the necrotic ulcers and surrounding inflammation in the upper respiratory tract, often with concurrent aspiration pneumonia. Histologically, a widespread vasculitis reflects the viral tropism for endothelial cells. Intracytoplasmic viral inclusion bodies may be seen in a variety of cells types.

Samples for Confirmation of Diagnosis

- **Histology**—formalin-fixed lesions from skin, alimentary and respiratory tissue, lymph node (LM)
- **Virology**—lymph node, skin lesion (ISO, EM)
- **Antigen detection**—affected tissue, blood, semen (PCR, antigen ELISA).

DIFFERENTIAL DIAGNOSIS

The rapid spread of the disease and the sudden appearance of lumps in the skin after an initial fever make this disease quite unlike any other disease of cattle.

Pseudolumpy skin disease (also known as Allerton virus infection and general infection of cattle with bovine herpesvirus-2), is associated with bovine herpesvirus-2, the agent of bovine mammillitis. It occurs primarily in southern Africa, although occasional cases occur in the United States, Australia, and the United Kingdom. Multifocal lesions are distributed over the body, are circular and up to 2 cm in diameter, and have an intact central area and raised edges, accompanied by loss of hair. Some lesions show a circular ring of necrosis around a central scab. The scabs fall off, leaving discrete hairless lesions that may be depigmented. The disease runs a course of approximately 2 weeks, and there is no mortality. Only the superficial layers of skin are involved. This is in contrast to the lesions of lumpy skin disease, which are often deep enough to expose underlying tissues. Herpesvirus can be isolated from the periphery of the lesions. Diagnosis can be made by polymerase chain reaction (PCR) on full-thickness skin biopsy.

TREATMENT

No specific treatment is available, but prevention of secondary infection with antibiotics or sulfonamides is recommended.

CONTROL

Lumpy skin disease moves into new territory principally by movement of infected cattle, and possibly by wind-borne vectors. Once in a new area, further spread probably occurs via insect vectors, and ticks have been implicated in maintaining the virus in between epidemics.[4,5] Control of cattle movement from uninfected to infected areas is an important measure to prevent the introduction of the virus. Once in an area, control is by vaccination.

Vaccination

Freeze-dried, live attenuated vaccines are commercially available and the most commonly used. There is antigenic homology between the *Capripoxviruses*, and thus vaccination of cattle with attenuated sheeppox virus has been used to protect against infection with LSD virus. This was used in countries previously free of LSD virus because it eliminated any risk of escape of attenuated live vaccine virus from vaccinated herds. However, incomplete protection with a vaccine based upon what was thought to be a Kenyan sheep and goatpox occurred during a 2006 outbreak of LSD in Egypt, and following the use of a sheeppox vaccine in Israel in 2006-2007 in which 11% of vaccinated cattle developed skin lesions.[3] Consequently, the attenuated Neethling strain vaccine of LSD virus was used in response to a serious outbreak of the disease in Israel during 2012. A battery of three molecular tests was able to differentiate infection with the vaccine strain, and a virulent virus was developed; no spread from vaccinated to nonvaccinated cattle was recorded.[9]

A small percentage of cattle vaccinated with the sheeppox virus do develop local granulomatous reactions, but there is no spread of the virus to sheep running with the cattle. However, the commonly used Kenyan sheeppox and goatpox vaccine virus (designated O-240) has been identified as an LSD virus; the low attenuation of this virus probably makes it unsafe for cattle because of its potential to cause clinical disease in vaccinated animals.[10] Other viruses capable of infecting sheep, goats, and cattle have been identified as potential candidates for vaccines against all capripox diseases.[10]

Vaccination of a herd at the start of an outbreak is of limited use. Most animals will already be incubating the disease, and poor needle hygiene in these circumstances may spread the disease. Slaughter of affected and in-contact animals, destruction of contaminated hides, and vaccination of at-risk animals is a common approach when the disease is introduced to a previously free country.

FURTHER READING

OIE Terrestrial Manual, Chapter 2.4.14. Lumpy skin disease. Accessed at: <http://www.oie.int/fileadmin/Home/eng/Animal_Health_in_the_World/docs/pdf/Disease_cards/LUMPY_SKIN_DISEASE_FINAL.pdf>. Accessed July 16, 2016.

Tuppurainen ESM, Oura CAL. Review: lumpy skin disease: an emerging threat to Europe, the Middle East and Asia. *Transbound Emerg Dis.* 2012;59:40-48.

REFERENCES

1. Fernandez P, et al. *Atlas of Transboundary Animal Diseases.* OIE; 2010.
2. EFSA Panel on Animal Health & Welfare. *EFSA J.* 2015;13:3986.
3. Tuppurainen ESM, Oura CAL. *Transbound Emerg Dis.* 2012;59:40.
4. Lubinga JC, et al. *Ticks Tick Borne Dis.* 2014;5:113.
5. Lubinga JC, et al. *Transbound Emerg Dis.* 2015;65:174.
6. Annadale CH, et al. *Transbound Emerg Dis.* 2015;61:443.
7. Shamsudeen F, et al. *J S Afr Vet Assoc.* 2014;85:1075.
8. Hailu B, et al. *Prev Vet Med.* 2014;115:64.
9. Menasherow S, et al. *J Virol Methods.* 2014;199:95.
10. Tuppurainen ESM, et al. *Antiviral Res.* 2014;109:1.

SHEEPPOX AND GOATPOX

SYNOPSIS

Etiology *Capripoxvirus.* Strains vary in virulence and host specificity.

Epidemiology Highly contagious, spread by aerosol, contact, and flies. Young and nonindigenous animals more susceptible. Morbidity and case-fatality rates are high.

Clinical findings Fever, generalized skin and internal pox lesions, lymphadenopathy, mucopurulent nasal discharge, high mortality.

Clinical pathology Fluorescent antibody and electron microscopy of biopsy material, serology, virus isolation.

Necropsy findings Pox nodular lesions in alimentary tract and respiratory tract.

Diagnostic confirmation Fluorescent antibody staining, virus isolation.

Control Vaccination.

ETIOLOGY

Sheeppox, goatpox and lumpy skin disease of cattle are members of the genus *Capripoxvirus*, one of six genera of poxviruses. The diseases produced by sheeppox and goatpox viruses are collectively called capripox infections. They are named on the basis of their host specificity in natural outbreaks and are usually highly host specific in natural infections, although exceptions exist. For example, Kenya sheeppox and goatpox viruses, and Yemen and Oman sheep isolates, infect both sheep and goats, although the disease caused by the same isolate can vary dramatically between the two hosts.[1] The viruses are closely related genetically, and hence they cross-react in serologic tests, and many can cross species barriers in experimental infections. Recombination may also occur naturally between isolates from different host species.

EPIDEMIOLOGY

Prevalence of Infection

Sheeppox and goatpox are prevalent in North and Central Africa north of the equator, the Indian subcontinent, the Middle East, China, Southwest Asia, and the former Soviet Union. Sporadic outbreaks occur in southern Europe, including Turkey, Greece, and Bulgaria, and elsewhere.[2] The *Capripoxvirus* infections of small ruminants are the most serious of all the pox diseases in animals, characterized by fever and skin lesions.[3] In susceptible flocks and herds morbidity is 75% to 100%, with outbreaks often causing death in 10% to 85% of affected animals depending on the virulence of the infecting strain.

Methods of Transmission

Sheeppox and goatpox are highly contagious. The virus enters via the respiratory tract, and transmission commonly is by aerosol infection associated with close contact with infected animals. The virus is present in nasal and oral secretions for several weeks after infection and can live in scabs that have fallen off the animal for several months. Spread can also occur from contact with contaminated materials and through skin abrasions produced iatrogenically or by insects. Capripox has been shown to spread via the bites of *S. calcitrans* and the tsetse fly.

Experimental Reproduction

The disease can be transmitted by intradermal, intravenous, and subcutaneous inoculation and by virus aerosols. Capripox antigen is detected 6 and 8 days postinfection in skin and lungs, respectively.[4]

Risk Factors

Animal Risk Factors

Both sheeppox and goatpox affect sheep and goats of all ages, all breeds, and both sexes, but young and old animals and lactating females are more severely affected. In areas where sheeppox is enzootic, imported breeds such as Merinos or some European breeds may show greater susceptibility than the native stock. Young animals are more susceptible.

Pathogen Risk Factors

The virus is resistant to drying and survives freezing and thawing. It is sensitive to extremes of pH and 1% formalin. Sensitivity to heat varies between strains, but most are inactivated at 60°C (140F) for 60 minutes. Isolates from most regions are host specific, but isolates from Kenya and Oman naturally infect both goats and sheep. Scabs shed by infected animals remain infective for several months.

Economic Importance

Loss is from mortality, abortions, mastitis, loss of wool, skin condemnation, and loss of exports. In ewes and does, severe losses may occur if the udder is invaded because of the secondary occurrence of acute mastitis. In some outbreaks, adult sheep are affected with the more severe form of the disease. Sheeppox is a potent threat to countries that have large sheep populations, and where the disease does not occur, because it is difficult to eradicate and has a high mortality rate.

In a natural outbreak in an intensive sheep dairy in Israel, losses accrued from acute illness, deaths, reduced milk production, and reduced fertility. Milk production declined for 8 weeks after the index cases and was accompanied by an increased somatic cell count.[5]

Zoonotic Implications

Human infections in people handling infected animals are not a consideration.

PATHOGENESIS

During an initial viremia, the virus is carried by infected monocytes/macrophages to many tissues, particularly the skin, respiratory tract, and gastrointestinal tract.[4] Syncytial cells are seen in skin, and these probably facilitate local spread of the virus. The development of typical pox lesions, as in vaccinia, is characteristic of the disease. The virus is present in greatest quantities from 7 to 14 days after inoculation. Passive protection by serum will protect against challenge. Circulating antibody limits spread of infection, but does not prevent replication of the virus at the site of inoculation.

CLINICAL FINDINGS

In sheep, sheeppox has an incubation period of 12 to 14 days, with the malignant form being the most common type in lambs. There is marked depression and prostration, a very high fever, and discharge from the eyes and nose. Affected lambs may die during this stage before typical pox lesions develop. When pox lesions develop, they appear on unwooled skin and on the buccal, respiratory, digestive, and urogenital tract mucosae. They commence as papules, then become nodular, occasionally vesicular, and pustular, then finally scab. Some progress from nodules to tumor-like masses. The mortality rate in this form of the disease may reach 50%. In the benign form, more common in adults, only skin lesions occur, particularly under the tail; there is no systemic reaction, and animals recover in 3 to 4 weeks. Abortion and secondary pneumonia are complications. In sheep, infection with goatpox is more severe than with sheeppox, with lesions on the lips and oral mucosa, teats, and udder.

Goatpox in goats is very similar clinically to sheeppox in sheep. Young kids suffer a systemic disease, with lesions spread generally over the skin and on the respiratory and alimentary mucosae. Adult goats may have systemic disease and extensive lesions, but in adult goats the disease is usually mild, and lesions are as described previously for the benign form in sheep. A flat hemorrhagic form of capripox is seen in some European goats, and this form has a high case-fatality rate.

CLINICAL PATHOLOGY

Antigen Detection

Diagnosis is based on typical clinical signs combined with laboratory confirmation of the presence of the virus or antigen. Using electron microscopy, large numbers of characteristic "sheeppox cells" containing inclusion bodies and typical capripox virions can be seen in biopsies of the skin. The virus can be cultured in tissue culture, but virus isolation as a method of rapid diagnosis is limited by the extended time it takes for virus cytopathic effects to develop and the need, with some strains, for several blind passages before this occurs. Direct fluorescent antibody testing is used to detect the presence of poxvirus in the edema fluid, and the antigen can be detected in biopsies of lymph glands by AGID using specific immune sera. An antigen detection ELISA is also available.

Serology

Serologic testing can be by virus neutralization, which is 100% specific, or by an indirect fluorescent antibody or an agar gel precipitation test (AGPT), both of which cross-react with antibody to orf virus. An indirect ELISA has a similar diagnostic sensitivity and slightly lower specificity than the virus neutralization assay.[6] Virus-specific analysis of antibody response by Western blot can differentiate the infections.

PCR and melt-point analyses for the detection of capripox antigen have been developed, some as duplex or multiplex assays to differentiate capripox infections from orf virus.[7] These are suitable for use in countries that do not have the disease and do not hold live capripox virus. Loop-mediated isothermal amplification (LAMP) assays are potentially a cost-effective test to rapidly differentiate sheeppox and goatpox during outbreaks.[8]

NECROPSY FINDINGS

In the malignant form, pox lesions extend into the mouth, pharynx, larynx, and vagina, with lymphadenopathy and a hemorrhagic spleen. Lesions may also appear in the trachea. Lesions in the lung are severe, manifesting as lentil-sized white pox nodules to a consolidating and necrotizing pneumonia. Lesions occasionally reach the abomasum and are accompanied by hemorrhagic enteritis.

Histologically, cells infected with capripox virus have a characteristic appearance with vacuolated cytoplasm and nuclei, marginated chromatin, and multiple inclusion bodies ("sheeppox cells"). With the use of double immunohistochemical labeling, the viral antigen appears in cells of the monocyte/macrophage lineage within 6 to 8 days of infection, and later in pneumocytes.[4]

DIFFERENTIAL DIAGNOSIS
Contagious ecthyma (orf)
Bluetongue

TREATMENT

No specific treatment is advised, but palliative treatment may be necessary in severely affected animals.

CONTROL

Control in countries or regions that are free of this disease centers around prohibiting the importation of live animals and unprocessed produce from infected areas and, if the infection is introduced, ring vaccination, the destruction of affected flocks, and the quarantine of infected premises.

Vaccination with natural lymph has been used in some affected areas, but it can spread the disease. Natural infection with one capripox strain imparts immunity to all capripox infections, and vaccination with a single capripox vaccine will give protection across all species and against all capripox infections.

A variety of commercial vaccines are available, and there is no easy basis for comparison. Killed virus vaccines elicit only temporary protection, but live attenuated vaccines protect against infection for more than 1 year. Colostral antibody can interfere with vaccination until 6 months of age. Vaccination programs in endemic areas recommend vaccination of lambs at 2 and 10 weeks, followed by an annual booster.[5] A subunit capripox virus vaccine has been developed.

Vaccination in the face of outbreak is unlikely to prevent deaths during the subsequent 2 weeks and, if needle hygiene is poor, may facilitate the spread of the disease.

FURTHER READING

Embury-Hyatt C, Babiuk S, et al. Pathology and viral antigen distribution following experimental infection of sheep and goats with *Capripoxvirus*. *J Comp Pathol*. 2012;146:106-115.

Radostits O, et al. Sheeppox and goatpox. In: *Veterinary Medicine: A Textbook of the Diseases of Cattle, Horses, Sheep, Goats and Pigs*. 10th ed. London: W.B. Saunders; 2007:1430-1431.

REFERENCES

1. Babiuk S, et al. *Transbound Emerg Dis*. 2008;55:263.
2. Bowden TR, et al. *Virol*. 2008;371:380.
3. Babiuk S, et al. *J General Virol*. 2009;90:105.
4. Embury-Hyatt C, et al. *J Comp Pathol*. 2012;146:106.
5. Yeruham I, et al. *Vet Rec*. 2007;160:236.
6. Babiuk S, et al. *Transbound Emerg Dis*. 2009;56:132.
7. Venkatesan G, et al. *J Virol Methods*. 2014;195:1.
8. Zhao Z, et al. *BMC Microbiol*. 2014;14:10.

CONTAGIOUS ECTHYMA (CONTAGIOUS PUSTULAR DERMATITIS, ORF, SCABBY MOUTH, SOREMOUTH)

SYNOPSIS

Etiology Orf virus. Genus *Parapoxvirus*. Family Poxviridae.

Epidemiology Primarily young lambs and kids. Morbidity may reach 100% and case-fatality rate 5% to 15%. Rapid spread in flock by contact or via inanimate objects such as feed troughs, eartag equipment, and emasculators. Scabs from lesions remain infective in the environment for a long time. Orf infections can cause considerable setback in young lambs and has economic importance as a result of restriction of movement and trade of affected sheep. May infect humans.

Signs Papules, pustules, scabs covering ulceration, granulation, proliferation, and inflammation. Lesions begin at oral mucocutaneous junction and oral commissures and spread to muzzle and oral cavity. Lambs cannot suck or graze. Malignant form occurs with invasion of alimentary tract. Severe systemic reaction can occur and lesions on coronets, ears, anus, and vulva. Lesions can be multifocal in goats.

Clinical pathology Electron microscopy, polymerase chain reaction (PCR)

Lesions Scabs, pustules, granulation tissue, and secondary lesions. Eosinophilic cytoplasmic inclusion bodies.

Diagnostic confirmation Clinical signs, differentiate virus by PCR.

Differential diagnosis list:

Ulcerative dermatosis

Proliferative dermatitis (strawberry footrot)

Blue tongue

Foot-and-mouth disease

Sheeppox and capripox

Treatment. Nothing specific; general care of lesions.

Control. Isolation of affected animals. Vaccination.

ETIOLOGY

Orf is associated with the orf virus, a type species of the genus *Parapoxvirus* (family Poxviridae). In addition to the orf virus (parapox ovis), the genus includes the viruses of bovine papular stomatitis (parapox bovis 1), pseudocowpox (parapoxvirus bovis 2), and a parapox virus of deer. The orf virus withstands drying and is capable of surviving at room temperature for at least 15 years. Restriction endonuclease digests of DNA shows considerable heterogeneity between different field isolates.

EPIDEMIOLOGY

Occurrence

The disease occurs worldwide in sheep and goats.[1] It causes unthriftiness, varying degrees of pain, and some economic loss. It occurs most commonly in 3- to 6-month-old lambs at pasture, although lambs 10 to 12 days of age and adult animals can be severely affected. Outbreaks involving the lips and face of young lambs and the udders of the ewes are common. This disease can occur at any time, but outbreaks are most common in grazing sheep during dry conditions, lambs in feedlots, and penned sheep being fed from troughs. The disease has occurred in musk ox, in which it causes heavy losses, and in reindeer, mountain goats and bighorn sheep, chamois, caribou, Dall sheep, buffalo, wild goats, and camels. The virus can be passaged in rabbits if large doses are placed on scarified skin or injected ID. Mild lesions develop on the chorioallantois of the 9- to 12-day-old chick embryo. Guinea pigs and mice are not susceptible.

The disease also occurs in humans working among infected sheep. In abattoir workers it is most common in those handling wool and skins.

Morbidity and Case Fatality

Outbreaks may occur in sheep and goats, with morbidity rates approaching 100% and case-fatality rates from 5% to 15%. The deaths that occur are a result of the extension of lesions in the respiratory tract, but the case fatality rate may reach 15% if severely affected lambs are not provided with adequate care and support, or if secondary infection and cutaneous myiasis (flystrike) are allowed to occur. In the rare outbreaks where systemic invasion occurs, the case-fatality rate averages 25% and may be as high as 75%. Under field conditions, recovered animals are immune for 2 to 3 years, but no antibodies appear to be passed in the colostrum, and newborn lambs of immune ewes are susceptible.

Methods of Transmission

Scabs that fall off from healing lesions contain the virus and remain highly infective for long periods in dry conditions, but survival of the disease in a flock may be the result of chronic lesions that exist for long periods on individual animals. Infection can be from environmental persistence of the virus or from infected sheep. Spread in a flock is very rapid and occurs by contact with other affected animals or by contact with contaminated inanimate objects, such as feed troughs or ear-tagging pliers. An outbreak of lesions on the tail has been recorded in association with the use of docking instruments.

It has been assumed that natural infections on pasture are the result of invasion of the virus after skin damage induced by prickly plants or stubble; application of a viral suspension to scarified skin is the established method of inducing orf. However, an outbreak has occurred in groups of lambs collected from several farms and transported in a vehicle over a period of 23 hours when there was no evidence of injury to their mouths.

Experimental Reproduction

The disease is readily reproduced by introduction of the virus onto scarified areas of skin. Immunity to reinfection is relatively solid at the site of initial infection, but shorter-duration lesions can be reproduced by rechallenge of these sheep at other sites.

Risk Factors

The primary risk factors are the presence of the virus and the immune status of the sheep. Mixing of sheep, such as occurs in a feedlot with sheep originating from several sources, allows transmission of the infection. Intercurrent infections may exacerbate the occurrence of disease on rare occasions. For example, the disease has spread from clinically normal ewes to susceptible 2- to 4-year-old ewes that were persistently infected with border disease virus. Lambs experimentally infected with *Ehrlichia phagocytophilia* and subsequently challenged with orf virus developed more severe lesions with a longer course than those in control lambs.

Economic Importance

The disease produces only a minor setback, except when it affects young sucking lambs with associated lesions on the teats and udders of their ewes. Loss from lamb mortality and secondary mastitis in these circumstances can be significant.

The disease assumed economic importance for Australia when shipments of sheep exported from Australia in 1989 to 1990 were rejected at some ports in the Middle East because of scabby mouth. Litigation is also a potential concern when zoonotic infections occur at petting zoos or fairs.

Zoonotic Implications

Orf virus is readily transmitted to humans and historically has been a risk for industrial workers handling raw wool.

Lesions occur at the site of infection, usually an abrasion infected while handling diseased sheep for shearing, crutching, or drenching, or by accidental inoculation with live scabby mouth vaccine. Lesions progress from macular to papular stages, are usually single, and are localized on the hands, arm, or face. The lesions are self-limiting and heal without scaring after 6 to 7 weeks. They are pruritic and respond poorly to local treatment. Orf is also a zoonotic consideration in petting zoos and fairs where children allow lambs to suck their fingers or otherwise become infected from handling sheep in interactive exhibits.

PATHOGENESIS

Damage to the skin is essential for the establishment of orf infection and the development of typical lesions. Following viral challenge of mildly abraded skin, the virus does not establish in the damaged epidermis, but instead replicates in the cells of an underlying replacement epidermal layer derived from the walls of the wool follicles. Following scarification of ovine skin and topical application of the orf virus, antigen cannot be detected in the skin during the period when the epidermis is being renewed. The virus can first be detected in the center of the newly differentiated epidermis immediately below the stratum corneum, 72 hours after infection. The location of the virus during the eclipse stage is unknown. The infection spreads laterally and uniformly from the new epidermis, initially in the outer stratum spinosum and subsequently throughout the entire depth of the epidermis. The skin reaction consists of a cellular response with necrosis and sloughing of the affected epidermis and underlying stratum papillare of the dermis. The cutaneous response to infection includes a delayed-type hypersensitivity reaction and an influx of inflammatory cells involving neutrophils, basophils, and possibly mast cells. Class II dendritic cells are also involved and appear to form the basis of a highly integrated local dermal defense mechanism. The lesions evolve through the stages of macule, papule, vesicle, pustule, scab formation, and resolution. The pustules develop within a few days and then rupture, resulting in ulcers and subsequently the formation of a thick overlying crust or scab that is shed within 3 to 4 weeks, leaving no scar. Immunity is solid but will last only about 8 months. Although there is an antibody immune response to the virus, recovery is the result of cell-mediated immune mechanisms. Experimentally, a secondary infection, following recovery from a primary infection, is milder and accelerated. During the secondary challenge, pustules and scabs develop earlier, the lesions resolve more rapidly, and no vesicular stage may occur.

CLINICAL FINDINGS

Sheep

Lesions develop initially as papules and then pustules, stages that are not usually initially seen, and progress to a raised and moderately proliferative area of granulation and inflammation covered with a thick, tenacious scab. Time from the initial lesions to the formation of scabs is approximately 6 to 7 days. New lesions will develop during the first 10 days of infection. The first lesions develop at the oral mucocutaneous junction, usually at the oral commissures, and are accompanied by swelling of the lips. From here they spread to the muzzle and nostrils, the surrounding haired skin, and, to a lesser extent, o the buccal mucosa. They may appear as discrete, thick scabs 0.5 cm in diameter, or coalesce and be packed close together as a continuous plaque. Fissuring occurs, and the scabs are sore to the touch. They crumble easily but are difficult to remove from the underlying granulation. Affected lambs suffer a severe setback because of restricted sucking and grazing. In benign cases the scabs dry and fall off, and recovery is complete in about 3 weeks.

Affected lambs sucking ewes may cause spread of the disease to the udder, where a similar lesion progression is seen on the teats (Fig. 16-6). Lesions on the teats predispose to mastitis, and secondary infection of the skin lesions by bacteria or fly larvae occurs in some cases. In rams, lesions on the scrotum may be accompanied by fluid accumulation in the scrotal sac and associated temporary infertility. A high incidence of infection can also occur where the dominant lesions are on the feet, occurring around the coronary band, the dew claws, and on the volar areas of the intervening skin.

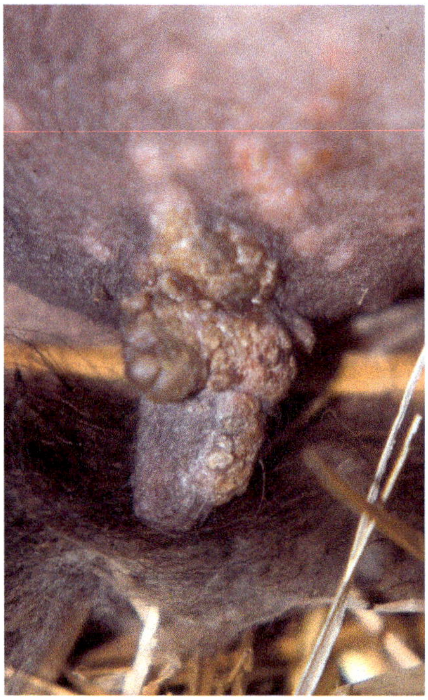

Fig. 16-6 Contagious ecthyma on the teat of an ewe. The ewe contracted the infection by being suckled by a lamb with orf lesions on the commissures of its mouth.

Occasionally severe edema of the face can occur in association with oral lesions. In a severe case, over 50% of 4-month-old Texel lambs grazing good-quality pastures in Ireland were affected.[2] The edema resolved after 10 days but appeared quite similar to that seen with experimental bluetongue infections.

Rarely, systemic invasion occurs and lesions appear on the coronets and ears, around the anus and vulva or prepuce, and on the nasal and buccal mucosae. There is a severe systemic reaction, and extension down the alimentary tract may lead to a severe gastroenteritis; extension down the trachea may be followed by bronchopneumonia. Lesions may also occur in the mouth, involving the tongue, gums, dental pad, or a combination of those sites. These are more commonly seen in outbreaks affecting lambs less than 2 months of age. In the mucosa of the mouth these lesions do not scab but are papular erosive and surrounded by an elevated zone of hyperemia. Extensive painful and proliferative lesions occur on the gingival margins of the incisor teeth.

In some outbreaks the lesions on the skin are highly proliferative and present as raw, raised, granulating lesions without an overlying scab. This manifestation appears more common in Suffolk sheep, and lesions are present on the lips, bridge of the nose, and around the eyes (Fig. 16-7). Cases of this proliferative form involving the feet are also recorded.

A malignant form of the disease has also been observed in sheep. It begins with an acute episode manifested by oral vesicles, followed by extension of these lesions down the gastrointestinal tract, followed later by granulomatous lesions and shedding of hooves.

An atypical case of the disease in sheep after extensive cutaneous thermal injury has been described. The virus was present in proliferative verrucous tissue lesions at the periphery of the original thermal injury. The lesions consisted of tightly packed 0.5-mm-diameter papillary projections.

Goats

An unusual case in a group of female goats has been described, with multifocal lesions over the head, neck, thorax, and flanks of each animal. The lesions developed approximately 2 weeks after the animals returned from a show at which the does were housed for 3 days in pens previously occupied by sheep. The lesions began as plaques, followed by epidermal proliferation and severe encrustation. Affected areas were discrete and approximately 2 to 7 cm in diameter. There were no lesions of the muzzle, lips, udders, or teats. Recovery occurred uneventfully within 3 to 6 weeks without treatment. The skin crusts gradually dried and fell off, leaving areas of alopecia and depigmented skin. Regrowth of hair followed.

Persistent orf occurred in a proportion of Boer goats following an outbreak. In most animals the disease ran a typical clinical course of 3 to 4 weeks, but in 2% of animals it persisted for several months, with lesions disseminated over the body. There were no particular distinguishing differences of the virus genome compared with those of other orf viruses, and the persistence was possibly a result of individual host-susceptibility factors.

CLINICAL PATHOLOGY

Electron microscopic identification of the virus is quick and generally reliable with multiple samples from an affected herd or flock. Viral DNA can also be detected by a number of PCR assays, including real-time PCR and a multiplex PCR to differentiate orf, sheeppox, and capripox viruses.[3] LAMP assays have also been developed.[4] These are comparable to a real-time PCR but require less sophisticated equipment and thus may be a suitable test where resources are limited but rapid differentiation of orf virus and poxviruses is necessary.

Recovered animals have elevated neutralizing antibodies in their serum that are detectable by a gel diffusion test. Other serologic tests have been developed but are not widely available and probably of little clinical value.

NECROPSY FINDINGS

In malignant cases there are irregularly shaped lesions with a hyperemic border in the oral cavity and the upper respiratory tract, with rare involvement of the mucosae of the esophagus, abomasum, and small intestine. Typical lesions are actually proliferative, with subsequent loss of centrally located cells creating an ulcer-like appearance. Microscopically, the hyperplastic epithelium contains swollen degenerate cells, some of which may house eosinophilic cytoplasmic inclusion bodies.

Samples for Confirmation of Diagnosis

- **Histology**—formalin-fixed lesions (LM)
- **Virology**—vesicle fluid, scraping from lesion (EM)

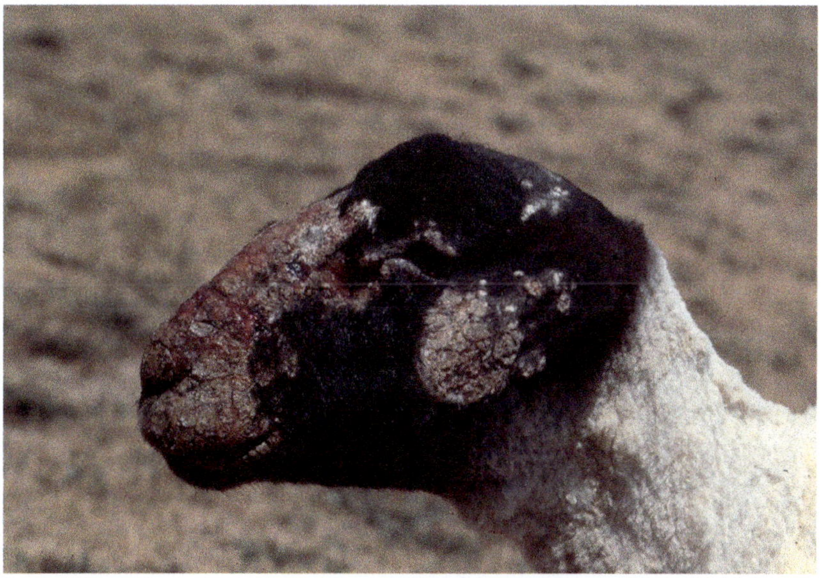

Fig. 16-7 **Extensive chronic lesions as a result of chronic orf infection in a Suffolk ewe lamb. These facial lesions are often accompanied by similar lesions on the distal limbs.**

DIFFERENTIAL DIAGNOSIS

In most outbreaks of ecthyma, the cases are sufficiently mild to cause no real concern about losses or about diagnosis.

Dramatic outbreaks of a very severe form of the disease may occur and may be confused with bluetongue. Very severe cases are also commonly seen in housed experimental sheep, especially colostrum-free lambs.

Ulcerative dermatosis is sufficiently similar to cause confusion in diagnosis, but this disease has not been reported for many years.

Mycotic dermatitis usually occurs on woolled skin, but lesions can occur on the lips and feet (strawberry footrot), have a thick dry asbestos-like scab, and are easily differentiated by laboratory culture.

Facial eczema is distinguished by diffuse dermatitis and severe edema and damage to the ears.

Papillomatosis (warts) need also to be considered in the differential diagnosis for the proliferative manifestations of contagious ecthyma, although warts are extremely uncommon in sheep.

Bluetongue is always accompanied by a high mortality rate and a severe systemic reaction, and lesions occur on the muzzle, the coronets, and extensively on the buccal mucosa. It is more common in adults than sucking lambs. Because it is transmitted by insect vectors, the morbidity rate is usually much less than the 90% commonly seen in contagious ecthyma.

Sheeppox may present a rather similar clinical picture, but the lesions are typical and there is a severe systemic reaction and heavy mortality rate.

Foot-and-mouth disease. The classic developed lesions of orf are easily differentiated from foot-and-mouth disease, but the papular and vesicular stages seen early in the course of orf, particularly lesions in the mouth, can be difficult to differentiate, especially when a prompt on-farm differentiation is required. The raised, firm, papular erosive nature of the lesion with the surrounding zone of hyperemia is a crucial differentiating feature in the field.

TREATMENT

Removal of the scabs and the application of ointments or astringent lotions are practiced but delay healing in most cases. Antiviral drugs have been combined with emollients in gels and sprays (e.g., cidofovir and sucralfate).[5] These formulations can decrease the time to healing and amount of virus shed in scabs, but will be impractical and not cost-effective in most flocks. Supportive treatment, such as providing soft, palatable food, may be helpful.

CONTROL

In the early stages of an outbreak, the affected animals should be isolated and the remainder vaccinated. Vaccination is of little value when a large number of animals are already affected. Persistence of the disease from year to year is common. If lesions are severe and consistently provide a setback, lambs should be vaccinated at 6 to 8 weeks of age. Vaccination when a few days old evokes a protective response. However, prelambing vaccination of the ewe is of no benefit for the lamb and so is not recommended. Vaccination of housed lambs should be given before the time that lesions have been observed in previous years.

Commercially available vaccines are typically a suspension of live tissue culture virus, often with a blue dye. An autogenous vaccine can also be prepared from a suspension of scabs in glycerol saline. The vaccine is scratched in a 5-cm line onto bare skin, usually the inside of the foreleg, brisket, or inner thigh. Alternative methods are to apply autogenous vaccine to a small area of scarified skin or to prick the ear with a needle dipped in the vaccine. Vaccination is effective for at least 2 years, but the lambs should be inspected 1 week after vaccination to check that a local reaction has occurred. A small proportion of vaccinated lambs may develop mild lesions around the mouth because of nibbling at the vaccination site. Absence of a local reaction signifies either a lack of viability of the vaccine or the existence of prior immunity. Immunity is not complete until 3 weeks after vaccination. As a further protective measure, removal of abrasive material from the environment is recommended but is not usually practicable. For the live-sheep export trade from Australia to the Middle East, sheep should be vaccinated at least 3 weeks before shipment to allow immunity to develop.

Because the vaccines are live virus vaccines and the shed scabs contain live virus, routine vaccination against orf in flocks that have not experienced the disease is not recommended. Outbreaks have occurred from vaccine virus.

FURTHER READING

Fleming SB, Wise LM, et al. Molecular genetic analysis of orf virus: a *parapox virus* that has adapted to skin. *Viruses*. 2015;7:1505-1539.

Radostits O, et al. Contagious ecthyma (contagious pustular dermatitis, orf, scabby mouth, soremouth). In: *Veterinary Medicine: A Textbook of the Diseases of Cattle, Horses, Sheep, Goats and Pigs*. 10th ed. London: W.B. Saunders; 2007:1418-1421.

REFERENCES

1. Nandi S, et al. *Small Rumin Res*. 2011;96:73.
2. Casey MJ, et al. *Vet Rec*. 2007;161:600.
3. Venkatesan G, et al. *J Virol Methods*. 2014;195:1-8.
4. Venkatesan G, et al. *Mol Cell Probes*. 2015;29:93.
5. Sonvinco F, et al. *AAPS J*. 2009;11:242.

ULCERATIVE DERMATOSIS OF SHEEP

Ulcerative dermatosis of sheep is an infectious disease characterized by the destruction of epidermal and subcutaneous tissues and the development of raw, granulating ulcers on the skin of the lips, nares, feet, legs, and external genital organs. The lesions on the lips occur between the lip and the nostril, those on the feet occur in the interdigital space and above the coronet, and the genital lesions occur on the glans and the external opening of the prepuce of rams and the vulva of ewes.

A virus, very similar to but antigenically different from the ecthyma virus, is the cause of the disease, which is likely to be confused with contagious ecthyma. However, the lesions are ulcerative and destructive, rather than proliferative as in ecthyma, and bleed easily. It is not highly infectious like bluetongue or sheeppox, and the "lip-and-leg" distribution of the lesions differentiates it from balanoposthitis of wethers, strawberry footrot (dermatophilosis), footrot, and interdigital abscess. The presence of lesions on the glans penis and their absence from mucosae, the typical ulcerative form of the lesion; the absence of pus; and the susceptibility of recovered animals to infection with ecthyma virus are diagnostic features of ulcerative dermatosis.

The typical morbidity rate is 15% to 20%, but up to 60% of a flock may be affected. Mortality is low if the sheep are in good condition and the lesions don't get secondary bacterial infection or flystrike. Physical contact at breeding time seems to be the most probable method of spread.

The lip cutaneous form of this disease is very rare and possibly has disappeared since its original description, or is very uncommon. A clinically similar disease to the genital infection of ulcerative dermatosis, with balanoposthitis and vulvovaginitis, is associated with *Mycoplasma mycoides*.

FURTHER READING

Radostits O, et al. Ulcerative dermatosis of sheep. In: *Veterinary Medicine: A Textbook of the Diseases of Cattle, Horses, Sheep, Goats and Pigs*. 10th ed. London: W.B. Saunders; 2007:1432.

POXVIRUS INFECTIONS IN HORSES (HORSEPOX, UASIN GISHU, VIRAL POPULAR DERMATITIS, EQUINE MOLLUSCUM CONTAGIOSUM)

Equids can be infected by horsepox virus or vaccinia virus. Infection is associated with classical horsepox, equine molluscum contagiosum, viral papular dermatitis, or Uasin Gishu disease and possibly a form of "greasy heel" in horses and donkeys. Classical horsepox, caused by infection of horses by a specific poxvirus (horsepox virus, HSPV), was common before the twentieth century and was considered a rare, if not extinct, disease of horses until it was again identified in Brazil in 2010.[1] The genome of HSPV has been determined and demonstrates that although it is closely related to vaccinia viruses, it contains additional genetic material that appears to confer some host specificity and pathogenicity.[2] HSPV, with cowpox virus, was used for vaccination of humans against smallpox before introduction of use of vaccinia virus.[3] Whereas most poxviruses are highly host adapted and do not cross species lines (e.g., variola virus causing smallpox in humans does not naturally infect animals), this is not the case with cowpox, horsepox, and vaccinia viruses, which can be zoonoses or anthroponoses. Widespread use of vaccinia virus live vaccines in humans was associated with a pox-like disease in horses.[3] This disease has largely not occurred since the cessation of the smallpox vaccination program, but other poxvirus diseases in animals are reported, and infection appears to have the potential to be zoonotic for horsepox and cowpox viruses, or anthroponotic (reverse zoonosis) for vaccinia viruses.[3-5]

The eradication of smallpox and the discontinuation of human vaccination in most countries were accompanied by a gradual reduction of the number of horse cases,[1-3] although the disease is not eradicated, and infections involving cattle, horses and humans occur in Brazil.[4] The virus isolated from horses (Pelotas 1 virus [P1V] and Pelotas 2 virus [P2V]) in Brazil is highly pathogenic in rabbits.[6,7] The source of the vaccinia virus in these outbreaks has not been determined (e.g., wildlife, rodents).[4]

Horses infected with the **vaccinia virus** used in human vaccine programs develop a transient and self-limiting disease characterized by pox-like lesions (papulopustular) in the mucous membranes of the mouth and in the skin of the lips and nose. Infection by particular strains of the vaccinia virus (P1V and P2V)) in Brazil causes papules and vesicles progressing to proliferative and exudative lesions on the muzzle, external nares, and external and internal lips (Fig. 16-8).[1] The vesicles erode, and the proliferative lesions progress to moist crusts and scars.

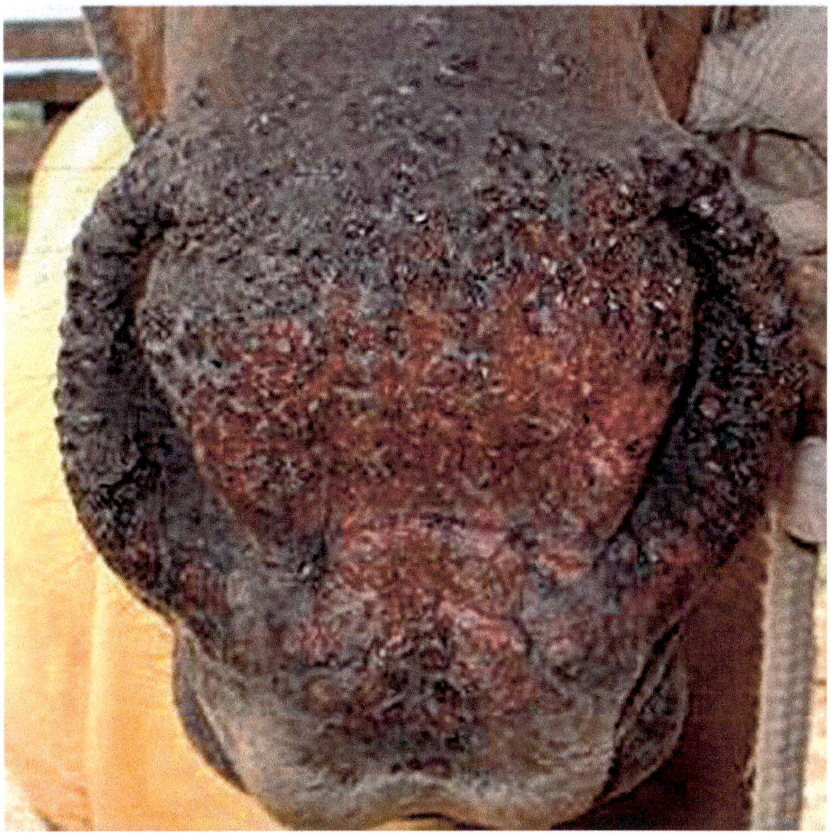

Fig. 16-8 **Muzzle of an affected mare during acute disease associated with infection by vaccinia-like virus. Multiple, confluent papules and proliferative lesions in the muzzle, between and surrounding the nares, and extending aborally.** (Reproduced with permission, Brum MCS et al. *J Vet Diagn Invest* 2010; 22:143.)

Clinical signs last approximately 6 to 12 days. The overall duration of the outbreak is 90 days.

Infection by classical HSPV causes either a relatively benign disease or a more severe, sometimes fatal, disease.[1,2] The benign or localized form (contagious pustular stomatitis) causes lesions in the muzzle and buccal cavity. The more severe form (equine papular stomatitis) is a generalized, highly contagious disease causing fever, skin lesions that can involve the udder, and death in some animals. Both adults and foals are susceptible.[2] Immunity after an attack is solid.

Typical pox lesions develop in a **leg form** or in a **buccal form.** In the **leg-form** nodules, vesicles, pustules, and scabs develop, in that order, on the back of the pastern and cause pain and lameness. There may be a slight systemic reaction, with elevation of temperature. In the **buccal form,** similar lesions appear first on the insides of the lips and then spread over the entire buccal mucosa, sometimes to the pharynx and larynx and occasionally into the nostrils. In very severe cases, lesions may appear on the conjunctiva, the vulva, and sometimes over the entire body. The buccal lesions cause a painful stomatitis, with salivation and anorexia as prominent signs. Most cases recover, with lesions healing in 2 to 4 weeks.

Uasin Gishu is a skin disease of nonindigenous horses of the Uasin Gishu plateau of Kenya and neighboring areas associated with a poorly documented poxvirus. The source of the virus, and its method of transmission, are unknown, although a wildlife host is presumed. Concerns have been raised of the potential for zoonotic spread or anthroponosis (reverse zoonosis) of horsepox viruses or vaccinia virus, respectively.[4,5] Lesions of Uasin Gishu occur on the head, neck, and flanks and resemble papillomas. Various stages of the lesions can be present in the same horse, and lesions can develop and regress intermittently for years. There is no specific treatment, and no control methods are reported.

Viral popular dermatitis is a disease of horses in the United States, the United Kingdom, and Australia. It is a contagious disease characterized by cutaneous lesions in the form of firm papules 0.5 to 2 cm in diameter. No vesicles or pustules are formed, but after 7 to 10 days a dry crust is detached, leaving small circumscribed areas of alopecia. The lesions are not itchy, there is no systemic disease, and the distribution of the lesions, and the way in which they can develop simultaneously in large numbers in introduced horses, is suggestive of an insect-borne disease.

The course of the disease varies between 10 days and 6 weeks. The disease is strongly suspected to be caused by a poxvirus.[1,2] A febrile reaction, up to 40.2° C (104.5° F), precedes the appearance of skin lesions by about 24 hours. There is no histologic description. Recovery is usually complete and uncomplicated. The disease is clinically similar to **molluscum contagiosum** in horses associated with poxvirus. This disease has similar papular lesions, which are hypopigmented and covered by tufts of raised hair, but the disease has a long clinical course. Histologically, these lesions show proliferation of keratinocytes containing large intracytoplasmic inclusions, known as molluscum bodies, which are composed of numerous pox virions.

Differential diagnoses include greasy heel, vesicular stomatitis, viral papular dermatitis, molluscum contagiosum, and Uasin Gishu. See Tables 16-3 and 16-4.

There is **no specific treatment**. Local wound care is indicated. Because of the contagious nature of the disease, rigid isolation and hygiene in the handling of infected horses is essential. No vaccine is available.

REFERENCES

1. Brum MCS, et al. *J Vet Diagn Invest*. 2010;22:143.
2. Tulman ER, et al. *J Virol*. 2006;80:9244.
3. Sanchez-Sampedro L, et al. *Viruses*. 2015;7:1726.
4. Campos RK, et al. *Arch Virol*. 2011;156:275.
5. Osadebe LU, et al. *Clin Infect Dis*. 2015;60:195.
6. Cargnelutti JF, et al. *Microb Pathogen*. 2012;52:192.
7. Cargnelutti JF, et al. *Res Vet Sci*. 2012;93:1070.

SWINEPOX

SYNOPSIS

Etiology Swinepox virus.

Epidemiology Widespread sporadic disease that is generally benign with low morbidity and low **mortality** in older pigs. High case fatality in congenitally infected and very young sucking piglets. Transmitted mechanically and by the hog louse.

Clinical findings Characteristic pox lesions mainly on skin of head, legs, and belly.

Clinical pathology Demonstration of typical lesions by histology and virus by electron microscopy.

Lesions Typical pox lesions.

Diagnostic confirmation Demonstration of typical lesions by histology and virus by electron microscopy.

Treatment None.

Control Control of hog louse.

Swinepox virus causes a mild, acute disease of swine characterized by typical poxvirus lesions of the skin. There are no public health concerns.

Table 16-3 Differential diagnosis of diseases of horses characterized by discrete lesions of the skin only

	EPIDEMIOLOGY			
Disease	**Method of spread**	**Behavior in herd**	**Lesions**	**Clinical pathology**
Horsepox	Extremely rare, usually benign. Can be severe. Spread by contact, rugs, grooming tools.	Solid immunity after attack. No recurrence. Lesions heal 2–4 weeks.	Typical pox lesions in mouth or behind pasterns. Rare cases have lesions in mouth, nostrils, vulva.	Electron microscopy of swab from lesion. Poxvirus present—horsepox virus or vaccinia virus. Polymerase chain reaction (PCR).
Vesicular stomatitis	Occurs in horses, cattle, and pigs. Spread by insert or contact. Clustered outbreaks summer and autumn.	Lesions last only 3–4 days. Solid immunity for 6 months.	On tongue and lips. Uncommon on udder or prepuce. Vesicles up to 2 cm rupture, leaving raw area; profuse ropey saliva. Heal quickly.	Virus isolation, PCR. Many serologic tests available.
Viral papular dermatitis	Insect vector. May affect many horses at one time. Local horses immune. Summer and autumn.	Recovered in 10 days to 6 weeks. Benign, disappears without trace.	Generalized cutaneous papules 0.5–2 cm in diameter, dry crust at 7–10 days, then spot of alopecia.	Assumed poxvirus.
Staphylococcal dermatitis	Sporadic. Lesions under harness suggest pressure or spread by contact. A common disease.	No information, does not spread much. Very difficult to cure in individual. Horse will not work under harness.	5-mm nodules then pustules. Slough, taking small scab and hair. Very painful to touch.	*Staphylococcus aureus* culture from swab of lesion.
Deep ringworm	Diffuse ringworm more common. Spread easily by direct contact or harness or tools.	Sporadic usually. Difficult to cure.	3-mm-diameter follicular nodule, hair loss leaving bald patch. No extensive lesions. Sore to touch, itchy. Spreads from axilla.	*Trichophyton* or *Microsporum* spp. on swab.
Demodectic mange	Spread via grooming tools and rugs. Rare.	Slow spread.	Lesions around face and eyes initially.	*Demodex* spp. in scraping.
Mycotic dermatitis	Wet, humid weather predisposes. Prolonged wetness. Mud leads to foot lesions. Biting flies may spread other forms.	May be number affected if weather conditions suitable.	Lesions commence on head at muzzle and around eyes, with lacrimation and mucopurulent nasal discharge, on lower legs or generalized. Not itchy; may be sore. Matted hair and scab can be lifted off an ovoid, slightly bleeding area.	Branching filamentous *Dermatophilus congolensis* on smear of lesion.
Tyroglyphosis	In horses fed recently harvested, infested grain, or at pasture.	Transient, self-limiting disease.	Dermatitis, itchy, scaly; with rubbing get alopecia and scab formation on muzzle and face, lower limbs at flexures.	Larvae of chigger mites *Pediculoides* and *Trombicula* spp. in scraping.
Photosensitization	Rare in horses. Feeding on St. John's wort or hepatotoxic plants; secondary to cholangiohepatitis or cholelithiasis.	Occurs only in sunlight. Disappears on removal from damaging feed and sun.	Extensive edema, weeping dermatitis, or skin sloughing on white parts. May also be signs of hepatic insufficiency.	Nil.
Queensland itch	Sporadic. During insect season. Only in horses outdoors.	Only hypersensitive horses affected. Disease persists as long as insects present. Interferes with work and grazing.	Intensely itchy. Lesions at tail butt, along back, withers, crest, poll, ears, down sides. Papules, hair rubs off. Pachydermia, no weeping.	Hypersensitivity indicated by eosinophilia in skin biopsy.
Ringworm	Ready transmission by contact and with equipment and premises. Most serious in winter.	Spontaneous recovery in about 3 months. Spread in herd can be very rapid.	Thick, dry, crumbly scab, 2-3 cm diameter, or diffuse alopecia with scaliness begin at girth or under head stall.	*Trichophyton* and *Microsporum* spp. on scraping.

Note: See also discussions of cutaneous globidiosis, multiple abscess caused by Corynebacterium pseudotuberculosis, anhidrosis, congenital absence of skin.

Table 16-4 Differential diagnosis of diseases of horses characterized by lesions of the skin of the lower limbs only

	EPIDEMIOLOGY			
Disease	**Method of spread**	**Behavior in herd**	**Lesions**	**Clinical pathology**
Glanders	Contact with infected horses. Ingestion from contaminated environment.	This is chronic form. Other cases of classical glanders with pulmonary and nasal mucosal involvement.	Nodules and ulcers on nasal mucosa, purulent discharge. Stellate scars on septum. Limb lesions mostly at hock (medial aspect): nodules 1–2 cm, discharge honey-like pus.	Mallein test. Complement fixation tests on serum. Transmission to guinea-pigs. *Burkholderia mallei* in smears.
Epizootic lymphangitis (equine blastomycosis)	Occurs in outbreaks. Spread by spores on contaminated bedding. May survive in soil. Entry through skin abrasions.	Horses cannot be worked. Common in large groups (e.g., military horses).	Ulcers at hocks, lymph nodes at hocks swell and discharge creamy pus. Lymphangitis. Some cases generalized with pulmonary abscesses.	*Histoplasma farciminosum* in smears of pus. Skin sensitivity test.
Sporotrichosis	Slow spread. Sporadic cases. Spread by contact and contamination.	Lesions heal 3–4 weeks, but new crops keep disease going.	Painless nodules at fetlocks ulcerate then heal. Lymphangitis in some animals.	*Sporotrichum schenckii* on smear.
Swamp cancer (pythiosis)	Sporadic. Infection or invasion of wound.	Does not spread.	On lower limbs, ventral abdomen, or below medial canthus of eye, lips. Papules to plaques 1 cm thick, connective tissue with ulcers up to 20 cm, with inspissated pus in pockets.	Biopsy and scrapings for hyphae of *Pythium insidiosum*, *Entomophthora coronata*, larvae of *Habronema megastoma*.
Greasy heel	Sporadic cases only. Horses standing in manure and urine.	Not contagious, but can be chronic and incapacitating.	Horizontal cracks and fissures behind pastern, very lame. Much sebaceous exudate. May develop cellulitis.	Nil.
Ulcerative lymphangitis	Infection of skin wounds in dirty stable.	Lesions heal in 1–2 weeks. New lesions develop for up to 12 months.	Painful nodules around pastern rupture; creamy green pus. Lame. Lymphangitis with ulcers.	No lymph node involvement. *Corynebacterium pseudotuberculosis* in pus. Other organism can cause similar disease.
Chorioptic mange	Widespread. Mostly draft and other working horses.	Most horses in group affected.	Violent stamping; rubs back of pasterns; swollen, scabby, cracked, greasy, painful to touch; lame.	Scrapings reveal mites, *Chorioptes equi*.

Note: See also horsepox (Table 16-3).

ETIOLOGY

The cause is swinepox virus, the sole member of the genus *Suipoxvirus* in the family Poxviridae.

EPIDEMIOLOGY

Occurrence

Swinepox (pigpox) occurs worldwide where swine are raised and is more common in swine units where there is poor sanitation.

Methods of Transmission

Transmission is not well understood. It is by contact transmission and mechanically by the pig louse (*Haematopinus suis*), and because these cannot always be found, it is suspected that possibly flies and other insects may also be involved. Young sucking pigs may have lesions on the face, with similar lesions on the udder of the sow, so there is evidence of spread by direct contact. Vertical transmission is also possible; there are reported cases of congenital infection. The virus can survive in scab material for several months and in dust and dried secretions.

Animal Risk Factors

The virus infects only swine and can infect all ages, but clinical disease is most commonly seen in young piglets. It is usually a sporadic disease, with occasional outbreaks affecting a cluster of litters within a herd, and of short duration. Some or all pigs in a litter may show clinical signs. The disease may appear apparently spontaneously or may occur only in pigs brought into the contaminated environment of a herd in which the indigenous pigs are immune.

The incidence in individual herds may be high. Mortality is usually low except in very young piglets and congenitally affected piglets, where mortality rates can be high. Congenital infection presents with low morbidity but high case fatality. Older animals seem to suffer few ill-effects.

PATHOGENESIS

The virus may enter the skin through preexisting skin lesions and then replicates in the keratinocytes of the stratum spinosum. It rarely affects other tissues. It can be isolated from the skin as soon as 3 days following intradermal inoculation. In field cases, the lesions progress through the classical phases of poxvirus infections but do not usually proceed past the pustular or vesicle stage. At this time there is rupture and the formation of scabs, which heal and drop off. Congenital infection is thought to occur when naïve pregnant sows become infected and develop viremia with infection of the fetal membranes. Not all fetuses are born affected, and compartmentalization of placentas may restrict further uterine spread as occurs with parvovirus infections.

CLINICAL FINDINGS

The morbidity may be high in individual herds where young pigs are affected, but the mortality is usually very low. The incubation period may be from 4 to 14 days. Small 1- to 1.5-cm-diameter papules develop first and may pass through the pustular and vesicular stage very quickly with the formation of red-brown, round scabs. In neonatal pigs, the rupture of many vesicles at one time may cause wetting and scab formation over the cheeks, and conjunctivitis and keratitis are present in many affected animals. In most cases the lesions are restricted to the belly and inside the upper limbs, but they may involve the back and sides and sometimes spread to the face. Lesions may coalesce. A slight febrile reaction may occur in the early stages in young animals, and in sucking pigs, deaths are observed. In adult pigs, detectable skin lesions are less well defined, restricted to the nonhaired softer skin areas, and frequently do not progress through the developmental stages to form scabs. Congenital swinepox is characterized by striking lesions present in piglets at birth, involving the skin and also commonly the tongue and hard palate. Affected piglets are born from healthy sows. Affected piglets may be stillborn or die within a few days after birth.

CLINICAL PATHOLOGY

The diagnosis is confirmed by examination of skin biopsies, which show hydropic degeneration of the stratum spinosum keratinocytes. Focal superficial erosions, marked epidermal hyperplasia with acanthosis, ballooning of epidermal cells, and occasional large eosinophilic intracellular inclusion bodies are present on histologic examination. Hydropic degeneration can also be seen in the outer sheaths of the hair follicles. There is no fluid accumulation between the keratinocytes. Necrosis may occur later. Inflammatory cells invade the underlying dermis. Electron microscopy can be used to detect the viral particles, and the virus can be cultivated in primary pig kidney cell tissue culture with at least seven passages. Crusts, papules, or pustules are best for this. Pigs will develop virus-neutralizing and virus-precipitating antibodies but not at high enough levels to make antibody tests reliable. There is strong immunity in recovered animals.

> **DIFFERENTIAL DIAGNOSIS**
>
> The distribution of the pox-like lesions and the association of the disease with louse infestations suggest the diagnosis. Swinepox may resemble swine vesicular disease, which is characterized by vesicles on the coronary bands, lips, tongue, and snout.
>
> Lesions associated with *Tyroglyphus* spp. mites are usually larger, occur anywhere on the body, and, like those of sarcoptic mange, are usually accompanied by itching. The causative mites are detectable in skin scrapings. Ringworm and pityriasis rosea have characteristic lesions that do not itch, occur in older pigs than typically does swinepox, and fungal spores are present in scrapings in the former disease.
>
> A vesicular disease with necrosis resembling swinepox has been attributed to infection with parvovirus, but there is little evidence that parvovirus is a primary skin pathogen.

TREATMENT

No specific treatment is available, and lesions cause so little concern to the pig, and heal so rapidly, that none is attempted.

CONTROL

Vaccination is not usually practiced, and control of the pig lice is the principal prophylactic measure attempted in most outbreaks.

Dermatomycoses

RINGWORM

> **SYNOPSIS**
>
> Invasion of cutaneous keratinized epithelial cells and hair fibers by dermatophytes.
>
> **Etiology** *Trichophyton, Microsporum* spp. fungi.
>
> **Epidemiology** Carrier animals are the source; spread is via direct contact or contact with infected inanimate objects. Housed animals most susceptible.
>
> **Clinical signs** Circumscribed areas of hairless skin; thick gray crumbly crusts (cattle) or shiny, bald areas (horses); heavy pityriasis; common locations where infection likely to contact (e.g., neck, sides).
>
> **Clinical pathology** Spores and mycelia in skin scraping, or in culture.
>
> **Necropsy lesions** Mycelia identifiable in skin sections.
>
> **Diagnostic confirmation** Laboratory typing of fungus in scraping or tissue.
>
> **Treatment** Spontaneous recovery usual. Topical ointments such as Whitfield's ointment, systemic griseofulvin. Vaccination widely used in European countries and supportive treatment.

ETIOLOGY

The associated fungi that grow on the hair, skin, or both are as follows:

- **Cattle:** *Trichophyton verrucosum* (most commonly), *T. mentagrophytes, T. megninii, T. rubrum, T. simii, T. verrucosum* var. *album, T. verrucosum* var. *discoides, Microsporum gypseum*
- **Sheep:** *T. verrucosum* var. *ochraceum, T. quinckeanum, T. mentagrophytes, M. gypseum* ("club lamb fungus" in show lambs in the United States), *Microsporum canis*
- **Goat:** *T. verrucosum*
- **Horse:** *T. equinum*, including a dark variant able to perforate hair in vitro (*T. equinum* var. *equinum*), *T. quinckeanum, T. mentagrophytes, T. verrucosum, Microsporum equinum* (syn. *M. canis*), *M. gypseum, Equicapillimyces hongkongensis*
- **Donkey:** *T. mentagrophytes, T. verrucosum*
- **Pig:** *T. mentagrophytes, T. rubrum, T. verrucosum* var. *discoides, M. canis, Microsporum nanum*

Uncommon dermatophytes also found in skin lesions in farm animals and horses include the following: *M. gypseum* and *Keratinomyces allejoi* in horses; *Malaessezia* spp. yeasts causing superficial mycoses in immunocompromised horses; *Scopulariopsis brevicaulis* in cattle; *M. nanum* in adult pigs, in which it is most common and in which the lesions are often so mild as to go unnoticed by the farmer; and *Alternaria alternata* in horses, goats, pigs, sheep and cattle.

A rare but similar disease is tinea versicolor, a fungal dermatomycosis associated with *Malassezia furfur* (syn. *Pityrosporum orbiculare*) on the teats of goats. The lesions are circular, discrete, slightly thickened, and scaly at the edges, but not painful. They are characterized by an alteration in the color of the surrounding skin, either darker or lighter. The infection persists on a patient for at least a year and in a flock for a longer period. Hyphae are distinguishable in sections of the lesions.

EPIDEMIOLOGY

Occurrence, Source of Infection, and Transmission

Ringworm occurs in all animal species in all countries but more commonly where animals are accommodated in dense groups, especially indoors.

Direct contact with infected animals is the common method of spread of ringworm, but indirect contact with inanimate objects, particularly bedding, harnesses, grooming kits, and horse blankets, is probably more important. Spores can exist on the skin without causing lesions, and up to 20% of normal animals in an infected group will act as carrier animals. Premises and harnesses may remain infective for long periods because fungal spores remain viable for years if they are kept dry and cool. Moderate heat and desiccation destroy them.

A dermatophytosis in lambs in the United States, called **club lamb fungus,** affects lambs during lamb show season. Approximately one-third of families reported that children or owners involved in showing these lambs developed skin lesions consistent with dermatophytosis.

Ringworm in yearling horses can interfere with training, causing economic losses because of the isolation required to prevent spread of infection to other horses and humans and to decrease environmental contamination.

Risk Factors

Pathogen Factors

M. gypseum, K. allejoi, and *M. nanum* are soil saprophytes, and the reasons for their assumption of pathogenicity are not understood.

Environment and Host Factors

A high incidence of clinical cases in the winter and of spontaneous recovery in the spring is common, but outbreaks also occur during the summer months, so that close confinement and possibly nutrition seem to be more important in the spread of the disease than other environmental factors such as temperature and sunlight. Humidity is known to be important, with high humidity being conducive to multiplication of the fungus. In calf-rearing and vealing units the prevalence is greater in units that continuously add or remove calves from the stock; an "all-in all-out" program is less conducive to spread of the disease.

Animal susceptibility is determined largely by immunologic status, and thus young animals are most susceptible.

Zoonotic Considerations and Economic Importance

Spread between species occurs readily, and in rural areas 80% of human ringworm may derive from animals. *Trichophyton* spp. infections are commonly contracted from horses and cattle[1] and *M. canis* infections from dogs. Ringworm of animal origin affects adult humans and children, and diagnosis and treatment are often very difficult.[2]

Injury to affected animals is of a minor nature, but sufficient damage to hides occurs to warrant some attempt at control of the disease.

PATHOGENESIS

Ringworm fungi chiefly attack keratinized tissues, particularly the stratum corneum and hair fibers, resulting in autolysis of the fiber structure, breaking off of the hair, and alopecia. Exudation from invaded epithelial layers, epithelial debris, and fungal hyphae produce the dry crusts that are characteristic of the disease. The lesions progress if suitable environmental conditions for mycelial growth exist, including a warm and humid atmosphere and a slightly alkaline pH of the skin. Ringworm fungi are all strict aerobes, and the fungi die out under the crust in the center of most lesions, leaving only the periphery active. It is this mode of growth that produces the centrifugal progression and the characteristic ring form of the lesions.

The significance of skin pH in the development of ringworm is widely known. The susceptibility of humans to ringworm infection is much greater before puberty than afterward, when the skin pH falls from about 6.5 to about 4.0. This change is largely attributable to excretion of fatty acids in the sebum, and these fatty acids are often highly fungistatic. Calves are more commonly infected than adult cattle, but whether this is a result of increased susceptibility in calves or the development of immunity in adults has not been determined.

There is some experimental evidence that traumatic injury of the skin is an important factor for the development of ringworm lesions in calves. Different numbers of microconidia of *T. verrucosum* are required to induce ringworm depending on the degree of shearing of the hair and scarification of the skin. *T. mentagrophytes* secretes a small peptide (hemolysin) that is suspected to result in cell-membrane damage and facilitate infection of the skin.[3]

Secondary bacterial invasion of hair follicles is common. The period after experimental infection before distinct lesions appear is about 4 weeks in calves, but considerably less in horses. Spontaneous recovery occurs in calves in 2 to 4 months, with the duration and severity of the disease often depending on the nutritional status of the host. A resistance to reinfection occurs after recovery from experimental or natural infection even though a local mycotic dermatitis may occur at the reinfection site. The immunity is specific to the fungal species concerned, and in horses immunity lasts up to 2 years.

CLINICAL FINDINGS

Cattle

The typical lesion is a heavy, gray–white crust raised perceptibly above the skin. The lesions are roughly circular and about 3 cm in diameter. In the early stages the surface below the crust is moist; in older lesions the scab becomes detached, and pityriasis and alopecia may be the only obvious abnormalities. Lesions are most commonly found on the neck, head, and perineum, but a general distribution over the entire body may occur, particularly in calves, and in severe cases the lesions may coalesce. Itching does not occur, and secondary acne is unusual.

Sheep

In sheep the lesions occur on the head and rarely in the fleeced areas, and although lesions usually disappear in 4 to 5 weeks, the disease may persist in the flock for some months. The lesions are discrete, round, nearly bald patches covered with a grayish crust. Similar lesions occur in goats, but they are distributed generally over all parts of the body. The exception to this description is a new ringworm associated with an unidentified *Trichophyton* that has appeared in sheep in the western U.S. states, plus Georgia and Kentucky, since 1989. Lesions occur extensively in fleeced areas and are characterized by shedding of the wool staple and exudation from the skin surface. Serious spread of the infection to human attendants occurs.

Outbreaks of ringworm in sheep flocks associated with *T. verrucosum* have been reported in Scotland. The outbreaks have been unusual because of the high morbidity rates and persistence of active lesions for up to 6 months. The presence of ringworm lesions precluded the sale of rams in affected flocks.

In club lamb fungus in show lambs in the United States, gross lesions typical of ovine dermatophytosis were located on all parts of the body and consisted of circular areas of matted wool, crusts, and discoloration.

Horses

The lesions may be superficial or deep. Superficial infections are more common. Lesions resulting from *T. equinum* commence as round patches of raised hair and soreness of the lesions to touch. This stage is followed about 7 days later by matting of the hair, which becomes detached, leaving a bald, gray, shining area about 3 cm in diameter. Fine scabs appear, and recovery with regrowth of hair commences in 25 to 30 days. Heavier scabs and larger lesions are usually a result of rubbing by the harness. Lesions associated with *M. gypseum* are smaller, about 10 mm in diameter, and are manifested either by the development of thick crusts or, more generally, a diffuse moth-eaten appearance with desquamation and alopecia. Less commonly, deeper structures are infected through the hair follicles, causing small foci of inflammation and suppuration. A small scab forms over the follicle and the hair is lost, but extensive alopecia and crust formation do not occur. Some irritation and itching may be caused by this type. The distribution of lesions in the horse differs from that in cows, with lesions usually appearing first on the axillary girth area and spreading generally over the trunk and over the rump; lesions may spread to the neck, head, and limbs. Some cases are clinically impossible to differentiate from dermatophilosis.

Chromoblastomycoses is a sporadic, slow-developing chronic granulatous fungal infection of skin following traumatic injury that has been reported occasionally in horses. Nodular granuloma-like nodules gradually appear that are clinically indistinguishable from habronemosis.

Brittle-tail syndrome of horses is a newly reported disease of horses in Hong Kong caused by a keratinolytic fungus, *Equicapillimyces hongkongensis*. Affected horses develop short, stumpy tails as a result of breakage of hairs in the dorsal layers of the tail.[4] The disease is contagious, and environmental or animal reservoirs (apart from horses) are unknown.

Pigs

Ringworm is not common in pigs. Regular ringworm lesions in pigs develop as a centrifugally progressing ring of inflammation surrounding a scabby, alopecic center. The lesion produced by *M. nanum* is different—there is no pruritus or alopecia and cutaneous reaction is minimal, but the centrifugal enlargement of each lesion may cause it to reach an enormous size.[5] Superficial, dry, brown crusts cover the affected area but are not obviously raised, except at the edges in some cases. The crusts are formed of flakes or dust composed of epithelial debris. Most lesions occur on the back and sides. Spontaneous recovery does not occur in adult pigs.

CLINICAL PATHOLOGY

Laboratory diagnosis depends on the demonstration of spores and mycelia in skin scrapings from the edge of the lesion and in culture. Skin scrapings should be made after decontaminating the skin with 70% ethyl alcohol, placing the scraping in a 10% solution of potassium hydroxide, and potentially adding lactophenol cotton blue before microscopic examination is performed. Spores are the diagnostic feature and appear as round or polyhedral, highly refractive bodies in chains (*Trichophyton* spp.) or mosaics (*Microsporum* spp.) in hair follicles, in epithelial scales, and in or on the surface of hair fibers. A hair perforation test, which measures the capacity of a fungal isolate to perforate human hair fibers in the laboratory, is used in the differentiation of dermatophytic species. Culture can take 2 to 6 weeks to provide a diagnosis; consequently, a PCR test using the primer pair for chitin synthase 1 (CHS1) gene has been developed for use in horses.[6] An ELISA for serodiagnosis has been developed for cattle, but it appears it will be most successful in monitoring response to vaccination and epidemiologic studies.[7]

The most useful technique for the early diagnosis of ringworm in cattle uses a small sterilized hairbrush. The skin lesion is first swabbed with a cotton swab containing 70% to 90% ethyl alcohol to remove environmental contaminants and allowed to dry. The lesion is then brushed; the brush is placed in a sterile plastic bag for immediate transportation to the laboratory[8] and subsequent culture within a few hours.

Examination of the skin of infected animals to detect the fluorescence associated with some fungal infections can also be a useful clinical aid, but many trichophyton fungi do not fluoresce, whereas petroleum jelly and other oily skin dressings may do so. Fungal hyphae in tissues can be identified, even down to the genus, by the use of immunofluorescent staining. The technique was devised for use on necropsy material but should have application for biopsy material and scrapings. Specimens to be sent for laboratory examination should be packed in envelopes because airtight jars and cans favor the growth of nonpathogenic fungi during transportation.

DIFFERENTIAL DIAGNOSIS

The diagnosis of ringworm depends on evidence of infectivity, the appearance of characteristic lesions, and the presence of fungal mycelia and spores. Diagnostic confirmation is by demonstration of fungal elements in a scraping or biopsy.

The differential diagnosis list of ringworm, which may be confused with diseases with similar clinical profiles, follows.

Cattle

- Mycotic dermatitis, which has tenacious scabs that cover a raw area of skin.
- Inherited parakeratosis, characterized by tenacious thick crusts that respond quickly and completely to dietary supplementation with zinc.
- Sarcoptic mange, in which mites can be demonstrated in scrapings; there is intense pruritus and a quick response to standard insecticides.
- Psoroptic mange, identifiable by the presence of mites in scrapings, pruritus, occurrence in housed cattle, and the location of the lesions over the hindquarter.

Horses

- Mycotic dermatitis, which is limited in its distribution to the back of the horse, and *Dermatonomus congolensis* can be cultured.
- Queensland itch diagnosable on its occurrence only in summer, only along the back, and the associated intense pruritus.
- Other equine dermatitides.

Pigs

- Pityriasis rosea, in which no mites can be demonstrated, and the disease is limited to a particular age group.
- Exudative epidermitis has extensive lesions with a characteristic greasy covering.
- Tyrogliphosis is self-limiting, associated with a new source of grain, and characterized by pruritus.
- Sarcoptic mange, identifiable by the mites in scrapings, the intense pruritus, and the prompt response to treatment with insecticide.

TREATMENT

Many recorded cures are no doubt a result of strategic treatment just before spontaneous recovery, but treatment is widely practiced and recommended because it greatly reduces contamination of the environment by infected animals. Local or systemic treatments are used, the latter when lesions are widespread. Gloves and protective clothing should be worn when treating affected animals because of the potential for zoonotic spread.[2] Administration of a live attenuated *T. verrucosum* vaccine to cattle with ringworm is effective in hastening the resolution of lesions.[9] Vaccination with an inactivated lyophilized *T. verrucosum* vaccine twice at a 14-day interval has been reported to be an effective treatment in horses with multiple ringworm lesions.[10]

Local Application

The crusts should be removed by scraping or brushing with a soft wire brush and burned; the selected medicament should be brushed on or rubbed in vigorously. Clipping of the hair may facilitate treatment application. Suitable topical applications include Whitfield's ointment (a mixture containing 6% benzoic acid and 3% salicylic acid);[11,12] propionic and undecylenic acid ointments; povidone–iodine, thiabendazole 1% to 5%, and captan ointments; ointments containing one of the azole compounds, such as imidazole, miconazole, or tioconazole (1%),[13] or enilconazole (0.2%),[5] and a 10% ammoniated mercury ointment; propolis (a resinous substance collected by honeybees from plants[11]); homeopathic remedies;[12] burnt motor oil;[14] a 10% solution of povidone–iodine; 5% to 10% copper sulfate solution;[14,15] solutions of quaternary ammonium compounds (1:200 to 1:1000); solutions of 0.25% hexadecamethylene-1, 16-bis-isoquinolinium chloride (Tinevet), and Hexetidine (bis-1,3 beta-ethylhexyl-5 methyl-5-amino-hexahydropyrimidine) borotannic complex; and ivermectin (SC, 200 μg/kg BW).[16] The long list of potential treatments indicates the lack of a definitive, large-population, randomized clinical trial using objective measures of treatment efficacy and a negative control group. Whitfield's ointment appears to have the strongest evidence of efficacy and is considered to have keratolytic, antimicrobial, and antifungal effects. Topical treatments are probably of greater value in the early stages of an outbreak when the lesions are small and few in number, and spontaneous resolution is likely in younger animals.

Sprays, Washes

When infection in a group is widespread, washes or sprays that can be applied over the entire body surface of all animals are used, although the efficacy of the preparations is less than that of ointments, and daily application for at least 5 days is required. Sprays have a big advantage if prophylactic treatment of all in-contact animals is recommended. Examples are agricultural Bordeaux mixture, 5% lime sulfur (20% w/v polysulfides diluted 1:20), captan (N-(trichloromethylthio)-cyclohex-4-ene-1, 2-dicarboxamide) 3%, N-trichloromethylthio-tetrahydrophthalimide, iodofors, 0.5% sodium hypochlorite, and natamycin (100 ppm). These treatments may not be available or permitted in every country.

Systemic Treatment

Systemic treatments recommended for use in farm animals include the IV injection of sodium iodide (1 g/14 kg body weight) as a 10% solution repeated on several occasions, and, if the high cost of the treatment can be overlooked, the oral administration of griseofulvin has been empirically recommended at 7.5 to 10 mg/kg BW once daily, with no strong evidence to support or refute this dosage protocol.

Spontaneous recovery is common in individual animals within 90 days, and careful appraisal of results in clinical trials is necessary. Many farmers overtreat their animals with irritant preparations administered daily for long periods. A crusty dermatitis, or even a neoplastic acanthosis, may result.

CONTROL

Hygiene

Failure to control an outbreak of ringworm is usually a result of the widespread contamination of the environment before treatment is attempted. Isolation and treatment of infected animals; the provision of separate grooming tools, horse blankets, and feeding utensils; and disinfection of these items after use on affected animals are necessary if the disease is to be controlled. All grooming equipment should be carefully washed and treated with a solution of enilconazole or 1:10 dilution of household bleach. Cleaning and disinfection of stables with a commercial detergent or a strong solution (2.5% to 5%) of phenolic disinfectant, 5% lime sulfur, 5% formalin, 3% captan, or 5% sodium hypochlorite is advisable where practicable. Good results are also claimed for the disinfection of buildings with a spray containing 2.0% formaldehyde and 1.0% caustic soda. Sunlight and a low stocking rate provide very effective control measures, which is why ringworm occurs at a much lower incidence in suckling beef calves in pasture than dairy calves raised in group housing with no direct sunlight.

Vaccination

A vaccine developed in the former Soviet Union has achieved a great deal of success in preventing infection in cattle and horses in most countries of Europe and Scandinavia. The nonadjuvanted vaccine includes lyophilized microconidia and hyphal elements of a highly immunogenic, nonvirulent strain of *T. verrucosum.* Small injection-site skin lesions are present for a few weeks in vaccinated calves.[17] Vaccination of all animals in the group is recommended, and isolation and treatment of infected animals and disinfection of premises and gear must be carried out at the same time.

The vaccine is almost totally without side effects except for very rare deaths as a result of anaphylaxis, apparently related to keeping reconstituted vaccine for too long a period. National vaccination campaigns have been successful in eradicating *T. verrucosum* from cattle herds.[17]

Nutrition

Although ringworm occurs in well-nourished and poorly fed animals, there does seem to be a tendency for the latter to become infected more readily and to develop more extensive lesions. Supplementation of the diet, particularly with vitamin A to young housed animals, should be encouraged as a preventive measure. The adequacy of dietary selenium and zinc intake should be determined.[18]

TREATMENT AND CONTROL

Treatment

Discrete lesions in calves or horses

Whitfield's ointment (6% benzoic acid, 3% salicylic acid) applied topically daily (R-2)

5% to 10% copper sulfate solution, daily for 15 days or 4 times at 5-day intervals (R-2)

1% tioconazole ointment, 2% miconazole ointment, 0.2% enilconazole solution (R-2)

Ivermectin (200 µg/kg BW, SC) (R-2)

Widespread multiple lesions

Topical 2% ketoconazole shampoo twice a week for 4 weeks in horses (R-2)

Consider oral griseofulvin (7.5 to 10 mg/kg BW once daily) in all species, but excessive cost and may not be permitted in many countries (R-2)

Control

Calves

Vaccinate with modified live *Trichophyton verrucosum.* (R-1)

All animals

Don't share grooming equipment between animals (R-1).

Ensure adequate sunlight and house on pasture with low stocking density. (R-2)

Ensure adequate vitamin A, selenium, and zinc status. (R-2)

FURTHER READING

Cafarchia C, Figueredo LA, Otranto D. Fungal diseases of horses. *Vet Microbiol.* 2013;167:215-234.

Chermette R, Ferreiro L, Guillot J. Dermatophytoses in animals. *Mycopathologia.* 2008;166:385-405.

Lund A, DeBoer DJ. Immunoprophylaxis of dermatophytosis in animals. *Mycopathologia.* 2008;166:407-424.

REFERENCES

1. Aghamirian MR, Ghiasian SA. *Mycoses.* 2009;54:e52-e56.
2. Agnetti F, et al. *Mycoses.* 2014;57:400.
3. Schaufuss P, et al. *Vet Microbiol.* 2007;122:342.
4. Wong SSY, et al. *Vet Microbiol.* 2012;155:399.
5. García-Sánchez A, et al. *Mycoses.* 2009;54:179.
6. Chung TH, et al. *Equine Vet J.* 2010;42:73.
7. Băgut ET, et al. *Clin Vaccine Immunol.* 2013;20:1150.
8. Papini R, et al. *Zoonoses Public Health.* 2009;56:59.
9. Arslan HH, et al. *Revue Med Vet.* 2007;10:509.
10. Ural K, et al. *J Equine Vet Sci.* 2008;10:590.
11. Cam Y, et al. *Vet Rec.* 2009;165:57.
12. Gupta VK, et al. *Intas Polivet.* 2013;14:333.
13. Kirmizigül AH, et al. *Kafkas Univ Vel Fak Derg.* 2013;19(suppl-A):A191.
14. Ghodasara SN, et al. *Intas Polivet.* 2013;14:336.
15. Kachhawaha S, et al. *Vet Practitioner.* 2011;12:106.
16. Kirmizigül AH, et al. *Kafkas Univ Vel Fak Derg.* 2012;18(3):523.
17. Lund A, et al. *Vet Immunol Immunopathol.* 2014;158:37.
18. Kojouri GA, et al. *Comp Clin Pathol.* 2009;18:283.

MUCORMYCOSIS

Mucormycosis is a rare disease of humans, horses, cattle, and pigs caused by coenocytic fungi of the order Mucorales. *Lichtheimia corymbifera* (formerly *Absidia corymbifera, Mycocladus corymbiferus*) causes severe disease and death of horses, abscessation of lymph nodes in pigs, and mastitis and abortion in cattle.[1,2] The disease is usually acute and progressive, and antemortem diagnosis is difficult. Clinical signs include fever, diarrhea, circling, convulsions, and acute death. Horses can have ulcerating skin lesions of the muzzle, nostrils, knees, and hocks, which can develop in animals that survive the acute disease. Necropsy examination reveals demarcated necrotic or hemorrhagic lesions in the respiratory and gastrointestinal mucosa, lungs, spleen, and brain. Thin-walled hyphae are visible in routine sections of tissue examined microscopically. There is no effective treatment or control. Zygomycotic lymphadenitis attributable to *Rhizomucor pusillus* or *Lichtheimia corymbifera* (formerly *Absidia corymbifera*) was detected in 0.04% of feedlot steers slaughtered in California. Lesions most commonly affected the mesenteric lymph nodes.[3]

REFERENCES

1. Piancastelli C, et al. *Repro Biol Endo.* 2009;7.
2. Zeeh F, et al. *Schweiz Arch Tierheilkd.* 2010;152:523.
3. Ortega J, et al. *Vet Pathol.* 2010;47:108.

MALASSEZIA SPP. DERMATITIS

Malassezia spp., formerly known as *Pityrosporum*, is a genus of fungi. Dermatitis associated with *Malassezia* spp. is described in goats and horses. A number of species of *Malassezia*, including *M. furfur*, *M. obtusa*, *M. globosa*, *M. pachydermatis*, *M. restricta*, *M. slooffiae*, *M. sympodialis*, and *M. equina*, are present on normal and abnormal skin of horses.[1,2] *Malassezia* spp. were cultured from 5 of 44 swabs and detected on microscopic examination in 40 of 44 swabs of preputial or mammary skin from 11 healthy horses, indicating the need for caution when ascribing etiologic importance to detection of this organism in samples of skin of horses with dermatitis.[1]

Lesions in a horse with alopecia areata included scaling and crusting dermatitis characterized histologically by mild to moderate hyperplasia, mild lymphocytic exocytosis, mild eosinophilic dermatitis, and diffuse parakeratosis with numerous budding yeasts. Alopecia areata might have predisposed the horse to infection, and disease caused by *Malassezia* spp., or the organism might have been an incidental finding.[2] The putative disease in goats is not well characterized.[3]

REFERENCES

1. White SD, et al. *J Vet Int Med*. 2006;20:395.
2. Kim DY, et al. *Vet Pathol*. 2011;48:1216.
3. Eguchi-Coe Y, et al. *Vet Dermatol*. 2011;22:497.

SPOROTRICHOSIS

Sporotrichosis is a contagious disease of horses, dogs, cats, cattle, and humans characterized by the development of **cutaneous nodules and ulcers** on the limbs that may be accompanied by lymphangitis.

ETIOLOGY

Sporotrichum schenckii (*Sporothrix beurmanii, S. schenckii, S. equi*) is a gram-positive dimorphic fungus that forms single-walled spores. The organism survives in a mycelial phase on living or decaying plant material but changes to a yeast phase when it enters a mammalian body through a puncture wound or bite.

EPIDEMIOLOGY

The disease is reported to occur in Europe, India, Africa, and the United States and likely occurs throughout the world.[1] The host range includes humans, horses, cattle, cats, camels, mice, rats, and chimpanzees. Economic loss caused by sporotrichosis is not great because the disease spreads slowly, the case fatality rate is low, and treatment is effective. Outbreaks of sporotrichosis in dairy cattle causes reduced milk production.

The causative agent persists in organic matter, and contamination of cutaneous wounds can occur either by contact with discharges from infected animals or from contaminated surroundings. The disease is readily spread from affected cats to humans. Transmission from horses to humans has not been reported.

Pathogenesis, Clinical Findings and Clinical Pathology

Local invasion through wounds results in the development of abscesses and discharging ulcers. Multiple, small, cutaneous nodules develop on the lower parts of the legs, usually near the fetlock. The nodules may follow lymphatics and extend to the proximal limb. The nodules are painless, develop a scab on the summit, discharge a small amount of pus, and heal in 3 to 4 weeks. Succeeding crops of lesions may cause the disease to persist in the animal for months. Lymphangitis, causing cording of the lymphatics, occurs.

Demonstration of gram-positive spores in discharges is diagnostic, but it is difficult because of their low number in horses and cattle, as opposed to the high number of spores present in lesions in cats. The organism can be demonstrated in air-dried smears of exudate stained with Wright stain or Romanowsky stain. The hyphal stage is rare in tissues. Injection of pus into rats or hamsters produces a local lesion containing large numbers of the yeast-like cells. The organism can be **cultured** on Sabourard agar.

DIFFERENTIAL DIAGNOSIS

Glanders
Epizootic lymphangitis
Ulcerative lymphangitis

TREATMENT AND CONTROL

Systemic treatment with **iodides** (potassium iodide orally or sodium iodide IV) is the most effective treatment. Local application of tincture of iodine daily to ulcers may suffice in mild cases. **Itraconazole** might be effective.

Prophylactic treatment of all cuts and abrasions, isolation and treatment of clinical cases, and disinfection of bedding, harnesses, and gear will prevent spread of the disease in enzootic areas. Thorough washing of hands and arms with povidone iodine or chlorhexidine is recommended for humans handling infected animals or plant material.

REFERENCE

1. Dalis JS, et al. *Vet Microbiol*. 2014;172:475.

EPIZOOTIC LYMPHANGITIS (PSEUDOGLANDERS, EQUINE BLASTOMYCOSIS, EQUINE HISTOPLASMOSIS)

SYNOPSIS

Etiology Histoplasma capsulatum var. farciminosum, a fungus.

Epidemiology Epizootic disease of low mortality of horses in Asia, Africa, and the Mediterranean. The disease has important adverse effects on the horse, the owner, and wider society in communities that rely on horses as draft animals.

Clinical signs Nodules, lymphadenopathy, and lymphangitis, usually of the hindlimbs. Nodules discharge creamy pus. Conjunctivitis and pneumonia may occur. Spontaneous resolution after a long course is usual.

Clinical pathology Organism in pus, fluorescent antibody test. Histofarcin skin test.

Lesions Lymphangitis, lymphadenitis.

Differential diagnosis Glanders (farcy), ulcerative lymphangitis, sporotrichiosis.

Diagnostic confirmation Demonstration of organism in pus. Clinical characteristics of the disease.

Treatment Parenteral iodides. Amphotericin.

Control Hygiene, slaughter, vaccination.

The disease is important in developing countries, such as Ethiopia, that have a dependence on use of equids as draft animals. In these communities, the disease has an adverse impact on affected equids beyond that caused by the lesions, because affected equids continue to be used as draft animals, because of lost utility of affected animals to owners, and because of the wider societal impact of the loss of availability of large numbers of draft animals.[1] Income generated from providing a cart-horse service is often the sole source of income for families in developing countries, and the presence of the disease reduces the utility of the equid and therefore the income of the family.[1,2]

ETIOLOGY

The cause is a fungus, *Histoplasma capsulatum* var. *farciminosum*, a dimorphic fungal soil saprophyte. The organism has also been classified by the genus name *Zymonema, Cryptococcus, Saccharomyces*, or *Blastomyces*.

The disease is listed by the OIE as a notifiable disease.

EPIDEMIOLOGY

The disease occurs as outbreaks in horses, donkeys, and mules in parts of Iran, Asia, India, northern Africa, and the Mediterranean littoral. Most outbreaks occur in autumn and winter or when large numbers of horses are gathered together for military or other purposes. The disease was detected 19% of cart horses in Ethiopia over an 18-month period, with the prevalence of the disease varying by geographic region from 0% to 39%.[3] The disease was more prevalent in areas with higher mean temperature.[3] The case-fatality rate is 10% to 15%, but the course is prolonged. Cattle and camels are rarely affected.

Fungal spores are carried from infected animals by direct contact or on bedding, grooming utensils, horse blankets, or harnesses, and gain entry through abrasions, usually on the lower limbs. A saprophytic stage in the soil has been suggested to account for the difficulty experienced in eradicating the disease. The organism has been isolated from the alimentary tract of biting flies, and they may play a role in the transmission of the disease.

Zoonotic Potential

Infection is reported in humans.

PATHOGENESIS

After gaining entry through wounds, the fungus invades subcutaneous tissue, sets up a local granuloma or ulcer, and spreads along the lymphatic vessels. The ocular form of the disease results from inoculation of the organism into the eye, likely by biting flies.

CLINICAL FINDINGS

The disease is primarily an ulcerating, suppurative, pyogranulomatous dermatitis, and, in most cases, lymphangitis. An ocular form of the disease is characterized by ulcerating conjunctivitis. Of 65 cases in cart mules in

Ethiopia, 92% had cutaneous lesions, 5% lung lesions, and 3% ocular lesions.[4] The incubation period in two horses experimentally infected varied from 4 weeks to 3 months.[5]

In the **cutaneous form** of the disease an indolent ulcer develops at the portal of entry, making its appearance several weeks to 3 months after infection occurs. The affected skin and subcutaneous tissues are thickened and firm.[4] Nodules that do not rupture are hairless. A spreading dermatitis and lymphangitis, evident as corded lymphatics with intermittent nodules, develops. Nodules rupture, discharging a thick, creamy pus. Local lymph nodes also enlarge and can rupture. Thickening of the skin in the area and general swelling of the whole limb are common. The lesions are painless.

The lesions usually develop on the limbs, particularly around the hocks, but may also be present on the back, sides, neck, vulva, and scrotum. Occasionally lesions appear on the nasal mucosa just inside the nostrils and do not involve the nasal septum. Ocular involvement is manifested by keratitis and conjunctivitis. Sinusitis and pneumonia occur in other forms of the disease.

The disease is chronic, persisting for 3 to 12 months. Spontaneous recovery occurs, and immunity is solid after an attack, but many animals are destroyed because of the chronic nature of the disease.

CLINICAL PATHOLOGY

Gram-positive, yeast-like cells, with a characteristic double-walled capsule, are easily found in discharges. The organisms are located both extracellularly and intracellularly in giant cells and macrophages. The agent can be cultured on special media, but the fungus dies quickly in specimens unless these are collected in antibiotic solutions, refrigerated, and cultured promptly. The specimen should be collected into a solution containing 500 units/mL penicillin.

The mallein test is negative, but a sterile filtrate of a culture of *H. capsulatum* var. *farciminosum* has been used in a cutaneous sensitivity test, and several serologic tests, including a fluorescent antibody test, are available. Antibodies to *H. capsulatum* var. *farciminosum* are detectable in serum before or at the time of development of lesions.

NECROPSY FINDINGS

Lesions are usually confined to the skin, subcutaneous tissues, and lymph vessels and nodes. In some cases, granulomatous lesions may be found in the lungs, liver, and spleen. Histologically, the lesion is quite characteristic and consists of pyogranulomatous inflammation with fibroplasia. Langerhans giant cells are common. The presence of numerous organisms, some of which show budding, in both intra- and extracellular tissue sections stained with H&E, Periodic acid–Schiff reaction, and Gomori methenamine–silver stain is of diagnostic value.

DIFFERENTIAL DIAGNOSIS

See Table 16-4.

Glanders (*Burkholderia mallei*)

Ulcerative lymphangitis (*Corynebacterium pseudotuberculosis*)

Sporotrichosis (*Sporothrix schenckii*)

Histoplasmosis (*Histoplasma capsulatum*)

TREATMENT AND CONTROL

Many treatments have been tried, largely without success. Parenteral iodides have been reported as effective in some cases, as has amphotericin. Sodium iodide is administered as a 10% solution at a dose of 1 mL per 5 kg IV once weekly for 4 weeks. Amphotericin is administered at a dose of 0.2 mg/kg body weight every 48 hours for three treatments, but it might not be economically feasible for use in developing countries.

Outbreaks in uninfected areas are probably best controlled by **slaughter of affected animals**. In enzootic areas, severe cases should be destroyed and less severe cases kept in strict quarantine while undergoing treatment; however, the high prevalence of the disease in some areas (39%) and economic importance to the horse owner of the animal continuing to work make this a difficult recommendation to enforce. All infected bedding, harnesses, and utensils should be destroyed or vigorously disinfected. Formalinized aluminum hydroxide adsorbed and heat-attenuated vaccines have been widely used, apparently with success.

FURTHER READING

Cafarchia C, et al. Fungal diseases of horses. *Vet Microbiol.* 2013;167:215-234.

Stringer AP. Infectious diseases of working equids. *Vet Clin Equine.* 2014;30:695.

REFERENCES

1. Scantlebury CE, et al. *Prev Vet Med.* 2015;120:265.
2. Nigatu A, et al. *6th Inter Coll Working Equines.* 2010:83.
3. Ameni G. *Vet J.* 2006;172:160.
4. Gobena A, et al. *J Equine Sci.* 2007;18:1.
5. Ameni G. *Vet J.* 2006;172:553.

EQUINE PHYCOMYCOSIS (SWAMP CANCER, PITHYOSIS, HYPHOMYCOSIS DESTRUENS, FLORIDA HORSE LEECH, BURSATTEE)

SYNOPSIS

Etiology Pithyium insidiosum, Basidiobolus haptosporus, or Conidiobolus coronatus

Epidemiology Tropical and subtropical areas of the world. Pythiosis occurs during the wet time of the year, but there is no seasonal distribution for B. haptosporus or C. coronatus.

Clinical signs All cause ulcerative granulomas. P. insidiosum causes lesions on the legs and ventral abdomen; B. haptosporus causes lesions on the side of the body, neck, and head; C. coronatus causes lesions in the oral, nasal, pharyngeal, and tracheal mucosae.

Clinical pathology Agar gel double diffusion test and histologic examination and immunohistochemical staining of tissue sections.

Lesions Ulcerative granulomas with sinus tracts containing yellow coagulated material.

Diagnostic confirmation Histologic examination of tissue.

Treatment Surgical excision. Sodium or potassium iodide. Vaccination.

Control None.

ETIOLOGY

The causes are fungi, including *Pythium insidiosum* (syn. *Hyphomyces destruens*), *Basidiobolus haptosporus* (syn. *B. haptosporus* var. *minor*), *Conidiobolus coronatus* (syn. *Entomophthora coronata*), and *Rhinosporidium* spp. *Pseudoallescheria boydii* causes granulomatous lesions of the nasal cavity. *Alternaria alternata* causes small granulomatous lesions on the head of horses, especially young horses.[1] *Scedosporium prolificans* has been associated with conjunctival lesions, arthritis, and osteomyelitis in horses.[2] Unidentified fungi also cause lesions containing black-colored granules or grains, the so-called "black-grain mycetomas."

Skin lesions in horses have been associated with infection by wide variety of fungi, including:[3] *Madurella mycetomatis, Curvularia erruculosa, Bipolaris speciferum, Cladosporium* spp., and *Exserohilum rostratum.* Nonpigmented fungi that cause localized fungal infections in horses include *P. boydii, Aspergillus versicolor, Alternaria tenuis,* and *Scedosporium apiospermum.*[3] *B. haptosporus* is a terrestrial fungus that lives in decaying vegetation.

EPIDEMIOLOGY

Occurrence

The disease occurs most commonly in **tropical and semitropical climates** but can occur in animals housed in temperate climates. Although the disease is recorded most commonly in horses, it does occur in young cattle, dogs, and humans.[4] Fungal disease, excluding that caused by the dermatophytes, accounted for 2.5% of nonneoplastic diagnoses of nodule skin lesions examined in Colorado and the prairie provinces of Canada.[5]

Pythiosis occurs mostly during the monsoon season in tropical areas, whereas infection by *B. haptosporus* and *C. coronatus* occurs year round. A survey in tropical northern Australia showed that granulomas of horses were caused by *P. insidiosum* in 77%, *B. haptosporus* in 18%, and *C. coronatus* in 5% of cases.

Animal Risk Factors

The fungi gain access to the subcutaneous tissues through wounds or other disruptions of the integrity of the skin or mucosa. A strong correlation between the occurrence of the lesions and frequent wetting and exposure to water is reported and is consistent with the concept of an aquatic life cycle and **motile zoospores** of *P. insidiosum*. There is no breed, age, or sex predilection. Multiple cases can occur in horses maintained in the same enclosure.

Zoonotic Potential

Many of these fungi cause disease in humans, for instance, *P. boydii* infection causes granulomas of the lower extremities of people in tropical regions and is referred to colloquially as Madura foot. However, there is no evidence of spread of infection from horses or other infected animals to humans, although appropriate caution should be exercised when handling infected tissues, especially by individuals with compromised immune function.

PATHOGENESIS AND CLINICAL FINDINGS

The **life cycle** of *P. insidiosum* involves colonization of leaves of aquatic plants where the organism undergoes sexual reproduction and produces sporangia. Motile zoospores, released from the sporangia, are attracted to plant and animal tissue, to which they adhere. Zoospores are attracted to damaged tissue, on which they encyst and develop germ tubes. The hyphae invade tissue and produce the granulomatous reaction and ulceration. Ejected kunkers (necrotic material infected with hyphae) may produce sporangia.

The large (20-cm), rapidly growing, circular, fibrotic, ulcerative granulomas caused by *P. insidiosum* usually develop on the lower limbs, ventral abdomen, or thorax and contain yellow concretions in sinus tracts (leeches or kunkers).[4,6,7] The lesions are pruritic and grow rapidly, often becoming greater 20 cm in diameter in 1 month. *P. insidiosum* lesions may involve underlying bone, and **osteomyelitis** may be a common feature of chronic pithyosis of the lower limbs. *Pithyium* spp. infection of the small intestine causes **eosinophilic enteritis** and granuloma formation, resulting in colic and the need for surgical resection. Dissemination of infection from subcutaneous sites to the liver, lung, and spleen occurs and results in a progressive weight loss and eventual death.

C. coronatus causes lesions similar to, but smaller than, those of pithyosis.[8] However, lesions are only on the nares, nasal passages, oral cavity, pharynx, or trachea. The lesions can be very slow growing and take 1 to 2 years to become invasive, whereas others grow rapidly. *P. boydii* causes granulomatous lesions of the nasal cavity in horses. *B. haptosporus* causes ulcerative, granulating lesions that have a hemorrhagic, edematous surface, in contrast to the fibrotic lesions caused by *Pithyium* spp., on the sides of the **trunk, thorax, neck, and head**. Lesions caused by *B. haptosporus* are pruritic.

A. alternata causes cutaneous nodules that are not painful or pruritic on the head of horses. The nodules may be solitary but are usually multiple and slowly progressive.[1]

S. prolificans causes infection of musculoskeletal structures, including joints and bone, usually secondary to puncture wounds or surgery. This organism causes disseminated lesions and a fatal disease in immunosuppressed humans.

CLINICAL PATHOLOGY

Culture of the causative fungus is a laborious task but is necessary to demonstrate presence of the organism, although PCR detection is becoming available and could replace culture as the definitive diagnostic test. A PCR test has been developed for the identification of *Pythium* spp., and this test also is useful for the detection of *C. coronatus*. Horses infected with *P. insidiosum* have a positive reaction to an **agar gel double-diffusion test**, and complement fixation and intradermal hypersensitivity tests are also of diagnostic value.

Examination of a biopsy specimen is also of value, but care is needed to include a portion of necrotic tissue in which hyphae are most likely to be found. *P. boydii* is indistinguishable from *Aspergillus* spp. on microscopic examination of tissue. **Immunohistochemical** staining methods, using indirect peroxidase techniques, are of value in distinguishing *Pythium* spp. from other fungi in swamp cancer lesions.

Necropsy examination of horses with disseminated pythiosis reveals small, firm, irregularly branched, yellow–white masses in the regional lymph nodes draining cutaneous lesions and in the liver, lungs and spleen. Histologically the masses are eosinophilic granulomas containing hyphal elements of *Pythium* spp.

DIFFERENTIAL DIAGNOSIS
Habronemiasis
Granulation tissue
Sarcoid
Fibrosarcoma
Amyloidosis of the nasal septum
Squamous cell carcinoma
Aspergillosis of the nasal septum
Osteomyelitis

TREATMENT

The most **efficacious treatment** for pythiosis and conidiobolomycosis is excision, although recurrence is common (30%) with larger lesions. Laser ablation of the bed of the granuloma may reduce the rate of recurrence. Larger lesions are usually treated medically. Fungal lesions respond to treatment of **sodium iodide** (20 to 40 mg/kg BW IV, q 24 h, as a 20% solution), followed by oral administration of **potassium iodide** (10 to 40 mg/kg po q 24h for 7 to 120 days). Potassium iodide can also be administered at a dose of 10 g/425 kg once daily, with the dose increasing by 2 g/day until the horse exhibits feed refusal or a dose of 20 g/day is achieved. Treatment should continue until signs of mycotic disease have resolved, which is often weeks to months. An alternative to potassium iodide is ethylenediamine dihydroiodide (1.3 mg/kg, oral q 12 hours for up to 4 months and q 24 hours for up to 1 year). Iodinism is a potential adverse effect of administration of sodium or potassium iodide, although this is rarely observed.

Amphotericin also gives good results as a systemic treatment (intravenously 0.4 mg/kg BW increasing to 1.5 mg/kg per day for 10 to 40 days) combined with local infiltration and after surgical excision in extensive lesions. Administration of amphotericin can be limited by its nephrotoxicity, which should be monitored during treatment. **Itraconazole** (3 mg/kg orally every 12 hours for 3 to 4 months) is effective in the treatment of *C. coronatus* infections of the nasal septum. **Fluconazole** (14 mg/kg oral loading dose followed by 5 mg/kg q 12 hours orally for 6 weeks) is effective in the treatment of nasal conidiobolomycosis in horses. The pharmacokinetics of fluconazole in horses have been determined, permitting rational dosing of this drug. Ketoconazole is not effective for the treatment of *C. coronatus* in horses.

Miconazole (5 grams of 2% solution) infused for 4 weeks into lesions in the nasal cavity, in combination with systemic administration of iodides, was effective in treatment of nasal lesions caused by *P. boydii*.

S. prolificans is resistant to commonly used antifungal drugs.

A **vaccine** composed of elements of *P. insidiosum* causes recovery or improvement in most cases. It also causes a severe reaction, sometimes a cold abscess, at the injection site. Other complications include osteitis and laminitis, which necessitate euthanasia.

REFERENCES

1. Dicken M, et al. *NZ Vet J.* 2010;58:319.
2. Berzina I, et al. *Vet Clin Pathol.* 2011;40:84.
3. Valentine BA, et al. *Vet Dermatol.* 2006;17:266.
4. Martins TB, et al. *J Comp Pathol.* 2012;146:122.
5. Schaffer PA, et al. *Can Vet J.* 2013;54:262.
6. Mosbah E, et al. *J Equine Vet Sci.* 2012;32:164.
7. Salas Y, et al. *Mycopathologia.* 2012;174:511.
8. Schumacher J, et al. *Equine Vet Educ.* 2007;19:405.

MADUROMYCOSIS

Maduromycosis is a skin disease of horses characterized by cutaneous granuloma caused by a variety of fungi, including *Helminthosporium spiciferum, Brachycladium spiciferum, Curvularia geniculate,* and *Monosporium apiospermum.* One or more lesions 1 to 2.5 cm in diameter appear anywhere on the skin but with a special frequency at the coronet. The incised lesion has a mottled appearance and drains pus containing the fungus.

Protozoal Diseases of the Skin

BESNOITIOSIS (ELEPHANT SKIN DISEASE)

SYNOPSIS

Etiology Intermediate host-specific tissue cysts of *Besnoitia besnoiti, B. caprae,* and *B. bennetti.*

Epidemiology Endemic disease in some tropical and subtropical areas, with high morbidity and low mortality. Rare disease elsewhere. Definitive host not known. Disease occurs in donkeys in the United States. Possible insect transmission of disease to cattle and goats.

Clinical findings Anasarca, alopecia, hyperpigmentation and scleroderma, and infertility.

Inspiratory dyspnea and loss of condition Pin-point nodules (cysts) on the scleral conjunctiva and nasal, pharyngeal, and/or laryngeal mucosa.

Lesions Parasitic cysts in dermis, subcutaneous, and other fascia.

Diagnostic confirmation Demonstration of bradyzoites in skin biopsy or scleral conjunctival scrapings.

Treatment and control Little information available.

Besnoitiosis is a parasitic disease of cattle, goats, horses, and certain wild animals. Infections in the chronic cystic stage can result in severe disease and/or production loss.[1-5]

ETIOLOGY

Besnoitia are cyst-forming coccidian (apicomplexan) parasites. The life cycle involves a definitive host and an intermediate host. There are seven classified species, of which three occur in domestic livestock. These are *B. besnoiti* in cattle, *B. caprae* in goats, and *B. bennetti* in horses, donkeys, and mules. The other four known *Besnoitia* species infect wildlife species. Cats are the definitive host for some *Besnoitia* infecting wildlife, but the definitive host(s) for the three domestic livestock species are unknown. Recent evidence suggests that *B. besnoiti* and *B. capri* are the same genetically, that they also have the same bradyzoite ultrastructure, and that they may not be separate species.[2,3]

EPIDEMIOLOGY

Occurrence

Besnoitiosis of livestock animals occurs as outbreaks in some tropical and subtropical regions, and sporadically in other areas. In endemic areas, the disease can affect a large proportion of the herd and cause significant economic loss.[1-3] **Bovine** besnoitiosis is recorded in the African continent, southern Europe,[1] South America, Israel, Asia, and the Russian Federation; **caprine** besnoitiosis in Kenya, Uganda, Iran, and Kazakhstan; and besnoitiosis is found in equids in Africa and has recently emerged in donkeys in the United States.[4,5]

Risk Factors

Besnoitia are relatively host specific. *B. besnoiti* infects cattle and in Africa also infects goats and wild ruminants. The Kenyan species of *B. caprae* does not infect cattle or sheep. The natural means of transmission is not known, but is presumed to be by ingestion of oocysts from the definitive host(s). Infection with *B. besnoiti* and *B. caprae* can be transmitted experimentally with endozoites and bradyzoites, and mechanically by infections or biting flies. Outbreaks of disease in cattle or goats occur in fly seasons, and it is postulated that biting insects may be important vectors. Transmission via semen from infected males is also suggested.

Economic Importance

B. besnoitia is an economically important parasite of cattle in Africa and Israel.[2,3] Although mortality is generally low, morbidity can approach 10% in the chronic stages. There is a loss of condition, and the fertility of male cattle and goats can be significantly impaired from chronic scrotal skin lesions. Skins have no value for tanning. Besnoitiosis in equids appears to have a rare occurrence, but there is evidence of an emergence in donkeys in the United States.[4,5]

PATHOGENESIS

Following infection of the intermediate host, the endozoites (tachyzoites) proliferate in macrophages, fibroblasts, and endothelial cells, causing **vasculitis** and thrombosis, particularly in capillaries and small veins of the dermis, subcutis, and testes. They then mature to form bradyzoite cysts (cystozoites) within fibroblasts. Replication is accompanied by cellular destruction and the release of inflammatory mediators, resulting in anorexia, lethargy, testicular degeneration, generalized edema of the skin, alopecia, and scleroderma.[2-5] *Besnoitia* cysts form in high numbers in the dermis and subcutaneous tissue. Inspiratory dyspnea is associated with infection in the upper respiratory tract.

CLINICAL FINDINGS

Bovine Besnoitiosis

Typical signs occur in two stages: the acute anasarca stage associated with the proliferation of endozoites and the chronic scleroderma stage associated with cyst formation.[2,3]

Acute Stage

In the acute stage there is fever and an increase in pulse and respiratory rates; warm, painful swellings appear on the ventral aspects of the body, interfering with movement. There is also generalized edema of the skin. The superficial lymph nodes are swollen, diarrhea may occur, and pregnant cows may abort. Lacrimation and an increased nasal discharge are evident; small, whitish, and elevated macules may be observed on the conjunctiva and nasal mucosa. The nasal discharge is serous initially, but it becomes mucopurulent later and may contain blood.

Chronic Stage

As the disease becomes chronic, the skin becomes grossly thickened and corrugated, and there is alopecia. A **severe dermatitis** is present over most of the body surface. Affected bulls often become sterile for long periods, particularly if the scrotal skin is affected. Cystic stages of the *Besnoitia* have been found in vascular lesions in the testes of affected animals and may be a major contributor to the sterility. **Cysts on the scleral conjunctiva** are considered to be of particular diagnostic importance.[3]

In endemic areas, the signs that attract clinical attention are alopecia and severely thickened and wrinkled skin, which is often thrown into folds around the neck, shoulder, and rump region and the carpal and tarsal areas. Small, subcutaneous, seed-like lumps can be palpated. In cattle, infections of the teat skin may result in lesions around the mouth in suckled calves. The case fatality rate can be ~10%, and the convalescence in survivors is protracted over a period of months.

Caprine Besnoitiosis

The acute stage is not commonly seen in goats; the disease presents like the chronic stage in cattle,[3] with dyspnea and cutaneous lesions. The cutaneous lesion is a chronic dermatitis of the legs, particularly the carpal and tarsal regions, and the ventral surface of the abdomen. It varies from mild thickening with superficial scaling, to marked thickening with hyperpigmentation and a serous discharge. The hair is sparse.

Equid Besnoitiosis

The clinical signs are similar for different species of equids (horses and donkeys).[4,5] Animals may show exercise intolerance, nasal discharge, and inspiratory dyspnea.

Skin lesions, like those in cattle and goats, are present on the ventral abdomen and legs or the whole body surface. Pin-point white nodules can be seen on the nares and sclera, and by endoscopy on the soft palate, pharynx, and/or larynx.[4,5]

CLINICAL PATHOLOGY

There is little information on hematology and blood chemistry. Hypergammaglobulinemia has been reported in one horse. Cysts containing a number of banana- or spindle-shaped zoites can be detected in scrapings or sections of skin or scleral conjunctival scrapings. Ear-tip biopsies are commonly used in surveys of goats, and many infected animals show no clinical signs of infection. Serum antibodies to *Besnoitia* spp. can be detected using an indirect immunofluorescence technique or ELISA, but such tests likely have inadequate sensitivity and specificity.

NECROPSY FINDINGS

At necropsy, apart from any lesions detected upon clinical examination, animals that die in the acute stage of disease usually have widespread petechiae and ecchymoses in the subcutis and edema in the lymph nodes and in the testis in males. In the chronic stage, small white granules (the size of sugar granules) may be found in multiple muscles, intermuscular fascia, and tendons, particularly in the limbs, neck, and nasal mucosa. Parasite stages are evident in lesions upon histologic examination, and they are found in endothelial cells and the intima of blood vessels, often associated with necrosis and a mild inflammatory reaction.

DIAGNOSTIC CONFIRMATION

The most efficient and cost-effective method of diagnosis of clinical disease is the demonstration of *Besnoitia* bradyzoites in skin biopsy smears or scleral conjunctival scrapings. PCR-based techniques might also be used.[5,6]

TREATMENT AND CONTROL

There is little information on treatment. Clinical cure of a donkey with a 9-month history of chronic skin disease is reported following prolonged oral administration of trimethoprim–sulfamethoxazole.[1] Animals should receive supportive therapy and be treated symptomatically for enteritis or dermatitis. A vaccine containing *Besnoitia besnoiti*, grown on tissue culture and originally isolated from blue wildebeest, has been used to vaccinate cattle. A durable immunity to the clinical form of the disease was reported, but low-level subclinical infection did occur.[1]

FURTHER READING

Bigalke RD, Prozesky L. Besnoitiosis. In: Coetzer JAW, Tustin RC, eds. *Infectious Diseases of Livestock*. Vol. 1. 2nd ed. Oxford: Oxford University Press; 2005:351.

REFERENCES

1. Radostits O, et al. *Veterinary Medicine: A Textbook of the Disease of Cattle, Horses, Sheep, Goats and Pigs*. 10th ed. London: W.B. Saunders; 2007:1517.
2. Olias P, et al. *Infect Genet Evol*. 2011;11:1564.
3. Jacquiet P, et al. *Vet Parasitol*. 2010;174:30.
4. Elsheikha HA. *Vet Parasitol*. 2007;145:390.
5. Ness SL, et al. *J Am Vet Med Assoc*. 2012;240:1329.
6. Schares G, et al. *Vet Parasitol*. 2011;178:208.

Nematode Infections of the Skin

SUMMER SORES IN HORSES (HABRONEMOSIS)

SYNOPSIS

Etiology Three nematode species, *Habronema muscae, H. majus* (syn. *H. microstoma*), and *Draschia megastoma*, infect the horse.

Epidemiology Larvae from eggs in the feces are ingested by fly larvae; adult flies deposit infective larvae on skin.

Signs Larvae deposited in wounds or in eye cause local inflammation and the development of extensive granulation tissue.

Clinical pathology Larvae may be found in skin scrapings, biopsies, or discharge; marked local eosinophilia.

Lesions Adult *D. megastoma* cause tumorlike lesions in stomach; other species cause a catarrhal enteritis.

Diagnostic confirmation *Gastric form:* eggs difficult to find in feces; *cutaneous form:* demonstration of larvae, eosinophils in biopsy or scraping.

Treatment Ivermectin.

Control Protect horses from flies; treat all skin wounds promptly.

ETIOLOGY

The various forms of cutaneous habronemosis, with local names such as "summer sores," "swamp cancer," and "bursattee," involve three nematode species, *Habronema muscae*, *Habronema majus* (syn. *microstoma*), and *Draschia megastoma*, the adults of which infest the stomach of horses.

LIFE CYCLE

Habronema spp. adults are larger (1 to 2.5 cm long) than those of *D. megastoma* (1.25 cm). The life cycles are indirect; all species use flies as their intermediate hosts. *H. muscae* and *D. megastoma* mainly use the housefly (*Musca domestica*)[1] but can use other muscid species, whereas *H. majus* usually passes through the stable fly (*Stomoxys calcitrans*),[2] although *Haematobia irritans exigua*, *Sarcophaga melanura*, and the housefly can also be used. The thin-walled larvated eggs hatch in the manure and are ingested by maggots, in which they develop. The infective form is reached at about the time the adult fly emerges from the puparium. Horses become infected by swallowing dead flies with feed or water, or, alternatively, infective larvae may pass through the proboscis of the fly when it is feeding on the lips or on wounds.[3] Larvae that are swallowed reach maturity in the stomach, whereas those deposited in wounds cause cutaneous habronemosis. Stray larvae may be found anywhere throughout the body but occasionally massive invasion of the lungs is seen.

EPIDEMIOLOGY

Habronema and *Draschia* have a worldwide distribution. They are of importance only in warmer climates, where they are commonly found, especially in wetter areas where the intermediate hosts are common.[4-6] Elsewhere they tend to be a sporadic nuisance. Gastric granulomas and most cutaneous lesions appear to be associated with *D. megastoma*, although typical cutaneous lesions do occur naturally and have been produced experimentally by the cutaneous implantation of *H. majus* or *H. muscae* larvae. The latter, however, only cause a transitory reaction. Horses of all ages are susceptible, but the disease is most common in adults.

PATHOGENESIS

Two types of gastric habronemosis occur. The more serious is associated with *D. megastoma*. Larvae invade the gastric mucosa and cause the development of large granulomatous masses that later fibrose. These tumors contain adult worms and have a central orifice through which eggs and larvae escape into the lumen. In many horses, the lesions cause only a mild chronic gastritis. In rare cases perforation occurs and is followed by a local peritonitis, which may involve the intestine, causing constriction, or the spleen, causing abscesses. *H. majus* and *H. muscae* do not cause tumors but penetrate the stomach glands and cause a catarrhal gastritis with the production of a thick tenacious mucus. Heavy burdens may cause ulceration. In donkeys, hyperoxemia, edema, erosions, and ulcers in addition to parasitic lesions have been observed.[7]

In cutaneous and conjunctival habronemosis, *Habronema* spp. larvae deposited in wounds cause local inflammation and the development of extensive granulation tissue.[5] Secondary bacterial or mycotic invasions may occur. In the eye, similar lesions form on the inner canthus, the nictitating membrane, or the eyelid. These can cause profuse lacrimation and other signs of local irritation.

CLINICAL FINDINGS

Gastric habronemosis does not usually provoke clinical signs, but affected animals may, on occasion, have a poor coat and a variable appetite. Large tumors may cause pyloric obstruction and gastric distension. When perforation occurs, there is depression, a fever of 39.5° to 40.5° C (103° to 105° F), and pain and heat on the left side just behind the costal arch. Mild to moderate colic may be evidenced when intestinal stenosis is present. If the spleen is involved, there is marked anemia and a gross increase in the total leukocyte count with a shift to the left.

Cutaneous habronemosis is manifested by the appearance of lesions on those parts of the body where skin wounds or excoriations are most likely to occur and where the horse cannot easily displace the vector flies. Thus they are most common on the face below the medial canthus of the eye and on the midline of the abdomen, extending in males onto the prepuce and penis. Less commonly, lesions may be found on the legs and withers, but those occurring in the region of the fetlocks and coronary band are especially serious. The cutaneous lesions commence as small papules with eroded, scab-covered centers. Development is rapid, and individual lesions may increase to 30 cm in diameter in a few months. The center is depressed and composed of coarse, red granulation tissue covered with a grayish necrotic membrane, and the edges are raised and thickened. Although the lesions do not usually heal spontaneously, they may regress in colder weather and recur the following summer. There is little discharge. The sores are unsightly, are inconvenient, and cause some irritation.

In **conjunctival habronemosis**, lesions on the nictitating membrane may be as large as 5 mm in diameter. The conjunctivitis is manifested by small, yellow, necrotic masses about 1 mm in diameter, accompanied by soreness and lacrimation, which do not respond to standard treatments for bacterial conjunctivitis.

CLINICAL PATHOLOGY

Diagnosis is difficult in the gastric form of the disease because the eggs and larvae are not easy to find in the feces. Biopsy of a cutaneous lesion reveals connective tissue containing small, yellow caseous areas up to 5 mm in diameter. Larvae may be found in skin scrapings or biopsies, and ocular lesions can be found in the conjunctival sac or discharge. A marked local eosinophilia occurs.

NECROPSY FINDINGS

Tumor-like lesions of *D. megastoma* bulge into the lumen of the stomach and may reach the size of a golf ball. Adult *Habronema* are stout worms, but their presence is often masked by a thick, tenacious layer of mucus. This is on the glandular part of the stomach and often close to the margo plicatus.

Granulomatous lesions may be found in all the sites mentioned in the description of clinical signs, and although varying in size, they are of essentially the same composition as described earlier under "Biopsy." Horses that have had the cutaneous form of the disease may have small nodules in the parenchyma of the lung. These are hard and yellowish and contain inspissated pus and larvae.

DIAGNOSTIC CONFIRMATION

A biopsy will confirm clinical diagnosis of the cutaneous and conjunctival forms of the condition. Experimentally, PCR assays targeting the application of the Internal transcribed spacer 2 (ITS2) of ribosomal DNA for specific identification of *Habronema* spp. in feces and biopsies have been developed.[8,9]

DIFFERENTIAL DIAGNOSIS

The gastric form of habronemosis is difficult to differentiate from infestation with stomach bot (*Gasterophilus*) larvae or *Trichostrongylus axei*. These parasites often coexist in the same animal. Cutaneous habronemosis must be distinguished from:

Fungal granulomata associated with *Hyphomyces destruens*

Overgrowth of granulation tissue following a wound

Equine sarcoids

TREATMENT

TREATMENT

Ivermectin (0.2 mg/kg SQ) (R-1)

Moxidectin (0.4 mg/kg) (R-1)

Fenbendazole (10 mg/kg, q.1d. for 5d) (R-2)

Few anthelmintics have been adequately tested against *Habronema* spp. and *D. megastoma*. Ivermectin 0.2 mg/kg will remove these species from the stomach with a single SC treatment,[10] but a second dose is sometimes necessary to promote healing in cutaneous lesions. Moxidectin (0.4 mg/kg) is active against adult *Habronema muscae*. Fenbendazole used at 10 mg/kg PO once daily for 5 days is reported to have high efficiency against *D. megastoma* and possibly *Habronema* spp.

CONTROL

Interruption of the life cycle by careful disposal of horse manure and control of the fly population are obvious measures. In enzootic areas all skin wounds and excoriations should be treated promptly to promote healing and protect them against flies.

FURTHER READING

Hodgikinson JE. Molecular diagnosis and equine parasitology. *Vet Parasitol.* 2006;136:109.

REFERENCES

1. Traversa D, et al. *Vet Parasitol.* 2007;150:116.
2. Traversa D, et al. *Vet Parasitol.* 2006;141:285.
3. Traversa D, et al. *Med Vet Entomol.* 2008;22:283.
4. Naem S. *Parasitol Res.* 2007;101:1303.
5. Yarmut Y, et al. *Isr J Vet Med.* 2008;63:87.
6. Schuster RK, et al. *Vet Parasitol.* 2010;174:170.
7. Teixeira WF, et al. *Rev Bras Parasitol Vet.* 2014;23:534.
8. Buzzell GR, et al. *Parasitol Res.* 2011;108:629.
9. Al-Mkaddem AK, et al. *Equine Vet J.* 2014;10(1111):doi.
10. Cutolo AA, et al. *Rev Bras Parasitol Vet.* 2011;20:171.

RHABDITID DERMATITIS

Pelodera is a subgenus of the soil nematode *Rhabditis*. Dermatitis associated with the larvae of *P. strongyloides* is rare. It is recorded most commonly in the dog,[1] but outbreaks have been observed in cattle, sheep, and horses. It has also been an incidental finding in other skin diseases associated with poor husbandry practices. Alopecia is marked, particularly on the neck and flanks. In moderate cases the skin on affected areas is thickened, wrinkled, and scurfy, and some pustules are present on the ventral abdomen and udder. Pustules are up to 1 cm in diameter and contain thick, yellow caseous material and worms. There is marked irritation and, in severe cases, affected areas are swollen and raw and exude serum.

Pelodera strongyloides is a free-living soil nematode found particularly in decaying leaf mold and similar material. When warm-blooded animals lie on its habitat for prolonged periods, it takes the opportunity to invade the skin. Thus infestation is encouraged by housing animals on warm, wet bedding. Under favorable conditions, the disease may spread rapidly. In these circumstances the lesions occur most commonly where the skin contacts the bedding. The nematodes are easily detected in skin scrapings or biopsy specimens and in samples of the bedding, preferably taken from the top few centimeters in the pen.

Control measures include the regular removal of soiled bedding and steps to ensure that the litter is kept dry. Spontaneous recovery usually occurs if these precautions are taken, but local application of a parasiticide and symptomatic therapy will speed recovery.

REFERENCE

1. Saari SA, Nikander SE. *Acta Vet Scand.* 2006;48:18.

ONCHOCERCIASIS (WORM NODULE DISEASE)

Onchocerca spp. are filamentous, thread-like nematodes found mostly as convoluted masses in fibrous tissues. They vary in length; those of the horse are 15 to 18 cm long, whereas bovine species may be as long as 75 cm. They are filarial worms, and the females produce motile embryos (microfilariae). These congregate in the skin and subcutaneous tissues at the favored feeding site of their intermediate host. Each *Onchocerca* species uses a particular biting fly, usually a species of *Culicoides* (midge) or *Simulium* (blackfly). Transmission takes place when infective larvae that develop in the fly are deposited on the skin of their host at a subsequent feed.

Infestation by adult worms is often symptomless, and prevalence tends to increase with age. Relatively nonpathogenic species of widespread occurrence in cattle include *O. gutturosa* in the ligamentum nuchae and *O. lienalis* in the gastrosplenic ligament, whereas horses often harbor *O. cervicalis* in the ligamentum nuchae and *O. reticulata* around the flexor tendons. In horses *O. cervicalis* can cause recurrent fluid-filled masses over the withers that lead to mild bone lysis of the dorsal spinous processes and mineralization within the soft tissue swelling.[1,2] Some cause rejection of meat for human consumption. *O. gibsoni* in Australian cattle, for example, provokes nodules up to 3 cm across in subcutaneous tissues, especially in the brisket. *O. ochengi* produces subcutaneous nodules in African cattle,[3,4] most commonly on the scrotum and udder. Other species may be more pathogenic, such as *O. armillata*, which lives in the aorta of cattle, buffalo, and goats in India and Iran.

Losses caused by adult worms are slight, although *O. gibsoni* in cattle causes unsightly lesions and rejection of beef carcasses from the high-class meat trade. The characteristic nodules of *O. gibsoni* are usually freely movable and consist of fibrous tissue canalized by the long body of the worms. With *O. armillata*, the inner wall of the aorta may be corrugated and swollen. In horses, new infections with *O. reticulata* may cause swelling of the suspensory ligament and a hot edematous swelling of the posterior part of the cannon that persists for 3 to 4 weeks. After the swelling subsides, the suspensory ligament remains thickened, and small caseated or calcified nodules may be palpated. Affected animals are lame while the area is edematous and swollen, but many recover when the swelling disappears. *O. cervicalis* causes fibrotic, caseous, and calcified lesions in the ligamentum nuchae, but clinical signs are not seen. The conditions known as "poll evil" and "fistulous withers" are no longer thought to be associated with this parasite.

Microfilariae may sometimes be damaging. Those of *O. cervicalis*, for example, are occasionally observed in the cornea of horses, but the proposed causal relationship with periodic ophthalmitis is no longer thought to be valid. They can, however, induce hypersensitivity reactions in the skin of some individuals. Lesions are characterized by alopecia, scaliness, and pruritus, particularly along the ventral abdomen. They may extend between the forelegs and backlegs to include the thigh, and in severe cases they may extend up the lower abdominal wall. Some horses have lesions on the face, neck, or thorax. The lesions may be confused with those associated with horn-fly feeding, but these are more likely to include crusting and ulcerating dermatitis. In onchocercosis, microfilariae are not detectable in the bloodstream but may be found in skin biopsies. *O. ochengi* in African cattle has been associated with a dermatitis resembling demodectic mange and pox, and in Turkey microfilariae of *O. gutterosa*, *O. lienalis*, and an unidentified species have recently been reported in association with teat lesions, including sores, chaps, and nodules.[5] In cattle, sheep, and horses common pathologic lesions that have been observed in muscle fasciae and connective tissues include greenish-gray coloration, edema, and small (3 to 10 mm) pale granulomatous nodules on fasciae. In the liver there are multifocal, small (2 to 6 mm), clustered pale or yellowish nodules. Histopathological examination of the nodules shows mild to intense infiltration with eosinophilic granulocytes and multifocal nodular lymphoplasmacytic aggregations.[5]

TREATMENT
Ivermectin (0.2 mg/kg, PO) (R2)
Moxidectin (0.4 mg/kg, PO) (R2)

Control of the intermediate hosts is virtually impossible, but valuable horses prone to hypersensitivity to *O. cervicalis* microfilariae can be partially protected by housing at night because most *Culicoides* species feed during twilight hours and/or at night. The use of insect repellents and avoidance, if possible, of grazing areas where the insects are likely to be in large numbers will also be beneficial. There is no specific treatment for the adult worms. A novel approach has been the experimental use of tetracycline to eliminate *O. ochengi* by killing the symbiotic bacterium *Wolbachia*, which is found in many, but not all, filarial species.[6,7] An experimental multivalent subunit vaccine based on recombinant proteins of *O. volvulus* has shown partial protection against patent *O. ochengi* infection in cattle.[8,9] Experimental treatment with three doses of 4 mg/kg melarsomine hydrochloride in aqueous solution by slow IV injection on alternate days has been shown to be macrofilaricidal in cattle with *O. ochengi* infection.[10] Oral ivermectin 0.2 mg/kg or moxidectin 0.4 mg/kg can be used to eliminate microfilariae in horses, but recurrence of microfilariae and lesions has been observed even after repeated treatment with ivermetin.[1,11] About 10% of treated horses develop an edematous reaction within 24 hours. This is usually restricted to the area of the lesion, but some may develop a pruritic ventral edema.

REFERENCES

1. Metry CA, et al. *J Am Vet Med Assoc.* 2007;231:39.
2. Hestvik G, et al. *J Vet Diagn Invest.* 2006;18:307.
3. Hildebrandt JC, et al. *Parasitol Res.* 2012;111:2217.
4. Eisenbarth A, et al. *Acta Trop.* 2013;127:261.
5. Solismaa M, et al. *Acta Vet Scand.* 2008;50:20.
6. Bah GS, et al. *Antimicrob Agents Chemother.* 2014;58:801.
7. Hoerauf A, et al. *Med Microbiol Immunol.* 2008;197:295.
8. Makepeace BL, et al. *PloS Negl Trop Dis.* 2009;3:10.
9. Achukwi MD, et al. *Parasite Immunol.* 2007;29:113.
10. Tchakoute VL, et al. *Proc Natl Acad Sci USA.* 2006;103:5971.
11. Katabarwa MN, et al. *J Parasitol Res.* 2013;2013:420928.

PARAFILARIOSIS

Horses in Europe, particularly eastern Europe, China, South America, and North Africa, are sometimes infected with *Parafilaria multipapillosa*, a 3- to 6-cm-long nematode. The female lives in a nodule in the skin, which it pierces to lay eggs on the surface. The subcutaneous nodules ulcerate, bleed, heal, and disappear spontaneously. The hemorrhagic exudate from the lesion attracts bloodsucking flies such as *Haematobia*, which ingest the eggs and act as the intermediate host. The condition is relatively benign, occurring in the spring, summer, and autumn. Many nodules may occur on a horse, but although unsightly, they do little harm unless they interfere with harness straps.

Similar lesions in cattle are associated with *P. bovicola*, which is endemic in eastern and some western European countries,[1-4] India, the Philippines, Japan, and South Africa. It has recently become established in Canada, Ireland, and Sweden, where it spread at a rate of 50 km/year. Muscid flies, for example, *Musca autumnalis* in Sweden and Belgium,[1] act as the intermediate host, and the prepatent period in cattle is 7 to 9 months.[1] The condition is seen mostly in late winter, spring, and summer and causes widespread economic losses as a result of carcass trimming and hide damage. The majority of lesions are superficial and localized, but sometimes they cover the whole carcass. In such cases intermuscular lesions will be found within the fascia of adjacent muscles. Subperitoneal, abdominal, subpleural, and thoracic lesions may also occur and cause condemnation of the whole carcass. *Suifilaria suis* causes similar lesions in the pig in South Africa.

Clinical signs are restricted to the presence of bleeding points, and a diagnosis may be made by examining a smear of the exudate microscopically for larvated eggs.[1]

DIFFERENTIAL DIAGNOSIS
• Insects bites (mainly tabanids)[1]
• Injuries[1]
• Warbles, bacterial or fungal granulomas[1]

TREATMENT
Ivermectin (0.2 mg/kg IM) (R-1)
Nitroxynil (20 mg/kg SQ q72 twice) (R-2)

Ivermectin markedly reduces the area of the lesions and the mass of affected tissue.[1] A control program for *P. bovicola* using ivermectin has been evaluated. Blood spots were dramatically reduced, but transmission was not stopped. Nitroxynil 20 mg/kg twice at 72-hour intervals is effective in reducing the number and area of lesions, but care must be taken to ensure accuracy of dosing or toxic signs of drug overdose may be seen.[5] Topical levamisole may also be effective.

REFERENCES

1. Caron Y, et al. *Vet Rec.* 2013;172:129.
2. Losson B, et al. *Vet Rec.* 2009;164:623.
3. Galuppi R, et al. *Vet Parasitol.* 2012;184:88.
4. Hamel D, et al. *Res Vet Sci.* 2010;89:209.
5. Borgsteede FH, et al. *Vet Parasitol.* 2009;161:146.

STEPHANOFILARIASIS

Stephanofilaria spp. are very small (up to 8 mm) filarial nematodes living in cysts at the base of hair follicles. They are associated with subcutaneous tissue lesions in cattle and buffalo. There are a number of species, including *S. dedoesi* (synonyms *S. assamensis*, *S. kaeli*, and *S. okinawaensis*), which provokes a dermatitis ("cascado") affecting the eyes, neck, withers, shoulders, and dewlap in cattle in parts of Asia, in addition to '"humpsore" in India, leg sores on cattle in Malaysia, and muzzle and teat lesions in Japan. *S. zaheeri* causes "earsore" in India, and *S. stilesi* is responsible for dermatitis of the ventral abdomen in parts of the United States and Russia. A similar species in Queensland, Australia, affects the head, neck, dewlap, and sternum. *S. boomkeri* has recently been described in pigs in Africa. The adult worms release microfilariae that later develop into flies that feed on the sores. The vector for *S. dedoesi* is *Musca conducens*, whereas the horn fly *Haematobia irritans* is the intermediate host for *S. stilesi* in the United States. The Australian species is probably spread by the buffalo fly, *Haematobia irritans exigua*.

Cutaneous stephanofilariosis starts with small papules that later coalesce to produce lesions varying from 3 to 15 cm in diameter. They are an extreme irritant, and evidence of rubbing is present. Part but not all of the hair is lost, and dried exudate forms a thick, crumbly scab that may crack to expose blood-stained fluid. Skin scrapings taken from beneath the scab may reveal worm fragments. If healing occurs, the scab disappears, leaving a scar. Infection does not affect growth rate, and treatment and control are required only in stud cattle in which lesions are esthetically undesirable.

TREATMENT
Levamisole (7.5 mg/kg PO) (R-2)

Ivermectin is an effective microfilaricide in buffaloes and reduces the number of adult worms. Oral levamisole 7.5 mg/kg once or twice at 3 -to 4-week intervals is reported to be effective. Ointments containing insecticides may aid control. The Asian species require a preexisting wound for infection to take place. Simple wound prevention and treatment would therefore reduce the risk of disease in this region.

Cutaneous Myiasis

Cutaneous infestation by fly larvae or maggots (known as myiasis) causes serious loss to the livestock industries across the world. Losses include mortality, increased morbidity, and reduced production of meat, milk, and fiber. The disease is associated with larvae of flies in two major dipteran families, Calliphoridae and Sarcophagidae.

Two types of cutaneous myiasis can be distinguished: primary, in which the fly larvae are obligate parasites feeding on living tissues, and secondary, in which the larvae feed primarily on necrotic tissues and only secondarily invade uninjured tissue. Clearly, primary myiasis is most significant to animal health and therefore the most costly, not only in terms of mortality, morbidity, and reduced productivity, but also in terms of cost of control. However, it may be difficult to differentiate primary from secondary myiasis because the larvae are superficially similar.

Three primary fly-strike disease states, resulting from the activities of different species, are well known and described. Blowfly strike by calliphorids such as *Lucillia cuprina* and *Lucillia sericata* is a major problem, particularly for sheep producers, in Australia, New Zealand, and Great Britain. The second group are the screwworms, *Cochliomyia hominivorax* (in the New World) and *Chrysomyia bezziana* (in southern Europe, Africa, and Asia), which are of importance across the livestock species and result in great costs for control. The sarcophagid (flesh fly) *Wohlfahrtia magnifica* causes traumatic myiasis in a wide range of livestock species, but has the greatest effect on goat and sheep production. This species occurs in southern Europe, particularly the Mediterranean and the steppe regions of the continent. Because of differences in the nature of the disease state and control practices for each of these three groups, they will be dealt with as separate entities.

BLOW-FLY STRIKE OF SHEEP

Blow-fly strike ("strike") is a very important cause of production and economic loss in most countries where large numbers of sheep are kept. In bad years many sheep may die (up to 30% of a flock), and the expense of controlling the flies and failure of wool to grow after recovery may be a serious cost, both for individual farmers and the overall industry. For example, in Australia the annual cost of blow-fly control and production losses in 2014 was estimated at around A$170 million.[1] Merino sheep, especially those with heavy skin wrinkles and fecal soiling, are by far the most susceptible breed.

SYNOPSIS

Etiology *Lucilia cuprina* and *L. sericata* are the most important primary flies; other calliphorids act as secondary invaders.

Epidemiology Fly numbers depend on temperature and moisture. Flies are attracted to wool that has been wetted or to areas affected by fleece rot, mycotic dermatitis, diarrhea, or urine staining. Incidence of strike is positively correlated with fly numbers, rainfall, humidity, cloud cover, and pasture growth. Covert (unnoticed) strikes provide larvae for future generations.

Clinical signs Sheep are restless, bite at the affected area, and wriggle their tails. Affected area is moist and malodorous, body temperatures may reach 42°C (107.6F), pulse and respiratory rates increase.

Clinical pathology A clinical examination is all that is necessary. The larvae of the primary and secondary flies can be differentiated, but this is of little use and rarely done.

Lesions Moist, malodorous areas containing active larvae. Predisposing diseases such as dermatophilosis, fleece rot, parasitic gastroenteritis, and footrot are easily identified.

Diagnostic confirmation Clinical signs are diagnostic.

Differential diagnosis Lice, sheep scab, screwworm fly infestations.

Treatment Insect growth regulators (principally cyromazine and dicyclanil), macrocyclic lactone endectocides, spinosad, or organophosphates (although the latter are restricted or no longer registered in many countries because of environmental and occupational health and safety concerns).

Control Dicyclanil protects from flystrike for up to 18 weeks, depending on the formulation; cyromazine and ivermectin for 10 to 12 weeks. Spinosad is an option for organic treatment and has short or no withholding period, but protects for only 2 to 3 weeks. The insect growth regulators do not kill existing larvae until they molt to the next stage; thus, ivermectin, spinosad, or an organophosphate (if permitted) need to be used if a rapid kill is desirable. Breeding and managing sheep to be less susceptible to strike, including the strategic or timely application of insecticide, form an integrated control program. For breech strike this is predominantly by genetic selection for decreased breech wrinkle and

Continued

reduced susceptibility to diarrhea, and control of predisposing diseases, especially gastrointestinal nematodes. The Mules operation reduces susceptibility by dramatically reducing breech wrinkle, but it remains controversial because of the pain and initial lost production associated with the procedure. Docking tails to the correct length and strategic timing of crutching and shearing are other important management factors. For body strike, reducing susceptibility of sheep to fleece rot by genetic selection and controlling mycotic dermatitis by appropriate management, such as not mustering or crowding wet sheep, are important.

ETIOLOGY

Despite there being a large number of species capable of causing the disease, there are two species that initiate most strikes and are of primary concern: *Lucilia cuprina* and *Lucilia sericata*. Locations of typical species are as follows:

- Australia: *L. cuprina*, *L. sericata* (secondary flies include *Calliphora stygia*, *Calliphora novica*, *Calliphora augur*, *Calliphora hilli*, *Calliphora albifrontalis*, *Chrysomyia rufifacies*, and *Chrysomyia varipes*)
- New Zealand: *L. sericata*, *L. cuprina* (*C. stygia*)
- Great Britain and northern Europe: *L. sericata* (secondary flies include *Calliphora erythrocephala*, *Calliphora vomitoria*, and *Phormia terra-novae*)
- North America: *Phormia regina*, *P. terra-novae*

LIFE CYCLE AND EPIDEMIOLOGY

The primary agents of flystrike are obligate parasites. *L. cuprina* is overwhelmingly important in the initiation of strike in sheep from Australia and South Africa. *L. cuprina* was confirmed to be present in New Zealand in 1988. and flystrike from this species is now a major disease in that country. In northern Europe the primary agent of flystrike is *L. sericata*, although there are some other minor species that have been reared from struck sheep.

The incidence varies widely, depending largely on the climate, with warm, humid weather being most conducive to a high incidence. In summer-rainfall areas flystrike may be seen most of the year, being limited only by dry winter conditions. In winter-rainfall areas it is usually too cold in the winter and too dry in the summer for outbreaks to occur.[2] Under these conditions abnormally heavy summer or autumn rains may be necessary before an outbreak will occur.

The Fly Population

Primary flies are of particular importance because they initiate the strike and provide suitable conditions for subsequent invasion by secondary flies. These latter flies are not of economic importance but may infest wool matted with dried exudate or feed on necrotic tissue surrounding a healing strike. In warm areas, pupal development may continue throughout the year, but as soil temperatures fall an increasing number of larvae fail to pupate, and larvae may overwinter until the following spring. Adult flies emerge in the spring, and after one to two breeding cycles, numbers increase to a peak in summer.[3] Numbers may remain high if climatic conditions are suitable, with adequate moisture being of prime importance, but fall dramatically in hot and dry conditions during the summer. An increase in numbers may occur again in the autumn.

All adult flies require carbohydrate and water, but females require protein for ovarian development. The flies are attracted to sheep that have undergone prolonged wetting such that bacterial growth and decomposition of the skin occurs. The association of breech strike with diarrhea and urine staining, and body strike with fleece rot, mycotic dermatitis, and footrot, is related to the excessive moisture deposited on the skin or to the production of serous exudates. Fleece-rot-affected wool with *Pseudomonas aeruginosa* has been shown to stimulate oviposition.

L. cuprina deposit eggs in batches of up to 300, the actual number depending on the fly's size and its ability to locate sufficient protein for egg development. Similarly, *L. sericata* deposit eggs in batches of approximately 200.

The average female longevity in the field in Australia is about 2 weeks, and females rarely live long enough to mature more than two or three batches of eggs. In the United Kingdom, mean female longevity is shorter at 5 days.

The eggs hatch in 12 to 24 hours, and the first instars feed on protein-rich serous exudate that has been provoked by bacterial damage or some other irritation. Larval mouth hooks and enzymes present in the saliva and excreta will further digestion of the skin. Large groups of larvae, particularly second and third instars, further damage of the skin, which extends the lesion and ensures a continuing supply of food. The second and third instars are 6 to 12 mm long, thick, and yellow and white in color, and they move actively. Larvae reach maturity after approximately 72 hours. They leave the feeding lesion, fall to the ground, wander briefly, and then burrow into the earth to pupate. The length of the life cycle is highly temperature dependent; it can be completed in as little as 8 days but may require up to 6 weeks in temperate regions such as the United Kingdom. Egg and larval stages are highly susceptible to desiccation, and mortality will be high if the relative humidity in the fleece falls below 60%. In temperate climates when the temperature declines in autumn, wandering larvae that have left the sheep will burrow into the ground but cease development, thereby overwintering as arrested mature larvae.

A few generations of primary flies are necessary before numbers are high enough to cause severe outbreaks, and so warm, humid weather must persist for a reasonable time before severe outbreaks occur. The incidence of body strike increases with the increase in the number of gravid flies and is positively correlated with rainfall, cloud cover, and rate of pasture growth. Other primary flies are not as effective as *L. cuprina* in initiating a strike, and in Australia and South Africa 85% to 90% of all primary strikes are a result of *L. cuprina*. Larvae of primary flies, other than *L. cuprina*, and secondary flies develop in carrion or in rotting vegetation, and their main role is to invade and extend the primary strike. *Ch. rufifacies* is the most important secondary fly in Australia. It requires higher temperatures than the other flies, is found later in the season, and is the first to disappear as temperatures fall.

Detailed population models have been developed for the strike by *Lucilia* spp. in Australia and northern Europe, and both have been used to predict onset of flystrike in sheep populations.[4,5] The latter model has been extensively validated and is sufficiently accurate to establish an early warning system for alerting producers of the impending onset of flystrike, and hence the optimum time for prophylactic treatment.

Distribution of flystrike in flocks is highly aggregated, with a small number of sheep having high numbers of larvae in lesions, a moderate number of sheep with low numbers of larvae, and the majority of sheep being unstruck. In part this is a result of the attractiveness of already-struck sheep to ovipositing flies, although other factors, such as innate attractiveness to flies, shown by the propensity of some sheep to be restruck within the same fly season, also play a role.

Susceptibility of Sheep

By far the most common site for flystrike is the breech, resulting from soiling and excoriation by soft feces and the urine of ewes. Lush pasture, parasitic gastroenteritis, and fleece length are predisposing factors, but individual sheep are predisposed because of their breech conformation. Excessive wrinkling of the skin on the back of the thighs and perineum, a narrow perineum and crutch, and an excessively long or short tail favor continuous soiling of the area and encourage "breech strike" or "tail strike."

"Body strike" occurs along the dorsum of the body, especially in young sheep in wet seasons when fleece rot or dermatophilosis is common. Less common sites for infestation are around the prepuce ("pizzle strike") and on the dorsum of the head when there is excessive folding of the skin ("poll strike"). Sheep grazing on tall, dense pasture are commonly affected by body strike because wet plants keep the fleece on the lower part of the body wet. Footrot lesions and wounds, especially castration incisions, docking wounds, and head wounds on rams caused by fighting, are also likely to provide good sites for blow-fly strike. Young sheep are more susceptible.

PATHOGENESIS

The first instars feed on the exudate produced by the bacterial infection on the skin, but the larvae also produce excretory/secretory enzymes that may cause some skin degradation after egg hatch and provide soluble molecules on which the first instars can feed. Later instars can cause severe skin damage when feeding. Larvae may also migrate from the original area of strike, along the surface of skin, to establish additional focal lesions.

Many primary strikes remain small and are unnoticed by the farmer. Such "covert" strikes may outnumber obvious strikes and are important as a source of future generations of flies. Once the initial strike is made, the site becomes suitable for the secondary flies, which invade and extend the lesion. The effects of strike include toxemia as a result of absorption of toxic products of tissue decomposition, loss of skin and subsequent fluid loss, and secondary bacterial invasion.

CLINICAL FINDINGS

Individual sheep may be struck at any time provided they are in a susceptible condition. Massive outbreaks tend to be confined to periods of humid, warm weather and are therefore in temperate areas usually limited in length to relatively short periods of 2 to 3 weeks, but in subtropical areas characterized by summer rainfall, severe strikes may occur over many months.

The clinical effects of blow-fly strike vary with the site affected, but all struck sheep have a basic pattern of behavior caused by the irritation of the larvae. The sheep are restless, moving about from place to place with their heads held close to the ground, and they become anorexic. They tend to bite or kick at the struck area and continually wriggle their tails.

If the area is large, there is an obvious odor, and the wool can be seen to be slightly lifted above the normal surrounding wool. The affected wool is moist and usually brown in color, although in wet seasons (when fleece rot is prevalent) other colors may be evident. In very early cases, the maggots may still be in pockets in the wool and not yet in contact with the skin. When they have reached the skin, it is inflamed and then ulcerated, and the maggots begin burrowing into the subcutaneous tissue.

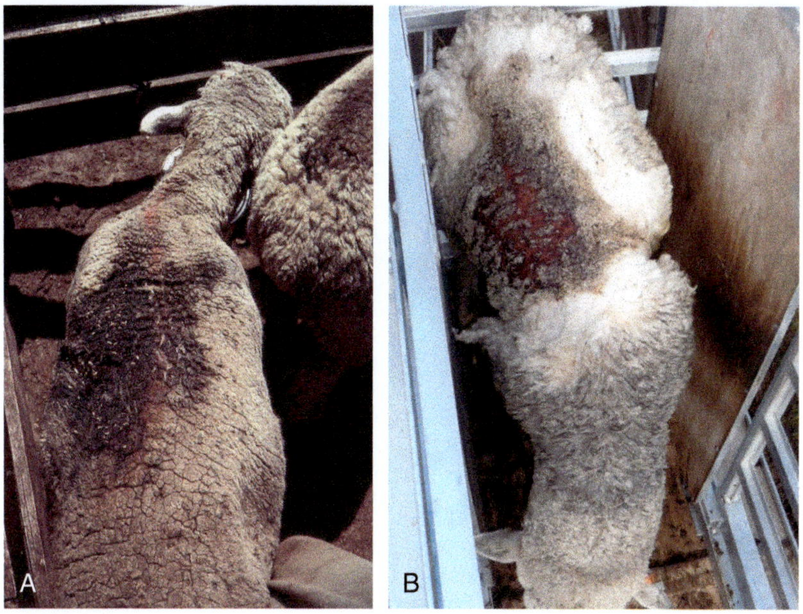

Fig. 16-9 **A, Body strike on a wether as viewed from above. The wether is depressed, and maggots (white) are visible on the surface of the struck area (blackened area of wool). B, Body strike on a weaned sheep as viewed from above. The wool has been clipped away from the edges of the lesion before application of treatment.**

Three days after the primary oviposition feed intake is reduced, rectal temperature rises to about 42°C (108°F), and pulse and respiratory rates increase. There is a reduction of feed intake and loss of body weight, and some sheep may die.[6] The wool may be too hot to handle as a result of the inflammation caused by the mass of maggots that can be seen when the wool over the strike is opened. When primary strikes are invaded by secondary flies, particularly *C. rufifacies*, the affected area is extended, and the maggots may burrow deeply into the tissues. Affected sheep may lose their fleece over the affected area (Fig. 16-9) and may suffer a break in the remaining fleece. Tracts of discolored wool may lead to other affected areas of skin. As the struck area extends, a scab forms over the center, the wool falls out, and the maggots are active only at the periphery.

CLINICAL PATHOLOGY AND NECROPSY FINDINGS

A clinical examination is all that is necessary to make the diagnosis, but identification of the flies responsible may be important if epidemiology is being considered. Identification of larvae should be carried out by a specialist. Molecular techniques for accurate identification are available but are a specialized research technique rather than routine diagnostic tool. Preservation of the larval stages is critical to these techniques, and larvae should be rapidly frozen or preserved in 70% ethanol. Fly trapping may not correlate with larval findings because not all flies are attracted equally by the commonly used baits.

DIFFERENTIAL DIAGNOSIS

Attention will be drawn to affected sheep by their foot stamping, tail twitching, and biting at the affected part. Affected sheep can easily be diagnosed by finding the moist, malodorous, maggot-infested area. Many covert strikes may be present without producing clinical signs. Predisposing diseases such as footrot, wound infections, dermatophilosis, and diarrhea resulting from parasitic gastroenteritis are usually easily detected, and fleece rot is indicated by matting of the wool and discoloration.

TREATMENT

Removal of wool from the surrounding area removes most of the maggots, and applying a dressing prevents reinfestation of the wound. Dressings containing cyromazine, spinosad, ivermectin, or an organophosphate such as diazinon, tetrachlorfenvinphos, or propetamphos (if permitted), are the most commonly used. Cyromazine is an insect growth regulator, and thus live larvae will be seen in the fleece for some days after treatment. Thus other chemicals need to be included in a dressing if immediate killing of larvae is desirable. Ivermectin at 0.3 mg/kg is highly effective in killing all larval stages, and no resistance has yet been reported. However, resistance to organophosphates is widespread in Australia; many products do not kill all the resistant larvae, with some performing poorly even against susceptible larvae. Preventing reinfestations is important, and thus application of the larvicide to the wool surrounding the treated area is essential.

CONTROL

In Australia, practical control of breech strike of Merino sheep in extensive farming areas has relied on the use of the Mules operation, which removes breech wrinkle and extends the bare areas around the perineum and tail. This has been integrated with other strategies to reduce the susceptibility of Merino sheep to strike, such as effective worm control to reduce diarrhea, and hence contamination of the perineal region with feces ("breech soiling"), correct tail length, strategic timing of crutching and shearing, and timely application of insecticides (an integrated pest management approach).[2,7] Control of strike in other situations is based on insecticidal treatment and treatment of wounds as they occur.

Under conditions of extensive sheep rearing, such as occur in Australia, New Zealand, and South Africa, and where climatic conditions are conducive to the development of the disease, the control of blow-fly strike is a major challenge. An extensive literature on the subject is available, so only a summary is given here.

Control programs can be thought of as having three components: reduction in fly numbers (mainly by strategic application of insecticide and fly trapping), prediction of risk periods (to most appropriately time activities such as crutching, shearing, or the application of insecticide), and reduction in susceptibility of sheep (mulesing of Merinos, genetic selection for plain breeches and/or reduced breech cover; control of predisposing factors, particularly diarrhea and fleece rot).

Reduction of Fly Numbers

Reducing the fly population has been of limited value because there are usually enough flies present to strike all susceptible sheep if suitable conditions are present. Nevertheless, if the primary fly responsible for initiating strikes can be controlled, the buildup of primary flies and involvement and importance of secondary flies is greatly reduced. Measures include early insecticide treatment, just before or after the first generation of primary flies emerge in areas that have a seasonal pattern of fly emergence; trapping of flies; early treatment of clinical cases; and the proper disposal of carcasses and wool waste. Biological control by the use of insects parasitizing blow flies has been proposed but has yet to be exploited.

A weather-driven model of flystrike risk in southeastern Australia predicted that strategic early treatment would reduce the number of treatments and have a positive cost-benefit outcome in high-risk areas where preventive treatments were routinely given, but there was less benefit for low-risk areas because treatments were not needed every year.[8] A large-scale field study comparing early strategic treatment of unmulesed Merino sheep with mulesed ones not given an insecticide found a similar prevalence of strike in both groups and concluded that this was a potential medium-term strategy for the control of strike in unmulesed Merinos in this area.[2,9]

Trapping, provided the traps are carefully tended and satisfactory baits are used, can reduce the number of blow flies. However, the benefits in reducing the prevalence of strike are mixed. The use of a trap designed specifically for *L. sericata*, the primary fly in the United Kingdom, reduced strikes by 55%.[10] However, despite reducing the numbers of *L. cuprina* by 60% to 80%, the use of a trap specific for this species (LuciTrap™) has not consistently reduced the prevalence of strikes in Australia or South Africa.[7,11] In addition, it is expensive and logistically difficult to use these traps in large flocks at the suggested distribution of 1 trap per 100 sheep. Nevertheless, trapping can still be useful to indicate the presence and abundance of blow flies and the most appropriate time to apply a strategic early treatment.[11]

It is also important to identify clinically affected sheep, particularly those affected early in the season, and to treat these infestations. If early-season strikes are not treated, they can propagate a larger second and third generation of flies on a farm, given that *L. cuprina* doesn't travel large distances. Thus large farms breed most of their own flies, and so outbreaks of strike will be potentially more problematic later in the season. When affected areas are clipped, the clippings should be treated with a suitable dressing to kill the larvae, then burned or buried.

Control by genetic manipulation of the fly offers some promise for long-term control, but this strategy has yet to be exploited with either *L. cuprina* or *L. sericata*. For example, reduced fertility in male flies and lethal mutants, such as flies that will be blind under field conditions and die, have been reported. The sequencing of the draft genome of *L. cuprina* may facilitate these and other developments, such as exploring genetic mechanisms of insecticide resistance, the design of novel insecticides, and other strategies.[12]

Prediction of Risk Periods

Flystrike results from a complex interaction between fly abundance and sheep susceptibility, both of which are directly related to weather, geography, and animal husbandry. Predictive models incorporating climatic and production components have been developed in the United Kingdom and are used to give producers warning of impending flystrike.[5] In Australia, models have been incorporated into tools on an advisory website for farmers and advisers (Flyboss), enabling them to compare management systems for flystrike risk.

Outbreaks of breech strike will occur if sheep have diarrhea or if ewes have urine wetting of the breech area because their tails are docked too short or too long. If an outbreak is routinely expected, such as during spring in a winter- or uniform-rainfall area, removal of breech wool by crutching or shearing, and/or the prophylactic application of insecticides, will largely eliminate or reduce the severity of strike. Crutching is routinely carried out before lambing or an expected increase in fly numbers and provides protection from strike for around 6 weeks in crossbreeds and mulesed Merinos but for a shorter period in unmulesed Merinos. It has a significant cost as a result of the labor and loss of wool involved, and thus many sheep farmers use prophylactic treatment with an insecticide.

Sporadic cases of body strike may occur in sheep at any time and cannot always be prevented, but if environmental circumstances conducive to high fly populations and high susceptibility of sheep are recognized, then short-term prophylactic measures can be taken. Warm, showery weather extending over several weeks allows several generations to be completed and sufficient flies to be available to cause an outbreak of strike. Once sufficient flies are present, an outbreak of flystrike may occur whenever the sheep become susceptible. Warm, humid weather, rain over 2 to 3 days, or grazing in long and wet grass may provide suitable conditions for the sheep to become susceptible to body strike. Sheep with poor physical conformation (e.g., high shoulder blades), fleece that is yellow with high suint and low wax content, and a wool staple structure more prone to wetting (pointed, thin staples that are less tightly packed) are most susceptible. The time of year when shearing is carried out also exerts a strong influence on the frequency and severity of outbreaks of body strike because the staple length when sheep are wetted determines the degree of wetting and rapidity of drying. It also influences susceptibility to breech strike, with a longer staple length usually facilitating a greater accumulation of feces ("dag").

Treatment and Prevention

Prophylactic treatment with insecticide has been a major part of blow-fly control for many years, and surveys in countries with significant sheep populations show that up to 90% of farmers in high-risk areas routinely treat their sheep. Currently available chemicals include the insect growth regulators (dicyclanil and cyromazine), macrocyclic lactones (ivermectin), and spinocyn (spinosad). Organophosphate chemicals have also been heavily used, but resistance is widespread, and thus the period of protection is reduced to as little as 3 to 5 weeks. There is also increasing concern over their environmental effects and occupational health and safety, and thus their use is restricted or prohibited in many jurisdictions. Resistance by *L. cuprina* to cyromazine has been detected in Australia, but application of this chemical at the recommended concentration is still effective in preventing reinfestations.[13]

Depending on the formulation used, the insect growth regulators can provide 10 to 12 (cyromazine) and 18 to 24 (dicyclanil) weeks of protection, and can be applied by high-volume jetting (cyromazine) or a low-dose spray (both). Their action is specific to dipteran larvae, although they inhibit chitin synthesis and thus larvae do not die until they molt.

The methods of application include dipping, jetting, and tip spraying. However, dipping requires specialized equipment, has higher labor costs, and is much slower and thus is not recommended unless lice are also present. Jetting is recommended for breech strike, and if the jetting piece is combed through the wool from the poll to the rump with the solution at high pressure (500 to 900 kPa), this method will also prevent body strike.

Reducing the Susceptibility of Sheep

The primary method for reducing the susceptibility of Merino sheep to breech strike has been the modified Mules and tail-strip operation.[14] Mulesing, originally developed to remove the wrinkled region of the breech, has been modified by incorporating pain relief to address concerns regarding animal welfare, which must be balanced against the effects of strike. Although still permitted by codes of practice in Australia, the technique remains controversial because of ongoing opposition from animal welfare activists and concern over production losses. The latter accrue following a significant growth setback when lambs are mulesed at a young age (6 to 10 weeks old), often leading to reduced weaning weights and higher mortality rates after weaning. The protection gained by mulesing surpasses that afforded by breeding and is immediate and permanent.

The Mules operation is often supplemented by a tail-strip operation, whereby a thin strip of woolled skin is removed from each side of the tail. This stretches the bare skin over much of the tail, reducing fecal and urinary contamination. Unfortunately, some contractors dock tails too short, leaving a "butted" tail that the sheep is unable to elevate when defecating, thereby increasing the degree of breech soiling (dag). When butted tails are combined with mulesing, there is often a high prevalence of squamous-cell carcinoma of the vulva. Consequently, docking tails to the correct length (tip of the vulva in ewes) and leaving a V-shaped flap of wool bearing skin on the tip of the tail is important.

Alternatives to mulesing have been developed and investigated in an ongoing research program funded by Australian woolgrowers.[15] These methods include plastic breech clips, applied to the breech of lambs at a similar age to mulesing, and the intradermal injection of compounds, such as sodium lauryl sulfate, into the breech area.[16] Unfortunately, to date no alternative has produced the degree of breech modification achieved by mulesing, nor have they significantly reduced the prevalence or risk of breech strike compared with unmulesed sheep. For example, in a field study involving over 6000 sheep there was a significant reduction in the breech wrinkle scores of hoggets and ewes that had clips applied as lambs, but these changes were only a fraction of the reduction seen in mulesed sheep. Compared with mulesed sheep, the clipped ones had from 3 to 27 times the risk of breech strike as hoggets, and 2 to 8 times the risk of strike as maiden ewes.[2,9]

Consequently, selective breeding to reduce the susceptibility of Merino sheep to breech strike is being recommended. This possibility was first noted in the 1930s, when sheep with certain breech characteristics were found to have a far higher risk of breech strike, whereas others were relatively immune.[14] However, these investigations were discontinued as a result of the effectiveness and widespread adoption of mulesing, plus the development of highly effective insecticides. Genetic selection offers cumulative and permanent chan ges, although not total reduction in risk. Several risk factors for breech strike were identified in a large-scale study in western Australia involving over 2800 unmulesed lambs sired by 49 rams.[17] The most important of these were breech soiling (dag), urine staining, and breech "cover" (the reverse of bare area), which had genetic correlations with breech strike of 0.64 to 0.81, 0.54, and 0.32, respectively. Breech wrinkle was not identified as a risk factor because these were a plain-bodied genotype of sheep. However, a similar study of typical wrinkly fine-woolled Merinos in a summer-rainfall area confirmed a strong relationship between breech strike and breech wrinkle.[18] This research has been summarized and published on an open-access website called Flyboss.[19] A similar genetic and phenotypic relationship of breech soiling with breech strike has been demonstrated for New Zealand Romney sheep and in the United Kingdom.[20]

Other good management practices are essential to prevention of flystrike. These include management of gastrointestinal nematodes to prevent diarrhea ("scouring"), docking of tails to the correct length, and crutching before a risk period (typically before lambing with ewes) to reduce breech soiling that predisposes animals to breech strike.

Pizzle strike can be dramatically reduced or eliminated by the use of testosterone implants to prevent posthitis ("pizzle rot"), and "ringing" (shearing of the pizzle area) provides 6 to 8 weeks of protection from strike. Pizzle dropping (the surgical separation of the preputial sheath from the belly) also provides good protection. However, treated sheep can be more difficult to shear, and it will no longer be an approved practice when draft Australian animal welfare standards are endorsed.[21] Fleece rot occurs most commonly on the withers of sheep, and the conformation that allows accumulation of moisture and the development of fleece rot and flystrike is heritable, so sheep with these faults should be culled. Although control is mainly centered on management, the application of an insecticide may be needed when weather conditions are particularly suitable for body strike, such as summer storms.

FURTHER READING

James PJ. Genetic alternatives to mulesing and tail docking in sheep: a review. *Aust J Exper Agric.* 2006;46:1-18.

Radostits O, et al. Blow fly strike. In: *Veterinary Medicine: A Textbook of the Diseases of Cattle, Horses, Sheep, Goats and Pigs.* 10th ed. London: W.B. Saunders; 2007:1590-1593.

Wall R. Ovine cutaneous myiasis: effects on production and control. *Vet Parasitol.* 2012;189:44-51.

REFERENCES

1. Report B. AHE.0010. *Meat and Livestock Australia.* Sydney: 2015.
2. Tyrell L, et al. *Aust Vet J.* 2014;92:348.
3. De Cat S, et al. *Aust J Entomol.* 2012;51:11.
4. Wardhaugh K, et al. *Med Vet Entomol.* 2007;21:153.
5. Wall R, et al. *Med Vet Entomol.* 2002;16:335.
6. Colditz I, et al. *Aust Vet J.* 2005;83:695.
7. Scholtz AJ, et al. *J S Afr Vet Assoc.* 2011;82:107.
8. Horton BJ. *Anim Prod Sci.* 2015;55:1131.
9. Larsen JWA, et al. *Aust Vet J.* 2012;90:158.
10. Broughan JM, Wall R. *Vet Para.* 2006;135:57.
11. Urech R, et al. *Aust J Entomol.* 2009;48:182.
12. Anstead CA, et al. *Nature Comms.* 2015;6:7344.
13. Levot GW. *Aust Vet J.* 2012;90:433.
14. James PJ. *Aust J Exper Agric.* 2006;46:1.
15. <http://www.wool.com/on-farm-research-and-development/sheep-health-welfare-and-productivity/sheep-health/breech-flystrike/>; Accessed 07.12.2015.
16. Colditz IG, et al. *Aust Vet J.* 2010;88:483.
17. Greef JC, et al. *Anim Prod Sci.* 2014;54:125.
18. Smith J, et al. *Proc Assoc Advanc Anim Breed Genet.* 2009;18:334.
19. <http://www.flyboss.com.au/breeding-and-selection.php>; Accessed 07.12.2015.
20. Pickering NK, et al. *New Zeal Vet J.* 2015;63:98.
21. <http://www.animalwelfarestandards.net.au/files/2011/02/Sheep-Standards-and-Guidelines-for-Endorsement-May-2014-080714.pdf>; Accessed 07.12.2015.

SCREWSWORM (*COCHLIOMYIA HOMINIVORAX* AND *CHRYSOMYIA BEZZIANA*)

Cutaneous myiasis associated with the screwworm maggots has been a cause of great financial loss in livestock in the western hemisphere, Africa, and Asia. Deaths may be heavy in groups of livestock that are at range and seen infrequently.

SYNOPSIS

Etiology *Cochliomyia hominivorax* in the New World (New World screwworm) and

Continued

Chrysomyia bezziana (Old World screwworm) in Africa and Asia.

Epidemiology Eggs laid in fresh wounds. Flies most active at 20° to 30° C (68 to 86 F). Disease spread by dispersal of flies or transport of infested animals.

Clinical signs Larvae invade the tissue, producing characteristic large lesions containing mature larvae and foul-smelling brown exudate.

Clinical pathology Not applicable.

Lesions Deep wound containing foul-smelling brown material and third instars.

Diagnostic confirmation Rows of spines are present on the anterior part of each segment of the third instar.

Differential diagnosis No other disease causes such lesions.

Treatment Ivermectin 0.2 mg/kg subcutaneously kills many larvae and provides protection for 16 to 20 days. Other insecticides used as gels or ointments twice weekly are also effective. Doramectin subcutaneously.

Control Eradication has been achieved in North and Central America by the mass release of sterile males. Chemical attractant baits will reduce the prevalence of flies and strikes. Breeding and management procedures such as castration and shearing should be carried out in the cold weather.

ETIOLOGY

Larvae of the flies *C. hominivorax* and *C. bezziana* cause myiasis or "screwworm disease" of animals. The flies are typically blowflies, *C. hominivorax* (New World screwworm), which is blue-green with an orange head, or *C. bezziana* (Old World screwworm), which is of similar coloring. *C. hominivorax* occurs in the Americas, and *C. bezziana* occurs in the Persian Gulf, Africa, and Asia. The occurrence of *C. bezziana* in Papua New Guinea provides a constant threat to livestock on the Australian mainland. A similar fly is *Callitroga* (*Cochliomyia*) *macellaria*, which is not a true "screw-fly" in that the larvae feed only on carrion or necrotic tissues.

EPIDEMIOLOGY

The screwworm maggots are obligatory parasites with no host specificity. Thus all domestic and wild mammals, marsupials, and birds are potential hosts. Females are attracted to fresh wounds, where they will oviposit. The navel of a newborn animal is a favored site, but fresh accidental or surgical wounds, such as those produced by castration, docking, and dehorning, are readily infested. Wounds that have already been infested are markedly attractive to the flies because of their odor. In bad seasons the flies will lay eggs on minor wounds such as areas of excoriation, tick bites, running eyes, peeling brands, and on the perineum soiled by vaginal and uterine discharges in animals that have recently given birth. Injury is not necessarily a prerequisite for screwworm strike in sheep, which can be struck in the intact infraorbital fossa and vulva. Wool loss and tenderness may occur, and the remaining fleece may be stained.

The development of the fly is favored by hot, humid weather. The optimum temperature range for *C. bezziana* is 20° to 30° C (68° to 86° F). Below this temperature, the flies become sluggish, and at 10° C (50° F) and below the flies will not move. Temperatures above 30° C (86° F) can be tolerated, provided shade is available. *C. hominovorax* is active all year in areas where temperatures exceed 16° C (61 F) and disperses rapidly from these areas as the temperature increases in the neighboring colder areas. The disease can be spread either by migration of flies or their carriage in livestock ships or commercial aircraft, by shipment of infested cattle or other livestock, and by movement of affected wildlife. The mean distance that *C. bezziana* can travel and deposit eggs is 11 km. The maximum distance is 100 km, but long distances are probably wind assisted. In the new environment the flies may die out if the climate is unsuitable or persist to set up a new enzootic area. Persistence of the fly in an area may depend on persistence in wildlife or in neglected domestic animals, although the latter do not usually survive unattended for more than about 2 weeks.

In many enzootic areas it is common for the fly to persist in neighboring warmer areas during winter, returning to its normal summer habitat as the temperature rises. This pattern is exemplified by the introduction of screwworms into the southeastern United States in 1933 where they had not previously occurred. The flies died out in most areas in winter but persisted in southern Florida. In succeeding summers migrations of flies northward caused outbreaks. The disease has since been eradicated from the area.

The disease is of importance in tropical and subtropical areas of Africa, Asia, North and South America, the Caribbean islands, Mexico, American states bordering on Mexico, and especially Central America. The prevalence of the fly in enzootic areas places severe restriction on the times when prophylactic surgical operations can be carried out.

The potential worldwide geographic distribution and abundance of *C. bezziana* has been assessed using a computer program. The differences in the observed global distribution and the potential predicted distribution indicate the areas at risk of colonization.

LIFE CYCLE

The screwworm flies have a typical fly life cycle with eggs, three larval instars, and a pupal stage. Females lay 150 to 500 white eggs in shingle-like clusters at the edges of fresh wounds. Larvae hatch in about 12 hours and penetrate the tissues surrounding the wound. The larvae preferentially feed on fresh, living tissue, which is digested by regurgitation of a wide variety of salivary enzymes. Oviposition by other screwworm flies is encouraged by the presence of larvae already in the wound. The larvae feed as a group and at their time of maturation will have created a deep lesion 10 to 12 cm in diameter. Larval development is complete in 5 to 7 days, after which they leave the wound and fall to the ground. These mature third instars burrow into the upper soil layers and pupate. On the ground, pupal development is highly temperature dependent, requiring from 3 to 60 days. Emerging flies commence egg-laying in about 1 week, having completed the life cycle, under optimum environmental conditions, in less than 3 weeks. There may be 15 or more generations per year.

The temperature sensitivity of the pupal stage, which is unable to survive freezing for more than short periods, limits the distribution of this parasite. As with all flies, pupal development is highly temperature regulated. The screwworm pupal development is inhibited at soil temperatures below 15° C (60° F). Temperatures below this point for more than 2 months cause death of the pupa. Thus the occurrence of the disease is limited to warm climates. Pupae are also affected by the moisture content of the soil. The emergence of adults is reduced when the moisture content is more than 50%, whereas temporary floods can drown pupae.

PATHOGENESIS

Following invasion of the wound a cavernous lesion is formed, characterized by progressive liquefaction, necrosis, and hemorrhage. Anemia and decreased total serum protein result from hemorrhage into the wound. Secondary bacterial infection, toxemia, and fluid loss contribute to the death of the animal. Surviving calves frequently develop infectious polyarthritis.

CLINICAL FINDINGS

The young larvae invade the nearby healthy tissues vigorously and do not feed on necrotic superficial tissue. A profuse brownish exudate, composed of larval excreta and host fluids, pours from the wound, and an objectionable odor is apparent. This is highly attractive to other flies, and multiple infestations of a single wound may occur within a few days. The resulting tissue damage may be so extensive that the animal is virtually eaten alive. Affected animals show irritation in the early phase of the infestation and by day 3 show pyrexia. Animals do not feed but wander about restlessly, seeking shade and shelter.

CLINICAL PATHOLOGY

It is imperative to differentiate screwworm infestation from infestation with other fly larvae. The appearance and smell of the wound are significant, but careful examination of the larvae is necessary to confirm the diagnosis. Mature larvae are 1 to 2 cm long and pink in color; they are pointed anteriorly and blunt posteriorly; two dark lines are visible reaching from the blunt posterior to the middle of the body, and they have rows of dark fine spines on the anterior part of each segment. Specimens forwarded to a laboratory for identification should be preserved in 70% alcohol.

NECROPSY FINDINGS

Superficial examination of infested wounds is usually sufficient to indicate the cause of death.

DIFFERENTIAL DIAGNOSIS

The presence of maggots in the wound is usually apparent. It is important to differentiate them from blow-fly larvae as described previously.

TREATMENT

Affected wounds should be treated with a dressing containing an efficient larvicide and preferably an antiseptic. The larvicide should be capable of persisting in the wound for some time to prevent reinfestation. An ointment or gel base is preferred so that as much of the active ingredient as possible is left in the site. It should be liberally and vigorously applied with a paint brush to ensure that larvae in the depths of the wound are destroyed. To avoid reinfestation in extensive lesions or in bad seasons, the treatment should be repeated twice weekly.

Thirteen acaricides, commonly used for *Boophilus microplus* control, have been tested against *C. bezziana* larvae. Although they are not sufficiently active to use as a primary treatment, their continued use for tick control would reduce screwworm populations.

Ivermectin 200 mcg/kg given subcutaneously kills all *C. bezziana* larvae up to 2 days old and many older larvae. It provides residual protection for 16 to 20 days. Bull calves treated with ivermectin at the time of castration were completely protected against strike. A preliminary study showed that closantel at 15 mg/kg body weight was effective, with a residual protection of 8 to 15 days. Doramectin 200 mcg/kg subcutaneously caused complete expulsion of *C. hominivorax* larvae within 8 days. Prophylactic use of ivermectin and doramectin significantly reduced occurrence of screwworm strike in cattle. Fipronil had a prophylactic effect, reducing occurrence of screwworm infestations in cattle and providing efficacious treatment in those that did become infested.[1]

CONTROL

In an enzootic area the incidence of the disease can be kept at a low level by the general institution of measures designed to break the life cycle of the fly. Surgical procedures should be postponed where possible until cold weather. In the warm months all wounds, including shearing cuts, must be immediately dressed with one of the preparations described under "Treatment." All range animals should be inspected twice weekly and affected animals treated promptly. Infestation of fresh navels is common, and newborn animals should be treated prophylactically. If possible, the breeding program should be arranged so that parturition occurs in the cool months. The routine use of ivermectin for internal parasite control provides protection for about 2 weeks.

In the United States, the Caribbean, and Central America, an eradication program has been successfully carried out against *C. hominivorax* using the sterile insect technique (SIT).[2] Huge numbers of pupae are mass reared on semiartificial media and exposed to the sterilizing effects of cobalt 60. The resulting sterile male flies are released over large areas, primarily by aerial drops, where they compete with wild males for available females, which mate only once. *C. hominivorax* has now been eliminated from the United States, the Caribbean, and all of Central America, up to the Darien Gap in Panama. *C. hominivorax* appeared in Libya in 1988, apparently with a load of sheep transported from South America, but has been eradicated using sterile male flies from the United States.[3]

Attractants may also be used to reduce the fly population. A chemical bait has been developed that, when combined with an insecticide, forms a screwworm adult suppression system (SWASS) that reduces the fly population and the incidence of strikes. An examination of the efficacy of various methods of baiting showed that polythene sachets containing sworm-lure 2, a pungent mixture of 11 chemicals, attracted flies (not *C. bezziana*) for at least 2 weeks and was as efficient as jar bait. This result needs confirming in a screwworm-endemic country.

REFERENCES

1. Lima WS, et al. *Vet Parasitol.* 2004;125:373.
2. Spradbery JP, Evans K. *Agric Zool Rev.* 1994;6:1.
3. Chaudhury MF. *Vet Parasitol.* 2004;125:99.

WOHLFAHRTIOSIS (FLESH FLY, *WOHLFAHRTIA MAGNIFICA*)

Cutaneous infestation by larvae of the sarcophagid fly, *Wohlfahrtia magnifica*, has become a major disease of domestic livestock, including birds managed extensively (e.g., geese) in the Mediterranean basin, eastern Europe, and western regions of China. The disease is particularly significant for sheep in these regions, where it is more prevalent than strike by the calliphorid fly, *L. sericata*.

Other species of this genus are known from North America, but they do not infest domestic species. They are predominantly reported in very young rodents and birds, although there are occasional reports in infants.[1] Mortality of infested hosts tends to be very high.

LIFE CYCLE AND EPIDEMIOLOGY

Larvae of this species are obligatory parasites developing only in the living flesh of warm-blooded vertebrates. They are not host specific. Adults are typical for this group of flies, being dark gray in color with three distinct black stripes on the thorax where the wings are attached.

Female flesh flies, which are active during the warm parts of the day, deposit first instars on the host, usually in small groups of 15 to 20. Each female may produce up to 170 larvae. Completion of the three larval stages takes from 5 to 7 days, after which the mature third instars leave the lesion and fall to the ground, where they pupate. Development of the fly within the pupa is regulated by temperature and may require between 7 and 21 days.

Larvae are usually deposited near small wounds (bites of blood-feeding arthropods are sufficient to attract the larvae), but the favored sites appear to be the genitalia.[2] Irritation of the vulva associated with the use of vaginal sponges for estrus synchronization may be a predisposing factor in sheep.

Flies are active between April and October, with several generations being produced. Little information is available on overwintering. Wildlife are suspected as being reservoir hosts, but little information is available on which are the most important.

PATHOGENESIS

Larvae have well-developed mouthhooks that are used to abrade the skin surface, and with the aid of a wide variety of salivary enzymes, they quickly produce a dramatic lesion. Lesions increase in size as the larvae grow and require additional fresh tissue. Each animal may have one or more focal lesions, each packed with larvae. In severe cases several lesions may coalesce into one larger site.

Animals are often struck multiple times during a season, suggesting the absence of protective immunity. This adds to the impact of this disease because animals must be constantly monitored.

CLINICAL PATHOLOGY AND NECROPSY FINDINGS

A clinical examination is all that is necessary to make the diagnosis. Larvae can be distinguished from those of the screwworm or strike flies by the presence of a large posterior cavity surrounded by a number of prominent tubercles. However, specific identification should be done by a specialist. Larvae should be preserved in 70% ethanol.

Affected animals are clearly stressed, showing restlessness and anorexia Lesions formed at the vulva or prepuce are the most significant, causing great discomfort and dysfunction. Lightly infested animals shown no impairment of productivity.[2] Infested animals develop strong antibody responses to salivary secretions, particularly of the third instars.[3]

TREATMENT

There are currently no products specifically registered for management of this disease. Evaluations of several drugs and treatment approaches have been made. Of particular interest is the equivocal results of trials with macrocyclic lactones. In sheep, ivermectin and moxidectin had no effect on existing infestations and no prophylactic effect or only short protection against early instars. In contrast, doramectin provided complete prophylactic protection for 21 days and significant reductions for 40 days.

The insect growth regulator dicyclanil has also been evaluated and shown to reduce prevalence of infestation in sheep. The reduction not only occurred in treated animals, but was seen in untreated herdmates, possibly as a result of the overall reduction in fly numbers.

RECOMMENDATION

Animals likely to be attractive to these flies should be checked weekly, and appropriate treatment should be applied as soon as fly larvae are detected.

REFERENCES

1. Colwell DD, O'Connor M. *J Med Ent.* 2000;37:854.
2. Sotiraki S, et al. *Vet Parasitol.* 2005;131:107.
3. Sotiraki S, et al. *Vet Parasitol.* 2003;116:327.

Mite Infestations

HARVEST MITES (CHIGGER MITES)

Infestations with trombidiform mites cause dermatitis in all species. Except for *Psorergates ovis*, *P. bos*, and *Demodex* spp., they are referred to as harvest or grain mites. These mites are primarily predatory on other arthropods associated with harvested grain and infesting animals only secondarily and usually transiently. It is usually the larval stages that are found feeding on animals, whereas the nymphs and adults are free-living. Hair loss and patchiness in cattle that are extremely well bedded often results from these mites but can be confused with louse infestations.

The larvae of *Pyemotes ventricosus*, *Neotrombicula autumnalis*, *Neotrombicula heptneri*, *Eutrombicula alfreddugesi*, *Eutrombicula splendens*, *Eutrombicula batatas*, *Trombicula* spp., and some species of *Leptotrombidium* and *Schoengastia* are parasitic on humans and most animals, causing dermatitis and, in humans, transmitting rickettsial diseases. Nymphs and adults are free-living predators feeding mainly on arthropods in grain and hay. The larvae are most active in the autumn at harvest time and may cause dermatitis in animals grazing at pasture or those confined in barns and being fed newly harvested grain.

Horses, cattle, and goats[1] are usually affected on the face and lips, which, in white-faced horses, may suggest a diagnosis of photosensitization, and around the feet and lower limbs, especially in the flexures. Affected areas are itchy and scaly, but with rubbing, small fragile scabs and absence of hair may become apparent. Infestation of horses with *Trombicula sarcina* causes a severe pruritus, and yearlings show irritation by lip-biting their legs and rubbing against stable walls. Stamping is uncommon and usually occurs when yearlings are stabled on fresh, contaminated bedding. Sheep, when first affected, stamp their feet repeatedly and bite their legs. The skin at the heels, coronet, and pasterns, and sometimes the shank, becomes erythematous and weeps fluid. The mites detach after 3 to 5 days and leave a small ulcerated area. In light infestations the mites may be confined to the area between the accessory digits, but in heavy infestations the skin over the whole of the lower limbs may be swollen and thickened. The infestation is self-limiting, and treatment is not usually necessary.

Infestation with *Tyroglyphus* spp. in pigs appears to be manifested by itchiness and the development of fragile scabs about 3 cm in diameter scattered over the body. Unlike the thick scabs of sarcoptic mange, the skin beneath appears normal. The infestations occur in pigs eating dry ground grain from automatic feeders, with lesions appearing several weeks after the dry feeding is begun and disappearing spontaneously about 3 weeks later. No treatment is necessary. Affected pigs show no ill-effects, but the lesions may be mistaken for those of swine-pox or sarcoptic mange. The ingestion of large numbers of mites appears to have no ill-effects.

Recent work on the role of *N. autumnalis* has suggested that these mites are capable of acting as reservoirs of *Borrelia burgdorferi*,[2] but this remains to be established.

RECOMMENDATIONS

No treatment is usually recommended, but a macrocyclic lactone will be effective if a treatment is required.

REFERENCES

1. Stelnikov AA, Kar S. *Acarologica.* 2015;55:355-359.
2. Kampen H, et al. *Exp App Acarol.* 2004;33:93-102.

ITCHMITES (*PSORERGATES OVIS, PSORERGATES BOS*)

The "itchmite," *Psorergates ovis*, has been recorded as a parasite of sheep in Australia, New Zealand, South Africa, the United States, Argentina, and Chile. *Psorergates bos* has also been recorded in cattle in the United Kingdom.

LIFE CYCLE AND EPIDEMIOLOGY

The entire life cycle of this mite—egg, larvae, two nymphal stages, and adult—takes place entirely on the host. In sheep the cycle takes 4 to 5 weeks. All stages occur in the superficial layers of the skin. The adults are extremely small and can be seen only with the aid of a microscope. Only the adults are mobile on the skin surface, and they spread infection by direct contact. In sheep this often occurs between recently shorn animals when contact is close and prolonged, such as when shorn sheep are packed in yards after shearing, or from ewe to lamb while suckling. Mite feeding activity, in addition to excreta, causes skin irritation, leading to rubbing and biting of the affected parts (principally the sides, flanks, and thighs) and raggedness, and sometimes shedding, of the fleece. Wool over these areas becomes thready and tufted and contains dry scales.

PATHOGENESIS

The skin shows no gross abnormality other than an increase in scurf. Histologically there is hyperkeratosis, desquamation, and increased numbers of mast cells. Irritation appears to be caused by hypersensitivity and results in biting and chewing of the fleece on the flanks and rump behind a line approximately from the elbow to the hips. In the individual sheep and in flocks, the disease spreads slowly, and thus it may be several years before clinical cases are observed and appreciable numbers are visibly affected. The incidence of clinical cases in a neglected flock may be as high as 15%. Sheep on poor nutrition have significantly higher mite populations, more scurf, and greater fleece derangement. Affected sheep may become tolerant after 1 to 2 years and show no signs, even though they remain infested.

Among sheep, Merinos are most commonly affected. The highest incidence is observed in this breed, particularly in areas where the winter is cold and wet. There is a marked seasonal fluctuation in the numbers of mites; the numbers are very low in summer, begin to rise in the autumn, and peak numbers are found in the spring. Spring or summer shearing exacerbates the decline in numbers. Clinically, the disease resembles louse infestation, but may be distinguished by the smaller proportion of the flock affected (10% to 15%), the less severe irritation, and the tendency of the sheep to bite those areas they can reach. Hence lesions are confined to parts of the flank and the hindquarters, and the wool tufts have a chewed appearance.

CLINICAL FINDINGS

Diagnosis depends on finding the mites in a skin scraping. The selection of sheep with excess scurf and fleece derangement increases the chance of finding mites, and in the absence of lice, ked, and grass seed infestation, about 75% of such sheep prove positive for *P. ovis*. The wool should be clipped as close as possible, the skin smeared lightly with oil, and then scraped over an area of about 25 cm^2. The mites have a seasonal incidence and may be very difficult to find in summer and autumn. For best results the scraping should be made on the ribs or shoulder in winter or spring. Scrapings are usually teased out in oil and examined microscopically without digestion. A number of scrapings may be needed from each sheep before mites can be demonstrated. Because of the difficulty of finding mites in summer and autumn, sheep dipped at that time cannot be said to be free of infestation until they prove negative on skin scraping in the following spring, when mite numbers should be at the highest levels.

TREATMENT AND CONTROL

There is no compound available that will eradicate itchmite after a single treatment. Arsenic, lime sulfur, and finely divided sulfur have been used and markedly reduce the number of mites. Because the mites are slow to build up, dipping every second year will mask the signs of infestation. However, arsenic is no longer used in most countries. Finely divided rotenone by itself or mixed with the synergist piperonyl butoxide reduces the mite population. It is usually combined with an organophosphate to include lice and ked control in the one product. Phoxim, an organophosphorous compound, has good activity, but two dippings 1 month apart are necessary to eradicate infestations. Amitraz causes a marked reduction in mites that will be maintained for some months.

A single subcutaneous injection of 0.2 mg/kg ivermectin freed sheep of mites for up to 56 days posttreatment. However, these sheep would have to be examined over a longer period to ensure eradication. Other macrocyclic lactone products, in various formulations, have been shown to have good efficacy. The absence of reports of itchmites over the last 15 years would suggest that the widespread use of macrocyclic lactone products has decreased the prevalence of infection.

DEMODECTIC MANGE (FOLLICULAR MANGE)

Mites of *Demodex* spp. infest hair follicles of all species of domestic animals. The disease causes little concern, but in cattle and goats there may be significant damage to the hide, and, rarely, death may result from a secondary bacterial invasion.

ETIOLOGY

Mites infesting the different host species are considered to be specific and are designated as *Demodex bovis* for cattle, *Demodex ovis* for sheep, *Demodex caprae* for goats, *Demodex equi* for horses, and *Demodex phylloides* for pigs.

Demodicosis may occur in farm animals of any age, especially those in poor condition, but most cases in cattle occur in adult dairy cattle in late winter and early spring. This differs from the well-known condition in the dog, which occurs in young, immunodeficient animals.

LIFE CYCLE AND EPIDEMIOLOGY

The entire life cycle is spent on the host. Adult mites invade the hair follicles and sebaceous glands, which become distended with mites and inflammatory material. The life cycle passes through the egg, larval, and two nymphal stages. The disease spreads slowly, and transfer of mites is thought to take place by contact, probably early in life. Calves can acquire mites from an infected dam in half a day. However, in horses, grooming instruments and rugs may transmit infection.

PATHOGENESIS

Invasion of hair follicles and sebaceous glands leads to chronic inflammation, loss of the hair fiber, and, in many instances, the development of secondary staphylococcal pustules or small abscesses. It is these foci of infection that cause the small pinholes in the hide that interfere with its industrial processing and limit its use. In most farm animals, the lesions are difficult to see externally, and only the advanced ones will be diagnosed.

CLINICAL FINDINGS

The important sign is the appearance of small (3-mm-diameter) nodules and pustules, which may develop into larger abscesses, especially in pigs and goats. The small lesions can be seen quite readily in short-coated animals and on palpation feel like particles of bird-shot in the hide. In severe cases there may be a general hair loss and thickening of the skin in the area, but usually there is no pruritus, and hair loss is insufficient to attract attention. The contents of the pustules are usually white in color and cheesy in consistency. In large abscesses the pus is more fluid. In cattle and goats the lesions occur most commonly on the brisket, lower neck, forearm, and shoulder, but also occur on the dorsal half of the body, particularly behind the withers. Larger lesions are easily visible, but very small lesions may only be detected by rolling a fold of skin through the fingers. In horses the face and around the eyes are predilection areas. Demodicosis in pigs usually commences on the face and spreads down the ventral surface of the neck and chest to the belly. There is little irritation, and the disease is observed mainly when the skin is scraped at slaughter. The disease may be especially severe in goats, spreading extensively before it is suspected and in some instances causing death. Severe cases in goats commonly involve several skin diseases, such as mycotic dermatitis, ringworm, besnoitiosis, and myiasis. Demodicosis is rare in sheep. In this species pustules and scabs appear on the coronets, nose, and tips of the ears, and around the eyes, but clinical signs are not usually seen, and mites may be found in scrapings from areas of the body not showing lesions.

CLINICAL PATHOLOGY

The characteristically elongated mites are usually easy to find in large numbers in the waxy material that can be expressed from the pustular lesions. They are much more difficult to isolate from squamous lesions. Lesions in hides can be detected as dark spots when a fresh hide is viewed against a strong light source. However, lesions may not be readily seen until the hair has been removed and the skin has been soaking for some time.

DIFFERENTIAL DIAGNOSIS

- The commonest error is to diagnose the disease as a nonspecific staphylococcal infection.
- In cattle and goats the disease often passes unnoticed unless the nodules are palpated.
- Deep-seated ringworm in horses has much in common with demodicosis.
- A satisfactory diagnosis can only be made by demonstration of the mite.

TREATMENT AND CONTROL

Repeated dipping or spraying with the acaricides recommended for other manges is usually carried out but is more to prevent spread than to cure existing lesions. Ivermectin, which does not eradicate the infection in dogs, possibly because of the difficulty in getting the acaricide to the mite, has been reported to cure 98% of beef bulls when used at 0.3 mg/kg. Recent developments in the development of diagnostics may allow newer techniques that will effectively detect infestations.[1]

REFERENCE

1. Wells B, et al. *Mol Cell Probes*. 2012;26:47-53.

SARCOPTIC MANGE (BARN ITCH)

Sarcoptic mange occurs in a wide variety of host species and causes a severe pruritic dermatitis. Although in most countries it has been a major problem and was a reportable disease, the advent of macrocyclic lactone endectocides has reduced the incidence of disease dramatically.

ETIOLOGY

The causative mite, *Sarcoptes scabiei*, is usually considered to have a number of varieties, each generally specific to a particular host species. Morphologic, immunologic, and molecular research confirms the close relationship among the varieties, but it does not explain the biological differences, particularly with respect to host specificity. Because host specificity is not strict and transference from one host species to another can occur, there is some concern when attempting to control the disease.

Animals in poor condition appear to be most susceptible, but conditions, especially overcrowding, in which sarcoptic mange occurs often go hand in hand with poor feeding and general poor husbandry. The disease is most active in cold, wet weather and spreads slowly during the summer months.

LIFE CYCLE AND EPIDEMIOLOGY

Female mites form shallow burrows in the lower stratum corneum of the skin, in which they deposit eggs. Development for both sexes includes a larval stage and two nymphal stages before molting to the adult. All life-cycle stages, except the eggs, can be found moving on the skin surface and are thus easily transferred to other hosts. The normal exfoliation of the skin eventually exposes the tunnels, exposing eggs as well. The life cycle, from egg to adult, takes 10 to 13 days.

Although direct contact between hosts is the most effective method of transmission, inert materials such as bedding, blankets, grooming tools, and clothing may act as carriers. Adult mites do not usually survive for more than a few days away from the host, but in optimum laboratory conditions they may remain alive for up to 3 weeks. In pigs, adult sows are often the source of infestation for young pigs even though they show no signs of the disease. Large numbers of mites can often be found in the ears of normal sows, and the mites are transmitted soon after farrowing. Significant scratching does not occur until a hypersensitivity develops some 8 to 10 weeks later and may continue until slaughter. A small proportion of young pigs do not develop a hypersensitivity, and these become chronically affected.

Among domestic species, pigs are most commonly affected, but it is an important disease in cattle and camels and occurs in sheep. It has been a notifiable disease in most countries, because of its severity, but a decline in prevalence accompanying the advent of new therapeutics has resulted in the removal of this requirement in some countries. People handling infested animals may become infected, but lesions will disappear if further contact is prevented.

Infested animals develop protective immunity and are able to clear challenge infestations rapidly. A proportion of infested hosts do, however, remain chronically infested, and mite populations may show a postpartum recrudescence, thereby facilitating transfer to the susceptible offspring.

PATHOGENESIS

Young animals, in particular piglets, become infected in the first few weeks of life and develop a hypersensitivity within 8 to 10 weeks. This allergic phase lasts for 8 to 9 months, and during this time affected animals are constantly itchy. The disease, if untreated, progresses to a localized crust formation characteristic of a chronic hyperkeratotic state.

Many infestations in pigs have little or no effect on weight gain, although there is some controversy, and treatments improve productivity (see following discussion). There are suggestions in other hosts of reduced feed efficiency. In some pigs, the loss of condition, production, and vitality may be severe, and the appearance of affected animals is esthetically displeasing. Erythema, papules, and intense pruritus may be seen. Few mites may be necessary to cause a reaction in a previously sensitized animal. A chronic condition is uncommon but is seen in pigs with an immunodeficiency.

In cattle and camels, severe hypersensitivity lesions occur and often lead to death. Sheep initially show an intense pruritus and rub the affected part against fences or bite at the skin. Later papules and vesicles occur and the skin becomes thickened, covered with pale scabs, and the hair is lost.

CLINICAL FINDINGS

Early lesions are characterized by the presence of small red papules and general erythema of the skin. The affected area is intensely itchy and frequently excoriated by scratching and biting. Loss of hair, thick brown scabs overlying a raw surface, and thickening and wrinkling of surrounding skin soon follow. In pigs the lesions commence on the trunk; in sheep and goats on the face; in cattle on the inner surface of the thighs, the underside of the neck and brisket, and around the root of the tail; and in horses and camels on the head and neck. Except in sheep, where the lesions do not spread to the woolled skin, lesions become widespread if neglected, and such animals may show systemic effects, including emaciation, anorexia, and weakness. In neglected cases, death may occur.

The course of sarcoptic mange is rather more acute than in the other forms of mange and may involve the entire body surface of cattle in a period as short as 6 weeks.

CLINICAL PATHOLOGY

Necropsy examinations are not usually undertaken. Deep scrapings that draw blood are required for accurate diagnosis and must be taken from the edges of any evident lesions (scrapings taken from the central portions of lesions are very often negative). Examination of scrapings either directly or after digestion in 10% potassium hydroxide will reveal mites and/or eggs. When practical, multiple scrapings from affected animals should be taken. Examination of the ear wax of pigs often shows mites when none can be seen in scrapings.

Change in behavior, a result of the intense pruritus, have been used in swine as an initial diagnostic tool. An increase in the rubbing index is indicative of infestation, but other clinical confirmation is required.

An ELISA for detection of antibodies to *Sarcoptes scabiei* has been developed. The test has high specificity and moderate sensitivity, being more sensitive in young animals undergoing their first infestation. It has been shown to work well in herd-level eradication programs and functions afterward as an effective surveillance tool.

Recent description of the genome of a canine variety has elucidated several aspects of the host response and biology of the mite.[1]

DIFFERENTIAL DIAGNOSIS

- Sarcoptic mange is the only mange that occurs in pigs. It can be confused with infestation with *Tyroglyphus* spp. mites or lice, or with swinepox, parakeratosis, infectious dermatitis, pityriasis rosea, and ringworm. In most of these diseases there are clinical features that are characteristic, and final diagnosis can be made on the presence or absence of the mite.
- The same comments apply to the differentiation in cattle of sarcoptic mange from chorioptic and psoroptic mange and from chlorinated naphthalene poisoning and ringworm.
- Horses may be affected by psoroptic or chorioptic mange, but the lesions are most common at the base of the mane and tail and at the back of the pastern, respectively.
- Infestation with the trombidiform mites and photosensitization may resemble sarcoptic mange.
- The disease is uncommon in sheep.

TREATMENT AND CONTROL

Macrocyclic lactone endectocides (including ivermectin, eprinomectin, moxidectin, and doramectin) are the preferred products for treatment of sarcoptic mange. Use of these products in pour-on or injectable formulations is highly efficacious when used at the label-recommended dose. Because of the residual activity of these compounds, retreatment is not usually necessary, although moxidectin given subcutaneously at 0.2 mg/kg to infested sheep resulted in a rapid clinical improvement but did not eliminate the mites. Two doses 10 days apart resulted in negative skin scrapings by 14 days posttreatment. A single injection to cattle eliminated the mites by day 14. The resolution of the lesions may take considerable time, but should not be misconstrued as product failure.

Prefarrowing treatment of sows with ivermectin to prevent transmission to the newborn piglets improves weight gain and early feed conversion.

If other treatments are used, they must be thoroughly applied so that all parts of the skin, especially under the tail, in the ears, and between the legs, are wetted by the acaricide. Although buildings, bedding, and other inert materials do not support the mite for more than a few days, they should also be treated unless they can be left in a dry state for 3 weeks.

RECOMMENDATION

Always treat affected animals. To control spread, animals should be isolated or quarantined.

REFERENCE

1. Rider SD, et al. *Parasites Vectors.* 2015;8:585.

PSOROPTIC MANGE (SHEEP SCAB, BODY MANGE, EAR MANGE)

Psoroptic mange is of greatest importance in sheep, in which it causes sheep scab, but it is also responsible for body mange in cattle and horses and ear mange in horses, sheep, goats, and rabbits. The disease is a major animal welfare concern.

ETIOLOGY

The various species of *Psoroptes* have now been reduced to two or three species. Based on molecular evidence, *Psoroptes ovis*, *Psoroptes cunilculi* and *Psoroptes cervinus* are identical despite differences in morphology and biology. It is clear that *P. ovis* from cattle and sheep are identical, although cross-transmission is not always successful. *P. equi* occurs on horses, donkeys, and mules in Great Britain and *P. natalensis* on cattle and the water buffalo. The ear mites are all *P. cuniculi*, and recent work has suggested this is a variant of *P. ovis* adapted to the aural environment. *P. cervinus* assumes a dual role, being an ear mite of the American bighorn and a body mite of the wapiti.

LIFE CYCLE AND EPIDEMIOLOGY

Psoroptic mange is a major disease in sheep that was once virtually eliminated in most progressive countries where wool production is an important industry. With the cessation of organophosphate dips in the United Kingdom there has been a resurgence of the problem. The disease in cattle was widespread in the United States but has now largely been brought under control. It can spread rapidly and cause serious losses in cattle if neglected, as shown by the serious losses that can occur in feedlots. The ear manges cause irritation and, in horses, a touchiness around the head.

Psoroptic mites abrade the surface and feed on lipid exudate, bacteria, and skin debris. Erythrocytes are not normally a constituent of the diet and may be accidentally ingested when host scratching results in skin breakage. They cause the formation of scabs, under which they live. The eggs are laid on the skin at the edge of a scab and hatch in 1 to 3 days, although this is prolonged if eggs are not in contact with the skin. There are the usual larval and nymphal stages, and the whole life cycle is complete in 10 to 11 days. All stages are capable of survival away from the host for up to 10 days, and under optimum conditions adult females may survive for 3 weeks.

Optimum conditions for development include high humidity and cool temperatures. Thus the disease is most active in autumn and winter months. This is a result of not only the increased activity of the mites but also the more rapid development in housed animals and the tendency for the disease to be most severe in animals in poor condition. When conditions are adverse, as in summer, mites survive in sheep in protected parts in the perineum, in the inguinal and interdigital regions, in the infraorbital fossae, and inside the ear and the scrotum. Spread occurs from sheep to sheep, but transmission from infected premises and by passive spread of pieces of wool also occurs.

The life cycle of the other species is thought to be similar. Spread of ear mite in horses can occur by grooming or by the use of infected harness.

PATHOGENESIS

The mite migrates to all parts of the skin and prefers areas covered with hair or wool. Salivary secretions and mite excreta contain proteinases that result in a severe allergic pruritus. The exudation of serum accumulates to form a crust. In cattle the mites are most active at the edge of the crust, and the lesion spreads peripherally. Infested calves have lower weight gains, lower feed conversion, and lower energy retention than noninfested calves. In sheep the mites are more generally distributed, and bacterial invasions of the skin are more common.

CLINICAL FINDINGS

Sheep

Cutaneous lesions may occur on any part of the body, but characteristically in badly affected sheep they are most obvious on the sides.[1] Very early lesions are small (6-mm-diameter) papules that ooze serum. Attention may be attracted to the area by raggedness of the wool caused by biting and scratching. In older lesions thin yellow crusts are present, and the wool commences to shed. The wool may contain large masses of scab material that binds the fibers together in a mat. Under suitable conditions the infestation spreads rapidly, and in 6 to 8 weeks three-quarters of the body may be affected.

In a typical outbreak of sheep scab many animals are affected and show itchiness and shedding of the fleece. Some become markedly emaciated and weak, and deaths may occur. However, it is possible to have the disease in a flock at a very low level of incidence and with minimal lesions. This usually occurs when the sheep are highly resistant because of good nutrition, climatic conditions are adverse for mite development, or treatment has been carried out but has been incomplete. In such cases there may be little or no clinical evidence of the disease, and a careful search for latent cases may be necessary. This is facilitated by packing the animals into a confined space, so that the mites become active, and watching for signs of itchiness.

Behavioral changes in infested sheep are dramatic, with sheep biting at the affected areas and rubbing or scratching. In addition, infested sheep exhibit stereotypic behaviors typical of animals under stress. These changes combine to reduce productivity. Animals exhibiting these changes should be carefully examined by palpating the surface of the skin in search of papules and scabs. Special attention should be paid to the ears, the base of the horns, the infraorbital fossa, and the perineal and scrotal areas in rams.

Goats

Lesions can vary from a dry crusty scab on the external ear canal with no clinical signs to severe lesions covering much of the body and causing death. However, it is commonly an ear mite, feeding on whole blood and causing the production of scabs that vary from a single layer lining the large sulcus at the base of the concha to abundant laminated scab formation occluding the meatus. In severe cases the poll may be affected, and scabs may also be found on the pasterns. Female goats serve as the source of infection for the kid; mites may be found by 5 days, and clinical signs are seen by the 3rd week of life. *Raillietia* may also be found in the ear of goats, but *Raillietia caprae* is easily differentiated microscopically because all legs are on the anterior part of the body.

Horses

P. equi causes the production of large, thick crusts on those parts of the body carrying long hair, such as the base of the mane and the root of the tail, and hairless areas such as the udder, prepuce, and axilla. Affected parts are itchy, the hair is lost, and with constant rubbing the surrounding skin becomes thickened. *P. cuniculi* infestations in horses cause severe irritation in the ear accompanied by discharge, shaking of the head, rubbing of the head, and tenderness of the poll.

Cattle

Typical lesions appear first on the withers, neck, and around the root of the tail. In severe cases they may spread to the rest of the body. The lesions are intensely itchy. They commence as papules but soon are covered with a scab, which enlarges peripherally and coalesces with other lesions so that very large areas of skin may become involved. The hair is lost and the skin becomes thickened, wrinkled, and covered with scabs. Badly affected animals becomes weak and emaciated and may die.

CLINICAL PATHOLOGY

The mites can be easily demonstrated in scrapings taken from the edges of the lesions. Examination is facilitated by prior digestion of the scraping in warm 10% potassium hydroxide solution.

An ELISA has been developed for diagnosis of Psoroptes infestation in sheep.[2] It has been applied to monitoring of infestations as part of efficient control programs.

DIFFERENTIAL DIAGNOSIS

- Severe cases of psoroptic mange in sheep are similar to mycotic dermatitis except that there is no itching in the latter. Diseases causing itchiness, such as scrapie, ked, and louse infestations and infestations with *Psorergates ovis* and harvest mites, do not have typical cutaneous lesions, and the latter group can usually be detected by examination for the causative parasites.
- In horses, attention is drawn to the condition because of the horse rubbing its head, by swelling around the base of the ear, or by resentment to the bridle passing over the ears. In some horses, the affected ear may droop.

TREATMENT AND CONTROL

Macrocyclic lactone endectocides are used most frequently for control of psoroptic scabies. Cattle treated with ivermectin must be separated from noninfested cattle for between 9 and 14 days; otherwise, spread and reinfection may occur. In sheep two treatments of ivermectin 0.2 mg/kg subcutaneously are necessary to eliminate infestations.

Moxidectin applied as a 0.5% pour-on at 0.5 mg/kg to cattle is effective against *P. ovis* lice, and *Chorioptes bovis*, and it was equally effective against *P. ovis* as 0.2 mg/kg by subcutaneous injection. In sheep, although a single subcutaneous dose of 0.2 mg/kg moxidectin gave a rapid clinical improvement, two doses 7 days apart were necessary to eliminate mites. In large-scale field use, sheep receiving a single injection in the autumn remained free of the infestation throughout the winter, and two injections 10 days apart were effective in treating outbreaks.

Doramectin injectable at 0.2 mg/kg SC was highly effective in eliminating mites in scrapings of infested cattle. The same treatment was found to protect cattle from infestation for up to 3 weeks.

If sheep are to be dipped, it is important to wet the skin thoroughly and pay special attention to severe cases where mites are likely to be present in inaccessible sites on the body. Thus a plunge dip is almost essential, and the sheep must be kept immersed in the dipping fluid for at least 1 minute. Prior shearing may be advisable but may lead to further spread of the infestation. Care must be taken to ensure that the concentration of the acaricide in the dip is maintained, especially when large numbers of sheep are being treated. Badly affected animals should be set aside, and inaccessible sites, including ears, horn bases, and perineum, should be treated manually with the dipping fluid. Dipped sheep should not be returned to their pastures or to the barn unless the latter has been thoroughly cleaned and sprayed with the dipping fluid.

The synthetic pyrethroids are variable in their efficacy. Flumethrin, used as a nonstripping dipping compound, eradicated *P. ovis* from sheep when used at 55 ppm and gave at least 7 weeks of protection.

In horses, affected ears should be cleaned of all wax, and ear preparations containing benzene hexachloride should be used at weekly intervals. Benzyl benzoate is a safe and effective treatment when given every 5 days for three treatments. Ivermectin is highly effective against *P. equi.*

Eradication of sheep scab on an area basis is usually undertaken by quarantine and compulsory treatment of all susceptible animals in the area at the same time. Now that there are effective treatments that do not require dipping, eradication of scab from areas should be more easily accomplished. The necessity to dip all animals in the area during a short period presents difficulties, and the cost of construction of dips and lack of desire to dip in cold climates are other obstructing factors. The use of pour-ons or injections is an attractive alternative to autumn dipping and has the added advantage of providing helminth control in late-season lambs and in ewes.[3] Further, even pregnant animals can be yarded and treated by subcutaneous injection or pour-on as long as care is taken in the yards. Where it is desired to keep the disease at a low level short of eradication, the disease is made notifiable, movement of stock is restricted, and infested farms are quarantined.

RECOMMENDATION

Treatment is absolutely necessary to keep this from becoming an animal welfare issue.

REFERENCES

1. Nunn FG, et al. *Mol Cell Probes*. 2011;25:212-218.
2. Losson BJ. *Vet Parasit*. 2012;189:24-43.
3. Wells B, et al. *Mol Cell Probes*. 2012;26:47-53.

CHORIOPTIC MANGE (TAIL MANGE, LEG MANGE, SCROTAL MANGE)

Chorioptic mange is the commonest form of mange in cattle and horses. Although the primary effect on cattle is esthetic damage, there are production effects in dairy animals. In horses, leg mange is a source of annoyance and inefficiency at work. In sheep, it affects the scrotum and may cause a decrease in fertility.

ETIOLOGY

Chorioptic mites were formerly named according to the host species, but those on cattle, horses, goats, and sheep are now considered to be one species, *Chorioptes bovis.* Another species, *Chorioptes texanus*, has been reported on goats, cattle, and Canadian reindeer.[1] In cattle, the mites are much more active in the latter part of the winter and tend to disappear in cattle at pasture. This diminution in activity is not noted in cattle kept housed in the summer.

LIFE CYCLE AND EPIDEMIOLOGY

C. bovis feed on the skin surface, abrading the upper layers with their mouthparts and contaminating the area with salivary secretions and excreta. Developmental stages are similar to that of *Psoroptes*, and a complete cycle, from egg to adult, requires approximately 3 weeks. The number of parasites is influenced by temperature and humidity, with the mite populations beginning to increase on sheep in early autumn and numbers reaching a peak in late autumn or early winter and declining in spring. In cattle the cycle is longer, with peak numbers occurring in late winter and early spring and declining in summer. Transmission is probably effected by direct contact in most instances, although in animals housed in barns, grooming tools may be an additional method of spreading the disease. Infestation of bedding is not a common method of transmission.

In horses, the parasites occur almost entirely in the long hair on the lower parts of the legs and are rarely found on other parts of the body. In cattle the disease is most evident in the winter, with lesions occurring most commonly on the perineum and back of the udder, extending in severe cases to the backs of the legs and over the rump. In the summer months, the mites persist in the area above the hooves, particularly the pasterns of the hind leg. In sheep, lesions are confined to the wool-less areas, chiefly the lower parts of the hindlegs and scrotum. Rams are more heavily infected than ewes and probably infect ewes while copulating. Lactating ewes probably act as the source of infection for lambs.

PATHOGENESIS

The mites cause an allergic exudative dermatitis; the yellowish serous exudate coagulates and breaks as the hair grows so that small scabby lesions are seen on the hair. In horses the mites cause severe irritation and itchiness. The initial lesion in cattle is a small nodule that exudes serum, causing matting of the hair. In severe cases these coalesce to form heavy scabs and cause thickening and wrinkling of the skin. Mites can be isolated from many animals that show no clinical evidence of the disease. Although most cases do not cause any symptoms, a rapidly spreading syndrome characterized by coronitis, intense irritation, and a marked fall in milk production has been reported.[2] *C. bovis* is a common parasite of sheep in the United States, New Zealand, and Australia, and causes an allergic exudative dermatitis on the scrotum of rams. This may cause a rise in temperature of the scrotal contents and severe testicular degeneration if the lesion has an area greater than 10 cm^2.

CLINICAL FINDINGS

The first sign in horses is usually violent stamping of the feet and rubbing of the back of the hind pasterns on wire, rails, or stumps. This is most evident during periods of rest and at night. Examination of the area is difficult because of the long hair present, and the horses may resent manipulation. In cases of long duration, the skin is seen to be swollen, scabby, cracked, and usually greasy; small amounts of serous exudate may be attached to most hair in the affected area.

Cattle show little evidence of cutaneous irritation, but the small crusty scabs (3 mm in diameter) on the escutcheon, udder, and thighs are unsightly. Although the mites appear to cause little trouble in the summer, occasional animals are seen that have thick, crusty scabs on the skin, just above the coronets and around the muzzle.

The main lesion in sheep is seen on the scrotum of rams, where an allergic dermatitis results in the production of a yellowish serous exudate over areas from a few millimeters to several centimeters.

CLINICAL PATHOLOGY

Scrapings from the affected areas usually contain large numbers of mites.

DIFFERENTIAL DIAGNOSIS

Greasy heel in horses resembles chorioptic mange except that pain is more evident in the former and itchiness in the latter. It has been suggested that the two diseases are etiologically related.

The lesions in cattle may go unnoticed but are not likely to be mistaken for those of any other disease, with the possible exception of other manges. The presence of chorioptic mites in footrot and mucosal disease lesions may be purely coincidental, but cases of chorioptic mange that have lesions around the coronet and muzzle may be mistaken for one of the erosive diseases.

Sheep with itchy, scabby legs may be infested with other forms of mange or have contagious ecthyma or strawberry footrot.

TREATMENT AND CONTROL

The macrocyclic lactone endectocides have shown efficacy against *Chorioptes* spp., but eradication of the parasites from a herd is difficult. Moxidectin 0.5 mg/kg applied as a pour-on eliminated *C. bovis* as well as sucking lice and *P. ovis*. When given as a single injection of 0.2 mg/kg, there was a marked decline in the number of mites, but few cattle were cleared of infection. Doramectin has high efficacy at the label rate in cattle, but a single treatment did not clear mites from all of the trial animals. Treatment with eprinomectin at recommended rates was completely effective, but mites persisted for at least 14 days.

Amitraz 0.05% removed 98% and phoxim 0.05% and 0.1% used twice at 10-day intervals has also eradicated the infection from cattle. Other compounds if used repeatedly will reduce mite numbers, but recrudescence may occur. Ivermectin 0.2 mg/kg given subcutaneously on two occasions reduced but did not eliminate the infestation on cattle. A single treatment of infested horses with ivermectin paste also did not remove all mites, but when combined with hair removal, washing encrusted areas with oil of salicylic acid, and the later removal of crusts with a stiff brush, eradication was achieved.

REFERENCES

1. Lusat J, et al. *Med Vet Entomol*. 2011;25:370.
2. Villarroel A, Halliburton MK. *Vet J*. 2013;197:233-237.

Ked and Louse Infestations

Ked and louse infestations cause irritation resulting in skin or wool damage. Blood loss may occur with some species.

SHEEP KED (*MELOPHAGUS OVINUS*)

Keds are flat, brown, wingless flies, about 6 to 7 mm in length, found on sheep throughout the world. Keds are now rarely reported in many countries because of good management and control. For example, it wasn't mentioned in a review of livestock ectoparasites of Europe and the Mediterranean,[1] although anecdotal evidence suggests it may be present in isolated pockets associated with organic production.[2] The ked can transmit *Trypanosoma melophagium* and *Rickettsia melophagi*, harmless blood parasites of sheep. Recent studies suggest that it may have more importance than otherwise indicated.[3] Staining of the wool by the feces of the ked reduces its value and gives it a peculiar musty odor. Heavy infestations cause skin blemishes, which are costly to the leather industry. Sheep in poor condition suffer most from infestations. Goats may also be infested.

LIFE CYCLE

Keds live their entire life cycle on the host. Adults of both sexes are blood feeders, and although the degrees of infestation usually encountered cause only irritation with resulting scratching, biting, and damage to the fleece, very heavy infestations may cause severe anemia. Spread is generally the result of direct contact between hosts. A recent review[2] suggests that this exchange is primarily between dams and their offspring and that it is predominantly the newly emerged adults that migrate to new hosts. Larvae develop within the female one at a time and are deposited on the host as mature third instars that pupate within a few hours. The female ked lives for 4 to 5 months and may lay up to 10 to 15 larvae, so buildup of infection is slow. The larvae are attached to the wool fiber some distance above, the skin and many larvae and pupae are removed at shearing. The young ked usually emerges in 20 to 22 days, but this period may be prolonged for up to 35 days in winter. The complete life cycle takes 5 to 6 weeks under optimal conditions. Heavy infestations usually occur in winter months, and they decline in the summer. The parasite is mainly seen in colder, wetter areas, and infestations may disappear when sheep are moved to hot, dry districts. Resistance is acquired in time, and resistant sheep grow better and produce more wool.

A seasonal pattern of infestation occurs. Keds are sensitive to hot, dry weather and numbers decrease markedly over the summer. Populations increase slowly over the autumn and winter. Although keds that have been dislodged from the host can live for up to 2 weeks if in mild moist conditions, most die in 3 to 4 days and probably do not play a part in reinfesting sheep.

Keds have recently been implicated in the transmission of *Anaplasma ovis* from infected sheep.[3] This potentially zoonotic disease can infect people, with important implications.

CONTROL

At shearing a large proportion of adults and pupae will be removed. This can provide effective control on adult sheep, particularly where a combination of hot conditions and a short fleece will kill most of the remaining keds. However, some may remain alive in protected places such as the ventral neck and breech regions and on younger stock. If treatment is carried out within the next 2 to 4 weeks, eradication will be achieved as long as all sheep are included and the insecticide used has a residual protection longer than the time taken for the last pupae to hatch.

Ivermectin and its analogs given at the standard anthelmintic dose will act to eliminate the ked populations. Closantel is also effective against keds.

REFERENCES

1. Wall R. *Vet Parasitol.* 2007;148:62-74.
2. Small RW. *Vet Parasitol.* 2005;130:141.
3. Hornock S, et al. *Vector Borne Zoonotic Dis.* 2011;11:1319-1321.

LOUSE INFESTATIONS (PEDICULOSIS)

Louse infestations are common throughout the world. The species are host specific and are divided into biting and sucking lice.

SYNOPSIS

Etiology Species-specific sucking and chewing lice affecting all animals.

Epidemiology Transmission from host to host. Lice show a marked seasonal periodicity, rising from low numbers after summer to a peak in the following late spring. Foot lice infested from pasture.

Clinical signs Irritation that causes rubbing, damage to the fleece or skin, and loss of milk production. Some species cause anemia. Foot lice cause stamping.

Clinical pathology Hair loss may result from hypersensitivity.

Lesions Skin lesions as a result of rubbing; fleeces have tufts protruding and lose their brightness.

Diagnostic confirmation Lice can be seen on careful inspection. Preferred site varies with host and species of louse.

Differential diagnosis In sheep, must be differentiated from *Psorergates*, ked, and *Psoroptes* infections. In other animals, separate from allergic dermatitis.

Treatment Macrocyclic lactones and synthetic pyrethroids (where available).

Control Pour-on and injectable treatments control lice on cattle, horses, sheep, and pigs. Good husbandry practices will reduce infestations. Plunge or shower dips used on sheep; all sheep should be treated, and sheep must be thoroughly wetted. Treatment should follow shearing, which removes many lice; sheep in short wool are also easier to wet.

ETIOLOGY

The important species are as follows:

- Cattle:
  Sucking lice—*Linognathus vituli* (long-nosed sucking louse), *Solenopotes capillatus* (small blue sucking louse), *Haematopinus eurysternus* (short-nosed sucking louse), *Haematopinus quadripertusus* (tail louse), *Haematopinus tuberculatus* (buffalo louse)
  Chewing lice—*Damalinia* (= *Bovicola*) *bovis*
- Sheep:
  Sucking lice—*Linognathus ovillus* (sucking face louse), *Linognathus africanus*, *Linognathus stenopsis* (goat sucking louse), *Linognathus pedalis* (sucking foot louse)
  Chewing lice—*Damalinia ovis*
- Goats:
  Sucking lice—*L.* (blue louse), *L. africanus*
  Chewing lice—*Damalinia caprae*, *Damalinia limbata*, *Damalinia crassiceps*
- Pigs:
  Sucking lice—*Haematopinus suis*
- Horses:
  Sucking lice—*Haematopinus asini*
  Chewing lice—*Damalinia equi*
- Donkeys:
  Chewing lice—*Werneckiella* (= *Bovicola*) *ocellatus*

LIFE CYCLE AND EPIDEMIOLOGY

Sucking Lice

All life-cycle stages of sucking lice are found on the host. Both sexes are obligate blood feeders, taking small meals from capillaries in the upper skin.[1] Survival off the host is limited, although some species, such as the foot lice of sheep, may survive away from the host for up to 2 weeks. Females lay 2 to 6 eggs per day, which are attached to individual hair shafts. Eggs complete embryo development and hatch within 5 to 11 days of deposition. Lice have three nymphal stages, which bear a morphologic similarity to the sexually mature adult stage. Each nymphal stage will take 2 to 4 days to complete. Louse development rate, at all stages, is highly temperature dependent and requires a narrow temperature range. Temperatures above 41°C (106 F) and 46°C (115 F) are lethal for eggs and adults, respectively, of *L. vituli.*[2] Optimal development takes place between 33°C and 37° C (91 F and 99 F). Lice therefore show a seasonal periodicity, with very low numbers in the summer when conditions are hot. Populations begin to increase with cooler fall temperatures, reaching maximum levels in late winter.[3]

Chewing Lice

All life-cycle stages of chewing lice are found on the host. Lice feed on dead skin cells, hair, and oil secretions, which they abrade from the surface using their chewing mouthparts. There may be some abrasion of the upper skin layers, and there has been demonstration that sheep develop antibodies to salivary sections of *Damalinia* (= *Bovicola*) *bovis.* Sex ratios are highly female biased, and there are suggestions that parthenogenesis occurs in some species. Females deposit less than 1 egg per day. Embryo development is completed in 7 to 10 days, producing nymphs that molt three times before reaching sexual maturity. As with the sucking lice, there is a strong temperature/development relationship that is highly regulated, with a narrow range for optimal development and survival. Chewing lice can survive off the host for up to 2 weeks.

Transmission of both types of lice occurs by direct contact, but inert objects such as blankets, grooming tools, and harnesses may remain infective for several days. Sheep may become infested with foot lice from the pasture. Young pigs may become infected some 10 hours after birth. Newborn calves rapidly acquire infestations from their dams.

CLINICAL FINDINGS AND DIAGNOSIS

Sucking Lice

All species cause irritation of the skin and stimulate scratching, rubbing, and licking, leading to restlessness, damage to hair coat or fleece and hides, and loss of milk production. These behavioral changes result in reduced efficiency, particularly in feedlot cattle.

Lice appear to be present on a large proportion of cattle, but measurement of their impact on productivity has produced equivocal results. It is often thought that infestation has little or no effect on weight gain and hematological values. However, there appears to be a synergistic effect between louse infestations and the presence of gastrointestinal nematodes that does have an influence on weight gain. Anemia is rare but has been described for heavy infestations of *L. vituli* and *H. eurysternus.* Treatment, however, may be warranted to reduce the damage to hides and prevent damage to fences and other fixtures. Hairballs may occasionally occur in calves as a result of continual licking. Cattle and pig lice have been reported as vectors of several rickettsial diseases, but this remains to be verified.[4]

The pig louse spreads swinepox, and although weight loss may not occur, even with heavy burdens, some pigs develop an allergic dermatitis, and the consequent rubbing leads to skin lesions.

Foot lice of sheep are thought to live on blood. Light infestations may not cause clinical signs, but moderate to severe infestations cause stamping and biting of the affected parts. Lice cause goats to rub or to bite their coats, which become matted and damaged. Angora goats can damage the hair shaft and lose their coats. Signs of infestation are restlessness, hair loss, and decreased milk production. In horses, *H. asini* is the more serious species because it removes blood and may cause some anemia.

Chewing Lice

Chewing lice cause irritation and rubbing. In sheep, the wool loses its brightness and may become matted and more yellow. There is evidence that a pelt defect called cockle is associated with infestation with body lice. The quantity and quality of the fleece is reduced, and losses up to AUS$3.20 per infested sheep have been measured.

Chewing lice on cattle also cause an increase in rubbing and licking, which contributes to reduction of efficiency and damage to facilities. Hair loss has been attributed to this infestation, but it is a controversial association because many other causes are likely. Lice have been implicated in the transmission of several bacterial pathogens, but this finding requires verification.[5]

Diagnosis of lice on cattle and horses requires close visual inspection, with particular attention being paid to known predilection sites. These include the head, the sides of the neck, the dewlap, the escutcheon, and tail switch. Effective diagnosis requires that hair be parted and skin examined at several locations at each of the predilection sites. Use of a supplementary light source and restraint of the animal are very helpful.

Chewing lice of cattle, sheep, and horses are recognized by their rounded heads and light brown color. These lice are highly mobile and will move away from inspection sites. Their eggs are difficult to see unless on dark-haired cattle or horses. Sucking lice are recognized by their gray or blue–gray color and their pointed heads. They tend to remain fixed to the skin.

Chewing lice may congregate on the dorsal surface and flanks, whereas sucking lice are found on the head and in the long hair of the mane and tail; in heavy winter infestations, however, lice may be found on any part of the body. In sheep with long wool, the greatest numbers of *D. ovis* may be seen on the midside, particularly the shoulders, from where they spread to the back and rump. After shearing, small residual infestations may be found on the ventral neck. Foot lice are usually found in clusters on those parts covered with hair, mainly on the lower limbs, but in heavy infestations they can be found in clusters above the hock, on the scrotum, in the belly wool, and, more rarely, on the face.

TREATMENT AND CONTROL

Self-grooming and grooming by herdmates effectively regulates louse populations on most hosts, but the effectiveness is limited when hair coat or fleece become too long for the tongue surface to effectively remove lice and eggs. Similarly, shearing is an important factor in reducing body lice populations on sheep. Between 30% and 50% of the population is removed with the fleece, and those remaining are subjected to a more variable microclimate. Populations are at their lowest 30 to 60 days after shearing. Reversing temperature gradients as sheep move in and out of shade, and very wet conditions, will also reduce lice numbers.

Body lice of sheep are relatively easy to eradicate if a clean muster is achieved, the sheep are thoroughly treated, and reinfestation is avoided. However, in practice, failure to eradicate commonly occurs as a result of the inability to thoroughly wet the fleece because of poor formulation of products or because the lice are resistant to the chemical used. The most difficult problem when attempting to eradicate lice from flocks over a large area is the diagnosis of lice in lightly infested flocks. Methods of detection of louse antibodies in fleece have been developed for use on the farm that give good results. Adoption has been limited, and in many cases the methods have been withdrawn from practice because the delay between testing and results has been too long. Similarly, techniques have been devised to test for lice by digesting the wool and examining the residue for lice, but the delays inherent in such a system often mean that by the time the farmer obtains the results, the optimum time to treat sheep has passed.

Affected sheep can be effectively treated with macrocyclic lactone or chitin synthesis inhibitors. An ivermectin 0.03% jetting fluid was reported to have high efficacy in treating lice in sheep with 3 to 9 months of wool, but failed to eradicate the lice. No treatment is known that can eradicate lice from long-woolled sheep under field conditions. Following treatment of foot lice, sheep should be moved to a paddock that has been free of sheep for a month.

Treatment of goats has not been studied extensively, and the treatments used on sheep and cattle are thought to be effective in goats. Lactating goats should not be treated.

Macrocyclic lactone-based products (ivermectin, moxidectin, doramectin, and eprinomectin) are available as pour-on or injectable formulations for cattle and have shown excellent efficacy against both sucking and chewing lice. Persistence of activity is one of the exceptional benefits of these products.

Essential oil treatments using a variety of products have been evaluated against *W. ocelatus* in donkeys and have been proven an effective alternative to synthetic chemicals.[4]

Sheep lice have been shown to quickly develop insecticide resistance, and strains of *D. ovis* that are resistant to the insecticides are common in the United Kingdom and Australia.[6] Tolerance has been reported in other species as well.[7] Resistance management strategies that use combination treatments are now considered the best approach to management of the problem.

Treatments should be timed to coincide with the beginning of louse population growth (i.e., autumn or early winter). Extremely early treatments often result in spring outbreaks that are caused by very small residual populations on a few animals.[8] Products with persistent activity, in excess of 21 days (e.g., macrocyclic lactones), do not require a second application.

Effective management of lice in a herd requires that new animals be isolated for a period of time sufficient for all lice to be eliminated by treatment. The introduction of one or two infested individuals, such as occurs when strays are allowed into a herd, leads to a slow buildup of infestation. In Australia, modeling approaches have been developed for the treatment of sheep.[9]

RECOMMENDATION

All animals in a herd should be treated for louse control to prevent the buildup of the louse population to a point that is damaging.

REFERENCES

1. Colwell DD. *Vet Parasitol.* 2002;104:319-322.
2. Colwell DD. *Vet Parasitol.* 2014;194:144-149.
3. Otter A, et al. *Vet Record.* 2003;153:176-179.
4. Ellse L, Wall RL. *Med Vet Entomol.* 2014;28:233-243.
5. Hornok S, et al. *Vet Parasitol.* 2010;174:355-358.
6. Sands B, et al. *Vet Rec.* 2014;doi:10.1136/vr.102777.
7. Ellse L, et al. *Vet Parasitol.* 2012;188:134-139.
8. James PJ, et al. *An Prod Sci.* 2011;51:753-762.
9. Lucas PG, Horton BJ. *Aust Vet J.* 2014;92:8-14.

Miscellaneous Skin Diseases Caused by Flies, Midges, and Mosquitoes

Although these insects differ quite markedly, they are dealt with together because they exert similar deleterious effects. Their activity causes stress and induces behavioral changes, and in many cases they are important vectors for a variety of parasites and infectious diseases.

STABLE FLIES (*STOMOXYS CALCITRANS*)

ETIOLOGY

The stable fly, *Stomoxys calcitrans*, has a cosmopolitan distribution. Other species, including *Stomoxys nigra*, occur in South Africa. *S. calcitrans* is a moderate-sized, gray to black fly about the size of a housefly. These are the most economically important species of fly affecting confined livestock in North America.

LIFE CYCLE AND EPIDEMIOLOGY

These insects have a typical fly life cycle, with eggs being deposited in high-organic-matter areas with an elevated moisture content, such as spilled feed and the edge of silage pits. The larvae grow in a temperature-dependent manner in the same high-organic-matter area through three larval stages. Pupae form in dry material at the edges of the areas where the larvae develop. Flies rest on fences and structural surfaces in a characteristic head-upward position and can readily be recognized by the prominent, forward-directed, pointed proboscis between short palps.

Stable flies of both sexes are blood feeders, attacking particularly cattle and horses, people, and, to a lesser extent, pigs. Bites are painful and often bleed freely when fresh. The flies are intermittent feeders, spending only short periods on the host; most of their time is spent resting on fences and building sides. Eggs are laid in high-moisture areas of rotting hay or straw, along the edge of silage pits, and on the edges of manure pack of feedlots and compost piles. Mature larvae leave the high-moisture sites to pupate in drier sites nearby. Development times are regulated by temperature, with higher temperatures resulting in more rapid development. A complete life cycle will require 3 to 4 weeks in summer. In temperate climates flies exhibit a distinct seasonality, with peak populations in middle to late summer. Larvae will overwinter in warmer areas of silage piles. The flies are highly mobile, traveling up to 20 km in search of suitable hosts. These flies have now moved onto pasture, where they can affect cattle that are fed from round bales left as a food source.[1]

Feeding activity by the flies results in stress to the animals and reduced efficiency through reductions in feeding time. When large numbers of flies are present, the animals will bunch to reduce biting rates. At high temperatures the bunching may result in cattle overheating.

PATHOGENESIS

S. calcitrans organisms are mechanical vectors for anthrax, infectious equine anemia, bovine virus, diarrhea virus, and surra. They are intermediate hosts for the nematode *Habronema majus*,[3] which is reputed to be a cause of allergic dermatitis in horses in Japan.

CLINICAL FINDINGS

A localized sensitivity of the forelimbs of cattle may develop and result in the formation of intradermal blisters that coalesce to form bleeding sores. With very heavy infestations some deaths may occur. Populations can be assessed by counting the number of flies on the front legs of cattle. When the average number exceeds 2 per leg, significant losses occur, and population management is required.

TREATMENT AND CONTROL

Effective management of stable flies requires removal of high-moisture, rotting organic matter from the environment.[2] Edges of silage pits, manure packs, and compost piles should be kept dry, and manure-contaminated bedding should be removed regularly. Insecticide treatments must be applied to all exterior surfaces (e.g., barn sides, fences, and exterior of feed bunks). Spraying of fixtures and walls, particularly sunlit walls where the flies often remain unnoticed, with long-acting compounds reduces infestations for 2 weeks or longer.

Application of insecticides or repellants directly on animals is generally impractical because of the short duration of efficacy. Low frequency of insecticidal application, when necessary, slows the development of insecticide resistance. Permethrin applied as a microencapsulated formulation gave longer protection than an emulsifiable concentrate. Affected horses can be treated locally with an analgesic cream, and if the irritation is severe they can be tranquilized with acetylpromazine.

RECOMMENDATION

Treatment is absolutely necessary to keep these flies from reaching population levels that are in excess of the economic threshold and from reaching levels where they are an animal welfare issue. Populations are also an issue for humans.

REFERENCES

1. Taylor DB, Berkebile DR. *Environ Entomol.* 2011;40:184.
2. Kneeland KM, et al. *USDA ARS.* Washington: 2012:173.
3. Amado S, et al. *Exp Parasitol.* 2014;136:35.

HORSE FLIES, MARCH FLIES OR BREEZE FLIES (*TABANUS* SPP.), AND DEER FLIES (*CHRYSOPS, HAEMATOPOTA,* AND *PANGONIA* SPP.)

Horse flies, march flies or breeze flies, and deer flies are large, robust, blood-feeding flies that are widespread in both temperate and tropical regions. Only the females take blood meals, but the bites are savage and cause significant distress to large animals, particularly horses and cattle. These flies can act as mechanical vectors of diseases caused by viruses (equine infectious anemia, bovine leukosis, vesicular stomatitis, hog cholera), bacteria (anthrax, tularemia), and trypanosomes (surra). Eggs are laid on the leaves of plants growing in or near standing water. The larval and pupal stages occur in the water or mud, and the life cycle takes 4 to 5 months to complete. The flies are active in summer and attack animals principally on the legs and ventral abdomen. Duration of activity can be relative short (i.e., 3 to 4 weeks), but stress on the animals can be very high during that time. Fly attacks lead to bunching of animals with the attendant likelihood of overheating and in some cases resulting in animals stampeding through fences. Adult flies are attracted to host volatiles, including components of host urine.[1] Control is difficult unless wet areas can be drained or livestock kept away from those areas where the flies are most active. Repellents have been used and are reasonably effective in horses subject to fly worry. The use of DEET affords protection for only a few days and is costly, but its use in milking cattle gives increased milk yield and butterfat. Synthetic pyrethroid-impregnated eartags give very little protection against these flies.

RECOMMENDATION

Control is extremely difficult for both larvae and adults but should be attempted for the purpose of reducing effects of adult flies on animal welfare.

REFERENCE

1. Mihok S, Mulye H. *Med Vet Entomol.* 2010;24:266-272.

HYPODERMA SPP. INFESTATION (WARBLE FLIES)

Infestations of cattle with the larvae of *Hypoderma* spp. cause serious damage to hides and carcasses, in addition to production losses. Occasional deaths result from anaphylactic shock or toxemia and damage to the central nervous system or esophagus. Several other flies with very similar life histories affect goats (*Przhevalskiana silenus*) and semidomestic reindeer (*Hypoderma tarandi*) in addition to affecting the well-being of wild ruminants. *Dermatobia hominis* larvae affect all species of ruminants and humans (tropical bot fly) in South America.

SYNOPSIS

Etiology *Hypoderma bovis* and *H. lineatum* in cattle, *H. sinense* in cattle and yaks, *H. diana* in deer, *H. tarandi* in reindeer and caribou, *Przhevalskiana silenus* in goats. Horses are occasionally affected.

Epidemiology Eggs attached to hair in spring to late summer, larvae penetrate skin and migrate to esophagus (*H. lineatum* and *H. sinense*) or spine (*H. bovis*), where they stay for 2 to 3 months; they then move to subdermal tissue along the back and after 2 to 3 months emerge from the breathing hole, fall to the ground, pupate, and emerge as adult flies 3 to 5 weeks later. Larvae of *P.* and *H. tarandi* do not undergo migration within deep tissues of their host.

Clinical signs Reduced growth and production. Larvae in the back cause obvious swellings; larvae in the spinal cord may cause posterior paralysis. Treatment of larvae while they are in the esophagus may cause serious edema, and edema and paraplegia may occur if animals are treated when larvae are in the spinal canal.

Clinical pathology An enzyme-linked immunosorbent assay (ELISA) is available.

Lesions Larvae are found in discolored tissue.

Diagnostic confirmation Swellings along back characteristic.

Differential diagnosis Traumatic injury to the spine; aberrant *S. vulgaris* larvae in the horse.

Treatment Macrocyclic lactone endectocides.

Control Treatments are given so as to *avoid* treating when larvae are in the esophagus or spinal canal. (Usually treated in autumn and spring, but varies with location.)

ETIOLOGY

There are two species that specifically parasitize cattle: *Hypoderma bovis* and *H. lineatum*. A third species, *H. sinense*, affects cattle and yaks in central Asia.[1,2] The adult flies are robust and hairy, are about the size of a bee (12 to 18 mm long), are yellow-orange in color, and have two wings. They are not easily seen because of the rapidity of their flight. Repeated infestation results in an acquired immunity that results in older animals being less severely affected than younger animals.

Horses are occasionally infected with *Hypoderma* species of cattle. The larvae are found in subcutaneous cysts on the back, but they have not been reported to complete development. This location causes problems if they are in the saddle region.

Losses to the cattle industry caused by warble fly have not been estimated recently, but in 1965 the loss was estimated to be US$192 million per annum in the United States, and in 1976 approximately $100 million. In 1982 the cost of warble fly was estimated as £35 million for Great Britain, but the parasite has now been eradicated from the United Kingdom and Ireland. Advent of the macrocyclic lactone endectocides has greatly reduced the prevalence of the cattle species in North America, but they persist in localized areas.[2]

Hypoderma tarandi, *H. acteon*, and *H. diana* infect reindeer/caribou and deer. *H. diana* is found throughout Europe in several deer species but may also occur in sheep. *H. actaeon*, also found throughout Europe, is known only from the red deer. These species do not undergo deep tissue migrations that characterize the life cycle of the cattle species.

Przhevalskiana silenus is similar to the previously described species and is a parasite of goats in the Mediterranean basin, parts of eastern Europe, Pakistan, and India. This species also does not have a deep tissue migration, and larvae tend to develop subcutaneously very near the site of initial skin penetration. The losses resulting from this parasite are significant and result from reductions in carcass quality and reduced animal health.

The larvae of *Dermatobia hominis*, a small (12 mm long) related fly, parasitize a wide variety of hosts and cause major economic losses to cattle production in South America. They also affect humans and are a major zoonosis for travelers in the region. Mature larvae are about 2.5 cm long and develop in a subcutaneous cyst that can be quite painful. Female *Dermatobia* oviposit on zoophilous, "porter" flies such as mosquitoes and stable flies, which they catch on the wing.[2] The eggs are transported to the mammalian host, and they hatch in response to increased temperature as the fly lands. Larvae penetrate the skin, but do not migrate. Treatment and control measures are the same as for *Hypoderma* spp. of cattle.

LIFE CYCLE AND EPIDEMIOLOGY

Warble flies historically were common parasites of cattle in the northern hemisphere, including North America and Europe, and are common in parts of Asia. The distribution of these parasites has been changing recently with the widespread use of macrocyclic lactone endectocides and the adoption of eradication programs in many European countries. Infestations south of the equator are rare and are the result of imported cattle, although endemic cases have occurred in Chile.

Adult flies are active in the spring to late summer, with *H. lineatum* usually appearing 3 to 4 weeks before *H. bovis*. *H. lineatum* attaches up 600 eggs, in strings of 5 to 25, to hairs on the legs or lower parts of the body, whereas *H. bovis* attaches eggs, one at a time, to hairs on the rump and upper parts of the hindleg. The oviposition flight of *H. bovis*, darting in to lay each egg, will terrorize cattle. Eggs hatch in 4 to 6 days. The larvae penetrate the skin using protease enzymes and migrate through connective tissues to reach the esophagus (*H. lineatum*) or the epidural fat in the spine (*H. bovis*), where they stay, feeding and growing, for 2 to 4 months. They subsequently continue their migration to reach the subdermal tissue of the back in the early spring. Here they make a breathing hole and become encased in a granulomatous cyst. They complete development in 1 to 2 months, passing through second and third instars, and emerge through the hole, fall to the ground, and pupate. Adult flies emerge some 3 to 5 weeks later. The fully developed larvae are thick and long (25 to 30 mm), light cream in color, but darkening to almost black as mature third instars. A single animal may have up to 300 larvae, each developing with granulomatous cysts, with breathing holes, under the skin of the back.

Hypoderma tarandi females deposit eggs on the hair of reindeer or caribou, and larvae hatch in approximately 7 to 10 days. Larvae penetrate the skin close to where the eggs are deposited and do not migrate into deep tissues. Flies are active during arctic summer, and larvae remain in the back until early spring.

Przhevalskiana silenus eggs are attached to host hairs, and the larvae hatch after 7 to 8 days. Larvae penetrate the skin in the area where they were deposited, where they remain throughout their development period. Flies are known to be active from May through June in southern Italy and can be found in host tissues from May through the following February.

The timing of the life cycle, that is, the period when grubs are present in the animals and the time at which the flies are present in large numbers, varies with the climate and is of importance in a control program. *H. lineatum* generally is 1 to 2 months ahead of *H. bovis*, and where the two flies are present, both "grub" and "fly" seasons may be very long. In the southern United States the fly season is February and March; in Canada it is June to August. The period when grubs are present in the back is December in the south and February to May in Canada. In Europe the larvae begin to move to the back from January to July.

PATHOGENESIS

Migrating first instars cause little damage as they use their proteolytic enzymes to migrate through connective tissue. The enzymes, however, have an antiinflammatory effect, partially through cleavage of complement components. Larvae maturing under the skin of the back form holes in the skin, and the reaction of the host encloses each grub within a granulomatous cyst. On rare occasions an anaphylactic reaction may occur in a sensitized animal as the result of death of migrating larvae; chance migration into the brain may also occur. Intracranial myiasis as a result of *H. bovis* has also been recorded in the horse. Treatment of animals when the first instars are in the esophagus may cause a massive inflammatory edema that may prevent feeding and swallowing of saliva; eructation may stop and bloating may occur. Treatment of *H. bovis* while it is in the spinal canal may also cause edema and mild to severe paraplegia.

CLINICAL FINDINGS

Cattle at pasture may be worried by adult fly attacks that disrupt grazing and breeding behavior, which are exacerbated when fly populations are large. Avoidance behavior, called gadding, may result in injury as cattle run into fences and other natural obstructions. Heavy infestations with larvae are commonly associated with poor growth, poor body condition, and production losses, but such heavy infestations are often complicated by other forms of mismanagement, including malnutrition and parasitic gastroenteritis. Immunosuppression results from the effect of larval secretions. Infected cattle milk poorly, and a considerable increase in milk production and milk fat occurs after treatment.

The presence of the subcutaneous larvae causes obvious swelling, with pain on touch. The swellings are usually soft and with an opening that is usually evident. There may be as many as 200 to 300 such lesions on the back of one animal.

With involvement of the spinal cord there is a sudden onset of posterior paralysis without fever and without other systemic signs. The suddenness of onset and the failure of the disease to progress usually suggest traumatic injury. A similar disease can occur in horses and is reputed to be more common in horses than in cattle.

CLINICAL PATHOLOGY

An ELISA that detects antibodies to the secreted enzymes of *H. lineatum* and *H. bovis* has been developed. It has been used in monitoring the eradication program in Great Britain and in France.[3] In addition, an antigen-capture ELISA, used to detect the presence of circulating quantities of the predominant larval enzyme, has been developed. This will be useful in differentiating active from cleared infestations and will be useful in detailed surveillance programs if used at the correct time in the life cycle.

NECROPSY FINDINGS

The first instars, migrating within connective tissue, are usually surrounded by a zone of yellow-green discoloration. Later larval stages lie in a subcutaneous, granulomatous cyst that may contain a pale fluid. Rarely the cyst will contain a large amount of purulent discharge. Other characteristic findings include the following:

- No other disease causes the characteristic swellings on the back.
- The differential diagnoses of posterior paralysis and anaphylaxis are discussed in detail under the respective headings of "Disease of the Spinal Cord" and "Anaphylaxis."
- The clinical signs of macrocyclic lactone poisoning have not been reported to cause these symptoms.
- Posterior paralysis as a result of destruction of the larvae in the epidural space usually occurs, but macrocyclic lactone products have not been reported to cause these symptoms.

TREATMENT

Macrocyclic Lactone Compounds

All larval stages of cattle grubs and other oestrid flies are very sensitive to macrocyclic lactone endectocides. Their widespread use in nematode control programs plays a major role in controlling warble flies. Their residual activity will persist for about 4 weeks.[4,5]

Treatment Recommendations

Treatment with a macrocyclic lactone-based product is strongly advised, both to increase productivity and to maintain population control.

Manual Removal

When small numbers of cattle are affected with relatively few warble grubs, manual removal of the larvae can be practiced. Incomplete removal or breaking the larvae during removal may cause a severe systemic reaction. This reaction and the one that sometimes occurs after systemic treatment of cattle infected with cattle grubs has been ascribed to anaphylaxis. However, there is evidence that it a direct result of toxins liberated from dead maggots and that phenylbutazone may control this toxin. The clinical signs include dullness, salivation, lacrimation, dyspnea, wrinkling of skin on the side of the neck, and edema under the jaw.

CONTROL

With the macrocyclic lactone endectocides, in general, systemic treatments are given at the end of fly activity and in the spring after first instars have left sensitive tissues. In those species that do not undergo deep tissue migration, treatment can be instituted anytime after the cessation of fly activity.

Cattle grub has been eradicated in Norway, Sweden, Denmark, Malta, Ireland, and Great Britain. Eradication programs were initiated in France.[3] Surveillance has decreased in most countries as a result of the excellent efficacy of the macrocyclic lactone products. However, evidence from Canada suggests that residual populations remain.[4] A joint Canadian–U.S. study using sterile male *Hypoderma* species eradicated these species from the test area, but the difficulty of mass producing flies, in the absence of an in vitro rearing system, makes this technique impractical for large-scale warble fly control.[6]

Vaccination of cattle using crude larval extracts has reduced both the number of warbles in the back and the number of larvae that could pupate.[7] Results of vaccination studies with recombinant antigens have been variable, and commercial development has ceased. Use of antigens derived from "hidden" sites such as the fatbody have produced excellent results,[5] and potential components have been identified, but further work has not been followed up.[8] Sequencing of the mitochondrial genome of *H. lineatum* has been completed.[9]

REFERENCES

1. Otranto D, et al. *J Parasitol.* 2004;90:958.
2. Colwell DD, et al., eds. *CABI Publishing.* 2006.
3. Boulard C, et al. *Vet Parasitol.* 2008;158:1-10.
4. Colwell DD. *Vet Parasitol.* 2013;197:297-303.
5. Rehbein S. *Vet Parasitol.* 2013;192:353-358.
6. Colwell DD. *Vet Parasitol.* 2011;175:313-319.
7. Dacal V, et al. *J Comp Path.* 2011;145(2-3):282-288.
8. Sandeman RM. *Parasite Immunol.* 2014;111:214-222.
9. Weigl S, et al. *Med Vet Entomol.* 2010;24:329-335.

HORN FLIES AND BUFFALO FLIES (*HAEMATOBIA* SPP.)

ETIOLOGY

The small (6-mm) grayish flies of the *Haematobia* species, known as horn flies and buffalo flies, have distinct geographic distributions, *H. irritans exigua* in Australia and South East Asia, *H. irritans irritans* throughout North and South America and Hawaii, and *H. minuta* in Africa. *H. irritans irritans* is common in Europe, where it causes few problems. This species was transported to North America in the late 1800s, where it rapidly established and spread. It has subsequently moved into South America, where it has also become a major problem. *Haematobia* species are known as vectors for the nematodes *Stephanofilaria stilesi*, but their impact is thought to be of little importance.

LIFE CYCLE AND EPIDEMIOLOGY

These insects have a typical fly life cycle and habits. Eggs are deposited away from the animal onto freshly deposited dung, where the larval stages develop in a highly temperature-regulated manner. The onset of diapause in the pupal stage is regulated at this stage and requires that the larvae be exposed to increased hours of low temperatures for the pupae to become diapause driven. Three larval stages are spent in the dung, with larvae feeding largely on bacteria. Pupae form in the dry regions outside of the dung pat. Both sexes of these flies are obligate blood feeders, primarily attacking pastured cattle and water buffalo. They do not survive off the host, other than for short periods. They are not known as vectors for any disease agents other than the nematodes *Stephanofilaria* spp. They cause significant reductions in productivity of pastured cattle through induction of stress, changes in grazing patterns, and, in extreme cases, blood loss. Burdens of 200 to 500 flies will reduce weight gains of beef cattle (up to 14% reduction) and milk yield of dairy cows. Heavy infestations (over 1000 flies) can cause serious loss of condition and, rarely, deaths. Control results in higher feed efficiency, increased growth rate, and increased calf-weaning weights.

The flies are easily recognized by the way in which the wings are held at rest, slightly divergent and angled upward, away from the body. Adult flies stay on the host most of the time, unless disturbed. Females leave the host, as feces are passed, to deposit eggs around edges of the freshly deposited dung. Larvae develop within the dung pat, feeding primarily on bacteria. Development is regulated by environmental temperatures, and the larvae are stimulated to enter diapause (arrested development) if temperatures become too low. Mature larvae exit the dung to pupate in the dry soil below and around the pat. A complete life cycle may require up to 3 weeks under optimal environmental conditions. Thus at higher temperatures in excess of 15 generations may be produced in a single season; in more temperate climates such Canada and the upper United States, only 5 generations may occur.

PATHOGENESIS

The flies congregate chiefly on the withers, shoulders, and flanks and around the horns and eyes. Flies take numerous (15 to 20) small blood meals per day. In North America feeding often takes place on the ventral midline and several 2- to 5-cm-diameter feeding lesions are often observed. Zebu cattle are less affected by the flies than British breeds, and although they may carry large populations of flies, they show fewer feeding lesions.

CLINICAL FINDINGS

Whereas adults rarely leave the host except for oviposition, the newly emerged flies of *H. irritans irritans* will travel up to 20 km in search of new hosts. They may be dispersed also by prevailing strong winds, and they are carried long distances by the movement of cattle to new pastures. The distribution of *H. irritans exigua* is controlled by environmental factors, particularly temperature and humidity. At temperatures below 21° C (70° F), the flies become sluggish, and at 5° C (41° F) they become comatose.

TREATMENT AND CONTROL

Infestations have been controlled by traps, insecticide sprays, back rubbers, dust bags, or eartags impregnated with insecticides. Traps have been designed for use with dairy cattle that walk through them on their way to and from the dairy. The flies are dislodged by gauze strips and are retained in the trap and killed when they rest on the insecticide-coated walls. Traps are rarely used today, but recent work with modified traps has given 80% to 90% control.

Back rubbers consist of absorbent material, impregnated with insecticide or oil, wrapped around a cable or chain suspended from a central pole and attached to ground-level supports or as a cable suspended a little over a meter above the ground between two posts 4 to 5 m apart. Cattle quickly learn to use rubbers to dislodge flies, and their coats become smeared with insecticide. Insecticidal-impregnated eartags attached to back rubbers and dust bags controlled horn fly for about 6 weeks, whereas fenvalerate tags were still effective 18 weeks after application.

Eartags impregnated with a mixture of organophosphorous compounds and synthetic pyrethroids have been widely used, but resistance has built up to levels that make this technique ineffective. Discontinuing the use of pyrethroid-impregnated eartags for one season does not allow substantial reduction in resistance to occur. Eartags impregnated with compounds of both classes have been effective in managing increases in pyrethroid resistance. Current recommendations for use of impregnated eartags note that tags should be applied to the cows (because they harbor the most flies and present the largest surface area for exposure to the insecticide) at the maximum recommended rate. Although this is less convenient, it helps to avoid one of the leading causes of insecticide resistance, which is the dilution of the insecticide as it spreads from calves to cows. Flies can also be controlled by dipping, but this technique is rarely used solely for flies. Current products are combined with synthetic pyrethroids to extend the protective period. In areas where cattle ticks require regular treatment, adequate control of flies may be gained incidentally, but if treatments are not effective cattle can be oversprayed with pyrethroids. Some research on control in North America[1] using essential oils has been conducted, and the microbiome[2] has been sequenced.

Macrocyclic lactone endectocides are highly effective against larval horn flies and the larvae of face flies, stable flies, and houseflies, often killing larvae for periods in excess of 8 weeks. However, in terms of practical control, where flies immigrate from surrounding herds, the duration of efficacy is not more than 2 weeks. In addition, the macrocyclic lactones generally cause significant reductions of nontarget insects in the dung community,[3] many of which are beneficial because they are natural enemies of the horn fly and buffalo fly. The various macrocyclic lactone products have differential effects on flies and other dung insects, and it appears that moxidectin has the least impact.[3] Virtually all of the cattle on pasture in North America are affected by horn flies, with the exception of those kept at higher elevations.[1] The effect will be altered by various factors, including both physical and biological characteristics of the flies and their hosts.

Pour-on formulations of pyrethroids are highly effective, as evidenced by application of 1% cyfluthrin. Insect growth regulators (e.g., Diflubenzuron) applied as a bolus gave 80% control of the immature stages of the face fly and horn fly in the manure for at least 20 weeks and reduced the number of dung beetles for 7 weeks. A 3% methoprene bolus was also active against flies but had no apparent effect on the dung beetles. The use of essential oils has been shown to have good fly control, but their use requires further testing.[1]

RECOMMENDATION

Treatment is necessary to keep populations below the economic threshold and to prevent this from becoming an animal welfare issue.

REFERENCES

1. Scasta JD. *J Int Pest Manage.* 2015;6:8.
2. LaChance S, Grange G. *Med Vet Entomol.* 2013;28:193-200.
3. Floate KD, et al. *Bull Entomol Res.* 2002;92:471-481.

BLACK FLIES, BUFFALO GNATS (SIMULIIDAE)

These small gray to black flies (5 mm) are members of the family Simuliidae and include a number of species and genera. The important flies appear to be *Cnephia pecuarum*, which is common in the southern states of the United States; *Simulium arcticum* and *Simulium luggeri* in Canada; *Austrosimulium pestilens* and *Austrosimulium bancrofti* in Australia; and *Simulium ornatum* in Great Britain. These very small flies occur in most parts of the world. With the exception of *S. arcticum* and two or three other species common in northern regions of North America, black flies are primarily a concern in tropical regions.

Female flies are voracious blood feeders. They are active in the summer months, when large numbers emerge from the streams and rivers where they have spent their larval and pupal stages.

A. pestilens has adapted to reach large numbers, mate, and oviposit within a very short time to utilize the flood situations that occur in northern Australia. The flies congregate in swarms and attack all animals, causing much worry and annoyance. They tend to bite animals around the legs, on the belly, and around the head, causing wheals and papules. The annoyance may be so intense that animals stampede or mill about, and young animals may be injured or even trampled to death and are frequently separated from their dams. Cattle may spend much of their time wallowing in mud or kicking up dust to keep the flies away. Herding of cattle onto bare areas reduces fly attacks because the flies commonly rest in tall grass, but this reduces feeding. The cause of death is unknown, although swelling of the throat causing suffocation, anaphylaxis, and direct toxicity are suspected. Filarid worms of *Onchocerca* spp. are transmitted by these flies, and their role as an intermediate host of nematodes has been discussed.

A similar situation occurs in northern Canada, where large numbers of *S. arcticum* have caused severe stress and occasional deaths of cattle introduced into the area of the Athabasca River and similar regions in the province of Saskatchewan. When black fly populations are extreme, previously unexposed cattle develop symptoms of shock resulting from blood loss and cumulative effects of the fly salivary secretions. In northern Saskatchewan, *S. luggeri* causes similar problems along major waterways.

Because the larval stages of these flies are passed in flowing streams where mouthparts are developed into fan-like structures for filtering out particles from water currents, large-scale control measures must be directed at killing the larvae at this stage. In the past, annual injection of methoxychlor upstream from major larval sites proved effective in reducing black fly populations, but off-target effects were undesirable. Repellents are of some use; alcoholic or aqueous solutions and dusts of permethrin, cypermethrin, and resmethrin can be applied to the whole body and will repel black flies for some days. Recently, toxins of *Bacillus thuringiensis* var. *israelensis* have been used in river injections in northern Saskatchewan, which has kept several species under control. An electrostatic sprayer that allows efficient application of repellents or insecticides to cattle under pasture conditions can be used. The insecticide or repellent solution is dispersed as charged droplets that are attracted to the hair of the animals.

HOUSEFLY (MUSCIDAE—*MUSCA DOMESTICA*)

The common housefly has a worldwide distribution and is of veterinary importance because it is capable of transmitting, in a mechanical manner, the causative bacteria of many infectious diseases. It is often cited as a means whereby anthrax, erysipelas, and brucellosis are spread, but its importance in this regard is largely unproven. Houseflies are intermediate hosts for the larvae of *Habronema muscae* and *Draschia megastoma*.

The eggs are laid in decaying organic matter of any kind. Larval development is temperature dependent, and a life cycle may be completed in 12 to 14 days so that in warm, wet summers the fly population may increase very rapidly, causing annoyance to livestock and farm workers.

Housefly population management requires frequent and thorough removal of manure and other rich organic matter. In dry weather the manure can be spread thinly on fields, but a more dependable method is to place it in a special fly trap (e.g., Baber's fly traps), from which larvae and adult flies cannot escape. Chemical treatments to control flies require application to resting sites on buildings and other facilities or the placement of baits containing methomyl, propoxur, naled, or dichlorvos at appropriate locations. Development of insecticide resistance can occur rapidly, and there are numerous examples of resistance to multiple classes of insecticide at a single location. Rotational use of insecticide classes is absolutely essential in the management of resistance.

Management of housefly populations can be augmented through release of parasitic wasps (family Pteromalidae) that kill pupae. These tiny wasps (1 to 2 mm long) actively search for the fly pupae and lay one or more eggs inside. The developing wasps devour the fly within the pupa. They have been found to be useful adjuncts to other fly control measures when used in confined facilities such as hog barns. Inundative releases at feedlots, where thousands of wasps are released at regular intervals throughout the fly season, have shown some efficacy but require an integrated approach with good manure management and selective application of insecticides.

Reducing the fly population in buildings is an important procedure in public health work, and many measures are recommended. It is not possible to give details of them here because so many factors have to be taken into consideration, including toxicity of the products used for humans and animals, development of resistance to the insecticides, and contamination of food products such as milk by the insecticides.

RECOMMENDATION

Fly control should always be attempted in an integrated manner with rational use of pesticides and other approaches.

BUSH FLIES (*MUSCA VETUSTISSIMA*)

Bush flies occur commonly in Australia in drier areas and are a cause of stress to livestock in the summer months. Bush flies die out in southern Australia each winter, but breeding continues in the north, and the regular northern winds that commence about September each year blow flies southward, which then repopulate the areas that are now suitable for reproduction. Larvae usually develop in fecal matter from several source animals. Adult *Musca vetustissima* occur in very large numbers and during the day congregate around the eyes, on the lips, on any visible mucous membrane, and on wounds to obtain moisture. They are thought to carry contagious ophthalmia of sheep, infectious keratoconjunctivitis of cattle, and contagious ecthyma of sheep; to delay the healing of wounds; to contribute to the lesions produced by buffalo flies (*Haematobia irritans exigua*); and to act as intermediate hosts for the larvae of *Draschia megastoma*, *Habronema muscae*, and *Thelazia* spp. Control of the fly population is virtually impossible in the areas where it occurs, but individual animals may be protected by repellents such as dimethyl phthalate or DEET. Sprays containing 1% of dichlorvos are effective but must be applied daily. Dung beetles, introduced from Africa, break up dung pats, which aids in control of larval stages and in reducing fly numbers. The bush fly has been implicated in the dissemination of several food-borne pathogens that can have serious concerns.[1]

RECOMMENDATION

Control of adults is recommended to alleviate animal welfare concerns.

REFERENCE

1. Vriesekoop F, Shaw R. *Foodborne Pathol Dis.* 2010;7:275-729.

FACE FLY (*MUSCA AUTUMNALIS*)

This medium-sized fly, indigenous to Europe and Asia, first appeared in North America in 1952 and is now present over large areas of Canada and the northeastern and north-central United States. The flies resemble the housefly but are slightly larger. They congregate on the face of cattle, feeding on nasal and lacrimal secretions and saliva. Very large numbers cause a certain amount of stress, cause petechiation in the eye, and are instrumental in transmitting infectious keratoconjunctivitis (pinkeye) of cattle. Face flies are vectors for the eyeworms, *Thelazia* spp., which infest the conjunctival sacs and lacrimal ducts of domestic animals.

Flies oviposit on fresh cattle manure, where larval development takes place. As with all flies, development is temperature dependent. In temperate latitudes the flies will overwinter as adults, resting inside homes and other farm structures.

Fly numbers are greatest in summer, and cattle are particularly troubled when outdoors. Repellents have been extensively used but are not highly successful. Self-applied or hand-applied dusts containing insecticides are extensively used. Reduction of face-fly populations on cattle can be achieved through use of synthetic pyrethroid-impregnated eartags, but their use is complicated by the presence of insecticide-resistant horn flies. Diflubenzuron boluses give 80% control of the immature stages of *M. autumnalis* in the manure for up to 20 weeks.

RECOMMENDATION

Control should be attempted but may be difficult in areas where resistance is a problem.

HEAD FLY (*HYDROTOEA IRRITANS*)

This medium-sized fly, similar in appearance to the housefly but having an olive abdomen and yellow wing bases, is found in the United Kingdom and Europe. It is a nonbiting muscid fly that swarms around animals and humans from late June to September. Larval development is in soil and litter, and generally there is only one life cycle per year. The lesions on sheep are self-inflicted trauma in attempts to alleviate fly irritation. Sores are often large and open, and they may be made more severe by bacterial invasion.[1] The wounds may predispose to blowfly strike by *Lucilia sericata*. The pathogens of summer mastitis of cattle can be spread mechanically by this fly as well as a number of related muscid flies, and *Trueperella (Actinomyces* or *Corynebacterium) pyogenes* has been shown to persist in *H. irritans* for up to 4 days.

Control is difficult and is similar to that used for the other nonbiting muscid fly, *M. autumnalis*. Eartags impregnated with 8.5% cypermethrin or 10% permethrin reduce the severity of fly damage in sheep, and tagged ewes give protection to their lambs. However, it is likely that resistance will quickly occur in the same manner as in the face fly. Head caps are most effective but are tedious to apply.

REFERENCE

1. Milne CE, et al. *Livestock Sci.* 2008;118:20-33.

BITING MIDGES (CERATOPOGONIDAE)

These tiny flies (1-3 mm long) are members of the family Ceratopogonidae, of which the most important genus is *Culicoides.* These flies are blood feeders and induce stress in hosts, and they can transmit infectious diseases such as bluetongue in sheep, horse sickness, and ephemeral fever in cattle.[1] They are also intermediate hosts for nematodes of the genus *Onchocerca.* Because of their importance as vectors of arboviruses, studies have been done on their feeding habits. Cattle and sheep are the most common hosts attacked, but some species also feed on birds or dogs. Hypersensitivity to the bites of *Culicoides* spp. results in an allergic dermatitis (sweet itch) in horses in Australia and North America and is discussed elsewhere. Cattle also show considerable irritation during attacks by large numbers of midges. They react with vigorous stamping of the feet, switching of the tail, and continuous movement.

The flies are plentiful in the warmer months and are most active at dawn and dusk. Because of their small size they are capable of being carried long distances by wind. Larvae develop in rich, high-organic-matter sites with high moisture content. Control of the larvae and of flies is virtually impossible, and most measures to reduce their importance are based on preventing access of the flies to the animals. Repellents, especially dimethyl phthalate or DEET, are effective on a short-term basis. Antihistamines can be used regularly but are too expensive for general use. Keeping horses away from areas where the flies are present in large numbers is advisable. Backline pour-on treatment of horses with 4 0mL of a 4% high-CIS permethrin 3 times weekly gave a good response in 86% of horses. Ivermectin at the recommended dose of 0.2 mg/kg would not produce the serum concentration that would have noticeable effects on blood-feeding *C. variipennis.* Recently, modeling of changing weather patterns indicates that such patterns may alter the distribution of important vectors and thus alter the influence of diseases.[2]

REFERENCES

1. Ruder MG, et al. *Vector Borne Zoonotic Dis.* 2015;15(6):348-363.
2. Zuliani A, et al. *PLoS ONE.* 2015;10(8):e0130294.

MOSQUITOES (CULICIDAE)

A number of mosquitoes, including *Psorophora, Aedes, Mansonia, Culex,* and *Anopheles* spp. are important parasites of domestic animals. When the blood-feeding females are present in large numbers, they cause stress to animals and have been known to kill young pigs and puppies by the severe anemia they produce. Although such occurrences are rarely recorded, the blood loss that can occur in severe infestations is surprising. The stress associated with mosquito attack is sufficient to cause reductions in efficiency, even in mature large animals.

Their most important role is as vectors of disease. *Culex tarsalis, Aedes dorsalis,* and *Aedes nigromaculis* transmit equine encephalomyelitis. *Culex tritaeniorhyncus* is the principal vector of Japanese B encephalitis in Japan. Various *Culex* species vector western equine encephalitis, eastern equine encephalitis, and West Nile virus. These viruses can have serious effects on unprotected horses and are transmissible to humans via mosquito bites. Vaccines are available to protect against all of these arboviruses. *Psorophora confinnis* is instrumental in spreading the eggs of *Dermatobia hominis,* the tropical warble fly; and *Mansonia* spp. transmit Rift Valley fever. The filarid worm *Setaria digitata* is also spread by mosquitoes.

Control over a large area must include drainage of collections of still surface water or destruction of the larvae by the addition of any one of a number of insecticides. For small groups of animals, protection from the attacks of mosquitoes can only be satisfactorily effected by mosquito-proof screens. Temporary protection by repellents such as dimethyl phthalate is only partial. Permethrin, 100 mL of a 0.5% emulsion, applied with an electrostatic sprayer provided greater than 70% protection for at least 72 hours.

Tick Infestations

SYNOPSIS

Etiology Many species of ticks act as vectors of disease or cause death from anemia; others cause paralysis. Heavy burdens cause loss of production.

Epidemiology Life cycles vary widely both in the number of hosts required and the host specificity. Animals are infested by larval or nymphal states on the ground.

Clinical signs Anemia, paralysis, tick fever, and tick worry.

Clinical pathology Ticks obvious on clinical examination. Blood smears for tick fevers (*Babesia, Theileria,* and *Anaplasma*).

Lesions Skin damage as a result of biting and rubbing; anemia. See other chapters for lesions as a result of diseases transmitted by ticks.

Diagnostic confirmation Ticks easily found, should be identified as to species.

Treatment Dipping, spraying, application of pour-ons and injectable acaricides.

Control Regular treatment at intervals dependent on the life cycle of the tick, pasture spelling to destroy free-living stages, the use of resistant cattle, and vaccination all play a part.

Tick infestations are of great importance in the production of animal diseases, particularly in livestock housed in tropical and subtropical areas. In addition to their role as vectors of infectious diseases, as outlined in the following discussion, heavy infestations can cause direct losses. Many ticks are active blood feeders and may cause death from anemia. Some species cause tick paralysis, and it is possible that other ticks may elaborate toxins other than those causing paralysis. Heavy tick burdens cause sufficient irritation and stress such that affected animals become anorexic, which may lead reduced productivity. One tick, *Boophilus microplus,* is reported to affect in excess of 75% of the world cattle population. The economic impact has been estimated at US$7 per animal per year, and in Brazil, which has the fifth largest cattle herd, the losses are estimated at US$2 billion per year.

Ticks are divided into two groups: Argasidae (soft-body ticks) and Ixodidae (hard-body ticks). The life cycles of the ticks vary widely. Some species pass their entire lives on one host, others pass different stages of the cycle on successive hosts, and others are parasitic only at certain stages. The eggs are laid in the soil, and larvae attach themselves to a passing host, on which they may develop through one or more nymphal stages before becoming adults. Adult females engorge on blood or lymph and drop to the ground to lay their eggs. One-host ticks are more easily controlled than those that pass part of their life cycles away from the host. A list of the single- and multiple-host ticks is shown in Table 16-5.

Although many ticks favor a particular host, they are usually not completely host-specific, and many parasitize a wide variety

TABLE 16-5 Single- and multiple-host ticks

One-host ticks
Boophilus spp.
Margaropus winthemi
Otobius megnini (adults are not parasitic)
Dermacentor albipictus
Two-host ticks
Rhipicephalus evertsi
Rhipicephalus bursa
Hyalomma spp. (most have two or three hosts)
Three-host ticks
Ixodes spp.
Rhipicephalus spp. (except *R. evertsi* and *R. bursa*)
Haemaphysalis spp.
Amblyomma spp.
Hyalomma spp. (most have two or three hosts)
Ornithodorus spp.—many hosts
Dermacentor spp.

of animals. In the limited space available here, the species are listed according to whether they transmit bacterial, viral, or rickettsial diseases of livestock or only cause worry. Ticks that transmit economically important protozoan diseases of livestock, such as babesiosis and theileriosis, are discussed in Chapter 11 (Table 11-7). Ticks that cause paralysis and other neurologic signs are discussed in Chapter 15.

Bacterial, Viral, and Rickettsial Diseases Transmitted by Ticks

The transmission of diseases associated with these agents may be effected by means other than ticks. *Anaplasma marginale* can be spread by biting flies if large numbers are present when the animals are experiencing a heavy parasitemia. Outbreaks of anaplasmosis can also occur following the use of unclean instruments for dehorning, vaccination, castration, or blood sampling, and anaplasmosis is easily caused by blood transfusions. The ticks involved more commonly in transmitting bacteria, viruses, and rickettsia are listed in Table 16-6. Transmission of *Anaplasma* may be transovarially, with one stage becoming infected and a subsequent stage passing the infection to a new host, or ticks may transmit infection within the one stage if they detach and feed on a new host.

Ticks That Cause Direct Losses

Ticks cause damage to hides and loss of production, anemia, and death when they are present in large numbers. They also cause greater morbidity and mortality during periods of drought, in addition to delays in fattening, resulting in animals held longer before they can be sold. Ticks that have this effect on production but are not known to cause paralysis or transmit infectious diseases in farm animals are as follows:

- *Otobius megnini*—the "spinose ear tick" of the United States and Canada
- *Amblyomma americanum*—the "Lone Star tick" of the United States
- *A. maculatum*—the "Gulf Coast tick" of the United States
- *Margaropus winthemi*—of South America and Africa
- *Ornithodorus moubata*—of Africa and Southeast Asia
- *O. savignyi*—of Africa and Southeast Asia
- *Haemaphysalis longicornis*—of Australia and New Zealand.

TREATMENT AND CONTROL OF TICK INFESTATIONS

Four methods are now available to treat and control tick infestations, with the primary role continuing to be played by chemical acaricides:

- Administration of acaricidal agents
- Pasture management
- Use of resistant cattle
- Vaccination

Acaricidal Agents

Individual animals can be effectively treated by the application of any one of a number of acaricides applied either as a spray or by dipping. The choice of acaricide for treatment depends largely on three factors:

- The persistence of the compound on the skin and hair coat
- The likelihood of residues toxic to humans appearing in the milk or meat
- Whether or not the ticks in the area have developed resistance to the particular acaricide

Arsenicals, in the form of water-soluble arsenic salts, have been widely used to treat tick infestations but are no longer used in many parts of the world because of resistance, toxicity, and environmental concerns.

Table 16-6 Diseases associated with bacteria, viruses, and rickettsia and reported to be transmitted by ticks

Disease	Causative agent	Vector ticks	Country
Tick pyemia (lambs)	*Staphylococcus aureus*	*Ixodes ricinus*	Great Britain
Tularemia (sheep)	*Francisella tularense*	*Haemaphysalis leporispalustris, H. otophila; Dermacentor andersoni, D. variabilis, D. pictus, D. marginatus; Ixodes luguri*	United States Norway, Europe, Russia, and states of the former USSR
Anaplasmosis			
Cattle	*Anaplasma marginale*	*Boophilus annulatus; Argas persicus; Dermacentor albipictus, D. andersoni, D. occidentalis, D. variabilis; Ixodes scapularis; Rhipicephalus sanguineus;*	North America
		Boophilus microplus,	Australia and South America
		B. decoloratus; Hyalomma excavatum; Rhipicephalus bursa, R. simus;	Africa
		Haemaphysalis punctata; Ixodes ricinus;	Europe
		Boophilus (annulatus) calcaratus	Russia, and states of the former USSR
Sheep and goats	*Anaplasma ovis*	*Dermacentor silvarum, Rhipicephalus bursa, Ornithodorus lahorensis*	Russia, and states of the former USSR
Brucellosis	*Brucella abortus* and *Br. melitensis*	Many ticks may be infected, but infection of host appears to occur only if ticks or their feces are eaten	Russia, and states of the former USSR
Heartwater	*Ehrlichia ruminantium*	*Amblyomma* spp.	Africa and Caribbean
African swine fever	Virus	*Ornithodous* spp.	Africa, Spain, Portugal
Louping-ill	Virus	*Rhipicephalus appendiculatus* (laboratory only) *Ixodes ricinus*	Africa England
Tick-borne fever	*Anaplasma phagocytophila*	*Ixodes ricinus* *Rhipicephalus haemaphysaloides*	Great Britain, Norway India
Caseous lymphadenitis of sheep	*Corynebacterium pseudotuberculosis*	*Dermacentor albipictus*	North America
Epizootic bovine abortion	*Spirochete*	*Ornithodorus coriaceus*	United States
Nairobi sheep disease	Virus	*Rhipicephalus appendiculatus*	Africa
Lyme disease	*Borrelia burgdorferi*	*Ixodes dammini, I. pacifieus, I. rieini*	United States, Europe, Australia

Chlorinated hydrocarbons replaced the use of arsenicals but have been withdrawn from most markets because of high toxicity and long duration of effect. Resistance to chemical acaricides, including macrocyclic lactones, has become a major issue for the effective management of one cattle tick, *Boophilus microplus*. In many cases cross-resistance between chemical families occurs, further complicating the use of rotational schemes aimed at managing the development and degree of resistance.

The same criteria apply in control as in treatment except that cost becomes a limiting factor when large numbers of animals require frequent treatments, and it is obvious in some circumstances that the effect of tick infestation on Brahman-cross steers is insufficiently great to warrant treatment. It is impossible to make specific recommendations on methods of application and the most efficient insecticide to use because these vary widely between species of ticks. However, whenever possible, treatment should be given systematically in a program based on the life cycle and epidemiology of the tick. A number of treatments may be used early in the tick season to prevent the increase in tick numbers. Care must be taken in areas where tick fevers also occur, so as not to disrupt the transmission of the tick-fever organisms and leave the cattle susceptible to later infection. Other special cases include *Otobius megnini*, the nymphs of which drop off to molt and lay eggs in protected spots, necessitating the spraying of buildings, fence posts, feed troughs, and tree trunks in feedlots where heavy infestations are most common. *Ornithodorus* spp. ticks are difficult to control because the nymphs and adults attach to feed for brief periods only. Where ticks that cause paralysis are common, it may be necessary to apply an insecticide as a dust and dip at short intervals.

Organophosphates

The organophosphates as a group are effective, but tick strains resistant to many of them have appeared. Other drugs in current use include dioxathion, diazinon, carbophenothion, coumaphos, ethion, bromophos-ethyl, chlorpyrifos, and phosmet. Pour-on applications of chlorpyrifos and phosmet have been tested but were not as effective as spray applications. Addition of acaricides to the feed has also been tried but has not been successful, whereas eartags impregnated with tetrachlorvinphos did not give satisfactory control and increased the risk of development of resistance to the drug.

Preparations vary in the duration of the protection they afford, and local conditions of rainfall and tick population must be taken into account when determining the time intervals between sprayings or dippings. A special case is that of young lambs that are exposed to tick pyemia. Sprays, dips, and ointments are too toxic, and the most effective procedure is the application of a liquid emulsion cream containing the insecticide to the wool-less parts of the body. Chlorpyrifos 0.48 kg/ha markedly reduces the number of ticks on the pasture, but it is too expensive for routine use.

Pyrethroids

Amitraz, a formamidine, and the synthetic pyrethroids have been used widely in Australia and have proved to be efficient, active against organophosphate-resistant strains, and safe. In a study in the United States, 0.025% amitraz applied as a whole-body spray or by dipping gave 86.0% or 99.8% control, respectively. Ticks resistant to DDT are also resistant to the synthetic pyrethroids, and to overcome resistance pyrethroids can be combined with an organophosphate. Successful combinations in Australia are cypermethrin plus chlorfenvinphos and deltamethrin plus ethion. A synthetic pyrethroid, flumethrin, has been marketed by itself at higher use concentrations for both plunge dipping and as a pour-on treatment. As a 1% pour-on, 1 mL per 10 kg body weight gave 97% efficacy, and 0.0033% as a spray gave 99% efficacy and acted more quickly. The efficacy of synthetic pyrethroid-impregnated eartags has been reported, but these are likely to lead to resistance. Cyhalothrin also controls multiresistant strains and is used in plunge dips.

Bioassay results show lambdacyhalothrin to be as effective as cyhalothrin as a whole-body spray, although the 1% pour-on was less than 50% effective. Resistance to all pyrethroids has been reported. Three pyrethroid acaricides have been shown to markedly reduce the hatching of eggs. Permethrin 0.1% or cypermethrin and cyfluthrin 0.05% could be useful in cleansing and disinfecting premises.

Macrocyclic Lactones

Ivermectin given subcutaneously gives satisfactory control of *Boophilus microplus* for 21 days following an initial lag period of 2 days. As little as 0.015 mg/kg per day gives complete control and raises the possibility of a slow-release subcutaneous implant. Two treatments of 0.2 mg/kg at 4-day intervals is considered satisfactory in cleansing cattle under field conditions. However, ivermectin may not be effective against *Ixodes ricinus*, but a slow-release bolus active for 90 days did give good control of a variety of ticks. If given topically, 0.5 mg/kg was required to reach the efficiency achieved by 0.2 mg/kg subcutaneously.

Moxidectin 0.2 mg/kg subcutaneously at 4-week intervals or 0.5 mg/kg as a pour-on along the back gives good protection against *B. microplus* resistant to organophosphorous insecticides and DDT, and each treatment has a rapid knockdown effect on populations of buffalo fly after treatment. Doramectin 0.2 mg/kg SC is highly efficacious in removing *B. microplus* and preventing reestablishment. Closantel 22.2 mg/kg orally to cattle (greater than the typical oral dose) was shown to disrupt the life cycle of *Rhipicephalus appendiculatus*; those that oviposited laid few eggs, and most of these did not hatch. Few larvae or nymphs molted.

Ticks in the ears of **horses** should be treated by the insertion of a few drops of an oily acaricidal preparation.

Use of Resistant Cattle

It is possible to reduce the impact of ticks and tick-borne diseases by the introduction of Brahman and Brahman-cross cattle, which are more resistant than British breeds and African cattle.[1] The resistance has been shown to be largely acquired, and it is mainly expressed against the larvae in the first 24 hours after attachment. In Australia the possibility that *B. microplus* might escape from its control area because of increased resistance to acaricides has been realized. For this reason a great deal of attention is being paid to the possibility of selecting cattle for tick resistance. In most tick-infested areas, cattle should have up to 50% *Bovis indicus* breeding because this allows for a reduction in the frequency of treatments. Penalties such as reduced live-weight gains, late maturity, and poor temperament become evident when cattle have more than 50% *B. indicus*. With successive infestations cattle differ in their response to *B. microplus*. Thus there is increased irritation and more licking and a decrease in the number of ticks carried. Resistance to ticks has been shown to be related to skin thickness and other factors and is heritable.[2] Selection for tick resistance does not affect milk production.

Pasture Management

Measures other than the application of acaricides used in the control of tick infestation include burning of pasture, removal of native fauna, and plowing of fields. So little is known of the bionomics of specific ticks in specific areas that these measures have been largely unsuccessful, and it is impossible to provide details for their proper implementation.

In contrast, pasture spelling and rotational grazing are capable of greatly reducing the tick population on farms in some areas. If cattle are placed on spelled pastures early in winter when the ticks are producing f ew or no progeny and then alternated at 4-month intervals, the tick population can be controlled with a markedly lower number of treatments. The practicability of the procedure depends on a full-scale financial assessment of the increased weight gains relative to the costs of management. Duration of the spelling period varies between 2 and 3 months in summer to 3 to 4 months in the winter, but these intervals need to be determined for each district. In practice, pasture spelling is rarely used.

In those areas where the epidemiology is known, it has been shown that in regions with a cold winter the females stop laying eggs, and the development of eggs is prolonged. This results in few larvae being available in the spring, and if repeated treatments are given at this time, pasture contamination will remain low for some months. In hot tropical areas where the required temperatures for tick breeding are always present, the dry period may cause mortality by desiccation.

Certain *Stylosanthes* spp., tropical legumes, can kill or immobilize larval ticks, and the use of these plants may simultaneously improve pasture quality and reduce the pasture contamination of larval ticks if high legume-to-grass ratios are achieved. *Brachiaria brizantha* has also been shown to be lethal to *Boophilus* larvae.

Vaccination

Crude vaccines made from extracts of semiengorged adult female *B. microplus* give effective immunity. The antibody destroys the cells lining the tick's midgut and allows blood to escape into the hemocele; some ticks die, and the fertility of those remaining is reduced by up to 70%. The fertility of males is also reduced. A recombinant vaccine based on a membrane-bound glycoprotein Bm86 from the tick's midgut has been isolated and was shown to be as effective as the native antigen in studies conducted between 1993 and 1997,[2] and to be effective against acaricidal-resistant ticks. Its major effect is a progressive control in tick numbers in successive generations through a decrease in their reproductive capacity.[2] Because the vaccine acts against an antigen in the tick's gut to which cattle are never exposed, they must be given booster injections at regular intervals. This was the first recombinant parasite vaccine sold commercially (TickGARD) and was initially marketed in 1994 in Australia.[3] A second antigen that significantly enhances efficacy and does not impair the response to Bm86has now been added to the vaccine,[4,5] which is currently available in one commercial formulation (Gavac) in North and South America.[3] Although vaccines offer long-term control, they need to be used with application of acaricides, use of tick-resistant cattle, and pasture management as part of an integrated pest management control system.

Integrated management of tick infestations requires the use of several complementary approaches to reduce populations below acceptable thresholds. One component of these strategies is the development of acaricidal pathogens that may augment other approaches such as vaccination and selective acaricide application. Fungal pathogens are under evaluation for use in this type of program, in particular *Metarhizium anisopliae* and *Beauvaria bassiana*.

ERADICATION

In most countries all that is attempted is reduction of the tick population by periodic dipping or spraying. Complete eradication is extremely difficult because of the persistence of ticks, especially multihost ticks, on wild fauna and the ability of adult ticks to live for very long periods away from a host. On the other hand, continuous treatment to restrain the tick population is highly conducive to the development of resistance, a problem that has become apparent in many tick areas.

Boophilus annulatus was eradicated from the southeastern United States by a program of continuous dipping at short intervals of all livestock in the area. *B. microplus* was also eradicated from Florida by a similar procedure, but 20,000 deer, the important alternate host in the area, had to be slaughtered. Concern has been expressed that deer and other wildlife species may threaten efforts to prevent *B. microplus* and *B. annulatus* from becoming reestablished in the southern United States after they are introduced from Mexico. Attempts to eradicate other single-host ticks in other countries generally have not been successful.

Although both dipping and spraying are recommended for the control of ticks, complete wetting of the animals, which can only be effected by dipping, is essential if eradication is to be undertaken. This adds another impediment to eradication plans because of the cost of constructing proper dips and yards. When one considers that dipping may have to be carried out every 14 days for 15 months, that every animal in the eradication area must be dipped, and that a strict quarantine of the area must be maintained, it is obvious that eradication cannot be undertaken lightly.

FURTHER READING

Ghosh S, Azhahianambi P, Yadav MP. Upcoming and future strategies of tick control: a review. *J Vector Borne Dis*. 2007;44:79-89.

REFERENCES

1. Shyma KP, et al. *J Parastit Dis*. 2015;39:1.
2. Canales M, et al. *BMC Biotechnol*. 2009;9:29.
3. Guerrero FD, et al. *Intern J Parasitol*. 2012;42:421.
4. de la Fuente J, et al. *Anim Health Res Rev*. 2007;8:23.
5. Domingos A, et al. *Rev Soc Bras Med Trop*. 2013;46:265.

Deficiencies and Toxicities Affecting the Skin

ZINC DEFICIENCY (PARAKERATOSIS)

SYNOPSIS

Etiology Dietary deficiency of zinc and factors that interfere with zinc absorption or utilization.

Epidemiology Growing pigs, cattle, and sheep. Excess of calcium favors disease in pigs.

Signs

Pigs Loss of body weight gain. Symmetric, crusty skin lesions (parakeratosis) over dorsum and ears, tail; become thick and fissured. No pruritus.

Ruminants Alopecia over muzzle, ears, tail head, hindlegs, flank, and neck. Stiff gait and swelling over coronets. Loss of wool and thickened skin in sheep. Infertility in rams. Poor growth in goats and skin lesions.

Clinical pathology Serum zinc concentrations lower than normal.

Necropsy findings Parakeratosis.

Diagnostic confirmation Histology of skin lesions and serum zinc levels.

Differential diagnosis list
Sarcoptic mange in cattle and pigs.
Exudative epidermitis in piglets.

Treatment Add zinc to diet.

Control Supplement zinc in diet.

ETIOLOGY

Pigs

A zinc deficiency in young, growing pigs can cause parakeratosis, but it is sometimes not a result of a simple zinc deficiency. Rapidly growing pigs have a high requirement for zinc in the diet.[1] The availability of zinc in the diet is adversely affected by the presence of phytic acid, a constituent of plant protein sources such as soybean meal. Much of the zinc in plant protein is in the bound form and unavailable to the monogastric animal such as the pig. The use of meat meal or meat scraps in the diet will prevent the disease because of the high availability of the zinc. Another unique feature of the etiology of parakeratosis in swine is that an excess of dietary calcium (0.5% to 1.5%) can favor the development of the disease, and the addition of zinc to such diets at levels much higher (0.02% zinc carbonate or 100 mg/kg zinc) than those normally required by growing swine prevents the occurrence of the disease. The level of copper in the diet may also be of some significance, with increasing copper levels decreasing the requirement for zinc. A concurrent enteric infection with diarrhea exacerbates the damage done by a zinc deficiency in pigs.

Weaning can induce transient declines in the serum zinc concentration of piglets, and this can be prevented by oral supplementation with zinc oxide.[2] The clinical importance of this decline is unclear.

Ruminants

A primary zinc deficiency resulting from low dietary zinc in ruminants is rare but does occur. Many factors influence the availability of zinc from soils, including the degree of compaction of the soil and the nitrogen and phosphorus concentration. The risk of zinc deficiency increases when soil pH rises above 6.5 and as fertilization with nitrogen and phosphorus increases. Some legumes contain less zinc than grasses grown on the same soil, and zinc concentration decreases with aging of the plant. Several factors may deleteriously affect the availability of zinc to ruminants and cause a secondary zinc deficiency. These include the consumption of immature grass, which affects digestibility; the feeding of late-cut hay, which may be poorly digestible; and the presence of excessive dietary sulfur. The contamination of silage with soil at harvesting can also affect the digestibility of zinc.

EPIDEMIOLOGY

Pigs

Parakeratosis in pigs was first recorded in North America in rapidly growing pigs, particularly those fed on diets containing growth promoters. The disease occurs most commonly during the period of rapid growth, after weaning and between 7 and 10 weeks of age. From 20% to 80% of pigs in affected herds may have lesions, and the main economic loss is a result of a decrease in growth rate. In general, the incidence is greater in pigs fed in dry lots on self-feeders of dry feed than in pigs with access to some pasture, which is preventive and curative.

A low level of dietary zinc intake during pregnancy and lactation of gilts can result in skin lesions, stressful parturition, and an increased incidence of intrapartum mortality of piglets and deleterious effects on neonatal growth.

It has been suggested that parakeratosis occurs because very rapidly growing pigs outstrip their biosynthesis of essential fatty acids, and when the diet is high in calcium the digestibility of fat in the diet is reduced at the same time. The net effect in rapidly growing pigs could be a relative deficiency of essential fatty acids.

Ruminants

There are naturally occurring cases in cattle, sheep, and goats. The disease is well recognized in Europe, especially in calves. It is common in some families of cattle, and an inherited increased dietary requirement for zinc is suspected. The inherited disease occurs in Friesian and Black Pied cattle and is known as lethal trait A46. Signs of deficiency appear at 4 to 8 weeks of age. The main defect is an almost complete inability to absorb zinc from the intestine; zinc administration is curative.

The disease in **cattle** has been produced experimentally on diets low in zinc, and naturally occurring cases have responded to supplementation of the diet with zinc. Calves remain healthy on experimental diets containing 40 mg/kg zinc, but parakeratosis has occurred in cattle grazing pastures with a zinc content of 20 to 80 mg/kg (normal 93 mg/kg) and a calcium content of 0.6%. There is also an apparently improved response in cattle to zinc administration if copper is given simultaneously. Parakeratosis has also been produced experimentally in goats and sheep.

Zinc nutrition may be involved in the immune responses of feedlot calves. When calves are stressed by transportation or challenged with the infectious bovine rhinotracheitis virus, they tend to have reduced fevers, higher dry matter intake, and less body weight loss when fed organic zinc and manganese sources than the corresponding oxide forms.

Outbreaks of the disease have occurred in **Sudanese Desert ewes** and their lambs fed on a zinc-deficient diet of Rhodes grass containing less than 10 mg/kg of zinc. The disease has also been diagnosed in **mature sheep and goats,** and the cause of the deficiency could not be determined. A marginal zinc deficiency, characterized by subnormal growth and fertility and low concentration of zinc in serum, but without other clinical signs, can occur in sheep grazing pastures containing less than 10 mg/kg zinc.

In Germany, skin lesions have occurred in alpacas and llamas with low-zinc and low-copper status. In the affected herd, the average serum zinc and copper levels were 0.17 and 0.49 μg/mL for alpacas and 0.22 and 0.38 μg/mL for llamas, respectively. The levels considered normal in llamas are 0.30 μg for zinc and 0.40 to 0.70 μg copper per mL.

PATHOGENESIS

The pathogenesis of zinc deficiency is not well understood. Zinc is a component of the enzyme carbonic anhydrase, which is located in the red blood cells and parietal cells of the stomach, and is related to the transport of respiratory carbon dioxide and the secretion of hydrochloric acid by the gastric mucosa. Zinc is also associated with RNA function and related to insulin, glucagon, and other hormones. It also has a role in keratinization, calcification, wound healing, and somatic and sexual development. Because it has a critical role in nucleic acid and protein metabolism, a deficiency may adversely affect the cell-mediated immune system.

Zinc and vitamin A deficiency can occur together, with complex interactions between the compounds affecting liver metabolism of vitamin A.[3] Zinc deficiency impairs vitamin A mobilization from the liver.

A zinc deficiency results in a decreased feed intake in all species and is probably the reason for the depression of growth rate in growing animals and body weight in mature animals. Failure of keratinization resulting in parakeratosis, loss and failure of growth of wool and hair, and lesions of the coronary bands probably reflects the importance of zinc in protein synthesis. There are lesions of the arteriolar walls of the dermis. The bones of zinc-deficient ruminants reveal abnormal mineralization and a reduction of zinc concentration in bones and cartilage and should be considered in animals with evidence of chondrodysplasia.[4] Retarded testicular development occurs in ram lambs, and complete cessation of spermatogenesis suggests impairment of protein synthesis.

CLINICAL FINDINGS

Pigs

A reduced rate and efficiency of body weight gain is characteristic. Circumscribed areas of erythema appear in the skin on the ventral abdomen and inside the thigh. These areas develop into papules 3 to 5 mm in diameter, which are soon covered with scales, followed by thick crusts. These crusts are most visible in areas about the limb joints, ears, and tail and are distributed symmetrically in all cases. The crusts develop fissures and cracks, become quite thick (5 to 7 mm), and are easily detached from the skin. They are crumbly and not flaky or scaly. No greasiness is present except in the depths of fissures. Little scratching or rubbing occurs. Diarrhea of moderate degree is common. Secondary subcutaneous abscesses occur frequently, but in uncomplicated cases, the skin lesions disappear spontaneously in 10 to 45 days if the ration is corrected. Affected boars have testicular abnormalities that impair fertility.[5]

Ruminants

In the naturally occurring disease in cattle, in severe cases, parakeratosis and alopecia may affect about 40% of the skin area. The lesions are most marked on the muzzle, vulva, anus, tailhead, ears, backs of the hindlegs, kneefolds, flank, and neck. Most animals have below-average body condition and are stunted in growth. After treatment with zinc, improvement is apparent in 1 week and complete in 3 weeks. Experimentally produced cases exhibit the following signs:

- Poor growth
- A stiff gait
- Swelling of the coronets, hocks, and knees
- Soft swelling containing fluid on the anterior aspect of the hind fetlocks
- Alopecia
- Wrinkling of the skin of the legs, scrotum, and neck and head, especially around the nostrils
- Hemorrhages around the teeth
- Ulcers on the dental pad

The experimental disease in cattle is manifested by parakeratotic skin, mainly on the hindlimbs and udder, and similar lesions on teats, which tend to become eroded during milking. The fetlocks and pasterns are covered with scabby scales. There is exudation first with matting of hair, then drying and cracking. The skin becomes thickened and inelastic. Histologically, there is parakeratosis. Clinical signs develop about 2 weeks after calves and lambs go onto a deficient diet so that there is no evidence of storage of zinc in tissues in these animals. In goats, hair growth, testicular size, and spermatogenesis are reduced, and growth rate is less than normal. Return to a normal diet does not necessarily reverse these signs, and the case-fatality rate is high. There is a marked delay in wound healing.

Zinc deficiency increases the risk of mastitis in dairy cows, potentially because of adverse alterations in mammary duct epithelium.[6] Deficiency is associated with increased somatic-cell numbers in milk, decreased thickness of stratum corneum in ductus papillaris, and increased leukocyte infiltration of udder parenchyma.[6]

Inherited zinc deficiency in cattle (lethal trait A46), which is caused in Holstein–Friesian cattle by a splice-site variant in SLC39A4, is described under the heading "Inherited Parakeratosis of Calves" later in this chapter.[7] An inherited syndrome in Fleckvieh cattle with similar phenotype is not a result of zinc deficiency, and it does not have the same genetic abnormality.[8]

Sheep

The natural disease in sheep is characterized by loss of wool and the development of thick, wrinkled skin. Wool-eating also occurs in sheep and may be one of the earliest signs noticed in lambs after being on a zinc-deficient diet for 4 weeks. Induced cases in lambs have exhibited reduced growth rate, salivation, swollen hocks, wrinkled skin, and open skin lesions around the hoof and eyes. The experimental disease in goats is similar to that in lambs.

One of the most striking effects of zinc deficiency in **ram lambs** is impaired testicular growth and complete cessation of spermatogenesis. Diets containing 2.44 mg/kg dry matter (DM) caused poor growth, impaired testicular growth, cessation of spermatogenesis, and other signs of zinc deficiency within 20 to 24 weeks. A diet containing 17.4 mg/kg DM of zinc is adequate for growth, but a content of 32.4 mg/kg DM is necessary for normal testicular development and spermatogenesis. On severely deficient experimental diets, other clinical signs in young rams are as follows:

- Drooling copious amounts of saliva when ruminating
- Parakeratosis around eyes and on nose, feet, and scrotum
- Shedding of the hooves
- Dystrophy and shedding of wool, which showed severe staining
- Development of a pungent odor

In naturally occurring cases in rams, the animals stood with their backs arched and feet close together.

A marginal zinc deficiency in ewes may be characterized by only a reduction in feed intake and a slightly reduced body weight, and no other external signs of disease. This is important because, in grazing ruminants, the lack of external signs indicates that zinc deficiency could easily pass undetected.

Infertility in Ewes

Infertility in ewes and a dietary deficiency of zinc have not been officially linked, but a zinc-responsive infertility has been described in ewes. Again, attention is drawn to the need for response trials when soil and pasture levels of an element are marginal.

An **experimental zinc deficiency in pregnant ewes** results in a decrease in the birth weight of the lambs and a reduced concentration of zinc in the tissues of the lambs; these effects are a result of the reduced feed intake characteristic of zinc deficiency. The zinc content of the diet did not significantly influence the ability of the ewes to become pregnant or maintain pregnancy. The combination of pregnancy and zinc deficiency in the ewe leads to highly efficient utilization of ingested zinc, and the developing fetus will accumulate about 35% of the total dietary intake of zinc of the ewe during the last trimester of pregnancy. The disease is correctable by the supplementary feeding of zinc.

Goats

Experimentally induced zinc deficiency in goats results in poor growth, low food intake, testicular hypoplasia, rough dull coat with loss of hair, and the accumulation of hard, dry, keratinized skin on the hindlimbs, scrotum, head, and neck. On the lower limbs the scabs fissure, crack, and produce some exudate. In naturally occurring cases in pygmy goats there was extensive alopecia, a kyphotic stance, extensive areas of parakeratosis, abnormal hoof growth, and flaky, painful coronary bands. A zinc-responsive alopecia and hyperkeratosis occurs in Angora goats. Affected animals had recurrent pruritus; hyperemia; exfoliation, fleece loss over the hindquarters, face, and ears; and a decline in reproductive performance. Zinc supplementation (40 or 80 mg/d) increases rate of fleece growth, plasma testosterone concentrations, and serum alkaline phosphatase activity in Cashmere goats.[9]

Immediately before parturition in cows, there is a precipitate fall in plasma zinc concentration, which returns to normal slowly after calving. The depression of zinc levels is greater in cows that experience dystocia. This has led to the hypothesis that dystocia in beef heifers may be caused in some circumstances by a nutritional deficiency of zinc and that preparturient supplementation of the diet with zinc may reduce the occurrence of difficult births. This phenomenon does not appear to occur in sheep. The level of serum zinc increases in cattle during the season of facial eczema when sporidesmin intoxication causes depletion of liver zinc.

CLINICAL PATHOLOGY

Skin Scraping

Laboratory examination of skin scrapings yields negative results, but skin biopsy will confirm the diagnosis of parakeratosis.

Zinc in Serum and Hair

Serum zinc levels may have good diagnostic value. Normal levels are 80 to 120 μg/dL (12.2 to 18.2 μmol/L) in sheep and cattle. Calves and lambs on deficient diets may have levels as low as 18 μg/dL (3.0 μmol/L). Dairy cattle with serum zinc less than 9.7 μmol/L are at increased risk of changes that predispose to mastitis.[6]

Normal serum zinc levels in sheep are above 78 μg/dL (12 μmol/L), and values below 39 μg/dL (6 μmol/L) or less are considered as evidence of deficiency. There is a general relationship between the zinc content of the hair and the level of zinc in the diet, but the analysis of hair is not considered to be a sufficiently accurate indicator of an animal's zinc status. In experimental disease in piglets, there is a reduction in serum levels of zinc, calcium, and alkaline phosphatase, and it is suggested that the disease could be detected by measuring the serum alkaline phosphate and serum zinc levels. Levels of zinc in the blood are very labile, and simple estimations of levels alone are likely to be misleading. For example, other intercurrent diseases commonly depress serum calcium and copper levels. In addition, zinc levels in plasma fall precipitately at parturition in cows; they are also depressed by hyperthermal stress. After 1 week on a highly deficient diet, serum zinc levels fall to about 50% of normal, or pretreatment, levels.

NECROPSY FINDINGS

Necropsy examinations are not usually performed, but histologic examination of skin biopsy sections reveals a marked increase in thickness of all the elements of the epidermis. Tissue levels of zinc differ between deficient and normal animals, but the differences are statistical rather than diagnostic.

> **DIFFERENTIAL DIAGNOSIS**
>
> Sarcoptic mange may resemble parakeratosis, but is accompanied by much itching and rubbing. The parasites may be found in skin scrapings. Treatment with appropriate parasiticides relieves the condition.
>
> Exudative epidermitis is quite similar in appearance, but occurs chiefly in unweaned pigs. The lesions have a greasy character that is quite different from the dry, crumbly lesions of parakeratosis. The mortality rate is higher.

TREATMENT

In outbreaks of parakeratosis in swine, zinc should be added to diet immediately at the rate of 50 mg/kg DM (200 mg of zinc sulfate or carbonate per kg of feed). The calcium level of the diet should be maintained at between 0.65% and 0.75%. The injection of zinc at a rate of 2 to 4 mg/kg BW daily for 10 days is also effective.

Zinc oxide suspended in olive oil and given IM at a dose of 200 mg of zinc for adult sheep and 50 mg of zinc for lambs will result in a clinical cure within 2 months. The oral administration of zinc at the rate of 250 mg zinc sulfate daily for 4 weeks resulted in a clinical cure of zinc deficiency in goats in 12 to 14 weeks.

CONTROL

Pigs

The calcium content of diets for growing pigs should be restricted to 0.5% to 0.6%. However, rations containing as little as 0.5% calcium and with normal zinc content (30 mg/kg DM) may produce the disease. Supplementation with zinc (to 50 mg/kg DM) as sulfate or carbonate has been found to be highly effective as a preventive, and there appears to be a wide margin of safety in its use, with diets containing 1000 mg/kg DM added zinc having no apparent toxic effect. Organic and inorganic zinc supplements are handled differently by pigs, with organic forms of zinc being more bioavailable.[1] Rapidly growing pigs require 75 mg/kg of organic zinc in a complex nursery diet to maximize growth, health, and well-being.[1] The standard recommendation is to add 200 g of zinc carbonate or sulfate to each ton of feed. Weight gains in affected groups are appreciably increased by the addition of zinc to the diet. The addition of oils containing unsaturated fatty acids is also an effective preventive. Access to green pasture, reduction in food intake, and the deletion of growth stimulants from rations will lessen the incidence of the disease but are not usually practicable.

Ruminants

For cattle, the feeding of zinc sulfate (2 to 4 g daily) is recommended as an emergency measure followed by the application of a zinc-containing fertilizer. As an alternative to dietary supplementation for ruminants, an intraruminal pellet has been demonstrated in sheep. It was effective for 7 weeks only and would not be satisfactory for long-term use. The creation of subcutaneous depots of zinc by the injection of zinc oxide or zinc metal dust has been demonstrated. The zinc dust offered a greater delayed effect. A soluble glass bolus containing zinc, cobalt, and selenium was able to correct experimentally induced zinc deficiency in sheep. The bolus supplied the daily requirement of the sheep for zinc with no detrimental effect on their copper status, although high-dose zinc supplementation does impair copper absorption in cattle that are provided additional copper in the diet.[10]

Zinc-methionine, an organic zinc supplement for dairy goats, improved udder health, an enhanced the absorption of nitrogen, and increased nitrogen retention. Recommended dietary intake of zinc for Cashmere goats is 86 mg/kg DM during the breeding season and cashmere-fiber growing period.[9]

REFERENCES

1. Hill GM, et al. *J Anim Sci.* 2014;92:1582.
2. Davin R, et al. *J Anim Physiol Nutr.* 2013;97:6.
3. Khakzad P, et al. *J Vet Res.* 2014;69:173.
4. Dittmer KE, et al. *Vet Pathol.* 2015;52:851.
5. Cigankova V, et al. *Acta Veterinaria Beograd.* 2008;58:89.
6. Davidov I, et al. *Rev Med Vet.* 2013;164:183.
7. Yuzbasiyan-Gurkan V, et al. *Genomics.* 2006;88:521.
8. Jung S, et al. *BMC Genomics.* 2014;15.
9. Liu HY, et al. *J Anim Physiol Nutr.* 2015;99:880.
10. Smith SL, et al. *New Zeal Vet J.* 2010;58:142.

PLANT POISONING ASSOCIATED WITH KNOWN TOXINS

DIANTHRONE DERIVATIVES

Hypericin, a complex derivative of dianthrone, is found in *Hypericum perforatum* (St. John's wort or Klamath weed) and *Hypericum triquetrifolium* and is the prototypical primary photosensitizing agent.[1] All parts of these plants are associated with photosensitive dermatitis when ingested by sheep and cattle, but they have to be eaten in large quantities. They are not very palatable, and most outbreaks occur when they are in the young stage and dominate the pasture. Narrow-leaf varieties contain 2 or 3 times as much hypericin as broadleaf varieties, and the flowering tops are 6 to 9 times as toxic as other parts. Clinical signs may appear within a few days of livestock going onto affected fields and usually disappear within 1 to 2 weeks after removal from them. Experimental production of poisoning with *H. perforatum* has shown that the plant contains a primary photodynamic agent. There is neither liver damage nor loss of hepatic function.

FAGOPYRIN

Fagopyrin, a red helianthrone pigment found in *Fagopyrum sagittatum* (buckwheat), is associated with primary photosensitization in all species.

FUROCOUMARIN

Plants containing furocoumarins (including psoralens) include the following:

- *Ammi majus*—bishop's weed, meadow sweet
- *Ammi visnaga*—visnaga
- *Cooperia pedunculata*—thunder lily
- *Cymopterus longipes*
- *Cymopterus watsonii*—wild or spring parsley
- *Heracleum mantegazzianum*—giant hogweed
- *Petroselinum* spp.—parsley
- *Thamnosma texana*—Dutchman's breeches, blister weed

Similar furocoumarins, identified as 4,5,8-trimethylpsoralen, 5-methoxypsoralen, and 8-methoxypsoralen, are also present in *Pastinaca sativa* (parsnip root) infested with the fungus *Ceratocystis fimbriata*, and *Apium graveolens* (celery) infested with *Sclerotinia* spp. (pink-rot fungus). These toxins have the particular characteristic of being photosensitizing by contact, without the need for ingestion, and are associated with serious lesions in humans. *A. majus* is most poisonous to livestock when there are ripe seeds in the seedheads. Its most serious occurrence is as a contaminant in hay. *C. pedunculata*, a perennial forb of western range country in the United States, occurs at times of high humidity or after rain has wet the foliage, and the live as well as dead leaves are toxic.

The clinical syndrome associated with plants containing furocoumarins is one of photosensitizing dermatitis. It includes severe cutaneous dermatitis, sometimes as severe as cutaneous gangrene, on the white parts of the skin on the dorsal and lateral sides of the body and edema of the head and ears, the lateral aspects of the teats, the unpigmented conjunctivae, the muzzle and the oral mucosa inside the lower lip, and the undersurface of the tip of the tongue. Photosensitive dermatitis in pigs may be associated with distinctive vesicles on the snout and raise a false alarm of viral vesicular disease. One serious international incident arose out of a feeding of moldy parsnips.

PLANT POISONINGS ASSOCIATED WITH UNIDENTIFIED TOXINS

DERMATITIS

- *Entandrophragma cylindricum*—redwood; shavings as bedding associated with balanoposthitis in rams
- *Excoecaria* spp.
- *Heracleum mantegazzianum*—cow parsnip
- *Vicia benghalensis*—popany vetch; associated with dermatitis, conjunctivitis, rhinitis, fever, and multiple eosinophilic granulomas in many organs[1]
- *Vicia dasycarpa*—woolly pod vetch; same symptoms as *V. benghalensis*
- *Vicia villosa*—hairy vetch; same signs as *V. benghalensis.*

PHOTOSENSITIZATION—PRIMARY; WITHOUT HEPATIC LESIONS

- *Echinochloa utilis*—Japanese millet
- *Erodium cicutarium*—storksbill
- *Froelichia humboldtiana*[2]
- *Holocalyx glaziovii*
- *Lachnanthes tinctoria*
- *Mentha satureioides*
- *Sphenosciadium capitellatum*
- *Medicago polymorpha*—burr trefoil
- *Verbena* spp.

Photodermatitis associated with *M. polymorphia* and *F. humboldtiana* occurs in all animal species on pasture dominated by the plant, usually in the spring. Lesions on the unpigmented parts of the skin disappear quickly when animals are taken off the pasture; there is no liver damage or permanent after-effects.[2] Aphids, which commonly infest the plant in very large numbers, contain large amounts of a photodynamic agent and may be important in some outbreaks of the disease.

REFERENCES

1. Soliva CR, et al. *J Anim Feed Sci.* 2008;17:352.
2. Souza PEC, et al. *Res Vet Sci.* 2012;93:1337.

SELENIUM TOXICOSIS

SYNOPSIS

Etiology Ingestion of plants or feed supplements or injection of pharmaceutical agents with excessive amounts of selenium.

Epidemiology Enzootic disease where soils and pasture contain toxic amounts of selenium; outbreaks after errors in feed supplementation or oral or injection doses.

Clinical pathology: Elevated concentration of selenium in body tissues and fluids.

Lesions:

Living Animals:

Acute: dyspnea, diarrhea, prostration, short course, death.

Chronic: emaciation, rough coat, stiff gait, lame, hoof deformity.

Postmortem:

Acute: evidence of cardiovascular compromise, hemorrhages.

Chronic: skeletal and cardiac myopathies.

Diagnostic confirmation: Elevated selenium levels in body fluids and tissues.

Treatment: None; avoid pastures with selenium-containing plants; take care with medication and feed additives containing selenium.

ETIOLOGY

Selenium toxicosis in animals is a worldwide problem, either as an acute or chronic poisoning. It is associated with the ingestion or injection of organic or inorganic selenium compounds as follows:

- Inorganic selenium compounds administered as feed supplements
- Organic selenocompounds (selenomethionine and methylselenocysteine) occurring in pasture plants[1-2]
- Pharmaceutical preparations administered orally or by injection, frequently combined with vitamin E[3]

Discrepancies exist in the toxic doses quoted in the literature, and the reasons for this are not fully understood. Identified animal factors include species, age, health, reproductive status, and nutritional status.[4] Other factors include dose, route of administration, and interactions with other dietary substrates.[3] The daily intake of a diet containing 2 mg/kg BW of selenium can be marginally toxic for sheep, yet pregnant and lactating ewes tolerated doses as high as 12 mg dietary selenium (as sodium selenite) per kilogram of BW for 72 weeks without developing any clinical or pathologic signs of selenium toxicosis.[5] Oral ingestion of 1 to 2.2 mg of Se/kg BW as sodium selenite caused mortality in lambs, but other lambs have survived doses of 4 mg/kg BW.[6,7] Feed containing 44 mg/kg selenium for horses and 11 mg/kg for pigs is associated with poisoning. Toxic single acute oral doses (as mg/kg BW) are 2.2 for sheep, 1.49 for horses,[3] 9 for cattle, and 15 for pigs.

EPIDEMIOLOGY

Occurrence

Pastoral

Selenium poisoning occurs in restricted areas in North America, Ireland, Israel, Canada, Australia, and South Africa where the soils are derived from particular rock formations containing a high content of selenium. The high level in these plants occurs from the high levels of selenium found naturally in the environment.

High levels of selenium in plants can also be found in areas where the soil is not naturally high in selenium. This is associated with industrial or commercial release of selenium into the water and soil.

Dosing Errors

Substantial losses as a result of selenium poisoning also occur because of misunderstanding about the dose rates of selenium compounds used therapeutically or prophylactically.

Risk Factors

Animal Risk Factors

Cattle are more tolerant than sheep. Pigs are unlikely to be exposed but can develop the disease in the field. Young animals are less tolerant than adults.

Dietary supplementation is used in the prevention of known deficiency syndromes such as white muscle disease in lambs, as a nonspecific growth stimulant, and as a prophylactic for a large number of other vague syndromes. The concurrent administration of monensin and selenium increases the toxicity of the selenium being fed. There are many case reports of unexpected illness and mortality in animals dosed with selenium preparations, and it is apparent that not all of the factors affecting selenium toxicity are known.

Organic selenium compounds, especially those occurring naturally in plants, may be more toxic than inorganic compounds, but this difference may not be apparent in ruminants because of alterations in ingested compounds produced by digestive processes in the rumen.[4] Selenite is more toxic than selenate, and both are more damaging than selenium dioxide.

Environmental Risk Factors

Industrial deposition (e.g., fly ash from soft coal deposited in fields) has been shown to be associated with increased selenium levels in tissues from sheep grazing there.

Farm Risk Factors

Selenium poisoning in animals grazing plants growing on seleniferous soils may be restricted to very distinct areas as small as individual fields. A low rainfall predisposes to selenium poisoning because soluble, available selenium compounds are not leached out of the topsoil, and lack of competing forage may force animals to eat large quantities of selenium-containing plants.

The effective selenium is contained in the top 60 to 90 cm of the soil profile, selenium at lower levels than this not being within reach of most plants. Selenium poisoning may occur on soils containing as little selenium as 0.01 mg/kg, but some soils may contain as much as 1200 mg/kg. Most pasture plants seldom contain selenium in excess of 100 ppm, but a number of species, the so-called converter or indicator plants, take up the element in such large quantities that selenium levels may reach as high as 10,000 ppm. Included in this category are *Acacia cana*; *Artemisia canescens*; *Aster* spp.; some of the *Astragalus*, *Atriplex*, and *Castilleja* spp.; *Comandra pallida*; *Descurainia pinnata*; *Grindelia* spp.; *Machaeranthera ramosa*; *Morinda reticulata*; *Neptunia amplexicaulis*; *Oonopsis*, *Penstemon*, and *Sideranthus* spp.; *Stanleya pinnata*; and *Xylorrhiza* spp.

These plants tend to grow preferentially on selenium-rich soils and are thus "indicator" plants. They are in general unpalatable because of a strong odor, and thus an acute syndrome is unlikely, but heavy losses have been attributed in the past to a chronic form of the disease known as alkali disease.

PATHOGENESIS

Ingested selenium compounds are absorbed primarily in the duodenum, with some absorption in the remainder of the small intestine. Little, if any, absorption occurs in the rumen. The mechanism of absorption varies depending on the specific form of selenium, with selenite absorption by passive transfer and selenomethionine and selenocysteine by active transport.[1,2] Tissue distribution also depends on the form of selenium, with the kidney and liver ultimately having the highest concentration of selenium. Placental transfer occurs, especially in the last trimester; little is excreted in the milk.[5] Metabolism occurs in the red blood cells and liver; excretion is primarily through urine, with a small amount of metabolized selenium excreted in the bile and feces.[1]

The mechanism of action is not well understood, and several different theories have been proposed.[3] Selenium occurs in plants in analogs of the sulfur-containing amino acids (e.g., selenocysteine), and a possible mechanism of intoxication is by interference with enzyme systems that contain these amino acids. Other proposed mechanisms include generation of free radicals, causing oxidative tissue damage, and incorporation into proteins, causing disruption of normal cell function.[3,4]

CLINICAL FINDINGS

Acute Poisoning

In naturally occurring and experimental poisoning there is severe respiratory distress, restlessness, complete anorexia, salivation, watery diarrhea, fever, tachycardia, abnormal posture and gait, prostration, and death after a short illness. Acutely poisoned horses showed marked central nervous system (CNS) signs, with ataxia and excitation, sweating, pyrexia, tachycardia, dyspnea, and death within 6 hours.[3] Mildly affected pigs show posterior ataxia, walking on tiptoe, difficulty in rising, sternal recumbency, tremor, and vomiting in some. Extreme cases assume a posture of lateral recumbency.

Chronic Poisoning

Chronic poisoning is manifested by dullness, emaciation, rough coat, lack of vitality, stiffness, and lameness. In cattle, horses, and mules the hair at the base of the tail and switch is lost, and in pigs, goats, and horses there may be general alopecia. There are hoof abnormalities, including swelling of the coronary band and deformity or separation and sloughing of the hooves, in all species. Lameness is severe. Congenital hoof deformities may occur in newborn animals. Hemorrhagic lesions on the proximal wall and soles of claws on all four feet may accompany these deformities. Chronic poisoning in pigs on rations containing 20 to 27 mg/kg is also associated with a syndrome of reduced feed intake and paraplegia and quadriplegia as a result of poliomyelomalacia. Pigs on marginal levels of intake of selenium (10 mg/kg) develop necrosis of the coronary band, low conception rates, and increased neonatal mortality.

CLINICAL PATHOLOGY

A moderate anemia occurs in acute and chronic poisoning, and a depression of hemoglobin levels to about 7 g/dL is one of the early indications of selenium poisoning. Selenium can be detected in the urine, milk, and hair of affected animals. Clinical illness is evident at blood levels of 3 mg/kg and at urine levels of more than 4 mg/kg of selenium. Normal serum levels of 140 to 190 ng/mL are elevated to the level of 1500 ng/mL.

Critical levels of selenium in hair include the following:

- Less than 5.0 mg/kg suggests that chronic selenosis is unlikely.
- From 5.0 to 10.0 mg/kg suggests borderline problems.
- More than 10 mg/kg is diagnostic of chronic selenosis.

NECROPSY FINDINGS

Acute

In confirmed cases of natural or experimentally produced acute selenium poisoning, most of the macroscopic findings can be attributed to cardiovascular compromise. There is pulmonary edema and congestion, petechiation of the thoracic viscera, and congestion of the liver, kidneys, and gastrointestinal tract. In parenterally overdosed lambs and piglets there is usually hydrothorax, hydropericardium, and ascites.

Histologic lesions may be minimal if the clinical course is brief. Changes that may be observed in animals surviving more than 24 hours include a serous effusion within pulmonary alveoli, mild hyaline or granular degeneration of skeletal muscle fibers, hydropic degeneration in renal tubular epithelial cells, and periacinar degeneration and necrosis of hepatocytes. Cardiac myocytes may appear swollen and contain areas of cytoplasmic granularity and lysis.

Chronic

In animals suffering from subacute to chronic selenium poisoning there is a skeletal and cardiac myopathy. Deformities of the feet and skin are usually apparent. Atrophy and dilatation of the heart and pulmonary edema, cirrhosis and atrophy of the liver, glomerulonephritis, mild gastroenteritis, and erosion of articular surfaces have also been recorded.

Symmetric poliomyelomalacia has been identified in both natural and experimental settings in pigs fed excessive selenium. The areas primarily affected are the ventral horns of the cervical and lumbar enlargements, with lesser damage in brainstem nuclei. The microscopic appearance of affected spinal cord includes vacuolation of the neuropil and sometimes of the cytoplasm of neurons. Neuronal chromatolysis, axonal swelling, and endothelial cell swelling and proliferation are consistently present.

Samples for Confirmation of Diagnosis

- **Toxicology**—50 g liver, kidney; 500 g of suspect feed (ASSAY [Se])
- **Histology**—formalin-fixed skeletal muscle, heart, liver, kidney, +/− spinal cord from cervical and lumbar enlargements (LM)

Selenium Levels in Tissue. In chronic selenosis in sheep, hepatic and renal levels of selenium are about 20 to 30 mg/kg, and levels in wool are in the range of 0.6 to 2.3 mg/kg. In horses, hair levels of more than 5 mg/kg are recorded.

The diagnosis of selenium poisoning rests largely on the recognition of the typical syndromes in animals in areas where the soil content of selenium is high or when there has been administration of selenium as medication or as a feed additive. The clinical and necropsy lesions associated with the poisoning cover a wide range of signs, and lesions and are not easily summarized. Diagnostic confirmation depends on an assay of toxic levels of selenium in body tissues or fluids.

DIFFERENTIAL DIAGNOSIS

Differential diagnostic list:

Acute poisoning
- Acute arsenic toxicosis
- Anaphylaxis
- Ionophores/tiamulin in swine
- Septicemia
- Toxemia

Chronic poisoning
- Hypovitaminosis A
- Laminitis
- Sodium chloride toxicosis

TREATMENT

A number of substances have been tried in the treatment of selenium poisoning, including potassium iodide, ascorbic acid, and beet pectin, but without apparent effect. The use of BAL is contraindicated.

CONTROL

Selenium in feeds should not exceed 5 mg/kg dry matter if danger is to be avoided, and feeding on pasture containing 25 mg/kg dry matter for several weeks can be expected to be associated with chronic selenium poisoning. Pasture may contain as much as 2000 to 6000 mg/kg of selenium and is associated with the acute form of the disease when fed for a few days.

Protection against the toxic effects of selenium in amounts up to 10 mg/kg in the diet has been obtained by the inclusion in the ration fed to pigs of 0.01% to 0.02% of arsanilic acid or 0.005% of 3-nitro-4-hydroxyphenyl arsonic acid. In cattle, 0.01% arsanilic acid in the ration or 550 mg/day to grazing steers gives only slight protection. The addition of linseed oil to the ration improves the efficiency of this protection. A high-protein diet also has a general protective effect.

When using selenium as a pharmaceutical agent, strict attention should be paid to the recommended dose and route of administration.

FURTHER READING

Blodgett DJ, Bevill RF. Acute selenium toxicosis in sheep. *Vet Hum Tox.* 1987;29:233-236.
Casteel SW, Osweiler GD, Cook WO, et al. Selenium toxicosis in swine. *J Am Vet Med Assoc.* 1985;186:1084-1085.

O'Toole T, Raisbeck MF. Pathology of experimentally induced chronic selenosis (alkali disease) in yearling cattle. *J Vet Diagn Invest.* 1995;7:364-373.

Perry TW, Beeson WM, Smith WH, et al. Effect of supplemental Se on performance and deposit of Se in blood and hair of finishing beef cattle. *J Anim Sci.* 1976;42:192-195.

Radostits O, et al. Selenium poisoning. In: *Veterinary Medicine: A Textbook of the Disease of Cattle, Horses, Sheep, Goats and Pigs.* 10th ed. London: W.B. Saunders; 2007:1811.

Raisbeck MF, Dahl ER, Sanchez DA, et al. Naturally occurring selenosis in Wyoming. *J Vet Diagn Invest.* 1993;5:84-87.

REFERENCES

1. Herdt TH. *Vet Clin North Am Food A.* 2011;27:255.
2. Nogueira CW, et al. *Arch Toxicol.* 2011;85:1313-1359.
3. Desta B, et al. *J Vet Diagn Invest.* 2011;23:623.
4. Kienzle E, et al. *Eur Eq Nutr Health Con.* 2006;3:1.
5. Davis PA, et al. *J Anim Sci.* 2006;84:660.
6. Faye B, et al. *Nutrients.* 2009;1:30.
7. Tiwary AK, et al. *J Vet Diagn Invest.* 2006;18:61.

IODINE TOXICOSIS

ETIOLOGY

Iodine is found in low concentrations in nature both as inorganic and organic forms. Common sources of iodine include iodized salt (100 ppm iodine), ethylenediamine dihydroiodide (EDDI), and iodine containing feed additives such as calcium iodate, potassium iodide, and sodium iodine.[1] Potassium iodide, the most water-soluble and chemically unstable form, is the least commonly used product in cattle feed; calcium iodate is the most stable product. Ethylenediamine dihydroiodide is often used to prevent or treat footrot in cattle but has been used in other countries to treat pythiosis in horses.[2]

Poisoning with inorganic iodine products is rarely associated with illness in animals. Excretion in milk and eggs is linear, and the toxic dose is large. As the amount of inorganic iodine ingested increases, so does the amount excreted in milk, with a fairly constant excretion ratio of 8% to 12% iodine.[3] Doses of 10 mg/kg BW daily are usually required to produce fatal illness in calves. There is a special occurrence of goiter in foals when the foal and the dam are fed excessive amounts of iodine, especially when kelp is fed as a dietary supplement. Intakes of 35 to 40 mg iodine/day in a mare can be associated with the development of goiter in her foal.

Toxicity with organic iodides has also occurred at much lower levels of intake (e.g., 160 mg/day per cow) and appears to be a practical risk when cows or calves are fed EDDI constantly as a prophylactic against footrot.

CLINICAL FINDINGS

Clinical signs vary depending on the species and form of iodine. Horses appear to be the most sensitive to iodine toxicosis, followed by ruminants and then pigs.[1,2] In cattle and sheep, signs include heavy dusting of the hair coat with large-sized dandruff scales, hair loss, dryness of the coat, coughing, and profuse nasal discharge.[1] Feed intake and milk production are often decreased. Other common signs in ruminants include lacrimation, hyperthermia, and hypersalivation. Exophthalmos occurs in some cases, and severely affected animals may die of bronchopneumonia. In horses, alopecia and heavy dandruff are characteristic. Anhidrosis, rhabdomyolysis, and exercise intolerance have also been reported.[2]

CLINICAL PATHOLOGY/NECROPSY

Serum iodine levels are elevated above the normal level[3] of 5 µg/100 mL up to 20 to 130 µg/mL.

Most of the postmortem lesions are associated with changes in the respiratory tract, with tracheitis, bronchopneumonia, and pleurisy reported in cattle. Lung tissue shows exudative inflammation, hypertrophy of the bronchial mucous membranes, bronchiole necrosis, and fibrinous exudate in the alveoli. Sheep with iodine toxicosis showed suppurative bronchopneumonia and fibrinous pneumonia.

FURTHER READING

Baker DH. Iodine toxicity and its amelioration. *Exp Biol Med.* 2004;229:473-478.

Paulikova I, Kovac G, Bires J, et al. Iodine toxicity in ruminants. *Vet Med Czech.* 2002;12:343-350.

Thompson LJ, Hall JO, Meerdink GL. Toxic effects of trace mineral excess. *Vet Clin North Am Food A.* 1991;7:277-306.

REFERENCES

1. Schone F, Rajendram R. Iodine in farm animals. In: Preedy VR, Burrow GN, Watson RR, Burlingham MA, eds. *Comprehensive Handbook of Iodine: Nutritional, Biochemical Pathologic and Therapeutic Aspects.* Academic Press; 2009:151.
2. Doria RGS, et al. *Arq Bras Vet Med Zootec.* 2008;60:521.
3. Norouzian MA, et al. *J Anim Vet Adv.* 2009;8:111.

Cutaneous Neoplasms

PAPILLOMA AND SARCOID

Sarcoid of horses and cutaneous papillomatosis of horses, goats, and cattle are specific diseases (see also "Sarcoid" and "Papillomatosis"). The lesions are characteristically nodular growths of viable tissue and, if there is no traumatic injury, with no discontinuity of the covering epidermis.

Aural flat warts (aural plaques) occur commonly in the horse and are caused by papillomavirus. Blackflies may serve as a vector. Lesions consist of one to several gray or white plaques involving the inner surface of the pinna. Similar lesions may occur around the anus, vulva, and inguinal regions. The lesions are usually asymptomatic, may persist indefinitely, may regress spontaneously, and are refractory to treatment.

SQUAMOUS-CELL CARCINOMA

Squamous-cell carcinoma can occur anywhere on the skin, and also in the mouth and maxillary sinus. Squamous-cell carcinoma in cattle and horses may develop as an uncommon complication of an infection with bovine papillomavirus type 1 and 2.[1] Common types are as follows:

- **Ocular squamous-cell carcinoma (cancer—eye)** is the commonest lesion, on the eyelids and the eyeball in horses and cattle (see also "Bovine Ocular Squamous-Cell Carcinoma" and "Equine Ocular Squamous-Cell Carcinoma")
- **Squamous-cell carcinomas in horses** are the second most common cutaneous neoplasia (after the equine sarcoid) in this species and primarily affect the glans penis and prepuce and the perianal region of aged horses.[2] Squamous-cell carcinoma can cause fatal metastases unless the primary tumor is resected in the early stages. Grossly similar lesions are caused by epithelial hyperplasia, habronemiasis, and squamous papillomata.
- **Vulvar squamous-cell carcinoma** appears frequently in Merino ewes as a result of excessive exposure of vulvar skin to sunlight after radical perineal surgery to help control blow-fly strike. Squamous-cell carcinomas also occur on the vulva of cattle, and a greater incidence has been observed on unpigmented than on pigmented vulvas.
- **Horn cancer** in cattle and rarely in sheep, goats, and buffaloes is a squamous-cell carcinoma arising from the pseudostratified columnar epithelium of the horn core mucosa; it is most prevalent in *Bos indicus* breeds. This tumor affects approximately 1% of the Indian cattle population and accounts for over 80% of reported tumors in Indian cattle. Steers have been reported to be affected more frequently than female animals. In the early stages, affected animals may rub the horns against a fixed object or shake the head frequently. A bloody discharge begins from the nostril on the affected side, or from the base of the horn, and the animal holds its head down and toward one side. The horn becomes loosened and falls off, leaving the tumor exposed to infection and fly infestation. Secondary metastases are common. The high prevalence of metastases in regional lymph nodes and internal organs discourages treatment, but a phenol extract of horn core tissue is immunogenic, and immunotherapy may be a successful treatment technique. Other forms of therapy are also practiced for squamous-cell carcinoma generally, including surgical excision,

preferably by cryotherapy, and radiofrequency hyperthermia.

- **Ear cancer** in sheep is in most cases a squamous-cell carcinoma. The lesion commences around the free edge of the ear and then invades the entire ear, which becomes a large, cauliflower-shaped mass. A high incidence may occur in some flocks. but the cause is not known; the presence of papillomavirus in many aural precancerous lesions suggests that the virus may participate in the etiology.
- **Ovine skin cancer**: A high incidence of epitheliomas has been recorded in some families of merino sheep in Australia. The lesions occur on the woolled skin and are accompanied by many cutaneous cysts. It has been suggested that predisposition to the neoplasm is inherited. Metastasis is common with both epitheliomas and squamous-cell carcinomas.
- "**Brand cancer**," which occurs as a granulomatous mass at the site of a skin fire or freeze brand, is usually considered to be of chronic inflammatory rather than neoplastic origin, but squamous-cell carcinomas are recorded at branding sites in sheep and cattle.
- **In goats**, the perineum is a common site for squamous-cell carcinoma. The udder, ears, and base of the horns may also be affected. Ulceration, flystrike, and matting of hair are unattractive sequelae. A bilaterally symmetric vulvar swelling as a result of ectopic mammary tissue that enlarges at parturition is likely to be confused with squamous-cell carcinoma. Milk can be aspirated from the swellings.

REFERENCES

1. Nasir L, Campo MS. *Vet Dermatol.* 2008;19:243-254.
2. Schaffer PA, et al. *J Am Vet Med Assoc.* 2013;242:99-104.

MELANOMA

Melanomas are skin neoplasias commonly occurring in pigs, horses, cattle, small ruminants, and camelids.[1] In horses, between 4% and 15% and in cattle approximately 6% of all tumors were reported to be melanomas.[1-3] In horses, melanomas primarily occur in mature gray- and white-coated horses, reaching a prevalence of over 80% in this subgroup of animals.[4] Although historically melanomas were considered to be benign skin proliferations, more recently the concept of melanoma as a neoplasia with malignant potential has become more accepted. Some sources claim that at least 66% of melanocytic tumors in horses eventually become malignant.[4]

Four types of melanocytic abnormalities are recognized in horses:[2,4]

- **Melanocytic nevi** are seen in younger horses independent of the coat color and are discrete and benign discolorations of the skin. Presence of several nevi is considered a predisposing factor for the development of dermal melanoma.[1]
- **Discrete dermal melanomas** present as single masses, most commonly in typical locations such as the tail, anal, perianal, perineal, and genital region. They are most common in mature gray horses with an average age of 13 years. Although dermal melanomas frequently are benign, malignant forms occur. Surgical excision at early stages is recommended and is curative in most cases.[1,4]
- **Dermal melanomatosis** refers to the occurrence of several dermal melanomas, and it has a high incidence of metastasis. Melanomatosis in general affects horses that are older than 15 years and is not amenable to surgical resection. Visceral metastasis is a not uncommon complication; this type of melanoma is considered to be potentially fatal.[4]
- **Anaplastic malignant melanomas** occur in older nongray horses, with a high incidence of metastasis.

The presentation of discrete dermal melanoma and dermal melanomatosis is referred to as **dermal melanoma.**

PATHOPHYSIOLOGY

Although the initiation of most animal melanomas is still poorly understood, the development of melanomas is epidemiologically linked to mutations generated by both UV-A and UV-B solar radiation. Malignant cells can infiltrate surrounding tissue and metastasize via lymphatic or blood vessels, with regional lymph nodes being the usual first target.[1] A genetic predisposition to the development of melanomas is recognized in Sinclair miniature pigs, Duroc pigs, and Angora goats, which have been proposed as potential models for human melanoma.[1] In horses, the well-recognized connection between gray coat color and the increased risk of melanoma has led to the assumption that specific genetic mutations in gray-coated horses may either predispose to or facilitate the development of melanoma. Presence of multiple melanocytic nevi is considered to increase the risk of melanoma. Melanocytic tumors can also be congenital (see also "Inherited Melanoma").

CLINICAL FINDINGS

Melanomas initially present as single, small, firm, raised nodule with a slow growth rate. They are frequently found incidentally during grooming or routine physical examination. Melanomas may be of any color, ranging from gray or brown to black, red, or even dark blue.[1] Typical locations for melanomas are the perineum, tail base, sheath, commissures of the lips, jugular furrow, and subauricular lymph nodes.[4] Although in many cases tumors may exist for many years without causing any clinical signs, the skin may ulcerate in rapidly growing tumors, leading to secondary bacterial infection. Large masses in the perianal region may impair defecation and result in fecal impaction. Similarly, large tumors in the neck area may impair head movement and the ability to eat, drink, and swallow. Visceral metastatic masses may occur in more advanced cases.[4]

CLINICAL PATHOLOGY

Although the location, appearance, and color of a mass can be highly suggestive, an excisional biopsy, which involves surgically removing small tumors integrally and submitting them to a diagnostic laboratory for histologic confirmation of the diagnosis, has been recommended whenever possible.[4]

TREATMENT

Single noninvasive tumors of small to moderate size have been surgically excised with good success and good prognosis. Surgical excision is unrewarding in cases with multiple tumors, infiltrating masses, or masses located around the parotid salivary gland, which complicate the surgical approach considerably.[4]

In horses, treatment with oral cimetidine, a histamine type 2 receptor antagonist, either at a dose of 2.5 mg/kg BW q8h or 7.5 mg/kg BW q24h p.os, for at least 60 days has yielded variable results.[3] Promising results were reported with the use of cisplatin, either as repeated intratumoral injection or as biodegradables beads in horses.[4]

FURTHER READING

Moore JS, Shaw C, Shaw E, et al. Melanoma in horses: current perspectives. *Equine Vet J.* 2013;25:144-151.

Smith SH, Goldschmidt MH, McManus MP. A comparative review of melanocytic neoplasms. *Vet Pathol.* 2002;39:651-678.

REFERENCES

1. Smith SH, et al. *Vet Pathol.* 2002;39:651-678.
2. Schaffer PA, et al. *J Am Vet Med Assoc.* 2013;242:99-104.
3. MacGillivray KC, et al. *J Vet Intern Med.* 2002;16:452-456.
4. Moore JS, et al. *Equine Vet J.* 2013;25:144-151.

LIPOMA

Lipomas are benign subcutaneous or submucosal tumors that can be locally extensive and consist of well-differentiated adipocytes. Lipomas are occasionally seen in horses but are rare in cattle. In horses, lipomas occur either as mesenteric or cutaneous lipomas. Mesenteric lipomas predominantly develop in older horses, presenting as pedunculated lipomas that may cause secondary complications such as intestinal strangulation.

Subcutaneous lipomas are the predominant form in young horses less than 2 years of age. The large majority of cutaneous lipomas are encapsulated and well demarcated from surrounding tissue, making them easily resectable, with minimal risk for recurrence. Occasionally lipomas may grow invasively, infiltrating surrounding tissue such as muscles, tendons, joints, and even bone. Despite their invasive growth, infiltrative lipomas are benign because they do not metastasize.[1] The invasive growth pattern makes integral resection of tumorous tissue impossible and results in high recurrence rates after surgical intervention.[1] Differentiating between lipomas and infiltrative lipomas is important to determine the eligibility for surgical resection and the prognosis but can be challenging under field conditions.[1]

In foals and calves, congenital external infiltrating lipomas have been reported.[2,3]

REFERENCES

1. Pease A. *Equine Vet Educ.* 2010;22:608-609.
2. Rebsamen E, et al. *Equine Vet Educ.* 2010;22:602-607.
3. Sickinger M, et al. *J Vet Diagn Invest.* 2009;21:719-721.

MAST CELL TUMORS

A mast cell tumor (mastocytoma) is a rare neoplasia primarily affecting the skin in cattle, horses, swine, and New World camelids. The large majority of mast cell tumors in cattle and horses are benign, but malignant forms have been described. Less than 6% of all equine and less than 1% of all bovine neoplasias have been identified as mastocytomas.[1-3] Incidental case of mast cell tumors have been reported in pigs, small ruminants, and New World camelids. Mast cell tumors in the species just mentioned are most frequently located in the skin, with no apparent site of predilection. Other than on the skin, mastocytomas in horses have also been identified in the gastrointestinal tract, salivary glands, eyes, testes, and spleen.[1] In cattle, apart from the cutaneous form, mast cell tumors have been found in spleen, lung, liver, lymph nodes, muscle tissue, omentum, abomasum, tongue, and uterus.

CLINICAL FINDINGS

Animals of all ages can be affected, and neither a gender nor a breed predilection has been reported.[2] Single lesions are the most common presentation, but cases of multicentric mastocytoma have been reported in different species.[1,4,5] In most instances a mastocytoma presents as slow-growing, indolent cutaneous or subcutaneous mass. Lesions typically are well demarcated and vary from 0.5 to 20 cm in diameter and feel firm or fluctuating on palpation. Masses located on the limbs are often firm and immovable.[1] The overlying skin is usually intact, although alopecia, hyperpigmentation, or ulceration may be present.[1]

CLINICAL PATHOLOGY

Diagnosis of cutaneous mastocytoma is either by fine-needle aspiration or excisional biopsy, removing the mass integrally. Histologically mast cell tumors are characterized by the predominance of well-differentiated mast cells. Mitotic figures are few in number, and eosinophilic infiltration of the mass is a consistent finding.[1] Older lesions may contain considerable amount of fibrosis, mineralization, and necrosis.[1]

TREATMENT

Cutaneous mastocytomas in cattle and horses in general are benign and indolent, but they rarely resolve spontaneously. Surgical excision may therefore be indicated for cosmetic reasons or when masses cause discomfort, and surgery is usually curative.

Other reported treatments include cryosurgery and the intra- or sublesional injection of corticosteroids (e.g., 10 to 20 mg methylprednisolone acetate).[1]

REFERENCES

1. Mair TS, Krudewig C. *Equine Vet J.* 2008;20:177-182.
2. Schaffer PA, et al. *J Am Vet Med Assoc.* 2013;242:99-104.
3. Tzu-Yin L, et al. *J Vet Diagn Invest.* 2010;22:808-811.
4. Martinez J, et al. *J Vet Diagn Invest.* 2011;23:1222-1225.
5. Millward LM, et al. *Vet Clin Pathol.* 2010;39:365-370.

LYMPHOMATOSIS

In cattle and horses, skin lesions occur as nodules in the subcutaneous tissue, most commonly in the paralumbar fossae and the perineum. In cattle, the lesions are associated with the virus of enzootic bovine leukosis (EBL) and are only one manifestation of the disease, usually being accompanied by lesions in other organs. In horses, there are no leukemic lesions in lymph nodes or visceral organs.

NEUROFIBROMATOSIS

This common lesion of nerves in cattle usually attracts attention only in abattoir specimens but can occur in a cutaneous form resembling a similar disease of humans; a particularly high prevalence of this benign disease is recorded in breeds of European pied cattle. Clinical cases are usually recorded in calves, in which there are cutaneous lesions that appear as tumor-like lumps between the eyes and on the cheeks. They are flat, round tumors up to 8 cm in diameter and of a lumpy, elastic consistency.

HISTIOCYTOMA

Histiocytomas originate from epidermal Langerhans cells of antigen-presenting lineage. This is a very rare benign neoplasm in farm animals but is recorded as cutaneous nodules or plaques, which bleed easily, in goats and cattle. The lesions regress spontaneously.

CUTANEOUS ANGIOMATOSIS

Angiomatosis is vasoproliferation originating from endothelial cells from blood vessels. The etiology of this condition that is rarely observed in horses, cattle, swine, small ruminants, and New World camelids is not yet understood. Causes discussed in the literature are inflammatory reactions, bacterial or viral infection, congenital abnormalities, and hyper- or neoplastic transformations.

In cattle, cutaneous angiomatosis most commonly presents as single or multiple cutaneous lesions situated most commonly along the dorsum of the neck characterized by recurrent profuse hemorrhage. The lesions consist of what appears to be protruding granulation tissue and are benign. Histologically angiomas are characterized by the nonencapsulated proliferation of vascular tissue that may or may not be infiltrated with inflammatory cells.

A juvenile version of angiomatosis in calves is characterized by similar lesions but in many organs, sometimes including the skin.

Surgical excision is effective.

HEMANGIOMA AND HEMANGIOSARCOMA

Benign vascular proliferations are occasionally encountered in most animal species. Cutaneous hemangiomas of young horses are morphologically the same as bovine cutaneous angiomatosis lesions. Young horses usually present with solitary lesions between 1 and up to 30 cm in diameter on distal parts of the limbs. The lesions can consist of nodules or plaques with firm to fluctuating consistency that bleed easily. The skin overlying the proliferation tends to be dark colored, hyperkeratotic, and associated with local alopecia.

Hemangiosarcomas (hemangioepithelioma) are malignant tumors recorded relatively frequently in older horses. They are large, highly vascular, subcutaneous masses, usually associated with one or more internal lesions. The primary lesion may be internal, commonly in the spleen, or cutaneous. Recurrence after excision, extensive local infiltration, and death as a result of anemia are common sequelae.

CONGENITAL SKIN TUMORS

Congenital tumors are defined as those existing at birth. A broader definition is that congenital tumors can be detected in fetuses and in newborns until 2 months of age. Embryonic tumors are those that arise during embryonic, fetal, or early postnatal development from a particular organ rudiment or tissue while it is still immature. Hamartomas are benign, tumor-like nodules composed of overgrowth of mature cells, which normally occur in the affected part but often with one element predominating. Hamartomas include hemangiomas, ameloblastomas, and rhabdomyomas. Teratomas are true neoplasms consisting of different types of tissue not native to the area in which they occur.

Cattle

Congenital skin neoplasms of cattle described include mast cell tumors, lymphosarcoma, myxoma, and vascular hamartoma. Benign melanomas, mastocytomas, hemangiomas and lymphangiomas, fibrosarcomas, neurofibromatosis, subcutaneous lipomas, multiple lipomas, and retroperitoneal lipomas have also been recorded in calves. The comparative aspects of tumors in calves have been described.

Pigs

The literature on congenital and hereditary tumors in piglets has been reviewed. Spindle-cell sarcoma, malignant melanoma, and papillomatosis are common congenital tumors of the skin of piglets. Congenital cutaneous papillomatosis of the head and neck of a newborn piglet has been described on a pig-breeding farm where sporadic cutaneous papillomatosis of the prepuce and scrotum had previously occurred in several boars.

Foals

Congenital tumors in foals are rare. Congenital skin tumors are of the papillomatous, vascular, and melanocytic types. The vascular tumors are capillary hemangiomas, cavernous hemangiomas, and hemangiosarcomas.

FURTHER READING

Misdorp W. Congenital tumours and tumour-like lesions in domestic animals. 1. Cattle: a review. *Vet Q*. 2002;24:1-11.
Misdorp W. Congenital tumours and tumour-like lesions in domestic animals. 2. Pigs: a review. *Vet Q*. 2003;25:17-30.
Misdorp W. Congenital tumours and tumour-like lesions in domestic animals. 3. Horses: a review. *Vet Q*. 2003;25:61-71.

Congenital and Inherited Defects of the Skin

Examples of common inherited skin defects that are present at birth are as follows:

- **Inherited parakeratosis** (lethal trait A46, adema disease, inherited nutritional zinc deficiency) occurs in cattle.
- **Dermatosis vegetans** of Landrace breed pigs is a hereditary skin disease characterized by well-demarcated, raised, roughened skin lesions; enlarged, ridged, discolored hooves; and characteristic giant-cell pneumonia.
- **Inherited congenital ichthyosis** (fish-scale disease) of calves is characterized by diffuse cutaneous hyperkeratosis, giving the skin an appearance of fish scale. Two forms, the more severe and lethal **ichthyosis fetalis** (bovine harlequin fetus) and the milder **ichthyosis congenitalis,** are recognized.[1]
- **Inherited hypotrichoses and alopecias** have been described in numerous cattle breeds. Inherited hypotrichosis is often associated with other congenital defects, such as dental anomalies, absent horn development, abnormal coat coloration, and others.
- **Epitheliogenesis imperfecta**, a rare congenital defect reported in calves, pigs, lambs, and foals, is characterized by a discontinuity of the squamous epithelium. There are sharply demarcated areas in which there is absence of epidermis. The condition is inherited as a single autosomal-recessive trait and is fatal if skin lesions are extensive.
- **Epitheliogenesis imperfect (aplasia cutis)** occurs in piglets as a result of ingestion of *Fusarium* spp. toxin.
- **Epidermolysis bullosa syndrome** is observed in calves, lambs, and foals (especially the Belgian breed) and is characterized by separation of the dermal–epidermal junction beneath the basal epithelium. Lesions involve the skin, mucocutaneous junctions, and oral mucosa. The defect is present at birth, but it may be several months before the disease is clinically apparent.
- **Hereditary equine regional dermal asthenia (hyperelastosis cutis)** is an inherited connective tissue disorder primarily seen in Quarter horses. The condition is characterized by sharply demarcated areas of loose skin, which is hyperfragile, tears easily, and exhibits impaired healing. The underlying cause is a faulty collagen fiber production.
- **Congenital dyserythropoiesis and dyskeratosis** of Polled Hereford calves is a congenital syndrome of alopecia and anemia. The condition is characterized by nonregenerative anemia that is accompanied by progressively worsening cutaneous lesions in the form of generalized alopecia and hyperkeratotic dermatitis.
- **Hair-coat-color-linked follicular dysplasia**
- **Familial acantholysis** in New Zealand Angus calves is characterized by defective cell-to-cell adhesion in the epidermis. The skin is normal at birth, but erosions and crusts develop on exposed skin. Partial separation of the hooves and skin shedding over the carpus may occur.
- **Cutaneous asthenia, dermatosparaxis,** and the **Ehlers–Danlos syndrome** are reported in cattle sheep, pigs, and horses and are characterized by faulty collagen production. Skin is fragile and hyperextensible from birth on, with disturbed wound healing.
- **Nevus** is an irregularly shaped, cutaneous defect, present at birth and originally covered with hair, but subsequently hairless. Depending on which cells are involved, a nevus is referred to as vascular, epidermal, connective tissue, or melanotic nevus. Individual lesions are 3 to 4 cm in diameter, bright pink, ulcerated, and inflamed. Vascular nevi consist of densely packed convoluted blood vessels, which bleed easily. Most lesions are on the lower limbs, especially at the coronet.
- **Dermoid cysts** are cystic structures occasionally observed in horses and other species containing hair, exfoliated skin, and glandular debris. Dermoid cysts are present at birth but may become apparent later in life as they grow in size.
- **Inherited epidermal dysplasia (baldy calf syndrome)** of Holstein–Friesian calves is an autosomal-recessive inherited lethal condition. Calves appear normal at birth but progressively loose hair and condition; they have elongated and narrow hooves and scaly skin. Secondary skin ulceration and failure of horn development occur.[2]

REFERENCES

1. Gentile A, Testoni S. *Slov Vet Res*. 2006;43:17-29.
2. Windsor PA, Agerholm JS. *Aust Vet J*. 2009;87:193-199.

INHERITED ALBINISM

Albinism is a congenital lack of melanin pigment in the skin, hair, and other normally pigmented structures such as the uveal tract. Albinism is classified as generalized or localized and as complete, partial, or incomplete. The affected skin in albinism is characterized microscopically as melanopenic rather than melanocytopenic, which distinguishes partial albinism from piebaldism. Most of the normal, inherited white markings that occur on horses are localized forms of piebaldism. Generalized and complete albino animals (oculocutaneous albinism) have white hair, white skin, and pink irides, and they usually exhibit photophobia. Generalized albinism in the horse is inherited as an autosomal-dominant trait that is only viable in the heterozygous states. These horses have incomplete albinism because there is some coloration to the iris.

DISORDERS OF COAT COLOR, PSEUDOALBINISM, AND LETHAL WHITES

There are a number of forms of pseudoalbinism and disorders of coat color in domestic animals that involve congenital systemic disease.[1-5] There is a nonlethal form in cattle and a lethal dominant form in horses in which 25% of conceptions produced by mating dominant white horses die in utero in early gestation. The only pigment in the affected foals is in the eyes.

The disease in **cattle** occurs in Angus, Brown Swiss, Holstein, and Hereford cattle. The Angus cattle have a brown coat and two-tone irises with an outer pale brown ring and an inner blue one. There appears to be no defect in digestion or metabolism. Hereford incomplete albinos have the Chediak–Higashi syndrome. The other breeds do not appear to have defects other than in pigmentation, and the defect in Angus is probably more accurately called "oculocutaneous hypopigmentation." They do have one problem; they are photophobic and prefer to be out of the sun.

A complete albinism in Icelandic **sheep** is manifested by white skin color, pink eyes, and impaired vision in bright light. It is an autosomal recessive. Albinism occurs in Karakul sheep. White lambs of an inbred flock of the Cameroon breed born with light blue eyes died within hours to days of birth, with signs of intestinal obstruction. Affected lambs had deletion of both copies of the gene for endothelin type-B receptor and deletion of a single copy of the gene in the phenotypically normal dams and several other unaffected sheep from the same flock.[6,7]

True albino **horses** rarely if ever occur in nature, but white horses with pigmented eyes do. They are more accurately called pseudo-albinos. See "Lethal White" for discussion of colonic aganglionosis caused by a mutation in the endothelin type-B receptor gene in overo white Paint horses.[5]

REFERENCES

1. Bettley CD, et al. *Anim Welfare.* 2012;21:59.
2. Charon KM, et al. *Annals Anim Welfare.* 2015;15:3.
3. Webb AA, et al. *Can Vet J.* 2010;51:653.
4. Bellone RR. *Anim Genet.* 2010;41:100.
5. Finno CJ, et al. *Vet J.* 2009;179:336.
6. Luehken G, et al. *PLoS ONE.* 2012;7.
7. Pauciullo A, et al. *Cytogen Genom Res.* 2013;140:46.

INHERITED SYMMETRIC ALOPECIA

Inherited symmetric alopecia is an inherited skin defect of cattle in which animals born with a normal hair coat lose hair from areas distributed symmetrically over the body. It has been observed in Holstein cattle as a rare disease, but its appearance among valuable purebred cattle has economic importance. It appears to be inherited as a single autosomal-recessive character. Loss of hair commences at 6 weeks to 6 months of age. The alopecia is symmetric and commences on the head, neck, back, and hindquarters, and progresses to the root of the tail, down the legs, and over the forelimbs. Affected skin areas become completely bald. Pigmented and unpigmented skin is equally affected; there is no irritation, and the animals are normal in other respects. Failure of hair fibers to develop in apparently normal follicles can be detected by skin biopsy.

INHERITED CONGENITAL HYPOTRICHOSIS

In inherited congenital hypotrichosis there is partial or complete absence of the hair coat with or without other defects of development. The main importance of the disease is in cattle, in which there are six syndromes, but it is also inherited in **pigs**, in which it is associated with low birth weight, weakness, and high mortality, and in Poll Dorset **sheep**, in which the face, ears, and lower legs are bald; there are no eyelashes; and the patient lacrimates excessively. The skin is thick, wrinkled, greasy, scaly, and erythematous. Hair fibers are completely absent from the follicles, but wool fibers and follicles are normal.

Viable Hypotrichosis

Viable hypotrichosis is recorded in North America in Guernsey and Jersey cattle. Calves are viable provided they are sheltered. They grow normally but are unable to withstand exposure to cold weather or hot sun. In most instances hair is completely absent from most of the body at birth, but eyelashes are present in addition to tactile hair around the feet and head. Occasionally hair may be present in varying amounts at birth but is lost soon afterward. There is no defect of horn or hoof growth. The skin is normal but has a shiny, tanned appearance and on sections no hair follicles are present in the skin. The condition is inherited as a single recessive character.

Congenital hypotrichosis has been reported in a Perheron draught horse. At birth there were circumscribed patchy areas of alopecia that was progressive, becoming almost complete by 1 year of age. Skin biopsy at 7 months of age revealed severe follicular hypoplasia, and the animal was still alive at 6 years of age.

Nonviable Hypotrichosis

Nonviable hypotrichosis is a complete hypotrichosis in which the thyroid is abnormally small and hypofunctional and the calves die shortly after birth.

Congenital Hypotrichosis and Anodontia (Anhidrotic Ectodermal Dysplasia)

Congenital X-linked hypotrichosis with missing teeth in bull calves is characterized by abnormal morphogenesis of the teeth, hair follicles, and eccrine sweat glands.[1-4] The disease has also been recognized in a cross-bred calf in Canada.[5] Two different forms can be distinguished according to the severity of the tooth defects: (1) congenital hypotrichosis with complete or almost complete anodontia, and (2) congenital hypotrichosis with completely missing incisors or defective incisors. Impaired body condition and growth of the affected animals result from missing teeth. In addition, animals with sparse hair are more susceptible to cold and more prone to skin lesions.

The phenotype and inheritance of hypotrichosis with nearly complete anodontia has been recorded in pedigreed Canadian and German Holstein calves. The phenotype is inherited as a monogenic X-linked recessive trait. An RT-PCR assay was used to identify the causative large genomic deletion in the bovine *EDA* gene. The bovine *EDA* gene encodes ectodysplasin A, a membrane protein expressed in keratinocytes, hair follicles, and sweat glands, which is involved in the interactions between cell and cell and/or cell and matrix.[1] A single-nucleotide polymorphism (SNP) at the 9(th) base of exon 8 in the EDA gene is located in the exonic splicing enhancers (ESEs) recognized by SRp40 protein. Consequently, the spliceosome machinery is no longer able to recognize the sequence as exonic and causes exon skipping.[1] The mutation determines the deletion of the entire exon (131 bp) in the RNA processing, causing a severe alteration of the protein structure and thus the disease. Analysis of the SNP allows the identification of carriers that can transmit the disease to the offspring.[1]

REFERENCES

1. Gargani M, et al. *BMC Vet Res.* 2011;7.
2. Karlskov-Mortensen P, et al. *Anim Genet.* 2011;42:578.
3. Ogino A, et al. *Hereditas.* 2011;148:46.
4. Ogino A, et al. *Anim Genet.* 2012;43:646.
5. Barlund CS, et al. *Can Vet J.* 2007;48:612.

Streaked Hairlessness

A sex-linked semidominant gene causes development of a streaked hairlessness in which irregular narrow streaks of hypotrichosis occur in female Holsteins.

Partial Hypotrichosis

Partial hypotrichosis has been recorded in polled and horned Hereford cattle. At birth there is a fine coat of short, curly hair that later is added to by the appearance of some very coarse, wiry hair. The calves survive but do not grow well. It is inherited as a simple recessive character. The disease in Poll Herefords results in the same short curly coat, but there is also a deficiency of hair in the switch and over the poll, brisket, neck, and legs in some cattle. Some have a much lighter hair-coat color. Histologically, there is a characteristic accumulation of large trichohyalin granules in the hair follicles.

Hypotrichosis and Coat-Color Dilution—"Rat-Tail Syndrome" in Calves

The abnormality is characterized by short, curly, malformed, sometimes sparse hair and lack of normal tail-switch development. Coat-color dilution and hypotrichosis occur when red animals, particularly of the Simmental breed and carrying the mutation responsible, are crossed with black or black-pied cattle.[1] Inherited as a dominant trait, 50% of progeny of such matings have black diluted to a charcoal- or chocolate-colored coat and variable degrees of hypotrichosis. This condition also occurs in offspring of Hereford–Friesian crosses and is evident as dilution of the dark coat color and hypotrichosis affecting particularly the tail switch when the hair of the tail is colored (hence "rat tail"). White hair is not affected.

The abnormality is in the premelanosome protein 17 gene (PMel17), and affected animals are heterozygous. Cattle that express the syndrome must have at least one dominant gene for black color and be heterozygous at the other locus.

A study of the inheritance of the abnormality found that all rat-tail calves were sired by Simmental bulls and were from cows with various percentages of Angus breeding. The abnormality had no effect on birth weight, weaning weight, or gain from birth to weaning. However, rat-tail calves had significantly lower rates of gain during the winter months from weaning to yearling than non-rat-tail calves. Histologically, there are enlarged, irregularly distributed, and clumped melanin granules in the hair shafts, which are asymmetric, short, curled, and small. The scale surface is rough and pitted, and scale fails to form in some areas.

REFERENCE

1. Jolly RD, et al. *New Zeal Vet J.* 2008;56:74.

INHERITED HAIR-COAT-COLOR-LINKED FOLLICLE DYSPLASIA

Some **"buckskin"-colored follicular dysplasia** occurs in so-called "Portuguese" Holstein cattle, a grade variant of Red Holsteins with a tan color instead of the red. This defect consists of a coat-color-linked hair follicle dysplasia, in which the colored hairs are shorter and less lustrous than the white hair, making the coat much finer and smoother. Test matings seem to confirm an autosomal-dominant inheritance.

A **black-hair-colored follicular dysplasia** is also recorded in Holstein cattle. Patches of hair loss varying from hypotrichosis to complete alopecia occur in a random fashion but only on black areas. Follicular dysplasia is evident in biopsy samples. The abnormality persists for the life of the animal and is of cosmetic importance only. An inherited etiology is assumed.

A follicular dysplasia in a mature Brangus-cross cow and a mature Angus cow has been described. Adult-onset alopecia occurred, and skin biopsy revealed follicular distortion and atrophy, with melanin clumping in follicular epithelium, hair bulb matrix cells, hair shafts, and infundibular keratin.

INHERITED BIRTHCOAT RETENTION

Inherited birthcoat retention is recorded in Merino and Welsh mountain sheep and characterized by a coat of hairy medullated fibers in contrast with the nonmedullated wool fibers of the normal sheep fleece.

INHERITED LEUKODERMA

The **Arab fading syndrome** commences in young horses, in particular families of Arab horses, as round, unpigmented patches of skin around the lips, eyes, perineum, and preputial orifice. Some cases recover spontaneously, but the blemish is usually permanent.

INHERITED EPIDERMAL DYSPLASIA (BALDY CALVES)

This is a lethal defect of Holstein–Friesian calves inherited as an autosomal-recessive character. The calves, most commonly heifers, are normal at birth but at 1 to 2 months of age begin to lose condition in spite of good appetites. The skin over most of the body is slightly thickened, scaly, and relatively hairless. There are also patches of scaly, thickened, and folded skin, especially over the neck and shoulders, and hairless, scaly, and often raw areas in the axillae and flanks and over the knees, hocks, and elbow joints. The skin over the joints is immovable. There is usually alopecia around the base of the ears and eyes. The tips of the ears are curled backward. The horns fail to develop, and there is persistent slobbering, although there are no mouth lesions. The hooves are long, narrow, and pointed because of gross overgrowth of the walls; these and stiffness of joints cause a shuffling, restricted gait. Calves assume a recumbent posture most of the time. Severe emaciation leads to destruction at about 6 months of age.

Histologic changes in the skin include acanthosis, hyperkeratosis, and patchy neutrophil invasion. The similarity of this condition to inherited parakeratosis and to experimental zinc deficiency suggests an error in zinc metabolism, but treatment with zinc had no effect on the course of the disease.

INHERITED PARAKERATOSIS OF CALVES (LETHAL TRAIT A46, ADEMA DISEASE)

See "Inherited deficiency of lymphocyte maturation in Chapter 11."

INHERITED DYSERYTHROPOIESIS–DYSKERATOSIS

See "Inherited Blood Diseases."

INHERITED CONGENITAL ABSENCE OF THE SKIN

Epitheliogenesis Imperfecta (Aplasia Cutis)

Absence of mucous membrane or, more commonly, absence of skin over an area of the body surface has been recorded at birth in pigs, calves, lambs, and foals. There is complete absence of all layers of the skin in patches of varying size and distribution. In **cattle** the defect is usually on the lower parts of the limbs and sometimes on the muzzle and extending onto the buccal mucosa. The disease is best known in Holstein–Friesians, but is also recorded in Japanese Black, Shorthorn, Sahiwal, and Angus cattle. In **pigs** the skinless areas are seen on the flanks, sides, back, and other parts of the body, and these areas develop into ulcers and are often secondarily infected, necessitating casualty slaughter.[1] The defect is usually incompatible with life, and most affected animals die within a few days. Inheritance of the defect in cattle is conditioned by a single autosomal-recessive gene, and pigs are thought to have the same genetic cause. Tissue-cultured fibroblasts from affected animals produce subnormal amounts of collagen and lipids.

REFERENCE

1. Benoit-Biancamano MO, et al. *J Vet Diagn Invest.* 2006;18:573.

Familial Acantholysis

Suspected of being an inherited disease, familial acantholysis in Angus calves is characterized by defective collagen bridges in the basal and prickle layers of the epidermis so that skin, normal at birth, is subsequently shed at the carpal and metacarpophalangeal joints and coronet, and there is separation of the horn at the coronet.

Epidermolysis Bullosa

Epidermolysis bullosa is a congenital disease of Suffolk and South Dorset Down sheep and Simmental and Brangus calves and is characterized by the formation of epidermal bullae in the mouth and on exposed areas of skin, such as the extremities of the limbs, muzzle, and ears, leading to shedding of the covering surface and separation of the horn from the coronet. Lesions may be present at birth. Simmental calves grow poorly, have hypotrichosis, and suffer repeated breaks in the skin, apparently as a result of an abnormal susceptibility to trauma. Most calves die, but some survive and the lesions subside. In Simmentals the disease is inherited as an autosomal-dominant trait. The disease in Brangus calves is very similar to familial acantholysis in Angus cattle.

The severe form of Herlitz junctional epidermolysis bullosa, which occurs in humans, has been recorded in foals of the French draft horse breeds. A mutation in the *LAMC2* gene is responsible for the defect. Affected foals were born with skin blistering and skin and buccal ulceration, followed by loss of hooves. In the affected skin, there was disjunction of the epidermis from the underlying dermis at the dermal–epidermal junction. Genomic DNA testing is used to determine the presence of the mutation in carrier animals.

Junctional Epidermolysis Bullosa (Hereditary Junctional Mechanobullous Disease)

Junctional epidermolysis bullosa (JEB) is inherited in Belgian foals; Danish Hereford, Belgian Blue, Charolais, Angus, and Simmental calves; and Suffolk, Churra, and South Dorset Down lambs.[1-4] The disease is inherited in an autosomal-recessive pattern.

JEB in horses is an autosomal-recessive trait affecting Belgians, other draft breeds, and American Saddlebred horses.[5,6] The heterozygous haplotype is common in draft breeds, with 17% of Belgian horses being carriers in North America and 8% to 27% of horses of the Breton, Comtois, Vlaams Paard, and Belgische Koudbloed Flander draft horse breeds being carriers in Europe.

The genetic defect responsible for JEB in the Belgian and European draft breeds is a cytosine insertion (1368insC) creating a premature stop codon in the *Lamc2* gene, which encodes the laminin γ2 subunit chain. The truncated laminin γ2 subunit chains lacks the C-terminal domain so it cannot interact with the other two subunits, thereby preventing the formation of laminin 5. The defect in Belgian Blue cattle is in the *LAMA3* gene, which encodes the alpha 3 subunit of the heterotrimeric laminin-332.[4] Laminin is widely distributed in the basement membrane of epithelial tissues, and lack of this family of proteins results in loss of cell adhesion between the dermis and epidermis.[4] The disease in Charolais calves is a result of a mutation in the integrin beta 4 gene (as for the disease in humans) and loss of function of this protein.[2] The disease in Hereford cattle is a result of a mutation in the *LAMC2* gene, encoding for laminin gamma 2 protein, which results in loss of function of the gene and lack of laminin gamma 2 protein.[3]

Foals are typically born alive, but irregular, reddened erosions and ulcerations develop in the skin and mouth over pressure points or after mild trauma. There are often extensive erosions along the coronary bands, with sloughing of hooves, and at mucocutaneous junctions of the mouth, rectum, and vulva. Dystrophic teeth that are visible at birth are white with irregular serrated edges and pitted enamel. Definitive diagnosis in draft horses requires DNA testing for JEB.

There is no treatment for affected foals, lambs, or calves, and they will eventually succumb to secondary infections or complete sloughing of the hooves.

Red Foot Disease of Sheep

Red foot disease of sheep is similar to junctional epidermolysis bullosa and occurs in Scottish Blackface and Welsh mountain sheep. The lesions are not present at birth but become apparent at 2 to 4 days of age when there is sloughing of skin of the limbs, the accessory digits, the ear pinna, and the epidermal layers of the cornea and buccal mucosa, especially the dorsum of the tongue. There is also an absence of head horn and a separation of hoof horn from the coronet. Pieces of horn become completely detached, exposing the red corium below, hence the term "red foot." The cutaneous and mucosal lesions often commence as blood-filled or fluid-filled blisters. The corneal lesions are similarly the result of sloughing of epidermal layers. Although the cause is unknown, there are indications that it is inherited.

FURTHER READING

Jolly RD, Blair HT, Johnstone AC. Genetic disorders of sheep in New Zealand: a review and perspective. *New Zeal Vet J.* 2004;52:52-64.

REFERENCES

1. Benavides J, et al. *Vet Dermatol.* 2015;26:367.
2. Michot P, et al. *Genet Select Evol.* 2015;47.
3. Murgiano L, et al. *BMC Vet Res.* 2015;11:334.
4. Sartelet A, et al. *Anim Gen.* 2015;46:566.
5. Finno CJ, et al. *Vet J.* 2009;179:336.
6. Cappelli K, et al. *BMC Vet Res.* 2015;11:374.

INHERITED HYPERBILIRUBINEMIA AND PHOTOSENSITIZATION

An inherited photosensitization with hyperbilirubinemia has been observed in Southdown sheep in New Zealand and the United States, and in Corriedales in California. It is inherited as an autosomal-recessive trait.

Liver insufficiency is present, but the liver is histologically normal. Phylloerythrin and bilirubin excretion by the liver is impeded, and the accumulation of phylloerythrin in the bloodstream causes the photosensitization. There is also a significant deficiency in renal function. Symptomatic treatment of photosensitization and confining the animals indoors may enable the lambs to fatten to market weight. The persistent hyperbilirubinemia is accompanied by an inability of the kidneys of these sheep to concentrate urine and the eventual death of the sheep from renal insufficiency.

Affected sheep live for several years if they are protected from sunlight and tend to die of renal failure associated with progressive fibrosis of the kidney.

A similar disease in Corriedale sheep in California is inherited as an autosomal-recessive trait. The functional defect is not in the uptake of unconjugated bilirubin and phylloerythrin, but rather its excretion from liver into bile. It affects lambs as they begin to eat pasture. Lambs live until 6 months of age if provided with some shade. There is also marked melanin-like pigmentation of the liver.

These two diseases are examples of the involvement of external environmental disease factors with a genetic disease: a diet of green forage (chlorophyll) and sunlight working in concert with the inborn error of metabolism to induce photosensitization.

INHERITED CONGENITAL ICHTHYOSIS (FISH-SCALE DISEASES)

Congenital ichthyosis is a disease characterized by alopecia and the presence of plates of horny epidermis covering the entire skin surface. It has been recorded only in Holstein and Norwegian Red Poll and probably in Brown Swiss calves among the domestic animals, although it occurs also in humans.

The newborn calf appears to be either partly or completely hairless, and the skin is covered with thick, horny scales separated by fissures that follow the wrinkle lines of the skin. These may penetrate deeply and become ulcerated. There are plenty of normal hair follicles and normal hairs, but these are lost in the areas covered by the growth of scales. A skin biopsy section will show a thick, tightly adherent layer of keratinized cells. The disease is incurable, and although it may be compatible with life, most affected animals are disposed of for esthetic reasons. The defect has been shown to be hereditary and to result from the influence of a single recessive gene.

INHERITED DERMATOSIS VEGETANS OF PIGS

Inherited dermatosis vegetans of pigs appears to be conditioned by the inheritance of a recessive, semilethal factor. Affected pigs may show defects at birth but in most instances lesions appear after birth and up to 3weeks of age. The lesions occur at the coronets and on the skin. Those on the coronets consist of erythema and edema with a thickened, brittle, uneven hoof wall. Lesions on the belly and inner surface of the thigh commence as areas of erythema and become wart-like and covered with gray-brown crusts.

Many affected pigs die, but some appear to recover completely. Many of the deaths appear to be a result of the giant-cell pneumonitis that is an essential part of the disease. The pathology of the disease indicates that it is the result of a genetic defect that selectively affects mesodermal tissue. It is known to have originated in the Danish Landrace breed.

DERMATOSPARAXIS (HYPERELASTOSIS CUTIS)

Dermatosparaxis is an extraordinary fragility of skin and connective tissue in general, with or without edema. It is probably inherited as a recessive character. It occurs in cattle, in horses (see "Hereditary Equine Regional Dermal Asthenia"), in Finnish and White Dorper sheep, and in a mild form in Merino sheep. The latter is inherited as a simple autosomal-recessive trait. The skin is hyperelastic, as are the articular ligaments; marked cutaneous fragility, delayed healing of skin wounds, and the development of papyraceous scars are also characteristic. Pieces of skin may be ripped off when affected sheep are being handled. In horses the skin in some parts of the body is thinner than elsewhere (e.g., the skin of the ventral abdomen) and the collagen bundles in the area are more loosely packed and are curved rather than straight. The proportion of acid-soluble collagen is also much higher in this abnormal skin. The disease involves a molecular defect of a collagen-binding protein and is related to a recognized problem in dogs and cats identified as "dominant collagen packing defect."

Hereditary equine regional dermal asthenia is discussed under that heading in the following section.[1] Ehlers–Danlos syndrome, recorded in Charolais and Simmental cattle, Quarter horses (cyclophilin-B gene independent),[2] Warmblood foals (cyclophilin-B gene independent),[3,4] and Rippolesa sheep, is also characterized by extreme fragility of the skin and laxness of joints in the newborn. There is a defect in collagen synthesis, and histopathological findings include fragmentation and disorganization of collagen fibers. The disease in Warmblood foals is well recognized and is caused by a defect in the equine procollagen-lysine, 2-oxoglutarate 5-dioxygenase 1 (PLOD1, or lysyl hydroxylase 1) gene.[5] Affected foals born at term have thin and friable skin, skin lesions on the legs and the head, and an open abdomen.[5] Histologic examination reveals abnormally thin dermis and markedly reduced amounts of dermal collagen bundles, with loose orientation and abnormally large spaces between deep dermal fibers. A genetic test is available and should be considered for Warmblood mares that abort, have stillborn foals, or have foals with characteristic lesions.[5] A case of dermal asthenia reported in a Warmblood in Australia was in a 6-week-old foal. Confirmatory genetic testing was not undertaken.[3]

The syndrome has also been recorded in lambs. The skin was loose and present in excessive amounts, with folds over the carpal joints and lower regions of the legs. In some lambs, there may be separation of the epidermis from the dermis with blood-filled cavitations and intact skin that can be easily torn.

REFERENCES

1. Rashmir-Raven AM, et al. *Equine Vet Educ.* 2015;27:604.
2. Steelman SM, et al. *J Equine Vet Sci.* 2014;34:565.
3. Marshall VL, et al. *Aust Vet J.* 2011;89:77.
4. Ruefenacht S, et al. *Schweiz Arch Tierheilkd.* 2010;152:188.
5. Monthoux C, et al. *BMC Vet Res.* 2015;11.

INHERITED MELANOMA

Inherited cutaneous malignant melanoma is found in National Institute for Health (NIH miniature) and Sinclair miniature swine. Its expression is associated with two genetic loci, one of which is associated with the swine major histocompatibility complex. Familial melanomas have also been recorded in members of successive litters from an individual Duroc × Slovak White sow.

INHERITED HYPERHIDROSIS

Inherited hyperhidrosis, a condition characterized by excessive sweating and thought to be inherited, is recorded in beef Shorthorn calves. The syndrome includes conjunctivitis, with some cases progressing to complete opacity of the cornea, heavy dandruff, and persistent wetness of the hair coat.

LAVENDER FOAL SYNDROME

Lavender foal syndrome is a congenital, inherited, autosomal-recessive disease of Egyptian Arab foals characterized by an unusual dilute coat color and signs of neurologic disease evident at birth. Additional details provided in Chapter 14 ("Diseases of the Nervous System").

HEREDITARY EQUINE REGIONAL DERMAL ASTHENIA (HYPERELASTOSIS CUTIS)

Hereditary equine regional dermal asthenia (HERDA) is a degenerative skin disease caused by an autosomal-recessive trait of Quarter horses and related breeds attributable to a mutation in *Equus caballus* chromosome 1 (ECA1).[1] The abnormality is a c.115G>A mutation in the peptidyl-propyl isomerase cis-trans B (PPIB) gene.[2] Resultant abnormalities in cyclophilin B cause a two- to threefold reduction in the tensile strength and elastic modulus of skin of affected horses.[3,4] The allele frequency in 651 elite performance American Quarter horses, 200 control (nonelite) American Quarter horses, and 180 control American Paint horses was 0.021, with cutting horses having a frequency of 0.142 and 28% of cutting horses being carriers.[5] The frequency of carriers is estimated to be 3.5% of Quarter horses in the United States and 1.6% in France.[1,6] Allele frequency is estimated at 2.9%, and carrier frequency at 5.8%, in American Quarter horses in Brazil.[2] A similar inherited disease of Warmbloods is reported, although the genetic basis has not been determined.[7,8] The disease can occur in Quarter horses without the PPIB mutation.[9]

Clinical signs typically appear at 1 to 2 years of age, at about the time of breaking for riding, and are evident as open wounds, sloughing of skin, hematomas, and seromas. Clinical signs can develop in foals. The skin of affected animals is "stretchy" and remains deformed for considerable periods of time when stretched. The lesions are most severe over the dorsum, although the mechanical abnormalities are present at all sites.[4] Horses with HERDA have a greater incidence of corneal ulcers than do unaffected horses.[10] The cornea of horses with HERDA is thinner than that of normal horses.[10]

Diagnosis is based on clinical signs, histologic examination of skin, and genetic testing. Histologic examination of skin of animals before the development of clinical signs is not conclusive in detecting the disease, although affected horses have thinner skin, on histologic examination, than do unaffected horses.[11,12] Measurement of skin thickness has sensitivity of 73% to 88% and specificity of 35% to 75%.[12] Skin thickness is not regionally distributed in affected horses. The genetic test is definitive.

There is no definitive treatment. Affected mares can carry foals to term and deliver safely.[11] Control involves the selective breeding of unaffected animals and those not carrying the disease, bearing in mind that it is an autosomal-recessive disease. However, the high prevalence of the disease in some uses of horses (cutting horses) suggests selection for the trait, perhaps because it is closely associated with a desired phenotype.

REFERENCES

1. Tryon RC, et al. *Genomics.* 2007;90:93.
2. Badial PR, et al. *Vet J.* 2014;199:306.
3. Bowser JE, et al. *Equine Vet J.* 2014;46:216.
4. Grady JG, et al. *Vet Dermatol.* 2009;20:591.
5. Tryon RC, et al. *J Am Vet Med Assoc.* 2009;234:120.
6. White SD, et al. *Vet Dermatol.* 2011;22:206.
7. Ruefenacht S, et al. *Schweiz Arch Tierheilkd.* 2010;152:188.
8. Marshall VL, et al. *Aust Vet J.* 2011;89:77.
9. Steelman SM, et al. *J Equine Vet Sci.* 2014;34:565.
10. Mochal CA, et al. *J Am Vet Med Assoc.* 2010;237:304.
11. White SD, et al. *Vet Dermatol.* 2007;18:36.
12. Badial PR, et al. *Vet Dermatol.* 2014;25:547.

DERMATOSIS VEGETANS

Dermatosis vegetans is a rare condition of pigs first described in 1967 and originating in the Swedish Landrace import to the United Kingdom. It is governed by a semilethal factor with autosomal-recessive inheritance. Often only two to three pigs per litter are affected. Pigs will often first show a decline in growth and then die after 7 to 8 weeks, but some occasionally recover. It is seen as three clinical conditions:

- There is an erythematous maculopapular dermatitis often present at birth or around 2 to 3 weeks of age. Lesions are found on the abdomen or inside of the thighs and may spread and pass through a Pityriasis-like phase. After 5 to 8 weeks the lesions become thickened and covered with crusts.
- The second group of lesions, usually present at birth, occur in the form of "clubfeet," with swelling and erythema and defective horn on the walls, sole, and bulb of the foot.

- The third major clinical condition is respiratory dysfunction, which is caused by a giant-cell pneumonitis. It is characteristic of the condition in pigs older than 1 week of age. There are granules present throughout the lung, and these heal by fibrosis. The differential diagnoses include pityriasis rosea, chronic exudative dermatitis, and vitamin deficiencies.

There is no treatment, and control is through culling of breeding stock that have been affected.

FURTHER READING

Done JT, et al. Dermatosis vegetans in the pig. *Vet Rec.* 1967;80:292.

PUSTULAR PSORIAFORM DERMATITIS (PITYRIASIS ROSEA)

The condition of pityriasis rosea in humans is not like the condition in pigs; thus, pustular psoriaform dermatitis (PPD) is a much better term for what is in fact a ring or rings of keratinized cells that are erythematous initially and raised surrounding a central crater. The condition occurs in young pigs, 3 to 14 weeks of age, is self-limiting, and is usually gone by 4 to 6 weeks following appearance.

The etiology is thought to be an autosomal-dominant gene with incomplete penetrance. It is definitely familial and may be more common in Landrace.

Clinically, there is a superficial accumulation of scales in a dry, lusterless coat.

Pityriasis scales are accumulations of keratinized epithelial cells, sometimes softened and made greasy by the exudation of serum or sebum. Overproduction, when it occurs, begins around the orifices of the hair follicles and spreads to the surrounding stratum corneum. The lesions are not itchy.

Diagnosis is based on age, clinical appearance, lack of itching and failure to demonstrate mites or ringworm on skin scrapings. Skin biopsy also helps in that there is an epidermal hyperplasia and superficial perivascular dermatitis.

Pityriasis is identified by the absence of parasites and fungi on skin scrapings.

DIFFERENTIAL DIAGNOSIS

Differential diagnosis of excessive bran-like scales on the skin, characterized by overproduction of keratinized epithelial cells, can be caused by deficiency of B vitamins, especially riboflavin and nicotinic acid, or linoleic acid and possibly other essential fatty acids, and poisoning by iodine. It can also be secondary to flea, louse, and mange infestations and ringworm infections. Also, hyperkeratosis and parakeratosis conditions should be considered.

TREATMENT

Treatment does not appear to have any effect, and self-cure is the norm. If there is secondary infection under conditions of bad hygiene, supportive therapy may help. Culling of the breeding stock producing the affected stock is advisable.

Eye and Conjunctival Diseases

CONJUNCTIVITIS AND KERATOCONJUNCTIVITIS

Conjunctivitis refers to inflammation of the covering membrane of the eye, including the orbit and the inner surface of the eyelids. The inflammation commonly extends to layers below the conjunctiva, referred to as keratoconjunctivitis.

ETIOLOGY

Causes of inflammation of the conjunctiva can be various and include bacterial, viral, parasitic, or mycotic infections; allergic and immune reactions; conjunctival foreign bodies; and trauma.

Specific Conjunctivitis

Cattle

- **Infectious bovine keratoconjunctivitis (IBK, pinkeye)** a common and highly contagious form of keratoconjunctivitis that is associated with *Moraxella bovis* (see also "Infectious Bovine Keratoconjunctivitis")
- **Listerial keratoconjunctivitis and uveitis (silage eye)** is associated with *Listeria monocytogenes*[1] (see also "Listerial Keratoconjunctivitis")
- **Ulcerative blepharitis and conjunctivitis** associated with *Moraxella bovoculi* in cattle[2,3]

Sheep and Goats

- **Infectious keratoconjunctivitis (pinkeye) of sheep and goats** associated with *Mycoplasma conjunctivae* and *Chlamydia psittaci.*

Pigs

- Chlamydial-associated conjunctivitis in pigs associated with *Chlamydia spp*[4]

Horses

- Eosinophilic keratoconjunctivitis of unknown etiology[5]
- Conjunctival habronemiasis caused by larval invasion of *Habronema spp.*
- Ocular onchocerciasis associated with microfilaria of *Omcocerca* spp. The causative association between these microfilaria and equine ocular disease is under debate.
- Fungal keratomycosis in foals and adult horses; *Aspergillus flavus* has been identified in some cases.

A. fumigatus is listed among the causes of mycotic keratitis in animals. Most cases begin as traumatic injuries with secondary infections or begin in eyes treated for long periods with broad-spectrum antibiotics.

Secondary Diseases in Which Conjunctivitis Is a Significant but Secondary Part of the Syndrome

Cattle

- Bovine viral diarrhea
- Malignant catarrhal fever
- Rinderpest
- Infectious bovine rhinotracheitis
- Viral pneumonia as a result of various viruses
- Bluetongue (specifically BTV-8)
- Besnoitiosis

Sheep

- Bluetongue

Pigs

- Swine influenza
- Inclusion-body rhinitis

Horses

- Equine viral arteritis
- Equine viral rhinopneumonitis

Nonspecific Conjunctivitis

Nonspecific conjunctivitis refers to inflammation caused by foreign bodies or chemicals, or secondarily as exposure keratitis, and conjunctivitis/keratitis in paralysis of eyelids as in listeriosis. Ant-bite conjunctivitis occurs in similar circumstances.

CLINICAL FINDINGS

Blepharospasm and weeping from the affected eye are the initial signs. Watery tears are followed by mucopurulent, then purulent ocular discharge if the lesion extends below the conjunctiva. Varying degrees of opacity of the conjunctiva may develop, depending on the severity of the inflammation. In the severest lesions there is underrunning of the conjunctiva with pus accompanied by vascularization of the cornea. During the recovery stage there is often long-lasting, diffuse opacity of the eye and terminally a chronic white scar in some cases.

CLINICAL PATHOLOGY

In herd or flock outbreaks, conjunctival swabs and/or scrapings should be taken for culture and examination of cells using special stains and histologic techniques.

REFERENCES

1. Erdogan HM. *Vet Clin North Am Food A.* 2010;26:505-510.
2. Angelos JA, et al. *Int J Syst Evol Microbiol.* 2007;57:789-795.
3. Galvao KN, Angelos JA. *Can Vet J.* 2010;51:400-402.

4. Becker A, et al. *J Vet Med A Physiol Pathol Clin Med.* 2007;54:307-313.
5. Wolfe JE, et al. *Equine Vet J.* 2010;22:375-381.

LISTERIAL KERATOCONJUNCTIVITIS AND UVEITIS (SILAGE EYE, BOVINE IRITIS)

SYNOPSIS

Etiology *Listeria monocytogenes* is the causative pathogen, presumably reaching the eye with contaminated feed particles. The condition is the result of a local listerial infection specifically affecting the eye and is not associated with systemic infection with *L. monocytogenes.* Cattle, sheep, and horses are affected.

Epidemiology Cattle fed poor-quality silage from round bales or ring feeders are at risk of developing the condition; allowing feed to fall on the cows' heads increases risk. In most cases individual animals are affected, but outbreaks have occurred. Incidence is highest in winter and early spring when animals are housed inside and fed silage.

Clinical findings Epiphora, conjunctivitis, blepharospasm, photophobia, corneal edema, uveitis. The condition is usually not associated with systemic disease.

Diagnostic confirmation Culture, polymerase chain reaction (PCR).

Treatment Self-limiting disease. Topical and systemic antibiotics.

Control Avoid feeding poor-quality silage, avoid feeding systems providing feed at or above the height of the animals' eyes.

ETIOLOGY

Listeria monocytogenes is the only causative agent associated with listerial conjunctivitis, which is a condition specifically affecting the eye.[1] It is unrelated to systemic infection with *L. monocytogenes* causing the classic forms of listeriosis (see also "Listeriosis"). Local uveitis associated with *L. monocytogenes* has been reported to occur in cattle, sheep, horses, fallow deer, and humans.[2]

Listeria is a ubiquitously occurring gram-positive, asporogenic bacterium easily surviving in organic material at temperatures between 3° and 45°C (37° to 113°F) and at pH as low as 3.8 in an aerobic environment. Silage of poor quality that is either not conserved anaerobically or not sufficiently acidic facilitates growth of *Listeria.* Listerial conjunctivitis is almost invariably associated with feeding poor-quality silage either directly as big bale or from ring feeders. With these feeding systems animals tend to burrow their heads into the bales, which not only exposes the eyes to the pathogen but also has the potential to mechanically damage the conjunctiva, thereby creating a portal of entry.[1]

EPIDEMIOLOGY

Occurrence

The disease has been reported to occur in different parts of the world, although most cases are recorded in the United Kingdom, probably because of greater awareness of the existence of this condition. The disease incidence is highest in **late fall, winter, and early spring** when animals are kept inside and fed silage. Frequently only individual cases occur, but outbreaks with morbidity rates far above 25% have been reported.[1,2] In the United Kingdom an overall animal incidence of 3.4% and an average incidence in affected herds of 66.5% was reported.[1]

Source of Infection

Because most cases of listerial keratoconjunctivitis have been linked to silage feeding, grass silage of poor quality contaminated with *L. monocytogens* is widely accepted as the primary source of infection.

Environmental Risk Factors

Feeding grass silage form big bales or ring feeders is considered a major predisposing factor. With cows starting to feed on the lower part of the bale, feed particles from the upper part continuously fall onto the head of the feeding animal, thereby increasing the risk of ocular contact with the pathogen.

CLINICAL FINDINGS

Although in most cases only one eye is affected, bilateral lesions can occur. Systemic disease is usually absent. First clinical signs include increased lacrimation and catarrhal conjunctivitis with photophobia and blepharospasm. Inflammation of the cornea, starting at the limbic border and spreading centripetally, results in a bluish-white opacity of the cornea. Corneal ulcers are uncommon.[1] In advanced cases focal aggregation of fibrin accumulating in the anterior eye chamber may become visible as white foci beneath the corneal surface. The course of the disease, which is considered to be self-limiting, is between 1 and 3 weeks when left untreated.[2]

CLINICAL PATHOLOGY

The tentative diagnosis can be made based on the clinical presentation in combination of the history (season and silage feeding) but should be confirmed by identifying *L. monocytogenes* from swab obtained from affected eyes. Cultures or PCR are used to identify the pathogen.

DIFFERENTIAL DIAGNOSIS

Infectious bovine keratoconjunctivitis (IBK) has a different seasonality (peaks occurring in the warm season of the year). Evaluation of housing and feeding system may provide further clues to differentiate between these conditions. Corneal ulceration is a common finding with IBK but not with listerial conjunctivitis.

Pasteurella multocida **(capsular type A)** has been isolated from the eyes of housed heifers that experienced outbreaks of severe keratitis with severe loss of corneal stroma within 72 hours of onset.

Mycoplasma bovis has been isolated from the eyes of steers with an outbreak of severe conjunctivitis with corneal opacity and ulceration, with disease being followed by serologic conversion in affected animals. Involvement of the eyelids with marked swelling was prominent. Conjunctivitis is prominent in other mycoplasmal infections that produce keratoconjunctivitis.

Chlamydial keratoconjunctivitis presents with identical clinical findings but has a protracted course despite treatment and a higher morbidity. *Chlamydophila* DNA can be detected by polymerase chain reaction (PCR) in conjunctival swabs. This disease is a possible zoonosis.

Infectious bovine rhinotracheitis

Bovine malignant catarrhal fever

Bovine viral diarrhea

Bluetongue (BTV-8)

Thelaziasis

Squamous-cell carcinoma

TREATMENT

A number of empirical treatment approaches have been reported, with variable outcome. Listerial keratoconjunctivitis is considered to be a self-limiting disease, and it is difficult to determine whether reported treatments were effective or if recovery was primarily a result of removing access to the primary cause.[3]

Proposed treatments include the topical use of eye ointments containing oxytetracycline or cloxacillin as well as the parenteral administration of repeated doses of oxytetracycline, procaine-penicillin, or ampicillin. The use of topical or subconjunctival dexamethasone application has been proposed, with variable outcome.[1-3]

TREATMENT

Topical treatment:

Benzathine cloxacillin eye ointment (250 mg q48) (R-2)

Oxytetracycline eye ointment (q24h) (R-2)

Systemic treatment:

Procaine-penicillin-G (40,000 IU/kg q24 IM) (R-3)

Oxytetracycline (10 mg/kg q24h IM) (R-3)

Ampicillin (10 mg/kg q24 SC) (R-3)

CONTROL

The most important control measures are to avoid feeding poor-quality silage and to use feeding systems that provide feed at a height that is below the animals' heads.

REFERENCES

1. Laven RA, Lawrence KR. *New Zeal Vet J.* 2006;54:151-152.
2. Staric J, et al. *Bull Vet Inst Pulawy.* 2008;52:353-355.
3. Erdogan HM. *Vet Clin North Am Food A.* 2010;26:505-510.

INFECTIOUS BOVINE KERATOCONJUNCTIVITIS OF CATTLE (PINKEYE, BLIGHT)

SYNOPSIS

Etiology *Moraxella bovis* is the primary infectious agent. Pili and hemolysin are the main virulence factors. Solar radiation, flies, and dust are contributing factors.

Epidemiology Cattle of all ages are susceptible. Source is asymptomatic carrier cattle, with transmission by mediate contagion and by flies. More common in summer months. Usually multiple cases in a herd.

Clinical findings Conjunctivitis, lacrimation, blepharospasm, photophobia, corneal edema, corneal ulceration.

Diagnostic confirmation Culture.

Treatment Self-limiting disease. Topical antibiotics, subconjunctival penicillin G, parenteral oxytetracyclines, florfenicol, tulathromycin. Protection of eye from sunlight.

Control Current vaccines have limited efficacy. Fly control.

ETIOLOGY

Hemolytic *Moraxella bovis* is the only infectious agent for which Koch's postulates have been established for infectious bovine keratoconjunctivitis (IBK), although other organisms, such as *Moraxella ovis, Moraxella bovoculi, Neisseria* spp., *Mycoplasma* spp., and *Chlamydia* spp. have been implicated.[1] Experimental infections in calves and studies on corneal tissue culture show a great variation in virulence between strains. Two virulence factors are determinants of cause in clinical disease. These are the **presence of fimbriae, so-called pili,** on the bacterial surface and the **production of β-hemolysin**. Other contributing virulence factors include phospholipases, iron acquisition systems, and hydrolytic and proteolytic enzymes.[1] *M. bovis* has serologically distinct shared and variable pilus epitopes, and strains can be distinguished by their pilus antigens into seven distinct **serogroups**. There are two distinct types of **pilus**, I and Q (formerly α and β). **Q pili mediate bacterial adhesion** to the cornea and the establishment of infection by preventing removal of the pathogen by the continual flushing effect of ocular secretions and the mechanical action of blinking. Beta-hemolysin is **cytotoxic** and produces corneal damage. In some outbreaks of pinkeye more than one serotype can be isolated from affected eyes.

In addition to *M. bovis*, other pathogens, such as *M. bovoculi, M. ovis, Chlamydia* spp., *Neisseria* spp., *Mycoplasma* spp., *Acholeplasma* spp., and viruses have been identified as common participants and are likely to contribute to the development of clinical disease. Infectious bovine rhinotracheitis virus causes ocular disease in its own right, but it may also be involved with *M. bovis* in causing the more severe disease. Clinical disease in experimentally induced IBK has been shown to be more severe when the calves are concurrently given a modified live infectious bovine rhinotracheitis virus vaccine.

Conjunctival infection with *M. bovoculi* has been proposed to play a role in the pathophysiology of IBK by some authors.[2-3] The evidence in support of this assumption is inconsistent. A clinical study consistently demonstrated the development of corneal ulcers after inoculation with hemolytic *M. bovis* but not with *M. bovoculi.*[3] *Branhamella ovis* causes a severe conjunctivitis in sheep and goats and is also recorded from outbreaks of keratoconjunctivitis in cattle in Israel; it may be a cause of vaccine breakdown in other countries.

Because the naturally occurring disease is usually much more severe than that produced experimentally, factors other than infectious agents have been examined. **Solar radiation**, **flies**, and **dust** have been shown to have an enhancing effect. Cultural characteristics of the organisms isolated from the conjunctiva can change with the level of solar ultraviolet radiation.

EPIDEMIOLOGY

Occurrence

The disease occurs in most countries of the world. Although it can occur in all seasons, it is most common in **summer and autumn**. The prevalence and severity of the disease vary greatly from year to year, and it may reach epizootic proportions in feedlots and in cattle running at pasture. There is no mortality, and cases in which there is permanent blindness or loss of an eye are rare. However, the morbidity rate can be as high as 80%, with the peak infection rate at weeks 3 to 4 of the outbreak. Severe outbreaks can be experienced in winter, especially if the cattle are confined in close quarters, such as barns or intensive feedlots.

Source of Infection

Cattle are the only known reservoir, and the organism is carried on the conjunctiva and also in the nares and vagina of cattle. Persistence of the disease from year to year is by means of infected but asymptomatic animals, which can act as carriers for periods exceeding 1 year. Receptors for I-pili may be found on tissues other than the cornea and facilitate colonization of noncorneal tissue and inapparent infection, and the organism can switch from expression of one pilus type to the other.

Environmental Risk Factors

The disease incidence shows a **clear seasonality,** with the highest incidence in the warmer months of the year. This seasonal expression has been associated with prolonged exposure of the eye to **UV radiation**, the increased **fly population,** and **long grass.**[1] The exposure of the eye to UV radiation increases the susceptibility to the disease and the severity of signs resulting from it. The face fly (*Musca autumnalis*) and Asian face fly (*Musca bezzii*), because of feeding preference for the area around the eyes, are important vectors.

Other environmental factors, such as dust, wind, and tall grass, can increase the disease incidence by causing mechanical irritation of the cornea.

Transmission

Transmission is thought to be by means of flies contaminated by the ocular and nasal discharge of infected cattle. Under experimental conditions, transmission is unusual in the absence of flies and occurs generally in their presence. *M. autumnalis* is known to remain infected for periods of up to 3 days. *M. bovis* can be isolated from the crops of *M. autumnalis* that have fed on the eyes of infected cattle.

Animal Risk Factors

Only cattle are affected, the young being most susceptible, but in a susceptible population, cattle of all ages are likely to be affected.

It is commonly observed that there is a much higher prevalence of the disease in *B. taurus* cattle as distinct from *B. indicus* cattle, and the severity and proportion of bilateral infections is much greater in *B. taurus* cattle than in crossbreeds. Hereford and Hereford crossbreed cattle have a significantly higher risk of developing IBK than other breeds or crossbreeds not containing Hereford.[1] This higher predisposition is thought to be based on a relationship between rate and severity of infection and the degree of **eyelid pigmentation**; eyes with complete pigmentation are less affected.

Immune Mechanisms

Previous infection appears to confer a significant immunity that lasts through to the next season, when further reinfection, usually with minimal clinical disease, confers further immunity. Lacrimal secretions contain antibody, and antibody directed against the **pilus antigens** of *M. bovis* will prevent adherence of the organism to the cornea. In experimental infections, significant protection against challenge can be achieved by prior vaccination with pilus antigens of the homologous strain.

However, there is antigenic diversity in pili from different strains of *M. bovis*, and vaccines composed of pili from one strain only confer protection to challenge with organisms of the same serogroup. Further, *M. bovis* in the eye can **switch** their pilus antigenicity in response to antibody presence and render monovalent vaccines ineffective. A polyvalent vaccine might provide protection, but polyvalent vaccines are less immunogenic than monovalent vaccines because of antigenic competition.

Economic Importance

Infectious bovine keratoconjunctivitis is a prominent disease in surveys of the predominant diseases in cattle and is considered the economically most important ocular disease of cattle. Losses result from reduced weight gain or loss of body condition; loss of milk production; costs of drugs, labor, and veterinary care; and loss of value of show animals. The conditions under which calves are reared can affect the importance of the disease. In veal calves, the disease may have no measurable effect on growth, but in calves running at pasture it can result in a significant reduction of weaning weight. Occasionally, animals become completely blind, and those at pasture may die of starvation. Animal welfare presents an increasing concern.

PATHOGENESIS

As mentioned, only piliated and hemolytic strains of *M. bovis* are pathogenic to cattle (determinant virulence factors). Attachment of *M. bovis* to the corneal epithelium requires the presence of pili and Q-piliated organisms that are more infectious than I-piliated strains. Hemolysins produced by these virulent strains are cytotoxic and cause the development of corneal ulcers by destroying corneal epithelial cells.

Microscopic corneal erosions are present within 12 hours of infection and occur at this time in the absence of a significant inflammatory response, indicating that the initial production of the corneal ulceration is a result of the direct cytotoxic activity of the organism. This is followed by focal loss of corneal epithelium, degeneration of keratocytes, and invasion of the corneal stroma with fibrillar destruction. An inflammatory reaction occurs several days postinfection and results in enlargement of the corneal ulcers with deeper stromal involvement, corneal edema, and corneal neovascularization. The lesions are localized in the eye, and there is no systemic infection.

CLINICAL FINDINGS

An incubation period of 2 to 3 days is usual, although longer intervals, up to 3 weeks, have been observed after experimental introduction of the bacteria. Injection of the corneal vessels and edema of the conjunctiva are the early signs and are accompanied by a copious watery lacrimation, blepharospasm, photophobia, and, in some cases, a slight to moderate fever with fall in milk yield and depression of appetite.

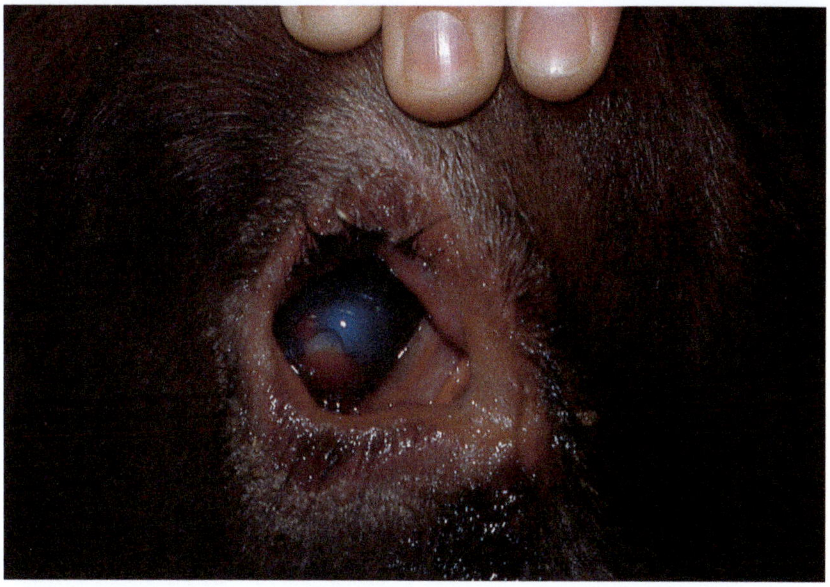

Fig. 16-10 Infectious bovine keratoconjunctivitis (IBK) in a beef steer. Note the extensive lacrimation and blepharospasm and the centrally located corneal ulcer with keratitis and conjunctivitis.

In 1 to 2 days, corneal edema presenting as a small opacity appears in the center of the cornea, and this may become elevated and ulcerated during the next 2 days, although spontaneous recovery at this stage is quite common. With progressive disease the opacity becomes quite extensive, and at the peak of the inflammation, about 6 days after signs first appear, it may cover the entire cornea. The color of the opacity varies from white to deep yellow (Fig. 16-10). As the acute inflammation subsides, the ocular discharge becomes purulent and the opacity begins to shrink, complete recovery occurring after a total course of 3 to 5 weeks.

One or both eyes may be affected. The degree of ulceration in the early stages can be readily determined by the infusion of a 2% fluorescein solution into the conjunctival sac, the ulcerated area retaining the stain.

About 2% of eyes have complete **residual opacity**, but most heal completely with a small, white scar persisting in some. In severe cases the cornea becomes conical in shape, there is marked vascularization of the cornea, and ulceration at the tip of the swelling leads to underrunning of the cornea with bright yellow pus surrounded by a zone of erythema. These eyes may rupture and result in complete blindness.

A proportion of cases will develop minimal clinical lesions and heal spontaneously, and the severity of clinical disease can also vary between outbreaks.

CLINICAL PATHOLOGY

The organism can be identified by culture or fluorescent antibody. The hemolytic form of the bacterium is noticeably more pathogenic than the nonhemolytic form. Serum agglutinins (1:80 to 1:640) are present 2 to 3 weeks after clinical signs commence, and a modified gel diffusion precipitin test is capable of detecting *M. bovis* antibodies. An ELISA test is also used for antibody detection in experimental studies; however, neither agglutinating antibody nor antibody detected by ELISA correlates well with individual animal resistance to infection. There is little indication for serologic examinations in clinical practice. Necropsy examinations are not usually necessary.

DIFFERENTIAL DIAGNOSIS

Traumatic conjunctivitis is usually easily differentiated because of the presence of foreign matter in the eye or the conjunctival sac or evidence of a physical injury.

***Pasteurella multocida* (capsular type A)** has been isolated from the eyes of housed heifers that experienced outbreaks of severe keratitis with severe loss of corneal stroma within 72 hours of onset.

Mycoplasma bovis has been isolated from the eyes of steers with an outbreak of severe conjunctivitis with corneal opacity and ulceration, with disease being followed by serologic conversion in affected animals. Involvement of the eyelids with marked swelling was prominent. Conjunctivitis is prominent in other mycoplasmal infections that produce keratoconjunctivitis.

Continued

Listerial keratoconjunctivitis and uveitis (silage eye) has a different seasonality and is associated with the use of specific feeding systems. Corneal ulcers are uncommon with listerial keratoconjunctivitis.

Chlamydial keratoconjunctivitis presents with identical clinical findings but has a protracted course despite treatment and a higher morbidity. *Chlamydophila* DNA can be detected by polymerase chain reaction (PCR) in conjunctival swabs. This disease is a possible zoonosis.

Infectious bovine rhinotracheitis

Bovine malignant catarrhal fever

Bovine viral diarrhea

Bluetongue (BTV-8)

Thelaziasis

Squamous-cell carcinoma

TREATMENT

Infectious bovine keratoconjunctivitis is frequently a **self-limiting disease**. Recovery commonly occurs without treatment, although early treatment will reduce the incidence of scarring of the eyes. Antibacterial treatment is commonly used, and mass treatment of the herd as opposed to just affected individuals may halt the occurrence of further cases. The route of administration is often determined by efficiency of the available treatment options, ease of access to the animals, availability of facilities to restrain animals for treatment, labor intensity of treatment, cost of the drug, and withhold times.

Topical Therapy

Early, acute cases respond to treatment with ophthalmic ointments and solutions containing antibiotics, but they need to be instilled in the conjunctival sacs at frequent intervals, which may be impractical under field conditions. The organism is **sensitive** to most antibiotics and sulfonamides but is resistant to erythromycin, lincomycin, and tylosin. The administration of an oil-based formulation of benzathine cloxacillin (250 to 375 mg per treatment dose) was found to be effective in therapy in controlled trials. Two doses, 72 hours apart, treating both eyes, even if only one eye is affected, is recommended. The use of the same ointment tube in affected and unaffected eyes is likely to present a risk for transmission of the pathogen.

Subconjunctival Therapy

The objective of subconjunctival treatment is to reduce the treatment dose and number of treatments while achieving higher antimicrobial tissue concentrations.[4] Although subconjunctival therapy with antibiotic was found to be effective in treating IBK in several studies, it is under contentious debate if the treatment effect is obtained through direct diffusion of the drug to the surrounding tissue or rather through continuous leakage of the antibiotic onto the conjunctiva from the injection site.[4] A small volume (1 to 2 mL) of procaine-penicillin G (300,000 IU/mL) is commonly injected under the scleral conjunctiva. Two treatments 48 to 72 hours apart were found to be equally effective as a single parenteral treatment with long-acting formulation of oxytetracycline (20 mg/kg).[4] Therapy must be administered under the bulbar conjunctiva but was found to be ineffective if given in the superior palpebral conjunctiva. A controlled trial found that subconjunctival penicillin was effective in treatment, but recurrence was higher than with treatment with parenteral oxytetracycline, and mass treatment of calves with subconjunctival penicillin does not eliminate infection.

The intrapalpebral injection of 2 mL of a 10% oxytetracycline formulation was found equally effective as the systemic treatment with oxytetracycline (20 mg/kg).[5] Transient swelling of the eyelids, leading to complete closure of the palpebral fissure, was observed in some cases after intrapalpebral injection of oxytetracycline. It was suggested that this transient closure of the eye may favor healing by protecting the cornea and conjunctiva.[5]

Another technique for prolonging the maintenance of high levels of antibiotic in the conjunctival sac is the use of collagen inserts impregnated with an antibiotic.

Parenteral Therapy

Parenteral treatment with two doses of long-acting oxytetracycline (20 mg/kg) 72 hours apart has been shown to ameliorate clinical signs of naturally occurring IBK.[4,5]

Recent studies have documented that florfenicol when administered either as a single subcutaneous dose of 40 mg/kg or two doses of 20 mg/kg administered 48 hours apart is effective for treatment of clinical IBK in calves. Healing times were shorter and relapses were fewer when using florefenicol instead of long-acting oxytetracycline for treatment of IBK in calves.

The use of tulathromycin, a macrolide antibiotic, was found to be effective to treat experimentally induced IBK in calves in one study.[6] A single dose of 2.5 mg/kg resulted in faster healing and higher bacteriologic cure compared with untreated control animals.

Tilmicosin administered at a dose of 5 or 10 mg/kg SC was found effective to treat IBK in one field study.[4]

The efficacy of a long-acting formulation of ceftiofur crystalline-free acid (CCFA) administered as a single subcutaneous dose at the base of the ear to treat naturally occurring IBK has been examined in one study. A dose of 6.6 mg of ceftiofur equivalents/kg was found to result in higher healing rates and faster healing times of naturally occurring IBK compared with untreated control animals.[7]

Ancillary Therapy

Severe cases should be placed in a dark shelter out of direct sunlight. If housing is not possible, eye flap **patches** are available and effective. They are glued on above the eye and can be flipped up for medication of the eye.

When corneal ulceration has occurred, recovery is always protracted. The use of topical ophthalmic anesthetics combined with atropine administration may be indicated to minimize ciliary spasm and pain. Severe cases may require that the third eyelid be temporarily sutured across the globe of the eye for several days to promote healing. The use of NSAIDs should be considered in more advanced and severe cases.

TREATMENT AND TREATMENT

Treatment

Topical treatment:

Benzathine cloxacillin ointment (250 to 375 mg topical q72h, 2 treatments) (R-1)

Subconjunctival injection:

Procaine-penicillin G (300,000 to 600,000 IU subconjunctival q48-72 h, 2 treatments) (R-1)

Intrapalpebral injection:

Oxytetracycline (treatment 1 to 2 mL of 10% solution intrapalpebral, single treatment) (R-2)

Systemic treatment:

Oxytetracycline long-acting formulation (20 mg/kg q48h IM, two treatments) (R-1)

Florfenicol (20 mg/kg q48 SC, 2 treatments or 40 mg/kg SC, single treatment) (R-1)

Tulathromycin (2.5 mg/kg SC, single treatment) (R-2)

Tilmicosin (5 mg/kg SC, single treatment) (R-3)

Treatment

Decrease exposure to dust and implement fly control, particularly against face flies (R-2)

Vaccination with commercially available or autogenous bacterins (R-3)

CONTROL

Eradication or prevention of the disease does not seem possible under extensive range conditions because of the method of spread, but if **fly control** can be fitted into the farm's management program this should significantly reduce the infection rate. Insecticide-impregnated eartags may help in the control of the disease but do not prevent it. In many herds the best that can be done is to keep animals under close surveillance and isolate and treat any cattle that show excessive lacrimation and blepharospasm. Cattle that have had the disease should not be mixed with those that have not until after the fly season.

Vaccination

There has been considerable effort to develop methods of immunoprophylaxis; however, the commercial bacterins, although available for over 30 years, have given inconsistent results, providing at best limited protection from subsequent infection and clinical disease. Killed, whole-cell vaccines require repeat injections, may be associated with anaphylactic reactions, and have not proven effective in the field. To avoid the need for repeated injections an adjuvant vaccine has been tested, but without apparent benefit.

Vaccines containing pilus antigens, with or without cornea-degrading enzyme antigens, protect against challenge with homologous strains of *M. bovis*, and some field trials report efficacy in naturally occurring outbreaks. However, others do not, and the results of field studies that have shown a beneficial effect from vaccination have been criticized on the basis of bias in the selection of controls. It is probable that currently available vaccines do not contain the diversity of antigens required to protect against the variety of strains that occur in natural outbreaks. Autogenous vaccines are a consideration in individual herds, but a recent controlled trial of an autogenous vaccine administered by subcutaneous or subconjunctival injection found no significant effect of either route or the vaccine on the incidence of disease.

Weekly treatment of both eyes of calves, but not the cows, with a furazolidone eye spray has been shown to be a more effective prophylaxis than vaccination with a commercial bacterin in some areas.

Total eyelid pigmentation may reduce the incidence of this disease, but the recorded differences are unlikely to arouse enthusiasm for a genetic approach to the problem.

FURTHER READING

Angelos JA. Infectious bovine keratoconjunctivitis (pinkeye). *Vet Clin North Am Food A.* 2015;31(1):61-79.

McConnel CS, Shum L, House JK. Infectious bovine keratoconjunctivitis antimicrobial therapy. *Aust Vet J.* 2007;85:65-69.

O'Connor AM, Brace S, Gould S, Dewell R, Engelken T. A randomized clinical trial evaluating a farm-of-origin autogenous *Moraxella bovis* vaccine to control infectious bovine keratoconjunctivitis (pinkeye) in beef cattle. *J Vet Intern Med.* 2011;25:1447-1453.

Postma GC, Carfagnini JC, Minatel L. *Moraxella bovis* pathogenicity: an update. *Comp Immunol Microbiol Infect Dis.* 2008;31:449-458.

REFERENCES

1. Postma GC, et al. *Comp Immunol Microbiol Infect Dis.* 2008;31:449-458.
2. Angelos JA. *Vet Clin North Am Food A.* 2010;29:73-78.
3. Gould S, et al. *Vet Microbiol.* 2013;164:108-115.
4. McConnel CS, et al. *Aust Vet J.* 2007;85:65-69.
5. Starke A, et al. *Dtsch Tierarztl Wochenschr.* 2007;114:219-224.
6. Lane VM, et al. *J Am Vet Med Assoc.* 2006;229:557-561.
7. Dueger EL, et al. *Am J Vet Res.* 2004;65:1185-1188.

OVINE AND CAPRINE CONTAGIOUS OPHTHALMIA (OVINE AND CAPRINE INFECTIOUS KERATOCONJUNCTIVITIS, CONTAGIOUS CONJUNCTIVO-KERATITIS, PINKEYE IN SHEEP AND GOATS)

SYNOPSIS

Etiology *Mycoplasma conjunctivae* is a significant cause, but other agents, in particular *Chlamydia pecorum*, *Moraxella ovis*, and other *Mycoplasma* spp., can produce clinically identical disease.

Epidemiology Rapid spread by contact with carrier animals. Usually occurs as outbreak in summer and when conditions are dry and dusty. Disease is most severe in weaned lambs.

Clinical findings Lacrimation, conjunctival hyperemia, pannus, neovascularization, iritis, keratitis in one or both eyes.

Diagnostic confirmation Clinical examination of the flock, exfoliative cytology, culture and polymerase chain reaction (PCR).

Treatment Topical or preferably parenteral tetracycline.

Control Avoid confinement and movement in dusty conditions. Fly control.

ETIOLOGY

A variety of organisms have been isolated from the eyes of sheep and goats with keratoconjunctivitis. Some are primary pathogens and others secondary invaders. It is difficult to attribute a primary etiological cause to a single agent because all the putative causal organisms have also been isolated from the eyes of normal sheep. Mixed infections occur during an outbreak, with potential synergism between *Mycoplasma* spp. and other infectious agents. The management circumstances that lead to outbreaks of disease with each agent, and the clinical syndromes that result, are not sufficiently distinct to allow the differentiation of the various etiologies on clinical or epidemiological grounds. There have been limited studies on the relative prevalence of flock outbreaks of disease associated with the various putative causes, but there is a strong evidence to incriminate *Mycoplasma* spp., particularly *M. conjunctivae*, as the major cause in domesticated sheep and goats, and wild ruminants such as chamois, Alpine ibex, European mouflon, and Bighorn sheep.

Mycoplasma conjunctivae

Mycoplasma conjunctivae is a common isolate in outbreaks of the disease. However, it is not present in all affected sheep and can also be isolated, with lesser frequency, from the eyes of clinically normal sheep. Disease can be reproduced with the inoculation of pure cultures of this organism into the eye of sheep and is then spread to other sheep by contact transmission. Consequently, it is thought to be a principal cause of pinkeye in sheep and goats.

Other Mycoplasmas

Other *Mycoplasma* spp. are frequently identified in the eyes of sheep and goats with pinkeye. *M. agalactiae* was considered a primary cause of an outbreak in Spain, whereas *M. arginini* and *Acholeplasma oculi* have been isolated from clinical cases of contagious ophthalmia. Infection with other mycoplasmas, such as *M. capricolum* subspp. *capricolum* and *M. mycoides* subspp. *capri*, can be accompanied by conjunctivitis, but other clinical signs, such as pneumonia, predominate.

Chlamydophila pecorum

Chlamydophila pecorum (*Colesiota conjunctivae*) was initially incriminated as a cause of contagious ophthalmia in sheep and goats in South Africa and Australia. It has been isolated from outbreaks of keratoconjunctivitis in sheep in the United States and the United Kingdom, and the disease has been reproduced experimentally. The strains are related to those associated with polyarthritis in sheep rather than abortion. A rickettsial agent, *Rupricapra rupricapae*, has been isolated from keratoconjunctivitis in chamois (*R. tragis*) and ibex (*Capra ibex*) in the French Alps. In Egypt, *Chlamydophila psittaci* was isolated at a higher rate from diseased eyes, compared with asymptomatic eyes, in both sheep (80% and 68%, respectively) and goats (92% and 76%, respectively).[1]

A number of bacteria, including *Branhamella* (*Neisseria*) *ovis*, *S. aureus* and *E. coli*, can be isolated from the eyes of animals with contagious ophthalmia, with rates of isolation from affected eyes higher than those from normal sheep. They have not always produced disease following experimental challenge. Consequently, they are considered to be secondary infections rather than having a primary causal role, exacerbating the lesions produced by the primary agent. *B. ovis* is considered a cause of follicular conjunctivitis. Similarly, *Moraxella bovis*, which is associated with contagious keratoconjunctivitis in cattle, has no apparent causal association with the disease in sheep, although it was isolated from clinical cases in goats in Nigeria.[2] *Listeria monocytogenes* may be a primary cause of keratoconjunctivitis and iritis in sheep.

EPIDEMIOLOGY

Occurrence

The disease is widespread in sheep of all breeds in most countries. Recently weaned animals are often the most severely affected.

Source of Infection and Transmission

The source of infection is infected or carrier animals. The disease is spread indirectly by flies, long grass, and dust contaminated by the tears of infected sheep, or directly by means of exhaled droplets or immediate contact. *M. conjunctivae* infects many wild small ruminant species and can be transmitted between domestic and wild animals.[3,4]

Risk Factors

The prevalence is highest during the warm, summer months and when conditions are dry and dusty and flies are abundant. The morbidity rate varies widely depending on seasonal conditions; it is usually about 10% to 15% but may be as high as 80%. Resistance to infection is reduced by other disease, poor nutrition, and adverse weather. Widespread outbreaks occur in some years where the disease contributes to poor growth and ill-thrift, presumably from reduce foraging ability, especially in young stock. Outbreaks during mating can reduce conception and lambing rates.

In many flocks at pasture the disease causes little disruption to grazing, and so only minor inconvenience. However, in other flocks, and in some years, higher morbidity, severe lesions, and detrimental effects on production occur. Clinical experience suggests that the incidence and the severity of the disease in an affected flock are increased by the stress, dust, and close contact associated with gathering and yarding of the flock. Thus a decision to treat during an outbreak can be associated with an apparent exacerbation of clinical disease.

PATHOGENESIS

Rapid onset of acute inflammation of the conjunctiva is followed by hyperemia of the sclera and pannus and opacity of the cornea.

CLINICAL FINDINGS

Clinical findings are similar with all agents associated with the disease. There is conjunctivitis, lacrimation, and blepharospasm, followed by keratitis with cloudiness of the cornea and some increase in vascularity. There is profuse lacrimation, and thus initial signs in the flock may be a brown discoloration below the eye associated with dust accumulating on lacrimal discharges.

Corneal opacity is initially most pronounced at the dorsal corneal–scleral junction. This is followed by vascularization, to produce a horizontal zone of opacity associated with an area of vertical-oriented vascularization in the upper area of the eye. In severe cases, the whole cornea is affected, and there may be corneal ulceration.

In flocks experiencing an outbreak, the disease in most sheep is mild if there are no complicating circumstances; the initial watery discharge from the eye becomes purulent, but recovery commences in 3 to 4 days and is complete at about 20 days. In some animals the cloudiness of the cornea may persist for several weeks or even permanently. Local ulceration of the cornea may cause collapse of the eyeball. One or both eyes may be affected, but many sheep have both eyes affected in outbreaks, and spread through the flock is rapid.

Conjunctivitis is followed by the development of granular lesions of follicular conjunctivitis on the palpebral conjunctiva and third eyelid, which are thought by some to be specific for infections involving *B. ovis*.

In goats, the disease is milder with little apparent ophthalmia or keratitis. A more severe keratoconjunctivitis than that associated with *M. conjunctivae*, and manifest with corneal edema, occurs in some outbreaks in goats, but its cause has not been established. All age groups are affected, and although the morbidity is usually 12% to 20%, it may reach 50%. Direct contact between animals appears to be necessary for spread of the infection, but the disease has not been transmitted experimentally. Conjunctivitis, opacity, vascularization, and sometimes ulceration of the cornea are accompanied by an ocular discharge and blepharospasm. In some goats there is severe corneal edema with intracorneal edema accumulating to a degree to produce corneal vesicles. In mildly affected goats, recovery begins in 4 to 7 days, but in severe cases, healing may not be complete for 2 to 4 weeks or longer.

CLINICAL PATHOLOGY

Scrapings can be taken for exfoliative cytology from the palpebral conjunctiva, preferably from early clinical cases. *Mycoplasma*, *Branhamella*, and *Chlamydophila* have characteristic morphology and can be demonstrated in Giemsa- or immunofluorescent-stained smears. Samples can also be submitted for culture identification, and paired serum samples can be submitted for examination for antibodies to *Chlamydophila*.

The determination of the etiologic agent currently has limited significance to the subsequent approach to the control and treatment of the disease, and so is largely academic. However, conventional and real-time PCR can be used to detect *M. conjunctivae* and *Moraxella* spp., and PCR is a more sensitive way of detecting of infection than culture.[5,6]

TREATMENT

A decision for treatment needs to be taken with consideration of the adverse effects on the disease of the associated movement and close yarding of the flock. Repeated treatments of sheep pastured under extensive grazing are impractical, and spontaneous recovery will occur within 3 weeks. Consequently, in extensive grazing conditions a decision for no treatment is often made.

A single intramuscular injection of long-acting tetracycline at 20 mg/kg halts further development of clinical conjunctivitis when given as clinical signs develop and results in rapid clinical cure in animals affected with keratoconjunctivitis produced by *M. conjunctivae*. Florfenicol readily penetrates tear fluid, with doses greater than 20 mg/kg needed to provide minimum inhibitory concentrations against most *Mycoplasma* spp.[7] However, neither parenteral or topical antibiotic treatment eliminates infection; thus, repeated infections in individual animals and recurrence of outbreaks in flocks are common. Where the etiology is not known and treatment is deemed desirable, tetracyclines administered either topically or parenterally, or topical treatment with cloxacillin or erythromycin ophthalmic ointments, have been shown to be of benefit.

CONTROL

Complete eradication of the disease is not attempted, but isolation of affected sheep and removal to grassier, less dusty pasture may reduce the rate of spread. Confinement of affected sheep should also be avoided.

FURTHER READING

Radostits O, et al. Ovine and caprine contagious ophthalmia (ovine and caprine infectious keratoconjunctivitis, contagious conjunctivo-keratitis, pinkeye in sheep and goats). In: *Veterinary Medicine: A Textbook of the Diseases of Cattle, Horses, Sheep, Goats and Pigs*. 10th ed. London: W.B. Saunders; 2007:1142-1143.

REFERENCES

1. Osman KM, et al. *Transbound Emerg Dis*. 2013;60:245.
2. Ojo OE, et al. *Niger Vet J*. 2009;30:56.
3. Jansen BD, et al. *J Wildl Dis*. 2006;42:407.
4. Fernandez-Aguilar X, et al. *BMC Vet Res*. 2013;9:253.
5. Vilei EM, et al. *J Microbiol Meth*. 2007;70:384.
6. Shen HG, et al. *J Appl Microbiol*. 2011;111:1037.
7. Regnier A, et al. *J Am Vet Med Assoc*. 2013;74:268.

DISEASES OF THE EYES ASSOCIATED WITH *MYCOPLASMA* SPP.

Mycoplasma conjunctivae is the etiologic agent causing **infectious keratoconjunctivitis of small and wild ruminants** (see also "Ovine and Caprine Infectious Keratoconjunctivitis").

In cattle *M. bovoculi* is frequently isolated from conjunctival swabs without necessarily being associated with clinical disease. The recovery rate of *M. bovoculi* from eye swabs obtained from clinically healthy cattle and animals with conjunctivitis was approximately 40% in both instances. *M. bovoculi* was isolated more frequently from animals younger than 2 years of age than from older animals, whereas the disease incidence of infectious keratoconjunctivitis was similar in both age groups. The higher recovery rate of *M. bovoculi* in younger animals was explained by the development of immunity after initial infection.

Other *Mycoplasma* spp. that have been isolated from cattle with keratoconjunctivitis are *M. bovis*, *M. bovigenitalium*, *M. bovirhinis*, *M. verecundum*, *Ureaplasma diversum*, *Acholeplasma laidlawii*, and *Acholeplasma oculi*, some of which have been incriminated as contributing to the development of **infectious bovine keratoconjunctivitis**.

THELAZIASIS (EYEWORM)

A number of species of the nematode genus *Thelazia* occur in the conjunctival sac and tear ducts of mammals throughout the world. *T. gulosa* and *T. skrjabini* are the main species in cattle in the New World, *T. rhodesi* is the commonest in the Old World, and *T. lacrymalis* is common in horses. They are thin worms up to 2 cm long. Infestation is often inapparent, but they may cause excessive lacrimation, photophobia, conjunctivitis,[1] corneal opacity,[2] keratitis, corneal ulceration, and abscess formation on the eyelids. In horses, this condition mainly occurs in young animals.[3] One U.S. survey in Kentucky found 43% of horses up to 4 years old to be infected. In those species that have been studied, the life cycles are indirect, with muscid flies, particularly the face fly *M. autumnalis*, being the intermediate hosts. These flies deposit larvae on the conjunctiva when feeding on fluid around the eye. The disease is mainly seen in summer and autumn when the flies are active. It is usually more common in cattle[1] and African buffalo[2] than horses, and worms may be more abundant in beef than in dairy cattle. Eyeworm in cattle is differentiated from infectious keratitis by observing the adult worm in the conjunctival sac or demonstrating first-stage larvae in eye washings. Ivermectin (0.2 mg/kg, repeated three times at 1-month intervals) is active against worms in African buffalo.[2] Ivermectin and doramectin are active against the adult worm in cattle, but anecdotal reports suggest that it may be less effective in horses.[3]

REFERENCES

1. Djungu DF, et al. *Trop Biomed.* 2014;31:844.
2. Munangandu HM, et al. *Korean J Parasitol.* 2011;49:91.
3. Lyons ET, et al. *Parasitol Res.* 2006;99:114.

"BRIGHT BLINDNESS" OF SHEEP CAUSED BY BRACKEN INGESTION

A progressive retinal degeneration associated with ptaquiloside was observed in sheep kept for more than 3 years on pastures heavily infested with bracken in the United Kingdom, and the disease has been produced experimentally in sheep fed bracken. Affected sheep are blind, reluctant to move, but bright and alert. The pupils are dilated and show poor light and menace reflexes, and on ophthalmoscopic examination there is retinal degeneration. This degeneration may be observable in many more sheep than the clinically blind ones. Leukopenia is a characteristic.

BOVINE OCULAR SQUAMOUS-CELL CARCINOMA

Bovine ocular squamous-cell carcinoma (BOSCC), often referred to as "cancer eye," is one of the most common neoplasms of cattle.

SYNOPSIS

Etiology Genetic–environmental interaction. Lack of pigmentation around the eye and solar radiation.

Epidemiology One of most common neoplasms of cattle; mostly in beef cattle breeds with white on their heads (Hereford, Simmental) and lacking pigment around the eye; animals over 5 years of age. Solar radiation is a major risk factor.

Signs Precursor lesions; single or multiple plaques on eyelid or conjunctiva, except the cornea or pigmented lid; may regress or lead to carcinomas of sclera resembling papillomas with crumbly, necrotic ulcerated mass attached to the eyelid, causing irritation to eye and conjunctiva and excessive lacrimation and pus. Invasion of surrounding tissues of eye and possibly to nearby lymph nodes.

Clinical pathology Histology of lesion.

Lesions Squamous-cell carcinoma.

Diagnostic confirmation Biopsy and histology.

Differential diagnosis list
Pinkeye
Lymphoma of periorbital tissues

Treatment Excision by cryosurgery. Radical surgery may be necessary. Immunotherapy with vaccines has been attempted.

Control Breeding program to increase degree of periocular pigmentation in white-faced beef cattle and remove genetically susceptible cattle from the breeding herd.

ETIOLOGY

A genetic–environmental interaction has been proposed as the cause. A relative **lack of circumocular and corneoscleral pigmentation**, both of which are highly heritable, increases the probability of lesion development when the animal is exposed to a carcinogenic agent such as the **ultraviolet component of sunlight**.[1] The carcinoma has been regarded as a papilloma-associated tumor because papillomavirus can be found in the precursor lesions, and papillomavirus DNA in the carcinomas. It is possible the papillomavirus infection predisposes to BOSCC by induction of precursor lesions, but papillomavirus does not appear to be needed for maintenance of the tumor. Moreover, advanced virological techniques have failed to reveal any association between the virus and the tumor.[2]

The *p53* gene product is highly expressed in bovine BOSCC, which provides support for its role in BOSCC tumor development.

EPIDEMIOLOGY

Occurrence

Bovine ocular squamous-cell carcinoma is a very common neoplasm of the eyelids and the eyeball of cattle and one of the most common neoplasms of cattle. The disease is most common in beef cattle, which are exposed to more sunlight than dairy cattle. Breeds affected most commonly are Hereford and Simmental, but BOSCC has also been recorded in Shorthorn, Holstein–Friesian, Guernsey, Jersey, Ayrshire, Brown Swiss, Normandy, Hollandensa, Javanese-Mongolian, and Brahman cattle.

The tumors are uncommon in cattle younger than 5 years and are almost never seen in cattle younger than 3 years. The condemnation rate at slaughter of cattle with ocular squamous-cell carcinoma in Canada is about 30% of cases. A squamous-cell carcinoma of the anal and perianal area of a 15-year-old bull has been recorded.

Risk Factors

The heritabilities and phenotypic and genetic correlations of eyelid and corneoscleral pigment and eye lesions associated with eye cancer were investigated in 2831 Herefords from 34 herds in 21 U.S. states and one Canadian province. The results indicated that periocular pigmentation and eyelid and corneoscleral pigment were highly heritable and genetically correlated. These findings lead to the general conclusion that the genetic effect on pigment determines to a large extent the degree to which the eye is susceptible to an environmental carcinogenic agent such as ultraviolet light. A very high heritability estimate ($h^2 = 0.79$) was reported for circumocular pigmentation in 3579 Simmental cattle in Germany.[1]

In Zimbabwe, ocular squamous-cell carcinoma was frequently observed in five breeding herds of Simmental cattle. In these herds, initial signs of the disease were evident in cattle of about 3 years of age, and gradually the prevalence increased to over 50% in animals over 7 years of age. It is suggested that because most cattle in Zimbabwe are slaughtered by 10 years of age, that more than 67% of cattle without periorbital skin pigmentation would develop the tumor. The tumors were multiple and commonly bilateral. Simmental cattle have a complete or partly white face, and the lack of facial pigmentation risks exposure to intense solar radiation when they are kept at a high altitude (1500 m) in a sunny and warm climate. The prevalence was much lower in white-faced Friesian cattle in the same environment, which indicates a genetic predisposition for the tumors in Simmental cattle, separate from periocular pigmentation. In Zimbabwe, the tumor is not recorded in fully pigmented cattle breeds.

The positive association between prevalence of BOSCC and various measures of solar radiation indicate a significant association between increasing risks of developing eye cancer and increasing levels of radiation. Ultraviolet light is generally regarded as an important risk factor. Most tumors are located only in the sun-exposed mucocutaneous areas not protected by hair. Tumors are predominantly localized in the third eyelid and the lateral limbus, and tumor growth usually starts at the outer edge, which receives the most sunlight. Cattle exposed to higher levels of ultraviolet radiation develop the disease at younger ages.

Economic Importance

The disease results in serious economic consequences through lessened productivity and carcass condemnations. Commercial cattle can be culled early without much loss, because only the head is condemned. Purebred cattle are more of a problem because of the difficulty of deciding when euthanasia must be the humane decision, rather than another attempted extirpation of the eye. An additional issue in purebred cattle is whether the bloodline of affected cattle should be preserved.

PATHOGENESIS

The initial lesion may be on the eyelid or any structure in the conjunctival sac, except the avascular cornea or pigmented eyelid. Lesions can encroach on these tissues from others nearby, carrying a blood supply with them.

The lesions develop through four stages. The first three, plaque, keratoma, and papilloma, are nonmalignant and have relatively high spontaneous regression rates. The fourth stage is the squamous-cell carcinoma, which does not regress. The tumor is located in the sclera adjacent to the lateral limbus, in the membrana nictitans (third eyelid), or in the lower eyelid (Fig. 16-11A-C). It is an invasive tumor, metastasizing along the draining lymphatics into cervical lymph nodes. Primary lesions of the lids are most likely to metastasize to these nodes.

Animals do not appear to develop resistance to the cancer; only a few cows with the disease develop measurable antibodies in their sera. It is one of the characteristics of this disease that the carcinomas appear to produce immunosuppressive substances, and removal of tumor mass reduces their blood concentrations.

In countries and in herds where ocular carcinoma is common, it is not unusual to encounter lesions on the labia of the vulva, especially if there are patches of unpigmented skin.

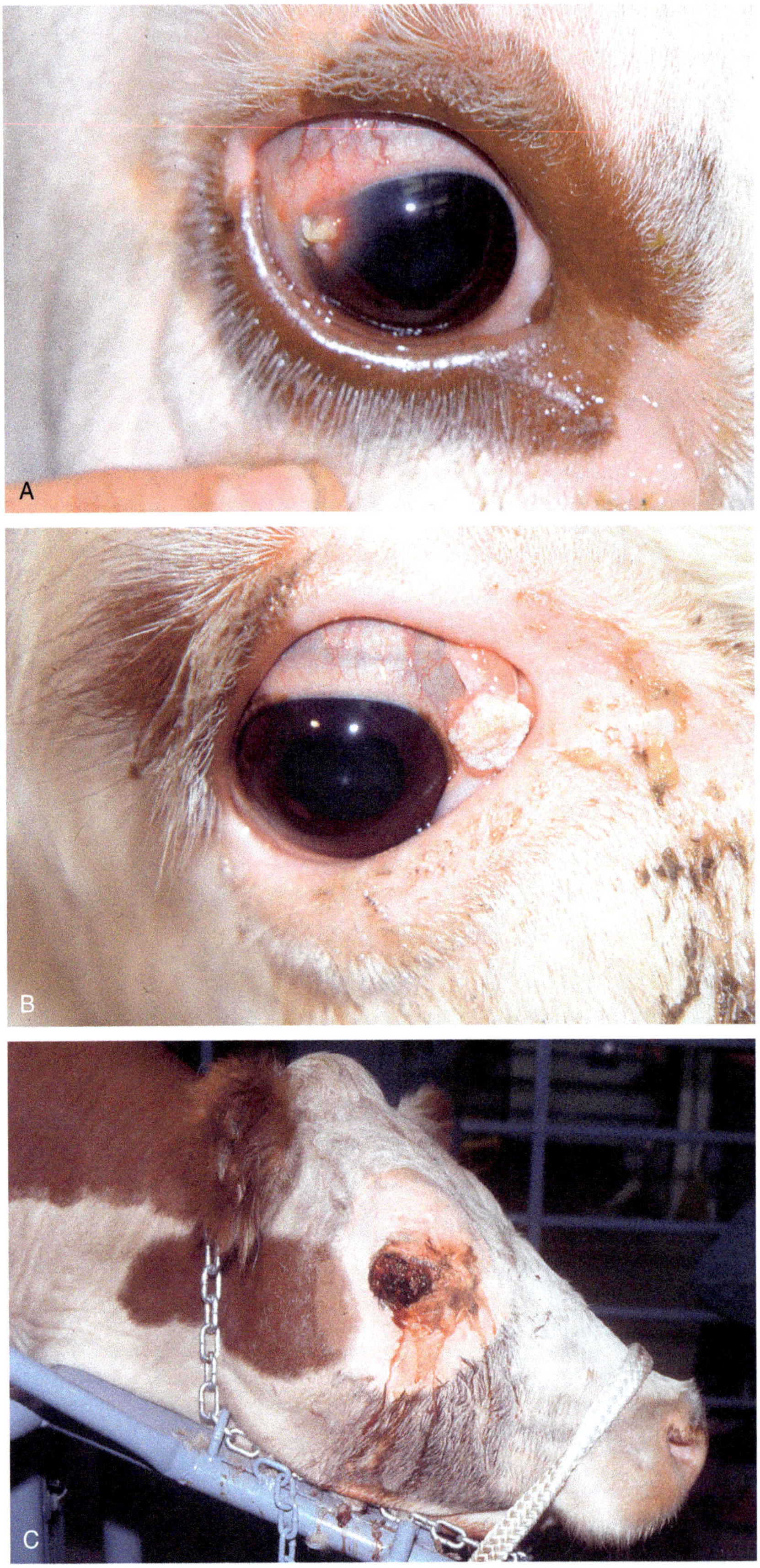

Fig. 16-11 A, Advanced plaque on the lateral limbus of the right eye from a Simmental cow. This is a precursor to ocular squamous-cell carcinoma. B, Advanced papilloma on the third eyelid of the right eye from a Simmental cow. This is a precursor to squamous-cell carcinoma. Note the small amount of periocular eyelid pigmentation. C, Advanced squamous-cell carcinoma of the right lower eyelid of a Simmental cow. The tumor mass is large enough that metastasis to the regional lymph node was likely.

CLINICAL FINDINGS

Typical precursor lesions are single or multiple plaques of gray–white, smooth or rough, hyperplastic to hyperkeratinized tissue anywhere in the conjunctiva (stage 1). Plaques may develop into keratoma or keratoacanthomas (stage 2) and papillomas (stage 3), which are also regarded as precursor lesions. Squamous-cell carcinomas (stage 4) may develop from any of these precursor stages, which may also regress spontaneously. **Classic ocular squamous-cell carcinoma lesions** resemble papillomas, with a fleshy, sometimes crumbly, often necrotic and ulcerated mass attached to the lid or the orbit by a wide base. They are visible even when the eyelids are closed, and they cause obvious irritation to the surrounding conjunctiva, resulting in increased lacrimation and sometimes in the discharge of pus. Invasion of surrounding tissues is common, but metastases to nearby lymph nodes and to viscera occur in only a few cases and then only late in the course of the disease. In general, all lesions with a dimension greater than 2 cm are cancerous (stage 4). The proportion of small precursor lesions that regress without specific treatment is up to 88%, which complicates evaluation of treatment efficacy.

The most common location for tumor development is the lateral corneoscleral junction (limbus), which usually accounts for three-fourths of all lesions. Other predilection sites are the nictating membrane (third eyelid) and middle to medial aspect of the lower eyelid. Tumors on the nictating membrane appear to grow more quickly than tumors located elsewhere.[3] Tumors in the eyelids have a higher frequency of metastasis than tumors of the cornea or limbus; this most likely reflects total tumor volume at diagnosis, with eyelid lesions typically being more extensive when the animal is first examined for treatment.

CLINICAL PATHOLOGY

Differentiation between carcinomas and precursor lesions is difficult clinically, and cytologic examination or biopsy is recommended for definitive diagnoses. The cytology of squamous-cell carcinomas in domestic animals has been described.

DIFFERENTIAL DIAGNOSIS

One of the difficulties encountered in the field is the clinical differentiation of benign precursor lesions from the malignant carcinomas; failure to do so may account for the high rates of spontaneous regression recorded, especially in Hereford cattle, where a spontaneous recovery rate of 88% has been recorded. To avoid this inaccuracy, exfoliative cytology by the examination of smears of lesions is helpful. Combined with a clinical assessment, this is the recommended method of confirming the diagnosis. Differentiation from similar lesions that are not BOSCC can only be achieved by proper laboratory examination of tissues.

BOSCC must be differentiated clinically from:

- Pinkeye and its complications, which result in excessive lacrimation and purulent material
- Lymphoma of the periorbital tissues, which usually manifests as exophthalmos

TREATMENT

Surgical excision of small lesions with a margin of 2 to 3 mm, accompanied by cryonecrosis (two freeze–thaw cycles) of the tumor site using appropriately sized copper probes placed in liquid nitrogen, is widely practiced in cattle. Results are good to excellent in cattle with small lesions (<2 cm in dimension). Enucleation (removal of the eye) and extirpation or exenteration (removal of the eye and para-orbital tissue) is commonly performed in animals with larger lesions (>2 cm in dimension) that indicate presence of carcinoma in situ that are locally invasive. The major challenges with enucleation are intraoperative hemorrhage and postoperative infection, which occurred in 19% of 53 cattle.[4] Radical surgery, including removal of the local lymph nodes and parts of the salivary gland, may be desirable in advanced cases of BOSCC.

Recurrence, or the development of new lesions at the same site, is common. Treatment can also be combined with immunotherapy, for example, with **bacillus Calmette–Guérin** (BCG) vaccine injected systemically or into the lesion, or with vaccination with BOSCC tumor material. There is a significant cell-mediated immune response in cattle with BOSCC, and it is thought that this immune process plays an important role in the rejection of the tumors. One controlled trial in cattle showed that intralesional injection of BCG vaccine can interrupt neoplastic progression and prevent malignant disease. A permanent regression after BCG vaccination can be expected in 37% of cases, recurrence at the same site in 26%, and continued growth in 37%.

A favorable response to a single injection of a saline phenol extract of fresh tumor tissue can induce a high rate of regression of ocular tumors, with a higher recovery rate after the use of 200 mg of lyophilized tumor extract compared with an injection of 100 mg. The injection may need to be repeated. Occasional tumors show enhancement of growth after vaccination, especially if it is repeated. The vaccine does not need to be autologous, and only one injection is required. A freeze-dried preparation of tumor antigen has been used successfully. In general, the use of a vaccine seems likely to provide a satisfactory method for controlling an esthetically distressing and financially important disease.

Reports on the effect of vaccination with a tumor vaccine on the vulvar form of squamous-cell carcinoma vary.

Daily peritumoral injections of BOSCC lesions up to 2.8 cm^2 in area with interleukin-2 for 10 days at 5000 to 1,000,000 U was effective in inducing complete tumor regression in 50% to 69% of tumors at 20 months, compared with 14% regression in control cattle injected with solvent.[3] Lower daily IL-2 doses (<200,000 U) were similarly effective as higher doses in inducing tumor regression at 9 months, but their effectiveness was not maintained at 20 months. Interleukin-2 is thought to induce tumor regression by initially inducing edema, then angiogenesis, recruitment of monocytes, and macrophage and lymphocyte activation. However, the tumor response rate to IL-2 treatment is lower than that achieved by surgery, which remains the preferred treatment for BOSCC.

Treatment by the use of radioactive implants or topically applied radiation has also been successful, but reduced availability and concerns about the use of radioactivity in a meat-producing animal has markedly decreased the application of localized radiation therapy. Other treatments that have received favorable comment, but need to be evaluated in the light of the known natural recovery rate of the benign precursor lesions, include radiofrequency hyperthermia and combinations of the previously described procedures.

TREATMENT AND CONTROL

Treatment

- Surgical excision of lesions > 2 cm in dimension (stage 4) (R-1)
- Surgical excision of lesions < 2 cm in dimension (stages 1, 2, 3, or 4) (R-1)
- Cryonecrosis (2 freeze–thaw cycles) (R-2)
- Intralesional BCG injection(s) (R-2)
- Intralesional IL-2 injections (200,000 to 2,000,000 U daily for 10 days) (R-2)
- Local radiofrequency hyperthermia (2 heating cycles) (R-2)
- Local radiation therapy (if available and permitted) (R-2)

Prophylaxis

- Decrease exposure to ultraviolet light (usually not practical) (R-1)
- Implement breeding program based on increasing periocular pigmentation (R-1)
- Remove direct descendants and sires and dams of cattle diagnosed with BOSCC (R-2)

CONTROL

Because of the strong correlation between absence of pigmentation of the eyelids and the occurrence of the disease, and because of the high heritability of this pigmentation in Hereford and Simmental cattle, it is suggested that a breeding program aimed at increasing the degree of pigmentation of eyelids could quickly reduce the incidence of the disease in this breed. A positive approach to the problem would be to crossbreed susceptible *B. taurus* cattle with *B. indicus* cattle, which always have pigmented eyelids and have much lower rates of eye cancer. In Ayrshires there is a corresponding predilection for squamous-cell carcinomata of the vulva, but the neoplasm does not occur on both sites in the same cow. Selection on the basis of the occurrence of lesions alone results in only limited reduction in incidence.

FURTHER READING

Tsujita H, Plummer CE. Bovine ocular squamous cell carcinoma. *Vet Clin North Am Food A.* 2010;26:511-529.

REFERENCES

1. Pausch H, et al. *PLoS ONE.* 2012;7:e36346.
2. Nasir L, Campo MS. *Vet Dermatology.* 2008;19:243.
3. Stewart RJE, et al. *Vet Rec.* 2006;159:668.
4. Schulz KL, Anderson DE. *Can Vet J.* 2010;51:611.

EQUINE OCULAR SQUAMOUS-CELL CARCINOMA

Squamous-cell carcinoma is one of the most common neoplasms of the horse and is the most common neoplastic tumor of the eye and orbit.

Equine ocular squamous-cell carcinoma (EOSC) is associated with a number of factors, including lack of pigmentation around the eye, exposure to solar radiation, mutations in the *p53* gene, and presence of equine caballus papillomavirus type 2 (EcPV-2) and bovine papillomavirus type 1 (BPV-1) DNA.[1,2] EcPV-2 is also found in squamous carcinoma of the penis of horses, but not in clinically normal nictitating membrane tissue (75 horses).[3] Although DNA of BPV-1 can be found in normal equine skin, there is increasing evidence of an etiologic link between mucocutaneous squamous-cell carcinoma (SCC) in horses and EcPV-2 infection. Approximately 25% of these tumors express cyclooxygenase-2 activity.[4-6]

The reported frequency has been highest in animals lacking periocular pigmentation and is more common in Appaloosa, albino, and color-dilute horses. An increased prevalence for ocular and adnexal SCC has been reported in Belgian draft horse breeds, Appaloosas, Paint horses, Thoroughbreds, and Quarter horses. A predisposition for the development of ocular and adnexal SCC has also been reported in geldings. The risk has been higher in draft breeds than in other pigmented breeds, probably related to the large expanses of white skin on the face and around the eye of the heavy draft breeds. The overall mean age range of affected animals is 8 to 10 years. In a series of limbal neoplasms in horses admitted to the Veterinary Teaching Hospital in the Netherlands, SCC was the most predominant tumor type, and Haflinger horses accounted for 69%, whereas their occurrence in the hospital population was 5%.

In a retrospective study of 50 cases submitted to the University of Florida Veterinary Medical Teaching Hospital, the Appaloosa accounted for the majority of cases, which may be a reflection of the high level of solar radiation in southeastern United States. The average age at which the tumor was diagnosed initially was 11.8 years; males accounted for 64% and females 36% of the cases. The rate of metastasis was 18%.

In the Florida study, higher cure rates were associated with surgical excision followed by radiation therapy for a cure rate of 75%, whereas with only surgical excision the cure rate was 55%. Best results with treatment are seen when surgical intervention is early. In horses, treatment is largely surgical, but all of the immunologic techniques developed for cattle have been used, including local irradiation therapy.

The most frequent site for ocular involvement is the nictitating membrane and conjunctiva, but the eyelids and cornea are also involved.

Treatment of ocular and adnexal SCC has included various types of therapy, with and without adjuvant radiation therapy. Types of treatment without adjuvant radiation therapy include excision, cryotherapy, radiofrequency hyperthermia, immunotherapy, chemotherapy with cisplatin, and carbon dioxide laser ablation. Treatment with adjuvant radiation therapy includes use of strontium 90 (Sr), cobalt 60 (Co), gold 198, iridium 192 (Ir), cesium 137, iodine 125 (I), and radon 222 (Rn). In a series of 157 cases of ocular and adnexa SCC, those treated with adjuvant radiation therapy had a significantly lower recurrence rate compared with those treated without adjuvant radiation therapy, independent of anatomic location.

Superficial keratectomy followed by cryosurgery is a simple and effective procedure for the treatment of small-sized limbal tumors (less than 2 cm) in horses. Sophisticated equipment is not required, and the legal restrictions associated with the use of radioactive substances in many countries are not a consideration.

Prevention is through reduction of exposure to sunlight through use of fly masks and tattooing of ocular tissue.

Ocular pseudotumors have been described in horses. They are proliferative inflammatory lesions involving the eye, adnexa, or orbit, which clinically mimic true neoplasms. Cases are characterized by a uniocular, pink, proliferative limbal or perilimbal lesion. Affected horses may be from 5 to 9 years of age. Most cases occurred during the summer months and none of the affected animals had a history of trauma or recent deworming. The dorsal bulbar conjunctiva was most commonly affected, followed by the third eyelid. Lesions were relatively flat with indistinct margins or discrete and nodular. Histologically, the lesion is inflammatory and characterized by predominantly lymphocytic infiltrates. The cause is unknown, but an immune-mediated pathogenesis is suspected based on the preponderance of immunocytes consisting primarily of lymphocytes. Treatment consists of surgical excision alone, partial resection with antiinflammatory therapy, or antiinflammatory therapy alone.

FURTHER READING

Dugan SJ, et al. Epidemiological study of ocular/adnexal squamous cell carcinoma in horses. *J Am Vet Med Assoc.* 1991;198:251-256.
Giuliano EA. Equine periocular neoplasia: current concepts and aetiopathogenesis and emerging treatment modalities. *Equine Vet J.* 2010;42:9-18.

REFERENCES

1. Kainzbauer C, et al. *Equine Vet J.* 2012;44:112.
2. Sykora S, et al. *Vet Microbiol.* 2012;158:194.
3. Knight CG, et al. *Vet Microbiol.* 2013;166:257.
4. McInnis CL, et al. *Am J Vet Res.* 2007;68:165.
5. Rassnick KM, et al. *J Vet Diagn Invest.* 2007;19:436.
6. Smith KM, et al. *Vet Ophthalmol.* 2008;11:8.

INHERITED EYE DEFECTS

Inherited eye defects of farm animals and horses are not uncommon and typically occur in breeds that originate from a small founder base, such as, for example, with the complex ocular abnormalities of "Rocky Mountain horses" (which actually originated in the Ohio Valley of the United States) or Texel sheep.[1,2] Abnormalities of the eyes include strabismus; microphthalmia; single, multiple, or complex intraocular abnormalities; cataracts; retinal abnormalities (night blindness); corneal lesions, including abnormal tissue on the surface of the cornea (dermoids) or corneal opacity; abnormal eyelid conformation (entropion); distichiasis; and absence of the nasolacrimal duct. The genetic basis for some of the more common lesions has been determined.[3-7]

Inherited convergent **medial strabismus with exophthalmos** occurs in German Brown, Jersey, Shorthorn, Ayrshire, Bulgarian Grey, Irish Friesian, German Fleckvieh, German Black and White, and Dutch Black Pied breeds.[7] The incidence of BCSE in German Brown cattle is 0.9% in adult cows and 0.1% in young animals. The disease appears to be inherited in an autosomal-dominant manner with incomplete penetrance, with a relative decrease in neurons in the nuclear region of the abducens nerve. This decrease in neurons induces paresis of the lateral rectus muscles and the lateral part of the retractor bulbi muscles, resulting in the clinical signs of exophthalmos and strabismus. Candidate genes for the defect are thought to be on bovine chromosomes 5 and 18.[8,9]

The disease is characterized by late onset (>1 year of age) of clinical signs that are

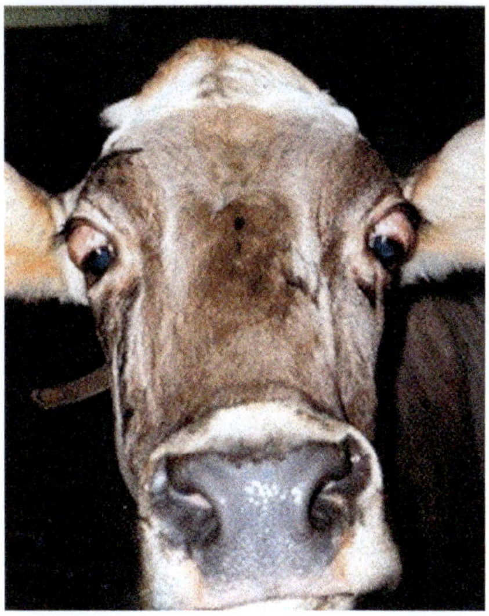

Fig. 16-12 Advanced case of bilateral convergent strabismus with exophthalmos in a German Brown cow. (Reproduced, with permission, from Mömke S, Distl O. Bilateral convergent strabismus with exophthalmus [BCSE] in cattle. An overview of clinical signs and genetic traits. *Vet J* 2007; 173:272-277.[7])

progressive, including bilateral, symmetric, permanent rotation of the eyeballs in an anterior-medial direction and slight to severe laterodorsal exophthalmos (Fig. 16-12).[7] Parts of the lateral rectus muscle or retrobulbar fat pad can become visible in severely affected animals. Epiphora is common in cattle with advanced BCSE. The sclera becomes darkly dark pigmented. Mildly affected animals compensate well and can be difficult to detect without close examination of the eyes, whereas more severely affected animals clearly have visual impairment up to and including blindness. There is no effective treatment.

An inherited, congenital **corneal opacity** occurs in Holstein cattle. The cornea is a cloudy blue color at birth, and both eyes are equally affected. Although the sight of affected animals is restricted they are not completely blind, and there are no other abnormalities of the orbit or the eyelids. Histologically there is edema and disruption of the corneal lamellae.

Lens dystrophy occurs in Brown Swiss cattle that are affected by an inherited congenital blindness. Japanese Black cattle also suffer from an inherited blindness caused by defects in the pupil, retina, and optic disk.

Congenital cataracts occur in a variety of breeds of cattle, and some have a suspected genetic component.[10] Multiple cataracts in a herd of Ayrshire cattle in Ireland were not clearly inherited, but the cause was not determined.[10] The condition of bilateral cataracts has been observed to be an inherited defect in Romney sheep. It is inherited as an autosomal-dominant trait and can be eradicated easily by culling. Congenital cataracts in Exmoor ponies in Canada are inherited in a sex-linked fashion, with the disease being significantly more common in females.[11]

Complete **absence of the iris** (aniridia) in both eyes is also recorded as an inherited defect in Belgian horses. Affected foals develop secondary cataracts at about 2 months of age. Total **absence of the retina** in foals has also been recorded as being inherited in a recessive manner.

Congenital stationary night blindness (CSNB) in Appaloosa horses is associated with homozygosity for the gene conferring the coat spotting pattern in horses, which itself is caused by a single incomplete dominant gene (LP).[5,12] LP maps to a 6-cM region on ECAl. Expression of transient receptor potential cation channel, subfamily m, member 1 (TRPM1) in the retina of homozygous Appaloosa horses is 0.05% the level found in non-Appaloosa horses. Decreased expression of TRPM1 in the eye and the skin may alter bipolar cell signaling and melanocyte function, thus causing both CSNB and LP in horses.[5]

Microphthalmia is reported to be an inherited defect in Texel sheep, but the incidence is low. It is a well-recognized genetic defect of Texel sheep in Europe. Following importation and "breeding up" of the breed in New Zealand in the 1990s, animals were released from quarantine for further expansion of the breed. The abnormality has occurred in a number of flocks in New Zealand, and an experimental breeding flock is maintained to study the molecular genetics. It is inherited as an autosomal-recessive trait. An outbreak in Texel sheep in New Zealand has been recorded. The optic globes are approximately one-half normal size, and the optic nerves at the chiasma are approximately one-half normal size. No other lesions are present in any organs. The retina is composed of an irregular mass attached to and continuous with the ciliary apparatus at one pole and connected to the optic nerve posteriorly by a short stalk. The morphology and morphogenesis of the defect has been followed in embryos at different ages from ewes known to be carriers of the microphthalmia factor. The primary event was abnormal development of the lens vesicle, with disintegration of the lens and subsequent overgrowth of mesenchymal tissue. The mesenchymal tissue later differentiated in various directions, whereas the epithelial structures found in the microphthalmic eyes at days 56 and 132 of gestation and in newborn lambs appeared to be remnants of the epithelial lens vesicle.

Typical colobomata, ophthalmoscopically visible defects of one or more structures of the eye, caused by an absence of tissue, have assumed a more prominent position than previously because of their high level of occurrence in Charolais cattle. The lesions are present at birth and do not progress beyond that stage. They affect vision very little, if at all. However, because they are defects they should be named in certificates of health, but they are not usually considered as being a reason for disqualification from breeding programs. In Charolais cattle the inheritance of the defect is via an autosomal-dominant gene with complete penetrance in males and partial (52%) penetrance in females. The prevalence may be as high as 6%, and in most cases both eyes are affected. The defect is a result of incomplete closure of one of the ocular structures at or near the line of the embryonic choroidal fissure. Failure of the fissure to close represents the beginnings of the coloboma. The retina, choroid, and sclera are usually all involved.

Entropion is inherited in a number of sheep breeds, including Oxfords, Hampshires, and Suffolks. Affected lambs are not observed until about 3 weeks of age when attention is drawn to the eyelids of the apparent conjunctivitis. A temporary blindness results, but even without treatment there is a marked improvement in the eyelids. Congenital entropion occurs in related Boer goat kids, but the mode of inheritance, if any, is unknown.[13]

Distichiasis, in which aberrant cilia are present at the eyelid margin, appears to occur with greater frequency in Friesian horses, in which rigid cilia cause corneal irritation or corneal ulceration. Although an inherited cause is suspected, the etiology is unclear.[14]

Ocular dermoids are recorded as genetically transmitted in Hereford cattle. They occur as multiple small masses of dystrophic skin complete with hair on the conjunctiva of both eyes of affected cattle. They can be anywhere on the cornea, on the third eyelid, or the eyelid, and they may completely replace the cornea; there may be a resulting marked dysplasia of the internal ocular structures.

Ocular dermoid cysts are single, solid, skin-like masses of tissue, adherent usually to the anterior surface of the eye, causing irritation and interfering with vision (Fig. 16-13). The eyelid, the third eyelid, and the canthus may also be involved, and the lesions may be unilateral or bilateral. When they occur at a high frequency in a population, it is likely they are inherited, as they can be in Hereford cattle. It is also recorded in foals. The defect is sometimes associated with microphthalmos. Surgical ablation is recommended.

Nasolacrimal duct fistulae, either unilateral or bilateral, occur in Brown Swiss cattle. The defect, evidenced by persistent epiphora and presence of a nasolacrimal fistula medial to the medial canthus of the eye, is inherited, although the mode of inheritance is unclear.[15,16]

Combined Ocular Defects

Although the vision appears unaffected, a large number of congenital defects of the eye

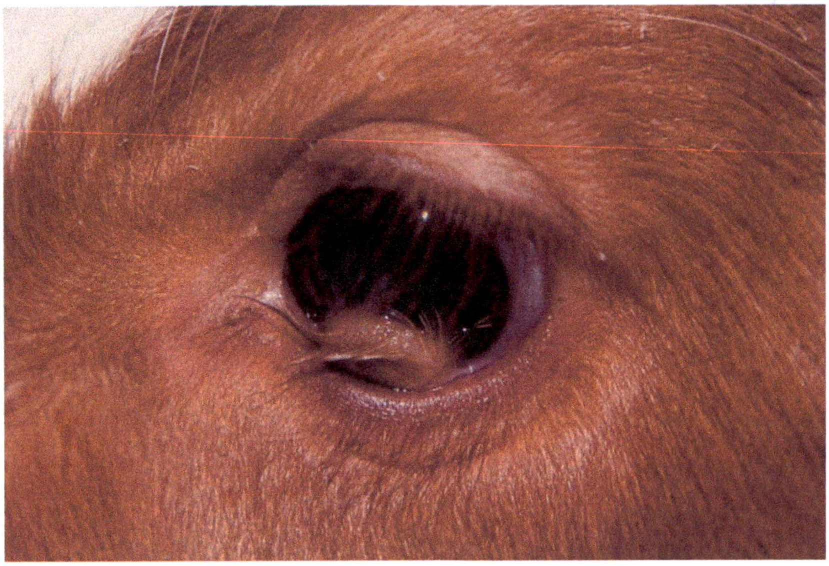

Fig. 16-13 Ocular dermoid cyst on the ventral corneal and limbus of the left eye of a Simmental calf.

have been observed in cattle, including Herefords, affected by partial albinism. The defects include iridal heterochromia, tapetum fibrosum, and colobomas. Congenital blindness is also seen in cattle with white coat color, especially Shorthorns. The lesions are multiple and include retinal detachment, cataract, microphthalmia, persistent pupillary membrane, and vitreous hemorrhage. Internal hydrocephalus is present in some, and hypoplasia of optic nerves also occurs.

A combination of **iridal hypoplasia, limbic dermoids, and cataracts** occurred in the progeny of a Quarter horse stallion, presumably as a result of a mutation in the stallion and transmission to the foals via an autosomal-dominant gene. The inheritance is simple autosomal recessive.

Irideremia (total or partial absence of iris), **microphakia** (smallness of the lens), ectopia lentis, and cataract have been reported to occur together in Jersey calves. The mode of inheritance of the characters is as a simple recessive trait. The calves are almost completely blind but are normal in other respects and can be reared satisfactorily if they are hand-fed. Although the condition has been recorded only in Jerseys, similar defects, possibly inherited, have also been seen in Holsteins and Shorthorns.

Multiple congenital ocular abnormalities occur with high frequency in Rocky Mountain horses and the closely related breeds Kentucky Mountain Saddle horse and Mountain Pleasure horse.[1,12,17,18] The cause is a missense mutation in the PMEL gene that has pleiotropic effects on the eye and coat color, causing a dilute or "silver" coat.[17] Similar to the silver mutation, MCOA is controlled by a dominant gene, with some reports demonstrating a codominant mode of inheritance and incomplete penetrance.[3,18] Homozygotes are thought to be more severely affected, having multiple abnormalities, whereas heterozygotes have cysts only, although this may not always be the case. Incomplete penetrance of this disorder has made studying the molecular mechanism behind these eye phenotypes difficult. Individuals carrying the causative mutation that are phenotyped as normal may either have cysts that were too small to detect or be true cases of nonpenetrance.[18] Equine MCOA is characterized by a diverse set of ocular phenotypes.[18] The predominant phenotype consists of large cysts, which are often bilateral, originating from the temporal ciliary body or peripheral retina, and additional phenotypes include abnormalities of the cornea, iris, lens, and iridocorneal angle.[18]

INHERITED NYSTAGMUS

Familial Undulatory Nystagmus

Familial undulatory nystagmus is an inherited defect of Finnish Ayrshire cattle characterized by a tremor-like, synchronous movement of the eyeballs. The tremor has small amplitude (1 to 2 mm) and fast (200/min) rate and is usually vertical. Nystagmus is present at all times, there is no sign of impaired vision, and the eye reflexes are normal. The condition is a blemish rather than a disease because there is no functional deficiency.

Pendular Nystagmus

Pendular nystagmus is an inherited defect of Holstein–Friesian cattle observed primarily in North America. A report from 1981 utilizing a convenience sample in New York state reported a prevalence of 0.51% in 2932 cattle from 62 herds. Affected cattle have a high-frequency (approximately 100 to 200 horizontal oscillations/minute) nystagmus of both eyes, with the eyes moving approximately 1 mm. Nystagmus has been observed shortly after birth in some calves, but the age of onset is not accurately known. Adult animals appear to be unaffected by the nystagmus and appear to have normal vision and balance and ocular reflexes. Pendular nystagmus is not thought to affect production and should not be mistaken as indicating the presence of a serious neurologic disease.

REFERENCES

1. Kaps S, et al. *Pferdeheilkunde*. 2010;26:536.
2. Tetens J, et al. *Tierarztl Prax Ausg G Grosstiere Nutztiere*. 2007;35:211.
3. Andersson LS, et al. *BMC Genet*. 2008;9.
4. Andersson LS, et al. *Mamm Genome*. 2011;22:353.
5. Bellone RR, et al. *Genetics*. 2008;179:1861.
6. Brunberg E, et al. *BMC Genet*. 2006;7.
7. Moemke S, et al. *Vet J*. 2007;173:272.
8. Fink S, et al. *Mol Vision*. 2012;18:2229.
9. Momke S, et al. *Anim Gen*. 2008;39:544.
10. Krump L, et al. *Irish Vet J*. 2014;67.
11. Pinard CL, et al. *Vet Ophthalmol*. 2011;14:100.
12. Bellone RR. *Anim Gen*. 2010;41:100.
13. Donnelly KS, et al. *Vet Ophthalmol*. 2014;17:443.
14. Hermans H, et al. *Equine Vet J*. 2014;46:458.
15. Braun U, et al. *BMC Vet Res*. 2014;10.
16. Braun U, et al. *Schweiz Arch Tierheilkd*. 2012;154:121.
17. Andersson LS, et al. *PLoS ONE*. 2013;8.
18. Grahn BH, et al. *Can Vet J*. 2008;49:675.

External Ear Diseases

OTITIS EXTERNA

Otitis externa, inflammation of the skin and external auditory canal, can affect cattle of all ages, in isolated cases, an entire herd, or in entire regions.

Arthropod parasites, foreign bodies, and sporadic miscellaneous infections may cause irritation in the ear, accompanied by rubbing of the head against objects and frequent head-shaking.

In tropical and subtropical regions, parasitic otitis is more important than in other more temperate regions. The mites *Raillietia auris* and *Dermanyssus avium*, the tick *Otobius magnini*, larvae (*Stephanofilaria zahaeeri*), free-living nematodes (*Rhabditis bovis*), and the blue fly (*Chrysomia bezziano*) are of importance in Europe, Africa, India, and America. *Malassezia* spp., *Candida* spp., *Rhodotorula mucilaginosa*, *Aspergillus* spp., and *Micelia sterilia* are common causes of otitis externa in cattle in Brazil.

When the syndrome occurs in a large number of animals in a herd, as it does in tropical countries, it is necessary to identify the specific causative agent. *R. bovis* is a common cause. Affected animals are depressed, eat little, and appear to experience pain when they swallow, and they shake their heads frequently. Both ears are affected in most cases, and there is a stinky, blood-stained discharge that creates a patch of alopecia below the ear. The area is painful when touched, the external meatus of the aural canal is obviously inflamed, and the parotid lymph nodes are enlarged. Extension to the middle ear is an unusual sequel. Topical treatment with ivermectin and a broad-spectrum antibiotic is effective.

Circumscribed ulcerative lesions on the ears with raised edges frequently associated with secondary bacterial or fungal infection are a common finding in cattle and buffaloes affected by buffalopox virus infection (see also "Coxpox and Bufallopox").

FURTHER READING

Duarte ER, Hamdan JS. Otitis in cattle, an aetiological review. *J Vet Med B Infect Dis Vet Public Health*. 2004;51:1-7.

EAR-TIP NECROSIS

Currently, ear-tip necrosis of pigs appears to be a more common condition.

ETIOLOGY

The condition may be associated with the presence of *Treponema pedis*. It can be cultured from the lesions and from the gingivae of pigs. It is anaerobic, fastidious, 4 mm to 6 mm in length, and 0.25 microns in diameter. There may be a sequence of infections when *Staphylococcus hyicus* is followed by the spirochetes and then infected with streptococci. In a recent study of putative agents, no single cause could be found, and it was suggested that the condition is multifactorial.[1]

EPIDEMIOLOGY

Ear-tip necrosis is usually seen in pigs at 1 to 16 weeks of age with a peak around 8 to 10 weeks. It may also occur in older pigs, when it is usually seen at the base of the ear. Typically it may occur in only one litter of pigs, and 80% may be affected. It may be associated with mixing and moving when a lot of pigs show ear biting.

Contributing factors are thought to include poor hygiene, high humidity, low air changes, overstocking, abrasions on feeders and pen divisions, and fighting associated with moving and mixing.

CLINICAL SIGNS

The affected pigs appear to show little evidence of distress and often recover spontaneously, and in these cases the only evidence of the condition is a crinkled edge to the ears. When it first appears, if the grease on the ear is removed you can see a crack in the skin, which obviously then allows bacterial penetration. Some persistent lesions may enlarge and spread. Occasionally, pigs show inappetence, unthriftiness, fever, or even death, often as a result of secondary infections.

PATHOLOGY

The lesions are black areas of necrosis with ulcers on the tips of the ears and the caudal edge of the ears. The lesions are dry and crusty, and in some cases there may be loss of the whole ear or part of the ear. This is caused by progressive thrombi formation leading to ischemia because there is a poor collateral circulation in the ear. In cases reported in Sweden, spirochetes were observed in silver-stained histologic sections, and a spirochete isolate was obtained and identified as a yet unnamed species of the genus *Treponema* closely resembling those found in digital dermatitis in cattle. The same organism was isolated from oral samples, along with *T. socranskii*.[2]

DIFFERENTIAL DIAGNOSIS

Simple ear biting is the main differential, but this usually starts at the base of the ear. Other septicemic causes of ear tissue loss, such as *H. parasuis*, *Salmonella*, or *S. suis*, may be suspected when ears are discolored, congested, or necrotic.

TREATMENT

Antibiotic sprays may or may not help.[2,3] A recent study has suggested that vaccination for PCV-2 infections may reduce the incidence of ear-tip necrosis.[4]

REFERENCES

1. Weissenbacher-Lang C, et al. *Vet J*. 2012;194:392.
2. Pringle M, et al. *Vet Micro*. 2010;139:279.
3. Pringle M, et al. *Vet Micro*. 2010;142:461.
4. Pejsak Z, et al. *Res Vet Sci*. 2011;91:125.

INHERITED CROP EARS

Inherited as a single autosomal-dominant incomplete character in Bavarian Highland cattle, the crop ear anomaly affects both ears, appears at birth, and varies from a minor trimming up to a complete deformity and reduction in size.

17 Metabolic and Endocrine Diseases

Introduction

Metabolic diseases are very important in dairy cows and pregnant ewes. In the other livestock species, metabolic diseases occur only sporadically. The high-producing dairy cow always verges on abnormal homeostasis, and the breeding and feeding of dairy cattle for high milk yields is etiologically related to metabolic disease so common in these animals. The salient features of the common metabolic diseases of farm animals are summarized in Table 17-1.

The term ***production disease*** includes those diseases previously known as ***metabolic diseases***, such as parturient paresis (milk fever), hypokalemia, hypomagnesemia, hyperketonemia and ketosis, hyperlipemia, and other conditions that are attributable to an imbalance between the rates of **input** of dietary nutrients and the **output** of production. When the imbalance is maintained, it may lead to a change in the amount of the body's reserves of certain metabolites and their "throughput." This generalization applies principally to energy balance (such as ketosis and hypoglycemia), in addition to hypomagnesemia, and to a lesser extent hypocalcemia. In these diseases output is greater than input, either because of the selection of cattle that produce so heavily that no naturally occurring diet can maintain the cow in nutritional balance or because the diet is insufficient in nutrient density or unevenly balanced. For example, a ration may contain sufficient protein for milk production but contains insufficient precursors of glucose to replace the energy excreted in the milk. Although we agree with the generalization on which the term *production disease* is based, we prefer to continue to use the expression *metabolic disease* because of common usage and the clinical focus that metabolism must match the level of production.

Metabolic Diseases of Ruminants

PERIPARTURIENT PERIOD IN CATTLE AND SHEEP

The incidence of metabolic disease in dairy cattle increases as milk production increases and, in particular, as the rate of increase in milk production increases (called **milk yield acceleration**). In dairy cows, the total disease incidence rapidly increases in the very late periparturient period, peaks on the day of parturition, and then rapidly declines until day 7 of lactation (Fig. 17-1). This critical 7-day window starting with parturition has a tremendous influence on morbidity, lactation production, reproductive performance, and mortality.

The susceptibility of dairy cows to metabolic disease appears to be related to the extremely high turnover of water, electrolytes, and soluble organic materials during the early part of lactation. With this rapid rate of exchange of water, sodium, calcium, magnesium, chloride, and phosphate, a sudden variation in their excretion or secretion in milk or by other routes, or a sudden variation in their intake because of changes in ingestion, digestion, or absorption, may cause abrupt, damaging changes in the internal environment of the animal. It is the volume of the changes in intake and secretion and the rapidity with which they can occur that affect the metabolic stability of the cow. In addition, if the continued nutritional demands of pregnancy are exacerbated by an inadequate diet in the dry period, the incidence of metabolic disease will increase. The effect of pregnancy is particularly important in ewes, especially those carrying more than one lamb.

Transition Period in Dairy Cows

The transition period is a crucial stage in the production cycle of the dairy cow; no other

Table 17-1 Salient features of metabolic diseases of farm animals

Disease	Etiology and epidemiology	Diagnosis	Treatment	Control
Milk fever of cattle	Hypocalcemia Occurs primarily in dairy cows after third lactation Also in beef cows 48 hours before or after calving and in midlactation	Low serum calcium concentration	Calcium salts IV, SC	Dietary management of anions–cations
Downer cow	Complication of milk fever; recumbent too long before treatment	Clinical findings Serum CK activity	Supportive therapy	Early treatment of milk-fever cases
Acute hypokalemia of cattle	In lactating dairy cows treated with corticosteroids for recurrent ketosis, and mastitis	Low serum potassium concentration	Potassium chloride IV	Avoid excessive use of isoflupredone for recurrent ketosis
Lactation tetany of mares	High-producing lactating mares being nursed by vigorous well-nourished foal a few weeks of age	Low serum calcium concentration	Calcium borogluconate	No reliable method available
Hypomagnesemic tetany (lactation tetany)	Lactating dairy cows on lush fertilized pastures Also in beef cows before and after calving	Low serum magnesium concentration	Magnesium salts IV	Supplementation of diets at strategic times with magnesium salts
Ketosis of cattle	Before and after parturition in cattle	Blood, urine, and milk levels of ketone bodies during the transition period 3 weeks before and after parturition	Glucose IV Propylene glycol and electrolyte solutions orally	Prepartum dietary management of energy intake
Pregnancy toxemia of sheep	Declining plane of nutrition in ewes in late pregnancy	Urinary ketones Hypoglycemia Metabolic acidosis and terminal uremia	Cesarean section or induction of parturition	Nutritional management of pregnant ewes to ensure a rising plane of nutrition in the second half of pregnancy
Fatty liver of cattle	High-producing dairy cows overfed during the dry period In well-conditioned beef cattle in late pregnancy when energy intake suddenly decreased	Ketonemia, ketonuria, hypoglycemia	Poor prognosis in severe cases Fluid and electrolyte therapy, glucose IV, propylene glycol orally and insulin	Nutritional management of pregnant cows to avoid excessive weight gain Avoid situations that reduce feed intake at time of parturition
Equine hyperlipidemia	Deranged fat metabolism Pregnant or lactating middle-aged ponies, donkeys, and American miniature horses worldwide Sporadic	Hyperlipidemia	Enteral or parenteral feeding, insulin, heparin Treat underlying disease	Maintain optimal body condition Prevent disease and nutritional stress in pregnancy
Postparturient hemoglobinuria	Dietary deficiency in high-producing dairy cows 2–4 weeks after calving Copper-deficient area Cruciferous crops	Low serum inorganic phosphorus concentration Low PCV Hemoglobinuria	Whole blood transfusion Sodium acid phosphate IV Dicalcium phosphate orally	Ensure adequate dietary phosphorous intake

period can affect subsequent production, health, and reproductive performance so greatly. The success of the transition period effectively determines the profitability of the cow during that lactation. Nutritional or management limitations during this time may impede the ability of the cow to reach maximal milk production. The primary challenge faced by cows is a sudden and marked increase of nutrient requirements for milk production, at a time when dry matter intake, and thus nutrient supply, lags far behind. Dry matter intake typically declines during the final week before parturition. This decline and changes in endocrine profiles contribute to elevated plasma nonesterified fatty acid (NEFA) concentrations, which have been related to the occurrence of fat-mobilization-related metabolic diseases such as fatty liver and ketosis. The magnitude of the decline in feed intake as parturition approaches may be a better indicator of metabolic health of postpartum cows than the actual level of feed intake. Diet, body-condition score, and parity influence dry matter intake and energy balance. The occurrence of diseases during the transition period results in lost milk production during the time of illness and often for the entire lactation.

A key area of the biology of transition cows is lipid metabolism. Excessive lipid metabolism from adipose tissue is linked with a higher incidence of periparturient diseases. Fatty livers were described in ketotic cows in the 1950s. Hepatic fat accumulation was then noted in normal cows during early lactation. This was followed by a description of a **fat-mobilization syndrome** in early lactation, in which cows mobilized body lipids from adipose tissue and deposited lipids in the liver, muscle, and other tissues. This was followed by descriptions of elevated nonesterified fatty acid concentrations during the last 7 days before calving being associated with a higher incidence of ketosis, displaced abomasum, and retained fetal membranes, but not associated with the incidence of milk fever. Understanding the metabolism of NEFA by the liver is a critical component of understanding the biology of the transition cow. Extreme rates of lipid

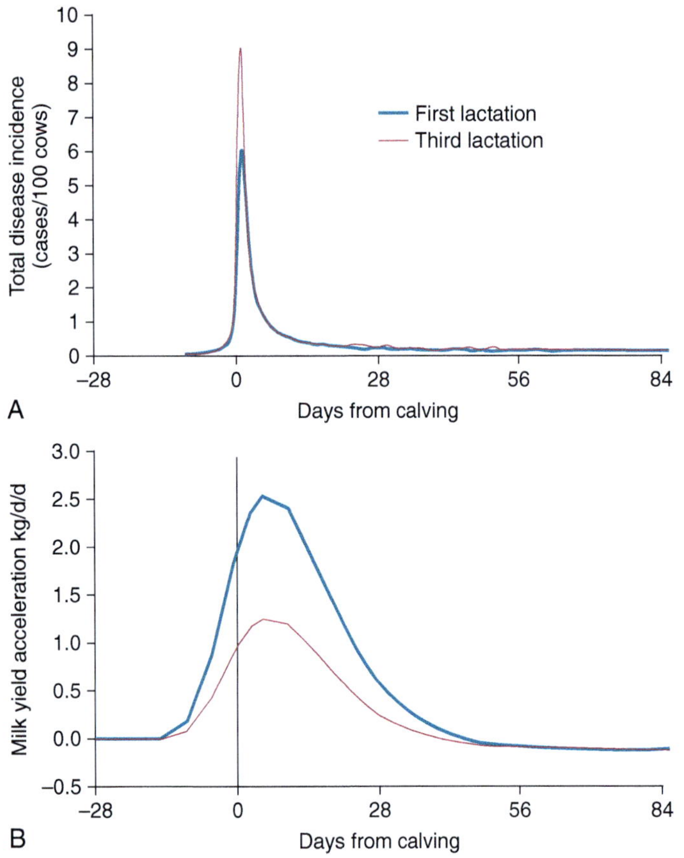

Fig. 17-1 **A,** Total disease incidence (sum of mastitis, ketosis, digestive disorders, and laminitis) relative to days from calving for first- and third-lactation cows in Danish dairy herds that calved in 1998. **B,** Acceleration in milk yield through lactation for cows peaking at 30 kg or 60 kg (bold line) of milk daily. (Reproduced with permission from Ingvartsen KL. Anim Feed Sci Technol 2006; 126:175-213.)

mobilization lead to increased uptake of NEFA by the liver and an increased rate of triglyceride accumulation in the liver. If this lipid infiltration becomes severe, the syndrome of hepatic lipidosis or fatty liver may result, which can then result in prolonged recovery from other diseases, increased incidence of other diseases, and increased susceptibility to induction of ketosis.

During the transition period, dairy cows undergo large metabolic adaptations in glucose, fatty acid, and mineral metabolism. The practical goal of nutritional management during this period is to support these metabolic adaptations. There are two different philosophic approaches for feeding transition cows in animals fed a total mixed ration. The first approach increases the energy density of the diet to "correct" for the anticipated decrease in dry matter intake in late gestation. Increasing the amount of energy supplied through dietary carbohydrate during the prepartum period results in generally positive effects on metabolism and performance of transition cows. In contrast, the second approach focuses on decreasing the energy density and increasing forage (by the daily provision of 2 to 4 kg of straw) in far-off cattle in an attempt to promote dry matter intake. Attempts to increase energy supply by feeding dietary fat sources or decrease energy expenditure by supplying specific fatty acids such as *trans*-10, *cis*-12conjugated linoleic acid to decrease milk-fat output during early lactation do not decrease the release of NEFAs from adipose tissue.

In addition to nutritional management strategies to optimize the health of the transition cow, certain feed additives are in use to reduce subclinical ketosis and reduce the incidence of displaced abomasum. **Monensin** is a carboxylic polyether ionophore produced by a naturally occurring strain of *Streptomyces cinnamonesis.* Monensin exerts its many effects by shifting the microbial populations in the rumen; this results in changes in the proportions of short-chain volatile fatty acids in the rumen, specifically increasing propionic acid and reducing the molar percentages of butyric acid and acetic acid. Increased rumen propionic acid concentrations directly lead to increased gluconeogenesis and should therefore decrease the incidence of ketosis and hyperketonemia in early lactation and improve energy balance. In Canada, monensin is approved to be administered as a controlled-release capsule (CRC) as an aid in the prevention of subclinical ketosis in lactating dairy cattle. The monensin CRC delivers 335 mg of monensin daily for 95 days, improves energy balance, and decreases the incidence of all three energy-associated diseases of lactating dairy cows: retained placenta, displaced abomasum, and clinical ketosis. Cows treated with the monensin CRC at 3 weeks before the anticipated calving date had decreased serum NEFA and β-hydroxybutyrate (BHB) concentrations and increased serum cholesterol and urea concentrations in the week immediately preceding precalving. Monensin has no effect on serum calcium, phosphorus, or glucose concentration in the precalving period. After calving, serum concentrations of BHB and phosphorus concentrations were lower and serum concentrations of cholesterol and urea higher in monensin-treated cows. The lower NEFA values indicate less fat mobilization, and the higher cholesterol suggests greater lipoprotein export from the liver. The higher urea levels are thought to result from a protein-sparing effect in the rumen, resulting in an increased supply of amino acids in the small intestine. There was no effect of treatment on serum NEFA, glucose, or calcium concentrations in the first week postcalving. Daily monensin ingestion starting before calving therefore improves indicators of energy balance in both the immediate precalving and postcalving periods.

Voluntary Dry Matter Intake in Periparturient Dairy Cattle

The factors affecting voluntary dry matter intake (DMI) of lactating cattle are extremely important and have received much attention for many decades. A substantial decrease in DMI is initiated in late pregnancy and continues into early lactation, with the lowest DMI occurring on the day of calving. Postpartum DMI is considerably higher in multiparous cows compared with primiparous cows and increases after lactation in both groups, but the rate of increases varies widely. In cows given diets of constant composition, the milk yield typically peaks at 5 to 7 weeks postpartum, and the maximum intake is reached between 8 and 22 weeks after calving. The increase in DMI from week 1 postpartum to time of peak intake is affected by the diet fed during lactation and also by prepartum feeding; the latter influences the amount of fat stored and therefore the body-condition score of the animal. The normal pattern of feed intake may be severely influenced by disease states because both clinical and subclinical infections are known to substantially reduce appetite and performance.

The decrease in DMI has traditionally been attributed to physical constraints such as the enlarging uterus, but this role may be overemphasized. The decrease in DMI coincides with changes in reproductive status, changes in fat mass, and metabolic changes in support of lactation. A number of metabolic signals may have a role in intake regulation. These signals include nutrients, metabolites, reproductive hormones, stress hormones, leptin, insulin, gut peptides, cytokines and neuropeptides such as neuropeptide Y, galanin, and corticotrophin-releasing factor.

Immunosuppression During the Transition Period

In addition to the adaptations in classical metabolism, cows during the transition period also undergo a period of reduced immunologic capacity during the periparturient period. The immune dysfunction is broad in scope, affects multiple functions of various cell types, and lasts from approximately 3 weeks before calving until approximately 3 weeks after calving. Cows during this period are more susceptible to mastitis. The etiology of periparturient immunosuppression is multifactorial and not well understood, but it seems to be related to physiologic changes associated with parturition and the initiation of lactation and to metabolic factors related to these events. Glucocorticoids are immunosuppressants, plasma cortisol concentration is increased at parturition, and endogenous glucocorticoids have been postulated to play a role in periparturient immunosuppression. Periparturient cattle have impaired expression of adhesion molecules and decreased migration capacity of blood neutrophils. Because the rapid recruitment of neutrophils into newly infected mammary tissue is the key immunologic defense against mastitis-causing pathogens in ruminants, periparturient neutrophil dysfunction may contribute to the increased susceptibility to mastitis at this time. Metabolic challenges around calving may also play in role in increased susceptibility, as non-esterified fatty acids significantly reduce the in vitro immunosuppressiveness of mononuclear cells of ewes, potentially resulting in impairment of cell-mediated and humoral immunity in sheep and cattle with ketosis.

Vitamin E is a fat-soluble membrane antioxidant that enhances the functional efficiency of neutrophils by protecting them from oxidative damage following intracellular killing of ingested bacteria. The parenteral administration of vitamin E has been investigated for the prevention of peripartum diseases such as retained placenta, metritis, and clinical mastitis. Only cows with marginal vitamin E status (serum α-tocopherol < 2.5 $\times 10^{-3}$) 1 week before calving will have a reduction in the risk of retained placenta following a subcutaneous injection of 3000 IU of vitamin E. In cows with an adequate serum vitamin E concentration there was no reduction, and primiparous animals were most likely to benefit from vitamin E 1 week before parturition. The associations between peripartum serum vitamin E, retinol, and β-carotene concentrations in dairy cattle and disease risk indicated that an increase in α-tocopherol of 1 μg/ML in the last week prepartum reduced the risk of retained placenta by 20%, whereas serum NEFA concentrations ≥ 0.5 mEq/L tended to increase the risk of retained placenta by 80%. In the last week prepartum, a 100-ng/mL increase in serum retinol was associated with a 60%decrease in the risk of early-lactation clinical mastitis.

Diseases of Lactation

Parturition is followed by the sudden onset of a profuse lactation, which, if the nutrient reserves have already been seriously depleted, may result in clinical metabolic disease. The essential metabolite that is reduced below the critical level determines the clinical syndrome that will occur. Most attention has been paid to variations in balances of calcium and inorganic phosphates relative to parturient paresis, magnesium relative to lactation tetany, and plasma glucose and ketone concentration and hepatic lipidosis relative to ketosis, but it is probable that other imbalances are important in the production of as yet unidentified syndromes.

The vast majority of production diseases of dairy cows occur very early in lactation. At this time, the cow is producing milk at a rate that is substantially less than her maximum. In terms of rate, high- and low-milk-yielding cows are producing rather similar amounts at this time. However, in terms of acceleration, the change in milk yield per day, it is highest immediately after calving. During the succeeding period of lactation, particularly in cows on test schedules and under the strain of producing large quantities of milk, there is often variable food intake, especially when pasture is the sole source of food, and instability of the internal environment inevitably follows. The period of early lactation is an unstable one in all species. Hormonal stimulation at this stage is so strong that nutritional deficiency often does not limit milk production, and a serious drain on reserves of metabolites may occur.

Recombinant bovine somatotrophin (rBST, sometribove zinc) is a synthetically derived hormone that may be identical to naturally occurring bovine growth hormone, or slightly modified by the addition of extra amino acids. The product was approved in the United States in 1993, and its use began commercially in 1994 in dairy herds to increase milk production. The product is a sterile, prolonged-release injectable formulation of rBST in single-dose syringes that each contain 500 mg of sometribove zinc. The recommended dosage protocol is one syringe injected subcutaneously (SC) in the postscapular region (behind the shoulders) or in the ischiorectal fossa (depression on either side of the tailhead) every 14 days beginning during the 9th week after calving and continuing until the end of lactation.[2] Approximately 15% of dairy herds in the United States used rBST in 2013. The product has been licensed for use in at least 20 other countries, including Argentina, Brazil, Chile, Colombia, Costa Rica, Ecuador, Egypt, Guatemala, Honduras, Jamaica, Lebanon, Mexico, Panama, Pakistan, Paraguay, Peru, Salvador, South Africa, South Korea, Uruguay, and Venezuela. In comparison, a number of countries, including Australia, Canada, Israel, Japan, New Zealand, and all European Union countries, have not approved its use.

A meta-analysis of the effects of rBST on milk production, animal health, reproductive performance, and culling was undertaken. Recombinant bovine somatotrophin was found to increase milk production by 11% in primiparous cows and 15% in multiparous cows, although there was considerable variation in the magnitude of the milk production increase between studies. Some statistically significant effects on milk composition (percentage of butterfat, protein, and lactose) were found; however, they were all very small. Treatment increased dry matter intake by an average of 1.5 kg/d during the treatment period, and dry matter intake remained elevated for the first 60 days of the subsequent lactation. Despite the increase in dry matter intake, treated animals had lower body-condition scores at the end of the treatment period, and the reduced scores persisted until the start of the subsequent lactation. Recombinant bovine somatotrophin increased the risk of clinical mastitis by approximately 25% during the treatment period, but there were insufficient data to draw firm conclusions about the effects of the drug on the prevalence of subclinical intramammary infections as assessed by somatic cell count. The increase in the incidence of clinical mastitis in cattle administered rBST appears similar to that expected from an increase in milk production alone using genetic selection and improved nutrition, milking frequency, and management practices. Use of rBST increased the risk of a cow failing to conceive by approximately 40%. For cows that did conceive, there was no effect on services per conception and only a small increase in average days open. Use of the drug had no effect on gestation length, but the information about a possible effect on twinning was equivocal. Cows treated with rBST had an estimated 55% increase in the risk of developing clinical signs of lameness. There appeared to be an increased risk of culling in multiparous cows. Use of the drug in one lactation period appeared to reduce the risk of metabolic diseases (particularly ketosis) in the early period of the subsequent lactation. It was found that the reproductive effects of the drug could be controlled by delaying its use until the cows were confirmed pregnant.

In 1998, an expert panel appointed by the Canadian Veterinary Medical Association at the request of Health Canada found a number of legitimate animal welfare concerns associated with the use of rBST. In 1999 Health Canada announced that it would not approve the use of rBST for sale in Canada on the basis of the health and welfare of cattle. The Royal College of Physicians and Surgeons of Canada's Expert Panel on Human Safety of rBST found no biologically plausible reason for concern about human safety if rBST were to be approved for sale in Canada. In 1999 a working group from within the Scientific Committee on Animal Health and Animal Welfare of the European Commission presented a more extensive report on rBST that summarized similar results and engaged substantive discussion of animal welfare issues. It concluded that rBST should not be used in dairy cattle in Europe. In October 1999, the European Commission banned the use and marketing of rBST in the European Union as of January 1, 2000.

Relationship Between Lactational Performance and Health of Dairy Cattle

There is little evidence that high-yielding cows have increased risk of dystocia, retained placenta, metritis, and left-side displacement of the abomasum. The association between high levels of production and periparturient diseases is inconsistent; in general, high levels of management (including nutrition and housing) are usually associated with high levels of production. Although no phenotypical relationship between milk yield and the risk of ketosis and lameness has been found, selection for higher milk yield will probably increase the lactational incidence risk for both diseases. Mastitis is the only disease for which a clear relationship between increased milk yield and increased risk of infection has been found. Continued selection for high milk yield should therefore be expected to increase the incidence of clinical mastitis in dairy cattle.

However, some authors have stated that "Reviewing existing literature, even with structured literature selection, is inadequate to the task of elucidating the relationship between the lactational performance and risk of production diseases."[3] The most notable feature of the literature evaluation is the large variability that exists between studies. This strongly suggests that there are important factors that need to be considered before meaningful conclusions concerning the relationship between lactational performance and risk of disease can be drawn.

Breed Susceptibility

The fact that some dams are affected much more by these variations than others is probably explainable on the basis of variations in internal metabolism and degree of milk production among species and among individuals. Among groups of cows, variations in susceptibility appear to depend on either genetic or management factors. Certainly, Jersey cows are more susceptible to parturient paresis than cows of other breeds. Even within breeds, considerable variation is evident in susceptibility between families. Under these circumstances, it seems necessary to invoke genetic factors as predisposing causes for metabolic diseases.

Management Practices

The management practices of most importance are nutrition and housing. In those sections of North America where cattle are housed during the winter and in poor pasture areas, ketosis is prevalent. In the Channel Islands, local cattle are unaffected by lactation tetany, whereas the disease is prevalent in the United Kingdom. In New Zealand, metabolic diseases are complex and the incidence is high, both of which are probably related to the practice of having the cows calve in late winter when feed is poor, the practice of depending entirely on pasture for feed, and the high proportion of Jerseys in the cattle population.

Detailed knowledge of the nutrition and housing factors is essential before any reasonable scheme of prevention can be undertaken. For example, knowledge of the complex behavioral needs of the dairy cow is essential to provide adequate housing during the transition period. In North American dairy herds, the flow of cows through the transition period often necessitates many changes of pens, which are disruptive to the social organization of cow groups. Stocking rates that exceed stall and feed bunk capacity place even greater challenges on the dairy cow at this time. Current free-stall recommendations include providing 75 cm (30 in.) of bunk space for close-up and fresh cows to ensure that overcrowding does not occur, moving preparturient cows to a new pen at least 8 to 10 days ahead of the anticipated calving date or when calving is imminent, adding cows to groups on a minimum of a weekly basis (it takes up to 1.5 days for a new social order to be determined after the addition of a new animal), and keeping a clean and comfortable environment.

The diagnosis and treatment of dairy cows with periparturient diseases requires a program suited to the particular herd. Particularly in large herds, there is a need for collaboration between the veterinarian, nutritionist, manager of the herd, and animal attendants. Specific procedures should be developed for each herd based on past experience with the problems of recently calved cows, the facilities, the skills of the workers, the priorities of management, and the flow patterns of the cows in the herd. Every effort must be made to prevent periparturient diseases in the cows. In general, diseases in the early postpartum period originate in the feeding and management of the dry cow. Important principles include a protocol of grouping parturient cows according to the feeding program and handling facilities on the farm. Groups of cows can be screened for mastitis, visual evidence of illness, daily milk yield, body temperature, and urine pH, and they can be palpated for evidence of metritis. Individual cows that have been identified by a screening method must be examined individually to make a diagnosis and decide on a treatment protocol based on the particular diagnosis.

Management and environmental factors can be manipulated to ease the transition into lactation. For example, the photoperiod, defined as the duration of light exposure an animal receives within a day, can be adjusted to produce clinically significant effects on periparturient health and subsequent lactational efficiency. Increasing the frequency of milking in the immediate postpartum period also produces persistent increases in milk yield and improvements in mammary health. In both techniques, evidence is emerging to support the concept that alteration of prolactin sensitivity is the mechanism underlying health and production responses. The reader is directed to publications related to production for more information on these and related topics.

Occurrence and Incidence of Metabolic Diseases

Knowledge of the etiologic and epidemiologic factors involved will help in understanding the occurrence and incidence of the various metabolic diseases. Largely because of variations in climate, the occurrence of metabolic disease varies from season to season and from year to year. In the same manner, variations in the types of disease occur. For example, in some seasons, most cases of parturient paresis will be tetanic; in others, most cases of ketosis will be complicated by hypocalcemia. Further, the incidence of metabolic disease and the incidence of the different syndromes will vary from region to region. Ketosis may be common in areas of low rainfall and on poor pasture. Lactation tetany may be common in colder areas and where natural shelter is poor. Recognition of these factors can make it possible to devise a means whereby the incidence of the diseases can be reduced.

The metabolic diseases, because of high prevalence and high mortality rate, are of major importance in some countries, so much so that predictive systems are being set up. Rapid analysis of stored feed samples, pasture, and soil is commonly used in Europe and North America, but the interesting development has been the recognition of "production diseases" and the consequent development of metabolic profile tests, particularly in the United Kingdom and Europe.

Record Keeping

The use of reliable records to monitor the health and production of dairy cows during the transition period is essential to evaluate the efficacy of programs at the farm level. Transition cow management programs will assist in determining how well cows are prepared for milk production and good health in the coming lactation. Appropriate monitoring should focus on three areas: **cows that die or are culled in early lactation, the productivity of the surviving cows in early lactation, and the rates of disease in the periparturient period.**

Cows that leave the herd in the first 60 days of lactation are usually culled because of disease or injury. Removal rates and their causes can be a critical monitor of the efficacy of transition cow management programs. Measuring productivity and health of cows in early lactation involves monitoring daily milk yields, first-test mature-equivalent 305-day projected milk, milk components at first Dairy Herd Improvement Association (DHIA) test day, milk-fat percentage, ratios of test-day components, somatic cell count at first DHIA test day, and peak milk (also called summit milk). DHIA records also allow comparison of the performance of each cow in early lactation to her performance in the prior lactation. Comparisons can be made of the changes in somatic cell count between the last test of the prior lactation and the first test of the current lactation and mature-equivalent 305-day difference from the prior lactation to the first test of the current lactation.

Health and production records in dairy herds have traditionally emphasized reproductive events and administered treatments for specific diseases. The records should capture the information about the common diseases that occur in most dairy herds. The record system should be set up to do the following:

- Monitor rates of well-defined disease events as a measure of the effectiveness of health and production programs and to aid in problem solving.
- Determine the clinical efficacy of treatments by monitoring retreatment rates for specific diseases.
- Maintain an individual cow history record for cow-side use to enhance treatment decisions.
- Measure compliance and consistency of implementation of the health program being used.
- Reconcile pharmaceutical purchases with treatment protocol entries and to meet regulatory requirements on the use of pharmaceuticals in food animals.
- Determine the costs of certain disease rates over achievable targets. The costs of specific diseases are compelling to most dairy herd producers. Good records can generate an incidence rate of common diseases. These costs include the immediate cost of treatment, the cost of the veterinarian's and herdsman's time. and the cost of milk withheld from the market. For the majority of diseases of recently calved cows, the cost per disease in the United States was estimated in 2001 at approximately US$320, with a range from $150 to $450.

An adequate record system will allow producers and veterinarians to determine the differences between actual performance and benchmark performance and then determine the causes of the shortfall. The most important determinants of profitability on dairy farms are milk income and feed cost, and the difference between milk income and feed costs is the **return-over-feed** index (**ROF**). Many factors affect the ROF index. These include three-times-daily milking, component percentages in the herd milk test, milk-fat and protein percentages, use of a core lipopolysaccharide antigen mastitis vaccine, and use of monensin in the lactating-cow diet (if permitted). One of the most important factors associated with profitability is milk production. From 80% to 95% of the income on dairy farms is derived from milk sales. Thus it is critical that the producer, the veterinarian, and other advisors collaborate to plan an animal health and production program that will result in the optimum ROF.

METABOLIC PROFILE TESTING

Methods are needed to monitor the nutritional and metabolic status of dairy herds. The most valuable methods will be those that are sensitive enough to detect change before clinical or economic consequences are manifested. A major challenge in the application of metabolic profile testing is dealing with extraneous sources of variation. Successful management of extraneous variation requires sampling strategies based on animal grouping and testing of multiple animals. Larger herds are more suitable for monitoring because they allow for better design sampling strategies and spread the costs of testing across more animals. Statistical process control methods offer a unique approach to interpretation that may increase the usefulness of metabolic profiles.

The traditional approach to herd-based assessment of metabolic status (also called the **Compton metabolic profile test**) is based on the concept that the laboratory measurement of certain components of plasma or serum of 7 to 10 cows per subgroup will reflect the nutritional status of the subgroup, with or without the presence of clinical abnormalities.[1] For example, a lower-than-normal mean plasma glucose concentration in a group of dairy cows in early lactation may indicate an insufficient intake of energy, which may or may not be detectable clinically. On a theoretical basis, the ability of the laboratory to make an objective assessment of the input–output (nutrient–productivity) relationships is an attractive tool for the veterinarian engaged in providing a complete health management service to a herd. The test would theoretically be able to detect the qualitative and quantitative adequacy of the diet of cows expected to produce a certain quantity of milk or return to estrus within a desirable length of time following parturition. A reliable test for the early diagnosis of nutritional deficiency or metabolic disease would therefore be a major step forward in attempting to optimize livestock production and obtain maximum yields at minimum costs.

There was considerable interest in metabolic profile testing following its earlier descriptions, which stimulated considerable field research. The results of the research have thus far indicated that the test may be useful only as an aid in the diagnosis of nutritional imbalance and production diseases. The results of metabolic profile testing are usually difficult to interpret without a careful conventional assessment of the nutritional status and reproductive performance of the herd, and it appears doubtful that such testing would reveal significant abnormalities that could not be detected using conventional clinical methods. Because of the cost of the test, the profile testing must be carefully planned with specific objectives. A regional diagnostic laboratory with automated analytical equipment should be available, and this is often a major limiting factor. The test should not be undertaken unless reference values for each laboratory measurement are available from the population within the area. The results from the groups within the herd are compared with local population means. Metabolic profiles have also been suggested as an aid in the selection of superior individuals.

The prediction of whether an individual cow is metabolically prepared to undergo a stressful lactation at a high level of production would seem to be a useful undertaking. This could be particularly important under management conditions of heavy concentrate feeding, lead feeding, zero grazing, or even indoor housing. There are no well-established, low-cost, practical protocols for conducting such profile tests.

Usefulness of Metabolic Profile Testing

Metabolic profiles in dairy cows were used initially in the United Kingdom in the 1960s. Success was limited primarily by the unjustified expectation that all biochemical concentrations in the blood of cows would reflect nutritional intake and status at all times. However, the practical value was found in the approach as an aid to nutritional management. In the 1970s the approach was reassessed and revised, culminating in a program for farmers evaluating health and productivity using metabolic profile testing as an integral part of a health management program involving a multidisciplinary approach. The UK Dairy Herd Health and Productivity Service (DHHPS) provides the opportunity for veterinarians to lead a multidisciplinary team that can monitor health, fertility, and production and can plan, when necessary, corrective action. Effectively the approach has been to **"ask the cows"** what they think of their nutrition by following a set of guidelines on timing, cow selection, and the use of background information. Metabolic profiling and body-condition scoring found that at least a third of the cows sampled were mobilizing excessive fat during the transition from the dry period to early lactation. Improving both health and nutrition, before and after calving, would improve reproductive performance in many herds. The DHHPS method now utilizes a team approach involving farmer, veterinarian, and agricultural advisor. If useful information is to be obtained, the blood-testing aspect depends critically on following a set of firm criteria for selection of small groups of typical cows within each herd; the timing of testing in relation to concentrate feeds, feed changes, and stage of lactation; and the collection of other data about the cows, such as body weight and condition, productivity, and feeding. The successful approach has been to look, following specific times of nutritional change, at metabolite levels in strictly defined small representative groups of cows within each herd in conjunction with information on body condition and weight, milk performance, and feeding. Comparison with optimum values, the degree of variation from them, and comparisons between groups within herds have allowed information about nutritional constraints on productivity to be made available to farmers more quickly and more specifically than by other means.

Biological and Statistical Basis for Herd Testing

The interpretation of herd-based tests for metabolic diseases is different from interpreting laboratory tests for metabolites from individual cows. Test results from individual cows are interpreted by comparing the value to a normal reference range established by the laboratory that did the testing. Normal ranges are often derived by calculating a 95% confidence interval (or a similar statistic) of test results from 100 or more clinically normal animals.

Herd test results for metabolic diseases can be interpreted as either the **mean test result of the subgroup** sampled or as the **proportion of animals above or below a certain cut-point within the subgroup**. There is a major philosophic difference and marked cost difference between the two approaches. At the moment, there does not appear to be a clear preference for either approach, and this area should be a focus of future investigation. An important difference in the approaches is that the cost of determining the mean value of a subgroup is very low if the samples from the subgroup are pooled and then analyzed. The only advantage of analyzing individual samples instead of pooled samples is that individual samples provide an estimate of the proportion of abnormal values. Whether knowing the proportion is worth the marked increased in analytical cost remains to be determined.

If a metabolite is associated with disease when it is above or below a biologic threshold (cut-point), then it should be evaluated as a proportional outcome. For example, hyperketonemia (subclinical ketosis) in dairy herds can be monitored by testing for β-hydroxybutyrate (BHB) or other ketone bodies in blood, plasma, serum, urine, or milk. Subclinical ketosis is a threshold disease, and cows are affected only when ketone concentrations are elevated. Plasma BHB concentrations above 1.0, 1.2, or 1.4 mmol/L (equivalent to 9.7, 11.7, or 14.4 mg/dL, respectively) are the most commonly used cut-points for detecting hyperketonemia (subclinical ketosis) in lactating dairy cattle. Early-lactation cows with plasma BHB concentrations above the selected cut-point have a four- to eightfold greater risk of developing displaced abomasum, a threefold greater risk of developing clinical ketosis, decreased 305-day milk production, increased severity of mastitis, a 50% increase in anestrus at 60 days in milk, and a 50% decrease in pregnancy at first insemination. NEFA concentrations in plasma are an indicator of negative energy balance in prepartum cows. Elevated plasma NEFA concentration before calving (>0.4 mEq/L for cows between 2 and 14 days before the anticipated calving date) is associated with a 4-fold increased risk for displaced abomasum, a 2- to 3-fold increase in the risk of subclinical ketosis, and 1.5-fold increased risk of retained placenta after calving.

It is also necessary to determine the alarm level for the proportion of animals above or below the described cut-point. The alarm level is determined from research results or clinical experience. The suggested alarm-level proportion for plasma BHB concentration with a cut-point of 1.4 mmol/L is greater than 10%; the proportion for plasma NEFA concentration with a cut-point of 0.4 mmol/L is greater than 10%.

Herd-based testing is useful only when a sufficient number of cows within the herd are tested, which gives reasonable confidence that the results truly represent the entire population of eligible cows in the herd. In the United States, the minimum sample size for herd-based tests with proportional outcomes has been estimated as 12 cows, based on 75% confidence intervals and a general detection cut-point of greater than 10%. Cows to be sampled need to be selected from the appropriate eligible or at-risk group. Obviously, measurement of a homogeneous group requires a large herd size; to sample 12 cows consistently between day 4 and day 14 of lactation requires a milking herd of at least 428 cows, assuming equal monthly calving rates. The subgroup size recommendation of 12 cows in the United States contrasts with the subgroup size recommendation of 7 to 10 cows in the United Kingdom. The difference in recommendations has not been reconciled.

The proper use of metabolic profiles depends on the timing of blood tests, the selection of cows to be included, and the collection and use of background information about the farm, feeding and feeding system, and physical state and performance of the cows.

Variables in Dairy-Herd Metabolic Profile Testing

There are five main areas of interest for metabolic profile testing:

1. Energy balance
2. Protein evaluation
3. Liver function
4. Macromineral evaluation
5. Urine evaluation

In general terms, measurement of analytes in urine has been greatly underutilized in metabolic profile testing, and it is clear that current testing protocols are not economically optimized.

Energy Balance

Strategic use of metabolic testing to monitor transition dairy cows should focus on measuring plasma NEFA concentration in the last week prepartum and plasma/serum BHB and urine acetoacetate concentration in the first and second weeks postpartum.

Nonesterified Fatty Acids

Plasma NEFA concentration provides the most sensitive indicator of energy balance, particularly in the last 2 weeks of gestation. Plasma NEFA concentration is useful for monitoring the energy status of dry cows in the last month of gestation, when rapid changes in energy-balance status may not be detectable from changes in body-condition score. Plasma NEFA concentrations start to increase 3 days before parturition and remain elevated for the first 9 days of lactation[7] (Fig. 17-2). High plasma concentrations of NEFAs indicate negative energy balance, which occurs in animals that are inappetent as a result of illness.

The serum concentrations of NEFAs have been monitored in dairy cows as predictors of displaced abomasum. In cows with left-displaced abomasum (LDA), mean NEFA concentration began to diverge from the mean in cows without LDA 14 days before calving, whereas mean serum BHB concentrations did not diverge until the day of calving. Prepartum, only NEFA concentration was associated with risk of LDA. Between day 0 and 6 days after calving, cows

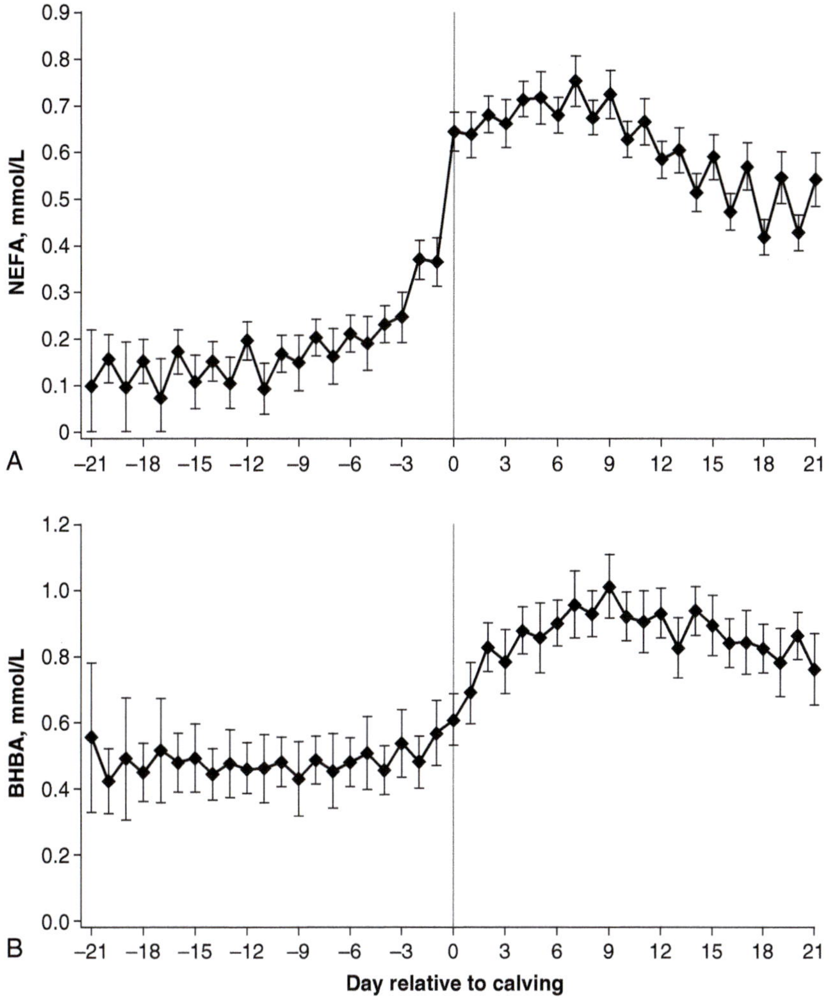

Fig. 17-2 Least-squares means and 95% confidence interval (error bars) for plasma nonesterified fatty acid concentration and β-hydroxybutyrate concentration in 269 multiparous Holstein–Friesian cows from 21 days prepartum to 21 days postpartum. (Reproduced with permission from McCarthy MM, Mann S, Nydam DV, Overton TR, McArt JAA. J Dairy Sci 2015; 98:6284-6290.)

with serum NEFA concentration of 0.5 mEq/L or greater were 3.6 times more likely to develop LDA after calving. In another study, cows with plasma NEFA greater than 0.3 mEq/L between 3 and 35 days before calving were twice as likely to subsequently have LDA. Strategic use of metabolic tests to monitor energy balance in prepartum dairy cows should therefore focus on measurement of plasma/serum NEFA concentration. There are three major drawbacks with this approach: the high cost of testing (US$8/test), the need to centrifuge blood to harvest serum or plasma, and the lack of a cow-side test. Until all three issues are satisfactorily resolved, plasma/serum NEFA testing will remain a research tool with minimal practical application.

β-Hydroxybutyrate

Plasma/serum BHB concentrations are affected by energy and glucose balance and are a less sensitive indicator of energy balance than plasma NEFA. High plasma BHB concentrations are associated with reduced milk production, increased incidence of clinical ketosis and LDA, and reduced fertility. The gold-standard test for hyperketonemia (subclinical ketosis) is plasma/serum BHB concentration, which is more stable after collection than plasma/serum acetone or acetoacetate concentrations. Prepartum BHB concentrations are relatively stable before parturition, but increase rapidly after parturition to peak at around 9 days in milk, after which time BHB concentration gradually declines (Fig. 17-2).

Subclinical ketosis may start at serum concentrations above 1.0 mmol/L. The alarm level for the proportion of cows above the cut-point of 1.0, 1.2, or 1.4 mmol/L has not been validated, but it is suggested that no more than 10% of early-lactation cows should have hyperketonemia (subclinical ketosis). In cows with serum BHB concentrations of 1.2 mmol/L or greater or 1.4 mmol/L or greater in the first week postpartum, the odds of LDA were three and four times greater, respectively, than in cows with BHB below the cut-points.[7]

Glucose

Plasma/serum glucose concentrations are usually lower in early lactation[4] and during the winter months; in early lactation, there is a heavy demand for glucose, and during the winter the energy intake is likely to be lower than necessary to meet requirements. One major cause of variation in blood glucose may be the major fluctuations in daily feed intake. Investigations of feed intake of dairy cows on commercial farms have shown that concentrate dispensers are commonly incorrectly adjusted, and errors of more than 50% in feed intake are sometimes found. In situations of marginal energy imbalance, glucose concentrations may be unreliable as an index of the adequacy of energy intake. Several factors may cause short-term changes in glucose concentration. Blood glucose may be influenced by the chemical nature of the carbohydrate and physical form of the feed and the roughage content of the feed. In addition, elevation of plasma glucose concentration has been associated with excitement and low environmental temperature.

There is some conflicting evidence about the relationship between the mean plasma glucose concentrations of a lactational group and insufficient energy intake and reproductive inefficiency. In some work, there is an expected relationship between low plasma glucose concentration and an increased incidence of ketosis. In others, the relationship is not clear; however, there was a more consistent relationship between the actual energy intake as a percentage of requirement and the plasma NEFA concentration, but this finding was not sufficiently reliable to be useful. The mean plasma glucose concentrations within 3 days before or after first service of cows that conceived on first service was higher than that of cows that returned, but the difference was only approaching significance at the 5% level, and it is doubtful whether this could be of practical value. Although plasma NEFA concentration is more sensitive than plasma glucose concentration as an indicator of energy status of the lactating cow, the excessive variability of this relationship during early lactation limits its usefulness. Plasma NEFA concentration begins to increase several weeks prepartum, peaks at parturition, and decreases gradually to normal concentrations after several weeks of lactation. Plasma glucose concentrations follow a similar pattern. The main disadvantage of using plasma glucose concentration as an index of metabolic balance is that glucose concentration is a tightly regulated variable, and marked metabolic imbalances need to be present before plasma glucose concentration is altered. However, this means that decreased plasma/serum glucose concentrations provide an unequivocal and specific indicator of negative energy balance.

Protein Evaluation

Currently, there is not a single biochemical factor that accurately reflects the protein status of dairy cattle. A number of indices have therefore been monitored, including milk urea nitrogen and plasma/serum urea nitrogen, creatinine, albumin, and total protein concentrations. Of these indices, milk urea nitrogen concentration in the bulk tank provides the best global picture of protein balance in a dairy herd.

Urea Nitrogen

Plasma urea nitrogen and milk urea nitrogen (MUN) concentration are useful indicators of protein status, particularly when the diet contains adequate energy.

Increases in plasma urea nitrogen concentration and ammonia occur primarily as a result of inefficient nitrogen utilization. An excess of rumen degradable protein results in an increase in the concentration of rumen ammonia, which is absorbed through the rumen wall and transported to the liver, where it is converted to urea. The catabolism of body protein for gluconeogenesis can also result in the production of ammonia, which is also converted to urea in the liver. Plasma urea nitrogen concentration has therefore been the most commonly used blood constituent for monitoring protein status and intake. Values greater than 19 mg/dL suggest excessive protein intake in the diet, whereas values less than 10 mg/dL suggest inadequate protein intake in the diet.

MUN concentration can be used as a management aid to improve dairy-herd nutrition and monitor the nutritional status of lactating dairy cows. Elevated MUN concentration indicates that excess protein has been fed to the dairy cow for a given level of production. Milk samples should be submitted to an accredited diagnostic laboratory for MUN analysis. The Azotest Strip, an on-farm dipstick test, lacks accuracy and is not recommended. The MUN target concentrations for lactating dairy cows fed according to National Research Council recommendations have been evaluated. The target MUN concentrations are 8.5 to 11.5 mg/dL for most dairy herds compared with the previous target concentrations of 12 to 16 mg/dL. MUN, together with percentage milk protein, is being used increasingly as an indicator of the dietary protein–energy balance. The time of sampling can have a significant effect on MUN concentrations; the highest concentration was found to occur in the morning, and the diurnal pattern was not influenced by intrinsic factors such as parity, days postpartum or daily milk yield. MUN concentration was significantly increased after refrigeration for 1 week.

Several reviews of the literature have examined the effect of protein nutrition on reproduction in dairy cows. The reported effect of high nitrogen intake on fertility is inconsistent. Experimentally, the ingestion of a high level of degradable protein commencing 10 days before insemination in lactating dairy cows had no effect on the reproductive performance of the lactating high-yielding dairy cow. The relationship between MUN concentration and the fertility of dairy cows from 250 herds in the United Kingdom found no relationship between bulk-tank MUN concentration and fertility, or between changes in bulk-tank MUN concentrations and fertility.

A meta-analysis of the literature evaluated the associations between dietary requirements for protein for dairy cattle, the metabolism of protein in cattle, factors influencing the degradability of protein in ruminant feeds, and factors influencing MUN concentrations. There are good correlations between dietary protein intake and rumen ammonia, blood urea, and milk urea concentrations. Ryegrass clover pastures provide feed in many of the temperate dairy regions of the world, and for much of the year pasture crude protein may exceed 30%, of which a high proportion is rapidly degradable. High dietary protein intakes may have a negative effect on reproductive performance in lactating dairy cows, but the role of milk urea as a predictor of fertility needs further definition given the high conception rates in many Australasian dairy herds. High intakes of dietary protein may induce adaptations in urea metabolism, and the negative relationship identified between high intakes of dietary protein and fertility for northern hemisphere dairy herds may not necessarily apply in Australasian dairy herds. Because of the potential for cows to adapt to high-protein diets, the use of a single MUN determination on a herd will have limited value as an indicator of nutritional status and little value as a predictor of fertility. The differing observations between various production systems indicate the need for careful consideration in applying recommendations for dietary protein management based on milk urea concentrations. MUN determinations may, however, have value, particularly when used in conjunction with other herd and nutritional data to assess the protein nutrition of dairy herds. It is unlikely that single or even serial determinations of MUN concentration in single cows or bulk-tank milk will have a high predictive value for determining the risk of conception in the cow or herd.

Albumin

Plasma/serum albumin concentration is related to the protein status of the animal and whether an acute-phase reaction has been induced. Lactation stage has a substantial effect on serum albumin concentration. Animals should be grouped into dry cows, early lactation (1 to 10 weeks), and later lactation. Minimal values for dry-cow means are from 2.9 to 3.1 g/dL, from 2.7 to 2.9 g/dL for recently calved cows, and from 3.0 to 3.2 g/dL for cows in later lactation.

Liver Function and Injury

The presence of liver injury can be evaluated by measuring plasma/serum aspartate amino-transferase (AST), sorbitol dehydrogenase (SDH), alkaline phosphatase, and gamma-glutamyl-transferase (GGT) activities. Of these enzyme activities, the plasma/serum AST activity is the most clinically useful, with plasma AST greater than 162 U/L being indicative of hepatic lipidosis. Because increased AST activity also reflects damaged skeletal muscle, AST activity is not a specific test for liver injury in cattle at calving or for a few days after calving because of the potential for parturition-related muscle damage.

Liver function can be assessed by measuring the plasma/serum total bilirubin, cholesterol, and albumin concentrations. Serum bile acid concentration is not a useful index of liver function in cattle. Calculation of the ratio of plasma NEFA to cholesterol on a molar basis appears to provide a clinically useful index to evaluate the degree of hepatic lipidosis and the liver's ability to export mobilized peripheral fat reserves, and has been able to predict the incidence of postpartum disease. The major drawback with measuring the NEFA:cholesterol concentration is the cost, in that each analysis costs approximately US$8/test, for a total test cost of US$16. Plasma/serum albumin concentrations are decreased for the first month after calving as a result of plasma volume expansion to accommodate the nutrient flow for milk production, loss into the uterine lumen associated with uterine involution, catabolism of body protein resulting from negative energy balance, and decreased hepatic function as a result of hepatic lipidosis. The major clinical utility of plasma/serum albumin concentration is therefore in the first 4 weeks of lactation.

Macromineral Evaluation

Abnormalities of the blood levels of the four macrominerals, calcium, phosphorus, magnesium, and potassium, in the cow during the transition period are involved in subclinical hypocalcemia, clinical milk fever, hypomagnesemia, and acute hypokalemia.

Calcium

Serum calcium concentrations are tightly regulated and are not sensitive indicators of input–output balance. Measurement of plasma/serum calcium concentrations during the first 24 hours after calving, particularly in multiparous dairy cows, can provide useful insight into the effectiveness of control programs for periparturient hypocalcemia.

Phosphorus

Serum inorganic phosphate concentrations tend to fall following long-term insufficient dietary intake.

Magnesium

Serum magnesium concentrations are usually low during the winter months, and subclinical hypomagnesemia exists in many herds, especially pregnant beef cattle. This can be converted into clinical hypomagnesemia with a sudden deprivation of feed or a sudden fall in environmental temperature. Supplementation of the diet with magnesium salts is protective.

Sodium

Low serum sodium concentrations occur in early lactation in cows grazing on summer pastures without supplementation with salt. Levels down to 135 mmol/L may be associated with depraved appetite and polydipsia and polyuria.

Potassium

Serum potassium concentrations have been difficult to interpret because the levels of the electrolyte in serum are not necessarily indicative of potassium deficiency. The normal serum potassium concentration is much more variable than that of sodium, and its average concentration in roughages of all kinds is nearly always in excess of requirements; any abnormalities are usually in the direction of excess.

Hematology

Hematocrit (Packed Cell Volume)

The hematocrit can be used as a general reflection of health. In most dairy herds, a low hematocrit may be a reflection of suboptimal energy and protein nutrition. Mean values of packed cell volume (PCV), hemoglobin, and serum iron are consistently higher in nonlactating cows than in lactating cows. Parasitism causing blood loss will result in a low hematocrit. The hematocrit varies with lactation stage, being highest in dry cows and lowest at peak (summit) milk. Cows should be grouped by lactation stage when evaluating hematocrit.

Urine Evaluation

Urine samples are easier to obtain than blood samples, although stimulation of the perineal area to induce urination is usually only 75% to 90% successful. Higher success rates in obtaining a urine sample are obtained in cattle that have been sitting down and that are encouraged to stand.

Urine appears to be the optimal fluid to monitor acid–base and calcium status in dairy cattle. The most accurate insight into acid–base homeostasis in healthy cattle is obtained by measuring urine net acid excretion (NAE) or net base excretion (NBE) (see Chapter 5). However, when urine pH is between 6.3 and 7.6, urine pH measured by urine dipsticks or pH papers provides an inexpensive and clinically useful insight into acid–base homeostasis in cattle.[5] This is because the change in urine pH over this pH range accurately reflects the change in NAE or NBE. Optimum target values for urine pH to decrease the incidence of milk fever in dairy herds have not been identified, and recommendations for optimal urine pH values vary widely.[5]

Feeding rations with low dietary cation-anion difference (DCAD) to dairy cows for at least 2 weeks before calving decreases the incidence of periparturient hypocalcemia. The most likely reason for this effect is that ingestion of a low-DCAD diet increases calcium (Ca) flux, which in nonlactating cows is most readily detected as an increase in urinary calcium excretion. Low urine pH decreases calcium uptake from the tubular lumen into the renal epithelial cell and therefore decreases calcium absorption in the distal convoluted tubule and connecting tubule, thereby directly resulting in hypercalciuria. It remains to be determined whether laboratory measurement of urinary calcium concentration is more accurate and cost-effective than cow-side measurement of urine pH or laboratory determination of urinary strong ion difference and NBE when evaluating the effectiveness of milk-fever control programs.

Timing of Blood Tests

In Relation to Feed Changes

Because changes in the diet of ruminants cause changes in the character of rumen activity, blood samples for metabolic profile testing should not be done until 2 weeks after a major dietary change. Minor changes such as an increase in the quantity of an existing component or in access to the same ration do not require a wait of more than 7 to 10 days. Changes in forage type, such as turnout to pasture, housing, or the introduction of silage, require the full 2 weeks. The same applies for introduction of concentrates or of a new type of concentrate.

In Relation to Feeding

There can be changes in biochemical values in blood associated with feeding. These are most marked in cows receiving their entire concentrate ration at milking time. In such cases, 2 hours should be allowed to elapse after milking before blood sampling. In circumstances where the major part of the concentrate input is mixed with the forages and is available for most of each 24 hours, the timing of tests in relation to feeding is less critical. If lower-yielding midlactation cows are included (see later discussion), their results can be used as a check to see if there is an effect of feeding on the biochemical values in the blood samples. Cows should not be separated at milking time and confined for hours without access to food while waiting for blood sampling because this can also affect the results.

The available recommendations regarding the timing of blood collection relative to feeding are somewhat confusing. A common recommendation is that blood samples should be obtained 5 hours after feeding if animals are fed a fresh total mixed ration once daily. This recommendation does not seem logical in that plasma BHB concentration is increased at this time in cattle fed rations based on corn (maize) silage because of the metabolism of absorbed butyrate by ruminal epithelial cells. In most nutritional studies, blood samples are collected in a preprandial state because this is most consistent, but this will give the highest plasma NEFA concentrations over a 24-hour period. On this basis, sampling should be done in the morning immediately before or at the time of feeding of a fresh total mixed ration.

In Relation to Calving Pattern and Seasonal Feeding Changes

The cow in early lactation is the most important because what happens to her in the first few weeks after calving has the major influence on her subsequent productivity, including her future fertility efficiency. Therefore blood sampling for metabolic profiles should be carried out at the beginning of each new calving season, with the first cows checked so that the majority can benefit from the information derived. Of equal importance is the need to test as soon as possible after the introduction of a new ration, so that evaluation of the cows' biochemistry can be made available as quickly as possible to determine **what the cows, the end users, think of the ration.** Therefore planning of metabolic profile tests needs to be done in advance and should take into account both expected calving pattern and feed changes. Without planning along these lines, time may be lost, and productivity with it.

Selection of Cows

Picking appropriate cows for blood sampling is very important. This is because some of the metabolites looked at, particularly those relating to energy balance, can quickly return to the optimum range as cows adapt themselves, including their productivity, to a nutritional constraint. It is possible for cows to experience a significant energy deficit in the first 2 to 3 weeks of lactation because of intake problems, lose excessive body condition, perhaps have their milk yield modified, and have their subsequent fertility efficiency suppressed, but yet still arrive at 4 weeks calved with all biochemical measurements within the optimum ranges. If blood is sampled at 4 weeks after calving or longer, a producer could see thin, underproducing cows with poor fertility but with nothing abnormal about their biochemistry. Thus the farmer would be entitled to feel the metabolic profile test was of no value. However, if those cows had been blood sampled at 14 days calved instead of 28 days, the blood results would have been quite different and would have identified the nutritional constraint on productivity.

The guidelines for metabolic profiling of dairy cattle recommend sampling from the following groups:

- Dry period (D): between 7 and 10 days before anticipated date of calving
- Early lactation (EL): between 3 and 14 days of lactation
- Midlactation (ML): between 50 and 120 days of lactation.

Individual variations in biochemical values are such that single cows should not be tested. **Groups of no less than five should be sampled.** They should not be picked at random, but rather should be typical, average cows of their stage of lactation. Cows with extremes of performance—either very high or very low—should not be selected. Cows with problems should also not be included because the type of analysis carried out is not designed to clarify individual problems. It is important to make all this clear to farmers in advance because they cannot be expected to appreciate the limitations of the analyses made. Experience in the Dairy Herd Health and Productivity Service in the United Kingdom suggests that selecting cows for metabolic profiles may be best done by the veterinarian in advance of the test after looking at the calving and production records. If there is a specific concern of poor conception rate, for example, farmers may expect only cows that failed to conceive to be sampled. This tactic hardly ever delivers helpful information because any nutritional constraints have by then been compensated for, and blood biochemical values are usually within optimum ranges. The best approach may be to include such cows as the midlactation group.

Dry-Cow Group

Because the dry period is so important to the success of the following lactation, blood sampling to make sure nutrition is adequate is essential. However, the nature of the measurements that can be made means that primarily **cows in the last 7 to 10 days of gestation should be sampled.** Blood sampling a group of dry cows with 1 month or longer to go to calving at the same time can sometimes provide a useful within-herd comparison with respect to energy balance. Such sampling may also identify the presence of dietary protein inadequacy—specifically, rumen degradable—in the early part of the dry period.

Early-Lactation Group

The definition used for the early-lactation group is most critical for the reasons given in the previous paragraph. Since the original Compton metabolic profile, in which a high-yielding cow was used as the definition, the importance of this group has become increasingly apparent. The definition also has had to be changed to take into account changes in farm practice. The way cows are fed now—total mixed rations, increased out-of-parlor concentrate feeding—has reduced the time after calving by when they can adapt themselves to an unsatisfactory diet. **To be sure of detecting the presence of an energy constraint in particular, blood sampling should be carried out between 3 and 14 days calved**—at less than 3 days, the metabolic impact of hypercortisolemia associated with parturition is still present; at more than 14 days, some cows will be thin, unproductive, and subfertile but may have compensated for their nutrition and thus have normal blood metabolite values.

Midlactation Group

Some cows that have past the period of peak yield and so past the greatest period of potential nutritional stress should always be included. **They should be between 50 and 120 days calved** so that they are still relatively high yielding. This group provides a within-herd comparison with the early-lactation cows. Without this it is very difficult to distinguish between problems caused by constraints on intake of food or protein and energy content; to identify changes in biochemical values caused by mistiming of tests in relation to feeding or by oddities in the diet, such as silage with a high butyric acid content; and to make judgments on concentrate/forage usage within the herd.

In the DHHPS program, a majority of farms do metabolic profiles three to four times a year at critical times as a check, or **"ask-the-cows-what-they-think"** exercise. Thus metabolic profiles are used as part of a proactive preventive health and productivity program. Some of the larger farms may do more than 10 tests a year to cover feed changes and to check on the success of any corrective action.

In the DHHPS program, a standard DHHPS metabolic profile includes analysis of plasma for NEFA, BHB, glucose, urea nitrogen (urea N), albumin, globulin, magnesium, and inorganic phosphate. Analyses for copper and glutathione peroxidase (GSHPx) are done on approximately one-third of samples received and thyroxine T4 on even fewer. Biochemical analysis is performed using two biochemical auto-analyzers, with standard internal controls. It also employs an independent, external quality control system. Derivation of optimum metabolite values are summarized in Table 17-2. They are BHB less than 0.6 mmol/L in dry cows and less than 1.0 mmol/L in cows in milk; glucose greater than 3.0 mmol/L; NEFA less than 0.5 mmol/L in dry cows and less than 0.7 mmol/L in cows in milk; urea N greater than 1.7 mmol/L; albumin greater than 30 g/L; globulin less than 50 g/L; magnesium greater than 0.7 mmol/L; phosphate greater than 1.3 mmol/L; copper greater than 9.2 µmol/L; glutathione peroxidase (GSHPx) greater than 50U/g HB; and thyroxine T4 greater than 20 nmol/L.

Table 17-2 Metabolic profile parameters in cattle—optimum values

Parameter	SI units
BHB	
Milkers	Below 1.0 mmol/L
Dry cows	Below 0.6 mmol/L
Plasma glucose	Over 3.0 mmol/L
NEFA	
Milkers	Below 0.7 mmol/L
Dry cows	Below 0.4 mmol/L
Urea nitrogen	1.7–5.0 mmol/L
Albumin	Over 30 g/L
Globulin	Under 50 g/L
Magnesium	0.8–1.3 mmol/L
Phosphate (inorganic)	1.4–2.5 mmol/L
Copper	9.4–19.0 µmol/L
Thyroxine T4 (iodine)	Over 20 nmol/L
GSHPx (selenium)	Over 50 units/g Hb

Energy. The data in Table 17-3 use only the cows fitting precisely the definitions of D, EL, and ML. The table shows that, overall, an average of 30% EL cows had metabolite results reflecting satisfactory energy status, as did 61% of ML cows and 43% of D cows. In both EL and ML groups, glucose is the metabolite most commonly outside its optimum range, followed by BHB and NEFA. The percentage of NEFA values above optimum is low in ML cows. The most common finding is high BHB and low glucose in the same cow. In tests showing most cows in an EL group having these results, there is usually one or two with high NEFAs as well. Some EL cows show only low glucose or only high NEFA. Where low glucose only predominates in EL cows, ML cows often show the same picture.

Protein. The plasma urea concentration results in Table 17-3 show that the EL stage is more vulnerable to low values than later in lactation, even though the cows would have been on the same diets in virtually every case. In fact, an even greater average percentage of the blood of 1361 cows sampled between 0 and 9 days after calving over the 5 years showed low urea concentration.

The proportion of low-urea-concentration results in D cows is high (Table 17-3). In addition to the category shown of 10 days or less before calving, 4335 cows were sampled at more than 10 days

Table 17-3 Annual (April–March) percentages outside optimum ranges of metabolite results in blood plasma in adult dairy cows[8]

	EARLY LACTATION (EL) (10–20 DAYS CALVED)					MID LACTATION (ML) (50–120 DAYS CALVED)					DRY (D) (7–10 DAYS PREPARTUM)				
	1999/00	2000/01	2001/02	2002/03	2003/04	1999/00	2000/01	2001/02	2002/03	2003/04	1999/00	2000/01	2001/02	2002/03	2003/04
β-hydroxybutyrate (BHB)	19.5	16.6	22.3	22.9	17.5	11.2	10.5	14.3	10.6	9.6	34.5	24.7	38.5	28.5	22.7
Glucose	46.0	48.7	43.1	49.0	59.3	21.8	25.9	14.5	22.5	25.4	23.9	27.3	21.7	27.3	33.8
Non-esterified fatty acid (NEFA)	19.1	22.2	24.9	27.4	28.0	0.6	2.1	1.8	2.7	3.1	10.8	15.0	14.2	13.0	14.8
One or more energy metabolite per cow	65	70	67	72	78	34	39	32	40	44	59	57	63	46	63
Urea-nitrogen (UreaN)	0.8	17.3	18.3	16.7	16.7	4.4	6.4	6.0	5.3	5.6	18.4	20.4	20.2	20.8	22.3
Number of cows	1295	1421	1248	1285	1530	914	1066	849	1179	1494	1160	1379	1253	1358	1543

prepartum, and 22% of them had low plasma urea concentrations.

Results outside the optimum ranges for albumin (0.6%), magnesium (2.5%), phosphate (1.0%), copper (10%), and GSHPx (3%) are relatively uncommon. Thyroxine T4 analysis was carried out in 836 samples on specific request, and only 3% were below optimum.

Background Information

So that full value can be obtained by the farmer from the metabolic-profile approach, information about the cows and the farm should accompany the blood samples to the laboratory. This should include cow identification; last calving date for milkers/expected for dry cows; body weight (calculation from heart-girth measurement with a weighband pulled to a constant 5-kg tension is the best because it is not affected by gutfill and usually most practical because no mechanical weighing device/crush is required); body-condition score by a palpation method; current daily milk yield; expected current daily milk yield; lactation number; daily supplementary feed intakes; daily estimated forage intakes; analytical description of feeds; and current herd milk solids percentages. It is useful to have information on herd size, breed, feeding systems, and health and fertility. A note of what concerns the farmer has, if any, should also be made.

Interpretation of Results at the Farm

Circumstances where the diagnosis of a nutritional constraint from blood samples is clearly correct, but the cause(s) are unclear from a distance and could be many, are common. Therefore it is very important that a final interpretation of what is not working and what are the best and most economic solutions ought to be made at the farm with the information from the laboratory in hand. Farm advisory visits should be made as soon as the results are available and discussions made, including farm staff and any other advisors involved. Experience in the DHHPS suggests that such a team approach produces a more balanced strategy and is more beneficial than each party working in isolation.

Written Advice

Any advice given should be recorded concisely in writing and copies given to all participants on the farm. This ensures that the agreed path is followed, creates a record, and ensures that the fee is for something tangible.

Milk Production, Activity Meters, and Rumination Monitors

The application of real-time monitoring of dairy cattle has great potential to provide low-cost and immediate insight into health and production. Of all potential indices, daily milk production (relative to previous production during the lactation or the previous lactation, or to peers) appears to provide the most sensitive and specific measure of dry matter intake and health. Milk production can be measured noninvasively and at very low cost using automated procedures at milking time. As diagnostic algorithms are refined, it is likely that monitoring of daily milk production will provide the most practical and low-cost method for evaluating health and production and for early disease detection.

Activity meters can detect standing and lying periods in cattle and from that information can infer time spent feeding in cows housed in free stalls or tie stalls. Rumination monitors detect the time spent ruminating each day, which is strongly associated with dry matter intake and health.

Body-Condition Score

Managing body reserves is critical for successful cow management and requires an accurate assessment of the cow's "condition." Body-condition scoring is an important aspect of metabolic diseases of farm animals. Body weight alone is not a valid indicator of body reserves because cows of a specific weight may be tall and thin or short and fat. The energy stores may vary by as much as 40% in cows of similar body weight, which emphasizes the futility and inaccuracy of relying on body weight alone as an index of cow condition. In addition, because tissue mobilization in early lactation occurs as feed intake is increasing, decreases in body-tissue weight can be masked by enhanced fill of the gastrointestinal tract, so that body-weight changes do not reflect changes in adipose tissue and lean-tissue weight.

There is a strong positive relationship (R^2 = 0.86) between BCS and the proportion of physically dissected fat in Friesian cows. Therefore the visual or tactile (palpation) appraisal of the cow's BCS provides a good assessment of body-fat reserves, ignoring—or minimizing the effect of—frame size and intestinal contents. Most animal and dairy scientists acknowledge the successful manipulation of BCS as an important management factor that influences or has a relationship to animal health, milk production, and reproduction in the modern dairy cow. For example, cows that lost 0.5 to 1.0 point in BCS between parturition and first service achieved a pregnancy-to-first-service rate of 53%, whereas those losing more than 1.0 point achieved a rate of 17%. In a seasonal pasture-based system for Holstein–Friesian cows, it is necessary to maintain the BCS at 2.75 or greater during the breeding season. BCS is important in achieving good reproductive performance. Loss of body condition between calving and first service should be restricted to 0.5 BCS to avoid a detrimental effect on reproductive performance.

BCS is a subjective method of assessing the amount of metabolizable energy stored

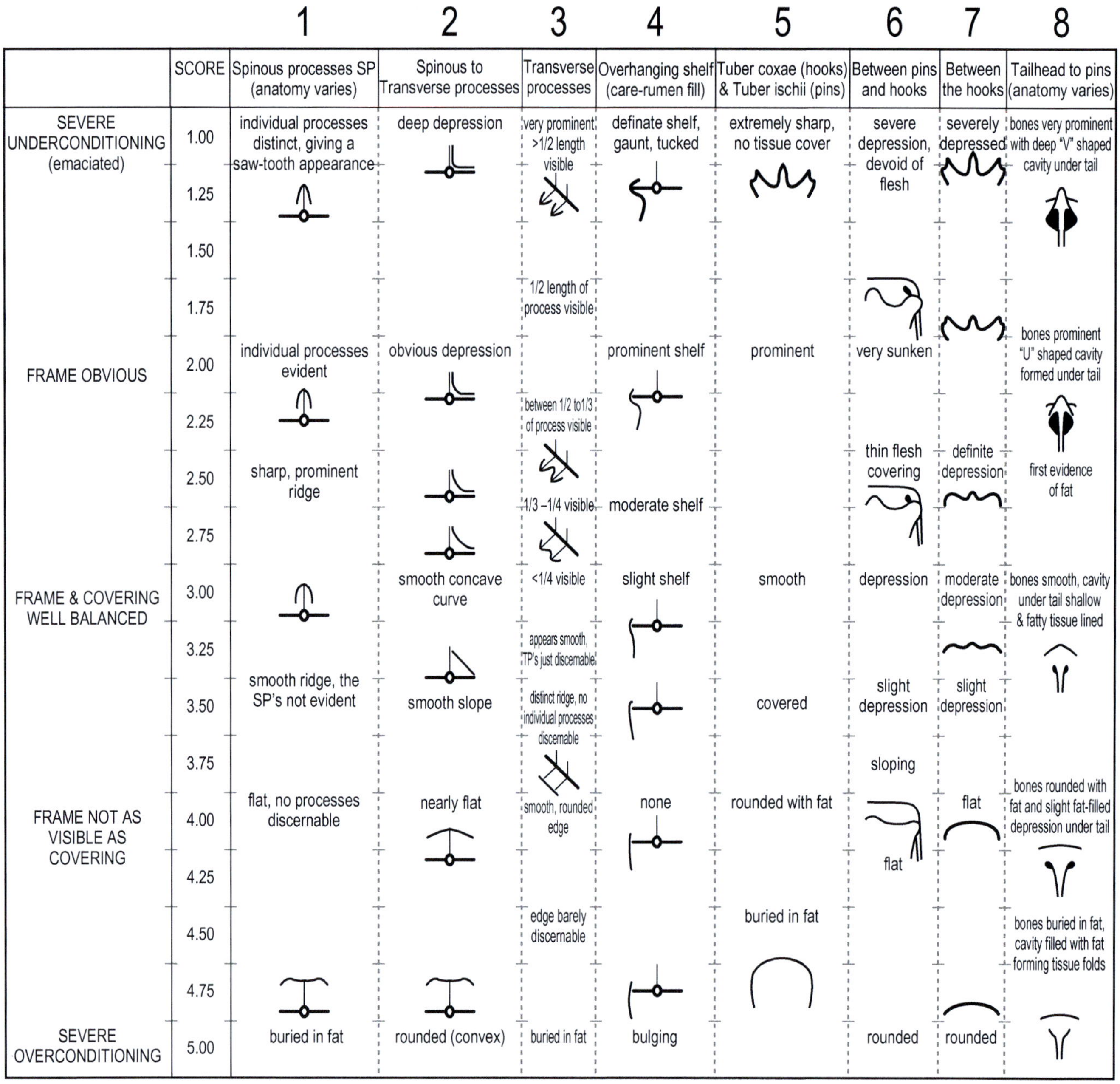

1
2
3
4
5
6
7
8
SCORE
Spinous processes SP (anatomy varies)
Spinous to Transverse processes
Transverse processes
Overhanging shelf (care-rumen fill)
Tuber coxae (hooks) & Tuber ischii (pins)
Between pins and hooks
Between the hooks
Tailhead to pins (anatomy varies)
SEVERE UNDERCONDITIONING (emaciated)
FRAME OBVIOUS
FRAME & COVERING WELL BALANCED
FRAME NOT AS VISIBLE AS COVERING
SEVERE OVERCONDITIONING
1.00
1.25
1.50
1.75
2.00
2.25
2.50
2.75
3.00
3.25
3.50
3.75
4.00
4.25
4.50
4.75
5.00
individual processes distinct, giving a saw-tooth appearance
individual processes evident
sharp, prominent ridge
smooth ridge, the SP's not evident
flat, no processes discernable
buried in fat
deep depression
obvious depression
smooth concave curve
smooth slope
nearly flat
rounded (convex)
very prominent; >1/2 length visible
1/2 length of process visible
between 1/2 to1/3 of process visible
1/3 –1/4 visible
<1/4 visible
appears smooth, TP's just discernable
distinct ridge, no individual processes discernable
smooth, rounded edge
edge barely discernable
buried in fat
definate shelf, gaunt, tucked
prominent shelf
moderate shelf
slight shelf
none
bulging
extremely sharp, no tissue cover
prominent
smooth
covered
rounded with fat
buried in fat
severe depression, devoid of flesh
very sunken
thin flesh covering
depression
slight depression
sloping
flat
rounded
severely depressed
definite depression
moderate depression
slight depression
flat
rounded
bones very prominent with deep "V" shaped cavity under tail
bones prominent "U" shaped cavity formed under tail
first evidence of fat
bones smooth, cavity under tail shallow & fatty tissue lined
bones rounded with fat and slight fat-filled depression under tail
bones buried in fat, cavity filled with fat forming tissue folds

Fig. 17-3 Body-condition scoring chart. (Adapted from Edmonson AJ, Lean IJ, Weaver LD, Farver T, Webster G. A body condition scoring chart for Holstein dairy cows. *J Dairy Sci.* 1989; 72:68–78.).

in fat and muscle (body reserves) in a live animal. BCS in dairy cows is done using a variety of scales and systems. This method involves palpating the cow to assess the amount of tissue under the skin. Scoring body condition and assessing changes in the body condition of dairy cattle have become strategic tools in both farm management and research. BCS is being researched worldwide. But international sharing, comparing, and use of generated data are limited because different BCS systems are used. There is difficulty in interpreting the literature because of variability in the way authors apply scoring methods. In the United States, Canada, and Ireland, a 5-point BCS system is used for dairy cows, whereas Australia and New Zealand use 8- and 10-point scales, respectively. The following scoring method is recommended for the 0-to-5 scale. A BCS chart[6] appears in Fig. 17-3.

Score: 1

- Condition: Poor.
- Tailhead area: Cavity present around tailhead. No fatty tissue felt between skin and pelvis, but skin is supple.
- Loin area: Ends of transverse processes sharp to touch and dorsal surfaces can be easily felt. Deep depression in loin.

Score: 2

- Condition: Moderate.
- Tailhead area: Shallow cavity lined with fatty tissue apparent at tailhead. Some fatty tissue felt under the skin. Pelvis easily felt.
- Loin area: Ends of transverse processes feel rounded, but dorsal surfaces felt only with pressure. Depression visible in loin.

Score: 3

- Condition: Good.
- Tailhead area: Fatty tissue easily felt over the whole area. Skin appears smooth, but pelvis can be felt.

- Loin area: Ends of transverse processes can be felt with pressure, but thick layer of tissue dorsum. Slight depression visible in loin.

Score: 4
- Condition: Fat.
- Tailhead area: Folds of soft fatty tissue present.
- Patches of fat apparent under skin. Pelvis felt only with firm pressure.
- Loin area: Transverse processes cannot be felt even with firm pressure. No depression visible in loin between backbone and hip bones.

Score: 5
- Condition: Grossly fat.
- Tailhead area: Tailhead buried in fatty tissue. Skin distended. No part of pelvis felt even with firm pressure.
- Loin area: Folds of fatty tissue over transverse processes. Bone structure cannot be felt.

Relationships Among International Body-Condition Scoring Systems

The New Zealand 10-point scale was compared with the scoring systems in the United States, Ireland, and Australia by trained assessors. Cows were assessed visually in the United States and Australia; in Ireland, cows were assessed by palpating key areas of the cow's body. Significant positive linear relationships were found between the New Zealand 10-point scale and the other scoring systems. The relationships between the 10-point BCS scale used in New Zealand and the scales used in Ireland and the United States are summarized in Table 17-4.

Table 17-4 Relationship between the 10-point BCS scale used in New Zealand and the 5-point BCS scale used in Ireland and the United States, and the 8-point scale used in Australia

New Zealand	USA	Ireland	Australia
1.0	1.83	1.21	2.74
1.5	1.98	1.41	3.01
2.0	2.14	1.61	3.28
2.5	2.30	1.81	3.55
3.0	2.46	2.01	3.82
3.5	2.62	2.21	4.09
4.0	2.78	2.41	4.36
4.5	2.94	2.61	4.63
5.0	3.10	2.81	4.90
5.5	3.26	3.01	5.17
6.0	3.42	3.21	5.44
6.5	3.58	3.41	5.71
7.0	3.74	3.61	5.98
7.5	3.90	3.81	6.25
8.0	4.06	4.01	6.52
8.5	4.22	4.21	6.79
9.0	4.38	4.41	7.06
9.5	4.54	4.61	7.33
10.0	4.70	4.81	7.60

FURTHER READING

Grummer RR. Nutritional and management strategies for the prevention of fatty liver in dairy cattle. *Vet J.* 2008;176:10-20.

LeBlanc S. Monitoring metabolic health of dairy cattle in the transition period. *J Reprod Dev.* 2010;56:S29.

Macrae AI, Whitaker DA, Burrough E, Dowell A, Kelly JM. Use of metabolic profiles for the assessment of dietary adequacy in UK dairy herds. *Vet Rec.* 2006;159:655.

REFERENCES

1. Borchardt S, Staufenbiel R. *J Am Vet Med Assoc.* 2012;240:1003.
2. <http://www.fda.gov/downloads/AnimalVeterinary/Products/ApprovedAnimalDrugProducts/FOIADrugSummaries/UCM050022.pdf>. Accessed June 18, 2016.
3. Ingvartsen KL, et al. *Prev Vet Med.* 2003;83:277.
4. Garverick HA, et al. *J Dairy Sci.* 2013;96:181.
5. Constable PD, et al. *Am J Vet Res.* 2009;70:915.
6. National Research Council. *Nutrient Requirements of Dairy Cattle.* 7th rev. ed. Washington DC: National Academy Press; 2001:13-27.
7. McCarthy MMM, et al. *J Dairy Sci.* 2015;98:6284.
8. Whitaker DA. *Cattle Pract.* 2005;13:27.

PARTURIENT PARESIS (MILK FEVER)

SYNOPSIS

Etiology Hypocalcemia just before, around, or after parturition.

Epidemiology Adult dairy cows in third parity and older; clinical case incidence of 4% to 9%, with low case fatality, but up to 50% of multiparous periparturient dairy cows affected subclinically. Most commonly occurs within 48 hours after calving, but also occurs several weeks before or after. Occurs in beef cattle in epidemics. Occurs in sheep and goats in epidemics, usually following stressors. Prepartum diets high in calcium.

Signs Three progressively worse stages including early signs such as restlessness, muscle fasciculation over shoulder and neck, cool skin, anorexia, rumen atony with mild bloat, and insecure gait. More advanced stages with general muscle weakness leading to sternal recumbency with head resting on the chest, mental depression, dilated pupils, weak heartbeat und pulse, increased heart rate, dry muzzle, dry feces, and hypothermia. Last stage characterized by lateral recumbency, severe obtundation, severe rumen bloat, barely audible heart, tachycardia, circulatory collapse, coma, and death.

Diagnostic confirmation Hypocalcemia and response to treatment with calcium borogluconate.

Treatment Calcium borogluconate IV, oral calcium salts.

Control Dietary management to reduce dietary potassium intake prepartum, while increasing the content of anions in the ration (low dietary cation–anion difference rations). Reducing dietary calcium content below requirements prepartum to prepare the organism for a negative calcium balance. Oral administration of calcium salts immediately before, at, and after calving. Oral or parenteral vitamin D and analogs before calving.

ETIOLOGY

A depression in the levels of ionized calcium in the extracellular space, including plasma, is the basic biochemical disturbance in milk fever. A transient period of subclinical hypocalcemia (total plasma calcium [Ca] < 2.0 mmol/L or 8 mg/dL) occurs at the onset of lactation caused by an imbalance between calcium influx to the extracellular pool from gut and bone and output in colostrum and milk. The sudden increase of Ca losses through the mammary gland at the onset of lactation presents a considerable challenge for the circuits regulating Ca homeostasis. With milk containing approximately 2 g of Ca per kg and colostrum approximately 2.3 g of Ca per kg, the production of 10 kg of milk or colostrum requires the equivalent of the entire amount of Ca available in the extracellular space of an adult cow. Calcium lost from the extracellular pool must be replaced by increasing intestinal absorption and bone resorption of calcium. Whereas the calcium requirements of a cow in late gestation are minimal at about 30 g/d, a dairy cow must mobilize an additional 30 g or more of calcium per day for milk production from parturition on. A certain degree of hypocalcemia around parturition is unavoidable and is a result of the lag time of counter-regulatory mechanisms reacting to the sudden imbalance of Ca homeostasis at the onset of lactation. Most cows adapt within 48 hours after calving by increases in plasma concentrations of parathyroid hormone (PTH) and 1,25-$(OH)_2D$, the biologically active form of vitamin D_3. The incidence of subclinical hypocalcemia, with serum Ca concentrations between 1.4 and 2.0 mmol/L (5.5 to 8.0 mg/dL) in multiparous periparturient cows has been estimated at 50%.[1] Clinical milk fever is estimated to occur in 5% of periparturient dairy cows in the United States.[2]

EPIDEMIOLOGY

Occurrence

Cattle

The disease occurs most commonly in high-producing multiparous lactating dairy cattle. Lactating beef cows also are affected, but less commonly.

Age. Hypocalcemia at calving is age related and most marked in cows at their third to seventh parturition, although rare cases have been observed at the first and second calvings.

Breed. Field observations have for many years suggested that Jersey, Swedish Red and White, and Norwegian Red breeds develop clinical milk fever more frequently than Holstein–Friesian cows.[3] The higher Ca concentration in milk from Jersey compared with Holstein cows has been proposed as possible explanation, although the absolute differences in Ca excreted through the mammary gland per day between breeds are negligible when considering the higher milk yield of Holstein–Friesian cows.[3] Differences in the number of intestinal vitamin D receptors regulating the intestinal Ca uptake have been reported in some studies.[3] The disease in beef cattle breeds occurs either in individual cows or in herd outbreaks.

Individual Cows. Individual cows, and to some extent families of cows, are more susceptible than others; the disease tends to recur at successive parturitions. The heritability of susceptibility to milk fever and hypocalcemia has been assessed as insignificant; different studies reported heritabilities of 0%, 4%, and 12.8%.[4] Complete milking in the first 48 hours after calving, as opposed to normal sucking by a calf, appears to be a precipitating factor. Several studies have reported that the incidence of milk fever is positively associated with the level of milk production.

Time of Occurrence. In cattle, milk fever occurs at three main stages in the lactation cycle. Most prepartum cases occur in the last few days of pregnancy and during parturition, but rare cases occur several weeks before calving. Some cases will occur a few hours before parturition or at the time of parturition when the attendant expects the cow to calve and the second stage of parturition does not occur because of uterine inertia resulting from hypocalcemia. Most cases occur within the first 48 hours after calving, and the danger period extends up to about the 10th postpartum day. Up to 20% of cases can occur subsequent to the 8th day after calving. In such cases the declines in serum Ca levels are smaller than in parturient cows. The clinical signs are also less severe, and there are fewer relapses after treatment. Occasional cases occur during mid- or even late lactation. Such cases are often recurrences of the disease in highly susceptible cows that were affected at calving. Undue fatigue and excitement may precipitate such attacks, and there is a special susceptibility at estrus. In the latter case, the depression of appetite by the elevation of blood estrogen levels may be a contributing factor.

Hypocalcemic episodes lasting 1 to 2 days may occur two or three times with a periodicity of about 9 days. Fluctuations in the intestinal absorption of Ca during this period may be the cause of Ca cycling. Subclinical hypocalcemia is of major significance because it inhibits reticulorumen motility, which affects appetite, delays intestinal absorption of nutrients, and exacerbates the negative energy balance already existing in the cow in the first month of lactation.

Stressors. Feed intake depression for 48 hours contributes to the depression of serum Ca levels, and this may be of importance in the production of hypocalcemic paresis in this species at times other than in the postparturient period. Pregnant beef cattle may develop hypocalcemic paresis during the winter months when they are fed on poor-quality roughage; within a group of such cows, lower-ranked individuals of the herd may suffer selective malnutrition. The disease has also occurred in beef cows affected with diarrhea of undetermined etiology. As another explanation of the heightened susceptibility of cows at estrus, a possible depression of the degree of ionization of calcium under the influence of estrogens has been proposed. Differences in total serum Ca or plasma ionized Ca values in cows during estrus, however, are not documented.

The intravenous administration of certain aminoglycosides, especially neomycin, elihydrostreptomycin, and gentamicin, may cause a reduction in the degree of ionization of serum calcium and a syndrome similar to milk fever. Oral dosing with zinc oxide (40 or 120 mg Zn/kg body weight [BW]) as a prophylaxis against facial eczema in ewes causes a serious drop in serum calcium levels 24 hours after treatment. Caution is recommended with the use of these drugs in parturient cows.

Sheep and Goats

In sheep, the disease commonly occurs in outbreaks in groups of ewes exposed to forced exercise, long-distance transport, sudden feed deprivation, and grazing on oxalate-containing plants or green cereal crops. These circumstances commonly precipitate outbreaks of hypocalcemic paresis in sheep; mature ewes are the most susceptible, particularly in the period from 6 weeks before to 10 weeks after lambing. Up to 25% of the flock may be affected at one time. The disease also occurs in young sheep up to about 1 year of age, especially when they graze green oats, but also when pasture is short in winter and spring, as in southeast Australia. The disease is manifested by paresis, but poor growth, lameness, and bone fragility can be detected in the rest of the flock. A sudden deprivation of feed or forced exercise of ewes can cause marked depression of the serum Ca levels. However, ewes are in a susceptible state in early lactation because they are in negative Ca balance. In late lactation a state of positive balance is a result of a low rate of bone resorption. There is an unexplained occurrence of hypocalcemia in sheep fed on hay when they are supplemented with an energy-rich concentrate, which increases their calcium intake. Another occurrence in ewes is at the end of a drought when the pasture growth is lush and very low in Ca content. The incidence may be as high as 10% and the case-fatality rate 20% in ewe flocks in late pregnancy or early lactation.

Hypocalcemia in sheep depresses endogenous glucose production and insulin release, and in late pregnancy in combination with hyperketonemia, it facilitates the development of pregnancy toxemia.

In does, a depression in serum levels of Ca and phosphorus occurs similar to that in cows, but in ewes no such depression occurs at lambing, and the intervention of a precipitating factor appears to be necessary to reduce the serum Ca level below a critical point.

Milking goats become affected mostly during the 4- to 6-year-old age group. Cases occur before and after kidding, some later than 3 weeks after parturition. Clinical syndromes are identical to those in cows, including the two stages of ataxia and recumbency. Serum Ca levels are reduced from normal levels for parturient does.

Morbidity and Case Fatality

Clinical Hypocalcemia

Several epidemiologic studies of milk fever have reported incidence rates between 5% and 10% for clinical milk fever in cattle, calculated either as the lactational incidence or incidence per cow year.[2,5] Overall clinical disease is sporadic, but on individual farms the incidence may occasionally reach 25% to 30% of high-risk cows. With early treatment mortality is low in uncomplicated cases, but incidental losses as a result of aspiration pneumonia, mastitis, and limb injuries may occur. From 75% to 85% of uncomplicated cases respond to parenteral Ca therapy alone. A proportion of these animals require more than one treatment, either because complete recovery is delayed or because relapse occurs. The remaining 15% to 25% are either complicated by other conditions or incorrectly diagnosed.

Subclinical Hypocalcemia

Subclinical hypocalcemia, defined as total plasma Ca between 1.4 and 2.0 mmol/L (5.5 and 8.0 mg/dL), is common in dairy cattle during the first few weeks of lactation. The incidence rates of subclinical postparturient hypocalcemia reported in the literature are in the range of 33% and may even increase to 50% in older cows.[1,5]

Risk Factors

Animal Risk Factors

Serum Ca levels decline in all adult cows at calving as a result of the Ca loss through the mammary gland at the onset of lactation. This decline is more pronounced in some cows than in others, and it is this difference that results in the varying susceptibility of animals to parturient paresis. First-calf heifers rarely develop milk fever because they are able to adapt more effectively to the high Ca demand at the onset of lactation. With increasing age, this adaptation process is hampered and results in moderate to severe hypocalcemia in older cows. The adaptation mechanism is directly related to the efficiency of intestinal absorption of Ca, which decreases with increasing age.

Calcium Homeostasis. The following three factors affect Ca homeostasis, and variations in one or more of them may contribute to the development of clinical disease in any individual:

1. Excessive loss of calcium in colostrum beyond the capacity of absorption from the intestines and mobilization from the bones to replace it. Variations in susceptibility between cows could be the result of variations in the Ca concentration in colostrum or milk and the volume of milk produced.
2. Impairment of absorption of Ca from the intestine at parturition.
3. Mobilization of Ca from storage in the skeleton may not be sufficiently rapid or efficient to maintain normal plasma Ca levels. The Ca mobilization rate is markedly reduced in cows in later pregnancy in response to the low requirements in the weeks before parturition. The lag time in reinitiating bone resorption at the moment Ca losses through the mammary gland suddenly begin contributes to the transient depression of the plasma Ca concentration. Bone resorption makes only a minor contribution to the total rate of Ca mobilization at parturition and is therefore of minor importance for the prevention of periparturient hypocalcemia. Osteoblasts are the only type of bone cell to express the 1,25-$(OH)_2D$ receptor protein, and the decrease in the numbers of osteoblasts with increasing age could delay the ability of bone to contribute Ca to the plasma Ca pool. Bone resorption shortly before and around calving can furthermore be hampered in states of metabolic alkalosis as it occurs in cows fed a ration with high potassium content. Animals with mild to moderate forms of compensated metabolic acidosis, in contrast, have enhanced bone-resorption activity, releasing additional Ca to the extracellular pool. Preventing alkalization by avoiding excessive dietary potassium and inducing mild to moderate acidosis by adding so-called anionic salts to the diet in late gestation are common strategies for prevention of milk fever in cattle (see also the discussion under "Control" in this chapter).

Historically it was proposed that failure to secrete sufficient levels of PTH or insufficient availability of 1,25-$(OH)_2D$ was the primary defect in cows that developed milk fever. More recent research has shown that the secretion of PTH and the production of 1,25-$(OH)_2D$ are similar in most cows with or without milk fever. However, about 20% of cows treated for parturient paresis experience relapsing episodes of hypocalcemia that require further treatment. These cows appear to be less efficient in producing adequate amounts of 1,25-$(OH)_2D$ at the onset of lactation. Both relapsing and nonrelapsing cows develop the same degree of hypocalcemia and secondary hyperparathyroidism, but production of 1,25-$(OH)_2D$ is about twofold greater in nonrelapsing cows than relapsing cows. Following treatment of parturient hypocalcemia with intravenous Ca salts and restoration of ruminal and intestinal motility, nonrelapsing cows establish Ca homeostasis over the next 3 to 4 days by increasing intestinal absorption of Ca, which is activated by a sufficient level of 1,25-$(OH)_2D$. In relapsing cows, even when rumen and intestinal motility are restored after treatment, hypocalcemia and paresis are likely to occur because of insufficient plasma 1,25-$(OH)_2D$. These cows may remain in this stage of prolonged hypocalcemia for several days, and only after a few days and several repeated treatments with Ca will the plasma levels of 1,25-$(OH)_2D$ increase to an adequate level to maintain Ca homeostasis. Tissue 1,25-$(OH)_2D$ receptor concentrations decline with age, which renders older cows less able to respond to the hormone; thus it will take longer for older cows to adapt intestinal Ca absorption mechanisms to meet lactational demands for Ca.

Body-Condition Score. A high BCS increases the risk of milk fever. The odds ratio of milk fever with a BCS greater than 4/5 on the first milk recording day after calving was 4.3, and cows with milk fever had a postpartum predisease body weight 12 kg higher compared with healthy cows, indicating an increased risk of milk fever as a result of higher body weight. Cows with subclinical hypocalcemia in the winter period had significantly higher mean body weight over the 60 days postpartum than normocalcemic cows, but the effect was not significant in cows calving during the summer months.

Dietary and Environmental Risk Factors

Several dietary factors of the pregnant cow during the prepartum period (last 4 weeks of gestation) can influence the incidence of milk fever in cattle.

Dietary Calcium. Feeding more than 100 g of calcium daily during the dry period is associated with an increased incidence of milk fever. The daily dietary Ca requirements of an adult cow in late gestation are in the range of 30 g Ca/d. When supplying Ca far in excess of the daily requirements (>100 g Ca/d), the active absorption of Ca from the digestive tract and mobilization from bone are homeostatically depressed and become quiescent. As a consequence, at calving when sudden changes of the Ca balance occur, the cow is unable to rapidly return to bone Ca stores or intestinal Ca absorption mechanisms and is susceptible to severe hypocalcemia until these mechanisms can be activated, which may take several days.

Feeding prepartum diets with a Ca concentration low enough to induce a negative Ca balance already before calving prevents milk fever by activating Ca transport mechanisms in the intestine and bone before parturition, thus allowing the animal to adapt more rapidly to the lactational drain of Ca. The challenge of this approach is to formulate a balanced dry-cow ration with a sufficiently low Ca concentration providing less than 20 g/d of absorbable Ca (see also the discussion under "Control" in this chapter).

Supplementing dietary Ca immediately before and around parturition may also lower the incidence of milk fever by providing additional dietary Ca at the moment intestinal Ca absorption is upregulated (see also the discussion under "Control" in this chapter).

Dietary Potassium. The dietary potassium content of the ration fed in late gestation is a major contributing factor to the risk of periparturient hypocalcemia. Positively charged electrolytes (cations) contained in the diet and absorbed from the digestive tract tend to alkalinize the organism, whereas electrolytes with a negative charge (anions) are acidifying.[6] Studies of the 1970s furthermore demonstrated that alkalization of the organism by increasing the amount of dietary cations increased the incidence of milk fever, whereas acidification by increasing the dietary anion content reduced the milk-fever incidence, which is the basis of the so-called dietary cation–anion difference (DCAD) concept (see also the discussion under "Control" in this chapter). With potassium being the quantitatively most important cation in a standard ruminant diet, it follows that high potassium concentrations (>2% of the ingested dry matter) in the ration fed to cows in their last weeks of gestation can considerably increase the incidence of periparturient hypocalcemia.

Dietary Magnesium. Magnesium deficiency during late gestation is a major risk factor for periparturient hypocalcemia, and hypomagnesemia is considered to be the most common cause of milk fever occurring in midlactating dairy cows.[3] Because magnesium is required for the release PTH from the parathyroid glands and furthermore influences the tissue sensitivity to PTH, the efficacy of PTH for the correction of hypocalcemia greatly depends on an adequate supply of magnesium.

Dietary Phosphorus. Prepartum diets high in phosphorus (P; > 80 g P/d) greatly increase the incidence of milk fever and the severity of hypocalcemia. High dietary levels of P increase the serum level of P, which is inhibitory to the renal enzymes that catalyze the conversion of vitamin D to its active form 1,25-$(OH)_2D$. Decreased amounts of 1,25-$(OH)_2D$ will not only reduce the intestinal absorption of P, but also of Ca, and thereby predispose to periparturient hypocalcemia.[7]

Dietary Cation–Anion Difference. Studies in the 1960s and 1970s showed that experimentally increasing the dietary cation concentration or decreasing the dietary anion concentration had an alkalinizing effect on the organisms, whereas feeding diets with a higher anion or lower cation concentration resulted in acidification. It was furthermore demonstrated that alkalization achieved through feeding high-cation/low-anion diets increased the incidence of milk fever, whereas acidification by increasing the ration of anions to cations caused the milk-fever incidence to decline.[6] Accordingly the basis of the DCAD concept is to modulate the ratio of cations to anions in the diet to reduce the risk of milk fever in cattle. The cation–anion difference of a diet is commonly given in milliequivalents (mEq) per kilogram of feed dry matter (DM; mEq/kg DM) or sometimes in mEq/100 g DM. Although several different equations have been proposed for the calculation of the DCAD, the most commonly used only considers the four quantitatively most important dietary ions: sodium (Na^+), potassium (K^+), chloride (Cl^-), and sulfur (S^{2-}). Other electrolytes, such as Ca, P, and magnesium, also affect the actual DCAD and thereby the effect on the acid–base status of the animal consuming the diet, and these compounds are included in some of the equations proposed in the literature to calculate the DCAD. However, because these minerals are present in relatively low amounts in the ruminant diet, their effect is considered to be minor. They are therefore commonly disregarded for practicability reasons.

The DCAD exerts a strong linear effect on the incidence of milk fever and is more important than the level of dietary Ca as a risk factor for milk fever. Prepartum diets high in cations such as potassium are associated with an increased incidence of milk fever, whereas diets high in anions, especially chloride and sulfur, result in a decrease in the incidence of the disease. Most forages, such as legumes and grasses, are high in potassium and are alkaline. The addition of anions, specifically chloride and sulfur, to the diet of dairy cows before parturition can effectively reduce the incidence of milk fever (see also the discussion under "Control" in this chapter).

Systemic acidification induced by anionic supplementation affects the function of PTH hormone, the major effect being an increased tissue response to PTH, which results in increased retention of Ca and enhanced mobilization of Ca from bone. A meta-analysis of 75 feeding trials designed to study the nutritional risk factors for milk fever in dairy cattle found that the prepartum dietary concentrations of S and dietary anion–cation balance ([Na + K]—[Cl + S]) were the two nutritional factors most strongly correlated to the incidence of milk fever. Dietary S acts as a strong anion and reduces the risk of milk fever, and increasing the dietary S concentrations lowers the odds ratio of developing milk fever.

ECONOMIC IMPORTANCE

Although economic losses from milk fever have decreased considerably since the introduction of intravenous treatment with Ca salts many years ago, the disease incidences reported in recent years remain similar to values reported decades ago.[2,5] The most obvious costs are associated with drugs, veterinary intervention, and losses resulting from complications in clinical cases. Costs associated with subclinical hypocalcemia are, however, considered to be far more important. Incidence rates between 3.5% and 7% for clinical disease and over 30% for subclinical hypocalcemia have been reported, and hypocalcemia is considered to be a so-called "gateway disease" that predisposes to a number of common fresh-cow disorders, such as dystocia, uterine prolapse, retained fetal membranes, mastitis, ketosis, abomasal displacement, ketosis, and immune suppression.[5] The costs per clinical case of milk fever have been estimated at US$300, whereas subclinical cases may cost around US$125 per case, based on estimates accounting for reduced milk production and increased risk of developing periparturient disorders such as ketosis or abomasal displacement.[8]

The literature on the effects of clinical and subclinical hypocalcemia is difficult to interpret because of the complex relationships between milk production, parity of lactation, breed of cattle, epidemiologic methods used, and management systems used, in addition to the reproducibility of the clinical observations and the accuracy of the recording systems used. In general, there is insufficient information available to document the consequences of milk fever and subclinical hypocalcemia. A summary of several consequences that have been examined follows here.

Milk Fever Relapses. Milk fever cases that need repeat treatment because of relapses increase the costs.

Downer-Cow Complications. The downer-cow syndrome associated with those milk fever cases that fail to respond to intravenous (IV) Ca treatment and remain recumbent for days before subsequently standing, those that die, or those that require destruction represents an important cause of economic loss. The literature reports incidence rates for the downer-cow syndrome ranging from 3.8% to 28.2% of milk-fever cows, with a case fatality rate of 20% to 67%.[9]

Dystocia and Reproductive Disease. Hypocalcemia at the time of parturition can result in uterine inertia, which may cause dystocia and uterine prolapse. In general, there is an increased risk of dystocia associated with milk fever, whether the farmer or the veterinarian attends to the dystocia.[5]

Retained Placenta. Several studies have found an increased risk of retained placenta following milk fever.

Metritis. A few studies have found an indirect relationship between milk fever and subsequent metritis.

Milk Production. There is no reliable evidence that the occurrence of milk fever or subclinical hypocalcemia in cows that recover following treatment affects milk production in the subsequent lactation. Some studies have found a limited effect, no effect, or even positive effect of milk fever on milk production.

Mastitis. Hypocalcemia not only impairs immune function but furthermore may weaken the tone of the teat sphincter, which has been proposed to facilitate intramammary infection, particularly in recumbent cows that are not milked or milked less frequently.[3] An odds ratio of 8.1 for mastitis has been estimated, for coliform mastitis the odds ratio is estimated at 9.0, and for acute clinical mastitis a relative risk of 1.5 following milk fever has been found.

Displacement of Abomasum. Odds ratios ranging from 2.3 to 3.4 for left-side displacement of the abomasum occurring in dairy cows with hypocalcemia at parturition have been estimated.

Ketosis. Studies on the occurrence of ketosis following milk fever have found relative risks or odds ratios ranging from 1.3 to 8.9; using all the confidence intervals, the relative risks/odds ratios range from 1.1 to 15.3.

Body Weight. A temporary drop in body weight occurs in cows with milk fever, but there is no long-term effect. In cows with subclinical hypocalcemia in early lactation, there may be some weight loss compared with cows with normal levels of calcium.

Culling. There may be an increased probability of culling cows that have had milk fever because of the complications or direct or indirect consequences associated with the disease. There is some evidence of culling cows in early lactation because of milk fever, but not in late lactation.

PATHOGENESIS

Hypocalcemia

Calcium has several functions relevant for the pathophysiology of periparturient hypocalcemia, which include the following:

- Cell membrane stability: Calcium bound to cell membranes contributes to the maintenance of adequate membrane stability. In excitable cells the decreased availability of ionized Ca results in higher cell membrane permeability, thereby altering the resting membrane potential and making nerve cells more excitable.
- Muscle contractility: Calcium is required to clear the binding site for myosin on the actin molecule inside the muscle fibers. The cross-bridging between actin and myosin is the basis for the contraction of muscle fibers. Decreased availability of Ca can therefore affect muscle contractility.
- Release of acetylcholine: Calcium is required for the neuronal release of the neurotransmitter acetylcholine into the synaptic cleft of the neuromuscular junctions. Calcium depletion can thus hamper the signal transmission at the level of the neuromuscular endplate.

Whereas decreased membrane stability and ensuing increased excitability are the probable underlying cause of hypocalcemic tetany of monogastric species and the muscle twitching observed in the early stages of milk fever in cattle, disturbed muscle fiber contractility and neurotransmitter release are considered the basis of the flaccid paresis observed in advanced stages of milk fever in ruminants.

The plasma Ca concentration is normally maintained between 2.1 and 2.6 mmol/L (8.4 to 10.4 mg/dL). Almost all multiparous dairy cows will experience at least transient and subclinical hypocalcemia, less than 1.8 mmol/L (7.5 mg/dL), within 24 hours after calving. In some cows, hypocalcemia is more pronounced, causing neuromuscular dysfunction resulting in clinical milk fever. Without treatment, levels may continue to decline to values as low as or even below 0.5 mmol/L (2 mg/dL), which is usually incompatible with life.

Hypocalcemia is the cause of the signs of typical milk fever. Atony of skeletal muscle and plain muscle are well-known physiologic effects of hypocalcemia in ruminants.

Experimental Hypocalcemia

Hypocalcemia can be induced experimentally by administering Na_2-EDTA intravenously, which results in the complex binding or chelation of ionized Ca. The IV infusion of Na_2-EDTA into cows over a period of 4 to 8 hours results in severe hypocalcemia and paresis and has been used extensively as a model for the reproduction of the disease. A standardized flow rate of 1.2 mL/kg per hour of a 5% solution of Na_2-EDTA until recumbency results in changes in plasma ionized Ca, total Ca, inorganic phosphate (Pi), and magnesium comparable to what is observed in spontaneous cases of milk fever. Induced hypocalcemia results in depression of the frequency and amplitude of rumen contractions as early as 1.0 mmol/L of ionized serum Ca, well before any clinical signs of hypocalcemia are detectable and while feeding behavior and rumination are still normal. The induction of subclinical hypocalcemia in cows results in a linear decrease in feed intake and chewing activity as the plasma ionized calcium decreases. Feed intake depression was observed with ionized Ca concentrations below 0.9 mmol/L and before other signs commonly associated with hypocalcemia were recorded. Feed intake approached zero when ionized Ca concentrations declined to 0.6 mmol/L. This suggests that hypocalcemia may contribute to the reduction in feed intake prepartum and depresses the rumination process, ultimately leading to anorexia. Experimental hypocalcemia in cattle furthermore resulted in a marked reduction in cardiac stroke volume, a 50% reduction in arterial blood pressure, and a significant reduction in ruminal and abomasal tone and motility.

In experimental hypocalcemia in sheep, blood flow is reduced by about 60% to all tissues except the kidney, heart, lung, and bladder, in which the reduction is not as high. During periods of prolonged hypocalcemia in cows and ewes, blood flow to skeletal muscles and the alimentary tract may be reduced to 60% to 70% of normal for a long period, which may present a predisposing factor for the downer-cow syndrome. Serum Ca and Pi levels are significantly lower in clinical cases than in comparable normal cows, and there is some relationship between the severity of the signs and the degree of biochemical change.

Signs of hypocalcemic tetany, presumably attributable the increased membrane instability, commonly recognized in nonruminant species are observed in the initial stages of milk fever in cattle:

- Nervousness and early excitement
- Muscle twitching
- Tetany, particularly of the hindlimbs
- Hypersensitivity and convulsive movements of the head and limbs

There are additional signs in the experimental disease, such as excessive salivation, excessive lip and tongue actions, and tail lifting. The serum muscle enzyme levels of creatine phosphokinase (CPK) and aminotransferase (AST) increase as a result of muscle injury associated with prolonged recumbency. Blood glucose levels increase, and serum Pi and potassium levels decrease.

The prolonged infusion of Na_2-EDTA in sheep over 18 hours at a rate to induce hypocalcemia and maintain recumbency resulted in prolonged periods of recumbency ranging from 36 to 64 hours before the animals were able to stand. There are also decreases in plasma sodium, plasma potassium, and erythrocyte potassium and prolonged increases in PCVs, suggesting that fluid replacement therapy may be indicated in cattle with prolonged recumbency associated with hypocalcemia. The activity of AST and CPK, the PCVs, and white blood cell (WBC) counts were elevated 24 hours later.

Hypomagnesemia

Hypomagnesemia is recognized as an importing contributing factor to periparturient hypocalcemia and has been proposed to be the major risk factor for milk fever occurring in cattle in mid- to late lactation.[3] The two mechanism through which Mg deficiency may predispose to hypocalcemia are an impaired release of PTH in response to hypocalcemia and decreased tissue sensitivity to PTH in hypomagnesemic states.[3] Hypomagnesemia can therefore predispose to clinical or subclinical milk fever by blunting the main counter-regulatory mechanism of hypocalcemia.

Hypophosphatemia

Low serum Pi concentrations are commonly observed in milk-fever cows, but also in healthy dairy cows, around parturition.[7] Although the clinical relevance of hypophosphatemia in recumbent cattle remains uncertain, empirical associations between hypophosphatemia and recumbency have been established.[9] Anecdotal reports from field veterinarians suggest that the numbers of recumbent periparturient dairy cows not responding to standard therapy with intravenous Ca salts and showing pronounced hypophosphatemia have increased in recent years. To date, however, there is no unequivocal evidence corroborating the hypothesis that hypophosphatemia plays a role in periparturient recumbency or confirming the treatment efficacy of oral or parenteral Pi supplementation to recumbent cattle.[7]

CLINICAL FINDINGS

Cattle

Three stages of milk fever in cattle are commonly recognized and described.

Stage 1

In the first stage, the cow is still standing. This is also the brief stage of nervousness, excitement, and tetany with hypersensitivity and muscle tremor of the head and limbs. The animal is disinclined to move and often has a decreased or no feed intake. There may be a slight shaking of the head, protrusion of the tongue, and grinding of the teeth. The rectal temperature is usually normal to slightly above normal; the skin may feel cool to the touch. The animal appears ataxic, with a stiff and insecure gait, and falls easily. Close examination reveals agalactia, rumen stasis, and scant feces. Heart rate and respirations may be within normal limits or slightly elevated.

Stage 2

The second stage is characterized by sternal recumbency with depressed consciousness; the cow has a drowsy appearance in sternal recumbency, usually with a lateral kink in the neck or the head turned into the flank (Fig. 17-4). When approached, some of these cows will open their mouths, extend the head and neck, and protrude their tongues, which may be an expression of apprehension and fear in an animal unable to stand. The tetany of the limbs present in the first stage is not present, and the cow is unable to stand. The muzzle is dry, the skin and extremities cool, and the rectal temperature subnormal (36 to 38°C, 97 to 101°F). There is a marked decrease in the absolute intensity of the heart sounds, whereas the heart rate is increased (about 80 bpm). The arterial pulse is weak and the venous pressure is also low, making it difficult to raise the jugular veins. The respirations are not markedly affected, although a mild forced expiratory grunt or groan is sometimes audible. Ruminal stasis and secondary bloat are common, and constipation is characteristic. There is also relaxation of the anus and loss of the anal reflex.

The eyes are usually dry and staring. The pupillary light reflex is incomplete or absent, and the diameter of the pupil varies from normal to maximum dilatation. A detailed examination of the pupils of cows with parturient paresis, nonparetic disorders, and nonparturient paresis found that the mean sizes of the pupils were not significantly different from one another. Rather, disparity of the size of the pupils was common. In cows that develop hypocalcemia a few hours before or at the time of parturition, the second stage of parturition may be delayed. Vaginal examination usually reveals a fully dilated cervix and normal presentation of the fetus. The cow may be in any stage of milk fever, and administration of Ca-salts IV will usually result in a rapid beneficial response and normal parturition.

Prolapse of the uterus is a common complication of milk fever, and often the Ca levels are lower than in parturient cows without uterine prolapse. Thus it is standard practice to treat cases of uterine prolapse with IV calcium salts.

Stage 3

The third stage is characterized by a severely obtunded or even comatose cow in lateral recumbency. There is complete flaccidity on passive movement, and the cow cannot assume sternal recumbency on its own. In general, the depression of temperature and the cardiovascular system are more marked. The heart sounds are almost inaudible, and the rate is increased up to 120 bpm; the pulse is almost impalpable, and it may be impossible to raise the jugular veins. Bloat is common because of prolonged rumen stasis and lateral recumbency. Without treatment, a few animals remain unchanged for several hours, but most become progressively worse during a period of several hours and die quietly from shock in a state of complete collapse.

Concurrent Hypomagnesemia. Mild to moderate tetany and hyperesthesia persisting beyond the first stage suggests a concurrent hypomagnesemia. There is excitement and fibrillary twitching of the eyelids, and tetanic convulsions are readily precipitated by sound or touch. Trismus may be present. The heart and respiratory rates are increased, and the heart sounds are much louder than normal. Without treatment, death occurs during a convulsion.

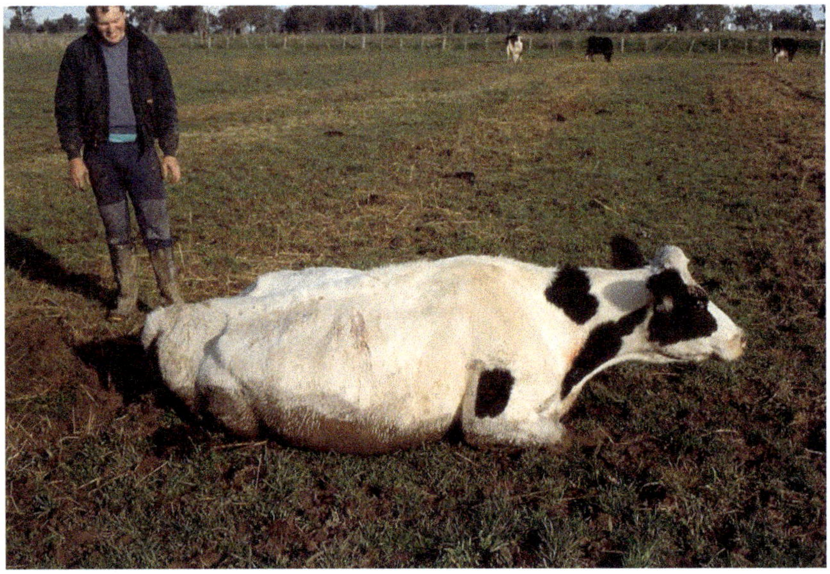

Fig. 17-4 Friesian cow with stage 2 periparturient hypocalcemia. The cow is unable to stand without assistance.

Sheep and Goats

The disease in pastured ewes is similar to that in cattle. The early signs include a stilty, proppy gait and tremor of the shoulder muscles. Recumbency follows, sometimes with tetany of the limbs, but the proportion of ewes with hypocalcemia that are recumbent in the early stages is much less than in cattle. A similar generalization applies to female goats. The characteristic posture is sternal recumbency, with the legs under the body or stretched out behind. The head is rested on the ground, and there may be an accumulation of mucus exudate in the nostrils. The venous blood pressure is low and the pulse impalpable. Mental depression is evidenced by a drowsy appearance and depression of the corneal reflex. There is loss of the anal reflex, constipation, tachycardia, hyposensitivity, ruminal stasis and tympany, salivation, and tachypnea. Response to parenteral treatment with Ca salts is rapid; the ewe is normal 30 minutes after an SC injection. Death often occurs within 6 to 12 hours if treatment is not administered. The syndrome is usually more severe in pregnant than in lactating ewes, possibly because of the simultaneous occurrence of pregnancy toxemia or hypomagnesemia. Fat late-pregnant ewes on high-grain diets indoors or in feedlots show a similar syndrome accompanied by prolapses of the vagina and intestine.

CLINICAL PATHOLOGY

Total serum Ca levels are reduced to below 2.0 mmol/L (8 mg/dL), usually to below 1.2 mmol/L (5 mg/dL), and sometimes to as low as 0.5 mmol/L (2 mg/dL). The reduction is usually, but not always, proportional to the severity of the clinical syndrome. Average figures for total serum Ca levels in the three species are as follows: cows, 1.30 ± 0.30 mmol/L (5.2 ± 1.2 mg/dL); ewes, 1.15 ± 0.37 mmol/L (4.6 ± 1.5 mg/dL); goat does, 0.94 ± 0.15 mmol/L (3.8 ± 0.6 mg/dL).

Although the concentration of ionized Ca, which is the biologically active fraction of the total Ca pool, is the factor determining the presence and severity of clinical signs in hypocalcemic animals, the total serum Ca concentration is commonly used for convenience. Measurement of ionized Ca concentration requires the use of ion-selective electrodes, which have become much more accessible in recent decades. Nonetheless, the association between ionized and total Ca in serum is tight, with excellent correlation between the two, which is why total Ca concentration in serum is considered clinically useful and sufficiently accurate in practice.[3] Between 42% and 48% of the total Ca content in the extracellular space is available as biologically active ionized Ca. A decrease in serum albumin or acidemia tends to increase the ionized Ca fraction, whereas alkalemia or an increase in serum albumin tends to decrease the proportion of ionized Ca.[3] Equine, bovine, and ovine blood may be stored for up to 48 hours without any clinically relevant alteration of blood Ca ion concentration.

Levels of ionized Ca in the venous whole blood of cows are as follows: normal, 1.06 to 1.26 mmol/L (4.3 to 5.1 mg/dL); slight hypocalcemia, 1.05 to 0.80 mmol/L (4.2 to 3.2 mg/dL); moderate, 0.79 to 0.50 mmol/L (3.2 to 2.0 mg/dL); severe hypocalcemia, less than 0.50 mmol/L (<2.0 mg/dL). Total serum Ca levels are reduced below normal in all cows at calving, whether they have milk fever or not, but not in ewes.

Serum **magnesium** levels are usually moderately elevated to 1.65 to 2.06 mmol/L (4 to 5 mg/dL), but in some areas low levels may be encountered, especially in cows at pasture.

Serum **inorganic phosphorus (Pi)** levels are usually depressed to 0.48 to 0.97 mmol/L (1.5 to 3.0 mg/dL).

Blood glucose levels are usually normal, although they may be depressed if ketosis occurs concurrently. Higher-than-normal blood glucose levels are likely to occur in cases of long duration and are presumable because Ca is required for the release of insulin from the pancreas.

Serum Muscle Enzyme Activity

Prolonged recumbency results in ischemic muscle trauma and necrosis and increases in the serum muscle enzyme activity of creatine kinase (CK) and aspartate aminotransferase (AST). During prolonged recumbency following treatment for milk fever, the levels of CK will remain elevated if muscle trauma is progressive in animals that are not rolled from side to side every few hours to reduce the effects of compression on the large muscle groups of the pelvic limbs (see also the discussion under "Downer-Cow Syndrome" in this chapter).

Hemogram

Changes in the leukocyte count include eosinopenia, neutrophilia, and lymphopenia suggestive of adrenal cortical hyperactivity, but similar changes occur at calving in cows that do not develop parturient paresis. High plasma cortisol levels and PCVs occur in cows with milk fever and are higher still in cows that do not respond to treatment. They are expressions of stress and dehydration. Clinicopathological findings in the other species are not described in detail except with regard to depression of total serum calcium levels.

NECROPSY FINDINGS

There are no gross or histologic changes unless concurrent disease is present.

DIFFERENTIAL DIAGNOSIS

A diagnosis of milk fever is based on the occurrence of paresis and depression of consciousness in animals following parturition. The diagnosis is supported by a favorable response to treatment with parenteral injections of calcium solutions and by biochemical examination of the blood. In ewes, the history usually contains some reference to recent physical stress, and the disease is more common in the period preceding lambing.

There are several diseases that cause recumbency in cows in the immediate postpartum period, and their differentiation is summarized in Table 17-5.

Several diseases that occur at the time of parturition must be differentiated from milk fever in cattle. These are grouped here according to the following categories:

- Other metabolic diseases
- Diseases associated with toxemia and shock
- Injuries to the pelvis and pelvic limbs
- Degenerative myopathy
- Downer-cow syndrome

Metabolic Diseases

Hypomagnesemia may occur as the sole cause of recumbency; it may accompany a primary hypocalcemia or result in secondary hypocalcemia so that the case presented is one of parturient paresis complicated by lactation tetany. Hyperesthesia, tetany, tachycardia, and convulsions are common instead of the typical findings of depression and paresis in milk fever.

Hypophosphatemia, which commonly accompanies milk fever, is suggested as a cause of continued recumbency in cows after partial response to Ca therapy; serum Pi levels are low and return to normal if the cow stands or following treatment with calcium salts. The role of hypophosphatemia in the etiology of periparturient recumbency in cattle is under contentious debate. Although there is no unequivocal evidence available supporting the role of P in the etiology of recumbency in cattle, cows not responding to IV Ca were found to have lower serum Pi levels.[7,9]

Severe hypokalemia (<2.5 mmol/L) in dairy cows is characterized by extreme weakness or recumbency, especially after treatment for ketosis with isoflupredone.[10] Clinical signs tend to resemble botulism rather than hypocalcemia, with flaccid paralysis of the tongue and masticatory muscles and the head resting on the ground rather than on the chest of the cow. The case-fatality rate is high in spite of therapy with potassium. Hypokalemic myopathy is present at necropsy.

Ketosis may complicate milk fever, in which case the animal responds to Ca therapy by standing but continues to manifest the clinical signs of ketosis, including in some cases the nervous signs of licking, circling, and abnormal voice.

Diseases Associated With Toxemia and Shock

During the immediate postparturient period, several diseases occur commonly and are characterized by toxemia.

Acute or peracute coliform mastitis is characterized by one or several obviously enlarged and inflamed mammary glands with watery and serouslike secretions that may be overlooked if the cow is recumbent. Other signs include fever in early stages that may be followed by hypothermia in advanced stages of toxemia or septicemia, tachycardia, dehydration, depression and weakness up to the point of recumbency, ruminal stasis, and frequently also watery diarrhea.

Aspiration pneumonia secondary to regurgitation and aspiration of rumen contents is a complication of third-stage milk fever, or accidental aspiration or fluid administration into the trachea of periparturient cattle that were meant to be drenched. Fever, dyspnea, expiratory grunt, severe depression, and anxiety are common. Auscultation of the lungs reveals the presence of abnormal lung sounds. Aspiration pneumonia should be suspected if the animal has been lying on its side, especially if there is evidence of regurgitation of ruminal contents from the nostrils, no matter how small the amount, or if there is a history of the animal having been drenched. Abnormal auscultatory findings may not be detectable until the second day. Early diagnosis is imperative if the animal is to be saved, and the mortality rate is always high.

Acute diffuse peritonitis resulting from traumatic perforation of the abomasum or uterus is characterized by severe depression, tachycardia, dehydration, rumen stasis, fever, weakness and recumbency, grunting or groaning with respiration, and possibly splashing sounds on ballottement of the abdomen.

Carbohydrate engorgement (grain overload) results in depression, dehydration, tachycardia, hypothermia, diarrhea, and weakness up to the point of recumbency. The rumen is atonic and mildly to moderately bloated. the rumen content is watery. and the fiber matt is absent. A positive steelband sound and splashing sounds may be audible over the rumen on auscultation and percussion of the left flank. Examination of the rumen fluid will reveal a sour smell with low pH (<5.0). Microscopic examination of a smear will reveal absence of living protozoa and a predominance of gram-positive microorganisms if a stain is performed.

Toxemic septic metritis occurs most commonly within a few days after parturition and is characterized by depression, anorexia, fever, tachycardia (100 to 120 bpm), ruminal stasis, and presence of foul-smelling uterine discharge found on vaginal examination. The fetal placenta may be retained. Some affected cows are weak and prefer recumbency, which resembles milk fever.

Prolapse and rupture of the uterus cause varying degrees of shock, with tachycardia, hypothermia and cool extremities, weakness and recumbency, and rapid death. A history of difficult parturition or assisted dystocia

Table 17-5 Parturient paresis: Differential diagnosis of common causes of recumbency in parturient adult cattle

Disease	Epidemiology	Clinical signs	Clinical pathology	Response to treatment
Milk fever (parturient paresis)	Mature cows, within 48 hours of calving, some in midlactation	Early excitement and tetany, then depression, coma, hypothermia, flaccidity, pupil dilatation, weak heart sounds No rumen movements HR increases as state worsens	Hypocalcemia, with total Ca < 5 mg/dL (1.25 mmol/L) calcium frequently combined with hypophosphatemia with low inorganic phosphate, < 3 mg/dL (0.9 mmol/L)	Rapid, characteristic response (muscle tremor, sweating on muzzle, defecation, urination, pulse amplitude and heart rate decrease and heart sound intensity improves after IV administration of Ca salt solutions)
Downer cows following milk fever	Most common in situation where milk fever and lactation tetany are common and intensity of treatment is lax; cows are left down too long before treatment	Moderately bright, active, eating Temp. slightly raised, HR 80–100 Unable to stand but tries—creepers or alert downer cows When dull and depressed—nonalert downers Long course, 1–2 weeks	Variable May be low inorganic phosphate, or potassium, or glucose Ketonuria, plasma CPK, and AST elevated	Variable response to calcium, phosphorus, and potassium salts Fluid therapy and provision of deep bedding and hourly rolling from side to side are necessary
Carbohydrate engorgement	Access to large amount readily fermentable carbohydrate when not accustomed Enzootic in high-grain rations in feedlots Intensive IV fluid and electrolyte therapy necessary for survival	Severe gastrointestinal atony with complete cessation of ruminal activity Fluid splashing sounds in rumen Severe dehydration, circulatory failure Apparent blindness, then recumbency and too weak to rise Soft, odoriferous feces	Hemoconcentration with severe acidosis, pH of rumen fluid below 5, serum calcium may be depressed No living protozoa in rumen	Rumenotomy or rumen lavage may be necessary Oral antibiotics, alkalinizing agents per os and IV
Hypomagnesemia (lactation, grass tetany)	All classes and ages of cattle, but most recently calved cows May occur in pregnant beef cattle	Excitement, hypersensitivity, muscle tremor, tetany Recumbent with tetanic convulsions, loud heart sounds, rapid rate Subacute cases remain standing	Low serum magnesium, < 1.2 mg/dL (0.5 mmol/L), low (undetectable) urine magnesium	Even after IV injection, response in a severe case may take 30 min, much slower than response to calcium in milk fever
Severe toxemia (acute diffuse peritonitis, coliform mastitis)	Sporadic only Mastitis most common where hygiene poor Peritonitis as a result of foreign body perforation of reticulum, perforation of abomasal ulcus, rupture of uterus or vagina	Recumbency, depression to coma, sleepy, dry nose, hypothermia, gut stasis, heart rate > 100 beats/min, may be grunting Examine mammary gland Examine abdomen for abdominal disease	Profound leukopenia Serum calcium may be as low as 7–8 mg/dL (1.75–2.0 mmol/L) Examine milk	Require supportive response for toxemia and shock Response is poor and temporary Prognosis very bad May die if treated IV with calcium or magnesium salts
Fat-cow syndrome	Fat dairy or beef cows in late gestation or at parturition Some predisposing cause precipitates illness in fat animals	Excessive body condition, anorexia, apathy, depression, recumbency that looks like milk fever, scant soft feces, ketonuria	Evidence of hepatic disease	Will recover if begin to eat Treat with fluids, glucose, insulin Provide good-quality palatable roughage
Physical injuries	Ruptured gastrocnemius, dislocation of hip, etc. Sporadic sequelae to milk fever, may be contributed to by osteoporosis, slippery ground surface, stimulating to rise too early	As for Maternal obstetric paresis with ruptured gastrocnemius, hock remains on ground when standing Excessive lateral mobility of limb with hip dislocation	Increase serum CK and AST activity	Supportive therapy, deep bedding, and frequent rolling
Acute hypokalemia	Dairy cattle treated for ketosis with isoflupredone acetate Calved within previous 30 days	Recumbent, very weak, appear flaccid, in sternal or lateral recumbency, unable to support head off ground, hold head in flank, anorexia; cardiac arrhythmia may present Most die or are euthanized	Serum potassium below 2.5 mEq/L Muscle necrosis at necropsy	Potassium chloride orally or very carefully IV (drip infusion)

AST, aspartate aminotransferase; CK, creatine kinase; IV, intravenous.

with fetotomy may be associated with rupture of the uterus. The administration of calcium salts may cause ventricular fibrillation and sudden death.

Although some elevation of the temperature may be observed in these severe toxemic states, it is more usual to find a subnormal temperature. The response to Ca therapy is usually a marked increase in heart rate, and death during the injection is common. Every case of recumbency must be carefully examined because these conditions may occur either independently or as complications of parturient paresis. In our experience, about 25% of cases of postparturient recumbency in cows are attributable primarily to toxemia or injury rather than to hypocalcemia.

Injuries to the Pelvis and Pelvic Limbs

Injuries to the pelvis and pelvic limbs are common at parturition because of the marked relaxation of the ligaments of the pelvic girdle. Seven types of leg abnormalities have been described in this group at an incidence level of 8.5% in 400 consecutive cases of parturient paresis. The described abnormalities include radial paralysis, hip dislocation, and rupture of gastrocnemius muscle. In most instances the affected animals are down and unable to stand, but they mentally alert; eat, drink, urinate, and defecate normally; have a normal temperature and heart rate; and make strong efforts to stand, particularly with the forelimbs.

Maternal obstetric paralysis is the most common injury. Although this occurs most frequently in heifers after a difficult parturition, it may also occur in adult animals following an easy birth and occasionally before parturition, especially in cows in poor body condition. The mildest form is evidenced by a frequent kicking movement of a hindleg, as though something was stuck between the claws. All degrees of severity—from the mild kicking through knuckling and weakness of one or both hindlegs, to complete inability to rise—may occur, but sensation in the affected limb is usually normal. There is traumatic injury to the pelvic nerves during passage of the calf. There are often gross hemorrhages, both deep and superficial, and histopathological degeneration of the sciatic nerves. In individual animals, injury to the obturator nerves is common and results in defective adduction of the hindlimbs. The position of the hindlimbs may be normal, but in severe cases, especially those with extensive hematoma along the sciatic nerve trunk, the leg may be held extended with the toe reaching the elbow as in a dislocation of the hip; however, in the latter case there is exaggerated lateral mobility of the limb. Additional injuries causing recumbency near parturition include those associated with degenerative myopathy, dislocation of the hip, and ventral hernia.

Dislocation of the coxofemoral joint can cause recumbency and inability to stand in some cows, whereas others can stand and move around. Recumbent cows are usually in sternal recumbency, and the affected limb is abducted excessively. In standing cows, the affected limb is usually extended, often difficult to flex, and often rotated about its long axis. The diagnostic criteria are as follows:

- Sudden onset of lameness with the affected limb extended and possibly rotated
- Displacement of the greater trochanter of the femur from its normal position relative to the ischiatic tuber and coxal tuber of the pelvis (compare left and right rear limb)
- Ability to abduct the limb manually beyond its normal range
- Crepitus in the hip on abduction and rotation of the limb
- Ability to palpate the femoral head per rectum or per vaginum against the cranial border of the ilium or pubis in cases of cranioventral dislocation, or in the obturator foramen in cases of caudoventral dislocation

Manual replacement by closed reduction is successful in 80% of cases of craniodorsal dislocation and in 65% of cases of caudodorsal dislocation; relapses are, however, common. The ability to stand before reduction is the most useful prognostic aid.

Degenerative Myopathy (Ischemic Muscle Necrosis)

Degenerative myopathy, affecting primarily the large muscles of the thighs, occurs commonly in cattle that have been recumbent for more than several hours. At necropsy, large masses of pale muscle are present, surrounded by muscle of normal color. Clinically it is indistinguishable from sciatic nerve paralysis. Markedly increased serum activities of CK occur in cows recumbent for several hours following the initial episode of milk fever as a result of ischemic necrosis. Persistent elevation of CK activity indicates progressive ischemic muscle necrosis as a result of continued compression of the large muscle masses of the pelvic limbs. Rupture of the gastrocnemius muscle or separation of its tendon from either the muscle or the tuber calcis may also cause myopathy.

Downer-Cow Syndrome

Downer-cow syndrome is a common sequel to milk fever in which postparturient cows that may initially have been hypocalcemic remain recumbent for unknown reason after repeated intravenous treatment with Ca salts. Following treatment, most of the clinical findings associated with milk fever resolve, but the animal remains unable to stand. Clinically, the animal may be alert with normal or slightly decreased appetite and will commonly recover and stand normally within several hours or a few days. The animal's vital signs are within the normal range, and its alimentary tract function is normal. However, some affected animals are anorexic, may not drink, exhibit bizarre movements of lying in lateral recumbency, dorsally extend the head and neck frequently, moan and groan frequently, assume a frog-legged posture with the pelvic limbs, and crawl or creep around the stall; these animals may die or are euthanized for humane reasons within a few days. The diagnostic dilemma with these cows is that, at least initially, they resemble cows with milk fever, and whether or not to treat them with additional amounts of calcium salts is questionable.

Nonparturient Hypocalcemia

Paresis with mental depression and associated with low total serum Ca levels can occur in cows at times other than at parturition. The cause is largely unexplained, but hypomagnesemia has been proposed as a major risk factor for this atypical form of clinical milk fever in cattle.[3] Hypocalcemia may also occur after gorging on grain and may be a significant factor in particular cases. Sudden rumen stasis as a result of traumatic reticulitis may rarely cause hypocalcemic paresis. Diarrhea, particularly when cattle or sheep are placed on new lush pasture, may also precipitate an attack. Access to plants rich in oxalates may have a similar effect, particularly if the animals are unaccustomed to the plants. Affected animals respond well to Ca therapy, but relapse is likely unless the primary cause is corrected. The differential diagnosis of diseases of nonparturient cows manifested principally by recumbency is also summarized in Table 17-5.

Hypocalcemic Paresis in Sheep and Goats

Hypocalcemia in sheep must be differentiated from pregnancy toxemia, in which the course is much longer, the signs indicate cerebral involvement, and the disease is restricted to pregnant ewes. There is no response to Ca therapy, and a positive test for ketonuria is almost diagnostic of pregnancy toxemia. At parturition, goats are susceptible to enterotoxemia and hypoglycemia (rarely), both of which present clinical signs similar to parturient paresis.

Hypocalcemia in Sows

Hypocalcemia is rare in sows. The disease must be differentiated from the mastitis, metritis, and agalactia complex, which is characterized by fever, agalactia, anorexia, toxemia, and enlarged and inflamed mammary glands.

Treatment

Every effort must be made to treat affected cows as soon as possible after clinical signs are obvious. Treatment during the first stage of the disease, before the cow is recumbent, is the ideal situation. The longer the interval between the time the cow first becomes recumbent and treatment, the greater the incidence of downer-cow syndrome as a result of ischemic muscle necrosis from prolonged recumbency. Complications of milk fever occur when cows have been in sternal recumbency for more than 4 hours. Farmers must be educated to appreciate the importance of early treatment. Cows found in lateral recumbency (third stage) should be placed in sternal recumbency until treatment is available. This will facilitate eructation and reduce the risk of aspiration if the cow regurgitates. Cows that have difficulty finding solid, nonslip footing beneath them will often not try to stand and may develop ischemic myonecrosis. Avoidance of this complication necessitates the placement of rubber or other mats under the cow or transportation of the cow to a piece of pasture with a dense sward on it.

Standard Treatment

IV with solutions containing Ca as Ca-gluconate, Ca-borogluconate, and—nowadays less commonly—as Ca-chloride is the treatment of choice. Most cows with milk fever can be treated successfully with Ca salt solutions providing 8 to 10 g of Ca (Ca-borogluconate is 8.3% Ca). The dose rate of Ca is frequently under discussion. A typical treatment for an adult lactating dairy cow with periparturient hypocalcemia is 500 mL of 23% Ca-borogluconate by slow IV injection with cardiac auscultation; this provides 10.7 g of Ca. Although the calculated Ca deficit in a recumbent periparturient dairy cow is 4 g Ca, additional Ca should be provided to overcome the ongoing losses in milk.[6] Underdosing increases the chances of incomplete response, with inability of the cow to rise, or of relapse, whereas considerable overdosing may result in potentially fatal cardiac toxicity. Additional subcutaneous administration of Ca-borogluconate (500 mL) markedly decreased the relapse rate in cattle receiving 500 mL of Ca-borogluconate IV for the treatment of hypocalcemia.[6]

The standard rate of administration is a rapid IV administration of the calculated dose of Ca-borogluconate over a period of 15 minutes. The maximum safe rate of Ca administration in cattle was determined to be 0.07 mEq of ionized Ca per kg body weight per minute, which is equivalent to 0.065 mL of a 23% Ca-borogluconate per kg body weight per minute.[6] An average nonhypocalcemic 600-kg cow could therefore safely be treated with intravenous Ca-borogluconate (23%) at an infusion rate of 39 mL/min. Immediately following IV administration of Ca-borogluconate over a period of 12 to 15 minutes, treated animals are commonly markedly hypercalcemic (up to 6 mmol/L or 24 mg/dL). The plasma Ca concentration will then gradually decline over a period of several hours. Although the direct effect of intravenously administered Ca does not last for more than 6 to 8 hours, this transient correction of hypocalcemia in most cases is not only associated with clinical recovery of recumbent animals, but also with improved feed intake and enhanced gastrointestinal motility, which will result in improved intestinal Ca absorption. This latter effect, which relies on the availability of adequate amounts of Ca for absorption in the digestive tract, is responsible for the sustained correction of hypocalcemia observed in most cases. However, in some cows, mechanisms regulating the Ca homeostasis are less effective or the oral Ca supply is insufficient, and subclinical or clinical hypocalcemia may recur. For this reason, it is astute to follow up on intravenously treated animals with oral supplementation of Ca salts for 1 to 2 days.

Because of concerns with these rapid and short-lived peaks in plasma Ca after rapid infusion of Ca salt solutions, it has been suggested that slower IV infusion might be safer and more effective. The slow infusion of a Ca solution via an IV indwelling catheter over 6 hours was compared with the conventional single IV administration of 600 mL of a 40% Ca-borogluconate and 6% Mg-hypophosphite solution over 15 minutes in cows recumbent with milk fever. Cows receiving the rapid infusion responded more quickly, stood sooner, and returned to normal demeanor more quickly. The slow infusion consisted of 200 ml IV over a 10-minute period, with the remaining 400 ml added to 10 L of a solution of 90 g sodium chloride and 500 g glucose and given via IV drip over a 6-hour period at a rate of 1.7 L/h. In cows treated rapidly, the serum Ca and magnesium levels increased rapidly compared with the infused cows. In sheep and goats, the recommended amount is 15 to 20 g IV with an optional 5 to 10 g SC. Sows should receive 100 to 150 mL of a similar solution IV or SC.

Routes of Administration

IV Route

The IV route is preferred because the response is rapid and obvious. The heart should be auscultated throughout the IV administration for evidence of gross arrhythmia, bradycardia, and tachycardia. Although bradycardia is a normal response to Ca administration in hypocalcemic animals and is of no concern, the IV administration should be interrupted in case arrhythmia or pronounced tachycardia is noticed. If the cardiac irregularity continues, the remainder of the solution can be given subcutaneously. The best recommendation is to give as much of the solution as possible intravenously and the remainder subcutaneously. The common practice of giving half the dose intravenously and half subcutaneously is a reasonable compromise because with this method there are fewer relapses. If a cow has been previously treated subcutaneously by the farmer, additional Ca given intravenously may cause toxicity if the improved circulation enhances the absorption of the subcutaneous Ca.

Toxemic cows are very susceptible to the IV administration of Ca-borogluconate, and death may occur. In such cases the heart rate increases markedly (up to 160 bpm); there is respiratory distress, trembling, and collapse; and the cow dies within a few minutes. SC or IV administration is preferred in cows with severe toxemia as a result of aspiration pneumonia, metritis, and mastitis.

Typical Response to Intravenous Ca-Borogluconate

Cows with milk fever exhibit a typical pattern of response to Ca-borogluconate IV if the response is favorable, including:

- Belching
- Muscle tremor, particularly of the flanks and often extending to the whole body
- Slowing and improvement in the amplitude and pressures of the pulse
- Decrease of the heart rate
- Increase in the intensity of the heart sounds
- Sweating of the muzzle
- Defecation

The feces are in the form of a firm fecal ball with a firm crust and covered with mucus. Urination usually does not follow until the cow stands. A slight transitory tetany of the limbs may also be observed. Many cows will eat and drink within minutes following successful treatment if offered feed and water.

In general, recovery can be expected in 75% of cases within 2 hours; in 10% recovery is complicated by one of the diseases discussed earlier, and 15% can be expected either to die or to require disposal. Of those that recover after one treatment, 25% to 30% can be expected to relapse and require further treatment.

Unfavorable Response to Intravenous Ca-Borogluconate

An unfavorable response is characterized by a marked increase in heart rate in cows affected with toxemia and bradyarrhythmia in animals developing an atrial block as a result of Ca overdosage. Overdosage may occur when a standard dose is administered to quickly, when an excessive dose is administered, when repeated doses are administered in excess of requirements, or when an individual with increased sensitivity to Ca is treated. Toxicity can, for instance, occur when farmers treat cases unsuccessfully by multiple SC injections and these are followed by an IV dose. When the peripheral circulation is poor, it is probable that the calcium administered subcutaneously is not absorbed until the circulation improves following the IV injection, and the large doses of Ca then absorbed cause acute toxicity.

Increased sensitivity to Ca has been reported in toxic animals with coliform mastitis or toxic metritis and in cows with severe ketosis or hepatic lipidosis. Hypokalemia that is common in anorectic animals may present a further factor predisposing to increased sensitivity of the heart muscle to excessive Ca doses. Sudden death may also occur after calcium injections if the cow is excited or frightened, which may be the result of an increased sensitivity to epinephrine. When affected cows are exposed to the sun or a hot, humid atmosphere, heatstroke may be a complicating factor. In such cases an attempt should be made to reduce the temperature to below 39.5°C (103°F) before the calcium is administered.

In all cases of IV treatment with Ca salts, the circulation must be monitored closely. If there is gross arrhythmia or a sudden increase in heart rate, the injection should be discontinued. In normal circumstances at least 15 minutes should be taken to administer the standard dose. The acute toxic effect of calcium salts seems to be exerted specifically on heart muscle, with a great variety of defects occurring in cardiac action; the defect type depends on the specific Ca salt used and the speed of injection. Electrocardiogram (ECG) changes after induced hypercalcemia show increased ventricular activity and reduced atrial activity. Atropine is capable of abolishing the resulting arrhythmia.

SC Route

The SC route is commonly used by farmers who treat affected cows at the first sign of hypocalcemia, preferably during the first stage when the cow is still standing. The SC route has also been used by veterinarians when the effects of IV administration of Ca are uncertain or if an unusual response occurs during IV administration. The main inconvenience of the SC route of administration is that the absorption is difficult to predict because of the often comprised blood flow to the periphery in affected animals.[11] Subcutaneous treatment with Ca solutions is inappropriate with severe hypocalcemia or dehydration because absorption in these animals is impaired, which may result in a markedly delayed treatment effect.[8] The amount of Ca administered per injection site should be limited to 1 to 1.5 g, which is equivalent to 50 to 75 mL of most commercial Ca infusion solutions.[11] Although most solutions containing Ca-gluconate or Ca-borogluconate are suitable for SC administration, the SC administration of salt solutions containing Ca-chloride should be avoided because these formulations are highly caustic. The SC administration of Ca solutions also containing glucose, particularly at higher concentrations, is discouraged because concentrated glucose can result in pronounced tissue irritation.[8] Administration of 500 mL of a 23% Ca-borogluconate solution over 10 injection sites was associated with an increase of the plasma Ca concentration of over 15% within 30 minutes; the plasma Ca concentration returned to baseline concentrations within 6 hours of treatment.[8]

Oral Route

Or administration of different Ca salts has been practiced for decades. Oral formulations are commonly based on Ca-chloride ($CaCl_2$) and Ca-propionate. Calcium chloride formulations have the advantage of low cost and a small volume required to administer an appropriate dose of 50 g Ca, but they are highly caustic and may cause severe damage of the digestive tract mucosa exposed to the concentrated formulation. Repeated treatment with $CaCl_2$ may furthermore result in uncompensated metabolic acidosis in treated animals.[11] In contrast, Ca-propionate formulations require a higher volume to provide the same amount of Ca and are absorbed at a slower rate but are less injurious to tissue and do not alter the acid–base equilibrium. In these formulations, the availability of propionate, which is a glucose precursor, has been marketed as a further potential advantage, but studies investigating the effect of the gluconate contained in these products failed to identify any positive effects on plasma glucose, insulin, or NEFA concentration in cows treated with Ca-gluconate.[12] Oral $CaCl_2$ formulations typically contain 50 g of Ca and increase the plasma Ca concentration within 30 minutes and for at least 6 hours.[6,8] Oral Ca formulations should only be administered to cattle with undisturbed swallowing ability, which precludes their use as first-line treatment in animals in an advanced stage of clinical hypocalcemia.

Failure to Respond to Treatment

A failure to respond favorably to treatment may be the result of an incorrect or incomplete diagnosis, or inadequate treatment. A poor response to treatment includes: (1) no observable changes in the clinical findings immediately following the calcium administration, or (2) the animal may respond to the calcium in all respects with the exception of being unable to stand for varying periods of time following treatment. An inadequate response also includes relapse after successful recovery, which usually occurs within 48 hours of the previous treatment. The needs of individual animals for Ca replacement vary widely depending on many factors, such as the body weight, milk yield, age, and degree of hypocalcemia. Incomplete responses may be more common in older cows and in cases of inability of the normal mechanisms to maintain serum Ca levels during the period of sudden changes in the equilibrium input and output of the extracellular Ca pool. The duration of the illness and the severity of clinical signs at the time of first treatment also affect the treatment response. In an extensive field study, there were no downer cows or deaths in cows still standing when first treated, 13% of downers and 2% of deaths occurred in cows in sternal recumbency when first treated, and 37% of downers and 12% of deaths occurred in cows in lateral recumbency when first treated. Therefore, in general, the longer the period from onset of milk fever to treatment, the longer the period of posttreatment recumbency and the higher the case-fatality rate. The best procedure to follow if response does not occur is to revisit the animal at 6- to 12-hour intervals and check the diagnosis. If no other cause of the recumbency can be determined, the initial treatment can be repeated on a maximum of three occasions. Beyond this point, further calcium therapy is seldom effective.

GENERAL MANAGEMENT AND CLINICAL CARE PROCEDURES

The care of the cow and the calf following milk fever is important. If the cow is recumbent for any length of time, she must be kept propped up in sternal recumbency and not left in lateral recumbency, which may result in tympany, regurgitation, and aspiration pneumonia. The cow should be rolled from side to side every few hours and provided with adequate bedding or moved to a suitable nonslip ground surface. In extreme climatic conditions, erection of a shelter over the cow is advisable if she cannot be moved to permanent shelter. If a cow is recumbent for more than 48 hours, occasional assisted lifting using appropriate cow lifters should be considered. However, heroic measures to get cows to stand should be avoided. Gentle nudging in the ribs or the use of an electric prod are the maximum stimulants advised. The best assistance that can be given to a cow attempting to stand is a good heave at the base of the tail when she is halfway up.

TREATMENT AND CONTROL

Treatment

Calcium gluconate (equivalent to 8 to 12 g Ca/cow IV or SC as single dose) (R-1)

Calcium borogluconate (equivalent to 8 to 12 g Ca/cow IV or SC as single dose) (R-1)

Calcium chloride (equivalent to 8 to 12 g Ca/cow IV as single dose) (R-2)

Calcium chloride (equivalent to 50 g Ca/cow) PO q12 for 48h (R-1)

Calcium propionate (equivalent to 50 g Ca/cow) PO q12 for 48h (R-2)

Control

Reduce dietary calcium intake 2 to 3 weeks before calving to less than 20 g Ca/cow/day (R-1)

Reduce dietary potassium content as much as possible in late gestation (in any case, below 2% in feed dry matter) (R-1)

Provide adequate dietary magnesium in late gestation (≈0.4% of feed dry matter) (R-1)

Anionic salts mixed into feed to obtain a dietary cation–anion difference of −100 to −150 mEq/kg of feed dry matter for at least 2 weeks before calving (R-1)

Zeolite A (250 to 500 g/cow/day) PO q24h for at least 2 weeks before calving (R-2)

Supplement diet in late gestation with vitamin D (R-1)

Vitamin D_3 (10 million IU/cow IM as single dose 3 to 7 days before expected calving) (R-2)

Vitamin D_2 (10 to 20 million IU/cow PO for at least 7 days before expected calving) (R-2)

Calcium chloride (equivalent to 50 g Ca/cow PO q12h for 48 hours from the time of parturition) (R-1)

Calcium propionate (equivalent to 50 g Ca/cow PO q12h for 48 hours from the time of parturition) (R-2)

Partial milking during the first days of lactation (R-3)

Udder insufflation in the first days of lactation (R-3)

CONTROL

When the incidence of milk fever increases to above 10% of high-risk cows (third or later lactations), a specific control program is necessary. When the incidence is low, a specific control program may not be economical, and the alternative is to monitor cows carefully at the time of parturition and for 48 hours after parturition and treat affected animals during the first stage of the disease if possible.

Strategies for prevention of periparturient hypocalcemia in general are based on one of following approaches:

- Reduction of dietary Ca available for intestinal absorption during the dry period
- Induction of mild to moderate acidosis during the last weeks of gestation
- Supplementation of vitamin D during the dry period
- Oral Ca supplementation around parturition
- Parenteral Ca administration around parturition
- Partial milking

For purposes of optimal nutritional management of dairy cows that are fed prepared feeds (not pasture based), the dry period is frequently divided into two distinct portions: cows in the early and middle part of the dry period (*far-off* or *regular* dry-cow group) and cows in the final 2 to 3 weeks before their calving date (*prefresh, transition, close-up, near, lead-feeding,* or *steam-up* group). Large herds may have additional subgroups of dry cows depending on management circumstances and facilities available. Special attention must be given to the mineral nutrition of the close-up group. Minerals should be provided to close-up cows in known quantities, either as part of a grain mixture or a total mixed ration (TMR).

Reduction of Dietary Calcium Available for Intestinal Absorption

Dietary Calcium Concentration in Late Gestation

Diets high in Ca during the prepartum period can result in a high incidence of milk fever, and diets low in Ca will reduce the incidence of milk fever in dairy cows. Feeding more than 100 g of Ca per cow per day during the dry period is associated with an increased incidence of milk fever. An adult cow requires only around 30 g/daily of Ca to meet maintenance and fetal demands in the last 2 months of late gestation. Low-Ca diets (<20 g [Ca/cow]/d) fed during the last 2 weeks before parturition are effective in reducing the occurrence of clinical milk fever. The low levels of dietary Ca push the organism into a negative Ca balance before calving, which activates the homeostatic mechanisms before the Ca losses through the mammary gland begin. These mechanisms include the secretion of PTH, which increases renal reabsorption of Ca within minutes, stimulates Ca resorption from bone within hours to days, and stimulates renal vitamin D metabolism to toward production of 1,25-$(OH)_2D$ within hours or days. The 1,25-$(OH)_2D$ stimulates the active transport of Ca across the intestinal epithelial cells. At the time of calving, the cow is more efficient in absorbing Ca from the digestive tract and mobilizing Ca from bone reserves. At least 14 days of a low-Ca diet are required to be effective in minimizing the incidence of milk fever.

Practicality of Feeding Diets Low in Calcium

There are practical problems with the implementation of the recommendation to feed diets low in Ca. Most farms utilizing homegrown forages, especially alfalfa, find it difficult to obtain forages that are low in Ca. A low-Ca diet can be achieved by replacing some or all alfalfa hay in the dry-cow diet with grass hay and using additional corn silage and concentrates. When feeding grass hay to dry cows, attention must be paid to the dietary potassium content of the dry-cow ration because high potassium intake tends to alkalinize the organism and thereby impair the efficacy of bone mobilization.

Binding Dietary Calcium

If formulating a diet low enough in Ca to induce a negative Ca balance is a problem, it is possible to reduce the digestibility of dietary Ca by adding a substance to the feed capable of binding dietary Ca and making it less available for intestinal absorption. The oral administration of sodium aluminum silicate or zinc oxide to cows in late lactation binds dietary Ca, thereby inducing a negative Ca balance. Supplementing the dry-cow ration with sodium aluminium silicate (zeolite A) at the rate of 1.4 kg of zeolite pellets per day (700 g of pure zeolite A) for the last 2 weeks of pregnancy results in a significant increase in plasma Ca and 1,25-$(OH)_2D$ around calving. It should, however, be noted that this amount of pellets is equivalent to over 10% of the dry matter feed intake of a dairy cow in the last days before calving. Plasma magnesium and inorganic phosphate levels also decrease, which has raised concerns with the use of these salts. Feed intake was decreased by over 20% in zeolite-treated cows compared with control cows, which was associated with significantly increased betahydroxybutyrate concentrations after calving.[13] Lower doses of zeolite A in the range of 250 g of pure zeolite A resulted in a less pronounced feed intake depression while significantly increasing the plasma Ca concentration around calving in cattle in third or higher lactation. This lower dose of zeolite A still was associated with decreased plasma inorganic phosphate concentrations, whereas plasma magnesium was unaffected.[13]

Feeding a vegetable oil supplement (soya bean oil) to pregnant pastured dairy cattle during the last 2 to 3 weeks of pregnancy is effective in preventing milk fever and increases milk solids production in early lactation. The same supplement has been used to stimulate Ca absorption and reduction in susceptibility to fasting-induced hypocalcemia in pregnant ewes. Following supplementation, the ewes are fasted overnight to challenge calcium homeostasis. Following fasting, there is a greatly increased capacity to absorb calcium.

Level of Phosphorus in Diet

Increased levels of dietary phosphorus, greater than 0.5% kg dry matter, can increase the incidence of milk fever. The increased intake increases the serum level of phosphorus, which has an inhibitory effect on renal enzymes catalyzing the activation of vitamin D_3. Decreased availability of bioactive vitamin D_3 results not only in reduced intestinal phosphate, but also reduced Ca absorption.

Calcium-to-Phosphorus Ratio in Diet

Although the ratio of Ca to phosphorus in the diet is of relevance in monogastric species, it is now recognized that this ratio is of little importance in ruminants, provided that the minimum requirements for both minerals are met. The presumable explanation for this difference from monogastric species is the high concentration of phosphorus in saliva in combination with the large volumes of saliva produced per day that are entering the rumen. The salivary P content will thus greatly distort the ratio of calcium to phosphate of the ingested diet.

Induction of Mild to Moderate Acidosis During Late Gestation: Cation–Anion Difference

A more reliable method of controlling milk fever in dairy cows is to manipulate the dietary cation–anion difference (DCAD) during the prepartum period. Diets high in cations, especially potassium and sodium, tend to induce milk fever compared with those high in anions, primarily chloride and sulfur, which can reduce the milk-fever incidence. When the dietary cation concentration is increased and these cations are absorbed from the digestive tract, they tend to increase the plasma strong ion difference (SID), thereby creating a metabolic (or strong ion) alkalosis. Conversely, dietary anions absorbed from the gut decrease the SID, which causes metabolic acidosis.[6] The feeding of diets containing an excess of anions relative to cations, thus with a low DCAD, will result in metabolic acidosis. Two PTH-dependent functions, bone resorption and renal production of 1,25-$(OH)_2D$, are enhanced in cows fed diets with added anions, and thus a low DCAD, which increases their resistance to milk fever and hypocalcemia.

The DCAD is expressed in milliequivalents per kilogram of dry matter (mEq/kg DM) or in some instances in mEq/100 g DM. Several different equations have been proposed for the calculation of the DCAD; for convenience, the most commonly used is $DCAD_4 = (Na^+ + K^+) - (Cl^- + S^{-2})$, which only considers the four (thus $DCAD_4$) quantitatively most important dietary ions. Other electrolytes, such as calcium, magnesium, and phosphorus, also affect the acid–base status and are included in some of the DCAD equations proposed in the literature. The impact of these minerals on the actual DCAD value is, however, considered to be minor because of the relatively low content of these elements in the ruminant diet.

The equation assigns the same acidification potency to each milliequivalent of Cl and S, although Cl is absorbed to a greater extent than S and thus has a higher potential of acidification. Such effects are considered in more developed DCAD equations that include a corrective factor for each element accounting for these differences in digestibility.

Calculation of the DCAD requires converting the dietary content of each mineral from g/kg or mg/kg to into charges per kg (equivalents/kg). The mass expressed in mmol/kg DM is equal to mEq/kg for all monovalent elements, with only one charge per molecule, such as Na^+, K^+, and Cl^-. Divalent elements, such as Mg^{+2}, Ca^{2+}, and S^{2-}, have two valences per molecule; thus 1 mmol is equivalent to 2 mEq. Table 17-6 provides reference values for determining the mEq of important electrolytes and converting from g/kg or percent diet dry matter (DM) to mEq/kg. Once milliequivalents are calculated, the DCAD can then be determined by subtracting the anions from the cations. The following equation can be used to calculate the DCAD from the percent element in the diet dry matter: mEq/100 g DM = [(%Na ÷ 0.023) + (%K ÷ 0.039)] − [(%Cl ÷ 0.0355) + (%S ÷ 0.016)].

Based on current evidence, the range that achieves the lowest incidence of milk fever is a DCAD of −10 to −15 mEq/100 g DM (−100 to 150 mEq/kg DM). Such a diet should be fed for 2 to 3 weeks before calving. This rate of supplementation is reported not to affect DM intake or energy balance before or after calving. A more moderate rate of supplementation to reduce the DCAD to 0 mEq/100 g dietary DM also did not decrease feed intake or energy status, but was less effective in preventing parturient hypocalcemia.

Most typical diets fed to dry cows have a DCAD of about +100 to +250 mEq/kg DM. Addition of a cationic salt such as sodium bicarbonate to the dry-cow diets increases the DCAD and thereby increases the incidence rate of milk fever. Decreasing the dietary potassium content, by choosing ration ingredients low in potassium or adding an anion source or a mixture of anionic salts containing Cl and S to the diet, lowers the DCAD and reduces the incidence of milk fever. Commonly used sources of anion salts include the Cl and SO_4 salts of calcium, ammonium, and magnesium. The phosphate salts have not been used because they are only weakly acidifying.

Table 17-6 Parturient paresis: Molecular weights, equivalent weights, and conversions from percent to milliequivalents (%–mEq) of anions and cations used in calculating dietary cation–anion difference

Element	Molecular weight (g/mol)	Valence	Equivalent weight (g/Eq)	To convert from % diet DM to mEq. Multiply by: (mEq/kg)
Sodium	23.0	1	23.0	434.98
Potassium	39.1	1	39.1	255.74
Chloride	35.5	1	35.5	282.06
Sulfur	32.1	2	16.0	623.75
Calcium	40.1	2	20.0	499.00
Magnesium	24.3	2	12.2	822.64
Phosphorus	31.0	1.8	17.2	581.14

The addition of anions to the diet to reduce dietary DCAD is limited in quantity because of problems with the palatability of the anionic salt sources commonly used. If the DCAD is greater than 250 mEq/kg, for instance, because of excessive amounts of dietary potassium, it is difficult to add enough anionic salts to lower the DCAD to the recommended −100 mEq/kg of the diet without affecting palatability. In these cases the first objective should be to reduce the dietary cation content as much as possible and only then determine the amount of anions required to achieve the proposed DCAD.

In one study, the incidence of milk fever was 47% when prepartum cows were fed a ration with a DCAD of +330.5 mEq/kg dietary DM and 0% when the prepartum ration had a balance of −128.5 mEq/kg dietary DM. The incidence of milk fever was reduced by the addition of chloride and sulfur in excess relative to sodium and potassium in the diet.

Although it has been proposed that dry cows on low-DCAD diets to control milk fever need to be supplemented with dietary Ca to compensate for increased renal Ca losses resulting from acidification, this recommendation is not undisputed. Several studies showed that the dietary Ca content of dry cows on a high-chloride diet had no effect on the occurrence rate of clinical hypocalcemia. Feeding rations with a dietary Ca between 0.5% and 1.5% did not alter the efficacy of low-DCAD diets, but high-Ca diets fed to dry cows were associated with slightly decreased feed intakes compared with control cows.[3] In any case, DCAD diets should not be combined with low-Ca diets or the use of Ca binding compounds in the feed before calving.

Monitoring the urine pH can be a useful aid to find the effective dose of anionic salts in the close-up ration. Adequate activation of mechanisms increasing Ca absorption from the gut and release from bone through mild to moderate acidification of the organism is associated with a decline of the urine pH below 7.0. Urine pH values of dry cows on a low-DCAD diet above 7.0 suggest that the degree of acidification may not be sufficient to effectively mobilize Ca through the mechanisms previously described. It is suggested that a urine pH between 6.0 and 7.0 is ideal.[3]

Anionic Salts for Acidification of Prepartum Diets for Dairy Cows

Several anionic salts are available for addition to the ration of prepartum dairy cows to prevent milk fever. Generally, acidification of the cows occurs within approximately 36 hours following addition of the anionic salts to the ration; it also takes less than 36 hours for the cow to return to an alkaline state following removal of the salts from the diet. The relative acidifying activity of anionic salts commonly used to prevent milk fever has been evaluated. Salts of chloride have about 1.6 times the acidifying activity of sulfate. Calcium and magnesium, which are usually not included in the DCAD equation, have a small but significant alkalinizing effect when accompanied by chloride or sulfate. The ranking of the anion sources tested at a dose of 2 Eq/day, from most to least potent urine acidifier, was **hydrochloric acid, ammonium chloride, calcium chloride, calcium sulfate, magnesium sulfate, and sulfur.** Magnesium sulfate is the most palatable of the anionic salts commonly supplemented, and calcium chloride is the least palatable. It is best to add the anionic salts to a total mixed ration. Because of the low incidence of milk fever in heifers, there is no need to feed anionic salts to heifers.

Anionic salts can reduce dry matter intake when more than 300 mEq of anions/kg diet DM are supplemented in the diet. The reductions in dry matter intake are commonly ascribed to decreased palatability, but they may represent a response to the metabolic acidosis induced by the salts. The duration of feeding anion salts ranges from 21 to 45 days before expected parturition. At least

5 days of consumption are necessary for maximal benefit.

Ammonium Chloride. Ammonium chloride is more effective than most other salts as an acidifier. The addition of ammonium chloride salts to prepartum diets offers considerable promise as a practical and reliable method of control of milk fever. Within the European Union, ammonium chloride is currently permitted as a pharmacologically active substance in veterinary medicinal products, but not as a zootechnical or feed additive in cattle.[14] Experimentally, the addition of ammonium chloride and ammonium sulfate, each at 100 g/head per day, to the prepartum diets 21 days before parturition decreased the incidence of milk fever from 17% in the unsupplemented group to 4% in the supplemented group.

Strategies for Supplementing Anion Sources

A systematic protocol for the addition of anions to a prepartum diet and monitoring of its effects is as follows:

1. perform macromineral analysis of all available forages for prepartum cows.
2. Select feed ingredients with a low DCAD, especially those low in potassium.
3. Calculate the DCAD of the diet without any supplemental anion sources. If the DCAD is more than +250 mEq/kg, then priority must be given to reduce this value by replacing some of the forage with a lower-DCAD forage.
4. Balance dietary magnesium at 0.40% DM by adding additional magnesium chloride or magnesium sulfate. Magnesium chloride is preferred.
5. Evaluate the feeding management of the prepartum cows. Ensure adequate feeding space and quality of feed.
6. Add supplemental chloride and/or sulfur to the prepartum cow diet to lower DCAD to about −150 mEq/kg DM.
7. Evaluate the dietary nonprotein nitrogen (NPN) and degradable intake protein (DIP) of the diet. If NPN is more than 0.50% of the diet DM or DIP is more than 70% of crude protein, then reduce the amount of ammonium salts or other NPN or DIP sources in the diet.
8. Monitor dry matter intake of the prepartum-cow group.
9. Consider more palatable anion sources or a reduced dose of anion sources if dry matter intake is depressed.
10. After 1 week of feeding anionic salts, monitor the pH of close-up dry cows. Urinary pH is an accurate indication of optimal dietary acidification. Collect urine from at least six cows at one time and average the urinary results. Adjust the dose of supplemental anions to achieve an average urinary pH of between 6.0 and 7.0.

DCAD and Acid–Base Balance of Dairy Cows on Pasture-Based Diets

The dairy industries of southern Australia and New Zealand are based largely on fresh pasture and pasture silage, and grazed pasture is the key determinant of the DCAD. The concentration of potassium is often in excess of 4%, and the DCAD greater than 500 mEq/kg DM, in pasture-based diets, yet the incidence risk of milk fever is not higher than those in other countries where dietary potassium is much lower. For a considerable part of spring and early summer, the DCAD of pasture in those countries may be in excess of +500 to +700 mEq/kg DM. The variation in the DCAD of pasture and the difficulty in accurately assessing dry matter intake make an accurate reduction in DCAD difficult to achieve practically. Pasture cation–anion difference in those conditions is not greatly influenced by stocking rate or associated management practices. The urine pH of grazing dairy cows in south eastern Australia remains relatively constant throughout the year despite changes in stage of lactation, management practices, season, weather, and large changes in DCAD. The DCAD of pasture throughout the year in south eastern Australia ranges from 0 to 800 mEq/kg DM and is often outside the levels previously recommended for optimal performance of lactating cows. For spring-calving herds on pasture, a high DCAD at the time of parturition presents practical problems in administering the large amounts of anionic salts required to lower urine pH and to decrease the incidence of hypocalcemia.

In these pasture-based systems, sulfur (S) is considered a more important dietary constituent in determining the risk of hypocalcemia than either chloride or potassium. The absorption efficiency of S is less than either Cl or K and would not be expected to incur the same change in systemic pH. Thus its importance in hypocalcemia prevention does not fit with the current understanding of how manipulation of DCAD influences calcium homeostasis. Studies indicate that precalving dietary S is more important in the control of hypocalcemia than either K or Cl concentration. Although the effects of a systemic acidosis on Ca absorption is accepted, the effect of S on periparturient Ca homeostasis when absorption of S is low in comparison to Cl, Na, or K suggest that there are mechanisms involved that are not related to acid–base balance. An increased incidence of milk fever may occur in pastured-based dairy when the diet is supplemented with Cl and S, even though calcium absorption, as indicated by urine calcium concentration, increases. The increased incidence may be a result of a greater demand for dietary calcium after calving following a reduction in the pH of body fluids precalving and the fact that pasture-based diets, as opposed to total mixed rations, are generally low in calcium. Supplementation of cows with calcium after calving increased plasma calcium concentration on the day of calving and during the subsequent 14 days. Milk production was not affected by pre- or postcalving treatments.

Experimentally, the application of potassium fertilizer on pasture resulted in a DCAD ranging from 350 to 535 mEq/kg DM, but calcium homeostasis in pasture-based dairy cows was not changed. Plasma concentrations were increased, and the risk of clinical periparturient hypocalcemia was reduced, by $MgCl_2$ and $MgSO_4$ delivered by 150 g $MgCl_2$, 200 g $MgSO_4$, and 35 g MgO/head daily for 21 days prepartum. After calving, cows were supplemented with 150 g $CaCO_3$/head per day for 4 days. Improvements in calcium homeostasis were not the result of an altered systemic pH.

The optimum DCAD for lactating cows grazing fresh pasture and the effect of deviating from the optimum on milk production have been examined under experimental manipulation of the dietary DCAD using a drench in early-lactation dairy cows in New Zealand. Dietary cation-anion differences ranged from +23 to +88 mEq/100 g of DM. As DCAD increased, there was a linear increase in blood pH and HCO_3 concentration and blood base excess. Plasma concentrations of Mg, K, and Cl declined as DCAD increased and Na increased. Urinary excretion of Ca decreased as DCAD increased. Increasing DCAD did not significantly affect milk yield or milk protein, but the concentration and yield of milk fat increased linearly. Milk production results suggest that DCAD for optimal production on pasture diets may be higher than the +20 mEq/100 g DM previously identified for total mixed rations.

Summary of Macromineral Nutritional Strategies for the Prevention of Hypocalcemia in the Soon-to-Calve or Transition Dairy Cow in Pasture-Based Systems

Circumstances and principles can be summarized as follows:

- When dairy cows are dried off, they are commonly moved onto nonirrigated pastures until calving. In the summer, dry cows would be put onto actively growing tropical pasture, whereas in autumn, winter, and spring, the pasture is most likely to be tropical pasture carried over from the previous summer. This carryover pasture is likely to be supplemented with medium-quality hay, silage, and grain or molasses 2 to 3 weeks before calving. Anionic salts have been added to these diets.
- The DCAD on a yearly basis ranges from 0 to 80 mEq/100 g DM.
- The incidence of milk fever in Australia ranges from 1.6% to 5.4%, but in some

years the incidence in individual herds may reach 20%. The incidence of subclinical hypocalcemia can range widely; up to 40% of apparently normal cows had subclinical hypocalcemia (total plasma calcium < 1.9 mmol/L during the first 12 days of lactation).
- In temperate climates, reducing dietary calcium to recommended low levels can be difficult to achieve, but in tropical pastures the levels are already low.
- Excessive levels of potassium may be the most important dietary risk factor for milk fever in Australian feeding systems. Potassium contents of pastures may be as high as 4% to 5% of DM. The use of potassium fertilizers exacerbates the problem. Potassium and consequently dietary DCAD peak in winter and are lowest in autumn. The majority of cows in Victoria, Australia, calve in winter to early spring when the potassium levels are high.
- Hypomagnesemia influences calcium homeostasis, and diets high in potassium reduce the concentration of plasma magnesium. Magnesium supplementation of the transition diet should be done to ensure that magnesium requirements are met (0.4% of DM).
- Excessive dietary phosphorus increases the concentration of phosphorus in plasma, which can induce hypocalcemia and increase the incidence of milk fever at calving. Supplements likely to increase the dietary intake of phosphorus above 40 g/day should not be fed to cows in the weeks before calving.

Supplementation of Vitamin D During the Dry Period

Parenteral Vitamin D_3 Application

In an attempt to reverse the negative Ca balance of susceptible cows at the onset of lactation, the administration of vitamin D_3 and its analogs has been used to increase intestinal Ca absorption. Vitamin D_3 is hydroxylated in the liver, and the resulting metabolite is 25-hydroxycholecalciferol. This is metabolized in the kidney to 1,25-dihydroxycholecalciferol, which has an active hypercalcemic effect but is difficult to synthesize. One of its analogs, 1-α-hydroxycholecalciferol, is as active, is easy to prepare, and is used pharmacologically. A single parenteral dose of 10 million IU per cow of intramuscular (IM) vitamin D_3 given 2 to 8 days before parturition is often recommended, although the dose recommendation based on body weight (1 million units per 45 kg BW) has given consistently better results. Two important inconveniences of the parenteral treatment with vitamin D_3 are the narrow time frame before calving during which vitamin D_3 must be administered to be effective and the narrow therapeutic range of the drug. If the cow fails to calve within 10 days of treatment, another 10 million units may need to be administered because cows treated more than 10 days before calving are at increased risk of developing clinical milk fever. Repeated treatment is associated with soft tissue calcification, particularly after repeated injections. Pregnant cows are more susceptible to calcification than nonpregnant animals. Whereas single doses below 10 million units to an adult cow were found to be considerably less effective in preventing clinical milk fever, a dose of 17 million units was lethal for 75% of treated animals.

Another disadvantage of using injectable vitamin D_3 is that although it is effective in preventing clinical milk fever, it tends to result in significantly lower plasma Ca concentrations between 3 and 14 days postpartum compared with untreated control cows. Cows treated with injectable vitamin D_3 therefore are at decreased risk of developing clinical milk fever around parturition but may be at increased risk of subclinical hypocalcemia during the first weeks of lactation. The problem appears to be that the effect of the exogenous metabolite on intestinal Ca absorption declines, whereas its inhibiting effect on the renal enzymes activating endogenous vitamin D_3 is more sustained. Treated cows therefore appear to be impaired in their ability to produce sufficient 1,25-$(OH)_2D$ to maintain enhanced intestinal absorption of calcium in the first weeks of lactation.

Oral Vitamin D Administration

Oral dosing with 20 million IU of vitamin D_2/d for 5 days to cows immediately before calving can markedly reduce the expected incidence of milk fever. Because the onset of action after oral treatment is more delayed than after injection, a cow must be treated for at least 5 days before calving for the treatment to be effective. The exact date of calving is often difficult to determine, and if the administration is discontinued for up to 4 days before calving, an unusually high incidence of the disease may follow, probably because of the depression of parathyroid activity that follows the administration. Toxicity of the oral treatment is considerably lower compared with injection. A dose of 30 million IU of vitamin D administered over 7 days was without obvious signs of toxicity. The danger of causing metastatic calcification, however, also exists; this has been produced with smaller doses (20 million IU daily for 10 days).

Oral Calcium Supplementation Around Parturition

The oral administration of easily absorbed Ca salts such as calcium chloride or calcium propionate providing the equivalent of 40 to 50 g calcium per dose as a bolus, gel, paste, or liquid, given in a single dose or repeated doses beginning 12 to 24 hours before calving and continuing to 24 hours after calving, is a common practice that will effectively increase the plasma Ca concentrations for at least 6 hours. Based on clinical studies, a treatment interval of 6 to 12 hours for the period around calving has been suggested. Depending on the type of formulation, its palatability, and the required treatment frequency, oral treatment can be more or less labor intensive, demanding, and invasive. Calcium chloride is highly soluble, resulting in a rapid increase of the plasma Ca concentration within 30 minutes, but it is also caustic and may result in epithelial lesions of the mucosa of the oropharyngeal region, esophagus, forestomaches, or abomasum. In contrast, Ca-propionate requires a larger volume to provide a similar amount of Ca and has a more delayed effect on the plasma Ca concentration, but it is less injurious and thus safer to administer. The combined administration of Ca together with propionate, which is a glucose precursor in the form of calcium propionate, has been used as a further supporting argument for the use of this compound around calving. However, studies investigating the effect of Ca-propionate on feed consumption, milk yield, plasma glucose, insulin, and NEFA concentration in periparturient cows failed to identify a beneficial effect.[12]

Prophylactic treatment with oral Ca formulations in contrast to parenteral Ca administration bears the advantage that it does not disturb mechanisms regulating the Ca homeostasis, but rather supports them by providing oral Ca while intestinal Ca absorption has been upregulated.[15]

Parenteral Calcium Supplementation Around Parturition

Intravenous or subcutaneous administration of Ca-gluconate or Ca-borogluconate solutions to cattle around parturition is sometimes practiced because this approach may be perceived as a convenient and inexpensive method to control milk fever.[15] However, increasing the plasma Ca concentration to supraphysiological levels, as often occurs after parenteral administration of therapeutic doses of Ca solutions, disturbs the endocrine circuits regulating calcium homeostasis by abruptly interrupting the PTH secretion that is essential to prevent excessive declines of the plasma Ca concentration around parturition. This disruption will result in a delay of the correction of the periparturient disequilibrium of the Ca balance, which has been documented in several studies. Cows treated prophylactically with Ca solutions parenterally have pronounced but transient hypercalcemia that is followed by decline of the plasma Ca concentration below pretreatment Ca concentrations within 12 hours. A recent study comparing IV Ca administration with oral Ca administration and no treatment in periparturient cows not showing clinical signs of milk fever revealed that plasma Ca concentrations were significantly higher than those in orally treated and control cows only for the first 4 hours posttreatment, but they were below the Ca concentrations of orally treated cows from 24 hours until at least 48 hours posttreatment and below the values of untreated cows from 36 hours until at least 48 hours posttreatment.[16] **Parenteral administration of Ca solutions should therefore be a tool reserved to rapidly correct clinical hypocalcemia and should never be a standard procedure at calving.**[8,15]

Partial Milking

Partial milking after calving has been proposed for decades as a strategy to decrease Ca losses through the mammary gland in early lactation. Although this practice evidently reduces the amount of Ca excreted through the mammary gland, studies investigating the effect of partial milk-out on the plasma Ca concentration in the first days of lactation failed to identify a beneficial effect.[6]

FURTHER READING

Block E. Manipulation of dietary cation–anion difference on nutritionally related production diseases, productivity and metabolic responses of dairy cows. *J Dairy Sci.* 1994;77:1437-1450.

Goff JP, Horst RL. Role of acid-base physiology on the pathogenesis of parturient hypocalcemia (milk fever)—the DCAD theory in principle and practice. *Acta Vet Scand.* 2003;97:51-56.

Houe H, et al. Milk fever and subclinical hypocalcemia—An evaluation of parameters on incidence risk, diagnosis, risk factors and biological effects as input for a decision support system for disease control. *Acta Vet Scand.* 2001;42:1-29.

Horst RL, Goff JP, Reinhardt TA. Role of vitamin D in calcium homeostasis and its use in prevention of bovine periparturient paresis. *Acta Vet Scand.* 2003;97:35-50.

Thilsing-Hansen T, Jorgensen RJ, Ostergard S. Milk fever control principles: a review. *Acta Vet Scand.* 2002;43:1-19.

REFERENCES

1. Reinhardt TA, et al. *Vet J.* 2011;188:122-124.
2. USDA. Dairy 2007, part I. Accessed February 15, 2014, at <http://www.aphis.usda.gov/animal_health/nahms/dairy/downloads/dairy07/Dairy07_dr_PartI.pdf>; 2007.
3. Goff JP. *Vet Clin North Am Food Anim Pract.* 2014;30:359-381.
4. DeGaris PJ, Lean IJ. *Vet J.* 2009;176:58-69.
5. Mulligan FJ, Doherty ML. *Vet J.* 2008;176:3-9.
6. Constable PD. *Proc XXVIII World Buiatrics Congress.* Cairns: 2014:59-63.
7. Grünberg W. *Vet Clin North Am Food Anim Pract.* 2014;30:383-408.
8. Oetzel GR. *Vet Clin North Am Food Anim Pract.* 2013;29:447-455.
9. Menard L, Thompson A. *Can Vet J.* 2007;48:487-491.
10. Constable PD, et al. *J Am Vet Med Assoc.* 2013;246:826-835.
11. Goff JP. *Vet J.* 2008;176:50-57.
12. Kara C. *J Biol Environ Sci.* 2013;7:9-17.
13. Grabherr H, et al. *J Anim Physiol Anim Nutr.* 2009;93:221-236.
14. EFSA. *EFSA J.* 2012;10:2738.
15. Martin-Tereso JM, Martens H. *Vet Clin North Am Food Anim Pract.* 2014;30:643-670.
16. Blanc CD. *J Dairy Sci.* 2014;97:6901-6906.

ACUTE HYPOKALEMIA IN CATTLE

SYNOPSIS

Etiology Sustained decrease in dry matter intake in lactating dairy cattle, abomasal disorder, alkalemia, two or more injections of isoflupredone acetate (corticosteroid/mineralocorticoid).

Epidemiology Most common in lactating dairy cattle with decreased appetite and high-milk-production potential and low muscle mass.

Clinical findings Generalized muscle weakness; depression; cardiac arrhythmias, particularly atrial fibrillation.

Clinical pathology Low serum/plasma potassium concentrations; alkalemia and hyperglycemia may be present.

Necropsy findings Multifocal myonecrosis with microphage infiltration and myofiber vacuolation, characteristic for hypokalemia myopathy.

Diagnostic confirmation Response to treatment, serum potassium concentration less than 2.5 mEq/L.

Treatment Potassium chloride administered orally, increased feed intake.

Control Maintain adequate dry matter intake, early detection and correction of abomasal disorders, no more than one treatment of isoflupredone acetate.

ETIOLOGY

Hypokalemia is most common in lactating dairy cattle and is secondary to the following:

- Anorexia resulting from clinical mastitis and retained placenta
- Upper gastrointestinal obstruction, particularly left-displaced abomasum, right-displaced abomasum, abomasal volvulus, and abomasal impaction
- Obligatory loss of potassium in milk (1.4 g potassium/L of milk)
- Hyperinsulinemia secondary to hyperglycemia and transcellular shift of extracellular potassium
- Sympathetic nervous system activation
- Aldosterone release in response to hypovolemia and the need for sodium retention
- Decreased whole-body potassium stores as a result of the relatively low muscle mass in dairy cows

In most cases, the hypokalemia is not severe enough to cause weakness and recumbency.

EPIDEMIOLOGY

Hypokalemia occurs commonly in lactating dairy cattle with prolonged inappetence (>2 days), but it is rare in adult ruminants with adequate dry matter intake and neonatal calves, lambs, and kids. Hypokalemia occurs more commonly in lactating dairy cows than beef cows or feedlot animals because of the additional loss of potassium in the milk, the lower muscle mass in dairy cows that results in decreased whole-body potassium stores, and the use of glycogen and skeletal muscle protein for energy in early lactation.

Milk typically has a potassium concentration of 36 mmol/L.[1] High-producing dairy cows are therefore at increased risk for hypokalemia, and the incidence of hypokalemia in the postparturient period increases as milk production increases. Early-lactation dairy cows are in a marked state of negative energy balance; catabolism of intracellular glycogen and protein leads to increased potassium excretion in urine and therefore whole-body potassium depletion because potassium is bound to glycogen.

Potassium excretion by the kidneys is via secretion by the distal tubular cells. Aldosterone or other steroids with mineralocorticoid activity enhance distal tubular secretion of potassium by increasing permeability of the tubular luminal membranes to potassium and increasing losses of potassium in the urine. Hypokalemia and whole-body potassium depletion is common in lactating dairy cattle receiving one or more injections of corticosteroids for ketosis that have mineralocorticoid activity, particularly isoflupredone acetate.[2,3] The hypokalemic effect occurs because the mineralocorticoid activity of isoflupredone enhances renal and gastrointestinal (saliva and colon) losses of potassium. Hypokalemia reaches its nadir of approximately 60% to 70% of the normal value by 72 hours after the first of two 10-mg injections. Exogenous or endogenous insulin release secondary to hyperglycemia following IV dextrose administration or corticosteroid administration can lead to hypokalemia associated with the intracellular movement of potassium accompanying glucose; this is a shift in potassium and not whole-body depletion.[4,5]

In general, alkalemia decreases serum potassium concentration, and acidemia increases serum potassium concentration. Hypokalemia therefore occurs commonly in ruminants with metabolic alkalosis. Experimental induction of metabolic alkalosis by oral administration of sodium bicarbonate in three Jersey cows caused marked metabolic (strong ion) alkalosis (base excess, 14 to 19 mEq/L), hypokalemia (2.6 to 3.1 mEq/L), and an increase in muscle potassium concentration of 6% to 10%, indicating an intracellular shift of potassium from the extracellular space to the intracellular space.

Whole-body depletion of potassium may be present in healthy dairy cattle immediately after calving, based on the results of potassium balance studies and studies documenting decreased skeletal muscle potassium content at calving and decreased urinary potassium concentrations immediately after calving.[2,6]

PATHOGENESIS

Potassium homeostasis in adult cattle is determined by the balance between absorption of potassium from the gastrointestinal (GI) tract and subsequent excretion by the kidneys and salivary glands. Transport of potassium is passive in the small intestine and active in the colon under the influence of aldosterone. The most important hormone affecting renal and salivary potassium excretion is aldosterone, which is released from the zona glomerulosa of the adrenal gland in response to hyperkalemia and other factors. At least 95% of whole-body potassium is intracellular, with skeletal muscle containing 60% to 75% of the total intracellular potassium. Total potassium losses in lactating cattle are 75% in urine, 13% in feces (mainly endogenous loss), and 12% milk, with urine, fecal, and milk losses being obligatory. Marked changes in serum or plasma potassium concentrations alter the resting membrane potential of cells because the potassium gradient generated by Na-K ATPase is the main cause for the negative electric potential across cell membranes. Hypokalemia therefore alters the resting membrane potential and leads to clinically significant changes in cellular and organ function. Hypokalemia indicates whole-body depletion of potassium unless induced by hyperglycemia and hyperinsulinemia.[4,5]

The potassium content of cattle has been estimated at approximately 2.2 g/kg BW. Lactating dairy cattle should be fed a diet containing at least 0.7% potassium on a dry-weight basis, although high-producing dairy cattle need a higher dietary potassium concentration, and potassium is frequently fed at 1.3% to 1.4% on a dry-weight basis. The absorption efficiency of potassium on a typical lactating dairy cow diet ranges from 74% to 88%, with potassium being absorbed in the small intestine and forestomach, with the former predominating. Rumen fluid in cattle usually has a potassium concentration of 24 to 85 mEq/L, and rumen fluid potassium concentration and potassium absorption are strongly dependent on intake. This indicates that increasing potassium intake (specifically, increasing rumen potassium concentration) will directly lead to increased potassium absorption. Studies in fed sheep have indicated a strong linear relationship between potassium absorbed from the rumen and rumen potassium concentration; however, it should be noted that the rate of potassium absorption depends also on whether the animal is fed or fasted. Fasting in sheep for 26 hours decreased rumen potassium concentration from 50 mmol/L to 24 mmol/L and decreased plasma potassium concentration from 4.2 to 3.7 mmol/L.

Potassium homeostasis is not considered to be under direct hormonal control in sodium-replete healthy lactating cattle because there is no association between plasma aldosterone concentrations and whole-blood or urine potassium concentrations.[3] Anorexia is thought to play an important role in the development of hypokalemia in cattle because 24 to 48 hours are needed for the mammalian kidney to adjust to a reduction in dietary potassium intake.[3] Dehydration also plays an important role in hypokalemia via aldosterone activation. There appears to be a gut or hepatoportal sensor that detects potassium intake and sends a signal to the kidney to increase potassium excretion in response to increased potassium ingestion, but the anatomic location of the sensor and the molecular pathway for signal transduction remain unknown.[7] Nevertheless, activation of the gut/hepatoportal sensor means that there is increased potassium excretion by the kidneys even before there is a detectable increase in serum potassium concentration following increased potassium intake.

Relative to an in vitro potassium concentration of 5 mmol/L, decreases in tissue bath potassium concentration decrease the amplitude of contraction of the circular muscle of the cow abomasal corpus; this smooth muscle is responsible for the propulsion of abomasal chyme.[8] Small, but nonsignificant, decreases in the force developed by abomasal smooth muscle from bulls is observed when in vitro potassium concentration is decreased from 5.4 to 2.0 to 3.0 mmol/L.[9] Hypokalemia may therefore result in decreased abomasal emptying rate and consequently an increased risk of developing left-displaced abomasum, abomasal volvulus, and potentially retained placenta and metritis in dairy cattle. The relationship between potassium concentration and skeletal muscle tone has not been determined for cattle, but studies in humans suggest hypokalemia must be marked (<2.0 to 2.5 mEq/L) to decrease skeletal muscle tone.

CLINICAL FINDINGS

Affected animals have generalized muscle weakness, decreased gastrointestinal motility, and depression. Severely affected animals are unable to stand or lift their heads from the ground. Cows with severe hypokalemia (<2.0 mEq/L) are usually recumbent and profoundly weak, appear flaccid, and lie in sternal or lateral recumbency. They are unable to support the weight of their heads off the ground and commonly hold their heads in their flanks. Profound weakness of the lateral cervical muscles may occur. Anorexia is common. Cardiac arrhythmias are often detectable on auscultation, and atrial fibrillation may be present on electrocardiography.

Cardiac arrhythmias are associated with abnormal serum potassium concentrations, both hypokalemia and hyperkalemia. In an unpublished study of 110 adult cattle with atrial fibrillation, hypokalemia was commonly present before the induction of atrial fibrillation. Although there do not appear to be any large-scale studies examining the association between hypokalemia and cardiac arrhythmias in adult cattle, hypokalemia, hypocalcemia, and alkalemia are commonly present in lactating dairy cattle with left-displaced abomasum and atrial fibrillation. In a recent study, 2/15 lactating dairy cows with experimentally induced hypokalemia and alkalemia developed atrial fibrillation that resolved within 24 hours of administration of KCl, accompanied by an increase in plasma potassium concentration and a decrease in blood pH.[6] Atrial fibrillation in other studies was diagnosed in 4/10, 2/14, and 5/17 cows with naturally acquired hypokalemia, and in 1/7 lactating dairy cows with experimentally induced hypokalemia following IM administration of two 20-mg doses of isoflupredone acetate at a 48-hour interval. Taken together, these findings suggest that hypokalemia plays an important role in the development of atrial fibrillation in adult cattle.

Signs of chronic potassium depletion in cattle include anorexia; pica characterized by hair licking, floor licking, and chewing of wooden partitions; rough hair coat; muscular weakness; irritability; paralysis; and tetany.

CLINICAL PATHOLOGY

The order of sensitivity/specificity in determining whole-body potassium depletion is as follows: skeletal muscle > serum/plasma > milk > erythrocyte/whole blood > urine > saliva.

Skeletal Muscle Potassium Content

Skeletal muscle potassium concentration is considered the most sensitive and specific method for assessing whole-body potassium status and therefore provides the gold-standard test. Skeletal muscle is considered the best tissue to sample because it contains approximately 75% of the whole-body stores of potassium. A standardized muscle should be evaluated in cattle because differences in potassium content of greater than 15% are present in individual animals, and this muscle-to-muscle variation is greater than that produced by breed.

Plasma Potassium Concentration

Determination of serum/plasma potassium concentration is required to confirm a suspected diagnosis of hypokalemia. A serum potassium concentration less than 2.5 mEq/L reflects severe hypokalemia, and most animals will be weak or recumbent. A serum potassium concentration of 2.5 to 3.5 mEq/L reflects moderate hypokalemia, and some cattle will be recumbent or appear weak, with depressed gastrointestinal motility. In addition to measurement of serum potassium concentration, determination of the serum concentrations of sodium, chloride, calcium, and phosphorus and the serum activities of creatine kinase and aspartate aminotransferase can be very helpful in guiding treatment of cattle with hypokalemia. Serum potassium concentration is usually a little higher than plasma potassium concentration because platelet activation releases potassium. In summary, a serum/plasma potassium concentration below the normal range provides unequivocal evidence of hypokalemia unless there is concurrent hyperinsulinemia or alkalemia.[4,5] However, because more than 95% to 98% of whole-body potassium stores are intracellular, it is likely that serum/plasma potassium concentration is not as sensitive as skeletal muscle potassium content in indicating whole-body potassium depletion.

Milk Potassium Concentration

Milk potassium concentration is theoretically more sensitive than serum/plasma potassium concentration in detecting whole-body potassium depletion in individual cows because the milk concentration of potassium is constant for an individual cow. Potassium depletion in lactating dairy cows caused milk potassium concentration to decrease from 1.45 g/L to 1.28 g/L; this was a greater percentage decrease than that in the plasma or whole blood of cattle with whole-body potassium depletion. However, there is marked individual variation in the milk concentration of potassium in healthy cattle, with variations of up to 50% occurring between cows. This variability appears to be a result of changes in milk fat, protein, and lactose percentage, with the highest correlation of milk potassium concentration being with milk lactose concentration ($R = -0.53$ or -0.74). The relationship between potassium and lactose is attributable to the fact that these are important contributors to milk osmolality, which is constant and isotonic. Milk potassium concentration also changes during lactation, being 42 mmol/L in early lactation, 40 mmol/L in midlactation, and 27 mmol/L in late lactation, with a mean bulk milk potassium concentration of 37 mmol/L. The large cow-to-cow variability in milk potassium concentration and dependence on milk lactose concentration make it difficult to produce a suitable cut-point for identifying whole-body potassium depletion in sick lactating dairy cows. However, milk potassium concentration has clinical utility in monitoring potassium homeostasis over time in an individual cow.

Erythrocyte Potassium Concentration

Erythrocyte potassium concentration is determined by measuring plasma potassium concentration and hematocrit, and then adding sufficient distilled water to hemolyze the erythrocytes followed by potassium measurement of the hemolyzed fluid and mathematical calculation. There is marked cow-to-cow variability in the erythrocyte potassium concentration (7 to 70 mmol/L) and sodium concentration (15 to 87 mmol/L) of healthy cattle that has a genetic basis with no breed influence. There are two main peaks of cellular potassium concentration, one at 20 mmol/L and a second at 50 mmol/L. In lactating dairy cattle with induced whole-body potassium deficiency, whole-blood potassium concentration changed similarly to plasma potassium concentration. However, in 180 cows, no relationship between plasma potassium concentration and erythrocyte potassium concentration was found. Measurement of erythrocyte or whole-blood potassium concentration is not currently recommended in evaluating whole-body potassium status.

Urine Potassium Concentration

Urine potassium concentrations are normally high (454 ± 112 mEq/L) but variable, with a mean fractional clearance of 82% and a coefficient of variation of 61%. The large variability in urine potassium concentration makes it difficult to produce a suitable cut-point for identifying whole-body potassium depletion. However, determination of urine potassium concentration has clinical utility in an individual cow ingesting a constant diet over time because it reflects potassium homeostasis. Urine pH may provide some value as a better screening test because aciduria may be present in response to a marked decrease in urine potassium concentration.[10]

Salivary Potassium Concentration

Salivary potassium concentrations are more influenced by aldosterone in the response to changes in serum sodium concentration, and salivary potassium concentration must therefore be compared with the salivary sodium concentration (one-for-one exchange), sodium homeostasis, and the ratio of serum sodium to potassium to have clinical utility. The normal saliva potassium concentration shows a large range of 4 to 70 mEq/L, with sodium homeostasis having the greatest effect. A study in cattle with left-displaced abomasum, right-displaced abomasum, or abomasal volvulus indicated no association between salivary potassium concentration and serum potassium concentration. Taken together, it appears that measurement of salivary potassium concentration provides minimal insight into whole-body potassium status.

NECROPSY FINDINGS

Necropsy of cattle with hypokalemia-induced recumbency reveals the presence of muscle necrosis in the pelvic limbs. Histologic examination of non-weight-bearing muscles reveals multifocal myonecrosis with microphage infiltration and myofiber vacuolation, which is characteristic of hypokalemic myopathy in humans and dogs. It is important to note that hypokalemic myopathy is also present in muscles not subject to ischemia of recumbency.

TREATMENT

Treatment of hypokalemia in lactating dairy cows should focus on surgical correction of abomasal displacement, increasing the potassium intake by increasing dry matter intake or the oral administration of KCl, and correction of hypochloremia, alkalemia, metabolic alkalosis, and dehydration.[2] Oral potassium administration is the method of choice for treating hypokalemia. Inappetent adult cattle should initially be treated with 120 g of KCl PO, followed by an additional oral treatment of 120 g KCl 12 hours later, for a total 24-hour treatment of 240 g KCl (0.4 g/kg BW).[6] Higher oral doses of KCl are not recommended because they can lead to diarrhea, excessive salivation, muscular tremors of the legs, and excitability.

Potassium is rarely administered intravenously; the IV route is used only for the initial treatment of recumbent ruminants with severe hypokalemia and rumen atony because it is much more dangerous and expensive than oral treatment. The most aggressive IV treatment protocol is an isotonic solution of KCl (1.15% KCl), which should be administered at less than 3.2 mL/kg/hr, equivalent to a maximal delivery rate of 0.5 mEq of potassium/kg BW per hour. Higher rates of potassium administration run the risk of inducing hemodynamically important arrhythmias, including ventricular premature complexes that can lead to ventricular fibrillation and death.

Palatable hay and propylene glycol orally are recommended. In a series of 14 cases, treatment consisted of potassium chloride given intravenously and orally at an average total daily dose of 0.42 g/kg BW (26 g orally and 16 g IV) for an average of 5 days, resulting in recovery in 11 cases after an average of 3 days. During recumbency, affected cattle require special attention to minimize ischemic necrosis of muscles of the pelvic limbs.

Glucocorticoids are often used to treat ketosis, and the most commonly used glucocorticoids are dexamethasone and isoflupredone acetate. Dexamethasone has little mineralocorticoid activity compared with prednisone and prednisolone, which are related chemically to isoflupredone. Dexamethasone is recommended for the treatment of ketosis in dairy cattle at a single dose of 10 to 20 mg IM, and repeated, if necessary, 12 to 24 hours later. Field observations indicate that repeated doses of isoflupredone acetate decrease plasma concentrations of potassium by 70% to 80%, which suggests a strong mineralocorticoid activity. It is recommended that isoflupredone acetate be used judiciously and animals be monitored for plasma potassium and any evidence of weakness and recumbency. Treatment with oral potassium chloride may be required, but treatment may be ineffective.

CONTROL

Oral administration of potassium is a mandatory component of fluid and electrolyte administration to inappetent lactating dairy cattle. Ensuring an adequate dry matter intake is the best method for preventing hypokalemia in lactating dairy cattle.

TREATMENT AND CONTROL

Treatment

KCl 120 g PO, followed by an additional oral treatment of 120 g KCl 12 hours later, for a total 24-hour treatment of 240 g KCl (0.4 g/kg BW) (R-1)

KCl 1.15% IV, less than 3.2 (mL/kg BW)/hour, equivalent to a maximal delivery rate of 0.5 mEq of potassium/kg BW per hour (R-2)

Isoflupredone acetate (R-4)

Control

Maintain adequate dry matter intake (R-1)

FURTHER READING

Constable PD. Fluids and electrolytes. *Vet Clin North Am Food Anim Pract.* 2003;19(3):1-40.

Sattler N, Fecteau G. Hypokalemia syndrome in cattle. *Vet Clin North Am Food Anim Pract.* 2014;30:351-357.

REFERENCES

1. Constable PD, et al. *J Dairy Sci.* 2009;92(1):296.
2. Constable PD, et al. *J Am Vet Med Assoc.* 2013;242:826.
3. Coffer NJ, et al. *Am J Vet Res.* 2006;67:1244.
4. Grünberg W, et al. *J Am Vet Med Assoc.* 2006;229:413.
5. Grünberg W, et al. *J Vet Intern Med.* 2006;20:1471.
6. Constable PD, et al. *J Dairy Sci.* 2014;97(3):1413.
7. Greenlee M, et al. *Ann Intern Med.* 2009;150:619.
8. Türck G, Leonhard-Marek S. *J Dairy Sci.* 2010;93(8):3561.
9. Zurr L, Leonhard-Marek S. *J Dairy Sci.* 2012;95:5750.
10. Constable PD, et al. *Am J Vet Res.* 2009;70(7):915.

DOWNER-COW SYNDROME

SYNOPSIS

Etiology Ischemic myopathy of large muscles of pelvic limbs and ischemic neuropathies of obturator or sciatic nerve or its branches secondary to prolonged recumbency associated with milk fever or dystocia; injury of bones, joints, and muscles; undetermined etiologies.

Epidemiology Most common in dairy cows with previous episodes of milk fever; in beef cows after prolonged or difficult calving. Delay of more than 4 hours in treatment for recumbent milk-fever cows. Hypophosphatemia and/or hypokalemia have been discussed as potential risk factors.

Signs Alert downer cows: Unable to stand following treatment for milk fever. Sternal recumbency; normal mental status, vital signs, and alimentary tract. Appetite and thirst normal or mildly decreased. Most will stand in few days if provided good clinical care and secondary muscle necrosis is minimized.

Nonalert downer cows: Persistent recumbency with altered mentation and vital signs; frequently unable to maintain sternal recumbency; abnormal position of legs; groaning; anorexia; die in several days.

Clinical pathology Increased serum activity of creatine kinase (CK) and aspartate aminotransferase (AST); serum phosphorus and potassium concentrations may be subnormal or elevated; proteinuria, myoglobinuria.

Necropsy findings Ischemic necrosis, edema and hemorrhage of large medial thigh muscles.

Diagnostic confirmation Increased serum activities of CK, AST, proteinuria; myoglobinuria necropsy lesions in cow unable to rise with no other lesions.

Treatment Provide excellent bedding or ground surface such as sand or dirt pack. Roll animal from side to side every few hours. Antiinflammatory therapy/pain management. Fluid and electrolyte therapy as necessary. Hoist cows making attempts to stand.

Control All recently calved dairy cows that are at high risk for milk fever must be observed closely 12 to 24 hours before and after calving for evidence of milk fever and while still standing; if recumbent, do not delay treatment for more than 1 hour. Can treat all high-risk cows with calcium salts orally to prevent clinical milk fever.

The term *downer cow* first appeared in the veterinary literature in the 1950s and referred to cattle that were too injured, weak, or sick to stand or walk without assistance.[1] In most of the early publications using this terminology a case definition was not provided or was imprecise, such as "cattle unable to rise" or "unable to stand without assistance," and did not make reference to possible etiologies, duration of recumbency, or outcome.[2] More recently the term *downer cow* was used to denote nonambulatory cattle recumbent for at least 24 hours without obvious reason.[1] A further classification of downer cows into mentally alert, nonambulatory cattle that are able to maintain themselves in sternal recumbency, so-called alert downer cows, and cows with moderate to severe mental obtundation and abnormal vital signs that frequently are unable to maintain sternal recumbency, the so-called nonalert downer cows, was proposed.[3] The term *creeper cows* is sometimes used to denote alert recumbent cows that are unable to bear weight on their hindlimbs but that use the forelegs to propel themselves over short distances.

ETIOLOGY

Alert downer cows are in most cases recumbent because of musculoskeletal or neurologic injuries such as lesions of the sciatic or obturator nerve secondary to dystocia (calving paralysis), fractures of long bones or the pelvis, hip luxation, or muscle injury as a result of primary trauma or secondary to prolonged recumbency. Nonalert downer cows comprise animals with systemic disease affecting mental status and general attitude, such as periparturient hypocalcemia, septicemia, hypovolemia, diffuse peritonitis, and severe hepatic lipidosis, or neurologic diseases affecting the brainstem or cortex.[3]

In most cases, the downer-cow syndrome is a complication of milk fever. Myopathies and neuropathies develop in nonambulatory cows secondary to prolonged periods of recumbency. Ischemic myopathy affecting the large muscles of the pelvic limbs and injuries to the tissues around the hip joint and of the obturator muscles are common in cows that do not fully recover and stand. Injuries to the musculoskeletal system are also common as a result of cows "spread-eagling" their hindlimbs if they are unsteady during parturition or forced to stand or walk on a slippery floor immediately before or following parturition.

A survey conducted among dairy operations in 21 U.S. states determined that the three most common causes for persistent recumbency were periparturient hypocalcemia (19%), calving-related injuries (22%), and injuries from slipping or falling (15%). Beef cattle operations reported calving paralysis as the single most common cause for downer-cow syndrome.[1]

EPIDEMIOLOGY

Occurrence

The disease is most common in dairy cows and typically occurs within the first 2 or 3 days after calving, often immediately following an episode of milk fever. Other debilitating conditions of periparturient cows that can be associated with persistent recumbency include acute coliform mastitis, septic metritis, and acute rumen acidosis (grain overload).

In the United States an estimated 270,000 cattle became nonambulatory on-farm in 2004, of which 57.4% were dairy and 31.5% beef cattle, corresponding to 1.2% of dairy cattle and 0.2% of beef cattle becoming persistently recumbent in 1 year.[4] An older survey conducted in 1986 in Minnesota that included data from 738 dairy operations and 34,656 cow years at risk reported incidences per herd and year between 0.4% and 2.1% (case definition in this study: "sternal recumbency for at least 24 h for no obvious reason"). The overall outcome was that 33% of downer cows recovered, 23% were slaughtered, and 44% died. The owners perceived that downer cows were high producers (48%) or average producers (46%), with only 6% being low producers. Approximately 58% of cases occurred within 1 day of parturition, and 37% occurred during the first 100 days of lactation. The incidence was highest (39%) during the three coldest months: December to February. A clinical survey conducted in New Zealand and including 433 periparturient recumbent cows reported a recovery rate of 39%, whereas 30% died, and 32% had to be destroyed. The case-fatality rate in this study was 11% higher in precalving recumbent cows than postcalving cows. A 2006 survey including dairy operations from 21 U.S. states reported that 78.6% of participating operations had at least one downer cow in 2006.[2] The case definition of a downer cow in this study was "nonambulatory cattle that were unable to stand for any length of time, including those that recovered."[2]

Because it is a syndrome lacking in clinical definition and includes all those "other cases" that cannot be otherwise classified, downer-cow incidence varies depending on the clinical acuity of the individual veterinarian and various environmental factors in different areas. In any case, the incidence seems to be increasing, particularly in intensive dairy farming areas, although this impression could arise from the increased necessity to effect a cure in valuable animals.

Risk Factors

Animal Risk Factors

Complication of Milk Fever. Prolonged recumbency after an episode of clinical milk fever either because of a delay in administration of proper treatment or delayed response to treatment is considered the most common primary cause of downer-cow syndrome. The incidences for downer-cow syndrome that is associated with milk fever reported in the literature range from 3.8% to 28.2% of all milk-fever cases.[5]

Prolonged recumbency, regardless of the primary cause, results in increased tissue pressure over a confined anatomic area, causing local ischemia and neuromuscular dysfunction. An insecure gait of a hypocalcemic periparturient cow presents an increased risk of injury from slipping or falling, such as muscle rupture, bone fractures, or hip luxation, that can result in downer-cow syndrome.

Traumatic Injuries to Pelvis and Pelvic Limbs. Traumatic injuries to bones, muscles, and nerves can be directly related to parturition (e.g. calving paralysis), be associated with muscle weakness and an insecure gait (e.g. in hypocalcemic cattle), or be the result of an inadvertent accident. **Calving paralysis** refers to a paresis or paralysis of one or both hindlimbs caused by a lesion of the obturator nerve and/or the lumbar root of the sciatic nerve inflicted during the calving process. Both nerves are vulnerable to compression between the bony birth canal and the calf at parturition; accordingly, nerve damage is most commonly diagnosed after dystocias, deliveries of large calves, or prolonged calvings. Calving paralysis is considered the most common cause for persistent recumbency in beef cattle.

Pressure injuries of the superficial nerves of the extremities may occur as secondary lesions in cows that are recumbent for an unrelated reason.

Serum Electrolyte Imbalances. Apart from hypocalcemia, hypophosphatemia, hypokalemia, and hypomagnesemia have been incriminated as potential factors contributing to downer-cow syndrome. **Hypophosphatemia** is a common finding in recumbent but also in healthy periparturient cows;[6] it is the mineral imbalance most commonly quoted as risk factor, especially in the so-called creeper cows, which are bright and alert and crawl about, but are unable to rise. The clinical relevance of hypophosphatemia in persistently recumbent animals has been debated contentiously, but an undisputed empirical observation is that hypophosphatemia is more common or more pronounced in recumbent periparturient cows that are unresponsive to intravenous calcium administration at least in very early stages of recumbency.[5,6] However, the mechanisms through which phosphate depletion may cause persistent recumbency are not well understood, and treatment response to oral or parenteral administration of phosphate salts is inconsistent.[6] Studies including cattle that were nonambulatory for longer than just a few hours, in contrast, found that low serum phosphorus levels are suggestive of a good prognosis, whereas nonsurvivors tend to have higher serum phosphorus concentrations.[3] A likely explanation for this finding is that cows recumbent for longer time periods may have developed more severe muscle damage that is associated with release of intracellular phosphorus into the circulation and thus an increase of the serum phosphorus concentration.

A long-term low-level **hypomagnesemia** has been associated with downer-cow syndrome, especially when it accompanies hypocalcemia. But it is usually manifested by a tetanic hyperesthetic state, which is not part of downer-cow syndrome.

Severe **hypokalemia** in cattle is associated with signs of depression and profound skeletal muscle weakness leading to recumbency.[7] Reports of pronounced hypokalemia in individual animals that were associated with persistent recumbency, with serum potassium concentrations below 2.0 mmol/L, have accumulated over the past decades. These cases have in most instances been traced back to the repeated use of isoflupredone, a mineral corticoid with strong kaliuretic effect that was commonly used for the treatment of ketosis in the United States.[7] Mild to moderate hypokalemia is known to occur in early lactating and anorectic cows, but the role of this mild form in the pathogenesis of downer-cow syndrome needs to be determined.[8]

The **age and stage of lactation** of a recumbent cow were found to be risk factors for nonrecovery. Recovery rates of nonambulatory cows were 10.1% for first-lactation cows, 17.7% for cows in their second to fourth lactation, and 22.2% for fifth-lactation cows.[2] Cows less than 15 days in milk had a recovery rate of 28.4%, whereas cows in later lactation had a 6.2% chance of making a full recovery.[2] Higher recovery rates in older cows and cows that were earlier in lactation have been attributed to an association between persistent recumbency and hypocalcemia. Cows that are older and earlier in lactation are more likely to be recumbent because of hypocalcemia as primary or contributing cause, which has a better prognosis than persistent recumbency for other reasons.

Duration of recumbency was also found to be associated with the likelihood of making a full recovery. Cows that were down for less than 24 hours recovered in 32% of the cases, whereas cows recumbent for longer periods had an 8.2% chance of recovery.[2]

A high **body-condition score** is a recognized risk factor for milk fever and therefore must also be considered as predisposing for downer-cow syndrome. Cows with a BCS above 4.0/5 around calving were found to be at 4.3 times higher risk to become nonambulatory than thinner cows. In contrast, cows in poor body condition, with a BCS below 2.5/5, recovered in 8.1% of all cases, whereas 16.6% of cows with a BCS of 2.75 or higher made a full recovery.[2]

Environmental and Management Risk Factors

A slippery ground surface is a major risk factor. Cattle that must walk across slippery floors, especially at the time of calving, may slip and fall and injure the large muscles of the pelvic limbs, resulting in an inability to stand.

PATHOGENESIS

In most cases downer-cow syndrome is a complication of an unrelated primary problem causing muscle weakness or persistent recumbency. Primary conditions that can lead to downer-cow syndrome have been grouped into four major categories: metabolic disorders (e.g., hypocalcemia, hypokalemia), acute systemic illness (e.g., coliform mastitis, toxic metritis), musculoskeletal disorders (e.g., fractures, joint luxation), and undetermined causes.[9]

Prolonged recumbency will result in secondary damage from excessive pressure on limbs squeezed between the body and the ground or from struggling to get up. If severe enough, these secondary lesions may prevent the affected cow from getting up, even though the primary cause of recumbency may in the meantime be resolved. Secondary damage can affect muscles, nerves, or other structural components such as bones or joints. Regardless of the initial cause, prolonged recumbency results in varying degrees of pressure damage predominantly affecting the hindlimbs. Based on the results of experimental studies, it has been suggested that 6 hours of recumbency is the time threshold, beyond which tissue damage as a result of excessive weight bearing must be expected. This underscores the importance of handling any persistently recumbent cow as a medical emergency.

Pressure damage in recumbent cattle primarily occurs in the major muscles of the hindlimbs, particularly the semitendinous muscle, muscles caudal to the stifle, and the peripheral sciatic nerve and its branches. The local tissue damage is referred to as **compartment syndrome**; systemic effects resulting from local tissue damage are summarized in the so-called **crush syndrome**.

Compartment Syndrome

A compartment of the body is composed of muscle and nerves within an anatomically defined area that is surrounded by a rigid muscle fascia layer. In a recumbent cow, the compartments of interest are the ones of the upper part and to a lesser extent the lower part of each hindlimb. The initial pressure acting on the hindlimb located underneath the body of a recumbent cow depends on the body weight resting on this limb and the rigidity of the ground on which the cow is lying. This pressure on the limb directly translates into increased pressure within the affected compartment and will result in partial or complete occlusion of venous blood flow before the arterial blood flow of the affected region is decreased. The mismatch between blood flow into and out of the compartment leads to a further pressure increase within the compartment. Impaired blood supply to muscles and nerves and ensuing tissue hypoxia will add to the direct damage from mechanical compression. The thick muscle-fascial boundaries surrounding the compartment prevent tissue expansion that would relieve the structures within the compartment from the excessive pressure. Cell damage and inflammation are associated with swelling, causing a further increase in pressure and contributing to a detrimental cascade of events.

Experimental external compression of the pelvic limb in goats, to simulate limb compression in recumbent cows, resulted in a marked reduction in the nerve conduction velocity of the peroneal nerve, which was associated with clinically evident limb dysfunction.

Crush Syndrome

Crush syndrome refers to the sum of the systemic effects of extensive muscle tissue injury and is attributed to the massive release of muscle-tissue breakdown products into the blood circulation. Notably, a large increase in the serum activity of muscle enzymes, such as aspartate aminotransferase (AST) or creatine kinase (CK); increases in serum concentration of predominantly intracellular electrolytes, such as potassium and phosphorus; and ultimately the appearance of myoglobin in urine are indicative of crush syndrome. Myoglobinuria is a potentially life-threatening complication of downer-cow syndrome that can lead to acute renal failure.

Experimental Sternal Recumbency

Experimentally induced sternal recumbency with one hindlimb positioned under the body to simulate prolonged recumbency will result in a swollen rigid limb within 6 to 9 hours. Following injury to the muscle cells, the serum activity of CK is markedly elevated at about 12 hours after the onset of recumbency. Proteinuria and in some severe cases myoglobinuria occur between 12 and 36 hours after the onset of prolonged recumbency, as a result the release of myoglobin from damaged muscles. In cows that make efforts to stand but cannot do so, continued struggling may result in rupture of muscle fibers and hemorrhage.

Acute focal myocarditis occurs in about 10% of cases, resulting in tachycardia, arrhythmia, and the unfavorable response to IV calcium salts observed in some cases. The cause of the myocardial lesion is unknown, but repeated administration of calcium salts has been suggested. The prolonged recumbency can result in additional complications, such as acute mastitis, decubitus ulcers, and traumatic injuries of the limbs.

The pathogenesis of the nonalert downer cow is not understood. Most such cows have had an initial episode of milk fever and did not respond satisfactorily. Within 1 or 2 days, affected cows have a preference for lateral recumbency and exhibit expiratory moaning and groaning. They represent about 2% of all cases of milk fever.

CLINICAL FINDINGS

Downer-cow syndrome may occur independently or follow apparent recovery after treatment for milk fever, except for the prolonged recumbency. In the typical case, affected cows either make no effort or are unable to stand following treatment for parturient paresis. About 30% of cows treated for milk fever will not stand for up to 24 hours following treatment. Affected cows are usually bright and alert with good or only mildly depressed feed intake and are thus classified as alert downer cows. The temperature is normal and the heart rate may be normal or elevated to 80 to 100 bpm. Tachycardia and arrhythmia occur in some cows, especially immediately following the administration of IV calcium, and sudden death has occurred. Respirations are usually unaffected. Defecation and urination are normal, but proteinuria is common and may indicate extensive muscle damage if marked.

Some affected cows may make no effort to stand. Others will make frequent attempts to stand but are unable to fully extend their pelvic limbs and lift their hindquarters more than 20 to 30 cm from the ground. On a nonslippery surface (bare ground, sand pack, or deep bedding) some cows are able to stand with some assistance by lifting on the tailhead or with the use of hip slings. Those cows that do not make an effort to stand usually cannot stand even with assistance, and if supported with cow slings, they will usually make no effort to bear weight with either the hindlimbs or the forelimbs. Their limbs appear stiff, painful, or numb, and they are unable or reluctant to bear weight. Damage to the peroneal nerve is usually present when there is hyperflexion of the fetlock joints, which is evident if and when the cow is able to stand and bear weight on the hindlimbs.

In some cases, the hindlimbs are extended on each side of the cow and reach up to the elbows on each side. In this position, the cow is bearing considerable weight on the medial thigh musculature and causing ischemic myopathy. This abnormal position of the legs may also result from dislocation of one or both hip joints or be associated with traumatic injuries surrounding the hip joints with or without rupture of the ligamentum teres. Regardless of the cause, the cow prefers this leg position and invariably will shift the legs back to the abnormal position if they are placed in their normal position.

In some cows, the signs may be more marked and bizarre, including a tendency to lie in lateral recumbency with the head drawn back. When placed and propped up in sternal recumbency, these cows appear almost normal, but when they are left alone, they revert to the position of lateral recumbency within a short period of time. Still more severe cases are hyperesthetic, and the limbs may be slightly stiff, but only when the cow is lying in lateral recumbency. These severe cases do not usually eat or drink and have been described as nonalert downers.

Complications in downer-cow syndrome are common and often result in death or the need for euthanasia. Coliform mastitis, decubitus ulceration, especially over the prominences of the hock and elbow joint, and traumatic injuries around the tuber coxae caused by the hip slings are common. When these complications occur in the early stages of the disease, they commonly interfere with any progress being made and become the focus of clinical attention.

The course of the disease is variable and dependent on the nature and extent of the lesions and the quality of the care and comfort that is provided for the cow during the first few days. About 50% of downer cows will stand within 4 days or less if cared for properly. The prognosis is poor for those that are still recumbent after 7 days, although some affected cows have been down for 10 to 14 days and subsequently stood up and recovered. Death may occur in 48 to 72 hours following the onset and is usually associated with myocarditis.

Clinical Examination of the Downer Cow

Clinical examination of the downer cow can be very difficult and challenging depending on the environmental circumstances and the physical size of the animal.[9] Causes of persistent recumbency in cattle include metabolic, musculoskeletal, neurologic, neoplastic, and inflammatory disease; accordingly, obtaining an adequate history and conducting a thorough physical examination are indispensable.[10] Key aspects of the history include age and stage of lactation of the animal, duration of recumbency, any previous clinical abnormalities before the recumbent stage, any previous treatments, diet and accidental access to new feeds, sudden unaccustomed exercise, and assessment of the management provided.

The environment and the ground surface surrounding the recumbent animal may provide clues about the possibility that the animal slipped, fell, and was injured.

A systematic physical examination of all accessible body systems is necessary. The animal should be examined visually from a distance for evidence of abnormalities of the carriage of the head and neck, to observe the position of the limbs, and to observe any attempts of the animal to stand or creep along the ground surface.

The details of the clinical examination are presented elsewhere in this book. The standard close clinical examination is necessary to determine body temperature, heart rate and pulse, respiratory rate, and the state of the major body systems, such as the respiratory tract, cardiovascular system, central nervous system for mental state, gastrointestinal tract, mammary gland, and reproductive tract, any of which may indicate the presence of abnormalities associated with shock that results in recumbency.

In the recently calved cow, particular emphasis must be given to adequate examination of the udder for mastitis, the uterus for metritis, and the gastrointestinal tract for diseases associated with toxemia, dehydration, and shock (abomasal volvulus, acute diffuse peritonitis, carbohydrate engorgement) that result in recumbency. A urine sample must always be obtained and tested for ketones and the presence of myoglobinuria. Careful systematic examination of the musculoskeletal system includes palpating the muscles, bones, joints, and feet of each limb, including passive flexion and extension of each limb. The coxofemoral joints are examined for evidence of dislocation. The vertebral column is examined for evidence of fracture or dislocation of vertebrae. It is important to examine both sides of the animal, which means rolling the cow over from side to side; often the animal may have to be rolled over more than once to repeat a particular examination.

A neurologic examination includes examination of the withdrawal reflexes, patellar reflexes, and sensation of all four limbs and the reflex arcs of the spinal cord; careful examination of lumbar and sacral areas, including sensation and tone in the tail; and examination of the cranial nerves.

The examination can be extended by lifting the downer cow with appropriate lifters and observing if the animal extends its limbs and attempts to bear weight. While the animal is being assisted to stand, additional examinations of other parts of the body can be made.

CLINICAL PATHOLOGY

The serum calcium and glucose concentrations are frequently within the normal range, whereas phosphorus and potassium concentrations may be decreased in cows with depressed feed intake or increased in animals with more pronounced muscle damage and/or dehydration. Results of hematologic examinations are usually unremarkable in early stages of the recumbency. The serum activity of CK and AST are usually markedly elevated by 18 to 24 hours after the onset of recumbency. Very high levels of serum CK activity shortly after the onset of recumbency that decline markedly within the following 24 to 48 hours are indicative of an acute muscle trauma (e.g., muscle rupture) that may be the cause of recumbency. More moderate elevation of the serum activity of CK with a tendency to slightly increase or remain constant over the following days is suggestive of continuous and ongoing muscle trauma resulting from prolonged muscle-tissue compression. Muscle tissue is rich in CK. and the plasma half-life of this enzyme in cattle is only about 8 to 9 hours; this parameter is therefore a sensitive but short-lived marker of muscle damage. When interpreting the serum CK activity of a recumbent cow, it is critical to consider the time of sample collection relative to onset of recumbency.

AST, in contrast, has a considerably longer half-life and remains elevated for several days after initial trauma. In a series of 262 recumbent dairy cows, serum samples were analyzed for CK, lactate dehydrogenase (LDH), and AST to evaluate the value of serum enzyme activities for predicting a failure to recover. The optimal cutoff points maximizing the sensitivity and specificity of the tests were 2330, 2225, and 171 U/L for CK, LDH, and AST, respectively. The predictive value of AST was significantly better, with optimal cutoff points of 128 and 189 U/L, respectively. AST provided the best predictive indicator of whether a recumbent cow would not recover, the best results being obtained with serum samples taken on the first day of recumbency.

In experimentally induced recumbency in cows, the CK activity remained within normal limits for the first 6 hours. However, by 12 hours there was a marked increase to mean values of 12,000 U/L rising to 40,000 U/L by 24 hours. There may be moderate ketonuria. A marked proteinuria is usually evident by 18 to 24 hours after the onset of recumbency. The proteinuria may persist for several days or be absent within a few days. In severe cases, the urine may be brown and turbid because of severe myoglobinuria.

Elevations of serum urea, muscle enzymes, and laboratory evidence of inflammation are considered the best prognostic indicators of an unfavorable recovery. The recovery rate was lower in cows with a total protein : fibrinogen ratio less than 10 : 1, and evidence of neutropenia and/or left shift. Cows with a serum urea level above 25 mmol/L and serum creatinine levels above 130 mmol/L had a poor prognosis.

NECROPSY FINDINGS

Hemorrhages and edema of the skin of traumatic origin are common. The major pathologic changes consist of hemorrhages and degeneration of the medial thigh muscles. Hemorrhages around the hip joint with or without rupture of the ligamentum teres are also common. Local areas of ischemic necrosis of the musculature (gracilis, pectineus, and adductor muscles) occur at the anterior edge of the pelvic symphysis. Eosinophilic infiltration of ruptured necrotic thigh muscles of downer cows has been described. Hemorrhages and edema of the nerves of the limbs (obturator, sciatic, peroneal, radial) are also common and usually associated with severe muscle damage. The heart is dilated and flabby; histologically, there is focal myocarditis. There is fatty degeneration of the liver, and the adrenal glands are enlarged. Histologically, there are also degenerative changes in the glomerular and tubular epithelium of the kidneys.

DIFFERENTIAL DIAGNOSIS

The diagnosis of downer-cow syndrome is typically made by exclusion of all other known causes of recumbency in a cow persistently recumbent for at least 24 hours while having received two courses of parenteral calcium treatment.

Differential diagnoses for alert downer cows:

- Hypocalcemia
- Calving paralysis
- Fractures of bone or pelvis
- Hip luxation
- Hypokalemia
- Botulism
- Spinal lymphosarcoma (BLV)

Differential diagnoses for nonalert downer cows:

- Hypokalcemia
- Hepatic lipidosis/puerperal liver coma
- Coliform mastitis
- Toxic metritis

- Hypomagnesemia
- Hypovolemic shock
- Septic shock
- Generalized peritonitis
- Acute rumen acidosis
- Right-displaced abomasum/abomasal volvulus
- Hypokalemia
- Botulism
- Meningoencephalitis
- Polioencephalomalacia

TREATMENT

Treatment of a nonambulatory cow evidently must focus on the primary cause of recumbency whenever it has been identified, but must also address secondary damage resulting from prolonged recumbency. The reader is referred to the corresponding chapter of this book for the treatment of primary cause of recumbency whenever it is known. Intensive supportive care is required for the treatment of secondary damage and prevention of further damage. The prognosis of a downer cow not only depends on the initial cause of the recumbency but to a large part also on the quality of the care provided during the recumbent period.

Antiinflammatory Therapy

Antiinflammatory therapy as part of pain management in ruminant production medicine has received increased attention over the past years because this is increasingly recognized as an essential aspect of animal welfare by veterinarians and owners alike.[11]

Although currently not much data are available to support the use of steroidal and nonsteroidal antiinflammatory drugs in downer cows, their use seems indicated not only to alleviate pain and discomfort of the sick, nonambulatory cow, but also to contain and control inflammation secondary to recumbency that is likely to exacerbate myopathy and neuropathy. Pain in cattle, as in other species, can occur as result of tissue damage, nerve damage, and inflammation, all factors considered to greatly contribute to downer-cow syndrome.[12] Repeated doses of nonsteroidal antiinflammatory drugs (NSAIDs) may be required for adequate control of pain and inflammation, which may put the treated animal at increased risk for adverse gastrointestinal effects, such as abomasal ulceration.[12] It is therefore advisable to instruct the patient owner to regularly check the produced feces for signs of melena.

A single but high dose of dexamethasone (0.2 to 0.3 mg/kg IV) early in the recumbent period has been advocated by some clinicians, based on clinical experience, to control and contain inflammatory neuropathy resulting from trauma or pressure. Because of the abortive effect of the treatment, this therapy in pregnant cows must be discussed with the animal owner.

Fluid and Electrolyte Therapy

Fluid and electrolyte therapy orally and if necessary parenterally is indicated in patients with inadequate water and feed intake. Multiple electrolytes can be added to the drinking water if the cow is drinking normally. The supplementation of minerals such as phosphates, magnesium, or potassium has been advocated, but they have been used without consistent success.

Oral fluid therapy by drenching is an effective way to maintain hydration in an alert animal. For a recumbent cow, drenching should only be considered in alert cows with a good swallowing reflex. Because the pressure on visceral organs is increased with recumbency, the amount of fluid administered per treatment should not exceed 40 L to prevent the risk of reflux as a result of increased intraruminal pressure.

Bedding and Clinical Care

The most important aspect of treatment is to provide the most comfortable bedding possible and to roll the cow from side to side several times daily to minimize the extent of ischemic damage and para-analgesia that results from prolonged recumbency. With conscientious care and the provision of good bedding, palatable feed, and liberal quantities of water, most cows will attempt to stand with some difficulty and assistance within 24 hours, and most will stand unassisted and normally 1 or 2 days later. A sand or dirt pack is the ideal ground surface to facilitate standing when downer cows attempt to stand. If affected cows are left on a slippery ground surface, they will not make an effort to stand and will become progressively worse. Cows should be milked normally and the udder kept clean by washing with germicide soap before milking, and postmilking teat dips should be applied.

Assisted Lifting to Aid Standing

The clinician and farmer are commonly faced with the questions of whether or not to lift a recumbent cow that has not attempted to stand within a few hours after treatment for milk fever. The guiding principle should be the behavior of the cow. If the cow makes an effort to stand on her own or by some coaxing such as a gentle nudge in the ribs, she should be assisted to stand by ensuring a good nonslip ground surface, providing deep bedding, and lifting up on the tailhead when she attempts to stand. The cow should be rolled from side to side every few hours and encouraged to stand a few times daily.

Several different kinds of **cow-lifting devices** have been used to assist downer cows to stand. Hip lifters, which fit and tighten over the tuber coxae, and body slings such as harnesses are designed to fit around the abdomen and thorax of the animal. These devices can assist a downer cow to stand if she makes some effort on her own. For those cows that make some effort to stand, the hip lifters or slings can be applied and the animal lifted to the standing position. If the animal bears weight on all four legs, she should be allowed to stand with the aid of the device for 20 to 30 minutes and then lowered down. This procedure can be repeated once or twice a day, provided the cow is able to support her own weight while standing. In most cases, such downer cows will stand on their own within a few days. While the cow is in the standing position, she can be milked, and other clinical examinations can be carried out.

The hip lifters can result in traumatic injuries to the tissues surrounding the tuber coxae if not used judiciously. Cows carrying their own weight after being lifted must not under any circumstances be left unattended while hoisted with the hip lifter because they could lose strength and hang in the device, which could result in severe trauma. Animals that make no effort to stand and bear weight on their own must not be left suspended in the lifter for more than a few minutes but lowered immediately. If the hip lifters are not applied carefully, the animal may slip out of the device while it is being lifted, which commonly results in tissue injury around the tuber coxae; fractures of the coxae have even occurred. These injuries are often unnoticed clinically, but contribute to persistent recumbency. Lifting devices must be used carefully by experienced personnel.

Body slings that fit around the abdomen and thorax of the animal are more suitable to lift down cows that will not readily bear weight after being hoisted, because they distribute the weight over several sites in contrast to the hip lifters, which concentrate the weight over the tuber coxae. However, the body slings are cumbersome to apply to a recumbent animal, and they require more time and experienced personnel to ensure proper application. When the slings are applied properly, they do appear to allow the lifted animal to stand comfortably for 30 minutes or more and promote recovery.

Lifting cows that make no effort to stand on their own is usually unsuccessful. When lifted, they usually do not bear any significant weight.

More recently, water flotation tanks have been used for the management of nonambulatory cows.[3] Proposed devices consist of a watertight metal tub with inside dimensions of approximately 234 cm long, 109 cm wide, and 130 cm high. The system can be mobile, and although the use is labor intensive, it can give good results when selecting suitable patients judiciously.[3] Depending on the system used the downer cow is either pulled into the tub on a mat and the ends of the tub closed to make a water-tight container with an open top like a bathtub or is fitted with a harness and lifted into the tub already filled with warm water. With the cow's head held up by a halter, the tub is filled with water at 37° C to 38° C (100° F to 102°F) as quickly as possible. Cows in lateral recumbency will roll into sternal recumbency when 40 to 50 cm of water are in the tub and will usually attempt to stand when the tub is one-half to two-thirds full. Cows are allowed to stand in the water for 6 to 8 hours, in some cases up to 24 hours. If the water temperature falls below 35° C (95°F), more hot water is added. When the decision is made to remove the cow, the water is drained and the end of the tub opened, or the cow is hoisted out of the tub on a sling. A recent retrospective study including 51 recumbent patients of a veterinary teaching hospital treated with flotation tank reported a success rate of this therapy of 37%.[3] The success rate could be higher if the selection of cases for flotation is more rigorous. Cows with ruptured tendons, fractures, luxated coxofemoral joints, septic polyarthritis, and other physical injuries of the musculoskeletal system are not good candidates for flotation. The most suitable case for flotation would appear to be the downer cow as a sequel to milk fever.

Handling, Transportation, and Disposition of Nonambulatory Cattle

There has been considerable controversy and disparity among veterinarians and livestock producers about the handling, transportation, and disposition of nonambulatory cattle. Economics has a major influence on decision making in these cases. There has been no common understanding of whether or not they are fit for transportation and which ones are fit for slaughter for salvage. When the owner and veterinarian are faced with a downer cow that is valuable and the cause of the recumbency is uncertain, the tendency is to either attempt to provide treatment for several days and assess the progress or consider slaughter for salvage. In the case of valuable breeding animals that are recumbent as a complication of milk fever, or a disease such as acute carbohydrate engorgement or peracute mastitis, supportive and specific therapies are commonly selected. In the case of downer cattle of commercial value, slaughter for salvage has been a common option. Cattle producers would like to obtain as much financial return as possible by slaughter for salvage. Cattle affected with complications of milk fever, traumatic injuries of the musculoskeletal system, and other diseases not associated with toxemia or septicemia are commonly submitted to slaughter for salvage. Transportation of these compromised animals has always been an animal welfare issue because of the difficulty of loading them humanely because of their size. The mere act of lifting, pulling, dragging, or by other means forcefully loading an animal weighing 500 to 800 kg onto a truck cannot be done without considerable pain and discomfort to the animal. However, beginning in the 1990s, worldwide concern emerged from the public about the handling and disposition of nonambulatory animals, particularly downer cows, regardless of the cause of their recumbency. Government animal health regulatory agencies, livestock associations, and veterinary associations began drafting regulations on the care and handling of nonambulatory recumbent animals such as the downer cow.

Downer-cow syndrome is an animal welfare issue, and the veterinarian should be proactive about the problem. Society is concerned about how downer animals are cared for and handled and the methods used for their disposition. If recovery does not occur within a few days, the prognosis is uncertain; the owner and veterinarian must decide whether to continue providing clinical care to the downer cow or whether the animal should be euthanized.

Euthanasia

The quality of care provided to a recumbent cow can easily become an issue of animal welfare, and humane euthanasia should always be considered, particularly in cases with poor prognosis or when the attending veterinarian can foresee that adequate supportive care cannot or will not be provided for whatever reason. Suggested "trigger points" for euthanasia suggested in the literature include the following:[10]

- Conditions with poor prognosis
- Pain and suffering that is unresponsive to treatment
- Anorexia over several days
- Nonalert downer cows not responding to treatment in due time
- Cows unable to maintain sternal recumbency
- Owner unable or unwilling to provide adequate care
- Complications such as pressure sore, mastitis, or other condition
- Deterioration despite adequate patient care
- Unresponsive to treatment for over 10 days

TREATMENT AND CONTROL

Treatment of primary cause as indicated

Supportive care

Move cow off concrete floor onto soft bedding (R-1)

Oral fluid therapy in dehydrated or anorectic cows (R-1)

Roll recumbent cow from one side to the other q4-8h (R-1)

NSAIDs (at label dose with label treatment interval) (R-2)

Dexamethasone (0.2 to 0.3 mg/kg IV as a single dose) (R-2)

Hoist cows that make attempts to stand (R-2)

Control

Close monitoring of periparturient cows for signs of milk fever (R-1)

Immediate and adequate treatment of cows with milk fever (R-1)

Provide comfortable calving area with soft bedding and nonslippery flooring (R-1)

Avoid moving pregnant cows too late to calving area (R-2)

Avoid moving fresh cows too early out of calving pen (R-2)

CONTROL

The early detection and treatment of milk fever will reduce the incidence and severity of downer-cow syndrome. Under ideal conditions, cows should be treated during the first stage of milk fever before they become recumbent. Once recumbent, cows should be treated as soon as possible and not delayed for more than 1 hour. Cows with milk fever should be well bedded with liberal quantities of straw or moved to a soft-ground surface. Recumbent cows should be coaxed and assisted to stand if possible after treatment for milk fever. If they are unable to stand, they should be rolled from one side to the other every few hours if possible. It is usually difficult to get owners to comply with this recommendation, but frequent rolling from side to side is necessary to minimize the ischemic necrosis. Dairy cows should be placed in a comfortable, well bedded box stall before calving and should be left in that box stall until at least 48 hours after partition in the event that milk fever develops.

FURTHER READING

Cox VS. Nonsystemic causes of the downer cow syndrome. *Vet Clin North Am Food Anim Pract.* 1988;4:413-433.

Grandin T. Welfare of cattle during slaughter and the prevention of non-ambulatory (downer) cattle. *J Am Vet Med Assoc.* 2001;219:1377-1382.

Green AI, et al. Factors associated with occurrence and recovery of nonambulatroy dairy cows in the United States. *J Dairy Sci.* 2008;91:2275-2283.

Poulton PJ. *Musculo-Skeletal Examination and Diagnosis of the Downer Cow.* Proc XXVIII World Buiatrics Congress. Cairns, Australia: 2014:212-218.

Poulton PJ. *Management of the Downer Cow.* Proc XXVIII World Buiatrics Congress. Cairns, Australia: 2014:219-222.

REFERENCES

1. Stull CL, et al. *J Am Vet Med Assoc.* 2007;231: 227-234.
2. Green AL, et al. *J Dairy Sci.* 2008;91:2275-2283.
3. Burton AJ, et al. *J Am Vet Med Assoc.* 2009;234: 1177-1192.
4. NASS. Accessed July 12, 2015, at <http://usda.mannlib.cornell.edu/usda/current/nacac/nacac-05-05-2005.pdf>; 2005.
5. Ménard L, Thompson A. *Can Vet J.* 2007;48: 487-4919.
6. Grünberg W. *Vet Clin North Am Food Anim Pract.* 2014;30:383-408.
7. Sattler N, Fecteau G. *Vet Clin North Am Food Anim Pract.* 2014;30:351-357.
8. Constable PD, et al. *J Am Vet Med Assoc.* 2013;242: 826-835.

9. Poulton PJ. Proc. XXVIII World Buiatrics Congress. 2014:212-218.
10. Poulton PJ. Proc XXVIII World Buiatrics Congress. 2014: 219-222.
11. Thomsen PT, et al. *Vet J.* 2012;194:94-97.
12. Coetzee JF. *Vet Clin North Am Food Anim Pract.* 2013;29:11-28.

HYPOMAGNESEMIC TETANIES

Tetany associated with a marked decrease in serum magnesium concentration is a common occurrence in ruminants. The syndrome associated with hypomagnesemia is relatively constant, irrespective of the cause, but the group of diseases in which it occurs has been divided into three groups:

- hypomagnesemic tetany of calves, which appears to result specifically from a deficiency of magnesium in the diet transport tetany
- a group of hypomagnesemias in ruminants characterized by lactation tetany, in which there may be a partial dietary deficiency of magnesium but in which nutritional or metabolic factors reduce the availability, or increase the body's loss, of the element so that serum magnesium levels fall below a critical point.

In general, the occurrence of hypomagnesemic tetany is related to three sets of circumstances. Most common is the occurrence in lactating cows turned out onto lush, grass-dominant pasture in the spring after wintering in closed housing—the classic lactation or grass tetany of Holland. Wheat pasture poisoning may occur when cattle or sheep are grazed on young, green cereal crops. The third occurrence is in beef or dry dairy cattle running at pasture in the winter, usually when nutrition is inadequate and where no shelter is provided in changeable weather rather than in severe, prolonged cold. Less common forms occur in housed animals on poor feed. Hypomagnesemia of sheep, although less common, occurs in the same general groups of circumstances as the disease in cattle. A chronic hypomagnesemia, without manifestations of tetany, can be a cause of suboptimal production efficiency and may predispose to hypocalcemia.

HYPOMAGNESEMIC TETANY (LACTATION TETANY, GRASS TETANY, GRASS STAGGERS, WHEAT PASTURE POISONING)

SYNOPSIS

Etiology The etiology is multifactorial, related to magnesium concentration in the diet and the presence of competing cations such as potassium and sodium that affect either herbage magnesium status or magnesium absorption.

Epidemiology Disease of all classes of ruminants, but reaches its highest incidence in older lactating cows exposed to bad weather or grazing green cereal crops or lush grass-dominant pasture.

Clinical findings Incoordination, hyperesthesia and tetany, tonic–clonic muscular spasms and convulsions. High case fatality without treatment.

Clinical pathology Serum, urine, vitreous humor, or cerebrospinal fluid (CSF) magnesium concentrations. Hypomagnesemia, and in some circumstances hypocalcemia.

Necropsy findings None specific.

Diagnostic confirmation Response to treatment, serum or urinary magnesium concentrations.

Treatment Magnesium or combined calcium/magnesium solutions administered IV or SC.

Control Magnesium supplementation, but a palatable and practical delivery method is a problem. Magnesium applied to pastures. Avoidance of movement and food deprivation at risk periods.

ETIOLOGY

Magnesium is the major **intracellular divalent cation** and is an essential element in a large number of enzymatic activities in the body. For this reason, it might be expected that hypomagnesemia would be rare. However, because of the peculiarities of absorption of magnesium in the ruminant forestomaches, and the use of animal and pasture management systems that can lead to marginal magnesium uptake, ruminants are at risk of hypomagnesemia.

Magnesium Homeostasis

There is **no feedback regulatory mechanism** to control concentrations of magnesium in the body of ruminants. As a consequence, magnesium concentrations in blood and extracellular fluid are essentially determined by the balance between dietary intake of magnesium, loss in feces and milk, and the modulating effect of magnesium **homeostasis by the kidney**.

Dietary Intake

In normal circumstances, magnesium absorbed from the diet is sufficient to meet the requirements of the body, and excess amounts are excreted in the urine.

Renal Excretion

The kidney is the major organ of homeostasis and can act to conserve magnesium. Magnesium is freely filtered across the renal glomerulus and is reabsorbed within the renal tubules, the degree of reabsorption acting in homeostasis. The endogenous daily urinary loss is typically 3 mg/kg BW, equivalent to 1.8 g/day for a 600-kg cow. When the dietary intake of magnesium is decreased, blood and interstitial fluid magnesium concentrations fall; excretion of magnesium in the urine will cease when **serum concentrations fall below 1.8 mg/dL**. The renal threshold for magnesium excretion is partially under the control of parathyroid hormone, and increased plasma concentrations of parathyroid hormone will act to conserve magnesium.

Magnesium Reserves

There are large stores of magnesium in the body, especially in bone. These are available to the young calf, but mobilization rate decreases with age, and in the adult ruminant there is little mobilization in response to short-term deficits of magnesium. In ruminants, this control mechanism for magnesium can maintain adequate concentrations of magnesium in bodily fluids in most production circumstances, but it can fail where there is a high requirement for magnesium coupled with a decreased intake. This combination leads to hypomagnesemia, and hypomagnesemic tetany is a possible outcome.

Lactation

Increased requirement for magnesium is almost always associated with the loss of magnesium in the milk during lactation. Whereas the amount of magnesium in milk is not high (14 mg/kg BW), the loss of magnesium to milk in high-producing animals (4.2 g of magnesium in 30 L of milk) represents a significant proportion of the dietary intake of magnesium. As a consequence of this drain, most instances of hypomagnesemia occur in lactating animals around the period of peak milk production, although in some circumstances the demands of late pregnancy are the cause of the increased requirement. The decreased intake of magnesium can result from an absolute deficiency of magnesium in the diet or because the availability or absorption of magnesium from the diet is impaired. These factors determine the circumstances of occurrence of the disease and are the **factors that can be manipulated for control**.

Factors Influencing Absorption of Magnesium

In the adult ruminant, magnesium absorption occurs in the forestomach with little absorption in the abomasum and small intestine. Some absorption occurs in the large intestine, particularly in sheep; however, it cannot compensate for malabsorption in the forestomach. Magnesium is absorbed from the small intestine of calves, lambs, and kids, but this ability appears to be lost when these animals become ruminants.

Na:K Ratio in Rumen

Magnesium is transported across the epithelium of the forestomaches by an active sodium-linked ATPase-dependent transport system. Absorption, and the serum magnesium concentration, is influenced by the

Na:K ratio in the rumen, which is determined by the dietary and salivary concentrations of sodium and potassium. Absorption of magnesium increases with an increasing Na:K ratio to plateau at a ratio of 5:1. Absorption is significantly impaired if the Na:K ratio is less than 3:1.

Young, rapidly growing grass that is low in sodium and high in potassium can result in **sodium deficiency** in grazing ruminants and can significantly depress the Na:K ratio in the rumen fluid, causing impaired magnesium absorption. Depression is observed at dietary potassium concentrations of greater than 22 g/kg dry matter.

Saliva normally has a high Na:K ratio, but where there is a deficit of sodium in the diet, a proportion of sodium in saliva may be replaced with potassium under the influence of aldosterone, which further negatively influences the uptake of magnesium.

Approximately 40% of the total magnesium available in extracellular fluid is secreted daily in saliva, and 20% of this is reabsorbed in the forestomach. When animals are on tetany-prone grass, forestomach absorption is impaired, which accounts for the susceptibility of ruminants to hypomagnesemia compared with monogastric animals.

Other Factors Influencing Absorption

Young grass fertilized with nitrogenous fertilizers has an increased crude protein content, which is readily fermentable and leads to increased ammonia concentrations. A sudden rise in ruminal concentrations of ammonia impairs magnesium absorption in the rumen. The uptake of magnesium is also influenced by the carbohydrate content of the diet; magnesium absorption is improved with increasing amounts of readily degradable carbohydrates. The mechanism of this action is not known, but low concentrations of readily degradable carbohydrate in tetany-prone pastures in combination with high concentrations of protein may be important to the occurrence of the syndrome. Volatile fatty acids provide the energy for the active transport of magnesium across the rumen wall and increase magnesium absorption.

Ruminal pH is thought to affect absorption efficiency by influencing magnesium solubility, which decreases markedly as ruminal pH increases above 6.5. Magnesium binders, such as fats, can form insoluble magnesium salts. Other dietary substances have been proposed to influence the absorption of magnesium, including calcium and phosphorus, organic acids such as citric acid and transaconitate, fatty acids, and aluminum, but the significance of their role is controversial.

Magnesium in Pastures and Tetany Hazard

The dietary intake of magnesium in grazing animals is directly related to the magnesium concentration in pastures, but other elements in pastures also influence magnesium absorption by the ruminant, as detailed earlier.

Required Magnesium Concentrations

Hypomagnesemia can result from the ingestion of pastures that have insufficient magnesium to meet dietary requirements. The estimated magnesium concentration in pasture required to meet the dietary requirement for pregnant or lactating cattle varies from 1.0 to 1.3 g/kg dry matter (DM) for pregnant cattle, depending on the stage of pregnancy, and from 1.8 to 2.2 g/kg DM for lactating cattle, with both estimates assuming minimal interference of absorption by other elements in the pasture.

The recommended minimal "safe" concentration of magnesium in pastures is 2 g/kg DM for lactating and pregnant cattle, with a preference for a concentration of 2.5 g/kg DM.

Magnesium Availability in Pastures and Hazard

Hypomagnesemia can also occur in animals grazing pastures with adequate concentrations of magnesium but that contain high concentrations of potassium and nitrogen, which, as detailed earlier, impair absorption of magnesium in the rumen. Pastures with concentrations of **potassium** of greater than 30 g K/kg DM and **nitrogen** greater than 40 g N/kg dry matter are considered hazardous.

An alternate method for estimating the potential **hazard of a pasture** is to calculate the **K/(Ca + Mg) ratio** using milliequivalent (mEq) values for this estimate. Pastures with ratios above 2.2 are considered a risk.

Winter Hypomagnesemia

The occurrence of hypomagnesemia is not restricted to cattle grazing lush pastures; it can also occur during winter. In **housed lactating dairy** cattle being fed conserved feeds, hypomagnesemia probably has the same genesis as that in grazing cattle, being associated with a high lactational drain of magnesium in combination with the feeding of conserved feeds prepared from pastures with marginal magnesium concentrations. Hypomagnesemia also occurs in **cattle outwintered** on poor-quality feed.

Hypomagnesemia and Hypocalcemia

In some outbreaks of hypomagnesemic tetany, there is also hypocalcemia, and although it is of less severe degree than in parturient paresis, there is increasing evidence that the actual onset of clinical tetany may be associated with a rapid fall in serum calcium levels superimposed on a preexisting hypomagnesemia. This is particularly true for wheat pasture poisoning but can also apply to outbreaks with different predisposing factors.

Chronic hypomagnesemia can have a profound effect on calcium homeostasis. Hypomagnesemia reduces the production and secretion of parathyroid hormone, reduces hydroxylation of vitamin D in the liver, and also causes target-organ insensitivity to the physiologic effects of parathyroid hormone and 1,25-dihydroxyvitamin D_3. Chronic subclinical hypomagnesemia can increase susceptibility to milk fever and can predispose to episodes of **milk fever and downer cows in lactating dairy cows** during the period of peak lactation.

Summary of Etiology

In summary, it appears that a number of factors are capable of causing hypomagnesemia in ruminants and that under particular circumstances one or other of them may be of major importance.

In lactation tetany of cows and ewes turned out onto lush pasture in the spring, a primary dietary deficiency of magnesium or the presence of high relative concentrations of potassium and nitrogen in the diet reduces the absorption of magnesium and possibly calcium.

In wheat (cereal) pasture poisoning, the ingestion of abnormally large amounts of potassium and low levels of calcium in the diet leads to hypomagnesemia and also hypocalcemia.

Hypomagnesemic tetany in cattle wintered at pasture and exposed to inclement weather is associated with low magnesium intake and inadequate caloric intake, and possibly to the resultant hyperactivity of the thyroid gland.

Although the suggestions as to the most important etiologic factors in each set of circumstances in which lactation tetany occurs may be valid, undoubtedly **combinations** of these and other factors have etiologic significance in individual outbreaks of the disease. The **worst combination** of causative factors, and the most common circumstances in which the disease occurs, is inadequate energy intake with a low dietary content of magnesium (grass pasture) in recently calved cows during a spell of cold, wet, and especially windy weather.

One other important factor is the **variation between individual animals in susceptibility** to hypomagnesemia and to the clinical disease. These variations are quite marked in cattle, and in intensively managed, high-producing herds it is probably worthwhile to identify susceptible animals and give them special treatment.

EPIDEMIOLOGY

Occurrence and Risk Factors for Lactation Tetany

Lactation tetany in dairy and beef cattle turned out to graze on lush, grass-dominant pasture after winter housing is common in northern Europe, the United Kingdom, and the northern parts of North America. Grass tetany also occurs in Australia and New Zealand, where the cows are not housed in winter but have access to a phenomenal flush of pasture growth in the spring. This also commonly occurs in beef cattle in all countries.

With housed cattle, or cattle fed conserved feed during the winter, most cases occur during the first 2 weeks after the cattle are turned out to **spring pasture**. Pasture that has been heavily top dressed with fertilizers rich in nitrogen and potash is potentially the most dangerous. The disease may also occur on this type of pasture even when the cattle have wintered on pasture in temperate regions. In regions where there is an autumn flush of pasture, a high incidence of hypomagnesemic tetany may occur in the **autumn** or early winter.

Cattle in the **first 2 months of lactation** and **4 to 7 years of age** are most susceptible, which probably reflects an increased risk because of a higher loss of magnesium in milk. **Friesian** cows have lower magnesium concentrations than Jerseys grazed under the same conditions.

In the northern parts of the United States, outbreaks commonly occur during periods of **low barometric pressure** when the **ambient temperature** ranges between 7°C (45°F) and 16°C (60°F) and **soil temperatures** are below 7°C (45°F). Outbreaks may be precipitated by inclement weather. In beef cattle there is commonly a history of poor nutrition and falling body condition in the past few weeks as a result of diminishing hay supplies.

Occurrence and Risk Factors for Wheat (Cereal) Pasture Poisoning

Wheat pasture poisoning is a misnomer because it can occur with grazing of any small-grain cereal pasture. It has been recorded in many countries, but it is most prevalent where **young cereal crops** are utilized for winter grazing. The southwestern United States has experienced heavy losses of cattle caused by this disease. This pasture can induce hypomagnesemia in **pregnant and lactating cattle and sheep**. The risk is with young, rapidly growing pasture, either in the **spring** or in the **autumn and winter** with pastures planted in late summer. The pasture is usually dangerous for only a few weeks, but heavy losses may occur in all classes of sheep and cattle. *Bos taurus* breeds are more susceptible to the development of hypomagnesemia than *Bos indicus*.

Occurrence and Risk Factors for Winter Hypomagnesemia

Hypomagnesemic tetany in cattle wintered in the open causes some losses in the United Kingdom, New Zealand, southern Australia, and the east-central states and Pacific slope of the United States. It occurs in cattle grazed on pasture in the winter with **minimal supplemental hay** and in cattle grazed on **aftermath crops** and corn stover. The disease occurs in regions with temperate climates, and risk is increased by **exposure to bad weather**, which is exacerbated by absence of trees or other **shelter** in fields and by failure to supply supplementary feed during these cold spells. The disease does not seem to occur in cattle kept outside in prolonged winters where environmental temperature is consistently very low and there is adequate feed. Hypomagnesemia, commonly presenting as chronic hypomagnesemia and sudden death, has been recognized as occurring in housed cattle in the winter in Europe for many years and recently has also been reported in the United States.

Morbidity and Mortality

In all of these forms of the disease, the morbidity rate is highly variable, reaching as high as 12% in individual herds and up to 2% in particular areas. The incidence varies from year to year depending largely on climatic conditions and management practices, and the disease is often limited in its occurrence to particular farms and even to individual fields.

Although an effective treatment is available, the **case-fatality rate is high** because of the short course. Because animals die before they are observed to be ill, there are not accurate figures on case fatality, but it is probably of the order of 30% in dairy cattle and considerably higher in beef cattle.

There have been few epidemiologic studies specifically addressing the importance of the syndrome. In Finland, a **lactational incidence** varying between 0.1% and 0.3% has been recorded, with an **increase in parity** to at least six for lactation tetany occurring on pasture but not for indoor tetany. No association with other diseases was found other than for milk fever. In Northern Ireland, approximately 10% of dairy cows and 30% of beef cows have subnormal or deficient blood magnesium concentrations during the grazing season, and hypomagnesemia is considered the cause of 20% of the sudden-death mortality in beef cattle. Surveys of beef cattle owners of the relative importance of different diseases invariably rate hypomagnesemia high in importance.

Pasture Risk Factors

In most areas of the world, there is a strong association between risk for hypomagnesemia and systems of pasture improvement and pasture fertilization to increase forage yield. There are a number of influences on the concentration of magnesium and other elements in pasture.

Pasture Species

Hypomagnesemia is a problem on grass-dominant pastures. Concentrations of calcium and magnesium are higher in legumes and forbs than in grasses. Within the grasses, different genotypes of the same species can differ markedly in calcium and magnesium concentrations, and most **cool-season grasses** have the potential to produce hypomagnesemia. However, there are some differences, and grasses with a high ratio of potassium to calcium and magnesium (e.g., *Dactylis glomerata*, *Lolium perenne*, *Phalaris arundinacea*) are more likely to cause grass tetany than those with low ratios (e.g., *Bromus inermis*, *Poa pratensis*, *Agrostis* spp.). On soil types where the disease is common, cool-season grass pastures top dressed with **nitrogenous fertilizers** are dangerous, and their toxicity may be increased by the **application of potash. Warm-season grasses** do not have the same risk, and grass tetany is not a problem in cattle grazing tropical grasses.

Cereal Pastures

The greater tendency of cereal grazing to cause hypomagnesemia is related to a high content of potassium and a low content of magnesium. The tetany hazard, in order of decreasing hazard, is wheat, oats, barley, rye.

Season

High concentrations of potassium and nitrogen and low concentrations of sodium and soluble carbohydrates occur in pastures during the early growing season and during rapid growth following cold, wet periods. Pasture magnesium concentrations may not be depressed, but the K/(Ca + Mg) ratio is increased.

Fertilization

Application of potash and nitrogenous fertilizers to pastures will decrease the concentration of calcium and magnesium in plants and will also increase the concentration of potassium and nitrogen. There is some evidence that nitrate sources of nitrogen depress magnesium less than ammonium sources of nitrogen.

Soil Type

The availability of magnesium to the plant is influenced by soil type, and some deficiencies in plant magnesium can be corrected by soil fertilization with magnesium. There is no strong association with any one soil type, but high potassium concentrations are consistently associated with increased risk for tetany.

Highly leached, acid, sandy soils are particularly magnesium deficient and the most likely to respond to liming and magnesium fertilization. In very acidic soils, high aluminum concentrations may depress magnesium uptake by plants.

A local knowledge of soil type and its influence on magnesium, potassium, calcium, and nitrogen uptake by pastures can allow the judicious selection or avoidance of the use of pastures for at-risk groups during periods of risk for hypomagnesemia.

Animal and Management Risk Factors

Dry Matter Intake

The dry matter and energy intake of ruminants can influence susceptibility to hypomagnesemia. A reduction in dry matter intake must reduce the magnesium intake; in situations where hypomagnesemia is already present, a further depression of serum magnesium levels can be anticipated when complete or partial starvation occurs. An insufficient intake of **fiber** in the winter months can precipitate hypomagnesemia in pastured cows and ewes, and lipolysis is accompanied by a fall in serum magnesium.

Period of Food Deprivation

Many outbreaks of hypomagnesemia are preceded by an episode of stress or temporary starvation. Whether chronic hypomagnesemia preexists or not, a period of starvation in lactating cows and ewes is sufficient to produce a marked hypomagnesemia, and the fall may be sufficiently great to cause clinical tetany. A period of **bad weather, yarding, transport, or movement** to new pastures or the introduction to **unpalatable pastures** may provide such a period of partial starvation.

Alimentary Sojourn

Diarrhea is commonly associated with lactation tetany on spring pasture and, by decreasing the alimentary sojourn, may also reduce magnesium absorption.

Climate

A close association between climatic conditions and serum magnesium levels has also been observed. Reduced levels occur in adult cattle and sheep exposed to cold, wet, windy weather with little sunshine and no access to shelter or supplementary feed. Supplementary feeding appears to reduce the effect of inclement weather on serum magnesium levels, and it is possible that failure to eat, or depression of appetite, and a negative energy balance during bad weather may be a basic contributing cause to hypomagnesemia in these circumstances.

Animal Movement

Epinephrine release will result in a precipitous fall in serum magnesium, and this may explain the common observation that clinical cases are often precipitated by excitement or movement of the herd.

Intensive Dairies

Intensive dairies that apply effluent on a limited land base can build soil potassium to high concentrations. Silage from these grounds can have a high risk for inducing hypomagnesemia.

Hypomagnesemia in Sheep

Hypomagnesemia occurs in sheep, particularly in Australia and the United Kingdom. The disease is not common, but it appears to be increasingly associated with pasture improvement practices, and it can cause heavy losses in individual flocks. It is more common in ewes bred for milk and lamb production. In outbreaks, **ewes with twins** are more liable to develop clinical disease than those with singles, and the main occurrence is in ewes **1 to 4 weeks after lambing,** with cases up to 8 weeks after lambing.

Disease is often precipitated by a **management procedure** involving movement and temporary food deprivation, and cases will occur within the first 24 hours following this and for a few days afterward. As in cattle, disease occurs when ewes are placed on lush grass pastures, but it is especially common where ewes in early lactation are placed on young cereal pastures. Losses usually cease when the flock is moved onto rough, unimproved pasture.

Cases also occur in sheep that are exposed to inclement weather when on low nutritive intake. Simultaneous hypomagnesemia and ketosis can occur in ewes after lambing if they are exposed to low feed availability. These cases do not respond well to treatment. Hypomagnesemia in ewes is predisposed by **prior pregnancy toxemia** in the flock.

PATHOGENESIS

Most evidence points to hypomagnesemia as the cause of the tetanic signs observed, but the concurrent hypocalcemia may have a contributory effect and in many instances may even be the dominant factor. Most clinical cases of the disease have serum magnesium concentrations below 1 mg/dL (0.4 mmol/L) compared with the reference range in cattle of 1.7 to 3.0 mg/dL (0.7 to 1.2 mmol/L), and there is a striking relationship between the incidence of the clinical disease and the occurrence of a seasonal hypomagnesemia.

The reduction in serum concentrations of magnesium is concurrent with a marked fall in the excretion of magnesium in the urine. In affected herds and flocks, many clinically normal cows and sheep have low serum magnesium concentrations. In some of these circumstances a concurrent hypocalcemia may be the precipitating cause.

Magnesium has many influences on impulse transmission in the neuromuscular system, including effects on the release of acetylcholine, on the sensitivity of the motor end plate, on the threshold of the muscle membrane, and on activation of the cholinesterase system. These offer an attractive hypothesis for the muscular irritability seen with the disease. However, it has also been established that magnesium concentrations in the cerebrospinal fluid (CSF) are more predictive of clinical disease than those in serum, which would indicate that alterations in central nervous system (CNS) function are more important than alterations in peripheral nerve function. It is also evident that CSF concentrations of magnesium in hypomagnesemic animals rise significantly after treatment with a magnesium salt. The need for this to happen would explain the delay of about 30 minutes after an IV injection before recovery occurs, because CSF volume turns over at approximately 1% per minute.

CLINICAL FINDINGS

For convenience, lactation tetany is described in acute, subacute, and chronic forms.

Acute Lactation Tetany

In acute lactation tetany, the animal may be grazing at the time and suddenly cease to graze, adopt a posture of **unusual alertness,** and appear uncomfortable; twitching of the muscles and ears is also evident. There is severe **hyperesthesia,** and slight disturbances precipitate attacks of continuous bellowing, frenzied galloping, and occasionally aggression. The gait becomes **staggering,** and the animal falls, with obvious tetany of the limbs, which is rapidly followed by **clonic convulsions** lasting for about a minute. During the convulsive episodes the following characteristics are common:

- Opisthotonos
- Nystagmus
- Champing of the jaws
- Frothing at the mouth
- Pricking of the ears
- Retraction of the eyelids

Between episodes, the animal lies quietly, but a sudden noise or touch may precipitate another attack.

The temperature rises to 40.0 to 40.5°C (104 to 105°F) after severe muscle exertion; the pulse and respiratory rates are also high. The absolute intensity of the heart sounds is increased so that they can be heard some distance away from the cow. Death usually occurs within 5 to 60 minutes, and the mortality rate is high because many die before treatment can be provided. The response to treatment is generally good if the animal is treated early.

Subacute Lactation Tetany

In subacute lactation tetany, the onset is more gradual. Over a period of 3 to 4 days, there is slight inappetence, **wildness of the facial expression,** and **exaggerated limb movements.** The cow often resists being driven and throws her head about as though expecting a blow. **Spasmodic urination** and frequent defecation are characteristic. The appetite and milk yield are diminished, and ruminal movements decrease. **Muscle tremor** and mild tetany of the hindlegs and tail with an unsteady, straddling gait may be accompanied by retraction of the head and trismus. Sudden movement or noise, the application of restraint, or the insertion of a needle may precipitate a violent convulsion.

Animals with this form of the disease may recover spontaneously within a few days or progress to a stage of recumbency with a similar but rather milder syndrome than in the acute form. Treatment is usually effective, but there is a marked tendency to relapse.

Chronic Hypomagnesemia

Many animals in affected herds have low serum magnesium levels but do not show clinical signs. There may be sudden death. A few animals exhibit a rather vague syndrome that includes dullness, unthriftiness, and indifferent appetite and may subsequently develop one of the more obvious syndromes. In lactating cows, this may be the development of paresis and a milk-fever-like syndrome that is poorly responsive to calcium treatment. Depressed milk production has also been attributed to chronic hypomagnesemia in dairy herds in New Zealand. The chronic type may also occur in animals that recover from the subacute form of the disease.

Parturient Paresis With Hypomagnesemia

This syndrome is described in the discussion of parturient paresis and consists of paresis and circulatory collapse in an adult cow that has calved within the preceding 48 hours but in which dullness and flaccidity are replaced by hyperesthesia and tetany.

CLINICAL PATHOLOGY

Serum or urinary magnesium concentrations can be used for clinical cases. Where an animal is dead and hypomagnesemia is suspect, a presumptive diagnosis can be made from samples taken from other at-risk animals in the group or from the **vitreous humor** of the dead animal. An acute-phase inflammatory response with leukocytosis and increased numbers of neutrophils and monocytes has been recorded in ruminants and laboratory animals fed magnesium-deficient diets.

Serum Magnesium Concentrations

Normal serum magnesium concentrations are 1.7 to 3.0 mg/dL (0.70 to 1.23 mmol/L). These levels in cattle are often reduced in seasonal subclinical hypomagnesemia to between 1 and 2 mg/dL (0.41 and 0.82 mmol/L), but risk for tetany is not present until the level falls to below 1.2 mg/dL (0.49 mmol/L).

The average concentration at which signs occur is approximately 0.5 mg/dL (0.21 mmol/L), and in sheep it is suggested that clinical tetany does not occur until the serum magnesium concentration is below 0.5 mg/dL (0.21 mmol/L).

Serum magnesium concentration in some animals may fall to as low as 0.4 mg/dL (0.16 mmol/L) without clinical illness. This may be a result of individual animal variation in the degree of ionization of the serum magnesium and in the difference between serum and CSF concentrations. A transitory elevation of serum magnesium concentration occurs after violent muscular exercise in cattle with clinical signs of hypomagnesemia.

Total serum calcium concentrations are often reduced to 5 to 8 mg/dL (1.25 to 2.00 mmol/L), and this may have an important bearing on the development of clinical signs. Serum inorganic phosphate concentrations may or may not be low.

In wheat pasture poisoning of cattle there is hypomagnesemia, hypocalcemia, and hyperkalemia. In acute tetany, serum potassium concentrations are usually dangerously high and may contribute to the high death rate.

Magnesium Concentrations in Cerebrospinal Fluid

Magnesium concentrations in CSF can be used as a diagnostic procedure, but CSF is not easily or safely collected in tetany cases. CSF collected up to 12 hours after death can be used diagnostically.

Magnesium concentrations in CSF of 1.25 mg/dL (0.51 mmol/L) were found in tetanic cows with hypomagnesemia (serum magnesium concentrations of 0.54 ± 0.41 mg/dL; 0.22 ± 0.17 mmol/L). In clinically normal cows with hypomagnesemia, comparable concentrations in CSF were 1.84 mg/dL (0.74 mmol/L) and 0.4 mg/dL (0.16 mmol/L) in serum. In normal animals CSF concentrations are the same as in plasma, that is, 2.0 mg/dL (0.82 mmol/L) and up. The magnesium content of ventricular CSF may be quite different from that of lumbar CSF. Ventricular CSF is also more responsive to changes in serum magnesium concentrations and is preferred for diagnosis at necropsy.

Vitreous Humor

Magnesium concentrations in vitreous humor (but not aqueous humor) can be measured because vitreous humor magnesium concentration remains stable for a longer period of time than magnesium concentrations in serum or CSF. In general, vitreous humor magnesium concentrations less than 0.55 mmol/L for cattle and less than 0.65 mmol/L for sheep up to 48 hours after death indicate the presence of hypomagnesemia, particularly at ambient temperatures of 4° C or 20° C.[1]

Vitreous humor is viscous and must be collected using a 14-gauge (preferably) or 16-gauge needle attached to a syringe. With the deceased animal placed in sternal recumbency, the needle is introduced vertically from a position caudal to the dorsal limbus of the eye parallel and caudal to the lens before aspiration (Fig. 17-5). The needle position should be altered to facilitate aspiration.[1] The aspirated sample should be placed in a plain tube and centrifuged, and the supernatant should be submitted for determination of the magnesium concentration. Aqueous humor should not be collected for analysis because it is readily contaminated by degenerating iris tissue and evaporation of free water across the cornea.

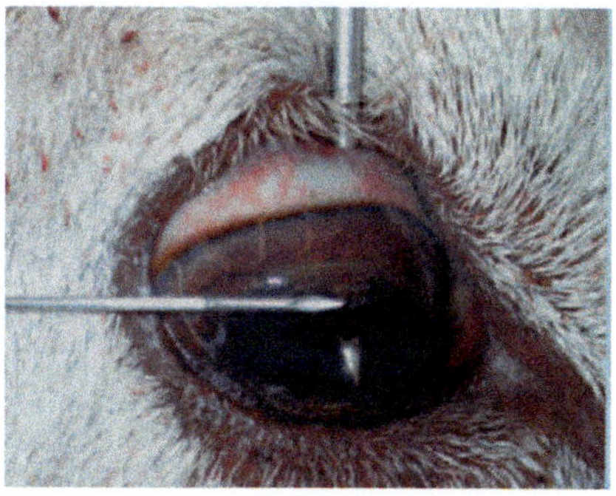

Fig. 17-5 Vitreous humor is sampled from a recently deceased animal by inserting a 14-gauge needle perpendicular and caudal to the limbus. The needle tip can be observed through the pupil. Aqueous humor is obtained by inserting a 21-gauge needle horizontally rostral to the limbus and into the anterior chamber. Vitreous humor is required to evaluate magnesium concentrations. (Reproduced, with permission, from Edwards G, Foster A, and Livesey C. *In Practice* 2009; 31:22-25.)

Urine Magnesium Concentrations

The occurrence of low urine magnesium levels is good presumptive evidence of hypomagnesemia; however, it is not the most sensitive test. Normalization of urine magnesium to simultaneously determine urine creatinine concentration will adjust urine magnesium concentration for animal-to-animal variability in urine concentration.[2] Further adjustment by calculating the fraction clearance of magnesium (requiring simultaneous determination of plasma/serum magnesium and creatinine concentrations) has not been shown to provide additional information beyond that provided by the concentration of urinary magnesium to creatinine alone.

Herd Diagnosis

The kidney is the major organ of homeostasis, and it has been argued that analysis of urine magnesium status is a more accurate method of assessing herd magnesium status than serum magnesium concentrations. The magnesium status of a herd, and the need to supplement the diet to prevent lactation tetany, can be established from the following values:

- serum magnesium concentrations
- urine magnesium concentrations
- urinary magnesium fractional clearance[2]
- creatinine-corrected urinary magnesium concentrations

Laboratory charges for urinary magnesium fractional clearance ratios are expensive. The determination of the **creatinine-corrected urinary magnesium concentration** from 10 cows in a herd has been found to be a more sensitive indicator of magnesium status of the herd than estimates from serum, and it is a better predictor of response to supplementation. Values of less than 1.0 mmol/L indicate that a positive response to supplementation is likely. **Urine**

magnesium concentrations below 1.0 mg/dL (0.4 mmol/L) indicate a danger for tetany.

NECROPSY FINDINGS

There are **no specific necropsy findings**. Extravasations of blood may be observed in subcutaneous tissues and under the pericardium, endocardium, pleura, peritoneum, and intestinal mucosa. Agonal emphysema may also be present.

The magnesium content of the bovine vitreous humor is considered to be an accurate estimate of magnesium status for 72 hours after death, provided the environmental temperature does not exceed 23°C (73°F) and there is not growth of bacterial contamination after sampling, which can result in a false low magnesium concentration. The addition of a small amount of 4% formaldehyde (3% of the vitreous humor volume) will allow accurate analysis for periods up to 72 hours after sampling.

Concentrations in the aqueous humor are not stable after death.

> **DIFFERENTIAL DIAGNOSIS**
>
> **Cattle**
> - Acute lead poisoning
> - Rabies
> - Nervous ketosis
> - Bovine spongiform encephalopathy
>
> **Sheep**
> - Hypocalcemia
> - Phalaris poisoning
> - "Stagger" syndromes

TREATMENT

IV administration of preparations containing magnesium or, more commonly, magnesium and calcium are used. The efficiency of the various treatments appears to vary from area to area, and even within areas under different conditions of management and climate. Response rates and recovery rates are much higher in cases treated early in the clinical course. IV chloral hydrate may be administered to reduce the severity of convulsions during treatment with magnesium. Case fatality, even with therapy, can be high, especially in advanced cases.

Combined Calcium/Magnesium Therapy

The safest general recommendation is to use a combined calcium–magnesium preparation (e.g., 500 mL of a solution containing 25% calcium borogluconate and 5% magnesium hypophosphite for cattle, 50 mL for sheep and goats) IV followed by an SC injection of a concentrated solution of a magnesium salt. The details and risks of administration of the type of solution are described in the section on parturient paresis. A combination of 12% magnesium adipate and 5% calcium gluconate at a dose rate of 500 mL is also used.

Magnesium Therapy

When magnesium solutions are used, 200 to 300mL of a 20% solution of magnesium sulfate may be injected **IV**; this is followed by a very rapid rise in serum magnesium concentration, which returns to preinjection levels within 3 to 6 hours. A much slower rise and fall occurs after **SC injection,** and for optimum results the SC injection of 200 mL of a 50% solution of magnesium sulfate has been recommended. A rise in serum magnesium of 0.5 mg/dL (0.21 mmol/L) occurs within a few minutes, and subsequent serum concentrations do not go above 5 mg/dL (2.06 mmol/L). In cases where serum magnesium concentrations are low because of seasonal hypomagnesemia, the injection of magnesium salts is followed by a rise and then a return to the subnormal preinjection levels.

The IV injection of magnesium salts is not without danger. It may induce cardiac dysrhythmia, or medullary depression may be severe enough to cause respiratory failure. If signs of respiratory distress or excessive slowing or increase in heart rate are noticed, the injection should be stopped immediately and, if necessary, a calcium solution injected.

The substitution of magnesium lactate for magnesium sulfate has been recommended to provide a more prolonged elevation of serum magnesium levels. A dilute solution (3.3%) causes minimal tissue injury and can be administered IV or SC. Magnesium gluconate has also been used as a 15% solution at dose rates of 200 to 400 mL. High serum magnesium concentrations are obtained more slowly and are maintained longer with magnesium gluconate than with magnesium sulfate. The feeding of magnesium-rich supplements, as described in the following section on control, is recommended after parenteral treatment.

Provision for Further Cases

The predisposing factors that lead to a case of hypomagnesemia apply to the herd as a whole, and it is probable that further clinical cases will occur before the effects of corrective strategies are observed. In extensive range situations, it is advisable to instruct the owner on how to treat cases because a delay in treatment can markedly increase the rate of treatment failures. SC treatment is within the realm of most, but successful therapy is also recorded by the rectal infusion of 30 g of magnesium chloride in a 100-mL solution; serum concentrations of magnesium return to normal levels within 10 minutes of administration.

CONTROL

Where possible, animals at high risk should be moved to low-risk pastures during the grass tetany season. High-risk pastures can be grazed by low-risk animals, steers, or yearling heifers, for example, during this period.

The occurrence of hypomagnesemia can be corrected by the provision of adequate or increased amounts of magnesium in the diet. A requirement as high as 3.0 g/kg DM diet may be required for lactating cows on spring pasture. The problem is in determining an **adequate delivery system,** and this will vary according to the management system. Thus blocked minerals containing magnesium or foliar dressing of magnesium may be adequate delivery systems where there is a high stocking density of cattle, but they are totally inadequate or economically unfeasible on range with one cow per 20 acres.

Magnesium oxide is commonly used for supplementation, but other magnesium salts can be used, and they have an approximate equivalent availability. The biological **availability** of magnesium from magnesium carbonate, magnesium oxide, and magnesium sulfate for sheep is influenced by particle size, but it has been determined as 43.8%, 50.9%, and 57.6%, respectively.

Feeding of Magnesium Supplements

The preventive measure that is now universally adopted is the feeding of magnesium supplements to cows during the danger period. The feeding of magnesite (containing not less than 87% magnesium oxide), or other sources of **magnesium oxide**, prevents the seasonal fall in serum magnesium concentrations. Daily administration by drenching, or in the feed, of at least 60 g of magnesium oxide per day is recommended to prevent the disease. This is not always completely effective, and in some circumstances large doses may be necessary. Daily feeding of 120 g is safe and effective, but 180 g daily may cause diarrhea. The dose for sheep and goats is 7 g daily or 14 g every second day. Magnesium phosphate (53 g/d) is also a safe and effective way of ensuring a good intake of magnesium. The protection afforded develops within several days of commencing administration and terminates abruptly after administration ceases.

Problems With Palatability

The problem with magnesium supplements is getting the stock to eat the required amount because they are unpalatable. This can be partially countered by mixing the supplement with molasses in equal parts and allowing free access to the mixture or feeding it in ball feeders, but uniform intake by all animals does not occur, and at-risk animals may still develop hypomagnesemic tetany. Similarly, magnesium blocks may have limited efficacy in preventing hypomagnesemia. **Salt blocks** can help repair the sodium deficiency associated with young spring grasses and improve the Na:K ratio in the rumen. If they also contain Mg they can be an aid in prevention, but usually, by themselves, they do not guarantee freedom from risk for tetany.

Spraying on Hay

One method of attempting to ensure an adequate intake of magnesium is to spray it on hay and to feed this hay as a supplement during periods of grass tetany risk. The common practice is as follows:

1. Mix magnesite with molasses.
2. Dilute mixture with water.
3. Spray mixture onto hay in the windrows when it is being made.
4. Inject mixture into the bales before feeding or spray onto the hay at feeding.
5. Tip bale of hay so that the cut side is uppermost and pour the mixture evenly over the entire surface area.
6. Determine the level of application by the amount of hay intended to be fed.

Depending on local circumstances, this method may or may not be effective because cattle and sheep will frequently not eat hay when on spring pasture unless they are confined for that purpose.

Pellets

Magnesium-rich pellets suggest themselves as a means of supplementation when the additional cost can be borne. Palatability is again a problem, and care needs to be taken to include palatable material in the pellets; alternatively, they may be mixed with other grain or molasses for feeding. Calves should be restricted from access because magnesium oxide at high levels of intake (2% and 4% of the ration) is toxic to calves and causes diarrhea with much mucus in the feces.

In some high-risk situations it may be advisable to provide magnesium in several forms to ensure adequate intake.

Routine Daily Drenching

A once-daily oral administration of magnesium oxide or magnesium chloride to lactating dairy cows (to provide 10 g magnesium per cow), administered with a drenching gun just before the cows leave the milking parlor, is used in New Zealand to ensure adequate supplemental magnesium during periods of high risk. The cows become used to the procedure (and the farmers adept at carrying it out), and it causes minimal disruption of management.

Heavy Magnesium "Bullets"

The use of heavy "bullets" of magnesium to prevent hypomagnesemia has been effective in laboratory trials, and they are available commercially in some countries. The objective is to place a heavy bullet of magnesium in the reticulum, from which it constantly liberates small amounts of magnesium—about 1 g/d. This objective is achieved, and the occurrence of the clinical disease is usually greatly reduced but not eliminated. In dangerous situations, it is customary to administer up to four bullets at a time. As with all bullets, there is a proportion lost by regurgitation and by passage through the gut. A special sheep-sized bullet is used in ewes, with similar results.

Top Dressing of Pasture

Top dressing of pasture, together with magnesium-rich fertilizers, raises the level of magnesium in the pasture and decreases the susceptibility of cattle to hypomagnesemia. For top dressing, calcined magnesite (1125 kg/ha) or magnesic limestone (5600 kg/ha) are satisfactory, with the former resulting in a greater increase in pasture magnesium.

Other magnesium-containing fertilizers can be used depending on cost. The duration of the improved magnesium status varies with the type of soil: it is greatest on light sandy loams, on which a dressing of 560 kg/ha of calcined magnesium can provide protection for 3 years. On heavy soils protection for only 1 year is to be expected. To avoid unnecessary expense, it may be possible to top dress one field with the magnesium fertilizer and keep this field in reserve for spring grazing. Fertilization with magnesium is expensive, and the response of pastures varies markedly with the soil type. It is advisable to seek agronomic advice.

Foliar Dusting and Spraying

The magnesium content of pastures can be raised much more quickly by spraying with a 2% solution of magnesium sulfate at fortnightly intervals or by application of very finely ground magnesium oxide to the pasture (30 kg/ha) before grazing commences. The technique is referred to as foliar dusting or spraying and has the advantage over feed supplementation that the intake is standard. It is very effective in cattle in maintaining serum magnesium concentrations and preventing the occurrence of the clinical disease.

Dusting with 20 to 50 kg MgO/ha can provide protection for up to 3 weeks, but the duration is adversely influenced by wind and rain. A MgO-bentonite-water slurry sprayed onto pastures (26 kg MgO and 2.6 kg bentonite/ha) is effective in providing protection in high-rainfall periods.

Provision in Drinking Water

The problem with water medication is that the water intake of the group to be treated is not known and may be minimal on rapidly growing pastures. However, water medication may provide a delivery system for magnesium on management systems such as extensive range pastures where other methods may have limited success. Water sources other than the medicated supply need to be fenced off or otherwise restricted. The addition of magnesium sulfate (500 g/100 L) or magnesium chloride hexahydrate (420 g/100 L) to the water supply during the risk period for hypomagnesemia has proved effective.

Management of Pasture Fields

The economics of dairy farming make it necessary to produce maximum pasture growth, and the development of tetany-prone pastures is unavoidable in many circumstances. In some areas it may be possible to reduce the danger of such pastures by encouraging the development of legumes. In other areas the period of legume growth does not coincide with the period of maximum risk for grass tetany.

Restricting the amount of potash added to pastures, especially in the period immediately preceding the risk period for tetany, or using potash fertilizers in the autumn or late spring after the period of risk can reduce risk of the disease. The grazing of low-risk animals on high-risk pastures is another strategy. Ensuring that ample salt is available during the danger period to counteract the high intake of potassium can also reduce risk of the disease.

Plant geneticists are developing cultivars of cool-season grasses with high magnesium content that could be used for grazing during the tetany season. Lactating sheep grazing a **high-magnesium cultivar** of perennial rye grass (*Lolium perenne* cv *Radmore*) in the spring have shown higher serum magnesium concentrations than sheep grazing control cultivar, and cultivars of tall fescue (*Festuca arundinacea*) with high magnesium and calcium concentrations and low tetany potential are also available.

Provision of Shelter

In areas where winter pasturing is practiced, the observation that serum magnesium levels fall during the winter and in association with inclement weather suggests that cattle and sheep should be provided with shelter at such times. If complete housing is impractical, it may be advisable to erect open-access shelters in those fields that have no tree cover or protection from prevailing winds. Fields in which lactating cows are kept should receive special attention in this regard. Unfortunately, the disease is most common on highly improved farms, where most natural shelter has been removed, and it is desired to keep the cows on the highly improved pasture to maintain milk production or fatten calves rapidly.

Time of Calving

In areas where the incidence of the disease is high, it may be advisable to avoid having the cows calve during the cold winter months when seasonal hypomagnesemia is most likely to develop. Unfortunately, it is often important to have cows calve in late winter to take advantage of the flush of spring growth when the cows are at the peak of their lactation.

Feeding on Hay and Unimproved Pasture

Because of the probable importance of lush, improved, grass pasture in producing the disease, the provision of some grain, hay, or rough grazing may reduce its incidence. It is most important that the periods of fasting, such as occur when cattle or sheep are yarded or moved or during bad weather, should be avoided, especially in lactating animals and when seasonal hypomagnesemia is likely to be present.

TREATMENT AND CONTROL

Treatment

IV administration of a solution containing 25% calcium borogluconate and 5% magnesium hypophosphite (500 mL for cattle, 50 mL for sheep and goats) (R-1)

SC administration of a 50% solution of magnesium sulfate (200 mL for cattle) (R-1)

IV administration of a 15% solution of magnesium gluconate (200 to 400 mL for cattle) or a 20% solution of magnesium sulfate (200 to 300 mL for cattle) (R-2)

Control

Magnesium oxide—daily administration by drenching or in the feed of 60 g (cattle) or 7 g (sheep and goats) (R-1)

Increase dietary magnesium intake at times of increased risk for hypomagnesemia (R-2)

Monitor urine magnesium-to-creatinine ratio of animals at increased for hypomagnesemia (R-2)

FURTHER READING

Brozos C, Mavrogianni VS, Fthenakis GC. Treatment and control of periparturient metabolic diseases: pregnancy toxemia, hypocalcemia, hypomagnesemia. *Vet Clin North Am Food Anim Pract.* 2011;27:105-113.

Foster A, Livesy C, Edwards G. Magnesium disorders in ruminants. *In Pract.* 2007;29:534-539.

Goff JP. Calcium and magnesium disorders. *Vet Clin North Am Food Anim Pract.* 2014;30:359-381.

Martin-Tereso J, Martens H. Calcium and magnesium physiology and nutrition in relation to the prevention of milk fever and tetany (dietary management of macrominerals in preventing disease). *Vet Clin North Am Food Anim Pract.* 2014;30:643-670.

Schonewille JT. Magnesium in dairy cow nutrition: an overview. *Plant Soil.* 2013;368:167-178.

REFERENCES

1. Edwards G, Foster A, Livesey C. *In Pract.* 2009;31: 22-25.
2. Schweigel M, et al. *J Anim Physiol Anim Nutr.* 2009;93:105-112.

HYPOMAGNESEMIC TETANY OF CALVES

SYNOPSIS

Etiology Hypomagnesemia, resulting from inadequate magnesium in the diet.

Epidemiology Most commonly calves 2 to 4 months of age, on whole milk or milk-replacer diets and poor or no roughage. Diarrhea and chewing of bedding or other coarse fiber may exacerbate the deficiency.

Clinical findings Apprehension, agitation, hypersensitivity to all external stimuli, fine muscle tremors progressing to spasticity and violent convulsions. Rapid course and high case-fatality rate.

Clinical pathology Serum magnesium concentrations below 0.8 mg/dL, bone calcium : magnesium ratio above 90 : 1.

Necropsy findings Calcification of the spleen, diaphragm, and endothelium of the aorta and endocardium. Enzootic muscular dystrophy is often concurrent.

Diagnostic confirmation Blood magnesium and response to treatment. Bone calcium : magnesium ratios.

Treatment and control Magnesium injection and dietary supplementation with magnesium compounds.

ETIOLOGY

The disease results when the dietary intake of magnesium is inadequate for the requirements of the calf. Affected animals may have concurrent hypocalcemia.

Magnesium Homeostasis in the Calf

Milk has low concentrations of magnesium. A milk diet provides adequate magnesium for the requirements of a growing calf up to a body weight of approximately 50 kg, but if milk is the sole diet, the intake of magnesium will be inadequate for requirements once this body weight is reached. The deficit will perpetuate if the other feeds that are fed are also low in magnesium.

In the young calf, magnesium is absorbed in the intestine; however, the efficiency of magnesium absorption decreases from 87% to approximately 30% at 3 months of age, when maximum susceptibility to the disease occurs. The efficiency of absorption is also decreased by a reduction in intestinal transit time caused by diarrhea.

In contrast to adult cattle, young calves can mobilize body stores of magnesium, which are principally located in the skeleton. Approximately 40% of the magnesium stored in the skeleton can be mobilized, which will protect against a short-term deficit.

Hypomagnesemic tetany in calves is often complicated in field cases by the coexistence of other diseases, especially enzootic muscular dystrophy.

EPIDEMIOLOGY

Occurrence

The disease is not common. Cases may occur sporadically, or a number of deaths may occur on one farm within a short period of time.

Risk Factors

The disease can occur under a number of different circumstances. Most commonly, hypomagnesemic tetany occurs in calves 2 to 4 months of age or older that are fed solely on a diet of whole milk, and calves receiving the greatest quantity of milk and growing most rapidly are more likely to be affected because of their greater need for magnesium for incorporation into developing soft tissues. It is most likely to occur in calves being fattened for veal. Those cases that occur in calves on milk replacer appear to be related to chronic scours and the low magnesium content of the replacer. This problem is less common than it once was because most modern commercial milk replacers have added adequate magnesium.

A significant loss of magnesium in the feces also occurs in calves allowed to chew fibrous material, such as bedding; the chewing stimulates profuse salivation and creates greater loss of endogenous magnesium. Peat and wood shavings are bedding materials known to have this effect.

Cases have also been reported in calves fed milk-replacer diets or milk, concentrates, and hay, and in calves running at pasture with their dams. Deaths resulting from hypomagnesemic tetany have also occurred in 3- to 4-month-old calves whose hay and silage rations were low in magnesium content.

Hypomagnesemia also occurs in young cattle, about 6 months of age, that are being fattened intensively indoors for the baby beef market. The phosphorus content of their diet is high, and a lack of vitamin D is probable. The situation is exacerbated by a shortage of roughage. The hypomagnesemia is accompanied by hypocalcemia.

Experimental Reproduction

A condition closely resembling the field syndrome has been produced experimentally by feeding an artificial diet with a very low content of magnesium and a high calcium content, and biochemical hypomagnesemia is readily produced in calves with a diet based on skim milk and barley straw. Hypomagnesemia has also been produced experimentally in very young foals by feeding a diet with a very low magnesium content. The clinical signs are similar to those in calves, and the calcification found in the walls of vessels of calves also occurs in foals.

PATHOGENESIS

On affected farms, calves are born with normal serum magnesium concentrations of 2 to 2.5 mg/dL (0.82 to 1.03 mmol/L), but the concentrations fall gradually in the succeeding 2 to 3 months, often to below 0.8 mg/dL (0.33 mmol/L). Tetany does not occur until the serum magnesium falls below this concentration and is most severe at concentrations below 0.6 mg/dL (0.25 mmol/L), although some calves in a group may have concentrations even lower than this and show few clinical signs.

Magnesium deficiency inhibits the release and action of parathyroid hormone, and this is thought to be the genesis of the concurrent hypocalcemia. It is probable that depression of the serum calcium level precipitates tetany in animals rendered tetany prone by low serum magnesium levels. Tetanic convulsions can occur in hypocalcemic calves in the absence of hypomagnesemia.

Hypomagnesemic tetany is not related in any way to enzootic muscular dystrophy, although the diseases may occur concurrently.

CLINICAL FINDINGS

The first sign in the experimental disease is constant movement of the ears. The temperature is normal and the pulse rate accelerated. Hyperesthesia to touch and grossly exaggerated tendon reflexes with clonus are present. Shaking of the head, opisthotonos, ataxia without circling, and a droopy, backward carriage of the ears are constant. There is difficulty in drinking because of the animal's inability to get to the bucket.

Initially, the calves are apprehensive, show agitation and retraction of the eyelids when approached, and are hypersensitive to all external stimuli, but they show no tetany. Later, fine muscle tremors appear, followed by kicking at the belly, frothing at the mouth, and spasticity of the limbs. Convulsions follow, beginning with stamping of the feet, head retraction, chomping of the jaws, and falling.

During the convulsions the following signs are present:

- Jaws are clenched.
- Respiratory movements cease.
- There are tonic and clonic movements of the limbs.
- There is involuntary passage of urine and feces.
- There are cycles of protrusion and retraction of the eyeballs.

The pulse rate rises to 200 to 250/min, and the convulsions disappear terminally. The pulse becomes impalpable, and cyanosis appears before death.

In field cases the signs are almost identical, but they are rarely observed until the terminal tetanic stage. Older calves usually die within 20 to 30 minutes of the onset of convulsions, but young calves may recover temporarily only to succumb to subsequent attacks. Cases that occur in young calves with scours, usually at about 2 to 4 weeks of age, show ataxia, hyperesthesia, opisthotonos, and convulsions as the presenting signs. The convulsions are usually continuous, and the calves die within 1 hour.

CLINICAL PATHOLOGY

Serum magnesium concentrations below 0.8 mg/dL (0.33 mmol/L) indicate severe hypomagnesemia, and clinical signs occur with levels of 0.3 to 0.7 mg/dL (0.12 to 0.29 mmol/L). Normal values are 2.2 to −2.7 mg/dL (0.9 to 1.11 mmol/L). Erythrocyte magnesium concentrations are also low, indicating a chronic deficiency. Serum calcium concentrations tend to fall when serum magnesium levels become very low and are below normal in most clinical cases.

The estimation of the magnesium in bone (particularly ribs and vertebrae) is a reliable confirmatory test at necropsy. Values below a ratio of 70 : 1 for calcium : magnesium may be regarded as normal, and those above 90 : 1 are indicative of severe magnesium depletion. In the normal calf the ratio is about 55 : 1.[1] Absolute bone calcium values are not decreased and are often slightly elevated. An incidental change is the marked increase in serum creatinine kinase activity in calves after an acute attack of hypomagnesemic tetany.

NECROPSY FINDINGS

There is a marked difference between the necropsy lesions of some natural cases and those in the experimental disease. In field cases, there is often calcification of the spleen and diaphragm, and calcified plaques are present in the aorta and endocardium, together with hyaline degeneration and musculature. In other cases necropsy lesions similar to those in enzootic muscular dystrophy occur.

In experimentally produced cases these lesions are not evident, but there is extensive congestion in all organs, and hemorrhages are present in unsupported organs, including the following:

- Gallbladder
- Ventricular epicardium
- Pericardial fat
- Aorta
- Mesentery wall
- Intestinal wall

The lesions are obviously terminal and are associated with a terminal venous necrosis. Some field cases present a picture identical to this.

DIFFERENTIAL DIAGNOSIS

- Acute lead poisoning
- Enterotoxemia caused by *Clostridium perfringens* type D
- Polioencephalomalacia
- Tetanus
- Vitamin A deficiency
- Meningitis

TREATMENT

Response to magnesium injections (100 mL of a 10% solution of magnesium sulfate) is only transitory because of the severe depletion of bone reserves of magnesium. This dose provides only a single day's requirements. A magnesium sulfate enema in warm water (containing 15 g of magnesium sulfate) was associated with a rapid response in hypomagnesemic 3-month-old calves.[2]

Follow-up supplementation of the diet with magnesium oxide or carbonate as described later is advisable. Chloral narcosis or tranquilization with an ataractic drug may be essential to avoid death as a result of respiratory paralysis during convulsions.

CONTROL

The provision of hay that is high in magnesium, such as alfalfa, helps to prevent the disease, as will well-formulated concentrates.

Supplementary Feeding of Magnesium

If begun during the first 10 days of life, supplementary magnesium feeding will prevent excessive drops in serum magnesium, but if begun after the calf is 7 weeks old, it may not prevent further depression of the levels. Supplementation should continue until at least 10 weeks of age. Daily feeding of the magnesium compound and fairly accurate dosing are necessary to avoid scouring or inefficient protection. For calves of average growth rate, appropriate dose rates are 1 g/d for calves to 5 weeks of age, 2 g/d for calves 5 to 10 weeks of age, and 3 g/d for calves 10 to 15 weeks of age of magnesium oxide or twice this dose of carbonate. Supplementation of the diet with magnesium restores serum calcium levels to normal and corrects the hypomagnesemia.

Magnesium Alloy Bullets

Two bullets of the sheep size (together releasing approximately 1 g/d of magnesium) per calf have shown high efficiency in preventing the clinical disease and also the hypomagnesemia that precedes it. Calves kept indoors and fed largely on milk should get adequate mineral supplement and vitamin D (70,000 IU vitamin D_3/d). Magnesium utilization will not be affected, but calcium absorption, which is often sufficiently reduced to cause a concurrent hypocalcemia, will be improved.

REFERENCES

1. Foster A, et al. *In Pract.* 2007;29:534.
2. Soni AK, Shukla PC. *Environ Ecol.* 2012;30:1601.

TRANSPORT RECUMBENCY OF RUMINANTS

Transport recumbency (tetany) occurs after prolonged transport, usually in cows and ewes in late pregnancy. It is also recorded in lambs transported to feedlots and in cows and sheep delivered to abattoirs. It is characterized by recumbency, alimentary tract stasis, and coma, and it is highly fatal. It occurs in most countries. Large losses can be encountered when cows and ewes in late pregnancy are moved long distances by rail, by truck, or on foot.

Although cows of any age in late pregnancy are most commonly affected, the disease has also been recorded in cows recently calved, bullocks, steers, dry cows, and lambs. Risk factors include the following:

- Heavy feeding before shipment
- Deprivation of feed and water for more than 24 hours during transit
- Unrestricted access to water
- Exercise immediately after unloading

There is an increased incidence of the disease during hot weather. The cause is unknown, although physical stress is an obvious factor. Lambs show the following characteristics:

- Restlessness
- Staggering
- Partial paralysis of hindlegs
- Early assumption of lateral recumbency

Death may occur quickly, or after 2 to 3 days of recumbency. There is mild hypocalcemia (7 to 7.5 mg/dL; 1.75 to 1.87 mmol/L). The recovery rate even with treatment is only fair.

Clinical signs may occur while the cattle are still on the transportation vehicle or up to 48 hours after unloading. In the early stages, animals may exhibit excitement and restlessness, trismus, and grinding of the teeth. A staggering gait with paddling of the hindlegs and recumbency occur, accompanied by stasis of the alimentary tract and complete anorexia. Animals that do not recover gradually become comatose and die in 3 to 4 days. There may be moderate hypocalcemia and hypophosphatemia in cattle. In sheep of various ages, some are hypocalcemic and hypomagnesemic, some are hypoglycemic, and some have no detectable biochemical abnormality. There are no lesions at necropsy other than those related to prolonged recumbency. Ischemic muscle necrosis is the most obvious of these lesions. The relationship of the disease to transport or forced exercise is diagnostic.

Some cases respond to treatment with combined calcium, magnesium, and glucose injections. Repeated parenteral injections of large volumes of electrolyte solutions are recommended. In lambs, the SC injection of a solution of calcium and magnesium salts is recommended, but the response is usually only 50%, due probably because of an intercurrent myonecrosis.

If prolonged transport of cows or ewes in advanced pregnancy is unavoidable, they should be provided with adequate food, water, and rest periods during the trip. The incidence of this condition after transportation appears to have been markedly reduced with increased monitoring and awareness of transportation-related morbidity and mortality.

KETOSIS AND SUBCLINICAL KETOSIS (HYPERKETONEMIA) IN CATTLE

SYNOPSIS

Etiology A multifactorial disorder of energy metabolism. Negative energy balance results in hypoglycemia, ketonemia (the accumulation in blood of acetoacetate, β-hydroxybutyrate [BHB] and their decarboxylation products acetone and isopropanol), and ketonuria.

Epidemiology Primary ketosis and subclinical ketosis occurs predominantly in well-conditioned cows with high lactation potential, principally in the first month of lactation, with a higher prevalence in cows with a higher lactation number. Loss of body condition in the dry period and immediately postpartum. Secondary ketosis occurs where other disease reduces feed intake.

Clinical findings Cattle show wasting with decrease in appetite, body condition, and milk production. Some have short periods of bizarre neurologic and behavioral abnormality (nervous ketosis). Response to treatment is good. Subclinical ketosis (hyperketonemia) is detected by tests for ketones, usually BHB in blood, plasma, or serum, and acetoacetate in urine.

Clinical pathology Hypoglycemia, ketonemia, ketonuria, or elevated ketones in milk.

Necropsy findings None specific. Varying degrees of hepatic lipidosis.

Diagnostic confirmation Ketonemia, ketonuria, or, less commonly, elevated ketone concentration in milk.

Treatment Intravenous glucose, parenteral corticosteroid, and oral glucose precursors such as propylene glycol. The disease responds readily to treatment in cattle with mild hepatic lipidosis and is self-limiting.

Control Correction of energy imbalance. Herd biochemical monitoring coupled with condition scoring. Daily monensin administration to late-gestation and early-lactation dairy cows.

ETIOLOGY

Glucose Metabolism in Cattle

The maintenance of adequate concentrations of glucose in the plasma is critical to the regulation of energy metabolism. The ruminant absorbs very little dietary carbohydrate as hexose sugar because dietary carbohydrates are fermented in the rumen to short-chain fatty acids, principally acetate (70%), propionate (20%), and butyrate (10%). Consequently, glucose needs in cattle must largely be met by gluconeogenesis. **Propionate and amino acids are the major precursors** for gluconeogenesis, with glycerol and lactate being of lesser importance.

Propionate is produced in the rumen from starch, fiber, and proteins. It enters the portal circulation and is efficiently removed by the liver, which is the primary glucose-producing organ. Propionate is the **most important glucose precursor**; an increased availability of propionate can spare the hepatic utilization of other glucose precursors, and production of propionate is favored by a high grain inclusion in the diet. The gluconeogenic effect of propionate should be contrasted to **acetate,** which is transported to peripheral tissues and to the mammary gland and metabolized to long-chain fatty acids for storage as lipids or secretion as milk fat.

Amino acids. The majority of amino acids are glucogenic and are also important precursors for gluconeogenesis. Dietary protein is the most important quantitative source, but the labile pool of body protein (particularly skeletal muscle) is also an important source; together they contribute to energy synthesis , milk lactose synthesis, and milk protein synthesis.

Energy Balance

In high-producing dairy cows there is always a negative energy balance in the first few weeks of lactation. The highest dry matter intake does not occur until 8 to 10 weeks after calving, but peak milk production is at 4 to 6 weeks, and energy intake may not keep up with demand. In response to a negative energy balance and low serum concentrations of glucose (and consequently low serum concentrations of insulin), cows will mobilize adipose tissue, with consequent increases in serum concentrations of **nonesterified fatty acids** (**NEFA**) and subsequent increases in serum concentrations of **β-hydroxybutyrate** (**BHB**), **acetoacetate,** and **acetone**. The hepatic mitochondrial metabolism of fatty acids promotes both gluconeogenesis and ketogenesis. Cows partition nutrients during pregnancy and lactation and are in a lipolytic stage in early lactation and at risk for ketosis during this period.

Hepatic Insufficiency in Ketosis

Hepatic insufficiency has been shown to occur in bovine ketosis, but it does not occur in all cases. Ketosis is defined as an increased plasma or serum concentration of ketoacids and is divided into three types. In **type I**, or "spontaneous" ketosis, the gluconeogenic pathways are maximally stimulated, and ketosis occurs when the demand for glucose outstrips the capacity of the liver for gluconeogenesis because of an insufficient supply of glucose precursors. Rapid entry of NEFAs into hepatic mitochondria occurs and results in high rates of ketogenesis and high plasma/serum ketone concentration. There is little conversion of NEFAs to triglycerides, resulting in little fat accumulation in the liver. In **type II** ketosis, manifest with **fatty liver**, gluconeogenic pathways are not maximally stimulated, and consequently mitochondrial uptake of NEFAs is not as active, and NEFAs become esterified in the cytosol, forming triglyceride. The capacity of cattle to transport triglyceride from the liver is low, resulting in accumulation and fatty liver. The occurrence of a fatty liver can further suppress hepatic gluconeogenic capacity. Hepatic insufficiency may occur more commonly in those cows predisposed to ketosis by overfeeding in the dry period. In **type III** ketosis, cattle are fed a diet (typically a high-maize ration) that results in a higher ruminal production of butyrate, which is directly metabolized by ruminal epithelial cells to butyrate.

Ketone Formation

Ketones arise from two major sources: butyrate in the rumen and mobilization of fat. A large proportion of butyrate produced by rumen fermentation of the diet is converted to BHB in the rumen epithelium and is absorbed as such. Free fatty acids produced from the mobilization of fat are transported to the liver and oxidized to produce acetyl-CoA and NADH.

Acetyl-CoA may be oxidized via the tricarboxylic acid (TCA) cycle or metabolized to acetoacetyl-CoA. Complete oxidation of acetyl-CoA via the TCA cycle depends on an adequate supply of oxaloacetate from the precursor propionate. If propionate, and consequently oxaloacetate, is deficient, oxidation of acetyl-CoA via the TCA cycle is limited, and acetyl-CoA is metabolized to acetoacetyl CoA and subsequently to acetoacetate and BHB.

The ketones BHB and acetoacetate can be utilized as energy sources. They are normally present in the plasma/serum of cattle, and their concentration is a result of the balance between production in the liver and utilization by the peripheral tissues. Acetoacetate can spontaneously convert to **acetone,** which is volatile and therefore exhaled in the breath; diffusion of acetone across the rumen epithelium into the rumen means that some acetone is eructated. Ruminal flora (most likely bacteria) can metabolize acetone to isopropanol, which can then be absorbed to increase plasma concentrations of **isopropanol**, a 3-carbon alcohol.[1]

Role of Insulin and Glucagon

The regulation of energy metabolism in ruminants is primarily governed by insulin and glucagon. Insulin acts as a glucoregulatory hormone stimulating glucose use by tissues and decreasing hepatic gluconeogenesis. Plasma insulin concentrations decrease with decreasing plasma concentrations of glucose and propionate. Insulin also acts as a liporegulatory hormone stimulating lipogenesis and inhibiting lipolysis. Glucagon is the primary counterregulatory hormone to insulin. The counteracting effects of insulin and glucagon therefore play a central role in the homeostatic control of glucose. A low **insulin : glucagon ratio** stimulates lipolysis in adipose tissue and ketogenesis in the liver. Cows in early lactation have low insulin : glucagon ratios because of low plasma glucose concentrations and are in a catabolic state. Regulation is also indirectly governed by **somatotropin**, which is the most important determinant of milk yield in cattle and is also lipolytic. Factors that decrease the energy supply, increase the demand for glucose, or increase the utilization of peripheral fat reserves as an energy source are likely to increase ketone production and ketonemia. There is, however, considerable cow-to-cow variation in the risk for developing clinical ketosis.

ETIOLOGY OF BOVINE KETOSIS

It is not unreasonable to view clinical ketosis as one end of a spectrum of a metabolic state that is **common in heavily producing cows** in the **postcalving period.** This is because high-yielding cows in early lactation are in negative energy balance and are subclinically ketotic as a result.

Cattle are particularly vulnerable to ketosis because, although very little carbohydrate is absorbed as such, a direct supply of glucose is essential for tissue metabolism, particularly the formation of lactose associated with milk production. The utilization of volatile fatty acids for energy purposes is also dependent on a supply of available glucose. This vulnerability is further exacerbated in the lactating dairy cow by the tremendous rate of turnover of glucose.

In the period between calving and peak lactation, the demand for glucose is increased and cannot be completely restrained. Cows will reduce milk production in response to a reduction of energy intake, but this does not follow automatically nor proportionately in early lactation because hormonal stimuli for milk production overcome the effects of reduced food intake. Under these circumstances, lowered plasma glucose concentrations result in lowered plasma insulin concentrations. Long-chain fatty acids are released from fat stores under the influence of both a low plasma insulin : glucagon ratio and the influence of high somatotropin concentration, and this leads to increased ketogenesis.

Individual Cow Variation

The rate of occurrence of negative energy status, and therefore the frequency of clinical ketosis cases, has increased markedly over the last 4 decades because of the increase in the lactation potential of the modern dairy cow. Because of the mammary gland's metabolic precedence in the partitioning of nutrients, especially glucose, milk production continues at a high rate, causing an energy drain. In many individual cows, the need for energy is beyond their capacity for dry matter intake, but there is between-cow variation in risk under similar nutritional stress. Clinical ketosis is easily produced in early-lactation dairy cows by reducing the daily feed intake.[2] Subclinical ketosis (hyperketonemia) in early-lactation dairy cows is associated with decreased dry matter intake and feeding time during the week before calving.[6]

Types of Bovine Ketosis

There are many theories on the cause and biochemical and hormonal pathogenesis of ketosis, in addition to the importance of predisposing factors. Reviews of these studies are cited at the end of this disease section. In general, it can be stated that clinical ketosis occurs in cattle when they are subjected to demands on their resources of glucose and glycogen that cannot be met by their digestive and metabolic activity.

A common classification of the disease based on its natural presentation in intensively and extensively managed dairy herds, and one that accounts for the early lactational demand for glucose, a limited supply of propionate precursors, and preformed ketones or mobilized lipids in the pathogenesis, has been developed. Such a classification scheme includes the following mechanisms for ketosis, which will be discussed in turn:

- Primary ketosis (production ketosis)
- Secondary ketosis
- Alimentary ketosis
- Starvation ketosis
- Ketosis resulting from a specific nutritional deficiency

Primary Ketosis (Production Ketosis)

This is the ketosis of most herds, the so-called estate acetonemia. Primary ketosis occurs in cows in good to excessive body condition that have high lactation potential and are being fed good-quality rations but that are in a negative energy balance. There is a tendency for the disease to recur in individual animals, which is probably a reflection of variation between cows in digestive capacity or metabolic efficiency. A proportion of primary ketosis cases appear as **clinical ketosis,** but a much greater proportion occurs as cases of **subclinical ketosis** in which there are increased concentrations of circulating ketone bodies but no overt clinical signs. Affected cattle recover with correct feeding and ancillary treatment.

Secondary Ketosis

Secondary ketosis occurs where the presence of **other disease** results in a **decreased food intake.** The cause of the reduction in food intake is commonly the result of abomasal displacement, traumatic reticulitis, metritis, mastitis, or other diseases common to the postparturient period. A high incidence of ketosis has also been observed in herds affected with fluorosis. An unusual occurrence reported was an outbreak of acetonemia in a dairy herd fed on a ration contaminated by a low level (9.5 ppm) of lincomycin, which caused ruminal microbial dysfunction. The proportion of cases of ketosis that are secondary and their diagnosis as such are both matters of great interest because a significant proportion of all cases of ketosis in lactating dairy cattle are secondary to other disease.

Alimentary Ketosis

Alimentary ketosis (also called type III in some classification systems) is a result of excessive amounts of **butyrate in silage** and possibly also a result of decreased food intake resulting from the poor palatability of high-butyrate silage. Silage made from succulent material may be more highly ketogenic than other types of ensilage because of its higher content of preformed butyric acid. Spoiled silage is also a cause, and toxic biogenic amines in silage, such as putrescine, may also contribute. This type of ketosis is commonly subclinical, but it may predispose to the development of production or primary ketosis.

Starvation Ketosis

Starvation ketosis occurs in cattle that are in poor body condition and that are fed poor-quality feedstuffs. There is a deficiency of propionate and protein from the diet and a limited capacity of gluconeogenesis from body reserves. Affected cattle recover with correct feeding.

Ketosis Resulting From Specific Nutritional Deficiency

Specific dietary deficiencies of **cobalt** and possibly phosphorus may also lead to a high incidence of ketosis. This may be in part a result of a reduction in the intake of total digestible nutrients, but in cobalt deficiency, the essential defect is a failure to metabolize propionic acid in the TCA cycle. The problem is restricted to the cobalt-deficient areas of the world, although the occurrence of cobalt deficiency in high-producing dairy cows in nondeficient areas has been described.

There is a marked nadir in food intake around calving, followed by a gradual increase. This increase is quite variable between cows, but in the great majority of cases does not keep pace with milk yield. The net result is that high-yielding dairy cows are almost certain to be in negative energy balance for the first 2 months of lactation.

EPIDEMIOLOGY

Occurrence

Ketosis is a very common disease of lactating dairy cattle and is prevalent in most countries where intensive farming is practiced. Ketosis occurs mainly in animals housed during the winter and spring months and is rare in cows that calve on pasture. In housed or free-stalled cattle, ketosis occurs year around. The occurrence of the disease is very much dependent on management and nutrition and varies between herds. As might be expected, **lactational incidence rates** vary between herds, and a review of 11 epidemiologic studies showed a lactation incidence rate for ketosis that varied from 0.2% to 10.0%.

The incidence of **subclinical ketosis** (more correctly called hyperketonemia) is influenced by the cut-point of plasma BHB used for definition, but it is much higher than the incidence of clinical ketosis, especially in undernourished herds, and can approach 40%. Incidence can be challenging and expensive to estimate because prevalence information is usually measured. In general, the incidence of subclinical ketosis is 1.8 times the prevalence.

Animal and Management Risk Factors

There are conflicting reports on the significance of risk factors for ketosis and subclinical ketosis, which probably reflect that the disease can be a cause or effect of a number of interacting factors. The disease occurs in the immediate postparturient period, with 90% of cases occurring in the first 60 days of lactation. Regardless of the specific etiology, ketosis occurs most commonly during the **first month** of lactation, less commonly in the second month, and only occasionally in late pregnancy. In different studies, the median **time to onset following calving** has varied from 10 to 28 days, with some recent studies showing a peak prevalence of subclinical ketosis in the first 2 weeks post-calving. A prolonged previous intercalving interval increases risk.

Age. Cows of any age may be affected, but the disease increases from a low prevalence at the first calving to a peak at the fourth calving, associated with the level of milk production. Lactational incidence rates of clinical ketosis of 1.5% and 9%, respectively, were found in a study of 2415 primiparous and 4360 multiparous cows. Clinical ketosis can also recur in the same lactation.

Herd differences in prevalence are very evident in clinical practice and in the literature, with some herds having negligible occurrence. Although apparent differences in breed incidence are reported, evidence for a heritable predisposition within breeds is minimal. Feeding frequency has an effect, with the prevalence of ketosis being much lower in herds that feed a **total mixed ration** (TMR) ad libitum compared with herds that feed roughage and concentrate separately fed twice a day (**component fed**).

Body-Condition Score. There are conflicting reports on the relation between BCS at calving and ketosis, but it is very likely that studies that have found no relationship have not had many fat cows in the herds examined. Fat body condition postpartum was observed to be associated with a higher first-test-day milk yield, milk-fat-to-protein ratio of greater than 1.5, increased body-condition loss, and a higher risk for ketosis. In another study, cows with a BCS greater than 3.25 at parturition and that lost 0.75 points in BCS in the first 2 months of lactation developed subclinical ketosis. Body-condition loss during the dry period also increases risk for ketosis in the following lactation.

Season. There is no clear association with season. In some but not all summer grazing areas, a higher risk is generally observed in cattle during the winter housing period. Higher prevalence has been observed in the late summer and early winter in Scandinavian countries.

Other Interactions. There is a **greater risk** for the development of ketosis in cows that have an extended long dry period;[3] those that develop milk fever, retained placenta, lameness, or hypomagnesemia; or those that have high milk production and high first milking colostrum volume.[3] Cows with twins are also at risk for ketosis in the terminal stages of pregnancy. There is a bidirectional relation between risk for displaced abomasum and risk for ketosis, but in a field study of 1000 cows in 25 herds, cows that had a serum BHB concentration greater than 1.4 mmol/L in the first 2 weeks of lactation had odds of 4:1 that a displaced abomasum would be diagnosed 1 to 3 weeks later. In another study of 1010 cows, a serum BHB concentration of 1.5 mmol/L or greater in the first 2 weeks of lactation was found to be associated with a threefold increase in ketosis or displaced abomasum. Interestingly, cows with increased blood BHB concentration immediately before surgical correction of left-displaced abomasum have increased longevity within the herd, compared with cattle with BHB concentrations within the reference interval.[7,8]

Economic Significance

Clinical and subclinical ketosis are major causes of loss to the dairy farmer. In rare instances the disease is irreversible and the affected animal dies, but the main economic loss results from the loss of production while the disease is present, the possible failure to return to full production after recovery, and the increased occurrence of periparturient disease. Both clinical and subclinical ketosis are accompanied by **decreased milk yields**; lower milk protein and milk lactose; **increased risk** for delayed estrus and lower first-service conception rates; lower pregnancy rates; increased intercalving intervals; increased risk of cystic ovarian disease, metritis, and mastitis; and increased involuntary culling.[4] The estimated economic loss from a single case of subclinical ketosis was US$117 in 2015, and the estimated average total cost per case of subclinical ketosis was $289 after considering the costs of displaced abomasum and metritis attributed to hyperketonemia.[5]

PATHOGENESIS

Bovine Ketosis

The principal metabolic disturbances observed, hypoglycemia and ketonemia, may both exert an effect on the clinical syndrome. However, in the experimental disease in cattle, it is not always clear what determines the development of the clinical signs in cases that convert from subclinical to clinical ketosis. In many cases, the severity of the clinical syndrome is proportional to the degree of hypoglycemia, and this, together with the rapid response to parenterally administered glucose in cattle, suggests **hypoglycemia as the predominant factor**. This hypothesis is supported by the development of prolonged hypoglycemia and a similar clinical syndrome to that of ketosis, after the experimental IV or SC injection of insulin (2 U/kg BW).

However, in most field cases the severity of the clinical syndrome is also roughly proportional to the degree of ketonemia. This is an understandable relationship because ketone bodies are produced in larger quantities as the deficiency of glucose increases. However, the ketone bodies are thought to exert an additional influence on the clinical signs observed; for instance, acetoacetic acid is known to be toxic and probably contributes to the terminal coma in diabetes mellitus in humans.

The **nervous signs** that occur in some cases of bovine ketosis are thought to be caused by the production of isopropanol, a breakdown product of acetone in the rumen,[1] although the requirement of nervous tissue for glucose to maintain normal function may also be a factor in these cases. A reasonable explanation for the development of nervous ketosis is that a rapid increase in plasma acetone concentration in an animal that has an active rumen flora leads to a rapid increase in ruminal acetone concentration. The acetone is metabolized by rumen microflora to isopropanol, which is then absorbed into the bloodstream, potentially leading to neurologic abnormalities. This mechanism is consistent with observations that nervous signs of ketosis are more common in cattle with severe ketosis that is rapidly induced.

Spontaneous ketosis in cattle is usually **readily reversible** by treatment; incomplete or temporary response is usually a result of the existence of a primary disease, with ketosis present only as a secondary development, although fatty degeneration of the liver in protracted cases may prolong the recovery period. Changes in ruminal flora after a long period of anorexia may also cause continued impairment of digestion.

Immunosuppression has been demonstrated with energy deficiency and ketosis. The higher susceptibility of ketotic postpartum cows to local and systemic infections may be related to impairment of the respiratory burst of neutrophils that occurs with elevated plasma concentrations of BHB.

CLINICAL FINDINGS

Two major clinical forms of bovine ketosis are described—wasting and nervous—but these are the two extremes of a range of syndromes in which wasting and nervous signs are present in varying degrees of prominence.

The **wasting form** is the most common of the two and is manifest with a gradual but moderate decrease in appetite and milk yield over 2 to 4 days. In component-fed herds, the pattern of appetite loss is often very specific in that the cow first refuses to eat grain, then ensilage, but may continue to eat hay. The appetite may also be depraved.

Body weight is lost rapidly, usually at a greater rate than one would expect from the decrease in appetite. Farmers usually describe affected cows as having a "woody" appearance because of the apparent wasting and loss of cutaneous elasticity presumably resulting from disappearance of subcutaneous fat. The feces are firm and dry, but serious constipation does not occur. The cow is moderately depressed and is quieter than usual. The disinclination to move and to eat may suggest the presence of mild abdominal pain, but localized pain cannot be detected via abdominal palpation.

The temperature and the pulse and respiratory rates are normal, and although the ruminal movements may be decreased in amplitude and number, they are within the normal range unless the course is of long duration, in which case they may virtually disappear. The characteristic sweet odor of ketones is detectable on the breath and often in the milk, but people vary in their ability to detect ketones on the breath (specifically the volatile ketone, acetone).

Very few affected animals die, but without treatment the milk yield falls; although spontaneous recovery usually occurs over about a month, as equilibrium between the drain of lactation and food intake is established, the milk yield is never fully regained. The fall in milk yield in the wasting form may be as much as 25%, and there is an accompanying sharp drop in the solids-not-fat content of the milk. In the wasting form, nervous signs may occur in a few cases, but they rarely comprise more than transient bouts of staggering and partial blindness.

In the **nervous form (nervous ketosis),** signs are usually bizarre and begin quite suddenly. The syndrome is suggestive of delirium rather than of frenzy, and the characteristic signs include the following:

- Walking in circles
- Straddling or crossing of the legs
- Head pushing or leaning into the stanchion
- Apparent blindness
- Aimless movements and wandering
- Vigorous licking of the skin and inanimate objects (Fig. 17-6)
- Depraved appetite
- Chewing movements with salivation

Hyperesthesia may be evident, with the animal bellowing on being pinched or stroked. Moderate tremor and tetany may be present, and there is usually an incoordinate gait. The nervous signs usually occur in **short episodes** that last for 1 or 2 hours and may recur at intervals of about 8 to 12 hours. Affected cows may injure themselves during the nervous episodes. Surgical correction of displaced abomasum in cows exhibiting some signs consistent with nervous ketosis should be delayed until their energy status has been evaluated and treatment instituted, if indicated.

Subclinical Ketosis (Hyperketonemia)

Subclinical ketosis is defined as an increase in blood/plasma/serum BHB above the normal reference range or ketonuria in a cow without detectable clinical signs of disease. Many cows that are in negative energy balance in early pregnancy will have ketonuria without showing clinical signs, but they

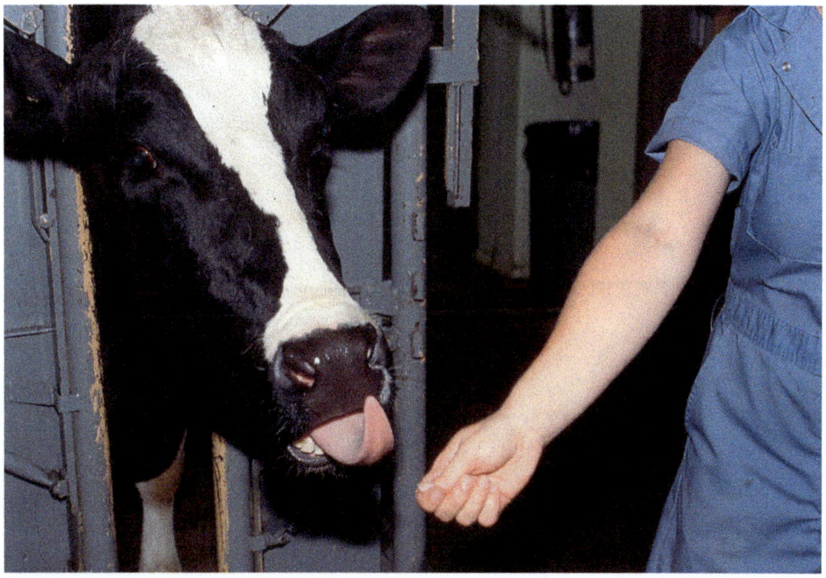

Fig. 17-6 Holstein–Friesian cow with nervous ketosis, manifest as excessive and sustained licking behavior.

will have diminished productivity, including depression of milk yield and a reduction in fertility. Clinical diagnosis is not effective, and in one study, diagnosis by routine urine testing at 5 to 12 days postpartum was considerably more efficient (15.6% detected) than diagnosis by the herdsman (4.4% detected). In a British study of 219 herds the annual mean rate of reported clinical ketosis was 0.5 per 100 adult cows, but the rate of subclinical ketosis, as defined by increased plasma concentrations of BHB and nonesterified fatty acids, was substantially higher. There is debate about whether subclinical ketosis is the correct term, with some support for replacing the term with *hyperketonemia*.

Potential milk production in cows with subclinical ketosis is reduced by 1% to 9%. Surveys of large populations show a declining prevalence of ketosis-positive cows after a peak in the period immediately after calving and a positive relationship between hyperketonemia and high milk yield. **Infertility** may appear as an ovarian abnormality, delayed onset of estrus, or endometritis resulting in an increase in the calving-to-conception interval and reduced conception rate at first insemination.[4]

CLINICAL PATHOLOGY

Hypoglycemia, ketonemia, and ketonuria are characteristic of the disease.

Glucose

Plasma glucose concentrations are reduced from the normal of approximately 50 to 65 mg/dL to 20 to 40 mg/dL. Ketosis secondary to other diseases is usually accompanied by plasma glucose concentrations above 50 mg/dL, and many cattle have much higher concentrations. Conversion factors are shown in Table 17-7.

Ketones

Most commonly, plasma or serum β-hydroxybutyrate (BHB) measured in SI units (mmol/L) is used for analysis of ketonemia. BHB is the quantitatively highest circulating ketone body in cattle. Plasma concentrations of BHB significantly correlate with plasma concentrations of acetoacetate, but acetoacetate is unstable in blood samples, whereas BHB is stable, particularly when samples are refrigerated or frozen. Normal cows have plasma BHB concentrations less than 1.0 mmol/L; cows with subclinical ketosis have blood or plasma/serum concentrations greater than 1.0, 1.2, or 1.4 mmol/L (the cut-point varies depending on the study, analytical method, and whether blood or plasma is analyzed).[9,10] Different cut-points have been proposed for serum BHB concentration in the first week postpartum (1.0 mmol/L) and the second week postpartum (1.4 mmol/L);[11] this may be attributable to blood BHB concentrations being highest at 8 days in milk.[12] In general, because the cut-point for the diagnosis of subclinical ketosis should be based on a detectable effect on decreasing milk production or an increased risk of adverse health events,[10] a consensus is developing around the use of serum/plasma BHB concentration greater than 1.0 mmol/L as the cut-point for subclinical ketosis based on the association with impaired reproductive performance[11] and increased risk of developing a displaced abomasum, puerperal metritis, or clinical ketosis.[13]

Cows with clinical ketosis usually have serum/plasma BHB concentrations in excess of 2.5 mmol/L, with values rarely reaching 10.0 mmol/L. Plasma BHB shows some diurnal variation in cows fed twice daily, with peak concentrations occurring approximately 4 hours after feeding and higher concentrations in the morning than in the afternoon. This diurnal variation is not as prominent in cows fed a total mixed ration ad libitum.

Measurement of blood or plasma/serum BHB concentration has recently become a cost-effective and convenient method for routine analysis and cow-side monitoring, with the introduction of low-cost point-of-care devices for measurement (US$2/test). The concentration of acetoacetate or BHB in urine and milk is also used for diagnostic purposes.[14] Concentrations of BHB and acetoacetate in urine and milk are less than those in plasma/serum, but the correlation coefficients for plasma/serum and milk BHB and plasma/serum and milk acetoacetate are 0.66 and 0.62, respectively. For cow-side use, urine acetoacetate concentration using the nitroprusside test and blood BHB concentration using a point-of-care device are currently the preferred tests for detecting subclinical or clinical ketosis in cattle.

Table 17-7 To convert from the SI unit to the conventional unit, divide by the conversion factor; to convert from the conventional unit to the SI unit, multiply by the conversion factor

Substrate	Conventional unit	Conversion factor	SI unit
β-hydroxybutyrate	mg/dL	0.0961	mmol/L
Acetoacetate	mg/dL	0.0980	mmol/L
Acetone	mg/dL	0.1722	mmol/L

Milk and Urine Cow-Side Tests

Cow-side tests have the advantage of being inexpensive and giving immediate results, and they can be used as frequently as necessary. A minor source of error is that the concentration of ketone bodies in these fluids will depend not only on the ketone concentration of the plasma, but also on the amount of urine excreted or on the milk yield. Milk concentration of ketones is less variable, easier to collect, and may give fewer false negatives in cows with subclinical ketosis.

Milk and urine ketone concentrations have been traditionally detected by the reaction of acetoacetate with **sodium nitroprusside** and can be interpreted in a semiquantitative manner based on the intensity of the reaction. The nitroprusside reaction detects both acetoacetate and acetone, but it is much more sensitive to acetoacetate than acetone; the latter is only detected when acetone concentrations are greater than 600 mmol/L, which represents a supraphysiologic concentration.[15] As a consequence, the nitroprusside test functions as a semiquantitative test of acetoacetate concentration and should be clinically regarded as a test of acetoacetate and not acetone. Several products are available commercially as strips or test powders and are commonly accompanied by a color chart that allows a classification of acetoacetate concentration in grades such as negative, trace (5 mg/dL; 0.5 mmol/L), small (15 mg/dL; 1.0 mmol/L), moderate (40 mg/dL; 2.0 mmol/L), or large (>80 mg/dL; 5 mmol/L), based on the intensity of the color of the reaction.[15] Milk powder tests are not sufficiently sensitive for detection of subclinical ketosis (report too many false negatives), and urine tests are not sufficiently specific (report too many false positives).

Milk Testing. The sensitivity and specificity of the nitroprusside powder test with milk in various studies is reported as 28% to 90% and 96% to 100%, respectively. Currently, a milk strip test detecting the concentration of BHB in milk is available and is graded on the concentration of BHB. In different studies, milk BHB has a reported sensitivity and specificity of 58% to 96% and 69% to 99%, respectively. These variations are in part a result of the use of different plasma BHB reference values (1.2 and 1.4 mmol/L) for designation of subclinical ketosis and different statistical methods for analysis. Somatic cell counts in milk greater than 1 million cells/mL will cause an elevation in reading of both the BHBA strip test and the nitroprusside tests.

Urine Testing. A nitroprusside tablet has a reported sensitivity and specificity of 100% and 59%, respectively, compared with serum BHB concentrations above 1.4 mmol/L; a nitroprusside strip test has a reported sensitivity and specificity of 78% and 96%, respectively, with a urine cut-point corresponding to "small" on the color chart or 49% and 99%, respectively, with a urine cut-point corresponding to "moderate" on the color chart. BHB test strips when used with urine have a reported sensitivity and specificity of 73% and 96%, respectively, at a urine cut-point of 0.1 mmol/L BHB and 27% and 99%, respectively, at a urine cut-point of 0.2 mmol/L BHB. Urinary ketone concentrations are more closely related to plasma ketone concentrations than are milk BHB and acetoacetate concentrations.[16,17] Moreover, urine acetoacetate concentration appears superior to milk BHB concentration in diagnosing ketosis.[17]

Milk-Fat-to-Protein Ratio. Milk-fat concentration tends to increase, and milk protein concentration tends to decrease, during postpartum negative energy balance. A **fat-to-protein ratio greater than 1.5** in first-day test milk is indicative of a lack of energy supply in the feed and of risk for ketosis and provides a similar test sensitivity (Se = 0.63) for detecting subclinical ketosis as does milk BHB concentration (Se = 0.58).[17] Milk production in multiparous animals is also separately associated with postpartum negative energy balance.[18]

Clinical Chemistry and Hematology. White and differential cell counts are variable and not of diagnostic value for ketosis. There are usually elevations of liver enzyme activity in plasma/serum, but liver function tests are within the normal range. Liver biopsy is the only accurate method to determine the degree of liver damage.

Plasma concentrations of NEFAs and total bilirubin are elevated in ketosis, with mean NEFA concentrations increasing above 0.3 mmol/L from 3 days before parturition to approximately 0.7 mmol/L from 0 to 9 days in milk, after which time plasma NEFA concentration gradually decreases.[12] The increase in bilirubin is attributed, in part, to hepatic dysfunction; however, bilirubin is not a sufficiently sensitive indicator to assess the extent of fat mobilization and liver function in cows with ketosis. Plasma cholesterol concentration is typically decreased for the stage of lactation; the decrease in cholesterol is a result of decreased hepatocyte secretion of very-low-density lipoproteins (VLDLs), which are cholesterol rich, or increased mammary uptake of cholesterol relative to cholesterol availability. After secretion, VLDLs are processed in plasma to intermediate-density lipoproteins by hydrolysis of triglycerides.[19] Intermediate-density lipoproteins are then metabolized in plasma to cholesterol-rich low-density lipoproteins that carry cholesterol to peripheral tissues, including the mammary gland.[19,20] A clinically significant proportion of lactating dairy cattle with ketosis have low plasma cortisol concentrations;[21] although the mechanism has not been determined, it is possible that decreased cholesterol availability negatively affects cortisol synthesis.

Liver glycogen levels are low, and the glucose tolerance curve may be normal. Volatile fatty acid levels in the rumen are much higher in ketotic than in normal cows, and the ruminal concentrations of butyrate are markedly increased relative to acetate and propionate acids. There is a small but significant drop in serum calcium concentrations (down to about 9 mg/dL [2.25 mmol/L]), probably as a result of decreased dry matter intake in lactating dairy cattle relative to the level of milk production.

Plasma and urine metabolic profiling shows promise as a means of differentiating cattle with clinical ketosis and subclinical ketosis from healthy cattle at the same stage of lactation. Twenty-five plasma metabolites[22,23] and 11 urine proteins[24] have been identified to differ between these three groups. Differences include changes in plasma amino acid concentrations that may reflect differences in feed intake relative to milk production or altered metabolic pathways and changes in urine polypeptide concentrations that may reflect decreased immune responsiveness.

NECROPSY FINDINGS

The disease is not usually fatal in cattle, but fatty degeneration of the liver and secondary changes in the anterior pituitary gland and adrenal cortex may be present.

DIFFERENTIAL DIAGNOSIS

Cattle

The clinical picture is usually too indefinite, especially in cattle, to enable a diagnosis to be made solely on clinical grounds. General consideration of the history, with particular reference to the time of calving, and the feeding program, and biochemical examination to detect the presence of hypoglycemia, ketonemia, and ketonuria are necessary to establish a diagnosis.

Wasting form:

- Abomasal displacement
- Traumatic reticulitis
- Primary indigestion
- Cystitis and pyelonephritis

Nervous form:

- Rabies
- Hypomagnesemia
- Bovine spongiform encephalopathy

TREATMENT

In cattle, a number of effective treatments are available for ketosis, but in some affected animals, the response is only transient; in rare cases, the disease may persist and cause death or necessitate slaughter of the animals. Most of these cases are secondary, and failure to respond satisfactorily to treatment is a result of the primary disease. Specific treatment for subclinical ketosis is usually not applied on an individual basis, but nutrition and management issues should be investigated whenever a large proportion of early-lactation cows are diagnosed with subclinical ketosis.

The rational treatment in ketosis is to relieve the need for glucose formation from tissues and allow ketone-body utilization to continue normally. Theoretically, the simplest means of doing this is by the administration of glucose replacement therapy. The effect of the administration of glucose is complex, but it allows the reversal of ketogenesis and the establishment of normal patterns of energy metabolism. Ideally, treatment should be at an early stage of the disease to minimize loss, and with subclinical ketosis this requires biochemical testing.

Replacement Therapy

Glucose (Dextrose)

The IV injection of 500 mL of a 50% solution of glucose results in transient hyperglycemia, increased insulin and decreased glucagon secretion, and reduced plasma concentration of NEFAs. Glucose administration effects a marked improvement in most cows, but relapses occur commonly unless repeated treatments are used. This is probably a result of the transience of the hyperglycemia (3 to 4 hours) or insufficient dosing—the dose required varies directly with the amount of lactose being lost in the milk. Contrary to widespread belief, **very little of the administered glucose is lost to urinary excretion** (<10%).[25,26] SC injections of hypertonic glucose prolong the response, but they are not recommended because they cause discomfort, and large unsightly swellings, which often become infected, may result. Intraperitoneal injections of 20% solution of dextrose have also been used, but they are not recommended because of the risk of infection.

Other Sugars

Other sugars, especially fructose, either alone or as a mixture of glucose and fructose (invert sugar), and xylitol, have been used in an effort to prolong the response, but idiosyncratic responses to some preparations, in the form of polypnea, muscle tremor, weakness, and collapse, can occur while the injection is being given.

Propylene Glycol and Glycerine/Glycerol

To overcome the necessity for repeated injections, propylene glycol can be administered as a drench. The traditional dose is 225 ml twice daily for 2 days, followed by 110 ml daily for 2 days to cattle, but higher volumes are also used for larger cattle (a typical treatment protocol in North America is 300 ml PO daily for 5 days). Some of the administered propylene glycol is metabolized to propionate in the rumen and absorbed, whereas some of the propylene glycol is absorbed directly across ruminal epithelium and metabolized by the liver. Propylene glycol (200 to 700 g daily), or **salts of propionate,** can be administered in the feed and give good results. Administration in feed is preferred by some because this method avoids dangers of aspiration with drenching; however, cows not used to its inclusion in the feed may show feed refusal. Studies also suggest that drenching of propylene glycol provides a more beneficial response than including the same amount in a total mixed ration; the bolus effect of propionate production appears to be more beneficial than a steady-state increase as a result of a bolus increase in plasma insulin concentration. It is recommended that for best results, dosing with propylene glycol should be preceded by an IV injection of glucose.

Parenteral infusions of glucose solutions and the feeding of glycerol depress the fat content of milk, and the net saving in energy may favorably influence response to these drugs. Glycerol and propylene glycol are not as efficient as glucose because conversion to glucose utilizes oxaloacetate. Propylene glycol is absorbed directly from the rumen and acts to reduce ketogenesis by increasing mitochondrial citrate concentrations; its metabolism to glucose occurs via conversion to pyruvate, with subsequent production of oxaloacetate via pyruvate carboxylase.

Other Glucose Precursors

Because of its glucogenic effect, sodium propionate is theoretically a suitable treatment, but when administered in 110- to 225-g doses daily, the response in cattle is often very slow. Lactates are also highly glucogenic, but both calcium and sodium lactate (1 kg initially, followed by 0.5 kg for 7 days) and sodium acetate (110 to 500 g/d) have given less satisfactory results than those obtained with sodium propionate. Ammonium lactate (200 g for 5 days) has, however, been used extensively, with reported good results. Lactose, in whey or in granular form in the diet, can increase dry matter intake, but it also increases ruminal butyrate concentration and plasma BHB concentrations.

Hormonal Therapy

Glucocorticoids. The efficiency of glucocorticoids in the treatment of bovine ketosis has been demonstrated in both experimental and field cases. The observation that a clinically significant proportion of lactating dairy cattle with ketosis have low plasma cortisol concentrations[21] provides support for glucocorticoid administration. Hyperglycemia occurs within 24 hours of glucocorticoid administration and appears to result from a repartitioning of glucose in the body rather than from gluconeogenesis.

Historically, many glucocorticoid preparations have been used successfully, but current drugs are more potent, require lower dosage, and have fewer side effects. A hyperglycemic state is produced for 4 to 6 days in ketotic cows given 10 mg of dexamethasone 21-isonicotinate, and other preparations that have a shorter duration of action, such as dexamethasone sodium phosphate (40 mg) and flumethasone (5 mg), are also used. Dexamethasone 21-isonicotinate (20 to 25 mg IM) decreases whole-body insulin sensitivity and affects glucose and lipid metabolism; it decreases liver fat content in early-lactating dairy cows with surgically corrected left-displaced abomasum.[27] Label regulations vary between countries; in general, the recommendations of the manufacturer with regard to glucorticoid use and dosage should be followed. Profound hypokalemia with high case fatality is a potential sequel to prolonged repeated therapy of ketosis with isoflupredone acetate, which has both glucocorticoid and mineralocorticoid activity. For this reason, only one treatment of isoflupredone acetate is recommended for cows with ketosis. Response of cows with primary ketosis to treatment with **corticosteroids and IV glucose is superior** to therapy with corticosteroids or IV glucose alone, with fewer relapses.

Insulin facilitates cellular uptake of glucose, suppresses fatty acid metabolism, and stimulates hepatic gluconeogenesis. Insulin is administered in conjunction with either glucose or a glucocorticoid and may be of particular value in early-onset cases of ketosis that are unresponsive to glucose or corticosteroid therapy, but it is not commonly used. The dose of protamine zinc insulin is 200 to 300 IU per animal (depending on body weight) administered SC every 24 to 48 hours as required. It should be recognized that endogenous insulin is released in all lactating dairy cattle administered 500 mL of 50% dextrose, although to a lower extent in ketotic cattle because they have a lower peak plasma glucose concentration following IV infusion of glucose or propionate;[28] consequently, IV dextrose administration should always be considered as a dual treatment of glucose and insulin.

Anabolic steroids have also been used for treatment of lactational ketosis and ketosis in late pregnant cows that are overfat, stressed, or have twin fetuses. Experimentally, 60 mg and 120 mg of trenbolone acetate are effective as single injections, but no extensive field trials are recorded, and the drug is banned for use in food animals in most countries.

Miscellaneous Treatments. Vitamin B_{12} and cobalt are indicated in regions where cobalt deficiency is a risk factor for ketosis. Cobalt is sometimes administered to cattle with ketosis in regions where cobalt deficiency does not occur, but the therapeutic value is not proven. Cyanocobalamin (vitamin B_{12}, 1 to 4 mg daily IV) in a combined formulation with butaphosphan has strong evidence supporting its role in normalizing energy status in early-lactation dairy cows when administered to dairy cattle before or around parturition.[29,30] Cyanocobalamin is essential for gluconeogenesis from propionate, and a theoretical argument can be made for the administration of cyanocobalamin for ketotic dairy cattle being treated for ketosis. It is also thought that high-producing dairy cows in early lactation have a relative or actual deficiency of cyanocobalamin.[30] Cysteamine (a biological precursor of coenzyme A) and also sodium fumarate have been used to treat cases of the disease. Reported results were initially good, but the treatment has not been generally adopted. The recommended dose rate of cysteamine is 750 mg IV for three doses at 1- to 3-day intervals.

Glucagon, although ketogenic, is strongly gluconeogenic and glycogenolytic, and glucagon concentrations are decreased in the plasma of fat cows at calving and cows with ketonemia. Glucagon could be of value in prevention and therapy, but it would require a prolonged delivery system because it has a very short physiologic half-life and its effects following a single injection are short-lived.

TREATMENT AND CONTROL

Treatment

- Propylene glycol (300 to 500 mL daily for 5 days, PO) (R-1)
- Dextrose (500 mL of 50% dextrose once, IV) (R-1)
- Dexamethasone, dexamethasone-21-isonicotinate or flumethasone, IM (R-1)
- Cyanocobalamin (vitamin B_{12}, 1 to 4 mg IV, daily for 2 to 6 treatments) (R-2)
- Isoflupredone (20 mg, IM, multiple injections) (R-3)
- Insulin (lente formulation, 200 IU SC daily for 3 days) (R-3)

Control

- Monensin (11 to 22 g/ton of total mixed ration on a 100% dry matter basis; oral administration of a controlled-release capsule delivers 335 mg/day for 95 days) (R-1)
- Propylene glycol (300 to 500 mL daily, PO) (R-1)
- Rumen-protected choline (15g daily, PO, from 25 days precalving to 80 days postcalving) (R-2)
- Cyanocobalamin (vitamin B_{12}, 1 to 4 mg IV, daily for 2 to 6 treatments before or at calving) (R-2)
- Isoflupredone (20 mg, IM, once), with or without insulin (100 U, SC) (R-3)

CONTROL

The control of clinical ketosis is integrally related to the adequate nutrition of the cow in the dry and lactating periods. This encompasses details such as the following:

- Dry matter intake
- Fiber digestibility
- Particle size distribution
- Energy density
- Fat incorporation in early lactation rations
- Protein content
- Feeding systems
- Rumen size
- Other factors better covered in texts on nutrition

It is difficult to make general recommendations for the control of the ketosis because of the many conditions under which it occurs, its probable multiple etiology, and feeding systems that vary from those that feed components separately to those that feed total mixed rations. Cows neither should have been starved nor be overfat at calving. Careful estimation of diets by reference to feed value tables is recommended, and detailed recommendations on diet and management are available, with the caveat that planned rations can deviate from feed bunk rations, and feed bunk dry matter and actual dry matter intake may not be the same. Too low a feeding frequency and the feeding of concentrates separate from roughage rather than as a total mixed ration can lead to an increase in rates of ketosis.

In the United States, dry cows are typically divided into two groups: far-off and close-up cows. Far off cows are generally fed to National Research Council (NRC) dry-cow feeding guidelines, and close-up cows are given an acidogenic ration that decreases the incidence of clinical milk fever (periparturient hypocalcemia) starting 3 weeks before the estimated calving date. Practical recommendations based on British feeding standards and units are also available.

In high-producing cows being fed stored feeds, poor-quality roughage commonly leads to ketosis. Wet ensilage containing much butyrate, and moldy or old and dusty hay, are the main offenders. In concentrates, it is the change of source that creates off-feed effects and precipitates attacks of ketosis.

Cows that are housed should get some exercise each day, and in herds where the disease is a particular problem during the stabling period, the cattle should be turned out to pasture as soon as possible in the spring.

The ration should contain adequate amounts of cobalt, phosphorus, and iodine.

If there is a high incidence of ketosis in a herd receiving large quantities of ensilage, reduction of the amount fed for a trial period is indicated.

Energy Supplements

Propylene glycol is used for the prevention of clinical and subclinical ketosis. Traditionally, propylene glycol has been drenched to cattle in early lactation at doses varying from 350 to 1000 mL daily for 10 days after calving. There is a linear effect of dose on plasma glucose. Propylene glycol can also be added to feed and is frequently present in commercial feed products, but a bolus dose of propylene glycol is more effective in raising blood glucose than incorporation in feed. A dose of 1 L per day given as an oral drench for 9 days before parturition has also been shown efficacious; however, it is important to note that at doses above 500 mL administered by drench or present in feed, some cows may develop rapid and shallow respiration, ataxia, salivation, and somnolence. For this reason, a maximum daily dose of 500 mL as a drench should considered.

Glycerol can be substituted for propylene glycol at equivalent dose rates, although most studies indicate that glycerol is inferior to propylene glycol. A preliminary report of a small experimental study with larger doses of glycerol showed that glycerol given orally at a dose of 1 L, 2 L, or 3 L elevated blood glucose concentrations to 16%, 20%, and 25%, respectively, of pretreatment values at 0.5 hours after treatment and that these concentrations remained elevated for 8 hours. Staggering, depression, and diuresis were observed in some cows given the 2-L or 3-L dose, but this could be prevented by administering the glycerol in a large (37-L) volume of water. It concluded that a dose of 1 L was effective in increasing milk production and reducing urinary ketones. Glycerol fed as a constant component in the transition dairy cow diet is not effective and possibly may be ketogenic when fed continually. Glycerol should only be used as drench in hypoglycemic cows and not fed as a component of the diet.

Propionic Acid and Its Salts

Propionic acid absorbed across the rumen wall is transported to the liver, where it is converted to glucose via gluconeogenesis to result in an increase in serum blood glucose levels. Older literature reports that 110 g/d fed daily for 6 weeks, commencing at calving, has given good results in reducing the incidence of clinical bovine ketosis and improving production, but is not palatable and has the risk of reducing feed intake. In controlled trials, feeding energy supplements containing propionic acid and/or its salts for 3 weeks prepartum and 3 weeks postpartum had a beneficial effect on milk production, but a variable effect on reducing subclinical ketosis.

Ionophores

Ionophores alter bacterial flora of the rumen, leading to decreases in gram-positive bacteria, protozoa, and fungi and increases in gram-negative bacteria. The net effect of these changes in bacterial flora is increased propionate production and a decrease in acetate and butyrate production providing increased gluconeogenic precursors. Field trials with monensin have consistently demonstrated a reduction in serum or blood BHB, acetoacetate, and HEFA concentrations. In addition, monensin increased serum or blood glucose, urea, and cholesterol concentrations, and decreased the prevalence of clinical ketosis, clinical mastitis, and displaced abomasum in dairy cattle.[31-33] Monensin also decreases methane production by cattle; methane production by ruminants has been considered as contributing to global warming. Although approved for administration to lactating dairy cows in more than 20 countries, ionophores are not labeled for inclusion in lactating-cow rations in a number of countries.

Monensin is approved for continuous administration (>14 days) to dairy cattle in the United States at 185 to 660 (mg/head)/day monensin to lactating cows or 115 to 410 (mg/head)/day monensin to dry cows. To accomplish this, monensin is approved to be fed at 11 to 22 g/ton of total mixed ration on a 100% dry matter basis, at a daily per-cow cost of about 2 to 4 cents. Monensin is also approved for use in the United States as part of a component feeding system at 11 to 400 g/ton (as is basis); this includes application as a "top dress," where a small amount of feed is added to a ration.

In some countries, monensin can be administered orally as a controlled-release capsule to cattle 2 to 4 weeks before calving. The capsule contains 32 g of monensin and releases approximately 335 mg monensin a day for 95 days. This product is effective and practical for a variety of feeding systems, and approximately 18% of dairy herds in Canada are administering monensin by controlled-release capsule.

Corticosteroids

Isoflupredone acetate (20 mg, IM, once) was not effective in preventing subclinical ketosis in early-lactation dairy cows, and it actually increased the likelihood of subclinical ketosis.[34]

Ancillary Agents

A commercially available injectable product containing **cyanocobalamin** (vitamin B_{12}, 1 to 4 mg daily IV) in a combined formulation with **butaphosphan** is effective in normalizing energy status when administered to dairy cattle 2 to 6 times before or around parturition.[29,30] The administration of cyanocobalamin and butaphosphan may be most beneficial in cows at increased risk of developing ketosis, such as older cows, overconditioned cows, or those experiencing dystocia or metritis.[29] Phosphorus may be limiting in early lactation, based on low liver phosphorus content in dairy cattle.[35] It is not clear whether additional phosphorus mitigates the reduction in hepatic phosphorus content.

Rumen protected choline (15 g/day) fed daily starting 25 days before calving and continuing to 80 days after calving decreased the incidence of clinical ketosis and improved the health of lactating dairy cows.[36] Choline is a precursor for phosphatidylcholine, which is thought to be rate limiting in early lactation; phosphatidylcholine deficiency is associated with impaired lipid metabolism.

Niacin is antilipolytic and induces increases in blood glucose and insulin, but there is conflicting evidence that **niacin** given in the feed has a beneficial effect on subclinical ketosis in cattle. It has been suggested that niacin should be supplemented from 2 weeks before parturition to 12 weeks postpartum.

General Control

Herd Monitoring. There is currently no consensus as to the optimal monitoring program for ketosis and subclinical ketosis in lactating dairy cattle, and consequently a variety of monitoring programs have been proposed. Challenges with developing optimal monitoring programs are the herd size (through the influence on the eligible numbers of animals available to be tested), ease of testing, cost of the test, and test sensitivity and specificity. In addition, the goals of the monitoring program need to be defined; typically they are either to monitor the adequacy of the diet relative to the level of milk production (i.e., the magnitude of negative energy balance in early lactation) or to identify animals to receive a standard treatment protocol, such as daily oral propylene glycol drenching. The optimal time for testing appears to be cows 3 to 9 days in milk because cows that are hyperketonemic at this stage of lactation are at highest risk for subsequent negative production and health effects, with the incidence and prevalence of subclinical ketosis occurring on day 5 of lactation.[37] A recent modeling approach utilizing 13,000 cows from 833 dairy farms in North America and Europe suggested that testing cows twice weekly from 3 to 9 days in milk was the most cost effective strategy when the subclinical ketosis incidence was between 15% and 50%; below an incidence of 15% it was not economical to test, and above 50% all cows should be treated without testing.[38] In addition, whenever the subclinical ketosis incidence increased to above 15%, a variety of testing and treatment protocols are economically beneficial.[38]

The six most valuable and practical indices for monitoring negative energy balance are urine acetoacetate concentration, blood BHB concentration, blood glucose concentration, body-condition score, back-fat thickness determined ultrasonographically, and milk-fat-to-protein ratio. The first five indices can be obtained cow side and at no cost or relatively low cost, although determining the blood BHB concentration costs approximately 5 to 10 times that of the first two tests and requires a blood sample. The milk-fat-to-protein ratio is readily obtained from individual monthly test data and is more highly correlated with energy balance than plasma BHB or glucose concentration.[39] This should be coupled with body-condition scoring or back-fat thickness to monitor the efficacy of the nutritional program. Plasma NEFA concentration is an excellent monitoring test of negative energy balance, but it is currently too expensive for routine herd monitoring, and an easy-to-use cow-side test is not available.

Urine testing using the nitroprusside test for acetoacetate is the simplest of the cow-side tests, and despite some reports that urine samples are difficult to obtain from all cattle, urine is easily obtained from more than 90% of cattle using the following standardized technique. First, stimulation of the perineum to obtain a urine sample must be the first part of the examination of the cow and ideally should be performed without the cow being aware that the veterinarian is present. Second, never hold the tail while stimulating the perineum because tail holding alerts the cow to the presence of the veterinarian, and it is not needed because cattle never urinate on their tails when posturing to urinate. Third, obtain urine samples in the normal environment of the animal; because cattle urinate on average five times per day, urine samples are easily obtained on recumbent cattle that are gently encouraged to stand.

Blood BHB testing has become very popular because of the availability of low-cost point-of-care meters. Despite this, it must be recognized that obtaining a blood sample is more complicated than obtaining a urine sample, and that the cost, although low, is much higher than that for urine acetoacetate or blood glucose testing. Moreover, serum BHB concentration is correlated with energy balance in a similar manner to plasma glucose concentration.[40] Automated monitoring by in-line measurements of ketone bodies in milk has been studied and may be of particular value in large dairies. BHB is proposed as the candidate because it is the more robust in milk, and where cows are fed a total mixed ration, it is not subject to significant diurnal variation. Milk BHB concentration can be measured in real-time with a fluorometric method that requires no pretreatment of the milk.

Biochemical monitoring of herds for subclinical ketosis and adequacy of periparturient feeding can be conducted using blood glucose estimations on a sample of cows in their second week of lactation. Plasma glucose concentrations below 45 mg/dL (2.4 mmol/L) suggest subclinical ketosis. For individual cows, blood glucose estimations should be done at about 14 days after calving. This method of monitoring is inexpensive using widely available point-of-care devices.

FURTHER READING

Gordon JL, LeBlanc SJ, Duffield TF. Ketosis treatment in lactating dairy cattle. *Vet Clin North Am Food Anim Pract*. 2013;29:433-445.

Ingvartsen KL. Feeding- and management-related diseases in the transition cow. Physiological adaptations around calving and strategies to reduce feeding-related diseases. *Anim Feed Sci Technol.* 2006;126:175-213.

McArt JAA, Nydam DV, Oetzel GR, Overton TR, Ospina PA. Elevated non-esterified fatty acids and β-hydroxybutyrate and their association with transition dairy cow performance. *Vet J.* 2013;198:560-570.

Opsina PA, McArt JA, Overton TR, Stokol T, Nydam DV. Using nonesterified fatty acids and β-hydroxybutyrate concentrations during the transition period for herd-level monitoring of increased risk of disease and decreased reproductive and milking performance. *Vet Clin North Am Food Anim Pract.* 2013;29:387-412.

Zhang Z, Liu G, Wang H, Li X, Wang Z. Detection of subclinical ketosis in dairy cows. *Pakistan Vet J.* 2012;32:156-160.

REFERENCES

1. Sato H. *Anim Sci J.* 2009;80:381.
2. Loor JJ, et al. *Physiol Genomics.* 2007;32:105.
3. Vanholder T, et al. *J Dairy Sci.* 2015;98:880.
4. Shin EK, et al. *Theriogenology.* 2015;84:252.
5. McArt JAA, et al. *J Dairy Sci.* 2015;98:2043.
6. Goldhawk C, et al. *J Dairy Sci.* 2009;92:4971.
7. Croushore WS, et al. *J Am Vet Med Assoc.* 2013;243:1329.
8. Reynen JL, et al. *J Dairy Sci.* 2015;98:3806.
9. Kessel S, et al. *J Anim Sci.* 2008;86:2903.
10. Borchardt S, et al. *J Am Vet Med Assoc.* 2012;240:1003.
11. Walsh RB, et al. *J Dairy Sci.* 2007;90:2788.
12. McCarthy MM, et al. *J Dairy Sci.* 2015;98:6284.
13. Opsina PA, et al. *J Dairy Sci.* 2010;93:546.
14. Denis-Robichaud J, et al. *Bovine Pract.* 2011;45:97.
15. Smith SW, et al. *Acad Emerg Med.* 2008;15:751.
16. Larsen M, Kristensen NB. *Acta Agric Scand Sect A.* 2010;60:239.
17. Krogh MA, et al. *J Dairy Sci.* 2011;94:2360.
18. Kayano M, Kataoka T. *J Vet Med Sci.* 2015;in press.
19. Kessler EC, et al. *J Dairy Sci.* 2014;97:5481.
20. Gross JJ, et al. *PLoS ONE.* 2015;10(6):doi:10.1371.
21. Forslund KB, et al. *Acta Vet Scand.* 2010;52:31.
22. Sun LW, et al. *J Dairy Sci.* 2014;97:1552.
23. Li Y, et al. *Vet Quart.* 2014;54:152.
24. Xu C, et al. *Vet Quart.* 2015;35:133.
25. Grunberg W, et al. *J Vet Intern Med.* 2006;20:1471.
26. Grunberg W, et al. *J Dairy Sci.* 2011;94:727.
27. Kusenda M, et al. *J Vet Intern Med.* 2013;27:200.
28. Djokovic R, et al. *Acta Vet Brno.* 2007;76:533.
29. Rollin E, et al. *J Dairy Sci.* 2010;93:978.
30. Furll M, et al. *J Dairy Sci.* 2010;93:4155.
31. Duffield TF, et al. *J Dairy Sci.* 2008;91:1334.
32. Duffield TF, et al. *J Dairy Sci.* 2008;91:1347.
33. Duffield TF, et al. *J Dairy Sci.* 2008;91:2328.
34. Seifi H, et al. *J Dairy Sci.* 2007;90:4181.
35. Grunberg W, et al. *J Dairy Sci.* 2009;92:2106.
36. Lima FS, et al. *Vet J.* 2012;193:140.
37. McArt JAA, et al. *J Dairy Sci.* 2012;95:5056.
38. McArt JAA, et al. *Prev Vet Med.* 2014;117:170.
39. Reist M, et al. *J Dairy Sci.* 2002;85:3314.

FATTY LIVER IN CATTLE (FAT-MOBILIZATION SYNDROME, FAT-COW SYNDROME, HEPATIC LIPIDOSIS, PREGNANCY TOXEMIA IN CATTLE)

Fatty liver (hepatic lipidosis) is an important metabolic disease of dairy cows in early lactation and is associated with decreased health status and reproductive performance.

SYNOPSIS

Etiology Mobilization of excessive body fat to liver during periods of negative energy balance at time of parturition or in early lactation of dairy cows and late pregnancy of beef cows.

Epidemiology High-producing dairy cows overfed during dry period may develop fatty liver syndrome just before or after calving precipitated by any factor or disease that interferes with feed intake. Occurs in well-conditioned beef cattle in late pregnancy when energy intake is suddenly decreased. Moderate and subclinical degrees of fatty infiltration may adversely affect reproductive performance of dairy cows.

Signs Inappetence to anorexia, ruminal atony, lethargic, inactivity, ketonuria, fat body condition, weakness and recumbency if worsens. Recover if continue to eat and appetite improves.

Clinical pathology Increase in plasma/serum nonesterified fatty acid, acetoacetate, β-hydroxybutyrate, and total bilirubin concentrations; increase in plasma/serum hepatic enzyme activity (particularly aspartate aminotransferase and ornithine carbamoyl transferase activity); increased fat content in liver biopsy.

Necropsy findings Fatty infiltration of liver, liver may appear yellow.

Diagnostic confirmation Liver biopsy.

Differential diagnosis list

- Left-sided or right-sided displacement of abomasum
- Milk fever
- Abomasal impaction
- Vagus indigestion
- Peritonitis

Treatment Fluid and electrolyte therapy including glucose IV (bolus infusion). Propylene glycol orally. Dexamethasone IM. Provision of palatable feed.

Control Avoid overfeeding during late lactation and dry period. Avoid situations that reduce feed intake at time of parturition.

ETIOLOGY

Fatty liver is caused by the mobilization of excessive quantities of fat from body deposits to the liver. It develops when the hepatic uptake of lipids exceeds the oxidation and secretion of lipids by the liver. Excess lipids are stored as triacylglycerol in the liver, and excessive lipid in hepatocytes is associated with decreased metabolic function of the liver. Fatty liver occurs because of a sudden demand of energy in the immediate postpartum period in well-conditioned lactating dairy cows. Fatty liver also occurs because of a sudden deprivation of feed in fat pregnant beef cattle, and is especially severe in those bearing twins. The disease is an exaggeration of what is a common occurrence in high-producing dairy cows that are in a state of negative energy balance in early lactation. A substantial drop in voluntary dry matter intake is initiated in late pregnancy and continues into early lactation. This decrease has traditionally been interpreted as caused by physical constraints in the abdomen as a result of the enlarging gravid uterus, but this purported mechanism appears to have been overemphasized. The decline in dry matter intake coincides with changes in reproduction status, changes in fat mass, and metabolic changes in support of lactation, and the associated metabolic signals are likely to play an important role in intake regulation. These signals include nutrients, metabolites, reproductive hormones, stress hormones, leptin, insulin, gut peptides, cytokines, and neuropeptides. Body fat, especially subcutaneous fat, is mobilized and deposited primarily in liver but also in muscle and the kidneys. Whether or not the cow is truly fat at parturition may not be important in determining the degree of fat mobilization, but the degree of negative energy balance in early lactation is critical.

EPIDEMIOLOGY

Occurrence and Incidence

Fatty infiltration of the liver is common in high-producing dairy cattle from a few weeks before and after parturition[1] and is associated with several periparturient diseases and an increase in the calving-to-conception interval. In dairy cows, fatty liver occurs primarily in the first 4 weeks after calving when up to 50% of all cows have some accumulation of triacylglycerol in the liver. A severe form of fatty infiltration of the liver immediately before or after parturition is known as the **fat-mobilization syndrome, fat-cow syndrome,** or **pregnancy toxemia** of cattle, and it can be highly fatal. In beef cattle, the disease occurs most commonly in late pregnancy when the nutrient intake is decreased in cattle that were previously well fed and in good body condition. In a field study, the percentage of cattle dying or being culled because of disease was affected by the amount of hepatic triglyceride: 15%, 31%, and 42% for cattle with mild, moderate, and severe hepatic lipidosis, respectively. **Outbreaks of the disease have occurred in dairy herds** in which up to 25% of all cows were affected, with a case-fatality rate of 90%.

Cattle have been classified into three groups on the basis of liver fat content determined histologically 1 week after parturition. Less than 20% lipid corresponds to less than 50 mg/g liver by weight; 20% to 40% lipid, 50 to 100 mg/g liver; and greater than 40% represents more than 100 mg/g liver. These concentrations correspond to mild, moderate, and severe cases of fatty infiltration, respectively. Cows with less than 20% lipid in the liver at 1 week after calving are considered normal, and those with more than 20% are considered to have a fatty liver. About 30% of high-yielding dairy cows in the United Kingdom are considered to have a fatty liver 1 week after calving. Clinical evidence of hepatic disease may not occur consistently until liver lipid concentrations are in the range of 35% to 45% or more.

Risk Factors

Host Factors

Fatty infiltration of the liver is part of a generalized fat-mobilization syndrome that occurs in early lactation, particularly in high-yielding dairy cows, as milk production outstrips appetite and body reserves are used to meet the energy deficit. In about 30% of high-producing cows, fatty infiltration in the liver is severe and is associated with reversible but significant effects on liver structure and function. In some populations of cows, the incidence of fatty liver is much lower and insignificant.

Diseases that occur commonly in early lactation predispose to fatty liver include **ketosis, left-side displacement of the abomasum, mastitis, retained fetal membranes, milk fever**, and **downer-cow syndrome.** Any disease of early lactation that affects appetite and voluntary intake can contribute to fatty liver.

The deficit occurs because dietary intake cannot meet the energy requirements for the high yield. Peak yields of milk are reached 4 to 7 weeks after calving, but the highest levels of voluntary feed intake are not reached until 8 to 10 weeks after calving. As a result of the energy deficit, the cow mobilizes body reserves for milk production and may lose a large amount of body weight.

The BCS at calving can have a direct effect on the health, milk yield, and fertility of cows. It represents the cumulative effects of the dry period, the BCS at drying off, and the loss of body condition during the dry period. The risk of retained placenta may be greater for cows underconditioned at drying, whereas cows that lost more body condition during the dry period may be more affected by both retained placenta and metritis; the two effects are independent of each other. The risk of ketosis is increased in cows overconditioned at calving, which may be a result of a long dry period. Cows calving at a higher BCS produced more milk, fat, and protein in the first 90 days of lactation, and the effect was most pronounced for milk-fat content. Cows with a higher BCS at calving were less prone to anestrus, but they did not conceive more successfully to first service. A reduction of 6 open days in primiparous cows was estimated for each additional unit of BCS at calving. Multiparous cows that lose more body condition during the dry period are more prone to inactive ovaries and are more likely to be open 150 days after calving in the next lactation.

Dairy cows with abnormally long dry periods also have a tendency to become obese and develop the fatty liver syndrome of parturition. The feeding of dairy cows in large groups, as in loose housing systems, has been associated with an increase in the incidence of the disease. The disease has occurred in pregnant heifers within 31 days after being turned out onto grass.

The disease can occur in **nonlactating dairy cows** by the imposition of a partial-starvation diet in late pregnancy in an attempt to reduce the body weight of cows that are considered to be too fat. Changing the diet of pregnant beef cows from silage to straw in an attempt to reduce their body weight and the incidence of dystocia has resulted in outbreaks of the disease.

In beef cattle in North America, the severe form of the disease, pregnancy toxemia, is seen most commonly in the last 6 weeks of pregnancy in cows that are fat and pregnant with twins. The affected cows are usually well fed until late pregnancy, when an unexpected shortage of feed occurs, or the cows are too fat and cannot consume sufficient low-energy feed to meet the demands of pregnancy. Under usual circumstances, the disease in beef cattle occurs sporadically: the morbidity is about 1%, but the mortality is usually 100%.

Pregnancy toxemia of cattle has occurred in pregnant beef cattle in Australia and the United Kingdom. First-calf heifers were more commonly affected than older cows, and most were in late pregnancy (7 to 9 months) or had just recently calved. Cows pregnant with twins are particularly susceptible.

Genetics of Lipid Mobilization

Cows generally mobilize body lipid reserves in early lactation and regain these reserves during subsequent pregnancy. Lipid mobilized from body reserves makes a substantial contribution to the energetic cost of milk production in early lactation. It is usually assumed that this mobilization of body energy reserves is entirely a response to a deficit in feed energy intake relative to milk energy output. This implies that increasing the energy content of the feed being offered would decrease body energy mobilization in early lactation. A number of studies indicate that this is not always the case. It has been proposed that mobilization of body reserves in early lactation and the subsequent gain in body reserves during pregnancy are to a large extent genetically driven. Genetically driven body-lipid change is defined as that which would occur in cows kept in an environment that was in no way constraining. It then follows that environmentally driven body-lipid change is defined as that which occurs in response to an environment that is constraining. The rationale and evidence for genetically driven body-lipid change have their basis in evolutionary considerations and in the changes in lipid metabolism throughout the reproductive cycle.

Environmental and Dietary Factors

In North America, the introduction of the system of **challenge feeding** of dairy cows was associated with an increased incidence of fatty liver. The overall effect of the system is to provide excess energy in the diet during late pregnancy or during the dry period generally. The diets fed may contain a high percentage of the cereal grains, corn ensilage, or brewer's grains. In this system, high-energy rations are fed beginning a few weeks before parturition. The total daily amount of feed is increased by regular increments to reach a high level at parturition and peak levels to coincide with the peak in the lactation curve several weeks after parturition. This resulted in some excessively fat cows at the time of parturition, when energy demands are high. The disease has also occurred in dairy cows that were fed excessive amounts of high-energy rations throughout the dry period. In dairy herds, fatty liver syndrome has also been associated with an increase in the incidence of milk fever, ketosis, and left-sided displacement of the abomasum, all of which are much more difficult to treat successfully because of the fatty liver.

Overfeeding during the dry period predisposes cows to accumulate fat in adipose tissue during the prepartum period. Before parturition, adipose tissue from overfed cows has higher rates of esterification than the adipose tissue of cows fed a restricted energy intake. In the fatty livers of these overfed cows, the rate of gluconeogenesis is not optimal, which results prolongation of lipolysis, particularly during the first few weeks after parturition. The increased lipolysis after parturition leads to a major increase in the hepatic triacylglycerol concentration and to a shift in hepatic fatty acid composition. Unrestricted feed intake during the dry period impairs postpartum oxidation and synthesis of fatty acids in the liver of dairy cows.

In Australia, only beef cattle have been involved in pregnancy toxemia; the fat and the obese are most commonly affected. The disease occurred most notably when there was a shift to autumn calving (February to April) when feed supplies were low because of low late-summer rainfall. The cows were in good to fat body condition because of lush pastures in the spring and early summer, but by autumn when the calving season approached, the feed supplies were low and the nutritive value of the pasture inadequate. The lack of feed combined with the expensive nature of supplementary feeding resulted in an inadequate level of nutrition during late pregnancy. The morbidity is usually from 1% to 3%, but may be as high as 10%, and the disease is usually fatal.

PATHOGENESIS

Fatty liver is associated with a negative energy balance that is essentially universal in dairy cows in the first few weeks of lactation. Most cows adapt to the negative energy balance through an intricate mechanism of metabolic adaptation. Fatty liver develops because of failure of these adaptive mechanisms. Under normal physiologic conditions, the total amount of fat increases in the liver beginning a few weeks before calving, rises to an average of about 20% (of wet-weight basis) 1 week after calving, and declines slowly to the normal level of less than 5% by 26 weeks after calving. However, the fat content varies from almost none to 70% among cows 1 week after calving. Fat mobilization begins about 2 to 3 weeks before calving and is probably induced by a changing hormonal environment before calving rather than an energy deficit. After calving, there is a larger increase in fat accumulation. The changes in the liver in dairy cows are functional and reversible and related to the metabolic demands of late pregnancy and early lactation.

The heavy demands for energy in the high-producing dairy cow immediately after parturition, or in the pregnant beef cow that may be bearing twins, result in an increased rate of mobilization of fat from body reserves, usually subcutaneous fat, to the blood that transports it to body tissues, particularly the liver but also muscle and the kidneys. Any decrease in energy intake caused by a shortage of feed or an inability of the cow to consume an adequate amount of feed during the critical periods of late pregnancy or early lactation results in the mobilization of an excessive amount of **nonesterified fatty acids** (**NEFAs**). This results in increased hepatic lipogenesis with accumulation of lipid in enlarged hepatocytes, depletion of liver glycogen, and inadequate transport of lipoprotein from the liver. Most of the lipid infiltration of the liver in dairy cows after calving is in the form of triacylglycerols because of the increased uptake of NEFAs and a simultaneous increase in diacylglycerol acyltransferase; the activity of this enzyme is activated by fatty acids. The gradual increase in plasma NEFA concentration during the final prepartum days may explain the gradual depression in dry matter intake and a contributing factor to triglyceride accumulation in the liver. During this period there is also an elevated concentration of plasma glucose and a lowered plasma BHB concentration. The serum lecithin : cholesterol acyltransferase activity in spontaneous cases of fatty liver in cows is also decreased, which may be associated with reproductive performance because cholesteryl esters are utilized for the synthesis of steroid hormones.

Cattle are prone to fatty liver because their hepatocytes have limited capacity to export VLDLs and therefore a limited ability to export accumulated fat in the hepatocytes. NEFAs transported to the liver are usually oxidized in the mitochondria and peroxisomes or secreted as VLDL particles into the blood. Fatty liver develops when the uptake of NEFAs by the liver exceeds the oxidation of NEFAs by the liver to CO_2, partial oxidation of NEFAs to form ketones, and export of phospholipids, cholesterol, and apoproteins from the liver as lipoproteins. For unknown reasons, the capacity for VLDL formation is low in cattle and further impaired in early-lactating cows a result of very low apoliprotein B100 (apoB100) availability, the main apolipoprotein of VLDL particles. Production of ketones in moderate levels is beneficial in that energy is exported from the liver to other tissues that can utilize ketones as an energy source. Excess lipids that cannot be exported are stored as triacylglycerol in the liver and are associated with decreased metabolic functions of the liver. Also, a prepartum surge of estrogen may contribute to the development of fatty liver in ruminants by increased fatty acid esterification along with limited export of triglyceride.

During fat mobilization, there is a concurrent loss of body condition and adipose tissue. The degree of mobilization will be dependent on the fatness of the cow and extent of the energy deficit. Fat and thin cows respond differently to the metabolic demands of early lactation. Fat cows appear less able to utilize mobilized fatty acids, and as a result they accumulate esterified fat in tissues. This can adversely influence susceptibility to disease, and the response of the cow to that disease imposes further metabolic demands, particularly on muscle and protein metabolism. Both fat and skeletal muscle mass are decreased after calving, and fat cows lose 2.5 times more muscle fiber area than thin cows. Thus the loss of body condition is a result of total tissue mobilization (protein and fat) rather than fat alone. There appears to be a higher rate of protein mobilization in fat cows than in thin cows.

Cows that are not fat initially do not develop fatty liver syndrome. Pregnant beef cows in thin body condition on pasture can become extremely emaciated and eventually recumbent and die of starvation, but they do not develop pregnancy toxemia.

CLINICAL FINDINGS

In dairy cattle, fat-cow syndrome occurs usually within the first few days following parturition and is commonly precipitated by any condition that interferes with the animal's appetite temporarily, such as the following:

- Parturient hypocalcemia
- Left-sided displacement of the abomasum
- Indigestion
- Retained fetal membranes
- Dystocia

Affected cows are usually excessively fat, with a BCS of 4/5 or higher. Excessive quantities of subcutaneous fat are palpable over the flanks, the shoulder areas, and around the tailhead. The affected cow usually does not respond to treatment for some of these diseases and becomes anorexic. The temperature, heart rate, and respiration are within normal ranges. Rumen contractions are weak or absent, and the feces are usually scant. Periods of prolonged recumbency are common, and affected cows may have difficulty in standing when they are coaxed to stand. A severe ketosis that does not respond to the usual treatment may occur. There is marked ketonuria. Affected cows will not eat and gradually become weaker and progress to totally recumbent, and they die in 7 to 10 days. Some cattle exhibit nervous signs consisting of a staring gaze, holding the head high, and muscular tremors of the head and neck. Some severe cases appear to develop hepatic failure, do not respond to therapy, and become weak and recumbent and die. Terminally there is coma, tachycardia, and marked hyperglycemia. The case-fatality rate in severe cases may reach 50% or more.

In fat beef cattle shortly before calving, affected cows are aggressive, restless, excited, and uncoordinated with a stumbling gait; sometimes have difficulty in rising; and they fall easily. The feces are scant and firm, and there is tachycardia. When the disease occurs 2 months before calving, the cows are depressed for 10 to 14 days and do not eat. Eventually they become sternally recumbent. The respirations are rapid, there may be an expiratory grunt, and the nasal discharge is clear, but there may be flaking of the epithelium of the muzzle. The feces are usually scant; terminally, there is often a fetid yellow diarrhea. The disease is highly fatal; the course is 10 to 14 days, and terminally there may be coma, with cows dying quietly.

In dairy cattle with moderately severe fatty liver, the clinical findings are much less severe, and most will recover within several days if they continue to eat even small amounts of hay. In dairy cattle, there is a relationship between the occurrence of a subclinical fatty liver within the first few weeks after parturition and inferior reproductive performance as a result of a delay in the onset of normal estrus cycles and a reduction in the conception rate that results in an increase in the average days between calving and conception. There may be differences in reproductive performance between cows with mild and moderate fatty livers early after calving. However, an examination of the postpartum hormone profiles of cows with fatty liver did not reveal the pathogenic mechanism of the reduced fertility. Fat-cow syndrome may also be associated with an increased incidence of parturient paresis and unresponsive treatment for ketosis in early lactation.

CLINICAL PATHOLOGY

Serum Biochemistry

The biochemical changes associated with fatty liver syndrome in cows depend on the severity of the fatty liver. There is a significant association between increasing serum biochemical abnormalities with increasing amounts of liver fat, although there may be considerable overlap in the distribution of individual test values in a population of animals with suspected fatty liver.

Increased plasma/serum nonesterified fatty acid, acetoacetate, BHB, and total bilirubin concentrations, and decreased serum fructosamine concentration,[2] are associated with increased liver fat percentage. Likewise, increased plasma/serum hepatic enzyme activity (particularly aspartate aminotransferase and ornithine carbamoyl transferase activity) is also associated with increased liver fat percentage. Other hepatic enzyme activities in plasma, such as alanine aminotransferase, sorbitol dehydrogenase, glutamate dehydrogenase, alkaline phosphatase, and gamma-glutamyl transferase activities, are poorly associated with liver fat percentage.[1] Possibly the most relevant biochemical index of the liver fat percentage is the **plasma NEFA : cholesterol** ratio. The rationale for using this ratio is that the plasma NEFA concentration reflects a metabolite that has not been cleared by the liver, whereas the plasma cholesterol concentration reflects the rate of hepatic reesterification and export as a VLDL. A high plasma NEFA : cholesterol concentration therefore is thought to indicate a high liver fat percentage. An increased concentration of plasma total bilirubin is also associated with increased liver fat percentage; competition between bilirubin and NEFA for the same binding site on hepatocytes decreases the hepatic uptake of bilirubin and therefore results in hyperbilirubinemia.[2] Serum fructosamine concentration provides a retrospective record of serum/plasma glucose concentrations over the previous 1 to 3 weeks and therefore provides a useful longer-term index of glucose availability. Serum fructosamine concentrations less than 213 μmol/L are predictive of hepatic lipidosis in dairy cattle.[2]

The plasma ammonia concentration in arterial or venous samples is poorly associated with liver fat percentage, but it is an excellent indicator of hepatic failure in severely affected cattle with hepatic lipidosis.[3] In cattle, ammonia in plasma is derived mainly from bacterial activity in the rumen and metabolism of tissue amino acids and is converted to urea by the liver or glutamine by the liver and other tissues. Consequently, severe liver dysfunction results in elevated plasma ammonia concentrations (>29 μmol/L), with higher ammonia concentrations in arterial samples than venous samples because of nonhepatic metabolism of ammonia.

Several cow-side blood, urine, and milk ketone tests are available for the detection of subclinical ketosis in postpartum dairy cows (see previous section on ketosis and subclinical ketosis). Metabolomic biomarkers show promise in identifying a typically pattern of changes in cattle with hepatic lipidosis; for example, plasma fibrinogen decreases inversely with the severity of hepatic lipidosis, presumably because of intracellular lipid accumulation interferes with fibrinogen synthesis.[4]

Hemogram

In cattle with subclinical fatty liver, there may be a leukopenia, neutropenia, and lymphopenia. Leukopenia has been observed in dairy cows with more than 20% liver fat in the second week after calving. This may be related to the increased incidence of postparturient diseases, such as mastitis and endometritis, observed in cows with subclinical fatty liver. In cows with fatty liver, there is decreased functional capacity of the polymorphonuclear cells. However, this is not necessarily a cause-and-effect relationship.

Liver Biopsy and Analysis

The severity of fatty liver has been arbitrarily classified into severe, moderate, and mild, based on the amount of triglyceride present in the hepatocytes.[1] In severe hepatic lipidosis, the accumulation of triglyceride in the cytoplasm is accompanied by disturbances in hepatic structure and function that may result in hypoglycemia and ketonemia; these signs are manifested as anorexia and depression, and there may be clinical evidence of nervous signs. A liver biopsy can be used to determine the severity of the fatty liver and the concentration of triglyceride and is the most reliable method of accurately estimating the degree of fatty infiltration of the liver.

The triglyceride concentration of liver in normal cows ranges from 10% to 15% on a wet-weight basis. Estimation of the lipid content of bovine liver samples obtained by biopsy may be made by biochemical or histologic methods. Both methods provide reasonable estimates of liver fat content over a wide range of values. The lipid content of bovine liver is highly correlated with its specific gravity and the submersion of needle biopsy specimens into water, and copper sulfate solutions with specific gravities of 1.025 and 1.055 can be used as a test to estimate lipid content. For routine clinical diagnosis, three solutions of specific gravities of 1, 1.025, and 1.055 can be used. Liver samples that float in all three solutions contain greater than 34% lipid, those that sink in water but float in solutions of 1.025 and 1.055 specific gravity contain less than 34% but greater than 25% lipid, whereas those that float only in solutions of 1.055 specific gravity contain less than 25% but greater than 13% lipid. Samples that sink in all three solutions contain less than 13% lipid. Some limited evidence indicates that cows with liver lipid concentrations above 34% are severely affected and can be expected to have clinical manifestations of hepatic insufficiency. Those with liver lipid levels between 34% and 25% are moderately affected and might have some clinical evidence of hepatic insufficiency. Those between 25% and 13% are mildly affected, which is the range of most postpartum dairy cows without any evidence of disease. Liver lipid concentrations below 13% are inconsequential.

Ultrasonography of the Liver

Ultrasonography of the liver has been used to evaluate fatty infiltration in dairy cattle with mixed results.[5,6] Two strategies have been employed: identification of hepatic enlargement by comparing liver position with published reference range relative to the ribs, and the echogenicity or brightness of the liver. In the normal cow, the hepatic ultrasonogram consists of numerous weak echoes distributed homogeneously over the entire area of the liver. The echo beam gradually attenuates as it passes through the normal liver tissue. The portal and hepatic veins can be seen within the normal echotexture, and the parenchymal edges are normally visible. In the fatty liver, there is a diffuse nature and echogenicity that are roughly proportional to the volume of fat vacuoles and the amount of triglyceride in the liver. Assessment of echogenicity is subjective and varies with equipment and settings on the ultrasonographic unit. Consequently, objective ultrasonographic indices of hepatic lipidosis are under investigation, such as spectral analysis and analysis of brightness (B)-mode image statistics and texture characteristics.[6] Technological challenges associated with digital processing of ultrasonographic images of the liver need to be resolved before the noninvasive measurement of liver fat percentage becomes a widely available diagnostic tool.

NECROPSY FINDINGS

In severe fatal cases, the liver is grossly enlarged, pale yellow, friable, and greasy. Mild and moderate cases are usually not fatal unless accompanied by another fatal disease, such as peracute mastitis. The degree of fatty infiltration in these instances is much less obvious. The histologic changes include the occurrence of fatty cysts or lipogranulomas, enlarged hepatocytes, compression of hepatic sinusoids, a decreased volume of rough endoplasmic reticulum, and evidence of mitochondrial damage. The latter two changes are reflected in reduced albumin levels and increased activities of liver enzymes in the blood. The proportions of the various fatty acids in the liver are altered considerably. Palmitic and oleic acid proportions are higher in fatty-liver cows than in normal cows, whereas stearic acid is lower.

> **DIFFERENTIAL DIAGNOSIS**
>
> In **dairy cows, fatty liver** must be differentiated from those diseases that occur commonly immediately following parturition.
>
> **Left-sided displacement of the abomasum** results in a secondary ketosis, inappetence, and pings over the left abdomen.
>
> **Retained placenta** and **metritis** may be accompanied by fever, inappetence to anorexia, ruminal atony, and a foul-smelling vaginal discharge. A degree of fatty liver may occur in these cows, making it indistinguishable from the effects of the retained placenta and metritis.
>
> **Primary ketosis** may occur immediately after parturition or within several days rather than at the most common time, at 6 to 8 weeks of lactation. Inappetence, ruminal hypotonicity, marked ketonuria, and a good response to glucose and propylene glycol are characteristic.
>
> In **beef cattle, pregnancy toxemia** before parturition must be differentiated from abomasal impaction, vagus indigestion, and chronic peritonitis.

TREATMENT

The prognosis for severe fatty liver is unfavorable. In general, cows with the severe fat-cow syndrome that are totally anorexic for 3 days or more usually die in spite of intensive therapy. The prognosis for cases with nervous signs is very poor. Liberal quantities of highly palatable good-quality hay and an ample supply of water should be provided. Cattle that continue to eat in increasing daily amounts will recover with supportive therapy and palatable feeds. The major prognostic factor is whether the cow will eat; failure of the appetite to return is usually a very poor prognostic sign.

Three treatment strategies for fatty liver are available. The most effective strategy is to decrease the rate of fat mobilization and therefore the plasma NEFA concentration; propylene glycol appears to act partly by this mechanism. The second strategy is to facilitate the complete oxidation of NEFAs in the liver. The third strategy is to increase the rate of export of VLDLs from the liver; choline is thought to act by this method. Because they address different mechanisms, combined treatment using propylene glycol and rumen-protected choline offers theoretical advantages. Several different therapeutic approaches have been tried and are discussed in detail in the previous section on ketosis and subclinical ketosis

Additional treatments that have been tried in cattle with fatty liver include intravenous fluids, ruminal transfaunation, and glucagon.

Fluid and Electrolyte Therapy. Intensive therapy directed at correcting the effects of the ketosis and the fatty liver is required. The recommended treatment includes continuous IV infusion of 5% **glucose and multiple electrolyte solutions** and the intraruminal administration of rumen juice (5 to 10 L) from normal cows in an attempt to stimulate the appetite of affected cows. Water and multiple electrolytes (10 to 30 L) can be administered intraruminally.

Glucagon. The subcutaneous injection of 15 mg/d of glucagon for 14 days beginning at day 8 postpartum decreases liver triglyceride concentrations in cows older than 3.5 years. Glucagon, containing 29 amino acids, is a pancreatic hormone that improves the carbohydrate status of cows by stimulating hepatic gluconeogenesis, glycogenolysis, amino acid uptake, and ureagenesis. The effect of glucagon on lipid metabolism is both direct and indirect because it directly increases lipolysis in adipose tissue but indirectly decreases lipolysis by increasing concentrations of plasma glucose and insulin. IV infusions of glucagon are not practical for on-farm use.

Glucocorticoids. Dexamethasone-21-isonicotinate (20 to 25 mg, IM) decreases hepatic total lipid and triglyceride content in cattle after surgical correction of left-displaced abomasum, which is a beneficial effect.[7]

Propylene glycol given orally at 300 mL/day for 5 days promotes gluconeogenesis and is used for the treatment of ketosis.

Insulin as zinc protamine at 200 to 300 SC twice daily promotes the peripheral utilization of glucose, but clinical results have been mixed. It is important to recognize that IV administration of glucose is always accompanied by insulin release, no matter the metabolic state of the cow. Consequently, IV glucose administration should be considered as a combined treatment with glucose and insulin.

Outbreaks in a Herd. When outbreaks of fat-cow syndrome occur in pregnant beef cattle, all remaining cows should be sorted into groups according to body condition and fed accordingly. Excessively fat cows should be fed the best-quality hay that is available along with a supplement. Fat cows should be exercised by feeding them on the ground and forcing them to walk.

TREATMENT AND CONTROL

Treatment

Propylene glycol (300 mL daily for 5 days, PO) (R-1)

Dextrose (500 mL of 50% dextrose once, IV) (R-1)

Dexamethasone, dexamethasone-21-isonicotinate, or flumethasone, IM (R-1)

Cyanocobalamin (vitamin B_{12}, 1 to 4 mg IV, daily for 2 to 3 treatments) (R-2)

Isoflupredone (20 mg, IM, multiple injections) (R-3)

Control

Monensin (controlled-release capsule, 335 mg/day) (R-1)

Propylene glycol (300 to 500 mL daily for 5 days, PO) (R-1)

Cyanocobalamin (vitamin B_{12}, 1 to 4 mg IV, daily for 2 to 6 treatments before or at calving) (R-2)

CONTROL

Control and prevention of fatty liver in cattle will depend on decreasing or eliminating most of the potential risk factors for the disease. Early recognition and treatment of diseases that affect the voluntary dietary intake in late pregnancy and immediately after parturition are necessary to minimize the mobilization of body-fat stores to meet the overall energetic requirements of the cow during the period of negative energy balance and to maintain or increase hepatic glucogenesis. Diseases such as ketosis, displaced abomasum, retained placenta, acute mastitis, milk fever, and downer-cow syndrome must be treated as early as possible to avoid varying degrees of hepatic lipidosis.

Dry Matter Intake and Energy Balance in the Transition Period

The literature on dry matter intake and energy balance in the transition period of the dairy cow has been reviewed.

The transition from late gestation to early lactation in the dairy cow is a critical period in the lactation–gestation cycle. During this period, feed intake is at the lowest level in the production cycle. In addition to the drop in feed intake, there is a concurrent transition from late gestation to lactation, with huge increases in energy demands. This leads to a negative energy balance that can result in ketosis or fatty liver. Voluntary dry matter intake (DMI) may decrease 25% and 52% during the final 14 days of gestation for first- and second-parity animals and aged (third and fourth or greater) cows, respectively. A negative energy balance can occur before parturition and is more likely to occur in heifers than cows because heifers have a lower DMI and an additional need for energy requirement for growth. The fall in DMI is the usual cause of a negative energy balance rather than an increase in energy requirements for fetal growth.

Metabolic Adaptations During the Transition Period

The primary goal of nutritional management strategies of dairy cows during the transition period should be to support the metabolic adaptations that occur. The hallmark of the transition period of dairy cattle is the dramatic change in nutrient demands that necessitates exquisite coordination of metabolism to meet requirements for energy, amino acids, and calcium by the mammary gland after calving. Estimates of the demand for glucose, amino acids, fatty acids, and net energy by the gravid uterus at 250 days of gestation and the lactating mammary gland at 4 days postpartum indicate approximately a tripling of demand for glucose, a doubling of demand for amino acids, and approximately a fivefold increase in demand for fatty acids during this period. In addition, the requirement for calcium increases approximately fourfold on the day of parturition. The literature on the integration of metabolism and intake regulation in periparturient animals has been reviewed.

Glucose Metabolism

The primary homeorhetic adaptation of glucose metabolism to lactation is the concurrent increase in hepatic gluconeogenesis and decrease in oxidation of glucose by peripheral tissues to direct glucose to the mammary gland for lactose synthesis. The major substrates for hepatic gluconeogenesis are propionate from ruminal fermentation, lactate from Cori cycling, amino acids from protein catabolism or net portal-drained visceral absorption, and glycerol released during lipolysis in adipose tissue.

Lipid Metabolism

The primary homeorhetic adaptation of lipid metabolism to lactation is the mobilization of body fat stores to meet the overall energetic requirements of the cow during a period of negative energy balance in early lactation. Body fat is mobilized into the bloodstream in the form of NEFAs that are used to make upward of 40% of milk fat during the first days of lactation. Skeletal muscle uses some NEFA for fuel, particularly as it decreases its reliance on glucose as a fuel during early lactation. Given that NEFA concentrations increase in response to increased energy needs accompanied by inadequate feed intake, and plasma NEFA concentrations usually are inversely related. The liver takes up NEFAs in proportion to their supply, but the liver typically does not have sufficient capacity to completely dispose of NEFAs through export into blood or catabolism for energy. Therefore cows are predisposed to accumulate NEFAs as triglycerides within liver when large amounts of NEFA are released from adipose tissue into the circulation.

Nutritional Management to Support Metabolic Adaptations During the Transition Period

Grouping Strategies

The primary goal of nutritional management strategies of dairy cows during the transition period should be to support the metabolic adaptations just described. Industry-standard nutritional management of dairy cows during the dry period consists of a two-group nutritional scheme. The National

Research Council (NRC) Nutrient Requirements of Dairy Cattle recommends that a diet containing approximately 1.25 Mcal/kg of NE_L should be fed from dry-off until approximately 21 days before calving, and that a diet containing 1.54 to 1.62 Mcal/kg of NE_L should be fed during the last 3 weeks before calving. The primary rationale for feeding a lower-energy diet during the early part of the dry period is to minimize BCS gain during the dry period. During the last 3 to 4 weeks prepartum, a diet higher in energy and protein concentration than current NRC recommendations should be fed so that adequate nutrient intake occurs within the limits of the reduced voluntary dry matter intake. Supplying excessive energy to dairy cows during the early dry period may have detrimental carryover effects during the subsequent early lactation. Managing cows to achieve a BCS of approximately 3.0 at drying off rather than the traditional 3.5 is now recommended.

Strategies to Meet Glucose Demands and Decrease NEFA Supply During the Transition Period

Carbohydrate Formulation of the Prepartum Diet. Feeding diets containing higher proportions of nonfiber carbohydrate (NCF) promotes ruminal microbial adaptation to NFC levels typical of diets fed during lactation and provides increased amounts of propionate to support hepatic gluconeogenesis and microbial protein (providing the diet contains sufficient ruminally degradable protein) to support protein requirements for maintenance, pregnancy, and mammogenesis.

Direct Supplementation With Glucogenic Precursors. Propylene glycol is a glucogenic precursor that has been used as an oral drench in the treatment of ketosis. Decreased concentrations of plasma NEFA and BHB follow oral administration of propylene glycol. The administration of an oral drench of propylene glycol for 2 days beginning at calving decreased concentrations of NEFA in plasma and increased milk yield during early lactation. However, in general, the lack of consistent production responses does not support a recommendation for routine use. Propionate supplements added to the diet to supply substrate for hepatic gluconeogenesis have also been used, but with inconsistent results.

Glycerol given orally is an effective treatment for lactational ketosis in dairy cattle. Feeding glycerol to dairy cows from 14 days prepartum to 21 days in milk did not have the glucogenic effect attributed to it when given orally as a drench to individual cows.

Monensin provided in controlled-release capsules (CRCs) administered 2 to 4 weeks prepartum has been shown to decrease the incidence of energy-associated diseases, subclinical ketosis, and left-side displaced abomasum by 40%, and a 25% reduction in retained placenta was found. The capsule delivers 335 mg/d of monensin for 95 days. The common mechanism for reduction of the incidences of these energy-associated diseases is likely to be improved energy metabolism during the transition period. The net effect of monensin within the rumen is to increase ruminal propionate production at the expense of ruminal acetate and methane production so that propionate supply is increased and the overall energetic efficiency of ruminal fermentation is increased.

Added Fat in Transition Diets. It has been proposed that dietary fat may partially decrease concentrations of NEFA and prevent the occurrence of ketosis. Dietary long-chain fatty acids are absorbed into the lymphatic system and do not pass first through the liver. The fat can provide energy for peripheral tissues and the mammary gland, and the increased energy availability would in turn decrease mobilization of body fat and decrease plasma NEFA concentrations. However, available evidence indicates that added fat fed to cows during the prepartum period does not decrease plasma NEFA concentrations.

Effects of Specific Fatty Acids on NEFA Supply. A substantial amount of research has examined the metabolic roles of individual fatty acids in transition-cow nutrition and metabolism. Feeding *trans*-10, *cis*-12 conjugated linoleic acid or transoctadecanoic acid experimentally may decrease the negative energy balance, but the ultimate metabolic effects in transition cows are as yet uncertain.

Because of the large economic losses associated with pregnancy toxemia in cattle, every economic effort must be made to prevent the disease. The principal method of control is to prevent pregnant cattle from becoming fat during the last trimester of pregnancy, particularly during the dry period in dairy cattle. During pregnancy, mature cattle should receive sufficient feed to meet the needs for maintenance and pregnancy, and the total daily nutrient intake must increase throughout the last trimester to meet the needs of the fetus. However, this increase is usually difficult to control without some cows getting fat and others losing weight. Sorting cows into groups on the basis of size and condition and feeding accordingly is recommended. Metabolic profiles may be used as a means of assessing energy status and, correspondingly, the likelihood of occurrence hyperketonemia or pregnancy toxemia. Both plasma glucose and BHB concentrations can be used.

Body-condition scoring of dairy cows at strategic times can be used to monitor the nutritional status of the herd and minimize the incidence and severity of fatty liver syndrome. The scoring should be done throughout the production cycle as part of a herd health program. Scoring done at calving, at 21 to 40 days, and 90 to 110 days postpartum can be used to monitor the nutritional status of the herd. Scoring done at 100 to 60 days before drying off provides an opportunity for management to make appropriate adjustments in the feeding program so that optimal body-condition goals are achieved. The optimum BCS of a cow at calving that will result in the most economical amount of milk has not yet been determined. On a scale of 5, the suggested optimum score at calving has ranged from 3 to 4. The optimum score will probably depend on the characteristics of the individual herd, which include type of cow, type of feedstuffs available, season of the year, environmental temperature, and the people doing the actual body-condition scoring.

FURTHER READING

Gordon JL, LeBlanc SJ, Duffield TF. Ketosis treatment in lactating dairy cattle. *Vet Clin North Am Food Anim Pract*. 2013;29:433-445.

Grummer RR. Nutritional and management strategies for the prevention of fatty liver in dairy cattle. *Vet J*. 2008;176:10-20.

Ingvartsen KL. Feeding and management related diseases in the transition cow. Physiological adaptations around calving and strategies to reduce feeding-related diseases. *Anim Feed Sci Technol*. 2006;126:175-213.

Ringseis R, Gessner CK, Eder K. Molecular insights into the mechanisms of liver-associated diseases in early-lactating dairy cows: hypothetical role of endoplasmic reticulum stress. *J Anim Physiol Anim Nutr*. 2015;99:626-645.

REFERENCES

1. Kalaitzakis E, et al. *J Vet Intern Med*. 2007;21:835.
2. Mostafavi M, et al. *Anim Prod Sci*. 2015;55:1005.
3. Mudron P, et al. *Vet Med Czech*. 2004;49:187.
4. Imhasly S, et al. *BMC Vet Res*. 2014;10:122.
5. Rafia S, et al. *Am J Vet Res*. 2012;73:830.
6. Starke A, et al. *J Dairy Sci*. 2010;93:2952.
7. Kusenda M, et al. *J Vet Intern Med*. 2013;27:200.

PREGNANCY TOXEMIA (TWIN LAMB DISEASE) IN SHEEP

SYNOPSIS

Etiology A multifactorial disorder of energy metabolism, with hypoglycemia and ketonemia (the accumulation in blood of acetoacetate, β-hydroxybutyrate, and their decarboxylation products acetone and isopropanol).

Epidemiology The disease in sheep is associated with a falling plane of nutrition, principally in the last month of pregnancy in ewes bearing twins and triplets, but can be induced by other stress at this time.

Clinical findings Encephalopathy with blindness, muscle tremor, convulsions, metabolic acidosis, and a clinical course of 2 to 8 days, usually terminating fatally unless treated early.

Clinical pathology Hypoglycemia, ketonemia, ketonuria.

Necropsy findings None specific. Twin lambs and fatty liver.

Diagnostic confirmation Ketonemia, ketonuria, or elevated ketones in milk. Elevated β-hydroxybutyrate (BHBA) in aqueous humor of dead sheep.

Treatment Parenteral glucose with corticosteroid and oral glucose precursors such as propylene glycol, occasionally insulin, or oral glucose and electrolyte therapy. Cesarean section or induction of parturition. Case fatality high.

Control Monitoring of condition score, pasture availability, feeding, and biochemical indicators of ketosis. Correction of energy imbalance if detected.

ETIOLOGY

Hypoglycemia and hyperketonemia are the primary metabolic disturbances in pregnancy toxemia. The precipitating cause is the energy demand of the conceptus in the latter part of pregnancy. However, there is a great deal of variation between sheep flocks in the prevalence of the naturally occurring disease under conditions that appear conducive to its development. The most important factor in pregnancy toxemia is a decline in the plane of nutrition during the last 4 to 6 weeks of pregnancy. This is the period when fetal growth is rapid and the demands for energy are markedly increased, particularly in ewes carrying twins or triplets. For example, the energy requirement for a 70-kg ewe carrying twins increases 36% in the last weeks of pregnancy, from 13.5 MJ (3.2 Mcal)/d midgestation to 18.3 MJ (4.4 Mcal)/d at term. The disease in goats during late pregnancy has the same initiating causes.

Pregnancy toxemia can be classified according to the underlying management cause that is critical to its control and prevention:

- Primary pregnancy toxemia
- Fat-ewe pregnancy toxemia
- Starvation pregnancy toxemia
- Secondary pregnancy toxemia
- Stress-induced pregnancy toxemia

EPIDEMIOLOGY

Primary Pregnancy Toxemia

Primary pregnancy toxemia is the most common. In most flocks it is a result of a declining plane of nutrition in the latter half of pregnancy, often exacerbated by a short period of food deprivation associated with a management procedure in late pregnancy, such as crutching, shearing, a change of environment, or drenching. In sheep grazing pastures the decreased plane of nutrition is often associated with inadequate pasture availability and/or overstocking. In sheep at pasture it occurs more frequently in early-lambing flocks, where there is insufficient supplement provided during autumn or winter. In some outbreaks ewes have been moved onto better pasture during late pregnancy specifically to prevent the occurrence of ketosis, but if ewes are unaccustomed to the new feed, their intake of metabolizable energy will be reduced.

For sheep that are housed in late pregnancy, the provision of poor-quality hay may predispose pregnancy toxemia. A change in feed type, feeding of moldy feed, or feed contaminated with manure can also lead to decreased intake, especially with goats. Competition for inadequate trough space can also be important. Goats exhibit greater dominant/submissive behavior than sheep, and this can result in lower food intake in submissive goats in groups that are being fed a partial supplement or total ration.

In all management systems, failing to identify and separate ewes bearing twins and triplets, and to feed them accordingly, or failing to increase the nutritional plane of mixed mobs of pregnant sheep during the last 6 weeks of pregnancy are important predisposing factors.

Fat-Ewe Pregnancy Toxemia

Fat-ewe pregnancy toxemia occurs without a specific stressor in ewes that are very well fed and are in an overfat condition in late pregnancy (a condition score of 4 or 5 on a scale of 1 [emaciated] to 5 [fat]). Fat ewes have a decreased food intake in late pregnancy when the volume of the rumen is reduced by the pressure of intraabdominal fat and the developing fetus. This can occur especially when feeds with high water content are being fed, such as silage or root crops. A lack of exercise is thought to predispose this type of pregnancy toxemia, and there is often concurrent hypocalcemia.

Starvation Pregnancy Toxemia

Starvation pregnancy toxemia occurs in ewes that are excessively thin. It is relatively uncommon, but it occurs in extensive grazing systems where there is prolonged drought and an inadequate alternative feed supply. It can occur in any production system where there is mismanagement and undernutrition.

Secondary Pregnancy Toxemia

Secondary pregnancy toxemia usually occurs as a sporadic disease as the result of the effect of an intercurrent disease, such as foot rot or foot abscess, that affects food intake. Heavy worm infestation, such as mixed infections of *Teladorsagia, Haemonchus*, or *Trichostrongylus* species, would add a similar drain on glucose metabolism and increase the chances of development of this condition.

Stress-Induced Pregnancy Toxemia

Stress-induced pregnancy toxemia is the least common variant of this condition, in which stress is the initiator. Examples are the close shepherding or housing of late-pregnant sheep of breeds not used to being housed, the transport of late pregnant sheep, and outbreaks following attack by dogs.

Occurrence

Pregnancy toxemia is seen primarily in ewes carrying triplet or twin lambs in the last 6 weeks of pregnancy, with the peak incidence in the last 2 weeks of pregnancy. It occurs wherever sheep are raised, but it is primarily a disease of sheep raised in intensive farming systems, either grazing or when housed during the winter. In part this is because the breeds of sheep used in intensive farming a re more likely to bear twins or triplets. In contrast, sheep breeds in extensive grazing systems commonly bear single lambs, and significant outbreaks of pregnancy toxemia are uncommon except where there is drought or insufficient pasture as a result of poor management. The attack rate in a flock varies with the nature and severity of the nutritional deprivation and the proportion of the flock at risk. It can be very high in starvation pregnancy toxemia, whereas fat-ewe pregnancy toxemia is generally sporadic. In outbreaks that follow management procedures or other stressors, clinical disease is not seen until 48 hours afterward, and new cases will develop over several days. Intercurrent disease in late-pregnant ewes, such as foot rot or foot abscess, may predispose pregnancy toxemia.

The natural incidence in intensively farmed sheep is approximately 2% of pregnant ewes, but where there are severe management deficiencies it may affect the majority of late-pregnant ewes. The proportion of flocks with cases varies by year, but in a study of sheep diseases in Canada, 19% of flocks reported cases of pregnancy toxemia. The case fatality is high unless treatment is initiated early in the clinical course, but even with early treatment many ewes will die.

Experimental Reproduction

Hypoglycemia and ketosis can be experimentally produced in pregnant sheep by undernourishment, but the resultant syndrome has biochemical and clinical differences from spontaneously occurring pregnancy toxemia. For example, loss of appetite is an early sign in the spontaneous disease, whereas starved experimental animals, even though hypoglycemic and ketotic, will eat feed when offered. Consequently, there is debate about whether hypoglycemia is the primary precipitating cause of the clinical signs in the naturally occurring disease.

There is a great deal of variation between sheep in the ease with which the hypoglycemia and ketosis can be produced experimentally and in the variation in incidence of the naturally occurring disease in conditions that appear to be conducive to it developing. It is likely that the difference between sheep depends on the metabolic efficiency of the liver.

Animal Risk Factors

Pregnancy

The disease occurs only in ewes in the last 6 weeks of pregnancy, with the peak incidence in the last 2 weeks. It occurs primarily in ewes carrying triplet or twin lambs, although ewes bearing a single, large lamb may also be affected.

Parity

The disease is uncommon in maiden ewes because of their lower fecundity, and then increases in prevalence up until 5 to 6 years of age.

Breed

Breed differences largely reflect differences in fecundity and differences in management systems. Thus the disease is more common in British lowland breeds and their crosses than the Merino. British hill-breeds are traditionally thought to be more resistant to the development of pregnancy toxemia in the face of nutritional deprivation of the ewe, but resistance is achieved at the expense of lamb birth weight and has the penalty of higher neonatal mortality. Differences in the susceptibility of individual sheep appear to be related to differences in rates of hepatic gluconeogenesis.

Economic Significance

The disease has considerable effect. Without treatment, the case-fatality rate can approach 100%, and in individual flocks the prevalence can be high enough to be classed as an outbreak. Treated ewes that recover may have dystocia and die during parturition or develop retained placenta and metritis. Flocks that experience pregnancy toxemia also have a significantly higher-than-normal mortality in neonatal lambs and often a severe decrease in wool quality. Often these flocks are also predisposed to hypomagnesemia during lactation.

PATHOGENESIS

Approximately 60% of fetal growth takes place in the last 6 weeks of pregnancy, and pregnancy toxemia results from inadequate energy intake during this time, usually in ewes with more than one fetus. Ewes that are predisposed to the disease have an ineffective gluconeogenic response to the continued preferential demands for glucose by the growing fetuses, resulting in hypoglycemia, lipid mobilization, and the accumulation of ketone bodies and cortisol. The reason for this predisposition is not precisely known, but the subsequent disease and metabolic changes are associated with excessive lipid mobilization. Elevated concentrations of BHB further suppress endogenous glucose production and exaggerate the development of ketosis. Thus the negative feedback of hyperketonemia on glucose production produces a self-perpetuating cycle.

An encephalopathy develops, thought to be a hypoglycemic encephalopathy from hypoglycemia in the early stages of the disease. The encephalopathy and the disease are frequently not reversible unless treated in the early stages. The onset of clinical signs is always preceded by hypoglycemia and hyperketonemia, although it is not related to the minimum blood glucose or maximum ketone levels, and thus hypoglycemia may not be the initial or precipitating cause of the syndrome. In affected ewes, there is an abnormally high level of cortisol in plasma, and adrenal steroid diabetes ("insulin resistance") may either contribute to or be a predisposing factor. For example, a comparison of ewes with a high risk of pregnancy toxemia (German Blackheaded Mutton) with a breed of lower risk (Finnish Landrace) found that the glucose elimination rate and glucose stimulated first-phase insulin secretion was lower and the basal rate of lipolysis significantly higher in the high-risk ewes. However, further investigation of insulin resistance and impaired insulin sensitivity, and the underlying cause of pregnancy toxemia, is needed.[1]

The increase in plasma concentrations of nonesterified fatty acids depresses cellular and humoral immune responses in the experimentally produced disease, but the clinical significance of this to naturally occurring disease is not clear.[2] Renal dysfunction is also apparent in the terminal stages of ovine ketosis and contributes to the development of clinical signs and the fatal outcome.

Those ewes that are carrying only one lamb and have been well fed before a short period of undernutrition may develop a subacute syndrome, both clinically and biochemically. In lines of ewe selected for increased fecundity, ewes bearing more than three fetuses have an increased susceptibility to pregnancy toxemia.[3]

CLINICAL FINDINGS

The earliest signs of ovine ketosis are separation from the group, altered mental state, and apparent blindness, manifested by an alert bearing but a disinclination to move. Sheep at pasture may fail to come up for supplementary feeding, and housed sheep may stand near the feed trough with other sheep but not eat. The ewe will stand still when approached by attendants or dogs and will turn and face them, but it will make no attempt to escape. If it is forced to move, it blunders into objects; when an obstacle is encountered, it presses against it with its head. Many affected ewes stand in water troughs all day and lap the water. Constipation with dry, scanty feces is common, and there is grinding of the teeth.

In later stages, marked drowsiness develops, and episodes of more severe nervous signs occur, but they may be infrequent and easily missed. In these episodes, tremors of the muscles of the head cause twitching of the lips, champing of the jaws, and salivation, and these are accompanied by a cog-wheel type of clonic contraction of the cervical muscles causing dorsiflexion or lateral deviation of the head, followed by circling. The muscle tremor usually spreads to involve the whole body, and the ewe falls with tonic-clonic convulsions. The ewe lies quietly after each convulsion and rises normally afterward, but is still blind.

Between the convulsions there is marked drowsiness that may be accompanied by head pressing; assumption of abnormal postures, including unusual positions of the limbs and elevation of the chin (the "stargazing" posture); and incoordination and falling when attempting to walk. A smell of ketones may be detectable on the breath.

Affected ewes usually become recumbent in 3 to 4 days and remain in a state of profound depression or coma for a further 3 to 4 days, although the clinical course is shorter in fat ewes. Terminally there may be a fetid diarrhea.

Fetal death often occurs and is followed by transient recovery of the ewe, but the toxemia caused by the decomposing fetus soon causes a relapse.

Affected ewes commonly have difficulty in lambing. Recovery may occur after the ewe lambs or if the lambs are removed by cesarean section in the early stages of the disease. In an affected flock, the disease usually takes the form of a slow, prolonged outbreak, with a few ewes affected each day over a period of several weeks. Recovered ewes may subsequently show a break in the wool.

CLINICAL PATHOLOGY

Hypoglycemia, ketonemia, and ketonuria are characteristic of the disease. The initial changes are similar to ketosis in cattle but the sequel is not. Hypoglycemia can be used as a diagnostic aid in the early stages of the disease, but is of limited value later on when the ewe becomes recumbent, when blood glucose levels may be normal or grossly elevated. This may follow fetal death, which has been shown to remove the suppressing effect of the fetus on hepatic gluconeogenesis.

Ketonemia and ketonuria are constant, with serum BHB concentrations greater than 3.0 mmol/L. Sheep develop a severe metabolic acidosis, develop renal failure with a terminal uremia, and become dehydrated. Liver function tests show liver dysfunction. Elevated plasma cortisol concentrations occur, with greater than 10 ng/mL indicative of pregnancy toxemia. However, elevated plasma cortisol can occur with other conditions, such as hypocalcemia.

NECROPSY FINDINGS

Without treatment, pregnancy toxemia in ewes is almost always fatal. At necropsy, there is severe fatty degeneration of the liver and usually constipation, although some cases have fetid, light-colored diarrhea. A large single or, more commonly. twin or greater number of fetuses are present. These may have died before the ewe and be in varying stages of decomposition.

Histopathologically there is hepatic lipidosis and a poorly defined renal lesion, and there may be evidence of neuronal necrosis. Hepatic glycogen concentrations are usually very low. Concentrations of BHB in the aqueous humor or the CSF greater than 2.5 mmol/L or 5.0 mmol/L respectively, are supportive of a diagnosis of pregnancy toxemia.

DIFFERENTIAL DIAGNOSIS

Pregnancy toxemia is usually suspected in late-pregnant ewes that show nervous signs and die within 2 to 7 days. There may be a history of exertion, stress, or sudden deprivation of food. **Hypocalcemia** can occur under similar circumstances, but the following help in differentiation:

1. The onset is within 12 hours of the stress.
2. A considerable proportion of the flock will be affected at the same time.
3. There is obvious myasthenia.
4. It has a much shorter course, 12 to 24 hours.
5. Affected animals respond well to treatment with solutions of calcium salts.

Differential diagnoses include

- Listeriosis
- Cerebral abscess
- Acidosis
- Uterine torsion or impending abortion
- Rabies

TREATMENT

Sheep treated very early in the course of the disease generally respond favorably,[4] but response to therapy is poor once sheep have become recumbent, and the IV administration of 50% dextrose at this time may hasten death. Optimum therapy requires the correction of fluid, electrolyte, and acid–base disturbances in addition to treating with glucose.

Parenteral Therapy

Ideally, individual sheep should be examined biochemically and the corrective therapy based on these results, with fluids, electrolytes, and glucose (dextrose) given over a prolonged period. A recommendation for glucose therapy is the administration of 5 to 7 g of glucose IV 6 to 8 times a day in conjunction with 20 to 40 units of zinc protamine insulin given IM every other day for 3 days. However, in many sheep-raising areas intensive laboratory monitoring and such intensive therapy is not possible because of lack of access, expense, or the number of sheep involved in an outbreak. In the absence of biochemical monitoring, therapy with glucose should be accompanied by the IV injection of isotonic sodium bicarbonate or lactated Ringer's solution, with additional fluids given by a stomach tube.

Standard doses of corticosteroids have little therapeutic effect in sheep, and thus treatment with these drugs is not recommended, although they are often used. Very large doses are effective in ewes still able to stand, but the success probably rests in the removal of the glucose drain by the induction of premature parturition.

Oral Therapy

Oral propylene glycol or glycerin (100 mL once daily) can be used to support parenteral glucose therapy. Less intensive therapy with propylene glycol or glycerin alone can give excellent results, especially with early treatment,[4] but is less successful with longer-standing cases. Oral drenching every 4 to 8 hours with 160 mL of a commercial calf scours concentrate (containing 28% glucose, 3.9% glycine, 5.3% sodium chloride, and other electrolytes) induces higher blood concentrations of glucose compared with drenching with glycerol or propylene glycol. Reported recovery rates are 90% in early and 55% in advanced cases. For the more intensive treatment of valuable ewes, insulin ([0.4 IU/kg]/d SC), combined with oral glucose precursors and electrolytes, may improve survival compared with treatment with oral glucose precursors and electrolytes alone.

Induction of parturition is an option, but it should only be used if the ewe is in the early stage of the disease because there is a delay in the delivery of the lambs (24 hours or more). If the ewe is unlikely to survive this period, cesarean section may be a better option. Induction can be achieved with dexamethasone 21-isonicotinate or the sodium phosphate form, at a dose rate of 16 to 25 mg per ewe, but dexamethasone trimethylacetate appears to be ineffective. Lambs will be born 24 to 72 hours after injection, with most born within 36 hours. Induction of parturition in normal sheep can be achieved with 10 mg of betamethasone or 2.5 mg of flumethasone, but there are no reports of their efficacy in sheep with pregnancy toxemia.

Cesarean Section

Cesarean section can be used as an alternate to glucose replacement, and provided that ewes are in the early stages of the disease, removal of the lambs by cesarean section probably has the greatest success. The demand for glucose by the lambs is immediately removed, and both the ewe and the lambs have a high chance of survival, provided that the cesarean section is conducted before there is irreversible brain damage in the ewe and the lambs are close to term. If the ewe is recumbent, then chances of survival, for both the ewe and the lamb, are reduced. The lamb may already be dead, and thus ultrasound examination will inform fetal age and condition and hence whether to undertake a cesarean section.

TREATMENT AND CONTROL

Treatment

Oral electrolyte and glucose (calf scours) concentrate solution (160 mL qid) (R-1)

OR Oral propylene glycol (60 mL bid or 100 mL/d for 3 days) (R-1)

For more intensive treatment, include: oral calcium (calcium lactate 12.5 g/d for 3 days); oral potassium (7.5 g KCl/d for 3 days); insulin 0.4 ([IU/kg]/d SC for 3 days) (R-2)

If hypoglycemia: Dextrose (60 to 100 mL IV) (R-2)

Abort fetus

Ewe: Dexamethasone (20 mg IV or IM) (R-2)

Doe: Dexamethasone plus prostaglandin F2α (10 mg IM) or synthetic analog (cloprostenol; 75 g/45 kg IM) (R-2)

Cesarean section if late-term fetus and valuable ewe/doe (R-2)

Control

Correct the contributing factors (e.g., insufficient feed or inadequate trough space, intercurrent disease such as foot rot or foot abscess) (R-1)

CONTROL

When clinical cases occur, the rest of the flock should be examined daily for evidence of ketosis, and affected animals should be treated immediately with oral glucose/glycine/electrolyte or propylene glycol/glycerol. Supplementary feeding of the flock should immediately be increased or started, with particular attention given to increasing in the intake of energy (carbohydrate). However, care is needed with cereal grains because rapid introduction can cause ruminal acidosis, and ewes may need from 0.25 to 1 kg/head per day (0.5 to 2.0 lb/head per day). Consequently, good-quality lucerne hay or legume grains, such as lupins or field peas, may be a safer option if ewes are not currently being fed a grain-based supplement, even though ewes do not need the higher protein content of these feeds.

Prevention

Ensure that the plane of nutrition is rising in the second half of pregnancy, even if it means restricting the diet in the early stages. An ideal condition score for ewes at 90 days of gestation is 2.75 to 3.0 on a scale of 1 to 5. If necessary, ewes with higher condition scores at the end of the first month of pregnancy can be fed to slowly lose 0.5 in condition score during the period to the third month of pregnancy without any detrimental effect on the ewe or the size or viability of the lamb. In many smaller flocks ewes tend to be in excessively high condition score early in pregnancy.

The last 2 months are important in the prevention of pregnancy toxemia because 70% of the lamb's birth weight is gained during the last 6 weeks of pregnancy. In intensively managed flocks the provision of cereal grain or a concentrate containing 10% protein during this period, at the rate of 0.25 kg/d, increasing to 1 kg/d in the last 2 weeks, provides adequate energy. During this period, there should be an increase in body weight of 10% for ewes with single lambs and 18% in those carrying twins, but the average condition score should remain around 3.0. Higher body-condition scores can result in higher birth weight of lambs, but this is usually not a financially viable strategy, and it increases the risk of fat-ewe pregnancy toxemia and dystocia. At the beginning of the fourth month of pregnancy, the flock can be divided into three groups by condition score, suboptimal, acceptable, and excess (overfat), and the groups are then fed accordingly. These can be monitored by condition scoring every 2 to 3 weeks during the fourth and fifth months of pregnancy. Maiden ewes should be fed as a separate group to provide for their growth in addition to pregnancy. Attention should also be given to broken-mouthed or older ewes to ensure that they maintain adequate body condition.

There are too many variations in flock structure and husbandry systems to discuss nutritional management in great detail here; readers should consult specialist texts appropriate to the system they work in.[5] However, in more intensive systems, especially prime lamb production, ewes can be pregnancy tested by ultrasound and divided into groups depending on whether they are barren or are carrying single or multiple fetuses. Account needs to be taken of those ewes (and does) that are timid and are thus, or for other reasons, slow feeders. If there is insufficient trough space or if the supplement is fed in small amounts and highly edible, a proportion may get little or no feed. The cost-effectiveness of a feeding program should be evaluated. In breeds with low twinning rates that are well managed, it is often more profitable to simply observe the flock and treat the occasional case.

Flock monitoring for latent pregnancy toxemia during the last 6 weeks of pregnancy can be conducted using serum BHB; concentrations of 0.8 mmol/L indicate adequate energy intake, 0.8 to 1.6 mmol/L indicate inadequate energy intake, and greater than 1.6 mmol/L indicate severe undernourishment. Pooled samples can reduce the cost of analysis, but serum glucose and BHB concentrations do vary significantly between flocks.

Ionophores are used in transition rations for dairy cows to prevent subclinical ketosis. There is some evidence that feeding monensin may have benefits for the energy metabolism of late pregnant ewes. Lower serum BHB, lowered feed intake, and improved feed efficiency have been observed, and thus further investigation of this strategy is warranted.[6]

FURTHER READING

Freer M, Dove H, Nolan JV. *Nutrient Requirements of Domesticated Ruminants*. Collingwood, Australia: CSIRO Publishing; 2007.

Radostits O, et al. Pregnancy toxemia in sheep. In: *Veterinary Medicine: a Textbook of the Diseases of Cattle, Horses, Sheep, Goats and Pigs*. 10th ed. London: W.B. Saunders; 2007:1668-1671.

REFERENCES

1. Duehlmeier R, et al. *J Anim Physiol Anim Nutr*. 2013;97:971.
2. Yarim GF, et al. *Vet Res Commun*. 2007;31:565.
3. Moallem U, et al. *J Anim Sci*. 2012;90:318.
4. Cal-Pereyra L, et al. *Ir Vet J*. 2015;68:25.
5. Freer M, Dove H. *Sheep Nutrition*. Collingwood, Australia: CABI and CSIRO; 2002.
6. Taghipoor B, et al. *Livestock Sci*. 2011;135:231.

STEATITIS, PANNICULITIS, AND FAT NECROSIS

Steatitis is inflammation of adipose tissue and can affect any fatty tissue. Clinical expression is usually because of inflammation of intraabdominal or subcutaneous fat (panniculitis). The disease can be relatively innocuous or fulminant and is reported for cattle, in which it is referred to as fat necrosis or bovine lipomatosis, and horses. The colloquial name is "yellow-fat disease" because of the color of affected tissues—a result of accumulation of lipofuscin and products of fat oxidation.[1-4] The disease is not neoplastic.

The **disease in cattle** is characterized by inflammation and necrosis of fat in the abdominal cavity. It can be clinically silent with lesions detected during rectal examination for pregnancy diagnosis or other reason. Clinical signs of the disease in cattle are usually attributable to space-occupying lesions (such as compression of the rectum) or intestinal obstruction as a result of constriction of the intestine by mesenteric accumulations of fat or fibrotic constriction of the lumen.[3] The lesions are firm masses present in any portion of the omental, mesenteric, or retroperitoneal fat or as mobile, free-floating structures in the abdomen.[2] The free-floating masses do not appear to originate from necrosis of fat.[2] The masses range from small nodules to large, solid, and irregularly shaped tumors. Unlike in horses, in which intraabdominal lipomas are often pedunculated (see Chapter 7) and cause acute intestinal obstruction when the peduncular stalk wraps and constricts the small intestine, the lesions in cattle are seldom pedunculated.[2]

The clinical disease in cattle can be variable and range from silent through inappetence, decreased milk production, persistent diarrhea, mild recurrent colic, acute colic, dystocia, urinary retention of feces, and decreased passage of feces. Masses can be detected on rectal examination or laparotomy. Ultrasonography (transcutaneous or transrectal) can be useful in detecting and characterizing the lesions.[3] The lesions are present as heterogenous hyperechoic masses in the retroperitoneal, omental, or mesenteric fat. A hyperechoic ring around the kidney is common.[3] Affected tissues can be biopsied with ultrasonographic guidance.

Abnormalities in the hemogram and serum biochemistry are confined to indicators of inflammation (neutrophilia), hypergammaglobulinemia, decreased concentrations of phospholipids and cholesterol, and an increase in concentration of free fatty acids.[3]

The disease must be differentiated from lymphosarcoma, adenocarcinoma, intraabdominal abscess, or dry fecal balls in the descending colon. The lesions are composed of necrotic fat embedded in normal adipose tissue with mild inflammatory infiltrates of neutrophils, lymphocytes, plasma cells, macrophages and giant cells, and fibrosis.[2] There is rarely evidence of pancreatitis in the disease in cattle.[2]

The cause of the disease is unknown, although a prevalence of 67% is reported in steers grazing tall fescue, in which serum cholesterol concentrations were abnormally low.

The **disease in horses** affects mostly foals and young animals and ponies. Older animals are less frequently affected.[1] Generalized steatitis can be a fulminant disease in horses, ponies, and foals.[1,4] Panniculitis, an unusual form of steatitis limited to the subcutaneous tissues, has been reported in an aged pony mare[5] and in perivaginal tissues after dystocia.[6] Perivaginal steatitis included involvement of the bladder ligament and subsequent rupture of the bladder.[6]

The clinical signs of generalized steatitis consist of anorexia and depression, fever, tachycardia, and subcutaneous edema.[1,4] Painful subcutaneous swellings can occur in the nuchal crest and inguinal and axillary regions. Affected horses often have mild to moderate colic and signs of abdominal tenderness. Rectal examination reveals painful masses in the mesentery of some horses.

Hematology and serum biochemical examination reveal mild to moderate leukocytosis, with occasional horses having leucopenia, hypoproteinemia, hypoalbuminemia, and increases in activity in serum of lactate dehydrogenase (LDH), aspartate aminotransferase (AST), GGT, and lipase and amylase.[1,4] Serum vitamin E concentrations are sometimes abnormally low.

Biopsy of some of the SC swelling reveals histopathological evidence of fat necrosis with mineralization. At necropsy, the fat is hard, dry, and yellow-white, with areas of necrosis forming abscess-like lesions up to 3 cm deep and 10 cm in diameter. The fat lining the abdominal wall may contain firm yellow-white and red tissue nodules up to 3 cm in diameter. Pancreatitis is evident in equids with systemic disease, and there is necrosis and inflammation in most fatty tissues (subcutaneous, retroperitoneal, mesenteric, and omental).[1]

Generalized steatitis with fat necrosis ("yellow-fat disease") has been recognized in many species at various ages and is thought to be related to a dietary deficiency of vitamin E and selenium and intake of unsaturated fatty acids.[1,5]

REFERENCES

1. de Bruijn CM, et al. *Equine Vet Educ.* 2006;18:38.
2. Herzog K, et al. *J Comp Pathol.* 2010;143:309.
3. Tharwat M, et al. *Can Vet J.* 2012;53:41.
4. Waitt LH, et al. *J Vet Diagn Invest.* 2006;18:405.
5. Radostits O, et al. Steatitis. In: *Veterinary Medicine: a Textbook of the Diseases of Cattle, Horses, Sheep, Goats and Pigs.* 10th ed. London: W.B. Saunders; 2006:1680.
6. Claes E, et al. *Vlaams Diergeneeskundig Tijdschrift.* 2014;83:36.

Inherited Metabolic Diseases of Ruminants

DEFICIENCY OF UMP SYNTHASE (DUMPS)

This is a partial deficiency of an enzyme that is involved in the conversion of orotate to uridine 5'-monophosphate (UMP) as a step in the synthesis of pyrimidine nucleotides. It is recorded at a high prevalence in Holstein–Friesian cattle in the United States and Japanese Black cattle and is characterized by an autosomal-recessive form of inheritance and the secretion of high levels of orotate in the milk.[1] Heterozygous animals have a partial deficiency of UMP synthase, but they have no individual or herd clinical abnormalities. Heterozygous animals can be detected biochemically by their half-normal levels of erythrocyte UMP synthase or by nested polymerase chain reaction (PCR) testing.[2,3] Bovine homozygotes die at about the 40th day of pregnancy. Embryonic mortality is the only form of loss.

REFERENCES

1. Ohba Y, et al. *J Vet Med Sci.* 2007;69:313.
2. Dai Y, et al. *China Anim Health Inspection.* 2014;31:76.
3. Paiva DS, et al. *Genet Mol Res.* 2013;12:3186.

HEPATIC LIPODYSTROPHY IN GALLOWAY CALVES

Hepatic lipodystrophy has been reported in Galloway calves on five farms in the United Kingdom over a 10-year period. Calves appear normal after birth but die by 5 months of age. Clinically there is tremor, opisthotonus, and dyspnea before affected calves become recumbent and die. At necropsy the liver is enlarged, pale, and mottled. Histologically there is evidence of hepatic encephalopathy. The cause is unknown, but limited evidence suggests a storage disease is possible.

Metabolic Diseases of Horses

EQUINE PITUITARY PARS INTERMEDIA DYSFUNCTION (FORMERLY EQUINE CUSHING DISEASE)

Equine pituitary pars intermedia dysfunction (PPID) is a slowly progressive neurodegenerative disease of older equids caused by nonmalignant hypertrophy and hyperplasia of melanotropes of the pars intermedia of the pituitary gland. It is characterized in its most severe form by hirsutism, laminitis, polyuria, and polydipsia.

ETIOLOGY

The pars intermedia of equids is composed of a single cell type—melanotropes—which are innervated by dopaminergic neurons of the periventricular nucleus. Innervation by these neurons is inhibitory on secretion by the melanotropes of proopiomelanocortin (POMC)-derived peptides. Thyrotropin-releasing hormone stimulates melanotropes.[1] The pars distalis of the pituitary of healthy horses releases adrenocorticotropic hormone (ACTH) in response to, among other stimuli, declines in plasma cortisol concentration. Cortisol exerts negative feedback on secretion of ACTH by the pars distalis, but not by the pars intermedia.[2]

The disease is attributable to degeneration of the periventricular hypophyseal dopaminergic neurons with subsequent development of a nonmalignant functional tumor comprised of melanotropes of the pars intermedia of the pituitary gland.

Cushing syndrome caused by adrenocortical tumors is exceedingly rare in equids.

EPIDEMIOLOGY

The disease is being diagnosed with increasing frequency.[3] The prevalence of the disease is not well documented, but surveys of owners indicate hair-coat abnormalities consistent with the disease in 15% to 39% of aged equids. Of 200 randomly selected equids 15 years of age or older in the United Kingdom, 22% had hair-coat abnormalities suggestive of PPID detected on clinical examination,[4] and owners of 12% of approximately ~980 aged equids in the United Kingdom reported hair-coat abnormalities and abnormal moulting.[5] Similarly, owners of 17% of 974 horses 15 years of age or older in Queensland, Australia, reported hirsutism.[6] Given that changes in hair coat are specific (95%) but of unknown sensitivity for the diagnosis of PPID,[7] these estimates likely provide the lower range for prevalence of the disease. Accordingly, 21% of 325 randomly selected horses 15 years of age or older in Queensland had PPID diagnosed based on measurement of plasma ACTH concentrations and using seasonally adjusted cutoff values.[8] This likely provides the best current estimate of the prevalence of PPID in mature and aged horses. Reports of prevalence of the disease provided in early studies likely were unreliable as indicators of disease frequency in the overall population of horses because of selective or nonrandom sampling of horses.

The disease occurs worldwide in all breeds of horses and ponies. Differences in geographic distribution are not reported.

The only well-recognized animal risk factor for the disease is increasing age (adjusted OR of 1.18 [95% CI, 1.1 to 1.25]) per year of age, and there is no apparent sex or breed predisposition.[8]

PATHOGENESIS

PPID is a neurodegenerative disease in which there is a loss of the inhibitory effect of dopamine with subsequent hypertrophy and hyperplasia of **melanotropes** of the pars intermedia of the pituitary gland with unchecked secretion of **proopiomelanocortin** and compression of the neurohypophysis, hypothalamus, and optic chiasma.[9] Production of proopiomelanocortin by melanotropes in the pars intermedia is not under the negative feedback control of glucocorticoids, and as a result, affected equids produce large quantities of POMC, melanocyte-stimulating hormone (α-MSH), β-endorphin, and smaller but still excessive quantities of ACTH. Production of ACTH results in loss of the normal circadian rhythm in serum cortisol concentration.[10] The space-occupying effects of the tumor can cause blindness because of compression of the optic chiasm. Polyuria and polydipsia are common and are probably related to neurohypophyseal dysfunction and compression of the pars nervosa, the source of antidiuretic hormone.[11]

Not all equids with PPID have **impaired glucose metabolism.**[12,13] A proportion of horses, estimated as ~40%, with PPID have evidence of abnormal glucose metabolism, including hyperinsulinemia, hyperglycemia, or both, although only 20% have evidence based on results of an IV glucose and insulin test.[12] Furthermore, horses with PPID do not have abnormalities in glucose metabolism detected during an isoglycemic clamp procedure.[13] It is unclear if the abnormal glucose metabolism and hyperinsulinemia are attributable to PPID or concurrent equine metabolic syndrome, but it is apparent that there should not be an assumption of abnormalities in glucose metabolism in all equids with PPID.

CLINICAL FINDINGS

Affected equids exhibit one or more findings of hirsutism, hyperhidrosis, polyuria, polydipsia, polyphagia, muscle atrophy (sarcopenia), laminitis, and docile demeanor.

Hirsutism is a clinical sign with high specificity (95%) for the disease,[7] meaning that aged equids with hirsutism are likely to have the disease and that there will be few false-positive diagnoses when hirsute aged equids are considered to have PPID. Equids with an owner-reported history of hirsutism are 7.8 times (95% CI, 3.7 to 16.6) more likely to have PPID than are nonhirsute equids of similar age.[8] Hirsutism is characterized by delayed or absent seasonal moulting resulting in a long, shaggy hair coat. There can be some lightening of the coat color. The changes in hair coat are a result of equids with PPID having a greater proportion of hair follicles in the anagen phase (95% of hair follicles on the neck) than healthy equids (15%).[14] Abnormalities of hair follicles resolve and resumption of moulting occurs with administration of pergolide.[14]

Polyuria and polydipsia are common clinical signs in equids with PPID and are likely secondary to diabetes insipidus and not to hyperglycemia.[11] Administration of desmopressin reduces polyuria and polydipsia.[11]

Hyperhidrosis is reported in affected equids, although it does not appear to have been quantified. Equids with PPID in hot environments can be anhidrotic, and this resolves with treatment of the PPID.[15]

Myopathy associated with PPID is characterized by atrophy of type 2 (slow-twitch) fiber types consistent with sarcopenia.[16] Plasma activity of muscle-derived enzymes is not greater in equids with PPID than in healthy aged-matched equids.[16] The molecular basis for muscle atrophy in equids with PPID has been investigated, but the mechanism remains unclear.[17]

There is often central obesity, characterized by excessive fat deposition in the crest of the neck and in the supraorbital fossae, but this is likely a reflection of comorbidity with equine metabolic syndrome rather than a characteristic of PPID. One report demonstrates insulin resistance in equids with PPID using the euglycemic-hyperinsulinemic clamp technique, but this is not a consistent finding.[13,18] However, equids were not screened for hyperinsulinemia before admission to the study and were selected from a population of equids referred for treatment of laminitis, among other diseases. These equids might well have had both equine metabolic syndrome (EMS) and PPID. Further evidence to support this comorbidity is that plasma fructosamine concentrations are not different between nonlaminitic equids with PPID and healthy controls (reference interval of 195.5 to 301.9).[19] Equids with PPID and laminitis have plasma fructosamine concentrations that are higher than those of animals with PPID but not laminitis.[19] Fructosamine is a reflection of average blood glucose concentrations over a period of weeks, and higher values are indicative of hyperglycemia.

Laminitis is common in equids with PPID (see "Laminitis of Horses," Chapter 15).[8] However, it is unclear if this is a result of PPID or comorbidity with EMS.

Rarely, affected equids are blind or have seizures. Affected equids are often infertile and heal poorly. Equids with PPID are considered immunosuppressed and susceptible to development of opportunistic infections and parasitism.[20,21]

Computed tomography allows measurement of the size of the pituitary gland of equids that correlates well with that measured postmortem.[22] The size of the pituitary gland can be evaluated antemortem.

The outcome is favorable in that 50% of equids are alive 4.6 years after diagnosis, most owners are satisfied with the equid's quality of life, and most (28/29; 97%) would treat a second equid with the disease.[3] In a study of cases diagnosed between 1993 and 2002, the cause of death among equids (15/20; 85%) was euthanasia, and 11/15 (73%) were euthanized because of conditions associated with PPID.[3]

CLINICAL PATHOLOGY

There are no characteristic findings on serum biochemical testing or hematology.[8] Resting serum cortisol concentrations of affected and healthy equids are similar and not useful in diagnosis.

DIAGNOSTIC CONFIRMATION

Antemortem diagnosis of PPID is not simple and is achieved on the basis of clinical signs and results of one or more of several diagnostic tests. It is important that testing be based on the presence of clinical signs compatible with the disease to minimize the frequency of false-positive diagnoses. Laboratory tests for the disease are not infallible, and the results of these tests should be viewed only in the context of the equid's clinical signs. Further complicating diagnosis of equine pars intermedia dysfunction is the slow and progressive onset of the disorder. It is therefore likely that attempting a definitive dichotomous answer (disease present or disease absent) based on laboratory testing is unreasonable—some mildly affected equids will test normal, and, less commonly, some apparently healthy equids with histologically normal pituitary glands will test positive. Repeated testing is warranted when test results are ambiguous or not consistent with clinical signs (primarily hirsutism).

Assessment of the utility of the various diagnostic tests is prevented by the lack of a gold-standard diagnosis, except for postmortem examination. Determination of sensitivity and specificity of laboratory tests, or clinical signs, is therefore difficult. Furthermore, antemortem testing is complicated by the seasonal and circadian variations in pituitary function with consequent changes in "resting" or basal serum or plasma concentrations of many analytes. Furthermore, plasma concentrations of some analytes, including ACTH, are affected by feeding.[23] The changes in pituitary function with season are a recognized physiologic phenomenon related to preparing or adapting physiologic functions to colder conditions and shorter days.[10,24-30] This phenomenon was not generally recognized before about 2005, and reports of the characteristics of diagnostics tests before that date should be interpreted with caution.

Laboratory tests used to diagnose pars intermedia dysfunction include measurement of serum or plasma cortisol, ACTH, glucose, or insulin concentrations; the ACTH stimulation test; the thyrotropin-releasing hormone stimulation test; administration of domperidone with subsequent measurement of plasma ACTH; measurement of urinary and salivary corticoid concentrations; and combinations of these tests (Table 17-8). The most widely accepted laboratory tests are the overnight dexamethasone suppression test and measurement of serum ACTH concentration. Other tests have been suggested, but either their sensitivity and specificity have not been determined or they involve measurement of multiple variables or of hormones for which assays are not readily commercially available. Measurement of basal serum insulin concentration is not a useful diagnostic test for equine pars intermedia dysfunction. Measurement of urine or salivary cortisol concentrations has been suggested as a means of diagnosing equine pars intermedia dysfunction, but neither has been validated in a sufficient number of equids to permit assessment of their clinical utility.[31]

One of the first diagnostic tests developed was the **overnight dexamethasone suppression test.**[31] After collection of a serum sample for measurement of cortisol, dexamethasone (40 µg/kg IM) is administered at about 5 p.m. A second blood sample is collected 15 hours later, with the option to collect a third sample 19 hours after dexamethasone administration. Normal horses will have a serum cortisol concentration of less than 1 µg/dL (28 nmol/L) in the second and third blood samples, whereas affected horses will not show a significant reduction in serum cortisol concentration from that of the initial sample. The sensitivity and specificity of this test are apparently high, with both reported in earlier studies to be approximately 100%.[31] However, recent studies of healthy horses demonstrate that there is considerable seasonal variation in the dexamethasone suppression test, with all of 39 healthy aged ponies and horses having normal tests in January (winter) but 10 of the same 39 (26%) having abnormal tests in September (autumn),[31] and that the test is specific but not sensitive.[32] These results suggest that these diagnostic tests should be interpreted with caution when conducted in the autumn.

Measurement of **plasma adrenocorticotropin (ACTH)** concentration has been widely accepted as a useful laboratory indicator of equine pars intermedia dysfunction. The plasma ACTH concentration varies with the age of the horse and with the season

Table 17-8 Diagnostic Testing Methods for Equine pituitary pars intermedia dysfunction (PPID)

Diagnostic test	Procedure	Sample	Interpretation	Comments (also see text)
Overnight DEX suppression	Collect serum between 4 and 6 p.m. Administer DEX at 40 μg/kg BW IM. Collect serum 19–20 hours later.	2 serum samples, 1 mL each; 1 pre-DEX administration and 1 post-DEX administration	Serum control of > μg/dL at 19 hours post-DEX administration suggests PPID.	A mildly decreased resting cortisol (pre-DEX administration) is typical of a PPID-affected horse. A resting cortisol of < 1.8 μg/dL is suggestive of iatrogenic adrenal insufficiency.
Endogenous plasma ACTH concentration	Collect EDTA plasma, preferably in plastic blood-collection tube. Separate plasma by centrifugation, and freeze for submission to laboratory. Avoid hemolysis and heat. Process sample within 8 hours of collection.	EDTA plasma sample, 1 mL	Normal reference range depends on methodology and laboratory. Typically an ACTH concentration < 35 pg/mL (chemiluminescent immunoassay) or < 45–50 pg/mL (radioimmunoassay) is considered normal.	ACTH is likely affected by many biologic events, all of which are not well documented at present. Seasons can have a profound effect, with higher concentrations seen in autumn.
Endogenous plasma α-MSH concentration	Collect EDTA plasma, preferably in plastic blood-collection tube. Separate plasma by centrifugation, and free for submission to laboratory. Avoid hemolysis and heat. Process sample within 8 hours of collection.	1 EDTA plasma sample, 1 mL	Nonautumn reference range: > 35 pmol/L suggests PPID.	Plasma α-MSH concentration is extremely seasonal. High concentrations are observed in autumn.
TRH stimulation assay	Collect serum. Administer TRH, 1 mg IV. Collect serum 30–60 minutes after TRH.	2 serum samples, 1 mL each: pre-TRH administration, 30 minutes post-TRH administration, and 24 hours post-DEX administration	30%–50% increase in serum cortisol 30 minutes after TRH administration suggests PPID.	Pharmaceutical TRH is expensive; TRH compounded for this use may be difficult to obtain. False-positive results may be common.
Combined DEX suppression/ TRH stimulation test	Collect plasma between 8 and 10 a.m. Administer DEX at 40 μg/kg BW IM. Administer TRH, 1 mg IV, 3 hours after DEX administration. Collect serum 30 minutes after TRH and 24 hours after DEX administration.	3 plasma samples, 1 mL each: pre-DEX administration, 30 minutes post-TRH administration, and 24 hours post-DEX administration	Plasma cortisol > 1 μg/dL at 24 hours post-DEX administration or ≥ 66% increase in cortisol levels 3 hours after TRH administration suggests PPID.	Some diagnostic laboratories prefer to use serum for measurement of cortisol levels. The effect of season on the combined test has not been assessed but would likely result in false-positive results as each of the component tests do.
Domperidone response test	Collect EDTA plasma at 8 a.m. Administer domperidone at 3.3 mg/kg BW po. Collect EDTA plasma at 2 and 4 hours after domperidone administration.	3 EDTA plasma samples, 1 mL each	A twofold increase in plasma ACTH concentration suggests PPID.	Higher doses (5 mg/kg po) may improve response. The 2-hour sample is more diagnostic in the summer and autumn, and the 4-hour sample is best in the winter and spring.

Abbreviations: ACTH, adrenocorticotropic hormone; BW, bodyweight; DEX, dexamethasone; IM, intramuscularly; IV, intravenously; THR, thyroid-releasing hormone. (Reproduced, with permission, from McFarlane, D. Vet Clin Equine *2011: 27;93-113. McFarlane D.* Vet Clin North Am Equine Pract. *2011;27:93.)*

of the year in both the northern and southern hemispheres, but not between ponies and horses.[33] The upper reference intervals of plasma ACTH for healthy horses in the United Kingdom in one report were 29 pg/mL between November and July and 47 pg/mL between August and October.[25] The reference intervals were obtained by sampling a convenience sample of hospitalised horses. A similar pattern is detected in the eastern and southern United States, with the autumnal peak in ACTH occurring earlier in horses in more northern locations.[1,24,29,30] This circannual variation in plasma ACTH occurs in both non-PPID and PPID horses, with PPID horses having higher concentrations than non-PPID horses at all times.[10,23,25,26,33,34] Furthermore, the increase in plasma ACTH concentrations stimulated by administration of thyrotropin-releasing hormone (1 mg, IV) to healthy horses is greater in autumn and summer than in late winter.[23,27] These results demonstrate the need for including consideration of season (photoperiod) and latitude when assessing the diagnostic importance of plasma ACTH concentrations in aged horses. It is prudent to use reference intervals developed in local laboratories or in distant laboratories with knowledge of the reference interval for the particular geographic location (latitude) and season of the horse.[30]

There is no circadian rhythm to ACTH concentrations in horses with PPID, but there is conflicting evidence of a circadian rhythm in healthy horses.[10,35,36] It appears that ACTH concentrations of horses are highest at 0800 hours and then decline over the day, although the changes are small and not likely to affect clinical interpretation of plasma ACTH concentrations.[35] There is not an ultradial rhythm (periodic changes during a 24-hour period) in plasma ACTH concentration, although measured concentrations do vary over brief periods of time (minutes) and to a greater extent in horses with PPID.[35]

Fasting and feeding affect plasma ACTH concentrations in healthy horses, with higher concentrations found 2 hours after feeding than after a 12-hour fast (46 vs. 17 pg/mL, respectively).[23]

Measurement of **plasma ACTH** combined with use of seasonally adjusted cutoffs provides good **sensitivity and specificity** for diagnosis of PPID, defined using the presence of hirsutism plus three or more clinical signs as the gold standard.[33] The referenced study was of 325 randomly selected horses 15 years of age or older in Queensland, Australia (approximate latitude 27.5°S). Cutoff values for diagnosis of PPID were 30 pg/mL (sensitivity and specificity of 80% and 82%, respectively) for nonautumn months and 77 pg/mL (sensitivity and specificity of 100% and 95%, respectively) during the autumn. It is important to note that the gold standard for determining the characteristics of the test was a clinical examination. Therefore the sensitivity and specificity reported for measurement of plasma ACTH concentration apply only for horses with characteristic clinical signs of the disease. The usefulness of measuring plasma ACTH concentration in horses that have milder, or nonexistent, clinical signs is unknown. Similarly, the clinical importance of elevated ACTH concentrations in younger horses is unclear, and such results should be considered cautiously and carefully before decisions regarding treatment are made.

Plasma concentrations of α-melanocyte-stimulating hormone (α-MSH) correlate well with plasma ACTH concentrations, and comments about seasonal and horse-related factors affecting ACTH concentrations also apply for α-MSH.[1,10,24,27,33,37]

Plasma ACTH concentrations can be measured before and after administration of **thyrotropin-releasing hormone** or **domperidone**.[37,38] The thyrotropin-releasing hormone test appears to have greater utility than administration of domperidone, with the latter having greater variation. These tests have not been adequately evaluated to recommend at this time.

The combined **dexamethasone suppression/thyroid-releasing hormone (TRH) stimulation** test has reported sensitivity and specificity of 88% and 76%, respectively.[7] The test is performed by administering 40 μg/kg of dexamethasone phosphate (or similar dexamethasone salt) intravenously between 8 a.m. and 10 a.m. Cortisol concentration in serum is then measured 3 hours later, and TRH (1 mg) is administered intravenously. Serum cortisol concentration is measured 30 minutes after TRH administration. Serum cortisol concentrations of healthy horses 30 minutes after TRH administration are unchanged from those at the time of TRH administration, whereas serum cortisol concentrations in horses with equine pars intermedia dysfunction increase by more than 66% of the baseline value.

Plasma **fructosamine** concentrations do not differ between healthy horses (range 195.5 to 301.9 mu mol/L) and horses with PPID.[39] **Plasma insulin** concentrations are increased in a proportion of horses with PPID and are suggested to be indicative of the risk of laminitis in these horses (see discussion of equine laminitis, Chapter 15).[40,41]

NECROPSY FINDINGS

The pituitary gland is usually enlarged as a result of the increased numbers of melanocortin cells comprising an adenoma of the pars intermedia. The adrenal cortices are usually of normal width, but they may be thickened in some cases. With the appropriate clinical history, the observation of a well-defined nodule within the pituitary gland is usually sufficient for confirmation of the diagnosis, but histology and immunohistochemical testing of the mass can be performed. There is only fair (kappa = 34%) agreement among pathologists for histologic diagnosis of the disease.

DIFFERENTIAL DIAGNOSIS

- Insulin resistance
- Diabetes insipidus (nephrogenic)
- Both of these diseases are exceedingly rare in horses
- Obesity
- Psychogenic polydipsia or salt eating
- Chronic renal failure

TREATMENT

Treatment is palliative and not curative in that clinical signs can be controlled by administration of pergolide, but the underlying neurodegenerative disease is not cured. The aim of treatment is to reduce secretion of the products of the melanotropes through the use of dopamine agonists or serotonin antagonists. Treatment must be continued for the life of the horse or pony.

The **treatment of choice** is administration of **pergolide mesylate**, a dopamine agonist, at 1.7 to 5.5 μg/kg orally every 24 hours. The recommended starting dose is 2.0 to 3.0 μg/kg once daily for 2 months, at which time clinical (hirsutism) and laboratory (plasma ACTH concentration) signs of the disease should be evaluated. The dose can be escalated by 1-μg/kg increments until control of clinical signs is achieved.

Pergolide mesylate is rapidly absorbed after oral administration to fasted mares with a time to maximum drug concentration in plasma of 0.4 hours, maximum concentration of 4 ± 2 ng/mL, and terminal elimination half-life estimated to be 5.9 ± 3.4 hours.[43]

Care should be exercised in the storage of pergolide mesylate compounded in an aqueous vehicle because it is susceptible to degradation if exposed to heat, light, or both.[44] Compounded pergolide formulations in aqueous vehicles should be stored in a dark container, protected from light, and refrigerated, and it should not be used more than 30 days after production. Formulations that have undergone a color change should be considered degraded and discarded.[44] A commercial form of pergolide mesylate formulated for use with horses and ponies (Prascend®, Boehringer Ingelheim) is available in some countries.

Cyproheptadine, a serotonin antagonist, is administered at 0.25 mg/kg orally every 24 hours for 1 month. If an acceptable response is achieved, then this dose is continued; if not, then the dose is increased to 0.25 mg/kg every 12 hours. This drug is now rarely used in the treatment of PPID.

Symptomatic treatment should include clipping of the hair coat in spring, treatment of laminitis and wounds, prevention of injuries and infection, and dietary management to reduce hyperglycemia in those animals with this abnormality documented (see "Equine Metabolic Syndrome"), in addition to maintenance of optimal body weight. Some equids with PPID lose weight and require careful nutritional management.

CONTROL

None.

FURTHER READING

Durham AE, McGowan CM, Fey K, Tamzali Y, van der Kolk JH. Pituitary pars intermedia dysfunction: diagnosis and treatment. *Equine Vet Educ.* 2014;26:216-223.

McFarlane D. Equine pars intermedia dysfunction. *Vet Clin North Am Equine Pract.* 2011;27:93-113.

McFarlane D. Pathophysiology and clinical features of pituitary pars intermedia dysfunction. *Equine Vet Educ.* 2014;26:592-598.

REFERENCES

1. McFarlane D, et al. *Dom Anim Endocrin.* 2006;30:276.
2. McFarlane D. *Equine Vet Educ.* 2014;26:592.
3. Rohrbach BW, et al. *J Vet Int Med.* 2012;26:1027.
4. Ireland JL, et al. *Equine Vet J.* 2012;44:101.
5. Ireland JL, et al. *Equine Vet J.* 2011;43:37.
6. McGowan TW, et al. *Aust Vet J.* 2010;88:465.
7. Frank N, et al. *J Vet Int Med.* 2006;20:987.
8. McGowan TW, et al. *Equine Vet J.* 2013;45:74.
9. McFarlane D. *Ageing Res Rev.* 2007;6:54.
10. Cordero M, et al. *Dom Anim Endocrin.* 2012;43:317.
11. Moses ME, et al. *Equine Vet Educ.* 2013;25:111.
12. Gehlen H, et al. *J Equine Vet Sci.* 2014;34:508.
13. Mastro LM, et al. *Dom Anim Endocrin.* 2015;50:14.
14. Innera M, et al. *Vet Dermatol.* 2013;24:212.
15. Spelta CW, et al. *Aust Vet J.* 2012;90:451.
16. Aleman M, et al. *Neuromuscul Disord.* 2006;16:737.
17. Aleman M, et al. *Am J Vet Res.* 2010;71:664.
18. Klinkhamer K, et al. *Vet Quart.* 2011;31:19.
19. Knowles EJ, et al. *Equine Vet J.* 2013;n/a.
20. McFarlane D, et al. *J Vet Int Med.* 2008;22:436.
21. McFarlane D, et al. *JAVMA.* 2010;236:330.
22. Pease AP, et al. *J Vet Int Med.* 2011;25:1144.
23. Diez de Castro E, et al. *Dom Anim Endocrin.* 2014;48:77.
24. Beech J, et al. *JAVMA.* 2009;235:715.

25. Copas VEN, et al. *Equine Vet J.* 2012;44:440.
26. Frank N, et al. *J Vet Int Med.* 2010;24:1167.
27. Funk RA, et al. *J Vet Int Med.* 2011;25:579.
28. Haritou SJA, et al. *J Neuroendocrin.* 2008;20:988.
29. McFarlane D, et al. *J Vet Int Med.* 2011;25:872.
30. Schreiber CM, et al. *JAVMA.* 2012;241:241.
31. Radostits O, et al. *Veterinary Medicine: a Textbook of the Diseases of Cattle, Horses, Sheep, Goats and Pigs.* London: Saunders; 2006:1686.
32. Beech J, et al. *JAVMA.* 2007;231:417.
33. McGowan TW, et al. *Equine Vet J.* 2013;45:66.
34. Lee Z-Y, et al. *Vet J.* 2010;185:58.
35. Rendle DI, et al. *Equine Vet J.* 2013;n/a.
36. Rendle DI, et al. *Equine Vet J.* 2014;46:113.
37. Beech J, et al. *JAVMA.* 2011;238:1305.
38. Beech J, et al. *J Vet Int Med.* 2011;25:1431.
39. Knowles EJ, et al. *Equine Vet J.* 2014;46:249.
40. Walsh D, et al. *J Equine Vet Sci.* 2009;29:87.
41. Durham AE, et al. *Equine Vet Educ.* 2014;26:216.
42. McFarlane D. *Vet Clin North Am Equine Pract.* 2011;27:93.
43. Wright A, et al. *J Vet Int Med.* 2008;22:710.
44. Davis JL, et al. *JAVMA.* 2009;234:385.

EQUINE METABOLIC SYNDROME

SYNOPSIS

Etiology Unknown, but likely involves genetic predisposition for insulin resistance with phenotypic expression permitted or induced by environmental factors that favor obesity.

Epidemiology Associated with obesity and particular breeds, especially ponies. Standardbreds appear to be at reduced risk. No sex predilection. Increasing incidence with age.

Clinical signs Obesity, regional adiposity including cresty neck, predisposition to laminitis.

Clinical pathology Hyperinsulinemia, hypertriglyceridemia, normal blood glucose concentration.

Diagnostic confirmation Demonstration of insulin resistance in presence of clinical signs of equine metabolic syndrome. Measurement of serum insulin and plasma or blood glucose concentrations. Requires validated insulin assay.

Treatment Weight loss, which can be difficult to achieve. Exercise. Potentially administration of insulin sensitizing drugs (metformin).

Control Maintenance of optimal body condition and prevention of obesity.

Equine metabolic syndrome (EMS) is a recently recognized condition of equids characterized by increased regional adiposity (localized deposition of fat) or generalized obesity, hyperinsulinemia, hypertriglyceridemia, insulin resistance, and a predisposition to laminitis that develops in the absence of other known inciting factors (such as colic, metritis, or acute carbohydrate overload).[1] Insulin resistance is defined as abnormally depressed insulin-mediated glucose transport into insulin-sensitive cells (adipose tissue, skeletal muscle). EMS is the clinical syndrome, whereas insulin resistance in an underlying metabolic abnormality.

ETIOLOGY

EMS likely has important genetic determinants, with manifestation of the syndrome when susceptible animals, by virtue of their genetic composition, are exposed to environmental conditions that favor or enable development of the disease. This is thought to be similar to the situation with human metabolic syndrome or type 2 diabetes. It is speculated that breeds of equids that evolved under conditions of frequent restriction of energy intake, such as during long winters, are genetically predisposed to have efficient energy metabolism that under modern management systems can result in obesity and development of insulin resistance.[1,2]

EPIDEMIOLOGY

The epidemiology of EMS is not well described, and there are few studies that have identified the frequency of the condition, using established case definitions, in large numbers of horses or ponies. Consequently, there is little evidence on outcome (morbidity, case-fatality rates, all-cause morbidity, specific-cause mortality) in horses and only anecdotal information on breed, age, and sex as risk factors. Twenty seven percent (51/188) of ponies of various breeds examined in Australia were hyperinsulinemic (>20 mu/mL) after ponies with documented PPID (see previous section) were excluded.[3] There is somewhat more information regarding the epidemiology of obesity in horses, but it should be recognized that not all obese horses are insulin resistant (and therefore do not fit the definition of EMS).[4,5] Similarly, there is information on the epidemiology of pasture-associated (endocrinopathic) laminitis (see "Laminitis of Horses," Chapter 15), and from this one can infer risk factors for insulin resistance and EMS.

Horses or ponies of different breeds but similar body weight differ in their insulin resistance, and there is consensus that particular **breeds** are at increased risk of EMS; these include ponies (of any of the common breeds), Morgan Horses, Paso Fino, Andalusian, Arabian, Saddlebred, Quarter Horses, Tennessee Walking Horses, and Warmblood Horses.[1,2] It appears that some light breeds such as Standardbreds and perhaps Thoroughbreds are at reduced risk. The frequency of the condition increases with age in ponies,[3] and sex does not appear to be a risk factor.

There is a **seasonality** to the occurrence of pasture-associated laminitis,[6] and this might represent seasonal changes in energy intake (from pasture) of susceptible animals rather than seasonal variations in severity of insulin resistance. However, there is evidence that measures of insulin resistance in horses and/or ponies vary depending on season, with declines in insulin sensitivity of ponies in summer.[7] Insulin sensitivity, defined using the combined insulin and glucose intravenous test, and serum insulin concentrations are not related to season in healthy, mature horses.[8,9]

Obesity is common in domestic horses, with studies in Scotland and the eastern United States finding that 45% and 19%, respectively, of horses were considered obese.[10,11] Although interpretation of both studies is limited by the localized nature of the sampling and restrictions on the types of horses included, these studies do support a wider consensus that obesity is common in horses. Chronic intake of energy in excess of maintenance needs (overeating) and insufficient exercise are thought to be risk factors, or inciting factors, for obesity.

PATHOGENESIS

EMS is primarily a manifestation of insulin resistance, and insulin resistance is often, but not always, associated with obesity. The syndrome likely includes abnormalities in energy metabolism, adipocyte function, hemostasis (thrombosis), inflammation, response to lipopolysaccharide (endotoxin) exposure, and oxidant stress.[1,12] The pathogenesis of laminitis associated with EMS ("endocrinopathic laminitis") is discussed elsewhere.

Insulin resistance is the decreased rate of transport of glucose into cells of glucose-sensitive tissues in response to exposure to insulin. Horses with insulin resistance have lesser reductions in blood glucose concentration in response to administration of insulin than do insulin-sensitive horses.[13,14] Insulin-stimulated glucose transport is achieved by GLUT-4 (glucose transporter protein 4, which is one of at least 12 glucose transporter proteins) when it is present on the surface of adipose or muscle tissue. Insulin causes the relocation of GLUT-4 within the cell to the cell plasma membrane and subsequent increases in rate of glucose transport into the cell. Horses with insulin resistance have abnormal glycemic and insulinemic responses to oral or IV administration of glucose or oral administration of sugar (see following discussion) and have reduced concentrations of GLUT-4 on the surface of skeletal muscle and adipose tissue.[15-17] Insulin resistance in horses is associated with an exaggerated response in plasma/serum insulin concentration after administration of glucose. This exaggerated response allows maintenance of resting blood glucose concentrations in the reference range in affected horses—so-called compensated insulin resistance.[1]

Insulin resistance in humans is currently thought linked to inflammation induced by macrophage activation in adipose tissue, and there is increasing evidence of a similar mechanism in equids.[18] The BCS of horses is also correlated with both plasma insulin concentration and serum amyloid A concentration (an acute-phase protein indicative of inflammation).[19] There are only minimal effects of insulin infusion (6-hour duration) on tumor necrosis factor alpha and interleukin(IL)-6 concentrations in the plasma of healthy horses,[20] and no association has been found between BCS or insulin concentration and plasma concentrations of tumor necrosis factor and IL-6.[19] Horses with EMS have prolonged inflammatory responses (evidenced by plasma IL-8, IL-10 and tumor necrosis factor concentrations) to infusion of endotoxin compared with healthy horses,[12] although the clinical importance of this observation is unclear. Horses with EMS have a marked increase in neutrophil reactive oxygen species production induced by phagocytosis that is strongly correlated to the blood insulin concentration.[21] In contrast, peripheral blood cells of obese hyperinsulinemic horses showed decreased endogenous proinflammatory cytokine gene expression (IL-1 and IL-6) and similar cytokine response following immune stimulation compared with that of control horses. The authors conclude that this could suggest that, unlike in people, cytokine-mediated inflammation does not increase in direct response to obesity or insulin resistance in horses.[21]

Mechanisms underlying obesity and regional adiposity are unclear, but at the most fundamental level involve an excess of energy intake over energy expenditure, with deposition of the net excess energy as fat. As discussed previously, some horses and ponies appear to be much more efficient at converting feed into energy, or at regulating energy use, with the result that it is challenging to achieve a reduction in the weight of these animals even with strict control of food intake.[22] The genetic or hormonal causes of this resistance to weight loss are unclear, although it is apparent that some horses and ponies have an exaggerated insulinemic response to ingestion of soluble carbohydrate.[2,17,23] This exaggerated response could be the underlying mechanism for hyperinsulinemia, obesity or regional adiposity, and endocrinopathic laminitis.[24]

Adipose tissue is an important source of hormones regulating energy metabolism and of inflammatory cytokines. Obesity, or "overconditioning," in horses (as assessed by BCS) is associated with higher plasma insulin and leptin concentrations than in optimally conditioned horses.[25,26] Obese horses also have higher triglyceride concentrations and lower red blood cell glutathione peroxidase activities (an indication of antioxidant capacity) than optimally conditioned horses.[27]

Regional obesity is an important risk factor in humans for metabolic syndrome and might be similarly so in horses and ponies. Visceral fat is important in humans, but it appears to be less so in horses, with nuchal ligament fat (which contributes to the cresty neck characteristic of affected horses and ponies) having greater proinflammatory gene expression (IL-1β and IL-6) in affected horses,[28] although others, using measurement of other markers of inflammation, find that the omental and retroperitoneal (visceral) fat of insulin-resistant horses have greater expression of markers of inflammation (Toll-like receptor 4 and suppressor of cytokine signaling 3 [SOCS-3]) than do insulin-sensitive horses.[18] Finally, there is evidence of regional differences in glucose transport by adipose tissue, with omental adipose tissue having the highest total GLUT content compared with subcutaneous and nuchal ligament fat in healthy horses, but having a reduced total GLUT4 content and cell surface expression in insulin-resistant horses.[16]

CLINICAL SIGNS

Equine metabolic syndrome is defined by obesity (with or without regional adiposity), insulin resistance, and increased susceptibility to laminitis. As such, only obesity and regional adiposity and clinical signs of active or past laminitis are physical evidence of the presence of metabolic syndrome. Affected ponies can be hypertensive.[5,7]

Clinical assessment of obesity/adiposity is achieved by use of body-condition scoring, measurement of subcutaneous or retroperitoneal fat by ultrasound, and grading of regional adiposity. Methods used for research studies include slaughter and dissection with proximate analysis of body constituents or measurement of the deuterium dilution space (volume of distribution) in living animals.[29,30] Bioelectrical impedance can be used to measure body-water content, but it has not achieved widespread clinical acceptance.[31] Measurement of body weight is not useful for assessment of obesity or adiposity because body weight is highly correlated with height and girth and does not provide an accurate indication of body fat.[32]

A number of body-condition scoring systems have been developed, and the two most commonly used are those of Henneke (later modified by various authors), which uses a 1-to-9 grading system (Table 17-9 and Fig. 17-7), and Carroll and Huntington, which uses a 1-to-5 grading system.[33,34] These grading systems were not developed to assess the fat content (proportion) of horses, but rather to assess "flesh" or the general body condition. Both systems have limitations, including their subjective nature and the fact that they have not been validated in all breeds and body types of horses (validation determines the relationship between BCS and a gold-standard measure of body fat, such as deuterium dilution space or carcass analysis), nor has their reliability (intrarater and interrater agreement/repeatability expressed as an intraclass correlation coefficient or, less optimally, a kappa or weighted-kappa statistic) been demonstrated over large numbers of raters. There are reports of an intraclass correlation coefficient (ICC) of 0.74 for four raters of 21 mares and 75 ponies, but details are not provided.[35] Another reports an ICC of 0.92, but without details to allow assessment of the methodology.[25] Additionally, body-condition scoring systems do not provide an assessment of regional adiposity, which might have greater clinical relevance.

BCS (1-to-9 scale) correlates well with percent body fat (TBF) when both are log transformed ($e^{TBF} = 0.006 + e^{1.56*BCS}$).[32] In practical terms, this means that the accuracy of this body-condition scoring system to predict the proportion of body fat declines as BCS increases—for example, the proportion of body fat varies from ~13% to 36% in horses with a BCS of 7 to 8/9.[32] The log-log BCS model correctly predicted body fat greater than 20% (BCS = 6.83) in 76% of horses and with sensitivity of 83% and specificity of 71%.[32] However, the need to use log-log transforms decreases the general utility of this technique.

Body-condition scoring is a demonstrably insensitive measure of changes in body fat—ponies subject to 11% reduction in body weight and a 45% reduction in body fat did not have a change in BCS.[36,37] This indicates that the BCS system (1-to-9 scale) has some utility in assessment of body-fat proportion in horses and ponies, but it should be used with a full awareness of its limitations.

The BCS correlates well with plasma concentrations of glucose tolerance, insulin sensitivity, and insulin, leptin, and triglyceride concentrations in horses or ponies,[5,19,35] all of which could be clinically important.

A grading system for assessment of regional adiposity evident as a "cresty neck" has been developed for use with ponies and horses.[35] The ICC (a measure of reliability between raters) is 0.70 for four raters of 21 mares and 75 ponies.[35] The "cresty neck score" correlates well with plasma insulin and glucose concentrations in pooled horse and pony data, and with insulin, leptin, glucose, and triglyceride concentrations when horses and ponies are considered separately. Additionally, ponies with a cresty neck score of 4 or greater are at increased risk of developing pasture-associated laminitis.[39] This scoring system therefore appears to be both reliable (good interrater agreement) and indicative of clinically meaningful variables and outcomes (Table 17-10).

Acute laminitis and residual signs of laminitis (sometimes call chronic laminitis) are common in animals with insulin resistance and provide the physical confirmation of EMS in these animals. Clinical signs of laminitis are described under that topic (Chapter 15).

Diagnosis

Definitive diagnosis of EMS of horses in the field is achieved by demonstration of insulin resistance in equids with appropriate clinical signs (obesity, regional adiposity, laminitis) and is confirmed by measurement of plasma concentrations of glucose and insulin.[1]

Table 17-9 Criteria for estimating body condition in light-breed horses

Score	Condition	Description
1	Poor	Animal is extremely emaciated. Spinous processes (parts of vertebrae that project upward), ribs, tailhead, hooks (tuber coxae; hip joints), and pins (tuber ischia; lower pelvic bones) projecting prominently. Bone structure of withers, shoulders, and neck easily noticeable. No fatty tissue can be felt.
2	Very thin	Animal is emaciated. Slight fat covering over base of the spinous processes, transverse processes (portions of vertebrae that project outward) of lumbar (loin area) vertebrae feel rounded. Spinous processes, ribs, tailhead, hooks, and pins are prominent. Withers, shoulders, and neck structures are faintly discernible.
3	Thin	Fat is built up about halfway on spinous processes; transverse processes cannot be felt. Slight fat cover over ribs. Spinous processes and ribs are easily discernible. Tailhead is prominent, but individual vertebrae cannot be visually identified. Hook bones appear rounded, but are easily discernible. Fat can be felt around tailhead (prominence depends on conformation). Hook bones are not discernible. Withers, shoulders, and neck are not obviously thin.
4	Moderately thin	Negative crease along back (spinous processes of vertebrae protrude slightly above surrounding tissue). Faint outline of ribs is discernible. Fat can be felt around tailhead (prominence depends on conformation). Hook bones are not discernible. Withers, shoulders, and neck are not obviously thin.
5	Moderate	Back is level. Ribs cannot be visually distinguished, but can be easily felt. Fat around tailhead begins to feel spongy. Withers appear rounded over spinous processes. Shoulders and neck blend smoothly into body.
6	Moderately fleshy	May have slight crease down back. Fat over ribs feels spongy. Fat around tailhead feels soft. Fat begins to be deposited along at sides of the withers, behind shoulders, and along neck.
7	Fleshy	May have crease down back. Individual ribs can be felt, but with noticeable filling of fat between ribs. Fat around tailhead is soft. Fat is deposited along withers, behind shoulders, and along neck.
8	Fat	Crease down back. Difficult to feel ribs. Fat around tailhead is very soft. Area along withers is filled with fat. Area behind shoulder is filled with fat and flush with rest of the body. Noticeable thickening of neck. Fat is deposited along inner thighs.
9	Extremely fat	Obvious crease down back. Patchy fat appears over ribs. Bulging fat around tailhead, along withers, behind shoulders, and along neck. Fat along inner thighs may rub together. Flank is filled with fat and flush with rest of the body.

Based on Henneke et al. (1983) Henneke DR, et al. Equine Vet J. *1983;15:371 and reproduced with permission. Carter RA, et al. In: Geor RJ, et al., eds.* Equine Applied and Clinical Nutrition. *W.B. Saunders; 2013:393.*

Table 17-10 Grading system for assessing regional adiposity in the neck of ponies and horses

Score	Description
0	No visual appearance of a crest (tissue apparent above the ligamentum nuchae). No palpable crest.
1	No visual appearance of a crest, but slight filling felt with palpation.
2	Noticeable appearance of a crest, but fat deposited fairly evenly from poll to withers. Crest easily cupped in one hand and bent from side to side.
3	Crest enlarged and thickened, so fat is deposited more heavily in middle of the neck than toward poll and withers, giving a mounded appearance. Crest fills cupped hand and begins losing side-to-side flexibility.
4	Crest grossly enlarged and thickened and can no longer be cupped in one hand or easily bent from side to side. Crest may have wrinkles/creases perpendicular to topline.
5	Crest is so large it permanently droops to one side.

Insulin resistance can be detected by use of measurement of insulin and glucose concentrations in a single blood sample (point testing) or by more sophisticated testing using measurement of these analytes on multiple occasions after administration of glucose and insulin to equids (dynamic testing)—either as the euglycemic clamp technique or the frequently sampled intravenous glucose and insulin test (minimal model).[40-42] The former has greater utility in clinical and field settings, although with the potential for reduced sensitivity and/or specificity, whereas the latter is useful for research or referral settings and is regarded as the gold standard for diagnosis.

Hyperglycemia is rarely detected in equids with insulin resistance, and measurement of blood glucose concentrations alone is not a useful test for detection of insulin resistance.[1] Detection of persistent, inappropriate hyperglycemia (i.e., that not associated with stress or ingestion of food) should prompt consideration of diabetes mellitus.[43]

Hyperinsulinemia in the absence of conditions that increase insulin secretion (stress, pain, feeding) is strong evidence of the presence of insulin resistance.[1] Interpretation of plasma or serum insulin concentration must include consideration of a number of factors that could affect the actual concentration reported by the laboratory. Physiologic factors that can increase serum insulin concentration include feeding, stress and pain, and administration of alpha-2 adrenergic agonists (xylazine, detomidine, romifidine, etc.). Feeding increases plasma insulin concentration in both healthy and insulin-resistant horses and confounds interpretation of the results of testing. Pain and stress increase both plasma glucose and insulin concentrations through increases in cortisol and epinephrine concentrations in blood, which decrease insulin sensitivity.[44] This could be important when testing equids with active laminitis or other causes of pain—evaluation should be delayed until the pain is resolved.[1]

Point testing of plasma glucose and insulin concentrations should be performed under controlled conditions and ideally after 6 hours of feed withholding and preferably with sampling between 8 and 10 a.m.[1] Horses can be fed a small amount of hay with a low content of nonstructural carbohydrates the night before testing (approximately 2 kg of hay per 500-kg horse) and then nothing immediately before testing.[1]

Laboratory factors can influence the insulin concentration reported for a blood sample. This is primarily a result of differences in testing methodology returning different concentrations for the same blood sample.[45] Until recently, most testing for equine insulin involved use of kits or testing methodology designed for use with human samples, taking advantage of the

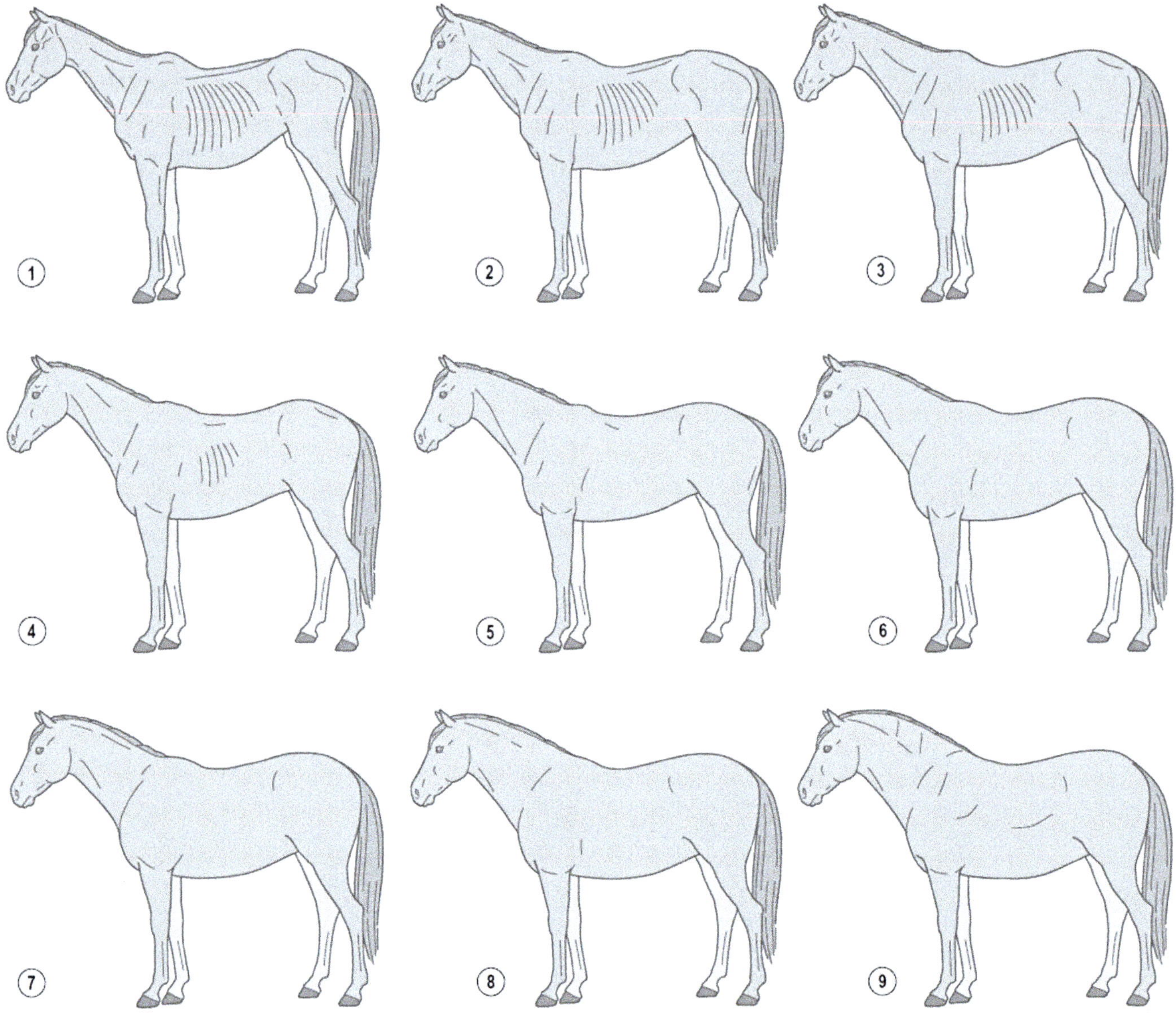

Fig. 17-7 Appearance of light-breed horses at each of the body-condition scores described by Henneke et al. (1983). Henneke DR, et al. *Equine Vet J.* 1983;15:371. (Reproduced with permission from Carter RA, et al. In: Geor RJ, et al., eds. *Equine Applied and Clinical Nutrition.* W.B. Saunders; 2013:393.)

considerable cross-reactivity between human and equine insulin. Equine-specific tests are now available, and their precision, accuracy, and specificity have been reported.[45] The gold-standard methodology is liquid chromatography–mass spectrometry (LC-MX), but this is expensive and has limited accessibility in laboratories processing large numbers of clinical samples. Analysis of six commonly used or available test kits for measuring plasma or serum concentrations of insulin demonstrated that none reflected concentrations measured by LC-MS and that only one provided reliable (valid) results—the Siemens Coat-a-Count Insulin Radioimmunoassay (RIA)—and only if samples with concentrations exceeding the highest standard were diluted with charcoal-stripped plasma and not the provided diluents.[45]

The effect of use of differing methods of measuring serum insulin concentration is that use of "cutoff" values for detecting insulin resistance provided by different laboratories is problematic. A value of 20 μU/mL is recommended as a cutoff, measured using the Siemens Coat-a-Count Insulin RIA, for defining insulin resistance.[1] However, this value should be interpreted with caution because the sensitivity (proportion of false negatives) and specificity (proportion of false positives) are not reported, and the test as a way of defining insulin resistance has not been well validated. It can be a useful screening test.[1] Local laboratories should be contacted before testing to determine the test used and whether the laboratory has determined reference ranges for its testing methodology.

Proxy indicators of insulin resistance, derived from measurement of plasma glucose and insulin concentrations, have been proposed and used to define insulin resistance and predict predisposition to laminitis in ponies.[7,40,41,46] A commonly used proxy is the RISQI:

$$RISQI = insulin\ concentration^{-0.5}$$

where lower values of the RISQI indicate lower insulin sensitivity.

Dynamic testing is usually achieved using combined glucose and insulin challenge tests of varying complexity.[1,41] One of these tests measures the insulin and glucose responses to IVs administration of glucose (150 mg/kg BW) and insulin (0.10 U/kg) with frequent sampling of blood (immediately before and at 1, 5, 15, 25, 35, 45, 60, 75,

90, 105, 120, 135, and 150 minutes after infusion).[1,5] Blood glucose concentrations of insulin-sensitive horses return to baseline values within 45 minutes of infusion of glucose. Insulin-resistant horses have a delayed decline of blood glucose concentrations and an exaggerated increase in plasma/serum insulin concentrations.[1,5] A more complex test, involving the frequent sampling of blood and delayed administration of insulin, is analyzed using the "minimal model" and yields four measures of insulin sensitivity, glucose disposal, and insulin secretion (pancreatic response).[41]

Dynamic testing can also involve the administration of insulin and monitoring of blood (plasma) glucose concentrations.[13,14] More complex testing involves the IV administration of increasing doses of insulin (either bovine or human recombinant) and measurement of blood glucose concentrations at defined times. The dose of insulin required to achieve a 50% reduction in blood glucose concentration is then used as the diagnostic index. This test is cumbersome and has a high risk of inducing hypoglycemia and is therefore of limited clinical utility.[13] A modified test involves administration of 0.1 U/kg IV of recombinant human insulin and measurement of blood glucose concentrations immediately before and 30 minutes after.[14] Insulin-sensitive horses (n = 6 in the study) all had a 50% or greater reduction in blood glucose concentrations 30 minutes after insulin administration, whereas none of the insulin-resistant horses (n = 6) had this response. The sensitivity and specificity of this test need to be determined in larger numbers of healthy and insulin-resistant horses for it to be clinically useful.

An oral sugar test (OST) provides results as reliable as the IV glucose tolerance test for detection of insulin resistance and hyperinsulinemia. The test involves oral administration of 0.15 mL/kg of corn syrup (approximately 150 mg/kg BW of dextrose-derived digestible sugars) to equids after an overnight fast. Plasma insulin and glucose concentrations are measured immediately before and 30, 60, and 90 minutes after administration of corn syrup. Equids with EMS have higher glucose and insulin concentrations than do unaffected horses.[17]

CLINICAL PATHOLOGY

Clinical pathology includes detection of hyperinsulinemia (as noted in the previous discussion), hyperleptinemia, hypertriglyceridemia, and normoglycemia. Plasma ACTH concentrations of horses with EMS are within the reference range for healthy horses, noting that horses with EMS might also have PPID.

NECROPSY

Affected horses are usually examined postmortem because of laminitis. Other than signs of laminitis and obesity/regional adiposity, there are no other characteristic lesions. The pancreas is normal.

> **DIFFERENTIAL DIAGNOSIS**
>
> - Obesity without insulin resistance
> - Pituitary pars intermedia dysfunction
> - Laminitis of cause other than EMS (systemic septic disease such as colitis or metritis)

TREATMENT

The objective of treatment is to improve the insulin sensitivity of affected equids. This can be achieved by reducing the proportion of the body made up of fat through careful dietary control. Administration of insulin-sensitizing drugs is attracting interest, but has yet to be of clearly demonstrated clinical utility.

Dietary Management

The fundamental aims of dietary management are as follows:

- Achieve and maintain an ideal BCS (body weight, noting earlier comments that body weight does not indicate body composition).
- Minimize intake of nonstructural carbohydrates because these induce an insulinemic and hyperglycemic response in EMS-affected equids and at-risk animals.[1]
- Ensure an adequate and balanced intake of essential nutrients.

The ideal BCS of ponies has been much mentioned, but little or seldom defined. The ideal body condition for a pony or horse would be one at which it has insulin sensitivity within the reference range (i.e., is not insulin resistant), has plasma triglyceride concentrations within the reference range, and is not at increased risk of laminitis. There is likely no one BCS that meets all of these criteria for all equids, and each animal must be considered in light of its own circumstances and physiology. Monitoring of measures of insulin resistance and plasma triglyceride concentration would provide guidance in achieving the animal's ideal, or acceptable, body weight.

Achieving and maintaining an acceptable BCS (as a proxy for proportion of body fat) is not easy.[47] Animals at most risk of obesity and regional adiposity are often metabolically equipped to maintain this body condition, and reducing body weight or BCS might not be as simple as just reducing feed intake.[22]

Recommendations for reduction in feed intake suggest that feeding 1.25% of body weight daily as hay is adequate to achieve a gradual reduction in body weight. However, planning a diet to provide a reduction in body weight while ensuring an adequate intake of essential nutrients and providing for the digestive and psychological health of the horse or pony can be challenging.

An initial step must be to eliminate or severely reduce access to pasture. Pasture provides unregulated access to fodder, and ponies can consume 2% to 5% of their body weight in pasture each day. This will result in weight gain. Additionally, pasture, and especially green pasture, has a high content of nonstructural carbohydrates (glucose, starch) that induces a glycemic and hyperinsulinemia response in ponies and susceptible horses. Access to pasture can be eliminated by housing animals on a dry lot or by fitting a grazing muzzle.

Hay can be fed as 1.25% to 1.5% of body mass as dry matter per day. The nonstructural carbohydrate content of the hay should be reduced by soaking it in cold water for 12 to 16 hours before feeding. The water used to soak the hay should not be provided to the horse or pony. Feeding this diet will induce a reduction in body weight and improvement in indices of insulin sensitivity.[22,37,48,49] Individual horses and ponies can be resistant to weight loss, and a reduction in daily dry matter intake to 1% of body weight might be needed to achieve loss of body weight. However, restriction of intake to this level can cause behavioral changes, such as eating bedding, chewing tails of companions, and other allotriophagia. An early example of dietary restriction inducing allotriophagia was that of Robert Falcon Scott's use of ponies in an expedition to reach the South Pole. The ponies displayed profound appetite for roughage as a consequence of their highly concentrated ration.

Supplements including chromium have been promoted as improving insulin sensitivity in horses. There is evidence that they are not effective, and there is no evidence of efficacy.[50]

Exercise

Exercise increases the insulin sensitivity of horses,[51] and it appears sensible to recommend an increase in the amount of exercise of obese ponies and horses.[1] However, moderate exercise training does not improve the insulin sensitivity of horses.[52] Moderate exercise by nonobese ponies previously affected with laminitis reduced serum amyloid A concentrations, heptoglobin concentrations, and postexercise serum insulin concentrations.[53] These results suggest a beneficial role for relatively low-intensity exercise (10 minutes enforced walking followed by 5 minutes of trotting) in reducing inflammation in ponies at risk of laminitis.

Medications

Administration of levothyroxine or metformin has been advocated for treatment of EMS.[1,54,55] Levothyroxine (0.1 mg/kg orally q24 h) causes weight loss and improves insulin sensitivity in obese horses and is recommended as an adjunct to dietary management.[55]

Metformin, which is used for treatment of type 2 diabetes in people, has been administered to horses in an attempt to improve insulin sensitivity. Although initial reports were favorable,[56] more recent pharmacologic investigation has not demonstrated its efficacy at a dosage of 15 mg/kg orally q12h in improving insulin sensitivity.[54,57-59] However, administration of metformin at 30 mg/kg q12h reduced glycemic and insulinemic responses of healthy horses and horses with dexamethasone-induced insulin resistance to administration of dextrose.[60] Whether this dosage will be effective in horses or ponies with naturally occurring insulin resistance remains to be determined.

Pioglitazone has been investigated in healthy horses, in which it does not improve insulin sensitivity (at 1 mg/kg q24h for 12 days) or attenuate the effects of endotoxin infusion on indicators of systemic inflammation.[61,62] The pharmacokinetics of pioglitazone in horses have been reported.[63]

FURTHER READING

Frank N, Tadros EM. Insulin dysregulation. *Equine Vet J.* 2014;46:103-112.

Frank N, et al. Equine metabolic syndrome. *J Vet Int Med.* 2010;24:467-475.

REFERENCES

1. Frank N, et al. *J Vet Int Med.* 2010;24:467.
2. Bamford NJ, et al. *Dom Anim Endocrin.* 2014;47:101.
3. Morgan RA, et al. *Aust Vet J.* 2014;92:101.
4. Treiber KH, et al. *JAVMA.* 2006;228:1538.
5. Frank N, et al. *JAVMA.* 2006;228:1383.
6. Menzies-Gow NJ, et al. *Vet Rec.* 2010;167:690.
7. Bailey SR, et al. *Am J Vet Res.* 2008;69:122.
8. Funk RA, et al. *J Vet Int Med.* 2012;26:1035.
9. Place NJ, et al. *J Vet Int Med.* 2010;24:650.
10. Thatcher CD, et al. *J Vet Int Med.* 2012;26:1413.
11. Wyse CA, et al. *Vet Rec.* 2008;162:590.
12. Tadros EM, et al. *Am J Vet Res.* 2013;74:1010.
13. Caltabilota TJ, et al. *J Anim Sci.* 2010;88:2940.
14. Bertin FR, et al. *Dom Anim Endocrin.* 2013;44:19.
15. Waller AP, et al. *J Vet Int Med.* 2011;25:315.
16. Waller AP, et al. *Biochim Biophys Acta.* 2011;1812:1098.
17. Schuver A, et al. *J Equine Vet Sci.* 2014;34:465.
18. Waller AP, et al. *Vet Immunol Immunopathol.* 2012;149:208.
19. Suagee JK, et al. *J Vet Int Med.* 2013;27:157.
20. Suagee JK, et al. *Vet Immunol Immunopathol.* 2011;142:141.
21. Holbrook TC, et al. *Vet Immunol Immunopathol.* 2012;145:283.
22. Argo CM, et al. *Vet J.* 2012;194:179.
23. Borer KE, et al. *J Anim Sci.* 2012;90:3003.
24. Bailey SR, et al. *Anim Prod Sci.* 2013;53:1182.
25. Carter RA, et al. *Am J Vet Res.* 2009;70:1250.
26. Ungru J, et al. *Vet Rec.* 2012;171:528.
27. Pleasant RS, et al. *J Vet Int Med.* 2013;27:576.
28. Burns TA, et al. *J Vet Int Med.* 2010;24:932.
29. Dugdale AHA, et al. *Equine Vet J.* 2011;43:552.
30. Dugdale AHA, et al. *Equine Vet J.* 2011;43:562.
31. Latman NS, et al. *Res Vet Sci.* 2011;90:516.
32. Dugdale AHA, et al. *Vet J.* 2012;194:173.
33. Carroll CL, et al. *Equine Vet J.* 1988;20:41.
34. Henneke DR, et al. *Equine Vet J.* 1983;15:371.
35. Carter RA, et al. *Vet J.* 2009;179:204.
36. Dugdale AHA. *Equine Vet J.* 2011;43:121.
37. Dugdale AHA, et al. *Equine Vet J.* 2010;42:600.
38. Carter RA, et al. In: Geor RJ, et al., eds. *Equine Applied and Clinical Nutrition.* W.B. Saunders; 2013:393.
39. Carter RA, et al. *Equine Vet J.* 2009;41:171.
40. Kronfeld D. *J Equine Vet Sci.* 2006;26:281.
41. Kronfeld DS, et al. *JAVMA.* 2005;226:712.
42. Firshman AM, et al. *Equine Vet J.* 2007;39:567.
43. Durham AE, et al. *Equine Vet J.* 2009;41:924.
44. Tiley HA, et al. *Am J Vet Res.* 2007;68:753.
45. Tinworth KD, et al. *Dom Anim Endocrin.* 2011;41:81.
46. Borer KE, et al. *Equine Vet J.* 2012;44:444.
47. Frank N, et al. *Equine Vet J.* 2014;46:103.
48. McGowan CM, et al. *Vet J.* 2013;196:153.
49. Schmengler U, et al. *Livestock Sci.* 2013;155:301.
50. Chameroy KA, et al. *Equine Vet J.* 2011;43:494.
51. Stewart-Hunt L, et al. *Equine Vet J.* 2010;42:355.
52. Carter RA, et al. *Am J Vet Res.* 2010;71:314.
53. Menzies-Gow NJ, et al. *Equine Vet J.* 2013;n/a.
54. Durham AE. *Vet J.* 2012;191:17.
55. Frank N, et al. *Am J Vet Res.* 2005;66:1032.
56. Durham AE, et al. *Equine Vet J.* 2008;40:493.
57. Tinworth KD, et al. *Vet J.* 2012;191:79.
58. Tinworth KD, et al. *Vet J.* 2010;186:282.
59. Tinworth KD, et al. *Am J Vet Res.* 2010;71:1201.
60. Rendle DI, et al. *Equine Vet J.* 2013;45:751.
61. Wearn JG, et al. *Vet Immunol Immunopathol.* 2012;145:42.
62. Suagee JK, et al. *J Vet Int Med.* 2011;25:356.
63. Wearn JMG, et al. *J Vet Pharmacol Ther.* 2011;34:252.

PHEOCHROMOCYTOMA (PARAGANGLIOMA)

Pheochromocytomas are unusual tumors of domestic animals and occur in cattle, sheep, and horses.[1-5] A pheochromocytomas is a neuroendocrine tumor of chromaffin cells of the adrenal medulla or extraadrenal chromaffin tissue. The tumor secretes catecholamines; in humans, clinical signs are related to elevated concentrations of circulating epinephrine or norepinephrine. The clinical presentation in horses usually involves intermittent or acute colic or hemoabdomen. Horses can die acutely of exsanguination into the abdomen from ruptured tumor.[2] Affected horses can be persistently or intermittently tachycardic with excessive or untimely sweating. The mass can be palpable near the left kidney or imaged by transrectal ultrasonography.[2,6] The normal right adrenal gland cannot be imaged transrectally in a horse.[6] The disease in cattle and sheep is usually detected at postmortem examination and has no real economic impact, with the exception of the rare valuable bull affected.[5] The disease can occur as part of multiple endocrine neoplasia, but is usually solitary, although gangliomas can metastasise.[7] Antemortem diagnosis can be confirmed by measuring high concentrations of metanephrine and vanillylmandelic acid, both of which are metabolites of catecholamines, in blood or urine. There is no effective treatment, nor are there control measures.

REFERENCES

1. Aydogan A, et al. *Rev Med Vet.* 2012;163:536.
2. Elsar N, et al. *Israel J Vet Med.* 2007;62:53.
3. Germann SE, et al. *Vet Rec.* 2006;159:530.
4. Nielsen AB, et al. *J Comp Pathol.* 2012;146:58.
5. Seimiya YM, et al. *J Vet Med Sci.* 2009;71:225.
6. Durie I, et al. *Vet Radiol Ultrasound.* 2010;51:540.
7. Herbach N, et al. *J Comp Pathol.* 2010;143:199.

GLYCOGEN BRANCHING ENZYME DEFICIENCY IN HORSES

Glycogen branching enzyme deficiency (GBED) is a fatal condition of fetuses and neonatal foals of the Quarter Horse, Paint Horse, and associated breeds.[1] The disease is caused by a nonsense mutation in codon 34 of the *GBE1* gene, which prevents the synthesis of a functional GBE protein and severely disrupts glycogen metabolism.[1] The mutant GBE1 allele frequency in registered Quarter Horse, Paint Horse, and Thoroughbred horses is reported as 0.041, 0.036, and 0.000, respectively.[2] Among 651 elite-performance American Quarter Horses, 200 control American Quarter Horses, and 180 control American Paint Horses, the GBED allele was detected with an overall frequency of 0.054.[3] GBED is inherited as a simple recessive trait from a single founder.[2] The disease is reported in North America and Germany.[4]

Affected foals are aborted, born dead, or affected at birth. It is estimated that up to 2.5% of fetal and early neonatal deaths in Quarter Horses and related breeds are associated with this defect.[2] Foals that are born alive are weak and hypothermic, some have flexural limb deformities, and all die usually within hours to days of birth.[5] Affected foals have refractory hypoglycaemia and minor elevations in serum activity of creatine kinase.

The disease is confirmed by detection of periodic acid–Schiff (PAS)-positive inclusions in the cardiac or skeletal muscle and genotype analysis. There is no effective treatment, and control is by selective and prudent breeding.

REFERENCES

1. Ward TL, et al. *Mamm Genome.* 2004;15:570.
2. Wagner ML, et al. *J Vet Int Med.* 2006;20:1207.
3. Tryon RC, et al. *JAVMA.* 2009;234:120.
4. Winter J, et al. *Pferdeheilkunde.* 2013;29:165.
5. Finno CJ, et al. *Vet J.* 2009;179:336.

LACTATION TETANY OF MARES (ECLAMPSIA, TRANSPORT TETANY)

Lactation tetany of mares is caused by hypocalcemia and is characterized by abnormal behavior progressing to incoordination and tetany. The precise cause of the hypocalcemia has not been determined, but the cause of the clinical signs is a marked reduction in serum concentration of ionized calcium. The effect of feeding diets high in calcium, such as alfalfa hay, during late pregnancy, and of abrupt changes in diet after parturition, have not been investigated in horses as they have in cattle (see discussion of milk fever).

The disease was most common when draft-horse breeding was widely practiced, but it is uncommon now.[1] The case fatality rate is high in untreated animals. Most cases occur in lactating mares, either at about the 10th day after foaling or 1 to 2 days after weaning. High-producing mares grazing on lush pasture are most susceptible and in many instances are engaged in hard physical work. The housing of wild ponies or prolonged transport can precipitate an episode. The latter has been a particularly important factor in the etiology of the disease in Britain and has been credited with precipitating it even in stallions and dry mares. Occasional cases occur without there being any apparent cause. The disease has occurred in a 20-year-old gelding pony. Hypocalcemia with clinical signs also occurs in horses used for prolonged exercise, such as endurance racing or 3-day events.

Hypocalcemia occurs in other diseases of horses, including colic and colitis, and as a result of hypoparathryoidism.[2,3]

Many mild cases of lactation tetany that recover spontaneously occur after transport, but the case fatality rate in some shipments can be greater than 60%. Mares that develop the disease at the foal heat or at weaning are usually more seriously affected, and the case fatality rate is high if mares are not treated in a timely fashion.

Severely affected animals sweat profusely and have difficulty moving because of tetany of the limbs and incoordination. The gait is stiff, and the tail is slightly raised. Rapid, labored respirations and wide dilatation of the nostrils are often accompanied by synchronous diaphragmatic flutter ("thumps") evident as a distinct thumping sound from the thorax. Muscular fibrillation, particularly of the masseter and shoulder region, and trismus are evident, but there is no prolapse of the membrana nictitans. Affected animals are not hypersensitive to sound, but handling can precipitate increased tetany. The temperature is normal or slightly elevated, and although the pulse is normal in the early stages, it later becomes rapid and irregular. The mare might make many attempts to eat and drink but appears to be unable to swallow, and passage of a stomach tube can be difficult. Urination and defecation are in abeyance, and peristalsis is reduced.

Within about 24 hours the untreated mare becomes recumbent; tetanic convulsions develop and become more or less continuous. The mare dies about 48 hours after the onset of illness. The tetany and excitement in the early stages suggest tetanus, but there is no prolapse of the third eyelid, and there is the usual relationship to recent foaling or weaning and physical exertion. The anxiety and muscle tremor of laminitis can be confused with those of lactation tetany, especially when it occurs in mares that have foaled and retained the placenta. Pain in the feet and bounding digital pulses are diagnostic features of this latter disease.

Hypocalcemia occurs with serum concentrations in the range of 4 to 6 mg/dL (1 to 1.50 mmol/L), and the degree of hypocalcemia has been related to the clinical signs. When serum calcium levels are higher than 8 mg/dL (2 mmol/L), the only sign is increased excitability. At levels of 5 to 8 mg/dL (1.25 to 2 mmol/L), there are tetanic spasms and slight incoordination. At levels of less than 5 mg/dL (1.25 mmol/L), there is recumbency and stupor. It is the concentration of ionized calcium that is important, and some animals, such as horses used for 3-day events, can have normal total calcium concentrations but abnormally low ionized calcium concentrations as a result of changes in acid:base status. If possible, serum concentrations of ionized calcium should be measured in horses with clinical signs suggestive of hypocalcemia. Hypomagnesemia with serum magnesium levels of 0.9 mg/dL (0.37 mmol/L) has been observed in some cases, but only in association with recent transport. Hypermagnesemia has been reported in other cases.

Treatment by IV administration of calcium borogluconate as recommended in the treatment of parturient paresis in cattle results in rapid, complete recovery. The dose for a 500-kg mare is 300 to 500 mL of a 25% solution of calcium borogluconate or gluconate administered slowly (over 15 to 30 min) intravenously. One of the earliest signs of recovery is the voiding of a large volume of urine. Occasional cases that persist for some days have been recorded.

REFERENCES

1. Radostits O, et al. Lactation tetany of mares. In: *Veterinary Medicine: a Textbook of the Diseases of Cattle, Horses, Sheep, Goats and Pigs.* 10th ed. London: W.B. Saunders; 2006:1651.
2. Borer KE, et al. *Equine Vet Educ.* 2006;18:320.
3. Durie I, et al. *J Vet Int Med.* 2010;24:439.

EQUINE HYPERLIPEMIA

SYNOPSIS

Etiology Abnormal energy metabolism secondary to inadequate caloric intake.

Epidemiology Pregnant or lactating middle-aged, overweight ponies, donkeys, and American miniature horses. Worldwide. Sporadic.

Clinical signs Depression, anorexia, weight loss, ventral edema, muscle fasciculation, mania, recumbency.

Clinical pathology Hypertriglyceridemia (triglyceride > 500 mg/dL, 5 mmol/L).

Necropsy findings Widespread lipidosis, swollen liver, hepatic rupture.

Treatment Increase energy intake through enteral or parenteral feeding. Treat underlying disease.

Control Maintain optimal body condition. Prevent disease and nutritional stress, including changes in diet and prolonged transportation.

ETIOLOGY

The potentially life-threatening disease hyperlipemia is associated with hyperlipidemia (an abnormal concentration of lipids in blood) in equids. The disease is a result of a derangement in fat metabolism secondary to nutritional stress and, in particular, inadequate energy intake.[1]

Hyperlipemia is the clinical syndrome of depression, weakness, and ventral edema with high blood concentrations of triglycerides and hepatic lipidosis. It carries a high case-fatality rate. A related condition is the detection of hypertriglyceridemia associated with an overt, severe, primary disease (colic, neoplasia, endocrine disease) in which the triglyceridemia likely has minimal clinical importance. Hyperlipemia has its greatest importance as a disease of ponies and donkeys in field situations and related to relatively minor inciting causes.

EPIDEMIOLOGY

Occurrence

Hyperlipemia occurs worldwide. Although its occurrence is sporadic, multiple cases can occur on a farm when there are a number of at-risk animals exposed to the same inciting factor, such as lack of adequate grazing or supplementary feeding. The annual incidence of the disease in ponies in southeastern Australia is 5%, and it is 2% to 10% in donkeys in the United Kingdom.[2] The case-fatality rate is 40% to 80%, although it appears to be less in hospitalized equids provided more focused care.[2,3] Incidence varies with season and locality; the disease in ponies in Europe occurs most commonly during late gestation (January–March), whereas in southern Australia, the disease is more common in ponies during early lactation (November–January).

Animal Risk Factors

Hyperlipemia can occur in any breed of horse or pony and in donkeys, but it is more common in ponies and donkeys.[2,3] Any breed of equid can develop hypertriglyceridemia as a result of a primary disease, but development to the clinical condition lipemia is most common in ponies, miniature horses, miniature donkeys, and donkeys. The disease is considered most common in females, uncommon in pony stallions and geldings, and rare in foals. Most affected ponies are more than 4 years old, and the peak incidence occurs in 9-year-olds. Hypertriglyceridemia occurs in foals secondary to other diseases.[3-5]

Risk factors for hyperlipemia (triglyceride concentration ≥ 4.4 mmol/L) in 449 donkeys with the disease from a population of 3829 donkeys included concurrent disease (odds ratio [OR] 77, 95% confidence interval [CI], 45 to 129), weight loss in previous month (OR = 6.4, 3.6 to 11.3), relocation to a new site (farm) (OR = 3.9, 1.3 to 12), dental disease (OR = 1.7, 1.1 to 2.8), history of inappetence (OR = 3.2, 1.3 to 7.9), and increasing age (OR = 1.26, 1.1 to 1.45).[2]

Horses and ponies with primary endocrine disease, including pituitary pars intermedia dysfunction (PPID) or suspected diabetes mellitus and conditions associated with insulin resistance, can have marked elevations in serum triglyceride concentrations (10.5 to 60.3 mmol/l) without evident clinical signs attributable to hypertriglyceridemia. The hypertriglyceridemia resolves with successful treatment of the underlying endocrine disease.[6]

Pregnancy and lactation increase the risk of the disease in ponies, but not in donkeys. The disease in miniature horses is always associated with underlying disease, such as colic, which is apparently an important risk factor. Underlying disease is identified in 50% of cases in ponies and 72% of affected donkeys;[2] however, many cases occur in pregnant or lactating pony mares without evidence of other disease.

Overweight ponies and donkeys are at increased risk, and insulin resistance is likely a risk factor for the disease.[7] Onset of disease is often preceded by some sort of stress, typically transport, lactation, food deprivation, or a combination of these factors. Characteristically the disease occurs in fat, middle-aged, pregnant, or lactating ponies that experience a decrease in feed intake. However, the disease is not restricted to this demographic, and horses or thin ponies can develop the disease.

Hypertriglyceridemia is detected in horses with evidence of systemic inflammatory response syndrome (severe illness associated with decreased feed intake). There is no opacity of the plasma or serum, and the hypertriglyceridemia has not been demonstrated to worsen the outcome of the underlying disease.

PATHOGENESIS

The combination of the innate insulin resistance of ponies and a nutritional stressor, such as disease, pregnancy, lactation, or food deprivation, results in excessive mobilization of fatty acids from adipose tissue at a rate that exceeds the gluconeogenic and ketogenic capacity of the liver.[1] Adipocytes of ponies, in response to norepinephrine, release fatty acids at a rate 6.5 times greater than those of horses, possibly providing at least a partial explanation for the difference in likelihood of differing breeds developing the disease. Lipolysis is mediated by β_2-adrenergic receptors in ponies and horses. The induction of excessive fat mobilization in ponies is likely associated with the well-characterized insulin resistance of this breed, especially in obese individuals. There is no difference between ponies and horses in the extent to which lipolysis is inhibited by insulin. The effect of insulin resistance on glucose uptake from the blood might be exacerbated in sick ponies by the increase in serum cortisol concentrations associated with stress or disease.

Equids have little propensity to produce ketones, and thus the excess fatty acids are reesterified in the liver to triglycerides and released into the circulation as very low-density lipoproteins (VLDLs). The **fundamental defect** in the disease is in the regulation of free fatty acid release from fat stores as a result of a defect in control of hormone-sensitive lipase, the enzyme responsible for hydrolysis of triglycerides to free fatty acids and glycerol in adipose tissue. Unchecked activity of this enzyme results in mobilization of fatty acids in hyperlipemic ponies that is 40 times the rate in normal ponies. There is no dysfunction of lipoprotein lipase, the enzyme mediating uptake of plasma free fatty acids by extrahepatic tissues, and its activity can be 300% of that of unaffected ponies.

Hyperlipidemia causes widespread lipidosis and organ dysfunction. Hepatic lipidosis compromises liver function, resulting in accumulation of toxic metabolites and derangement in coagulation.

CLINICAL FINDINGS

The clinical course varies between 3 and 22 days but is generally 6 to 8 days. The unchecked disease progresses from mild depression and inappetence; through profound depression, weakness, and jaundice; to convulsions or acute death in 4 to 7 days. Depression, weight loss, and inappetence are the initial signs in 90% of cases. Approximately 50% of cases have fasciculation of muscles of the limb, trunk, or neck. Ventral edema unrelated to parturition occurs in approximately 50% of cases. Inappetence progresses to anorexia and depression, which is followed by somnolence and hepatic coma. Compulsive walking or mania develops in 30% of cases. Signs of mild colic, including flank watching, stretching, and rolling, are evident in 60% of cases. The incidence of jaundice is variable. Many animals show a willingness to drink, but they are unable to draw water into the mouth and swallow. Others continually lap at water. The temperature is normal or moderately elevated, and heart rate and respiratory rates are increased above normal. Diarrhea is an almost constant feature in the terminal stages.

Visual examination of the plasma or serum phase of a blood sample collected from an affected animal reveals cloudy, milky, mildly opalescent plasma.

CLINICAL PATHOLOGY

There is usually leukocytosis with neutrophilia. Hyperlipidemia is a consistent feature of the disease. Serum triglyceride concentrations will be at least 5 mmol/L (500 mg/dL) and can be much higher. Serum cholesterol and free fatty acid concentrations are also increased, although less so than triglycerides. The plasma triglyceride concentration is of minimal prognostic use in ponies, but most American miniature horses with triglyceride concentrations above 1200 mg/dL (12 mmol/L) die.

Plasma glucose concentration is usually low. Ketonemia and ketonuria do not occur. Biochemical evidence of liver disease is characteristic of the advanced disease. Serum activity of gamma-glutamyltransferase (GGT) can be elevated before clinical signs of disease are apparent. Serum creatinine and urea nitrogen concentrations increase as renal function declines. Blood clotting time increases. Metabolic acidosis develops terminally. Hematologic and biochemical variables can also be affected by any underlying disease.

Diagnostic confirmation of hyperlipemia is achieved by demonstration of hyperlipidemia (plasma triglyceride concentrations above 5 mmol/L [500 mg/dL]) in a horse with appropriate clinical signs.

The utility of point-of-care (stall-side) analyzers has been investigated, and both units performed adequately, although not perfectly.[8,9] The upper operating range of both units (~6.0 mmol/L) was lower than values for triglycerides in severely affected animals, which limits their usefulness, although it does allow identification of equids with very high concentrations. The instruments have coefficients of variation for measurement of the same sample of 10% to 16%, which limits their usefulness in monitoring responses to treatment. These analyzers are useful for field measurement of triglyceride concentrations in equids, but care should be taken in evaluating values that exceed the range of the instrument.

NECROPSY FINDINGS

Extensive fatty change is present in most internal organs, but especially in the liver, which is yellow to orange, swollen, and friable. Liver rupture with intraabdominal hemorrhage may be present. Tissue pallor as a result of lipid accumulation is also prominent in the kidney, heart, skeletal muscle, and adrenal cortex. Serosal hemorrhages of the viscera reflect disseminated intravascular coagulation. The necropsy should also include an examination for lesions that might predispose the animal to hyperlipidemia, such as pancreatic damage or laminitis. Histologically, widespread microvascular thrombosis and intracellular lipid in various tissues are evident.

Samples for Postmortem Confirmation of Diagnosis

Samples for postmortem diagnosis include formalin-fixed liver, kidney, heart, adrenal, skeletal muscle, and pancreas for light microscopic examination.

> **DIFFERENTIAL DIAGNOSIS**
>
> - Parasitism
> - Anemia
> - Liver disease, including pyrrolizidine toxicosis
> - Serum hepatitis
> - Aflatoxicosis
>
> Hyperlipemia should be considered in any pony with a history of weight loss, inappetence, and progressive somnolence, especially in late pregnancy or early lactation.

TREATMENT

- The principles of treatment are as follows:
- Treatment of the underlying or inciting disease
- Restoration and maintenance of a positive energy balance
- Correction of any defects in hydration, acid–base, and electrolyte status
- Reduction of the hyperlipidemia

Every effort should be made to determine whether there is an underlying disease, and if so, it should be treated aggressively. Parasitism is a common inciting disease, as are equine Cushing's disease and neoplasia (lymphosarcoma, gastric squamous cell carcinoma) in older ponies.

The negative energy balance must be corrected. A mature, nonpregnant, and nonlactating 200-kg (440-lb) pony has energy requirements (digestible energy intake) of 9.3 Mcal/d (38 mJ/d), whereas a lactating pony has energy requirements of 13.7 Mcal/d (57.2 mJ/d). Affected animals should be encouraged to eat and must be supplemented either orally or intravenously if they will not eat a sufficient quantity. Supplements, either oral or IV, are unlikely to meet all the animal's energy requirements, but normalization and stabilization of blood glucose concentrations, and the apparent consequent changes in hormonal milieu, inhibit lipolysis and enhance clearance of triglycerides from plasma and hepatic and renal tissues.

Oral supplementation using commercial equine or human enteral nutrition preparations has been successful for treatment of the disease in American miniature horses and donkeys. If these products are not available, a homemade gruel consisting of alfalfa pellets and cottage cheese can be used. These preparations are administered every 6 hours through a nasogastric tube. Alternatively, glucose can be given orally (1 g/kg, as 5% solution every 6 hours, about 5 L to a 250-kg pony) or intravenously (5% solution, 100 mL/kg per day as a continuous IV infusion). As noted earlier, this dose of glucose will not meet the energy needs of the pony, but it might be sufficient, along with treatment of the underlying disease and supportive care, to restore normal fat metabolism. Provision of parenteral nutrition is feasible and apparently effective, but expensive and technically demanding, thereby restricting its use to veterinary hospitals.[10,11]

Mares in late pregnancy can be aborted, and lactating mares should have the foal removed.

Dehydration and abnormalities in electrolyte and acid–base status should be corrected by oral or IV administration of isotonic fluids (lactated Ringer's solution) and, if necessary, sodium bicarbonate.

Encephalopathy associated with liver failure should be treated with oral neomycin (20 mg/kg, every 6 hours) or lactulose (1 mL/kg, every 6 hours).

Hyperlipidemia should be reduced by minimizing free fatty acid production by adipose tissue and enhancing triglyceride removal from plasma. Free fatty acid production is minimized by ensuring adequate energy intake and normal plasma glucose concentrations. Use of insulin and heparin has been recommended for reduction of plasma free fatty acid concentration. However, the efficacy of these treatments is not clear, and the emphasis should be placed on provision of adequate energy intake rather than administration of these hormones. Insulin (protamine zinc insulin) is administered at 0.1 to 0.3 IU/kg SC every 12 to 24 hours. Blood glucose concentrations should be monitored, and the insulin dose may need to be adjusted. Heparin (40 to 100 IU/kg SC every 6 to 12 hours) can be given to increase lipoprotein lipase activity and promote the clearance of triglycerides from plasma. It should be noted that lipoprotein lipase activity is not deficient in affected ponies, and therefore the administration of heparin to ponies with hyperlipemia is not recommended. Severely affected ponies may have an increase in clotting time that could be exacerbated by heparin.

Corticosteroids and adrenocorticotropic hormone are contraindicated in treatment of this disease.

CONTROL

A mature, nonpregnant, and nonlactating 200-kg (440-lb) pony has energy requirements of 9.3 Mcal/d (38 mJ/d), whereas a lactating pony has energy requirements of 13.7 Mcal/d (57.2 mJ/d), and every effort should be made to meet these requirements. This might require dietary supplementation during periods of nutritional stress, such as drought, late pregnancy, peak lactation, or transportation. Ponies should be maintained in optimal body condition, and nutritional stress should be avoided. A parasite and disease control program should be instituted. Transport of pregnant and lactating ponies should be avoided.

FURTHER READING

Hughes KJ, et al. Equine hyperlipemia: a review. *Aust Vet J.* 2004;82:136.

McKenzie HA. Equine hyperlipidemias. *Vet Clin North Am Equine Pract.* 2011;27:59.

REFERENCES

1. Radostits O, et al. Equine hyperlipemia. In: *Veterinary Medicine: a Textbook of the Disease of Cattle, Horses, Sheep, Goats and Pigs.* 10th ed. London: W.B. Saunders; 2006:1678.
2. Burden FA, et al. *J Vet Int Med.* 2011;25:1420.
3. Waitt LH, et al. *JAVMA.* 2009;234:915.
4. Armengou L, et al. *J Vet Int Med.* 2013;27:567.
5. Ollivett TL, et al. *Equine Vet J.* 2012;(suppl):96.
6. Dunkel B, et al. *Equine Vet J.* 2014;46:118.
7. Oikawa S, et al. *J Vet Med Sci.* 2006;68:353.
8. Naylor RJ, et al. *Vet Rec.* 2012;170:228B.
9. Williams A, et al. *Equine Vet Educ.* 2012;24:520.
10. Durham AE. *Vet Rec.* 2006;158:159.
11. Magdesian KG. *Equine Vet Educ.* 2010;22:364.

Disorders of Thyroid Function (Hypothyroidism, Hyperthyroidism, Congenital Hypothyroidism, Thyroid Adenoma)

Disorders of thyroid function as a result of abnormalities in the thyroid gland, pituitary gland, or hypothalamus are uncommon in the domestic species and are best documented for the horse. Thyroid disorders secondary to excessive or inadequate intake of iodine or selenium deficiency are discussed under those headings. Animals with low concentrations of thyroid hormones, usually total T3 and total T4, in blood could have nonthyroidal illness syndrome, which is well described in humans and dogs.[1] Furthermore, neonates have lower concentrations of thyroid hormones in blood than do adults, and premature neonates have even lower concentrations.[2]

ETIOLOGY

Disorders of thyroid function result in hypothyroidism or hyperthyroidism.[3] Hypothyroidism can result from diseases of the thyroid gland (primary hypothyroidism), pituitary gland (secondary hypothyroidism as a result of reduced secretion of thyroid-stimulating hormone), or hypothalamus (tertiary hypothyroidism, decreased thyrotropin [thyroid-releasing hormone] secretion). Autoimmune thyroiditis has not been described in horses. Lymphocytic thyroiditis occurs in goats. Consumption of propylthiouracil (4 mg/kg body weight orally once daily for 4 to 6 weeks) induces hypothyroidism in adult horses. Administration of trimethoprim-sulfadiazine (30 mg/kg orally q24 h for 8 weeks), which can induce hypothyroidism in humans and dogs, does not impair thyroid function of most horses. Systemic illness, such as sepsis, or starvation can alter function of the hypothalamic–pituitary–thyroid axis, resulting in euthyroid sick syndrome, more recently termed nonthyroidal illness syndrome. The syndrome has been documented in adult horses[1] and in foals with septic and nonseptic illnesses.[2,4,5]

Hereditary congenital hypothyroidism secondary to defects in thyroglobulin production occurs in sheep, goats, and Afrikander cattle. The disease is inherited as an autosomal-recessive trait. The cause of congenital hypothyroidism in foals is uncertain, although ingestion of nitrates by the pregnant dam is strongly suspected. Partial thyroidectomy of equine fetuses results in birth of foals with clinical and pathologic characteristics similar to those in the spontaneous disease.

Hyperthyroidism in horses is attributable to functional adenocarcinoma or adenoma of the thyroid gland, but most thyroid tumors are not functional.[6-8]

EPIDEMIOLOGY

The frequency with which hypothyroidism occurs in adult horses is unknown. It is relatively common practice to administer thyroid hormone or iodinated casein to fat horses; to those with laminitis, rhabdomyolysis, or anhidrosis; or to enhance fertility, but documentation of abnormal thyroid function in these animals is rare. None of 79 clinically normal brood mares had an abnormal response to thyroid-stimulating hormone administration, indicating that hypothyroidism is uncommon in this type of animal. Importantly, horses with nonthyroid-related illness often have low concentrations of thyroid hormones in the blood without evidence of thyroid dysfunction—this is referred to as the euthyroid sick or nonthyroidal illness syndrome and is not indicative of thyroid disease.

Abnormalities of the thyroid gland were detected in 12% of 1972 **goats** examined in India. Of thyroid glands examined from 1000 goats in India, 2.4% had colloid goiter, 39% had parenchymatous goiter, 1.8% had lymphocytic thyroiditis, and 2.1% were fibrotic.

Congenital hypothyroidism in foals occurs in western Canada and the western and northern United States. One survey of necropsy records of almost 3000 equine fetuses and neonatal foals in western Canada found that 2.7% had histologic evidence of thyroid and musculoskeletal abnormalities consistent with congenital hypothyroidism. Congenital hypothyroidism occurs in Dutch goats, Merino sheep, and Afrikander cattle. Hypothyroidism is reported in an East Friesian ram.

Hyperthyroidism is a sporadic disease of older horses for which other risk factors are not identified.

Exercise and participation in endurance racing or competitive show jumping usually, but not always, influences serum concentrations of thyroid hormones, but is not considered a pathologic process.[9,10] The response depends on the type and intensity of exercise—endurance exercise (40 to 420 km) reduces plasma concentrations of T3 and T4 at the end of the race, with return to basal concentrations by 24 hours.[11] Serum T4 concentrations are lower in overtrained or malconditioned young Standardbred horses.[12]

Thyroid tumors are common in older horses, with ~50% having adenomas evident on histologic examination of the thyroid gland. The clinical course of such tumors is benign, although their size can be quite impressive. Thyroid adenocarcinoma is much less common but has a malignant course.[6-8]

Fetal undernutrition of lambs during late gestation adversely affects postnatal thyroid function and causes hyperthyroidism as adult sheep.[13]

CLINICAL FINDINGS

Clinical characteristics of hypothyroidism in adult horses are poorly defined, largely because of the difficulty of confirming the diagnosis and the pharmacologic effect of exogenous thyroid hormones. Clinical abnormalities anecdotally attributed to hypothyroidism include exercise intolerance, infertility, weight gain, maldistribution of body fat, agalactia, anhidrosis, and laminitis, among others. Peripheral neuropathy and keratitis sicca (secondary to facial nerve dysfunction) responsive to levothyroxine administration has been reported in a horse.[14] Definitive association of these clinical syndromes with abnormalities of thyroid function is lacking.

Thyroidectomy of horses causes a reduction in resting heart rate and body temperature, docility, decreased food intake, increased cold sensitivity, dull hair coat, and delayed shedding of hair. Blood and plasma volumes of horses increased after removal of the thyroid glands. Effects of thyroidectomy were reversed by administration of thyroxine, with the exception of blood and plasma volume that did not return to euthyroid values. Thyroidectomized horses did not become obese or develop laminitis.

Induced hypothyroidism in goats is evident as a loss of body weight, facial edema, weakness, profound depression, and loss of libido.

Congenitally hypothyroid foals have a prolonged gestation but are born with a short and silky hair coat, soft and pliable ears, difficulty in standing, lax joints, and poorly ossified bones. The foals are referred to as dysmature. Characteristic musculoskeletal abnormalities include inferior (mandibular) prognathism, flexural deformities, ruptured common and lateral extensor tendons, and poorly ossified cuboidal bones.

Horses with **hyperthyroidism** are tachycardic, display cachexia, and have hyperactive behavior. There is usually detectable enlargement of the thyroid gland both on physical examination and on scintigraphic imaging.

Thyroid adenomas are evident as a unilateral nonpainful enlargement of the thyroid gland of older (>15 years) horses and are detectable on scintigraphic examination.[15] Ultrasonographic and scintigraphic imaging of the thyroid gland of healthy horses is described.[16] Thyroid adenocarcinoma presents as metastatic disease with both local and distant spread. Some affected horses have signs of hyperthyroidism, although this is unusual.[6]

Anhidrosis in horses is not associated with abnormal thyroid function.[17]

CLINICAL PATHOLOGY

Hematologic abnormalities in hypothyroid horses are not well documented. Induced hypothyroidism in horses causes increases in serum concentrations of VLDLs, triglycerides, and cholesterol, and decreased concentrations of NEFAs. Induced hypothyroidism in goats caused hypoglycemia, hypercholesterolemia, and anemia. Hypothyroidism in a ram caused hypercholesterolemia.

Thyroid Hormone Assays

Assays are available for measurement of serum concentrations of T3, T4, free T4 (fT4), free T3 (fT3; radioimmunoassay or equilibrium dialysis), and/or TSH in various species.[18-20] Values of each of these analytes vary depending on the method of analysis, physiologic status of the animal, and administration of other compounds (Table 17-11). Serum concentrations of thyroid hormones are high at birth and decline with age in ruminants and nonruminants.[5,21,22] For example, serum T3 concentrations of weaned Thoroughbred foals declined from 2.89 to 0.29 nmol/L at 7 and 9 months of age, serum T4 concentrations from 100.17 to 21.77 nmoL at 1 month and at 10 months, serum fT3 concentrations were 6.96 and 1.50 pmol/L at 1 month and 4 months of age, and serum fT4 concentrations were 31.40 and 4.93 pmol/L at 1 month and 9 months of age.[22]

There are statistically significant **diurnal variations** in serum concentrations of T3 and T4 in adult horses, with the lowest concentrations observed during the early morning hours, likely coincident with the time at which metabolic rate is lowest (Table 17-8). There is not a seasonal variation in thyroid hormone concentrations in horses.[23] **Feed restriction** for 3 to 5 days lowers serum concentrations of T3, T4, and fT4 in horses by 24% to 42%. Administration of **phenylbutazone** decreases concentrations of fT4 (measured by equilibrium dialysis) and T4 by 4 days of treatment, which can persist for up to 10 days after discontinuation of phenylbutazone. The decrease in T4 is suggested

Table 17-11 Serum or plasma concentrations of thyroid hormones and thyroid-stimulating hormone in foals, horses, donkeys, and cattle

Physiologic status	Serum or plasma tT3	Serum or plasma tT4	fT4	TSH
Age				
Birth (<10 hours)	991 ng/dL 12.8 ± 7.4 mmol 366 ± 222 ng/L	28.8 µg/dL 493 ± 58 nmol/L 13.3 ± 5.1 µg/dL	12.1 ng/dL	
1–3 days	940 ng/dL	28.0 µg/dL	12.1 ng/dL	
4 days	935 µg/dL 7.8 ± 4.2 mmol	11.2 µg/dL 232 ± 61 nmol/L	5.9 ng/dL	
5–11 days	631 µg/dL	7.45 µg/dL	3.30 ng/dL	
20 days	4.2 ± 0.9 mmol	36.7 ± 17.4 nmol/L		
22–90 days	192 µg/dL	2.57 µg/dL	1.76 µg/dL	
28 days	3.1 ± 0.4 mmol	30.6 ± 17.4 nmol/L		
1.5–4 months	193 ± 9 ng/dL	4.02 ± 0.19 µg/dL		
2–5 years	120 ± 8 ng/dL	2.9 ± 0.1 µg/dL		
6–10 years	86 ± 7.5 ng/dL	1.7 ± 0.1 µg/dL		
11–25 years	84 ± 9 ng/dL	1.6 ± 0.1 µg/dL		
Adult mares and geldings	0.99 ± 0.51 nmol/L	12.9 ± 5.6 nmol/L	12.2 ± 3.5 pmol/L (RIA)	0.39 ± 0.30 ng/mL
Adult mares and geldings		19 (17.6–22.1) nmol/L	11 (10.5–11.8) pmol/L (RIA)	
Adult mares and geldings		19 (17.6–22.1) nmol/L	22 (20.9–25.1) pmol/L (ED)	
Adult geldings, 16.00 hours	53.2 ± 12.4 ng/dL	2.43 ± 0.81 µg/dL		
Adult geldings, 04.00 hours	42.0 ± 11.5 ng/dL	1.79 ± 0.63 µg/dL		
Adult horses	1.02 ± 0.16 nmol/L	19.9 ± 1.7 nmol/L	11.6 ± 0.7 pmol/L	
Adult horses[25]	47.7 (32.7–62.8) pg/mL (mean, range)	1.64 (0.37–3.2) ug/dL (mean, range)	0.23 (0.12–0.34) ng/dL (mean, range)	
Sex				
Mare	89.9 ± 7.9 ng/dL	1.7 ± 0.1 µg/dL		
Gelding	92.9 ± 9.7 ng/dL	1.69 ± 0.1 µg/dL		
Stallion	123 ± 9.7 ng/dL	1.97 ± 0.2 µg/dL		
Broodmare (not pregnant)	62 ± 2.7 ng/dL	1.47 ± 0.47 µg/dL		
Donkeys[25]	67 (40–130) pg/mL (mean, range)	3.5 (.057–8.1) ug/mL (mean, range)	0.44 (0.14–0.85) ng/dL (mean, range)	
Adult cattle		64 (31–97) nmol/L		
Beef cattle[18]		Mean ± 2 SD		
Dairy cattle[18]		56 (25–91) nmol/L Mean ± 2 SD		1.3–15.5 µU/mL (2.5%–97.5% range) 1.3–9.2 µU/mL (2.5%–97.5% range)
Calves[18]	5.06 (2.02–16.1) nmol/L Mean ± 2 SD	241 (84–283) nmol/L Mean ± 2 SD		7.3 (1.3–19.7) µU/mL (2.5–97.5% range)
Disease				
Calves				
Goiter	0.43 (0.65–17.3) nmol/L (2.5%–97.5% range)	13 (13–348) nmol/L (2.5%–97.5% range)		47.4 (25.3–80.0) nmol/L (2.5%–97.5% range)
Horses				
Induced hypothyroidism (PTU)		4 (1–10) nmol/L	4.5 (1.5–13) pmol/L (RIA)	
Induced hypothyroidism (PTU)			8 (1–20) pmol/L (ED)	
Euthyroid sick horses		2 (2–24) nmol/L	5 (2–13) pmol/L (RIA)	
Euthyroid sick horses			19 (4–48) pmol/L (ED)	

ED, equilibrium dialysis; fT4, free T4; RIA, radioimmunoassay; SD, standard deviation; TSH, thyroid-stimulating hormone; tT3, total T3; tT4, total T4.
Mean ± SD or median (95% confidence interval).
To convert µg/dL to nmol/L for T4 or fT4, multiply by 12.87.
To convert ng/dL to nmol/L for fT3 or T3, multiply by 0.0154.
fT4 determined by RIA or ED. PTU, propylthiouracil

to be attributable to displacement of T4 from protein binding sites by phenylbutazone, but this does not explain the decrease in fT4. Topical application twice daily of 50 g of an ointment containing 17 mg/100g of **dexamethasone-21-acetate** (daily application of 17 mg dexamethasone) suppressed serum T3 and T4 concentrations during 10 days of treatment and for at least 20 days after cessation of treatment.[24] The clinical significance of phenylbutazone-induced decreases in thyroid hormones is uncertain, but should be considered when assessing thyroid function in horses.

Plasma concentrations of fT3, tT3, rT3, fT4, and tT4 of **donkeys** differs with the age of the donkey and from that of adult horses (Table 17-11).[25] Donkeys less than 5 years of age have higher serum fT3, tT3, rT3, fT4, and tT4 than older donkeys.[25]

Because of the number of analytical and physiologic factors that affect serum thyroid hormone concentrations, values considered normal vary considerably, as illustrated by the finding that 44 of 79 clinically normal nonpregnant broodmares had serum T4 concentrations below the reference range, although responses to TRH were normal. This example illustrates the need to determine reference ranges based on the methodology used and with well-defined definition of the physiologic state of the animals being tested.

Diagnosis of hypothyroidism is aided by demonstration of inappropriate responses of the thyroid gland to administration of TSH or TRH,[17,26] although the use of these tests depends on determining the increase in serum T3 and/or T4 that is expected in normal horses and in horses with thyroid disease. Of 79 clinically normal mares, all had some increase in T3, and 77 had an increase in T4, 2 hours after IV administration of 1 mg of TRH intravenously. The mean increase in serum T3 concentration was 4.5 times that of resting values (from 0.62 ng/mL to 2.44 ng/mL), whereas serum T4 concentration increased to a mean of 2.1 times that of resting value (from 14.7 ng/mL to 28.6 ng/mL). Although responses to administration of TSH have been reported, responses indicative of abnormal thyroid function—other than complete lack of response—have not been determined, and the utility of the test has been questioned.

The TSH response test involves administration of 5 IU of TSH intravenously. Blood samples are collected before administration and 30 minutes after, 2 hours after, and 4 hours after administration. Serum concentrations of T3 and T4 in healthy horses double after administration of TSH. An alternative involves administration of 5 IU IM and collection of blood before and 3 and 6 hours after TSH administration. TSH is often unavailable.

The TRH response test requires administration of 0.5 to 1 mg of TRH IV. Serum concentrations of T3 and T4 at 2 and 4 hours are double those before TRH administration in horses with normal thyroid function.

Measurement of fT4 in serum is useful for assessment of thyroid function. fT4 concentrations can be normal in horses with low concentrations of T3 and T4, and in this situation are likely indicative of normal thyroid function.

Measurement of serum concentrations of TSH is useful in determining thyroid responsiveness to endogenous TSH. Elevated TSH concentrations in horses with low serum concentrations of T3, T4, or fT4 is indicative of thyroid dysfunction.

Diagnosis of hypothyroidism in horses should be based on the presence of compatible clinical signs, low serum concentrations of thyroid hormones (T3, T4, fT4), elevated concentrations of TSH, lack of an increase in serum concentrations of thyroid hormones in response to administration of TRH, and increased TSH concentration in serum in response to TRH administration. Diagnosis of hypothyroidism should not be based solely on clinical signs or on the measurement of resting (unstimulated) serum T3 or T4 concentrations. At a minimum, appropriate clinical signs and documentation of an abnormal response to stimulation testing (TSH or TRH) are essential for diagnosis of hypothyroidism in horses. Measurements of fT4 concentrations determined by equilibrium dialysis are useful in determining thyroid function in sick horses in which T3 and T4 concentrations are low because fT4 concentrations will be normal in horses without thyroid disease.

Foals with congenital hypothyroidism have abnormally low concentrations of T3 and T4 and less-than-expected increases in serum concentrations of these hormones in response to TSH administration.

Horses with hyperthyroidism have markedly elevated concentrations of T3 and T4. Concentrations of T4 do not decline in response to administration of T3. T3 (2.5 mg) is administered intramuscularly twice daily for 3 days and serum concentrations of T3 and T4 measured. T4 concentrations in the serum of healthy horses decline by approximately 80%, whereas those of horses with hyperthyroidism do not decline.

NECROPSY FINDINGS

Findings on necropsy examination of hypothyroid horses have not been reported. Foals with congenital hypothyroidism have histologic evidence of thyroid hyperplasia, but no gross signs of goiter.

TREATMENT

Treatment of confirmed hypothyroidism in horses is achieved by administration of levothyroxine (20 µg/kg PO q24h). Serum T3 concentrations peak in 1 hour and then decline, whereas concentrations of T4 peak in 2 hours and persist for 24 hours. Administration of levothyroxine to healthy (euthyroid) horses resulted in 3.7- to 5.4-fold increases in pretreatment total T4 concentrations in serum.[27] The clinical status of horses treated for hypothyroidism should be monitored during treatment and serum concentrations of T3 and T4 measured every several months. Iodinated casein, which is no longer readily available in the United States, is administered at 5 g/450 kg body weight orally once daily. Administration of thyroxine or iodinated casein for treatment of low serum thyroid hormone concentrations in horses with nonthyroidal illness syndrome (euthyroid sick syndrome) should be done judiciously, if at all.

A response to thyroxine administration is not necessarily confirmation of hypothyroidism because thyroxine can have marked effects in horses with normal thyroid function.[27] Administration of thyroxine (up to 96 mg/470-kg horse, orally once daily) increases serum concentrations of T4 and, to a lesser extent, fT4, and decreases concentrations of TSH. The increases in T4 are associated with a loss of body weight; decreases in serum concentrations of triglycerides, cholesterol, and VLDLs; and an increase in whole-body insulin sensitivity. Thyroxine should be administered with caution to horses with normal thyroid function.

CONTROL

There are no recognized control measures for hypothyroidism in adult horses. Minimizing intake of nitrates by pregnant mares appears warranted, but definitive proof of the efficacy of this practice is lacking. Pregnant mares should not be fed fodder or supplements that interfere with thyroid function.

The inherited disorder in sheep, cattle, and goats can be prevented by selective breeding.

FURTHER READING

Breuhaus BA. Disorders of the equine thyroid gland. *Vet Clin North Am Equine Pract.* 2011;27:115.

REFERENCES

1. Hilderbran AC, et al. *J Vet Int Med.* 2014;28:609.
2. Breuhaus BA. *J Vet Int Med.* 2014;28:1301.
3. Radostits O, et al. *Veterinary Medicine: a Textbook of the Diseases of Cattle, Horses, Sheep, Goats and Pigs.* 10th ed. London: W.B. Saunders; 2006:1688.
4. Himler M, et al. *Equine Vet J.* 2012;44:43.
5. Pirrone A, et al. *Theriogenology.* 2013;80:624.
6. Tan RHH, et al. *J Vet Int Med.* 2008;22:1253.
7. Tucker RL, et al. *Equine Vet Educ.* 2013;25:126.
8. Ueki H, et al. *J Comp Pathol.* 2004;131:157.
9. Fazio E, et al. *Vet Rec.* 2008;163:713.
10. Ferlazzo A, et al. *Equine Vet J.* 2010;42:110.
11. Graves EA, et al. *Equine Vet J.* 2006;(suppl):32.
12. Leleu C, et al. *Equine Vet J.* 2010;42:171.
13. Johnsen L, et al. *J Endocrinol.* 2013;216:389.
14. Schwarz BC, et al. *JAVMA.* 2008;233:1761.
15. Saulez MN, et al. *Equine Vet Educ.* 2013;25:118.
16. Davies S, et al. *Vet Radiol Ultrasound.* 2010;51:674.
17. Breuhaus BA. *J Vet Int Med.* 2009;23:168.
18. Guyot H, et al. *J Vet Diagn Invest.* 2007;19:643.
19. Breuhaus BA, et al. *J Vet Int Med.* 2006;20:371.
20. Kasagic D, et al. *Acta Veterinaria (Beograd).* 2011;61:555.
21. Paulikova I, et al. *Acta Veterinaria (Beograd).* 2011;61:489.
22. Fazio E, et al. *Livestock Sci.* 2007;110:207.
23. Place NJ, et al. *J Vet Int Med.* 2010;24:650.
24. Abraham G, et al. *Vet J.* 2011;188:307.
25. Mendoza FJ, et al. *Equine Vet J.* 2013;45:214.
26. Breuhaus BA. *Vet Clin North Am Equine Pract.* 2011;27:115.
27. Frank N, et al. *Am J Vet Res.* 2008;69:68.

IODINE DEFICIENCY

SYNOPSIS

Etiology Primary dietary deficiency of iodine or secondary to conditioning factors such as calcium, *Brassica* plants, or bacterial pollution of water.

Epidemiology In all species, most common in continental landmasses. Neonatal animals. Diets of dams deficient in iodine as a result of abundant pasture growth or leaching of iodine from soil in years of unusually high rainfall, or diets containing conditioning factors such as certain plants.

Signs Goiter as palpable enlargement of thyroid gland. Neonatal mortality as a result of stillbirths or weak neonates not able to suck that die in few days, alopecia at birth, myxedema.

Clinical pathology Serum total iodine concentration.

Necropsy findings Thyroid enlargement, alopecia, myxedema.

Diagnostic confirmation Goiter and iodine deficiency.

Differential diagnosis list
- Weak-calf syndrome
- Abortion
- Congenital defects
- Hypothyroidism

Treatment During an outbreak, oral administration of 280 mg/head potassium iodide to pregnant ewes and provision of iodized salt licks. Lambs with goiter can be administered 20 mg potassium iodide per os, once.

Control Ensure adequate dietary intake of iodine in pregnant animals.

Iodine metabolism is influenced by physiologic and environmental factors, making assessment of thyroid status, and the need for supplementation, challenging. See previous section for a discussion of hypothyroidism.

ETIOLOGY

Iodine deficiency can be a result of deficient iodine intake or secondarily conditioned by a high intake of calcium, diets consisting largely of *Brassica* spp., or gross bacterial pollution of feedstuffs or drinking water. A continued intake of a low level of cyanogenetic glycosides (e.g., in white clover) is commonly associated with a high incidence of goitrous offspring. Linamarin, a glycoside in linseed meal, is the agent producing goiter in newborn lambs born from ewes fed the meal during pregnancy. A continued intake of the grass *Cynodon aethiopicus*, which has low-iodine and high–cyanogenetic glucoside content, can cause goiter in lambs. Rapeseed and rapeseed meal are also goitrogenic. Presence of abundant pasture after unusually high rainfall and a "seasonal break" (marked increase in pasture growth in the weeks after end of summer) is associated with clinical iodine deficiency in newborn lambs.[1]

Goiter or hypothyroidism in newborn lambs occurs when pregnant ewes have a low iodine intake or ingest goitrogens.

EPIDEMIOLOGY

Occurrence

Goiter caused by iodine deficiency occurs in all of the continental landmasses. It is not of major economic importance because of the ease of recognition and correction, but if neglected it can cause heavy mortalities in newborn animals. Stillbirth or death of newborns reduced a pregnancy rate at midterm (number of fetuses detected by ultrasonographic examination/number of ewes) of 130% to a marking rate at ~2 weeks of age to 70%.[1] The most common cause of iodine deficiency in farm animals is the failure to provide iodine in the diet. The sporadic occurrence of the disease in marginal areas attracts most attention. An epidemiologic survey in Germany found that up to 10% of cattle and sheep farms and 15% of swine herds were affected with iodine deficiency, which included both primary and secondary conditions as a result of the presence of nitrates, thiocyanates, or glucosinolates in the diet.

The importance of subclinical iodine deficiency as a cause of neonatal mortality could be much greater than that of clinical disease. For example, in southern Australia, ewes supplemented with iodine by a single injection of iodine in oil have shown lower mortality in the lambs, have grown larger lambs, or performed the same as controls. In New Zealand, subclinical iodine deficiency has been recognized in a sheep flock in which fertility and lamb perinatal mortality occurred and was corrected by supplementation of the ewes with iodine. The annual cost associated with iodine deficiency in one Manawata Romney flock was conservatively estimated at $6.00 per ewe. Iodine supplementation reduces perinatal mortality and increases lambing percentage by 14% to 21% in pasture-fed ewes. Thus subclinical iodine deficiency can affect reproductive performance and perinatal lamb mortality.

Young animals are more likely to bear goitrous offspring than older ones, and this may account for the apparent breed susceptibility of Dorset Horn sheep, which mate at an earlier age than other breeds.

A survey of crossbred cows in the Punjab of India found that 36% of cows were iodine deficient, with considerable geographic variation from 0% to 86% within Punjab. The cardinal clinical signs of iodine deficiency were absent, and basal plasma T3 (triiodothyronine) and T4 (plasma thyroxine) concentrations and their ratios did not differ between deficient and control cows. The response to injection of 1 mL of 78% ethiodized oil can prevent the deficiency for more than 70 days.

Risk Factors

Dietary and Environmental Factors

A simple deficiency of iodine in the diet and drinking water can occur and is related to geographic circumstances. Areas where the soil iodine is not replenished by cyclical accessions of oceanic iodine include large continental landmasses and coastal areas where prevailing winds are offshore. In such areas, iodine deficiency is most likely to occur where rainfall is heavy and soil iodine is continually depleted by leaching. Iodine ingested in the diet comes largely from ingestion of soil, either directly or on pasture. Consequently, abundant pasture growth can reduce intake of soil and lead to iodine deficiency in sheep.[1]

Soil formations rich in **calcium** or lacking in humus are also likely to be relatively deficient in iodine. The ability of soils to retain iodine under conditions of heavy rainfall is directly related to their humus content, and limestone soils are, in general, low in organic matter. A high dietary intake of calcium also decreases intestinal absorption of iodine, and in some areas, heavy applications of lime to pasture are followed by the development of goiter in lambs. This factor can also be important in areas where drinking water is heavily mineralized.

There are several situations in which the relationship between iodine intake and the occurrence of goiter is not readily apparent. Goiter may occur on pastures containing adequate iodine; it is then usually ascribed to a secondary or conditioned iodine deficiency. A diet rich in plants of the ***Brassica* spp.**, including cabbages and brussels sprouts, may cause simple goiter and hypothyroidism in rabbits, which is preventable by administered iodine. Severe iodine deficiency can occur when ewes are fed *Brassica* crops for long periods. Brassicas such as swedes, turnips, and kale have low iodine content and contain goitrogens, and they may result in weak newborn lambs with enlarged thyroid glands. Goiter occurred in 85% of lambs examined at necropsy that born from ewes fed on the *Brassica* crop and not supplemented with iodine.

Diffuse hyperplastic goiter has occurred in calves in beef cows in Japan that were on pasture or being fed feed containing *Rorippa indica*, Hiern, genus *Brassica*, family Crucifera, Inugarash, which contains thiocyanate. The iodine content of the waters on affected farms was low at 0.361 μg/L and 0.811 μg/L and that of the pastures, 87 μg/kg and 121 μg/kg, on two different farms.

Hypothyroidism has also been produced in rats by feeding rapeseed and in mice by feeding rapeseed oil meal. Feeding large quantities of kale to pregnant ewes causes a high incidence of goiter and hypothyroidism, also preventable by administering iodine in the newborn lambs. The goitrogenic substance in these plants is probably a glucosinolate capable of producing thiocyanate in the rumen. The thiocyanate content, or potential content, varies between varieties of kale, being much less in rape-kale, which also does not show the twofold increase in thiocyanate content other varieties show in autumn. Small young leaves contain up to five times as much thiocyanate as large, fully formed leaves. Some of these plants are excellent sources of feed, and in some areas, it is probably economical to continue feeding them, provided suitable measures are taken to prevent goiter in the newborn. Although kale also causes mild goiter in weaned lambs, this does not appear to reduce their rate of gain.

A diet high in linseed meal (20% of ration) given to **pregnant ewes** may result in a high incidence of goitrous lambs, which is preventable with iodine or thyroxine. Under experimental conditions, groundnuts are goitrogenic for rats, the goitrogenic substance being a glycoside-arachidoside. The goitrogenic effect is inhibited by supplementation of the diet with small amounts of iodine. **Soybean by-products** are also considered to be goitrogenic. **Gross bacterial contamination of drinking water** by sewage is a cause of goiter in humans in countries where hygiene is poor. There is a record of a severe outbreak of goitrous calves from cattle running on pasture heavily dressed with crude sewage. Prophylactic dosing of the cows with potassium iodide prevented further cases. Feeding sewage sludge is also linked to the occurrence of goiter.

Goiter in lambs may occur when permanent pasture is plowed and re-sown. This may be a result of the sudden loss of decomposition and leaching of iodine-binding humus in soils of marginal iodine content. In subsequent years the disease may not appear. There may be some relation between this occurrence of goiter and the known variation in the iodine content of particular plant species, especially if new pasture species are sown when the pasture is plowed. The maximum iodine content of some plants is controlled by a strongly inherited factor and is independent of soil type or season. Thus in the same pasture, perennial rye grass may contain 146 µg iodine per 100 g dry matter (DM) and Yorkshire grass only 7 µg/100 g DM. Because goiter has occurred in lambs when the ewes are on a diet containing less than 30 µg iodine per 100 g DM, the importance of particular plant species becomes apparent. A high incidence of goiter associated with heavy mortality has been observed in the newborn lambs of ewes grazing on pasture dominated by white clover and by subterranean clover and perennial rye-grass.

Thyroid-weight : birth-weight ratios greater than 0.8 g/kg in lambs are indicative of iodine deficiency and should be considered a risk factor for iodine deficiency in lambs. Ratios less than 0.4 g/kg rarely occur among deficient flocks.[2]

Congenital goiter has been observed in foals born to mares on low iodine intake, but also to mares fed an excessive amount of iodine during pregnancy.

PATHOGENESIS

Iodine deficiency results in a decreased production of thyroxine and stimulation of the secretion of thyrotropic hormone by the pituitary gland. This commonly results in hyperplasia of thyroid tissue and a considerable enlargement of the gland. Most cases of goiter of the newborn are of this type. The primary deficiency of thyroxine is responsible for the severe weakness and hair abnormality of the affected animals. Although the defect is described as hairlessness, it is truly hypoplasia of the hairs, with many very slender hairs present and a concurrent absence and diminution in the size of hair follicles. A hyperplastic goiter is highly vascular, and the gland can be felt to pulsate with the arterial pulse; a loud murmur may be audible over the gland. Colloid goiter is less common in animals and probably represents an involutional stage after primary hyperplasia.

Other factors, particularly the ingestion of low levels of cyanide, exert their effects by inhibiting the metabolic activity of the thyroid epithelium and restricting the uptake of iodine. Thiocyanates and sulfocyanates are formed during the process of detoxication of cyanide in the liver, and these substances have a pronounced depressing effect on iodine uptake by the thyroid. Some pasture and fodder plants, including white clover, rape, and kale, are known to have a moderate content of cyanogenetic glucosides. These goitrogenic substances may appear in the milk and provide a toxic hazard to both animals and humans. The inherited form in cattle is a result of the increased activity of an enzyme that deiodinates iodotyrosines so rapidly that the formation of thyroxine is inhibited.

Iodine is an essential element for normal fetal brain and physical development in sheep. A severe iodine deficiency in pregnant ewes causes reduction in fetal brain and body weight from 70 days of gestation to parturition. The effects are mediated by a combination of maternal and fetal hypothyroidism, the effect of maternal hypothyroidism being earlier than the onset of fetal thyroid secretion. There is also evidence of fetal hypothyroidisms and absence of wool growth and delayed skeletal maturation near parturition.

CLINICAL FINDINGS

Goiter is an unambiguous indicator of iodine deficiency in lambs and calves,[2] but clinically important increases in thyroid size might be easily missed unless careful attention is paid to assessment of the thyroid gland in newborns.[3] Thyroid volume can be estimated in calves by ultrasonographic examination.[4] It is important to recognize that ingestion of excessive iodine also can result in goiter in neonates and adults.[5]

A high incidence of **stillbirths and weak, newborn animals** is the most common manifestation of iodine deficiency.[3] Partial or complete **alopecia** and palpable enlargement of the thyroid gland are other signs that occur with varying frequency in the different species. Affected foals have a normal hair coat and little thyroid enlargement, but they are very weak at birth. In most cases, they are unable to stand without support, and many are too weak to suck. Excessive flexion of the lower forelegs and extension of lower parts of the hindlegs has also been observed in affected foals. Defective ossification occurs in foals and lambs (Fig. 17-8), and in foals the manifestation is collapse of the central and third tarsal bones, leading to lameness and deformity of the hock. Enlargement of the thyroid also occurs commonly in adult horses in affected areas, with Thoroughbreds and light horses being more susceptible than draft animals.

In **cattle**, the incidence of thyroid enlargement in adults is much lower than in horses, and the cardinal manifestations are gross **enlargement of the thyroid gland and weakness in newborn calves**. If they are assisted to suck for a few days, recovery is usual, but if they are born on the range during inclement weather, many will die. In some instances, the thyroid gland is sufficiently large to cause obstruction to respiration. Affected calves have a thick neck and appear to be suffocating. Lethargy, weakness, and difficulty in consuming colostrum are common. Partial alopecia is a rare accompaniment.

In **pigs**, the characteristic findings are birth of **hairless, stillborn, or weak piglets, often with myxedema** of the skin of the neck. The hairlessness is most marked on the limbs. Most affected piglets die within a few hours of birth. Thyroid enlargement may be present, but it is never sufficiently great to cause visible swelling in the live pig. Survivors are lethargic, do not grow well, and have a waddling gait and leg weaknesses as a result of weakness of ligaments and joints.

Adult **sheep** in iodine-deficient areas can show a high incidence of thyroid enlargement, but are clinically normal in other respects. Newborn lambs manifest weakness, extensive alopecia, and palpable, if not visible, enlargement of the thyroid glands (Fig. 17-9). The gestation length of ewes may be increased, and there is increased perinatal mortality, especially in inclement weather. Marginal iodine deficiency can result in nonspecific production losses from embryonic mortality or high perinatal lamb death and reduced lamb growth rates and is difficult to diagnose.[3]

Goats present a similar clinical picture, except that all abnormalities are more severe than in lambs. Goat kids are goitrous and alopecic. The degree of alopecia varies from complete absence of hair, through very fine hair, to hair that is almost normal.

Animals surviving the initial danger period after birth may recover, except for partial persistence of the goiter. The glands may pulsate with the normal arterial pulse and may extend down a greater part of the neck and cause some local edema. Auscultation and palpation of the jugular furrow may reveal the presence of a murmur and thrill,

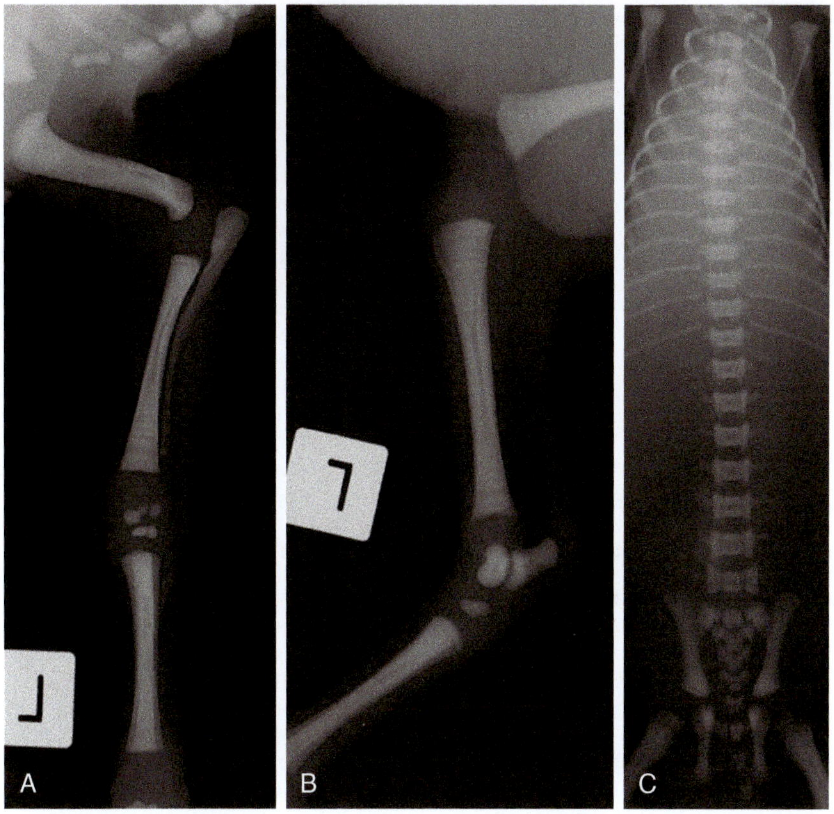

Fig. 17-8 Radiographs of a stillborn lamb from a flock with severe iodine deficiency revealing lack of mineralization of the epiphyses of long bones and vertebral bodies and presence of incompletely ossified cuboidal bones of the carpus and tarsus. (Reproduced with permission from Campbell AJD, et al. *Aust Vet J.* 2012;90:235.)

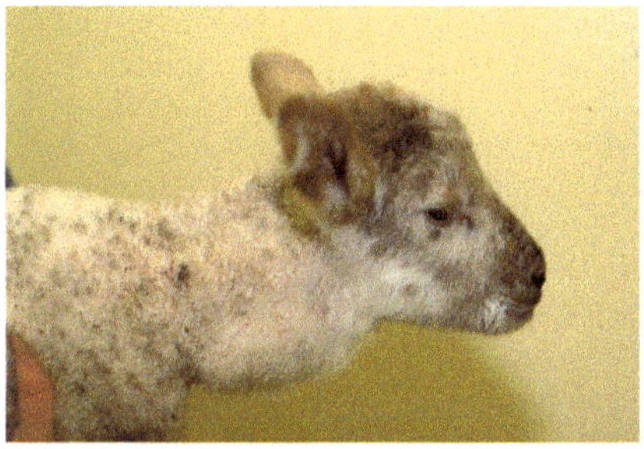

Fig. 17-9 Marked goiter in a neonatal lamb as a result of in utero iodine deficiency. A palpable thrill was present in the ventral cervical region.

the "thyroid thrill," as a result of the increased arterial blood supply of the glands. Calves that had larger goiter and were hairless (n = 8) died within the first day of life, whereas four others with moderate goiter and normal hair lived.[6]

Although loss of condition, decreased milk production, and weakness might be anticipated, these signs are not usually observed in adults. Loss of libido in the bull, failure to express estrus in the cow, and a high incidence of aborted, stillborn, or weak calves have been suggested as manifestations of hypothyroidism in cattle, whereas prolonged gestation is reported in mares, ewes, and sows. As noted previously, pathognomonic changes in production indices are not available for diagnosis of iodine deficiency.[2]

Goiter has occurred in newborn foals whose mares were supplemented with excess iodine during the last 24 hours of pregnancy.

CLINICAL PATHOLOGY

There are no wholly satisfactory indices of the severity of iodine deficiency, and biochemical markers of iodine metabolism, such as serum iodine or thyroxine (T4) and triiodothyronine (T3) concentrations, have not been shown to accurately and reliably reflect an animal's iodine status, identify marginal deficiency, or predict the production response of a flock to iodine supplementation.[2] Thyroid-related hormones often do not discriminate between adequate and marginal iodine status in pasture-fed livestock during supplementation trials, probably a result of the complex, adaptive systems maintaining homeostasis of these important regulators of cell growth and metabolic rate.[7] Knowles and Grace (2007) think that data are inadequate to quantify the relationship between iodine status and an economically relevant measure of animal performance, and this has hindered the setting of laboratory reference ranges for biomarkers.[2] However, measurement of serum total iodine concentration, which is an elemental determination that comprises the iodinated hormones plus various chemical forms of serum inorganic iodine, might be more effective in diagnosing iodine deficiency than measurement of serum iodine concentration or biochemical markers (see following "Control" section).[7]

Several criteria have been used for the laboratory diagnosis of iodine deficiency in sheep, including T3 and T4 and related hormones. They include thyroid weight, lamb thyroid-to-body-weight ratio, and comparison of serum T4 (serum thyroxine) concentrations in lamb and dam. However, concentrations of biochemical and hormonal markers are variable and difficult to compare among reports because of, among other factors, differing assay methodologies.[8]

Measurement of thyroid-stimulating hormone concentrations (TSH, thyrotropin) appears to be useful in detection of hypothyroidism attributed to iodine deficiency in calves.[6] TSH is significantly higher in goitrous calves compared with healthy calves, whereas plasma iodine concentrations do not differ. Concentrations, and ratios, of T4, T4/T3 ratio, T4/TSH ratio, rT3, and T3 are higher in healthy calves than in calves with goiter. Calves with goiter that die have higher TSH values; lower T4, T3, T4/TSH, and rT3; but similar T4/T3 ratio ($P > 0.1$) than calves with goiter that live. In the absence of TSH assay, the T4/T3 ratio can be used to diagnose hypothyroidism in newborn calves.[6] Feed iodine concentration was 175 mg/kg DM (reference range > 1200 mg/kg DM) in a herd of cattle with 10% incidence of stillbirth and death of newborns as a result of iodine deficiency.[9]

Thyroid-weight : birth-weight ratios greater than 0.8 g/kg in newborn lambs are indicative of iodine deficiency. Ratios less than 0.4 g/kg rarely occur in lambs of flocks deficient in iodine. Intermediate ratios are ambiguous.[2] The relationship between thyroid and body weight is not linear and is best defined by a probit plot (Fig. 17-10), and this nonlinear relationship should be considered when interpreting these ratios for diagnosis of iodine deficiency and need for supplementation.[2]

Other tests are concentrations of iodine in plasma, milk, and urine, all of which reflect current iodine status rather than revealing a profile or providing indications of previous iodine status.

Estimations of iodine levels in the blood and milk are reliable indicators of the iodine status of the animal. There may be between-breed differences in blood iodine levels, but levels of 2.4 to 14 μg of protein-bound iodine per 100 mL of plasma appear to be in the normal range. In ewes, an iodine concentration in milk of below 8 μg/L indicates a state of iodine deficiency. Bulk-tank milk iodine content should be greater than 300 μg/L.

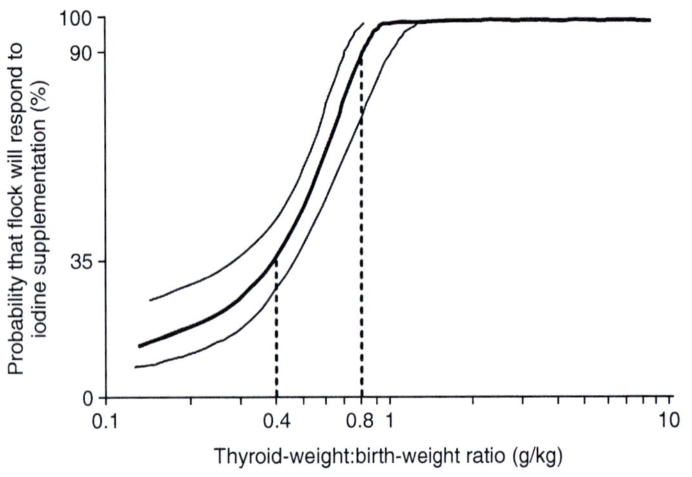

Fig. 17-10 Plot of probability that a flock of ewes will respond to iodine supplementation based on lamb thyroid-weight: body-weight ratios. A ratio of 0.40 g/kg (95% confidence interval [CI] = 0.29 to 0.47) predicted with 35% probability, and a ratio of 0.80 g/kg (95% CI = 0.70 to 0.99) predicted with 90% probability, that a lamb came from an unsupplemented (i.e., iodine-deficient) flock. (Reproduced with permission from Knowles SO, et al. *N Z Vet J.* 2007;55:314.)

Changes in serum thyroid hormone levels in newborn calves have been used as a diagnostic index in endemic goiter, but their high variation has been unreliable. The T4/T3 ratio of calves with goiter was lower than in healthy calves and adult cows, and it may be a useful diagnostic aid.

In determining the iodine status of an area, iodine levels in soil and pasture should be obtained, but the relationship between these levels, and between them and the status of the grazing animal, may be complicated by conditioning factors.

NECROPSY FINDINGS

Macroscopic thyroid enlargement, alopecia, and myxedema may be evident. The weights of thyroid glands have diagnostic value. In full-term normal calves the average fresh weight is 6.5 g; in lambs 2 g is average. Newborn lambs from ewes unsupplemented with iodine had a mean ratio of thyroid weight (g) to body weight (kg) of 0.40 g/kg or greater. In calves with severe thyroid hypertrophy, the gland may be heavier than 20 g.

The iodine content of the thyroid will also give some indication of the iodine status of the animal. At birth, a level of 0.03% of iodine on a wet-weight basis (0.1% on dry weight) can be considered to be the critical level in cattle and sheep. On histologic examination, hyperplasia of the glandular epithelium may be seen. Follicles depleted of colloid, infolded, and lined by columnar epithelium are indicative of hypothyroidism in lambs born from ewes unsupplemented with iodine.

The hair follicles will be found to be hypoplastic. Delayed osseous maturation, manifested by absence of centers of ossification, is also apparent in goitrous newborn lambs.

Samples for Confirmation of Diagnosis

- **Toxicology**—1 thyroid gland (assay [iodine])
- **Histology**—skin, thyroid (LM)

DIFFERENTIAL DIAGNOSIS

Iodine deficiency is easily diagnosed if goiter is present, but the occurrence of stillbirths without obvious goiter may be confusing. Abortion as a result of infectious agents in cattle and sheep must be considered in these circumstances. In stillbirths resulting from iodine deficiency, gestation is usually prolonged beyond the normal period, although this may be difficult to determine in animals bred at pasture. Inherited defects of thyroid hormone synthesis are listed under the heading of inherited diseases. Hyperplastic goiter without gland enlargement has been observed in newborn foals in which rupture of the common digital extensor tendons, forelimb contracture, and mandibular prognathism also occur. The cause of the combination of defects in unknown.

TREATMENT

When outbreaks of iodine deficiency occur in neonates, the emphasis is usually on providing additional iodine to the pregnant dams. The recommendations for control can be adapted to the treatment of affected animals. During an outbreak, oral administration of 280 mg/head potassium iodide to pregnant ewes and provision of iodized salt licks is advisable.[1] Lambs with goiter can be administered 20 mg potassium iodide per os, once.[1]

CONTROL

The recommended dietary intake of iodine for cattle is 0.8 to 1.2 mg/kg DM of feed for lactating and pregnant cows and 0.1 to 0.3 mg/kg DM of feed for nonpregnant cows and calves. Monitoring of lamb thyroid: body-weight ratios in areas at risk for iodine deficiency can be useful in determining the need for supplementation before and/or during pregnancy.[2] Thyroid-weight: birth-weight ratios greater than 0.8 g/kg are indicative of iodine deficiency, and ewes should be supplemented premating or during pregnancy to prevent goiter the following year. Ratios less than 0.4 g/kg rarely occurred among deficient flocks, so the probability of benefit from supplementation is low. Intermediate ratios are ambiguous, and individual-farm supplementation trials might be required to detect and manage the risks of marginal deficiency.

Pastures in New Zealand that contain 0.24 mg iodine/kg DM provide an adequate intake for dairy cows. The injection of iodine (iodized oil) IM three times at a dose of 2370 mg iodine/dose at the start of lactation and at 100-day intervals increased iodine concentrations in milk to 58 µg/L for at least 98 days after each treatment. Two iodine injections at 100-day intervals increased milk iodine concentrations to 160 µg/L and 211 µg/L at least 55 days after each treatment, but had no effect on serum thyroid hormone concentrations. Iodine supplementation had no effect on milk, milk fat, or milk protein yield. Increasing iodine concentration in milk by IM injection of iodine could provide a method for increasing iodine intakes of humans, especially children.

Iodine can be provided in salt or a mineral mixture. The loss of iodine from salt blocks may be appreciable, and an iodine preparation that is stable but contains sufficient available iodine is required. Potassium iodate satisfies these requirements and should be provided as 200 mg of potassium iodate per kilogram of salt. Potassium iodide alone is unsuitable, but when mixed with calcium stearate (8% of the stearate in potassium iodide) it is suitable for addition to salt—200 mg/kg of salt.

Individual dosing of pregnant ewes, on two occasions during the fourth and fifth months of pregnancy, with 280 mg potassium iodide or 370 mg potassium iodate has been found to be effective in the prevention of goiter in lambs when the ewes are on a heavy diet of kale. For individual animals, weekly application of tincture of iodine (4 mL for cattle; 2 mL for pigs and sheep) to the inside of the flank is also an effective preventive. The iodine can also be administered as an injection in poppy seed oil (containing 40% bound iodine): 1 mL given IM 7 to 9 weeks before lambing is sufficient to prevent severe goiter and neonatal mortality in the lambs. Control of goiter can be achieved for up to 2 years. The gestation period is also reduced to normal. A similar injection 3 to 5 weeks before lambing is less efficient.

The administration of long-acting injectable iodine (iodized oil) at a dose of 390 mg iodine to ewes, 5 weeks premating, prevented goiter in newborn lambs from ewes fed swedes or swedes/turnips/kale as winter supplement. Administration of ~400 mg iodine per ewe increased serum iodine concentrations from 41 (standard deviation [SD] 12.2) µg iodine/L ($n = 54$) to 109 (SD 18.5) µg/L ($n = 20$; $p < 0.001$) at lambing ~99 days later, regardless of forage fed. High serum iodine concentrations persisted for 127 to 206 days after supplementation.[2] Diet did not affect iodine concentrations in ewe serum or milk. Responses of serum total iodine concentration (an elemental determination that comprises the iodinated hormones plus various chemical forms of serum inorganic iodine[7]) to injection of iodized oil to sheep are proportional to dose level increasing from 42 µg/L to approximately 150 and 240 mu g/L for sheep administered either 300 mg or 400 mg of iodine, remaining elevated for 161 days.[2] Milk concentrations of iodine were 26, 271, and 425 µg/L for sheep administered no supplemental iodine or 300 mg or 400 mg, respectively. Mean serum iodine concentrations of lambs from supplemented ewes with 300 mg or 400 mg iodine were 237 and 287 mu g I/L at birth, and by weaning were similar (62 ± 3 mu g/L). Concentrations in lambs born of ewes that were not supplemented were less than ~140 µg/L and were markedly affected by the diet of the ewe.[7]

Administration of 0.45 mg or 0.90 mg of potassium iodide orally daily to crossbred dairy goats increased mean milk iodine concentrations from 60.1 ± 50.5 (unsupplemented goats) to 78.8 ± 55.4 and 130.2 ± 62.0 mu g/L (mean ± SD), respectively. Milk production was not affected.[10]

A device to release iodine slowly into the forestomaches, while still retaining its position there, has given good results in preventing congenital goiter in lambs when fed to ewes during late pregnancy.

A recommended approach for iodine supplementation in sheep is as follows:[2]

1. If feeding *Brassica* crops, then supplement ewes.
2. If any lamb thyroid-weight : birth-weight ratio is greater than 0.8 g/kg, then supplement ewes. The relationship between thyroid weight and body weight is not linear and is best defined by a probit plot (Fig. 17-10), and this nonlinear relationship should be considered when interpreting these ratios for diagnosis of iodine deficiency and need for supplementation.[2]
3. If all or most thyroid-weight : birth-weight ratios are less than 0.4 g/kg, there is probably no need to supplement ewes because the probability of benefit is low.
4. If many thyroid-weight : birth-weight ratios fall between 0.4 and 0.8 g/kg, then the iodine status of the flock is unclear and can be impossible to determine from biomarkers.
   Supplement the ewes if other evidence is persuasive, such as occurrence of iodine deficiency in the district. An on-farm supplementation trial might be required to detect marginal deficiency on these properties.

REFERENCES

1. Campbell AJD, et al. *Aust Vet J.* 2012;90:235.
2. Knowles SO, et al. *N Z Vet J.* 2007;55:314.
3. Robertson SM, et al. *Aust J Exp Agr.* 2008;48:995.
4. Metzner M, et al. *Vet Radiol Ultrasound.* 2015;56:301.
5. Ong CB, et al. *J Vet Diagn Invest.* 2014;26:810.
6. Guyot H, et al. *Cattle Pract.* 2007;15:271.
7. Knowles SO, et al. *J Anim Sci.* 2015;93:425.
8. Todini L. *Animal.* 2007;1:997.
9. Annon. *Vet Rec.* 2011;169:461.
10. Nudda A, et al. *J Dairy Sci.* 2009;92:5133.

INHERITED GOITER

Inherited goiter is recorded in Merino sheep, Afrikaner cattle, crossbred Saanen dwarf goats, Boer goats, possibly Poll Dorset sheep, and pigs, and it appears to be inherited as a recessive character. The essential defect is in the synthesis of abnormal thyroid hormone, leading to increased production of thyrotropic factor in the pituitary gland, causing in turn a hyperplasia of the thyroid gland. In Afrikaner cattle the defect stems from an abnormality of the basic RNA, and heterozygotes can be identified by blot hybridization analysis.

Clinically in **sheep,** there is a high level of mortality, enlargement of the thyroid above the normal 2.8 g (but varying greatly up to 222 g), and the appearance of lustrous or silky wool in the fleeces of some lambs. Other defects that occur concurrently are edema and floppiness of ears, enlargement and outward or inward bowing of the front legs at the knees, and dorsoventral flattening of the nasal area. The thyroglobulin deficiency in the neonatal lamb may result in defective fetal lung development and the appearance of neonatal respiratory distress syndrome; there is dyspnea at birth.

The clinical picture in **goats** is the same as for lambs. It includes retardation of growth, sluggish behavior, rough and sparse hair coat that worsens as the goats get older, and thick and scaly skin.

In Afrikaner **cattle,** most of the losses are from stillbirths or from early neonatal deaths. Some are caused by tracheal compression from the enlarged gland. It is the calves with the largest glands that have the greatest mortality. In these cattle there may be a concurrent inherited gray coat color, a defect in a red breed.

In **pigs,** hairless and swollen piglets with enlarged thyroid glands occur, in the proportions with normal piglets consistent with an autosomal-recessive mode of inheritance.

Diseases Caused by Nutritional Deficiencies

INTRODUCTION

Three criteria are suggested for the assessment of the importance of nutrition in the etiology of a disease state in a single animal or in a group of animals:

- Is there evidence from an examination of the diet that a deficiency of a specific nutrient or nutrients may be occurring?
- Is there evidence from an examination of the animals that a deficiency of the suspected essential nutrient or nutrients could cause the observed disease?
- Does supplementation of the diet with the essential nutrient or nutrients prevent or cure the condition?

The difficulties encountered in satisfying these criteria, and making an accurate and reliable diagnosis of a nutritional deficiency, increase as investigations progress into the area of trace element and vitamin nutrition. The concentration of these micronutrients in feedstuffs and body tissues are exceedingly small, and assays are often difficult and expensive. Because of these difficulties it is becoming more acceptable to describe individual syndromes as "responsive diseases"—that is, the investigation satisfies only the third of the previously listed three criteria. This practice is not ideal, but has advantages in that it is more a more cost-effective approach, and relevant control measures are directly assessed.

EVIDENCE OF A DEFICIENCY AS THE CAUSE OF THE DISEASE

Evidence of a deficiency as the cause of the disease will include evidence of a deficiency in the diet or an abnormal absorption, utilization, or requirement of the nutrient under consideration. Additional evidence may be obtained by chemical or biological examination of the feed.

Diet

The diet for a considerable period before the occurrence of the disease must be considered because body stores of most dietary factors may delay the appearance of clinical signs. Specific deficiencies are likely to be associated with particular soil types, and in many instances national or local soil and geological maps may predict the likely occurrence of a nutritional disease. Diseases of plants may also indicate specific soil deficiencies, such as "reclamation disease" of oats, which indicates copper deficiency. The predominant plant species in the pasture sward may also be important; subterranean clover selectively absorbs copper, legumes selectively absorb molybdenum, and *Astragalus* spp. accumulate selenium.

Farming practices can have a strong influence on the concentration of specific nutrients in livestock feed. For example, heavy applications of nitrogen fertilizer can reduce the copper, cobalt, molybdenum, and manganese content of pasture. On the other hand, many applications of lime will reduce the concentration of copper, cobalt, zinc, and manganese in plants, but increase molybdenum. These effects are significant enough to influence the trace-element nutrition of grazing livestock. Modern hay-making methods, with their emphasis on the artificial drying of immature forage, tend to conserve vitamin A, but may result in a gross deficiency of vitamin D. Improved pasture species and increased applications of fertilizer can exaggerate the depletion of trace elements from marginally deficient soil, giving rise to overt deficiency disease in previously marginal or unaffected areas. Thus local knowledge of farming and feeding practices in a particular area is of primary importance in the diagnosis of nutritional deficiency states.

Abnormal Absorption

Although a diet may contain adequate amounts of a particular nutrient, some other factor, by decreasing its absorption, may induce a deficiency. For example, excess phosphate reduces calcium absorption, excess calcium reduces the absorption of iodine, and the absence of bile salts prevents proper absorption of the fat-soluble vitamins. Chronic enteritis reduces the absorption of most essential nutrients. The list of antagonisms that exist between elements continues to grow, most being an interference with absorption. For example, excess calcium in the diet interferes with the absorption of fluorine, lead, zinc, and cadmium, such that it may cause nutritional deficiencies of these elements, but it also reduces their toxic effects when they are present in the diet in excessive amounts.

Abnormal Utilization of Ingested Nutrients

Abnormal utilization of ingested nutrients may also have an effect on the development of conditioned deficiency diseases. For example, molybdenum and sulfate reduce copper storage, vitamin E has a sparing effect on vitamin A, and thiamine reduces the dietary requirement for essential fatty acids.

Abnormal Requirement

An enhanced growth rate of animals, either by improved nutrition or genetic selection, may increase their requirement for specific nutrients to the point where deficiency disease occurs. There seems to be little doubt that there is a genetic variation in mineral metabolism, and it has been suggested that it may be possible to breed sheep to "fit" deficiency conditions. The significance of the inherited component of an animal's nutritional requirement is unknown, but should not be overlooked when policies to upgrade livestock in deficient areas are being planned.

EVIDENCE OF A DEFICIENCY ASSOCIATED WITH THE DISEASE

Evidence of a deficiency associated with the disease is usually available from experimental work that demonstrates the clinical signs and necropsy findings produced by each deficiency. Several modifying factors may confuse the issue. Under natural circumstances, nutritional deficiencies may not be a single entity, and thus clinical and necropsy findings will often be complicated by deficiencies of other factors and intercurrent infections. Most syndromes are variable and insidious in their onset, and clinical signs and gross necropsy lesions in many nutritional deficiency diseases are either minimal or nonspecific. This increases the challenge of making a definitive diagnosis.

Consequently, laboratory examination of blood and animal tissues is an essential diagnostic aid in many instances. However, the normal range of blood or tissue concentrations of minerals and vitamins, or their biochemical markers, and those values that indicate deficiency, are often not well established. Experimentally induced and naturally occurring nutritional deficiencies provide an indication of the changes that occur in the concentrations of a particular nutrient, but variations resulting from age, genotype, production cycle, length of time on the inadequate diet, previous body stores of the element, and intercurrent disease and stressors can complicate the results, making them difficult to interpret.

In most cases, nutritional deficiencies affect a proportion of the herd or the flock at the same time. The clinicopathological examination should include a selection of both normal and clinically affected animals because the comparison of results from these groups allows a more accurate and reliable interpretation of laboratory tests, facilitating a diagnosis.

EVIDENCE BASED ON CURE OR PREVENTION BY CORRECTION OF THE DEFICIENCY

The best test of the diagnosis of a suspected nutritional deficiency is to observe the effect of supplementing that nutrient, either directly to the animal or via the ration. Confounding factors can occur, such as spontaneous recovery; hence, adequate controls and a sufficient sample size are essential. Curative responses may be poor because of an inadequate dose or advanced tissue damage. Alternatively, the abnormality may have only been a predisposing or secondary factor to another factor that is still present. A common cause of confounding in therapeutic trials is the impurity or bioactivity of the preparations used, particularly with trace elements and vitamins. The preparations used may also have some intrinsic pharmacologic activity and hence partially or temporarily ameliorate the condition without a deficiency actually having been present.

Monitoring of Nutritional Status

On breeding farms, there are several different age groups of animals at different levels of growth and production. This requires close surveillance to avoid either a deficiency or overnutrition in each class of animal. Scoring of the body condition of dairy and beef cattle, sheep, and pigs is commonly used as an indicator of the adequacy of the diet leading to the present time (termed *prior nutrition*).

The feeds and feeding program have a major influence on reproductive performance, and hence growth and milk production and must be monitored regularly. The veterinarian must be aware of any changes in the feeding program that have occurred since the last farm visit or that are intended in the near future. Veterinary clinical nutrition is now a specialty that should provide new and useful information for the practitioner working with a particular species or class of food animals. An experienced and competent nutritionist should be consulted to assist with complex nutritional problems.

Nutritional Management in Dairy Herds

Advising farms about nutrition is a key activity for dairy cattle practitioners. Feed costs are approximately 60% of the total cost of producing milk, so even minor improvements in feeding efficiency can be profitable.

Some dairy practitioners function as the nutritional specialist for the dairy farms they serve, collecting feed samples for nutrient analysis, formulating rations, and advising on crop and harvesting conditions. These veterinarians often devote a considerable amount of their professional time to nutritional management. Nevertheless, it is common for farms to employ a professional nutritionist or to use a nutritionist employed by a feed company or local cooperative. These professionals generally formulate the rations and submit feed samples for nutrient analysis. For these herds, the veterinarian can have an important role in ensuring that the diet described on paper is adequately formulated and delivered to the cows. Routine scheduled activities, such as measuring the dry matter of forages, hand-mixing of total mixed ration (TMR) for one cow and comparing it with the machine-mixed TMR (termed the TMR test mix), and scoring the feed bunk to assess feed sorting and dry matter intake are important procedures that help to ensure the successful delivery of a nutritional program. Assessing pasture conditions by periodic inspection of pasture is an important component of managing the nutritional program of herds that use management-intensive grazing. These quality control activities should be conducted routinely as part of the health and production management program.

There is probably no aspect of a dairy enterprise that has a wider impact than the feeding program, which has direct effects on production and growth. Many health problems on a dairy farm relate in some way to the feeding program, and a significant portion of the farm's labor is spent planting, growing, harvesting, mixing, and feeding rations. Investment in equipment used in feeding programs is also an important capital cost. Small changes in feeding programs may bring about large changes in productivity, health, income, feed costs, labor allocation, cash flow, and debt. Thus the total savings from these small changes can be substantial, with one study showing that routine nutritional consultation by a veterinarian can save 14% of total feed costs even without accounting for improved production or health effects.

For these reasons, veterinarians who wish to serve their dairy clients on a whole-farm basis must become actively involved in the herd's feeding program. Dairy herds are often fed unbalanced, expensive rations, but as a consultant independent from the feed company, a veterinarian can provide unbiased advice about the feed program. For example, a recumbent, hypocalcemic cow raises questions about dry-cow feeding, whereas an anestrous, thin cow with smooth ovaries raises questions about energy and dry matter intake (DMI) during early lactation. If the average mature equivalent milk production for the herd falls by 220 kg (500 lb), this generates the same sense of urgency as a cow with a prolapsed uterus. A dairy veterinarian cannot truly serve a client's needs by practicing therapeutic medicine in isolation from the nutrition of the herd and thus must acquire skills to directly deal with nutrition problems.

As the average size of dairy herds increases, many dairy farmers now rely on a team of advisors rather than just one or two. Consequently, a nutritional consultant, local veterinarian, and remote specialist consultant may all be providing advice to a dairy farm, and thus awareness of and communication about the feeding program, and the indicators of performance of the farm, are critical. It imperative that, as part of the advisory team, the dairy veterinarian knows about dairy nutrition and is aware of, but preferably involved in, the ration formulation.

Levels of Nutritional Service

Having decided to be involved in a dairy's feeding program, a first step is for the client and veterinarian to discuss and agree on the level of nutritional advice that is to be provided. This varies from herd to herd, depending on the veterinarian's expertise, the client's ability and interest, and the role of other consultants. There are essentially four levels of service that might be provided, as described next.

Level 1: Problem Identification and Analysis

At level 1, the veterinarian takes on the task of monitoring the dairy herd for indicators of nutrition-related problems. Many areas need to be monitored: production, milk composition, DMI, body scores, disease rates, heifer management and growth, and feed costs. Based on these measures, the veterinarian can identify problems as they arise, form and test hypotheses about likely causes, and interact with the client and other advisors as the problems are prioritized and addressed.

Level 2: Ration Analysis

Level 2 requires assessment of the adequacy of diets that are actually being fed to the cows. Problems of balance or economics are referred to the appropriate person, for example, if reformulation of a specific diet is needed. This involvement may be difficult to sustain if the person formulating the ration resents being "second-guessed," but it can work well if a functional team approach is in place.

Level 3: Ration Formulation

If a dairy veterinarian takes responsibility for ration formulation, the veterinarian will need considerably enhanced skills in dairy nutrition, far beyond those traditionally taught at veterinary colleges. Typically, this involves using a computer program to formulate a balanced, least-cost ration for each class of animal. It requires expertise in the mechanics of how feeds are handled and fed to cows on a daily basis, and hence an intimate knowledge of the farm and its personnel and daily trends in the price and availability of feed components.

If not well managed, this level of service has several pitfalls because it lacks the on-farm follow-up, supervision of implementation, and monitoring of results that are included in level 4. There is a truism about feeding dairy cows that every cow has three rations: the one formulated, the one delivered, and the one actually eaten. The best feeding programs minimize the difference among these three rations. If the veterinary consultant's role stops at formulation, then mistakes can occur in delivery and feedbunk management that can doom the program to failure. However, if the program fails, it is the ration formulation that is most likely to be blamed.

Level 4: Total Program Consulting

Level 4 service includes the critical aspects missing from level 3 because the veterinarian plays an active role in implementing the feeding recommendations. Attention is paid to areas such as bunk management, cow comfort, feeding frequency and scheduling, quality control, and consistency of feeding management. Working closely with the producer, plans for future forage production can be generated, including attention to factors such as timing the harvest for maximum feed value. The monitoring described in level 1 is sustained, and timely adjustments and feedback are provided to ensure that the rations are accomplishing the desired ends. In the long term, this is the level of service that is most desirable for both the specialist dairy veterinarian and client. The producer benefits from the added supervision and support, and the veterinarian can assure the client that the program is implemented as it is intended. If it is not working, the total program can be modified, often with the veterinarian as a part of a team that includes a nutritionist. When multiple consultants are used in larger herds, this team approach provides the owner with the best opportunity for expert advice, and the specialist dairy veterinarian is often best suited to be the "team leader."

Nutritional Management of the Beef Breeding Herd

Good nutrition provides the essential basis for optimum productivity in cattle-breeding operations. Despite this, nutritional expertise has not been a traditional strength of many food-animal veterinarians.

Throughout the world, beef-breeding operations are generally range or pasture based. These operations are conducted in diverse environments, with great variation in nutritional management. In many countries, the area of pasture or rangeland required to maintain a cow–calf unit may vary from 0.5 to 1 ha (1 or 2 acres) in intensive high-rainfall regions to many square kilometers in remote dryland areas. However, in general, the land area or amount of pasture necessary for production is related to local economic realities. This, in turn, is related to levels of managerial and resource inputs that differ markedly between regions, markets, and enterprises. Notwithstanding this variation, there are a number of principles of good nutritional management that can be universally applied to cattle breeding operations. Regardless of region, an important consideration is that of maintaining or improving production (increasing income) while reducing costs per unit of production. In simple terms, financial return from a beef-breeding operation is a function of number of calves, their weaning weight, and price. On the cost side is the cost of maintaining the breeding females. This varies considerably between farms, both within and between regions. Although it can be influenced, the price received is generally not significantly controlled by the farm business. However, both the number of calves born and their weaning weights are strongly influenced by an appropriate management calendar that matches nutritional demand with the supply of pasture. For example, good nutritional management helps to ensure that as many females as possible are cycling at the start of the breeding season. This, combined with good bull management, helps to ensure that calves are born early and that they are older and heavier at weaning than later-born calves.

In general, nutrition is the most important limiting factor of beef-breeding performance, and thus an understanding of the principles underlying the nutritional management of breeding females is essential. Effective monitoring does not necessarily require a higher degree in nutrition, although it should include sufficient knowledge and wisdom to know when additional expertise is needed. A starting point is to have a working knowledge of the different energy measuring systems (total digestible nutrients [TDN], metabolizable energy [ME], and net energy, NE) that are commonly used and their applications for different classes of animals, activities, and feedstuffs, and to identify one with which the veterinarian can work best. The Nutrient Requirements of Beef Cattle from the National Research Council (NRC) in the United States is a useful document, with the 7th edition published in 2000. This is packaged with a computer program that includes ration formulators and a library of feeds and feedstuffs. A number of programs for least-cost-ration formulation in beef herds are also available from Departments of Agriculture or commercial suppliers.

Nutritional Advice for Beef Feedlots

Beef feedlots frequently consult a qualified nutritionist to assist in the formulation of cost-effective rations. In this case the veterinarian should communicate regularly with the nutritionist to be aware of the composition of the diets and any changes that are planned. Because feed is the major portion of the cost per unit of body weight gain, it is imperative that the diet be the lowest-cost diet possible while providing nutrients that allow optimum growth and finishing. Most of the emphasis in feedlot nutrition has been on the development of cost-effective diets that support a maximum growth rate without any deleterious effects. Considerable information is available on the nutrient requirements for feedlot cattle and on the feeds and feeding systems used.

The precise specifications of the diets are the responsibility of the nutritionist, but the feedlot veterinarian is often able to evaluate the quality of the feed delivery system. This includes whether cattle are fed on time, whether the feed delivered to troughs is properly mixed, and whether feed intake is intermittent as a result of insufficient trough space, poor trough and pen design, inclement weather, and muddy or slippery ground. Any deviations should be discussed with feedlot managers and the consulting nutritionist, similar to the team approach suggested for large dairy herds.

Nutritional deficiency diseases are uncommon in feedlot cattle because cattle usually receive a diet that contains the nutrients required for maintenance and promotion of rapid growth. Diets prepared according to the Nutrient Requirements of Beef Cattle should meet all the requirements under most conditions.

Specific nutrient deficiencies are extremely rare because diets are prepared every few days or daily, and it would be highly unusual for a feedlot to use a feedstuff deficient in a specific nutrient for a prolonged period. However, such a situation may occur on a small farm or opportunistic feedlot that prepares its own diet with little or no attention to the need to supplement homegrown feeds. Thus there are only a few nutrition-related diseases that may affect a well-managed feedlot, but these diseases may cause large economic losses when they occur. They include the following:

- Carbohydrate engorgement (grain overload or lactic acidosis)
- Feedlot bloat or ruminal tympany
- Feeding errors, including accidental incorporation of an excessive amount of feed additives, such as monensin or urea; sudden unintended changes in the composition of the diet; and accidental feeding of the wrong dietary mix

Nutritional Advice for Swine-Herds

Veterinarians involved in health management of swine-herds must be well informed about the nutrient requirements of the different age groups of pigs. Feed constitutes 60% to 80% of the cost of producing a market pig, so every effort is needed to increase the efficiency of feed use. Surveys of well-managed pig farms in Alberta, Canada, found a 20% difference in feed costs, and it is estimated that in the industry the range in feed costs is likely to be near 50%. Reduction of the feed cost of the highest-costing farm to that of the lowest-costing farm would save that farm more than US$23,000 annually, a reduction in the cost of production of $6.80/pig. The trend is to use complete feeds formulated by feed company nutritionists familiar with the nutrient composition of local feedstuffs. With complete diets, specific nutrient deficiencies are uncommon.

The major problem is the efficiency of utilization of the different feeds throughout the life cycle of the pig. The nutrient requirements of the pig at various phases of growth, from birth to market weight and of breeding stock, are well established. The remaining questions relate to the amount of feed provided during the different growth phases of the pig to achieve optimum production and yield the best carcass. The following are some recommended practices for increasing efficiency of feed utilization:

- Provide well-balanced diets with adequate levels of amino acids, energy, vitamins, and minerals necessary to meet the particular demands of the pig at each stage of its life cycle. The diet depends on the demands, usually characterized as the growth rate or lean deposition, with feed intake being the supply function. Feed intake is limited by appetite, and thus other nutrients are matched to expected energy intake and subsequent growth.
- Use least-cost formulation to the extent that it is feasible. The least-cost energy source in most of the pig-rearing areas is corn, and the most common protein source is soybean meal.
- Restrict the level of a properly balanced diet for sows during gestation to avoid overfeeding. Sows that have lost excessive body weight in the previous lactation need supplemental feed during the dry period to avoid thin-sow syndrome.
- Ad-lib feeding for growing pigs is usually optimal unless the genotype deposits excess fat during the latter stages of growth.
- Market pigs as close to optimum slaughter weight as possible to maximize margin over feed costs.
- Avoid feed wastage by using well-designed feeding systems and proper adjustment of feeders.
- Use pelleting of diets to increase digestibility, especially of small grains, and to decrease feed wastage. However, pelleting does predispose pigs to gastroesophageal ulcers.

The feed efficiency of the pigs from weaning to market should be monitored regularly. It is often difficult to obtain accurate data for a specific group of pigs because a common feeding system for multiple groups is often used. However, the total amount of feed used and the total weight of pigs marketed will give an estimate of feed efficiency.

Although the nutrient requirements of pigs are well known, they do continue to change because of changes in growth and production characteristics. Pigs with high lean-growth rates require higher levels of amino acids to support their increased rate of body protein deposition. Similarly, high-milk-producing sows nursing large litters have increased amino acid requirements. The NRC in the United States provides an important service in establishing the nutrient requirements of swine and other species. The 10th edition of the Nutrient Requirements of Swine was published in 1998, and it includes areas such as modeling nutrient requirements and reducing nutrient excretion, particularly nitrogen and phosphorus, which can contribute to environmental pollution.

The approach used to produce estimates of nutrient requirements account for the pig's body weight and the accretion of lean (protein) tissue, gender, health status, and various environmental factors. To accurately estimate nutrient needs of gestating and lactating sows, there is a need to account for body weight, weight gain during gestation, weight loss during lactation, number of pigs in the litter, weight gain of the litter (a reflection of milk yield), and certain environmental factors. A series of integrated equations is used to account for the many factors known to influence nutrient requirements. These provide the framework for modeling the biological basis of predicting requirements. The NRC models predict the levels of nutrients (outputs) needed to achieve a certain level of production under a given set of environmental conditions (inputs).

Five principles were used to develop the models: (1) ease of use by people with varying levels of nutritional expertise; (2) continued relevance; (3) structural simplicity; (4) transparency, so that all equations are available to the user; and (5) empirical data at the whole-animal level was used rather than data based on theoretical values. Three independent models were developed for growth, gestation, and lactation. The growth model estimates amino acid requirements of pigs from weaning to market weight, and the gestation and lactation models estimate energy and amino acid requirements of gestating and lactating sows.

Few revisions were needed from the previously published mineral requirements; higher dietary requirements for sodium and chloride in the young pig were established, and manganese requirements were increased from 10 to 20 ppm for gestating and lactating sows.

Feed composition tables are built from multiple databases on the nutrient composition of feeds, including the feed industry and datasets outside the United States and Canada.

The information on water was expanded, with more detailed information on the factors that influence water intake. Information on nonnutritive feed additives, such as antimicrobial agents, anthelmintics, microbial supplements, oligosaccharides, enzymes, acidifiers, flavors, odor-control agents, antioxidant pellet binders, flow agents, high-mineral supplements, and carcass modifiers, is also included.

Nutritional Advice for Sheep Flocks

The influence of nutrition on the reproductive performance of ewes has been a matter of concern for many years. Clearly, the relationship between the provision of nutrients and requirements for optimum reproductive performance is seldom ideal because of the wide range of environmental conditions and the seasonal breeding patterns of most sheep breeds. Prolonged periods of undernutrition often occur during midpregnancy, partly the result of the decline in feed availability and quality over that stage of the reproductive cycle and partly from the seasonal variability in pasture growth.

Prolonged moderate to severe undernutrition of ewes bearing twins in midpregnancy reduces placental development and can cause a significant reduction in lamb birth weight and increased lamb mortalities. Considerable progress has been made in understanding the principles of nutrition of sheep and in defining their nutrient requirements for maintenance, pregnancy, and lactation. It has been established that mortality rates are high in lambs with birth weights below the breed norm, and that after birth the absolute growth rates are lower in surviving light lambs than in heavier lambs of the same breed. The plane of nutrition and the size of the placenta have been recognized as major determinants of the fetal growth rate. Fetal growth retardation in undernourished ewes has a placental component, and thus factors that affect placental growth are highly relevant.

The 21-week gestation can be divided into a number of periods to consider the effects of nutrition on reproduction within each period. In the first 4 weeks of gestation, embryonic loss is the main sequelae of inadequate nutrition. During this period, it is generally recommended that the body-condition score (BCS) of the ewe be maintained at an average of 3.0, on a scale of 1 (emaciated) to 5 (very fat), to minimize embryonic and early fetal loss. This is followed by a period of 2 months in which there is rapid growth of the placenta, but during which growth of the fetus in absolute terms is still small. Over this period, losses in body weight should not exceed 5%, and BCS should be maintained at 2.7 to 3.0. Finally, there is the phase from 90 days to parturition, in which gain in the mass of the fetus amounts to 85% of its birth weight, during which time nutrient intake must be increased if excessive weight loss in the ewe and light-birth-weight lambs are to be avoided.

Placental and Fetal Growth

Placental development in the pregnant ewe begins about 30 days after conception. The number of placentomes associated with each fetus is fixed at this time, but the total weight of the placentomes increases until about 90 days of gestation, after which there is little change. The factors that influence the ultimate size of the placenta and its weight include hormonal and nutritional factors, prolonged environmental heating of pregnant ewes, parity, and possibly genotype. However, by far the most important determinant is nutrition of the ewe. Moderately severe undernutrition during early and midpregnancy significantly reduces placental weight at term and causes chronic intrauterine growth retardation.

The size of the placenta is a major determinant of fetal growth. In well-fed ewes, the fetal growth rate until 120 days (17 weeks) of gestation is not positively correlated with placental weight, but fetal growth rate is limited by the size of the placenta during the last 3 to 4 weeks of pregnancy. However, when ewes are underfed, the influences of a lighter placenta on fetal growth rate are evident sooner, with placental weight and fetal growth positively correlated from as early as 90 days (13 weeks) of gestation. During the first 90 days of pregnancy, placental growth is reduced when ewes are moderately underfed. Light fetuses in ewes with placenta weights near the bottom of the normal range suffer chronic and progressive hypoxemia and hypoglycemia. This affects fetal metabolism, causing fetal death during late pregnancy, fetal hypoxemia during parturition, premature birth, and a high perinatal mortality rate from hypoglycemia and hypothermia, the latter being more severe in lighter lambs.

The extent to which ewes maintained on a fixed ration draw on their own body reserves in an attempt to meet the energy costs of pregnancy is determined by fetal weight. In well-fed ewes, fetal growth rate remains constant until at least 120 days of gestation and then decreases. However, the absolute growth rate increases markedly during the last 8 weeks of gestation, when fetal growth is most rapid, exceeding 100 g/day near birth. The growth rate among fetuses is highly variable, which accounts for birth weights ranging from 2 kg to over 7 kg. When ewes that have previously been well fed are severely underfed at any stage during the last 40 to 50 days of pregnancy, fetal growth rate decreases by 30% to 70% within 3 days. This demonstrates that mobilization of maternal reserves is substantially less than fetal requirements, emphasizing the importance of a continuous supply of good-quality feed during late pregnancy. The larger the fetal burden, the more susceptible an ewe is to hypoglycemia during underfeeding.

Refeeding after severe underfeeding can reverse the reduced growth rate of fetuses, but the response depends on the duration of the underfeeding. If the period of underfeeding is 16 days or less, the growth rate increases when ewes are refed, but there is no change when refeeding occurs after 21 days of severe underfeeding. Moderate underfeeding of pregnant ewes for 85 days reduces the fetal growth rate irreversibly. Refeeding them in late pregnancy does not cause fetal growth rate to increase, but it does prevent further decreases after 120 days.

Lamb Losses

The major consequences of prenatal growth retardation are on lamb survival. Neonatal mortality increases markedly in many environments when the birth weight falls below 3 to 3.5 kg. Compared with normal lambs, low-birth-weight animals have reduced insulation because of the smaller number of wool fibers, greater relative heat loss because of their larger surface area per unit of body weight, and a reduced capability to maintain heat production because of their lower fat and energy reserves. All of these factors increase their susceptibility to environmental stress and reduce their ability to compete with normal-sized siblings.

Underfeeding during pregnancy reduces available body lipids in lambs by about 47%, and it also decreases the lactose, lipid, and protein available in colostrum during the first 18 hours after birth by about 50%. Newborn lambs have to draw on body reserves of glycogen to maintain heat production during the first 18 hours after birth. Consequently, they depend heavily on colostrum and supplements, when these are provided, to avoid hypoglycemia and hypothermia.

The effects of maternal nutrition on udder development and on the production and yield of colostrum and milk in ewes have also been examined. In the 30 days before birth, there is a marked increase in the rate of mammary tissue growth in the ewe. In well-fed ewes with one or two lambs, large volumes of colostrum accumulate in the mammary glands during the last few days of pregnancy, and copious milk secretion begins soon after birth, with averages of 1800 to 2800 mL of colostrum and milk being produced during the first 18 hours. Udder growth rates show a similar pattern to fetal growth rates, such that the greatest increase in udder weight occurs in the last 30 days of gestation, and the weight of udder tissue is 30% to 40% of the total weight of the litter. Colostrum production is proportional to udder weight, but refeeding ewes a few days before lambing fills the udder tissue present rather than increasing udder tissue weight. In underfed ewes, accumulation of colostrum before birth is reduced markedly, lactogenesis is delayed, and the total production of colostrum and milk during the first 18 h averages only 1000 mL. Subsequently, for ewes on both planes of nutrition, milk production increases, reaching a peak about 1 to 2 weeks after birth. Underfeeding ewes from 105 days (15 weeks) of gestation can reduce the total yield of colostrum during the first 18 hours after birth by decreasing mammary tissue growth. Thus the prepartum accumulation of colostrum and its subsequent rates of secretion are reduced. Improving the ewe's nutrition from 1 hour after birth can increase the secretion rates of colostrum between 10 and 18 hours.

The growth rate of lambs during the first few weeks of life is positively correlated with birth weight. Low planes of maternal nutrition during late pregnancy and early lactation are generally associated with low birth weights, milk yields, and postnatal growth rates, and high planes of nutrition are associated with the opposite effects. A marked increase in the plane of maternal nutrition at birth can overcome the inhibitory effects on lactation and lamb growth rate of underfeeding in late pregnancy.

Ewe Body-Condition Score

Target condition scores for ewes at different stages of their reproductive cycle have been developed by research groups and departments of agriculture in many countries. These vary according to the predominant breeds and production systems in each country, and they can be quite different for a Merino, Dorset, or Friesian ewe used for wool, meat, or dairy production versus a dual-purpose enterprise producing both meat and wool. Consequently, readers should directly access information appropriate to the production systems of their clients. However, in general, the aim at breeding time is to have ewes with a BCS of 3.0 to 3.5, which ensures maximum ovulation rate. Ewes with a BCS of 3.5 at breeding can be allowed to lose no more than 5% of their body weight, steadily, during the second and third months of pregnancy, equivalent to approximately 0.5 to 1 BCS units. This mild degree of undernutrition enables good placental growth, establishing the basis for maximum fetal growth in the fourth and fifth months of pregnancy, during which the fetus achieves over 80% of its growth. During these final 2 months of pregnancy, there is a limit to the extent to which body-fat reserves can be used because excessive mobilization of fat deposits as a consequence of inadequate dietary energy supply leads to pregnancy toxemia. Ewes with a BCS below 3.0 should be managed to maintain that score.

In late gestation, the optimum BCS ranges from 2.75 to 3.0. In contrast, early lactation is a period in which body fat can be safely used to meet some of the high-energy demands of lactation. During this period, a loss of BCS of from 0.5 to 1.0 (equivalent to 5 kg of fat for a 70-kg ewe at mating) may occur. However, replacement of body fat, to increase the BCS to 3.0 to 3.5 before the next mating, is important to maximize ovulation rate and achieve optimum reproductive performance.

Winter shearing of pregnant ewes during the final 10 weeks of pregnancy can cause a significant increase in lamb birth weight by stimulating ewe appetite. However, this also increases the base energy requirements of the ewe at a feed-limiting time of the year in many production systems (e.g., winter for a spring-lambing flock). Thus it is not always an optimum or profitable system, but this will vary between production systems and different countries.

The nutrient requirements for maintenance, breeding, pregnancy, and lactation of ewes have been cataloged, and optimum feeding strategies for the breeding ewe can be formulated. The evaluation of the ewes' ration during late gestation by monitoring plasma concentrations of the BHB has been described, and these evaluations have been used to provide nutritional advice in intensively managed flocks during late gestation.

In more intensively managed flocks, achieving optimum reproductive performance requires adjusting feeding strategies and the nutrient value of the diet to meet the needs of each stage of the reproductive cycle. Requirement for metabolizable energy increases above maintenance levels from 8 to 12 weeks of pregnancy, increasing further in late pregnancy and lactation. During early lactation, when the energy requirements of prolific ewes exceed the voluntary intake from all but the highest-quality diets, body-fat reserves are used and then replenished toward the end of lactation, when milk yield declines, and in the period leading up to rebreeding.

The rapid growth of the fetus after 90 days of pregnancy and increased energy demand may require the feeding of cereal or legume concentrates, rather than hay, which has far lower metabolizable energy content. This is particularly true for ewes carrying twins or triplets.

In contrast to the ability of the ewe to use body reserves when the intake of energy fails to meet her needs, particularly in early lactation, there is little scope for sustaining production by drawing on body protein. For example, lactating ewes can lose up to 7 kg of body fat during a 4-week period in early lactation, when energy intake is below requirements. For ewes on a low-protein intake, the maximum daily loss of protein is around 26 g. Therefore it is important to meet the protein needs of the ewe during pregnancy, but especially during late pregnancy, to ensure adequate fetal growth, udder development, and colostrum production.

The estimates for the minimum protein requirements of the animal are based on distinguishing between the needs of the rumen microflora for rumen-degradable protein and of the host animal for additional undegraded dietary protein when rumen-degradable protein fails to meet those requirements. In practice, the dietary allowances for late pregnancy and early lactation are higher than the sum of the rumen-degradable protein and undegradable protein.

FURTHER READING

Freer M, ed. *Nutrient Requirements of Domesticated Ruminants [eBook]*. Melbourne: CSIRO Publishing; 2007.

Freer M, Dove H, eds. *Sheep Nutrition*. Wallingford, Oxon, UK: CSIRO and CABI Publishing; 2002.

Hayton A, Husband J, Vecqueray R. Nutritional management of herd health. In: Green M, ed. [eBook]. *Dairy Herd Health*. Wallingford, Oxon, UK: CAB International; 2012.

Herring AD. *Beef Cattle Production Systems*. Wallingford, Oxon, UK: CAB International; 2014.

Subcommittee on Dairy Cattle Nutrition, Committee on Animal Nutrition, Board on Agriculture, National Research Council Subcommittee on Dairy Cattle Nutrition. *Nutrient Requirements of Dairy Cattle*. 7th ed. Washington, DC: National Academy Press; 2000.

Subcommittee on Beef Cattle Nutrition, Committee on Animal Nutrition, Board on Agriculture, National Research Council. *Nutrient Requirements of Beef Cattle*. 7th rev. ed. Washington, DC: National Academy Press; 2000.
Subcommittee on Horse Nutrition, Committee on Animal Nutrition, Board on Agriculture, National Research Council. *Nutrient Requirements of Horses*. 6th rev. ed. Washington, DC: National Academy Press; 2007.
Subcommittee on Sheep Nutrition, Committee on Animal Nutrition, Board on Agriculture, National Research Council. *Nutrient Requirements of Sheep*. 6th rev. ed. Washington, DC: National Academy Press; 1985.
Subcommittee on Swine Nutrition, Committee on Animal Nutrition, Board on Agriculture, National Research Council. *Nutrient Requirements of Swine*. 10th rev. ed. Washington, DC: National Academy Press; 1998.

Deficiencies of Energy and Protein

DEFICIENCY OF ENERGY

ETIOLOGY

Insufficient quantity or quality of feed is a common nutritional deficiency and practical problem of feeding livestock. The term *protein-energy malnutrition* is used to describe a form of incomplete starvation in which a suboptimal amount of energy and protein is present in the diet. Such deficiencies typically occur when livestock are underfed, and often the two scenarios cannot be separated.

EPIDEMIOLOGY

A deficiency of energy is the most common production-limiting nutrient deficiency of farm animals. There may be inadequate amounts of feed available, or the feed may be of low quality (low digestibility). The availability of pasture may be inadequate because of overgrazing, drought, or snow covering. Alternatively, it may be too expensive to provide enough supplementary feed of the required quality, or the available feed may be of such low quality and poor digestibility that animals cannot consume enough to meet energy requirements. In some cases, forage may contain a high concentration of water, which limits total energy intake.

CLINICAL FINDINGS

The clinical findings of an energy deficiency depend on the age of the animal, whether or not it is pregnant or lactating, concurrent deficiencies of other nutrients, and environmental factors. In general, an insufficient supply of energy in young livestock causes decreased growth and delayed onset of puberty. In mature animals, there is reduced milk production and a shortened lactation. A prolonged energy deficiency in pregnant beef heifers will result in a failure to produce adequate quantities of colostrum at parturition. In mature animals, there is also a marked loss of body weight, especially when demand for energy increases in late pregnancy and early lactation. There are prolonged periods of anestrus, which reduces the reproductive performance of the herd. Primigravid females are particularly susceptible to protein-energy malnutrition because of their requirements for growth and maintenance. A deficiency of energy during late gestation can produce undersized, weak neonates with a high mortality rate, whereas abomasal impaction is associated with energy deficiency during prolonged cold weather, especially in pregnant beef cattle and ewes being wintered on poor-quality roughage. Heat loss from the animal to the environment increases considerably during cold weather, and when ambient temperatures are below the critical temperatures, the animal responds by increasing metabolic rate to maintain normal body core temperature.[1] If sufficient feed is available when temperatures are below the lower critical temperature, ruminants will increase their voluntary feed intake to maintain body temperature. If sufficient feed is not available, the animal will mobilize energy stored as fat or muscle to maintain body temperature and thus lose body weight. In the case of ruminants and horses, if the feed is of poor quality, for example, poor-quality roughage, the increased feed intake may result in impaction of the abomasum and forestomaches in cattle and of the large intestine in the horse.

Cold, windy, and wet weather will increase the needs for energy, and the effects of a deficiency are exaggerated, often resulting in weakness, recumbency, and death. A sudden dietary deficiency of energy in fat, pregnant beef cattle and ewes can result in starvation ketosis and pregnancy toxemia. Hyperlipemia occurs in fat, pregnant or lactating ponies that are on a falling plane of nutrition.

Protein-energy malnutrition occurs in neonatal calves fed inferior-quality milk replacers that may contain insufficient energy or added nonmilk proteins, which may be indigestible by the newborn calf. A major portion of the body fat present at birth can be depleted in diarrheic calves deprived of milk and fed only fluids and electrolytes for 4 to 7 days. Feeding only fluids and electrolytes to normal, healthy newborn calves for 7 days can result in a significant loss of perirenal and bone-marrow fat and depletion of visible omental, mesenteric, and subcutaneous fat stores. The amount of body fat present in a calf at birth is an important determinant of the length of time an apparently healthy calf can survive in the face of malnutrition. Calves born from dams on an adequate diet usually have sufficient body fat to provide energy for at least 7 days of severe malnutrition. The absence of perirenal fat in a calf at 2 to 4 days of age suggests inadequate reserves of fat at birth and chronic fetal malnutrition.

DEFICIENCY OF PROTEIN

A deficiency of protein commonly accompanies a deficiency of energy. However, the effects of the protein deficiency, at least in the early stages, are usually not as severe as those of energy deficiency. Insufficient protein intake in young animals results in reduced appetite, lowered feed intake, inferior growth rate, lack of muscle development, and a prolonged time to reach maturity. In mature animals, there is loss of weight and decreased milk production. In both young and mature animals, there is a drop in hemoglobin concentration, packed cell volume, total serum protein, and serum albumin. In the late stages, there is edema associated with the hypoproteinemia. Ruminants do not normally need a dietary supply of essential amino acids, in contrast to pigs, which need a natural protein supplement in addition to the major portion of total protein supplied by the cereal grains. The amino acid composition of the dietary protein for ruminants is not critical because the ruminal flora synthesize the necessary amino acids from lower-quality proteins and nonprotein sources of nitrogen.

CLINICAL FINDINGS

The clinical findings of a protein deficiency are similar to those of an energy deficiency, and the clinical findings of both resemble those of many other specific nutrient deficiencies and subclinical diseases. Protein-energy malnutrition in beef cattle occurs most commonly in late gestation and is characterized clinically by weakness, clinical recumbency, marked loss of body weight, a normal mental attitude, and a desire to eat. Cows with concurrent hypocalcemia will be anorexic. If the condition occurs at the time of parturition, there will be an obvious lack of colostrum. Calves of these cows may attempt to vigorously suck their dams, attempt to eat dry feed, drink surface water or urine, and bellow continuously. Affected cows and their calves may die within 7 to 10 days.

Protein-energy malnutrition is less common in dairy cattle because they are usually fed to meet the requirements of maintenance and milk production. Dairy calves fed inferior-quality milk replacers during periods of cold weather will lose weight, become inactive and lethargic, and may die within 2 to 4 weeks. Affected calves may maintain their appetites until just before death. Diarrhea may occur concurrently and be confused with acute undifferentiated diarrhea as a result of the enteropathogenic viruses or cryptosporidiosis. Affected calves recover quickly when fed cow's whole milk.

Protein-energy malnutrition also occurs in sheep and, less commonly, in goats. Excessive dental attrition is a common cause in grazing sheep, which is exacerbated by the excessive ingestion of soil.

DIFFERENTIAL DIAGNOSIS

The diagnosis will depend on an estimation of the concentration of energy and protein in the feed, or a feed analysis, and comparing the results with the estimated nutrient requirements of the class of affected animals. In some cases, a sample of feed used several weeks earlier may no longer be available, or the daily feed intake may not be known. Marginal deficiencies of energy and protein may be detectable with the aid of a metabolic profile test. Specific treatment of livestock affected with protein-energy malnutrition is usually not undertaken because of the high cost and prolonged recovery period. Oral and parenteral fluid and electrolyte therapy can be given as indicated. The provision of high-quality feeds appropriate to the species is the most cost-effective strategy.

PREVENTION

The prevention of protein-energy malnutrition requires the provision of the nutrient requirements of the animals according to age, stage of pregnancy and production, the environmental temperature, and the cost of the feeds. Body-condition scoring of cattle and sheep can be used as a guide to monitor body condition and nutritional status. Regular analysis of feed supplies will assist in the overall nutritional management program. The published nutrient requirements of domestic animals are only guidelines to estimated requirements because they were determined in experimental animals selected for uniform size and other characteristics. Under practical conditions, all of the common factors that affect requirements must be considered.

FURTHER READING

Freer M, ed. *Nutrient Requirements of Domesticated Ruminants [eBook]*. Melbourne: CSIRO Publishing; 2007.

Freer M, Dove H, eds. *Sheep Nutrition*. Wallingford, Oxon, UK: CSIRO and CABI Publishing; 2002.

Hayton A, Husband J, Vecqueray R. Nutritional management of herd health. In: Green M, ed. [eBook]. *Dairy Herd Health*. Wallingford, Oxon, UK: CAB International; 2012.

Herring AD. *Beef Cattle Production Systems*. Wallingford, Oxon, UK: CAB International; 2014.

REFERENCE

1. Grazfeed v 5.04, CSIRO. Accessed at <http://www.hzn.com.au/grazfeed.php>; June 18, 2016.

LOW-MILK-FAT SYNDROME

In low-milk-fat syndrome, the concentration of fat in milk is reduced, often to less than 50% of normal, while milk volume is maintained. This syndrome is a significant cause of wastage in high-producing cows. Low concentration of fat in milk occurs with ruminal acidosis in cattle.[1] The cause appears to be an increase in concentrations of conjugated linoleic acid in the diet, with subsequent reduction in lipogenesis in the udder.[2] A supply of polyunsaturated fatty acids in the cows' ration and alteration in fermentation in the rumen results in biohydrogenation of linoleic acid (abundant in oils and seeds) and formation of intermediate fatty acids in the rumen. These incompletely hydrogenated fatty acids are absorbed into the blood and have an inhibitory effect on lipogenesis.[3] This syndrome occurs most commonly in cows on low-fiber diets, for example, lush, irrigated pasture or grain rations that are ground very finely or fed as pellets. Treatment is achieved by administration of sodium bicarbonate or magnesium oxide, which increase fiber digestibility and hence the propionate : acetate ratio. Magnesium oxide also increases the activity of lipoprotein lipase in the mammary gland and increases uptake of triglycerides by the mammary gland from the plasma.[4]

REFERENCES

1. Atkinson O. *Cattle Pract*. 2014;22:1.
2. Gulati SK, et al. *Can J Anim Sci*. 2006;86:63.
3. Dubuc J, et al. *Point Veterinaire*. 2009;40:45.
4. Radostits O, et al. *Veterinary Medicine: a Textbook of the Diseases of Cattle, Horses, Sheep, Goats, and Pigs*. 10th ed. London: W.B. Saunders; 2006: 1686.

Diseases Associated With Deficiencies of Mineral Nutrients

There is an enormous literature about mineral nutrient deficiencies in livestock, and thus it is not possible to comprehensively review it here, but some general comments are appropriate. In developed countries, severe deficiencies of single elements affecting very large numbers of animals now seldom occur. The diagnostic research work has been done, the guidelines for preventive programs have been outlined, and these have been applied in the field. Thus the major contributions to knowledge have already been made, and what remains is essentially applying and extending that knowledge. Some loose ends remain, including preventing the overzealous or unnecessary application of minerals, which can produce toxicoses or is simply not cost-effective; sorting out the relative importance of the constituent elements in combined deficiencies, characterized by incomplete response to single elements; and devising better ways of detecting marginal deficiencies.

At least 15 mineral elements are essential nutrients for ruminants. The macrominerals, required daily in gram amounts, are calcium, phosphorous, potassium, sodium, chlorine, magnesium, and sulfur. The trace elements, or microminerals, are copper, selenium, zinc, cobalt, iron, iodine, manganese, and molybdenum. Improving trace-element nutrition of grazing livestock, in a way that is cost-effective and that meets consumer perceptions and preferences, is a continuing challenge.[1]

PREVALENCE AND ECONOMIC IMPORTANCE

Despite experimental evidence that deficiencies or excesses of trace elements can influence growth, reproductive performance, or immunocompetence of livestock, there is often a lack of information on the prevalence and economic significance of such problems. Most published reports of trace-element-related diseases are case reports and thus provide insufficient information to assess prevalence and economic impact on a regional or national scale. Many reports are also compromised by commercial bias. Despite this, Food and Agriculture Organization/World Health Organization (FAO/WHO) Animal Health Yearbooks show that of the countries providing information on animal diseases, 80% report nutritional diseases of moderate or high incidence, and trace-element deficiencies or toxicities are involved in more than half of those whose causes were identified. As a specific example, in the United Kingdom it has been estimated that despite the activities of its nutritional and veterinary advisory services, and extensive supplementation, clinical signs of copper deficiency occur annually in approximately 1% of the cattle population. Copper deficiency can also predispose to increased mortality as a result of infectious diseases in lambs, and so it is likely that the economic losses from copper deficiency may be considerably underestimated even in developed agricultural economies.

DIAGNOSTIC STRATEGIES

In developed countries with more advanced livestock industries, the emphasis is on disease prevention rather than therapy, and the cost-effective control of trace-element deficiencies is a matter of ongoing farmer education rather than research. Copper, cobalt, selenium, and iodine deficiencies can affect reproductive performance, appetite, early postnatal growth, and immunocompetence on a herd or flock basis, and thus emphasis is placed on identifying the risk of deficiency before clinical signs appear.

Monitoring the trace-element status of livestock is typically done by blood, saliva, or tissue analysis, or less commonly by measuring the concentration of the trace element in the diet. An alternative way of monitoring preclinical stages of a trace element deficiency is to identify and measure a biochemical indicator that reflects changes in the activity of an enzyme involved in a key metabolic pathway, such as vitamin B_{12} or glutathione peroxidase, which are indirect measures of cobalt and selenium nutrition in sheep, respectively. To be useful, techniques should be able to predict the likely pathologic outcome of different suboptimal concentrations of a particular measure, and hence when it is clinically and economically justifiable to apply treatments or interventions. For example, a high proportion of grazing cattle become hypocupremic if maintained on pasture forage, but they don't develop clinical signs of deficiency, and only a small percentage exhibit any physiologic response to the administration of copper. This illustrates the variation in the development of clinical signs of copper deficiency, which can be induced by a simple dietary deficiency or by interactions between copper and other elements in the diet, such as molybdenum, sulfur, and iron. There is also evidence that genetic variation influences the utilization of trace elements by livestock. For example, there are differences in dietary requirements for copper between some breeds of sheep. Sheep can also be selected for a high or low concentration of plasma copper, which can have profound physiologic consequences in the low-copper group.

Thus although it is known from soil maps and local knowledge where trace-element deficiencies occur, their prevalence and importance may be underestimated because subclinical deficiency may go unnoticed for prolonged periods.

DEFICIENCIES IN DEVELOPING COUNTRIES

In developing countries, deficiencies of trace elements are often hidden or confounded by gross nutritional deficiencies of energy, protein, phosphorus, and water, which affect postnatal growth and reproductive performance. Undernutrition is the most important limitation to herbivore livestock production in tropical countries, but mineral deficiencies or imbalances in soils and pasture forages, particularly of phosphorus, cobalt, or copper, are also responsible for poor reproductive performance and low growth rates.

PATHOPHYSIOLOGY OF TRACE-ELEMENT DEFICIENCY

The physiologic basis of trace-element deficiency is complex.[1] Some trace elements are essential for the function of a single enzyme, whereas others are involved in multiple metabolic pathways. Consequently, a deficiency of a specific element may affect one or more metabolic processes and produce a variety of clinical signs in different classes of livestock. Furthermore, there is a wide variation in the clinical response to decreased blood or tissue concentrations of a trace element between individuals. For example, two animals in a herd or flock with the same concentration of copper in their blood may be in different body condition. Their susceptibility to clinical disease will also be influenced by their age, physiologic status (pregnant, lactating, or dry), genetic differences, and interactions with other trace elements. For example, there is good evidence that whereas dietary copper may be adequate for some breeds of sheep, such concentrations may be deficient, or even toxic, for others.

Dietary deficiency does not inevitably lead to clinical disease, but several factors interact and predispose the animal to clinical disease, including the following:

- Age—for example, late-term fetal lambs are highly susceptible to demyelination as a result of copper deficiency, which produces "swayback."
- Genetic differences and individual variation in response to deficiency.
- Fluctuating demand for trace elements because of changes in growth, physiologic status (especially lactation), and diet.
- Substitution—the use of alternative metabolic pathways in response to a deficiency, such as selenium, which may incompletely protect sheep from white-muscle disease when the diet is deficient in vitamin E.
- Size of the functional reserves.

The trace elements are component parts of many tissues and are often involved in metabolic pathways, either as a single key enzyme or in many interacting components. Consequently, their deficiency leads to a variety of pathologic consequences, metabolic defects, and clinical signs. These are summarized in Table 17-12.

The soil and its parent materials are the primary sources of trace elements from which soil–plant–animal relationships are built. Soil maps created from geochemical surveys can help identify areas in which livestock are exposed to excessive ingestion or deficiencies of trace elements. Variations in the concentration of most trace elements in soils are quite wide, ranging from soils that are grossly deficient to those that are potentially toxic. The availability of trace elements to plants is controlled by their total concentration in the soil and their chemical form. Certain species of plants take up more trace elements than others, and the ingestion of soil can also have a profound effect on the nutrition and metabolism of some trace elements.

It is often difficult to determine the role of individual trace elements in deficiency states because many trace-element

Table 17-12 Principal pathologic and metabolic defects in essential trace-element deficiencies

Deficiency	Pathologic consequence	Associated metabolic defect
Copper	Defective melanin production	Tyrosine/DOPA oxidation
	Defective keratinization; hair, wool	–SH oxidation to S–S
	Defective cross linkages in connective tissue, osteoporosis	Lysyl oxidase
	Ataxia, myelin aplasia	Cytochrome c oxidase
	Growth failure	Decreased biogenic molecules such as gastrin
	Anemia	Ceruloplasmin (ferroxidase)
	Uricemia	Urate oxidase
Cobalt	Anorexia	Methyl malonyl CoA mutase
	Impaired oxidation of propionate	Tetrahydrofolate methyl transferase
	Anemia	
Selenium	Myopathy; cardiac/skeletal	Peroxide/hydroperoxide destruction
	Liver necrosis	Decreased glutathione peroxidase
	Defective neutrophil function	OH; O_2 generation
Zinc	Anorexia, growth failure	Multifactorial; increased expression of leptin (satiety signal) and cholecystokinin (appetite regulation), reduced pyruvate kinase
	Parakeratosis	Polynucleotide synthesis, transcription, translation?
	Perinatal mortality	
	Thymic involution	
	Defective cell-mediated immunity	
Iodine	Thyroid hyperplasia	Decreased thyroid hormone synthesis
	Reproductive failure	
	Hair, wool loss	
Manganese	Skeletal/cartilage defects	Chondroitin sulfate synthesis
	Reproductive failure	

deficiencies produce nonspecific and specific clinical signs, especially when complex interactions occur. Consequently, the dose–response trial still has a significant role to investigate complex or marginal deficiencies and whether a cost-effective response will occur on a particular farm.[2] A properly conducted dose–response trial requires comparison of the response to treatment, typically a biochemical indicator and a measure of production, such as body weight, in a supplemented and control group. Ideally, animals should be randomly selected and allocated to groups, and the groups should be of sufficient size to reliably detect an economically significant difference (e.g., have a 95% chance of detecting a 1-kg difference in body weight). Where appropriate, the control (unsupplemented) group should be treated with the vehicle or inactive portion of the substance given to the supplemented group (a placebo). Additional requirements for a reliable dose–response trial include a careful appraisal of the reasons for conducting the trial, a suitable form of treatment, and a reliable biochemical method for monitoring the response to the trace element. Dose–response trials establish a link between a trace element and certain clinical signs. They can also identify factors that modify the response to a trace element and, importantly, provide some indication of the economic response to supplementation.

The ad hoc field observations made by veterinarians who make a diagnosis of a trace-element deficiency, followed by treatment or dietary changes, are subjective and usually lack controls. Nevertheless, they are useful in that they indicate the magnitude and variability of response that might be expected in future studies.

There are major challenges in predicting and diagnosing trace-element deficiencies in grazing livestock, including complex interactions between dietary constituents and the homeostatic mechanisms of the animal. Thus it is usually impossible to predict from the composition or analysis of the diet whether clinical signs of deficiency will occur. Consequently, assessment of the absorbable, rather than the total, concentration of elements in the diet is now considered to be more important in understanding the nutritional basis for the deficiencies, but tests of the livestock are a more definitive assessment of deficiency.

LABORATORY DIAGNOSIS OF MINERAL DEFICIENCIES

The diagnosis of mineral deficiencies, particularly trace-element deficiencies, relies heavily on the interpretation of the biochemical tests. This is because deficiencies of any one or more of several trace elements can result in nonspecific clinical abnormalities, such as loss of weight, growth retardation, anorexia, and inferior reproductive performance.

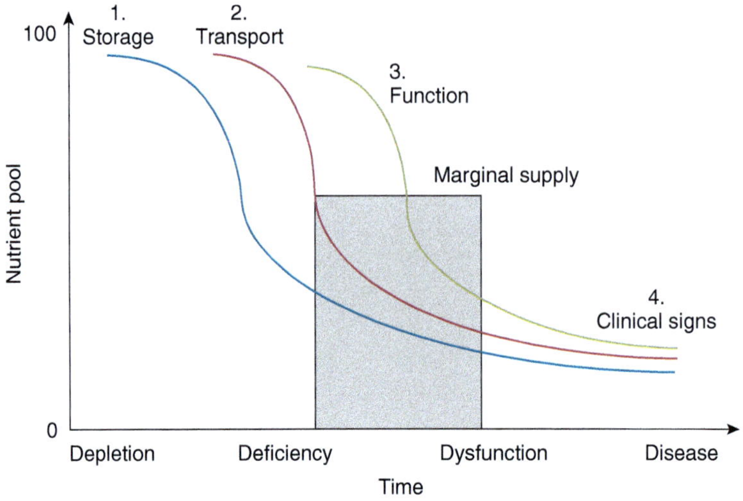

Fig. 17-11 The sequence of pathophysiological changes that can occur in mineral-deprived livestock, commencing with depletion and ending with clinical disease, and their relation to the body pools of that nutrient. (Reproduced with permission from Suttle NF. *Mineral Nutrition of Livestock*. 4th ed. Wallingford, Oxon, UK: CAB International; 2010 [Chapter 1].)

The interpretation of biochemical criteria of trace-element status is governed by three important principles: **relationship with intake, time, and function**. These are further explained as follows:

1. Relationship between the tissue concentrations of a direct marker and the dietary intake of the element will generally be sigmoid in shape (a dose–response curve). The important point on the curve is the intake at which the requirement of the animal is passed, which is the intake of the nutrient needed to maintain normal physiologic concentrations of the element and/or avoid impairment of essential functions. For several markers of trace-element status, the position on the *x*-axis at which the requirement is passed coincides with the end of the lower plateau of the response in marker concentration. Under these conditions, the marker is an excellent index of sufficiency and body reserves, but an insensitive index of a deficiency. If requirement is passed at the beginning of the upper plateau, the marker is a poor index of sufficiency, but a good index of deficiency. This principle allows direct markers to be divided into storage and nonstorage types corresponding to the former and latter positions on the *x*-axis.
2. Nonstorage criteria can be divided into indicators of acute and chronic deficiency, and two types of relationships can be distinguished: a rapid, early decline in marker concentration followed by a plateau; and a slow, linear rate of decline. Markers with a slow, linear response will be good indices of a chronic deficiency, but unreliable indices of acute deficiency, because they cannot respond quickly enough. Conversely, the marker with a rapid, early decline will be a good index of acute deficiency, but an unreliable indicator for chronic deficiency if the low plateau is reached before functions are impaired. Those biochemical criteria that are based on metalloenzyme or metalloprotein concentrations in erythrocytes are of the slow type because the marker is incorporated into the erythrocyte before its release into the bloodstream, and thereafter its half-life is determined by that of the erythrocyte, which is 150 days or more. Metalloenzymes or metalloproteins in the plasma with short half-lives provide markers of the rapid type.
3. A deficiency can be divided into four phases: depletion, deficiency (marginal), dysfunction, and clinical disease. During these phases there are progressive changes in the body pools of mineral that serve as storage (e.g., liver for copper, bone for Ca and P), transport (e.g., plasma), and function (e.g., muscle enzymes) (Fig. 17-11).[3]

Depletion is a relative term describing the failure of the diet to maintain the trace-element status of the body, and it may continue for weeks or months without observable clinical effects when substantial body reserves exist. When the net requirement for an essential element exceeds the net flow of the absorbed element across the intestine, then depletion occurs. The body processes may respond by improving intestinal absorption or decreasing endogenous losses. During the depletion phase, there is a loss of trace element from any storage sites, such as the liver, during which time the plasma concentrations of the trace element may remain constant. The liver is a common store for copper, iron, and vitamins A and B_{12}.

If the dietary deficiency persists, eventually there is a transition from a state of depletion to one of deficiency, which is marked by biochemical indications that the homeostatic mechanisms are no longer maintaining a constant level of trace elements necessary for normal physiologic function. After variable periods of time, the concentrations or activities of trace-element-containing enzymes will begin to decline, leading to the phase of dysfunction. There may be a further lag period, the subclinical phase, before the changes in cellular function are manifested as clinical disease. The biochemical criteria can be divided, according to the phase during which they change, into indicators of marginal deficiency and dysfunction. The rate of onset of clinical disease will depend on the intensity of the dietary deficiency, the duration of the deficit, and the size of the initial reserve. If reserves are nonexistent, as with zinc metabolism, the effects may be acute, and the separate phases become superimposed. The application of these principles to the interpretation of biochemical criteria of trace-element status is presented elsewhere where applicable, in the discussion of each mineral nutrient.

The definitive etiologic diagnosis of a trace-element deficiency will depend on the response in growth and health obtained following treatment or supplementation of the diet. The concurrent measurement of biochemical markers will aid in the interpretation and validation of those markers for future diagnosis. The strategies for anticipating and preventing trace-element deficiencies include regular analysis of the feed and soil, which is not highly reliable, and monitoring samples from herds and flocks to prevent animals from entering the zone of marginal trace-element deficiencies that precedes the onset of functional deficiency. The decision to intervene can be safely based on the conventional criteria of marginal trace-element status.

FURTHER READING

Lee J, Masters DG, White CL, Grace ND, Judson GJ. Current issues in trace element nutrition of grazing livestock in Australia and New Zealand. *Aust J Agric Res.* 1999;50:1341-1364.

Suttle NF. *Mineral Nutrition of Livestock*. 4th ed. Wallingford, Oxon, UK: CAB International; 2010.

REFERENCES

1. Suttle NF. *Mineral Nutrition of Livestock*. 4th ed. Wallingford, Oxon, UK: CAB International; 2010 [Chapter 1].
2. Ibid., [Chapter 19].
3. Ibid., [Chapter 3].

18 Diseases Primarily Affecting the Reproductive System

Infectious Diseases Primarily Affecting the Reproductive System

This chapter presents information related to important and selected livestock pathogens that affect not only the fertility but also the health of animals, and in some cases, such as bovine brucellosis, the health of humans. It is worth noting that national control and eradication campaigns against *Brucella abortus* infection in cattle played, and continue to play, an important global role in expanding the veterinary profession. More recently, the worldwide spread of porcine reproductive and respiratory syndrome (PRRS) virus during the last 20 years has had a marked economic impact on the swine industry. As a consequence, PRRS is currently one of the most intensively researched diseases of livestock.

Readers seeking detailed information related to reproductive performance, the estrous cycle, conception, pregnancy, and parturition are directed to the many excellent textbooks that address these subjects.

INDUCTION OF PARTURITION

CALVES

The induction of parturition in pregnant cows during the last 6 weeks of gestation by the parenteral injection of corticosteroid with or without prostaglandin F2α (PGF2α) has raised the question of animal welfare and of the possible effects of prematurity on the disease resistance of the newborn calf. The induction of premature parturition in cattle has found application in the following areas:

- With pastoral-based dairy production, synchronization of the calving period has allowed maximal utilization of seasonally available pastures by the synchronization of peak demand for dry matter intake with spring flush in pasture growth. In pastoral-based herds with breeding for seasonal calving, late-calving cows will be induced and these average approximately 8% of the herd.
- Ensuring that calving coincides with the availability of labor to facilitate observations and management of calving and to overcome the inconvenience caused by late-calving cows.
- Minimizing dystocia in small heifers and animals with exceedingly long gestation periods (past due).
- The therapeutic termination of pregnancy for various clinical reasons.
- As an aid in the control of milk fever in combination with parenteral administration of vitamin D analogs.

A variety of short-acting and long-acting corticosteroids have been used. A single injection of a short-acting formulation is used when it is desirable to induce calving within the last 2 weeks of gestation. Earlier in pregnancy short-acting corticosteroids were found to be insufficiently reliable to induce parturition, which has led to the common use of long-acting corticosteroid formulations. A variety of protocols to induce premature parturition (3–6 weeks before due date) are used in practice; the main issue is the poor predictability of the time of calving relative to treatment when using long-acting corticosteroids. Common protocols use a second treatment with short-acting corticosteroids or the administration of PGF2α 50 to 10 days after the initial treatment. The use of PGF2α at least 9 days after treatment with long-acting corticosteroids was found to reliably narrow down the calving time, with the great majority of all cows calving within 72 hours of PGF2α treatment.[1] The use of PGF2α did not improve the viability of the premature neonates or their survival rate.

For cattle near term (within 2 weeks of due date) the use of short-acting corticosteroid formulation is more appropriate with parturition generally occurring within 2 to 4 days posttreatment.[2]

The **mortality rate** of induced calves is considerable and can exceed 30%, particularly when dams are induced at or before the eighth month of gestation.[2] Mortality in calves born as a result of induced parturition is primarily a result of prematurity, and calf mortality is generally low when calving is induced within 12 days of parturition, although there are welfare concerns. The calves born earlier in pregnancy after using long-acting corticosteroid are usually lighter in weight, lethargic, and slow to stand and to suck properly. The serum immunoglobulin concentration was found to be lower in calves born from dams induced with long-acting corticosteroids because of interference with intestinal absorption by the corticosteroid. Up to 60% of calves born following induction with long-acting corticosteroids are at risk for failure of transfer of passive immunity. The colostrum available to such calves also has a reduced immunoglobulin content, and there may also be a reduction in the total volume of colostrum available from the induced-calving cows. Immunoglobulin absorption rates were not impaired when short-acting corticosteroids are used to induce calving close to term.

Artificial induction of parturition is an important risk factor for retention of the placenta, and the incidence is reported to vary from 20% to 100%. Subsequent reproductive performance of induced cows can be impaired. A risk for acute gram-negative bacterial infections is reported in a low (0.3%) proportion of cows following induction with dexamethasone. The use of long-acting corticosteroids was also associated with a higher incidence of photosensitization in treated heifers.[2]

In a study where partus induction was systematically used in cows that exceeded a gestation length of 282 days, no detrimental effects on calf viability, cow health, and productive and reproductive performance during lactation were found compared with untreated control animals. The incidence of retained fetal membranes in untreated animals was not recorded in this study and could thus not be compared with treated animals.[2]

When parturition is induced in large herds of beef cattle, particularly with a high percentage of heifers, increased surveillance will be necessary after the calves are born to avoid mismothering. Every attempt must be made to establish the cow–calf pair (neonatal bond) and move them out of the main calving area. Heifers that disown their calves must be confined in a small pen and be encouraged to accept the calf and let it suck, which is sometimes a very unrewarding chore. Calf mortality can be very high where calving is induced earlier than 35 weeks of pregnancy.

LAMBS

The induction of parturition in sheep is not a common practice, but it can be used to synchronize lambing in flocks where there are accurate dates of mating for individual ewes. Unless accurate dates are available, there is risk of prematurity. Also, ewes that are more than 10 days from their normal parturition date are unlikely to respond.

Induction of parturition is also used as a therapeutic ploy to terminate pregnancies in sheep with pregnancy toxemia. Induction is usually performed with dexamethasone and less commonly with betamethasone or flumethasone, which is more expensive. Lambing occurs 36 to 48 hours later, and there may be breed differences in response. Variability in lambing time can be reduced by the use of clenbuterol and oxytocin.

FOALS

The induction of parturition in mares for reasons of economy, management convenience, concern for prolonged gestation, or clinical conditions such as prepubic tendon rupture or research and teaching is now being practiced.

Foaling can be induced with oxytocin, ideally administered as an intravenous (IV) drip over 15 to 30 minutes, and occurs within 15 to 90 minutes of its administration. High doses of oxytocin are potentially dangerous to the foal and low doses (10–20 IU) are preferred. Glucocorticoids, and antiprogestagens that are effective in inducing pregnancy in other species, are either ineffective in the mare or capricious in their efficacy and can also be associated with adverse effects on the foal.

Prostaglandin F2α and its analogs have been used for partus induction in the mare and low doses (5–12 mg intramuscularly [IM]) may be effective at term, but repeated treatments may be required. The time interval between treatment and delivery is difficult to predict and can range from 1 to 48 hours. The use of PGF2α for partus induction in mares has been discouraged because considerable risks such as premature placental separation and foal death that have been associated with this treatment.[3]

Induction of parturition in the mare is not without risk and has been associated with the birth of foals that are weak, injured, or susceptible to perinatal infections. The period of fetal maturation is relatively short in the horse and is considered to be the last 2 to 3 days' gestation. Because spontaneous parturition in healthy mares can occur between 320 and 360 days, there is the risk of delivering a foal that is premature and nonviable. Fetal maturity is the major prerequisite for successful induced parturition, and the three essential criteria are

- A gestational length of more than 330 days
- Substantial mammary development and the presence of colostrum in the mammary gland with a calcium concentration greater than 10 mmol/L
- Softening of the cervix

The rise in calcium concentration is the most reliable predictor of fetal maturity and milk calcium concentrations above 10 mmol/L, in combination with a concentration of potassium that is greater than sodium, are indicative of fetal maturity. Commercial milk test strips are available for estimating mammary secretion electrolyte concentrations; however, it is recommended that testing be done in an accredited laboratory.

In mature foals, head lifting, sternal recumbency, and evidence of suck reflex occurs within 5 minutes of spontaneous full-term deliveries. The foal can stand within 1 hour and suck the mare within 2 hours. The behavior and viability of the premature foal after induced parturition have been described. The overall survival rate of foals delivered from induced parturition before 320 days' gestation was 5%. Four patterns of neonatal adaptation were observed on the basis of righting, sucking, and standing ability. If the suck reflex was weak or absent and the foals were unable to establish righting reflexes, the prognosis of survival was poor. Foals born before 300 days' gestation did not survive for more than 90 minutes; foals born closer to 320 days' gestation had a better chance of survival and exhibited behavioral patterns of adaptation.

In addition to the potential delivery of a premature or weak foal, other adverse effects of induction can be dystocia, premature placental separation, and retained placenta.

PIGLETS

The induction of parturition of gilts and sows on days 112, 113, or 114 of gestation is highly reliable and can be achieved by a single IM injection of 175 μg of cloprostenol or 5 to 10 mg of PGF2α. The sows farrow approximately 20 to 36 hours later. Synchronization of farrowing can be improved by administration of oxytocin (5–30 IU) 20 to 24 hours after injection of PGF2.

Induction of parturition has been used on large-scale farms to allow a concentration of labor, to improve supervision and care at the time of farrowing, to reduce the incidence of the mastitis/metritis/agalactia syndrome, and to reduce the percentage of stillborn piglets. The end day of a batch farrowing system can be fixed and weekend farrowing avoided. The subsequent fertility of the sows is not impaired. Induction on day 110 may be associated with a slight increase in perinatal mortality.

TREATMENT

Premature partus induction cattle (>2 weeks before due date):

Dexamethasone trimethyl-acetate (or other long-acting formulation) (25–30 mg/animal IM as single dose) (R-1)

Dinoprost (or other PGF2α-analogon) (25 mg/animal IM as a single dose 5–10 days after dexamethasone treatment) (R-2)

Partus induction cattle (<2 weeks before due date):

Dexamethasone sodium-phosphate (or other short-acting formulation) (40 mg/animal IM as a single dose) (R-1)

Continued

Cloprostenol (500 μg/animal IM 36–48 h after dexamethasone treatment) (R-1)

Dinoprost (25 mg/animal IM as a single dose 36–48 h after dexamethasone treatment) (R-2)

Partus induction mare:

Oxytocin (10–20 IU/animal as IV drip over 15–30 min, several repetitions possible) (R-1)

Prostaglandin F2α (or analogon) (R-3)

Partus induction sow:

Prostaglandin F2α (or analogon) (10–25 mg/animal IM) (R-1)

Cloprostenol (175 μg/animal IM) (R-1)

Oxytocin (5–30 IU/animal IM 20–24 h after treatment with PGF2α) (R-1)

Partus induction ewe:

Dexamethasone (15–20 mg/animal IM) (R-1)

IM, *intramuscularly;* IV, *intravenously.*

FURTHER READING

Ingoldby L, Jackson P. Induction of parturition in sheep. *In Pract.* 2001;23:228231.

MacDiarmid SC. Induction of parturition in cattle using corticosteroid: a review. Part 1. Reasons for induction, mechanisms of induction and preparations used. *Anim Breed Abstr.* 1983;51:40319.

MacDiarmid SC. Induction of parturition in cattle using corticosteroid: a review. Part 2. Effects of induced calving on the calf and cow. *Anim Breed Abstr.* 1983;51:499508.

Pressing AL. Pharmacologic control of swine reproduction. *Vet Clin North Am Food Anim Pract.* 1992;8:70723.

REFERENCES

1. Mansell PD, et al. *Aust Vet J.* 2006;84:312.
2. Villarroel A, Lane VM. *Can J Vet Res.* 2010;74:136.
3. Olsey J. *Equine Vet Educ.* 2003;15:164.

FREEMARTINISM IN CALVES

A freemartin is defined as a sterile female partner of a pair of heterosexual twins. In cattle, 92% of females born cotwins to males are freemartins.

In normal calves, the chromosomal identification of females is 60,XX (60 chromosomes, both X chromosomes) and of males is 60,XY (the Y being smaller and not readily paired with its opposite X chromosome).

The freemartin is the classical example of the chimera in cytogenetics. They are the individuals that contain two or more cell types that originated in separate individuals. The only way in which a chimera can develop is via the fusion of circulations or zygotes in utero. Sex chromosome chimerism is also reported in goats, sheep, and pigs, and, although the male partners of female twins are usually anatomically normal, they often have reduced fertility. Bulls born cotwin with freemartin females may also be chimeric and have low reproductive efficiency.

The diagnosis of freemartinism has been based on physical examination, karyotyping, or blood typing, and each has its limitations. There is variation in the degree of reproductive tract abnormalities in freemartins. The external genitalia may appear normal, the vulval hair may be coarser than usual, or the clitoris may be enlarged. The vagina is generally expected to be shorter than normal. The cervix, uterus, uterine tubes, and ovaries may be absent, present in underdeveloped form, or may appear normal on rectal palpation.

Special cytogenetic techniques are also available that facilitate the diagnosis of freemartinism in a female calf of a male–female twinning. In freemartins (phenotypically female, but also carrying male cells) there is a mixture of mostly 60,XX chromosomes to a cell and a small proportion of 60,XY cells. A large number of cells need to be analyzed if only the freemartin calf is available, because the proportion of abnormal cells present may be as low as 2%. It is, however, possible to make a diagnosis on the examination of 10 to 20 cells, provided the male twin is also analyzed; the female may have very few XY chromosomes, but the male will have a very high proportion of XX chromosomes. This technique is much more accurate than blood group analysis or clinical observations of a short vagina, enlarged clitoris, and the presence of a vulval tuft of hair. Karyotyping is a definitive method of freemartin diagnosis, but it is tedious, time-consuming, and expensive. Blood typing analysis may be performed on both the male and female cotwins to demonstrate two blood group populations, but it is expensive and requires blood samples from both cotwins.

The **polymerase chain reaction** (PCR) method of freemartin diagnosis using sex-specific DNA sequences is rapid, accurate, relatively simple, and inexpensive to perform, and a blood sample is required only from the female cotwins. It allows for the accurate decision of freemartinism down to a level of 0.05% of male chimeric cells present.

FURTHER READING

Padula AM. The freemartin syndrome: An update. *Anim Reprod Sci.* 2005;87:93-109.

BULLER STEER SYNDROME

SYNOPSIS

Etiology Unknown. Behavioral problem of steers in feedlots.

Epidemiology Prevalence varies and increases with increasing age and weight at entry.

Clinical findings and lesions Areas of denuded hair, subcutaneous hematomas, and other traumatic injuries.

Treatment Symptomatic.

Control Removal from pen.

ETIOLOGY

The buller steer syndrome is a **behavioral** problem in cattle confined in feedlots[1] of unknown etiology. Within a pen of cattle, one or more cattle persistently ride a particular individual or individuals of the group. The ridden animals are referred to as bullers. There have been several suspect etiologies. Improper placement of hormonal growth implants has been suspected as being associated with this behavioral problem.

EPIDEMIOLOGY

Occurrence

The syndrome occurs only in cattle in feedlots. A recent survey conducted among U.S. feedlots revealed a feedlot prevalence of 68.8% of all surveyed feedlots and an animal level prevalence of 2.8%.[1] The prevalence increases with increasing weight and age. The case fatality has been estimated at 1%. The incidence of occurrence is higher in the summer and the fall and during the first 30 days of the feeding period.

Epidemiologic studies indicate that bullers occur as a point source epidemic with the cause occurring soon after cattle arrive in the feedlot and mingle into pen groups. The peak incidence of bullers occurs much sooner after arrival and declines much quicker in older cattle. Bullers occur significantly sooner after mixing in older cattle than in younger cattle. The pen prevalence also increases as cattle become older on arrival at the feedlot and are more aggressive. As the prevalence of intact bulls increases in pens of cattle, so does the prevalence of bullers, presumably caused by more aggressiveness in the bulls.

Risk Factors

Postulated causative and risk factors include the incorrect timing and administration of hormonal growth implants, reimplantation and double dosing, estrogenic substances in feeds, pheromones in the urine of certain cattle, improper or late castration of young cattle, daily feedlot management, weather and seasonal factors, disease, group size, and dominance behavior. However, these factors have not been well substantiated, and controlled studies have found little influence of implant type and implant timing on buller incidence.

The mixing and confinement of **unfamiliar cattle** into pen groups, with subsequent agonistic interactions because these cattle established a social hierarchy, are considered as important risk factors. Both riding behavior and antagonistic behavior cease once cattle establish a stable social hierarchy. This suggests that riding behavior and subsequent identification of bullers is associated with this dominance behavior. It is possible that when a dominant animal becomes ill in a pen, other more subordinate animals in the pen that were previously subdued in dominance contests may want to fight the sick animal to achieve higher social status.

Economic Importance

The syndrome has been ranked along with acute undifferentiated bovine respiratory disease and foot rot as **one of the three most important disease syndromes** in beef feedlots in North America. In addition to the economic loss from decreased weight gain, injury, treatment, death, and carcass condemnation, there are economic losses associated with extra handling necessary to accommodate affected cattle, the disruption of uniform marketing of cattle, especially in custom feedlots, and the need for extra pens in which to house the bullers. The importance of the syndrome includes animal welfare aspects.

Bullers may be at significantly greater risk of illness and mortality (from bacterial pleuropneumonia) than other steers. The association between illness, mortality, and bullers among individuals was greatest among the oldest yearling steers.

CLINICAL FINDINGS

Two types of bullers are identified. **Type 1 or true bullers** stand as if they were a heifer in estrus and do not move away or show agonistic behavior when being mounted by rider cattle. There can be several rider cattle in a pen and type 1 bullers are rapidly damaged. **Type 2 bullers** are animals that appear low in social dominance. They use aggression to discourage riders and will lie down to avoid being ridden.

Affected animals show areas of denuded hair and have extensive subcutaneous hemorrhage. The hematomas may become infected and develop to subcutaneous pockets of pus and gas. Other traumatic injuries, such as limb fractures, also occur.

CONTROL

Management of the syndrome has usually involved identification and removal from the pen to prevent injury and even death from riding-related injuries. The high rate of risk of illness and mortality in bullers relative to other feedlot steers suggests that bullers should always be checked for evidence of illness in addition to their removal from their designated pen to prevent severe riding-related injuries. Treating sick bullers may improve the chance of settling them back into their designated pen by allowing them to resume their original position in the social hierarchy.

FURTHER READING

Blackshaw JK, Blackshaw AW, McGlone JJ. Buller steer syndrome review. *Appl Anim Behav Sci*. 1997;54:97.

REFERENCE

1. USDA-APHIS. Feedlot 2011.Part IV. 2014. <http://www.aphis.usda.gov/animal_health/nahms/feedlot/downloads/feedlot2011/Feed11_dr_PartIV.pdf>; Accessed 20.01.2014.

Infectious Diseases Primarily Affecting the Reproductive System

BRUCELLOSIS ASSOCIATED WITH *BRUCELLA ABORTUS* (BANG'S DISEASE)

SYNOPSIS

Etiology *Brucella abortus*

Epidemiology Major cause of abortion in cattle in countries without a national control program. Undulant fever in humans; is an important zoonosis. Sexually mature animals susceptible; outbreaks occur in first-calf heifers, older cows are infected but do not abort. Transmitted directly from the infected animal to the susceptible animal by uterine discharges. Congenital infection occurs. Infection in wildlife species but significance to domestic animals unknown. Infection introduced into herd by unknown infected carrier animal. Natural infection and vaccination result in immunity to abortion but not infection, and infected animals remain serologically positive for a long time.

Signs Abortion epidemics in first-calf unvaccinated heifers after fifth month of pregnancy. Subsequent pregnancies carried to term. Orchitis and epididymitis in bulls. Synovitis (hygroma) occurs. Fistulous withers in horses.

Clinical pathology Serology. Serum agglutination test is standard test. Rose Bengal test (rapid screening test). Complement fixation test. ELISA test. Milk ring test. False-positive reactors are a major problem.

Lesions Necrotizing placentitis, inflammatory changes in fetus.

Diagnostic confirmation Culture organism from fetus. Positive serologic test in unvaccinated animal.

Treatment No treatment.

Control Test and reduce reservoir of infection. Quarantine. Depopulation. Vaccination to reduce incidence of abortion and percentage of infected animals. Eradication on herd and area basis by test and cull.

ELISA, *enzyme-linked immunosorbent assay.*

ETIOLOGY

Brucella abortus, a gram-negative, facultative intracellular coccobacillus of the family Brucellaceae, is the organism responsible for **bovine brucellosis**. *B. abortus* is one of 10 species with validly published names, including *B. melitensis, B. abortus, B. suis, B. ovis, B. neotomae, B. canis, B. ceti, B. pinnipedialis, B. microti,* and *B. inopinata,* each of which has specific host preferences.[1] *B. abortus* is responsible for bovine brucellosis, *B. melitensis* is the main causative agent of brucellosis in small ruminants and men, *B. suis* for brucellosis in swine, and *B. ovis* in sheep. *B. abortus* has eight recognized biovars (1–7, 9) of which the most prevalents are 1–4, and 9.[2] Approximately 5% of infections are from biovar 1. Biovar 2 was isolated in an outbreak of brucellosis in cattle in Canada in 1986. In the United States, biovars 1 to 4 are found.

EPIDEMIOLOGY

Occurrence and Prevalence of Infection

Bovine brucellosis has a worldwide occurrence and, according to the Food and Agriculture Organization (FAO), the World Health Organization (WHO), and the World Organization for Animal Health (OIE), is still one of the most important and widespread bacterial zoonoses in the world. The prevalence of infection varies considerably among herds, areas, and countries. Many countries have made considerable progress with their eradication programs, and some have eradicated the disease. However, in other countries brucellosis is still a serious disease facing the veterinary and medical professions. Currently, Australia, New Zealand, Canada, Japan, and 16 member states of the European Union (EU) have a status as officially brucellosis free.[2,3] Bovine brucellosis remains prevalent in several southern European countries and the Mediterranean basin. The seroprevalence of bovine brucellosis in the Kars district of Turkey between 2004 and 2006 was determined to be around 34%.[4] In Greece 0.97%, in Italy 0.51%, in Portugal 0.19%, in Spain 0.07%, and in the UK 0.09% of all cattle herds were positive for brucellosis in 2012.[3] Although bovine brucellosis has been reported from Egypt (biovar 1), Iran (biovar 2), and Sudan (biovar 6), little is known about the infection prevalence in the region.[5]

In the United States, the entire country is classified as class free for bovine brucellosis. Notwithstanding, infection remains highly prevalent in the wildlife population in the Greater Yellowstone area, with occasional spread to cattle. Repeated incidents of brucellosis-infected cattle in Montana, Idaho, and Wyoming have been reported in recent years.[2] Bovine brucellosis remains an important bacterial disease in Mexico, with biovars 1–6 the most prevalent. Although limited epidemiologic data are available for Central America, the disease seems to prevail widely, with an estimated animal prevalence of between 4% and 8% and a (dairy) herd prevalence between 10% and 25%.[5] In South America Chile made great progress toward eradicating the disease, but it remains prevalent in Venezuela (animal seroprevalence 3%–4%), Argentina (animal seroprevalence 2%–3%), and Brazil.[5]

The livestock prevalence was estimated at 8.2% in East Africa, 15.5% in West Africa,

14.2% in South Africa, and 13.8% in North Africa.[6]

Cattle

Infection occurs in cattle of all ages but is most common in sexually mature animals, particularly dairy cattle. **Abortions are most common during outbreaks and primarily occur in unvaccinated heifers over 5 months pregnant.** Bulls are affected with orchitis, epididymitis, and seminal vesiculitis.

Camelids

Brucellosis has been reported in the one-humped (*Camelus dromedaries*) and two-humped camel (*C. bactrianus*) and New World camelids such as llama (*Lama glama*), alpaca (*lama pacos*), guanaco (*lama guinicoe*), and vicuña (*Vicugna vicugna*) and was related to contact with small and large ruminants infected with either *B. abortus* or *B. melitensis.*[7]

Wildlife Species

The infection has been observed in American and European bison (*Bison bison, B. bonasus*); domestic buffalo (*Bubalus bubalus*); elk (*Cervus elaphus canadensis*); deer; coyotes; wild opossums; and raccoons, moose, and other wild and domesticated ruminants. Infection of moose with *B. abortus* biovar 1 is highly fatal, and it is likely that the moose is a dead-end host for brucellosis. Experimental inoculation of the organism into badgers results in the development of antibodies and elimination of the organism, which indicates that the badger is relatively resistant to infection and unlikely to be a reservoir of the organism.

Bison and elk are potential reservoirs of bovine brucellosis and have been associated with recurrence of bovine brucellosis in the Greater Yellowstone area in the United States. Brucellosis associated with *B. abortus* was first detected in bison (*B. bison*) in Yellowstone National Park in 1917 and has been present ever since. Bison can remain latently infected with virulent *B. abortus* until attainment of reproductive age despite extensive use of vaccination and serologic testing.

Cattle and bison appear to maintain *B. abortus* at higher seroprevalence than other ungulate species. The seroprevalence in the Yellowstone bison and elk population is estimated with 40% to 60% and 22%, respectively.[8,9] This has been associated with physiologic and immunologic characteristics common to bovine species but is probably also caused by typical behavioral patterns of large social groups and the periparturient behavior of bison dams that tend to calve within groups that facilitate disease transmission through direct contact around parturition.[10] In contrast elk dams segregate themselves during the periparturient period and meticulously clean the birthing site, considerably reducing the risk of disease transmission through direct contact.[11] Disease transmission may, however, be common during the abortion period in the last trimester of pregnancy from February to April, when many elk congregate in large groups on lower elevation winter habitat that overlaps with cattle-grazing areas.[11] From 2009 to 2011 eight infected cattle or captive bison herds were detected in Wyoming and Montana and all episodes were genetically or epidemiologically linked to elk, suggesting that spillover transmission from elk to cattle is epidemiologically more important than transmission from bison to cattle.[11] This has been explained with the continuously increasing elk population, which is currently above management target values in many areas of the Greater Yellowstone area and the greater mobility of free-ranging elk.[10]

Horses

In horses the organism is often found in chronic bursal enlargements as a secondary invader rather than a primary pathogen. It is commonly present with *Actinomyces bovis* in fistulous withers and poll evil. It has also been identified as a cause of abortion in mares. A serologic survey of horses over a period of 8 years revealed that 8% to 16% of serum samples were positive. However, experimentally infected horses do not excrete the organism in sufficient numbers to infect susceptible in-contact cattle.

Pigs and Sheep

The organism can be recovered from naturally infected pigs and, although not normally pathogenic in this species, may occasionally cause abortion. The disease occurs naturally in sheep exposed to infected cattle, which has significant implications for brucellosis eradication.

Dogs

Naturally acquired *B. abortus* infection can occur in dogs associated with infected cattle. Although farm dogs are not generally considered to be a major reservoir of *B. abortus,* the organism has been isolated from dogs on a farm in which several cattle were serologically positive for brucellosis, and dogs should be included in any investigation and eradication of the disease.

Methods of Transmission

Parturition/Abortion

The **risk posed to susceptible animals** following parturition or abortion of infected cattle depends on three factors:

- Number of organisms excreted
- Survival of these organisms under the existing environmental conditions
- Probability of susceptible animals being exposed to enough organisms to establish infection

The organism achieves its greatest numbers in the contents of the pregnant uterus, the fetus, and the fetal membranes, all of which must be considered as major sources of infection. The numbers of organisms in the tissues of two naturally infected cows and their fetuses were as follows: umbilicus $2.4 \times 10^8 - 4.3 \times 10^9/g - 1.4 \times 10^{13}/g$. This illustrates the potentially large numbers of organisms that can be shed and to which other animals and humans are potentially exposed. However, the numbers of organisms decrease when uterine discharges are cultured at sequential parturitions, and a substantial number of uterine samples from infected cows are culture negative at the second and third parturition following challenge.

Transmission

The disease is transmitted by ingestion, penetration of the intact skin and conjunctiva, and contamination of the udder during milking. The organism does not multiply in the environment but merely persists, and the viability of the organism outside the host is influenced by the existing environmental conditions. Grazing on infected pasture, or consuming feedstuffs or water supplies contaminated by discharges and fetal membranes from infected cows, and contact with aborted fetuses as well as infected newborn calves are the most common methods of spreading the disease.

Intraherd spread occurs by both vertical and horizontal transmission. **Horizontal transmission is usually by direct contamination** and, although the possibility of introduction of infection by flies, dogs, rats, ticks, infected boots, fodder, and other inanimate objects exists, it is not significant relative to control measures. The organism is ingested by the face fly but is rapidly eliminated, and there is no evidence for a role in natural transmission. Evidence exists for horizontal, dog-to-dog, cattle-to-dog, dog-to-cattle, and dog-to-human transfer of infection. The most likely and effective means of cattle-to-dog transfer is exposure to aborted fetuses or infected placental membranes, because dogs commonly ingest the products of parturition.

Spread Between Herds

Movement of an infected animal from an infected herd to a susceptible noninfected herd is a common method of transmission. The rate of spread will depend on the level of surveillance testing. In Great Britain, which is officially brucellosis free, 20% or more of both beef and dairy cattle more than 24 months old are tested routinely. A simulation model indicates that reducing the level of testing would have a major effect on the rate of spread of infection, should it be imported.

Spread Between Countries (Breach of Biosecurity)

A quantitative risk assessment model to determine the annual risk of importing brucellosis-infected breeding cattle into Great

Britain from Northern Ireland and the Republic of Ireland, which are not brucellosis free, was developed. Predictions estimated that brucellosis could be imported from Northern Ireland every 2.63 years and from the Republic of Ireland every 3.23 years. Following this assessment, the Department of Environment, Food, and Rural Affairs introduced postcalving testing for all imported breeding cattle. Under this system, all imported animals are issued a passport that records their age and pregnancy status. This information enables identification of animals that require testing and provides an additional safeguard in maintaining official brucellosis status.

Congenital Infection

Congenital infection may occur in calves born from infected dams but its frequency is low. The infection occurs in utero and may remain latent in the calf during its early life; the animal may remain serologically negative until its first parturition, when it then begins to shed the organism. Calves born from reactor dams are serologically positive for up to 4 to 6 months because of colostral antibodies and later become serologically negative even though a latent infection may exist in a small proportion of these calves. The **frequency of latent infections** is unknown, but may range from 2.5% to 9%. Latent infections in serologically negative animals are of some concern because they remain unnoticed and can potentially serve as a source of infection later. However, latent infections in calves born from infected cows are infrequent. The organism could not be isolated from any of 150 calves born to infected cows, 135 of which were experiencing their first pregnancy after infection. In one report, a heifer from a herd affected with widespread infection with *B. abortus* biotype 2 was moved to a brucellosis-free herd and remained apparently free from brucellosis until 9 years later, when the same animal produced a strongly positive serologic reaction and the same biotype was isolated from its milk. Such observations have resulted in the recommendation that calves from seropositive dams should not be used for breeding. Even vaccinated heifers from seropositive dams can harbor a latent infection. There is a risk that 2.5% of heifer calves born from serologically positive dams will react in early adulthood and constitute a threat to a reestablished herd.

Survival of Organism

The organism can survive on grass for variable periods depending on environmental conditions. In temperate climates, infectivity may persist for 100 days in winter and 30 days in summer. The organism is susceptible to heat, sunlight, and standard disinfectants, but freezing permits almost indefinite survival. The activity of several disinfectants against *B. abortus* has been examined, and representatives of the phenolic, halogen, quaternary ammonium, and aldehyde groups of disinfectants at 0.5% or 1.0% concentrations in the absence of serum generally inhibited a high concentration of the organism.

Uterine Discharges and Milk

A cow's tail heavily contaminated with infected uterine discharges may be a source of infection if it comes in contact with the conjunctiva or the intact skin of other animals. In the same way that the more common forms of mastitis can be spread during milking, *B. abortus* infection can be spread from a cow whose milk contains the organism to an uninfected cow. This may have little significance in terms of causing abortion, but it is of particular importance in its effects on agglutination tests on milk and the presence of the organism in milk used for human consumption.

Bulls and Semen

Bulls do not usually transmit infection from infected to noninfected cows mechanically. Infected bulls may discharge semen containing organisms but are unlikely to transmit the infection. The risk of spread from the bull is much higher, however, if the semen is used for artificial insemination. Some infected bulls are negative on serum agglutination tests and their carrier status can only be detected by the isolation of organisms from the semen or agglutination tests on seminal plasma.

Carrier Cows

Few infected cows ever recover from infection completely and should be considered as permanent carriers whether or not abortion occurs. Excretion of the organism in the milk is usually intermittent, is more common during late lactation, and can persist for several years. In cattle vaccinated before infection, the degree of excretion of *B. abortus* in the milk is less than in nonvaccinated animals. Embryo transfer from infected donors may be achieved without transfer of infection, and superovulation is unlikely to reactivate the release of *Brucella* into the uterus during the period when embryos are normally collected. Thus embryo transfer is a safe procedure for salvaging genetic material from infected animals.

The herd characteristics and the results of the first herd test may be used as predictors of the potential presence or absence of *B. abortus* in herds with reactors to the tube agglutination test. The presence of only single suspicious reactors on the first test is a reliable predictor of lack of infection. The presence of one or more positive reactors on the first herd test is a reliable predictor of the presence of infection.

Risk Factors

The risk factors that influence the initiation, spread, maintenance, and/or control of bovine brucellosis are related to the animal population, management, and the biology of disease. The variables that contribute significantly to seropositive animals are

- Size of farm premises
- Percentage of animals on a premises that are inseminated artificially
- Size of investment in livestock
- Number of cows that aborted in the previous year, whether or not dairying is the major agricultural activity of the premises
- Policy of the owner regarding disposal of reactor animals

The longer infected animals are in contact with the remainder of the herd, the greater will be the ultimate number of seropositive animals. In a defined geographic area in northern Mexico where a brucellosis control program did not exist, the greatest percentage of seropositive animals was related to larger farms, poor artificial insemination technique, and small financial investment in the farm.

From a practical viewpoint, the factors influencing the transmission of brucellosis in any given geographic region can be classified into two fundamental categories: those associated with the transmission of disease between herds and those influencing the maintenance and spread of infection within herds. Factors influencing interherd transmission include the purchase of infected replacement animals, which is influenced by frequency of purchase, source of purchase, and brucellosis test history of purchased animals. The proximity of infected herds to clean herds is an important risk factor. Cattle contacts at fence lines, sharing of pastures, and strays of infected animals into clean herds are common methods by which transmission occurs to adjacent herds.

The risk factors associated with spread of the disease within a herd include unvaccinated animals in infected herds, herd size, population density, method of housing, and use of maternity pens. Large herd sizes are often maintained by the purchase of replacement cattle, which may be infected. It is also more difficult to manage large herds, which may lead to managerial mistakes that allow the disease to spread. There is a positive association between population density (number of cattle to land area) and disease prevalence, which is attributed to increased contact between susceptible and infected animals. The use of maternity pens at calving is associated with a decrease in the prevalence of infection, presumably from decreasing the exposure of infected and susceptible animals.

Animal Risk Factors

Susceptibility of cattle to *B. abortus* infection is influenced by the age, sex, and reproductive status of the individual animal. **Sexually mature, pregnant cattle are more susceptible to infection with the organism than sexually immature cattle of either sex.** Natural exposure to field strains occurs primarily at the time of parturition of infected cows. The greater the number of infected cows that abort or calve, the greater the exposure risk to the other cattle in the herd. An important application of this observation is that infected cows need to be removed from the herd before parturition. Young cattle are less susceptible to *B. abortus* than older, sexually mature cattle. Susceptibility appears to be more commonly associated with sexual maturity than age. Young, sexually immature cattle generally do not become infected following exposure, or recover quickly. Susceptibility increases with pregnancy and as the stage of gestation increases. The probability of isolation of the organism at parturition increased from 0.22 to 0.90 as fetal age at exposure of nonvaccinated heifers increased from 60 to 150 gestation days.

Management Risk Factors

The spread of the disease from one herd to another and from one area to another is almost always caused by the movement of an infected animal from an infected herd into a noninfected susceptible herd. The unregulated movement of cattle from infected herds or areas to brucellosis-free herds or areas is the major cause of breakdowns in brucellosis eradication programs. A case-control study of brucellosis in Canada indicated that herds located close to other infected herds and those herds whose owners made frequent purchases of cattle had an increased risk of acquiring brucellosis. Once infected, the time required to become free of brucellosis was increased by large herd size, by active abortion, and by loose housing.

Pathogen Risk Factors

Brucella spp., in contrast to other pathogens, do not possess typical virulence factors such as a capsule, flagella, exotoxins, or inducers or host cell apoptosis. They express a **lipopolysaccharide (LPS)** that, in contrast to LPS from other gram-negative pathogens, is nonendotoxic but is important for the protection from complement-mediated bacterial killing and the resistance against antimicrobial peptides such as defensins and lactoferrin.[12]

Brucella spp. possess a number of **outer membrane proteins (OMPs)**, some of which are required for full virulence, and that are recognized as antigen by immunity receptors such as Toll-like receptors (TLRs), triggering proinflammatory cytokine release.[13] Certain mutants of *B. abortus* lack a major 25-kDa OMP (Omp25), which renders them unable to replicate efficiently in bovine phagocytes and chorionic trophoblasts. Expression of OMPs is regulated through **the BvrR/BvrS two-component regulatory system**, which also modulates the host cell cytoskeleton on invasion, contributing to pathogen virulence.[12] The BvrR/BvrS two-component regulatory system furthermore regulates the expression of the **type IV secretion system (T4SS)**, which is crucial for intracellular survival in host cells and virulence in vivo. T4SS is required for *Brucella* spp. to reach their intracellular replication niche.[12]

Immune Mechanisms

Brucellas are able to survive within host leukocytes and may use both neutrophils and macrophages for protection from humoral and cellular bactericidal mechanisms during the periods of hematogenous spread.

Immunity against brucellosis is principally mediated by cellular immune responses because it is an intracellular pathogen. *B. abortus* is an efficient inducer of type 1 cellular immune responses, and interferon gamma (IFN-γ) is crucial for control of brucellosis. Infections are chronic and often lifelong. The bovine T lymphocyte in brucellosis is a critical component of host defense based on mononuclear phagocyte activation by IFN-γ. The killing of *Brucella*-infected mononuclear phagocytes and IFN-γ–mediated activation of mononuclear phagocytes are the major mechanisms of host defenses against brucellosis in cattle.

The antibody response to *B. abortus* in cattle consists of an early IgM isotype response, the timing of which depends on the route of exposure, the dose of the bacteria, and the health status of the animal. The IgM response is followed almost immediately by production of IgG_1 antibody and later by small amounts of IgG_2 and IgA. Most cross-reacting antibody from exposure to bacteria other than *Brucella* spp. or environmental antigens consists mainly of IgM. Serologic tests that measure IgM are therefore not desirable, because false-positive results occur. Because IgG_2 and IgA antibodies accumulate later after exposure and are usually present in small and inconsistent amounts, the main isotype for serologic testing is IgG_1.

Naturally infected animals and those vaccinated as adults with strain 19 remain positive to the serum and other agglutination tests for long periods. The serum of infected cattle contains high levels of IgM, IgG_1, IgG_2, and IgA isotypes of antibody. Most animals vaccinated between 4 and 8 months of age return to a negative status to the test within a year. All are considered to have a relative immunity to infection. Calves from cows that are positive reactors to the test are passively immunized via the colostrum. The half-life of colostral antibodies to *B. abortus* in calves that have received colostrum from either vaccinated noninfected or infected dams is about 22 days. It is possible that some calves remain immune sufficiently long to interfere with vaccination. After vaccination of cattle with strain 19 of the organism, IgM antibodies appear after about 5 days, reaching peak values after 13 days. IgG_1 antibodies appear a little later or simultaneously with IgM, and peak values are reached at 28 to 42 days, after which they decline. The same general pattern follows experimental infection with virulent strains and also in chronic field cases, except that IgM antibody declines to low levels and residual activity resides in IgG_1 and IgG_2 as well as in IgA, which remain at higher levels.

Economic Importance

Losses in animal production caused by this disease can be of major importance, primarily because of decreased milk production in aborting cows. The common sequel of infertility increases the period between lactations, and in an infected herd the average intercalving period may be prolonged by several months. In addition to the loss of milk production, there is the loss of calves and interference with the breeding program. This is of greatest importance in beef herds where the calves represent the sole source of income. A high incidence of temporary and permanent infertility results in heavy culling of valuable cows, and some deaths occur as a result of acute metritis following retention of the placenta.

Zoonotic Implications

According to the Food FAO, the WHO, and OIE, brucellosis is still one of the most important and widespread zoonoses in the world. Of the six *Brucella* spp. known to cause human disease (*B. melitensis, B. abortus, B. suis, B. canis, B. ceti,* and *B. pinnipedialis*), *B. melitensis* is the one with the largest public health impact because it is the most virulent species and has the highest prevalence in small ruminant populations in many areas of the world. *B. abortus* and *B. suis* serovars 1, 3, and 4 are also important human pathogens; *B. suis* serovar 2 and *B. canis* are uncommon human pathogens. Most cases in humans are occupational and occur in farmers, veterinarians, and slaughterhouse personnel after direct contact with infected animals or animal material contaminated with the pathogen. The organism can be isolated from many organs other than the udder and uterus, and the handling of a carcass of an infected animal may represent severe exposure. Brucellosis is also one of the most easily acquired laboratory infections.[15] Infection can also occur after ingestion of raw milk or raw milk products. Officially approved methods of commercial pasteurization render naturally *Brucella*-contaminated raw milk safe for consumption.

In endemic regions, the reported incidences of human brucellosis range from less than 0.01 per 100,000 population to more than 200 per 100,000 population.[15] In the United States, where approximately 100 cases of human brucellosis are reported annually, the incidence rate is less than 0.05 per 100,000 population.[15] In Europe the highest incidences were reported from Greece (1.09 per 100,000 population), Portugal (0.36 per 100,000 population), and Spain (0.13 per 100,000 population), which together accounted for 67.7% of all confirmed cases of human brucellosis in member states of the EU in 2012.[14] Of the human cases reported within the EU in 2012 where species information was available 83.9% were caused by *B. melitensis,* 10.1% *B. abortus,* 3.0% *B. suis,* and 3.0% by other *Brucella* spp.[14] The importance of the disease in humans is an important justification for its eradication. The cost-effectiveness to human health and the potential net economic benefits of a nationwide mass vaccination program for livestock over a period of 10 years has been evaluated using Mongolia as the model. If the costs of vaccination of livestock against brucellosis were allocated to all sectors in proportion to the benefits, the intervention would be cost-effective and would result in net economic benefits.

PATHOGENESIS

The successful coexistence of *Brucella* spp. with its preferred host is the outcome of coevolutionary relationships and selection pressures, which result in a stalemate where the pathogen has evolved to survive within the biologic system of the host, and the host has evolved innate and acquired immune systems that allow controlled survival of infection by the pathogen, ultimately supporting the survival of the host–pathogen system.

Following ingestion most commonly through the digestive or respiratory tract *Brucella* spp. can invade epithelial cells of the host, allowing infection though intact mucosal surfaces. Once invasion successfully occurs the organism may be phagocytized by host immune cells and may also invade nonphagocytic host cells through a mechanism that is not entirely understood. Following cell invasion the organism is contained in a membrane-bound modified phagosome, the *Brucella*-containing vacuole (BCV), and interferes with intracellular trafficking, preventing fusion of the BCV with lysosome markers and directing the BCV to the rough endoplasmic reticulum, which is highly permissive for intracellular replication of *Brucella.*[12] Invaded polymorphonuclear leukocytes then transport the pathogen to regional lymph nodes, other sites such as the reticuloendothelial system, and organs such as the udder and when present the fetal placenta. In the draining lymph node, *Brucella* infection causes cell lysis and eventual lymph node hemorrhage 2 to 3 weeks following exposure. Because of vascular injury, some of the bacteria enter the bloodstream and subsequent bacteremia occurs, which disseminates the pathogen throughout the body.

B. abortus has a predilection for the placenta; udder; testicle; and accessory male sex glands, lymph nodes, joint capsules, and bursae. Erythritol, a substance produced by the fetus and capable of stimulating the growth of *B. abortus,* occurs naturally in greatest concentration in the placental and fetal fluids and is responsible for localization of the infection in these tissues. Invasion of the gravid uterus results in a severe ulcerative endometritis of the intercotyledonary spaces. The allantochorion, fetal fluids, and placental cotyledons are invaded, and the villi are destroyed. The organism has a marked predilection for the ruminant placenta. In acute infections of pregnant cows, up to 85% of the bacteria are in cotyledons, placental membranes, and allantoic fluid. The resulting tissue necrosis of the fetal membranes allows transmission of the bacteria to the fetus. The net effect of chorionic and fetal colonization is abortion during the last trimester of pregnancy. The characteristic pneumonia in aborted fetuses is caused by localization of perivascular foci in the interlobular septa of the lung, indicative of hematogenous spread in the fetus rather than aspiration of contaminated fetal fluids. Fetuses inoculated with sufficient numbers of *B. abortus* will abort 7 to 19 days postinoculation. With experimental conjunctival exposure of pregnant heifers with the organism, the numbers of infected animals and the number of tissue samples positive for the organism are increased as fetal age at exposure increases from gestation days less than 127 to more than 157. **Abortion occurs principally in the last 3 months of pregnancy**, and the incubation period is inversely proportional to the stage of development of the fetus at the time of infection.

Congenital infection can occur in newborn calves as a result of in utero infection, and the infection may persist in a small proportion of calves, which may also be serologically negative until after their first parturition or abortion.

In the adult, nonpregnant cow, localization occurs in the udder, and the uterus, if it becomes gravid, is infected from periodic bacteremic phases originating in the udder. Infected udders are clinically normal, but they are important as a source of reinfection of the uterus, as a source of infection for calves or humans drinking the milk, and because they are the basis for the agglutination tests on milk and whey. Variable disease expression may occur in the male reproductive tract and musculoskeletal system, particularly affecting large joints, of either sex.

CLINICAL FINDINGS

Abortion

The clinical findings are dependent on the immune status of the herd. In highly susceptible nonvaccinated pregnant cattle, abortion after the 5th month of pregnancy is a typical feature of the disease in cattle. In subsequent pregnancies, the fetus is usually carried to full term, although second or even third abortions may occur in the same cow. Retention of the placenta and metritis are common sequelae to abortion. Mixed infections are usually the cause of the metritis, which may be acute, with septicemia and death following, or chronic, leading to sterility.

The history of the disease in a susceptible herd can usually be traced to the introduction of an infected cow. Less common sources are infected bulls, or horses with fistulous withers. In a susceptible herd, it is common for the infection to spread rapidly and for an abortion "storm" to occur. The storm might last for a year or more, at the end of which time most of the susceptible cows are infected and have aborted and then carry their calves to full term. Retained placentae and metritis could be expected to be common at this time. As the abortion rate subsides, the abortions are largely restricted to first-calf heifers and new additions, because other animals of the herd acquire partial resistance.

In recent years, particularly in areas where vaccination is extensively practiced, an insidious form of the disease may develop, which spreads much more slowly and in which abortion is much less common.

Orchitis and Epididymitis

In the bull, orchitis and epididymitis occur occasionally. One or both scrotal sacs may be affected, with acute, painful swelling to twice normal size, although the testes may not be grossly enlarged. The swelling persists for a considerable time, and the testis undergoes liquefaction necrosis and is eventually destroyed. The seminal vesicles may be affected and their enlargement can be detected on rectal palpation. Affected bulls are usually sterile when the orchitis is acute but may regain normal fertility if one testicle is undamaged. Such bulls are potential spreaders of the disease if they are used for artificial insemination.

Synovitis

B. abortus can often be isolated from the tissues of nonsuppurative synovitis in cattle. Hygromatous swellings, especially of the knees, should be considered with suspicion. Progressive and erosive nonsuppurative arthritis of the stifle joints has occurred in young cattle from brucellosis-free herds that had been vaccinated with strain 19 vaccine. The calves may or may not be serologically positive, but synovial fluid and joint tissue samples contain immunologic evidence of strain 19 *B. abortus* antigenic material. The synovitis has been reproduced by intraarticular injection of the vaccine.

Fistulous Withers

In horses, the common association of *B. abortus* is with chronic bursal enlargements of the neck and withers, or with the navicular bursa, causing intermittent lameness, and the organism has been isolated from mares that have aborted. When horses are mixed with infected cattle, a relatively high proportion can become infected and develop a positive reaction to the serum agglutination test without showing clinical illness. Some horses appear to suffer a generalized infection with clinical signs including general stiffness, fluctuating temperature, and lethargy.

CLINICAL PATHOLOGY

The major objective in the laboratory diagnosis of brucellosis is to identify animals that are infected and potentially shedding the organism and spreading the disease. Most infected animals are identifiable using the standard serologic tests, but latent infection occurs in some animals that are serologically negative. Furthermore, vaccinated animals may be serologically positive and uninfected, and transitory titers occur sporadically in a small percentage of animals, for which there is no clear explanation. These diagnostic problems make control and eradication programs difficult to administer and difficult to explain to animal owners.

The collection and submission of samples to the laboratory must be done with care, and careful attention must be given to recording the identity of the animal and the corresponding sample, which should be uniquely identified. For blood samples, it is recommended that silicone-coated evacuated glass tubes without additives be used to collect the blood sample, because they ensure effective clotting and clot retraction, to provide an easy source of serum without the need for centrifugation. Clotting is also aided by maintaining the sample at 25°C to 37°C for 1 to 2 hours.

Laboratory tests used in the diagnosis of brucellosis include isolation of the organism and serologic tests for the presence of antibodies in blood, milk, whey, vaginal mucus, and seminal plasma. The organism may be present in the cervical mucus, uterine flushings, and udder secretions of experimentally infected cows for up to 36 days after abortion.

Identification of *Brucella* spp.

Staining

The appearance of specifically stained smears and the colonial morphology can lead to a presumptive diagnosis of brucellosis. *Brucella* bacteria are not really acid-fast but are resistant to decolonization by weak acids, and the presence of a weakly acid-fast intracellular organism, stained with the Stamp-modified Ziehl–Neelsen method may be suggestive for the presence of *Brucella* spp. in the smear. However, staining has a very limited sensitivity because of the low number of organisms present that may be present in some tissues and body fluids of infected animals. Positive results must be interpreted carefully because of the morphologic similarities of *Brucella* organisms with other pathogens associated with abortion, such as *Coxiella burnetii* or *Chlamydia abortus*.[7] Results, positive or negative, should only be considered presumptive and always need to be confirmed ideally by culture.

Culture

The gold standard diagnostic test continues to be based on isolation and characterization of the organism from the organs and lymph nodes of the fetus, the placenta, milk, vaginal mucus, or uterine exudate. Bacteriologic methods detect the organism directly and thus limit the possibility of false-positive results. Isolation of the organism from the udder secretion of a cow is conclusive evidence of infection. Culture methods are reliable and usually definitive. A range of specific culture media are commercially available. A disadvantage is the long time required for definitive identification. Most culture results are positive between the 7th and 21st day and rarely become positive before the 4th day of culture.[16] Incubation for at least 45 days has been advised before declaring a blood sample negative for *Brucella* spp.[16] Furthermore *Brucella* organisms are among the most dangerous bacteria with which to work in terms of the risk of producing laboratory-acquired infections.[7]

Detection by Polymerase Chain Reaction (PCR)

The PCR-based assays for *Brucella* spp. have been developed and are simple. PCR has been applied to tissues such as aborted fetuses and associated maternal tissues, blood nasal secretions, semen, and food products such as milk and soft cheeses. *Brucella* spp. can be detected in the milk of naturally infected cattle, sheep, goats, and camels using a PCR assay that is more sensitive than the culture method. A further diagnostic advancement of recent years is the Bruce-ladder PCR, which is a multiplex PCR assay that helps to identify and differentiate several *Brucella* spp., including vaccine strains, in a single step.[17]

Serologic Tests

In the absence of a positive culture of *B. abortus*, a presumptive diagnosis is usually made based on the presence of antibodies in serum, milk, whey, vaginal mucus, or seminal plasma.

The antibody response following infection depends on whether or not the animal is pregnant and on the stage of gestation. On average, the agglutinins and complement fixation antibodies become positive 4 weeks following experimental infection during the fourth to sixth months of gestation and not until about 10 weeks if experimental infection occurs 2 months before or after insemination. The serologic diagnosis is considered to be unreliable when applied 2 to 3 weeks before and after abortion or calving.

Any of the currently available serologic tests or combination of tests measures the response of a single animal at one point in time and does not describe the status of the herd. When the tests are used in the recommended sequence and in combination, along with a consideration of accurate epidemiologic data, the limitations of each test can be minimized. None of the tests is absolutely accurate, and there are varying degrees of sensitivity. The result has been the development of a very extensive range of tests, each of which has its own special applicability. The salient features are as follows.

Agglutination Tests

Serum Agglutination Test

The serum (tube) agglutination test (SAT) or microtiter plate variants of it are some of the traditional standard tests, which are widely used, but are not recognized as prescribed or alternative tests. The main limitations are

- Detect nonspecific antibodies as well as specific antibodies from *B. abortus* infection and vaccination
- During the incubation stage of the disease these tests are often the last to reach diagnostically significant levels
- After abortion caused by *B. abortus* they are often the last tests to reach diagnostically significant levels
- In the chronic stage of the disease, the serum agglutinins tend to wane, often becoming negative when the results of some other tests may be positive.

Rose Bengal Test (Buffered Plate Antigen or Card Test)

The rose Bengal test (RBT) is a simple, rapid spot-agglutination test using antigen stained with rose Bengal and buffered to low pH. The test detects early infection and can be used as an initial screening test. False-positive reactions are caused by residual antibody activity from vaccination, colostral antibody in calves, cross-reaction with certain bacteria such as *Yersinia enterocolitica,* and laboratory error. False-negative reactions are observed during early incubation of disease and immediately after abortion. However, the RBT is an excellent test for the large-scale screening of sera. The application of the RBT as a screening test, followed by a confirmatory or complementary test, can markedly increase the proportion of infected cattle that test positive.

For **beef cattle**, screening of herds can be achieved by collecting blood at abattoirs and submitting it to the RBT or tube agglutination test. Reactors are traced back to the herd of origin, and the herd is tested. In heavily infected herds, it is best to remove all cows positive to the RBT even though it is highly sensitive and there will be a small percentage of false-positive cows. In herds where the prevalence of infection is low and where vaccination has been used, this procedure will eliminate too many false-positive cows. In this situation the sera positive to the RBT are submitted to a more definite confirmatory test such as the complement fixation test (CFT), and only those animals reacting to the test are discarded.

Complement Fixation Test

The CFT is one of the prescribed tests for international trade and is widely accepted as a confirmatory test. It rarely exhibits nonspecific reactions and is useful in differentiating titers of calfhood vaccination from those caused by infection. The reactions to the CFT recede sooner than those to the serum agglutination test after calfhood vaccination with the strain 19 vaccine. The CFT titers do not wane because the disease becomes chronic and often the CFT reaches diagnostic levels sooner than the serum tube agglutination test following natural infection. In addition, recent technical laboratory advances have allowed much greater speed and accuracy in doing the CFT and it is now considered to be the nearest approach to a definitive test for infection. Nonetheless, because of its complexity the CFT requires good laboratory facilities and skilled laboratory personnel.

Enzyme-Linked Immunosorbent Assays

Two main types of immunosorbent assay have been used: the indirect and competitive formats.

Indirect Enzyme-Linked Immunosorbent Assay

The indirect enzyme-linked immunosorbent assay (iELISA) has been a useful test during an eradication program, after vaccination has ceased; for screening; or as a supplementary test to the CFT. Several variations of the assay using either whole-cell, smooth lipopolysaccharide (sLPS), or O-polysaccharide (OPS) as an antigen have been validated.[7] The iELISA has gained wide acceptance for serologic diagnosis of bovine brucellosis because of its ability to detect antibody of all isotopes, unlike the conventional tests. The iELISA can be useful in conjunction with the CFT during the later stages of an eradication program, when it is important to reduce the number of false-negative serologic reactions that contribute to the persistence of problem herds. The iELISA has an excellent sensitivity and specificity but cannot distinguish between the antibody response induced by vaccination with *B. abortus* strain 19 and natural infection.

The iELISA has also been developed and validated for milk, and several different variations of this assay are currently commercially available.

Competitive Enzyme-Linked Immunosorbent Assay

The competitive ELISA (C-ELISA) uses monoclonal antibody specific for one of the epitopes of the *Brucella* spp., which makes it more specific than assays using cross-reacting antibody. The C-ELISA is thus more specific but less sensitive than the iELISA. It eliminates most but not all reactions caused by cross-reacting organisms and in most but not all cases, eliminates reactions with residual antibody in animals vaccinated with strain 19.[7] The OIE therefore recommends the further investigation of positive reactors with the C-ELISA using appropriate complementary or confirmatory diagnostic tests.[7]

Fluorescence Polarization Assay

This test can be done outside the diagnostic laboratory, allowing for rapid and accurate diagnosis. The fluorescence polarization assay (FPA) can be done almost anywhere using a portable analyzer, which receives power from a laptop computer, using serum, milk, or ethylenediaminetetraacetic acid (EDTA) anticoagulated blood. The FPA technology has been developed and validated for the serologic diagnosis of brucellosis in cattle, pigs, sheep, goats, bison, and cervids. Sufficient cross-reactivity of the common epitopes of *B. abortus, B. melitensis,* and *B. suis* OPS has allowed for the use of a single antigen for all species of smooth *Brucella* and animals. The FPA was initially developed for testing serum; however, the technology has been extended to testing whole blood and milk from individual animals or bulk tank samples pooled from 2000 or fewer animals. The accuracy results of the FPA equals or exceeds those obtained using other serologic tests such as the buffered antigen plate agglutination test, the milk ring test, the CFT, the IELISA, and the C-ELISA. Validation of studies of the FPA and the C-ELISA for the detection of antibodies to *B. abortus* in cattle sera and comparison to the standard agglutination test, the CFT, and the iELISA, found that the FPA is highly superior. It offers a clear advantage because it is easy to use. Full implementation and acceptance of FPA methods for the diagnosis of brucellosis will necessitate the use of an International Standard Serum panel containing at least a low titer-positive sample and a negative sample.

Brucellin Skin Test

The brucellin skin test presents an alternative immunologic test that can be used to test unvaccinated animals. Tested animals are injected intradermally with 0.1 mL of a standardized brucellin preparation consisting of purified, sLPS-free *Brucella* antigen. The skin thickness at the injection site is measured with Vernier calipers before and 48 to 72 hours after injection. Skin thickening of at least 1.5 to 2 mm at the injection site are considered a positive reaction. This test is among the most specific brucellosis tests available, provided it is conducted with a purified, standardized antigen preparation; serologically negative unvaccinated animals with a positive reaction to the skin test are therefore considered as infected.[7] Because not all infected animals show a positive reaction the test is not recommended as a stand-alone test for the purpose of international trade.

Sensitivity and Specificity of Serologic Tests

Serologic tests must have high sensitivity to ensure that all true serologic reactors are detected. However, with a high sensitivity, a high rate of false-positive reactions may be expected and hence the need for the use of a confirmatory test to identify false-positive reactors. Confirmatory tests must therefore demonstrate a high level of diagnostic specificity and yet maintain an effective diagnostic sensitivity.

It has been recommended to use a buffered *Brucella* antigen test, such as the buffered plate antigen test or the RBT as a screening test. Either the CFT or the indirect enzyme immunoassay is appropriate for use as a confirmatory test in situations requiring a high specificity. The relationships between the quantitative serology and infection status of brucellosis in bison in Yellowstone National Park have been evaluated and found to be similar to those in chronically infected cattle.

Antibodies in Milk

The **milk ring test** is a satisfactory inexpensive test for the surveillance of dairy herds for brucellosis. A small sample of pooled fresh milk or cream, from no more than 25 cows, is tested and the herd is classified only as suspicious or negative. Final determination of the status of a suspicious herd and each animal in it is accomplished by blood testing. The more frequently a herd is tested with the milk ring test, the more effective the test becomes as a method to detect early infections, preventing serious outbreaks in susceptible herds. At least three tests done annually are now required by some regulatory agencies. The major limitation of the test is the dilution factor, which occurs in large dairy herds where large quantities of milk are stored in bulk tanks. To adjust for this dilution effect, larger sample volumes are used with increasing herd size. Although 1 mL of bulk milk is required for herds with up to 150 head, the use of 2 mL for herds between 150 and 450 head and 3 mL for herds with 450 to 700 head has been advised.[7] False-positive reactions have been observed with cattle vaccinated less than 4 months before testing and in samples containing colostrum or mastitic milk.

The milk iELISA test is a sensitive, specific, and inexpensive method for screening large numbers of individual or bulk milk samples for the antibody to *B. abortus*. An ELISA using potassium chloride extract of the organism used on bulk tank milk samples of dairy herds was highly specific and is considered as a highly reliable test for monitoring brucellosis control programs. The combined use of an ELISA and PCR on milk samples gives a sensitivity of 100%.

False-Positive Reactors

A major problem in brucellosis eradication programs has been the false-positive animals or singleton reactor, which may remain persistently suspicious or positive in a herd that is otherwise considered to be free of brucellosis. It is of some concern because of the unnecessary slaughter of uninfected animals.

Cross-reacting antibodies usually result from exposure to antigen(s) that share antigenic determinants with *Brucella* spp., which are found in a large number of bacteria. The most prominent cross-reaction is with *Yersinia enterocolitica* O:9, which shares the major OPS almost completely with *B. abortus*. Serologic cross-reactions have also been demonstrated between smooth *Brucella* spp. and *Escherichia coli* O116:H21 and *E. coli* O157:H7, *Francisella tularensis, Salmonella* serotypes of Kauffman–White group N, *Pseudomonas maltophilia, Vibrio cholerae,* and *Y. enterocolitica* serotype O:9. Only rarely will naturally occurring *E. coli* O157:H7 infections cause false-positive reactions with standard serologic tests for bovine brucellosis. The standard serologic tests are unreliable in differentiating between *Y. enterocolitica* and *Brucella*-infected cows, but both the lymphocyte transformation and brucellin skin tests could be used to differentiate them.

Other causes of false positives include a *B. abortus*-infected animal, strain 19 residual vaccination titer, and naturally occurring nonspecific agglutinins, which may occur in some cattle populations. These agglutinins are EDTA labile and can be differentiated from agglutinating antibodies by the addition of EDTA to the diluent used in the standard serum agglutination test. The serologic cross-reactions are of major significance when the prevalence of infection has decreased to a very low level. At this stage it becomes much more important to correctly identify the status of animals reacting to the serologic tests for brucellosis.

The incorrect attribution of such reactions to factors other than *Brucella* infection is likely to result in herd breakdowns and failure to control the disease. On the other hand, the misinterpretation of cross-reactions as evidence of brucellosis results in the imposition of unnecessary restrictions and waste of resources. The problem of serologic cross-reactions has resulted in considerable research and an investigation to find laboratory tests, which will accurately distinguish positive, infected animals from positive, noninfected animals. Differentiation of cross-reacting antibodies can be difficult to achieve, especially in the case of *Y. enterocolitica* O:9 antigen, but immunodiffusion, immunoelectrophoresis, and primary binding tests and cross-absorption procedures are useful. The DNA homology of *B. abortus* strains 19 and 2308 has been examined using restriction enzyme analysis. Strain 19 is the official U.S. Department of Agriculture (USDA)-attenuated *Brucella* vaccinal strain for cattle, and strain 2038 is a virulent laboratory-adapted strain that is pathogenic to cattle. The DNA differences between the two strains are small and will require analysis at the DNA sequence level.

The serologic assay of choice for screening samples for antibody to *B. abortus* is the FPA. It is robust, very rapid, and field-adaptable, without subjective results. The C-ELISA is a useful confirmatory assay. The sera from cattle naturally infected with *B. abortus,* vaccinated with *B. abortus* S19, or immunized with *Y. enterocolitica* O:9 or *E. coli* O157:H7, were compared for antibody content to the same bacteria by iELISA, FPA, and C-ELISA. The serologic assay of choice for screening samples for antibody to *B. abortus* is the FPA. Between the two tests, nearly all reactivity to *E. coli* O157:H7 and more than one-half of the sera with antibody to *Y. enterocolitica* O:9 could be eliminated as *Brucella* reactors. These assays, perhaps in combination with a brucellin skin test, may be capable of distinguishing virtually all reactions caused by *Y. enterocolitica* O:9.

NECROPSY FINDINGS

The host responses at the organ and tissue levels have been described and are summarized here. Lymph nodes draining the sites of the early stages of infection have marked germinal center hyperplasia and hypertrophy, accompanied by acute neutrophilic and eosinophilic lymphadenitis. In the later stages of the infection, lymph nodes draining mammary gland, head, and reproductive tract develop chronic granulomatous lymphadenitis, which is usually associated with cortical and paracortical T-cell–dependent lymphoid depletion, germinal center expansion, and deep histiocytic expansion. The spleen may develop lymphoid hyperplasia and histiocytic and plasmacytic expansion in the germinal centers, and the mammary gland usually has a pronounced interstitial lymphoplasmacytic mastitis. In the uterus, there is usually an endometritis, fibrosing mural lymphocytic metritis, and caruncular necrotizing vasculitis, whereas the placenta is colonized with *B. abortus* and has extensive desquamation of fetal chorioallantoic trophoblasts with subsequent hematogenous spread to villous trophoblastic epithelium, and **necrotizing fibrinopurulent cotyledonary placentitis of the placental arcades** accompanied by granulation and intercotyledonary inflammation exudation. The placenta is usually edematous. There may be leathery plaques on the external surface of the chorion, and there is necrosis of the cotyledons. The key microscopic feature of this inflamed chorioallantois is the presence of **intracytoplasmic coccobacilli within chorionic trophoblasts**. The use of modified Ziehl–Neelsen stains on impression smears from fresh placentas can provide a rapid presumptive diagnosis. The fetal lesions consist of marked fibrinopurulent necrotizing bronchopneumonia; monocytic and neutrophilic alveolitis; thromboembolic necrotizing arteritis and lymphangitis; fibrinopurulent pleuritis; and granulomata of the liver, spleen, kidney, and lymph nodes. In **fetuses naturally and experimentally infected** with *B. abortus*, the tissue changes include lymphoid hyperplasia in multiple lymph nodes, lymphoid depletion in the thymic cortex, adrenal cortical hyperplasia, and disseminated inflammatory foci composed mainly of large mononuclear leukocytes.

The affected joints usually develop a fibrinous and granulomatous synovitis with proliferative villous projection formation, proliferative tendovaginitis with lymphoplasmacytic nodule formation, and arthritis with articular erosions, which may be associated with suppurative, granulomatous bursitis. In the testes there are unilateral or bilateral visceral to parietal tunica adhesions, interstitial lymphocyte orchitis with seminiferous tubular degeneration, necrotizing intratubular orchitis, and acute fibrinopurulent periorchitis with infarction. The ampulla may have a unilateral or bilateral granulomatous epididymitis with focally necrotic purulent and calcified sperm granulomata, and the seminal vesicles have unilateral or bilateral necrotizing fibrinopurulent seminal vesiculitis and interstitial lymphocytic, plasmacytic seminal vesiculitis with necrosis.

The distribution of *B. abortus* in experimentally and naturally infected cattle has been examined. In experimentally infected pregnant cows, the most frequently infected specimen was the mammary lymph node; the organism could also be found in other lymph nodes, uterine caruncles, cotyledons, or fetal tissues. In naturally infected heifers, the most frequently infected specimen was the mandibular lymph node. In bulls, the most frequently infected tissues were the mandibular, caudal superficial cervical, subiliac, and scrotal lymph nodes.

The lesions in *Brucella*-positive aborted fetuses and placentas in bison are similar to those in experimental infections of *B. abortus* in bison and cattle. Both *B. abortus* biovar 1 and *B. abortus* biovar 2 were isolated from specimens collected from aborted bison fetuses or stillborn calves and their placentas. The infection can also be associated with death in calves at least 2 weeks of age.

Samples for Confirmation of Diagnosis

- Bacteriology: maternal caruncle; placenta, fetal stomach content, lung (culture, has special growth requirements; cytology, Stamp's or Koster's stain on placental smears)
- Histology: fixed placenta, lung, spleen, brain, liver, kidney; maternal caruncle (light microscopy, immunohistochemistry)

Note the zoonotic potential of this organism when handling carcasses and submitting specimens.

DIFFERENTIAL DIAGNOSIS

The diagnosis of the cause of abortion in a single animal or in a group of cattle is difficult because of the multiplicity of causes that may be involved. When an abortion problem is under investigation, a systematic approach should be used. This includes a complete laboratory evaluation and follow-up inquiries into each herd.

The following procedure is recommended:

- Ascertain the age of the fetus by inspection and from the breeding records.
- Take blood samples for serologic tests for brucellosis and leptospirosis.
- Examine uterine fluids and the contents of the fetal abomasum at the earliest opportunity for trichomonads, and subsequently by cultural methods for *B. abortus, Campylobacter fetus,* trichomonads, *Listeria* spp., and fungi.
- Supplement these tests by examination of urine for leptospires, and of the placenta or uterine fluid for bacteria and fungi, especially if the fetus is not available.
- Examine placenta fixed in formalin for evidence of placentitis.

It is most important that all examinations are done in all cases because coincident infections with more than one agent are not uncommon.

In the early stages of the investigation, the herd history may be of value in suggesting the possible etiologic agent. For example, in brucellosis, abortion at 6 months or later is the major complaint, whereas in trichomoniasis and vibriosis, failure to conceive and prolongation of the diestrual period is the usual history.

Of special interest is epizootic bovine abortion, which is a major disease of rangeland cattle in the western United States. A spirochete has been isolated from the soft tick *Ornithodoros coriaceus* and from the blood of fetuses with lesions of epizootic bovine abortion. The disease occurs at a very high level of incidence but only in cattle introduced to a certain area; resident cattle are usually unaffected. Cattle returned to the area each winter are unaffected after the first abortion. The cows are unaffected systemically. Aborted fetuses show characteristic multiple petechiae in the skin, conjunctiva, and mucosae; enlargement of lymph nodes; anasarca; and nodular involvement of the liver.

In most countries where brucellosis is well under control and artificial insemination limits the spread of vibriosis and trichomoniasis, leptospirosis may be the most common cause of abortion in cattle.

However, surveys in such countries reveal that in about two-thirds of the abortions that occur no causative agent is detectable with routine laboratory techniques. In only 35% of cases was the cause determined, and brucellosis accounted for less than 1% of the total. In an Australian experience, the cause of abortion was determined in only 37% of cases in spite of the submission of the fetus, placenta, and maternal serum. The general procedures for submission of specimens to the laboratory and laboratory methods are available.

Bulls

Infected bulls may be serologically positive or negative, and their semen may be culturally positive or negative, but the organism may be isolated at slaughter. Clinical examination may reveal the presence of epididymitis, orchitis, seminal vesiculitis, and ampullitis. All bulls from known infected herds should therefore be considered as suspicious, regardless of their serologic status, and not be used for artificial insemination.

TREATMENT

Treatment is unsuccessful because of the intracellular sequestration of the organisms in lymph nodes, the mammary gland, and reproductive organs. *Brucella* spp. are facultative intracellular bacteria that can survive and multiply within the cells of the macrophage system. Treatment failures are considered to be caused by the inability of the drug to penetrate the cell membrane barrier instead of the development of antimicrobial resistance.

CONTROL AND ERADICATION

Most countries with brucellosis have programs designed to control and ultimately eradicate the infection in cattle to reduce economic losses and protect the public from the disease. These programs usually have several components, and to ensure effectiveness each component needs to be scientifically sound and accepted by all concerned. The major components of a control and eradication program are as follows.

Test and Reduction of Reservoir of Infection

All breeding cattle in the herd are tested, and those that are positive are culled and sent for slaughter. This removes infected cows from the herd and reduces exposure and transmission within the herd. Of particular importance is the detection and removal of infected cows before parturition.

Quarantine

This is a period of time during which cattle movement is restricted and the cattle are tested. This will prevent interherd transmission by infected cattle, especially those that are test negative and incubating the disease. The quarantine period should be sufficiently long that all cattle have had sufficient time to develop brucellosis and ensure that the remaining cattle will not be a source for interherd transmission. The time will usually range from 120 days to 1 year, or until all breeding animals have completed a gestation without test evidence of infection.

Depopulation

Depopulation is slaughter of all cattle in a herd when all animals have been exposed and are capable of becoming infected and acting as a source of new infection.

Vaccination

Properly vaccinated cattle are less likely to be infected and, therefore, are less likely to shed field strains of the organism. Vaccination strategies will be discussed in more detail below.

Education

All participants in a program must understand and adopt the scientific basis for the program. This includes livestock producers, veterinarians, and regulatory officials.

Guidelines

To be successful, any program needs guidelines and policies, which must be followed and modified to meet the needs of certain areas or herds.

Apart from the question of human exposure to infection, the cost and economic benefits of an eradication program must be assessed against the costs and benefits from a vaccination control program. Certain basic considerations apply to all programs aimed at the eradication of brucellosis.

- The control programs indigenous to any given area must receive primary recognition, and any plan or plans must be adapted to that area
- Cooperation at all levels of government from local to the national is essential for the success of a program. This is attained only after an intensive program of education has been performed. The individual owner of an infected herd must recognize the problem of brucellosis and express a willingness to cooperate. Experience has shown that the owner must be impressed with the hazards of the disease for human health and with the economic losses in the herd
- A reliable and uniform diagnostic procedure must be generally available.
- If disease is detected in a herd, established procedures should be available for handling the disease. If immunization is to be used, a standardized and effective vaccine must be readily available. The disposal of infected animals may create a serious economic threat for the owner and the possibilities of financial compensation must be explored
- Finally, and of major importance, the movement of animals from one area to another must be controlled at a high level, because a rigid eradication program in one area may be nullified by neglect in a neighboring area.

Sufficient information exists about bovine brucellosis that it can be eradicated. The disease was considered to have been eradicated from Great Britain in 1981; in 1985, having met certain European Community criteria for national surveillance and with over 99.8% of the cattle herds free from brucellosis, all herds within the country not under restrictions were designated as being officially brucellosis free for trade purposes. However, small foci of infection persisted, and following the prohibition of the use of *Brucella* vaccines the national herd was becoming fully susceptible to brucellosis. This was followed by outbreaks of brucellosis in southwest England from 1984 to 1986. The movement of cattle through premises owned by dealers who specialized in the purchase and sale of newly calved cattle was a significant epidemiologic feature of these herd breakdowns.

Control by Vaccination

Because of the serious economic and medical consequences of brucellosis, efforts have been made to prevent the infection through the use of vaccines. Historically brucellosis vaccines were composed of attenuated strains of *B. abortus* and *B. melitensis.* These vaccines were shown to be effective in reducing pathogen transmission and production loss, but were less effective in preventing infection. Another inconvenience of these whole-cell vaccines was that they interfere with diagnostic assays detecting antibody against the O-side chain of the *Brucella* LPS.[18] Currently vaccines used to protect livestock against infection with *B. abortus* contain one of three attenuated live strains of *B. abortus:* strain 19, RB51, and strain 82.

Brucella abortus Strain 19 Vaccine

Vaccines containing the live *B. abortus* strain 19 are the most widely used vaccines to prevent bovine brucellosis and are considered the reference vaccines to which any other vaccine is compared.[7] The vaccine protects uninfected animals living in a contaminated environment, enabling infected animals to be disposed of gradually. This overcomes the main disadvantage of the test and disposal method of eradication, in which infected animals must be discarded immediately to avoid spread of infection. *B. abortus* strain 19 has a low virulence and is incapable of causing abortion except in a proportion of cows vaccinated in late pregnancy. Strain 19 is a smooth *B. abortus* strain expressing the O-antigen on its LPS. Antibody produced in response to vaccination will interfere with diagnostic assays identifying this antigen, which is a major problem with the use of these vaccines. Another weakness of the vaccines is that it cannot completely prevent infection.[18]

Strain 19 vaccines are normally administered to female calves between 3 and 8 months old as a single subcutaneous dose of 5 to 8 × 10^{10} organisms (**calfhood vaccination**). There is no significant difference between the immunity conferred at 4 and at 8 months of age. Calves vaccinated with strain 19 at 2 months of age have resistance comparable to those vaccinated at 4 to 8 months of age. However, generally, calves under 75 days of age are immunologically immature in response to strain 19 vaccine. Vaccination of calves with a single dose at 3 to 5 weeks of age does not provide protection compared with vaccination at 5 months of age.

In calves vaccinated between the recommended ages, the serum agglutination test returns to negative by the time the animals are of breeding age, except in a small percentage (6%) of cases. The LPS with an O-chain on *B. abortus* strain 19 explains the appearance and persistence of antibodies in serum following vaccination. These antibodies are detectable in the serologic assays used for the diagnosis of brucellosis and are the major problem with strain 19 vaccination, because they prevent easy differentiation of vaccinated from infected cattle. The appearance and persistence of these antibodies depends on age, dose, and route of vaccination. This situation makes the continued use of the vaccine incompatible with simultaneous application of test and slaughter procedures for the control of brucellosis.

In brucellosis-free herds where heifers are vaccinated between 4 and 9.5 months of age, positive titers may persist for up to 18 months if they are tested with screening tests such as the RBT. This supports the official policy in some countries not to test vaccinated heifers before 18 months of age and to retest positive cases with the CFT.

In most control programs, vaccination is usually permitted up to 12 months of age, but the proportion of persistent postvaccinal serum and whey reactions increases with increasing age of the vaccinates. Such persistent reactors may have to be culled in an eradication program unless the reaction can be proved to be the result of vaccination and not due to virulent infection.

Vaccination of adult cattle is usually not permitted if an eradication program is contemplated, but it may be of value in reducing the effects of an abortion storm. Under specific circumstances vaccination of adult cattle with a reduced single subcutaneous dose of 3 × 10^8 to 3 × 10^9 viable organisms can be used but will result in persistent antibody titers in some animals. Furthermore, the risk of abortion when vaccinating pregnant animals and the risk of excretion of the vaccine strain in milk has been reported.[7] An alternative vaccination protocol for adult cattle consists in the single or repeated subconjunctival administration of a dose of 5 × 10^9 living organisms. This latter protocol was reported to reduce the risk of abortion and shedding in milk while providing similar protection.[7]

Vaccination of bulls is of no value in protecting them against infection and has resulted in the development of orchitis and the presence of *B. abortus* strain 19 in the semen. For these reasons the vaccination of bulls is discouraged.

Efficiency of Brucella abortus Strain 19 Vaccine

Calfhood Vaccination. This can be assessed by its effect on both the incidence of abortion and the prevalence of infection as determined by testing. Field tests show a marked reduction in the number of abortions that occur, although the increased resistance to infection, as indicated by the presence of *B. abortus* in milk, may be less marked. Vaccinated animals have a high degree of protection against abortion and 65% to 75% are resistant to most kinds of exposure. The remaining 25% to 35% of vaccinated animals may become infected but usually do not abort. Experimentally, 25% of cattle vaccinated with strain 19 will become infected following challenge. Vaccinated animals continually exposed to virulent infection may eventually become infected and act as carriers without showing clinical evidence of the disease.

In summary, vaccination with a single dose of *B. abortus* strain 19 vaccine given subcutaneously at 3 to 8 months of age confers adequate immunity against abortion for five or more subsequent lactations under conditions of field exposure. Multiple or late vaccinations have no appreciable advantage and increase the incidence of postvaccinal positive agglutination reactions. When breakdowns occur, they are caused by excessive exposure to infection and not by enhanced virulence of the organism. In herds quarantined for brucellosis, calfhood vaccination reduces reactor rates, duration of quarantine, and the number of herd tests.

Adult Vaccination. Vaccination of adult cows with strain 19 vaccine is highly successful in reducing the number of infected cows in large dairy herds in which it is impossible to institute management procedures for the ideal control of brucellosis.

The vaccination of adult cattle with a reduced dose of vaccine is efficacious and results in an agglutinin response that declines more rapidly after vaccination than when the full dose is used. The reduced dose also provides protection comparable to the standard dose. Vaccination eliminates clinical disease and reduces exposure of infection to susceptible cattle. The reduction of infected adult cattle may vary from 60% to 80% in 6 to 9 months following vaccination. The CFT becomes negative sooner than the standard tube agglutination test following vaccination and can be used to distinguish postvaccine titers from culture-positive cows. The use of reduced doses of strain 19 vaccine in adult cows will also help to eliminate the problem of postvaccine titers.

The protection provided by **subcutaneous and conjunctival routes of vaccination** is the same but the subcutaneous route may result in a persistent serologic response, which requires complement fixation testing and milk culture to identify infected animals.

The principal advantages of adult vaccination include the following:

- An effective method of control of abortion
- Reduction in the reactor losses in herds
- Reduction of the number of tests required to eliminate brucellosis from infected herds

The major disadvantages of adult vaccination are

- Residual vaccine titers
- Persistent positive milk ring test
- Persistent strain 19 infection in a small percentage of adult vaccinates
- The stigma attached to adult vaccinates, which identifies them with infected herds, even though brucellosis has been eliminated and the herd released from quarantine

B. abortus strain 19 has been recovered from the supramammary lymph nodes of cattle at slaughter that were vaccinated with a low dose of the vaccine 9 to 12 months previously and had persistent titers to the CFT. The stage of gestation affects the immune responses of cattle to strain 19 vaccination. Cattle that are late in the first or early in the second trimester of gestation (84 to 135 days) at the time of administration of a low dose of strain 19 are at greater risk of being positive by official tests for brucellosis. Vaccination of cattle during the third trimester with a low dose of the vaccine is not as efficacious as when performed earlier. Although reduced-dose strain 19 vaccination is a possible alternative to the total depopulation of problem herds, its use during pregnancy should be avoided because of the risk of abortion and positive serologic titers and positive bulk milk ring tests.

The results expected following adult vaccination depend on the disease situation. In herds vaccinated in the acute phase of the disease, abortion may continue for 60 to 90 days but the incidence begins to decline by 45 to 60 days. A large number of serologic reactors will be present for the first 120 days following vaccination, and testing is usually not done for the first 60 days. The rate of reactors declines rapidly after 120 days and with good infected herd management most adult vaccinated herds can be free of brucellosis 18 to 24 months following vaccination.

The prevalence of *B. abortus* strain 19 infection in adult vaccinated cattle is low and is often not permanent. The prevalence is lower among cattle given the reduced dose of the vaccine subcutaneously. Bacteriologic examination of the milk and serologic examination of the infected cattle are necessary to identify strain 19 infected cattle, which can be retained for milk production because the infections are temporary.

Adult vaccination, even with a low dose, should **not be used in uninfected herds** because of persistent titers, which may last for more than 12 months in up to 15% of vaccinated animals, and because of the potential for abortion. The illegal or unintentional use of the standard dose of strain 19 vaccine in adult cattle will result in a sudden steep antibody titer response in the CFT, which declines in 6 to 11 months. In herds where adult vaccination with a reduced dose of vaccine is used, blood samples should be collected about 4 months after vaccination and subsequently at intervals of 2 months. Those positive to the CFT should be culled. In one study of three large dairy herds in California, the CFT at 2 and 4 months after vaccination was used to identify and cull pregnant reactor cows that were at risk of aborting or calving. The prevention of parturition of infected cows is an effective management technique.

Systemic Reactions to Vaccination With Strain 19

These occur rarely in both calves and adults, and may be more severe in Jersey calves than in other breeds. A local swelling occurs, particularly in adult cattle, and there may be a severe systemic reaction manifested by high fever (40.5–42°C; 105–108°F) lasting for 2 to 3 days, anorexia, listlessness, and a temporary drop in milk production. An occasional animal goes completely dry. The swellings are sterile and do not rupture, but a solid, fibrous mass may persist for many months.

Deaths within 48 hours of vaccination have been recorded in calves after the use of lyophilized vaccine.

B. abortus strain 19 vaccine has been associated with lameness in young cattle with synovitis following vaccination. Experimentally, the intraarticular injection of the vaccine strain can produce synovitis similar to that which occurs following vaccination.

Septicemia due to *B. abortus* may cause some deaths but in most cases the reaction is anaphylactic, and vaccinated calves should be kept under close observation. Immediate treatment with epinephrine hydrochloride (1 mL of 1:1000 solution subcutaneously) or antihistamine drugs is recommended and is effective provided it can be administered in time.

Cows in advanced pregnancy may abort if vaccinated, but the abortion rate is only about 1%; although *B. abortus* strain 19 organisms can be recovered from the fetus and placenta, their virulence is unchanged and they do not cause further spread of infection. Vaccination with strain 19 does not have a deleterious effect on the subsequent conception rate.

Brucella abortus Strain RB51 Vaccine

Brucella abortus strain RB51 (SRB51) is a live, stable, rough mutant of *B. abortus* strain 2308 that lacks much of the LPS O-side chain, therefore, it does not interfere with serologic surveillance tests. Since 1996 vaccines containing SRB51 have become the official vaccines for prevention of brucellosis in several countries.[7] The results of studies comparing the efficacy of SRB51 and strain 19 vaccines in the literature are inconsistent. Generally, SRB51 vaccines are administered subcutaneously to female calves between 4 and 12 months old with a dose of 1 to 3.4 × 10^{10} living organisms.[7] Heifer calves vaccinated at 3 months, 5 months, or 7 months of age with the SRB51 vaccine were protected when challenged against infection and abortion during their first pregnancy. None of the heifers developed antibodies that reacted in the standard agglutination test. A reduced dose of 1 × 10^9 viable organisms administered as calfhood vaccine does not protect against *B. abortus* infection.

Vaccination of cattle over 12 months of age may be permitted under some circumstances and is performed by subcutaneous administration of a single dose of 1 to 3 × 10^9 viable organisms. The use of SRB51 vaccines in pregnant cows is discouraged. The strain RB51 has a tropism for the bovine placental trophoblast and has been associated with placentitis and abortion under field conditions.[7] A reduced dose of an SRB51 vaccine containing 1 × 10^9 viable organisms given to pregnant cattle was protective against infection with *Brucella abortus* without causing placentitis or abortion but resulted in shedding of the vaccine strain in a significant proportion of vaccinated animals.[7] Vaccination of mature sexually intact bulls and heifers with a standard calfhood dose of SRB51 is not associated with shedding or colonization in tissues, and does not appear to cause any reproductive problems when administered to sexually mature cattle. Use of the vaccine in cattle already vaccinated with strain 19 vaccine will not cause positive responses on confirmation tests and does not interfere with brucellosis surveillance.

Studies with strain RB51 vaccine indicate that it is as efficacious as *B. abortus* strain 19 vaccine but is much less abortigenic in cattle. It does not produce any clinical signs of disease after vaccination and does not produce a local vaccination reaction at the injection site. The organism is cleared from the bloodstream within 3 days and is not present in nasal secretions, saliva, or urine. Immunosuppression does not cause recrudescence, and the organism is not spread from vaccinated to nonvaccinated cattle. The vaccine is safe in all cattle over 3 months of age.

In the United States, strain RB51 vaccine was licensed by the USDA's Animal and Plant Health Inspection Service (APHIS) in 1996 for use in cattle and was approved for use in the Cooperative State–Federal Brucellosis Eradication Program. Strain RB51 vaccine must be administered by an accredited veterinarian or by a state or federal animal health official. Calves must be vaccinated with the calf dose (1–3.4 × 10^{10} organisms) between 4 and 12 months of age. Only animals in high-risk areas should be vaccinated over 12 months of age.

Vaccinates must be identified with the standard metal vaccination eartag and a vaccination tattoo. The tattoo will be the same as the tattoo for *B. abortus* strain 19 vaccination except the first digit for the quarter of the year will be replaced with an R to distinguish animals vaccinated with RB51 from those vaccinated with strain 19. Recording and reporting are the same as with strain 19 vaccine. The diagnosis requires special diagnostic tests that are not routinely available in most hospitals. Both strains are sensitive to a range of antimicrobials. Physicians deciding to initiate a metaphylactic treatment in a human patient exposed to the RB51 vaccine strain must be advised that this strain is resistant to rifampin, one of the antimicrobials of choice for the treatment of human brucellosis.

Brucella Vaccines in Wildlife

A reservoir of *B. abortus*-infected bison in the Greater Yellowstone area in the United States is an obstacle in the effort to eradicate brucellosis from the United States and a source of potential reinfection for livestock in the states of Wyoming, Idaho, and Montana. The free-ranging and infected bison in the area migrate from public land on to private lands and may come into contact with cattle. *Brucella*-induced abortions in bison have occurred under experimental and field conditions, and infected bison can transmit brucellosis under range conditions. Wild and free-ranging bison in parts of western Canada have also been shown to be infected with bovine brucellosis. Therefore a safe and effective vaccine suitable for delivery to free-ranging bison in the Greater Yellowstone area and in Canada is considered useful in reducing the risk of transmission and an aid in the prevention and control of the disease.

Brucella abortus Strain 19 in Bison

The use of strain 19 vaccine has been evaluated in pregnant bison and 10-month-old calves, and the results have been unsatisfactory. In adult bison, strain 19 was found to be highly abortigenic, and animals vaccinated as calves were not protected from infection after experimental inoculation in later life.[18]

Brucella abortus Strain RB51 in Bison

The vaccine is safe for vaccination in herds of naive and previously exposed bison calves, young growing bison, adult males, and adult pregnant and nonpregnant females. Fetal lesions do not appear to be significant with bison cows vaccinated with RB51 in early gestation, but placentitis and abortion have occurred incidentally in advanced stages of pregnancy. Limited data from efficacy studies indicate that booster vaccination with strain RB51 vaccines may increase the protection after experimental challenge.[18]

Calfhood vaccination of bison with SRB51 vaccines is efficacious in protecting against intramammary, intrauterine, and fetal infection following exposure to a virulent strain of *B. abortus* during pregnancy. However, these vaccines appear to be less effective in bison than in cattle in protecting from experimental infection. Limited data from efficacy studies indicate that booster vaccination with strain RB51 vaccines may increase the protection after experimental challenge.[18] Calfhood vaccination with SRB51 would be beneficial in a program to reduce the prevalence of *B. abortus* field stains in American bison. As with cattle, SRB51 calfhood vaccination provides a method to prevent transmission and reduce the numbers of susceptible individuals in a bison herd without interfering with serologic identification of *Brucella*-infected animals. Brucellosis management programs in bison and elk are unlikely to be successful if capture and hand vaccination is necessary. The effect of hand vaccination versus ballistic vaccination for vaccination of bison and elk on the immunologic responses to SRB51 has been evaluated. Ballistic delivery may require a greater dose of SRB51 to induce cell-mediated immune responses in bison that are comparable to those induced by hand injection.

Brucella abortus Strain RB51 in Elk (Cervus elaphus canadensis)

Several studies conducted in elk using strain 19 and SRB51 vaccines have yielded disappointing results with poor or no protection against experimental infection. Neither single nor repeated doses provided significant protection against *B. abortus*–induced abortion. Following vaccination, elk remain bacteremic for a prolonged period of time, rapidly develop high antibody titers while the cellular immune response is poor or lacking.[18]

Control Programs on a Herd Basis

The following recommendations are based on the need for flexibility depending on the level of infection that exists and the susceptibility of the herd and the disease regulations in effect at the time.

During an Abortion Storm

Test and disposal of reactors may be unsatisfactory during an outbreak because spread occurs faster than eradication is possible. Vaccination of all nonreactors is recommended in some countries or, if testing is impracticable, vaccination of all cattle. It is preferable to retest the herd before the second vaccination and to cull cows with a threefold rise in agglutination titer.

Heavily Infected Herds in Which Few Abortions Are Occurring

These do not present an urgent problem because a degree of herd resistance has been reached. All calves should be vaccinated immediately, and positive reactors among the remainder should be culled as soon as possible. Periodic milk ring tests (preferably at 2-month, and no more than 3-month, intervals) on individual cows are supplemented by complement fixation and culture tests.

Lightly Infected Herds

These present a special problem. If they are situated in an area where infection is likely to be introduced, calfhood vaccination should be implemented and positive reactors immediately culled. If eradication is the goal in the area, culling of reactors will suffice, but special market demands for vaccinated cattle may require a calfhood vaccination policy. When a herd is declared free of brucellosis on the basis of serum agglutination tests, its status can be maintained by introducing only negative-reacting animals from brucellosis-free herds and annual blood testing. In areas where dairying predominates, semiannual testing of milk may be substituted for blood testing.

In all of the previously mentioned programs, the careful laboratory examination of all aborted fetuses is an important and necessary corollary to routine testing. There are many difficulties achieving control and eventual eradication on a herd basis. These relate mainly to the failure of owners to realize the highly infectious nature of the disease and to cooperate fully in the details of the program. Particularly, they may fail to recognize the recently calved cow as the principal source of infection. In a herd control program, such cows should be isolated at calving and blood tested at 14 days, because false-negative reactions are not uncommon before that time.

Hygienic Measures

These include the isolation or disposal of infected animals; disposal of aborted fetuses, placentas, and uterine discharges; and disinfection of contaminated areas. It is particularly important that infected cows be isolated at parturition. All cattle, horses, and pigs brought on to the farm should be tested, isolated for 30 days, and retested. Introduced cows that are in advanced pregnancy should be kept in isolation until after parturition, because occasional infected cows may not show a positive serum reaction until after calving or abortion. Chlorhexidine gluconate is an effective antiseptic against *B. abortus* and is recommended for washing the arms and hands of animal attendants and veterinarians who come into contact with contaminated tissues and materials.

Eradication on an Area Basis by Test and Slaughter and Cessation of Calfhood Vaccination

Following a successful calfhood vaccination program, eradication on an area basis can be considered when the level of infection is below about 4% of the cattle population. Brucellosis control areas must be established and testing and disposal of reactors and their calves at foot is performed. Financial compensation is paid for disposal of reactors. Infected herds are quarantined and retested at intervals until negative; in heavily infected herds complete depopulation is often necessary. Brucellosis-free areas are established when the level of infection is sufficiently low, and the movement of cattle between areas is controlled to avoid the spread of infection.

Farms with a low incidence may find it possible to engage in an eradication program immediately provided the incidence on surrounding farms is low. Breakdowns may occur if there are accidental introductions from nearby farms, and in these circumstances it is hazardous to have a herd that is not completely vaccinated. When the area incidence is low enough (about 5%) that replacements can be found within the area or adjoining free areas, and immediate culling of reactors can be performed without crippling financial loss, compulsory eradication by testing and disposal of reactors for meat purposes can be instituted. Compensation for culled animals should be provided to encourage full participation in the program.

The work of testing can be reduced by using screening tests to select herds for more intensive epidemiologic and laboratory investigation. In dairy herds, the milk ring test conducted on bulk milk samples is useful. In beef herds, the favored procedure is the collection of blood from drafts of cattle at the abattoir and use of the RBT. The same technique has also been used to screen shipments of beef destined for countries with an aversion to meat infected with *B. abortus*. An additional means of reducing labor costs in an eradication program is the use of automated laboratory systems such as the one available for the RBT and the one based on agglutination and CFT. An educational program to promote herd owners to voluntarily submit all aborted fetuses to a laboratory for bacteriologic examination is also deemed necessary in any eradication scheme. When an area or country is declared free, testing of all or part of the population needs to be performed only at intervals of 2 to 3 years, although regular testing of bulk milk samples (milk ring test) and of culled beef cows in abattoirs and examination of fetuses should be maintained as checks on the eradication status. In all eradication programs, some problem herds will be encountered in which testing and disposal do not eliminate the infection. Usually about 5% of such herds are encountered and are best handled by a "problem herd" program. Fifty percent of these herds have difficulty because of failure to follow directions. The other half usually contain infected animals that do not respond to standard tests. Supplementary bacteriologic and serologic tests as set out previously may occasionally help these spreader animals to be identified and the disease to be eradicated.

United States

Efforts to eradicate brucellosis associated with *B. abortus* in the United States began in 1934 as an economic recovery program to reduce the cattle population because of the Great Depression. Brucellosis was considered the most significant livestock disease at that time, with a reactor rate of 11.5%. In 1954, a cooperative federal and state program was launched based on calfhood vaccination and test and slaughter with compensation. Two very effective surveillance programs for detecting brucellosis were the market cattle testing and milk ring testing of dairy herds. On July 10, 2009, all 50 states, Puerto Rico, and the U.S. Virgin Islands were officially classified as class free for bovine brucellosis.[19] The number of human cases of brucellosis declined with the decline in number of cases in animals. As of 2013, about 100 human cases per year are reported of which most cases are associated with consumption of unpasteurized milk and milk products of goat origin infected with *B. melitensis.*

Bison and elk in the Greater Yellowstone area are the last known remaining reservoir of *B. abortus* in the United States. Control of brucellosis in these species on public lands requires special consideration to preserve the largest wild, free-ranging population of bison in the United States. Vaccination trials are under way.

The primary surveillance methods for testing eligible cattle in the United States have been the **market cattle testing** program in the beef industry and the **milk ring testing** in the dairy industry. In 2009, the National Surveillance Unit USDA-APHIS identified considerable redundancies in bovine brucellosis surveillance in regions classified as class free for bovine brucellosis for at least 5 years.[19] Consequently, slaughter surveillance was reduced, and brucellosis milk surveillance was eliminated in 2011.

Market Cattle Testing

Surveillance by this method is part of the marketing process. Testing is done at livestock markets, slaughterhouses, livestock buying stations, or dealer premises. This type of testing is very effective, especially if required at the first point of assembly of cattle after leaving the farm of origin. Until 2011 95% or more of cows and bulls 2 years of age or older were required to be tested for brucellosis at slaughter in the United States. As of 2011 the number of slaughter plants participating in slaughter surveillance testing was reduced to 13 of the 40 top establishments and two bison slaughter plants. These slaughter plants are located in 13 states, representing all regions of the country.

Milk Ring Testing

Surveillance by this method involves the regular, periodic testing of milk or cream from commercial dairy herds. Milk ring testing is required twice annually in commercial dairy herds in states officially declared free of brucellosis, and four times annually in states not officially free of brucellosis. This test is very sensitive and is done on a small sample of milk from the entire herd. The milk ring test itself is simple and inexpensive. A well-managed testing program is important to public health and can reduce the exposure potential of contaminated dairy products to humans by quickly identifying affected herds. Routine brucellosis ring testing was discontinued in the United States in 2011, following the recommendation of the National Surveillance Unit of the USDA-APHIS that had identified redundancies in the diagnostic surveillance of bovine brucellosis in regions free of brucellosis for over 5 years.[19]

Australia

In Australia, under range conditions, considerable progress toward eradication of brucellosis in large beef herds has been possible. Management must be motivated and confident that the disease can be permanently eradicated. All cattle should be permanently identified, security between subherds must be good, vaccination histories must be accurate, and accurate round-up (mustering) of cattle must be possible. Quarantine facilities for infected subherds must be strict and absolutely reliable, and fence lines must be impenetrable. The development of a two-herd system, based on segregation of weaned heifer calves from adult cows and maintenance of testing pressure on the adults, will reduce the chance of infection of heifers. All calves from reactor dams are discarded, which necessitates positive identification. Only bulls or semen from brucellosis-free herds should be used in clean herds. In some situations, a laboratory is established on the ranch and equipped to do RBT and CFT. This increases the efficiency of the testing program and creates an excellent team effort between management, laboratory personnel, and the field veterinarian.

New Zealand

In New Zealand, the brucellosis status of accredited herds is monitored by a triennial CFT with a sensitivity of greater than 95%. Slaughterhouse surveillance, as performed in Australia, has a low probability of identifying infected herds. A skin test for brucellosis is attractive because it could be used at the same time as routine tuberculin testing.

Canada

In Canada, the bovine brucellosis eradication program is a success story that began in 1950 when the national prevalence of infection was about 9%. With the cooperative Federal–Provincial Calfhood Vaccination Program, the prevalence of infection was reduced to 4.5% by 1956. In 1957, a test and slaughter program was begun in which brucellosis control areas were established and mandatory testing of all cattle was done using the tube agglutination test. Reactors were identified and ordered to be slaughtered, and compensation was paid. Infected herds were quarantined and retested until negative or in some cases completely depopulated. When the infection rate was reduced to below 1% of the cattle population and 5% of the herds, the area was certified for a period of 3 years. When the infection rate was reduced to below 0.2% of the cattle in the area and 1% of the herds, the area was designated brucellosis free and certified for a period of 5 years. In the 1960s, the milk ring test and the market cattle testing programs were introduced as surveillance procedures. These are done on a continuing basis, are effective in locating infected herds, and have reduced the volume of on-farm testing required to recertify areas.

When the national level of infection was reduced to below 0.2%, calfhood vaccination was deemphasized to overcome the problem of distinguishing between persistent vaccination titers and titers caused by natural infection. Thus all seropositive animals could be disposed of and no vaccination privileges allowed. In 1973, an increase in the incidence of brucellosis occurred, which necessitated some modifications in the eradication program. The intensity of milk ring testing was increased, herds adjacent to infected herds were tested, the length of quarantine of infected herds was increased, and calves from reactor dams were ordered to be slaughtered. In heavily infected herds and in those in which it is not possible to maintain effective quarantine, it was preferable to completely depopulate a herd rather than conduct tests and successive retests. In the Canadian experience, brucellosis-free herds usually became infected when the owner unknowingly purchased an infected animal. The uncontrolled movement of infected animals from infected herds to brucellosis-free herds was a major obstacle in the final stages of the eradication.

The rate of progress in an eradication program is determined mainly by the rate at which herds that are accredited free of the infection become reinfected. The severity of reinfection (or **breakdown**) is dependent on the proportion of the herd that has been vaccinated as calves. The cessation of compulsory calfhood vaccination results in a large proportion of cattle that are fully susceptible to *B. abortus* infection. The prevention of reinfection requires a constant surveillance system.

Canada was declared free of bovine brucellosis in 1985. In 1997, a comprehensive review of Canada's bovine brucellosis surveillance program was undertaken. As a result of the findings of this review, a number of modifications to the surveillance program were introduced in 1999. The routine serologic testing of market and slaughter cattle and the routine milk ring testing of all dairy cattle were discontinued in 1999. However, auction market testing of cattle 24 months and older continues in the five markets in northern Alberta and British Columbia in response to the disease risk associated with the infected free-roaming bison herds in and around Wood Buffalo National Park.

In April 2000, the vaccination of calves with reduced dosage strain 19 *B. abortus* vaccine was discontinued. Strain RB51 *B. abortus* vaccine is not licensed for use in Canada.

Bovine brucellosis in wildlife is restricted to free-roaming bison in and around Wood Buffalo National Park in northern Canada. Information on this occurrence is found in Canada's report to the OIE Wildlife Diseases Working Group.

FURTHER READING

DelVecchio VG, Wagner MA, Eshenbrenner M, et al. *Brucella* proteomes: a review. *Vet Microbiol.* 2002;90:593-603.

Ragan VE. The Animal and Plant Health Inspection Service (APHIS) brucellosis eradication program in the USA. *Vet Microbiol.* 2002;90:11-18.

Lapaque N, Moriyon I, Moreno E, Gorvel J-P. *Brucella* lipopolysaccharide acts as a virulence factor. *Curr Opin Microbiol.* 2005;8:60-66.

OIE. Bovine brucellosis. OIE Terrestrial Manual. At: <http://www.oie.int/fileadmin/Home/eng/Health_standards/tahm/2.04.03_BOVINE_BRUCELL.pdf>; 2009 Accessed 25.01.14.

WHO. Brucellosis in humans and animals. At: <http://www.who.int/csr/resources/publications/Brucellosis.pdf>; 2006 Accessed 27.01.14.

REFERENCES

1. Scholz HC, Vergnaud G. *Rev Sci Tech.* 2013;32:149.
2. Díaz-Apparicio E. *Rev Sci Tech.* 2013;32:53.
3. EFSA. *EFSA J.* 2014;12(3547):175.
4. Otlu S, et al. *Acta Vet Brno.* 2008;77:117.
5. Lopez LB, et al. *Open Vet Sci J.* 2010;4:72.
6. McDermott J, et al. *Rev Sci Tech.* 2013;32:249.
7. OIE 2009. At: <http://www.oie.int/fileadmin/Home/eng/Health_standards/tahm/2.04.03_BOVINE_BRUCELL.pdf>; 2014 Accessed 25.02.14.
8. White PJ, et al. *Biol Conserv.* 2011;144:1322.
9. Scurlock BM, Edwards WH. *J Wildl Dis.* 2010;46:442.
10. Cross PC, et al. *Rev Sci Tech.* 2013;32:79.
11. Schumaker B. *Rev Sci Tech.* 2013;32:71.
12. Poester FP, et al. *Rev Sci Tech.* 2013;32:105.
13. Baldi PC, Giambartolomei GH. *Rev Sci Tech.* 2013;32:117.
14. EFSA. *EFSA J.* 2014;12:3547.
15. The Center for Food Security and Public Health 2007. At: <http://www.cfsph.iastate.edu/Factsheets/pdfs/brucellosis.pdf>; 2014 Accessed 27.01.14.
16. WHO 2006. At: <http://www.who.int/csr/resources/publications/Brucellosis.pdf>; 2014 Accessed 27.01.14.
17. McGiven JA. *Rev Sci Tech.* 2013;32:163.
18. Olsen SC. *Rev Sci Tech.* 2013;32:207.
19. USDA. At: <http://www.aphis.usda.gov/animal_health/animal_diseases/brucellosis/downloads/natl_bruc_surv_strategy.pdf>; 2010 Accessed 27.01.14.

BRUCELLOSIS ASSOCIATED WITH *BRUCELLA OVIS*

SYNOPSIS

Etiology *Brucella ovis.*

Epidemiology Organism carried by sexually mature rams with spread by direct contact or passive venereal infection. Predominantly a disease of sheep, but red deer stags can be naturally infected.

Clinical findings Complete or partial infertility in rams caused by epididymitis. Epididymal abnormality can be detected by palpation in some affected rams. Occasionally abortion in ewes and neonatal mortality in lambs.

Clinical pathology Serology of most value including complement fixation, gel diffusion, and ELISA; semen examination.

Diagnostic confirmation Physical palpation of scrotal contents; serology; culture or PCR of semen, testes, and seminal vesicles, aborted material.

Treatment Oxytetracycline in valuable rams.

Control Total segregation of normal and young rams. Initial culling of rams with palpable scrotal abnormality and subsequent repeated serologic testing and culling of seropositive rams. Where permitted, vaccination with live *B. melitensis* strain Rev. 1 is an alternative.

ETIOLOGY

Brucella ovis has significant DNA homology with other members of the *Brucella* genus and shares antigenic and other characteristics. However, it has a permanently rough phenotype, whereas *B. melitensis* and *B. abortus* colonies are smooth.[1]

EPIDEMIOLOGY

Geographic Occurrence

Brucellosis of sheep associated with *B. ovis* has been reported in most of the major sheep-producing regions of the world, including Australia, New Zealand, North and South America, Central Asia, Russia, South Africa, and Europe, but is not a major cause of ram wastage in Great Britain. When the disease is first diagnosed in a country, and before control procedures are established, the flock prevalence of infection can be as high as 75% and as many as 60% of rams may be infected. The prevalence of infection is generally much lower in countries and in flocks that have established control programs.

Host Occurrence

In nature mainly sheep are affected, with the ram more susceptible than the ewe. A small number of natural cases occur in farmed red deer (*Cervus elaphus*) in New Zealand, but most infections resolve after 340 days and it is regarded as a self-limiting disease.[2] It is difficult to establish infection in laboratory animals. However, white-tailed deer and goats can be infected experimentally and develop epididymitis. There is no evidence of natural infection in goats, even in those that graze with infected sheep.

The Merino breed and Merino-derived crossbreeds show a much lower incidence of the disease than do British breeds. The disease is most important in large flocks where there is multisire breeding.

Source of Infection

The infected ram is the source of infection and perpetuates the disease in a flock. The majority of infected rams excrete the organism in semen, and in most rams the active excretion in semen probably persists indefinitely. Ewes are more resistant to infection, but the organism can be isolated from them in infected flocks. After being bred by an infected ram, the majority will not carry infection for more than one or two heat cycles. Infection may result in early embryonic death and occasionally abortion or the birth of weak and poorly viable lambs. In ewes where the infection does persist to produce abortion, the organism is present in the placenta, vaginal discharges, and milk.

Transmission

Transmission between rams occurs via passive venereal infection and by direct ram-to-ram transfer. Passive venereal infection occurs from ewes that have been bred by an infected ram in the same heat cycle. Under natural conditions, this may be the major form of transmission from ram to ram during the breeding season. Infection can also be transmitted between rams in the nonbreeding season when housed or grouped together on pasture. This occurs as they sniff and lick each other's prepuce and by homosexual activity. Submissive rams may lick the prepuce of dominant rams as a trait in the dominance hierarchy. Spread of infection in a group of virgin rams is recorded. Lambs born from infected ewes and drinking infected milk do not become persistently infected.

The organism can survive on pasture for several months, but transmission by fomites appears to have no practical significance. However, transmission from infected rams to infection-free red deer stags grazed on the same pasture can occur, and it is not known if this results from direct contact between the animals or indirectly via environmental and pasture contamination.

Host Risk Factors

All postpubertal rams are susceptible to infection, but disease is more common in adult rams and disease prevalence increases with age, probably because of greater exposure to infection. Differences between flocks in the prevalence of disease suggest that environmental factors and stress may modulate susceptibility, but the risk factors are poorly defined. When the number of affected rams in a flock is greater than about 10%, the fertility of the flock is appreciably decreased.

Experimental Reproduction

Experimentally, rams can be infected by the IV, subcutaneous, intratesticular, oral, conjunctival, and preputial routes, but the latter two are the most effective. The first observable abnormality is the presence of inflammatory cells in the semen, which appear at 2 to 8 weeks. *B. ovis* appears in the ejaculate at approximately 3 weeks, but it is not always present in an infected ram after that.[3] Testicular and epididymal lesions can be palpated at about 9 weeks after infection but may occur earlier in some rams. A significant proportion of infected rams have no palpable lesions but still excrete the organism.

Ewes in early pregnancy can also be infected by the oral and IV routes, but many of these infections are transient and do not result in abortion. Abortion caused by placentitis has been produced experimentally. Intrauterine infection produced experimentally also causes lesions in and death of the fetus, but the significance of this to natural cases is undetermined.

Economic Importance

The economic effects of the disease are subtle but significant. The effect of the disease on ram fertility can influence the number of rams that are required in a flock, with the required ram to ewe ratio significantly reduced in *B. ovis*–free flocks. The percentage of lambs born early and within the first 3 weeks of the lambing period is also markedly increased. Lambing percentage may be reduced by 30% in recently infected flocks and by 15% to 20% in those where the infection is endemic. The loss of rams of high genetic potential and the need for repeat serologic testing are additional costs. In the United States, the advantage in a control program has been calculated as an additional return of $12 per ewe mated.

Zoonotic Implications

B. ovis is not a zoonosis, but live *Brucella* vaccines used for prevention of this infection in some countries, such as Rev. 1 *B. melitensis* vaccine, are pathogenic to humans and should be handled and used with care.

PATHOGENESIS

There is an initial bacteremia, often with a mild systemic reaction, and the organism can be isolated from the internal organs of animals slaughtered after experimental infection. However, systemic disease is not a feature of the natural disease, and clinical disease results from localization and inflammation in the epididymides, typically in the tail. Inflammation in this area results in sperm stasis and extravasation with a subsequent immunologic reaction that is often unilateral, causing a spermatocele and reduced fertility. Not all infected rams have palpable lesions in the epididymis, and infection can also establish in the seminal vesicles and ampullae. In either case the organism is shed in the ejaculate.

Generally, *B. ovis* has low pathogenicity for ewes. The primary effect is a placentitis, which interferes with fetal nutrition, sometimes to the point of causing fetal death, but more commonly producing lambs of low birth weight and poor viability.

Analysis of the immune response by microarray hybridization and reverse transcription (RT)-PCR found that infection with *B. ovis* causes upregulation of genes involved in phagocytosis and downregulation of host defense mechanisms, both of which probably contribute to the chronic nature of the infection.[4]

CLINICAL FINDINGS

The first reaction in rams is a marked deterioration in the quality of the semen together with the presence of leukocytes and *Brucella*. Acute edema and inflammation of the scrotum may follow. A systemic reaction, including fever, depression, and increased respiratory rate, accompanies the local reaction.

Regression of the acute syndrome is followed, after a long latent period, by the development of palpable lesions in the epididymis and tunicae of one or both testicles.

The palpation of both testicles simultaneously is the best method of examination. The epididymis is enlarged and hard, more commonly at the tail; the scrotal tunics are thickened and hardened; and the testicles are usually atrophic. The groove between the testis and epididymis may be obliterated.

The abnormalities are often detectable by palpation, but many affected rams show no acute inflammatory stage and others may be actively secreting *Brucella* and poor-quality semen in the chronic stage in the absence of palpable abnormalities. Palpable abnormality of the scrotal contents may be present in less than 50% of serologically positive rams. Affected rams have normal libido.

There are usually no clinical signs in the ewe but in some flocks infection causes abortion or the birth of weak or stillborn lambs, associated with a macroscopic placentitis.

In red deer, only a small proportion of stags infected with *B. ovis* develop epididymitis detectable by scrotal palpation.[5] In contrast to rams, in most stags the infection resolves within 12 months following infection.[2]

CLINICAL PATHOLOGY

Semen examination, including culture of the ejaculate, and serologic tests are used in suspect individuals and in groups of rams. The complement fixation and ELISA tests are by far the most useful; many infected rams have palpably normal scrotal contents and microbiologically negative semen. Ultrasound examination of the scrotal contents can reveal anechoic areas that correspond to foci of fibrosis, but these appear no earlier and are nonspecific, offering no real advantage over scrotal palpation.

Multiplex PCRs to differentiate *B. ovis* from *Actinobacillus seminis* and *Histophilus ovis* have been described for use on semen or urine.[6,7] Real-time PCR has also been used to type *Brucella* from field material, such as ovine placenta, without the need for culture.[8]

Semen Examination

A combination of semen examination and palpation of the testicles for abnormalities will identify approximately 80% of infected rams. In affected animals the findings are a general reduction in semen quality, a reduced total sperm output, poor motility, and a high proportion of spermatozoa with secondary morphologic abnormalities.

Culture

B. ovis is fastidious in its growth and requires special cultural techniques. The examination of the semen for the presence of leukocytes has been used to determine those sheep that should be cultured for *B. ovis,* but it is not a highly sensitive screening test. PCR for detection of *B. ovis* in semen has an equivalent sensitivity to culture.

Serology

The CFT, the standard test in many countries, is the prescribed test for international trade, and when used in conjunction with genital palpation has allowed the eradication of *B. ovis* from flocks. However, a small proportion of infected rams are negative to CFT, which can compromise or delay eradication programs. The sensitivity and specificity of the various serologic tests depend mainly on the antigens used and the serologic cut points, which may vary between countries and laboratories. A UK study reported the sensitivity of an ELISA, gel diffusion, and CFT as 97.6, 96.4, and 92.7%, respectively, with all tests 100% specific. Studies in other countries support this ranking, but others suggest that the ELISA has no advantage over the classic complement and gel diffusion tests. A combination of serologic tests may increase the sensitivity closer to 100%, but will obviously increase testing costs. Seroconversion occurs slightly earlier with the ELISA, compared with the complement fixation and gel diffusion tests, so it may be useful in situations where infection is rapidly spreading within a group of rams.[9]

Serologic tests will not differentiate vaccinated from infected sheep or sheep infected with *B. melitensis.*

NECROPSY FINDINGS

In the acute stage, there is inflammatory edema in the loose scrotal fascia, exudate in the tunica vaginalis, and formation of granulation tissue. In the chronic stage, the tunics of the testes become thickened and fibrous and develop adhesions. There are circumscribed indurations in the epididymis and these granulomata may also be present in the testicle. In advanced stages, they undergo caseation necrosis. As the epididymis enlarges the testicle becomes atrophied. *B. ovis* can usually be isolated from the genital organs, especially the tail of the epididymis, and rarely from internal organs and lymph nodes. Similar lesions are described in red deer stags.[5]

The abortus is characterized by thickening and edema, sometimes restricted to only a part of the placenta, with firm, elevated yellow-white plaques in the intercotyledonary areas and varying degrees of cotyledonary necrosis. Microscopically, organisms are visible within the cytoplasm of trophoblasts of the inflamed placenta. A vasculitis is often present. The organism can be isolated from the placenta and the stomach and lungs of the lamb.

Samples for Confirmation of Diagnosis

- Bacteriology and PCR: epididymal granuloma, seminal vesicle, inguinal lymph node/fetal lung, stomach content, placenta (culture, has special growth requirements; cytology, Stamp's or Koster's stain on placental smear; PCR)
- Histology: formalin-fixed epididymis, testicle, seminal vesicle, inguinal lymph node from rams; in abortions placenta, fetal lung, liver, spleen, kidney, heart, brain

DIFFERENTIAL DIAGNOSIS

Infection with *Actinobacillus seminis* and *Histophilus ovis* can cause similar scrotal lesions, although many rams with abnormalities of intrascrotal tissues do not have brucellosis or infectious epididymitis.

Abortion in ewes may be associated with a number of infectious diseases, which are summarized in Table 18-1.

TREATMENT

Treatment of naturally occurring cases is rarely undertaken. IM administration of long-acting oxytetracycline at 20 mg/kg body weight (BW), given every 3 days for 24 days, along with the daily IM administration of 20 mg/kg of dihydrostreptomycin sulfate, resulted in bacteriologic cure of 90% of experimentally infected rams. Oxytetracycline alone is less effective, but the use of dihydrostreptomycin is prohibited in food-producing animals in many countries. Treatment is economically feasible only in valuable rams and must be instituted before irreparable damage to the epididymis has occurred. The treatment of rams that are infected but without palpable lesions results in a significant improvement in breeding soundness classification on examinations subsequent to treatment.

CONTROL

Control is by preventing the spread of infection between rams and detecting and culling infected rams. In small flocks, culling of all rams and replacement with *B. ovis*–free rams may be the most cost-effective approach. Some control can be achieved using scrotal palpation to detect infected rams, but this must be combined with repeated serologic testing if eradication is the goal. Vaccination may be the most economical and practical means of controlling the disease in areas with a high incidence of infection and in regions of the world where eradication by test and slaughter is impractical.

Eradication

In a flock where the diagnosis has been confirmed all rams are palpated and those with scrotal abnormalities are culled. The remaining rams are tested serologically and reactors culled. Serologic tests are repeated at monthly intervals, with culling of reactors, until all rams are serologically negative. Further tests, 6 and 18 months later, are used to confirm eradication.

Infection spreads rapidly during the mating season, so eradication should be delayed until after the breeding season. During breeding it may be wise to run two breeding flocks, with virgin rams and rams known to be free of infection separated from older or suspicious rams (seropositive and/or those with scrotal lesions). Strict separation of the two ram flocks must be maintained at all times, and the clean group must not mate ewe flocks that have been mated to the suspect rams.

Several countries have voluntary accreditation schemes based on inspection of boundary fencing, restricting the introduction of new rams to those from accredited flocks and serologic testing.

Vaccination

A number of vaccines have been used, but none is fully effective. In some countries, vaccination is not permitted and eradication by test and slaughter is the only method of control.

Table 18-1 Diagnostic summary of infectious abortion in ewes

		Epidemiology and diagnosis			Laboratory findings	
Disease	*Transmission*	*Time of abortion*	*Clinical data*	*Fetus*	*Serology*	*Vaccination*
Brucellosis (*Brucella ovis*)	Passive venereal, ram to ram	Late or stillbirth, weak lambs	Abortion in ewes, epididymitis in rams	Organisms in fetal stomach and placenta	CFT or ELISA	In some countries simultaneous *B. abortus* strain 19 and killed *B. ovis* vaccine, or *B. melitensis* Rev. 1 vaccine
Campylobacter fetus or *C. jejuni*	Ingestion High stocking rate, intensive grazing, and supplementary feeding on the ground increases risk	Mainly young ewes; last 6 weeks of pregnancy, stillbirths, weak lambs	Metritis in ewes after abortion	*Campylobacter* in stomach, large necrotic foci in liver	Agglutination test, flock only	Formalin-inactivated bivalent vaccine can increase live lambs by around 10%; variable efficacy depending on which strains are present
Enzootic abortion of ewes (*Chlamydophila abortus*)	Ingestion	Last 2–3 weeks. Stillbirths, weak lambs	No sickness in ewes, neonatal mortality	*Chlamydophila* in fetal cotyledons Degenerative changes in placenta	ELISA, CFT, PCR	Killed vaccine gives moderate immunity. Live attenuated vaccine
Listeriosis (*Listeria monocytogenes*)	Probably ingestion	After 3 months	Retained placenta and metritis Septicemia in some ewes	Organisms in fetal stomach Autolysis, necrotic foci in liver	Agglutination and complement fixation of doubtful value	In some countries killed or live attenuated vaccines
Salmonellosis (*Salmonella abortusovis*)	Probably ingestion Carrier sheep	Last 6 weeks	Metritis after abortion	Organisms in fetal stomach Not in the United States	Agglutination test	Doubtful efficacy
Salmonellosis (*S. dublin, S. montevideo, S. typhimurium*)	Ingestion	Last month	Abortion: fetal metritis, neonatal mortality	Organisms in stomach	Agglutination test	—
Toxoplasmosis	Ingestion	Late or stillbirths Live-born weak lambs	Abortion, stillbirths, and neonatal mortality; no illness in ewe	Multiple small necrotic foci in fetal cotyledons Toxoplasma in cells of trophoblast epithelium	Modified agglutination test, ELISA of limited value in adult; test pleural fluid of fetus PCR	Live S48 tachyzoite in some countries (e.g., UK, New Zealand); single dose 3 weeks before mating
Rift Valley fever	Insects	—	Important cause of abortion in all species in Central Africa Heavy mortality in young animals	Acidophilic inclusions hepatic cells	Hemagglutination inhibition and ELISA Fluorescent antibody for tissues	Available in endemic countries
Coxiellosis (Q-Fever)	Inhalation, ingestion	Later term and weak lambs	No illness in ewe, neonatal mortality	Fetus fresh, Intercotyledonary necrotizing placentitis	Fluorescent and PCR; serology of limited value	Vaccine available in Europe but not in most other countries
Tick-borne fever	Ticks	Late, following systemic disease	Fever and abortion	None specific	Giemsa smear of blood, PCR Counterimmunoelectrophoresis	None
Border disease	Ingestion	All stages, stillbirth	Infertility in ewes, hairy shaker lambs	Virus isolation	See text description	None that are specific for sheep strains

CFT, *complement fixation test;* ELISA, *enzyme-linked immunosorbent assay;* PCR, *polymerase chain reaction.*

Killed *B. ovis* vaccines, even with adjuvants, have poor efficacy. The use of a killed vaccine may be inadvisable in flocks where eradication is being attempted, because it may protect against clinical disease but allow a carrier state in some rams in which there is excretion of the organism in animals that become seronegative. An experimental vaccine prepared from enriched OMPs and rough LPS of *B. ovis* gave equivalent protection in challenge studies to that given by *B. melitensis* Rev. 1 vaccine.

A combined vaccine containing killed *B. ovis* in an adjuvant and *B. abortus* strain 19 also provided durable immunity but had several disadvantages. Vaccinated animals become seropositive, which compromises the subsequent use of serologic tests for eradication. Strain 19 also can cause epididymitis, and vaccinated rams may excrete strain 19 in their semen.

Live *B. melitensis* strain Rev. 1 has been found to be most effective and is the most widely used vaccine, where permitted. This strain was developed in the 1950s from a virulent isolate that had become streptomycin dependent. It is avirulent for rams, and subcutaneous or conjunctival vaccination provides protection against experimental and field challenge. Vaccinated animals become positive to the complement fixation and ELISA tests, but titers are low and can be minimized by using the conjunctival route for vaccination. However, vaccinated animals can excrete *B. melitensis* strain Rev. 1, and it can cause abortions, so alternative vaccine candidates are being evaluated. These include an OMP extracted from *B. melitensis* (Omp31) and an attenuated strain of *B. ovis* (Delta abcBA). The latter protects against experimental challenge with virulent *B. ovis* and is considered a potential vaccine strain for rams.[10]

If vaccination is used there should also be a program of culling clinically abnormal rams, and ram replacements should be yearlings vaccinated at 4 to 5 months.

FURTHER READING

Ridler AL, West DM. Control of *Brucella ovis* infection in sheep. *Vet Clin North Am Food Anim Pract.* 2011;27:61-66.

REFERENCES

1. Whatmore AM. *Infect Genet Evol.* 2009;9:1168.
2. Ridler AL, et al. *New Zeal Vet J.* 2006;54:85.
3. Carvalho Júnior CA, et al. *Small Rumin Res.* 2012;102:213.
4. Galindo RC, et al. *Vet Immunol Immunopathol.* 2009;127:295.
5. Ridler AL, et al. *New Zeal Vet J.* 2012;60:146.
6. Saunders VF, et al. *Aust Vet J.* 2007;85:72.
7. Moustacas VS, et al. *BMC Vet Res.* 2013;9:51.
8. Gopaul KK, et al. *Vet Rec.* 2014;175:282.
9. Ridler AL, et al. *New Zeal Vet J.* 2014;62:47.
10. Silva AP, et al. *PLoS ONE.* 2015;10:e0136865.

BRUCELLOSIS ASSOCIATED WITH *BRUCELLA SUIS* IN PIGS

Brucella suis infection may be inapparent or may result in stillbirths, abortion, and infertility in both sexes. In boars it causes infection of the testicles and accessory sex glands. It will cause disease in man[1].

SYNOPSIS

Etiology Disease in pigs is caused by *Brucella suis* biovars 1–3. Biovars 1–4 cause rare disease in cattle.

Epidemiology Disease in pigs is transmitted by contact, ingestion, and venereally.

Clinical findings
Sows: Infertility, irregular estrus, small litters, and abortion.
Boars: Orchitis, lameness, incoordination, and posterior paralysis.
Piglets: Mortality.

Clinical pathology Isolation of organism. Several serologic tests available but none with good sensitivity.

Necropsy Metritis, orchitis, osteomyelitis. Granulomatous inflammation and foci of caseous necrosis.

Diagnostic confirmation Isolation of *B. suis* and herd serology tests.

Treatment None satisfactory.

Control Serologic testing and disposal of reactors. No effective vaccine. Humans, and occasionally cattle. Transmission congenital or by ingestion or contact with infected placenta, vaginal discharge, or milk.

Clinical findings Abortion storms, abortions often in last 2 months of pregnancy. Weak-born lambs.

Clinical pathology Culture of organism. Serologic tests and skin hypersensitivity testing for herd diagnosis.

Necropsy findings Placentitis.

Diagnostic confirmation Only by isolation of the organism.

Control Slaughter eradication. Vaccination with Rev. 1 vaccine, which will produce abortion in pregnant animals.

ETIOLOGY

It is a small, aerobic, gram-negative *Bacillus*. Remember that *B abortus* and *B. melitensis* will also occasionally infect the pig, however, only *B. suis* will cause systemic and generalized infections in pigs. The other species will infect pigs, but the infection is self-limiting and the infection is usually restricted to the local lymph nodes. There are five biovars.

EPIDEMIOLOGY

Geographic Occurrence

Biovar 1

Biovar 1 is important in pigs and occurs worldwide, but the disease has not been recorded in the UK, Canada is disease free, and the prevalence is very low in the United States. It is particularly important in the Philippines and the Pacific islands and Africa.

Biovar 2

Biovar 2 occurs in pigs in west central Europe, particularly Croatia and Czechoslovakia, and also in hares. There appears to be a close relationship between pigs and wildlife in this strain and wild boar in particular.[2] Occasionally it appears in cattle, dogs, and horses.

Biovar 3

Biovar 3 has a close similarity to *B. melitensis* biovar 2 and requires phage typing, oxidative metabolic testing, or PCR for differentiation. It also occurs in pigs in the United States, South America, and southeast Asia. It is a problem in wild boar where it may reach 8% to 32% prevalence,[3,4] and particularly in Italy[5] and Spain[6] the spill over from wild boar to domestic pigs is a particular problem.[7]

Biovar 4

Biovar 4 is a cause of rangiferine brucellosis (reindeers, caribou, bison, moose, etc.) and can transmit to cattle but does not appear to be a disease of pigs. It will transmit to humans.

Biovar 5

Biovar 5 is murine brucellosis. It may also include *B. microti,* which has been isolated from voles and wild rodents in Russia.[8]

Host Occurrence

Domestic, wild, or feral pigs are the host for biotypes 1 and 3, and widespread infection in feral pigs is recorded in Queensland, Australia, and the southern states of the United States. Bison may remain reservoirs. Incursion to domestic pigs from wild boar is an increasing problem.

Cattle and horses may be infected, especially if they share a range with feral pigs, and this association adversely affects the status of cattle herds undergoing brucellosis eradication programs. Cattle are noncontagious hosts, but an outbreak in Switzerland where the disease had not appeared since 1946 has been attributed to a spread of infection from horses.

Biovar 1

Biovar 1 has been isolated from the semen of a ram. Infection in dogs, usually symptomless but occasionally producing orchitis or epididymitis, or granulomas can result from eating raw pig meat.

Biovar 2

In addition to the pig, the European hare (*Lepus capensis*) is also a major host for biovar 2, and this biovar is common in central Europe. Some studies have suggested that the type found in hares in Europe is a different strain from the wild boar.[9]

Biovar 4

Biovar 4 can transmit to cattle in contact with infected reindeer. Wild canids can also be naturally infected with biovar 4, presumably by ingestion.

Source of Infection

Infected boars can shed 10^4 to 10^7 colony-forming units (CFU) of *B. suis* per milliliter of semen. The bacterium is also shed in the milk.

The introduction of infected pigs, usually a boar or the communal use of an infected boar, is the common means of introduction of the bacterium into a pig unit. Artificial insemination using noncertified or untreated semen can also spread the disease as can ova. Transmission usually requires direct or close contact and is usually oral. Discharges in milk and uterine secretions are infectious. Sows may be carriers and piglets can spread the disease horizontally. It is thought that infection through the conjunctiva is also a possibility. It probably does not survive in the environment unless contained in organic matter under cold conditions. Within a piggery the disease is spread by ingestion and by coitus. The ingestion of food contaminated by infected semen and urine and discharges from infected sows are also important methods of spread. Dried secretions, if frozen, may remain infective. Most disinfectants and sunshine kill the virus.

The feeding of kitchen waste containing raw pig meat also presents a risk. Domestic herds are also at risk when they are kept under extensive husbandry methods in areas where there is a high prevalence of infection in feral pigs. Cattle infected with biovar 1 are noncontagious to other livestock and can have normal pregnancies and give birth to uninfected calves.

Wild animals, including hares and rats, may provide a source of infection with biovar 2, and ticks are also suspected of transmitting the disease.

Host and Pathogen Risk Factors

The fact that *B. suis* survives so well in raw meat, e.g., 128 days in sausage meat, means that prepared pork products are always a source of infection. They can survive freezing for over 2 years. Environments and pastures can be infected for a long period of time.

B. suis is more resistant to adverse environmental conditions than *B. abortus,* although its longevity outside the body has not been fully examined. It is known to survive in feces, urine, and water for 4 to 6 weeks. As the environmental temperature rises, the survival in the environment decreases. It is also deactivated by bright sunlight. It has also been known to survive desiccation.

Among pigs, susceptibility may vary with age. The prevalence of infection is much higher in adults than in young pigs, although this may represent an exposure risk rather than an age-related risk. Susceptibility is much greater in the postweaning periods and is the same for both sexes, but there may also be genetically determined differences in susceptibility. Some piglets acquire infection from the sow, either from the ingestion of infected milk or by congenital infection.

Lateral spread through a herd is rapid because of the conditions under which pigs are kept. No durable herd immunity develops and, although a stage of herd resistance is apparent after an acute outbreak, the herd is again susceptible within a short time and the bacteria can spread rapidly on entry to a herd. Within a few months 50% may be infected and 70% to 80% may be involved at the start of the outbreak. Further outbreaks may occur if infection is reintroduced.

In an enzootic area, the proportion of herds infected is usually high (30%–60%). The prevalence of seropositivity in an infected herd varies but can be as high as 66%. Seroprevalence in feral pigs is also high, is higher in adult pigs than pigs under 6 months of age, and varies between populations of feral pigs.

Economic Importance

The disease is economically important because of infertility and reduction in numbers of pigs weaned per litter. Mortality in live-born piglets, which occurs during the first month of life, may be as high as 80%. The mortality rate is negligible in mature animals, but sows and boars may have to be culled because of sterility, and occasionally pigs are culled because of posterior paralysis. In addition, eradication involves a great deal of financial loss if complete disposal of a registered herd is undertaken.

Zoonotic Implications

Biovar 2 is not a zoonosis, but biovars 1, 3 (as pathogenic as *B. melitensis*), and 4 have considerable significance for public health and are very pathogenic to humans. In countries where pigs are a significant part of animal farming and the human diet, *B. suis* is the major cause of human brucellosis (e.g., South America).[10,11]

B. suis presents an occupational hazard, particularly to abattoir workers, and to a lesser extent to farmers and veterinarians and hunters.[12] *B. abortus* and *B. melitensis* may also be found in pig carcasses and present similar hazards. *B. suis* can be widespread in the carcass of infected pigs, and undercooked meat can be a source of human infection. This is particularly true for wild boar and feral pig meat. A recent experiment described infection with biovar type 1 and its transmission to negative pigs after 4 to 6 weeks. Antibody was detected in blood samples from farmers and abattoir workers.

In infected cattle, *B. suis* localizes in the mammary gland without causing clinical abnormality and, where cattle and pigs are run together, the hazard to humans drinking unpasteurized milk may be significant. Biovar 4 causes human disease associated with consumption of caribou.

Human brucellosis at a pig slaughterhouse in Argentina has been described.[13] The median age of the slaughterhouse workers was 40 (23–65) and they had worked for 1 to 9 years in the slaughtering or butchery part of the plant. A systemic or localized disease with recurrent episodes was described. The chronic disease may be progressive. The patients' serum antibody titers (SAT) titers ranged from 1 : 25 to 1 : 12.800 and CFT from 1 : 10 to 1 : 1280. Of the pigs tested, 11% of the males (7/62) and 18% of the females (25/138) were positive. It is suggested that the swine keepers did not send infected animals for incineration but sent them to slaughter. Diagnoses are rarely made on farms that breed pigs. Such pigs arriving at packing plants have high levels of organisms but rarely have lesions and genital infections that may be a major source of infection. Protective clothing, such as gloves, protective clothing, eye protection, and protection of any bare skin, is essential.

PATHOGENESIS

Infection is followed by multiplication in the local lymph nodes. Only 10^{4-7} organisms will produce an experimental infection, but the severity of the infection is not correlated with either the dose or the route of infection. As for the other species, *B. suis* requires the *vir*B operon-encoded T455 for intracellular invasion and multiplication within host cells. The T455 mutants are not able to survive and multiply in macrophages or epithelial cells.

As in brucellosis associated with *B. abortus,* there is initial systemic invasion possibly through the M cells of the lymphoid tissue in the gut, but also possibly the oral, nasopharyngeal, conjunctival, or vaginal mucosa. There is generally a long period of incubation before clinical signs appear. In young animals these are not necessarily visible and will depend mainly on the age, sex, and physiologic state of the animals at the time they are infected. The organism then appears in the bloodstream, usually within 1 to 7 weeks, and often lasts for 5 weeks but can persist for up to 34 weeks. However, infection with *B. suis* differs from that associated with *B. abortus* in that localization occurs in several organs in addition to the uterus and udder, and the organism is found in all body tissues and produces a disease similar to undulant fever in humans. The organisms persist in lymph nodes, joints, bone marrow, and the genital tract. The more common manifestations of localization are abortion and infertility caused by localization in the uterus; lymphadenitis, especially of the cervical lymph nodes; arthritis and lameness caused by bone and joint localization; and posterior paralysis caused by osteomyelitis. In boars, involvement of the testicles often leads to clinical orchitis, and the boars are probably infected for life. Widespread infection makes handling of the freshly killed carcass hazardous and creates a risk for brucellosis in humans eating improperly cooked pork.

CLINICAL FINDINGS

Do not forget that clinical signs in pigs may also be produced by *B. abortus* and *B. melitensis*. Porcine brucellosis is usually a more generalized and chronic disease than bovine brucellosis.[14]

The clinical findings in swine brucellosis vary widely, depending on the site of localization. The signs are not diagnostic, and in many herds a high incidence of reactors is observed with little clinical evidence of disease. Reproductive inefficiency is the common manifestation.

Sows

Infection at service usually results in early abortion, sometimes as early as 17 days after natural service with infected boars, with return to estrus at 5 to 8 weeks after service, which may be the only sign that infection has taken place.

Infertility, irregular estrus, small litters, and abortion occur. Later infection will give rise to mummification and stillbirths. The incidence of abortion varies widely between herds but is usually low and is usually early. Infection of the fetus may lead to abortion. As a rule, sows abort only once in a lifetime, and this is most common during the third month of pregnancy. Affected sows usually breed normally thereafter. Sows may remain carriers and may shed organisms in milk and uterine discharges, which may be extremely bloody and may be accompanied by endometritis and retained fetal membranes.

Boars

Orchitis with testicular swelling, epididymitis, and necrosis of one or both testicles is followed by sterility usually within 7 weeks of infection. Lameness, incoordination, and posterior paralysis are fairly common. The onset is gradual, and signs may be caused by arthritis or, more commonly, osteomyelitis of lumbar and sacral vertebral bodies. Testicular atrophy may result at around 19 weeks. Boars have a low rate of recovery (less than 50%). After infection, enough animals remain infected to perpetuate the disease.

In both sows and boars, the bones and joints may be involved, and in these cases there may be posterior paralysis and lameness. Nodules may be seen in the spleen and liver and abscesses may be seen in boars.

Piglets

A heavy mortality in piglets during the first month of life is sometimes encountered, but most piglet loss results from stillbirths and the death of weak piglets within a few hours of birth. Up to 10% may contract infection when they are young and retain the infection until adulthood.

CLINICAL PATHOLOGY

Culture

Laboratory identification of the disease is difficult. It should be routine to use more than one culture method.[15] Isolation of the organism should be attempted if suitable material is available. Such material for culture includes aborted fetuses, testicular lesions, abscesses, blood and lymph nodes (particularly the submandibular, gastrohepatic, and external iliac nodes).[16] The organism is a small, slender, aerobic gram-negative organism that produces 1- to 2-mm colonies on blood agar after 2 to 4 days. A new method of culture has been described for *B. suis* called LNIV-M.[17] Interestingly, in a study of wild boar the organism was isolated from 93% of males but only 61% of females.[18]

PCRs using the *omp* 2b gene or RT-PCR may be more reliable.[19] *B. suis* can be differentiated from the other species by PCR,[20-22] although it may be less successful than culture.[23]

A fingerprinting technique based on a PCR method for multilocus variable number tandem repeat analysis (MLVA) has been developed.[24]

There is no PCR test for differentiating the five biovars from each other.[25]

Serology

Antibodies are usually developed 6 to 8 weeks after infection. These tests are only useful on a herd basis. There is no satisfactory serologic test. Some animals remain seronegative to all tests. Recently indirect or competitive ELISAs have been developed and may be 98% and 100% specific.[26]

An ELISA compared with complement fixation was found to be just as sensitive and as specific a test for both pigs and hares for *B. suis* infections. A meat juice ELISA has also been shown to be a valuable method for testing both hares and wild boars. There is considerable individual variation in the antibody response of pigs following infection, and some may be culture positive but have negative or indefinite titers to the common tests. Pigs under 3 months of age have a poor antibody response to infection.

Serologic tests in common use include the rose Bengal plate agglutination test, Rivanol test, rose Bengal card test, complement fixation, agar gel immunodiffusion, and tube agglutination. The preferred test varies between countries but most use the rose Bengal plate or card test. *B. abortus* antigens are used for diagnosis because *B. suis* has the same surface LPS antigens. Estimates of the sensitivities of the complement fixation and tube agglutination tests range from 40% to 51%, and they range from 62% to 79% for the rose Bengal plate test. The immunodiffusion test has poorer sensitivity than the standard serologic tests. The sensitivity and specificity of all the tests have been shown to vary with the stage of infection in the experimental disease, and it has been recommended that more than one test should be used for diagnosis. A recent study showed a range of sensitivity from 84% to 100% with the CFT low at 84% and the serum agglutination test high at 100%. The sensitivities ranged from 79.7% to 100%, with the serum agglutination test low at 79.7% and iELISA and C-ELISA high at 100%. A recent validation of the polarization assay as a serologic test for the presumptive diagnosis of porcine brucellosis has shown promise. Tests have been reviewed,[26,27] and both authors say that the problem is cross-reaction with *Yersinia* O9.

NECROPSY FINDINGS

On necropsy, there may be arthritis, posterior paralysis, spondylitis, and abscess formation in both sexes. The lesions are usually granulomatous as a result of persistent cytokine release, and these may be in the liver, kidney, spleen, and reproductive tracts.

Many organs may be involved in chronic cases. Chronic metritis manifested by nodular, white, inflammatory thickening, 2 to 5 mm in diameter, and abscessation of the uterine wall is characteristic with or without hemorrhage and necrosis. Arthritis may be purulent, and necrosis of vertebral bodies in the lumbar region may be found in lame and paralyzed pigs. The clinical orchitis of boars is revealed as testicular enlargement or atrophy and testicular necrosis, often accompanied by lesions in the epididymis and seminal vesicles. Splenic enlargement and pronounced lymphadenopathy, caused by hyperplasia of mononuclear phagocytes, occur in some cases. Typical histologic changes consist of granulomatous inflammation with neutrophils, macrophages, and giant cells and hyperplasia of reticular tissues and foci of caseous necrosis in the liver, kidney, spleen, and reproductive tract.

DIAGNOSIS

Diagnosis is suggested by the clinical signs, the necropsy findings, clinical pathology, and epidemiologically by the presence of wild boar locally. None of the tests is capable of diagnosing disease in the individual animal. The real problem of diagnosis is the cross-reactions with *Y. enterocolitica* O:9 infection.[28] In a survey of slaughter pigs in the UK 10% were found to have *Y. enterocolitica* in their gut.[29] There are false positives caused by this organism in initial screenings as the antibody lasts 2 to 9 weeks following *Y. enterocolitica* infection. They can be eliminated by testing for cellular immunity by measuring the IFN-γ generation by leukocytes.

Internationally accepted tests for swine brucellosis include ELISAs, FPA, RBT, buffered plate agglutination test, and the CFT.

Samples for Confirmation of Diagnosis

- Bacteriology: *adults,* culture swab from joint, lymph nodes, spleen, uterus, epididymis, or other site of localization; *fetus,* lung, stomach content, placenta (has special growth requirements)
- Histology: formalin-fixed samples of above tissues (light microscopy)

Note the zoonotic potential of this organism when handling carcasses or submitting specimens.

> **DIFFERENTIAL DIAGNOSIS**
>
> The protean character of this disease makes it difficult to differentiate. Syndromes that need differentiation include:
> - Abortion and infertility in sows
> - Posterior paresis diseases of spinal cord
> - Mortality in young pigs is also caused by many agents, and the important entities are listed in Chapter 19 in the section on Perinatal Disease—General Epidemiology.

TREATMENT

Treatment with a combination of streptomycin parenterally and sulfadiazine orally, or with tetracycline, is ineffective, although combinations of oxytetracycline, streptomycin, and possibly gentamicin have been used.[30] It is unlikely that treatment will ever be attempted on a commercial scale.

CONTROL

Vaccination

No suitable vaccine is available.[31] Strain 19 *B. abortus, B. abortus* "M" vaccine, living attenuated *B. suis* vaccines, and phenol and other extracts of *B. suis* are all ineffective. In a recent study, a natural rough mutant of *B. suis* that does not induce adverse clinical effects or tissue localization but does induce significant humoral and cellular immune responses after vaccination in swine has been observed.[32] The antibody responses to infection in any case are often not powerful enough to eliminate infection.

Test and Disposal

In herds where the incidence of reactors is high, complete disposal of all stock as they reach marketing age is by far the best procedure because of the difficulty in detecting individual infected animals. This is most practicable in commercial pork-producing herds. Restocking the farm should be delayed for 6 months after thorough disinfection is complete. The existing serologic tests can be used for certifying herds free of infection that can then provide replacement stock. Repopulation programs can also use specific pathogen-free pigs.

The alternative is to commence a two-herd segregation program, and this is recommended for purebred herds that supply pigs for breeding purposes. Total disposal is not usually economical in these herds. Once a herd diagnosis has been established, all the breeding animals must be considered to be infected; all piglets at weaning are submitted to the serum agglutination, Rivanol, or other test and, if negative, go into new quarters to start the nucleus of a free herd. It is probably safer to wean the pigs as young as possible and test again before mating. If complete protection is desired, these gilts should be allowed to farrow only in isolation, should then be retested, and their piglets used to start the clean herd. A modified scheme based on the previously mentioned method of weaning and isolating the young pigs as soon as possible but without submitting them to the serum agglutination test has been proposed, but its weakness is that infections may occur and persist in young pigs.

After eradication is completed, breakdowns are most likely to occur when infected animals are introduced. All introductions should be from accredited free herds, should be clinically healthy, and be negative to the serum agglutination test twice at intervals of 3 weeks before introduction.

Eradication of swine brucellosis from an area can only be achieved by developing a nucleus of accredited free herds and using these as a source of replacements for herds that eradicate by total disposal. Sale of pigs for breeding purposes from infected herds must be prevented.

With the advent of infection in wild boar and feral pigs, it is essential to maintain an effective separation from them when there are domestic pigs, and this is especially true where there are outdoor pig units. Recently contaminated wood has been shown to be a problem.[33]

REFERENCES

1. Meirelles-Bartolli RB, et al. *Trop Anim Health Prod.* 2012;44:1575.
2. Wu N, et al. *J Wildl Dis.* 2011;47:868.
3. Koppel C, et al. *Eur J Wildl Dis.* 2007;53:212.
4. Munoz PM, et al. *BMC Infect Dis.* 2010;10:46.
5. Bergagna S, et al. *J Wildl Dis.* 2009;45:1178.
6. Closa-Sebastia F, et al. *Vet Rec.* 2010;167:826.
7. Cvetnic Z, et al. *Rev Sci Tech.* 2009;28:1057.
8. Audic S, et al. *BMC Genomics.* 2009;10:352.
9. Lavin S, et al. *Informacion Veterinaria.* 2006;10:18.
10. Lucero N, et al. *Epidem Infect.* 2008;136:496.
11. Ariza J, et al. *PLoS Med.* 2007;4:e317.
12. Irwin MJ, et al. *N S W Public Health Bull.* 2009;20:192.
13. Escobar GL, et al. *Comp Immunol Microbiol Infect Dis.* 2013;36:575.
14. Megid J, et al. *Open Vet Sci.* 2010;4:119.
15. De Miguel MJ, et al. *J Clin Microbiol.* 2011;49:1458.
16. Abril C, et al. *Vet Microbiol.* 2011;150:405.
17. Ferreira AC, et al. *Res Vet Sci.* 2012;93:565.
18. Stoffregen WC, et al. *J Vet Diagn Invest.* 2007;19:227.
19. Hinic V, et al. *BMC Vet Res.* 2009;5:22.
20. Garin-Bastuji B, et al. *J Clin Microbiol.* 2008;46:3484.
21. Lopez-Goni I, et al. *J Clin Microbiol.* 2008;46:3484.
22. Mayer-Scholl A, et al. *J Microbiol Methods.* 2010;80:112.
23. Bounaadja L, et al. *Vet Microbiol.* 2009;137:156.
24. Garcia-Yoldi D, et al. *J Clin Microbiol.* 2007;45:4070.
25. Ferrao-Beck L, et al. *Vet Microbiol.* 2006;115:269.
26. McGiven JA, et al. *Vet Microbiol.* 2012;160:378.
27. Praud A, et al. *Prev Vet Med.* 2010;104:94.
28. Jungersen G, et al. *Epidemiol Infect.* 2006;134:347.
29. Milnes A, et al. *Epidemiol Infect.* 2008;136:739.
30. Grillo MJ, et al. *J Anim Chemother.* 2006;58:622.
31. Stoffregen WC, et al. *Am J Vet Res.* 2006;67:1802.
32. Stoffregen WC, et al. *Res Vet Sci.* 2013;95:451.
33. Calfee MW, Wendling M. *Lett Appl Microbiol.* 2012;54:504.

BRUCELLOSIS ASSOCIATED WITH *BRUCELLA MELITENSIS*

> **SYNOPSIS**
>
> **Etiology** *Brucella melitensis.*
>
> **Epidemiology** Disease of goats, sheep, humans, and occasionally cattle. Transmission congenital or by ingestion or contact with infected placenta, vaginal discharge, or milk.
>
> **Clinical findings** Abortion storms, abortions often in last 2 months of pregnancy. Weak-born lambs. Important zoonotic disease in humans.
>
> **Clinical pathology** Polymerase chain reaction (PCR) and culture of organism. Serologic tests and skin hypersensitivity testing for herd diagnosis.
>
> **Necropsy findings** Placentitis.
>
> **Diagnostic confirmation** Isolation of the organism, PCR.
>
> **Control** Slaughter eradication. Vaccination with *B. melitensis* Rev. 1 vaccine, but this can cause abortion in pregnant animals.

ETIOLOGY

B. melitensis causes brucellosis in goats and sheep, is capable of infecting most domestic animal species, and is the primary cause of brucellosis of humans (Malta fever) in many countries. There are three biovars of the organism that have differing geographic distribution, but no difference in pathogenicity or animal species affected. There is a close relationship to other members of the genus, which currently has 10 species but is expanding with the advent of molecular typing.[1]

EPIDEMIOLOGY

Geographic Occurrence

The distribution of *B. melitensis* is more restricted than that of *B. abortus* and its primary area of occurrence is in the Mediterranean region, including southern Europe. Infection is also present in west and central Asia, Mexico, countries in Central and South America, and in Africa. Northern Europe is free of infection, except for periodic incursions from the south, as are Canada, the United States, southeast Asia, Australia, and New Zealand.

The prevalence of infection varies between countries and regions, but in many countries the prevalence has declined in the past 20 years in association with mandatory vaccination policies. However, in many others it is not effectively controlled because of the low incomes or nomadic nature of those who farm small ruminants. Hence it is regarded as a neglected but very important disease of livestock and humans in developing countries.[2,3]

Host Occurrence

Goats and sheep are highly susceptible. Susceptibility in sheep varies with the breed, with Maltese sheep showing considerable resistance. The organism is capable of causing disease in cattle and has been isolated from buffalo, yaks, camels, and pigs.

Source of Infection

The source of infection is the infected carrier animal. Introduction to a naive herd or flock occurs with the introduction of an infected animal, and persistence results from sheep or goats that are prolonged excreters. Excretion is from the reproductive tract and in milk.

Reproductive Tract

Infected does and ewes, whether they abort or give birth normally, discharge many brucellas in their uterine exudates and placenta. The organism can be present in uterine discharge for at least 2 months following parturition in infected goats. The vaginal exudate of infected virgin or open animals may also contain the bacteria, but transmission between animals is most likely from the massive exposure provided by an infected placenta.

Milk

The majority of goats infected during pregnancy will excrete the organism in milk in the subsequent lactation and many will excrete it in all future lactations. In sheep, the period of excretion of the organism from the uterus and in milk is usually less than in goats, but the organism can be present in milk throughout lactation. The duration of excretion in cattle is not known.

Transmission

Routes of infection for both adults and young are via ingestion, by nasal or conjunctival infection, and through skin abrasions, with infected placenta and uterine discharge as a major source.

In Utero Infection

Infection of the fetus during pregnancy does not necessarily result in abortion: infected kids and lambs may be born alive but weak, or they may be quite viable. In some cases the infection persists in a latent form until sexual maturity, when pregnant animals may abort the first pregnancy. However, others, if weaned early from their dams and from the infected environment, become free from the infection as adults.

Colostrum and Milk

Latent infection can also be acquired from the ingestion of infected colostrum and milk. This is a major route of transmission and perpetuation of infection in a herd or flock.

Host and Pathogen Risk Factors

The organism is reasonably resistant to environmental influences and under suitable conditions can survive for over 1 year in the environment. *B. melitensis* is susceptible to disinfectants in common use at recommended concentrations.

In goats and sheep, the infection of a naive herd or flock will produce an abortion storm, following which most animals are infected but immune, and further abortions are usually limited to young or introduced animals. Because of the limited periods of excretion in sheep the disease tends to be self-limiting in small flocks that have few new introductions. It can be a continuing problem in large flocks because of massive environmental contamination of areas used for pregnant and lambing ewes. In some areas the prevalence of brucellosis associated with *B. melitensis* is linked to the practice of animal movement to summer and mountain pastures in which there is commingling of sheep and goats from a variety of sources on the same pasture.[3]

Spread in beef cattle is slow, presumably because they are usually farmed at lower stocking rates, whereas spread in dairy herds can be more rapid and extensive.

Economic Importance

Brucellosis has major veterinary and human importance in affected countries. Costs include production loss associated with infection in animals, the considerable cost of preventive programs, and human disease. There is further loss from restriction in international trade in animals and their products.

The occurrence of *B. melitensis* in the sheep and goat population of countries that have eradicated *B. abortus* poses a threat for the continuing occurrence of brucellosis in cattle herds.

Zoonotic Implications

B. melitensis is the most invasive and pathogenic for humans of the three classical species of the genus, and is the cause of Malta or Mediterranean fever in humans, which is an extremely debilitating disease. It is an important zoonosis in areas of the world in which *B. melitensis* is enzootic in goats and sheep. The disease in humans is severe and long-lasting and often occurs in communities with limited access to antimicrobial therapy. Control and eradication of the infection in animal populations has high priority in all countries.

Large numbers of organisms are excreted at and following parturition, providing a source of infection for humans managing the herd or flock and also for people in the immediate vicinity from aerosol infection with contaminated dust. The risk of infection is high in cultures that cohabit with their animals or when weak, infected newborn animals are brought into the house for warmth and intensive care. Milking of sheep and goats is usually manual, often with poor sanitation and milking-time hygiene. Raw milk and cheese products from infected goats, sheep, or cattle also provide a risk and were the mechanism for the occurrence of Malta fever that initiated the definition of the disease.

Abattoir workers, shearers, and people preparing goat and sheep skins are also at risk. The risk for veterinarians is primarily from assisting birthing in infected animals and herds, but is also the examination of any animal that is subclinically infected. There is also the risk of accidental self-inoculation with live vaccine.

Vaccination of small ruminants with *B. melitensis* Rev. 1 vaccine is a primary method in controlling the human disease. In Greece, a 15-year period of vaccination was associated with a drop in the incidence of human brucellosis, but when this program was stopped the prevalence of abortions in animals and the incidence if brucellosis in humans increased dramatically, only to be controlled by the reinstitution of vaccination of animals as an emergency mass vaccination program. However, although the Rev. 1 vaccine is attenuated compared with field strains, it retains some virulence and incorrect selection from the seed stock can result in vaccines with considerable virulence for both vaccinated animals and in-contact humans.

Because of its pathogenicity to humans and animals, *B. melitensis* is listed as an agent of bioterrorism and agroterrorism. It is thought that fewer than 10 CFU are capable of infecting humans via aerosols. This would require mass therapy of human populations and destruction of animal populations.

PATHOGENESIS

The organism is a facultative intracellular parasite. As in other forms of brucellosis, the pathogenesis depends on localization in lymph nodes, udder, and uterus after an initial bacteremia. In goats, this bacteremia may be sufficiently severe to produce a systemic reaction, and blood culture may remain positive for a month. Localization in the placenta leads to the development of placentitis, with subsequent abortion. After abortion, uterine infection persists for up to 5 months, and the mammary gland and associated lymph nodes may remain infected for years. Spontaneous recovery may occur, particularly in goats that become infected when they are not pregnant. In sheep, the development of the disease is very similar to that in goats. In cattle, *B. melitensis* has a similar pathogenesis and produces a persistent infection in the mammary gland and the supramammary lymph node, with obvious significance for public health.

CLINICAL FINDINGS

Abortion during late pregnancy is the most obvious sign in goats and sheep, but as in other species there may be a storm of abortions when the disease is introduced, followed by a period of flock resistance during which abortions do not occur. Abortion is most common in the last 2 months of pregnancy. The excretion of the organism in milk is not accompanied by obvious signs of mastitis. Infection in males may be followed by orchitis, which is frequently unilateral.

In experimental infections, a systemic reaction occurs with fever, depression, loss of weight, and sometimes diarrhea. These signs may also occur in acute, natural outbreaks in goats and may be accompanied by mastitis, lameness, and hygroma; however, they are uncommon in the natural disease and their occurrence in the experimental disease reflects a massive challenge dose. Osteoarthritis, synovitis, and nervous signs may occur in sheep.

In pigs, the disease is indistinguishable clinically from brucellosis associated with *B. suis.*

In many instances, *B. melitensis* infection reaches a high incidence in a group of animals without signs of obvious illness, and its presence may be first indicated by the occurrence of disease in humans infected from the herd or flock. This is so in cattle where the infection is subclinical and does not produce abortion, but the organism is shed in milk.

CLINICAL PATHOLOGY

Culture and Molecular Tests

Positive blood culture soon after the infection occurs and isolation of the organism from the aborted fetus, vaginal mucus, or milk are the common laboratory procedures used in diagnosis. The organism is moderately acid fast, and staining smears from the placenta and fetus with a modified Ziehl–Neelsen method may give a tentative diagnosis; however, this does not distinguish this infection from *B. ovis* or the agent of enzootic abortion (*Chlamydia abortus*), and culture is required.

The organism can be detected by PCR in the abomasal fluid of aborted fetuses and, compared with culture, PCR has a sensitivity and specificity of 97.4% and 100%, respectively. PCR can also be used to detect the organism in tissues, semen, and milk. A real time RT-PCR has been used to type Brucella from field samples, such as ovine placenta, without the need for culture.[4]

Multilocus variable-number tandem repeats analysis (MVLA) is an alternative to classical biotyping and may be useful in analyzing the epidemiology and source of outbreaks. For example, in 2011 a strain of *B. melitensis* in a single infected flock in Sardinia, a region of Italy free from this disease since 1998, was confirmed as being a rare America lineage and probably originating from Spain.[5] Multiplex PCR and high-resolution melt point analysis has also been used to differentiate *Brucella* spp.

Serology

The conventional serologic tests for the diagnosis of *B. melitensis*—agglutination, CFT, and the rose Bengal or card test—use the same antigens that are used for the diagnosis of *B. abortus* infections (either whole cells or sLPS).

The RBT and CFT are the most widely used. These, plus iELISA and FPA are prescribed tests for international trade.[6] The RBT is not 100% specific, but is typically used as a screening test with the CFT applied in series or parallel. RBT or CFT is not sufficiently sensitive to accurately detect infection in an individual animal. Nevertheless, they can be used to detect infected herds for slaughter eradication of the disease. They can be used for test and slaughter programs within an infected herd, but their reduced sensitivity makes this strategy less effective in sheep and goats compared with cattle. A combination of these tests and tests performed on several occasions may increase the accuracy of detection of infected animals. If only one test is possible, the CFT is recommended, but it suffers from the requirement for a sophisticated laboratory, which is not always available in affected areas.

Conventional serologic tests will not differentiate infection with different species of *Brucella* and will not differentiate infection associated with *Y. enterocolitica* type O:9.

Several ELISA tests have been evaluated for use in small ruminants, some using recombinant antigens such as Omp31 and others using whole-cell antigens. These include indirect, competitive, and blocking ELISAs. A C-ELISA had a diagnostic sensitivity ranging from 74% to 89%, depending on cutoff values, and a specificity from 93% to 97%.[7] Comparisons of the FPA and commercial ELISA tests with the RBT and CFT have shown no great advantages over the older tests, with the iELISA often having a slightly greater sensitivity. Overall testing sensitivity may be improved if these tests are used in parallel.[7,8]

Brucella-free animals are serologically positive for long periods following vaccination with *B. melitensis* Rev. 1, with varying persistence in different serologic tests. The period of seropositivity is shorter in animals vaccinated conjunctivally.

Milk Tests

The milk ring test used for testing pooled (bulk) milk in cattle is not useful in small ruminants. Other tests include whey CFTs, whey Coombs or antiglobulin test, whey agglutination tests, and a milk ELISA. They have no apparent advantage over serologic tests, and in many cases they are less sensitive, hence, they are not suitable as screening tests using pooled milk samples.

Allergic Tests

An intradermal allergic test using 50 mg of brucellin INRA (purified and free from LPS) can be used for diagnosis. The injection sites in goats are the neck or caudal fold and in sheep the lower eyelid, with reactions read in 48 hours. The test has high specificity in flocks that are free of infection and not vaccinated. However, it has little advantage over conventional serologic tests in infected herds, and Rev.-1-vaccinated animals can react for at least 2 years. It has particular value in identifying some animals that are false-positive reactors, differentiating infections with *Y. enterocolitica* but not *B. ovis.* Anergy occurs between 6 and 24 days after injection.

NECROPSY FINDINGS

There are no lesions that are characteristic of this form of brucellosis. The causative organism can often be isolated from all tissues but the spleen, lymph nodes, and udder are the most common sites for attempted isolation in chronic infection.

Samples for Confirmation of Diagnosis

- Bacteriology: *adults,* spleen, lymph node, udder, testicle, epididymis; *fetus,* lung, spleen, placenta (culture: has special growth requirements; cytology: Stamp's or Koster's stain on placental smear; PCR); *fetus,* PCR of fetal abomasal fluid
- Histology: formalin-fixed samples of the previously listed tissues

The zoonotic potential of this organism means care needs to be taken when handling potentially infected material, and specimens should be properly packaged when submitted to a laboratory.

> **DIFFERENTIAL DIAGNOSIS**
>
> The primary differential is from other forms of brucellosis (seen in this chapter) and other causes of abortion in small ruminants.

TREATMENT

Treatment is unlikely to be undertaken in most animals because it is unlikely to be economically feasible or therapeutically effective. For example, a dose of 1000 mg per animal of long-acting tetracycline given every 3 days for 6 weeks achieved a cure rate of 75%.

CONTROL

Hygiene

Control measures must include hygiene at kidding or lambing and the disposal of infected or reactor animals. Separate pens for kidding does that can be cleaned and disinfected, early weaning of kids from their does and their environment, and vaccination are recommended. In endemic areas, all placentas and dead fetuses should be routinely buried.

Eradication

Where a group is infected for the first time it may be most economical to dispose of the entire herd or flock, because eradication by test and slaughter is prolonged by the lack of sensitivity of the serologic tests.

Many countries that have this disease have statutory control measures and the disease can be eradicated, such as from Cyprus. *B. melitensis* also can be eradicated, with difficulty, from dairy cattle. However, vaccination may be the only practical method of control in areas in which there is a high prevalence of the disease, extensive management systems, communal and nomadic grazing, and a low socioeconomic level.

Rev. 1 Vaccination

Rev. 1 vaccine is a live, attenuated *B. melitensis* strain derived from a virulent *B. melitensis* isolate that is resistant to dihydrostreptomycin. It is the reference vaccine strain that provides protection against infection with *B. melitensis* in sheep and goats and against infection with *B. ovis* in rams. However, this vaccine has significant disadvantages, including persistent serologic response and, although attenuated compared with field strains, it retains some virulence. Incorrect selection from the seed stock can result in vaccines with considerable virulence for both vaccinated animals and in-contact humans.

Vaccination with Rev. 1 produces a bacteremia that is cleared by 14 weeks in goats and a shorter time in sheep. Vaccination at 3 to 8 months of age confers a high degree of immunity that lasts for more than 4 years in goats and 2½ years in sheep. The initial recommendations were to vaccinate replacement animals with the expectation that herd/flock immunity would develop over time. However, this has proved ineffective in some regions, and whole-flock/herd vaccination is now recommended in certain countries.

Vaccination of pregnant goats and sheep, especially in the second and third month of pregnancy, will result in abortion and the excretion of the living *B. melitensis* vaccine organism in the vaginal discharge and the milk. Consequently, the vaccine should not be used in pregnant animals or for 1 month before breeding. Vaccination of lactating animals may be followed by excretion of the organism in the milk for a short time. Reduced dose vaccination or conjunctival vaccination does not significantly reduce the risk of vaccine-induced abortions in pregnant animals, although reduced-dose Rev. 1 vaccination has been shown to provide protection for at least 5 years in endemically infected areas.

Conjunctival vaccination does decrease the period of seropositivity following vaccination. Vaccine efficacy and safety can vary with the manufacturer. National policies promoting widespread vaccination of sheep and goats with Rev. 1 vaccine have resulted in a significant reduction in the prevalence of small ruminant brucellosis and in the incidence rates of human brucellosis. However, Rev. 1 vaccine is also pathogenic to humans and its excretion, and persistence in milk following vaccination can result in human infection.

The general approach in endemically infected countries is to institute a whole-flock vaccination scheme followed by a young-stock vaccination until the prevalence of the disease is reduced, at which time test and slaughter can be implemented to eradicate the disease. This ignores the risk of adverse disease in the vaccinated animals and the risk for human infection from the vaccine strain. There is an urgent need for a nonvirulent vaccine that induces seropositivity that can be differentiated from the seropositivity resulting from natural infection.

Other Vaccines

To circumvent the problem of persistent serologic response, ongoing efforts have been made to develop defined rough mutant vaccine strains that would be more effective against *B. melitensis.* Various studies have examined cell-free native and recombinant proteins as candidate protective antigens, with or without adjuvants. However, limited success has been obtained in experimental models with these, or with DNA vaccines encoding known protective antigens.[9]

B. abortus strain 19 has been used for vaccination and appears to give protection that is as good as that achieved with the attenuated *B. melitensis* vaccine.

FURTHER READING

Blasco JM, et al. Control and eradication of *Brucella melitensis* in sheep and goats. *Vet Clin North Am Food Anim Pract.* 2011;27:95-104.

Whatmore AM. Current understanding of the genetic diversity of *Brucella,* an expanding genus of zoonotic pathogens. *Inf Genet Evol.* 2009;9:1168-1184.

REFERENCES

1. Whatmore AM. *Inf Genet Evol.* 2009;9:1168.
2. Ducrotoy MJ, et al. *PLoS Negl Trop Dis.* 2014;8(7):e3008.
3. Kasymbekov J, et al. *PLoS Negl Trop Dis.* 2013;7(2):e2047.
4. Gopaul KK, et al. *Vet Rec.* 2014;175:282.
5. De Massi F, et al. *Transbound Emerg Dis.* 2015;62:463.
6. OIE. Terrestrial Manual. 2012 Ch 2.7.2; 968.
7. Minas A, et al. *Vet J.* 2008;177:411.
8. Fiasconaro M, et al. *Small Rumin Res.* 2015;130:252.
9. Da Costa Martins R, et al. *Expert Rev Vaccines.* 2012;11:87.

ABORTION IN EWES ASSOCIATED WITH *SALMONELLA ABORTUSOVIS*

Salmonella abortusovis (*S. enterica* serovar Abortusovis) is a gram-negative rod-shaped aerobic bacterium of the family Enterobacteriaceae. The pathogen is highly adapted to sheep and is considered to be host specific for this species in which it can cause abortion. S. Abortusovis infection has a worldwide occurrence with a generally low prevalence. The infection appears to be more common in some European and Western Asian countries.

Transmission and spread of the infection occurs through infected animals that are introduced to flocks naive to the pathogen. The reservoir of infection is infected animals that do not abort. The organisms persist in internal organs of the **asymptomatic carriers** for up to 6 months and are excreted in the feces and vaginal mucus for periods up to 4 months. Infection can occur through the oral, conjunctival, or respiratory route, but oral ingestion is thought to be the main mode of infection. Venereal spread has been postulated, and rams certainly become infected, but all the evidence is against spread at coitus. Intrapreputial inoculation results in infection of rams and the passage of infected semen for up to 15 days.

The only significant clinical sign of S. Abortusovis infection is abortion, which is common during the second half to last third of gestation. Lambs may also be stillborn or die within the first day of life. Mortality in lambs is common from either weakness and ensuing hypothermia and hypoglycemia or to the development of acute pneumonia in previously healthy lambs up to 2 weeks old.

In flocks naive to the infection, introduction of the pathogen can cause abortion storms, with up to 60% of ewes aborting generally in the last trimester of gestation. Ewes rarely develop clinical signs, although some may transiently have a fever or develop postabortive endometritis with vaginal discharge. Septic metritis and peritonitis in dams has been associated with deaths among ewes. Spread of the disease is strongly associated with the presence of aborting ewes and subsequent heavy environmental contamination. In flocks where the pathogen is endemic, abortion occurs sporadically, mainly affecting primiparous and newly introduced ewes. The infection appears to induce a strong immune response preventing abortion during the following pregnancies.[1]

Identification of the disease depends on isolation of the organism, which is present in large numbers in the fetus, placenta, and uterine discharges. Use of PCR to identify S. Abortusovis is feasible because the organism has an IS200 element in a distinct chromosomal location. The resulting PCR assay has high specificity for S. Abortusovis, effectively discriminating it from other *S. enterica* serovars. The disease can be diagnosed in fetuses by using a coagulation test on fetal stomach contents. The test had a sensitivity and specificity of 100% and 90% in a small number of samples.

Serologic tests to detect antibody to *S. abortusovis* include the SAT, hemagglutination inhibition, complement fixation, indirect immunofluorescence, gel immunodiffusion, and ELISA.

A strong immunity develops after an attack, and an autogenous vaccine has shown good results in the control of the disease.[1] The results of vaccination need to be very carefully appraised because flock immunity develops readily and the disease tends to subside naturally in the second year.

The clinical findings in S. Dublin infections in ewes are very similar, and infection has become more important as a cause of abortion in ewes in the UK than S. Abortusovis. S. Ruiru has also been recorded as a cause of abortion in ewes, and ewes with salmonellosis associated with *S. typhimurium* may also lose their lambs. S. Brandenburg is a cause of illness and abortion in sheep, horses, calves, goats, and humans in New Zealand. Other **differential diagnoses** for abortion in ewes include chlamydiosis, brucellosis, campylobacteriosis, listeriosis, coxiellosis (Q-fever), and toxoplasmosis.

The administration of broad-spectrum antibiotics might aid in controlling an outbreak, but available reports are not generally encouraging. Chloramphenicol and the trimethoprim and sulfadiazine combination are considered effective for treatment, but use of chloramphenicol in animals intended for human food production is not permitted in many countries. A live *S. typhimurium* vaccine with optimal level of attenuation for sheep constructed by means of "metabolic drift" mutations was highly effective in preventing S. Abortusovis–induced abortions under field trial conditions. Subcutaneous and conjunctival vaccination with a live attenuated strain of S. Abortusovis confers immunity for at least three lambing periods. More recent vaccines, including those containing plasmid-cured strains of S. Abortusovis, are effective in preventing pregnancy loss in response to experimental challenge with wild-type S. Abortusovis.

To contain the spread of the infection during an outbreak aborted ewes should be isolated and abortion products that contain large amounts of bacteria must be destroyed. Disinfection of stalls and fomites with an agent with proven efficacy against *Salmonella* spp. is important.

FURTHER READING

Jack EJ. *Salmonella* abortion in sheep. *Vet Annu.* 1971;12:57.

REFERENCE

1. Cagiola M, et al. *Vet Microbiol.* 2007;121:330.

ABORTION IN MARES AND SEPTICEMIA IN FOALS ASSOCIATED WITH *SALMONELLA ABORTUSEQUI (ABORTIVOEQUINA)* (EQUINE PARATYPHOID)

This is a specific disease of Equidae characterized by abortion in females, testicular lesions in males, and septicemia in the newborn.

ETIOLOGY

Salmonella abortusequi (*abortivoequina*) (also known as *Salmonella enterica* serovar Abortusequi) is a host-adapted serovar causing abortion in mares and donkeys. S. Abortusequi strains vary in virulence, with more virulent strains having greater in vitro cytotoxigenicity. It is possible to determine the origin and progression of outbreaks of the disease by determining pulsed-field gel electrophoretic patterns of S. Abortusequi.

EPIDEMIOLOGY

The infection appears to be limited to horses and donkeys. Although widely reported in the early 1900s, this disease is rarely encountered and is one of the less common causes of either abortion or septicemia in horses. Recent reports of the disease are from Austria, Brazil, Croatia, Japan, and India, although the disease occurs in other countries. However, in the early 1990s, an outbreak of abortion occurred in a herd of 38 horses, in which 21 mares aborted between 5 and 10 months of gestation.

Natural infection may be caused by the ingestion of foodstuffs contaminated by uterine discharges from carriers or mares that have recently aborted. Transmission from the stallion at the time of service is also thought to occur. The infection may persist in the uterus and cause repeated abortion or infection of subsequent foals. Transmission from a female donkey to mares is reported with abortion a result in both species.

PATHOGENESIS

When infection occurs by ingestion, a transient bacteremia without marked systemic signs is followed by localization in the placenta, resulting in placentitis and abortion. Foals that are carried to term probably become infected in utero or soon after birth by ingestion from the contaminated teat surface or through the umbilicus.

CLINICAL FINDINGS

Abortion usually occurs at about the seventh or eighth month of pregnancy. The mare can show signs of impending abortion followed by difficult parturition, but other evidence of illness is usually lacking. Retention of the placenta and metritis are common sequels and may cause serious illness, but subsequent sterility is unusual. A foal that is carried to term by an infected mare may develop an acute septicemia during the first few days of life or survive to develop polyarthritis 7 to 14 days later. Polyarthritis has also been observed in foals from vaccinated mares that showed no signs of the disease.

Infection in the stallion has also been reported with clinical signs including fever, edematous swelling of the prepuce and scrotum, and arthritis. Hydrocele, epididymitis, and inflammation of the tunica vaginalis are followed by orchitis and testicular atrophy.

CLINICAL PATHOLOGY

The organism can be isolated from the placenta, the uterine discharge, the aborted foal, and the joints of foals with polyarthritis. A high titer of *Salmonella* agglutinins in the mare develops about 2 weeks after abortion. Vaccinated mares will give a positive reaction for up to a year.

NECROPSY FINDINGS

The placenta of the aborted foal is edematous and hemorrhagic and may have areas of necrosis. The nonspecific changes of acute septicemia will be manifested in foals dying soon after birth; polyarthritis is found in those dying at a later stage.

Samples for Confirmation of Diagnosis

- Bacteriology: placenta, fetal stomach content, lung, culture swabs of joints (culture)
- Histology: formalin-fixed placenta, various fetal tissues including lung, liver (light microscopy)

TREATMENT

The antimicrobials recommended in the treatment of salmonellosis should also be effective in this disease.

CONTROL

Careful hygiene, including isolation of infected mares and disposal of aborted material, should be practiced to avoid spread of the infection. Infected stallions should not be used for breeding. In the past, when this disease was much more common than it is now, great reliance was placed on vaccination as a control measure. An autogenous or commercial bacterin, composed of killed S. Abortusequi organisms, was injected on three occasions at weekly intervals into all mares on farms in which the disease was enzootic, commencing 2 to 3 months after the close of the breeding season. A smaller dose (5 mL) of vaccine of higher concentration is as effective as a larger dose (20 mL) of vaccine of lower concentration. A formol-killed, alum-precipitated vaccine is considered to be superior to a heat-killed, phenolized vaccine. In China, a virulent strain vaccine is credited with effective protection after two injections 6 months apart.

The widespread use of vaccines and hyperimmune sera is credited with the almost complete eradication of the disease in developed countries.

CHLAMYDIAL ABORTION (ENZOOTIC ABORTION OF EWES, OVINE ENZOOTIC ABORTION)

SYNOPSIS

Etiology *Chlamydia abortus.*

Epidemiology Prevalence varies within regions and between countries. Oral route of infection, with the placenta and uterine discharge of aborting ewes the major source of infection. Pregnant sheep infected by contact with aborting ewes usually do not abort until the next lambing season. Zoonotic.

Clinical findings Abortion, stillborn and weak-born lambs.

Necropsy findings Necrotic and hemorrhagic placental cotyledons, intercotyledonary areas thickened, edematous, and leathery.

Diagnostic confirmation Demonstration of the organism in the placenta by polymerase chain reaction, rising titer in paired serum samples.

Control Isolation of aborting ewes. Killed vaccine with adjuvant gives short-term protection and can be used in pregnant ewes during an outbreak in an attempt to reduce the number of abortions. Live attenuated vaccines may be more effective but cannot be used during pregnancy.

ETIOLOGY

Chlamydia abortus (previously known as *Chlamydophila abortus* and *Chlamydia psittaci* biotype 1/serotype 1) has a tropism for ruminant placenta and causes the disease commonly referred to as ovine enzootic abortion (OEA). The organism causes a similar disease in goats, and although this organism also can produce abortion in cattle, pigs, and horses, abortion associated with this organism is not common in these species. There is considerable genetic diversity among strains that cause abortion.

EPIDEMIOLOGY

Occurrence

The disease is one of the most common causes of diagnosed abortion in sheep and goats in the UK, Europe, Asia, the United States, and other countries. In the UK, it accounts for approximately 45% of abortions, and it is particularly common in lowland flocks that are intensively managed at lambing. However, its importance varies from country to country. It is an uncommon cause of abortion in Northern Ireland, and the disease does not occur in Norway, Australia, or New Zealand.

There have been several studies of seroprevalence in Europe that show a high seroprevalence in both domestic and wild ruminants but, until recently, most surveys have used the complement fixation test (CFT), which is not specific for *C. abortus;* therefore, the true seroprevalence of *C. abortus* in many countries is not well established.

Source of Infection and Transmission

Infection is introduced into a flock by the purchase of latently infected replacements that usually abort at the end of their first pregnancy. Within a flock, the major source of infection is the placenta and the uterine discharge of aborting ewes. The main routes of transmission of *C. abortus* are oral or nasal: either ingestion of organisms shed in vaginal fluids and placental membranes at the time of abortion or lambing, or the inhalation of aerosols from contaminated areas. Pasture and the environment are contaminated by vaginal discharges, placenta, and aborted fetuses, and infected ewes shed the organism for a week before aborting and 2 weeks afterward. The elementary body of *C. abortus* is resistant to both physical and chemical influences, because it is metabolically inactive and the rigid cell envelope is osmotically stable and poorly permeable. Consequently, the organism is thought to survive for several days on pasture and longer in cold weather.

Infection of the ewe lamb may occur at birth, shortly following, or at subsequent lambing periods. Infection of pregnant ewes in early or midgestation results in either abortion in the final 2 to 3 weeks of gestation or the birth of stillborn or weak lambs that frequently die in the first few days of their life. Abortion always appears in the last weeks of gestation regardless of the time of infection. Infection of ewes in the last 5 to 6 weeks of pregnancy usually leads to the development of a latent infection, in which ewes appear to be uninfected until the next lambing season, when they abort. Thus late pregnant sheep may be infected by contact with aborting ewes, but usually do not abort until the next lambing season.

The common pattern of infection and disease is the small number of abortions in year 1 following the introduction of infected replacement ewes and then an epidemic abortion storm, in which up to 35% of ewes abort in the last 3 weeks of gestation or give premature birth to weak or dead lambs. After aborting, ewes develop a protective immunity and, in endemically infected flocks, 5% to 10% of the ewes abort annually. Surviving lambs born to infected mothers may be affected by enzootic abortion in ewes (EAE) in their first pregnancy.

Sheep that have aborted, subsequently rebreed successfully, do not have further abortions, and the organism is not present in the placenta or vaginal discharge of subsequent pregnancies. However, levels of immunity vary and some may excrete organisms at estrus or seasonally for up to 3 years.

In chronically infected sheep, persistent infection can be demonstrated in the endometrial cells of the reproductive tract, and the organism is excreted in vaginal fluids during estrus.

Vaginal challenge of ewes at breeding time will result in infection and subsequent abortion. Thus venereal or passive venereal transmission is a possible route of infection but is not common. Chronic infection of the male genital tissues has been recorded, and infection may impair fertility in both rams and bulls.

The epidemiology of abortion with this agent in cattle is unknown, but it may transmit to cattle from infected sheep on the same farm.

Experimental Reproduction

The disease is readily reproduced experimentally. Following subcutaneous injection there are no signs of clinical disease other than a modest increase in rectal temperature for 2 days after infection. There is a systemic antibody response that peaks 2 weeks after infection and then decreases until just before abortion or parturition, during which there is a second increase in antibodies to *C. abortus.* Experimental infection at 70 to 75 days pregnancy can cause abortion in the last 2 to 3 weeks of pregnancy or the birth of stillborn or live lambs. There is variation in the severity of the placental lesions in experimental infections. Abortion is associated with severe placental lesions, but the reason for the variation in severity and fetal manifestations is not known.

Economic Importance

In the UK, enzootic abortion is the most common infectious cause of abortion in lowland flocks that are intensively managed at lambing time and has a major economic impact on agricultural industries worldwide. There are no recent estimates, but losses in the UK were estimated in the early 1990s at £15 to £20 million per annum.

Zoonotic Implications

There is some risk for people working with livestock, such as shepherds and abattoir workers, for respiratory infection with this organism. However, the major zoonotic risk is to pregnant women because of the ability of *C. abortus* to colonize the human placenta. Human infection in early pregnancy results in abortion, whereas later infection can result in stillbirth or preterm labor. Infection is probably oral, from infected hands or food following handling of infected sheep or goats, or contaminated fomites such as clothing. Practices at lambing, such as mouth to mouth resuscitation of weak lambs or bringing weak lambs into the house to be warmed, promote zoonotic spread. Consequently, infected placentas and dead lambs should be handled using gloved hands and disposed of by burning or burial. The organism can be detected in the milk of both sheep and cattle, so consuming raw milk also poses a risk for zoonotic infection.

PATHOGENESIS

Following infection, it is thought that the organism resides first in the tonsil and is then disseminated by blood and lymph to other organs, although the site of latent infection is not definitely known. Release from the latent state during pregnancy is thought to be caused by immune modulation and leads to bacteremia and infection of the placenta. Despite being a key feature of infection with *C. abortus,* little is understood about the underlying mechanisms that result in latent infections. However, experimental intranasal infection of nonpregnant ewes with a low or moderate dose of organisms induced latent infection and subsequent abortion, whereas a higher dose stimulated protective immunity.[1]

The organisms invade the trophoblast cells of the fetal cotyledon then spread to the intercotyledonary regions of the chorion, producing a necrotic suppurative placentitis and impairment of the maternal–fetal exchange of nutrients and oxygen, hence, fetal death and abortion. An inflammatory response in the fetus may also contribute to fetal death.

It is not known why, regardless of the time of infection, pathologic changes in the placenta do not commence before 90 days' gestation, or even as late as 120 days, although this coincides with the commencement of rapid fetal growth.

CLINICAL FINDINGS

There are generally no premonitory indications of the impending abortions, which occur in late pregnancy. Ewes suffer no obvious systemic effects, but retained placenta and metritis can occur in goats. A vaginal discharge, lasting up to 3 weeks following the abortion, is common. Additional losses are caused by stillbirths and weak-born lambs and kids that die soon after birth.

In cattle, the infection causes abortion in the last third of pregnancy. Infected calves born alive may show lethargy, depression, and may be stunted. Mixed infections with *C. abortus, C. suis* and Chlamydia-like organisms (*Parachlamydia* and *Waddlia* spp.) are recorded in cattle and associated with abortions featuring necrotic placentitis, but the true prevalence and significance of these infections is not clear.[2,3]

CLINICAL PATHOLOGY

If the flock history and placental lesions suggest OEA, smears from affected and adjacent chorionic villi of the placenta can be appropriately stained (e.g., Giemsa or modified Ziehl–Neelsen) and examined under high magnification. Single or clumps of small, coccoid elementary bodies (300 nm) will stain red compared with blue cellular debris. Vaginal swabs from recently aborted ewes and smears of the fleece of uncleaned lambs or fetal abomasal contents can also be examined but contain fewer organisms. The organisms appear similar to *Coxiella burnetii,* the agent of coxiellosis (Q fever), so this is not a definitive test.

Commercial antigen detection kits (fluorescent antibody test [FAT] and ELISA) are available but do not discriminate between Chlamydial species.

Chlamydial DNA can be amplified by conventional or real time RT-PCR. These are highly sensitive, but can result in false positives if samples are cross-contaminated or false negatives if samples contain PCR-inhibitory substances. RT-PCR is rapid and relatively easily standardized and can demonstrate the DNA of *C. abortus* in tissues and swabs, such as of vaginal fluid, conjunctivae, and fetal membranes.[4,5] A number of multiplex PCR tests are described and can differentiate between Chlamydial species and other agents of infectious abortion, such as *Toxoplasma gondii* and *C. burnetii.*[6]

C. abortus can be isolated in embryonated chicken eggs or cell culture, but most diagnostic laboratories do not do this because of the zoonotic risk and requirement for level 2 biocontainment.

Infection in aborting animals can be demonstrated by rising serologic titers in paired serum samples collected 3 weeks apart. The CFT is commonly used but has only moderate sensitivity and is not specific because of common antigens shared with other Chlamydiae and some gram-negative bacteria. It will also be positive in vaccinated animals. Ambiguous results, such as suspected false-positive tests in flock accreditation programs or export testing, can be analyzed further by a Western blot using specific antigens.

A number of research and commercial ELISA tests have been developed. Those based on whole-cell or extracts of chlamydial elementary bodies have better specificity than the CFT but are less sensitive. Those based on segments of the outer membrane protein (OMP) or synthetic peptide antigens have greater sensitivity and specificity and are now more frequently used in diagnostic, epidemiologic, and seroprevalence studies.[7]

Vaccinated animals will react to the currently used serologic tests, but wild-type and vaccine strains of *C. abortus* can be differentiated by PCR-restriction fragment length polymorphism (RFLP).[8] This has provided evidence that the temperature sensitive mutant strain 1B used in vaccines is associated with ovine abortions in Scotland.[9,10]

NECROPSY FINDINGS

Aborted fetuses typically have no gross abnormalities. Fetal fluid may contain chlamydial antibody and, although less sensitive than either isolation in McCoy cells or detection of chlamydial LPS antigen, can be useful when placenta is not available. Histologically, there may be mononuclear cell infiltration of hepatic portal areas and multifocal areas of hepatitis. The placenta is critical for diagnosis of chlamydial abortion in both cattle and sheep.

Placental cotyledons are necrotic and hemorrhagic, and the intercotyledonary areas are thickened, edematous, and leathery. This is in direct contrast to the targeting of cotyledons seen with toxoplasmosis. Chlamydial organisms can be seen in tightly packed sheets within the cytoplasm of swollen trophoblasts in formalin-fixed tissues or in direct placental smears using modified Gimenez, Koster's, or other appropriate stains. Well-preserved, fresh placenta should be examined because the organisms are difficult to demonstrate in the fetus. Immunohistochemical stains perform well on formalin-fixed specimens. Most laboratories are reluctant to culture *Chlamydia* spp. because of their zoonotic potential.

Samples for Confirmation of Diagnosis

- **Bacteriology:** chilled liver, lung, placenta (cytology, PCR, ELISA)
- **Histology:** fixed placenta, liver (light microscopy, IHC)

The zoonotic potential of this organism means care needs to be taken when handling potentially infected material, and specimens should be properly packaged when submitted to a laboratory.

> **DIFFERENTIAL DIAGNOSIS**
>
> Other causes of abortion in cattle and ewes are given in Tables 18-1 and 18-2.

CONTROL

Ewes that have aborted should be isolated from the rest of the flock. There should be proper hygiene of the lambing areas, including disposal of bedding and aborted materials, and disinfection of pens with intensive lambing systems. Long-acting oxy tetracycline has been used at 20 mg/kg IM in early pregnant sheep within an aborting flock to reduce subsequent abortions. However, treated ewes still shed the organism in vaginal discharges, and treatment at 10-day intervals may be needed.

Vaccines

Killed and live attenuated vaccines are available, but none are fully protective. **Killed vaccines,** composed of egg-derived or tissue culture organisms of one or two strains have been used for several decades. They are variably effective, but can reduce the frequency of abortion and shedding of the organism. However, outbreaks have occurred in vaccinated sheep, with strain variation a possible

Table 18-2 Diagnostic summary of causes of abortion in cattle

				Field examination		Laboratory diagnosis	
Epidemiology disease	*Clinical features*	*Abortion rate*	*Time of abortion*	*Placenta*	*Fetus*	*Isolation of agent*	*Serology*
Brucellosis (*Brucella abortus*)	Zoonotic disease, chronic infection, abortion, retained placenta, and metritis	High, up to 90% in susceptible herds	5 months +	Severe placentitis, thickened placenta with surface exudate	Possibly pneumonia	Culture of fetal stomach, placenta, uterine fluid, milk, and semen	Serum and blood agglutination test, milk ring test, whole milk plate agglutination test; whey plate agglutination, semen plasma, and vaginal mucous agglutination test
Trichomoniasis (Trichomonas *foetus*)	Venereally transmitted disease resulting in early embryonic loss with occasional abortion and pyometra	Moderate, 5%–30%	Primarily first 5 months	Flocculent material and clear, serous fluid in uterine exudate	Usually no gross lesions, histologically fetal giant cell pneumonia may occur	Hanging drop or culture examination of fetal stomach and uterine exudate within 24 hours of abortion; isolation, best source in female pyometra fluid if pyometra exists; best method is InPouch; in male bull's preputial smegma with InPouch	Cervical mucous agglutination test; serology rarely performed, mucus agglutination or complement fixation hemolytic assay
Neosporosis (*Neospora caninum*)	Worldwide distribution of infection in both dairy and beef cattle, most abortions reported in dairy cattle In addition to abortion, mummification and birth of full-term infected calves can occur with or without clinical signs Chronic infection in which congenital transmission commonly occurs during pregnancy, acquired postnatal infection may also occur	Sporadic or outbreaks common (20%–40%) Repeat abortions from same cows can occur	3–8 months of gestation (mean 5.5 months)	No characteristic gross lesions in placenta Parasite may be present	Autolyzed midgestation fetus, widespread histologic inflammatory lesions in fetus including nonsuppurative necrotizing encephalitis and myocarditis	Identify parasite in fetal tissues by immunohistochemistry stain or PCR	Antibodies in fetus and cow IFAT and ELISA antibodies used for serologic detection Positive result supports infection in cow and/or fetus but is not causal proof; negative result in dam strong evidence that neosporosis not involved in abortion; serologic comparison of groups of aborting and nonaborting herdmates useful in establishing the role in herd outbreaks of abortion
Vibriosis (*Campylobacter fetus* subsp. *venerealis*)	Venereally transmitted, resulting in infertility, irregular, moderately prolonged diestrus with occasional abortion Epidemiology similar to trichomonosis except for a longer vaginal carrier state (up to 4 months after uterus has cleared organism) Significance: fertility returns but is still a threat to any uninfected bull	Low, up to 5%, may be up to 20%	46 months	Semiopaque, little thickening Petechiae, localized avascularity and edema	Flakes of pus on visceral peritoneum Fibrin may be present in serosal cavities Usually associated with suppurative pneumonia in fetus	Culture of fetal stomach, placenta, and uterine exudate Sporadic abortion, not venereally transmitted, can be associated with *C. fetus* subsp. *fetus* and *C. jejuni*, which need to be differentiated from *C. fetus* subsp. *venerealis*	Blood agglutination after abortion (at 3 weeks) Cervical mucous agglutination test at 40 days after infected service

Table 18-2 Diagnostic summary of causes of abortion in cattle—cont'd

				Field examination		Laboratory diagnosis	
Epidemiology disease	*Clinical features*	*Abortion rate*	*Time of abortion*	*Placenta*	*Fetus*	*Isolation of agent*	*Serology*
Leptospirosis (*Leptospira interrogans* serovar pomona and *Leptospira hardjo*) *L. borgpetersenii* serovar hardjo (formerly serovar hardjo-*bovis*) occurs worldwide; *L. interrogans* serovar hardjo (formerly hardjo-prajitno) primarily in the UK	Abortion may occur at acute febrile stage, later, or unassociated with illness	25%–30%	Abortions may occur throughout gestation; Late, 6 months +	Avascular placenta, atonic yellow-brown cotyledons, brown gelatinous edema between allantois and amnion	Fetus usually autolyzed, occasional icterus Fetal death common	Fluorescent antibody stain of smears of fetal kidney or PCR Direct examination of urine of cow by dark-field or fluorescent antibody stain	Positive serum agglutination test 14–21 days after febrile illness Titers usually at or near maximum at time of abortion Chronically infected *L. hardjo* dams may have low or negative titers
Infectious bovine rhinotracheitis (IBR)	Abortion storms in inadequately vaccinated animals. May be associated with upper airway disease in one or several animals	Variable	Most in second half of gestation	No significant gross lesions	Autolyzed fetus, rarely may have pale foci of hepatic necrosis Histopathology characteristic with multifocal necrosis	Virus isolation or PCR on placenta or fetal tissues Immunohistochemistry or fluorescent antibody stain on fetal tissues	Acute and convalescent sera
Mycoses (*Aspergillus, Absidia*)	Variable incidence, more common in cooler moist climates, retained placenta may occur	Unknown. 6%–7% of all abortions encountered	3–7 months	Necrosis of maternal cotyledon, adherence of necrotic material to chorionic cotyledon causes soft, yellow, cushion-like structure Small yellow, raised, leathery lesions on intercotyledonary areas	Minority of fetuses have skin lesions May be small raised, gray-buff, soft lesions, or diffuse white areas on skin Resemble ringworm	Direct examination of cotyledon and fetal stomach for hyphae, suitable cultural examination Histopathology on placenta	

Continued

Table 18-2 Diagnostic summary of causes of abortion in cattle—cont'd

				Field examination		Laboratory diagnosis	
Epidemiology disease	*Clinical features*	*Abortion rate*	*Time of abortion*	*Placenta*	*Fetus*	*Isolation of agent*	*Serology*
Listeriosis (*Listeria monocytogenes*)	May be an associated septicemia (Cows that abort may die of septicemia near term.) Retained placentas and metritis may also occur	Low, rare abortion storms related with poorly fermented silage	About 7 months	—	Autolysis Foci of necrosis in liver and other organs	Organisms in fetal stomach, liver, and throughout fetus placenta and uterine fluid	Agglutination titers higher than 1:400 in contact animals classed as positive
Epizootic bovine abortion	Tick-transmitted bacterial infection, occurs in dry foothill pastures in the western United States in which tick vector resides No clinical signs in aborting cattle Herd immunity develops Incubation period ≈3 months after exposure to agent	Abortion storms may occur, usually in heifers and newly introduced cattle High, 30%–40%	Third trimester abortion or birth of premature weak calves	Negative	Fresh fetus with petechiae in mucosa, enlarged lymph nodes and spleen, subcutis edema, ascites, nodular swollen liver	Diagnosis based on typical histologic lesions, etiologic bacterial agent has been identified by DNA analysis but is not culturable on artificial media Bacterial rod can be detected with special stains (Steiner silver stain and immunohistochemistry)	No serology test, elevated fetal IgG levels
Bovine viral diarrhea (BVD)	Variable outcome of fetal infection depending on timing of infection and other factors. Persistent bovine viral diarrhea virus infection in full-term live calves a significant problem for exposure of other animals	Less than 10%	Any time during gestation Most common in first trimester	No obvious gross lesions	Mummification, variable fetal lesions possible including deformities (cerebellar, pulmonary, or renal hypoplasia), myocardial lesions with congestive heart failure, thymic depletion or no lesions	Immunohistochemical or fluorescent antibody examination of tissues to detect virus Virus isolation or PCR also available Animals affected early with congenital lesions may no longer be positive for virus at time of abortion	Fetal antibody, evidence of seroconversion in dam and/or herd

Nutritional: *Ingestion of excessive amounts of performed estrogens in the diet may cause abortion. There are usually accompanying signs due to increased vascularity of the udder and vulva. Possible dietary factor in so-called lowlands abortion.*
Isoimmunization: *Has not been observed to occur naturally in cattle. It has been produced experimentally by repeated IV injections of blood from the one bull of pregnancy. Intravascular hemolysis occurs in the calves.*
Unknown: *30%–75% of most abortions examined are undiagnosed. The ingestion of large quantities of pine needles is suspected as a cause of abortion in range cattle in the United States. Infection with* Ureaplasma *and* Mycoplasma *spp. are other causes of undetermined relative importance.*
ELISA, *enzyme-linked immunosorbent assay;* IFAT, *indirect fluorescent antibody test;* PCR, *polymerase chain reaction.*

explanation when using monovalent vaccines. The addition of Freund's incomplete adjuvant provides better protection, and some other adjuvants may improve the efficiency of killed vaccines against naturally occurring enzootic abortion. Killed vaccines can be used in pregnant ewes and have been used in the face of an outbreak in an attempt to reduce the prevalence of abortion.

A live vaccine containing a temperature-sensitive attenuated strain of *C. abortus* (strain 1B) provides reasonable, but not complete, protection against *C. abortus*. It is registered for use in sheep (not goats). Live attenuated vaccines should not be used in pregnant ewes because they may pose a risk of zoonotic infection and have been associated with abortions.[8-10]

Recombinant and DNA vaccines have shown little protection against experimental challenge with *C. abortus*.

FURTHER READING

Radostits O, et al. Chlamydophila abortion (enzootic abortion of ewes, ovine enzootic abortion). In: *Veterinary Medicine: A Textbook of the Diseases of Cattle, Horses, Sheep, Goats and Pigs*. 10th ed. London: W.B. Saunders; 2007:1435-1437.

Stuen S, Longbottom D. Treatment and control of *Chlamydial* and *Rickettsial* infections in sheep and goats. *Vet Clin North Am Food Anim Pract*. 2011;27:213-233.

REFERENCES

1. Longbottom D, et al. *PLoS ONE*. 2013;8(2):e5790.
2. Ruhl S, et al. *Vet Microbiol*. 2009;135:169.
3. Reinhold P, et al. *Vet J*. 2011;189:257.
4. Sachse K, et al. *Vet Microbiol*. 2009;135:2.
5. Gutierriez J, et al. *Vet Microbiol*. 2011;147:119.
6. Gutierriez J, et al. *J Vet Diagn Invest*. 2012;24:846.
7. Wilson K, et al. *Vet Microbiol*. 2009;135:38.
8. Laroucau K, et al. *Vaccine*. 2010;28:5653.
9. Wheelhouse N, et al. *Vaccine*. 2010;28:5657.
10. Sarginson N, et al. *New Zeal Vet J*. 2015;63:284.

COXIELLOSIS (Q-FEVER)

SYNOPSIS

Etiology *Coxiella burnetii*.

Epidemiology High seroprevalence in ruminants. Latent infection with recrudescence and excretion at parturition. Infection by direct contact and inhalation. Persists in the environment. Important zoonotic disease.

Clinical findings Infection in ruminants is common. Clinical disease is less common and presents mainly as abortion in sheep and goats.

Necropsy findings Placentitis. Organisms demonstrable in placental trophoblast cells by fluorescent antibody.

Diagnostic confirmation Fluorescent antibody staining and PCR of aborted material and vaginal discharge. Acid-fast rodlike organisms in stained impression smear of placenta. Serology (ELISA, CFT, immunofluorescent antibody) or bulk tank milk test to establish herd infection status.

Control Vaccination possible in many countries. Isolation of aborting ruminants. Destruction of bedding and straw contaminated with birth fluids.

Zoonotic aspects Infection of humans can vary from asymptomatic to severe and even fatal. Presents mainly as a mild influenza-like illness with pneumonia, but chronic infections can have serious outcomes, including endocarditis and osteoarticular disease. Mainly follows contact with sheep and goats around parturition rather than cattle.

CFT, *complement fixation test;* ELISA, *enzyme-linked immunosorbent assay;* PCR, *polymerase chain reaction.*

ETIOLOGY

Coxiellosis (Q) fever is a zoonosis associated with *C. burnetii*, which is an obligate intracellular parasite classified within the family Coxiellaceae (formerly Rickettsiaceae). It can be divided into six genotype clusters on the basis of RFLP, although different methods can be used such as multispacer sequence typing (MST) or MLVA, which can identify up to 17 different microsatellite markers.[1] The presence or absence of specific genotypes could explain inconsistencies in reports on the effects of coxiellosis, particularly on reproduction in cattle. Coinfection with multiple genotypes can occur, although a large study of milk samples in the United States identified predominantly genotype ST20 in bovine milk and mainly ST8 in caprine milk,[2] whereas ST20 was associated with an abortion storm in a goat dairy in the UK[3] and ST33 with the large outbreak in the Netherlands.[4] Unlike other rickettsiae, *C. burnetii* it is quite resistant to environmental influences and is not dependent on arthropod vectors for transmission. It displays two antigenic phases or phenotypes: Phase 1 is more infectious and able to replicate in the host, and Phase 2, which is unable to replicate (these phases correspond to the smooth and rough phases of other gram-negative bacteria, respectively).

EPIDEMIOLOGY

Occurrence

The organism has worldwide distribution, although serologic surveys have found no evidence of infection in New Zealand.

C. burnetii cycles in a wide variety of wildlife species and their ectoparasites. The infection also cycles in domestic animals; cattle, sheep, and goats are the main livestock reservoirs of infection for humans. Rates of infection in farm animals vary considerably between locations, between countries, and with time, because there appears to be cycles of infection within regions.[5]

There can be a wide range in the seroprevalence of Q fever within regions and within individual herds or flocks. In cattle, from 4% to 100% of herds have been reported as positive (either seropositive or bulk milk test), and the within-herd prevalence varies from 0% to 49%.[6] The flock and within-flock prevalence in sheep and goats shows similar ranges and, as for cattle, varies according to year and region.[5,6] There is little information on management or other factors that might influence this variation in prevalence, but one study found a significantly higher prevalence in housed cattle compared with cattle kept on pasture. Analysis of data from 69 publications found the overall mean prevalence to be slightly higher in cattle (estimate of 20% and 38% for herd and within-herd prevalence, respectively) than for small ruminants (sheep and goat; 15% and 25% for flock and within-flock prevalence, respectively).[6] The prevalence in flocks of dairy goats and dairy sheep is much higher than in nondairy flocks.

Source of Infection and Transmission

Infection and transmission is by direct contact and by inhalation. Infection of non-pregnant animals is clinically silent and is followed by latent infection until pregnancy, at which time there is recrudescence with infection in the intestine, uterus, placenta, and udder and excretion from these sites at parturition. The organism is present in high concentration in the placenta and fetal fluids and subsequent vaginal fluids, is also excreted in urine, and is present in the feces of sheep from 11 to 18 days postpartum. In a longitudinal study in a naturally infected sheep flock in France, the number of *C. burnetii* was higher in vaginal mucus and feces compared with milk, peaked 3 weeks after abortion or birth, and was highest in primiparous and aborting ewes.[7] Shedding of *C. burnetii* in the feces can be persistent, so this can contribute significantly to environmental contamination with the organism. Infection can result in abortion, stillbirths, or poorly viable lambs, but the neonates of infected, excreting ewes are often born clinically normal.

Abortion usually does not occur at successive pregnancies. However, there can be recrudescence of infection and excretion at these pregnancies, especially the one immediately following, and reproductive failure at a second consecutive pregnancy is recorded in goats.[8] Goats excrete the organism in vaginal discharges for up to 2 weeks, it is present in milk for up to 52 days after kidding, and is also found in the feces. It also strongly adheres to the zona pellucida not removed by standard washing procedures. Thus the possibility of transfer of *C. burnetii* by embryo transfer cannot be ruled out.[9]

In cattle, maximum shedding also occurs at and 2 weeks following parturition, the organism is excreted in milk for at least several months and can be detected for up to 2 years in bulk tank milk. Abortion in cattle is less common than in goats and sheep and is sporadic rather than occurring as abortion storms like occur with sheep and goats. The organism is present in the semen of seropositive bulls, and venereal transmission is suspected.

There is a significant contamination of the environment of infected animals at the time of parturition and abortion. This is a major risk period for transmission of the disease within herds and flocks and presents a significant zoonotic risk. The organism is still present in large concentrations in soil 12 months after outbreaks of coxiellosis on goat farms.[10]

Pathogen Risk Factors

C. burnetii is very resistant to physical and chemical influences and can survive in the environment, manure, and soil for several months. It can resist common chemical disinfectants but is susceptible to sodium hypochlorite, 1:100 Lysol solution, and formalin fumigation provided a high humidity is maintained.

There is strain variation in the organism, and differences in genotypes and DNA sequences have been correlated with differences in the type of disease occurring in humans and domestic ruminants. The organism is highly infectious, with the infective dose for humans estimated to be one organism.

Zoonotic Implications

In humans infection is primarily by inhalation. Sources of infection include such diverse materials as soil; airborne dust; wool, bedding; and other materials contaminated by urine, feces, or birth products of animals. The potential for human infection from these sources is substantial (e.g., ovine manure used as a garden fertilizer has been incriminated).

Sheep and goats have traditionally been identified as the major reservoir of infection for humans, and the location of urban populations in proximity to large dairy goat herds was a significant reservoir in the Dutch outbreak from 2007 to 2010.[1]

The organism is present in the milk of infected cattle, sheep, and goats. A significant proportion of seropositive cattle excrete the organism in milk, and periods and duration of excretion are variable but may persist at least 2 years. *C. burnetii* is destroyed by pasteurization but there is a risk for people who consume raw milk, particularly unpasteurized milk from sheep and goat.

Rates of seropositivity in humans vary markedly between surveys, but there is a higher rate of seropositivity in people that are associated with domestic animals and their products and with farm environments (such as farm workers, veterinarians, livestock dealers, dairy plant and slaughterhouse workers, and shearers).[5]

Many instances of infection in humans have been linked to exposure to parturient sheep and goats. A spectacular example is the 2007 to 2010 epidemic in the Netherlands, in which over 3000 notifications of human disease were analyzed and only 3.7% of people had worked in agriculture or slaughterhouses.[11] This outbreak was attributed to airborne transmission of contaminated dust originating from dairy goat farms located in densely populated areas. The number of human cases abruptly declined after control measures were implemented on the goat and sheep farms, including vaccination, the mass culling of more than 50,000 pregnant does and ewes on infected farms to reduce shedding of the organism, and mandatory PCR testing of bulk tank milk for *C. burnetii*.[11] Living close (<2 km) to a large dairy goat farm that had an abortion storm caused by *Coxiella burnetii* was identified as the major risk factor for human cases during the Netherlands epidemic.[12]

Coxiellosis in humans is referred to as Q-fever and is often asymptomatic, but can result in acute disease characterized by fever, general malaise, headache, and less commonly, pneumonitis, hepatitis, and meningoencephalitis. Endocarditis, hepatitis, and osteoarticular diseases are manifestations of chronic disease in around 2% of human infections.[11] Those at most risk of chronic disease are immunocompromised individuals and pregnant women. There is a concern that the prevalence of infection in farm animals is increasing and spreading geographically, so that there is a greater risk for human infection, particularly when dairy farms are located near urban populations. Epidemics of human infection have been documented in several countries including Australia, France, Germany, the United States, Bulgaria, the UK, and the Netherlands.[11]

C. burnetii is considered a potential agent for bioterrorism because of its survival in the environment, the ease with which it can be transmitted by aerosol and wind, and the very low infectious dose.

CLINICAL FINDINGS

Infection of ruminants can occur at any age and is usually clinically inapparent. In the experimental disease in cattle, anorexia is the only consistent clinical finding. *C. burnetii* is a cause of abortion storms and sporadic abortion in sheep and goats but only rarely associated with sporadic abortion in cattle.[13] Abortion occurs during the latter part of pregnancy in individual does or ewes, usually with no sign of impending abortion.

In the 2007 to 2010 epidemic in the Netherlands, abortion storms were reported on 28 dairy goat and 2 sheep dairy farms, with up to 60% of goats aborting compared with an average of 5% abortions on the sheep farms.[11]

CLINICAL PATHOLOGY

There are a number of serologic tests, including complement fixation, microagglutination, ELISA and indirect immunofluorescence, and PCR (both conventional and quantitative real-time PCR). A comparison of these tests concluded a combination tests was preferable, such as ELISA for serology and PCR for detection of DNA of the organism.[14]

The immunofluorescence assay is used as the seroreference test for the serodiagnosis of coxiellosis. It can detect antibody to phase variants and can provide epidemiologic information because Phase 1 antibody is associated with recent and acute infections and Phase 2 antibody with chronic infections.

Conventional and quantitative real-time PCR tests can be conducted on bulk tank milk and are a useful means of monitoring herd or flock prevalence within regions and outbreaks within herds or flocks.[15,16]

NECROPSY FINDINGS

There are seldom gross lesions in aborted fetuses, but foci of necrosis and inflammation are occasionally seen in the liver, lung, and kidney microscopically.[13] The placenta from aborting animals is usually thickened and a purulent exudate or large, red-brown foci of necrosis is typically seen in the thickened intercotyledonary areas. Microscopically, large numbers of necrotic neutrophils are usually visible on the chorionic surface, and swollen trophoblasts filled with the organisms can also be found in well-preserved specimens. This is consistent with bacterial replication occurring only in the trophoblasts of placenta, and not in other organs, of experimentally infected pregnant does and their kids.[17] Examination of placental impression smears stained with Gimenez, Koster's, or other appropriate techniques provides a means of rapid diagnosis. However, care must be taken to avoid confusing *Coxiella*-infected trophoblasts with cells containing *Chlamydophila* organisms. Coxiellosis can be confirmed by PCR, fluorescent antibody staining of fresh tissue, or immunohistochemical staining of formalin-fixed samples. In most laboratories, culture is not attempted because of the zoonotic potential of this agent.

Samples for Confirmation of Diagnosis

- **Bacteriology and detect DNA:** chilled placenta (fetal liver and spleen) (cytology, FAT, PCR)
- **Histology:** fixed placenta and fetal lung, liver, kidney (light microscopy, immunohistochemistry)

Note the zoonotic potential of this agent when handling aborted material and packaging and submitting specimens.

DIFFERENTIAL DIAGNOSIS

- Other causes of abortion in sheep and goats (*Campylobacter, Chlamydophila,* and *Toxoplasma*, Table 18-1).
- The diagnosis of the disease in farm animals, other than abortion, suspected as associated with this agent is difficult and relies on the detection of the organism.
- A positive serologic test in an animal or herd is indicative of infection at some time but does not indicate an association with the problem at hand.
- PCR or PCR-ELISA has been used for detection of the organism in milk.

ELISA, *enzyme-linked immunosorbent assay;* PCR, *polymerase chain reaction.*

CONTROL

Aborting animals should be isolated for 3 weeks and aborted and placenta-contaminated material burnt. Ideally, manure should be composted for 6 months before application to fields to inactivate the organism, and closed composting with CaO or $CaCN_2$ has been practiced following outbreaks in the Netherlands, France, and Germany.[5] Feed areas should be raised to keep them free from contamination with feces and urine.

Although Q fever has significant implications for human health, until recently it has not been regarded as important enough to justify national or regional control strategies based on control in the animal population. In the Netherlands, a seasonal epidemic of animal and human *C. burnetii* infections occurred in 2007, but was no different from several previous isolated outbreaks in Europe. Subsequently, the unexpected scale of the outbreak in 2008 meant that national and regional public health authorities were largely unprepared for the expanding epidemic.[5,18]

The response in the Netherlands was to cull all pregnant dairy goats on affected farms before the 2010 kidding season, without reference to individual testing, and to vaccinate dairy goats and dairy sheep.[18,19] A retrospective analysis identified that testing pregnant goats by PCR or ELISA, followed by culling only the positive goats, would not have effectively reduced the massive bacterial shedding on these farms because many infected goats would not have been detected.[20]

Inactivated Phase 1 vaccines show a good and persistent antibody response, suggesting that vaccination should limit the excretion of the organism. However, there is little economic incentive for vaccination of livestock when an outbreak of coxiellosis is not occurring, and a vaccine for livestock is not available in many countries. A systematic review and meta-analysis of investigations into the use of inactivated Phase 1 vaccines, such as used in the Dutch outbreak, found a significantly reduced risk of shedding in vaginal mucus, uterine fluids, milk, and feces of vaccinated goats exposed to infection compared with controls. However, it was concluded that there was no reduction in the risk or amount of shedding in vaccinated ewes compared with unvaccinated ones.[21]

Vaccination of humans has reduced infection rates in high-risk groups and is used in the appropriate circumstances in Australia, such as workers on goat and sheep dairy farms, abattoir workers, veterinarians, and veterinary students.

During a natural outbreak of coxiellosis in a dairy flock, two treatments with oxytetracycline at days 100 and 120 of pregnancy failed to reduce shedding of the organism in vaginal fluids, milk, or feces compared with untreated ewes.[22] In this flock, vaccination for three consecutive seasons reduced the proportion of ewes shedding the organism to around 4%.

Pasteurization of milk that is consumed fresh is preferable, but veterinarians dealing with herds that provide raw milk should ensure that these herds are seronegative or bulk tank milk is PCR negative for *C. burnetii.* In a study of manufactured dairy products in France (mainly cheese, but also yogurt, cream, and butter), the DNA of *C. burnetii* was detected in 64%, but no viable organisms were recovered. A greater proportion of food products from large-scale manufacturers were positive compared with artisan food.[23]

FURTHER READING

Agerholm JS. *Coxiella burnetii* associated reproductive disorders in domestic animals—a critical review. *Acta Vet Scand.* 2013;55:13.

Georgiev M, et al. Q fever in humans and animals in four European countries, 1982 to 2010. *Euro Surveill.* 2013;18:pii 20407.

Hogerwerf L, et al. Reduction of Coxiella burnetii prevalence by vaccination of goats and sheep, the Netherlands. *Emerg Infect Dis.* 2011;17:379-386.

O'Neil TJ, et al. A systematic review and meta-analysis of phase I inactivated vaccines to reduce shedding of Coxiella burnetii from sheep and goats from routes of public health importance. *Zoonoses Public Health.* 2014;61:519-533.

Roest HIJ, et al. The Q fever epidemic in the Netherlands: history, onset, response and reflection. *Epidemiol Infect.* 2011;139:1-12.

REFERENCES

1. Roest HIJ, et al. *Emerg Infect Dis.* 2011;17:668.
2. Pearson T, et al. *BMC Microbiol.* 2014;14:41.
3. Reichel R, et al. *Res Vet Sci.* 2012;93:1217.
4. Tilburg JJHC, et al. *Emerg Infect Dis.* 2012;18:887.
5. Georgiev M, et al. *Euro Surveill.* 2013;18:pii 20407.
6. Guatteo R, et al. *Vet Microbiol.* 2011;149:1.
7. Joulié A, et al. *Appl Environ Microbiol.* 2015;81: 7253.
8. Berri M, et al. *Res Vet Sci.* 2007;83:47.
9. Alsaleh A, et al. *Theriogenology.* 2013;80:571.
10. Kersh GJ, et al. *Appl Environ Microbiol.* 2013;79:1697.
11. Djikstra F, et al. *FEMS Immunol Med Microbiol.* 2012;64:3.
12. Schimmer B, et al. *BMC Infect Dis.* 2010;10:69.
13. Agerholm JS. *Acta Vet Scand.* 2013;55:13.
14. Niemczuk K, et al. *Vet Microbiol.* 2014;171:147.
15. Garcia-Pérez AL, et al. *J Dairy Sci.* 2009;92:1581.
16. Bauer AE, et al. *BMC Vet Res.* 2015;11:186.
17. Roest H-J, et al. *PLoS ONE.* 2012;7:e48949.
18. Roest HIJ, et al. *Epidemiol Infect.* 2011;139:1.
19. Hogerwerf L, et al. *Emerg Infect Dis.* 2011;17:379.
20. Hogerwerf L, et al. *Vet J.* 2014;200:343.
21. O'Neill TJ, et al. *Zoonoses Public Health.* 2014;61:519.
22. Astobiza I, et al. *Vet J.* 2013;196:81.
23. Eldin C, et al. *Am J Trop Med Hyg.* 2013;88:765.

DISEASES OF THE GENITAL TRACT ASSOCIATED WITH *MYCOPLASMA* SPP.

Vulvovaginitis in cattle, sheep, and goats may be associated with ***Mycoplasma agalactiae* var. *bovis.*** The same infection, when introduced with semen into the uterus, can cause endometritis and salpingitis, resulting in temporary infertility and failure to conceive. Persistent infection of the genital tract of bulls has also been produced experimentally.

Although **ureaplasmas** and ***M. bovigenitalium*** are considered to pertain to the normal flora of the lower urogenital tract of ruminants, these organisms have also been associated with reproductive disease.[1] In healthy individuals *Ureaplasma diversum* is usually limited in its distribution to the vestibule and vulva. Both microorganisms have been isolated from the vulva of animals with granular vulvovaginitis, and the disease could be transmitted experimentally. *M. bovigenitalium* infection has further been associated with infertility, abortion, and birth of weak calves.[1] These infections adversely affect reproduction when they are either acute or chronic; along with producing granular vulvovaginitis, some strains can, if introduced to the upper reproductive tract, cause transitory endometritis and salpingitis. Because *U. diversum* is a normal inhabitant of the upper respiratory tract and the lower urogenital tract of ruminants, contamination of fetal membranes or fetal tissue submitted to the diagnostic laboratory should be considered.[2] The diagnosis of *U. diversum* as a causative agent for abortion should therefore ideally be based on isolation of the pathogen from fetal lung tissue, stomach content, or placenta, coupled with the presence of compatible lesions in the lung and placenta.[2]

Ureaplasmas, *M. bovis,* and *M. bovigenitalium* have been found in the reproductive tract of bulls and their semen. Using PCR for the detection of mycoplasma in semen, *M. mycoides* subsp. *mycoides* SC (the causative agent of the contagious bovine pleuropneumonia) has been found in semen of yearling bulls with seminal vesiculitis. Mycoplasmas in semen can be transmitted through in vitro fertilization (IVF) and infect embryos, and supplementation of culture media with standard antibiotics and washing embryos as recommended by the International Embryo Transfer Society are not effective in making IVF embryos free from *M. bovis* and *M. bovigenitalium. M. bovis* in frozen semen can survive the antibiotic combination of gentamicin, tylosin, and lincomycin and spectinomycin.

In horses, ***M. equigenitalium, M. subdolum***, and ***Acholeplasma* spp**. have been associated with infertility, endometritis, vulvitis, and abortion as well as with reduced fertility and balanophostitis in stallions.[3] Notwithstanding, these microorganisms are also commonly isolated from clinically healthy horses, which has raised questions about their direct association with genital disease. Two microorganisms frequently isolated from the upper respiratory tract of horses, ***M. equirhinis*** and ***M. felis,*** have also been isolated from the genital tract of stallions but have not been associated with any clinical disease.[3]

In pigs infection with ***M. suis,*** the causative agent of eperythrozoonosis, has also been associated with infertility, abortion, stillbirth, and birth of weak piglets.[1]

REFERENCES

1. Given MD, Marley MSD. *Theriogenology.* 2008;70:270.
2. Anderson ML. *Theriogenology*. 2007;68:474.
3. Spergser J, et al. *Vet Microbiol.* 2002;87:119.

EQUINE COITAL EXANTHEMA

Equine coital exanthema is a **venereal disease** associated with infection of equids by equine herpesvirus-3 (EHV-3). The genome of EHV-3 has been sequenced.[1] The disease is highly contagious and has economic importance because of disruptions to breeding programs on stud farms when stallions have clinical signs or there is an outbreak of disease among mares. The economic impact is greatest in those breeds or studbooks, such as Thoroughbreds, that do not permit artificial insemination of mares.[2]

Transmission is usually venereal from affected or clinically normal carrier animals in which the infection is thought to be latent in sciatic ganglion.[3] The virus is highly contagious, and outbreaks among mares in an embryo transfer facility in which both donor and recipient mares were affected is strongly suggestive of iatrogenic spread by personnel or on equipment such as ultrasound probes.[2] Inapparent or latent infection is apparently common, with 14% of 220 Thoroughbred mares on a stud farm having EHV-3 genome detectable by PCR in swabs of the perineum and vagina and 48% having serum antibodies to the virus.[3] The virus can be excreted intermittently by infected mares, although the factors determining reactivation have not been determined.[3] Efforts to demonstrate that administration of corticosteroids induces reactivation of EHV-3 shedding are inconclusive.[4]

The disease can be reproduced experimentally with more severe disease and longer shedding of the virus in mares that are seronegative at the time of infection than in seropositive mares.[5]

The disease is relatively mild and causes only local signs manifested by papular, then pustular, and finally **ulcerative lesions** of the vaginal mucosa, which is generally reddened. The ulcers can be as large as 2 cm in diameter and 0.5 cm deep and are surrounded by a zone of hyperemia. In severe cases the lesions extend onto the vulva and the perineal skin to surround the anus. There can be pain on passage of feces, and the anorectal lymph nodes are enlarged.[2] In the male, similar lesions to those on the perineum of the mare are found on the penis and prepuce. Many mild cases are unobserved because there is no systemic disease and affected horses eat well and behave normally. The effect on fertility is equivocal although there might be a loss of libido during the active stage of the disease in stallions. The **incubation period** is 2 to 10 days and the course up to complete healing of ulcers is about 14 days, although depigmented lesions on the perineum can persist for months.[3]

EHV-3 has been associated with **unilateral rhinitis** in adult horses examined with the same endoscope. All horses were affected unilaterally and in the nostril through which the endoscope was passed.[6]

Diagnosis can be achieved by use of virus isolation or demonstration of viral DNA in skin lesions or swabs of the vaginal or perineal regions.[3] Secondary bacterial infection can lead to suppurative discharge and a longer course. In some outbreaks lesions occur on the skin of the lips, around the nostrils, and on the conjunctiva and can also be present on the muzzle of the foal. Ulcerative lesions of the pharyngeal mucosa also occur in infections with EHV-2 and with equine adenovirus. Ulcerative lesions of the oral mucosa are of great importance because of the necessity to diagnose vesicular stomatitis early.

Treatment is symptomatic and can include cleaning of lesions, although this might not be necessary in uncomplicated disease. Mares with severe inflammation of the perianal tissues with or without enlargement of the anorectal lymph nodes and signs of pain on defecation might benefit from administration of fecal softening agents (mineral oil) or diets.

Control can be achieved by use of artificial insemination, but careful attention must be paid to biosecurity measures that minimize the opportunity for iatrogenic spread on stud farms or embryo transfer facilities. Recommendations for control in embryo transfer facilities and stud farms include the following[2,7]:

- Strict adherence to hygiene procedures designed to prevent both the direct and indirect transmission of the virus.
- Personnel with direct contact with mares should wear long, disposable examination sleeves and short latex gloves, which should be changed between subsequent inspections.
- Ultrasonography probe should be covered with a disposable glove or be carefully disinfected before the inspection of each mare.
- All instruments and other devices used during the inspection procedure, artificial insemination, and embryo collection must be either disposable or washed and sterilized between uses.

FURTHER READING

Barrandeguy M, Thiry E. Equine coital exanthema and its potential economic implications for the equine industry. *Vet J.* 2012;191(1):35-40.

REFERENCES

1. Sijmons S, et al. *Genome Announc.* 2014;2:e00797.
2. Barrandeguy M, et al. *J Equine Vet Sci.* 2010;30:145.
3. Barrandeguy M, et al. *Theriogenology.* 2010;74:576.
4. Barrandeguy M, et al. *Equine Vet J.* 2008;40:593.
5. Barrandeguy M, et al. *Vet Microbiol.* 2012;160:319.
6. Barrandeguy M, et al. *Vet Rec.* 2010;166:178.
7. Barrandeguy M, et al. *Vet J.* 2012;191:35.

PORCINE REPRODUCTIVE AND RESPIRATORY SYNDROME (PRRS)

SYNOPSIS

Etiology Porcine reproductive and respiratory syndrome virus belonging to the Arteriviridae family.

Epidemiology Highly contagious disease of swine manifested by reproductive failure, and respiratory disease in young pigs. Worldwide occurrence; spreads rapidly in swine-raising areas during the last 20 years. Subclinical infection endemic in most swine herds; incidence of clinical disease lower but causes severe economic losses. Pigs become infected in nursery from older infected pigs; persistent infection for several months is common. Different antigenic strains with variable virulence. Natural infection or vaccination results in immunity, but viremia still common. Infection with virus may predispose to secondary infections of respiratory tract. Transmitted by direct contact, feces and discharges, importation of infected pigs into herds, aerosol infection, and semen.

Signs Highly variable clinical syndrome.

Reproductive failure Outbreaks of late gestation abortions, stillbirths, mummified fetuses, weak neonates, and high rate of return to estrus. Problem may persist and recur for many months.

Respiratory form Anorexia, fever, dyspnea, polypnea, coughing, unthriftiness, high mortality in young pigs and low in older pigs and breeding stock. Deaths occur in acute phase.

Lesions Interstitial pneumonia with reduction in alveolar macrophages. Aborted and mummified fetuses, stillbirths, and weak neonates with pulmonary lesions.

Diagnostic confirmation Serologic testing for viral antibody titers. Detection of virus in tissues and alveolar macrophages using immunofluorescent microscopy and other techniques.

Differential diagnosis list Major differential is porcine circovirus infections

Respiratory disease:

Pneumonia caused by

- *Mycoplasma hyopneumoniae*
- *Actinobacillus pleuropneumoniae*
- *Pasteurella multocida*
- Glasser's disease (*Haemophilus parasuis*)
- *Streptococcus suis*

Reproductive failure

- Leptospirosis
- Parvovirus
- Brucellosis
- Aujeszky's disease
- Hog cholera virus

Treatment Must clinically manage outbreak to minimize mortality in young pigs.

Control Segregation and off-site rearing of recently weaned pigs. Nursery depopulation and clean up protocol. Import only virus-free breeding stock into breeding herds. Both live attenuated and dead vaccines available for sows and piglets.

INTRODUCTION

PRRS is a significant cause of respiratory disease in its own right but is also a significant contributor to the porcine respiratory disease complex (PRDC).[1] The ever-expanding diversity of porcine reproductive and respiratory syndrome virus (PRRSV) infections has been emphasized.[2] This agent is one of the three major contributors to the continuing evolution of respiratory disease in pigs (swine influenza virus [SIV], PRRS, and porcine circovirus type 2 [PCV2]).

ETIOLOGY

PRRS is caused by an RNA virus morphologically, structurally, and genomically similar to members of the genus *Arterivirus* of the family **Arteriviridae** belonging to the Order Nidovirales[3] including equine arteritis virus. The virus was first isolated in Lelystad in the Netherlands in 1991 (it was initially called the "Lelystad virus"). The mystery swine disease in North America was then shown to be a similar virus. These two strains are considered to be one virus but differ genetically and antigenically. The North American and European strains are only 60% identical at the nucleotide level.[4]

In terms of evolution, it is possible that lactic dehydrogenase virus of mice infected wild boar in Central Europe and became adapted. It then went to North Carolina in the United States possibly in wild boar. It is thought that the most likely date for a common isolate of the European strains is before 1981. The two species of PRRSV then developed separately on the two continents. Some evidence of this comes from a study of the number of nucleotides in open reading frame 7 (ORF7) of the virus from the United States (372 nucleotides), and the European virus (Lelystad types) had 387 nucleotides, but the Lithuanian strains that were collected had 378 nucleotides.

The European viruses (Lelystad type) have become known as type 1, and the North American viruses as type 2 viruses (ATC-2332 was the first).

There is the implied existence of two distinct genotypes derived from a common ancestor.[5] New clinical cases may occur because of other microbes interacting with the virus but also because new viral variants escape the neutralizing responses of pigs to the previous pig strains of PRRSV.[6]

Genome

The virus has a genome of approximately 15.4 kb consisting of 10 ORFs. ORF1a and ORF1b comprise 80% of the genome and encode polyproteins that are processed to 14 nonstructural proteins (nsps)[7] by viral proteases. ORF 2a, ORF2b, ORF3, ORF4, ORF5a, and ORF5-7 encode eight structural proteins: GP2a, GP2b, GP3, GP4, ORF5a, GP5, matrix protein (M), and nucleocapsid (N).[8,9]

All of these structural proteins have been shown to be important for virus infectivity because of their critical roles in virion assembly and/or interaction with cell-surface receptors.[8] N-linked glycosylation of GP5 is critically important for virus replication.[10] The heterodimer consisting of the GP5 and M proteins is required for infectivity of arteriviruses. GP5 plays a key role in viral entry by interacting with the host cell receptor.[11] ORF2b is also essential for virus infectivity and is likely to function as an ion channel to facilitate uncoating of the virus.[12,13] GP3 is found in type 1 and 2 viruses.[14]

One other protein, (N) or nucleocapsid, synthesized by ORF7 is highly immunogenic and has been used for most antibody studies. It is found in the cytoplasm and the nucleus in which it has an important role in antagonizing cellular gene function. The more recent type 2 strains still exhibit variability in sequence and pathogenicity.[15]

A novel structural protein in PRRSV has been discovered to be encoded by an alternative ORF5, and this protein is referred to as ORF5a and is expressed in infected cells. Pigs infected also express ORF5a antibodies. It is found in all PRRSV subgenomic RNA5 genes as an alternative reading frame and in all other arteriviruses, which suggests that it may play an important role.[16]

There is evidence of recombination between vaccine and wild-type PRRSV strains.[17] There is an exceptional diversity in PRRSV strains in Eastern Europe,[18] which is developed from European viruses and the use of attenuated virus vaccines (containing North American viruses) and these are associated with new genetic subtypes.

GP4-specific neutralizing antibodies might be a driving force in PRRSV evolution.[19] Amino acid substitutions in the GP4 neutralizing epitope may abrogate antibody recognition and favor the development of neutralizing antibody-resistant variants.

The genetic and antigenic characterization of the complete genomes of type 1 PRRSV isolated in Denmark over a period of 10 years have been described. In Denmark, more than 50% of the herds are affected[20] by type 1 and/or type 2.[20] The study showed that there were two major clusters within the type 1 genotype. The differences from the original Lelystad virus varied from 84.9% to 98.8% for ORF5 and 90.7% to 100% for ORF7 for the nucleotide identities. The results strongly suggest that there have been at least two independent introductions of type 1 PRRSV into Denmark with significant drift in several regions of the virus. The genetic dissection of complete genomes of type 2 PRRS viruses isolated in Denmark over 15 years has been described.[21] The virus arrived at the same time as Ingelvac PRRS-MLV, and since then the viruses were found to be 94.0% to 99.8% identical to the vaccine strain. The nucleotide identity was 90.9% to 100% for ORF5 and 93.0% to 100% for ORF7. There was wide diversity in the nsp2 with some deletions in the NSP2 region. The analysis showed that all Danish isolates belonged to a single cluster (sublineage 5.1) resembling the type 2 prototype isolate VR-2332.

North American Viruses (Type 2 Porcine Reproductive and Respiratory Syndrome Virus)

The North American genotype PRRSVs in China have evolved independently from those in other countries, suggesting that geographic separation might be one factor influencing the molecular evolution of PRRSV.[22]

There is an exceptional diversity of North American type 1 PRRSV[4,5] in China.[23]

Korean strains have evolved from North American strains imported some years earlier and have evolved separately from other Asian countries, suggesting that geographic separation may influence the molecular evolution.[24]

European Viruses (Type 1 Porcine Reproductive and Respiratory Syndrome Virus)

In a study of over 100 new PRRSV UK isolates, all type 1, in the period from 2003 to 2007, it was found that some strains were similar to those found in the early 1990s.[25] It was also found that the diversity is greater now than it was then.[26]

The evolution of Spanish strains of PRRSV from 1991 to 2005 has been studied from 1991 to 2005 using the ORF5 of the virus.[27,28]

The emergence of PRRSV in Sweden was described in 2007 when it was detected through a national surveillance program.[29]

In a study in Thailand, European isolates seem to have evolved from the Lelystad virus, whereas the Thai U.S. isolate may have come from vaccine strains that were not available in Thailand so they may have been imported in pigs or semen and later spread.[30]

High Pathogenicity Viruses

In June 2006, an unknown disease characterized by high fever, high morbidity, and high mortality was seen in many areas of China. It was highly pathogenic and characterized by a unique discontinuous deletion of 30 amino acids in the nsp2 protein with extensive substitutions in the GP5 sequence from the ORF5 gene. This epidemic has affected over 2 million pigs in China, with over 400,000 deaths.[31] A further 140,000+ pigs with 40,000 deaths occurred between January and July 2007.[32] A similar outbreak in Vietnam caused huge losses in 2007.[33,34] The genetic variation and pathogenicity of a highly virulent PRRSV has been described.[35] The genomic diversity of Chinese PRRSV isolates from 1996 to 2009 has been described.[36] They are divided into four highly diverse groups, and it is suggested that they developed from the domestic Chinese viruses by gradual variation and evolution. A new variant has since been described.[37] The complete genome sequences of two other variant PRRSVs isolated from vaccinated pigs have been described.[38] The high pathogenicity (HP)-PRRSV strain has become the predominant strain in China.[39] This virus has undergone rapid evolution and can circumvent immune responses induced by currently used vaccines.

A 1-year study of dynamics and evolution of type 1 and 2 PRRSV in a swine farm in Korea[40] showed the farm was first infected with a type 2 virus and then with a type 1 virus of unknown etiology. The type 1 virus has undergone further change.[41]

The magnitude of differentially expressed gene profiles in HP-PRRSV–infected pigs compared with the original VR-2332–infected pigs is consistent with the increased pathogenicity of HP-PRRSV in vivo.[42]

Spread of High Pathogenicity Porcine Reproductive and Respiratory Syndrome

Highly pathogenic strains of PRRSV have been identified within both genotypes[43-45] and have been isolated in China and Southeast Asia.[31,34,45] A 59 amino acid discontinuous deletion has been found in an HP-PRRSV Chinese virus,[46] whereas most of the previous HP-PRRSVs have had a 30 amino acid deletion.[47] Six different subgenotypic isolates have been found in pigs in China from 2006 to 2008.[48] New genomic characteristics of HP-PRRSV do not lead to significant changes in pathogenicity.[49] High pathogenicity strains have been described in Vietnam.[50] These have been found to be different from the Chinese strains and cause different pathogenic outcomes in American high-health swine.[51]

A highly pathogenic PRRSV virus isolated from a piglet stool in North America was sequenced.[52]

Experimental Infections With High Pathogenicity Porcine Reproductive and Respiratory Syndrome

Experimental infection with a Chinese HP-PRRSV in American swine showed that it replicated in swine with at least a 100-fold increased kinetic activity over VR-2332, which is the American reference strain. It caused significant weight loss, exacerbated disease because of bacterial sepsis, and had more severe histologic lesions. It rapidly transmitted between animals. It also greatly increased serum cytokine levels associated with innate (IFN-α and IFN-β; TNF-α;, and IL-1β, IL-6, and IL-8) and adaptive immunity (IL-2, IL-4, IL-10, IL-12, and IFN-γ) in bronchoalveolar lavage fluid and most of them in serum and tracheobronchial lymph node homogenates.[53] These included IFN-α, IL-1β, IL-2, IL-10, and IFN-γ. In addition, IL-12 was also elevated 11 days postexposure. None of the pigs inoculated with VR-2332 had significant elevations in the serum levels of the 10 cytokines. It may be that this represents a severe cytokine release syndrome or cytokine storm, as has been suggested for humans.[54-56] These conditions share many features including massive inflammatory responses, elevated serum cytokine levels, and multiorgan disease often with death.[57]

ECONOMIC LOSS

A recent study of economic loss caused by PRRSV was made in the Netherlands, and it was found that the loss varied between €59 and €379 per sow per 18-week period of the outbreak. The mean loss was €126. The costs after the outbreak varied from €3 to €160 per sow.[58]

EPIDEMIOLOGY

Occurrence

PRRSV was first reported as a new disease in swine-raising areas in North America in 1986 to 1987, and in 1991 it was recognized in, and spread rapidly across, Western Europe. The disease was first recognized in Germany in 1990 and in the Netherlands in 1991 and then spread rapidly. Based on serologic surveys, there is no evidence of infection in swine herds in Switzerland[59] and Australia.

The introduction of legislation in some countries to restrict the movement of pigs from affected farms slowed the spread of the disease, but the rapid spread of the disease initially to the southwest of Europe and then to the north, paralleled the direction of the wind. Airborne spread was also suspected because even well-managed and isolated herds became infected, but airborne spread over distances of a few kilometers continued to occur, particularly in areas with high pig population density.

The terms ***mystery pig disease*** and ***blue-eared pig disease*** were used because the etiology was unknown and the skin of the ears of affected pigs commonly appeared blue. The disease affects pregnant gilts and sows, unweaned and recently weaned pigs, and growing–finishing pigs. Outbreaks of late-term abortions, high numbers of stillbirths and mummified or weak newborn piglets, and respiratory disease in young unweaned and weaned pigs are common. After 10 or more years of acceptance and relief that the European virus was not as pathogenic as the North American virus, it is now accepted in Europe that the recent evolution of the virus may now be causing as many problems as the North American virus always has done.

A high seroprevalence of PRRSV and SIV on Spanish farms was found to be over 85% for sows, around 80% for finishers, and around 50% for boar studs.[60]

It has also been studied in wild boars in Germany and 15.9% of 531 examined were found to be positive.[61] The genetic diversity of PRRSV in selected herds in the pig-dense region of northwestern Germany showed that of 65 samples tested 5 were the North American type and 60 were the European type 1.[62] Of the original 18 herds visited only 2 reported clinical signs 2 years later.

Both the European genotype (type 1) and the North American (type 2) genotype now circulate globally.[63]

Strains within the genotype may differ by as much as 20% with the GP5 protein showing the widest heterogeneity with 50% to 55% difference between types 1 and 2.[5]

The distribution of genotypes of PRRSV in Ontario from 2004 to 2007 and the association between genotype and clinical signs of disease have been described,[64] and four RFLP types were recognized. In a further study, it was suggested that the diversity in Canada is not described adequately by RFLP typing.[65]

Prevalence of Infection

In endemic herds 30% to 70% of pigs may be seropositive to the virus and about 60% of herds have some seropositive pigs. Although the seroprevalence may be high in herds in some regions, the incidence of clinical disease is lower and variable. Although the number of herds with the acute form of the disease has been decreasing, the infection is now **endemic** in many herds, characterized by increased mortality and suboptimal performance in nursery pigs, with active spreading of the virus mainly in nurseries. In endemically infected herds, **subpopulations of infected animals** may exist consisting of a low prevalence (<10%) of seropositive animals in the breeding animals and a high prevalence (>50%) of seropositive nursery piglets. The elimination of these susceptible subpopulations, by exposing all members of a population to the virus, is used as a control strategy in large herds in which there may be subpopulations of highly susceptible breeding females. The virus can persist in nonpregnant sows and be transmitted to naive in-contact sows. A PRRSV strain may persist in a herd for up to 3.5 years displaying as little as 2% variation in ORF5 during this period. In 78% of herds with multiple submissions, genetically different strains were identified within 1 year of the original identification. Virulent PRRSV isolates exhibit longer viremias but not more elevated levels; they induce higher death rates and cause more severe clinical signs in a respiratory disease model. More virulent strains grew to significantly higher levels in pigs than did cell culture–adapted isolates. Pathogenic consequences and immunologic responses of pigs to PRRSV are closely related to viral load in acute infections as reflected in viral titers in blood.

On some farms in Great Britain, PRRSV fails to persist indefinitely on some infected farms, with fade-out more likely in smaller herds with little or no reintroduction of infectious stock. Persistence of infection may be associated with large herds in pig-dense regions with repeated introductions.[66]

In a study of 33 sites established as PRRSV free, it was found that 40% became positive within 1 year of establishment.[67]

Morbidity and Mortality

The morbidity rate in young pigs may be up to 50%, and mortality in nursery piglets can reach 25%. Death is usually associated with secondary bacterial infections such as *Salmonella* Choleraesuis, *Streptococcus suis, Actinobacillus pleuropneumoniae,* and *Haemophilus parasuis.* Major losses occur in reproductive failure, but figures for the magnitude of reproductive losses during an outbreak are not readily available. Generally, the reproductive performance of positive herds is significantly lower than negative herds.

Risk Factors

The severity and duration of outbreaks following infection are variable. Some herds may be devastated by high production losses, whereas other herds may have almost no losses. Differences in morbidity and mortality may be caused by dose of virus at exposure, differences in host susceptibility, differences in strain virulence, environmental or housing differences, or the production practices in the herd.

A study of risk factors in Quebec[68] suggested that the transmission of PRRSV is likely to occur through the sites belonging to the same owner or through a 5-km area.

In a study of risk factors for PRRSV infection, it was found that there was a higher proportion of infected farms in areas of high pig density (more than 15,000 pigs within a 10-km radius from the farm), if they used live virus vaccines, if they were located in a high-density pig area, or if dead pigs had been collected. Farms weaning at 28 days or more had lower odds of being PRRSV positive compared with those weaning at 21 to 27 days.[69]

Animal Risk Factors

Nursing piglets lacking maternal immunity, young growing and finishing pigs, and sows lacking acquired immunity from natural infection or vaccination are highly susceptible to infection and clinical disease. Severe disease appears to be more likely in large herds that have a large turnover of pigs, purchase replacements from other herds, and do not use a quarantine system. Introduction of the virus to previously virus-naive herds may cause severe economic losses. In the recent outbreaks in Denmark, the study of 107 herds showed that a variety of hazards were identified including close neighboring herds, increasing herd size, and purchase of semen from infected studs used for artificial insemination.

There is a within-breed genetic variation for commercially relevant traits that could be exploited in future breeding programs.[70] A significant line difference in growth in two genetically diverse commercial pig lines was seen during infection with PRRSV.[71]

One study has shown that the number of piglets per litter infected by PRRSV was lower for the Landrace breed than for Large White, Duroc, and Pietrain breeds.[72]

In a study of 316 herds in Canada, it was found that the three most important factors for the spread of PRRSV RFLP 1-18-4 were sharing the same herd ownership, gilt source, and market trucks.[73] Spatial proximity could not be identified as a contributor to the spread.

Environmental and Management Risk Factors

Housing of all age groups in one building, introduction of new animals, housing on slatted floors, storage of slurry under floors, exposure to transport vehicles, and lack of disinfection procedures have been suggested as factors that increase the probability of herd infection. Lack of quarantine facilities for recently imported pigs is a major risk factor. There appears to be infrequent spread during warm weather compared with cold weather.

Pathogen Risk Factors

PPRS virus strains have many identical properties with some antigenic differences. Strains of the virus from the United States and Canada are antigenically similar but different from the European Lelystad virus isolate. All the strains appear to be highly infectious. There are serologic differences between the European and American strains, and the antigenic and genomic differences between the North American and European isolates suggest the existence of two genotypes. There are different genotypes and at least three minor genotypes within the major U.S. genotype. The simultaneous coexistence of the strains has been shown, but the significance of the observation is not understood. Genetic variations exist not only between European and U.S. strains but also among the U.S. isolates, indicating the heterogeneous nature of the virus. Antigenic variation may affect the accuracy of diagnostic tests and the efficacy of vaccines. The North American strains have been called type 2 virus, and they are continually varying. The European type 1 virus was thought to be less virulent and less likely to change, but this may not be so because recent isolations show that it is also continuing to change.

Infection with the virus does not always result in clinical disease, and the detection of high levels of serum antibody in many herds without history of clinical disease suggests that the consequences of natural and experimental infection depend on a complex of factors associated with host susceptibility and virus virulence. From 2000 to 2001, there were severe outbreaks in the United States associated with new isolates. There are now both European and U.S. strains originating from viral vaccines in Poland. The effects of the virus on reproductive performance are strain dependent. Strains of the virus cross the placenta when given to pregnant sows, and most sows will remain clinically normal and farrow normally. However, depending on the strain used, the number of late-term dead fetuses from gilts infected experimentally at 90 days' gestation may vary widely, and all gilts become viremic and develop antibodies. There are also marked differences in pathogenicity for the respiratory tract between U.S. strains of the virus compared with the Lelystad virus when inoculated experimentally into 4-week-old cesarean-derived colostrum-deprived pigs. Some strains cause severe lesions of the lymphoid and respiratory systems, which appear to be the major sites of viral replication. The difference in pathogenicity may explain the variation in severity of clinical disease observed in field outbreaks.

Field observations have suggested that the presence of the virus in a herd may increase the susceptibility of animals to other infections. However, studies with sequential infection of the virus followed by experimental inoculation with *H. parasuis, Pasteurella multocida,* or *A. pleuropneumoniae* have failed to demonstrate increased severity of disease. There is, however, strong evidence to say that PRRSV predisposes to *S. suis.* It may also predispose to *Salmonella* Choleraesuis, *Bordetella bronchiseptica,* or *M. hyopneumoniae.* This view is not universal in that infection with the virus did not increase the severity of experimental *M. hyopneumoniae* (MH) infection in young piglets. However, in the laboratory investigation of PRDC the most potent combination of agents is PRRSV and MH. A model of the dual infection has recently been described in which MH was shown to predispose to PRRSV infection. Based on diagnostic submissions, however, concurrent pulmonary bacterial infections may occur in up to 58% of cases in which the virus was also isolated.

There is also the possibility that many strains may be found in the same herd, e.g., three strains were found in one herd. Several viruses have been found in the same pig, and one great authority has expressed the view that each virus in each pig may be different from every other virus.

A syndrome was described in neonatal pigs marked by neurovirulence. Replication in the brain was verified by IHC in brain sections. Meningoencephalitis induced by the virus was unusually severe.

Methods of Transmission

Virus is produced rapidly after infection, probably within 12 hours. The virus was shown to evolve continuously in infected pigs with different genes of the viral genome undergoing various degrees of change.

There are unlikely to be any wildlife reservoirs (except for feral and wild pigs), although infected mallard can still excrete the virus 39 days later. Most pigs clear PRRSV within 3 to 4 months but some may remain persistently infected for several months. The antibody response does not reflect the carrier status. It is possible that cytokines can switch the balance from a subclinical infection to disease manifestation. There is no evidence that PRRSV is found in the tonsils as a representative tissue.

The virus spreads rapidly within herds when infected pigs are housed in confinement. Up to 90% of sows may seroconvert within 3 months of the virus being introduced into a closed breeding herd. The mode of spread is presumed to be by direct contact, probably nose to nose. The virus generally requires close pig-to-pig contact to achieve an exposure dose.

Presence Within the Herd

The virus is present in a variety of biologic fluids; nasal discharge (positive 21 days later); oropharyngeal scrapings (158 days later); possibly mammary secretions, although this is probably uncommon as previous vaccination does appear to prevent shedding; urine (28 days) and feces (28 days); and intranasal inoculation has been used to reproduce the disease experimentally. The feces may be an intermittent source, a usual source, or not a source. The virus is present in saliva and, considered in the context of the **social behavior** of pigs, may play an important role in transmission.

The virus may persist in, and circulate between, different age groups and locations in a herd for several months despite the absence of clinical disease and may be transmitted by contact to replacement animals or to uninfected farms. Infected pigs may remain carriers of the virus for up to 15 weeks. Persistent and contact infection can be maintained in a nursery if uninfected pigs are continuously exposed to infected pigs. Pigs in the nursery become infected through contact with older infected pigs and not by in utero or postpartum exposure to infected sows. Long-term surveys of farrow-finish herds reveal that isolation rates of the virus reach highest level of 70% to 100% of pigs, 6 to 8 weeks of age, which coincided with the lowest level of maternal immunity. If you rely on infected nursery pigs to transmit infection to incoming gilts in acclimatization studies, then nursery pigs may only be viremic for a maximum of 60 days. There is no association between lymphadenopathy and PRRSV viremia in nursery pigs 4 and 6 weeks postweaning. Viremia cannot be predicted solely on the basis of clinical signs. Large finishing enterprises purchasing pigs of variable infection and immune status provide ideal conditions for persistent virus circulation. Breeding herd subpopulations of infected pigs may exist and perpetuate and enhance the infection in a herd. The inability to control such subpopulations may reduce opportunities for successfully controlling the disease.

Infection may **persist** for an extended period of time because of the following:

- Incomplete infection of the susceptible population during the acute phase
- Introduction of susceptible breeding stock
- A persistent viral infection in individual pigs with the potential of shedding virus under certain conditions, such as grouping for weaning or farrowing
- A rapid decline in passive immunity in young pigs and variable periods of active immunity

Genetic randomness of isolates does not correlate with geographic distance. Movement on to the farm of PRRSV does not generally occur by distance-limited processes, such as the usual wildlife vectors, but more typically occurs because of long-distance transport of animals or semen.

It is likely that piglets born with infection from in utero exposure probably may remain viremic for life, even in the face of antibody formation. Neonatal infection is probably cleared slowly, but infection in the older animal may be cleared much more quickly.

Experimental infection suggests that PRRSV infection is eventually cleared from the host and persistent infection rarely lasts more than 200 days.

In a study in France, a semiquantitative real time RT-PCR was developed to assess the evolution of the viral genome in blood and nasal swabs from inoculated and contact pigs with time. Viral genome was detected from 7 to 77 days postinfection (DPI), whereas viral genome shedding was detectable from nasal swabs from 2 to 48 DPI. The infections increased from 7 to 14 days and then decreased slowly to 42 DPI. The evolution of infectiousness was mainly correlated with the time course of viral genome in the blood, whereas the decrease of infectiousness was strongly related to the increase in total antibodies.[74]

A mathematical model of within-herd transmission dynamics of PRRSV, fade-out and persistence, has been described.[75] It was found that fade-out was likely to occur when breeding females failed to pass the virus on to the piglets. Persistence was more likely to occur once infection was present in piglets, which in turn infected rearing pigs. The probability of persistence was higher in large herds, increased contact between different age groups, and increased reintroduction of infectious gilts.

Possible routes of transmission include introduction of vaccinated animals, use of semen from vaccinated artificial insemination boars, and aerosol spread.

Introduction of Vaccinated Animals

The disease has occurred in PRRSV-seropositive herds in Denmark with no previous clinical evidence of PRRSV. These herds were then vaccinated with a modified live virus vaccine licensed for use in pigs 3 to 18 weeks of age. Boars entering artificial insemination units were also vaccinated. Following vaccination, a large number of herds experienced an increased number of abortions and stillborn piglets and an increasing mortality in the nursing period. The problems occurred mainly in herds without clinical signs among sows and with sows with low antibody titers in the period immediately before vaccination. The PRRSV was isolated from fetuses and identified as the vaccine virus. The evidence suggested that the vaccine virus had spread to nonvaccinated sows followed by transplacental infection of the fetuses. Spread of the vaccine virus was also demonstrated in a nonvaccinated and previously virus-free breeding herd. There are three main methods of spread:

1. Introduction of infected animals: Spread between herds is associated with the introduction of infected carrier pigs.
2. Use of semen from vaccinated or infected boars: Infected boars may shed the virus in their semen for up to 40 days after experimental infection. In boars, the virus can be found in semen by PCR for much longer periods than

can be found in the blood by virus isolation or antigen detection, and the likelihood is that monocytes enter the bulbourethral glands, which then contaminate the semen. Following experimental infection of sexually mature boars the virus was present in the semen 3 to 5 days after infection and on days 13, 25, 27, and 43. Using a PCR assay the virus can be detected in semen for up to 92 days after experimental infection. The insemination of gilts with semen from experimentally infected boars resulted in clinical signs of disease and failure to conceive. Following artificial insemination of gilts with semen from experimentally infected boars, the gilts will seroconvert. The use of the modified-live PRRS virus vaccine in boars is controversial because some boars may still shed wild-type virus in semen after challenge exposure 50 days after vaccination. The inoculation of PRRSV-negative replacement gilts with serum from nursery pigs presumed to be viremic resulted in seroconversion of all 50 gilts tested.

Exposure of pregnant gilts to either attenuated (vaccine) or virulent (field) strains of the virus can result in congenital infection. Congenitally infected pigs can support virus replication for a long period of time during which the viral replication is confined to the tonsils and lymph nodes. After 260 days there were no serum antibodies, and between 63 and 132 days there was no evidence of virus in the lung. Vaccine and field strains can be transmitted postnatally from infected to noninfected littermates. Pigs infected with field strains have an inferior rate of survival and growth than do noninfected pigs. This suggests that use of attenuated virus vaccine during gestation is questionable.

3. Aerosol spread: Airborne spread across regions and between countries was suspected in Europe during the winter of 1990 to 1991. The infection appeared to spread by the airborne route from Germany, across the Netherlands, and into Belgium. Low temperatures, low sunlight, and high humidity may have facilitated airborne spread. Airborne spread up to 20 km has been suggested, but most airborne spread is probably limited to less than 2 km. Usually it is difficult to transmit the agent 1 m. Although an experiment failed to transmit infection from pig to pig in a trailer parked 30 m away, there is a suggestion that it is transmitted for a short distance, but this possibly only occurs intermittently. Aerosol infection might be responsible in the absence of any other means of spread.[76,77] The effect of temperature and relative humidity on an aerosol of PRRSV has been calculated, and it is more stable at lower temperature and/or lower humidity.[78]

In a study of aerial transmission,[79] it was found that 21/21 aerial samples were positive from exhaust gases from an experimentally infected pig group. Five of 114 long-distance samples were positive and were collected 2.3, 4.6, 6.6, and 9.1 km from the experimentally infected herd. Interestingly, only PRRSV variant 1-8-4 was detected, whereas 1-18-2 and 1-26-4, the other two strains given to the source pigs, were not detected. A production region model to assess the airborne spread of PRRSV has been produced by the same team.[80] Animal age, MH coinfection, and PRRSV isolate pathogenicity did not significantly influence the concentration of aerosol shedding. The shedding of PRRSV in aerosols may be isolate dependent.[81]

A production region model has been used to assess the airborne spread of PRRSV.[82]

The median infectious dose of PRRSV via aerosol exposure has been described.[83] The MN-184 isolate was far more infectious than the VR-2332 isolate.

Long-distance transmission of PRRSV was confirmed in a study where 1.3% of 306 samples were positive. These samples were positive 4.7 km away from the source population.[84]

Other Sources

Fomites

Fomites and infected personnel were shown to be capable of transmitting the virus following contact with infected material. Infected hands, boots, and protective clothing can transmit it.[85] Needles will transmit the virus. People do not usually act as vectors.

Meat

Pig meat does not retain detectable amounts of the virus, and it is unlikely that the transmission through meat occurs. PRRSV can survive in fresh pork at refrigerator temperatures, and the moving of meat juice may increase the risk of viral spread from personnel to pigs.[86] In a study of PRRSV in muscle it was found that 13/89 samples between 28 and 202 days after inoculation were found to be positive by quantitative RT-PCR, but if fed to pigs there was no evidence of infection, suggesting that the test detected noninfectious PRRSV in pig meat.[87]

Insects

Mosquitoes were not seen in one study to be a likely vector for PRRSV. Houseflies may pose some level of risk for the transport and transmission of PRRSV between pig populations under field conditions.[88] The intestinal tract of houseflies will support infectious PRRSV for up to 12 hours following feeding on an infected pig but only for a short period of time on the surface of the fly.

Virus Survival

The PRRS virus is fairly labile and does not survive for more than 1 day on solid fomites, but does survive for several days in well and city water. It may survive for several years in deep frozen tissues, but only 1 month at 4° C (39° F), 48 hours at 37° C (99° F), and less than 45 minutes at 56° C (133° F). There appears to be a low risk from contaminated lagoon water, and the viability of PRRSV in swine effluent is relatively short (18 days), although this is very temperature dependent.

Economic Importance

The export market for pork from a country can be seriously affected when a disease such as PRRSV occurs. When the disease was recognized in the United States, countries such as Mexico, Japan, Canada, and South Korea banned the importation of pork from the United States or required certification that the swine originated from premises where, within the 30 days before the issuance of the health certificate, no swine were introduced from a municipality in which a premises infected with the virus is located.

The economic losses may be very high because of stillbirths, abortions, small litter sizes, and birth of weak pigs, which increases preweaning mortality and increased nonproductive days. In weaned pigs, losses are associated with respiratory disease. In addition, there are the costs of control, which may be high, dependent on the control strategies undertaken. Typically, about 20% loss in annual production can be expected from a severe outbreak.

Negative weaned pigs had an increased margin per pig of $2.12 over the pigs minimally affected by PRRSV in the nursery but which seroconverted in the finishing herd and $7.07 over the pigs with persistently circulating PRRSV in the nursery.

PATHOGENESIS

Effects on Macrophages and Dendritic Cells

PRRSV has a very restricted tropism for porcine alveolar macrophages (PAMs) and some peripheral blood monocytes.[63]

Replication of PRRS in the PAMs directly impairs their basic functions including phagocytosis, antigen presentation, and production of cytokines.[89,90] The virus undergoes a productive replication in these cells leading to cell death via both apoptosis and necrosis mechanisms. In addition, there is also a reduced expression of major histocompatibility complex (MHC) class I and MHC class II, CD14, and CD11 cells.

PRRSV also induces necrosis or apoptosis of macrophages and lymphocytes in the lung and lymphoid organs, impairing the host response.[91]

In eukaryocytes, autophagy is a widely found mechanism that transports damaged cell organelles and long-lived proteins to lysosomes for degradation.[92] The autophagy induced by PRRSV infection plays a part in sustaining replication in host cells.[93]

PRRSV causes a massive increase in the number of B cells, resulting in lymphoid hyperplasia, hypergammaglobulinemia, and autoimmunity in neonatal piglets. There is a preferential expansion of certain clones bearing certain H chain third complementary lengths. The same dominant B-cell type clones occur throughout the body. The authors believed that hypergammaglobulinemia results from the products of these cells.[94]

Many piglets are probably infected in utero. PRRSV infection modulates the leukocyte subpopulations in peripheral blood and bronchoalveolar fluids. Following infection the number of CD8+ cells increased in systemic lymphoid tissue, whereas numbers of B cells increased in mucosal associated lymphoid tissue. Virus infection induces a simultaneous polyclonal activation of B cells mainly in the tonsils and an exaggerated and prolonged specific humoral immune response caused by persistent viral infection in lymphoid organs. Piglets surviving in utero infections have a high count of CD8+, CD2 +, CD4+, and SLA-class II cells in the peripheral blood.

Persistent infection occurs in these pigs. Virus appears to persist in the lymphatic organs and particularly the tonsils and the lungs. Lymphoid tissue tropism occurs during persistent infection when the piglets have been exposed in utero.

Neonatal or nursery infection is probably through the virus reaching the nasopharyngeal epithelium following inhalation from the nose-to-nose contact with other pigs. It is then probably removed to the tonsils in which they are internalized into cells of the macrophage/monocyte series.

Initially, a viremia occurs, with subsequent distribution and multiplication of the virus in multiple body systems and organs causing interstitial pneumonia, vasculitis, lymphadenopathy, myocarditis, and encephalitis. Alveolar macrophages are primary targets for virus multiplication, but this does not fully explain the pathogenesis. Multiple glycoproteins appear to be involved in infection of pulmonary alveolar macrophages. Possibly up to 40% of alveolar macrophages are destroyed. Whether it is a particular group that is damaged or all the alveolar macrophages are damaged is not known, but after about 28 days there is a resumption of normal alveolar macrophage function. PRRSV causes the apoptosis of alveolar macrophages and pulmonary intravascular macrophages. The increase in IFN-γ–positive cells correlated well with the severity of the lung lesions, which may be because of the presence of PRRSV in the lung. IFN-γ markedly inhibits the replication of PRRSV in macrophages.

RECEPTORS

As few as 10 or even fewer virus particles inoculated into the nose or given IM will infect a pig. The virus may enter the cell through an endocytic pathway or through a virus receptor. A third possibility is that the virus may enter the cell through an antibody-dependent enhancement with virus–antibody complexes entering the cell through Fc receptors on the cell surface.

There may be a PRRSV ligand for a cell-surface heparin-like receptor on pulmonary alveolar macrophages.

Several receptors have been described including heparin sulfate, sialoadhesin,[95] and vimentin.[96] The interaction of PRRSV with sialoadhesin inhibits alveolar macrophage phagocytosis.[97] Recently, CD163, a molecule that is expressed solely on the monocytic lineage,[98] has been identified as a possible cellular receptor for PRRSV.[99] This is a receptor that allows previously nonpermissible cells to become susceptible to PRRSV. It is a hapten/hemoglobin scavenger in the scavenger receptor cysteine-rich superfamily. Other factors also appear to be necessary for PRRSV permissiveness.[100] The initial step in infection involves heparin sulfate glycosaminoglycans as an initial attachment receptor and subsequent engagement of the Siglec sialoadhesin resulting in a virus internalization via clathrin-mediated endocytosis. The viral membrane M and the M/GP5 complex were identified as ligands for the initial attachment receptor. Sialic acids present on the surface of the PRRS virions have been shown to play an essential role in PRRSV infection. Recently CD163 was identified as a key receptor and involved in the entry into macrophages.[101] In a recent study,[102] it was suggested that expression of CD163 on macrophages in different microenvironments in vivo possibly may determine the replication levels of PRRSV and the virus pathogenicity.

VIRUS ENTRY

For productive infection, viruses need to enter the target cell and release their genome.[103,104] It has been shown that PRRSV entry into the alveolar macrophage involves attachment to a specific virus receptor followed by a process of endocytosis by which virions are taken into the cell within vesicles by a clathrin-dependent pathway.

It has recently been shown that PRRSV enters early endosomes after internalization but does not continue through the endocytic pathway to late endosomes. It colocalizes with its internalization receptor sialoadhesin on the cell surface and beneath the plasma membrane.[105] Sialoadhesin downregulates phagocytosis in PAMs (not CD163).[97]

There is a significant role for IL-10 in the CD163 and PRRSV susceptibility during the differentiation of macrophages. Possibly the internalization of PRRSV via CD163 in the target cells may induce the expression of IL-10, which in turn induces the expression of CD163 on neighboring cells.

Virus entry into the porcine macrophage has been reviewed[106] as has the virus structural and nonstructural proteins in viral pathogenesis.[107]

REPLICATION

The primary targets for replication are alveolar macrophages of the lung and other cells of the monocyte/macrophage lineage including pulmonary intravascular macrophages, subsets of macrophages in lymph nodes, and spleen and intravascular macrophages of the placenta and umbilical cord. A highly pathogenic strain may possess an expanded tropism to include epithelial cells.

The virus can persist in the pig for up to 132 days after birth in tonsil and lymph nodes infected in utero and from 105 to 157 days from pigs infected in postnatal infection. Over time the initial levels of viral load may decrease 10,000-fold in the tonsil or lymph nodes. The wild-type virus is capable of inducing a higher level of viral load than the mutations.[108-111]

The high pathogenicity strains from China in 2006 contain a unique 30 amino acid deletion in the nsp2 coding region, but this is not associated with virulence of these strains but nsp2 can attenuate replication and virulence.[112] The virus can cross the placenta at about 90 days' gestation and infect the fetus and can use the thymus as the principal site of replication and induce antiviral cytokines.[113]

Macrophages are activated by endogenous danger signals.[114]

There are mitogen-activated protein kinase cascade pathways, which are essential building blocks in the intracellular signaling systems. There are four of these pathways that have been identified, and one of these is the extracellular signal-regulated kinase (ERK) signaling pathway. This has been shown to play an important role in the postentry steps of PRRSV replication cycle and contributes to viral infection.[115]

PRRSV E protein is likely to be an ion-channel protein embedded in the viral envelope and facilitates uncoating of the virus and release of the genome in the cytoplasm.[116] This E protein is probably nonessential for virus infectivity but promotes growth of the virus.[117]

PRRSV can infect and replicate in monocyte and bone marrow–derived dendritic cells.[90,118,119] The exposure of bone marrow–derived immature dendritic cells to PRRSV produced a downregulated expression of MHC class I.

The monocytes and macrophages are the main cellular target for PRRSV replication, particularly the alveolar macrophages. It also replicates in vitro in dendritic cells and bone marrow-derived monocytes.[118-121] It has a higher predilection for PAMs than septal macrophages.[122] PAMs phagocytose whereas septal cells may modulate immune responses. There is a complex viral replication mechanism in immune cells such as alveolar macrophages for PRRSV.[123]

General Effects of Porcine Reproductive and Respiratory Syndrome Virus on the Immune System

Generally, both innate and adaptive immune responses to PRRSV are suppressed. It produces modest levels of IFN-α and proinflammatory cytokines.[120] In addition, the response is weak and slow. Neutralizing antibodies are slow to be produced. Cell-mediated responses in the form of IFN-γ producing cells can take 4 to 8 weeks to develop. The virus produces an increase in IL-10, which is possibly immunosuppressive because it suppresses antigen-presenting cell activities such as processing and presenting antigen and expression of IL-1, IL-12, IL-18, TNF-α, and type I IFN expression.[119]

Macrophage Damage

The PRRSV nucleocapsid protein regulates alveolar macrophages and, in a study of infected macrophages, 23 protein spots were found that were differentially expressed. Of these, 15 had a statistically significant alteration including 4 upregulated and 11 downregulated[124] spots. Individual mature nsps are found in virus-infected cells.[125]

The alveolar macrophages when infected round up, show bleb formation, and eventually rupture. TNF-α released from damaged macrophages after PRRSV infection may induce apoptosis in uninfected lymphoid cells. In a study of cells in the lungs, it was found in both noninfected and infected cells. The majority of the apoptotic cells were noninfected. The peak of apoptosis was at 14 days and was preceded by a peak of IL-1 and IL-10 production at 9 DPI. The PRRSV infection directly interferes with type I IFN transcriptional activation.

Toll-Like Receptors

PRRSV inhibits TLR expressions in PAMs at 6 hours postinfection and it is then restored at 24 DPI when the cells showed upregulated IL-12.[126]

The possibility of increased expression of TLR mRNA and cytokines in pigs with PRRSV has been shown.[127] In these experiments there was an upregulation of TLR 2, 3, 4, 7, and 8 in at least one of the lymphoid tissues and cells.

Modulation of Immune Responses

Cellular Changes (Natural Killer, T-Regulatory, etc.)

The original VR-2332 prototype North American strain of the virus induces immune modulatory changes at mucosal tissues. Peak antibody response and cytokine IFN-γ were detected at PID30 with increased TGF-β until PID60. Populations of CD4+, CD8+, CD4+ CD8+ T cells, natural killer (NK) cells, and γδ T cells in the lungs and lymphoid tissues were significantly modulated favoring PRRSV persistence. The NK-cell–mediated cytotoxicity was significantly reduced in infected pigs. In addition, increased populations of immunosuppressive T-regulatory cells (T-regs) and associated cytokines were also observed in infected pigs.[128] These results suggest that both innate (γδ T cells and NK cells) and adaptive immune cell subsets were modulated in mucosal tissues in which the virus persists for a long time. IL-10 and TGF-β are immunosuppressive in nature produced by T-regs and are upregulated in PRRSV-infected pigs.[129] Although wild-type parenteral strain VR-2332 is avirulent it dampens the most essential immune components at the site of replication, which are the lung parenchyma and lymphoid tissue, resulting in weak and delayed anti-PRRSV immunity.

NK cells are only a small fraction of circulating lymphocytes that are not B or T cells. Cytokines IL-2 and IFN-α are activators of T cells.[130] PRRSV is a poor inducer of IFN-α. These cells early in infections kill infected cells and produce cytokines.[131] PRRSV-infected macrophages are less susceptible to NK cells. This reduced activity begins at 6 hours postinfection and coincides with the detection of observable PRRSV structural proteins.[132] It is likely that the transcription of viral genes and proteins also contributes to the resistance of PRRSV-infected macrophages toward NK cells. PRRSV infection inhibits both NK and cytotoxic T-cell activity via a common mechanism.[133] It might be that during PRRSV infection the virus may modulate the ligands for the NK receptors on the surface of pulmonary alveolar macrophages, leading to insufficient NK cytotoxicity.

The PRRSV has a suppressive effect on the NK cells, which are part of the innate immune response. They are usually activated by IL-2, IL-12, IL-15, IL-18, and IFN-α and by the interaction between NK activating receptors and their ligands on target cells.[134] One of the components of reduced NK cell activity is the possibility that there is incomplete activation of NK cells by a lower level of activating cytokines.[135] PRRSV-infected pulmonary alveolar macrophages showed a reduced susceptibility toward NK cytotoxicity, and this may represent one of the multiple evasion strategies of PRRSV.[133]

Replicating PRRSV in both infected and contact pigs was responsible for rapid modulation in NK cell–mediated cytotoxicity and alteration in the production of important immune cytokines. These changes produce a delay in adaptive immunity. At 2 DPI 50% of viremic pigs had a greater than 50% reduction in NK cell–mediated cytotoxicity, and nearly a onefold increase in IFN-α was found in the blood of some pigs. Enhanced secretion of IL-4 was found in 90% of pigs and IL-10 and IL-12 in a few pigs. IFN-γ was not enhanced. There was a reduced frequency of myeloid cells, CD4+ CD8+ T cells, and CD4– CD8+ T cells, and upregulated frequency of lymphocytes bearing natural T-reg cell phenotype were detected in viremic pigs.[136]

This is associated with a decrease in cytotoxicity but not the number of NK cells (increased IL-4, IL-10, and IL-12).[136] Regulatory T cells (induced by type 2 but not type 1 PRRS) also impair the host.[137-140]

There is a decrease in the number of antigen-presenting cells and T cells in the tonsil and lymph nodes of PRRSV-infected pigs, suggesting a modulation of the host immune response.[141]

CD14 + monocytes may also infiltrate the interstitial tissue in the lung and develop into interstitial macrophages. The early development of subneutralizing or nonneutralizing antibody may have a significant effect on the development of PRRS by antibody-dependent enhancement, which can facilitate the attachment and internalization of the virus onto host cells through Fc receptor-mediated endocytosis.[142]

A higher expression of proinflammatory cytokines is also expressed in septal macrophages in pigs.[122,143] T-regs[143] control the immune response and maintain homeostasis and are natural or induced. Induction of T-regs during the early stage of PRRSV infection is one of the ways pathogens escape the immune response.[138,139,144-147]

Cytokines

Many cytokines influence the immune response to PRRSV infection (Table 18-3). TNF-α may act as an antiviral cytokine protecting cells from infection by an IFN-independent mechanism, and several strains of PRRSV have a low ability to induce the expression.

The cytokines IL-10 and IL-12 are expressed in inflammatory lesions in the lung and play an important role in the defense against PRRSV. In some PRRSV infections, there was no change in the levels of IL-10, IL-12, and IFN-γ in PRRSV infections. It also induces minimal levels of T-helper-1 (Th1) cytokines (IL-12 and IFN-γ).[90]

In utero–infected pigs showed significantly increased IL-6, IL-10, and IFN-γ mRNA expression (IL-2, IL-4, and IL-12 remained the same) and this was concurrent with a significant decrease in the number of CD4+ CD8+ T cells. The cell-mediated and cytokine message profiles returned to normal.

The increased expression of IL-1α, IL-6, and TNF-α in the lungs of pigs with PRRSV is correlated with the development of interstitial pneumonia.[122] Different isolates induce

Table 18-3 Cytokines and porcine reproductive and respiratory syndrome[159]

Cytokine	Function
IL-1	Attracts macrophages, monocytes, polymorphs
IL-6	Induces acute phase proteins Upregulates CD163 receptor
IL-10	Upregulates CD163 receptor Upregulates in the lung
TNF-α	Inhibits replication of PRRSV Induces acute phase proteins Downregulated in PRRSV-infected macrophages Downregulates CD163 receptor
IFN-α	Interferes with replication of PRRSV Downregulated in PRRSV-infected macrophages
IFN-γ	Inhibits replication of PRRSV Enhanced by vaccination with IL-12/IFN-α Downregulates CD163 receptor
IL-10	Correlates with expression in the lung Inhibits IFN-γ in the lung
TGF-β	Induces T-regs after PRRSV infection Correlates with expression in the lung Downregulates CD163 receptor

IFN, *interferon;* PRSSV, *porcine reproductive and respiratory syndrome virus.*

different patterns of IL-10 and TNF-α. Four possible phenotypes were identified, but different cells had different capabilities. In addition, cytokine-release profiles on antigen-presenting cells could induce different expressions of cell markers.[121]

Certain regions of nsp2 also downregulate IL-1β and TNF-α.[148] The inhibition of early cytokine production contributes to the weak innate immune response, delayed neutralizing antibody, slow IFN-γ response, and a depressed cytotoxic T-cell response.[149]

In PRRSV infections, the production of proinflammatory cytokines is limited.[150] The nsps may downregulate TNF-α.[151,152]

IL-10 inhibits the synthesis of proinflammatory cytokines as well as inhibiting the production of IFN-α, and may also suppress the proinflammatory response to PRRSV-infected pigs. There is a significant correlation between the response to PRRSV antigen expression and the expression of regulatory cytokines, such as IL-10 and TGF-β in the lungs but not in the lymph nodes.[153,154]

There may be, as a result of the cytokine expression, a reduction of the infiltration and proliferation of inflammatory cells.[155] IL-10 is expressed mainly by septal macrophages and TGF-β mainly by PAMs. There may be different expressions of different cytokines by different subsets of the lung cells. TGF-β production may be dependent on the PRRSV strain.[156] CD163 is one component of a complex of receptors required for entry of PRRSV entry into the cell including heparin sulfate and sialoadhesin. It is upregulated by IL-10 and IL-6 promoting PRRSV entry into the cell and replication but downregulated by TNF-α, TGF-β, and IFN-γ.[102,157]

The induction of the IL-10 response may be one of the strategies used by PRRSV to modulate the host immune responses.[158] Increases in IL-4, IFN-γ, and TNF-α were found in the lymphocytes of infected piglets, but IL-8 showed a decrease. Other authors have the opposite view, which suggests that T cells showed an increase in CD8+ CD4+ and CD4– CD8+ subsets within activated cells, whereas CD4+ CD8– cells decreased with time. T cells responding to the virus showed a Th1 type cytokine production pattern. These authors[158] also reported a decrease in TNF-α and a decrease of IL-1α and macrophage inflammatory protein.

Perhaps this is the key to PRRSV infections in that all pigs may respond differently. There may be either depressive or stimulatory effects. The imbalance of IL-12 and IL-10 produced in PRRSV-infected pigs may favor the humoral responses and suppress cell-mediated immune responses for the first 2 weeks of life.

PRRSV was detected in the cytoplasm of macrophages at two peaks, 3 to 7 DPI and second at 14 DPI. IFN-α increased at 3 DPI, and IFN-γ and IL-12 were increased at 3 to 7 DPI and 14 to 17 DPI, but IL-10 was lower than the others suggesting that other factors also play a part.[153]

Interferons

PRRSV is able to downregulate the production of inflammatory cytokines such as type I interferons (IFN-α, IFN-β, TNF-α, and IL-1). Pigs that can clear PRRSV early have early expression of these cytokines.[160] Five of the 13 nsps were found to inhibit IFN-β promoter activation, particularly nsp1β[161] as well as TNF-α promoter activity.[162] One of the mechanisms to suppress the immune response would be to suppress several key immune regulatory cytokines, such as type IFN, IL-1, TNF-α, IL-12, and IL-6, and upregulate to aberrant levels the antiinflammatory cytokines IL-10.[162]

IFN-α is an early response to PRRSV, but the virus circumvents the host innate response with an inadequate production of type I IFNs, resulting in a delayed IFN-γ production, cellular immunity, and neutralizing antibodies and a delayed viral clearance.[163]

PRRSV is able to suppress the transcription of key antiviral genes, TNF-α and IFN-β, when infection was antibody-dependent enhanced. This pathway of infection allows PRRSV to specifically target antiviral genes and alters the innate intracellular immune responses in macrophages.[164]

The proposed model of how PRRSV nsp1 negatively regulates IFN-β has been shown.[165] Plasmacytoid dendritic cells are not present in large numbers in blood but, when exposed to viruses, usually morph into dendritic cells but not when exposed to PRRSV and may help in the persistence of the virus.[166]

In the bone marrow–derived monocyte cells, there was also a significantly increased secretion of IL-1, IL-6, IL-8, IL-10, and IFN-γ but not IL-12 or TNF-α.[167]

Infection with PRRSV increased serum levels of IL-1β, IL-6, TNF-α and IFN-γ. It also increased mRNA for the proinflammatory cytokines as well as the mRNA for TLR3, LR4, and TLR7 in the tracheobronchial tree. Most of the proinflammatory genes were also upregulated in the discrete brain areas.[168]

PRRSV does not elicit a specific IFN-γ response in nonadult animals, and IFN-γ cells may be present in similar numbers in both infected and control animals.[169] PRRSV suppresses T-cell recognition of infected macrophages.[170]

The ORF1a and ORF1b are translated to generate polyproteins, which are processed by viral proteases to form 14 different nsps.[7] Several of the nsps have been identified as integral members of viral replication and transcription machinery, whereas others might be involved in these processes through their interaction with host cell factors.[7,171] The nsps are also likely to regulate viral pathogenesis through their involvement in modulation of host innate immune responses. The nsp1β-mediated subversion of the host innate response plays an important role in PRRSV pathogenesis.[172]

The type I IFNs constitute a major player of the host innate immune system Viral replication intermediates like double-stranded RNA (dsRNA) are sensed by cytoplasmic (RIG-1–like helicases) as well as endosomal (TLR3) sensors, which trigger a complex signaling cascade.[173,174] These signaling events result in an activation of several transcription factors including interferon regulatory factor 3 (IRF3), nuclear factor kappa B ($NF\text{-}_{\kappa\beta}$) and activating transcription factor-2. These factors drive expression of type I IFN genes. Once secreted, they bind to receptors on the cell surface, which ultimately leads to the synthesis of IFN-stimulated genes.[175] Viruses have produced several measures to counteract the IFN production,[176] and PRRSV infection results in poor type I IFN production. The nsps of PRRSV inhibit IFN-dependent transcription. The nsp1α and nsp1β proteins suppress both IRF3 and $NF\text{-}_{\kappa\beta}$–mediated IFN gene induction.[148,177,178] The nsp1β also interferes with IFN signaling.[148,179] The nsp2 is likely to play an important role in the subversion of innate antiviral defenses and provides a basis for elucidating the mechanisms underlying

PRRSV pathogenesis.[180] The PRRSV nsp2 has a cysteine protease domain at its N terminal, which belongs to the ovarian tumor protease family and which appears to antagonize the type I IFN induction.[181]

It also interferes with the activation and signaling pathway of type I IFNs by blocking nuclear translocation.[179] Certain regions of nsp2 are nonessential for PRRSV replication but may play an important part in modulation of the host immunity.[148] PRRSV nsp2 interferes with NF-$_\kappa\beta$ signaling, which is important for its activation.[181] The virus lasts up to 5 months after infection in some lymphoid tissues. The levels of proinflammatory cytokines are also low, and the development of other effector components is slow (neutralizing antibodies and antigen-specific T cells). Therefore there is an inappropriate suboptimal initial innate response to PRRSV.[182] A nonsuppressive PRRSV virus could therefore be expected to stimulate a strong adaptive immune response.[183] The IFN inhibitory nature of PRRSV nsp1 in the context of virus infection was confirmed.[175,184,185] The nsp1 is cleaved into nsp1α and nsp1β, and the nsp1β has the ability to inhibit IFN synthesis and signaling.[186]

Type I IFNs (IFN-α and IFN-β) promote production of antiviral mediators and elicit NK-cell activity for killing viral-infected cells. They also induce the maturation of dendritic cells into antigen presenting cells, macrophage development, and maturation and together with IL-6 convert B cells into plasma cells.[187] How this might be achieved by the PRRSV has been suggested.[178,181,188] Increased levels of IFN-α at the time of challenge delays PRRSV viremia[189] and lessens the severity of the disease. That the presence of IFN-α at the time of infection can alter the innate and adaptive immune responses was confirmed.[190]

PRRSV encodes viral products that are able to suppress type I IFN production in different ways by interfering with the various transcription factors in the regulation of IFN expression.[172,180,181,190-192] The impairment of type I IFN induction seems to be linked to a weak adaptive immunity, which includes a delayed or slow development of humoral and cellular immunity responses leading to viral persistence in infected pigs.[193,194] Pigs infected with PRRSV had moderate interstitial pneumonia, and the virus was found in all tested tissues. Peak antibody response and IFN-γ occurred at 30 DPI with increased TGF-β until 60 DPI.[128]

The nsp2 inhibits the antiviral function of IFN-stimulated gene (ISG) 15.[195] IFN-stimulated genes are the ISGs of which ISG15 is one of the most highly expressed proteins that functions as an effector molecule in the host cell response to viral infection.

The induction of the IL-10 response may be one of the strategies used by PRRSV to modulate the host immune responses.[158] Increases in IL-4, IFN-γ, and TNF-α were found in the lymphocytes of infected piglets, but IL-8 showed a decrease. It has been shown that T cells show an increase in CD8+ CD4+ and CD4− CD8+ subsets within activated cells, whereas CD4+ CD8− cells decreased with time. T cells responding to the virus showed a Th1-type cytokine production pattern. There is also a reported decrease in TNF-α and a decrease of IL-1α and macrophage inflammatory protein. Perhaps this is the key to PRRSV infections in that all pigs may respond differently. There may be either depressive or stimulatory effects. The imbalance of IL-12 and IL-10 produced in PRRSV-infected pigs may favor the humoral responses and suppress cell-mediated immune responses for the first 2 weeks of life.

DIFFERENTIAL EFFECTS IN DIFFERENT PARTS OF THE BODY

The differential expression of proinflammatory cytokines in the lymphoid organs of PRRSV-infected pigs has been described.[196] The expression was different in the different body compartments. IL-1α and TNF-α were the most highly expressed in the mediastinal lymph nodes. IL-6 was most expressed in the retropharyngeal lymph nodes, but none was expressed in the tonsil. Proinflammatory cytokines are able to modulate the expression of CD163, a hemoglobin scavenger receptor that also acts as a PRRSV receptor and is involved in viral uncoating.[197] Whereas IL-6 can upregulate this receptor expression, TNF-α can downregulate it, inhibiting PRRSV replication. The imbalance in cytokines may play a role in the susceptibility to PRRSV replication.

Recombinant porcine IFN-α given to cells before infection reduced the cytopathogenicity of PRRSV, and viral propagation and antibody responses were delayed. It might be that the IFN alleviated damage to the immune system or enhanced the propagation of host cytotoxic T lymphocytes.[198]

Cytokine expression by macrophages in the lungs of pigs infected with PRRSV has been described.[122] Expression of IL-1α, IL6, and TNF-α correlated with the severity of pulmonary pathology and the numbers of pulmonary macrophages. Significant correlations were found between PRRSV infection and the expression of IL-12p40 and IFN-γ and between the expression of TNF-α and IFN-γ. These findings suggest that PRRSV modulates the immune response by the upregulation of IL-10, which may in turn reduce the expression of cytokines involved in viral clearance (IFN-α, IFN-γ, IL-12p40, and TNF-α). The results also suggest that expression of IFN-γ is stimulated by IL-12p40 and TNF-α but not IFN-α. All of these cytokines were expressed mainly by septal macrophages with weaker expression by alveolar macrophages, lymphocytes, and neutrophils. There appears to be a differential activation of septal and alveolar macrophages in PRRSV infection, with septal macrophages as the major source of cytokines.

There is probably a regulatory role of PRSSV ORF1A on porcine alveolar gene expression.[199]

The expression of PRRSV antigens is correlated with the expression of regulatory cytokines such as IL-10 and TGF-β in the lungs of pigs.[122,154] There are no substantial changes in the level of serum proinflammatory cytokines. Expression of proinflammatory cytokines were increased in mediastinal lymph nodes, but there was little increase in the tonsils and retroperitoneal lymph node.[196]

DIFFERENTIAL EFFECTS OF DIFFERENT STRAINS

There is a differential expression of cytokines by different PRRSV isolates[121] and within different lymphoid organs.[196]

The virulence of these strains may be caused by the impairment of TNF-α by inhibiting the ERK signaling pathway.[200] The limited expression of TNF-α with some strains of PRRSV may be a mechanism in which some are able to impair the host immune response and prevent viral clearance. These downregulations have been associated with nsps1α and 1β and 2.[148]

TGF-β and IL-10 are immunomodulatory cytokines that are able to downregulate the host response. An increased mRNA and protein expression of TGF-β has been observed in PRRSV infection with the North American type II PRRSV.[122,138,201] There is an enhanced expression of TGF-β protein in lymphoid organs and the lung following PRRSV, and this may be important because it is an immunomodulatory cytokine.[202]

In some cases new strains can induce a preferential cytokine profile,[203] and the experimental results show a defective pattern of both innate and adaptive immunity that underlies the long-term persistence of PRRS-infected pigs. Both serum-neutralizing antibody and IFN-γ secreting cells were defective in experimental infections.[204]

On the other hand, in the field, there are complex interactions of virus/host further complicated by interactions with bacterial agonists such as LPS. Under field conditions there was poor or no development of a specific IFN-γ response rather than a delayed one.[170,205] Type 2 isolates are more pneumovirulent than type 1 isolates as seen by clinical signs and macroscopic and microscopic lesions.[206]

Genotype 2 strains of PRRS are more efficient at escaping the intrinsic antiviral activity induced by type I and type II IFNs. Monocyte-derived macrophages can be used by the virus instead of alveolar macrophages.[207]

In a study comparing 39 isolates, there were different effects depending on the strain and the host cell infected.[121] All strains produced high levels of IL-1 and IL-8 in macrophage cultures but could be differentiated in their responses with IL-10 and TNF-α.

STRAIN VARIATIONS

A comparative analysis of the immune response in experimental infections with three strains of PRRSV showed that although the outcome of infection was similar with clearance at 33 DPI, there were differences in the immune response to the viruses. The "Lena" strain produced fever and clinical signs, whereas the Lelystad virus and Belgium strain A did not. It also resulted in high virus titers in serum, low numbers of IFN-γ secreting cells, a change in leukocyte populations, and a delayed antibody response to immunization with Aujeszky's disease virus. Levels of IL-1β, IFN-α, IL-10, IL-12, TNF-α, and IFN-γ mRNA of the Lena-infected pigs were also increased but not in the other two infections.[208]

The phenotypic modulation and cytokine profiles of antigen presenting cells infected with European type subtype 1 and 3 PRRSV strains in vitro and in vivo was described.[209] The subtype 3 strains (largely Eastern European, e.g., the Lena strain) are more virulent than the type 1 strains. Bone marrow–derived dendritic cells and alveolar macrophages were infected. The Lena strain caused more apoptosis and a higher level of infectivity and some downregulation of the cell-surface molecules. These facts may have explained the increased pathogenicity of the Lena strain and have dampened the specific immune responses. This could explain the delayed and decreased adaptive immune responses observed after infections with this strain.

The effect of genotypic and biotypic differences among PRRS viruses on the serologic assessment of pigs for virus infection has shown that[210] all of the pigs inoculated with field virus became seropositive (indirect fluorescent antibody [IFA] and ELISA). There was a great deal of variation in the onset and level of serum virus neutralization antibody in individual pigs and with each virus. The authors concluded that biotype differences may affect the kinetics of humoral immune response.

Recent studies have suggested that the new strain (Lena) replicates more efficiently than the old Lelystad virus in nasal mucosal explants. This is probably caused by the use of a broader population of entry receptor cells.[211]

HIGH PATHOGENICITY PORCINE REPRODUCTIVE AND RESPIRATORY SYNDROME PATHOGENESIS

Classical PRRS produces apoptosis in a variety of organs including lungs, testes, lymph nodes, and thymus. Apoptotic changes in peripheral immune organs and lungs, following experimental infection of piglets with highly pathogenic and classical PRRS, have been described.[212] Previous reports have suggested that HP-PRRS induces thymic atrophy with related thymocyte apoptosis, but there have been no reports in other tissues. The HP-PRRS exhibited much greater cell tropism than the usual PRRS and led to serious injury in tonsil, spleen, and lymph nodes. There were large numbers of apoptotic cells in the organs examined. In HP-PRRS alone, in comparison with vaccinated pigs receiving HP-PRRS, piglets showed thymus atrophy, decreased serum levels of IL-4, and increased serum levels of IL-10 and IFN-γ. The results suggested that elevated IL-10 levels at the early stage of infection may enhance viral survival and delay the onset of protective immunity.[213] The HP-PRRSV affects all stages of production. Pregnant sows manifest abortion and give birth to weak and stillborn piglets, and there are morbidity and mortality rates of 50% to 100%.

DEVELOPMENT OF LESIONS

There was also a temporary immunosuppression in piglets at about 4 weeks postinfection. Vascular lesions associated with PRRSV infection are analogous to those observed in horses with equine arteritis virus, which is also a member of the Arteriviridae family, and the renal lesions of equine viral arteritis infection correspond to those of PRRSV. Inflammatory infiltrates are seen at the junction of the renal cortex and medulla, with vascular changes associated with the muscular tunics of small arterioles.

The characteristic lesions can be reproduced in conventional pigs at 1 week, 4 weeks, or 10 weeks of age, and the variation in severity of clinical disease can be attributed to differences in strain virulence. The effects of the virus on reproductive performance are also strain dependent. There is no evidence that virus will grow in the ovarian tissues but may be taken into them by circulating macrophages. PRRSV can replicate in the testicular germ cells, but there is no evidence that there is any PRRSV in ova, indicating that the female gonad is resistant to persistent infection. Some strains are of low pathogenicity, whereas others are highly pathogenic. The reproductive disease has been reproduced experimentally, and the effects on the fetus are dependent on the stage of gestation. Aerosol exposure of nonimmune pregnant gilts to the Lelystad virus in late gestations (84 days) results in clinical disease. After an incubation period of 4 to 7 days, all sows are inappetent and listless for 6 to 9 days. Some sows develop blue-colored ears accompanied by abdominal respirations. Sows may farrow at days 116 and 117 of gestation, giving birth to dead, mummified, and live piglets. Many of the live-born piglets are pale, listless, and weak, and some are in respiratory distress and exhibit varying degrees of splayleg or muscular tremors. The virus may be isolated from stillborn piglets or those born alive. Antibody is present in precolostral serum samples or ascitic fluids of piglets, which demonstrates transplacental passage of the virus.

The gross and microscopic lesions in the fetuses from sows experimentally infected oronasally with the virus at 90 days' gestation consist of hemorrhage of the umbilicus and necrotizing umbilical arteritis with periarterial hemorrhage. Severe pulmonary lesions are present in fetuses inoculated in utero with the virus between 45 and 49 days' gestation. Even the lowest PRRSV exposure dose caused reproductive failure in naive, unvaccinated animals. When sows are inoculated oronasally with the virus in midgestation, the virus does not readily cross the placenta but replicates in fetuses that are inoculated directly in midgestation. It is suggested in prenatal piglets that PRRS replicates primarily in lymphoid tissues, having gained access to them from the placenta via the bloodstream. Thus the fetuses are more susceptible in late gestation than earlier in midgestation, or there is greater likelihood of transplacental infection during late gestation. Experimentally, the intrauterine inoculation of the virus into gilts on the day after natural breeding may have little or no effect on their reproductive performance. There appears to be no direct or indirect effect on luteal function contributing to PRRSV-induced abortion. The virus may cause cell death directly, such as the alveolar macrophages, or in lymphoid tissues. PRRSV affects Marc 145 cells, which undergo necrosis at a much higher rate than apoptosis, and increases with virus levels used to infect the cells. Apoptosis does occur in PRRSV-infected cells, but it is a late event during PRRSV replication and rapidly results in a necrotic-like death. Lesions have been seen in the placenta and in the vessels of the umbilical cord, but these are rarely reported with European strains, although they may be more common with the North American strains.

The original descriptions of porcine necrotizing pneumonia (PNP) were associated with swine influenza, but more recent research has shown that PRRSV is consistently and predominantly associated with PNP and should be considered the key etiologic agent for PNP together with PCV2.

The pathogenesis of a Korean type 1 PRRSV in experimentally infected pigs has been described.[214] Infected pigs developed multifocal, tan-mottled areas of lung. Microscopic lesions were multifocal, mild to moderate, and generally most extensive at 5 to 7 DPI and were nearly resolved by 28 DPI. PRRSV nucleic acid was detected in cytoplasm of macrophages and type 1 and II pneumonocytes.

HIGH PATHOGENECITY PROCINE REPRODUCTIVE AND RESPIRATORY SYNDROME RESPONSES

HP-PRRSV infection could impair TNF-α production by inhibiting the ERK signaling pathway.[215]

In HP-PRRS the marked inappetence and severe respiratory signs are related to the severe interstitial pneumonia and high levels of expression of IL-1α in the lungs compared with other PRRSV strains.[215]

High pathogenicity PRRSV displays an expanded tissue tropism in vivo suggesting that this may contribute to its high pathogenicity. Positivity was recorded in macrophages in lymphoid organs but also in the epithelium including gastric mucous membrane and mucous glands.[216]

The HP-PRRS epidemic in China, the so-called high fever disease with nervous signs, has been on the increase in China since 2009. There was a nonsuppurative encephalitis with lymphohistiocytic perivascular cuffing and infiltration of leukocytes into the neuropil. The electron microscope showed that the virus that infected the endothelial cells crossed the blood-brain barrier into the central nervous system (CNS) and then induced cellular damage to the neurons and neuroglial cells.[217]

An HP-PRRSV strain (HuN4) was shown to produce a loss of appetite, decrease in BW, raised body temperature, and respiratory signs. Lesions were of multifocal interstitial pneumonia with macrophage infiltration. The lesions in the lymph nodes were characterized by collapsed follicles, depletion of germinal centers, and reduction in lymphocytes. Perivascular cuffing and glial nodules were observed in some brains. PRRSV was detected in macrophages, alveolar epithelial cells, and vascular endothelial cells in the tonsil and lymph nodes. It is more pathogenic than some strains because of its higher replication rate.[218]

Chinese and Vietnamese strains of HP-PRRSV cause different outcomes in U.S. swine.[53,218] The Vietnamese virus replicated in an approximately 10-fold lower level in serum than did the Chinese virus. It also produced a lower temperature response and resulted in a lower mortality. The cytokine responses in a 9-plex panel varied between the strains, between the tissues examined, and by the inoculum dose. In this study, also using the U.S. prototype strain VR-2332, all three produced detectable levels of TNF-α, IL-1β, IFN-γ, IL-10, and IL-12p70, but the levels and the kinetics also differed. There was also a high sustained level of IL-10 and IFN-γ, and these might impair effective immune clearance.[53,219,220] Polyclonal B-cell activation can result in IL-10 producing B cells.[221] PRRSV produces a polyclonal activation of B cells accompanied by a hypergammaglobulinemia.[222-224] This leads to deregulated cytokine production.

IMMUNOLOGY

The immune responses generated by PRRSV and control of the disease by immune mechanisms are not yet completely understood.

There are highly conserved T-cell epitopes on nsps9 and 10 of type 2 PRRSV,[225] and these may be important in the formulation of immunogens to provide broad cross-protection against diverse strains of PRRSV.

Inoculation with different PRRSV strains results in different virologic and immunologic outcomes and in different degrees of homologous and heterologous protection.[156] The core effect of the virus is to infect and cause abnormalities in the macrophages. Disturbed macrophages may fail to present antigen successfully. More important, whatever cytokines are present in the pig or are induced by the PRRSV in that particular host may determine the outcome. It was shown that PRRSV is slow to produce both neutralizing antibodies and cell-mediated immunity, but it does produce an IFN response in PRRSV-infected lymphoid tissue.

Following natural infection, most pigs are resistant to subsequent infection, but the mechanisms of protective immunity are not understood. It has been suggested that the immune response to PRRSV has some degree of strain specificity. Indeed, it has also been suggested that the ability to cross the placenta is also strain specific and that although maternal immunity may not prevent transplacental infection, it may exert additional selection pressure. Circulating antibodies to the virus are detectable within 14 and 21 DPI based on indirect immunofluorescence test or ELISA, and 15-kDa protein is the most immunogenic of the viral proteins and may provide the antigenic basis for the development of improved diagnostic tests. However, this response is not of neutralizing antibodies. These may take a long time to develop. At the same time the occurrence of IFN-γ–producing cells is initially weak, but this becomes much stronger from 3 to 6 months after infection. This response may be enhanced by the use of IL-12. Several structural, functionally distinct, and specific antibodies to the virus are generated following infection or vaccination. Cell-mediated immune responses specific to the virus also occur. The relative role of humoral and cell-mediated immunity in providing protection against disease is unknown.

A unique feature of infection is that viremia and circulating antibodies may exist together; the antibodies protect pigs from reinfection and reduce or eliminate shedding of the virus in the semen of boars. Sows are immune to further disease associated with the virus following recovery from acute infection. Following an outbreak of reproductive disease the level of performance will return to normal, suggesting that immunity develops following natural exposure. Protection against subsequent reproductive losses is of long duration in individual animals. However, cross-protection to different strains may not occur. Experimentally infected sows are protected against reproductive losses when challenged with homologous virus over 300 days after initial exposure. Extended studies against homologous infection found that the duration of protection was at least 604 days, which is essentially lifelong protection. Protective immunity was based on two criteria: the absence of transplacental transfer of challenge virus and the apparent lack of virus replication in the dam 21 days following inoculation.

Piglets born from seropositive sows acquire **colostral antibodies** that decline at highly variable rates from 3 to 8 weeks after birth. Passive immunity provides effective immunity for the piglets, but loss of passive immunity at various ages results in susceptible pigs and infection that results in persistence of the virus in pigs 6 to 9 weeks of age, which are considered as the major reservoir of the virus in farrow-finish herds. In the absence of natural infection, maternal antibodies become undetectable between 6 and 10 weeks of age. Some litters do not have maternal antibodies and may not have detectable antibodies until 4 weeks of age, and clinical disease may occur at 2 weeks of age. By 8 weeks of age, antibodies are usually detectable in all pigs and they persist for several months. However, there may be a large variation in the levels of antibodies in piglets at 10 to 12 weeks of age when they are moved to the finishing units. In longitudinal surveys, the seroprevalence of the virus in the 4- to 5-week-old pigs was higher than in the 8- to 9-week-old pigs, and most pigs were negative when they entered the finishing units. In herds where the virus persists, sows did not suffer repeated reproductive losses, indicating that some form of protective immunity develops.

The virus has a predilection for immune cells, and disease manifestations can be linked directly to changes in the immune system. The replication of the virus in the cells of the immune lineage, especially macrophages, may lead to immunosuppression and predispose to secondary infections. Thus immunity to the virus may be a double-edged sword; the virus attacks the immune system, which may cause immunosuppression, while inducing protective antibodies.

Antibody-dependent enhancement of infection may also occur, because low levels of antibody enhance the ability of the virus to enter the pulmonary alveolar macrophage cells and replicate and destroy the cells. This may be important in sucking and nursery pigs exposed to the virus during a period of declining maternal antibody.

PRRSV complicates the ability of the host to respond to infection through several immune evasion mechanisms.[63,226] PRRSV infection is characterized by a delayed appearance of neutralizing antibodies (3–4 months) and a slow development of virus-specific IFN responses. PRRSV nsp2 is increasingly emerging as a multifunctional protein possibly with a profound impact on PRRSV replication and viral pathogenesis.[227] Acquired immunity has been reviewed.[63,184,204,226] After infection, most antibodies are nonneutralizing and are principally targeted to N and nsp2 proteins. Neutralizing antibodies appear from 2 to 4 weeks but do not peak until several weeks to months later. Virus persists in the presence of neutralizing antibody. It is possible that PRRSV produces "decoy" epitopes that produce nonneutralizing antibodies.[228]

The T-cell responses to PRRSV are induced 2 to 8 weeks postinfection and are detected against all structural proteins encoded by ORFs 2 to 7 but are considered to be weak, transient, and highly variable.

GP5 and M are the major proteins of the envelope of PRRSV, and the GP5/M ectodomain peptide epitopes are available for host antibody recognition but are not associated with antibody-mediated virus neutralization.[229]

CLINICAL FINDINGS

The main feature of clinical disease associated with this virus was the extreme variability of the clinical signs. Generally, signs associated with PRRSV appear to result from a combination of genetic factors and herd management characteristics. The relative influences of these two factors differ depending on the specific clinical signs in question. These may vary from inapparent infection to sudden death and abortion storms (the sow abortion and mortality syndrome).

The condition continues to evolve from the first descriptions of mystery swine disease in the United States and Canada and blue-eared pig disease in Europe. The swine mortality and abortion syndrome was then described in the United States. Then, there have been the high pathogenicity cases in China ("high fever disease") characterized with greater than 20% mortality[230-232] and the highly virulent 1-18-2 strain that occurred in the north central United States in 2007.[233]

Concurrent Infections

The increased secondary bacterial infection has been linked to an upregulation of CD14 and LPS-binding protein in PAMs.[234] The effects of the virus on the immune system may explain the suspected immunosuppression and secondary infections, which are recognized clinically but have not been reproduced experimentally.

Its synergism with PCV2 is in doubt. It does not seem to be potentiated by the other great pig pathogen PCV2 virus, but it has been proposed that it may increase the severity of PRRSV-induced interstitial pneumonia. PRRSV infection may enhance PCV2 replication. It is predisposed by MH, and this can be reduced by vaccination for MH. In turn, PRRSV predisposes to *B. bronchiseptica*. Both may interact to reduce the efficiency of lung defense mechanisms and facilitate infection with *P. multocida*. There is little effect on *H. parasuis* secondary infection with a slight increase in macrophage uptake of *H. parasuis* during the early infection, which is reduced after 7 days. There is evidence that concurrent infection with transmissible gastroenteritis virus and PRRSV is likely to have little or no effect on subsequent shedding or persistence of infection. Infection with PRRSV is common in pigs with postweaning multisystemic wasting syndrome (PMWS), but there is no evidence that PRRS is necessary for the development of it. PRRSV has been seen in a swine herd with porcine cytomegalovirus. Synergism between PRRSV and S. Choleraesuis has been described with unthriftiness, rough hair coats, dyspnea, and diarrhea. Pigs that received dexamethasone were the most severely affected and half died, but they also shed significantly more organisms in feces and also had significantly higher PRRSV titers. Simultaneous infection between PRRSV and *S. suis* is much more severe than with either agent on its own. PRRSV-induced suppression of pulmonary intravascular macrophage function may in part explain PRRSV associated susceptibility to *S. suis* infection.

There is also a clear synergism between PRRSV and LPS in the exhibition of respiratory signs in conventional pigs. In these infections with the virus and bacteria, the rise in TNF-α, IL-1, and IL-6 was 10 to 100 times higher than in the single infections. Reproductive failure and respiratory disease are the major clinical findings that are also highly variable between herds. All age groups in a herd may be affected within a short period of time.

Pigs infected with both PRRSV and MH had a greater percentage of pneumonic lung, increased clinical disease, and lower viral clearance than pigs with single infections. There were also increased levels of IL-β, IL-8, IL-10, and TNF-α in lung lavage fluid, and this may be the way that the combined infection increases the pulmonary response.

Clinical disease is often more severe when accompanied by infection with PCV2[1] and is associated with other conditions in the field that often appear as indicators of the underlying PRRSV infection.[135,235] These are mainly caused by the pneumovirulence of the virus and its persistence in lymphoid organs. There is a decrease in NK cell cell–mediated activity caused by a decreased expression of IFN. The adaptive immune response is also impaired, leading to an increased apoptosis of PAMs caused by increased IL-6 and IL-10.[135,236]

Pigs with PRRSV and subsequently exposed to porcine respiratory coronavirus (PRCV) had reduced weight gains, higher incidence of fever, and more severe pneumonia compared with either single infection.[236] This was caused by reduced IFN-α in the lungs and reduced NK cells, and it coincided with the pneumonia. The subsequent PRCV enhanced the level of PRRSV replication in the lung and a tendency to increased serum Th1 activity (IFN-γ) but decreased type II activity (IL-4) responses, further exacerbating the PRRSV pneumonia. More severe alveolar macrophage apoptosis then occurred.

Pulmonary function has been studied in PPRRS-affected pigs.[237] Infected pigs developed fever, reduced appetite, respiratory distress, and dullness within 9 DPI. The noninvasive pulmonary tests revealed airway obstruction, reduced lung compliance, and reduced lung gas transfer. The effects were worst at 9 to 18 DPI in which they were accompanied by an increased respiratory rate and decreased tidal volume. Expiration was affected more than inspiration, and this is caused by airflow limitation predominantly in the peripheral airways. Pigs have both obstructive and restrictive disorders and have shorter breathing cycles and shallower respiration. The energy requirement for breathing increases because of the increased effort.

Infection with the European PRRSV causes CNS disorders in the suckling pig.[238] PRRSV was detected in the macrophages in the cerebrum by IHC.

Reproductive Failure

If 90-day gestational gilts are given vaccine or field strains of PRRSV then some pigs are born dead, most pigs survive, and some pigs are infected in utero. Vaccine strains did not affect postnatal growth, but field strains reduced growth. It may be that the virus entered the reproductive tract through the viremia and then the seeded tissues may release the virus back into the serum at low levels.

The infection of fetuses with an attenuated virus shows the same immune dysfunction as in wild-type infections in piglets kept in isolators.[224]

All sows given IM injections of a mild strain of PRRSV at 90 days' gestation showed transmission of the virus in utero. The proportion of virus-positive pigs and their level of viremia were higher at 4 days of age than at birth or weaning. The findings suggest that monitoring piglets in late lactation will enable assessment of the shedding of the virus from sows.[239]

Landrace gilts when given PRRSV had a significantly reduced number of fetuses but a similar effect in crossbred pigs was not found. The Landrace had less weight loss during pregnancy, suggesting greater tolerance of PRRSV infection. Breeds do differ in phenotypic impacts of PRRSV.[240]

Anorexia, lethargy, depression, and mild fever in pregnant gilts and sows are common initial clinical findings affecting 5% to 50% of animals. This is commonly followed by a sudden increase in early farrowings at 108 to 112 days' gestation, late-term abortions, stillborn and mummified fetuses, partially autolyzed fetuses, weak neonates with high mortality within a few hours or days after birth, late returns to estrus, and repeat breeders. This is generally followed by midgestation abortions and marked increases in the percentage of mummified fetuses, early embryonic death, and infertility. In large herds, successive groups of 10% to 20% of gilts and sows may become anorexic over a period of 2 to 3 weeks. Cyanosis of ears, tails, vulvas, abdomens, and snouts may occur in a small number of sows, which is more common in European outbreaks and uncommon in North America. Following the initial outbreak, a storm of reproductive failure may occur consisting of premature farrowings, late-term abortions, an increase in stillbirths, mummified fetuses, and weak neonates. This second phase of reproductive failure may last 8 to 12 weeks. Stillbirths may reach 35% to 40%. Weak-born piglets die within 1 week and contribute to a high preweaning mortality.

The interaction between PRRSV and the late gestation pig fetus has been described.[113] The major site of replication was the thymus. There were elevated IFN-γ and TNF-α in tissues from infected piglets. The hyperplastic fetal lymph nodes had large numbers of B cells. Fetal infection can alter the selection of PRRSV variants and may represent a source of PRRSV genetic diversity.

The pathogenesis of PRRSV in experimentally infected pregnant gilts has been described.[241] There was a significant increase in apoptotic cells in lung, heart, thymus, liver, adrenal gland, and spleen of stillborn fetuses compared with live-born piglets. The majority of cells were either full of PRRSV or apoptotic but not both. Apoptotic cells outnumbered PRRSV cells. PRRSV may replicate in the fetal implantation sites and cause apoptosis of infected macrophages and the surrounding cells.[242] In a review of the pathogenesis and prevention of placental and transplacental PRRSV infection, it was found that the virus replicates in the endometrium and placenta in late gestation, and this is responsible for the range of PRRSV-related reproductive problems.[243]

PRRSV is shed in the milk of infected sows, and the antigen is present in the in the mammary glands of experimentally infected sows.[244]

Today with the original European strains there may be just outbreaks of rolling inappetence or occasional early farrowings. However, there are serious clinical outbreaks in Italy, Poland, and the UK associated with new variants.

Reproductive disease may be preceded by, or follow, respiratory disease in the breeding herd, finishing pigs, or younger pigs. The reproductive aspect of the disease typically lasts from 4 to 5 months, occupying an entire reproductive cycle within a herd. This is followed by a return to normal performance. Repeated incidents of reproductive failure in individual gilts and sows are unusual, but recurrent episodes may occur in herds purchasing replacement gilts that do not have sufficient immunity.

Vaccinating sows with the North American PRRSV-based modified live vaccine does not prevent reproductive failure after insemination with European PRRSV-spiked semen.[245]

Outbreaks of the disease are characterized by a period of severe reproductive problems in the breeding herd, followed by a return to near normal reproductive performance, punctuated by recurrent episodes of reproductive failure. Most herds eventually return to preoutbreak levels of reproductive performance, but some herds never achieve preoutbreak performance levels.

Boars may also be affected with anorexia, fever, coughing, lack of libido, and temporary reduction in semen quality. PRRSV infection affects seminal quality for a limited period only. The virus can be transmitted to sows through insemination.[238]

Boars naturally coinfected with PRRSV and PCV2 can be found, and at least two different strains of virus from serum and semen can be detected.[246] A group of spontaneously infected boars seroconverted 4 weeks postinfection. There was an increase in the acrosome-defective spermatozoa and sperm motion patterns.[247]

Respiratory Disease

The most important problem facing many of the larger pig industries in the world is PRDC. The most important contributor to this syndrome is PRRSV. The generation of immunity capable of protecting pigs by mediating virus inhibition through virus-neutralizing antibodies or IFN takes time.

Disease occurs in pigs of any age, but especially in nursing and weaned pigs, and is characterized by anorexia, fever, dyspnea, polypnea, coughing, and subnormal growth rates. A bluish discoloration of the ears, abdomen, or vulva may also occur (blue-eared disease). Death may occur in the acute phase. In some herds, up to 50% of pigs are anorexic, up to 10% may have a fever, up to 5% are cyanotic, and up to 30% have respiratory distress. In weanling pigs, the morbidity may be as high as 30%, with a mortality of 5% to 10%. Nursery pigs exhibit respiratory distress and growth retardation. Conjunctivitis, sneezing, and diarrhea are common. All of these signs may appear to move through the various age groups in the herd over several days and a few weeks. The course of the disease in a herd may last 6 to 12 weeks. In gilts and sows of any parity, anorexia and fever, lasting for several days, are noted initially. The acute-phase respiratory disease may last several months but is often followed by a long period of postweaning respiratory disease, which may last up to 2 years. This long course is often accompanied by secondary infections in successive batches of weaned pigs. Unthriftiness may persist throughout the finishing period with an ineffective response to antibiotics and vaccines.

Preweaning morbidity and mortality is a major feature of the disease. Litters are often unthrifty, and many deaths occur within the first week of age.

In a study of a newly established farrow-to-finish farm in Poland that was negative for PRRS on establishment but positive for PCV2, it was found that the conception rate dropped from 89% to 51% and the abortion rate increased from 0.5% to 11.0% with the onset of PRRS infection. Then the mortality was elevated, and clinical disease typical of PMWS occurred. The abortion level returned to normal 4 months later, and the conception rate returned to normal 4 months after that.[248]

CLINICAL SIGNS IN HIGH PATHOGENICITY PORCINE REPRODUCTIVE AND RESPIRATORY SYNDROME VIRUS

Infection with these signs is associated with severe clinical signs, pulmonary lesions, and aberrant host responses.[249,250]

CLINICAL PATHOLOGY

Acute Phase Proteins

Acute phase proteins (APPs) are synthesized by the liver hepatocytes in response to proinflammatory cytokines. They induce inflammatory reactions and fever, but overproduction may produce an antiinflammatory state. PRRSV may not produce an APP response caused by a poor preinflammatory cytokine response. There is an early expression of haptoglobin (modulates immune response and interacts with CD163), which is the receptor for PRRSV, increasing expression of IL-10 (antiinflammatory), and pig major acute protein, but the response of C-reactive protein (CRP; activates complement and opsonization) and serum amyloid A (chemoattractant for monocytes, T cells, and polymorphs) is delayed and variable.[201] The haptoglobin may modulate the immune response and induce the antiinflammatory IL-10.

The CD163 removes the hemoglobin–haptoglobin complexes circulating in the blood and decreases the amount of iron available for bacteria and reduces oxidative stress.

Haptoglobin levels and pig major acute proteins were increased at 10 DPI, but CRP and serum amyloid showed a delayed and highly variable increase. All three proinflammatory cytokines (IL-1β, IL-6, and TNF-α) were poorly expressed, and only a mild increase in IL-1β was observed at 7 DPI. The increased expression of haptoglobin coincided with the light enhancement observed in both IL-6 and TNF-α and might be related with an increased expression of IL-10. The low expression of TNF-α may point to a possible mechanism of viral evasion of the host immune response.[201]

An 8-plex Luminex assay has been developed to detect swine cytokines after vaccination. It will detect innate (IL-1β, IL-8, IFN-α, TNF-α, and IL-12), regulatory (IL-10), Th1 (IL-4), and Th2 (IL-4) cytokines.[251]

PRRSV infection significantly increases the number of alveolar macrophages in bronchoalveolar lavage fluid approximately 10-fold between day 10 and day 21 of infection. Approximately 63% of the cells were cytotoxic T cells (CTLs) and NK cells. Serum haptoglobin levels were increased from 7 to 21 DPI.

Piglets also become anemic in PRRSV infections, and the most highly pneumovirulent strains induced the most severe anemia. This is probably caused by a direct or indirect effect on the erythroid precursor cells of the bone marrow.

A definitive diagnosis requires detection of virus in infected animals and detection of antibodies in fetal fluid or in precolostral blood of stillborn and weak-born piglets. Detection of antibodies in sera of groups of pigs of different ages is also necessary. The most suitable body fluid and tissue samples and diagnostic tests for the etiologic diagnosis of PRRS are dependent on several variables including:

- Age of pigs from which samples are collected
- Stage of infection (acute or persistent)
- Available complement of diagnostic reagents
- Urgency of obtaining results

When congenitally or neonatal pigs are affected, both serum and alveolar macrophages are reliable samples. For older pigs, alveolar macrophages are more reliable than serum.

Detection or Isolation of Virus

The gold standard is the isolation of the virus. A PAM cell line has been developed for the growth of PRRSV.[252]

In an interlaboratory ring trial in Europe to test the real-time RT-PCR tests it was found that there were great differences in the qualitative diagnostics as well as analytical sensitivity. False negatives were a problem, and to achieve maximum safety in the results it was suggested that different assays or kits should be used.[253]

Boars

Serum is the best method to detect PRRSV during an acute infection in boars.[254] Semen samples failed to detect the virus in most cases. Pooling of samples resulted in a decline of sensitivity.

In a study of commercial tests (RT-PCRs) for diverse strains of PRRSV in boars, in serum, semen blood swabs, and oral fluids[255] from experimentally infected animals, it was found that serum and blood swabs had the best performance and highest detection rates. These were at their highest between 3 and 5 DPI. Oral fluids had the lowest detection rates. The virus can be demonstrated by isolation using cell cultures, by direct detection of viral antigen in tissue sections, or by the detection of virus-specific RNA. Two commercial ELISAs and an in-house florescent microbead immunoassay were tested to detect IgG antibodies in serum and oral fluids for both type 1 and type 2 virus. The tests were similar in sensitivity and specificity but the commercial test kit IDEXX Se detected positive animals earlier than the test kit HIPRA Se. The oral fluid and serum had similar detection rates.[256]

Samples used for virus isolation include serum, thoracic fluid, spleen, and lung. Porcine pulmonary alveolar macrophages are used for isolation of virus. Alveolar macrophages using immunofluorescence microscopy can be used for detection of virus during acute infections. The PCR assay is a reliable, sensitive, and rapid test for the detection of virus in boar semen. It can also be used to determine whether suckling piglets are infected with PRRSV before vaccination and for determining the relationship between parity and shedding of virus. It can also be used to obtain PRRSV piglets. PCR followed by RFLP analysis using several restriction enzymes provides a good genetic estimate for isolate differentiation. A reverse transcription and PCR, coupled with a microplate colormetric assay, is an automated system that is a reliable and easy test for the routine detection of the virus in semen samples from seropositive boars. Multiplex RT-nested PCR can be applied to formalin-fixed tissues.

A nested PCR has been described that is 100 to 1000 times more sensitive than the usual PCR. An assessment of the viral load can possibly be made by using the quantitative competitive RT-PCR. A quantitative TaqMan RT-PCR is time-saving, easy to handle, less likely to be cross-contaminated, and highly sensitive and specific. Immunohistochemical techniques are available for the detection of virus in formalin-fixed tissues. The virus was detected in 11% to 23% of animals with interstitial pneumonia. It was found in 21% to 31% of animals less than 3 months of age but in only 6% to 17% of those more than 4 months of age. The immunogold silver staining i s superior to the immunoperoxidase staining systems for detection of virus in formalin-fixed tissues. RT-PCR is also available and can distinguish between North American and European strains.

A double in situ hybridization (ISH) technique has been developed that can show both PRRSV and PCV2 and a small number of alveolar macrophages stain for both antigens.

A rapid detection method using RT-loop mediated isothermal amplification assay has been described.[257,258]

RT-PCRs have been developed for the detection and differentiation of European and U.S. PRRSV.[259,260] These cannot differentiate U.S. and HP-PRRS, but the duplex real-time RT-PCR test developed[261] will do this. The test was also compared with standard single PCRs, and the results were found to be in 98.7% agreement.

A method using phages harboring specific peptides that recognize the N protein of PRRSV has been used to distinguish it from other viruses.[262]

Serology

A recent study has described the production of GP3, GP5, and N-specific hybridomas and an extensive collection of monoclonal antibodies that may help in diagnosis because they reacted with a range of genetically different PRRS viruses.[263] ELISAs differ in their sensitivity, and those that showed higher sensitivity could be used for early detection in individual pigs, especially in PRRSV-free herds.[264]

In a study of the humoral responses in boars measured in serum samples and oral fluid specimens, it was found that IgM, IgA, and IgG were first detected in serum samples collected on DPI 1, 7, and 10, respectively, and in oral fluids from 3 to 7 DPI for IgM, 7 to 10 DPI for IgA, and 8 to 14 DPI for IgG, respectively.[265]

Serologic tests have good sensitivity and specificity for diagnosis on a herd level but less so on the individual animal. The tests in common usage are described below. One of the problems is that the serologic response to a nonvirulent strain is the same as it is to a virulent strain. It is also important to realize that although a positive result for antibody indicates exposure to virus, a negative test does not necessarily mean that the pig is free from PRRSV or has not been in contact with the virus.

Immunoperoxidase Monolayer Assay Test

The immunoperoxidase monolayer assay (IPMA) is often the first test used. Approximately 75% of sows infected with the virus seroconvert to the Lelystad virus. However, the IPMA does not allow for large-scale surveys.

Indirect Enzyme-Linked Immunosorbent Assay (iELISA)

The iELISA is used for the routine serodiagnosis; it is simple, inexpensive, effective, and a better alternative to the indirect immunofluorescent assay or the immunoperoxidase assay. It is suitable for the screening of large numbers of samples and is best used as a herd test. Because of marked differences between and within North American and European virus isolates, serologic tests using only one antigenic type of the virus may potentially yield false-negative results with antisera against diverse antigenic types of the virus. A mixture of ELISA antigens from North American and European strains gives superior results when both types of viruses are known to exist.

A meat juice ELISA has been developed that gives complete agreement with the serum ELISAs.

Unexpected positives have been shown following the use of commercial ELISA testing kits, and these results can be improved by using competitive and blocking ELISA.[266]

A multiplex method for simultaneous serologic detection of PRRS and PCV2 has been described.[267]

Indirect Florescent Antibody Assay (IFAT)

The IFAT is a highly sensitive test. Antibody titers are detectable in infected pigs 8 days after inoculation. The IgM IFAT is also a rapid and simple test for diagnosing recent infection as early as 5 to 28 DPI in 3-week-old piglets, and 7 to 21 DPI in sows.

Modified Serum Neutralization Test

This test is useful for the detection of later and higher levels of antibody when the conventional methods cannot detect antibody. The test can differentiate between strains. The serum neutralization test is not used for routine diagnosis because neutralizing antibodies do not appear early in the infection.

Herd Diagnosis

The serologic diagnosis must be used and applied on a herd basis and acute and convalescent sera submitted for optimal results. A baseline herd sampling is necessary to evaluate the status of a herd and to determine whether and in which groups the virus is circulating. In large herds of over 500 sows, samples are taken from 30 animals in each breeding, gestation, and farrowing group, with representation from all parties. In addition, 10 nursery pigs (5 weeks old), 10 pigs at the end of the nursery period, and 10 pigs in the late finishing stage constitute a **herd profile**. Thus serologic monitoring can be used to monitor the circulation of virus within a closed herd and to determine infection status of breeding animals that are to be introduced into seronegative herds. Results from the sow sera indicate whether the sow herd is virus negative, stable, or has an active virus circulation. Comparison of the early and late nursery pigs indicates if the virus is circulating in the nursery. Comparing the nursery results with the end of the finishing period indicates if the virus is circulating in the finishing groups of pigs. IFAT titers in pigs range from 1:256 to 1:1024 by 2 to 3 weeks after infection. Titers decline over 3 to 4 months unless reintroduced by exposure to circulating virus. Uninfected nursing pigs are negative or have maternal antibody. Seropositive 9- to 10-week-old pigs leaving the nursery indicate virus circulation in the nursery. If pigs leaving the nursery are negative and positive later in the finishing unit, virus circulation is occurring in the finishing unit.

Sera from outbreaks of the disease in the United States, Canada, and Europe have been compared, and although the isolates from both continents are closely related, the strains isolated in the United States and Canada are more closely related serologically than they are to the European strains.

Oral Fluids

Saliva has also been used for haptoglobin and CRP estimations in PRRS-affected pigs under field conditions.[268,269] The values were higher in a conventional herd with chronic PRRS than a specific pathogen-free herd. Increases were also found independently with age. The use of preweaning oral fluid samples detects the circulation of wild-type PRRSV.[270] Overall, preweaning litter oral fluid samples could provide a sensitive approach to surveillance for PRRSV in infected, vaccinated, or presumed negative pig breeding herds.

Antigen Detection

PCR reactions were partially inhibited in the oral fluid matrix compared with RNA extraction, and it should not be assumed that methods designed for use in serum would perform as well in oral fluid.[271-275] Oral fluid testing was found to be useful for virus detection[276] and superior to serum for the detection of PRRSV using PCR over the 21-day observation period of their study. Individually penned oral-fluid sampling could be an efficient, cost-effective way to maintain surveillance in a boar stud.

Serology

An assay was developed and validated for use in oral fluids.[277] A titer of 1:8 in oral-fluid samples was considered to be virus specific and could be detected 28 days after vaccination or infection. It had 94.3% specificity and 90.5% repeatability. The levels were correlated with serum levels.

The IgG oral fluid ELISA can provide efficient, cost-effective PRRSV monitoring in commercial herds and be used in elimination programs.[278] In a study of 100 oral-fluid samples from pens containing positive pig at five levels of PRRSV prevalence tested at six laboratories, it was found that the mean positivity for PRRSV RNA was 62% and for antibodies it was 61%. The study supported the use of pen-based oral-fluid sampling for PRRSV surveillance.[279] An oral fluid assay was ring tested in the United States [280] in 12 laboratories and was found to be highly repeatable and reproducible.

NECROPSY FINDINGS

There is a high level of viremia for 102 weeks, then a lower level for another 2 to 3 weeks, and subsequently low levels of virus may persist for several months, but finally PRRSV is eliminated after 2 to 4 months. PRRSV-specific nonneutralizing antibodies arise quickly from 7 DPI, but low titers of neutralizing antibody are only detected from 25 to 35 DPI. In some pigs, both low levels of replicating virus are found in the presence of neutralizing antibodies. The adaptive cell-mediated immune response is exerted by CTLs and Th cell lymphocytes in cooperation with Th1-activated NK and macrophages. The CTLs may reduce viral replication in the lungs and lymphoid tissue after 2 weeks DPI and in the complete clearance of virus in 2 to 4 months. It was shown that peripheral blood monocytes fail to exert CTL activity toward PRRSV-infected macrophages.[281]

Type 2 PRRSV is more virulent than type 1in the experimental setup with higher mean viral titers and greater macroscopic and microscopic lesions at the same points on a timescale similar to a type 1 virus. Mean numbers of PRRSV-positive cells in lungs and lymph nodes were also higher for the type 2 virus.[282]

Type 2 PRRSV infection mediates apoptosis in B- and T-cell areas in lymphoid organs of experimentally infected pigs, and the increased apoptosis may play a part in the impairment of the host immune response during PRRSV infection.[283]

In a study of three European viruses it was shown that a Belgian strain was more highly pathogenic than the Lelystad virus and a British field strain, not because of increased viral load and better replication but because of an enhanced inflammatory immune response.[284]

A series of postmortem examinations of different aged pigs from different stages of production will reveal what is going on over time. A series of such examinations will probably show more than any other investigations.

No characteristic gross lesions are present in sows, aborted fetuses, or stillborn piglets. Microscopic lesions that may be present in aborted fetuses include vasculitis of the umbilical cord (not recorded in European strain infections) and other large arteries, myocarditis, and encephalitis. Unfortunately, none of these changes is present consistently, and the majority of fetuses and placentas are histologically normal. These lesions are all more common in the North American virus infections.

In suckling and grower pigs, infection with the PRRSV is usually characterized by an interstitial pneumonia. The PRRSV affects both pulmonary intravascular macrophages, which may be important as a replication site, and alveolar macrophages. Loss of bactericidal function in pulmonary intravascular macrophages may facilitate hematogenous bacterial infections. When Danish isolates were injected into piglets, PRRSV was isolated from the lungs and/or tonsillar tissues from both dead and culled piglets under 14 days of age. Tracheobronchial and mediastinal lymph nodes are usually enlarged and firm. The gross pulmonary changes vary from lungs that appear normal but fail to collapse, to lungs that are diffusely red, meaty, and edematous. Porcine proliferative and necrotizing pneumonia has been linked to infection with PRRSV, although the involvement of an unidentified copathogen cannot yet be discounted. Grossly, this form of pneumonia appears as confluent consolidation of the cranial, middle, and accessory lobes, together with the lower half of the caudal lobe. Affected lobes are red-gray, moist, and firm (meaty) in consistency. On cross-section, the affected lobes are bulging and dry, and the pulmonary parenchyma appears similar to thymic tissue.

Generally, histologic lesions in piglets are focal nonsuppurative inflammatory conditions particularly in the lung and heart. Most of the cells undergoing apoptosis do not have markers for PRRSV, which suggests that there is an indirect mechanism for the induction of apoptosis.

Multifocal areas of interstitial pneumonia (more extensive at 10 DPI rather than 21 DPI) were regarded as the structural basis for reduced lung compliance and gas exchange disturbances.[237] There was a cough that the authors interpreted as caused by bronchospasm because there was no evidence of tracheitis, bronchiolitis, or airway mucus, and this was supported by the presence of peripheral airway obstruction. Cell death occurs through both apoptosis and necrosis.[285]

Histologically, in addition to marked proliferation of type II pneumocytes in alveoli, there is severe necrosis of bronchiolar epithelium, with necrotic cellular debris plugging the airway lumina.

In pigs infected with HP-PRRSV, there was a distinct thymus atrophy. The lesions in the thymus were found to have severe cortical depletion of thymocytes. There was a 40-fold increase in apoptosis of thymocytes compared with piglets infected with non–HP-PRRSV at 7 DPI.[286]

In the less severe and more common forms of PRRSV pneumonia, the alveoli contain protein-rich fluid and large macrophages, some of which may appear degenerate. There is patchy thickening of the alveolar septa caused by infiltrating mononuclear leukocytes and mild, type II pneumocyte hyperplasia. Lymphoplasmacytic cuffing of arterioles is common, and syncytial cells are occasionally seen. In field outbreaks, it is usual for the lung pathology to be complicated by concurrent respiratory pathogens.

Microscopic lesions may be found in many other tissues and include multinucleate cell formation within lymph nodes; infiltrates of lymphocytes and plasma cells in the heart, the brain, and the turbinates; and a lymphocytic perivasculitis in various sites. Thymic lesions include severe cortical depletion of thymocytes. An ISH technique is a rapid, highly specific, and sensitive detection method for the diagnosis of PRRS virus in routinely fixed and processed tissues. Immunohistochemical techniques can also be used to detect the virus in neurovascular lesions. PRRSV and reovirus 2 have been found in brain, lung, and tonsil by inoculation into Marc 145 and CPK cells. IHC on one section would give a positive in 48% of cases, but if five sections were studied then there are positives in >90% of PRRSV-infected pigs. If the animals are vaccinated then the positives fall to 14%.

PNP is a common finding in Spain and is characterized by hypertrophy and proliferation of type 2 pneumonocytes and the presence of necrotic cells in the alveolar lumina. PCV2 was found in 85.1% of the cases by ISH and IHC and PRRSV was found in 44.6% of the cases; 39.1% had PCV2 as the sole agent and only 4.1% had PRRSV as the sole agent.[287]

Samples for Confirmation of Diagnosis

Lung appears to be the best tissue for identification of the virus in various ages of the pig and at various times following infection. Thymus is probably the best choice for aborted fetuses.

- **Histology:** lung, tonsil thymus, thoracic lymph node, brain, kidney, heart, (umbilicus from fetus) (light microscopy, immunohistochemistry (IHC)); a monoclonal antibody-based IHC method for the detection of European and U.S. PRRSV was shown to be useful in detecting both types.[288]
- **Virology:** lung, thoracic lymph node, tonsil (virus isolation, fluorescent antibody test (FAT), PCR).

DIFFERENTIAL DIAGNOSIS

Respiratory disease must be differentiated from the following:

- Swine influenza
- Porcine respiratory coronavirus
- Enzootic pneumonia (*Mycoplasma hyopneumoniae*)
- *Actinobacillus pleuropneumoniae*
- *Pasteurella multocida*
- Glasser's disease (*Haemophilus parasuis*)
- *Streptococcus suis*.

Reproductive disease must be differentiated from other causes of abortion, stillbirths, and weak neonates in pigs:

- Leptospirosis
- Encephalomyocarditis virus
- Hog cholera virus
- Pseudorabies virus
- Parvovirus
- Fumonisin, which is a recently identified mycotoxin produced by *Fusarium moniliforme*, has been associated with the appearance of PRRS in swine herds in the United States

A definitive diagnosis requires a detailed epidemiologic investigation of the epidemic including a detailed analysis of the breeding and production records for the previous several months, and the submission of tissue and serum samples for laboratory investigation.

TREATMENT

There is no specific treatment against the virus. In outbreaks of respiratory disease, mortality can be reduced by ensuring that the environmental conditions in the barns and pens are adequate, the stocking density is kept low, and the feeds and feeding programs are monitored. Routine procedures such as tail docking, iron injections, castrations, teeth clipping, and cross-fostering should be delayed or not done during the acute phase of the disease. Supplemental heat for neonatal pigs should be provided if necessary. Sows that have aborted their litters should not be bred until the normal time of weaning. This will reduce the incidence of infertility common at the first estrus after the abortion or premature farrowing. Culling of sows should be minimized and weekly breedings increased by 10% to 15%. Replacement gilts may be introduced into the premises for exposure to infection before breeding. The consequences of boar infertility and low libido may be minimized by use of artificial insemination or by using multiple sires on each sow. Recurrent illness and secondary infections in weaner and growing pigs can be continuing problems for a few months after an acute outbreak. Reducing the stocking density and an all-in/all-out strategy have been successful in reducing the chronic problem. If there is the possibility of treating secondary infections, then this should be undertaken. Serum inoculation of naive gilts has been described, and this was shown to be capable of stabilizing sow herds, as shown by the production of negative weaned pigs.

Tylvalosin, a macrolide antibiotic, and to some extent tilmicosin inhibit the in vitro replication of European and American PRRSV possibly by raising the endosomal pH (PRRSV requires a low endosomal pH).[289]

A report has suggested that *N*-acetylpenicillamine will inhibit PRRSV replication.[290]

CONTROL

It is the stealthy nature of PRRSV infection and its efficient transmission that has prevented elimination.[291] The challenges of control have resulted in the development of regional control systems.[292,293] These involve cooperation in a region, new technologies, and the demonstration that PRRSV has been eliminated.

The potential role of noncommercial swine populations in the United States in the spread of PRRSV have been highlighted.[294] They comment on the lack of knowledge of biosecurity in this group of swine herders, the practice of showing pigs at many events, evidence that exposure to PRRS is very frequent, and close interactions with commercial herds and that these facts make it necessary to involve these groups in regional control.

Control of PRRSV is difficult, unreliable, and frustrating because of the complexity of the disease; the uncertainty of some aspects such as immunity, persistence, diagnosis, and the lack of published information based on control programs have been evaluated under naturally occurring field conditions. Much of the information available on control is anecdotal and not based on well-designed control programs that can be compared and evaluated. A major problem is the difficulty of obtaining a definitive etiologic diagnosis when presented with young growing pigs with respiratory disease and the possibility that other pathogens could be involved. The diagnosis of reproductive failure in gilts and sows is also commonly uncertain.

Some characteristics of the disease are important in planning control programs for individual herds:

- Infection is highly contagious and is transmitted by direct contact. Nonimmune pregnant gilts and sows and young pigs are highly susceptible to infection, resulting in large economic losses.
- Infection of breeding stock results in immunity. The efficacy of vaccination is not well established.
- Maternal immunity is present in piglets born from seropositive sows.
- Infection can persist for many weeks and months in individuals and in subpopulations of animals.
- Infections are usually introduced into a herd by the introduction of infected pigs.

There are two main options for control: eradication of the virus from individual swine herds and controlling the disease in individual herds to create a stable positive system that allows to live with the disease. Controlling the disease requires developing strategies to make pigs immune to the infection by controlling infection pressure in the herd and inducing naturally acquired immunity in the herd or inducing acquired immunity through vaccination. The recommendations for control set out here are guidelines that can be applied and modified to meet different circumstances.

Dietary plant extracts (capsicum, garlic, and turmeric) improve immune responses and growth efficiency of pigs experimentally infected with PRRSV.[295]

FILTRATION SYSTEMS

A production region model was used to assess the spread of PRRSV[296] and showed the importance of aerosol spread. More than 30 swine systems in the Midwest have remained free from PRRSV for 2 to 3 years following implementation of an air-filtration system using MERV 16 filters, and this system should be regarded as the gold standard.[297-299]

Retrograde air movement is a real risk for PRRSV introduction into filtered airspaces in animal houses, and different treatments have been investigated.[300]

In a study of before and after filtration it was found that outbreaks occurred at a rate of 0.5 outbreaks a year before filtration, but after the risk was reduced by introducing air filtration the outbreaks were reduced to 0.06 to 0.22 outbreaks a year.[301]

The financial implications of air-filtration systems have been studied.[302] Model outputs suggested that the filtered farm produced 5927 more pigs on a 3000-sow farm and paid for the installations within 5.35 to 7.13 years, depending on the sow herd productivity. If there was a premium of $5 per PRRS-negative piglet, then the payback period was reduced to 2.1 to 2.8 years.

Eradication of the Virus From the Herd

Depopulation and Repopulation

Eradication of the virus from the herd by depopulation of the entire herd followed by repopulation with virus-free breeding stock is biologically possible, but in most cases it is impractical and too expensive. Obtaining virus-free breeding stock is usually not possible and, if possible, the herd is highly susceptible to accidental reinfection.

Control in Infected Herds

Nursery Depopulation

Control within a breeding herd is based on the observation that pigs commonly seroconvert to the virus during the nursery period. Pigs are seronegative shortly after weaning, but 80% to 100% are seropositive at 8 to 10 weeks of age. A control program based on **nursery depopulation** consists of emptying the nurseries and moving **all of the pigs** to off-site finishing facilities or selling them as feeder pigs. Test and removal has been described. This is combined with batch farrowing and weaning at intervals of at least 3 weeks. The nurseries are completely emptied, cleaned three times with hot water and disinfectant, the slurry pits are pumped out after each cleaning, and the facilities are kept empty for 14 days, during which time all pigs weaned are moved to off-site nurseries and after which the conventional flow of pigs into the cleaned facilities is resumed. The control program can result in significant improvements in both average daily gain and percentage mortality, but it will not eliminate the virus from the herd. Using a partial budget model to measure the profitability of nursery depopulation, the financial consequences indicate that it is a profitable strategy to improve pig performance in herds affected with the virus. Additional income is generated by the increased number and weight of marketable pigs, as a result of their increased growth rate and decreased mortality. Lower treatment costs reduce overall expenses, but there are additional costs because of the extra feed necessary to raise the additional pigs and the costs required to house the depopulated pigs. However, it is possible that the economic benefits are from the control of other pathogens and not merely the PRRS virus.

Table 18-4 Nursey depopulation and cleanup protocol for elimination of PRRS

Day	Procedure
1	Empty all nurseries, off-site wearing, pump out slurry pits, clean and wash rooms with hot water (>95° C, 203° F), and disinfect with formaldehyde-based product; allow disinfectant water to remain in pits overnight
2	Pump out pits, repeat washing procedure, and disinfect in phenol-based product; allow disinfectant to remain in pits
311	Allow facility to remain vacant
12	Pump out slurry pits, repeat washing procedure, and disinfect with formaldehyde-based product
13	Allow facility to remain vacant
14	Resume conventional flow of pigs into clean nurseries

The details for nursery depopulation and cleanup protocol for the elimination of the virus are shown in Table 18-4.

In an experimental infection with PRRSV, it was found that the infected pigs had greater serum concentrations of IL-1β, TNF-α, IL-12, IFN-γ, IL-10, and haptoglobin than sham controls. The results indicated that PRRSV-stimulated secretion of cytokines involved in innate, Th1, and T-reg immune responses. Mannan oligosaccharides regulated the expression of nonimmune and immune genes in pig leukocytes[303] and were able to enhance the immune response without overstimulation. Mannan oligosaccharide-containing compounds were found to decrease the levels of the serum TNF-α. The levels of IL-1β and IL-12 may help to promote innate and T-cell immune functions.[304]

Management of the Gilt Pool

Management of the gilt pool is the single most important strategy for long-term effective control. Controlling the infection in the breeding herd is a prerequisite to controlling infection in the nursery and finishing pig groups. Strategies like partial depopulation and piglet vaccination are ineffective unless the breeding herd is first stabilized, preventing piglets from becoming infected before weaning. Replacements are a major source of introduction of the virus and activating existing virus in the breeding herd. They also initiate the formation and maintenance of breeding herd replacements.

Subpopulations are subsets of naive or recently infected gilts or sows that coexist within chronically infected herds. These subpopulations perpetuate viral transmission in the breeding herd and farrowing units, which ultimately produces successions of infected piglets before weaning. Modifications in gilt management that may minimize subpopulations include ceasing introduction of replacement animals for a 4-month period, beginning to select replacements from the finishing unit, or introducing a 4-month allotment of gilts at one time.

Exposure to the virus in the breeding herd can be controlled by managing the gilt pool using two strategies. In one strategy, herds may be closed to outside replacements, and replacement males and females are raised on the farm. In the other strategy, replacement gilts are held in an off-site holding facility from 9 to 12 weeks of age until breeding age at 7 to 7.5 months, or even much earlier. This is combined with nursery depopulation as described earlier. Before entry of the gilts into the herd, they are serologically tested for evidence of seronegativity or a declining titer, which is required for entry into the herd. The gilts are isolated and quarantined for acclimatization for 45 to 60 days. This may be combined with two vaccinations, 30 days apart, after entering quarantine. This method reduces the risk of introducing potentially viremic animals into the existing population. The method selected will depend on the production system, management capabilities, and facilities available on each farm. The introduction of younger gilts, in larger groups, less frequently throughout the year, is being recognized as the most effective method for introducing replacement stock to virus-infected herds and long-term control of the disease.

Controlled Infection of Breeding Herd

The presence of subpopulations of highly susceptible breeding animals in the herd can be a major risk factor for maintaining viral transmission within problem herds and may explain recurrent outbreaks of reproductive failure. By intentionally exposing all members of a population to the virus, it may be possible to eliminate subpopulations and produce consistent herd immunity. In endemic herds, exposure of gilts to the virus before breeding is critical for prevention of reproductive failure. Seronegative replacement gilts can be introduced into seropositive herds at 3 to 4 months of age to allow for viral exposure before breeding. If the status is uncertain, quarantine and exposure to nursery pigs of the importing unit is a suitable policy if replacement gilts are bought in before they are bred. It is possible to convert a PRRS-positive unit to a negative herd by managing the gilt pool and regulating the pig flow. It appears that PRRSV infection eventually either disappears or becomes inactive in the donor gilt population. Similarly, serum from nursery pigs (thought to be PRRSV viremic) given to negative replacement gilts resulted in seroconversion of all 50 gilts receiving the serum.

Control of Secondary Infections

When outbreaks of the disease occur in nursing piglets, and virus circulation is occurring continuously in the farrowing facility, the following are recommended:

- Cross-foster piglets only during the first 24 hours of life
- Prevent movement of pigs and sows between rooms
- Eliminate the use of nurse sows
- Euthanize piglets with low viability
- Minimize injections of suckling pigs
- Stop all feedback of pig and placental tissues
- Follow strict all-in/all-out pig flow in the farrowing and nursery rooms.

These are similar to the system developed in the United States called the McRebel system. This was a method of control showing that cross-fostering of piglets should be minimal within the first 24 hours and banned after this time.

Feedback has been tried, although there are a lot of reasons not to do so. Minced whole piglets were fed to sows and the herd then closed for 23 weeks. No clinical signs were observed. One-third of the sows present at the time of the outbreak were still seropositive 20 months after the deliberate infection. Disinfection at cold temperatures was described.

Biosecurity

Standard methods, such as quarantining and serologic screening of imported breeding stock and restrictions on visitors, are recommended to keep units free of infection. Control of infection between herds depends on restricting the movement of pigs from infected herds to uninfected herds. If pigs have to be bought in, then seropositive animals should be imported into seropositive herds. Only seronegative boars should be allowed entry into artificial insemination units.

Biosecurity practices regarding PRRSV have been investigated in Quebec in two areas of different swine density. A questionnaire was sent to 125 breeding sites and 120 growing sites. The frequency of biosecurity practices ranged from 0% to 2% for a barrier at the site entrance, 0% to 19% for showering, 20% to 25% for truck washing between loads, 51% to 57% for absence of rendering or rendering without access to the site, and 26% to 51% for absence of gilt purchase or purchase with quarantine. Better practices were found in the breeding herds. In the high-density area, there was a lower level of biosecurity on the growing sites. There were two patterns of biosecurity, a low one and a high one. For the breeding sites the higher pattern was observed when the site was away from other pig sites, more than 300 m from a public road, with a higher number of sows or being part of integrated production.[305] In a second part of the study, on prevalence and risk factors, it was found that the overall prevalence of PRRS was 74.0%. Four main factors were associated with PRRS positivity, and these were large pig inventory, proximity to closest site (16%), absence of shower (27%), and free access to the site by the rendering truck (10%).[305] Boar studs that are free should only import boars that are certified free from tested herds. The status of the boar stud should be tested every 2 weeks with a combination of ELISA and PCR.

Testing protocols that used PCR on serum detected the PRRSV introduction earlier than the protocols that used PCR on semen, and these were earlier than those that used ELISA on serum. The most intensive protocol (testing 60 boars three times a week by PCR on serum) would need 13 days to detect 95% of the PRRSV introductions.[306]

A vaccination study using a modified live PRRSV vaccine on European and North American PRRSV shedding from boars showed that boar vaccination decreased the shedding of U.S. PRRSV but not the European strain.[307]

Vaccine and Vaccination

The inefficiency of current vaccines to cross-protect against all strains of PRRSV may be caused by variability within GP5.[2]

Adjuvants for use in PRRSV vaccines have been reviewed.[308] Of 11 adjuvants tested 5 enhanced cell-mediated immunity to PRRSV. In particular, IL-12 and CpG ODN significantly enhanced the protective efficacy of PRRSV vaccines in challenge models. The immunostimulatory oligodeoxynucleotides have been used previously.[309]

TLR ligands enhance the protective effects of vaccination against PRRS syndrome in swine using killed vaccines.[310]

Vaccination with a combined PRRSV/MH vaccine did not differ in protective efficacy compared with the protective efficacy of the two single vaccines. This indicates that neither vaccine interfered with each other.[311]

Vaccine efficacy of PRRSV chimeras has been described,[312] and the study suggested that only specific chimeras can attenuate clinical signs in swine and that attenuation cannot be directly linked to primary virus replication.

Pigs infected with PRRSV at the time of vaccination for swine influenza had an increased level of macroscopic and microscopic pneumonia, suggesting that there was a reduced SIV vaccine efficiency.[313] In addition, there was also increased clinical disease and shedding of SIV during the acute phase of SIV infection.

Immunologic solutions for the treatment and prevention of PRRSV have been reviewed.[314] No differences were found between intradermal and IM vaccinated pigs and those subsequently exposed to a heterologous Italian strain.[315]

The antibody response and the maternal immunity when PRRSV-immune sows were boosted with experimental farm-specific and commercial PRRSV vaccines has been described.[316] The study was designed to boost PRRS-immune sows against circulating viruses. Three PRRSV isolates were taken. Booster vaccinations used either commercial vaccines or inactivated farm-specific isolate vaccines. A boost was found in all three farm-specific vaccinations. The commercial attenuated vaccine boostered immunity in 2/3 herds but the commercial nonattenuated dead vaccine did not affect the immunity on any of the three farms. In a second part of the study, similar vaccines were given at 60 days' gestation. The farm-specific vaccines produced a significant increase in farm-specific neutralizing antibodies in all sows. Virus-neutralizing antibodies were also transferred to the piglets via colostrum and were detectable in the serum of these animals until 5 weeks after parturition. Not all sows vaccinated with the commercial attenuated vaccine showed an increase in the farm-specific virus-neutralizing antibodies, and the piglets in this group received a lower level of colostral antibodies. The number of viremic animals was significantly lower in the piglets of both groups of vaccinated animals than among mock vaccinated animals until at least 9 weeks of age.

Vaccination of Gilts

The two commercial modified live virus vaccines against PRRSV in pregnant gilts were shown to replicate in pregnant gilts and to cross the placenta.[317] It was concluded that the vaccines had no marked detrimental effects in pregnant gilts but that they could cross the placenta and lead to the birth of congenitally affected piglets.

Intranasal delivery of PRRS-MLV with a potent adjuvant (from *M. tuberculosis* whole-cell lysate) to elicit cross-protective immunity to a heterologous strain of PRRSV generated effective cross-immunity. There was reduced lung pathology, enhanced neutralizing antibodies, and reduced viremia. There was a reduced secretion of immunosuppressive cytokines (IL-10 and TGF-β) and an upregulation of the Th-1 cytokine IFN-γ in blood and lungs.[318]

The ORF5a antibody response is neither neutralizing nor protective.[319]

Vaccination is an aid to management in developing effective immunity. The goal is to produce a constant level of immunity across a defined population. This effectively immunizes the entire population and eliminates the nonimmune, susceptible subpopulations. Vaccination is most effective when used in replacement gilts combined with adequate isolation and acclimatization and in sows after farrowing and prebreeding. The routine vaccination of sows is not economically viable in herds affected with PRRSV. The vaccine is best suited for stabilizing the herd and is a necessity before nursery depopulation or commingling segregated early weaning piglets from virus-positive herds. Vaccination is also intended to produce protective immunity in weaned and growing pigs. The PRRS virus exists in many forms and therefore the closer the genetic makeup between the immunizing virus and the challenge virus the better.

Both inactivated and modified live virus vaccines are available.

Previous vaccination with a live attenuated strain produced an increase in proinflammatory cytokines and proimmune cytokine gene expression. In addition, a higher level of cortisol production suggested that there was an activation of the hypothalamus-pituitary-adrenal axis response. Vaccination produces an early immune response in pigs and a more efficient control of inflammation.[320]

Inactivated Vaccines

Immunization of pigs with a genotype I attenuated vaccine provided partial protection against challenge with a highly virulent genotype II strain. There was a lower mortality, fewer days of fever, lower frequency of catarrhal bronchopneumonia, higher weight gains and lower viremia compared with unvaccinated control pigs.[321]

Killed vaccines that are inactivated using methods that preserve the PRRSV entry-associated domains are most useful for the development of effective inactivated vaccines because they facilitate internalization into macrophages.[322] An experimental inactivated PRRSV vaccine that induces virus-neutralizing antibodies has been described.[323] The vaccine uses an optimized inactivation procedure and a suitable adjuvant, and by using these methods it was shown that inactivated PRRS vaccines can be developed that induce virus-neutralizing antibodies and offer partial protection on challenge.

Killed vaccines may not produce a measurable antibody response stimulation, but activation of lymphocytes does occur and any subsequent exposure with vaccine or field virus increases that response. There is no possibility of producing a viremia and no chance of producing shedding, and there are no detrimental effects on the host. However, there is no evidence that killed vaccines protect against heterologous challenge.

A killed, oil-adjuvanted vaccine based on a Spanish isolate of the virus is intended for protection against reproductive disease in gilts and sows. Initial vaccination involves 2 vaccinations, 21 days apart, with the second vaccination at least 3 weeks before breeding and with booster vaccinations recommended during subsequent lactations. Experimental challenge provides 70% protection based on pigs born alive and surviving to 7 days.

An autogenous inactivated vaccine was compared with commercial vaccines against homologous and heterologous challenge.[324] In this study the experimental inactivated homologous vaccines shortened the viremia on challenge, but the experimental heterologous and commercial inactivated vaccine had no or only a limited effect on the viremia.

Live Vaccines

A study in China[325] on farms with a complex microbial ecology showed that mass vaccination with an attenuated virus vaccine can improve health status and production performance of sows and their offspring.

Modified live vaccines do give a safe and efficacious protection against a wide variety of heterologous challenge strains. The vaccine virus can be transmitted from vaccinated to naive pigs and to naive herds. Vaccination of boars causes the virus to be shed, but if they have been previously exposed and then are vaccinated then there is no release of virus.

The live vaccine given to finishing pigs will protect against respiratory infections. A modified live virus vaccine given once is safe for use in pregnant sows, and vaccine virus is not transmitted to susceptible contact pigs. In growing pigs vaccinated at 3 to 18 weeks of age, the vaccine elicits protective immunity within 7 days and lasts 16 weeks. Compared with controls, vaccinated animals have a reduced level of viremia, their growth rates are superior, and they have a reduced number of lung lesions. Field trials suggest that the vaccine provides protection to nursery pigs in units with endemic infection. Live viral vaccines in sows may or may not be a good idea because they demonstrated that reduced numbers of pigs were born alive and there were increased numbers of stillborn piglets to vaccinated sows irrespective of the stage of vaccination. Both single-strain and multi-strain vaccines can be attenuated and be useful immunogens, but additional studies are needed to make sure that the multistrain vaccines can be recommended for routine field use.

In Denmark in 1996, the use of a modified live virus vaccine licensed for use in pigs 3 to 18 weeks of age was used in a large number of PRRSV seropositive herds. Following vaccination, a large number of herds experienced an increased incidence of abortions, stillbirths, and poor performance during the nursery period. The vaccine virus was isolated from fetuses, and it was concluded that the virus was transmitted to seronegative nonvaccinated pregnant gilts and sows (see the section Methods of

Transmission). The viruses were collected and sequenced and shown to have only a 60% homology to Lelystad virus, the European type strain, but a 98.5% homology to strain ATC-2332, which is the North American reference strain. It was therefore thought that the vaccine viruses were reverting to their natural antecedents and their virulence. Describing the vaccine virus it was shown that given to piglets it could infect nonvaccinated sows. Given to sows it can produce congenital infection, fetal death, and an increased preweaning mortality.

The vaccine virus can be maintained in the population where it may undergo considerable genetic change and then lead to the establishment of new variants. Vaccination with the U.S. type vaccine produces little effect on viremia with EU PRRSV. Vaccination with EU type vaccines produced complete suppression of EU PRRSV isolates.

A modified live virus vaccine has been evaluated in pigs vaccinated at 3 weeks of age and challenged at 7 weeks of age. Efficacy was evaluated using homologous and heterologous strains of virus known to cause respiratory and reproductive disease. The vaccine controlled respiratory disease but did not prevent infection and viremia. There are no published reports of randomized clinical trials evaluating the vaccines under naturally occurring conditions. In many cases of PRDC, vaccination fails simply because it was given too late or because there was no cross-protection to heterologous strains.

DNA vaccination is said to produce both humoral and cellular responses and neutralization epitopes on the viral envelope glycoproteins encoded by ORF4. Possibly recombinants can be used as vaccines.

In a survey in Germany, 18.5% of the samples were positive for the EU wild-type virus, EU genotype vaccine virus was detected in 1.3%, and the North American genotype vaccine virus was found in 8.9% of all samples. North American vaccine virus was frequently detected in nonvaccinated animals.[326]

The first modified-live vaccine was first released in 1994 and since then a number of other modified live and killed-virus vaccines have been developed. Vaccines should induce rapid immunity, have no adverse reactions, and be able to differentiate vaccinated from naturally infected animals (DIVA vaccine).[308,327,328]

Mass vaccination using modified live virus against homologous infection was shown to be effective in reducing economic losses from PRRSV. It did not eliminate the virus but it did reduce viral shedding 97 DPI.[329] Two vaccines were compared (one inactivated and one modified live), and the modified live virus was the only type of vaccine capable of establishing protective immunity as measured by viral load in blood and tissues. The inactivated vaccine evoked no measurable protective immunity. The modified live vaccine seemed to be based on cell-mediated immunity.[330]

A modified live vaccine partially protected a group of pigs given a heterologous virus vaccine; intervention reduced the duration of shedding but did not reduce the viral load in tissues or the proportion of persistently infected pigs. When the pigs were subsequently given the highly virulent virus, infection and shedding were not prevented.[331]

The modified live vaccines for PRRSV have been reviewed.[332] None of the vaccines studied (Ingelvac PRRS MLV, Amervac PRRS, Pyrsvac-183, and Porcilis PRRS by the IM route) caused detectable clinical signs in vaccinated pigs, although lung lesions were found. Neither Pyrsivac-183 nor Porcilis PRRS could be detected in the pulmonary alveolar macrophages or in lung sections by IHC, suggesting that these viruses may have lost their ability to replicate in PAM. In these pigs, there was also a lower transmission rate and a delay in the onset of viremia, which may be explained by the lack of infection and therefore replication in the alveolar macrophage.

Novel strategies for the next generation of vaccines have been described[333] and stress the future importance of reverse genetics system-based vaccine development. Serologic marker candidates have been identified.[334,335] Vectored vaccines may have a place in the future.[336-338]

Recombinant fowlpox virus-based virus with coexpression of GP5/GP3 proteins of PRRSV and swine IL-18 has been described[339] as potential vaccines.

The fusion of the heat shock protein (HSP70) of *H. parasuis* with GP3 and GP5 of PRRSV enhanced the immune responses and protective efficacy of a vaccine.[340] The strategy of coexpressing GPGP-linked GP5 and M fusion protein may be a promising approach for future PRRSV vaccine development.[341] A canine adenovirus has also been used as a vehicle.[342]

Overattenuation of an HP-PRRSV (over 100 passages) was used to produce a possible vaccine[343] suggesting that loss of pathogenicity has to be balanced with loss of antigenicity.

Vaccination against PRRSV resulted in significantly lower viral loads of PCV2 in animals over 13 weeks compared with nonvaccinated animals but it had no effect on quantitative PCR results for PRRSV in 4- to 12-week-old pigs. PRRS vaccinates had significantly lower levels of PCV2 viral loads when peak wasting disease was seen.[344]

Concurrent PRRSV and PCV2 vaccination produced no interference with the development of the specific humoral and cell-mediated immunity and is associated with clinical protection on natural challenge.[345] PRRSV vaccine induced a low but significant virus-specific response IFN-γ secreting cell response on stimulation with both the vaccine strain and two heterologous PRRSV isolates.[346]

An isolate of PRRSV has been shown to produce IFNs and may be useful for the development of vaccines.[347]

Vaccination Against High Pathogenicity Porcine Reproductive and Respiratory Syndrome

A live attenuated vaccine was successfully produced from an HP-PRRSV strain TJ and the attenuation produced a further 120 amino acid deletion as well as the 30 amino acid deletion found in these HP-PRRSV strains.[348] The pigs were protected from the lethal challenge and did not develop fever and clinical disease. The vaccinated pigs also gained more weight and had milder pathologic lesions. The effective protection lasted at least 4 months.

A live attenuated vaccine has been used against HP-PRRSV.[349]

Vaccination of Boars

The use of an attenuated virus vaccine in boars resulted in a marked reduction in viremia and shedding of the virus in semen compared with nonvaccinated control animals. Introducing a vaccination program using the live virus vaccine may be considered as a potential method to reduce the risk of transmission of virus by artificial insemination. In contrast, no changes in onset, level, and duration of viremia, or shedding of virus in semen, were observed using the inactivated virus vaccine.

FURTHER READING

Dee S, et al. Use of a production region model to assess the efficacy of various air filtration systems for preventing airborne transmission of PRRS and *M. hyopneumoniae:* Results from a 2 year study. *Virus Res.* 2010;154:177-184.

Dokland T. The structural biology of PRRSV. *Virus Res.* 2010;154:86-97.

Frossard J-P. Porcine reproductive and respiratory syndrome virus evolution and its effect on control strategies. *Pig J.* 2013;68:20-25.

Gomez-Laguna J, et al. Immunopathogenesis of PRRSV in the respiratory tract of pigs. *Vet J.* 2013;195: 148.

Karniychuk UU, Nauwynck HJ. Pathogenesis and prevention of placental and transplacental porcine reproductive and respiratory syndrome virus infection. *Vet Res.* 2013;44:95.

Murtaugh MP, Genzow M. Immunological solutions for treatment and prevention of PRRS. *Vaccine.* 2011;29:8192-8204.

Murtaugh MP, et al. The ever-expanding diversity of PRRSV. *Virus Res.* 2010;154:18-30.

Nauwynck HJ, et al. Microdissecting the pathogenesis and immune response of PRRSV infection paves the way for more efficient PRRSV vaccines. *Transboundary Emerg Dis.* 2012;59(suppl 1):50-54.

Sang Y, et al. Interaction between innate immunity and PRRSV. *Anim Health Res Rev.* 2011;12:149-167.

Shi M, et al. Molecular epidemiology of PRRSV: A phylogenetic perspective. *Virus Res.* 2010;154:7-17.

Thanawongnuwech R, Suradhat S. Taming PRRSV: Revisiting the control strategies and vaccine design. *Virus Res.* 2010;154:133-140.

Yoo D, et al. Modulation of host cell responses and evasion strategies for PRRSV. *Virus Res.* 2010;154:48-60.

Zhou L, Yang H. PRRSV in China. *Virus Res.* 2010;154:31-37.

REFERENCES

1. Opriessnig T, et al. *Anim Health Res Rev.* 2011;12:133.
2. Murtaugh MP, et al. *Virus Res.* 2010;154:18.
3. Gorbalenya AE, et al. *Virus Res.* 2006;117:17.
4. Fang Y, et al. *Arch Virol.* 2007;152:1009.
5. Shi M, et al. *Virus Res.* 2010;154:7.
6. Martinez-Lobo FJ, et al. *Vaccine.* 2011;29:6928.
7. Fang Y, Snijder EJ. *Virus Res.* 2010;154:61.
8. Firth AE, et al. *J Gen Virol.* 2011;92:1097.
9. Johnson CR, et al. *J Gen Virol.* 2011;92:1107.
10. Wei Z, et al. *J Virol.* 2012;86:9941.
11. Xia Pa, et al. *Vet Microbiol.* 2009;138:297.
12. Lee C, Yoo D. *Virology.* 2006;346:238.
13. Kim W-I, et al. *Vet Microbiol.* 2013;162:10.
14. de Lima M, et al. *Virology.* 2009;390:31.
15. Brockmeier S, et al. *Virus Res.* 2012;169:212.
16. Johnston CR, et al. *J Gen Virol.* 2011;92:1107.
17. Wenhui L, et al. *J Virol.* 2012;86:9543.
18. Stadejek T, et al. *J Gen Virol.* 2006;87:1835.
19. Costers S, et al. *Virus Res.* 2010;154:104.
20. Kvisvgaard LK, et al. *Virus Res.* 2013;178:197.
21. Kvivsgaard LK, et al. *Vet Microbiol.* 2013;167:334.
22. Zhu L, et al. *Vet Microbiol.* 2011;147:274.
23. Li Y, et al. *Vet Microbiol.* 2009;138:150.
24. Cha S-H, et al. *Vet Microbiol.* 2006;117:248.
25. Frossard J-P, et al. *Vet Microbiol.* 2012;158:308.
26. Frossard J-P, et al. *Vet Microbiol.* 2013;162:507.
27. Mateu E, et al. *Virus Res.* 2006;115:198.
28. Prieto C, et al. *Vet J.* 2009;180:363.
29. Carlsson U, et al. *Transbound Emerg Dis.* 2009;56:121.
30. Amonsin A, et al. *Virol J.* 2009;6:143.
31. Tian K, et al. *PLoS ONE.* 2007;2:3526.
32. Xiao XL, et al. *J Virol Methods.* 2008;149:49.
33. Normile D. *Science.* 2007;317:1017.
34. Feng Y, et al. *Emerg Infect Dis.* 2008;14:1774.
35. Wu J, et al. *Arch Virol.* 2009;154:1589.
36. Li B, et al. *Vet Microbiol.* 2010;146:226.
37. Wang L, et al. *J Virol.* 2012;86:13121.
38. Zhang G, et al. *J Virol.* 2012;86:11396.
39. Li B, et al. *J Clin Microbiol.* 2011;49:3175.
40. Kim HK, et al. *Vet Microbiol.* 2011;150:230.
41. Kim S-H, et al. *Vet Microbiol.* 2010;143:394.
42. Miller LC, et al. *Vet Res.* 2012;8:208.
43. Xiao S, et al. *BMC Genomics.* 2010;11:544.
44. Hu SP, et al. *Transbound Emerg Dis.* 2012;60:351.
45. Lv J, et al. *J Gen Virol.* 2008;89:2075.
46. Shen J, et al. *Genome Announc.* 2013;1:e00486-13.
47. Zhou L, et al. *Virus Res.* 2009;145:97.
48. Zhou Y-J, et al. *Virus Res.* 2009;144:136.
49. Yu X, et al. *Vet Microbiol.* 2012;158:291.
50. Metwally S, et al. *Transbound Emerg Dis.* 2010;57:315.
51. Guo B, et al. *Virology.* 2013;446:238.
52. Song T, et al. *J Virol.* 2012;86:4040.
53. Guo B, et al. *Virology.* 2013;435:372.
54. Descotes J, Gourand A. *Expert Opin Drug Metab Toxicol.* 2008;4:1537.
55. Tarrant JM. *Toxicol Sci.* 2010;117:4.
56. Sun Y, et al. *Viruses.* 2012;4:424.
57. Behrens EM, et al. *J Clin Invest.* 2011;121:2264.
58. Nieuwehhuis N, et al. *Vet Rec.* 2012;170:225.
59. Corbellini LG, et al. *Vet Microbiol.* 2006;118:267.
60. Lopez-Soria S, et al. *Transbound Emerg Dis.* 2010;57:171.
61. Reiner G, et al. *Vet Microbiol.* 2009;136:250.
62. Greiser-Wilke I, et al. *Vet Microbiol.* 2010;143:213.
63. Kinman TG, et al. *Vaccine.* 2009;8:2704.
64. Rosendal T, et al. *Can J Vet Res.* 2010;74:118.
65. Brar MS, et al. *J Gen Virol.* 2011;92:1391.
66. Evans CM, et al. *Vet Res.* 2008;4:48.
67. Holtkamp DJ, et al. *Prev Vet Med.* 2010;96:186.
68. Lambert M-E, et al. *Vet Res.* 2012;8:76.
69. Velasova M, et al. *Vet Res.* 2012;8:184.
70. Lewis CRG, et al. *J Anim Sci.* 2009;87:876.
71. Doeschl-Wilson AB, et al. *J Anim Sci.* 2009;87:1638.
72. Badaoui B, et al. *BMC Vet Res.* 2013;9:58.
73. Kwong GPS, et al. *Prev Vet Med.* 2013;110:405.
74. Charpin C, et al. *Vet Res.* 2012;43:69.
75. Evans CM, et al. *Prev Vet Med.* 2010;93:248.
76. Dee S, et al. *Can J Vet Res.* 2006;69:64.
77. Pitkin A, et al. *Vet Microbiol.* 2009;136:1.
78. Hermann J, et al. *Vet Res.* 2007;38:81.
79. Otake S, et al. *Vet Microbiol.* 2010;145:198.
80. Pitkin A, et al. *Vet Microbiol.* 2009;136:1.
81. Cho JG, et al. *Can J Vet Res.* 2006;70:297.
82. Pitkin A, et al. *Vet Microbiol.* 2009;136:1.
83. Cutler TD, et al. *Vet Microbiol.* 2011;151:229.
84. Dee S, et al. *Vet Res.* 2009;40:39.
85. Pitkin A, et al. *Can J Vet Res.* 2009;73:298.
86. Cano JP, et al. *Vet Rec.* 2007;160:907.
87. Molina RM, et al. *Transbound Emerg Dis.* 2008;56:1.
88. Pitkin A, et al. *Can J Vet Res.* 2009;73:91.
89. De Baere MI, et al. *Vet Res.* 2012;43:47.
90. Wang X, et al. *Arch Virol.* 2007;152:289.
91. Gomez-Laguna J, et al. *Transbound Emerg Dis.* 2012;10:1865.
92. Klionsky DJ. *Nat Rev Mol Cell Biol.* 2007;8:931.
93. Liu Q, et al. *Virology.* 2012;429:136.
94. Butler JE, et al. *J Immunol.* 2007;178:6320.
95. An T-Q, et al. *Vet Microbiol.* 2010;143:371.
96. Kim JK, et al. *J Virol.* 2006;80:689.
97. De Baere MI, et al. *Vet Res.* 2012;43:47.
98. Welch S-K, Calvert JG. *Virus Res.* 2010;154:98.
99. Calvert JG, et al. *J Virol.* 2007;81:7371.
100. Cafruny WA, et al. *Virol J.* 2007;3:90.
101. Lee YJ, Lee C. *Vet Immunol Immunopathol.* 2012;150:213.
102. Patton JB, et al. *Virus Res.* 2009;140:161.
103. Gruenberg J, van der Goot FG. *Nat Rev Mol Cell Biol.* 2006;7:495.
104. Misinzo GM, et al. *Vet Res.* 2008;39:55.
105. Van Gortp H, et al. *Arch Virol.* 2009;154:1939.
106. Van Breedam W, et al. *J Gen Virol.* 2010;91:1659.
107. Music N, Gagnon CA. *Anim Health Res Rev.* 2010;11:135.
108. Lee C, et al. *Virology.* 2006;346:238.
109. Pei Y, et al. *Virus Res.* 2008;135:107.
110. Kwon B, et al. *Virology.* 2008;380:371.
111. Wang C, et al. *Vet Microbiol.* 2008;131:339.
112. Faaberg KS, et al. *Virus Res.* 2010;154:77.
113. Rowland RR. *Virus Res.* 2010;154:1.
114. Zhang X, Moser DM. *J Pathol.* 2008;214:161.
115. Lee YJ, Lee C. *Virus Res.* 2010;152:50.
116. Lee C, Yoo D. *Virology.* 2006;355:30.
117. Du Y, et al. *Virus Res.* 2010;147:294.
118. Chang HC, et al. *Vet Microbiol.* 2008;129:281.
119. Flores-Mendoza L, et al. *Clin Vaccine Immunol.* 2008;15:720.
120. Loving CI, et al. *Immunology.* 2007;120:217.
121. Gimeno M, et al. *Vet Res.* 2011;42:9.
122. Gomez-Laguna J, et al. *J Comp Pathol.* 2010;142:51.
123. Zhang Y, et al. *Vet Microbiol.* 2012;160:473.
124. Sagong M, Lee C. *Virus Res.* 2010;151:88.
125. Li Y, et al. *J Gen Virol.* 2012;93:829.
126. Chaung H-C, et al. *Comp Immunol Microbiol Infect Dis.* 2010;33:197.
127. Liu C-H, et al. *Vet Microbiol.* 2009;136:266.
128. Manickam C, et al. *Vet Microbiol.* 2013;162:68.
129. Silva-Campo E, et al. *Virology.* 2012;430:73.
130. Pintaric M, et al. *Vet Immunol Immunopathol.* 2008;121:61.
131. Lodoen MB, Lainier LL. *Curr Opin Immunol.* 2006;18:391.
132. Costers S, et al. *Arch Virol.* 2008;153:1453.
133. Cao J, et al. *Vet Microbiol.* 2013;164:261.
134. Caliguri MA. *Blood.* 2008;112:461.
135. Renukaradhya GJ, et al. *Viral Immunol.* 2010;23:457.
136. Dvivedi V, et al. *Virol J.* 2012;9:45.
137. Cecere TE, et al. *Vet Microbiol.* 2012;160:233.
138. Silva-Campo E, et al. *Virology.* 2009;387:373.
139. Silva-Campo E, et al. *Virology.* 2010;396:264.
140. Silva-Campo E, et al. *Virology.* 2012;85:23.
141. Rodriguez-Gomez IM, et al. *Transbound Emerg Dis.* 2013;60:425.
142. Halstead SB, et al. *Lancet Infect Dis.* 2010;10:712.
143. Belkaid Y. *Nat Rev Immunol.* 2007;7:875.
144. Dwivedi V, et al. *Vaccine.* 2011;29:4067.
145. LeRoith T, et al. *Vet Immunol Immunopathol.* 2011;140:312.
146. Wongyanin P, et al. *Vet Immunol Immunopathol.* 2010;132:170.
147. Silva-Campo E, et al. *Virology.* 2012;430:73.
148. Chen Z, et al. *J Gen Virol.* 2010;91:1047.
149. Costers S, et al. *Vet Res.* 2009;40:46.
150. Gomez-Laguna J, et al. *Comp Immunol Microbiol Infect Dis.* 2011;34:143.
151. Subramaniam S, et al. *Virology.* 2010;406:270.
152. Subramaniam S, et al. *Virology.* 2012;432:241.
153. Barranco I, et al. *Vet Immunol Immunopathol.* 2012;149:262.
154. Gomez-Laguna J. *Vet Microbiol.* 2012;158:187.
155. Backus GS, et al. *Environ Health Perspect.* 2010;118:1721.
156. Diaz I, et al. *Vet Res.* 2012;43:30.
157. Weaver LK, et al. *J Leucocyte Biol.* 2007;81:663.
158. Hou J, et al. *Virol J.* 2012;9:165.
159. Gomez-Laguna J, et al. *Vet J.* 2013;195:148.
160. Lunney JK, et al. *Virus Res.* 2010;154:185.
161. Beura LK, et al. *J Virol.* 2010;84:1574.
162. Subramaniam S, et al. Proc 90th Meet Conf Res Work Anim Dis, Chicago 2009; Abstr. 176.
163. Overend C, et al. *J Gen Virol.* 2007;88:925.
164. Bao D, et al. *Vet Immunol Immunopathol.* 2013;156:128.
165. Shi X, et al. *Virus Res.* 2010;153:151.
166. Calzada-Nova G, et al. *Vet Immunol Immunopathol.* 2010;135:20.
167. Peng Y-T, et al. *Vet Microbiol.* 2009;136:359.
168. Miguel JC, et al. *Vet Immunol Immunopathol.* 2010;135:314.
169. Klinge KL, et al. *Virol J.* 2009;6:177.
170. Dotti S, et al. *Res Vet Sci.* 2013;94:510.
171. Beura LK, et al. *J Virol.* 2011;85:12939.
172. Beura LK, et al. *J Virol.* 2010;84:1574.
173. Bowie AG, Unterholzer L. *Nat Rev Immunol.* 2008;8:911.
174. Kawai T, Akira S. *Int Immunol.* 2009;21:317.
175. Beura LK, et al. *Virology.* 2012;433:431.
176. Versteeg GA, GarciaSastre A. *Curr Opin Microbiol.* 2010;13:508.
177. Beura LK, et al. *J Virol.* 2010;84:1574.
178. Song C, et al. *Virology.* 2010;407:268.
179. Patel D, et al. *J Virol.* 2010;84:11405.
180. Li H, et al. *J Gen Virol.* 2010;81:2947.
181. Sun Z, et al. *J Virol.* 2010;84:7832.
182. Kimman TG, et al. *Vaccine.* 2009;27:315.
183. Nan Y, et al. *Virology.* 2012;43:261.
184. Yoo D, et al. *Virus Res.* 2010;154:48.
185. Zhou Y, et al. *Can J Vet Res.* 2012;76:255.
186. Chen Z, et al. *Virology.* 2010;198:87.
187. Huber JP, Farrar JD. *Immunology.* 2011;132:446.
188. Luo R, et al. *Mol Immunol.* 2008;45:2839.
189. Brockmeier SL, et al. *Viral Immunol.* 2009;22:173.
190. Brockmeier SL, et al. *Clin Vaccine Immunol.* 2012;19:508.
191. Kim O, et al. *Virology.* 2010;402:315.

192. Sagong M, Lee C. *Arch Virol.* 2011;156:2187.
193. Lee YJ, Lee C. *Virology.* 2012;427:80.
194. Ait-Ali T, et al. *Immunogenetics.* 2011;63:437.
195. Sun Z, et al. *J Virol.* 2012;86:3839.
196. Barranco I, et al. *Transbound Emerg Dis.* 2012;59:145.
197. Van Gorp H, et al. *J Gen Virol.* 2008;89:2943.
198. Dong S, et al. *Res Vet Sci.* 2012;93:1060.
199. Gudmundsdottir I, Risatti GR. *Virus Res.* 2009;145:145.
200. Hou J, et al. *Virus Res.* 2012;167:106.
201. Gomez-Laguna J, et al. *Comp Immunol Microbiol Infect Dis.* 2010;33:51.
202. Gomez-Laguna J, et al. *Vet Microbiol.* 2012;158:187.
203. Darwich L, et al. *Vet Microbiol.* 2011;150:49.
204. Mateu E, Diaz I. *Vet J.* 2008;177:345.
205. Dotti S, et al. *Res Vet Sci.* 2011;90:218.
206. Martinez-Lobo FJ, et al. *Vet Microbiol.* 2011;154:58.
207. Garcia-Nicolas O, et al. *Virus Res.* 2014;179:204.
208. Weesendorp E, et al. *Vet Microbiol.* 2013;163:1.
209. Weesendorp E, et al. *Vet Microbiol.* 2013;167:638.
210. Kim W-I, et al. *Vet Micrbiol.* 2007;123:10.
211. Frydas IS, et al. *Vet Res.* 2013;44:73.
212. Wang G, et al. *Virol J.* 2014;11:2.
213. Wang G, et al. *Vet Immunol Immunopathol.* 2011;142:170.
214. Han K, et al. *J Comp Pathol.* 2012;147:275.
215. Hou J, et al. *Virus Res.* 2012;167:10.
216. Li L, et al. *Virol J.* 2012;9:203.
217. Cao J, et al. *J Vet Diagn Invest.* 2012;24:767.
218. Guo B, et al. *Virology.* 2013;435:372.
219. Mege JL, et al. *Lancet Infect Dis.* 2006;6:557.
220. Borghetti P, et al. *Comp Immunol Microbiol Infect Dis.* 2011;34:143.
221. Parcina M, et al. *J Immunol.* 2013;190:1591.
222. Butler JE, et al. *J Immunol.* 2007;178:6329.
223. Butler JE, et al. *J Immunol.* 2008;180:2347.
224. Sun XZ, et al. *Vaccine.* 2012;30:3646.
225. Parida R, et al. *Virus Res.* 2012;169:13.
226. Diaz I, et al. *Virus Res.* 2010;154:61.
227. Han J, et al. *J Virol.* 2010;84:10102.
228. Kinman TG, et al. *Vaccine.* 2009;27:3704.
229. Li J, Murtaugh MP. *Virology.* 2012;433:367.
230. Tong GZ, et al. *Emerg Infect Dis.* 2007;13:1434.
231. An T-Q, et al. *Emerg Infect Dis.* 2010;16:365.
232. Li L, et al. *Virus Res.* 2010;154.
233. Murtaugh M Proc 40th Ann Meet Am Assoc Swine Vet, Dallas, TX, 459.
234. Qiao S, et al. *Vet Microbiol.* 2011;149:213.
235. Diaz I, et al. *Vet Res.* 2012;43:30.
236. Jung K, et al. *J Gen Virol.* 2009;90:2713.
237. Wagner J, et al. *Vet J.* 2011;187:310.
238. Beilage EG, et al. *Tierartzl Prax.* 2007;35:294.
239. Cano JP, et al. *Can J Vet Res.* 2009;73:303.
240. Lewis CRG, et al. *Anim Prod Sci.* 2010;50:890.
241. Han K, et al. *J Comp Pathol.* 2013;148:396.
242. Karniychuk U, et al. *Microb Pathog.* 2011;51:194.
243. Karniychuk U, Nauwynck HJ. *Vet Res.* 2013;44:95.
244. Kang I, et al. *Res Vet Sci.* 2010;88:304.
245. Han K, et al. *Clin Vaccine Immunol.* 2012;19:319.
246. Burgara-Estrella A, et al. *Transbound Emerg Dis.* 2012;59:532.
247. Schulze M, et al. *Acta Vet Scand.* 2013;55:16.
248. Stadejek T, et al. *Vet Rec.* 2011;169:441.
249. Xiao S, et al. *BMC Genomics.* 2010;11:544.
250. Hu SP, et al. *Transbound Emerg Dis.* 2012;10:1865.
251. Lawson S, et al. *Vaccine.* 2010;28:5356.
252. Lee YJ, et al. *J Virol Methods.* 2010;163:410.
253. Wernike K, et al. *J Vet Diagn Invest.* 2012;24:855.
254. Rovira A, et al. *J Vet Diagn Invest.* 2007;19:502.
255. Gerber PF, et al. *J Clin Microbiol.* 2013;51:547.
256. Gerber PF, et al. *J Virol Methods.* 2014;197:63.
257. Li Q, et al. *J Virol Methods.* 2009;155:55.
258. Rovira A, et al. *J Vet Diagn Invest.* 2009;21:350.
259. Lurchachaiwong W, et al. *Lett Appl Microbiol.* 2008;46:55.
260. Balka G, et al. *J Virol Methods.* 2009;115:1.
261. Chen N-H, et al. *J Virol Methods.* 2009;161:192.
262. Ren X, et al. *J Clin Microbiol.* 2010;48:1875.
263. Van Breedam W, et al. *Vet Immunol Immunopathol.* 2011;141:246.
264. Diaz I, et al. *J Vet Diagn Invest.* 2012;24:344.
265. Kittawornrat A, et al. *Vet Res.* 2013;9:61.
266. Okinaga T, et al. *Vet Rec.* 2009;164:455.
267. Lin K, et al. *J Clin Microbiol.* 2011;49:3184.
268. Gutierrez AM, et al. *Vet Immunol Immunopathol.* 2009;132:218.
269. Gomez-Laguna J, et al. *Vet J.* 2010;85:83.
270. Kittawornrat A, et al. *Vet Microbiol.* 2014;168:331.
271. Chittick WA, et al. *J Vet Diagn Invest.* 2011;23:248.
272. Prickett JR, et al. *J Swine Health Prod.* 2008;16:86.
273. Prickett JR, et al. *J Vet Diagn Invest.* 2008;20:156.
274. Prickett JR, Zimmerman JJ. *Anim Health Res Rev.* 2010;10:1.
275. Ramirez A, et al. *Prev Vet Med.* 2012;104:292.
276. Kittawornrat A, et al. *Virus Res.* 2010;154:1700.
277. Ouyang K, et al. *Clin Vaccine Immunol.* 2013;20:1305.
278. Kittawornrat A, et al. *J Vet Diagn Invest.* 2012;24:262.
279. Olsen C, et al. *J Vet Diagn Invest.* 2013;25:328.
280. Kittawornrat A, et al. *J Vet Diagn Invest.* 2012;24:1057.
281. Costers S, et al. *Vet Res.* 2009;40:46.
282. Han K, et al. *Vet J.* 2013;195:313.
283. Gomez-Laguna J, et al. *Transbound Emerg Dis.* 2013;60:273.
284. Morgan SB, et al. *Vet Microbiol.* 2013;163:13.
285. Lee S-M, Kleiboeker SB. *Virology.* 2007;365:419.
286. He Y, et al. *Vet Microbiol.* 2012;160:455.
287. Grau-Roma L, Segales J. *Vet Microbiol.* 2007;119:144.
288. Han K, et al. *J Vet Diagn Invest.* 2012;24:719.
289. Stuart AD, et al. *Pig J.* 2008;61:42.
290. Jiang Y, et al. *Vet Res Commun.* 2010;34:607.
291. Rowland RR. *Sci Direct.* 2007;174:451.
292. Rowland RR, Morrison RB. *Transbound Emerg Dis.* 2012;59(suppl 1):55.
293. Mondaca-Fernandez E, Morrison RB. *Vet Rec.* 2007;161:137.
294. Wayne SR, et al. *J Am Vet Med Assoc.* 2012;240:876.
295. Liu Y, et al. *J Anim Sci.* 2013;91:5668.
296. Pitkin A, et al. *Vet Microbiol.* 2009;136:1.
297. Dee S, et al. *Vet Microbiol.* 2009;138:106.
298. Dee S, et al. *Vet Rec.* 2010;167:976.
299. Spronk G, et al. *Vet Rec.* 2010;166:758.
300. Alonso C, et al. *Vet Microbiol.* 2012;157:304.
301. Alonso C, et al. *Prev Vet Med.* 2013;112:109.
302. Alonso C, et al. *Prev Vet Med.* 2013;111:268.
303. Che TM, et al. *J Anim Sci.* 2011;89:3016.
304. Che TM, et al. *J Anim Sci.* 2012;90:2784.
305. Lambert M-E, et al. *Prev Vet Med.* 2012;104:74.
306. Rovira A, et al. *J Vet Diagn Invest.* 2007;19:492.
307. Han K, et al. *Clin Vaccine Immunol.* 2011;18:1600.
308. Charerntantanakul W. *Vet Immunol Immunopathol.* 2009;129:1.
309. Linghua Z, et al. *Vaccine.* 2007;25:1735.
310. Zhang L, et al. *Vet Microbiol.* 2013;164:253.
311. Drexler CS, et al. *Vet Rec.* 2010;166:70.
312. Thanawongnuwech R, Suradhat S. *Virus Res.* 2010;154:133.
313. Kitikoon P, et al. *Vet Microbiol.* 2009;139:235.
314. Murtaugh MP, Genzow M. *Vaccine.* 2011;29:8192.
315. Martelli P, et al. *Vaccine.* 2007;25:3400.
316. Geldhof MF, et al. *Vet Microbiol.* 2013;167:260.
317. Scortti M, et al. *Vet J.* 2006;172:506.
318. Dwivedi V, et al. *Vaccine.* 2011;29:4058.
319. Robinson SR, et al. *Vet Microbiol.* 2013;164:281.
320. Borghetti P, et al. *Comp Immunol Microbiol Inf Dis.* 2011;34:143.
321. Roca M, et al. *Vet J.* 2012;193:92.
322. Delrue I, et al. *Vet Res.* 2009;40:62.
323. Vanhee M, et al. *Vet Res.* 2009;40:63.
324. Geldof MF, et al. *BMC Vet Res.* 2012;8:182.
325. Zhao Z, et al. *Vet Microbiol.* 2012;155:247.
326. Beilage EG, et al. *Prev Vet Med.* 2009;92:31.
327. de Lima J, et al. *Vaccine.* 2008;26:3594.
328. Fang Y, et al. *J Gen Virol.* 2008;89:3086.
329. Cano JP, et al. *Am J Vet Res.* 2007;68:565.
330. Zuckerman FA, et al. *Vet Microbiol.* 2007;123:69.
331. Cano JP, et al. *Vaccine.* 2007;25:4382.
332. Martinez-Lobo F, et al. *Vet Res.* 2013;44:115.
333. Huang YW, Meng XJ. *Virus Res.* 2010;154:141.
334. de Lima M, et al. *Virology.* 2006;353:410.
335. Vu HLX, et al. *Vaccine.* 2013;31:4330.
336. Cruz JLG, et al. *Virus Res.* 2010;154:150.
337. Pei Y, et al. *Virology.* 2009;389:91.
338. Huang Q, et al. *J Virol Methods.* 2009;160:22.
339. Guoshan S, et al. *Vaccine.* 2007;25:4193.
340. Li J, et al. *Vaccine.* 2009;27:825.
341. Chia M-Y, et al. *Vet Microbiol.* 2010;146:189.
342. Cai J, et al. *J Vet Med Sci.* 2010;72:1035.
343. Yu X, et al. *Clin Vaccine Immunol.* 2013;20:613.
344. Genzow M, et al. *Can J Vet Res.* 2009;73:87.
345. Martelli P, et al. *Vet Microbiol.* 2013;162:358.
346. Ferrari L, et al. *Vet Immunol Immunopathol.* 2013;151:193.
347. Nan Y, et al. *Virology.* 2012;432:261.
348. Leng X, et al. *Clin Vaccine Immunol.* 2012;19:1199.
349. Tian Z-J, et al. *Vet Microbiol.* 2009;138:34.
350. Hu SP, et al. *Transbound Emerg Dis.* 2013;60:351.

MENANGLE

This causative virus was first identified in a three-farm disease outbreak in New South Wales in 1997. It causes reproductive problems in pigs and congenital defects and has the fruit bat as an asymptomatic reservoir. It can cause a flu-like disease in man. Only one outbreak has been described. It normally lives asymptomatically in fruit bats.

ETIOLOGY

The causative agent is an RNA virus in the family Paramyxoviridae in the genus *Rubulavirus.* It is closely related to Tioman virus found in fruit bats on Tioman Island, Malaysia.

EPIDEMIOLOGY

A variety of fruit bats are seropositive, including the gray-headed flying fox, black fruit bat, and spectacled fruit bat, but the virus has not been isolated from them. These fruit bats have been found in other areas of Australia as well as the original area around Menangle, New South Wales.

Bat feces and urine are probably the source of infection. Transmission from pig to pig is slow and probably requires close contact. In one building, it took a long time for the sows to become affected. It probably spreads from farm to farm via infected animals. There is no sign of persistent infection and no evidence of long-term virus shedding. Present evidence suggests that virus survival in the environment is short because sentinel pigs placed in an uncleaned area did not seroconvert.

CLINICAL SIGNS

There is no knowledge of the incubation period as yet. In the initial outbreak, clinical signs were seen only on the farrow-to-finish farm but infected pigs were found in all three farms.

The disease was an outbreak of reproductive disease with fetal death; fetal abnormalities including congenital defects, such as skeletal and neurologic defects[1]; mummified fetuses; stillborn fetuses; smaller litters with fewer live piglets; and a reduced farrowing rate. The farrowing rate fell from over 80% to around a low of 38% reaching an average of 60%. Many sows returned to estrus 28 days after mating, which suggests that there has been an early death of the litter. Some sows remain in pseudopregnancy for more than 60 days. It probably crosses the placenta and spreads fetus to fetus. Once the infection became endemic in the farrow-to-finish herd the reproductive failures ceased.

PATHOLOGY

The mummified fetuses vary in size and are 30 days or older. The virus causes the degeneration of brain and spinal cord. In particular, the cerebral hemispheres and cerebellum are smaller. Occasionally there may be effusions and pulmonary hypoplasia. Eosinophilic inclusions are found in the neurons of the cerebrum and spinal cord. Sometimes there is a nonsuppurative meningitis, myocarditis, and hepatitis. Experimental infections show shedding 2 to 3 days after infection in nasal and oral secretions. A tropism for secondary lymphoid tissues and intestinal epithelium has been demonstrated.[2] No lesions have been seen in piglets born alive or other postnatal pigs.

DIAGNOSIS

The diagnosis is suspected when the reproductive parameters change very suddenly, as shown earlier.

Diagnosis is confirmed by virus culture, and electron microscopy and virus neutralisation tests confirm the identity of the virus. Serologic tests include ELISAs, and the best way to test the herd is to use this for the sows for antibody.

DIFFERENTIAL DIAGNOSIS

The differential diagnosis includes porcine parvo virus (PPV), classical swine fever (CSF), porcine reproductive and respiratory syndrome (PRRS), encephalomyocarditis virus (EMCV), pseudorabies virus (PRV), Japanese encephalitis, swine influenza virus (SIV), and blue eye. Noninfectious causes such as toxins or nutritional deficiencies should also be considered.

TREATMENT

It seems likely that young pigs are infected by the virus when the maternal antibody concentration declines at 14 to 16 weeks of age. By the time they enter the breeding herd their immunity is quite strong.

CONTROL

The best advice is to avoid contact with all fruit bats.

FURTHER READING

Philbey AW, et al. An apparently new virus (family *Paramyxoviridae*) infection for pigs, humans and fruit bats. *Emerg Infect Dis*. 1998;4:269.

REFERENCES

1. Philbey AW, et al. *Aust Vet J*. 2007;85:134.
2. Bowden TR, et al. *J Gen Virol*. 2012;93:1007.

JAPANESE ENCEPHALITIS (JE; JAPANESE B ENCEPHALITIS)

Japanese encephalitis is an infectious disease primarily affecting horses and to a lesser extent pigs, with important zoonotic potential. It causes in excess of 50,000 human cases a year, with a case mortality rate of 25%. The condition in equides is associated with encephalitis and is covered in detail in Chapter 14 under Japanese encephalitis. In pigs the condition is associated with reproductive failure, whch is covered hereunder.

ETIOLOGY

The causative agent is the Japanese encephalitis virus of the family Flavivirdae, genus *flavivirus*. Based on the phylogenetic analysis of the viral envelope "E" gene, 5 different genotypes have been identified.

EPIDEMIOLOGY

The natural distribution range of the virus is southeast Asia and Australasia. The vectors are *Culex* spp and in particular *C. tritaeniorhynchus*. The virus activity is naturally maintained through bird–mosquito cycles with the heron family in particular. The night herons, little egrets and plumed egrets are particularly active as a reservoir. Pigs are important "amplifying hosts." Pigs and these birds may allow the overwintering of the virus when mosquitoes are absent.

PATHOGENESIS

Viremia results from the mosquito bite and usually nothing is seen. Occasionally there may be a mild fever. but quite often the virus goes straight to the testicles and causes an orchitis.

CLINICIAL SIGNS

Fetal death is common with mummified fetuses as well as stillborn and weak pigs. Boars undergo reproductive failure.

PATHOLOGY

Largely related to the abnormal fetuses.

DIAGNOSIS

RT-PCR and nested RT-PCR can be used to detect the virus when virus isolation is negative. Antibody can be detected by haemagglutination inhibiton, ELISAs (IgM capture ELISA), and latex agglutination tests.

CONTROL

Live attenuated vaccines should be given to breeding stock 2 to 3 weeks before the start of the mosquito season. Attenuated and adjuvanted vaccines are also available.

FURTHER READING

Mackenzie JS, Williams DT. The zoonotic flaviviruses of southern, southeastern and eastern Asia and Australasia: The potential for emergent viruses. *Zoonoses Public Health*. 2009;56:338.

NEOSPOROSIS

SYNOPSIS

Etiology The protozoan parasite *Neospora caninum;* the dog is identified as the definitive host of *N. caninum,* but the main route of infection in cattle appears to be by vertical transmission.

Epidemiology An infection of cattle worldwide and associated with epidemic and endemic abortion. Point source and congenital infections occur.

Clinical findings Abortion in cows and perinatal mortality and encephalomyelitis in congenitally infected calves.

Clinical pathology Serologic testing of maternal serum and fetal fluids.

Necropsy findings Fetal lesions of multifocal nonsuppurative encephalitis, myocarditis, and/or periportal hepatitis. Infection confirmed by immunohistochemistry or polymerase chain reaction-based tools.

Diagnostic confirmation A presumptive diagnosis can be based on the fetal histologic lesions and seropositivity of the dam, but the definitive diagnosis requires the demonstration of the parasite in fetal tissues by immunohistochemical labeling, coupled with serologic examinations.

Control Feed hygiene and calving hygiene. Cull congenitally infected cattle.

ETIOLOGY

Neospora caninum is a cyst-forming coccidial (apicomplexan) parasite with an indirect life cycle.[1-9] *N. caninum* primarily infects dogs and cattle; however, it has a **wide host range** and infects all major domestic livestock species as well as companion animals and some wildlife animals. Dogs are the definitive host and cattle the major intermediate host. Natural infection is infrequently reported in sheep, goats, and deer.[1-3] *N. caninum* is a sporadic cause of encephalomyelitis and myocarditis in several species, but its principal importance is its association with **endemic and epidemic abortion in cattle.** It is now the most common diagnosis for abortion in cattle in most countries.

EPIDEMIOLOGY

Occurrence

N. caninum was initially associated with abortion in the early 1990s in pastured cattle in Australia and New Zealand and as a major cause of abortion in dairies in the United States. Since then, abortion associated with *N. caninum* has been reported in many countries in cattle under varying management conditions and has a **worldwide occurrence.**[2,3]

Abortion may be **epizootic or sporadic.** In epizootic abortion, the number of cows aborting varies. It is usually between 5% and 10%, but up to 45% of cows may abort within a short period. The period of abortion may be a few weeks to a few months. There is no major seasonal occurrence, and abortion occurs in both beef and dairy cows. Sporadic abortions occur mainly in cows that have been infected congenitally, and seropositive cows have greater risk for repeat abortions. Seropositivity in herds can be high but varies considerably. Seropositive dams have a 3- to 7-fold greater risk of abortion than seronegative dams.

Methods of Transmission

There are two routes of infection of cattle. The dog is the definitive host of *N. caninum.* Infection of cattle can occur via the ingestion of oocytes from dog feces contaminating feed or water. However, vertical (i.e., congenital) transmission occurs in both cattle and dogs, and vertical transmission appears the major route for infection in most cattle.[1-3] Live-born calves from congenitally infected cows are themselves congenitally infected; the infection is thought to be **persistent and lifelong**. A study conducted on two dairies found 81% of seropositive cows gave birth to congenitally infected calves.[1] Seroprevalence did not increase with cow age and was stable through the study period. The probability of a calf being congenitally infected was not associated with dam age, dam lactation number, dam history of abortion, calf gender, or length of gestation. Other studies have shown that this route of transmission is highly efficient, resulting in infection of 50% to 95% of the progeny of seropositive dams.

Congenital infection can result in abortion or the birth of a "normal," infected calf, and an infected cow can give birth to a clinically normal, infected calf at one pregnancy and abort in the subsequent pregnancy.[2,3] The occurrence of infection in some herds can be associated with specific family lines.

Although vertical transmission is the major route of infection that leads to sporadic abortions in cattle associated with *N. caninum,* epidemiologic evidence suggests that postnatal (point) infection is often the cause of outbreaks of abortion. Where dog feces are the source of infection, many cattle are often exposed, and this point source of infection commonly results in outbreaks of abortion. Farm dogs have been shown to have a higher seroprevalence to *N. caninum* than urban dogs, suggesting that neosporosis cycles between cattle and dogs in rural environments.[4]

The importance of postnatal infection versus vertical infection in the genesis of abortion may vary among countries, and be associated with differences in farm management systems.[4]

Experimental Studies

Abortion has been produced by experimental challenge of fetuses and pregnant cattle with culture-derived tachyzoites of *N. caninum.*[1] Fetal death and resorption or abortion has been reproduced in ewes challenged at 45, 65, and 90 days' gestation, but not 120 days, and lesions resemble those of ovine toxoplasmosis.[2] The disease has also been reproduced experimentally in goats,[1] but the importance and prevalence of this infection in naturally occurring abortions in small ruminants remains to be determined. Contaminated placenta, milk, and colostrum can result in infection of calves less than 1 week of age.

Risk Factors

Outbreaks of abortion often appear to be point source infections, but the risk factors, other than probable mass exposure to dog feces containing sporulated *N. caninum* oocysts, are not known. Neosporosis in dairy herds often occurs as an epizootic, with multiple abortions occurring in a 1- to 2-month period. Severely autolytic fetuses are aborted between 5 and 7 months of pregnancy in most reports, but earlier or later abortions can occur (range is between 3 and 8.5 months of pregnancy).

Endemic abortion is more likely associated with the presence of **congenitally infected** cattle in the herd, which are at **high risk of aborting**, particularly in the initial pregnancy and in the pregnancy during the first lactation.[2,3] Cows that have aborted have a higher risk for abortion in subsequent pregnancies, but this risk decreases with each subsequent pregnancy. It has been postulated that immunosuppression resulting from concurrent infection with other agents, such as bovine viral diarrhea virus (BVD) , may increase the risk for infection with *N. caninum* and precipitate abortion outbreaks.

Economic Importance

Economic losses relate to abortion and costs associated with establishing the diagnosis and rebreeding or replacement costs.[5] Seropositivity is also associated with increased risk of stillbirth and increased risk of retained placenta. Losses associated with epidemic abortion have been estimated at tens (20–85) of millions of dollars to the dairy or beef industries in Australasia and the United States.

Although seropositive heifers have been reported to produce less milk than seronegative herdmates, this difference in milk production between seropositive and seronegative animals is not necessarily apparent in herds unaffected by an abortion problem. Study of beef cattle has suggested that seropositivity might be associated with reduction in average daily weight gain, but production performance and carcass measures are not consistently reported to be affected.

PATHOGENESIS

N. caninum has a predilection for fetal chorionic epithelium and fetal placental blood vessels, producing a fetal vasculitis and inflammation and degeneration of the chorioallantois, and widespread necrosis in the placentome.[6] Tachyzoites penetrate host cells and are located in a parasitophorous vacuole. They can be found in macrophages, monocytes, vascular endothelial cells, fibroblasts, hepatocytes, renal tubular cells, and in the brain of infected animals. With neuromuscular disease, cranial and spinal neural cells are infected. Cell death is caused by the replication of tachyzoites (during endodyogeny).

CLINICAL FINDINGS

Abortion is the cardinal clinical sign observed in infected **cows.**[2,3] Fetuses may die in utero, or can be reabsorbed, mummified, stillborn, born alive but diseased, or born clinically normal but infected. Cows that are infected can have **decreased milk production** in the first lactation, producing approximately 1 L less of milk per cow per day than uninfected cows, are prone to abort, and have a higher risk of being culled from the herd at an early age.

In addition to the occurrence of early abortion, the disease in beef herds is associated with the birth of live-born, premature, **low birthweight** calves. Depending on the degree of prematurity, these calves can be kept alive with intensive care during the neonatal period.

Most congenitally infected calves are born alive without clinical signs. Occasionally, congenital infection can be manifest with ataxia, loss of conscious proprioception, paralysis, and/or other **neurologic deficits** in new-born calves,[2] but most congenitally infected calves appear as clinically normal and, surprisingly, some evidence suggests that congenital infection does not necessarily have a detrimental effect on calf health and survival.[3]

N. caninum infection has been demonstrated in the nervous system of a **horse** with progressive debilitation, followed by a sudden onset of neurologic disease with paraplegia. It appears to be a rare cause of neurologic disease in horses, but should be considered in the differential diagnosis of equine protozoal myeloencephalitis.

CLINICAL PATHOLOGY

Serologic testing can be conducted using IFAT or ELISA, and there appears to be good agreement in results between the two tests. ELISA using recombinant protein appears to have a higher diagnostic specificity and sensitivity than using whole-tachyzoite lysates.[7] IFAT is commonly used and achieves a relatively high diagnostic specificity and sensitivity for the detection of maternal infection.[7] The persistence of serum antibody titers following infection is uncertain, and they might fluctuate during pregnancy. A positive titer in a cow that has aborted indicates exposure but not causality. IgG avidity patterns have been used to predict the duration of infection. Diagnosis can also be conducted by detecting anti-*N. caninum* antibody or genomic DNA of *N. caninum* in **fetal pleural fluid or sera.**[7]

NECROPSY FINDINGS

Gross findings are not specific and the fetus may be fresh, autolyzed, or in early stages of mummification; in the placenta, the cotyledons are usually necrotic.[10] The brain may be autolyzed, but should still be submitted for examination as well as the heart, liver, and placenta, if available. Histologic findings commonly relate to **multifocal nonsuppurative encephalitis, myocarditis hepatitis, and/or placentitis** Liver lesions may be more prominent in epizootic abortions. IHC or PCR can be used to detect tachyzoites or their DNA in tissues (particularly in the brain).[7] IHC can be specific, but insensitive for identifying *Neospora* in the placenta; therefore, maternal serology should be used in conjunction.

TREATMENT

There is no treatment that can be used to curtail an ongoing abortion epidemic. Possible drug therapies are generally not considered an option because of likely unacceptable milk and meat residues and withdrawal problems.

DIFFERENTIAL DIAGNOSIS

Serology and/or polymerase chain reaction can confirm infection in individual cows.

Because of the high prevalence of infection, and the occurrence of congenital infection, care must be taken in extrapolating the results of a single positive diagnosis to problems of abortion. The high rate of natural congenital infection means that evidence of infection in an aborted fetus is not proof of causation of abortion, and fetal examination should be coupled to serologic examination of aborting and nonaborting animals in the herd to assess statistical differences.

- Other causes of abortion in cattle
- Weak calf syndrome

CONTROL

All efforts should be made to exclude the possibility of dog **fecal contamination** of cattle feed and water and of the grazing environment.[4] **Placentas, aborted fetuses, and dead calves** should be removed immediately and disposed of so that the definitive host and cattle cannot gain access to them.

Congenitally infected cows are at high risk of abortion, and abortion rates in infected herds can be substantially reduced by **culling** infected animals.[2-4] Congenitally infected calves can be identified by testing precolostral blood samples using a specific and sensitive serologic test and culled at a young age. If precolostral blood sampling is not feasible, examination of sera at 6 months of age should identify infected calves, with positive titers indicating either congenital infection or postnatal infection. Calves introduced into a herd should be seronegative.

It is possible that strategic therapy of pregnant cows with an appropriate antiprotozoal drug could abort the infection. This could be effective in beef cattle, but would probably not be legal or appropriate in lactating dairy cattle.

Although evidence for increased risk for *Neospora* abortion caused by immunosuppression resulting from concurrent infection with BVD virus is equivocal, control of BVD infections should be a component of antineosporosis control.

There has been a considerable effort to develop vaccines against neosporosis.[8,9] An inactivated tachyzoite vaccine was approved in the United States for use in pregnant cows. There are no controlled studies on its efficacy in mitigating the effects of bovine neosporosis in dairy cattle. Vaccination of dairy cattle may interfere with a herd test and cull policy.

FURTHER READING

Goodswen SJ, Kennedy PJ, Ellis JT. A review of the infection, genetics, and evolution of Neospora caninum: from the past to the present. *Infect Genet Evol.* 2003;13:133-150.

Gondim LF. *Neospora caninum* in wildlife. *Trends Parasitol.* 2006;22:247-252.

Hemphill A, Vonlaufen N, Naguleswaran A. Cellular and immunological basis of the host-parasite relationship during infection with *Neospora caninum. Parasitology.* 2006;133:261-278.

Innes EA. The host-parasite relationship in pregnant cattle infected with *Neospora caninum. Parasitology.* 2007;134:1903-1910.

Innes EA, Bartley PM, Maley SW, Wright SE, Buxton D. Comparative host-parasite relationships in ovine toxoplasmosis and bovine neosporosis and strategies for vaccination. *Vaccine.* 2007;25:5495-5503.

Williams DJ, Hartley CS, Björkman C, Trees AJ. Endogenous and exogenous transplacental transmission of *Neospora caninum*—how the route of transmission impacts on epidemiology and control of disease. *Parasitology.* 2009;136:1895-1900.

REFERENCES

1. Radostits O, et al. Diseases associated with protozoa. In: *Veterinary Medicine: A Textbook of the Disease of Cattle, Horses, Sheep, Goats and Pigs.* 10th ed. London: W.B. Saunders; 2007:1509.
2. Dubey JP, Lindsay DS. *Vet Clin North Am Food Anim Pract.* 2006;22:645.
3. Dubey JP, Schares G. *Vet Parasitol.* 2011;180:90.
4. Dubey JP, et al. *Clin Microbiol Rev.* 2007;20:323.
5. Reichel MP, et al. *Int J Parasitol.* 2013;43:133.
6. Dubey JP, et al. *J Comp Pathol.* 2006;134:267.
7. Dubey JP, Schares G. *Vet Parasitol.* 2006;140:1.
8. Innes EA, Vermeulen AN. *Parasitology.* 2006;133(suppl):S145.
9. Reichel MP, Ellis JY. *Int J Parasitol.* 2009;39:1173.
10. Schlafer DH, Miller RB, Maxie MG, eds. Female genital system. In: *Jubb, Kennedy and Palmer's Pathology of Domestic Animals.* Vol. 3. 5th ed. Edinburgh, UK: Saunders; 2007:429.

DOURINE (*MALADIE DU COIT*)

SYNOPSIS

Etiology *Trypanosoma equiperdum.*

Epidemiology Venereal disease of horses, mules, and donkeys, endemic in southern and northern Africa, Asia, and possibly South and Central America.

Clinical signs Primary genital signs, secondary cutaneous signs, and tertiary nervous signs and emaciation.

Lesions Edematous swelling and later, depigmentation of external genitalia, emaciation, anemia, and subcutaneous edema.

Differential diagnosis list

- Nagana
- Surra
- Coital exanthema
- Equine infectious anemia.
- Purulent endometritis

Treatment Chronic cases unresponsive to trypanocides and may become carriers. Treatment is thus not recommended.

Control Elimination of reactors, control of breeding and movement of animals in affected regions or countries.

ETIOLOGY

Trypanosoma equiperdum belongs to the *brucei* group, subgenus *Trypanozoon,* but occurs only as long, slender, and monomorphic form. It may be more appropriately referred to as *T. brucei equiperdum.* Unlike *T. brucei. brucei,* it has lost part of its kinetoplast DNA (hence dyskinetoplastic). The parasite is morphologically indistinguishable from *T. evansi* in blood smears. *T. equiperdum* is the only pathogenic trypanosome that does not require an arthropod vector for its transmission. It resides more in extra vascular tissue fluid than in blood.

EPIDEMIOLOGY

Occurrence

Dourine is endemic in Asia, Africa, southeastern Europe, and Central America. It has been eradicated from North America, and strict control measures have reduced the incidence to a low level in most parts of Europe. It occurred in Italy in 2011.[1] The disease is endemic in parts of Ethiopia and Namibia and is rarely reported in other parts of sub-Saharan Africa. It has not been reported in Latin America for over 20 years. It is possible that lack of reporting in some countries may be caused by very strict international regulations that tend to discourage official notification of the disease. All Equidae are susceptible, and natural infection is known to occur only in horses, mules, and donkeys. In Ethiopia, the disease is more prevalent during the breeding season from June to September.[2]

Measures of Disease Occurrence

In most countries, dourine now occurs only sporadically; its prevalence has declined generally because the horse is no longer that important militarily, economically, and agriculturally, and because of strict control measures in many countries. A recent survey of 237 horses from an endemic area of Ethiopia showed that infection rates varied with the method of examination.[3] The rates were 4.6% based on standard parasitologic methods, 27.6% on serology, and up to 47.6% on DNA detection by PCR. This was the first time in more than 30 years that a fresh strain of *T. equiperdum* was isolated from clinical cases of dourine. Case mortality varies; in Europe, it may be as high as 50% to 70%, but it is much lower elsewhere, although many animals may have to be destroyed as a means of control.

Methods of Transmission

Natural transmission occurs only by coitus, but infection can also be acquired through intact oral, nasal, and conjunctival mucosae in foals at birth. The source of infection may be an infected stallion or mare actively discharging trypanosomes from the urethra or vagina, or an uninfected male acting as a physical carrier after serving an infected mare. The trypanosomes inhabit the urethra and vagina but disappear periodically so that only a proportion of potentially infective matings result in infection. Invasion occurs through intact mucosa, and no abrasion is necessary.

Risk Factors

T. equiperdum is incapable of surviving outside the host. Like other trypanosomes, it also dies quickly in cadavers. Some animals, especially donkeys and mules, may be clinically normal but act as carriers of the infection for many years. Because the disease does not require an arthropod vector for its transmission, and in view of the extensive movement of horses across continents that now takes place, the risk of infection, though small, is present in every country, as with any other venereal disease. Thoroughbred horses are more susceptible than indigenous horses, and donkeys tend to show more chronic signs.

Immune Mechanisms

Infected animals produce antibodies to successive antigenic variants, as in *T. brucei.* Recovered animals often become carriers. Blood from infected horses is rarely infective to other horses, and the disease is not easily transmitted to ruminants under experimental conditions. Humans are not affected.

Biosecurity Concerns

There are none except when animals have to be moved internationally.

PATHOGENESIS

T. equiperdum shows a remarkable tropism for the mucosa of genital organs, the subcutaneous tissues, and the peripheral and CNSs. Trypanosomes deposited during coitus penetrate the intact genital mucosa, multiply locally in the extracellular tissue space, and produce an edematous swelling that may later undergo fibrosis. Subsequent systemic invasion occurs, and localization in other tissues causes vascular injury and edema, manifested clinically by subcutaneous edema. Invasion of the peripheral nervous system and the spinal cord leads to incoordination and paralysis.

CLINICAL FINDINGS

The severity of the clinical syndrome varies depending on the strain of the trypanosome and the general health of the horse population. The disease in Africa and Asia is much more chronic than in South America or Europe and may persist for many years, often without clinical signs, although these may develop when the animals' resistance is lowered by other disease or malnutrition.

The incubation period varies between 1 and 4 weeks, but could extend to more than 3 months in some animals. Initial signs may not be recognized until the breeding season. The ensuing disease will manifest genital signs in the primary stage, cutaneous signs in the secondary stage, and nervous signs in the tertiary stage.

In stallions, the **initial signs** are swelling and edema of the penis, scrotum, prepuce, and surrounding skin, extending as far forward as the chest. Paraphimosis may occur, and inguinal lymph nodes are swollen. There is a moderate mucopurulent urethral discharge. In mares, the edema commences in the vulva and is accompanied by a profuse fluid discharge, hyperemia, and sometimes ulceration of the vaginal mucosa. The edema spreads to the perineum, udder, and abdominal floor. In Europe, the disease is more severe; genital tract involvement is often accompanied by sexual excitement and more severe swelling.

In the **secondary stage**, cutaneous urticaria-like plaques, 2 to 5 cm in diameter, develop on the body and neck and disappear within a few hours up to a few days. These so-called silver dollar spots are pathognomonic for dourine but are not always present and are uncommon in endemic areas. Succeeding crops of plaques may result in persistence of the cutaneous involvement for several weeks.

Progressive anemia, emaciation, weakness, and nervous signs that appear at a variable time after genital involvement characterize the **tertiary stage.** Stiffness and weakness of the limbs are evident and incoordination develops, progressing terminally to ataxia and paralysis. Marked atrophy of the hindquarters is common, and in all animals there is loss of condition, in some to the point where extreme emaciation necessitates destruction. Lack of coordination of the hind legs, swelling of the external genitalia, and emaciation were the most common clinical signs in horses suspected to have dourine in Ethiopia.

CLINICAL PATHOLOGY

Trypanosome detection is difficult, but should be attempted in edema fluid, subcutaneous plaques, and vaginal or urethral washings or blood in early stages. Inoculation of blood into laboratory rodents is not as helpful as with other members of the *brucei* group.

An efficient CFT is available and was the basis for a successful eradication program in Canada. However, the test does not distinguish between members of the *brucei* group. Other serologic tests that can be used include the IFAT, the capillary agglutination test for trypanosomes, and the ELISA, but the CFT remains the most reliable. Serologic tests do not distinguish between members of the *brucei* group; hence they are of limited value in areas where *T. brucei* or *T. evansi* is endemic, even when monoclonal antibodies are used. In recent interlaboratory ring trials to evaluate serologic methods for dourine diagnosis, 9 out of 22 laboratories observed a false-positive result with a known *T. evansi*-positive serum, whether by CFT or IFAT.[4] However, diagnosis can be made based on serologic tests and characteristic clinical signs under the right epidemiologic setting.[2]

PCR has been used to detect trypanosome DNA and is an indication of an active infection, unlike serologic tests that detect past and current infections. Still, the PCR test cannot yet distinguish *T. equiperdum* from *T. evansi* or *T. brucei.*[5,6]

With the recent isolation of new strains of *T. equiperdum* from clinical cases in Ethiopia,[3] the first in 4 decades worldwide, there is hope that new internationally recognized tests for the diagnosis of dourine will be developed soon.

NECROPSY FINDINGS

Emaciation, anemia, and subcutaneous edema are always present, and edema of the external genitalia may be evident or the external genitalia may have healed, leaving the characteristic depigmented scars of permanent leukodermic patches. Lymph nodes are enlarged, and there is softening of the spinal cord in the lumbosacral region.

Histologic lesions consist of lymphoplasmacytic infiltration in the spinal nerves, ganglia, and meninges of the lumbar and sacral regions and in affected skin and mucosa. Trypanosomes can be found in sections of the skin and genital mucosa during the primary and secondary phases of the infection. Affected lymph nodes show nonspecific lymphoid hyperplasia.

DIFFERENTIAL DIAGNOSIS

The full clinical syndrome is diagnostic, when present, because no other disease has the clinical and epizootiologic characteristics of dourine. However, when the full clinical picture is not developed, other diseases like nagana, surra, coital exanthema, equine infectious anemia, and purulent endometritis should be considered. With one exception, all recent reports of the disease have been based on clinical signs, serology, and detection of trypanosome DNA, but not on parasitologic detection.

TREATMENT

TREATMENT AND CONTROL

None is recommended.

Many trypanocidal drugs have been used in the treatment of dourine, but results are variable, chronic cases in particular are unresponsive to treatment. The main drawback is that treated animals may remain inapparent carriers and could continue to spread the disease or complicate serologic tests. Nevertheless, in Ethiopia, treatment of experimentally infected horses with Cymelarsan at 0.25 mg/kg BW was found to be effective for both acute and chronic cases.[7]

Berenil (diminazene) at 7 mg/kg BW as a 5% solution injected IM, with a second injection of half the dose 24 hours later, or suramin (10 mg/kg IV for two to three treatments at weekly intervals), or quinapyramine sulfate (3–5 mg/kg in divided doses injected subcutaneously) have been tried in the past.

CONTROL

In dourine-free countries, an embargo should be placed on the importation of horses from countries in which the disease is endemic, unless the animals have been properly tested and found negative. Eradication on an area or herd basis is by the application of the CFT, along with strict control of breeding and movement of horses. Positive reactors are disposed of, and two negative tests not less than a month apart can be accepted as evidence that the disease is no longer present. Castration or neutering of infected animals is not adequate because mating can still occur.

FURTHER READING

Abebe G. Trypanosomosis in Ethiopia. *Ethiopia J Biol Sci.* 2005;4:75-121.

Barrowman P, et al. Dourine. In: Coetzer JAW, Thomson GR, Tustin RC, eds. *Infectious Diseases of Livestock With Special Reference to Southern Africa.* Vol. 1. Cape Town: Oxford University Press; 1994:206-212.

Desquesnes M. *Livestock Trypanosomoses and Their Vectors in Latin America.* Paris: OIE (World Organization for Animal Health); 2004.

Hunter AG, Luckins AG, Trypanosomosis. In: Sewell MMH, Brocklesby DW, eds. *Handbook on Animal Diseases in the Tropics.* 4th ed. London: Baillière Tindall; 1990:204-226.

Luckins AG, et al. Dourine. In: Coetzer JAW, Tustin RC, eds. *Infectious Diseases of Livestock.* Vol. 1. 2nd ed. Cape Town: Oxford University Press; 2004:297-304.

OIE. *Manual of Diagnostic Tests and Vaccines for Terrestrial Animals.* Vol. 2. 6th ed. 2008:845-851.

Stephen LE. *Trypanosomiasis: A Veterinary Perspective.* Oxford: Pergamon Press; 1986.

REFERENCES

1. Pascucci I, et al. *Vet Parasitol.* 2013;193:30.
2. Hagos A, et al. *Proceedings of ISCTRC.* Kampala, Uganda: 2009:317.
3. Gari FR, et al. *Trop Anim Health Prod.* 2010;42:1649.
4. Cauchard J, et al. *Vet Parasitol.* 2014;205:70.
5. Li FJ, et al. *Mol Cell Probes.* 2007;21:1.
6. Tran T, et al. *Parasitology.* 2006;133:613.
7. Hagos A, et al. *Vet Parasitol.* 2010;171:200.

Toxic Agents Primarily Affecting the Reproductive System

ESTROGENIC SUBSTANCES

ETIOLOGY

Poisoning occurs either accidentally or intentionally from administration of a number of different products. Supplementation may be by addition to the feed, but is usually by subcutaneous implants. Many of them are used as growth promotants to increase weight gain and feed efficiency in animals.[1] Estrogen in some form can be found in the following four categories of growth promotants:

- Endogenous hormones (estradiol-17-β, progesterone, testosterone)[1,2]
- Synthetic hormones (ethinylestradiol, others)[1]
- Xenobiotics (zearalenone [α-zearalanol; zeranol], trenbolone)[1,3]
- Miscellaneous (diethylstilbestrol and related compounds such as hexestrol and dienestrol)[1]

EPIDEMIOLOGY

Occurrence

Poisoning by estrogenic substances occurs in the following circumstances:

- Natural substances such as genistein present in plants and as zearalenone in fungi[1,3]
- Dietary supplements for fattening cattle[1]
- Overdosage of medications used in clinical infertility cases
- Pigs fed hexestrol implants in capon necks
- Cattle fed on chicken litter from farms on which estrogens are used as supplements.

Risk Factors

Animal Risk Factors

Steers implanted with an estrogen at a standard dose rate may respond in an exaggerated manner and show signs of toxicity. Estradiol implants are reputed to be associated with more of these problems than zeranol.

Environmental Risk Factors

Estrogens from treated animals are found in the environment in water and animal manure and may act as endocrine disrupters. Water treatment plants are able to remove most of the estrogens, but animal manure is not regulated in the many parts of the world unless it is discharged into a water supply.[4-6]

Farm Risk Factors

Pasture may be contaminated by manure from cattle treated orally or by subcutaneous implants with estrogenic substances that pass significant amounts in the feces.[2,6] Ensilage made from the pasture may also be contaminated.

Human Risk Factors

Estrogenic substance administration as a management tool is regarded unfavorably in many countries because of the risk of intoxication occurring in humans eating contaminated meat. Their use is banned in some and strictly controlled in others. In one small study, a palpable mammary tumor was observed in a rat implanted with a 12-mg zeranol pellet.[3] The presence of environmental zearalenone has been proposed as a link to early puberty and anabolic growth effects in young girls.[7]

PATHOGENESIS

Signs and lesions are the direct result of amplification of the pharmacologic effects of the substances.

CLINICAL SIGNS

Idiopathic Female Estrogenism

In addition to the toxic effects associated with estrogens in specific plants, increased estrogenic activity is also encountered in mixed pasture, generally only at certain times and on particular fields. Clinically the effects are those of sterility, some abortions, swelling of the udder and vulva in pregnant animals and virgin heifers, and endometritis with a slimy, purulent vaginal discharge in some animals. Estrous cycles are irregular. In milking cows, there is depression of the milk yield, reduction in appetite, and an increase in the cell count of the milk.

Male Estrogenism

Steers in feedlots may exhibit excessive mounting by other steers, sometimes to the point of causing death. Head injuries caused by head-to-head butting, frequent bawling, stampedes, and pawing the ground to the point of hole-digging are other reported signs. These problems tend to pass off after a short time. Preputial prolapse may be a problem in *Bos indicus* cattle. Experimental feeding of zeranol to young bulls is associated with retardation of testicular and epididymal development.

Nymphomania in Cows

Larger doses of stilbestrol, usually administered accidentally to cows, may be associated with prolapse of the rectum and vagina and elevation of the tail head caused by relaxation of the pelvic ligaments. Susceptibility to fracture of the pelvic bones and dislocation of the hip are common sequelae. Nymphomaniac behavior in such animals results in other skeletal injuries, especially fracture of the wing of the ilium.

Swine Estrogenism

Common clinical signs include weight loss, decreased feed efficiency, straining, prolapse of the rectum, incontinence of urine, anuria, and death.[8] Estrogens such as zearalenone ingested by sows after day 11 to 13 of the estrous cycle can be associated with retention of corpora lutea and a syndrome of anestrus or pseudopregnancy, which typically persists for 45 to 60 days postestrus. This effect may occur at zearalenone concentrations of 3 to 10 ppm in the diet. Pregnant sows given zearalenone postbreeding may have failure of implantation and early fetal abortion.

Urethral Obstruction

Heavy mortalities have occurred in feeder lambs after the use of implants of estrogens as a result of prolapse of the rectum, vagina, and uterus, together with urethral obstruction by calculi. The calculi consist largely of desquamated epithelial and inflammatory cells that form a nidus for the deposition of mineral; the desquamation is probably stimulated by the estrogen. Also, urethral narrowing caused by the estrogen facilitates complete obstruction by the calculi.

CLINICAL PATHOLOGY

High blood levels of estrogens are characteristic. In swine, the syndrome of anestrus associated with zearalenone will be accompanied by elevated progesterone concentrations caused by the retention of corpora lutea.

NECROPSY FINDINGS

Enlargement and vascular engorgement of accessory sex organs, especially in neutered animals, are characteristic. Uterine enlargement and keratinization of vaginal epithelium may be detected, and in mature female swine there may be persistent multiple retained corpora lutea. Swine also show inflammation and necrosis of the rectal wall, enlargement of the kidneys, thickening of the ureters and distension of the bladder, and gross enlargement of the prostate and seminal vesicles. Histopathology on jejunum obtained from pigs treated with low doses of zearalenone and T-2 toxin showed normal crypts and villi but decreased numbers of goblet cells and acidophilic granulocytes in the mucous membrane and numerous plasma cells in the intestinal epithelium.[8]

FURTHER READING

Adams NR. Detection of the effects of phytoestrogens on sheep and cattle. *J Anim Sci.* 1995;73:1509-1515.

Burnison BK, Hartman A, Lister A, et al. A toxicity identification evaluation approach to studying estrogenic substances in hog manure and agricultural runoff. *Environ Toxicol Chem.* 2003;22:2243-2250.

Leffers H, Naesby M, Vendelbo B, et al. OEstrogenic potencies of zeranol, oestradiol, diethylstiboestrol, bisphenol-A and genistein; implications for exposure assessment of potential endocrine disruptors. *Hum Reprod.* 2001;16:1037-1045.

Soto AN, Calabro JM, Prechtl NV, et al. Androgenic and estrogenic activity in water bodies receiving cattle feedlot effluent in Eastern Nebraska, USA. *Environ Health Persp.* 2004;112:346-352.

REFERENCES

1. Biswas S, et al. *J Soil Water Con.* 2013;66:325.
2. Khanal SK, et al. *Environ Sci Technol.* 2006;40: 6537.
3. Zhong S, et al. *Anticancer Res.* 2011;31:1659.
4. Chen TS, et al. *Sci Total Environ.* 2010;408:3223.
5. Alvarez DA, et al. *Water Res.* 2013;47:3347.
6. Gadd JB, et al. *Environ Pollut.* 2010;158:730.
7. Massart F, et al. *J Pediatr.* 2008;152:690.
8. Andretta I, et al. *Arch Zootech.* 2010;59:123.

PHYTOESTROGEN TOXICOSIS

SYNOPSIS

Etiology Ingestion of plants that produce estrogen (phytoestrogens) resulting in a number of reproductive problems.

Epidemiology Pastures dominated by specific strains of legumes, in lush growth mode, or hay or silage made from such pasture, are associated with problems if exposure is prolonged. Sheep are much more susceptible than cattle.

Clinical pathology Positive estrogen assay in blood.

Lesions

Live animals: Severe flock infertility in sheep; prolongation of estrus periods, interestrus periods shortened.

Postmortem: Ewes show cystic endometrial degeneration.

Diagnosis confirmation Laboratory assay of feed, blood, and tissue; the appearance of genital pathology at necropsy, or with a uterine biopsy or laparoscopy.

Treatment None.

Control Grazing management, use of low-phytoestrogen cultivars.

ETIOLOGY

Important estrogenic substances found in plants and fungi include the following:

- Plants
  - Coumestans (coumestrol, 4-methoxycoumestrol, repensol, trifoliol)[1]
  - Isoflavones (daidzein, formononetin, genistein, biochanin A, glycitein)[2,3]
  - Isoflavan (equol, a metabolite of daidzein)[3]
- Fungi (resorcylic acid lactones [zearalenone])[4]

Compared with pharmaceutical agents, these substances have low estrogenic activity, but they are associated with serious clinical effects because of the high concentrations they reach in some plants and daily intake over long periods. The coumestans are most common in plants of the *Medicago* genus; isoflavones are most common in the *Trifolium, Baptisia,* and *Cytisus* genera. Only *Medicago* and *Trifolium* spp. are of any importance to animals. Those likely to contain sufficient amounts to be associated with disease are

Fusarium (variety of species); contains zearalenone[4]
Glycine max (soybean; contains coumestans and isoflavones; affects pigs)
Medicago sativa (alfalfa, lucerne; contains coumestans; affects cattle, sheep)
Trifolium alexandrinum (isoflavones)
T. alpestre (alpestrine clover; contains isoflavones)
T. pratense (red clover; contains isoflavones; affects sheep)[1]
T. repens (white clover, Ladino clover; contains coumestans)[1]
T. subterraneum (subterranean clover; contains isoflavones; affects sheep).

EPIDEMIOLOGY

Occurrence

Animals on pasture are at the greatest risk, but poisoning can also occur on diets containing prepared feeds such as soybean (*Glycine max*) meal, or moldy feed containing *Fusarium* fungi.

Risk Factors

Animal Factors

Phytoestrogen toxicosis is clinically important only in sheep. Cattle are generally considered to be less sensitive than sheep.[1,5,6] For example, cows can ingest large amounts of estrogens (over 40 g per day per cow) in red clover without showing any reduction in reproductive efficiency. Horses usually graze the toxic pasture without ill effects.

Massive reproductive wastage has been experienced in sheep on pastures dominated by such plants as *Trifolium subterraneum,* and the death rate from dystocia and prolapse of the uterus can also be high. The most common abnormality is a failure to conceive, even with multiple matings, and the flock breeding status worsens progressively, with the lambing percentage falling from a normal 80% down to 30%. Sheep eating a lot of estrogenic clover in the spring can become temporarily infertile, but are normally fertile again by the usual breeding season in the autumn. However, ingestion of the plant in several successive years is associated with "permanent clover disease"—infertility from which ewes do not recover. Under these conditions sheep farming becomes unprofitable, and large areas of country have been made unsuitable for sheep raising because of this disease.

Human Factors

Various phytoestrogens have been found in foods of animal origin (eggs, milk, meat, fish, and seafood). Equol was found in several foods, including eggs, milk, and meat.[7] Not all phytoestrogens are harmful and many of them are have known human health benefits.[8] Many, however, are endocrine disruptors, which means that they can produce adverse health effects as well.

Plant Factors

The estrogenic activity of pastures depends on the degree of domination of the pasture by the toxic plants, the variety of the plant species, and the duration of the animal's exposure to them. Newly sown pastures are usually most toxic because of domination by the sown legume. Pastures deficient in phosphorus are also likely to be clover dominant. High nitrogen fertilizer applications reduce phytoestrogen content. Varieties of *Trifolium subterraneum,* e.g., Yarloop, Dwalganup, Dinninup, and Geraldton, are much more toxic than Bacchus Marsh and Daliak. Pastures containing more than 30% of the first four varieties are likely to be unsafe. In some clovers, e.g., red clover, the estrogen content varies with the season, and is high in early spring, low in midsummer, and high again in the autumn after the hay has been taken off. Insect damage to pasture can increase the estrogen content 10-fold, and bacterial infection (e.g., by *Pseudopezzia medicaginnis,* a leaf-spotting organism on alfalfa) and fungal infection by 100-fold. Plants that have matured in the field and set seed have no estrogenic potency, but the making of potent fodder into hay causes little depression of estrogen content. Clover ensilage can contain high levels of estrogens, and the ensiling process is considered to increase the estrogenic effect of clover 3- to 5-fold.

Trifolium repens (white clover, in contradistinction to Ladino clover), does not have a high content of estrogens.[1] However, when heavily infested with fungi it can contain significant amounts. It is thought that the production of estrogens is a byproduct of the plant's mechanism of resistance to the fungal infection. Ladino clover, a large-growing variety of white clover, may contain large quantities of a highly active estrogen (coumestrol), and when it dominates a pasture and is grazed when the pasture is lush, it may be associated with the cornification of vaginal epithelium and functional infertility in ewes. Three estrogenic compounds have been isolated from *T. pratense* (red clover), and where this plant dominates the pasture a clinical syndrome similar to that associated with subterranean clover may be observed. Ewes grazing on red clover pasture, especially a toxic cultivar of the plant, may have their conception rate at the first mating cycle reduced from 75% to as low as 25%.

PATHOGENESIS

Much of the metabolism of phytoestrogens in ruminants occurs in the rumen as well as in the liver.[1] The differences between sheep and cattle in the ruminal metabolism of these compounds are thought to be the reason for the comparative freedom of cattle from the clinical disease.

The amount of phytoestrogen ingested by a ewe on a highly poisonous pasture may equal her daily estrogen secretion at the peak of her estrous cycle. The effect of the phytoestrogens is exerted mainly on the uterus and ovaries. Structurally, there is hyperplasia and hypertrophy of the epithelium of the uterus, vagina, and cervix, and dysplasia of the granulosa cells of the ovary, with a consequent reduction in secretion of estradiol. Increases in teat size and milk secretion are additional, secondary effects.

The functional abnormality is not one of estrus; in sheep the demonstration and duration of estrus may be normal or depressed, and the defect is one of sperm transport because of changes in the composition of cervical mucus and the structure of cervical glands. The change is to more watery mucus, and this is the basis of a test in affected sheep in which the watery mucus is more readily absorbed by a cottonwood plug inserted in the vagina. The increased weight of the plug is a positive test.

It is possible that a good deal of the infertility seen in ewes on improved clover pasture may be associated with its high estrogen content, in spite of the absence of the more dramatic evidence of hyperestrogenism described earlier. Because it is necessity to use this pasture, a great deal more needs to be known about the seasonal occurrence of the estrogenic substances and the management of sheep grazing the pasture so that the effects of the disease can be minimized.

CLINICAL FINDINGS

Ewes

Clover disease, the severe clinical manifestation of phytoestrogen poisoning, and rarely seen today, includes dystocia, prolapse of the uterus or vagina, severe infertility, and death. The more common and less severe field expression of phytoestrogen poisoning is a significant decrease in fertility rate. It may be temporary with normal reproductive efficiency returning soon after the ewes are moved to clover-free pasture. In ewes exposed to a low level intake of estrogens over a long period, e.g., in excess of two grazing seasons, a process of irreversible "defeminization" may occur. This is a state of permanent subfertility. The estrous cycle is normal, but an abnormally large number of ewes fail to conceive. In affected flocks, there may also be a high incidence of maternal dystocia caused by uterine inertia, or failure of the cervix or vagina to dilate. Affected ewes show little evidence of impending parturition and many full-term fetuses are born dead.

Male Castrates

Wethers may secrete milk, and metaplasia of the prostate and bulbourethral glands is evident. These can be detected at an early stage of development by digital rectal palpation. Continuing hyperplasia and cystic dilatation of these glands is associated with their prolapse in a subanal position, followed by rapid weight loss and fatal rupture of the bladder. Rams usually show no clinical abnormality, and their fertility is not impaired.

Cattle exhibit clinical signs less often than sheep, with experimental reports of decreases in conception and fertilization caused by prolongation of oocyte maturation and decreased sensitivity of the corpus luteum to luteolytic agents.[5,6] Temporary infertility; discharge of cervical mucus; and swelling of the mammary gland, vulva, and uterus have all been recorded in cattle.

Gilts exposed to genistein may develop structural changes and abnormalities in the cervix and uterus.[9]

CLINICAL PATHOLOGY

Laboratory assays are available and essential to diagnosis and monitoring of feed contents of phytoestrogens.[7] Chemical assays are not as sensitive as biologic assessments based on increased size of genitalia in subject animals.

NECROPSY FINDINGS

Severe cystic degeneration of the endometrium is present in the most severe cases. Similar clinical and histopathologic changes have been produced by the daily injection of 0.03 mg of diethylstilbestrol per ewe for a period of 6 months. There is also a long-term change in the cervix with an increased incidence of cervicitis and a histologically observable transformation to a uterine-like appearance. In ewes on a long-term intake of toxic pasture, the lesions include elevation of the tail head, partial fusion of the vulvar labia, and clitoral hypertrophy.

Diagnostic confirmation of phytoestrogen poisoning requires laboratory assay of feed, blood, and tissue, and the appearance of genital pathology at necropsy, or with a uterine biopsy, or laparoscopy.

DIFFERENTIAL DIAGNOSIS

Differential diagnosis list
- Overdose of pharmaceutical preparation as part of a program to improve fertility in a herd.
- Overdose of an implant or feed additive with a growth stimulant that has estrogenic capability.

TREATMENT

Administration of testosterone is a logical response to poisoning but appears to be an unlikely commercial proposition.

CONTROL

Avoidance of high estrogenic activity strains of the respective plants, grazing management to avoid dangerous pasture at the most toxic part of the season, and dilution of the estrogen intake by providing additional and alternative feeds, are all used to control the disease. Prevention of clover disease can only be achieved by proper management of sheep and pasture to avoid ingestion of excessive amounts of estrogens. Vaccination with a phytoestrogen-immunogenic protein conjugate has produced good levels of antibodies, but has not been successful in preventing the problem. Careful management of flocks on estrogenic pasture can significantly improve reproductive output.

FURTHER READING

Adams NR. Detection of the effects of phytoestrogens on sheep and cattle. *J Anim Sci*. 1995;73:1509-1515.

Hughes CL. Phytochemical mimicry of reproductive hormones and modulation of herbivore fertility by phytoestrogens. *Environ Health Persp*. 1988;78:171.

Kuiper G, et al. Interaction of estrogenic chemicals and phytoestrogens with estrogen receptor β. *Endocrinology*. 1998;139:4252-4263.

Radostits O, et al. Phytoestrogen poisoning. In: *Veterinary Medicine: A Textbook of the Disease of Cattle, Horses, Sheep, Goats and Pigs*. 10th ed. London: W.B. Saunders; 2007:1873.

REFERENCES

1. Steinshamn H, et al. *J Dairy Sci*. 2008;91:2715.
2. Hoikkala A, et al. *Mol Nutr Food Res*. 2007;51:782.
3. Jackman KA, et al. *Curr Med Chem*. 2007;14:2824.
4. Zinedine A, et al. *Food Chem Toxicol*. 2007;45:1.
5. Borzym E, et al. *Med Weter*. 2008;64:1107.
6. Piotrowska KK, et al. *J Reprod Dev*. 2006;52:33.
7. Kuhnle GGC, et al. *J Agric Food Chem*. 2008;56:10099.
8. Patisaul HB, et al. *Front Neuroendocrinol*. 2010;31:400.
9. Ford JA, et al. *J Anim Sci*. 2006;84:834.

ZEARALENONE TOXICOSIS

SYNOPSIS

Etiology Zearalenone is an estrogenic mycotoxin produced primarily by fungus in the genus *Fusarium*, which is the causative agent. *F. graminearum* is the species most responsible for animal reproductive problems, but *F. cerealis, F. culmorum, F. cookwellense, F. equiseti*, and *F. semitectum* are contaminants of moldy maize, wheat, oats, and barley grain and cause issues as well.

Epidemiology Global issue with zearalenone found in a variety of cereals and foodstuffs in many countries.

Clinical pathology None in particular; progesterone levels may be decreased.

Lesions Associated with hyperestrogenism and include abortions, stillbirths, mammary gland enlargement and secretions, vulvar edema, and vaginitis in females as well as testicular atrophy and mammary gland enlargement in males.

Diagnostic confirmation Presence of zearalenone and/or metabolites in feces, urine, and serum; presence in feedstuffs.

Treatment Remove animals from contaminated feed and correct prolapses.

Control Keep moisture content of stored grain below 15%–16%; feed contaminated grains to less susceptible animals.

ETIOLOGY

Zearalenone is a nonsteroidal estrogenic mycotoxin produced primarily by fungi in the genus *Fusarium. F. graminearum* is the species most responsible for animals' reproductive problems, but *F. cerealis, F. culmorum, F. cookwellense, F. equiseti*, and *F. semitectum* are contaminants of moldy maize, wheat, oats, and barley grain and are associated with toxicosis.[1,2] Swine are most commonly affected, but cases have occurred in sheep and cattle[3,4] and more rarely in horses.[5]

EPIDEMIOLOGY

Occurrence

The fungi that produce zearalenone primarily colonize corn, but they also infect other cereal grains such as barley, wheat, and oats.[1,2] Zearalenone has also been detected in a number of other plants including rice, sorghum, millet, and soybeans. Most typically, contamination occurs from high moisture during storage; field contamination has been reported but occurs less often. Zearalenone has been detected in pastures in New Zealand, which has been associated with infertility in ewes.[6] Contamination of food and animals is considered a global problem because zearalenone has been found in Africa, Asia, Australia, Europe, North America, and South America.[2]

Risk Factors

Animal Risk Factors

Swine of all ages, but especially prepubertal gilt, are the most sensitive to the effects of zearalenone. The primary effects are reproductive and depend on the dose and time of administration in relationship to the animal's estrous cycle.[5,6]

Farm Risk Factors

Elevated levels of zearalenone in the feed are primarily associated with improper storage and not contamination in the field.[2]

Human Risk Factors

There is considerable concern that humans, especially young girls, will be adversely affected by zearalenone in cereal products, milk and milk-based products, and meats. In Europe, 32% of mixed cereal samples from nine countries were found to be contaminated with zearalenone. Zearalenone is excreted in milk and present in some concentration in meats in animals with high intake, but currently the risk to humans is thought to be low.[2]

PATHOGENESIS

Zearalenone is rapidly absorbed following an oral exposure, with an estimated uptake of 80% to 85%.[1,2] In swine, it can be detected in the serum within about 30 minutes after ingestion.[2] Distribution is primarily to the adipose tissue and the ovary and uterus. The liver is the main site of metabolism, but other tissues such as the intestine, kidney, ovary, and testis are metabolic sites.[1] Two different biotransformation pathways have been proposed and likely play a role in the susceptibility `of different species.[1,5] Zearalenone is either conjugated with glucuronic acid or hydroxylated to α- and β-zearalenol.[1,5] In swine, the preferred route is conjugation with conversion to primarily α-zearalenol.[1,4,5] Sheep are similar to swine but cattle convert to β-zearalenol, a less estrogenic metabolite.[4] Excretion is biliary in most species with significant enterohepatic recirculation occurring.[1]

Zearalenone crosses cell membranes and binds to cytosolic 17β-estradiol receptors. Once this occurs, it is translocated into the nucleus where it binds to estrogen-responsive elements and stimulates mRNA synthesis resulting in estrogen-like effects.[1,3]

CLINICAL FINDINGS

Swine

Pigs of all ages are affected, including piglets nursing on sows, which themselves show no signs of estrogenism. The most significantly affected are the 6 to 7-month-old gilts. Vulvovaginitis, including swelling of the vulva to three to four times normal size, enlargement of mammary glands, a thin catarrhal exudate from the vulva, and increased size and weight of the ovaries and uterus, is the severest form of the poisoning.[3,6] Prolapse of the vagina is common (up to 30% of affected pigs) and there is prolapse of the rectum in some pigs (5%–10%). The toxin reduces serum progesterone levels in sows, but the administration of progesterone to affected gilts does not counteract the estrogenic effects. The syndrome is indistinguishable from that produced by long-term overdosing with diethylstilbestrol. Signs appear 3 to 6 days after feeding of moldy grain commences and disappear soon after the feeding stops. The mortality rate is high because of the secondary development of cystitis, uremia, and septicemia.

The more important manifestation of the poisoning may be infertility, including absence of estrus, high levels of stillbirth, neonatal mortality, and reduced litter size. Small fetal size, fetal malformations, splayleg and hindlimb paresis, pseudopregnancy, and constant estrus are also recorded.[3]

Zearalenone in male pigs can induce feminizing characteristics; suppress libido; and decrease spermatogenesis, testicular weights, and serum testosterone concentrations.[2]

Ruminants

In cattle, the effect of zearalenone is largely on conception rate, and the rate of services per conception may rise, but the overall effect is less than in sows. Milk production may be decreased.[2] Behavioral estrus occurs at times unrelated to ovarian cycles and in late pregnant cows. There is idiopathic vaginitis. Symmetric enlargement of the mammary glands is recorded in prepubertal dairy heifers feeding on fungus-infected corn. Estrogenic disturbances are also suspected in sheep. Abortion is suspected to occur, and mild vulvovaginitis and hypertrophy of the uterus are recorded. Experimental feeding of zearalenone to lactating cows and ewes does result in minor contamination of their milk sufficient to produce hyperestrogenism in a lamb sucking a poisoned ewe.

Horses

Zearalenone toxicosis is rarely reported in horses.[1] A recent study using equine ovarian cultured granulosa cells demonstrated that zearalenone may play a role in some equine reproductive disorders.[5]

CLINICAL PATHOLOGY

Zearalenone and its metabolites can be identified in urine, plasma, and feces by high-performance liquid chromatography[7] and in feedstuffs by liquid chromatography mass spectrometry and a rapid immunoassay.[8,9] In 2003, 16 countries limited the amount of allowable zearalenone in maize and cereals; the allowable concentration varies from 50 to 1000 μg/kg depending on the country.[5]

NECROPSY FINDINGS

On necropsy, there are nonspecific findings other than expected changes associated with estrogen-related reproductive tract abnormalities. These include changes in ovarian weight with decreased numbers of corpora lutea, increased dead piglets, vaginal and rectal prolapses, vulvar edema and vaginitis in females, and testicular atrophy and mammary gland enlargement in males.[10]

DIFFERENTIAL DIAGNOSIS

Differential diagnosis list
- Accidental overdose of synthetic estrogen substances
- Estrogenic substances
- Phytoestrogens

TREATMENT

Complete recovery follows when the feeding of the affected grain is stopped and no treatment other than surgical repair of the prolapsed organs is attempted.

CONTROL

The moisture content of grains should be kept below 15% to 16% during storage. If contaminated feeds must be used, they should be fed to animals less susceptible to toxicosis. The 2006 EU guidelines for zearalenone in feeds recommend that piglets and gilts do not receive more than 0.1 mg zearalenone/kg BW; sows and fattening pigs no more than 0.25 mg zearalenone/kg BW; and sheep, goats, calves, and dairy cows no more than 0.5 mg zearalenone/kg BW.[10]

FURTHER READING

Etienne M, Jemmali M. Effects of zearalenone (F2) on estrous activity and reproduction in gilts. *J Anim Sci.* 1982;55:1-10.

Tanaka T, Hasegawa A, Yamamoto S, et al. Worldwide contamination of cereals by the *Fusarium* mycotoxins nivalenol, deoxynivalenol, and zearalenone. Survey of 19 countries. *J Agric Food Chem.* 1988;36:979-983.

Radostits O, et al. Zearalenone. In: *Veterinary Medicine: A Textbook of the Disease of Cattle, Horses, Sheep, Goats and Pigs.* 10th ed. London: W.B. Saunders; 2007:1911.

REFERENCES

1. Minervini F, et al. *Int J Mol Sci.* 2008;9:2570.
2. Zinedine A, et al. *Food Chem Toxicol.* 2007;45:1.
3. Kanora A, et al. *Vet Med-Czech.* 2009;12:565.
4. Malekineja HR, et al. *Vet J.* 2006;172:96.
5. Minervini F, et al. *Reprod Biol Endocrinol.* 2006;4:62.
6. Upadhaya SD, et al. *Asian-Aus J Anim Sci.* 2010;23:1250.
7. Songsermsakul P, et al. *J Chromatography B.* 2006;843:252.
8. Tanaka H, et al. *Rapid Commun Mass Spectrom.* 2006;20:1422.
9. Kolosova AY, et al. *Anal Bioanal Chem.* 2007;389:2103.
10. Tiemann U, et al. *Food Addit Contam.* 2007;24:306.

MARE REPRODUCTIVE LOSS SYNDROME (EARLY FETAL LOSS, LATE FETAL LOSS, FIBRINOUS PERICARDITIS, AND UNILATERAL UVEITIS)

SYNOPSIS

Etiology Exposure to Eastern tent caterpillars (ETCs; *Malacosoma americanum*), in particular during the spring when the caterpillars are most active.

Epidemiology Occurs primarily in the Ohio River valley, but reported in other states. Risk factors are the presence of black cherry trees on pasture, ETC, and feeding hay on the ground.

Clinical pathology Culture of fetal and placental tissue most commonly results in growth of non–β-hemolytic streptococci and/or *Actinobacillus*.

Lesions Inflammation of the intraamniotic umbilical cord (funisitis), premature placental separation, placental edema, placentitis, diffuse alveolitis, and hemorrhage in a variety of organs.

Diagnostic confirmation Based on the presence of appropriate clinical signs with a history of exposure of affected horses to ETCs.

Treatment Supportive care only.

Control Removal of cherry trees from pasture, spraying ETC nests and pastures with pyrethrin pesticides, keeping horses off pasture or muzzling mares on pasture during active ETC months.

ETIOLOGY

In 2001 an epidemic of early fetal loss (40–80 days; range 40–140 days) and late fetal loss (about 340 days) was recognized in north central Kentucky, southern Ohio, and Tennessee affecting over 3500 mares.[1,2] It occurred again in 2002 but far fewer horses were affected. The epidemic was termed mare reproductive loss syndrome (MRLS). At the same time there was also a marked increase in incidence of birth of weak foals and fibrinous pericarditis and unilateral uveitis in adult horses in the same region.[1-3] Research in horses and pigs confirmed the causative agent as *Malacosoma americanum*, the Eastern tent caterpillar (ETC). Similar episodes of equine abortions, now referred to as equine amnionitis and fetal loss (EAFL), occurred in Australia and have been associated with the *Ochrogaster lunifer*, the processionary caterpillar.[4,5]

EPIDEMIOLOGY

Historically, many epidemiologic studies were performed to determine the source of the epidemic. Several toxins such as fescue, nitrate/nitrite, phytoestrogens, and mycotoxins were examined and ruled out leaving a strong association between the presence of ETCs (*M. americanum,* black cherry trees (*Prunus serotina*), and feeding horses hay off the ground. Black cherry trees were involved because they are the preferred host tree for ETC and may be a source of cyanide. Black cherry trees (i.e., cyanide) were ruled out as a cause of MRLS, and an association with ETC was examined experimentally. In several different experiments, pregnant horses (50 to 200 days' gestation) were exposed to various forms of ETC and only those mares exposed to live ETC larvae aborted. These were the first studies to reproduce MRLS and demonstrate that ETC could cause pregnancy loss in mares. Further studies demonstrated that the cuticle (setae; hairs) is the structure responsible for the abortigenic activity.[1,2] Culture of the placental fluid or fetal tissues in both early and late losses showed non–β-hemolytic streptococci and *Actinobacillus,* which are bacteria routinely found in the oral cavity of horses.[2,6] Finally, the syndrome was reproduced in pigs with abortions occurring 13 to 16 days after first ingestion.[1] More important, histopathologic examination showed ETC setae imbedded in the gastrointestinal mucosa that were surrounded by microgranulomatous lesions.[1,2,6] A similar pattern was subsequently confirmed in pregnant and nonpregnant mares.

Occurrence

The first well-studied and documented outbreak of abortions occurred from April 26 through mid-June of 2001, with a lower incidence of disease during the same months in 2002. An abortion storm, which may have been related, occurred in Kentucky in 1991 and 1982, but no epidemiologic studies were performed.[1] In 2006, a similar syndrome associated with large numbers of ETC was reported in Florida.[2]

The 2001 to 2002 outbreak caused early fetal loss in 25% to 63% of mares on one-third of farms, 14% to 24% on another third, and 2% to 13% on the remaining one-third. Approximately 21% of mares pregnant at 42 days' gestation were not pregnant when examined at 70 to 90 days' gestation. The expected pregnancy loss rate between 42 days and parturition is 12%. Over 3500 mares (3000 early fetal losses; 500 late fetal losses) aborted during the outbreak.[1,3] The economic losses incurred because of MRLS during 2001 and 2002 are estimated to be $500 million.[1]

Risk Factors

Animal Risk Factors

Risk factors for the disease are the presence of black cherry trees, exposure to ETC (especially the presence of large numbers of caterpillars on pasture), and pasturing or feeding hay to horses at pasture.

For late-term abortion the risk factors include increased amount of time at pasture, less time in stall, feeding concentrate on the ground, increased proportion of feed obtained from pasture, and being fed exclusively in pasture during the final 4 weeks of gestation. All of these factors favor exposure to ETC.

Risk factors for pericarditis include presence of mares or foals with MRLS on the farm, grazing, and exposure to ETC. Risk factors for uveitis have not been defined.

Farm Risk Factors

ETCs are endemic to the eastern United States including the Ohio River valley. Egg masses are laid on many trees in the Rosaceae family including black cherry trees, which are the preferred host. Eggs hatch in the early spring when the cherry trees bud. Local populations of the caterpillars fluctuate dramatically from year to year, but mares are likely exposed to small numbers of the caterpillars every spring. Climatic conditions that favor survival of ETC and synchronize their maturation result in simultaneous hatching of large numbers of eggs. The rapid emergence of large numbers of caterpillars results in abrupt and heavy exposure of horses and consequent development of MRLS. Weather conditions thought to contribute to the 2001 outbreak include a period of low temperatures in March, above normal temperatures in April, and a frost and freeze in late April immediately followed by several warm days.

PATHOGENESIS

The pathogenesis of the diseases associated with MRLS has not been well defined. Based on experimental studies and natural cases, ETC setae are likely involved in the pathophysiology. Two different hypotheses have been proposed:

- Setae lodged in the gastrointestinal submucosa causes inflammation, form microgranulomas, and disrupt the mucosal barrier. Resident bacteria such as *Actinobacillus* spp. penetrate the barrier, resulting in bacteremia and hematogenous spread to the placenta, fetus, pericardium, uvea, and meninges.[1,6]
- Setae or parts of the exoskeleton contain an as yet unidentified toxin that is toxic to the placenta and fetus.[1]

CLINICAL FINDINGS

Early Fetal Loss

This is detected by per rectum uterine examination, either manual or using ultrasonographic visualization of uterine contents, during early pregnancy. Fetal loss occurs after 35 days, conception not being affected, and affected mares do not come into estrus because of the presence of endometrial cups, which do not regress until 100 to 180 days after ovulation.[3]

Mares have no clinically detectable premonitory signs of fetal loss.[1,2] Ultrasonographic examination of the uterus of pregnant mares reveals that the allantoic fluid of fetuses <80 days of age has increased echogenicity on the day of fetal death. Allantoic fluid increases in echogenicity with increasing fetal age, and care should be taken when interpreting this observation.

Late Fetal Loss

Late fetal loss occurs as a late-term abortion (final several weeks of gestation), birth of a stillborn foal at full term, and the birth of a foal that is weak and of reduced viability. The birth of an affected foal is associated with premature placental separation ("red bag" deliveries), foaling while standing, and explosive expulsion of the fetus and placenta. Foals born alive are weak, have sunken eyes, progressive neurologic signs consistent with hypoxia, and have a high death rate (50%) despite intensive care. Severe leukopenia at birth often progresses to leukocytosis at 24 to 48 hours of age. Serum biochemical abnormalities include elevated serum creatinine concentrations, hypoglycemia, and increased serum creatine kinase activity. Bacteria isolated from stillborn foals at necropsy or on culture of blood samples from sick foals are nonspecific organisms, including nonhemolytic streptococci and *Actinobacillus* spp.

Fibrinous Pericarditis

Clinical signs in horses of both genders include tachycardia, pleural effusion, pericardial effusion, ascites, fever, abdominal pain, and sudden death.[1,2] Younger horses (<2 years of age) may be more susceptible to developing pericarditis. There is accumulation of large quantities of pericardial fluid and fibrin deposition on the parietal and visceral pericardial surfaces evident on ultrasonographic examination of the chest. The lungs have ultrasonographic evidence of consolidation consistent with pneumonia in approximately 50% of cases. Pericardiocentesis yields abundant fluid that is light yellow and has a low white blood cell count ($<5 \times 10^9$/L) characterized by well-preserved neutrophils. Horses with a prolonged course of the disease (>2 weeks) can have elevated white cell counts in pericardial fluid secondary to opportunistic infection, usually with *Actinobacillus* spp.[6] Hematologic abnormalities are minimal and characterized by a slight leukocytosis in approximately 50% of cases. Azotemia occurs in horses with severe cardiac tamponade.

Unilateral Uveitis

Clinical signs are acute and unilateral and include corneal edema, exudates in the anterior and posterior chambers, and iris hemorrhage.[1] Progression of the syndrome leads to blindness and global atrophy. There is no age predilection and no organisms have been found on culture.

CLINICAL PATHOLOGY

Culture of fetal and placental tissue most commonly results in growth of non–β-hemolytic streptococci and/or *Actinobacillus*. *Actinobacillus* spp., along with several other bacteria, has been isolated from fibrinous pneumonia.

Diagnostic confirmation is based on the presence of appropriate clinical signs with a history of exposure of affected horses to ETCs.

DIFFERENTIAL DIAGNOSIS

Differential diagnosis list:
Cyanide toxicosis
Ergot/fescue
Infectious causes of placentitis
Mycotoxicosis
Nitrate toxicosis
Phytoestrogens

NECROPSY FINDINGS

Examination of the placenta, stillborn foals, and foals that die after birth reveals inflammation of the intraamniotic umbilical cord (funisitis), premature placental separation, placental edema, placentitis, diffuse alveolitis, and hemorrhage in a variety of organs. Horses with pericarditis have impressive accumulation of hairy fibrin in the pericardial space with marked thickening of the visceral and parietal pericardium (a hoary heart).

TREATMENT

Treatment of affected foals is primarily supportive in nature. Horses with pericarditis should have the fluid drained to relieve or prevent cardiac tamponade and to minimize the accumulation of fibrin. Pericardial fluid may need to be drained several times, and its accumulation should be monitored ultrasonographically. Administration of broad-spectrum antibiotics should be based on culture and sensitivity of pericardial fluid. Treatment for uveitis is standard and includes atropine, antiinflammatory agents, topical and systemic antibiotics (culture and sensitivity as indicated), and other agents such as cyclosporin or tissue plasminogen activator.

CONTROL

This is based on prevention of ingestion of ETC by horses. Preventing horses from ingesting caterpillars by minimizing access to pasture and feeding hay in stalls is likely to be beneficial.

Other control measures include removing wild or black cherry trees, the favored host species for ETCs, from pastures, hedges, and fence rows; applying pesticides to trees to kill over wintering eggs or, after hatching, caterpillars; installation of barriers to caterpillar migration onto pasture; manual removal of egg tents; installing pheromone traps; and restricting access of mares to pasture.[7,8]

Application of bifenthrin or permethrin, but not 3% horticultural oil, to egg masses (tents) during the winter prevents emergence of caterpillars in the spring. Insecticidal soap or oils sprayed on neonatal caterpillars is minimally effective. Bifenthrin or spinosad are effective against all instars for 7 days when sprayed on foliage. Injection of trunks of cherry trees with dicrotophos or emamectin is effective against all instars, but injection with milbemectin or avermectin is not effective. A spray of 50 mL of 39% permethrin diluted in 4 L of water and applied to a 2-m wide band of pasture outside the fence line kills migrating caterpillars and prevents them obtaining access to pasture. This solution can also be sprayed on the trunks of trees to kill caterpillars as they leave the tree.

FURTHER READING

Cohen ND, Donahue JG, Carey VJ, et al. Case-control study of late-term abortions associated with mare reproductive loss syndrome in central Kentucky. *J Am Vet Med Assoc.* 2003;222:199-209.

Cohen ND, Carey VJ, Donahue JG, et al. Descriptive epidemiology of late-term abortions associated with the mare reproductive loss syndrome in central Kentucky. *J Vet Diagn Invest.* 2003;15:295-297.

Dwyer RM, Garber LP, Traub-Dargatz JL, et al. Case-control study of factors associated with excessive proportions of early fetal losses associated with mare reproductive loss syndrome in central Kentucky during 2001. *J Am Vet Assoc.* 2003;222:613-619.

Sebastian MM, Gantz MG, Tobin T, et al. The mare reproductive loss syndrome and the eastern tent caterpillar: a toxicokinetic/statistical analysis with clinical, epidemiologic, and mechanistic implications. *Vet Ther.* 2003;4:324-339.

REFERENCES

1. Sebastian MM, et al. *Vet Pathol.* 2008;45:710.
2. McDowell KJ, et al. *J Anim Sci.* 2010;88:1379.
3. Volkmann D, et al. *Reprod Domest Anim.* 2008;43:578.
4. Perkins NR, et al. Pregnancy loss in mares associated with exposure to caterpillars in Kentucky and Australia. In: Panter KE, Wierenga TL, Pfister JA, eds. *Poisonous Plants: Global Research and Solutions.* Wallingford, UK: CAB International; 2007:165.
5. Cawdell-Smith AJ, et al. *Equine Vet J.* 2012;44:282.
6. Donahue JM, et al. *Am J Vet Res.* 2006;67:1426.
7. Townsend L, et al. *J Equine Vet Sci.* 2007;27:249.
8. Haynes KF, et al. *Envrion Entomol.* 2007;36:1199.

EQUINE AMNIONITIS AND FETAL LOSS

EAFL is the name given to a syndrome of abortions that occurred in horses in New South Wales between April and October 2004.[1] Mares from 4 months to term aborted fetuses with signs of inflammatory changes primarily involving the amnion (amnionitis) and amniotic portion of the umbilical cord (funisitis).[2,3] Clinical signs in mares before abortion were minimal.

The syndrome, while occurring several years after the epidemic of MRLS in the United States, had some similarities and caterpillars were looked at as a possible source of the problem. Several caterpillars were examined with the *O. lunifer* (the processionary caterpillar) ultimately causing abortion in two different experimental studies involving early pregnancy and midlate pregnancy.[3,4]

There are some differences between the two syndromes. An infectious agent has been identified in both EAFL and MRLS, but they are not the same bacteria. The predominant bacteria isolated from EAFL cases were environmental coryneforms and gram-negative rods, whereas *Actinobacillus* and non–β-hemolytic streptococci were common isolates from MRLS cases.[2,5] Fibrinous pericarditis and unilateral uveitis affected a number of horses in the MRLS epidemic but did not occur with EAFL.[1] Finally, although devastating, the number of horses involved in the 2004 EAFL outbreak was considerably less than the 2001 to 2002 MRLS epidemic.

REFERENCES

1. Todhunter KH, et al. *Aust Vet J.* 2009;87:35.
2. Cadwell-Smith AJ, et al. *Equine Vet J.* 2012;44:282.
3. Caldwell-Smith AJ, et al. *Proceedings Australian College of Veterinary Science Annual Conference.* 2009:31.
4. Cadwell-Smith AJ, et al. *J Equine Vet Sci.* 2013;33:321.
5. Todhunter K, et al. *Aust Vet J.* 2013;91:138.

PLANTS AND FUNGI (UNKNOWN TOXINS) AFFECTING THE REPRODUCTIVE SYSTEM

PLANTS

Plants Associated With Abortion

- *Iva angustifolia* (narrow-leafed sumpweed)
- *Salvia coccinea* (red salvia)
- *Tanacetum vulgare* (tansy)
- *Verbena bonariensis* (purple top)

Plants Associated With Prolonged Gestation

- *Lysichiton americanus* (skunk cabbage)
- *Salsola tuberculatiformis* (cauliflower saltwort; in ewes it is associated with atrophy of the pituitary, adrenal, and thymus glands of the fetus and prolongation of pregnancy to as long as 213 days).

Plants Associated With Congenital Defects

- *L. americanus* (skunk cabbage; is associated mostly with craniofacial deformity).

FUNGI

Fungi Associated With Reproductive Dysfunction

- *Penicillium roqueforti,* growing on moldy mixed grain and ensilage, is suspected of causing bovine abortion and retained placenta.

- *T. repens* (white clover) does not normally contain estrogens, but when heavily infested with fungi it may contain significant amounts.
- *Ustilago hordei* (barley smut) fungus is thought to be toxic to farm animals; feeding it to experimental animals has been associated with infertility and stillbirths.
- In southeastern Australia a common infertility syndrome, including abortion and fetal mummification, has been ascribed to an onion-like weed, *Romulea rosea*. There is a suspicion that the disease may be caused by a toxin produced by a fungus, *Helminthosporium biseptatum*, which grows on the weed.

Congenital and Inherited Diseases Primarily Affecting the Reproductive System

CHROMOSOMAL TRANSLOCATIONS IN CATTLE

A chromosomal translocation is a mutation occurring when two nonhomologous chromosomes exchange parts, which results in a chromosomal rearrangement. The most common type or translocation is the **reciprocal translocation** (RCP) in which a segment from one chromosome is exchanged with a segment of another nonhomologous chromosome, creating a pair of translocation chromosomes. A particular form of reciprocal translocation is the **Robertsonian translocation (ROB)**. During a ROB participating chromosomes break at their centromeres (center pieces) and the long arms of the two chromosomes merge to form a single chromosome with one centromere and two long arms. At the same time, a new chromosome containing both short arms is also created, which typically only contains nonessential genetic information and is lost during following cell divisions. Chromosomal translocations are identified by the chromosomal series involved. Thus a 1/29 translocation represents a fusion between a chromosome of each of the pairs numbered 1 and 29.

A number of chromosomal rearrangements have been identified in different livestock species over the years and have been associated with clinical conditions such as intersexuality, congenital malformations, and reproductive dysfunction.[1] Some of the translocations that occur endemically in certain regions have been associated with significant economic losses.[2] Several European countries have established cytogenic screening programs to monitor the occurrence of chromosomal translocations in the livestock population.[1] In Italy the incidence of RCP in cattle determined in an official cytogenic screening program was 0.3%, whereas 7.1% of studied animals were carriers of a ROB.[2] By far the most common ROB identified was the so-called translocation 1/29, which is endemic in the region, accounting for 99.6% of all ROBs.[2]

Translocation 1/29 has been identified in many breeds of cattle and has been associated with significant reductions in the fertility of cows bred by artificial insemination services. Early embryonic death occurs in embryos produced by fertilization of affected gametes or fertilization of normal gametes by spermatozoa carrying the 1/29 translocation. There is no abnormality of serving behavior or semen quality. The translocation has been shown to be inherited in most European beef breeds including the Blonde d'Aquitaine, Swedish Red and White, Charolais, Danish Limousin, British Friesian and Red Poll breeds, and in the wild British White cattle. In Bolivian Creole cattle breeds, in the Creole-like cattle, the average frequency was 10.42% with a variation from 0% to 28.2%. In contrast, Yacumeño and Creole-type cattle did not show the centric fusion. The highly significant differences between Creole cattle breeds in relation to the 1/29 translocation could be the consequence of factors such as founder group, genetic drift, and selection. The low frequency observed in the Saavendreño Creole dairy cattle might be caused by breeding under a more intensive system and selection according to milk yield and fertility traits. The frequency of affected animals in a breed may vary between 1% and 20%. Karyotyping and culling of abnormal bulls in most artificial breeding centers has reduced the impact of the defect.

Translocations 1/21, 2/4, 14/20, and **13/2** have also been identified in bulls, the 1/21 in Holstein Friesian cattle, and the latter two seem to be widespread in Simmental cattle. None of them has been linked with a disease, but it is becoming accepted practice not to use such animals for artificial insemination and in some countries to refuse their importation.

A cytogenetic survey of Holstein bulls at a commercial artificial insemination unit to determine the prevalence of bulls with centric fusion and chimeric anomalies found that chimeric fusion is extremely rare in Holstein bloodlines available by artificial insemination in the United States. However, chimeric bulls are more common and reportedly have decreased reproductive performance. Because of the possibility of de novo onset of chimeric fusion at any time, early cytogenetic screening should be encouraged for prospective bulls intended for artificial insemination programs.

Translocation 27/29 is suspected of being associated with reduced fertility in Guernsey cattle. These and other abnormalities of chromosomal structure were detected in an examination of a large number of infertile dairy heifers.

REFERENCES

1. Ducos A, et al. *Cytogenet Genome Res*. 2008;120:26.
2. DeLoreni L, et al. *J Anim Breed Genet*. 2012;129:409.

INHERITED PROLONGED GESTATION (ADENOHYPOPHYSEAL HYPOPLASIA)

Prolonged gestation occurs in cattle and sheep in several forms and is usually, although not always, inherited.[1]

The forms of the disease are prolonged gestation with fetal gigantism or prolonged gestation with deformed or normal or small size fetuses. Differential diagnoses include: mistaken breeding date, intrauterine death and fetal mummification, and pituitary abnormalities in the fetus caused by infection by BVD virus, Akabane virus or bluetongue virus, ingestion of *Veratrum californicum*, and genetic abnormalities.[1]

The disease is caused by lack of a functioning fetal hypothalamic-pituitary axis and consequent inability of the fetus to initiate parturition. The result is prolonged gestation and continued growth of the fetus. The hypothalamic-pituitary axis is also critical for survival of the newborn and affected animals are not viable.

PROLONGED GESTATION WITH FETAL GIGANTISM

The inherited disease is recorded in Holstein,[2] Ayrshire, and Swedish cattle with prolongation of pregnancy from 3 weeks to 5 months. The cows may show marked abdominal distension, but in most cases the abdomens are smaller than one would expect. Parturition, when it commences, is without preparation. Udder enlargement, relaxation of the pelvic ligaments, and loosening and swelling of the vulva do not occur, and there is also poor relaxation of the cervix and a deficiency of cervical mucus. Dystocia is usual and cesarean section is advisable in Holstein cattle, but the Ayrshire calves have all been reported as having been born without assistance. The calves are very large (48 to 80 kg BW) and show other evidence of postterm growth, with a luxuriant hair coat and large, well-erupted teeth that are loose in their alveoli, but the birthweight is not directly related to the length of the gestation period.

The calves exhibit a labored respiration with diaphragmatic movements more evident than movements of the chest wall. They invariably die within a few hours in a hypoglycemic coma. At necropsy there is adenohypophyseal hypoplasia and hypoplasia of the adrenal cortex and the thyroid gland. The progesterone level in the peripheral blood of cows bearing affected calves does not fall before term as it does in normal cows.

PROLONGED GESTATION WITH CRANIOFACIAL DEFORMITY

This form of the disease has been observed in Guernsey, Jersey, and Ayrshire cattle. It differs from the previous form in that the fetuses are dead on delivery, show gross deformity of the head, and are smaller than the normal calves of these breeds born at term. In Guernsey cattle the defect has been shown to be inherited as a single recessive character, and it is probable that the same is true in Jersey cattle. The gestation period varies widely with a mean of 401 days.

Clinical examination of the dams carrying defective calves suggests that no development of the calf or placenta occurs after the seventh month of pregnancy. Death of the fetus is followed in 1 to 2 weeks by parturition unaccompanied by relaxation of the pelvic ligaments or vulva or by external signs of labor. The calf can usually be removed by forced traction because of its small size. Mammary gland enlargement does not occur until after parturition.

The calves are small and suffer varying degrees of hypotrichosis. There is hydrocephalus and in some cases distension of the gut and abdomen caused by atresia of the jejunum. The bones are immature and the limbs are short. Abnormalities of the face include cyclopian eyes, microphthalmia, absence of the maxilla, and the presence of only one nostril. At **necropsy** there is partial or complete aplasia of the adenohypophysis. The neural stalk is present and extends to below the diaphragm sellae. Brain abnormalities vary from fusion of the cerebral hemispheres to moderate hydrocephalus. The other endocrine glands are also small and hypoplastic.

The disease has been produced experimentally in ewes by severe ablation of the pituitary gland, or destruction of the hypothalamus, or section of the pituitary stalk in the fetus and by adrenalectomy of the lamb or kid. Infusion of adrenocorticotropic hormone into ewes with prolonged gestation caused by pituitary damage produces parturition but not if the ewes have been adrenalectomized beforehand.

PROLONGED GESTATION WITH ARTHROGRYPOSIS

A form of prolonged gestation, which occurs in Hereford cattle and is thought to be inherited, is accompanied by arthrogryposis, scoliosis, torticollis, kyphosis, and cleft palate.

Prolonged gestation is also reported in **Belgium Blue cattle** and appears to have a genetic component. Affected calves were not grossly abnormal.[1]

REFERENCES

1. Cornillie P, et al. *Vet Rec.* 2007;161:388.
2. Buczinski S, et al. *J Vet Med A.* 2007;54:624.

INHERITED INGUINAL HERNIA AND CRYPTORCHIDISM

Inguinal hernias and cryptorchidism in pigs have been considered to be inherited defects for many years, but the evidence is uncertain.

INGUINAL HERNIAS

Inguinal hernias of pigs have been shown to be inherited in some breeds (e.g., Duroc and Landrace), but not in others (e.g., Yorkshires). The genetic basis has been investigated in Large White pigs and Landrace pigs and the candidate genes narrowed to a region on SSC13 (Sus scrofa chromosome) between 34 and 37 Mb.[1] In Pietrain pigs, genes involved in collagen metabolism (homeobox A10 [HOXA10] and matrix metalloproteinases 2 [MMP2]) and one gene encoding zinc finger protein multitype 2 (ZFPM2; important in the development of diaphragmatic hernia) were significantly associated with hernias.[2]

Cryptorchidism

Evidence suggesting the inheritance of cryptorchidism in swine, sheep, horses, and Hereford cattle and hermaphroditism in swine is also available.

Cryptorchidism is a common congenital anomaly in pigs, and a genome-wide association study of Large White and Landrace pigs localizes the associated gene or genes to candidate genes to SSC8 (Sus scrofa chromosome) between 65 and 73 Mb.[1]

Cryptorchidism is common in equids, and there is concern that it might be hereditary.[3] Unilateral cryptorchidism is overrepresented in Percherons, American Saddle Horses, and American Quarter Horses among hospital admissions for cryptorchid castration and has an incidence of 15% among Friesian colt foals.[4] Approximately 9% of the ~600 Icelandic Horse yearling stallions did not have both testes in the scrotum.[5] The likelihood of cryptorchidism in yearlings was significantly influenced by farm and time period of birth. Heritability estimates for cryptorchidism ranged from 0.12 to 0.32 (standard error [SE] 0.08–0.12) on the observable scale, and from 0.35 to 0.96 (SE 0.24–0.40) when transformed to the underlying continuous scale.[5] Cryptorchidism in horses appears to be inherited with a polygenic pattern of transmission, although analysis of microsatellite markers of 24 affected horses did not reveal significant associations with allelic or genotypic frequencies.[6]

REFERENCES

1. Sevillano CA, et al. *Genet Sel Evol.* 2015;47:18.
2. Zhao X, et al. *Am J Vet Res.* 2009;70:1006.
3. Hartman R, et al. *J Am Vet Med Assoc.* 2015;246:777.
4. Stout TAE. *Equine Vet J.* 2013;45:531.
5. Eriksson S, et al. *Livestock Sci.* 2015;180:1.
6. Diribarne M, et al. *J Equine Vet Sci.* 2009;29:37.

19 Perinatal Diseases

Introduction

This chapter considers the principles of the diseases that occur during the first month of life in animals born alive at term. Diseases causing abortion and stillbirth are not included. The specific diseases discussed are presented separately under their own headings.

The inclusion of a chapter on diseases of the newborn, and at this point in the book, needs explanation. The need for the chapter arises out of the special sensitivities that newborns have:

- Their immunologic incompetence
- Their dependence on adequate colostrum containing adequate antibodies at the right time
- Their dependence on frequent intake of readily available carbohydrate to maintain energy
- Their relative inefficiency in maintaining normal body temperature, upward or downward

All of these points require emphasis before proceeding to the study of each of the body systems.

There are no particular aspects of a clinical examination that pertain only to or mostly to neonates. The same clinical examination as is applied to adults is used, with additional, careful examination for congenital defects and diseases, which may involve the umbilicus, the liver, the heart valves, the joints and tendon sheaths, the eyes, and the meninges, and for birth-related trauma (e.g., rib fracture, joint luxation, distal limb fracture).

Because there is a much greater susceptibility to infectious disease, dehydration, and death, diagnosis and treatment must be reasonably accurate and rapid. Supportive therapy in the form of fluids, electrolytes and energy, and nursing care are especially important in the newborn to maintain homeostasis.

Perinatal and Postnatal Diseases

One of the difficulties in the study of perinatal and postnatal diseases is the variation in the type of age classification that occurs between publications, which makes it difficult to compare results and assessments. The term *perinatal* is usually used to describe morbidity or mortality that occurs at birth and in the first 24 hours of life. The term *neonatal* is usually used to describe morbidity or mortality between birth and 14 days. However, there is variation in the use of these terms. To ensure that our meanings are clear, we set out in the following section what we think is the most satisfactory classification of all the diseases of the fetus and the newborn, which is adapted from a scheme proposed for lambs. The importance of this type of classification is in the assessment of risk for a given type of disease and in the prediction of likely causes that should be investigated by further examinations. This approach is not of major importance in the assessment of disease in an individual animal, although it is of importance in helping establish the priority in diagnostic rule-outs. The classification is, however, of considerable value in the approach to perinatal morbidity and mortality in large flocks or herds, where an assessment of the age occurrence of morbidity and mortality can guide subsequent examinations to the probable group of cases, with optimal expenditure of investigative capital.

GENERAL CLASSIFICATION

FETAL DISEASES

Fetal diseases are diseases of the fetus during intrauterine life, for example, prolonged gestation, intrauterine infections, abortion, fetal death with resorption or mummification, and goiter.

PARTURIENT DISEASES

Parturient diseases are diseases associated with dystocia, causing cerebral anoxia or fetal hypoxemia, and their consequences and predispositions to other diseases; injury to the skeleton or soft tissues and maladjustment syndrome of foals are also included here.

POSTNATAL DISEASES

Postnatal diseases are divided into early, delayed, and late types:

- **Early postnatal disease** (within 48 hours of birth). Deaths that occur during this period are unlikely to be caused by an infectious disease unless it has been acquired congenitally. Most diseases occurring in this period are noninfectious and metabolic (e.g., hypoglycemia and hypothermia as a result of poor mothering, hypothermia as a result of exposure to cold, low vigor in neonates as a result of malnutrition). Congenital disease will commonly manifest during this period but may sometimes manifest later. Infectious diseases are often initiated during this period, but most manifest clinically at a later age because of their incubation period; some (e.g., navel infection, septicemic disease, and enterotoxigenic colibacillosis) have a short enough incubation to occur during this period.
- **Delayed postnatal disease** (2 to 7 days of age). Included in this category are desertion by the mother, mammary incompetence resulting in starvation, and diseases associated with increased susceptibility to infection as a result of failure in the transfer of colostral immunoglobulins (the predisposing causes to these occur in the first 12 to 24 hours of life). Examples include colibacillosis, joint ill, lamb dysentery, septicemic disease, and most of the viral enteric infections in young animals (e.g., rotavirus and coronavirus).
- **Late postnatal disease** (1 to 4 weeks of age). There is still some influence of hypogammaglobulinemia, with late-onset enteric diseases and the development and severity of respiratory disease in this period, but other diseases not directly associated with failure of transfer of immunoglobulins, such as cryptosporidiosis, white muscle disease, and enterotoxemia, start to become important.

PERINATAL DISEASE—GENERAL EPIDEMIOLOGY

Diseases of the newborn and neonatal mortality are a major cause of economic loss in livestock production. In cattle, sheep, and pigs, the national average perinatal mortalities exceed by far the perinatal mortality experienced in herds and flocks with good management. In these species the identification of the management deficiencies that are the cause of a higher-than-acceptable mortality in a herd or a flock is a most important long-term responsibility of the practicing veterinarian and, in most instances, is more important than the identification of the causal agent or the short-term treatment of individual animals with neonatal disease. In contrast, in horses, the individual is of extreme importance, and the primary thrust is in the treatment of neonatal disease.

All animals must be born close to term if they are to survive in a normal farm environment. Minimal gestational ages for viability (in days) for each of the species are as follows:

- Calf—240
- Foal—311
- Lamb—138
- Piglet—108
- Cria—295

LAMBS

Mortality Rates

Neonatal lamb mortality is one of the major factors in impairment of productivity in sheep-raising enterprises around the world, and nearly half of all preweaning lamb deaths occur on the day of birth.[1] Mortality can obviously vary with the management system (intensive versus extensive lambing, highly supervised versus minimally supervised, variations in the provision of shelter, etc.) and according to whether there is a particular disease problem in a given flock. Nonselective mortality surveys have shown population mortality rates in lambs, from birth to weaning, that vary from 10% to 30%, and there are flocks that may exceed this upper figure in the face of a major problem. In well-managed flocks, neonatal mortality is less than 10% and in some is below 5%.

Major Causes

The major cause of neonatal mortality in lambs is noninfectious disease. Many studies have explored the causes for neonatal lamb mortality, which are broadly categorized as follows:[2]

- Death related to birth process
- Failure of neonatal adaptation to postnatal life
- Infectious disease
- Functional disorders
- Predation

Fetal Disease

Infectious abortion can cause considerable fetal, parturient, and postnatal mortality in infected flocks, but it is a relatively minor cause of perinatal mortality overall. In contrast to other large animal species, abortion storms in sheep are often accompanied by significant mortality in liveborn animals. Many agents associated with abortion in ewes produce placentitis and cause abortion in late pregnancy. This frequently results in the birth of liveborn growth-retarded and weak lambs that die during the first few days of life. Any investigation of perinatal mortality in sheep should also consider the presence of agents causing abortion, although abortion and the birth of dead lambs is always prominent in abortion outbreaks.

Parturient Disease

Stillbirth occurs largely as a result of prolonged birth and fetal hypoxemia. Prolonged birth and dystocia are particular problems in large single lambs. Higher rates of stillbirth can also occur in flocks that are in poor condition. Prolonged birth is a major risk factor for subsequent postnatal disease.

Postnatal Disease

Starvation and hypothermia are common causes of death of neonatal lambs that can result from decreased vigor, pain or trauma after a difficult delivery, failure to adapt to postnatal life, or infectious disease. A number of studies have consistently identified **low birth weight** as the single most important factor associated with lamb mortality.[1,2] Other common factors associated with the mortality rates of neonatal lambs are litter size (which cannot entirely be attributed to lower birth weight of twins), lamb sex (with males having higher mortality than females), and lamb behavior.[1] Management practices that have been found to reduce lamb mortality include winter feeding of pregnant ewes and housing at lambing.[2]

Birth Weight

Birth weight is determined by the nutrition and genetics of the ewe and by litter size, which is also determined by the parity and genetics of the ewe. Reflecting these influences, most surveys of neonatal mortality in lambs show the following characteristics:

- A significant association between the body condition score or **nutrition of the late pregnant ewe** and perinatal mortality
- A relation between **birth weight** and mortality (depending on the breed, a birth weight of less than 2.5 to 3.0 kg has increased risk for death)
- A higher mortality in lambs from **primiparous ewes**[1]
- A pronounced effect of **litter size**, with mortality in lambs born as triplets being higher than in those born as twins, which in turn is higher than that in lambs born as singles

Lambs with low birth weight are born with fewer body reserves, are less vigorous at birth, and take longer to stand (and thus to reach the teat and ingest colostrum). They are also more susceptible to hypothermia because of higher body surface relative to body mass, lower body fat content, and lower thermogenic capacity as a result of lower muscle mass.

The association between birth weight and lamb mortality has a U-shaped pattern, with the lowest mortality rates with normal birth weight and increasing mortality rates with both decreasing and increasing birth weight. An increase in mortality in large-birth-weight lambs born as singles has been associated with increased risk for dystocia.

Environmental Factors

Environmental factors of temperature, wetness, and wind can greatly affect lamb mortality rates; their influence varies according to the management system.

The identification of the determinants of mortality just described is of more than academic value because almost all can be modulated by the identification of **at-risk groups** and the adjustment of management procedures or by the identification and mitigation of adverse environmental factors.

Infectious Disease

Infectious disease can be important in some flocks but commonly contributes to lamb mortality from 2 days of age on. The major infectious diseases of lambs that cause mortality are enteritis and pneumonia. Their prevalence varies with the management system—enteric disease and liver abscess are more common in shed lambing systems than with lambing at pasture. Risk for pneumonia is greatest in very light or heavy lambs and in lambs from maiden ewes and ewes with poor milk production.

Other Factors

Other factors can be important in individual flocks or regions. Lambs found dead or missing may account for significant losses in some conditions, such as mountain or hill pastures. **Predation**, or predation injury, is an important cause of loss in some areas of the world and, depending on the region, can occur from domestic dogs, coyotes, birds, or feral pigs. **Poor mothering** and an inability of the ewe to gather and bond to both lambs in the case of twins can be a problem in Merinos and can cause permanent separation of lambs from the ewe and subsequent death from starvation.

Management at lambing can also influence the patterns of mortality. Intensive stocking at the time of lambing allows increased periparturient supervision and tends to reduce the incidence of stillbirths and lamb mortality related to parturition. It can furthermore ensure the early feeding of colostrum to weak lambs. On the other hand, it can result in a greater occurrence of mismothering associated with the activities of "robber" ewes and may increase lamb mortality related to infectious disease.[3] Mortality rates can differ between breeds, and lambs from crossbred dams may have higher survival rates.

Recording Systems

Simple systems for recording, determining, and evaluating the major causes of lamb mortality in a flock, for determining the time of death in relation to birth, and for relating the deaths to the weather and management system are available. These systems of examination are effective in revealing the extent of lamb losses and the areas of management that require improvement, and they are much more cost-effective than extensive laboratory examinations, which may give little information on the basic cause of the mortality. More intensive examination systems that combine these simple examinations with selected biochemical indicators of determinant factors are also available.

DAIRY CALVES

Mortality Rates

Mortality rates of neonatal calves reported in the literature are often subdivided into **perinatal mortality,** which frequently—but not consistently—includes stillborn calves, and **postnatal mortality,** which in most cases includes calf mortalities occurring from 48 or 72 h onward to several months of age. Comparing numbers from different studies is difficult not only because of different definitions of the perinatal and postnatal periods, but also because some studies include all births, whereas others only include births of heifer calves.

Perinatal Mortality Rates

Perinatal mortality rates for dairy calves reported from countries with a developed dairy industry range from 2% to 10%, with a consistently increasing trend over the past decades.[4,5] The majority of perinatal deaths, approximately 75%, are considered to occur in the first hour of life, with the remainder occurring either before parturition (approximately 10%) or between 1 and 72 h after birth (approximately 15%).[4] Mortality rates in dairy calves in the first 24 h of life are between 6.5% and 9.7%.[6,7]

Neonatal Mortality Rates

Studies reporting neonatal mortality rates in calves, defined as mortality from day 3 of life on, are difficult to compare because different time ranges are considered, and some studies include all calves, whereas others only include heifer calves. In a recent U.S. study including 1138 births, a mortality rate of 4.6% for the period until 135 days of life was reported; a French study based on over 3 million calvings determined a mean mortality rate of 4.2% for the period between 3 and 30 days for the years 2005/2006.[8,9] In general, mortality rates for the perinatal period (0 to 48 h) tend to be higher than mortality rates for neonatal calves (from 3 days on), which underscores how critical the perinatal period is for the newborn calf.

Mortality rates for unweaned dairy heifers in the United States were surveyed repeatedly between 1996 and 2007 and were found to have declined from 10.8% in 1996 to 7.8% in 2007.[10]

Fetal Disease/Abortion

Abortion is a term generally used to describe the expulsion of a dead fetus from 45 to 265 days of gestation. A large dairy survey conducted in the United States in 2007 estimated that approximately 4.5% of all pregnant dairy heifers and cows had aborted in 2006.[13] The majority of these have no diagnosed cause.

Major Causes

Perinatal Mortality

The exact cause of death in the perinatal period, which often includes stillborn and weakborn calves, frequently remains undetermined. Epidemiologic studies investigating the risk factors for perinatal mortality in dairy calves have identified a number of genetic and nongenetic factors that are consistently associated with perinatal mortality.[4,7,11,12] Dystocia has consistently been identified as the single most important factor associated with perinatal mortality. Reported odds ratios (ORs) vary widely (2.7 to 14.6), but suggest that calves requiring assisted delivery have a 2.7 to 14.6 higher risk of death in the perinatal period than spontaneously born calves.[4] Other factors contributing to perinatal mortality include **lactation number** (calves born from heifers being more likely to die in the first hours of life than calves from multiparous cows), **birth weight** (calves with a birth weight of less than 20 kg and over 60 kg being at increased risk),[7] and **days of gestation** (calves born before 272 days of gestation being 6.7 times more likely to die than calves born between 272 and 302 days of gestation).[7] The OR for the death of a **twin calf** in the perinatal period was estimated at 13.4 times greater compared with singleton calves.[4]

Calving-associated anoxia may be an important contributing factor in these deaths.

Postnatal Mortality

Mortalities of neonatal dairy calves in the first days and weeks of life are attributable in large part to diarrheal disease. In a large survey conducted in the United States in 2007, diarrhea was by far the most common cause of death in unweaned dairy heifers, accounting for 56.5% of all deaths in that age category.[13] Other causes included respiratory problems (22.5%), undetermined causes (7.8%), lameness or injury (1.7%), and navel or joint infections (1.6%).[13]

Postnatal Disease

Calves are at highest risk for death in the first 2 weeks of life and especially in the first week. Septicemic and enteric diseases are most common during this period, with respiratory disease being more common after 2 weeks of age. **Failure of transfer of passive immunity** is a major determinant of this mortality.[14] The economic significance of neonatal disease can be considerable, and the occurrence of disease as a calf can also subsequently affect days-to-first-calving intervals and long-time survival in the herd. Death also causes a loss of genetic potential, both from the loss of the calf and the reluctance of the farmer to invest in higher-priced semen in the face of a calf mortality problem.

Meteorologic or **seasonal influences** may have an effect on dairy calf mortality rate, and this can vary with the region.[4,7] In cold climates during the winter months, an increase in mortality may be associated with the effects of cold, wet, and windy weather, whereas in hot climates there may be an increase in mortality during the summer months in association with heat stress.

Management

Management is a major influence, and in well-managed dairy herds, calf mortality usually does not exceed 5% from birth to 30 days of age. Risk factors for disease morbidity and mortality in dairy calves relate to the **infection pressure** to the calf and factors that affect its **nonspecific** and **specific resistance** to disease. It is generally recognized that mortality is associated with the **type of housing** for calves, calving facilities, the person caring for the calves, and attendance at calving.[4] Thus calves that are born in separate calving pens have a lower risk of disease than those born in loose housing or stanchion areas, and the value of good colostrum feeding practices is apparent. Studies on the role of calf housing and the value of segregated rearing of calves in reducing infection pressure generally show beneficial health results.

The quality of management will be reflected in rates of failure of transfer of passive immunity and will also affect the infection pressure on the calf during the neonatal period. Quality of management is very hard to measure but is easily recognized by veterinary practitioners.

The epidemiologic observations that calf mortality is lower when females or family members of the ownership of the farm manage the calves, rather than when males or employees perform these duties, is probably a reflection of this variation in quality of management and suggests that owner managers and family members may be sufficiently motivated to provide the care necessary to ensure a high survival rate in calves. Even so, calf health can be excellent with some hired calf-rearers and very poor with some owner calf-rearers.

BEEF CALVES

Mortality Rates

Mortality in beef herds is usually recorded during the period from birth to weaning and has ranged from 3% to 7% in surveys, with higher rates in calves born to heifers; significantly higher mortality can occur in herds with disease problems. In a survey conducted in the United States in 2007, a perinatal mortality rate (including stillbirths) of 2.9% and a postnatal mortality rate (for the period from birth to weaning) of 3.5% was determined.[15] The majority of this mortality occurs within the first week of life, and most of it occurs in the parturient or immediate postnatal period as a result of prolonged birth or its consequences.

Major Causes

Dystocia resulting in death is common, and dystocial calves, twin-born calves, and calves born to heifers are at greater risk for postnatal disease. Enteric and respiratory diseases occur in outbreaks in some years, and very cold weather can result in high loss from hypothermia. In a 2007 survey conducted in the United States, beef calf mortality before weaning was found to be attributable to birth-related problems in 25.7%, to weather-related causes in 25.6%, to undetermined causes in 18.6%, to digestive tract problems (including diarrhea) in 14.0%, and to respiratory tract problems in 8.2% of all deaths.[15] Diarrhea and other infectious diseases become the most important cause of death in calves from their third day of life on.

Fetal Disease

Abortion rates appear to be lower than in dairy cattle, usually less than 1%. The majority of these are not diagnosed as to cause, but of those that are, infectious abortion is the most common diagnosis.

Parturient Disease

Accurate prospective and retrospective studies have shown that 50% to 60% of the parturient deaths in beef calves are associated with slow or difficult birth and that the mortality rate is much higher in calves born to heifers than from mature cows. **Dystocial birth** can lead to injury of the fetus and to hypoxemia and may not necessarily be associated with fetal malposition. **Birth size** is highly heritable within all breed types of cattle, and perinatal mortality will vary between herds depending on their use of bulls with high ease-of-calving ratings in the breeding of the heifer herd. Milk fever and overfatness at calving are other preventable causes of mortality. Selective intensive supervision of calving of the heifer herd can also result in a reduction of perinatal mortality.

Postnatal Disease

Scours and pneumonia are the next most important causes of mortality in beef calves, followed by exposure to extremely cold weather or being dropped at birth into deep snow or a gully.[15] The incidence of diarrhea is greatest in the first 2 weeks of life, and there is considerable variation in incidence between herds. However, explosive outbreaks of diarrhea or exposure chilling can be significant causes of mortality in certain years. The purchase of a calf for grafting, often from a market, is a significant risk for introduction of disease to a herd.

The **body-condition score** of the dam can influence calf mortality; dams with high condition scores have a higher risk for dystocial mortality, and those with low scores have a higher risk for infectious disease. Mortality from diarrhea is often higher in calves born to heifers, possibly because heifers are more closely congregated for calving supervision or because of a higher risk for failure of transfer of passive immunity in this age group. Congenital abnormalities can be an occasional cause of mortality in some herds.

PIGLETS

Mortality Rates

Preweaning mortality rates in commercial pig farms reported from different parts of the world range between 11% and 20%, with more than 30% of the mortality occurring in the first 24 hours and more than 50% in the first 4 days of life.[16-18] Mortality increases as the mean litter size increases and as the mean birth weight of the piglets decreases. In most herd environments, the minimal **viable weight** is approximately 1 kg. The mean number of piglets weaned is related to the size of the litter up to an original size of 14 and increases with parity of sows up to their fifth farrowing. Preweaning mortality is negatively correlated with herd size and farrowing crate utilization, and it is positively correlated with the number of farrowing crates per room. The use of farrowing crates was found to reduce neonatal mortality by 50% in some studies, mainly as a result of decreased frequency of crushing of piglets by the sow.

Major Causes

Surveys of neonatal mortality in piglets have repeatedly indicated that the most important causes of death in piglets from birth to weaning are noninfectious in origin.[16,17,19] The major causes are **starvation and crushing** (75% to 80%; although these may be secondary to, and the result of, hypothermia), congenital abnormalities (5%), and infectious disease (6%). The major congenital abnormalities are congenital splayleg, atresia ani, and cardiac abnormalities. Infectious diseases may be important on certain individual farms but do not account for a major cause of mortality.

Fetal Disease

Fetal disease rates in most herds are low unless there is an abortion storm or poor control of endemic infections such as parvovirus. In contrast to other species, the majority of abortions are diagnosed and are infectious.

Parturient Disease

Stillbirths account for 4% to 8% of all deaths of piglets born, and 70% to 90% are type II or intraparturient deaths, in which the piglet was alive at the beginning of parturition.[16] The viability of newborn piglets can be accurately evaluated immediately after birth by scoring skin color, respiration, heart rate, muscle tone, and ability to stand. Stillbirths are more commonly born in the later birth orders of large litters, and it is a relatively common practice for sows to be routinely given oxytocin at the time of the birth of the first piglet to shorten parturition. Controlled trials have shown that although oxytocin administration at this time will result in a significant decrease in farrowing time and expulsion intervals, there is a significant increase in fetal distress, fetal anoxia, and intrapartum death and an increase in piglets born alive with ruptured umbilical cords and meconium staining.

Postnatal Disease

The large percentage of mortality caused by **crushing** and trampling likely includes piglets that were starved and weak and thus highly susceptible to being crushed. The estimated contribution of crushing and starvation to neonatal mortality varies from 19% to 58% of liveborn mortality.[16] The body-condition score of the sow at the time of farrowing, the nursing behavior of the sow, the sow's ability to expose the teats to all piglets, and the sucking behavior of the piglets also have a marked effect on survival.

Cold stress is also an important cause of loss, and the provision of a warm and comfortable environment for the newborn piglet in the first few days of life is critical.[17] The lower critical temperature of the single newborn piglet is 34°C (93°F). When the ambient temperature falls below 34°C (93°F), the piglet is subjected to cold stress and must mobilize glycogen reserves from the liver and muscles to maintain deep body temperature. The provision of heat lamps over the creep area and freedom from draughts are two major requirements.

Management

Minimizing the mortality rate of newborn piglets will depend on management techniques, which include the following:

- Proper selection of the breeding stock for teat numbers, milk production, and mothering ability
- The use of farrowing crates and creep escape areas to minimize crushing injuries
- Surveillance at farrowing time to minimize the number of piglets suffering from hypoxia and dying at birth or a few days later
- Batch farrowing, which allows for economical surveillance
- Fostering to equalize litter size
- Cross-fostering to equalize nonuniformity in birth weight within litters
- Improvement in the thermal comfort of the piglets
- Supplemental iron
- Artificial rearing with milk substitutes containing purified porcine gammaglobulin to prevent enteric infection

FOALS

Mortality Rates

Foals are usually well supervised and cared for as individual animals. Neonatal death is less frequent than in other species, but equivalent rates of morbidity and mortality occur on some farms. Infectious disease is important, along with structural and functional abnormalities that are undoubtedly better recognized and treated than in any of the other large animal species. In a large survey of thoroughbred mares in the United Kingdom, only 2% of newborn foals died, only 41% of twins survived, and 98% of singles survived. In contrast, a mortality rate of 22% between birth and 10 days was recorded in an extensively managed system. A recent retrospective study from Ireland determined a foal mortality rate of 5% during the first 12 months; 64.7% of deaths occurred during the first 30 days, and 82% of all deaths occurred within the first 6 months of life.[20]

Major Causes

Fetal Disease

Fetal disease is a major cause of loss; in one study, infections accounted for approximately 30% of abortions. In a retrospective study of 1252 fetuses and neonatal foals submitted for postmortem examination over a 10-year period in the United Kingdom, equine herpes virus and placentitis accounted for 6.5% and 9.8% of the diagnoses, respectively. The placentitis occurred in late gestation, was concentrated around the cervical pole and lower half of the allantochorion, and was associated with ascending chronic infections of bacteria or fungi resident in the lower genital tract.

Parturient Disease

Neonatal asphyxia, dystocia, umbilical cord abnormality, congenital abnormalities, and musculoskeletal trauma are important causes of foal mortality. A retrospective study from Ireland found that 45.5% of all deaths that occurred in the first 30 days of life were attributable to congenital abnormalities, 18.2% to the perinatal asphyxia syndrome, and 18.2% to musculoskeletal trauma.[20] In a UK study, umbilical cord disorders accounted for 38.8% of the final diagnoses. Umbilical cord torsion usually resulted in death of the fetus in utero, but the long cord/cervical pole ischemia disorder resulted in intrapartum death and a fresh fetus with lesions consistent with acute hypoxia.

Twins are at higher risk for spontaneous abortion.

Postnatal Disease

Postnatal disease causing mortality from birth to 2 months of age includes lack of maturity (36%), structural defect (23%), birth injury (5%), convulsive syndrome (5%), alimentary disorder (12%), generalized infection (11%), and other (miscellaneous; 9%). Of the **infectious diseases**, gastrointestinal and septicemic diseases have the greatest importance. Whereas in the past many of these conditions would have been fatal, significant advances in the science of equine perinatology were made in the 1980s and 1990s, and protocols for the treatment of neonatal disease have been developed that are based on equivalents in human medicine. These have proved of value in the management and treatment of prematurity, immaturity, dysmaturity, and neonatal maladjustment syndromes in newborn foals and in enteric and septicemic diseases. Different levels of intensive care have been defined, starting from those that can be applied at the level of the farm and increasing in sophistication, required facilities, and instrumentation to those that are the province of a specialized referral hospital. Early follow-up studies indicate that this approach is of considerable value in foals with neonatal disease and that most surviving foals become useful athletic adults.

NEW WORLD CAMELID CRIAS

Mortality Rates

Mortality of newborn llamas and alpacas is low compared with other production animal species, which in part because New World camelids (NWCs) are frequently kept as companion animals and receive better attention and more intensive treatment in cases of disease. Preweaning mortality rates for llama and alpaca crias are in the range of 2% to 6%, with the great majority of deaths occurring in the first week of life.[21,22]

Major Causes

Fetal Disease

Abortion and fetal loss after 100 days of gestation have been estimated to occur in 5% of all pregnancies in NWCs.[23] Common noninfectious causes for abortion include stress (e.g., related to transport), nutritional deficiencies, and iatrogenic administration of PGF2α or glucocorticoids. Documented infectious causes for abortion include toxoplasmosis, brucellosis, chlamydiosis, listeriosis, leptospirosis, and neosporosis.[23]

Parturient Disease

Perinatal mortality of crias is strongly associated with the course of parturition and the age of the dam at birth. Dystocia and assisted birth clearly increase the risk for postnatal morbidity and perinatal and postnatal mortality in NWC crias, as in other species.[21]

Postnatal Disease

The great majority of preweaning mortality occurs in the first week of life, and hypothermia and starvation were determined to be the most common causes of death. Low birth weight was found to considerably increase the risk of perinatal death, as was young age of the dam. Primiparous dams 2 to 3 years old give birth to lighter calves than do older dams and are considered to produce less colostrum, and of inferior quality, than their multiparous herd mates. Small crias have more difficulties standing and getting sufficient amounts of colostrum and lose more body heat because of greater body surface relative to body mass, and thus they are at increased risk of starving to death or of developing perinatal or postnatal diseases.[21] A difficult parturition negatively affects perinatal vitality and thereby considerably increases the risk for postnatal morbidity and mortality.[22]

FURTHER READING

Dwyer CM. The welfare of neonatal lambs. *Small Rumin Res.* 2008;76:31-41.

Mee JF, Berry DP, Cromie AR. Prevalence of, and risk factors associated with, perinatal calf mortality in pasture based Holstein-Friesian cows. *Animal.* 2008;2:613-620.

REFERENCES

1. Dwyer CM. *Small Rumin Res.* 2008;76:31-41.
2. Dwyers CM. *J Anim Sci.* 2008;86:E246-E258.
3. Holmøy IH, et al. *Prev Vet Med.* 2012;107:231-241.
4. Mee JF, et al. *Animal.* 2008;2:613-620.
5. Bicalho RC, et al. *J Dairy Sci.* 2007;90:2797-2803.
6. Lombard JE, et al. *J Dairy Sci.* 2007;90:1751-1760.
7. Bleul U. *Livest Sci.* 2011;135:257-264.
8. Linden TC, et al. *J Dairy Sci.* 2009;92:2580-2588.
9. Raboisson D, et al. *J Dairy Sci.* 2013;96:2913-2924.
10. USDA. 2007. (Accessed 10.01.14, at <http://www.aphis.usda.gov/animal_health/nahms/dairy/downloads/dairy07/Dairy07_dr_PartII.pdf>).
11. Gundelach Y, et al. *Theriogenology.* 2009;71:901-909.
12. Guliksen SM, et al. *J Dairy Sci.* 2009;92:2782-2795.
13. USDA. 2007. (Accessed 10.01.14, at <http://www.aphis.usda.gov/animal_health/nahms/dairy/downloads/dairy07/Dairy07_ir_CalfHealth.pdf>).
14. Stilwell G, Carvalho RC. *Can Vet J.* 2011;52:524-526.
15. USDA APHIS. 2010. (Accessed 10.01.14, at <http://www.aphis.usda.gov/animal_health/nahms/beefcowcalf/downloads/beef0708/Beef0708_is_Mortality.pdf>).
16. KilBride AL, et al. *Prev Vet Med.* 2012;104:281-291.
17. O'Reily KM, et al. *Vet Rec.* 2006;159:193-196.
18. Li YZ, et al. *Can J Anim Sci.* 2012;92:11-22.
19. Weber R, et al. *Livest Sci.* 2009;124:216-222.
20. Galvin NP, Corley KTT. *Ir Vet J.* 2010;63:37-43.
21. Bravo PW, et al. *Anim Reprod Sci.* 2009;111:214-219.
22. Sharpe MS, et al. *Aust Vet J.* 2009;87:56-60.
23. Vaughan JL, Tibary A. *Small Rumin Res.* 2006;61:259-281.

PERINATAL DISEASE—SPECIAL INVESTIGATION OF ANY NEONATAL DEATHS (ILLNESS)

The following protocol is a generic guide to the investigation of deaths of newborn animals. It will require modification according to the species involved.

1. Determine the duration of pregnancy to ensure that the animals were born at term.
2. Collect epidemiologic information on the problem. Where possible, the information should include the following:
   - What is the abnormality?
   - What are the apparent age at onset and the age at death?
   - What clinical signs are consistently associated with the problem?
   - What is the prevalence and proportional risk in particular groups (maternal, paternal, nutritional, vaccinated, etc.)?
   - What is the parity of the dam that gave birth to the animal, and what proportional risk does this reflect within the group?
   - What is the birth history of affected animals? Are births supervised, and if so, what is the frequency of observation and what are the criteria for intervention? What is the proportional risk associated with prolonged birth?
   - Is there an effect of litter size, and what is the health of the other littermates?
   - Was there any difference in management of the dams of the affected animals compared with the group as a whole?
   - What is the farm policy for feeding colostrum?
   - What were the environmental conditions during the past 48 hours? (In housed animals, the quality of the environment should be measured objectively.)
3. Conduct a postmortem examination of all available dead neonates. The determination of body weight is essential, and measures of **crown–rump length** can also give an indication of gestational age. In order of precedence, the purpose of the postmortem examination is to determine:
   - The time of death in relation to parturition (e.g., fetal disease, parturient disease, early or delayed postnatal death). This can be determined from the state of the lungs, the nature of the severed end of the umbilical artery and the presence of a clot, the state of the brown-fat deposits, whether the animal has walked, and whether it has suckled before death.
   - The possibility that animals born alive have died because of cold stress, hypoglycemia, and starvation. An indication can be obtained from an examination of the brown-fat reserves and observation of the presence or absence of milk in the gastrointestinal tract and fat in the intestinal lymphatics. The presence of subcutaneous edema in the hind limbs is also relevant.
   - The possible presence of birth injury or trauma. In addition to examination of the ribs and liver for trauma and the presenting areas for subcutaneous edema, the brain should be examined for evidence of hemorrhage.
   - The presence of infectious disease. If necessary, samples can be submitted for examination.
   - The presence of congenital disease
4. If abortion is suspected, specimens of fetal tissues and the placenta are sent for laboratory examination. Examinations requested are pathologic and microbiological for known pathogens for the species of animal under consideration.
5. A serum sample should be collected from the dam for serologic evidence of teratogenic pathogens, followed by another sample 2 weeks later. Samples from unaffected dams should also be submitted. A precolostral serum sample from affected animals may assist in the diagnosis of intrauterine fetal infections.
6. Investigate management practices operating at the time, with special attention to clemency of weather, feed supply, maternalism of dam, and surveillance by the owner—all factors that could influence the survival rate. Where possible, this should be performed using objective measurements. For example, in calf-rearing establishments, the efficacy of transfer of colostral immunoglobulins should be established by the bleeding of a proportion of calves and actual measurement, food intake should be established by actual measurement, and so forth.

FURTHER READING

English PR, Morrison V. Causes and prevention of piglet mortality. *Pig News Info.* 1984;4:369-376.

Haughey KC. Perinatal lamb mortality: its investigation, causes and control. *J S Afr Vet Assoc.* 1991;62:78-91.

Kasari TR. Wikse SE. Perinatal mortality in beef herds. *Vet Clin North Am Food Anim Pract.* 1994;10:1-185.

Mellor DJ, Stafford KJ. Animal welfare implications of neonatal mortality and morbidity in farm animals. *Vet J.* 2004;168:118-133.

Randall GCB. Perinatal mortality. Some problems of adaptation at birth. *Adv Vet Sci.* 1978;22:53.

Rook JS, Scholman G, Wing-Procter S, Shea M. Diagnosis and control of neonatal losses in sheep. *Vet Clin North Am Food Anim Pract.* 1990;6:531-562.

Rossdale PD, McGladdery AJ. Recent advances in equine neonatology. *Vet Annu.* 1992;32:201-208.

Perinatal Disease—Congenital Defects

SYNOPSIS

Etiology Genetic, infectious, toxic, and physical causes are recognized for some defects, but the etiology of most is not known.

Continued

Epidemiology Low but significant incidence in all animals; epidemiology depends on cause.

Clinical findings Congenital defects can be structural or functional; clinical signs depend on organ system(s) affected.

Clinical pathology Specific serologic and biochemical tests can be used in the diagnosis and control of some congenital disease and, if available, are detailed under specific disease headings.

Necropsy findings Specific to the particular problem.

Diagnostic confirmation Abnormalities of structure or function that are present at birth are obviously congenital defects; they may or may not be inherited, and inherited defects may or may not be manifest at birth; genome analysis for inherited defects.

Control Avoidance of exposure to teratogenic agents; vaccination for some teratogenic infections; identification of carriers for genetic defects.

ETIOLOGY

Congenital disease can result from defective genetics or from an insult or agent associated with the fetal environment. A neonate with a congenital defect is an adapted survivor from a disruptive event of a genetic or environmental nature or of a genetic–environmental interaction at one or more of the stages in the sequences of embryonic and fetal development.

Genetic abnormalities may result in a wide spectrum of disorders that can vary from severe morphologic malformations to the presence of inborn errors of metabolism in animals that may be born apparently normal and develop disease later in life.

Susceptibility to injurious **environmental agents** depends on the nature and the severity (dose size and duration of application) of the insult and decreases with fetal age. Before attachment, the zygote is resistant to teratogens but susceptible to chromosomal aberrations and genetic mutations. Agents that disrupt blastula and gastrula stages and that interfere with normal apposition of the uterine mucosa are usually embryotoxic and induce early embryonic death.

The period during which an **organ system** is being established is a particularly critical period for that system, and different teratogens, if applied at that time, can produce similar defects. One example is the complex of arthrogryposis and cleft, which can occur in the calves of cattle grazing certain species of lupine, in calves infected in utero with Akabane virus, and as an inherited disease in Charolais calves.

Many noninherited congenital defects in animals occur in **"outbreaks,"** which is a reflection of the exposure of the pregnant herd to a virus, poisonous plant, or other teratogen during a period of fetal susceptibility. Because this occurs in early pregnancy, it is often very difficult to determine the nature of this exposure at the time the animals are born.

Some teratogens are quite **specific** in the defect that they produce, and their action may be limited to a single species; a tentative diagnosis as to cause can be based on this association. Others produce a wide variety of abnormality that may also occur with other teratogens, and cause is less obvious.

The exact etiology of most congenital defects is unknown. Influences that are known to produce congenital defects are presented here.

Chromosomal Abnormality and Inheritance

Most chromosomal abnormalities are associated with poor fertility and early embryonic death. A few are structural or numerical aberrations of chromosomes. The importance of chromosomal abnormality to congenital defects in farm animals has not been studied extensively, but a study of 55 aborted and stillborn calves found 6 with an abnormal chromosome component. Chromosomal abnormality is usually associated with multiple deformations. Most chromosomal abnormalities are mutant genes, and the majority are inherited as recessive traits. There are many examples among domestic animals.

Viral and Other Infections

Members of the Bunyaviridae (Akabane virus, Cache valley virus, and Rift Valley fever virus), *Orbivirus* (bluetongue virus, epizootic hemorrhagic disease virus, and Chuzan virus), and *Pestivirus* (bovine virus diarrhea virus, border disease virus, and hog cholera virus) families; Japanese B encephalitis virus; and Wesselsbron virus are recognized teratogens. Other viruses also can result in fetal death without malformation. Examples are as follows:

- Akabane virus—this infection of pregnant cattle, sheep, and goats causes arthrogryposis, microencephaly, and hydrocephalus. Infection of, and disease of, the fetus depends on the stage of pregnancy and the fetus's immunologic status. In cattle infected between 76 and 104 days of pregnancy, hydranencephaly predominates; arthrogryposis predominates with infections between 104 and 173 days of gestation, and poliomyelitis predominates after 173 days. In sheep the window of susceptibility for congenital defects is between 30 and 50 days.
- Cache valley virus—congenital infection of lambs with Cache valley virus produces disease very similar to that produced by Akabane virus in cattle. The period of susceptibility for congenital defects is 36 to 45 days of pregnancy.
- Rift Valley fever virus infection of pregnant sheep results in placentitis and abortion, but attenuated vaccine strains produce arthrogryposis and brain defects.
- Bluetongue virus—vaccination of ewes with attenuated vaccine virus between days 35 and 45 of pregnancy causes a high prevalence of porencephaly in lambs. Natural infections of sheep (50 to 80 days of gestation) and cattle (60 to 120 days of gestation) can result in fetal death and resorption or the birth of stillborn animals, weakborn animals, and animals with hydrocephalus, hydranencephaly, and, occasionally, arthrogryposis. Similar defects are produced by Chuzan, Aino, and Kasba virus infections.
- Bovine viral diarrhea—infection with cytopathogenic strains before 100 days can result in abortion and mummification, cerebellar hypoplasia, and optic defects, including cataracts, retinal degeneration, and hypoplasia and neuritis of the optic nerves. Other defects are brachygnathia, curly coats, abortion, stillbirth, and mummification. Infection of the bovine fetus between 45 and 125 days of gestation with a noncytopathic biotype of the virus can result in the development of a persistently viremic and immunotolerant calf that is carried to term, is born alive, remains persistently viremic, and may later develop mucosal disease.
- Border disease virus—the window of susceptibility is from 16 to 90 days of gestation, and, depending on the fetal age at infection and the presence of a fetal immune response, fetal infection may result in fetal death, growth retardation, the birth of persistently infected lambs, or lambs born with hypomyelinogenesis, hydranencephaly, and cerebellar dysplasia. Coat defects may also be seen.
- Hog cholera virus—vaccination of sows with modified vaccine virus between days 15 and 25 of pregnancy produces piglets with edema, deformed noses, and abnormal kidneys. Natural infection with field virus can cause reproductive inefficiency and cerebellar hypoplasia in piglets.
- An unidentified virus is associated with the AII type of congenital tremor in pigs.
- Congenital infection with Wesselsbron virus and with Rift Valley fever is

recorded as producing central nervous system disease in cattle and sheep.
- Japanese B encephalitis virus in pigs can result in abortion or in the birth of weak, mummified, or stillborn piglets and live piglets with neurologic abnormalities. The window of susceptibility is from 40 to 60 days of gestation.
- Pseudorabies virus infection of the pregnant sow can result in myoclonia congenita in piglets.
- Viral, bacterial, and protozoal agents that produce abortion in animals can also produce intrauterine growth retardation and the birth of weakborn neonates that are highly susceptible to mortality in early life.

Nutritional Deficiency

Many congenital defects in animals are known to be caused by deficiencies of specific nutrients in the diet of the dam. Examples are as follows:
- Iodine—goiter and increased neonatal mortality are caused in all species; prolonged gestation occurs in horses and sheep. Congenital musculoskeletal lesions are seen in foals (congenital hypothyroid dysmaturity syndrome). Deficiency may result from a primary deficiency or be induced by nitrate or *Brassica* spp. Syndromes are also produced by iodine excess, often associated with feeding excess seaweed or seaweed products.
- Copper—enzootic ataxia in lambs can result from either to a primary copper deficiency or a secondary deficiency in which the availability of copper is interfered with by other minerals (e.g., molybdenum and iron).
- Manganese—chondrodystrophy and limb deformities in calves
- Vitamin D—neonatal rickets
- Vitamin A—eye defects, harelip, and other defects in piglets
- Vitamin E and/or selenium—congenital cardiomyopathy and muscular dystrophy
- Congenital cobalt deficiency is reported to reduce lamb vigor at birth and to increase perinatal mortality because of impaired immune function in the lamb. A similar effect on immune function in neonatal lambs and calves has been proposed with copper deficiency.
- Malnutrition of the dam can result in increased neonatal mortality and is suspected in the genesis of limb deformities and in congenital joint laxity and dwarfism in calves.
- Vitamin A deficiency induced by feeding potato tops or water with high nitrate content has been associated with congenital blindness in calves.

Poisonous Plants

The teratogenic effects of poisonous plants have been reviewed in detail. Some examples are as follows:
- *Veratrum californicum* fed to ewes at about the 14th day of pregnancy can cause congenital cyclopia and other defects of the cranium and brain in lambs, in addition to prolonged gestation. When fed at 27 to 32 days of pregnancy, it can produce limb abnormalities. Tracheal stenosis has been produced by feeding at 31 to 33 days of gestation. The alkaloid cyclopamine is the teratogenic substance.
- "Crooked-calf disease" is associated with the ingestion of *Lupinus* sp. during pregnancy. This is a major problem on some rangelands in western North America. There are approximately 100 species of *Lupinus* in Canada and the United States, but the disease has been mainly associated with *L. sericeus*, *L. leucophyllus*, *L. caudatus*, and *L. laxiflorus*. These species are thought to be toxic because of their content of anagyrine, but some piperidine alkaloids may also produce the disease. The disease has been reproduced by feeding anagyrine-containing lupines to pregnant cattle between 40 and 90 days of gestation, but it can occur with later feeding in natural grazing. The syndrome is one of arthrogryposis, torticollis, scoliosis, and cleft palate.
- *Astragalus* and *Oxytropis* spp. locoweeds cause limb contracture in calves and lambs, in addition to fetal death and abortion.
- Tobacco plants—ingestion of *Nicotiana tabacum* (burley tobacco) and *Nicotiana glauca* (tree tobacco) by sows between 18 and 68 days of gestation, with peak susceptibility between 43 and 55 days, can cause limb deformities in their piglets. The teratogen is the piperidine alkaloid anabasine. Cleft palate and arthrogryposis have also been produced experimentally in the fetuses of cattle and sheep fed *N. glauca* during pregnancy, but the plant is not palatable, and thus this is an unlikely cause of natural disease.
- *Conium maculatum*, poison hemlock, fed to cows during days 55 to 75 of pregnancy, to sheep in the period of 30 to 60 days of pregnancy, and to sows in the period of 30 to 62 days of pregnancy will cause arthrogryposis, scoliosis, torticollis, and cleft palate in the fetuses. Cattle are most susceptible. The piperidine alkaloids coniine and coniceine are responsible.
- *Leucaena leucocephala* (or mimosine, its toxic ingredient) causes forelimb polypodia (supernumerary feet) in piglets when fed experimentally to sows.
- Fungal toxicosis from the feeding of moldy cereal straw has been epidemiologically linked to outbreaks of congenital spinal stenosis and bone deformities associated with premature closure of growth plates in calves.

Farm Chemicals

Certain farm chemicals are associated with teratogenic effects, including the following:
- Some benzimidazoles (parbendazole, cambendazole, oxfendazole, albendazole netobimin) are important teratogens for sheep, producing skeletal, renal, and vascular abnormality when administered between 14 and 24 days of pregnancy.
- Methallibure, a drug used to control estrus in sows, causes deformities in the limbs and cranium of pigs when fed to sows in early pregnancy.
- Apholate, an insect chemosterilant, is suspected of causing congenital defects in sheep.
- The administration of trichlorfon to pregnant sows can result in the birth of piglets with cerebellar hypoplasia and congenital trembles.
- Organophosphates have been extensively tested and found to be usually nonteratogenic. A supposed teratogenic effect is probably more a reflection of the very common usage of these substances in agriculture (see the discussion in the section on poisoning by organophosphates).
- Griseofulvin given to a mare in the second month of pregnancy is suspected of causing microphthalmia and facial bone deformity in a foal.

Physical Insults

Physical insults can also result in fetal abnormalities; examples are as follows:
- Severe exposure to beta or gamma irradiation (e.g., after an atomic explosion) can cause a high incidence of gross malformations in developing fetuses.
- Rectal palpation of pregnancy using the amniotic slip method between 35 and 41 days of pregnancy in Holstein Friesian cattle is associated with atresia coli in the calf at birth, but there is also a genetic influence. It is probable that the cause is palpation-induced damage to the developing colonic vasculature.
- Hyperthermia applied to the dam experimentally causes congenital deformities, but this appears to have no naturally occurring equivalent. The most severe abnormalities occur after exposure during early pregnancy (18 to 25 days in ewes). Disturbances of central nervous system development are the most common. Defects of the spinal

cord manifest themselves as arthrogryposis. and exposure of ewes to high temperatures (42°C, 107.5°F) causes stunting of limbs; the lambs are not true miniatures because they have selective deformities, with the metacarpals selectively shortened. The defect occurs whether nutrition is normal or not. Hyperthermia between 30 and 80 days of pregnancy in ewes produces growth retardation in the fetus. Developmental abnormalities have been reproduced experimentally in explanted porcine embryos exposed to environmental temperatures similar to those that may be associated with reproductive failure resulting from high ambient temperatures in swine herds.

Environmental Influences

Currently, there is considerable interest in the possible teratogenic effects of human-caused changes in the environment. The concern is understandable because the fetus is a sensitive biological indicator of the presence of noxious influences in the environment. For example, after an accidental release of polybrominated biphenyls, much of the angry public commentary related to the probable occurrence of congenital defects. The noxious influences can be physical or chemical. In one examination of the epidemiology of congenital defects in pigs, it was apparent that any environmental causes were from the natural environment; human-caused environmental changes, especially husbandry practices, had little effect. A current concern in some regions is an apparent increase in congenital defects thought to be associated with exposure to radiofrequency electromagnetic fields associated with mobile telephone networks, but there are few hard data.

EPIDEMIOLOGY

Individual abnormalities differ widely in their spontaneous occurrence. The determination of the cause of congenital defects in a particular case very often defies all methods of examination. Epidemiologic considerations offer some of the best clues, but they are obviously of little advantage when the number of cases is limited. The possibility of inheritance playing a part is fairly easily examined if good breeding records are available. The chances of coming to a finite conclusion are much less probable. The determination of the currently known teratogens has mainly been arrived at following epidemiologic studies suggesting possible causality followed by experimental challenge and reproduction of the defect with the suspected teratogen.

An expression of the **prevalence** of congenital defects is of very little value unless it is related to the size of the population at risk, and almost no records include this vital data. Furthermore, most of the records available are retrospective and based on the number of cases presented at a laboratory or hospital.

Reported prevalence rates of 0.5% to 3.0% for calves and 2% for lambs are comparable with the human rate of 1% to 3%. A much higher rate for animals of 5% to 6% is also quoted. A study of over 3500 cases of abortion, stillbirth, and perinatal death in horses found congenital malformations in almost 10%. A very extensive literature on congenital defects in animals exists, and a bibliography is available.

Some breeds and families have extraordinarily high prevalence rates because of intensive inbreeding. The extensive use, by artificial insemination, of certain genetics can result in a significant increase in the occurrence and similar nature of congenital defects when the bulls are carriers of genetic disease. The use of bulls that were carriers for complex vertebral malformation syndrome, for example, resulted in an approximately threefold increase in the presence of arthrogryposis, ventricular septal defect, and vertebral malformations in Holstein Friesian calves submitted to diagnostic laboratories in the Netherlands between 1994 and 2000.

Checklists of recorded defects are included in the Further Reading section.

PATHOGENESIS

The pathogenesis of many of the congenital defects of large animals is poorly understood, but it is apparent that the disease produced by each teratogen is likely to have its own unique pathogenesis. Congenital defects in large animals include defects induced from structural malformations, from deformations, from the destruction of tissue by extraneous agents, and from enzyme deficiencies, or from a combination of these.

Structural Malformations and Deformations

Structural malformations result from a localized error in morphogenesis. The insult leading to the morphogenic error takes place during organogenesis and thus is an influence imposed in early gestation. **Deformations** occur where there is an alteration in the shape of a structure of the body that has previously undergone normal differentiation. Deforming influences apply later in the early gestational period, after organogenesis.

Deformation is the cause of arthrogryposis and cleft palate produced by the piperidine alkaloids from *Conium maculatum* and *Nicotiana* spp. and by anagyrine from *Lupinus* spp., which produce a chemically induced reduction in fetal movements. Ultrasound examination of the normal fetus shows that it has several periods of stretching and vigorous galloping during a 30-minute examination period. In contrast, the fetus that is under the influence of anagyrine has restricted movement and lies quietly, often in a twisted position. Restricted fetal limb movement results in arthrogrypotic fixation of the limbs, and pressure of the tongue on the hard palate when the neck is in a constant flexed position inhibits closure of the palate. In experimental studies there is a strong relation between the degree and duration of reduced fetal movement, as observed by ultrasound, and the subsequent severity of lesions at birth.

Restriction in the movement of the fetus, and deformation, can also result from teratogens that produce damage and malfunction in organ systems, such as the primary neuropathy that occurs in the autosomal-recessive syndrome in Charolais cattle and the acquired neuropathy in Akabane infection, both of which result in arthrogryposis through absence of neurogenic influence on muscle activity.

It has been suggested, with some good evidence, that the etiology and pathogenesis of congenital torticollis and head scoliosis in the equine fetus are related to an increased incidence of transverse presentation of the fetus. Flexural deformities of the limbs are also thought to be a result of errors in fetal positioning and limited uterine accommodation, which may be further complicated by maternal obesity. Abnormal placental shape may also be important in the genesis of skeletal deformations.

Viral Teratogenesis

Viral teratogenesis is related to the susceptibility of undifferentiated and differentiated cells to attachment, penetration, and virus replication; the pathogenicity of the virus (cytopathogenic versus noncytopathogenic strains of bovine viral diarrhea); the effects that the virus has on the cell; and the stage of maturation of immunologic function of the fetus at the time of infection. Viral infections can result in prenatal death, the birth of nonviable neonates with severe destructive lesions, or the birth of viable neonates with growth retardation or abnormal function (tremors, blindness). The gestational age at infection is a major influence. In sheep infected with border disease virus between 16 and 90 days of gestation, the occurrence of the syndromes of early embryonic death, abortion, and stillbirth and the birth of defective, small, and weak lambs are related to the fetal age at infection. Certain viruses cause selective destruction of tissue and of organ function late in the gestational period, and the abiotrophies are examples of selective enzyme deficiencies. The pathogenesis of the viral diseases is given under their specific headings in later chapters.

Inherited Congenital Defects

A number of **inherited congenital defects**, some of which are not clinically manifest until later in life, are associated with specific enzyme deficiencies. Examples are maple syrup urine disease (MSUD), citrullinemia, factor XI deficiency in cattle, and the lysosomal storage diseases. Inherited lysosomal storage diseases occur when there is excessive accumulation of undigested substrate in cells. In mannosidosis, the disease occurs as a result of an accumulation of saccharides caused by a deficiency of either lysosomal α-mannosidase or β-mannosidase. In GM_1 gangliosidosis, disease is caused by a deficiency of β-galactosidase; in GM_2 gangliosidosis, the cause is a deficiency of hexosaminidase.

The age at development of clinical signs and their severity are dependent on the importance of the enzyme that is deficient, the biochemical function and cell type affected, and, in storage disease, the rate of substrate accumulation. Factor XI deficiency is manifest with bleeding tendencies, but the condition is not necessarily lethal. In contrast, calves with citrullinemia and MSUD develop neurologic signs and die shortly after birth, whereas the onset of clinical disease can be delayed for several months with α-mannosidosis.

CLINICAL AND NECROPSY FINDINGS

The intention is to give details of the clinical signs of all the congenital defects here, but some general comments are necessary. Approximately 50% of animals with congenital defects are **stillborn**. The defects are usually readily obvious clinically. Diseases of the nervous system and musculoskeletal system rate high in most published records, which may be related to the ease with which abnormalities of these systems can be observed. For example, in one survey of congenital defects in pigs, the percentage occurrence rates in the different body systems were as follows:

- Bones and joints, 23%
- Central nervous system, 17%
- Special sense organs, 12%
- Combined alimentary and respiratory tracts (mostly cleft palate and atresia ani), 27%
- Miscellaneous (mostly monsters), 9%
- Genitourinary and abdominal wall (hernias), each 5%
- Cardiovascular system, 3%

In a survey of congenital defects in calves, the percentage occurrence rates were as follows:

- Musculoskeletal system, 24%
- Respiratory and alimentary tracts, 13%
- Central nervous system, 22%
- Abdominal wall, 9%
- Urogenital, 4%
- Cardiovascular, 3%
- Skin, 2%
- Others, 4%
- (Anomalous-joined twins and hydrops amnii accounted for 20%.)

In a survey of foals, the approximate percentage occurrence rates were as follows:

- Musculoskeletal system, 50%
- Respiratory and alimentary tracts, 20%
- Urogenital, 9%
- Abdominal wall, 6%
- Cardiovascular, 5%
- Eye, 5%
- Central nervous system, 5%

Contracted foal syndrome and craniofacial abnormalities were the most common congenital defects in a study of stillbirth and perinatal death in horses.

Many animals with congenital defects have more than one anomaly. In pigs, for example, the average is two, and considerable care must be taken to avoid missing a second and third defect in the excitement of finding the first. In some instances, the combinations of defects are repeated often enough to become specific entities. Examples are microphthalmia and cleft palate, which often occur together in piglets, and microphthalmia and patent interventricular septum in calves.

There are a number of defects that cannot be readily distinguished at birth and others that disappear subsequently. It is probably wise not to be too dogmatic in predicting the outcome in a patient with only a suspicion of a congenital defect or one in which the defect appears to be causing no apparent harm. A specific instance is the newborn foal with a cardiac murmur.

Sporadic cases of congenital defects are usually impossible to define etiologically, but when the number of affected animals increases, it becomes necessary and possible to attempt to determine the cause.

CLINICAL PATHOLOGY

The use of clinical pathology as an aid to diagnosis depends on the disease that is suspected and its differential diagnosis. The approach varies markedly with different causes of congenital defects: **specific tests** and procedures are available for some of the viral teratogens, for congenital defects associated with nutritional deficiencies, and for some enzyme deficiencies and storage diseases, and the specific approach for known teratogens is covered in the individual diseases section.

When an unknown viral teratogen is suspected, precolostral blood samples should be collected from the affected neonates and also from normal contemporaries that are subsequently born in the group. Precolostral serum can be used for investigating the possible fetal exposure of the group to an agent, and the buffy coat or blood can be used for attempted virus isolation. IgG and IgM concentrations in precolostral serum may give an indication of fetal response to an infecting agent even if the agent is not known and there is no serologic titer to known teratogenic agents.

Enzyme-based tests have been used to virtually eradicate carriers of α-mannosidosis in cattle breeds in Australia and New Zealand, and DNA-based tests are used to detect and eliminate the carriers of such diseases as generalized glycogenosis in cattle.

DIFFERENTIAL DIAGNOSIS

- The diagnostic challenge with congenital defects is to recognize and identify the defect and to determine the cause.
- Syndromes of epidemic disease resulting from environmental teratogens are usually sufficiently distinct that they can be diagnosed on the basis of their epidemiology combined with their specific clinical, pathologic, and laboratory findings and on the availability of exposure.
- Congenital defects occurring sporadically in individual animals pose a greater problem. There is usually little difficulty in defining the condition clinically, but it may be impossible to determine the cause. With conditions where there is not an obvious clinical diagnosis, an accurate clinical definition may allow placement of the syndrome within a grouping of previously described defects and suggest possible further laboratory testing for further differentiation.

The examination for cause of an unknown congenital defect is usually not undertaken unless more than a few newborn animals in a herd or area are affected in a short period of time with similar abnormalities. A detailed epidemiologic investigation will be necessary, which will include the following:

- Pedigree analysis. Does the frequency of occurrence of the defect suggest an inherited disease, or is it characteristically nonhereditary?
- Nutritional history of dams of affected neonates and alterations in usual sources of feed
- Disease history of dams of affected neonates
- History of drugs used on dams
- Movement of dams during pregnancy to localities where contact with teratogens may have occurred
- Season of the year when insults may have occurred
- Introduction of animals to the herd

The major difficulty in determining the cause of nonhereditary congenital defects is the long interval of time between when the causative agent was operative and when the animals are presented, often 6 to 8 months. Detailed clinical and pathologic examination of affected animals offers the best opportunity in the initial approach to determine the etiology based on the presence of lesions that are known to be caused by certain teratogens.

FURTHER READING

Angus K. Congenital malformations in sheep. *In Pract.* 1992;14:33-38.

De Lahunta A. Abiotrophy in domestic animals: a review. *Can J Vet Res*. 1990;54:65-76.
Dennis SM. Congenital abnormalities. *Vet Clin North Am Food Anim Pract*. 1993;9:1-222.
Dennis SM, Leipold HW. Ovine congenital defects. *Vet Bull*. 1979;49:233.
Leipold HW, Huston K, Dennis SM. Bovine congenital defects. *Adv Vet Sci Comp Med*. 1983;27:197-271.
Panter KE, Keeler RC, James LF, Bunch TD. Impact of plant toxins on fetal and neonatal development. A review. *J Range Manag*. 1992;45:52-57.
Parsonson IM, Della-Porta AJ, Snowdon WA. Development disorders of the fetus in some arthropod-bovine virus infection. *Am J Trop Med Hyg*. 1981;30:600-673.
Rousseaux CG. Congenital defects as a cause of perinatal mortality of beef calves. *Vet Clin North Am Food Anim Pract*. 1994;10:35-45.
Rousseaux CG. Developmental anomalies in farm animals. I. Theoretical considerations. *Can Vet J*. 1988;29:23-29.
Rousseaux CG, Ribble CS. Developmental anomalies in farm animals. II. Defining etiology. *Can Vet J*. 1988;29:30-40.
Whitlock BK, Kaiser L, Maxwell HS. Heritable bovine fetal abnormalities. *Theriogenology*. 2008;70:535-549.

INTRAUTERINE GROWTH RETARDATION

Intrauterine growth retardation is a special form of congenital defect. It is a failure to grow properly, in contrast to a failure to gain body weight, and occurs when the developmental age is less than the chronologic (gestational) age. **Runt** is a common colloquial agricultural term. Normal fetal growth rate is determined by genetic and epigenetic factors, and cross-breeding experiments suggest that fetal size is regulated by the embryonic/fetal genotype and also is an effect of maternal genotype. Litter size has an effect on birth weight in all species, most likely through effects on the placental delivery of nutrients and removal of waste products relative to total fetal mass. A **genetic** association with intrauterine growth retardation has been shown in Japanese Black calves.

There is a strong positive association between placental mass and fetal size at birth in all species, and the majority of cases of growth retardation result from inadequate placentation, disturbance in utero of placental blood flow, or placental pathology.

ETIOLOGY

There are a number of different etiologies.

Heat stress to ewes in the final third of pregnancy will result in intrauterine growth retardation, but the condition is not as severe as when ewes are exposed in the second third of pregnancy, which is the period of placental growth. Hyperthermia results in a redistribution of blood away from the placental vascular bed and a decrease in cotyledon mass, with consequent reduction in birth weight. The degree of growth restriction is directly related to the degree of hyperthermia to which the ewe is exposed and her heat tolerance. The growth retardation affects fetal weight more than fetal length, and although there is some reduction in the growth of the brain, it is relatively less than that of the internal organs, resulting in an increased brain : liver weight ratio at birth.

Viral infections, such as border disease and bovine virus diarrhea in ruminants and parvovirus in pigs, produce growth-retarded neonates, as do bacterial and other infections that result in placentitis.

Inadequate placentation is the cause of runt piglets. Runts are smaller and thinner and have disproportionately larger, domed heads compared with normal pigs. A deficiency in specific **trace elements** is suspect in some field cases of growth retardation in ruminants, but there is no evidence for deficient trace-element nutrition in runt pigs.

Inadequate nutrition can result in growth retardation in utero. Growth retardation can be produced in fetal pigs, lambs, and calves by **maternal caloric undernutrition**. Nutritional restriction in ewes reduces the number of placental lactogen receptors that mediate amino acid transport in fetal liver and glycogen synthesis in fetal tissue, leading to depletion of fetal liver glycogen stores. This has been postulated as a possible cause of the fetal growth retardation that accompanies maternal caloric undernutrition; runt pigs have a reduced metabolic rate and lower skeletal muscle respiratory enzyme activity. This deficiency persists after birth; runt pigs have a lower core temperature and a lessened ability to increase their metabolic rate and heat production in response to cold.

Paradoxically, **overnourishing the adolescent ewe** will also result in placental growth restriction and in utero growth retardation. This effect is most evident in the second third of pregnancy. This syndrome is accompanied by the birth of lambs with a shorter gestational age, commonly reduced by 3 days. It is thought that the fetal hypoxia and hypoglycemia that accompany placental insufficiency might stimulate the maturation of the fetal hypothalamic–pituitary–adrenal axis, initiating early parturition. The growth of those lambs that survive initially lags behind that of normal lambs, but there is compensatory growth and no difference in weight at 6 months of age.

Measurements that can be used to determine the presence of growth retardation in a **dead fetus** include crown–rump (anal) length, brain weight, body weight, ratios of brain to body weight, long-bone weight, and appendicular ossification centers. Formulas are available to determine the degree of growth retardation.

In the **live animal** the presence of radiodense lines in long bones and the examination of closure of ossification centers can provide evidence for prior stressors in pregnancy that induce fetal growth retardation, such as malnutrition or infection of the dam, that may not be found by other examinations.

Intrauterine growth retardation is accompanied by an impaired cellular development of tissues, such as the small intestine and skeletal muscle, and disproportionately large reductions in the growth of some organs, such as the thymus, spleen, liver, kidney, ovary, and thyroid. There is an associated impairment of thermogenesis, immune function, and organ function at birth. In lambs there is impaired development of secondary wool follicles.

The **survival** of fetuses with growth retardation requires special nutritional care and the provision of adequate heat; this topic is discussed in the section on critical care for the newborn. In large piggeries that practice batch farrowing, the survival of runts can be significantly improved by the simple practice of fostering them together in one litter on one sow so that they do not have to compete with larger-birth-size and more vigorous pigs, by ensuring adequate colostrum intake and adequate environmental warmth, and by feeding using a stomach tube in the first few hours of life, if indicated.

FURTHER READING

Ferenc K, Pietrzak P, Godlewski MM, et al. Intrauterine growth retarded piglet as a model for humans—studies on the perinatal development of the gut structure and function. *Reprod Biol*. 2014;14(1):51-60.
Wu G, Bazer FW, Wallace JM, et al. Board-invited review: intrauterine growth retardation: implications for the animal sciences. *J Anim Sci*. 2006;84(9):2316-2337.

Physical and Environmental Causes of Perinatal Disease

Neonatal animals are newborns. The definition of a neonate is not precisely defined in terms of age of the animal and likely will vary from species to species dependent on the ability of the newborn to survive relatively independently and on the maturity or degree of postnatal development. Most farm mammals can be considered neonates until they are 2 weeks of age.[1]

The health of neonates is determined by factors that influence their growth and development in utero and their capacity to adapt to extrauterine life. Neonates affected by intrauterine conditions that impede their normal development (intrauterine growth retardation or premature birth) might not be prepared for the rapid and extensive physiologic changes needed to survive after birth. Furthermore, conditions experienced by the newborn can adversely affect its health and well-being; key among these factors are adequate nutrition, transfer of passive immunity from the dam, a thermoneutral environment or protection from the adverse effects of excessive cold or heat, and protection from risk of injury.

PERINATOLOGY

Clinical care of the newborn animal in large animal veterinary medicine has traditionally started at the time of birth, but there is a growing recognition of the importance of antenatal and parturient events to the subsequent viability of the neonate.[2] This has been particularly recognized by equine clinicians and has led to the clinical concept of perinatology. One purpose of perinatology is to expand the care of the neonate into the antenatal and parturient period through the use of measurements that reflect fetal health or that can predict risk to fetal viability. Measures that can be used are still being developed and evaluated, but the following discussion includes those that have apparent value.

HEART RATE

Fetal heart rate recorded by electrocardiography (ECG) or by ultrasound can be used as a measure of fetal viability, for the detection of twins, and as a monitor for fetal distress during parturition.[3] The fetal heart rate of foals declines during gestation (Fig. 19-1) to approximately 60 to 80 beats/min near to term, and that of fetal calves is approximately 110 beats/min during the final 2 weeks of gestation.[4]

It has been suggested that a base heart rate of 80 to 92 beats/min with baseline variations of 7 to 15 beats/min and occasional accelerations above this is normal for the fetal heart rate of equids, and that bradycardia is evidence of abnormality. Continued monitoring traces may be needed to assess fetal distress.

Cardiac arrhythmia is common at the time of birth and for the first few minutes following and is thought to result from the transient physiologic hypoxemia that occurs during the birth process.

An alternative to fetal ECG monitoring is use of per rectum or percutaneous

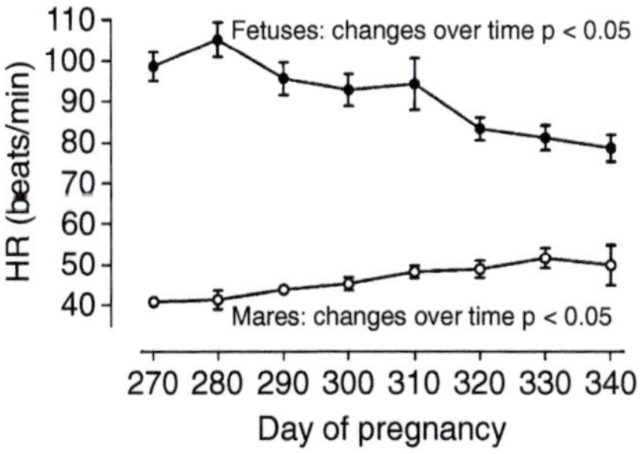

Fig. 19-1 Heart rate of mare and fetus from 270 days of gestation until foaling. The heart rate of the mare increases, whereas that of the foal declines, as the duration of gestation increases. (Reproduced from Nagel et al., 2011.[16])

ultrasonography to detect carotid or peripheral pulse rates in foals and calves.[4,5]

ULTRASOUND EXAMINATION

The fetus can be examined by **ultrasound** to establish the presentation, the presence of twins, the heart rate, the presence and quality of fetal movement, the presence of placentitis, placental thickness, the presence of echogenic particles in the amniotic fluid, the depth of allantoic and amniotic fluid, and an estimate of body size from the measurement of the aortic and orbit diameters.[3,5-8] Measurements of fetal heart rate, fetal aortic diameter (an indicator of fetal size and, if measured near parturition, fetal birth weight),[8] uteroplacental contact, maximal fetal fluid depths, uteroplacental thickness, and fetal activity have allowed the development of objective measures to assess fetal well-being (Fig. 19-2).[6]

Clinicopathologic examination of samples of the **amniotic fluid** for the determination of pulmonary maturity and other measures of foal health is limited because there is a considerable risk for abortion and placentitis, even with ultrasound-guided amniocentesis, and the technique is not recommended for routine clinical use.

PREMATURITY

The average gestational length for mares is 343 days (range, 307 to 381), with the duration of gestation being longer for mares foaling later in the spring and for mares giving birth to a male foal (344 versus 341 days for a filly foal, respectively). There is no effect of breed of the mare or her age on gestational length.[9] Approximately 95% of mares were found to foal between 320 and 360 days of gestation, with 1.1% foaling at less than 320 days. Death rates were 8.3%, 3.6%, and 4.8% for foals born at less than 320 days, 320 to 360 days, and more than 360 days of gestation, respectively.[9] The difference was not statistically significant, but the number of foals born at less than 320 days was small (12), and this could have masked a statistical difference in case fatality rates. No foal lived if it was born at less than 311 days of gestation. Foals born at less than 320 days of gestational age are considered premature, and those born at less than 310 days are at significant risk for increased rate of death.[10]

Dystocia is associated with increased morbidity and case fatality rate in foals. Stage II labor lasting longer than 40 minutes is associated with increased risk of stillbirth (16×), death after birth (8×), and illness in the foal (2×).[9]

Similar data are available for cattle. For instance, in 41,116 calvings of Japanese Black cattle, there were 1013 stillbirths (2.46%) and 3514 dystocias (8.55%). Stillbirth rates were greater for those born at 301 or more days of pregnancy (OR: 1.049 [1.035 to 1.062]) and at 270 or fewer days of pregnancy (OR: 2.072 [2.044 to 2.101]) compared with those at between 281 and 290 days of pregnancy.[11] Among Holsteins, Jerseys, and crossbreds, gestation length was ~275 days, with male calves having a gestation length 1.2 days longer. The percentage of stillbirths was 6.6% across all observations, with 9.6% among first-parity dams and 5.1% among multiparous dams.[12]

Traditionally, external signs have been used to predict a premature foaling, and the common signs used are the enlargement of the udder, milk flow, and the occurrence of vaginal discharge. Causes of early foaling include bacterial or fungal placentitis and twin pregnancy. Several **assays** are used as alternate methods of determining whether foaling is imminent and if problems are present.

Plasma **progestogen** concentrations in mares decline in pregnancy to reach a low around 150 days of gestation. Plasma progestogen cannot be used to accurately predict the time of foaling, and a single sample is not diagnostic. There is a strong correlation between the presence of plasma progestogen concentrations above 10 ng/mL before a gestational age of 310 days and the presence of placental lesions, and a rapid drop in concentration to below 2 ng/mL that persists for more than 3 days indicates impending abortion. Current research is examining the profiles of individual progestogens during pregnancy to determine whether the profile of any progestogen can be used as a predictor of fetal distress.

There is considerable interest in predicting the time of parturition in mares. Recognition that significant changes occur in udder secretions during the last week of gestation, including a drop in pH on the day of foaling and increases in concentrations of calcium and potassium and declines in levels of sodium and chloride, has led to the development of several relatively simple tests.[13] These tests include measurement of the refractive index, pH, and calcium concentration of udder secretions during the week before anticipated parturition. Samples can be analyzed for calcium carbonate concentration using a water hardness kit, for pH with pH test paper, and for refractometry index with a Brix or similar refractometer. The positive predictive value (PPV) of parturition occurring within 72 hours and the negative predictive value (NPV) within 24 hours for calcium carbonate concentration (≥400 μg/g) were 94% and 98%, respectively.[14,15] The PPV within 72 hours and the NPV within 24 hours for the pH test (≤6.4) were 98% and 99%, respectively. The PPV within 72 hours and the NPV within 24 hours for the Brix test (≥20%) were 73% and 97%, respectively. The high negative predictive value of measurement of calcium concentrations (by either method) and pH provides a way of determining when the mare is not likely to foal within the next 24 hours.[14]

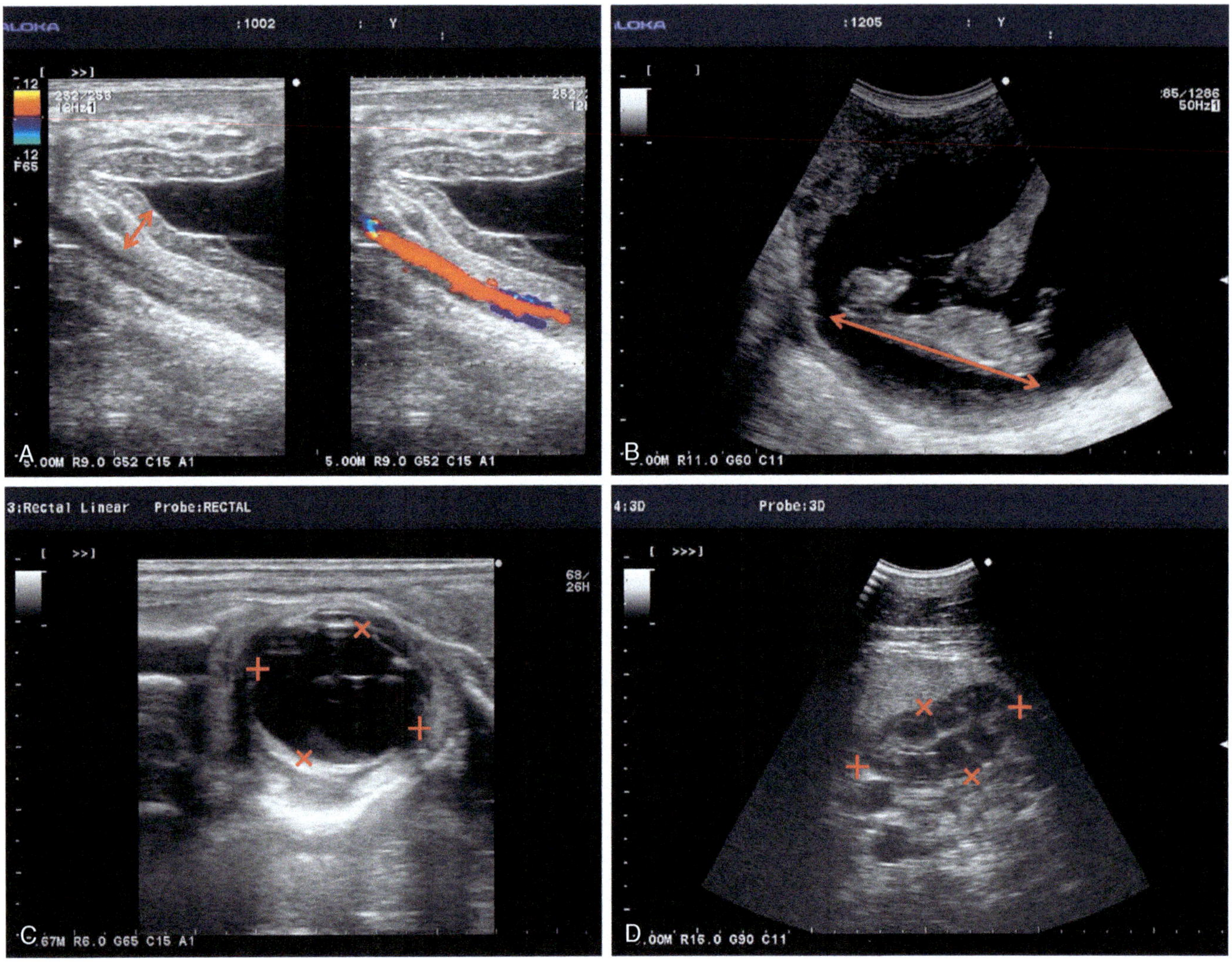

Fig. 19-2 Measurement of ultrasonographic indices of pregnant mare. **A,** Transrectal images in the ventral part of the uterine body, near the cervix. Headers show the combined thickness of the uterus and placenta (CTUP). **B,** Transrectal image of crown rump length (CRL) (header). **C,** Transrectal image of fetal eye orbit. Eye length (=) and width (×) measurements are shown. Eye length is measured from the maximum length of the inner margins of the vitreous body, and eye width is measured from the margin of the anterior portion of the capsule of the lens to the inner margin of the optic disc. **D,** Transabdominal image of the fetal abdomen at the level of the kidney. Kidney cross-sectional length (=) and width (×) measurements are shown. (Reproduced with permission from Murase et al., 2014.[6])

FURTHER READING

Satue K, et al. Factors influencing gestational length in mares: a review. *Livest Sci.* 2011;136:287-294.

REFERENCES

1. Studdert VP, et al. *Comprehensive Veterinary Dictionary*. London: Elsevier; 2012.
2. Foote AK, et al. *Equine Vet J.* 2012;44:120.
3. Gargiulo GD, et al. *BMC Vet Res.* 2012;8:1.
4. Breukelman S, et al. *Theriogenology*. 2006;65:486.
5. Bucca S, et al. *Proc Amer Assoc Equine Pract.* 2007:335.
6. Murase H, et al. *J Vet Med Sci.* 2014;76:947.
7. Ferrer MS, et al. *Theriogenology*. 2014;82:827.
8. Buczinski S, et al. *Can Vet J.* 2011;52:136.
9. McCue PM, et al. *Equine Vet J.* 2012;44:22.
10. Satue K, et al. *Livest Sci.* 2011;136:287.
11. Uematsu M, et al. *Vet J.* 2013;198:212.
12. Dhakal K, et al. *J Dairy Sci.* 2013;96:690.
13. Canisso IF, et al. *Vet Rec.* 2013;173:218.
14. Korosue K, et al. *J Am Vet Med Assoc.* 2013;242:242.
15. Korosue K. *Vet Rec.* 2013;173:216.
16. Nagel C, et al. *Reprod Domest Anim.* 2011;46:990.

PREMATURITY AND DYSMATURITY OF FOALS

Foals that are born before 300 days are unlikely to survive, and foals born between 300 and 320 days of gestation are considered premature but can survive (see earlier discussion).[1] **Premature foals** are characterized clinically by low birth weight, generalized muscle weakness, poor ability to stand, lax flexor tendons, weak or no suck reflex, lack of righting ability, respiratory distress, short and silky haircoat, pliant ears, soft lips, increased passive range of limb motion, and sloping pastern axis. Radiographs may show incomplete ossification of the carpal and tarsal bones and immaturity of the lung, and there may be clinical evidence of respiratory distress. **Full-term foals** born after 320 days of gestation but exhibiting signs of prematurity are described as **dysmature.**

Premature foals have hypoadrenal corticalism. They are neutropenic and lymphopenic at birth and have a narrow neutrophil-to-lymphocyte ratio. In premature foals older than 35 hours the neutrophil count can be used to predict survival, and foals that remain neutropenic after this time have a poor prognosis. Premature foals also have low plasma glucose, low plasma cortisol, and a blood pH of less than 7.25. An extensive collaborative investigation of equine prematurity has been conducted, and information on foal metabolism and guidelines for laboratory and clinical assessment of maturity are available.[2] Foals that are born with clinical abnormalities suggestive of intrauterine growth retardation, prematurity, or dysmaturity are more likely to have an abnormal placenta and have higher serum concentrations of creatinine.[3]

The **placenta** is critical to the fetus in the antenatal period, and pregnancies involving placental lesions commonly result in foals that suffer premature-like signs at whatever stage they are delivered.[3,4] Placental edema, placental villous atrophy, and premature separation of the placenta are significant causes of fetal ill-health and delayed development.[5]

Precocious lactation of the mare can be associated with placentitis. The examination of the placenta for evidence of placentitis and for the presence of larger-than-normal avillous areas should be part of normal foaling management. There is a high correlation between both allantochorionic weight and area and foal weight in normal placentas. Normal placentas had a low association with subsequent perinatal disease in the foals.[3,4] In contrast, abnormal placental histology was associated with poor foal outcome (three normal foals from 32 abnormal placentas). Edema, sacculation, and strangulation are other abnormalities and can be associated with microscopic deposits of minerals within the lumen of placental blood vessels.

REFERENCES

1. Satue K, et al. *Livest Sci*. 2011;136:287.
2. Dunkel B, et al. *Equine Vet J*. 2012;44:1.
3. Pirrone A, et al. *Theriogenology*. 2014;81:1293.
4. Bianco C, et al. *Theriogenology*. 2014;82:1106.
5. Wilsher S, et al. *Equine Vet J*. 2012;44:113.

PARTURIENT INJURY AND INTRAPARTUM DEATH

During parturition extreme mechanical forces are brought to bear upon the fetus, and these can result in direct traumatic damage or can impair fetal circulation of blood by entrapment of the umbilical cord between the fetus and the maternal pelvis, which can lead to hypoxemia or anoxia and death of the fetus during the birth process. Neonates that suffer birth trauma and anoxia but survive are at risk for development of signs of neurologic disease, have reduced vigor, are slower to suck, and are at increased risk for postnatal mortality.[1]

In all species, but in ruminants in particular, the **condition of the dam** can have a marked influence on the prevalence of birth injury and its consequences. The effect is well illustrated in sheep, where the two extremes of condition can cause problems. Ewes on a high plane of nutrition produce a large fetus and also deposit fat in the pelvic girdle, which constricts the birth canal, predisposing to dystocia. Conversely, thin ewes may be too weak to give birth rapidly. **Pelvic size** can influence the risk of birth injury, and ewe lambs and heifers mated before they reach 65% of mature weight are at risk. **Pelvimetry** is used to select heifers with adequate pelvic size for breeding, but the accuracy and validity of this method are seriously questioned. **Breed** is also a determinant of length and ease of labor and the subsequent quickness to time to first suckle.

TRAUMA AT PARTURITION

Traumatic injuries can occur in apparently normal births, with prolonged birth, and as a result of dystocia, which may or may not be assisted by the owner. Incompatibility in the sizes of the fetus and the dam's pelvis is the single most important cause of dystocia, and birth weight is the most important contributing factor. In cattle, expected progeny difference (EPD) estimates for calf birth weight are good predictors of calving ease. In foals, calves, and lambs the chest is most vulnerable to traumatic injury, but there is the chance of vertebral fracture and physical trauma to limbs with excessive external traction.[2]

Fractured ribs are common in foals and can lead to laceration of the lungs and heart and internal hemorrhage.[3] **Rupture of the liver** is common in some breeds of sheep and can also occur in calves and foals. A retrospective study of rib and vertebral fractures in calves suggests that most result from excessive traction and that, as a result, smaller dystocial calves are more at risk. **Vertebral fractures** occur as the result of traction in calves with posterior presentations and in calves with hip lock. Trauma is a major cause of neonatal mortality in piglets, but it occurs in the postparturient phase and is associated with being overlain or stepped on by the sow. It is possible that the underlying cause of crushing mortality in piglets is hypothermia.

Intracranial hemorrhage can result in damage to the brain. A high proportion (70%) of nonsurviving neonatal lambs at birth or within 7 days of birth have single or multiple intracranial hemorrhages, with the highest incidence being in lambs of high birth weight.[4] Similar lesions have been identified in foals and calves, but they are not a common finding in foals with neonatal maladjustment syndrome. Experimentally controlled parturition in ewes showed that duration and vigor of the birth process affected the severity of intracranial hemorrhages, and further studies indicated that these birth-injured lambs had depressed feeding activity and that they were particularly susceptible to death from hypothermia and starvation.

Birth anoxia associated with severe dystocia in cattle can result in calves with lower rectal temperatures in the perinatal period than normal calves and a decreased ability to withstand cold stress. Intracranial hemorrhage, especially subarachnoid hemorrhage, occurs in normal full-term deliveries as the result of physical or asphyxial trauma during or immediately following delivery.

In a prolonged birth, **edema** of parts of the body, such as the head and particularly the tongue, may also occur. Edema occurs particularly in the calf and the lamb, possibly because of less close supervision at parturition, and also because the young of these species can sustain a prolonged birthing process for longer periods than the foal without their own death or death of the dam. The edema can interfere with subsequent sucking, but the principal problem relative to neonatal disease is the effect of the often prolonged hypoxia to which the fetus is subjected. There is interference with the placental circulation and failure of the fetus to reach the external environment. The hypoxia may be sufficient to produce a stillborn neonate, or the neonate may be alive at birth but not survive because of irreparable brain damage. Intrapartum deaths resulting from prolonged parturition occur in piglets.

REFERENCES

1. Murray CF, et al. *Vet J*. 2013;198:322.
2. Barrier AC, et al. *Vet J*. 2013;197:220.
3. Jean D, et al. *Equine Vet J*. 2007;39:158.
4. Dutra F, et al. *Aust Vet J*. 2007;85:405.

FETAL HYPOXIA

Hypoxemia and hypoxia can occur as a result of influences during the birth process or because of pulmonary immaturity in premature births. The most common causes are dystocia, interrupted or restricted blood flow through the umbilical vein (carrying oxygenated blood to the fetus) and artery, and placental lesions, including premature separation of the placenta during labor, that reduce the effective surface area of the placenta in contact with the endometrium.[1] Intrapartum hypoxemia of the fetus resulting from **prolonged parturition** is common, particularly in calves born to first-calf beef heifers, and is presumed to be associated with the greater case fatality rate and morbidity in foals born after stage 2 labor of greater than 40 minutes.[2] Prolonged duration of parturition in ewes increases the risk of asphyxia (90× for each 10-min increase), decreases the viability score of lambs, and increases the latency to suckle the udder. Twin-born lambs were found to have a 16-fold greater risk of asphyxia.

Transient tachypnea occurs immediately after birth and is normal. **Prolonged tachypnea**, with flaring of the nostrils, open-mouth breathing, exaggerated rib retraction, and paradoxical breathing patterns, is highly suggestive of primary pulmonary abnormality. Failure of respiration can occur at this stage and creates an urgent need for resuscitation measures. In the foal, **body position** can have a major effect on arterial oxygen tension. A foal that is unable to stand or to right itself from lateral recumbency is at risk from atelectasis and should be assisted to lie in sternal recumbency to stand. Hypoxia and hypercapnia resulting from mismatching of ventilation and perfusion are accentuated by prolonged recumbency.

Placental dysfunction or restriction of blood flow in the umbilical vessels during the second stage of labor can result in fetal hypoxia and death. Blood flow in umbilical vessels is reduced during uterine contractions and ceases during stage 2 labor in cattle as the calf's head appears at the vulva and just before delivery of the calf.[1] Before this stage, blood flow in the umbilical vein is significantly lower in acidotic than in nonacidotic calves, indicating impairment of oxygen delivery to the fetus and development of increased blood lactate concentrations.[1]

Fetal capillary blood pH and oxygen and carbon dioxide tensions can be measured during parturition, as is common practice in human obstetrics.[3] Fetal blood is collected from capillaries in the front feet as they project from the vulva by making a small incision (nick) in the skin and collecting blood into a capillary tube, which is then sealed before blood-gas analysis.[3] In 38 calves, some of which were born as a result of relieved dystocia or cesarean section, fetal capillary blood-gas values and pH (mean ± standard deviation [SD]) during the final 30 minutes of stage 2 labor were as follows: pH = 7.30 ± 0.10 (min 6.99, max 7.43), Po_2 = 19.5±9.4 mm Hg, Pco_2=55.9±26.0 mm Hg, HCO_3^- = 26.0 ± 4.4 mm Hg, base excess = −0.9 ± 5.3 mM/L, and oxygen saturation = 21.9 ± 16.6.[3] These compare with the following values in capillary blood obtained after recovery from birth in healthy calves: pH = 7.37 ± 0.11, Po_2 = 58.4 ± 17.0 mm Hg, Pco_2 = 38.1 ± 13.2 mm Hg, HCO_3^- = 20.8 ± 4.9 mm Hg, base excess = −3.2 ± 4.4 mM/L, and oxygen saturation = 82.4 ± 14.9%.[3] Similarly, jugular vein blood collected from 79 **lambs** immediately after birth (before onset of regular breathing) had the following values: pH = 7.21 ± 0.09 (range, 6.99 to 7.41), Po_2 = 18.4 ± 9.8 mm Hg (4 to 53), Pco_2 = 65.4 ± 12.5 mm Hg (29.6 to 103.7), HCO_3^- = 26.5 ± 4.0 mm Hg (13.9 to 35.4), base excess = −1.3 ± 5.1 mM/L (−16 to 9), and oxygen saturation = 21.2 ± 16.6% (0 to 85).[4] Both normal calves and lambs are acidotic, hypoxemic, and hypercapnic during birth as a result of impaired placental blood flow, and prolonged duration of stage 2 of parturition likely exacerbates this hypoxia and increases morbidity and fatality rate.[1]

A similar syndrome has been produced experimentally by clamping the umbilical cord of the bovine fetus in utero for 6 to 8 minutes, followed by a cesarean section 30 to 40 minutes later. Calves born following this procedure may die within 10 to 15 minutes after birth or survive for up to 2 days. During the experimental clamping of the umbilical cord, there is a decline in the blood pH, Po_2, and standard bicarbonate levels and an increase in Pco_2 and lactate levels. There is also increased fetal movement during clamping and a release of meconium, which stains the calf and the amniotic fluid. Those that survive for a few hours or days are dull and depressed, cannot stand, and have poor sucking and swallowing reflexes, and their temperature is usually subnormal. They respond poorly to supportive therapy. A slight body tremor may be present, and occasionally tetany and opisthotonus occur before death. Calves that are barely able to stand cannot find the teats of the dam because of uncontrolled head movements. At necropsy of these experimental cases, there are petechial and ecchymotic hemorrhages on the myocardium and endocardium, there is an excess of pericardial fluid, and the lungs are inflated. When the experimental clamping lasts only 4 minutes, the calves usually survive.

Meconium staining (brown discoloration) of the coat of the newborn at birth is an important indicator that it has suffered hypoxia during or preceding the birth process,[5,6] and such neonates merit close supervision in the early postnatal period. In lambs, severe hypoxia during birth results in death within 6 days of birth. **Neurologic lesions** in lambs that died between birth and 6 days of age include hemorrhages in the meninges, brain congestion and edema, neuronal ischemic necrosis, intraparenchymal hemorrhages in the medulla oblongata and cervical spinal cord, parasagittal cerebral necrosis, and periventricular leukomalacia.[7] Edema was more severe in the brain than in other regions of the central nervous system. Ischemic neurons first appeared 24 hours postpartum, increased linearly in number between 48 hours and 5 days postpartum, and had a laminar distribution in the cerebral cortex, indicating a hypoxic-ischemic encephalopathy.[7] No significant lesions were found in antepartum deaths or in those aged between 7 and 16 days. Lesions in the central nervous system can explain most deaths at birth and within 6 days of birth. The lesions were hypoxic-ischemic and appeared to be related to birth injury in some cases.[7] Similar lesions are not found in foals with neonatal maladjustment syndrome (see page 1871).

Fetal anoxia associated with **premature expulsion** of the **placenta** occurs in all species. Anoxia occurs in all parities of cow and with little relation to calving difficulty, although malpresentation is a predisposing factor. Prepartum diagnosis in cattle is hindered by the low prevalence of prepartum vaginal hemorrhage, and the majority of fetuses die during the birth process. The placenta is expelled with the fetus. **Premature separation** of the placenta ("red bag") occurs in foals and is an emergency that requires immediate attention. Premature placental separation occurs in approximately 1.6% of births and is associated with a case fatality rate of 18% in the foals.[2]

In all species the prevention of intrapartum hypoxia depends on the provision of surveillance. Universal surveillance is usually not practical for species other than the horse, and in cattle, for example, it tends to concentrate on the group at most risk so that surveillance, and assistance if necessary, is provided for first-calf heifers at the time of calving. Heifers that do not continue to show progress during the second stage of parturition should be examined for evidence of dystocia, and obstetric assistance should be provided if necessary.

The treatment and care of foals with this syndrome is described in the section on critical care of the newborn later in the chapter. The monitoring, treatment, and care of agricultural animals with this syndrome should follow the same principles but is usually limited by the value of the animal and the immediate access to a laboratory. Measures such as the time from birth to sternal recumbency, the time from birth to standing, and the time from birth to first suckle have been used to grade calves and identify those that might require intervention and treatment, but the best method of evaluation is an assessment of muscle tone. There is no effective practical treatment for calves affected with intrapartum hypoxia other than the provision of ventilation, as for the foal, and the correction of the acidosis. The airway should be cleared, and if physical stimulation of ventilation gives no response, then mechanical ventilation should be attempted. The practice of direct mouth-to-mouth ventilation assistance should be strongly discouraged, especially in lambs, because of the risk from zoonotic disease agents. Doxapram hydrochloride has been used in calves to stimulate respiration, but without demonstrated efficacy.

REFERENCES

1. Bleul U, et al. *Theriogenology*. 2007;67:1123.
2. McCue PM, et al. *Equine Vet J*. 2012;44:22.
3. Bleul U, et al. *Theriogenology*. 2008;69:245.
4. Dutra F, et al. *J Anim Sci*. 2011;89:3069.
5. Mota-Rojas D, et al. *Livest Sci*. 2006;102:155.
6. Castro-Najera JA, et al. *J Vet Diagn Invest*. 2006;18:622.
7. Dutra F, et al. *Aust Vet J*. 2007;85:405.

HYPOTHERMIA IN NEWBORNS

The environment of the neonate has a profound effect on its survival. This is especially true for lambs and piglets, in which hypothermia and hypoglycemia are common causes of death. Hypothermia can also predispose to inadequate milk intake, including colostrum, and increase the risk and severity of infectious disease. A fuller description, including hypothermia affecting adults, is provided under "Hypothermia" in Chapter 5.

LAMBS

Cold stress and resultant death rates of lambs is an important animal welfare issue.[1] Lambs are very susceptible to cold, and hypothermia is an important cause of mortality in the early postnatal period.[2] **Cold stress** to neonatal lambs is attributable to heat loss resulting from one or more of the factors of low ambient temperature, wind, and evaporative cooling. The healthy newborn lamb has a good ability to increase its metabolic rate in response to a cold stress by shivering and nonshivering thermogenesis (brown adipose tissue). The energy sources in the neonatal lamb are liver and muscle glycogen, brown adipose tissue, and, if it nurses, the energy obtained from colostrum and milk. The ingestion of colostrum can be essential for early thermogenesis in lambs, especially twin lambs.

The **critical temperature** (the ambient temperature below which a lamb must increase metabolic heat production to maintain body temperature) for light-birth-weight lambs is 31° C to 37° C (88°–99° F) in the first days of life.

The risk of death from hypothermia is highest in lambs of small birth size. **Heat production** is a function of body mass, whereas **heat loss** is a function of body surface area. Large-birth-size lambs have a greater body mass in relation to surface area and are thus more resistant to environmental cold stress. In contrast, small-birth-size lambs, with a smaller body mass relative to surface area, are more susceptible to chilling. The dramatic nature of this relationship was shown in early studies on cold stress and survival in lambs many years ago. Birth weight is lower in twins and triplets and in the progeny of maiden ewes. Susceptibility is also influenced by maternal nutrition in pregnancy (see the next section) because this can both influence placental mass, birth weight, and the energy reserves of the neonate and also affect the activity of the ewe at parturition, and the resultant poor mothering behavior and mismothering can result in starvation in the lamb.

Lambs are particularly susceptible to cold stress during the first 5 days of life. During this period hypothermia can result from heat loss in excess of summit metabolism or from depressed heat production caused by intrapartum hypoxia, immaturity, and starvation.

Heat loss is a function of the surface area available for convective, conductive, and evaporational heat loss; ambient temperature; wetness of the skin (fleece); and wind speed. These factors can be described mathematically as follows:

$$\text{Chill index } (kJ/m^2/hr) = 481 + (11.7 + 3.1 * V) * (40 - T) - (418 * [1 - e^{-0.04Ra}]),$$

where temperature (T), rain (Ra), and wind speed (V) are considered and are related to mortality rate in newborn lambs (Fig. 19-3).

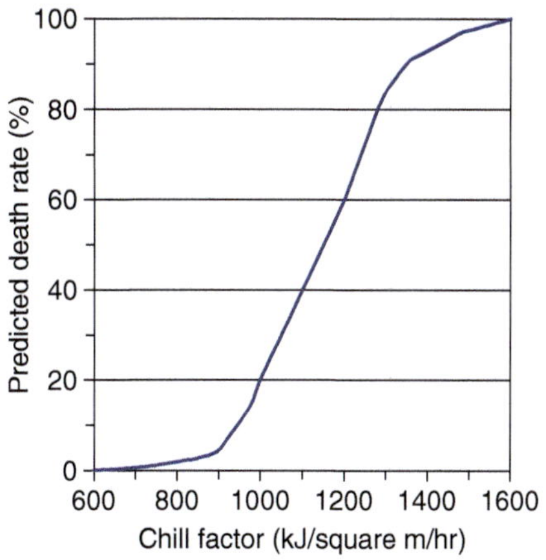

Fig. 19-3 Predicted death rate for neonatal lambs as a function of wind chill. (Data generated from LambAlive. Horizon Agriculture [www.hzn.com.au/lambalive.php] and courtesy of Dr. John Larsen, University of Melbourne.[6,7])

Heat Loss in Excess of Summit Metabolism

Low-birth-weight lambs born into a cool environment where there is wind are especially susceptible because of the evaporative cooling of fetal fluids on the fleece. For a small newborn lamb, the evaporative cooling effect of a breeze of 19 km/h (12 mph) at an ambient temperature of 13° C (55° F), common in lambing seasons in many countries, can be the equivalent of a cold stress equivalent to 25° C (77° F). The heat loss in these circumstances can exceed the lamb's ability to produce heat (summit metabolism), and progressive hypothermia and death result. Hypothermia as a result of heat loss in excess of summit metabolism can also occur when there is rain or just with cold and wind. Death occurs primarily in the first 12 hours of life.

Hypothermia From Depleted Energy Reserves

Hypothermia occurring in lambs after 12 hours of age is usually a result of depletion of energy reserves in periods of cold stress; milk is the sustaining energy source. There are three major causes of hypothermia from depleted energy reserves.

One of the early manifestations of developing hypothermia is the **loss of sucking drive**; severe cold stress and developing hypothermia can result in behavioral changes that cause low milk intake and subsequent depletion of energy reserves.

The second important cause is **mismothering**; the third is related to **birth injury**. Most researched measures of maternal behavior, temperament, and lambing difficulty are poorly correlated genetically with lamb survival.[3] Dystocia-related hypoxia is associated with acidemia, a reduction in summit metabolism, and disturbance in thermoregulation and can result in hypothermia. Birth-injured lambs, usually large single-born lambs, have depressed sucking and feeding activity, and actions to increase the birth weight of lambs above a certain point are likely to be counterproductive.[4] The relationship between mortality of lambs and birth weight is a U-shaped curve, with smaller and larger lambs at increased risk of death.[2]

In lambs that have hypothermia associated with heat loss in excess of summit metabolism, heat is required for **therapy**, but in lambs with starvation hypothermia the administration of glucose is also necessary. Glucose is administered intraperitoneally at a dose of 2 g/kg body weight using a 20% solution. Following the administration of the glucose, the lambs should be dried with a towel if wet and rewarmed in air at 40° C (104° F). This can be done in a warming box using a radiant heater as the heat supply. Care should be taken to avoid hyperthermia. Careful attention must be given to the nutrition of the lambs after rewarming; otherwise, relapse of hypothermia will occur. A feeding of 100 to 200 mL of colostrum will also be beneficial, but lambs should not be fed before they are normothermic because aspiration pneumonia is a risk. Experimental hypothermia in lambs has shown little direct long-term pathologic effect.

In most countries the selection of time of lambing is dictated by nutritional considerations and the seasonality of the ewes' sexual behavior, and lambing occurs at a time of year when cold stress is likely. The **control** of loss from hypothermia in newborn lambs requires supervision at lambing and protection from cold. Shed lambing will reduce cold-stress loss. The provision of shelter in lambing paddocks is effective at reducing mortality rate and in increasing profitability.[5] The site is important because birth sites in lambing paddocks are not randomly distributed, and there is variation in the preferred sites between breeds. Some ewes will seek shelter at lambing, but many ewes in wool will not. In some flocks, sheep are shorn before lambing in an attempt to force this shelter-seeking trait.

Experimentally, there is a strong relationship between breed and the degree of hypothermia produced. There is also convincing evidence that rearing ability is heritable in sheep, that some of this relates to traits within the newborn lamb, and that a significant reduction in neonatal mortality associated with susceptibility to hypothermia could be achieved with a genetic approach.

Lambs are also susceptible to **hyperthermia**, and thermoregulation is not efficient at high environmental temperatures. Heat prostration and some deaths can occur in range lambs when the environmental temperature is high, especially if lambs have to perform prolonged physical exercise and if there is an absence of shade.

CALVES

Hypothermia as a result of environmental influence is less common in full-term healthy calves than in lambs, but mortality rates have been shown to increase with decreasing ambient temperature and increasing precipitation on the day of birth. The **critical temperature** for neonatal calves is much lower than that for lambs, approximately 13°C (55°F), and *Bos taurus* calves are more resistant to cold stress than are *Bos indicus*.

Experimentally produced hypothermia in calves causes little overt injury except for peripheral damage to exterior tissues. During cooling there can be significant peripheral hypothermia before any marked reduction in core body temperature. Calves have a remarkable ability to resist and overcome the effects of severe cold temperatures. However, there is a relationship between the occurrence of cold weather and calf deaths, including those resulting from "weak-calf syndrome," and deficiencies in thermoregulation occur in animals born prematurely and in dystocial calves. As in lambs, dystocia will reduce teat-seeking activity and sucking drive, and dystocial calves have lower intakes of colostrum, lower body temperatures, and decreased ability to withstand cold stress.

Rewarming of hypothermic calves can be by radiant heat, but immersion in warm water produces a more rapid response and with minimal metabolic effort. The prevention of hypothermia requires the provision of shelter from wet and wind for the first few days of life. Cows can be calved in a shed; alternatively, sheds for calves can be provided in the fields. Beef calves will use shelters in inclement weather; these may not improve their health status, although they are in common use.

PIGLETS

Hypothermia from heat loss and hypothermia/hypoglycemia from starvation are major causes of loss in neonatal pigs. Newborn piglets have a reasonably good ability to increase their metabolic rate in response to cold stress, but they have limited energy reserves, especially limited brown adipose tissue, and they consequently rely on a continual intake of milk for their major energy source, sucking approximately every hour. Young pigs have a good ability for peripheral vasoconstriction at birth, but surface insulation is deficient because at this age there is no subcutaneous layer of fat. The **critical temperature** for young pigs is 34°C (93°F).

Thermoregulation is inefficient during the first 9 days of life and is not fully functional until the 20th day. Newborn piglets must be provided with an external heat source in the first few weeks of life. The body temperature of the sow cannot be relied upon for this, and the preferred air temperature for neonatal pigs is 32°C (89.5°F) during the first day and 30°C (86°F) for the first week. In contrast, the preferred temperature for the sow is about 18°C (64°F). A **separate environment** (creep area) must be provided for the piglets. Provided that there is an adequate ambient temperature to meet the requirements of the piglets and good floor insulation, hypothermia will not occur in healthy piglets of viable size unless there is a failure of milk intake.

Birth anoxia, with resultant reduced vigor, reduced teat-seeking activity, and **risk for hypothermia**, occurs particularly in later-birth-order pigs in large litters from older sows. Failure of milk intake can also occur with small-birth-size piglets and is influenced by litter size, low number of functional teats relative to litter size, and teat-sucking order.

FOALS

There have been few studies on thermoregulation in foals, but the large body mass in relation to surface area renders healthy newborn foals, like healthy calves, relatively resistant to cold. Also, foals are less likely to be born in a hostile environment than are other farm animals. Significant foal mortality from hypothermia as a result of starvation and exposure can occur in extensively managed herds, and dystocia, low birth weight, and poor mothering are contributing factors.

Sick and **premature foals** can have difficulty in maintaining body temperature in normal environments, and the metabolic rates of sick foals and premature foals are approximately 25% lower than those of healthy foals.

The relatively larger ratio of surface area to mass, lower energy reserves, and lower insulation of the coat of premature foals, coupled with the lower metabolic rate, place them at particular risk for hypothermia. **Dystocial foals** also have lower metabolic rates, but dysmature foals appear to thermoregulate normally. Methods of investigation that allow postmortem differentiation of placental insufficiency, acute intrapartum hypoxemia, inadequate thermogenesis, and starvation as causes of mortality in foals are available.

Hypothermia should be suspected in premature foals when the rectal temperature falls below 37.2°C (99°F) and should be corrected with external warmth, rugging, or moving to a heated environment. If fluids are being administered, they should be heated to normal body temperature.

REFERENCES

1. Dwyer CM. *Small Rumin Res.* 2008;76:31.
2. Hinch GN, et al. *Anim Prod Sci.* 2014;54:656.
3. Brien FD, et al. *Anim Prod Sci.* 2014;54:667.
4. Hatcher S, et al. *J Anim Sci.* 2009;87:2781.
5. Young JM, et al. *Anim Prod Sci.* 2014;54:773.
6. Lamb Alive. Horizon Agriculture. (Accessed June 15, 2016, at <http://www.hzn.com.au/lambalive.php>).
7. Nixon-Smith WF. The forecasting of chill risk ratings for new born lambs and off-shears sheep by the use of a cooling factor derived from synoptic data. Working Paper No. 150. Commonwealth Bureau of Meteorology, Melbourne, Vic.; 1972.

MATERNAL NUTRITION AND THE NEWBORN

There is increasing evidence that the maternal environment for a fetus affects lifelong characteristics of offspring and the subsequent generation of offspring ("grandchildren"). Although the effects of the maternal environment on the development of offspring are complex and involve factors such as maternal nutrition and health during gestation, birth weight of the fetus, sex of the fetus, quality of lactation by the dam, and environmental conditions, there is now solid evidence of epigenetic effects ("programming") in determining the growth and productivity of offspring in domestic species, and reviews are available.[1-4] It is now well understood that factors such as maternal nutrition can have long-lasting effects on an animal's health and productivity and that these effects can be transmitted to progeny separate from changes in the genotype (DNA composition).[2] This phenomenon, recognized in human medicine,[5] is well documented in pigs and cattle[6,7] and has risen to have considerable economic importance as part of the Australian Lifetime Wool project.[8-10] The concept is that early life (including in utero) environmental conditions cause epigenetic changes that can persist for the life of the individual and that can be transmitted to offspring.

Epigenetic changes involve methylation of cytosine in cytosine-guanine dinucleotides and alteration of histones in genetic material such that the accessibility of DNA for transcription is reduced or eliminated. The result is that methylated genes are silenced and not transcribed. Methylation of DNA and histones thereby affects the phenotype of the animal because the changes are transmitted during mitosis to daughter cells. Epigenetic effects can be cell and organ specific and can be transmitted to offspring.

An associated phenomenon important to animal breeding is the concept of imprinted genes. Genomic imprinting is a phenomenon in mammals in which the father and mother contribute different epigenetic patterns to the fetus. A limited number of monoallelic expressed genes exert their effect in a parent-of-origin-specific manner through specific genomic loci in the parents' germ cells. For these genes, expression is restricted to one of the two parentally inherited chromosomes. Imprinted chromosomes are silenced, allowing the other chromosome to be expressed, which is referred to as maternally expressed/paternally imprinted or paternally expressed/maternally imprinted.[1] Although the number of genes that can imprint is limited, many of these genes encode for proteins that regulate a wide variety of biological processes, including embryonic and neonatal growth, metabolism, and behavior.[1] Understanding of this process has followed observations on abnormalities in animals born as a result of assisted reproductive technologies (including in vitro fertilization and somatic-cell nuclear transfer cloning) that alter methylation of chromosomes in gametes.[1,11] (See "Disorders of Cloned Offspring," page 1870).

Fetal programming describes the lifelong effects of in utero exposure of the fetus to various conditions.[2] Experimental maternal undernutrition during gestation adversely affects intermediate energy metabolism in lambs tested at ~20 weeks of age, evident as lower insulin secretory capacity and greater tissue insulin sensistivity.[12] Some of the effects of in utero exposure to the fetus could have lifelong effects on attributes important for agricultural productivity. This has been demonstrated for sheep in the Lifetime Wool project, in which numerous studies have revealed the importance of providing optimal nutrition and body condition for ewes for both the ewes' productivity and the lifetime productivity of their lambs.[13,14] The body weight profile of Merino ewes determines the fleece weight and fiber diameter of their progeny, with an optimal weight profile of the ewe resulting in higher fleece weight and finer wool in the progeny.[8] It does not appear that nutrition of the ewe affects milk production by her daughter and, therefore, live weight at weaning of the ewe's daughter's progeny.[15]

There is interest in fetal programming and epigenetics for horses, but currently there are no practical implications, although these can be anticipated.[3,4]

Effects on both the dam and the fetus can occur from overfeeding or underfeeding of the dam,[9] and there can be effects from the influences of trace-element deficiencies or toxic substances. Severe **undernutrition** of the dam can affect fetal size and its thermogenic rate, with consequences as described earlier. Prepartum protein restriction has the greatest effect. Severe undernutrition of the dam can also lead to weak labor and increased rates of dystocia and can limit the development of the udder. Colostrogenesis may be impaired, with a greater risk of infectious disease in the neonate, and milk production may be significantly reduced or delayed, with a risk of starvation.

Most information is available for the effects of nutrition of the pregnant ewe on fetal growth rate, udder development, the availability of energy in the body reserves of fetuses at term, and the amount and energy content of colostrum. In sheep, maternal nutrition can have a significant influence on fetal growth rate and placental size.[16] The underfeeding of hill sheep in late pregnancy markedly reduces the term weight of the udder and the prenatal accumulation and subsequent rates of secretion of colostrum. A low plane of nutrition in late pregnancy results in a marked decrease in fetal body-lipid and brown-fat reserves, a marked reduction in the total production of colostrum, and a reduction in the protein concentration in colostrum during the first 18 hours after parturition. However, exposure of late pregnant ewes to cold by shearing increases lamb birth weight and lamb brown-fat reserves.

Inadequate nutrition can also result in in utero growth retardation. Growth retardation can be produced in fetal pigs, lambs, and calves by **maternal caloric undernutrition**. Nutritional restriction in ewes reduces the number of placental lactogen receptors that mediate amino acid transport in fetal liver and glycogen synthesis in fetal tissue, leading to depletion of fetal liver glycogen stores. This has been postulated as a possible cause of the fetal growth retardation that accompanies maternal caloric undernutrition. Runt pigs have a reduced metabolic rate and lower skeletal muscle respiratory enzyme activity. This deficiency persists after birth; runt pigs have a lower core temperature and a lessened ability to increase their metabolic rate and heat production in response to cold. Paradoxically, **overnourishing the adolescent ewe** will also result in placental growth restriction and in utero growth retardation. This effect is most evident in the second third of pregnancy. This syndrome is accompanied by the birth of lambs with a shorter gestational age, commonly reduced by 3 days. It is thought that the fetal hypoxia and hypoglycemia that accompany placental insufficiency might stimulate the maturation of the fetal hypothalamic–pituitary–adrenal axis, initiating early parturition.

Maximum lamb survival is achieved at intermediate lamb birth weights, and the **nutritional management** of the pregnant ewe in fecund flocks is very important. Ewes with multiple lambs can be selected using ultrasound and fed separately from those with singles. Pregnant maiden ewes should also be fed to their separate requirements. The recommendation is for a body-condition score of 3.0 to 3.5 at mating, with a fall of 0.5 in score during the second and third months of pregnancy and a subsequent rise in score to 3.55 to the point of lambing, and with a distinct weight gain in late pregnancy. Equivalent condition scores are also appropriate for other species.

Toxic substances and trace-element deficiencies can result in increased risk for fetal and neonatal mortality and are discussed under those headings. Of particular significance is the agalactia, prolonged gestation, and fetal distress at birth seen in mares fed grain contaminated with ergot (*Claviceps purpurea*) and in mares grazing tall fescue (*Festuca arundinacea*) containing the endophyte fungus *Acremonium coenophialum*.

FURTHER READING

Kenyon PR, Blair HT. Foetal programming in sheep—effects on production. *Small Rumin Res.* 2014;118:16-30.

O'Doherty AM, et al. Genomic imprinting effects on complex traits in domesticated animal species. *Front Genet.* 2015;6:156.

REFERENCES

1. O'Doherty AM, et al. *Front Genet.* 2015;6:156.
2. Kenyon PR, et al. *Small Rumin Res.* 2014;118:16.
3. Fowden AL, et al. *J Equine Vet Sci.* 2013;33:295.
4. Dindot SV, et al. *J Equine Vet Sci.* 2013;33:288.
5. Heijmans BT, et al. *Proc Natl Acad Sci USA.* 2008;105:17046.
6. Altmann S, et al. *J Nutr Biochem.* 2013;24:484.
7. Micke GC, et al. *Reproduction.* 2011;141:697.
8. Thompson AN, et al. *Anim Prod Sci.* 2011;51:794.
9. Oldham CM, et al. *Anim Prod Sci.* 2011;51:776.
10. Lifetime Wool project—more lambs, better wool, healthy ewes. Department of Agriculture and Food Western Australia. (Accessed 06.15, at <http://www.lifetimewool.com.au/>).
11. Tian X. *Annu Rev Anim Biosci.* 2014;2:23.
12. Husted SM, et al. *Am J Physiol.* 2007;293:E548.
13. Ferguson MB, et al. *Anim Prod Sci.* 2011;51:763.
14. Behrendt R, et al. *Anim Prod Sci.* 2011;51:805.
15. Kenyon PR, et al. *Anim Prod Sci.* 2014;54:1465.
16. Gardner DS, et al. *Reproduction.* 2007;133:297.

POOR MOTHER–YOUNG RELATIONSHIP

Any examination of neonatal mortality suspected of being caused by hypothermia, starvation, or infection as a result of failure of transfer of passive immunity, and even trauma by crushing in piglets, must take into account the possibility that poor mothering and a poor mother–young bond could be the primary cause. Inadequate maternal care leads to rapid death of the newborn under extensive conditions where there is no human intervention to correct the problem.[1] The defect is most likely to be on the side of the dam, but it may originate with the offspring, especially in those that are hypothermic.[2] A poor relationship may be genetic or nutritional, and, on the part of the offspring, it may be the result of birth trauma.

For both the dam and the young, there is a much greater chance of establishing a good bond if the animal has been reared in a group rather than as an individual. Because sight, smell, taste, and hearing are all important in the establishment of seeking and posturing to suckle activity by the dam and seeking, nuzzling, and sucking activity by the offspring, any husbandry factor that interferes with the use of these senses predisposes to mortality. Weakness of the offspring as a result of poor nutrition of the dam, harassment at parturition by overzealous attendants, and high growth of pasture are obvious examples. Poor mother–young relationship can be a problem in cattle, pigs, and sheep, and occasionally in horses, especially with extensive foaling practices. In pigs a poor mother–young relationship may be developed to an intense degree in the form of farrowing hysteria, which is dealt with under that heading. In sheep a poor mother–young relationship can be a significant contributor to neonatal death from starvation, especially

Table 19-1 Scoring system for assessing vigorousness of newborn lambs[2]

Score	Description
1	Does not stand for at least 40 min; little or no teat-seeking drive; does not appear alert or active
2	Attempts to stand after 30 min; low teat-seeking drive and tendency to follow ewe; shows some alertness but not very active; does not appear coordinated in attempts
3	Shakes head within 30 s; attempts to stand within 15 min; seeking teat within 10 min of standing; follows ewe but distracted by other moving objects; generally alert and active; coordination may be lacking
4	Attempts to stand within 10 min of birth; seeking teat within 5 min of standing; strong tendency to follow ewe; alert and active and well-coordinated movements
5	Attempts to stand within 5 min of birth; follows ewe closely; very alert and active

Table 19-2 Definitions for lamb behaviors[2]

Behavior	Definition
Shakes head	Lamb raises and shakes head
To knees	Lamb rolls onto chest, gathers legs under it, and pushes front half of the body up off the ground
Attempts to stand	Lamb supports bodyweight on at least one foot
Stands	Lamb stands unsupported on all four feet for > 5 s
Reaches udder	Lamb approaches ewe and nudges her in the udder region
Unsuccessful suck	Lamb places head under ewe in contact with the udder, but either fails to grasp the teat or releases it without sucking
Sucks	Lamb hold teat in its mouth and appears to be sucking with appropriate mouth and head movements, may be tail-wagging, remains in this position for > 5 s

in highly strung breeds such as the Merino, which have a higher mismothering rate than do Romney ewes.[2,3]

Bonding occurs rapidly after birth, although there is some minor variation between species, with bonding starting within a few minutes of birth in sheep but taking up to 2 to 3 hours in some horses, for example. The strength of bonding also appears to vary between species. The bonding of the dam to the neonate is usually quite specific, although this can be modulated by management systems, and the neonate may be less selective and will often attempt to suck other dams. With sheep lambed under intensive lambing practices, this can lead to high rates of mismothering and subsequent abandonment, when preparturient "robber" ewes adopt lambs from multiple births. A high degree of shepherding is required to minimize loss in these management systems, whereas in extensive systems a strong bonding is established if the ewe and lamb are allowed to remain relatively undisturbed on the lambing site for 6 hours. A scoring system is available to allow objective assessment of the vigor of newborn lambs (Tables 19-1 and 19-2).

There is evidence of genetic and parental (sire) effects on the ability of lambs to follow the dam and to avoid mismothering. These effects appear to be modest.[2,4,5]

Vaginal cervical stimulation and the central release of oxytocin are thought to be important in initiating maternal behavior, although caudal epidural anesthesia for delivery does not effect mothering or bonding. Sucking is also a major determinant. Recognition is olfactory and auditory and mediated by the release of neurotransmitters.

Bonding is often slower with primiparous dams and is also delayed where there is postpartum pain. A failure of bonding leads to rejection and abandonment of the neonate.

Maternal care is also important to neonatal survival, and there is significant difference in litter mortality from crushing and injury among sows related to sow behavior and their response to piglet distress calls. A description of normal and abnormal behavioral patterns of the mare and foal is available, and techniques for fostering have been described.

REFERENCES

1. Bickell SL, et al. *Anim Prod Sci.* 2010;50:675.
2. Hergenhan RL, et al. *Anim Prod Sci.* 2014;54:745.
3. Plush KJ, et al. *Appl Anim Behav Sci.* 2011;134:130.
4. Brien FD, et al. *Anim Prod Sci.* 2014;54:667.
5. Hinch GN, et al. *Anim Prod Sci.* 2014;54:656.

TEETH CLIPPING OF PIGLETS

It is necessary to shorten the needle teeth of the upper and lower jaw of the newborn pig using a clean pair of sharp nail clippers or a grinding wheel. It is essential to practice good hygiene or infection of tooth roots can occur, leading to local inflammation and infection with the possibility of abscessation associated with *Fusobacterium* and *Trueperella.* It is not done before 6 hours of age because it will interfere with the absorption of colostrum. It is done to prevent damage to the sow's teats or to other piglets before 7 days after birth. Damage to the sow's teats will cause pain and reluctance to allow suckling. Damage to other piglets may interfere with the establishment of the "pecking order" in the litter.

Failure of Transfer of Passive Immunity (Failure of Transfer of Colostral Immunoglobulin)

The acquisition and absorption of adequate amounts of colostral immunoglobulins is essential to the health of ruminant, porcine, and equine neonates because they are born virtually devoid of circulating immunoglobulin. **Failure of passive transfer** (FPT) has been a commonly used term to describe the transfer of passive immunity (immunoglobulins, specifically IgG1 in colostrum) from the dam to the neonate. The process by which colostral immunoglobulin is absorbed is far from passive; it is an active and focused activity. Accordingly, FPT provides an incorrect summary of this process, and **failure of transfer of passive immunity** (**FTPI**) provides a more accurate descriptive term. Adequate antibody transfer is the cornerstone of all neonatal preventive health programs, but FTPI remains an important problem particularly affecting the dairy industry. Educational campaigns targeting dairy producers have been launched in the past decades, and, encouragingly, the prevalence of FTPI in dairy heifers in the United States decreased from over 40% in 1992 to 19% in 2007.[1]

Much of the description that follows refers to the calf because more studies on transfer of passive immunity have been conducted in calves. However, most of the information is applicable to the other species; where there are differences, these are mentioned.

NORMAL TRANSFER OF IMMUNOGLOBULINS

Immunoglobulins in colostrum are present in different concentrations. The major immunoglobulin in colostrum is IgG. IgG consists of two fractions, IgG_1 and IgG_2, which contribute 80% and 5% to 10%, respectively, to the total colostral immunoglobulin concentration. IgM and IgA each account for approximately 5% of the colostral immunoglobulin content. IgG is concentrated in colostrum by an **active, selective, receptor-mediated transfer** from the blood of the dam across the mammary secretory epithelium. This transfer to colostrum begins approximately 4 to 6 weeks before parturition and results in colostral IgG concentrations in first milking colostrum that are several-fold higher than maternal serum concentrations. This active IgG transfer ceases suddenly at the onset of lactation, presumably in response to increased prolactin secretion around parturition.[2] IgA and IgM are largely derived from local synthesis by the mammary gland rather transfer from plasma.

Following ingestion by the newborn, a significant proportion of these immunoglobulins is transferred across the epithelial cells of the small intestine during the first few hours of life and transported via the lymphatic system to the blood. Immunoglobulins in blood are further varyingly distributed to extravascular fluids and to body secretions depending on the immunoglobulin class.

These absorbed immunoglobulins protect against systemic invasion by microorganisms and septicemic disease during the neonatal period. Unabsorbed immunoglobulins and immunoglobulins resecreted into the gut play an important role in protection against intestinal disease for several weeks following birth. FTPI has unequivocally been associated with increased morbidity and mortality and reduced growth rates of neonates. Adequate immunoglobulin supply at birth is associated with higher first- and second-lactation milk production and decreased risk of culling during the first lactation.[5]

In foals, FTPI presents a significant risk for the development of illness during the first 3 months of life.

Lactogenic Immunity

The IgG concentration in milk falls rapidly following parturition in all species, and immunoglobulin concentrations in milk are low (Table 19-3). In the sow, the concentration of IgA falls only slightly during the same period, and it becomes a major immunoglobulin of sows' milk. IgA is synthesized by the mammary gland of the sow throughout lactation and serves as an important defense mechanism against enteric disease in the nursing piglet. IgA in milk is an important mucosal defense mechanism in piglets, whereas in the calf there is little IgA in milk, but some enteric protection is provided by colostral and milk IgG and IgG derived from serum that is resecreted into the intestine.

FAILURE OF TRANSFER OF PASSIVE IMMUNITY

FTPI is the major determinant of septicemic disease in most species. It also modulates the occurrence of mortality and severity of enteric and respiratory disease in early life and performance at later ages.

In terms of the modulation of disease, there can be no set cut-point for circulating immunoglobulins because this cut-point will vary according to the farm, its environment, infection pressure, and the type of disease. Values are given as guidelines. **FTPI in calves** has been defined as a **serum IgG concentration below 1000 mg/dL (10 mg/mL)** when measured between 24 hours and 7 days of age. With **foals**, the equivalent IgG cutoff concentrations **for FTPI** and **partial FTPI are given as 400 mg/dL** and **800 mg/dL**, respectively. Although a serum IgG concentration above 400 mg/dL might be adequate for healthy foals kept in a clean environment with minimal pathogen exposure, a concentration above 800 mg/dL is considered optimal.[6] For **New World camelid crias,** a cut-point value for the serum IgG concentration **of 1000 mg/dL** measured at around 36 hours of life has been recommended.[7]

Rates of FTPI in dairy calves can vary widely between farms, but they were estimated to be in the range of 20% in a recent nationwide survey conducted in the United States.[1] In beef calves FTPI rates tend to be lower; a recent Canadian study reported the incidence of FTPI, defined as serum IgG concentrations below 800 mg/dL, of 6% and a rate of marginal transfer of passive immunity (800 mg/dL < IgG < 1600 mg/dL) of 10%.[8] Failure rates in foals reported in the literature are approximate 13% to 16%. Rates in lambs are also comparatively low, and the incidence of FTPI in crias has been estimated to be around 10%.[7]

In animals that are **fed colostrum artificially**, risk for FTPI is primarily dependent on the amount or mass of immunoglobulin present in a feeding of colostrum, the time after birth that this is fed, the efficiency of its absorption from the digestive tract, and possibly also the degree of bacterial contamination.[1] The mass of immunoglobulins fed is determined by the concentration of immunoglobulin in the colostrum and the volume that is fed. Feeding trials with calves suggest that a **mass of at least 150 g** of IgG is required in colostrum fed to a 45-kg calf to obtain adequate (≥1000 mg/dL IgG) colostral immunoglobulin concentrations in serum.

In animals that **suck colostrum naturally**, such as foals, risk for FTPI is primarily dependent on the concentration of immunoglobulin in the colostrum, the amount that is ingested, and the time of first suckling. Inadequate colostral immunoglobulin concentration and delay in ingestion of colostrum are the two important factors in FTPI in foals.

DETERMINANTS OF TRANSFER OF COLOSTRAL IMMUNOGLOBULINS

1. Amount of immunoglobulin in colostrum fed:
   a. *Volume* of colostrum fed
   b. *Concentration* of immunoglobulins in colostrum
2. Amount of colostrum actually suckled or fed
3. Rate of abomasal or gastric emptying after colostrum ingestion
4. Efficiency of absorption of immunoglobulins by neonate
5. Time after birth of suckling or feeding
6. Time of collection of colostrum after calving (with artificial colostrum feeding)
7. Degree of bacterial contamination of colostrum

Table 19-3 Failure of transfer of passive immunity;[1] concentrations and relative percentage of immunoglobulins in serum and mammary secretions of cattle and pigs

		CONCENTRATION (mg/ml)			TOTAL IMMUNOGLOBULIN (%)		
Animal	**Immunoglobulin**	**Serum**	**Colostrum**	**Milk**	**Serum**	**Colostrum**	**Milk**
Cow	IgG_1	11.0	75.0	0.59	50	81	73
	IgG_2	7.9	2.9	0.02	36	5	2.5
	IgM	2.6	4.9	0.05	12	7	6.5
	IgA	0.5	4.4	0.14	2	7	18
Sow	IgG	21.5	58.7	3.0	89	80	29
	IgM	1.1	3.2	0.3	4	6	1
	IgA	1.8	10.7	7.7	7	14	70

Determinants of Immunoglobulin Concentration in Colostrum

Nominal concentrations of immunoglobulin in the first milking colostrum of cows and sows are shown in Table 19-4.[1] Current conventional wisdom posits that **high-quality bovine colostrum** should contain **at least 50 g/L IgG,**[2] and that 3 L of high-quality colostrum should be fed as soon as possible after birth.[3,4] This strategy will provide the needed 150 g of colostral IgG. There can be substantial variation in the concentration of immunoglobulin in colostrum in all species, and the ingestion of a "normal" amount of colostrum that has low immunoglobulin concentration may provide an insufficient amount of immunoglobulin for protection. In a study of over 900 first-milkings colostrum from Holstein Friesian cows, only 29% of the colostrum samples contained a sufficiently high concentration of immunoglobulin to provide 100 g IgG in a 2-L volume. The equivalent percentages for 3- and 4-L volume feedings were 71% and 87%, respectively.

It is apparent that variation in colostral immunoglobulin concentration can be a cause of FTPI. Some causes of this variation are the following:

- The concentrations of immunoglobulin in colostrum fall dramatically after parturition. The concentrations in second-milking colostrum are approximately half those in the first milking, and by the fifth postcalving milking, concentrations approach those found during the remainder of lactation. A similar situation exists with **horses**. The mean concentrations of IgG in colostrum of mares 3 to 28 days before foaling is greater than 1000 mg IgG/dL, whereas at parturition the mean concentrations may vary from 4000 to 9000 mg/dL. The concentrations decrease markedly to 1000 mg/dL in 8 to 19 hours after parturition.
- The immunoglobulin concentration of colostrum decreases after calving even when the cow is not milked. It is important that this colostrum be **milked as soon as possible after parturition.** Colostrum that is collected 6 hours or later after calving has a significantly lower concentration than that collected 2 hours after calving. In a study documenting the effect of time since parturition on colostral IgG concentration, it was observed that colostral IgG concentration decreased by 3.7% during each subsequent hour after calving because of postparturient secretion of IgG-poor milk by the mammary glands.
- Colostrum from cows or mares that have been **premilked** to reduce udder edema or from dams that **leaked colostrum** before parturition have low immunoglobulin concentrations, and alternate colostrum should be fed for immunoglobulin transfer.
- In cattle, **dry periods** of less than 30 days may result in colostrum of lower immunoglobulin concentration.
- **Premature foaling** or the **induction of premature parturition** using long-acting corticosteroids in cattle can result in colostrum with low immunoglobulin concentration and/or low volume.
- In cattle, average colostral immunoglobulin concentrations are higher in cows in third or higher **lactation groups** compared with younger cows. However, colostrum from all lactation numbers can produce adequate immunoglobulin mass. There is no scientific basis for not feeding first-milking colostrum from first-lactation cows.
- Larger-volume first-milking colostrum tends to have lower immunoglobulin concentrations than smaller-volume colostrum, presumably as a result of dilution.
- Immunoglobulin concentrations were found to be higher in the early temporal fractions of a single milking of first-milking colostrum. This might suggest that segregation of the first portion of the first-milking colostrum could provide colostrum with higher immunoglobulin concentration for feeding.
- There are **breed differences** in the concentration of immunoglobulins in first-milking colostrum. In **cattle**, beef breeds have higher concentrations. Many dairy breeds, including Holstein Friesian, produce colostrum of relatively low immunoglobulin concentration, and a significant proportion of calves that suckle cows of these breeds ingest an inadequate mass of immunoglobulin. Channel Island breeds have a greater concentration of immunoglobulin in colostrum that Holstein Friesians. **Breed differences** are also seen in **horses**, with Arabian mares having higher colostral immunoglobulin concentrations than Standardbreds, which in turn are higher than those of Thoroughbreds. Breed differences also occur in **sheep**, with higher concentrations in meat and wool breeds than dairy breeds.
- Heat **stress** to cattle in the latter part of pregnancy results in lower colostral immunoglobulin concentrations.
- Colostral volume but not colostral immunoglobulin concentration is reduced in mastitic quarters, and it is unlikely that mastitis is a major determinant of the high rate of FTPI in dairy calves. Colostrum from cows with clinical mastitis should nonetheless not be fed because it may contain pathogens in large amounts and has unphysiologic composition.
- The **pooling of colostrum** in theory could avoid the variation in immunoglobulin concentration of individually fed colostrum and could provide a colostrum that reflects the antigenic experience of several cattle. In practice, colostrum pools from Holsteins invariably have low immunoglobulin concentrations because high-volume, low-concentration colostrum dilutes the concentration of the other samples in the pool. If pools are used, the diluting influence of low-immunoglobulin-concentration, high-volume colostrum should be limited by restricting any individual cow's contribution to the pool to 9 kg (20 lb) or less. However, pooling increases the risk of disease transmission because multiple cows are represented in a pool and the pool is fed to multiple calves. This can be important in the control of Johne's disease, bovine leukosis, *Mycoplasma bovis*, *E. coli*, and *Salmonella* spp.
- **Bacterial contamination** of colostrum can have a negative effect on transfer of passive immunity. The current recommendation is that fresh colostrum should contain less than 100,000 cfu/mL total bacteria count and less than 10,000 cfu total coliform count.[2] One study found that 85% of colostrums sampled from 40 farms in the United States exceeded this threshold. Colostrum that is to be fed or stored should be collected with appropriate preparation and sanitation of the cow and of the milking equipment used on fresh cows.
- **Pasteurization of colostrum** either at 63°C (145°F) for 30 min or 72°C (162°F) for 15 s was shown to reduce colostrum IgG concentration by at least 30% and to thicken or congeal the colostrum. In contrast, **pasteurization at 60°C (140°F) for 60 min** was found to affect neither colostral IgG concentration nor fluid characteristics while eliminating or at least significantly decreasing the content of major pathogens, including *Mycobacterium avium subps. paratuberculosis, M. bovis, E. coli*, and *Salmonella* spp.
- **Old mares** (older than 15 years) may have poor colostral immunoglobulin concentration.

Volume of Colostrum Ingested

Dairy Cows

The volume of colostrum that is fed has a direct influence on the mass of immunoglobulin ingested at first feeding. The average volume of colostrum ingested by nursing Holstein Friesian calves in the first 24 hours of life is reported as 2.4 L, but there is wide variation around this mean. In **natural suckling** situations, calves may fail to ingest adequate colostrum volumes before onset of the closure process and therefore absorb insufficient colostral immunoglobulin. Early assisted suckling may help avoid this. In dairy calves the volume of colostrum that is ingested can be controlled in **artificial feeding systems** using nipple bottle feeders or esophageal tube feeders. **Bucket feeding** of colostrum is not recommended because training to feed from a bucket can be associated with erratic intakes.

The **traditional recommendation** for the volume of colostrum to feed at first feeding to calves is 2 L (2 quarts). However, only a small proportion of first-milking colostrum from Holsteins contains a sufficiently high concentration of immunoglobulin to provide 100 g IgG in a 2-L volume, and higher volumes of colostrum are required to achieve this mass intake. Some calves fed with a **nipple bottle** will drink volumes greater than 2 L, but others will refuse to ingest even 2 L of colostrum in a reasonable period of time, and calf rearers may lack the time or patience to persist with nipple bottle feeding until the required volume has been ingested by all calves.

Larger volumes of colostrum can be fed by an **esophageal feeder,** and single feedings of large volumes of colostrum (3.5 to 4.0 L per 45 kg of body weight) result in the lowest percentage of calves with FTPI by allowing calves fed colostrum with relatively low immunoglobulin concentrations to receive an adequate immunoglobulin mass before closure. Feeding this volume by an esophageal feeder causes no apparent discomfort to a minimally restrained calf and was not found to negatively affect intestinal IgG absorption compared with voluntary intake of the same (large) volume.[10] There is nonetheless some debate around the recommendation to systematically tube feed neonatal calves because of animal welfare concerns. In several European countries animal welfare legislation prohibits force-feeding of animals without medical indication.[20]

Beef Cows

With beef breeds very effective colostral immunoglobulin transfer is achieved with natural sucking. This is thought to be a result of the greater vigor at birth exhibited by these calves and the higher immunoglobulin concentrations in beef colostrum, requiring a smaller volume intake to acquire an adequate mass. **Natural sucking** will give an adequate volume intake, and there is no need to artificially feed colostrum unless the dam is observed to refuse nursing or the calf's viability and sucking drive are compromised. The **yield of colostrum** and colostral immunoglobulins in beef cows can vary widely, and range beef heifers may produce critically low volumes of colostrum. Differences in yield can be attributed to breed or to nutritional status, although undernutrition is not an effect unless it is very severe.

Ewes

Colostrum yield is high in ewes in good condition at lambing, but it may be low in ewes with condition scores of 1.5 to 2.0.

Sows

In sows there is also very effective colostral immunoglobulin transfer with natural sucking, and piglets average an intake of 5% to 7% of body weight in the first hour of life. There is between-sow variation in the amount of colostrum, and there can be a large variation in colostrum supply from teat to teat, which may explain variable health and performance. During farrowing and for a short period following, colostrum is available freely from the udder, but thereafter it is released in ejections during mass suckling. A strong coordinated sucking stimulus is required by the piglet for maximum release of colostrum, and this requires that the ambient temperature and other environmental factors be conducive to the optimum vigor of the piglets. Small-birth-weight piglets, **late-birth-order** piglets, and piglets sucking posterior teats obtain less colostrum.

All Species

In all species a low-volume intake may also occur because of the following factors:

- Poor **mothering behavior,** which may prevent the newborn from sucking; occurrence of disease; or milk fever
- Poor **udder and/or teat conformation** so that the newborn cannot suck normally or teat seeking is more prolonged. Udder-to-floor distance is most critical, and low-slung udders can account for significant delays in intake. Bottle-shaped teats (35-mm diameter) also significantly reduce intake.
- Delayed and **inadequate colostral intake** frequently accompanies perinatal asphyxia or acidemia because of the greatly decreased vigor of the calf in the first few hours of life. Perinatal asphyxia can occur in any breed and is greatly increased by matings resulting in fetal–maternal disproportion and dystocia.
- The newborn may be weak, traumatized, or unable to suck for other reasons; a **weak sucking drive** can be a result of congenital iodine deficiency, cold stress, or other factors.
- Disease of the periparturient dam, such as clinical hypocalcemia in cattle or the mastitis metritis agalactia complex in sows, may preclude adequate colostrum intake by offspring.
- Failure to allow newborn animals to ingest colostrum may occur under some management systems.

Efficiency of Absorption

After ingestion of colostrum by the newborn, colostral immunoglobulins are absorbed from the small intestine, by a process of pinocytosis, into the columnar cells of the epithelium. In the newborn calf this is a very rapid process, and immunoglobulin can be detected in the thoracic duct lymph within 80 to 120 minutes of its being introduced into the duodenum. The **period of absorption** varies between species and with immunoglobulin class. The mechanism by which absorption ceases is not well understood, but it may be related to replacement of the fetal enterocyte. The region of maximum absorption is in the lower small intestine, and peak serum concentrations are reached by 12 to 24 hours in all species. Absorption is not limited to immunoglobulin, and **proteinuria** during the first 24 hours of life is associated with the renal excretion of low-molecular-weight proteins such as β-lactoglobulin.

Feeding Methods, "Closure of the Gut," and Immunoglobulin Absorption

Under normal conditions complete loss of the ability to absorb immunoglobulin (closure of the gut) occurs by 24 to 36 hours after birth in all species, and there is a significant reduction in absorptive ability (as much as 50% in some studies but minimal in others) by 8 to 12 hours following birth. The **time from birth to feeding** is a crucial factor affecting the absorption of colostral immunoglobulin in all species, and any delay beyond the first few hours of life, particularly after 8 hours, significantly reduces the amount of immunoglobulin absorbed.

The recommendation is that all neonates should be fed colostrum within the first 2 hours of life.

Natural Sucking

Natural sucking is the desired method of intake of colostrum and is the most efficient, but it is influenced by the sucking drive and **vigor** of the neonate at birth. Newborns that suck colostrum can achieve very high concentrations of colostral immunoglobulin, and the efficiency of absorption is best with this feeding method. However, in dairy calves natural sucking is commonly associated with a high rate of FTPI because of **delays in sucking** coupled with low intake. Rates of FTPI in calves allowed to obtain colostrum via voluntary nursing reported in the literature can be as high as 40% to 60%.[1] Many factors influence the occurrence of delayed sucking, but calf vigor and birth-related asphyxia are the most important. Parity of the dam, conformation of the udder, and breed were also found to be significantly associated with the rate of FTPI. One older study reported that 46% of all calves born to multiparous cows had failed to nurse within 6 hours of birth compared with 11% of calves of primiparous cows.[11] Jersey calves have better rates of successful transfer of passive immunity with natural sucking than do Holsteins Friesians.

Artificial Feeding

In contrast, when calves are **fed colostrum artificially**, minimal delays from birth to the time of colostrum feeding occur, and maximal colostrum immunoglobulin absorption results. In breeds such as Holstein Friesians, where colostral immunoglobulin concentrations tend to be low and maximal efficiency of absorption is necessary, the logical way to minimize risk of FTPI is to feed the maximum volume of colostrum that is well tolerated within the first few hours of life. The published literature consistently reports higher calf serum IgG concentrations and a lower rate of FTPI in response to larger colostrum feeding volumes.[2,10,12]

Other Influences

Even with the best available on-farm colostrum-selection methods, **large colostrum-feeding volumes are essential** to minimize the risk of FTPI in breeds with relatively low colostral immunoglobulin concentrations. The method is particularly advantageous where time constraints of other farm activities limit the time available for calf feeding. The major detrimental influence on absorptive efficiency of immunoglobulin is **delayed feeding after birth**. Other factors that may affect absorptive efficiency include the following:

- **Perinatal asphyxia or acidemia** may have both direct and indirect effects on colostral immunoglobulin transfer. Asphyxia has a major effect on subsequent sucking drive, and acidemic calves ingest far less colostrum than calves with more normal acid–base status at birth. In carefully controlled colostrum feeding studies, a significant negative correlation between the degree of hypercapnia and the efficiency of absorption of colostral immunoglobulin in the first hours of life was demonstrated. However, this effect was only transient because there was no difference in serum IgG concentration at the time of gut closure between normoxic and hypoxic calves.
- In one early study, a **mothering effect** was reported in which calves remaining with their dams absorbed colostral immunoglobulin more efficiently than calves removed immediately to individual pens. However, other studies have shown much smaller or no effects of mothering using similar experimental designs. The different results of these studies have not been reconciled.
- There can be **seasonal** and **geographic** variations in transfer of immunoglobulin in calves, although these are not always present on farms in the same area, and their cause is unknown. Where seasonal variation occurs in temperate climates, the mean monthly serum IgG concentrations are lowest in the winter and increase during the spring and early summer to reach their peak in September, after which they decrease. The cause is not known, but a decrease in sucking drive is observed in colder months and may contribute. In subtropical climates, peak levels occur in the winter months, and low levels are associated with elevated temperatures during the summer months. **Heat stress** in late pregnancy will reduce colostral immunoglobulin concentration, but high ambient temperature is a strong depressant of absorption, and the provision of shade will help to obviate the problem.
- The efficiency of absorption may be decreased in **premature calves** that are born following induced parturition using long-acting corticosteroids; in contrast, medical **induction of parturition** with short-acting corticosteroids in cattle does not interfere with the efficiency of absorption of immunoglobulins in calves.
- The absorption of small volumes (1 to 2 L) fed by an esophageal feeder is usually suboptimal and inferior to the absorption after sucking the same small volume.[10] This effect may at least in part be attributable to retention of some colostrum in the immature forestomaches for several hours. The calf will feel satiated and not inclined to suck naturally for the next few hours.
- A **trypsin inhibitor** in colostrum may serve to protect colostral IgG from intestinal degradation. It varies in concentration between colostrums. The addition of a trypsin inhibitor to colostrum improves immunoglobulin absorption.
- In a study of **mare-associated determinants of FTPI** in foals (based on serum Ig measurements), there was a trend to increase rates of FTPI in foals from mares aged over 12 years, but no significant association with age, parity, or gestational age of foals over 325 days was found. There was an association with season, with a lower incidence in the late spring compared with foals born earlier in the year and with a foal score based on a veterinary score of foal health and "fitness."

Traditionally it has been considered that the **movement** of animals, either the dam just **before parturition** or the newborn animal during the first few days of life, is a special hazard for the health of the calf. The postulated reason is that the dam may not have been exposed to pathogens present in the new environment and thus not have circulating antibodies against these pathogens. The newborn animal may be in the same position with regard to both deficiency of antibodies and exposure to new infections. Although this may be the case in some situations, the developing practice of contract-rearing of dairy heifers away from the farm to be brought back as close-up springers and the practice of purchase of close-up heifers on the farm are not associated with appreciable increase in mortality in their calves.

Decline of Passive Immunity

Colostral antibody concentrations in blood fall quickly after birth and have usually disappeared by 6 months of age. In the **foal**, they have fallen to less than 50% of peak level by 1 month of age and to a minimum level between 30 and 60 days. This is the point at which naturally immunodeficient foals are highly susceptible to fatal infection.

In **calves**, the level of IgG declines slowly and reaches minimum values by 60 days, in contrast to IgM and IgA, which decline more rapidly and reach minimum values by approximately 21 days of age. The half-lives for IgG, IgM, and IgA in calves are approximately 20, 4, and 2 days, respectively, and the half-lives of IgGa, IgGb, IgG(T), and IgA in foals are approximately 18, 32, 21, and 3.5 days, respectively.

Immunologic competence is present at birth, but endogenous antibody production does not usually reach protective levels until 1 month, and maximum levels are not reached until 2 to 3 months of age. The endogenous production of intestinal IgA in the piglet begins at about 2 weeks of age and does not reach significant levels until 5 weeks of age.

Foals that acquire low concentrations of immunoglobulins from colostrum may experience a transitory hypogammaglobulinemia at several weeks of age as the levels fall and before autogenous antibodies develop. They are, as expected, more subject to infection than normal.

OTHER BENEFITS OF COLOSTRUM

In addition to its immunoglobulin content, colostrum contains considerably more protein, fat, vitamins, and minerals than milk and is especially important in the transfer of fat-soluble vitamins. It has **anabolic effects,** and lambs that ingest colostrum have a higher summit metabolism than colostrum-deprived lambs. Colostrum also contains growth-promoting factors that stimulate DNA synthesis and cell division, including high concentrations of insulin-like growth factor (IGF)-1.

Colostrum contains approximately 1×10^6 leukocytes/mL, and several hundred million are ingested with the first feeding of colostrum. In calves, 20% to 30% of these are lymphocytes and cross the intestine into the circulation of the calf. It is postulated that they have importance in the development of neonatal resistance to disease, but there is little tangible evidence. Calves fed colostrum depleted of leukocytes are thought to be more poorly protected against neonatal disease than those fed normal colostrum.

ASSESSMENT OF TRANSFER OF PASSIVE IMMUNITY

Because of the importance of transfer of colostral antibodies to the health of the neonate, it is common to quantitatively estimate the levels of immunoglobulins, or their surrogates, in colostrum and in serum to predict risk of disease and to take preventive measures in the individual or to make corrective management changes where groups of animals are at risk.

Assessment in the Individual Animal

When samples are taken from an individual animal to determine the risk for infection, sampling is undertaken early so that replacement therapy can be given promptly if there has been inadequate transfer. IgG is detectable in serum 2 hours following a colostrum feeding and **sampling at 8 to 12 hours** after birth will give a good indication of whether early sucking has occurred and has been effective in transfer. This type of monitoring is commonly performed in foals and camelid crias.[7,13] There are a number of different tests that can be used; some are quantitative and others semiquantitative. In calves, sampling may be undertaken for similar reasons, but the cost of replacement therapy is limiting.

Assessment Tests on Serum

Sampling to **monitor** the efficacy of a farm policy for feeding and handling colostrum, to evaluate the passive immunity status in **calves to be purchased,** or to determine the **rates of FTPI** in investigations of neonatal disease can be conducted at any time in the first week of life after 24 hours with most tests. Numerous tests are currently available, some of which directly measure serum IgG concentration and some of which estimate the IgG concentration based on the serum concentration of the total globulin or other protein fractions.

Radial Immunodiffusion

The radial immunodiffusion (RID) is based on the precipitation of antigen and antibody to an insoluble precipitin complex and thus directly measures IgG concentration in serum or plasma. The RID is considered the reference method to measure serum/plasma IgG, but it takes at least 24 h to perform and thus longer than is desirable for most clinical purposes. In a recent study two commercial RID test kits for calves were compared, and a large bias and wide limits of agreements between the two tests were found, which has raised questions about the reliability of the results.[21]

Lateral-Flow Immunoassay

The lateral-flow immunoassay is a calf-side test directly measuring IgG in serum or plasma with reportedly high sensitivity and specificity. Although the test can be performed on-site and results are available within 20 min, it only provides a pass/fail result using a cutoff value of 10 mg/mL.[2]

Turbidimetric Immunoassay

The turbidimetric immunoassay (TIM) is commercially available and can be run on a handheld chemistry analyzer to be used with bovine serum. In a preliminary study conducted at the University of Minnesota, the test was found to be more accurate than indirect tests such as serum refractometry.

Zinc Sulfate Turbidity Test

The zinc sulfate turbidity test is based on a selective precipitation reaction of the salt with high molecular weight proteins such as immunoglobulin (not specifically IgG). The test is commonly used with a test solution containing 200 mg/L zinc sulfate but was found to have poor specificity and would only classify 69% of tested calves correctly. Increasing the zinc sulfate concentration from 200 to 350 mg/L considerably improved the specificity and positive predictive values of the test, but this test modification is not widely used.[15] Another inconvenience is that hemolyzed blood samples will give artificially high readings, and the reagent must be kept free of dissolved carbon dioxide.

Sodium Sulfite Precipitation Test

The sodium sulfite precipitation test is based on the selective precipitation of high-molecular-weight proteins with sodium sulfate at different concentrations. Test solutions of 14%, 16%, and 18% sodium sulfite are commonly used, and the development of turbidity at a certain concentration allows for a crude estimate of the serum immunoglobulin concentration; the lower the concentration at which turbidity occurs, the higher is the concentration of immunoglobulin. Particularly the use of the 14% and 16% sodium sulfite solutions was found to result in an unacceptably high percentage of calves being misclassified as FTPI while having adequate serum immunoglobulin concentrations.[15]

Serum γ-Glutamyltransferase Activity

Serum γ-glutamyltransferase (GGT) activity has been used as a surrogate for determining the efficacy of transfer of passive immunity in calves and lambs (not in foals). GGT activity is high in the colostrum of ruminants (but not horses), and serum GGT activity in calves and lambs that have sucked or been fed colostrum is 60 to 160 times greater than normal adult serum activity and correlates moderately well with serum IgG concentrations. The half-life of GGT from colostrum is short, and serum GGT activity falls significantly in the first week of life. Serum GGT values equivalent to a serum IgG concentration of 10 mg/mL are 200 IU/L on day 1 of life and 100 IU/L on day 4. Serum GGT concentrations less than 50 IU/L indicate FTPI.

Serum Total Protein

Measuring total protein concentrations in serum or plasma with a refractometer is a practical, rapid, and inexpensive method to estimate the immunoglobulin concentration by extrapolating it from the total protein concentration. Despite the indirect nature of the test, there is a reliable correlation between the refractometer reading and total immunoglobulin concentration measured by RID. In healthy calves a serum total protein of 5.5 g/dL or greater is associated with adequate transfer of passive immunity.

Serum total protein has a good predictive value for fate of the newborn, and the facile and practical nature of the test and its predictive ability commend it for survey studies in calves and lambs but not foals. Cut-points will vary with the environment and the infection pressure to the calves. The sensitivity of the test is maximal using a cut-point of 5.5 g/dL, and the specificity is maximal at a cut-point of 5.0 g/dL. Because serum total protein concentration measured by refractometry can result in an incidental misclassification of an individual calf, this test is primarily recommended as a screening tool to assess the colostrum management on a herd level, but not as diagnostic tool for an individual animal. Herd screening could be conducted by testing a minimum of 12 calves on a farm between 24 hours and 7 days old. At least 80% of tested calves should have serum protein concentrations above 5.5 g/dL to consider the colostrum management satisfactory at the herd level.

Serum total protein concentration can also be estimated using the same Brix refractometer used for measuring colostral IgG concentration, with an appropriate adjustment factor.[14]

Glutaraldehyde Coagulation Test

The glutaraldehyde test was initially introduced to identify hypergammaglobulinemia in adult cattle with chronic inflammatory disease. The semiquantitative test is based on a clotting reaction of glutaraldehyde in the presence of high immunoglobulin concentration, where the time to clot formation is negatively correlated with the serum IgG.[16] A modified glutaraldehyde coagulation test is also available for the detection of hypogammaglobulinemia in neonatal calves, but it is less accurate.[15] The test may yield false-positive results with hemolysis and is difficult to quantitate.

Latex Agglutination Test

A commercial latex agglutination test is available for horses. It is rapid and provides semiquantitative results, but results were reported to be inconsistent.

ELISA Snap-Test

ELISA snap-tests are foal-side immunologic tests directly measuring IgG in a semiquantitative manner. Test kits are commercially available for foals and have been available for calves. In foals the available snap-tests were found to be rapid and accurate.

Monitoring Colostrum

Brix Refractometry

The most accurate and practical way to ensure that an adequate colostral mass is fed is to test the colostrum using a Brix refractometer (the digital version is preferred). This instrument was designed for use in food processing but was adapted in the late 1970s to provide a low-cost test of colostrum quality. A Brix refractometer value of 21% or 22% or higher indicates acceptable colostrum (same value for fresh or frozen samples; approximately equivalent to a colostral IgG concentration of 50 g/L); colostrum with a value below 21% or 22% should be discarded.[17,18]

Specific Gravity

Specific gravity, determined by refractometry, can be used as a measure of the immunoglobulin content of colostrum. In **mares** the concentration of immunoglobulin in colostrum is highly correlated with the specific gravity of the colostrum, which in turn is highly correlated with the serum immunoglobulin levels achieved in foals. Temperature-corrected measurements are most accurate. Measurement of colostrum specific gravity provides a rapid and easy method of identifying foals likely to be at a high risk for FTPI and the need to provide them with colostrum of a higher Ig content. To prevent FTPI, it is recommended that the colostral specific gravity should be equal to or greater than 1.060, and the colostral IgG concentration should be a minimum of 3000 mg/dL.

In **cattle** the relation of specific gravity of colostrum to colostral immunoglobulin concentration is linear but is better in Holstein Friesian than in Jersey cows. The measurement is simple, but there is a correction for temperature, and air trapped in colostrum taken by a milking machine can give a false reading if the measurement is taken too quickly after milking. The cut-point recommended to distinguish moderate from excellent colostrum has been set at 1.050, approximating an IgG concentration of 50 g/L, and is based on the amount of immunoglobulin required for a 2-L (2-quart) feeding. Specific gravity is not a perfect surrogate for immunoglobulin concentration with cattle colostrum. It has good negative prediction, but it will falsely pass 2 out of 3 colostrums that have unacceptably low immunoglobulin concentrations. An analysis of first-milking colostrum in midwestern U.S. dairies found that specific gravity differed among breeds and was influenced by month of calving, year of calving, lactation number, and protein yield in previous lactation and that it was more closely associated with colostrum protein concentration ($r = 0.76$) than IgG_1 concentration ($r = 0.53$).

Glutaraldehyde Test

This test for mare colostrum is available commercially and is reported to have a high predictive value for colostrums that contain more than 38 mg/mL of IgG and have a specific gravity greater than 1.060.

ELISA

Recently a cow-side immunoassay kit has become available commercially in the United States. The kit provides a positive or a negative response, with the cut-point being a concentration of 50g/L of IgG in colostrum, and has accuracy sufficient to recommend its use for rejection of colostrums with low immunoglobulin concentration.

CORRECTION OF FAILURE OF TRANSFER OF PASSIVE IMMUNITY

Oral Therapy

Oral therapy can be considered in individual animals (generally foals and crias), provided that FTPI—or the risk thereof—is diagnosed and the treatment is administered before gut closure (i.e., not later than 18 h of life). For foals, oral administration of at least 0.5 L frozen equine colostrum of good quality (specific gravity > 1.060) that has been properly stored and thawed is recommended. Alternatives include colostrum substitutes containing lyophilized IgG or good-quality bovine colostrum. The latter option is probably the least effective and requires at least 4 L of good-quality (specific gravity >1.050) colostrum.

Parenteral Immunoglobulins

Blood transfusion is commonly used in food animal practice, and the method is described elsewhere in this text. Fresh plasma from a random donor or purified hyperimmune plasma that is commercially available for foals and crias in some countries are alternatives. Large amounts are required to obtain the required high serum concentrations of immunoglobulins, and intravenous infusion can be accompanied by transfusion-type reactions.

AVOIDANCE OF FAILURE OF TRANSFER OF PASSIVE IMMUNITY

With all species, with the exception of dairy calves, the common practice is to allow the newborn to suck naturally. The policy for avoidance of FTPI with naturally sucking herds should be to provide supplemental colostrum by artificial feeding of those neonates with a high risk for FTPI, based on the risk factors detailed earlier. In the dairy calf, rates of FTPI with natural sucking are so high that many farms opt to remove the calf at birth and feed colostrum by hand to ensure adequate intake.

Colostrum

Colostrum can be stripped from the dam and fed fresh, or the neonate can be fed stored (banked) colostrum.

Colostrum for Banking

With **dairy cows**, first-milking colostrum from a cow with a first-milking yield of less than 10 kg should be used. The temptation for the farmer is to store the leftover from the feeding of large-volume colostrum. The leftover colostrum should not be used because it has a high probability of containing a low immunoglobulin concentration.

Colostrum from **mares** should have a specific gravity of 1.060 or more, and 200 mL can be milked from a mare before the foal begins sucking.

Storage of Colostrum

Colostrum can be kept at **refrigerator temperature** for approximately 1 week without significant deterioration in immunoglobulins; bacteria counts, however, may reach unacceptably high levels (above 100,000 cfu/mL) after 2 days in refrigerated milk.[2] Addition of potassium sorbate in a 0.5% final solution impairs bacterial growth for several days.[2] The addition of 5 g of propionic or lactic acid per liter extends the storage life to 6 weeks, but, more commonly, colostrum is frozen for storage. **Frozen colostrum**, at −20°C (−4°F), can be stored for at least 1 year, and there is no impairment in the subsequent absorption of immunoglobulins. Frozen colostrum should be stored in flat plastic bags in the amount required for a feeding, which facilitates thawing. **Thawing** should be at temperatures below 55°C (131°F). Higher temperatures and microwave thawing result in the deterioration of immunoglobulins and antibodies in frozen colostrum and frozen plasma.

Pasteurization of Colostrum

There are several indications for pasteurization of colostrum. This procedure can be a suitable instrument in a program for the control of specific infectious diseases, such as paratuberculosis, salmonellosis, or *M. bovis* infection, but it can also be useful to ameliorate calf health by improving colostrum quality and reducing the exposure of the neonate to pathogens. On-farm pasteurization of bovine colostrum for 60 min at 60°C (140°F) results in elimination or at least significant reduction of bacterial contamination without impairing fluid characteristics or availability of IgG for intestinal absorption.[9] One recent study reported significantly higher serum IgG concentrations at 24 h of life when calves were fed pasteurized colostrum compared with calves receiving the same quality and amount of raw colostrum.[19] The authors attributed this effect to reduced bacterial interference with intestinal IgG absorption. Pasteurization extends the shelf life of refrigerated colostrum without additives to 8 to 10 days when stored in clean, sealed containers.

Cross-Species Colostrum

Colostrum from another species can be used to provide immunologic protection when same-species colostrum is not available. Bovine colostrum can be fed to a number of different species. Although absorption of immunoglobulin occurs and significant protection can be achieved, the use of cross-species colostrum is not without risk, and the absorbed immunoglobulin has a short half-life. Bovine colostrum has been successfully used for many years to improve the survival rate of hysterectomy-produced artificially reared pigs. It has also been used as an alternate source of colostral antibody for rearing goats free of caprine arthritis–encephalitis (CAE). Colostrum from some cows can result in the development of hemolytic anemia, occurring at around 5 to 12 days of age, in lambs and kids because the IgG of some cows attaches to the red cells and their precursors in bone marrow, resulting in red cell destruction by the reticuloendothelial system. Bovine colostrum can be tested for "antisheep" factors by a gel precipitation test on colostral whey, but this test is not generally available. Bovine colostrum can provide some protection to newborn foals against neonatal infections, and protection appears to result from factors in addition to the immunoglobulins, which have a short half-life in foals.

Colostrum Supplements

In recent years there has been a move to develop supplements or even replacements for colostrum to feed calves. These have been attempted using IgG concentrated from bovine colostrum, milk whey, eggs, or bovine serum. The search for colostrum substitutes or colostrum replacers has been prompted by the problem of the variability of IgG concentration in natural colostrum. It has also been prompted by possible limitations of availability of high-quality colostrum on dairy farms as a result of discarding colostrum from cows that test positive for diseases that can transmit through colostrum, such as paratuberculosis, bovine leukosis, and *M. bovis.*

There is evidence that the inclusion of **colostrum replacer (CR)** or **colostrum supplement (CS)** products can impair the efficiency of colostral immunoglobulin, and if they are fed, they should be fed after normal colostrum rather than mixed into the colostrum. It has been proposed that the distinction between a colostrum supplement and a colostrum replacer should be the immunoglobulin mass contained in the product, with a colostrum supplement containing less than 100 g IgG per dose and a colostrum replacer having sufficient immunoglobulin mass in a dose to result in a serum IgG concentration greater than 10 mg/mL following a feeding. Furthermore, CR products are formulated to provide adequate protein, energy, minerals, and vitamins to completely replace colostrum, which is not the case for CS supplement products. When fed as the sole source of immunoglobulin to colostrum-deprived calves, CS products achieve circulating concentrations of immunoglobulin that are lower than those achieved by natural colostrum containing equivalent amounts of immunoglobulin.

A large mass of immunoglobulin is required for acquisition of adequate serum immunoglobulin concentrations. Calves fed a colostrum replacement containing a high mass (250 g) of an IgG derived from bovine serum and fed at 1.5 and again at 13.5 hours after birth achieved equivalent serum IgG concentrations to calves fed normal colostrum and showed no difference in gain or health parameters during the first 4 weeks of life. However, the performance of commercially available products for IgG supplementation varies greatly, with many of them faring badly. The choice of a specific product should therefore be based on the availability of convincing data supporting the efficacy of the product in question.

The use of colostrum replacers should be limited to situations where sufficient amounts of colostrum of adequate quality are unavailable. There can be little justification for more widespread use, particularly because there are limited independent health-related publications documenting their efficacy. Also, as mentioned earlier, in addition to immunoglobulin, natural colostrum contains various substances important to neonatal physiology.

Lacteal-Secretion-Based Preparations

Colostrum supplements prepared from whey or colostrum are available commercially in many countries. Depending on the manufacturer, they contain varying amounts of immunoglobulin, but significantly less than first-milking colostrum. The amount of immunoglobulin contained varies, but the recommendations for feeding that accompany these products indicate that they will supply approximately 25% or less of the immunoglobulin required to elevate calf serum IgG concentrations above 1000 mg/dL. There is a further problem in that the immunoglobulins in products made from colostrum or whey are poorly absorbed, and trials assessing their ability to increase circulating immunoglobulins when fed with colostrum have generally shown little improvement and no improvement in health-related parameters.

Bovine-Serum-Based Preparations

Colostrum supplements prepared from bovine serum are also available commercially, but regulations governing the feeding of blood or blood products to calves (risk reduction for bovine spongiform encephalopathy) may limit their availability in some countries. The absorption of immunoglobulin from these bovine-serum-derived commercial products appears better than from milk-protein-derived products, and consequently they are also marketed as colostrum replacers.

The IgG in a commercially available bovine serum colostrum replacer has been shown to be effectively absorbed when fed to newborn lambs. The feeding of 200 g of IgG in the first 24 hours of life resulted in a mean plasma concentration of 1800 mg/dL.

Administration of Colostrum

Foals

Foals should be allowed to suck naturally. The specific gravity of the mare's colostrum can be checked at foaling; if this is less than 1.060, supplemental colostrum may be indicated. Foals that do not suck, or that have serum IgG concentrations less than 400 mg/dL at 12 hours of age, or that require supplementation for other reasons, should be fed colostrum with a specific gravity of 1.060 or more at an amount of 200 mL at hourly feedings.

Dairy Calves

Assisted Natural Sucking

Leaving the newborn dairy calf with the cow is no guarantee that the calf will obtain sufficient colostrum, and a high proportion of dairy calves fail either to suck early or to absorb sufficient immunoglobulins from ingested colostrum. This problem can be alleviated to some extent by **assisted natural sucking,** but this can fail because not all calves requiring assistance are detected. An alternate approach is to milk 2 L of colostrum from the dam, bottle feed each calf as soon after birth as possible, then leave the calf with the cow for 24 hours and allow it to suck voluntarily. Although this will not be as effective as a system based entirely on artificial feeding of selected colostrum, it is an approach that is suitable for the smaller dairy farm.

Artificial Feeding Systems

With **artificial feeding systems**, the calf is removed from the dam at birth and fed colostrum by hand throughout the whole absorptive period. Nipple bottle feeding can be used, with 2 L of colostrum given every 12 hours for the first 48 hours of life. The first feeding is usually milked from the cow by hand, and the remaining feedings are from the colostrum obtained from the cow after the first machine milking. With care and patience, this system can result in good transfer of passive immunity in all calves except those born to dams that have very low concentrations of immunoglobulin in their colostrum. Unfortunately, with Holstein Friesians this can be a significant percentage. An extension of this system is to bottle feed at the same frequency but to feed stored colostrum selected for its superior immunoglobulin content. Bottle feeding of newborn calves requires considerable **patience**, and its success is very much dependent on the calf feeder and on the availability of the feeder's time when faced with a calf that has a slow intake.

Where the diligence of the calf feeders is poor, or where there is a time constraint on their availability, the feeding of a large volume of colostrum (4 L to a 45 kg calf) by **esophageal feeder** at the initial feeding immediately after birth can be a successful practice. The **large-volume feeding** also allows the delivery of an adequate mass of immunoglobulin with colostrum that has low immunoglobulin concentrations without impairing the intestinal IgG absorption rate compared with voluntary intake of the same large amount of colostrum.[10] The practice usually uses stored colostrum, and the feeding can be achieved within a few minutes. It can be supplemented by bottle feeding of a second feeding at 12 hours of life.

The practice of feeding stored colostrum as the sole source of colostrum is limited to larger dairy herds, but it does allow the selection of superior colostrum for feeding, with selection based on weight and specific gravity as detailed earlier.

Beef Calves

Beef calves should be allowed to suck naturally, and force-feeding of colostrum to beef breeds should not be practiced unless there is obvious failure of sucking. Where colostrum is required, as with weak beef calves, calves with edematous tongues, and calves that have been subjected to a difficult birth, it can be administered with an esophageal feeder or a stomach tube.

Lambs

Lambs are allowed to suck naturally, but there can be competition between siblings for colostrum; one large single lamb is capable of ingesting, within a short period of birth, all the available colostrum in the ewe's udder. Lambs require a total of 180 to 210 mL colostrum/kg body weight during the first 18 hours after birth to provide sufficient energy for heat production. This amount will usually provide enough immunoglobulin for protection against infections. **Supplemental feeding** of colostrum may be advisable for lambs from multiple birth litters, lambs that lack vigor, and those that have not nursed by 2 hours following birth. This can be done with a nipple bottle or an esophageal feeder.

Piglets

Colostral supplementation is not commonly practiced with piglets. An immunoglobulin dose of 10 g/kg body weight on day 1 followed by 2 g/kg on succeeding days for 10 days is sufficient to confer passive immunity on the colostrum-deprived pig.

FURTHER READING

Barrington GM, Parish SM. Bovine neonatal immunology. *Vet Clin North Am Food Anim Pract.* 2001;17:463-476.

Black L, Francis ML, Nicholls MJ. Protecting young domestic animals from infectious disease. *Vet Annu.* 1985;25:46-61.

Godden S. Colostrum management for dairy calves. *Vet Clin North Am Food Anim Pract.* 2008;24:19-39.

McGuirk SM, Collins M. Managing the production, storage, and delivery of colostrum. *Vet Clin North Am Food Anim Pract.* 2004;20:593-603.

Mellor D. Meeting colostrum needs of lambs. *In Pract.* 1990;12:239-244.

Norcross NL. Secretion and composition of colostrum and milk. *J Am Vet Med Assoc.* 1982;181:1057.

Quigley JD, Drewry JJ. Nutrient and immunity transfer from cow to calf pre- and postcalving. *J Dairy Sci.* 1998;81:2779-2790.

Rooke JA, Bland IM. The acquisition of passive immunity in the newborn piglet. *Livest Prod Sci.* 2002;78:13-23.

Staley TE, Bush LJ. Receptor mechanism of the neonatal intestine and their relationship to immunoglobulin absorption and disease. *J Dairy Sci.* 1985;68:184-205.

Weaver DM, Tyler JW, VanMetre D, Hoetetler DE, Barrington GM. Passive transfer of colostral immunoglobulins in calves. *J Vet Intern Med.* 2000;14:569-577.

REFERENCES

1. Beam AL, et al. *J Dairy Sci.* 2009;92:3973-3980.
2. Godden S. *Vet Clin North Am Food Anim Pract.* 2008;24:19-39.
3. Morin DE, et al. *J Am Vet Med Assoc.* 2010;237:420-428.
4. Mokhber-Dezfooli MR, et al. *J Dairy Sci.* 2012;95:6740-6749.
5. Faber SN, et al. *Prof Anim Sci.* 2005;21:420-425.
6. McCue PM. *Am J Vet Res.* 2007;68:1005-1009.
7. Whitehead CE. *Vet Clin North Am Food Anim Pract.* 2009;25:353-366.
8. Waldner CL, Rosengren LB. *Can Vet J.* 2009;50:275-281.
9. Godden S, et al. *J Dairy Sci.* 2006;89:3476-3482.
10. Godden SM, et al. *J Dairy Sci.* 2009;92:1758-1765.
11. Edwards SA, Broom DM. *Res Vet Sci.* 1979;26:255-256.
12. Godden SM, et al. *J Dairy Sci.* 2009;92:1750-1757.
13. Austin SM. *Equine Vet Educ.* 2013;25:585-589.
14. Deelen SM, et al. *J Dairy Sci.* 2014;97:1-7.
15. Weaver DM, et al. *J Vet Intern Med.* 2000;14:569-577.
16. Metzner M, et al. *J Vet Med A Physiol Pathol Clin Med.* 2007;54:449-454.
17. Bielmann V, et al. *J Dairy Sci.* 2010;93:3713-3721.
18. Quigley JD, et al. *J Dairy Sci.* 2013;96:1148-1155.
19. Johnson J, et al. *J Dairy Sci.* 2007;90:5189-5198.
20. Lorenz I, et al. *Ir Vet J.* 2011;64:10.
21. Ameri M, Wilkerson MJ. *J Vet Diagn Invest.* 2008;20:333-336.

Clinical Assessment and Care of Critically Ill Newborns

The following discussion focuses on care and treatment of critically ill foals, although the principles are applicable to any species. The increasing availability of secondary and tertiary care for ill newborns has allowed the development of sophisticated care for newborns of sufficient emotional or financial value.[1] This level of care, at its most intensive, requires appropriately trained individuals (both veterinarians and support staff) and dedicated facilities. True intensive care of newborns requires 24-hour monitoring. The following discussion is not a comprehensive guide to intensive care of newborns, but is rather an introduction to the general aspects of advanced primary or basic secondary care. Sophisticated interventions, such as mechanical ventilation and cardiovascular support, are mentioned but not discussed in detail.

CLINICAL EXAMINATION

Initial assessment of an ill newborn should begin with collection of a detailed history, including length of gestation, health of the dam, parturition, and behavior of the newborn after birth, including the time to stand and to commence nursing activity. Physical examination should be thorough, with particular attention to those body systems most commonly affected. A form similar to that in Figure 19-4 is useful in ensuring that all pertinent questions are addressed and that the physical examination is comprehensive.

Examination of ill neonates should focus on detection of the common causes of disease in this age group: sepsis, either focal or systemic; prematurity or dysmaturity; metabolic abnormalities (such as hypoglycemia or hypothermia); birth trauma; diseases associated with hypoxia; and congenital abnormalities. Detailed descriptions of these conditions are provided elsewhere in this chapter.

Sepsis

Sepsis is an important cause of illness in neonates that can manifest as localized infections without apparent systemic signs, localized infections with signs of systemic illness, or systemic illness without signs of localized infection.[2]

Localized infections without signs of systemic illness include septic synovitis or osteomyelitis and omphalitis. Signs of these diseases are evident on examination of the area affected and include lameness, distension of the joint, and pain on palpation of the affected joint in animals with synovitis or osteomyelitis and an enlarged external umbilicus with or without purulent discharge in animals with infections of the umbilical structures. Specialized imaging and hematologic and serum biochemical examinations (see following discussion) are useful in confirming the infection.

Systemic signs of sepsis include depression, failure to nurse or reduced frequency of nursing, somnolence, recumbency, fever or hypothermia, tachypnea, tachycardia, diarrhea, and colic, in addition to any signs of

Foal Examination Protocol (age< 1mon)

The Ohio State University Veterinary Teaching Hospital

Special considerations: ______________________

Clinician: ______________

Student: ______________

Date: __________ Time: ______ AM/PM

History

Mare

Age: ____ No of previous foals: ____ Problems with previous foals? __No __Yes ____________

Uterine infections/Vaginal discharge? __No __Yes ____________

liiness during pregnancy? __No __Yes ____________

Milk dripping? __No __Yes How long? ____________

Vaccinations? __ No __Yes What/When? ____________

Deworming?__No__Yes When? ____________

Feeding: ____________

Breeding date: ________ Duration of prenancy: ________ → __on term __early __overdue (____days)

Dystocia? __No __Yes ____________

Early cord rupture? __No__Yes ________ Premature placental separation?__No__Yes ________

Placenta completely passed? __No__Yes Condition of placenta: ____________

Meconium staining? __No__Yes ____________

Udder: __ Normal __ Abnormal ____________

Colostrum quality: __ Normal __Low-quality ________ Amount: __Normal __Reduced ________

Foal

Spontaneous breathing?__No__Yes ________ Time to stand: ______ Time to nurse: ______

Nursing normally?__No__Yes ________ Colostrum/Milk given? ________

Behavior normal? __No__Yes ________ IgG tested?__No__Yes ________

Urination?__ No __Yes ______ Meconium passed?__No__Yes ______ Enema given?__No__Yes ______

Medications given?__ No __Yes ____________

Umbilicus treated?__ No __ Yes ____________

Presenting complaint: ____________

Previous treatment: ____________

The Ohio State University
Form-209046

Foal Examination Protocol

Fig. 19-4 Examples of forms used to document and record historical aspects and findings on physical examination of foals less than 1 month of age.

Continued

Physical Examination Date: ______________ Time: ______AM/PM

Temperature: _____ºF Pulse rate: _____/min Respiratory rate: _____ /min Body weight: _____ kg / _____ lb

Inspection:

Behavior: ____________________

Signs of prematurity? __no __yes (__Haircoat __Forehead __Ears __Joints __Tendons ____________)

Skin and haircoat: ____________________

Body condition: ____________________

Suckle reflex: __good __moderate __weak __none ____________________

Eyes: __normal __Entropion (L)(R) __Uveitis (L)(R) __Corneal ulcer (L)(R) ____________________

Cardiovascular

Pulse quality: __strong __moderate __weak / __regular __irregular ____________________

Mucous membranes: ______________ CRT: ___ sec. Skin turgor: ____________

Jugular veins: __normal __collapsed __distended ______________ Catheter __left __right

Cardiac auscultation: HR: _____ Intensity: _________ Rhythm: __regular __irregular ____________

Murmurs: __no __yes ____________________

Respiration

Nasal discharge: __no __yes ______________ Cough: __no __yes ______________

Lymph nodes: __normal:______________ Auscultation: __normal: ______________

GI tract

Colic: __no __yes ____________ GL sounds: ____________ Abd. distention: __no __yes ____________

Fecal consistency: ______________ Digital palpation/Meconium: ______________

Urogenital

Umbilicus: __normal ____________________

Urination: __no __yes __straining ____________ Scrotum/Testes – Vulva/Vagina:___normal ____________

Musculoskeletal

Joints: __normal ____________________

Lameness: __ no __yes ____________________

Deformations/Angular limb deformities: _____ no __yes ____________________

Neurologic:

__normal ____________________

Seizures: __ no __ yes ____________________

Senior Student: ______________ Attending Clinician: ______________

Foal Examination Protocol

Fig. 19-4, cont'd

localized disease. Fever is a specific, but not sensitive, sign of sepsis in foals. The presence of petechia in oral, nasal, ocular, or vaginal mucous membranes, the pinna, or coronary bands is considered a specific indicator of sepsis, although this has not been documented by appropriate studies. A similar comment applies for injection of the scleral vessels. A scoring system (the sepsis score) has been developed to aid in the identification of foals with sepsis.

The **sepsis score** was developed with the intention of aiding identification of foals with sepsis, thereby facilitating appropriate treatment. A table for calculation of the sepsis score (the modified sepsis score) is provided in Table 19-11. Foals with a score of 12 or greater are considered to be septic, with a sensitivity of 94% in the original report. However, more recent studies, including one of 1095 foals, have found the sensitivity and specificity of the sepsis score to be less than the original report. The modified sepsis score detected sepsis with a sensitivity of 56% and a specificity of 73% using a cutoff value of 11 or more. A cutoff value of 7 yielded a sensitivity of 84% and specificity of 42%.[3] These recent studies are broadly consistent with earlier studies that demonstrate that the sepsis score has limited sensitivity (67%, 95% CI 59% to 75%) and specificity (76%, 95% CI 68% to 83%) in foals less than 10 days of age. Similarly, 49% of 101 foals with positive blood cultures had a sepsis score of 11 or less, indicating a low specificity of the test. The low to moderate sensitivity of the sepsis score for detection of sepsis or bacteremia means that many foals with sepsis are incorrectly diagnosed as being nonseptic (i.e., a high false-negative rate), whereas a moderate to low specificity means that the false-positive rate might be excessive, with a number of foals being considered septic when they are not. This is an important shortcoming of the test because accurate and prompt identification of foals with sepsis is assumed to be important for both prognostication and selection of treatment. The sepsis score might be useful in some situations, but its shortcomings should be recognized when using it to guide treatment or determine prognosis.

Prematurity and Dysmaturity

Detection of **prematurity** is important because it is a strong risk factor for development of other diseases during the immediate postpartum period. The detection of prematurity is often based on the length of gestation. However, the duration of gestation in Thoroughbred horses varies considerably, with 95% of mares foaling after a gestation of 327 to 357 days. The generally accepted "average" gestation is 349 days, with fillies having shorter gestations than do colts (348 versus 350 days) and gestation length declining by approximately 20 days, from 360 to 340 days, in Standardbred mares in New Zealand.[4] Ponies have a shorter gestation (333 days, range 315 to 350 days). Therefore a diagnosis of prematurity should be based not just on gestational age but also on the results of physical, hematologic, and serum biochemical examination of the newborn. Factors helping in the determination of prematurity are listed in Table 19-4. Foals that are immature (premature) at birth typically have low birth weight and small body size, a short and silky hair coat, and laxity of the

Table 19-4 Criteria to assess stage of maturity of the newborn foal

Criterion	Premature	Full term
Physical		
Gestational age	320 d	Normally > 330 d
Size	Small	Normal or large
Coat	Short and silky	Long
Fetlock	Overextended	Normal extension
Behavior		
First stand	>120 min	<120 min
First stand	>3 h	<3 h
Suck reflex	Poor	Good
Righting reflexes	Poor	Good
Adrenal activity		
Plasma cortisol values over first 2 h postpartum	Low levels (<30 ng/mL)	Increasing levels (120–140 ng/mL) at 30–60 min postpartum
Plasma ACTH values over first 2 h postpartum	Peak values (≈650 pg/mL) at 30 min postpartum and declining subsequently	Declining values from peak (300 pg/mL at birth)
Response to synthetic ACTH1-24 (short-acting Synacthen), dose 0.125 mg IM	Poor response shown by a 28% increase in plasma cortisol and no changes in neutrophil: lymphocyte ratio	Good response shown by a 208% increase in plasma cortisol and widening of neutrophil : lymphocyte ratio
Hematology		
Mean cell volume (fl)	>39	<39
White blood cell count ($\times10^9$/L)	6.0	8.0
Neutrophil : lymphocyte ratio	<1.0	>2.0
Carbohydrate metabolism		
Plasma glucose levels over first 2 h postpartum	Low levels at birth (2–3 mmol/L), subsequently declining	Higher levels at birth (4.1 mmol/L), maintained
Plasma insulin levels over first 2 h postpartum	Low levels at birth (8.6 μU/mL), declining	Higher levels at birth (16.1 μU/mL), maintained
Glucose tolerance test (0.5 mg/kg body weight IV)	Slight response demonstrated by a 100% increase in plasma insulin at 15 min postadministration	Clear response demonstrated by a 250% increase in plasma insulin at 5 min postadministration
Renin–angiotensin–aldosterone system		
Plasma renin substrate	Higher and/or increasing levels during 15–60 min postpartum	Low (<0.6 μg/mL) and declining levels during 15–30 min postpartum
Acid–base status (pH)	<7.25 and declining	>7.3 and maintaining or rising

IM, intramuscularly; IV, intravenously.

flexor and extensor tendons. The cranium is rounded, and the pinnae lack tone (droopy ears). The foals are typically weak and have trouble standing, which is exacerbated by laxity of the flexor tendons and periarticular ligaments. **Dysmature** (postmature) foals are typically large, although they can be thin, and have a long hair coat and flexure tendon contracture. These signs are consistent with prolonged gestation combined with inadequate intrauterine nutrition. Healthy foals stand approximately 65 min (interquartile range, 45 to 100 minutes) after birth.[4] Examination of the placenta, either by ultrasonographic examination before birth or by direct examination, including histologic and microbiologic testing, after birth is useful in identifying abnormalities that have significance for the newborn.

Hypoxia

Hypoxia during late gestation, birth, or the immediate postpartum period has a variety of clinical manifestations depending on the tissue or organ most affected. Signs of central nervous system dysfunction are often assumed to be a result of cerebral hypoxia during birth, although neonatal maladjustment syndrome does not appear to be related to hypoxia (see "Neonatal Maladjustment Syndrome," page 1871). Other signs suggestive of peripartum hypoxia include colic and anuria.

Hypoglycemia

Foals that are hypoglycemic because of inadequate intake, such as through mismothering, congenital abnormalities, or concurrent illness, are initially weak, with rapid progression to somnolence and coma.

Endocrine Abnormalities

Abnormalities in endocrine function of foals are common and often associated with risk of death.[1,5-10] Septic foals have higher serum ACTH, cortisol, and ACTH : cortisol ratios, and higher serum parathyroid hormone concentrations (but not calcitonin concentrations) than do healthy foals of the same age.[5,6] Septic foals have lower insulin and IGF-1 and higher ghrelin, growth hormone, and glucagon concentrations than do healthy foals.[7,8] Arginine vasopressin concentrations are higher in septic foals.[9] Plasma adrenomedullin concentrations are highest in sick foals (both septic and nonseptic) and might be a useful marker of foal health.[10] Critically ill foals may also have evidence on nonthyroidal illness syndrome (see "Diseases of the Thyroid," Chapter 17).[11]

DIAGNOSTIC IMAGING

Radiographic and ultrasonographic examination of neonates can be useful in determining maturity and the presence of abnormalities. Prematurity is evident as failure or inadequate ossification of cuboidal bones in the carpus and tarsus. Radiographs of the thorax should be obtained if there is any suspicion of sepsis or pneumonia because thoracic auscultation has poor sensitivity in detecting pulmonary disease in newborns. The severity of abnormalities in the lungs of foals detected by radiographic examination is related to prognosis, with foals with more severe disease having a worse prognosis for recovery. Abdominal radiographs may be useful in determining the site of gastrointestinal disease (see discussion of foal colic).

Ultrasonography is a particularly useful tool for examination of neonates, in large part because their small size permits thorough examination of all major body cavities. Ultrasonography of the umbilical structures can identify omphalitis and abscesses of umbilical remnants and, when available, is indicated as part of the physical examination of every sick neonate.

Examination of the **umbilical structures** can reveal evidence of infection, congenital abnormalities, and urachal tears. Examination of the umbilicus can be achieved using a 7.5-mHz linear probe (such as that commonly used for reproductive examination of mares), although sector scanners provide a superior image. Examination of the umbilical structures should include examination of the navel and structures external to the body wall, the body wall, the umbilical stump as it enters the body wall and separates into the two umbilical arteries, the urachus and apex of the bladder, and the umbilical vein. The size and echogenicity of each of these structures should be determined. For foals less than 7 days of age, the intraabdominal umbilical stump should be less than 2.4 cm in diameter, the umbilical vein less than 1 cm, and the umbilical arteries less than 1.4 cm (usually < 1 cm). Examination of these structures should be complete: the umbilical vein should be visualized in the umbilical stump and then followed as it courses along the ventral abdominal wall and into the liver; the umbilical arteries should be visualized in the umbilical stump and then as they separate from that structure and course over the lateral aspects of the bladder; the urachus should be visualized from the external umbilical stump through the body wall and as it enters the bladder.

Abnormalities observed frequently in the umbilical structures include overall swelling, consistent with omphalitis; gas shadows in the urachus or umbilical stump, which are indicative of either a patent urachus allowing entry of air or growth of gas-producing bacteria; and the presence of flocculent fluid in the urachus, vein, or artery, which is consistent with pus. Urachal tears can be observed, especially in foals with uroperitoneum.

Ultrasonographic examination of the **abdomen** is useful in identifying abnormalities of gastrointestinal function and structure, including intestinal distension or thickening of the intestinal wall. Thickness of the wall of the intestinal tract of healthy Standardbred foals of less than 5 days of age are as follows (95% predictive interval): 1.6 to 3.6 mm for the stomach, 1.9 to 3.2 mm for the duodenum, 1.9 to 3.1 mm for the jejunum, 1.3 to 2.2 mm for the colon, and 0.8 to 2.7 mm for the cecum.[12] Intussusceptions are evident as "donut" lesions in the small intestine, but evaluation of the clinical importance of these findings should be considered in the context of the foal. Intussusceptions are detected in a large proportion of healthy neonatal foals as incidental findings.[12] Gastric outflow obstruction should be suspected in foals with a distended stomach evident on ultrasonographic examination of the abdomen. Herniation through the umbilicus or inguinal ring can be confirmed by ultrasonographic examination.[13] Uroperitoneum is readily apparent as excessive accumulation of clear fluid in the abdomen. Hemorrhage into the peritoneum can be detected as accumulation of echogenic, swirling fluid. Accumulation of inflammatory fluid, such as in foals with ischemic intestine, is detected by the presence of flocculent fluid.

Ultrasonographic examination of the **chest** can reveal the presence of pleural abnormalities, consolidation of the lung (provided that the consolidated lung is confluent with the pleura), accumulation of fluid in the pleural space (hemorrhage secondary to birth trauma and fractured ribs, inflammatory fluid in foals with pleuritis), pneumothorax (usually secondary to lung laceration by a fractured rib), or congenital abnormalities of the heart.

Advanced imaging modalities, such as **computed tomography (CT) and magnetic resonance imaging (MRI)**, are available at referral centers and are practical in foals and other neonates because of the small size of the animals. These modalities are useful in detection of intrathoracic and intraabdominal abnormalities, including abscesses, gastrointestinal disease, and congenital abnormalities. MRI is particularly useful for diagnosis of diseases of the brain and spinal cord.

CLINICAL PATHOLOGY

Serum Immunoglobulin Concentration

Serum or plasma immunoglobulins are associated with the risk of death in hospitalized foals. Foals with serum IgG concentration less than or equal to 4.0 g/L were 4.7 (95% CI 2.6 to 8.5) times as likely to die as were foals with a concentration greater than 8 g/L. Foals with an IgG of greater than 4 g/L and less than 8 g/L were 3.7 (2.0 to 6.8) times as likely to die as were foals with concentrations above 8 g/L.[14]

Serum immunoglobulin G (IgG) concentration, or its equivalent, must be measured in every ill or at-risk newborn and should be repeated every 48 to 96 hours in critically ill neonates. A variety of tests are available for rapid detection of FTPI in foals and calves. Although measurement of serum IgG concentration is ideally performed by the gold standard test, a radial immunodiffusion, this test requires at least 24 hours to run, whereas the stall-side or chemistry analyzer tests can be run in a few minutes. The sensitivity and specificity have been determined for a number of these rapid tests. Overall, most tests have high sensitivity (>80%), meaning that the few foals that have low concentrations of IgG are missed, but poor specificity (50% to 70%), meaning that many foals that have adequate concentrations of immunoglobulin are diagnosed as having inadequate concentrations. The exact sensitivity and specificity depend on the test used and the concentration of immunoglobulin considered adequate. The high sensitivity and low specificity of most of the available rapid tests result in a number of foals that do not need a transfusion receiving one. However, this error is of less importance than that of foals that should receive a transfusion not receiving one.

Serum or plasma concentrations of IgG should be measured after approximately 18 hours of age, and preferably before 48 hours of age—the earlier FTPI is recognized, the better the prognosis for the foal. Foals that ingest colostrum within the first few hours of birth have minimal increases in serum IgG concentration over that achieved at 12 hours of age, suggesting that measurement of serum IgG concentration as early as 12 to 18 hours after birth is appropriate. This early measurement of serum IgG concentration could be especially important in high-risk foals. The oldest age at which measurement of serum IgG is useful in foals is uncertain, but depends on the clinical condition of the foal. Typically, immunoglobulin concentrations of foals that have adequate concentrations of IgG within the first 24 hours reach a nadir at about 6 weeks of age and then rise to concentrations similar to adults over the next 2 to 3 months.

Hematology

It is important to recognize that the hemogram of neonates differs from that of older animals (Table 19-5) because these differences can affect the clinical assessment of the animal. The hematologic and serum biochemical values of foals and calves can vary markedly during the first days and weeks of life, and it is important that these maturational changes are taken into account when assessing results of hematologic or serum biochemical examination of foals. Hematologic examination can reveal evidence of hemolytic disease, bacterial or viral infection, or prematurity/dysmaturity (Table 19-4). Repeated hemograms are often necessary to monitor for development of sepsis and responses to treatment.

Foals with **sepsis** can have a leukocyte count in the blood that is low, within the reference range, or high. Approximately 40% of foals with sepsis have blood leukocyte counts that are below the reference range. Most foals with sepsis (approximately 70%) have segmented neutrophil counts that are below the reference range, with fewer than 15% of foals having elevated blood neutrophil counts. Concentrations of band cells in blood are above the reference range in almost all foals with sepsis. Some foals born of mares with placentitis have a very pronounced mature neutrophilia without other signs of sepsis; these foals typically have a good prognosis. Lymphopenia is present in foals with equine herpervirus-1 septicemia or Arabian foals with severe

Table 19-5 Hematologic values of normal foals and calves

	FOALS			CALVES		
Variable	*<12 h*	*1 week*	*1 month*	*24 h*	*48 h*	*3–4 weeks*
PCV (%)	42.5 ± 3.4	35.3 ± 3.3	33.9 ± 3.5	34 ± 6	32 ± 6	35 ± 3
(L/L)	0.43 ± 0.03	0.35 ± 0.03	0.33 ± 0.04	0.34 ± 0.06	0.32 ± 0.06	0.35 ± 0.03
Plasma protein (g/dL)	6.0 ± 0.8	6.4 ± 0.6	6.1 ± 0.5	6.4 ± 0.7	6.4 ± 0.7	6.4 ± 0.3
(g/L)	60 ± 8	64 ± 6	61 ± 5	64 ± 7	64 ± 7	64 ± 3
Fibrinogen (mg/dL)	216 ± 70	290 ± 70	400 ± 130	290 ± 105	335 ± 120	285 ± 145
(g/L)	2.16 ± 0.7	2.90 ± 0.7	4.00 ± 1.30	2.90 ± 1.05	3.35 ± 1.20	2.85 ± 1.45
Hemoglobin (g/dL)	15.4 ± 1.2	13.3 ± 1.2	12.5 ± 1.2	10.9 ± 2.1	10.5 ± 1.8	11.3 ± 1.02
(g/L)	154 ± 12	130 ± 12	125 ± 12	109 ± 21	105 ± 18	113 ± 10
Red blood cells ($\times 10^6$/μL)	10.7 ± 0.8	8.8 ± 0.6	9.3 ± 0.8	8.17 ± 1.34	7.72 ± 1.09	8.86 ± 0.68
(10^{12}/L)	10.7 ± 0.8	8.8 ± 0.6	9.3 ± 0.8	8.17 ± 1.34	7.72 ± 1.09	8.86 ± 0.68
MCV (fL)	40 ± 2	39 ± 2	36 ± 1	41 ± 3	41 ± 3	39 ± 2
MCHC (g/dL)	36 ± 2	38 ± 1	37 ± 1	32.1 ± 0.8	32.6 ± 1.0	32.8 ± 1.6
(g/L)	360 ± 20	380 ± 10	370 ± 10	320 ± 8	326 ± 10	328 ± 16
MCH (pg)	14 ± 1	15 ± 1	14 ± 1			
Nucleated cells (10^6/μL)	9500 ± 2500	9860 ± 1800	8150 ± 2030	9810 ± 2800	7760 ± 1950	8650 ± 1690
(10^9/L)	9.5 ± 2.5	9.86 ± 1.80	8.15 ± 2.03	9.81 ± 2.80	7.76 ± 1.95	8.65 ± 1.69
Neutrophils (10^6/μL)	7950 ± 2200	7450 ± 1550	5300 ± 200	6500 ± 2660	4110 ± 2040	2920 ± 1140
(10^9/L)	7.95 ± 2.20	7.45 ± 1.55	5.30 ± 0.20	6.50 ± 2.66	4.11 ± 2.04	2.92 ± 1.14
Band neutrophils (10^6/μL)	24 ± 40	0	4 ± 13	310 ± 460	210 ± 450	10 ± 30
(10^9/L)	0.02 ± 0.04	0	0.00 ± 0.01	0.31 ± 0.46	0.21 ± 0.45	0.01 ± 0.03
Lymphocytes (10^6/μL)	1350 ± 600	2100 ± 630	2460 ± 450	2730 ± 820	2850 ± 880	5050 ± 800
(10^9/L)	1.35 ± 0.6	2.10 ± 0.63	2.46 ± 0.45	2.73 ± 0.82	2.85 ± 0.88	5.05 ± 0.80
Thrombocytes (10^3/μL)	266 ± 103	250 ± 70	300 ± 80			
(10^9/L)	266 ± 103	250 ± 70	300 ± 80			
Serum Fe (μg/dL)	380 ± 60	175 ± 80	138 ± 60		71 ± 60	127 ± 60
(mg/L)	3.80 ± 0.6	1.75 ± 0.8	1.38 ± 0.6		0.7 ± 0.6	1.27 ± 0.6
TIBC (μg/dL)	440 ± 50	385 ± 80	565 ± 65		420 ± 67	
(mg/L)	4.40 ± 0.5	3.85 ± 0.8	5.65 ± 0.65		4.2 ± 0.7	
UIBC (μg/dL)	55 ± 40	210 ± 100	430 ± 85			
(mg/L)	0.55 ± 0.4	2.10 ± 1.00	4.30 ± 0.85			
Iron saturation (%)	87 ± 9	46 ± 20	25 ± 12			

Sources: Harvey JW et al. Equine Vet J *1984; 16:347; Adams R et al.* Am J Vet Res *1992; 53:944; Tennant B et al.* Cornell Vet *1975; 65:543.*

combined immunodeficiency. Thrombocytopenia occurs in some foals with sepsis. Hyperfibrinogenemia is common in foals that have sepsis, although the concentration might not be above the reference range in foals examined early in the disease.

Hyperfibrinogenemia is common in foals born of mares with placentitis and reflects systemic activation of the inflammatory cascade even in foals that have no other evidence of sepsis. Serum amyloid A concentrations are above 100 mg/L in foals with sepsis. Septic foals also have blood concentrations of proinflammatory cytokines, and of plasma C-reactive protein,[15] that are higher than those in healthy foals. Plasma haptoglobin concentrations are not different between surviving and nonsurviving foals and are only minimally lower in foals with sepsis than in nonseptic hospitalized foals.[15] Indices of coagulation are prolonged in foals with sepsis, and concentrations of antithrombin and protein C antigen in plasma are lower than in healthy foals. These abnormalities indicate that coagulopathies are common in septic foals.

Prematurity is associated with a low neutrophil:lymphocyte ratio (<1.5:1) in blood and red cell macrocytosis (Table 19-4). A neutrophil:lymphocyte ratio above 2:1 is considered normal. Premature foals that are not septic can have low blood neutrophil counts but rarely have immature neutrophils (band cells) or toxic changes in neutrophils.

Serum Biochemistry

Care should be taken in the interpretation of the results of serum biochemical examinations because normal values for newborns are often markedly different from those of adults, and they can change rapidly during the first days to weeks of life (Table 19-6). Serum biochemical examination can reveal electrolyte abnormalities associated with renal failure, diarrhea, and sepsis. Elevations in serum bilirubin concentration or serum enzyme activities may be detected. As a minimum, blood glucose concentrations should be estimated using a chemical strip in depressed or recumbent newborns.

Markedly elevated serum **creatinine** concentrations are not uncommonly observed in foals with no other evidence of renal disease. The elevated serum creatinine in these cases is a consequence of impaired placental function during late gestation, with the consequent accumulation of creatinine (and probably other compounds). In foals with normal renal function, which most have, the serum creatinine concentration should decrease to 50% of the initial high value within 24 hours. Other causes of high serum creatinine concentration that should be ruled out are renal failure (dysplasia, hypoxic renal failure) and postrenal azotemia (uroperitoneum).

Blood or plasma **L-lactate concentrations** are useful indicators of the presence and severity of systemic disease that impairs oxygen delivery to tissue (hypoxemia, poor perfusion, anemia) or use by tissue (endotoxemia), but it is not specific for any one disease or group of diseases, with the exception that septic foals have higher concentrations than do nonseptic foals.[16-19] However, the difference between septic and nonseptic foals (4.8 [range, 0.6 to 37) and 3.3 [range, 0.3 to 21] mmol/L) is not sufficiently different to make it useful in an individual animal.[20] Blood lactate concentrations of healthy foals are greatest at birth to 12 hours of age and then decline.[16] Blood lactate concentrations of foals that do not survive their acute illness do not decline in response to therapy,[16] and risk of death increases by 1.1 for each mmol/L increase in blood lactate concentration of foals at time of admission to a veterinary hospital.[17,20] Serial measurement of blood lactate concentrations and calculation of an "area-under-the-curve" measure also provides useful information related to risk of death, but not the cause of the disease.

Sepsis is usually associated with hypoglycemia, although septic foals can have normal or elevated blood glucose concentrations. Hypoglycemia is attributable to failure

Table 19-6 Serum biochemical values of normal foals and calves

	FOALS			CALVES		
Variable	*<12 h*	*1 week*	*1 month*	*24 h*	*48 h*	*3 weeks*
Na^+ (mEq/L) (mmol/L)	148 ± 8	142 ± 6	145 ± 4	145 ± 7.6	149 ± 8.0	140 ± 6
K^+ (mEq/L) (mmol/L)	4.4 ± 0.5	4.8 ± 0.5	4.6 ± 0.4	5.0 ± 0.6	5.0 ± 0.6	4.9 ± 0.6
Cl (mEq/L) (mmol/L)	106 ± 6	102 ± 4	103 ± 3	100 ± 4	101 ± 5.0	99 ± 4
Ca^{2+} (mg/dL)	12.8 ± 1	12.5 ± 0.6	12.2 ± 0.6	12.3 ± 0.2	12.3 ± 0.3	9.4 ± 0.6
(mmol/L)	3.2 ± 0.25	3.1 ± 0.15	3.05 ± 0.15	3.1 ± 0.1	3.1± 0.1	2.3 ± 0.2
PO_4^- (mg/dL)	4.7 ± 0.8	7.4 ± 1.0	7.1 ± 1.1	6.9 ± 0.3	7.6 ± 0.2	7.1 ± 6.4
(mmol/L)	1.52 ± 0.26	2.39 ± 0.32	2.29 ± 0.36	2.3 ± 0.1	2.5 ± 0.1	2.3 ± 1.8
Total protein (g/dL)	5.8 ± 1.1	6.0 ± 0.7	5.8 ± 0.5	5.6 ± 0.5	6.0 ± 0.7	6.5 ± 0.5
(g/L)	58 ± 11	60 ± 7	58 ± 5	56 ± 5	60 ± 7	65 ± 5
Albumin (g/dL)	3.2 ± 0.3	2.9 ± 0.2	3.0 ± 0.2			
(g/L)	32 ± 3	29 ± 2	30 ± 2			
Creatinine (mg/dL)	2.5 ± 0.6	1.3 ± 0.2	1.5 ± 0.2			
(μmol/L)	221 ± 53	115 ± 18	133 ± 18			
Urea nitrogen (mg/dL)	19.7 ± 4.4	7.8 ± 3.4	9.0 ± 3.0	12.6 (7.1–21.2)		
(mmol/L)	3.4 ± 1.6	1.6 ± 0.6	1.7 ± 0.5	2 (1.5–3.6)		
Glucose (mg/dL)	144 ± 30	162 ± 19	162 ± 22	130 ± 27	114 ± 19	70 (52–84)
(mmol/L)	8.0 ± 1.6	9.0 ± 1.0	9.0 ± 1.2	7.23 ± 1.5	6.34 ± 1.1	3.9 (2.9–4.7)
Total bilirubin (mg/dL)	2.6 ± 1.0	1.5 ± 0.4	0.7 ± 0.2	<2.5	<0.9	<0.6
(μmol/L)	45 ± 17	26 ± 6	12 ± 4	<42	<15	<10
Direct bilirubin (mg/dL)	0.9 ± 0.1	0.5 ± 0.2	0.3 ± 0.2	<0.6	<0.3	<0.3
(μmol/L)	15 ± 2	8.5 ± 3	5 ± 3	<10	<5	<5
GGT (IU/L)	47.5 ± 21.5	49.1 ± 21.2		890 ± 200	600 ± 180	70 ± 10
ALK (IU/L)	3040 ± 800	1270 ± 310	740 ± 240	<1150	<1000	<770
AST (IU/L)	199 ± 57	330 ± 85	340 ± 55	<60	<33	<32

Values are mean ± standard deviation.
ALK, alkaline phosphatase; AST, aspartate aminotransferase; GGT, gammaglutamyl transpeptidase.
Sources: Bauer JE et al. Equine Vet J *1984; 16:361; Pearson EG et al.* J Am Vet Med Assoc *1995; 207:1466; Jenkins SJ et al.* Cornell Vet *1982; 72:403; Dalton RG.* Br Vet J *1967; 123:48; Wise GH et al.* J Dairy Sci *1947; 30:983; Diesch TJ et al.* New Zeal Vet J *2004; 52:256; Patterson WH, Brown CM.* Am J Vet Rev *1986; 47:2461; Thompson JC, Pauli JV.* New Zeal Vet J *1981; 29:223*

to nurse, whereas hyperglycemia indicates loss of normal sensitivity to insulin. Indicators of renal, hepatic, or cardiac (troponin) damage can increase in foals with sepsis, causing organ damage or failure. Foals with sepsis tend to have elevated concentrations of cortisol in serum.

Prematurity is associated with low concentrations of cortisol in plasma or serum and minimal increase in response to intramuscular administration of 0.125 mg of exogenous ACTH (corticotropin). Plasma cortisol concentration of normal full-term foals during the first 24 hours of life increases from a baseline value of approximately 40 ng/mL to over 100 ng/mL 60 minutes after ACTH administration, whereas plasma cortisol concentrations in premature foals do not increase from values of slightly less than 40 ng/mL. At 2 and 3 days of age, plasma cortisol concentrations of full-term foals increase twofold after ACTH administration, albeit from a lower resting value, but do not increase in premature foals. Blood glucose concentrations of premature foals are often low, probably because of inability to nurse.

Blood Gas

Arterial blood pH, Pco_2, and Po_2 should be measured to determine the newborn's acid–base status and the adequacy of respiratory function. Foals with hypoxemia are five times more likely to have pulmonary radiographic abnormalities. Prolonged lateral recumbency of foals compromises respiratory function, and arterial blood samples should be collected with the foal in sternal recumbency. Repeated sampling may be necessary to detect changes in respiratory function and to monitor the adequacy of oxygen supplementation or assisted ventilation.

Blood Culture

Identification of causative organisms of sepsis in foals can aid in prognostication and potentially in selection of therapy, although there does not appear to be a relation between antimicrobial sensitivity of organisms isolated from blood, as determined by Kirby–Bauer testing, and survival of foals. Anaerobic and aerobic blood cultures should be performed as early in the disease process as possible, and preferably before initiation of antibiotic treatment, although antimicrobials should not be withheld from a newborn with confirmed or suspected sepsis to obtain a result from blood culture. Strict aseptic technique should be used when collecting blood for culture. Blood cultures should also be collected if there is a sudden deterioration in the newborn's condition.

Gram-negative enteric bacteria are the most common isolates from blood of newborn foals, with *E. coli* the most common isolate. *A. equuli* is also a common isolate from foals. There are important differences in diseases produced by the various organisms, with foals with *A. equuli* septicemia being twice as likely to die, seven times more likely to have been sick since birth, six times more likely to have diarrhea, five times more likely to have a sepsis score of more than 11, and three times more likely to have pneumonia than foals with sepsis associated with other bacteria.

A problem with blood culture is the time needed to obtain either interim or final results because this can delay detection of infection or decisions to use focused antimicrobial therapy. Use of real-time polymerase chain reaction (PCR) to detect bloodstream infection of foals will likely supplement conventional blood culture in foals.[21]

Other Body Fluids

Synovial fluid should be submitted for aerobic and anaerobic culture, Gram stain, and cytologic examination when signs of synovitis, such as lameness, joint effusion, or joint pain, are present.

Analysis of cerebrospinal fluid (CSF) is indicated in newborns with signs of neurologic disease. Samples of CSF should be submitted for cytologic examination, measurement of total protein concentration, Gram stain, and bacterial culture.

Urinalysis may provide evidence of renal failure (casts) or urinary tract infection (white blood cells).

Abdominal fluid should be collected in foals with abdominal pain or distension and should be submitted for cytologic examination and, if uroperitoneum is suspected, measurement of creatinine concentration.

TREATMENT

The principles of care of the critically ill newborn farm animal are as follows:

- The newborn should be kept in a sanitary environment to minimize the risk of nosocomial infections.
- Systemic supportive care should be provided to maintain homeostasis until the newborn is capable of separate and independent existence.
- There should be frequent and comprehensive reevaluations of all body systems to detect signs of deterioration and allow early correction.
- Provision should be made to ensure adequate passive immunity (serum or plasma IgG concentration > 8 g/L) to reduce the risk of secondary infections or to treat existing infections. Transfer of passive immunity should be evaluated using laboratory methods that measure serum or plasma IgG concentration.

The level of care provided depends on the value of the animal and the available facilities, personnel, and expertise. Newborns of limited financial worth are usually treated on the farm, whereas valuable foals and calves can be referred for specialist care. Referral of sick neonates to institutions and practices with expertise in provision of critical care to newborns should be timely and prompt and, when necessary, should be recommended on the first visit.

Nursing Care

The sophistication of care for critically ill newborns depends on the facilities and personnel available, with intensive management requiring dedicated facilities and trained personnel available 24 hours a day. The minimum requirement for providing basic care of ill newborns is a sanitary area in which the newborns can be protected from environmental stress. Often this means separating the newborn from its dam.

Excellent nursing care is essential for maximizing the likelihood of a good outcome. Critically ill animals might benefit from constant nursing care. Strict attention must be paid to maintaining the sanitary environment to minimize the risk of nosocomial infections. The newborn should be kept clean and dry and at an ambient temperature in its thermoneutral zone. Bedding should prevent development of decubital ulcers. Foals should be maintained in sternal recumbency, or at least turned every 2 hours, to optimize their respiratory function.

Correction of Failure of Transfer of Passive Immunity

Colostral Immunoglobulin

Ideally, adequate transfer of passive immunity is achieved by the newborn nursing its dam and ingesting an adequate amount of colostrum containing optimal concentrations of immunoglobulins, principally IgG (IgGb) in foals. Foals need approximately 2 g of IgG per kilogram of body weight to achieve a plasma concentration of 2000 mg/dL (20g/L); therefore a 45-kg foal needs approximately 90 g of IgG to attain a normal serum IgG concentration (or approximately 40 g to achieve a serum IgG concentration of 800 mg/dL [8 g/L]). Assuming that colostrum contains on average 10,000 mg/dL (100 g/L), foals must ingest at least 1 L of colostrum to obtain sufficient immunoglobulin. Because colostral IgG concentration varies considerably (from 2000 to 30,000 mg/dL), specific recommendations regarding the quantity of colostrum to be fed to neonatal foals cannot be made with certainty. However, colostrum with a specific gravity of more than 1.060 has an IgG concentration of more than 3000 mg/dL (30 g/L), suggesting that foals should ingest at least 1.5 L to achieve serum IgG concentrations above 800 mg/dL (8 g/L).

Critical Plasma IgG Concentrations in Foals

There is some debate as to what constitutes a critical serum or plasma IgG concentration. Foals that ingest an adequate amount of colostrum typically have serum immunoglobulin concentrations during the first week of life greater than approximately 2000 mg/dL (20 g/L). Both 400 mg/dL

(4 g/L) and 800 mg/dL (8 g/L) have been recommended as concentrations below which foals should be considered to have increased likelihood of contracting infectious disease, but recent evidence strongly supports the use of 800 mg/dL (8 g/L) as the minimal concentration in hospitalized foals. However, on a well-managed farm the serum IgG concentration was not predictive of morbidity or mortality among foals, suggesting that serum immunoglobulin concentration in some populations of foals is not an important risk factor for infectious disease. The foals in this study were from an exceptionally well-managed farm. Other researchers have found that foals with serum IgG concentration below 800 mg/dL (8 g/L) are at markedly increased risk of subsequent development of infectious disease, including sepsis, pneumonia, and septic arthritis. It is likely that there is no single concentration of IgG in serum that is protective in all situations, and the concentration of IgG in serum that is desirable in an individual foal depends on the risk factors for infectious disease of that foal. Our opinion is that a minimum serum IgG in foals free of disease and housed in closed bands on well-managed farms is 400 mg/dL (4 g/L). For foals at increased risk of disease—for instance, those on large farms with frequent introduction of animals and foals that are transported or housed with foals with infectious disease—the minimum advisable serum IgG concentration is 800 mg/dL (8 g/L). Foals that have infectious disease should have serum IgG concentrations of at least 800 mg/dL, and it might be advantageous for these foals to have even higher values, as indicated by the enhanced survival of foals with septic disease administered equine plasma regardless of their serum IgG concentration. This therapeutic advantage could be because of the additional IgG or because of other factors included in the plasma. Transfusion of plasma to sick foals improves neutrophil function, an important advantage given that oxidative burst activity of neutrophils from septic foals is reduced compared with that in healthy foals.

Plasma Transfusion

The ability of foals to absorb macromolecules, including immunoglobulins, declines rapidly after birth, being 22% of that at birth by 3 hours of age and 1% of that at birth by 24 hours of age. Consequently, by the time that FTPI is recognized, it is no longer feasible to increase serum IgG concentrations by feeding colostrum or oral serum products. Foals should then be administered plasma or serum intravenously. The **amount of plasma** or serum to be administered depends on the target value for serum IgG concentration and the initial serum IgG concentration in the foal. For each gram of IgG administered per kilogram of body weight of the foal, serum IgG concentration increases by approximately 8.7 mg/dL (0.87 g/L) in healthy foals and 6.2 mg/dL (0.62 g/L) in sick foals. To achieve serum IgG concentrations above 800 mg/dL (8 g/L) in foals with serum IgG concentrations below 400 mg/dL (4 g/L), they should be administered 40 mL/kg of plasma containing at least 20 g/L of IgG. Similarly, foals with serum IgG concentrations above 400 mg/dL (4g/L) but below 800 mg/dL (8 g/L) should be administered 20 mL/kg of plasma. For 45-kg foals, these recommendations translate to administration of 1 or 2 L of plasma, respectively.

The ideal product for transfusion into foals with FTPI is **fresh frozen plasma** harvested from horses that are Aa and Qa antigen-negative and that do not have antibodies against either or both of these red blood cell antigens (see the discussion of neonatal isoerythrolysis). The donor horses should have been vaccinated against the common diseases of horses and have tested negative for equine infectious anemia. Good-quality commercial products specify the minimum concentration of IgG in the plasma. Concentrated serum products that do not need to be frozen until use are available. These are much more convenient for field use than are plasma products that must be frozen until immediately before transfusion. However, the IgG concentration of these products is often not specified, and the manufacturer's recommendations for dosing often result in administration of inadequate amounts of immunoglobulin. Serum products can produce adequate concentrations of IgG in foals, but the dose is usually two to three times that recommended by the manufacturer. An adequate dose of concentrated serum products is approximately 1 L for some products. The crucial point is that it is not the volume of plasma or serum that is administered that is important, but rather the quantity of immunoglobulin delivered to the foal. A total of 20 to 25 g of IgG is required to raise the serum IgG concentration of a 50-kg foal by 400 mg/dL (4 g/L).

Plasma should be administered intravenously; oral administration is likely to be wasteful, especially in foals more than a few hours old. Frozen plasma should be thawed at room temperature or by immersion in warm (<37° C, 100° F) water. Thawing by immersion in water at temperatures higher than body temperature can cause denaturation and coagulation of proteins, with loss of efficacy of transfused immunoglobulins. Plasma should never be thawed or warmed using a microwave because this denatures the proteins.

Administration of plasma should be intravenous; intraperitoneal administration, such as used in pigs or small ruminants, has not been investigated in foals. The thawed plasma should be administered through a jugular catheter using a blood administration set containing a filter (160- to 270-µm mesh) to prevent infusion of particulate material. Strict asepsis should be used. The foal should be adequately restrained for the procedure, with some active foals needing moderate tranquillization. Premedication with antihistamines or nonsteroidal antiinflammatory drugs is usually not necessary. The plasma should be infused slowly at first, with the first 20 to 40 mL administered over 10 minutes. During this period the foal should be carefully observed for signs of transfusion reaction, which is usually evident as restlessness, tachycardia, tachypnea, respiratory distress, sweating, or urticaria. If these signs are observed, the transfusion should be stopped, and the foal should be reevaluated and treated if necessary. If no transfusion reactions are noted during the first 10 minutes, the infusion can then be delivered at 0.25 to 1.0 mL/kg/min (i.e., about 1 L/h for a 50-kg foal). Rapid infusion can result in acute excessive plasma volume expansion, with the potential for cardiovascular and respiratory distress.

Serum IgG concentration should be measured after the infusion to ensure that an adequate concentration of IgG has been achieved. Serum IgG can be measured as early as 20 minutes after the end of the transfusion.

Nutritional Support

Provision of adequate nutrition is essential to the recovery of ill newborns. Healthy newborn foals have estimated energy requirements of 500 to 625 kJ/kg/d (120 to 150 kcal/kg/d) and consume approximately 20% of their body weight as milk per day. Measurements of foal energy expenditure using indirect calorimetry reveal expenditure of ~60 to 80 kcal/kg/d in healthy foals, which is reduced to ~50 kcal/kg/d for critically ill foals.[22]

The best food for newborns is the dam's milk, and newborns that are able to do so should be encouraged to nurse the dam. However, if the foal is unable to nurse or the dam is not available, then good-quality milk substitutes should be used. Soy and other plant-protein-based milk replacers are not suitable for newborns. Commercial products formulated for foals, calves, and lambs are available. Human enteral nutrition products supplying 0.7 to 1 kcal/mL (2.8 to 4.1 kJ/mL) can also be used for short-term (several days to a week) support of foals.

It is preferable to provide enteral, rather than parenteral, nutrition to ill newborns with normal or relatively normal gastrointestinal function. Sick neonatal foals should initially be fed 10% of their body weight as mare's milk, or a suitable replacer, every 24 hours, divided into hourly or 2-hour feedings. If the foal does not develop diarrhea or abdominal distension, then the amount fed can be increased over a 24- to 48-hour period to 20% to 25% of the foal's body weight (or 150 kcal/kg/day; 620 kJ/kg/day). Newborns can be fed by nursing a bottle or bucket or via an indwelling nasogastric tube such as a foal feeding tube, stallion catheter, human feeding tube, or enema tube. Every attempt should be made to encourage the newborn to nurse its dam as soon as the newborn can stand. Adequacy of nutrition can be monitored by measuring blood glucose concentrations and body weight.

Parenteral nutrition (PN) can be provided to newborns that are unable to be fed by the enteral route. This can be achieved by administration of various combinations of solutions containing glucose (dextrose), amino acids, and fat. A commercial product that does not include lipid has been used successfully for up to 12 days in foals. One product that has been used successfully for foals is a solution of amino acids (5%), dextrose (25%), and electrolytes (Clinimix E; Baxter Healthcare Corporation, Deerfield, IL). Lipid emulsion is not added to the preparation. Additional multivitamin supplements including calcium gluconate (provided 2.5 mmol/L), magnesium sulfate (6 mEq/L), B-vitamin complex (thiamine 12.5 mg/L; riboflavin 2 mg/L; niacin 12.5 mg/L; pantothenic acid 5 mg/L; pyridoxine 5 mg/L; cyanocobalamin 5 μg/L), and trace elements (zinc 2 mg/L; copper 0.8 mg/L; manganese 0.2 mg/L; chromium 8 μg/L) are added. Administration is through a catheter, a single-lumen 14-gauge over-the-wire catheter (Milacath), inserted in the jugular vein with its tip placed in the cranial vena cava. A double-T extension set is used to allow concurrent constant-rate infusion of isotonic crystalloid fluids and intravenous administration of medication in one line and PN solution in the other. An infusion pump is used for continuous-rate infusion of the solutions. The PN solution should be prepared under aseptic conditions just before administration and used for only a period of 24 hours after preparation. A 0.22-μm filter is included in the administration line to remove all bacteria, glass, rubber, cellulose fibers, and other extraneous material in the PN solution. The filters and administration sets are changed with each new bag of PN solution.

The rate of PN infusion is determined based on the weight and physical and metabolic condition of the foal. The general protocol is based on the assumption that sick foals expend approximately 50 kcal/kg body weight per day (basal rate).[22] The PN is started at half the basal rate for 12 hours, increasing to the basal rate over 24 to 48 hours, and then in some foals increased slowly to 75 kcal/kg/d if tolerated by the foal. The clinical condition of the foal is assessed frequently. Blood glucose concentrations should be measured every 6 to 8 hours during the introduction and weaning of PN until the blood glucose concentration is stabilized. Insulin can be administered during hyperglycemic crises ($\gg$250 mg/dL) at a dose of 0.1 to 0.4 U/kg regular insulin intramuscularly, but this is rarely needed. When a constant rate of PN is achieved, glucose concentrations should be measured every 8 to 12 hours, depending on the clinical condition of the foal. Foals are weaned off the PN as their clinical condition improves, and enteral feeding is gradually increased. The rate of PN is halved every 4 to 12 hours if blood glucose concentration is stable until half the basal rate is obtained, at which time the infusion is discontinued if the foal is bright, alert, and nursing well.

PN is supplemented with isotonic fluid therapy administered intravenously. The fluid rate and composition are determined based on clinical condition, packed cell volume, total protein, and serum electrolyte concentrations (Na, Cl, Ca, K and HCO_3). The composition and rate are adjusted to maintain normal hydration and electrolyte and acid–base status. During the period that foals receive PN, enteral feeding is initially withdrawn, and the foals are muzzled or separated from the mare. Beginning 24 hours after the institution of PN, 20 to 40 mL of mare's milk ("trophic" feeding) is administered enterally every 4 hours. The trophic feeding provides nutrition to enterocytes and stimulates production of lactase in the small intestine in preparation for resumption of enteral feeding. As the foals are weaned off the PN, enteral feedings are gradually increased from small trophic feeding every 4 hours to allowing the foal to nurse from the mare for 2 to 5 minutes every 2 hours and eventually unrestricted nursing from the mare.

Antimicrobial Treatment

Normal newborns are at risk of acquiring life-threatening bacterial infections, and the risk increases when they do not ingest adequate colostrum in a timely fashion or are subjected to environmental stresses (see the discussion on neonatal infection). Newborns in which bacterial infection is suspected and those at high risk of developing an infection, such as sick newborns with FTPI, should be administered antimicrobials. Antimicrobial therapy should not be delayed pending the results of bacterial culture and antimicrobial sensitivity testing.

The choice of antimicrobial is determined by the likely infecting agent and clinical experience with antimicrobial susceptibility of local strains of pathogens. In general, broad-spectrum antimicrobials are chosen because it is almost impossible to predict, based on clinical signs, the nature of the infecting agent and its antimicrobial susceptibility. Although *Streptococcus* spp. were historically reported to be the cause of most infections in neonatal foals, currently infections of neonatal foals are usually a result of gram-negative organisms, including *E. coli*, *Klebsiella* spp., and *Salmonella* spp. Because of the wide variety of infecting agents and their varying antimicrobial susceptibility, it is possible to make only general recommendations for antimicrobial therapy of neonates. A frequently used antimicrobial regimen is an aminoglycoside (gentamicin or, more commonly, amikacin) and penicillin. Some commonly used drugs and their doses are listed in Table 19-7. Dosage of antimicrobials in foals differs somewhat from that of adults, and the pharmacokinetics of drugs in normal foals are often different from those of the same drug in sick foals. Consequently, higher dosages administered at prolonged intervals are often indicated in sick foals, especially when concentration-dependent drugs such as the aminoglycosides are used.

The response to antimicrobial therapy should be monitored, using physical examination and clinical pathology data, on at least a daily basis. Failure to improve should prompt a reconsideration of the therapy within 48 to 72 hours, and a worsening of the newborn's condition may necessitate changing the antimicrobial sooner than that. The decision to change antimicrobial therapy should be guided, but not determined, by the results of antimicrobial sensitivity testing of isolates from the affected newborn. These antimicrobial susceptibility patterns should be determined locally because the results can vary geographically, although results of studies are published.[23,24] The utility of antimicrobial sensitivity testing in determining optimal antimicrobial therapy for foals has not been determined, although it is likely that, as with mastitis in cows, sensitivity to antimicrobials determined by the Kirby–Bauer method will not be useful in predicting efficacy.

Fluid Therapy

Fluid therapy of newborns differs from that of adult animals because of important differences in fluid and electrolyte metabolism in newborns. The following guidelines are suggested:

- **Septic shock**—sequential boluses of 20 mL/kg delivered over 5 to 20 minutes with reevaluation after each bolus. Usually, 60 to 80 mL/kg is the maximum dose before use of pharmacologic support of blood pressure is considered. Care should be taken to avoid fluid overload, and the foal should be reevaluated after each bolus and the need for continued fluid therapy determined. Continuous infusion of fluid is not indicated.
- **Maintenance support**—this should be determined based on the ongoing losses and the clinical status of the animal. However, general recommendations are as follows:
  - First 10 kg of body weight—100 mL/kg/d
  - Second 10 kg of body weight—50 mL/kg/d

Table 19-7 Antimicrobials used in neonatal foals

Antimicrobial	Dose and route	Frequency	Comments
Amikacin sulfate	25 mg/kg, IM or IV	24 h	Excellent Gram-negative activity, potentially nephrotoxic. Use with a penicillin.
Amoxicillin trihydrate	25 mg/kg, PO	6–8 h	Variable absorption decreasing with age. Limited Gram negative spectrum.
Amoxicillin–clavulanate	15–25 mg/kg, IV	6–8 h	Enhanced Gram-negative spectrum.
Amoxicillin sodium	15–30 mg/kg, IV or IM	6–8 h	Limited Gram-negative spectrum. Use with an aminoglycoside. Safe.
Ampicillin sodium	10–20 mg/kg, IV or IM	6–8 h	Limited Gram-negative spectrum. Use with an aminoglycoside. Safe.
Ampicillin trihydrate	20 mg/kg, PO	6–8 h	Limited Gram-negative spectrum. Variable absorption decreasing with age.
Cefotaxime sodium	15–25 mg/kg, IV	6–8 h	Use for bacterial meningitis. Expensive.
Cefoperazone sodium	20–30 mg/kg, IV	6–8 h	Use for *Pseudomonas* spp. infections.
Cefpodoxime proxetil	10 mg/kg PO	8–12 h	Broad spectrum and well absorbed by foals after oral administration.
Ceftazidime sodium	20–50 mg/kg, IV	6–8 h	Third-generation cephalosporin. Save for refractory infections.
Ceftiofur sodium	10 mg/kg, IV over 15 min	6 h	Broad spectrum. Note higher dose than used in adults.
Chloramphenicol palmitate	50 mg/kg, PO	6–8 h	Broad spectrum, bacteriostatic. Human health risk. Restricted use.
Chloramphenicol sodium succinate	50 mg/kg, IV	6–8 h	Broad spectrum, bacteriostatic. Human health risk. Restricted use.
Ciprofloxacin	5 mg/kg, IV	12 h	Broad spectrum. Potentially toxic to developing cartilage.
Enrofloxacin	5–7.5 mg/kg, PO or IV	12–24 h	Broad spectrum. Potentially toxic to developing cartilage.
Gentamicin sulfate	12 mg/kg, IV or IM	36 h	Good Gram-negative spectrum. Nephrotoxic. Use with a penicillin. Dose should be decreased to 6.6 mg/kg IV or IM every 24 hours for foals > 2 weeks of age.
Metronidazole	15–25 mg/kg, IV or PO	8–12 h	Active against obligate anaerobes and protozoa only.
Oxytetracycline	5 mg/kg, IV	12 h	Variable Gram-negative activity. Safe. Cheap. High and prolonged dose protocols have the potential to result in discoloration of the teeth.
Procaine penicillin G	20,000–40,000 IU/kg, IM	12 h	Very limited Gram-negative activity. Muscle soreness. Cheap.
Sodium or potassium penicillin G	20,000–40,000 IU/kg, IV or IM	6 h	Limited Gram-negative activity. Use with an aminoglycoside.
Pivampicillin	15–30 mg/kg, IV or IM	8 h	Ampicillin prodrug.
Ticarcillin sodium	50 mg/kg, IV	6 h	Active against Gram-negative organisms. Expensive.
Ticarcillin-clavulanate	50 mg ticarcillin/kg, IV	6 h	Extended activity. Expensive.
Trimethoprim-sulfonamide	15–30 mg/kg, PO, IV	12 h	Cheap. Broad spectrum. Limited efficacy in treating septicemia in foals.

- Weight in excess of 20 kg—25 mL/kg/d

Neonates with high ongoing losses, such as those with diarrhea or gastric reflux, can have higher fluid requirements.

Care should be taken to prevent administration of **excess sodium** to foals because they have a limited ability to excrete sodium. The recommended intake is 2 to 3 mEq/kg/d, and this includes sodium administered in parenteral fluids. One liter of isotonic sodium chloride provides a 50-kg foal's sodium requirements for 1 day.

A suitable maintenance fluid for foals is isotonic dextrose (5%) with supplemental potassium (10 to 40 mEq/L).

Respiratory Support

Respiratory failure, evidenced by elevated arterial Pco_2 and decreased Po_2, may be a result of depressed central activity, weakness of respiratory muscles, or lung disease. Regardless of the cause, should the hypoxemia become sufficiently severe, oxygenation must be improved by increasing respiratory drive, increasing the inspired oxygen tension, or employing mechanical ventilation. Foals should always be maintained in sternal recumbency to allow optimal respiratory function.

Provision of respiratory support should be considered when the arterial Po_2 is less than 60 mm Hg (8 kPa) and the arterial Pco_2 is more than 60 mm Hg (8 kPa) in a foal in sternal recumbency. Pharmacologic respiratory stimulants have only a very short duration of action and are of limited use. Nasal insufflation of oxygen is achieved by placing a nasopharyngeal tube and providing oxygen at a rate of 5 L/min.

Mechanical ventilation is useful for maintaining oxygenation in foals with botulism, with more than 80% of foals surviving in one small study. However, this intervention requires considerable expertise and sophisticated equipment. The prognosis is much worse for foals with diseases of the lungs that require mechanical ventilation.

Gastroduodenal Ulcer Prophylaxis

Ill neonatal foals are often treated with antacid drugs in an attempt to prevent the development or progression of gastroduodenal ulcers, although the efficacy of this approach is unproven. There is a trend toward not administering antiulcer medications to foals except for those with demonstrated gastric ulceration, in part because of the recognition that critically ill foals often have gastric pH above 7.0, and administration of ranitidine does not affect this pH. (See "Gastric Ulcers in Foals" for further discussion.)

COMMON COMPLICATIONS

Complications of the neonate's disease or its treatment occur frequently:

- Entropion is common in critically ill foals and, although readily treated, can cause corneal ulceration if undetected.
- Aspiration pneumonia occurs in weak foals, often as a result of aggressive bottle feeding or regurgitation of milk around a nasogastric tube.
- Nosocomial infections can be severe and life-threatening and are best prevented by strict hygiene and asepsis.
- Septic synovitis/arthritis occurs as a consequence of bacteremia and should be treated aggressively.
- Omphalitis and omphalophlebitis occur and can be an undetected cause of fever and relapse. These are best detected by ultrasonographic examination of the abdomen.
- Patent urachus, evident as urine at the navel, usually resolves with time and local treatment.
- Uroperitoneum as a result of urachal rupture occurs in critically ill foals and should be suspected in any ill foal that develops abdominal distension.
- Angular limb deformities and excessive flexor tendon laxity occur frequently in ill neonatal foals but usually resolve with minimal symptomatic treatment as the foal recovers its strength.

PROGNOSIS

The prognosis for critically ill neonates depends on many factors, including the nature and severity of the disease, facilities available for care, and the expertise of the personnel caring for the neonate. There is a consensus that the recovery rate for severely ill foals has improved over the last decade because of provision of better care. There are reports of survival rates of around 80% for foals treated at a specialized intensive care unit. However, the high cost of providing care for these animals has prompted studies to determine outcome, as a means of deciding whether, financially, treatment is warranted. Surviving Thoroughbred foals do not differ from siblings with regard to percentage of starters, percentage of winners, or number of starts, but surviving foals achieve significantly fewer wins and total earnings.[25]

The increased number of foals being treated intensively has resulted in prospective studies of outcome. The prognosis for athletic activity for foals with septic arthritis is poor. Thoroughbred foals with **septic arthritis** have odds of 0.28 (95% CI 0.12 to 0.62; roughly one-quarter of the likelihood) for racing compared with a cohort of healthy foals. Multisystemic disease, in addition to the presence of septic arthritis, decreased the likelihood of racing to one-tenth that of healthy foals (OR 0.12, 95% CI 0.02 to 0.90). Affected foals that survive take almost 40% longer to race for the first time. Approximately 30% to 48% of affected Thoroughbred foals eventually race, compared with approximately 65% of normal foals.

Attempts to determine prognostic indicators for survival of foals have been partially successful, but they tend to be most applicable to the intensive care unit in which they were developed. The common theme is that sicker foals are less likely to be discharged from the hospital alive.

Characteristics of foals that are more likely to survive include ability to stand when first examined, normal birth, white blood cell (WBC) count in blood that is within or above the reference range, lack of dyspnea, normal plasma fibrinogen concentration, and short duration of disease. The odds of a hospitalized neonatal foal surviving can be calculated using the following formula:

$$\begin{aligned}&\mathit{Logit}\ (\mathit{Probability\ of\ survival})\\&\quad = -0.3072 - 2.0115\ (\mathit{Cold\ extremities})\\&\quad\quad - 0.8166\ (\mathit{Prematurity})\\&\quad\quad - 0.7685\ (\geq 2\ \mathit{Infection}/\\&\quad\quad \mathit{inflammation\ sites}) + 0.9877\ (\mathit{IgG})\\&\quad\quad + 1.1331\ (\mathit{Glucose}) + 0.9043\ (\mathit{WBC})\end{aligned}$$

In addition, the survival odds can be summarized in a much more useful form by the methods shown in Tables 19-8 and 19-9. An app to calculate survival probabilities is available for Android phones.[26]

Table 19-8 Method for calculating survival score in hospitalized neonatal foals[1]

Variables	Score	
Cold extremities	No	Yes
	2	0
Prematurity (<320 days)	No	Yes
	1	0
≥2 infection/ inflammation sites	No	Yes
	1	0
IgG (mg/dL)	<400	≥400
	0	1
Glucose (mg/dL)	<80	≥80
	0	1
WBC × ($10^3/\mu L$)	≤4	>4
	0	1
TOTAL SCORE		

Table 19-9 Probability of survival for hospitalized neonatal foals with survival scores calculated according to table 19-8

Total foal survival score	Probability of survival
0	3%
1	8%
2	18%
3	38%
4	62%
5	82%
6	92%
7	97%

FURTHER READING

Austin SM. Assessment of the equine neonate in ambulatory practice. *Equine Vet Educ.* 2013;25:585-589.

Toribio RE. Endocrine dysregulation in critically ill foals and horses. *Vet Clin North Am Equine Pract.* 2011;27:35.

REFERENCES

1. Dembek KA, et al. *PLoS ONE.* 2014;9.
2. Taylor S. *Equine Vet Educ.* 2015;27:99.
3. Weber EJ, et al. *Equine Vet J.* 2015;47:275.
4. Dicken M, et al. *N Z Vet J.* 2012;60:42.
5. Gold JR, et al. *J Vet Intern Med.* 2007;21:791.
6. Hurcombe SDA, et al. *J Vet Intern Med.* 2009;23:335.
7. Barsnick RJIM, et al. *J Vet Intern Med.* 2011;25:123.
8. Barsnick RJ, et al. *Equine Vet J.* 2014;46:45.
9. Borchers A, et al. *Equine Vet J.* 2014;46:306.
10. Toth B, et al. *J Vet Intern Med.* 2014;28:1294.
11. Himler M, et al. *Equine Vet J.* 2012;44:43.
12. Abraham M, et al. *J Vet Intern Med.* 2014;28:1580.
13. Bodaan CJ, et al. *Equine Vet Educ.* 2014;26:341.
14. Liepman R, et al. *Equine Vet J.* 2015;47:526-530.
15. Zabrecky KA, et al. *J Vet Intern Med.* 2015;29:673.
16. Castagnetti C, et al. *Theriogenology.* 2010;73:343.
17. Borchers A, et al. *Equine Vet J.* 2012;44:57.
18. Tennent-Brown B. *Vet Clin North Am Equine Pract.* 2014;30:399.
19. Pirrone A, et al. *Theriogenology.* 2012;78:1182.
20. Borchers A, et al. *Equine Vet J.* 2013;45:2.
21. Pusterla N, et al. *Vet Rec.* 2009;165:114.
22. Jose-Cunilleras E, et al. *Equine Vet J.* 2012;44:48.
23. Russell CM, et al. *Aust Vet J.* 2008;86:266.
24. Theelen MJP, et al. *Equine Vet J.* 2014;46:161.
25. Sanchez LC, et al. *J Am Vet Med Assoc.* 2008;233:1446.
26. <https://play.google.com/store/apps/details?id=edu.ohio_state.org.foalscore.foalscore>.

STILLBIRTH/PERINATAL WEAK-CALF SYNDROME

SYNOPSIS

Etiology Uncertain; probably multiple etiologies and multifactorial.

Epidemiology Most commonly several cases on a farm; several farms affected in a geographic region in a single season; problem may not occur for several years and then occur as "epidemic" in a region.

Clinical findings Calves may be born weak and unable to stand. More commonly, they are born apparently normal and stand but subsequently collapse with hypothermia and die within a few hours of birth.

Lesions Petechial hemorrhages, subcutaneous edema, and hemorrhage commonly in the subcutaneous tissue of the carpal and tarsal joints.

Diagnostic confirmation Specific to cause.

Treatment Supportive.

Control Specific to cause.

HISTORICAL ASPECTS

A syndrome of newborn calves called *weak-calf syndrome* was first recognized in Montana in 1964. It has been recognized throughout the United States and other countries since then, and it is considered a major economic loss in beef cattle herds. In the earlier descriptions of the syndrome, calves were affected by 10 days of age, and approximately 20% were affected at birth. Morbidity ranged from 6% to 15%. In some herds, sporadic abortions occurred before calving season of the herd began. In some cases, affected calves died within minutes after being born with varying degrees of obstetric assistance.

In calves that survived for a few days, clinical findings included lassitude, depression, weakness, variable body temperature, a reddened and crusty muzzle, lameness, reluctance to stand, enlargement of the carpal and tarsal joint capsules along with periarticular subcutaneous swellings, and a hunched-up back if they stood. Diarrhea occurred in some calves after a few days of illness, but it was not a major clinical finding. Treatment was ineffective, and the case fatality rates ranged from 60% to 80%.

At necropsy, the prominent lesions were hemorrhage and edema of the subcutaneous tissues over the tarsal and carpal joint regions and extending distally. Polysynovitis with hemorrhagic synovial fluid often containing fibrin was also common. Erosive and hemorrhagic lesions of the forestomaches and abomasum also occurred. Several different pathogens were isolated from these calves, but no consistent relationship between the pathogens and the lesions was ever determined.

In retrospect, the case definitions were not well described, and it is probable that several different diseases of newborn calves were lumped into the enigma of weak-calf syndrome. As more detailed clinical and laboratory examinations of sick newborn calves have been done over the years, some of the causes of the original syndrome have been identified as specific diseases of newborn calves.

Widely ranging clinical and pathologic findings have been associated with weak-calf syndrome. In the most common situation, calves are born weak and die within 10 to 20 minutes after birth; sometimes they live for up to a few days. At necropsy there are no obvious or only few lesions to account for the illness. Calves that are weak after birth because of traumatic injuries associated with dystocia or other significant lesions can be accounted for according to the nature and severity of the lesions. Reports from Northern Ireland in recent years indicate that in dairy herds the incidence of weak-calf syndrome has ranged from 10% to 20% of all calves born. Field observations in problem herds found that the gestation period is of normal duration, but parturition is usually prolonged, with the first and second stages of labor lasting 24 hours. Affected calves usually are born alive but are unable to sustain breathing following birth. Despite resuscitation efforts, they commonly die within 10 minutes, often accompanied by prominent uncoordinated movements of the limbs. Some calves are stillborn, and whether or not this is a variation of the syndrome is uncertain. In a report from the United Kingdom, the syndrome occurred in calves born from heifers and was characterized by failure to breathe at birth or breathing with difficulty, and/or failing to move after birth, and failure to suck. The term *stillbirth/perinatal weak-calf syndrome* has been suggested as more appropriate.

Dummy-Calf Syndrome

A variation of weak-calf syndrome is dummy-calf syndrome, which has been reported in the southern United States. Affected calves appear normal at birth and are generally alert, but they lack the instinct or the desire to seek the teat or suck after birth and for up to several hours later. The syndrome may occur in calves of any birth weight. The incidence has been highest in purebred Brahman females, but it has also occurred in Aberdeen Angus, Hereford, Chianina, and Brown Swiss breeds of cattle. Field observations indicate that affected calves did not stand for up to 1 to 2 hours after birth to initiate teat-seeking behavior. Dummy calves appear to lack the sensitivity to teat-seek, and if they fail to locate a teat by about 4 to 5 hours after birth, they commonly lose the sucking reflex and then require intensive nursing care by bottle feeding to initiate sucking. In calves that fail to suck and ingest colostrum, hypothermia, hypoglycemia, and neonatal infections are common complications. Concurrently, the dam loses interest in the calf and may abandon it.

ETIOLOGY AND EPIDEMIOLOGY

The etiology of weak-calf syndrome is unclear, but several epidemiologic observations have suggested some possible causes. These include the following:

- Fetal infection near term
- Underdevelopment because of nutritional inadequacy of the maternal diet during pregnancy
- Placental insufficiency
- Maternal dietary deficiencies of selenium and vitamin E
- Hypothyroidism
- Traumatic injuries associated with dystocia and excessive force during obstetric assistance
- Fetal hypoxia from prolonged parturition

Fetal Infections

Fetal infections in the last few days before term can result in stillbirth or weak calves that may die within hours or days after birth. In one series of 293 weak calves in Northern Ireland, **leptospiral infection** was present in 25% of the calves. Calves in which leptospiral antigen was detected in the placenta were significantly lighter by an average of 6 kg to 10 kg than calves with no antigen in the placenta. Calves infected with *Leptospira* in utero were more likely to be infected by *T.* (formerly *Arcanobacterium) pyogenes* or *Bacillus* species, and infection of the placenta is associated with a lower body weight. The adrenal gland, lung, and placenta are the most useful tissues to examine for leptospiral antigen.

Bovine viral diarrhea (BVD) virus infection has been identified in several herds with high occurrence rates of weak-calf syndrome. Effects of intrauterine infection with this virus will depend on the stage of pregnancy at which infection occurs, but birth of stillborn, weak, or dummy calves certainly warrants taking this differential into consideration (see also "Bovine Viral Diarrhea").

An unidentified type of adenovirus has been associated with weak-calf syndrome on a large dairy farm in Israel. At birth the calves were reluctant to suck or drink colostrum and were force-fed colostrum with an orogastric tube. Affected calves were weak at birth and unable to rise without assistance; when forced to move they walked stiffly, suggestive of polyarthritis. An adenovirus was detected in the feces, synovial fluid, and aqueous humor of affected calves.

Maternal Nutritional Deficiency Causing Fetal Underdevelopment

Hypothyroidism as a result of iodine deficiency in the pregnant dam has been considered on the basis of thyroid hyperplasia in some calves. Analysis of the laboratory data from 365 calves that died from the stillbirth/perinatal weak-calf syndrome in Ireland found some differences between calves with abnormal versus normal thyroid glands. Glands weighing more than 30 g were probably abnormal. Abnormal glands were heavier, constituted a greater percentage of the calf's body weight, and had a lower iodine concentration. A higher proportion of calves with an abnormal thyroid gland had uninflated lungs and pneumonia. Abnormal thyroid glands had a lower selenium concentration in the kidneys.

Hypothyroidism as a result of iodine deficiency can be caused by either inadequate dietary iodine supply or the presence of goitrogens in feed. Goitrogens are substances that impair thyroid hormone synthesis, either by inhibiting iodine uptake (cyanogenic goitrogens) or by inhibiting organic binding of iodine by the thyroid glands (goitrogens of the thiouracil type).[1]

However, the experimental reproduction of iodine deficiency in pregnant heifers by feeding an iodine-deficient diet over the last 4 to 5 months of pregnancy resulted in clinicopathologic changes and pathologic changes in the thyroid glands of both the heifers and their calves, but all calves in the iodine-deficient group were born clinically normal.

Because selenium plays a role in the function of the thyroid glands, selenium deficiency can cause hypothyroidism despite adequate dietary iodine supply. **Maternal dietary deficiency of selenium** in pregnant cattle has also been examined, but field trials have failed to show any protective effect from the parenteral administration of pregnant cattle with selenium. The parenteral administration of both selenium and iodine to pregnant cattle did not have any effect on the incidence of the syndrome between treated and untreated herds; the incidences were 7.9% and 7.4%, respectively.

A general nutritional inadequacy in the maternal diet can result in underdevelopment of the fetus and the birth of smaller-than-normal calves, but the deficiency usually must be grossly inadequate. A clinical trial showed that feeding a protein-restricted ration (7% crude protein) during the last trimester of pregnancy resulted in 11.4% lower birth weights than in control animals and in compromised thermogenic ability of the newborn calves, which has been proposed as a contributing factor to perinatal mortality of calves.[2] Another study reported a selective decrease in absorption of colostral IgG_1 and IgG_2 from the gut in calves from heifers fed protein-deficient diets during the last trimester of pregnancy, which implies a higher risk for FTPI in these calves.[3]

Placental Insufficiency

Intrauterine growth retardation associated with feto-placental dysfunction has been described in Japanese Black beef calves.[4] Affected calves were weak when born at term and were underweight compared with normal calves. Anemia as a result of bone marrow dysfunction was present in affected calves and presumably was associated with intrauterine growth retardation. Thymic hypoplasia is another common finding in Japanese Black calves that died during the perinatal period, which also has been attributed to intrauterine growth retardation and is thought to contribute to perinatal weak-calf syndrome, which has a high occurrence rate in this breed.[4,5] There is some evidence that an immune inadequacy based on T-lymphocyte function may be associated with weak-calf syndrome in Japanese Black calves, which could be related to the thymic hypoplasia because the thymus is the site of T-cell maturation.

Dams delivering weak calves also had lower serum concentrations of estrone sulfate during late pregnancy than those of normal calves, suggesting a feto-placental dysfunction. The dysfunction was influenced by sires and maternal families.

Fetal Hypoxemia

Fetal hypoxemia resulting from prolonged parturition or dystocia may be a cause or contributing factor to weak-calf syndrome. Various predisposing factors can cause prolonged interference with fetal blood or oxygen supply, which can result in death during delivery or shortly after.

Examination of blood-gas values in newborn calves has shown that a prolonged parturition or delivery terminated by forced extraction results in a severe acidemia as a result of oxygen deprivation and ensuing anaerobic glycolysis with lactate accumulation in combination with hypercapnia, resulting in respiratory acidosis. As blood pH drops, first vitality is reduced, subsequently vital organs such as the brain are damaged, and ultimately the fetus dies.

The bovine fetus appears relatively susceptible to hypoxia and hypercapnia, which has been studied experimentally by clamping the umbilical cords of fetuses for 4 to 8 minutes, at 24 to 48 hours before expected birth, followed by a cesarean section 30 to 40 minutes later. Calves born following this procedure may die in 10 to 15 minutes after birth or survive for only up to 2 days. Under these experimental conditions, fetuses can survive anoxia for 4 minutes, but most will die following 6 or 8 minutes of anoxia.[6] During the clamping there is also increased fetal movement and a release of meconium that stains the calf and the amniotic fluid. Those that survive for a few hours or days are dull and depressed, cannot stand, and have poor sucking and swallowing reflexes, and their temperatures are usually subnormal. They respond poorly to supportive therapy. Some calves whose umbilical cords were clamped for 4 minutes were born weak and made repeated efforts to raise their heads and move onto the sternum, but they were unable to maintain an upright position for long. These calves become hypothermic and dull, and their sucking and swallowing reflexes are present but weak. These calves are usually too weak to suck the cow even when assisted, and they commonly develop diarrhea and other complications.

Dystocia and Traumatic Injuries at Birth

Over 50% of perinatal mortality is generally attributed to dystocia, and dystocia may be an important contributing factor to weak-calf syndrome because of fetal hypoxia or traumatic injuries associated with obstetric assistance.[7] In a study of 13,296 calvings over a period of 15 years in two research herds in Montana, calf mortality as a result of dystocia accounted for the single largest loss category through the first 96 hours postpartum. Reported ORs vary widely (2.7 to 14.6), but they suggest that calves requiring assisted delivery had a 2.7 to 14.6 higher risk of death in the perinatal period than spontaneously born calves.[8] At necropsy of the calves that died as a result of dystocia, the findings included a froth-filled trachea, nonfunctional lungs, bruises, contusions, hemorrhages, bone fractures, and joint dislocations. It was concluded that the provision of adequate obstetric assistance at the right time could have reduced the mortality associated with dystocia.

Traumatic injuries of calves at birth are caused primarily by the mechanical influence of traction during delivery and can result in asphyxia and a high perinatal mortality rate. Excessive traction is the most important cause of rib and vertebral fractures in the calf during dystocia. A series of 235 calves that died perinatally were examined by necropsy to determine the possible causes of death related to dystocia. Most of the parturitions were protracted and needed veterinary assistance, and 58% of the calves had pathologic evidence of asphyxia. Calves delivered by extraction had pathologic evidence of asphyxia more often than those born unassisted or delivered by cesarean section. Intrapulmonary amniotic material may be present in the lungs, representing evidence of perinatal respiratory distress. The aspiration of small amounts of amniotic fluid with or without meconium is common in calves and is not associated with hypoxemia, respiratory acidosis, or failure of passive transfer.

Premature Expulsion of Placenta

Premature expulsion of the placenta has been associated with perinatal calf mortality. Field observations indicate that the majority of affected fetuses die of fetal hypoxia during stage 2 of calving. The most significant risk factor associated with premature expulsion of the placenta was fetal malpresentation and malposture. Prolongation of the second stage of parturition allows for sufficient detachment of the placenta for it to occupy the posterior part of the genital tract. The placenta is frequently expelled together with the calf. In one series of cases, there was no significant relationship between the occurrence of premature expulsion of the placenta and parity, calving difficulty, previous calving history, or sex of the calf.

NECROPSY FINDINGS

All calves that die should be examined by necropsy to identify possible causes. It is important to establish if there is one disease complex or several different diseases of newborn calves.

In the weak-calf syndrome described in Northern Ireland, at necropsy many calves had petechial hemorrhages in the thymus gland, on the ventricular epicardium, and in the parietal pleura and endocardium. These lesions were similar to those present in animals that died of acute terminal asphyxiation. The gasps made in response to asphyxia in utero result in amniotic fluid being inhaled into the respiratory tract. In one study, 84% of stillborn calves had these lesions of asphyxia. It is well established that asphyxiation during birth is a major factor in intrapartum stillbirth in piglets and contributes to early postnatal mortality. Froth may be present in the caudal trachea of some calves that die within 10 to 20 minutes after birth.

Varying degrees of subcutaneous edema of the head and/or bruising of the rib cage are also common. Fractures of the ribs are common, accompanied by intrathoracic hemorrhage. Vertebral body fractures occur commonly at the thoracolumbar region and may be accompanied by intraabdominal hemorrhage. The lungs may be inflated normally, partially inflated, or not inflated. Severe bruising and hemorrhage occur around the costochondral junctions, at the sternal extremities of the costal cartilages, and over the sternum and shoulder regions. In some cases, the traumatic lesions are severe and may involve primarily the right side of the rib cage. Severe subcutaneous hemorrhage and edema may be present over the carpal and fetlock joints as a result of the pressure applied by the obstetric chains or ropes.

In the syndrome described in the United States, the lesions either appeared at birth or developed in the first few weeks of life. At necropsy the prominent lesions are marked edema and hemorrhages of the subcutaneous tissues over the carpal and tarsal joints and extending distally down the limbs. The synovial fluid may be tinged with blood and contain fibrinous deposits. Erosions or ulceration of the gastrointestinal tract, petechial hemorrhage of internal organs, involution of the thymus gland, and hemorrhages in skeletal muscle have also been present.

The weak-calf syndrome described in Japanese Black calves was associated with atrophy of the red bone marrow and thymic hypoplasia.[9] Degeneration of brainstem nerve cells, attributed to protracted hypoxia, was also noticed.

Samples for confirmation of diagnosis include the following:

- Bacteriology—fetal liver, lung, stomach content, adrenal gland; placenta (culture); special detection techniques for *Leptospira* antigens
- Histology—fixed placenta, lung, spleen, brain, liver, kidney; maternal caruncle (light microscopy, Immunohistochemistry)

DIFFERENTIAL DIAGNOSIS

Determination of the cause of weak-calf syndrome in a herd is often difficult because the limits of the case definition cannot be determined. Several risk factors may interact to contribute to the disease. The most common definition is a calf that is alive at birth, appears normal otherwise, but either fails to breathe or breathes for less than approximately 10 minutes and then dies. If they survive for several hours or a few days, affected calves are usually in sternal recumbency, depressed, reluctant to stand unassisted, reluctant to walk, and not interested in sucking. They may not respond favorably to supportive therapy.

Case definition

When an epidemic of the disease is encountered, an epidemiologic investigation of the herd is necessary in an attempt to identify possible risk factors.

The patterns of occurrence should be determined:

- Is the problem more common in calves born to heifers than cows? In some situations, the owner may provide more surveillance for the calving heifers and less for the mature cows, with a consequent greater incidence of weak calves born from the cows.
- Is there any evidence that parturition is prolonged in the heifers or the cows? If so, what are the possible reasons?
- How long are heifers and cows in the herd allowed to calve unassisted before obstetric assistance is provided?
- Is it possible that some nutritional, management, or environmental factor is interfering with normal parturition?
- Is the condition more common in male or female calves, and what are the relative birth weights?
- How soon after birth are the calves affected?
- What is the course of the illness after the first clinical abnormalities are noted?
- Is the serologic herd status regarding specific infectious diseases known (e.g., *leptospirosis*, BVD, bluetongue)?
- The veterinarian should make every effort to clinically examine a representative number of affected calves.

TREATMENT

Calves born weak, unable to stand, lacking the instinct to seek the teat, or lacking a suck reflex need intensive care, including force-feeding of colostrum and the provision of warm surroundings to prevent hypothermia and other complications. Affected calves must be assisted to suck the dam normally. Bottle feeding for a few days may be necessary until the calf becomes strong enough to suck the dam on its own.

CONTROL AND PREVENTION

Control and prevention of weak-calf syndrome is based on empirical observations, beginning with insuring **adequate nutrition of the dam** to avoid any possible nutritional factors affecting neonatal calf vitality. The provision of **adequate surveillance at calving time** and competent obstetric assistance when necessary is also crucial to avoid prolonged parturition and fetal hypoxia in calves.

When epidemics of the disease are occurring, the surveillance of calving must be intensified, and it may be necessary to intervene with obstetric assistance earlier than usual. Determination of the cause may require that the veterinarian attend several calvings, make detailed clinical examinations of the length of parturition, and observe the parturition process and the health of the calves at birth.

FURTHER READING

Mee JF. The role of micronutrients in bovine periparturient problems. *Cattle Pract.* 2004;12:95-108.

Meijering A. Dystocia and stillbirth in cattle—a review of causes, relations and implications. *Livest Sci.* 1984;11:143-177.

Randall GCB. Perinatal mortality: some problems of adaptation at birth. *Adv Vet Sci Comp Med.* 1978;22:53-81.

REFERENCES

1. Tripathi MK, et al. *Anim Feed Sci Tech.* 2007;132:1-27.
2. Cartsens GE, et al. *J Anim Sci.* 1987;65:745-751.
3. Blecha F, et al. *J Anim Sci.* 1981;53:1174-1180.
4. Uematsu M, et al. *Vet J.* 2013;198:212-216.
5. Takasu M, et al. *J Vet Med Sci.* 2008;70:1173-1177.
6. Dufty JH, et al. *Aust Vet J.* 1977;53:262-267.
7. Mee JF, et al. *Vet J.* 2014;199:19-23.
8. Mee JF, et al. *Animal.* 2008;2:613-620.
9. Ogata Y, et al. *J Vet Med A.* 1999;46:327-334.

DISEASES OF CLONED OFFSPRING

The successful cloning of domestic animals using somatic-cell nuclear transfer has resulted in birth of offspring with a high frequency of clinical abnormalities. Cloning of livestock and horses is achieved by transfer of nuclear material from the cell of an adult animal to the enucleated egg of an animal of the same species (somatic-cell nuclear transfer), with subsequent implantation of the resulting embryo in a surrogate dam and birth of a live, viable offspring. However, the use of nuclear material from somatic cells of adult animals, and from fetal cells, frequently does not result in normal development of the embryo and placenta.

The abnormal development in cloned embryos is a consequence of altered methylation of the genome in transferred nuclear material. This applies particularly for imprinted genes, which are those genes for which only one copy is expressed in the embryo, compared with nonimprinted genes for which both parental copies of the gene are expressed. The lower frequency of expression of imprinted genes (i.e., only one copy, paternal or maternal) is a result of methylation of DNA or chromatin proteins that makes the DNA inaccessible for transcription.[1] Imprinting is a form of epigenetic control of gene expression. To date, 132 imprinted genes have been identified in mice, but only 25, 21, and 14 in cattle, pigs, and sheep, respectively.[1] Imprinted genes encode proteins involved in regulation of many cell processes, including embryonic and neonatal growth and development.[1,2]

In normal reproduction, the paternal genome is demethylated during passage through the oocyte and fusion with the maternal genome. Consequently, the methylation marks of the two genomes (paternal and maternal) are different at the end of the cleavage process. Transfer of somatic nuclear material into an enucleated oocyte results in exposure of both genomes to the active demethylating process in the cytoplasm of the oocyte and uniform or variable demethylation of both genomes. The loss of these parent-specific epigenetic markers results in widespread dysregulation of imprinted genes and subsequent abnormalities in the placenta, fetus, and newborn. Imprinting marks (methylation) are erased during early development, and reprogramming of somatic-cell nuclei used in cloning and these abnormalities in epigenetic control of expression of imprinted genes result in biallelic expression of imprinted genes.[3] The loss of epigenetic control of imprinted genes causes at least some of the abnormalities common in cloned ruminants, including large-offspring syndrome (LOS).[3]

A small proportion of transferred blastocysts develop in viable animals. For cattle, of 134 recipients that received blastocysts, 50 were pregnant 40 days after blastocyst transfer, and 23 had full-term pregnancies. For all species studied, fewer than 3% of cloned embryos result in birth of viable animals. Abnormalities in the placenta and newborn cloned animals are reported for cattle and sheep, but are less frequently reported, if at all, for pigs and equids (horses and mules). Factors influencing the risks of abnormalities in newborns include the source of the nuclear material, type of in vitro culture media, coculture with somatic cells, hormonal treatments, and manipulation of the embryo.[1,4] The frequency of birth of live animals born after somatic-cell nuclear transfer from well-differentiated tissue (e.g., fibroblasts) or fetal somatic cells is lower than after nuclear transfer from embryonic cells (7%, 15%, and 34%, respectively).

The cause of placental, fetal, and neonatal abnormalities is abnormal expression of imprinted genes as a consequence of transfer of nuclear material from differentiated somatic cells,[5] conditions and media used for maintenance and culture of cytoplasts and blastocysts, and techniques used for handling cells.[3,6-8] The key abnormality is loss of methylation of imprinted genes contributed by each parent, with subsequent biallelic expression of these genes. There is debate about which epigenetic or genetic abnormalities underlay the development of placental and fetal abnormalities. Aberrant hypomethylation of IGF-2 and CDKC1C genes has been identified in calves with LOS and results in biallelic expression in the liver and placenta of affected animals.[1] Abnormalities in embryologic development of vasculature is identifiable early during embryogenesis in calves and might be the defect underlying pulmonary, circulatory, and umbilical abnormalities in cloned calves.[9] Furthermore, there is decreased expression of genes in the lungs of cloned goats that do not survive compared with those of healthy kids. Compared with normal goats of the same age from conventional reproduction, expression of 13 genes (BMP4, FGF10, GHR, HGFR, PDGFR, RABP, VEGF, H19, CDKNIC, PCAF, MeCP2, HDAC1, and Dnmt3b) decreased in transgenic cloned goats that died at or shortly after birth.[6] Expression of eight genes (FGF10, PDGFR, RABP, VEGF, PCAF, HDAC1, MeCP2, and Dnmt3b) decreased in fetal death of transgenic cloned goats.[6] A comprehensive list of genes known to be involved in embryogenesis and fetal and placental growth and a description of the effect of decreased expression of these genes are available.[10]

Clinical findings in cloned calves and lambs include abortion, placental abnormalities, large birth size, poor extrauterine viability, respiratory disease, cardiovascular abnormalities, and neurologic disease compatible with neonatal encephalopathy. LOS is confined to ruminants and is characterized by overgrowth, evident as abnormally high birth weight, enlarged tongue, umbilical hernias, and hyporglycemia.[3] Abortion occurs after day 90 of gestation in 30% to 50% of pregnancies in cattle, resulting from transfer blastocysts containing transferred nuclear material. Abnormalities, including hydroallantois, are present in approximately 25% of advanced pregnancies. **Placental abnormalities** include hydroallantois, a reduction in the number of placentomes (from a normal value of approximately 100 to as few as 26 to 70 in cloned calves), abnormally large placentomes (140 g in cloned calves versus 33 g in conventional calves), and edema of the placenta.[10] Maternal retention of the placenta is common and occurs in most cows. Duration of gestation is probably longer in cloned calves, although the frequent delivery of cloned calves by cesarean section makes assessment of gestational duration difficult. Cloned calves are heavier than conventional calves, often by as much as 25%, a well-recognized part of the **large-offspring syndrome** that affects calves born as a result of reproductive manipulation, including in vitro fertilization. Viability of cloned calves that are born alive (commonly by cesarean section) is less than that of conventional calves; only approximately two-thirds of cloned calves born alive survive more than 1 month, although others have reported better survival. Similar results are reported for horses.

A high proportion of cloned calves have **clinically detectable abnormalities** at or soon after birth, including sepsis, neonatal encephalopathy, respiratory failure, umbilical abnormalities, anemia, flexure contracture, abdominal distension, and renal dysfunction. Respiratory failure is a common finding and might reflect persistent fetal circulation or inadequate surfactant production, as evidenced by the high pulmonary artery pressures and signs consistent with patent ductus arteriosus.[11] Left heart failure, which can also cause pulmonary hypertension, is reported in cloned calves. Umbilical abnormalities are evident as abnormal umbilical cord structure (multiple arteries and veins) and large size, with a high risk of hemorrhage from the umbilical cord after birth. Cloned calves have higher body temperatures than do conventional calves.

Of 27 cloned calves delivered alive, 7 were bradypneic or apneic at birth, 5 had flexural limb deformities, and at least 23 had enlarged umbilical cords. The calves were acidotic at birth as a result of both respiratory and lactic acidosis. Calves had normocytic hypochromic anemia, stress leukogram (leukocytosis, neutrophilia, and lymphopenia), and hypoproteinemia (with both hypoalbuminemia and hypoglobulinemia) and had increased serum creatinine concentration.[12] Three of the calves did not develop other clinical signs and were considered healthy after birth, whereas 22 had at least one important clinical abnormality detected during the week after birth. Twelve of the calves developed omphalitis. Fourteen of the calves died or were euthanised.[12]

Hematologic abnormalities include anemia and decreased mean corpuscular volume. Biochemical abnormalities include hypoxemia, azotemia, and hypoglycemia. Plasma leptin and IGF-2 concentrations are higher, and thyroxine lower, in cloned calves. Serum cortisol and adrenocorticotropic hormone (ACTH) stimulation tests do not differ between cloned and conventional calves. Cloned calves can mount normal immune responses.[13] Failure of transfer of passive immunity can occur if calves are unable to suckle or are not administered colostrum or plasma.[12]

Necropsy examination reveals placentomegaly, presence of excess pleural and peritoneal fluid, hepatomegaly, interstitial pneumonia or pulmonary consolidation and alveolar proteinosis, right ventricular dilation, and hepatocellular vacuolation.

Treatment is supportive and directed toward correcting hypoxemia and providing nutritional, fluid, and environmental support (see earlier discussion).

There are currently no recognized methods for preventing these abnormalities, but incremental improvements in methodology and culture techniques will continue to result in fewer cloned offspring with these abnormalities.

FURTHER READING

Hill JR. Incidence of abnormal offspring from cloning and other assisted reproductive technologies. *Annu Rev Anim Biosci*. 2014;2:307-321.

O'Doherty AM, et al. Genomic imprinting effects on complex traits in domesticated animal species. *Front Genet*. 2015;6:156.

Smith LC, et al. Developmental and epigenetic anomalies in cloned cattle. *Reprod Domest Anim*. 2012;47:107-114.

REFERENCES

1. O'Doherty AM, et al. *Front Genet*. 2015;6:156.
2. Tian X. *Annu Rev Anim Biosci*. 2014;2:23.
3. Smith LC, et al. *Reprod Domest Anim*. 2012;47:107.
4. Hill JR. *Annu Rev Anim Biosci*. 2014;2:307.
5. Liu J, et al. *Reprod Domest Anim*. 2013;48:660.
6. Meng L, et al. *Theriogenology*. 2014;81:459.
7. Smith LC, et al. *Anim Reprod*. 2010;7:197.
8. Su J, et al. *Livest Sci*. 2011;141:24.
9. Maiorka PC, et al. *PLoS ONE*. 2015;10:e0106663.
10. Palmieri C, et al. *Vet Pathol*. 2008;45:865.
11. Brisville AC, et al. *J Vet Intern Med*. 2011;25:373.
12. Brisville AC, et al. *J Vet Intern Med*. 2013;27:1218.
13. Chavatte-Palmer PM, et al. *Cloning Stem Cells*. 2009;11:309.

EQUINE NEONATAL MALADJUSTMENT SYNDROME (NEONATAL ENCEPHALOPATHY, DUMMY FOAL, BARKERS, AND WANDERERS)

This is a syndrome of foals less than 36 hours of age characterized by a spectrum of changes in mentation ranging from failure to suckle, abnormal behavior, and seizures through coma in otherwise apparently healthy foals. The syndrome is defined by the clinical abnormalities and not by a common etiology.

ETIOLOGY

The clinical signs associated with this syndrome can be produced by a number of diseases, each of which has its particular etiology. Diseases that contribute to this syndrome include antenatal, natal, or postnatal hypoxia;[1] a range of congenital abnormalities (hydrocephalus, hydrencephalus,[2] and such); metabolic disorders;[3] placental abnormalities;[4] intracranial hemorrhage; prematurity; and thoracic trauma. Fetal or perinatal hypoxia has achieved some prominence as a cause of neonatal maladjustment syndrome in the absence of consistent demonstration of lesions of hypoxia on histopathologic examination of foals. There are isolated cases in which histologic evidence of hypoxia exists, but these are the exception rather than the rule. Finally, most foals with neonatal maladjustment syndrome improve rapidly and completely recover within several days—a clinical course not expected with neonatal or perinatal asphyxia in other species.

Recent evidence implicates a role of neuroactive progestagen derivatives in the etiopathogenesis of neonatal maladjustment syndrome.[5,6] Plasma concentrations of these neuroactive steroids in foals are high immediately after birth and decline rapidly in healthy foals, but not in foals with neonatal maladjustment syndrome.[5] Foals with neonatal maladjustment syndrome and foals with other illness have higher concentrations of progestagen derivatives than do healthy foals.[5] Plasma concentrations of progestagen derivatives decline in sick foals that do not have neonatal maladjustment syndrome, but not in foals with the syndrome.[5] Progestagen derivatives include progesterone, pregnenolone, androstenedione, dehydroepiandrosterone, and epitestosterone.[5] Evidence from other species and limited experimental evidence in foals indicate that allopregnanolone infusion induces changes in mental status that mimic those seen in foals with neonatal maladjustment syndrome.[6] It is proposed that a subset of foals with signs of neonatal maladjustment syndrome have disease attributable to persistence of the fetal hypothalamic–pituitary–adrenal axis after birth.

EPIDEMIOLOGY

The disease is sporadic and occurs worldwide, with an annual **incidence** in foals of less than 1%.[7] Foals of either sex and of any breed born to mares of any age or reproductive history can be affected. The **case fatality rate** is very low for appropriately treated foals without other systemic illness.

PATHOGENESIS

Hypoxia resulting from intracranial vascular accidents, asphyxia at birth, or placental insufficiency before birth damages the central nervous system, causing a wide variety of signs of neurologic dysfunction.

A proposed pathogenesis for foals with persistently high plasma concentrations of progestagen derivatives after birth is failure of the foal's hypothalamic–pituitary–adrenal axis to rapidly adjust to extrauterine life.[6] In utero, foal movement and activity is suppressed, presumably at least in part by high concentrations of neuroactive progestagens. At birth in healthy foals there is a rapid reduction in concentration of these hormones coincident with increases in activity of the foal. Progestagen derivatives, some of which can cross the blood–brain barrier, modulate the activity of the $GABA_A$ receptor and at high concentrations completely inhibit its activity, providing a potential explanation for the somnolence and other signs displayed by foals with neonatal maladjustment syndrome and high plasma progestagen concentrations.[5]

Neurologic abnormalities and a failure to nurse result in a failure of the transfer of maternal immunoglobulins, which predisposes the foal to septicemia and hypoglycemia. Failure to nurse also results in hypoglycemia and malnutrition.

CLINICAL SIGNS

Foals that are abnormal at birth can display a range of behavioral abnormalities, from lack of suckle reflex to convulsions with extensor rigidity. The placenta of affected foals is often abnormal, or there is a history of prolonged parturition. Affected foals either do not develop or lose the suck reflex, have no affinity for the mare, and are unable to locate the udder or teat. Aimless wandering and a characteristic "barking" vocalization are sometimes present. Recumbent foals struggle wildly and in an uncoordinated fashion to stand. Convulsing foals usually display opisthotonos with extensor rigidity. Other signs of convulsive activity include facial twitching and grimacing, nystagmus, rapid blinking, sucking, chewing, and drooling. Between episodes foals are usually depressed or somnolent. Affected foals display little or no interest in the mare. Convulsing foals are tachypneic, tachycardic (>180 bpm), and hyperthermic (>39°C, 102°F) during and immediately after convulsions. It is important to recognize that the severity of clinical signs varies from very mild (foals are often described by owners as being a bit slow or dimwitted) through to grand mal seizures.

Foals that are normal at birth can develop signs by 24 hours of age. The signs are similar to those described previously, with the exception that the foals are initially able to ambulate. It is important to realize that healthy newborn foals lack a menace reflex, have a hypermetric gait and intention tremor, and become flaccid when restrained. The reflex response of healthy foals to restraint by a handler placing one arm under the foal's neck and another around the buttocks and squeezing is to become "floppy" and somnolent.[6] Foals restrained in this way become immobile, lie down, and have an increased pain threshold during restraint.[6]

Affected foals can take days to weeks to recover completely. Blind foals that do not have ocular lesions can take as long as 4 to 6 weeks to regain vision.

Ancillary testing is not usually indicated unless the foal fails to respond after approximately 7 days. At that time, CT or MRI examination of the brain might be indicated to detect congenital anomalies such as hydrocephalus. Examination of CSF should be performed in any foal with signs of central nervous system dysfunction in the presence of fever or other signs of sepsis.

CLINICAL PATHOLOGY

There are no routine hematologic or serum biochemical abnormalities characteristic of the disease, although it is prudent to conduct such examinations to eliminate other diseases; common characteristics are as follows[3]:

- Affected foals usually have **failure of transfer** of maternal immunoglobulins (serum IgG < 400 mg/dL).
- They may be **hypoglycemic** (<80 mg/dL, 4 mmol/L).
- **Cerebrospinal** fluid is often normal, although it may contain red blood cells or appear xanthochromic as a result of bleeding.

Detection of **biomarkers of brain injury** has been investigated. Plasma concentrations of **ubiquitin C-terminal hydrolase** (UCHL1) are higher (6.57, range 2.35 to 11.9 ng/mL) in foals with signs of neonatal maladjustment syndrome (defined as neonatal hypoxic-ischemic encephalopathy in the study) than in healthy foals (2.52, range 1.4 to 4.01 ng/mL).[8] The sensitivity and specificity for diagnosis of neonatal maladjustment syndrome based on a cutoff of ubiquitin C-terminal hydrolase concentrations in plasma of 4.01 ng/mL were 70% and 94%, respectively.[8]

Measurement of **plasma progestagen concentrations** of foals with signs of neonatal maladjustment syndrome might prove to be useful in diagnosis of the disease. Foals with high concentrations of progestagens could be treated appropriately, and those with low or normal concentrations could be further investigated for other diseases such as intracranial hemorrhages or hydrocephalus.

DIAGNOSTIC CONFIRMATION

Definitive diagnosis of the disease is difficult and is based on exclusion of other diseases that can cause similar signs and, at necropsy, demonstration of intracranial lesions consistent with the disease.

NECROPSY FINDINGS

Gross changes are typically limited to diffuse pulmonary congestion with a variable degree of atelectasis. In cases in which dystocia has been a contributing factor, fractured ribs and foci of subcutaneous edema and hemorrhage are sometimes noted. Occasionally, macroscopic cerebral hemorrhages are visible. Histologically, the key findings are hemorrhagic foci within the brain and areas of ischemic necrosis in the cerebral cortex. Meconium and other components of aspirated amniotic fluid accompanied by atelectasis and a mild inflammatory response may be present within the lung. In less affected foals the brain lesions are restricted to hemorrhage, cerebral swelling, and edema. Some affected foals subject to necropsy examination have evidence of intracranial vascular accidents, but it must be recognized that this is a biased sample; many foals recover from the disorder. Affected foals that are euthanized for financial or management reasons often have no detectable lesions in the brain.

Samples for Postmortem Diagnostic Confirmation

Samples for postmortem diagnostic confirmation include formalin-fixed brain, including cerebral cortex, cerebellum, and brainstem, and lung for light microscopic examination.

> **DIFFERENTIAL DIAGNOSIS**
>
> The disease must be differentiated from other diseases that cause neurologic or behavioral abnormalities in foals, including sepsis; renal, hepatic, or gastrointestinal disease, which can occur secondary to fetal hypoxia; hydrocephalus; hypoglycemia; meningitis; neonatal isoimmune hemolytic anemia; and prematurity, dysmaturity, or immaturity (Table 19-10).

TREATMENT

The principles of treatment are as follows:

- Control of convulsions
- Treatment of cerebral edema and hemorrhage
- Correction of FTPI
- Nutritional support and general nursing care

The management of affected foals is mainly supportive and is a time-consuming and labor-intensive endeavor. Provision of nutritional support, treatment of failure of transfer of maternal immunoglobulins, and nursing care are discussed in detail in the section "Principles of Care of the Critically Ill Neonate."

For other than emergency treatment of seizures, in which **diazepam** (0.1 to 0.4 mg/kg, intravenously, as required) or **midazolam** (0.05 to 0.1 mg/kg IV, as required) are useful, **phenobarbital** (phenobarbitone), **phenytoin,** and **primidone** are the drugs of choice for long-term control of seizure activity. Phenobarbital is administered initially at a dose of 9–20 mg/kg intravenously in 30 mL of isotonic saline infused over 15 to 30 minutes. Maintenance therapy is a similar dose intravenously (7–9 mg/kg IV over 20 min every 8–12 hours) or a lower dose (1–5 mg/kg) orally, every 8 hours, and the dose is adjusted

Table 19-10 Differential diagnosis of comatose ("sleeper") neonatal foals

Disease	Epidemiology	Clinical findings	Clinical pathology	Lesions	Treatment and prognosis
Septicemia	*E. coli, Klebsiella* spp., *Streptococcus* spp., *Salmonella* spp., *Actinobacillus suis,* Equine herpesvirus-1. Failure of transfer of passive immunity.	Abrupt onset of depression, fever, failure to nurse, and recumbency. Later diarrhea, pneumonia, and joint distension.	Culture of organism from blood or lesions (joints, lungs, feces).	Consistent with septicemia. Pneumonia. Septic synovitis, arthritis, and osteomyelitis.	Broad-spectrum antibiotics, supportive care (see "Principles of Providing Care to the Critically Ill Neonates"). Guarded to poor prognosis.
Isoimmune hemolytic anemia	Incompatible mating of Aa + or Qa + stallion with negative mare.	Normal at birth. Subsequent depression, cessation of nursing, exercise intolerance, icterus, and anemia. Hemoglobinuria in severe cases.	Positive Coombs' test to demonstrate immunoglobulin on foal's red cells. Dam's colostrum agglutinates or lyses foal red cells.	Anemia, icterus. Death from anemic hypoxia.	Transfusion of washed dam's red blood cells or of compatible donor (check dam's plasma with donor's red cells). Fair prognosis.
Uroperitoneum	Ruptured bladder, urachus or ureteral defect. Colts 1–3 days of age. Foals of either sex with other systemic diseases.	Normal at birth. Onset of abdominal distension, mild colic, depression, and recumbency. May urinate small volumes.	Peritoneal fluid has high creatinine concentration. Hyperkalemia, hyponatremia, and hypochloremia.	Uroperitoneum. Rupture bladder, urachus or ureter.	Surgical correction AFTER drainage of abdomen and resolution of hyperkalemia with intravenous dextrose or 0.9% NaCl. Good prognosis with appropriate care.
Hypoglycemia	Failure to nurse. Rejection by mare. Mare has no milk (agalactia).	Normal at birth, repeated attempts to nurse. Gradual onset (hours) of weakness and depression.	Low blood glucose concentration (<60 mg/dL, 3 mmol/L).	None. No food in stomach.	Excellent response to feeding or intravenous glucose.
Neonatal maladjustment syndrome	Sporadic.	Onset of abnormal behavior, recumbency, failure to nurse or orient to mare. Aimless wandering and vocalization.	None characteristic. Frequently failure of transfer of passive immunity.	Usually none apparent. Occasional intracranial vascular accidents.	Supportive care (see "Principles of Providing Care to Critically Ill Neonates"). Good prognosis.
Congenital defects	Sporadic.	Depends on nature of cardiac, gastrointestinal, or central nervous system defect.	None.	Consistent with defect.	Usually no treatment. Poor prognosis depending on defect.

to provide control of seizures while minimizing the degree of sedation. Because of the long elimination half-life of phenobarbital in foals (~200 hours) and the transient nature of the disease, once seizure control is achieved, administration of phenobarbital can be discontinued. Drug concentrations will be at or above the target concentration (5 to 30 µg/mL) for several days after the final dose. **Phenytoin** (5 to 10 mg/kg intravenously or orally initially, then 1 to 5 mg/kg every 4 hours) or **primidone** (20 to 40 mg/kg orally every 12 to 24 hours, to effect) are also used to control convulsions.

Definitive demonstration of the presence of cerebral edema or intracranial hemorrhage is impossible without sophisticated imaging devices, such as MRI or CT. However, treatment is often initiated on the basis of clinical signs. None of the treatments has demonstrated efficacy, and some are controversial. **Dimethyl sulfoxide** (DMSO) is given intravenously at 0.5 to 1 mg/kg once or twice daily for 3 days as a 10% solution. **Mannitol** (0.25 g/kg, intravenously as a 20% solution) may be effective in treating cerebral edema, but it is contraindicated if intracranial hemorrhage is present. **Glucocorticoids** (dexamethasone, 0.2 to 1 mg/kg, or prednisone, 1 to 2 mg/kg) might reduce intracranial inflammation and swelling. They might be contraindicated in foals with sepsis.

Magnesium sulfate (0.05 mg/kg per hour for 1 hour, then 0.025 mg/kg/h intravenously for up to 48 hours) is often administered to foals with suspected hypoxic encephalopathy in an attempt to minimize neuronal damage. There is no objective evidence of its efficacy in foals.

Foals with respiratory depression can be administered **caffeine** (10 mg/kg orally once and then 3.0 mg/kg orally q 24 hours). There is objective evidence of the lack of efficacy of this treatment in improving survival or decreasing arterial carbon dioxide tension in foals with a diagnosis of neonatal hypoxia-ischemia.[9] Adverse effects include agitation, hyperesthesia, tachycardia, and convulsions.

Good nursing care is critical in affected foals, and a concerted and persistent effort should be made to encourage the foal to nurse the mare. Encouraging the foal to nurse can be frustrating for the handler and mare, but should be done regularly, about every 4 hours, and preferably when the foal is hungry. Affected foals often begin to nurse quite suddenly. Foals should be provided with nutritional support, such as with mare's milk administered by indwelling nasogastric tube, until they are able to suckle.

Affected foals can require up to 4 to 6 weeks to recover completely, although most do so within 1 week of birth, and hasty decisions regarding euthanasia should not be made without recognition of the sometimes long time required for complete recovery.

CONTROL

Prevention of hypoxia in neonates by close monitoring of the health of the mare and of parturition may reduce the incidence of the disease.

FURTHER READING

Diesche TJ, Mellor DJ. Birth transitions: pathophysiology, the onset of consciousness and possible implications for neonatal maladjustment syndrome in the foal. *Equine Vet J.* 2013;45:656-660.

REFERENCES

1. Dickey EJ, et al. *J Vet Intern Med.* 2011;25:1231.
2. Baiker K, et al. *Equine Vet Educ.* 2010;22:593.
3. Johnson AL, et al. *Equine Vet Educ.* 2012;24:233.
4. Wilcox AL, et al. *Vet Pathol.* 2009;46:75.
5. Estell KE, et al. *J Vet Intern Med.* 2013;27:663.
6. Madigan JE, et al. *Equine Vet J.* 2012;44:109.
7. Wohlfender FD, et al. *Equine Vet J.* 2009;41:179.
8. Ringger NC, et al. *J Vet Intern Med.* 2011;25:132.
9. Giguere S, et al. *J Vet Intern Med.* 2008;22:401.

Neonatal Infectious Diseases

SYNOPSIS

Etiology Common infections for each animal species are listed under "Etiology" in the discussion. Most etiologies are bacterial, but some are viral.

Epidemiology Commonly predisposed by management and environmental factors and difficult delivery that increase the exposure risk and load and decrease the resistance of the neonate.

Clinical findings Depending on the pathogen and portal of entry, local infection or septicemia with following localization can occur; signs can be specific for the agent and the affected organ(s).

Clinical pathology White blood cell and differential counts, toxic change, serum immunoglobulin concentrations, blood gas analysis, acute-phase protein concentrations, blood culture.

Necropsy findings Specific to disease.

Diagnostic confirmation Specific to disease.

Treatment Treatment may include antimicrobial therapy, correction of acid–base disturbance, fluid and electrolyte therapy, blood or plasma transfusion, antiinflammatory therapy, and other supportive treatment.

Infection is a common cause of morbidity and mortality in neonates. There are a number of specific infectious pathogens that can cause disease. Other microorganisms normally present in the neonate's environment can become opportunistic pathogens whenever the immunologic status of the neonate is impaired. Maternal immunoglobulins are not transferred transplacentally in ungulates, and the newborns rely on the acquisition of immunoglobulins from colostrum for passive antibody protection.

ETIOLOGY

In domestic farm animals the common infections that can produce disease during the neonatal period are described in the following subsections. (Relative importance and prevalence statistics are not given because these vary from area to area and with differing management systems.)

Calves

- Enteritis associated with enterotoxigenic *Escherichia coli*; *Salmonella* spp.; rotavirus and coronavirus; *Cryptosporidium parvum*; *Clostridium perfringens* types A, B, and C; and occasionally by the virus of infectious bovine rhinotracheitis and bovine viral diarrhea
- Bacteremia and septicemia associated with *E. coli*, *Listeria monocytogenes*, *Pasteurella* spp., streptococci, or *Salmonella* spp.

Pigs

- Septicemia with or without localization in joints, endocardium, and meninges associated with *Streptococcus suis*, *Streptococcus equisimilis*, *Streptococcus zooepidemicus*, and *L. monocytogenes*
- Bacteremia, septicemia, and enteritis associated with *E. coli*
- Transmissible gastroenteritis, Aujeszky's disease, swine pox, enterovirus infections, and vomiting and wasting disease associated with viruses
- Enteritis associated with *C. perfringens*, *Campylobacter* spp., rotavirus, and *Coccidia* spp.
- Arthritis and septicemia associated with *Erysipelothrix rhusiopathiae*

Foals

- Septicemia with localization associated with *E. coli*, *Actinobacillus equuli*, *Klebsiella pneumoniae*, α-hemolytic streptococci, *S. zooepidemicus*, *L. monocytogenes*, *Rhodococcus equi*, and *Salmonella typhimurium*
- Enteritis associated with *C. perfringens* types A, B, and C; *Clostridium difficile*; *R. equi*; *Salmonella spp.*; *Strongyloides westeri*; *C. parvum*; and rotavirus.

Lambs

- Septicemia or bacteremia with localization in joints and/or synovia and/or leptomeninges associated with *E. coli*, *L. monocytogenes*, streptococci, micrococci, *E. rhusiopathiae*, and *Chlamyodophila* spp.
- Enteritis associated with enterotoxigenic *E. coli*, *Salmonella* spp., rotavirus and coronavirus, and *C. parvum*
- Lamb dysentery associated with *C. perfringens* types B and C

- Gas gangrene of the navel associated with *Clostridium septicum, Clostridium novyi*, and *Clostridium chauvoei*
- Pyemia associated with *Staphylococcus aureus, Fusobacterium necrophorum*, and *Trueperella* (formerly *Arcanobacterium) pyogenes*
- Pneumonia, polyserositis, and peritonitis associated with *Pasteurella multocida* and *Mannheimia hemolytica*

The agents listed in the following subsections are recorded as causing neonatal infections but are less common than those listed in the previous subsections and not of as great importance.

Calves

Pseudomonas aeruginosa, *Streptococcus pyogenes, Streptococcus faecalis, S. zooepidemicus, Pneumococcus* spp.; enteritis resulting from *Providencia stuartii, Chlamydophila* spp., *A. equuli.*

Lambs

S. aureus (tick pyemia); enteritis resulting from *E. coli*, rotavirus; pneumonia resulting from *Salmonella abortus–ovis.*

Foals

Enterobacter cloacae, *S. aureus, Pasteurella multocida, P. aeruginosa, T. pyogenes, Serratia marcescens.*

All Species

Nonspecific infections are associated with pyogenic organisms, including *T.* (formerly *Arcanobacterium) pyogenes* and *Fusobacterium necrophorum; S. faecalis, S. zooepidemicus, Micrococcus* spp., and *Pasteurella* spp. occur in all species.

EPIDEMIOLOGY

The occurrence of neonatal disease is broadly influenced by two main factors: the exposure or infection pressure of the infectious agent to the neonate and the ability of the neonate to modulate the infection so that disease does not occur. Some agents are sufficiently virulent in their own right that an exposure can lead to disease. With others, the majority, the defenses of the host must be compromised or the infection challenge must be very high before clinical disease occurs. Management of the neonate has a great influence on both of these factors, and the recognition and correction of these risks is the key to the prevention of neonatal disease in both the individual and the group.

Sources of Infection

Postnatal Infection

The vast majority of infections are acquired by the neonate after birth, directly from the environment into which it is born. The source of infection can be any adult animal present in the maternity area, an infected neonate housed in close proximity, contamination of the environment, or an animal caretaker functioning as mechanical or biological vector. Details for the common neonatal diseases are given under the individual disease headings.

Prenatal Infection

Some bacterial and viral infections that manifest with neonatal disease are acquired in utero and are associated with bacteremia/viremia in the neonate.[1] The majority of these are agents that cause abortion, and neonatal septicemia is only part of the disease spectrum associated with these pathogens. Examples include many of the agents producing abortion in sheep.

Some septicemic infections in **foals**, particularly those associated with *A. equuli, S. zooepidemicus, Salmonella abortusequi*, and possibly some *E. coli* septicemic infections, are acquired by prenatal infection. If the disease is intrauterine in origin, it reaches the foal's organism via the placenta, probably by means of placentitis resulting from a bloodborne infection or endometritis of the mare.

Viral infections that are acquired in utero are listed in the section on congenital disease.

Routes of Transmission

The **portal of infection** is commonly by oral ingestion, but infection may also occur via aerosol inhalation. Invasive organisms capable of producing bacteremia and septicemia invade through the nasopharynx or through the intestinal epithelium. An alternate route of infection and invasion is via the umbilicus. Routes of **excretion** are via the feces in enteric disease and the nasal secretions, urine, and sometimes the feces in septicemic disease, resulting in contamination of the neonatal environment.

Where neonates are in groups or in close contact, direct transmission by fecal, respiratory secretion, and urine aerosols are common routes for transmission of infection. Neonatal bull calves that are group-housed and that suck one another's navels can transmit infection by this activity.

Risk Factors and Modulation of Infection

Immunity

Neonates are generally more susceptible to infection than their adult counterparts. The calf, lamb, piglet, and foal are born without significant levels of immunoglobulins and possess almost no resistance to certain diseases until after they have ingested colostrum and absorbed sufficient quantities of immunoglobulins from the colostrum. **Failure of transfer of passive immunity** is a major determinant and is discussed under that heading.

Immune Responsiveness

All components of the immune system are present in foals and calves at birth, but the immune system of the newborn animal is less mature than its adult counterpart, at least for the first 30 days of life, and does not respond as effectively to an antigen stimulus.

Immune responsiveness is age-dependent but also varies with the antigen. In colostrum-fed animals, part of the inefficiency of the newborn to produce humoral antibodies following exposure to antigens is the interference from circulating colostral antibody and the downregulation by colostrum of endogenous immunoglobulin production.

Colostrum-deprived calves respond actively to injected antigens and are thought to be immunologically competent at birth with respect to most antigens. Immune competence begins during fetal life, and the age of gestation at which this occurs varies according to the nature of the antigen. The bovine fetus will produce antibodies to some viruses, beginning at 90 to 120 days, and by the third trimester of gestation it will respond to a variety of viruses and bacteria. The lamb will respond to some antigens beginning as early as 41 days and not until 120 days for others. The piglet at 55 days and the fetal foal also respond to injected antigens.

The presence of high levels of antibodies in the precolostral serum of newborn animals suggests that an in utero infection was present, which is useful for diagnostic purposes. The detection of immunoglobulins and specific antibodies in aborted fetuses can be a useful aid in the diagnosis of abortion in cattle.

Exposure Pressure

The exposure pressure is a factor of the cleanliness of the environment of the neonate. The phenomenon of a "buildup of infection" in continual-throughput housing for neonatal animals has been recognized for decades and has been translated to many observations of risk for neonatal disease associated with suboptimal hygiene and stocking density in both pen and paddock birthing areas. Details for the individual species are provided in the section on perinatal disease.

Age at Exposure

With several agents that produce neonatal disease, the age of the neonate at infection and the infecting dose have a significant influence on the outcome. Examples are the importance of age with respect to susceptibility to disease associated with some enteric infections. Disease associated with enteropathogenic *E. coli* and with *C. perfringens* types B and C occurs only in young animals, and if infection can be avoided by hygiene in this critical period, disease will not occur regardless of subsequent exposure. Colostrum-deprived calves show significant resistance to challenge at 7 days of age with strains of *E. coli* that invariably produce septicemic disease if challenged at the time of birth, and isolation of an immunocompromised neonate is an important factor in its survival. Thus the management of the neonate and its environment is a critical determinant of its health. Age at exposure also varies with the epidemiology of the pathogen, and segregated early weaning is used to reduce transmission of and infection with certain pathogens in pigs.

Animal Risk Factors

Animal risk factors that predispose to infection include those that interfere with sucking drive and colostral intake, such as cold stress and dystocia. These are detailed in the preceding section on perinatal disease.

PATHOGENESIS

The pathogenesis varies with the neonatal infectious disease under consideration and is given for each of these in the special medicine section.

An infection can remain localized at the initial site of infection, as is the case with uncomplicated omphalitis or enterotoxigenic *E. coli* infection, or it can spread by invading the organism (e.g., via the nasopharynx, the gastrointestinal tract, or the umbilical vein or urachus). In the latter case the usual pattern of development is bacteremia followed by **septicemia** with severe systemic signs, or **bacteremia** with few or no systemic signs followed by **localization** in various organs.[2] **Localization** is most common in the joints, producing a suppurative or nonsuppurative arthritis. Less commonly there is localization in the eye to produce panophthalmitis, in the heart valves to cause valvular endocarditis, or in the meninges to produce meningitis.

Secondary lesions often take time to develop, and signs usually appear at 1 to 2 weeks of age. This is especially true with some of the streptococcal infections, in which bacteremia may be present for several days before localization in the joints and meninges produces clinical signs. Bacterial meningitis in newborn ungulates is preceded by bacteremia followed by a fibrinopurulent inflammation of the leptomeninges, choroid plexuses, and ventricle walls, but it does not affect the neuraxial parenchyma. It is proposed that the bacteria are transported in monocytes, which do not normally invade the neuraxial parenchyma.

Dehydration and acid–base and electrolyte imbalance can occur very quickly in newborn animals, whether diarrhea and vomiting (pigs) are present or not, but obviously are more severe when there is fluid loss into the gastrointestinal tract. In gram-negative sepsis the prominent signs are those of endotoxemia.

CLINICAL FINDINGS

The clinical findings depend on which organ systems are affected, the rapidity of growth of the organism, its propensity to localize, and its potential to produce toxemia. Clinical signs are often vague and unspecific in the initial phase of septicemia until the infection localizes and affects one or several organs.[1,2] Organisms that have a low propensity for toxemia present with fever, depression, anorexia, and signs referable to localization. These include endocarditis with a heart murmur; panophthalmitis with pus in the anterior chamber of the eye; meningitis with rigidity, pain, and convulsions; and polyarthritis with lameness and swollen joints. With more virulent organisms there are clinical signs of toxemia and bacteremia, including fever, and advanced stages result in hypothermia, severe depression, obtundation, coma, petechiation of mucosae, dehydration, acidemia, and rapid death.

The clinical and clinicopathologic characteristics of the septicemic foal were detailed in an outbreak of septicemia in colostrum-deprived foals and in the clinical records of 38 septicemic foals admitted to a referral clinic. The major clinical findings included lethargy, unwillingness to suck, inability to stand without assistance but remaining conscious, unawareness of environment and thrashing or convulsing, diarrhea, respiratory distress, joint distension, central nervous system abnormalities, uveitis, and colic. Fever was not a consistent finding.

A **sepsis score** has been developed for foals based on 14 measures related to historical, clinical, and laboratory data (Table 19-11). The score derived from the collective differential scoring of these data has been found to be more sensitive and specific for infection than any parameter taken individually. However, a subsequent study of 168 foals presented to a university hospital found that the sepsis score correctly predicted sepsis in 58 out of 86 foals and nonsepsis in 24 out of 45 foals, resulting in a sensitivity of 67%, a specificity of 75%, a positive predictive value of 84%, and a negative predictive value of 55%, and it was suggested that the score system should be used with care because the low negative predictive value limited its clinical utility.

A sepsis score for calves, based on fecal consistency, hydration, behavior, ability to stand, state of the umbilicus and degree of injection of scleral vessels, and presence of hypoglycemia and abnormal neutrophil cell count, was found to have reasonable predictive value.[3]

The clinical findings specific to individual etiologic agents are given under their specific headings in the special medicine section of this book.

CLINICAL PATHOLOGY

Clinical pathology is used as an integral part of the evaluation of a sick neonate and to help formulate a treatment plan. A major evaluation is to attempt to confirm the presence or absence of sepsis, and this type of evaluation has been developed most successfully in the foal. **Blood culture** is part of this examination, but the time for a positive result limits its value in the acutely ill neonate. Laboratory findings in foals with neonatal sepsis are variable and depend on the severity, stage, and site of infection. **Serial examinations** are commonly used. In examinations relating to the possible presence of septicemia, particular emphasis is placed on the results of the white blood cell and differential counts, the presence of toxic change (toxic granulation and vacuolization), serum immunoglobulin concentrations, arterial oxygen concentrations, the presence of metabolic acidosis, abnormal blood glucose concentrations, and elevated fibrinogen levels.[1,4]

DIFFERENTIAL DIAGNOSIS

- The principles of diagnosis of infectious disease in newborn animals are the same as for older animals. However, in outbreaks of suspected infectious disease in young animals, there is usually a need for more diagnostic microbiology and pathology.
- With outbreaks, owners should be encouraged to submit all dead neonates as soon as possible for a meaningful necropsy examination.
- In addition to postmortem examination, it is necessary to identify the factors that may have contributed to an outbreak of disease in newborn calves, piglets, or lambs, and only detailed epidemiologic investigation will reveal these.

TREATMENT

The first principle is to obtain an etiologic diagnosis if possible. Ideally a drug sensitivity of the causative bacteria should be obtained before treatment is given, but this is not always possible. It may be necessary to choose an **antibiotic** based on the tentative diagnosis and previous experience with treatment of similar cases.

Outbreaks of infectious disease are common in litters of piglets and groups of calves and lambs, and individual treatment is often necessary to maximize survival rate. Supportive fluid and electrolyte therapy and correction of acid–base disturbances are described in detail under "Disturbances of Free Water, Electrolytes, and Acid–Base Balance."

The provision of **antibodies** to sick and weak newborn animals through the use of blood transfusions or serum is often practiced, especially in newborn calves in which the immunoglobulin status is unknown. Whole blood given at the rate of 10 to 20 mL/kg body weight, preferably by the intravenous route, will often save a calf that appears to be in shock associated with neonatal diarrhea. The blood is usually followed by fluid therapy. Serum or plasma can also be given at half the dose rate. The blood should not be taken from a cow near parturition because the circulating immunoglobulins

Table 19-11 Worksheet for calculating a sepsis score for foals less than 12 days of age[1]

	NUMBER OF POINTS TO ASSIGN					
Variable	*4*	*3*	*2*	*1*	*0*	**Score for this case**
1. Historical data						
a. Placentitis, vulvar discharge before delivery, dystocia, sick dam, induced parturition		Present			Absent	
b. Gestation length (days)		<300	300–310	311–330	>330	
2. Clinical examination						
a. Petechiation or scleral injection (nontraumatic)		Marked	Moderate	Mild	None	
b. Rectal temperature (° C)			>38.9	<37.8	37.9–38.7	
c. Hypotonia, convulsions, coma, depression			Marked	Moderate	Mild	
d. Anterior uveitis, diarrhea, respiratory distress, swollen joints or open wounds		Present			Absent	
3. Hemogram						
a. Neutrophil count (cells × 10^9/L)		<2.0	2.0–4.0 or 8.0–12.0 >12	4.0–8.0		
b. Band neutrophils (cells × 10^9/L)		>0.2	0.05–0.2		<0.05	
c. Toxic changes in neutrophils	Marked	Moderate	Slight		None	
d. Fibrinogen concentration (g/L)			>6.0	4.1–6.0	4.0	
4. Laboratory data						
a. Blood glucose (mmol/L)			<2.7	2.7–4.4	>4.4	
b. IgG concentration (g/L)	<2.0	2.0–4.0	4.1–8.0		>8.0	
c. Arterial oxygen tension (Torr)		<40	40–50	51–70	>70	
d. Metabolic acidosis (base excess < 0)				Present	Absent	
Total points for this foal						

To calculate the sepsis score, assign foal a score corresponding to the historical physical examination and laboratory data included in the table. A score of 11 or less predicts the absence of sepsis correctly in 88% of cases, whereas a score of 12 or higher predicts sepsis correctly in 93% of cases. For foals less than 12 hours of age that have nursed or received colostrum, assign a value of 2 for the serum immunoglobulin score. If the foal has not nursed, assign a value of 4.

will be low from the transfer into the mammary gland.

Plasma is often incorporated into the therapeutic regimen in foals, both for its immunoglobulin content and for its effect on blood volume and osmotic pressure. Stored plasma can be used. A dose of 20 mL plasma/kg body weight given slowly intravenously is often used, but significantly higher doses are required to elevate circulating immunoglobulins by an appreciable amount. Blood may be collected, the red blood cells allowed to settle, and the plasma removed and stored frozen. The donor plasma should be prescreened for compatibility. Lyophilized hyperimmune equine serum as a source of antibodies may also be fed to foals within 4 hours after birth. Good nursing care is also essential.

Further information on treatment is given in the section on critical care for the newborn later in this chapter.

CONTROL

Methods for avoidance of failure of transfer of passive immunity and the principles for prevention of infectious disease in newborn farm animals follow in this chapter. The control of individual diseases is given under specific disease headings elsewhere in this book.

REFERENCES

1. Sanchez LC. *Vet Clin North Am Equine Pract.* 2005;21:273-293.
2. Fecteau G, et al. *Vet Clin North Am Food Anim Pract.* 2009;25:195-208.
3. Biolatti C, et al. *Schweiz Arch Tierheilkd.* 2012;154:239-246.
4. Holis AR, et al. *J Vet Intern Med.* 2008;22:1223-1227.

PRINCIPLES OF CONTROL AND PREVENTION OF NEONATAL INFECTIOUS DISEASES

The four principles of control and prevention of infectious diseases of newborn farm animals are as follows:

- Reduction of risk of acquisition of infection from the environment
- Removal of the newborn from the infectious environment if necessary
- Increasing and maintaining the nonspecific resistance of the newborn
- Increasing the specific resistance of the newborn through the use of vaccines

The application of each of these principles will vary depending on the species, the spectrum of diseases that are common on that farm, the management system, and the success achieved with any particular preventive method used previously.

REDUCTION OF RISK OF ACQUISITION OF INFECTION FROM THE ENVIRONMENT

The animal should be born in an environment that is clean, dry, sheltered, and conducive for the animal to get up after birth, suck the dam, and establish bonding.[1,2] Calving and lambing stalls or grounds, farrowing crates, and foaling stalls should be prepared in advance for parturition. No conventional animal area can be sterilized, but it can be made reasonably clean to minimize the infection rate before colostrum is ingested and during the first few weeks of life when the newborn animal is very susceptible to infectious disease.

With seasonal calving or lambing there can be buildup of infection in the birth area, and animals born later in the season are at greater risk of disease. In these circumstances it may be necessary to move to secondary lambing or calving areas. In northern climates snow may constrict the effective calving area and result in a significant buildup of infection. Buildup of infection pressure must be minimized by a change to a fresh calving/lambing area and by the frequent movement of feed bunks or feed areas. Any system that concentrates large numbers of cattle in a small area increases environmental contamination, and close confinement of heifers and cows around calving time is a known risk factor for calf mortality. With large herds both the cow herd and heifer herd should be broken into as many subgroups as is practical. Extensive systems where cows calve out over large paddocks are optimal, and with more intense systems a group size no larger than 50 has been suggested.

Lambing sheds and calving areas for beef cattle should be kept free of animal traffic during the months preceding the period of parturition. In dairy herds, maternity pens separate from other housing functions should be provided and cleaned and freshly bedded between calvings. Certainly they should not also be used as hospital pens.

In swine herds, the practice of batch farrowing, with all-in all-out systems of management and disinfection of the farrowing rooms, is essential. Sows should be washed before entry to the farrowing area, and the floor of the farrowing crate should be of the type that minimizes exposure of the piglet to fecal material at birth.

The swabbing of the **navel** with tincture of iodine or chlorhexidine solutions to prevent entry of infection is commonly practiced by some producers and seldom by others. In a heavily contaminated environment it is recommended, although hard evidence supporting the efficacy of this procedure is currently lacking.[1] Severance of the umbilical cord too quickly during the birth of foals can deprive the animal of large quantities of blood, which can lead to neonatal maladjustment syndrome.

When deemed necessary, some **surveillance** should be provided for pregnant animals that are expected to give birth, and assistance provided if necessary. The major objective is to avoid or minimize the adverse effects of a difficult or slow parturition on the newborn and the dam. Physical injuries, hypoxia, and edema of parts of the newborn will reduce the vigor and viability of the newborn and, depending on the circumstances and the environment in which it is born, may lead to disease or even death soon after birth.

When possible, every effort should be made to minimize exposure of the neonate to extremes of temperature (heat, cold, snow). Shelter sheds should be built if necessary.

In beef herds, the practice of purchasing male dairy calves to foster on to cows whose calves have died should be discouraged. If calves are purchased, they should be from a herd whose health status is known to the veterinarian and certainly never through a market. Similarly, colostrum should be obtained from cows within the herd and stored frozen for future use. Colostrum obtained from a different herd presents a biosecurity risk because it can transmit diseases such as bovine enzootic leukemia or Johne's disease. Furthermore, purchased dairy colostrum is commonly second- or third-milking colostrum and of limited immunologic value. The use of a commercial colostrum supplement or replacer is possible, although they have significant limitations.

REMOVAL OF THE NEWBORN FROM THE INFECTIOUS ENVIRONMENT

In some cases of high animal population density (e.g., a crowded dairy barn) and in the presence of known disease, it may be necessary to transfer the newborn to a noninfectious environment temporarily or permanently. Adult cows shedding enteric pathogens are a risk for calf infection. Thus dairy calves are often removed from the dam at birth and placed in individual pens inside or outdoors in hutches and reared in these pens separately from the main herd. This reduces the severity of neonatal diarrhea and pneumonia and risk for mortality compared with calves allowed to remain with the dam. **Individual housing** in hutches is preferred because this avoids navel sucking and other methods of direct-contact transmission of disease. Humans entering these hutches should also practice interhutch hygiene. The prevalence of disease is higher in enclosed artificially heated barns than in hutches. However, despite the well-established value of individual rearing of calves, animal welfare regulations in several countries require that there be visual and tactile contact between calves. The removal of the cow–calf pair from the main calving grounds to a "nursery pasture" after the cow–calf relationship (neonatal bond) is well established, at 2 to 3 days of age, has proved to be a successful management practice in beef herds. This system moves the newborn calf away from the main calving ground, which may be heavily contaminated because of limited space. It necessitates that the producer must plan the location of the calving grounds and nursery pastures well in advance of calving time. Calves that develop diarrhea in the calving grounds or nursery pasture are removed with their dams to a **"hospital pasture"** during treatment and convalescence. The all-in all-out principle of successive population and depopulation of farrowing quarters and calf barns is an effective method of maintaining a low level of contamination pressure for the neonate.

INCREASING THE NONSPECIFIC RESISTANCE OF THE NEWBORN

Following a successful birth, the next important method of preventing neonatal disease is to ensure that the newborn ingests colostrum as soon as possible. With natural sucking the amount of colostrum ingested by the neonate will depend on the amount available, the vigor of the animal, the acceptance by the dam, and the management system used, which may encourage or discourage the ingestion of liberal quantities of colostrum. Beef cows that calve at a condition score lower than 4 (out of 10) are at higher risk of having calves that develop failure of transfer of passive immunity, and the ideal condition score at calving is 5 to 6.

The method of colostrum delivery that is needed to optimize transfer of passive immunity to the dairy calf will vary with the breed of cow, the management level of the farm, and the priority given to calf health. Owner acceptance of alternate feeding systems to natural sucking also is a consideration. The success of the farm policy for the feeding of colostrum is easily monitored by one of the tests described earlier, as is the effect of an intervention strategy.

Newborn male dairy calves are commonly assembled and transported to market or to calf-rearing units within a few days of birth. Studies have repeatedly shown high rates of FTPI in this class of calf. The high rates occur either because the original owner does not bother to feed colostrum to the calf, knowing it is to be sold, or because calves are purchased off the farm before colostrum feeding is completed. The effects of the transportation can have a further deleterious effect on the defense mechanism of the calves, and they are at high risk of disease.

Calf-rearing units should preferably purchase calves directly from a farm with an established policy of feeding colostrum before the calf leaves the farm, and every effort should be made to reduce the stress of transportation by providing adequate bedding, avoiding long distances without a break, and attempting to transport only calves that are healthy. In some countries there is now legislation requiring the feeding of colostrum and limiting the transport of newborn calves.

The honesty of the stated farm colostrum feeding policy can be monitored by testing the calves for their immunoglobulin concentration in serum. Where this is not possible and market calves must be used, the entry immunoglobulin concentration should be tested; the incidence of infectious disease in low-testing calves will be high unless hygiene, housing, ventilation, management and nutrition are excellent. The entry immunoglobulin concentration of calves entering veal or other calf-rearing units is a prime determinant of subsequent health and performance. The "alert" cut-point can be established for an individual farm by monitoring of individual immunoglobulin concentrations and subsequent calf fate.

Following the successful ingestion of colostrum and establishment of the neonatal bond, emphasis can then be given to provision, if necessary, of any special nutritional and housing requirements. Newborn piglets need supplemental heat, and attention must be given to the special problems of intensive pig husbandry. Orphan and weak piglets can now be reared successfully under normal farm conditions with the use of milk replacers containing added porcine immunoglobulins. Heat is often provided to lambs for the first day in pen lambing systems.

Milk replacers for the newborn must contain high-quality ingredients. Calves younger than 3 weeks are less able to digest nonmilk proteins, and the fats best used by the calf are high-quality animal source fats and slightly unsaturated vegetable oils. A 22% crude protein is recommended for milk replacers comprised only of milk proteins and 24% to 26% in replacers that contain nonmilk protein sources. The level of fat should be at least 15%; higher fat concentration will provide additional energy, which may be required in colder climates. Feeding utensils must be cleaned and disinfected between each feeding if disease transmission is to be minimized.

With animals at pasture, the mustering and close contact associated with management procedures such as castration and docking pose a risk for disease transmission. These procedures should be performed in yards prepared for the purpose—preferably temporary yards erected for this sole purpose in a clean area.

INCREASING THE SPECIFIC RESISTANCE OF THE NEWBORN

The specific resistance of the newborn to infectious disease may be enhanced by vaccination of the dam during pregnancy to stimulate the production of specific antibodies that are concentrated in the colostrum and transferred to the newborn after birth. Vaccination of the dam can provide protection for the neonate against enteric and respiratory disease. Details are given under the specific disease headings in this text. The vaccination of the late fetus in utero stimulates the production of antibody but its practical application has yet to be determined.

FURTHER READING

Black L, Francis ML, Nicholls MJ. Protecting young domestic animals from infectious disease. *Vet Annu.* 1985;25:46-61.

Brenner J. Passive lactogenic immunity in calves: a review. *Israel J Vet Med.* 1991;46:1-12.

Dwyer CM. The welfare of the neonatal lamb. *Small Rumin Res.* 2008;76:31-41.

Godden S. Colostrum management for dairy calves. *Vet Clin North Am Food Anim Pract.* 2008;24:19-39.

Larson RL, Tyler JW, Schultz LG, Tessman RK, Hostetler DE. Management strategies to decrease calf death losses in beef herds. *J Am Vet Med Assoc.* 2004;224:42-48.

Mee JF. Newborn dairy calf management. *Vet Clin North Am Food Anim Pract.* 2008;24:1-17.

REFERENCES

1. Mee JF. Newborn dairy calf management. *Vet Clin North Am Food Anim Pract.* 2008;24:1-17.
2. Dwyer CM. The welfare of the neonatal lamb. *Small Rumin Res.* 2008;76:31-41.

COLIBACILLOSIS OF NEWBORN CALVES, PIGLETS, LAMBS, KIDS, AND FOALS

SYNOPSIS

Etiology Pathogenic serotypes of *Escherichia coli:* septicemic, enterotoxigenic (ETEC); enteropathogenic (EPEC); enterohemorrhagic (EHEC), also referred to as verocytotoxigenic (VTEC) or Shiga-toxin-producing (STEC); and necrotoxigenic *E. coli* (NTEC).

Epidemiology Affects newborn calves, piglets, lambs, and goat kids. Risk factors include colostrum deprivation, overcrowding, adverse climatic conditions, and inferior milk replacers. Prevalence of ETEC varies between herds. EHEC (O157:H7) in cattle is not normally associated with clinical disease, but it presents a major zoonotic concern.

Signs Weakness and collapse (septicemia), diarrhea, and dehydration; complications such as meningitis or polyarthritis.

Clinical pathology Isolation of organism from feces or blood; hematology and serum biochemistry to evaluate inflammation and acid–base and electrolyte imbalance.

Lesions Septicemic lesions, dehydration, enteritis.

Diagnostic confirmation Culture of organism and serotyping.

Treatment Antimicrobials, antiinflammatory drugs, fluid and electrolyte therapy.

Control Reduce infection pressure on neonates. Ensure adequate transfer of passive immunity, and vaccinate pregnant dams to induce specific colostrum antibody. Minimize stressors and their effect on neonates.

ETIOLOGY

Colibacillosis is associated with pathogenic serotypes of *E. coli*. For the most part, *E. coli* is a group of harmless bacteria that serve as indicator organisms for fecal contamination and breaches in hygiene. However, several strains have acquired virulence factors, turning them into potentially dangerous pathogens.[1] The prevalence of the different pathogenic serotypes of *E. coli* in farm animals has remained relatively constant for many years. Certain serotypes cause diarrhea and others cause septicemia. Serotypes include the following:

- **Enterotoxigenic *E. coli*** (ETEC) is the most common enteropathogen that causes diarrhea in newborn farm animals. The bacteria cause diarrhea by adhering to enterocytes, colonizing the intestinal mucosa, and **producing enterotoxins**. Enterotoxins cause hypersecretion of electrolytes and water into the small intestine without causing significant morphologic damage or invading tissue.[2]
- **Enteropathogenic *E. coli*** (EPEC) are the **"attaching and effacing"** strains that colonize the small intestine, where they attach tightly to the epithelial cells of the villus and cause typical **attaching and effacing lesions**. They do not produce toxins and seldom invade the intestinal mucosa.
- **Enterohemorrhagic *E. coli*** (EHEC) also cause attaching and effacing lesions and are among the *E. coli* strains capable of producing toxins similar to the one produced by *Shigella dysenteriae* type I. They are therefore also referred to as **Shiga-toxin-producing *E. coli*** (STEC). Because Shiga toxins are detected with the Vero cell-toxicity test, STEC are also known as **verotoxin or verocytoxin-producing *E. coli*** (VTEC). Shiga toxins may cause anything from mild diarrhea to severe hemorrhagic colitis. In humans EHEC is responsible for the highly fatal hemolytic–uremic syndrome in children.[3] **EHEC are highly prevalent in cattle** but in general do not cause clinical disease in this species, although some Shiga-toxin-producing *E. coli* have been associated with diarrhea in calves. Cattle are the main reservoir of ***E. coli*** O157:H7, one of the important EHEC strains, causing a broad range of clinical disease in humans (see the section on enterohemorrhagic *E. coli* in farm animals and zoonotic implications). Shiga-toxin-producing *E. coli* strains have been associated with edema disease in swine.[2]
- **Necrotoxigenic *E. coli*** (NTEC) strains produce cytotoxic necrotizing factor (CNF)1 or 2. NTEC2 isolates are restricted to ruminants, particularly calves and lambs with diarrhea and septicemia.
- **Septicemic *E. coli*** strains of serogroup 078 are invasive and cause septicemia in calves, piglets, and lambs. Their powerful endotoxins cause endotoxic shock, with a high case fatality rate.

EPIDEMIOLOGY

Occurrence and Prevalence of Infection

The prevalence of colibacillosis has increased in recent years. There are several possible reasons for this, including size of herds, shortage of qualified labor, automated livestock-rearing systems, and increased population density.

Colibacillosis occurs most commonly in newborn farm animals and is a significant cause of economic loss in raising livestock. It is a complex disease in which several different risk factors interact with certain pathogens, resulting in the disease. There are at least two different types of the disease: **enteric colibacillosis** is characterized by varying degrees of diarrhea, dehydration, acidosis, and death in a few days if not treated; **coliform septicemia** is characterized by severe illness and rapid death within hours.

Cattle and Calves

The infection prevalence of **enterohemorrhagic *E. coli***, particularly the *E. coli* O157:H7 strain, has been studied extensively because of concerns with beef and raw milk as source of foodborne disease in humans. In the United States *E. coli* O157:H7 infection prevalence rates based on positive fecal samples were between 0.2% and 8.4% for cows, 1.6% and 3.0% for heifers, and 0.4% to 40% for calves. Infection prevalence rates reported from Canada, Italy, Japan, and the United Kingdom were 0.3% to 16.1% for cows, 10.0% to 14.1% for heifers, and 1.7% to 48.8% for calves.[4] These numbers underscore the obvious effect of animal age on the epidemiology of infection with *E. coli O157:57.* The **considerable prevalence of this EHEC strain** in cattle has little impact on animal health because EHEC infection in this species is normally not associated with clinical disease, but it presents a **serious public health concern.**

The prevalence of **enterotoxigenic *E. coli*** (ETEC) in diarrheic calves varies widely geographically, between herds, and depending on the age of the animals. The prevalence can be as high as 50% to 60% in diarrheic calves under 3 days of age and only 5% to 10% in diarrheic calves 8 days of age. In some countries the prevalence is only 5% to 8% in diarrheic calves under 3 days of age. Thus **enterotoxigenic colibacillosis is a major cause of diarrhea in calves less than 3 days of age** and is not associated with outbreaks of diarrhea in calves older than 3 days. ETEC infection in calves older than 2 to 3 days will in most cases be associated with a viral infection. The prevalence of ETEC infection is very low or nil in clinically normal calves in herds that have not had a problem with diarrhea. In some beef herds affected with diarrhea in young calves there may be little evidence of infection with enterotoxigenic *E. coli,* and other factors need to be examined.

Piglets

The prevalence of ETEC in diarrheic piglets varies geographically and with herds. In some areas the F5 (K99) pilus was found more frequently than F4 (K88) or F6 (987P), whereas in other regions the F4 pilus is more common. The F4 and F18 pilus adhesins are most commonly associated with postweaning diarrhea of pigs.

Morbidity and Mortality Rates

Calves

In dairy calves raised under intensive and poorly managed conditions the morbidity rate of infection with ETEC may reach 75%, but it is usually about 30%. Case fatality rates vary from 10% to 50% depending on the level of clinical management.

In beef calves the morbidity rates vary from 10% to 50% and the case fatality rates from 5% to 25% or even higher in some years. The population mortality rate in both beef and dairy calves can vary from a low of 3% in well-managed herds to a high of 60% in problem herds in certain years.

Piglets

In piglets the morbidity rate of preweaning diarrhea varies widely between herds, but it averages about 6% of litters, mostly in the first week of life. The morbidity rates increase with increased litter size and decrease with increasing parity of the sow. Losses as a result of stillbirths, traumatic injuries, starvation, and undersize at birth account for a much greater combined total preweaning loss, but colibacillosis accounts for approximately 50% of the gastroenteropathies encountered during the preweaning period.

Postweaning diarrhea (PWD) occurring in the 2 weeks following weaning is one of the economically most important diarrheal diseases in piglets in which colibacillosis plays an important etiologic role.[5] ETEC associated PWD commonly occurs in the immediate postweaning period. Outbreaks can occur suddenly, with mortality rates of 50% and higher. Affected animals can die acutely or show profuse diarrhea for up to 4 days. In uncomplicated cases mortality rates rarely exceed 10%.[5] Postweaning diarrhea of pigs is covered in detail under this heading.

Risk Factors

Several risk factors influence the occurrence of the disease, each one of which must be considered, evaluated, and modified or removed if necessary when investigating the cause of an outbreak so that effective clinical management and control of the disease may be achieved.

Animal Risk Factors

Animal Species

The pathogenesis of colibacillosis involves a number of host factors, of which the presence of specific receptors for adhesins and enterotoxins is probably among the most important.[6] Clinical disease associated with *E. coli* infection is largely dependent on the presence of specific receptors that usually only occur in one or few animal species. because of this receptor specificity of adhesins and enterotoxins, **ETEC strains have considerable species specificity.**[7]

Age and Birth Weight

Diarrhea associated with ETEC occurs in **calves** mainly during the first few days of life, rarely in older calves, and never in adults. Epidemiologic studies of both beef and dairy calves indicate that more than 80% of clinical cases associated with ETEC F5 (K99) occur in calves younger than 4 days of age. The ability of the F5 ETEC to adhere to the small intestinal epithelium of calves decreases continuously from 12 hours of age to 2 weeks of age.[8] The mechanism of this age-related resistance is not well understood, but it may be related to development of resistance to colonization of the small intestine as the calf becomes older. This could be associated with the replacement of villous epithelial cells that occurs in the first few days after birth.

The disease is more common in **piglets** born from gilts than from sows, which suggests that immunity develops with developing age in the sow and is transferred to the piglets. In a survey of approximately 4400 litters of piglets over a period of 4 years in a large piggery, 64% of the litters were treated for diarrhea before weaning, and piglets born to sows under parity 2 were 1.7 times more likely to develop diarrhea before weaning than litters born to sows over parity 3. The susceptibility or resistance to *E. coli* diarrhea in piglets has an inherited basis. The cell surface receptor for the F4 (K88) antigen is inherited in a simple mendelian way, with adherence (*S*) dominant over nonadherence (*s*). Homozygous dominants (*SS*) and heterozygotes (*Ss*) possess the receptor and are susceptible, whereas in the homozygous recessive (*ss*) the receptor is absent and the pigs are resistant. The highest incidence of diarrhea occurs in susceptible progeny born from resistant dams and sired by susceptible sires. Most if not all pigs have intestinal receptors for F5 ($K99^+$) pili and an inheritance pattern similar to F4 (K88) receptors does not exist for F5 receptors.

Immunity and Colostrum

Newborn farm animals are agammaglobulinemic and must ingest colostrum and absorb colostral immunoglobulin within hours of birth to obtain protection against septicemic and enteric colibacillosis. The transfer of immunoglobulin from the dam to the neonate is termed *transfer of passive immunity*. **Failure of transfer of passive immunity** predisposes the neonate to development of infectious diseases (see also the section "Failure of Transfer of Passive Immunity").

Transfer of maternal immunoglobulin to calves depends on three successive processes:

- Formation of colostrum with a high concentration of immunoglobulin by the dam
- Ingestion of an adequate volume of colostrum by the calf
- Efficient absorption of colostral immunoglobulin by the calf

Colostral immunoglobulin is absorbed for up to 24 hours after birth in calves and up to 48 hours in piglets. However, in calves the maximum efficiency of absorption occurs during the first 6 to 12 hours after birth and decreases rapidly from 12 to 24 hours after birth. Following absorption, transfer to the intestinal lumen is a major means of IgG clearance in calves, and this transfer results in antigen-binding antibody in the intestinal lumen. Both blood-derived antibody and lactogenic antibody are significant sources of passive antibodies in the intestinal lumen of the neonatal calf. Maintenance of high concentrations of milk-derived antibodies in the small intestinal lumen may require more than twice-a-day feedings because antibodies derived from a milk diet are predominantly cleared from the intestinal lumen by 12 hours after feeding. Transfer of passively acquired antibodies from the circulation to the small intestinal lumen is therefore a reasonable hypothesis to explain the strong association between high serum passive immunoglobulin concentrations and reduced morbidity in neonatal calves.

Newborn dairy calves should ingest 80 to 100 g of colostral IgG, and ideally up to 150 g, within a few hours after birth to achieve serum immunoglobulin of 1000 mg/dL.

Environmental and Management Risk Factors

Meteorologic Influences

Although few epidemiologic data are available to support the claim, many veterinarians have observed a relationship between adverse climatic conditions and colibacillosis in both calves and piglets. During inclement weather, such as a snowstorm, a common practice in beef herds is to confine the calving cows in a small area, where they can be fed and watered more easily. The overcrowding is commonly followed by an outbreak of acute calf diarrhea. There is evidence that cold, wet, and windy weather during the winter months and hot, dry weather during the summer months have a significant effect on the incidence of dairy calf mortality.

The risk factors for mortality from diarrhea in beef calves in Alberta, Canada, have been examined. The odds of mortality were increased when the cows and heifers were wintered on the same grounds, when the herd was wintered and calved on the same grounds, and if the cows and heifers were calved on the same grounds. The morbidity and mortality rates from diarrhea during the first 30 days of life increased with an increasing percentage of heifers calving in the herd. Heifers are commonly more closely confined during the calving season for more effective observation and assistance at parturition. This may lead to increased contamination of the environment and the abdominal wall and udder of the heifers. Additional factors in heifers include a higher incidence of dystocia and maternal misbehavior and lower volume and quality of colostrum, all of which can result in weak calves that may not acquire sufficient colostral immunity.

Nutrition and Feeding Methods

Dairy calves fed milk substitutes may be more susceptible to acute undifferentiated diarrhea, some of which may be a result of enteric colibacillosis, compared with those fed cows' whole milk. Extreme heat treatment of the liquid skim milk in the processing of dried skim milk for use as milk substitutes for calves results in denaturation of the whey protein, which interferes with digestibility of the nutrients and causes destruction of any lactoglobulins that are present and may have a protective effect in the young calf.

Irregular feeding practices resulting in dietetic diarrhea may contribute to a higher incidence of enteric colibacillosis in calves. The person feeding and caring for the calves is an important factor influencing calf mortality a result of diarrhea. Although it is generally thought that general or specific nutritional deficiencies, such as a lack of energy, protein, or vitamin A, in the maternal diet predispose to colibacillosis, particularly in calves and piglets, there is no direct evidence that specific nutritional deficiencies are risk factors. However, they probably are, at least in indirect ways, for example, by having an effect on the amount of colostrum available at the first milking after parturition in first-calf heifers underfed during pregnancy.

Standard of Housing and Hygiene

Housing and hygienic practices are probably the most important environmental risk factors influencing the incidence of colibacillosis in calves and piglets, but they have received the least amount of research effort compared with other aspects, for example, control of the disease through vaccination. As the size of herds has increased, and as livestock production has become more intensified, the quality of hygiene and sanitation, particularly in housed animals, has assumed major importance. The disease is much less common when calves are run at pasture or are individually tethered, or penned, on grass.

Source of the Organism and Its Ecology and Transmission

Ingestion is the most likely portal of infection in calves, piglets, and lambs, although infection via the umbilical vessels and nasopharyngeal mucosa can occur. It has been suggested that certain serotypes of *E. coli* may enter by the latter route and lead to the development of meningitis.

In most species, it is assumed that the primary source of the infection is the feces of infected animals, including the healthy dams and neonates, and diarrheic newborn animals, which act as multipliers of the organisms. In some cases, the organism may be cultured from the vagina or uterus of sows whose litters become affected. In pig herds the total number of organisms on each sow is highest in the farrowing barn, decreases when the sow is returned to the breeding barn, and is lowest when the sow is in the gestation barn.

Calves acquire the infection from contaminated bedding and calf pails, dirty calf pens, nearby diarrheic calves, overcrowded calving grounds, and the skin of the perineum and udder of the cow. The organism is spread within a herd through the feces of infected animals and all the inanimate objects that can be contaminated by feces, including bedding, pails, boots, tools, clothing, and feed and water supplies. The organism is one of the first encountered by newborn farm animals, usually within minutes after birth. In cattle, the tonsil can be a reservoir for STEC in healthy animals. It is possible that virulent *E. coli* can be present and may be transferred to calves when they are licked by their dams at birth. The high population density of animals that occurs in overcrowded calving grounds in beef herds and heavily used calving pens in dairy herds and the continuous successive use of farrowing crates without a break for cleanup contribute to a large dynamic population of *E. coli*. The population of bacteria in an animal barn will continue to increase with the length of time the barn is occupied by animals without depopulation, clean-out, disinfection, and a period of vacancy. In some countries where lambing must be done in buildings to avoid exposure to cold weather, the lambing sheds may become heavily contaminated within a few weeks, resulting in outbreaks of septicemic and enteric colibacillosis.

Infected animals are the main reservoir for ETEC, and their feces are the major source of environmental contamination with the bacteria. Passage of the *E. coli* through animals causes a "multiplier effect"; each infected animal excretes many more bacteria than it originally ingested. Diarrheic calves are the most extreme multipliers because they often pass 1 L or more of liquid feces containing 10^{10}/g ETEC within 12 hours, and recovered calves can continue to shed bacteria for several months.

Normal calves and adult cows can serve as reservoirs of infection, and the bacteria can persist in a herd by circulating through animals of all ages. Carrier animals introduced to an uninfected herd are thought to be one of the main causes of natural outbreaks. The duration and amount of shedding probably depend on the degree of confinement, resulting population density, herd immunity, environmental conditions, and perhaps the serotype of the organism.

Pathogen Risk Factors

Virulence Factors of E. coli

Virulence factors of *E. coli* include *pili (fimbriae), enterotoxins (exotoxins), endotoxins,* and *capsules.* The adhesins in the pili of ETEC allow them to adhere to intestinal villous epithelial cells and prevent peristaltic elimination by the gut and to produce enterotoxins.

The virulence factors are relevant to vaccine efficacy. The species-specific adhesin antigens must be identified and incorporated into vaccines, which are given to pregnant females in an attempt to stimulate the production of specific antibody in the colostrum, which will provide protection against enterotoxigenic colibacillosis. An essential element of vaccine development is the detection of common fimbrial antigens occurring among most pathogenic isolates and able to induce antibodies that block bacterial adhesion. The great diversity of potential pathogenic serotypes encountered in colisepticemia and the failure of serotype-specific antibody to cross-protect against a heterologous challenge in experimental infection have made it difficult to develop vaccines against septicemic colibacillosis.

The major virulence factors of ETEC in calves are the F5 (K99) adhesin antigen and the heat-stable enterotoxin (ST). The colonization in the small intestine of calves by F5 ETEC appears to be site specific, having a predilection for the ileum. Some serogroups also elaborate the F41 adhesin to the F5. Other surface-adhesive antigens, such as Att 25 and F17, have been identified on bovine enteropathogenic and septicemic *E. coli*. The F17a-positive ETEC strains are no longer isolated from diarrheic calves in some countries. It is postulated that the use of a vaccine including O101, K32, and H9 antigens in addition to F5 explains the strongly reduced incidence of the O101:K32:H9, F5 *E. coli* clone. A F4-related fimbrial antigen occurs on some enterotoxigenic and septicemic strains.

Enterotoxins are plasmid-regulated secreted peptides of ETEC bacteria that affect the intestinal epithelium. Two types of enterotoxins are differentiated, large-molecular-weight (88 kDA) heat-labile enterotoxins (LT) and small-molecular-weight heat-stable enterotoxins (ST).[7] LT enterotoxins are predominantly produced by human and porcine ETEC strains, whereas ST enterotoxins are produced by human, porcine, and bovine ETEC strains. The heat-stable enterotoxin from bovine ETEC has been purified and characterized. There is evidence of a form of ST enterotoxin that is common to bovine, porcine, and human strains of ETEC.

Most strains of **septicemic *E. coli*** belong to certain serogroups with virulence properties that enable them to resist the defense mechanisms that would normally eliminate other *E. coli*. **Septicemic strains produce endotoxin**, which results in shock and rapid death, usually in calves that are less than 5 days of age and with FTPI. Isolates of *E. coli* from the blood of critically ill bacteremic calves on a calf-rearing farm in California constituted a heterogeneous group and were found to be aerobactin positive and often resistant to the bactericidal effects of serum. The relative importance of individual serogroups varies between countries. However, it has been established that typeable isolates of *E. coli* from septic calves belong to a relatively small number of serogroups.[9] Strains commonly isolated from calves with septicemia belong to serogroups O78 and O15.[9,10]

Enterohemorrhagic *E. coli* (EHEC) and Shiga-toxin-producing *E. coli* (STEC) are recognized in humans and animals with increased frequency and constitute a major zoonotic concern (see the discussion of enterohemorrhagic *E. coli* in farm animals and zoonotic implications). These organisms are members of O111, O103, O5, and O26 serogroups, and none produces enterotoxin, nor do they possess the F5 pili. They produce the potent Shiga toxins or verotoxins SLT1 and SLT2; and some strains, the **attaching and effacing *E. coli* (AEEC)**, attach to and efface the microvilli of the enterocytes, causing diarrhea and dysentery as a result of hemorrhagic colitis in calves 2 to 5 weeks of age. The effacing (*eae*) gene and the gene coding for the Shiga toxin 1 (*SLT1*) are associated with most isolates of AEEC in cattle. They have been isolated from both diarrheic and healthy sheep and goats.

A study of the onset and subsequent pattern of shedding of STEC O26, O103, O111, O145, and O157 in a cohort of beef calves on a mixed cattle and sheep farm in Scotland found that O26 was shed by 94% of the calves and that 90% of the O26 isolates carried the *vtx1*, *eae*, and *ehl* genes. *E. coli* O103 was the second most commonly shed serogroup of the tested calves, and the pattern of shedding was sporadic and random. There was an absence of shedding of *E. coli* O111, and the prevalence of shedding of O145 was low. Although some shedding of O157 occurred, shedding in calves was sporadic and infrequent. For O26, O103, and O157, there was no association between shedding by calves and shedding by dams within 1 week of birth. For O26 and O103, there was no association between shedding and diarrhea and no significant change in shedding following housing. In a sample of Australian dairy farms, calves as young as 48 to 72 hours had evidence of fecal excretion of STEC, indicating that dairy cattle are exposed to STEC from birth. Calves at weaning are most likely to shed STEC O26 or *E. coli* O157, similar to the prevalence surveys in the northern hemispheres.

Naturally occurring cases of attaching and effacing lesions of the intestines in calves with diarrhea and dysentery and infected with *E. coli* O126:H11, the predominant *STEC* strain in humans, have been described in the United Kingdom. STEC and *eae*-positive non-STEC have been isolated from diarrheic dairy calves 1 to 30 days of age.

E. coli O157 has been isolated from neonatal calves and has been implicated as a cause of diarrhea in calves. The isolates carried various virulence genes, such as *Ehly*, *eae*, *stx1*, and *stx2*. The *Ehly* gene may be a virulence marker for bovine enterohemorrhagic *E. coli* O157 strains. Similar findings have been reported in dairy cattle herds in Brazil. Strains of *E. coli* possessing a subtype beta intimin, normally found in human enteropathogenic *E. coli*, have been found in diarrheic calves in Brazil.

Non-O157 STEC have been isolated from diarrheic calves in Argentina, and the serotypes carried virulence traits associated with increased pathogenicity in humans and cattle. Severe clinical syndromes associated with non-O157 STEC are common in children under 4 years of age and may be associated with diarrheic calves, which shed highly virulent STEC strains and could act as a reservoir and contamination source in these areas.

E. coli O116, a serogroup previously associated with cases of hemolytic–uremic syndrome in humans, has been associated with an outbreak of diarrhea and dysentery in 1- to 16-week-old calves in India. *E. coli* O103:H2, an STEC strain causing disease in humans, has been isolated from calves with dysentery and from a sheep in Australia.

Necrotoxigenic *E. coli* (NTEC), which produce **cytotoxic necrotizing factor (CNF)**, have been isolated from cattle in Northern Ireland and Spain and from diarrheic piglets in England. NTEC1 strains from cattle, pigs, and humans can belong to the same serogroups/biogroups, carry genes coding for adhesions belonging to the same families, and possess other identical virulence-associated properties, and they therefore do not exclude the possibility of cross-infection between humans and farm animals in some cases. In Spain NTEC were detected by tissue culture and PCR in 15.8% of diarrheic dairy calves from 1 to 90 days of age; the majority were NTEC producing CNF2, and the risk increased with age. There was also a strong association between CNF2 and F17 fimbriae. The NTEC, with their associated adhesins and toxins, were present in diarrheic and septicemic calves as early as 1958, and their prevalence seems to be increasing. Their role in causing disease needs further examination.

Most ETEC from **neonatal pigs** belong to the so-called "classical serogroups": O8:K87, O45, O138:K81, O141:K85, O147:K89, O149:K91, and O157:KXVX17. Strains of these serogroups usually express and produce F4 (K88), F5 (K99), F6 (987P), F18 and F41 pilus antigens. With the exception of F18, these pilus antigens mediate adhesion of *E. coli* to ileal villi in neonates, causing profuse diarrhea in unweaned pigs. The F4 and F5 piliated strains are the most common cause of enteric disease in piglets under 2 weeks of age. ETEC strains that produce F6 pili colonize the small intestines and cause diarrhea in neonatal pigs under 6 days of age, but not older pigs. F18, in contrast, is not associated with neonatal colibacillosis in piglets, but together with F4 is the most common adhesin associated with postweaning colibacillosis. There are also some ETEC strains that produce none of the antigens mentioned previously.

F4 produces heat-labile enterotoxin (LT), F5 and F6 do not produce LT, and all three types produce heat-stable enterotoxin STa in infant mice. Some isolates produce neither LT nor STa but produce enterotoxin in ligated intestinal loops of pigs (STb). Other "nonclassical" strains colonize the small intestine to a certain extent, do not strongly adhere to the intestinal epithelium, and produce enterotoxin and diarrhea in neonatal piglets.

The porcine ETEC strains that induce diarrhea in piglets less than 2 weeks of age but not in older pigs are designated class 2, whereas those strains that induce diarrhea in older pigs are class 1 ETEC. The bovine ETEC strains have several features in common with the porcine class 2 organisms, which include the possession of the 0 antigens 8, 9, 20, or 101; characterization as mucoid colonies; possession of F5 pili; and production of heat-stable enterotoxin. Most ETEC strains of pigs belong to a restricted number of serogroups.

Lambs

Enterotoxigenic strains of *E. coli* can be isolated from the feces of approximately 35% of diarrheic lambs. ETEC strains have also been isolated from the blood of a small percentage of diarrheic lambs. F5 (K99) piliated *E. coli* are associated with outbreaks of diarrhea in lambs under a few days of age. F17 fimbriae *E. coli* have been isolated from diarrheic lambs and kids, but none of the isolates produced any of the toxins normally associated with ETEC strains. Attaching and effacing *E. coli* negative for Shiga toxin but positive for *eae* have been isolated from goat kids affected with severe diarrhea, with a high case fatality rate.

Zoonotic Implications of *E. coli*

Cattle are a major source of EHEC strain O157:H7, which is associated with foodborne disease in humans. (See "Enterohemorrhagic *Escherichia coli* in Farm Animals and Zoonotic Implications.")

PATHOGENESIS

The factors important in understanding the pathogenesis of colibacillosis are the affected species, the age and the immune status of the animal, and the virulence factors of the strain of *E. coli,* particularly its capacity to invade tissues and produce septicemia or to produce an enterotoxin. Diarrhea, dehydration, metabolic acidosis, bacteremia, and septicemia are the major pathogenetic events in the various forms of colibacillosis.

Septicemic Colibacillosis (Coliform Septicemia)

Septicemic colibacillosis occurs in all species as a result of invasive strains of *E. coli* invading the tissues and systemic circulation via the intestinal lumen, nasopharyngeal mucosa, and tonsillar crypts, or umbilical vessels. The intestinal permeability to macromolecules in the newborn piglet may predispose to the invasion of septicemia-inducing *E. coli.* These strains are able to invade extraintestinal tissues, to resist the bactericidal effect of complement in blood, to survive and multiply in body fluids, to escape phagocytosis and intracellular killing by phagocytes, and to induce tissue damage by the release of cytotoxins. Calves and piglets that are deficient in colostral immunoglobulins are highly susceptible to septicemia. Colostrum provides protection against colisepticemia, but it may not prevent diarrhea associated with *E. coli.* Also, colostrum-fed calves are much more resistant to endotoxin than colostrum-deprived calves. Calves, piglets, and lambs that have normal levels of serum immunoglobulins are generally protected from septicemia. The clinical findings and lesions in septicemic colibacillosis are attributable to the effects of endotoxin, which causes shock. The general effects of endotoxin in cattle include hypothermia, decreased systemic blood pressure, tachycardia and decreased cardiac output, changes in WBC counts, alterations in blood coagulation, hyperglycemia followed by hypoglycemia, and depletion of liver glycogen. Animals that recover from septicemia may later develop lesions as a result of local infection of other organs at varying periods of time. Arthritis is a common associated finding in calves, foals, and lambs. Meningitis is common in calves and piglets. Polyserositis as a result of *E. coli* has been recorded in pigs.

Enteric Colibacillosis

Enterotoxigenic Colibacillosis

Enterotoxigenic strains of *E. coli* (ETEC) colonize and proliferate in the upper small intestine and produce enterotoxins, which cause an increase in net secretion of fluid and electrolytes into the gut lumen. The adhesion of *E. coli* to the intestinal epithelial cells is mediated by bacterial pili. The enterotoxigenic form of colibacillosis occurs most commonly in calves and piglets and less commonly in lambs and kids.

The factors that allow or control the colonization and proliferation of these strains and their production of enterotoxin are not well understood. The bacterial fimbriae attach to specific receptor sites on villous epithelial cells, following which the bacteria multiply and form microcolonies that cover the surface of the villi. The capsular polysaccharide of *E. coli* may also be involved in adhesion and colonization. The fimbriae of *E. coli* are strongly immunogenic, a factor that is utilized in the production of vaccines. Because the F5 antigen is only expressed at an environmental pH above 6.5, colonization of the mucosa of the small intestinal tract starts in the ileum, where the intraluminal pH is the highest, and progresses proximally from there.[8] Once established in the gut, ETEC strains start producing and secreting a heat-stable enterotoxin. Similar to the expression of F5, production of enterotoxin is pH dependent, with very limited production at an environmental pH below 7.0.[8] Although this does not appear to have been studied specifically, it can be hypothesized that any factor resulting in an increase of the pH in the gut lumen will facilitate the proliferation of the organism; conversely, lowering the pH may reduce the severity of colibacillosis.

Diarrhea, Dehydration, Metabolic Acidosis, and Electrolyte Imbalance

The production of the enterotoxin results in net secretion of fluid and electrolytes from the systemic circulation into the lumen of the intestine, resulting in varying degrees of diarrhea, dehydration, electrolyte imbalances, acidemia, circulatory failure, shock, and death. The hyperkalemia that is observed in a subset of calves with severe dehydration and acidemia has been associated with cardiac arrhythmias, including bradycardia and atrial standstill.

The effect of the enterotoxin on the gut of calves, piglets, and other species is similar to the effect of cholera enterotoxin in humans and takes place through an intact mucosa. Enterotoxin stimulates mucosal adenylcyclase activity, leading to an increase in cyclic adenosine monophosphate (AMP), which increases intestinal chloride secretion. The increased intraluminal chloride content osmotically drags water into the gut to an amount that exceeds the absorptive capacity of the intestinal mucosa, thereby causing diarrhea. The secretion originates primarily in the intestinal crypts, but the villous epithelium also has a secretory function. The mucosal membrane colonized by ETEC remains morphologically intact. The fluids secreted are alkaline and, in comparison to serum, isotonic, low in protein, and high in sodium and bicarbonate ions. Distension of the abdomen of diarrheic calves may occur, which may be associated with fluid distension of the abomasum and the intestines.

When the disease is confined to the intestine, it responds reasonably well to treatment in the early stages. If death occurs, it is a result of acidemia, electrolyte imbalance, and dehydration. The acid–base and electrolyte changes in piglets 1 to 3 days of age infected naturally and experimentally with ETEC reveal severe dehydration, acidemia, and metabolic acidosis.

Severe metabolic changes can occur in calves with diarrhea. If the disease is progressive, acidemia and metabolic acidosis become more severe as lactic acidosis develops, and severe hypoglycemia may occur. If large amounts of fluid are lost, hypovolemia and shock occur.

Historically, conventional wisdom held that **metabolic acidosis** in diarrheic calves is the result of fecal bicarbonate loss and formation of L-lactate as a result of increased anaerobic glycolysis in dehydrated animals with decreased tissue perfusion. However, accumulation of L-lactate in neonatal diarrheic calves only appears to occur in calves in their first week of life. Because the relationship between L-lactic acid accumulation and the severity of metabolic acidosis could not be confirmed in clinical cases, it was proposed that exogenous acid supply to the organism must be the major contributor to the so-called **anion-gap acidosis** typically observed in diarrheic calves.[12] The anion gap, defined as the sum of the major cations minus the sum of the major anions, is a measure of "unspecified organic and inorganic acids," of which lactic acid forms a considerable part. It was not until the end of last century that **D-lactic acid accumulation** was first identified as a major contributor to elevated anion gaps in diarrheic calves. In the meantime, several studies confirmed that D-lactic but not L-lactic acidosis is a common occurrence in diarrheic calves. Furthermore D-lactic acidosis was identified as a major contributory factor in calves with high anion-gap acidosis.[12] It is currently assumed that D-lactic acidosis is caused by increased intestinal absorption of this compound in diarrheic calves, where malabsorption results in bacterial fermentation of unabsorbed carbohydrates to D-lactate.[12] Recent retrospective studies suggested that the major driving factor of the acidemia of diarrheic calves was an increase in unmeasured anions, of which lactic acid forms a considerable part. The loss of fluid through the intestinal tract with high sodium and low chloride content is likely to contribute to the so-called strong-ion acidosis. The increase of the total plasma protein concentration that is commonly observed with marked dehydration and resulting in a so-called weak-acid acidosis was found to be a minor contributor to acidemia in diarrheic calves.[13]

The severity and nature of the acidosis in diarrheic calves vary with the age of the calf. Younger calves tend to dehydrate more rapidly and severely than older calves, which may be related to the greater incidence of enterotoxigenic colibacillosis in the young age group. The severity of dehydration, hypothermia, and acidemia is associated with the level of obtundation. Accordingly, the degree of deterioration of the patient's demeanor in combination with the age of the calf are used to predict the severity of acidemia; the more severe the acidemia, the greater the depression.

Conventional wisdom posits that neurologic effects such as ataxia, somnolence, or even coma are primarily caused by severe acidemia or metabolic acidosis, but a series of recent studies unequivocally demonstrated that disturbed neurologic function can better be explained by the frequently observed increase in plasma D-lactate concentration than acidemia/metabolic acidosis per se.[14,15] Experimental studies conducted on euhydrated calves showed that neurologic signs similar to the ones observed in severely diarrheic calves can be reproduced by inducing hyper–D-lactatemia without concomitant acidosis. In contrast, experimentally inducing severe hyperchloremic acidosis in calves did not result in noteworthy effects on the demeanor of treated calves.[16,17]

Hyperkalemia in the Diarrheic Calf

Hyperkalemia is the most prominent electrolyte disturbance recognized in dehydrated diarrheic calves that are severely acidemic. It occurs despite significant net losses of potassium into the gut in diarrheic animals. A recent retrospective study conducted on patients of a teaching hospital revealed an incidence of hyperkalemia in diarrheic calves of 34%.[18] The predominant clinical finding associated with hyperkalemia is bradycardia and arrhythmia that can lead to atrial standstill, with fatal outcome. Although the association between hyperkalemia and acidemia is well established, the underlying mechanism is poorly understood.[19] The long-held mechanism responsible for hyperkalemia in diarrheic calves is directly associated with extracellular acidosis and the electrochemical exchange of K^+ for H^+ across the cell membrane, leading to a shift of potassium from the extracellular to the intracellular space in exchange for H^+ that tends to shift into the opposite direction with increasing extracellular H^+ concentrations. Although widely accepted, this proposed mechanism lacks a sound physiochemical basis because a decrease in plasma pH from 7.4 to 7.0 would increase the extracellular H^+ concentration from 0.000,040 mmol/L to 0.000,100 mmol/L. An equimolar exchange of K^+ for H^+ can therefore only account for an increase of the serum potassium concentration of 0.000,06 mmol/L, an effect that not only is not measurable with current laboratory equipment but also is physiologically irrelevant.[19] An alternative mechanism that has been proposed is impaired activity of Na/K-ATPase in states of acidemia, resulting in impaired transport of potassium into the intracellular space.[19] The previously mentioned retrospective study found the occurrence and the degree of hyperkalemia to be more closely associated to the degree of dehydration than to the decrease in venous blood pH or base excess, suggesting that the impaired ability to excrete potassium through the urinary tract may play a more important role than metabolic acidosis/acidemia in the etiology of hyperkalemia in dehydrated calves.[18]

Hypernatremia in the Diarrheic Calf

Hypernatremia is uncommon in diarrheic calves generally suffering from isotonic or mildly hypotonic dehydration. However, incidental cases of hypernatremia have been reported. It is presumed that mixing errors in the preparation of oral electrolyte solutions to treat diarrhea rather than diarrhea itself is the cause. The experimental oral administration of 1 L of electrolyte concentrate containing 2750 mEq sodium found that calves would willingly consume the solution mixed with milk, and developed signs of hypernatremia within 6 hours of administration.

Effect of Colostral Immunoglobulin Status

An adequate level of serum immunoglobulin can protect calves from death as a result of the effects of diarrhea, but not necessarily from diarrhea. The best protection is provided if both the immunoglobulin levels in the serum and the levels in the colostrum and milk during the first week after birth are high. The immunoglobulin subclasses in the plasma of calves that have received sufficient colostrum are IgG, IgM (and IgM is probably the more important of the two for the prevention of septicemia), and IgA. The serum IgG concentrations of calves under 3 weeks of age dying from infectious disease were much lower than those in normal calves. Of the dead calves, 50% had serum IgG levels that were more than 2 standard deviations below the normal mean, and an additional 35% had concentrations greater than 1 standard deviation below the normal mean. In the intestine, no single subclass of immunoglobulin is known to be responsible for protection against the fatal effects of diarrhea. Individually, each immunoglobulin subclass can prevent death from diarrhea even though calves may be affected with varying degrees of diarrhea. In contrast to the situation in the pig, IgA appears to be least effective.

In pigs, IgA becomes the dominant immunoglobulin in sow colostrum after the first few days of lactation, and this is the immunoglobulin that is not absorbed but is retained in, and reaches a high level in, the gut and plays a major role in providing local protection against enteric colibacillosis in piglets. Porcine colostral IgA is more resistant to gastrointestinal proteolytic enzymes than IgG_2 and IgM. On the other hand, IgG is at a peak concentration in colostrum in the first day after parturition, is readily absorbed by the newborn piglet, and is vital in providing protection against septicemia. Lysozyme in sows' milk may assist in the control of the bacterial population in the gut of the unweaned piglet.

Intestinal Mucosa

In general, ETEC exert their effects by the enterotoxin causing hypersecretion through an intact intestinal epithelium. However, the intraluminal exposure of the jejunum of 3-week-old pigs to sterile crude-culture filtrates from strains of *E. coli* known to produce two types of ST will induce microscopic alterations of the villous epithelium. Focal emigration of neutrophils, especially through the epithelium above aggregated lymphatic follicles; stunting of jejunal and ileal villi; and adherence of bacteria to jejunal and ileal mucosae are the most consistent findings. These changes are useful in making the diagnosis of enterotoxigenic colibacillosis in calves. Although enterotoxigenic strains are considered to be noninvasive, this does not preclude the possibility that invasion into the systemic circulation may occur, resulting in septicemia, or that septicemic strains may not also be present.

Enzyme histochemistry studies of the small intestinal mucosa in experimental infections of calves with rotavirus and ETEC indicate a marked decrease in enzyme activity in dual infections and a lesser decrease in monoinfections. Increased enzyme activity occurred in parts of the intestinal mucosa that were not affected or only slightly affected by the enteropathogens, which may be an adaptation of the mucosa to maintain absorptive function. Lactose digestion is slightly impaired in calves with mild diarrhea. Calves with acute diarrhea are in a catabolic state and respond with a larger increase of plasma glucose concentration to a given amount of absorbed glucose than do healthy calves.

Fat and carbohydrate malabsorption frequently occurs in diarrheic calves over 5 days of age and contributes to the development of D-lactic acidosis, which has been associated with a strong neurotoxic effect that is presumably responsible for the impaired demeanor of diarrheic calves.

Attaching and Effacing Colibacillosis

Attaching and effacing enteropathogenic *E. coli* can cause naturally occurring diarrhea and dysentery in calves at 18 to 21 days. They do not produce enterotoxin but adhere to the surface of the enterocytes of the large intestine. Affected calves pass bright red blood in the diarrheic feces. The lesions in experimentally infected calves are indistinguishable from those produced by some *E. coli* that are enteropathogenic for humans, rabbits, and pigs. The bovine O118:H16 EHEC strain is able to colonize the intestine of newborn calves, inducing diarrhea 24 hours after challenge and producing attaching and effacing lesions in the small and large intestines.

Synergism Between Enteropathogens

Enterotoxigenic colibacillosis occurs naturally and can be reproduced experimentally using ETEC in calves less than 2 days of age but not in calves 1 week of age. Diarrheic calves older than 3 days of age may be infected with enterotoxigenic F5 (K99) *E. coli* and rotavirus. There is evidence that prior or simultaneous infection of the intestine with rotavirus will enable the *E. coli* to colonize in older calves. Thus there may be synergism between rotavirus and ETEC in calves older than 2 days; this may explain the fatal diarrhea that can occur in calves at 1 week of age, which normally would not be fatal with a single infection. The rotavirus may enhance the colonization of *E. coli*.

The simultaneous experimental infection of neonatal gnotobiotic calves at 24 hours of age with rotavirus and ETEC results in a severe diarrheal disease. The same situation occurs in piglets. However, in both species the effect was considered to be additive rather than synergistic.

Summary of Pathogenesis

Septicemic colibacillosis occurs in newborn animals, and FTPI is the major predisposing factor. Enteric colibacillosis occurs in colostrum-fed animals and is associated with the colonization and proliferation of ETEC, which produce enterotoxin and cause varying degrees of diarrhea, acidemia, and dehydration. Although single infections occur commonly, as in piglet diarrhea, and what was previously described as enteric–toxemic colibacillosis in calves, multiple infections with ETEC and viruses and other agents are more common.

CLINICAL FINDINGS

Calves

Coliform Septicemia

Coliform septicemia is most common in calves during the first 4 days of life and is described as the systemic inflammatory response syndrome (SIRS) to an active infectious process.[20] Most affected calves have low levels of serum IgG because of inadequate transfer of colostral immunoglobulin.[21] The illness is peracute, with the course varying from 24 to 96 hours, with a survival rate of less than 12%. Early clinical signs are vague and nonspecific. Affected animals are weak and obtunded, commonly recumbent, and dehydrated; tachycardia is present, and although the temperature may be high initially, it falls rapidly to subnormal levels when the calf becomes weak and moribund. The suck reflex is weak or absent, the oral mucous membranes are dry and cool, and the capillary refill time may be prolonged. Cold extremities, weak peripheral pulse, and prolonged capillary refill time are common. Scleral injection is common. Diarrhea and dysentery may occur but are uncommon.

The involvement of multiple body systems and organs is characteristic of neonatal septicemia, and careful clinical examination is required to detect abnormalities. If a calf survives the septicemic state, clinical evidence of postsepticemic localization may appear in about 1 week. This includes arthritis, meningitis, panophthalmitis, and, less commonly, pneumonia. In a series of 32 cases of meningitis in neonatal calves, the most frequent clinical findings were lethargy, anorexia, recumbency, loss of the suck reflex, stupor, and coma. Opisthotonos, convulsions, tremors, and hyperesthesia were seen less frequently. The case fatality rate was 100% in spite of intensive therapy, and lesions of septicemia were present at necropsy.

Predictors of Septicemia

The early clinical findings of septicemia in neonatal calves are vague and nonspecific and are often indistinguishable from the findings of noninfectious diseases or those of focal infections such as diarrhea. Positive blood cultures are required for a definitive diagnosis of septicemia, but results are not usually available for 48 to 72 hours, and false negatives are common. Laboratory parameters that have been proposed to identify potentially septic calves include hypoglycemia, left shift of neutrophils, and signs of toxicity of neutrophils.[20]

No single laboratory test has emerged as being completely reliable for the early diagnosis of septicemia in farm animal neonates, and therefore scoring systems and predictive models using obtainable historical, clinical, and clinicopathologic data have been developed.[20] The goal of these mathematical models is to identify septicemic neonates early in the course of disease when appropriate therapy would be most likely to result in a favorable outcome. In a study of diarrheic calves under 28 days of age submitted to a referral clinic for treatment, 31% of the calves were septicemic, based on blood culture. Two models to predict septicemia were used. Clinicopathologic variables associated with an increased risk of septicemia were moderate (1.99 to 5.55 mg/dL) and marked (>5.66 mg/dL) increases in serum creatinine (OR 8.63), moderate to marked toxic changes in neutrophils (OR 2.88), and FTPI (IgG concentrations β 800 mg/dL, globulin β 2 g/dL [OR 2.72], and total serum protein β 5 g/dL). The clinical variables associated with an increased risk of septicemia were age under 5 days (OR 2.58), focal infection (OR 2.45), recumbency (OR 2.98), and weak suck reflex (OR 4.10).

Enteric Colibacillosis

Enteric colibacillosis is the most common form of colibacillosis in newborn calves, primarily 3 to 5 days of age. It may occur in calves as early as 1 day of age and only rarely up to 3 weeks. The clinical severity will vary depending on the number and kind of organisms causing the disease. The presence of a single ETEC may cause a state of collapse usually designated as **enteric toxemia**. In this form of the disease the outstanding clinical signs include severe weakness, coma, subnormal temperature, cold and clammy skin, pale mucosae, wetness around the mouth, collapse of superficial veins, slowness and irregularity of the heart, mild convulsive movements, and periodic apnea. Diarrhea is usually not evident, although the abdomen may be slightly distended, and succussion and auscultation may reveal fluid-splashing sounds suggesting a fluid-filled intestine. The prognosis for these calves is poor, and they commonly die 2 to 6 hours after the onset of signs.

In the more common form of the disease in calves, there is diarrhea in which the feces are profuse and watery to pasty, usually pale yellow to white in color, and occasionally streaked with blood flecks and very foul-smelling. The dry-matter content of the feces is commonly below 10%. Defecation is frequent and effortless, and the tail and perineum are soiled with feces. The temperature is usually normal in the initial stages but becomes subnormal as the disease worsens. Affected calves may or may not suck or drink depending on the degrees of acidosis, dehydration, and weakness. Calves under 8 days of age may be weak, primarily from the effects of rapid and severe dehydration; in calves older than 8 days the acidemia and metabolic acidosis, a considerable part of which is a result of the accumulation of D-lactic acid, tend to be more severe and make a greater contribution to obtundation and weakness. In the early stages of the disease, the abdomen may be slightly distended as a result of distension of fluid-filled intestines, which can be detected by succussion and auscultation of the abdomen. In some of these calves the diarrhea is not yet obvious but is delayed for several hours, when it can become quite profuse. Mildly to moderately affected calves may be diarrheic for a few days and recover spontaneously with or without treatment. However, 15% to 20% of calves with enteric colibacillosis become progressively worse over a period of 3 to 5 days, gradually become more weak, lose the desire to suck, and progressively appear more obviously dehydrated.

Throughout the course of the diarrhea the degree of dehydration will vary from just barely detectable clinically (4% to 6% of body weight [BW]) to up to 10% to 16% of body weight. The degree of dehydration can be estimated by "tenting" the skin of the lateral portion of the cervical region and measuring the time required for the skin fold to return to normal. In calves with 8% dehydration, 5 to 10 seconds will be required for the skin fold to return to normal; in 10% to 12% dehydration, up to 30 seconds will be required. Recession of the eyeball (enophthalmos) is an alternative method validated to reliably estimate the degree of dehydration in diarrheic calves. Slight sinking of the eyeball without an obvious space between the eyeball and the orbit represents 6% to 8% dehydration, moderate separation of the eyeball from the orbit represents 9% to 12% dehydration, and marked separation of the eyeball from the orbit represents over 12% and up to 16% dehydration. A summary of the relationship between degree of dehydration (% BW), depth of enophthalmos (mm), cervical skin tent duration in seconds, and the state of the mucous membranes and extremities in calves with experimentally induced diarrhea is set out in Table 19-12.[1]

Affected calves can lose 10% to 16% of their original body weight during the first 24 to 48 hours of the diarrhea. The hyperkalemia in calves with neonatal diarrhea has been associated with cardiac rate and rhythm abnormalities, including bradycardia and atrial standstill. Herd outbreaks of the disease in beef calves may last for several weeks, during which time almost every calf will be affected within several days after birth.

Veal calf hemorrhagic enteritis is a fatal syndrome of veal calves characterized by anorexia, fever, diarrhea with mucus-containing feces that become bloody in the later stages, and hemorrhagic diathesis on the conjunctivae and mucous membranes of the mouth and nose. The etiology is unknown; the *E. coli* strains isolated from the feces of affected calves produced enterotoxins and Shiga toxins, but their significance is uncertain.

In some calves between 10 and 20 days of age with a history of diarrhea in the previous several days, from which they have recovered, there will be metabolic acidosis without clinical signs of dehydration. Affected calves are depressed, weak, ataxic, and sometimes recumbent, and they appear comatose. Affected calves respond quickly to treatment with intravenous sodium bicarbonate. A similar syndrome occurs in goat kids.

Lambs and Goat Kids

Although some cases manifest enteric signs, and chronic cases may occur, colibacillosis in lambs is commonly septicemic and peracute. Two age groups appear to be susceptible: lambs 1 to 2 days of age and lambs 3 to 8 weeks old. Peracute cases are found dead without premonitory signs. Acute cases show collapse and occasionally signs of acute meningitis manifested by a stiff gait in the early stages, followed by recumbency with hyperesthesia and tetanic convulsions. Chronic cases are usually manifested by arthritis. The disease in goat kids is similar to that in lambs.

Table 19-12 Degree of dehydration in calves with experimentally induced diarrhea

Degree of dehydration (% BW)	Depth of enophthalmos (mm)	Cervical skin-tent duration (s)	Mucous membranes and extremities
0	None	Less than 2	Moist
2	1	3	Dry
4	2	4	Dry
6	3	5	Dry
8	4	6	Cool extremities
10	6	7	Cool extremities
12	7	>8	Cool extremities
>14	>8	>10	White mucous membranes

Piglets

Coliform Septicemia

Coliform septicemia is uncommon but occurs in piglets within 24 to 48 hours of birth. Some are found dead without any premonitory signs. Usually more than one piglet, and sometimes the entire litter, will be affected. Severely affected piglets seen clinically are weak and almost comatose, appear cyanotic, feel cold and clammy, and have a subnormal temperature. Usually there is no diarrhea. The prognosis for these piglets is poor, and most will die in spite of therapy.

Edema disease is unique form of colibacillosis occurring in piglets between a few days after birth to well after weaning. It is caused by Shiga-toxin-producing *E. coli* strains that induce degenerative angiopathy of small arteries and arterioles.

Enterotoxigenic Colibacillosis

Newborn Piglet Diarrhea

Newborn piglet diarrhea, a form of colibacillosis in piglets, occurs from 12 hours of age up to several days of age, with a peak incidence at 3 days of age. As with the septicemic form, usually more than one pig or the entire litter is affected. The first sign usually noticed is the fecal puddles on the floor. Affected piglets may still nurse in the early stages, but they gradually lose their appetite as the disease progresses. The feces vary from a pasty to watery consistency and are usually yellow to brown in color. When the diarrhea is profuse and watery, there will be no obvious staining of the perineum and hindquarters with feces, but the tails of the piglets will be straight and wet. Sick piglets occasionally vomit, although vomiting is not as prominent as with transmissible gastroenteritis. The temperature is usually normal or subnormal. The disease is progressive; diarrhea and dehydration continue, and the piglets become very weak and lie in lateral recumbency and make weak paddling movements. Within several hours they appear very dehydrated and shrunken, and they commonly die within 24 hours after the onset of signs if not treated. In severe outbreaks the entire litter may be affected and die within a few hours of birth. The prognosis is favorable if treatment is started early, before significant dehydration and acidosis occur.

Postweaning Diarrhea

The postweaning diarrhea (PWD) form of colibacillosis in piglets presents an economically important cause of death of weaned piglets. It is commonly seen within days of weaning. In peracute cases piglets are found dead with an obviously dehydrated appearance, deeply sunken eyes, and cyanotic extremities. In less acute cases the first sign may be a loss in condition that is largely a result of dehydration. Diarrhea may not be apparent in all cases because fluid may just accumulate in the gut in some animals. If present, diarrhea can be watery to pasty, may contain blood in some instances, and may last between 1 and 5 days (see also "Post-weaning Diarrhea of Pigs").

CLINICAL PATHOLOGY

Culture and Detection of Organism

If septicemia is suspected, blood should be submitted for isolation of the organism and determination of its drug sensitivity. Blood for culture must be taken aseptically and inoculated directly into brain–heart infusion broth. Because of the limited sensitivity to detect bacteremia by a single culture, the blood sample should be repeated a few hours later to enhance recovery rate and confirm septicemia.

The **definitive etiologic diagnosis of enteric colibacillosis** depends on the isolation and characterization of *E. coli* from the intestines and the feces of affected animals. The best opportunity of making a diagnosis is when untreated representative affected animals are submitted for pathologic and microbiological examination. The distribution of the organism in the intestine; determination of the presence of F4 (K88), F5(K99), or F6 (987P) antigens; and the histopathologic appearance of the mucosa contribute to the diagnosis.

The routine culture of feces and intestinal contents for *E. coli* without determining their virulence determinants is of limited value. The laboratory tests used to identify enterotoxigenic F4 (K99) *E. coli* include a direct fluorescent antibody technique with conventional culturing methods and the ELISA, with or without monoclonal antibody, to detect the organism or the enterotoxin in the feces. DNA gene probes specific for genes encoding enterotoxin and adhesins are available and are being used to evaluate *E. coli* isolated from diarrheic animals. Isolates of the organism can also be examined for the presence of toxins using an enzyme immune assay test and latex agglutination test.

Detection of STEC in feces has relied on cytotoxicity testing and DNA hybridization. Several ELISAs are available, and monoclonal antibodies to the Shiga toxins ST1 and ST2 have been used to examine feces from animals. The isolation of *E. coli* O157:H7 has relied on its ability to ferment sorbitol. A sandwich ELISA using monoclonal antibodies to *E. coli* Shiga toxins 1 and 2 for capture and detection is available for detection of STEC in animal feces. A PCR test is also available for detection of ST genes in *E. coli* isolated from cattle, sheep, and pigs affected with diarrhea.

The determination of drug sensitivity of the *E. coli* isolated from the feces of diarrheic calves and piglets is commonly done, but it is of limited value without determining which isolate is enteropathogenic.

Hematology and Serum Biochemistry

A total and differential leukocyte count and remarkable changes in the fibrinogen concentration may indicate the presence of septicemia or severe intestinal infection. However, severely affected calves may not have grossly abnormal hemograms.[21] In enteric disease, the major changes in plasma composition are dehydration, electrolyte imbalance, and metabolic acidosis/acidemia. The total plasma osmolality tends to be decreased.

The packed cell volume and the total protein concentration of the blood will indicate the degree of dehydration, although the increase of total protein in calves with FTPI may underestimate the degree of dehydration. The blood urea nitrogen (BUN) concentration may be increased in severe cases because of inadequate renal perfusion. The blood bicarbonate concentration is markedly reduced, indicating the presence of metabolic acidosis. Decreased blood pH values represent acidemia. Calves with a venous blood pH below 7.0 require immediate parenteral therapy for acidemia. Other serum electrolytes are variable, but there may be a slight decrease in serum sodium and a slight increase in serum chloride. In severely dehydrated animals hyperkalemia may occur, which may result in bradyarrhythmia.[18]

Hematologic abnormalities associated with **septicemia** vary with the stage and severity of the disease. Abnormal neutrophil counts (neutrophilia or neutropenia), a left shift of neutrophils, and signs of toxicity in neutrophils are commonly seen in septic animals.[11,20,21] Hypoglycemia is another common, although certainly not pathognomonic, finding in septic calves.

NECROPSY FINDINGS

In **coliform septicemia** there may be no gross lesions, and the diagnosis may depend on the isolation of the organism from the filtering organs. In less severe cases there may be subserosal and submucosal hemorrhages. A degree of enteritis and gastritis may be present. Occasionally, fibrinous exudates are found in the joints and serous cavities, and there may be omphalophlebitis, pneumonia, and meningitis. The histologic features of such presentations of colibacillosis are those of septicemia and toxemia.

In **enteric colibacillosis** of piglets and calves the carcass appears dehydrated, but the intestine is flaccid and filled with fluid. In calves, the abomasum is usually distended with fluid and may contain a milk clot. Clots are typically absent in calves fed whey milk replacers that do not contain casein. The abomasal mucosa may contain numerous small hemorrhages. In both calves and pigs, the intestinal mucosae may appear normal or hyperemic, and there may be edema of the mesenteric lymph nodes. Mild atrophy or even fusion of jejunal and ileal villi is often seen, but the key microscopic observation is the **presence of bacilli adherent to the brush borders of enterocytes**. Ultrastructurally, there is increased epithelial cell loss from the villus about 12 hours after experimental inoculation of calves with an ETEC.

In calves affected with attaching and effacing *E. coli* there is pseudomembranous ileitis, mucohemorrhagic colitis, and proctitis. Microscopic examination of well-preserved gut segments reveals bacterial adherence, atrophy of ileal villi, and erosion of enterocytes.

In addition to traditional bacteriologic culture techniques, the ETEC may be identified by several tests, including indirect fluorescent antibody (IFA) tests specific for F4 (K88), F5 (K99), and F6 (987P) pilus antigens. The IFA tests can be performed on impression smears or frozen sections of ileal tissue, and the results are available within a few hours. Newer techniques such as DNA gene probes, enzyme immune assays, and latex agglutination tests are now available to identify those isolates that are enterotoxin producers and have adhesin properties.

During severe disease outbreaks it is often necessary to conduct the necropsy examination on diarrheic animals that have been killed specifically for the purpose of obtaining a definitive etiologic diagnosis. The combined use of bacteriologic, parasitologic, and virological methods, together with histologic and immunofluorescent studies of fresh intestinal tissue, will provide the most useful information about the location of the lesions and the presence of enteropathogens. Postmortem autolysis of the intestinal mucosae and invasion of the tissues by intestinal microflora occurs within minutes after death, so gut samples should be collected immediately following euthanasia of the animal.

Samples for Confirmation of Diagnosis

Coliform Septicemia

- Bacteriology—chilled spleen, lung, liver, culture swabs of exudates, umbilicus, meninges (culture)
- Histology—fixed samples spleen, lung, liver, kidney, brain, and any gross lesions

Enteric Colibacillosis

- Bacteriology—chilled segments of ileum and colon (including content; culture and/or FAT, latex agglutination, PCR)
- Histology—fixed duodenum, jejunum, ileum, colon, and mesenteric lymph node

Table 19-13 Possible causes of bacteremia/septicemia and acute neonatal diarrhea in farm animals

Calves	Piglets	Lambs and kids	Foals
Bacteremia/septicemia			
Escherichia coli *Salmonella* spp. *Listeria monocytogenes* *Pasteurella* spp. *Streptococcus* spp. *Pneumococcus* spp.	*E. coli* *Streptococcus* *L. monocytogenes*	*E. coli* *Salmonella* spp. *L. monocytogenes* *Erysipelothrix rhusiopathiae*	*E. coli* *Actinobacillus equuli* *Salmonella abortivoequina* *Salmonella typhimurium* *Streptococcus pyogenes* *L. monocytogenes*
Acute neonatal diarrhea			
Enteropathogenic and enterotoxigenic *E. coli* Rotavirus Coronavirus Bovine torovirus (Breda virus) Bovine calicivirus Bovine norovirus *Cryptosporidium* spp. *Giardia* spp. *Salmonella* spp. *Eimeria* spp. (calves at least 3 weeks old) *C. perfringens* type C	Enteropathogenic *E. coli* *Salmonella* spp. Transmissible gastroenteritis virus *C. perfringens* type C (rarely A) *Clostridium difficile* Rotavirus PRRSV *Isospora* spp.	*Clostridium perfringens* type C *C. perfringens* type B (lamb dysentery) Rotavirus Caprine herpesvirus	Foal-heat diarrhea Rotavirus *C. perfringens* type B

PRRSV, porcine reproductive and respiratory syndrome virus.

DIFFERENTIAL DIAGNOSIS

The definitive etiologic diagnosis of septicemic colibacillosis is dependent on the laboratory isolation of the causative agent, which is usually a single species or organism. The septicemias of the newborn cannot be distinguished from one another clinically. The definitive etiologic diagnosis of enteric colibacillosis in newborn calves and piglets may be difficult and often inconclusive because the significance of other organisms in the intestinal tract and feces of diarrheic animals cannot be easily determined.

Table 19-13 lists the possible causative agents of diarrhea and septicemia in newborn farm animals. Using the combined diagnostic approach of detection of enteropathogens in the feces before death and in the intestinal mucosa after death, it is possible to identify where ETEC, rotavirus, coronavirus, *Salmonella* spp., and *Cryptosporidium* spp. appear to be the only or principal causative agents. However, mixed infections are more common than single infections.

Every effort that is economically possible should be made to obtain an etiologic diagnosis. This is especially important when outbreaks of diarrhea occur in a herd or when the disease appears to be endemic. The use of an interdisciplinary approach will increase the success of diagnosis. This includes making a visit to the farm or herd and making a detailed epidemiologic investigation of the problem. The diagnosis depends heavily on the epidemiologic findings, the microbiological and pathologic findings, and sometimes on the results of treatment.

The major difficulty is to determine whether or not the diarrhea is infectious in origin and to differentiate it from dietetic diarrhea, which is most common in hand-fed calves and in all newborn species that are sucking high-producing dams. In dietetic diarrhea the feces are voluminous and pasty to gelatinous in consistency; the animal is bright and alert and is usually still sucking, but some may be inappetent.

TREATMENT

Coliform Septicemia

Intensive critical care is required for the treatment of neonatal coliform septicemia. Early identification of animals suspected of being septicemic and early therapeutic intervention are important determinants of the treatment success. Evidence from human medicine indicates that the survival rate must be expected to decrease by 10% for every hour antimicrobial therapy is delayed in patients in septic shock.[22] A recent consensus statement in human medicine recommends initiation of intravenous antimicrobial therapy within the first hour after having recognized severe septicemia.[23] Thus, in most cases antimicrobial therapy has to be initiated before confirmatory culture results are available.

Although *E. coli* may be cultured from the blood of septicemic foals and calves, a significant percentage of isolates are gram-positive, which justifies the use of antimicrobials that have a broad spectrum. Antimicrobials are given parenterally and may be given continuously intravenously, more than once daily and daily until recovery is apparent. Isolation of the organisms from blood and determination of drug sensitivity constitute the ideal protocol. Intravenous fluid and electrolyte therapy are administered continuously until recovery is apparent (see "Principles of Fluid and Electrolyte Therapy"). Whole blood transfusions are used in calves and foals, especially when immunoglobulin deficiency is suspected from the history or is determined by measurement of serum immunoglobulins of blood. In one series on neonatal septicemia in calves, in which *E. coli* accounted for 50% of the bacterial isolates, the survival rate was only 12%.

Enteric Colibacillosis

The considerations for treatment of enteric colibacillosis include the following:

- Fluid and electrolyte replacement
- Antimicrobial and immunoglobulin therapy
- Antiinflammatory therapy
- Antimotility drugs
- Intestinal protectants
- Alteration of the diet
- Probiotics
- Clinical management of outbreaks

Fluid and Electrolyte Replacement

The dehydration, acidosis, and electrolyte imbalance are corrected by the parenteral and oral use of simple or balanced electrolyte solutions. The provision of fluid therapy in diarrheic dehydrated calves under field conditions in veterinary practice has been described. It is important to obtain an adequate history of the case, including age of the calf, duration of the diarrhea, and all treatments already given by the owner. The physical examination of the calf includes a standard clinical examination with emphasis on evaluating the degree of dehydration and acidosis.

Dehydration is evaluated by two clinical observations:

- **Skin elasticity**. The skin of the middle of the neck is better than the eyelid. A portion of the skin is tented and twisted for 1 second, and then the time to return to the initial position is measured—less than 2 seconds in the normal calf, 6 seconds in moderate (8%) dehydration, and more than 8 seconds in severe (12%) dehydration (Table 19-12).
- **Position of eyeball in the orbit and extent of enophthalmos**. This is determined by measuring the distance between the globe and the orbit. The eyeball is not sunken in healthy calves. Degrees of dehydration of 4%, 8%, and 12% are represented by 2-mm, 4-mm, and 7-mm enophthalmos, respectively (Table 19-12).

The degree of metabolic acidosis can be evaluated by determining the degree of obtundation, muscular tone, ability to stand, intensity of the sucking reflex, temperature of the inside of the oral cavity, and age of the calf that correlate with an estimate of the **base deficit**. The following categories for diarrheic calves are being used under field conditions:

1. Calves with good muscular tone and the ability to stand, strong suck reflex, and warm oral cavity have no base deficit if younger than 8 days of age and up to 5 mEq/L if older than 5 days.
2. Calves that can stand, have a slightly cool oral cavity, and have a weak suck reflex have a base deficit of 5 mEq/L if under 8 days of age and 10 mEq/L if older than 8 days.
3. Calves in sternal recumbency with a cool oral cavity and no suck reflex have a base deficit of 10 mEq/L if under 8 days of age and 15 mEq/L if older than 8 days.
4. Calves in lateral recumbency that lack a suck reflex and have a cold oral cavity have a base deficit of 10 mEq/L if under 8 days of age and 20 mEq/L if older than 8 days.

Categorizing Diarrheic Calves Into Treatment Groups

Based on the history and clinical findings, affected calves can be divided into the following categories according to the type of therapy required and which is most economical:

1. **Oral fluid therapy**—calves with a history of acute diarrhea, less than 7% dehydrated, slightly dry oral mucosa, good suck reflex, good muscle tone, alert, able to stand, and warm mouth. These can be treated with oral fluids and electrolytes.
2. **Oral fluid therapy and hypertonic saline solution**—calves with 7% to 9% dehydration and slight acidosis, weak suck reflex, good muscular tone, and warm mouth. Administer hypertonic saline solution (7.5% NaCl) intravenously at 3 to 4 mL/kg BW in 5 minutes. Assure voluntary intake of oral fluids, or administer oral fluids and electrolytes by stomach tube at 40 to 60 mL/kg BW. Reevaluate in 6 to 8 hours.
3. **Intravenous fluid therapy with alkalinizing agents**—calves that are more than 9% dehydrated, have dry and cool oral mucous membranes, are recumbent, have no suck reflex, and are very depressed. Provide intravenous replacement and maintenance fluid and electrolyte therapy including an alkalinizing agent for a period of 6 to 8 hours and up to 24 to 36 hours if necessary.

The details for parenteral and oral fluid and electrolyte therapy are described under "Principles of Fluid and Electrolyte Therapy."

Antimicrobial Therapy

Antimicrobials have been used extensively for the specific treatment of colibacillosis in calves and piglets because it was assumed that an infectious enteritis was present. It has been difficult to evaluate the efficacy of antimicrobials for the treatment of enteric colibacillosis because of the complex nature of the interactive factors that affect the outcome in naturally occurring cases. These include the presence of mixed infections, the effects of whether or not milk is withheld from the diarrheic calves, the effects of the immune status of individual calves, the variable times after the onset of diarrhea when the drugs are given, the possible presence of antimicrobial resistance, and the confounding effects of supportive treatment such as electrolyte and fluid therapy.

Change in Small Intestinal Bacterial Flora in Calves With Diarrhea

There has been a paradigm shift in the last 40 years toward categorizing an episode of calf diarrhea as being the result of a specific etiologic agent, such as rotavirus, coronavirus, cryptosporidia, *Salmonella* spp., or ETEC. Although the etiologic approach has correctly focused attention on preventive programs, including vaccination and optimizing transfer of colostral immunity, the approach has diverted attention from the universal finding of all studies, which is that calves with diarrhea of whatever etiology have coliform bacterial overgrowth of the small intestine.

Studies completed more than 70 years ago documented increased numbers of *E. coli* bacteria in the abomasum, duodenum, and jejunum of scouring calves. Moreover, calves severely affected with diarrhea had increased numbers of *E. coli* bacteria in the anterior portion of their intestinal tracts compared with mildly affected animals. More recent studies have consistently documented the fact that calves with naturally acquired diarrhea, regardless of age and the etiologic cause for the diarrhea, have altered small intestinal bacterial flora. Specifically, *E. coli* bacterial numbers were increased 5- to 10,000-fold in the duodenum, jejunum, and ileum of calves with naturally acquired diarrhea, even when the diarrhea was not attributable to ETEC, and where rotavirus and coronavirus were identified in the feces. The largest increase in *E. coli* bacterial numbers occurs in the distal jejunum and ileum, whereas the *E. coli* or coliform bacterial numbers in the colon and feces are similar or higher for calves with diarrhea than calves without diarrhea, with *E. coli* being more numerous in the feces of colostrum-deprived than colostrum-fed calves. Small intestinal overgrowth with coliform bacteria can persist after departure of the initiating enteric pathogen.

In calves with naturally acquired diarrhea, increased small-intestinal colonization with *E. coli* has been associated with impaired glucose, xylose, and fat absorption.

Mixed infections with enteric pathogens are commonly diagnosed in calves with naturally acquired diarrhea, and the clinical signs and pathologic damage associated with rotavirus infection are more severe when *E. coli* is present than when it is absent. Primary viral morphologic damage to the small intestine also facilitates systemic invasion by normal intestinal flora, including *E. coli*.

In calves with experimentally induced ETEC diarrhea, colonization of the small intestine by *E. coli* has been associated with impaired glucose and lactose absorption, decreased serum glucose concentration, and possibly increased susceptibility to cryptosporidial infection.

In summary, calves with diarrhea have increased coliform bacterial numbers in the small intestine, regardless of etiology, and this colonization is associated with altered small-intestinal function, morphologic damage, and increased susceptibility to bacteremia. It therefore follows that administration of antimicrobials that decrease small-intestinal coliform bacterial numbers in calves with diarrhea may prevent the development of bacteremia, decrease mortality, and decrease morphologic damage to the small intestine, thereby facilitating digestion and absorption and increasing growth rate.

Incidence of Bacteremia in Calves With Diarrhea

Calves with diarrhea are more likely to have FTPI, and this group of calves, in turn, is more likely to be bacteremic. Colostrum-deprived calves that subsequently developed diarrhea were frequently bacteremic, whereas bacteremia occurred much less frequently in colostrum-fed calves that developed diarrhea.

Based on field studies of diarrheic calves, it can be assumed that, **on average, 30% of**

severely ill calves with diarrhea are bacteremic, with *E. coli* being the predominantly isolated pathogen. The risk of bacteremia is higher in calves with FTPI than in calves with adequate transfer of passive immunity, and the risk of bacteremia is higher in calves 5 days of age or younger. Veterinarians should also assume that 8% to 18% of diarrheic calves with adequate transfer of passive immunity and systemic illness are bacteremic. The prevalence of bacteremia is sufficiently high in systemically ill calves that effective antimicrobial treatment for potential bacteremia should be routinely instituted, with emphasis on treating potential *E. coli* bacteremia, regardless of transfer of passive immunity status and treatment cost. Withholding an effective treatment for a life-threatening condition, such as bacteremia in calves with diarrhea, cannot be condoned on animal welfare grounds.

Antimicrobial Susceptibility of Fecal *Escherichia coli* Isolates

The most important determinant of antimicrobial efficacy in calf diarrhea is obtaining an effective antimicrobial concentration against bacteria at the sites of infection (small intestine and blood). The results of fecal antimicrobial susceptibility testing have traditionally been used to guide treatment decisions; however, susceptibility testing in calf diarrhea probably has clinical relevance only when applied to fecal isolates of ETEC or pathogenic *Salmonella* spp. and blood culture isolates from calves with bacteremia. Validation of susceptibility testing as being predictive of treatment outcome for calves with diarrhea is currently lacking.

The ability of fecal bacterial culture and antimicrobial susceptibility testing using the Kirby–Bauer technique to guide treatment in calf diarrhea is questionable when applied to fecal *E. coli* isolates that have not been identified as enterotoxigenic. There do not appear to be any data demonstrating that fecal bacterial flora is representative of the bacterial flora of the small intestine, which is the physiologically important site of infection in calf diarrhea. Marked changes in small-intestinal bacterial populations can occur without changes in fecal bacterial populations, and the predominant strain of *E. coli* in the feces of a diarrheic calf can change several times during the diarrhea episode. Furthermore, and most importantly, 45% of calves with diarrhea had different strains of *E. coli* isolated from the upper and lower small intestine, indicating that fecal *E. coli* strains are not always representative of small-intestinal *E. coli* strains. Marked discrepancies in antimicrobial resistance among *E. coli* strains isolated from different segments of the upper and lower intestinal tract of healthy veal calves at slaughter have also been reported in a more recent study.[24]

An additional bias present in most antimicrobial susceptibility studies conducted on fecal *E. coli* isolates is that data are frequently obtained from dead calves, which are likely to be treatment failures. The time since death is also likely to be an important determinant of the value of fecal culture because such a rapid proliferation of bacteria occurs in the alimentary tract after death that the results of examinations made on dead calves received at the laboratory can have little significance. Calves that die of diarrhea are likely to have received multiple antimicrobial treatments, and preferential growth of antimicrobial-resistant *E. coli* strains starts within 3 hours of antimicrobial administration. A further concern with fecal susceptibility testing is that the Kirby–Bauer breakpoints (minimum inhibitory concentration [MIC]) are not based on typical antimicrobial concentrations in the small intestine and blood of calves. Studies documenting the antimicrobial susceptibility of *E. coli* isolates from the small intestine of untreated calves, based on achievable drug concentrations and dosage regimens, are urgently needed. Until these data are available, it appears that antimicrobial efficacy is best evaluated by the clinical response to treatment, rather than the results of in vitro antimicrobial susceptibility testing performed on fecal *E. coli* isolates. Thus, the value of antimicrobial susceptibility testing as a tool to guide the choice of an antibiotic to treat enterotoxigenic colibacillosis must currently be considered as very limited. Nonetheless, antimicrobial susceptibility testing presents an important tool to monitor the development of resistances not only of pathogens, but also of so-called indicator bacteria normally isolated in healthy animals in the field.[25,26] Because antimicrobial resistance can be transferred via plasmids from apathogenic bacteria to pathogens, monitoring trends in resistance patterns in the field is of critical importance.

Surveillance for Antimicrobial Resistance in *Escherichia coli* Isolates

The purpose of monitoring antimicrobial resistance through so-called indicator bacteria is to avoid misjudgment (overestimation) of resistance levels that would be extrapolated from resistance of pathogenic bacteria.[24] As mentioned earlier, pathogens isolated from sick or deceased animals have frequently been exposed to antimicrobial therapy, which is likely to alter resistance patterns. A comparison of antibiotic resistance for *E. coli* populations isolated from groups of diarrheic and control calves in the United Kingdom found a higher incidence of antibiotic-resistant *E. coli* in samples obtained from farms with calf diarrhea than from farms without the disease. Considering all samples, bacterial colonies in 84% were resistant to ampicillin, in 13% to Apramycin, and in 6% to nalidixic acid. Antibiotic resistance among ETEC from piglets and calves with diarrhea in a diagnostic laboratory survey of one geographic area in Canada over a 13-year period found that the least resistance occurred against ceftiofur for all isolates, followed by apramycin and gentamicin for porcine and florfenicol for bovine isolates.

In a UK study over a 5-year period, *E. coli* isolates from calves with diarrhea became more resistant to furazolidone, trimethoprim-potentiated sulfonamide, clavulanic-acid-potentiated amoxicillin, and tetracycline. *E. coli* strains from outbreaks of diarrhea in lambs in Spain became increasingly resistant to nalidixic acid, enoxacin, and enrofloxacin. Some antimicrobial-resistant *E. coli* strains from diarrheic calves in the United States may possess a chromosomal *flo* gene that specifies cross-resistance to both florfenicol and chloramphenicol, and its presence among *E. coli* isolates of diverse genetic backgrounds indicates a distribution much wider than previously thought. In Spain, 5.9% of *E. coli* strains from cattle were resistant to nalidixic acid, and 4.9% were resistant to enrofloxacin and ciprofloxacin. In sheep and goats, only 0.5% and 1.4%, respectively, of the strains were resistant to nalidixic acid, and none was resistant to fluoroquinolones. Most of the quinolone-resistant strains were nonpathogenic strains isolated from cattle. Susceptibility data obtained from 10 European countries for the years 2002 to 2004 revealed that although there was a generally high prevalence of resistance of *E. coli* isolated from diarrheic calves, resistance patterns varied considerably between countries.[25] Generally high resistance of *E. coli* in the range of 50% or higher was reported from most countries for ampicillin, streptomycin, sulfonamides, trimethoprim, combinations of trimethoprim and sulfonamides, and tetracyclines.[25] Although resistance of *E. coli* isolated from diarrheic calves against fluoroquinolones was rare in several countries, resistance rates at or above 20% were reported from Spain, Belgium, and France.[25] In certain regions of Italy the incidence of enrofloxacin-resistant *E coli* strains was reported to have increased from 14.2% in 2002 to over 40% in 2008.[27]

The CTX-M-14-like enzyme has been detected in *E. coli* recovered from the feces of diarrheic dairy calves in Wales. The enzyme is an extended-spectrum beta-lactamase (ESBL), which confers resistance to a wide range of beta-lactam (penicillin and cephalosporin) compounds. Organisms possessing ESBLs are considered to be resistant to second-, third-, and fourth-generation cephalosporins, and in vitro resistance to amoxicillin/clavulanate among producers is variable, reflecting the amount of beta-lactamase produced. In addition to this enzyme, the isolates produced a TEM-35 (IRT-4) beta-lactamase that conferred resistance to the amoxicillin/clavulanate combination. These two enzymes confer resistance to all the beta-lactamase compounds approved for veterinary use in the United

Kingdom. Thus their occurrence in animals may be an important development for both animal and public health. ESBLs in human infections have emerged as a significant and developing problem, occurring in patients in the community and in those with recent hospital contact. Spread of this form of resistance in bacteria affecting the animal population could have serious implications for animal health, rendering many therapeutic options redundant.

Antimicrobial resistance to intestinal bacteria also occurs in dairy calves fed milk from cows treated with antibiotics and has been associated with the prophylactic administration of medicated milk replacer.[28] The resistance increases with higher concentrations of antibiotics in the milk. Susceptibility of fecal and environmental *E. coli*, *Salmonella* spp., and *Campylobacter* spp. to tetracyclines was monitored on farms during use of medicated milk replacer and after discontinuation of this practice. Discontinuing the use of medicated milk replacer resulted in increased susceptibility of these organisms to tetracyclines within 3 months, without causing an increase of disease occurrence.[28]

Antimicrobial Susceptibility of Blood *Escherichia coli* Isolates

The Kirby–Bauer technique for antimicrobial susceptibility testing has more clinical relevance for predicting the clinical response to antimicrobial treatment when applied to blood isolates rather than fecal isolates. This is because the Kirby–Bauer breakpoints (MICs) are based on achievable antimicrobial concentrations in human plasma and MIC_{90} values for human *E. coli* isolates, which provide a reasonable approximation to achievable MIC values in calf plasma and MIC_{90} values for bovine *E. coli* isolates. Unfortunately, susceptibility results are not available for at least 48 hours, and very few studies have documented the antimicrobial susceptibility of blood isolates in calves with diarrhea. In a 1997 study of dairy calves in California, the antimicrobial susceptibility of isolates from the blood of calves with severe diarrhea or illness produced the following results: ceftiofur, 19/25 (76%) sensitive; potentiated sulfonamides, 14/25 (56%) sensitive; gentamicin, 12/25 (48%) sensitive; ampicillin, 11/25 (44%) sensitive; tetracycline, 3/25 (12%) sensitive, although there was a clinically significant year-to-year difference in the results of susceptibility testing that may have reflected different antimicrobial administration protocols on the farm.

Evidence-Based Recommendations for Antimicrobial Treatment of Diarrheic Calves

The four critical measures of success of antimicrobial therapy in calf diarrhea are as follows (in decreasing order of importance): (1) mortality rate, (2) growth rate in survivors, (3) severity of diarrhea in survivors, and (4) duration of diarrhea in survivors.

In his review of the literature on the use of antibiotics for the treatment of calf diarrhea, Constable concluded that the statement that oral or parenteral antimicrobials should not be used is not supported by a critical evidence-based review of the literature.[29] The arguments used to support a nonantimicrobial treatment approach have included the following:

- Orally administered antimicrobials alter intestinal flora and function and thereby induce diarrhea, which has been documented on more than one occasion with chloramphenicol, neomycin, and penicillin.
- Antimicrobials harm the "good" bacteria in the small intestine more than the "bad" bacteria (an undocumented claim in the calf).
- Antimicrobials are not effective (a statement that is clearly not supported by the results of some published peer-reviewed studies).
- Antimicrobial administration promotes the selection of antimicrobial resistance in enteric bacteria.

In calves with diarrhea and moderate to severe systemic illness, the positive predictive value (0.65) of clinical tests (sensitivity = 0.39, specificity = 0.91) and the positive predictive value (0.77) of laboratory tests (sensitivity = 0.40, specificity = 0.95) for detecting bacteremia are too low, assuming reasonable estimates for the prevalence of bacteremia (30%). Accordingly, it is recommended that clinicians routinely assume that 30% of ill calves with diarrhea are bacteremic and that bacteremia constitutes a threat to the life of the calf. Antimicrobial treatment of diarrheic calves should therefore be practiced and focused against *E. coli* in the small intestine and blood because these constitute the two sites of infection. In addition, the antimicrobial must reach therapeutic concentrations at the site of infection for a long enough period (the treatment interval) and, ideally, have only a narrow gram-negative spectrum of activity to minimize collateral damage to other enteric bacteria. Fecal bacterial culture and antimicrobial susceptibility testing is not recommended in calves with diarrhea because fecal bacterial populations do not accurately reflect small-intestinal or blood bacterial populations, and the breakpoints for susceptibility test results have not been validated. Antimicrobial efficacy is therefore best evaluated by the clinical response to treatment.

The efficacy of antimicrobial therapy can vary with the route of administration and when given orally, whether the antimicrobial is dissolved in milk, oral electrolyte solutions, or water. Oral antimicrobials administered as a bolus or contained in a gelatin capsule are deposited into the rumen and therefore have a different serum concentration–time profile than antimicrobials dissolved in milk replacer that are suckled by the calf. Antimicrobials that bypass the rumen are not thought to alter rumen microflora, potentially permitting bacterial recolonization of the small intestine from the rumen. Finally, when oral antimicrobials are administered to calves with diarrhea, the antimicrobial concentration in the lumen of the small intestine is lower and the rate of antimicrobial elimination faster than in healthy calves.

In the United States parenterally administered oxytetracycline and sulfachloropyridiazine and orally administered amoxicillin, chlortetracycline, neomycin, oxytetracycline, streptomycin, sulfachloropyridazine, and sulfamethazine are currently labeled for the treatment of calf diarrhea. Unfortunately, there is little published data supporting their efficacy in treating calves with diarrhea. Extralabel antimicrobial use (excluding prohibited antimicrobials) is therefore justified in treating calf diarrhea because of the apparent lack of published studies documenting clinical efficacy of antimicrobials with a label claim and because the health of the animal is threatened; suffering or death may result from failure to treat systemically ill calves.

Administration of Oral Antimicrobials to Treat *Escherichia coli* Overgrowth of the Small Intestine

Based on published evidence for the oral administration of these antimicrobial agents, only amoxicillin can be recommended for the treatment of diarrhea; dosage recommendations are amoxicillin trihydrate (10 mg/kg every 12 h) or amoxicillin trihydrate–clavulanate potassium (10 mg/kg amoxicillin trihydrate and 2.5 mg/kg clavulanate potassium every 12 h) for at least 3 days; the latter constitutes extralabel drug use. Concurrent feeding of milk and amoxicillin does not change the bioavailability of amoxicillin, although amoxicillin is absorbed faster when dissolved in an oral electrolyte solution than in milk replacer, and absorption is slowed during endotoxemia, presumably because of a decrease in abomasal emptying rate. Amoxicillin trihydrate is preferred to ampicillin trihydrate for oral administration in calves because it is labeled for the treatment of calf diarrhea in the United States and is absorbed to a much greater extent. However, a field study comparing oral amoxicillin (400 mg every 12 h) and ampicillin (400 mg every 12 h) treatments for diarrhea reported similar proportions of calves with a good to excellent clinical response (79%, 49/62 for amoxicillin bolus; 80%, 59/74 for amoxicillin powder; 65%, 47/65 for ampicillin bolus; $p > 0.30$ for all comparisons). The addition of clavulanate potassium to amoxicillin trihydrate is recommended because clavulanate potassium, although not having a direct antimicrobial effect, is a potent irreversible inhibitor of beta-lactamase, increasing the antimicrobial spectrum of activity.

Oral administration of potentiated sulfonamides is not recommended for treating calf diarrhea because of the lack of efficacy studies. Gentamicin (50 mg/calf orally every 12 h) markedly decreased *E. coli* bacterial concentrations in the feces of healthy calves, and treatment with gentamicin has been shown to improve stool consistency in calves with experimentally induced *E. coli* diarrhea. However, oral administration of gentamicin is not recommended because antimicrobials administered to calves with diarrhea should have both local and systemic effects, and orally administered gentamicin is poorly absorbed.

Colistin administered orally is frequently used in calves in piglets to treat enterotoxic colibacillosis. Oral colistin will decrease the number of *E. coli* bacteria in the intestinal lumen and thereby the amount of enterotoxin affecting the intestinal mucosa and can present an effective treatment of uncomplicated cases of enteric colibacillosis. Because colistin is poorly absorbed from the alimentary tract, this treatment is not indicated in cases of suspected septicemia.

Oxytetracycline and chlortetracycline are not recommended for the oral treatment of bacteremia, although tetracyclines may have some efficacy for treating *E. coli* bacterial overgrowth of the small intestine. Tetracyclines are bound to calcium, and oral bioavailability when administered with milk is 46% for oxytetracycline and 24% for chlortetracycline.

Florfenicol achieves high concentrations in the lumen of the small intestine and is 89% absorbed when orally administered to milk-fed calves; however, florfenicol does not provide the most appropriate antimicrobial for treating calf diarrhea, because the MIC_{90} for *E. coli* is very high at 25 μg/mL and florfenicol (11 mg/kg orally) was shown to fail to reach the MIC_{90} value in plasma.

Fluoroquinolones clearly have proven efficacy in treating calf diarrhea, and a label indication exists in Europe for oral and parenteral enrofloxacin and oral marbofloxacin for the treatment of calf diarrhea. Oral fluoroquinolones have a high oral bioavailability. However, it must be emphasized that extralabel use of the fluoroquinolone class of antimicrobials in food-producing animals in the United States is illegal and obviously not recommended. Also, in other countries it may be illegal to use some of the antimicrobials mentioned here because of the regulations regarding their use in food-producing animals.

The indiscriminate use of antibiotics in milk replacers for the treatment of newborn calves and piglets is widespread and must be viewed with concern when the problem of drug-resistance transfer from animal to animal and to humans is considered.

In calves with diarrhea and no systemic illness (normal appetite for milk or milk replacer, no fever), it is recommended that the clinician should monitor the health of the calf and should not administer oral antimicrobials.

Administration of Parenteral Antimicrobials to Treat *Escherichia coli* Bacteremia

A common and widely recommended treatment is ceftiofur (2.2 mg/kg intramuscularly/subcutaneously every 12 h) for at least 3 days. Ceftiofur is a broad-spectrum third-generation cephalosporin and beta-lactam antimicrobial that is resistant to the action of beta-lactamase; the MIC_{90} for *E. coli* is less than 0.25 μg/mL, the recommended dosage schedule maintains free plasma antimicrobial concentrations at the desired value of four times the MIC_{90} value for the duration of treatment in 7-day-old calves, and 30% of the active metabolite of ceftiofur (desfuroylceftiofur) is excreted into the intestinal tract of cattle, providing antimicrobial activity in both the blood and the small intestine. Parenteral (2 mg/kg, intramuscularly once) administration of ceftiofur hydrochloride decreased mortality rate and the severity of diarrhea in pigs with experimentally induced enteric colibacillosis, although these pigs were not suspected to be bacteremic. The beneficial effects of parenteral ceftiofur in these pigs was attributed to decreasing intestinal luminal concentration of pathogenic *E. coli*. Administration of ceftiofur to treat bacteremia and diarrhea in calves constitutes extralabel drug use.

In those countries where the use of fluoroquinolones in food-producing animals is permitted for this indication, parenteral administration to calves with diarrhea has been recommended because of their broad-spectrum bactericidal activity, particularly against gram-negative bacteria. It must be emphasized that extralabel use of the fluoroquinolone class of antimicrobials in food-producing animals in the United States and other countries is illegal and obviously not recommended.

Cephalosporins and fluoroquinolones are among the most commonly used antimicrobials to treat colibacillosis in farm animals because of their proven efficacy and because they have largely maintained their activity against *E. coli*. Recent trends of decreasing susceptibility of *E. coli* and other pathogens mainly to fluoroquinolones and to a lesser degree to third- and fourth-generation cephalosporins have, however, been reported and present a serious public health issue (see following discussion under "Use of Antimicrobials That Are of Critical Importance for Human and Veterinary Medicine").[25-27]

Another recommended treatment is parenteral amoxicillin trihydrate or ampicillin trihydrate (10 mg/kg intramuscularly every 12 h) for at least 3 days. Although parenteral ampicillin has proven efficacy in treating naturally acquired diarrhea, whereas ceftiofur has unproven efficacy, the broad-spectrum beta-lactam antimicrobials amoxicillin and ampicillin are theoretically inferior to ceftiofur because parenterally administered ampicillin and amoxicillin reach lower plasma concentrations and require a higher MIC than ceftiofur, and they are not beta-lactamase-resistant. The intramuscular administration of amoxicillin and ampicillin is preferable over subcutaneous administration because the rate and extent of absorption are superior after intramuscular injection.

Parenteral treatment with potentiated sulfonamides (20 mg/kg sulfadiazine with 5 mg/kg trimethoprim, intravenously or intramuscularly depending on the formulation characteristics, every 24 h for 5 d) is also widely used. The efficacy of potentiated sulfonamides has only been proved when treatment commenced before clinical signs of diarrhea were present. It is therefore unknown whether potentiated sulfonamides are efficacious when administered to calves with diarrhea and depression, although it is likely that potentiated sulfonamides are efficacious in the treatment of salmonellosis.

Parenteral administration of gentamicin and other aminoglycosides (amikacin, kanamycin) cannot currently be recommended as part of the treatment for calf diarrhea because of the lack of published efficacy studies, prolonged slaughter withdrawal times (15 to 18 months), potential for nephrotoxicity in dehydrated animals, and availability of amoxicillin, ampicillin, and ceftiofur.

Chloramphenicol had proven efficacy in treating calf diarrhea resulting from *Salmonella enterica* serotypes Bredeney and Dublin, but it is now illegal for use in food-producing animals in the United States and in many other countries. The related antimicrobial florfenicol (20 mg/kg intramuscularly) failed to reach the MIC_{90} value in plasma and only exceeded the MIC_{90} value for less than 60 minutes when administered intravenously (11 to 20 mg/kg IV).

In calves with diarrhea and no systemic illness (normal appetite for milk or milk replacer, no fever), the clinician should monitor the health of the calf and refrain from administering oral or parenteral antimicrobials.

Use of Antimicrobials That Are of Critical Importance for Human and Veterinary Medicine

Antimicrobials commonly used for the treatment of colibacillosis in food-producing animals include third- and fourth-generation cephalosporins and fluoroquinolones, some of which have a label for the treatment of septicemia caused by *E.coli* in calves in some European and other countries and some of which can be used in an extralabel manner in certain countries.[30] These classes of antimicrobials are considered to be **critically important for human and animal health,** and thus recent reports of increasing prevalence of resistance of *E. coli*, *Salmonella* spp., and *Enterobacter* spp. against these classes of antimicrobials are very concerning.[25-27] Although there appears to be general consensus that these antimicrobials should be used restrictively in veterinary medicine, there is currently no harmonized approach on prudent use of cephalosporins and fluoroquinolones in animals. Guidance on prudent use of antimicrobials for animals have been published in many countries, but most are on a general level, and cephalosporins and fluoroquinolones are not always specially addressed.[30]

The World Organization for Animal Health (OIE) issued the following recommendations for these classes of antimicrobials:[31]

- They are not to be used as preventive treatment applied by feed or water in the absence of clinical signs.
- They are not to be used as first-line treatment unless justified. When used in a second-line treatment, such use should ideally be based on the results of bacteriologic tests.
- Extralabel/off-label use should be limited and reserved for instances in which no alternatives are available. Such use should be in agreement with the national legislature in force.

Immunoglobulin Therapy

One of the important factors determining whether or not an animal will survive enteric colibacillosis is the serum immunoglobulin status of the animal before it develops the disease. The prognosis is unfavorable if the level of immunoglobulin is low at the onset of diarrhea, regardless of intensive fluid and antimicrobial therapy. Most of the literature on therapy omits this information and is therefore difficult to assess. There is ample evidence that the mortality rate will be high in diarrheic calves that are deficient in serum immunoglobulin, particularly IgG, in spite of exhaustive antimicrobial and fluid therapy. This has stimulated interest in the possible use of purified solutions of bovine gammaglobulin in diarrheic calves that are hypogammaglobulinemic. However, they must be given by the intravenous route and in large amounts, the cost of which would be prohibitive. In addition, they are unlikely to be of value once the calf is affected with diarrhea; they are protective and probably not curative. Whole blood transfusion to severely affected calves may be used as a source of gammaglobulin, but unless given in large quantities will not significantly elevate serum immunoglobulin concentrations in deficient calves. Limited controlled trials indicate that there is no significant difference in the survival rate of diarrheic calves treated with either a blood transfusion daily for 3 days; fluid therapy given orally, subcutaneously, or intravenously, depending on the severity of the dehydration; or fluid therapy with antibiotics. Those calves that survived, regardless of the type of therapy, had high immunoglobulin concentrations before they developed diarrhea. This emphasizes the importance of the calf ingesting liberal quantities of colostrum within the first few hours after birth.

Analgesic and Antiinflammatory Therapy

Pain in sick farm animals has become an important issue for veterinarians and producers and is perceived as important animal welfare issue by the public. Adequate pain management should be part of any state-of-the-art treatment approach.

Diarrhea can be accompanied by abdominal pain as a result of intestinal inflammation and cramping. In addition to controlling pain, the main objectives of antiinflammatory therapy in animals with colibacillosis are to control the inflammatory process in the intestinal tract and to ameliorate the effects of endotoxemia and septicemia.[32] Several field studies reported that diarrheic calves receiving nonsteroidal antiinflammatory drugs (NSAIDs) in conjunction with fluid therapy showed less signs of pain, made a faster recovery, and had better weight gains in the reconvalescent period.[33] Although the underlying mechanisms do not appear to have been studied in detail, the proven beneficial effects of several NSAIDs have been attributed to their analgesic, antiinflammatory, antipyretic, and antisecretory properties.

Two broad categories of antiinflammatory agents that are available are the corticosteroids and the NSAIDs. Little evidence documenting the efficacy of corticosteroids for the treatment of calf diarrhea is available, but the use of this class of antiinflammatory drugs has been discouraged on the theoretical grounds that diarrheic calves already tend to have higher concentrations of plasma cortisol of endogenous origin and because of the immunosuppressive effect of these compounds.[32]

The efficacy of different NSAIDs such as meloxicam, ketoprofen, or flunixin meglumine in diarrheic calves that were systemically ill has been investigated in several studies.[32] A single treatment with meloxicam (0.5 mg/kg intravenously [IV]) and treatment with ketoprofen (6 mg/kg IV) twice, 4 hours apart, were both found to improve general attitude, the fecal score, and the feed intake of systemically affected calves with diarrhea.[32] Flunixin meglumine (2.2 mg/kg IV) hastened clinical recovery, but only for animals that had visible amounts of blood in feces.[34]

Because treatment with NSAIDs in diarrheic animals bears the risk of causing renal damage by further decreasing renal perfusion in already dehydrated animals, adequate oral and/or parenteral fluid therapy must be assured. An empirical guideline posits that treatment with NSAIDs should be limited to a single treatment whenever possible but should not exceed three treatments, a recommendation that has been justified by the risk of abomasal ulceration that is associated with prolonged use of these antiinflammatory agents.[32]

Antimotility Drugs

Administration of substances reducing intestinal motility to treat diarrhea in farm animals is advocated by some veterinarians. Compounds such as hyoscine-N-butylbromide and atropine have a proven inhibitory effect on intestinal motility, which undisputedly results in a rapid decrease of the fecal output in diarrheic patients. Although reducing fecal production may be interpreted as positive treatment outcome, it can also be seen as sequestration of gut fluid in the intestinal tract. Delaying the excretion of intestinal contents in patients suffering from malabsorptive diarrhea bears the risk of enhanced fermentation of unabsorbed carbohydrates and other nutrients. This could not only exacerbate enteral dysbiosis, but also the accumulation of D-lactic acid, which was found to markedly contribute to the clinical symptoms observed in diarrheic calves.[12] There does not appear to be any hard evidence in favor or against the use of antimotility drugs in diarrheic animals. Their use is nonetheless discouraged based on the possible negative effects that certainly outweigh the subjective perception of clinical improvement that is based on the apparent reduction of feces production.[32,35]

Intestinal Protectants

Intestinal protectants such as kaolin and pectin are in general use for diarrheic animals; however, as with antimotility drugs, their value is uncertain. When they are used, the feces become bulky, but intestinal protectants do not have any known effect on the pathogenesis of the disease.

Alteration of the Diet

Whether or not diarrheic newborn animals should be deprived of milk during the period of diarrhea is under controversial debate. Diarrheic piglets are usually treated with an antimicrobial orally and left to nurse on the sow. Diarrheic beef calves are commonly treated with oral fluids and electrolytes and left with the cow. However, in dairy calves it is a common practice to reduce the milk intake of diarrheic animals for up to 24 hours or until there is clinical evidence of improvement. The withholding of milk from diarrheic calves has been advocated based on the consideration that lactose digestion is impaired and that "resting" the intestine for a few days will consequently minimize additional osmotic diarrhea caused by fermentation of undigested lactose in the large intestine. In contrast, the argument in favor of continuous feeding of milk is that the intestinal tract requires a constant source of nutrition, which it receives from the ingesta in the lumen of the intestine. To date, there is no scientific evidence available confirming that transiently starving diarrheic animals has any beneficial effects on the clinical outcome. Studies exploring the effect of continuous milk feeding in diarrheic calves failed to confirm any deleterious effect, such as prolonged morbidity time, higher mortality rate, or higher treatment frequency. To the contrary, calves kept on milk had higher weight gains during the period of reconvalescence.[32,36] Although diarrheic animals clearly should be supplemented with oral electrolyte solutions to assist the compensation of excessive fluid and electrolyte loss, the currently available evidence is clearly in favor of maintaining the animal on milk or milk replacer. Calves should be offered reduced quantities of whole milk per feeding with higher feeding frequency. Milk should not be diluted with water because this may interfere with the clotting mechanism in the abomasum. In contrast to oral electrolyte solutions, milk should not be force-fed with an esophageal tube feeder because this will prevent closure of the reticular groove and thus foster accumulation of milk in the rumen, where it would be subject to bacterial fermentation.

Probiotics

The use of so-called probiotics for treatment and prevention of diarrhea has become increasingly popular over the past decades. Probiotics are defined as live microorganisms that, when administered in adequate amounts, confer a beneficial effect on the health of the host.[37] Most probiotics intended for veterinary use belong to the broad class of lactic acid bacteria, which include *Lactobacillus*, *Bifidobacterium*, *Enterococcus*, and *Streptococcus* spp. Probiotics have been claimed to promote gastrointestinal health and immunity, to reduce the shedding of potential pathogens in feces, and to reduce the need for therapeutic intervention.[38] Most importantly, probiotics are widely considered not to be present any health risk for the patient. Unfortunately, to date there are no published clinical data obtained in animals supporting any of these claims. Of particular concern is that the use of probiotics in humans has been associated with *Lactobacillus* bacteremia in several immunocompromised patients, and deleterious effects with some commercial products have been observed in neonatal foals.[39] In veterinary medicine concerns have been voiced about the uncritical use of probiotics, particularly in neonates with systemic disease or with a compromised intestinal mucosa.[40,41] With the current knowledge, the use of probiotics cannot be recommended for treatment or prevention of neonatal diarrhea.

Clinical Management of Outbreaks

Veterinarians should consider the following principles when outbreaks of colibacillosis in neonatal farm animals are encountered:

- Visit the farm and conduct an epidemiologic investigation to identify risk factors.
- Examine each risk factor and how it can be minimized.
- Examine affected animals.
- Identify and isolate all affected animals if possible.
- Treat all affected animals as necessary.
- Take laboratory samples from affected and normal animals.
- Make recommendations for the control of diarrhea in animals to be born in the near future.
- Prepare and submit a report to the owner describing the clinical and laboratory results and how the disease can be prevented in the future.

TREATMENT

Calf enterotoxic colibacillosis
Fluid therapy (highest priority)
Parenteral fluid therapy to correct acid–base and water and electrolyte imbalances* (R-1)
Oral rehydration solution* (R-1)

Antimicrobial therapy
Amoxicillin (10 mg/kg IM/PO every 12h for at least 3 days) (R-2)
Amoxicillin-clavulanate (12 mg combined/kg PO/IM every 12h for at least 3 days) (R-2)
Ampicillin (10 mg/kg PO/IM every 12h for at least 3 days) (R-2)
Colistin (100,000 IU/kg PO every 24h for at least 3 days) (R-2)
Enrofloxacin (2.5 to 5 mg/kg IV/IM/SC/PO every 24h for at least 3 days) (R-2)
Neomycin (10 mg/kg PO q12h) (R-2)
Trimethoprim-sulfonamide (25 mg combined/kg IV/IM/PO every 12h for at least 3 days (R-2)

Antiphlogistic therapy
Flunixin meglumine (2.2 mg/kg IV once) (R-2)
Ketoprofen (6 mg/kg IM once) (R-2)
Meloxicam (0.5 mg/kg IV/SC once) (R-2)

Antimotility drugs (R-3)

Probiotics (R-3)

Calf septicemic colibacillosis
Antimicrobial therapy
Amoxicillin-clavulanate (25 mg/kg IV/IM every 6–8h) (R-2)
Ampicillin-sodium (10 mg/kg IV/IM every 8h) (R-2)
Cefquinome (2 mg/kg IM every 24h) (R-2)
Ceftiofur (2.2 mg/kg IM/SC every 12 h) (R-2)
Enrofloxacin (5 mg/kg IV/IM every 24 h) (R-2)
Florfenicol (20 mg/kg IM every 24h) (R-2)
Trimethoprim-sulfonamide (25 mg combined/kg IV every 8–12h) (R-2)

Piglet enterotoxic colibacillosis
Fluid therapy (highest priority)
Oral rehydration solution* (R-1)
Amoxicillin (10 mg/kg PO/IM every 12h for at least 3 days) (R-2)
Amoxicillin-clavulanate (12 mg combined/kg PO/IM every 12h for at least 3 days) (R-2)
Ampicillin (10 mg/kg PO/IM every 12h for at least 3 days) (R-2)
Ceftiofur (1.1 to 2.2 mg/kg IM every 24h for at least 3 days) (R-2)
Chlortetracycline (20 mg/kg PO every 24h for at least 3 days) (R-2)
Enrofloxacin (2.5 to 5 mg/kg IV/IM/SC/PO every 24h for at least 3 days) (R-2)
Colistin (100,000 IU/kg PO every 24h for at least 3 days) (R-2)
Oxytetracycline (10 mg/kg IM every 24h for at least 3 days) (R-2)
Neomycin (10 mg/kg PO every 12h for at least 3 days) (R-2)
Trimethoprim-sulfonamide (25 mg combined/kg IV/IM/PO every 12h for at least 3 days (R-2)

*See "Principles of Fluid and Electrolyte Therapy."

CONTROL

Because of the complex nature of the disease, it is unrealistic to expect total prevention, and control at an economical level should be the major goal. Effective control of colibacillosis can be accomplished by the application of three principles:

- Reduce the degree of exposure of the newborn to the infectious agents.
- Provide maximum nonspecific resistance with adequate colostrum and optimum animal management.
- Increase the specific resistance of the newborn by vaccination of the dam or the newborn.

Reduction of the Degree of Exposure of the Newborn to the Infectious Agents

The emphasis is on ensuring that newborns are born into a clean environment. Barns, confinement pens, and paddocks used as parturition areas must be clean and should preferably have been left vacant for several days before the pregnant dams are placed in them.

Dairy Calves

The following comments are directed particularly at calves born indoors, where contamination is higher than outdoors:

- Greatest attention must be paid to maternity pen hygiene. Calves should be born in well-bedded clean and dry box stalls.
- Obstetric intervention and assistance to calving should be provided by adequately trained personnel in a calm and hygienic manner.

- Immediately after birth the umbilicus of the calf should be swabbed or dipped 2% iodine tincture or chlorhexidine solution.
- In herds with high disease incidence the residence time of calves in the maternity pen should be kept as short as possible and calves moved to clean, dry, and well-bedded individual calf pens or hutches as soon as possible after birth.
- Calves affected with diarrhea should be removed from the main calf barn if possible and treated in isolation.

Beef Calves

Beef calves are usually born on pasture or on confined calving grounds, and the following guidelines apply:

- Calving grounds should have been free of animals previous to the calving period; the grounds should be well drained, dry, and scraped free of snow if possible. Each cow–calf pair should be provided with at least 2000 sq ft of space. Calving on pasture with adequate protection from wind is ideal. Covering the calving grounds with straw or wood shavings provides a comfortable calving environment.
- In large beef herds, in a few days following birth when the calf is nursing successfully, the cow–calf pair should be moved to a nursery pasture to avoid overcrowding in the calving grounds.

In beef herds, breeding plans should ensure that heifers calve at least 2 weeks before the mature cows. Limiting the breeding and therefore the calving season to 45 days or less for heifers also offers several advantages. A short calving season allows the producer to more effectively and economically concentrate personnel resources on calving management compared with a longer calving season. Calving heifers earlier allows them additional time required before the next breeding season to be on an increasing plane of nutrition necessary to maintain a high conception rate. The earlier calving of heifers also provides less exposure of their calves to infection pressure from the mature animals in the herd.

The incidence and severity of neonatal disease will typically increase, and the age at disease onset will decrease, as the calving season progresses. This phenomenon is common in beef herds because of the effect of the calf as a biological amplifier. The more the calving season is shortened, the more the biological amplification effect is negated.

For beef herds, it is necessary to have a plan for cattle movement throughout the calving season. This requires a minimum of four or five separate pastures: a gestation pasture, a calving pasture, and a series of nursery pastures. To ensure that beef calves are born in a sanitary environment, the herd should be moved from the gestation pasture to the calving pasture 1 to 2 weeks before calving. One day after birth, the cow or heifer and her calf should be moved to a nursery pasture. Cow–calf pairs should be added to a single nursery pasture until the appropriate number of pairs has been reached. Thereafter, cow–calf pairs can be added to a second nursery pasture. The difference in age between the oldest and youngest calf in a nursery pasture should never exceed 30 days, and smaller differences are preferable. This negates the biological amplification effect. The longer the calving season, the greater the need for a large number of nursery pastures. Calves that develop diarrhea should be removed immediately to an area away from healthy calves, treated, and not returned until all calves in the group are at low risk for developing diarrhea (>30 days of age).

The nutrition of the pregnant cows, and particularly the first-calf heifers, must be monitored throughout gestation to ensure an adequate body condition and sufficient resources to provide an adequate supply of good-quality colostrum.

Veal Calves

Veal calves are usually obtained from several different sources, and 25% to 30% or higher may be deficient in serum immunoglobulin. The following guidelines apply to veal calves:

- On arrival, calves should be placed in their individual calf pens, which were previously cleaned, disinfected, and left vacant to dry.
- Feeding utensils are a frequent source of pathogenic *E. coli* and should be cleaned and air-dried daily.
- Calves affected with diarrhea should be removed and isolated immediately.

Lambs and Kids

The principles described earlier for calves apply to lambs and kids. Lambing sheds can be a source of heavy contamination and must be managed accordingly to reduce infection pressure on newborn lambs.

Piglets

Piglets born in a total-confinement system may be exposed to a high infection rate. The following guidelines apply to piglets:

- The all-in/all-out system of batch farrowing, in which groups of sows farrow within a week, is recommended. This system will allow the herdsman to wean the piglets from a group of sows in a day or two and clean, disinfect, and leave vacant a battery of farrowing crates for the next group of sows. This system will reduce the total occupation time and the infection rate. The continuous farrowing system without regular breaks is not recommended.
- Before being placed in the farrowing crate, sows should be washed with a suitable disinfectant to reduce the bacterial population of the skin.

Provision of Maximum Nonspecific Resistance With Adequate Colostrum and Optimum Animal Management

The first step of fostering maximum nonspecific resistance is the provision of optimal nutrition to the pregnant dam, which will result in a vigorous newborn animal and adequate quantities of colostrum. At the time of parturition, surveillance of the dams and the provision of any obstetric assistance required will ensure that newborns are born with as much vigor as possible. Parturition injuries and intrapartum hypoxemia must be minimized as much as possible.

Colostrum Management

The next most important control measure is to ensure that liberal quantities of good-quality colostrum are available and ingested within minutes and no later than a few hours after birth. Although the optimum amount of colostrum that should be ingested by a certain time after birth is well known, the major difficulty with all species under practical conditions is to know how much colostrum a particular neonate has ingested. Because modern livestock production has become so intensive, it is imperative that the animal attendants make every effort to ensure that sufficient colostrum is ingested by that particular species. In a recent national survey in the United States, the estimated prevalence of failure of passive immunity transfer in female dairy calves was 19.2%.[41]

Failure of transfer of passive immunity (FTPI), as determined by calf serum immunoglobulin IgG_1 concentration below 1000 mg/dL at 48 hours of age, occurred in 61.4% of calves from a dairy in which calves were nursed by their dams, 19.3% of calves from a dairy using nipple bottle feeding, and 10.8% of calves from a dairy using tube feeding. A higher prevalence of FTPI in dairy calves can occur because an insufficient volume of colostrum is ingested by the calf. When artificial feeding is used, inadequate immunoglobulin concentration in the colostrum fed is the most important factor resulting in FTPI. The prevalence of FTPI in dairy herds can be minimized by artificially feeding all newborn calves large volumes (3 to 4 L) of fresh or refrigerated first-milking colostrum from cows that had nonlactating intervals of normal duration. This volume is considerably greater than the intake that Holstein calves usually achieve by sucking and also exceeds the voluntary intake of most calves fed colostrum by nipple bottle.

Calves need to ingest at least 100 g of IgG_1 in the first colostrum feeding to ensure adequate transfer of passive immunity. Thus the routine force-feeding of a sufficient amount of pooled colostrum immediately after birth results in high serum levels of colostrum immunoglobulin in dairy calves and is becoming a common practice in dairy herds.

Encouraging and assisting the calf to suck within 1 hour after birth is also effective. The provision of early assisted sucking of colostrum to satiation within 1 hour after birth will result in high concentrations of absorbed immunoglobulin in the majority of calves. The ingestion of 100 g or more of colostral immunoglobulin within a few hours after birth is more effective in achieving high levels of colostral immunoglobulin in calves than either leaving the calf with the cow for the next 12 to 24 hours or encouraging the calf to suck again at 12 hours, which will not result in a significant increase in absorbed immunoglobulin.

Despite early assisted sucking, a small proportion of calves will remain hypogammaglobulinemic because of low concentrations of immunoglobulin in their dams' colostrum, usually associated with leakage of colostrum from the udder before calving.

In large herds where economics permit, a laboratory surveillance system may be used on batches of calves to determine the serum levels of immunoglobulin acquired. An accurate analysis may be done by electrophoresis or an estimation using the zinc sulfate turbidity test. Blood should be collected from calves at 24 hours of age. Samples taken a few days later may not be a true reflection of the original serum immunoglobulin concentrations. The information obtained from determination of serum immunoglobulin in calves at 24 hours of age can be used to improve management practices, particularly the early ingestion of colostrum.

Quality of Colostrum

Specific Gravity

Differentiating high-immunoglobulin-concentration colostrum from low-immunoglobulin-concentration is problematic. Measurement of the specific gravity of the colostrum of dairy cows with a commercially available hydrometer (Colostrometer) has been explored. Originally it was claimed that measurement of specific gravity provided an inexpensive and practical method for estimating colostral immunoglobulin concentration. However, the specific gravity of colostrum is more correlated with its protein concentration than immunoglobulin concentration and varies with colostral temperature, thus limiting the predictive accuracy of the test. In addition, different relationships between specific gravity and immunoglobulin concentration of colostrum have been observed for different populations of Holstein Friesian and Jersey cows and between herds. Specific gravity may also vary considerably according to season of the year. Specific gravity was measured in 1085 first-milking colostrum samples from 608 dairy cows of four breeds on a single farm during a 5-year period. The specific gravity more closely reflected protein concentration than IgG concentration and was markedly affected by month of calving. Colostral specific gravity values were highest for Holstein and Jersey cows, cows in third or later lactation, and cows calving in autumn. They were lowest in Brown Swiss and Ayrshire cows, cows in first or second lactation, and cows calving in summer. Thus using the specific gravity of colostrum as an indicator of IgG concentration has potential limitations.

Frozen and Thawed Colostrum

Colostrum can be banked as frozen colostrum for future use. Excess colostrum can be stored frozen and thawed as necessary to provide an IgG source when administration of dam colostrum is impractical or insufficient. Experience has shown that the composition of frozen colostrum remains constant throughout storage. No significant changes in pH, percentage acidity, milk fat, total solids, total nitrogen, or nonprotein resulted from colostrum being stored. Feeding 4 L of frozen thawed colostrum (which had been frozen at −20°C (−4°F) for 24 h) to calves by orogastric tube at 3 hours after birth did not result in a significant difference in IgG absorption compared with calves receiving fresh colostrum.

Pasteurization of Colostrum

There are several indications for pasteurization of colostrum. This procedure can be a suitable instrument in a program for the control of specific infectious diseases, such as paratuberculosis, salmonellosis, or *M. bovis* infection, but it can also be useful to ameliorate calf health by improving colostrum quality and reducing the exposure of the neonate to pathogens. On-farm pasteurization of bovine colostrum for 60 min at 60°C (140°F) results in elimination or at least significant reduction of bacterial contamination without impairing fluid characteristics or availability of IgG for intestinal absorption.[7] One recent study reported significantly higher serum IgG concentrations at 24 hours of life when calves were fed pasteurized colostrum compared with calves receiving the same quality and amount of raw colostrum.[42] The authors attributed this effect to reduced bacterial interference with intestinal IgG absorption. Pasteurization extends the shelf life of refrigerated colostrum without additives to 8 to 10 days when stored in clean, sealed containers.

Colostrum Supplements and Replacers

Some colostrum-derived oral supplements containing immunoglobulin are available for newborn calves in which colostrum intake is suspected or known to be inadequate. **Colostrum supplement** products have been developed to provide exogenous IgG to calves when the dam's fresh colostrum is of low IgG concentration. Many producers also use these products to replace colostrum when it is unavailable as a result of maternal agalactia, acute mastitis, or other causes of inadequate colostrum supply. However, they contain low immunoglobulin concentrations compared with those found in high-quality first-milking colostrum. Most colostral supplements provide only 25 to 45 g of IgG/dose of 454 g, which is reconstituted in 2 L of water. Feeding one or even two doses of such supplements is insufficient to provide a mass of 100 g of IgG within the first 12 hours after birth. **Colostrum replacers** are intended to provide the sole source of IgG and thus must provide at least 100 g of IgG. Newborn colostrum-deprived dairy calves fed spray-dried colostrum containing 126 g of immunoglobulin in 3 L of water as their sole source of immunoglobulin achieved normal mean serum immunoglobulin concentrations. Whey protein concentrate as a colostrum substitute, administered to calves as a single feeding, was ineffective in preventing neonatal morbidity and mortality compared with a single feeding of pooled colostrum.

The IgG derived from bovine serum or immunoglobulin concentrates from bovine plasma are well absorbed by neonatal calves when given in adequate amounts. The serum concentration of IgG in calves at 2 days of age force-fed a colostrum supplement containing spray-dried serum (total of 90 g immunoglobulin protein) within 3 hours after birth was much lower than in calves fed 4 L of fresh colostrum. The mass of IgG and the method of processing are critical. Products providing less than 100 g of IgG/dose should not be used to replace colostrum.

To be successful, colostral supplements and replacers must provide enough IgG mass to result in 24-hour calf serum IgG concentrations of more than 10 g/L.

Purified Bovine Immunoglobulin

The administration of purified bovine gammaglobulin to calves that are deficient appears to be a logical approach, but the results have been unsuccessful. Large doses (30 to 50 g) of gammaglobulin given intravenously would be required to increase the level of serum gammaglobulin from 0.5 g/dL to 1.5 g/dL of serum, which is considered an adequate level. The cost would be prohibitive. The administration of gammaglobulin by any parenteral route other than the intravenous route does not result in a significant increase in serum levels of the immunoglobulin.

To be effective, infusion of immunoglobulin derived from blood must increase serum IgG concentrations and reduce morbidity and mortality before weaning without affecting later production. Parenteral infusions of immunoglobulin will increase the concentrations of serum IgG in calves, but may not necessarily have an effect on morbidity or mortality. High levels of specific circulating immunoglobulin can serve as a reservoir of antibodies to move into the intestine and prevent enteric infection. Thus immunoglobulin sources other than colostrum may not provide immunoglobulins that are specific for antigens present in the environment or might be insufficient when calves are exposed to a heavy infection pressure.

Beef Calves

The management strategies to decrease calf death losses in beef herds have been described. The role of management intervention in the prevention of neonatal deaths includes measures to improve host defenses and environmental hygiene to minimize outbreaks of neonatal disease. Specific attention is centered on preventing dystocia, improving transfer of colostral immunoglobulin, and limiting environmental contamination.

The following practices should be implemented:

- Management of the beef herd must emphasize prevention of dystocia, which involves limiting calf size and ensuring adequate pelvic area of the dams.
- Beef calves should be assisted at birth, if necessary, to avoid exhaustion and weakness from a prolonged parturition.
- Normally beef calves will make attempts to get up and suck within 20 minutes after birth, but this may be delayed for up to 8 hours or longer. Beef calves that do not suck within 2 hours should be fed colostrum by nipple bottle or stomach tube. Whenever possible, they should be encouraged and assisted to suck to satiation within 1 hour after birth. The dam can be restrained and the calf assisted to suck. If the calf is unable or unwilling to suck, the dam should be restrained and milked out by hand, and the calf should be fed the colostrum with a nipple bottle or stomach tube. The mean volume of colostrum and colostral immunoglobulin produced in beef cows and the absorption of colostral immunoglobulin by their calves can vary widely. Beef calves deserted by indifferent dams need special attention. FTPI is common and estimated at 10% to 40% of beef calves.
- Constant surveillance of the calving grounds is necessary to avoid overcrowding, to detect diarrheic calves that should be removed, to avoid mismothering, and to ensure that every calf is seen to nurse its dam. Although up to 25% of beef calves may not have sufficient serum levels of immunoglobulin, the provision of excellent management will minimize the incidence of colibacillosis. The recently developed practice of corticosteroid-induced parturition in cattle may result in a major mismothering problem if too many calves are born too quickly in a confined space. Every management effort must be used to establish the cow–calf herd as soon as possible after birth. This will require high-quality management to reduce the infection rate even further and minimize any stressors in the environment.

Lambs

Lambs require 180 to 210 mL of colostrum/kg BW during the first 18 hours after birth to provide sufficient energy for heat production. Such an intake will usually also provide enough colostral immunoglobulin. Early encouragement and assistance of the lambs to suck the ewe is important. Well-fed ewes usually have sufficient colostrum for singletons or twins. Underfed ewes may not have sufficient colostrum for one or more lambs, and supplementation from stored colostrum obtained by milking other high-producing ewes is a useful practice.

Piglets

The following practices should be implemented for piglets:

- Every possible economical effort must be made to ensure that each newborn piglet obtains a liberal supply of colostrum within minutes of birth. The farrowing floor must be well drained, and it must be slip-proof to allow the piglets to move easily to the sow's udder. Some herdsmen provide assistance at farrowing, drying off every piglet as it is born and placing it immediately onto a teat.
- The washing of the sow's udder immediately before farrowing with warm water and soap will reduce the bacterial population and may provide relief in cases of congested and edematous udders.
- The piglet creep area must be dry, appropriately heated for the first week, and free from drafts. During farrowing, colostrum is released in discrete ejections, possibly by discrete release of oxytocin associated with parturition. Therefore, as the piglets are born they must be as close to the udder as possible to take advantage of these discrete ejections.

Increasing Specific Resistance of the Newborn by Vaccinating the Pregnant Dam or the Newborn

The immunization of neonate farm animals against colibacillosis by vaccination of the pregnant dam or by vaccination of the fetus or the neonate has received considerable research attention in recent years, and the results appear promising.

Such vaccines are practical and effective for the following reasons:

- Most fatal ETEC infections in farm animals occur in the early neonatal period when antibody titers in colostrum and milk are highest.
- More than 90% of the ETEC in farm animals belong to a small family of fimbrial antigens.
- Fimbriae consist of good protein antigens on the bacterial surface, where they are readily accessible to antibodies.
- Fimbriae are required for a critical step (adhesion–colonization) early in the pathogenesis of the disease.
- Novel or previously low-prevalence fimbrial antigens have not emerged to render the vaccines ineffective.

The pregnant dam is vaccinated 2 to 4 weeks before parturition to induce specific antibodies to particular strains of enteropathogenic *E. coli*, and the antibodies are then passed on to the newborn through the colostrum. The mechanism of protection is the production of antibodies against the pilus antigens, which are responsible for colonization of *E. coli* in the intestine.

Vaccination is an aid to good management and not a replacement for good management practices. Vaccines to prevent ETEC diarrhea in calves and piglets are based on the prevailing fimbrial antigens for colonization by ETEC in calves (F5) and newborn pigs (F4, F5, and F6). Reliable data on the efficacy of the commercial vaccines based on randomized clinical field trials are not available, but most animal health professionals perceive that the vaccines are effective and that disease occurs primarily in unvaccinated herds. There are unpublished anecdotal reports that use of the vaccine in cattle has shifted the peak occurrence of diarrhea in calves from the first week to the third and fourth week after birth. The extensive use of fimbria-based vaccines can select against the prevailing fimbrial antigen types as reflected in the vaccines, and emergence of new or previously low-prevalence fimbrial antigens may occur. Fimbriae antigenically distinct from F1, F4, F6, F41 occur among ETEC. However, these antigen types are less prevalent than those currently used in commercial vaccines. There is no evidence that ETEC with novel colonization mechanisms or new fimbrial antigens have emerged under the selection pressure of vaccination. Nor is there evidence that previously "low-prevalence" fimbrial antigen types of ETEC, not represented in the vaccines, have emerged as "common pathogens" filling an ecological niche left by the fimbrial antigen types targeted by the vaccines.

Calves

Vaccination of pregnant cattle with either purified *E. coli* F5 (K99) pili or a whole-cell preparation containing sufficient F5 antigen can significantly reduce the incidence of enterotoxigenic colibacillosis in calves. Good protection is also possible when the dams are vaccinated with a four-strain *E. coli* whole-cell bacterin containing sufficient F5 pilus antigen and the polysaccharide capsular K antigen. Colostral antibodies specific for F5 pilus antigen and the polysaccharide capsular K antigen on the surface of the challenge exposure strain of ETEC are protective. There is a highly significant correlation between lacteal immunity to the F5 antigen and the prevention of severe diarrhea or death in calves challenged with enterotoxigenic *E. coli.* The colostral levels of F5 antibody are highest during the first 2 days after parturition, which is the most susceptible period for enterotoxigenic colibacillosis to occur in the newborn calf. The continuous presence of the F5 antibody in the lumen of the intestine prevents adherence of the bacteria to the intestinal epithelium. The F5 antibody is also absorbed during the period of immunoglobulin absorption and may be excreted into the intestine during diarrhea. This may be one of the reasons that mortality is inversely proportional to serum immunoglobulin levels. The pregnant dams are vaccinated twice in the first year, 6 and 2 weeks before parturition. Each year thereafter they are given a single booster vaccination. An oil-emulsion *E. coli* F5 bacterin given once or twice to pregnant beef cows 6 weeks before calving elicited high levels of serum antibodies that provided protection against experimental infection of newborn calves for up to 87 weeks after vaccination.

Vaccines containing both the F5 antigen of ETEC and rotavirus, and in some cases coronavirus, have been evaluated, with variable results. The colostral antibodies to the F5 antigen are higher in vaccinated than unvaccinated dams, but the colostral antibodies to rotavirus and coronavirus may not be significantly different between vaccinated and unvaccinated dams. In these field trials vaccination had no effect on the prevalence of diarrhea, calf mortality, or the presence of the three enteropathogens. In other field trials the combined vaccine did provide some protection against outbreaks of calf diarrhea. The use of an inactivated oil-adjuvanted rotavirus *E. coli* vaccine given to beef cows in the last trimester of pregnancy decreases the mortality from diarrhea and has a positive influence on the average weight gains of the calves at weaning. To be effective the rotavirus and coronavirus antibodies must be present in the postcolostral milk for several days after parturition, during the period when calves are most susceptible to the viral infection. Vaccination of pregnant cows twice during the dry period at intervals of 4 weeks can increase the colostral antibody levels to *E. coli* F5 by 26 times on day 1 compared with controls. Much lower increases occur at the levels of coronavirus and rotavirus.

A commercially inactivated vaccine containing bovine rotavirus (serotype G6 P5), bovine coronavirus (originally isolated from a calf with diarrhea), and purified cell-free *E. coli* F5 (adsorbed on to aluminum hydroxide gel), formulated as an emulsion in a light mineral oil, has been evaluated in a herd of Ayrshire/Friesian cows vaccinated once at 31 days before the first expected calving date. Compared with control cows, a significant increase in the mean specific antibody titer against all three antigens occurred in the serum of vaccinated animals (even in the presence of preexisting antibodies), which was accompanied by increased levels of protective antibodies to rotavirus, coronavirus, and *E. coli* F5 in their colostrum and milk for at least 28 days.

Because naturally acquired antibodies to the **J5 antigen** may have an important role in the control of neonatal disease caused by bacterial infections with associated pathogens that share antigens with *E. coli* (J5 strain), vaccination of calves with an *E. coli* O111:B4(J5) vaccine at 1 to 3 days of age and 2 weeks later has been evaluated to control morbidity and mortality in dairy calves up to 60 days of age. The use of either a killed *E. coli* O111:B4(J5) bacterin or a modified live, genetically altered (aro-) *Salmonella dublin* vaccine, or both, in neonatal calves was effective in reducing mortality resulting from colibacillosis and salmonellosis. Such a vaccine may be beneficial in controlling mortality in well-managed herds, but it is contraindicated in poorly managed herds.

Passive immunotherapy of calves under 2 days of age with J5 *E. coli* hyperimmune plasma given subcutaneously at a dose of 5 mL/kg BW has been examined. The plasma was found to be safe and potent. It was not superior to control plasma or to no treatment for calf morbidity and mortality.

The oral administration of a F5-specific monoclonal antibody to calves during the first 12 hours after birth may be an effective method of reducing the incidence of fatal enterotoxigenic colibacillosis, particularly when outbreaks of the disease occur in unvaccinated herds. Clinical trials indicate that the severity of dehydration, depression, and weight loss and the duration of diarrhea were significantly reduced in calves that had received the F5-specific monoclonal antibody. In experimentally challenged calves the mortality was 29% in the treated calves and 82% in the control calves.

The decision to vaccinate in any particular year will depend on the recognition of risk factors. Such risk factors include the following:

- A definitive diagnosis of ETEC F5 in the previous year
- A population density in the calving grounds that is conducive to the disease
- Calving during the year when the environmental conditions are wet and uncomfortable for the calves
- A large percentage of primiparous dams that do not have protective levels of F5 antibody in their colostrum

Piglets

Piglets born from gilts are more susceptible than those from mature sows, which suggests that immunity improves with parity. On a practical basis this suggests that gilts should be mixed with older sows that have been resident on the premises for some time. The length of time required for such natural immunization to occur is uncertain, but 1 month during late gestation seems logical.

Naturally occurring enteric colibacillosis in newborn piglets can be effectively controlled by vaccination of the pregnant dam. Field trials in large-scale farm conditions indicate that the vaccines are efficacious. Partial budget analysis of vaccinating pregnant sows with *E. coli* vaccines revealed an economic return on investment of 124% because of the decrease in morbidity and mortality resulting from diarrhea in piglets at 1 to 2 weeks of age. Three antigen types of pili, designated F4, F5, and F6, are now implicated in colonization of the small intestine of newborn piglets by ETEC. The vaccination of pregnant sows with oral or parenteral vaccines containing these antigens will provide protection against enterotoxigenic colibacillosis associated with *E. coli* bearing pili homologous to those in the vaccines. The parenteral vaccines are cell-free preparations of pili, and the oral vaccines contain live enteropathogenic *E. coli.* The oral vaccine is given 2 weeks before farrowing and is administered in the feed daily for 3 days as 200 mL per day of a broth culture containing 10^{11} *E. coli.* A simple and effective method of immunization of pregnant sows is to feed live cultures of ETEC isolated from piglets affected with neonatal colibacillosis on the same farm. The oral vaccine can be given in the feed, beginning about 8 weeks after breeding and continued to parturition. The oral vaccine results in the stimulation of IgA antibody in the intestinal tract, which is then transferred to the mammary gland and into the colostrum. A combination of oral and parenteral vaccination is superior to either route alone. The parenteral vaccine is given about 2 weeks after breeding and repeated 2 to 4 weeks before parturition. The parenteral vaccination results in the production of high levels of IgM antibody for protection against both experimental and naturally occurring enterotoxigenic colibacillosis. This vaccination also reduces the number of *E. coli* excreted in the feces of vaccinated sows, which are major sources of the organism. Immunization of pregnant sows with an *E. coli* bacterin enriched with the F4 antigen results in the secretion of milk capable of preventing adhesion of F4 *E. coli* to the gut for at least 5 weeks after birth, at which time the piglet becomes naturally resistant to adhesion by the organism.

The possibility of selecting and breeding pigs that may be genetically resistant to the disease is being explored. The highest incidence of diarrhea occurs in progeny of resistant dams sired by susceptible sires. The homozygous dominants (SS) and the heterozygotes (Ss) possess the receptor and are susceptible, whereas it is absent in the homozygous recessives (ss) and the pigs are resistant. Sows that are genetically resistant may not be able to mount an immune response to the F4 antigen because of the inability of the organism to colonize the intestinal tract.

Competitive Exclusion Culture

An alternative method of control is the use of competitive exclusion cultures. The theory of competitive exclusion technology is to colonize the neonatal gastrointestinal tract with beneficial/commensal bacteria considered to be the normal flora of the healthy animals of a particular species. The mechanism of action is not known, but hypotheses include the following: exclusion of enteropathogens by competitive attachment sites and/or for nutrients; stimulation of the local immune mechanisms, which precludes colonization/invasion by enteric pathogens; and the production of various antimicrobial substances that either have direct action on pathogenic bacteria or produce conditions within the intestine that are unfavorable for the growth and colonization by pathogens. Experimentally, the oral administration of a porcine competitive exclusion culture to piglets within 12 hours after birth resulted in significant reductions in mortality, incidence of fecal shedding, and intestinal colonization by *E. coli* compared with control values. Mortality decreased from 23% in the control group to 2.7% in the treated group.

Lambs and Kids

Vaccination of pregnant ewes with F5 antigen will confer colostral immunity to lambs challenged with homologous ETEC. The pregnant ewes are vaccinated twice in the first year, at 8 to 10 weeks and 2 to 4 weeks before lambing; in the second year, one vaccination 2 to 4 weeks before lambing is adequate.

Immunization of pregnant goats has been used to stimulate the development of lacteal immunity against naturally occurring colibacillosis in kids. Vaccination of pregnant does 1 month before parturition with a subunit vaccine containing F4, F5, and F6 fimbrial antigens of *E. coli* and *C. perfringens* types B, C, and D toxins in an aluminum hydroxide adjuvant, along with improved management conditions, was highly successful in reducing neonatal morbidity and mortality resulting from diarrhea. Compared with two control groups, one in which no improvement in management was made and the second in which improvements were made without vaccination, in the vaccinated group with improved management conditions, neonatal morbidity and mortality were both reduced by a factor of 3 in group 1 and by factors of 9.5 and 12.5 in groups 2 and 3, respectively. Also, the duration of diarrhea was 3.7 and 12 times shorter in the kids of groups 2 and 3, respectively.

FURTHER READING

Acres SD. Enterotoxigenic *Escherichia coli* infections in newborn calves: a review. *J Dairy Sci.* 1985;68:229-256.

Constable PD. Antimicrobial use in the treatment of calf diarrhea. *J Vet Intern Med.* 2004;18:8-17.

DebRoy C, Maddox CW. Identification of virulence attributes of gastrointestinal *Escherichia coli* isolates of veterinary significance. *Anim Health Res Rev.* 2001;1:129-140.

Gyles CL, Prescott JF, Songer JG, Thoen CO. *Pathogenesis of Bacterial Infections in Animals.* 3rd ed. Ames, IA: Blackwell; 2004.

Larson RL, Tyler JW, Schultz LG, et al. Management strategies to decrease calf death losses in beef herds. *J Am Vet Med Assoc.* 2004;224:42-48.

Moxley RA. *Escherichia coli* O157H:7: an update on intestinal colonization and virulence mechanisms. *Anim Health Res Rev.* 2004;5:15-33.

Renter DG, Sargeant JM. Enterohemorrhagic *Escherichia coli* O157H:7: epidemiology and ecology in bovine production environments. *Anim Health Res Rev.* 2002;3:83-94.

REFERENCES

1. Farrokh C, et al. *Int J Food Microbiol.* 2013;162:190-212.
2. Mainil J. *Vet Immunol Immunopathol.* 2013;152:2-12.
3. ECDC/EFSA. 2011. (Accessed 10.01.16, at 2014 <http://www.ecdc.europa.eu/en/publications/Publications/1106_TER_EColi_joint_EFSA.pdf>).
4. Hussein HS, Sakuma T. *J Dairy Sci.* 2005;88:450-465.
5. Laine TM, et al. *Acta Vet Scand.* 2008;50:21.
6. Duan Q, et al. *Ann Microbiol.* 2012;62:7-14.
7. Nagy B, Fekete PZ. *Int J Med Microbiol.* 2005;295:443-454.
8. Foster DM, Smith GW. *Vet Clin North Am Food Anim Pract.* 2009;25:13-36.
9. Fecteau G, et al. *Vet Microbiol.* 2001;78:241-249.
10. Ghanbarpour R, Oswald R. *Trop Anim Health Prod.* 2009;41:1091-1099.
11. Corley KTT, et al. *Equine Vet J.* 2007;39:84-99.
12. Lorenz I. *Vet J.* 2009;179:197-203.
13. Gomez DE, et al. *J Vet Intern Med.* 2013;27:1604-1612.
14. Abeysekara S, et al. *Am J Physiol Endocrinol Metab.* 2007;293:E356-E365.
15. Lorenz I. *Vet J.* 2004;168:323-327.
16. Lorenz I, et al. *Vet Rec.* 2005;156:412-415.
17. Gentile A, et al. *J Vet Intern Med.* 2008;22:190-195.
18. Trefz FM, et al. *Vet J.* 2013;195:350-356.
19. Constable PD, Grünberg W. *Vet J.* 2013;195:217-272.
20. Biolatti C, et al. *Schweiz Arch Tierheilkd.* 2012;154:239-246.
21. Fecteau G, et al. *Vet Clin North Am Food Anim Pract.* 2009;25:195-208.
22. Kumar A. *Curr Infect Dis Rep.* 2010;12:336-344.
23. Dellinger RP, et al. *Crit Care Med.* 2004;32:853-873.
24. Catry B, et al. *Microb Drug Resist.* 2007;13:147-150.
25. Hendriksen RS, et al. *Acta Vet Scand.* 2008;50:28.
26. Hendriksen RS, et al. *Acta Vet Scand.* 2008;50:19.
27. Manchese A, et al. *Microb Drug Resist.* 2012;18:94-99.
28. Kaneene JB, et al. *J Clin Microbiol.* 2008;46:1968-1977.
29. Constable PD. *J Vet Intern Med.* 2004;18:8.
30. Scientific Advisory Group on Antimicrobials of the Committee for Medicinal Products for Veterinary Use. *J Vet Pharmacol Ther.* 2009;32:515-533.
31. World Organization for Animal Health. OIE list of antimicrobial agents of veterinary importance, 2013. (Accessed 15.12.13, at <http://www.oie.int/fileadmin/Home/eng/Our_scientific_expertise/docs/pdf/OIE_List_antimicrobials.pdf>).
32. Constable PD. *Vet Clin North Am Food Anim Pract.* 2009;25:101-120.
33. Todd CG, et al. *J Anim Sci.* 2007;85(suppl 1):369.
34. Barnett SC, et al. *J Am Vet Med Assoc.* 2003;223:1329-1333.
35. Lorenz I, et al. *Ir Vet J.* 2011;64:9.
36. Garthwaite BD, et al. *J Dairy Sci.* 1994;77:835-843.
37. Nomoto K. *J Biosci Bioeng.* 2005;100:583-592.
38. Senok AC, et al. *Clin Microbiol Infect.* 2005;11:956-966.
39. Wynn SG. *J Am Vet Med Assoc.* 2009;5:606-613.
40. Weese JS, Rousseau J. *J Am Vet Med Assoc.* 2005;226:2031-2034.
41. Beam AL, et al. *J Dairy Sci.* 2009;92:3973-3980.
42. Godden SM, et al. *J Dairy Sci.* 2012;95:4029-4040.

WATERY MOUTH OF LAMBS (RATTLE BELLY, SLAVERS)

SYNOPSIS

Etiology Nonenteropathogenic *E. coli* endotoxemia predisposed by failure of passive transfer.

Epidemiology Higher risk with intensive housing with poor hygiene.

Clinical findings Loss of sucking reflex, retention of meconium or feces, excessive mucoid saliva, abomasal distension.

Lesions None specific.

Diagnostic confirmation Nothing pathognomonic.

Treatment Fluids and energy via stomach tube; antimicrobials.

Control Antimicrobials at birth, pen hygiene, ensure adequate colostral transfer.

ETIOLOGY

Watery mouth of lambs is thought to be the result of endotoxemia in young lambs. It is postulated that the neutral pH of the abomasum in newborn lambs coupled with low concentrations of colostral immunoglobulin in the gut allow rapid multiplication of nonenteropathogenic strains of *E. coli* in the gut, and to some extent systemically, which results in endotoxemia.

EPIDEMIOLOGY

Occurrence

The syndrome is primarily reported in lambs in Great Britain but has also been reported in New Zealand and in goat kids in Spain and North America. A related but perhaps separate entity, termed *salivary abomasum disease*, has been reported as common in 3- to 17-day-old lambs and kids in Greece.[1]

Animal and Environmental Risk Factors

Lambs 12 to 72 hours of age are affected. The disease is seen under all management systems, but it is rare in pastured flocks and occurs most commonly in lambs kept in intensive housing where there is poor hygiene of the lambing environment. Lambs from prolific ewes are at risk, and the disease is more common in triplets than twins or singles.

Delayed or poor colostral intake is a major risk factor, and situations that predispose this may lead to outbreaks. A high prevalence has occurred in ram lambs castrated by the use of an elastic band at a very young age, and the resulting pain may have dissuaded them from feeding.

Other risk factors, all of which reduce sucking by the lamb, are inclement weather, mismothering, maternal agalactia, competition between twins or triplets, low vitality, and ewes in poor condition.

Experimental Disease

An equivalent clinical syndrome is reproducible by administering nonenterotoxic strains of *E. coli* by mouth to colostrum-deprived lambs, all of whom died within 24 hours.

Economic Importance

Watery mouth disease is a major cause of mortality of housed newborn lambs in Great Britain and is reported to be the cause of approximately 25% of all deaths of lambs in indoor intensive lambing systems. Where conditions allow, morbidity rates may approach 24%; without early treatment, case fatality rates are high.

PATHOGENESIS

Gram-negative bacteria, nonenterotoxigenic and nonenteropathogenic *E. coli*, in the environment are ingested as a result of a contaminated environment, or from a contaminated fleece, and survive passage through the neutral pH of the abomasum to be absorbed into the systemic circulation by the natural pinocytosis that occurs in the intestinal epithelium of newborn ruminants, producing endotoxemia.

CLINICAL FINDINGS

Affected lambs are normal at birth but become sick at 24 to 48 hours and up to 72 hours old. The disease is characterized by dullness, lethargy, a complete failure to suck, and excessive mucoid saliva around and drooling from the mouth. As the disease progresses there is hypothermia, failure to pass feces, cold extremities, depression to the point of coma, anorexia, and, in the late stages, abdominal distension and recumbency, but rarely diarrhea. The alimentary tract is full of fluid, and the lamb rattles when it is shaken. Some lambs are hypothermic, but the temperature is normal at the onset of the condition and falls to subnormal as the disease progresses. Progress is rapid, with death 6 to 24 hours after the first signs of illness. Salivary abomasum disease is reported in flocks that vaccinate against clostridial disease.[2]

CLINICAL PATHOLOGY

Total protein concentrations and base excess values are significantly elevated compared with normal lambs. Blood glucose concentrations are normal but may be low in the terminal phase of the disease.

NECROPSY FINDINGS

There are no findings specific to watery mouth syndrome. The abomasal contents are fluid and mucoid and contain small milk curds, and the intestine is filled with gas. A case series of lambs with salivary abomasum disease found pale kidneys and acute tubular necrosis in 90%. *E. coli* was cultured from only 6 of 37 abomasa in this study.[2]

TREATMENT

Treatment with intramuscular amoxillin and clavulanic acid, intravenous flunixin meglumine, and oral rehydration fluid, when administered early in the clinical course, has resulted in a high recovery rate in field cases. Dextrose solution should also be given to those lambs that are hypoglycemic, and external warming should be provided. Other recommended treatments include emptying the alimentary tract by purgation or enema.

> **DIFFERENTIAL DIAGNOSIS**
>
> Most neonatal disease of lambs is manifest with diarrhea, which is not present in watery mouth. The early stages of *Colisepticemia* and *Clostridium perfringens* type B or C present with similar clinical signs, but they are easily differentiated later in the clinical course or at postmortem examination. Hypothermia/starvation/cold stress can present with similar clinical findings, but the history and environmental circumstances of occurrence differ.

CONTROL

In outbreaks the administration of antibiotics to all newborn lambs within 15 minutes to 2 hours of birth dramatically reduces the occurrence of further cases. Fresh or frozen sheep or cow colostrum should be supplemented to lambs at risk. The provision of ewe colostrum at 50 mL/kg BW within 6 hours of birth prevents the disease.

Lambing areas and associated pens and yards should be kept clean and freshly bedded. Contaminated fleece should be removed from around the udder of the ewe before lambing, and every effort should be made to ensure early and adequate colostral intake by newborn lambs, especially for twins and triplets.

REFERENCES

1. Christodoulopoulos G. *Vet Rec.* 2008;162:732.
2. Christodoulopoulos G, et al. *Vet Rec.* 2013;172:100.

OMPHALITIS, OMPHALOPHLEBITIS, AND URACHITIS IN NEWBORN FARM ANIMALS (NAVEL ILL)

Infection of the umbilicus and its associated structures occurs commonly in newborn farm animals and appears to be particularly common in calves. The umbilical cord consists of the amniotic membrane, the umbilical veins, the umbilical arteries, and the urachus. The amniotic membrane of the umbilical cord is torn at birth, and gradually the umbilical vein and the urachus close, but they remain temporarily outside the umbilicus. The umbilical arteries retract as far back as the top of the bladder.

In many countries regulations govern the minimal age at which neonatal calves can be shipped or sent to market and slaughter. The wetness or dryness of the umbilicus is used as a surrogate measure of age in welfare regulations, and the requirement is that the umbilical cord at the junction with the abdominal skin should be dry and shriveled. The drying time varies from 1 to 8 days, with variation between breeds and a longer drying period in bull calves. As might be expected, this measure is only an approximate surrogate for age, but approximately 90% of calves have dry navels by 4 days of age.[1]

Incidence of the disease is scarcely reported. The 30-day incidence of clinically apparent omphalitis in Thoroughbred foals in the United Kingdom was 0.7%, which was not reduced by administration of antimicrobials prophylactically.[2] Omphalitis was considered the cause of death in 23% of 247 calves 4 to 7 days of age that died during the preslaughter period (12 to 18 hours) at abattoirs in New Zealand.[1] The death rate was 0.7%, of which 23% was attributable to omphalitis. Omphalitis was the cause of wastage (condemnation of the carcass) in 54% of calves examined after slaughter.[1]

Infection of the umbilicus occurs **soon after birth** and can result in omphalitis, omphalophlebitis, omphaloarteritis, or infection of the urachus, with possible extension to the bladder, causing cystitis. There is usually a **mixed bacterial flora** including *E. coli*, *Proteus* spp., *Staphylococcus* spp., *T. pyogenes*, *Bacteroides* spp., *F. necrophorum*, and *Klebsiella* spp. The most common, and presumed clinically important, infections in foals are by *E. coli* and *S. zooepidemicus*. Infection of umbilical remnants in foals by *Clostridium sordelli* causes peritonitis, urachitis, omphalophlebitis, and omphaloarteritis.[3]

Bacteremia and localization with infection may occur in joints, bone, meninges, eyes, endocardium, and end-arteries of the feet, ears, and tail. The navel can also be the source of infection, leading to septicemia, arthritis, and fever of unknown origin in neonates with FTPI. The incidence of abnormalities of the umbilicus and consequent rate of umbilical infection is high in cloned calves.[2-5]

OMPHALITIS

Omphalitis is inflammation of the external aspects of the umbilicus and occurs commonly in calves and other species within 2 to 5 days of birth and often persists for several weeks. The umbilicus is enlarged, is painful on palpation, and can be closed or draining purulent material through a small fistula. The affected umbilicus can become very large and cause subacute toxemia. The calf is moderately depressed, does not suck normally, and is febrile. Treatment consists of surgical exploration and excision. A temporary drainage channel may be necessary.

OMPHALOPHLEBITIS

Omphalophlebitis is inflammation of the umbilical veins. It can involve only the distal parts or extend from the umbilicus to the liver. Large abscesses can develop along the course of the umbilical vein and spread to the liver, with the development of a hepatic abscess that can occupy up to one-half of the liver. Affected foals and calves are usually 1 to 3 months of age and are unthrifty because of chronic toxemia. The umbilicus is usually enlarged with purulent material; however, in some cases the external portion of the umbilicus appears normal-sized. Placing the animal in dorsal recumbency and deep palpation of the abdomen dorsal to the umbilicus in the direction of the liver might reveal a space-occupying mass. **Ultrasonographic** examination, including measurement of the size of umbilical structures, allows detection of omphalophlebitis, including any extension along the vein to the liver.

Affected calves and foals are inactive, inappetent, and unthrifty and may have a mild fever. Parenteral therapy with antibiotics is not uniformly successful and may need to be administered for prolonged times. Exploratory laparotomy and **surgical removal** of the abscess is often necessary. Large hepatic abscesses are usually incurable unless surgically removed, but the provision of a drain to the exterior and daily irrigation may be attempted if resection is not feasible.

OMPHALOARTERITIS

In omphaloarteritis, which is less common, the abscesses occur along the course of the umbilical arteries from the umbilicus to the internal iliac arteries. The clinical findings are similar to those in omphalophlebitis: chronic toxemia, unthriftiness, and failure to respond to antibiotic therapy. An unusual presentation is that of distal aortic aneurysm secondary to ascending infection of the umbilical artery.[6] The affected foal was 3 months of age and was examined because of colic and frequent urination. Treatment of omphalophlebitis consists of surgical removal of the abscesses.

URACHITIS

Infection of the urachus may occur anywhere along the urachus, from the umbilicus to the bladder. The umbilicus is usually enlarged and draining purulent material, but it can appear normal. Deep palpation of the abdomen in a dorsocaudal direction from the umbilicus may reveal a space-occupying mass. Extension of the infection to the bladder can result in cystitis and pyuria.[5] **Contrast radiography** of the fistulous tract and the bladder will reveal the presence of the lesion. The treatment of choice is exploratory laparotomy and surgical removal of the abscesses. Recovery is usually uneventful.

CONTROL

The control of umbilical infection depends primarily on **good sanitation and hygiene** at the time of birth. The application of drying agents and residual disinfectants such as tincture of iodine is widely practiced. However, there is limited evidence that chemical disinfecting is of significant value. Chlorhexidine is more efficient in reducing the number of organisms than 2% iodine or 1% povidone iodine. High concentrations of iodine (7%) are most effective, but these are damaging to tissue and should not be used.

REFERENCES

1. Thomas GW, et al. *N Z Vet J*. 2013;61:127.
2. Wohlfender FD, et al. *Equine Vet J*. 2009;41:179.
3. Ortega J, et al. *Vet Pathol*. 2007;44:269.
4. Brisville AC, et al. *J Vet Intern Med*. 2013;27:1218.
5. Lores M, et al. *Can Vet J*. 2011;52:888.
6. Archer RM, et al. *N Z Vet J*. 2012;60:65.

NEONATAL STREPTOCOCCAL INFECTION

SYNOPSIS

Etiology Various *Streptococcus* spp.

Epidemiology Neonatal foals, calves, lambs, piglets.

Signs Acute painful swelling of joints, lameness, fever; signs of meningitis, omphalophlebitis, ophthalmitis; sudden death.

Clinical pathology Culture organism from joint fluid.

Necropsy findings Fibrinopurulent synovitis, purulent meningitis and omphalophlebitis.

Diagnostic confirmation Recovery of organism from joint fluid.

Differential diagnosis Other infectious causes of arthritis, meningitis, and omphalophlebitis.

Treatment Antimicrobials, usually penicillin.

Control See "Principles of Control and Prevention of Infectious Diseases of Newborn Farm Animals" in Chapter 3.

ETIOLOGY

Streptococci are an important cause of septicemia, polyarthritis, meningitis, polyserositis, endocarditis, and unexpected death in the neonates of all farm animal species. Meningitis associated with streptococcal infection is restricted to the neonate in all species except piglets, in which outbreaks can occur in pigs after weaning, and lambs infected with *S. suis*, in which meningitis can occur as a sporadic disease at 3 to 5 months of age. Historically, there are reports of isolates of most of the Lancefield groups of beta-hemolytic streptococci, of nonbeta-hemolytic streptococci, and of viridans group streptococci from neonatal disease in farm animals. Commensal skin streptococci can occasionally cause disease in presumably immunocompromised neonates. However, the majority of neonatal disease is associated with a limited number of streptococcal species, although there can be geographic variation in their relative prevalence within animal species.

In **foals,** *S. zooepidemicus* (*S. equi* subsp. *zooepidemicus*) is the most common streptococcal species recovered from septicemic disease and polyarthritis and is also a cause of placentitis and abortion in mares.[1,2] *S. equisimilis* (*S. dysgalactiae* subsp. *equisimilis*) is a less common isolate.[2]

S. suis and *S. equisimilis* are the most common species incriminated in **piglets**. *S. suis* is especially important and is presented separately in the next section. Other Lancefield groups have been associated with sporadic disease. In **calves,** *S. dysgalactiae* and *S. uberis* are the common streptococcal isolates from synovial fluid of neonatal calves with arthritis. Beta-hemolytic streptococci are isolated from approximately 16% of septicemic calves in South Africa.[3] *Streptococcus pluranimalium* infection is reported in a single premature calf.[4]

S. dysgalactiae is also reported to be the most common cause of outbreaks of arthritis in neonatal lambs in Great Britain. *Streptococcus bovis* biotype 1 is reported to cause meningoencephalitis in llama cria.[5] *Streptococcus agalactiae* causes periarticular abscesses in camel foals in Africa.[6]

Streptococci can also contribute to purulent infections at local sites, such as navel ill of all species or otitis media in neonatal calves, although the latter is more commonly caused by *M. bovis.*[7]

EPIDEMIOLOGY

Occurrence and Prevalence

The importance and relative prevalence of streptococcal infections in neonatal disease varies among countries and with surveys.

Streptococci are a common cause of postnatal infections of **foals,** representing 50% of such cases in some surveys, but with a lower prevalence in others. Up to 20% of abortions in mares are a result of placentitis from streptococcal infection. Streptococcal septicemia as a result of beta-hemolytic streptococci may occur in foals under 5 days of age that have been stressed and have FTPI.

In **calves,** neonatal infections with streptococci are usually sporadic and less common than infections with gram-negative bacteria and may be predisposed by FTPI. In **lambs,** *S. dysgalactiae* is associated with outbreaks with high morbidity, and in Great Britain *S. dysgalactiae* is reported to be the cause of over 70% of cases of polyarthritis in lambs during their first 3 weeks of life. Despite the high attack rate in these outbreaks, it is rare for more than one of twins or triplets to have disease. Streptococcal arthritis associated with *S. suis* infection in piglets is a common disease and is covered in a separate section.

Source of Infection

The source of the infection is usually the environment, which may be contaminated by uterine discharges from infected dams or by discharges from lesions in other animals. *S. dysgalactiae* is reported to survive for up to a year on clean straw, as opposed to wood shavings, which do not support the persistence of the organism.

The portal of infection in most instances appears to be the umbilicus, and continued patency of the urachus is thought to be a contributing factor in that it delays healing of the navel. In piglets there can be high rates of infection associated with infection entering through skin abrasions such as carpal necrosis resulting from abrasive floors or facial lesions following fighting. Contaminated knives at castration and tail docking, or contaminated ear taggers, can result in infection and disease. Other mechanical vectors include the screwworm fly (*Cochliomyia americana*).

The organism can be isolated from the nasopharynx of the sow, and direct infection from the sow to the piglet is suggested by some epidemiologic data.

Economic Importance

Affected foals and other species may die or be worthless as working animals because of permanent injury to joints. There is also loss resulting from condemnation at slaughter.

Zoonotic Implications

S. zooepidemicus is associated with human infections,[8] particularly nephritis, and many human infections can be traced back to the consumption of contaminated animal food products. Some strains of *S. equisimilis* can also infect humans.

PATHOGENESIS

The infection spreads from the portal of entry to produce a bacteremia that is not detectable clinically. The period of bacteremia is variable but it may last several days in piglets. A terminal acute fatal septicemia is the common outcome in animals under 1 week of age; in older animals, suppurative localization in various organs is more common. Arthritis is the most common manifestation, with synovitis and invasion of medullary bone of the epiphysis with microabscessation and ischemic necrosis of bone. Other manifestations of infection include ophthalmitis in foals and calves, meningitis and endocarditis in piglets, meningitis in calves, and endocarditis and sudden death in lambs. Streptococcal endocarditis can be produced by the intravenous inoculation of group L *Streptococcus*. Lesions are well established within 5 days, the left heart is most commonly affected, and myocardial and renal infarction occur.

CLINICAL FINDINGS

Foals

The disease is one of septicemia, often with localization of infection in joints (septic arthritis) or an eye (hypopyon), and is described in detail under "Neonatal Infection" (page 1874). Infection of the umbilicus can cause omphalitis and omphalophlebitis.

Piglets

Arthritis and meningitis may occur alone or together and are most common in the 2- to 6-week age group. More commonly, several piglets within a litter are affected. The arthritis is identical to that previously described in foals. With meningitis there is a systemic reaction comprising fever, anorexia, and depression. The gait is stiff, the piglets stand on their toes, and there is swaying of the hindquarters. The ears are often retracted against the head. Blindness and gross muscular tremor develop, followed by inability to maintain balance, lateral recumbency, violent paddling, and death. In many cases there is little clinical evidence of omphalophlebitis. With endocarditis the young pigs are usually found comatose or dead, without premonitory signs having been observed.

Lambs

Lameness in one or more limbs of lambs up to 3 weeks of age is the common presenting sign of infection with *S. dysgalactiae*, but approximately 25% of lambs can be initially recumbent. With this infection there is not major joint swelling in the early stages, and myopathy or delayed swayback may be initial considerations. In contrast with outbreaks that occur following docking, the incubation period is short, usually 2 to 3 days, and there is intense lameness, with swelling of one or more joints appearing in a day or two. Pus accumulates, and the joint capsule often ruptures. Recovery usually occurs with little residual enlargement of the joints, although there may be occasional deaths as a result of toxemia.

Calves

Calves show polyarthritis, meningitis, ophthalmitis, and omphalophlebitis. The ophthalmitis may appear very soon after birth. The arthritis is often chronic and causes little systemic illness. Calves with meningitis show hyperesthesia, rigidity, and fever.

CLINICAL PATHOLOGY

Pus from any source may be cultured to determine the organism present and its sensitivity to the drugs available. Bacteriologic examination of the uterine discharges of the dam may be of value in determining the source of infection. The success rate with blood cultures is not very high, but an attempt is worthwhile. The identification of the causative bacteria is important, but the sensitivity of the organism may mean the difference between success and failure in treatment. The specific identity of the streptococcus should be determined.

NECROPSY FINDINGS

Suppuration at the navel and severe suppurative arthritis affecting one or more joints are usual. Abscesses may also be present in the liver, kidneys, spleen, and lungs. Friable tan masses of tissue are common on the heart valves of affected piglets, and this valvular endocarditis may also be observed in other species. Peracute cases may die without suppurative lesions having had time to develop. Necropsy findings in the meningitic form in pigs include turbidity of the CSF, congestion of meningeal vessels, and the accumulation of white, purulent material in the subarachnoid space. Occasionally this exudate blocks the flow of CSF in the ventricular system, causing internal hydrocephalus. Histologically there is infiltration of the affected tissue by large numbers of neutrophils, usually accompanied by fibrin deposition.

Samples for Confirmation of Diagnosis

Confirmation of diagnosis is made with the following samples:

- Bacteriology—culture swabs from joints, meninges, suppurative foci; tissue pieces of valvular lesions, lung, spleen, synovial membrane (culture)
- Histology—formalin-fixed samples of a variety of organs, including brain, lung, spleen, liver (light microscopy)

DIFFERENTIAL DIAGNOSIS

Omphalophlebitis and suppurative arthritis in foals may result from infection with *Escherichia coli, Actinobacillus equuli*, or *Salmonella abortusequi*, but these infections tend to take the form of a fatal septicemia within a few days of birth, whereas streptococcal infections are delayed in their onset and usually produce a form of polyarthritis. In pigs there may be sporadic cases of arthritis as a result of staphylococci, but the streptococcal infection is the common one. Arthritis as a result of *Mycoplasma hyorhinis* is less suppurative, but it may require cultural differentiation. Glasser's disease occurs usually in older pigs and is accompanied by pleurisy, pericarditis, and peritonitis. Erysipelas in very young pigs is usually manifested by septicemia. Nervous disease of piglets may resemble arthritis on cursory examination, but there is an absence of joint enlargement and lameness. However, the meningitic form of the streptococcal infection can easily be confused with viral encephalitides. Meningitis in young calves may also be associated with *Pasteurella multocida*. Polyarthritis in calves, lambs, and piglets may also be associated with infection with *Trueperella pyogenes* and *Fusobacterium necrophorum*. *S. suis* type 2 can also be the cause of meningitis in older pigs at 10 to 14 weeks of age.

The response of streptococcal infections to treatment with penicillin may be of value in the differentiation of the arthritides, and the microscopic and histologic findings at necropsy enable exact differentiation to be made. In lambs, suppurative arthritis occurs soon after birth and after docking. The other common arthritis in the newborn lamb is that associated with *Erysipelothrix rhuriophiae*, but this usually occurs later and is manifested by lameness without pronounced joint enlargement. Calves may also develop erysipelatous arthritis.

TREATMENT

Penicillin is successful as treatment in all forms of the disease if irreparable structural damage has not occurred. In newborn animals, the dosage rate should be high (20,000 IU/kg BW) and should be repeated at least once daily for 3 days. If suppuration is already present, a longer course of antibiotics will be necessary, preferably for 7 to 10 days. Piglets treated early in the course of the disease will survive but may runt. Because of the common litter incidence in piglets and the occurrence of subclinical bacteremia, it is wise to also treat all littermates of affected piglets. Benzathine or benethamine penicillins can be used in conjunction with shorter-acting penicillins.

CONTROL

The principles of control of infectious diseases of the newborn are described elsewhere. Because the most frequent source of infection in foals is the genital tract of the dam, some attempt should be made to treat the mare and limit the contamination of the environment. Mixed bacterins have been widely used to establish immunity in mares and foals against this infection, but no proof has been presented that they are effective. On heavily infected premises the administration of long-acting penicillin at birth may be advisable. A major factor in the control of navel and joint ill in lambs is the use of clean fields or pens for lambing because umbilical infection originating from the environment seems to be more important than infection from the dam in this species. Docking should also be done in clean surroundings; if necessary, temporary yards should be erected. Instruments should be chemically sterilized between lambs. Regardless of species and where practicable, all parturition stalls and pens should be kept clean and disinfected, and the navels of all newborn animals should be disinfected at birth. Where screwworms are prevalent, the unhealed navels should be treated with a reliable repellent.

REFERENCES

1. Russell CM, et al. *Aust Vet J*. 2008;86:266.
2. Erol E, et al. *J Vet Diagn Invest*. 2012;24:142.
3. Kirecci E, et al. *J S Afr Vet Assoc*. 2010;81:110.
4. Seimiya YM, et al. *J Vet Med Sci*. 2007;69:657.
5. Twomey DF, et al. *Vet Rec*. 2007;160:337.
6. Younan M, et al. *J Camel Pract*. 2007;14:161.
7. Gosselin VB, et al. *Can Vet J*. 2012;53:957.
8. Pelkonen S, et al. *Emerg Infect Dis*. 2013;19:1041.

Neonatal Neoplasia

Congenital neoplasia is rare, occurring at a substantially lower rate than in adults, and accounts for a minor percentage of findings in surveys of neonatal mortality. It is probable that genetic rather than environmental factors influence its development.

Clinical signs depend on the type of neoplasm and its site, and they can result in dystocia or abortion. A variety of tumors have been recorded in all large animal species and are predominantly of mesenchymal origin.

In calves, malignant lymphoma is most commonly reported. It is usually multicentric and also affects the skin. Sporadic bovine leukosis of young calves may also be present at birth. Other tumors reported predominant in calves include diffuse peritoneal mesothelioma, mixed mesodermal tumor, mast cell tumor, hemangiomas, and cutaneous melanoma.

Melanomas (both benign and malignant) also occur in foals and piglets. Duroc Jersey, Vietnamese pot-bellied pigs, and Sinclair miniature pigs have a high incidence of congenital malignant melanoma, which is fatal in approximately 15% of affected pigs but regresses spontaneously, and without recurrence, in the remainder.

A breed predisposition to cardiac rhabdomyoma is recorded in Red Wattle pigs.

Papillomatosis is rare, but **lingual papillomatosis** is reported as a cause of enzootic disease of piglets in China.

20 Diseases of the Mammary Gland

Introduction

Mastitis is inflammation of the parenchyma of the mammary gland regardless of the cause. Mastitis is therefore characterized by a range of physical and chemical changes in the milk and pathologic changes in the glandular tissue. The most important changes in the milk include discoloration, the presence of clots, and the presence of large numbers of leukocytes. There is **swelling**, **heat**, **pain**, and **edema** in the mammary gland in many clinical cases. However, a large proportion of mastitic glands are not readily detectable by manual palpation or by visual examination of the milk using a strip cup; these quarters represent subclinical infections. Because of the large numbers of subclinical cases, the diagnosis of mastitis depends largely on indirect tests, which depend, in turn, on the somatic cell concentration or electrolyte (sodium or chloride) concentration of milk. It seems practicable and reasonable to define mastitis as a disease characterized by the presence of a significantly increased somatic cell concentration in milk from affected glands. The increased somatic cell concentration is, in almost all cases, caused by an increased neutrophil concentration, which represents a reaction of glandular tissue to injury and is preceded by changes in the milk that are the direct result of damage to glandular tissue. However, the exact clinical and laboratory changes that occur in the udder as a result of infection can also be caused by other factors in the absence of infection. Until it becomes common usage to define mastitis in terms of the sodium or chloride concentration of the milk (as measured by electrical conductivity) or increased permeability of the blood-milk barrier (as measured by albumin concentration), there appears to be no point in changing the current definition of mastitis based on an abnormal-looking secretion or an increased somatic cell concentration. Characterization of mastitis depends on the identification of the causative agent whether it be infectious or physical.

Most of the information presented here deals almost entirely with bovine mastitis because of its economic importance, but small sections on ovine, caprine, porcine, and equine mastitis are included at the end of the chapter.

Bovine Mastitis

GENERAL FEATURES

A total of about 140 microbial species, subspecies, and serovars have been isolated from the bovine mammary gland. Microbiological techniques have enabled precise determination of the identity of many of the mastitis pathogens. Based on their epidemiology and pathophysiology, these pathogens have been further classified as causes of **contagious**, **teat skin opportunistic** or **environmental** mastitis.

SYNOPSIS

Etiology
- **Contagious pathogens**: *Staphylococcus aureus, Streptococcus agalactiae, Corynebacterium bovis,* and *Mycoplasma*
- **Teat skin opportunistic pathogens**: Coagulase-negative staphylococci
- **Environmental pathogens**: Environmental *Streptococcus* spp. including *Streptococcus uberis* and *S. dysgalactiae*, which are the

most prevalent; less prevalent is *S. equinus* (formerly referred to as *S. bovis*). Environmental coliforms include the gram-negative bacteria *Escherichia coli, Klebsiella spp.,* and *Enterobacter* spp., and *Trueperella* (formerly *Arcanobacterium,* or *Actinomyces,* or *Corynebacterium*) *pyogenes.*
- **Uncommon pathogens**: Many, including *Nocardia* spp., *Pasteurella* spp., *Mycobacterium bovis, Bacillus cereus, Pseudomonas* spp., *Serratia marcescens, Citrobacter* spp., anaerobic bacterial species, fungi, and yeasts

Epidemiology
- Incidence of clinical mastitis ranges from 10%-12% per 100 cows at risk per year. Prevalence of intramammary infection is about 50% of cows and 10%-25% of quarters. Case–fatality rate depends on cause of mastitis.
- Contagious pathogens are transmitted at time of milking; teat skin opportunistic pathogens take any opportunity to induce mastitis; environmental pathogens are from the environment and induce mastitis between milkings.
- Environmental pathogens are the most common cause of clinical mastitis in herds that have controlled contagious pathogens.
- Prevalence of infection with contagious pathogens ranges from 7%–40% of cows and 6%–35% of quarters.
- Prevalence of infection with environmental pathogens: coliforms 1%–2% of quarters; streptococci less than 5%

Risk factors
- **Animal risk factors**: Prevalence of infection increases with age. Most new infections occur in the dry period and in early lactation. Highest rate of clinical disease occurs in herds with low somatic cell counts (SCCs). Morphology and physical condition of the teat are risk factors. Selenium and vitamin E status influence incidence of clinical mastitis. High-producing cows are more susceptible.
- **Environmental risk factors**: Poor quality management of housing and bedding increases infection rate and incidence of clinical mastitis caused by environmental pathogens.
- **Pathogen risk factors**: Ability to survive in the environment, virulence factors (colonizing ability and toxin production), susceptibility to antimicrobial agents
- **Economics**: Subclinical mastitis is a major cause of economic loss caused by loss of milk production, costs of treatment, and early culling.

Clinical signs
- **Gross abnormalities in secretion** (discoloration, clots, flakes, and pus)
- **Physical abnormalities of udder**: Acute, diffuse swelling and warmth, pain, and gangrene in severe cases; chronic, local fibrosis and atrophy
- **Systemic response**: May be normal or mild, moderate, acute, peracute with varying degrees of anorexia, toxemia, dehydration, fever, tachycardia, ruminal stasis, and recumbency and death

Clinical pathology
- **Detection at the herd level**: Bulk tank milk SCCs. Culture of bulk tank milk
- **Detection at the individual cow level**: Abnormal looking milk, culture of composite or quarter milk samples. Indirect tests include SCCs of composite or quarter milk samples, California mastitis test of quarter milk samples, and in-line milk conductivity tests of quarter milk samples.
- **Use of selective media to differentiate gram-positive and gram-negative pathogens** in cases of clinical mastitis
- **Differential diagnosis list**: Other mammary abnormalities include periparturient udder edema, rupture of the suspensory ligament, and hematomas; blood in the milk of recently calved cows.

Treatment
- **Clinical mastitis in lactating cow**: Mild cases of clinical mastitis (abnormal secretion only) may not require treatment; however, all clinical mastitis episodes accompanied by an abnormal gland or systemic signs of illness should be treated with antimicrobial agents given by intramammary infusion (all cases) and parenterally (selected cases). Acute and peracute mastitis cases also require supportive therapy (fluid and electrolytes) and nonsteroidal antiinflammatory agents. Culture milk of representative clinical cases but antimicrobial susceptibility testing has not been validated.
- **Dry cow therapy**: Intramammary infusion of long-acting antimicrobial agents at drying off provides the best treatment for subclinical mastitis caused by contagious pathogens. Must adhere to milk withholding times after treatment with antimicrobial agents to prevent milk drug residues, which is a major public health issue. Currently available cowside antimicrobial residue tests are not reliable.

Control
- Principles of control:
  1. Eliminate existing infections
  2. Prevent new infections
  3. Monitor udder health status
- Components of a mastitis control program:
  1. Use proper milking management methods.
  2. Proper installation, function, and maintenance of milking equipment
  3. Dry cow management
  4. Appropriate therapy of mastitis during lactation
  5. Culling chronically infected cows
  6. Maintenance of an appropriate environment
  7. Good record keeping
  8. Monitoring udder health status
  9. Periodic review of the udder health management program
  10. Setting goals for udder health status

Contagious Mastitis Pathogens

There are many contagious mastitis pathogens. The most common are *Staphylococcus aureus* and *Streptococcus agalactiae.* The usual source of contagious pathogens is the infected glands of other cows in the herd; however, the hands of milkers can act as a source of *S. aureus.* The predominant method of transmission is from cow to cow by contaminated common udder washcloths, residual milk in teat cups, and inadequate milking equipment. Programs for the control of contagious mastitis involve improvements in hygiene and disinfection aimed at disrupting the cow-to-cow mode of transmission. In addition, methods to eliminate infected cows involve antimicrobial therapy and the culling of chronically infected cows.

Generally, a conscientious mastitis control program will eradicate *S. agalactiae* from most dairy herds. It is much more difficult to deal with a herd that has a high prevalence of *S. aureus,* but it can be eradicated from low-prevalence herds.

Mycoplasma bovis is a less common cause of contagious mastitis; it causes outbreaks of clinical mastitis that do not respond to therapy and are difficult to control. Most outbreaks of *M. bovis* are associated with recent introductions of new animals into the herd. Characteristically, clinical mastitis occurs in more than one quarter, there is a marked drop in milk production, and there is little evidence of systemic disease. The laboratory diagnosis of mycoplasmal mastitis requires specialized media and culture conditions. Antimicrobial therapy is relatively ineffective, and culling is the predominant strategy.

Teat Skin Opportunistic Mastitis Pathogens

The incidence of mild clinical mastitis associated with bacterial pathogens that normally reside on the teat skin is increasing, particularly in herds that have controlled major contagious mastitis pathogens. Teat skin opportunistic pathogens have the ability to create an intramammary infection via ascending infection through the streak canal. Accordingly, their epidemiology of infections differs from those of contagious and environmental pathogens, and it is useful to consider them in a separate category. Coagulase-negative staphylococci (CNS) are the most common teat skin opportunistic mastitis pathogens.

Environmental Mastitis Pathogens

Environmental mastitis is associated with three main groups of pathogens, the coliforms (particularly *Escherichia coli* and *Klebsiella* spp.), environmental *Streptococcus* spp., and *Trueperella pyogenes.* The source of these pathogens is the environment of the cow. The major method of transmission is from the environment to the cow by inadequate management of the environment. Examples include wet bedding, dirty lots, milking wet udders, inadequate premilking udder and teat preparation, housing systems that allow teat injuries, and poor fly control. Control strategies for environmental mastitis include improved sanitation in the barn and yard areas, good premilking udder preparation so that teats are clean and dry at milking time, and fly control. Special attention is necessary during the late dry period and in early lactation.

Coliform organisms are a common cause of clinical mastitis, occasionally in a severe peracute form. Clinical cases of coliform infection are generally found in low levels in most herds and do not routinely result in chronic infections. There is increasing evidence that, as the contagious pathogens are progressively controlled in a herd, the incidence of clinical cases associated with coliform organisms increases. The pathogenesis, epidemiology, predisposing risk factors, diagnostic problems, therapy, and control methods have been the subject of extensive, worldwide research efforts.

Environmental streptococci have become a major cause of mastitis in dairy cattle. Streptococcal infections are associated with many different species; however, the most prevalent species are *Streptococcus uberis* and *Streptococcus dysgalactiae.* Infections with these organisms can cause clinical mastitis that is commonly mild to moderate in nature. More frequently, these organisms cause a chronic subclinical infection with an increased milk somatic cell concentration. Many herds that have implemented the five-point program for mastitis control have found that environmental streptococci represent their most common mastitis problem.

T. pyogenes is an important seasonal cause of mastitis in dry cows and late pregnant heifers in some parts of the world. Intramammary infections with *T. pyogenes* are severe, and the gland is almost always lost to milk production.

Several other pathogens are included in the environmental class of infections. These pathogens invade the mammary gland when defense mechanisms are compromised or when they are inadvertently delivered into the gland at the time of intramammary therapy. This group of opportunistic organisms includes *Pseudomonas* spp., yeast agents, *Prototheca* spp., *Serratia marcescens,* and *Nocardia* spp. Each of these agents has unique microbiological culture characteristics, mechanisms of pathogenesis, and clinical outcomes. These infections usually occur sporadically. However, outbreaks can occur in herds or in an entire region and are usually the result of problems with specific management of hygiene or therapy. For example, mastitis associated with *Pseudomonas aeruginosa* has occurred in outbreaks associated with contaminated wash hoses in milking parlors. Iodide germicides used in wash lines are often at too low a concentration to eliminate *Pseudomonas* spp. Outbreaks of clinical mastitis associated with *Nocardia* spp. have been associated with the use of blanket dry cow therapy and the use of a specific neomycin-containing dry cow preparation.

The mastitis pathogens, and their relative importance, continue to evolve as new management methods and control practices are developed. Thus there is an ongoing need for epidemiologic studies to characterize the pathogens and describe their association with the animals and their environment. Improved control methods can develop only from investigations into the distribution and pathogenic nature of the microorganisms isolated.

ETIOLOGY

Bovine mastitis is associated with many different infectious agents, commonly divided into those causing **contagious mastitis,** which are spread from infected quarters to other quarters and cows, those that are normal teat skin inhabitants and cause **opportunistic mastitis,** and those causing **environmental mastitis,** which are usually present in the cow's environment and reach the teat from that source. Pathogens causing mastitis in cattle are further divided into **major pathogens** (those that cause clinical mastitis) and **minor pathogens** (those that normally cause subclinical mastitis and less frequently cause clinical mastitis).

Major Pathogens

Contagious Pathogens

- *S. agalactiae*
- *S. aureus*
- *M. bovis*

Environmental Pathogens

Environmental *Streptococcus* species include *S. uberis* and *S. dysgalactiae,* which are the most prevalent; less prevalent is *S. equinus* (formerly referred to as *S. bovis*). The environmental coliforms include the gram-negative bacteria *E. coli, Klebsiella* spp., and *Enterobacter* spp. *T. pyogenes* mastitis can be an important problem in some herds.

Minor Pathogens

Several other species of bacteria are often found colonizing the teat streak canal and mammary gland. They rarely cause clinical mastitis and are known as **minor pathogens.** They include the **coagulase-negative *Staphylococcus* spp.** such as *S. hyicus and S. chromogenes,* which are commonly isolated from milk samples and the teat canal. *S. xylosus* and *S. sciuri* are found free living in the environment; *S. warneri, S. simulans,* and *S. epidermidis* are part of the normal flora of the teat skin (and therefore are teat skin opportunistic pathogens). The prevalence of coagulase-negative *Staphylococcus* spp. is higher in first-lactation heifers than in cows and higher immediately after calving than in the remainder of lactation. In recent studies, they have been found as teat canal and intramammary infections in nulliparous heifers.

Corynebacterium bovis is also a minor pathogen; it is mildly pathogenic and the main reservoir is the infected gland or teat duct. However, in some herds, *C. bovis* appears to be a common cause of mild clinical mastitis. *C. bovis* spreads rapidly from cow to cow in the absence of adequate teat dipping. The prevalence of *C. bovis* is low in herds using an effective germicidal teat dip, good milking hygiene, and dry cow therapy. The presence of *C. bovis* in a gland will reduce the likelihood of subsequent infection with *S. aureus.*

Uncommon Mastitis Pathogens

Many other bacteria can cause severe mastitis, which is usually sporadic and usually affects only one cow or a few cows in the herd. These include *Nocardia asteroides, N. brasiliensis,* and *N. farcinica, Histophilus somni, Pasteurella multocida, Mannheimia* (formerly *Pasteurella*) *haemolytica, Campylobacter jejuni, Bacillus cereus,* and other gram-negative bacteria including *Citrobacter* spp., *Enterococcus faecalis, E. faecium, Proteus* spp., *Pseudomonas aeruginosa,* and *Serratia* spp. Anaerobic bacteria have been isolated from cases of mastitis, usually in association with other facultative bacteria, e.g., *Peptostreptococcus indolicus, Prevotella melaninogenica* (formerly *Bacteroides melaninogenicus*), *Eubacterium combesii, Clostridium sporogenes,* and *Fusobacterium necrophorum.*

Fungal infections include *Trichosporon* spp., *Aspergillus fumigatus, A. nidulans,* and *Pichia* spp.; yeast infections include *Candida* spp., *Cryptococcus neoformans, Saccharomyces* spp., and *Torulopsis* spp. Algal infections include *Prototheca trispora* and *P. zopfii.*

Leptospiras, including *Leptospira interrogans* serovar Pomona, and especially *Leptospira interrogans* Hardjo, cause damage to blood vessels in the mammary gland and gross abnormality of the milk. They are more correctly classified as systemic diseases with mammary gland.

Some viruses may also cause mastitis in cattle, but they are of little importance.

EPIDEMIOLOGY

This section deals with the general aspects of epidemiology of bovine mastitis. For information about the epidemiology of mastitis in the other animal species see the appropriate sections at the end of this chapter.

Occurrence and Prevalence of Infection

Occurrence refers to the location of the disease and the kinds of animals affected. **Prevalence** is the percentage of the population affected with a specific disease in a given population at a certain point in time. The **incidence** is a rate, such as the total number of new cases of clinical mastitis, and is a percentage of the animals at risk that develop a specific disease during a certain period of time. Prevalence is a function of the incidence and the duration of infection.

Prevalence

In most countries, surveys in dairy herds indicate that the **prevalence of infection** of mastitis pathogens is approximately 50% of cows and 10% to 25% of quarters. The prevalence of infection in dairy heifers of breeding age and in pregnant dairy heifers varies widely from 30% to 50% of heifers and 18% of quarters to as high as 97% of heifers and 75% of quarters.

Incidence

The **average annual incidence of clinical mastitis**, calculated as the number of clinical quarter cases per 100 cows at risk per year, including the dry period, in individual herds ranges from 10% to 12% in most herds, but higher incidences, ranging from 16% to 65%, occur in some herds. The greatest risk of first acquiring mastitis occurs early in lactation, usually in the first 50 days. The risk of clinical mastitis also increases with increasing parity. In beef herds, 32% to 37% of cows and 18% of quarters may have intramammary infection, which has a significant negative effect on calf weaning weights.

Case-fatality rates vary widely depending largely on the identity of the causative organism. For example, *S. agalactiae* mastitis is not a fatal disease, but peracute staphylococcal mastitis in a recently calved cow often may be fatal. Details of the occurrence of the different types of mastitis are presented in their individual sections in this chapter.

Relative Prevalence of Infection With Intramammary Pathogens

The prevalence of infection with intramammary pathogens in cattle with clinical mastitis differs from country to country, primarily based on whether cows are pasture based or confinement fed, and whether cattle were housed in free stalls or tie stalls. For example, in the United States, coliform bacteria are most frequently isolated from cows with clinical mastitis. The most frequently isolated bacteria from cattle with clinical mastitis in Canada are *S. aureus, E. coli, S. uberis*, and CNS.[1] In Europe, clinical mastitis caused by *Klebsiella* spp. occurs less frequently than *E. coli* mastitis, whereas the two pathogens are of equal importance in the United States because of the more frequent use of sawdust and wood shavings for bedding. In Norway, *S. aureus* is the predominant pathogen, followed by *S. dysgalactiae.* In Sweden, *S. aureus* is the predominant pathogen, followed by *E. coli, S. dysgalactiae, S. uberis*, CNS, *T. pyogenes*, and *Klebsiella* spp.[2] In Finland, *S. aureus* is also the predominant pathogen from clinical mastitis cases, followed by CNS, *S. uberis, S. dysgalactiae*, and *E. coli.*[3] *S. uberis* was the most common cause of clinical mastitis in Belgium, followed by *E. coli.*[4] In comparison, *S. uberis* is the most common cause of clinical mastitis in New Zealand,[1] and *S. aureus* is the predominant pathogen in Ireland, followed closely by *S. uberis*, coliform bacteria, environmental streptococci, and finally CNS.[5]

The bacteriologic identification of mastitis pathogens is important because optimal control and eradication procedures depend on the prevalent pathogens in the herd. In addition, the validity of epidemiologic investigations aimed at determining transmission patterns or the impact of environmental and managemental factors to a large extent depends on exact bacteriologic diagnosis.

Contagious Pathogens

The prevalence of infection with *S. aureus* in cows ranges widely, usually from 7% to 40%, but it is higher in some herds. A survey of Danish dairy herds found that 21% to 70% of all cows and 6% to 35% of all quarters were infected. *S. aureus* was isolated from 10% of quarter samples and was the most common species isolated. The prevalence of streptococci, including *S. agalactiae*, ranges from 1% to 8% of cows. A relative incidence of *S. agalactiae*, other streptococci and *S. aureus* of 1 : 1 : 2 is a common finding. *S. aureus* may still assume some importance as a cause of subclinical mastitis, but its prevalence has been reduced by modern mastitis control programs, leading to a higher proportion of culture-negative mastitic quarters and a corresponding, and perhaps consequent, increase in infections by *E. coli* and *Klebsiella* spp. The prevalence of infection caused by *Mycoplasma* spp. varies widely.

The prevalence of infection caused by an individual pathogen, and therefore the ratio between its incidence and that of other pathogens, depends on several risk factors such as size of herd and quality of management, especially milking parlor hygiene and cleanliness of accommodation, and parity of animal (heifer or cow). For example, large, zero-grazed herds kept in drylot conditions are likely to encounter more hygiene problems than conventionally housed herds mainly because of constant soiling of the udder by inadequate or improper bedding in larger units. In those circumstances there is likely to be a much higher prevalence than usual of mastitis associated with *E. coli* and *S. uberis.*

Teat Skin Opportunistic Pathogens

Coagulase-negative staphylococcal species were found in 4.1% of samples; the most frequently isolated were *S. epidermidis* (1.3%), *S. chromogenes* (1.0%), and *S. simulans* (0.7%).

Environmental Pathogens

The prevalence of intramammary coliform infections in a dairy herd seldom exceeds 1% to 2%; the prevalence of intramammary environmental streptococci is less than 5% in well-managed herds but may exceed 10% in some problem herds. A characteristic of intramammary coliform infections is the short duration, with 40% to 50% persisting less than 7 days. The majority of environmental streptococci infections last less than 30 days. In a survey of Danish dairy herds, *S. dysgalactiae* (1.6%) and *S. uberis* (1.4%) were the second and third most common species isolated.

Heifers

Surveys of intramammary infection of heifers in regions such as Louisiana indicate variability in prevalence and duration of intramammary infection according to species of bacteria present around the time of parturition. About 20% of heifers were infected with *S. aureus* and 70% with CNS, the minor pathogens that are part of the normal teat skin flora of heifers. *S. chromogenes* was isolated from 15% of all quarters of heifers before parturition but decreased shortly after parturition to 1%. Up to 97% of breeding age and pregnant dairy heifers and 75% of their quarters may be infected with *S. aureus, S. hyicus*, and *S. chromogenes.* Infections with *S. simulans* and *S. epidermidis* occurred in 1% to 3% of quarters both before and after parturition. *S. dysgalactiae* was isolated from 4% to 6% of quarters before and immediately after parturition. Intramammary infections with *S. aureus* rarely occurred before parturition but increased during the first week after parturition. There was no association between the prevalence of *S. aureus* in heifers before parturition and the prevalence in lactating cows.

Distribution of Pathogens in Clinical Mastitis

The distribution of pathogens isolated from cases of clinical mastitis has changed with the adoption of control programs from a high frequency of isolation of *S. aureus* and *S. agalactiae* to a higher isolation rate of other pathogens, particularly environmental pathogens. For example, in 171 randomly selected dairy herds, the average annual incidence of clinical mastitis was 13 quarter cases per 100 cows per year. The most frequent isolates from clinical cases were *E. coli* (16%), *S. aureus* (14%), *S. uberis* (11%), and *S. dysgalactiae* (8%). In another survey, the most common isolates from clinical cases were CNS and *E. coli*, each at 15% of samples taken. In a 2-year observational study of 65 dairy herds in Canada, there was considerable variation in the incidence of clinical mastitis among farms. Overall, 20% of cows experienced one or more cases of clinical mastitis during lactation. The pathogens isolated were coliforms (17%), other *Streptococcus* spp. (14%), *S. aureus* (7%), gram-positive bacilli (6%), *C. bovis* (2%), *S. agalactiae* (1%), and other *Staphylococcus* spp. (29%). There was no growth in 18% of samples, and 8% were contaminated. Clearly the main difference is that the rate of *S. aureus* in clinical cases is higher in continental Europe and lower in England and North America.

Source of Infection

Contagious Pathogens

S. agalactiae and *S. aureus* reside primarily in the udder of infected cows; the source of infection is other infected cows and exposure to uninfected quarters is limited to the milking process.

Teat Skin Opportunistic Pathogens

A number of species of coagulase-negative staphylococcus reside primarily on the teat skin of cattle.

Environmental Pathogens

S. uberis, S. dysgalactiae, and coliforms are common inhabitants of the cow's environment such as bedding. The exposure of uninfected quarters to environmental pathogens can occur at any time during the life of the cow, including milking time, between milkings, during the dry period, and before first calving in heifers.

Methods of Transmission

Infection of each mammary gland occurs via the teat canal, with the infection originating from either an infected udder or the environment; in dairy cattle the infection originating from infected udders is transmitted to the teat skin of other cows by milking machine liners, milkers' hands, washcloths, and any other material that can act as an inert carrier.

Risk Factors

Risk factors that influence the prevalence of infection and the incidence of clinical mastitis are outlined here. Individual factors that are of particular importance in the individual types of mastitis are described under those headings.

Animal Risk Factors

Age and Parity

The prevalence of infected quarters increases with age, peaking at 7 years. Surveys of the prevalence of intramammary infection in dairy heifers a few days before their first parturition reveals that 45% are infected, and the quarter infection rate may be 18%. Some studies found intramammary infections in 97% of heifers and 74% of quarters.

Stage of Lactation

Most **new infections** occur during the **early part of the dry period** and in the **first 2 months of lactation**, especially with the environmental pathogens. In heifers, the prevalence of infection is often high in the last trimester of pregnancy and several days before parturition, followed by a marked decline after parturition. In dairy heifers, most of these prepartum infections are associated with the minor pathogens, but some surveys have found evidence of infection by the major pathogens.

Some of these differences may be related to changes in the milk as a medium for bacterial growth. For example, bacteria such as *C. bovis* grow best in milk secreted in the middle of lactation, whereas dry period secretion inhibits its growth. During the dry period the quarter's capacity to provide phagocytic and bactericidal activities diminishes.

Season of Year

The relationship between the incidence of mastitis and season of the year is variable, depending on geographic and climatic conditions. In subtropical and tropical areas the incidence may be higher during winter or spring calvings from the increase in infection pressure associated with increased humidity. In temperate climates and confined dairy herds, the incidence of mastitis is typically higher in summer; this has been attributed to ambient temperatures facilitating the growth of mastitis pathogens in bedding.[6]

Somatic Cell Count

The highest average incidence of clinical mastitis caused by environmental bacteria may occur in herds with the lowest bulk tank milk somatic cell count (SCC; <150,000 cells/mL) and a low prevalence of subclinical infection.[6]

Breed

Generally, the incidence of mastitis is greater in Holstein Friesians than in Jerseys, but this may reflect differences in management rather than a true genetic difference. Valid comparisons between breeds have not been reported.

Milking Characteristics and Morphology of Udder and Teat

High milking rate and large teat canal diameter have been associated with increased SCC or risk of intramammary infection. Milk leaking in cows in herds with a low bulk tank milk SCC has also been associated with an increased rate of clinical mastitis. Decreasing teat-end-to-floor distance is also a risk factor for clinical mastitis and may be associated with an increased incidence of teat lesions.[7] Heritability estimates of teat-end-to-floor distance or udder height range from 0.2 to 0.7, which may be a consideration in the selection indices of bulls. Periparturient udder edema is also be a risk factor for clinical mastitis.[7]

Physical Condition of Teat

The teat end is the first barrier against invading pathogens, and the efficiency of teat defense mechanisms depends on the integrity of teat tissue; its impairment leads to an increase in the risk of intramammary infection. Teat thickness is an aid to evaluating teat tissue status. Milking machine characteristics can induce a decrease or increase in teat thickness after milking compared with premilking values. Increases in teat thickness of more than 5% are significantly associated with infection and new infection, but the association was not significant when teat thickness decreased by more than 5%. Coagulase-negative staphylococcal infections are significantly associated with both increases and decreases in teat thickness numerically greater than 5%, but there is no association between teat thickness and *S. aureus* infections. In a longitudinal study of 135 dairy cows teat condition, as assessed immediately after milking, did not appear to be associated with the risk of new intramammary infections, inflammatory response, or mastitis.[8]

Hyperkeratosis of the teat orifice is a commonly observed condition in the dairy cow because of machine milking; the degree of hyperkeratosis may be increased by a poor milking system. There is wide variation in the degree of hyperkeratosis between herds; the score increases with lactational age and peaks, for any lactation, and at 3 to 4 months after parturition, and declines as the cows dry off. There is no significant relationship between mean SCC and the degree of hyperkeratosis at the herd level. However, there is an association between higher hyperkeratosis scores and higher microbial teat canal load, particularly for two common environmental mastitis pathogens, *E. coli* and *S. uberis,* but surprisingly not for *S. aureus* teat canal load.[9] Severe hyperkeratosis of the teat end is associated with an increased risk of clinical mastitis in the UK, but moderate hyperkeratosis was not predictive of clinical mastitis incidence.[10] Together, these data indicate that only severe disruption of the normal anatomy of the teat orifice is associated with an increased risk of developing clinical mastitis.[10]

Udder Hygiene

Dirty udders are associated with increased SCC and an increased prevalence of intramammary infection caused by contagious and environmental pathogens.[7] It makes sense that an increased bacterial challenge of the teat and udder is associated with an increased risk of mastitis (Fig. 20-1). Udder hygiene could be a proxy for general mastitis management skills, because good mastitis control programs result in a low prevalence of infection with contagious and environmental pathogens.

Nutritional Status

Vitamins E and A as well as selenium may be involved in resistance to certain types of mastitis. Early reports found that supplementation with antioxidants such as selenium and vitamin E had a beneficial effect on udder health in dairy cattle by decreasing the incidence and duration of

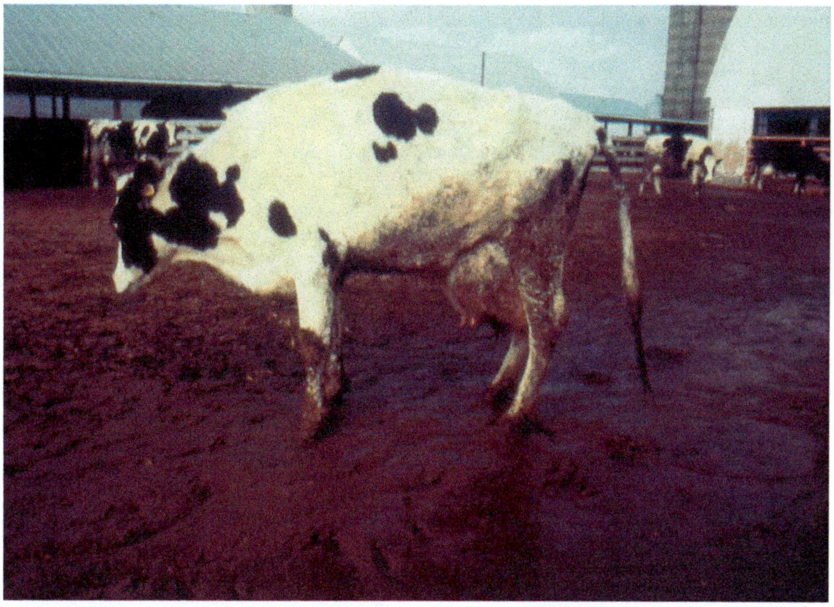

Fig. 20-1 The environmental bacterial challenge can be formidable in confinement dairy operations, as demonstrated from a Midwest dairy in the United States.

clinical mastitis. An increase in selenium concentration in whole blood was associated with a decrease in all infections, including *S. aureus, T. pyogenes,* and *C. bovis.* There was no association between different infections or SCC and concentrations of vitamin E, vitamin A, or β-carotene, but an association existed between vitamin A concentration and SCC. There may an association between feed intake and risk of clinical mastitis: milk fat to protein ratios <1.0 (typically indicating the presence of subacute ruminal acidosis) or >1.5 (typically indicating the presence of excessive fat mobilization) predicts an increased likelihood of clinical mastitis within the following week.[8]

Genetic Resistance to Mastitis

A variety of morphologic, physiologic, and immunologic factors contribute to a cow's resistance or susceptibility to mastitis, and each of these factors is influenced to some extent by heredity.[7] Differences in udder depth, teat length, teat shape, and teat orifice morphology are thought to be associated with differences in mastitis occurrence. The production of keratin in the streak canal and the physical and biochemical characteristics of keratin are important contributors to mastitis resistance. Many of the defense mechanisms of the udder, including lysozyme, lactoferrin, immunoglobulins, and leukocytes, are direct products of genes and have a genetic basis. For dairy cattle, heritability estimates for clinical mastitis average about 0.05. These low heritability estimates indicate that there is very little genetic influence on clinical mastitis but a very strong environmental influence.

Somatic Cell Count. Differences in heritability between herds with high and low SCCs are not significant. However, differences among bulls' daughter groups for both clinical mastitis and SCC are reasonably large, suggesting that selection of sires can be important in mastitis control. An analysis of the disease and breeding records of a large number of Swedish bulls siring daughters whose milk had a low SCC count found genetic correlations from 0.71 to 0.79 between SCC and clinical mastitis. It was concluded that it is possible to improve resistance to clinical mastitis by selecting for a low SCC.

The strong phenotypic and genetic association between SCC and mastitis indicates that breeding programs based on SCC may be effective as an indirect means of improving mastitis resistance. However, greater emphasis on SCC may decrease genetic gain in yield traits, which are economically more important.

Milk Yield

The genetic correlation between milk yield and mastitis is about 0.2 to 0.3, which suggests that animals genetically above average for milk yield are more susceptible to mastitis and that low-yielding cows tend to be more resistant. However, the low correlation value suggests that this relationship is not a strong tendency. The positive correlation implies that genetic improvement for milk yield is accompanied by a slow decline in genetic resistance to mastitis. Examination of the association between milk yield and disease in a large number of dairy cows found that higher milk yield was not a factor for any disease except mastitis. However, the association between milk yield and mastitis does not imply causation. At least two biological explanations are plausible: increased injury and leaking of milk between milkings. Improved mastitis control efforts have offset the genetic trend for increased susceptibility to mastitis. The low heritability for mastitis indicates the great importance of environmental factors in causing differences in the prevalence of infection and the incidence of clinical mastitis.

In summary, selection for milk yield alone results in increased incidence of mastitis. The positive genetic correlation between milk yield and mastitis suggests that genes that increase milk yield tend to increase susceptibility to mastitis. Selection indices that maximize genetic improvement for net economic benefit will not decrease the incidence of mastitis, but indices that include SCC, udder depth, or clinical mastitis will diminish the rate of increase in mastitis by 20% to 25%. Using **predicted transmitting ability** (PTA), an estimate of genetic merit, it has been found on average that daughters of bulls with high PTAs for SCC have a higher incidence of mastitis; sires with low PTA for somatic cell scores (SCSs) should therefore be selected. All of the economically important traits are weighted into a selection index for the selection of bulls, which will improve net income over cost of production.

Dairy cattle with enhanced and optimally balanced antibody and cell-mediated immune responses are known as **high immune responders**. These adaptive immune responses are separate to innate immunity and are heritable, with heritability estimates of 0.25 to 0.35. These estimates are similar in magnitude to those for milk production traits, indicating that an appropriately weighted selection index would improve overall cow health and production.[11]

Other Concurrent Diseases

These may be important risk factors for mastitis. Retained placentas, teat injuries, and teat sores may be associated with a higher incidence of mastitis. Sole ulceration of any severity occurring in more than one digit has been associated with an approximately threefold higher risk of *S. aureus* infections in the first lactation. It is suggested that sore feet could increase the risk of teat lesions, presumably as a result of difficulty in standing.

Immunologic Function of Mammary Gland

The immune function of the mammary gland is impaired during the periparturient period; it is susceptible to mastitis during transition periods, such as drying off and colostrogenesis. As a result, the **incidence of new intramammary infections is highest during the early nonlactating period and the periparturient period.**

Innate immunity plays an important role in maintaining a healthy mammary gland.[12] **Pattern recognition receptors** (PRRs) recognize well-conserved patterns on the surface of microbes called **pathogen-associated molecular patterns** (PAMPs).

The initial interaction between PAMPs and PRRs plays an important role in the subsequent inflammatory response.[13,14] Lactoferrin is another component of innate immunity. It reaches high concentrations in the glandular secretions during the dry period, particularly during involution of the mammary gland. Because of its high secretion concentration and ability to bind iron, lactoferrin provides important innate antimicrobial activity against new intramammary infections in the dry period, particularly coliform bacteria.[14,15]

The most important components of the defense against common bacterial pathogens are blood-derived **neutrophils** and **opsonizing antibodies**. An inadequate rate of neutrophil recruitment to combat a new intramammary infection has a profound effect on the outcome of infection, because cows with a rapid and massive recruitment of neutrophils to an infected gland clear an intramammary infection within 12 to 18 hours postinfection.

It is also important that an early inflammatory response in the infected mammary gland enables leakage of IgG_2 (opsonizing antibodies) because this facilitates neutrophil phagocytosis of bacteria. The **staggered one-two punch** of **peak IgG_2 concentrations** within 4 hours of infection and **peak neutrophil response** within 6 to 12 hours of infection greatly facilitates clearance of new intramammary infections.

Blood-derived neutrophils must undergo **margination**, **adherence,** and **migration** to arrive in the mammary gland, in which they perform **phagocytosis**, **respiratory burst,** and **degranulation**. Margination is via expression of three adhesion molecules from the selectin family, specifically L-selectin (also called CD62L) on neutrophils, E-selectin (also called CD62E), and P-selectin (also called CD62P) on vascular endothelial cells. Neutrophil L-selectin makes the initial contact between "streaming" neutrophils in the bloodstream and the vascular wall; this contact slows neutrophil movement and allows them to "roll" along the endothelium while surveying for the presence of proinflammatory mediators at the sites of tissue infection. When the rolling neutrophils detect the presence of one or more proinflammatory mediators, they immediately shed surface L-selectin (CD62L) adhesion molecules and upregulate and activate Mac-1 (CD11b/CD18) adhesion molecules, stopping neutrophil rolling and permitting tight adherence of the neutrophil to the endothelium. Once adhered, neutrophils commence diapedesis by migrating between endothelial cells to the site of infection. Neutrophil migration therefore has three components: hyperadherence (cessation of rolling), diapedesis, and chemotaxis. Any delay or inhibition in this process can lead to peracute mastitis and severe clinical disease. This is best illustrated by bovine leukocyte adhesion deficiency in Holstein Friesian cattle; affected calves cannot produce Mac-1 molecules and have a prominent neutrophilia because streaming neutrophils cannot migrate to the site of infection. Migration of neutrophils is slow during the first few weeks of lactation, and this delay in neutrophil migration is thought to be responsible for the increased incidence and severity of intramammary infections during early lactation.

Previous Mastitis

Cows with a history of mastitis in the preceding lactation may be almost twice as susceptible to clinical mastitis in the current lactation as those without mastitis in the preceding lactation.

Preexisting Intramammary Infections

Existing intramammary infections with minor pathogens has a **protective effect** against infections with major pathogens that is prominent in experimental infection studies that involve a large inoculum that bypasses the teat canal.[16] The observed protective effect of minor pathogen infection may not occur under commercial dairy conditions. The strongest protective effect was observed with coagulase-negative staphylococci, whereas intramammary infection with *C. bovis* did not provide protection against intramammary infection by a major pathogen.[16] Elimination of minor pathogens with postmilking teat disinfection may therefore result in an increase in the incidence of subclinical and clinical mastitis. Discontinuation of teat dipping may be associated with an increase in the prevalence of minor pathogens, increase in the incidence of *S. aureus* infections, and decrease in the incidence of *E. coli* infections.

Use of Recombinant Bovine Somatotropin

Because the risk of clinical mastitis increases as milk production increases, there has been considerable scientific and public controversy over the potential effects that the use of recombinant bovine somatotropin (bST) might have on the incidence of clinical mastitis and the subsequent use of antimicrobials from therapy. In some field trials, the use of bST did not result in an increase in the incidence of clinical mastitis compared with controls. In other trials, a significant increase in the incidence of clinical mastitis occurred in treated cows compared with controls. However, the incidence of clinical mastitis was greater in treated cows compared with controls before bST was used. In trials done on well-managed farms that had controlled contagious mastitis and had low rates of clinical mastitis caused by environmental pathogens, the use of bST was not associated with an increase in clinical mastitis, discarded milk because of therapy, or culling for mastitis. Interpretation of a direct effect of bST on mastitis incidence is confounded by the higher incidence of mastitis in cows of higher milk production.

Environmental and Management Risk Factors

Quality and Management of Housing

Factors such as climate, housing system, type of bedding, and rainfall interact to influence the degree of exposure of teat ends to mastitis pathogens. Because dairy cattle spend 40% to 65% of their time lying down, **the quality and management of housing for dairy cattle has a major influence on the types of mastitis pathogen that infect the mammary gland, as well as the degree of infection pressure.**

The major sources of environmental pathogens are the cow's environment, including bedding, soil, feedstuffs, and water supplies. Environmental pathogens multiply in bedding materials, with which the cow's teats are in close and prolonged contact. Bacterial growth in bedding depends on temperature, amount of moisture and nutrients available, and the pH. Fresh bedding can be a source of contamination even before it is used: *Klebsiella pneumoniae* can be present in green, hardwood sawdust in higher numbers than in other types of bedding, and major outbreaks of environmental mastitis caused by *K. pneumoniae* have occurred following the use of contaminated wood products in bedding, described in detail in that section. Dry, unused bedding contains few pathogens, but after being used it becomes contaminated and provides a source in which pathogens multiply to high numbers in 24 hours. Organic bedding materials such as straw, sawdust, wood shavings, and paper support the growth of pathogens. Inorganic materials such as sand retain less moisture and do not provide a supply of nutrients for the pathogens; bacterial counts in these materials are usually lower than in organic materials. Housing lactating cattle on sawdust leads to six times more *Klebsiella* bacteria and twice as much coliform bacteria on the teat ends compared with housing cattle on sand. In contrast, there were 10 times more environmental streptococci bacteria on teat ends when cows were housed on sand, compared with housing on sawdust. Surveys indicate that herds using wood chips or sawdust as bedding material have higher rates of clinical mastitis compared with those using straw bedding.

High humidity and high ambient temperatures favor growth of pathogens. Cows in confinement housing with organic bedding materials have the highest incidence of environmental mastitis in the warm, humid months of the year. Pasturing herds during the summer months usually reduces the incidence of coliform mastitis, although rates of environmental streptococci may remain high. In drylot systems the incidence of coliform mastitis may be associated with periods of high rainfall. Herds with more months on pasture may have a higher incidence of clinical mastitis, which may be associated with factors such as sanitation and the stress of transition between pasture and confinement housing.

The **management and design of housing systems** influence the prevalence of intramammary infection and the incidence of clinical mastitis. Any housing factor or management system that allows cows to become dirty or damage teats or that causes overcrowding will result in an increase in clinical mastitis. This includes the size and comfort of free stalls, the size of the alleyways, ease of movement of cattle, and the cleaning system. Failure to keep alleyways, cow stalls and bedding clean and dry will increase the level of contamination of the teats. Overcrowding, poor ventilation, and access to dirty ponds of water and muddy areas in which cows congregate are major risk factors.

The **size of the milking cowherd** may be positively associated with an increased incidence of clinical mastitis, because it can be more difficult to control contagious mastitis in a herd with a greater prevalence of infection and a larger number of cow-to-cow contacts. As herd size increases, manure disposal and sanitation problems may increase exposure to environmental pathogens. However, regional and management differences may confound the association of size with infection status. Some recent data suggest lower SCC in large herds. The use of designated maternity areas providing an isolated and clean environment for parturition may be associated with a lower incidence of clinical mastitis.

If hygiene and bedding maintenance are neglected in the housing accommodation the prevalence of environmental forms of mastitis may increase markedly. Periodic inspection of dry cows is an essential part of mastitis control.

Milking Practices

The failure to use established and reliable methods of mastitis control is an important risk factor. This is a major subject, which includes efficiency of milking personnel, milking machines, high milking speed, and especially hygiene in the milking parlor. Wet teats and udders are a risk factor for increased SCC, especially in the presence of teat impacts from liner slippage. The use of a separate drying cloth for each cow is associated with a lower SCC. Effective use of a postmilking germicidal teat dip is critical for the control of contagious mastitis. Increasing person-hours spent milking per cow may be associated with a higher rate of clinical mastitis. Contaminated milking equipment—including milk hoses, udder wash towels, and teat dip products—has been associated with outbreaks of environmental mastitis from *S. marcescens* and *P. aeruginosa*. Drying off procedures at the end of lactation and an active policy on drying off treatment are equally important.

The **absence of milk quality regulations that place emphasis on SCC is also a risk factor.** Conversely, the presence of strict regulations with penalties for high SCC is an important incentive to institute mastitis control programs that improve the quality of milk. The absence of a health management program consisting of regular farm visits by the veterinarian may also be a risk factor for mastitis, which may be associated with a relative lack of awareness by the producer of the importance of the principles of mastitis control.

Pathogen Risk Factors

Viability of Pathogens

The ability of the pathogen to survive in the cow's immediate environment (resistance to environmental influences including cleaning and disinfection procedures) is a characteristic of each pathogen. The causes of contagious mastitis are more susceptible to disinfection than the causes of environmental mastitis.

Virulence Factors

There is a wide variety of virulence factors among the mastitis pathogens. These are described under specific mastitides. The influence of many bacterial virulence factors depends on the stage of lactation and severity of the intramammary infection and the effects elicited by the virulence factors on bovine mammary tissue. A few examples of the common virulence factors are noted here.

Colonizing Ability

The ability of the pathogens to colonize the teat duct, then to adhere to mammary epithelium, and to initiate mastitis is a major characteristic of the major bacterial causes of mastitis. *S. aureus* strains that cause mastitis can bind to ductular udder epithelial cells and to explant cultures of bovine mammary glands. There are differences in the adhesion characteristics among strains of the organism, which may explain the different epidemiologic characteristics of the organisms in some herds. Comparison of strains isolated from different *S. aureus* mastitis cases between herds reveals that only a limited number of genotypes of *S. aureus* are most prevalent.

Toxins

E. coli isolates that cause mastitis produce lipopolysaccharide endotoxin, which is responsible for many of the inflammatory and systemic changes observed during acute coliform mastitis. *S. aureus* isolated from intramammary infections produces many potential virulence factors, including enterotoxins; coagulase and alpha-, beta-, and delta-toxins; hemolysin; hyaluronidase; and leukocidins, which are considered to be involved in the varying degrees of inflammation characteristic of staphylococcal mastitis from subclinical to peracute gangrenous mastitis. Virulence factors of *S. uberis* include hyaluronidase and the hyaluronic capsule.

Production and Economic Losses

Although mastitis occurs sporadically in all species, it assumes major economic importance in dairy cattle and may be one of the most costly diseases in dairy herds. Mastitis results in economic loss for producers by increasing the costs of production and by decreasing productivity. The premature culling of potentially profitable cows because of chronic mastitis is also a significant loss. Because of the large economic losses, there is a potential for high returns on investment in an effective control program. The component economic losses can be divided into the following:

- Loss of milk production
- Discarded milk from cows with clinical mastitis and treated cows
- Replacement cost of culled cows
- Extra labor required for treatment and monitoring
- Veterinary service for treatment and control
- Cost of first trimester abortions caused by clinical mastitis
- Cost of decreased conception rate caused by clinical mastitis 1 week before or 2 weeks after artificial insemination[17]
- Cost of control measures

There are additional costs such as antimicrobial residues in milk from treated cows, milk quality control, dairy food manufacturing, nutritional quality of milk, degrading of milk supplies caused by high bacteria or SCC, and interference with the genetic potential of some cows from early involuntary culling because of chronic mastitis.[18] The total annual cost of mastitis in the dairy cattle population is estimated to be 10% of the total value of farm milk sales, and about two-thirds of this loss is caused by reduced milk production in subclinically affected cows. The production and economic losses are commonly divided into those associated with subclinical and clinical mastitis.

Subclinical Mastitis

Total milk losses from quarters affected with subclinical mastitis have been estimated to range from 10% to 26%. Lower SCCs are associated with higher milk production, and rolling herd average milk production has been estimated to decrease by 190 kg per unit increase of linear SCS. Most estimates indicate that on average an affected quarter results in a 30% reduction in productivity, and an affected cow is estimated to lose 15% of its production for lactation. This loss is sometimes expressed as a loss of about 340 kg of saleable milk, which is caused by the loss of production and the value of milk that has to be withheld from sale. The loss in production by an infected quarter may be largely compensated by increased production in the other quarters so that the net loss from the cow may be less than expected. In addition to these losses, there is an added loss of about 1% of total solids by changes in composition (fat, casein, and lactose are reduced and glycogen, whey proteins, pH, and chlorides are increased), which interferes with manufacturing processes, and other losses include increased culling rates and costs of treatment. Comparisons between low- and high-prevalence herds always show a financial advantage of about 20% to the low-prevalence herds, with the gain varying with the local price of milk or butter fat. In beef herds the losses are in the form of rare deaths of cows and failure of the calves to gain weight.

Approximately 75% of the economic loss from subclinical mastitis is attributable to loss of milk production. Other costs include discarding milk from treated cows, drug costs, veterinary costs, labor, and loss of genetic potential of culled cows.

Clinical Mastitis

Clinical mastitis results in marked decreases in milk production, which are much larger in early than late lactation.[19] Milk production losses are also greater in cows with multiple lactations than first-lactation cows[19] and vary with pathogen type. Generally, gram-negative clinical mastitis cases have a greater milk loss than gram-positive and other cases.[20] In primiparous cattle, the greatest production losses were associated with *E. coli* and "untreatable" mastitis pathogens including *T. pyogenes*, *Mycoplasma* spp., *Prototheca*, and yeast.[21] In multiparous cattle, the greatest production losses were associated with *Klebsiella* spp. and untreatable mastitis pathogens. Clinical mastitis episodes caused by CNS were not associated with a detectable production loss.[21]

Clinical mastitis also decreases the duration of lactation and increases the likelihood of culling. Clinical cases of brief duration that occur after the peak of lactation affect milk production very little but can induce abortion during the first 45 days of gestation. Clinically affected quarters may not completely recover milk production in subsequent lactations, but these carry-over losses are not as large as the losses from acute mastitis.

The **costs of clinical mastitis** in dairy herds have been estimated in a number of countries. In a large 5-herd study in New York state in 2008 each clinical mastitis case cost $71 per cow-year, with a mean cost per clinical episode of $179. The latter estimate was based on $115 for milk yield loss, $14 for increased mortality, and $50 for treatment-associated costs.[22] These estimates did not include the cost of control programs.

The component causes of economic loss associated with mastitis outlined previously vary according to the causative pathogen and are described under specific mastitides. In general terms *S. aureus* and *E. coli* may cause death from peracute mastitis; *T. pyogenes* causes complete loss of quarters; staphylococci and streptococci cause acute clinical mastitis, but their principal role is in causing subclinical mastitis, resulting in a reduction of milk produced and a downgrading of its quality. Of these, *S. agalactiae* causes the greatest production loss, whereas *S. aureus* has the higher infection rate, greater resistance to treatment, and longer duration of infection. At one time *S. aureus* represented the impassable barrier to mastitis control programs.

Other factors that affect the magnitude of the loss associated with mastitis include age (the loss is greatest in mature cows) and when the attack occurs in the first 150 days of lactation.

Zoonotic Potential

With mastitis there is the danger that the bacterial contamination of milk from affected cows may render it unsuitable for human consumption by causing food poisoning, or interfere with manufacturing processes or, in rare cases, provide a mechanism of spread of disease to humans. Tuberculosis, listeriosis, salmonellosis, and brucellosis may be spread in this way. Raw (unpasteurized) milk can be a source of food-borne pathogens, and consumption of raw milk can result in sporadic disease outbreaks. For instance, sampling bulk tank raw milk in Ontario revealed the presence of *Listeria monocytogenes, Salmonella* spp., *Campylobacter* spp., or verocytotoxigenic *E. coli* in 2.7, 0.2, 0.5, and 0.9% of milk samples, respectively. These findings emphasize the importance of continued diligence in the application of hygiene programs within dairies and the separation of raw from pasteurized milk and milk products.

PATHOGENESIS

Infection of the mammary gland always occurs via the teat canal and on first impression the development of inflammation after infection seems a natural sequence. However, the development of mastitis is more complex than this and can be most satisfactorily explained in terms of three stages: **invasion, infection**, and **inflammation.** Of the three phases, prevention of the invasion phase offers the greatest potential for reducing the incidence of mastitis by good management, notably in the use of good hygienic procedures.

Invasion is the stage at which pathogens move from the teat end to the milk inside the teat canal.

Infection is the stage in which the pathogens multiply rapidly and invade the mammary tissue. After invasion the pathogen population may be established in the teat canal and, with this as a base, a series of multiplications and extensions into mammary tissue may occur, with infection of mammary tissue occurring frequently or occasionally depending on its susceptibility. Multiplication of certain organisms may result in the release of endotoxins, as in coliform mastitis, which causes profound systemic effects with minimal inflammatory effects.

Inflammation follows infection and represents the stage at which clinical mastitis occurs with varying degrees of clinical abnormalities of the udder and variable systemic effects from mild to peracute; gross and subclinical abnormalities of the milk appear. Abnormalities of the udder include marked swelling, increased warmth and, in acute and peracute stages, gangrene in some cases and abscess formation and atrophy of glands in chronic stages. The systemic effects are caused by the mediators of inflammation. Gross abnormalities of the milk include a decrease in milk yield, the presence of the products of inflammation, and marked changes in the composition of the milk.

The most significant subclinical abnormality of the milk is the increase in the **SCC**, the most common measurement of milk quality and udder health. Milk somatic cells in a healthy gland consist of several cell types, including neutrophils (<11%), macrophages (66%–88%), lymphocytes (10%–27%), and a smaller percentage of epithelial cells (0%–7%). Neutrophils are the predominant cell type found in mammary tissues and secretions during inflammation, and in mastitis they constitute more than 90% of total mammary gland leukocytes. Once at the site of infection, neutrophils phagocytose and kill pathogens. Neutrophils exert their bactericidal effect through a respiratory burst that produces hydroxyl and oxygen radicals, which are important components of the oxygen-dependent killing mechanism.

In the healthy lactating mammary gland, the SCC is less than 100,000 cells/mL of milk. During intramammary infection, the glandular SCC can increase to more than 1,000,000 cells/mL of milk within a few hours because of the combined effect of an increased number of neutrophils (numerator) and a decreased glandular secretion volume (denominator). **The severity and duration of mastitis are critically related to the promptness of the neutrophil migratory response and their bactericidal activity at the site of infection.** As they colonize and multiply in the mammary gland, some bacteria release metabolic by-products or cell-wall components (endotoxin if a gram-negative bacteria) that serve as chemoattractants for leukocytes. If neutrophils move rapidly from the bloodstream and are able to eliminate the inflammatory stimuli (bacteria), then recruitment of neutrophils ceases and the SCC returns to normal levels. If bacteria are able to survive this immediate host response, then the inflammation continues, resulting in neutrophil migration between adjacent mammary secretory cells toward the alveolar lumen. Prolonged diapedesis of neutrophils damages mammary tissue, resulting in decreased milk production. The duration and severity of the inflammatory response therefore has a major impact on the quantity and quality of milk produced.

The major factor affecting the SCC at the herd and individual cow level is the prevalence of intramammary infection at a glandular level. Because marked increases in SCC are a result of cells being attracted to the mammary tissue because of the mediators produced during a local infection, events that do not affect udder health are unlikely to have a direct or dramatic effect on SCC. Little evidence exists that any factor other than normal diurnal variation has a major influence on SCC in the absence of intramammary infections.

The effects of mastitis on milk yield are highly variable and depend on the severity of the inflammation, the causative agents and the lesions produced, the efficiency of treatment, the production level, and the stage of lactation. Mastitis in early lactation causes a larger decrease in milk yield with long-term effects than mastitis in late lactation. Mastitis caused by *S. aureus* generally evolves into persistent but moderate infections, unlike those associated with coliforms. Mastitis associated with *T. pyogenes* results in suppurative lesions, poor response to treatment, and culling. *M. bovis* causes chronic induration and almost complete loss of milk production without recovery.

CLINICAL FINDINGS

Details of the clinical findings are provided under each specific type of mastitis. The clinical findings should be used only as a guide because different pathogens can cause chronic, subclinical, subacute, acute, and peracute forms of the disease, and clinical differentiation of the different causes of mastitis is difficult. The greatest clinical accuracy achievable, even in a specialist hospital environment and after adaptation to suit local conditions, is about 70%, which is not sufficiently accurate to be clinically useful. In other words, bacteriologic culture of milk from an affected gland is required before specific pathogen-directed treatment can be implemented.

Clinical mastitis is detected using only the results of the physical examination, and a useful definition of clinical mastitis is a negative answer to the question: Would you drink this? In other words, "undrinkable" is a simple and generalizable concept for defining clinical mastitis, because milk from cows with clinical mastitis is not suitable for drinking. New cases of clinical mastitis are defined as being separated by at least 14 days.

The clinical findings in mastitis include abnormalities of secretion, abnormalities of the size, consistency and temperature of the mammary glands and, frequently, a systemic reaction. In other words, there are **three categories of clinical mastitis**: **abnormal secretion**, **abnormal gland,** and an **abnormal cow** (systemic disease). Abnormal secretion is visibly abnormal (i.e., is not drinkable). An abnormal gland is larger and firmer than other quarters. An abnormal cow is pyrexic, depressed, or has decreased appetite or milk production. This three-part categorization scheme has excellent clinical utility, is readily understood by everyone, and provides a sound pathophysiological basis for treatment. In particular, it is likely that optimal treatment protocols can be developed for the three levels of clinical mastitis. Other categorization systems have been developed, but they lack the simplicity and generalizability of the secretion, gland, and cow system.

Clinical mastitis episodes are also categorized according to their severity and duration.

Severity is characterized as follows:

- **Peracute:** severe inflammation with swelling and heat and pain of the quarter with a marked systemic reaction, which may be fatal
- **Acute:** severe inflammation without a marked systemic reaction
- **Subacute:** mild inflammation with persistent abnormality of the milk

Duration is characterized as follows:

- **Short-term** (as in *E. coli* and *Klebsiella* spp.)
- **Recurrent** (as in *S. aureus* and *S. dysgalactiae*)
- **Persistent** (as in *S. agalactiae* and *M. bovis*)

Abnormal Secretion

Proper examination of the milk requires the use of a **strip cup**, preferably one with a **shiny, black plate** that permits the detection of discoloration as well as clots, flakes, and purulent material. Milk is drawn on to the black plate in pools, and comparisons are made between the milk of different quarters. Because the herdsman frequently has little time to examine milk for evidence of mastitis, it is customary to milk the first few streams onto the floor; in some parlors black plates are set in the floor. The practice does not appear to be harmful if the floor is kept washed down.

Discoloration may be from blood staining or wateriness, with the latter usually indicating chronic mastitis when the quarter is lactating. Little significance is attached to barely discernible wateriness in the first few streams but, if this persists for two to three streams or more, it is an abnormality. One of the major unresolved issues in bovine mastitis is how to treat a cow with abnormal secretion on the first one to two streams that subsequently has normal-looking milk. Clots or flakes are usually accompanied by discoloration and they are always significant, indicating a severe degree of inflammation, even when small and present only in the first few streams. Blood clots are of little significance in a mastitis case, and neither are the small plugs of wax that are often present in the milk during the first few days after calving, especially in heifers. Flakes at the end of milking may be indicative of mammary tuberculosis in cattle.

During the **dry period** in normal cows, the secretion changes from normal milk to a clear watery fluid, then to a secretion the color and consistency of honey, and finally to colostrum in the last few days before parturition. Some variation may occur between individual quarters in the one cow; if this is marked, it should arouse suspicion of infection.

The **strip cup** provides a valuable tool for detecting clinical mastitis and constitutes part of the routine physical examination of the lactating cow. The most sensitive use of the strip cup is to observe the ability of milk from one quarter to mix with milk from another quarter; incomplete mixing (evidence of streaming) indicates that secretions from the two quarters differ and suggests the presence of an intramammary infection in one of the quarters. However, it should be remembered that the strip cup can only detect clinical mastitis, and detection of subclinical mastitis requires use of indirect tests such as SCC of composite milk samples from individual cows, or application of the California mastitis test (CMT) to quarter samples or measuring the electrical conductivity of quarter samples.

Abnormal Gland

Abnormalities of size and consistency of the quarters may be seen and felt. Palpation is of greatest value when the udder has been recently milked, whereas visual examination of both the full and empty udder may be useful. The udder should be viewed from behind, and the two hindquarters should be examined for symmetry. By lifting up the hindquarters, the forequarters can be viewed. A decision on which quarter of a pair is abnormal may depend on palpation, which should be performed simultaneously on the opposite quarter of the pair. Although in most forms of mastitis the observed abnormalities are mainly in the region of the milk cistern, the whole of the quarter must be palpated, particularly if tuberculosis is suspected. The teats should be inspected and palpated for skin lesions, especially around the teat end. The supramammary lymph nodes should also be palpated for evidence of enlargement.

Palpation and inspection of the udder are directed at the detection of fibrosis, inflammatory swelling, and atrophy of mammary tissue. Fibrosis occurs in various forms. There may be a diffuse increase in connective tissue, giving the quarter a firmer feel than its opposite number and usually a more nodular surface on light palpation. Local areas of fibrosis may also occur in a quarter; these may vary in size from pealike lesions to masses as large as a fist. Acute inflammatory swelling is always diffuse and is accompanied by heat and pain and marked abnormality of the secretion. In severe cases there may be areas of gangrene, or abscesses may develop in the glandular tissue. The terminal stage of chronic mastitis is atrophy of the gland. On casual examination an atrophied quarter may be classed as normal because of its small size, whereas the normal quarter is judged to be hypertrophic. Careful palpation may reveal that, in the atrophic quarter, little functioning mammary tissue remains.

Abnormal Cow (Systemic Response)

A systemic response including toxemia, pyrexia, tachycardia, tachypnea, ruminal hypomotility, depression, recumbency, and anorexia may or may not be present, depending on the type and severity of the infection.[23] The hock-to-hock distance is increased in cattle with clinical mastitis (Fig. 20-2), reflecting a change in stance caused by the presence of localized pain in the udder.[23] The mechanical threshold to pain of cows with clinical mastitis is lower than that of control cows.[23] Daily feed intake is decreased by approximately 1.2 kg during the 5 days before clinical mastitis is detected, and cows eat more slowly and are less competitive at the feed bunk when they have clinical mastitis.[24-26] Cows with clinical mastitis also spend more time standing and less time lying with affected quarter(s) on the down side.[25,26]

A systemic response is usually associated with severe mastitis associated with *E. coli*, *Klebsiella* spp., or *T. pyogenes* and occasionally with *Streptococcus* spp. or *Staphylococcus* spp. Clinical mastitis episodes caused by *T. pyogenes* produces the greatest decrease in milk production. In contrast, clinical mastitis caused by environmental streptococci and CNS is associated with the smallest decrease in milk production. Clinical mastitis episodes caused by *S. aureus* are associated with the highest risk of culling.

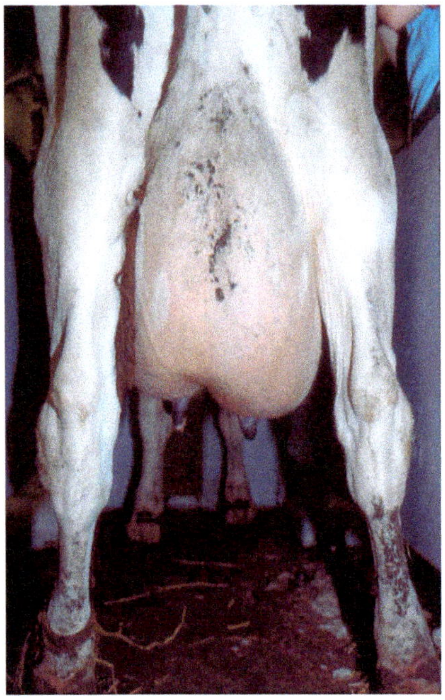

Fig. 20-2 Increased hock-to-hock distance in a Holstein Friesian cow with clinical mastitis in the right rear quarter.

FURTHER READING

Pyörälä S. Mastitis in post-partum dairy cows. *Reprod Domest Anim.* 2008;43(suppl 2):252-259.

REFERENCES

1. Riekerink RGMO, et al. *J Dairy Sci.* 2008;91:1366.
2. Unnerstad HE, et al. *Vet Microbiol.* 2009;137:90.
3. Koivula M, et al. *Acta Agr Scand Sect A.* 2007;57:89.
4. Verbeke J, et al. *J Dairy Sci.* 2014;97:6926.
5. Keane OM, et al. *Vet Rec.* 2013;173:17.
6. Elghafghuf A, et al. *Prev Vet Med.* 2014;117:456.
7. Compton CWR, et al. *J Dairy Sci.* 2007;90:4171.
8. Zoche-Golob V, et al. *Prev Vet Med.* 2015;121:64.
9. Paduch JH, et al. *Vet Microbiol.* 2012;158:353.
10. Breen JE, et al. *J Dairy Sci.* 2009;92:2551.
11. Thompson-Crispi K, et al. *Front Immunol.* 2014;5:493.
12. Oviedo-Boyso J, et al. *J Infect.* 2007;54:399.
13. de Souza FN, et al. *Am J Immunol.* 2012;8:166.
14. Aitken SL, et al. *J Mammary Gland Biol Neoplasia.* 2011;16:291.
15. Adlerova L, et al. *Vet Med (Praha).* 2008;53:457.
16. Reyher KK, et al. *J Dairy Sci.* 2012;95:6483.
17. Hertl JA, et al. *J Dairy Sci.* 2014;97:6942.
18. Petrovski KR, et al. *Tydskr S Afr Vet Ver.* 2006;77:52.
19. Hagnestam C, et al. *J Dairy Sci.* 2007;90:2260.
20. Schukken YH, et al. *J Dairy Sci.* 2009;92:3091.
21. Hertl JA, et al. *J Dairy Sci.* 2014;97:1465.
22. Bar D, et al. *J Dairy Sci.* 2008;91:2205.
23. Kemp MH, et al. *Vet Rec.* 2008;163:175.
24. Sepúlveda-Varas P, et al. *Appl Anim Behav Sci.* 2014 DOI: 10.1016/j.applanim.2014.09.022.
25. Siivonen J, et al. *Appl Anim Behav Sci.* 2011;132:101.
26. Fogsgaard KK, et al. *J Dairy Sci.* 2015;98:1730.

Diagnosis of Bovine Mastitis

Detection of Clinical Mastitis

The initial diagnosis of clinical mastitis is made during routine physical examination. Laboratory culturing of milk samples for bacteria and *Mycoplasma* spp., and for determining the antimicrobial susceptibility of *S. aureus* (specifically whether it produces β-lactamase), is very useful for instituting optimal treatment protocols for cows with clinical mastitis and for instituting appropriate control measures. However, because subclinical mastitis has the greatest influence on the cost of mastitis to the producer, it is also advantageous to diagnose subclinical mastitis on a cow and quarter level.

Detection of Subclinical Mastitis

Culturing large numbers of milk samples, although the gold standard for diagnosing intramammary infection, is too expensive and impractical for routine use. Much attention has therefore been given to the development of indirect inexpensive tests to predict the presence of an intramammary infection. Currently available indirect tests detect only the presence of inflammation (subclinical mastitis) and not intramammary infection, but are of value as screening tests; milk from quarters or cows with a positive screening test are then submitted to bacteriologic culture. **Subclinical mastitis can only be detected by laboratory examination** and cannot, by definition, be detected during routine physical examination. In other words, the secretion from a quarter with subclinical mastitis appears drinkable.

Detection at the Herd Level

The prevalence of intramammary infection or subclinical mastitis is monitored by determining the **bulk tank milk SCC,** and the most likely mastitis pathogens are identified by **culturing bulk tank milk**. These two methods are recommended for diagnosing the presence and prevalence of mastitis pathogens on a herd basis.

Bulk Tank Milk Somatic Cell Counts

The SCC of bulk tank milk is an indirect measure of the prevalence of mastitis within a dairy herd. The SCC is increased primarily, but not exclusively, because of subclinical mastitis associated with gram-positive bacterial intramammary infections. There is a good correlation between the number of streptococci (*S. agalactiae, S. dysgalactiae,* and *S. uberis*) colony forming units (CFUs) found in bulk tank milk and its SCC. The number of CFUs of *S. aureus* is moderately correlated to the bulk tank milk SCC. As contagious mastitis has become more effectively controlled, environmental mastitis pathogens have become a relatively more important cause of high SCC in bulk tank milk, especially in herds with moderate (<400,000 cells/mL) to low (<150,000 cells/mL) bulk tank milk SCC.

The **SCC of bulk tank milk** has become a widely used test because it provides a sensitive and specific indicator of udder health and milk quality. The sample for analysis is obtained by agitating the milk for 5 to 10 minutes and collecting a sample from the top of the bulk tank milk using a clean dipper. The sample should not be collected near the outlet valve because this varies from that in the rest of the tank. The SCC of bulk tank milk is widely used to regulate whether milk may be legally sold and to determine the price paid for raw milk. Premium and penalty payments are calculated on the basis of a 3-month geometric mean of weekly bulk milk tank SCC measurements. Milk processing plants in most developed countries use automatic electronic somatic cell counters routinely to provide a monthly report of the bulk tank milk SCC. The test requires only that the sample for examination be taken randomly and not frozen, that it be prepared

Table 20-1 Estimated prevalence of infection and losses in milk production associated with bulk tank milk somatic cell count

Bulk tank milk somatic cell count (cells/mL)	Infected quarters in herd (%)	Production loss (%)
200,000	6	0
500,000	16	6
1,000,000	32	18
1,500,000	48	29

with the correct reagent, that the laboratory counter be set at the right calibration, and that the sample be examined quickly or preserved with formalin to prevent cell losses during storage. The bulk tank milk SCC is extremely useful in creating awareness of the existence of a mastitis problem, so that when the SCC of bulk tank milk exceeds permissible limits further investigation of the herd is indicated. In a seasonal herd in which all cows are at the same stage of lactation, the bulk milk cell count will normally be high in early lactation and just before drying off. To overcome these and other factors that are likely to transiently influence bulk tank milk SCC, it is recommended that correction factors be introduced into the estimation or that a rolling SCC, in which monthly data are averaged for the preceding 3 months, be used. Consideration of this figure will avoid too hasty conclusions on one high count caused by an extraneous factor.

It is not possible to use the bulk tank milk SCC to determine the number of cows in a herd affected by mastitis, but it is possible to estimate fairly accurately the number of infected quarters. Generally, as the bulk tank milk SCC increases, the prevalence of infection increases and losses in production increase. Production losses calculated as a percentage of production expected with a count of 200,000 cells/mL are shown in Table 20-1. A bulk tank milk SCC of more than 300,000 cells/mL is considered to indicate a level of mastitis in the herd that warrants examination of individual cows. Herds with a high bulk tank milk SCC have significantly lower production levels and are less likely to use a postmilking teat dip or to have a regular program of milking machine maintenance or automatic cluster removal.

Culture of Bulk Tank Milk

Bacteria present in bulk tank milk may originate from infected udders, from teat and udder surfaces, or from a variety of other environmental sources; however, despite the large number of potential sources for bacteria, culture of bulk tank milk is a useful technique for screening for major mastitis pathogens. The culture of *S. aureus* and *S. agalactiae* from bulk tank milk is a reliable indicator of infection by those pathogens in the herd. The number of those pathogens found on culture is determined by the number of bacteria shed, the number of infected cows, the milk production level of infected cows relative to herd mates, and the severity of infection. A single culture of bulk tank milk has low sensitivity but high specificity for determining the presence of *S. agalactiae* or *S. aureus* in the herd. Thus many infected herds will be called negative, but very few uninfected herds will be called positive. Pathogens such as *Nocardia* spp. and *Mycoplasma* spp. have also been identified by culture of bulk tank milk. Generally, the sensitivity of a single bulk tank milk culture to detect the presence of intramammary infections caused by *S. agalactiae* ranges from 21% to 77%, for *S. aureus* it ranges from 9% to 58%, and for *M. bovis* it is 33%.

Environmental bacteria such as *S. uberis, S. dysgalactiae,* and coliforms may enter milk from intramammary infections, but also from nonspecific contamination. The presence of these organisms in bulk tank milk may relate to the general level of environmental contamination and milking hygiene in the herd. Udder infections with these environmental pathogens are predominantly of short duration and characterized by clinical disease, which makes their inadvertent introduction to the bulk tank less likely.

String sampling or milk line sampling from the positive pressure side of the milking system is the collection of milk samples from a group of cattle instead of the entire herd, as in bulk tank milk sampling. String sampling may have some merit in identifying subgroups of cattle with the highest prevalence of infection. It is thought to be more sensitive in monitoring herds for contagious pathogens than bulk tank milk sampling. If a production group tests positive on a string culture, then individual composite milk cultures can be performed to identify individual animals. Information of the culture results from string sampling should assist development of control programs; however, milk samples left in the pipeline from one string can confound the culture results of subsequent strings.

Numerous bacteriologic techniques have been used to isolate and identify pathogens in bulk tank milk, but none has been established as the gold standard method for the culture of milk from bulk tanks. The most suitable laboratory medium for growth and classification of the pathogens from bulk tank milk needs to be determined. Sampling strategies have included weekly and monthly samples, but it remains to be determined which strategy is optimal relative to herd size and management, disease characteristics, and practicality.

Detection at the Individual Cow Level

Abnormalities of the udder and **gross abnormalities of milk** in cattle with clinical mastitis have been described earlier. In individual cows with clinical mastitis, culture of the secretion from an infected quarter can be done. In animals without clinical mastitis, culture of the secretion represents a direct test for intramammary infection. The objective is to identify cows with contagious mastitis so that they can be treated or culled, or to identify the nature and source of environmental mastitis pathogens. Fulfillment of these requirements requires bacteriologic culture of milk samples so that the pathogens can be named; this is because **identification of mastitis pathogens is central to the development of effective treatment and control programs**. Detection of infected cows requires an individual cow examination and application of an indirect (screening) test for subclinical mastitis, such as the SCC of a composite milk sample, followed by culture of a representative subset of cows to determine the most prevalent pathogen. **Indirect tests estimate the prevalence of infection,** and **microbiological examination identifies the mastitis pathogens;** from this information an appropriate control plan can be formulated.

Culture of Individual Cow Milk

Individual cow milk can be cultured as part of a herd examination for mastitis, or on individual **quarter samples**, or on **composite samples** including milk from all four quarters. A variety of definitions have been used for diagnosing the presence of an intramammary infection in research studies, such as the presence of the same pathogen in duplicate samples collected immediately after each other, or the presence of the same pathogen in two of three consecutive cultures obtained on different sampling dates. These definitions are too expensive and impractical for clinical practice. **Individual quarter samples are preferred** by some at dry off because the costs of treatment dictate that the least possible number of quarters be treated. With this technique only affected quarters are treated at dry off; if the quarter infection rate is low the saving in treatment costs is relatively large if the cost of culturing is low. A full economic comparative analysis of the balance between the cost of diagnosis versus the cost of treatment on a quarter or cow basis does not appear to have been performed. A confounding issue is that within a cow the four quarters are not independent in relationship to intramammary infection or subclinical mastitis; if one quarter is infected then there is an increased probability that one or more of the remaining quarters are infected or have subclinical mastitis.[1] On this basis, when treating subclinical intramammary infection at dry off, it makes more sense to treat the cow (i.e., all four quarters) and not specific quarters within a cow.

A consensus has been reached as to how best to interpret a single milk culture from a quarter (Table 20-2).[2-4] A reasonable

Table 20-2 Sensitivities and specificities for diagnosing an intramammary infection based on the culture of a single milk sample from a quarter using a 10-μL volume

	SENSITIVITY (%)/SPECIFICITY (%)			
Threshold for detection (CFU/10 μL)	**CNS[a]**	***Staphylococcus aureus***	***Streptococcus* spp.[b]**	***Escherichia coli***
≥1	61.2/84.3	90.4/99.8	29.1/94.8	76.5/99.9
≥10	26.0/98.1	72.0/100.0	6.9/99.9	47.1/100.0

[a]*CNS, coagulase-negative staphylococci.*
[b]*Primarily S. uberis.*
Source: Data are categorized by pathogen type and two different detection thresholds. (Reprinted, with permission, from the National Mastitis Council [www.nmconline.org].)

definition of an intramammary infection is ≥1 CFU/10 μL. Culturing duplicate milk samples from the quarter (at the same milking or close together in time) can improve the sensitivity or specificity definition, but not both.

Milk sampling for culture must be performed with due attention to cleanliness because samples contaminated during collection are worthless. The technique of cleaning the teat is of considerable importance. If the teats are dirty, they must be washed and then properly dried or water will run down the teat to the teat end and infect the milk sample. The end of the teat is cleaned with a swab or gauze dipped in 70% alcohol, extruding the external sphincter by pressure to ensure that dirt and wax are removed from the orifice. Brisk rubbing is advisable, especially of teats with inverted ends. The first two or three streams are rejected because their cell and bacterial counts are likely to be a reflection of the disease situation within the teat rather than within the udder as a whole. The next few streams, the premilking sample, are the approved ones because of their greater accuracy. For complete accuracy a premilking and a postmilking sample are taken. Indirect and chemical tests for mastitis can be performed more accurately on foremilk as on later milk, partly because the strippings have a higher fat concentration that alters the water compartment of milk on a volume basis.

If individual quarter samples are collected, screw-cap vials are most satisfactory. During collection the vial is held at an angle to the ground to avoid as much as possible the entrance of dust, skin scales, and hair. If there is delay between the collection of samples and laboratory examinations, the specimens should be refrigerated or frozen. Freezing of milk samples appears to have variable effects on bacterial counts, depending on the bacteria. *T. pyogenes* and *E. coli* counts are decreased by freezing, coagulase-negative *Staphylococcus* spp. counts are increased, and *Streptococcus* and *S. aureus* counts are either unaffected or increased.

The laboratory techniques used vary widely and depend to a large extent on the facilities available. Incubation on blood agar is most satisfactory, because selective media for *S. agalactiae* have the disadvantage that other pathogens may go undetected. Smears of incubated milk are generally unsatisfactory because not all bacteria grow equally well in milk, and the bacterial count has to be high for microscopic detection. Augmented systems of culturing milk samples, which can provide superior results in terms of the number of infected quarters detected depending on the pathogen, include a variety of approaches, such as preculture incubation,[5] centrifugation,[6] freezing of the milk sample at −20 or −196°C (−4 or −321°F),[7,8] and inoculation of the medium with a larger inoculum volume (100 μL) than the standard inoculum volume of milk.[9] The concern with augmented culture methods is that they may amplify contaminants obtained during sampling and therefore decrease the specificity of milk culture. Laboratory culturing techniques can be very time-consuming and expensive unless modern, prepackaged identification systems are used that provide the speed needed to make the examination a worthwhile one.

A milk sample is considered contaminated when three or more species of bacteria are isolated. A quarter is considered to be cured when bacteria, isolated at initial sample, are not present in any samples 14, 21, or 28 days later. An uninfected quarter at the initial sampling time that is infected when resampled at 14, 21, or 28 days indicates a new intramammary infection. A quarter that is infected at initial sampling but infected with another bacteria 14, 21, or 28 days later also indicates a new intramammary infection.

Selective culture media plates, such as biplates (MacConkey agar and blood agar with 1% esculin), triplates (MacConkey agar, blood agar, and TKT agar [thallium, crystal violet, and staphylococcal toxin] in 5% blood agar with 1% esculin), AccuMast, Minnesota Easy Culture System II, Petrifilm, and Veto-Rapid plates can be used to differentiate between gram-positive and gram-negative pathogens and no growth, and they may aid in the rational and targeted use of antimicrobial agents for clinical cases of mastitis.[10–14] A major advance in mastitis pathogen identification is the use of an automated mass spectrometry (MS) system that uses matrix-assisted laser desorption ionization time-of-flight (**MALDI-TOF**) technology. MS of representative bacterial colonies provides species information on bacterial isolates, particularly CNS.

There is interest in developing other cowside tests to determine whether the causative pathogen is gram-negative or gram-positive. One such approach uses dilution of the milk sample, filtration through a membrane with a pore size that retains bacteria, and staining of the bacteria with specific stains. The filtration procedure takes 5 minutes, but the need for microscopic examination decreases the utility of this as a cowside test. A commercially available cowside test for endotoxin (Limast-test), which indicates the presence of gram-negative bacteria, was used in Scandinavia but appears to be no longer available.

A common diagnostic problem is a bacteriologically negative culture in cows with clinical mastitis. Even when milk samples are collected appropriately and bacteriologic culture is done using routine laboratory methods, 15% to 40% of samples from clinical mastitis episodes are bacteriologically negative (yield no growth). Failure of these samples to yield a mastitis pathogen may be the result of spontaneous elimination of infection, a low concentration of pathogens in the milk, intermittent shedding of the pathogen, intracellular location of the pathogens, or the presence of inhibitory substances in the milk. Augmented culture techniques may reduce, but do not eliminate, negative culture results and may facilitate growth of contaminant organisms. Dairy producers and veterinarians therefore face a dilemma when no bacteria or bacteria commonly regarded to be of minor pathogenicity, such as *C. bovis* or coagulase-negative *Staphylococcus* spp., are cultured from the milk of cows with clinical mastitis, particularly if clinical signs persist. Most bacteriologically negative cases of clinical mastitis appear to be caused by low-grade infections with gram-negative bacteria. When no bacterial pathogen can be isolated from cases of clinical mastitis using standard culture techniques, enzyme-linked immunosorbent assays (ELISAs) may be used to detect antigens against *S. aureus, E. coli, S. dysgalactiae,* and *S. agalactiae.* Antigens to these pathogens may be detectable using an ELISA in up to 50% of quarter samples from cows with clinical mastitis in which no pathogens were isolated but in which the SCC was more than 500,000 cells/mL. Despite these promising findings, ELISAs are not widely used in the identification of mastitis pathogens.

A real-time commercially available multiplex polymerase chain reaction (PCR) test (**PathoProof**) was globally launched in 2008 for the diagnosis of mastitis pathogens. The test has potentially valuable advantages of greater sensitivity and faster time to produce a definitive result. The major disadvantages are cost (typically more expensive than routine milk culture), the inability to determine whether bacterial remnants detected by PCR in a milk sample reflect the presence of viable bacteria, and the lack of susceptibility testing results.[15-19] The bacterial remnant versus viability issues is particularly problematic when low amounts of pathogenic DNA have been detected, and a consensus on the economic value of PCR testing has not been reached.[20,21] In 2015, more than 80% of quarter milk samples in Finland were diagnosed using PCR.[16] Currently, PCR tests appear to provide their greatest value in the routine testing of bulk tank milk for pathogen surveillance, for research studies related to clinical mastitis episodes with no bacterial growth on culture, and for investigating mastitis epidemics caused by an unusual pathogen.

Indirect Tests for Subclinical Mastitis

Indirect tests include **SCCs** using automated electronic counters, the **CMT**, increases in **electrical conductivity** of milk, and increases in the activity of cell associated enzymes (such as **NAGase**) in milk. ELISA tests to detect neutrophil components have been developed but are not commercially available. Of these indirect tests, only the CMT and electrical conductivity can be used cowside, with CMT providing a more accurate screening test than electrical conductivity. It is important to understand that these indirect tests detect the presence of inflammation (subclinical mastitis) and not the presence of intramammary infection, although the vast majority of subclinical mastitis episodes are caused by intramammary infection.

The Somatic Cell Count of Composite or Quarter Samples

There is a strong relationship between the SCC of quarter samples of milk and the milk yield, with SCC increasing slightly as milk production decreases but increasing markedly with intramammary infection of the quarter. The distribution of SCC in a herd reflects the distribution of subclinical mastitis and therefore the likely distribution of intramammary infections. The most important factor affecting SCC in an individual cow is the number of quarters infected with a major or minor pathogen. In most herds, the prevalence of infection will increase through a lactation and will also increase with the age of the cow. Cell counts in the first few days of the lactation are often exceptionally high and unreliable as indicators of intramammary infection, and in uninfected cows the counts will drop to a low level within 2 weeks of calving and remain low throughout the lactation unless an intramammary infection occurs. The SCC of a cow that remains free of infection

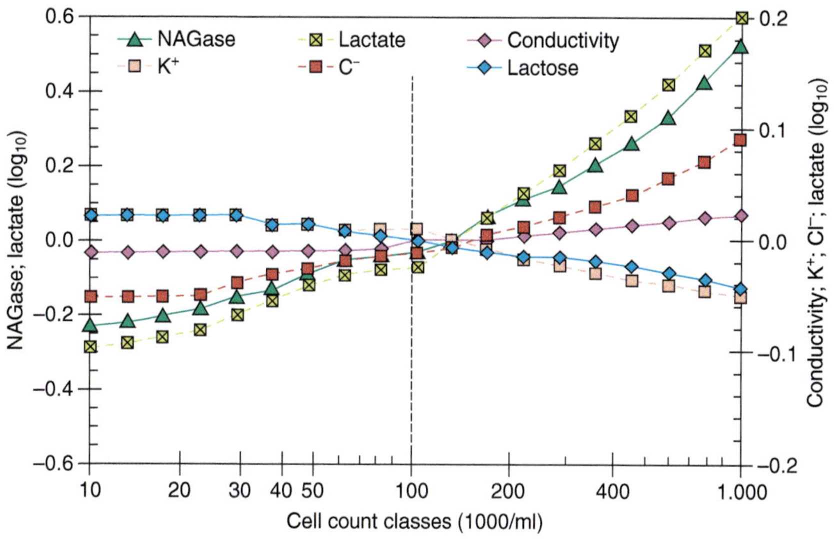

Fig. 20-3 Mean deviation (in log10) of selected milk constituents from the overall means in relation to somatic cell count ($n = 9326$ quarter milk samples). (Reproduced with permission from Hamann J. *XXII World Buiatrics Congress*, Hannover, August 18-23, 2002, 334-345.)

throughout her life will remain very low. However, older cows may have higher counts because the prevalence of infection is higher with age, and older cows are more likely to have had previous infections with residual lesions and leaking of somatic cells into the milk. There are also consistent and significant differences in actual SCC between cows, with individual cows tending to maintain the same class of count throughout their lives. Cows that have consistently low SCC do not seem to be more susceptible to mastitis than others. Attempts to base a breeding program to reduce the prevalence of mastitis on the selection of cows with an innately low composite SCC have been discarded because of fluctuations in numbers within cows.

Healthy quarters have an SCC below 100,000 cells/mL, and **this cut point should be used to indicate the absence or presence of intramammary infection on a gland basis.** This cut point looks very solid for a gland, because many milk components differ from normal values whenever the SCC exceeds 100,000 cells/mL (Fig. 20-3). Moreover, mean SCC counts for bacteriologically negative quarters, quarters infected with minor pathogens, and quarters infected with major pathogens were 68,000, 130,000, and more than 350,000 cells/mL, respectively.

Because of the time and labor saved it is now customary to do automated electronic cell counts on **composite milk samples** that have already been collected for butterfat testing. Regular reports of individual cow SCCs are therefore widely available in herds that routinely test production parameters of their cattle. An exciting new development in mastitis control is the **portable somatic cell counter**, which was designed for on-farm use, providing targeted and immediate SCC information for quarter or composite milk samples. Using the composite sample technique does distort the SCC; for example, the dilution of high-SCC milk from a bad quarter by low-SCC milk from three normal quarters could mean that a cow with one infected quarter might not be detected. Composite SCCs of less than 200,000 cells/mL are considered to be below the limit indicative of inflammation, even though uninfected quarters have an SCC of less than 100,000 cells/mL. Factors that affect the composite milk SCC include the number of quarters infected, the kind of infection (*S. agalactiae* is a more potent stimulator of cellular reaction than *S. aureus*), the strictness with which milk from cows with clinical mastitis is kept out of the bulk tank, the age of the cows (older cows have higher counts), the stage of lactation (counts are highest in the first days after calving and toward the end of lactation), and the herd's average production with the cell count reducing as milk yield increases.

An SCC scoring system that divides the SCC of composite milk into 10 categories from 0 to 9, known as the somatic cell score (**SCS**) (originally called the linear score), is becoming more widely used. The SCS is a base 2 logarithm of the SCC (in cells/mL), in which $SCS = \log_2(SCC/100{,}000) + 3$. Likewise, to calculate SCC (in cells/mL) from the SCS, the following formula is used: $SCC = 100{,}000 \times 2^{(SCS-3)}$. An SCC of 100,000 cells/mL therefore converts to an SCS of 3. Each 1-unit increase (or decrease) in SCS is associated with a doubling (or halving) of the SCC. For example, score 2 is equivalent to an SCC of 50,000 cells/mL, and scores of 4 and 5 correspond to 200,000 and 400,000 cells/mL. Conversion of SCC to SCS values is performed as shown in Tables 20-3 and 20-4. The principal reason for using the SCS is to achieve properties that are required to use conventional statistical methods: mean equal to median, normal distribution, and uniform variance among samples within lactation, among cows within herd or among daughters within sire.

The proportion of neutrophils in the SCC is very low (<11%) in healthy quarters but is markedly increased in quarters with intramammary infection (to >90%). Accordingly, the percentage of neutrophils in the SCC may provide a useful indication of intramammary infection, but it is not currently performed.

SCSs can also be determined for colostrum, in which they are useful in indicating the presence of intramammary infection (Table 20-5).

Table 20-3 Calculating somatic cell score (previously called linear score) from the somatic cell count

Example: SCC = 200,000 cells/mL

a. Divide the SCC by 100,000 cells/mL (200,000/100,000 = 2)
b. Determine the natural log (ln) of the results of step 1 (ln 2 = 0.693)
c. Divide this value by 0.693 (i.e., 0.693/0.693 = 1)
d. Add 3 to the result of step **c** = 1 + 3 = 4 (SCS)

SCC, *somatic cell count;* SCS, *somatic cell score.*

California Mastitis Test of Quarter Samples

The CMT **is the most reliable and inexpensive cowside test for detecting subclinical mastitis.** It is also known as the rapid mastitis test, Schalm test, or the Mastitis-N-K test, which was developed in 1957 and constituted a modification of the Whiteside test. The CMT reagent contains a detergent that reacts with DNA of cell nuclei and a pH indicator (bromocresol purple) that changes color when the milk pH is increased above its normal value of approximately 6.6 (mastitis increases pH to 6.8 or above). The CMT is mixed with quarter milk samples that have been previously collected into a white container, and the sample is gently swirled; the result is read within 15 seconds as a negative, trace, 1, 2, or 3 reaction depending on the amount of gel formation in the sample. Maximum gel formation actually occurs from 1 to 2.5 minutes, depending on the quarter SCC, and continued swirling of the mixture after the time of peak viscosity produces an irreversible decrease in viscosity. Cows in the first week after calving or in the last stages of lactation may give a strong positive reaction.

The close relationships between the CMT reaction and the SCC of milk, and the reduced productivity of affected cows, are shown in Tables 20-4 and 20-5, respectively. If the CMT is used to minimize the false-negative rate (produce the highest sensitivity), then the test should be read as negative (CMT = negative) or positive (CMT = trace, 1, 2, or 3). If the CMT is used to minimize the false-positive rate (produce the highest specificity) for culling decisions, then the test should be read as negative (CMT = negative or trace) or positive (CMT = 1, 2, or 3).

CMT scores can also be determined for colostrum, in which the score is useful in indicating the presence of intramammary infection (see Table 20-5). The equivalent SCC for CMT scores of negative or trace are different for colostrum and milk, but the SCC for CMT scores of 1, 2, and 3 are similar for colostrum and milk.

Table 20-4 Conversion of somatic cell scores (previously called linear scores) to somatic cells counts (cells/mL) and predicted loss of milk

		POUNDS OF MILK LOST PER LACTATION	
SCS	**Somatic cell count midpoint (cells/mL)**	**First lactation**	**Second lactation**
0	12,500	0	0
1	25,000	0	0
2	50,000	0	0
3	100,000	200	400
4	200,000	400	800
5	400,000	600	1,200
6	800,000	800	1,600
7	1,600,000	1,000	2,000
8	3,200,000	1,200	2,400
9	6,400,000	1,400	2,800

SCS, *somatic cell score.*

NAGase Test of Composite or Quarter Samples

The NAGase test is based on the measurement of the activity of a cell-associated enzyme (*N*-acetyl-β-D-glucosaminidase) in

Table 20-5 California mastitis test reactions and equivalent somatic cell counts and somatic cell scores for bovine milk and somatic cell counts for bovine colostrum

Test result	Reaction observed	Equivalent milk SCC	Equivalent SCS	Colostrum geometric mean SCC
Negative	The mixture remains fluid without thickening or gel formation.	0–200,000 cells/mL	0–4	500,000 cells/mL
Trace	A slight slime formation is observed. This reaction is most noticeable when the paddle is rocked from side to side.	150,000–500,000 cells/mL	5	670,000 cells/mL
1+	Distinct slime formation occurs immediately after mixing solutions. This slime may dissipate over time. When the paddle is swirled, fluid does not form a peripheral mass, and the surface of solution does not become convex or "domed up."	400,000–1,500,000 cells/mL	6	890,000 cells/mL
2+	Distinct slime formation occurs immediately after mixing solutions. When the paddle is swirled the fluid forms a peripheral mass, and the bottom of the cup is exposed.	800,000–5,000,000 cells/mL	7–8	3,400,000 cells/mL
3+	Distinct slime formation occurs immediately after mixing solutions. This slime may dissipate over time. When the paddle is swirled the surface of the solution becomes convex or domed up.	>5,000,000 cells/mL	9	6,260,000 cells/mL

SCC, *somatic cell count;* SCS, *somatic cell score.*

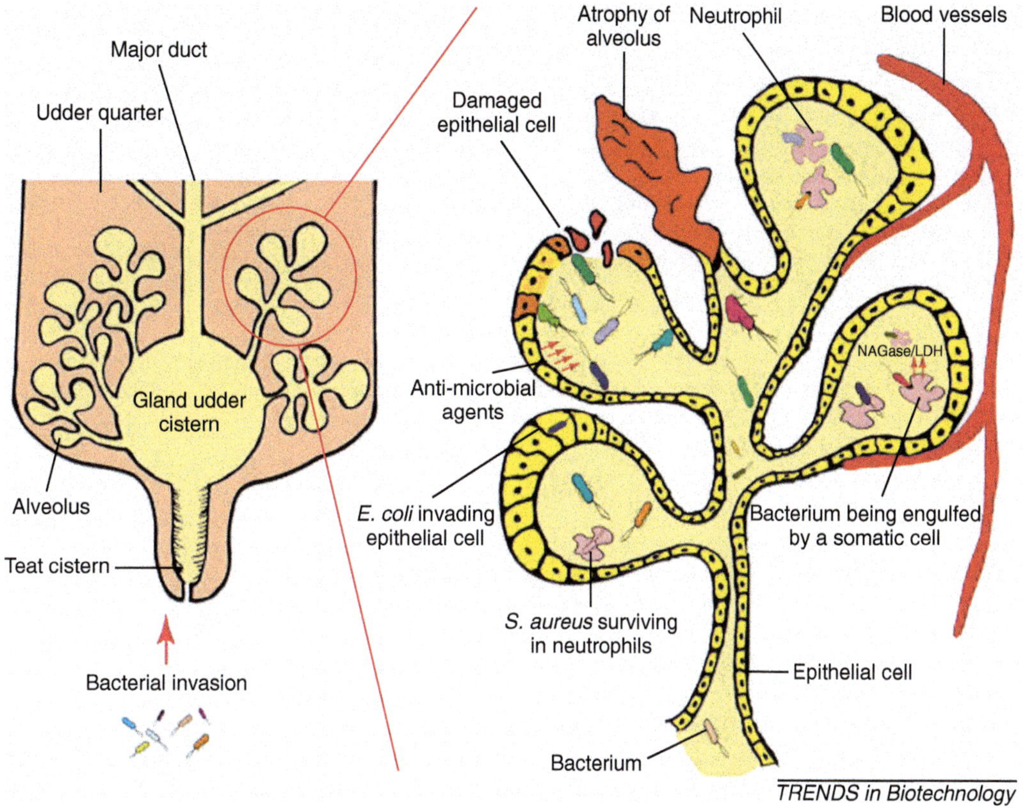

Fig. 20-4 Schematic representation of the development of mastitis in an infected udder. Contagious and environmental pathogens invade the udder via the streak canal and teat cistern. The pathogens then multiply in the udder in which they are attacked by neutrophils. Epithelial cells lining the alveoli are damaged during bacterial multiplication and subsequent immunologic response, with release of enzymes such as NAGase and lactate dehydrogenase (depicted). The tissue response to infection varies based on pathogen, infective dose, immunologic state, and response of the cow, as well as other factors. (Reproduced with permission from Viguier C, Arora S, Gilmartin N, Welbeck K, O Kennedy R (2009) Mastitis detection: current trends and future perspectives. *Trends Biotechnol* 27:486-493.)

the milk, with a high enzyme activity indicating a high cell count (Fig. 20-4). NAGase is an intracellular lysosomal enzyme derived primarily from damaged mammary epithelial cells with a small contribution from neutrophils.[22] The test is suited to the rapid handling of large numbers of samples because of the ease of its automation, and the test can be done on fresh milk and read on the same day. However, because most of the NAGase activity is intracellular, samples should be frozen and thawed before analysis to induce maximal NAGase activity. The NAGase test is reputed to be the most accurate of the indirect tests and as good as SCC in predicting the infected status of a quarter.[23,24] It uses a less sophisticated reading instrument than the average automatic cell counter. If all tests are available it is best to consider the NAGase test and SCC as complementary tests and perform both of them. Milk NAGase levels are high at the beginning and the end of lactation, as with cell counts. The test has also been validated for use with goat milk.

Related tests that have not been studied as extensively as NAGase but show promise in the detection of subclinical mastitis are milk lactate dehydrogenase (LDH) and alkaline phosphatase (ALP) activity.[24–29] Both enzymes are cytoplasmic constituents of cells, and an increase in milk activity of LDH or ALP indicates the presence of cellular injury.

Electrical Conductivity Tests of Quarter Samples

A test that has received a great deal of attention because it can be used in robotic milking systems is based on the increase in concentration of sodium and chloride ions, and the consequent increase in electrical conductivity, in mastitic milk. The electrolyte changes in milk are the first to occur in mastitis, and the test is attractive for this reason. A number of factors affect these characteristics; however, and to derive much benefit from the test it is necessary to examine all quarters and use differences between the quarters to indicate affected quarters. For greater accuracy all quarters need to be monitored each day. An experimental unit that takes all these factors into consideration has been fitted to a milking machine and, by a computer-prepared analysis, monitors variations in electrical conductivity in each quarter every day. Electrical conductivity is attractive as a test because it measures actual injury to the udder rather than the cow's response to the damage like SCC and NAGase activity do. However, a meta-analysis indicated that using an absolute threshold for conductance did not provide a suitable screening test, because both sensitivity and specificity were unacceptably low. In addition, in a study of 173 dairy cows in South Africa, the CMT was more accurate than electrical conductivity for identifying quarters having an intramammary infection or an SCC > 200,000 cells/mL.[30] The use of differential conductivity (within cow quarter comparison) results in improvement in test sensitivity and specificity and is currently the only recommended application of this indirect test.

The most commonly promoted method for measuring electrical conductivity is a handheld device with a built-in cup into which milk is squirted (foremilk is preferred). Experimentally induced clinical mastitis caused by *S. aureus* and *S. uberis* was detectable by changes in electrical conductivity of foremilk: 90% of cases were detectable when clots first appeared and 55% of cases were detectable up to two milkings before the appearance of clots. This suggests that clinical mastitis associated with these two major pathogens may be able to be detected earlier by electrical conductivity than by waiting for milkers to detect visible changes in the milk.

Changes in electrical conductivity reflect changes in secretion Na, K, and Cl concentration, and it is likely that measurement of Na and K ion concentrations in milk will provide a low-cost clinically useful diagnostic test for subclinical mastitis.[30,31]

L-lactate, glucose, lactose, and haptoglobin concentration in quarter samples. L-lactate concentration is markedly increased in the milk of cows with clinical mastitis, and is mildly to moderately increased in cows with subclinical mastitis.[29,31] The magnitude of the increase appears to be correlated with the leukocyte count in milk and the number of CFUs.[32] Glucose concentration is decreased in the milk of cows with clinical mastitis and subclinical mastitis through a yet to be determined mechanism.[31] Milk lactose percentage is decreased in cows with subclinical mastitis because milk is isotonic and inflammation increases the secretion concentration of Na, K, and Cl. Because milk is isotonic and lactose is the predominant osmotic agent in milk, the increase in electrolyte concentrations directly leads to a decrease in lactose concentration, measured on a percentage basis.[22]

The concentration of serum amyloid A and haptoglobin, which are acute phase reactants, increases in the secretion from glands with subclinical mastitis.[28] Skim milk haptoglobin concentration can discriminate between mastitis episodes caused by major or minor pathogens,[27] although this is most likely an indirect association, because major pathogens, by definition, cause greater injury to the mammary gland.

Comparison of Indirect Methods

The effects of subclinical intramammary infection on several parameters in foremilk from individual quarter milk samples have been compared. The SCC, electrical conductivity, pH, NAGase activity, and the concentrations of sodium, potassium, lactose, and α-1-antitrypsin were measured from individual quarters. The SCC, NAGase activity, electrical conductivity, and concentrations of sodium, α-1-antitrypsin, and lactose were all useful indirect indicators of infection. The SCC was able to discriminate between infected and uninfected quarters in cows better than electrical conductivity, pH, and NAGase activity.

Hematology and Serum Biochemistry

In severe clinical mastitis there may be marked changes in the leukocyte count, packed cell volume, and serum creatinine and urea nitrogen concentration because of the effects of severe infection and toxemia. In particular, clinical mastitis episodes associated with gram-negative bacteria frequently cause a profound leukopenia, neutropenia, lymphopenia, and monocytopenia as a result of the endotoxemia, as well as an increased packed cell volume. In contrast, the leukogram in cattle with clinical mastitis associated with gram-positive bacteria is normal or mildly increased.

Ultrasonography of the Mammary Gland

Two-dimensional (2D) ultrasonographic images of the gland cistern, parenchymal tissue, and teat are easily obtained using a 5-, 7.5-, or 8.5-MHz linear array transducer, and ultrasonography is becoming more widely used to guide treatment of teat and gland cistern abnormalities. However, there are few reports of the use of ultrasonography to diagnose or prognose clinical mastitis episodes, although this is likely to be a fruitful area for investigation.

The best 2D images of the udder parenchyma are obtained by clipping the hair on the udder and applying a coupling gel. This minimizes the air between the transducer face and skin. Imaging the normal adjacent quarter is very helpful in identifying abnormalities. Imaging should be performed in two planes, sagittal to the teat (and therefore perpendicular to the ground), and transverse to the teat (and therefore horizontal to the ground). The injection of sterile 0.9% NaCl through a teat cannula into the gland provides a practical contrast agent that can help further define the extent of any abnormalities. The superficial supermammary lymph nodes can be seen on ultrasound using a 7.5-MHz linear transducer, and the lymph node is well demarcated from the surrounding tissues. Mean lymph node length was 7.4 cm (range 3.5–15.0 cm) and mean depth was 2.5 cm (range 1.2–5.7 cm). Lymph node size increased with age and is predictive of the presence of subclinical intramammary infection in cattle.[33] Similarly, superficial inguinal lymph node size is predictive of SCC in sheep.[34]

Mastitis produces an increased heterogeneous echogenicity to the milk in the gland cistern, compared with an uninfected quarter.[35] It is important to make this visual comparison without altering the contrast and brightness setting on the ultrasonographic unit.

Infrared Thermography of the Mammary Gland

Infrared thermography shows promise for the real-time noninvasive diagnosis of mastitis in dairy cattle. This will be particularly valuable in cattle that are robotically milked, in which the diagnosis of clinical mastitis remains problematic.

Methodology for infrared thermography has been developed for the mammary gland.[36] Thermograms should be obtained with the animal in an environment to which it has been adapted for 30 minutes and out of direct sunlight and wind. The udder should be free from moisture, dirt, and foreign material; this is usually accomplished by brushing the hair on the udder or washing and drying the udder. Thermography is effective for the early diagnosis of clinical mastitis.[37-39] There have been mixed reports regarding the accuracy of thermography to detect subclinical mastitis in dairy cattle[40,41] using mean quarter temperature and maximum quarter temperature.[36,39]

Biopsy of Mammary Tissue

A biopsy of mammary tissue can be used for histologic and biochemical evaluation in research studies. The use of a rotating stainless steel cannula with a retractable blade at the cutting edge has been described for obtaining biopsy material from cows. Despite some postoperative bleeding, milk yield and composition in the biopsied gland were affected only transiently.

NECROPSY FINDINGS

Necropsy findings are not of major interest in the diagnosis of mastitis and are omitted here but included in the description of specific infections.

DIFFERENTIAL DIAGNOSIS

The diagnosis of clinical mastitis is not difficult if a careful clinical examination of the udder is performed as part of the complete examination of a cow with systemic clinical findings. Examination of the udder is sometimes omitted in a recumbent animal only for severe mastitis to be discovered later. The diagnosis of mastitis depends largely on the detection of clinical abnormalities of the udder and gross abnormalities of the milk or the use of an indirect test like the California mastitis test to detect subclinical mastitis.

Other mammary abnormalities that must be differentiated from clinical mastitis include **udder edema**, **rupture of the suspensory ligament**, and **hematoma**. These are not accompanied by abnormalities of the milk unless there is hemorrhage into the udder. The presence of stray voltage in the milking plant should not be overlooked in herds in which the sudden lowering of production arouses an unfounded suspicion of mastitis. Differentiation of the different causes of mastitis is difficult on the basis of clinical findings alone but must be attempted, especially in peracute cases in which specific treatment must be given before results of laboratory examinations are available. A pretreatment sample of milk from the affected glands for culture and antimicrobial sensitivity may provide useful information about the health record of the cow and the need to consider alternative therapies, and could provide information on new infections in the herd.

FURTHER READING

Brandt M, Haeussermann A, Hartung E. Technical solutions for analysis of milk constituents and abnormal milk. *J Dairy Sci.* 2010;93:427-436.

Franz S, Floek M, Hofmann-Parisot M. Ultrasonography of the bovine udder and teat. *Vet Clin North Am Food Anin Pract.* 2009;25:669-685.
Gurjar A, Gioia G, Schukken Y, et al. Molecular diagnostics applied to mastitis problems on dairy farms. *Vet Clin North Am Food Anim Pract.* 2012;28:565-576.
Lam TJGM, Riekerink O, Sampomon OC, Smith H. Mastitis diagnostics and performance monitoring: a practical approach. *Ir Vet J.* 2009;62(suppl 4):S34-S39.
Pyörälä S. Indicators of inflammation in the diagnosis of mastitis. *Vet Res.* 2003;34:565-578.
Viguier C, Arora S, Gilmartin N, et al. Mastitis detection: current trends and future perspectives. *Trends Biotechnol.* 2009;27:486-493.

REFERENCES

1. Berry DP, Meaney WJ. *Prev Vet Med.* 2006;75:81.
2. Dohoo IR, et al. *J Dairy Sci.* 2011a;94:250.
3. Dohoo IR, et al. *J Dairy Sci.* 2011b;94:5515.
4. Reyher KK, Dohoo IR. *J Dairy Sci.* 2011;94:3387.
5. Artursson K, et al. *J Dairy Sci.* 2010;93:1534.
6. Punyapornwithaya V, et al. *J Dairy Sci.* 2009;92:4444.
7. Petzer IM, et al. *Onderstepoort J Vet Res.* 2012;79:343.
8. Pehlivanoglu F, et al. *Vetrinarski Arhiv.* 2015;85:59.
9. Walker JB, et al. *J Vet Diagn Invest.* 2010;22:720.
10. Royster E, et al. *J Dairy Sci.* 2014;97:3648.
11. McCarron JL, et al. *J Dairy Sci.* 2009;92:5326.
12. Cameron M, et al. *Prev Vet Med.* 2013;111:1.
13. de Vries EMM, et al. *Prev Vet Med.* 2014;113:620.
14. Viora L, et al. *Vet Rec.* 2014;10.1136/vr.102499.
15. Keane OM, et al. *Vet Rec.* 2013;173:268.
16. Hiitiö H, et al. *J Dairy Res.* 2015;82:200.
17. Koskinen MT, et al. *J Dairy Sci.* 2010;93:5707.
18. Taponen S, et al. *J Dairy Sci.* 2009;92:2610.
19. Cantekin Z, et al. *Kafkas Univ Vet Fak Derg.* 2015;21:277.
20. Murai K, et al. *Prev Vet Med.* 2014;113:522.
21. Mahmmod YS, et al. *Prev Vet Med.* 2013;112:309.
22. Zhao X, Lacasse P. *J Anim Sci.* 2008;86(suppl 1):57.
23. Nielsen NI, et al. *J Dairy Sci.* 2005;88:3186.
24. Mizeck GG, et al. *J Dairy Res.* 2006;73:431.
25. Babaei H, et al. *Vet Res Commun.* 2007;31:419.
26. Kalantari A, et al. *Ann Biol Res.* 2013;4:302.
27. Hiss S, et al. *Vet Med (Praha).* 2007;52:245.
28. Åkerstedt M, et al. *J Dairy Res.* 2011;78:88.
29. Lehmann M, et al. *J Dairy Res.* 2015;82:129.
30. Fosgate GT, et al. *Vet J.* 2013;196:98.
31. Silanikove N, et al. *J Dairy Res.* 2014;81:358.
32. Lindmark-Månsson H, et al. *Int Dairy J.* 2006;16:717.
33. Khoramian B, et al. *Iran J Vet Res.* 2015;16:75.
34. Hussein HA, et al. *Small Rumin Res.* 2015;129:121.
35. Santos VJC, et al. *Reprod Domest Anim.* 2015;50:251.
36. Metzner M, et al. *Vet J.* 2014;199:57.
37. Hovinen M, et al. *J Dairy Sci.* 2008;91:4592.
38. Pezeshki A, et al. *Vet Res.* 2011;42:15.
39. Metzner M, et al. *Vet J.* 2015;204:360.
40. Polat B, et al. *J Dairy Sci.* 2010;93:3525.
41. Colak A, et al. *J Dairy Sci.* 2008;91:4244.

TREATMENT OF BOVINE MASTITIS

The treatment of the different causes of clinical and subclinical mastitis may require specific protocols, which are described under specific mastitis pathogens later in the chapter. The general principles of mastitis treatment are outlined here.

Historical Aspects of Antimicrobial Therapy for Clinical and Subclinical Mastitis

Between about 1950 and 1990, on a worldwide basis, all forms of both clinical and subclinical bovine mastitis were treated with a wide variety of antimicrobial agents either by intramammary infusions or parenterally and commonly by both routes in acute and peracute cases. Most veterinarians treated clinical mastitis and evaluated the response on the basis of clinical outcome. Generally, it was thought that antimicrobial agents were effective for the treatment of clinical and subclinical mastitis in lactating cows. However, there are very few scientific publications based on randomized clinical trials in which the efficacy of intramammary antimicrobial agents for treatment of clinical mastitis was compared with untreated controls. If antimicrobial agents were used and the animal recovered, it was assumed that treatment was efficacious. If the cow did not respond favorably, several reasons were usually enumerated for the treatment failure. However, most of these reasons, although biologically attractive, are hypothetical and have not been substantiated scientifically. Gradually, over the years, veterinarians began to doubt the efficacy of antimicrobial agents for the treatment of all cases of clinical mastitis. In addition, and of major importance, milk from treated cows had to be discarded for up to several days after the last day of treatment because of antimicrobial residues; this was a major expense. Currently, optimized treatment strategies focus on efficacy, economics, animal welfare aspects, and the milk withhold time of antimicrobial treatment.

Efficacy is assessed on the basis of **clinical cure** or **bacteriologic cure**. Most producers are interested in the return to normal milk (clinical cure) and are much less interested in the return to a sterile quarter (bacteriologic cure). Because clinical mastitis is defined as abnormal milk, the return to normal (drinkable) milk represents a clinical cure. Bacteriologic cure represents the inability to isolate the initial pathogen 14 to 28 days after the start of treatment. Other important indicators of efficacy are milk production, dry matter intake, the amount of saleable milk, and mortality or culling rates after treatment.

Some examples of the efficacy or inefficacy of antimicrobial agents illustrate the controversy. It is well accepted that the cure rate following intramammary treatment of clinical or subclinical mastitis caused by *S. agalactiae* in the lactating cow is high (80%–90%). In contrast, the cure rate of clinical and subclinical mastitis caused by *S. aureus* in the lactating cow is considerably lower (40%–50%), but certainly not 0%. In herds with a low prevalence of contagious mastitis, most cases of mild clinical mastitis (abnormal secretion only) in lactating cows are caused by environmental streptococci and coliforms and may recover without antimicrobial therapy, although antimicrobial administration increases the clinical and bacteriologic cure rate. Antimicrobial agents may be ineffective for the treatment of clinical mastitis associated with *M. bovis, T. pyogenes, Nocardia* spp., and *P. aeruginosa.*

In the 1970s dairy processing plants, veterinarians, consumer advocates, public health authorities, and milk-quality regulating agencies began to express concern about antimicrobial residues in milk from cows treated for mastitis. The public health and milk industry concerns about residues combined with the controversy about the efficacy of antimicrobial agents for clinical mastitis has also provided a stimulus to evaluate the efficacy and consequences of using antimicrobial agents. Since the early 1990s, much emphasis has been placed on alternative methods of treating clinical mastitis, leading to a reduction in the use of antimicrobial agents during the lactating period. Such strategies have been defended based on a lack of information concerning the efficacy and economics of antimicrobial therapy associated with pathogens other than *S. agalactiae,* and by the need to reduce the risk of residue violation. However, a recent study concluded that not administering antibiotics to cows with clinical mastitis was imprudent and unethical.

There is a need for additional randomized controlled field trials to evaluate the use of antimicrobial agents for the treatment of clinical mastitis. Well-conducted clinical mastitis treatment trials represent an invaluable, although difficult and expensive, effort to evaluate efficacy of antimicrobial agents under field conditions. In should be noted that the use of antimicrobial agents for the treatment of **subclinical mastitis** at the end of lactation, known as **dry cow therapy**, is accepted worldwide and is based on scientific evidence using randomized clinical trials. Dry cow therapy is one of the principles applied in the effective control of bovine mastitis, in which much progress has been made since the early 1970s.

Treatment Strategy

The treatment strategy will depend on whether the mastitis is **clinical** or **subclinical** and the health status of the herd, including its mastitis history. Clinical mastitis is further categorized as **abnormal secretion**, **abnormal gland,** or **abnormal cow**, as described previously. If treatment is indicated, the major decision is whether to administer antimicrobial agents parenterally or by intramammary infusion.

An important aspect of treatment is the accurate positive identification of the animal(s) to be treated, the recording of the relevant clinical and laboratory information, the treatments being used, and monitoring the response. Useful information would include:

- Cow identification
- Quarters affected
- Date of mastitis event
- Lactation number
- Date of calving
- Identification of pathogen(s)
- Treatment used, including dose, route, and duration
- Milk withholding time and time when returned to the milking string
- Most recent level of milk production

Options for treating cows with clinical mastitis include treating all cows with antimicrobial agents, treating none of the cows with antimicrobial agents, or treating only specific cows with antimicrobial agents. Treating all cows results in increased costs for those cows with clinical mastitis associated with pathogens not susceptible to the antimicrobial agent used, especially if the signs are likely to resolve before the milk withholding period has expired. Treatment of all cows is also associated with increased risk of violative residues in the bulk milk. Treating none of the cows with antimicrobial agents has animal welfare implications, because an effective treatment is not administered to some cattle with clinical mastitis, and nontreatment allows gram-positive pathogens to persist, increasing the probability of a recurrence of clinical mastitis or causing a herd epidemic of mastitis. Accordingly, **nontreatment of all cases of mastitis is not a viable option**. Treating only specific cows with antimicrobial agents requires an accurate method of determining which animals should be treated. However, clinical judgment and predictive models are too inaccurate to distinguish between clinical mastitis associated with gram-negative and gram-positive pathogens. To select cows for antimicrobial therapy on the basis of bacteriologic culture is costly and delays treatment; clinical judgment would still be necessary because bacteria are not isolated from 15% to 40% of milk samples from cows with clinical mastitis.

Veterinarians should always ask and answer four questions related to antimicrobial therapy in bovine mastitis:

1. Is antimicrobial therapy indicated?
2. Which route of administration (intramammary, parenteral, or both) should be used?
3. Which antimicrobial agent should be administered?
4. What should be the frequency and duration of treatment?

Is Antimicrobial Therapy Indicated?

The first decision is **whether to treat** a particular case with antimicrobial agents and whether supportive therapy is required. Therapy decisions should be made in context with the overall objectives of the lactating cow treatment protocol. The availability of approved, effective treatment products is an essential component of the program. A number of factors are important in determining which cases of mastitis should be treated during lactation. These factors include the type of pathogen involved, the type and severity of the inflammatory response, the duration of infection, the stage of lactation, and the age and pregnancy status of the cow.

Type of Pathogen Involved

There are marked differences in the bacteriologic cure rates of the various major mastitis pathogens after therapy during lactation. The outcome of treatment during lactation is poor for cases of *S. aureus* mastitis. On the other hand, *S. agalactiae* responds extremely well to lactating cow therapy, and all infected cows should be treated. Cases of mastitis associated with environmental organisms have reasonable, but variable, cure rates.

Type and Severity of the Inflammatory Response

The predominant type of inflammatory process involved influences the objectives of the therapy program. Herds with clinical mastitis problems will aim at reducing clinical signs, returning the milk to saleable quality and avoiding residue violations. Herds with a predominance of subclinical mastitis are concerned with avoiding the spread of infection and reducing the prevalence of the major pathogens involved. Both types of herd have the primary objective of restoring the production potential.

The severity of the inflammatory response is also important in the selection of cases for mastitis therapy during lactation. Heat, pain and swelling of the quarter (abnormal gland) are clinical signs that indicate the need for antimicrobial therapy. Many producers, however, will treat any cow that shows clots in the milk (abnormal milk). There are no reports to verify that treatment of cows exhibiting abnormal milk only is efficacious and economically justifiable, although it is probable that treatment of clinical mastitis episodes of abnormal milk but normal gland caused by *S. agalactiae* is efficacious and economic. Treatment success is lower in cows with high NAGase concentrations in milk compared with cows with low NAGase concentrations.

Duration of Infection

For the contagious organisms, especially *S. aureus*, the duration of infection is an important determinant of its susceptibility to therapy during lactation. In chronic *S. aureus* mastitis, the organism survives intracellularly in leukocytes, becomes walled off in small abscesses of mammary ducts, and has the ability to exist in the L-form state. At this point *S. aureus* is virtually incurable during lactation. With new methods of automated detection of subclinical intramammary infection such as in-line electrical conductivity measurement, new infections may be detected much earlier. The cure rate of *S. aureus* during lactation needs to be reevaluated when treatment is administered early in the course of infection.

Stage of Lactation

The stage of lactation is an important determinant of the benefit : cost ratio of mastitis therapy during lactation. It may be uneconomical to treat even cases with a high probability of cure during late lactation.

Age and Pregnancy Status of Cow

The probability of a cure is greater in young cows, and age should be considered in selecting cases for mastitis therapy during lactation.[1] The economic aspects of treatment for late-lactation, nonpregnant cows are obviously different from those for midlactation pregnant cows.

A mastitis therapy program for lactating cows should be based on a complete understanding of the mastitis status of the herd, and individual cow treatment decisions should be consistent with the overall herd mastitis therapy program.[2] A record system for treatment should be established so that it is possible to monitor the efficacy of the mastitis treatment program.

The udder health status in a particular herd will determine whether the lactating cow mastitis therapy strategy should be targeted at the individual cow level or at the herd level. The level of emphasis should clearly reflect the objectives of the therapy program. For example, a herd with low bulk tank milk SCC and sporadic cases of environmental mastitis should target the lactating cow therapy strategy at the cow level. The primary objectives would be to alleviate clinical signs, to achieve a bacteriologic cure, and to restore the cow's production. On the other hand, a herd with moderate to high bulk tank milk SCCs and a significant prevalence of contagious organisms should aim the program at the herd level. In this case the objective would be to limit the spread of infection, markedly reduce or eradicate a specific pathogen, and increase herd production. A clear statement of treatment philosophy (individual cow level or herd level) in a particular herd is needed to direct establishment of well-defined treatment protocols for mastitis in lactating cows.

Intramammary infection (mastitis) is identified by the presence of clinical signs or the results of a direct test (culture of milk) or indirect tests such as SCC, CMT, or electrical conductivity. The detection of clinical or subclinical mastitis does not necessarily indicate that therapy should be administered, although animal welfare issues dictate that treatment must be administered to cattle with an abnormal gland or systemic signs (abnormal cow) because these animals are undergoing pain and discomfort. A decision to use treatment during lactation should be based on the likelihood of achieving the objectives of the therapy program. Several factors are important in the selection of cows for treatment. These factors can significantly influence the cure rate achieved with therapy or the economic benefit realized.

The herd history of udder health will indicate the probable cause of clinical mastitis. Cows with mild cases of clinical mastitis (abnormal secretion only) in herds with a low prevalence of contagious mastitis pathogens are likely to be affected with environmental pathogens and commonly return to clinically normal milk in four to six milkings. This has led to the development of treatment algorithms based on the results of culturing clinical cases using selective media. Using this approach, milk cultures are obtained from all cattle with clinical mastitis and plated using biplates or triplates. All cattle with abnormal glands or signs of systemic illness (abnormal cow) are immediately treated with antimicrobial agents and appropriate ancillary treatment, with subsequent antimicrobial treatment based on the preliminary culture results at 18 to 24 hours or the final culture results at 48 hours. In contrast, treatment is initially withheld from all cattle demonstrating abnormal secretion only; antimicrobial treatment is instituted based on the culture results. One such scheme recommends using intramammary antibiotics to treat affected quarters with *S. aureus*, CNS, and environmental streptococci, infusing intramammary antibiotics into all quarters of cows with one or more quarters infected with *S. agalactiae* and not administering antibiotics to cows with coliform bacteria or no growth. When using this delayed approach to antimicrobial treatment, it is important that cattle with abnormal milk only are closely monitored, and that antimicrobial treatment is immediately instituted when signs of an abnormal gland or abnormal cow are present. The major difficulty with implementing the delayed approach is the difficulty in transporting the milk sample to and receiving the results from the diagnostic laboratory in a time-effective manner. For practical reasons, this approach works only if on-farm culturing is performed.

An 8-herd study involving 422 cows with clinical mastitis in the Great Lakes region of North America was conducted to investigate the effectiveness and safety of selective treatment of clinical mastitis using on-farm culture results. The secretion from affected quarters was cultured for 18 to 24 hours using a biplate. Quarters with a gram-positive or mixed growth were treated with intramammary cephapirin sodium. Quarters with a gram-negative or no growth were not treated. Unfortunately, the study design enrolled cattle with clinical mastitis and abnormal secretion (72% of total), or abnormal secretion and abnormal gland (28% of total); as discussed previously the latter group should not have an effective treatment withheld for 24 hours, because an abnormal gland is associated with pain and discomfort. Use of selective antibiotic treatment based on 24-hour culture results reduced intramammary antibiotic use by half without impacting days to clinical cure, bacteriologic cure risk, and treatment failure risk within 21 days.[3] Selective treatment also had no impact on long-term outcomes, such as recurrence of clinical mastitis in the same quarter, increased SCS, decreased milk production, or cow survival for the remainder of the lactation.[4] This study supports the selective treatment of clinical mastitis episodes using intramammary cephapirin and an on-farm culture system for those mastitis episodes that have abnormal secretion.

A decision tree analysis of treatment strategies, including selective treatment of clinical mastitis using on-farm culture results, indicated that the optimal economic strategy was to treat clinical mastitis episodes caused by gram-positive organisms for 2 days (compared with a 5-day or 8-day treatment protocol) and to not treat mild clinical mastitis episodes caused by gram-negative organisms or associated with no bacterial growth.[1] This economic analysis needs to be updated based on recent studies with naturally occurring mastitis documenting improved efficacy with extended treatment durations.[5,6]

Table 20-6 Summary of three-compartment model for anatomic location of infection caused by mastitis pathogens in cattle

	PHARMACOLOGIC COMPARTMENT		
Mastitis pathogen	**Milk and ducts (abnormal secretion)**	**Parenchyma (abnormal gland)**	**Systemic (abnormal cow)**
Contagious pathogens			
Staphylococcus aureus	+	++	–
Streptococcus agalactiae	++	+	–
Mycoplasma bovis	+	+	++
Corynebacterium bovis	++	–	–
Teat skin opportunistic pathogens			
Coagulase-negative staphylococci	++	–	–
Environmental pathogens			
Escherichia coli	+	–	++
Klebsiella pneumoniae	+	–	++
Environmental streptococci	++	+	–
Trueperella pyogenes	+	++	–
Antimicrobial therapy			
Intramammary	Good to excellent	Moderate	Poor
Parenteral	Poor to moderate	Moderate to excellent	Good to excellent

Antimicrobial therapy is categorized on the basis of route of administration and likely efficacy when treating a susceptible infection.
++, extensive infection; +, moderate infection; –, minimal or no infection
Source: Adapted from Erskine RJ et al. Vet Clin North Am Food Anim Pract 2003;19:109.

Which Route of Administration (Intramammary, Parenteral, or Both?)

The second decision is the route of administration. The goal of antimicrobial treatment is to attain and maintain an effective concentration at the site of infection. Three pharmacologic compartments are recognized for infection by mastitis pathogens:

- Milk and epithelial lining of the ducts and alveoli
- Parenchyma of the mammary gland
- The cow (Table 20-6)

Generally, infections confined primarily to the milk and ducts (such as *C. bovis* and CNS) are easily treated with intramammary antibiotics. In contrast, infections caused by mastitis pathogens with the potential for systemic infection (such as *E. coli, K. pneumoniae,* and *M. bovis*) are best treated with parenteral antibiotics. Mastitis pathogens that are the most difficult to treat are those that are principally infections of parenchymal tissue (such as *S. aureus* and *T. pyogenes*); this is because it is more difficult to attain and maintain an effective antibiotic concentration at this anatomic site when administering antibiotics by the intramammary or parenteral routes.

Which Antimicrobial Agent Should Be Administered?

The third decision is the antimicrobial agent. The selection of the antimicrobial class for the particular mastitis pathogen has traditionally been based on culture and susceptibility testing and, although some in vivo data are now available, the choice is still largely dependent on case studies rather than on controlled experiments. Culture and antimicrobial susceptibility testing of the pathogen is not necessarily a justifiable basis for selecting the antimicrobial agent to be used in individual cows, and the response to treatment of clinical mastitis in two recent studies was unrelated to the results of in vitro susceptibility tests.

Antimicrobial agents are usually selected based on availability of labeled drugs, clinical signs in the cow, milk culture results for previous mastitis episodes in the herd, experience of treatment outcome in the herd, treatment cost and withdrawal times for milk, and slaughter. Many veterinarians and researchers have also recommended the routine use of susceptibility testing to guide treatment decisions. Susceptibility testing for guiding treatment of clinical mastitis should not be a routine recommendation for a number of reasons. First, the cost of susceptibility testing and a minimum 2-day delay in obtaining the results makes susceptibility testing irrelevant to the initial treatment protocol. Second, the medical profession does not routinely apply susceptibility testing to the initial treatment of a non–life-threatening illness; it is therefore difficult to understand why treatment of bovine mastitis should be held to a higher standard. Third, and most importantly, the validity of agar diffusion susceptibility breakpoints derived from humans in the treatment of bovine mastitis has not been established and is extremely questionable because bovine mastitic milk pH, electrolyte, fat, protein, and neutrophil concentrations; growth factor composition; and pharmacokinetic profiles differ markedly from those of human plasma. Moreover, antibiotics are distributed unevenly in an inflamed gland, and high antibiotic concentrations can alter neutrophil function in vitro, having the potential to inhibit bacterial clearance in vivo.

Adequate databases of in vitro minimum inhibitory concentration (MIC) values for clinical mastitis pathogens are currently unavailable, although adequate databases are available for subclinical mastitis isolates. Although we have a good knowledge of the pharmacokinetics of many parenteral antibiotics used to treat clinical mastitis, most pharmacokinetic data have been obtained in healthy cattle, and it has become increasingly clear that the pharmacokinetic values in healthy cows are different to those in cows with clinical mastitis. In addition, pharmacokinetic values for many of the intramammary antibiotics used to treat clinical mastitis are unknown, and there is a limited understanding of the pharmacodynamics of antibiotics in treating mastitis. More importantly, the breakpoints currently recommended for all parenterally and almost all intramammarily administered antibiotics used to evaluate susceptibility or resistance[7-10] are based on achievable serum and interstitial fluid concentrations in humans after oral or intravenous antibiotic administration. The relevance of these breakpoints to achievable milk concentrations in lactating dairy cows after intramammary, subcutaneous, intramuscular, or intravenous administration is dubious at best.

Results from field studies are available to evaluate the validity of susceptibility breakpoints in guiding treatment of cows with clinical or subclinical mastitis. The results from these field studies suggest that the following antibiotics may have valid (but not necessarily optimal) breakpoints for treating clinical or subclinical mastitis associated with specific bacteria: parenteral penicillin G for subclinical *S. aureus* infections, intramammary cephapirin for clinical *Streptococcus* spp. infections, and parenteral trimethoprim-sulfadiazine for clinical *E. coli* infections. Of these three antibiotics, the breakpoints for penicillin G and cephapirin have only been validated for bacteriologic cure, whereas the breakpoint for trimethoprim-sulfadiazine is validated for clinical cure. Because duration of infection before treatment, antibiotic dosage, dosage interval, and duration of treatment influence treatment outcome, many more field studies must be completed to validate the currently assigned antibiotic breakpoints for pathogens causing clinical mastitis.

To properly use the known pharmacokinetics of parenterally and intramammarily administered drugs, it is necessary to know something about their diffusion into mammary tissue, the degree of binding of a drug to mammary tissues and secretions, the ability to pass through the lipid phase of milk, and the degree of ionization. All of these factors influence the level of the antibiotic in the mammary gland.[11] Major challenges with modeling the milk concentration–time relationship exist for antibiotics administered parenterally or by the intramammary route. As a consequence, a new pharmacokinetic modeling approach for the treatment of mastitis has been developed.[12] Much of the published pharmacokinetic data are based on foremilk concentration, which is not representative of the antibiotic concentration in quarter milk[13,14] and has been conducted in healthy cows without clinical mastitis. The latter issue is of great importance because clinically important differences in pharmacokinetic values have been identified for ruminants with and without experimentally induced mastitis.[15] For lactating cows the preferred treatment is one that maintains an MIC for 72 hours without the need for multiple infusions and without prolongation of the withdrawal time. The most successful antimicrobial agents for dry period treatment are those that persist longest in the udder, preferably as long as 8 weeks. These characteristics depend on the release time from the transport agent in the formulation and the particle size and diffusion capabilities of the antibiotic.

The formulation of the preparation will affect the duration of the maintenance of the MIC. The third-generation cephalosporins (such as ceftiofur) and fluoroquinolones are the drugs of choice for use in cases in which the infection may be associated with either a gram-positive or gram-negative organism; however, these antimicrobial agents may not be able to be used to treat mastitis in some countries. Mixtures of penicillin and an aminoglycoside are also in common use for this purpose. Penicillin G and penethamate are favored for gram-positive infections. Of special importance are the β-lactamase–producing strains of *S. aureus,* against which β-lactam penicillins are ineffective; cloxacillin is a commonly used and effective intramammary formulation for these strains of *S. aureus.* The drugs that have the best record of diffusion through the udder after intramammary infusion are penethamate, ampicillin, amoxicillin, erythromycin, and tylosin. Those of medium performance are penicillin G, cloxacillin, and tetracyclines. Poor diffusers, which have a longer half-life in the udder because they bind to protein, include streptomycin and neomycin. Streptomycin is not used much now because of the high level of resistance to it, especially by *S. uberis* and *E. faecalis.*

In summary, treatment of clinical mastitis should be based on bacteriologic diagnosis or assessment of the likely causative agent and take current guidelines on the prudent use of antimicrobials into account. The initial treatment of clinical mastitis episodes should be based on herd data and personal experience for the geographic region[16] or the results of on-farm culture for clinical mastitis episodes with only abnormal secretion.[3,4] The treatment of subclinical mastitis during lactation is rarely economical.

What Should Be the Frequency and Duration of Treatment?

The fourth decision is the **frequency and duration of treatment**. The frequency of administration for parenterally administered antimicrobial agents is dependent primarily on their pharmacokinetics and pharmacodynamics. Fluoroquinolones and aminoglycosides are **concentration-dependent** antimicrobial agents in which increasing concentrations at the site of infection increase the bacterial kill rate. Macrolides, β-lactams, and lincosamides are **time-dependent** antimicrobial agents in which exceeding the MIC at the site of infection for a prolonged percentage of the interdosing interval correlates with improved efficacy. In contrast, the frequency of administration for intramammary formulations is dependent primarily on the milking schedule, because these agents are primarily cleared by milk removal. For example, the clearance of pirlimycin is strongly and positively correlated ($r = 0.97$) to 24-hour milk production at the time of dosing. With all intramammary formulations being licensed based on the results of studies of twice-daily milking, the recent industry trend in some parts of the world toward thrice-daily milking has created uncertainty as to whether intramammary treatment should be repeated after every milking or even whether once-a-day intramammary administration is as efficacious as twice- or thrice-daily administration.[13,17,18]

Recent studies have confirmed long-held beliefs that **appropriate antimicrobial therapy** (commonly called **extended or aggressive antimicrobial therapy**) for 5 to 8 days is more effective in treating intramammary infections than label intramammary therapy (2–3 days).[5,6,19] In other words, increasing the duration of antimicrobial administration increases treatment efficacy. Extended antimicrobial therapy is opposed by some producers because such treatment may be off-label and results in a longer milk withhold time and, consequently, the amount of milk that has to be discarded. In contrast, extended therapy of clinical mastitis episodes that have been treated for 2 to 3 days but the secretion remains abnormal is perceived by some producers as part of the social norm of "being a good farmer."[20] Extended therapy is opposed by dairying administrators because of the inevitable increase in the number of infringements of health regulations relating to antibiotic residues in milk. The inappropriately short treatment duration for most intramammary products has been a major hindrance to developing effective antimicrobial treatment protocols.

Intramammary Antimicrobial Therapy

For reasons of convenience and efficiency, antimicrobial udder infusions are in common use for the treatment of certain causes of mastitis in lactating cows and for dry cow therapy. For example, the cure rate of *S. agalactiae* using intramammary infusions in lactating cows exceeds 95%. Disposable tubes containing suitable antimicrobials in a water-soluble ointment base are ideal for dispensing and for the treatment of individual cows. Multiple-dose bottles containing aqueous infusions are adequate and much cheaper per dose when large numbers of quarters are to be treated, but repeated use of the same container increases the risk of contamination. The degree of diffusion into glandular tissue is the same when either water or ointment is used as a vehicle for infusion; the duration of retention within the gland depends on the vehicle.

Most antimicrobial agents currently available in the United States in commercial intramammary infusion products are active against the staphylococci and streptococci, with cephapirin (a first-generation cephalosporin) having good activity against coliform bacteria, and ceftiofur (a third-generation cephalosporin) having excellent activity against coliform bacteria. Until recent years the emphasis was on the elimination of gram-positive cocci from the udder, but gram-negative infections, especially *E. coli*, have increased in prevalence to the point where a broad-spectrum preparation is almost essential for both lactation and dry period treatments. Generally, antimicrobials administered by the intramammary route for the treatment of clinical mastitis should be bactericidal because neutrophil phagocytosis of bacteria is impaired in milk.

The choice of antimicrobial agents for intramammary infusion should be based on the following:

- Mechanism of antimicrobial action and spectrum of bacteria controlled
- Diffusibility through mammary tissue
- Cost

Strict hygiene is necessary during treatment to avoid the introduction of bacteria, yeasts, and fungi into the treated quarters; the use of a short cannula that just penetrates the external sphincter is preferred because it is less likely to introduce bacteria and leaves more of the keratin plug in place in the streak canal. This is important because the keratin plug has antimicrobial properties. Care must be taken to ensure that bulk containers of mastitis infusions are not contaminated by frequent withdrawals and that individual, sterilized teat cannulas, usually part of commercial, single-dose ointment tubes, are used for each quarter. Bulk treatments are best avoided because of the high risk of spread of pathogens.

Infusion Procedure

The teats must be cleaned and sanitized before infusing the quarter to avoid introduction of infection. The following steps are recommended:

- Clean and dry the teats.
- Dip teats in an effective germicidal product. Allow 30 seconds' contact time before wiping teats with an individual disposable towel (one towel per cow, use one corner of the towel for each teat).
- Thoroughly clean and disinfect each teat end with cotton soaked in 70% alcohol. Use a separate piece of cotton for each teat.
- Prepare teats on the far side of the udder first, followed by teats on the near side.
- Treat quarters in reverse order: near side first, far side last.
- Insert only the tip of the cannula into the teat end (**partial insertion**). Do not allow the sterile cannula to touch anything before infusion. Most approved dry cow infusion products (and lactating tubes) are marketed with a dual cover that can be used for partial or full insertion.
- Dip teats in a germicidal product after treatment.
- Identify treated cows and remove them from the milking herd to prevent antimicrobials from entering the milk supply.

Diffusion of infused intramammary drugs is often impeded by the blockage of lactiferous ducts and alveoli with inflammatory debris. Complete emptying of the quarter by the parenteral injection of oxytocin (10–20 IU intramuscularly) followed by hand stripping of affected quarters before infusion has been recommended in cases of clinical mastitis, but efficacy studies are lacking, the volume stripped is usually small, and the procedure is painful to the cow. If stripping is performed, the intramammary infusion is given after the last stripping of the day has been done, avoiding any further milking of the gland until the next milking.

Parenteral Antimicrobial Therapy

This should be considered in all cases of mastitis in which there is an abnormal gland and is preferred in all cases of mastitis in which there is an abnormal cow (fever, decreased appetite, or inappetence). The systemic reaction can usually be brought under control by standard doses of antimicrobial agents, but a bacteriologic cure of the affected glands may not be achieved because of the relatively poor diffusion of the antimicrobial from the blood into the milk. However, the rate of diffusion is greater in affected than in normal quarters. Parenteral treatment is also recommended when the gland is markedly swollen and intramammary infusions are unlikely to diffuse to all parts of the glandular tissue.[19] To achieve adequate therapeutic levels of an antimicrobial in the mammary gland by parenteral treatment it is necessary, for the above reasons, to use higher than normal dose rates daily for 3 to 5 days.[19] Milk from treated cows must be withheld from the bulk tank for the stated period of time of that antimicrobial following the date of last treatment.

Treatment of Lactating Quarters

There are three situations to consider: the emergency single case of clinical mastitis requiring immediate treatment; the herd with a problem of too many clinical cases or intractable cases, but where the identity of the pathogen is known; and the cow with subclinical mastitis.

Emergency Treatment When the Type of Infection Is Unknown

Cases of acute and peracute mastitis (abnormal cow) in lactating cows, and in dry cows close to calving, are serious problems for the field veterinarian. The need for treatment is urgent; it is not possible to wait for the results of laboratory tests to guide the selection of the most appropriate antibiotic. Clinical findings, season of the year; and management practices may give a broad hint as to the specific bacterial cause, but in most such circumstances it is necessary to use a broad-spectrum approach to treatment. Parenteral therapy with oxytetracycline (administered intravenously to increase bioavailability and therefore plasma and milk concentrations), penethamate hydriodide, a potentiated sulfonamide or similar broad-spectrum antimicrobial agent should be supplemented with intramammary infusion with a β-lactamase–resistant antimicrobial such as a first-generation cephalosporin (cephapirin), a third-generation cephalosporin (e.g., ceftiofur), penicillin G–neomycin combination, or other approved broad-spectrum intramammary infusion. Parenteral ceftiofur is not effective in clinical mastitis episodes that have abnormal secretion or abnormal gland and secretion.

A consensus is developing that clinical mastitis episodes that manifest as abnormal secretion or abnormal secretion and gland should be treated only by the intramammary route, and that clinical mastitis episodes that manifest as abnormal secretion, gland, and cow should be treated by both the intramammary and parenteral routes. The latter group would also benefit from the administration of antiinflammatory agents and intravenous fluid therapy, depending on the severity of the systemic signs. A consensus is also developing that extended intramammary therapy (effectively more appropriate duration therapy) beyond the traditional 2- to 3-day treatment regimen is preferred when permitted by label directions and country recommendations[5,6]; however, the optimal duration of intramammary therapy remains to be determined.

In a multicenter study in Europe comparing three β-lactam–based intramammary products for the treatment of 491 clinical mastitis episodes, the bacteriologic cure rate for intramammary administration of a combination of cephalexin (200 mg, first-generation cephalosporin) and kanamycin (133 mg) or cefquinome (75 mg, fourth-generation cephalosporin) were similar but higher than that for intramammary infusion of cefoperazone (100 mg, third-generation cephalosporin).[16] In a multifarm (n = 28) study in New Zealand comparing three cephalosporin-based intramammary products for the treatment of 1462 clinical mastitis episodes, the bacteriologic cure rates were similar for intramammary administration of procaine penicillin (1 g), cefuroxime sodium (250 mg, second-generation cephalosporin), or a combination of procaine penicillin G (1,000,000 U) and dihydrostreptomycin (0.5 g).[21] However, quarters treated with cefuroxime were more likely to be retreated within 30 days than quarters receiving either of the other two treatments.[21]

Field studies show that, in herds in which clinical mastitis is often caused by environmental pathogens, intravenous administration of oxytetracycline, intramammary infusion of cephapirin, and supportive therapy (including intravenous administration of flunixin meglumine or fluids) produce a higher rate of clinical and bacteriologic cure than supportive treatment alone. In addition, antimicrobial treatment is more effective than supportive treatment alone. In cows with clinical mastitis caused by *E. coli* the use of procaine penicillin G intramuscularly was no more effective than not using antimicrobial agents; this result is expected based on penicillin's gram-positive spectrum of activity. Knowledge of the likely causative agent is therefore helpful when making decisions about therapy of clinical mastitis episodes during lactation.

Provision of other supportive therapy, such as fluids and electrolytes, is also crucial to the survival of the cow and minimization of the severity of the mastitis and extent of permanent injury to the udder. The efficacy of frequent stripping, with or without intramammary infusion, is uncertain. Nonsteroidal antiinflammatory drugs (NSAIDs) decrease pain associated with an abnormal gland; in addition, they enhance recovery and reduce fever in severe cases.

Treatment When the Infecting Organism Is Known

A common situation encountered by a bovine practitioner is the dairy herd that has had an outbreak of clinical mastitis or has received a warning notice from the milk processor that the bulk milk SCC or bacterial count is above acceptable limits. The situation calls for a complete mastitis control program, including conducting an investigation to determine the causative bacteria present, the source of the infection, hygiene in the milking parlor, and the importance of risk factors such as milking machine management, plus recommended antimicrobial preparations selected on the basis of the causative agent. Treatment of a number of identified subclinical cases at the commencement of the program, and of individual cases subsequently, can be based on the known common infection in the herd. Among gram-positive cocci, the response to antimicrobial agents is excellent for streptococci. For staphylococci a cure rate of 65% is about the best that can be expected, and unless there are good reasons for doing otherwise it is recommended that treatment be postponed until the cow is dry. Standard treatments for lactating cows include penicillin alone (100,000 units) or in combination with streptomycin (1 g) or neomycin (500 mg), and a combination of ampicillin (75 mg) and sodium cloxacillin (200 mg). Acid-resistant penicillins, e.g., phenoxymethylpenicillin, are probably best not used as mammary infusions because of their ability to pass through the human stomach, thus presenting a more serious potential threat to humans drinking contaminated milk. Because of the widespread and often indiscriminate use of penicillin, a large part of the mastitis that occurs is associated with penicillin-resistant bacteria, especially *S. aureus*. Treatment programs need to take this into account when recommendations are made about the antibiotic to be used.

Intramammary infections associated with **environmental streptococci** that manifest signs of clinical mastitis are usually acute but only moderately severe. In most of these cases the streptococci are sensitive to antimicrobial agents, and they often recover spontaneously with good management and nursing care. If not, they usually respond well to therapy.[22] Bacteriologic cure rates of 60% to 65% can be expected following a single intramammary infusion of a cephalosporin product.

In one randomized controlled field trial of clinical mastitis associated with *Streptococcus* spp. or coliform bacteria, the clinical cure rate by the 10th milking was significantly higher when intramammary cephapirin, intravenous oxytetracycline, or both were used along with supportive therapy (oxytocin and stripping of affected glands and, in severely affected cows, the use of flunixin meglumine and fluids) compared with supportive treatment alone. These results indicate that, in herds in which clinical mastitis is often associated with environmental pathogens, antimicrobial therapy and supportive therapy may result in a better outcome than supportive therapy alone.

Treatment of Subclinical Mastitis

It is generally considered not advisable to treat subclinical mastitis during lactation.[23,24] However, it is important to consider the causative organism, the age of the cow, the number of intramammary infections for the cow, and the udder health status of the herd.[25] There are several situations in which lactational therapy of subclinical mastitis is indicated; for example, herds with *S. agalactiae* infections should consider several approaches to therapy during lactation. *S. agalactiae* infections respond well to therapy during lactation, with cure rates of 80% to 100% expected. All approved intramammary therapy preparations are efficacious, including penicillin, cephalosporins, cloxacillin, and erythromycin. In herds with a high prevalence of *S. agalactiae* mastitis, **blitz therapy** can be used for eradication of the pathogen, increased milk production, and reduced penalties for high SCCs. There is, however, a risk of residue violation, problems with disposal of milk from treated cows, and considerable costs involved. It is also important to ensure that standard mastitis control procedures, such as postmilking teat disinfection and blanket dry cow therapy, have been implemented. The benefit:cost ratios for various approaches to blitz therapy of *S. agalactiae*–infected herds have been studied. The prevalence of infected cows, and their stage of lactation, are important determinants of the type of program selected.

Therapy of cows with subclinical mastitis caused by *S. aureus* during lactation is much less rewarding. Under field conditions, cases of *S. aureus* are difficult to cure during lactation. Reported cure rates following intramammary therapy are between 15% and 60%. Lactational therapy of subclinical *S. aureus* mastitis using intramuscular penicillin along with intramammary amoxicillin infusion, compared with the intramammary infusion alone, increased the cure rate to 40%, which represented a doubling of the cure rate with intramammary therapy alone. Improvements in the cure rate of subclinical gram-positive intramammary infections have also been obtained with parenteral penethamate hydroiodide.[25] If treatment by this method is used in combination with data on the age of cow, stage of lactation, duration of infection, and level of SCC, the economic benefit of treating some cases of *S. aureus* mastitis during lactation may be attractive.

Subclinical infections associated with environmental streptococci, and occasionally by coliform organisms, can be found in moderate numbers in some herds. Although spontaneous cure rates are higher with these environmental infections, individual cows may merit treatment during lactation. In these cases, the previously listed factors should be used and are important in the selection of cases to be treated.

Prepartum antibiotic treatment of heifers is of benefit in herds experiencing a high incidence of clinical mastitis in recently calved heifers. CNS are frequently isolated from late-gestation heifers, and intramammary treatment with sodium cloxacillin (200 mg) or cephapirin sodium (200 mg) 7 days before expected parturition is highly effective and economically beneficial.

Antiinflammatory Agents

NSAIDs have been evaluated for the treatment of field and experimental cases of acute and peracute mastitis. They have beneficial effects on decreasing the severity of clinical signs based on changes in rectal temperature, heart rate, rumen motility, and pain associated with the mastitis and are routinely administered as part of the initial treatment of cattle with severe clinical mastitis and marked systemic signs (pyrexia, tachycardia, tachypnea, and ruminal hypomotility). On the basis of one comparative study, NSAIDs appear to ameliorate systemic abnormalities to a greater degree than corticosteroids. The strongest evidence to support the administration of NSAIDs is available for meloxicam, ketoprofen, and phenylbutazone.

Administration of meloxicam (250 mg subcutaneously once) to dairy cows in New Zealand with acute clinical mastitis being treated with three daily intramuscular injections of penethamate hydriodide (5 g) decreased posttreatment SCC and decreased culling from the herd from 28% to 16%.[26] Ketoprofen at 2 g intramuscularly once daily combined with sulfadiazine and trimethoprim intramuscularly given daily to cows with acute clinical mastitis, and complete milking of affected quarters several times daily, significantly improved survival and milk production compared with cows not receiving the NSAID. A reanalysis of the published results indicated that phenylbutazone at 4 g intramuscularly once daily combined with sulfadiazine and trimethoprim intramuscularly given daily to cows with acute clinical mastitis significantly improved the percentage of cows with milk production returning to more than 75% of previous levels compared with cows not receiving the NSAID. However, intramuscular administration of phenylbutazone is not currently recommended because of the potential for myonecrosis. Moreover, phenylbutazone is not permitted to be administered to dairy cattle greater than 20 months of age in the United States. Dipyrone (20 g, intramuscularly) administered once daily in the same study was not effective. It is not permitted to be administered to food-producing animals in some countries, including the United States.

There is minimal evidence that treatment of clinical cases with NSAIDs alters the inflammatory response in the udder, although pretreatment of cattle with experimentally induced mastitis does alter the local (glandular) inflammatory response to infection. Flunixin meglumine concentrations are low in milk, which is consistent with its properties as a weak acid that has difficulty crossing the blood-milk barrier. Flunixin meglumine (2 mg/kg, intravenously, twice 24 hours apart) did not alter the survival rate of dairy cows with severe *E. coli* or *S. uberis* mastitis compared with intravenous administration of 45 L of isotonic crystalloid fluids. Flunixin meglumine is often administered as part of the initial treatment of clinical mastitis in cows manifesting systemic signs of illness, and flunixin residues are being detected in milk from dairy cattle being sent for human consumption. This may reflect the markedly slower clearance of flunixin in cows with clinical mastitis.[27] The one-time administration of 1 g of flunixin meglumine intravenously or 4 g of phenylbutazone intravenously, along with intramammary infusion of gentamicin (150 mg) at 12-hour intervals for four treatments, had no significant beneficial effect in cows with acute toxic mastitis associated with *E. coli* and *Klebsiella* spp. However, the results of this study do not indicate a lack of effectiveness of flunixin meglumine or phenylbutazone, because it is difficult for one dose of any NSAID to have a detectable effect on clinical signs in naturally occurring mastitis cases.

Supportive Therapy

Supportive treatment, including the intravenous administration of large quantities of isotonic crystalloid fluids, is indicated in cattle with severe systemic illness. Large volumes of isotonic crystalloid fluids can be rapidly administered under pressure at 0.5 L/min through a 12-gauge catheter in the jugular vein, using a 7.5-L garden weed killer spray pump. The administration of hypertonic saline followed by immediate access to drinking water is a practical method of providing fluid therapy to cows with severe mastitis, especially peracute coliform mastitis. A dose of 4 to 5 mL/kg body weight (BW) of 7.5% saline is given intravenously over 4 to 5 minutes. This is usually followed by the animal consuming large quantities of water. Circulating blood volume is increased and there is mild strong ion (metabolic) acidosis, improved renal function, and changes in calcium and phosphorus homeostasis compared with cows given a similar volume of 0.9% NaCl. Fluid therapy is covered extensively in Chapter 5.

Adjunctive Therapy

Cytokines may be useful as adjunctive therapy with existing antimicrobials to improve therapeutic efficacy, particularly in lactating cows. Cytokines are natural regulators of the host defense system in response to infectious diseases. The combination of a commercial formulation of cephapirin with recombinant interleukin (IL)-2 consistently improved the cure rate of treating *S. aureus* mastitis by 20% to 30% compared with use of the antimicrobial alone.

Ozone is a gas (O_3) that rapidly inactivates bacteria and viruses. It was prepared with a commercially available ozone therapy device and administered to cattle with clinical mastitis. The administration of 100 mL of 70% ozone decreased SCC over 1 week, suggesting that ozone may be an effective adjunct therapy.[28]

Magnitude of Response to Therapy

The treatment of some causes of mastitis can be highly effective in removing infection from the quarter and returning the milk to normal composition. However, the yield of milk, although it can be improved by the removal of congestion in the gland and inflammatory debris from the duct system, is unlikely to be returned to normal in severe clinical cases, at least until the next lactation. The degree of response obtained depends particularly on the causative agent, the speed with which treatment is commenced, and other factors described earlier. A "cure" may mean disappearance of clinical signs, elimination of the infectious cause, or both of those plus return to normal function and productivity. Which of these is the objective in any particular case or herd will influence the decisions to be made about treatment in an individual case of the disease.

Failure to respond to therapy of the lactating cow may be caused by the following:

- The presence of microabscesses and inaccessibility of the drug to the pathogen
- Ineffective drug diffusion
- Inactivation of the antimicrobial by milk and tissue proteins

- Inefficient killing of the bacteria and intracellular survival of bacteria
- Increased antimicrobial resistance
- The development of L-forms of bacteria

Dry Cow Therapy

Dry cow therapy is the use of intramammary antimicrobial therapy immediately after the last milking of lactation and is an important component of an effective mastitis control program. Intramammary infusions at drying off **decrease the number of existing infections** and **prevent new infections during the early weeks of the dry period.** Dry cow therapy should be routinely administered and remains one of the cornerstones of an effective mastitis control program. **Blanket dry cow therapy** is treatment of all four quarters at drying off, compared with **selective dry cow therapy** based on treatment of only those quarters that are infected. When subclinical mastitis is very low in some herds, selective dry cow therapy can be considered, but nearly all herds use blanket dry cow therapy. The problem with selective dry cow therapy is the accuracy of available indirect tests to "select" cows for treatment or nontreatment. Currently available indirect tests are not sufficiently accurate (the exception being quarter milk cultures) to be used as a basis for selective dry cow therapy.

Intramammary infusions approved for dry cow therapy contain high levels of antimicrobial agents in a slow-release base that maintains therapeutic levels in the dry udder for long periods of time. Most dry cow therapy infusion products are intended to eliminate existing infections caused by *S. aureus* and *S. agalactiae* at drying off and to prevent new infections caused by the same pathogens and environmental streptococci in the early dry period.

In herds with a high prevalence of contagious mastitis, dry cow therapy has been efficacious and economically beneficial in reducing the prevalence of intramammary infections. The consistent application of effective mastitis control procedures has reduced the prevalence of contagious pathogens and the bulk tank milk SCC (<300,000 cells/mL), and owners of these herds questioned dry cow therapy because of the economics and the concerns of residues in the milk. Field trials in herds with a low prevalence of contagious mastitis indicate that dry cow therapy at the end of lactation increased 17-week milk production during the subsequent lactation and was economically beneficial compared with not treating them. However, in the subsequent lactation, the incidence of clinical mastitis was not reduced and the SCCs were not significantly different from those of cows not treated at the end of lactation.

The most effective time to treat subclinical intramammary infections is at drying off. Dry cow therapy has the following advantages over lactation therapy:

- The cure rate is higher than that achieved by treatment during lactation.
- A much higher dose of antimicrobial can be used safely.
- Retention time of the antimicrobial in the udder is longer.
- The incidence of new infections during the dry period is reduced.
- Tissue damage by mastitis may be regenerated before parturition.
- Clinical mastitis at calving may be reduced.
- The risk of contaminating milk with antimicrobial residue is reduced.

Selection of a suitable dry period treatment should take into account the fact that gram-negative infections are not common at that time because of the high concentration of lactoferrin in the dry secretions. Accordingly, attention should be directed at the inclusion of a potent antibiotic against *Streptococcus* spp., β-lactamase–producing *S. aureus,* and *T. pyogenes.* Cloxacillin and cephalosporins are popular for the purpose; for example, a recommended treatment is cephapirin or sodium cloxacillin in a slow-release base with an expected cure rate of 80% against streptococci and 60% against *S. aureus.* A large North American trial involving 6 dairy herds and 1091 cows identified no difference in the risk of cure between dry off and calving, and no effect of treatment on the risk for the presence of a new intramammary infection for the first 6 days in milk after calving, for cattle treated at dry off with intramammary procaine penicillin G (1,000,000 U) and dihydrostreptomycin (1 g), ceftiofur hydrochloride (500 mg), or cephapirin (300 mg) dry cow formulations.[29] In contrast, a study in Central Florida involving 2 dairy herds and 402 cows identified that cattle treated at dry off with intramammary ceftiofur hydrochloride (500 mg) had lower odds of having clinical and subclinical mastitis in the early part of the subsequent lactation than cows treated with intramammary procaine penicillin G (1,000,000 U) and dihydrostreptomycin (1 g).[30]

Most dry cow preparations maintain an adequate minimum concentration in the quarter for about 4 weeks, but some persist for 6 weeks. There is little, if any, value in treating cows again before the due calving date. There is always a possibility of introducing infection while infusing an intramammary preparation and farmers are reluctant to break the teat canal seal, but it may be necessary to do so if summer mastitis is prevalent in the area.

Prepartum Antimicrobial Therapy in Heifers

Intramammary infusion of a cephapirin dry cow therapy preparation into pregnant heifers 10 to 12 weeks prepartum eliminated over 90% of the intramammary infection caused by *S. aureus, Streptococcus* spp., CNS spp., and coliforms. The SCCs of cured quarters were comparable to uninfected control quarters after parturition. At parturition, 24% of treated quarters were positive for the antimicrobial; however, no quarters were positive at 5 days postpartum.

Treatment of Mastitis on Organic Dairy Farms

The sale of organic dairy products is increasing worldwide, and the common occurrence of mastitis in dairy cattle provides an animal welfare challenge about how to appropriately treat clinical mastitis episodes in organic dairy farms. In the United States, use of antimicrobials to treat dairy cattle results in permanent loss of organic status for that animal,[31] whereas organic dairy farms in the European Union and Canada are permitted limited use of antimicrobials for emergency treatments per year.[32] Consequently, organic farmers use a variety of treatments for clinical mastitis, including homeopathy, vitamin supplements, and botanicals.[31] They also use veterinarians less frequently than similarly sized conventionally managed dairy herds.[33]

Treatment with a botanical preparation containing extracts of *Thymus vulgaris, Gaultheria procumbens, Glycyrrhiza uralensis, Angelica sinensis,* and vitamin E did not affect the resolution of clinical mastitis at day 4 of treatment, but it decreased the time to clinical recovery in cattle with clinical mastitis in Colorado.[32] This botanical formulation contained chemicals with documented antiinflammatory, antiseptic, or nutritional effects. Intramammary infusion of a live culture of *Lactococcus lactis* may be efficacious in the treatment of subclinical and clinical mastitis in dairy cattle.[34]

Antimicrobial Residues in Milk and Withholding Times

Label instructions must be followed to ensure that drug residues do not occur, especially from cows with a shorter than normal dry period. Antibiotic residue testing of the milk of a recently calved cow can be done if there is a suspicion of residues, but this is a misuse of a test designed for bulk tank milk testing and therefore suffers from problems with sensitivity and specificity.

Treatment and control of mastitis accounts for the largest percentage of antimicrobial use on dairy farms. Following treatment by the intramammary or parenteral route, the concentration of antimicrobial agents in the milk declines over time to levels that are considered safe and tolerable for humans. The duration of time for the concentrations to decline to acceptable limits is known as the **withholding time** or the **withdrawal period** during which the milk cannot be added to the bulk tank supply but must be withheld and discarded. The presence of residues in milk is a major public health concern that adversely affects the dairy industry, the practicing veterinarian, and the perception the public has of the safety of milk for human consumption. The public perception of the safety of milk is crucial, and veterinarians have a responsibility to respond to these concerns through public education and quality control of milk production.

Other serious consequences of antimicrobial residues in milk are their effect on the manufacture of dairy products and the potential development of antimicrobial sensitivity syndromes in humans. In most countries the maximum intramammary dose of antimicrobial agents is limited by legislation, and the presence of detectable quantities of antimicrobial agents in milk constitutes adulteration. Attention has also been directed to the excretion of antimicrobial agents in milk from untreated quarters, after treatment of infected quarters, and after their administration by parenteral injection or by insertion into the uterus. The degree to which this excretion occurs varies widely between animals and in the same animal at different points in the lactation period, and it differs from one antibiotic to another. Milk from cows subjected to dry period treatment is usually required to be withheld for 4 days after calving. The use of any dry period treatments in lactating cows causes prolonged retention of the antimicrobial in milk and is a most serious violation of the legislation.

Veterinarians have the responsibility to warn farmers of the need to withhold milk, and both should be aware of the withholding times of each product, the details of which are usually required to be included on its label. Marking the cow in some way to remind the farmer, by application of a leg band or placing dye on the udder, is advisable.

Antimicrobial Residue Tests

Several cowside tests are available to detect antimicrobial residues in the milk of cows that have been treated for mastitis. The goal of cowside testing is to assist in the production of high-quality, antimicrobial-residue–free milk from dairy herds. To be consistent with the intent of a quality assurance program, cowside testing would be used only on cows recently treated with antimicrobial agents and only after appropriate milk withholding times had been followed. The ideal test would have a high sensitivity and high specificity.

Most of the cowside screening tests for antimicrobial residues are imperfect because of a high rate of false-positive results when used on field samples. The direct costs to producers can be high because of the unnecessary disposal of milk and imposition of fines and penalties. False-positive results also cause the unnecessary culling of some cows, and concern about the interpretation of positive assay results, the appropriateness of withholding periods, and the safety of milk creates mistrust among consumers, producers, veterinarians, and regulatory personnel. The specificity of four commercially available tests ranged from 0.78 to 0.95. None of the test kits has been validated to meet performance standards for sensitivity and specificity. This applies to individual cow samples, bulk tank milk samples, and tanker truck samples.

The presence of naturally occurring bactericidal products in the milk of cows with acute and convalescent mastitis is the most likely cause of the false-positive results of the tests (such as Delvotest) that are based on bacterial growth inhibition of β-lactam antimicrobial agents. Immunoglobulins, complement, lysozyme, lactoferrin, and phagocytic cells are products of inflammation in the milk of cows with mastitis that can inhibit bacterial growth. The milk from cows with experimental endotoxin-induced mastitis is at increased risk for false-positive assay results using commercial residue tests. The incidence of false-positive results is very low in milk from cows that have not had a history of mastitis or antimicrobial therapy. Naturally occurring bactericidal products in mastitic milk can be removed by heating at 82°C (180°F) for 5 minutes; this temperature does not denature antimicrobial agents present in milk. Heat treatment therefore appears to provide a very practical way to reduce false-positive results on milk from individual cows.

A sample of milk can be submitted for antimicrobial residue testing up to three times. First, a producer may test a sample from a specific cow at the end of her withdrawal period. Second, milk is sampled at the tanker truck level. Third, should the tanker truck sample have positive results, bulk tank milk samples from each dairy herd that contributed to that tanker truck are tested.

There is a need for validation of the diagnostic assays used to detect antimicrobial residues in milk. Acceptance of assays for regulatory purposes must be based on protocols that include field estimates of assay performance before the assays are used by the public. Three strategies have been suggested to balance public health concerns with economic concerns of dairy producers caused by false-positive results:

1. Retest samples that yield positive results with a confirmatory assay of specificity close to 100%. Only those samples that also yield positive results on the second assay are considered to be positive for violative residues.
2. Recalibrate the assay to increase specificity. This will usually result in loss of sensitivity.
3. Use an alternative assay of higher specificity.

It is suggested that regulatory monitoring of residues at a national level will be best served by use of a combination of at least two assays: initial screening with a highly sensitive and inexpensive assay followed by confirmation testing with an assay of high specificity (>99%) that can quantify the concentration of the antimicrobial residue. All tanker samples that yield positive results with a screening assay should be rechecked with a quantitative assay. If the quantitative assay detects a concentration greater than the safe level, safe concentration, or tolerance level, only then would the milk be deemed to have violative residue and fines and penalties be imposed. The complex dynamics of current milk residue tests discourage practitioners from recommending testing procedures to dairy producers.

As an approximate guide, the recommended periods for which milk should be withheld from sale after different methods of antimicrobial administration are (in times after last treatment)

- Udder infusion in a lactating cow (72 hours)
- Parenteral injection, one only (36 hours)
- Parenteral injections, series of (72 hours)
- Antimicrobial agents parenterally in long-acting bases (10 days)
- Intrauterine tablet (72 hours)
- Dry cow intramammary infusion (to be administered at least 4 weeks before calving and the milk withheld for at least 96 hours afterward)

Permanently Drying Off Chronically Affected Quarters

If a quarter does not respond to treatment and is classified as incurable, the affected animal should be isolated from the milking herd, or the affected quarter may be permanently dried off by inducing a chemical mastitis. Historically used methods, arranged in decreasing order of severity, are infusions of

- 30 to 60 mL of 3% silver nitrate solution
- 20 mL of 5% copper sulfate solution
- 100 to 300 mL of 1 : 500, or 300 to 500 mL of a 1 : 2000 acriflavine solution

If a severe local reaction occurs, the quarter should be milked out and stripped frequently until the reaction subsides. If no reaction occurs, the quarter is stripped out 10 to 14 days later. Two infusions of these solutions may be necessary.

The **best method for permanently drying off a quarter is infusion of 120 mL of 5% povidone iodine solution (0.5% iodine)** after complete milk out and administration of flunixin meglumine (1 mg/kg BW, intravenously). This causes permanent cessation of lactation in the quarter but does not alter total milk production by the cow. If the goal is chemical sterilization, then three daily infusions of 60 mL of chlorhexidine suspension should be administered after complete milk out. The majority of treated cows (5/7) returned to milk production in the quarter in the subsequent lactation. The infusion of 60 mL of chlorhexidine, followed by milking out at the next subsequent milking and repeat of the infusion 24 hours after the initial treatment, is also effective in making infused quarters nonfunctional within 14 to 63 days. Histologic evaluation of the infused quarters revealed that secretory tissues had involuted to a nonsecretory state and appeared similar to blind or nonfunctional quarters. However, as noted earlier, milk production may return in the gland in the subsequent lactation. Studies have demonstrated that the intramammary infusion of 10 mL of a peptide concentrate of casein hydrolysate is efficacious in drying off a quarter for the remainder of the lactation, but the quarter recovers over the dry period and milk production returns to similar levels the following lactation.[22,35] The infusion of casein induces an accelerated involution of the mammary gland. The effectiveness of this approach in drying off infected quarters does not appear to have been evaluated.

TREATMENT AND CONTROL OF CLINICAL MASTITIS IN LACTATING DAIRY COWS[a]

Treatment

Abnormal secretion

Perform on-farm culture and treat gram-positive isolates 18–24 hours later with an intramammary formulation that has proven efficacy against common gram-positive mastitis pathogens per label directions (R-1).

Administer broad-spectrum intramammary formulation per label directions (R-2).

Abnormal secretion and abnormal gland

Administer broad-spectrum intramammary formulation per label directions (R-1)

Administer extended duration of intramammary therapy (R-2).

Abnormal secretion, abnormal gland, and abnormal cow

Administer broad-spectrum intramammary formulation per label directions (R-1).

Administer extended duration of intramammary therapy (R-2).

Parenteral cefquinome, ceftiofur, fluoroquinolones, penethamate hydriodide, or oxytetracycline per label directions (R-1)

Intravenous fluid therapy with low-volume hypertonic saline or high-volume isotonic crystalloids (R-2)

Antiinflammatory agents, including meloxicam (250 mg, subcutaneously, once) (R-2)

Control

See extensive section on control of mastitis later in this chapter.

[a]*Causative agent unknown. If the causative agent is known, then refer to specific treatment and prophylaxis recommendations for the etiologic agent in this chapter.*

FURTHER READING

Constable PD, Morin DE. Treatment of clinical mastitis: using antimicrobial susceptibility profiles for treatment decisions. *Vet Clin North Am Food Anim Pract.* 2003;19:139-156.

Leslie KE, Petersson-Wolfe CS. Assessment and management of pain in dairy cows with clinical mastitis. *Vet Clin North Am Food Anim Pract.* 2012;28:289-305.

Pyörälä S. Treatment of mastitis during lactation. *Ir Vet J.* 2009;62(suppl 4):S40-S44.

Roberson JR. Treatment of clinical mastitis. *Vet Clin North Am Food Anim Pract.* 2012;28:271-288.

Royster E, Wagner S. Treatment of mastitis in cattle. *Vet Clin North Am Food Anim Pract.* 2015;31:17-46.

REFERENCES

1. Pinzón-Sánchez C, et al. *J Dairy Sci.* 2011;94:1873.
2. Oliveira L, Ruegg PL. *J Dairy Sci.* 2014;97:5426.
3. Lago A, et al. *J Dairy Sci.* 2011;94:4441.
4. Lago A, et al. *J Dairy Sci.* 2011;94:4457.
5. Swinkels JM, et al. *Vet J.* 2013;197:682.
6. Truchetti G, et al. *Can J Vet Res.* 2014;78:31.
7. Petrovski KR, et al. *Aust Vet J.* 2015;93:227.
8. Lindeman CJ, et al. *J Vet Diagn Invest.* 2013;25:581.
9. Bengtsson B, et al. *Vet Microbiol.* 2009;136:142.
10. Cortinhas CS, et al. *Am J Vet Res.* 2013;74:683.
11. Gehring R, Smith GW. *J Vet Pharmacol Ther.* 2006;29:237.
12. Whittem T, et al. *J Vet Pharmacol Ther.* 2012;35:460.
13. Stockler RM, et al. *J Dairy Sci.* 2009;92:4262.
14. Stockler RM, et al. *J Vet Pharmacol Ther.* 2009;32:345.
15. Badawy SA, et al. *Small Rumin Res.* 2015;133:67.
16. Bradley AJ, Green MJ. *J Dairy Sci.* 2009;92:1941.
17. Gordon PJ, et al. *J Dairy Sci.* 2013;96:4455.
18. Lindquist DA, et al. *J Dairy Sci.* 2015;98:1856.
19. Kalmus P, et al. *J Dairy Sci.* 2014;97:2155.
20. Swinkels JM, et al. *J Dairy Sci.* 2015;98:2369.
21. McDougall S, et al. *New Zeal Vet J.* 2007;55:161.
22. Pinzón-Sánchez C, Ruegg PL. *J Dairy Sci.* 2011;94:3397.
23. Sandgren CH, et al. *Vet J.* 2008;175:108.
24. Leitner G, et al. *Israel J Vet Med.* 2012;67:162.
25. Steele N, McGougall S. *New Zeal Vet J.* 2014;62:38.
26. McDougall S, et al. *J Dairy Sci.* 2009;92:4421.
27. Kissell LW, et al. *J Am Vet Med Assoc.* 2015;246:18.
28. Enginler SO, et al. *Acta Scientiae Veterinariae.* 2015;43:1260.
29. Arruda AG, et al. *J Dairy Sci.* 2013;96:4419.
30. Pinedo PJ, et al. *J Dairy Sci.* 2012;95:7015.
31. Ruegg PL. *J Anim Sci.* 2009;87(suppl 1):43.
32. Pinedo P, et al. *Can Vet J.* 2013;54:479.
33. Richert RM, et al. *J Am Vet Med Assoc.* 2013;242:1732.
34. Klostermann K, et al. *J Dairy Res.* 2008;75:365.
35. Leitner G, et al. *Livestock Sci.* 2007;110:292.

Mastitis Pathogens of Cattle

In the following sections, the special features of each mastitis associated with one or a group of pathogens will be described using the usual format of the book. Mastitis in cattle is categorized as being associated with contagious, teat skin opportunistic or environmental pathogens, and as being common (**major pathogen**) or less common (**minor pathogen**). The features that are unique to the diagnosis, treatment, and control of each mastitis pathogen will be outlined, but details applicable to all causes of mastitis were presented earlier.

Mastitis of Cattle Associated With Common Contagious Pathogens

STAPHYLOCOCCUS AUREUS

SYNOPSIS

Etiology *Staphylococcus aureus* is a major pathogen of the mammary gland and a common cause of contagious bovine mastitis. *S. aureus* also causes mastitis in sheep and goats.

Epidemiology Major cause of mastitis in dairy herds without an effective mastitis control program. Prevalence of infection 50%–100%; prevalence of 1%–10% in herds with low bulk tank milk SCCs, 50% in high-SCC herds, quarter infection rate 10%–25% in high-SCC herds. Source of infection is infected udder; infection transmitted at milking. Chronic or subclinical *S. aureus* mastitis is of major economic importance.

Clinical findings

- Chronic *S. aureus* mastitis is most common and is characterized by high SCC and gradual induration of udder, drop in milk yield, and atrophy with occasional appearance of clots in milk or wateriness.
- Acute and peracute *S. aureus* mastitis most common in early lactation. Acute swelling of gland with fever; milk is abnormal with thick clots and pus; gangrene of gland and teat in peracute form. Systemic reaction with anorexia, toxemia, fever, ruminal stasis

Clinical pathology Culture individual cow milk sample (composite or quarter) or polymerase chain reaction (higher sensitivity); indirect tests are high SCC and California mastitis test results.

Necropsy findings Peracute, acute, and chronic (recurrent) clinical mastitis, subclinical mastitis common

Diagnostic confirmation Culture milk for pathogen

Differential diagnosis

- Peracute mastitis
- Peracute coliform mastitis
- *Trueperella* (formerly *Arcanobacterium* or *Corynebacterium*) *pyogenes* mastitis
- Parturient paresis
- Acute and chronic mastitis. Not clinically distinguishable from other causes of mastitis. Must culture milk

Treatment

- **Lactating cows:** Cure rates for lactating cows with subacute staphylococcal mastitis less than 50%. Intramammary infusions daily for at least 3 days, preferably 5–8 days

- **Peracute mastitis:** Antimicrobial agents parenterally and intramammary that are β-lactamase resistant, fluid and electrolyte therapy
- **Dry cow therapy:** Chronic or subclinical mastitis best treated at drying off with long-acting intramammary antimicrobial infusions that are β-lactamase resistant

Control

- Prevent new infections by early identification, culling infected cows, and good milking procedures, including hygienic washing and drying of udders and teats before milking and postmilking germicidal teat dips. Regular milking machine maintenance. Consider segregation of infected cows.
- Eliminate existing infections by dry cow therapy.
- Immunization with vaccines may be possible in future.

SCC, somatic cell count.

ETIOLOGY

Coagulase-positive *S. aureus* is a major pathogen of the bovine mammary gland and a common cause of contagious mastitis in cattle. It also causes mastitis in sheep and goats.

EPIDEMIOLOGY

Occurrence and Prevalence of Infection

Coagulase-Positive Staphylococci

Historically, *S. aureus* was one of the most common causes of bovine mastitis in dairy cattle worldwide. In the last 25 years, the prevalence of infection and the occurrence of clinical mastitis caused by *S. aureus* has decreased in herds using effective mastitis control measures. However, surveys indicate that 50% to 100% of herds may be infected. In low-SCC herds, the prevalence of infection in cows ranges from 1% to 10%. In other herds, especially those with high SCCs, up to 50% of cows may be infected with *S. aureus,* with quarter infection rates ranging from 10% to 25%. The prevalence of infection of *S. aureus* in heifers at parturition can range from 5% to 15%. **The majority of intramammary infections caused by *S. aureus* are subclinical.** The incidence of clinical mastitis caused by *S. aureus* is dependent on its prevalence of infection in the herd. With an effective mastitis control program, the most common causes of clinical mastitis are the environmental pathogens. However, in some herds with a low rolling SCC, incidence of clinical mastitis caused by *S. aureus* ranges from 190 to 240 cases per 100 cows per year, with about 47% of the clinical cases being *S. aureus.*

Source of Infection and Method of Transmission

S. aureus is ubiquitous in the environment of dairy cattle. The infected mammary gland of lactating cows is the major reservoir and source of the organism. The prevalence of intramammary infection in primiparous heifers at parturition ranges from 2% to 50% and may represent an important reservoir of infection in herds with a low prevalence of infection. The organism may be present on the skin of the teats and external orifices of heifers, bedding materials, feedstuffs, housing materials, nonbovine animals on the farm, and equipment. In herds with a high prevalence of infection (>10% of cows), the organism was present in bedding, the hands and noses of dairy herd workers, insects, and water supplies. Transmission between cows occurs at the time of milking by contaminated milkers' hands and teat cup liners. Although *S. aureus* can multiply on the surface of the skin and provide a source of infection for the udder, the teat skin lesions are usually infected originally from the udder, and teat skin is a minor source of infection. In herds with a low prevalence of infection, most new cases of *S. aureus* mastitis may be from extramammary sources rather than indicating cow-to-cow transmission.[1]

The horn fly (*Hameotobia irritans*) is an important vector for transmitting *S. aureus* mastitis in heifers, particularly in heifers with scabs on the teat ends. Prevention of high populations of flies in heifers is therefore needed to decrease new infections in this group.[2]

Risk Factors

Animal Risk Factors

Several animal risk factors influence the prevalence of infection and the occurrence of clinical mastitis caused by *S. aureus.*

Local Defense Mechanisms

Abrasions of the teat orifice epithelium are an important risk factor for *S. aureus* mastitis. In experiments, teat canal infection or colonization may develop in 93% of experimentally abraded teat canal orifices compared with 53% in control quarters. Chapping of the teats and thickness of the teat barrel are correlated and significantly influence recovery of *S. aureus* from the skin.

Colonization With Minor Pathogens

The presence of minor pathogens such as CNS protects against new intramammary infections associated with the major pathogen *S. aureus.* This may be the result of an elevated SCC or an antimicrobial-like substance provided by the CNS that inhibits the growth of *S. aureus.* Conversely, quarters infected with CNS may be more susceptible to new infections with *S. agalactiae.* Quarters that are infected with *C. bovis* are protected against *S. aureus* infection but not against most streptococcal species.

Parity of Cow

The prevalence of intramammary infection and subclinical infection caused by *S. aureus* increases with the parity of the cow. This is probably from the increased opportunity of infection with time and the prolonged duration of infection, especially in a herd without a mastitis control program.

Presence of Other Diseases

The presence of periparturient diseases such as dystocia, parturient paresis, retained placenta, and ketosis has been identified as a risk factor for mastitis. The occurrence of sole ulcers in multiple digits may be associated with *S. aureus* in the first lactation.

Heredity

Experimentally, the presence of certain bovine lymphocyte antigens increased the susceptibility to *S. aureus* infection, but heritability estimates of susceptibility after experimental challenge were low and unstable.

Immune System

The infection rate of *S. aureus* is dependent on the ability of the immune system to recognize and to eliminate the bacteria. Staphylococcal antibodies are present in the blood of infected cows, but they appear to afford little protection against mastitis associated with *S. aureus.* This may be because of the low titer of the antibodies in the milk. Antibody titers in the serum rise with age and after an attack of mastitis.

The development or persistence of *S. aureus* mastitis depends on the interaction between invading bacteria and the host's defense system, principally the somatic cells in an infected gland, which are more than 95% polymorphonuclear cells. The number of bacteria isolated from milk samples of *S. aureus*-infected mammary glands is characterized by a cyclic increase and decrease concomitant with an inverse cycling of the SCC. This relationship between SCC and numbers of bacteria indicates that the cells within the mammary gland have a central role in the pathogenesis of *S. aureus* infection. There appear to be qualitative changes in the ability of the animal's somatic cells to phagocytose the bacteria. During the period of high SCC, the cells are able to kill bacteria 9000 times more efficiently than during the low-SCC period. The relative inability of the polymorphonuclear cells to kill bacteria during the low-SCC period may explain the source of reinfection. Phagocytosis and killing of the bacteria may also be inefficient because of low concentrations of opsonins, a lack of energy source, and the presence of casein and fat globules in the milk. The function of the intramammary polymorphonuclear cell (somatic cells) may also be affected by immunosuppression induced by cortisol and dexamethasone in treated cows.

Environmental and Management Risk Factors

Several herd-level management risk factors are important for the spread of *S. aureus.*

Poor teat and udder cleaning can allow spread of the organism among quarters of the same cow, and can allow contamination of milking units, which are commonly transferred among cows without washing or rinsing. The use of high-line parlors is a risk; this may be caused by the greater fluctuation in vacuum, especially when units are removed, leading to a greater occurrence of teat-end impacts in which bacteria in the milking unit may enter the teat canal to establish a new udder infection.

Extensive surveys reveal that management procedures that are most effective in reducing infection rates and cell counts associated with infections with *S. aureus* are

- Postmilking teat dipping
- Maintaining a good supply of dry bedding for housed cows
- Thorough disinfection of the teat orifice before infusing intramammary preparations
- Milking clinical cases last

Failure to use these management techniques will increase the risk of intramammary infection with *S. aureus*.

Pathogen Risk Factors

Virulence Factors

It has been known since 1961 that a variety of strains of *S. aureus* associated with clinical mastitis exist and that some of these strains appear to be more infectious within a herd, differing in the severity of clinical signs and persistence of infection.[3–9] *S. aureus* has several virulence factors that account for its pathogenicity and persistence in mammary tissue in spite of adequate defense mechanisms and antimicrobial therapy. **Most isolates from cattle appear to be host adapted and different from human *S. aureus* isolates.** *S. aureus* has the ability to **colonize the epithelium** of the teat and the streak canal and can adhere and bind to epithelial cells of the mammary gland. The specific binding is to the extracellular matrix proteins fibronectin and collagen, which can induce the epithelial cell to internalize the organism, protecting it from both exogenous and endogenous bactericidal factors. Some strains of *S. aureus* are capable of **invading bovine mammary epithelial cells** in culture, and the invasion process requires eukaryotic nucleic acid and protein synthesis as well as bacterial synthesis.

Some strains of *S. aureus* produce **toxins**, some of which may cause **phagocytic dysfunction**. The β-toxin, or a combination of α- and β-toxins, is produced by most pathogenic strains isolated from cattle, but its pathogenic significance is uncertain. The β-toxin damages bovine mammary secretory epithelial cells, increases the damaging effects of α-toxin, increases the adherence of *S. aureus* to mammary epithelial cells, and increases the proliferation of the organism. All strains produce **coagulase** (hence the term coagulase-positive *S. aureus*), which converts fibrinogen into fibrin; this appears to assist the invasion of tissues. **Leukocidin** produced by *S. aureus* may inactivate neutrophils. There is one report in a small number of cases that the presence of small colonies on bacterial culture (reflecting a slower rate of growth) is associated with chronic mastitis in cattle.[10]

Many staphylococcal strains (coagulase negative and coagulase positive) are able to produce an **extracellular exopolysaccharide layer** surrounding the cell wall called a **biofilm**. This capsular structure and its production of slime have been associated with virulence against host defense mechanisms because it facilitates bacterial adherence and colonization on mammary glandular epithelial cells and provides a protective "blanket" against immunologic attack and barrier to antibiotic diffusion. In addition, bacteria contained in a biofilm can have a low metabolic rate and therefore be less susceptible to antibiotic activity.[11–14] Biofilm-forming ability has been identified in 36% to 38% of cows with subclinical *S. aureus* mastitis.[12,14]

A major pathogenic factor is the ability of the organism to colonize and produce microabscesses in the mammary gland so that it is protected from normal defense mechanisms, including phagocytic activity from neutrophils. The difficulty in removing staphylococci from an infected quarter is largely caused by the bacteria's ability to survive in intracellular sites. There is also an ability to convert to a **nonsusceptible L-form** when exposed to antimicrobial agents and to return to standard forms when the antimicrobial is withdrawn.

Genotype of Strains

Phage typing and ribotyping can be used to classify strains from clinical and subclinical *S. aureus* mastitis. **DNA fingerprinting techniques,** using PCR, are also being used to differentiate various strains of the organism. A large number of different types of *S. aureus* can be isolated from cases of bovine mastitis, but a few types predominate within different countries. Surveys have found that only a small number of genotypes cause most cases of *S. aureus* mastitis, which may be useful information in determining the dynamics of infection in a herd and how infection spreads from cow to cow. Fine-structure molecular epidemiologic analysis of *S. aureus* recovered from cows in the United States and Ireland indicates that only a few specialized clones of *S. aureus* are responsible for the majority of cases of bovine mastitis and that these clones have a broad geographic distribution. **A predominant strain is usually responsible for most clinical and subclinical *S. aureus* infections in a herd**, and it is currently thought that *S. aureus* is a clonal organism that spreads from cow to cow.[3,5,6] Moreover, most strains isolated from milk are different from strains isolated from the teat skin. In other words, most *S. aureus* strains isolated from mastitis demonstrate both host and site specificity. This has important implications in the control of mastitis associated with *S. aureus*, because a rational and effective strategy for control of intramammary infections should be directed against clones that commonly cause disease.

Methicillin-Resistant Staphylococcus Aureus

The increased concern about nosocomial **methicillin-resistant *S. aureus* (MRSA)** infections in human medicine and small animal practice[15] has led to surveys of MRSA prevalence in cattle with mastitis. In a study of 207 clinical mastitis cases in Iran, 20% were caused by *S. aureus* and 2.4% were caused by MRSA.[16] In 36 cows with subclinical mastitis in Brazil, 11% of infections were caused by MRSA,[17] and in Serbia 5% of 213 *S. aureus* isolates were identified as MRSA.[18] There are no data available indicating that the clinical course of MRSA mastitis episodes in cattle differs from episodes caused by methicillin-susceptible strains of *S. aureus;* however, MRSA isolation in Italian herds was more likely to be isolated in herds with low *S. aureus* prevalence, with 9% of *S. aureus* isolates being MRSA.[19]

Economic Importance

The overall prevalence of mastitis caused by *S. aureus* is much higher than for *S. agalactiae,* and the need for culling causes much greater economic consequences. The risk of new infections is a continuing concern. Response to treatment is comparatively poor, and satisfactory methods for the eradication of staphylococcal mastitis from infected herds have yet to be devised.

Zoonotic Implications

The presence of *S. aureus* in market milk may present a degree of risk to the consumer because of the organism's capacity to produce enterotoxins and a toxic shock syndrome toxin, which cause serious food poisoning. Mastitic milk does not constitute any large risk for *S. aureus* enterotoxin food poisoning.

PATHOGENESIS

The disease can be reproduced experimentally by the injection of *S. aureus* organisms into the udder of cattle and sheep, but there is considerable variation in the type of mastitis produced. This does not seem to be caused by differences in virulence of the strains used, although strain variations do occur, but may be related to the size of the inoculum used or, more probably, to the lactational status of the udder at the time of infection. It is possible to induce *S. aureus* infection in the bovine teat cistern; the teat tissues are able to mount a marked local inflammatory response, but in spite of large numbers of neutrophils that invade the teat they are unable to control the infection, except when the numbers of bacteria are low.

Infection during early lactation may result in the peracute form of mastitis, with gangrene of the udder. During the later stages of lactation or during the dry period new infections are not usually accompanied by a systemic reaction but result in the chronic or acute forms. Chronic *S. aureus* mastitis in cows has been converted to the peracute, gangrenous form by the experimental production of systemic neutropenia.

In the **gangrenous form** the death of tissue is precipitated by thrombosis of veins causing local edema and congestion of the udder. *S. aureus* is the only bacteria that commonly causes this reaction in the udder of the cow, and the resulting toxemia is caused by bacterial toxins and tissue destruction. Secondary invasion by *E. coli* and *Clostridium* spp. contributes to the severity of the lesion and production of gas.

The pathogenesis of acute and chronic *S. aureus* mastitis in the cow is the same; the variation occurs only in degree of involvement of mammary tissue. In both forms each focus commences with an acute stage characterized by proliferation of the bacteria in the collecting ducts and, to a lesser extent, in the alveoli. In **acute** mastitis the small ducts are quickly blocked by fibrin clots, leading to more severe involvement of the obstructed area.

In the **chronic** form there are fewer foci of inflammation, and the reaction is milder; the inflammation is restricted to the epithelium of the ducts. This subsides within a few days and is replaced by connective tissue proliferations around the ducts, leading to their blockage and atrophy of the drained area. The leukocyte infiltration into the stroma, the epithelial lining, and the lumina indicate an obvious deficiency of secretory and synthesizing capacity caused by limitation of the alveolar lumina and the distension of the stroma area.

A characteristic of chronic *S. aureus* mastitis that is important in its diagnosis is the cyclical shedding of the bacteria from the affected quarter. Paralleling this variation is a cyclical rise and fall in the number of polymorphonuclear cells in the milk and their capacity to phagocytose bacteria. In some cases abscesses develop and botryomycosis of the udder, in which granulomata develop containing gram positive cocci in an amorphous eosinophilic mass, is also seen.

CLINICAL FINDINGS

Chronic *Staphylococcus aureus* Mastitis

The most important losses are caused by the chronic form or subclinical form of mastitis. Although 50% of cattle in a herd may be affected, only a few animals will have abnormalities recognizable by the milker. Many cases are characterized by a slowly developing induration and atrophy with the occasional appearance of clots in the milk or wateriness of the first streams. The SCC of the milk is increased, as well as the CMT results of infected quarters, but the disease may go unnoticed until much of the functional capacity of the gland is lost. The infection can persist and the disease may progress slowly over a period of many months.

Acute and Peracute *Staphylococcus aureus* Mastitis

Acute and peracute staphylococcal mastitis are rare but do occur and can be fatal, even if aggressively treated. **Acute *S. aureus* mastitis** is most common in early lactation. There is severe swelling of the gland, and the milk is purulent or contains many thick clots. Extensive fibrosis and severe loss of function always result.

Peracute *S. aureus* mastitis occurs usually in the first few days after calving and is highly fatal. There is a severe systemic reaction with elevation of the temperature to 41°C to 42°C (106°F–107°F), rapid heart rate (100–120 beats/min), complete anorexia, profound depression, absence of ruminal movements, and muscular weakness, often to the point of recumbency. The onset of the systemic and local reactions is sudden. The cow may be normal at one milking and recumbent and comatose at the next. The affected quarter is grossly swollen, hard and sore to touch, and causes severe lameness on the affected side.

Gangrene is a constant development and may be evident very early. A bluish discoloration develops that may eventually spread to involve the floor of the udder and the whole or part of the teat, or may be restricted to patches on the sides and floor of the udder. Within 24 hours the gangrenous areas become black and ooze serum and may be accompanied by subcutaneous emphysema and the formation of blisters. The secretion is reduced to a small amount of bloodstained serous fluid without odor, clots, or flakes. Unaffected quarters in the same cow are often swollen, and there may be extensive subcutaneous edema in front of the udder caused by thrombosis of the mammary veins. Toxemia is profound, and death usually occurs unless early, appropriate treatment is provided. Even with early treatment the quarter is invariably lost and the gangrenous areas slough. Separation begins after 6 to 7 days, but without interference the gangrenous part may remain attached for weeks. After separation, pus drains from the site for many more weeks before healing finally occurs.

CLINICAL PATHOLOGY

Culture of Individual Cow Milk

Bacteriologic culture of milk is the best method for identifying cows with *S. aureus* intramammary infection. A problem in the laboratory identification of *S. aureus* is that **bacteria are shed cyclically from infected quarters, thus a series of samples are necessary to increase overall test sensitivity when culture is used**. The sensitivity of a composite (4-quarter) sample may be as low as 53%, but it is higher when performed on a quarter basis.[20] Factors that have the greatest impact on the sensitivity of culture, in order of importance, are the

- Type of milk sample
- Volume of milk cultured
- Time interval between repeated milk sample collection strategies

Quarter samples taken on day 1 and repeated either on day 3 or day 4, and cultured separately using 0.1 mL of milk for culture inoculum, were predicted to have sensitivities of 90% to 95% and 94% to 99%, respectively. Repeated quarter samples collected daily and cultured separately gave a sensitivity of 97% and a specificity from 97% to 100%. Culturing of composite milk samples instead of individual quarter samples increases the number of false-negative results in diagnosing *S. aureus* mastitis, but the sensitivity of composite samples can be increased by using 0.05 mL of milk for inoculation instead of 0.01 mL, which is the volume recommended by the National Mastitis Council (NMC). Freezing of milk samples before processing either does not affect the bacterial count or enhances it by about 200%; the latter response is attributed to fracturing of cells containing viable *S. aureus* bacteria. Bacterial counts of more than 200 CFU/mL are commonly used as a criterion for a positive diagnosis of infection.

Milk is typically plated onto sheep blood agar plates to facilitate the growth of a large range of potentially pathogenic microorganisms, but this does not facilitate the growth of all known pathogens. Biochemical tests such as a positive coagulase test and a positive catalase test are routinely used to differentiate *S. aureus* from other gram-positive cocci. *S. aureus* grows very well on sheep blood agar and typically produces a zone of incomplete lysis of erythrocytes around the colony, which may contain an inner zone of complete lysis called double hemolysis.[21] The presence of double hemolysis is diagnostic for *S. aureus*, but colony types that do not demonstrate this morphology need a tube coagulase test to be positive to make a diagnosis of *S. aureus* mastitis with 100% specificity. However, it needs to be recognized that not all coagulase-positive staphylococci are *S. aureus*. Differentiation is best performed by subculturing colonies on sheep blood agar with complete hemolysis at 24 hours' incubation onto CHROMagar plates; *S. aureus* isolates grow on this media as mauve to rose colonies.[21]

MALDI-TOF MS shows great promise as a rapid method for accurately differentiating *S. aureus* from the other seven staphylococcal spp. that are coagulase positive by analyzing the metabolic signature of a bacterial colony in under 4 hours.[22]

The Pathoproof Mastitis **PCR assay** has the highest test sensitivity (91%) and specificity (99%) from cow-level composite samples,[20] and it may provide the preferred test method for composite milk samples when the trade-off between test cost, sensitivity, and specificity is evaluated.

Numerous immunodiagnostic tests have been developed to diagnose *S. aureus* mastitis, with an emphasis on rapid cowside diagnostic tests, but none of these tests has been able to achieve the appropriate balance between sensitivity, specificity, and cost.[23] Increased concentrations of haptoglobin and mammary-associated serum amyloid A occur in the milk of cows with *S. aureus* mastitis, accompanied by increases in serum concentrations of haptoglobin and serum amyloid A.[24]

Culture of Bulk Tank Milk

The culture of 0.3 mL of bulk tank milk for *S. aureus* using special Baird–Parker culture media is a practical method for detecting the organism in bulk tank milk and monitoring its spread in dairy herds; the sensitivity and specificity for detection of the bacteria ranged from 90% to 100%.

Somatic Cell Counts and California Mastitis Test

In an attempt to decrease the cost of sampling all quarters for culture, an alternative strategy is to use the SCC as a screening test to identify which cows to culture for *S. aureus*. For all intramammary infections, the sensitivity and specificity of SCC range from 15% to 40% and 92% to 99%, respectively. Composite milk sample SCCs have a low sensitivity, ranging from 31% to 54% for detecting cows with *S. aureus*. Individual quarter SCCs have a higher sensitivity, ranging from 71% to 95% depending on the study and cut point chosen, but quarter sampling is impractical because SCC is usually performed on a composite sample. Both composite and quarter milk SCC testing result in an unacceptably high proportion of infected cows being missed, and are therefore not currently recommended as a screening test if the goal is to identify all cows with an *S. aureus* intramammary infection in the herd.

CMT has also been used as a screening test to identify quarters or cows to culture. Using a CMT trace, 1, 2, or 3 to indicate the presence of an intramammary *S. aureus* infection produced a range of sensitivities from 0.47 to 0.96 and specificities of 0.41 to 0.80.[20]

In summary, culture of quarter milk samples (preferably) or a composite milk sample is superior to a quarter SCC or CMT for the diagnosis of *S. aureus* intramammary infection. Culture is strongly preferred if it is important to identify all positive cows in a herd because the sensitivity of indirect tests (such as SCC and CMT) is inadequate.

Enzyme-Linked Immunosorbent Assays for Antibody in Milk

ELISA tests for detecting *S. aureus* antibody in milk have been developed but are not widely used. Rapid laboratory tests incorporating these ELISAs, including the Staph-Zym test, have demonstrated 84% to 90% accuracy in identifying staphylococci.

Acriflavine Disk Assay

The acriflavine disk assay is a practical, accurate method for differentiating *S. aureus* isolates from non–*S. aureus* staphylococci.

NECROPSY FINDINGS

In peracute staphylococcal mastitis, the affected quarter is grossly swollen and may contain bloodstained milk dorsally but only serosanguineous fluid ventrally. There is extreme vascular engorgement and swelling, often progressing to moist gangrene of the overlying skin. Bacteria are not isolated from the bloodstream or tissues other than the mammary tissue and regional lymph nodes. Histologically, there is coagulation necrosis of glandular tissue and thrombosis of veins.

In milder forms of staphylococcal mastitis the invading organisms often elicit a granulomatous response. Microscopically, such "botryomycotic" cases are characterized by granulomas with a central bacterial colony and by progressive fibrosis of the quarter.

Samples for Confirmation of Diagnosis

- Bacteriology: chilled mammary tissue, regional lymph node
- Histology: fixed mammary tissue

DIFFERENTIAL DIAGNOSIS

Because of the occurrence of the peracute form in the first few days after parturition, the intense depression, and inability to rise, the dairy producer may conclude that the cow has **parturient paresis**, which is characterized by weakness, recumbency, hypothermia, rumen stasis, dilated pupils, tachycardia with weak heart sounds, and a rapid response to intravenous calcium gluconate. The mammary gland is usually normal in parturient paresis.

Peracute *S. aureus* mastitis is characterized by marked tachycardia, fever, weakness, and evidence of severe clinical mastitis with swelling, heat, abnormal milk with serum and blood, and sometimes gas in the teat and often with gangrene of the teat up to the base of the udder. Other bacterial types of mastitis, particularly *Escherichia coli* and *Trueperella pyogenes,* may cause severe systemic reactions, but gangrene of the quarter is less common.

Peracute coliform mastitis is a much more common cause of severe mastitis than *S. aureus* mastitis. The chronic and acute forms of staphylococcal mastitis are indistinguishable clinically from many other bacterial types of mastitis, and bacteriologic examination is necessary for identification.

TREATMENT

The bacteriologic cure rates for the treatment of *S. aureus* mastitis with either intramammary infusion or parenteral antimicrobial administration are notoriously less than satisfactory, particularly in the lactating cow. Bacteriologic cure rates after antimicrobial treatment seldom exceed 50%, and infections commonly persist throughout the lifetime of the cow. There are three likely reasons: inadequate penetration of the antimicrobial agent to the site of infection, formation of L-forms of *S. aureus,* and β-lactamase production.

Inadequate Penetration of Antimicrobial Agent

There is **inadequate penetration of the antimicrobial agent** into the site of intramammary infection in the lactating cow, and the organism survives in phagocytes that are inaccessible. There may also be inactivation of the antimicrobial by milk and serum constituents, and the formation of L-forms of the organism during treatment, varying between 0% and 80% of bacteria.

Antimicrobial Resistance

Antimicrobial-resistant strains of *S. aureus* occur in specific geographic regions because of predominant *S. aureus* clones and are often β-lactamase producers; the enzyme confers resistance to β-lactam antimicrobial agents such as penicillin G, penethamate hydriodide, ampicillin, and amoxicillin.[25] This emphasizes the need for knowledge of local epidemiologic factors when determining treatment in cases in which the results of culture and susceptibility testing are not available. Cloxacillin and nafcillin are effective, but only against gram-positive bacteria; they are less effective against nonlactamase staphylococci. Clavulanic acid added to amoxicillin overcomes this β-lactamase resistance as does **cloxacillin** added to ampicillin, and this is made use of in a popular intramammary formulation. First- and third-generation cephalosporins and erythromycin are effective against β-lactamase–producing staphylococci, and first- and third-generation cephalosporins are also effective against gram-negative bacteria. A cephapirin dry cow product administered to heifers with *S. aureus* infections resulted in bacteriologic cure and left the quarters clear well into their first lactation. Intramammary cloxacillin and ampicillin is generally considered to be the preferred initial treatment for *S. aureus* mastitis because β-lactamase production by *S. aureus* is sufficiently common.

Antimicrobial therapy for *S. aureus* subclinical mastitis during the lactating period is not economically attractive because of low bacteriologic cure rates, discarding of milk during the withholding period, and the lack of an economically beneficial increase in production following treatment. Dry cow treatment at the end of lactation is much more effective, being successful in 40% to 70% of cases, although treatment should be attempted in heifers infected early in lactation. Cows that are infected with *S. aureus* should be appropriately identified, segregated if possible, and milked last or with separate milking units. Culling of infected cows is also an option for consideration, but a detailed economic analysis of this popular recommendation is lacking.

Lactating Cow Therapy

The treatment of clinical cases of *S. aureus* mastitis using intramammary antimicrobial infusions is less than satisfactory but is often done. However, clinical recovery following therapy does not necessarily eliminate the infection, and some of the published literature on cure rates has not made the distinction between clinical and bacteriologic cure rates. Generally, the cure rate depends on the duration of infection, the number of quarters infected, whether it is a hindquarter or front quarter, whether the strain of *S. aureus* is a β-lactamase producer, the immune status of the cow, the antimicrobial agent administered, and the duration of treatment. Current recommendations to ensure the best treatment success rate are to combine intramammary and parenteral antimicrobial treatment or **use extended intramammary treatment alone for 4 to 8 days**. Penicillin G is regarded as the antimicrobial agent of choice for *S. aureus* strains that are penicillin sensitive. Intramammary pirlimycin also has good clinical efficacy when administered as extended therapy for 8 days.[1] An additional advantage of extended therapy with pirlimycin is decreased transmission of *S. aureus* infection within the herd and decreased incidence of strain-specific clinical mastitis within the herd.[1]

The following intramammary infusions, given daily at 24-hour intervals for 3 treatments (unless stated otherwise), have been used for the treatment of clinical cases of *S. aureus* mastitis, with expected clinical cure rates of about 27% to 60% in lactating cows. Subclinical cases are left until the cow is dried off:

- Sodium cloxacillin (200–600 mg for three infusions)
- Tetracyclines (400 mg)
- Penicillin-streptomycin combination (100,000 units, 250 mg)
- Penicillin-tylosin combination (100,000 units, 240 mg)
- Novobiocin (250 mg per infusion for three infusions)
- Cephalosporins (most strains of *S. aureus* are sensitive to cephapirin)
- Cefquinome (75 mg per infusion for three infusions; fourth-generation cephalosporin)
- Pirlimycin-extended therapy (eight 50-mg doses, 24 hours apart, for 8 days)

In a study of 184 cases of subclinical *S. aureus* mastitis in New York, commercially available intramammary infusions were not significantly more effective than untreated controls (43% bacteriologic cure), with the following bacteriologic cure rates: erythromycin (65%), penicillin (65%), cloxacillin (47%), amoxicillin (43%), and cephapirin (43%). In a multicentered randomized clinical trial in Europe, extended intramammary treatment with cefquinome improved clinical cure in lactating dairy cattle from 60% (three infusions 12 hours apart) to 84% (additional three infusions 24 hours apart), but did not alter bacteriologic cure.[26]

A slightly more effective treatment for subclinical *S. aureus* intramammary infection, with a cure rate of 50%, is simultaneous intramammary infusion of amoxicillin (62.5 mg) and intramuscular injection of procaine penicillin G (9,000,000 units). This study was the first to demonstrate that combined parenteral and intramammary therapy was more effective than intramammary infusion alone. Because of the persistence of the infection in each herd, the final choice of the antimicrobial to be used should be based on a culture and susceptibility test; the latter is to determine whether the predominant *S. aureus* strain in the herd is a β-lactamase producer; this is because **β-lactamase–producing strains are harder to cure and require a specific antibiotic protocol**. The bacteriologic cure rate for penicillin-sensitive infections treated with parenteral and intramammary penicillin G was 76%, compared with β-lactamase–producing strains treated with parenteral and intramammary amoxicillin-clavulanic acid (29%).

The application of cytokines as an adjunct to antimicrobial therapy may help to increase the number of phagocytes in the mammary gland and enhance cell function. The experimental intramammary infusion of recombinant interleukin into infected or uninfected mammary glands elicited an influx of polymorphonuclear leukocytes exhibiting subsequent enhanced activity and increased the cure rate 20% to 30% in quarters infected with *S. aureus*.

A novel method for decreasing the transmission of *S. aureus* within a herd is to **selectively cease lactation in infected quarters of lactating cattle**. The best method for permanently drying off a quarter is infusion of 120 mL of 5% povidone iodine solution (0.5% iodine) after complete milk out and administration of flunixin meglumine (1 mg/kg BW, intravenously). Therapeutic cessation of milk production in one quarter does not alter daily milk production but does decrease individual cow SCC and its contribution to the bulk tank milk SCC. The final outcome of selectively drying off infected quarters is a decrease in the rate of new intramammary infections in the herds and a lowering in the bulk tank milk SCC.

Peracute Mastitis

Early parenteral treatment of peracute cases with adequate does of antimicrobials such as trimethoprim-sulfonamide or penicillin is deemed necessary to improve the survival rate. When penicillin is used the initial intramuscular injection should be supported by an intravenous dose of crystalline penicillin, with subsequent intramuscular doses to maintain the highest possible blood level of the antimicrobial over a 4- to 6-day period; tamethicillin or penethamate hydriodide are preferred to achieve this. Intramammary infusions are of little value in such cases because of failure of the drugs to diffuse into the gland. The intravenous administration of large quantities of electrolyte solutions is also recommended. Hypertonic saline, as recommended for peracute coliform mastitis, has not yet been evaluated but may be indicated. Frequent massage of the udder with hot wet packs and milking out the affected gland is recommended. Oxytocin is used to promote letdown but is relatively ineffective in severely inflamed glands. Surgical amputation of the teat may be indicated to promote drainage of the gland, but only in cows with necrotic teats.

Dry Cow Therapy

It has become a common practice to leave chronic *S. aureus* cases until they are dried off before attempting to eliminate the infection. The material is infused into each gland after the last milking of the lactation and left in situ. The major benefits of dry cow therapy are the **elimination of existing intramammary infections** and **prevention of new intramammary infections during the dry period**. In addition, milk is not discarded and bacteriologic cure rates are superior to those obtained during lactation.

The factors associated with a bacteriologic cure after dry cow therapy of subclinical *S. aureus* mastitis have been examined. The probability of cure of an infected quarter *decreased* when

- SCC increased (>250,000 cells/mL)[26]
- Age of cow increased
- Another quarter was infected in the same cow
- Infection was in a hindquarter
- The percentage of samples that were positive for *S. aureus* was higher before drying off

Cows with more than one infected quarter were 0.6 times less likely to be cured than cows with one infected quarter. The cure rate of quarters affected with *S. aureus* can be predicted using a formula that considers several cow factors and quarter factors. The prediction of the probability of cure in an 8-year-old cow with three quarters infected with the organism and an SCC of 2,300,000 is 36%. In a 3-year-old cow with one quarter infected and an SCC of 700,000, the probability of cure is 92%. This information is often available at drying off and can be used to select cows that are unlikely to be cured to be removed from the herd by designating them as "do not breed" and culling when it is economically opportune.

Most intramammary antimicrobial infusions are satisfactory for dry cow therapy provided they are combined with slow-release bases. Bacteriologic cure rates vary between herds from 25% to 75% and average about 50%. The use of parenteral antimicrobials such as oxytetracycline along with an intramammary infusion of cephapirin did not improve the cure rate for *S. aureus.*

CONTROL

Because of the relatively poor results obtained in the treatment of staphylococcal mastitis, any attempt at control must depend heavily on effective methods of preventing the transmission of infection from cow to cow. *S. aureus* is a contagious pathogen, the udder is the primary site of infection, and hygiene in the milking parlor is of major importance. To reduce the source of the organism, a program of early **identification, culling, and segregation** is important to control *S. aureus* mastitis in a dairy herd, although successful implementation of all three aspects is challenging. Satisfactory control of *S. aureus* mastitis has historically been difficult and unreliable; however, at the present time the quarter infection rate can be rapidly and profitably reduced from the average level of 30% to 10% or less.

The strategies and practices described under the control of bovine mastitis later in this chapter are highly successful for the control of *S. aureus* mastitis when applied and maintained rigorously. The control program includes the following:

- Ensure optimal teat condition, particularly around the teat orifice.
- Hygienic washing and drying of udders before milking, wearing disposable gloves during milking
- Regular milking-machine maintenance
- Teat dipping after milking. Teat dipping in 1% iodine or 0.5% chlorhexidine, either in 5% to 10% glycerin, is effective against *S. aureus* mastitis. In vitro studies have demonstrated that bacteria can grow at concentrations of iodine at ≤0.1% and chlorhexidine at ≤0.0002%.[27] Teat dipping helps to eliminate infected quarters and reduces the new infection rate by 50% to 65% compared with controls, and the addition of glycerin to the teat dip improves teat and teat-orifice condition. The disinfection of hands or use of rubber gloves provides additional advantages.
- Dry cow treatment on all cows
- Culling cows with chronic mastitis
- Milking infected cows last (very difficult to implement in free-stall housing or pasture feeding)

An alternative but radical control strategy when all else has failed is to permanently dry off the infected quarter using a povidone iodine infusion.

Vaccination

Immunization against *S. aureus* mastitis has been widely researched for 100 years. Different vaccines based on cellular or soluble antigens with and without adjuvants have been given to dairy cows, but protection against infection and clinical disease has been unsatisfactory when used in the field. Currently available vaccines are autogenous bacterins (made to order using isolates from clinical cases on the farm), recombinant protein, DNA-recombinant protein, or contain one or more *S. aureus* strains that are thought to provide good cross-protection.[28] The goals of such vaccines are to decrease the severity of clinical signs and increase the cure rate, particularly when administered to heifers before they calve. Vaccination has also been used simultaneously with antimicrobial therapy during lactation or at dry off in an attempt to augment the cow's immune response, with mixed success. For example, combined administration of 3 doses of a polyvalent *S. aureus* bacterin over 21 days and intramammary administration of pirlimycin in all 4 quarters once daily for 5 days (days 16–20) eliminated *S. aureus* infection at a higher rate (40%) than untreated controls (9%).[29]

Based on published efficacy studies, currently available vaccines cannot be recommended as part of the routine measures for controlling *S. aureus* mastitis. Challenges with developing an effective vaccine include the intracellular location of infection, ability to produce a biofilm, and insufficient vaccine-induced opsinizing antibody in milk to facilitate phagocytosis and clearance of *S. aureus* from infected mammary gland tissue.[30,31]

Development of an effective *S. aureus* vaccine remains one of the most important issues confronting the control of infectious diseases in cattle.

TREATMENT AND CONTROL

Treatment

Treat mild to moderate clinical cases during lactation with penicillin G formulation if susceptibility is known, otherwise administer β-lactamase–resistant intramammary formulation; consider using extended therapy (R-1).

Treat moderate to severe clinical cases during lactation with parenteral β-lactamase antimicrobial (such as penethamate hydriodide) and intramammary formulation; consider using extended therapy (R-1).

Treat subclinical infections in freshly calved heifers with penicillin G formulation if susceptibility is known, otherwise administer β-lactamase–resistant intramammary formulation; consider using extended therapy (R-1).

Treat subclinical infections during lactation (R-3).

Control

Implement 10-point mastitis control plan (R-1).

Cull chronically infected *S. aureus* mastitis cows (R-1).

Blanket dry cow therapy with β-lactamase–resistant intramammary formulation (R-1)

Milk *S. aureus*-infected cows last (R-2).

Eradicate infection from herd (R-2).

Vaccinate using *S. aureus* bacterins (R-3).

FURTHER READING

Barkema HW, Schukken YH, Zadoks RN. Invited Review: the role of cow, pathogen, and treatment regimen in the therapeutic success of bovine *Staphylococcus aureus* mastitis. *J Dairy Sci.* 2006;89:1877-1895.

Keefe G. Update on control of *Staphylococcus aureus* and *Streptococcus agalactiae* for management of mastitis. *Vet Clin North Am Food Anim Pract.* 2012;28:203-216.

Scali F, Camussone C, Calvinho LF, et al. Which are important targets in development of *S. aureus* mastitis vaccine? *Res Vet Sci.* 2015;100:88-99.

Zecconi A. *Staphylococcus aureus* mastitis: what we need to know to control them. *Israel J Vet Med.* 2010;65:93-99.

REFERENCES

1. Barlow JW, et al. *BMC Vet Res.* 2013;9:28.
2. Ryman VE, et al. *Res Vet Sci.* 2013;95:343.
3. Anderson KL, et al. *Am J Vet Res.* 2006;67:1185.
4. Fournier C, et al. *Res Vet Sci.* 2008;85:439.
5. Graber HU, et al. *J Dairy Sci.* 2009;92:1442.
6. Capurro A, et al. *Vet J.* 2010;185:188.
7. Oliveira L, et al. *Am J Vet Res.* 2011;72:1361.
8. Piccinini R, et al. *J Dairy Res.* 2012;79:249.
9. Lundberg A, et al. *Acta Vet Scand.* 2014;56:2.
10. Atalla H, et al. *Foodborne Pathog Dis.* 2008;5:785.
11. Melchior MB, et al. *J Vet Med B.* 2006;53:326.
12. Oliveira M, et al. *Vet Microbiol.* 2006;118:133.
13. Oliveira M, et al. *Vet Microbiol.* 2007;124:187.
14. Snel GGM, et al. *Vet Microbiol.* 2014;174:489.
15. Middleton JR, et al. *J Clin Microbiol.* 2005;43:2916.
16. Jamali H, et al. *J Dairy Sci.* 2014;97:2226.
17. Silva NCC, et al. *Lett Appl Microbiol.* 2014;59:665.
18. Savic NR, et al. *Acta Vet Beograd.* 2014;64:115.
19. Luini M, et al. *Vet Microbiol.* 2015;178:270.
20. Mahmmod YS, et al. *Prev Vet Med.* 2013;112:309.
21. Graber Hu, et al. *Res Vet Sci.* 2013;95:38.
22. Motta CC, et al. *African J Microbiol Res.* 2014;8:3861.
23. Febres-Klein MH, et al. *Eur J Clin Microbiol Infect Dis.* 2014;33:2095.
24. Eckersall PD, et al. *J Dairy Sci.* 2006;89:1488.
25. Sakwinska O, et al. *Appl Environ Microbiol.* 2011;77:3428.
26. Swinkels JM, et al. *J Dairy Sci.* 2013;96:4983.
27. Azizoglu RO, et al. *J Dairy Sci.* 2013;96:993.
28. Pereira UP, et al. *Vet Microbiol.* 2011;148:117.
29. Smith GW, et al. *J Am Vet Med Assoc.* 2006;228:422.
30. Middleton JR, et al. *J Dairy Res.* 2006;73:10.
31. Middleton JR, et al. *Vet Microbiol.* 2009;134:192.

STREPTOCOCCUS AGALACTIAE

SYNOPSIS

Etiology *Streptococcus agalactiae* is a major pathogen of the mammary gland and a common cause of contagious bovine mastitis in some countries.

Epidemiology Major cause of mastitis in dairy herds without an effective mastitis control program. Prevalence of infection 10%–50% of cows and 25% of quarters. In herds with an effective control program there is a prevalence of less than 10% of cows. Has been eliminated from many herds with treatment and control. Highly contagious obligate pathogen. Infection is transmitted at milking.

Clinical findings Individual repeated episodes of subacute to acute mastitis are most common. Gland is swollen and warm, and milk is watery and contains clots. Gradual induration of udder if not treated

Clinical pathology Culture of individual cow milk samples or bulk tank milk samples. Latex agglutination test

Necropsy findings Not important

Diagnostic confirmation Latex agglutination test for specific identification of organism

Differential diagnosis Cannot differentiate clinically from other causes of acute and chronic mastitis. Must culture milk

Treatment Mastitis associated with *S. agalactiae* in lactating cows is sensitive to intramammary therapy with a wide variety of antimicrobial agents resulting in a high rate of clinical and bacteriologic cures. Blitz therapy (simultaneous treatment of all positive cows in a herd) is commonly used to reduce prevalence of infection in herd.

Control Eradication is possible. Identify and treat infected quarters, cull incurable cows. Premilking teat and udder sanitation, postmilking teat dipping, and dry cow therapy

ETIOLOGY

Streptococcus agalactiae infections with environmental streptococci are described in the next section.

EPIDEMIOLOGY

Occurrence and Prevalence of Infection

S. agalactiae was the major cause of mastitis before the antimicrobial era and is still a significant cause of chronic mastitis in which control procedures for contagious mastitis are not used. Herd prevalence rates of infection range from 11% to 47%. Typically, in a herd infected with the pathogen, the prevalence of infection could be as high as 50% of cows, but more recent surveys indicate much lower within-herd prevalences, ranging from 8% to 10%. Where good hygienic measures and the efficient treatment of clinical cases are in general use, the prevalence of infection within a herd will be less than 10% of cows. Following the use of antimicrobial agents, *S. agalactiae* was superseded by *S. aureus* and coagulase-negative *Staphylococcus* spp. as the major cause of bovine mastitis. In herds with a high bulk tank milk SCC, the probability is high that *S. agalactiae* infection is the most prevalent pathogen.

Source of Infection

S. agalactiae is a highly contagious obligate parasite of the bovine mammary gland. The main source of infection is the udder of infected cows, although when hygiene is poor contamination of the environment may provide an additional source. The teats and skin of cattle, milkers' hands, floors, utensils, and clothes are often heavily contaminated. Sores on teats are the most common sites outside the udder for persistence of the organism. The infection may persist for up to 3 weeks on hair and skin and on manure and bricks. The importance of environmental contamination as a source of infection is given due recognition in the general disinfection technique of eradication. Spread of infection between herds is most often associated with purchase of infected cows and heifers but can also result from hiring of relief milkers.[1]

Transmission of Infection

Transmission from animal to animal is most common from the medium of milking machine liners, hands, udder cloths, and possibly bedding.

The streak canal is the portal of entry, although there is doubt as to how invasion into the teat canal and then gland occurs. Suction into the teat during milking or immediately afterward does occur, but growth of the bacteria into the canal between milking also appears to be an important method of entry. It is difficult to explain why heifers that have never been milked may be found to be infected with *S. agalactiae,* although suckling between calves after ingestion of infected milk or contact with infected inanimate materials may be sources of infection.

Risk Factors

There is no particular breed susceptibility, but infection does become established more readily in older cows and in the early part of lactation. Poor hygiene, incompetent milking personnel, and faulty or maladjusted machinery are important risk factors. **The most important risk factors are the failure to use postmilking teat dip and the selective or nonuse of dry cow therapy**. The use of a common washrag or sponge is also a risk factor. Inadequate treatment of clinical cases of mastitis is also a frequent risk factor in infected herds.

S. agalactiae has the ability to adhere to the mammary gland tissue, and the specific microenvironment of the udder is necessary for growth of the organism. The virulence of various strains of the organism is related to differences in their ability to adhere to the mammary epithelium. Bacterial ribotyping has been used to characterize strains of the organism to determine their geographic distribution. The physical characteristics of the teat canal may influence the susceptibility to streptococcal infection. The mechanisms used by *S. agalactiae* to penetrate the teat canal are influenced more by the diameter of the teat canal lumen, as reflected by the peak flow rate, than by teat canal length.

Economic Importance

The disease is of major economic importance in milk production. In individual cows, the loss of production associated with *S. agalactiae* mastitis is about 25% during the infected lactation, and in affected herds the loss may be of the order of 10% to 15% of the potential production. Reduction of the productive life represents an average loss of one lactation per cow in an affected herd. Deaths caused by *S. agalactiae* infection rarely if ever occur, and complete loss of productivity of a quarter is uncommon; the losses are incurred in the less dramatic but no less important fashion of decreased production per cow.

PATHOGENESIS

When the primary barrier of the streak canal is passed, if bacteria are not flushed out by the physical act of milking they proliferate and invasion of the udder tissue follows. There is considerable variation between cows in the developments that occur at each of the three stages of invasion, infection, and inflammation. The reasons for this variation are not clear, but resistance appears to depend largely on the integrity of the lining of the teat canal. After the introduction of infection into the teat, the invasion, if it occurs, takes 1 to 4 days and the appearance of inflammation 3 to 5 days. Again there is much variation between cows in the response to tissue invasion, and a balance may be set up between the virulence of the organism and undefined defense mechanisms of the host so that very little clinically detectable inflammation may develop despite the persistence of a permanent bacterial flora.

The **development of mastitis** associated with *S. agalactiae* is essentially a process of invasion and inflammation of lobules of mammary tissue in a series of crises, particularly during the first month after infection. Each crisis develops in the same general pattern. Initially there is a rapid multiplication of the organism in the lactiferous ducts, followed by passage of the bacteria through the duct walls into lymphatic vessels and to the supramammary lymph nodes, and an outpouring of neutrophils into the milk ducts. At this stage of initial tissue invasion, a short-lived systemic reaction occurs, and the milk yield falls sharply as a result of inhibition and stasis of secretion caused by damage to acinar and ductal epithelium.

Fibrosis of the interalveolar tissue and involution of acini result even though the tissue invasion is quickly cleared. Subsequently, similar crises develop and more lobules are affected in the same way, resulting in a stepwise loss of secretory function with increasing fibrosis of the quarter and eventual atrophy.

The **clinicopathologic findings** vary with the stage of development of the disease. Bacterial counts in the milk are high in the early stages but fall when the SCC rises at the same time as swelling of the quarter becomes apparent. In some cases bacteria are not detectable culturally at this acute stage. The SCC rises by 10 to 100 times normal during the first 2 days after infection and returns to normal over the next 10 days. The febrile reaction is often sufficiently mild and short-lived to escape notice. When the inflammatory changes in the epithelial lining of the acini and ducts begin to subside, the shedding of the lining results in the clinical appearance of clots in the milk. Thus the major damage has already been done when clots are first observed. At the stage of acute swelling, it is the combination of inflamed interalveolar tissue and retained secretion in distended alveoli that causes the swelling. Removal of the retained secretion at this stage may considerably reduce the swelling and permit better diffusion of drugs infused into the quarter. Inflammatory reactions also occur in the teat wall of affected quarters.

The variations in resistance between cows and the increased susceptibility with advancing age are unexplained. Hormonal changes and hypersensitivity of mammary tissue to streptococcal protein have both been advanced as possible causes of the latter. Local immunity of mammary tissue after an attack probably does not occur, but there is some evidence to suggest that a low degree of general immunity may develop. The rapid disappearance of the infection in a small proportion of cows in contrast to the recurrent crises that are the normal pattern of development suggests that immunity does develop in some animals. The antibodies are hyaluronidase inhibitors and are markedly specific for specific strains of the organism. A nonspecific rise in other antibodies may occur simultaneously, and this is thought to account for the field observations that coincident streptococcal and staphylococcal infections are unusual and that the elimination of one infection may lead to an increased incidence of the other.

CLINICAL FINDINGS

In the experimentally produced disease, there is initially a sudden episode of acute mastitis, accompanied by a transient fever, followed at intervals by similar attacks, which are usually less severe. In natural cases fever, lasting for a day or two, is occasionally observed with the initial attack, but the inflammation of the gland persists and the subsequent crises are usually of a relatively mild nature. These degrees of severity may be classified as **abnormal cow** when the animal is febrile and off its feed; **abnormal gland** when the inflammation of the gland is severe, but there is no marked systemic reaction; and **abnormal secretion** when the gland is not greatly swollen, pain and heat are absent, and the presence of clots in watery foremilk may be the only apparent abnormality. Induration is most readily palpable at the udder cistern and in the lower part of the udder and varies in degree with the stage of development of the disease.

The milk yield of affected glands is markedly reduced during each crisis but, with proper treatment administered early, the yield may return to almost normal. Even without treatment the appearance of the milk soon becomes normal, but the yield is significantly reduced and subsequent crises are likely to reduce it further.

CLINICAL PATHOLOGY

The **CAMP test**, which has served as the universally used means of identifying *S. agalactiae* for many years, has been displaced by a commercial **latex agglutination test**, which contains specific reagents necessary for the identification of *S. agalactiae* and is suitable for general laboratory use. When used on isolates of samples from bulk tank milk, the sensitivity and specificity are 97.6% and 98.2%, respectively. An ELISA test correlates well with the bulk tank milk SCC and provides a suitable alternative.

The critical judgment to be made is deciding when the quarter infection rate is so high that control or eradication measures are necessary. A decision can be made on the basis of the bulk tank milk SCC as an indicator of the prevalence of mastitis on a quarter basis and on culture of the bulk tank milk sample to indicate that *S. agalactiae* is the important pathogen, but this approach is too inaccurate to be recommended. There seems to be no alternative to performing bacteriologic culture and determining SCC on milk samples from individual cows or quarters. Milk samples collected for bacteriologic examination for the presence of *S. agalactiae* can be stored in the frozen state. The number of samples that will be culturally positive when the stored frozen samples are thawed will either be unchanged or enhanced up to 200%; the latter response is attributing to fracturing of cellular debris containing *S. agalactiae*.

Culture From Bulk Tank Milk Samples

The presence of the organism in bulk tank milk is caused by shedding of bacteria from infected quarters, and cyclic shedding is typical. The specificity of culture from bulk tank milk is very high; the sensitivity is more variable and typically much lower but can be increased by using selective media. A rapid, real-time quantitative PCR assay, the PathoProof mastitis PCR, provides a useful herd test when performed on bulk tank milk, because the test detects both growth-inhibited and nonviable bacteria.[2] When used at a cycle threshold of <40 this PCR test can be considered as a positive; however, for cycle thresholds >40 bacteriologic culture is recommended to confirm the presence of infection. A quantitative PCR assay specific for *S. agalactiae* has been developed.[3]

Total Bacterial Count

The total bacterial count in bulk tank milk can be markedly increased because of the presence of *S. agalactiae* mastitis in the herd. Samples of bulk tank milk from infected herds commonly contain bacterial counts in the range of 20,000 to 100,000 CFU/mL, because a cow in the early stages of infection can shed up to 100,000,000 bacteria/mL. The standard plate count can drop from 100,000 to 2,000 CFU/mL after implementation of a modified blitz therapy and control program to control *S. agalactiae.*

Culture From Individual Cow Samples

Composite milk samples are satisfactory, because the number of cows identified as positive does not increase by quarter sampling. The sensitivity and specificity of a single culture from individual cows ranges between 95% and 100%.

Somatic Cell Count

S. agalactiae produces high SCC in individual cows, which has a significant influence on the bulk tank milk SCC.

NECROPSY FINDINGS

The gross and microscopic pathology of mastitis associated with *S. agalactiae* are not important in the diagnosis of the disease.

DIFFERENTIAL DIAGNOSIS

The clinical diagnosis of *S. agalactiae* mastitis depends entirely on the isolation of *S. agalactiae* from the milk. Differentiation from other types of acute and chronic mastitis is not possible clinically.

TREATMENT

S. agalactiae is **very sensitive to intramammary therapy** using a wide variety of commercially available intramammary infusion preparations. Systemic therapy is also effective but offers no advantages over the intramammary route. Clinical cases should be treated whenever they occur because of the need to prevent transmission to uninfected quarters and cows. Subclinical cases identified at any stage of lactation should be treated immediately because of the excellent response to treatment. Treatment of *S. agalactiae* mastitis with intramammary infusions will result in a high percentage of infections being eliminated economically and with few residual concerns, provided the milk withholding times are observed.

Infections at all stages of lactation have 90% to 100% cure rates with penicillin, erythromycin, cloxacillin, and cephalosporins. Gentamicin, neomycin, nitrofurazone, and polymyxin B have poor activity. Procaine penicillin G is universally used as a mammary infusion at a dose rate of 100,000 units. Higher dose rates have the disadvantage of increasing penicillin residues in the milk. A moderate increase in efficiency is obtained by using procaine penicillin rather than the crystalline product, and by using 100,000 units of penicillin in a long-acting base the cure rate (96%) is significantly better than with quick-acting preparations (83%).

To provide a broader spectrum of antimicrobial efficiency penicillin is often combined with other drugs that are more effective against gram-negative organisms. A mixture of penicillin (100,000 units) and novobiocin (150 mg) provides a cure rate ranging from 89% to 98%. It is necessary to maintain adequate milk levels for 72 hours: three infusions at intervals of 24 hours are recommended, but dosing with two infusions 72 hours apart, or one infusion of 100,000 units, in a base containing mineral oil and aluminum monostearate, gives similar results. As a general rule clinical cases should be treated with three infusions, and subclinical cases, particularly those detected by routine examination in a control program, with one infusion. Recovery, both clinically and bacteriologically, should be achieved in at least 90% of quarters if treatment has been efficient. Intramuscular administration of ceftiofur is not efficacious as a treatment to eliminate the organism, compared with intramammary infusion of penicillin (100,000 units) and novobiocin (150 mg) daily for two treatments. Likewise, intramuscular administration of penethamate hydriodide (5 g) was not as effective as a treatment to eliminate *S. agalactiae* compared with intramammary infusion of ampicillin (75 mg) and cloxacillin (200 mg) twice daily for 3 days.[4]

Other antimicrobial agents used in the treatment of *S. agalactiae* infections include the tetracyclines and cephalothin, which are as effective as penicillin and have the added advantage of a wider antibacterial spectrum, an obvious advantage when the type of infection is unknown. Neomycin is inferior to penicillin in the treatment of *S. agalactiae* mastitis, whereas tylosin and erythromycin appear to have equal efficacy. A single treatment with 300 mg of erythromycin is recommended as curing 100% of quarters infected with *S. agalactiae*. Lincomycin (200 mg) combined with neomycin (286 mg) and administered twice at 12-hour intervals also has good efficacy. In a study of 1927 cases of subclinical *S. agalactiae* mastitis in New York, all commercially available intramammary infusions were more effective than untreated controls (27% bacteriologic cure), with the following bacteriologic cure rates: amoxicillin (86%), erythromycin (81%), cloxacillin (77%), cephapirin (66%), penicillin (63%), hetacillin (62%), pirlimycin (44%).

In dry cows, one infusion is sufficient, and milk concentrations of penicillin remain high for 72 hours. Cloxacillin eliminated the organism from 98% and 100% of infected cows in two different studies.

Blitz Therapy

The prevalence of subclinical mastitis caused by *S. agalactiae* can be reduced more rapidly by treatment of infected cows during lactation than by dry cow therapy and postmilking teat dipping. *S. agalactiae* is one of the few pathogens causing subclinical mastitis that can be treated economically during lactation and can be eliminated from herds with **blitz antimicrobial therapy followed by good sanitation procedures**. All cows are sampled, and those that are positive are treated simultaneously with penicillin and novobiocin. Cows not responsive to the first treatment are identified and retreated or culled. Failure to institute sanitation procedures for the control of the pathogen may result in subsequent outbreaks of mastitis.

If blitz therapy of all infected cows is not possible because of the short-term effect of lost milk production on income, a modified treatment protocol is recommended. The herd is divided into two groups, based on a composite milk SCC of 500,000. Those cows in the high category are treated with 300 mg of erythromycin, intramammarily. When lactating cow numbers reach their lowest point, all animals are treated with the same product. At drying off, cows are treated with 500 mg of cloxacillin and 250 mg of ampicillin.

CONTROL

Eradication on a herd basis of mastitis associated with *S. agalactiae* is an accepted procedure and has been undertaken on an area scale in some countries. The control measures as outlined later in this chapter are designed especially for this disease and should be adopted in detail. If suitable hygienic barriers against infection can be introduced and if the infection can be eliminated from individual quarters by treatment, the disease is eradicable fairly simply and economically.

The control program consists of

- Identifying infected quarters
- Treating infected quarters on two occasions if necessary
- Culling incurable cows

The control program is particularly applicable in herds in which an unacceptable level of clinical cases is backed by a high incidence of subclinical infections. **Premilking teat and udder sanitation, postmilking teat dipping, and dry cow therapy** are vital aspects of the control program.

Vaccination

Vaccination against *S. agalactiae* has been attempted and elicits systemic hyperimmunity but no apparent intramammary resistance. Development of an effective vaccine will be difficult because of the multiplicity of strains involved and the known variability between animals in their reaction to intramammary infection.

Biosecurity

As with any eradication program a high degree of vigilance is required to maintain a "clean" status. This is particularly so with mastitis caused by *S. agalactiae*. Breakdowns are usually caused by the introduction of infected animals, even heifers that have not yet calved, or the employment of milkers who carry infection with them. Most dairy farms in the United States are in an ongoing process of herd expansion or replacement acquisition by the addition of purchased animals. Introduction of contagious mastitis associated with *S. agalactiae, S. aureus,* and *M. bovis* is a common result. It has been recommended that herd additions should be screened for these important pathogens; however, currently available screening tests do not have perfect sensitivity.

TREATMENT AND CONTROL

Treatment

Treat clinical cases during lactation with penicillin G formulation (R-1).

Consider blitz therapy of herd using intramammary formulation during lactation (R-2).

Treat clinical cases during lactation with parenteral antimicrobial (such as penethamate hydriodide) (R-3).

Control

Implement 10-point mastitis control plan, including postmilking teat dip or spray (R-1).

Blanket dry cow therapy with intramammary formulation (R-1)

Eradicate infection from herd (R-1).

Vaccinate against *S. agalactiae* (R-3).

FURTHER READING

Keefe G. Update on control of *Staphylococcus aureus* and *Streptococcus agalactiae* for management of mastitis. *Vet Clin North Am Food Anim Pract.* 2012;28:203-216.

REFERENCES

1. Mweu MM, et al. *Prev Vet Med.* 2012;106:244.
2. Mweu MM, et al. *Vet Microbiol.* 2012;159:181.
3. de Carvalho NL, et al. *Curr Microbiol.* 2015;71:363.
4. Reyes J, et al. *J Dairy Sci.* 2015;98:5294.

CORYNEBACTERIUM BOVIS

ETIOLOGY

Corynebacterium spp. are a common contagious cause of subclinical mastitis in dairy cows, and 89% of isolates are *C. bovis*.[1] For this reason, mastitis isolates identified as *Corynebacterium* spp. are frequently termed *C. bovis*. It has been cultured from dairy cattle with clinical mastitis in 1.7% of cases and, in a herd that had controlled contagious mastitis pathogens, *C. bovis* was the only pathogen isolated in 22% of clinical mastitis episodes. There is considerable debate about the significance of *C. bovis* infections for mammary gland health and cow productivity. For this reason, *C. bovis* is classified as a **minor pathogen**.

EPIDEMIOLOGY

The main reservoir of infection appears to be the teat canal region, but *C. bovis* is also isolated from the teat cistern, gland cistern, and mammary parenchyma.[2] *C. bovis* spreads rapidly from cow to cow in the absence of adequate teat dipping. It is extremely contagious, and the duration of intramammary infection is long (many months). The prevalence of *C. bovis* is typically low in herds using an effective germicidal teat dip, good milking hygiene, and dry cow therapy.

In vivo and in vitro studies have demonstrated that the bacteria has a predilection for the streak canal, and this predilection has been associated with a requirement for lipids (possibly in the keratin plug) for growth. It is possible that *C. bovis* infection in the streak canal may compete with ascending bacterial infections for nutrients, decreasing the new intramammary infection rate. Alternatively, the mild increase in SCC associated with *C. bovis* infection might increase the ability of the quarter to respond to a new intramammary infection. The *C. bovis* genome has been sequenced, and this indicated a bacteria that is well equipped to reside in the bovine udder, particularly the streak canal. The genome contains a number of genes related to lipolysis, including metabolism of glycerols and phosphoacylglycerols, and utilization of casein and lactose.[3]

Intramammary infection with *C. bovis* induces a higher than normal SCC,[2] increasing the resistance of the colonized quarter to invasion by a major pathogen. In particular, the lowest rate of intramammary infection with major pathogens is observed in quarters infected with *C. bovis*.

CLINICAL FINDINGS

An intramammary infection with *C. bovis* is infrequently associated with clinical disease but usually causes a mild to moderate increase in the SCC and a small increase in the CMT score.[4] Milk production losses are usually not detectable, and the mastitis is typically a thicker than normal milk (abnormal secretion); occasional cases also have a large firm gland (abnormal gland), with systemic signs of illness being unusual (abnormal cow). There are clear herd-to-herd differences in the apparent clinical pathogenicity of *C. bovis*, suggesting that strains of different virulence are present.

TREATMENT

C. bovis is very susceptible to penicillin, ampicillin, amoxicillin, cephapirin, and erythromycin and most other commercially available intramammary infusions. There is no need for parenteral treatment. The duration of infection is prolonged (months) in animals not treated with antimicrobial agents.

CONTROL

Long-term intensive programs of teat dipping and dry cow therapy will markedly reduce the prevalence of *C. bovis*. Because of its status as a minor pathogen, specific control measures (such as vaccination) are not indicated.

> **TREATMENT AND CONTROL**
>
> **Treatment**
> Treat *Corynebacterium bovis* clinical mastitis episodes during lactation with an intramammary formulation (R-1).
>
> **Control**
> Implement 10-point mastitis control plan, with particular emphasis on teat dipping/spraying and blanket dry cow intramammary treatment (R-1).

REFERENCES

1. Gonçalves JL, et al. *Vet Microbiol*. 2014;173:147.
2. Blagitz MG, et al. *J Dairy Sci*. 2013;96:3750.
3. Schröder J, et al. *J Bacteriol*. 2012;194:4437.
4. Madut NA, Gadir AEA. *J Cell Anim Biol*. 2011;5:6.

M. BOVIS AND OTHER *MYCOPLASMA* SP.

ETIOLOGY

A number of species of *Mycoplasma*, especially *M. bovis* and occasionally *Mycoplasma* species group 7, *Mycoplasma* F-38, *M. arginini, M. bovirhinis, M. canadensis, M. bovigenitalium, M. alkalescens, M. capricolium, M. californicum*, and *M. dispar*, have been isolated from clinical cases. Other mycoplasmas, not usually associated with the development of mastitis, also cause the disease when injected into the udder. There is also evidence of mastitis associated with *Ureaplasma* spp. A striking characteristic of the mycoplasmas is that they seem to be able to survive in the presence of large numbers of leukocytes in the milk. Antibodies to the bacteria have not been detectable in sera or whey from animals infected with some strains, but complement-fixing antibodies are present in the sera of animals recovered from infection with other strains.

> **SYNOPSIS**
>
> **Etiology** *Mycoplasma bovis*, other *Mycoplasma* spp.
>
> **Epidemiology** A highly contagious mastitis causing outbreaks of clinical mastitis. Most common in large herds with recent introductions. Transmitted within herds by bulk mastitis treatments and poor milking hygiene. Cows of all ages and any stage of lactation but those in early lactation are most severely affected.
>
> **Clinical findings** Sudden onset of clinical mastitis in many cows, usually all four quarters, marked drop in milk production and may stop lactating, swelling of the udder and gross abnormality of the milk without obvious signs of systemic illness, eventually udders atrophy and do not return to production. Can cause clinical, subclinical, and chronic intramammary infections. Calves suckling milk from infected cows may develop otitis media/interna.
>
> **Clinical pathology** Special culture and staining of milk techniques
>
> **Necropsy findings** Purulent interstitial mastitis
>
> **Diagnostic confirmation** Identification of pathogen in milk
>
> **Differential diagnosis** Epidemiology and clinical findings are characteristic of *Mycoplasma* mastitis. May resemble other causes of chronic mastitis unresponsive to treatment
>
> **Treatment** Not responsive to commonly used mastitis treatments protocols. Identify and cull affected cows for slaughter.
>
> **Control** Prevent entry of infected cows into herd. Eradicate infection by culling affected cows.

Acholeplasma laidlawii is not a mastitis pathogen, but it has been observed that a high proportion of bulk tanks will give positive cultural tests for it, especially during wet, rainy weather. This increase is accompanied by an increase of clinical mycoplasmal mastitis caused by pathogenic mycoplasma. *A. laidlawii* is considered to be a milk contaminant in these circumstances.

The group of diseases, including mastitis, that are associated with *Mycoplasma* spp. in sheep and goats are dealt with separately.

EPIDEMIOLOGY

Occurrence and Prevalence of Infection

The disease was first reported in 1961 in the United States and since then has been recorded in Canada, Europe, Israel, and Australia. The quarter infection rate in infected herds varies widely.

Source of Infection

The epidemiology of the disease has been incompletely characterized. *Mycoplasma* mastitis is most common in large herds and in herds in which milking hygiene is poor and when cows are brought in from other farms or from public saleyards. *Mycoplasma* mastitis usually breaks out subsequently after a delay of weeks or even months. The delay in development of an outbreak may be related to the long-term persistence of the organism (more than 12 months) in some quarters, and some cows become shedders of the organism without ever exhibiting signs of severe clinical mastitis.

M. bovis is capable of colonizing and surviving in the upper respiratory tract and the vagina, and extramammary colonization explains many of its epidemiologic paradoxes. An interesting epidemiologic observation is the detection of mycoplasmas and infectious bovine rhinotracheitis virus in affected udders at the same time. The virus could be the much sought after unknown factor in the etiology of the disease. Outbreaks of mastitis are recorded concurrently with outbreaks of vaginitis and otitis media/interna vestibulitis.

Transmission

Entry of the disease to a herd is usually by the purchase of animals and their introduction without quarantine. Transmission within a herd is most common at milking via machine milking or the hands of milkers.[1] Transmission can also be through the use of bulk mastitis treatments administered through a common syringe and cannula. Although the disease occurs first in the inoculated quarter, there is usually rapid spread to all other quarters.

Hematogenous spread of *M. bovis* has been demonstrated. Colonization of body sites other than the mammary gland is common, and *M. bovis* isolates from the respiratory and urogenital systems are frequently the same *M. bovis* subtypes that cause mastitis.

Mycoplasma spp. group 7 has also been isolated from cases of pneumonia and polyarthritis in calves fed milk from cows with mycoplasmal mastitis.

Risk Factors

Cows of all ages and at any stage of lactation are affected, and cows that have recently calved show the most severe signs and dry cows the least severe signs. There are several recorded outbreaks in dairy herds in dry cows, and one of them is immediately after mammary infusions of dry period treatment that affected all quarters of all cows.

Experimental production of the disease with *M. bovis* causes severe loss of milk production, a positive CMT reaction, and clots in the milk. Experimental infection produces little tissue necrosis, but *Mycoplasma* are detectable in many tissues, including blood, vagina, and fetus, indicating that hematogenous spread has occurred. It is also apparent that spread of infection between quarters in one cow can be hematogenous. There are no significant pathologic differences between mastitis produced by *M. bovigenitalium* and *M. bovis;* however, *M. bovis* remains the most common cause of mycoplasmal mastitis in dairy cattle.

Economic Importance

The disease is a disastrous one because of the high incidence in affected herds and the almost complete cessation of lactation. Many cows fail to ever return to milking; as many as 75% of affected cows may have to be culled.

PATHOGENESIS

This is a purulent interstitial mastitis. Although infection probably occurs via the streak canal, the rapid spread of the disease to other quarters of the udder and occasionally to joints suggests that hematogenous spread may occur. The presence of the infection in heifers milked for the first time also suggests that systemic invasion may be followed by localization in the udder.

M. bovis appears to have a number of virulence attributes, with **variable surface lipoproteins** (Vsps) an important virulence factor. Some of these surface antigens are involved in the adherence of *M. bovis* to epithelial cells; adherence is important because the small genome of *M. bovis* means that the organism is dependent on the host for essential biosynthetic pathways, such as amino acids, lipids, and nucleotides. The Vsps also play an important role in interacting with the cow's immune system.

CLINICAL FINDINGS

In lactating cows, there is a sudden onset of swelling of the udder, a sharp drop in milk production, and grossly abnormal secretion in one or more quarters. In most cases all four quarters are affected, and a high-producing cow may fall in yield to almost zero between one milking and the next. Dry cows show little swelling of the udder. Although there is no overt evidence of systemic illness, and febrile reactions are not observed in most field cases in lactating cows, those that have recently calved show the most obvious swelling of the udder and may be off their feed and have a mild fever. However, cows infected experimentally show fever up to 41°C (105.5°F) on the third or fourth day after inoculation, which is at the same time the udder changes appear. The temperature returns to normal in 24 to 96 hours. In some cases the supramammary lymph nodes are greatly enlarged. **The classic clinical presentation is severe clinical mastitis in multiple quarters of multiple cows with minimal systemic signs of disease.** A few cows, with or without mastitis, develop arthritis in the knees and fetlocks. The affected joints are swollen, with the swelling extending up and down the leg. Lameness may be so severe that the foot is not put to the ground.[2] *Mycoplasma* may be present in the joint.

The secretion from affected quarters is deceptive in the early stages because it appears fairly normal at collection; on standing, however, a deposit, which may be in the form of fine, sandy material, flakes, or floccules, settles out leaving a turbid whey-like supernatant. Subsequently the secretion becomes scanty and resembles colostrum or soft cheese curd in thin serum. The secretion may be tinged pink with blood or show a gray or brown discoloration. Within a few days the secretion is frankly purulent or curdy, but there is an absence of large, firm clots. This abnormal secretion persists for weeks or even months.

Affected quarters are grossly swollen. Response to treatment is very poor, and the swollen udders become grossly atrophied. In infection with one strain of the *Mycoplasma,* many cows do not subsequently come back into production, although some may produce moderately well at the next lactation. With other strains there is clinical recovery in 1 to 4 weeks without apparent residual damage to the quarter.

Mycoplasmal mastitis caused by *M. bovigenitalium* may be very mild and disappear from the herd spontaneously and without loss of milk production.

CLINICAL PATHOLOGY

The causative organism can be cultured without great difficulty by a laboratory skilled in working with *Mycoplasma.* Samples for culture should be freshly collected and transported at 4°C (39°F), and concurrent infection with other bacteria is common. Diagnosis at the herd level can be made by culturing bulk tank milk or milk from cows with clinical mastitis or increased SCC. However, the sensitivity of bulk tank milk culturing is poor (33%–59%). A marked leukopenia, with counts as low as 1,800 to 2,500 cells/μL, is present when clinical signs appear and persists for up to 2 weeks. SCCs in the milk are very high, usually over 20,000,000 cells/mL. In the acute stages the organisms may be able to be visualized by the examination of a milk film stained with Giemsa or Wright–Leishman stain. Species identification of *Mycoplasma* isolates is usually done using immunofluorescence and homologous fluorescein-conjugated antibody or an indirect immunoperoxidase test (immunohistochemistry). Speciation of the causative *Mycoplasma* species is recommended.

NECROPSY FINDINGS

Grossly, diffuse fibrosis and granulomatous lesions containing pus are present in the mammary tissue. The lining of the milk ducts and the teat sinus is thick and roughened. On histologic examination the granulomatous nature of the lesions is evident. Metastatic pulmonary lesions have been found in a few longstanding cases.

Samples for Confirmation of Diagnosis

- Mycoplasmology: chilled mammary tissue, regional lymph node (special media)
- Histology: fixed mammary tissue

DIFFERENTIAL DIAGNOSIS

A presumptive diagnosis can be made based on the clinical findings, but laboratory confirmation by culture of the organism is desirable. Because the organism does not grow on standard media and other pathogenic bacteria are commonly present often lead to errors in the laboratory diagnosis unless attention is drawn to the characteristic field findings.

TREATMENT

The majority of *M. bovis* strains isolated from cattle are susceptible in vitro to fluoroquinolones, florfenicol, and tiamulin. Approximately half of the isolates are susceptible to spectinomycin, tylosin, and oxytetracycline, and very few isolates are susceptible in vitro to gentamicin, tilmicosin, ceftiofur, ampicillin, or erythromycin. The clinical relevance of these in vitro susceptibility data to treating mycoplasmal mastitis remains questionable.

Cows diagnosed with mycoplasmal mastitis should be considered to be infected for life. None of the common antimicrobial agents appear to be effective and oil–water emulsions used as intramammary infusions appear to increase the severity of the disease. Parenteral treatment with oxytetracycline (5 g intravenously, daily for 3 days) has been shown to cause only temporary improvement. A mixture of tylosin 500 mg and tetracycline 450 mg used as an infusion cured some quarters. Unless treatment is administered very early in the course of the disease, the tissue damage has already been done.

A puzzling observation in one study was that identification of infected cows and preferential culling of these cows was not associated with eliminating the infection from the herd, provided that good milking practices were followed.[3] Infection was eliminated from most herds in that study within 1 month of the initial diagnosis.[3]

CONTROL

Prevention of introduction of the disease into a herd appears to depend on avoidance of introductions, or isolating introduced cows until they can be checked for mastitis. A popular biosecurity recommendation is to culture the milk of all replacement cows for *M. bovis,* but the sensitivity and specificity of milk culture in cows with subclinical infections appears to be low. The disease spreads rapidly in a herd, and affected animals should be culled immediately or placed in strict isolation until sale. Eradication of the disease can be achieved by culling infected cows identified by culturing milk and nasal swabs, especially at drying off and calving. When eradication is completed the bulk tank milk SCC is the best single monitoring device to guard against reinfection. An alternative program recommended for large herds is the creation of an infected subherd that is milked last. There appears to be merit in the frequent culturing of bulk milk samples as a surveillance strategy for problem herds and areas. Frequent culturing overcomes the poor sensitivity of bulk tank milk culturing. Cows with infected quarters are segregated into the subherd, and cows developing clinical illness or decreased milk yield are culled.

Intramammary infusions must be performed with great attention to hygiene and preferably with individual tubes rather than multidose syringes. Most commercial teat dips are effective in control. Use of disposable latex gloves with disinfection of the gloved hands between cows may minimize transmission at milking.

Vaccination is a possible development but is unlikely to be a satisfactory control measure because the observed resistance of a quarter to infection after a natural clinical episode is less than 1 year. This may be because of the presence of variable surface proteins that enable the pathogen to evade host immunity or because mycoplasmas appear to activate the host immune system via secreted secondary metabolites.[4] An *M. bovis* bacterin is commercially available in the United States that contains multiple strains of *M. bovis.* Autogenous bacterins have also been made for specific herds; however, no vaccine has proven efficacy for preventing, decreasing the incidence of, or decreasing the severity of clinical signs of mycoplasmal bovine mastitis.

Mycoplasma are sensitive to drying and osmotic changes but more resistant than bacteria to the effects of freezing or thawing. Amputating the teats of affected quarters may result in heavy contamination of the environment and is not recommended. Because *M. bovis* can cause respiratory disease, otitis media/interna, and arthritis in calves, all colostrum and waste milk fed to calves should be pasteurized.

TREATMENT AND CONTROL

Treatment

Identify, segregate, but do not treat infected cattle with confirmed subclinical or clinical mastitis caused by *Mycoplasma bovis* mastitis (R-1).

Control

Implement 10-point mastitis control plan (R-1).

Eradicate infection from herd as soon as practical (R-1).

Pasteurize waste colostrum or milk fed to suckling calves (R-2).

Screen purchased cows for intramammary infection with *M. bovis* (R-2).

Vaccinate using *M. bovis* bacterins (R-3).

FURTHER READING

Burki S, Frey J, Pilo P. Virulence, persistence, and dissemination of *Mycoplasma bovis. Vet Microbiol.* 2015;179:15-22.

REFERENCES

1. Aebi M, et al. *Vet Microbiol.* 2012;157:363.
2. Wilson DJ, et al. *J Am Vet Med Assoc.* 2007;230:1519.
3. Punyapornwithaya V, et al. *Can Vet J.* 2012;53:1119.
4. Zbinden C, et al. *Vet Microbiol.* 2015;179:336.

Mastitis of Cattle Associated With Teat Skin Opportunistic Pathogens

COAGULASE-NEGATIVE STAPHYLOCOCCI

Because of the intense investigation of coagulase-positive staphylococcal mastitis (*S. aureus*), coagulase-negative staphylococcal intramammary infections have come under closer scrutiny and are now among the most common bacteria found in milk, especially in herds in which the major pathogens have been adequately controlled. There is considerable debate about the significance of these pathogens for the mammary gland and for cow productivity.[1-3] For this reason, these pathogens continue to be classified as **minor pathogens**.

ETIOLOGY

CNS are common but minor contagious pathogens that include *S. epidermidis, S. hyicus, S. chromogenes, S. simulans,* and *S. warneri* that are normal teat skin flora, and *S. xylosus* and *S. sciuri* that come from an uncertain site. At least 10 different species of CNS have been isolated from cattle with mastitis. *S. simulans, S. chromogenes,* and *S. epidermidis* are the predominant CNS species in bovine mastitis and are associated with persistent intramammary infection[4]; *S. simulans* is a common isolate from older cows, whereas *S. chromogenes* is most frequently isolated from heifers before calving and during their first lactation.

EPIDEMIOLOGY

CNS are predominantly **teat skin opportunistic pathogens** and cause mastitis by ascending infection via the streak canal. They appear to have a protective effect against colonization of the teat duct and teat skin by *S. aureus* and other major pathogens, with the exception of *E. coli* and the environmental streptococci. Sources of CNS, other than the mammary gland and teat skin, are suspected to be in the dairy environment for some species, and it is likely that further investigation on a species level will identify species that are predominantly found in the environment[5] or have close human contact.[6] Preliminary findings indicate that *S. chromogenes* and *S. epidermidis* may be more host adapted to the bovine mammary gland and therefore have contagious characteristics. In comparison, *S. simulans* and *S. haemolyticus* may have environmental reservoirs; therefore their epidemiology may be more similar to that of environmental mastitis pathogens.[5] Large differences from farm to farm have been reported.[7]

Studies in the United States found that 20% to 70% of heifer quarters are infected before parturition with CNS, but these infections are usually eliminated spontaneously or with antimicrobial therapy during early lactation. A survey of the prevalence and duration of intramammary infection in heifers in Denmark in the peripartum period found *S. chromogenes* in 15% of all quarters before parturition, but this decreased to 1% of all quarters shortly after parturition. In Finland, CNS are the most commonly isolated bacteria from milk samples of heifers with mastitis. Infections with *S. simulans* and *S. epidermidis* occurred in 1% to 3% of quarters both before and after parturition. Infection with *S. simulans* persisted in the same quarter for several weeks, but intramammary infections with *S. epidermidis* were transient.

Coagulase-positive *S. hyicus* and *S. intermedius* have been isolated from some dairy herds and can cause chronic, low-grade intramammary infection and be confused with *S. aureus*. The prevalence of infection with *S. hyicus* was 0.6% of all cows and 2% of heifers at parturition; the prevalence of infection of *S. intermedius* was less than 0.1% of cows.

The major economic impact of CNS infection is that the mild to moderate increase in SCC, when coupled with a moderate to high prevalence of infection, may discount the price paid for milk.[8] *S. simulans, S. chromogenes,* and *S. xylosus* appear to increase SCC to a much greater degree during subclinical infection than other CNS.[7,9] Intramammary infection with CNS does not appear to have an effect on milk yield or composition.[3] For heifers, the presence of a CNS intramammary infection at calving was associated with fewer cases of clinical mastitis and higher milk yield in their first lactation.[1] Based on these findings, the authors concluded that CNS intramammary infection around calving should not be a cause of concern.[1]

CLINICAL FINDINGS

CNS are usually associated with mild clinical disease (abnormal secretion only and occasionally abnormal gland) and are commonly isolated from mild clinical cases of mastitis and subclinical infections. For example, *Staphylococcus* spp. have been cultured from dairy cattle with clinical mastitis in 29% of cases, and subclinical infections usually induce a moderate increase in SCC.

CLINICAL PATHOLOGY

Intramammary infections by minor pathogens such as CNS result in a higher than normal SCC, increasing the resistance of the colonized quarter to invasion by a major pathogen. Although these bacteria are capable of causing microscopic lesions, they are not nearly as pathogenic as *S. aureus,* and necropsy reports are lacking.

A small number of CNS isolates are methicillin resistant,[10] and 54% of CNS in one study were identified to have slime-producing ability.[11] The epidemiologic or clinical relevance of these observations are not known.

A major challenge with research into the role of CNS in bovine mastitis has been the lack of a sufficiently accurate but low-cost method for identifying CNS on the species level. Commercially available test kits that use biochemical tests do not appear to be sufficiently accurate to be used for research purposes, whereas analytical methods using MALDI-TOF technology and molecular methods involving PCR show promise.[9]

TREATMENT

Spontaneous cure is common. CNS, including *S. chromogenes, S. hyicus,* and others, are very susceptible to ampicillin, amoxicillin, clavulanic acid, cephapirin, erythromycin, gentamicin, potentiated sulfonamides, and tetracyclines, with some studies reporting resistance to penicillin. In a study of 139 cases of subclinical coagulase-negative staphylococcal mastitis in New York, the bacteriologic cure rates of commercially available intramammary infusions were similar to that of untreated controls (72% bacteriologic cure), with the following bacteriologic cure rates: cephapirin (89%), amoxicillin (87%), cloxacillin (76%), and penicillin (68%). The current consensus view is that an intramammary treatment duration of 2 to 3 days should be used for cows with clinical signs of mastitis caused by CNS, because the mastitis usually responds well to treatment. Subclinical CNS infections usually do not need treatment because spontaneous elimination is common, and the presence of bacteria in a milk sample may reflect contamination of the sample with teat skin flora.

The use of a combination of novobiocin and penicillin, and cloxacillin as dry cow therapy for CNS gave cure rates of over 90%.

CONTROL

Implementation of a mastitis control program will be very effective in decreasing intramammary infection and clinical mastitis episodes caused by CNS. Because of its current categorization as an opportunistic teat skin bacteria that can cause milk mastitis, attention should be focused on postmilking test dipping and optimizing teat skin condition, particularly around the teat orifice. Specific control measures (such as vaccination) are not indicated because of its status as a minor pathogen.

TREATMENT AND CONTROL

Treatment

Treat clinical coagulase-negative staphylococci mastitis episodes during lactation with an intramammary formulation per label directions (R-1).

Treat subclinical coagulase-negative staphylococci intramammary infections during lactation with an intramammary formulation (R-3).

Control

Implement 10-point mastitis control plan, with particular emphasis on postmilking teat dipping/spraying and optimizing teat condition, particularly around the teat orifice (R-1).

FURTHER READING

Pyörälä S, Taponen S. Coagulase-negative staphylococci—emerging mastitis pathogens. *Vet Microbiol.* 2009;134:3-8.

Taponen S, Pyörälä S. Coagulase-negative staphylococci as cause of bovine mastitis—not so different from *Staphylococcus aureus*? *Vet Microbiol.* 2009;134:29-36.

REFERENCES

1. Piepers S, et al. *J Dairy Sci.* 2010;93:2014.
2. Pate M, et al. *J Dairy Res.* 2012;79:129.
3. Tomazi T, et al. *J Dairy Sci.* 2015;98:3071.
4. Thorberg BM, et al. *J Dairy Sci.* 2009;92:4962.
5. Piessens V, et al. *Vet Microbiol.* 2012;155:62.
6. Schmidt T, et al. *J Dairy Sci.* 2015;98:6256.
7. De Visscher A, et al. *J Dairy Sci.* 2015;98:5448.
8. Schukken YH, et al. *Vet Microbiol.* 2009;134:9.
9. Supré K, et al. *J Dairy Sci.* 2011;94:2329.
10. Febler AT, et al. *J Antimicrob Chemother.* 2010;65:1576.
11. Bochniarz M, et al. *Polish J Vet Sci.* 2014;17:447.

Mastitis of Cattle Associated With Common Environmental Pathogens

Environmental mastitis is associated with bacteria that are transferred from the environment to the cow rather than from other infected quarters. ***E. coli, Klebsiella* spp.**, and **environmental streptococci** are the major pathogens causing environmental mastitis.

COLIFORM MASTITIS ASSOCIATED WITH *ESCHERICHIA COLI, KLEBSIELLA* SP., AND *ENTEROBACTER AEROGENES*

ETIOLOGY

Many different serotypes of *E. coli,* numerous capsular types of *Klebsiella* spp. (most commonly *K. pneumoniae*), and *Enterobacter aerogenes* are responsible for coliform mastitis in cattle. *E. coli* isolated from the milk of cows with acute mastitis cannot be distinguished as a specific pathogenic group on the basis of biochemical and serologic test reactions. The incidence of antimicrobial resistance is also low in these isolates because they are opportunists originating from the alimentary tract, from which antimicrobial resistant *E. coli* are rarely found in adults. Other gram-negative bacteria that are not categorized as coliforms but can cause mastitis include *Serratia, Pseudomonas,* and *Proteus* spp.

SYNOPSIS

Etiology Many different serotypes of *Escherichia coli,* numerous capsular types of *Klebsiella* spp., and *Enterobacter aerogenes.* These are commonly called coliform bacteria; other gram-negative bacteria (such as *Pseudomonas aeruginosa*) can cause environmental mastitis but are not categorized as coliform bacteria.

Epidemiology Dairy cattle housed in total confinement or drylot; uncommon in pastured cattle. Most important mastitis problem in well-managed, low-SCC herds. Quarter infection rate low at 2%-4%. Incidence highest in early lactation. Eight percent to 90% of coliform infections result in clinical mastitis; 8%-10% are peracute. Causes clinical mastitis rather than subclinical mastitis. Source of infection is environment between milkings, during dry period and prepartum in heifers. Isolates of *E. coli* are opportunists. Sawdust and shavings bedding contaminated with *E. coli* and *Klebsiella* spp. (particularly *K. pneumoniae*) are a major source of bacteria; much worse when wet (rainfall or high humidity). Coliform intramammary infection highest during 2 weeks following drying off and in 2 weeks before calving. Animal risk factors include:

- Low SCC
- Decrease of neutrophil function in periparturient cow
- High susceptibility in early lactation
- Contamination of teat duct
- Selenium and vitamin E status

Outbreaks of coliform mastitis do occur, and are commonly associated with major change in management of the environment (introduction of sawdust for bedding may result in outbreaks of *Klebsiella* mastitis).

Clinical findings

Acute: Swelling of gland, watery milk with small flakes, mild systemic response, recovery in a few days

Peracute: Sudden onset of severe toxemia, fever, tachycardia, impending shock; cow may be recumbent. Quarter may or may not be swollen and warm, secretions thin and serous and contain very small flakes. May die in few days

Clinical pathology Culture milk. Somatic cell count. Marked leukopenia, neutropenia, and degenerative left shift. Bacteremia may occur, particularly in severely affected cattle.

Necropsy findings Edema, hyperemia, hemorrhages and necrosis of mammary tissue. Major changes in teat and lactiferous sinuses and ducts; invasion of organism into parenchyma is not a feature of *E. coli.*

Diagnostic confirmation Culture of organism from milk and high SCC

Differential diagnosis:

- Parturient hypocalcemia paresis
- Carbohydrate engorgement lactic acidosis

Other causes of acute and severe mastitis (must culture milk):

- Environmental streptococci
- *Staphylococcus aureus* and *Streptococcus agalactiae*

Treatment Must consider status and requirements for each case based on severity. Use of antimicrobial agents is indicated in moderately to severely affected animals; efficacy uncertain in mild cases. Some infections become persistent if antibiotics are not administered. Severely affected cattle also need supportive fluid and electrolyte therapy (such as hypertonic saline), and possibly NSAIDs for endotoxemia.

Control Manage outbreaks by examination of environment. Improve sanitation and hygiene. Regular cleaning of barns. Dry bedding. Avoid crowding. Keep dry cows on pasture if possible. Replace sawdust and shavings with sand for bedding. Emphasize premilking hygiene, including premilking germicide teat dipping and keep cows standing for at least 30 minutes after milking. Core lipopolysaccharide antigen vaccine in dry period and early lactation to reduce incidence of clinical mastitis caused by gram-negative bacteria

EPIDEMIOLOGY

Occurrence of Clinical Mastitis

The occurrence of coliform mastitis has increased considerably in recent years and is a cause for concern in the dairy industry and among dairy practitioners. Coliform mastitis occurs worldwide and is most common in dairy cattle that are housed in total confinement during the winter or summer months. Where cows are kept in total confinement in a drylot, outbreaks of coliform mastitis may occur during wet, heavy rainfall seasons. The disease is uncommon in dairy cattle that are continuously in pasture, but it has been reported in pastured dairy cattle in New Zealand.

In contrast to contagious mastitis, environmental mastitis associated with coliform bacteria is primarily associated with clinical mastitis rather than subclinical mastitis. Clinical mastitis associated with environmental pathogens (including the environmental streptococci) is now the most important mastitis problem in well-managed, low-SCC herds. In a survey of the incidence of clinical mastitis and distribution of pathogens in dairy herds in the Netherlands, the average annual incidence was 12.7 quarter cases per 100 cows per year. The most frequent isolates from clinical cases were *E. coli* (16.9%), *S. aureus* (14.4%), *S. uberis* (11.9%), and *S. dysgalactiae* (8.9%).

The incidence of clinical coliform mastitis is highest early in lactation and decreases progressively as lactation advances. The rate of intramammary infection is about four times greater during the dry period than during lactation. The rate of infection is also higher during the first 2 weeks of the dry period and during the 2 weeks before calving. Eighty percent to 90% of coliform infections results in varying degrees of clinical mastitis in the lactating cow; approximately 8% to 10% of coliform infections result in peracute mastitis, usually within a few days after calving. The disease also is common in herds that concentrate calving over a short period of time.

Prevalence of Infection

The prevalence of both intramammary infection and the incidence of clinical mastitis caused by coliform bacteria has increased, particularly in dairy herds with a low prevalence of infection and incidence of clinical mastitis caused by *S. aureus* and *S. agalactiae* as a result of an effective mastitis control program. Compared with other causes of mastitis, coliform infections are relatively uncommon and, in databases on herd surveys, the percentage of quarters infected with these pathogens is low. The percentage of quarters infected at any one time is generally low, at about 2% to 4%.

In the UK, about 0.2% of quarters of cows may be infected at any one time. Surveillance of a dairy herd in total confinement in the United States indicated that infection with coliform bacteria by either day of lactation or day of the year never exceeded 3.5% of quarters, and this maximum was reached on the day of calving. However, coliform infections may cause 30% to 40% of clinical mastitis episodes. In herds with a problem, up to 8% of cows have been infected with coliform bacteria, and 80% of the cases of clinical mastitis may be caused by coliform infections.

Duration of Infection

Coliform intramammary infections are usually of short duration. Over 50% last less than 10 days; about 70% less than 30 days; and only 1.5% exceed 100 days in duration.

Source of Infection and Mode of Transmission

The primary reservoir of coliform infection is the dairy cow's environment (environmental pathogen); this is in contrast to the infected mammary gland, which is the reservoir of major contagious pathogens (*S. aureus* and *S. agalactiae*) and the main reservoir of infection in cattle with *M. bovis.* Exposure of uninfected quarters to environmental pathogens can occur at any time during the life of the cow, including during milking, between milkings, during the dry period, and before calving in heifers.

Morbidity and Case Fatality

In dairy herds with low bulk tank milk SCCs the average herd incidence of clinical mastitis is 45 to 50 cases per 100 cows annually, with coliforms isolated from 30% to 40% of the clinical cases. This is similar to an average incidence of 15 to 20 cases of coliform mastitis per 100 cows in herds with low bulk tank milk SCCs. Other observations indicate that the number of clinical cases of coliform mastitis varies from 3 to 32 per 100 cows per year, but the average incidence in dairy herds can be as low as 6 to 8 per 100 cows per year.

Coliform mastitis is one of the most common causes of fatal mastitis in cattle. The case–fatality rate from peracute coliform mastitis is usually high and may reach 80% in spite of intensive therapy. Outbreaks of the disease can occur with up to 25% of recently calved cows affected within a few weeks of each other.

Risk Factors

Pathogen Risk Factors

The isolates of *E. coli* from bovine mastitic milk are simply opportunist pathogens and represent a number of different strains that mostly lack known *E. coli* virulence factors.[1-3] This finding suggests that specific cow factors probably play a more important role in determining the severity of clinical signs after intramammary infection.[3] The isolates that cause coliform mastitis possess lipopolysaccharides (endotoxin), which form part of the outer layer of the cell wall of all gram-negative bacteria. Coliform bacteria isolated from the milk of cows or from their environment have different degrees of susceptibility to the bactericidal action of bovine sera, and the majority of isolates that cause severe mastitis are serum resistant in some, but not all studies.[4,5] Serum-sensitive organisms are unable to multiply in normal glands because of the activity of bactericidins reaching milk from the blood. Of the strains of *E. coli* isolated from cases of mastitis in cattle in England and Wales, only those that were serum resistant were reisolated from expressed milk following intramammary inoculation of lactating cows. Other observations indicate that serum-resistant coliforms have no selected advantage over serum-susceptible coliforms in naturally occurring intramammary infections. Strains of *Klebsiella* that cause mastitis were resistant to bovine serum in one study.

There are also somatic and capsular factors of coliforms that affect resistance to bovine bactericidal activity. The presence of long polar fimbriae and an enteroaggregative heat-stable enterotoxin are also prevalent in the majority, but not all, of the strains isolated from cattle with clinical *E. coli* mastitis.[5] The fibronectin binding property of *E. coli* from bovine mastitis may be an important virulence factor that allows the organism to adhere to the ductular epithelium. *E. coli* isolates from clinical mastitis cases were able to resist phagocytosis by neutrophils, multiply faster, and ferment lactose more quickly than environmental *E. coli* isolates from the environment.[4]

A minority of *E. coli* intramammary infections result in persistent infection. *E. coli* strains that are more likely to result in persistent infections are better able to invade and replicate within mammary epithelial cells than strains that do not result in persistent infections and were more likely to be resistant to multiple antibiotics.[6,7]

Environmental Risk Factors

All the environmental components that come in contact with the udder of the cow are considered potential sources of the organisms. The coliform bacteria are opportunists, and contamination of the skin of the udder and teats occurs primarily between milkings when the cow is in contact with contaminated bedding rather than at the time of milking. Feces, which are a common source of *E. coli,* can contaminate the perineum and the udder directly or indirectly through bedding, calving stalls, drylot grounds, udder wash water, udder wash sponges and cloth rags, teat cups, and milkers' hands. Cows with chronic coliform mastitis also provide an important source of bacteria, and direct transmission probably occurs through the milking machine. Inadequate drying of the base of the udder and the teats after washing them before milking can lead to a drainage of coliform-contaminated water down into the teat cups and subsequent infection.

Bedding

Sawdust and shavings used as bedding that are contaminated and harbor *E. coli,* and particularly *K. pneumoniae,* are major risk factors for coliform mastitis. Cows bedded on sawdust have the largest teat-end population of total coliforms and klebsiellae; those bedded on shavings have an intermediate number, and those on straw have the least. Experimentally, the incubation of bedding samples at 30°C to 44°C (86°F–111°F) resulted in an increase in the coliform count; at 22°C (71°F) the count was maintained, and at 50°C (122°F) the bacteria were killed. Wet bedding, particularly sawdust and shavings, promotes the growth of coliform bacteria, especially *Klebsiella* spp.

The relationship between the bedding populations of Enterobacteriaceae was studied over a 12-month period in a dairy herd. The analyses revealed that rainfall bedding populations of *E. coli* and coliform mastitis incidence were statistically independent, whereas there was a strong association between rainfall and *K. pneumoniae* bedding populations and the incidence of *K. pneumoniae* mastitis. The lack of an association between bedding population of *E. coli* and coliform mastitis, along with the observation that cows are most susceptible immediately after parturition, suggest that the ability of the bacteria to penetrate the streak canal may be a factor of resistance in the cow and not a characteristic of the organism. Also, it appears that the cow in early lactation is not as susceptible to *K. pneumoniae* as to *E. coli.*

The ability of several different bedding materials to support the growth of environmental pathogens has been outlined under controlled conditions. Bedding materials vary in their ability to support growth of different pathogens, and under barn conditions it appears that high bacterial counts are influenced by factors more complex than the type of bedding alone. Even clean damp bedding may support bacterial growth.

High populations of coliform bacteria on the teat end, unless accompanied by actual chronic quarter infection, are probably transitory and represent recent environmental contamination that would usually be eliminated by an effective sanitation program at milking time. However, any teat skin population, whether associated with infection in another quarter, from contaminated teat cup liners or from other environmental sources, must be considered as a potential source of new infection.

Animal Risk Factors

Factors that influence the susceptibility of cows to coliform mastitis include the SCC of the milk, the stage of lactation, and the physiologic characteristics and defense mechanisms of the udder (particularly the speed of neutrophil recruitment), teat characteristics, and the ability of the cow to counteract the effects of the endotoxins elaborated by the organisms.

Somatic Cell Count

Experimentally, an SCC of 250,000 cells/mL in the milk of a quarter may limit significant growth of bacteria and development of mastitis when small inocula of coliform organisms are experimentally introduced into the gland. SCCs of 500,000 cells/mL provided complete protection. Thus cows in herds with a low incidence of streptococcal and staphylococcal mastitis have a low milk SCC and are more susceptible to coliform mastitis. Dairy herds with low herd bulk tank milk SCCs may have a greater incidence of severe toxic mastitis than herds with higher counts.

Neutrophil Recruitment and Function

Increased susceptibility to coliform mastitis in the periparturient cow is primarily caused by impaired neutrophil recruitment to the infected gland. In fatal cases of peracute mastitis in cows within 1 week after parturition there may be large numbers of bacteria in mammary tissues and an absence of neutrophilic infiltration. Other observations indicate a high correlation between poor preinfection chemotactic activity of blood neutrophils and susceptibility to intramammary *E. coli* challenge exposure. Experimentally, in periparturient cows the inability to recruit neutrophils rapidly into the mammary gland following intramammary infection is associated with an overwhelming bacterial infection and peracute highly fatal mastitis. The periparturient cows are unable to control bacterial growth during the first few hours after bacterial inoculation and, consequently, the bacterial load is much higher when neutrophils finally enter the milk. The lack of neutrophil mobilization could be caused by

- Failure to recognize bacteria
- Lack of production of inflammatory mediators
- A defect in the ability of the cells to move into the milk compartment

In ketonemic cows, experimental *E. coli* mastitis is severe, regardless of preinfection chemotactic response.

High levels of cytokines are present in the milk of cows that lack the ability to recruit leukocytes, which is evidence that the cells recognized the bacteria. All of this suggests that the critical defect is in the neutrophils of the periparturient cow. Certain cell-surface receptors on leukocytes may be important defense mechanisms against *E. coli* polysaccharides. Bovine mammary neutrophils possess cell surface C14 and C18 and lectin—carbohydrate interactions mediating nonopsonic phagocytosis of *E. coli*—which may be important in controlling these infections.

Selenium and Vitamin E Status

The positive effects of supplemental vitamin E and selenium on mammary gland health are well established. An adequate dietary level of selenium enhances the resistance of the bovine mammary gland to infectious agents. Experimentally induced intramammary *E. coli* infections are significantly more severe, and of longer duration, in cows whose diets have been deficient in selenium than in cows whose diets were supplemented with selenium. The enhanced resistance is thought to be associated with a more rapid diapedesis of neutrophils into the gland of cows fed diets supplemented with selenium, which limits the numbers of bacteria in the gland during infection.

Vitamin E is especially important to mammary gland health during the peripartum period. Plasma concentrations of α-tocopherol begin to decline at 7 to 10 days before parturition, reach nadir at 3 to 5 days after calving, and then start increasing. When plasma concentrations are maintained during the peripartum period by injections of α-tocopherol, the killing ability of blood neutrophils is improved. The supplementation of the diets of dry cows receiving 0.1 ppm of selenium in their diets with vitamin E at 1000 IU/day reduced the incidence of clinical mastitis by 30% compared with cows receiving 100 IU/day. The reduction was 88% when cows were fed 4000 IU/day of vitamin E during the last 14 days of the dry period.

There are also marked effects of dietary selenium on milk eicosanoid concentrations in response to an *E. coli* infection, which may be associated with the altered pathogenesis and outcome of mastitis in a selenium-deficient state.

Stage of Lactation and Defense Mechanism

Coliform mastitis occurs almost entirely in the lactating cow and rarely in the dry cow. The disease can be produced experimentally in lactating quarters much more readily than in dry quarters. The difference in the susceptibility may be caused by the much higher SCCs and lactoferrin concentrations in the secretion of dry quarters than in the milk of lactating quarters. Cows with known uninfected quarters at drying off may develop peracute coliform mastitis at calving, suggesting that infection occurred during the dry period. New intramammary infections can occur during the nonlactating period, especially during the last 30 days, remain latent until parturition, and cause peracute mastitis after parturition.

The **rate of coliform intramammary infection** is highest during the 2 weeks following drying off and in the 2 weeks before calving. The fully involuted mammary gland appears to be highly resistant to experimental challenge by *E. coli*, but it becomes susceptible during the immediate prepartum period. More than 93% of *E. coli* intramammary infection associated with the nonlactating period originated during the second half of that period.

Several physiologic factors may influence the level of resistance of the nonlactating gland to coliform infection. The rate of new intramammary infection is highest during transitions of the mammary gland from lactation to involution and during the period of colostrum production to lactation. There can be a sixfold increase in coliform infections from late lactation to early involution, but 50% of these new infections do not persist into the next lactation. Also, the rate of spontaneous elimination of minor pathogens is high during the nonlactating period. The difference in susceptibility or resistance to new intramammary infection may be due, in part, to changes in concentration of lactoferrin, IgG, bovine serum albumin, and citrate, which are correlated with in vitro growth inhibition of *E. coli, K. pneumoniae,* and *S. uberis.*

There is also a slower increase in polymorphonuclear neutrophils in milk after new intramammary infection in early lactation than in mid and late lactation. These conditions may explain the occurrence of peracute coliform mastitis in early lactation. This suggests latent infection or, more likely, that infection occurred at a critical time just a few days before and after calving, when the streak canal became patent and the population of coliform bacteria on the teat end was persistently high because the cow was not being milked routinely and thus would not be subjected to udder washing and teat dipping. Coliform bacteria can pass through the streak canal unaided by machine milking; this may be associated with the high incidence of coliform mastitis in high-yielding older cows, which may have increased patency of the streak canal with age.

Newly calved cows can be classified as moderate or severe responders to experimentally induced coliform mastitis. Following infection there is a diversity of responses varying from very mild to very acute inflammation of the gland and evidence of systemic effects such as fever, anorexia, and discomfort. Losses in milk yield and compositional changes are most pronounced in inflamed glands and, in severe responders, milk yield and composition did not return to preinfection levels. It is proposed that the severe and long-lasting systemic disturbances in severe responders can be attributed to absorption of endotoxin.

In summary, coliform mastitis is more severe in periparturient cows because of the inability to slow bacterial growth early after infection. This inability is associated with low SCC before challenge and slow recruitment of neutrophils. There may also be deficits in the ability of leukocytes to kill bacterial pathogens.

Contamination of Teat Duct

The sporadic occurrence of the disease may be associated with the use of contaminated teat siphons and mastitis tubes and infection following traumatic injury to teats or following teat surgery. Several teat factors are important in the epidemiology of *E. coli* mastitis. It is generally accepted that *E. coli* is common in the environment of housed dairy cows and that mastitis can be produced experimentally by the introduction of as few as 20 organisms into the teat cistern via the teat duct. However, the processes by which this occurs under natural conditions are unknown. *E. coli* does not colonize the healthy skin of the udder or the teat duct.

The teat duct normally provides an effective barrier to invasion of the mammary gland by bacteria. As a result of machine milking there is some relaxation of the papillary duct, followed by gradual reduction in the duct lumen diameter in the 2 hours following milking. This period of relaxation after milking may be a risk factor predisposing to new intramammary infection.

Experimental contamination of the teat ends with a high concentration of coliform bacteria by repeated wet contact; however, this does not necessarily result in an increase in new intramammary infection. The experimental application of high levels of teat-end contamination with *E. coli* after milking repeatedly led to high rates of intramammary infection, which suggests that penetration of the teat duct by *E. coli* occurs in the period between contamination and milking. Milking machines that produce cyclic and irregular vacuum fluctuations during milking can result in impacts of milk against the teat ends, which may propel bacteria through the streak canal and increase the rate of new infections caused by *E. coli* and outbreaks of peracute coliform mastitis.

Downer Cows

Cows affected with the downer cow syndrome following parturient paresis, or recently calved cows that are clinically recumbent for any reason, are susceptible to coliform mastitis because of the gross contamination of the udder and teats with feces and bedding.

Other Defense Factors

Lactoferrin and Citrate. The failure of lactoferrin within mammary secretions to prevent new infections and mastitis near and after parturition may be caused by a decrease in lactoferrin before parturition. Lactoferrin normally binds the iron needed by iron-dependent organisms; these multiply excessively in the absence of lactoferrin. Also, citrate concentrations increase in mammary secretions at parturition and may interfere with iron binding by lactoferrin.

Serum Antibody to *E. coli.* The serum IgG_1 ELISA titers recognizing core lipopolysaccharide antigens of *E. coli* J5 in cattle are associated with a risk of clinical coliform mastitis. Titers less than 1:240 were associated with 5.3 times the risk of clinical coliform mastitis. Older cattle in the fourth or greater lactations were also at greater risk, even though titers increased with age. There is a titer-independent age-related increase in clinical coliform mastitis. Active immunization of cattle with an Rc-mutant *E. coli* (J5) vaccine resulted in a remarkable decrease in the incidence of clinical coliform mastitis.

PATHOGENESIS

After invasion and infection of the mammary gland, *E. coli* proliferates in large numbers and releases endotoxin on bacterial death or during rapid growth when excess bacterial cell wall is produced. Endotoxin causes a change in vascular permeability, resulting in edema and acute swelling of the gland and a marked increase in the number of neutrophils in the milk. The neutrophil concentrations may increase 40 to 250 times and strongly inhibit the survival of *E. coli.* This marked diapedesis of neutrophils is associated with the remarkable systemic **leukopenia** and **neutropenia** that occurs in peracute coliform mastitis. Large numbers of epithelial cells are sloughed into the glandular secretion very early in infection before the influx of immune cells into the affected gland and probably contribute to the breakdown in the blood-milk barrier.[8] The severity of the disease is influenced by the

- Degree of the preexisting neutrophils in the milk
- Rate of invasion and total number of neutrophils that invade the infected gland
- Susceptibility of the bacteria to serum bactericidins that are secreted into the gland
- Amount of endotoxin produced[9]

Stage of Lactation

The severity of disease is dependent on the stage of lactation. Experimental infection of the mammary gland of recently calved cows with *E. coli* produces a more severe mastitis compared with animals in midlactation. This may be caused by a delay in diapedesis of neutrophils into the mammary gland of recently calved cows. Furthermore, because of this delay there may be no visible changes in the milk for up to 15 hours after infection, but the systemic effects of the endotoxin released by the bacteria are evident in the cow (fever, tachycardia, anorexia, rumen hypomotility or atony, and mild diarrhea). The net result is endotoxemia, which persists as long as bacteria are multiplying and releasing endotoxin. This persistent endotoxemia is probably a major cause of failure to respond to therapy compared with the transient endotoxemia in the experimental inoculation of one dose of endotoxin.

Neutrophil Response

The final outcome is highly dependent on the degree of neutrophil response. If the neutrophil response is delayed and growth of the organisms is unrestricted, the high levels of toxin produced could cause severe destruction of udder tissue and general toxemia. If the animal responds quickly there is often little effect on milk yield because the injury is confined to the sinuses without involvement of secretory tissues. The ability of the neutrophils to kill *E. coli* varies among cows. Experimental infection of the mammary gland of cows with *E. coli* results in the stimulation of a long-lasting opsonic activity for the phagocytosis and killing of the homologous strain of the organism by neutrophils. Thus it is not opsonic deficiency that is the problem in early lactation; rather, it is a **failure of rapid migration of neutrophils into the gland cistern.**

The rapidity and efficiency of the neutrophil response are major factors in determining the outcome. If the neutrophil response is rapid, clinical disease will be mild or go undetected, self-cure will occur, and the cow returns to normal; the milk may be negative for the bacteria. This may be one important cause of an increase in the percentage of clinical mastitis cases in which no pathogens can be isolated from the milk. Failure of the cow to mount a significant neutrophil response results in the multiplication of large numbers of bacteria, the elaboration of large amounts of endotoxin, and severe highly fatal toxemia. In these cases, bacteria are readily cultured from the milk. In less serious and nonfatal cases, the recruitment of neutrophils does not fail but is delayed; this results in acute clinical mastitis with progressive inflammation and permanent loss of secretory function. The bacteria are not always readily eliminated from the infected gland by the neutrophils. Coliform bacteria may remain latent in neutrophils and, in naturally occurring cases, it is not uncommon to be able to culture the organism from the mammary gland during and after both parenteral and intramammary antibacterial therapy.

Numbers of Bacteria in Milk

The numbers of bacteria in the milk also influence the outcome. If bacterial numbers exceed 10^6 CFU/mL, the ability of the neutrophil to phagocytose is impaired. If the bacterial count is less than 10^3 CFU/mL at 12 hours postinfection, the bacteria will be rapidly eliminated and the prognosis will be favorable. This response is seen as a subacute form of the disease with spontaneous self-cure. If the neutrophil response is slow or delayed, the cow will exhibit more severe signs of coliform mastitis caused by toxemia. This is most common in recently calved cows and is characterized clinically by a serous secretion in the affected quarter that later becomes watery along with fever, depression, ruminal hypomotility, and mild diarrhea. The prognosis in these cases is unfavorable. These more severe forms of coliform mastitis usually occur after calving and in the first 6 weeks of lactation. Cows with coliform mastitis in mid to late lactation generally generate a rapid neutrophil response rate, and their prognosis is likely to be favorable.

Experimental Endotoxin-Induced Mastitis

In an attempt to further understand the pathogenesis of coliform mastitis, the effect of experimentally introducing *E. coli* endotoxin into the mammary gland has been examined. The intramammary infusion of 1 mg *E. coli* endotoxin induces acute mammary inflammation and transient, severe shock from which cows recover within 48 to 72 hours. Udder edema is apparent within 2 hours but begins to subside in 4 to

6 hours. The SCC increases within 3 to 5 hours, and at 7 hours the count is 10 times normal. A mild systemic reaction with a transient fever occurs in some cows. High concentrations of IL-1 and IL-6 are detectable in the milk of infused glands, beginning 3 to 4 hours after infusion. Milk concentrations of bovine serum albumin are increased from baseline levels to peak levels within 2 hours, indicating increased vascular permeability induced by inflammatory mediators. The infusion of endotoxin into the teat cistern of cows induces a rapid local inflammatory response of short duration with an influx of neutrophils into the teat cistern.

The intramammary infusion of endotoxin results in a sequential increase of immunoglobulin in milk whey and of phagocytosis of staphylococci by milk polymorphonuclear cells. This is consistent with spontaneous recovery of cows with acute coliform mastitis. Endotoxin infusion can also result in increases in arachidonic acid metabolites such as thromboxanes, and cytokines, which may be involved in mediation of local quarter inflammation, and the systemic signs observed in acute coliform mastitis. Histamine, serotonin, leukotrienes, and arachidonic metabolites are also released following experimental *K. pneumoniae* mastitis. There is also a marked increase in prostaglandin concentrations, which indicates that they may play a role in the pathogenesis of endotoxin-induced mastitis and that the use of NSAIDs may be of value therapeutically.

In **peracute coliform mastitis**, severe toxemia with fever, shivering, weakness leading to recumbency in a few hours, and mild diarrhea are common and probably caused by the absorption of large quantities of endotoxin. For many years it was thought that bacteremia did not occur in severe cases of coliform mastitis. However, **bacteremia is present in 32% to 48% of naturally occurring cases of coliform mastitis**. In experimental endotoxemia in cattle there is profound leukopenia (neutropenia and lymphopenia), a mild hypocalcemia, and elevation in plasma cortisol concentration. Hypocalcemia also occurs in naturally occurring cases and is thought to be caused by a decreased abomasal emptying rate associated with the endotoxemia. Experimentally infused endotoxin is detoxified very rapidly after absorption into the circulation.

In the acute form, the systemic changes are usually less severe than in the peracute form. However, in both forms, there is marked agalactia and the secretions in the affected quarter become serous and contain small flakes. Coliform organisms are not active tissue invaders, and in affected cattle that survive the systemic effects of the endotoxin the affected quarter(s) will usually return to partial production in the same lactation, and even full production in the next. However, in some cows that survive the peracute form, subsequent milk production in the current lactation is inadequate and cows are commonly culled.

A retrospective analysis of cows with clinical and laboratory features of coliform mastitis revealed that 60% returned to produce a milk-like secretion in the affected quarters in the current lactation and 40% did not. However, only 63% of the former group and 14% of the latter group remained in the herd and produced milk in the next lactation. Some cows were culled during the current lactation for low milk production and other reasons, some died, and others were culled for mastitis. Of the original 88 cows with coliform mastitis, only 38 (43%) remained in the herd and produced milk in the next lactation.

CLINICAL FINDINGS

Peracute coliform mastitis in the cow is a severe disease characterized by a sudden onset of agalactia and toxemia. The cow may be normal at one milking and acutely ill at the next. Complete anorexia, severe depression, shivering and trembling, cold extremities (particularly the ears), and a fever of 40°C to 42°C (104°F–108°F) are common. Within 6 to 8 hours after the onset of signs the cow may be recumbent and unable to stand. At that stage, the temperature may be normal or subnormal, all of which may superficially resemble parturient paresis. The heart rate is usually increased up to 100 to 120 beats/min, the rumen is static, there may be a mild watery diarrhea, and dehydration is evident. Polypnea is common, and in severe cases an expiratory grunt may be audible because of pulmonary congestion and edema.

The **affected quarter**(s) is usually swollen and warm but not remarkably so, and for this reason coliform mastitis may be missed on initial clinical examination. The cow may be severely toxemic, febrile, and have cold extremities before there are visible changes in the mammary gland or the milk. The mammary secretion is characteristic, and there are changes from the consistency of watery milk initially to a thin, yellow serous fluid containing small meal-like flakes that are barely visible to the naked eye; these are best seen on a black strip plate used for gross examination of milk. Additional quarters may become affected within a day or two of the initial infection.

The course of peracute coliform mastitis is rapid. Some cows will die in 6 to 8 hours after the onset of signs, and others will live for 24 to 48 hours. Those that survive the peracute crisis will either return to normal in a few days or remain weak and recumbent for several days and eventually develop the complications associated with prolonged recumbency. Intensive intravenous fluid therapy may prolong the life of the cow for up to several days, but significant improvement may not occur and eventually euthanasia may appear to be the desirable course of action.

Acute coliform mastitis is characterized by varying degrees of swelling of the affected gland and variable systemic signs of fever and inappetence. The secretions of the gland are watery to serous in consistency and contain flakes. Recovery with appropriate treatment usually occurs in a few days. During the first day of infection affected cows spend approximately 10% less time lying than when they were healthy. This small difference would not be clinically detectable unless the animal was monitored with an activity monitor.[10,11]

A clinically useful disease severity scoring system is helpful in directing treatment protocols.[12] The most useful and easily understood system uses three easily identified categories of clinical mastitis: (1) abnormal secretion only, (2) abnormal secretion combined with abnormal gland (such as swelling, heat, erythema, pain, and decreased quarter milk production), and (3) abnormal cow (systemic signs of illness, such as fever, tachycardia, decreased rumen contraction rate, and depression) combined with abnormal secretion and abnormal gland.

Accuracy of Clinical Diagnosis

Various diagnostic schemes that use clinical parameters to differentiate cows with clinical mastitis caused by gram-negative bacteria from those with clinical mastitis associated with gram-positive bacteria have been developed. Generally, all these schemes predict gram-negative bacteria as the cause if the milk is watery or yellow, if the mastitis episode occurs in summer, and if rumen motility is decreased or absent. Experienced clinicians are not much better at predicting the causative agent than inexperienced clinicians. The conclusion from all of these studies is that **clinical observations do not allow sufficiently accurate prediction of clinical mastitis pathogens** and should not be used as the sole criteria for deciding whether cows are treated with antibiotics, or even the class of antibiotic to be administered. Even the best predictive algorithm was wrong 25% of the time if the prevalence of gram-negative mastitis was 50%, which is too high an error rate to be used to guide treatment. In comparison, flipping a coin to attribute the causative agent as being gram-positive or gram-negative is wrong only 50% of the time.

An increase in the ability of a positive test to predict a gram-negative bacterial infection as the cause for a clinical mastitis episode is provided by examining for the presence of endotoxin in milk (sensitivity [Se] = 0.72; specificity [Sp] = 0.95), whether the **segmented neutrophil count** is less than 35% of the total leukocyte count (Se = 0.87; Sp = 0.71), whether the segmented neutrophil count is less than 3200 cells/μL (Se = 0.93; Sp = 0.89; Fig. 20-5), and by culturing

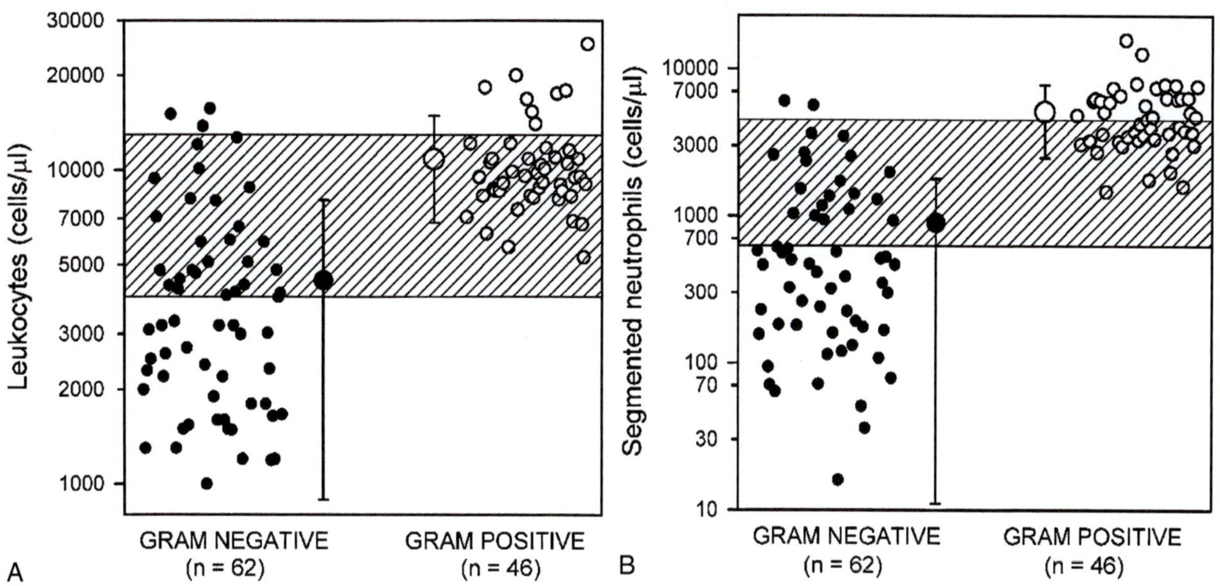

Fig. 20-5 Scatter plot of blood leukocyte count (left panel) and segmented neutrophil count (expressed on a logarithmic scale; right panel) for 108 lactating dairy cattle with acute clinical mastitis caused by Gram-negative bacteria or Gram-positive bacteria. The hatched area represents the reference range, and data are expressed as mean ± standard deviation. Cattle with acute Gram-negative mastitis are much more likely to be leukopenic and neutropenic. (Reproduced with permission from Smith GW, Constable PD, Morin DE. *J Vet Intern Med* 2001;15(4):394-400.)

on selective media (Se = 0.60; Sp = 0.98). The **endotoxin test** is a cowside test (Limast-test) that was commercially available in Scandinavia. Assessment of the white blood cell count and differential count is widely available in veterinary practice but is not a cowside test and is therefore not ideal. Both the milk endotoxin test and blood neutrophil count have adequate sensitivity and specificity for use to guide treatment decisions.

Chronic coliform mastitis is characterized by repeated episodes of subacute mastitis, which cannot be readily clinically distinguished from other common causes of mastitis.

Subclinical coliform mastitis is characterized by the presence of coliform organisms in the milk samples of cows without clinical evidence of mastitis. The prevalence of intramammary infection in quarters with coliform bacteria is low relative to contagious mastitis pathogens, ranging from 0.9 to 1.2%.

CLINICAL PATHOLOGY

Culture of Milk

Milk samples should be submitted for culture to identify the causative agent, but antimicrobial susceptibility testing has not been validated and is currently not recommended to guide treatment decisions. In the peracute case, the milk samples will yield a positive culture. In less acute cases, the milk sample may be negative because the neutrophils have cleared the bacteria.

Application of newer methods for bacterial identification suggest that *K. variicola* may be misidentified as *K. pneumoniae* in dairy cattle with clinical mastitis culture using routine procedures.[13]

Somatic Cell Count and California Mastitis Test Scores

In the experimental disease the SCC of milk from the inoculated quarter ranges from 14,000,000 to 25,000,000 cells/mL at 5 hours after inoculation. The CMT on secretions from affected quarters is usually +3.

Hematology

In peracute coliform mastitis there is hemoconcentration, a marked leukopenia, neutropenia, and a degenerative left shift caused by the margination of large numbers of neutrophils in response to endotoxin. There is also a moderate lymphopenia, monocytopenia, and thrombocytopenia (see Fig. 21-5). If the degenerative left shift, leukopenia, neutropenia, and thrombocytopenia become worse on the second day after the onset of clinical signs, the prognosis is unfavorable.[14] An improvement in the differential white count on the second day is a good prognostic sign.

Endotoxin Presence in Milk and Plasma

A commercially available cowside test (Limast-test) for endotoxin was available in Scandinavia. The test required at least 10^4 to 10^5 CFU of gram-negative bacteria for a positive test result. The test took 15 minutes to run on milk samples and was able to detect the presence of endotoxin and therefore gram-negative bacteria, but it did not differentiate between *E. coli* and *K. pneumoniae*.

Serum Biochemistry

The biochemical abnormalities observed in naturally occurring cases include uremia, high aspartate aminotransferase activity, and strong ion (metabolic) acidosis in fatal cases, whereas in surviving cases there were decreased concentrations of sodium, potassium, and chloride, and strong ion (metabolic) alkalosis.[14,15] In acute cases there is a transient early hyperglycemia.[16]

NECROPSY FINDINGS

There is edema and hyperemia of the mammary tissue. In severe cases hemorrhages are present and are accompanied by thrombus formation in the blood and lymphatic vessels; there is necrosis of the parenchyma.

A study of the progressive pathologic changes in experimental and natural cases of *E. coli* mastitis in cows reveals that damage is most marked in the epithelium of the teat and lactiferous sinuses and diminishes rapidly toward the ducts. In hyperacute cases, the organisms are largely confined to the ductular and secretory lumen and there is little invasion of the parenchyma, despite the presence of large numbers of organisms. In some cases there may be intense neutrophil infiltration, subepithelial edema, and epithelial hyperplasia of the sinuses and large ducts. In hyperacute cases in the immediate postpartum period, infiltration of neutrophils may be negligible. Bacteremia can occur in dairy cattle with coliform mastitis.

Samples for Confirmation of Diagnosis

- Bacteriology: chilled mammary tissue, regional lymph node
- Histology: formalin-fixed mammary tissue

DIFFERENTIAL DIAGNOSIS

- **Peracute coliform mastitis** in cattle is characterized clinically by a sudden onset of toxemia, weakness, shivering, often recumbency, fever in the early stages followed by a normal temperature or hypothermia in several hours, and characteristic gross changes in the milk, which usually is watery and contains some particles barely visible to the unaided eye. The peracute form of the disease is most common in recently calved cows.
- **Parturient hypocalcemia paresis** occurs in recently calved cows. The weakness and recumbency resembles peracute coliform mastitis but the marked increase in heart rate, and dehydration and mild diarrhea if present, are not characteristic of parturient paresis and should prompt further clinical examination, particularly of the udder. In the early stages of coliform mastitis the changes in the milk may be just barely visible. Those clinical findings that are most useful to predict peracute coliform mastitis include watery consistency of milk, shivering, firmness of udder, tachycardia, polypnea, fever, weakness, and mastitis of less than 24 hours' duration. A marked leukopenia and neutropenia are characteristic of coliform mastitis, whereas in parturient paresis there is usually a neutrophilia and stress leukon (neutrophilia, no left shift, lymphopenia, monocytosis, and eosinopenia). The differential diagnosis of recumbency in the immediate postpartum period is discussed under parturient paresis.
- **Carbohydrate engorgement lactic acidosis** causes rapid onset of weakness, recumbency, diarrhea, dehydration, and ruminal stasis and resembles the clinical findings of shock in peracute coliform mastitis. However, the rumen contains an excess of watery fluid, and the pH is below 5.0
- **Acute coliform mastitis** cannot be accurately differentiated from all other common causes of acute mastitis with abnormal gland and abnormal milk, including the environmental streptococci *S. uberis and S. dysgalactiae,* and the contagious pathogens *S. aureus* and *S. agalactiae.* Culture of the milk is necessary.

TREATMENT

The treatment of coliform mastitis in cattle has been controversial, but recent studies have clarified the **important role that antimicrobial agents play in treating severely affected cattle.** Historically, the treatment of coliform mastitis was based on the principles of treating a bacterial infection with varying degrees of inflammation. A combination of broad-spectrum antimicrobial agents administered parenterally and by intramammary infusion, fluid and electrolyte therapy, frequent stripping out of the affected glands with the aid of oxytocin, and antiinflammatory drugs have been used with varying degrees of success based on empirical and anecdotal experience. Only a handful of clinical trials have evaluated the efficacy of therapeutic agents used in naturally occurring cases of coliform mastitis, especially for the peracute form of the disease.

Most of the controversy has centered on the rational use of antimicrobial agents. The use of antimicrobial agents for the treatment of coliform mastitis has been questioned for several reasons:

- Clinical signs are primarily caused by the effects of endotoxin in the mammary gland, with formation of endogenous inflammatory mediators within the udder and their subsequent release into the systemic circulation.
- The severity of clinical signs is correlated with the number of bacteria in the affected gland.
- Most mild cases of coliform mastitis (abnormal milk but normal gland and cow) are self-limiting and resolve without antimicrobial therapy. However, a small percentage of these mild clinical cases develop persistent infection.
- There is speculation that the use of bactericidal antimicrobial agents may result in the bolus release of large quantities of lipopolysaccharides in the mammary gland associated with a rapid kill of bacteria, but this has not been observed in any study. In contrast, endotoxin release occurs from rapid bacterial growth alone, which will be prevented by administration of an effective antibiotic.
- Many, but not all, of the broad-spectrum antimicrobial agents currently approved for use in lactating cattle do not result in high enough concentrations in the milk when given parenterally.

Most of the antimicrobial agents currently used for the treatment of coliform mastitis in lactating dairy cows are not approved for use in food-producing animals. Because of this extralabel use and the lack of pharmacokinetic data for adequate withholding times, the risk of drug residues in milk and meat is increased.

The prognosis in the peracute form of the disease is unfavorable if severe clinical toxemia is present. Severe depression, weakness, diarrhea and dehydration, recumbency, and a heart rate over 120 beats/min are indicators of an unfavorable prognosis. The successful treatment of peracute coliform mastitis requires the earliest possible action and clinical surveillance until recovery is apparent.

Treatment Trials Using Antimicrobial Agents and Untreated Controls

Treatment trials with **experimentally induced** coliform mastitis in cattle during lactation have failed, for the most part, to demonstrate efficacy of antimicrobial therapy. This is because all experimental models do not accurately reproduce the naturally occurring disease, and not because antibiotics are ineffective. Accordingly, treatment efficacy should be based on the results of randomized field trials. The major considerations for antimicrobial use in coliform mastitis include:

- Early administration to decrease the exposure of the cow to endotoxin
- The severity of clinical signs are positively associated with the bacterial and endotoxin concentration in the affected quarter.[9]
- Ensuring appropriate withholding periods for milk and meat
- The benefit: cost ratio

The antimicrobial susceptibilities of *E. coli* isolates from coliform mastitis vary considerably; drug susceptibility determination is not routinely recommended because the breakpoints have not been validated and the bacteria come from diverse sources in the environment.

Parenteral Antimicrobial Agents

Broad-spectrum antimicrobial agents should be administered parenterally to cattle with systemic signs of disease (abnormal cow), preferably by the intravenous route initially, followed by intramuscular administration to maintain appropriate plasma concentrations. The first reason to administer parenteral antibiotics is that the **severity of clinical signs is correlated with the numbers of bacteria in milk from the affected gland.** The second main reason to administer parenteral antibiotics is to **combat bacteremia, which is present in 32% to 48% of severely affected cattle.** Based on pharmacokinetic/pharmacodynamic values, the results of experimentally induced and naturally acquired infections, and in vitro antimicrobial susceptibility testing (if this has any relevance to in vivo susceptibility), most *E. coli* isolated from the mammary glands of cattle are theoretically susceptible to third-generation cephalosporins (such as ceftiofur), fourth-generation cephalosporins (such as cefquinome), fluoroquinolones, gentamicin, amikacin, trimethoprim-sulfonamide, and oxytetracycline. Of these antimicrobials, third-generation cephalosporins, fourth-generation cephalosporins, fluoroquinolones, and potentiated sulfonamides have documented efficacy in naturally acquired or experimentally induced cases of acute *E. coli* mastitis, with moderate evidence supporting the efficacy of intravenous oxytetracycline.

- **Ceftiofur** is a third-generation cephalosporin that is resistant to β-lactamases and has excellent in vitro activity against *E. coli.* When given parenterally to cows with experimental coliform mastitis, ceftiofur did not produce drug concentrations in milk above the reported MICs for coliform bacteria. However, when administered to cows with naturally occurring coliform mastitis, ceftiofur-treated cows (2.2 mg/kg BW intramuscularly every 24 hours) were three times less likely to die or be culled from the herd and had more saleable milk than nontreated cattle.

- **Cefquinome** is a fourth-generation cephalosporin that is resistant to β-lactamases and has excellent in vitro activity against *E. coli.* Parenteral cefquinome therapy (1 mg/kg BW intramuscularly twice at 24 hours apart), with or without intramammary cefquinome (75 mg, three times at12-hour intervals), increased the bacteriologic cure rate and significantly improved clinical recovery and return to milk production in experimentally induced *E. coli* mastitis.
- **Danofloxacin**, a fluoroquinolone with excellent in vitro activity against *E. coli,* given intravenously once at 6 mg/kg BW was effective in treating experimentally induced *E. coli* mastitis.[17]
- **Enrofloxacin**, a fluoroquinolone with excellent in vitro activity against *E. coli,* given intravenously initially then subcutaneously once (5 mg/kg BW) was effective in treating experimentally induced *E. coli* mastitis, but had minimal efficacy in treating naturally acquired *E. coli* mastitis in a randomized clinical trial.[18] Generally, parenterally administered enrofloxacin increased the rate of initial *E. coli* clearance from the infected mammary gland. In a randomized clinical trial, a lower dose of enrofloxacin (2.5 mg/kg intramuscularly daily for 3 days) did not improve the survival rate of cows with *E. coli* mastitis, but it did result in a lower SCC at the first monthly herd recording after treatment.[19]
- **Gentamicin** has been used on an extralabel basis for the treatment of acute and peracute coliform mastitis because more than 90% of isolates from milk from affected cows are susceptible in vitro. However, the parenteral administration of gentamicin at 2 g intramuscularly every 12 hours until the appetite improved to dairy cows with mastitis predicted to be associated with gram-negative bacteria did not result in significant improvement compared with cows with similar mastitis that did not receive an antimicrobial or received erythromycin.
- **Trimethoprim-sulfadiazine** (trimethoprim 4 g, sulfadiazine 20 g, intramuscularly every 24 hours for 3–5 days) is efficacious in treating naturally acquired cases of coliform mastitis. The recovery rate of cows with clinical mastitis caused by coliform bacteria susceptible to sulfonamide-trimethoprim was 89% compared with 74% in cows infected with coliforms resistant to the combination given parenterally, combined with NSAIDs and complete milking of affected quarters several times daily. Sulfadiazine or sulfamethazine (sulfadimidine) are preferred to sulfadoxine because the latter produces much lower milk concentrations after parenteral administration.
- **Oxytetracycline** (16.5 mg/kg BW intravenously every 24 hours for 3–5 days), combined with intramammary cephapirin (200 mg) and supportive care (intravenous or oral fluids, flunixin meglumine, and stripping of the mammary gland) was more effective in treating coliform mastitis than similar treatment without antibiotics in cattle with naturally acquired mastitis.

Intramammary Antimicrobial Agents

Intramammary preparations of antimicrobial agents can be infused into the affected quarters after they have been stripped out completely at the start and end of the day. Evidence supporting the use of intramammary treatment for naturally acquired mild to moderate cases of *E. coli* mastitis (abnormal secretion and abnormal gland) is available for ceftiofur (125 mg daily for 5 consecutive days)[20] and cephapirin (200 mg per treatment). On theoretical grounds mild to moderate *Klebsiella* spp. mastitis episodes should also respond to intramammary ceftiofur or cephapirin treatment, because the spontaneous cure rate appears to be lower than that for *E. coli.*[20] The initial choice of antimicrobial will depend on previous experience of treatment efficacy in the herd.

- **Ceftiofur**: Based on clinical response and the results of antimicrobial susceptibility testing of coliform isolates from cows with naturally occurring mastitis (if relevant to in vivo performance), ceftiofur is an excellent choice for intramammary infusion in suspected cases of coliform mastitis.
- **Cephapirin**: Based on clinical response in lactating dairy cattle with experimentally induced *E. coli* mastitis, intramammary infusion of cephapirin (300 mg per quarter) at 4-, 12-, 24-, and 36-hour postinfection inhibited bacterial growth in milk decreased the inflammatory response.[21] The relevance of these findings to the treatment of naturally occurring cases of *E. coli* mastitis remains to be determined. This is because treatments were applied 4 hours after intramammary inoculation of *E. coli* when clinical signs of mastitis are usually not evident or are very mild.
- **Gentamicin**: The intramammary infusion of 500 mg of gentamicin did not affect the duration or severity of experimentally induced coliform mastitis. The numbers of *E. coli* in the milk after intramammary inoculation were not affected by the intramammary infusion of gentamicin, despite maintaining a mean minimal gentamicin concentration in milk of 181 μg/mL between dose intervals. The infusion did not affect the body temperature or the magnitude and duration of the inflammatory process in the glands as measured by the SCCs and peak albumin and immunoglobulin concentrations in the milk. It should be noted that gentamicin is not approved for use in the treatment of bovine mastitis, and in some jurisdictions it is not approved for any use.

A study of the efficacy of intramammary antibiotic therapy for the treatment of naturally occurring clinical mastitis associated with environmental pathogens found no difference in the short-term clinical or bacteriologic cure rates between quarters infused with 62.5 g of amoxicillin every 12 hours for three milkings or 200 mg of cephapirin every 12 hours for two milkings and those treated with 100 units of oxytocin intramuscularly every 12 hours immediately before milking for two or three milkings alone. However, the cost per episode of mastitis associated with the use of cephapirin was higher than the other two treatments, partly because of the longer milk withdrawal time (96 hours) associated with the drug. The percentage of relapses was higher for cows in the oxytocin treatment group, especially when the mastitis-associated pathogen was an environmental *Streptococcus* sp.

Stripping of the Affected Quarter

An artificial intramammary environment has shown that milking 12 times daily could lead to elimination of *E. coli,* suggesting that frequent stripping would be an effective treatment. Indeed, stripping (augmented by oxytocin) is a popular but largely unsubstantiated recommendation for treating severe cases of coliform mastitis. There is one report of cattle with acute coliform mastitis that suggests irrigation of the affected quarter with 1 to 3 L of 0.9% NaCl resulted in a higher recovery rate 30 days later.[22]

Oxytocin at 10 to 20 units per adult cow given intramuscularly, followed by vigorous hand massage and hourly stripping of the affected quarter, may assist in removing inflammatory debris. Oxytocin doses higher than this are not needed, and intravenous administration is not needed because oxytocin is rapidly absorbed when injected intramuscularly. Oxytocin can be repeated and used as long as an effect is obtained.

Effective removal of coliform bacteria and endotoxin will minimize their local effects in the mammary gland and decrease the systemic signs of endotoxemia. The main problems with stripping are the labor involved, the small volumes produced, the potential for creating additional pain and discomfort for the cow (and the producer when the cow kicks), and potential contamination of the environment if the secretion is stripped onto the ground. The role of frequent stripping, if any, in the treatment of clinical mastitis remains to be determined.

Fluid and Electrolyte Therapy

Fluid and electrolyte therapy are essential for the treatment of acute and peracute coliform mastitis to counteract the effects of the endotoxemia. Isotonic polyionic electrolyte solutions (such as Ringer's solution) are given at 80 mL/kg BW for the first 24 hours by continuous intravenous infusion and at a slower rate than that over the following days. For a mature dairy cow (400–600 kg) a total of 32 to 48 L is therefore needed in the first 24-hour period, with 20 L given during the first 4 hours and the remainder over the next 20 hours. A favorable response is usually clinically evident in 6 to 8 hours. If the animal has not improved after 5 days of intensive fluid therapy (the 5-day rule for clinical improvement), the prognosis for survival is poor.

The large amounts of isotonic fluids and electrolytes that have been advocated and used are expensive to administer by continuous intravenous infusion and require monitoring over many hours. A possible alternative is the use of small volumes of hypertonic saline, which can be transported easily and administered rapidly. **Hypertonic saline** can be safely administered to cattle with endotoxin-induced mastitis. Hypertonic saline (7.2% NaCl) is given intravenously at 4 to 5 mL/kg BW intravenously over 4 to 5 minutes followed by immediate access to drinking water. The changes following administration of hypertonic saline include transient expansion of the plasma volume, hypernatremia, and hyperchloremia. The intravenous administration of hypertonic saline to clinically normal cows with access to water increases circulatory volume rapidly, induces slight strong ion (metabolic) acidosis, and increases glomerular filtration rate. Fluid therapy is covered in detail in Chapter 5.

Antiinflammatory Agents

NSAIDs are frequently administered as adjunctive therapy in coliform mastitis, particularly in the peracute form of the disease. **Ketoprofen**, a cyclooxygenase type 1 and type 2 inhibitor and lipoxygenase inhibitor, is the only currently available NSAID with documented efficacy in naturally acquired cases of coliform mastitis.

Ketoprofen has been evaluated as adjunctive therapy for the treatment of acute clinical mastitis in dairy cows, most cases of which were associated with gram-negative pathogens. All cases were treated with 20 g of sulfadiazine and 4 g of trimethoprim intramuscularly followed by one-half dose daily until recovery. Ketoprofen was given at 2 g intramuscularly daily for the duration of the antimicrobial therapy. Recovery rates for the nonblind contemporary controls and the blind placebo controls were 84% and 71%, respectively. In the nonblind controlled ketoprofen and placebo-controlled ketoprofen treatment groups, recovery rates were 95% and 92%, respectively. The odds ratio (OR) of recovery was significantly high in the placebo-controlled study (OR = 6.8), and high but not significant in the nonblind controlled study (OR = 2.6). It was concluded that ketoprofen significantly improved recovery rate in clinical mastitis. Oral ketoprofen (4 mg/kg in 500 mL of water and administered orally) was similarly effective in lactating dairy cattle to intramuscular ketoprofen (3 mg/kg) administered 2 hours after intramammary endotoxin infusion.[23] This does not necessarily translate to efficacy in the treatment of field cases of acute *E. coli* mastitis because bacterial multiplication is not present following endotoxin infusion, and overt clinical signs were not apparent when treatments were applied.

A similar clinical field trial evaluating the efficacy of phenylbutazone and dipyrone for the treatment of mastitis caused mostly by coliforms revealed a beneficial effect but no difference between the efficacies of the two drugs. Neither phenylbutazone nor dipyrone is permitted for use in lactating dairy cattle in the United States, but their use is permitted in some countries.

A single administration of flunixin meglumine (2.2 mg/kg, intravenously) to lactating dairy cattle when clinical mastitis was evident after intramammary infusion of *E. coli* increased dry matter intake on day 1 and milk yield on days 3 and 4 after treatment.[24] The antiinflammatory effect of either flunixin meglumine or dexamethasone was evaluated compared with controls in experimentally induced coliform mastitis. Dexamethasone at 0.44 mg/kg intravenously and flunixin meglumine at 1.1 mg/kg intravenously were both given 2 hours after inoculation of the quarter with *E. coli,* which is essentially a pretreatment administration because clinical signs are not evident at this time. Flunixin meglumine was also administered once 8 hours after the initial dose. Dexamethasone reduced the rectal temperature and the mammary surface temperatures and prevented further increase in rectal temperature above 39.2°C (102.5°F). The response to flunixin meglumine was less than expected, which suggested that a higher dose of 2.2 mg/kg may be necessary in lactating dairy cattle. The administration of flunixin meglumine at 2.2 mg/kg intramuscularly or flurbiprofen at 2 mg/kg intravenously before clinical signs appeared in experimental *E. coli* mastitis abolished the febrile response during the first 9 hours after infection and lessened the decrease in rumen motility. In a separate study flunixin meglumine at 1.1 mg/kg intravenously 4 hours after inoculation of the *E. coli* mitigated the small reduction in lying time seen with acute *E. coli* mastitis;[11] this finding has minimal clinical relevance because this protocol is effectively a pretreatment administration because clinical signs of mastitis are usually not evident or very mild at this time.

The intramammary administration of prednisolone (20 mg) in conjunction with intramammary cephapirin (300 mg) had an antiinflammatory effect in cattle with experimental *E. coli* mastitis, as indicated by lower density of leukocytes in mammary tissue, lower IL-4 concentration in the glandular secretion of infected quarters, and a faster restoration of milk quality.[21] The relevance of these findings to the treatment of naturally occurring cases of *E. coli* mastitis is questionable because treatments were applied 4 hours after intramammary inoculation of *E. coli* when clinical signs of mastitis are usually not evident or very mild.

Carprofen, a long-acting NSAID, reduced the fever, tachycardia, and udder swelling associated with *E. coli*-endotoxin–induced mastitis. The long-acting properties of carprofen may be considered a therapeutic advantage over flunixin meglumine, which requires frequent dosing.

Combination Therapy

Fluid and electrolyte therapy and flunixin meglumine, in combination and individually, have been evaluated in a 3-year study of a large number of cows with toxic mastitis. Cows were allotted to one of three groups:

- Fluid therapy (45 L of intravenous isotonic electrolyte solution) and flunixin meglumine at 2 g
- Fluid therapy intravenously only
- Flunixin meglumine only

All cases were treated with parenteral and intramammary antimicrobial agents, oxytocin, and calcium borogluconate. There was no significant difference in the rate of survival between the treatment groups, and 54% of the cows survived.

CONTROL

The control of coliform mastitis is characteristically difficult, unreliable, and frustrating. Several cases of fatal peracute coliform mastitis may occur in a herd of 100 cows during a period of a year, in spite of the existence of apparently excellent management. The general principles of mastitis control that have been effective for the control of *S. aureus* and *S. agalactiae* mastitis have been unsuccessful for the control of coliform mastitis because infection of the mammary gland occurs by direct contact with the environment, usually between milkings. For the control of coliform mastitis, the emphasis is on the prevention of new infection. Core lipopolysaccharide antigen vaccines are useful and are discussed later.

Management of Outbreaks

When an outbreak of peracute coliform mastitis is encountered the following procedures are recommended in an attempt to prevent new cases:

- Culture milk samples and obtain a definitive etiologic diagnosis (in other words, **put a name to the causative pathogen**).
- Examine the bedding for evidence of heavy contamination with coliform bacteria. If sawdust or wood shavings are being used, replace with sand, if possible, or change more frequently.
- Conduct a general clean-up of the stall and lounging areas.
- Improve premilking hygiene.
- Examine milking machine function.
- Allow cows access to fresh feed immediately after milking to ensure that they remain standing for at least 30 minutes to allow time for the streak canal to close.

Housing and Environment

The normal presence of coliform bacteria in every aspect of the cow's environment must be recognized, but every effort must be made to avoid situations that allow a buildup of bacterial numbers. This is especially important in dairy herds that have been on an effective mastitis control program, resulting in a high percentage of cows with low SCCs in their milk, which increases their susceptibility to coliform mastitis. The overall level of sanitation and hygiene must be improved and maintained in these herds.

Bedding

Dairy cows lay down for 12 to 14 hours each day, and during this time their teats are in direct contact with a contaminated environment. The key to control is to minimize the number of bacteria in the bedding environment that are mastitis pathogens. Most coliform infections in periparturient cows occur very early in the dry period or just before calving, so efforts to prevent infection should be centered on these periods. Management of the dry cow environment may provide the best opportunity for prevention of infection. Although no reliable recommendations are available, cows that are housed during part or all of the day or night should be bedded on **clean** and **dry** bedding and not overcrowded to prevent heavy fecal contamination. When possible, dry and preparturient cows are best maintained on pasture. There remains an urgent need for the determination of optimum space and bedding requirements for the lounging areas of dairy cows kept under loose housing. Bedding should be kept as dry as possible. Excessively wet bedding should be removed from the back one-third of the stalls daily and replaced with fresh bedding. The addition of lime may decrease bacterial growth. Sawdust and shavings harbor more coliform bacteria than straw and require special attention. The buildup of high numbers of coliform bacteria in the bedding of cow cubicles can be controlled by the daily removal of the sawdust from the rear of the cubicle and rebedding with clean sawdust, which is usually of low coliform count. The use of a paraformaldehyde spray on sawdust bedding reduced the coliform count for 2 to 3 days, but it returned to its predisinfection level in 7 days. When outbreaks of coliform mastitis are encountered that are possibly associated with heavily contaminated sawdust or shavings, the bedding should be removed immediately and replaced with clean, fresh, dry straw. The use of sawdust or shavings as bedding should be avoided if possible. Sand is now considered to be the "gold standard" and the most suitable alternative.

Regular Daily Cleaning of Barns

This is necessary to minimize contamination of teats. In free-stall and loose-housing dairy barns, every management technique available must be used to ensure that cows do not defecate in their stalls and increase the level of contamination. This requires daily raking of the bedding in free-stall barns and adjusting head rails to ensure that cows do not lie too far forward in the stall and to ensure that they defecate in the alleyway.

In dairy herds that are confined for all or part of the year, the level of contamination usually increases as herd size increases; and usually the ventilation is inadequate. This leads to excessively humid conditions, which promote the development of coliform bacteria in wet bedding. This will require increased attention to sanitation and hygiene.

Milking Procedures

Postmilking teat dipping with a disinfectant has little effect on reducing the incidence of coliform mastitis because contamination of the teats occurs between milkings rather than at milking. Thus one logical approach to the control of coliform mastitis is to reduce environmental contamination. In the event of gross fecal contamination of the udder and teats, additional time and care will be required at milking time. Premilking udder preparation can significantly influence milk quality. Lowest bacterial counts in milk are observed when the teats of cows are cleaned with water followed by thorough drying with paper towels, or when a teat disinfectant is applied to the teats followed by drying with paper towels. In addition, premilking teat disinfection in association with good udder preparation reduces the rate of intramammary infections by environmental pathogens by about 51% compared with good udder preparation only.

Premilking Teat Disinfection

Many dairy producers have now incorporated premilking teat disinfection into their mastitis control strategy, and many different teat dips are used. Premilking teat dips containing 0.25% iodine, 0.1% iodophor, 0.25% iodophor, and 0.55% iodophor with 1.9% linear dodecyl benzene sulfonic acid (LDBSA) have been evaluated and have provided consistent results. Premilking and postmilking teat disinfection, in association with good udder preparation, are significantly more effective in prevention of environmental pathogen intramammary infection than good udder preparation and postmilking teat disinfection. No chapping or irritation of teats was observed. However, premilking teat disinfection has not been shown to decrease the incidence of clinical mastitis.

Postmilking Barrier Teat Dips

Barrier test dips include latex, acrylic, and polymer-based products that create a physical seal between the teat and the environment and theoretically decrease the exposure of the teat end to environmental mastitis pathogens, decreasing the incidence of new coliform intramammary infections during lactation. The efficacy of this barrier product was thought to be caused by the persistency of the dip on teats between milkings; however, barrier dips were not consistently successful. In summary, barrier teat dips with germicidal agents are no more effective in decreasing the incidence of environmental mastitis than postmilking germicidal teat dips.

Nutrition

Vitamin E or selenium deficiency decreases neutrophil chemotaxis into the mammary gland and decreases the intracellular killing of bacteria by neutrophils. It is therefore important to ensure that vitamin E and selenium intakes are adequate; this is best achieved by daily ingestion of 1000 IU of vitamin E and 3 mg of selenium for dry cows and daily ingestion of 400 to 600 IU vitamin E and 6 mg of selenium for lactating cows.

Vitamin C is the most important water-soluble antioxidant in mammals and, consequently, plasma vitamin C concentration may impact neutrophil function.[25] Daily ingestion of Vitamin C (30 g/day orally) had no effect on neutrophil phagocytosis, bacterial killing, or the severity of mastitis in dairy cattle following intramammary infusion of endotoxin.[25] The current data do not support the administration of Vitamin C in the diet as part of the control measures for *E. coli* mastitis.

Prevention of Infection During Dry Period

Considerable movement of coliform bacteria can occur from the teat apex into the teat sinus in cows that are not being milked, so cows that are ready to calve should be kept on grass or moved into a clean area at least 2 weeks before calving, their udders and teats washed daily if necessary, and teat dipping with a teat disinfectant begun 10 days before calving. This is particularly necessary for older cows and those that are known to be easy milkers. The teats of those cows that are "leakers" just before calving may have to be sealed with a barrier teat dip or collodion to minimize the chance of infection.

Recumbent Cows

Cows that are recumbent and unable to stand (e.g., the downer cow) should be well bedded on clean dry straw; their udders should be kept clean and dry, and the teats should be dipped with a teat disinfectant. Strict hygiene must be practiced when using teat siphons and teat creams, and strict asepsis should be observed when doing teat surgery.

Milking Machine

Irregular vacuum fluctuations in the milking machine may induce coliform mastitis in quarters exposed to a high level of contamination. The operation and sanitation of the milking machine, especially those parts in direct contact with the teats, must therefore be examined.

Vaccination

Core Lipopolysaccharide Antigen Vaccine

The vaccination of cows during the dry period and early lactation with core lipopolysaccharide antigen vaccine (such as the Re mutant *Salmonella typhimurium* or the Rc mutant *E. coli* O111:B4, named the J5 vaccine) provides one tool to reduce the incidence and severity of clinical coliform mastitis. These vaccines are available in the United States and are based on mutated gram-negative bacteria with exposed core antigens of lipopolysaccharide. The core antigen (lipid A component) is uniform between bacterial species possessing lipopolysaccharide and is immunogenic. On theoretical grounds, the Re mutant (*S. typhimurium*) should provide better protection than the Rc mutant (*E. coli* J5) because the lipid A component is more accessible to the immune system; however, comparative studies of vaccine efficacy have not been performed. Generally, core lipopolysaccharide vaccines are weakly immunogenic, and frequent dosing (hyperimmunization) appears to increase vaccine efficacy. However, the economic benefits of hyperimmunization have not been determined.

The Re and Rc mutant vaccines are protective against natural and experimental challenge to gram-negative bacteria, and in most, but not all studies, **reduce the incidence and severity of clinical gram-negative bacterial mastitis in lactating dairy cows.**[26–29] In a prospective cohort study in two commercial dairy herds, during the first 90 days of lactation, cows vaccinated with *E. coli* J5 vaccine were at five times lower risk of developing clinical coliform mastitis than unvaccinated cows. This is corroborated with the observation that cows with naturally occurring serum IgG ELISA titers higher than 1:240 against the gram-negative core antigen of *E. coli* J5 had 5.3 times lower risk of developing clinical coliform mastitis than cows with lower titers. Vaccination reduced the severity of clinical signs following intramammary experimental challenge with a heterologous *E. coli* strain. In cows vaccinated with the J5 bacterin at drying off, at 30 days after drying off and within 48 hours after calving, and challenged 30 days after calving with a strain of *E. coli* known to cause mild clinical mastitis, the duration of intramammary infection and local signs of mastitis were reduced compared with controls. Also, the concentrations of bovine serum albumin in milk 24 hours after challenge were greater in control cows than in vaccinated cows.

A partial budget analysis of vaccinating dairy cattle with one core lipopolysaccharide antigen vaccine (the Rc mutant of *E. coli* or J5 strain) indicated that herd vaccination programs were predicted to be profitable when more than 1% of cow lactations resulted in clinical coliform mastitis and predicted to be profitable at all herd milk production levels.

Core lipopolysaccharide antigen vaccines have the potential to have deleterious effects because of their endotoxin content. For instance, vaccination of late lactation and dry cattle with the *S. typhimurium* Re mutant transiently decreased leukocyte and blood-segmented neutrophil concentration, but the decrease is probably clinically insignificant. This response is typical for endotoxin administration. Vaccination of lactating dairy cattle with the *E. coli* Rc mutant decreased milk production by 7% at the second and third milkings after vaccination. These two studies indicate that core lipopolysaccharide antigen vaccines should not be administered to diseased cattle or to healthy cattle in hot and humid weather because of their decrease in cardiovascular reserve. Moreover, to minimize the total bolus exposure to endotoxin, core lipopolysaccharide vaccines should not be administered at the same time as other gram-negative vaccines.

TREATMENT AND CONTROL

Treatment

Treat mild and moderate *Escherichia coli*, *Klebsiella* spp., and *Enterobacter aerogenes* clinical mastitis episodes (abnormal secretion and abnormal gland) during lactation with a β-lactamase–resistant intramammary formulation with activity against gram-negative bacteria per label directions (R-1).

Treat severe *E. coli*, *Klebsiella* spp., and *E. aerogenes* clinical mastitis episodes (abnormal secretion, abnormal gland, and abnormal cow) during lactation with parenteral third- or fourth-generation cephalosporins, fluoroquinolones, potentiated sulfonamides, or intravenous oxytetracycline per label directions, in conjunction with intramammary treatment that may be extended to 5 days or 8 days per label directions (R-1).

Administer intravenous small-volume hypertonic saline or large-volume isotonic crystalloid solutions to severe clinical mastitis episodes (R-1).

Administer nonsteroidal antiinflammatory agents (ketoprofen, possibly flunixin meglumine) to cattle with systemic signs of illness (R-2).

Treat subclinical intramammary infections during lactation with an intramammary formulation (R-3).

Control

Implement 10-point mastitis control plan, with particular emphasis on ensuring cows are housed in a clean dry environment and that clean dry teats are milked (R-1).

Ensure cows remain standing for at least 30 minutes after milking (R-1).

Ensure adequate vitamin E and selenium intake in periparturient dairy cattle (R-1).

Consider implementing premilking teat disinfection (probably with 0.1%–0.5% iodophor formulation) (R-2).

Administer core-lipopolysaccharide antigen vaccine (Re mutant *Salmonella typhimurium* or Rc mutant *E. coli* O111:B4) at least every 6 months in herds with a high incidence of coliform mastitis (R-2).

FURTHER READING

Hogan J, Smith KL. Managing environmental mastitis. *Vet Clin North Am Food Anim Pract.* 2012;28:217-224.

Schukken Y, Chuff M, Moroni P, et al. The "other" Gram-negative bacteria in mastitis. *Vet Clin North Am Food Anim Pract.* 2012;28:239-256.

Suojala L, Kaartinen L, Pyorala S. Treatment for bovine *Escherichia coli* mastitis—an evidenced-based approach. *J Vet Pharmacol Ther.* 2013;36:521-531.

REFERENCES

1. Silva VO, et al. *Can J Microbiol.* 2013;59:291.
2. Blum SE, et al. *PLoS ONE.* 2015;10(9):30136387.
3. Wenz JR, et al. *J Dairy Sci.* 2006;89:3408.
4. Blum S, et al. *Vet Microbiol.* 2008;132:135.
5. Blum SE, Leitner G. *Vet Microbiol.* 2013;163:305.
6. Dogan B, et al. *Vet Microbiol.* 2006;116:270.
7. Fairbrother JH, et al. *Vet Microbiol.* 2015;176:126.
8. Wagner SA, et al. *Am J Vet Res.* 2009;70:796.
9. Jacobsen S, et al. *Vet Res.* 2005;36:167.
10. Cyples JA, et al. *J Dairy Sci.* 2012;95:2571.
11. Zimov JL, et al. *Am J Vet Res.* 2011;72:620.
12. Wenz JR, et al. *J Am Vet Med Assoc.* 2006;229:259.
13. Podder MP, et al. *PLoS ONE.* 2014;9(9):e106518.
14. Hagiwara S, et al. *J Vet Med Sci.* 2014;76:1431.
15. Bleul U, et al. *Vet Rec.* 2006;159:677.
16. Moyes KM, et al. *J Anim Sci Biotechnol.* 2014;5:47.17.
17. Poutrel B, et al. *J Dairy Res.* 2008;75:310.
18. Suojala L, et al. *J Dairy Sci.* 2010;93:1960.

19. Persson Y, et al. *Vet Rec.* 2015;176:673.
20. Schukken YH, et al. *J Dairy Sci.* 2011;94:6203.
21. Sipka A, et al. *J Dairy Sci.* 2013;96:4406.
22. Shinozuka Y, et al. *J Vet Med Sci.* 2009;71:269.
23. Banting A, et al. *Vet Rec.* 2008;163:506.
24. Yeiser EE, et al. *J Dairy Sci.* 2012;95:4939.
25. Weiss WP, Hogan JS. *J Dairy Sci.* 2007;90:731.
26. Gurjar AA, et al. *J Dairy Sci.* 2013;96:5053.
27. Erskine RJ, et al. *J Am Vet Med Assoc.* 2007;231:1092.
28. Wilson DJ, et al. *J Dairy Sci.* 2007;90:4282.
29. Wilson DJ, et al. *J Dairy Sci.* 2008;91:3869.

ENVIRONMENTAL STREPTOCOCCI

SYNOPSIS

Etiology *Streptococcus uberis, S. dysgalactiae,* other *Streptococcus* spp. are most common; occasionally *Enterococcus* spp.

Epidemiology Common cause of subclinical and clinical mastitis in herds and countries that have controlled contagious mastitis. Responsible for approximately one-third of all cases of clinical mastitis in herds without contagious pathogens. Rate of infection high during first 2 weeks following drying off and 2 weeks before calving. Duration of infection usually short (<8 days). Prevalence of infection at calving: 11% of cows and 3% of quarters. Bedding materials (high in straw bedding) most important source of environmental streptococci; bacteria can be isolated from many different feedstuffs and several locations on cow (teats, rumen, feces, saliva, lips, and nares). Bacterial numbers low in sand, which is bedding of choice

Clinical findings Abnormal secretion, abnormal gland, usually no systemic signs. Recovery in two to three milkings with intramammary treatment

Clinical pathology Culture of milk

Necropsy findings Not applicable

Diagnostic confirmation Culture bacteria from milk and milk somatic cell count

Differential diagnosis Cannot differentiate from other causes of subacute and acute mastitis without culture of milk

Treatment Antimicrobial intramammary infusions increase bacteriologic cure rate and decrease percentage of relapses. Intramammary antibiotics should be routinely administered to all clinical cases of mastitis caused by environmental streptococci.

Control Decrease exposure of teat end to pathogens by attention to environment, dry bedding, sand for bedding, premilking hygiene, and premilking germicide teat dipping. Dry cow therapy with penicillin G, cloxacillin, erythromycin, and first-generation (cephapirin) or third-generation (ceftiofur) cephalosporins. Application of an internal teat sealant of bismuth subnitrate at dry off may decrease new infection rate in dry period.

ETIOLOGY

S. uberis and *S. dysgalactiae* and the enterococci are the most commonly isolated environmental streptococci from intramammary infections. Other uncommon environmental streptococci involved in bovine mastitis include *S. equi* var. *zooepidemicus, S, viridans, S. equinus* (*S. bovis*), *Streptococcus* spp. group G, *S. pyogenes,* and *S. pneumoniae.* Both *S. uberis* and *S. dysgalactiae* are widespread in the animal's environment and on the skin of the teats. *Enterococcus* spp. are also a common cause of environmental intramammary infections.

EPIDEMIOLOGY

Occurrence and Prevalence of Infection

In countries in which the prevalence of intramammary infections caused by the contagious pathogens *S. agalactiae* and *S. aureus* has been reduced or eradicated, the proportion of intramammary infections associated with **environmental streptococci** has increased markedly; in some areas these organisms are the leading or second leading cause of both subclinical and clinical mastitis in dairy cattle. *S. uberis* is now a common cause of intramammary infection occurring during the dry period, with most clinical cases occurring during the first part of lactation. Many infections acquired during the dry period persist to lactation and contribute to the incidence of clinical mastitis in early lactation. *S. uberis* has become the most commonly isolated pathogen from clinical mastitis episodes in grazing dairy cattle in Australia and is present in 33% of submitted samples in southeast Australia.[1]

The rate of new infection caused by environmental streptococci is elevated during the first 2 weeks following drying off and the 2 weeks before calving; the rate of new infections is greater during the first month of lactation than during the remainder of the lactation. Approximately 50% of new infections occur during the dry period and 50% in the early part of lactation. The rate of new infections during the dry period is about five times greater than during lactation. Based on data from surveys of milk samples over a 10-year period, the point prevalence of infection of environmental streptococci was 4% of quarters and 12% of cows. The percentage in heifers at calving is similar to that in cows. The prevalence of environmental streptococci isolation at drying off and calving was 2.5% and 3.0%. Environmental streptococcal intramammary infections are usually short-lived (<28 days), with only a small percentage becoming chronic.

The most important change in the epidemiology of bovine mastitis over the past decade has been the rise in the importance of environmental pathogens, mainly causing clinical mastitis, relative to contagious pathogens. Remarkable increases in both the coliforms and environmental streptococci as causes of clinical mastitis have occurred. The percentage of clinical cases of mastitis from which environmental streptococci can be isolated ranges from 14% in Ontario to 26% in the UK. When expressed as a percentage of clinical cases from which a major pathogen was isolated, environmental streptococci are isolated in 37% to 45% of cases.

Source of Infection

The environmental streptococci, especially *S. uberis,* have been isolated from bedding materials and the lips and tonsils of cows, with the abdominal skin of cows often harboring the largest population. Some cows are permanently colonized with *S. uberis* and may pass large numbers of the bacteria in the feces. Fecal shedding is thought to play an important role in the maintenance of *S. uberis* populations on dairy farms, and is the likely source of large numbers of the organism in straw bedding on farms in which this form of mastitis persists. The numbers of environmental streptococci in organic bedding materials vary with the type of bedding. Large numbers of *S. uberis* are found in straw bedding and much lower numbers in sawdust and wood shavings. The numbers of streptococci recovered from the teats of cows bedded on sawdust are lower than those bedded on straw. Long straw used in calving box stalls or as bedding in loose housing can be a source of considerable exposure to environmental streptococci.

S. dysgalactiae can also be found in the environment of dairy cattle and has been isolated from the tonsils, mouth, vagina, and the mammary glands. It has characteristics of both a contagious and an environmental pathogen, and some categorization schemes place it in the contagious category, although it is primarily an environmental pathogen. *S. dysgalactiae* is also associated with summer mastitis, which affects dry cows and heifers during the summer months. It has been isolated from the common cattle fly *Hydrotoea irritans,* which may be involved in the establishment and maintenance of bacterial contamination of teats. *S. dysgalactiae* may colonize the teat before infection with *T. pyogenes* and anaerobic bacteria such as *P. indolicus* and *F. necrophorum.*

Risk Factors

Environmental Risk Factors

The major risk factor for environmental streptococci infection is **exposure of the teat end to mastitis pathogens in the environment**. Transmission is predominantly from the environment. Exposure of uninfected teats to environmental streptococci can occur during the milking process, between milkings, during the dry period, and before parturition in first-lactation heifers. The rate of new infections is greatest during the summer months in North America.

Housing and management practices on dairy farms may contribute to contamination of bedding materials and exposure of teats to environmental streptococci. Housing facilities that predispose to the accumulation of feces on cows will increase the rate of exposure of the teat end to the pathogens. Straw bedding appears to increase the risk of *S. uberis* mastitis, and an increase in *S. uberis* mastitis cases occurs when cows are housed in deep straw pack.

Pastured cattle are generally at reduced risk for environmental streptococcal mastitis compared with cows in confinement housing. However, certain pasture conditions, such as areas under shade trees, poorly drained ground surfaces, ponds and muddy areas, may result in a high rate of exposure to the pathogens, particularly to *S. uberis.* The environmental streptococci are the most significant environmental pathogen in New Zealand dairy herds in which cows spend almost 100% of their time on pasture.

S. dysgalactiae is commonly isolated from heifers and cows in the dry period and is one of the most prevalent pathogens isolated from cases of summer mastitis. The spread of *S. dysgalactiae* between cows within dairy herds may occur directly or by way of the milking machine or environment.

Animal Risk Factors

S. uberis is the most common cause of clinical mastitis at calving in cattle in pasture-based dairy systems.[2] The risk of new infections is influenced by the stage of lactation and parity of the cow. The **rate of new infection is highest during the 2 weeks following drying off and the 2 weeks before calving.** The high rates of new infection following drying off may be associated with the lack of flushing action of milking, changes in the composition of the mammary secretion, which may enhance the growth of the pathogens, and the lack of a keratin plug in the streak canal. The primary defense mechanisms for *S. uberis* are the length of the teat canal and the amount of keratin in the lining. Antimicrobial dry cow therapy reduces the infection rate in the early part of the dry period but has little or no effect on preventing infection with *S. uberis* at the end of the dry period. The increase in susceptibility to infection just before parturition may be associated with the lack of milking when the gland is accumulating fluid, loss of keratin plugs from streak canals, or immunosuppression of the periparturient period. The **rate of infection is also higher in older cows** than for either heifers or cows in second lactation, and highest during the summer months for both cows in lactation and cows in the dry period. This is in contrast to contagious pathogens, in which exposure occurs primarily during the milking process. A small percentage of animals have highly resistant phenotypes for *S. uberis* infection.[2]

Pathogen Risk Factors

S. uberis is ubiquitous in the cow's environment with multiple environmental habitats. Consequently, the mammary gland is exposed continuously to the pathogen during lactation and the dry period, and infections are associated with a large variety of strains, some of which are not capable of inducing clinical mastitis or prolonged infections of subclinical mastitis.[3] Several virulence factors of *S. uberis* have been identified that are important in the pathogenesis of environmental mastitis. Antiphagocytic factors allow *S. uberis* to infect and multiply in the gland and to adhere to and invade the mammary tissue. Bovine mammary macrophages are capable of phagocytosis of the organism, but certain strains of *S. uberis* are capable of resisting phagocytosis by neutrophils because of their **hyaluronic acid capsule.** The ability of *S. uberis* to invade the bovine mammary epithelial cells could result in chronic infection and protection from host defense mechanisms and the action of most antimicrobial agents, which may explain the intractable response to therapy in some cases. However, most apparently "intractable" infections are caused by an inappropriately short duration of treatment.

S. dysgalactiae behaves like both a contagious and an environmental pathogen[4] and can invade bovine mammary epithelial cells, which may explain the persistence of infection. Different biotypes of *S. dysgalactiae* have been identified, and strains can possess several antiphagocytic factors, including M-like protein, α-2-macroglobulin, capsule and fibronectin binding, and virulence factors, including hyaluronidase and fibrinolysin.

An existing intramammary infection caused by *C. bovis* is a risk factor for environmental streptococcal infection through an unidentified mechanism.

Economic Importance

The major economic losses associated with environmental streptococcal mastitis are caused by clinical mastitis resulting in lost production, milk withholding, premature culling, increased labor, and costs of therapy and veterinary services. Eighty-eight percent of the loss associated with clinical mastitis is attributed to loss of milk production and milk withholding. Pluriparous cows lost 2.6 times as much as first-calf heifers, and cows less than 150 days in milk lost 1.4 times more than cows more than 150 days in milk. Intramammary infection with *S. uberis* at calving in heifers resulted in a decreased lactational milk yield, even with subclinical infections, which means that *S. uberis* infections at calving should be routinely treated.[5]

PATHOGENESIS

The current consensus is that environmental streptococci (with the possible exception of *S. dysgalactiae*) are not contagious pathogens.[4]

In experimental infection of dairy cows with *S. uberis* there is acute inflammation, resulting in the accumulation of large numbers of neutrophils in the secretory acini in 24 hours. Adherence to mammary epithelial cells followed by internalization appears to be important in the establishment of infection.[6,7] Infection also leads to the recruitment of activated T cells that are able to kill *S. uberis* and appear to play an important role in an effective immune response.[8] After 6 days of infection, the neutrophil response is still evident, but there is cellular infiltration, septal edema, extensive vacuolation of secretory cells, focal necrosis of alveoli, small outgrowths of the secretory and ductular epithelium, and widespread hypertrophy of the ductular epithelium. The organism is present free or phagocytosed, in macrophages in the alveolar lumina, adherent to damaged secretory or ductular epithelium, in the subepithelium and septal tissue, and in lymphatic vessels and lymph nodes. The macrophage and activated T cells are important as the primary phagocytic cells,[7,8] but the marked neutrophil response may be ineffective as a defense mechanism. It is hypothesized that the marked neutrophil response following infection with *S. uberis,* rather than the organism, may be responsible for most of the effects of the mastitis. At least 11 virulence-associated genes have been identified in *S. uberis,* but it is not clear which are of major importance.[9]

CLINICAL FINDINGS

Approximately 50% of environmental streptococcal intramammary infections cause clinical mastitis during lactation. Clinical abnormalities occur in 42% to 68% of these infections in the same herd in different years. The clinical findings are usually limited to abnormal secretion or abnormal gland. In about 43% of cases the findings are limited to abnormal milk, 49% involve abnormal secretion and an enlarged (abnormal) gland, and in only 8% of cases do systemic signs include a fever and anorexia (abnormal cow). Clinical recovery commonly occurs in 24 to 48 hours. Natural infections with *S. uberis* appear to be more severe than natural infections with *S. dysgalactiae,* based on higher milk SCC for *S. uberis* mastitis episodes during the 4-month period after treatment.[4]

CLINICAL PATHOLOGY

The laboratory diagnostic tests for these pathogens are the same as for *S. agalactiae.* All the environmental streptococci except *S. dysgalactiae* hydrolyze esculin on blood agar. Species can be differentiated with reasonable success using a variety of biochemical tests, such as the API20 Strep and serologic grouping using specific antisera of Lancefield groups; however, this approach is laborious, time-consuming, and does not accurately differentiate every streptococcal mastitis pathogen. Biophysical analytical techniques have recently been applied with success to accurately differentiate streptococcal mastitis pathogens, including MALDI-TOF MS, which is mainly based on ribosomal proteins, and Fourier transform infrared spectroscopy, which covers the entire biochemical composition of a bacterial cell.[10]

> **DIFFERENTIAL DIAGNOSIS**
>
> *Streptococcus uberis* mastitis in dry cows may be sufficiently severe to resemble mastitis associated with *Trueperella pyogenes*. Diagnosis depends on cultural examination of the milk.

TREATMENT

Antimicrobial Agents

The in vitro susceptibility of environmental streptococci to antimicrobial agents is high. Most isolates of *S. uberis* and *S. dysgalactiae* are susceptible to penicillin, novobiocin, amoxicillin, and cephapirin. A high percentage (96%) are also susceptible to tetracycline, but susceptibility to aminoglycosides is much lower. Most cases of clinical mastitis associated with *S. uberis* and *S. dysgalactiae* respond well to intramammary infusions of penicillin, cephalosporins, cloxacillin, erythromycin, and tetracyclines. Spontaneous cures can also occur. Clinical cases in lactating cows should be treated by at least two intramammary infusions 12 hours apart; this may produce a clinical cure but fail to produce a bacteriologic cure. Subclinical infections in **late lactation** may be left until the dry period. For clinical cases in the first 100 days of lactation there is substantial economic benefit from intramammary treatment. Some cases associated with strains of *S. uberis* appear intractable to treatment; extended treatment is necessary in these animals. Failure of treatment may be caused by epithelial cell invasion and movement of the bacteria into subepithelial layers, possibly reducing the effectiveness of the antimicrobial. Apparently recurrent episodes of clinical mastitis caused by *S. uberis* despite adequate treatment are more likely from a subsequent infection with a new strain, rather than ineffective treatment.[1] Parenteral treatment is rarely needed to treat cattle with confirmed *S. uberis* clinical mastitis.

Extended therapy (for 5 days or 8 days) with intramammary ceftiofur (125 mg), pirlimycin (50 mg), or penethamate hydriodide, dihydrostreptomycin sulfate, and framycetin sulfate, every 24 hours, increases the bacteriologic cure rate for cattle with experimentally induced *S. uberis* mastitis. In a study of 1148 cases of subclinical environmental streptococci mastitis in New York, commercially available intramammary infusions were more effective than untreated controls (66% bacteriologic cure), with the following bacteriologic cure rates: amoxicillin (90%), penicillin (82%), and cloxacillin (79%).

Treatment using oxytocin and frequent stripping of the affected glands without intramammary antibiotic administration is not recommended because cure rates are much lower. Moreover, not administering antimicrobial agents results in a higher relapse rate. Many of the relapses were associated with the environmental streptococci; therefore **intramammary antimicrobial treatment should be routinely performed.** In particular, because clinical mastitis with an abnormal gland or abnormal cow induces some pain and discomfort in the cow, **withholding an effective treatment (intramammary antimicrobials) cannot be condoned on animal welfare grounds.**

Meloxicam (250 mg subcutaneously once) was administered to dairy cows in New Zealand with mild clinical mastitis receiving three daily intramuscular injections of penethamate hydriodide (5 g). In this population, *S. uberis* was the most common isolate, and the addition of meloxicam to the treatment protocol decreased the posttreatment SCC and decreased culling from the herd from 28% to 16%.[11]

CONTROL

The control of mastitis caused by environmental streptococci is achieved by **decreasing the exposure of pathogens to the teat end** and by increasing the resistance to intramammary infections. A specific control recommendation for environmental streptococci mastitis is **not to bed on straw**, but this may not be a practical or economic recommendation for some producers. If straw bedding is used, a reduction in the teat-end exposure to *S. uberis* can result from frequent (daily) replacement of bedding. The key factor promoting environmental streptococci mastitis is bedding on wet or damp straw.

Reducing the exposure of the teat end to manure and dirt depends on **maintenance of a clean and dry environment.** The alleys and holding pens should be frequently scraped, and places in which cows lie down should be dry. Special attention must be directed to the dry cow and close-up heifer housing, the calving area, lactating cow housing, and the milking parlor and milking hygiene. Organic bedding materials such as straw that support large numbers of environmental pathogens when wet should be kept dry. Sand is the ideal bedding material because it has the lowest number of coliform and environmental pathogens. Milking time hygiene should emphasize milking of clean, dry teats and udder, with a properly functioning milking machine. Predipping with a teat dip germicide may reduce environmental mastitis by as much as 50%, but this reduction does not occur in all herds.

Dry cow therapy to prevent new infections has not been as successful for the control of all causes of environmental mastitis as it has been for contagious mastitis. However, dry cow therapy is more effective against the environmental streptococci than against coliform bacteria. Application of an **internal teat sealant** of bismuth subnitrate at dry off is effective in preventing infections associated with *S. uberis* during the dry period. Combined administration of a dry cow intramammary formulation and an internal teat sealant has become routine in Australia as a fundamental plank in dairy herds with endemic *S. uberis* mastitis.[12]

A long-acting intramammary infusion dry cow therapy containing 250 mg of cephalonium administered after the last milking of lactation reduced the incidence of new infections caused by *S. uberis* from 12.3% to 1.2%. Clinical infections during the dry period were most prevalent in quarters identified as having open teat canals. Fewer open teat canals were observed among treated quarters over the first 4 weeks of the dry period. It is proposed that the teat canal of treated quarters closed earlier than those of untreated quarters. Most of the new infections in the untreated controls occurred within the first 21 days of the dry period. Normally, the teat canal is dilated for up to 7 days after drying off, with a keratin plug then forming over the following 14 to 21 days. It is suggested that once a physical keratin seal has formed in the teat canal after drying off, an uninfected quarter has a very low risk of infection over the remainder of the dry period. Treated quarters had a lower incidence of new clinical infections during the next lactation and lower SCCs.

Vaccination

Experimentally, multiple intramammary vaccinations with whole killed *S. uberis* cells resulted in complete protection against experimental infection in cattle. Bacteria could not be isolated from the quarters after challenge, and protection occurred in the absence of a marked neutrophil response. Preparations containing plasminogen activator or recombinant *S. uberis* adhesion molecule may form the basis of a vaccine against *S. uberis*.[13]

Vaccines are presently commercially unavailable, and vaccination is not currently recommended as part of the control program for mastitis caused by environmental streptococci.

> **TREATMENT AND CONTROL**
>
> **Treatment**
>
> Treat clinical mastitis episodes during lactation with an intramammary formulation that is effective against gram-positive bacteria per label directions; consider extended

Continued

intramammary therapy in chronic cases (R-1).

Treat subclinical *S. uberis* intramammary infections at calving with an intramammary formulation that is effective against gram-positive bacteria per label directions (R-1).

Administer nonsteroidal antiinflammatory agents (meloxicam) to cattle with clinical mastitis that is predominantly caused by environmental streptococci (R-2).

Control

Implement 10-point mastitis control plan, with particular emphasis on ensuring cows are housed in a clean dry environment and that clean dry teats are milked (R-1).

Ensure cows remain standing for at least 30 minutes after milking (R-1).

Administer a long-acting intramammary formulation with activity against gram-positive bacteria at dry off to all cows, followed by infusion of an intramammary teat sealant (R-1).

REFERENCES

1. Abureema S, et al. *J Dairy Sci.* 2014;97:285.
2. Turner SA, et al. *J Dairy Res.* 2013;80:360.
3. Tassi R, et al. *J Dairy Sci.* 2013;96:5129.
4. Lundberg A, et al. *Acta Vet Scand.* 2014;56:80.
5. Pearson LJ, et al. *J Dairy Sci.* 2013;96:158.
6. Almeida RA, et al. *Vet Microbiol.* 2015;179:332.
7. Tassi R, et al. *Vet Res.* 2015;46:123.
8. Denis M, et al. *Vet Res Commun.* 2011;35:145.
9. Reinoso EB, et al. *FEMS Microbiol Lett.* 2011;318:183.
10. Schabauer L, et al. *BMC Vet Res.* 2014;10:156.
11. McDougall S, et al. *J Dairy Sci.* 2009;92:4421.
12. Runciman DL, et al. *J Dairy Sci.* 2010;93:4582.
13. Prado ME, et al. *Vet Immunol Immunopathol.* 2011;141:201.

TRUEPERELLA PYOGENES

SYNOPSIS

Etiology *Trueperella pyogenes*, formerly known as *Arcanobacterium pyogenes, Actinomyces pyogenes,* or *Corynebacterium pyogenes*

Epidemiology Important cause of sporadic suppurative mastitis, most common in dry cows or pregnant heifers. Outbreaks occur in Europe in summer (called summer mastitis) associated with seasonally active biting flies, such as *Hydrotoea irritans*. Other bacteria (*Streptococcus dysgalactiae* and *Peptostreptococcus indolicus*) may be required to initiate clinical mastitis.

Clinical findings Gland is severely swollen and hard, usually only one quarter affected. Secretion from infected quarters is initially watery with clots and later purulent. Initially severe systemic signs including fever, inappetence, tachycardia, depression, and mortality rate up to 50%. In cattle surviving the initial infection, the affected quarter becomes abscessed, with drainage of purulent material at the base of the teat.

Clinical pathology Culture of milk

Necropsy findings Abscesses in one gland and severe systemic reaction are strong presumptive necropsy findings of *T. pyogenes* mastitis.

Differential diagnosis Cannot definitively differentiate from other causes of acute mastitis without culture of milk; however, the presence of abscesses in mastitis is strongly suggestive of *T. pyogenes.*

Treatment Responds poorly to treatment with parenteral procaine penicillin G or oxytetracycline and intramammary penicillin. Affected quarter is almost always lost for milk production.

Control Intramammary infusion with dry cow preparation every 3 weeks during the dry period. Control fly populations. Isolate cows with draining abscesses.

ETIOLOGY

T. pyogenes (formerly *Arcanobacterium pyogenes, Actinomyces pyogenes,* and *Corynebacterium pyogenes*) causes two forms of severe clinical mastitis: sporadic cases of suppurative mastitis, mostly in housed cattle, referred to as **pyogenes mastitis**, and a clinically similar disease that occurs in outbreaks in cattle during the summer months in Europe and Scandinavia and is referred to as **summer mastitis**. Successful transmission of infection has been performed, but the bacteria is rarely present in pure culture in the naturally occurring disease and is not the specific cause of summer mastitis. When the organism is applied to the teat skin at the end of the teat, infection of the quarter does not occur unless the teat end is injured, which is when anaerobic bacteria are also involved in the infection.

In summer mastitis the purulent material in the quarter usually contains *T. pyogenes* as a primary pathogen, but the severity of the disease is determined by the presence of anaerobes such as *P. indolicus; S. dysgalactiae; F. necrophorum; P. melaninogenica; Fusobacterium* spp.; a microaerophilic, gram-positive coccus (Stuart–Schwan coccus); and other Bacteroidaceae and *Micrococcus* spp. are also found. These bacterial species are found on the teats and conjunctiva and in the oral cavity of healthy cattle. *F. necrophorum* was recovered almost exclusively from the oral cavity, *P. indolicus* and *T. pyogenes* most frequently from teat skin, and isolates of *P. melaninogenica* subsp. *levii* were evenly distributed between conjunctiva and teat tip samples. There is also a distinct seasonal pattern of the isolation of the pathogens, which corresponds closely to the seasonal activity of the fly *H. irritans.*

It has also been proposed that *S. dysgalactiae* is the primary cause, and the others secondary invaders, but all these bacteria are capable of causing suppurative mastitis when infused into the udder. *T. pyogenes* alone establishes itself readily in mammary tissue after experimental introduction but causes only a subclinical disease, but inclusion of summer mastitis exudate provokes the classical syndrome of summer mastitis. Experimental infections with *T. pyogenes* and *P. indolicus* cause a much more serious disease, and are less responsive to treatment if the infection is introduced into a dry quarter instead of into a lactating one. The bacterial flora in cases of summer mastitis is quite variable. In some years in the UK, many cases are apparently caused by pure infections of *M. haemolytica*. In pyogenes mastitis, *T. pyogenes* is often found in pure culture, but the other bacteria listed in summer mastitis are also common accompaniments. *A. ulcerans* is an uncommon cause of a subacute mastitis.

EPIDEMIOLOGY

Occurrence and Prevalence of Infection

Bovine mastitis associated with *T. pyogenes* occurs sporadically and is most common in dry cows or pregnant heifers, although lactating cows may also be affected. A high prevalence is also recorded in heifer calves as young as 2 months. In the UK, Japan, northern Europe, Florida, and infrequently in a group of countries scattered all over the world, there is a much higher incidence of suppurative "summer mastitis" during the summer months when nonlactating females are left at pasture and not kept under close observation. In the UK 20% to 60% of farms are affected, the same herds are affected each year, and about 40% of farms never experience the disease.

Source of Infection and Mode of Transmission

The portal of infection is unknown, although it is presumed to be via the streak canal. The method of spread is uncertain in sporadic cases but insects, especially biting ones such as *H. irritans,* appear to play an important role in outbreaks of summer mastitis in northern Europe. The prevalence of the disease is related to the peaks of the fly populations and the prevailing climate, especially the wind force and direction.

Risk Factors

The incidence is much higher in wet summers and on heavily wooded and low-lying farms when the fly population is high. Dairy breeds are the predominant target, mostly at the end of gestation or in the first few days of the lactation. Heavy fly populations are a common accompaniment of an outbreak. It has been suggested that some triggering mechanism is needed before contamination of the teat and invasion and infection of the gland can occur. The infection rate of *T. pyogenes* in udders is much less in housed cattle than in the same cattle at pasture. In Australia the disease occurs mostly in lactating cows and usually after injury or the development of black spot on the teat. Outbreaks are also recorded in association with outbreaks of foot-and-mouth disease and herpes mammillitis virus damage to the teats.

Economic Importance

Summer mastitis is a serious disease because the mortality rate without adequate treatment is probably about 50%, and the affected quarters of surviving cows are always totally destroyed. In pyogenes mastitis the mortality rate is much less, but the loss of the quarter means that the cow is culled.

PATHOGENESIS

It is suggested that the infection is carried from udder to udder by flies and that massive invasion of the mammary tissue occurs via the teat canal that is damaged. The greater part of the gland is affected at the first attack, causing a severe systemic reaction and loss of function of the entire quarter. The disease has been reproduced by inoculation of the mammary gland of pregnant heifers with *T. pyogenes, F. necrophorum,* and *P. indolicus.* All animals developed moderate to severe clinical mastitis: 4 out of 10 animals recovered completely and had a normal lactation after calving. In 6 of 10 animals, the course of the disease was severe and affected quarters failed to produce milk after calving.

CLINICAL FINDINGS

Mastitis associated with *T. pyogenes* is usually peracute with a severe systemic reaction, including fever (40°C–41°C; 105°F–106°F), rapid heart rate, complete anorexia, and severe depression and weakness. Abortion may occur during this stage. In almost all cases only one quarter is affected, most commonly a front one. The teat is swollen and inflamed and the quarter is very hard, swollen, and sore; the secretion is watery with clots early and later purulent, with a typical putrid odor. The SCC from the secretion of affected cows is extremely high, and the secretion resembles a purulent process more than milk.[1] Affected cows usually carry a large fly population. If the cow survives the severe toxemia, the quarter becomes extremely indurated and abscesses develop, later rupturing through the floor of the udder, commonly at the base of the teat. These may be presented as chronic cases, but they are usually residual after an acute episode. True gangrene, such as occurs in staphylococcal mastitis, rarely if ever occurs in uncomplicated infections with *T. pyogenes,* but quarters may be so severely affected that sloughing occurs. Lameness in the hindlimb on the affected side occurs in some cases, and the limb joints may be swollen. The function of the quarter is permanently lost, and cows that have calved recently may go completely dry. Severe thelitis with extreme thickening and obstruction of the teat is a common sequel. Partial or complete obstruction of the teat and damage to the teat cistern can also occur independently of an acute attack of mastitis. Fetal growth retardation is thought to be a feature of calves born to cows affected by summer mastitis during pregnancy.

CLINICAL PATHOLOGY

Isolation of the bacteria is required. Freezing of milk samples reduces the number of samples giving a positive cultural result. MALDI-TOF MS provides a promising tool for the rapid identification of *T. pyogenes.*[2]

NECROPSY FINDINGS

Details of the pathology of the disease are not available.

> **DIFFERENTIAL DIAGNOSIS**
>
> The seasonal incidence of the disease in some areas, the acute inflammation of the quarter, the suppurative nature of the mastitis, the development of abscesses, and the severe systemic reaction make this form of mastitis one of the easiest to diagnose clinically in cattle.

TREATMENT

Summer mastitis normally responds extremely poorly to treatment, and the affected quarter is almost always lost for milk production. Failure of therapy is caused by the extensive purulent processes in the udder and not to antimicrobial resistance. Bacterial isolates from cases of summer mastitis are susceptible to penicillin G and other β-lactam antimicrobials. However, penicillin G has limited distribution throughout the inflamed udder. Given parenterally to experimental cases of summer mastitis, it was effective in about 40% of cases if treatment was initiated within 32 hours after inoculation. In peracute cases parenteral treatment with sodium sulfadimidine or one of the tetracyclines is preferable and should be accompanied by repeated stripping of the quarter. Broad-spectrum antimicrobial agents are usually given by intramammary infusion, but the quarter is almost always rendered functionless.

Affected quarters can also be treated by permanently drying the quarter off. The best method for permanently drying off a quarter is infusion of 120 mL of 5% povidone iodine solution (0.5% iodine) after complete milk out and administration of flunixin meglumine (1 mg/kg BW, intravenously). This causes permanent cessation of lactation in the quarter but does not alter total milk production by the cow.

Clearing of proteinaceous debris from the affected quarter may be aided by the intramammary application of proteolytic enzymes, but the outcome as far as the quarter is concerned is unlikely to be much altered and amputation of the teat to facilitate drainage is a common treatment. Even with intensive therapy, at least 80% of quarters are rendered useless and many of those that respond are greatly reduced in productivity.

CONTROL

The question of control of this form of mastitis centers largely on summer mastitis. Many prophylactic measures, including infusion of the quarter when the cow is dried off, sealing the teat ends with collodion, and vaccination with toxoid, have been tried but with inconclusive results. The most favored technique is intramammary infusion with a dry cow preparation (e.g., cloxacillin 500 mg and ampicillin 250 mg in a long-acting base) at 3-week intervals during the dry period. Less frequent administration offers less protection. An alternative intramammary infusion procedure is to use cephalonium at 4-weekly intervals.

Repeated spraying of the udder, for example automatically at watering points, with a contact insecticide is commonly performed during the fly season and is thought to be effective. An alternative to spraying is the use of insecticide-impregnated ear tags, or pour-ons. Careful daily examination of dry cows during the summer may enable affected quarters to be identified, the cows to be isolated, and the quarters treated at an early stage, limiting the spread of infection. In particular, cows with purulent material draining from an affected quarter need to be isolated from other cattle. Early treatment of teat lesions to limit bacterial colonization by bacteria, possibly transported by flies, is recommended. The known susceptibility of particular farms, and particular paddocks on those farms, demands proper care in planning the pasturing of dry cows during the danger period.

> **TREATMENT AND CONTROL**
>
> **Treatment**
>
> Treat clinical mastitis episodes immediately with intravenous oxytetracycline (R-1).
>
> Permanently dry off affected quarters if cow is to remain in the herd (R-2).
>
> **Control**
>
> Isolate cow from the rest of the herd if spontaneous purulent discharge from udder is present (R-1).
>
> Fly control during summer months for pastured cattle (R-1).

FURTHER READING

Egan J. *Actinomyces pyogenes* mastitis with particular emphasis on summer mastitis. *Ir Vet J.* 1994;47:180-186.

REFERENCES

1. Zastempowska E, Lassa H. *Vet Microbiol.* 2012;161:153.
2. Nagib S, et al. *PLoS ONE.* 2014;9:e104654.

Mastitis of Cattle Associated With Less Common Pathogens

PSEUDOMONAS AERUGINOSA

Mastitis in cattle and sheep associated with *P. aeruginosa* is rare and occurs usually as sporadic cases after intramammary infusion with contaminated material.

ETIOLOGY

P. aeruginosa is the most common cause, although other *Pseudomonas* spp. can cause disease. *P. aeruginosa* produces a number of extracellular toxins; hemolysin is cytotoxic for most cells and is considered the most potent toxin produced, lecithinase (phospholipase) can destroy cell membranes, and protease degrades proteins. In 25 *P. aeruginosa* isolates from the milk of cattle with mastitis in Egypt, 80% carried the hemolysin virulence factor, whereas 72% were lecithinase positive and 16% were protease positive.[1]

EPIDEMIOLOGY

P. aeruginosa is common in the environment of cattle because of its innate ability to survive for long periods in dry and moist conditions. Occasionally a number of animals in the herd are affected with *P. aeruginosa* mastitis; the infection usually originates in contaminated water used for washing udders. The organism has the capacity to colonize inert materials such as loops of hose and the interior surface of water heaters, so that high bacterial concentrations may be in the water left in the hose between milkings. It may be an advantage in these circumstances to flush out the udder washing system before commencing each milking. Once the teats are contaminated, the entry of the organisms to the teats is facilitated by overmilking and by putting the milking cups on while the udder is still wet. Serious outbreaks in cows have also occurred in association with the use of a suspected contaminated mastitis infusion used as a dry period treatment. The cows became affected soon after calving. Prolonged herd outbreaks are rare.

Rarely, strains of this organism are highly virulent and cause fatal mastitis with generalized lesions. Less commonly there is a high level of infection in a herd caused by a contaminated water supply but with no clinical cases. Reinfection is common unless the source of infection is removed.

CLINICAL FINDINGS

The mastitis in cattle is usually mild, subacute, or chronic, but can be clinically severe with a mortality rate as high as 17% of affected cows. Clinically, there is a severe systemic reaction and acute swelling of the gland with the appearance of clotted, discolored milk; the function of the gland is usually completely lost at the first attack, but recurrent crises may occur.

CLINICAL PATHOLOGY

Culture of the organism in milk is necessary to confirm the diagnosis.

NECROPSY FINDINGS

The disease can be fatal, and the gross and histologic findings are similar to other causes of clinical mastitis in cows.

> **DIFFERENTIAL DIAGNOSIS**
>
> Bovine mastitis associated with *Pseudomonas aeruginosa* must be differentiated from the many other forms of acute mastitis associated with this species; this can be done only by bacteriologic examination of the milk.

TREATMENT

Treatment with antimicrobial agents is generally unsuccessful. *P. aeruginosa* is an intrinsically multidrug-resistant bacteria because it has decreased outer membrane permeability, efflux systems, and produces β-lactamase.[2,3] Most bovine mastitis strains are also strong biofilm producers that further decrease antimicrobial effectiveness.[4] However, *P. aeruginosa* isolates from cattle with mastitis are susceptible to a wider variety of antimicrobials than similar isolates from humans.[2] This has been attributed to a lack of selection pressure in the cow's environment.[2] Third-generation cephalosporins such as ceftiofur, aminoglycosides such as gentamicin and amikacin, and fluoroquinolones are most likely to be efficacious in treating affected animals,[4] but susceptibility testing may be helpful in identifying which antimicrobials not to administer on the basis of a very high MIC.

CONTROL

The standard control program described later in the chapter should control the disease in cows. The oral administration of an organic iodine compound and vaccination with a killed autogenous vaccine are credited with bringing the disease under control in one herd.

REFERENCES

1. Younis G, et al. *Adv Anim Vet Sci.* 2015;3:522.
2. Ohnishi M, et al. *Vet Microbiol.* 2011;154:202.
3. Ghazy AE, et al. *Alexandria J Vet Sci.* 2015;44:80.
4. Park HR, et al. *Acta Vet Hung.* 2014;62:1.

MANNHEIMIA (PASTEURELLA) SPECIES

Mastitis associated with *Mannheimia* (formerly *Pasteurella*) *haemolytica* and *Pasteurella multocida* is common in ewes, occurring in a peracute gangrenous form, but is comparatively rare in cattle and goats.

ETIOLOGY

In cattle *M. haemolytica* and *P. multocida* are the causative organisms; *M. haemolytica* has also been isolated from many cases of **summer mastitis** in the UK.

EPIDEMIOLOGY

In cattle the disease is encountered rarely, and usually sporadically, but it may be a problem in individual herds, particularly in which calves are reared by nurse cows.

CLINICAL FINDINGS

In cattle the mastitis is severe with fever, profound toxemic shock, weak pulse, tachycardia, and recumbency. The affected quarter is very swollen and the milk is watery, red-tinged, and contains flakes. Disseminated intravascular coagulopathy may cause internal bleeding at many sites. All four quarters may be affected. There is complete cessation of milk flow in affected and unaffected quarters and subsequent fibrosis and atrophy. Newborn calves allowed to suck colostrum from affected cows may die of pasteurellosis.

Clinical Pathology

Culture of the organism in the milk is necessary to confirm the diagnosis.

NECROPSY FINDINGS

The disease is not fatal in cows.

> **DIFFERENTIAL DIAGNOSIS**
>
> Bovine mastitis associated with *Pasteurella multocida* must be differentiated from the many other forms of acute mastitis associated with this species; this can only be done by bacteriologic examination of the milk.

TREATMENT

In cattle, streptomycin administered by intramammary infusion is effective, but tetracycline is preferred. Recurrence in quarters that appear to have recovered is not infrequent, and response to treatment is often poor.

CONTROL

The standard control program described later in the chapter should control the disease in cows.

NOCARDIA SP.

Nocardial mastitis is an uncommon occurrence in cattle and is manifested as an acute or subacute mastitis accompanied by extensive granulomatous lesions in the udder.

ETIOLOGY

Nocardia are aerobic, gram-positive, filamentous, branching rods.[1] *Nocardia* spp. are ubiquitous environmental saprophytes with more than 30 named species.[2] *N. asteroides* can be cultured from the milk of affected quarters, and the disease can be produced experimentally by this organism. The most common species isolated from bovine mastitis are *N. nova* and *N. farcinica*.[3] Occasional cases of chronic mastitis associated with *N. africana, N. arthritidis, N. asteroides, N. brasiliensis, N. cyriacigeorgica, N. neocaledoniensis,* and *N. puris* have also been recorded.[3]

EPIDEMIOLOGY

Occurrence

With rare exceptions, nocardial mastitis in cattle has been recorded as a sporadic infection affecting only one or two cows in a herd. Accidental introduction of the causative bacteria into udders when infusions are being administered may create a herd problem. A large number of cases occurred in Canada from 1987 to 1989 because of intrinsic contamination of a neomycin-containing dry cow formulation with an amikacin-resistant strain of *N. farcinica*.[4,5] *N. neocaledoniensis* was isolated from the quarters of nine dairy cattle in Italy with chronic mastitis; intramammary infection was attributed to inadequate hygiene procedures during administration of intramammary therapy.[2] *Nocardia* is recorded as being a relatively common chronic mastitis in Cuba. Confinement of dairy cattle in muddy pens has been associated with an increased incidence of nocardial mastitis.

Source of Infection and Mode of Transmission

The bacteria is a common soil contaminant and probably gains entrance to the udder when udder washing is ineffective or udder infusion is not performed aseptically. *Nocardia* can survive in ineffective teat dips and may be spread by their use. The disease is most common in freshly calved adult cows, particularly if infusion of the udder with contaminated materials is performed in the dry period. *N. farcinica* is capable of surviving in mixtures used for intramammary infusion for up to 7 weeks. There is one record of a massive outbreak with many deaths in dairy cattle that was probably caused by the use of a contaminated homemade udder infusion.

Risk Factors

A sharp increase in isolations of *N. farcinica* in milk samples at veterinary diagnostic laboratories in Canada was related to the extensive use of a particular dry period treatment. Teat dips containing recommended concentrations of iodine or dodecylbenzene are effective against *Nocardia*, whereas those containing chlorhexidine acetate are not effective. When the dip is contaminated during use it may spread the organism to other quarters and other cows.

Economic Importance

The disease is a serious one because there is extensive destruction of tissue, loss of production, and occasionally death of a cow. Also, there is a possibility that human infection may occur, because the organism may not be destroyed by usual pasteurization procedures.

PATHOGENESIS

The inflammation of the teat sinus and lower parts of the gland suggests invasion via the teat canal. Infection of mammary tissue results in the formation of discrete granulomatous lesions and the development of extensive fibrosis, and the spread of inflammation occurring from lobule to lobule. Infected animals are not sensitive to tuberculin.

When infection occurs early, in the first 15 days of lactation, the reaction is systemic with fever and anorexia. At other times the lesions take the form of circumscribed abscesses and fibrosis. There may also be infected foci in supramammary and mesenteric lymph nodes.

CLINICAL FINDINGS

Affected animals may show a systemic reaction with high fever, depression, and anorexia, but an acute or subacute inflammation is more usual. Fibrosis of the gland and the appearance of clots in a grayish, viscid secretion that also contains small, white particles is the usual clinical picture. The fibrosis may be diffuse but is usually in the form of discrete masses 2 to 5 cm in diameter. Badly affected glands become grossly enlarged and may rupture or develop sinus tracts to the exterior. None of these cases recovers sufficiently to justify retention, and all are eventually culled.

Laboratory examinations of herds in which cases occur may also reveal subclinical cases that have intermittent flare-ups.

CLINICAL PATHOLOGY

The bacteria can be detected on culture of the milk. Small (1-mm diameter) specks are visible in the milk and, on microscopic examination, these prove to be felted masses of mycelia. Herds containing infected cows have been readily identified by culture of bulk milk samples. A gentamicin–blood culture medium has good selectivity. The normal blood agar plates need to be kept for an extended period of time to detect growth. Colonies may not appear until 72 hours.

NECROPSY FINDINGS

Grossly, diffuse fibrosis and granulomatous lesions containing pus are present in the mammary tissue. The lining of the milk ducts and the teat sinus is thick and roughened. On histologic examination the granulomatous nature of the lesions is evident. Metastatic pulmonary lesions have been found in occasional longstanding cases.

Samples for Confirmation of Diagnosis

- Bacteriology: mammary tissue, regional lymph node
- Histology: formalin-fixed mammary tissue for light microscopy

> **DIFFERENTIAL DIAGNOSIS**
>
> The appearance of the milk is distinctive, but cultural examination is necessary for positive identification.

TREATMENT

The disease does not respond well to treatment because of its chronic granulomatous nature. In vitro susceptibility tests suggest amikacin, gentamicin, and neomycin should be effective but will probably need to be administered for 1 to 2 weeks.

CONTROL

Invasion probably occurs via the teat canal from a soil-borne infection; proper hygiene at milking and strict cleanliness during intramammary infusion are therefore necessary on farms in which the disease is enzootic. Treatment in late cases is unlikely to be of value because of the nature of the lesions, and in affected herds particular attention should be given to the early diagnosis of the disease.

REFERENCES

1. Rieg S, et al. *BMC Microbiol.* 2010;10:61.
2. Pisoni G, et al. *J Dairy Sci.* 2008;91:136.
3. Condas LAZ, et al. *Vet Microbiol.* 2013;167:708.
4. Brown JM, et al. *Vet Microbiol.* 2007;125:66.
5. Kogure T, et al. *Antimicrob Agents Chemother.* 2010;54:2385.

BACILLUS SP.

Bacillus spp. are considered part of the normal microflora of the bovine teat.[1] *Bacillus cereus* and *B. subtilis* are saprophytic organisms and only chance mastitis pathogens; they have been known to cause an acute hemorrhagic mastitis in cattle. *B. cereus* cases are often associated with contamination associated with teat injuries or surgery. The mastitis may also occur in cows at the time of calving and is associated with the feeding of brewers' grains in which the spores of *B. cereus* are present. Some strains of *Bacillus* spp. appear nonpathogenic and the strain isolated from the teat of clinically healthy cattle can change rapidly over time.[1]

The infection is thought to occur during the dry period following the use of dry cow therapy preparations that may have been contaminated with the organism. Infection probably occurs at the time of infusion, but the acute mastitis does not occur until after parturition. *B. cereus* is a spore former and may remain dormant in the mammary gland for long periods, unaffected by the presence of the antibiotic. In one outbreak, 62 of 67 cows infused with a dry cow infusion product contaminated with the organism developed acute hemorrhagic mastitis. Six cows died; the remainder survived but were subsequently culled and slaughtered because of recurrent mastitis, inadequate milk production, and loss of weight.

Clinically, there is peracute to acute mastitis affecting one or more quarters. There is severe swelling and pain and the secretions are red-tinged and serous in consistency. Initially there is a high fever (40°C–41°C; 104°F–106°F) and severe toxemia. Affected cows are weak and quickly become recumbent; death may occur in 24 to 36 hours. Gangrene may occur and, in cows that survive, portions of affected gland will slough out and a chronic relapsing mastitis will persist. Experimentally produced mastitis caused by *B. cereus* causes toxemia, acute swelling of the quarter, and clots in the milk. The mastitis persists in a chronic form, and the quarter eventually dries up.

The organism can be usually cultured from milk samples from affected quarters. At necropsy there is focal hemorrhagic necrosis of the mammary tissue, acute lymphadenitis, and disseminated intravascular coagulation.

Treatment consists of intensive fluid therapy, a broad-spectrum antibiotic intravenously, and vigorous massage and stripping of the affected gland. Intramammary infusion of the most suitable antibiotic determined by culture and sensitivity is indicated, but the results are often not good because of the presence of severe hemorrhage and necrosis and plugging of the lactiferous ducts. Prevention depends on the use of sterile techniques during teat surgery and the use of sterile intramammary infusions and instruments. In problem herds, autogenous bacterins have been prepared but not extensively evaluated. If *B. cereus* infection is identified in the mammary glands of dry cows the recommended prevention program is infusion of each quarter with 750 mg of neomycin and 375 mg of framycetin.

B. subtilis is recorded less frequently as a cause of acute mastitis. Infection is characterized by yellow or bloody milk, sometimes with clots, and the cow is febrile.

CAMPYLOBACTER JEJUNI

Only one case of clinical mastitis has been recorded, but the incident is of some importance because of its zoonotic impact. Infection of the udder by the organism is easy to establish, and the infection is persistent but subclinical for the most part. Other experimental cases have been recorded, and campylobacters that have not been further identified have also been observed in naturally occurring cases. These are characterized by fine granular clots in the milk, very high cell counts, and a transient episode of fever and swelling of the quarter.

CLOSTRIDIUM PERFRINGENS TYPE A

This is a rare form of mastitis characterized by high fever, swelling, and superficial hyperemia of the affected quarter, followed later by gangrene, enlargement of the supramammary lymph nodes, a thin brown secretion containing gas, and subcutaneous emphysema. Early treatment with a broad-spectrum antibiotic can be successful, but advanced cases are uniformly fatal.[2]

FUSOBACTERIUM NECROPHORUM

This is a rare type of mastitis but is likely to have a high incidence in the herd when it occurs. Mixed infections of *F. necrophorum* appear to play an important role in summer mastitis caused by *T. pyogenes* (see section earlier this in chapter). Affected quarters have a viscid, clotty, stringy secretion but there is little fibrosis. No systemic reaction occurs, but treatment with a variety of antibiotics is unsuccessful.

HISTOPHILUS SOMNI

Histophilus somni (formerly *Haemophilus somnus*) has caused mild, chronic mastitis, including an acute form with high fever and bloodstained milk and a gangrenous form.

LISTERIA MONOCYTOGENES

Udder infection with *L. monocytogenes* is reported more often in sheep and goats than cattle.[3] However, it is a gram-positive facultative anaerobe that is being recorded with increasing frequency as a cause of bovine mastitis because of the zoonotic importance of the organism in dairy products. Most cases in cattle are subclinical and abnormal milk is rare.[3,4] The SCC is usually greater than 10^7 cells/mL milk. An ELISA and PCR have been used to detect antibody or bacterial antigen, respectively, in milk. One cow in Ireland with clinically normal milk was persistently infected for 6 months with a serotype 1/2b strain.[3] The milking system can be exposed to a variety of *L. monocytogenes* strains, but only a small percentage of these strains are able to persist within the milking system, suggesting that these strains possess factors that promote survival in this ecological niche.[5] Culture of bulk tank milk samples is an adequate means of locating herds with infected cows. Over a 23-year period in Denmark, the percentage of cows infected with the organism varied from 0.01% to 0.1% and that of herds with an infected cow from 0.2% to 4.2%.

Identifying listeriosis-infected cows is not easy because most infections are subclinical and clinical mastitis is usually mild; the milk is often normal in appearance, but the quarter does lose productivity and the milk carries a high SCC. The disease is characteristically unresponsive to treatment with penicillin, although the organism may be sensitive to the antibiotic in in vitro tests. The persistence of the clinical signs should arouse suspicion of *L. monocytogenes* as a cause.

MYCOBACTERIUM SP.

Tuberculous mastitis is described under tuberculosis. Other mycobacteria, especially *M. lacticola,* have been isolated from cases of mastitis in cattle that occur after the intramammary infusion of therapeutic agents in oils. The disease can be reproduced by the intramammary injection of the organism in oil but not when it is in a watery suspension. Subsequent oily infusions exacerbate the condition. Clinically, there is tremendous hypertrophy of the quarter with the appearance of clots in discolored milk, but there is no systemic reaction. Affected animals do not show sensitivity to avian or mammalian tuberculin. No treatment is effective. It is suggested that the treatment of injured teats and quarters with oil-based intramammary preparations is inadvisable because of the risk of them already being infected with mycobacteria.

A mild, acute mastitis, self-terminating and unresponsive to treatment, has occurred in outbreak form. It may be unassociated with intramammary infusion but is apparently predisposed because of stress and associated with an unidentified mycobacterium.

M. fortuitum is encountered rarely as a cause of a severe outbreak of bovine mastitis. Infected quarters are seriously damaged and do not respond to treatment, and affected cows die or are salvaged. The disease can be reproduced experimentally, and affected animals show positive reactions to mammalian and avian tuberculosis and some sensitivity to johnin. Similar experiences are recorded with *M. smegmatis* and *M. cheloane.* The mammary secretion of affected quarters varies from pus to a watery fluid containing flakes, and there is a high milk loss and irreparable damage to quarters. *M. smegmatis* causes hypertrophy of the gland of such proportions that all cases need to be culled. At least 15 different unique mycobacterial species have been cultured from unpasteurized bovine milk in Brazil.[6]

SERRATIA SP.

S. marcescens is the most common *Serratia* species causing mild chronic mastitis in cattle in which swelling of the quarters with clots in the milk appear periodically.[7] *Serratia* mastitis occurs naturally and has been produced experimentally.[7] *S. liquefaciens* has caused a similar mastitis. Most cases are sporadic, but herd outbreaks caused by the use of contaminated sawdust as bedding and inadequate cleaning of the teats before milking may occur. An epidemic in New York state was associated with the use of a chlorhexidine-containing teat disinfectant that permitted the growth of *Serratia* spp.[8,9] Generally, *Serratia* mastitis is not as severe as that caused by *E. coli* or *Klebsiella* spp.

S. marcescens is susceptible to a large number of antimicrobials in vitro with the exceptions being penicillin, ampicillin, and cephapirin.[10] Neomycin (2 g initially followed by 3 daily doses of 1 g by intramammary infusion) has provided a satisfactory treatment.

FUNGI AND YEASTS

A larger variety of fungi and their unicellular form (yeasts) have been isolated from the glands of cattle with clinical mastitis, but the true pathogenic potential of a number of these isolates has yet to be determined.

Cryptococcus neoformans, the yeast that causes human cryptococcosis, has caused acute mastitis in cattle and buffaloes. Contaminated infusion material and spread from other infected quarters are the probable sources of infection. Infection in humans drinking the milk is unlikely to occur because the yeast does not withstand pasteurization, but there may be some hazard to farm families. Although there is no systemic reaction, the mastitis may be acute, with marked swelling of the affected quarter and the supramammary lymph node; a severe fall in milk yield; and the appearance of a viscid, mucoid, gray-white secretion. Clinical mastitis persists for some weeks and, in many cases, subsides spontaneously, but in others the udder is so severely damaged that the cow has to be slaughtered. Systemic involvement occurs rarely. At necropsy, there is dissolution of the acinar epithelium and in chronic cases a diffuse or granulomatous reaction in the mammary tissue and lymph node. Similar lesions have been found in the lungs.

Many other fungi, including *Candida* spp., *Saccharomyces* spp., *Pichia* spp., and *Torulopsis* spp. have also caused mastitis in cattle. A survey of 91 bovine cases of fungal/yeast mastitis in the United States showed that 78% belonged to *Candida* spp.; this genus contains at least seven different species that have been isolated from the bovine mammary gland.[11] Infection is probably introduced by contaminated intramammary infusions or teat cup liners. Establishment of the infection is encouraged by damage to the mammary epithelium and stimulated by antibiotic therapy; for example, *Candida* spp. use penicillin and tetracyclines as sources of nitrogen.

A fever (41°C; 106°F) is accompanied by a severe inflammation of the quarter, enlargement of the supramammary lymph nodes, and a marked fall in milk yield. The secretion consists of large, yellow clots in a watery supernatant fluid. Lesions are limited to the walls of the milk cistern, and there is no invasion of the mammary gland itself. Usually the disease is benign and spontaneous recovery follows in about a week.

Trichosporon spp. can cause mastitis in cattle and is manifested clinically by swelling of the gland and clots in the milk. The infection rate is low, and the fungi disappear spontaneously. Experimental transmission of the disease has been effected. In cases of infection by *Aspergillus fumigatus* or *A. nidulans* there are multiple abscesses in the quarter. These are surrounded by granulation tissue, but the milk ducts are generally unaffected.

None of these infections responds well to antimicrobial therapy but treatment with iodides, either sodium iodide intravenously, organic iodides by mouth, or iodine in oil as an intramammary infusion, might be of value. A number of drugs, including cycloheximide, nystatin, polymyxin B, neomycin, and isoniazid, have been tested for efficiency against mastitis in cattle produced experimentally by the infusion of *C. neoformans* but did not alter the clinical course of the disease. Merthiolate (20 mL of a 0.1% solution) as an infusion daily for 2 to 3 days is reported to have a beneficial effect if administered early in the course of the disease. Actinomycotic agents tested in vitro against fungi, mostly *Candida* spp., from cases of mastitis showed sensitivity to clotrimazole, nystatin, polymyxin, miconazole, and amphotericin B, and least sensitivity to 5-fluorocytosine. Miconazole (200 mg as an intramammary infusion administered a total of 8 times at 12-hour intervals) was not effective in treating dairy cows with moderate to severe clinical mastitis.[12] Sulfamethoxypyridazine given parenterally (22 mg/kg BW for 2–3 days) has resulted in more than 50% clinical cures in quarters infected with *C. krusei*. A case of mastitis caused by *A. fumigatus* has been successfully treated by concurrent intraarterial injection and intramammary infusion of 100 mg of miconazole at each site. Clinical signs included fever, anorexia, and depression; a hard, swollen, hot gland with clots in the milk; and a negative response to treatment with intramammary antibiotics.

ALGAE

The only known plants that cause infectious diseases in animals are unicellular round to ovoid colorless algae in the genus *Prototheca*, which lack chlorophyll.[13] *Prototheca* is ubiquitous in the environment. It is a zoonotic disease that can be transmitted to humans when they ingest milk from infected cows.

P. zopfii and *P. blaschkeae* have been identified as causes of chronic bovine mastitis.[14,15] *P. zopfii* consists of different biotypes based on biochemical and serologic grounds, and all clinical and subclinical mastitis isolates are genotype 2,[13,16–19] or genotype 3, now renamed *P. blaschkeae*. Extremely strong herd-level risk factors identified associated with the presence of *Prototheca* in composite milk samples were intramammary infusions with a nonintramammary formulation (OR = 136.8), the use of a dry cow internal teat sealant (OR = 34.2), or the use of a dry cow external teat sealant (OR = 80.0).[20] These high OR estimates support the presence of a causal effect between poor teat hygiene practices and intramammary infection with *Prototheca* spp. Reduced milk yield, large white clots in watery milk, and induration of the affected quarter may be the only clinical signs. Cases of this disease are usually sporadic, but one severe outbreak is recorded. Experimental transmission of the disease causes a progressive pyogranulomatous lesion in the gland, and the organism can be isolated from draining lymph nodes. *Prototheca* spp. are commonly isolated from animal environments, particularly mud and standing water.

P. zopfii strains isolated from mammary glands are resistant to many antimicrobials, but are susceptible to kanamycin, gentamicin, amphotericin, and ketoconazole.[19] Treatment is usually unsuccessful, and affected cows should be culled; because of a high prevalence rate in many affected herds the loss to the farmer can be considerable.

Control measures should focus on implementing good hygiene practices at milking and identifying environmental sources for contamination. Iodine teat dip concentrations (0.16%–0.63%) and sodium hypochlorite teat dip concentrations (0.04%–0.16%) were effective in killing *Prototheca* in one study[21]; another study identified minimal microbiocidal concentrations of 0.3% to 1.3% for iodine and 0.005% to 0.020% for chlorhexidine.[22] *Prototheca* can form biofilms, even on stainless steel, and this may facilitate their persistence in the dairy environment.[23] Bedding type appears to impact growth of *Prototheca* spp.,[24] but the recommended strategy of housing cattle on clean dry bedding should decrease the risk of mastitis caused by *Prototheca* spp.

TRAUMATIC MASTITIS

Injuries to the teats or udder that penetrate to the teat cistern or milk ducts, or involve the external sphincter, are commonly followed by mastitis. Any of the organisms that cause mastitis may invade the udder after such injury, and in such cases mixed infections are usual. All injuries to the teat or udder, including surgical interference, **should be treated prophylactically with broad-spectrum antibiotics.**

REFERENCES

1. Al-Qumber M, Tagg JR. *J Appl Microbiol.* 2006;101:1152.
2. Osman KM, et al. *Comp Immunol Microbiol Infect Dis.* 2010;33:505.
3. Hunt K, et al. *Ir Vet J.* 2012;65:13.
4. Rawool DB, et al. *Int J Food Microbiol.* 2007;113:201.
5. Latorre AA, et al. *Appl Environ Microbiol.* 2011;77:3676.
6. Franco MMJ, et al. *BMC Vet Res.* 2013;9:85.
7. Harp JA, et al. *Vet Immunol Immunopathol.* 2006;109:13.
8. Muellner P, et al. *Spat Spatiotemporal Epidemiol.* 2011;2:159.9.
9. Schukken Y, et al. *Vet Clin North Am Food Anim Pract.* 2012;28:239.
10. Ohnishi M, et al. *Vet Microbiol.* 2011;154:202.
11. Dworecka-Kaszak B, et al. *Scientific World J.* 2012;196347.
12. Roberson JR, Kalck KA. *Bovine Pr.* 2010;44:52.
13. Möller A, et al. *Vet Microbiol.* 2007;120:370.
14. Marques S, et al. *J Clin Microbiol.* 2008;46:1941.
15. Osumi T, et al. *Vet Microbiol.* 2008;131:419.
16. Ricchi M, et al. *Vet Microbiol.* 2013;162:997.
17. Cremonesi P, et al. *J Dairy Sci.* 2012;95:6963.
18. Sobukawa H, et al. *J Dairy Sci.* 2012;95:4442.
19. Jagielski T, et al. *J Antimicrob Chemother.* 2012;67:1945.
20. Pieper L, et al. *J Dairy Sci.* 2012;95:5635.
21. Salerno T, et al. *Res Vet Sci.* 2010;88:211.
22. Krukowski H, et al. *Turk J Vet Anim Sci.* 2013;37:106.
23. Goncalves JL, et al. *J Dairy Sci.* 2015;98:3613.
24. Adhikari N, et al. *J Dairy Sci.* 2013;96:7739.

Control of Bovine Mastitis

Improvement in udder health has been a major initiative of the dairy industry for over 50 years. The thrust of these efforts has been on the implementation and use of management techniques to limit the spread of major mastitis pathogens, reducing the quarter infection rate. Detailed mastitis control strategies have been outlined and promoted by the National Institute for Research in Dairying (NIRD) and the NMC (www.nmconline.org/). With proper implementation, these programs result in a dramatic decrease in the prevalence of common contagious mastitis pathogens. Herds that have successfully implemented a comprehensive mastitis control program also need to develop strategies to control infection with environmental organisms, as well as using an effective monitoring system for new infections. Achievement of excellent udder health for the production of high-quality milk is a realistic and important goal for all aspects of the dairy industry.

The adoption of effective mastitis control programs has often been less than desirable, even with extensive research validation of the recommended control practices and with major extension efforts at both national and local levels. The reasons for this slow adoption of proven mastitis control strategies are not well documented, even though producers look to the veterinary profession for information on mastitis and its control. Veterinarians usually become involved in mastitis control in one of the following circumstances:

- The herd is experiencing a higher than normal incidence of clinical cases.
- The milk processing plant reports a higher than permissible total bacterial count or bulk tank milk SCC.
- A farmer who is not performing the standard program of postmilking teat dipping and dry period treatment asks for advice—either as a single mastitis control program or, more probably, as part of a herd health management program.

The procedure is the same in all these situations, and any variation is in terms of speed and intensity. It consists of an assessment of the herd's mastitis status and the implementation of a recommended mastitis control program.

Udder Health Improvement

The benefit of an integrated mastitis program is improved udder health; this improvement is progressive and can usually be observed within a few years after implementation at the herd level. Methods now exist to control contagious pathogens and reduce the bulk tank milk SCCs to below 400,000 cells/mL. With good management, the incidence of clinical mastitis can be kept low (7–21 cases per 100 cows per year) by culling any cow with chronic or recurrent mastitis and paying great attention to housing and management standards.

Although the rate of contagious mastitis has been decreased with implementation of an integrated mastitis program, the rate of infections and the incidence of mastitis associated with environmental pathogens such as *S. uberis* and the coliform bacteria have not decreased. Approximately 65% of clinical cases are now caused by environmental pathogens. Organisms prevalent in the cow's environment currently cause the most costly types of mastitis in the United States.

Economic Benefits, Incentives, and Penalties

Mastitis is one of the most costly diseases in dairy herds. Some surveys indicate that the cost incurred by producers because of clinical mastitis is much higher than the cost of prevention. An integrated mastitis control program has always been an excellent investment for the dairy farmer, with a revenue to cost ratio of approximately 6 : 1; most of the additional revenue is from increased milk production.

Differential payments to farmers for milk quality are also an **economic** incentive to adopt a control program. The widespread adoption of bulk tank milk SCCs as a measure of milk quality, and the adoption of payment schemes of increasing severity, has stimulated farmers to reduce their cell count. Many milk marketing cooperatives have established both penalty and incentive programs based on bulk tank milk SCC and total bacterial counts as global measures of milk quality.

Requirements

The requirements for a successful mastitis control program include a willing farmer, a capable diagnostic laboratory, an enthusiastic and knowledgeable veterinarian, a record keeping system, adequate milking machinery, and adequate housing facilities.

The farmer must have health and production goals and be willing to achieve them by making a commitment to invest the resources to control mastitis. Wide variations in the costs of controlling and monitoring mastitis in herds are evident because of lack of client compliance with accepted recommendations for mastitis control. There are also variations in the level of mastitis control procedures adopted by producers that affect the success of a program. Lack of adoption may result from a lack of awareness of the economic returns from a complete program, adoption of a new practice only in response to a problem, or competition for liquid financial resources from other aspects of the enterprise.

The veterinarian must be knowledgeable about all aspects of mastitis and be willing to invest the time and effort required to provide sound advice based on the health and production information obtained from monitoring the herd. A data recording system that records all the udder health and production data and the milk quality of each cow and the herd on a regular basis is a vital requirement. A diagnostic laboratory or milk recording agency that provides regular SCCs of individual cows is necessary to monitor udder health. The milking machine and the housing facilities must be adequate for the size of the herd. Farmworkers must be aware of the health and production goals of the herd and adhere to the principles of mastitis control.

OPTIONS IN THE CONTROL OF MASTITIS

The broad options for control are either eradication or decreasing the infection rate, either by legislative control or implementing a voluntary program.

Eradication

Complete eradication of bovine mastitis from a herd or geographic region is not a practicable target in most circumstances. The exception is mastitis caused by *S. agalactiae*, which can be eradicated from individual herds by a blitz antibiotic technique. The difficulty in attempting to eradicate mastitis is that the contagious causes of mastitis, *S. agalactiae* and *S. aureus,* are so contagious, and the sources of infection so widespread, that adequate quarantine would be very difficult to maintain. In the case of *S. aureus* there is the additional difficulty of eliminating the infection from its intracellular sites in mammary tissue. The environmental infections, especially *E. coli,* pose an even greater problem. They are so ubiquitous that reinfection would be almost immediate in cows housed in economically practicable surroundings.

Decreasing the Infection Rate

This is a practicable proposition; the degree of limitation is dependent on the need to maintain cost-effectiveness. One of the virtues deriving from this necessity is the concept that subclinical mastitis causes a continuous low-level leukocytosis in the milk that acts as a protective mechanism against other infections. Present-day knowledge about immunity in the mammary gland suggests that control programs that reduce milk SCCs to unrealistically low concentrations may reduce the gland's resistance to clinical mastitis. Correspondingly, the complete elimination of common udder pathogens such as *S. agalactiae* and *S. aureus* is thought to increase the susceptibility of the udder to environmental pathogens, especially coliform bacteria. Another relevant example is the commonly encountered minor pathogen *C. bovis,* which may be a significant microbial agent in maintaining the resistance of udders. The mastitic effect of this organism is too low to warrant specific action, but the infection rate with major pathogens is significantly lower in quarters that harbor *C. bovis* than in those that do not. An intensive program to disinfect udders could well eliminate *C. bovis* and increase susceptibility to other pathogens. *C. bovis* is likely to be more important where cows are housed, or confined in straw yards, and therefore more exposed to teat contamination with coliforms. The question of whether it is better practice to maintain some level of bacterial infection with innocuous organisms in the udder as a protection against more damaging pathogens, rather than to attempt complete bacterial sterilization, is still unresolved. For now it is generally agreed that decreasing the infection rate is the appropriate target.

Legislative Control

Mastitis does not lend itself to eradication (as set out under the section Eradication), so legislative control of the disease is not widely implemented. Norway has implemented national control of mastitis, starting with a requirement in 1975 that records of mastitis treatments were to be maintained. This was followed by implementation of the Norwegian Mastitis Control Program in 1982.[1]

A Voluntary Program

Most of what is done in mastitis control in dairy herds is through voluntary involvement by producers in programs aimed at reducing the incidence of mastitis and maintaining the infection rate at a low level. The justification for control of the disease is purely economic, and a control program must therefore be based on its applicability on each individual farm. Area or national control can only be in the form of providing incentives by educational and laboratory assistance to individual farmers who wish to participate. The value of a mastitis awareness program, and the part played by the two-way flow of information between farmers and the program operators, is most apparent when an area campaign is conducted by a government or industrial sponsor. Once a control program is in place it is customary for milk processors, aided in some places by government agencies, to encourage participation by paying incentives for bulk tank milk with low SCCs or bacteria counts, or refusing to accept milk for processing or, in some cases, refusing to transport milk that does not satisfy statutory requirements. This could be the first step in incorporating the program into planned health and production programs that promote mastitis control and maintenance of milk production at financially optimal levels.

Mastitis infections in beef cattle herds are currently at too low a level for a mastitis control program to be financially advantageous.

PRINCIPLES OF CONTROLLING BOVINE MASTITIS

DYNAMICS OF INFECTION

The principles of a bovine mastitis control program are based on changing the dynamics of infection, which are as follows:

- **Prevalence of infection is a function of the rate of new infection minus the rate of elimination**
- **Rate of new infection is a function of the level of exposure times the number of susceptible quarters**
- **Rate of elimination is a function of the number of infections times the efficacy of treatment plus spontaneous cure**

Successful control occurs when the level of infection is held low or is decreased, either by preventing new infections or eliminating existing infections.

The dynamics are not, however, so simple in reality. They vary with the susceptibility of the individual animal, which changes with **age** and **stage of lactation** (Fig. 20-6) and is **season dependent.** The dynamics may vary with the pathogens involved, and the relative importance between herds can be very considerable and also vary with time. The duration of infection may be extremely different for different pathogens. *E. coli* causes mild to severe acute clinical disease but usually self-eliminates quickly; it is rarely found in subclinical infections. *S. agalactiae* and *S. aureus* are very persistent, and *S. aureus* responds poorly to treatment. The rate of elimination and the persistency of these pathogens are highly variable. Similarly, there can be large variations in the rate of new infections, which is closely related to the identifiable risk factors, including rate of teat contamination, mechanisms aiding teat penetration, and effectiveness of establishment and growth of bacteria in the mammary gland.

The success of a control program can be measured by the decrease in level of infection and the speed with which this is achieved. The farmer must be able to appreciate progress within a year to remain enthusiastic about application of the methods. The level of infection can be controlled significantly by lowering the rate of new infections, but the speed of change really depends on the duration of the infection and is thus related more to the rate of elimination. No control procedures are available to prevent all new infections, and only culling of chronically infected cows is absolutely successful in eliminating infections. Control schemes therefore require both prevention and elimination to give optimal effect, and that optimum will vary with each pathogen.

The specific components of a mastitis control program must be devised to fulfill three basic principles: (1) **eliminate existing infections**, (2) **prevent new infections,** and (3) **monitor udder health.**

1. ELIMINATE EXISTING INFECTIONS

The control program must reduce the duration of infection in the cows. Antimicrobial therapy during the dry period remains the best method of achieving this objective (Fig. 20-7). Treatment during lactation can be useful to eliminate some existing infections, depending on the causative agent, and is often effective in resolving clinical mastitis episodes. Culling of chronic cases that are not eliminated with dry period treatment is also used to remove the most persistent existing infections. Further study needs to focus on development of treatment protocols and on cowside identification of the causative bacterial agent.

2. PREVENT NEW INFECTIONS

The control program must reduce the rate at which new infections occur. The dipping of all teats in an effective teat dip after each milking is the best method to reduce the new infection rate. Ensuring that the milking machine is functioning properly and used correctly will result in less spread of infection. The dry period is the time of greatest risk of new infection, and blanket dry cow

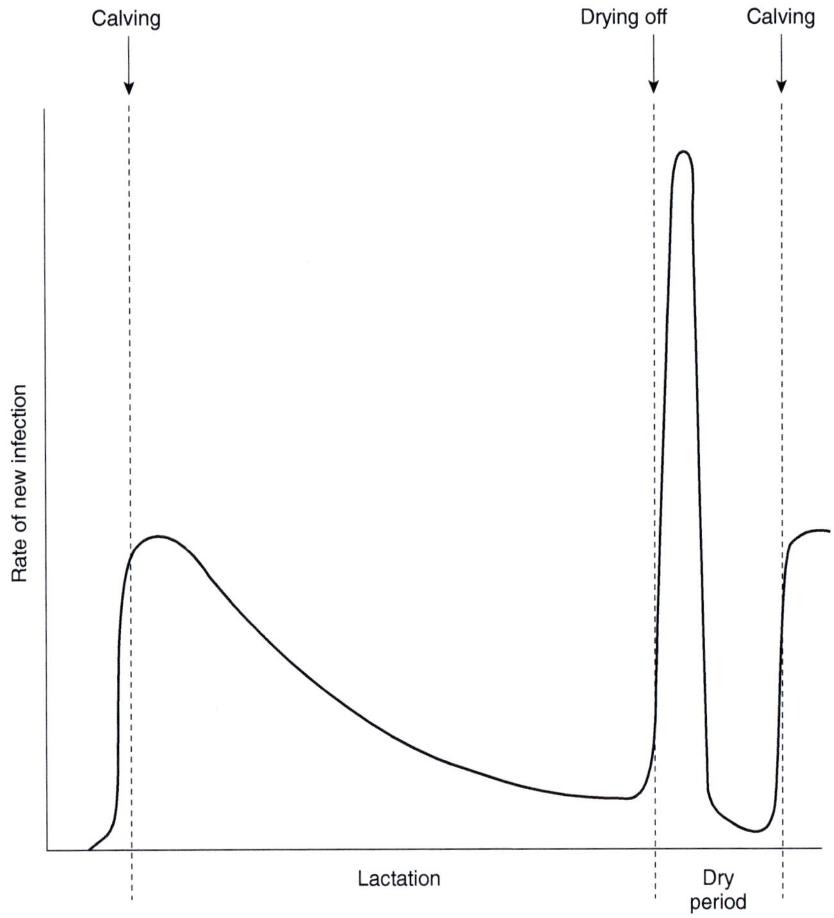

Fig. 20-6 New infection rate in cows by stage of lactation. (Reproduced with permission from Natzke RP. *J Dairy Sci* 1981;64:1431-1441.)

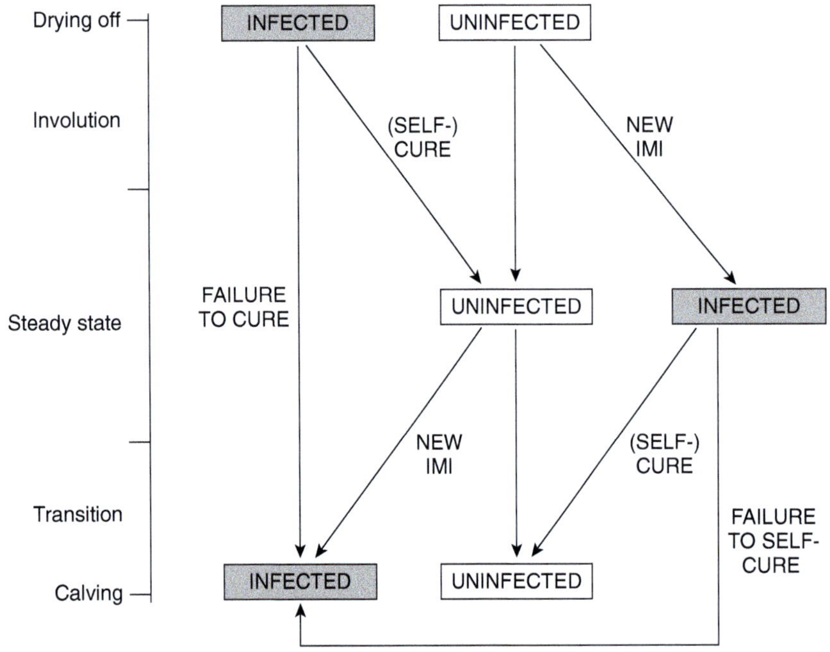

Fig. 20-7 A summary of the possible outcomes for individual quarters during the dry period. IMI, intramammary infection. (Reproduced with permission from Bradley A, Barkema H, Biggs A, et al. *Dairy Herd Health,* Wallingford, UK: CAB International 2012;144.)

therapy or application of an internal teat sealant is efficacious in preventing new infections during the dry period. Environmental and nutritional management have also become important for the prevention of new infections. Specific recommendations for methods of reducing new infection rate depend on the predominant pathogen in the herd.

A novel method for preventing new infections during the second half of the dry period and the start of lactation is to administer polyethylene glycol–conjugated **bovine granulocyte colony-stimulating factor** (**bG-CSF**) subcutaneously approximately 7 days before the anticipated calving date followed by a second injection immediately after calving. Administration of **bG-CSF** markedly increased the blood neutrophil count and decreased the number of clinical mastitis episodes caused by environmental pathogens.[2]

3. MONITOR UDDER HEALTH STATUS

An ongoing program to monitor the udder health status of individual cows as well as the herd is needed to evaluate the effectiveness of the control efforts. Monitoring methods should also assist with specific decision making, such as optimized treatment protocols or culling. In the five-point mastitis control programs recommended by the NIRD and the NMC, monitoring was not emphasized. As udder health status improves, and as milk quality premiums and penalty programs become meaningful, there is a need to continuously monitor udder health.

MASTITIS CONTROL PROGRAMS

A major step forward in mastitis control occurred in 1970 with the publication of the results of controlled field studies performed by the NIRD. The **five-point control plan** was based on attacking the key areas in the dynamic processes of mastitis, and the individual components of the plan were evaluated as efficacious by field testing in dairy herds. Its success has been well documented. **The five-point plan has been highly successful for the control of contagious mastitis but is not adequate for the control of environmental mastitis.** The plan depends heavily on the motivation, education, and financial commitment of the milkers and the herd owner to achieve good and consistent results.

The five-point mastitis control program is as follows:

1. Udder hygiene and proper milking methods
2. Proper installation, function, and maintenance of milking equipment
3. Dry cow management and therapy
4. Appropriate therapy of mastitis cases during lactation
5. Culling chronically infected cows

Five additional management practices are recommended to make a **10-point mastitis control program,** which includes emphasis on an appropriate environment, particularly for the control of environmental mastitis, and the keeping of records, monitoring udder health, and setting goals for udder health status.

6. Maintenance of an appropriate environment
7. Good record keeping
8. Monitoring udder health status
9. Periodic review of the udder health management program
10. Setting goals for udder health status

The 10-point mastitis control program satisfies the basic needs of the farmers, which is an essential prerequisite in the implementation of a voluntary program. The program is profitable, within the scope of the producer's technical skill and understanding, capable of being introduced into current management systems, and encourages farmers to continue the program by rapidly reducing the occurrence of clinical mastitis and the rejection of milk by milk processors on the grounds of quality. Very helpful checklists that include all components of the recommended mastitis control program are available for North America and international dairy enterprises (www.nmconline.org; accessed July 2016).

The components of the recommended 10-point mastitis control program are the same for all situations. The exact level of severity at which it will be implemented depends on its cost-effectiveness; higher milk and cattle prices will justify higher financial inputs. The program has the virtues of simplicity, profitability, and widespread applicability, and most countries with a significant dairy industry have devised their own variant of it to suit their own local needs, especially the targets of freedom from infection and other quality-control criteria. The 10-point program was designed primarily for the control of the common contagious mastitis pathogens and may encounter difficulties unless measures to control the environmental infections receive special attention.

TEN-POINT MASTITIS CONTROL PROGRAM

1. UDDER HYGIENE AND PROPER MILKING METHODS

The principles of a proper milking procedure include:

- Premilking udder hygiene
- Stimulation of milk letdown
- Efficient removal of the milk
- Postmilking teat disinfection

These principles are important for controlling the spread of contagious pathogens and for preventing new intramammary infections associated with environmental organisms. There is much farm-to-farm and region-to-region variation in how these milking procedures are applied. Milking methods are often taught to milkers by observation of the current methods used on the farm, and milkers are seldom objectively evaluated, especially in family farm operations with only one or two farm employees.

Several important steps are necessary in establishing a milking management routine, including the following.

Establish and Maintain a Regular Milking Schedule in a Stress-Free Environment

A management routine using twice-daily milking should strive for a 12-hour interval. In the same way, an 8-hour interval between milkings is necessary for thrice-daily milking. The milking schedule is obviously less important with robotic milking. Consistency is as important as maintaining these exact intervals. Any influence that may add stress to the milking environment is to be avoided. For example, harsh crowd gates, rough handling, barking dogs, and people shouting can be associated with epinephrine release, which will counteract the effect of oxytocin for efficient milk letdown.

Ensure That Teats Are Clean and Dry Before Milking

The major objective of premilking udder preparation and teat sanitation is to reduce the microbial population of teat skin, particularly at the teat end. The aim of these techniques is to minimize the probability of new intramammary infection and have good milking performance. Milking time hygiene is extremely important because of the potential interaction between milking machine function and the microflora of teat skin. The incidence of intramammary infection is highly correlated with the number of mastitis pathogens on the teat end at milking.

Udder Hygiene Score

An udder hygiene scoring system has been developed, with the udder viewed from behind. Score 1 is an udder free of dirt, score 2 has 2% to 10% of the surface area dirty, score 3 has 10% to 30% of the surface area covered with dirt, and score 4 has more than 30% of the surface area covered with caked-on dirt. A hygiene scoring system is repeatable and easy to use, but only hygiene scores for the udder and hindlimbs are associated with cow composite milk SCCs.

Premilking Cow Preparation

Premilking cow preparation is a step in milking management in which there is considerable variability between what is recommended and what is actually practiced. **The goal is to milk clean and dry teats.** Current recommended procedures for premilking udder preparation range from water hose washing and manual drying of teats, to washing teats with a paper towel wetted in warm sanitized solution plus drying with a single service paper towel, to the use of premilking teat dipping in germicide plus paper towel drying. The additional step of premilking teat disinfection (predipping) has been incorporated as part of the milking routine on many dairy farms. It is argued that manual teat washing improves stimulation and the release of oxytocin for milk letdown, in addition to cleaning debris from the teats and teat ends. However, with properly functioning milking equipment, there is little evidence that the manual massage is necessary for good milk letdown. In milking parlors in which handheld spray washers are used, it is important to avoid wetting the udder. Excessive water use can lead to bacterial contamination of the teat cups and to an increase in the incidence of mastitis. In addition to individual paper towels, the use of disposable latex or nitrile gloves is also recommended to minimize the transfer of mastitis pathogens from the milkers' hands to the teats. Gloves that become soiled with organic and fecal material should be replaced.

Check Foremilk and Udder for Mastitis

Early clinical mastitis can be detected by physical examination of the udder for swelling, heat, or pain, and by using a strip cup or black plate to examine foremilk from each quarter of each cow before every milking. This step has been a standard NMC management recommendation, but the supporting evidence has been inconsistent. The rate of implementation of foremilk stripping (forestripping) is widely variable and depends on the management system used. Forestripping is more common in milking parlor situations.

Checking foremilk has three major advantages:

1. Detection of clinical mastitis (such as the presence of clots and stringy or watery milk), as early as possible: Detection of abnormalities is enhanced if the milk is evaluated against a dark surface such as a black strip plate.
2. Forestripping: This theoretically aids in preventing new infections of the mammary gland by flushing pathogens from the teat streak canal before milking. Bacterial colonization of the teat canal may not represent a problem until the organisms gain access to the teat sinus beyond the rosette of Furstenburg.
3. Stimulation of the milk letdown process: This could be helpful in systems in which minimal cow preparation is used, such as a premilking program consisting of only a dry wipe.

In tie-stall barns, a strip cup is necessary to avoid contaminating the stall bedding or the cow herself. In milking parlors, it is common to use the concrete floor surface for detection of abnormalities in the milk. In either case it is important to recognize the potential for cow-to-cow transmission of pathogens by milk contact from one teat to another. For this reason, forestripping must be done before the predipping or udder washing step.

Foremilk stripping is often not done in pasture-based dairy industries, such as Australia and New Zealand, because it takes time and slows down the milking process. Moreover, if the clinical mastitis incidence is 2 cases per month per 100 lactating dairy cattle, then in herds milking twice a day, milkers have to forestrip 12,000 teats to identify one clinical case of mastitis. Despite the very low incidence of clinical mastitis detected by foremilk stripping, in seasonal calving herds that are pasture based it is probably helpful to examine the foremilk for the first 2 to 4 weeks after calving, because this is the highest incidence of clinical mastitis in this dairy system.

Premilking Teat Disinfection

Premilking teat disinfection, more commonly referred to as **predipping**, is used by some dairy producers as a component of a mastitis control program. Premilking teat disinfection in association with good udder preparation and postmilking teat disinfection can further reduce the occurrence of new intramammary infections during lactation. The use of predipping is increasing as the predominant cause of mastitis shifts from contagious pathogens to environmental pathogens. Controlled studies on the effectiveness of predipping indicate significant merit in the use of iodine predipping for the reduction of udder infections caused by environmental pathogens in some, but not all studies. Some studies found that premilking teat dipping with 0.25% iodophor did not reduce the incidence of clinical mastitis caused by environmental pathogens, and the use of 0.5% iodophor plus good udder preparation did not affect the prevalence of infection of coagulase-negative *Staphylococcus* spp., but the rate of clinical mastitis in the control group was 1.38 cases per 1000 cow-days compared with 1.06 cases per 1000 cow-days in the predipped group. The benefit: cost ratio of 0.37 indicated that the benefit of reduced incidence of clinical cases of mastitis did not justify the added expense required to predip the herd. A study in New Zealand with pasture-based dairy cattle found that the addition of premilking chloramine-T teat disinfection provided no benefit to that obtained by postmilking chloramine-T teat disinfection applied as a spray.[3]

Although premilking teat dipping with iodine-based sanitizers may play a role in reducing new intramammary infections, there are some precautions that should be taken. The major concern is the potential for increased iodine residues in milk. Predipping with either 0.5% or 1% iodophor does not significantly increase milk iodine residues if a paper towel is used to dry the teats. Without drying, iodine residues are significantly increased. In addition, predipping in combination with postmilking teat disinfection may increase the potential for residues.

Implementation of predipping into the cow preparation methods may require significant management changes, such as the drying of teats. Some, or possibly all, of the improvement in udder health associated with the implementation of a predipping program may be attributable simply to the milking of clean, dry teats. Before the commencement of predipping, attaching the unit to wet or dirty teats may have been common. Whatever management methods are adopted on a particular farm, premilking hygiene and udder preparation can have a significant effect on milk bacterial counts and on the incidence of mastitis. In summary, the current evidence supports the use of premilking teat disinfection as a routine procedure in dairy herds in which environmental pathogens are the predominant cause for mastitis. A 2008 survey in the United States indicated that the most commonly used germicidal predip formulations were iodine (60%), chlorhexidine (12%), unspecified (8%), chlorine (7%), fatty-acid based (2.5%), and quaternary ammonium (0.3%).

Attach the Milking Unit Properly

The milking unit teat cups should be carefully attached to the udder within 90 seconds of starting udder preparation. The milk letdown process that follows the release of oxytocin after udder stimulation is at maximum for 3 to 5 minutes. Some effects of the oxytocin may last up to 8 minutes. It is important to use this physiologic event to its maximum for the most efficient removal of the milk. The proper timing of attaching the milking unit has been shown to shorten milk-out time and increase lactation productivity. However, consistency in the time interval from stimulation to attachment of the unit is as important as the exact time.

When attaching the teat cups, it is imperative to minimize the amount of air drawn into the system. Excessive air inlet could result in vacuum fluctuations, which may predispose to milk aerosol impacts of the teat end and machine-induced infections.

The machine position and support should be adjusted as necessary during milking. This will ensure that quarters milk out properly. The milking unit should hang on the cow as straight and level as possible. Improperly adjusted support could contribute to uneven milk out and to an unbalanced udder on some cows; in addition, there is an increased probability of liner slips and squawking, which in turn will increase the risk of new intramammary infections. The mechanics and importance of liner slips will be discussed with milking machine function later in this chapter.

The use of proper milking machine attachment and adjustment methods affects the number of milker units that can be efficiently handled per person. With a tie-stall barn pipeline milking system it is recommended that a maximum of three units per person be used. It is unlikely that producers who milk with more than three units in a tie-stall barn are using appropriate cow preparation and milking machine attachment methods.

Minimize Machine Stripping and Avoid Liner Slips

The majority of milking-machine-induced intramammary infections occur near the end of milking. Liner slips occur with a greater frequency near the end of milking. During a liner slip, air sneaks in between the teat and liner (heard as a squawk), increasing the potential for small droplets of contaminated milk to be propelled backward against the end of the other teats (**teat-end impacts**). Over a sustained period of time, liner slips and milk impacts may result in an intramammary infection.

Machine stripping is the act of putting hand pressure on the milker unit at the end of milking to remove extra milk. Machine stripping is habit forming, and will eventually lead to increased milking time. It also increases the risk of squawking, liner slips, and milk impacts.

Avoid Overmilking or Removing the Unit Under Vacuum

As soon as a cow is milked out, the vacuum to the milker unit should be shut off, and the teat cups should be removed. The milker unit should gently "fall off" the teats, causing no irritation. This is best performed using automatic take-offs that detect a low flow of milk from the teat end and automatically detach the milking cluster from the udder. Removing the unit under vacuum will cause milk and air to impact onto the teat ends. Overmilking should be avoided to prevent teat-end irritation. The unit should be removed as soon as the first quarter is milked out. The risk of liner slip is also increased during overmilking, but there is little evidence that overmilking will result in an increased rate of intramammary infection, unless liner slips and teat-end impacts occur. The practice of removing teat cups individually is also discouraged.

Use an Effective and Safe Postmilking Teat Germicide (Teat Dip) After Every Milking

Teat dipping or spraying with a germicidal solution immediately after every milking is an effective milking management practice to reduce the rate of new intramammary infections. **Postmilking teat antisepsis is regarded as the single most effective mastitis control practice in lactating dairy cows.** The prevalence of *C. bovis* in milk cultures usually reflects inadequate teat disinfection, because spread of *C. bovis* is easily controlled by postmilking test disinfection. Quarters colonized with *C. bovis* usually remain so until treated with an effective dry-cow intramammary formulation. In other words, the prevalence of *C. bovis* infection will usually not decrease for approximately a year after implementing an optimal postmilking disinfection protocol.

Teat dipping or spraying is a simple, effective, and economical means to reduce bacterial populations on teat skin. There is general agreement that the numbers and types of bacteria on teat skin have a direct relationship to the incidence and types of intramammary infections that develop in a herd. An effective teat dip, correctly used, will reduce the incidence of new udder infections by 50% to 90%.[3]

There are several major classes of postmilking teat sanitizer and many available products within each class. The classes of product vary widely in their composition, formulation, and mode of action. Each product should be evaluated for its safety, efficacy, advantages, and disadvantages. The most commonly used teat dips fall into several major classes, with geographic differences in availability. A 2008 survey in the United States indicated that the most commonly used germicide postdip formulations were iodine (69%), chlorhexidine (13%), fatty-acid based (7%), unspecified (4%), chlorine (2%), and quaternary ammonium (0.6%).

Iodine Formulations

Iodine teat dips are used extensively and marketed in a variety of formulations, ranging from 0.1% to 1.0% available iodine. Iodine formulations are active against bacteria, viruses, and fungi, and ideally they should be used at a minimum 0.5% available iodine concentration. The safety and efficacy of these products are well established, and it is difficult to identify a reason why iodine formulations should not be the preferred choice for postmilking teat antisepsis. They were historically called iodophor teat dips because many contained phosphoric acid, which is no longer the case.

Chlorhexidine

Chlorhexidine teat dips are also widely used and effective for reducing new infections. They are more efficacious in the presence of organic material than other classes of product. Chlorhexidines have a broad spectrum of antimicrobial activity and excellent persistence on teat skin, but they are minimally effective against viruses and fungi. Commercial preparations are formulated with a dye to make the product visible and with glycerin to minimize teat skin irritation.

Linear Dodecyl Benzene Sulfonic Acid Products

LDBSA teat dips contain an organic acid and are formulated with emollients. They are generally nonstaining, tolerant of organic matter, and less irritating than most other products; their efficacy against major mastitis organisms is well established.

Quaternary Ammonium Compounds

A variety of quaternary ammonium chemicals, in combination with lanolin or glycerin, are available as teat dip germicides and are safe and effective. They are readily broken down in the environment and depend heavily on proper formulation for effectiveness.

Sodium Hypochlorite

Many dairy farmers prepare their own teat dip by dilution of commercial laundry bleach to a final concentration of 4% sodium hypochlorite. It is effective and extremely low cost. However, these dips are not government approved, have a strongly disagreeable odor, and can be inactivated by organic material. There is also a risk of mixing errors, resulting in the potential for irritation of teats and milkers' hands.

External Teat Sealants (Barrier Teat Dips)

A goal that has yet to be achieved is development of a barrier teat dip that provides an effective teat sealant for use in lactating cows and withstands environmental contamination but is easily removed with minimal premilking udder preparation. Latex and acrylic latex-based products have been developed to act as a physical barrier to the entrance of mastitis pathogens into the udder. These products were aimed at the prevention of coliform mastitis. However, it has proved to be difficult to remove the residual product from teats. Furthermore, the barrier product alone is not intended to be effective against other major mastitis organisms.

External teat sealants have been formulated in combination with disinfectants to provide protection as both a barrier and a germicide. A postmilking teat disinfectant containing 0.64% sodium hypochlorite in a gel formulation was an effective and safe teat dip preparation. However, in experimental studies, barrier teat dips were no more efficacious in preventing new intramammary infections caused by *S. aureus* and *S. agalactiae* than no teat dip or the use of a nonbarrier product. In contrast to their current use in lactating dairy cows, external and internal teat sealants are increasingly applied at dry off (see the section Dry Cow Management and Therapy).

Selection and Use of Teat Disinfectants

With the extensive array of commercially available postmilking teat germicidal preparations, producers need some guidelines to make an appropriate selection for use on their farms. Manufacturers of teat dips should provide the producer with documentation of the efficacy and safety of each product. In the United States, teat dip products must be listed with the Food and Drug Administration (FDA). The FDA regulates teat dips for compliance with label accuracy and manufacturing quality, but efficacy data are not required for registration. In Canada, teat dips must be approved by the Bureau of Veterinary Drugs. This approval process requires extensive data on human safety, animal safety, and the efficacy of each new teat dip submission. Standard protocols have been endorsed for the evaluation of teat dip efficacy under conditions of experimental challenge with mastitis pathogens, as well as under conditions of natural exposure in commercial dairy herds.

In the United States, iodine-based teat dips are the most commonly used product for postmilking disinfection, and an **iodine-based teat dip in 10% glycerin is generally regarded as the gold standard teat dip** against which all other teat dips are compared. Dairy producers should request information on effectiveness when selecting a teat dip. Veterinarians should assist producers with interpretation of the data. There is no evidence that changing teat dips on a regular basis is necessary to prevent the development of resistant mastitis bacteria. Monitoring several measures of udder health status will signal the need for a change in teat dip product. The teat dip selected must be compatible with other chemical preparations used in the milking management system.

Postmilking teat dips can be applied by dipping or spraying. In North America, **dipping has been the most popular method**. However, with the increase in herd size and parlor automation, there is an increase in the use of teat spraying because it is quicker and easier. Spray and dip application of the same product result in equal efficacy, when done appropriately; however, it is easier to do a bad job of teat coverage with spraying than dipping. Under field conditions, the effectiveness of either method will depend on adequate coverage of each teat. A general recommendation is that **as much of each teat should be covered as is possible and no less than the lower half**.

Teat dips should be stored in a cool dry place and not be allowed to freeze. Contamination should be prevented and expiry dates observed. For economic reasons, producers are tempted to dilute commercially available products; however, their effectiveness and safety may not be maintained. **At the end of milking, unused teat dip solution should *not* be poured back into the original container.** Dipping devices should be cleaned regularly.

In cold weather conditions, precautions should be taken with respect to teat dipping. A high emollient concentration product should be used. Dipped teats should be allowed to dry before cows are exposed to cold and windy conditions. This may be accomplished by allowing the dip 30 minutes of contact time, followed by removal of excess disinfectant with a laundered dairy cloth or a single-use paper towel. Windbreaks should be provided for cows that have access to outside areas. These combined strategies will minimize the occurrence of frostbite of wet teats.

Establish Milking Order and Segregation Programs

In herds with a significant prevalence of contagious pathogens, such as *S. aureus,* establishing a specific milking order may be helpful to limit the rate of new infections. This is a popular veterinary recommendation that is **difficult to implement** because it usually requires massive disruption of the milking procedure. Generally, first-lactation heifers and fresh cows should be milked first. Cows with high SCCs, chronic clinical mastitis, and current clinical cases should be milked last. The maintenance and management of both SCCs and clinical mastitis records becomes important to make milking order programs work.

In larger herds, cows are usually grouped according to stage of lactation and production level. For nutritional management reasons, it is often suggested to have high-, medium-, and low-production groups. In herds with a high prevalence of *S. aureus* mastitis, it has been suggested that the problem of spread would be stopped by simply isolating infected cows and milking them last. In theory, segregation combined with culling and effective dry cow management should allow the prevalence of *S. aureus* to approach zero. However, the change in prevalence of *S. aureus* infection in unsegregated herds compared with herds using a segregated program indicates no significant difference. A more significant decrease in prevalence of *S. aureus* mastitis was found in herds that gave priority to a full milking hygiene program in combination with dry cow therapy and culling. Segregation is not a simple, stand-alone solution to a contagious mastitis problem.

Disinfect Teat Liners

Disinfection of the milking machine teat cup liners between cows has the potential of limiting the spread of contagious organisms from cow to cow because bacterial populations in liners can be greatly reduced by sanitization. However, there is considerably less documentation that flushing liners will result in major reductions in contagious mastitis problems.

In tie-stall milking barns, **liner disinfection** is a laborious process that involves dipping the claw in a series of solutions. Liners must be put through a rinse, a disinfectant, and another rinse to remove the germicide. The solutions should be kept hot and replaced when they become overly contaminated. Only two liners can be dipped at one time if the milk hose remains connected to the pipeline to avoid an air lock in the claw, which will reduce the disinfection process. However, if the milk hose is disconnected from the milk pipeline, then all four liners can be dipped at one time. Even with these limitations, dairy herds with intensive management, utilizing individual cow SCCs and culture information, can effectively use liner sanitization to limit the spread of contagious pathogens. Electric hot pails are commercially available to maintain the disinfection solution at a sterilization temperature.

In large milking parlor operations, automatic **backflushing** of milking units between cows is commercially available but expensive to install. In conjunction with automatic take-offs, the claw is flushed with rinse water, followed by disinfectant, and again rinsed, immediately after the unit detaches from a cow. An alternative procedure (**cluster dunking**) involves backflushing the milking units with water until a clear stream is obtained and then dunking the milking units in a bucket containing disinfectant while avoiding trapping of air in the dunking process. Large numbers of pathogens can be removed from teat cups by the backflushing process, but documented reductions in the new intramammary infection rate are not available. For instance, backflushing decreased the numbers of staphylococci and gram-negative bacteria on liners by 98.5% and 99.5%, respectively and caused a small decrease in the number of new infections by *C. bovis* but had no effect on the incidence of new infections by staphylococci, streptococci, or coliforms. Until backflushing has been demonstrated to decrease the new infection rate, the procedure cannot be a routine recommendation.

2. PROPER INSTALLATION, FUNCTION, AND MAINTENANCE OF MILKING EQUIPMENT

The milking machine plays an integral role in the efficiency of the operation of a dairy farm, and it has direct contact with teat tissue. It must perform properly and consistently, two or three times a day (or much more frequently in robotic milkers), day after day, year after year. For these reasons, it is important that the milking system is installed according to approved guidelines. Regularly scheduled maintenance should be performed, and machine function should be evaluated by periodic analysis of the system. All persons in the milking management process should thoroughly understand the basic components, function, and operation of the milking equipment. They should also be aware of the significance of regular equipment maintenance and of the importance of good milking techniques.

Milking System Function and Objectives

The milking system performs several basic functions to achieve its objectives:

- Causing milk to flow from the teat by exposing the teat ends to a partial vacuum
- Massaging the teat in an effort to relieve the effects of a continuous milking vacuum
- Protecting the milk from contamination while it is transported to a storage device, which cools and stores the milk until it can be transported to the processing plant

Components of a Milking System

To perform the basic functions and to achieve the objective of efficient removal of the milk with minimal opportunity for intramammary infection, milking and milk handling equipment requires three basic components:

- Vacuum system
- Milk pipeline system
- Bulk milk tank for milk cooling and storage

Considerable engineering expertise goes into the proper design, installation, and function of milking equipment. For the purposes of understanding the basic principles of machine milking, a brief description of these three components will be provided.

Vacuum System

Vacuum Pump

The function of milking equipment depends on the creation of a partial vacuum. A **vacuum pump** is used to continuously remove some of the air from the various lines in the milking system. The amount of air removed determines the system vacuum level, which is important for proper function. The vacuum level is monitored using a gauge that is read in either kilopascals (kPa), millimeters of mercury (mm Hg), or inches of mercury (in.Hg). If one-half of the air is removed from the system, then the vacuum gauge will read 50 kPa (15 in.Hg) vacuum. Vacuum pumps are rated on the basis of the volume of air they can move when the intake vacuum is at 50.7 kPa (15.0 in.Hg). Cubic feet per minute (CFM) is the standard air flow measurement used. The CFM rating of a vacuum pump determines the number of milking units that can be used on the system. For example, to operate 6 units, the minimum vacuum pump capacity is 52 CFM.

Vacuum Reserve Tank

Because the vacuum pump continuously removes a constant amount of air from the system, a **vacuum reserve tank** is placed between the pump and the vacuum supply line. The purpose of this tank is to provide a common site for connecting the vacuum header lines and to provide a reserve of vacuum to help buffer the sudden admission of air into the system. For example, when a milking unit falls off a cow, there should be enough reserve vacuum to maintain the system function. The amount of reserve vacuum needed in a system is a function of pump capacity, pump performance, regulator operation, and the degree of system leakage. Vacuum reserve tanks are usually constructed of PVC plastic and should not be less than a 75-L capacity.

Vacuum Regulator

A **vacuum regulator** or controller is an important component of the vacuum system. The function of the regulator is to keep the vacuum of the milking system at a preset level by responding to changing air admissions into the system. The regulator should be located in proximity to, or directly on, the vacuum reserve tank. It should be sensitive to handle a rapid response to changes in vacuum. Servo-diaphragm regulators are the most sensitive style available and are highly recommended. An increase in vacuum pump capacity cannot compensate for poor regulator function. Likewise, a sensitive regulator cannot compensate for a deficiency in pump capacity. The two components must work well together.

It is recommended that two vacuum gauges be installed in the system to monitor the system vacuum. One gauge should be located on the milking vacuum supply line near the regulator. A second gauge is best situated at the far end of the vacuum pulsation line. A portable mercury manometer should be used on a regular basis to calibrate the accuracy of the system vacuum gauges and to make adjustments to the vacuum regulator. The preferred vacuum system installation consists of two header lines from the vacuum reserve tank, continuing to form a completely looped pulsation line. The recommended vacuum lines are 76-mm diameter PVC pipe, adequately supported, and slightly sloped in the direction of air flow and with automatic drain valves. This line allows for attachment of the milking unit pulsators.

Pulsation System

A properly functioning pulsation system is critical to teat and udder health. The pulsator causes the chamber between the teat cup shell and the liner to alternate regularly from vacuum to air source. Pulsators are either electromagnetic or pneumatic. In an electromagnetic system, all pulsators function together off an electrical signal. An electronic control circuit turns current on and off to the electromagnet. Pneumatic pulsators run off the vacuum system and use air to move a plunger or slide valve to cover and uncover the air passage, producing the pulsating action.

An understanding of the dynamics within the teat cup and the characteristics of pulsation is crucial to ensuring that the objectives of mechanical milking are achieved. The chamber between the teat cup shell and the liner is regularly subjected to a vacuum source, whereas the inside of the liner is under stable milking vacuum at all times. The pulsation cycle involves a milk phase and a rest or massage phase. When air is admitted between the shell and the liner, the liner collapses around the cow's teat. The collapsed liner has a massaging action on the teat, which is called the **rest** or **massage phase**. Milk does not flow from the teat during this phase. When the pulsator opens, the space between the liner and the shell is exposed to system vacuum. This creates equal pressure on both sides of the liner, causing it to open. The cow's teat end is now exposed to the milking vacuum. This vacuum, in combination with the internal pressure of milk letdown within the cow's udder, causes milk to be drawn out through the teat streak canal. This component of pulsation is called the **milk phase**. The process of milking involves repeatedly opening (milk phase) and closing (rest phase) the teat cup liner.

The **pulsation cycle** is measured by the time, in seconds, for the completion of one milk phase and one rest phase. The **pulsation rate** refers to the number of cycles completed by a pulsator in 1 minute. Pulsation rates range from 45 to 60 cycles per minute. The **pulsation ratio** is the length of time in each cycle that the pulsator is in its milk phase compared with its rest phase. A common pulsation ratio is 60:40, indicating that in each pulsation cycle the teat cup chamber will be milking 60% of the time and massaging the teat 40% of the time. Wide pulsation ratios can speed up milking time but can put undue stress on the teats and teat ends from insufficient rest, predisposing to new intramammary infections.

Pulsation phase refers to the method of pulsation for the whole milking unit and is either simultaneous or alternating. In simultaneous pulsation all four teat cups milk at the same time and rest at the same time. With alternating pulsation, two teat cups milk while two teat cups rest, then alternate to complete the pulsation cycle. The alternating action may be from side to side or from front to rear. Alternating pulsation has several advantages. It allows a more uniform milk flow into and out of the claw, which helps to minimize flooding of the claw, resulting in fluctuations in the teat-end vacuum. In addition, front/rear alternating pulsation allows for a wider pulsation ratio on the rear quarters, which encourages a more uniform and timely milk out of all four quarters. For alternating pulsation systems with two different ratios, care must be taken to ensure that air hoses are not reversed when attached to the claw.

Electromagnetic pulsators are unaffected by environmental temperature and can function at a constant preset pulsation rate and ratio. Pneumatic pulsators can be greatly affected by changes in temperature and system vacuum. They require more maintenance and constant checking of the settings. Thus **electromagnetic pulsators using alternating pulsation are most recommended**, particularly for high-producing cows with fast milk letdown.

If a teat cup is not positioned properly on a teat, the liner may slip down the teat and produce a squawking sound. As this is happening, air is entering around the teat into the liner. The entrance of this air changes the system of stable milking vacuum within the claw and the other teat cups. These changes lead to droplets of milk being driven in a reverse direction back at the teat ends of the other teats. These are referred to as **milk impacts**. Repeated teat-end milk impacts, particularly with milk contaminated by mastitis pathogens, can result in new intramammary infections.

Milk Transport System

Milking parlors and stanchion barn pipelines have similar systems for transporting milk from the cow to the bulk tank. The components of the transport system will be described in the direction of milk flow. The rubber or silicone insert in each teat cup is referred to as a **liner** or **inflation**. The liner should milk cows safely, with a minimal number of squawks from downward slippage, and without the teat cup crawl action of riding up on the teats to the base of the udder. Liner performance depends on many interrelated characteristics of the milking system. **Narrow bore liners are recommended**. Liners must be compatible with the teat cup shell. The most important management consideration with respect to teat cup liners is to **ensure regular replacement, as recommended by the manufacturer.** As a general guideline, natural rubber liners last 500 to 700 cow milkings, synthetic rubber liners 1000 to 1200 cow milkings, and silicone liners 5000 to 10,000 cow milkings. The desired milking inflation replacement interval (in days) can be calculated using the following formula:

$$\begin{aligned}&\textit{Number of days between changes}\\&\quad=((\textit{number of cow milkings/set of liners})\\&\qquad\times(\textit{number of units}))/\\&\qquad\quad((\textit{number of cows milking})\\&\qquad\times(\textit{number of milkings/day}))\end{aligned}$$

Other rubber parts of the unit, such as the short air tubes on the claw, should be constantly checked for cracks or signs of wear. These problems could seriously affect air flow and liner pulsation. Proper storage in dark, cool conditions, as well as the correct use of cleaners and sanitizers, can affect the life of rubber parts.

Milk Claw

The **milk claw** is an important component of the milking unit. The claw is the collection point for milk from the four teat cups and should have adequate capacity to handle peak milk flow without flooding. Each claw should have a means of shutting off the vacuum to the teat end, so that the unit is not removed under vacuum. Most claws have an air vent in the upper half to allow a predetermined quantity of air into the unit to facilitate milk flow away from the cow and into the pipeline. Claws should routinely be **inspected for cleanliness, plugged air vents, and dented liner connectors**.

A long milk hose is used to carry milk from the claw to the pipeline. The hoses can be made of plastic, rubber, or silicone. **They should be as short as possible,** with an appropriate hose hanger. If the milk hose is crimped or allowed to loop, milk flows will be interrupted, which leads to irregular fluctuations in teat-end vacuum. The milk hose should attach to an inlet located in the top third of the milk pipeline, at the 11 o'clock or 12 o'clock position. Inlets should be self-draining, self-closing, and should not cause milk flow restrictions that would result in irregular teat-end vacuum fluctuations.

Milk Pipeline

The **milk pipeline** serves two important functions: transporting milk from the cow to the receiver jar and carrying air flow to provide milking vacuum to the teat end. Either glass or stainless steel can be used for milk pipeline construction. The milk line should form a complete circuit and must be rigidly supported from the floor to maintain the appropriate slope. It is generally recommended that **milk lines be installed as low as is practical**. In milking parlors, low pipelines are installed below udder level. In stall barns, high pipelines are used, but they should be no higher than 2 m above the cow platform. Milk moves by gravity through the pipeline to the receiver jar. The milk line must be self-draining and should have a continuous slope from the high point toward the milk receiver jar. The **correct slope** is important for the movement of milk and air during milking and for proper cleaning of the system. In the construction of new tie-stall barns, it is recommended that the foundation, floor, and gutter be sloped toward the milk house end. This will help to minimize pipeline height and to ensure that line slope will facilitate drainage during milking and washing.

Line diameter is another important feature of milk pipeline design. In addition to line slope and the level of herd production, pipeline diameter will determine the number of milking units that a system can handle. Too many units will lead to milk line flooding and a reduction in air flow rate. Slugs of milk moving through the line is an obvious sign of milk line flooding. This problem will have a negative impact on milking time, herd production, and udder health. The recommended minimum pipeline diameter is 51 mm (2.0 in.). At this pipeline size, high-producing herds should not use more than three milking units per pipeline slope. Thus larger pipeline sizes are often recommended for new installations. Pipeline couplers or welds must prevent air leakage into the system.

Milk should flow into the receiver jar in a continuous, unimpeded fashion. When sufficient milk has accumulated, an electronic probe triggers the milk pump to transfer milk from the receiver jar to the bulk tank. A milk filter is inserted into the transfer system to remove coarse impurities that may have entered the line. The receiver jar is connected to the main vacuum supply. A device called a sanitary trap is used to separate the "air-only" portion of the milking system from the "milk-handling" side of the system. The sanitary trap is designed to protect the vacuum supply from potential damage caused by the chemical cleaning and sanitizing solutions used to clean milk pipelines.

A milking system should have the capability of measuring the amount of milk from each cow. In older milking parlor systems, weight jars were often used for this purpose. They allowed for a quick visual means of monitoring individual cow production at each milking, as well as providing vacuum stability to the cow. However, they were expensive and represented a challenge to clean. More recently, milk metering systems have been developed that give an **electronic digital readout of the milk volume produced** at each parlor station. These systems can often be adapted to provide automatic data recording in an on-farm computer system. In stall barn pipeline installations, several types of mechanical milk meters are in use. It is important that any metering system should not be restrictive to the flow of air and milk. These restrictions can cause a drop in teat-end vacuum and the occurrence of irregular teat-end vacuum fluctuations. Increased milking time, incomplete milk out, and new intramammary infections can result.

Bulk Milk Tank

The bulk milk tank is the vessel used to cool and store raw milk until it is picked up by the bulk milk transport truck. All tanks must be of an approved sanitary design and construction. They must be of sufficient capacity to cool and store up to 3 days of milk production. The cooling capabilities of bulk milk tanks are clearly specified. Appropriate cleaning and sanitizing procedures for bulk tanks are critical to prevent bacterial growth and contamination of raw milk.

Relationship of Milking Equipment to Udder Health

The milking machine can influence new intramammary infection rates in several ways:

- It may be a carrier of mastitis pathogens from one cow to the next.
- It may serve as a pathway of cross-infection within cows.
- Malfunctioning or improperly used equipment may result in failure to relieve congestion in teat tissue. Eventually, teat-end damage and intramammary infection can occur.
- Abrupt loss of milking vacuum may create changes in air movement of sufficient force to move pathogens past the streak canal defenses. This phenomenon, known as the impact mechanism, was described earlier.

The pathogenesis of new infections related to machine milking probably involves all four of these factors. However, even though the milking system becomes the focus of many herd udder health investigations, there is little evidence that machine factors are of primary importance in most problem herds. It has been difficult to link milking machine factors and prevalence of herd infection, with the clear exceptions being **pulsation failure** and the **impact mechanism.** Mastitis has been difficult to produce experimentally by altering machine function.

Appropriate pulsation is important for sufficient teat-end massage. Although continuous vacuum will remove milk from cows' teats, eventually it will result in excessive congestion, edema, and teat-end damage. An adequate compressive load by the liner on the teat tissue is necessary to relieve the congestion. Mechanical failure of the pulsator, shortness of the liner barrel. and a too-short liner rest phase are the most common examples of pulsation problems. The impact mechanism results from an abrupt loss of milking vacuum. Poor liner design has been shown to increase the frequency of liner slips. During a liner slip, a reverse pressure gradient occurs across the streak canal of the other three teats. Liner design has been shown to be very important in reducing the amount of slippage. In combination with liner slips, the vacuum fluctuations that result from pulsation problems can lead to new intramammary infection.

Even with the myriad of potential machine problems, milking equipment is not usually the major risk factor for poor udder health.

Maintenance and Evaluation of Milking Equipment

The most important aspect of udder health management related to milking equipment is the establishment of an appropriate evaluation, maintenance, and service schedule. Farm personnel should incorporate an inspection of the equipment into their regular milking process. Many of the problems discussed in conjunction with the description of milking system components can be discovered during this daily inspection. In addition, the producer should have milking equipment serviced on a regular basis. Items such as the vacuum pump, regulator, pulsators, and sanitary trap would be included in this check list. Also included in this inspection will be regular changing of the teat cup liners and other rubber parts. It is common for equipment dealers to schedule a regular visit to each farm client for the purpose of conducting this periodic maintenance schedule and for dispensing chemical cleaners and disinfectants used in the udder health management program.

A complete milking system analysis should be conducted on a regularly scheduled basis. This regular analysis is perhaps just as important as the initial design and installation of the system. Many dairy cattle specialists believe that a regular independent analysis will ensure proper equipment function. Milking system analysis can be conducted by equipment dealers, government extension staff, veterinarians, or independent technicians. All these individuals need the appropriate knowledge and training. It is essential to use some type of systematic milking system analysis worksheet to record various performance measurements and to identify components requiring service or upgrading. A complete system analysis should be conducted at least once a year, and records should be kept for future reference.

Robotic Milking

Mastitis control in robotic milking systems has specific challenges related to ensuring that clean dry teats are milked, diagnosing clinical mastitis, and the treatment of cows with clinical mastitis. Additional information is provided in a review article by Edmondson listed in additional reading.

3. DRY COW MANAGEMENT AND THERAPY

The proper management of dry cows and late-gestation heifers is an important component of a mastitis control program. The dry period offers a valuable opportunity to improve udder health while cows are not lactating. However, the beginning and the end of the dry period represent periods of increased risk of infection. **The objective of udder health management during the dry period is to minimize the number of infected quarters at calving.** Two of the three major principles of udder health management must be met to achieve this objective. **Infections present at the time of drying off should be eliminated,** and **the rate of new intramammary infections during the dry period must be minimized.** Thus dry cow therapy has a dual role in eliminating existing infections and preventing new infections during the dry period and has been widely adopted by dairy farmers. If these two principles are followed, udders will be free of infection at calving and can be expected to produce a maximum amount of low-cell-count milk in the subsequent lactation. Intramammary administration of long-acting antimicrobial agents to all cows at drying off remains a routine recommendation.

Epidemiology of Intramammary Infection During the Dry Period

The development of effective udder health management strategies for the dry period requires an understanding of the epidemiology of intramammary infections in dry cows. This in turn requires an understanding of the incidence of new infections during the dry period and the types of pathogen involved. Risk factors that affect the susceptibility of dry cows should also be understood.

Incidence of New Infections

The rate of new intramammary infections is significantly higher in the dry period than during lactation. The greatest increase in susceptibility is during the first 3 weeks of the dry period. In this period, the new infection rate is many times higher than during the preceding lactation as a whole. A second period of heightened susceptibility occurs just before parturition. The reported rates of new intramammary infection in the dry period vary widely. Reasons for these differences include the diagnostic criteria used and the types of organism considered to be major pathogens. There are also important herd-level effects, such as the prevalence of existing infections at drying off and the method of dry off. The average rate of new infections in untreated dry cows is expected to be between 8% and 12% of quarters.

Types of Pathogen Causing New Infections During the Dry Period

Contagious pathogens are transmitted among cows and quarters in association with the milking process. **Environmental pathogens** are primarily contracted from contamination with organisms in manure and bedding. **Teat skin opportunistic pathogens** are present on the teat, particularly the teat end. Contagious, environmental, and teat skin opportunistic pathogens need to be considered in designing mastitis control schemes for the dry period.

Exposure to environmental pathogens is likely to continue throughout the dry period; thus prevention of new dry period infection with environmental agents represents a considerably greater challenge. Herds that have implemented a basic mastitis control program still need to be aware of the importance of preventing environmental infections in the dry period. There are different rates of infection by the various environmental agents as the dry period progresses. For example, infections with environmental streptococcal species, *Klebsiella* spp., and *Enterobacter* spp. occur more frequently early in the dry period. On the other hand, *E. coli* infections tend to occur immediately before calving. Dry cow management strategies need to account for the risk of infection during the entire period from last milking until the next calving.

Risk Factors That Affect Susceptibility in Dry Cows

Several factors contribute to the variation in susceptibility during the dry period. These factors are included in the following sections.

Teat-End Protection

The cessation of routine milking-time hygienic practices such as teat dipping allows bacterial subpopulations on teat skin to increase in number and diversity. *S. aureus* numbers are high immediately after drying off, and environmental pathogens are more prevalent on teat skin late in the dry period and at calving time. Teat-end lesions increase the likelihood of intramammary infections during the dry period. A plausible mechanism to explain this association is that teat-end lesions increase the surface area available for bacterial colonization while presenting a variety of environmental niches. For instance, quarters with cracked teat ends were 1.7 times more likely to develop a new intramammary infection during the dry period than unaffected quarters.

The streak canal of the teat is more penetrable by bacteria during the early dry period. The **keratin plug** in the streak canal must form early and completely in the early dry period to prevent penetration and growth of bacteria and decrease the incidence of new intramammary infections. However, this natural internal teat sealant does not form in some cows, and delay in formation is common. For instance, in cows in New Zealand, 45% of teats are open on day 7 of the dry period, and 25% are still open on day 35 of the dry period. Similar results were obtained in North American dairy cows. Quarters that remain open during the dry period are 1.8 times more likely to develop a new intramammary infection than quarters that have developed an effective keratin plug. Internal and external teat sealants are discussed later in this chapter.

Swelling of the mammary gland, an increasing volume of secretion, and leaking colostrum contribute to the high risk of new infection during the prepartum period.

Resistance Mechanisms Within the Mammary Gland

Throughout the dry period there are marked changes in the composition of mammary gland secretions and in the concentration of protective factors such as leukocytes, immunoglobulins, and lactoferrin. These changes probably influence the variation in susceptibility to both environmental and contagious pathogens.

Substantial evidence exists that innate and acquired defense mechanisms are lowest from 3 weeks precalving to 3 weeks postcalving. This lowered responsiveness includes aspects of systemic and mammary gland immunity that may account, in part, for the increased incidence of peripartum disease. Polymorphonuclear neutrophil function is impaired during the peripartum period and may contribute to the increased incidence of mastitis following calving. Diminished lymphocyte responsiveness around calving has also been observed. The role of the cow in effectively transferring antibodies and cells to the mammary gland before parturition to ensure high-quality colostrum is also an important function, and this may be affected by prepartum vaccination schedules and the ability of the animal to respond effectively.

Milk Production at Dry Off

A high level of milk production at dry off increases the incidence of new intramammary infections at calving. It is reasonable to assume that high milk production at dry off will produce a higher intramammary pressure, increasing the likelihood of an open streak canal early in the dry period. High milk production at dry off will also decrease the concentration of protective fractions such as phagocytic cells, immunoglobulin, and lactoferrin, decreasing resistance within the mammary gland. The finding that cows leaking milk following dry off are four times more likely to develop clinical mastitis in the dry period supports the concept that **increased milk production at dry off increases the rate of new intramammary infections**.

Method of Drying Off

The industry standard method for cessation of lactation (drying off) is abrupt cessation of milking, in which milking stops on the day scheduled for dry off (all cows are usually scheduled to "go dry" on the same day each week) to facilitate administration of dry cow intramammary antibiotics, vaccinations, and vitamin E/selenium injections.

The large increase in milk production over the past 50 years has led to a new challenge; producers are forced to dry off dairy cattle at the end of lactation that have high milk production (>15–20 kg/day). Abrupt drying off high-producing dairy cattle leads to rapid mammary distention and the leakage of milk that appears to be associated with an increased incidence of environmental intramammary infection. Abrupt drying off of high-producing dairy cattle also results in stress (based on increased fecal corticosteroid concentrations)[4] and behavioral changes, including bellowing, increased standing time looking at the milking parlor (indicating a preference to be milked), and reduced number of lying bouts.[5] Consequently, abrupt dry off of high-producing dairy cattle is increasingly viewed as an animal welfare and mastitis problem, and many producers are interested in effective and practical methods that alleviate stress at dry off.

For decades, the standard recommendation to decrease mammary distention and therefore stress when abruptly drying off high-producing dairy cattle has been to decrease energy intake over 1 to 2 weeks before dry off. In North America in component fed systems, this recommendation is implemented by decreasing the amount of grain fed. In total mixed ration systems, this recommendation is implemented by decreasing the total amount fed when cows are individually housed; however, this recommendation is impractical in free-stall systems. Other approaches have been a gradual cessation of milking (such as once a day for the last 5 days).[5] Generally, gradual cessation of milking has not provided any significant production advantages, and as a result, abrupt cessation of milking remains the industry standard at dry off, coupled with an immediate change in diet.

A longstanding recommendation has been to decrease water intake at dry off, because this decreases milk production. This practice is rarely undertaken in northern Germany,[6] and it has been discouraged by the New Zealand dairy industry to comply with animal welfare codes. However, water intake is likely to be decreased at abrupt dry off because drinking behavior appears to be closely coupled with milking in dairy cattle and is also dependent on dry matter intake.[7]

Parity

Older cows are more likely to develop new intramammary infections during the dry period. This increased predilection may be caused by increased milk production at dry off, increased prevalence of abnormal teat placement (increasing exposure of the teat end to pathogens), or increased prevalence of open streak canals because older cows have higher milk production.

Risk Factors That Affect Susceptibility in Heifers

An increased risk for intramammary infection in the preparturient period in heifers is associated with the presence of *S. aureus* or *M. bovis* in the herd, calving in summer, high herd bulk tank milk SCCs, poor fly control, mastitic milk fed to calves, and contact with adult cows. Other risk factors are increased age at first calving, prepartum milk leakage, blood in milk, and udder edema.

Udder Health Management Strategies for Dry Cows

Antimicrobial Therapy (Dry Cow Therapy)

Antimicrobial therapy at the end of lactation (dry cow therapy) has been one of the key steps in mastitis control programs and has become the most effective and widely used control method for dry cows. The efficacy and advantages of antimicrobial therapy are well known. A meta-analysis concluded that the use of effective dry cow products resulted in a 78% increase in the elimination of existing infections,[8] with no detectable difference for pathogen type, including *S. aureus*. An accompanying meta-analysis indicated that dry cow therapy provided significant protection against new intramammary infections caused by *Streptococcus* spp. during the dry period and the first 21 days of lactation, but no protection was observed for new coliform or *Staphylococcus* spp. intramammary infection.[9]

Long-acting antimicrobial preparations have been formulated to **eliminate existing infections** and to **prevent new infections**. These preparations include benzathine cephapirin, benzathine cloxacillin, and sustained-release formulations of erythromycin, novobiocin, and penicillin. The withholding period for milk from animals treated with these dry cow formulations ranges from 30 to 42 days after treatment. It is important that the label directions are followed carefully for the recommended dosage level, required withdrawal period, storage guidelines, and expiry dates. A general recommendation is that dry cow treatment should never be administered within 1 month of the expected calving date. Single-dose syringe preparations of dry cow antibiotic treatment are recommended. The risk of contamination by environmental bacteria and yeast is much higher for multiple-dose bottles than for single-dose syringes. If bulk containers are used, great attention should be paid to maintaining sterility.

The use of long-acting and short-acting antimicrobial intramammary infusions at dry off have been compared. In some cases, short-acting antimicrobial agents were more effective than long-acting ones in eliminating infections caused by *S. aureus* or treating cows infected with major pathogens diagnosed twice before drying off. Intramammary infusion of cephapirin sodium 15 days prepartum in heifers was effective in reducing intramammary infections during late gestation and reduced the occurrence of residues in milk during early lactation. The milk of heifers that calve less than 15 days after treatment may contain antimicrobial residues.

Intramammary infusion is a widely used and highly recommended procedure for mastitis therapy; however, there is a potential for the introduction of pathogens during the infusion process. Insanitary infusion practices can introduce antibiotic-resistant environmental organisms into the udder. Infection with opportunistic microorganisms, such as yeast or *Nocardia* spp., may cause more extensive udder damage than the original organism for which treatment was being administered. Adequate teat-end preparation and careful dry cow treatment procedures can reduce this risk. Dry cow treatment procedures should be performed as follows:

- Milk out the udder completely.
- Immediately following teat cup removal, dip all teats in an effective teat dip.
- Allow the teat dip to dry. If necessary, remove excess dip from teat ends with a clean single-service paper towel.
- Disinfect each teat end by scrubbing for a few seconds with a separate alcohol-soaked cotton swab. Start with the teats on the far side of the udder and work to the near side.
- Infuse each quarter with a single-dose syringe of a recommended dry cow treatment. Start with the teats on the near side of the udder. Use the partial insertion method of administration into

the teat streak canal. Preferably, a modified infusion cannula should be provided with the treatment product.
- Dip all teats in an effective teat dip immediately following treatment.

The necessity of using appropriate dry cow treatment procedures cannot be overemphasized. An increased incidence of *Nocardia* spp. mastitis has been associated with blanket dry cow therapy, especially neomycin-containing products. However, *Nocardia* spp. were not found as a contaminant of the suspected products. Teat-end preparation by scrubbing with an alcohol-soaked cotton swab was protective against the occurrence of *Nocardia* spp. infection when teats were experimentally contaminated with organisms immediately before drying off. Most commercial dry cow treatment products provide individually wrapped alcohol-soaked cotton swabs for use with each syringe. The use of good teat-end preparation before intramammary infusion needs to be continually emphasized.

The method of intramammary infusion may be important. Partial insertion of the infusion cannula (up to 4 mm) results in fewer new intramammary infections and improved cure rates. The improvement with a short cannula is attributed to fewer organisms being delivered beyond the streak canal and decreased physical trauma to the streak canal. In addition, antimicrobial agents that are deposited within the streak canal should control local infections. Modified infusion cannulas for the convenient use of a partial insertion method of administration are now available for commercial dry cow products.

Another approach to preventing the problems associated with intramammary infusion would be the development of an effective systemically administered dry cow treatment. Preliminary results have indicated improved efficacy against *S. aureus* infections using a systemically administered fluoroquinoline antibiotic (norfloxacin nicotinate).

Blanket Versus Selective Dry Cow Therapy

Three strategies for intramammary antimicrobial treatment of dry cows are available, although the current recommendation for all herds is blanket therapy:
- **Blanket therapy** (treat all quarters of all cows)
- **Selective cow therapy** (treat all quarters of any cow infected in one or more quarters)
- **Selective quarter therapy** (treat infected quarters only).

Although blanket dry cow therapy is a cornerstone of any mastitis control program, there is some controversy concerning the need to treat all quarters of all cows (**blanket therapy**) or only those quarters or cows requiring treatment. The controversy has gained momentum because the implementation of udder health management practices has reduced the prevalence of infection and global interest in decreasing the use of antibiotics. As a result, Nordic countries have implemented selective dry cow therapy as part of their national mastitis control program.[10] The major reasons for selective therapy are to
- Avoid the elimination of minor pathogens, which may make cows more susceptible to environmental agents
- Reduce the expense of treatment
- Address increasing consumer concern regarding the routine administration of antibiotics to food-producing animals
- Avoid the possible emergence of antibiotic-resistant organisms

Each of these reasons should be carefully considered in making a decision between blanket and selective dry cow therapy. Selective dry cow therapy is preferable provided that an accurate, practical, and inexpensive method for selecting infected cows is available. This is the major problem with selective dry cow therapy because in most herds the sensitivity and specificity of the test used for selection is not adequate. The majority of economic analysis studies indicate that the optimum return on investment is provided by treating every quarter of every cow at drying off.

As general udder health improves and bulk tank milk SCC remains low, producers question the need to continue dry treatment on all cows and are attracted by a potential reduction in costs for the purchase of dry cow treatment. However, selective therapy requires a decision as to which cows or quarters are to be treated. The sensitivity and specificity of currently available screening tests are inadequate as a basis for decisions concerning selective therapy. The history of the number of episodes of clinical mastitis, lactation number, individual cow composite SCC during lactation and at dry off, CMT results during lactation or at dry off, and even bacteriologic culture toward the end of lactation all result in leaving some infected cows untreated; conversely these result in the treatment of many uninfected cows. An important requirement for large-scale implementation of selective dry cow therapy is the development of a cheap, practical, sensitive, and specific test to identify infected cows. The failure to prevent new intramammary infections during the dry period with the selective approach must also be considered. New infections in the dry period will become increasingly important as contagious pathogens are eliminated from herds. Finally, blanket dry cow therapy reduces new infection rates for quarters from approximately 14% to 7%. The increase in milk production alone resulting from prevention of these new infections provides enough return to offset the cost of treatment for all cows.

The most practical method currently available for implementing selective dry cow treatment appears to be a low SCC on a cow basis at the last milk recording before drying off, with a low SCC defined as <150,000 cells/mL for primiparous and <250,000 cells/mL for multiparous cows.[10] In a split udder study of 1657 low-SCC cows in the Netherlands, the incidence of clinical mastitis in untreated quarters in the first 100 days of lactation was 70% higher than in quarters infused with a dry cow intramammary product containing 314 mg of potassium benzylpenicillin, 1000 mg of procaine benzylpenicillin, and 500 mg of neomycin sulfate. Clinical mastitis was most commonly caused by *S. uberis*. The SCC at calving and 14 days in milk were also higher in quarters dried off without antibiotics.[10] Despite increased antibiotic use for treating additional cases of clinical mastitis, total antibiotic use was decreased by 85% in low-SCC cows not administered an intramammary dry cow antibiotic.[10] This study highlights the balance the veterinarian must reach between increased incidence of clinical mastitis (and therefore more pain and discomfort) and overall reduction in antibiotic use when a selective dry cow therapy approach is applied using the most practical test.

Information presently available indicates that the general recommendation should be for **routine treatment of all quarters of all cows at the time of drying off (blanket dry cow therapy)**. There is a need to identify important management practices to limit new infections in untreated dry cows and to develop new screening tests to determine which cows should be treated. New environmental management methods and modern information processing capabilities may lead to the development of better selective dry cow treatment programs. These may include the administration of ancillary therapeutic agents. For instance, the intramammary infusion of recombinant bovine IL-2 along with cephapirin sodium at drying off marginally increased the cure rate of intramammary infections associated with *S. aureus*, but not other pathogens, during the dry period compared with the administration of cephapirin only. Interleukin did not affect the incidence of new intramammary infections for any pathogen group. However, the intramammary infusion of interleukin at drying off was associated with an increased incidence of abortion in dairy cows 3 to 7 days after the infusion.

Factors Affecting the Success of Antimicrobial Treatment of Dry Cows

Despite blanket dry cow therapy, some cows calve with infected quarters and some with clinical mastitis. Several risk factors affecting the results of dry cow treatment have been evaluated. Some of these factors are
- **Number of quarters infected.** With *S. aureus* infections, there is a significant decrease in cure rate as the number of quarters infected per cow increases. Quarters from cows with either three or four of their quarters infected have a very poor cure rate.

- **Age of the cow**. As the age of the cow increases, the probability of *S. aureus* infections being cured by dry cow therapy decreases.
- **SCC before drying off**. The cure rate of *S. aureus*–infected quarters diminishes as the SCC before treatment increases. Controlling for age and number of quarters infected, there was a significantly lower cure rate in quarters with an SCC of more than 1,000,000 cells/mL.
- **Herd of origin**. There is a distinct herd effect on the success of dry cow therapy. The cure rate of *S. aureus* has been shown to be higher in herds with good hygiene and with a low prevalence of *S. aureus* infections at drying off.

There is considerable potential in using individual cow and herd-level information to predict the likelihood of a cure with dry cow therapy. For example, an older cow with three quarters infected with *S. aureus* and a persistently high SCC has a low probability of a cure. Continued development of information management systems to assist with therapy and culling decisions will clarify the expectations of dry cow treatment.

Persistent *S. aureus* infections represent only one of the shortcomings of antibiotic treatment for dry cows. Most dry cow products are formulated for efficacy against gram-positive cocci. These antibiotics are of limited usefulness against gram-negative bacteria. In other words, new coliform infections would not be prevented by this therapy.[11] Even though dry cow products are formulated for sustained activity, the provision of adequate protection during the critical prepartum period is questionable. The persistence of effective levels of antimicrobial agents has been evaluated for various dry cow treatments and depends on the formulation; very few products have persistent activity until the time of calving.

Internal Teat Sealants

As discussed previously in risk factors for infection in the dry period, **the keratin plug is a natural internal teat sealant** that provides an effective barrier to new intramammary infections. High milk production at dry off increases the likelihood that the streak canal remains open and presumably compromises formation of the keratin plug, increasing the risk of intramammary infection.

A recent promising development in mastitis control has been **exogenous internal teat sealants** that are applied at dry off. The teat sealant product most extensively evaluated contains a heavy inorganic salt (**bismuth subnitrate**) in a paraffin wax base; this product does not have antibacterial properties but acts as a **physical barrier** to ascending intramammary infections. Because it is not an antibiotic use of the product may be permitted on organic dairies in some countries. The formulation of bismuth subnitrate used has a higher density than milk causing it to sink to the bottom of the teat canal in which it creates a physical barrier. Administration of internal teat sealants alone requires meticulous attention to aseptic technique because it is easy to facilitate transfer of bacteria on the teat end into the gland during infusion.[12]

A meta-analysis of 18 publications concluded that internal teat sealants decreased new intramammary infections by 73% compared with untreated cows and decreased the risk of clinical mastitis after calving by 48% compared with untreated cows.[13] The same meta-analysis also concluded that internal teat sealants combined with antibiotic dry cow therapy decreased new intramammary infections by 25% compared with cows treated with antibiotic dry cow therapy alone and further decreased the risk of clinical mastitis after calving by 29%. The addition of an antimicrobial agent is a logical addition to the bismuth subnitrate internal teat sealant and has been a routine addition to the teat sealant for some years in Ireland. An experimental challenge study in New Zealand indicated that the addition of 0.5% chlorhexidine to the internal teat sealant at dry off increased the protection against intramammary infection after calving.[14]

Dry period length may be a factor to consider when deciding whether to use internal teat sealants, which persist for at least 100 days in treated cattle. As such, internal teat sealants are theoretically more likely to prevent new intramammary infections in cows with long dry periods than infusion of a long-acting intramammary antibiotic because an effective antibiotic concentration after infusion rarely persists longer than 70 days in glandular secretions.[15] However, study results have been mixed on this topic, with dry period length having no impact on the new infection rate or incidence of clinical mastitis in New Zealand dairy cattle administered an internal teat sealant. In contrast, a UK study found in cattle with a dry period length >70 days that the new infection rate was 11% in quarters treated with cephalonium compared with 4% in cows receiving combined cephalonium and internal teat sealant.[16]

Insertion of an internal teat sealant before calving shows promise as a control measure for heifer mastitis. In a New Zealand study of first-calf heifers, infusion of an internal teat sealant at approximately 30 days before calving decreased the incidence of *S. uberis* intramammary infection by 84% and the incidence of clinical mastitis by 68% in the first 14 days of lactation.[17]

Bismuth subnitrate internal teat sealants clearly show promise for the prevention of new intramammary infections during the dry period. However, because **bismuth subnitrate teat sealants do not eliminate existing intramammary infections**, and an accurate method for determining the infection status of a quarter is unavailable (the exception being milk culture), the recommended application of internal teat sealants requires combined application with intramammary dry cow therapy, with the teat sealant infused immediately after infusion of the intramammary dry cow antibiotic. The teat sealant should not be massaged upward after infusion. This combined therapy is more effective than either treatment alone but may be uneconomical; however, a study conducted on grazing dairy cattle in Australia concluded that the use of combined therapy was likely to be of benefit in herds that had a clinical mastitis incidence of 6% or more in the first 3 weeks of lactation.[18] Widespread adoption of internal teat sealants will be facilitated by development of an accurate low-cost test for determining intramammary infection status at dry off.

It is important that the internal teat sealant does not reach the bulk milk tank. At the first milking after calving, each quarter should be stripped 10 to 12 times and colostrum should be withheld for a minimum of 4 days.

External Teat Sealants

A longer-standing approach to providing a physical barrier to ascending infections is the use of external teat sealants, which were originally developed for use in lactating cows. The major problem with external teat sealants is the duration of adherence, which is too long for lactating cow use and too short for dry cows. Teat-end lesions and teat length influence the adherence of external teat sealants. Widespread adoption of external teat sealants will require a product that provides prolonged protection but is easily removed at calving.

Teat Disinfection

Postmilking teat disinfection is a very effective means of reducing new infections in lactating cows. However, the efficacy of teat disinfection in decreasing the incidence of new intramammary infections in the dry period has been discouraging. Daily teat dipping for the first week of the dry period is not effective in reducing *S. uberis* infections. The lack of efficacy of teat disinfection needs to be contrasted to the efficacy of internal teat sealants.

Intramammary Devices

Intramammary devices have been developed for use in preventing new infections in both lactating and dry cows. However, there is conflicting evidence as to the reduction in infection rate in quarters fitted with these devices, and such devices are no longer being investigated. The incidence of clinical mastitis may be less in cows fitted with these devices compared with control cows, but the prevalence of subclinical infection is unaffected. Intramammary devices induce a significant increase in postmilking SCC compared with control cows, and test-day SCCs may be higher than in control cows.

Vaccination of the Dry Cow

Immunization and immunotherapy for the control and prevention of mastitis have been active areas of research. Effective vaccines would have to eliminate chronic intramammary infections, prevent new intramammary infections, or decrease the incidence or severity of clinical mastitis. Currently available mastitis vaccines may reduce the incidence and severity of clinical mastitis but have not eliminated chronic intramammary infections or prevented new intramammary infections. The inability of vaccines to prevent infection may be caused by the wide variety of pathogens, inadequate specific antibodies, or the failure of antibodies to enter the mammary gland before infection. Currently available vaccines should be used as adjuncts to other more effective control strategies.

Vaccines have been developed to reduce the incidence and severity of clinical mastitis associated with gram-negative pathogens. R-mutant bacteria have an exposed inner wall structure (core lipopolysaccharide antigens) that is highly uniform, even among diverse and distantly related gram-negative bacteria. Vaccines containing killed R-mutant bacteria provide broad-spectrum immunity against a wide variety of unrelated gram-negative bacteria. The most commonly used coliform mastitis vaccines are the Rc-mutant *E. coli* O111:B4, known as the J5 vaccine, and the Remutant *S. typhimurium*, both of which are commercially available in the United States. R-mutant vaccines have been efficacious in reducting the incidence and severity of clinical mastitis caused by gram-negative bacteria. More than 50% of large (>200 cows) dairy herds and more than 25% of all dairy herds in the United States are using core lipopolysaccharide antigen vaccines. No protection is provided against environmental streptococci and staphylococci, or the contagious pathogens.

No effective vaccines are currently available for the control of mastitis caused by *S. aureus, S. agalactiae,* environmental streptococci, and *M. bovis*.

The use of recombinant bovine cytokines as adjuvants to enhance specific immunity in the mammary gland of cows after primary immunization indicate an enhancement of specific immunity in the mammary gland, which may be effective in mastitis immunization protocols.

Management of the Environment for Dry Cows

Dry cows should be provided with an environment that is as clean and dry as possible. If this is not feasible in confinement housing, it is probably better to maintain dry cows on pasture. Variations in the load of coliforms and environmental streptococci in the environment are important predictors of new infection rates. Minimizing the exposure to environmental bacteria will reduce the new infection rate. However, some pasture conditions promote the crowding of cows under shade trees. In hot, humid, and muddy conditions, heavy contamination of such a small area can result in a significant risk of new environmental infections in the dry period. In good weather, it is ideal to hold parturient cows in a clean, grassy area in which they can be observed and assisted if necessary.

In confinement housing systems for dry cows, it is important to provide adequate space, ventilation, bedding, and lighting to ensure cleanliness and comfort. Maternity (calving) stalls should be bedded with clean straw, sawdust, or shavings. Other important procedures for managing the environment for dry cows include adopting an effective fly control program. Clipping the hair on the udders, flanks, and inside the hind legs will help reduce contamination. **The words clean, dry, cold, and comfortable summarize the ideal environment for dry cows.** The words clean and dry also summarize the goal for the teat before attachment of the inflation during milking.

Nutritional Management of Dry Cows

A nutritionally balanced dry cow feeding program is important to ensure udder health. A role has been suggested for specific nutritional factors in resistance to mastitis, especially over the dry period. Adequate levels of vitamin E and selenium in dry cow rations appear to be important for udder health at calving and in early lactation. This effect may be mediated through enhanced resistance mechanisms. Other vitamins and minerals may be important in udder health, but their role is less well substantiated.

Nutritional management of dry cows is also important for reducing the risk of milk fever, which is an important predisposing factor to mastitis in fresh cows. Appropriate body condition can be achieved by good nutritional management in late lactation. The association between body condition, energy metabolism, and udder health needs further clarification.

4. APPROPRIATE THERAPY OF MASTITIS DURING LACTATION

The early recognition and treatment of clinical cases remains an important part of a mastitis control program. Improvements in understanding of the epidemiology, pathophysiology, and response to therapy of various mastitis pathogens have clarified the role of intramammary and parenteral antimicrobial agents for of the treatment of clinical and subclinical mastitis during lactation. This was covered extensively earlier in this chapter.

5. CULLING CHRONICALLY INFECTED COWS

The final step of the five-point mastitis control program is the selective removal of cows with chronic intramammary infection from the herd. Most producers have interpreted this recommendation to mean that cows with recurrent episodes of clinical mastitis should be eliminated. For example, some herds have established that cows having three or more clinical cases of mastitis in a lactation will be culled (**the popular three strikes and out approach**). However, very little research has been conducted to determine the effect of various culling strategies on herd udder health status and on the incidence of clinical cases.

Nevertheless, culling chronically infected cows meets one of the three guiding principles of mastitis control, namely the elimination of existing intramammary infections. Through the use of available monitoring techniques and the establishment of a defined culling program, a valuable opportunity exists to improve udder health by culling.

Generally, a record of chronic mastitis and severe fibrosis detected on deep udder palpation should be the basis of a recommendation to cull. Culling is an effective and documented mastitis control measure for some specific mastitis pathogens. For example, the removal of infected cows is a key element of the recommended mastitis control program for herds with a high prevalence of *S. aureus* infection. Removal of cows found to be infected with *S. aureus* accounted for more than 80% of the costs involved in the control program. Culling is also important in the control of other mastitis pathogens that respond poorly to antimicrobial therapy. Herds with mastitis cases associated with *M. bovis, Nocardia* spp., and *P. aeruginosa* should be aware of the benefits of culling infected cows.

A dairy herd culling program should be based on consideration of the net present value of each cow in the herd compared with the value of a replacement heifer. The net present value depends on the age of the cow, her potential for milk production, the stage of lactation, and her pregnancy status. Factors that determine the likelihood of treatment success, such as pathogen and duration of mastitis, as well as the cost of treatment, also need to be considered in calculating the net present value of the cow with mastitis. After consideration of the relative importance of udder health in the overall herd health management program, additional economic pressure may be applied to cows with a specific udder health status. For example, if an *S. aureus* control program is a major priority in the health management program, additional economic pressure should be applied in removal decisions of cows with known *S. aureus* infections. As health management data collection and analysis improve in sophistication, decision analysis methods and expert computer models will be used to provide this information automatically.

Biosecurity for Herd Replacements

Replacement animals may be purchased to increase herd size or to maintain cow numbers following culling. Biosecurity measures must be used to ensure that herd replacements are not infected with contagious mastitis pathogens (specifically *S. aureus, S. agalactiae,* and *M. bovis*). However, an economic analysis of the different components of a biosecurity program has not been performed, and it is likely that some components of currently used programs are not cost-effective.

An optimal biosecurity program includes knowing the herd of origin, knowing the cows, and protecting the home herd.

Know the Farm of Origin

- Request a bulk tank milk culture from the farm of origin
- Request the following data: 6 to 12 months of bulk tank milk SCC, bulk tank milk bacterial counts, and 6 to 12 months of records for clinical mastitis

Know the Cows

When purchasing single or small groups of animals the following prepurchase procedures are recommended:

- SCC and clinical mastitis records for each cow to be purchased
- Results of bacteriologic culturing of quarter milk samples from each cow on arrival (if lactating) or at calving (if late gestation) for *S. aureus, S. agalactiae,* and *M. bovis.* Generally, the sensitivity of a single milk culture to detect the presence of intramammary infections caused by *S. agalactiae* is approximately 95%, for *S. aureus* it ranges from 30% to 86%, and for *M. bovis* it is 24%.
- A physical examination of each cow, including udder, milk quality, and teat ends

Protect the Home Herd

Consider all purchased animals as potential health risks to the home herd by doing the following:

- Maintain all newly purchased animals in separate or isolated facilities until diagnostic tests for udder health have been completed and there is no evidence of infection that may spread to the rest of the herd (usually <14 day quarantine).
- Evaluate all herd replacements for evidence of antimicrobial residues in milk.
- Milk all purchased animals last or with separate milking equipment until it is determined that they are free of infection.
- Obtain results of bacteriologic culturing of bulk tank milk samples or string samples for *S. aureus, S. agalactiae,* and *M. bovis;* culturing should be done on more than one occasion because the sensitivity of bulk tank milk culturing is not 100%, and is less than 50% for *M. bovis.*

6. MAINTENANCE OF AN APPROPRIATE ENVIRONMENT

The multifactorial nature of mastitis has been emphasized throughout this chapter. Intramammary infection results from a complex interaction between the cow, the mastitis pathogens, and the environment. Thus the control of unfavorable environmental influences is extremely important in dairy herd udder health management programs.

Intramammary infection involves exposure of the teat surface to potentially pathogenic microorganisms, entry of the pathogens into the gland via the teat duct, and establishment of the pathogens in the mammary tissue, producing an inflammatory response. Many environmental factors can influence this process of exposure, bacterial entry, and establishment of infection. For example, the type of bedding and manure management can have a great impact on the contamination of teat skin with microorganisms. Housing design can have an impact on the prevalence of teat injuries, which will influence intramammary invasion by mastitis pathogens. Extreme climatic conditions, poor nutritional management, and cow stocking densities will influence the immune system and the establishment of intramammary infection. A comprehensive udder health management program should involve steps to minimize the detrimental influences of the environment.

Global Environmental Influences

Worldwide, there are major differences in dairy herd health and production systems. For example, the type of animal used, economics of production, climatic conditions, housing structures, and management methods are widely variable. These differences greatly affect the interaction of cows with their environment, even though the predominant causative organisms are the same under different systems. Thus there are major variations in the relative incidences of different pathogens and in the importance of various approaches to mastitis control.

Classification of Environmental Influences

The influences of the total environment can be divided into the following:

- **External environment.** All aspects of the environment outside the housing facilities make up the external environment. This includes the regional differences in climate, geography, and agricultural tradition. There are also local factors within a region that can have an important influence. These local factors include the topographic features of the land, natural shelters from the climate, and the availability of pasture.
- **Internal environment.** All environmental conditions inside the cow buildings make up the internal environment. The general internal environment includes the type of housing system, temperature, humidity, and air quality. There are also specific internal environmental influences such as stall design, type of bedding, nutritional management, and manure disposal. The milking environment has a major influence through the equipment, cow preparation methods, and approach to general hygiene.

External Environmental Influences on Mastitis Control

There is minimal evidence that external environmental factors directly influence the incidence of mastitis; however, the external environment determines the way in which cows are housed, fed, and milked. Through these associations, the external environment can be an important risk factor in problems with udder health in dairy herds.

Regional Environment

The climate and geographic features of a region have implications for the prevalence of mastitis. The ambient temperatures and amount of rainfall often determine the types of housing and nutritional program used. Extremely hot or cold conditions interact with other predisposing management factors. In areas prone to severe rainstorms, teats may be exposed to wet or muddy conditions. The soil type, cropping policy, and presence of other industries can also have an indirect impact on the prevalence of mastitis; for example, regions suitable for growing cereal grains will commonly use straw as a bedding material, which may favor the growth of environmental streptococcal organisms. In contrast, dairying areas close to the forestry industries may favor sawdust or shavings as bedding. The use of these materials may influence the incidence of coliform mastitis.

The socioeconomic structure and agricultural policy of a particular region can affect management factors known to influence udder health. These factors determine herd size and labor costs. Large herd sizes necessitated by economic conditions will dictate the housing, feeding, and milking management practices used. More recently, regional policy toward regulation of bulk tank milk SCC levels has had a profound impact on udder health status.

Local Environment

The local environmental factors such as the topography of the land, the presence of natural shelters, and the type of pasture grown are thought to influence udder health status. However, direct scientific evidence is lacking. One important exception is summer mastitis, which affects nonlactating heifers and cows. This udder infection with *T. pyogenes* is greatly affected by the local environment, probably through the propagation of insects important in its transmission. Protected pastures increase insect populations and can result in a high incidence of infection.

Internal Environmental Influences on Mastitis Control

The incidence of new intramammary infections can be greatly affected by the management and facilities used in confinement dairying systems. General aspects of the internal environment exert their influence on all cows in the herd, such as the type of housing and milking system. Tie-stall barns pose different environmental stresses from a free-stall system. The air quality and noise levels can have an impact on animal health. The nutrient content of component feedstuffs can affect disease resistance.

Specific internal environmental factors exert their influence on an individual cow basis. For example, the stall design and tying system affect individual cows differently. Many epidemiologic studies have revealed interactions between udder disease and internal environmental conditions. Most of these studies relate to European tie-stall and seasonal grazing systems. However, the results are generally relevant to most housing and management systems. Some of the most important general and specific influences of the internal environment are as follows.

Housing

Housing factors account for a great deal of the variation in udder health status between herds. In both tie-stall and free-stall barns, short and narrow stalls are associated with increased incidence of teat tramps and mastitis. An appropriate partition between stalls is beneficial. Stanchions or neck straps with chains can restrict the movement of the cow and increase the risk of teat injury. This occurs especially as cows are rising. In addition, the use of electrical cowtrainers has been associated with an increase in the rate of subclinical mastitis. The use of adequate amounts of a good bedding material will reduce mastitis incidence in both tie-stall and free-stall housing systems. Even though there are reports of specific bedding materials being associated with certain mastitis problems, the use of adequate amounts of properly maintained bedding is beneficial. Straw, shavings, sawdust, sand, shredded newspaper, and other cushion systems have all been used effectively.

The climate and air quality maintained within a building can have a major influence on udder health. Draughty conditions, high relative humidity, and marked changes in indoor temperature over a 24-hour period are factors that contribute to higher mastitis rates. Adaptation to adverse internal environmental conditions may cause stress, which can reduce the cow's defense mechanisms. Indoor climate, especially temperature and humidity, can also account for differences in the concentration of pathogenic organisms to which cows are exposed.

Nutritional Management

A complex relationship exists between the quantity and quality of feed and udder health status. Improper nutritional management can result in an increase of new intramammary infections, the exacerbation of preexisting chronic infections, and an increase in clinical mastitis. Several mechanisms have been suggested for this association. An improper anion to cation balance in the dry cow ration is a predisposing factor for periparturient hypocalcemia, which in turn increases the risk of new intramammary infections. Feeding programs that result in excessively fat or abnormally thin cows may affect resistance to disease. Also, there is some evidence that feeds high in estrogenic substances may be detrimental to udder health status.

The dietary concentration of some vitamins and minerals may have an important relationship to udder health. Studies have shown that intramammary infection is related to plasma concentrations of vitamin E and blood concentrations of selenium. Dietary supplementation of vitamin E and selenium improved the natural resistance of the mammary gland to infection. Associations between udder health and the levels of vitamin A, β-carotene, zinc, and other nutrients have been proposed but are not well documented.

Management Approach

Cow supervision, decision making, and general animal care by dairy herd managers may be important epidemiologic factors in the relationship between environment and udder health. For example, lack of consistency in the performance and timing of various herd activities results in decreased udder health status. Irregular intervals between milkings should be avoided.

General Hygiene

Even outside the milking environment, general hygiene can greatly influence the exposure of the udder and teats to pathogenic bacteria. The degree of hygiene achieved is directly related to the type of housing, the amount of bedding, and the efficiency of manure removal. Worldwide trends toward increasing herd sizes and decreasing labor force necessitate more emphasis on the importance of cow hygiene.

Udder Singeing

Hair on the udder facilitates the accumulation of fecal material and other organic material that, when wet, can contaminate the teat orifice and result in new intramammary infections, or enter the bulk tank milk vat. Udder hair can be removed by clipping or more quickly by "udder singeing" every 2 to 3 months, which has become popular in parts of North America. A soft yellow flame from a handheld propane torch is held about 15 to 20 cm below the udder to singe the udder hair and the ash brushed away using a gloved hand. Studies have demonstrated that udder singeing results in cleaner udders, but a beneficial effect on decreasing herd SCC, milk bacterial count, or the incidence of clinical mastitis does not appear to have been reported. Appropriate clinical studies documenting the pain and discomfort associated with the procedure do not appear to have been conducted.

Use of Recombinant Bovine Somatotropin

It has been suggested that the use of bST may increase the incidence of clinical mastitis by an indirect mechanism that acts through increased milk production. Controlled field studies have shown that the use of bST is not associated with an increase in the incidence of clinical mastitis, milk discarded because of therapy for clinical mastitis, or culling for mastitis.

Environmental Control in an Udder Health Management Program

There is a strong association between herd udder health status and the number of stress factors operating within the herd. It has been proposed that mastitis occurs when stress factors exceed the cow's ability to adapt. It follows that a major objective of an udder health management program should be to limit the number and severity of environmental stress factors.

Veterinarians responsible for udder health management programs should have a good understanding of the importance of environmental management. The three major objectives of environmental control for improvement of udder health are to prevent

- Contamination of the teat end
- Invasion of mastitis pathogens
- Pathogens from establishing in the mammary gland

The important steps in achieving these three objectives have been discussed. For example, an adequate housing system and manure handling are important to limit bacterial contamination of the teats. The prevention of environmentally induced teat injuries will aid in preventing invasion of pathogens into the gland. The producer's approach to cow management, control of the nutritional program, and ensuring that the internal environment is appropriate will all greatly improve host defense mechanisms and prevent intramammary pathogens from establishing within the gland.

7. GOOD RECORD KEEPING

Good record keeping involves the collection of useful data to monitor performance, calculation of appropriate indices, and decision making based on comparison to target levels. For acceptable performance the monitoring process is repeated and the cycle continues. If performance is not acceptable, further evaluation and analysis is performed, and a plan of action is instituted. Once again, the monitoring process carries on and the cycle continues. For many of the health management programs in food animal practice, a limiting factor is the availability of accurate and objective data. With respect to udder health, data have been readily available. Bulk tank milk SCC, individual cow composite SCC, and bacteriologic culture results are all accessible and useful. These data provide the information necessary to monitor udder health status and to make specific health management decisions. However, problems can still exist. Herds with a low prevalence of infection and very low bulk tank milk SCC can still have a high incidence of environmental infections and clinical mastitis cases. Thus an important step in an effective udder health management program is the maintenance and use of mastitis records. The increasing adoption of computerized dairy health management record systems provides an opportunity to make effective use of a clinical mastitis episode and therapy data. Even without a computerized system, manual records for clinical mastitis are easy to implement and use.

Objectives and Uses of Clinical Mastitis Records

The objective of maintaining computerized or manual records of clinical mastitis episodes is to complete the decision-making capabilities of a mastitis control program. The availability of this information will allow completion of the health management cycle over the entire spectrum of herd udder health situations.

There are several important uses of clinical mastitis records:

- To assess the risk factors associated with clinical mastitis episodes
- To evaluate lactational and dry cow therapy programs

To provide information useful in the evaluation of net present value of individual cows for the purposes of culling decisions. Without the ready availability of accurate data surrounding mastitis events, decisions associated with therapy, culling, and the removal of risk factors are difficult to make.

Recording Clinical Mastitis Data

There is a limited amount of specific data necessary to make effective use of mastitis records as a health management tool. The cow identification, date of the clinical episode occurrence, type of therapy used, and the date that milk withholding will be complete are the essential pieces of information. If a manual record system is used, it will be important to add the lactation number, the date of calving, and the most recent test date production. A standard form that calculates the distribution of clinical episodes by lactation number and by stage of lactation is desirable. These are the same distributions often provided with an individual cow SCC report.

Using Clinical Mastitis Monitoring Systems

Because clinical mastitis is a common event in dairy production, it is ironic that these records have not traditionally been kept. The key to overcoming this hurdle is the regular use of this information for health management decisions. Some of these uses and decisions are as follows.

Cow Versus Herd Clinical Mastitis Problems

Calculation of the percentage of cows affected in the herd and the average number of clinical episodes per affected cow will aid in determining whether the clinical mastitis is more of an individual cow problem or a herd-level issue.

Probability of Recurrence of Clinical Mastitis in the Same Lactation

The number of animals with repeat cases of mastitis divided by the total number of clinical cases gives an estimate of the likelihood of recurrence. The same calculation can be made for specific parity groups. This information can be useful to characterize the problem, and for culling decisions.

Stage of Lactation and Seasonal Profile

If clinical mastitis data are collected consistently over a considerable period of time, potentially useful problem-solving information can be derived. For example, calculating days in lactation at first occurrence can help to identify specific risk factors for new intramammary infections. There is a higher proportion of clinical occurrences during the first few weeks after calving. However, analysis of clinical mastitis records might yield a different stage-of-lactation profile. In these cases, the evaluation of potential nutritional, environmental, or other stress factors would be indicated. There may be different immediate and long-term solutions that should be implemented.

Analysis of clinical mastitis records over several years may identify a significant seasonal pattern, such as the documented seasonal pattern for bulk tank milk SCC data and antibiotic residue violations. Action may be necessary to deal with seasonal environment and housing problems that impact new infection rates.

Days of Discarded Milk

It is very common for producers to have an aggressive attitude toward the treatment of clinical mastitis. This approach may result in huge economic losses if waste milk is not fed to calves. These losses are largely the result of discarded milk during the clearance of antibiotic residues from treated cows. Calculating the days of discarded milk may suggest that the mastitis therapy program during lactation should be evaluated. Establishment of an appropriate treatment program and careful selection of cows for therapy might significantly decrease the need for discarding milk. In addition, cows that are responsible for a large percentage of the discarded milk should be identified for selective removal. The calculations from mastitis records that can help to clarify these issues include:

- Total days of discarded milk for the herd
- Days of discarded milk per episode
- Days of discarded milk by lactation number
- Accrued days of discarded milk for individual cows

8. MONITORING UDDER HEALTH STATUS

An important step missing from early mastitis control programs was the monitoring of udder health status. Although intuitively it appears necessary to chart the progress of any program, it is only quite recently that monitoring has been included as an integral component of udder health management. **Monitoring is now recognized as the third key principle of mastitis control.** The development of objective, inexpensive, and efficient methods of monitoring udder health has made it much easier to complete the health management cycle for this component of herd programs.

The implementation of SCC measurement on bulk tank milk and on individual cow samples has been widespread throughout the major dairy regions of the world. Because SCC is objective and standardized, it can be used to evaluate the progress of regional control programs. This has allowed rapid improvement in udder health compared with most of the other components of dairy health management programs. Regional authorities have established new regulatory limits and targets for milk quality performance.

Implementing an effective system of monitoring udder health involves:

- Monitoring udder health at the herd level
- Monitoring udder health of individual cows
- Use of cowside diagnostic tests

This discussion will emphasize the use of monitoring methods for decision making and problem solving in udder health management programs. Monitoring of udder health should be done at the **herd level** and **individual cow level**.

Monitoring Udder Health at the Herd Level

The monitoring of bulk tank milk provides the best method to evaluate the overall udder health status of dairy herds and the effectiveness of mastitis control programs. **Herd-level monitors of udder health include bulk tank milk SCC, bulk tank milk bacteriologic culture, and herd summaries of individual cow SCC data.** Analysis of clinical mastitis records is also useful for monitoring udder health at the herd level.

Bulk Tank Milk Somatic Cell Counts

Most milk marketing organizations and regional authorities regularly measure SCC on bulk tank milk as a monitor of the milk quality and udder health status of each herd. Many of these agencies use bulk tank milk SCC for penalty deductions or incentive payments. Improvement in bulk tank milk SCC is associated with improvement in other measures of milk quality such as bacterial counts, inhibitor test violations, and milk freezing point. Countries and regions set milk quality targets using this SCC data, with milk being rejected from processing plants when the bulk tank milk SCC exceeds 400,000 to 1,000,000 cells/mL, depending on the country.

Several management practices are associated with low, medium, and high SCC in bulk tank milk. Postmilking teat disinfection and dry cow therapy are most frequently associated with herds with a low bulk tank milk SCC. In herds with a low bulk milk SCC, more attention is given to hygiene than in herds with a medium or high bulk tank milk SCC. Cubicles, drinking buckets, and cows are cleaner in herds with a low bulk tank milk SCC. Cleaner calving pens and cubicles for herds with low bulk tank milk SCC coincide with the observations that bedding for lactating cows and in maternity pens is drier for herds with a low bulk tank milk SCC. In herds with a high bulk tank milk SCC, a higher percentage of cows are culled because of a high SCC.

The incidence of clinical mastitis in dairy herds may not be different among those with low, medium, and high bulk tank milk SCC. However, clinical mastitis associated with gram-negative pathogens such as *E. coli, Klebsiella* spp., or *Pseudomonas* spp. occurs more commonly in herds with a low bulk tank milk SCC. Clinical mastitis associated with *S. aureus, S. dysgalactiae,* and *S. agalactiae* occurs more often in herds with a high bulk tank milk SCC. Systemic signs of illness associated with clinical mastitis occur more often in herds with a low bulk tank milk SCC. In herds with a high bulk tank milk SCC, more cows with a high milk SCC were culled. In herds with a low bulk tank milk SCC, more cows were culled for teat lesions, milkability, udder shape, fertility, and character than in herds with a high bulk tank milk SCC. In herds with a low bulk tank milk SCC, cows were culled more for export and production reasons.

Herd Average of Weighted Individual Cow Somatic Cell Count

The arithmetic mean of individual cow SCC values, weighted by the cow's milk production, is also a good measure of the general udder health status of the herd. It should be noted that the high degree of variability of SCC measurements makes it inappropriate to compare this mean directly with the bulk tank milk SCC.

Other Herd-Level Somatic Cell Count Monitors

There are several other calculations using individual cow SCC data that are useful for monitoring herd udder health. Generally, these indices attempt to use mathematical calculations to reduce the impact of individual cows and to measure the change over time. These summaries are used to assist producers in the use of individual cow SCC information at the herd level. These indices include the following.

Herd Average Somatic Cell Score

The use of the somatic cell score (SCS, linear score; Tables 20.4 and 20.5) can simplify SCC interpretation and buffer the effects of individual cows with very high values. Thus the herd average of SCS is a very useful monitor of herd udder health status. A realistic goal for most dairy herds is an average SCS of less than 3.0, equivalent to fewer than 100,000 cells/mL. It is not correct to estimate herd production loss from the average linear score using the individual cow linear score–production loss relationship developed for bulk tank milk SCC.

Percentage of Herd Over Somatic Cell Count Threshold

Interpretation of SCC and SCS requires the choice of a threshold value for classification of cows as positive and negative. The threshold value used ranges from 200,000–400,000 cells/mL (SCS, 4 to 5). A useful herd goal for subclinical mastitis is to have less than 15% of cows with SCC values greater than 200,000–250,000 cells/mL (prevalence). A second goal is to have fewer than 5% of cows developing new subclinical infections each month (incidence).

Percentage of Herd Changing Somatic Cell Count to Over Threshold

Most uses of SCC data focus on the determination of current udder health status. In other words, SCC is used as an estimate of the prevalence of existing infections in the herd; however, an important objective of a mastitis control program is to minimize the number of new intramammary infections. The change in the SCC of individual cows from month to month can be used as an estimate of the rate of new infections, and the use of SCC data in this way has been evaluated. Using SCC changes from month to month as a test for the rate of new infections has low sensitivity and high specificity. More research is needed on the usefulness of SCC to monitor the occurrence of new infections.

A popular way to represent these data graphically is to plot the SCC value (or linear score) for the current month on the *y*-axis and the SCC value (or linear score) for the preceding month on the *x*-axis. This graphing arrangement is preferred because the current SCC value is dependent, in part, on the previous SCC value. Using this graphical approach, individual SCC values in the upper left quadrant are new infections, values in the upper right quadrant are persistent infections, and values in the lower right quadrant are resolved infections.

Bacteriologic Culture of Bulk Milk

Although SCC is widely used for monitoring udder health status in dairy herds, decision making often requires information about the prevalence of specific pathogens. With the regular collection of bulk tank milk samples for the purposes of quality monitoring programs, culturing of the bulk tank milk is an attractive alternative to culturing milk from individual cows. Bulk tank milk culture has been formally evaluated as a mastitis screening test. For the major mastitis pathogens, bulk milk culture had a low sensitivity. Even in herds infected with *S. agalactiae,* repeated bulk milk cultures were necessary to detect positive herds. Mastitis pathogens of greatest interest are contagious pathogens, such as *S. agalactiae, S. aureus, M. bovis,* and *C. bovis.*

The **standard plate count** (plate loop count) provides an estimate of the total numbers of aerobic bacteria in bulk tank milk and is an important measure of milk quality and udder health. It is most commonly used to evaluate the efficiency of cleaning the milking system. **A standard plate count of less than 10,000 CFU/mL can be achieved on most farms, and less than 5,000 CFU/mL should be the goal.** Standard plate counts higher than 10,000 CFU/mL indicate milking of cows with dirty teats or mastitis, poorly sanitized milking equipment, or delayed cooling of milk in the bulk tank. Many herds routinely have bacteria counts of 1,000 CFU/mL or less. Total bacterial counts have some value as an early warning system because up to 50% of violations of the standard are associated with mastitis-related bacteria. For example, bacterial counts in the milk of acute clinical cases may be as high as 10,000,000 CFU/mL. Milk from subclinically infected quarters may contain 1,000 to 10,000 CFU/mL, and normal quarters yield less than 1000 CFU/mL. In nonmastitic cows, higher counts (up to six times higher) are seen in housed cows than in pastured cows.

The **preliminary incubation count** is an estimate of the total number of cold-loving bacteria. As such, the preliminary incubation count provides an index of milk production on the farm. A preliminary incubation count below 50,000 CFU/mL can be achieved on most farms, with less than 10,000 CFU/mL being the goal. The preliminary incubation count should be less than 3 to 6 times the standard plate count.

Herd-Level Measures of Clinical Mastitis

The incidence of clinical mastitis, calculated as cases per 100 cows per year, can provide a rough assessment of new intramammary infections. The goal is less than 2 new cases per 100 cows each month (equivalent to <24% of cows affected each year). Calculation of the total treatment days can provide a herd-level assessment of the approach to therapy of clinical mastitis, as well as an estimate of the economic losses.

In a random sample of dairy herds in the Netherlands, the following risk factors were associated with a higher incidence of clinical mastitis: one or more cows leaking milk, one or more cows with trampled teats, no disinfection of the maternity area after calving, consistent use of postmilking teat disinfection, Red and White cattle as the predominant breed, and an annual bulk tank milk SCC of less than 150,000 cells/mL. Factors associated with a higher rate of clinical mastitis caused by *E. coli* included cows with trampled teats, no disinfection of the maternity area after calving, consistent use of postmilking teat disinfection, use of a thick layer of bedding in the stall, and the stripping of foremilk before cluster attachment. Factors associated with a higher rate of clinical mastitis caused by *S. aureus* included Red and White cattle as the predominant breed, cows with trampled teats, stripping of foremilk before cluster attachment, no regular disinfection of the stall, no regular replacement of stall bedding, and an annual bulk tank milk SCC of less than 150,000 cells/mL. Teat disinfection appeared to increase the incidence of clinical mastitis associated with *E. coli*, which may be explained by the higher incidence around calving and during early lactation, when the resistance of cows is low combined with an increase in the numbers of environmental bacteria associated with maternity pens.

Monitoring Udder Health of Individual Cows

Earlier in this chapter, one direct test (culture) and several indirect tests for intramammary infection were described. Currently, four methods are widely used to detect subclinical mastitis: culture of composite or quarter samples, SCC values of composite or quarter samples, and CMT and electrical conductivity of quarter samples. Currently, cow-level data (culture or SCC) are the most commonly used of these four monitoring tools, but the usefulness of these tests varies depending on their cost, sensitivity, specificity, convenience, and availability.

Bacteriologic Culture of Milk

Culture of aseptically collected milk samples has been a cornerstone of mastitis control programs. Extensive diagnostic laboratory systems have been developed for the culture of milk. For many years, milk bacteriology has been recognized as the gold standard of mastitis diagnostic tests. The sensitivity and specificity of milk bacteriology are now being examined and, as the costs of laboratory procedures have risen, there is an increasing need to justify diagnostic expenses. However, there is still an important need for information concerning the predominant types of mastitis organism active in a herd.

Several schemes have been proposed for obtaining a pathogen profile of the mastitis pathogens in a herd. The following suggestions are offered as the most appropriate times to collect samples for milk bacteriology:

- **Pretreatment milk samples from clinical cases**. Samples should be frozen, collected at a herd visit, and submitted for culture.
- **Cows that have an increased SCC**. At each scheduled herd visit, each cow that has an increase in SCC over a preset threshold is sampled, and the sample is submitted for culture.
- **A composite milk sample from each lactating cow in the herd**. This whole-herd culture would be conducted annually, or more frequently, depending on the herd situation. This method is most appropriate for herds having problems with contagious pathogens, but the economics of this approach have not been evaluated.
- **Culture of cows at a specific management event.** One example is milk culture at drying off and at the first milking after calving. This can be useful for assessment of the dry cow management program.

The cost-effectiveness of any one or a combination of these methods of obtaining a bacteriologic profile of a herd's milk will depend on the current situation in the herd. For the vast majority of dairy herds, the routine culture of cows for subclinical mastitis diagnosis is not cost-effective. Herds with a low bulk tank milk SCC and a low incidence of clinical mastitis episodes can conduct an efficient udder health management program without culturing milk. It is very wise, however, to collect pretreatment milk samples from clinical mastitis cases. These samples can be frozen without significant alterations of the culture results for most pathogens. The samples are collected at a scheduled herd visit and submitted to the laboratory. In most herds, this approach will give a meaningful bacteriologic profile of the herd and assist in assessment of the treatment protocol.

C. bovis is not a common cause of clinical mastitis on most farms but is frequently found in random milk samples. Because *C. bovis* is highly infectious and susceptible to teat disinfection, it has been suggested that its prevalence could be used as an indicator of teat-dipping efficiency in a herd, either of the intensity of the dipping or of the efficacy of the dip. Because *C. bovis* is limited in its colonization to the streak canal, it is valuable as a monitor of teat disinfection.

Somatic Cell Counts

Several management decisions can be based on individual cow composite SCCs. Before any decisions can be made using SCC, criteria must be established to categorize cows based on their SCC results. This involves establishing threshold values or other criteria. The **recommended threshold is 250,000 cells/mL in herds with a low prevalence (<5%) of subclinical mastitis**, providing a sensitivity of 0.55 and specificity of 0.96. In comparison, the **recommended threshold is 200,000 cells/mL in herds with a high prevalence (40%) of subclinical mastitis**, providing an apparent sensitivity of 0.73 to 0.89 and a specificity of 0.86. A clinically more appropriate approach is to calculate likelihood ratios using test sensitivity and specificity, estimated herd prevalence, and a spreadsheet. Cows are identified for further investigation based on their SCC, using three different methods:

- **Change in SCC to over the threshold**. A cow with a marked increase in SCC from one month to the next would be identified as potentially being infected.
- **Persistently elevated SCC**. Cows with a persistently elevated SCC month after month would be identified for management intervention. The lactation average linear score and the lifetime linear score are also useful in this respect. This information is especially useful if dry period therapy has already been unsuccessful for the cow in question.
- **Percentage contribution to herd average**. An estimate of the percentage of the SCC in bulk tank milk contributed by each problem cow can be calculated using individual cow test-day milk weights and SCC data. It should be noted that cows with high milk production and intermediate SCC levels can make a significantly higher

contribution to SCC than some cows with a very high SCC but low production. It is not uncommon for a few problem cows to be responsible for more than 50% of the cells in the bulk tank, particularly in small herds. In most circumstances, the cows with the highest percentage contribution merit immediate action.

With these methods of identifying individual cows based on SCC results, several udder health management decisions can be made, including:

- **Selection of cows for milk bacteriologic culture**. The importance of having a good bacteriologic profile of the intramammary infections in the herd has been emphasized. Several lactation events are suggested as useful times to collect milk for bacteriology. One such event is a clinical mastitis episode. Selection of cows for culture can also be based on an elevated SCC.
- **Selection of cows for dry cow treatment**. Blanket dry cow therapy is currently recommended for most herds. However, herds that use selective dry cow therapy need a suitable screening test to make therapy decisions; such a test is currently unavailable, although individual cow SCCs may be of some help in this decision-making process. Cows with a very high SCC have significantly lower cure rates after dry cow treatment than cows that are infected but have a lower SCC. The SCC can be used as a general indicator of the expected success of dry cow treatment.
- **Treatment during lactation**. The development of a treatment protocol and the criteria for selecting cows to treat during lactation were presented earlier. Treatment on the basis of a change in individual cow SCC from month to month is not economically justifiable. Many other factors need to be considered for a cost-effective treatment decision, and SCC could be one of these criteria.
- **Evaluation of the response to treatment**. Individual cow SCC data can be used as a preliminary evaluation of the mastitis therapy program. With good records on clinical cases and the treatment administered, individual cow SCC data in the months following treatment can be used as a general indicator of the response to therapy. Spontaneous cures and new infections will confound this evaluation, but with data from multiple farms and over a considerable time period a low-cost preliminary evaluation can be achieved.
- **Culling decision**. The lifetime average SCC or linear score of an individual cow is useful additional information in making specific culling decisions. In conjunction with milk culture results, the SCC data are useful to help establish a cow's net present value. An elevated SCC month after month serves to emphasize that culling is the only method of elimination of some chronic cases of mastitis. Removal of these cows eliminates a source of infection for the rest of the herd, as well as assisting in general improvement in the quality of the bulk tank milk.
- **Alter the milking order**. It is generally recommended that infected cows be milked last, although this is often impractical for free-stall and pasture-based dairy enterprises. Individual cow SCC can be used to establish a milking order in tie-stall barns. Alternatively, some large herds establish a special milking string for infected cows. These milking order and segregation programs can be based on SCC results, but cows with an elevated SCC but no intramammary infection may be incorrectly classified. In segregation programs these false-positive cows may be at increased risk.
- **Management procedures to limit the effect of individual cows**. There is some evidence that machine disinfection after milking infected cows may limit the spread of contagious pathogens. In an intensively managed tie-stall herd, it is possible to manually disinfect the milking unit between cows. To maximize the efficiency of this labor-intensive step, individual cow SCC can be used to identify the cows after which machine disinfection would be useful. Another management method involves using the milk from specific cows for feeding calves. In situations in which there are significant financial incentives for low SCC bulk milk, removal of the milk from one or two cows can have an impact on the amount of premium received. Individual cow SCC values can be used to identify specific cows that should be eliminated from the bulk tank. Precautions need to be taken to prevent intersucking between calves receiving this high-SCC milk.
- **Use of individual cow SCC in economic decision analysis**. The relationship between individual cow SCC and milk production losses has been well established. SCC values can be used to estimate the economic losses from subclinical mastitis. This information may be extremely useful in calculating the potential economic benefit of implementing a new udder health management strategy.

Problem Solving Using Individual Cow Somatic Cell Counts

A simple approach to problem solving involves defining the problem by **answering the questions: who, when, where, and what is involved** in the situation. Individual cow SCCs provide an inexpensive consistent source of information to answer these questions. This process is completed by dividing the herd into subgroups and calculating the percentage of cows with SCCs over a threshold (250,000 cells/mL) in each group.

- **Who is affected?** The herd can be subdivided based on several defining characteristics. These include production level, genetic factors (sire), and other characteristics such as having a previous clinical mastitis episode. A gradual increase in the proportion of elevated SCC would normally occur as lactation number increases. Thus a higher percentage of older cows are expected to have elevated SCCs than first-lactation and second-lactation animals. A high proportion of elevated SCC values in heifers would suggest a problem in the replacement program or a breakdown of hygiene in the immediate periparturient period for first-calf heifers. A markedly elevated percentage of high-SCC cows in older animals suggests that infections have become chronic and that the culling strategy should be reevaluated.
- **When does high SCC occur?** It is appropriate to examine SCC distributions according to stage of lactation and season of the year. Normally there is a gradual increase in the prevalence of elevated counts as the lactation progresses. If the prevalence of cows with elevated SCCs is high in early lactation, it suggests a problem with dry cow management or with new infections occurring around the time of calving. If the distribution of cows over threshold shows a dramatic increase during lactation, cow-to-cow transmission of contagious organisms is suspected. Measures of new infection rate are also helpful in solving these problems. The percentage of cows over threshold in the herd can be charted over time. It is expected that this indicator will indicate the same seasonal trends as found in bulk tank milk SCC in the population. For example, the percentage of the herd over threshold should be highest in the fall and lowest in the spring. An increase in this index in the spring would contradict the population trend and should be investigated.
- **Where are the affected cows located?** The distribution of cows with elevated SCC according to their location in the tie-stall barn, in milking strings, or according to milking order may provide evidence for some risk factors for new infections. A mastitis problem caused by environmental pathogens in a free-stall operation can be difficult to solve. Calculating the percentage of cows with

an SCC greater than 250,000 cells/mL for each milking group can help to determine where the problem is most severe. If a specific milking order is followed, as is the case in most tie-stall systems, the distribution of cows with elevated counts according to milking order can demonstrate weaknesses in milking hygiene.

- **What is the problem and why has it occurred?** The information obtained by answering the questions **who, when,** and **where** in the problem-solving process can go a long way toward defining **what** the problem is. Prevalence distributions can be combined with the incidence of clinical mastitis, information from milk cultures, and an estimate of the financial losses to complete the picture. Subsequently, specific solutions will be aimed at **why** this problem might exist.

With the development of computerized dairy health management records systems, the epidemiologic analysis of udder health information can be greatly simplified. Ultimately, specific risk factors would be automatically tested for statistical significance. In addition, the relative importance of many potential risk factors would be evaluated.

9. PERIODIC REVIEW OF THE UDDER HEALTH MANAGEMENT PROGRAM

Many aspects of mastitis control, such as milking management and therapy of clinical cases, become routine practices. However, changes continue to occur in the udder health status of the herd, environmental conditions, and available technology. With these changes, the current udder health management program may no longer be appropriate. New employees may be introduced, and it is possible that various steps are not being appropriately implemented. In some dairy herds, management practices are passed on from previous generations without critical examination. Mastitis results from a continually evolving relationship between microorganisms, the cow, and the environment. Any program intended to limit problems from these relationships needs to be reevaluated on a regular basis.

An effective udder health management program should undergo regular periodic review. The review process should involve the producer and the herd veterinarian, although input may be sought from various farm management advisors. The review should be objective and thorough, but simple and easy to conduct. The use of a standard investigation form structured on the 10 steps of the mastitis control program is recommended. The same standard form can be used for the investigation of problem herds.

10. SETTING GOALS FOR UDDER HEALTH STATUS

The establishment of realistic targets of performance for various udder health parameters is the final component in an udder health management program. These goals are important to determine whether there have been shortfalls in the milk quality and udder health performance. The goals should be realistic and achievable, as well as having economic significance. In addition, the targets must be easily measured and should be accepted by all members of the farm management and labor team.

The setting of appropriate goals for mastitis control efforts is crucial for completion of the health management cycle. In some cases, the target will be the industry reference value; however, in most situations it will be a farm-specific level of performance.

Relationship of Udder Health to Productivity and Profitability

Mastitis is generally considered to be the most costly disease facing the dairy industry. The reduced profitability is caused by two major factors:

- Reduced milk production associated with subclinical mastitis accounts for approximately 70% of the economic loss.
- The treatment costs, culling, and reduced productivity associated with clinical mastitis are responsible for the remaining losses.

Production Losses From Increased Somatic Cell Count

It is well accepted that milk production decreases as SCC increases, but the relationship between SCC and milk production is curvilinear for individual cattle but approximates a straight line when a logarithmic transformation (such as somatic cell score) is used. Estimates of the milk production losses range from 3% to 6% with each one unit increase of somatic cell score (SCS) above 3. The loss in first-lactation heifers is greater than that in older cows. A general rule of thumb would suggest that there is 5% loss for each unit of SCS increase above a linear score of 3.

There is also a relationship between bulk tank milk SCC and milk production because there is a linear decrease in herd milk production with an increase in bulk tank milk SCC. Estimates of the production loss range from 1.5% to 3.0% for each increase of 100,000 cells/mL over a baseline of 150,000 cells/mL. Using an average of these estimates, daily milk and dollar losses can be calculated from bulk tank milk SCC and herd production levels.

Clinical Mastitis and Lost Productivity

Economic losses associated with the treatment of clinical mastitis arise from the cost of drugs, veterinary services, and milk discarded. In addition, decreased milk production, premature culling, and replacement heifer costs are also significant. However, more than 80% of the loss attributed to a clinical episode involves the discarding of nonsaleable milk and decreased milk production.

ASSESSMENT OF THE COST-EFFECTIVENESS OF MASTITIS CONTROL

Dairy producers look to their veterinarian for information and services related to mastitis and its control. With this motivation, veterinarians should be able to implement comprehensive udder health management programs on the majority of dairy farms. To achieve a high rate of implementation of mastitis control strategies, it may be necessary to demonstrate the cost:benefit ratio of the suggested practices before they are adopted. A reassessment of their impact over time may also be useful. A 2008 study in the Netherlands estimated that a single episode of clinical mastitis cost €210, with subclinical and clinical mastitis costing an estimated €140 per cow per year, and found that the majority of farmers underestimated the cost of mastitis.[19]

Mastitis control is feasible, practical, and cost-effective. The economics of the efforts of a mastitis control program in a herd can be estimated. There are several steps necessary to complete this assessment.

1. Programs for monitoring udder health and for establishing achievable goals must be in place for an economic assessment.
2. The losses resulting from mastitis must be quantified. The amount of reduced milk production resulting from increased SCC is calculated. In addition, costs associated with the discarded milk and treatment of clinical cases must be estimated.
3. The udder health management program to be implemented must be described. An accounting system should be established to calculate the costs associated with this program.
4. Using an estimate of the potential loss for a hypothetical herd with no mastitis control efforts, the profitability of the herd's current udder health management program is determined.
5. By estimating the costs of implementing new udder health management measures, the remaining potential profits from mastitis control can be calculated.

This economic assessment is done using a computer spreadsheet program. With such a computer program, veterinarians can simply and rapidly input actual values for a particular farm and assess the economic circumstances. The impact of each element of control can be considered from the point of view of a cost:benefit ratio. The results of economic assessment will vary widely from farm to farm, but usually the following conclusions are made:

- Mastitis will remain a costly disease, even with implementation of properly applied, effective control programs.
- Loss of milk production attributable to subclinical infection will remain a major cause of economic loss because of mastitis in most herds.
- Proper application of simple, inexpensive mastitis control procedures will have a significant impact on profitability and will bring higher returns on investment.

FURTHER READING

Bradley A, Barkema H, Biggs A, et al. Control of mastitis and enhancement of milk quality. In: Green M, ed. *Dairy Herd Health*. Wallingford, UK: CAB International; 2012:117-168.

Edmondson P. Mastitis control in robotic milking systems. *In Pract*. 2012;34:260-269.

Mein GA. The role of the milking machine in mastitis control. *Vet Clin North Am Food Anim Pract*. 2012;28:307-320.

Nickerson SC. Control of heifer mastitis: antimicrobial treatment—an overview. *Vet Microbiol*. 2009;134:128-135.

REFERENCES

1. Østerås O, Sølverød L. *Ir Vet J*. 2009;62(suppl 26):S26.
2. Hassfurther RL, et al. *Am J Vet Res*. 2015;76:231.
3. Williamson JH, Lacy-Hulbert SJ. *New Zeal Vet J*. 2013;61:262.
4. Bertulat S, et al. *J Dairy Sci*. 2013;96:3774.
5. Zobel G, et al. *J Dairy Sci*. 2013;96:5064.
6. Bertulat S, et al. *Vet Rec*. 2015;2:e000068.
7. Cardot V, et al. *J Dairy Sci*. 2008;91:2257.
8. Halasa T, et al. *J Dairy Sci*. 2009b;92:3150.
9. Halasa T, et al. *J Dairy Sci*. 2009a;92:3134.
10. Scherpenzeel CGM, et al. *J Dairy Sci*. 2014;97:3606.
11. Bradley AJ, et al. *J Dairy Sci*. 2011;94:692.
12. Bradley AJ, et al. *J Dairy Sci*. 2010;93:1566.
13. Rabiee AR, Lean IJ. *J Dairy Sci*. 2013;96:6915.
14. Petrovski KR, et al. *J Dairy Sci*. 2011;94:3366.
15. Laven RA, et al. *New Zeal Vet J*. 2014;62:214.
16. Berry EA, Hillerton JE. *J Dairy Sci*. 2007;90:760.
17. Parker KI, et al. *J Dairy Sci*. 2007;90:207.
18. Runciman DJ, et al. *J Dairy Sci*. 2010;93:4582.
19. Huijps K, et al. *J Dairy Res*. 2008;75:113.

Miscellaneous Abnormalities of the Teats and Udder

Several diseases are characterized clinically by lesions of the skin of the teats and udder. These diseases are most common in dairy cattle and are of economic importance because teat lesions cause pain and discomfort during milking, and udder edema and udder cleft dermatitis are very common in heifers at calving.

The skin of the wall of the teat and the skin surrounding the teat canal orifice must be inspected closely to observe lesions and palpated to detect lesions covered by scabs. It may be necessary to superficially irrigate and gently wash teat lesions with warm 0.9% NaCl solution to see the morphology and spatial arrangement of the lesions. The entire skin of the cranial, lateral, and posterior aspects of the udder should be examined by inspection and palpation. Lesions may be restricted to the lateral aspects of the udder and teats, as in photosensitization, or completely surround the teats, as in pseudocowpox.

In North America, the most common viral diseases of the teats of cattle, which result in vesicles or erosion of the teats, include pseudocowpox and bovine herpes mammillitis, with vesicular stomatitis occurring occasionally. The vesicular diseases of the teats are particularly important because they require differentiation from the exotic vesicular diseases such as foot-and-mouth disease. The appearances of the lesions of each of these diseases are similar, which makes clinical diagnosis difficult. However, in most cases, the morphologic and epidemiologic differences in the lesions in groups of animals aid in the diagnosis.

In pigs, **necrosis of the skin of the teats of newborn piglets** may occur in outbreak form. Abrasion of the nipples of baby pigs raised on rough nonslip concrete may be observed as acute lesions or be apparent only when the piglets mature and are found to have deficient teat numbers, as described under agalactia.

The skin of the mammary gland and teats of lactating ewes may be affected by the lesions of **contagious ecthyma**, which are transmitted from the lips of suckling lambs. **Ulcerative dermatosis** of the teats in lactating ewes has lesions similar to those of herpes mammillitis in cows. It is a disease of housed ewes and may be initiated by bedding on infected straw. Mastitis and teat deformity are common sequels. The etiology varies from *S. aureus* to CNS or *Pasteurella* spp.

LESIONS OF THE BOVINE TEAT

Traumatic injuries to teats are very common and range from superficial lacerations to deep lacerations into the teat cistern with the release of milk through the wound. Accidental trampling of a teat by a cow may cause amputation of the teat.

Chapping and cracking of the skin of the teats is common in dairy and beef cattle. The cracks in the skin are often linear and multiple and are painful when palpated or when the milking machine teat cups are applied to the affected teats. Cracks of the skin of the teats initiated by milking machine action can be aggravated by environmental factors to create chapping of the teats. The condition is common when adverse weather conditions follow turn out in spring. Linear lesions appear on the teat wall near the teat–udder junction and extend transversely around the teat. The addition of **10% glycerin** to the teat dip provides an excellent method of improving teat skin condition.

Frostbite of teats occurs in dairy cows housed outdoors during severely cold weather without adequate bedding. The skin of the teats is cold, necrotic, and oozes serum. Usually the front teats are more severely affected than the rear teats because the latter are less exposed to adverse ambient temperatures.

Teat-end lesions are common in dairy cattle. Lesions include teat canal eversion, teat canal prolapse, prolapse of the meatus, eversion of the meatus, and teat orifice erosion. Limited information is presently available about the mechanism of development for these lesions and their clinical significance; one study found no association between the presence or absence of a teat-end lesion and intramammary infection.

It is normal to see a 2-mm wide white ring around each teat orifice of machine milked cows. The first stage of a teat orifice abnormality occurs when this ring undergoes hypertrophy, keratinization, and radial cracking. Progression leads to increased hypertrophy, secondary bacterial infection, scab formation, eversion of the distal teat canal, and eventually teat orifice erosion. Improper milking machine function can produce teat orifice abnormalities. Excessive or fluctuating vacuum levels, faulty teat cup liners, incorrect pulsation ratios, and other faults attributed to inadequate maintenance and careless use of milking machines have been shown to cause teat injury. A high milking vacuum combined with a relatively low pulsation chamber vacuum can result in bruising and hemorrhage of the teat-end teat wall by the slapping action of the liner.

Black spot (black pox) is a sporadic lesion of the teat tip characterized by a **deep, crater-shaped ulcer** with a **black spot** in the center. Black spot lesions occurring at the ends of the teats commonly involve the teat sphincter and are responsible for a great deal of mastitis. This abnormality is caused in most cases by excessive vacuum pressure or overmilking in teats that are naturally firm and have pointed ends. There is no specific bacteriology, although *F. necrophorum* is commonly present, and *S. aureus* is frequently isolated from the lesions. Lesser lesions of teat sphincters are listed under vacuum pressure in bovine mastitis control. The lesions are painful, leading to kicking by the cows, sometimes to repeated kicking off of the teat cups, and to blockage of the sphincter. *T. pyogenes* mastitis is a common sequel. Black spot lesions are poorly responsive to treatment, even if the machine error is corrected.

Treatment of black spot is usually by topical application of ointments: Whitfield's, 10% salicylic acid, 5% sulfathiazole and 5% salicylic acid, and 5% copper sulfate are all recommended. An iodophor ointment, or iodophor teat dip with 35% added glycerol, is also effective, but treatment needs to be thorough and repeated and milking machine errors need to be corrected.

Thelitis or inflammation of the tissues of the teat wall leading to gangrene is a common complication of gangrenous mastitis, and is most commonly associated with peracute *S. aureus* mastitis. The skin of the teats is cold, edematous, and oozes serum. The subcutaneous aspects are commonly distended with gas. The skin is commonly dark-red to purple-black. Sloughing of the skin may be evident.

Inflammation of the wall of the teat (thelitis) is a nonspecific lesion usually associated with traumatic injury to the lining of the teat cistern. The wall of the cistern is thickened, hardened, painful, and, in chronic lesions, irregular in its internal lining. The lesion can be felt as a dense, vertical cord in the center of the teat tip. The lesions have historically been intractable to treatment, which usually consists of intramammary antibiotics and refraining from milking. The recent application of teat endoscopy has assisted in identifying cattle that are most likely to respond to medical or surgical treatment.

Bovine nodular thelitis was first described in France in 1963, with subsequent reports in Japan and Switzerland. The disease is characterized by nodular lesions in the teat wall and ventral portion of the udder. The lesions are multicentric nodules containing atypical acid-fast mycobacteria, including *M. terrae* and undescribed *Mycobacterium* species that are related to *M. leprae* and *M. lepromatosis*.[1] Some nodules evolve to ulcers, demonstrating cicatrization and fibrosis.

Photosensitization of the teats (photosensitive thelitis) is a local manifestation of generalized photosensitization, but occasionally photosensitive thelitis is the first clinical abnormality detected by the producer. There is a characteristic erythema and hardness of the unpigmented or white parts of the lateral aspects of each teat. The medial aspect is soft and cool. The teats are also painful and in the early stages apparently irritable, because affected cows will also stand in ponds or waterholes in such a way that the teats are immersed, and then rock backward and forward. They will also brush the sides of the udder with the hind feet in a way that could suggest the stamping movements of abdominal pain. In cases in which the photosensitization is related to the induction of parturition by the administration of corticosteroids, the skin lesions are usually restricted to the teats. In cases due to other causes there are usually obvious lesions of photosensitive dermatitis on the dorsal aspects of the body but confined to the white parts.

Corpora amylacea are inert concretions of amyloid that may become calcified and detached from the mammary tissue so that they cause blockage of the teat canal and cessation of milk flow. They are formed as the result of stasis caused by blocked mammary tissue ducts and resorption of the milk fluids.

Papillomatosis of the teats is caused by bovine papillomavirus and is characterized clinically by small, white, and slightly elevated nodules with a 0.3-cm diameter or elongated tags 1 cm long that are removable by traction. This is covered more extensively in Chapter 16.

Pseudocowpox is characterized clinically by painful localized edema and erythema with a thin film of exudate over the edematous area. Vesicle formation is uncommon. Within 48 hours of onset of signs, a small orange papule develops, shortly followed by the formation of an elevated, small, and dark-red scab. The edges of the lesion then extend and the center becomes umbilicated; at 1 week the lesion measures approximately 1 cm in diameter. By 10 days the central scab tends to desquamate, leaving a slightly raised circinate scab commonly termed a "ring" or "horseshoe" scab. One teat may have several such lesions, which coalesce to form linear scabs. The majority of lesions desquamate by 6 weeks without leaving scars, although occasionally animals develop chronic infection.

REFERENCE

1. Pin D, et al. *Emerg Infect Dis*. 2014;20:2111.

LESIONS OF THE BOVINE TEAT AND UDDER

Thermal burns of the skin of the udder and teats may occur in mature cattle exposed to grass fires. The hairs of the udder and base of the teats are singed black. Thermal injury to the skin varies from marked erythema of the teats to blistering and necrosis and weeping of serum.

BOVINE HERPES MAMMILLITIS

SYNOPSIS

Etiology Bovine herpesvirus-2, rarely bovine herpesvirus-4

Epidemiology Occurs as an outbreak in cows, particularly heifers, usually within 2 weeks after calving. Commonly followed by persistent infection in the herd

Clinical findings Lesions confined to teats and udder. Vesicles leading to sloughing of skin and necrotic ulceration. Prolonged clinical course

Clinical pathology Virus isolation and electron microscopy on fresh lesions and serology

Treatment Antiseptic and emollient ointments

Control Isolation and milking hygiene, but not effective. Control of periparturient udder edema

ETIOLOGY

The causative virus, **bovine herpesvirus-2** (BHV-2), is an α-herpesvirus. Infection with BHV-2 can produce two distinct syndromes in cattle, **bovine herpes mammillitis,** in which there are vesicular and erosive lesions with necrotic ulceration on the skin of the udder and teats, and **pseudolumpy skin disease** (Allerton virus), which manifests with generalized superficial skin lesions over the body. Pseudolumpy skin disease is uncommon. The difference in clinical manifestations between the two diseases may be caused by the strain of the virus or the method of infection. **BHV-4** (DN599 strain), which is usually associated with respiratory disease in cattle, is also capable of causing mammary pustular dermatitis.

EPIDEMIOLOGY

Occurrence

Herpes mammillitis is recorded in North America, Australia, Europe, and Africa, but probably has **widespread occurrence**. Herds infected for the first time have a high morbidity rate; subsequently, the incidence is low and is limited to fresh heifers. The **morbidity** rate varies between 18% and 96%, with susceptible herds recording more than 30% affected. The **mortality** rate is negligible.

ORIGIN OF INFECTION AND TRANSMISSION

Introduction of bovine ulcerative mammillitis into a herd may occur with the introduction of infected animals, but outbreaks have been observed in self-contained herds. Spread within a herd is consistent with the presence of carrier animals, which may shed virus during times of stress, particularly in the periparturient period. Latent infection is an intrinsic trait of herpesvirus infections, and BHV-2 has been isolated from the trigeminal ganglion of healthy cattle.[1] It is presumed that the virus also remains latent in inguinal nerves but this has not been verified in cattle. However, BHV-2 has been demonstrated in lumbar ganglia of ewes experimentally inoculated with BHV-2; these ganglia are sensory to the ovine udder.[2] There is a seasonal incidence of clinical disease that has been related to the activity and presence of insect vectors. Experimental studies indicate that transmission requires virus inoculation at or below the level of the stratum germinativum of the teat or udder skin; therefore trauma associated with milking, teat cracks, or biting flies is a requirement for infection to be transferred. Milking machine liners, hands, and udder cloths may act as carriers of virus when a large amount of it is being released.

Seasonal and circumstantial evidence in the **UK** and **Australia** suggest an insect vector, but this has not been confirmed by attempts at transmission with the stable fly (*Stomoxys calcitrans*), and in the Midwest of the **United States**, the disease is more common in the winter months between November and April.

Survival of the virus for long periods in carrier animals occurs, and it is thought that this may be the means of survival of the virus within a herd that has become immune. Infection in some cows is suspected to result in chronic infection at the teat end with the cows becoming **hard milkers** and **carriers** of the disease.

Animal and Pathogen Risk Factors

Lesions are most common in animals within the **first 2 weeks after calving**, particularly in **heifers**, and the disease is more severe in heifers. Heifers that have **udder edema** at calving are particularly prone to develop severe lesions. Occasionally, lesions may be seen on the teats of replacement heifers, and calves suckling infected dams often develop mouth lesions.

The disease is **usually self-limiting**, persisting in a herd for 6 to 15 weeks, and the severity of the lesions decrease as the outbreak progresses. Immunity appears to last about a year; herds infected naturally can suffer recurrences a year later. **Large herds** may have **persisting** disease, particularly in heifers.

The virus is relatively resistant to environmental influences and can survive freezing. It is susceptible to **iodophor disinfectants** and less so to hypochlorites.

Economic Importance

Forms of loss include a much higher incidence of mastitis, reduction in milk in affected herds by up to 20%, the **culling** of some cows because of severe mastitis and of heifers because of intractable ulcers, and a great deal of interference with normal milking procedure.

Zoonotic Implications

There are anecdotal reports of herpetic lesions in farmers exposed to infected cattle.

PATHOGENESIS

Typical clinical lesions and histopathological changes can be produced locally by introduction of the virus into scarifications of the skin of the teat and the oral mucosa and by intradermal and intravenous injection. There is no viremia, and spread is by local extension. In contrast to the poxes, the characteristic lesion in mammillitis is destructive. The higher incidence of the disease and the greater severity of the lesions close to calving are thought to be from the immunosuppression caused by parturition and to a greater predisposition from periparturient udder edema.

CLINICAL FINDINGS

There is an **incubation period** of 5 to 10 days. There is no systemic illness, and lesions are confined to the teats and udder. When the disease occurs in a herd for the first time the first case is usually in a cow that has calved during the previous 2 to 3 days. Rapid lateral spread then occurs to other cows.

Bovine herpes mammillitis is characterized by the formation of variable-sized vesicles, severe edema, and erythema of the teat with subsequent erosion of the teat epithelium. The vesicles rupture within 24 hours, and copious serous fluid often exudes from the dermis. Scabs form over the lesions by the fourth day, and the epithelium is reestablished under the scab by the third week, although the trauma of milking may delay healing, especially when secondary infection occurs. Scar formation on recovery is uncommon. Lesions may be present on several teats and the base of the udder.

In cows calved more than a few weeks previously, the characteristic lesions are almost entirely confined to the skin of the teats; in recently calved cows they are restricted to the skin of the teats and the udder. The severity of the disease in recently calved cattle appears to be directly proportional to the degree of postparturient edema which is present. **Vesicles** occur but are not commonly seen. They are characteristically thin walled, 1 to 2 cm in diameter, variable in outline, and often commence at the base of the teat and spread over much of the udder surface (Fig. 20-8). Rupture and confluence of vesicles leads to weeping and extensive **sloughing** of the skin.

In the most **severe cases**, the entire teat is swollen and painful, the skin is bluish in color, and it exudes serum and sloughs, leaving a raw ulcer covering most of the teat. In less severe cases, there are raised, deep red to blue, circular plaques, 0.5 to 2 cm in diameter, which develop shallow ulcers. In most cases, scab formation follows, but machine milking causes frequent disruption of them, resulting in frequent bleeding. The least severe lesions are in the form of lines of erythema, often in circles and enclosing dry skin or slightly elevated papules, which occasionally show ulceration. Mild lesions tend to heal in about 10 days, but severe ulcers may persist for 2 or 3 months. The severity of lesions on the teats on longer-calved cows varies, but in all cases the lesions are sufficiently painful to make milking difficult. Lesions on the skin of the udder heal more rapidly because of the absence of trauma.

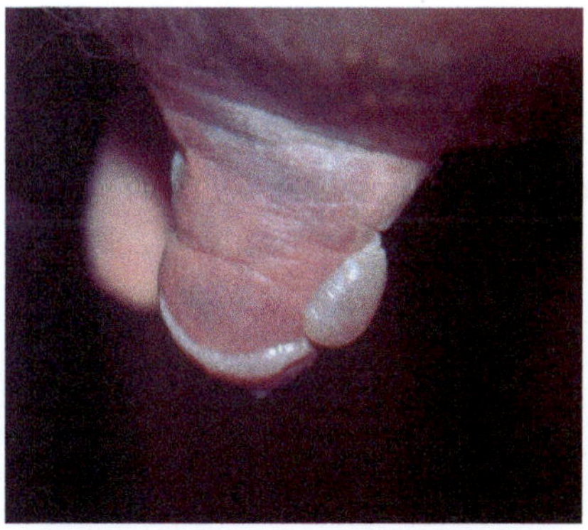

Fig. 20-8 Vesicles on the left foreteat of a Holstein heifer with acute herpes mammillitis infection. The vesicles are fragile and appear as the first sign of infection.

Ulcers in the mouth of affected cows have been observed rarely, and calves suckling affected cows develop lesions on their oral mucosae and muzzles. Ulcerative lesions on the vaginal mucosa have been recorded rarely. During the recovery phase there is obvious scar formation and depigmentation. Infrequently, secondary infections are severe and animals are euthanazed.[3]

CLINICAL PATHOLOGY AND NECROPSY FINDINGS

Material for tissue culture, electron microscopy, or cutaneous transmission tests is best obtained by syringe from early vesicles, or as swabs from early ulcers or oral lesions. The virus may be difficult to demonstrate if the lesions are as old as 7 days and if there has been intensive application of teat disinfectants such as iodophors.

Serology is more commonly used for diagnosis. The presence of high virus-neutralizing antibody titers in serum taken during the acute phase of the disease, and a fourfold increase or decrease in titer in paired samples, are all supportive for diagnosis. Titers of 1:16 or higher for BHV-2 and 1:20 for BHV-4 indicate exposure. Antibody to both viruses should be tested for diagnostic purposes.

Necropsy is not commonly performed, and no necropsy reports of cases of bovine ulcerative mammillitis are available.

DIAGNOSIS

DIFFERENTIAL DIAGNOSIS

Diagnosis is made on the basis of clinical signs in multiple animals. Virus may be isolated from aspirating the fluid from vesicles before they rupture. Serology has been performed to identify a threefold to fourfold rising titer but it is not widely available, and many animals seroconvert early in the disease process.

Differentiation of other diseases of the skin of the teat and udder is dealt with in the section on cowpox.

TREATMENT

There is no specific treatment, and the aim should be to develop scabs that can withstand machine milking. This is most easily effected by the application of a water-miscible, antiseptic ointment just before putting the cups on, followed by an astringent lotion, such as triple dye, immediately after milking. Crystal violet dyes have an excellent reputation as treatments. Cattle that develop a thickened teat caused by secondary bacterial infections are likely to develop clinical mastitis, and treatment success of affected quarters is poor.

CONTROL

Isolation of affected animals and strict hygiene in the milking parlor are practiced but have little effect on the spread of the disease. Milking heifers first also has minimal impact on disease spread. An **iodophor** disinfectant is recommended for use in the dairy to prevent spread because it has good virucidal activity. Reducing the incidence and severity of **periparturient edema** in heifers may reduce the severity of herpes mammillitis. Inoculation of the natural virus away from the teats produces a local lesion and good immunity, but the method has not been tested as a control procedure.

REFERENCES

1. Campos FS, et al. *Vet Microbiol.* 2014;171:182.
2. Torres FD, et al. *Res Vet Sci.* 2009;87:161.
3. Kemp R, et al. *Vet Rec.* 2008;163:119.

LESIONS OF THE BOVINE UDDER OTHER THAN MASTITIS

Udder Impetigo

Udder impetigo associated with *S. aureus* is characterized by small, 2- to 4-mm diameter pustules at the base of the teats that may spread to involve the entire teat and the skin of the udder. This disease is important because of the discomfort it causes, its common association with staphylococcal mastitis, the occasional spread to milkers' hands, and the freq uency with which it is mistaken for cowpox. The lesions are usually small pustules (2- to 40-mm diameter), but in occasional animals they extend to the subcutaneous tissue and appear as furuncles or boils. The most common site is the hairless skin at the base of the teats, but the lesions may spread from here on to the teats and over the udder generally. Spread in the herd appears to occur during milking, and a large proportion of a herd may become affected over a relatively long period. The institution of suitable sanitation procedures, such as dipping teats after milking, washing of udders before milking, and treatment of individual lesions with a suitable antiseptic ointment, as described earlier, usually stops further spread. An ancillary measure is to vaccinate all cows in the herd with an autogenous bacterin produced from the *S. aureus* that is always present. Good immunity is produced for about 6 months, but the disease recurs unless satisfactory sanitation measures are introduced.

Sores of bovine teat skin in Norway, characterized by the presence of *S. aureus* and referred to as **"bovine teat skin summer sore"** are thought to be caused by cutaneous invasion by *Stephanofilaria* spp. nematodes. The differential diagnosis of discrete lesions on bovine teat skin is dealt with in the subject of cowpox.

Udder Cleft Dermatitis

Severe clinical disease caused by **udder cleft dermatitis (udder rot, flexural seborrhea)** of cattle is most common in dairy heifers that have calved recently. Lesions are present in three locations on the udder: between the halves of the udder (udder cleft dermatitis), on the ventral midline immediately cranial to the udder, and on the caudodorsolateral aspect of the udder in which it comes into contact with the medial aspect of the thigh. Lesions are usually detected during foot trimming or milking and are clearly underdiagnosed—cross-sectional studies in Sweden and the Netherlands identified a prevalence of lesions in the cranial udder of 18% in 1084 cows in 30 dairy herds, and 5% in 948 cows in 20 dairy herds, respectively.[1,2] Udder cleft dermatitis occurs is most common in older dairy cattle; higher producing dairy cattle; and cows with a deep udder relative to the hock, large front quarters, and a small angle between the udder and the abdominal wall.[1,2] Although the etiology remains uncertain, there is speculation that bacteria associated with digital dermatitis may be associated with the development of udder cleft dermatitis.[3]

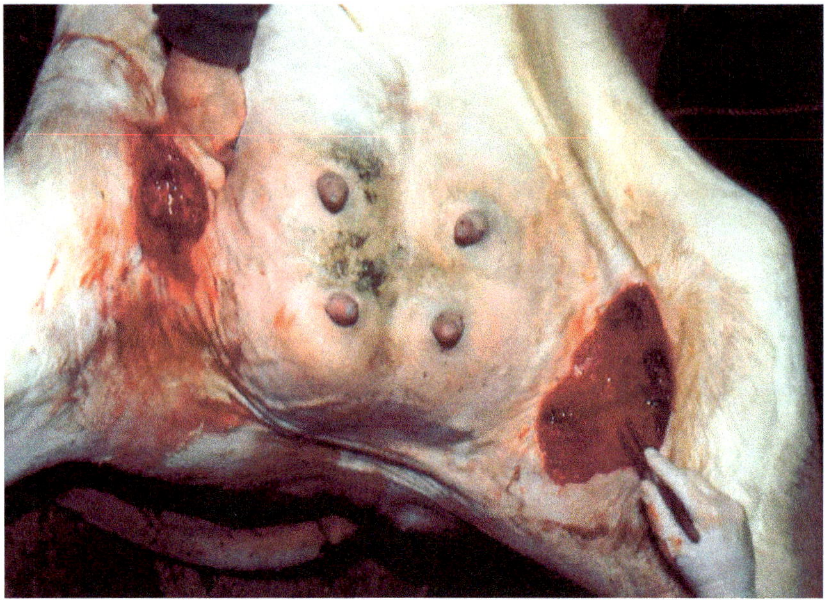

Fig. 20-9 Healing udder cleft dermatitis in the caudodorsolateral aspect of the udder of a Holstein Friesian heifer. The heifer is in dorsal recumbency. Smooth beds of granulation tissue are developing 1 week after aggressive debridement of the focal areas of dermatitis.

Udder edema is thought to play an important role in development of lesions on the caudodorsolateral aspect of the udder, because these are most common in periparturient dairy heifers and typically are more severe. The etiology of caudodorsolateral lesions in heifers may be different to that of cranial lesions in older cows.

In lesions of all three anatomic sites, there is variable inflammation and outpouring of sebum. Extensive skin necrosis may develop in a small number of cases, characterized by a prominent odor of decay. The irritation and pain of the caudodorsolateral lesion may cause the animal to appear lame when walking, and the animal may attempt to lick the affected part. Shedding of the oily, malodorous skin leaves a raw surface beneath, which heals in 3 to 4 weeks. Anecdotal reports exist of extension of infection into the subcutaneous veins resulting in severe hemorrhage and death.[2]

Freshly calved heifers with lesions on the caudodorsolateral aspect of the udder benefit from resolution of udder edema and mechanical debridement using a towel drawn repeatedly across the inguinal area. In advanced cases, a soft tissue curette is used to facilitate debridement of necrotic material after casting the cow in dorsal recumbency, or in lateral recumbency and elevating the upper hindlimb, so that the inguinal area can be adequately visualized (Fig. 20-9).

The efficacy of topical treatment is unknown. Lesions in the other two sites are usually asymptomatic and treatment efficacy is unknown.

Blood in the Milk (Mammary Gland Hematoma)

Blood in the milk is usually an indication of a rupture of a blood vessel in the gland by direct trauma (such as getting caught on top of a wooden fence or the result of a kick) or more commonly by capillary bleeding in heifers with udder edema. Although in the latter circumstance the bleeding usually ceases in 2 to 3 days, it may persist beyond this period and render the milk unfit for human consumption. The discoloration varies from a pale pink to a dark chocolate brown and may still be present 7 to 8 days after parturition. Rarely, the blood loss may be sufficiently severe to require treatment for hemorrhagic shock (see Chapter 4). Cases of blood in the milk are usually sporadic in occurrence, but there are records of herds with over 50% of cows affected; clotting defects were not detected in these herds.

Treatment is often requested, although the cow is clinically normal in all other respects. Intravenous administration of calcium borogluconate or parenteral coagulants such as intravenous formaldehyde (see Chapter 5) is widely practiced, but efficacy studies are lacking and it is difficult to believe that either treatment has therapeutic value. Difficulty may be experienced in milking the clots out of the teats, but they will usually pass easily if they are broken up by compressing them inside the teat. The presence of bloodstained milk in all four quarters at times other than immediately postpartum should arouse suspicion of leptospirosis or diseases in which extensive capillary damage occurs.

UDDER EDEMA

Edema of the udder at parturition is physiologic, but it may be sufficiently severe to cause edema of the belly, udder, and teats in dairy cows and occasionally in mares. In most cases the edema disappears within a day or two of calving, but if it is extensive and persistent it may interfere with suckling and milking. Udder edema is symmetric and extends cranially to the udder along the ventral abdomen (Fig. 20-10). The presence of an asymmetric ventral edema should alert the veterinarian to a mammary vein hematoma or thrombophlebitis of the mammary vein secondary to intravenous injection. The tissue feels colder to the touch than surrounding skin and pits on finger pressure. In severe cases, it extends caudodorsally in the perineal region. A 10-level scale of severity has been devised for dairy cattle and could be applied in assessing the effects of treatment (Table 20-7). Edema is a prominent sign in inherited rectovaginal constriction of Jersey cows, and is described under that heading.

Table 20-7 Scale used in rating udder edema

Score	Definition
0	No edema apparent
1	Edema in the base of the udder around one or two quarters
2	Edema in the base of the udder around two or three quarters
3	Edema covering the lower half of the udder
4	Edema beginning to show in the midline and umbilicus
5	Extensive fluid accumulation along the midline and umbilicus
6	Edema covering entire udder. Median suspensory ligament crease has disappeared.
7	Midline fluid accumulation extended to the brisket
8	Midline fluid accumulation extended dorsally; the subcutaneous abdominal vein is indistinguishable.
9	Fluid accumulation extended to the thighs
10	Severe edema; marked fluid accumulation in the vulva; edema extensive in all of the areas mentioned earlier

Source: From Tucker WB et al. J Dairy Sci 1992; 75:2382.

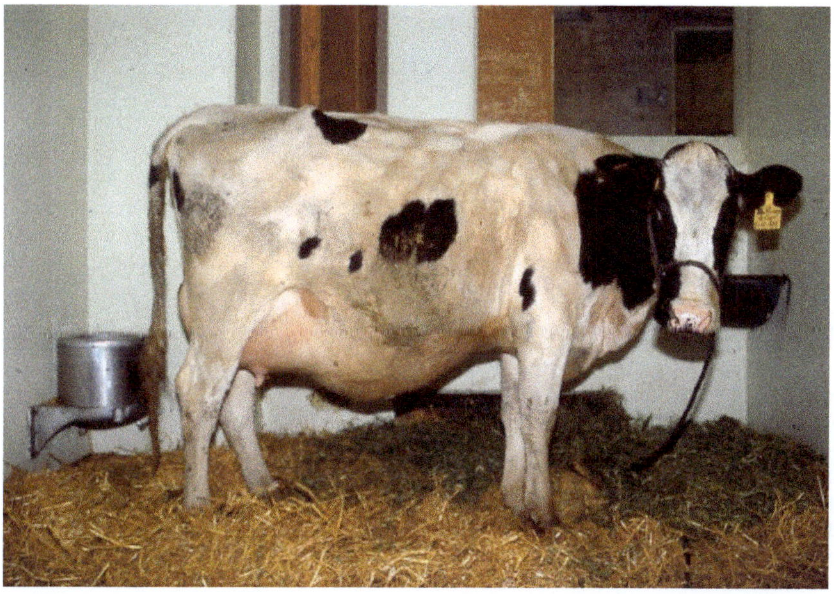

Fig. 20-10 Udder edema in a 2-year-old Holstein Friesian heifer that calved a few days previously. Note the extension of edema cranial to the udder. This is a grade 5/10 udder edema score.

Udder edema is most severe in periparturient dairy heifers, and the mechanism for its development is not well understood. Hypoproteinemia is not a precursor of udder edema. One epidemiologic study identified an increased risk of udder edema in dairy heifers if calving was in winter, the heifer was taller at the withers, and a bull calf was born.[4]

It is a common recommendation that the amount of grain fed in the last few weeks of pregnancy be limited, and there is evidence that heavy grain feeding predisposes to the condition, at least in heifers. High sodium or potassium intakes increase the incidence and severity of udder edema, especially in housed cattle; the disease often disappears when cows are turned out to pasture. The tendency for udder edema may be heritable in some herds and selection against bulls that sire edematous daughters is thought to be worthwhile. Such a tendency could be mediated through a complex interaction between sex steroids, which are thought to play a role in the etiology. There is also a reduction in blood flow through, and an increase in blood pressure in, the superficial epigastric or milk veins of cows with chronic edema, through an unidentified mechanism.

A mild form of udder edema is the presence of a hard localized plaque along the ventral abdomen immediately cranial to the udder after parturition in heifers. This is common and relatively innocuous but may interfere with milking or ventral abdominal surgical repair of a left displaced abomasum. If the mild udder edema occurs repeatedly over a number of lactations it may result in permanent thickening of the skin (scleroderma) of the lateral aspect of the udder. Hot fomentations, massage, and the application of liniments are of value in reducing the hardness and swelling. A chronic form of the disease is recorded from New Zealand, but no credible etiologic agent has been proposed.

If udder edema is severe, one or more of the following empirical treatments is recommended. Milking should be started some days before parturition, but colostrum from heifers should be discarded because it is likely to be of poor quality. After parturition, frequent milking and the use of diuretic agents is recommended. Corticosteroids appear to exert no beneficial effect. Acetazolamide (1–2 g twice daily orally or parenterally for 1–6 days) gives excellent results in a high proportion of cases, with the edema often disappearing within 24 hours. Chlorothiazide (2 g twice daily orally or 0.5 g twice daily by intravenous or intramuscular injection, each for 3–4 days) is also effective. Furosemide is the most potent diuretic agent and should be administered parenterally (1 mg/kg BW, intramuscularly or intravenously; 5 mg/kg BW orally) in severe cases of udder edema, but prolonged use can result in hypokalemia, hypochloremia, and metabolic alkalosis. The use of diuretics before calving may be dangerous if considerable fluid is lost. When there is a herd problem, detection of the cause is often difficult.

An outbreak of udder edema in ewes has been recorded. Affected animals were afebrile, bright, and clinically normal except for the udder, which within 24 hours of lambing was white, cool, and firm, with edema. The milk was normal grossly and laboratory tests detected no abnormalities. Most ewes recovered within 5 to 10 days of lambing.

Hard udder or indurative mastitis in goats is described under the heading of caprine arthritis–encephalitis, and that in ewes under maedi.

RUPTURE OF THE SUSPENSORY LIGAMENTS OF THE UDDER

Rupture of the suspensory ligaments is most common in adult cows and develops gradually over a number of years. The cause is thought to be severe udder edema at calving, with excessive weight on the udder causing breakdown of the udder attachments, particularly the median suspensory ligament. The result is that the teats on affected cows are not vertically aligned but point more laterally. When rupture of the suspensory ligament occurs acutely, just before or after parturition, the udder drops markedly and is swollen and hard, the teats point laterally, and serum oozes through the skin. Severe edema occurs at the base of the udder. The condition may be confused with gangrenous mastitis or abdominal rupture caused by hydrops allantois on cursory examination. Partial relief may be obtained with a suspensory apparatus, but complete recovery does not occur.

AGALACTIA

The most important cause of agalactia in farm animals is postpartum dysgalactia syndrome (PPDS) in sows, formerly named mastitis-metritis-agalactia (MMA) syndrome, which is addressed later in this chapter. The general principles that apply to PPDS also apply to the less common cases of agalactia that occur in all species. There is partial or complete absence of milk flow, which may affect one or more mammary glands. The condition is of major importance in gilts and sows, although it occurs occasionally in cattle. The importance of the disease in gilts and sows derives from the fact that piglets are very susceptible to hypoglycemia. The condition may be caused by failure of letdown or absence of milk secretion.

The causes of **failure of letdown** include painful conditions of the teat; sharp teeth in the piglets; inverted nipples that interfere with suckling; primary failure of milk ejection, especially in gilts; and excessive engorgement and edema of the udder. In many sows the major disturbance seems to be hysteria, which is readily cured by the use of tranquilizing drugs. Treatment of the primary condition and the parenteral administration of oxytocin, repeated if necessary, is usually adequate.

Ergotism may be a specific cause of agalactia in sows and has been recorded in animals fed on bullrush millet infested with ergot.

Apparent **hormonal defects** do occur, particularly in cattle. Sporadic cases occur in which cows calve normally and have a normal udder full of milk but fail to let it down when stimulated in the normal way. A single injection of oxytocin is often sufficient to start the lactation. In rare cases repeated injections at successive milkings are required. There is one report of a number of cows in a herd being affected. The cows were under severe stress for a number of reasons and had depressed serum cortisol levels. In heifers and gilts there may be complete absence of mammary development and, in such cases, no treatment is likely to be of value. In animals that have lactated normally after previous parturitions, the parenteral administration of chorionic gonadotrophin has been recommended but often produces no apparent improvement.

Mares grazing fescue may fail to lactate after parturition because of inhibition of prolactin release.

Milk Drop Syndrome

This is a herd syndrome in which the milk yield falls precipitately without there being any clinical evidence of disease, especially mastitis, or obvious deprivation of food or water. Heat stress (particularly the combination of heat and humidity), summer fescue toxicosis, and leptospirosis caused *Leptospira hardjo* are among the more common causes.

Low Milk Fat Syndrome

In this syndrome the concentration of fat in milk is reduced, often to less than 50% of normal, although milk volume is maintained. This syndrome is a significant cause of wastage in high-producing cows. Low concentration of fat in milk occurs with ruminal acidosis in cattle.[5] The cause appears to be an increase in concentrations of conjugated linoleic acid in the diet, with subsequent reduction in lipogenesis in the udder.[6] A supply of polyunsaturated fatty acids in the cows' ration and alteration in fermentation in the rumen results in biohydrogenation of linoleic acid (abundant in oils and seeds) and formation of intermediate fatty acids in the rumen. These incompletely hydrogenated fatty acids are absorbed into the blood and have an inhibitory effect on lipogenesis.[7] It is most common in cows on low-fiber diets, for example, lush, irrigated pasture, or grain rations that are ground very finely or fed as pellets. Treatment is achieved by administration of sodium bicarbonate or magnesium oxide, which increase fiber digestibility and hence the propionate : acetate ratio. Magnesium oxide also increases the activity of lipoprotein lipase in the mammary gland and increases uptake of triglycerides by the mammary gland from the plasma.[8]

REFERENCES

1. Persson Waller K, et al. *J Dairy Sci.* 2014;97:310.
2. Olde Riekerink RGM, et al. *J Dairy Sci.* 2014;97:5007.
3. Stamm LV, et al. *Vet Microbiol.* 2009;136:192.
4. Melendez P, et al. *Prev Vet Med.* 2006;76:211.
5. Atkinson O. *Cattle Pract.* 2014;22:1.
6. Gulati SK, et al. *Can J Anim Sci.* 2006;86:63.
7. Dubuc J, et al. *Point Veterinaire.* 2009;40:45.
8. Radostits O, et al. Low milk fat syndrome. In: *Veterinary Medicine: A Textbook of the Diseases of Cattle, Horses, Sheep, Pigs, and Goats.* 10th ed. London: W.B. Saunders; 2006:1686.

"FREE" OR "STRAY" ELECTRICITY AS A CAUSE OF FAILURE OF LETDOWN

Free electrical current is common in dairies, especially recently built ones. The problem is most common when a herd moves into a new shed, but it also occurs with alterations to electrical equipment and wiring or with ordinary wear and tear. The stray current is present in the metallic part of the building construction, much of which is interconnected. Cows are very sensitive to even small amperages and are highly susceptible because they make good, often wet contact with the metal and with wet concrete on the floor. People working in the dairy are not likely to notice the electrical contact because they are usually wearing rubber boots. The voltage present would be too low to be of much interest to the local power authority, and an independent technician may be necessary to perform the examination, which should be performed while the milking machine is working. The effects of free electricity in the milking shed may be as follows:

- Fatal electrocution, stunning causing unconsciousness, frantic kicking, and bellowing, which are all manifested when the animal contacts the electrified metal, as set down under the heading of electrocution
- Restlessness, frequent urination, defecation, failure to let milk down, and in tie-stalls frequent lapping at the water bowl but refusing to drink; the abnormal behavior may be apparent only when the cow is in a particular position or posture.
- Startled, alert appearance with anxiety, baulking, and refusal to enter the milking parlor
- Failure of letdown leads to lower milk production and recrudescence of existing subclinical mastitis leading to appearance of clinical signs.

Table 20-8 Diagnosis of free electricity problems based on voltage difference between two points that can be accessed by an animal with resultant current flow

Normal	0–0.5 V
Suspicious as possible cause for abnormal behavior	1.0–2.0 V
Moderate behavioral reactions possible	1.5–3.0 V
Behavioral reactions likely	>3.0 V

The estimates are guidelines and there is marked individual animal variability.

In spite of the many field observations of these abnormalities experimental application of AC current up to 8 mA causes changes in behavior but not in milk yield or letdown. Additional information on stray voltage is provided in Chapter 4.

Recommended guidelines for a diagnosis of free electricity problems are set out in Table 20-8. For simplicity it can be assumed that cows will behave abnormally if the free voltage exceeds 1 V AC, although 2 V and a current of 3.6 to 4.9 mA does not reduce milk production. A safer threshold is 0.35 V AC as a maximum. A proper voltmeter is necessary to make a diagnosis, and in most circumstances a qualified electrician is necessary for the exercise.

The development of voltages in the metalwork of the milking shed can arise from many factors. Obvious short circuits from faulty wiring are the least common cause. Most cases are caused by accumulation of relatively low voltages because of increased resistance in the earth or ground system, thus neutral to earth voltages. Reasons for the accumulation include a poor earthing or grounding system, grounding rods that are too short to reach the water table, insufficient grounding rods, or dry seasons lowering the water table. The problem may be intermittent and even seasonal, depending on climatic conditions that facilitate the passage of current through the cow as an alternative grounding system.

NEOPLASMS OF THE UDDER

The most common neoplasm of cows' teats is viral papillomatosis. It is esthetically unattractive and may play a part in harboring mastitis organisms on the teat skin. It is dealt with in detail under the heading of papillomatosis. Similar papillomata occur on the teat and udder skin of lactating Saanen goats. Rarely, these lesions may develop a squamous cell carcinoma lesion of low malignancy.

Neoplasms of the bovine udder are extraordinarily rare. In a report by the United States Department of Agriculture in 1945, 13 million bovine udders were inspected and none were found to have gross evidence of cancer. There are a handful of isolated reports of fibrosarcoma, carcinoma, and fibroadenoma of the mammary gland in cattle.[1] Carcinomas are rarely reported in goats, and adenoma and carcinoma are very rare in sheep.[1,2] Malignant mammary carcinoma occurs occasionally in mares. The extremely low rate of mammary gland neoplasia in female ruminants is primarily attributed to their herbivore diet and because many ruminants are slaughtered before reaching middle age.[1] An additional reason for the low rate is that female ruminants that are retained in the herd or flock have an extremely low lifetime exposure to estrogen as they spend most of their reproductive life being pregnant or not cycling.

TEAT AND UDDER CONGENITAL DEFECTS

The common sporadic defects in cows are supernumerary teats, fused teats with two teat canals opening into one teat sinus, hypomastia, absence of a teat canal and sinus, and absence of a connection between the teat sinus and the udder sinus; in sows insufficient and inverted teats are the common errors. Supernumerary teats are common (up to 33%) in Simmental and Brown Swiss heifers and are removed surgically. A high prevalence of defects is recorded in Murrah buffaloes and inheritance of hypomastia, rudimentary teats, and angulation of teats is suspected in cows.

Traditionally sows are required to have at least 12 functional teats and sows deficient in this regard are likely to be culled. Reasons for the deficit include inherited shortage (teat number is highly heritable), misplaced teats (usually too far posteriorly to be accessible to the piglets), or unevenly placed, inverted teats, either congenital or acquired as a result of injury; vestigial nipples that do not acquire a lumen, cistern, or gland; and normal-sized teats that are occluded. Inverted teats in sows may be this way because they lack a teat upturn, which is the teat duct opening directly into the mammary gland cistern.

FURTHER READING

Reinemann DJ. Stray voltage and milk quality. A review. *Vet Clin North Am Food Anim Pract.* 2012;28:321-345.

REFERENCES

1. Mihevc SP, Dovc P. Mammary tumors in ruminants. *Acta Argic Slovenica.* 2013;102:83.
2. McElroy MC, Bassett HF. *J Vet Diagn Invest.* 2010;22:1006.

MILK ALLERGY

Signs of allergy, principally urticaria, are often manifested by cows during periods of milk retention. Most of these occur as the cow is being dried off. The Channel Island breeds of cattle are most susceptible, and the disease is likely to recur in the same cow at subsequent drying off periods; it is almost certainly inherited as a familial trait.

The important clinical signs relate to the skin. There is urticaria, which may be visible only on the eyelids or be distributed generally. Local or general erection of the hair may also be seen. A marked muscle tremor, respiratory distress, frequent coughing, restlessness to the point of kicking at the abdomen and violent licking of themselves, and even maniacal charging with bellowing may occur. Other cows may show dullness, recumbency, shuffling gait, ataxia, and later inability to rise. The temperature and pulse rates are usually normal or slightly elevated, but the respiratory rate may be as high as 100 beats/min.

Diagnosis of milk allergy can be made by the intradermal injection of an extract of the cow's own milk. A positive reaction occurs with milk diluted as much as 1 in 10,000, and edematous thickening is present within minutes of the injection. Other clinicopathologic observations include the development of eosinopenia, neutrophilia, and hyperphosphatemia during an attack.

Spontaneous recovery is the rule, but antihistamines are effective, especially if administered early and repeated at short intervals for 24 hours. Prevention is usually a matter of avoiding milk retention in susceptible cows, but in many cases it is preferable to cull them.

Mastitis of Sheep

ETIOLOGY

Most cases of clinical mastitis are caused by *S. aureus* or *Mannheimia* spp. (predominantly *M. haemolytica* and *M. glucosida*, but also *M. ruminalis*). Each is responsible for around 40% of cases in ewes suckling lambs for meat or wool production, whereas in dairy sheep *S. aureus* has a higher prevalence, and is responsible for around 80% of clinical cases.[1,2] *S. agalactiae* is also important, with other agents including CNS (often associated with persistent subclinical infections and elevated SCCs), *E. coli*, *H. somni* (formerly *H. ovis*), *Clostridium perfringens* type A, *Pseudomonas* spp., *C. pseudotuberculosis*, or *E. faecalis*. *Acholeplasma oculi* is predominantly isolated from cases of contagious ophthalmia but can cause mastitis and agalactia.

Another important cause is *M. agalactiae*, the agent of contagious agalactia, which is described under that syndrome.

EPIDEMIOLOGY

Occurrence

Most cases of clinical mastitis in ewes occur up to 4 to 8 weeks after parturition or immediately after weaning. Compared with housed ewes, those grazing pasture have a lower prevalence with cases predominantly caused by *M. haemolytica* or *Staphylococcus* spp.

Many cases are associated with teat injury from any cause, such as when ewes are housed on abrasive floors.

Clinical mastitis in grazing ewes averages only about 2% per year, but mastitis can be responsible for up to 10% of all ewe deaths. More than 30% of dairy ewes can have subclinical mastitis.

The forms of loss in milk sheep are the same as those for dairy cattle: reduced milk production, reduced milk quality, which can negatively affect cheese production, and the culling of affected ewes. In meat and fiber sheep the most obvious losses are deaths, usually from gangrenous mastitis, and decreased growth and deaths in lambs. Where suckling lambs have access to supplemental feed the effect of subclinical mastitis on lamb performance is negligible.

The sheep dairy industry in many countries is developing, so anything that adversely affects the quantity and quality of ovine milk, especially for the production of cheese, will cause financial loss. In Greece, where ewe milk is used to produce feta cheese, the prevalence of subclinical mastitis in flocks varies from 29% to 43%, with CNS and *S. aureus* isolated from 44% and 33% of the positive milk samples, respectively.

Staphylococcal Mastitis

The most prevalent mastitis pathogen of the ewe is *S. aureus*. The incidence of clinical mastitis may be as high as 20%, with ewe mortality rates of from 25% to 50%. The affected halves in surviving ewes are usually necrotic and destroyed. Chronic mastitis can cause a 25% to 30% reduction in milk yield from the affected udder halves. Consequently, this disease is very important in countries, such as Greece, in which ewes' milk is an important component of the human diet. The disease is probably spread from infected bedding grounds, with the infection gaining entry through teat injuries caused by suckling lambs. Intensive housing can be associated with an increased prevalence of lesions, probably caused by cross-suckling by lambs with oral or nasal infections.[3]

Other staphylococcal mastitides in ewes include *S. epidermidis;* many clinically normal quarters show a high rate of infection with coagulase-negative staphylococcus. Experimental infection with *S. chromogenes* causes clinical mastitis, *S. simulans* causes subclinical mastitis, and *S. xylosus* causes a transient increase in the SCC.

Mannheimia Mastitis

Peracute, gangrenous mastitis associated with *Mannheimia* spp. is a common mastitis. *M. haemolytica* and *M. glucosida* can be isolated from affected halves, and the disease can be reproduced experimentally by the intramammary infusion of cultures of the organism. *S. aureus, T. pyogenes,* and streptococci are often present as secondary invaders.

Mannheimia mastitis occurs sporadically in the western United States, Australia, and Europe in ewes kept under systems of husbandry varying from open pasture to enclosed barns. Mastitis is most common in ewes suckling large lambs up to 3 months old. Infection is thought to occur through injuries to teats, perhaps caused by over vigorous suckling. Occurrence is not related to hygiene, and many outbreaks occur in grazing sheep. However, because of sheep's behavior (using "sheep camps" at night), it is possible that these areas become contaminated and facilitate transmission by contact with infected soil or bedding. There is a high diversity among *Mannheimia* isolates, and horizontal transmission by lamb suckling probably occurs.[4]

Streptococcal Mastitis

Streptococcal mastitis can be reproduced by the introduction of *S. agalactiae* into the mammary glands and occurs naturally in dairy ewes. The infection originates from an infected udder and is transmitted to the teat skin of other ewes by milking machine liners, milkers' hands, washcloths, and any other material that can act as an inert carrier. *S. dysgalactiae* and *S. uberis* are also occasionally isolated.

PATHOGENESIS

The mechanisms of pathogenesis are similar to those for bovine mastitis.

CLINICAL FINDINGS

In milking ewes clinical mastitis is similar to that in cows, with acute and subacute forms manifested by swelling of the gland and wateriness and clots in the milk. Most clinical cases occur with 2 to 3 weeks of parturition or at weaning, and take the form of gangrenous mastitis, affecting one or both halves.

Staphylococcal Mastitis

In sheep there is a strong similarity between this form of mastitis and that associated with *M. haemolytica*. They are both peracute, gangrenous infections. The ewe is usually recumbent and profoundly toxic, and the affected gland and the surrounding area of belly wall are blue-green in color and cold to the touch. A few drops of clear, bloodstained liquid is all that can be expressed from the udder. A fatal clinical course of 1 to 2 days is usual.

Mannheimia Mastitis

Mannheimia mastitis is an acute systemic disturbance, with a high fever (40°C–42°C; 105°F–107°F), anorexia, dyspnea, and profound toxemia, with acute swelling of the gland and severe lameness on the affected side. This lameness is an important early sign and is useful in locating affected animals in a group. The udder is at first hot, swollen, and painful and the milk watery, but within 24 hours the half is discolored blue-black and cold, with a sharp line of demarcation from normal tissue. The secretion is watery and red and contains clots. The temperature subsides in 2 to 4 days, the secretion dries up entirely, and the animal either dies of toxemia in 3 to 7 days or survives with sloughing of a gangrenous portion of the udder. This is followed by the development of abscesses and the continual draining of pus. Usually only one side is affected. Cases of pneumonia caused by the same organism may occur in lambs in flocks in which ewes are affected.

Clostridial Mastitis

C. perfringens A is a rare and highly fatal cause of acute mastitis in ewes. Clinical signs of infection are principally hemolytic and are characterized by hemoglobinuria, jaundice, and anemia, plus fever, anorexia, and recumbency. The affected half is swollen, painful, and hot and contains watery, brown, flocculent secretion.

Caseous Lymphadenitis and Mastitis

Suppurative lesions associated with *C. pseudotuberculosis* are common in ovine mammary glands, but they usually involve only the supramammary lymph nodes and are not true mastitis. However, the function of the mammary gland may be lost when the infection spreads from the lymph node to mammary tissue.

Pseudomonal Mastitis

Naturally occurring pseudomonal mastitis in ewes is likely to be gangrenous and lethal, as well as accompanied by severe lameness in the hindlimb on the affected side. Infected intramammary infusions or milking machine malfunction are the usual means of introducing the infection.

CLINICAL PATHOLOGY

The SCC is a useful predictor of mammary gland infection of individual dairy ewes, although thresholds are not as uniform or as widely accepted as for dairy cows.[5,6] The SCC in normal ewe milk ranges from 0.5 to 1.0×10^6 cells/mL, with 95% of samples having counts $<0.5 \times 10^6$ cells/mL. Ewe milk SCC tends to increase more in later lactation compared with the cow, but consecutive testing when counts range from 0.5 to 1.0×10^6cells/mL will improve its diagnostic accuracy. In bulk milk samples, counts of 0.65×10^6 cells/mL indicate that from 10% to 15% of ewes in a flock have subclinical mastitis.[5]

Other tests include the California Milk Test, a reliable indicator of SCC, and staining milk films with Giemsa or May-Grunwald stains to detect what type and proportion of cells are present. Early mammary gland infections change the proportion of ions in milk; thus measuring electrical conductivity can indicate mastitis. However, there are large interanimal and intraanimal variations, so specific algorithms that account for this daily variation are required.[7] Ultrasound examination of the udder and supramammary lymph nodes and infrared thermography of the udder are potentially rapid and sensitive tests for subclinical mastitis in specialist dairy flocks.[8,9] Infection of ewes with maedi-visna virus does not alter their SCC.

NECROPSY FINDINGS

The gross appearance of the affected glands varies with the agent involved and the duration of the process. Generally, the swollen, hemorrhagic, and/or gangrenous nature of fatal acute ovine mastitis is obvious. A purulent exudate is sometimes present, especially in the case of chronic *C. pseudotuberculosis* infection.

Samples for Confirmation of Diagnosis

- Bacteriology: chilled mammary gland for aerobic culture; anaerobic culture if *Clostridium* sp. is suspected.

> **DIFFERENTIAL DIAGNOSIS**
>
> *Mannheimia* mastitis is peracute and resembles mastitis associated with *Staphylococcus aureus*. A similar disease in ewes has been ascribed to *Actinobacillus lignieresii*. Suppurative mastitis associated with *Corynebacterium pseudotuberculosis* is chronic, and no systemic signs occur.

TREATMENT

Broad-spectrum parenteral and intramammary antimicrobial agents are effective. Although ewes probably require smaller doses of intramammary infusions than cows, it is customary to use ordinary cow-type mammary infusion treatments. However, this results in a much longer period during which the milk in the half has a level of antibiotic greater than acceptable limits for human consumption (the "withhold period"). The treatment of ewes with peracute gangrenous mastitis requires systemic treatment, but this is often not successful and the affected half sloughs after several weeks.

CONTROL

Control programs for milking sheep flocks are less well defined, but principles similar to those outlined for dairy cows apply. This requires early detection and prompt treatment of affected ewes with an effective antimicrobial. Results of culture and sensitivity testing will not be immediately available, but milk samples should be collected aseptically from affected and nonaffected ewes to inform future treatment options, with the aim of testing up to 10 isolates of each species present.[2] Dry treatment with intramammary infusions into both halves of dairy ewes has been shown to reduce subclinical infections and/or SCC during the next lactation.[10] Selective treatment of ewes with a consistently high SCC, rather than treatment of all ewes, will be a more cost-effective strategy, but this information will only be available within well-developed dairy operations. For flocks of suckling ewes with a high prevalence of mastitis the use of dry period treatment at weaning may be useful, but care and aseptic technique is required to prevent iatrogenic infections.

Phenotypic culling of affected dairy or suckling ewes is often undertaken, although this will not reliably prevent further clinical or subclinical infections in the flock. Genetic selection of dairy ewes with a reduced SCC is an indirect way of reducing susceptibility to mastitis infections and may offer a longer-term option for the control of subclinical mastitis. However, to have the most chance of success this needs reliable pedigree information, performance recording, and estimates of breeding values.[6]

Staphylococcal Mastitis

Two multivalent bacterins have been released for use against staphylococcal mastitis in dairy cattle, Lysigin (United States) and Startvac (Europe and Canada), but as yet they have not been systematically evaluated in sheep. The former, a multivalent whole-cell lysed bacterin, did not prevent infections but reduced the severity of mastitis after experimental challenge of heifers with *S. aureus*. Vaccination did not lower SCC, increase milk yields, or reduce the staphylococcal infection rate.[10] The second product includes an inactivated *E. coli* strain. It does not eliminate new staphylococci infections, but field studies in dairy cattle show a reduced time and transmissibility of infections.[11]

For dairy ewes, frequent changing of pasture areas and culling of affected ewes may help reduce environmental contamination and control the spread of infection.

Mannheimia Mastitis

In older studies polyvalent hyperimmune serum and an autogenous vaccine of killed *M. haemolytica* were shown to prevent intramammary infections with *Mannheimia* spp. More recently, *M. haemolytica* serotype 1 has been used in vaccines in an attempt to control respiratory disease in cattle and pasteurellosis in sheep. However, a primary virulence factor of *Mannheimia* spp. isolates is leukotoxin A (LktA), and this may have an important role in immunity to disease caused by *Mannheimia* spp. A comparison of the similarity of the LktA of *Mannheimia* spp. isolated from clinical cases of mastitis found that the LktA from *M. glucosida* may be more suitable for a monovalent vaccine than the LktA from *M. haemolytica*.[12]

FURTHER READING

Arsenault J, et al. Risk factors and impacts of clinical and subclinical mastitis in commercial meat-producing sheep flocks in Quebec, Canada. *Prev Vet Med*. 2008;87:373.

REFERENCES

1. Omaleki L, et al. *J Clin Microbiol*. 2010;48:3419.
2. Mavrogianni VS, et al. *Vet Clin North Am Food Anim Pract*. 2011;27:115.
3. Mørk T, et al. *Vet Microbiol*. 2012;155:81.
4. Omaleki L, et al. *J Vet Diagn Invest*. 2012;24:730.
5. Fragkou IA, et al. *Small Rum Res*. 2014;118:86.
6. Riggio V, et al. *Small Rum Res*. 2015;126:33.
7. Romero G, et al. *Small Rum Res*. 2012;107:157.
8. Hussein HA, et al. *Small Rum Res*. 2015;129:121.
9. Martins RFS, et al. *Res Vet Sci*. 2013;94:722.
10. Spanu C, et al. *Small Rum Res*. 2011;97:139.
11. Middleton JR, et al. *Vet Microbiol*. 2009;134:192.
12. Schukken YH, et al. *J Dairy Sci*. 2014;97:5250.

Mastitis of Goats

S. aureus and *E. coli* are the most common causes of clinical mastitis. Other infectious agents include *Pseudomonas* spp., *S. hyicus* (much less pathogenic than *S. aureus*), *S. dysgalactiae*, *S. pyogenes*, *S. intermedius*, *A. pyogenes*, and *Bacillus* spp. and, more rarely, *K. pneumoniae*, *C. pseudotuberculosis*, *M. haemolytica*, and *Actinobacillus equuli* causes a systemic reaction and granulomatous lesions in the udder and lungs. The gland prevalence of subclinical mastitis *N. asteroides* in goats, caused predominantly by infection with CNS, can range from 9% to 65%, although these organisms are often present in clinically normal halves.[1]

Goats have intrinsically higher SCCs than cows or sheep, which increase with age and stage of lactation, so goat milk can often exceed legal thresholds for human consumption mandated in some jurisdictions in the absence of a high prevalence of clinical or subclinical mastitis.[2]

Mastitis is also an important sign in the infectious diseases associated with *M. agalactiae* and *M. mycoides* var. *mycoides*.

Staphylococcal Mastitis

This is the most common cause of mastitis in goats and the same CNS can persist in subclinical infections for up to 7 months.[1] A New Zealand study of over 600 does from 18 herds found bacteria in 23.3% of glands, and CNS (13.4%) and *Corynebacterium* spp. (7.3%) were the most common isolates.[3] The incidence of new infections was highest in early lactation, and prevalence of infections increased with age.

S. aureus is commonly isolated from clinical mastitis but at a much lower prevalence than CNS. Experimentally produced *S. aureus* mastitis in goats has a similar pathogenesis to that in the cow except for a marked tendency for the staphylococci to invade and persist in foci in the interacinar tissue. As in cattle, some staphylococci in goats' milk produce enterotoxins and the toxic shock syndrome toxin, so these can cause food poisoning in humans. Latex agglutination tests are available for the identification of the enterotoxins.

Streptococcal Mastitis

Goats are susceptible to *S. agalactiae* and *S. uberis,* and sporadic cases or outbreaks of mastitis associated with these and other streptococci do occur. In flocks of milking goats the infection is passed from infected quarters to others by means of the milkers' hands, the teat cups of milking machines, and washcloths used to disinfect the udder before milking. *S. zooepidemicus* causes chronic suppurative mastitis in does, and artificially induced infections with *S. dysgalactiae* are indistinguishable from mastitis associated with *S. agalactiae.* The pathogenesis is probably similar in all streptococcal mastitides.

Pseudomonas Mastitis

Experimental pseudomonas mastitis in goats is acute, with extensive necrosis and fatal septicemia. As for dairy cattle, infection is often introduced through contaminated water.[1]

Summer Mastitis

Summer mastitis associated with *T. pyogenes* has been produced experimentally in goats with udder lesions typical of acute suppurative mastitis. Nonlactating goats developed a severe mastitis, whereas lactating animals were less severely affected.

Other Infections

Mastitis in goats is associated with an organism tentatively identified as *M. haemolytica. Yersinia pseudotuberculosis* has caused mastitis in an aborting goat doe that probably experienced a bout of systemic yersiniosis. This infection would be a potential zoonosis. Granulomatous lesions in the mammary glands and in internal organs have been observed in goats experimentally infected with *Cryptococcus neoformans.*

CLINICAL FINDINGS

Clinical mastitis in goats is similar to that in cattle, with subclinical, chronic, acute, and peracute gangrenous forms occurring. Particular care is needed in the clinical examination of goat's milk because of its apparent normality when there are severe inflammatory changes in the udder.

SCCs in milk of goats are higher than in cattle or sheep but vary widely because of the apocrine nature of milk secretion.[2] The counts increase with stage of lactation, lower milk production, and increased parity, and goats without intramammary infection may have an SCC of more than 1×10^6 cells/mL, which is the mandated limit of goat milk for human consumption in some jurisdictions.[4] These variations make the value of SCC as a guide to diagnosis in goats controversial.

In staphylococcal mastitis, infected halves have higher NAGase and CMT than normal halves. However, they and the LDH and antitrypsin tests give variable results, thus they are still not considered to be as reliable as in dairy cows.[5]

Treatment and Control

Treatment and control of mastitis techniques to be used in goat does have been adapted from those used for cattle, with the details of dry period and lactational treatments informed by laboratory culture. If cow dose rates are used, retention of the antibiotic in the udder of goats will be prolonged, even for short-acting products such as ampicillin, so withholding periods need to be increased.[6]

For treatment of acute cases, intravenous flunixin meglumine is an effective antipyretic and leads to clinical improvement in the mammary gland when combined with intravenous dextrose and electrolytes. The preferred antimicrobials to achieve therapeutic tissue concentrations in the mammary gland include macrolides, trimethoprim, tetracyclines, and fluoroquinolones.[7]

Vaccination using killed bacterins has been investigated for a number of years, and two multivalent bacterins are available for use against staphylococcal mastitis in dairy cattle, Lysigin (United States) and Startvac (Europe and Canada). The effect of the former on the prevalence of staphylococcal mastitis and SCC in a 30-doe U.S. dairy goat herd was evaluated over 18 months.[8] The average SCC of vaccinates was lower (1.3 versus 1.5×10^6 cells/ mL for controls), which reduced the milk below the mandated level for human consumption, and they had more spontaneous cures (1.28 versus 0.6 per doe for controls).

REFERENCES

1. Contreras A, et al. *Small Rum Res.* 2007;68:145.
2. Leitner G, et al. *Vet Immunol Immunopathol.* 2012;147:202.
3. McDougall S, et al. *New Zeal Vet J.* 2014;62:136.
4. Paape MJ, et al. *Small Rum Res.* 2007;68:114.
5. McDougall S, et al. *J Dairy Sci.* 2010;93:4710.
6. Ferrini AM, et al. *J Agric Food Chem.* 2010;58:12199.
7. Mavrogianni VS, et al. *Vet Clin North Am Food Anim Pract.* 2011;27:115.
8. Kautz FM, et al. *Res Vet Sci.* 2014;97:18.

Contagious Agalactia in Goats and Sheep

SYNOPSIS

Etiology Classic disease caused by *Mycoplasma agalactiae* in sheep and goats; also *M. agalactiae, M. mycoides* subsp. *capri* (formerly *M. mycoides* large colony type), and *M. capricolum* subsp. *capricolum* in goats

Epidemiology Outbreaks and severe disease are especially problematic in the Mediterranean area of Europe and Africa. Introduction of infected animals. Direct spread by infected milk and ocular discharge to suckling young and to adults by contamination of bedding, feed, and milking equipment

Clinical findings Triad of mastitis, arthritis, and ocular disease. Sometimes accompanied with respiratory disease, abortion, and diarrhea

Lesions Indurative mastitis with abscessation, polyarthritis

Diagnostic confirmation Culture, polymerase chain reaction, serology

Treatment Antimicrobials may mitigate disease severity but not achieve a bacteriologic cure.

Control Flock/herd biosecurity, milking-time hygiene. Test and slaughter eradication. Vaccines have poor efficacy.

ETIOLOGY

Contagious agalactia is a disease of sheep and goats, particularly those used for milk production. *M. agalactiae* is the main causal agent in sheep and goats, but *M. mycoides* subsp. *capri* and *M. capricolum* subsp. *capricolum* produce a similar if not identical clinical presentation. There is apparent variation in virulence between isolates from different regions and countries. The situation in goats is quite complex, and frequently more than one of these agents can be isolated from the same outbreak.

M. putrefaciens, first isolated from the joints of arthritic goats in California, has been isolated and implicated in some outbreaks of contagious agalactia, but experimental challenge with this organism does not produce classical contagious agalactia. *M. putrefaciens* can cause septicemia, pneumonia, and mastitis in small ruminants that are predisposed by other diseases.

EPIDEMIOLOGY

Occurrence

Contagious agalactia is endemic in most European countries and Africa and occurs in many other areas of the world including Asia and the Indian subcontinent, the Middle East, and North and South America. The disease is common in Mediterranean countries, and is particularly widespread and problematic in Spain.

Prevalence

In endemic areas the disease is cyclic in occurrence with periods of outbreaks of severe disease interspersed with periods of chronic or mild disease.

Peak rates of clinical disease occur after parturition in both the dams and their young with another peak occurring in association with the onset of machine milking after the young are removed from suckling. The mortality rate can be high (10%–30%), and many adult females are culled because the udder is permanently damaged.

Transmission

The organisms are present in the milk and ocular secretions of infected animals and in respiratory secretions in which the pulmonary form of the disease is present. Transmission is by direct contact, aerosol transmission, ingestion, and by contact with infected fomites. The young are infected through the ingestion of infection present in colostrum and milk. Infected milk can also contaminate bedding, feed and dairy equipment, and spread occurs with machine milking. The organisms reside in the ear canal of asymptomatic carrier sheep and goats, and are thought to be transmitted by ear mites. Venereal transmission is also thought to occur.

The common practice of transhumance and communal grazing in endemic areas promotes transmission between herds and flocks, either from direct contact or grazing over infected pastures. The organisms have been isolated from outbreaks of disease in a range of wild ruminants, but the role of these in the epidemiology of contagious agalactia in domestic small ruminants is unclear.[1] Illegal importation of animals from an endemically infected area can introduce the disease to disease-free areas.

Experimental Reproduction

Contagious agalactia can be reproduced experimentally and reflects the natural disease with acute and chronic multifocal necrotizing mastitis, acute arthritis, conjunctivitis, and subacute enteritis. Shedding of the organism precedes the onset of clinical disease by 1 to 10 days. The experimentally produced disease is much more severe in pregnant animals.

Host Risk Factors

The relative severity of clinical disease in sheep versus goats depends on the infecting mycoplasma and varies with region. There are also breed and age differences in susceptibility. Septicemia and acute disease is more common in young lambs and kids and lactating females, with less severe disease in adult males and nonlactating nonpregnant females. Asymptomatic carriers are important in transmission of the organisms.

Pathogen Risk Factors

There is regional variation in the virulence of isolates; *M. agalactiae, M. mycoides* subsp. *mycoides* subsp. *capri, M. capricolum* subsp. *capricolum*, and *M. putrefaciens* have all been isolated from goats in Australia and the United States over several decades, but clinical disease in these countries associated with these organisms is extremely rare.

Molecular studies show a high genetic diversity of *M. agalactiae* isolates from goats in Spain compared with relatively low diversity from sheep isolates in France and Spain.[2,3] This has implications for vaccines developed to control the disease in goats.

CLINICAL FINDINGS

The classical signs of contagious agalactia include septicemia, arthritis, mastitis, conjunctivitis, and localization in abscesses, but these are not all consistently present in outbreaks.

In acute cases the onset is sudden with pyrexia, abrupt and complete agalactia, and unilateral or bilateral swelling of the udder with enlargement of the mammary lymph nodes and the development of multiple abscesses in the mammary gland. Induration of the udder may result in culling. In animals that survive, mycoplasma are excreted in the milk for several months and will persist in the udder to subsequent lactations.

Arthritis may be manifested by lameness or recumbency and its presence detected in the carpal and tarsal joints by the occurrence of heat and palpable joint fluid and confirmed by aspiration and examination of joint fluid. Conjunctivitis progresses to keratitis with corneal revascularization in one or both eyes. Some cases have diarrhea.

In less acute cases, there is a long period of illness of from one to several months. Abortion may also occur and genital disease with vulvovaginitis and metritis occurs in some outbreaks.

CLINICAL PATHOLOGY

Herd diagnosis is possible by the isolation of the organism *M. agalactiae* from the bloodstream, joint fluid, and mammary tissue. A multiplex real-time PCR on a range of samples, including bulk milk, can be used to identify the disease if the causative *Mycoplasma* spp. are present.[4]

Herd diagnosis can also be made serologically. The complement fixation (CFT) test becomes positive soon after clinical signs, although commercial ELISA kits can have variable sensitivity and specificity depending on the strain of *M. agalactiae* and cross-reactions with nonpathogenic *Mycoplasma* spp.[5]

NECROPSY FINDINGS

Lesions are indicative of indurative mastitis with abscessation, lymphadenopathy, arthritis, and ocular disease.

Samples for Confirmation of Diagnosis

- **Bacteriology (aerobic culture) and PCR:** milk, ocular fluid, joint fluid aspirate, nasal swabs, ear swabs, lung lesions, brain
- **Serology:** CFT, ELISA

TREATMENT

Antimicrobial therapy can reduce the severity of disease and mortalities and is an alternative to culling, especially for animals of high genetic merit. The preferred antibiotics are fluoroquinolones, tetracyclines, and macrolides. Antibiotic resistance to tetracyclines, or an intrinsic lack of efficacy, is a problem as is the cost and practicality of therapy in many endemic areas. In vitro sensitivity testing of field isolates of *M. agalactia* found enrofloxacin most effective, followed by tylosin, tetracycline, lincomycin, and spectinomycin, with high cure rates reported with lincomycin, spectinomycin, and tylosin. However, treatment of bucks with marbofloxacin did not eliminate *Mycoplasma* from the ear canal of goat bucks, so it would have little impact on eliminating carriers in chronically affected herds.[6]

CONTROL

The majority of infections in healthy flocks come from introduction of carriers or contact with infected animals. Thus isolation from infected flocks and herds and a closed herd policy are important control measures. Where disease is restricted to a small number of flocks in a geographically isolated area, slaughter of serologically or culturally positive flocks can be an effective control method. In endemic areas disease is common, so eradication by slaughter is not an option and control relies on biosecurity, hygiene, antibacterial therapy, and the use of killed monovalent and polyvalent vaccines.

The efficacy and duration of immunity to vaccines is relatively poor, but they do reduce excretion of mycoplasma and clinical disease. Vaccination of sheep and goats with either an attenuated live vaccine or a killed adjuvant vaccine of *M. agalactiae* gives mixed results; in late pregnant ewes the former is too virulent, and the latter insufficiently so unless it is used in ewes before mating, when efficiency is good. Early vaccination is recommended because of the susceptibility of young animals but should not be performed before 10 weeks of age. Extensive use of both vaccines over a period of 13 years resulted in almost complete disappearance of the disease from Romania, but live attenuated vaccines are not permitted in many countries.

Comparison between commercial vaccines shows that a saponified vaccine gives better results than a live, egg-cultured vaccine, and saponin and phenol inactivated vaccines show better efficacy against experimental disease than do vaccines killed by heat or formalin. An *M. agalactiae* bacterin combined with a mineral oil adjuvant has given good results when three doses are given before, and one dose after, each parturition, and the herd is kept isolated. Intramammary vaccination provides the highest level of antibody.

Autogenous vaccines prepared from milk, brain, and mammary gland homogenates from infected sheep have been used for many years in parts of Europe but have been linked to outbreaks of scrapie.

In infected herds, hygiene at milking time is important in limiting the spread of disease. Pasteurization of colostrum (60 minutes at 60°C; 140°F) eliminates *M. mycoides* subsp. *capri*, but *M. agalactiae* can survive for 120 minutes at 60°C (140°F).[7]

FURTHER READING

Gómez-Martin A, Amores J, et al. Contagious agalactia due to *Mycoplasma* spp. in small ruminants: epidemiology and prospects for control. *Vet J.* 2013;198:48-56.

Radostits O, et al. Contagious agalactia of sheep and goats. In: *Veterinary Medicine: A Textbook of the Diseases of Cattle, Horses, Sheep, Pigs, and Goats.* 10th ed. London: W.B. Saunders; 2007:1138-1139.

REFERENCES

1. Chazel M, et al. *BMC Vet Res.* 2010;6:32.
2. De la Fe C, et al. *BMC Vet Res.* 2012;27:146.
3. Nouvel LX, et al. *Microbiol Infect Dis.* 2012;35:487.
4. Becker CA, et al. *J Microbiol Methods.* 2012;90:73.
5. Poumarat F, et al. *BMC Vet Res.* 2012;8:109.
6. Gómez-Martin A, et al. *Small Rum Res.* 2013;112:186.
7. Paterna A, et al. *Vet J.* 2012;196:263.

Mastitis of Mares

Mastitis in mares is generally regarded as rare, but it might be more common in breeding animals than has previously been recognized. The percentage of mastitis in breeding mares is about 5% and is most common during udder involution, but lactating and juvenile mares as well as suckling foals are also affected.[1] *C. pseudotuberculosis, P. aeruginosa, S. zooepidemicus, S. equi, S. pyogenes, S. aureus, E. coli, Klebsiella* spp., and *Neisseria* spp. can cause the disease. β-Hemolytic streptococci have been found in the milk of many normal, just-foaled mares. Mastitis in nonlactating mares can be caused by *S. aureus* and evident as chronic, draining abscessation (botryomycosis).[2] Predisposing factors, other than lactation, are not identified. Mastitis can be traumatic (as a result of a kick), extension of an abdominal incision into the mammary gland, secondary to teat suckling of nonlactating mares, and in filly foals.[3]

Other causes of mammary gland enlargement in mares include fungal infection, neoplasia (lymphoma, adenocarcinoma), and idiopathic causes.[4,5]

Clinical cases occur at any time during the lactation and many occur in nonlactating mares. Many mares with typical signs of severe swelling and soreness of the udder, but without abnormal milk, are first observed when a sick foal has not suckled for 24 hours. In streptococcal mastitis there may be severe local pain and moderate systemic signs. In most cases both halves are affected.

The milk, or udder secretions, are usually abnormal. Cell counts exceeding 100,000 cells/mL during lactation and 400,000 cells/mL during involution are regarded as abnormal.[1]

Severe cases, sometimes accompanied by fever, depression, and anorexia, show swelling, pain, and heat in the affected half, and ventral edema and clots in the milk; the mare is lame in the leg on the affected side. Gangrene and sloughing of the ventral floor of a gland can occur.

Because of the high frequency of gram-negative bacteria as causative agents in mares, treatment should include a broad-spectrum antibiotic in an intramammary infusion plus parenteral antibacterial treatment such as with gentamicin-penicillin or trimethoprim-sulfonamide combinations. Hot packs and frequent milking are also recommended.

REFERENCES

1. Boehm KH, et al. *Praktische Tierarzt.* 2009;90:842.
2. Smiet E, et al. *Equine Vet Educ.* 2012;24:357.
3. Gilday R, et al. *Can Vet J.* 2015;56:63.
4. Brendemuehl JP. *Equine Vet Educ.* 2008;20:8.
5. Brito MdF, et al. *Ciencia Rural.* 2008;38:556.

Postpartum Dysgalactia Syndrome of Sows

PPDS is a failure to provide sufficient colostrum and milk to piglets during the early stages of lactation. It is usually not accompanied by inflammatory lesions. A whole variety of names have previously been given to this complex syndrome including the mastitis-metritis-agalactia (MMA) syndrome. (The term mastitis-metritis-galactia was originally developed to describe sows with agalactia that had swollen udders, assumed to be caused by mastitis, and the appearance of a vulval discharge, assumed to be caused by metritis.) Progress in this field has only been made possible by the efforts of Guy-Pierre Martineau and Chantal Farmer and their colleagues. Most practicing veterinarians might now recognize MMA as the most serious version of PPDS in which there is clinical mastitis or metritis or recognizable toxemia, but there are many more cases of PPDS than there are MMA.

ETIOLOGY

The etiology is unclear and complex. Lactation is a very complex physiologic process. Many factors are involved, but they all result in a disturbed gilt or sow that is unable to deliver a proper colostrum/milk supply through adverse hormonal, biochemical, (collectively been called dys-homeorhesis), farrowing, and nursing responses (collectively called behavioral responses). There are four main areas that are involved in the PPDS syndrome:

- Toxemia: The sow may contribute toxins from the gut following constipation, from the bladder following cystitis, from the mammary gland following mastitis, and from the uterus following endometritis postfarrowing.[1] The levels of toxins may also be affected by low feed intake, low water intake, stress, lack of exercise, overfeeding in late gestation, and inadequate vitamin E levels.
- Bad management of the gilt in preparation for farrowing by incorrect feeding: This happens by moving at the wrong time and because of new social groupings. This may be complicated by the effects of moving sows into crates from loose housing, etc., and poor environment (too hot for sows, rarely too cold). These factors distress the sow, cause stress, and affect lactation through neurophysiologic mechanisms.
- The sow may be too fat, over muscled, or undergoing inflammation as a result of disease or toxemia or be in pain or suffering from anorexia as a result of a multitude of factors. She may not have developed the normal mammary development to sustain the required level of lactation, which may in part be from genetics.
- Colostrum and milk production may be faulty for a whole variety of reasons that lead to the individual piglet not receiving sufficient colostrum and/or milk. A major problem in the determination of the etiology is the difficulty of being precise in the description of the clinical findings of the abnormal mammary glands of affected sows. The common clinical findings are swelling of the glands, agalactia, toxemia, and fever. There is a very considerable farm effect in the appearance of the condition because sow care and management are so individual and important. There is considerable overlap in the clinical findings from one affected sow to another, but the lesion present in the mammary glands may vary from uncomplicated physiologic congestion and edema to severe necrotizing mastitis.

Ringarp published the classic work on this disease based on 1180 cases of postparturient illness in sows in which agalactia was present. At least five causes of agalactia or hypogalactia were recognized, which are as follows (the incidence of each group as a percentage of the total cases is given in parentheses):

- Eclampsia (0.6%), usually of older sows, responding to calcium and magnesium therapy
- Failure of milk ejection reflex (3.3%), affecting primarily first-litter gilts and usually treated satisfactorily with oxytocin
- Mammary hypoplasia (1.5%) in gilts, resulting in deficient milk secretion
- Primary agalactia (6%), in which reduced milk supply is the only abnormality
- Toxic agalactia (88.6%), the most important numerically and economically. It is characterized by

anorexia, depression, fever, swelling of the mammary glands, and a course of 2 to 4 days. Mastitis was commonly present, but there was no evidence of metritis.

Mastitis

Postweaning mastitis is not uncommon after drying off. Chronic mastitis as a result of traumatic contact between udders and dirty infected floors or traumatic piglets' teeth resulting in abscesses, granulomas, and fibrous udders at weaning or after are also common. Where there are damaged glands sows are not usually agalactic but they may be producing less.

In many instances, traumatic injury from unclipped piglets' teeth and infected sawdust bedding are factors in mastitis in sows. Quite often, the condition occurs in the first 3 days postpartum and in many cases, if severe and untreated, will lead to the death of sows. Infectious mastitis is suggested as a major cause in many clinicopathologic investigations, and there is a greater incidence of intramammary infection in PPDS-affected sows compared with normal sows. Peracute mastitis in sows is readily recognized as a clinical entity, but less severe infections may result in small foci of inflammation within the gland that cannot be detected on clinical examination. Single gland mastitis is uncommon except when there are particularly vindictive piglets causing severe teat trauma. Glands may then become unusable, and this may cause more piglet pressure on available teats and functional glands, which may in turn increase the trauma to the remaining glands and accelerate the process. Mastitis is recognizable clinically by inflammation, edema, skin congestion, pyrexia, and inappetence in the sow and failing piglets. Gram-negative organisms predominate (*E. coli*, *Enterobacter*, and *Klebsiella* spp.), but there are also gram-positive organisms (streptococci and staphylococci).[2] *E. coli* and *K. pneumoniae* have been recovered from the mammary glands of naturally affected cases, and both bacterial species are associated with histopathological changes of mastitis. Experimental intramammary inoculation of sows with field isolates of *E. coli* and *K. pneumoniae* has resulted in cases of lactation failure and mastitis that closely resemble naturally occurring cases. Unfortunately, they cannot always be demonstrated. *Streptococcus* spp. and *Staphylococcus* spp. have also been isolated, but these are frequently isolated from healthy glands not associated with pathologic changes. It is unlikely that *Mycoplasma* spp. are important.

Coliforms are the most significant pathogens isolated from sows with mastitis. Coliform mastitis is often the most visible of the disorders involved in this syndrome.[3,4] In the second study, there were no differences in virulence genes demonstrated in the *E. coli* from healthy sows and sows with mastitis. Pathologic examination of affected sows that were euthanized within 3 days after parturition revealed the presence of varying degrees of mastitis, and *E. coli* and *Klebsiella* spp. were the most common organisms recovered. A recent study has shown that *E. coli* strains from mastitis in sows are highly variable in serotype, biochemical profile, virulence factors, and random amplified polymorphic DNA (RAPD) type. No relationship between serotypes, virulence factors, and RAPD types was found. Toxic agalactia can be produced experimentally by the introduction of *E. coli* endotoxin into the mammary gland of sows at parturition. The clinical, hematologic, and serum biochemical changes are similar to those that occur in naturally occurring cases of toxic agalactia. *E. coli* endotoxin acting at the level of the hypothalamus can suppress prolactin release, which results in a pronounced decline in milk production. Experimental *Klebsiella* mastitis in sows is an excellent model for the study of toxic agalactia because of infectious mastitis.

Agalactia may also be the result of a deficiency of prolactin. Prolactin levels may be dramatically reduced by even the smallest amounts of endotoxin. Any factor that interferes with the release of prostaglandin from the uterus may affect the increase in prolactin that must occur to stimulate lactogenesis immediately before parturition.

In summary, field observations have suggested many different causes and predisposing factors, including infectious mastitis, nutritional disturbances, metabolic disorders, and the stress of farrowing in total confinement in a crate. Based on the examination of spontaneously occurring cases, infectious mastitis appears to be a major cause. Both prolactin and oxytocin release can be stopped by stressors and toxins from bacteria such as *E. coli*.

EPIDEMIOLOGY

Occurrence

PPDS is most common in sows at farrowing or within the first 48 hours after parturition, and in sows that farrow in crates indoors. A peak incidence during the summer months has also been observed. The disease will often occur in one batch and then disappear again for months.

Morbidity and Case Fatality

Morbidity and mortality data are not readily available or precise because of the difficulty of making a reliable clinical diagnosis. Epidemiologic observations indicate that the risk of sows developing toxic mastitis increases with increasing age up to the third or fourth litter. The population incidence of toxic agalactia ranges from 4% to 10% of all farrowings, whereas the herd incidence may vary from 0% to 100%. A recent study in Denmark[5] suggested that 32.5% of sows on the first day of farrowing, 31.5% on the second day, and 10.1% on the third day after farrowing were affected (using the criteria of inappetence, reddened or swollen mammary glands, and temperature over 39.4°C; 102.9°F).

The fatality rate in sows is usually less than 2%, but piglet losses caused by starvation and crushing may be as high as 80%. The disease does not usually recur in the same animal, and this suggests that immunity develops and sows should not necessarily be culled.

RISK FACTORS

Feed

The risk factors that have been proposed based on field observations include overfeeding during pregnancy and a drastic change of feed at farrowing.

Reduced feeding on the day of farrowing followed by an increase over the first week of lactation reduces PPDS,[6] and a fish diet before farrowing improves feed intake after farrowing.[7] It is best to switch diets 7 days before farrowing.

Constipation of the sow at farrowing[8] has been suggested as a cause of PPDS. Higher rates of PPDS do occur in constipated sows, which may be associated with pain.[9] However, clinical and pathologic examinations of both spontaneously occurring cases of agalactia and experimental agalactia induced by the introduction of *E. coli* endotoxin into the mammary gland have been unable to support the observation of constipation. Both sick and normal sows defecate less frequently from 1 day before farrowing until 2 days later. There is no difference in the weight of feces in the terminal colon and rectum between sick and normal sows.

Digestive disturbances and certain feeding practices have been associated with the disease. Sows that have been on high-level feeding during pregnancy appear to be susceptible to the disease, especially if they are subjected to a change of feed immediately before parturition. Also, any management practice that results in a marked change in feed intake at or near farrowing may appear to precipitate the disease. A sudden change of feed severe enough to result in gastrointestinal stasis has been used to reproduce the condition experimentally.

The effects of different feed allowances during late pregnancy may affect the incidence rate of the disease. Feeding sows during the last 15 days of gestation a diet at a level of 3.4 kg daily compared with 1.0 kg daily resulted in an incidence rate of 26.6% and 14.0%, respectively. The explanation for the effects of feeding is unknown. It has been proposed that intense feeding may promote toxin production in the alimentary tract, but how this is related to mastitis is unknown. Another hypothesis suggests that increased feeding in late gestation may intensify the initiation of lactation and result in udder engorgement and increased susceptibility to intramammary infection. A further suggestion is that moldy food may play a part, but this has never been proven.

The clinical status of the mammary glands, the bacteriologic findings, and the total cell count and its percentage of polymorphonuclear leukocytes and pH in colostrum and milk secretion during the first 3 weeks of lactation of sows on high- or low-feeding regimes during late pregnancy have been examined. *E. coli* infection was present in 80% of the sows affected with toxic agalactia and 30% of the healthy sows. The *E. coli* were eliminated at between 3 and 8 days of lactation and were not isolated from sows examined at the time of weaning. The different feeding regimes did not influence the total cell count, the polymorphonuclear cells, or the pH in milk from bacteriologically negative glands or glands with *E. coli* mastitis. The two feeding regimes had no influence on total cell count, the percentage of polymorphonuclear cells, or the pH of colostrum and milk of healthy sows.

The only mycotoxin found to be important in PPDS was shown to be ergot,[10] which probably affects prolactin production. Insufficient water may also be a factor. Omega 3 reduces inflammation and omega 6 increases inflammation.

A variety of ingredients may influence PPDS; probiotics reduce PPDS, as do formic acid, lactulose, and fermented potato protein.

Housing

Moving sows only 4 days before farrowing has been associated with more PPDS than moving them at 7 days.[6] Housing sows so that they can in fact nest rather than placement in crates may reduce PPDS.[8] Houses that are too hot encourage sows not to eat.

Management

Insufficient time for the sow to adjust to the farrowing crate after being transferred from the gestation unit is thought to be an important factor, as is the induction of farrowing.[7] Frequent supervision of farrowing sows may reduce the problems of PPDS. Cross-fostering may also help.[11]

The disease occurs under management, environmental, and sanitation conditions ranging from very poor to excellent; however, the possible relationship between the level of bacterial contamination in the farrowing barn and on the skin of the sow and the incidence of the disease has apparently not been examined. Dirty conditions greatly increase the bacterial contamination of the udder. Environmental or other animal noises and disturbances and uncomfortable farrowing crates are potential PPDS factors.

Animal Factors

The initiating factors have not been identified. The incidence of the disease may be higher in sows with larger litters than sows in the same herd that remain healthy and in those with a higher number of stillbirths and pigs found dead after birth. Long gestation and long farrowing times increase the incidence of PPDS. It is more common in young sows and relatively rare in older sows. Low exercise has also been suggested as a cause, and this also contributes to constipation. The role of water intake or lack of it and stress or disturbance during parturition has also not been investigated. This may also contribute to the fat sow and the over muscled sow syndrome,[12,13] which may also contribute to PPDS.

The nursing behavior of the sow and the suckling behavior of the piglets may provide an explanation for the pathogenesis and clinical findings of some cases of agalactia in sows. Successful ejection of milk by the sow is dependent on proper stimulation of the sow's udder by the piglets followed by a complex response by the sow. A period of time ranging from 15 to 45 minutes must elapse from the last successful milk ejection to the next. Failure of milk ejection may occur in up to 27% of sows that attempt to suckle their piglets within 40 minutes after the previous milk ejection. The failure of milk ejection in sows within the first few crucial adjustment days after farrowing might possibly contribute to the cause of mastitis and engorgement of the mammary glands.

The over fat sow has a lower glucose tolerance postpartum with a lower appetite, and drinks less and lies down more. The sow may have already switched to a catabolic state at or before farrowing using body reserves to produce milk.[14] Just before farrowing the circulating levels of nonesterified fatty acids also rise,[8] which indicates a catabolic state. There may also be a resistance to insulin at farrowing if there have been high levels of energy fed in late pregnancy.[15]

Microorganisms

Each section of the mammary gland of the sow is divided into a separate rostral and caudal section, each with its own teat cistern and teat canal. In a sow with 14 teats there are 28 potential portals of entry, so mastitis is common immediately after parturition when the teat canals have become patent. Bacteria in the gut and in endometritis have been proposed as a source of endotoxin, particularly as β-hemolytic streptococci and coliforms have been associated with the condition.

Some clinicopathologic examinations of affected sows have revealed the presence of a slightly enlarged, flaccid uterus from which coliform and streptococcal organisms can be recovered. However, pathologic evidence of metritis in affected sows is uncommon; the organisms that can be recovered are common in the reproductive tract of normal sows after parturition, and their recovery from vaginal mucus is difficult to interpret.

PATHOGENESIS

The pathogenesis of infectious mastitis caused by *E. coli* or *Klebsiella* spp. is probably similar to that of bovine mastitis in which the infection gains entry through the teat canal and invades the mammary tissue causing mastitis. Endotoxemia accounts for the fever initially as well as for the depression, anorexia, and agalactia, even in glands that are unaffected. The lipopolysaccharide endotoxins acting at the level of the hypothalamus and hypophysis suppress the release of prolactin, which results in a marked decline in milk production. The endotoxin may also have a direct inhibitory effect on the mammary gland. There is a higher prevalence of bacterial endotoxin in the blood of affected sows compared with control animals. The endotoxin can be detected in the blood of about 33% of sows affected with coliform mastitis. However, the oral administration of endotoxin daily to prepubertal gilts did not result in any clinical abnormalities. Experimentally, mastitis can be produced in sows by contamination of the skin of the teats with *K. pneumoniae* either shortly before or after parturition. The clinical signs are similar to those described for MMA; mastitis is present in more than 50% of the mammary gland subsections, and a marked leukopenia and degenerative left shift occurs. A total of 120 organisms is sufficient to produce the mastitis when the organisms are inoculated into the teats. In recent experimental infections with *E. coli* it was shown that the time of infection of the mammary gland relative to parturition and the number of circulating neutrophils at the time of infection influenced the development of clinical coliform mastitis in the sow. Similarly, parturition allows the penetration of vaginal organisms into the reproductive tract, and the absorption of endotoxin reduces F2α in the uterus. This stimulates prolactin, which may contribute to the hypogalactia and agalactia.

CLINICAL FINDINGS

At one extreme is the sow that has no signs but has poor growth in piglets,[16] and this may have meant that colostrum provision has failed and not been noticed until the piglets begin to fade away. At the other extreme is a severely affected sow with high mortality in piglets.

PPDS occurs in sows between 12 and 48 hours (sometimes 72 hours) after farrowing and is characterized clinically by anorexia, lethargy, restlessness, lack of interest in the piglets, fever, swelling of the mammary glands (udder edema), and agalactia. Most affected animals respond to therapy within 12 to 24 hours. Pathologically, there are varying degrees of mastitis. In some sows the level of oxytocin may be half the level in unaffected sows. The disease is of major economic importance when outbreaks occur because the inadequate milk production leads to high piglet mortality from starvation and secondary infectious diseases. In cases of subclinical MMA there is often a failure to achieve weaning weights (<4 kg at 24 days).

Necropsy of spontaneously occurring cases has frequently confirmed the presence of mastitis, but the incidence of metritis has been insignificant.

The prevalence of the condition appears to have reduced recently with the increased attention to hygiene in the farrowing house and the use of more porous and less traumatic floorings. When it does occur it can be quite common, with up to 11% to 58% of the sows affected. A recent case definition suggests that the pathognomonic signs are poor piglet growth and sow rectal temperatures greater than 39.5°C (103.1°F).

Sometimes there may be a delay in parturition of more than 5 hours. The sow is usually normal, with a normal milk flow, for the first 12 to 18 hours after farrowing. Normally, the sow will suckle her piglets for about 20 seconds once an hour. One of the first indications of the disease is the failure of the sow to suckle her piglets. She is uninterested in the piglets, generally lies in sternal recumbency, and is unresponsive to their squealing and suckling demands. Litters of affected sows are noisier and are generally scattered around the pen searching for an alternative food supply. Such piglets may drink surface water or urine in the pen and infectious diarrhea may occur. If suckling is permitted, it does not progress from the vigorous nosing phase to the quiet letdown stage, and it is accompanied by much teat-to-teat movement by the piglets. Many piglets may die of starvation and hypoglycemia. A failure to grow at more than 105 g per day is a sure sign of piglet problems. Some sows are initially restless and stand up and lie down frequently, which contributes to a high mortality from crushing and trampling.

Affected sows do not eat, drink very little, and are generally lethargic. The body temperature is usually elevated and ranges from 39.5°C to 41°C (103.1°F to 105°F), especially if there is mastitis. However, there is a wide range of "normal temperatures" in newly lactating sows from 38.4°C to 40.5°C (101.1°F to 104.9°F),[17] but this may be lactational hyperthermia. Mild elevations in body temperatures of sows in the first 2 days after parturition are difficult to interpret because a slight elevation occurs in normal healthy sows. This is known as uncomplicated farrowing fever. However, temperatures above 40°C (104°F) are usually associated with acute mastitis that requires treatment. One detailed investigation of the disease in Sweden concluded that 78% of sows with a temperature exceeding 39.5°C (103.1°F) had clinical evidence of mastitis. It is suggested that a temperature of 39.4°C (102.9°F) at 12 to 18 hours after farrowing is an appropriate threshold at which to give preventive treatment for the disease. The heart and respiratory rates are usually increased.

Initial temperatures greater than 40.5°C (104.9°F) are usually followed by severe illness and toxemia. Normally, the sows get better within 3 days, but not always if the temperature is very high.

Characteristic findings are present in the mammary glands including varying degrees of swelling and inflammation. In most cases, several glands are affected, which may appear as diffuse involvement of the entire udder. Individual sections (half glands) are enlarged, warm, and painful, and may feel "meaty" and lack the resilience of normal mammary tissue. There may be extensive subcutaneous edema around and between each section, which results in a ridge of edema on the lateral aspects of the udder extending for its entire length. The skin overlying the sections is usually reddened and is easily blanched by finger pressure. The teats are usually empty and may be slightly edematous. A few drops of milk may be expressed out of some teats after gentle massage of the section or the administration of oxytocin but rarely can a normal stream of milk be obtained. In severe cases of mastitis the milk contains flakes and pus or is watery.

The feces are usually scant and drier than normal, but whether or not constipation is present in most cases is uncertain. The inappetence and anorexia and failure to drink normally could account for the reduced volume of feces. Constipation with impaction of the rectum with large quantities of feces is uncommon in sows, and when it does occur as the only abnormality it has little effect on appetite and milk production.

A vaginal discharge is normal following parturition, and normal sows frequently expel up to 50 ml of a viscid, nonodorous, and clear mucus that contains variable amounts of white material within the first 3 days following farrowing. Tenacious strands of this discharge may also be observed within the vagina. The presence of this discharge has been misleading and has been interpreted as evidence of the presence of metritis. Necropsy examination after euthanasia of affected sows has failed to reveal evidence of significant metritis. The clinical diagnosis of metritis in sows is difficult, but generally large quantities of dark-brown, foul-smelling fluid are expelled several times daily, accompanied by severe toxemia. This is uncommon in sows. Diagnosis is usually made on clinical signs.

CLINICAL PATHOLOGY

Examination of Milk

The number of somatic cells in the milk from sows with mastitis will range from 2 to 20 × 10^9 cells/mL compared with the normal of less than 2 × 10^9 cells/mL. Significant numbers of bacteria are present in the milk of more than 80% of sows with toxic agalactia. Milk obtained for laboratory examination and culture should be taken after thorough cleaning and disinfection of the teats to minimize contamination by skin flora. However, because mastitis may be present in only one or a few of the mammary gland subsections in the sow and because it is often impossible to clinically identify affected subsections and distinguish them from unaffected adjacent glands, which may be swollen and agalactic because of continuous swelling, a valid assessment of intramammary infection is not possible unless milk samples are obtained from each subsection. Subclinical mastitis may not be easy to detect with cells not reaching 2 × 10^9 cells/mL but 75% may be polymorphs. Normally, milk is around 1 × 10^9 cells/mL.

Hematology and Serum Biochemistry

Some hematologic and biochemical changes are present in affected sows but may not be marked enough to be a routine reliable diagnostic aid. In severe cases of infectious mastitis, a marked leukopenia with a degenerative left shift is common. In moderate cases there is a leukocytosis and a regenerative left shift. The serum biochemical changes that occur in naturally occurring cases and in the experimental disease are recorded. The plasma cortisol levels are commonly elevated, which may be caused by a combination of the stress of parturition and infectious mastitis. The plasma protein-to-fibrinogen ratio is lower than normal, and the plasma fibrinogen levels are commonly increased in severe cases that occur 8 to 16 hours after parturition.

NECROPSY FINDINGS

Lesions in the udder and the reproductive tract are not consistent. If they are found, the most important lesions are in the mammary gland. There may be extensive edema and some slight hemorrhage of the subcutaneous tissue. Grossly, on cross-section of the mammary tissue there is focal to diffuse reddening and often only one subsection of a mammary gland may be affected. Histologically, the mastitis may be focal or diffuse in distribution, and the intensity of the lesion varies from a mild catarrhal inflammation to a severe purulent and necrotizing mastitis usually involving more than 50% of all the mammary glands. There are no significant lesions of the uterus compared with the state of the uterus in normal healthy sows immediately after parturition. The adrenal gland is enlarged and heavier than normal, presumably caused by adrenocortical hyperactivity. In a series of spontaneous cases, *E. coli* and *Klebsiella* spp. were most commonly isolated from the mammary tissues. The abscesses of the mammary glands of sows examined at slaughter are not sequelae to coliform mastitis but rather probably caused by injuries and secondary infection.

Samples for Confirmation of Diagnosis

- Bacteriology: mammary gland, regional lymph node
- Histology: formalin-fixed mammary gland

DIFFERENTIAL DIAGNOSIS

The characteristic clinical findings in toxic mastitis and agalactia are a sudden onset of anorexia and lack of interest in the piglets, acute swelling of the mammary gland, hypogalactia or agalactia, a moderate fever, and a course of about 2 days. The mammary secretion from mastitic glands may be watery or thickened and contain pus, and the cell count will be increased up to 20 × 10^9 cells/mL. The acute swelling and agalactia of infectious mastitis must be differentiated from other noninfectious causes of acute swelling or "caking" of the mammary glands, which also results in agalactia as follows:

- Agalactia caused by a failure in milk letdown is most common in first-litter gilts and is characterized by a fullness of the mammary glands but an inability of the gilt to suckle her piglets in spite of her grunting at them. The gilt is usually bright and alert and systemically normal. The response to oxytocin is dramatic, and repeat treatment is rarely necessary.
- Farrowing fever is characterized clinically by loss of appetite, inactivity, and a body temperature of 39.3°C–39.9°C (102.7°F–103.8°F) with minimal detectable changes of the mammary gland.
- Parturient psychosis of sows is characterized by aggressive and nervous behavior of the sow after the piglets are born. The sow does not call the piglets, and does not allow them to suck. When the piglets approach the sow's head, she will back away, snap, and make noisy staccato nasal expirations. Some sows will bite and kill their piglets. The mammary gland is usually full of milk, but the sow will not let it down. Ataractic drugs and/or short-term general anesthesia are indicated, and the response is usually excellent. Some sows need repeated tranquilization or sedation for the first few days until the maternal–neonatal bond is established.
- Other causes of agalactia accompanied by enlargement of the mammary gland include inherited inverted teats and blind teats caused by necrosis of the teats occurring when the gilt was a piglet. These are readily obvious on clinical examination. The sharp needle teeth of piglets may cause the sow to refuse to suckle her piglets. The sow attempts to suckle but leaps up suddenly, grunting and snapping at the piglets. The piglets squeal and fight to retain a teat, thus causing more damage to the teats, which is obvious on clinical examination. Other causes of agalactia accompanied by systemic illness include retained piglets and infectious disease such as outbreaks of transmissible gastroenteritis and erysipelas. The common causes of agalactia in pigs in which there is lack of mammary development include ergotism, immature gilts, and inherited lack of mammary development.

TREATMENT

Most affected sows will recover within 24 to 48 hours if treated with a combination of antimicrobials, oxytocin, and antiinflammatory agents. The treatment should begin when the temperature reaches 39.4°C (102.9°F).

Antimicrobials are indicated in most cases because infectious mastitis and metritis are two common causes of the disease. The choice is generally determined by previous experience in the herd or region, but broad-spectrum antimicrobials are indicated because *E. coli* and *Klebsiella* spp. are the most common pathogens involved. They should be given daily for at least 3 days. Usually ampicillin, tetracyclines, trimethoprim-sulfonamide, or enrofloxacin is used.

As soon as possible after the disease is recognized every effort must be made to restore normal mammary function through the use of oxytocin and warm water massaging of the affected mammary glands.

Oxytocin 30 to 40 U intramuscularly or 20 to 30 U intravenously is given, frequently, to promote the letdown of milk. If there is a beneficial response the piglets should be placed on the sow if she is willing to allow them to suck. This will assist in promoting milk flow. Massage of the mammary glands with towels soaked in warm water and hand milking for 10 to 15 minutes every few hours may assist in reducing the swelling and inflammation and promote the flow of milk. It will also relieve the pain and encourage the sow to suckle her piglets. Intramuscular injections of oxytocin may be repeated every hour, along with massaging of the glands with warm water. Failure of milk letdown or a low response following the use of oxytocin may be caused by a reduced sensitivity of the sow to oxytocin during the first week of lactation. In the normal, healthy sow the peak response to oxytocin occurs in the second week of lactation and gradually decreases to a low response by the eighth week.

Oxytocin has an effect for about 14 minutes, whereas the long-acting analog has an effect for about 6 hours. Preliminary results of its use in agalactic sows indicate superior results compared with oxytocin.

Antiinflammatory agents are commonly used for their antiinflammatory effect but are rarely used on their own; flunixin meglumine has been shown to be beneficial as well as ketoprofen[18] to alleviate pyrexia and endotoxemia. Recently meloxicam and oxytocin were shown to reduce mortality compared with flunixin. Plasma cortisol levels are increased in the experimental disease and for this reason may be contraindicated. However, field reports suggest that their use along with antimicrobials and oxytocin provides a better response than when they are not used. Corticosteroids used alone do not appear to prevent the disease or enhance recovery. To be effective they must be used in combination with antimicrobials and oxytocin. Dexamethasone at the rate of 20 mg intramuscularly daily for 3 days for sows weighing 150 to 200 kg has been recommended.

Sows with toxemia almost invariably dehydrate, so fluid therapy is essential.[19]

Supplementation of Piglets

The hypoglycemic piglets must be given a supply of milk and/or balanced electrolytes and dextrose until the milk flow of the sow is resumed, which may take 2 to 4 days, and most importantly they must be kept warm until body reserves are reestablished. Piglets should receive 300 to 500 mL of milk per day divided into hourly doses of 40 to 50 mL given through a 12- to 14-French plastic tube passed orally into the stomach. A solution of balanced electrolytes containing 5% glucose can also be given for 1 to 2 days if a supply of cows' milk is not available. Intraperitoneal injection of 15 ml of 5% glucose will prevent starvation. Condensed canned milk diluted with water 1:1 is a satisfactory and readily available supply of milk. In severe cases in which the return to milk production and flow are unlikely, the piglets should be fostered onto other sows. If these are unavailable, the use of milk substitute fortified with porcine gamma globulin is recommended to prevent the common enteric diseases. This is discussed under colibacillosis. Many more piglets are treated for diarrhea when the sows are treated for MMA, perhaps up to 19% compared with up to 9% normally.

CONTROL

It is necessary for modern pig farms to develop control measures[6,20] and to assess the six major areas outlined previously.[21] It has been difficult to develop a rational approach to control because the disease has been considered to be a complex syndrome caused by several different factors. However, the control of infectious mastitis would seem to be of major importance. The routine use of antibiotics and oxytocin without indication does not appear to be helpful. Farrowing crates should be vacated, cleaned, disinfected, and left vacant for a few days before pregnant sows are transferred from the dry sow barn and placed in the crates. Pregnant sows should be washed with soap and water before being placed in the crate. Farrowing crates must be kept clean and hosed down if necessary, particularly a few days before and after farrowing to minimize the level of intramammary infection. In problem herds, it may be necessary to wash and disinfect the skin over the mammary glands immediately after farrowing. All-in/all-out in the farrowing area with proper cleaning and disinfection facilitated by batch farrowing will reduce the disease. An opportunity for exercise will help, because under outdoor conditions (sows in paddocks) the condition is rare.

To minimize the stress to the sow of adjusting to the farrowing crate and the farrowing facilities, the sow should be placed in the crate at least 1 week before the expected date of farrowing.

The nature and composition of the diet fed to the sow while in the farrowing crate should not be changed. To minimize the risk of toxic agalactia, it is recommended that the daily feed allowance be related to body condition score. It may be necessary to reduce the feed to 1 kg/day (from 100 days' gestation) before farrowing. The daily intake (compared with the intake during the dry period) may be increased on the day after the sow has farrowed and in increments thereafter as the stage of lactation proceeds. The inclusion of bran at the rate of one-third to one-half of the total diet for 2 days before and after farrowing has been recommended to prevent constipation. In some herds the use of lucerne meal or other vegetable protein at the rate of 15% of the diet may help control the disease. However, under intensified conditions it may be impractical to prepare and provide these special diets on a regular basis. Although field observations suggest that a bulky diet at the time of farrowing will minimize the incidence of toxic agalactia, there is little scientific evidence to support the practice.

Antimicrobial agents used prophylactically have apparently been successful in controlling some outbreaks. A trimethoprim-sulfadimidine and sulfathiazole combination at 15 mg/kg in feed from day 112 of gestation to day 1 after farrowing may reduce the prevalence. Using oxytocin early may also help. In a recent study where *E. coli*, streptococci, and staphylococci were the most cultured pathogens, marbofloxacin (10% solution) was found to be superior to amoxicillin. All *E. coli* were susceptible to the former, but 32% were resistant to the latter antibiotic.

The use of prostaglandins for the induction of parturition in sows has not been associated with a marked consistent change in the incidence of the disease. Some field trials have shown a reduction, whereas others have had no effect.

FURTHER READING

Martineau G-P, et al. Postparturient dysgalactia syndrome: a simple change in homeorhesis. *J Swine Health Prod.* 2013;21:85-95.

Ringarp N. A post-parturient syndrome with agalactia in sows. *Acta Vet Scand Suppl.* 1960;7:1-153.

REFERENCES

1. Foisnet A, et al. *J Rech Porcine France.* 2010;42:15.
2. Foisnet A. PhD thesis Univ. Rennes France. 2010; 250.
3. Gerjets I, Kemper N. *J Swine Health Prod.* 2009;17:97.
4. Gerjets I, et al. *Vet Microbiol.* 2011;152:361.
5. Larsen I, Thorup R. *Proc Int Pig Vet Soc.* 2006;256.
6. Papadopoulos GA. PhD thesis Ghent Univ. 2008; 229.
7. Papadopoulos GA, et al. *Vet J.* 2010;184:167.
8. Oliviero C, et al. *Anim Reprod Sci.* 2009;119:85.
9. Cowart RP. Parturition and dystocia in swine. In: Youngquist RS, Threlfall WR, eds. *Large Animal Theriogenology.* St. Louis: Saunders; 2007:778.
10. Kopinski J, et al. *Aust Vet J.* 2007;85:169.
11. Martel G, et al. *Livestock Sci.* 2008;116:96.
12. Solignac T. *Porc Mag.* 2008;424:133.
13. Solignac T, et al. *Proc Int Cong Pig Vet Soc.* 2010;124.
14. Van den Brand H. *Proc 7th Int Cong Pig Vet Soc.* 2006;177.
15. Boren CA, Carlson MS. *Arbeitar.* 2006;100:14.
16. Foisnet A, et al. *J Anim Sci.* 2010;88:1672.
17. Bories P, et al. *J Rech Porcine France.* 2010;42:233.
18. Sabatate D, et al. *Pig J.* 2012;67:19.
19. Reiner G, et al. *Tierarztl Praxis.* 2009;37:305.
20. Maes D, et al. *Tierarztl Praxis.* 2010;1:15.
21. Martineau G-P, Morvan H. *Les Mal Prod.* 2010;18:514.

21 Systemic and Multi-Organ Diseases

Diseases of Complex or Undetermined Etiology

COLD COW SYNDROME

Cold cow syndrome is a herd disease problem reported only from the United Kingdom in the early 1980s in cows freshly turned out onto lush pasture with a high (27% to 43%) soluble carbohydrate content. There is a high morbidity (up to 80%) and a large number of outbreaks in an area. The syndrome includes hypothermia, dullness, inappetence, agalactia, and profuse diarrhea. Affected cows feel cold to the touch. Some have perineal edema; some collapse. The herd milk yield falls disastrously, but there is a quick return to normal if the cows are moved to a different field. The problem may occur on the same pasture each year and recur if the cows are returned to the same pasture. There is no obvious clinicopathologic abnormality. It is postulated that the syndrome might be a result of zearalenone or related metabolites produced by microfungi in the pasture.

RECUMBENCY IN HORSES OF UNDETERMINED ETIOLOGY

Diagnosis and management of adult horses that are recumbent can be challenging. The large size of adult horses, the variety of conditions that can cause recumbency, the difficulty in performing a thorough clinical examination, and the need for prolonged and intensive care all present formidable obstacles to management of recumbent horses. Causes of prolonged (>8 h) recumbency in horses are listed in Table 21-1. Other causes of acute recumbency of shorter duration are usually obvious on initial examination.

EPIDEMIOLOGY

The epidemiology of recumbent horses is covered in detail in the sections dealing with each of the specific diseases, and information on large series of recumbent horses is sparse. Overall, for 148 horses treated in a referral veterinary hospital with excellent resources and expertise to manage recumbent horses, there were 109 nonsurvivors and 39 survivors (case-fatality rate of 74%). Odds of death within the first 3 days of hospitalization increased with longer duration of clinical signs before presentation, with horses showing clinical signs for over 24 hours being 4.16 (95% confidence interval [CI] 1.04 to 16.59) times more likely to die; presence of band neutrophils (odds ratio [OR] 7.9, 95% CI 1.39 to 45.5); not using the sling (OR 4, 95% CI 1.1 to 15.7); and horses that were unable to stand after treatment (OR 231, 95% CI 23 to 2341). Increasing cost was associated with lower odds of death (OR 0.96, for each additional $100 billed, 95% CI 0.93 to 0.99), likely because of greater financial resources increasing the chance of success.[1]

There does not appear to be any breed, age, or sex distribution beyond that anticipated for the specific diseases.

EXAMINATION OF THE RECUMBENT HORSE

History

Careful questioning of the horse's attendants can reveal valuable information regarding the cause of recumbency. Causes such as observed trauma, foaling, and excessive unaccustomed exercise are readily determined from the history. In addition to inquiries about the cause of the recumbency, estimates of the duration of recumbency should be obtained from the attendants. This can often be best elicited by asking when the horse was last observed to be standing. A history of recent illness, abnormal behavior or unusual use immediately before the horse became recumbent is useful. The horse's age, sex, breed, and use should be determined. Information regarding management, vaccination and deworming status, feeding, and health of other horses can be revealing. Outbreaks of recumbency suggest either an infectious (equine herpesvirus-1) or toxic (botulism, ionophore) cause. Questions should be directed toward discerning the cause of the horse's recumbency rather than collecting information.

Physical Examination

Physical examination of recumbent horses is challenging but should be as complete as practical and safe. The examination should begin with a general assessment of the horse and its surroundings and can be directed at answering a series of questions:

- Are the surrounding conditions safe for the horse and people? Is the footing sound?
- Is there evidence of the horse struggling or thrashing?
- Has the horse defecated and urinated recently?
- Is there evidence of exposure to toxins or physical evidence of the reason for recumbency?

Examination of the horse should begin with measurement of heart rate, respiratory rate and temperature (rectal temperature might not be accurate if there is dilation of the anus), examination of mucous membranes and an assessment of its hydration, body condition and level of consciousness. The horse should be thoroughly examined for evidence of trauma. Although the examination should be complete, initial examination of cases for which the cause of recumbency is not immediately obvious should focus on the nervous and musculoskeletal systems.

- Is the horse alert and able to sit in sternal recumbency, or is it unconscious and in lateral recumbency? Can the horse rise with assistance?
- Is the horse's mentation normal?
- Are there any spontaneous voluntary or involuntary movements?
- Can the horse eat and drink?
- Are the cranial nerves normal?
- Is there evidence of trauma to the head or neck?
- Is there evidence of paresis or paralysis? Are only the hindlimbs involved, or are both the hindlimbs and forelimbs involved?
- Are the peripheral reflexes normal (withdrawal, patellar, cervicofacial, cutaneous, anal, penile)?
- Is cutaneous sensation present in all regions? If not, what are the anatomic boundaries of desensitized areas?
- Is the position of the limbs normal? Is there evidence of crepitus, swelling, or unusual shape of the limbs or axial skeleton?
- Are the horse's feet normal? Does it have laminitis? What is the response to application of hoof testers?
- Are abnormalities detected on rectal examination (fractured pelvis, distended bladder, fecal retention, pregnancy), provided that it is safe to perform one?

Other body systems should be evaluated as indicated or necessary. The heart and lungs should be auscultated, although detecting abnormal lung sounds in a recumbent horse is difficult. The horse should be rolled and thus a complete examination can be performed. Assisting the horse to stand using a rope tied to the tail and thrown over a rafter, or preferably using a sling, can be useful in assessing the severity of the horse's illness (i.e., can it stand at all?) and in facilitating a complete physical examination. If there is a suspicion that the horse has colic, a nasogastric tube should be placed to check for accumulation of liquid gastric contents, a rectal examination performed, and peritoneal fluid collected.

Ancillary diagnostic testing includes radiography of limbs and/or axial spine as indicated by the history or physical examination, myelography if a compressive lesion of the cervical spinal cord is suspected, endoscopic examination of the pharynx and guttural pouches (especially in horses with a history of falling; see section on rupture of the longus capitus muscle), ultrasonography of the chest and abdomen, collection of cerebrospinal fluid, and electromyography.

Hematologic abnormalities are sometimes reflective of the causative disease. Serum **biochemical abnormalities** are reflective of the causative disease and in addition are influenced by muscle damage caused by the horse being recumbent (increased creatine kinase and aspartate aminotransferase activity), inappetent (increased total and indirect bilirubin and triglyceride concentrations), and unable to drink or gain access to water (increased serum urea nitrogen, creatinine, sodium, chloride, total protein, and

Table 21-1 Causes and diagnostic features of recumbency of more than 8 hours in duration in adult horses

Cause	Clinical signs and diagnosis	Treatment	Prognosis and comments
Neurologic disease			
Botulism[3]	Horse alert. Flaccid paralysis, dysphagia, weak corneal or palpebral reflex.	Administration of specific antitoxin or multivalent antitoxin.	Can require prolonged treatment. Prognosis poor for recumbent horses.
	Often multiple animals affected. Toxin isolation in mice.	Supportive care.	
Tetanus	Horse alert. Rigid paralysis. Signs worsened by stimuli. Often history of recent wound and lack of vaccination.	Tetanus antitoxin (IV or intrathecally). Penicillin. Wound debridement. Sedation (acepromazine, chloral hydrate). Minimize stimulation (dark, quiet stall).	Guarded prognosis.
Trauma—vertebral	Alert horse. Signs depend on site of lesion. Can be difficult to detect vertebral fractures in adult horses. Radiography.	None specific.	Poor prognosis.
Trauma—cranial	Unconscious or severely altered mentation. Seizures. Head wounds. Blood from ears and nostril. Imaging (radiography, CT, MRI).	Antiinflammatory drugs including flunixin meglumine, phenylbutazone, corticosteroids. Drugs to reduce swelling (mannitol and hypertonic saline). Control of seizures (diazepam, midazolam, barbiturates). Heroic craniotomy.	Very poor prognosis.
Cervical vertebral instability	Alert horse. Acute-onset ataxia and recumbency. Young horse (<4 years old). Radiography and myelography.	Antiinflammatory drugs. Rest. Surgical vertebral stabilization.	Poor prognosis.
Vestibular disease	Normal to depressed, depending on cause. Signs of vestibular disease include circling and falling to one side, head tilt, and nystagmus. Diagnosis by endoscopic examination of guttural pouches, radiography of skull, and examination of CSF.	Antibiotics, antiinflammatory drugs. Surgical or medical treatment of guttural pouch disease.	Poor to guarded prognosis.
Equine herpesvirus-1 myoencephalopathy	Usually alert horse. Recumbency follows period of posterior ataxia with fecal and urinary incontinence. Fever in early stages of disease. CSF xanthochromic. Viral isolation or detection of virus by PCR. Serology. Often multiple horses affected.	Supportive care. Valacyclovir or similar drug in early stages.	Guarded prognosis. Affected horses can be infectious.
Arboviral encephalitis (Eastern, Western, West Nile, Japanese B encephalitis)	Alert horse or altered mentation, depending on the disease. CSF consistent with inflammation. Viral isolation or detection by PCR. Serology.	Supportive care. Dexamethasone for West Nile encephalitis.	Epidemiology is characteristic. Prognosis is poor for recumbent horses. Vaccines available.
Migrating parasite larvae	Mentation depends on anatomic site of parasite. Eosinophils in CSF.	Ivermectin 400 μg/kg orally. Corticosteroids.	Sporadic disease.
Neoplasia (melanoma, lymphosarcoma, cholesterol granuloma)	Alert horse. Signs of spinal cord compression. Diagnosis by imaging (radiography, myelography, CT). CSF usually normal.	No specific treatment.	Hopeless prognosis.
Equine motor neuron disease	Alert horse. Good appetite. Profound muscle weakness and atrophy. Prolonged periods of recumbency but usually able to stand when stimulated.	Supportive care. Vitamin E.	Guarded to poor prognosis. Lifelong disease.
Equine protozoal myeloencephalitis	Variable mentation and signs of neurologic disease. Diagnosis based on neurologic examination and results of Western blot of CSF or serum.	Antiprotozoal medications.	Guarded to fair prognosis.
Rabies	Variable mentation. Protean signs of neurologic disease. Important zoonosis. Diagnosis by immunofluorescent antibody testing of brain.	No treatment. If suspected, then appropriate barrier isolation measures must be instituted until the horse dies or recovers, or another diagnosis is confirmed.	Rare cause of recumbency in horses.
Postanesthetic myelopathy	Acute-onset posterior paresis evident on recovery from general anesthesia.	Supportive care.	Poor to hopeless prognosis.
Musculoskeletal disease			
Acute rhabdomyolysis (exertional, atypical)	Alert horse. History of unaccustomed or strenuous exercise. Painful. Sweating. Firm painful muscles. Pigmenturia.	Fluid diuresis. Pain control. Supportive care.	Guarded to fair prognosis. Can recur. Can progress to acute renal failure.
	High CK and AST activity in serum.		

Table 21-1 Causes and diagnostic features of recumbency of more than 8 hours in duration in adult horses—cont'd

Cause	Clinical signs and diagnosis	Treatment	Prognosis and comments
Laminitis	Alert horse. Assumes sternal recumbency easily. Bounding digital pulses. Pain on application of hoof tester to feet.	Pain control. Corrective shoeing.	Guarded to poor prognosis for long-term care.
Fracture of long bone or pelvis	Horse usually able to stand on three legs. Bilateral fracture of femurs. Diagnosis by physical examination and radiography.	Euthanasia.	
Foaling paralysis (obturator nerve paresis)	Dystocia. Mare unable to stand after difficult foaling. Legs excessively abducted.	Supportive care. Antiinflammatory drugs. Sling horse.	Guarded prognosis.
Bilateral femoral nerve paresis	Occurs in horses suspended by the hind limbs during anesthesia.	Supportive care.	Guarded prognosis.
Hyperkalemic periodic paralysis	Alert horse. Anxious. Muscle fasciculations. Muscle weakness. High serum potassium concentration. Electromyography. Unusual for recumbency to persist for < 1–2 hours. Diagnosis by detection of appropriate genome.	Administration of dextrose or calcium solutions. Prevention by administration of acetazolamide, feeding low-K^+ diet and selective breeding.	Guarded to good prognosis. Lifelong care needed.
Environmental			
Heat stress/exhaustion	Depressed mentation. Compatible history of exercise in hot and humid conditions or exposure to extreme heat. Hyperthermia.	Rapid cooling. Administration of fluids.	Guarded to poor prognosis. Death often associated with DIC.
Hypothermia	Depressed mentation. History of exposure to extreme cold. Hypothermia.	Warming. Prolonged care necessary.	Guarded to poor prognosis.
Lightning strike	Horses at pasture. History of electrical storm activity. One or more horses can be affected. There can be evidence of burns, fractures of long bones or the axial skeleton, or vestibular disease.	Supportive care. Euthanasia for animals with severe disease.	
Gunshot wounds	Horses at pasture. Often during hunting season. Can be malicious. Physical examination variable. Entry hole and exit hole can be difficult to identify.	Supportive care, depending on site of wound.	Horses that have been shot and are recumbent have a poor prognosis.
Metabolic			
Starvation, inanition	Alert horse. Grade 1 or 2 of 9 body condition score.	Careful refeeding and supportive care.	Poor to fair prognosis.
Hypocalcemia, hyponatremia	Depressed mentation. Seizures. Confirmed by measurement of serum electrolyte concentrations. Unusual cause of recumbency in adult horses.	Correction of electrolyte deficit. Gradual correction of hyponatremia.	Good prognosis.
Liver disease	Depressed, seizures, head pressing. Jaundice. Elevated serum concentrations of bilirubin, ammonia, and bile acids and increased activity of gammaglutamyl transpeptidase and sorbitol dehydrogenase.	Supportive care. Provision of hydration and nutrition. Correction of hypoglycemia. Administration of lactulose.	Poor prognosis. History of exposure to hepatotoxins.
Hypoglycemia	Seizures. Measurement of blood glucose concentrations. Iatrogenic or malicious, associated with insulin administration. Unusual cause in adult horses.	Administration of glucose intravenously.	
Water deprivation	Variable mentation from normal to seizures. Associated with inadequate water intake (e.g., broken bore or dry tank supplying horses at pasture).	Judicious rehydration. Provision of unrestricted access to water can result in water intoxication.	Cause is usually obvious (lack of access to water). Guarded prognosis.
Senile collapse	Alert horse. Old horse. History of progressive weakness. No other causes of recumbency identified.	Supportive care. Correction of metabolic abnormalities. Provision of good-quality nutrition.	Poor prognosis.
Intoxications			
Ionophores (monensin, salinomycin, etc.)	Alert. Acute-onset colic and muscle weakness. Recumbency. Diagnosis is based on history of exposure and measurement of drug concentrations in blood or tissues, and feed.	Supportive. No specific treatment.	Poor to guarded. Horses surviving the acute episode can have exercise intolerance as a result of persisting myocardial disease.

AST, aspartate transferase; CK, creatine kinase; CSF, cerebrospinal fluid; CT, computed tomography; DIC, disseminated intravascular coagulation; IV, intravenously; MRI, magnetic resonance imaging; PCR, polymerase chain reaction.

albumin concentrations). Cerebrospinal fluid is reflective of any inciting disease but is usually normal.

MANAGEMENT AND CARE

The principles of care are treatment of the primary disease, prevention of further illness or injury, assisting the horse to stand, and provision of optimal nutrition and hydration. Median duration of hospitalization in one report of 148 horses treated at a referral hospital was 2.8 days (interquartile range of 1.5 to 8 days).[1]

Treatment of the primary disease is covered in other sections of this book. Similarly, maintenance of hydration and electrolyte status is covered elsewhere. Maintenance of normal hydration is sometimes problematic in recumbent horses because of limited access to water and unwillingness to drink. Provision of fresh, palatable water is essential. Intravenous or enteral (nasogastric intubation) administration of fluids and electrolyte solutions might be necessary in some recumbent horses, especially early in their illness.

Horses with diseases that cause recumbency often have problems with fecal and urinary incontinence or retention. Catheterization of the urinary bladder might be necessary to relieve distension in horses with neurogenic upper motor bladder or lower motor bladder dysfunction, or in male horses that are reluctant to urinate when recumbent. Catheterization of the bladder is often repeated. To minimize the risk of iatrogenic cystitis, the procedure should be performed aseptically. Administration of bethanechol might increase detrusor muscle tone and aid urination, and phenoxybenzamine (0.5 mg/kg intravenously over 15 minutes) might decrease sphincter tone in horses with upper motor neurone bladder.

Horses that can eat should be fed a balanced, palatable, and nutritious diet. Tempting horses with reduced appetite with treats such as apples, carrots, and horse treats might stimulate appetite for hay and grain. Horses that are unable to eat should be fed through a nasogastric tube. Slurries of alfalfa pellets or commercial diets can be administered through nasogastric tubes. The maintenance needs of a sedentary 425-kg horse are approximately 15 to 18 Mcal/d. The maintenance needs of a recumbent horse are unknown, but are probably less than that of normal sedentary horses.

COMPLICATIONS—PREVENTION

A major challenge in managing recumbent horses is preventing further injury. Abnormalities caused by recumbency include abrasions and lacerations, gastric ulceration, corneal ulceration, pneumonia, cystitis, pigmenturia, muscle hemorrhage and tearing, impaction colic, laminitis, and catheter-site infection or inflammation.[1]

Recumbent horses often make repeated efforts to stand, which, although encouraging to all involved, can result in further injury. An attempt to stand can injure the horse's head, especially the periorbital regions, and skin over bony prominences such as over the wing of the ilium. Minimization of further injury is achieved by use of a sling or tail rope to assist horses to stand; housing in a padded stall with deep, soft bedding (although this can interfere with the horse's ability to stand); and protection of the head and distal limbs with a helmet and bandages, respectively. Recumbent horses kept in well-grassed pasture often do well and have minimal self-inflicted trauma.

Decubital ulcers occur over pressure points, such as the wing of the ilium, point of the shoulder, and zygomatic arch, and can become severe. Recumbent horses that paddle can abrade the skin over limb joints, with subsequent increased risk of septic arthritis. Bandages, helmets, ointments such as silver sulfadiazine paste, and soft bedding minimize but do not eliminate these abrasions. Recumbent horses that cannot or do not voluntarily move from side to side should be rolled every 2 to 4 hours.

Peripheral pressure neuropathy can occur in recumbent horses. The radial nerve and facial nerve are most often affected. Prevention is achieved by use of padded bedding, slings, frequent rolling, and a helmet.

Recumbent horses can sustain muscle damage from pressure on large muscle groups. For large or well-muscled horses this can result in large increases in serum creatine kinase activity and myoglobinuria. Myoglobinuria can cause acute renal failure, although this degree of myoglobinuria in recumbent horses is unusual.

Pneumonia can occur as a result of recumbency. Horses that are dysphagic are at increased risk of aspiration of feed material and saliva, and hence development of aspiration pneumonia. Horses receiving corticosteroids are at increased risk of bacterial and fungal (*Aspergillus* spp.,) pneumonia. Although not every recumbent horse should be administered antimicrobials, this is indicated in horses at increased risk of developing pneumonia. Antimicrobials should have a broad spectrum, including activity against *Streptococcus* spp., such as a combination of penicillin and an aminoglycoside.

Slinging of horses is labor intensive and requires a sling that is designed for use with horses. Horses that accept being supported by a sling have increased chances of survival (OR of 4 for death for horses not using a sling [1.1% to 16%, 95% CI)] than do horses that cannot or will not use a sling.[1] Horses should not be lifted using hip slings intended for use with cattle. Use of these slings to lift horses by grasping over the wing of each ilium is inhumane and unsuccessful. There are slings designed specifically for use with horses (e.g., Anderson Sling Support Device).[2]

Horses in slings should be closely monitored and not allowed to hang in the sling. The horses should be assisted to stand in the sling every 6 or 8 hours. The sling should be used to help the horse to get up and provide some support while it is standing, but the horse should not have all its weight borne by the sling for more than a few minutes. Horses that have an excessive amount of weight borne by the sling for a prolonged period of time have trouble breathing and might develop colic, rupture of the urinary bladder, diaphragmatic hernia, or rectal prolapse.

Potentially catastrophic complications include septic arthritis, radial nerve injury, bladder rupture, diaphragmatic hernia, rectal prolapse, colon torsion, and long bone fracture. The risk of these complications can be minimized by the practices detailed previously, but they cannot be eliminated.

FURTHER READING

Gardner R. Evaluation and management of the recumbent adult horse. *Vet Clin North Am.* 2011;27:527-534.

Pusterla N, et al. How to lift recumbent equine patients in the field and hospital with the UC Davis large animal lift. *AAEP Proceedings.* 2006;52:87-92.

REFERENCES

1. Winfield LS, et al. *Equine Vet J.* 2014;46:575.
2. Pustera N, et al. *AAEP Proceedings.* 2006;52:87.

THIN SOW SYNDROME

SYNOPSIS

Etiology The syndrome is the result of inadequate nutrition and unbalanced nutrition in pregnancy and lactation but may also result from parasitic or chronic infectious disease.

Epidemiology Loss of weight to the point of inanition, particularly in first- and second-litter gilts.

Clinical findings Inanition.

Control Recognition of the relation between voluntary feed intake in pregnancy and lactation; feeding based on condition scores.

Thin cow syndrome is a condition of sows, particularly sows at the end of lactation or in the early dry period where there has been tremendous lactational weight loss and this has not been regained. It was formerly common in outdoor or yard systems, particularly in the United Kingdom, but currently is rarely seen because management practices and nutritional knowledge have advanced markedly. There are a number of causes of wasting and the occurrence of thin sows.

ETIOLOGY

Historically, the major cause of thin sow syndrome was the complete lack of awareness that sows needed to be fed correctly in pregnancy to prepare for farrowing and in lactation to provide milk for 9 or more piglets consuming 800+ ml of milk per piglet per day.

EPIDEMIOLOGY

It emerged as a problem in the 1970s as a result of poor understanding of the interrelation between feed intake in pregnancy and that in lactation. The syndrome is most common in first- and second-litter gilts but can affect all parities when nutrition is inadequate. The voluntary intake of food by sows during lactation is inversely related to the intake in pregnancy. Consequently, sows that are fed at high levels during pregnancy will gain excessive weight during pregnancy but will voluntarily restrict feed intake during lactation and lose excessive weight during lactation. In contrast, sows that are fed what is basically a maintenance ration 2.0 to 2.5 kg (4.5 to 5.5 lbs) of a balanced sow ration during pregnancy will gain adequate weight for conceptus and body growth and during lactation will consume adequate feed for lactation requirements and loose minimal weight in this period. Knowledge of sow nutrition has improved such that major problems with this syndrome should not occur, but there is still a risk of inadequately feeding sows selected for lean genotype and high litter size and weaning weights. First- and second-litter gilts may require more feed to provide for body growth. This was combined with the move to intensive indoor housing of pregnant sows. Penning of sows exacerbated social dominance/submissive relationships.

Modern commercial highly bred sows do not have the subcutaneous fat reserves necessary for outdoor production and thus are prone to body-weight loss in exposed fields and yards. The second major group of causes is environmental. Often sows are kept in yards or arks with minimum straw for bedding, which alleviates to some extent low environmental temperatures. Environmental causes include cold or drafty housing, fluctuating temperatures, too high a temperature in the farrowing house, wet bedding, and lack of drinking water.

Early weaning increases the risk of thin sow syndrome, especially if the nutrition is inadequate. Afflicted animals were often on low-level feeding to avoid obesity.

Parasitic disease, particularly associated with infestation with *Oesophagostomum* spp. and *Hyostrongylus* spp., contributes to wasting in sows and the occurrence of thin sow syndrome.

Thin sows can be a component of the syndrome of infectious diseases such as cystitis and pyelonephritis.

CLINICAL FINDINGS

Within a herd, thin sow syndrome develops over a period of months and often one or two pregnancy cycles, with a gradually decline in the body condition of the group until 20% to 30% of sows have a low body-condition score. No abnormalities are evident on clinical examination, but the sows fail to regain weight after weaning, particularly sows after their first litter. The most critical period for weight loss is the first 2 weeks after weaning. Affected sows have a poor appetite but often show pica and excessive water intake and may be anemic.

CONTROL

Feeding During Pregnancy

Currently the risk for thin sow syndrome exists where it is assumed that all pregnant sows can be fed a standard amount of ration. Problems are likely to occur when sows are run in groups and fed as a group, where timid sows are likely to be bullied out of their required share of food. Individual feeders or stall feeding, and particularly electronic feeders, will prevent this.

Feeding During Lactation

The critical issue is to ensure adequate feed and energy intake during lactation. This can be achieved by not feeding to excess during pregnancy, restricting the feed intake of sows in the first few days after farrowing to encourage better feed intake in later lactation, ensuring an adequate and constant supply of water, ad lib feeding during lactation, and providing a high-energy-density lactation diet.

In addition, enclosing the creep with heat for the piglets and thus the farrowing house can be kept at a lower temperature for the sow and controlling parasitic disease will help.

Condition scoring is a valuable guide to the feeding of individual sows and for a judgment of feeding practices in the herd as a whole. On a score of 1 to 5, it should be very rare to find sows with condition scores of 1 or 5. The optimum is to have sows entering the farrowing house between condition score 3 and 4 and not less than 2.5 at weaning. First- and second-parity sows in poor condition at weaning are best "skipped" at the first heat and mated on the second heat.

Methods for condition scoring and guidelines can be found at http://www.defra.gov.uk/animalh/welfare/farmed/pigs/pb3480/pigsctoc.htm.

WILD BOAR AS VECTORS FOR INFECTIOUS DISEASE

There is an increasing worldwide focus on wild boar and escaped domesticated (feral) pigs as a reservoir of infection for pig diseases of epizootic nature,[1-3] particularly in Europe and the United States, where the hunting fraternity has a vested interest in these animals. Wild animals have great potential as a source of both viral and parasitic diseases, and the wild boar (*Sus scrofa*) is no exception. In many cases, they are shy and retiring, frequently inhabiting woodland, where their numbers are not really appreciated. Where there is a high density, there is a high transmission rate of infection.[4]

There is wide variation in populations in different countries in Europe. It is the second most important wild ungulate in Europe and is important in Germany, France, Spain, Poland, and the Czech Republic; in the United States, they are found in 39 of 50 states.

Wild boar have become increasingly common across Europe because they free range. In Switzerland, the population of wild boar has shown a steady increase over the last 15 years.[5] Commercial pigs have also become increasingly reared outside, so the possibility of disease transmission has increased rapidly. To illustrate this, a recent study in Switzerland of contacts between piggeries and wild boar[6] showed that 5% of the piggeries recorded the presence of crossbred pigs on their premises. The pigs of the Mangalitza breed were the most at risk of such matings. A study of the risk of such happenings was made,[7] and it showed that the risk was highest when the disease under consideration was spread by aerosol (e.g., African swine fever, classical swine fever) rather than those spread by venereal means (e.g., brucellosis). They can also possibly be a hazard to humans as well.[8]

There is a technique for assessing relative abundance and aggregation.[9]

Overall, the disease situation in the wild boar is not well understood. Various diseases are outlined in the following discussion; the diseases are arranged alphabetically.

RISK FACTORS

The greater the distance between the outdoor pigs and the managing homestead, the greater the risk of intrusion by wild boar. Unsupervised units are definitely at risk. Close proximity to forest also increases the risk of disease. Piggeries with pasture paddocks are also at considerable risk from wild boar. Commercial hunting sites maintain an overabundant wild boar population.[9,10] The role of fences has been discussed.[11] Concentrated feed sources are a high point of contact, and these fields for outdoor pigs should be effectively fenced. Feral swine require dense vegetation for thermoregulation. They also require areas of surface water and moist areas in which to wallow.

DISEASE IN GENERAL

Generally, if wild boar are farmed, then the diseases are the same as for domestic pigs.[12] A large study of wild boar in Campania in southern Italy[13] showed that 4.4% were positive for *Brucella* spp., 2.6% for *Leptospira interrogans,* 19.3% for *Salmonella* spp., 30.7% for Aujesky's disease, 7.9% for porcine parvovirus, and 37.7% for porcine reproductive and respiratory virus, but all were negative for African swine fever, classical swine fever. Thus the wild boar does provide a challenge to the domestic pig if there is contact between the two groups.

AFRICAN SWINE FEVER

Wild boar are natural hosts for African swine fever (ASF), but a survey in Spain in an area previously infected showed neither virus nor antibody,[14] suggesting that permanent recovery of freedom is possible. The outbreak was extremely expensive in Spain and took 30 years to eradicate. This was because of poor biosecurity, *Ornithodorus* ticks, and the presence of wild boar. The study suggested that even in highly dense wild boar populations, such as in the natural parks, ASF circulation cannot be maintained in the absence of other sources of infection. The recent incursion into Russia has shown wild boar affected in Russia, Ukraine, and Lithuania.

ASTROVIRUSES

Astroviruses were found in the feces of wild boar in Hungary.[15]

AUJESKY'S DISEASE

Aujesky's disease virus (ADV) has been found in wild boar in Switzerland.[16,17] Culling of wild boar appeared to have no effect on the presence of ADV.[18] It has now largely disappeared from domestic pigs in Europe.[17,19] However, it was found recently in wild boar in Austria.[20] In Germany, two cases of ADV were reported in 2010 and had central nervous system (CNS) signs and nonsuppurative panencephalitis.[21] It is quite a widespread infection in wild boar in some regions. In wild boar, ADV virus is relatively attenuated, and it may have adapted to coexistence with the specific host population. There is also a wide diversity in the wild boar population. It is probably spread by direct contact and not aerosols, especially over long distances. Currently, oral vaccination for wild boar is not an option, but it has been successful experimentally.[22] Fencing is the main control method. Adequate monitoring is the only real control.

BRUCELLOSIS

The most commonly isolated strain from wild boar in central, eastern, and western Europe is *Brucella suis* biovar 2. It has been found in the Czech Republic, Hungary, Poland, Slovakia, Slovenia and Switzerland,[16,23] and Germany.[24] *B. suis* was found in 28.8% of wild boar, and antibodies were found in 35.8%.[5]

In Croatia, 424 sera from wild boar were looked at in 2003 to 2004,[25] and 27.6% were shown to have seropositivity.

In northeastern Spain, the presence of *Brucella* was studied in wild boar because in Spain the presence of fencing, supplemental feeding, and illegal restocking of wild boar have become common management practices to increase the number of wild boar in an area. They have been bred illegally, crossbred to domestic pigs, or imported, particularly from France.[26] *Brucella* antibodies were detected in 28/256 samples (10.9%).[27] In the United States, spillover from wild boar to domestic pigs has been suspected but never been confirmed (in the United States, there are also bison and elk as a possible source), but strain analysis can help in this situation.[28] In this study, *Brucella* isolates were found in 77% of pigs, and 68% had *B. suis* isolates that were biovar 1, with 92% in males and only 34% in females. The authors also pointed out that wild boar could also be a reservoir for *Brucella abortus* in addition to *B. suis*. In the southeastern United States (South Carolina), wild boar have antibodies to porcine parvovirus (PRV), *B. suis,* and porcine circovirus type 2 (PCV2), but not to Swine Influenza virus (SIV) or porcine reproductive and respiratory syndrome virus (PRRS). In North Carolina there was no PRV or *B. suis,* but 1/20 had PRRS, 86/120 had PCV2, and 9/19 had SIV. In other words, infection in wild and feral pigs can be highly local.

CAMPYLOBACTER SPP.

Campylobacter strains were isolated from feral swine in California following an *Escherichia coli* O157:H7 outbreak associated with spinach. Of the swine samples, 40% were positive, and six species were isolated: *coli, fetus, hyointestinalis, jejuni, lanienae,*[29] and *sputorum.* The study highlighted the need to keep wild animals clear of vegetable crops and highlighted the potential of infecting humans, particularly hunters.

CHLAMYDIAE

A high seroprevalence of Chlamydiaceae has been demonstrated in Spain,[30] but until the report of conjunctivitis and ocular lesions,[31] it was not possible to show diseases related to *Chlamydia.* The affected pig had ulcerations and corneal opacities. The lesions in the wild boar were similar to those seen in experimental infections of commercial pigs.

CLASSICAL SWINE FEVER

In Germany, classical swine fever (CSF) has been present for several decades. The reverse transcription polymerase chain reaction (RT-PCR) has been used to study the evolution to CSF in wild boar.[32] Wild boar were an important source of outbreaks for domestic pigs. Many of the animals were less than 1 year old; thus, the removal of young animals, particularly boar, by hunting reduces the risk of infection. Oral immunization for wild boar was begun in 1993[33] (C-strain bait vaccine[34]) and does help in the control effort.[35] Younger animals are less efficiently vaccinated and are more frequently affected than older boar.[36] Baits may more attractive to older pigs. The optimal vaccination time for pigs is October/November.[37] Increasing the level of baiting does not seem to improve the situation. Baiting is not of great usage in controlling CSF because of low bait usage (62%); however, it does help to describe patterns of feral swine movement, facilitate observation, and improve efficacy.[38]

Most of the previous outbreaks in the wild boar population with high-pathogenicity CSF were largely self-limiting,[39] but morbidity and mortality rates in outbreak regions are high. Recent outbreaks have involved the less damaging genotype 2.3 strains. The change from high to moderate virulence prolonged the virus circulation. It is also possible that monitoring and detection have improved, leading to declining severity following an outbreak rather than selection against a highly virulent virus.

The multiplex RT-PCR can be used to differentiate natural CSF from vaccinated animals,[40] and the marker vaccine is safe.[41] The three outbreaks in northeastern France, between 2002 and 2011, occurred in wild boar and a pig herd in Moselle, and the third occurred in wild boar in the Bas-Rhin area. All were genotype 2.3 and were derived from lineages from the Rhineland–Palatinate lineages in Germany. The Bas-Rhin outbreak lasted until 2007, and the virus evolved slightly over this period.[83]

CRYPTOSPORIDIA

Two species of *Cryptosporidia, C. suis* and *C. scrofarum,* were described in wild boar in central Europe (Austria, Czech Republic, Poland, and the Slovak Republic). In none of the detected cases was clinical disease found. In most cases the infections were single, but in some both species were found together. The PCR was a better detection method than the microscopic.[81]

ESCHERICHIA COLI

E. coli O157:H7 was found in feral swine in central California near spinach fields responsible for disease outbreaks.[42] Not much is known about *E. coli* in wild boar, but it appears to be individual and diverse. In a study in central Europe, it was found that wild boar carried antimicrobial-resistant *E. coli* in their feces. In the wild boar, the level of resistance was 6%. Five multiresistant isolates producing extended-spectrum beta-lactamase (ESBL) were recovered from the wild boar.[89] The detection and characterization of O157:H7 and non-O157 Shiga-toxin-producing *E. coli* in wild boars have been described in wild boar in Spain.[90]

ERYSIPELAS

In Iberian wild boar the prevalence was 15%,[18] and infection has been described in Spain.[27]

FASCIOLA HEPATICA

The *Fasciola hepatica* parasite has recently been found in a feral wild boar in Scotland,[43] although it has been described previously in feral Nebrodi black pigs in Sicily, Italy.[44] Occasionally the flukes are found to be adults in the liver, although the pig is considered resistant to the development of liver fluke.

FOOT-AND-MOUTH DISEASE

Contact with the virus in cattle occurs most commonly at water courses for feral and wild boar.[45]

HEPATITIS E

Hepatitis E (Hep E) in humans is thought to be associated with eating raw pig meat or wild boar, particularly liver. Hunting is associated with a higher prevalence[46-48] of antibodies in humans. Wild boars in southeastern France may be a source of infection for humans.[46]

There is a high seroprevalence of antibodies to Hep E in forestry workers (31%) and wild boars (14%) in France[49] and in Iberian wild boars.[50] The wild boar prevalence is related to the geographic location. In Italy, there were seropositive wild boar.[51] In Germany, the prevalence in wild boars was studied using liver samples from wild boar, and 14.9% were found to be positive.[52,53] A further study in Germany showed a 29.9% prevalence, but it varied considerably between the regions that were analyzed. All the isolates were genotype 3 (3i, 3h, 3f, and 3e), but the type depended on the hunting spot.[54] It was found in all areas and all regions but more frequently in rural areas. There were three sources of infection: hunting, wild boar meat, and fecal contamination. Even in Japan there is a risk from wild boars.[55] In Spain, 28% of wild boar tested were found to be positive[56] and 12% in the Netherlands.[57] It was found in Croatia,[58] Czechoslovakia,[59] and Sweden.[60] Within these overall prevalence rates, there is evidence of quite high local prevalence rates.[61] The suspicion is that wild boar infection may spill over into the domestic pig population and then into the human population, but there is no proof that this happens.[62] Several studies in Germany have shown hepatitis E virus (HEV) genotype 3 within the wild boar population and in domestic pigs.[52-54,96,97]

LEPTOSPIRA SPP.

In wild boar, antibodies to *Leptospira* spp. and leptospiral cells have been seen,[63] and they have been detected in Japan.[64,65] Wild boars (15.2%) were found to carry *Leptospira* more commonly than deer, although cases in both have increased rapidly in Japan in recent years. The supposition is that they wallow in the mud to keep cool and can get infected under these conditions. The suggestion is that wild boar leptospires may prove a hazard to hunters, meat-processing workers, and hunting dogs in Japan. A study in Swedish wild boar suggested that the infection was much less common than in the rest of Europe.[66] In Poland, the level of antibodies detected was 25%, in Germany it was 18%, and in Italy it was 12%.

LYMPHADENITIS

In a study of lymphadenitis in wild boar in Brazil, β-hemolytic streptococci (10%), *Mycobacterium* spp. (8.4%), and *Rhodococcus equi* (6.6%) were the most common cause of lesions.[67]

MYCOBACTERIUM BOVIS

The risk of infection in wild boar is age dependent and correlates with abundance and spatial aggregation.[9] In some parts of Spain, the wild boar is a maximum risk for domestic pigs.[1] In south-central Spain, wild boar tuberculosis (TB) may be the main driver of bovine TB. Culling of 50% of the population of European wild boar (*Sus scrofa*) in south-central Spain showed that *M. bovis* reduced by 21% to 48%. In Portugal, in the 2005 to 2006 hunting season, 18/162 wild boars from 3/8 study areas were positive for *M. bovis.*[68] Detection of *M. bovis* was most consistently associated with variables linked to the wild ungulate's relative abundance; thus, wild boar may be a reservoir for *M. bovis.*

In New Zealand, the transmission of *M. bovis* to cattle occurs through the reservoir of the bush-tailed possum. In those areas where control of the possum was carried out, the level of *M. bovis* in the feral pigs was reduced. The feral pigs do not seem to pass the disease to other pigs.[69] Data from Corsica suggest that wild and domestic animals are in an epidemiologic bovine tuberculosis (bTB) transmission cycle.[70]

Experimental infection of wild boar with *M. avium* subsp. *avium* has been carried out and was similar to the natural disease.[71] The lesions in wild boar are frequently in the thoracic lymph nodes and lungs, suggesting that respiratory infection occurs. In the Iberian Peninsula, it may well be that the wild boar contribute to the persistence of the infection in domestic pigs, depending on the size of the local population.[82] *M. bovis* was first isolated from a feral wild boar in the United Kingdom in 2010,[86] although it had been isolated from farmed wild boar previously; there are now several pockets of wild boar in the United Kingdom countryside. Many lymph nodes, particularly the mandibular, retropharyngeal, and mesenteric, were affected. There was a granulomatous lymphadenitis with small numbers of acid-fast bacteria. Spoligotype 17 was identified and is also found in other wildlife in the area.

The immunopathology of granulomas in naturally infected wild boar has been described.[87] In wild boar, the pattern of infection is contained, not generalized. The majority of granulomas did not have any acid-fast bacteria, and only a few had multinucleate giant cells.

There was a large presence of T cells and macrophages exhibiting a high level of interferon gamma (IFN-γ) activity at all stages of granuloma development. A high level of nitric oxide production from macrophages was also found.

The influence of PCV2 on bTB in wild boar populations has been studied.[88] In Spain, two of the risk factors for TB in wild boar include the density of the population and the age of the boar. The role of other pathogens has not been investigated. The presence of bTB in 551 hunted wild boar from southwestern Spain was studied. A statistical relationship was found between the prevalence rates of bTB and PCV2. Where PCV2 was highest, so was the occurrence of bTB. Wild boar with PCV2 were also more likely to have generalized lesions.

In a recent study in the United Kingdom of the hotspots for *M. bovis* infections, it was found that infected pigs were found on farms where there was poor biosecurity or where the animals were raised outdoors. In some cases, the strains found in pigs correlated better with the strains found in badgers rather than in cattle, suggesting that pigs could be a sentinel for detecting *M. bovis* in wildlife.[91]

In Spain, the intradermal bovine tuberculin test in wild boar was only approximately 77.4% effective (24/31). The enzyme-linked immunoabsorbent assay (ELISA) has been used more recently and may give a better result in wild boar.[98] Wild boar can act as maintenance hosts,[99] but they are usually regarded as a "dead-end" host.[100] A number of other species of *Mycobacteria* other than *M. bovis* and *M. avium* have been found in domestic pigs and wild boar in Brazil.[101]

MYCOPLASMA HYOPNEUMONIAE

Mycoplasma hyopneumoniae (MH) is common in Swiss wild boar,[72] as detected by RT-PCR. There was little information on enzootic pneumonia (EP) in wild boar until the study in Spain in 2010,[102] which showed that antibodies were detected in 21% of 428 serum samples and in 20% of nasal swabs. MH was detected by nested polymerase chain reaction (nPCR) and in 8% (of 156) of lung samples. No gross lesions were seen in any of the pigs, but histologic lesions were seen in 18 of 63 (29%) of lung samples. The conclusion was that the EP lesions were likely to be subclinical.

PARASITES

Over 30 species of parasites have been found in wild boars (in particular, flukes, tapeworms, and nematodes are included in this list).

PORCINE CIRCOVIRUS TYPE 2

PCV2 has a variable prevalence in Europe, but there is a high prevalence in Spain in Iberian wild boar[50] and in Romania.[73,92-94] In Germany, only 0.3% of wild boar were positive compared with 8.7% of domestic pigs.[74] The wild boar had much lower levels of PCV2 load than domestic pigs.

In a study in Korea, the prevalence of PCV2 infection was found to be 4.98% (91/1825).[95] The PCV2 ORF2 sequences belonged solely to subgroups 1A/B and 1C of the PCV2b genotype.

PORCINE PARVOVIRUS

Porcine parvovirus (PPV) is widespread in wild boar (14% to 77%) depending on the country but does not seem to cause lesions, although it may cause problems to wild boar sows in their first pregnancy in midgestation. The forces that drive the evolution of PPV are unknown. However, it appears that in the presence of antibodies, the neutral selection seems to be more important than adaptive evolution.[103] In wild boar populations, phylogenetic analysis has revealed that PPV is more diverse than in domestic pigs.[104] Thus, wild boar populations may have played a vital part in the emergence of new PPV phenotypes.

PORCINE REPRODUCTIVE AND RESPIRATORY SYNDROME

In Spain there was a low prevalence of porcine reproductive and respiratory syndrome (PRRS) in wild boar,[18] whereas in Italy[13] and Germany it was quite high,[61] but it is probably not a reservoir status.[27] In China, high-pathogenicity PRRS may be transmitted in hybrid wild boar.[6]

PORCINE SAPELOVIRUS

Porcine sapelovirus type 1 (PSV1) has recently been isolated from a wild boar in Japan. It was formerly known as porcine enterovirus A.[105]

SALMONELLA SEROTYPES

Wild boar in northern Italy[75] (1313 boars) were examined, and 326 salmonellae were isolated (24.8%). Thirty different serovars were isolated from three different *Salmonella enterica* spp.

In a study of wild boars in the Latium region of Italy, 10.8% were positive; many serovars were, found but *S. typhimurium* was only found in 1.8%. The most important point was that most of these salmonellae carried resistance genes, particularly to sulfonamides (92.5%) sulfonamide–trimethoprim (14.8%), colistin (14.8%), and streptomycin (18.5%), with the others at much lower levels.[85]

Wild boars may act as healthy carriers of a wide range of *Salmonella* species.[76] In a study in Australia of an isolated wild boar population, it was found that there were *Salmonella* spp. in 36.3% of fecal samples and 11.9% of mesenteric lymph nodes.[77] Thirty-nine serovars were found (29 in feces and 24 in the lymph nodes). The transmission is from old to young pigs, possibly through the water features.

Wild boar in Spain, northern Italy, Portugal, and Slovenia[84] have also been found to be seropositive or have had the organism isolated from wild boar populations.

SWINE INFLUENZA

A survey in the United States showed wide state-to-state variation, with up to 14.4% positive for H3N2 inTexas[106] and with higher prevalence levels in the Carolinas.[107] In a recent survey, 2% were positive for H1 and 40% for H3.[108] In Germany, 5.2% of pigs had antibodies to both H1N1 and H3N2.[109]

TOXOPLASMA

A case of congenital toxoplasmosis has been described in a wild boar from Spain.[79] The histopathologic results suggest that the shot sow and her three fetuses all had toxoplasmosis. Myositis was found in many samples and interstitial pneumonia in the fetuses. The absence of cysts is consistent with the experimental infection reported in pigs.[80] The parasite was detected by PCR in nearly all the tissues.

TRICHINELLA

Trichinella has been found in wild boar in Corsica,[78] where the muscle antibody ELISA was positive. It necessitates proper veterinary controls on wild boar meat and proper cooking of meat.

CONTROL

Tight biosecurity to separate wild boar from domestic pigs is essential to prevent the incursion of disease into the domestic pig herds. Fencing of water tanks is something that is not normally considered, but it should be with wild boar. You can raise water tanks and thus cattle can drink but wild pigs cannot. Similarly, feeding deer with corn also attracts feral pigs.

REFERENCES

1. Naranjo V, et al. *Vet Microbiol.* 2008;127:1.
2. Ruis-Fons F, et al. *Eur J Wildl Dis.* 2008;54:549.
3. Munoz P, et al. *BMC Infect Dis.* 2010;10:46.
4. Ruis-Fons F, et al. *Vet J.* 2008;176:158.
5. Wu N, et al. *J Wildl Dis.* 2011;47:868.
6. Wu J, et al. *J Virol.* 2012;86:13882.
7. Hartley M, et al. *Eur J Vet Res.* 2010;56:401.
8. Meng XJ, Lindsay DS. *Philos Trans R Soc Lond B Biol Sci.* 2009;364:2697.
9. Acevedo P, et al. *Epidemiol Infect.* 2007;135:519.
10. Gortazar C, et al. *PLoS ONE.* 2010;3:7.
11. Lavelle MJ, et al. *J Wildl Manage.* 2012;75:1200.
12. Halli O, et al. *Vet J.* 2012;194:98.
13. Montagnaro S, et al. *J Wildl Dis.* 2010;46:316.
14. Mur L, et al. *Transbound Emerg Dis.* 2012;59:526.
15. Reuter G, et al. *Arch Virol.* 2012;157:1143.
16. Koppel C, et al. *Eur J Wildl Res.* 2007;58:212.
17. Muller T, et al. *Arch Virol.* 2011;156:1691.
18. Boadella M, et al. *Prev Vet Med.* 2012;107:214.
19. Muller T, et al. *Epidemiol Infect.* 2010;138:1590.
20. Steinriel A, et al. *Vet Microbiol.* 2012;157:276.
21. Schultze C, et al. *Berl Munch Tierartzl Wschr.* 2010;123:359.
22. Maresch C, et al. *Vet Microbiol.* 2012;161:20.
23. Leuenberger R, et al. *Vet Rec.* 2007;160:362.
24. Metzel E, et al. *Eur J Wildl Res.* 2007;58:153.
25. Wu N, et al. *J Wildl Dis.* 2011;47:868.
26. Cvetnic Z, et al. *Rev Sci Tech Off Int Epiz.* 2009;28:1057.
27. Closa-Sebastia F, et al. *Eur J Wildl Res.* 2011;57:977.
28. Stoffregen WC, et al. *J Vet Diag Invest.* 2007;19:227.
29. Scweitzer N, et al. *Foodborne Pathogen Dis.* 2011;8:615.
30. Salinas J, et al. *Vet Microbiol.* 2009;135:46.
31. Riso D, et al. *J Zoo Wildl Med.* 2013;44:159.
32. Depner K, et al. *J Vet Res B.* 2006;53:317.
33. Ballesteros C, et al. *Prev Vet Med.* 2011;98:198.
34. Kaden V, et al. *Rev - Off Int Epizoot.* 2008;25:989.
35. Rossi S, et al. *Vet Microbiol.* 2010;142:99.
36. Rossi S, et al. *Vet Microbiol.* 2010;142:99.
37. Ruden S, et al. *Vet Microbiol.* 2008;132:2938.
38. Campbell TA, et al. *Prev Vet Med.* 2012;104:249.
39. Lange M, et al. *Prev Vet Med.* 2012;106:185.
40. Blome S, et al. *Vet Microbiol.* 2011;153:373.
41. Koenig P, et al. *Vaccine.* 2007;25:3391.
42. Jay MT, et al. *Emerg Infect Dis.* 2008;13:1908.
43. Thompson H, et al. *Vet Rec.* 2009;165:697.
44. Capucchio MT, et al. *Vet Paras.* 2009;159:37.
45. Cooper SM, et al. *J Wildl Dis.* 2010;46:152.
46. Kaba M, et al. *Vet J.* 2010;186:259.
47. Kim Y, et al. *J Clin Virol.* 2011;50:253.
48. Mansuy JM, et al. *J Clin Virol.* 2009;44:74.
49. Carpentier A, et al. *J Clin Path.* 2012;50:2888.
50. Boadella M, et al. *Transbound Emerg Dis.* 2012;58:39549.
51. Martelli P, et al. *Vet Microbiol.* 2008;126:74.
52 Schielke A, et al. *Virology J.* 2012;6:58.
53. Kaci S, et al. *Vet Microbiol.* 2008;128:380.
54. Adlhoch C, et al. *Vet Microbiol.* 2009;139:270.
55. Toyoda K, et al. *Jap J Gastro Hepat.* 2008;23:1885.
56. de Deus N, et al. *Vet Microbiol.* 2008;129:163.
57. Rutjes SA, et al. *J Virol Methods.* 2010;168:197.
58. Jemersic L, et al. *Ecohealth.* 2011;7(suppl 1):S144.
59. Sedlak K, et al. *J Wildl Dis.* 2008;44:777.
60. Widen F, et al. *Epidemiol Infect.* 2011;139:361.
61. Reiner GC, et al. *Vet Microbiol.* 2009;145:1.
62. Wichmann O, et al. *J Infect Dis.* 2008;198:172.
63. Jansen A, et al. *Emerg Infect Dis.* 2007;13:739.
64. Koizumi N, et al. *Jap J Infect Dis.* 2008;61:465.
65. Koizumi N, et al. *J Vet Med Sci.* 2009;71:797.
66. Boqvist S, et al. *J Wildl Dis.* 2012;48:492.
67. Lara GH, et al. *Res Vet Sci.* 2011;90:185.
68. Santos N, et al. *J Wildl Dis.* 2009;45:1048.
69. Nugent G, et al. *Epidemiol Infect.* 2012;140:1036.
70. Richomme C, et al. *J Wildl Dis.* 2010;46:627.
71. Garrida JM, et al. *Vet Microbiol.* 2010;144:240.
72. Kuhnert P, et al. *Vet Microbiol.* 2009;152:191.
73. Turcitu MA, et al. *Res Vet Sci.* 2011;91:e103.
74. Reiner G, et al. *Vet Microbiol.* 2010;145:1.
75. Chiari M, et al. *Acta Vet Scand.* 2013;55:42.
76. Wachek S, et al. *Foodborne Pathog.* 2010;7:307.
77. Ward MP, et al. *Vet Microbiol.* 2013;162:921.
78. Richomme C, et al. *Vet Parasitol.* 2010;172:150.
79. Calero-Bernal R, et al. *J Wildl Dis.* 2013;49:1019.
80. Garcia JL, et al. *Exp Parasitol.* 2006;113:267.
81. Nemejc K, et al. *Vet Parasitol.* 2013;197:504.
82. Gortazar C, et al. *Mammal Rev.* 2012;42:193.
83. Simon G, et al. *Vet Microbiol.* 2013;166:631.
84. Vengust G, et al. *J Vet Med B.* 2006;53:24.
85. Zottola T, et al. *Comp Immunol Microbiol Infect Dis.* 2013;36:161.
86. Foyle KL, Delahay RJ. *Vet Rec.* 2010;doi:10.1136/vr.c2681.
87. Garcia-Jiminez WL, et al. *Vet Immunol Immunopathol.* 2013;156:54.
88. Risco D, et al. *Transbound Emerg Dis.* 2013;60(suppl 1):121.
89. Literak I, et al. *J Appl Microbiol.* 2009;108:1702.
90. Sanchez S, et al. *Vet Microbiol.* 2010;143:420.
91. Bailey SS, et al. *Vet J.* 2013;198:391.
92. Cadar D, et al. *Acta Vet Hung.* 2010;58:475.
93. Cadar D, et al. *Virus Genes.* 2011;43:376.
94. Cadar D, et al. *Infect Genet Evol.* 2012;12:420.
95. An D-J, et al. *Vet Microbiol.* 2014;169:147.
96. Baechlein C, et al. *Berl Munch Tierartzl Wschr.* 2013;126:25.
97. Wenzel JJ, et al. *J Clin Virol.* 2011;52:50.
98. Boadella M, et al. *J Vet Diag Invest.* 2011;23:77.
99. Naranjo V, et al. *Vet Microbiol.* 2008;127:1.
100. Corner LA. *Vet Microbiol.* 2006;112:303.
101. Lara GH, et al. *Res Vet Sci.* 2011;90:185.

102. Sibila M, et al. *Vet Microbiol.* 2010;144:214.
103. Streck AF, et al. *J Gen Virol.* 2013;94:2050.
104. Cadar D, et al. *Infect Genet Evol.* 2012;12:1163.
105. Abe M, et al. *Virus Genes.* 2011;doi:10.1007/s11262-011-0628-2.
106. Hall JS, et al. *J Wildl Dis.* 2008;44:362.
107. Corn JL, et al. *J Wildl Dis.* 2009;45:713.
108. Baker SR, et al. *Vet Rec.* 2011;168:564.
109. Kaden V, et al. *Vet Microbiol.* 2008;131:123.

Multi-Organ Diseases Due to Bacterial Infection

ANTHRAX

SYNOPSIS

Etiology *Bacillus anthracis.*

Epidemiology Global occurrence and often occurs as outbreaks. Spores survive in soil for many years and disease is enzootic in certain areas. Pastoral outbreaks associated with periods of climatic extremes. Outbreaks also associated with infected feedstuffs.

Clinical findings Ruminants and horses—acute/peracute disease characterized by fever, septicemia, and sudden death. This may be accompanied by subcutaneous edematous swellings in horses. More prolonged disease with cellulitis of the neck and throat in swine.

Clinical pathology Because of risk for human exposure hematology and blood chemistry are not performed. Demonstration of organism in blood or subcutaneous fluid.

Necropsy findings Carcass should not be opened if anthrax suspected; the diagnosis is made from the examination of aspirated carcass blood. Exudation of tarry blood from the body orifices of the cadaver, failure of the blood to clot, absence of rigor mortis and the presence of splenomegaly.

Diagnostic confirmation Identification of organism in blood or tissues by polychrome methylene blue stain of smear or by monoclonal antibody-fluorescent conjugates. Culture, Ascoli test, polymerase chain reaction (PCR).

Treatment Antibiotics, antiserum.

Control Prevention of further spread. Vaccination.

ETIOLOGY

Bacillus anthracis, a gram-positive, rod-shaped, aerobic, immobile, capsulated, spore-forming bacterium belonging to the family Bacillacae is the causative agent of the disease.[1] Although the vegetative form of *B. anthracis* is not very robust, the spores persist in the environment for decades, easily withstand cold temperatures, and even survive in dried and salted hides. Sporulation occurs with exposure of the bacillus to free oxygen, which is the case when it is shed from the host organism into the environment. Although ingested spores readily return to the vegetative state once the host organism is infected, the vegetative form is practically not encountered in the environment. Sporulation of *B. anthracis* requires an environmental temperature range between 12° and 42° C (53–107° F) and does not occur at temperatures below 9° to 12° C (48–53° F).[2]

EPIDEMIOLOGY

Occurrence

Anthrax is a disease known since ancient times. It probably originated in sub-Saharan Africa and has spread to have a worldwide distribution. During the late nineteenth and early twentieth centuries, anthrax was the infectious disease with the highest case-fatality rate in domestic and wild animals. For instance, in 1923 an anthrax outbreak in South Africa was responsible for the death of an estimated 60,000 animals. The development of the so-called **Sterne vaccine** and the discovery of antibiotics in the middle of the last century provided effective tools to control the disease, which has lost its importance in large parts of the world since then. In recent years, anthrax received increased attention because it is a **potential agent of bioterrorism**. The reality of this threat became apparent after a bioterrorist attack in the fall of 2001 in the United States, when five letters sent by mail containing small amounts anthrax spores contaminated more than 30,000 people, killed 5 people, and infected 17.[3]

Currently anthrax is a sporadic disease in western Europe, North America, and Australia, although there are regions in these parts of the world where the disease remains enzootic. Such areas include specific zones in the North-Western Territories and Alberta in Canada and in eastern North and South Dakota, northwest Minnesota, and southwest Texas in the United States.[1] Anthrax is essentially absent from northern and central **Europe** but remains enzootic in Greece, Turkey, Spain, southern Italy, and Albania. The disease also persists in certain countries of **Latin America,** such as Bolivia, Peru, and Mexico, and is enzootic in Haiti. Endemic regions of **Asia** include the Philippines, South Korea, eastern India, the mountainous region of western China, and Mongolia.[1]

In tropical and subtropical climates with high annual rainfalls, the infection persists in the soil, and thus frequent, serious outbreaks of anthrax are commonly encountered. In some **African countries** the disease occurs every summer and reaches a devastating occurrence rate in years with a heavy rainfall. Wild fauna—including hippos, cape buffalo, and elephants—die in large numbers.

In **temperate, cool climates** only sporadic outbreaks derive from the soil-borne infection. Accidental ingestion of contaminated bone meal or pasture contaminated by tannery effluent are more common sources. In this circumstance outbreaks are few, and the number of animals affected is small.

Source of the Infection

Infection can occur directly from the soil or from fodder grown on infected soil, from contaminated bone meal or protein concentrates, or from infected excreta, blood, or other discharges from infected animals. The initial source is often from old anthrax graves where the soil has been disturbed.

Spread of the organism within an area may be accomplished by streams, insects, dogs, feral pigs, and other carnivores, and by fecal contamination from infected animals and birds. Avian scavengers such as gulls, vultures, and ravens can carry spores over considerable distances, and the feces of carrion-eating birds can contaminate waterholes. Infected wildlife is also a source for domestic animals on common grazing land. Water can be contaminated by the effluent from tanneries, from infected carcasses, and by flooding and the deposition of anthrax-infected soil.

Introduction of infection into a new area is usually through contaminated animal products, such as bone meal, fertilizers, hides, hair, and wool, or by contaminated concentrates or forage. This form of transmission presents a particular danger because it can cause clinical disease silently anywhere, even where anthrax is unknown, and at any time of the year.[1] In recent years as many as 50% of consignments of bone meal imported into the United Kingdom have been shown to be contaminated with the anthrax bacillus. Outbreaks in pigs can usually be traced to the ingestion of infected bone meal or carcasses.

Transmission of the Infection

Infection gains entrance to the body by ingestion, inhalation, or through the skin. Although the exact mode of infection is often in doubt, it is generally considered that most animals are infected by the ingestion of contaminated food or water. Microwounds of the mucous membrane of the digestive are thought to serve as portal of entry for *B. anthracis.* The increased incidence of the disease on sparse pasture is thought to be attributable to both the ingestion of contaminated soil and to injury to the oral mucosa facilitating invasion by the organism.

Inhalation infection is thought to be of minor importance in animals, although the possibility of infection through contaminated dust must always be considered.[2] It has been proposed that inhalation of spores can lead to some sort of chronic carriage, with onset of disease any time after inhalation.[2] "Woolsorter's disease" in humans is a result of the inhalation of anthrax spores by workers in the wool and hair industries, but even in these industries cutaneous anthrax is much more common.

Biting flies, mosquitoes, ticks, and other insects have often been found to harbor anthrax organisms, and the ability of some to transmit the infection has been demonstrated experimentally. However, there is little evidence that they are important in the spread of naturally occurring disease, with the exception of tabanid flies. The transmission is mechanical only, and a local inflammatory reaction is evident at the site of the bite. The tendency, in infected districts, for the heaviest incidence to occur in the late summer and autumn may be a result of the increase in the fly population at that time, but an effect of higher temperature on vegetative proliferation of *B. anthracis* in the soil is more likely.

An outbreak of anthrax has been recorded following the injection of infected blood for the purpose of immunization against anaplasmosis. There have been a number of reports of the occurrence of anthrax after vaccination, probably as a result of inadequately attenuated spores. Wound infection with *B. anthracis* occurs occasionally.

Risk Factors

Host Risk Factors

The disease occurs in all vertebrates but is most common in cattle and sheep and less frequent in goats and horses. Humans occupy an intermediate position between this group and the relatively resistant pigs, dogs, and cats. In farm animals, the disease is almost invariably fatal, except in pigs, and even in this species the case-fatality rate is high.

Algerian sheep are reported to be resistant and, within all species, certain individuals seem to possess sufficient immunity to resist natural exposure. Whether or not this immunity has a genetic basis has not been determined. The most interesting example of natural resistance is the dwarf pig, in which it is impossible to establish the disease. Spores remain in tissues ungerminated, and there is complete clearance from all organs by 48 hours. The ability to prevent spore germination appears to be inherited in this species.

Pathogen Risk Factors

Pathogenic strains of *B. anthracis* possess two important virulence factors: the **capsule** and the **toxin complex,** consisting of **three proteins known as protective antigen (PA), lethal factor (LF),** and **edema factor (EF).** These virulence factors are encoded in two plasmids, pXO1 (encoding PA, LF and EF) and pXO2 (encoding the capsule). Both plasmids are required for full virulence.

The ability of the bacillus to establish itself in the tissues of the host was found to be inherently dependent on the possession of a capsule. Variants of *B. anthracis* having lost the capsule were also found to have lost their virulence.[4] Although the presence of this polypeptide capsule was found to be an important factor allowing the bacterium to multiply within the host, its precise mechanism of action is not entirely understood.[2] It was long held that its primary function was to discourage the phagocytic activity of lymphocytes and to neutralize anthracidal substances normally present in tissue, but this is not supported by results of more recent in vitro studies.[2] In any case, the capsule appears to facilitate the evasion of the bacillus from the host's immune system, possibly also by protecting surface antigens of the bacterium from exposure to antibodies.

As noted, the **anthrax toxin complex** consists of three synergistically acting proteins: **PA**, **LF**, and **edema factor (EF)**. Whereas independently each of these proteins is innocuous, the combination of them provokes death in infected animals. PA appears to be important for the binding to specific target cells and the introduction of LF and EF into these target cells. EF is an adenylate cyclase that triggers the abnormal production of cyclic-AMP, causing altered ion and water movement and thereby resulting in the edema formation that is characteristic of anthrax.[2] Alteration of the c-AMP signaling pathways was shown to disturb activation of immune cells. LF is a zinc-dependent protease that disrupts regulatory pathways in eukaryotic cells associated with phosphorylation. The mechanism through which this disruption leads to the known effects of LF remains to be fully determined.

Environment Risk Factors

Outbreaks originating from a soil-borne infection always occur after a major climate change, for example, heavy rain after a prolonged drought or dry summer months after prolonged rain, and always in warm weather when the environmental temperature is over 15°C (60°F). Sporulation of the vegetative state of *B. anthracis* shed into the environment rapidly occurs with environmental temperatures above 12°C (53°F), and thus vegetative bacilli are practically not found in the environment.[5] It has been proposed that spores may collect and concentrate in so-called storage areas. Spores have a high surface hydrophobicity, giving them a tendency to clump, become concentrated, and remain suspended in standing water, with f urther concentration on the soil surface as the water evaporates. This relationship to climate has made it possible to predict "anthrax years."

Other risk factors in the environment include close grazing of tough, scratchy feed in dry times, which results in abrasions of the oral mucosa, and confined grazing on heavily contaminated areas around water holes. Some genotypes appear to persist better in calcium-rich soils and organic soils, and poorly drained soils have risk in endemic areas.

Economic Importance

In most developed countries, vaccination of susceptible animals in enzootic areas has reduced the prevalence of the disease to negligible proportions on a national basis, but heavy losses may still occur in individual herds. Loss occurs as a result of mortality but also from withholding of milk in infected dairy herds and for a period following vaccination.

Zoonotic Potential

Anthrax has been an important cause of fatal human illness in most parts of the world, but in developed countries it is no longer a significant cause of human or livestock wastage because of appropriate control measures. However, it still holds an important position because of its potential as a zoonosis, and it is still an important zoonosis in developing countries. It is a **major concern as an agent of bioterrorism** and is listed as a category A agent by the U.S. Centers for Disease Control and Prevention.

An account of an outbreak in a piggery in the United Kingdom should be compulsory reading for veterinary students as an example of the responsibilities of veterinarians in a modern public-health-conscious and litigation-minded community.[6,7] In developing countries, anthrax can still be a major cause of livestock losses and a serious cause of mortality among humans who eat meat from infected animals and develop the alimentary form of this disease, or those who handle infected carcasses.

Cutaneous anthrax has occurred in veterinarians following postmortem examination of anthrax carcasses. The areas at particular risk for infection are the forearm above the glove line and the neck. Infection begins as a pruritic papule or vesicle that enlarges and erodes in 1 to 2 days, leaving a necrotic ulcer with subsequent formation of a central black eschar.

PATHOGENESIS

Upon ingestion of the spores, infection may occur through defects or microwounds of the mucosa of the digestive tract. Alternatively, infection can occur through skin abrasions or skin lesions (e.g., from biting flies) or inhalation of spores.

From the site of entry spores are transported by macrophages to the regional lymph nodes, where they can enter the bloodstream and spread throughout the rest of the organism; septicemia, with massive invasion of all body tissues, follows.

The severity of the clinical signs depends on the infectious dose, the quality of the bacillary capsule, the amount of toxin produced, and the susceptibility of the host species. The previously mentioned toxin complex produced by *B. anthracis* causes edema and tissue damage, acute renal failure, terminal anoxia, and death resulting from shock. The characteristic terminal hemorrhage to the exterior from orifices of the animal at death is caused by the action of the toxin on the endothelial cell lining of blood vessels, resulting in breakdown and bleeding.[2]

In pigs, localization occurs in the lymph nodes of the throat after invasion through the upper part of the digestive tract. Local lesions usually eventually lead to a fatal septicemia.

CLINICAL FINDINGS

The incubation period after field infection is not easy to determine but is probably 1 to 2 weeks.

Cattle and Sheep

The disease occurs in a peracute and acute form in cattle and sheep.

The **peracute** form of the disease is most common at the beginning of an outbreak. The animals are usually found dead without premonitory signs, the course being probably only 1 to 2 hours, but fever, muscle tremor, dyspnea, and congestion of the mucosae may be observed. The animal soon collapses, and it dies after terminal convulsions. After death, discharges of blood from the nostrils, mouth, anus, and vulva can occur.

The **acute** form runs a course of about 48 hours. Severe depression and listlessness are usually observed first, although they are sometimes preceded by a short period of excitement. The body temperature is high, up to 42°C (107°F), the respiration rapid and deep, the mucosae congested and hemorrhagic, and the heart rate much increased. No food is taken, and ruminal stasis is evident. Pregnant cows may abort. In milking cows, the yield is very much reduced, and the milk may be bloodstained or deep yellow in color. Alimentary tract involvement is usual and is characterized by diarrhea and dysentery. Local edema of the tongue and edematous lesions in the region of the throat, sternum, perineum, and flanks may occur.

Pigs

In pigs, anthrax may be acute or subacute. There is fever, with dullness and anorexia, and a characteristic inflammatory edema of the throat and face. The swellings are hot but not painful and may cause obstruction to swallowing and respiration. Bloodstained froth may be present at the mouth when pharyngeal involvement occurs. Petechial hemorrhages are present in the skin, and when localization occurs in the intestinal wall, there is dysentery, often without edema of the throat. A pulmonary form of the disease has been observed in baby pigs that inhaled infected dust. Lobar pneumonia and exudative pleurisy were characteristic. Death usually occurs after a course of 12 to 36 hours, although individual cases may linger for several days.

Horses

Anthrax in the horse is always acute but varies in its manifestations with the mode of infection. When infection is by ingestion, there is septicemia with enteritis and colic. When infection is by insect transmission, hot, painful, edematous, subcutaneous swellings appear about the throat, lower neck, floor of the thorax and abdomen, prepuce, and mammary gland. There is high fever and severe depression, and there may be dyspnea as a result of swelling of the throat or colic as a result of intestinal irritation. The course is usually 48 to 96 hours.

CLINICAL PATHOLOGY

Hematology and blood chemistry examinations are not conducted because of the risk for human exposure. In the living animal the organism may be detected in a stained smear of peripheral blood. The **reference standard** for diagnosis is the detection, by **microscopic examination**, of a clearly defined metachromatic capsule on square-ended bacilli (often in chains) in a blood smear stained with polychrome methylene blue. The blood should be carefully collected in a syringe to avoid contamination of the environment. When local edema is evident, smears may be made from aspirated edema fluid or from lymph nodes that drain that area. For a more certain diagnosis, especially in the early stages when bacilli may not be present in the bloodstream in great numbers, blood culture or the injection of syringe-collected blood into guinea pigs is satisfactory.

Fluorescent antibody techniques are available for use on blood smears and tissue sections. Monoclonal antibodies are also used to provide specific identification of anthrax organisms.

The Ascoli test can be used to demonstrate antigen in severely decayed tissue samples, and a nested PCR technique has been used to demonstrate antigen in environmental samples; PCR methods can also be used to confirm the identity of bacterial isolates. If other detection methods fail, experimental animal inoculation can be attempted.

As the carcass decomposes and the vegetative forms of *B. anthracis* die, diagnosis by smear is more difficult; an immunochromatographic test for antigen has been developed that has high specificity and does not give positive results in recently vaccinated cattle. In cases where antibiotic therapy has been used, the identification from blood smears or culture may be difficult, and animal passage may be necessary.

Because antibodies develop in the late stage of disease serology will be of use only for retrospectives studies and only in species with low susceptibility to *B. anthracis,* such as pigs. In these cases acute and reconvalescent sera can be assayed for their antibody titer by means of an ELISA.

Shipping infectious material presents risk for spread of the pathogen and human exposure. Before planning to ship infectious material to a diagnostic laboratory, local authorities and the diagnostic laboratory should be consulted. The reader is furthermore referred to the guidelines of the World Health Organization (WHO) for the transport of infectious substances.[8]

NECROPSY FINDINGS

There is a striking absence of rigor mortis, and the carcass undergoes gaseous decomposition, quickly assuming the characteristic "sawhorse" posture. All natural orifices usually exude dark, tarry blood that does not clot. **If there is a good reason to suspect the existence of anthrax, the carcass should not be opened.** If a necropsy is carried out, the failure of the blood to clot, widespread ecchymoses, bloodstained serous fluid in the body cavities, severe enteritis, and splenomegaly are strong indications of the presence of anthrax. The enlarged spleen is soft, with a consistency likened to blackberry jam. Subcutaneous swellings containing gelatinous material and enlargement of the local lymph nodes are features of the disease in horses and pigs. Lesions are most frequently seen in the **soft tissues of the neck and pharynx** in these species.

To confirm the diagnosis on an **unopened carcass**, peripheral blood or local edema fluid should be collected by needle puncture. Because the blood clots poorly, jugular venipuncture may permit sample collection. Smears prepared from these fluids should be stained with polychrome methylene blue and examined. These fluid samples can also be used for bacteriologic culture if smear results are equivocal. The smears should be prepared and interpreted by an experienced and qualified microbiologist.

If decomposition of a carcass is advanced, a small quantity of blood may be collected from the fresh surface of an amputated tail or ear. A portion of spleen is the specimen of choice for bacteriologic culture if the carcass has been opened.

Anthrax is a **reportable disease** in many countries, requiring the involvement of government regulatory agencies when the disease is suspected or when the diagnosis is confirmed. Representatives of these agencies can often facilitate sample collection and transportation to an appropriate laboratory. **If anthrax is suspected, then shipping diagnostic samples via the mail or courier systems is strongly discouraged** (see previous discussion).[8]

Samples for Confirmation of Diagnosis

- Bacteriology—unopened carcass: blood or edema fluid in sealed, leakproof container; opened carcass: previously described samples plus spleen (local lymph nodes in horses, pigs) in sealed,

leakproof containers (direct smear, culture, bioassay)
- Histology—formalin-fixed spleen/local lymph nodes if carcass has been opened (light microscopy)

Note the zoonotic potential of this organism when handling the carcass and submitting specimens.

DIFFERENTIAL DIAGNOSIS

There are many causes of sudden death in farm animals, and differentiation is often difficult. Diseases where there can be multiple deaths suggestive of anthrax include the following:
- Lightning strike
- Peracute blackleg
- Malignant edema
- Bacillary hemoglobinuria
- Hypomagnesemic tetany

TREATMENT

Severely ill animals are unlikely to recover, but in the early stages, particularly when fever is detected before other signs are evident, recovery can be anticipated if the correct treatment is provided. Penicillin (20,000 IU/kg BW twice daily) has had considerable vogue, but concerns have been raised in recent years because of the occasional appearance of β-lactamase-producing strains that were thus resistant to penicillin. The range of occurrence rates of penicillin-resistant strains reported in the literature is broad, ranging from 0% to 11.5%.[2] Reports of naturally occurring resistance to penicillin among fresh animal isolates are exceedingly rare.[2] Penicillin has remained the recommended antibiotic in both animals and humans, at least in developing countries, where it is affordable and available almost everywhere. Because of the susceptibility of *B. anthracis* to a broad range of antimicrobials, a wide range of alternative choices exists among them tetracyclines, aminoglycosides, macrolides, and chinolones. It is desirable to prolong treatment to at least 5 days to avoid a recrudescence of the disease.

Antibiotics are effective against *B. anthracis,* but there are currently no effective therapeutic options against toxemia, which persists even after antimicrobial therapy may have eliminated the bacteria.[1]

The treatment of anthrax in livestock is legally prohibited in certain countries. In those countries the destruction of animals with clinical signs of anthrax without spilling of blood is required. Some countries even require the slaughter of the entire herd following a case of anthrax, a procedure that is considered unnecessary and wasteful.[2]

TREATMENT AND CONTROL

Treatment

Penicillin G sodium/potassium (20,000 IU/kg IV every 12h at least as loading dose IV) (R-2)

Procaine penicillin (22,000 IU/kg IM every 12h or 44,000 IU kg IM q24h) (R-2)

Oxytetracycline (10 mg/kg IV or IM every 24h) (R-2)

Anthrax hyperimmune serum (R-2)

Control

Anthrax vaccine (R-1)

Anthrax hyperimmune serum to animals at risk (R-2)

Procaine penicillin (44,000 IU/kg every 24h to animals at risk) (R-2)*

Oxytetracycline (long-acting formulation 20 mg/kg every 72h to animals at risk) (R-2)*

**Antibiotics administered within 7 to 10 days of vaccination with anthrax vaccine will impair efficacy of vaccine.*[2]

CONTROL

The control of meat- and milk-producing animals in infected herds in such a way as to avoid any risk to the human population is a special aspect of the control of anthrax. When an outbreak occurs, the placing of the farm in quarantine, the destruction of discharges and cadavers, and the vaccination of survivors are part of the animal disease control program and indirectly reduce human exposure. Prohibition of movement of milk and meat from the farm during the quarantine period should prevent entry of the infection into the human food chain.

Disposal of infected material is most important, and hygiene is the biggest single factor in the prevention of spread of the disease. Infected carcasses should not be opened but immediately burned in situ together with manure, bedding, and soil contaminated by discharges. Deep burial, with an ample supply of quicklime, may also be used but is less desirable because it bears the risk of groundwater contamination. If the carcass and infectious material cannot be disposed of immediately, a liberal application of 5% formaldehyde on the carcass and its immediate surroundings will discourage scavengers.

All suspected cases and in-contact animals must be segregated until cases cease, and for 2 weeks thereafter the affected farm must be kept in quarantine to prevent the movement of livestock. The administration of hyperimmune serum to in-contact animals may prevent further losses during the quarantine period, but prophylactic administration of a single dose of long-acting tetracycline or penicillin is a much commoner tactic. Because currently used anthrax vaccines contain live attenuated bacteria, they should not be used in combination with antimicrobial therapy.

Disinfection of premises, hides, bone meal, fertilizer, wool, and hair requires special care. When disinfection can be carried out immediately, before spore formation can occur, ordinary disinfectants or heat (60° C [140° F]) for a few minutes) are sufficient to kill vegetative forms. This is satisfactory when the necropsy room or abattoir floor is contaminated. When spore formation must be expected to have begun (i.e., within a few hours of exposure to the air), disinfection is almost impossible by ordinary means. Strong disinfectants such as 5% Lysol require being in contact with spores for at least 2 days. Strong solutions of formalin or sodium hydroxide (5% to 10%) are probably most effective. Peracetic acid (3% solution) is an effective sporicide; if applied to the soil in appropriate amounts (8 L/m^2), it is an effective sterilant. Infected clothing should be sterilized by soaking in 10% formaldehyde. Shoes may present a difficulty, and sterilization is most efficiently achieved by placing them in a plastic bag and introducing ethylene oxide. Contaminated materials should be damp and left in contact with the gas for 18 hours. Hides, wool, and mohair are sterilized commercially by gamma-irradiation, usually from a radioactive cobalt source. Special care must be taken to avoid human contact with infected material; if such contact does occur, the contaminated skin must be thoroughly disinfected. The source of the infection must be traced and steps taken to prevent further spread of the disease. Control of the disease in a feral animal population presents major problems.

Immunization

Immunization of animals as a control measure is extensively used. Veterinary anthrax vaccines contain spores from attenuated strains of *B. anthracis* and are classified into two categories:
- **Live attenuated vaccines, capsulated and nontoxigenic (cap +/tox–).** Strains used in these vaccines are devoid of the plasmid pX01 that encodes the toxin complex of *B. anthracis* (e.g., Pasteur vaccine).
- **Live attenuated vaccines, noncapsulated and toxigenic (cap–/tox +).** Strains in these vaccines lost the plasmid pXO2 encoding the capsule antigen (e.g., Sterne vaccine).

The sporulation character of both vaccine classes has the advantage of keeping the live vaccine viable over long periods. The **Pasteur vaccines** have the disadvantage that the various animal species show varying susceptibility to the vaccines, and anthrax may result from vaccination in some cases. This has been largely overcome by preparing vaccines of differing degrees of virulence for use in different species and in varying circumstances. Another method of overcoming the virulence is the use of saponin or saturated saline solution in the vehicle to delay absorption. This is the basis of the carbozoo vaccine.

The **Sterne vaccine** has overcome the risk of causing anthrax by vaccination and produces a strong immunity. It is the vaccine used in most countries. Although only one dose was originally thought to be necessary, with cases ceasing about 8 days after vaccination, it now appears that two vaccinations are necessary in some situations.

Currently only a few countries use Pasteur vaccines, whereas the Sterne vaccine is widely used because it is characterized by its elevated protective capacity and very low residual residence.[1]

A febrile reaction does occur after vaccination; the milk yield of dairy cows will be depressed, and pregnant sows will probably abort.

When the disease occurs for the first time in a previously clean area, all in-contact animals should either be treated with hyperimmune serum or be vaccinated. The measures used to control outbreaks, and the choice of a vaccine depend largely on local legislation and experience. Ring vaccination has been used to contain outbreaks of the disease, and in enzootic areas annual revaccination of all stock is necessary. Surface contamination of a pasture (as opposed to deep soil contamination) can persist for 3 years, and cattle grazing these pastures should be revaccinated annually for this period. In endemic areas cattle are routinely vaccinated yearly.

Milk from vaccinated cows is usually discarded for 72 hours after the injection in case the organisms in the vaccine should be excreted in the milk. Ordinarily the organisms of the Sterne vaccine do not appear in the milk and cannot be isolated from the blood for 10 and 7 days, respectively, after vaccination. Vaccinated animals are usually withheld from slaughter for 45 days.

Deaths as a result of anthrax have occurred in 3-month-old llamas after vaccination with a Stern vaccine and may occur in goats. Older crias and adults were unaffected. It was assumed that the dose of vaccine was excessive for such young animals. In these species two vaccinations 1 month apart with the first dose one-quarter of the standard dose can be used.[1]

FURTHER READING

Dragon DC, Rennie RP. The ecology of anthrax spores: tough but not invincible. *Can Vet J.* 1995;36: 295-301.

World Health Organization (WHO). Anthrax in humans and animals. 4th ed. 2008 at: <http://www.who.int/csr/resources/publications/anthrax_webs.pdf>; Accessed 20.01.14.

REFERENCES

1. Fasanella A, et al. *Vet Microbiol.* 2010;140:318.
2. World Health Organization (WHO). Anthrax in humans and animals. 4th ed. 2008 at: <http://www.who.int/csr/resources/publications/anthrax_webs.pdf>; Accessed 20.01.14.
3. Jernigan JA, et al. *Emerg Infect Dis.* 2001;7:933.
4. Schwartz M. *Mol Asp Med.* 2009;30:347.
5. Hugh-Jones M, Blackburn J. *Mol Asp Med.* 2009;30:356.
6. Edginton AB. *Vet Rec.* 1990;127:321.
7. Williams DR, et al. *Vet Rec.* 1992;131:363.
8. WHO. 2013 at: <http://apps.who.int/iris/bitstream/10665/78075/1/WHO_HSE_GCR_2012.12_eng.pdf>; Accessed 20.01.14.

BOVINE TUBERCULOSIS

SYNOPSIS

Etiology Mycobacterium bovis and, to a lesser extent, Mycobacterium caprae.

Epidemiology All age groups and species are susceptible, but infection is predominantly in cattle and pigs. Infected cattle are the main source of infection, but wildlife reservoirs are important in some regions and preclude the eradication of bovine tuberculosis in some countries. Inhalation is the major method of transmission between cattle. Pigs get primarily infected orally. Zoonosis, with most common route of infection through consumption of unpasteurized dairy products; other routes of infection include inhalation and direct contact.

Clinical findings Progressive emaciation, capricious appetite, and fluctuating temperature with signs referable to localization, such as respiratory disease, pharyngeal obstruction, reproductive disorder, and mastitis. In pigs, the disease is subclinical, but tuberculous lesions in cervical lymph nodes.

Clinical pathology Tuberculin testing. Single intradermal test is the official test in most countries, with the single intradermal comparative test for cattle suspected as false-positive reactors; interferon-gamma testing.

Necropsy findings Tuberculous granulomas may be found in any of the lymph nodes, or there may be generalized tuberculosis.

Diagnostic confirmation Culture of organism or identification by polymerase chain reaction (PCR) or other molecular techniques.

Control Test and slaughter. Most countries have official eradication programs.

ETIOLOGY

Bovine tuberculosis is defined as infection of any bovide with disease causing mycobacterial species within the ***Mycobacterium* tuberculosis complex (MTC)**.[1] The MTC comprises a range of mycobacterial species, including *Mycobacterium tuberculosis, M. bovis, M. africanum, M. microti, M. canettii, M. pinnipedii* and *M. caprae,* but the most common etiologic agents of bovine tuberculosis are ***M. bovis*** and to a lesser extent to ***M. caprae***. *M. caprae* was previously considered to be a subspecies of *M. bovis* but is now recognized as genetically distinct species within the MTC.[2]

Mycobacteria are acid-fast gram-positive bacteria of the family Mycobacteriaceae. These organisms can survive for months outside the animal host, particularly in a cold, dark, and moist environment. At temperatures between 12° and 24°C (54–75°F), survival times between 18 and 332 days have been reported.[2]

M. bovis is the mycobacterial species most commonly associated with tuberculosis in cattle. A wide range of species, including humans, are susceptible to *M. bovis* infection, but only cattle and in certain geographic regions some wildlife species function as maintenance hosts for *M. bovis*. Cattle, goats, and pigs are most susceptible to infection, whereas sheep and horses show a high natural resistance. *M. caprae,* formerly designated as *M. tuberculosis* subsp. *caprae* and later as *M. bovis* subsp. *caprae,* was initially only recognized as the main etiologic agent of caprine tuberculosis, but is currently also recognized as a common etiologic agent of tuberculosis in cattle, domesticated pigs, wild boar, wild and farmed red deer, and camelids in many Central and western European countries.[3]

EPIDEMIOLOGY

Occurrence

During the first part of the twentieth century, bTB was widespread and present in most parts of the world, with herd prevalence rates of up to 63% and animal prevalence rates in the range of 20% to 45%. With the introduction of rigorous bTB control programs in many developed countries during the second half of the twentieth century, the occurrence of bTB in the cattle population of these countries decreased dramatically, and many countries were able to virtually eradicate the disease and are now classified as officially bTB free (OTF). bTB is a disease notifiable to the World Organization of Animal Health (OIE) and is included in the so called OIE List A, comprising "transmissible diseases that are considered to be of socioeconomic and/or public health importance within countries and that are significant in the international trade of animals and animal products."[2] Clinical tuberculosis in animals is now a rarity in countries with eradication programs in place; occasional smaller outbreaks affecting one or few herds, however, occur regularly even in countries recognized as OTF. The presence of the disease is usually signaled by detection in carcasses at abattoirs.

Within the European Union, where all member states have TB eradication programs in place, the herd prevalence of bTB has been relatively stable in recent years, with rates between 0.37% and 0.67% from 2007 to 2012.[4] Thirteen member states of the European Union, including France, Germany,

Belgium, Poland, and Sweden, in addition to Norway and Switzerland, have the status of OTF, nonofficially free member states are, among others, the United Kingdom (Great Britain and Ireland), Italy, Greece, Spain, and Portugal.[4] A slight increase in the herd prevalence in nonofficially TB-free member states from 0.46% to 1.26% was recorded between 2007 and 2012.[4] The highest herd prevalence rates in 2012 were reported from Great Britain (10.40%), Ireland (4.37%), Spain (1.18%), and Greece (0.41%).[4] Herd outbreaks of *M. bovis* infection were recorded in several OTF member states in 2012, including France (169 herds), Germany (23 herds), Poland (7 herds), the Netherlands (2 herds), and Belgium and Slovenia (1 herd each). Three herds infected with *M. caprae* were identified in Austria.[4] With the national herd prevalence remaining below 0.1%, the OTF status of affected countries is not suspended.

In the United States, all states with exception of Michigan and California only have cattle herds certified as officially free of bTB. *M. bovis* infection of white-tailed deer, which is a maintenance host, remains a significant barrier to the U.S. bTB eradication program. *M. bovis* is still endemic in the white-tailed deer population in northeastern Michigan and northern Minnesota, presenting a potential source of infection for the local cattle population in that region. The number of confirmed cases of TB in Michigan livestock could, however, be reduced to single-digit figures since 2005.[5]

Australia obtained OTF status in 1997 after nearly 30 years of sustained bTB eradication. In New Zealand, where the eradication is complicated by the presence of the possum, also functioning as maintenance host for *M. bovis,* the implemented eradication program was highly successful in reducing the number of infected herds from 1700 in the mid-1990s to 66 in 2012.[5]

Source of Infection

Cattle

Infected cattle are the main source of infection for other cattle. Organisms are excreted as aerosol in exhaled air and in sputum, feces (from both intestinal lesions and swallowed sputum from pulmonary lesions), milk, urine, vaginal and uterine discharges, and discharges from open peripheral lymph nodes. Animals with gross lesions that communicate with airways, skin, or intestinal lumen are obvious disseminators of infection. Cattle in the early stages of the disease, before any lesions are visible, may also excrete viable mycobacteria in nasal and tracheal mucus. In experimentally infected cattle, excretion of the organism commences about 90 days after infection.

Wildlife Reservoirs

A large number of wildlife and feral species can be naturally infected with *M. bovis* or *M. caprae.* Although most wildlife and feral animals are unimportant as sources for infection to cattle, in some areas of the world certain species function as significant maintenance hosts and reservoirs for infection in cattle. These reservoirs escape traditional test and slaughter control programs and result in regions where the disease remains endemic in cattle herds.

- In areas of southwestern **England** and the Republic of **Ireland,** infected **badgers** (*Meles meles*) are significant in the epidemiology of the disease in cattle, and infection of cattle is thought to be from badger urine contamination of pastures. Badgers have also been found to make nocturnal visits to farm buildings and cattle troughs to feed, during which they defecate and urinate directly onto the cattle feed.
- In **New Zealand** infection occurs in the **brush-tail possum** (*Trichosurus vulpecula*) and produces lesions in peripheral lymph nodes with discharging sinuses. Much of New Zealand's residual problem with bTB is in cattle running on the pasture–bush margin, where there is ample opportunity for cattle–possum contact. Infection of cattle is thought to occur when curious cattle sniff moribund possums.
- Mule **deer** (*Odocoileus hemionus*), white-tailed deer (*O. virginianus*), elk (*Cervus elaphus canadensis*), and **bison** (*Bison bison*) in **North America** and red deer in Great Britain and Ireland can all act as maintenance hosts and in some regions spread infection to cattle through comingling or sharing of winter feed, resulting in foci of herd infections.
- **Buffaloes** (*Syncerus caffer*) in **South Africa** and water buffaloes (*Bulbalis bulbalis*) in the Northern Territory of **Australia** can also act as maintenance hosts.
- High infection rates approaching 50% have been reported in the **wild boar** (*Sus scrofa*) population of the **Iberian Peninsula**, where this species is regarded as maintenance host for *M. bovis.*[6] In northwestern Italy, wild boar are considered as spillover hosts that are unable to maintain infection without continued introduction from other species.[7]

Methods of Transmission

In most cases infection occurs through inhalation or ingestion and, to a lesser degree, contact through penetration of the agent through breaks in the skin. Inhalation is the almost invariable portal of entry in housed cattle, and even in those at pasture it is considered to be the principal mode of transmission.

Ingestion

Infection by ingestion is possible at pasture when feces contaminate the feed and communal drinking water and feed troughs, but a large infective dose is required. Under natural conditions, stagnant drinking water containing the pathogen may cause infection up to 18 days after its last use by a tuberculous animal, whereas a running stream does not represent an important source of infection to cattle in downstream fields.

The survival of the organism in the environment is influenced by temperature, moisture, exposure to the desiccating effect of sunlight, and ultraviolet light. The organism can survive for long periods in feces and soil, but most studies show that survival on pasture is measured in weeks rather than months and that environmental contamination of pasture is not of major importance in the epidemiology of the disease in cattle.

Other Routes

The drinking of infected milk by young animals is a common method of transmission where the disease is endemic, but mammary infection occurs late in the course of the disease and is less common in countries with advanced control programs. Other uncommon routes of infection include intrauterine infection at coitus, by the use of infected semen or of infected insemination or uterine pipettes, and intramammary infection by the use of contaminated teat siphons or by way of infected cups of milking machines. The feeding of tuberculous cattle carcasses to pigs has also caused a severe outbreak of the disease. Unusual sources of infection are infected cats, goats, and even humans. Stockmen with genitourinary infections have transmitted infection to cattle through urinating in the cattle environment.

Risk Factors

Environment Risk Factors

Housing predisposes to the disease, as do high stocking intensity and a large number of animals on a farm, and thus the disease is more common and serious where these forms of husbandry are practiced. The closer the animals are in contact, the greater is the chance that the disease will be transmitted.

Among beef cattle the degree of infection is usually much lower because of the open-range conditions under which they are kept. However, individual beef herds may suffer a high morbidity if infected animals are introduced and large numbers of animals have to drink from stagnant water holes, especially during dry seasons.

Host Risk Factors

Zebu (*Bos indicus*) type cattle are thought to be much more resistant to tuberculosis than European cattle, and the effects on these cattle are much less severe, but under intensive feedlot conditions a morbidity rate of 60% and a depression of weight gain can be experienced in tuberculous Zebu cattle.

Pigs are susceptible to infection with *M. bovis,* and disease levels in general reflect those in the local cattle population from which the infection derives, either by the ingestion of dairy products or by grazing over the same pasture as cattle. The lower relative prevalence in pigs is attributable to a number of factors, particularly the tendency of the disease to remain localized in this species and the early age of slaughter. Prevalence is higher in older pigs. When the disease is common among dairy cattle in an area, 10% to 20% of the local pigs are likely to be infected. Tuberculosis in pigs is now rare in countries with bTB control programs in place, but reports from Portugal and Spain showing that *M. bovis* strains can circulate in cattle, pigs, and wild boar indicate that infection of domesticated and feral pigs can be of epidemiologic relevance under certain circumstances.[8]

Infection of **goats** with *M. bovis* or *M. caprae* has a worldwide occurrence and is well recognized in many European countries with a large small ruminant population, such as the United Kingdom, Italy, Portugal, Spain, and Greece. In countries that are not officially free of bTB, infection can circulate between cattle and goats, particularly if these species are kept in close proximity to each other and share pastures or water sources. This underscores the importance to include caprine flocks in the TB surveillance in these countries, which, however, is not done in most cases.[8]

Sheep have historically been considered to be resistant. However, the increasing number of reports of TB infection in this species either with *M. bovis* or *M. capra,* particularly in non-TB-free countries, suggests that the prevalence of infection in sheep may have been underestimated.[8] Experience in New Zealand has shown that the disease can be quite prevalent in this species, with up to 5% of flocks being infected, probably as a result of a high prevalence in local cattle and possums.

In **horses** the disease occurs rarely, largely as a result of limited exposure to infection, but natural resistance also appears to play a part.

Over the past decades, infection with *M. bovis* and also with *M. microti* has been diagnosed with increased frequency in **New World camelids (NWCs)**, particularly in regions that are not free of bTB.[8] NWCs are highly susceptible to infection with *M. bovis* and *M. microti,* and they may function as reservoir of the disease for cattle and wildlife.[8] A complicating factor is that antemortem diagnosis of infection with *M. bovis* is difficult in NWC. Diagnostic tests successfully used to control and eradicate tuberculosis in cattle were found to have a low sensitivity and specificity in NWC.[8]

Tuberculosis can be a problem in **farmed deer** and may also be encountered in elk, wild deer of various species, water buffalo, camels, bison, elephants, wild carnivores, monkeys and other wild fauna, and birds. Most are dead end-hosts, but some may act as important reservoirs of infection for cattle, as mentioned earlier. Infection with *M. bovis* in **zoo animals** may present a particular problem because of the longer life expectancy of potentially infected animals and the relatively close contact with other species, including humans.

Pathogen Risk Factors

The causative organism is moderately resistant to heat, desiccation, and many disinfectants. It is readily destroyed by direct sunlight unless it is in a moist environment. In warm, moist, protected positions, it may remain viable for weeks.

Economic Importance

bTB is a serious infectious disease of cattle and other ruminant species and has been classified as disease of socioeconomic and public health importance that is significant in the international trade of animals and animal products by the World Organization for Animal Health (OIE). bTB is under strict control in most developed countries but still has important economic and social implications in the beef and dairy cattle industry of countries affected by the disease. Incurred costs not only result from losses of cattle because of tuberculosis, decreased productivity, and losses of carcass value, but also from control and eradication measures. On a national level, costs are incurred for increased regulation, animal movement control, and enforcement of compliance and indemnification programs. Trade restrictions for farms, regions, or countries that are not certified as OTF will add to the economic damage.

Zoonotic Importance

Historically, bTB was an important zoonotic disease transmitted from cattle to humans through the consumption of unpasteurized dairy products and to a lesser extent through direct animal contact when the organism is inhaled or penetrates the body through a break in the skin. In countries where bTB is still endemic, it presents an occupational hazard for farmers, veterinarians, workers in the meat industry and slaughterhouse, and hunters. The widespread occurrence of tuberculosis in exotic animals maintained in captivity adds to the public health importance of these infections.

With introduction of pasteurization of dairy products as standard procedure and intensive veterinary surveillance of the cattle population, in many countries the diseases has lost its importance as zoonotic disease. Whereas over 30% of all human TB cases were attributable to infection with *M. bovis* before introduction of pasteurization, this number has plummeted to less than 2% of all confirmed cases today.[9] Nonetheless, in regions of the world where bTB control programs have not been implemented and the disease in cattle remains endemic, this condition is still an important zoonotic disease. In these countries, between 10% and 20% of all human cases of tuberculosis are associated with infection with *M. bovis.*[10] The currently increasing incidence of tuberculosis in humans, particularly in immunocompromised humans, has led to a renewed interest in the zoonotic importance of *M. bovis.*

In the United States, the Centers for Disease Control and Prevention (CDC) records approximately 220 cases of tuberculosis in humans associated with *M. bovis* every year, which is equivalent to less than 2% of all human cases of tuberculosis.[11] The highest percentage levels on a national basis are recorded in Mexico with 13.8%, Uganda with 7%, and Nigeria with 5% of all human TB cases caused by *M. bovis.*[10]

Within the European Union, a total of 125 confirmed cases of human *M. bovis* infections were recorded in 2012. Most cases were reported from Germany (44 cases), followed by the United Kingdom (35 cases), Spain (15 cases), Italy (9 cases), and the Netherlands (8 cases); Switzerland, a non-EU member state, reported 5 confirmed cases in that year.[4]

PATHOGENESIS

Tuberculosis spreads in the body by two stages, the primary complex and postprimary dissemination. The **primary complex** consists of the lesion at the point of entry and in the local lymph node. A lesion at the point of entry is common when infection is by inhalation. When infection occurs via the alimentary tract, a lesion at the site of entry is unusual, although tonsillar and intestinal ulcers may occur. More commonly the only observable lesion is in the pharyngeal or mesenteric lymph nodes.

A visible primary focus develops within 8 days of entry being effected by the bacteria. **Calcification** of the lesions commences about 2 weeks later. The developing necrotic focus is soon surrounded by granulation tissue, monocytes, and plasma cells, and the pathognomonic "tubercle" is established. Bacteria pass from this primary focus, which is in the respiratory tract in 90% to 95% of cases in cattle, to a regional lymph node and cause the development of a similar lesion there. The lesions in the lungs in cattle occur in the caudal lobes in 90% of cases. In calves fed tuberculous milk, the primary focus is likely to be in the pharyngeal or mesenteric lymph nodes, with hepatic lesions as the major manifestation of postprimary spread.

Postprimary dissemination from the primary complex may take the form of acute miliary tuberculosis, discrete nodular lesions in various organs, or chronic organ tuberculosis caused by endogenous or exogenous reinfection of tissues rendered allergic to tuberculoprotein. In the latter case, there may be no involvement of the local lymph node. Depending on the sites of localization of infection, clinical signs vary, but because the disease is always progressive, there is the constant underlying toxemia, which causes weakness, debility, and the eventual death of the animal.

In cattle, horses, sheep, and goats, the disease is progressive; although generalized tuberculosis is not uncommon in pigs, localization as nonprogressive abscesses in the lymph nodes of the head and neck is the most common finding.

CLINICAL FINDINGS

Cattle

Although signs referable to localization in a particular organ usually attract attention to the possible occurrence of tuberculosis, some general signs are also evident. Some cows with extensive miliary tubercular lesions are clinically normal, but in most cases progressive emaciation unassociated with other signs occurs, which should arouse suspicion of tuberculosis. A capricious appetite and fluctuating temperature are also commonly associated with the disease. The hair coat may be rough or sleek. Affected animals tend to become more docile and sluggish, but the eyes remain bright and alert. These general signs often become more pronounced after calving.

Lungs

Pulmonary involvement is characterized by a chronic cough as a result of bronchopneumonia. The **cough** is never loud or paroxysmal, occurring only once or twice at a time, and is low, suppressed, and moist. It is easily stimulated by squeezing the pharynx or by exercise and is most common in the morning or in cold weather. In the advanced stages when much lung has been destroyed, dyspnea with increased rate and depth of respiration becomes apparent. At this stage, abnormalities may be detected by auscultation and percussion of the chest. Areas with no breath sounds and dullness on percussion are accompanied by areas in which squeaky crackles are audible, often most audible over the caudal lobes. Tuberculous pleurisy may occur but is usually symptomless because there is no effusion. Involvement of the bronchial lymph nodes may cause dyspnea because of constriction of air passages, and enlargement of the mediastinal lymph node is commonly associated with recurrent and then persistent ruminal tympany.

Intestine

Rarely, tuberculous ulcers of the small intestine cause diarrhea. Retropharyngeal lymph node enlargement causes dysphagia and noisy breathing as a result of pharyngeal obstruction. Pharyngeal palpation, or endoscopy, reveals a large, firm, rounded swelling in the dorsum of the pharynx. Chronic, painless swelling of the submaxillary, prescapular, precrural, and supramammary lymph nodes is relatively rare.

Uterus

Reproductive disorders include uterine tuberculosis, which is uncommon with bovine strains except in advanced cases. Spread by contiguity from the uterus causes peritonitis, bursitis, and salpingitis, with the lesions in the salpinx taking the form of small enlargements containing a few drops of yellow fluid. In tuberculous metritis, there may be infertility, or conception may be followed by recurrent abortion late in pregnancy, or a live calf is produced that in most cases dies quickly of generalized tuberculosis. Lesions similar to those of brucellosis occur on the placenta.

In cows that fail to conceive, there may be a chronic purulent discharge heavily infected with the organism, and the condition is very resistant to treatment. A number of cows will have an associated tuberculous vaginitis affecting chiefly the ducts of Gartner. Rare cases of tuberculous orchitis are characterized by the development of large, indurated, painless testicles.

Mastitis

Tuberculous mastitis is of major importance because of the danger to public health, risk of spread of the disease to calves, and the difficulty of differentiating it from other forms of mastitis. Its characteristic feature is a marked induration and hypertrophy, which usually develops first in the upper part of the udder, particularly in the rear quarters. Palpation of the supramammary lymph nodes is essential in all cases of suspected tuberculous mastitis. Enlargement of the nodes with fibrosis of the quarter does not necessarily indicate tuberculosis, but enlargement without udder induration suggests either tuberculosis or lymphomatosis. In the early stages, the milk is not macroscopically abnormal, but very fine floccules appear later and settle after the milk stands, leaving a clear, amber fluid. Later still, the secretion may be an amber fluid only.

Pigs

Pigs get infected through oral ingestion of the pathogen, leading to primary lesions in the oropharyngeal lymph node and the digestive tract. Tuberculous lesions in cervical lymph nodes usually cause no clinical abnormality unless they rupture to the exterior. Generalized cases present a syndrome similar to that seen in cattle, although tuberculous involvement of the meninges and joints is more common.

Horses

As in pigs, infection in horses commonly occurs through the digestive route, again leading to primary lesions in the oropharyngeal lymph node and the digestive tract.[12] The commonest syndrome in horses is caused by involvement of the cervical vertebrae in which a painful osteomyelitis causes stiffness of the neck and inability to eat off the ground. Less common signs include polyuria, coughing as a result of pulmonary lesions, lymph node enlargement, nasal discharge, and a fluctuating temperature.

Sheep and Goats

Bronchopneumonia is the commonest form of the disease in these species and is manifested by cough and terminal dyspnea. In some goats, intestinal ulceration, diarrhea, and enlargement of the lymph nodes of the alimentary tract occur. In both species the disease is only slowly progressive, and in affected flocks many more reactors and necropsy-positive cases are often found than would be expected from the clinical cases that are evident. In kids the disease may be more rapidly progressive and cause early death.

New World Camelids

Infection of a camelid herd with either *M. bovis* or *M. microti* may go unnoticed until one or several animals die, presenting suspicious lesions at necropsy. Affected animals may either be found dead or show signs of general distress with weight loss and respiratory symptoms before dying.[13]

CLINICAL PATHOLOGY

The antemortem diagnosis of bovine tuberculosis still presents a challenge because all available and routinely employed tests suitable for antemortem diagnosis have limitations regarding sensitivity and specificity.[14] Diagnostic tests for bTB can broadly be classified into direct and indirect diagnostic tests, with direct tests identifying the presence of the causative agent in the host and indirect tests using immunologic markers to determine whether an infection had occurred in an individual animal. Current bTB eradication programs are based on a screening and slaughter policy, and all use indirect tests determining the presence of a cellular or humoral immune response to a challenge with bovine tuberculin. Knowledge of the various tests used, including their deficiencies and advantages, is essential.

Direct Tests

Direct tests targeted at directly identifying the agent in postmortem specimens include microscopic examination, culture, and nucleic acid recognition methods. Direct tests targeted at identifying the causative agent in an animal form part of the passive abattoir surveillance that is an integral part of all bTB eradication programs and can be applied on samples collected during postmortem examination. All carcasses of slaughtered cattle are visually screened for characteristic gross pathologic findings that may be indicative of infection. Histopathology, culture, and molecular methods are then used to identify bacteria in abnormal tissue. Passive abattoir surveillance is considered highly cost effective but has the major drawback of lack of sensitivity. Extensive lesions are present in advanced stages of tuberculosis only, which have become a rarity in regions with ongoing bTB surveillance; small organ lesions are easily missed during abattoir meat inspection.[2]

The collection and pooling of samples from several grossly unremarkable lymph nodes from the head and thorax has been suggested as suitable material for bacteriologic culture.

Microscopic Examination

Mycobacteria can be demonstrated microscopically in smears and tissue material from clinical samples. Special stains such as the Ziehl-Neelsen or fluorescent acid-fast stain are used to determine the presence of acid-fast bacteria, which, together with the characteristic histologic lesions, can lead to a presumptive diagnosis; however, the diagnosis requires further confirmation.[2] Particularly in ruminants, histologic lesions contain few bacteria which may lead to a negative result, although *M. bovis* can be isolated in cultures.,

Culture

Specimens for culture are first homogenized following decontamination and are then centrifuged. The sediment is used for microscopic examination and culture. Cultures are incubated on specific media at 37°C (99°F) for at least 8 weeks, but preferably 10 to 12 weeks. If growth occurs, smears are prepared using specific acid-fast stains. Growth of *M. bovis* is generally observed between 3 and 6 weeks of culture.[2] Because *M. bovis* must be differentiated from other species of the *M. tuberculosis* complex, further testing is required. The major disadvantage of cultures is the long turnaround time, and the primary limitation results from the poor quality of samples often submitted to the diagnostic laboratory.

Nucleic Acid Recognition Methods

The polymerase chain reaction (PCR) is a laboratory technique for identifying the presence of bacteria-specific DNA that has been extensively evaluated for the detection of *M. tuberculosis* complex in specimens of human and, more recently, also of animal origin. In principle, the PCR presents an attractive diagnostic procedure allowing for the identification and differentiation of specific pathogens. The method is rapid, cost effective, and easy to standardize. For the diagnosis of tuberculosis in animals, however, commercial kits and in-house methods have been evaluated with unsatisfactory results.[2] The reasons why the PCR does not yet fulfill its diagnostic potential as diagnostic test for tuberculosis are various. False-positive and false-negative results have not only been attributed to the low number of bacteria often present in samples, but also to difficulties with the decontamination methods, the presence of polymerase enzyme inhibitors in the samples, and difficulties in extracting DNA from mycobacteria that possess a robust cell wall.[15] Current molecular methods are therefore not yet considered adequate for direct detection of *M. bovis*, either from ante- or postmortem samples.[15]

Indirect Tests

Indirect tests can again be subdivided into cellular-immunity-based and humoral-immunity-based diagnostic tests. Cellular-immunity-based tests determine the occurrence of a delayed hypersensitivity reaction in general in the form of swelling after intradermal application of tuberculin protein. These so-called intradermal tuberculin tests are the standard diagnostic tools of bTB eradication programs used for antemortem diagnosis of *M. bovis* infection.

Blood-based cellular immunity tests include the interferon-γ test, which is now accepted as complementary test in many national bTB eradication programs and is recognized as alternative test of international trade, and the lymphocyte proliferation assay. Humoral-immunity-based tests are serologic diagnostic tools that determine the presence of specific antibody indicating prior exposure to antigen of *M. bovis*.

Intradermal Tuberculin Test

The intradermal tuberculin test is the standard diagnostic tool for detection of bTB and consists of the intradermal injection of **bovine tuberculin purified protein derivate (PPD)** into a skin fold of a specific location of the body and the subsequent detection of swelling as a result of delayed hypersensitivity 72 hours later.[2] Because of differences in sensitivity of the skin of different body parts, different approaches for the intradermal tuberculin test are in use. The **caudal skin fold** at the base of the tail (**caudal fold test [CFT]**) is used primarily for practicality reasons in the United States, Canada, and New Zealand, and formerly also in Australia, whereas in Europe and the United Kingdom a **cervical skin fold** of the lateral aspect of the neck is used for the so-called **single intradermal test (SIT)**. Applying the intradermal test in the cervical region results in higher sensitivity and specificity compared with the caudal skin fold but is more labor intensive because it requires better restraint of the animal and clipping of the skin.[16] Whereas the interpretation of the CFT consists of manual palpation to determine swelling approximately 72 hours after injection, the interpretation of the SIT and SICT (described in the following discussion) is done by measuring the thickness of the skinfold before and 72 hours after injection using calipers.

Where the presence of paratuberculosis (Johne's disease), avian tuberculosis, or a high prevalence of infection with environmental mycobacteria is suspected, nonspecific sensitization must be considered. In these cases, the **single intradermal comparative test (SICT),** consisting of the simultaneous intradermal administration of bovine and avian tuberculin on two different injection sites of the neck, either one on each side or both on the same side approximately 12 cm apart and one above the other, is administered. The test is read 72 hours later and the reaction to both tuberculins compared with each other. The greater of the two reactions indicates the organism responsible for the sensitization. This test is not generally intended for primary use in detecting reactors but only to follow up known reactors to determine the infecting organism. Its use as a primary test is recommended when a high incidence of avian tuberculosis or Johne's disease is anticipated or when vaccination against Johne's disease has been carried out. The comparative test is adequate to differentiate between vaccination against Johne's disease and tuberculosis, and the distinction is easier the longer the time between vaccination and testing.

Historically, other tests using bovine tuberculin to determine hypersensitivity—such as the vulvar, ophthalmic, or palpebral test; the short thermal test; and the Stormont test—have been used but are now obsolete.

Special Aspects of Sensitivity to Tuberculin

- Potency and standardization of tuberculins: Modern-day tuberculin used for diagnostic purposes is a purified protein derivative (PPD) of bovine or avian tuberculin that is prepared from the heat-treated products of growth and lysis of *M. bovis* (or *M. avium* in the case of avian tuberculin). Production methods have in the meantime largely been standardized, and with PPD being a licensed product, it requires production under good manufacturing practice conditions that comply with official requirements of the World Organization for Animal Health (OIE).[2] The standardized preparation is meant to ensure that the final product contains a precise concentration of standardized quality; nevertheless, the protein content of tuberculin does not precisely predict its biological activity or potency, which is a critical parameter strongly affecting the outcome of the test.[14] Potency testing is therefore required as further step in the manufacturing process to standardize product quality, which is done by comparing the potency to a reference standard in guinea pigs. It must, however, be noted that the clinical potency determined in tuberculous guinea pigs is not necessarily representative of the clinical potency in cattle.[16] A bovine tuberculin is considered adequate for diagnosis as part of an official test program when providing a minimum of 2000 IU PPD per dose, with an estimated potency of between 66% and 150%.[14]

- Dose: The dose of tuberculin must be at least 2000 IU of bovine (or avian for the SCIT) tuberculin; in cattle with diminished allergic sensitivity, higher doses of up to 5000 IU may be required. In any case the injection volume should not exceed 0.2 mL.[2] The exact dose for the particular tuberculin that is officially prescribed must be strictly adhered to when the cervical skin test is used. In the United States 0.1 mL is recommended for herds of unknown status and 0.2 mL in known infected herds when cases with low sensitivity are to be carefully sought. The method of injection of tuberculin also has some importance when the cervical site is used. A careful intradermal injection produces the largest swelling, and a quick thrust produces the least.
- Desensitization during tuberculin testing: When a suspicious reactor is encountered, the question of when to retest is complicated by the phenomenon of desensitization caused by the absorption of tuberculin and other foreign proteins. Desensitization is more marked and of longer duration after an (accidental) subcutaneous than after an intradermal injection. After an SID test the period of desensitization is short, but as a practical procedure, it is recommended that animals giving a suspicious result to an SID test not be retested before 60 days.

  The desensitization phenomenon can be used to obscure a positive reaction. If tuberculin is injected and thus the test is made in the desensitized period, no reaction will occur in infected animals.
- Postparturient desensitization: Tuberculous cattle go through a period of desensitization immediately before and after calving, and as many as 30% give false-negative reactions returning to a positive status 4 to 6 weeks later. The loss of sensitivity is probably a result of the general immunologic hyporeactivity that occurs associated with parturition. Calves drinking colostrum from infected dams give positive reactions for up to 3 weeks after birth even though they may not be infected.
- Anergy: Anergic animals are those with visible lesions of tuberculosis but that do not react to a cutaneous delayed hypersensitivity test. The number of these can be reduced by being careful to inject sufficient tuberculin (2000 IU) at the right site and to read the test at 72 hours. There is still a residuum of cases that do not respond, especially those with extensive pulmonary involvement.

Summary of Testing Procedures in Cattle

In summary, it is usual to use the single intradermal test as a routine procedure.

Annual testing of all cattle, quarantine of test-positive herds, and a movement ban into TB-free areas have historically been effective in TB control schemes. The sensitivity and specificity of the skin test are moderately high, but false-positive and false-negative reactions occur.

False-positive reactions (no gross lesion reactors) may be given by the following:

- Animals sensitized to other mycobacterial allergens, including those of human or avian tuberculosis or paratuberculosis (Johne's disease); relatively nonpathogenic mycobacteria (e.g., skin tuberculosis); and, by ingestion, nonpathogenic mycobacteria in permanent waters inhabited by birds, or poultry litter fed to cattle when the birds are infected with *M. avium*
- Animals sensitized to other allergens (e.g., *Nocardia farcinicus*)
- Animals injected with irritants at the injection site before reading of the tuberculin test, when compensation rates for reactors exceed true cattle prices

The proportion of false-positive reactions is likely to increase as control programs progress toward eradication and can undermine farmers' confidence in the control program. Reactors that are thought to be nonspecific should be retested by the comparative test in the cervical region 7 days after the response to the SID or CFT. Alternatively, cattle can be retested using the whole-blood interferon-gamma assay 8 to 28 days after the skin test.

False-negative reactions may be given by the following:

- Advanced cases of tuberculosis
- Early cases until 6 weeks after infection
- Cows that have calved within the preceding 6 weeks
- Animals desensitized by tuberculin administration during the preceding 8 to 60 days
- Old cattle
- Low-potency tuberculin or bacterial contamination of the tuberculin
- Variable dose with multidose syringes

Tuberculin Testing in Other Species

Pigs

The most generally used method is the SID test, injecting 0.1 mL of standard-potency mammalian tuberculin into a fold of skin at the base of the ear, but the test is relatively inaccurate in this species. The test is read 24 to 48 hours later; an increase in skin thickness of 5 mm or more constitutes a positive reaction. In positive animals the skin thickening often exceeds 10 mm and shows superficial necrosis and sloughing.

If the animal is infected with *M. avium*, the maximum skin thickening may not occur until 48 hours after injection. When no attempt is being made to determine the type of infection, mixed avian and mammalian tuberculins may be used and the test read at 24 to 48 hours. If avian tuberculin alone is used, the test should be read at 48 to 72 hours, and an increase in skin thickness of 4 mm is classed as positive.

Many suspicious reactions occur in pigs because of the tendency of lesions to regress and the sensitivity to tuberculin to diminish, with maximum sensitivity occurring 3 to 9 weeks after infection. A retest in 6 to 8 weeks should determine whether or not the disease is progressing. Although positive reactors may in time revert to a negative status, there may be macroscopic lesions in these animals at necropsy. However, viable organisms are not usually recoverable from the lesion, the infection apparently having been overcome.

Some decrease in skin sensitivity after parturition occurs in sows infected with *M. bovis* but may not occur when the infection is associated with *M. avium*. Comparative tests work efficiently in this species, with little or no reaction to heterologous tuberculin.

Horses

The results obtained with subcutaneous and intradermal tuberculin tests are very erratic and must be assessed with caution, especially when the test is positive because many false-positives occur. The horse appears to be much more sensitive than cattle to tuberculin, and much smaller doses of standardized tuberculin are required. As little as 0.1 mL of PPD tuberculin is sufficient to elicit a positive reaction, and testing may provoke an anaphylactic reaction. No safe recommendations can be made on tests in this species because of lack of detailed information, but the occurrence of a systemic reaction with a positive cutaneous test can be accepted as indicating the presence of infection.

Sheep and Goats

The single intradermal test is relatively inaccurate, with some tuberculous animals giving negative reactions, although on the basis of results achieved in experimentally infected goats, it is adequate. The test injection is usually given in the caudal fold as in cattle, but injection into the skin of the inside of the thigh of sheep is also satisfactory. An increase in thickness of 5 mm in the fold constitutes a positive reaction.

New World Camelids

Diagnostic tests used for in vivo identification of cattle infected with *M. bovis* are considered highly unreliable in NWCs because they have demonstrated a lack of sensitivity and specificity when applied according to the protocol used in cattle.[8] In dromedaries the diagnostic performance of the SCIT was found to be improved somewhat when the test was performed on the axillar skin and read after 5 days, although a considerable number of animals also reacted to avian tuberculin.[15]

Interferon-γ Assay (IFN-γ)

An in vitro assay of cell-mediated reactivity by detection and quantitation of γ-interferon known as the interferon-γ assay (IFN-γ) is licensed and commercially available in some countries. It is based on the detection of IFN-γ liberated from white blood cells in whole-blood cultures incubated with PPD tuberculin and has the advantage that tested cattle need only be handled once. It can detect infected cattle as early as 3 to 5 weeks after infection even with low exposure level. It also has value in retesting skin-test-positive cattle that may be false-positive reactors, but for this purpose it should be used between 8 and 28 days after skin testing because assay reactions are diminished if conducted on samples taken at the 3-day reading revisit after skin testing. Ideally, the test should be set up in the laboratory on the same day as sampling or, at the most, after overnight storage of the blood. Current testing is with *M. bovis* PPD, which can contain cross-reacting antigens to other mycobacterial species, and more specific and sensitive tests using antigens specific to *M. bovis* are being evaluated.

A recent meta-analysis reported an estimated sensitivity of 67%, which is superior to the SCIT, and a specificity of 96%, which is inferior to the SCIT, for the IFN-γ.[16] The IFN-γ is available as commercial test kit and is now approved as official diagnostic test in several national bTB eradication and control programs, including programs in the European Union, the United States, New Zealand, and Australia.

Lymphocyte Proliferation Test

Like the IFN-γ test, the lymphocyte proliferation test is an in vitro test that is conducted either on whole blood or purified lymphocytes and determines and compares the reactivity of peripheral lymphocytes to avian and bovine tuberculin. The test result is the difference in reactivity of lymphocytes to bovine (B) and avian (A) tuberculin; the B–A value is calculated and compared with a cutoff value. The test is not used for routine diagnostics because it requires the handling of radioactive material and long incubation periods.[2]

Serologic Tests for Diagnosis of Tuberculosis

In the final stages of a tuberculosis eradication program, the percentage of reactors, which are not in fact tuberculous, increases to the point where a more discerning test than the one based on cutaneous hypersensitivity is required. Most of the tests tried so far have been serologic ones. Their aim is to identify anergic animals and cases sensitized by some other bacteria.

Serologic tests, including complement fixation, fluorescent antibody, direct bacterial agglutination, precipitin, and hemagglutination tests, have been developed but have little potential value for the routine diagnosis of tuberculosis.

Early enzyme-linked immunosorbent assay (ELISA) tests to crude mycobacterial antigens had limited value, but an ELISA that examines antibody to defined antigens of *M. bovis* before and after skin testing appears useful in detecting nonspecific reactors.

Serologic tests may, however, be of some value for the diagnosis of tuberculosis in domestic animal and wildlife species such as farmed deer, NWCs, badgers, nonhuman primates, or elephants, where cellular-immunity-based diagnostic tests are not available and intradermal tuberculin test have been proven unreliable.[2]

NECROPSY FINDINGS

Cattle, Sheep, and Goats

These show similar lesions with a standard distribution. Tuberculous granulomas may be found in any of the lymph nodes, but particularly in bronchial, retropharyngeal, and mediastinal nodes. In the lung, miliary abscesses may extend to cause a suppurative bronchopneumonia. The pus has a characteristic cream to orange color and varies in consistency from thick cream to crumbly cheese. Tuberculous nodules may appear on the pleura and peritoneum.

All localized lesions of tuberculosis tend to stimulate an enveloping fibrous capsule, but the degree of encapsulation varies with the rate of development of the lesion. Generalized cases are denoted by the presence of **miliary tuberculosis,** with small, transparent, shot-like lesions in many organs, or by pulmonary lesions that are not well encapsulated and caseated. The presence of bronchopneumonia or hyperemia around pulmonary lesions is highly suggestive of active disease. Cases with tuberculous mastitis or discharging tuberculous metritis must also be considered as likely to be potent spreaders of the infection.

Chronic lesions are characteristically discrete and nodular and contain thick, yellow to orange, caseous material, often calcified and surrounded by a thick, fibrous capsule. Although such lesions are less likely to cause heavy contamination of the environment than open lesions, affected animals are important as sources of infection. It should be noted that suspect cattle slaughtered as part of bovine tuberculosis eradication programs may be culture-positive and yet have no typical gross or microscopic lesions.

Pigs

Generalized tuberculosis, with miliary tubercles in most organs, is seen in pigs, but the common finding is localization in the tonsils and the submaxillary, cervical, hepatic, bronchial mediastinal, and mesenteric lymph nodes. The nodes are markedly enlarged and consist of masses of white, caseous, sometimes calcified, material, surrounded by a strong, fibrous capsule and interlaced by strands of fibrous tissue. Because of the regressive nature of the disease in pigs, these lesions are often negative on culture.

Horses

The characteristic distribution of tubercles in horses includes the intestinal wall, mesenteric lymph nodes, and spleen. The cut surface of these firm nodules has a fleshy appearance similar to that of neoplastic tissue. There is also a tendency for lesions to develop in the skeleton, particularly the cervical vertebrae.

Histologically, there is some variation between the domestic species with regard to features such as mineralization and the degree of tissue necrosis. In some cases acid-fast bacilli may be difficult to demonstrate using conventional stains. A comparison of the infection in cattle and cervid species suggests that tuberculosis should be considered in cervids even when the lesions have a suppurative and necrotizing character, with a minimal granulomatous component. Culture of *M. bovis* is difficult and time consuming, and it poses a considerable public health risk. Methods such as immunoperoxidase staining and PCR can permit detection of the organisms while minimizing public health risks.

Samples for Confirmation of Diagnosis

- Bacteriology—affected lymph nodes, lung, granulomas from viscera (culture [has special growth requirements], PCR)
- Histology—formalin-fixed samples of these tissues (light microscopy, immunohistochemistry, PCR)

Note the zoonotic potential of this organism when handling the carcasses and submitting specimens.

DIFFERENTIAL DIAGNOSIS

Because of the chronic nature of the disease and the multiplicity of signs caused by the variable localization of the infection, tuberculosis is difficult to diagnose on clinical examination. If the disease occurs in a particular area, it must be considered in the differential diagnosis of many diseases of cattle. In pigs, the disease is usually so benign that cases do not present themselves as clinical problems and are found only at necropsy. The rarity of the disease in horses, sheep, and goats makes it an unlikely diagnostic risk, except in groups that have

Continued

had abnormally high exposure to infected cattle. Differential diagnoses include the following:

- Mycobacteriosis associated with the *M. avium–intracellulare* complex and atypical
- Mycobacteria and *M. tuberculosis* in particular in pigs
- Lung abscess as a result of aspiration pneumonia
- Pleurisy and pericarditis following traumatic reticulitis
- Chronic contagious bovine pleuropneumonia
- Upper respiratory disease
- Actinobacillosis
- Bovine leukosis
- Lymphadenopathy
- Other causes of mastitis

TREATMENT

Treatment of tuberculosis in cattle is not permitted in countries with an established bTB eradication program, requiring removal of reactors from the herd. Treatment may, however, be permitted in some cases, such as in valuable zoo animals.

Because of the progress being made in the treatment of human tuberculosis with such drugs as isoniazid, combinations of streptomycin and *para*-aminosalicylic, and other acids, the treatment of animals with tuberculosis has undergone some examination, and claims have been made for the efficiency of long-term oral medication with isoniazid both as treatment and as control. It is not a favored option in eradication-conscious countries.

CONTROL

Eradication of bTB has been virtually achieved in many countries. The methods used have depended on a number of factors, but ultimately the **test and slaughter policy** has been the only one by which effective eradication had been achieved.

Control on a Herd Basis

Control in a herd rests on removal of the infected animals, prevention of spread of infection, and avoidance of further introduction of the disease.

Tuberculin Testing

Detection of infected animals depends largely on the use of the intradermal tuberculin test. All animals over 3 months of age should be tested and positive reactors disposed of according to local legislation. Suspicious reactors are retested at intervals appropriate to the test used. At the initial test, a careful clinical examination should be conducted on all animals to ensure that there are no advanced clinical cases that will give negative reactions to the test. Doubtful cases and animals likely to have reduced sensitivity, particularly old cows and those that have calved within the previous 6 weeks, may be tested by one of the special sensitivity or serologic tests described previously or retested subsequently. The single comparative intradermal test (SCIT) should be used where infection with *M. avium* is anticipated or where a high incidence of reactors occurs in a herd not showing clinical evidence of the disease.

Retesting

Until recently, if the incidence of reactors was high at the first test or if "open" lesions were found at necropsy in culled animals, emphasis was placed on repeat testing at short intervals to avoid the situation in which the spread of the disease might overtake the culling rate. It is now thought that all animals with tuberculosis should be regarded as equally potent disseminators of the infection. Retests of the herd should be carried out at 3-month intervals until a negative test is obtained. A further test is conducted 6 months later, and if the herd is again negative, it may be classed as free of the disease. Subsequent check tests should be carried out annually.

Prevention of Spread

Hygienic measures to prevent the spread of infection should be instituted as soon as the first group of reactors is removed. Feed troughs, water troughs, and drinking cups should be cleaned and thoroughly disinfected. Suspicious reactors being held for retesting should be isolated from the remainder of the herd. Separation of infected and susceptible animals by a double fence provides practical protection against spread of the disease.

It is important that calves being reared as herd replacements be fed on tuberculosis-free milk, either from known free animals or pasteurized. Rearing calves on skim milk from a communal source is a dangerous practice unless the skim milk is sterilized. All other classes of livestock on the farm should be examined for evidence of tuberculosis. Farm attendants should be checked because they may provide a source of infection.

If a number of reactors are culled, attention must be given to the possibility of infection being reintroduced with replacements, which should come from accredited herds. Failing this, the animals should be tested immediately, isolated, and retested in 60 days. Infection from other herds should be addressed by preventing communal use of watering facilities or pasture and by maintaining adequate boundary fences.

It is inadvisable to attempt a control program until it can be guaranteed that all animals can be gathered, identified, tested, and segregated, a difficult proposition in cattle run on extensive range country with little manpower and few fences.

Control on an Area Basis

The method used to eradicate bovine tuberculosis from large areas will depend on the incidence of the disease, methods of husbandry, attitude of the farming community, and the economic capacity of the country to stand losses from a test and slaughter program.

Education

An essential first step is the prior education of the farming community. Livestock owners must understand the economic and public health significance of the disease, its manifestations, and the necessity for the various steps in the eradication program. Eradication must also be compulsory because voluntary schemes always leave foci of infection. Adequate compensation must be paid to encourage full cooperation by way of payment for animals destroyed or bonuses for disease-free herds or their milk or beef.

Staging

It is essential at the beginning of a program to determine the incidence and distribution of the disease by tuberculin testing of samples of the cattle population and a meat inspection service. Eradication can commence in herds and areas that have a low incidence of the disease. These will provide a nucleus of tuberculosis-free cattle to supply replacements for further areas as they are brought into the eradication scheme.

Vaccination

Vaccination may offer a major alternative to test and slaughter in the control of bovine tuberculosis but currently suffers from both lack of efficacy and the problem of vaccinated cattle reacting to current tests for TB. Vaccination may be used as a temporary measure when the incidence of tuberculosis is high and a routine test and slaughter program may be economically impossible until it is lowered, or when an eradication program cannot be instituted for some time but it is desired to reduce the incidence of the disease in preparation for eradication.

Bacillus Calmette–Guérin (BCG) vaccination is the only method available for field use. Vaccination must be repeated annually, and the vaccinated animal remains positive to the tuberculin test. Calves must be vaccinated as soon after birth as possible and do not achieve immunity for 6 weeks. The immunity is not strong, and vaccinated animals must not be submitted to severe exposure. In field circumstances where the disease is prevalent, only modest results, if any, can be expected.

There are a number of newer, prospective vaccines, including subunit and synthetic peptide vaccines, antigenically improved BCG, attenuated mutants of *M. bovis*, and protective antigens expressed in attenuated live vaccine vectors. Detection of vaccinated cattle from naturally infected cattle could be possible with vaccine-specific antigens in the interferon-gamma assay.

Test and Slaughter

When the overall incidence of tuberculosis is 5% or less, compulsory testing and the slaughter of reactors is the only satisfactory method of eradication. A combination of lines of attack is usually employed.

Accredited areas are set up by legislation, and all cattle within these areas are tested and reactors removed. Voluntary accreditation of individual herds is encouraged outside these areas. In some countries, focal points of extensive infection outside accredited areas have been attacked under special legislation.

When an area or country has been freed from the disease, quarantine barriers must be set up to avoid its reintroduction. Within the area, the recurrent cost of testing can be lessened by gradually increasing the interest period to 2 and then to 3 or even 6 years as the amount of residual infection diminishes. Meat inspection services provide a good observation point should any increase in incidence of the disease occur. Among range beef cattle it is usual to check samples of animals at intervals rather than the entire cattle population.

Problems in Tuberculosis Eradication

Complete eradication of tuberculosis has not really been achieved in any country. In many, a state of virtual eradication has been in existence for years, but minor recrudescences occur. In the final stages of an eradication program a number of problems achieve much greater importance than in the early stages of the campaign. The major problems that arise are as follows.

No-Visible-Lesion Reactors

The percentage of reactors with no gross lesions or no visible lesions (NVL) at slaughter rises steeply as the disease prevalence decreases. In part this occurs because gross examination has poor sensitivity for detection of infection, but it is also inevitable given the falling prevalence of disease and the specificity of the tuberculin test. NVL reactors create administrative and public relations difficulties. Resolution of this problem awaits the validation of the interferon-gamma assay or other accepted serologic tests.

"Breakdowns"

Individual herds that have been accredited after a number of free tests may be found to have the disease again, often with a very high incidence. This may be because an anergic carrier has been left in the herd and tests have been too far apart or because of a break in the security of the herd, with infection from purchased cattle or transmission between cattle in neighboring herds.

"Traceback"

A principal source of information on the location of infected herds in the final stages of a program could be a traceback originating from infected animals at packing plants. It is often impossible, and a major advance would be a suitable method of identifying individual animals that could be utilized up to the killing floor. The two most popular methods are fabric labels stuck on the rump with skin contact glue and wraparound plastic or metal tail-tags bearing an identification number for the farm of origin. They have two problems. They can be removed at the abattoir and reused; they fall off if the tail is docked, a popular practice in some areas. Electronic identification might solve this problem but meets political and other resistance in many countries. Recent experience with bovine spongiform encephalopathy and other concerns for food safety will likely remove this resistance, and most countries have or are developing effective traceback programs.

Large Herds

Another kind of difficulty in eradication is where cattle are run under very extensive conditions on large ranches or stations as in North America, South America, and Australia. There can be difficulty in ensuring a complete muster, and there is a great need for a test that does not require that cattle be held in a mustering site for 3 days before the test is read. Problems with continuing infection also occur in large intensive dairies where the policy is test and cull, and the whole dairy cannot be depopulated at one time.

Wildlife Reservoirs

Spread to cattle from wild fauna is a major problem in the United Kingdom, where badgers and deer are important sources of infection; in New Zealand, where the brush-tailed possum plays the same role; and a risk from deer exists in several countries. In New Zealand, the possum is considered a pest and does considerable damage to the ecosystem; possum control programs are accepted. However, the badger in Britain, and deer in most countries, are protected species and suitable control programs, acceptable to animal protectionists, are difficult to negotiate in this sensitive area of public relations. DNA fingerprinting can establish sources of infection and the importance of wildlife reservoirs to cattle.

Control of Tuberculosis in Pigs

M. bovis infection in pigs usually results from the feeding of infected milk, skim milk, or whey to pigs or allowing cattle and pigs to graze the same pasture. The first step in the control of tuberculosis in a pig herd is to remove the source of infection, and then to test and remove the reacting animals, which is not an efficient procedure because of the relative inaccuracy of the tuberculin test in this species. The nonprogressive nature of the disease means that transmission between pigs is unlikely to occur to a significant extent, except perhaps in breeding animals.

FURTHER READING

Cousins DV. *Mycobacterium bovis* infection and control in domestic livestock. *Rev Sci Tech Off Int Epiz.* 2001;20:71-85.

Good M, Duignan A. Perspectives on the history of bovine TB and the role of tuberculin in bovine TB eradication. *Vet Med Int.* 2011;410-470.

Pérez-Lago L, Navarro Y, García de Viedma D. Current knowledge and pending challenges in zoonosis caused by *Mycobacterium bovis:* a review. *Res Vet Sci.* 2014;97:S94-S100.

Pesciaroli M, Alvarez J, Boniotti MB, et al. Tuberculosis in domestic animal species. *Res Vet Sci.* 2014;97:S78-S85.

Pritchard DG. A century of bovine tuberculosis 1888–1988: conquest and controversy. *J Comp Pathol.* 1988;99:357-399.

Wood PR, Monahan ML, eds. Bovine tuberculosis. *Vet Microbiol.* 1994;40:1-205.

REFERENCES

1. European Commission Health, Consumer Protection Directorate-General. 2013 at: <http://ec.europa.eu/food/animal/diseases/eradication/tb_workingdoc2006_en.pdf>; Accessed 03.03.15.
2. OIE. 2009 at: <http://www.oie.int/fileadmin/Home/eng/Health_standards/tahm/2.04.07_BOVINE_TB.pdf>; Accessed 03.03.15.
3. Rodriguez-Campos S, et al. *Res Vet Sci.* 2014;97:S5.
4. EFSA. *EFSA J.* 2014;12(2):3547.
5. DEFRA. 2014 at: <https://www.gov.uk/government/uploads/system/uploads/attachment_data/file/300447/pb14088-bovine-tb-strategy-140328.pdf>; Accessed 02.03.15.
6. Palmer MV. *Transbound Emerg Dis.* 2013;60:1.
7. Hardstaff JL, et al. *Res Vet Sci.* 2014;97:S86.
8. Pesciaroli M, et al. *Res Vet Sci.* 2014;97:578.
9. Pérez-Lago L, et al. *Res Vet Sci.* 2014;97:S94.
10. Bezos J, et al. *Res Vet Sci.* 2014;97:S3.
11. CDC. 2011 at: <http://www.cdc.gov/tb/publications/factsheets/general/mbovis.pdf>; Accessed 03.03.15.
12. Domingo M, et al. *Res Vet Sci.* 2014;97:S20.
13. Twomey DF, et al. *Vet J.* 2012;192:246.
14. Bezos J, et al. *Res Vet Sci.* 2014;97:S44.
15. Wernery U, et al. *Vet Microbiol.* 2007;192:246.
16. Downs S, et al. *Proc Soc Vet Epidemiol Prev Vet Med.* 2011;139.

TUBERCULOSIS ASSOCIATED WITH *MYCOBACTERIUM TUBERCULOSIS*

Mycobacterium tuberculosis is occasionally isolated from cattle or pig livestock with tuberculous lesions, but this is rare. Outbreaks of tuberculosis in animals associated with *M. tuberculosis* of human origin are transitory, and removal of tuberculous humans from the environment usually results in the disappearance of positive reactors in cattle.

In recent years a considerable increase in the occurrence rate of tuberculosis associated with *M. tuberculosis* was noticed among the wildlife population of South African zoos.[1] The considerable genetic diversity of strains involved in cases of TB in wild animals suggests that animals contracted the infection from human visitors to the zoos rather than from an internal source. This development is considered to be the result of the human tuberculosis epidemic in South Africa spilling over to wild animals.[1]

M. tuberculosis has been isolated from a subset of pig carcasses that have been condemned because of the presence of tuberculous lesions at two slaughterhouses in Ethiopia.[2] The presence of *M. tuberculosis* in pig carcasses suggests transmission of the pathogen between both species and supports the idea that pigs may indeed not be dead-end hosts for mammalian tuberculosis.[2]

In cattle herds, the reactors and necropsy lesions are most common in the young stock. Many reactors have no visible lesions; those that do occur are small and confined to the lymph nodes of the digestive and respiratory systems. Pigs may develop minor lesions in lymph nodes, but sheep, goats, and horses appear to be resistant. *M. tuberculosis* infections in pigs are usually the result of feeding offal from a tubercular household or contact with a tuberculous attendant.

REFERENCES

1. Michel AL, et al. *Transbound Emer Dis.* 2013;6046-6052.
2. Arega SM, et al. *BMV Vet Res.* 2013;9:97.

MYCOBACTERIOSIS ASSOCIATED WITH *MYCOBACTERIUM AVIUM INTRACELLULARE* COMPLEX AND WITH ATYPICAL MYCOBACTERIA

SYNOPSIS

Etiology *Mycobacterium avium–intracellulare* complex and other mycobacteria.

Epidemiology Ubiquitous in nature. Infection by ingestion. High concentration can build up in animal bedding of various types. Domestic or wild birds are a source of classic avian tuberculosis serovars. Can cause disease in humans particularly when immunocompromised.

Clinical findings Most infections are of the draining lymph nodes of the alimentary tract and are subclinical, but they can result in carcass condemnation. Generalized cases manifest with chronic weight loss and diarrhea.

Clinical pathology Tuberculin testing in cattle and swine. Culture, polymerase chain reaction (PCR).

Necropsy findings Microgranulomas, with or without caseation, in lymph nodes.

Control Reduction of environmental contamination.

ETIOLOGY

The *M. avium-intracellulare* complex (MAC) comprises two mycobacterial species: *M. avium* and *M. intracellulare. M. avium* is further subdivided into four subspecies: *M. avium* subsp. *avium, M. avium* subsp. *paratuberculosis, M. avium* subsp. *sylvaticus,* and *M. avium* subsp. *hominissuis.* The classical *M. avium* serovars are the cause agents of tuberculosis in poultry, whereas *M. avium* subsp. *hominissuis* is an opportunistic pathogen primarily infecting swine and humans. *M. avium* subsp. *pararuberculosis* is the causative agent of paratuberculosis in cattle and small ruminants (Johne's disease) and is discussed in the corresponding chapters of this book.

The MAC comprises ubiquitous opportunistic pathogens of a large range of species, and in livestock these pathogens have the most importance in swine. Tuberculosis associated with these organisms in livestock is usually not manifest clinically and is not a major disease problem, but infected animals react to the intradermal tuberculin test, creating difficulty in *M. bovis* tuberculosis eradication programs. Outbreaks in pig herds can cause significant losses because of carcass condemnation. In pigs, a significant proportion of reactors to tuberculin are attributable to infection with organisms of this complex, and infected cattle and pigs are potential sources of infection for the increasing number of MAC (particularly *M. avium* subsp. *hominissuis*) infections in humans.

EPIDEMIOLOGY

Occurrence

Lymphadenitis in pigs associated with these organisms is reported from all continents.

Source and Transmission

Organisms of the MAC are ubiquitous in nature and can be isolated from soil, plants, water, and animal feed and animal bedding. Infected birds nesting in animal or feed buildings are the most common source of *M. avium* subsp. *avium* and contaminate feed and water supplies. In contrast, isolates of *M. avium* subsp. *hominissuis* are commonly isolated from the environment and can be isolated from various species of flies and beetles that inhabit the ground, bedding, and feed in farm environments. Several studies have confirmed the role of peat that is used for bedding or as feed additive as source of infection with *M. avium* subsp. *hominissuis* for piglets.[1] The organisms are resistant to acidic environments, which allows them to survive in the acidic, humid environments of peat bogs and decomposed feces, and the lipopolysaccharide bacterial wall promotes survival in environments inside and outside barns for extended periods of time.[2]

Ingestion appears the normal route of infection, and pigs infected with *M. avium* subsp. *homonissuis* excrete the organism m in **feces.**[3] In pigs the use of dirt **floors** or deep litter, rather than bare concrete or slats, increases the risk of infection and the development of macroscopic lymphadenitis in large numbers of pigs. The length of time that pigs are kept on the litter is also important, and severe outbreaks can occur in pigs kept on litter for the entire period from weaning to slaughter. Sawdust, straw, peat, and wood shavings have all been found to be highly contaminated. Sphagnum moss contaminated with *M. cookii* and environmental exposure to other mycobacteria may result in sensitization of cattle to bovine tuberculin.

M. avium subsp. *avium* is the cause of tuberculosis in domestic and wild birds, which are infected by ingestion of contaminated feed or soil and excrete large numbers of organisms in feces. Although infection in domestic livestock is commonly contracted from domestic poultry, from soil-borne infection, or from pen floors or feeds contaminated by wild birds, pig-to-pig transmission can also occur.

Economic Importance

Clinical disease is not important, but at slaughter organs with tuberculous lesions are discarded, and the entire carcass may be condemned or require heat treatment before being released for human consumption.

Zoonotic Importance

Infections with atypical mycobacteria are not uncommon in humans and have higher prevalence in immunocompromised humans. Members of the MAC, in particular *M. avium* subs. *hominissuis,* cause both pulmonary infections in immunocompetent individuals and disseminated diseases in acquired immunodeficiency syndrome. Another typical manifestation of *M. avium* infection is lymphadenitis in the head and neck region of children.[4]

Animals, or animal products, may be a source for human infection, but direct associations are difficult to prove. Although not clinically ill, human workers have been found to be infected on farms when the disease occurred in pigs. It is likely that infections in humans and animals on the one farm come from the one source, but it is also possible that spread from animals to humans occurs.

CLINICAL AND NECROPSY FINDINGS

Cattle

With classic avian tuberculosis, sensitivity to tuberculin may disappear soon after cattle are removed from contact with infected birds. Infection with this group of organisms produces microgranulomas in lymph nodes. Local lesions may persist in the mesenteric lymph nodes, the meninges, and in the uterus and udder, and occasional cases of open pulmonary tuberculosis have been observed. In uterine infections recurrent abortion may occur, and mammary localization causes induration and involvement of lymph nodes, similar to the lesions associated with *M. bovis.* Generalized tuberculosis can occur in up to 50% of cases.

Goats and Sheep

Goats and sheep appear to have a strong natural resistance to infection with *M. avium* complex. A high incidence of avian tuberculosis has been observed in a herd of goats, and although the disease progresses slowly, this species may act as reservoirs for other species. Animals with progressive disease show anorexia and chronic diarrhea and wasting.

Deer

Infection in wild and farmed deer occurs and may serve as a source of infection for carrion-eating birds.

Horses

Horses are resistant to infection with *M. avium* complex, although rare, generalized cases of tuberculosis have been reported in this species. It is possible that disease occurs only in horses that are immunosuppressed by other factors. A common history is chronic diarrhea and weight loss. Less common manifestations include dermatitis, alopecia, and skin ulceration. Granulomatous enteritis is commonly present at necropsy. Two cases have been recorded in which the lesions in the cervical lymph nodes were accompanied by lesions in cervical vertebrae. The lesions were similar to those seen in cervical vertebral osteomyelitis associated with *M. bovis.*

Pigs

Infection is usually sporadic in pigs in herds but in some herds can be enzootic.[5] The naturally occurring disease is nonprogressive and usually restricted to the lymph nodes of the head and neck and the mesenteric lymph nodes. Occasional generalized cases with involvement of liver, lungs, and kidneys occur; an outbreak of pulmonary tuberculosis associated with *M. avium* and clinical symptoms such as wasting and abortion has been reported in pigs. The lesions may be free of suppuration and resemble neoplastic tissue, but granulomatous and occasionally caseous lesions in lymph nodes also occur. Similar lesions are associated with *Rhodococcus equi.* Granulomatous lesions that develop in the tonsils and intestinal wall result in the passage of organisms in the feces for at least 55 days, and transmission to in-contact pigs occurs readily.[1]

Tuberculosis produced experimentally in pigs by the oral administration of *M. avium* is generalized, provided the inoculation dose is sufficiently large. Transmission from these pigs to contact pigs occurs. Vaccination of pigs with BCG vaccine provides partial protection against experimental infection with *M. avium.*

CLINICAL PATHOLOGY

The lesions at postmortem or slaughter inspection are characteristic, but culture and identification of the organism is required for confirmation. Growth is slow, and PCR technologies offer faster diagnosis, with some ability to distinguish between individual species and serovars. Smears of lesions associated with some of these agents do not stain positive with acid-fast stains.

Tuberculin Testing

With infections in cattle, sensitivity to tuberculin occurs to both avian and bovine tuberculin, but is greater to avian tuberculin. With atypical mycobacteria the response is also short-lived, with significant changes in sensitivity occurring between successive tests. The comparative tuberculin test is becoming more widely used because of the growing importance of these infections. It is not uncommon to have more than one species of mycobacteria causing disease in a herd at the one time.

The single intradermal comparative tuberculin (SCIT) test consisting of the simultaneous intradermal injection of bovine and avian tuberculin has been used to differentiate between infections with MAC and *M. bovis,* which pertains to the *M. tuberculosis* complex (MTC) in swine. Animals infected with mycobacteria of the MTC tend to show a stronger reaction to bovine than to avian tuberculin, whereas animals previously exposed to organisms of the MAC show a reverse reaction.[3]

Tuberculin skin testing in horses is not conducted because 70% of clinically normal horses show positive reactions.

TREATMENT AND CONTROL

Treatment is not usual, except possibly in horses. Antimicrobial treatment in humans for this complex of organisms includes amikacin, ciprofloxacin, rifampin, and the macrolide azithromycin.

In swine herds with enzootic infection, culling on the basis of skin sensitivity is usually not practical because of the high prevalence of infection and high environmental contamination. Control procedures concentrate on the reduction of environmental contamination by a change from bedding to solid or slatted floors, frequent washing and disinfection of pen floors, separate weaner and grower facilities, and exclusion of wild birds from buildings and feed areas.

FURTHER READING

Thorel MF, Huchzermeyer HF, Michel AL. *Mycobacterium avium* and *Mycobacterium intracellulare* infection in mammals. *Rev Sci Tech Off Int Epiz.* 2001;20:204-218.

REFERENCES

1. Johansen TB, et al. *Biomed Res Int.* 2014;189649.
2. Biet F, et al. *Vet Res.* 2005;36:411.
3. Agdelstein A, et al. *Vet Res.* 2014;46.
4. Jarzembowski JA, Young MB. *Arch Pathol Lab Med.* 2008;132:1333.
5. Alvarez J, et al. *Epidemiol Infect.* 2011;139:143.

YERSINIOSIS

ETIOLOGY

There are pathogenic and nonpathogenic strains of *Yersinia pseudotuberculosis* and *Yersinia enterocolitica.* The pathogenic strains of both organisms possess chromosomal and plasmid-mediated virulence determinants.

Y. pseudotuberculosis can be divided into 15 major serogroups, based on O-antigens, some of which can be further divided into subgroups on the basis of type-specific somatic and flagellar antigens. There is variation in animal and human pathogenicity between the serogroups.

Y. enterocolitica is divided into six major biotypes, designated as 1A (generally regarded as nonpathogenic), and 1B, 2, 3, 4, and 5. It is serologically heterogeneous, with 54 serotypes originally identified on the basis of somatic antigens, which was subsequently simplified to 18 serogroups.[1] Bioserotypes may be host-specific. Serotypes O:2, O:3, O:5, O:8, and O:9 have been most often associated with infection in farm animals and humans. Other serotypes appear to be largely nonpathogenic, although virulence factors have recently been detected in some biotypes previously regarded as nonpathogenic. Serotype O:9 is antigenically very similar to *Brucella* spp., and infection with this serotype is a cause of false-positive reactions to *Brucella* agglutination and complement fixation tests.

EPIDEMIOLOGY

Occurrence

Yersiniosis has worldwide occurrence, although there appear to be regional differences in the species of animal infected, the prevalence of disease, and the organism involved. *Y. pseudotuberculosis* has historically been associated with sporadic pyemic disease in sheep manifest with extensive abscessation of internal organs such as liver and spleen. Subsequently, *Y. pseudotuberculosis* and *Y. enterocolitica* have been associated with enterocolitis in cattle, sheep, pigs, goats, buffalo, and farmed and feral deer. Enteric disease in ruminants has been most reported from Australia, New Zealand, and the United States.[2]

Yersinia pseudotuberculosis

Y. pseudotuberculosis is a common inhabitant of the intestine in a wide variety of domestic and wild mammals. Wild birds and rodents are also reservoirs of the organism, and fecal–oral spread on pastures and in water is a major method of transmission. Spring migratory birds can spread pathogenic types over long distances, although these are usually not associated with disease in ruminants.

There may be differences in the host specificity of different serotypes and strains. Rodents and birds may be the major reservoirs for serotypes I and II, which infect deer and goats, whereas sheep and cattle may be maintenance hosts for serotype III.

In an Australian study, *Y. pseudotuberculosis* serotype III was isolated from the feces of healthy sheep in 5% of flocks examined, although the prevalence was probably much higher because only a small number of sheep were sampled in each flock. Infection was more common in young sheep and occurred during the winter and spring months, and excretion of the organism persisted for 1 to 14 weeks. A 23-year retrospective study of disease caused by *Y. pseudotuberculosis* in goats in California found that cases occurred predominantly in winter and spring and were clustered in certain years. The most common syndromes were enteritis and/or typhlocolitis (64%), abscessation (14%), and abortion (12%).[2]

In cattle, the organism has been found without disease in up to 26% of normal cattle and on 84% of farms tested. The fecal excretion that occurs in clinically normal sheep and cattle possibly results from a subclinical infection of the intestine; experimental challenge of ruminants can result in the establishment of the organism in the intestine, with the presence of microscopic abscessation in the lamina propria and serologic conversion in the absence of clinical disease.

Enteric disease associated with this organism in both cattle and sheep appears to occur as the result of a heavy infection pressure in animals that are debilitated from other influences. These include cold wet weather, inanition and starvation, trace-element deficiency, change of diet, management procedures such as marking, and, in farmed deer, procedures such as capture, yarding, and recent transport.

In sheep, attack rates in the flock for clinical disease have ranged from 1% to 90%, with a mean of 18% and a population mortality varying from 0% to 7%. *Y. pseudotuberculosis* may also cause sporadic abortion in cattle, goats, and sheep. In sheep, abortion rates of 1% to 9% are recorded, with abortion occurring in the latter part of pregnancy and without clinical illness in the ewes. The organism is the cause of occasional cases of bovine caprine mastitis, epididymitis, and orchitis in rams, and it may be found in sporadic cases of abscessation and lymphangitis in ruminants.

Yersinia enterocolitica

Y. enterocolitica is less commonly associated with clinical disease in farm animals, although apparently healthy animals can excrete strains that are potentially pathogenic for humans for much of the year. Diarrhea associated with this organism can occur in sheep, and the organism can be isolated from affected lambs. However, harmful strains of Y. *enterocolitica* tend to be less pathogenic to sheep and goats than pathogenic strains of *Y. pseudotuberculosis.*

Enterocolitis is recorded in sheep and goats. Biotype 5, serotype O:2,3 has been isolated from some of these. In an Australian survey in the early 1990s this organism was detected in 17% of flocks and was isolated from young sheep at all seasons of the year. In a study of goat flocks in New Zealand, 80 of 82 *Y. enterocolitica* isolated from 18 flocks were biotype 5 O:2,3.[3] Young goats (those < 1 year old) had from 2.2 to 12.9 times the risk of shedding potentially pathogenic isolates than older goats. Clinical disease appears to be predisposed by the same stress factors as apply with disease associated with *Y. pseudotuberculosis.* For example, *Y. enterocolitica* was isolated from the caecum of lambs with severe diarrhea grazing fodder beet in the United Kingdom.[4] The weather at the time of the outbreak was cold and wet, and the yearling sheep were seen congregating around pools of water in the paddock. Parasitism and poor nutrition were also thought to be contributing factors. Disease is typically recorded in sheep less than 1 year of age, with attack rates varying from 2% to 55% and population mortalities ranging from 0.3% to 17%. *Y. enterocolitica* is also an occasional cause of abortion in sheep, and this has been reproduced experimentally.

Whereas *Y. enterocolitica* is commonly isolated from pigs, and pigs are a major reservoir for human disease, it is a rare cause of clinical disease in pigs, although clinical enteric disease can be produced by experimental challenge of colostrum-deprived pigs. Normal pigs challenged with serotype 0:3 excreted the organism in feces but were fecal-culture-negative 10 weeks after challenge and at slaughter, even though the organism could be isolated from the tonsils at slaughter. Pigs seroconverted 19 days after challenge and remained seropositive until slaughter 70 days later.

Zoonotic Implications

Yersinia pseudotuberculosis

Human infection with *Y. pseudotuberculosis* is primarily manifest with septicemia, and renal failure is a sequela. In addition to food-borne infection, the consumption of water contaminated by animal feces appears to be a major risk factor. Raw milk consumption is also a risk. Human cases are usually sporadic, although outbreaks have been reported from Finland and Russia.[5]

Yersinia enterocolitica

Gastrointestinal disease associated with *Y. enterocolitica* appears to have increasing prevalence in humans, being the third most commonly reported zoonosis in Europe, and can be associated with a reactive arthritis as a sequela. Septicemia does occur but is largely limited to those with other underlying disease. The bioserotype most often associated with human disease is 4/O:3, with other bioserotypes including 2/O:5,27, 1B/O:8, and 2/O:9.[1] Pigs are a major reservoir for *Y. enterocolitica,* and pork and pork products are sources for human infection.[6] Bioserotype 4/O:3, in particular, is commonly isolated from the tonsils and pharynx of pigs at slaughter and less commonly from feces. The rate of isolation varies geographically and with farm source, and it has been suggested that pathogen-free breeding is a method for control. A high rate of biotype 1A, which is a common isolate from livestock and generally thought to be non-pathogenic for humans, was isolated from sheep feces, but not tonsil, from sheep at slaughter in Gotland, Sweden.[6] Recently, the virulence gene *ail* (adhesion invasion locus) has been identified in some strains of *Y. enterocolitica* biotype 1A, and thus a more thorough examination of these biotypes may be justified.[7-9]

In contrast to Australia and New Zealand, it is thought that in Europe the pig is the only domestic animal consumed by humans that regularly harbors pathogenic *Yersinia.* There is an apparent increasing prevalence of bioserotype 4/O:3 infections in humans in the Northern Hemisphere, and pigs and pork products are considered to be important sources. A survey in Great Britain comparing isolates of *Y. enterocolitica* from cattle, sheep, and pigs with those from humans over a 2-year period did not find a strong correlation between pathogenic serotypes isolated from the two groups, with the exception of isolates from pigs. The importation of meat products has been incriminated as the vehicle of introduction of pathogenic serotypes into Japan. There would appear to be an increased risk for infection in humans handling pigs at slaughter and in veterinarians in pig practice.

Bioserotype 3/O:5,27 is common in animals in the United Kingdom, but not isolated from humans. This bioserotype increased the secretion of the cytokines IL-6 and IL-8 from macrophages infected in vitro, compared with other biotype 3 and 4 isolates.[10] It was proposed that these differences in the interaction of the bacteria with the host immune system may explain why this bioserotype is not pathogenic for humans.

PATHOGENESIS

Invasion of the intestinal epithelium is followed by inflammation in the mucosa and the formation of microabscesses in the lamina propria and mesenteric lymph nodes. Ulcers and disruption of the intestinal mucosa lead to loss of fluid and function. The intestinal lesions are accompanied by villous atrophy and lead to malabsorption and ill-thrift, diarrhea, or a combination of the two.

CLINICAL FINDINGS

Affected animals may present with a syndrome of chronic ill-thrift and in a wasted condition with or without diarrhea. Where diarrhea is present, the feces are watery, foul-smelling, and black in color, but occasionally they also contain mucus and blood. Diarrhea persists for 2 to 3 weeks in an individual animal and may require the removal of soiled wool ("crutching" or "dagging") to reduce the risk of fly strike.

CLINICAL PATHOLOGY

There is a neutrophilia with a left shift. Affected animals are often hypoproteinemic and anemic, although this may be a reflection of the underlying malnutrition. In experimental infections antibody develops by 9 to 19 days after infection and may be an aid to diagnosis. The organism can be isolated from the feces. Multiplex PCR, capable of detecting 10 pathogenic serobiotypes of *Y. enterocolitica*, and real-time PCR have been developed to discriminate pathogenic *Y. enterocolitica* from other members of this genus.[11]

NECROPSY FINDINGS

There are liquid intestinal contents but usually no gross findings. Some sheep may have thickening of the mucosa of the small intestine and the cecum and colon, and the mesenteric lymph nodes may be enlarged and edematous.

The characteristic findings on histopathology consist of a segmental suppurative erosive enterocolitis. Microabscesses, consisting of aggregations of neutrophils with prominent colonies of gram-negative coccobacilli, are present in the mucosa. Lesions are most prevalent in the jejunum and ileum and are accompanied by atrophy of villi and hyperplasia of cryptal epithelium. Microabscesses may coalesce to produce extensive erosions, and there may be microabscesses in the liver.

The placenta from sheep that have aborted in association with *Y. pseudotuberculosis* is thickened and edematous, with necrotic debris in the intercotyledonary zone, and must be differentiated from enzootic abortion.

Samples for Confirmation of Diagnosis

- Bacteriology—jejunum, ileum, colon, mesenteric lymph node (culture—sometimes requires cold enrichment)
- Histology—formalin-fixed jejunum, ileum (several sections), colon, mesenteric lymph node (light microscopy)

Note the zoonotic potential of this organism when handling the carcasses and submitting specimens.

DIFFERENTIAL DIAGNOSIS

The major differential is the syndrome of weaner ill-thrift, caused mainly by undernutrition and gastrointestinal parasitism, and other agents that cause diarrhea, such as salmonellosis.

TREATMENT AND CONTROL

Isolates vary in their sensitivity to antibiotics, and a sensitivity test is advisable. Most isolates show in vitro sensitivity to the aminoglycosides, to tetracyclines, and to sulfonamides or a combination of sulfonamides and trimethoprim. Sulfonamides and trimethoprim are reported not to be effective in the treatment of yersiniosis in cattle; long-acting tetracyclines are recommended for the treatment of both infections, in combination with supportive therapy.

A vaccine is available for deer in New Zealand, but in other countries there is no specific control for ruminants and pigs. Live attenuated oral vaccines have been evaluated in laboratory animals and afforded good cross-protection against heterologous strains of *Y. pseudotuberculosis.*[12] In grazing animals mitigating the effects of parasitism, particularly during winter, and maintenance of good nutrition are thought to be important factors in avoiding clinical disease.

FURTHER READING

Bergsbaken BT, Cookson T. Innate immune response during *Yersinia* infection: critical modulation of cell death mechanisms through phagocyte activation. *J Leuk Biol.* 2009;86:1153-1158.

Fredriksson-Ahomaa M, et al. Molecular epidemiology of *Yersinia enterocolitica* infections. *FEMS Immunol Med Microbiol.* 2006;47:315-329.

Laukkanen-Ninios R, et al. Population structure of the *Yersinia pseudotuberclosis* complex according to multilocus sequence typing. *Env Microbiol.* 2011;13:3114-3127.

Radostits O, et al. Yersiniosis. In: *Veterinary Medicine: A Textbook of the Diseases of Cattle, Horses, Sheep, Goats and Pigs.* 10th ed. London: W.B. Saunders; 2007:954-956.

Slee KJ, Skilbeck NL. The epidemiology of *Yersinia pseudotuberculosis* and *Y. enterocolitica* infections in sheep in Australia. *J Clin Microbiol.* 1992;30:712-715.

REFERENCES

1. Drummond N, et al. *Food Path Dis.* 2012;17:179.
2. Giannitti F, et al. *J Vet Diag Invest.* 2014;26:88.
3. Lănada EB, et al. *Aust Vet J.* 2005;83:563.
4. Otter A, Callaghan G. *Vet Rec.* 2008;162:699.
5. Laukkanen-Ninios R, et al. *Env Microbiol.* 2011;13:3114.
6. Söderquist K, et al. *Acta Vet Scand.* 2012;54:39.
7. Kraushaar B, et al. *J Appl Microbiol.* 2011;111:997.
8. Sihvonen LM, et al. *Food Path Dis.* 2011;8:455.
9. Kumar P, Virdi JS. *J Appl Microbiol.* 2012;113:1263.
10. McNally A, et al. *J Med Microbiol.* 2006;55:725.
11. Lambertz ST, et al. *Appl Environ Microbiol.* 2008;74:6060.
12. Quintard B, et al. *Comp Immunol Microbiol Infect Dis.* 2010;33:e59.

TULAREMIA

SYNOPSIS

Etiology *Francisella tularensis* subsp. *tularensis* in North America; *Francisella tularensis* subsp. *holarctica* in Asia, Europe, and North America.

Epidemiology Primarily wild animal disease with wide occurrence in the Northern Hemisphere. Among domesticated animals, cats and lambs are most, and pigs less, susceptible; seasonal, associated with heavy tick infestation. Tabanidae, rodents, and lagomorphs function as hosts and vectors. Zoonosis, potential bioterrorist agent.

Clinical findings Tick infestation. Fever, stiffness of gait, diarrhea, weight loss, recumbency. Wool break.

Clinical pathology None specific.

Necropsy findings Subcutaneous swellings at site of tick attachment, lymphadenitis, and septicemia in sheep. Pigs have pleuritis, pneumonia, and abscessation of submaxillary and parotid lymph nodes.

Diagnostic confirmation Identification of agent by immunohistochemistry, polymerase chain reaction (PCR) or culture; serology in survivors.

Treatment Tetracyclines, streptomycin.

Control Tick control, repellents.

ETIOLOGY

Francisella tularensis, the causative organism of tularemia is a gram-negative, nonspore-forming coccobacillus pertaining to the family Francisellaeceae. The bacterium survives in the environment for prolonged periods. Viable bacteria can be found after weeks and months in the carcasses and hides of infected animals and in fomites, which include grain, straw, dust and water. It is highly resistant to freezing and can survive in meat of infected animals stored at −15° C (5° F) for 3 years.[1]

Currently, four subspecies with different animal hosts and different geographic distribution are recognized:[2]

- *F. tularensis* subsp. *tularensis* (type A): This is the most virulent subspecies; it is found in North America and associated with rabbits, ticks, and sheep.
- *F. tularensis* subsp. *holarctica* (*palaearctica,* type B): This subspecies is less virulent and is found in Asia, Europe and North America. It is often isolated in association with streams, ponds, lakes, and rivers. Beavers and muskrats in North America and lemmings and beavers are presumably responsible for maintaining the water association of this bacterium. There is evidence suggesting that the pathogen can persist in water (possibly associated to protozoa) for prolonged periods of time.
- *F. tularensis* subsp. *mediasiatica:* This serotype has only been isolated in Kazakhstan and Turkmenistan. Little is known about its virulence, but is considered to comparable to that of subsp. *holarctica.*
- *F. tularensis* subsp. *novicida:* This strain has thus far only been isolated from humans; it has been linked to waterborne transmission in Australia,

Spain, and the United States. The strain of subsp. *novicida* isolated in Australia is the only one identified in the Southern Hemisphere thus far.

EPIDEMIOLOGY

Tularemia is a highly contagious disease occurring principally in wild animals, but it may transmit to farm animals and cats, causing septicemia and high mortality. It can occur either as epizootics or as sporadic disease. It is a zoonosis that is responsible for approximately 100 clinical cases in humans every year in the United States.

Occurrence

Tularemia is primarily restricted in its occurrence to countries in the **Northern Hemisphere** and occurs in most of them. In the United States tularemia is recognized in all states except Hawaii. It is most prevalent in the central-western states of the United States, including Missouri, Arkansas, Oklahoma, South Dakota, and Kansas.[3] In Europe, the disease is more prevalent in eastern European countries and less common in continental western Europe.[2] Epidemics affecting the human population have occurred in Spain, Portugal, Sweden, and Kosovo.

Risk Factors

Animal Risk Factors

F. tularensis has a wide host range and is recorded in over 100 species of bird and wild and domestic animals. Common wild animal hosts include rabbits, muskrats, beavers, and a variety of rodents, including voles, squirrels and lemmings. Disease in domesticated animals most commonly occurs in **cats and sheep** and to a lesser extent in pigs, dogs, and horses; cattle appear to be relatively resistant but can be infected in association with heavy tick infestation. Sheep and pigs of all ages are susceptible, but most losses occur in lambs; in pigs, clinical illness occurs only in piglets. There is a sharp seasonal incidence, with the bulk of cases occurring during the spring months. The morbidity rate in affected flocks of sheep is usually about 20% but may be as high as 40%, and the mortality rate may reach 50%, especially in young animals.

Transmission

The **major reservoirs** and transmitters of the infection are rabbits, hares, wild rodents, **ticks**, and flies. The principal mammalian target host in North America is the cottontail rabbit (*Sylvilagus* spp.). With sheep, transmission occurs chiefly by the bites of the wood tick, *Dermacentor andersoni*, and from *Haemaphysalis otophila*, with the ticks becoming infected in the early part of their life cycle when they feed on rodents. In Europe, *Ixodes ricinus* and *Dermacentor reticulatus* are vectors. Transmission to pigs and horses is thought to occur chiefly by tick bites, but **mechanical transmission** to laboratory animals does occur with tabanid and blackflies. In the former Soviet Union and northern Europe, the bacterium has been demonstrated to be transmitted by mosquitoes.[2] Tabanid flies, which include the horsefly and the deerfly, have been implicated as vectors in the western United States and northern Europe.[1] At least 20 flea species were identified as potential vectors, although their role in the spread of the disease is uncertain. Neither in flies nor mosquitoes the pathogen was confirmed to reside in the salivary glands, suggesting that they may function as mechanical rather than biological vectors.

In contrast, **transstadial** and **transovarial transmission** occurs in the tick. The adult ticks infest sheep, and pastures bearing low shrubs and brush are particularly favorable to infestation. The ticks are found in greatest numbers on the sheep around the base of the ears, top of the neck, throat, axillae, and udder.

Pathogen Risk Factors

There is little information concerning virulence mechanisms of *F. tularensis*. The capsule appears to be a necessary component for expression of full virulence and protects against serum-mediated lysis. The lipopolysaccharide has unusual biological and structural properties and low toxicity in vitro and in vivo.

Pronounced differences in virulence between subtypes are well established. *F. tularensis* subsp. *tularensis* is by far the most virulent subspecies for all affected species and is associated with the highest mortality rates in animals and humans.

Zoonotic Implications

Humans can acquire *F. tularensis* from various sources. Most exposures appear to result from the handling of infected rabbits and other wildlife (e.g., during hunting activities), but infections can arise from **bites** of ticks and haematophagus flies, from the **ingestion** of contaminated meat and water, and from the bite or scratch of infected cats. Inhalation of aerosolized bacteria appears to be a less common route of infection but is associated with respiratory tularemia, which has the highest fatality rate of all clinical presentations of tularemia.[2] The disease is an occupational hazard to hunters and workers in the sheep industry in areas where the disease occurs. Spread of the disease to humans may also occur in abattoir workers who handle infected sheep carcasses. Person-to-person transmission has not been documented.

F. tularensis is one of the most infectious pathogens known in human medicine, with an extremely low infectious dose (10 bacteria when injected subcutaneously and 25 bacteria when inhaled as aerosol). Because of its high infectivity, the fact that it causes infection through inhalation in combination with its stability in aerosols, *F. tularensis* is recognized as **potential bioterrorist agent**.

PATHOGENESIS

Tularemia is an acute septicemia, but localization occurs, mainly in the parenchymatous organs, with the production of granulomatous lesions.

CLINICAL FINDINGS

Sheep

The incubation period has not been determined. A heavy tick infestation is usually evident.

The **onset** of the disease is slow with a gradually increasing stiffness of gait, dorsiflexion of the head, and a hunching of the hindquarters; affected animals lag behind the group. The pulse and respiratory rates are increased, the temperature is elevated up to 42°C (107°F), and a cough may develop. There is diarrhea, the feces being dark and fetid, and urination occurs frequently, with the passage of small amounts of urine. Body weight is lost rapidly, and progressive weakness and recumbency develop after several days, but there is no evidence of paralysis, with the animal continuing to struggle while down. Death occurs usually within a few days, but a fatal course may be as long as 2 weeks. Animals that recover commonly shed part or all of the fleece but are solidly immune for long periods.

Pigs

The disease is latent in adult pigs, but young piglets show fever up to 42°C (107°F), accompanied by depression, profuse sweating, and dyspnea. The course of the disease is about 7 to 10 days.

Horses

In horses, fever (up to 42°C [107°F]) and stiffness and edema of the limbs occur. Foals are more seriously affected and may show dyspnea and incoordination in addition to the previously mentioned signs.

CLINICAL PATHOLOGY

Isolation of the pathogen can be attempted from impression smears or fixed specimens of organs such as liver, spleen, bone marrow, kidney, or lung and from blood smears. Immunologic methods such as the fluorescent antibody test are considered most reliable to identify the agent.[4] Polymerase chain reaction (PCR) protocols are now widely used to confirm the presence of bacterial DNA.

Serologic tests are the standard tests used for the diagnosis of tularemia in humans. In veterinary medicine serology may be employed for epidemiologic surveys of animal species resistant to the infection, but it is of limited value in susceptible species that commonly die before seroconversion occurs. The agglutination test is the most commonly used test for the diagnosis of tularemia, with a titer of 1:50 being regarded as a positive test in pigs. Serum from pigs affected with brucellosis does not agglutinate tularemia antigen, but serum from pigs affected with tularemia agglutinates brucellosis antigen. Cross-agglutination between *F. tularensis* and *Brucella abortus* is less common in sheep, and an accurate diagnosis can be made on serologic grounds because of the much greater agglutination that occurs with the homologous organism. Titers of agglutinins in affected sheep range from 1:640 to 1:5000 and may persist at levels of 1:320 for up to 7 months. A titer of 1:200 is classed as positive in sheep. In horses the titers revert to normal levels in 14 to 21 days.

Enzyme-linked immunosorbent assays (ELISAs) are available to identify either IgM, IgA, or IgG in infected animals. Because IgM levels are sustained for prolonged periods after infection, a high titer cannot be used as an indication for recent infection.[4]

NECROPSY FINDINGS

In sheep, large numbers of ticks may be present on the hides of fresh carcasses. In animals that have been dead for some time, dark-red subcutaneous areas of congestion up to 3 cm in diameter are found and may be accompanied by local swelling or necrosis of tissues. These lesions mark the attachment sites of ticks. Enlargement and congestion of the lymph nodes draining the sites of heaviest tick infestation are often noted. Pulmonary edema, congestion, or consolidation are inconstant findings.

In pigs the characteristic lesions are pleuritis, pneumonia, and abscessation of submaxillary and parotid lymph nodes. The organisms can be isolated from the lymph nodes and spleen and from infected ticks. Isolation can also be effected by experimental transmission to guinea pigs. Techniques such as immunoperoxidase staining of fixed specimens and PCR of fresh tissues can circumvent the need for culture of this zoonotic agent.

Samples for Confirmation of Diagnosis

- Bacteriology—lung, liver, lymph node, spleen, kidney, bone marrow, blood (immunohistochemistry, PCR, culture—requires cystine-enriched media)
- Histology—previously mentioned tissues fixed in formalin (light microscopy, immunohistochemistry)

Note the zoonotic potential of this organism when handling the carcasses and submitting specimens.

DIFFERENTIAL DIAGNOSIS

The occurrence of a highly fatal septicemia in sheep during spring months when the sheep are heavily infested with *Dermacentor andersoni* should suggest the possibility of tularemia, especially if the outbreak occurs in an enzootic area.

Tick paralysis. This occurs in the same area and at the same time of the year as tularemia but is not accompanied by fever, and there is marked flaccid paralysis. Recovery from tick paralysis occurs commonly if the ticks are removed.

Other septicemias include *P. trehalosi* in sheep and *Haemophilus* spp. in sheep and cattle. These are unusual in the age group in which tularemia occurs and are not associated with tick infestation. In pigs, local lesions can resemble tuberculosis.

Anthrax.

TREATMENT

Streptomycin, gentamicin, tetracyclines, and fluorochinolones are effective treatments in humans and companion animals. Oxytetracycline (10 mg/kg body weight [BW] IV or IM every 24 hours).

TREATMENT AND CONTROL

Treatment

Streptomycin (10 mg/kg IM every 24h) (R-2)

Oxytetracycline (10 mg/kg IV or IM every 24h) (R-2)

Enrofloxacin (2.5 mg/kg IM/SC every 24 hours for 3 to 5 days) (R-2)

Control

Tick control

Repellents

CONTROL

An outbreak of tularemia in sheep can be rapidly halted by spraying or dipping with an insecticide to kill the vector ticks. In areas where ticks are enzootic, sheep should be kept away from shrubby, infested pasture or sprayed regularly during the months when the tick population is greatest. An experimental live attenuated vaccine has been developed, but there is no routine vaccination of livestock.

FURTHER READING

Feldman KA. Tularemia. *J Am Vet Med Assoc.* 2003;222:725-730.

Petersen JM, Schriefer ME. Tularemia: emergence/re-emergence. *Vet Res.* 2005;36:455-467.

Tarnvik A, Priebe HS, Grunow R. Tularaemia in Europe: an epidemiological overview. *Scand J Infect Dis.* 2004;36:350-355.

World Health Organization (WHO). WHO guidelines on tularemia. 2007 at: <http://www.cdc.gov/tularemia/resources/whotularemiamanual.pdf>; Accessed 01.02.14.

REFERENCES

1. The Center for Food Security and Public Health. 2009 at: <http://www.cfsph.iastate.edu/Factsheets/pdfs/tularemia.pdf>; Accessed 01.02.14.
2. WHO. 2007 Available at: <http://www.cdc.gov/tularemia/resources/whotularemiamanual.pdf>; Accessed 01.02.14.
3. Anon. *MMWR.* 2013;62:963.
4. OIE. Terrestrial manual. 2008 at: <http://www.oie.int/fileadmin/Home/eng/Health_standards/tahm/2.01.18_TULAREMIA.pdf>; Accessed 01.02.14.

MELIOIDOSIS

SYNOPSIS

Etiology *Burkholderia pseudomallei.*

Epidemiology Ubiquitous soil saprophyte endemic to Southeast Asia, northern Australia, and the South Pacific. Occurs primarily 20° north and south of the equator. Transmission is by inhalation of contaminated dust and cutaneous abrasion. Primarily a disease of sheep and goats and humans, occasional disease in horses, and subclinical infection in pigs.

Clinical findings Septicemia, weakness, recumbency, and death in sheep. Septicemia, pneumonia, and lymphangitis in horses.

Clinical pathology Culture, serology, allergic skin test.

Necropsy findings Abscessation of internal organs.

Treatment and control General hygienic procedures. Little specific information available.

ETIOLOGY

Burkholderia pseudomallei is the sole cause. There is considerable genetic variability, and strains vary in pathogenicity. The organism causes latent (asymptomatic), acute, or chronic disease, depending largely on the host resistance to the organism.[1]

EPIDEMIOLOGY

Occurrence

The disease occurs almost exclusively in tropical countries 20° north and south of the equator and is endemic in Southeast Asia, Asia, and northern and subnorthern areas of Australia. Disease occurs in rodents, rabbits, pigeons, humans, animals in zoologic gardens, dogs, cats, horses, pigs, sheep, goats, alpacas, reptiles, and camels, but rarely in cattle.[2-6] In domestic animals the disease has occurred in outbreak form in pigs, goats, and sheep in Australia; in the Caribbean area and in Cambodia; in horses in Malaysia and Iran; in pigs and cattle in Papua New Guinea and Australia; in horses in France in 1976 to 1978; and in cattle in Argentina. Goats appear to be more susceptible than cattle or horses.[4]

The incidence rate in Thailand during 2006 to 2010 was 1.6 cases per 100,000 goats, 0.02 cases per 100,000 pigs, and 0.01 cases per 100,000 cattle. There were reports of the disease in a single camel, crocodile, deer, horse, monkey, and zebra. However, incidence rates varied considerably with region of the country, with rates as high as 101 cases per 100,000 goats and 19 cases per 100,000 people.[4] The estimates for animals are likely an underrepresentation of the actual incidence of the disease because not all dead animals are subject to postmortem examination.

Risk Factors

The risk factors for occurrence of melioidosis on small ruminant farms in Malaysia include the following: bush clearing around farms (odds ratio [OR] = 661, 95% confidence interval [CI] = 112-3884, *P* = 0037), *B. pseudomallei* present in the soil (OR = 623, 95% CI = 103-3768, *P* = 0046), other animal species present (OR = 796, 95% CI = 114-5599, *P* = 0037), and flooding or waterlogging conditions (OR = 1195, 95% CI = 139-1026, *P* = 0024).[7]

Source and Methods of Transmission

In endemic areas the organism is a ubiquitous soil saprophyte and is present in moist soil and waterholes which are the primary reservoirs from which most infections are acquired. A variety of free-living amoebae, including *Acanthamoeba* and *Hartmannella* spp., are potential hosts to *B. pseudomallei.* The majority of cases in livestock are associated with the "wet season" and exposure to surface water and mud. Infection occurs through inhalation, ingestion, in association with skin wounds via contaminated dust particles or water, or by insect bites. Infected animals pass the organism in their feces, and the disease in rodents runs a protracted course, making these animals important reservoirs of infection.

Pathogen Risk Factors

B. pseudomallei is very hardy and can survive in water at room temperature for up to 10 years, in muddy water for up to 7 months, and in soil in the laboratory for up to 30 months.[1] The organism can survive in contaminated injectable drugs and has ability to survive for some time in cetrimide 3% and chlorhexidine 0.3% solution. Varying degrees of virulence are observed in different strains of the organism, but starvation or other conditions of stress appear to increase the susceptibility of experimental animals to infection.

Experimental Production

The disease can be produced experimentally in goats, sheep, rats, mice, hamsters, and pigs.

Zoonotic Implications

Humans are at risk for infection within endemic areas, and although this can be zoonotic, it can also occur without direct animal contact through inhalation. The disease of humans presents with various clinical pictures ranging from asymptomatic state, to localized infection such as pneumonia, to acute fatal septicemia.

Veterinarians and animal owners are at risk from localized or generalized infection from infected animals. Pregnant women handling goats aborting with this infection have risk for infection and abortion. Infected areas are often rural in nature, and pasteurization of commercially sold milk should be ensured, as should condemnation of infected carcasses at abattoirs.

Pathogenesis

The pathogenesis of melioidosis involves infection of animals by *B. pseudomellia* in the environment, with subsequent transepithelial spread in infected macrophages. There is initial bacteremia or septicemia and subsequent localization in various organs. Experimentally induced melioidosis in goats induced by percutaneous administration of the organism is characterized by septicemia with undulating fever, wasting, anorexia, hindlimb paresis, mastitis, and abortion.[8] Necropsy lesions include widely scattered microabscesses after intraperitoneal injection and a chronic disease with abscesses in the lungs and spleen when the infection is administered subcutaneously. In pigs, experimental infection results in a generalized chronic infection.

CLINICAL FINDINGS

Sheep

Signs consist mainly of weakness, respiratory disease, and recumbency, with death occurring in 1 to 7 days. In experimentally infected sheep, a severe febrile reaction occurs and is accompanied by anorexia, lameness, and a thick, yellow exudate from the nose and eyes. Some animals show evidence of central nervous system involvement, including abnormal gait, deviation of the head and walking in circles, nystagmus, blindness, hyperesthesia, and mild tetanic convulsions. The disease is usually fatal. Skin involvement is not recorded.

Goats

The syndrome may resemble the acute form as seen in sheep, but it more commonly runs a chronic course with abscessation. Mastitis is common in infected goats, with one study finding mammary infection in 35% of infected goats.

Pigs

Disease is usually chronic and manifested by cervical lymphadenitis, but in some outbreaks there are signs similar to those in other species. In such outbreaks slight posterior paresis, mild fever, coughing, nasal and ocular discharge, anorexia, abortion, and some deaths may occur.

Horses

The syndrome is one of an acute metastatic pneumonia with high fever and a short course. Cough and nasal discharge are minimal, and there is a lack of response to treatment with most drugs. Other signs in horses include colic, diarrhea, and lymphangitis of the legs. Subacute cases become debilitated and emaciated and develop edema. Affected horses may survive for several months. A case of acute meningoencephalitis is described in a horse. The onset was sudden and manifest with violent convulsions.

CLINICAL PATHOLOGY

The organism is easily cultured and may be isolated from nasal discharges. The organism can be differentiated from *B. mallei* on multiplex quantitative PCR (qPCR) or using a PCR allelic discrimination assay.[9,10] Injection into guinea pigs and rabbits produces the typical disease. An allergic skin test using melioidin as an antigen, a complement fixation test (CFT), and an indirect hemagglutination (IHA) test are available. An ELISA is available that can detect antibodies to *B. pseudomallei* in goats.[11] The IHA test is recommended for screening and the CFT for confirmation in cases of active melioidosis in goats and pigs. Affected horses can give a positive reaction to the mallein test.

NECROPSY

Multiple abscesses in most organs, particularly in the lungs, spleen, and liver, but also in the subcutis and the associated lymph nodes, are characteristic of the disease in all species. In sheep respiratory infection is common, and these abscesses in the lung contain thick or caseous, green-tinged pus similar to that found in *Corynebacterium pseudotuberculosis* lesions. Lesions in the nasal mucosa proceed to rupture, with the development of ragged ulcers. An acute polyarthritis, with distension of the joint capsules by fluid containing large masses of greenish pus, and acute meningoencephalitis have been observed in experimental cases.

A high incidence of lesions in the aorta of goats is reported in Australia. Nine out of 43 (21%) goats had aortic lesions at autopsy. Seven of these goats died as a result of a ruptured aortic aneurysm.

DIAGNOSTIC CONFIRMATION

Culture of the organism confirms the diagnosis.

DIFFERENTIAL DIAGNOSIS

Sheep
Caseous lymphadenitis
Actinobacillosis

Horses
Glanders
Strangles

Pigs
Tuberculosis

TREATMENT

Treatment is unlikely to be undertaken in farm animals because of the nature of the disease and the risk of exposure to humans. Little information is available on satisfactory treatments of melioidosis in farm animals, but recommendations for humans are available. Penicillin, streptomycin, chlortetracycline, and polymyxin are ineffective, but in vitro tests suggest that oxytetracycline, novobiocin, chloramphenicol, and sulfadiazine are most likely to be valuable, with oxytetracycline the preferred drug. In horses, chloramphenicol is an effective treatment.

CONTROL

There is currently no vaccine for melioidosis.[12]

Prevention involves removing animals from the contaminating source. Water supplies can be chlorinated. This and the elimination of infected animals and the disinfection of premises should be the basis of control procedures. Housed animals can be removed from soil by raising them from the ground on wooden slats or with concrete or paved floors. Treatment of soil with lime reduces the risk (OR = 0.028) of animals developing melioidosis.[7]

FURTHER READING

Adler NRL, et al. The molecular and cellular basis of pathogenesis in melioidosis: how does *Burkholderia pseudomallei* cause disease? *FEMS Microbiol Rev.* 2009;33:1079-1099.

REFERENCES

1. Adler NRL, et al. *FEMS Microbiol Rev.* 2009;33:1079.
2. Hampton V, et al. *Emerg Infect Dis.* 2011;17:1310.
3. Johnson CH, et al. *Comp Med.* 2013;63:528.
4. Limmathurotsakul D, et al. *Emerg Infect Dis.* 2012;18:325.
5. Parkes HM, et al. *J Fel Med Surg.* 2009;11:856.
6. Zehnder AM, et al. *Emerg Infect Dis.* 2014;20:304.
7. Musa HI, et al. *J Appl Micro.* 2015;119:331.
8. Soffler C, et al. *Int J Exp Pathol.* 2014;95:101.
9. Janse I, et al. *BMC Infect Dis.* 2013;13.
10. Bowers JR, et al. *PLoS ONE.* 2010;5.
11. Mekaprateep M, et al. *J Microbiol Meth.* 2010;83:266.
12. Choh L-C, et al. *Front Cell Inf Micro.* 2013;3.

HEARTWATER (COWDRIOSIS)

SYNOPSIS

Etiology *Ehrlichia (Cowdria) ruminantium,* a rickettsial organism.

Vectors *Amblyomma variegatum* and *Amblyomma hebraeum.*

Epidemiology Endemic disease of cattle, sheep, goats and wild ruminants in Africa and the Caribbean; high mortality in exotic animals.

Clinical signs High fever, nervous signs, diarrhea, and death if acute; may be mild and inapparent.

Clinical pathology Nonspecific.

Diagnostic confirmation Rickettsial colonies in capillary endothelium (brain preparations), polymerase chain reaction (PCR).

Lesions Ascites, hydrothorax, hydropericardium, and severe pulmonary edema.

Differential diagnosis list Anthrax, rabies, cerebral babesiosis, cerebral theileriosis, meningitis or encephalitis.

Treatment Short- and long-acting tetracyclines.

Control Vaccination based on infection and treatment methods, tick control, and chemoprophylaxis.

ETIOLOGY

Ehrlichia (*Cowdria*) *ruminantium* is a gram-negative, intracellular rickettsial organism in the order of Rickettsiales. It occurs in colonies or morulae with a predilection for the vascular endothelium and stains blue with Giemsa stain. The organism is coccoid, 0.2 to 0.5 microns in diameter. It can now be cultivated in vitro, and it can also grow in mice. Cyclical development takes place in intestinal and salivary epithelia of ticks. Widely ranging *E. ruminantium* genotypes with differing cross-protection capacities usually circulate simultaneously in the same region, leading to a poor vaccine efficacy.[1] However, all isolates obtained at different geographic levels (village, region, and continent) possess a major antigenic protein 1 (MAP1) that is conserved.[2] This protein is used for serologic diagnosis, but the antigen cross-reacts with other *Ehrlichia* spp., including *E. equi,* the cause of equine granulocytic ehrlichiosis. Variants of *E. ruminantium* that do not cause disease in livestock have also been reported from South Africa.[3]

EPIDEMIOLOGY

Occurrence

Heartwater was first recognized in South Africa in the nineteenth century.[4] The disease is limited in its occurrence to sub-Saharan Africa, including the islands of Madagascar, Sao Tome, Reunion, Mauritius, Zanzibar, and Mayotte in the Indian Ocean. It is also present on the three Caribbean islands of Guadeloupe, Marie-Galante, and Antigua, where it threatens the American mainland because of the risk of spread of its tick vector by migratory birds or by uncontrolled movement of animals.[5] Heartwater is one of the main causes of death in imported breeds of cattle, sheep, and goats in endemic areas.

Measures of Disease Occurrence

In endemic areas, morbidity and mortality rates are low, but the percentage of serapositive titers for heartwater could be as high as 100% in adult cattle, depending on the abundance of tick vectors. In Tanzania, antibodies to *E. ruminantium* were found in 68.6% of the sheep and 64.7% of the goats examined by ELISA, but the infection was unevenly distributed within districts.[6] Case mortality can be as high as 100% in peracute cases in sheep and goats and as low as 0 to 10% in cattle. The disease is less severe in indigenous breeds and related game animals reared in enzootic areas, some of which may become symptomless carriers. The N'Dama breed in West Africa is reported to be well adapted to heartwater, partly because it can resist tick burdens under traditional farming system. Conversely, the Angora goat is highly susceptible, and Merino sheep are moderately so.

Method of Transmission

Heartwater is transmitted by many ticks of the *Amblyomma* genus, especially by *A. variegatum* (the tropical bont tick) mostly in western, central, and eastern Africa and the Caribbean, and by *A. habraeum* mostly in southern Africa. The geographic distribution of the ticks appears to be spreading. Infection in ticks is transmitted transstadially and possibly transovarially. A single infected tick can transmit the disease to the host, and this can occur 1 to 2 days after attachment as nymph or 2 to 3 days as adult. Vertical transmission to calves and lambs in utero and in colostral milk has been reported. Several wild ruminants can be infected and become subclinical carriers and reservoirs. Tick feeding on them can transmit the disease to domestic ruminants. In the Caribbean, cattle egrets are suspected to spread *A. variegatum* between islands. However, recent molecular studies of isolates from the Caribbean and Africa would suggest that there was a simultaneous introduction of several strains of *E. ruminantium* from Africa into the Caribbean.[7] Nevertheless, heartwater is considered to be a threat to the American mainland, where potential vectors such as *A. maculatum* are present but do not harbor the disease or where the vector may be introduced by migratory birds and become established. Similarly, southern Italy is considered at risk of introduction and establishment of infected *Amblyomma* ticks through migratory birds.[8] The organism does not infect humans.

Risk Factors and Immune Mechanisms

Animals at greatest risk are exotics imported into endemic areas and at times when the vector population is high, usually during the rains. Angora goats are also highly susceptible and therefore difficult to immunize by the current method of infection and treatment. Cattle and sheep recovering from the disease are immune for 6 months to 4 years but may be carriers for 8 months or longer. Immunity is related to the ability of lymphocytes in infected animals to produce interferon gamma (IFN-γ).[9] An age-dependent resistance has long been recognized, and young animals were thought to have innate resistance. This was later shown to be attributable to low-grade infection of the young in colostral cells or following intrauterine transmission. In small ruminants, the resistance begins to wane at the age range of 4 and 12 weeks when they are most susceptible.[10]

ECONOMIC IMPORTANCE

Heartwater is the most important rickettsial infection of ruminants in Africa and the second most important tick-borne disease after East Coast fever. In southern Africa, it is regarded as the most important disease of ruminants. In general, heartwater is a more serious problem where *A. habraeum* is the vector. In countries or regions where there is endemic stability, losses from heartwater are minimal until new animals are introduced or moved from nonendemic to endemic areas. On the other hand, because most losses are in exotic animals, heartwater is a major constraint to livestock improvement in sub-Saharan Africa. Furthermore, it has the potential to spread from North Africa to Europe and from the Caribbean to the American mainland.

Biosecurity Concerns

Heartwater requires the vector tick to get established in any community. Therefore there is concern about possible illegal importation of infected animals or ticks to the southern United States where potential vectors exist. Migratory birds can also introduce infected ticks to parts of the Mediterranean countries where the environment is suitable for the establishment of *Amblyomma*.

PATHOGENESIS

There is limited new information on the pathogenesis of heartwater. The rickettsial organisms are introduced into the host in the saliva of an infected tick. They multiply in reticuloendothelial cells of the local lymph node, rupture the cells, and are released into the circulation, where they invade endothelial cells of blood vessels in all organs, where further multiplication takes place. Organisms can be found in phagosomes of circulating neutrophils but are more abundant in endothelial cells. Invasion of vascular endothelium causes increased vascular permeability, leading to edema, especially in the lungs, body cavities, and the brain, by mechanisms that are not understood because infected endothelial cells show minimal cytopathic effects. Brain edema is responsible for the nervous signs, severe hydropericardium will impair cardiac function, and severe pulmonary edema with hydrothorax would lead to death from asphyxia. In goats, renal ischemia and nephrosis have been described, and irreversible kidney damage may be the cause of death in such cases.

CLINICAL FINDINGS

The incubation period is 1 to 3 weeks after transmission in tick saliva. Depending on the susceptibility of individual animals and the virulence of the infecting organism, the resulting disease may be peracute, acute, subacute, or mild and inapparent. Peracute cases show only high fever, prostration, and death with terminal convulsions in 1 to 2 days. Acute cases are more common and have a course of about 6 days. A sudden febrile reaction is followed by inappetence, listlessness, and rapid breathing, followed by the classical nervous syndrome that is characteristic of heartwater. It comprises ataxia, chewing movements, twitching of the eyelids, circling, aggression, apparent blindness, recumbency, convulsions, and death. Profuse, fetid diarrhea is frequent.

Subacute cases are less severe but may terminate in death in 2 weeks or the animal may gradually recover. The mild form is often subclinical and is seen mainly in indigenous animals and wild ruminants with high natural or induced resistance. The case-mortality rate in peracute cases is 100%; in acute cases, 50% to 90%; and in calves at less than 4 weeks of age, it is 5% to 10%; most animals recover in mild cases.

CLINICAL PATHOLOGY

Hematologic changes in heartwater are not specific, but there may be thrombocytopenia, neutropenia, eosinopenia and lymphocytosis. Confirmatory diagnosis is based on identifying the rickettsia in capillary endothelial cells using a Giemsa-stained squash preparation of brain tissue at postmortem. The rickettsiae occur as blue to reddish-purple colonies or morulae of five to several hundred coccoid organisms (0.2 to 0.5 microns in diameter) in the cytoplasm of the cells close to the nucleus. An immunohistochemical staining technique has also been described. Injection of blood into sheep may also be used as a diagnostic procedure because sheep are highly susceptible.

The polymerase chain reaction (PCR) assay is preferred for confirmatory diagnosis in a sick animal. To this end, a quantitative pCS20 real-time PCR has been developed and can be performed within 2 hours in live animals; it is also an effective assay for epidemiologic surveillance and monitoring of infected animals, and it can be used by paraveterinary staff.[11-12] However, it cross-reacts with at least two other *Ehrlichia* spp. Nested pCS20 PCR is highly sensitive and can be used to detect infected ticks.[13] A more sensitive and highly specific new test has been reported. It is the loop-mediated isothermal amplification (LAMP) assay, in which DNA amplification is completed in 1 hour.[14] Assays using two sets of LAMP primers designed from the pCS20 and sodB genes were more sensitive than conventional pCS20 PCR assay. LAMP detected 16 different isolates from geographically distinct countries, and no cross-reaction was observed with genetically related Rickettsiales. Because of its simplicity and specificity, LAMP also has the potential for use in clinical laboratories in resource-poor countries where heartwater is endemic and for active screening in areas under threat of introduction of the disease.

Serologic tests are used for surveys, and the two tests recommended are indirect fluorescent antibody (IFA) and ELISA. The close antigenic relationship between *E. ruminantium* and other *Ehrlichia* spp. often leads to false positives. The ELISA based on recombinant MAP1 protein of *E. ruminantium* is more sensitive, but all serologic assays have poor sensitivity and specificity.

NECROPSY FINDINGS

Standard lesions are ascites, hydrothorax, and hydropericardium. Pulmonary edema is often severe, accompanied by copious froth in the tracheobronchial airways. There may be subserosal hemorrhages in most cavities. Lymph nodes are swollen and wet, and the spleen is markedly enlarged. In goats with nephrosis, the kidneys will be soft. Although hemorrhages have been described in the brain, this organ often has no remarkable gross lesions; microscopically, there is perivascular mononuclear infiltration and edema along with presence of rickettsial colonies in capillary endothelial cells. The colonies disappear quickly as autolysis sets in. Foci of malacia may be present. Tissues for histopathology should include brain, lungs, lymph nodes, spleen, and kidneys. In addition, squash preparations of brain should be submitted for direct staining with Giemsa of for PCR detection.

DIFFERENTIAL DIAGNOSIS

In endemic areas, heartwater should be suspected in susceptible animals infected with *Amblyomma* and having a fever of unknown origin, especially when accompanied by nervous signs. The clinical and pathologic findings are not specific, and the diagnosis must be based on detection of rickettsial organisms.

The peracute form should be differentiated from anthrax and the acute form from rabies, sporadic bovine encephalomyelitis, tetanus, cerebral forms of theileriosis, babesiosis, trypanosomosis, meningitis, listeric or other encephalitis, hypomagnesemia, and poisoning with strychnine, lead and organophosphates. Appropriate laboratory tests are utilized to eliminate these differentials.

TREATMENT

TREATMENT AND CONTROL

Treatment

Oxytetracycline (10–20 mg/kg IM in early stages) (R-1)

Sulfamethazine (55 mg/kg SC) (R-2)

Hyperimmune serum (R-4)

Control

Infection and treatment with tetracycline IM or with doxycycline implant SC (R-1)

Attenuated vaccine from cell culture (R-1)

Vector control (R-1)

Field cases of heartwater are difficult to treat successfully because available drugs are effective only in early febrile stages before neurologic signs develop. In the early stages, short-acting tetracyclines (oxytetracycline at 10 to 20 mg/kg BW or doxycycline at 2 mg/kg) and long-acting forms at reduced doses are effective. Sulfonamides (e.g., sulfamethazine) were also used in the early stages but are less effective. Hyperimmune serum is reported to be of no curative value. Supportive therapy to reduce either the pulmonary edema or the neurologic signs or to stabilize membranes in general is being investigated, but with little success.

Chemoprophylaxis involves administration of tetracyclines or subcutaneous implantation of doxycycline in susceptible animals when they are introduced into an endemic area. Results are not always predictable.

CONTROL

Heartwater has traditionally been controlled by four different approaches: controlling the tick vector by dipping, establishing endemic stability, performing immunization by infection and treatment, and preventing the disease by regular administration of prophylactic antibiotics.[15] Control efforts have been hindered by abundance of ticks in endemic areas, by high rate of the carrier state following infection, and by lack of efficient vaccine in the field as a result of the high genetic diversity of strains circulating in any given area.[16]

Past efforts to control heartwater were based on intensive acaricide treatment to control ticks in endemic areas. It involved frequent use of acaricides (plunge dipping) up to 52 times a year. This has now been shown to be environmentally unfriendly and economically unsustainable, and it would invariably lead to animals that remained always susceptible. For example, it was observed in Zimbabwe that large farms applying acaricides very frequently (more than 30 times per annum) had higher morbidity and mortality than farms applying acaricides less frequently.

Long-acting acaricides have largely replaced the earlier ones applied frequently. Apart from being more environmentally friendly, occasional use of acaricides helps in the establishment of endemic stability in treated animals because they can still be exposed to low levels of infection. For example, flumenthrin 1% pour-on at 45-day intervals was found to provide effective protection of Friesian–Zebu crossbred cattle against important ticks, but it must be applied correctly at the recommended dose. Pure Zebu and N'Dama cattle would probably require less frequent applications. Flumenthrin pour-on is gradually replacing plunge dipping for the control of ticks and tickborne diseases in general.

Vaccination is based on infection and treatment regimen that was first developed more than 50 years ago. It involves an intravenous injection of virulent organisms in cryopreserved sheep blood, followed by treatment with tetracyclines at the first indication of fever. The exposure of calves and lambs up to 3 weeks of age, without treatment, is considered optimal for the development of resistance, but kids may still be susceptible. Vaccination may lead to some deaths, the immunity may wane in absence of reinfection, and animals may become carriers. Nevertheless, the use of inactivated vaccines from cell-cultured *E. ruminantium* combined with an adjuvant led to a reduction in mortality from heartwater in cattle, sheep, and goats exposed to field challenges in Botswana, Zambia, Zimbabwe, and South Africa. Recently, an attenuated vaccine from *E. ruminantium* (Welgevonden) stock given intramuscularly was found to provide protection against virulent homologous needle challenge in Merino and Angora goats; injection did not produce disease, and protection was for at least 12 months after immunization.[17] In the Gambia, an attenuated vaccine was found to be superior to an inactivated vaccine for sheep.[18] Mass production of *E. ruminantium* variants from different regions of sub-Saharan Africa is one of the difficulties that must be overcome in producing a heartwater vaccine from cell culture.[19] Recently, a process for the large-scale production of a ready-to-use inactivated vaccine against heartwater was described.[20]

Experimental studies using DNA recombinant vaccines so far have met with only limited success, and none has been as effective as immunization with live organisms.[9,21] The development of a universal recombinant vaccine would require increased knowledge of *E. ruminantium* biology, including virulence mechanisms.[5] So far, the goal of producing an effective vaccine against the disease in the field still remains frustratingly just beyond reach.[4]

What is advocated today is integrated control based on the establishment of endemic stability by vaccination or natural challenge and general reduction in tick infestation through periodic application of long-acting insecticides when warranted.

FURTHER READING

Bezuidenhout JD, et al. Heartwater. In: Coetzer JAW, Thomson GR, Tustin RC, eds. *Infectious Diseases of Livestock With Special Reference to Southern Africa.* Vol. 1. Cape Town: Oxford University Press; 1994:351.

Bigalke RD. Heartwater: past present and future. *Onderstepoort J Vet Res.* 1987;54:163.

OIE. *Manual of Diagnostic Tests and Vaccines for Terrestrial Animals.* Paris: OIE; 2008 chapter 2.01.06:217.

Scott GR. Cowdriosis. In: Sewell MMH, Brocklesby DW, eds. *Handbook on Animal Diseases in the Tropics.* 4th ed. London: Baillière Tindall; 1990:234.

REFERENCES

1. Nakao R, et al. *Parasite Vectors.* 2011;4:137.
2. Railiniaina M, et al. *Vet Parasitol.* 2010;167:187.
3. Allsopp BA, et al. *Vet Microbiol.* 2007;120:158.
4. Allsopp BA. *Vet Parasitol.* 2010;167:123.
5. Vachiery N, et al. *Dev Biol (Basel).* 2013;135:191.
6. Swai ES, et al. *Trop Anim Health Prod.* 2009;41:959.
7. Vachiery N, et al. *Ann NY Acad Sci.* 2008;1149:191.
8. Pascucci I, et al. *Vet Ital.* 2007;43:655.
9. Liebenberg J, et al. *Vet Immunol Immunopathol.* 2012;145:340.
10. Faburay B, et al. *BMC Infect Dis.* 2007;7:85.
11. Stein HC, et al. *J S Afr Vet Assoc.* 2010;81:160.
12. Steyn HC, et al. *Vet Microbiol.* 2008;131:258.
13. Kelley PJ, et al. *J Med Entomol.* 2011;48:485.
14. Nakao R, et al. *BMC Microbiol.* 2010;10:296.
15. Allsopp BA. *Onderstepoort J Vet Res.* 2009;76:81.
16. Adakal H, et al. *Infect Genet Evol.* 2009;9:1320.
17. Zweygarth E, et al. *Vaccine.* 2008;26(suppl 6):G34.
18. Feburay B, et al. *Vaccine.* 2007;25:7939.
19. Pedregal A. *Ann N Y Acad Sci.* 2008;1149:286.
20. Marcelino I, et al. *Vaccine.* 2015;33:678.
21. Pretorius A, et al. *Vaccine.* 2007;25:2316.

HISTOPHILUS SEPTICEMIA OF CATTLE (*HISTOPHILUS SOMNI* OR *HAEMOPHILUS SOMNUS* DISEASE COMPLEX)

SYNOPSIS

Etiology *Histophilus somni* (formerly *Haemophilus somnus*)

Epidemiology High prevalence of infection in cattle population; low incidence of disease. Occurs in North American feedlot cattle, in the United Kingdom, and in some European countries. Young growing cattle are most commonly affected. Originally, thrombotic meningoencephalitis (TME) was most common lesion, but pleuropneumonia and myocarditis are more common now. Several virulence factors of organism may account for different forms of disease. Organism resides in respiratory and reproductive tracts of both females and males.

Signs Thrombotic meningoencephalitis with fever, ataxia, joint swellings, weakness, recumbency, and death in 12 to 24 hours; pleuropneumonia and myocarditis with rapid death; reproductive failure with abortion.

Clinical pathology Marked changes in leukon. Demonstrate and culture organism from cerebrospinal fluid, joint fluid, pleural cavity, and myocardium.

Lesions Meningoencephalitis, hemorrhagic infarcts in brain, retinal hemorrhages,

Continued

pleuropneumonia, myocarditis. Vasculitis in infected tissue.

Diagnostic confirmation Culture, polymerase chain reaction (PCR).

Treatment Antimicrobials.

Control *H. somni* bacterin vaccines are available but unreliable; metaphylactic treatment with antimicrobials at time of placement in feedlot is frequently used.

ETIOLOGY

Histophilus somni (formerly *Haemophilus somnus*) is a gram-negative, fastidious pleomorphic coccobacillus of the family Pasteurellaceae. Earlier investigations have shown that *H. somni, Haemophilus agni,* and *Histophilus ovis* represent the same species, and recent analysis of genes of strains supports the allocation of this species to a novel genus within the family Pasteurellaceae as *Histophilus somni.*[1] *H. somni* causes a variety of diseases in cattle, including septicemia, thrombotic meningoencephalitis (TME), pleuropneumonia, myocarditis, reproductive failure with abortion, polyarthritis, and, in sheep, mastitis, septicemia, and epididymitis.

EPIDEMIOLOGY

Prevalence of Infection

H. somni is an obligate inhabitant of mucosal surfaces of bovines, ovines, and related ruminants with worldwide occurrence. It is frequently found as an asymptomatic commensal in the male prepuce, the female vagina, and occasionally in the upper respiratory tract.[1] More than 50% of normal bulls, 8% to 10% of normal cows, and 10% of normal rams have *H. somni* in the reproductive tract. Among those that have had the disease and survived, the serologic reactor rate varies from 50% to 100%. Some surveys found more positive reactors in beef cattle and dairy cattle from infected herds than in dairy cattle from herds without clinical disease.

Occurrence of Disease

H. somni is responsible for a variety of clinical syndromes in cattle, most of which occur in feedlot and dairy calves, although disease was also observed in grazing cattle.[2] Infection of cattle with *H. somni* may cause septicemia, thrombotic meningoencephalitis (TME), polysynovitis, pleuritis, suppurative bronchopneumonia, myocarditis, otitis media, mastitis, and reproductive tract diseases. When infection of cattle with the organism was first described in 1956, the primary form of the disease was TME. Since then, many different clinical forms of the infection have been described. Suppurative bronchopneumonia, fibrinous pleuritis, and myocarditis are now being recognized with increased frequency in feedlot cattle and are being attributed to *H. somni* infection. Based on necropsy examinations over a 20-year period in a Saskatchewan diagnostic laboratory, there has been an increasing percentage of cattle with pneumonia and myocarditis associated with the organism and a decreasing percentage with TME. However, because of the practical difficulties in making a specific clinical, pathologic, and microbiological diagnosis in situations where the disease complex occurs, there is some uncertainty about the relative importance of the organism in causing certain diseases, such as pneumonia of feedlot cattle. For example, because of the variability of nature and extent of the lesions in bovine respiratory disease and the common occurrence of mixed infections, it is difficult to determine whether *H. somni* or *M. haemolytica* is the primary pathogen.

The disease occurs most commonly in **feedlot cattle** in North America after they have been commingled from different sources. The disease has also been recognized in the United Kingdom, Germany, Switzerland, and Israel. The organism has been found in the tonsillar tissues of American bison (*Bison bison*) and has been the cause of bronchopneumonia in bison.

The incidence rate of TME in a susceptible group of calves is low, averaging about 2%, but may be up to 10% in some outbreaks. The case-fatality rate, however, is 90% if affected animals are not identified and treated early in the course of the disease.

TME was historically a disease of feedlot cattle from 6 to 12 months of age with highest occurrence during the fall and winter months. In Canada TME occurred most commonly in cattle about 4 weeks after arrival in the feedlot, with a range of 1 week to 7 months. It also occurred in feedlot cattle in Argentina.

The disease complex that is encountered more commonly now is characterized by **pleuritis, pneumonia, and myocarditis** and can be the most significant cause of mortality in feedlot calves. Death from pneumonia attributable to the infection occurs mainly during the first 5 weeks in the feedlot; death from myocarditis, pleuritis, TME, septicemia, and euthanasia because of polysynovitis occurs mainly after the third week. This disease complex is occurring despite routine vaccination of calves on arrival in the feedlot. A history of respiratory tract disease preceding the outbreak is common, and in some cases TME had occurred in the same herd in the previous year.

H. somni also causes various forms of reproductive failure in cattle. The importation of infected young rams into a flock can have a deleterious effect on the percentage of ewes that lamb. Purchasing replacement animals and having cattle on the same farm were risk factors for infection in the flock. The possibility of interspecies transmission between cattle and sheep requires further study.

Risk Factors

Animal Risk Factors

Thrombotic meningoencephalitis, pleuropneumonia, and myocarditis occur most commonly in feedlot calves 6 to 12 months of age.

Pathogen Risk Factors

The literature on the virulence factors of the organism has been reviewed.[2,3] Several virulence factors have been identified, including adherence, synthesis of lipooligosaccharide (LOS) and LOS phase variation, antigen variation of surface proteins, synthesis of immunoglobulin binding proteins, or the production of histamine and hemolysin.

Adherence. *H. somni* colonizes the surface of mucous membranes. In the asymptomatic carrier state the organism remains at the mucosal surface without invading cells; it attaches to nonepithelial cells, as has been documented in the example of bovine aortic endothelial cells. It is assumed that nonpilus adhesins are involved in the adherence of the organism to the cell surface.[2] *H. somni* attaches in large numbers to bovine vaginal epithelial cells, and attachment may be all that is necessary to produce infertility as a result of endometritis or degeneration of embryos during early gestation. The organism is able to persist in the lungs of calves for 6 to 10 weeks in the presence of specific antibody and in the absence of clinical abnormalities other than sporadic coughing.

Lipooligosaccharides (LOS or Endotoxin). Endotoxin produced by *H. somni* lacks the long, repeated polysaccharide chains that are characteristic for some gram-negative bacteria and is thus more appropriately designated as lipooligosaccharide (LOS) rather than lipopolysaccharide. The microorganism can vary the structure of the LOS by switching on and off specific genes encoding individual glycosyltransferases that are responsible for attaching individual glycoses to the oligosaccharide molecule, a phenomenon termed as **LOS phase variation**. The structure of the LOS outer core oligosaccharides of some strains mimics that of host glycosphingolipids, which may allow the organism to evade the host's immune system by camouflaging bacterial antigen.[1] LOS specifically triggers bovine platelet aggregation and may thereby contribute to adherence and colonization of respiratory epithelial cells and bovine endothelial cells. LOS was furthermore found to mediate apoptosis of bovine endothelial cells; the cytotoxic properties and the serum resistance of some strains have also been proposed to be associated with the production of LOS.[4]

Antigen Variation of Surface Proteins. Surface proteins or outer membrane proteins (OMPs) are important immunologic structures accessible for the host's immune system.

Strains of *H. somni* are diverse in molecular mass and antigenic reactivity. Although the precise role of OMPs in the pathogenesis of histophilosis is not yet understood, they may play an important role in the ability of the organism to evade the host's immune system and cause disease.[2]

Immunoglobulin-Binding Proteins. Immunoglobulin-binding proteins (IgBPs) are characterized by their affinity to IgG_2 immunoglobulin and are thought to enable *H. somni* to evade antibody defense. Although it is well accepted that IgBPs are important determinants of serum resistance of pathogenic *H. somni* strains, the underlying mechanism is not yet well explained.[3] Some isolates of the organism are indeed able to multiply in vivo because they are resistant to complement, and bovine leukocytes are incapable of destroying the organism in the absence of specific antibody.

Transferrin-Binding Proteins. *H. somni* is inherently dependent on the availability of iron and in absence of available iron produces transferrin-binding proteins (TBPs) that specifically bind bovine transferrin but not transferrin of other species.[3] This was proposed as one of the underlying causes for the host specificity of *H. somni.*

Biofilm Synthesis. *H. somni* was found to produce biofilm in vitro and in vivo, which is a virulence factor likely contributing to the pathogenesis of histophilosis. Strains of *H. somni* isolated from diseased tissue often have the greatest capacity to form a biofilm.[5] Furthermore, different strains were found to produce biofilm with different structures, and difference in biofilm architecture may correlate with resistance to the host's immune defense mechanisms.[1]

Some strains are serum resistant and others serum sensitive, which may explain the ability of certain strains to invade beyond mucous membrane surfaces. Virulence differences also exist between *H. somni* strains following intratracheal challenge of bovine lungs. Those strains isolated from encephalitic lesions, or from the prepuce, will not produce the same degree of experimental pneumonia as those strains isolated from lung lesions. Preputial and septicemic isolates of ovine *H. somni* are similar to bovine *H. somni* in pathogenicity and in surface antigens. Ovine isolates given by intracisternal inoculation to 2- to 3-month-old lambs caused fatal meningoencephalitis and myelitis.

In summary, many virulence factors are involved in several steps of pathogenesis. Adherence is likely to be important in colonization, complement resistance in survival in the circulation or inflammatory sites, and cytotoxicity in evading killing by phagocytes and in initiation of vasculitis, and invasion through the endothelium. The host damage that occurs as a result may be further exacerbated by inflammatory mediators released by the host in response to *H. somni.*

Methods of Transmission

The method of transmission and portal of entry are unclear. A feature of infections with this organism is its persistence at mucosal sites in both subclinical and diseased animals. The organism can be isolated from the respiratory and reproductive tracts of normal animals.

In bulls, the organism has been isolated from semen and the preputial orifice, preputial cavity, urinary bladder, accessory sex glands, ampulla of the ductus deferens, and the preputial washings of steers. Most bulls harbor the organism in the prepuce. Thus the potential exists for venereal transmission of *H. somni,* for lateral spread from the genital tract, and for environmental contamination by the organism.

The organism has also been isolated from the vagina, vestibular gland, cervix, uterus, and bladder of cows. The prevalence of infection in normal cows varies depending on the herd and geographic location, but 10% to 27% can harbor the organism. The organism can colonize the vagina of cows without causing disease, and it is thought to have a primary etiologic role in vaginitis and cervicitis in cows.

The organism has been isolated from the udder secretions of cattle with naturally occurring mastitis.

Urine is also a source of the organism. The young beef calf in a cow–calf herd can become infected as early as 1 month of age and become a nasal carrier of the organism without showing any signs of clinical disease. The mature cow is considered to be a major source of infection for the calf. The method of transmission is presumed to be by contact with infective respiratory and reproductive secretions or by aerosol transmission, especially in close-contact feedlots.

The organism can survive more than 70 days when it is mixed with cerebrospinal fluid, whole blood, blood plasma, vaginal mucus, or milk and frozen at −70° C (−94° F). At 23.5° C (73.5° F) it can survive beyond 70 days when mixed with whole blood and nasal mucus. The viability of the organism in urine at all temperatures is less than 24 hours and less than 15 minutes at 20° C (68° F) and 37° C (98° F). It survives for less than 1 day in milk at room temperature or when incubated at 37° C (98° F) and should be considered as a possible cause of mastitis in cases that are negative on routine bacteriologic culture.

Immune Mechanisms

Serum antibody titers do not correlate with susceptibility to clinical disease. Naturally acquired humoral immunity does not influence the outcome of experimental intravenous inoculation of the organism. Also, the role of naturally acquired antibody in protecting cattle from disease is uncertain. The levels of naturally occurring serum bactericidal activity to *H. somni* are low or absent in calves at 4 to 6 months of age, when they are most susceptible to TME. The levels increase with age and are high in mature cows; yearlings have intermediate levels.

Convalescent sera from calves with experimental *H. somni* pneumonia protect calves against acute *H. somni* pneumonia. Marked serum exudation characterizes the early stages of experimental pneumonia, and antibody should be involved in protection. The specificity of this protection is directed primarily against outer-membrane proteins (OMPs) of the organism. These antigens may also be useful in serologic diagnosis because convalescent calves have high IgG_1 and IgG_2 titers to *H. somni* for several weeks. The measurement of serum IgG_1 is a more reliable test to detect a current or recently active infection. Later, there is a sustained increase in IgG_2. The development of a systemic IgG_2 antibody response is the basis for local immunologic protection in the bovine reproductive tract.[3]

The immune response in cattle to the major outer membrane proteins during infection is weak and directed to antigenically variable determinants in a strain specific manner that may have important implications in protective immunity. Vaccination of 1- to 2-month-old calves with commercial aluminum-hydroxide-adjuvanted *H. somni* bacterins elicits an ELISA-detectable IgE response 14 days after injection, which may be associated with severe clinical disease associated with type I hypersensitivity.

PATHOGENESIS

H. somni first establishes itself in the host by colonizing the surface of the mucous membranes. It is not known if strains harbored in the respiratory tract or the genital tract invade the circulatory system to cause septicemia with ensuing localization in many tissues and organs. Although respiratory disease preceding TME has been described, experimental intratracheal inoculation resulted in colonization of the upper and lower respiratory tract without concomitant septicemia.[2]

The ability of *H. somni* to survive in both mononuclear phagocytes and neutrophils may be important in the establishment of the chronic multisystemic infection characteristic of bovine histophilosis. With TME the sequence of events may be initiated by adhesion of the bacterium to vascular endothelial cells. The organism's LOS induces endothelial cell apoptosis and contraction and desquamation of cells, with exposure of subendothelial collagen; thrombosis and vasculitis is followed by ischemic necrosis of adjacent parenchyma. The common site of localization is the brain. Multifocal areas of hemorrhagic necrosis occur throughout the brain, resulting in TME and causing the typical clinical findings of depression, paresis, and recumbency. Localization in synovia results in polysynovitis. Fibrin thrombi occur in the small vessels and capillaries of the liver, spleen, kidney, lung, heart, and brain, which suggests that **disseminated intravascular coagulation** may be a feature of the pathogenesis of *Histophilus* septicemia. Myocarditis has been recognized with increased frequency and is characterized by acute or chronic heart failure.[6]

The pathogenesis of *Histophilus* pneumonia is not clear. Although *H. somni* has been isolated from cattle with bronchopneumonia and fibrinous pneumonia in pure culture and in combination with *Pasteurella* spp., the lungs of cattle dying of TME are not usually affected with a fibrinous pneumonia. The pneumonia that is attributed to the organism is characteristically subacute or chronic, and it is probable that the portal of entry is via the upper respiratory tract. However, it is difficult to reproduce the disease by aerosol challenge with *H. somni*. The organism produces and secretes histamine, which may be enhanced by carbon dioxide concentrations that approximate those in the bronchial tree.

The microscopic lesions in the lungs of cattle with pneumonia from which *H. somni* is isolated consist of suppurative to necrotizing bronchiolitis, particularly in calves with subacute to chronic pneumonia. The experimental pneumonia is characterized by purulent to fibrinopurulent bronchiolitis accompanied by alveolar filling with fibrin, neutrophils, and macrophages. Laryngitis and polypoid tracheitis have also been attributed to *H. somni*, but the evidence for a cause and effect relationship is limited.

Hemorrhagic necrotic lesions also occur in the spinal cord, which contribute to the muscular weakness, recumbency, and paralysis encountered in some cases with or without brain lesions. Lesions in the esophagus, forestomaches, and intestines may account for the bloat and alimentary tract stasis that occurs in the experimental disease.

The septicemia usually causes marked leukopenia, neutropenia, and degenerative left shift.

Cattle dying of experimentally induced and naturally occurring disease have high levels of agglutinating *H. somni* antibody, but not of complement-fixing antibody. Because septicemia can occur even with high levels of serum antibody, it is hypothesized that the formation of antigen–antibody complexes may contribute to the development of vasculitis. It is possible that previous exposure to *H. somni* infection is necessary for typical TME to occur. Inoculation of colostrum-deprived calves with *H. somni* causes septicemia but does not produce lesions typical of TME. This suggests that the disease may be an example of a type III hypersensitivity reaction or serum sickness.

The organism can cause inflammatory disease in the genital tract of cows or may merely colonize the healthy genital mucosa. Vaginitis, cervicitis, and endometritis have been associated with infection by *H. somni*. Experimentally, the organism can be embryocidal, which indicates a possible role in early embryonic mortality. Sporadic abortions have been reported following septicemia and placentitis, the latter being characterized by thrombosis and vasculitis as observed with TME and *Histophilus* pneumonia.[3]

CLINICAL FINDINGS

The range of clinical findings associated with *H. somni* infection in cattle has changed remarkably over the last decades. Historically, TME was the major form of the disease. However, fewer cases of this presentation are being diagnosed now, whereas many more cases of other forms of the disease are becoming prevalent.

Thrombotic Meningoencephalitis (TME)

In the typical nervous form of the disease, thrombotic meningoencephalitis (TME), it is common for several animals to be affected within a few days or at one time, but single cases do occur. Some affected animals may be found dead without any premonitory signs, and often this may be the first sign of disease in the group.

In the more common acute form, in which there is usually neurologic involvement, cattle may be found in lateral or sternal recumbency and may or may not be able to stand. The temperature is usually elevated up to 41 to 42°C (105.8–107.6°F) but may be normal in some cases. Depression is common, the eyes are usually partially or fully closed, and unilateral or bilateral blindness may be present. Originally the disease was called the **"sleeper syndrome"** because the eyes were partially closed. Recumbent cattle that attempt to stand may have considerable difficulty and exhibit obvious ataxia and weakness. Others that are able to stand, when attempting to walk, knuckle over on the hind fetlocks, are grossly atactic, and usually fall after walking a short distance. In the recumbent position, opisthotonos, nystagmus, muscular tremors, hyperesthesia, and occasionally convulsions will occur, but the emphasis is on muscular weakness and paralysis rather than signs of irritation. Otitis media with concurrent meningitis may also occur.

TME is rapidly fatal in 8 to 12 hours if not treated when signs are first noticed. Affected cattle that are treated before becoming recumbent commonly recover in 6 to 12 hours, which is an important clinical characteristic of the disease. Once recumbent, particularly with obvious neurologic involvement, the affected animal will either die in spite of treatment or remain recumbent and deteriorate over a period of several days. Secondary complications, such as pneumonia and decubitus ulcers, usually result.

The **ocular lesions** consist of foci of retinal hemorrhages and accumulations of exudate that appear like "cotton tufts." Although these fundic lesions are not present in all cattle affected with *H. somni*, they are a valuable aid to the diagnosis. The organism has been isolated from the conjunctival sacs of feedlot cattle affected with conjunctivitis.

Otitis in feedlot cattle has also been attributed to the organism. The ears are commonly drooping, and affected animals appear depressed. A combination of otitis and meningitis in young cattle associated with the organism has been described.

The **synovitis** is characterized by distension of the joint capsules, usually the major movable joints such as the hock and stifle joints, but any joint may be involved. Pain and lameness are only mild; when treated early, the synovitis usually resolves in a few days. In a few cases there is marked lameness and a preference for recumbency associated with hemorrhages in muscle. The organism has been isolated from a calf with a urachal abscess.

Respiratory Disease

The clinical findings of the respiratory form of the disease, which has been diagnosed with increased frequency in the last decades, have not been clearly described. It is unlikely that there are any distinctive clinical features. Most feedlot calves with pleuritis attributable to *H. somni* die in the pen without ever having been treated.

Epidemiologic surveys of weaned beef calf mortality attributable to pneumonia and pleuritis associated with *H. somni* suggest that death from pneumonia occurred during the first 5 weeks after arrival in the feedlot. The median fatal disease onset for pneumonia was day 12, and for myocarditis and pleuritis, day 22. It is suggested that pneumonia and pleuritis should be suspected in feedlot cattle that have been treated unsuccessfully for bovine respiratory disease in the previous several days. Laryngitis, tracheitis, pleuritis, and pneumonia can occur alone or in combination with the acute neurologic form of the disease. The laryngitis is characterized clinically by severe dyspnea, mouth-breathing, and stertor. Conjunctivitis similar to that seen in infectious bovine rhinotracheitis (IBR) may occur, and isolation of the organism from ocular swabs is necessary to make the definitive diagnosis. Chronic suppurative orchiepididymitis in a calf from which *H. somni* was isolated has been described.

Myocarditis

In the myocardial form of the disease, affected animals may be found dead without any previous illness having been recorded or they may have been treated for respiratory disease within the previous few weeks with a variable response. If seen early in the course of the myocarditis, the most common clinical findings are a fever and depression. With advanced stages of myocarditis, exercise intolerance, mouth-breathing, and protrusion of the tongue occur. Affected animals may collapse and die while being moved from their home pen to the hospital pen in the feedlot. Most animals with myocarditis have a previous history of being treated for an undifferentiated fever and depression within the previous 10 to 14 days. When returned to their home pens, they may be found dead or in severe respiratory distress.

Chronic free-gas bloat is a not uncommon finding in naturally occurring cases and occurs frequently in the experimental disease.

CLINICAL PATHOLOGY

Hematology

In most cases there are changes in the total and differential leukocyte count. Leukopenia and neutropenia may be present in severe cases, whereas in less severe cases a neutrophilia with a left shift is more common. In the cerebrospinal fluid, the total cell count is markedly increased, and neutrophils predominate. The Pandy globulin test on cerebrospinal fluid is usually strongly positive. In the synovial fluid the total cell count is also increased, and neutrophils predominate.

Culture of Organism

The organism can be cultured from blood, cerebrospinal fluid, synovial fluid, urine, brain, kidney, and liver, less commonly from pleuritic fluid and tracheal washings. In vivo *H. somni* was isolated more often from bronchioalveolar lavage fluid than from nasopharyngeal swabs.[3] Culture of *H. somni* is poorly sensitive because the organism is fragile and fastidious. Collected samples must be shipped in a timely manner using special transport media and under refrigeration. Growth of *H. somni* is slow, requiring at least 48 to 72 hours on selective culture media and incubated on presence of 10% CO_2. Previous antimicrobial therapy may further decrease the chances of successful recovery of the germ from an infected animal. The PCR technique is a more sensitive method for detection of the organism than bacterial culture and immunochemistry. The interpretation of a culture positive result is complicated by the common occurrence of asymptomatic carriers. Only large numbers of *H. somni,* ideally in pure culture obtained from a lesion, are considered confirmatory.[3]

Serology

Cattle with experimental or naturally occurring disease have high levels of agglutinating anti–*H. somni* antibody. Recovered animals are positive to the complement fixation test (CFT) within 10 days following infection, and titers begin to decline to low levels 30 days after infection.

A microagglutination test is available, but this test preferentially detects IgM antibody, an antibody class commonly cross-reacting with other members of the family Pasteurellaceae. Immunologic cross-reaction may explain why most cattle are positive on microagglutination in the absence of a history of *H. somni* disease or related clinical signs. ELISAs identifying the presence of IgG_2 are more specific; however, there is no significant difference in serum IgG_2 titers between culture-negative and culture-positive but asymptomatic animals. It was proposed that seroconversion could also occur in asymptomatically infected carrier animals.[3]

An immunoblot test can detect an immune response after experimental abortion, experimental pneumonia, or vaccination with a killed vaccine. It is also able to distinguish between animals with an immune response as a result of disease or vaccination with the organism and those animals that are asymptomatic carriers, culture negative, or infected with closely related bacteria.

Paired serum samples obtained during acute and convalescence phase can be useful retrospectively.

NECROPSY FINDINGS

The characteristic lesions of TME are hemorrhagic infarcts in any part of the brain and spinal cord. These are usually multiple and vary in color from bright red to brown and in diameter from 0.5 to 3 cm. Cerebral meningitis may be focal or diffuse, and the cerebrospinal fluid is usually cloudy and slightly yellow-tinged. Hemorrhages may also be present in the myocardium, skeletal muscles, kidneys, and serosal surfaces of the gastrointestinal tract.

There may be petechiation and edema of the synovial membranes of joints. There is an excessive quantity of synovial fluid, which is usually cloudy and may contain fibrinous flecks. The articular cartilage is usually not affected.

Pulmonary involvement is characterized by a fibrinopurulent bronchopneumonia, although the posterior aspects of the lung may be edematous and have a rubbery consistency. Histologically, there is fibrinosuppurative bronchiolitis accompanied by filling of the alveoli with fibrin, neutrophils, and macrophages. Peribronchiolar fibrosis and bronchiolitis obliterans, interlobular fibrosis and thrombosis of interlobular and pleural lymphatics develop in chronic cases. Fibrinous or serofibrinous inflammation of the peritoneum, pericardium, or pleura is found in more than 50% of cases. There may be focal ulceration and fibrinonecrotizing inflammation extending from the pharynx down into the trachea. Polypoid tracheitis has also been reported.

Histologically, vasculitis and thrombosis with or without infarctions and a cellular component composed almost entirely of neutrophils may be seen in all tissues where localization occurs, especially the heart but also the placenta in case of abortion.[3] Myocardial abscesses may develop and are most common in the left ventricular free wall, particularly in the papillary muscles.

Samples for Confirmation of Diagnosis

- Bacteriology—culture swabs from brain/meningeal and joint lesions; lung, spleen, heart (culture, PCR)
- Histology—formalin-fixed brain, lung, heart, kidney, synovial membrane (light microscopy, immunohistochemistry)

DIFFERENTIAL DIAGNOSIS

Thrombotic meningoencephalitis attributable to *Histophilus somni* is characterized by sudden onset of weakness, ataxia, depression, fever, enlarged joints, and rapid death within 12 to 24 hours. There are marked changes in the cell count of the cerebrospinal fluid and the leukogram. There is a rapid response to treatment in the early stages.

In **polioencephalomalacia**, blindness, normal temperature, nystagmus, opisthotonos, and convulsions are common.

In ***Listeria* meningoencephalitis,** there is unilateral facial paralysis with deviation of the head and neck and a normal or slightly increased temperature. The cerebrospinal fluid in listeriosis usually contains an increased number of mononuclear cells.

***Mycoplasma bovis* infection** can cause polyarthritis, otitis media in calves, and, in rare instances, meningoencephalitis.

Hypovitaminosis A in young cattle 6 to 12 months of age is characterized by sudden onset of short-term convulsions and syncope lasting 10 to 30 seconds, during which they may die but from which they more commonly recover to appear normal. Exercise such as walking from pasture to the farmstead will commonly precipitate the seizures. Eyesight may be slightly impaired, but the menace reflex is usually present.

Pneumonia and pleuritis associated with *H. somni* cannot be distinguished clinically from the other common causes of pneumonia in cattle, and the diagnosis is usually made at necropsy.

Myocarditis attributable to *H. somni* may cause sudden death or congestive heart failure, which will require a necropsy examination for a diagnosis.

TREATMENT

Cattle with TME must be treated with antimicrobials as soon as clinical signs are obvious. Florfenicol, an analog of thiamphenicol, at a dose of 20 mg/kg BW intramuscularly and repeated 48 hours later, is effective for the treatment of acute undifferentiated fever in feedlot calves and may be the antimicrobial of choice if *H. somni* infection is a major cause of mortality in feedlot calves. Oxytetracycline at 20 mg/kg BW intravenously daily for 3 days is effective when treatment is begun within a few hours after the onset of clinical signs. The prognosis in recumbent cattle is unfavorable, but treatment for 2 to 4 days may be attempted. A failure to respond after 3 days of treatment usually indicates the presence of irreversible lesions. The MICs of 33 antimicrobial agents for *H. somni* indicated high in vitro susceptibility to penicillin G, ampicillin, colistin, and novobiocin; oxytetracycline also revealed high activity. Once the disease has been recognized in a group, all in-contact animals should be observed closely for the next 7 to 10 days to detect new cases in the initial stages so that early treatment can be given. The treatment of pneumonia and pleuritis attributable to *H. somni* is the same as for acute undifferentiated bovine respiratory disease.

TREATMENT AND CONTROL

Treatment

Oxytetracycline (20 mg/kg IV every 24h for at least 3 days) (R-2)

Florfenicol (20 mg/kg IM every 48h) (R-2)

Control

H. somni bacterin vaccine

Florfenicol (40 mg/kg IM as single treatment)

Oxytetracycline (long acting formulation 20 mg/kg IM as single treatment)

CONTROL

Satisfactory control procedures are not available because the pathogenesis and epidemiology of the disease are not well understood. When an outbreak of the nervous form of the disease is encountered, the provision of constant surveillance and early treatment is probably the most economical and effective means of control.

Metaphylactic Antimicrobial Therapy

Postarrival metaphylactic treatment with antibiotics is widely used in feedlots to control undifferentiated bovine respiratory disease (UBRD) and was shown to reduce morbidity and mortality associated with this disease complex.[7,8] Evidence supporting the metaphylactic or prophylactic use of antimicrobials to reduce occurrence rate and mortality directly associated with *H. somni* infection is scant. Mass medication with long-acting oxytetracyclines did not reduce the risk of histophilosis mortality, but it reduced the risks of bovine respiratory disease morbidity and mortality by 14% and 71%, respectively.[2]

Vaccination

Vaccines have been available for use in North America and are mainly labeled for protection from TME but not the other forms of histophilosis; their efficacy is uncertain.[9] One bacterin is immunogenic and will protect vaccinated cattle against the nervous form of the infection produced by intravenous and intracisternal inoculation of the organism. Two injections of the bacterin given subcutaneously 2 to 3 weeks apart are recommended. Controlled field trials indicate that the bacterin reduces the morbidity and mortality rates of nervous system disease in vaccinated cattle compared with nonvaccinated animals. However, the efficacy of the bacterin has been difficult to evaluate because the incidence of naturally occurring disease in nonvaccinated control animals is usually low and may not be significantly greater than in vaccinated animals.

The efficacy of a *H. somni* bacterin to reduce mortality was evaluated in auction-market-derived beef calves vaccinated immediately upon arrival at the feedlot. The vaccine had no significant effect on overall crude mortality but appeared to reduce the incidence rate of fatal disease during the first 2 months in the feedlot when the risk of fatal disease onset was highest. When mortalities unlikely to be associated with *H. somni* were removed from the analysis, the mortality rate in male calves was reduced by about 17% in the vaccinated group. A second vaccination 2 weeks after arrival did not reduce the mortality risk.

Vaccination of feedlot calves on arrival with a genetically attenuated leukotoxin of *M. haemolytica* combined with bacterial extracts of *H. somni* increased serum antibody titers to both organisms and reduced acute undifferentiated bovine respiratory disease. However, it is not known what proportion of the respiratory disease was attributable to *H. somni.*

Vaccinating calves twice with a killed whole-cell bacterin reduced the clinical and pathologic effects of experimentally induced *H. somni* pneumonia. Calves vaccinated once were incompletely protected.

There is no published evidence to indicate that vaccination of feedlot calves before or after entry into the feedlot with any of the available *H. somni* vaccines will provide protection against the various forms of clinical disease, particularly the respiratory and myocardial types described earlier.[9] The disease complex is occurring in feedlot calves in spite of vaccination. A rational vaccination program would consist of vaccinating calves at least twice, 2 to 4 weeks apart, with the second vaccination occurring at least 2 weeks before entry into the feedlot.

FURTHER READING

Corbeil LB. *Histophilus somni* host-parasite relationships. *Anim Health Res Rev.* 2008; 8:151-160.

Kwiecien JM, Little PB. *Haemophilus somnus* and reproductive disease in the cow: a review. *Can Vet J.* 1991;32:595-601.

Miller RB, Lein DH, McEntee KE, et al. *Haemophilus somnus* infection of the reproductive tract: a review. *J Am Vet Med Assoc.* 1983;182:1390-1392.

Pérez DS, Pérez FA, Bretschneider G. *Histophilus somni*: pathogenicity in cattle. An update. *An Vet (Murcia).* 2010;26:5-21.

Sandal I, Inzana TJ. A genomic window into the virulence of *Histophilus somni. Trends Microbiol.* 2009;18:90-99.

Siddaramppa S, Inzana TJ. *Haemophilus somnus* virulence factors and resistance to host immunity. *Anim Health Res Rev.* 2004;5:79-93.

REFERENCES

1. Sandal I, Inzana TJ. *Trends Microbiol.* 2010;18:90.
2. Pérez DS, et al. *An Vet (Murcia).* 2010;26:5.
3. Corbeil LB. *Anim Health Res Rev.* 2007;8:151.
4. Elswasifi SF, et al. *Vet Res.* 2012;43:49.
5. Sandal I, et al. *J Bacteriol.* 2007;189:8179.
6. O'Toole D, et al. *Vet Pathol.* 2009;46:1015.
7. Nickel JS, White BJ. *Vet Clin North Am Food A.* 2010;26:285.
8. Taylor JD, et al. *Can Vet J.* 2010;51:1351.
9. Larson RL, Step DL. *Vet Clin North Am Food A.* 2012;28:97.

SEPTICEMIA AND THROMBOTIC MENINGOENCEPHALITIS IN SHEEP ASSOCIATED WITH *HISTOPHILUS SOMNI*

SYNOPSIS

Etiology *Histophilus somni* (formerly *Haemophilus agni, Histophilus ovis*)

Epidemiology Worldwide occurrence but not a common disease. In affected flocks, cases occur over several weeks to result in a significant population mortality.

Clinical findings Acute disease and affected sheep commonly found dead. Septicemia, polyarthritis, and occasionally meningitis primarily in lambs 4 to 7 months of age.

Necropsy findings Multiple hemorrhages throughout the carcass. Focal hepatic necrosis. Polyarthritis, meningoencephalitis.

Diagnostic confirmation Isolation of the organism.

Treatment and control Oxytetracycline.

ETIOLOGY

Histophilus somni falls within the family Pasteurellaceae. This organism, previously known as *Haemophilus agni* and *Histophilus ovis,* has been isolated from sheep, bighorn sheep, and bison with a number of different pyogenic conditions, including septicemia, polyarthritis, thrombotic meningoencephalitis, general pyemia, metritis, mastitis, abortion, neonatal mortality, and epididymitis.[1]

EPIDEMIOLOGY

Disease associated with *H. somni* in sheep has worldwide occurrence but is not common.

The most common presentation is lameness and septicemia in lambs aged 4 to 7 months, but infection with this organism can also result in polyarthritis in lambs 1 to 4 weeks of age. The morbidity rate varies between outbreaks, but the case-fatality rate is likely to be 100% unless treatment is undertaken, and the population mortality rate can approach 10%. Outbreaks may last several weeks;, within a flock, cases of the disease occur sporadically but over a long period.

In some outbreaks, both in lambs and adult sheep, meningoencephalitis is the primary presentation, and the clinical and pathologic findings are similar to those of thromboembolic meningoencephalitis in cattle. The method of transmission is unknown, but the disease does not appear to spread by pen contact and cannot be produced by oral, nasal, or conjunctival exposure to the organism. Environmental or other stress may be a predisposing factor. *H. somni* has been isolated from the genital mucosa of goats that are in contact with sheep flocks, but their role in transmission of this organism is not clear.[2]

PATHOGENESIS

The organism colonizes the respiratory and reproductive tract mucosa and invades to produce septicemia and disseminated bacterial thrombosis, leading to a severe focal vasculitis.

CLINICAL FINDINGS

Affected sheep are often found dead. Depression, high fever (42°C [107°F]), disinclination to move, and collapse with movement are the obvious clinical signs, and affected lambs may die within 12 hours of becoming ill. Lambs that survive more than 24 hours develop a severe arthritis with a palpable increase in joint fluid and heat in the joints. They are usually recumbent, and those with meningoencephalitis show hypersalivation, convulsions, and opisthotonos. The clinical course is short.

CLINICAL PATHOLOGY

Hematology and blood chemistry are not commonly conducted because of the acute nature of the disease and the availability of carcasses for postmortem. Initially there is leukopenia and neutropenia, with neutrophilia and left shift in more prolonged cases. Total cell count is elevated in cerebrospinal fluid and joint fluid, and these also can be cultured for the organism. Antibody detected by complement fixation persists for about 3 months in animals that survive.

NECROPSY FINDINGS

At necropsy the most striking feature is the presence of multiple hemorrhages throughout the carcass. Focal hepatic necrosis surrounded by a zone of hemorrhage is also a constant finding. Lambs that die in the early stages of the disease show minimal joint changes, but those that survive for more than 24 hours develop fibrinopurulent arthritis. Histologically, the disease is a disseminated bacterial thrombosis leading to a severe focal vasculitis. This change is most apparent in the liver and skeletal muscles. More protracted cases can have hemorrhages in the leptomeninges and foci of liquefactive necrosis at the gray–white junction of cerebral hemispheres, basal gray nuclei, and thalamus. Microscopically, these foci exhibit suppurative necrosis and vascular thrombosis, with bacterial colonies inside the abscesses.[3]

Samples for Confirmation of Diagnosis

- Bacteriology—swabs from joint fluid, liver, meningeal fluid for culture and PCR
- Histology—formalin-fixed liver and brain for histology and immunochemistry

DIFFERENTIAL DIAGNOSIS

Because of the acute nature of the clinical disease, the disease is likely to be confused with acute septicemia associated with *E. coli* or *P. trehalosi,* and with enterotoxemia. The characteristic hepatic lesions and histology serve to identify the disease, and final diagnosis depends on isolation of the organism.

TREATMENT AND CONTROL

Antimicrobials, such as tetracyclines or tilmicosin,[4] need to be given very early in the course of the disease if they are to be effective. Because of the acute nature of the disease, vaccination is likely to be the only satisfactory method of control. Although there is no label, vaccine immunity after a field attack seems to be solid. Mass treatment of the group of sheep at risk with long-acting tetracyclines is a possible strategy to reduce the occurrence of further cases.

FURTHER READING

Corbeil LB. *Histophilus somni* host–parasite relationships. *Anim Health Rev.* 2008;8:151-160.
Radostits O, et al. Focal symmetrical encephalomalacia. In: *Veterinary Medicine: A Textbook of the Diseases of Cattle, Horses, Sheep, Goats and Pigs.* 10th ed. London: W.B. Saunders; 2007:997-998.

REFERENCES

1. Corbeil LB. *Anim Health Rev.* 2008;8:151.
2. Janosi K, et al. *Vet Micro.* 2009;133:383.
3. Romero A, et al. *Veterinaria.* 2013;49:38.
4. Blackall PJ, et al. *Aust Vet J.* 2007;85:503.

TICK PYEMIA OF LAMBS (ENZOOTIC STAPHYLOCOCCOSIS OF LAMBS)

SYNOPSIS

Etiology Infection with *Staphylococcus aureus* predisposed by infection with *Anaplasma* (formerly *Ehrlichia*) *phagocytophila.*

Epidemiology Disease of young lambs that occurs in areas that are habitats for *Ixodes Ricinus.*

Clinical and necropsy findings Septicemia and subsequent abscessation in internal organs.

Diagnostic confirmation Isolation of organism.

Treatment Long-acting antimicrobials.

Control Tick control.

ETIOLOGY

The disease has a complex causality and results from a septicemia produced by *Staphylococcus aureus* predisposed by infection with *Anaplasma* (formerly *Ehrlichia) phagocytophila,* which is transmitted by *Ixodes ricinus.*

EPIDEMIOLOGY

Enzootic disease has been recorded only in the United Kingdom and occurs only in the hill areas that are habitats for the tick *I. ricinus.* The disease occurs in the spring and early summer. The annual incidence varies with the year and between farms. On average, 5% of lambs at risk are affected, but on some farms the incidence may be as high as 29% in certain years.

In enzootic areas the disease has considerable economic importance and has been stated to affect as many as 300,000 lambs every year, the majority of which die or fail to be profitable.

PATHOGENESIS

Experimental and epidemiologic studies have established a clear relationship between infection with *A. phagocytophila,* the agent of tick-borne fever, and susceptibility to infection with *S. aureus.* The role of the tick is in the transmission of *A. phagocytophila,* which produces waves of bacteremia detectable by quantitative PCR as early as 1 day following experimental infection.[1]

Infection with *A. phagocytophila* produces a significant lymphocytopenia that develops 6 days after infection and affects all subsets of T- and B-lymphocytes, and also a prolonged neutropenia lasting for 2 to 3 weeks combined with a thrombocytopenia. Up to 70% of the neutrophils are parasitized from the onset of the parasitemia and have impaired function, and lambs with tick-borne fever have a much higher susceptibility to experimental infection with *S. aureus* than noninfected lambs. The ticks are not thought to necessarily provide portals of entry for, nor to be the primary carriers of, the infection with *S. aureus,* although they are important in this respect. *S. aureus* can gain entry through a variety of sources, and in affected flocks there is a high incidence of lambs carrying the same infection on their nasal mucosa.

CLINICAL AND NECROPSY FINDINGS

Lambs aged 2 to 10 weeks are affected. They may die quickly of septicemia or show signs of localization of infection. Clinically, this is most evident by infections that localize in joints or the meninges to manifest as arthritis or meningitis, but on postmortem examination abscesses can be found in any organ, including the skin, muscles, tendon sheaths, joints, viscera, and brain.

TREATMENT AND CONTROL

Treatment of the established disease has limited value, and efforts should be directed at prevention or mitigation of early infection during the bacteremic phase.

The strategic use of long-acting antibiotics has shown success in this respect. On farms with enzootic disease, benzathine penicillin administered at 3 weeks of life has been shown to result in a marked decrease in the incidence of subsequent clinical disease. The use of long-acting tetracyclines has the additional advantage of protecting against infection with the agent of tick-borne fever and *S. aureus* infection; two treatments of lambs, the first between 1 and 3 weeks of age and the second between 5 and 7 weeks, has been shown to result in a significant reduction in morbidity and mortality. In addition, the treatment has been accompanied by increased weight gain.

Tick control by dipping lambs or using a pour-on insecticide significantly reduces the incidence of clinical disease and increases weight gain of clinically normal lambs. Separation of the lambs for dipping has not been associated with problems of mis-mothering. A combination of antibiotic and acaricide treatment may be the most effective and in one trial reduced losses from 10.3% to 0.6%. Dipping the whole flock in an acaricide in spring, although it will not completely eradicate tick infestation, will reduce the incidence of tick pyemia.

Pyemic infection with *S. aureus* is also recorded in association with tick infestation in camels in Saudi Arabia.

FURTHER READING

Woldehiwet Z. The natural history of *Anaplasma phagocytophilum*. *Vet Parasitol*. 2010;167:108-122.

REFERENCE

1. Thomas RJ, et al. *J Comp Path*. 2012;147:360.

SEPTICEMIC PASTEURELLOSIS OF CATTLE (HEMORRHAGIC SEPTICEMIA)

ETIOLOGY

Hemorrhagic septicemia (HS) is mainly associated with two specific serotypes of *P. multocida*, a gram-negative, aerobe coccobacillus of the family Pasteurellaceae. The Asian serotype is designated B:2 and the African serotype is E:2 by the Carter–Heddlestone system, corresponding to 6:B and 6:E by the newer Namioka–Carter system. The letter denotes the capsular antigen and the cipher the somatic antigen. Other serotypes—namely, A:1, A:1,3, A:3, A:4, B:1, B:2,5, and others—have occasionally been isolated from HS outbreaks.[1] Serotype E:2 has thus far only been retrieved in Africa, whereas serotype B:2 was isolated from cases on other continents but also from Egypt and Sudan.

Although *P. multocida* does not readily survive in the environment, it is thought that it can survive for hours and probably days in moist soil and water.

EPIDEMIOLOGY

Occurrence

Hemorrhagic septicemia is a highly fatal acute septicemic disease predominantly affecting **water buffaloes and cattle**. Occasional outbreaks among pigs and less frequently among sheep, goats and bison have been reported. Incidental cases have been reported in horses, donkeys, elephants, yaks and camels.[2]

HS is considered economically important in Asia, Africa, and the Middle East, with highest incidences in Southeast Asia. Cases have also been reported form countries in southern Europe and the United States, where outbreaks among bison were reported. In regions where the disease is endemic it causes heavy death losses and has emerged as the economically most important bacterial disease following the successful eradication of rinderpest and the continued low mortality of food-and-mouth disease.[1] HS is listed on list B of the World Organization for Animal Health (OIE), which includes "transmissible diseases that are considered to be of socioeconomic and/or public health importance within countries, and that are significant in the international trade of animals and animal products."[3]

Both morbidity and case-fatality rates vary between 50% and 100%, and animals that recover require a long convalescence. Morbidity will depend on the immune status of the herd, either acquired naturally or induced by vaccination. The greater the percentage of immune to nonimmune animals, the lower will be the morbidity. In endemic areas, adult animals develop a naturally acquired immunity, and large outbreaks no longer occur in these areas. The incidence of disease is reduced significantly in areas where the vaccine is used.

Risk Factors

Animal Risk Factors

The disease predominantly affects water buffaloes and cattle, but buffaloes are considered to be more susceptible to clinical disease. These species also present the most important host reservoir for the pathogen. It is estimated that in endemic areas up to 5% of water buffaloes and cattle are carriers and thus potential shedders of the pathogens.[1]

All age groups are susceptible to infection, but in endemic regions, older animals previously exposed to the pathogen may have antibodies providing some protection. In these regions the most susceptible age group is 6 months to 2 years of age. Colostral immunity of calves from cows vaccinated against hemorrhagic septicemia peaks at 8 to 16 weeks of age and then declines. There is no difference in susceptibility between breeds.

The immune status and health of the individual animal and the herd are considered important factors in the epidemiology of HS. Stress resulting from inadequate feed supply, disease, or exhaustion is considered an important predisposing factor for clinical disease.[2]

Pathogen Risk Factors

P. multocida possesses a number of virulence factors, which include the capsule, fimbriae, and adhesins; outer membrane proteins (OMPs); endotoxin (lipopolysaccharide [LPS]); siderophores; and a number of extracellular enzymes.[1] Endotoxin appears to be the most important virulence factor responsible for clinical disease. LPS of serogroups B and E were found to be identical, and intravenous inoculation with LPS from these strains allowed for reproduction of clinical disease and death within hours, consistent with severe endotoxemia in water buffaloes.[1] Synthesis of the extracellular enzyme hyaluronidase appears to be a specific feature of serotype B:2, but the significance of the enzyme for the virulence of the pathogen is not known.[1]

Environmental Risk Factors

Although clinical disease can occur at any time of the year, close herding and wet conditions clearly contribute to the spread of the disease. Outbreaks of the disease are often associated with wet, humid weather during the rainy season.

Stressors such as inadequate feed supply or exhaustion are considered important predisposing factors that not only increase the susceptibility to clinical disease, but also stimulate shedding of the bacterium from subclinically infected animals.

During intervening periods the causative organism persists on the tonsillar and nasopharyngeal mucosae of carrier animals.

Transmission

Transmission of *P. multocida* occurs either through oral ingestion or inhalation, either during direct contact between infected und susceptible individuals or via fomites such as contaminated feed or water. The saliva of affected animals contains large numbers of *Pasteurella* during the early stages of the disease. Although infection occurs by ingestion, the organism does not survive on pasture for more than 24 hours. Biting insects to not seem to be significant vectors.[2]

PATHOGENESIS

The portal of entry of infection is thought to be the tonsils. A fulminating septicemia occurs, which is associated with the capsular material of the organism and its endotoxin. In acute and peracute cases death ensues within 8 to 24 hours of appearance of the first clinical signs. The effects of the septicemia are most severe in the respiratory tract, heart, and gastrointestinal tract. In cattle and buffalo there is rapid translocation of bacteria from the respiratory tract to the blood, liver, and spleen, suggesting that the bacteria are able to invade via the mucosal epithelial layers.

CLINICAL FINDINGS

The disease is an acute septicemia and is clinically characterized by a sudden onset of fever (41 to 42°C [106–107°F]), followed by profuse salivation, submucosal petechiation, severe depression, and death in about 24 hours. On range lands, animals may be found dead without any clinical signs having been observed. Localization may occur in subcutaneous tissue, resulting in the development of warm, painful swellings about the throat, dewlap, brisket, or perineum, and severe dyspnea may occur if the respiration is obstructed. In the later stages of an outbreak, some affected animals develop signs of pulmonary or alimentary involvement. *P. multocida* may be isolated from the saliva and the bloodstream. The disease in pigs is identical to that in cattle.

CLINICAL PATHOLOGY

Culture and Detection of Bacteria

Laboratory diagnosis is by isolation and identification of the causative agent. The organism can be cultured from blood or a nasal swab from an animal within a few hours of death. Blood or a nasal swab during the clinical phase of the disease is not reliable because the septicemia is a terminal event.[2] From older carcasses, a long bone is used for culture from the bone marrow. Biochemical and serologic tests are used for identification and serotyping of *P. multocida*. Serotyping can be done by rapid slide agglutination, indirect hemagglutination, agar gel immunodiffusion, and counterimmunoelectrophoresis.[4] DNA fingerprinting and other molecular techniques are suitable for epidemiologic studies to trace an outbreak back to its origin.

Serology

Serology is not normally used for diagnosis because of the peracute and highly fatal course of disease; however, high titers (1:160 or higher) by indirect hemagglutination (IHA) in surviving in-contact animals are suggestive of disease.[2]

NECROPSY FINDINGS

At necropsy, the gross findings are usually limited to generalized petechial hemorrhages, particularly under the serosae, and edema of the lungs and lymph nodes. Subcutaneous infiltrations of gelatinous fluid may be present, and in a few animals there are lesions of early pneumonia and a hemorrhagic gastroenteritis. Varying degrees of lung involvement range from generalized congestion to patchy or extensive consolidation. Thickening of the interlobular septa may be prominent. Lymph nodes in the thoracic region are enlarged and hemorrhagic. Isolation of the causative bacteria is best attempted from heart, blood, and spleen samples.

DIFFERENTIAL DIAGNOSIS

The differential diagnoses for hemorrhagic septicemia include many other conditions causing peracute death, sometimes without specific clinical signs:

- Blackleg
- Anthrax
- Rinderpest
- Lightning strike
- Acute salmonellosis

More protracted cases with signs of respiratory distress:

- Pneumonic pasteurellosis (shipping fever, enzootic calf pneumonia)
- Atypical interstitial pneumonia
- Mycoplasmosis

TREATMENT

Treatment is of little use once clinical signs have become apparent because of the acute/peracute course of disease.[2] Various antimicrobials have been used to treat HS in cattle and other species, including tetracyclines, penicillin, and sulfonamides, but monitoring of antimicrobial susceptibility of *P. multocida* strains associated with HS revealed a gradual development of in vitro resistance, particularly against sulfonamides.[1] Treatments described in the section on pneumonic pasteurellosis of cattle should also be effective in this disease. Whatever antimicrobial is chosen, an initial intravenous loading dose is required to reach bactericidal concentrations in blood as fast as possible.

TREATMENT AND CONTROL

Antimicrobial therapy

Penicillin G sodium/potassium (22,000 IU/kg initial IV then IM every 12h) (R-2)

Procaine penicillin (22,000 IU/kg IM every 12h or 44,000 IU/kg IM every 24h after initial IV loading dose of penicillin G sodium/potassium) (R-2)

Oxytetracycline (10 mg/kg initial IV then IM every 24 for 4 days) (R-2)

Trimethoprim ([2.66 mg/kg] + sulfadoxine [13.33 mg/kg] initial IV then IM every 12h) (R-2)

Enrofloxacin* (2.5-5 mg/kg SC q24h)

Ceftiofur sodium* (1.2–2.2 mg/kg IV every 24h)

Ceftiofur hydrochloride* (2.2 mg/kg SC every 24 after initial IV loading dose of ceftiofur sodium)

Metaphylaxis

Tulathromycin (2.5 mg/kg SC as single dose)

Florfenicol (40 mg/kg SC as single dose)

Tilmicosin (10 mg/kg SC as single dose)

Gamithromycin (6 mg/kg SC/IM as single dose)

Oxytetracycline long-acting formulation (20 mg/kg IM as a single dose)

Enrofloxacin* (7.5–12.5 mg/kg SC/IM as single dose) (R-3)

Danofloxacin* (8 mg/kg SC as single dose) (R-3)

Ceftiofur* crystalline acid free (6.6 mg/kg SC posterior pinna as single treatment) (R-3)

Vaccination

Vaccination with inactivated HS vaccine (R-1)**

Vaccination with modified live vaccine (intranasal) (R-1)**

**Classified as critically important antimicrobials in human and veterinary medicine. Use as first-line treatment is discouraged.[5]*

***Colostral antibody interferes with vaccine efficacy in calves.*

CONTROL

Hemorrhagic septicemia can be eradicated from nonendemic areas by animal movement control, quarantines, tracing of contacts, culling of infected and exposed animals, and disinfection of the premise. Although treatment may be successful when initiated early in the course of the disease, up to 20% of surviving animals are estimated to become clinically unapparent shedders, thereby creating a host reservoir.[2]

In endemic areas the condition is mainly controlled by vaccination. Removing identified carrier animals, avoiding stress by providing adequate feed supply, and avoiding overcrowding, particularly during the rainy season, can further reduce the risk of clinical disease and transmission of the infection.

Treatment of animals that were in contact with clinical herdmates may be suitable to limit morbidity and mortality rates during an outbreak.[2]

Antimicrobial Metaphylaxis

Although the metaphylactic use of antimicrobials as disease control is debatable from the point of view of prudent antimicrobial use, the treatment of clinically still healthy in-contact animals during an outbreak may be indicated and justified by the high case-fatality rate that is largely attributable to the peracute course of disease.[2]

Vaccines

Vaccines against HS are widely used in endemic areas and are the only practical approach to prevent HS.[1] Initially, inactivated vaccines based on plain bacterins of *P. multocida* were used, to which various adjuvants were added later to enhance immune response. The commonly used vaccines are alum precipitated vaccines, aluminium hydroxide gel vaccines, oil-adjuvant vaccines (OAVs), and multiemulsion vaccines (MEVs), which vary considerably in the duration of immunity induced and in side effects. Alum-precipitated vaccines are widely used. Plain broth bacterins, or alum-precipitated and aluminum hydroxide gel vaccines, are administered twice a year because these vaccines offer immunity of 4 to 6 months. OAVs give both a higher degree and a longer duration of immunity, up to 1 year, but have not been popular because they are difficult to inject and because of local tissue reactions and abscess formation at the site of injection. To overcome this issue, an (MEV of a thinner viscosity has been developed that provide immunity parallel to the OAV.

Generally, inactivated vaccines are widely used in endemic areas and are effective in reducing the disease incidence. Disadvantages of these vaccines are the short duration of immunity they provide and the high costs of production.[2]

A fallow deer strain aerosol vaccine (strain B:3,4) developed in Myanmar is currently the only available modified live (MLV) HS vaccine. The safety, efficacy, and cross-protectivity of this vaccine has been tested in young cattle and buffaloes in Myanmar, where more than 1.5 million animals were inoculated with the vaccine between 1989 and 1999. A recommended dose of 2×10^7 viable organisms was used for the efficacy test. The administration of 100 times the recommended dose to 50 cattle and 39 buffalo calves was innocuous. Three out of three buffaloes were protected 7 months after they were vaccinated, and 12 months after they were vaccinated, 3 out of 4 buffaloes were protected against a subcutaneous challenge with serotype B:2, which killed 3 of 3 unvaccinated buffaloes; 12 months after they were vaccinated, 8 out of 8 cattle survived a serotype B:2 challenge that killed 4 out of 4 unvaccinated controls. The vaccinated cattle had developed serum antibodies detectable by the passive mouse protection test. Indirect hemagglutination tests on sera taken from cattle 10 days and 5 weeks after they were vaccinated showed high titers on antibodies. The serum of vaccinated cattle cross-protected passively immunized mice against infection with *P. multocida* serotypes E:2, F:3,4, and A:3,4. The intranasal aerosol vaccination is safe, even at very high dose levels, and does not induce anaphylactic shock even after repeated vaccinations. The freeze-dried live vaccine is stable for at least 3 years at room temperatures of 30 to 36°C (86 to 97°F), and thus a "cold chain," which is impracticable for many hemorrhagic-septicemia-endemic areas, is not necessary for the storage and transport of the vaccine.

The Food and Agriculture Organization (FAO) of the United Nations has reviewed development and use of this MLV vaccine in Myanmar and has commended the intranasal use of live B:3,4 vaccine as safe and potent and has suggested that the technology be transferred to other countries. Nevertheless, no other country is currently using the MLV vaccine.[2]

FURTHER READING

Shivachandra SB, Viswas KN, Kumar AA. A review of hemorrhagic septicemia in cattle and buffalo. *Anim Health Res Rev.* 2011;12:67-82.

Verma R, Jaiswal TN. Hemorrhagic septicemia vaccines. *Vaccine.* 1998;16:1184-1192.

REFERENCES

1. Shivachandra SB, et al. *Anim Health Res Rev.* 2011;12:67.
2. OIE. 2009 at: <http://www.oie.int/fileadmin/Home/eng/Animal_Health_in_the_World/docs/pdf/HAEMORRHAGIC_SEPTICEMIA_FINAL.pdf>; Accessed 20.01.14.
3. OIE. 2014 at: <http://www.oie.int/en/animal-health-in-the-world/the-world-animal-health-information-system/old-classification-of-diseases-notifiable-to-the-oie-list-b/>; Accessed 20.01.14.
4. OIE. 2008 at: <http://www.oie.int/fileadmin/Home/eng/Health_standards/tahm/2.04.12_HS.pdf>; Accessed 20.01.14.
5. World Organization for Animal Health. OIE list of antimicrobial agents of veterinary importance. 2013 <http://www.oie.int/fileadmin/Home/eng/Our_scientific_expertise/docs/pdf/OIE_List_antimicrobials.pdf>; Accessed 14.12.13.

PASTEURELLOSIS OF SHEEP AND GOATS

Mannheimia (Pasteurella) haemolytica and *Bibersteinia trehalosi* are the main causes of pasteurellosis in sheep and goats. Under the old classification system, *M. haemolytica* was classified into two biotypes, A and T, which were then subdivided into serotypes based on antigenic differences in capsular polysaccharide.

- The serotypes within biotype A are now classified as *Mannheimia haemolytica* with the exception of serotype A11, which is a separate species, *Mannheimia glucosida*.
- The most common manifestation of *M. haemolytica* in sheep is pneumonic pasteurellosis, which occurs in all ages.
- *M. haemolytica* is a secondary invader, and a cause of death, in chronic enzootic pneumonia in sheep and goats that is initiated by *Mycoplasma ovipneumoniae*.
- *M. haemolytica* infections in sheep also cause septicemic pasteurellosis in young suckling lambs, which often occurs in association with pneumonic pasteurellosis in the same flocks, and mastitis in ewes.[1,2]
- Palpable lesions in the testicles of rams have also been associated with heavy pure growth of organisms from the *Pasteurella* cluster.[3] Lesions include epididymitis, spermatic granulomas, testicular atrophy, and adhesions between the vaginal tunic and scrotum.
- *M. glucosida* comprises a heterogeneous group of organisms that cause opportunistic infections of sheep, especially mastitis.[1,2]
- Biotype T of *M. haemolytica* contains four serotypes and is now classified as *Bibersteinia trehalosi.* Isolates of *B. trehalosi* that are leukotoxin A (LktA) positive are associated with septicemic disease in weaned sheep.
- Genetic analyses show that bovine and ovine strains of *M. haemolytica* represent genetically distinct subpopulations that are specifically adapted to, and elicit disease in, either cattle or sheep.
- These analyses also demonstrate that traditional classification based upon metabolic characteristics lack the resolution and accuracy to reliably classify isolates. Consequently, for reliable epidemiologic investigations they should be augmented by molecular techniques such as 16s rRNA and LktA screening using PCR assays.[4]
- *P. multocida* is an uncommon respiratory pathogen in sheep in temperate areas but may be of greater importance in tropical areas.

SEPTICEMIC PASTEURELLOSIS OF SUCKLING LAMBS

Septicemic pasteurellosis is a disease of young lambs typically associated with *M. haemolytica* biotype A. It occurs in lambs from 2 days to 2 months of age but presents most commonly at 2 to 3 weeks of age. The young lamb is highly susceptible to biotype A infections, which progress rapidly from the tonsils and lungs to a fatal septicemia. The organism is also a primary pathogen in goat kids. Septicemic pasteurellosis in suckling lambs may occur as an isolated disease but more commonly occurs in conjunction with pneumonic pasteurellosis, with younger lambs succumbing to the former and ewes and older lambs to the latter. This disease probably does not warrant a separate classification but is kept separate because some outbreaks are manifest only by septicemia in lambs.

There is a significant difference in the incidence of death from septicemic pasteurellosis in lambs between flocks that are infested with *Ixodes ricinus* and flocks that are *Ixodes* free. It is thought that immune suppression from tick-borne fever caused by *A. phagocytophilum* can predispose to septicemic pasteurellosis. Lambs that die are usually 4 to 8 weeks of age. *B. trehalosi* can also cause of this condition.[5]

A single subcutaneous injection of 10 mg/kg tilmicosin or intramuscular injection of 20 mg/kg oxytetracycline is effective in preventing disease. Tulathromycin (2.5 mg/kg, SC), a semisynthetic macrolide, may also be an effective treatment.[6]

P. multocida is a rare cause of septicemic disease in neonatal lambs but can occur with a high morbidity and high case-fatality rate. Clinically, it presents with a syndrome resembling watery mouth with marked salivation, abdominal distension, and a short clinical course. On postmortem examination, there is excess peritoneal and pleural pericardial fluid. Prophylactic long-acting tetracycline at a dose of 100 mg per lamb has prevented further cases.

MANNHEIMIA MASTITIS IN SHEEP

M. haemolytica, M. glucosida, and *M. ruminalis* have been isolated from cases of peracute, gangrenous acute mastitis in sheep.[1] *M. haemolytica* is the most common cause of mastitis in meat-producing flocks. It occurs in the Canada, United States, Australia, New Zealand, and Europe in ewes kept under systems of husbandry that vary from open pasture to enclosed barns, and is a major cause of mastitis in ewes in Britain. A variety of typed and untyped strains within biotype A are isolated, with serotype A2 most common from cases of acute mastitis. Mastitis is most common in ewes suckling large lambs up to 3 months old. There is a high diversity among *Mannheimia* isolates. Horizontal transmission by lamb suckling probably occurs, supported by the observation that the prevalence of mastitis associated with this organism is less in dairy sheep than in meat flocks.[7]

PNEUMONIC PASTEURELLOSIS AFFECTING WILDLIFE

Pasteurella and *Mannheimia* spp. have been isolated from a number of different species of wildlife, but there has been particular concern with outbreaks of acute fatal pneumonic pasteurellosis that have occurred in Rocky Mountain and desert bighorn sheep (*Ovis canadensis*) following commingling with domestic sheep or feral goats. This appears to be a complex polymicrobial disease, with *M. ovipneumoniae, M. haemolytica,* LktA-positive *B. trehalosi, P. multocida,* respiratory syncytial virus, and parainfluenza-3 virus isolated from natural cases, and some argument over which agent is the primary cause.[8] Experimental challenge with *M. haemolytica* will induce disease, and bighorn sheep are particularly susceptible to pathogenic (LktA positive) biotype A strains acquired from commingling with domestic sheep. This, coupled with the stress of high densities and food shortage, was thought to be important in the epidemiology of this disease. However, bighorn sheep are not naturally infected with *M. ovipneumoniae,* and spread of this agent from domestic sheep to susceptible populations of bighorn sheep, which then increases their susceptibility to *M. haemolytica,* has been proposed as an alternative explanation.[8] If this is the case, vaccinating domestic sheep against *M. ovipneumoniae* may be an effective way to reduce exposure and disease in bighorn sheep.

Nevertheless, whereas previous vaccines were not effective, repeated doses of an experimental multivalent vaccine containing *M. haemolytica* serotypes A1 and A2 and *B. trehalosi* serotype 10 did protect bighorn sheep against experimental challenge with a pathogenic *M. haemolytica.*[9] A commercial multivalent killed vaccine (OviPast Plus™) with five strains of *M. haemolytica* (A1, 2, 6, 7, 9) and four strains of *B. trehalosi* (T3, 4, 10, 15) is available in the United Kingdom for the reduction of mortalities as a result of pneumonic pasteurellosis in sheep. However, this vaccine did not increase weight gain or reduce lung scores in a study in seven flocks in New Zealand.[10] A primary virulence factor of *Mannheimia* spp. isolates is leukotoxin A (LktA), which are toxic to ruminant leukocytes and probably have an important role in immunity to disease caused by *Mannheimia* spp. A comparison of the similarity of the LktA of *Mannheimia* spp. isolated from clinical cases of mastitis found that the LktA from *M. glucosida* may be a more suitable candidate for a monovalent vaccine than the LktA from *M. haemolytica.*[11]

REFERENCES

1. Omaleki L, et al. *J Clinic Microbiol.* 2010;48:3419.
2. Omaleki L, et al. *J Vet Diag Invest.* 2012;24:730.
3. Garcia-Pastor L, et al. *Small Rumin Res.* 2009;87:111.
4. Miller MW, et al. *J Wildlife Dis.* 2013;49:653.
5. Daniel R, et al. *Vet Rec.* 2015;177:24.
6. Clothier KA, et al. *Vet Microbiol.* 2012;156:178.
7. Omaleki L, et al. *J Vet Diag Invest.* 2012;24:730.
8. Besser TE, et al. *Prev Vet Med.* 2013;108:85.
9. Subramaniam R, et al. *Clin Vaccine Immunol.* 2011;18:1689.
10. Goodwin-Ray KA, et al. *Vet Rec.* 2008;162:9.
11. Omaleki L, et al. *Vet Micro.* 2014;174:172.

PASTEURELLOSIS OF SWINE

Pasteurella multocida (PM) is an important pathogen of pigs. Toxigenic strains, in conjunction with *Bordetella bronchiseptica,* are recognized as the etiologic agents of atrophic rhinitis described under that heading. Pneumonic pasteurellosis and septicemic pasteurellosis are also manifestations of infection with *P. multocida* in pigs. *P. multocida* capsular type A can cause pneumonia in growing pigs but also septicemia and arthritis. It has been consistently isolated from skin lesions in sporadic cases of porcine dermatitis and nephropathy syndrome. Strains from pigs may be found in nasal passages of pig workers, and pig strains have been found in bronchopneumonia in humans. There is therefore the possibility of occupational exposure. Some forms are very similar to pleuropneumonia, with dyspnea, cyanosis, and sudden death.

PNEUMONIC PASTEURELLOSIS

Etiology

P. multocida is commonly isolated from the lungs of pigs with chronic pneumonia, purulent bronchopneumonia, and pleurisy. Isolates are predominantly capsular serotype A strains with some serotype D strains. It is possible to serotype *P. multocida* and of the 16 serotypes, serotypes 3 and 5 are the predominant isolates.[1] In most herds, there is a single isolate, and this is usually A3. In one study, 88% of the lung strains were type A (OMP strains 1:1, 2:1, 3:1, 5:1, and type 6:1). It may be a primary pathogen with a relatively high degree of virulence and a considerable transfer of capsular biosynthesis and *tox*A genes between strains of both type A and type D. Virulence genotypes have also been studied.[2] It may be that most *P. multocida* strains have the *tox*A gene, which suggests widespread genetic diversity in the capsular type A strains[3] and that a single clone might be more predominant in a particular pig population. For many years it was thought that toxigenic strains were not found in the lung, but in three surveys, 25% to 90% of the pneumonic strains were toxigenic. A study looked at 230 isolates from 250 pigs and found that 200 (88%) were A, 4% were D, and 9% were untypeable. The *tox*A gene was found in 13%, of which 11% belonged to A, 1% to D, and 1% could not be typed. Serotype D strains were specifically associated with abscesses in the lung. A wide diversity is found in the lung.

P. multocida is a common secondary infection in the lungs of pigs with enzootic pneumonia associated with *M. hyopneumoniae.* The pneumonic lesions from dual infections are more severe than those from *M. hyopneumoniae* alone. The organism is also commonly associated with *A. pleuropneumoniae.*

Epidemiology

In the microbiome of the soft palate of swine it was found that members of the Pasteurellaceae predominate.

Although found in other species, it is generally assumed that there is little interspecies transfer. The tonsils of the pig are an important site of colonization of many pathogenic and commensal organisms. In a study of the microbiome of the tonsils in 12 healthy pigs from two herds, it was found that Pasteurellaceae dominated the tonsillar biome of all the pigs, comprising 60% of the total.

It is generally considered that *P. multocida* is not a primary pathogen of the lower respiratory tract and that its involvement in pneumonia is secondary to infection with other respiratory pathogens. A large-scale survey in Germany of 6560 postmortem examinations found that pneumonia was present in 24.4% of cases. In 49.3% of these *P. multocida* was found, and with increasing age there was an increasing rate of recovery of *P. multocida*. Most of the lung cultures (54.2%) showed multiple infections. Pneumonic pasteurellosis cannot be reproduced by the intranasal or intratracheal challenge of healthy pigs with *P. multocida* but can be reproduced by challenge to pigs whose pulmonary clearance mechanisms have been compromised by infections with *M. hyopneumoniae*, pseudorabies virus, or by anesthesia and other stresses, and also lungworms. Although atmospheric ammonia may predispose to nasal attachment of *P. multocida* type D, it seems unlikely that this applies to pulmonary infection. The organism is carried in the nasal cavity and tonsils of pigs, and carriage rates are higher in herds with a history of chronic respiratory disease.

Transmission is by aerosol and more probably by direct nose-to-nose contact and thence by inhalation or ingestion. The bacterium has a short-term survival in aerosols, particularly of low humidity (less than 1 hour), but it survives for longer at high humidity and lower temperature. Heating to 60°C (140°F) will kill it, but it can survive for up to 14 days in water, 6 days in slurry, and up to 7 weeks in nasal washings at room temperature. There is always the feeling that the condition is most common under conditions where mycoplasmosis is common and where there is poor husbandry, notable overcrowding, and poor hygiene and where environmental stress is high. As a result, it is often seen after transport, mixing, or moving groups of pigs.

Pathogenesis

Pneumonic pasteurellosis results from the colonization of existing lung lesions by inhaled organisms, often from reservoirs in the nasopharynx and tonsil, and the major virulence mechanisms are unknown. It is suspected that they may attach particularly to the alveoli by means of fimbriae or pili. Serotype A strains are resistant to phagocytosis, which has been attributed to the presence of capsular hyaluronic acid and might allow their colonization of lung lesions. Isolates from lung lesions are not invariably toxigenic. A recent study has shown that there is a change in the functional capabilities of the blood cells, with oxygen radical formation and phagocytosing neutrophils elevated after infection. The disease is difficult to produce experimentally, and large volumes of inoculum mist be used in the trachea together with other infectious agents or their toxins to produce pathology. It has been reproduced when nontoxigenic strains are given repeatedly by intrabronchial injection following *A. pleuropneumoniae* or *M. hyopneumoniae* infections Strains vary in their ability to produce secondary pneumonia and pleuritis in these experimental models, suggesting the existence of specific pneumotropic and pleurotropic strains, which is supported by epidemiologic studies that have found that a single strain predominates in problem herds.

Clinical Findings

There is a possibility of a hyperacute condition in which the only sign is sudden death.

Pneumonic pasteurellosis is a common cause of sporadic cases of acute bronchopneumonia in grower–finisher pigs. Affected pigs have fever of up to 41°C (106°F), are anorectic and disinclined to move (lethargic), and show significant respiratory distress with labored respiration and increased lung sounds, often breathing through the mouth. Cyanosis may occur. Without treatment, death is common after a clinical course of 4 to 7 days. There is a marked tendency for the disease to become chronic, resulting in reduced weight gain and frequent relapses, and real recovery seldom occurs. It can occur as an outbreak, spreading to affect several pigs within a group. The first indication of disease within a group and of an impending outbreak may be the finding of a pig dead with a peracute infection. In an intermediate stage there may be fever, coughing, and poor growth rate for about 3 to 5 weeks before recovery. The disease may also exist in a chronic form as part of the porcine respiratory disease complex, with little evidence of overt clinical disease but with an adverse effect on growth rate and food-conversion efficiency.

Necropsy Findings

At necropsy the lesions are considered to be typical of what is normally called enzootic pneumonia—a chronic bronchopneumonia with abscessation. Pleuritis is common, and there may also be pericarditis. In some instances, there may be carcass congestion, and the trachea may be full of frothy fluid. Experimental infections have caused between 15.5% and 39.4% of lung tissue to be affected with pneumonia. Histologically, the airways are filled with degenerate leukocytes, but the overall lung pathology is often complicated by other pathogens. Peracute fatalities show an acute necrotizing and fibrinous bronchopneumonia reminiscent of bovine pneumonic pasteurellosis. There is edema, congestion, and hemorrhage with bronchiolar exudation containing bacteria, neutrophils, and macrophages, which are also present in the alveoli. Small bronchi and bronchioles may be completely occluded by the exudates.

Diagnosis

Diagnosis is through the clinical signs (fever, dyspnea, cyanosis, sudden death), lesions at gross postmortem, histopathology, and isolation of *P. multocida*. Aerobic culture from these cases usually produces a pure culture of the organism.

DIFFERENTIAL DIAGNOSIS

The disease must be differentiated from other causes of respiratory disease in pigs.

Enzootic pneumonia of pigs, unless accompanied by pasteurellosis, is not manifested by a marked systemic or pulmonary involvement.

Dyspnea is a prominent sign in **Glässer's disease,** but there is obvious arthritis; at necropsy the disease is characterized by arthritis, a general Serositis, and meningitis.

Pleuropneumonia associated with *A. pleuropneumoniae* causes a severe pneumonia with rapid death, and differentiation from pasteurellosis is necessary at necropsy.

The septicemic and acute enteric forms of salmonellosis in pigs are often accompanied by pulmonary involvement, but these are usually overshadowed by signs of septicemia or enteritis. Chronic pasteurellosis has to be differentiated from lungworm infestations and ascariasis.

Treatment

The animals are usually severely ill, and therefore treatment is first by parenteral injection and then by water medication; once they start to eat, medication should continue with in-feed antibiotics.

Treatment is with antibiotics, commonly with tetracyclines. There is also a case for using ceftiofur, penicillin, streptomycin, trimethoprim/sulfonamides, ampicillin, spiramycin, and spectinomycin for 3 to 5 days. Tilmicosin and telithromycin would also be suitable antibiotics. There is significant variation in the antibiotic sensitivity of isolates, and the choice of antibiotic should be based on a sensitivity established for the organism for that farm. In a recent survey in the United Kingdom, 15% of *P. multocida* isolates were resistant to tetracyclines, and it was also reported that resistance to trimethoprim/sulfonamides, Apramycin, and neomycin was found in some isolates. A German survey showed that 55% were resistant to sulfonamides.

Control

Vaccination is ineffective, although autogenous vaccines have been produced that are effective (need to be certain that you have the strain causing the problem). Control depends on management of the risk factors, which are described under enzootic pneumonia of swine because pasteurellosis is often secondary to that condition. In particular, all-in, all-out management with vaccination for enzootic pneumonia is essential. Tiamulin at 40 ppm in the feed has also been used strategically at the time of stress, for example, over mixing and moving.

SEPTICEMIC PASTEURELLOSIS

Septicemic disease with death occurring within 12 hours and without signs of pneumonia is occasionally observed in neonatal pigs. They are associated with *M. haemolytica* infection (occasionally *P. trehalosi* that is untypeable), and in many cases there is an association with sheep. Septicemic disease is also recorded in India in association with infection with capsular serotype B. The disease occurs in all ages of pigs, including adults, and is manifest with fever, dyspnea, and edema of the throat and lower jaw. A population mortality of 40% in a group of pigs is recorded. Clinical signs are rarely seen. Acute septicemic disease in grower pigs aged 14 to 22 weeks and associated with serotype D has been recorded in Australia. Cases can be confused with those caused by taxon 15 of APP.

An outbreak of hemorrhagic septicemia was reported from Australia associated with *P. multocida* subsp. *gallicida* in a large pig herd. Affected pigs were found dead, with swelling of the pharyngeal region and blue discoloration of the ventral abdomen and ears. On gross postmortem there was hemorrhage and congestion on serosal surfaces. The postmortem picture is reported to resemble that seen in *A. suis* infection with a superimposed pneumonic pasteurellosis. Histologic examination of the viscera showed widespread vascular damage with thrombus formation and intravascular colonies of bacteria.

Samples for Confirmation of Diagnosis

- Bacteriology—lung, bronchial node (plus liver, spleen, kidney for septicemic form). Culture produces large mucoid colonies 3 mm to 5 mm in diameter on blood agar. In the past the recovered organisms were rarely toxigenic. Some isolates did have fimbriae. On a smear gram-negative coccobacilli may be seen. In early cases aerobic cultures of heart blood and lung lesions will give a pure culture. Anaerobic cultures often yield *Bacteroides* spp. as well, and if *Haemophilus* cultures will also often prove positive. Further identification using electrophoretic typing may be necessary, as in the case of secondary infection in sporadic cases of porcine dermatitis and nephropathy syndrome. Here a high proportion had a single electrophoretic type (01) isolated from a range of tissues. In the septicemic form the organism was readily cultured from the liver, spleen, and lymph nodes.
- Histology—formalin-fixed lung (variety of organs for septicemic form) (light microscopy)

REFERENCES

1. Garcia N, et al. *Vet Rec.* 2011;169:362.
2. Ewers C, et al. *Vet Microbiol.* 2006;114:304.
3. Berthe A, et al. *Vet Microbiol.* 2009;139:97.

STREPTOCOCCUS SUIS INFECTION OF YOUNG PIGS

There are three organisms that infect the neonatal pig quite commonly—*Haemophilus parasuis, S. suis,* and *Actinobacillus suis,* which have been dubbed the "suis-cides." *S. suis* (SS) is therefore one of the early colonizers of the pig; by the end of the nursery period, most pigs are infected. Virulence may be an attribute of strains that colonize the young pig poorly but infect older animals more easily, in the absence of maternal antibody. They also have public health importance.

SYNOPSIS

Etiology *Streptococcus suis;* 35 capsular serotypes exist if you include 1/2. Worldwide, type 2 is probably the most common, and types 1 through 9 are more frequent than types 10 to 34.

Epidemiology - Occurs principally in piglets under 12 weeks of age

Signs Septicemia, arthritis, meningitis, pericarditis, endocarditis, polyserositis, and pneumonia.

Clinical pathology Culture organism.

Lesions Fibrinous polyserositis, purulent meningitis, myocarditis, vegetative endocarditis, fibrinous arthritis, or fibrinous or hemorrhagic pneumonia may be a secondary problem.

Diagnostic confirmation Culture organism from body tissues and blood.

Differential diagnosis Arthritis as a result of the following:

Mycoplasma hyorhinis
Erysipelas
Glässer's disease

Meningitis as a result of the following:

Escherichia coli
Trueperella pyogenes
Pasteurella multocida

Treatment Antimicrobials based on culture and sensitivity.

Control Provision of optimum environment (temperature and relative humidity). Avoid overcrowding in nursery pens. Age spread of pigs in pens should not exceed 2 weeks. Use all-in, all-out pig flow. Control of other common infectious diseases. Avoid nutritional deficiencies. Consider mass medication of feed with antimicrobials. Possible use of autogenous vaccines.

ETIOLOGY

The streptococci are gram-positive, encapsulated, facultative anaerobes; are coccoid or ovoid; and occur singly or in pairs or in chains. *S. suis* (SS) type 1 (SS1) and *S. suis* type 2 (SS2) were the original capsular types of the organism, which appeared to account for most epidemics of the disease. SS types are related to Lancefield's group D. The Lancefield's groups R, S, RS, and T are no longer used.[1] There are now 35 known SS capsular types. Even now, new species of *Streptococcus,* such as *S. ferus,* are being isolated from pigs. The important species of *Streptococcus* that have been isolated in the pig are shown in Table 21-2.[2,3]

At least 40% of the genome of SS is distinct from the other species of *Streptococcus.*[4,5] The strains within each capsular serotype are also very diverse genetically.[6-8]

EPIDEMIOLOGY

The epidemiology of SS is very complex. The isolation of different strains within the same herd and the predominance of particular strains within some herds are evidence that infection by SS is a dynamic process and reinforce the idea that the epidemiology is complex.

The distribution of the serotypes varies widely across the world. In general, SS1-9 is the most commonly found type and likely to cause disease.[9,10] SS9-34 will colonize, but this type is less likely to cause disease. There may be one, two, or even more serotypes in a single pig. In some countries one serotype is more important (e.g., SS14 in Scotland or SS7 in Scandinavia).[11] The position is complicated because a certain serotype in one

Table 21-2 Species of streptococci isolated from the pig with principal locations

Intestine	Tonsils	Oral cavity	Vagina
hyointestinalis	*suis*	*orisuis*	*hyovaginalis*
suis	*porcinus*	*mutans*-like	*thoraltensis*
alactolyticus	*dysgalactiae* ssp. *equisimilis*		
bovis			

country is not necessarily of the same virulence and importance in another because the genetic makeup of the strains varies geographically. It is further complicated in that, following culture, the strains may lose their capsules and become untypeable.[9,10] Again, in general, in Eurasia, SS2 is the most common,[12] and in North America it is SS2 and SS3, but SS2 is not necessarily the most prevalent.[9,10] There are considerable differences between the SS2 in Europe and the SS2 in North America.

Occurrence

Diseases associated with SS occur worldwide, generally affecting pigs 2 weeks to 22 weeks of age but capable of causing disease in any age of susceptible pig. Most cases occur just after weaning and are associated with weaning stressors such as moving, mixing, overcrowding, and inadequate ventilation. SS2 causes outbreaks of meningitis in young pigs 10 to 14 days after weaning. The disease occurs most commonly in intensive systems of high population density, such as flat-deck rooms and early (grower) finishing pens. Sporadic cases occur in older pigs, including adults, depending on immunity.

The organism has also been isolated from cattle, sheep, goats, a horse with meningitis, fallow deer, and cats and increasingly from other species. It has also been isolated from wild boar.[13]

Prevalence of Infection

SS2 is the most prevalent serotype. Types 3, 4, 7, 8, and 14 have been isolated from affected pigs in the United Kingdom. In Australia, SS2 was detected in 58% of the palatine tonsils, in 66% of the pneumonic lungs, and in 28% of the healthy lungs. Overall, the carrier rate in piggeries was 60%. The organism was also present in the blood of 3% of apparently normal pigs at slaughter. It could also be cultured from many other tissues, including the vagina of sows, and it is possible that piglets are infected during birth. Specific pathogen-free herds are free of the organism, and hysterectomy-derived piglets are born SS free.

The rate of infection of the environment of the pigs can also be very high. In Canada, all 35 serotypes have been isolated, with SS2 being the most prevalent of all isolates. The other capsular types in decreasing order were 3, 7, 1/2, 8, 23, and 4. Over a period of several years, more than 60% of isolates belong to capsular types 2, 1/2, 3, 4, 7, and 8. In a survey of clinically healthy piglets 4 to 8 weeks of age in Quebec, the organism could be isolated from 94% of piglets and 98% of farms. The typeable isolates of the organism are more frequently recovered from pigs between 5 and 10 weeks of age, whereas untypeable isolates are most frequently found in animals more than 24 weeks old. In the United States, serotype 3 was most prevalent (26.1%), followed by serotypes 8 (17.4%), 2, 4, and 7 (15.2%). There were no significant differences in the epidemiologic features, clinical signs, or lesions in pigs infected with multiple serotypes compared with a single serotype of SS.

Only some Scandinavian countries reported a higher incidence of type 7 over type 2. In Denmark, SS2 accounted for 29% of the isolates; SS7 for 17%; and 3, 4, and 8 for a further 9% to 10%. SS7 was isolated more frequently than reported in other countries, causing septicemia, arthritis, and meningitis. In Finland, the most common types isolated from dead pigs were 7, 3, and 2, respectively, and they were most frequently isolated from cases of pneumonia. In the Netherlands, SS2 was most frequently isolated from pigs with meningitis. SS9 and SS2 have been isolated as the cause of septicemia and meningitis in weaned pigs in Australia.

Morbidity and Case Fatality

The incidence of clinical disease ranges from 0% to 15%. In a 3-year survey of a breeding herd, the combined morbidity and mortality rates attributable to meningitis from SS2 were 3%, 8%, and 9.1%, respectively.

Methods of Transmission

The organism is usually transmitted by healthy carriers. The organism is carried in the tonsils and occasionally in the nose of healthy pigs[14,15] of all ages, and transmission to uninfected pigs can occur within 5 days of mixing. In a herd where there are no clinical signs there is usually a low carriage of SS. There is a higher carriage in herds where there is clinical disease.[16] The introduction of breeding gilts from infected herds results in disease appearing subsequently in weanlings and growing pigs in the recipient herds. The detectable carrier rates in different groups of pigs can vary from 0% to 80% and are highest in weaned pigs aged 4 to 10 weeks. Over 80% of the sows in an individual herd may be subclinical carriers. They do not normally carry the organism in the nasal cavity but in the vagina. Based on the results of sampling of sows and piglets at parturition, and being able to culture multiple serotypes of the organism from the sow's vaginal secretions and oropharyngeal samples of piglets, it is highly probable that the newborn piglet is infected during birth by the organism, which is transferred from the sow's vagina to the dorsal surface and oral cavity of the piglet. However, even though most pigs are colonized by weaning age, colonization by the virulent strains of SS2 takes longer and usually does not occur before 15 days of age. This could constitute a risk factor for developing disease later when maternal immunity has waned.

Weaned carrier pigs transmit the infection to previously uninfected pigs after mixing following weaning. The organism can persist in the tonsils of carrier pigs for more than 1 year, and in the presence of circulating opsonic and binding antibodies, and in pigs receiving penicillin-medicated feed. Thus the organism can be endemic in some herds without causing recognizable clinical disease. House flies can carry the organism for at least 5 days and can contaminate feed for at least 4 days.

The carrier rate in some surveys of slaughter pigs ranges from 32% to 50% of pigs 4 to 6 months of age. Sporadic cases of SS2 have also been found in pigs with bronchopneumonia (secondary to enzootic pneumonia), pleuropneumonia, arthritis, vaginitis, and aborted fetuses and in neonatal piglets 1 to 2 days of age affected with fatal septicemia. It appears that the organism is found in the lungs of pigs affected with pneumonia more frequently in North America than in other countries. Although airborne infection of type 2 has been described, it is thought that indirect transmission is a much better way to infect piglets because it is easily transmitted via fomites. It can survive in feces for 104 days at 0° C (32° F) and for 10 days at 9° C (48° F) and in dust for 54 days at 0° C and 25 days at 9° C. Experimentally, pure cultures of the organism placed on rubber and plastic surfaces, especially when protected by swine manure, are viable up to 55° C (131° F) and can survive if kept frozen for up to 10 days. In the summer, at a temperature in the middle range, it may survive for about 8 days. The organism is readily destroyed by disinfectants. It can be spread by contaminated pig nose snares and needles used for blood sampling. SS can also be transmitted by flies.

Risk Factors

Animal Risk Factors

The host factors that render pigs susceptible to clinical disease are uncertain. Over 30 different gram-positive bacterial organisms may occur in the nasal cavities and tonsils of unweaned pigs between 2 weeks and 6 weeks of age. It is suggested that strains of SS2 vary in pathogenicity and that the occurrence of disease is dependent on both exposure to a pathogenic strain and undetermined secondary factors. The peak incidence of SS from 5 to 10 weeks of age suggests that the stressors of weaning may render pigs susceptible to clinical disease and certainly to the horizontal spread of the infection. At this point any infected pig may be shedding large numbers of organisms. Most weaned pigs carry SS, but few appear to carry virulent strains.[16] In an outbreak, one strain of SS usually predominates. The presence of other infectious diseases, such as porcine reproductive and respiratory syndrome (PRRS) and *Actinobacillus pleuropneumoniae,* may be associated with a higher-than-average prevalence of infection with SS. PRRS certainly increases susceptibility to SS infection experimentally. In utero infection with PRRS makes pigs more susceptible to subsequent neonatal SS infections. Infection of specific-pathogen-free pigs with PRRS virus may be a risk factor for infection and disease associated with SS. Similarly, the pseudorabies virus may enhance clinical disease associated with SS. In addition, faulty teeth clipping may be associated with the condition in young pigs.

Environmental and Management Factors

The incidence of clinical disease appears to depend on environmental factors (which may be important in the spread of SS), such as inadequate ventilation, high population density, and other stressors. Several environmental and management risk factors have been associated with a high prevalence of pigs harboring SS in swine herds. Excessive environmental temperature fluctuation in the nursery pig facilities was the most common factor. Nursery pig environmental temperatures should not fluctuate more than 1.1° to 1.7°C (34° to 35° F) over a 24-hour period to prevent chilling of pigs. Fluctuations in temperature are caused by drafts, inadequate heaters, or poorly insulated buildings. Excessive relative humidity was also a factor; the recommended range for nursery pigs is 55% to 70%. The third and fourth most common factors were age spread of more than 2 weeks for pigs in the same room and crowding (both increasing SS transmission rates). The fifth most common factor was the use of continuous flow facilities, which allows for build-up of dust and manure (and therefore SS) and increased infection pressure. An unusual case where SS was isolated from the lumen of the small intestine occurred when a feed was formulated with no salt and 58.5 kg instead of 3.5 kg of vitamin premix. Once the ration was corrected, the problem disappeared.

SS2 can survive in feces for 104 days at 0°C (32°F), up to 10 days at 9°C (48°F), and up to 8 days at 22 to 25°C (71 to 77°F). It can survive in dust for up to 25 days at 9°C (48°F) but could not be isolated from dust stored at room temperature for 24 hours. The organism is rapidly inactivated by disinfectants commonly used on farms. Liquid soap inactivates SS2 in less than 1 minute at a dilution in water of 1 in 500. The organism can survive in pig carcasses at 40°C (104°F) for 6 weeks and may therefore be an important source of the organisms for infection in humans.

Pathogen Risk Factors

Most studies of virulence have been associated with studies on SS2. Some have proved to be virulent, others not so.[11] New factors are being discovered all the time. For example, a new virulence gene virA was discovered that only occurs in virulent strains.[17] Many other secreted substances, important as virulence factors, are probably awaiting discovery.

Colonization of piglets occurs very early in life, with most pigs being colonized by weaning age; virulent strains of SS2 may not colonize until later. Early colonization reduces the subsequent clinical signs. Despite the association of bacteria with disease, they may also be recovered from the nasal cavities and tonsils of healthy pigs. High numbers of organisms were isolated from the cerebrospinal fluid of clinically normal pigs. A study also showed that a persistent epidemic strain of SS was consistently isolated from the brains of pigs over a 2-year period.

There are differences in pathogenicity between serotypes and between strains of the same serotype. In the United Kingdom there are differences in pathogenicity between types 1 and 2; type 1 causes less severe disease in piglets, whereas type 2 causes a more severe and acute disease in older and growing pigs. Highly virulent and completely avirulent type 2 strains exist. Different strains of SS2 vary in their ability to cause meningitis. Streptococci require manganese but not iron as a growth factor, which affects the activity of superoxide dismutase in cell cultures.

Capsules

One of the main virulence factors is the presence of the capsules, which are powerfully antiphagocytic. The organism is classified into serotypes on the antigenic specificity of its capsular polysaccharide. The capsule, certainly for SS2, plays an important role in pathogenesis. It is an important antiphagocytic factor.[18] Because many nonpathogenic strains are capsulated, there are probably many other interrelating factors.

There are also modifications of the cell wall, such as lipoteichoic acids and peptidoglycans.[11,19,20-22]

Proteins

The virulence markers of the organism include the structural proteins muramidase-related protein (MRP) and extracellular factor (EF). There are virulence differences between strains of the same serotype based on the presence or absence of muramidase-released proteins. It has also been reported that some of these proteins are not essential for virulence; on the other hand, there is sometimes a strong association between proteins and strain virulence.[12,23] Most Canadian field isolates of SS2 do not produce these virulence-related proteins.

Fibronectin and fibrinogen-binding protein played a role in the colonization of specific organisms involved in a SS infection.[24] An IgG binding protein in the 60-kDa range has been shown to bind IgG in a nonimmune way. A 44-kDa protein has been isolated as a virulence marker of SS2, and the presence of antibodies against this protein appears to be necessary to obtain complete protection against the disease.

Recently, 36 environmentally regulated genes have been identified. Strains of SS2 from Europe are genotypically different from those of North America. A serum opacity-like factor has also been identified as a novel virulence determinant.[11]

Suilysin

Suilysin, an extracellular protein with hemolytic properties, has been described, and it is cytotoxic.[25] In one study most SS2 field strains from four different European countries produced this hemolysin. Between 58% to 90% of strains from the Netherlands, Denmark, France, England, and Italy produced the suilysin but only 1% of Canadian strains. A total of 164 field isolates from diseased pigs in four countries were serotyped and tested for suilysin. SS2 was the most prevalent type isolated from all four countries. After SS2, SS9 was most prevalent in the Netherlands and France and SS7 in Denmark. All the English isolates were SS2. No nonvirulent suilysin-producing SS2 strains have been reported.

Hemolysin

The hemolysin gene was found in over 80% of the strains that were associated with meningitis, septicemia, and arthritis but in only 44% of pneumonia isolates.

Other Properties

The organism bears fimbriae and pili, and the capsular materials from different serotypes have distinct morphologies. Certain strains possess hemagglutinating properties.

Glutamine synthetase is required for the full expression of virulence in SS2.[26] Recently glutamate dehydrogenase, glyceraldehyde 3-phosphate dehydrogenase, and a secreted nuclease have been suggested as aiding the virulence of SS2.[27]

Adhesion

There are also adhesins.[5,21,28] SS2 isolates possess a factor that allows them to adhere to porcine lung. Australian isolates of SS are genetically very diverse, which suggests that serotyping is not a reliable technique for identifying specific strains and not a good predictor of the genetic background of a given isolate.

Zoonotic Implications

Splenectomized humans are particularly at risk from certain infections, including streptococci, and should not handle or come into contact with pigs in particular. Death is not common in humans in North America but does occur in Europe and is much more common in Asia,[29] which may be a feature of greater contact with SS2. It has been identified as an important emerging zoonotic agent,[30] particularly in the East.

Infections with SS2 are the most common infections in humans (from pigs or raw pork). The Chinese outbreaks may be associated with undercooked or raw pork.[28,31] A high percentage of pork in Asian markets is contaminated with SS.[32] It is possible that many human cases are misdiagnosed, such as in those that were described in Southeast Asia, where 5 of 8 cases of SS were described as *S. viridans*. SS in humans is associated with the nasopharynx[33] and the gastrointestinal tract; diarrhea is often a prominent feature,[34] but SS can produce very variable clinical signs in humans. The clinical manifestations in humans include meningitis and septicemia, which may be accompanied by arthritis, endophthalmitis, and disseminated intravascular coagulation. Endocarditis and acute gastroenteritis have also been reported. Deafness occurred in 50% to 60% of cases and is a result of cochlear sepsis following invasion of the organism from the subarachnoid space into the perilymph of the inner ear. Vertigo and ataxia occurred in 30% and arthritis in 53% of patients. There was a case-fatality rate of 13%. The organism invades the cerebrospinal fluid within monocytes, an example of the "Trojan horse" mechanism of entry.

A truck driver has recently been described with septic shock. It is thought that SS25 has evolved to become the highly pathogenic SS1, which has in turn evolved to become epidemic strain SS7, which in turn stimulates the production of large amounts of proinflammatory cytokines, leading to streptococcal shock syndrome.[35]

In the United Kingdom, the highest incidence of meningitis attributable to SS2 is in butchers and abattoir workers; transmission is thought to be mainly via minor skin abrasions, and often there is no visible point of entry. Subclinical infection in pigs sent to slaughter represents a potential source of infection for abattoir workers; eviscerators who remove the larynx and lungs have a significantly higher risk of exposure to the organism than other abattoir workers.

Within infected herds in New Zealand, up to 100% of pigs are carriers, and SS2 infection may be one of the most infectious potentially zoonotic pathogens present in New Zealand, although very rarely resulting in clinical disease. The annual incidence of subclinical infection and seroconversion in pig farmers in New Zealand is close to 28%.

PATHOGENESIS

Streptococci exist in extremely different phenotypes with regard to adhesion, invasion, and cytotoxicity. These features depend on the state of encapsulation and environmental growth conditions.

The crypts of the tonsils are a site of persistence, multiplication, and portal of entry of a variety of pathogens, including SS. Invasive disease occurs in a minority of infected pigs. It is not clearly known how SS travels from the mucosal surfaces to the blood and produces a bacteremia, then septicemia, and finally meningitis. Most bacteria remain extracellular, with fewer than 2% of monocytes containing bacteria.[36,37] Persistent bacteremia is an important phase in the pathogenesis of SS2 meningitis. There is a high level of adhesion of bacteria to phagocytic cells. SS adheres to brain microvascular endothelial cells, and suilysin can damage these. It has been shown that SS capsular strains stimulate tumor necrosis factor alpha (TNF-α) and interleukin (IL)-6, but the suilysin and the extracellular protein do not do so on their own. It is likely that the enhanced production of inflammatory cytokines contributes to the more severe signs and an early death.[38,39] A terminal acute fatal septicemia is the common outcome in young animals, but in older animals localization can occur in synovial cavities, endocardium, eyes, and meninges. Virulent isolates of SS2 possess capsules and are relatively resistant to phagocytosis. Isogenic mutants defective in capsule production were not virulent. SS is able to adhere to but not to invade epithelial cells, and the adhesins are partially blocked by the capsule and are part of the cell wall. The highly virulent isolates possessed the suilysin, muramidase-releasing protein, and extracellular protein factor phenotype.[40] SS are able to survive and replicate within macrophages, and the bacteria enter the cerebrospinal fluid space in association with migrating monocytes, which move through choroid plexuses. They therefore enter the cerebrospinal fluid by a "Trojan horse" mechanism similar to that used by some viral pathogens of the central nervous system (CNS). The predominant lesions are suppurative or fibrinopurulent inflammation in brain, heart, lungs, and serosae. SS9 may produce a different distribution of lesions compared with SS2. The disease has been reproduced experimentally in pigs and laboratory animals by intravenous, intranasal, and subarachnoid routes. Certain strains of streptococci can cause vascular lesions, with the development of fibrinohemorrhagic pneumonia and septal necrosis. Of importance in the pathogenesis of SS infections is the predisposing role of PRRS. This effect of PRRS has still only been experimentally demonstrated with SS.

CLINICAL FINDINGS

Multiple *Streptococcus* spp. are implicated in lameness and CNS signs in piglets and sows. There is significant variation of carrier states and clinical signs with the individual serotypes. Although morbidity is usually less than 5% in an endemic infection, the case-mortality rate may be as high as 20%. The earliest clinical sign is often a raised temperature, followed by reduced appetite, depression, shifting lameness. In a new infection on a premises, only sudden death may be seen at first. It does occur as hyperacute, acute, subacute, and chronic pictures, with the basic difference being the time scale of events.

Arthritis and meningitis may occur alone or together and are most common in the 2- to 6-week age group. More commonly several piglets within a litter are affected. Meningitis is particularly associated with serotypes 1, 2, 1/2, 3, 4, 8, 9, 14, and 16; septicemia with 2; arthritis with 7 and 14; abscesses with 2; bronchopneumonia with 2, 3, 7, 10, 15, and 27; and reproductive damage with 2, 13, and 22; 14 can be associated with any clinical condition.

An experimental infection with SS9 in SPF pigs produced meningitis, arthritis, and serositis.[41]

The arthritis is characterized by enlarged and distended joint capsules, lameness, and pain on palpation of the affected joints. Fever, depression, reluctance to move, and inactivity are common.

Meningitis is characterized by fever, anorexia, and depression. The gait is stiff, the piglets stand on their toes, and there is swaying of the hindquarters. The ears are often retracted against the head. Blindness and gross muscular tremor develop, followed by inability to maintain balance, lateral recumbency, violent paddling, and death. In many cases there is little clinical evidence of omphalophlebitis.

In epidemics of meningitis attributable to SS2, sudden death in one or more pigs may be the first sign. The eyes may stare. Affected pigs found alive are uncoordinated and rapidly become recumbent. There is opisthotonos, paddling, and convulsions and death in less than 4 hours. A fever of up to 41°C (105°F) is common. In the United Kingdom, meningitis of recently weaned pigs is the most striking feature of SS2 infection.

Otitis interna is a common sequela to many cases of SS meningitis. Arthritis is common in younger pigs.

In endocarditis, which is a relatively rare clinical sign (except in North America), and in septicemia the piglets are usually found comatose or dead without premonitory signs having been observed.

Valvular endocarditis attributable to SS2 has also been reported in a 13-week-old finishing pig in a breeding herd that had a long history of SS meningitis. Occasionally, the infection results in conjunctivitis, rhinitis abortion, and vaginitis.

CLINICAL PATHOLOGY

Culture or Detection of Organism

The organism can be cultured from joint fluid, cerebrospinal fluid, blood, and the brain at necropsy. Often the lungs will yield SS, but the role of SS in primary lung disease is not understood. The tonsils of live pigs may be swabbed and cultured for the organism. Improved and selective media are available for the isolation and serotyping of the organism. An indirect fluorescent antibody test can be used to identify the organism on tonsillar swabs of live pigs. Because of multiple antimicrobial resistance among strains of the organism, drug sensitivity testing on a routine basis is recommended. Highly virulent strains of SS2 and SS1 were detected in tonsillar specimens using a PCR. Rapid serotype-specific PCR assays have been developed. A multiplex PCR for identifying four capsular types and four associated virulence markers was described.[23]

Serology

The specific serotype of SS should be determined. A simplified laboratory method is available for the identification of SS strains associated with different animal hosts or located in different body regions. An ELISA using monoclonal antibodies directed against virulence markers of SS can distinguish between virulent and avirulent strains of the organism. A rapid and specific double-sandwich ELISA is available for the detection and capsular typing of the organism, with a specificity of 97.6% and sensitivity of 62.5%. However, many laboratories are not readily equipped to identify the numerous serotypes of the organism.

NECROPSY FINDINGS

In pigs dying from SS2 infection, the gross and microscopic findings are usually found in the brain, heart, and joints and include one or more of fibrinopurulent polyserositis, fibrinous polyarthritis, fibrinous or hemorrhagic bronchopneumonia, suppurative meningitis, hemorrhagic necrotizing myocarditis, and vegetative valvular endocarditis. Gross myocardial lesions cannot be distinguished from those of mulberry heart disease. In cases with meningitis, there is turbidity of the cerebrospinal fluid, congestion of meningeal vessels, and variable amounts of white exudate in the subarachnoid space. The brain may be so swollen that the cerebellum herniates into the foramen magnum. Suppuration is usually most evident along the ventral aspect of the brain, and the meninges may appear grayish as a result of neutrophilic inflammation.

The typical histologic picture is one of acute inflammation—neutrophils and fibrin dominate the response. There is a choroiditis, encephalitis, and meningitis. Other changes that may be observed in SS infections of the central nervous system include internal hydrocephalus, foci of liquefaction necrosis, subacute (mononuclear cell-rich) meningoencephalitis, or meningoencephalomyelitis with bilateral subacute optic perineuritis and Gasserian ganglioneuritis. In the tonsils, SS organisms can be seen in the subepithelial lymphoid tissue and in the crypt lumen and crypt epithelium. SS9 is more prone to cause bronchopneumonia than the spectrum of lesions typical of SS.

Samples for Confirmation of Diagnosis

- Bacteriology—spleen; culture swabs from serosal surfaces, joints, and meninges are best. The significance of SS-positive lungs is not yet resolved. Biochemical tests can be used (Amylase and Vosges-Proskauer tests are positive for SS). Cerebrospinal fluid is the material for the best diagnosis. Bacterial culture is difficult if the animals have been treated, and this is so even when they receive growth-promoting antibiotics. Immunomagnetic isolation of SS2 and SS1/2 from swine tonsils has been described, and it is better than the standard procedure.
- PCRs have been used in human medicine but not in veterinary medicine.[1]
- Histology—formalin-fixed samples of a variety of organs, including lung, brain, heart, liver (light microscopy) are best. Immunohistochemistry 42 and in situ hybridization have been described for use on formalin-fixed tissue and are able to detect single infected cells. Using immunohistochemistry (IHC) the bacteria can be seen in the cytoplasm of the neutrophils and macrophages, and the IHC may be positive even though culture is negative following antibiotic or growth promotant administration.

Note the zoonotic potential of this organism when handling the carcass and submitting specimens.

DIAGNOSIS

Diagnosis is often possible based on clinical signs, gross pathology, histopathology, and culture if the carcasses are fresh and the correct sites are examined. A colloidal gold-based immunodiagnostic assay has been described for SS2 and SS1/2 43. Serotyping by coagglutination will enable the SS strain to be identified. The genetic diversity within and between strains is increasing.[6] The same SS isolated from different geographic regions may be genetically and phenotypically very different.[42]

Serologic tests are generally not very useful because of the diversity of the strains involved, but an ELISA has been developed for human exposure.[33]

DIFFERENTIAL DIAGNOSIS

In pigs, there may be sporadic cases of arthritis attributable to staphylococci but the streptococcal infection is the common one. Arthritis attributable to *M. hyorhinis* is less suppurative but may require cultural differentiation. Glässer's disease occurs usually in older pigs and is accompanied by pleurisy, pericarditis, and peritonitis. Erysipelas in very young pigs is usually manifested by septicemia. Nervous disease of piglets may resemble arthritis on cursory examination, but there is an absence of joint enlargement and lameness. However, the meningitic form of the streptococcal infection can easily be confused with viral encephalitides. Meningitis in young pigs may also be associated with *P. multocida* and *E. coli*. Polyarthritis in calves, lambs, and piglets may also be associated with infection with *T. pyogenes* and *F. necrophorum*. SS2 can also be the cause of meningitis in older pigs of 10 to 14 weeks of age.

TREATMENT

Antimicrobials

In summary, there has been an increasing level of resistance to tetracyclines and erythromycin and a variable resistance to ciprofloxacin and penicillin.[43] Most SS are resistant to tetracyclines.[44] If treatment is based on serotyping and sensitivity testing, then there is much less chance of treating or creating resistant organisms.

In Denmark, over the last 15 years there has been an increase in resistance of SS isolates to the two most commonly used antibiotics, tylosin and tetracyclines. The strains show a varying pattern of resistance dependent on to which of the 21 ribotype profiles they belong. For example, strains causing meningitis were more resistant to sulfamethoxazole, but those causing pneumonia were more resistant to tetracyclines. Tilmicosin has been used successfully to remove clinical signs of streptococcal meningitis from a herd.

Penicillin has been the treatment of choice, but penicillin-resistant isolates have emerged. Penicillin sensitivity can no longer be assumed for all strains of SS, and the routine use of penicillin must be reevaluated. In one study, more than 50% of isolates of SS were not susceptible to penicillin. Penicillin did not eliminate the organism from the tonsils of carrier pigs treated daily for several days. In some surveys, the antimicrobial sensitivity of SS indicates a high degree of sensitivity to ampicillin, cephalothin, and trimethoprim–sulfamethoxazole, and resistance to the aminoglycosides gentamicin and streptomycin. It is recommended that trimethoprim–sulfamethoxazole be used for the treatment of affected pigs and be given daily for 3 days. An occasional strain may be resistant to trimethoprim–sulfamethoxazole.

None of the resistant strains produced beta-lactamase. Conjugation of antibiotic resistance in SS has been reported, which may explain the multiple antimicrobial resistance. The genes responsible for resistance appear to be homologous to genes found in many other species of bacteria. Treatment of pigs affected with meningitis attributable to SS2 with either trimethoprim–sulfadiazine or penicillin reduced the case-fatality rate from 55% to 21%. Cefquinome has been shown to improve cure rates (67%) compared with ampicillin (55%) and to reduce mortality from 35% with ampicillin to 24% with cefquinome.

Passive immunization against SS2 has been described.

CONTROL

At the present time there are no known specific methods for the prevention of the disease complex associated with SS2. The recommendations are based on empirical field observations. Regular isolation of the agent from any clinical cases will confirm the continuation of a strain or the arrival of a new strain and hopefully differentiate virulent from nonvirulent.[15]

It has been suggested that ceftiofur administered by injection for 3 consecutive days following SS challenge is the most effective regimen for minimizing disease associated with PRRS virus and SS infection. The use of potassium penicillin G in drinking water for several days was reported as being successful[45] and will reduce mortality. A combination of medication and vaccination was seen to remove SS from the tonsils of carrier sows.[47]

Environment and Management

Good management and hygiene techniques should be emphasized. Based on observations of the effects of management practices on SS carrier rate in nursery pigs, excessive temperature fluctuations, high relative humidity, crowding, and an age spread exceeding 2 weeks of pigs in the same room were associated with a higher-than-average percentage of carrier pigs.

Nursery pig environmental temperature should not fluctuate more than 1.1° to 1.7°C (34° to 35°F) over a 24-hour period.

Excessive relative humidity must be avoided; the recommended range of relative humidity for nursery pigs is 55% to 70%.

The age spread between pigs in the same room should not exceed 2 weeks. Young, potentially naive piglets raised in the same air space as older animals may be exposed to high concentrations of the organism.

Adequate space to avoid crowding is also necessary. Crowding occurs when less than 0.18 m^2 is provided for each 22.7 kg of pig. The use of an all-in, all-out production system is recommended, compared with a continuous flow system, which allows for a build-up of pathogens. The control of the most commonly encountered infectious diseases is also important. A well-fortified nutritional program may also aid in the control of SS infection and the carrier state in a swine herd.

Segregated early weaning programs have been used in an attempt to control the disease but appear to be unsuccessful in reducing the carrier state. Pigs are weaned at an early age and moved to a separate site in an effort to separate the piglets from the sows, which are the primary source of the organism. Carrier pigs readily transmit the infection to uninfected pigs, and the main method of spread between herds is the movement of infected breeding stock or weaner pigs. In herds that are free of the infection, it is necessary to avoid the importation of infected pigs. Eradication of SS2 infection can be attempted by depopulation of suspected carrier sows and replacement with noninfected breeding stock.

Mass Medication of Feed

Mass medication of individual pigs or medication of the feed during periods of high risk may control the incidence of clinical disease. Outbreaks in sucking piglets have been controlled by a single injection of benethamine penicillin to all piglets given 5 days before the average age of onset of clinical signs. The feeding of oxytetracycline (400 g/ton) for 14 days immediately before the usual onset may control the occurrence of the disease at a low level in weaned pigs, although there is increasing evidence of resistance. The use of a medicated feed containing trimethoprim–sulfadiazine (1:5) at a rate of 500 g/ton for the first 6 weeks after weaning did not significantly reduce the incidence of disease. Oral prophylactic medication with either procaine penicillin G or a mixture of chlortetracycline, sulfadimidine, and procaine penicillin G reduced the incidence of meningitis. Penicillin V administered orally provided higher plasma concentrations of drug. The inclusion of penicillin V potassium (10%), at a rate of 2 kg/ton of feed, significantly reduced the incidence of streptococcal meningitis when fed to the pigs for a total of 6 weeks from 4 to 10 weeks of age.

Tiamulin in the drinking water at 180 mg/L of water for 5 days significantly reduced the effects of experimentally induced SS infections.

Vaccination

Most vaccination studies have been carried out with piglets.[46] Either commercial or autogenous bacterins are available. Autogenous vaccines need to use strains from systemic sites such as the meninges, spleen, liver, and joints, nasal cavity, or tonsils, but not the lungs because they are more likely to be the nonvirulent SS. A study showed that SS9 bacterin produced a much lower level of efficacy than a SS2 vaccine.[47] Homologous protection is always more successful than for heterologous strains, which is why it is essential to continually monitor the strains in an endemically affected herd. A commercial vaccine reduced mortality from 17% to 2.6%. What constitutes an effective antigen is still a matter of conjecture. High levels of antibody against MRP and EF proteins did not confer protection.[48]

Studies are being conducted on the use of vaccines containing the immunogenic polysaccharide from SS2. However, the protection provided by whole-cell vaccines is probably type specific, which suggests that such vaccines should contain many serotypes if broad protection is desired. A trial minimizing variation in weaning age to achieve a uniform size with a combination of an autogenous vaccine and ceftiofur sodium has been reported. The protective levels of antibody did not prevent the survival of the organism in either tonsils or joints. An ELISA can be used to evaluate the antibody response in pigs vaccinated with SS2.

Different components of the organism are being examined to identify possible fractions for the preparation of a subunit vaccine. A subunit vaccine containing both MRP and EF, formulated with an oil/water adjuvant, that protected pigs against challenge with a virulent SS2 has been proposed. Vaccination of sows with 2 mL of bacterin prevented neurologic signs but not lameness, bacteriuria, or mortality in their progeny from challenge at 13 to 21 days of age. Immunization of experimental mice with a live avirulent strain of SS2 provided protection, which may be extrapolated for consideration in pigs. A vaccine containing purified suilysin protected mice against a lethal homologous challenge and induced protection against clinical signs in pigs after homologous challenge. Pigs vaccinated with a vaccine containing purified suilysin were protected from challenge with the homologous strain of the organism, whereas pigs vaccinated with a vaccine containing most of the extracellular antigens, and the placebo pigs, developed clinical disease. Suilysin is produced by most of the field strains tested and could be an important cross-protection factor.

Medicated early weaning does not produce eradication. The establishment of a new herd by hysterectomy and artificial rearing will allow this, and freedom can only be maintained by intense 24/7 biosecurity. Complete degreasing, cleaning, disinfection, and drying and letting a building rest before repopulating with SS-free stock from a known SS-free pyramid is the only way to get rid of a persistent infection.

REFERENCES

1. Gottschalk M, et al. *Future Microbiol.* 2010;5:371.
2. Takada K, Hirasawa M. *Int J Syst Evol Microbiol.* 2007;57:1272.
3. Takada K, et al. *Microbiol Immunol.* 2008;52:64.
4. Chen C, et al. *PLoS ONE.* 2007;2:e315.
5. Holden M, et al. *PLoS ONE.* 2009;4:e6072.
6. Blume V, et al. *Int Microbiol.* 2009;12:161.
7. Luey C, et al. *J Microbiol Method.* 2007;68:648.
8. Marois C, et al. *Canad J Vet Res.* 2006;70:94.
9. Fittipaldi N, et al. *Vet Microbiol.* 2009;139:320.
10. Messier S, et al. *Can Vet J.* 2008;49:461.
11. Baums CG, et al. *Infect Immunol.* 2006;74:6154.
12. Wei Z, et al. *Vet Microbiol.* 2009;137:196.
13. Baums C, et al. *Appl Environ Microbiol.* 2007;73:711.
14. Luque I, et al. *Vet J.* 2010;186:396.
15. MacInnes J, et al. *Canad J Vet Res.* 2008;72:242.
16. Marois C, et al. *Canad J Vet Res.* 2007;71:14.
17. Li P, et al. *Microbiol Pathog.* 2010;49:305.
18. van Calsteren MR, et al. *Biochem Cell Biol.* 2010;88:513.
19. Chabot-Roy G, et al. *Microbiol Pathog.* 2006;41:121.
20. Fittipaldi N, et al. *Mol Microbiol.* 2008;70:1120.

21. Fittipaldi N, et al. *PLoS ONE*. 2010;5:e8426.
22. Takamatsu D, et al. *Vet Microbiol*. 2009;138:132.
23. Silva L, et al. *Vet Microbiol*. 2006;115:117.
24. Essglass M, et al. *Microbiol*. 2008;154:2668.
25. Lecours MP, et al. *J Infect Dis*. 2011;204:919.
26. Si Y, et al. *Vet Microbiol*. 2009;139:80.
27. Zhang X-H, et al. *Microbiol Pathog*. 2009;47:267.
28. Ye C, et al. *Emerg Infect Dis*. 2006;12:1203.
29. Gottschalk M, et al. *Anim Hlth Res Rev*. 2007;8:29.
30. Lun Z-R, et al. *Lancet Infect Dis*. 2007;7:201.
31. Tang J, et al. *PLoS ONE*. 2006;3:e151.
32. Cheung P, et al. *Int J Food Microbiol*. 2008;127:316.
33. Smith T, et al. *Emerg Infect Dis*. 2008;14:1925.
34. Wertheim H, et al. *Clin Infect Dis*. 2009;48:617.
35. Ye C, et al. *J Infect Dis*. 2009;199:97.
36. Tenenbaum T, et al. *Brain Res*. 2006;1100:1.
37. Tenenbaum T, et al. *Cell Biol*. 2009;11:323.
38. Dominguez-Punaro M, et al. *J Immunol*. 2007;179:1842.
39. Feng Y, et al. *Trends Microbiol*. 2010;18:124.
40. Vanier G, et al. *Microbiol Pathog*. 2009;46:13.
41. Beineke A, et al. *Vet Microbiol*. 2008;128:423.
42. Rehm T, et al. *J Med Microbiol*. 2007;56:102.
43. Hendriksen R, et al. *Acta Vet Scand*. 2008;50:19.
44. Wisselink H, et al. *Vet Microbiol*. 2006;113:73.
45. Byra C, et al. *Can Vet J*. 2011;52:272.
46. Swilders B, et al. *Vet Rec*. 2007;160:619.
47. Buttner N, et al. *Vet Immunol Immunopathol*. 2012;146:191.
48. Kock C, et al. *Vet Immunol Immunopathol*. 2009;132:135.

STREPTOCOCCAL LYMPHADENITIS OF SWINE (JOWL ABSCESSES, CERVICAL ABSCESSES)

Cervical or "jowl" abscess of pigs is observed mainly at slaughter. Clinically, there is obvious enlargement of the lymph nodes of the throat region, particularly the mandibular and the retropharyngeal. It is of considerable importance because of the losses resulting from rejection of infected carcasses at meat inspection.

The condemnation rate of pig heads at slaughter was as high as 78% to 94% in some herds in the 1960s. However, since then, the incidence of jowl abscesses in pigs has declined steadily. This may be a result of changes in management of pig herds and the use of antibiotic feeding.

Most jowl abscesses in swine are associated with beta-hemolytic streptococci of Lancefield's group E type IV, although *P. multocida, E. coli,* and *T. pyogenes* may also be present. Some additional serotypes have been isolated. Jowl abscessation occurs primarily in postweaning and finishing pigs. Piglets under 28 days of age are relatively resistant, and even colostrum-deprived piglets are resistant to clinical disease following experimental infection.

The disease has been produced by feeding or the intranasal or intrapharyngeal instillation of streptococci, and they are thought to be the cause, with infection occurring through the tonsil or pharyngeal mucosa from contaminated food and water. The contamination occurs from abscess material leaking into food or water. In herds where cervical abscess is a problem, streptococci can commonly be isolated from the vaginas of pregnant sows and the pharynges of normal young pigs. The persistence of the infection in herds is thought to depend on the presence of carrier animals. Transmission occurs via feed and drinking water. After infection has occurred, bacteremia develops, and abscesses are initiated in the cervical lymph nodes in a high proportion of pigs. Infrequently, abscesses occur in atypical sites other than the head and neck. Pigs that have recovered from the natural disease are immune to experimental challenge. A microtitration agglutination test is available to detect infections associated with type IV streptococci.

Vaccination of pregnant sows with an autogenous or commercial bacterin containing streptococci and staphylococci is thought to be of value in protecting the litters of the vaccinated sows. Vaccination of young pigs with a whole-culture bacterin has provided some protection. The use of an oral vaccine prepared from an avirulent strain of group E streptococci and sprayed into the oropharynx is highly effective as a preventive measure. None of these vaccines is widely used because the condition is very sporadic. A number of prophylactic regimens based on the feeding of antibiotics have been proposed and generally give good results. Chlortetracycline fed to young pigs at the rate of 220 g/ton for 1 month is an example. Treatment of breeding pigs at the same time is likely to have a beneficial effect in reducing the severity of exposure of the young pigs to infection. A similar advantage can be gained by keeping the treated groups isolated from untreated groups of older pigs. Because piglets under 28 days of age are relatively resistant to clinical disease, the weaning and isolation from older pigs is a successful control program.

ERYSIPELAS IN SWINE

Erysipelas of pigs is the major disease of animals associated with *Erysipelothrix rhusiopathiae,* and it can occur in all stages of pig production. The condition is seen as sudden death; as an acute disease, possibly with diamond-shaped skin lesions; and also as a chronic disease with arthritis and vegetative endocarditis and reproductive failure in adults. In many minimal-disease herds they have tended not to vaccinate, and then the epizootics have occurred as a result of an increasing lack of immunity. It is zoonotic, most commonly causing erysipeloid in the fingers.

SYNOPSIS

Etiology *Erysipelothrix rhusiopathiae.*

Epidemiology Pigs worldwide. Common in unvaccinated pigs raised outdoors. High case-fatality rate if not treated. Organism in environment and transmitted by carrier pigs. Important zoonosis.

Clinical signs Hyperacute sudden death. Sudden onset of acute disease, fever, anorexia, typical diamond-shaped skin lesions. Arthritis, endocarditis in chronic form.

Clinical pathology Organism in blood. Hemogram and serology.

Necropsy findings Skin lesions, widespread ecchymotic hemorrhages (kidney, pleura, peritoneum), venous infarction of stomach. Nonsuppurative proliferative arthritis. Vegetative endocarditis.

Diagnosis Culture and isolate organism from blood in acute case and then tissues.

Differential diagnosis Other septicemias of pigs:

- Septicemic salmonellosis
- Hog cholera and African swine fever
- Streptococcal septicemia and arthritis
- Streptococcal endocarditis

Other arthritides of pigs:

- Glässer's disease
- Mycoplasma synoviae and hyorhinis arthritis
- Rickets and chronic zinc poisoning
- Foot rot of pigs
- Leg weakness

Treatment Penicillin.

Control Vaccination, with at most 6 month-interval until new and improved vaccines appear.

ETIOLOGY

Erysipelothrix rhusiopathiae (formerly insidiosa) (ER) is the causative bacterium, and the disease can be produced in hyperacute, acute, and subacute septicemic and chronic forms by the injection of cultures of the organism. The organism occurs as rough and smooth strains; the smooth are more virulent. At least 29 antigenic types have been identified, and usually types 1 and 2 are isolated from the septicemic forms.[1] The species has recently been divided into two species on the basis of the DNA tests that reflect biochemical and serologic characteristics. Many of the serotypes have been regrouped and called *Erysipelothrix tonsillarum* (ER), which is nonpathogenic.[2] This is found in the tonsil and is morphologically and biochemically similar to ER but has a very distinctive genetic profile. However, some species identified as ET on serology have been shown to be ER on multilocus enzyme electrophoresis. In addition, the restriction fragment length polymorphism (RFLP) typing using the PCR products of the Spa A gene have been used to subdivide the serotypes.[3] Recently. a new classification has been put forward based on Spa genes.[4,5] These are proteins, and at least three genes are known (Spa1, Spa2 and Spa3).[6,7]

Erysipelas rhusiopathiae now contains the former serotypes 1, 2, 4, 5, 6, 8, 9, 11, 12, 15, 16, 17, 19, 21, and N.

Erysipelas tonsillarum now contains serotypes 3, 7, 10, 14, 20, 22, and 23. Serotypes 13 and 18 are intermediate and called *Erysipelas* species strains 1 and 2 (also contains a few 9 and 10), respectively, and strain 3, which contains some strains of 7 and is as yet untypeable.[3] The identification and characterization of *E. inopinata* has not yet been determined.[8]

EPIDEMIOLOGY

Occurrence

Erysipelas in pigs occurs worldwide and causes serious economic loss, substantially as a result of deaths, morbidity and devaluation of pig carcasses because of arthritis. However, because the indoor confinement of swine and no contact with contaminated soil has followed, the occurrence of the disease has decreased markedly. The exception to this would be outdoor units where no regular vaccination is practiced. The other major exceptions are those parts of the world where the backyard or enthusiast's pigs are still found and where hygiene and biosecurity are usually nonexistent. Historically, the disease occurred most commonly in unvaccinated growing pigs over 3 months of age and adults. This is primarily because the maternal antibody is thought to last up to 3 months. The infection, usually with serotypes 1a or 2, has also been demonstrated in wild boars, so these should not be forgotten as a reservoir. Perhaps more important, these strains were resistant to oxytetracycline and/or dihydrostreptomycin.

Prevalence of Infection

The prevalence of infection with ER in carrier pigs ranges from 3% to 98%, with most surveys indicating that 20% to 50% of pigs are carriers, particularly in the tonsils. Carriers occur among vaccinated and unvaccinated pigs. The organism has been isolated from 10% of apparently healthy slaughter pigs and may explain its wide prevalence. In addition, the organism has been isolated from over 30 species of wild birds and 50 species of wild animals.

Morbidity and Case Fatality

Morbidity and case-fatality rates in pigs vary considerably from area to area, largely because of variations in virulence of the particular strain of the organism involved. On individual farms or in particular areas the disease may occur as a chronic arthritis in finishing pigs or as extensive outbreaks of the acute septicemia, or both forms may occur together. In unvaccinated pigs, the morbidity in the acute form will vary from 10% to 30%; the case-fatality rate may be as high as 75%.

Methods of Transmission

Soil contamination occurs through the feces of affected or carrier pigs. Other sources of infection include infected animals of other species, mouse contamination, open muck heaps and effluent on the soil, and birds. Straw-based systems are often highly contaminated. The clinically normal carrier pig is the most important source of infection, with the tonsils being the predilection site for the organism. Young pigs in contact with carrier sows rapidly acquire the status of carriers and shedders. Because the organism can pass through the stomach without loss of viability, carrier animals may reinfect the soil continuously, and this appears to be the main cause of environmental contamination. The organism can survive in feces for several months. All effluent contains species of *Erysipelothrix* but not necessarily ER. However, its persistence in soil is variable and may be governed by many factors including temperature, pH, and the presence of other bacteria. The organism can be isolated from the effluent of commercial piggeries and from the soil and pasture of effluent disposal sites for up to 2 weeks after application of the effluent containing the organism. Although the environment is considered to be secondary to animals as a reservoir of infection, the survival of the organism in the environment could create an infection hazard. Flies are known to transmit the disease, and a lowered prevalence has been attributed to the use of insecticides.

Under natural conditions, skin abrasions and the alimentary tract mucosa are considered to be the probable portals of entry, and transmission is by ingestion of contaminated feed. Occasional outbreaks occur after the use of virulent and incomplete avirulent cultures as vaccines. Abortion storms in late pregnant sows with septicemic death in sucklers may be the first indication of the disease in specific-pathogen-free herds.

Spread of the infection can also occur to most other species. The organism has been recovered from sylvatic mammals in northwestern Canada. It has been isolated from a horse affected with vegetative endocarditis. It has, at times, been found in fish meal, but this is now less used in pig diets. It is possible that other species, such as cattle, may harbor strains that are pathogenic for swine.

Risk Factors

It may be that some serotypes are resident in a single farm, and an outbreak may represent the arrival of a new serotype on that farm.

There is considerable variation in the ease with which the disease can be reproduced and in its severity. Many factors, such as age, health and intercurrent disease, exposure, and heredity, influence both natural and artificial transmission. Stress may predispose to the condition, but virulence of the strain is probably the most important factor. Smooth strains can be used successfully to produce the disease experimentally, but rough strains appear to be nonpathogenic. This variation in virulence between strains of the organism has been utilized in the production of living, avirulent vaccines.

Animal Risk Factors

Infected pigs probably shed the agent in feces and oronasal secretions and also in urine, and direct contact is probably the most usual method.

Pigs of all ages are susceptible. Recently farrowed sows seem to be particularly susceptible. This suggests that fatigue may be a factor. Sudden diet changes have also predisposed, as have heat and cold stress. When the strain is virulent, pigs of all ages, even sucklers a few weeks old, develop the disease. Almost entire litters under 2 weeks of age may be affected. Piglets from an immune sow may get sufficient antibodies in the colostrum to give them immunity for some weeks. It is likely that the animals are immune to the strains that are normally found in their particular environment. Possibly the arrival of new serotypes through new pig arrivals or the turning over of previously contaminated land together with an increase in stress are the main factors. It is known that ER from bovine tonsils is pathogenic for mice and pigs and possibly pathogenic for other animals and humans.

Pathogen Risk Factors

At least 32 serotypes are known to exist and many strains; however, 15 probably commonly affect pigs. Serotypes 1 and 2 are the most common types isolated from swine affected with clinical erysipelas and are generally thought to be the only serotypes that cause the acute disease. The other serotypes are relatively uncommon, and none of them has yet been a cause of acute epidemics, but some have been isolated from lesions of chronic erysipelas. Serotypes 1a, 3, 5, 6, 8, 11, 21, and type N have been isolated from pigs with chronic erysipelas, mainly arthritis and lymphadenitis.

Not all serotypes isolated from pigs are virulent. In a survey in Japan, the organism was found in 10% of the tonsils of healthy slaughter pigs: 54% were serotype 7, 32% serotype 2, 9.5% serotype 6, and 1.6% each of serotypes 11, 12, and 16. All serotype 2 isolates were highly virulent for pigs, whereas the other serotypes were only weakly virulent. Members of the other nonvirulent or weakly virulent group, mainly serotype 7 strains, are considered to be resident in porcine tonsils. Serotypes 1a or 2 were found most commonly in pigs in Australia, less commonly in sheep, and infrequently in other animals. Serotypes 1a and 1b accounted for 79% of the isolates from diseased pigs. The genetic diversity of Australian field isolates of ER and ET indicates widespread diversity. Those recovered from sheep or birds were more diverse than those isolated from pigs, and isolates of serovar 1 were more diverse than those of serovar 2. The diversity indicated that serotyping of ER is unreliable as an epidemiologic tool.

The serotype antigens of ER are immunologically distinct, and commercial bacterins prepared from the common serotypes will not provide protection against other pathogenic serotypes. This may be an explanation for the epidemics that may occur in vaccinated pigs. The 64 to 66 kDa protein appears to be most immunogenic. Also, a variety of serotypes may be recovered from pigs affected with the septicemic and arthritic forms of the disease.

The organism is resistant to most environmental influences, and to heat (15 minutes at 60°C [14° F]), and can survive in animal tissues at 40°C (105° F) and frozen tissues and is not readily destroyed by chemical disinfection, including 0.2% phenol and by drying agents. It can survive for 60 months in frozen or refrigerated media, 4 months in flesh, and 90 days in highly alkaline soil and is resistant to drying. It will also resist salt preparations and other food preservatives.

Zoonotic Implications

Because of human susceptibility, swine erysipelas has some public health significance. Veterinarians in particular are exposed to infection when vaccinating with virulent cultures. It commonly contaminates pig products and therefore is quite a common infection in abattoir workers or butchers or those employed in similar trades. It usually produces a swollen finger and is known as erysipeloid. In this context, there have been recent advances in slide agglutination and latex agglutination tests for rapid diagnosis, which have a good correlation with each other and subsequent culture. Now a PCR identifying four species has been described, principally for use in the abattoir. Recently a case of endocarditis and presumptive osteomyelitis has been described, so care is needed. Type 21 is recorded as having produced a septicemia in humans.[1]

PATHOGENESIS

The invasion of the susceptible pig by ER can occur under particular circumstances, for example, if weather conditions are hot and humid or in particular fields or buildings. Experimentally, it is often easier to infect the pig through scarified wounds than through intravenous infusions, through the gut, or through intravenous injections. There are marked differences in virulence between strains.

There is the presence in the pathogenic serotypes of a capsule that resists phagocytosis. Some virulent strains also produce a phosphorylcholine which resists phagocytosis. Some others may produce a neuraminidase, which may cleave the mucopolysaccharides in cell walls and cause vascular damage leading to hemorrhage and thrombosis. The surface protective antigen, a protein, Spa is also important in pathogenesis. There is also the possibility of novel adhesins called RspA and RspB. Apparently, avirulent strains do not have these four important features. Invasion of the bloodstream occurs in all infected animals in the first instance. Septicemia results within 1 to 7 days. The subsequent development of either an acute septicemia or a bacteremia with localization in organs and joints is dependent on undetermined factors. Virulence of the particular strain may be important, and this may depend on the number of recent pig passages experienced. Coagulase activity is a possible virulence factor. Concurrent viral infection, especially hog cholera, may increase susceptibility of the host.

Localization in the chronic form is commonly in the skin, joints, and other heart valves, with probable subsequent bacteremic episodes, and it may start from as early as 4 days after initial infection, although the cartilage lesions may be delayed until about 8 months, and they can then continue to progress for at least 2 years. Selective adherence of some strains of ER to heart valves may be a factor in the pathogenesis of endocarditis. In joints, the initial lesion is an increase in synovial fluid and hyperemia of the synovial membrane, followed in several weeks by the proliferation of synovial villi (really a synovitis), thickening of the joint capsule, and enlargement of the local lymph nodes. Diskospondylitis also occurs in association with chronic polyarthritis attributable to erysipelas. Amyloidosis may occur in pigs with chronic erysipelas polyarthritis. The heart lesions may begin with early inflammatory changes associated with emboli.

There has been some controversy over whether the arthrodial lesions result from primary infection or whether they result from hypersensitivity to the *Erysipelothrix* or other antigens. Current opinion suggests that the former is the case but that the lesions are enhanced by immunologic mechanisms to persistent antigen at the site. There are increased levels of immunoglobulins IgG and IgM in the synovial fluids of pigs with polyarthritis attributable to ER, and the levels are considered to be only partly a result of serum and increased permeability. The presence of antibody does not remove the organism from the joints.

Abortion is thought to occur as a result of high fever, but the organism has been isolated from the fetus. Congenital erysipelas has also been recorded. In these cases, the organism can be recovered from the anterior vagina.

CLINICAL FINDINGS

There are several forms of disease. These include hyperacute, acute, subacute, and chronic.

Hyperacute Form

Quite often the disease is seen for the first time in pigs approaching market weight. The animal is usually found dead or is dull, is depressed, has a temperature of 42°C (106–109° F), and dies quickly; it usually occurs in finishing pigs and is uncommon in sows.

Acute and Subacute Forms

This form is uncommon in adults. The signs vary with age and immune status. The acute usually die within 12 to 48 hours of the onset of signs. After an incubation period of 1 to 7 days, there is a sudden onset of high fever (up to 42°C [108°F]), which is followed some time later by severe prostration, complete anorexia, thirst, and occasional vomiting. Initially, affected pigs may be quite active and continue to eat even though their temperatures are high. However, generally in an outbreak one is initially presented with one or two dead or severely affected pigs showing marked red (scarlet flush) to purple discoloration of the skin of the jowl and ventral surface (may even be whole-body cyanosis), with others in the group showing high fever, reluctance to rise, and some incoordination while walking. Dyspnea is a common feature. Conjunctivitis with ocular discharge may be present.

Skin lesions are almost pathognomonic but may not always be apparent. These may take the form of the classical diamond-shaped, red, urticarial plaques about 2.5 by 5 cm square that occur within the 24 to 48 hours of the onset of clinical signs, or a more diffuse edematous eruption with the same appearance. These lesions can also be palpated as raised patches. In the early stages the lesions are often palpable before they are visible. The lesions are most common on the belly, inside the thighs, and on the throat, neck, and ears, and usually appear about 24 hours after the initial signs of illness. Sometimes they can be felt rather than seen. After a course of 2 to 4 days the pig recovers or dies, with diarrhea, dyspnea, and cyanosis evident terminally. The mortality rate may reach 75%, but wide variation occurs. Pregnant animals may abort, and it is thought that this is a result of the fever, but it may be that there is a direct fetal action because congenital infections and isolations of the organism from the fetus have occurred. There may occasionally be waves of returns to service and abortion storms. Inflected boars recover but may be infertile for 6 to 8 weeks.

The so-called "skin" form is usually the acute form with more prominent skin localization but less severe signs of septicemia and with a low mortality. The skin lesions disappear in about 10 days without residual effects. In the more serious cases the plaques spread and coalesce, often over the back, to form a continuous deep-purple area extending over a greater part of the skin surface. The affected skin becomes black and hard, and the edges curl up and separate from an underlying, raw surface. The dry skin may hang on for a considerable time and rattle while the pig walks, or it may slough off.

Chronic Form

Many of the chronic cases require euthanasia because they deteriorate rapidly.

Signs are vague and indistinct except for the joint lesions characteristic of this form of the disease. Bacteria may localize in the joints. There may be alopecia, sloughing of the tail and tips of the ears, and dermatitis in the form of hyperkeratosis of the skin of the back, shoulders, and legs; growth may be retarded. Joint lesions are most common in the elbow, hip, hock, stifle, and knee joints and cause lameness and stiffness. The joints are obviously enlarged and are usually hot and painful at first but in 2 to 3 weeks are quite firm and without heat. This is especially the case when the arthritis has been present for some time, allowing healing and ankylosis to develop. Paraplegia may occur when intervertebral joints are involved or when there is gross distortion of limb joints.

A subclinical form of synovitis may occur that affects feed intake and results in a reduced rate of growth.

Endocarditis also occurs as a chronic form of the disease with or without arthritis. Suggestive clinical signs are often absent, with the animals dying suddenly without previous illness, especially at times of exertion, such as mating, or movement between pens. In others there is progressive emaciation and inability to perform exercise. With forced-exercise dyspnea, cyanosis and even sudden death may occur. The cardiac impulse is usually markedly increased, the heart rate is faster, and a loud murmur is audible on auscultation if the valves are badly damaged. Cyanosis, tachycardia and tachypnea, and heart murmurs may feature in these cases.

In Switzerland, chronic swine erysipelas is suspected where there is vegetative endocarditis, arthritis, and the culture of ER from vulval discharges. These signs are also accompanied by poor fertility and increased prevalence of abortions, stillbirths, and small litter size. Vaccine was used to control an outbreak of purulent periparturient vulval discharge in which ER was the only organism isolated. In one study anterior vaginal samples from 64 sows all yielded ER.

CLINICAL PATHOLOGY

Detection of Organism

In the acute form, examination of blood smears may reveal the presence of the bacteria, particularly in the leukocytes, but blood culture is likely to be more successful as a method of diagnosis. Repeated examinations in the chronic forms of the disease may by chance give a positive result during a bacteremic phase. Final identification of the organism necessitates mouse or pigeon inoculation tests and protection tests in these animals using antierysipelas serum.

Hematology

In the early stages of the acute form there is first leukocytosis, followed by leukopenia and monocytosis. The leukopenia is of moderate degree (40% reduction in total leukocyte count at most) compared with that occurring in hog cholera. The monocytosis is quite marked, varying from a 5-fold to a 10-fold increase (2.5% to 4.5% normal levels rise to 25%).

Serology

The efficiency of agglutination tests for ER is not clear. They appear to be satisfactory for herd diagnosis but not sufficiently accurate for identification of individual affected pigs, particularly clinically normal carrier animals. A more accurate and reliable complement fixation test is available, but an enzyme immunoassay test is much quicker, easier, and more economical to perform. An ELISA test has been used.

NECROPSY FINDINGS

Experimentally the disease can be produced by oral dosing; by intradermal, intravenous, and intraarticular injection; and by application to scarified skin, conjunctiva, and nasal mucosa. The arthritic form of the disease can be reproduced by multiple intravenous inoculations of ER.

The microscopic lesions include vasculitis in capillaries and venules in many sites, including glomeruli, pulmonary capillaries, and the skin. Sometimes, it is possible to see emboli of bacteria without specific stains to demonstrate bacteria.

Acute and Subacute Forms

In the hyperacute cases, all that may be seen is a congested carcass with discoloration of the skin. The degree of skin discoloration may provide a clue to prognosis, in that it is said that if the skin lesions are pink to light purple, then resolution will often occur within 4 to 7 days, but the dark angry black/purple lesions have a grave prognosis.

Classic "diamond skin" lesions may be present. They are almost pathognomonic. However, the diffuse, purplish discoloration of the belly and cyanosis of the extremities common to other septicemic diseases of pigs is a more reliable finding. Internally, petechial and ecchymotic hemorrhage occurs, mainly on the pleura and peritoneum and beneath the renal capsule but also on the heart, kidney, pleura, liver, and spleen. Venous infarction of the stomach is accompanied by swollen, hemorrhagic mesenteric lymph nodes, and there is congestion of the lungs and liver. Infarcts may be present in the spleen and kidney and the former much enlarged. Histologic changes in all tissues are those of toxemia and thrombosis. Large numbers of intravascular organisms are often visible. There are no specific histologic changes.

Chronic Form

There may be necrotic skin lesions and embolic lesions in organs and the enlarged joints,

A nonsuppurative proliferative arthritis involving limb and intervertebral joints is characteristic. Synovitis, with a serous or serofibrinous amber-colored intraarticular effusion, occurs first ; degenerative changes in the subendochondral bone, cartilage, and ligaments follow. When the synovial changes predominate, the joint capsule and villi are thickened. There are enlarged, dark-red pedunculations or patches of vascular granulation tissue, which spread as a pannus onto the articular surface. When bony changes predominate, the articular cartilage is detached from the underlying bone, causing abnormal mobility of the joint. Ulceration of the articular cartilage may also be present. Local lymph node enlargement is usual. With time, the joint lesions often repair by fibrosis and ankylosis sufficiently to permit use of the limb.

Endocardial lesions, when present, are large, friable vegetations on the valves, often of sufficient size to block the valvular orifice. Occasionally, endocarditis may be the only lesion seen, but this is a rare occurrence. Erysipelas is often said to rank below *S. suis* as a cause of endocarditis in growing pigs, but ER was the most frequent isolate from cases of endocarditis seen in slaughtered pigs. Infarcts occur in the kidney, and these may also yield pure cultures of the organism. Chronic joint lesions are often sterile, but bacteriologic culture should nevertheless be attempted. The probability of positive isolation increases with the number of joints sampled, and isolations are more frequent from the smaller, distal joints.

DIAGNOSIS

Clinical signs (fever, lameness, and skin lesions) and the absence of respiratory signs and anorexia are suggestive and confirmed by isolation of the agent from blood in the acute stages. Diagnosis from joints in chronic stages is more difficult. Postmortem examination of the acute case cases will usually allow culture from the heart, blood, spleen, and bone marrow, particularly the long bones.

Samples for Confirmation of Diagnosis

With acute cases, the tests are more successful. Bacteriologic examination of subacute cases is less successful, and chronic cases often not successful.

- Bacteriology—culture swabs from joints; synovial membranes in culture media; heart valve masses, spleen, kidney, skin and bone marrow, particularly from a long bone. Smears of heart blood are particularly useful in the first 1 to 2 days of the acute diseases. The organism is a slender, facultative anaerobe and gram-positive rod that produces a 1-mm gray colony after 24 hours of incubation on blood agar. It may be observed singly, in short chains, or as a palisade.

There are a variety of short gram-positive rods that can be confused with *Erysipelas* organisms.[9] Different morphologic types (rough and smooth colonies), exist and the rough are considered less virulent. Enrichment techniques and the use of selective media will also increase the frequency of isolation.[9]

- Florescent techniques have been developed to show antigen in joints. New PCR techniques have also been used.
- Histology—formalin-fixed synovial membranes, heart valve masses, spleen, kidney, and skin lesions (light microscopy) are useful. There may be granulation tissue on the heart valves. The synovial lesions are characterized by macrophages and lymphocytes with synoviocyte proliferation. The vasculitis is extensive, and thrombi and bacterial colonies may be seen. Immunohistochemistry aids in the differential diagnosis from the other bacteria (*Mycoplasma, S. suis,* and *H. parasuis*).[10]

Antigen detection has helped greatly in detection. PCR and RT-PCR have been developed. A multiplex PCR has been developed to differentiate ER and ET11, and strain 2 was then added.[11] A qRT-PCR has been described for ER and ET13 and for differentiating vaccine strains from field strains.[12]

Note the zoonotic potential of this organism when handling the carcass and submitting specimens.

DIFFERENTIAL DIAGNOSIS

Erysipelas in pigs is not ordinarily difficult to diagnose because of the characteristic clinical and necropsy findings. In the occasional situation in which anthrax may have occurred in the past, it is worth testing a smear of edema fluid taken by a needle from the jowl or ear region for this pathogen before opening of the carcass. The acute disease may be confused with the other septicemia affecting pigs, but pigs with erysipelas usually show the characteristic skin lesions and are less depressed than pigs with hog cholera or salmonellosis. Rarely, *A. pleuropneumoniae* and *H. parasuis* may also appear similar.

Other septicemias of pigs:

- Septicemic salmonellosis is characterized by gross bluish-purple discoloration of the skin, especially the ears, some evidence of enteritis, and polypnea and dyspnea.
- Hog cholera is characterized by large numbers of pigs affected quickly, weakness, fever, muscle tremors, skin discoloration and rapid death; convulsions are also common.
- Streptococcal septicemia and arthritis are almost entirely confined to suckling pigs in the first few weeks of life as is septicemia associated with *Actinobacillus suis.*
- Streptococcal endocarditis has a similar age distribution to erysipelas endocarditis and bacteriologic examination is necessary to differentiate them.

Other arthritides of pigs:

The chronic disease characterized by joint disease occurs in pigs of all ages but less commonly in adults and must be differentiated from the following conditions:

- Glässer's disease in pigs is accompanied by a severe painful dyspnea. At necropsy there is serositis and meningitis
- Mycoplasma hyorhinis arthritis generally affects pigs less than 10 weeks of age and produces a polyserositis and polyarthritis. However, *Mycoplasma hyosynoviae* can produce simple polyarthritis in growing pigs. In general, the periarticular, synovial, and cartilaginous changes are less severe in these infections compared with erysipelas; however, cultural differentiation is frequently necessary.
- Rickets and chronic zinc poisoning produce lameness in pigs, but they occur under special circumstances and are not associated with fever, and rickets is accompanied by abnormalities of posture and gait that are not seen in erysipelas.
- Foot rot of pigs is easily differentiated by the swelling of the hoof and the development of discharging sinuses at the coronet.

Leg weakness. In recent years there has been a marked increase in chronic osteoarthritis and various forms of "leg weakness" in growing swine, probably related to the increased growth rate resulting from modern feeding and management practices.

TREATMENT

Antimicrobial Therapy

Penicillin and antierysipelas serum (available only in some countries) comprise the standard treatment, often administered together by dissolving the penicillin in the serum. The antiserum lasts about 2 weeks. Penicillin alone is usually adequate when the strain is mildly virulent. Standard dose rates give a good response in the field, but experimental studies suggest that 50,000 IU/kg BW of procaine penicillin intramuscularly for 3 days and preferably 5 days is required for complete chemotherapeutic effect. Most animals are significantly improved within 2 days. Oxytetracycline is also useful, but in a Japanese study, over 70% of the strains were resistant. Chronic cases do not respond well to either treatment because of the structural damage that occurs to the joints and the inaccessibility of the organism in the endocardial lesions. Most strains are susceptible to ampicillin, cloxacillin, benzylpenicillin, ceftiofur, tylosin, enrofloxacin, and danofloxacin. Most strains are resistant to apramycin, neomycin, streptomycin, and spectinomycin and also to sulfonamides and polymyxins.

CONTROL

Successful control depends on good hygiene (cleaning, disinfection, and separation from feces and contaminated fields); biosecurity (other pigs and other species); reduction of stress, an effective 6-month vaccination policy, preferably two doses, for all animals over 3 months of age, including boars; and rapid diagnosis, quarantine, and treatment. The organism is inactivated by most disinfectants but is never completely eliminated. Effective bird and rodent control is important, especially if they are near feed such as in outdoor herds. Where there are scrape-through systems, there is never complete control. Do not forget that sheep and turkeys may also be a source of infection.

Eradication

Eradication is virtually impossible because of the ubiquitous nature of the organism and its survival in suitable environments. Complete removal of all pigs and leaving the pens unstocked is seldom satisfactory. Eradication by slaughter of reactors to the agglutination test is not recommended because of the uncertain status of the test.

General hygienic precautions should be adopted. Clinically affected animals should be disposed of quickly, and all introductions should be isolated and examined for signs of arthritis and endocarditis. This procedure will not prevent the introduction of clinically normal carrier animals. All animals dying of the disease should be properly incinerated to avoid contamination of the environment. Although thorough cleaning of the premises and the use of very strong disinfectant solutions is advisable, these measures are unlikely to be completely effective. The organism is susceptible to all the usual disinfectants, particularly caustic soda and hypochlorites. Whenever practicable, contaminated feedlots or paddocks should be cultivated for a spell before repopulating.

Specific-pathogen-free piggeries established on virgin soil may remain clinically free of erysipelas for several years. However, because of the high risk of introduction of the organism, it is advisable to vaccinate routinely.

Immunization

Because of the difficulty of eradication, biological prophylactic methods are in common use. Immunizing agents available include hyperimmune serum and vaccines.

Antierysipelas Serum

The parenteral administration of 5 to 20 mL of serum, with the amount depending on age, will protect in-contact pigs for a minimum of 1 to 2 weeks, possibly up to 6 weeks, during an outbreak. Suckling pigs in herds where the disease is endemic should receive 10 mL during the first week of life and at monthly intervals until they are actively vaccinated, which can be done as early as 6 weeks, provided the sows have not been vaccinated. Repeated administration of the serum may cause anaphylaxis because of its equine origin. For this reason, it has been withdrawn from sale in many countries.

Vaccination

There is no fully satisfactory vaccine available for erysipelas because of the strain variation and short duration of immunity, but vaccines have reduced the occurrence of clinical disease. Regular administration at 6-month intervals overcomes this to some extent, but there is always the possibility of a new strain appearing. Most vaccines are formalized whole cultures. Most bacterins are serotype 215, and most of the attenuated live vaccines (only available in some countries, such as the United States and Japan) contain 1a. Vaccines containing serotypes 2 and 10 protect against both *Erysipelothrix* species. Serum-simultaneous vaccination has been largely replaced by the use of bacterins, for which lysate and absorbate preparations are available, or by the use of attenuated or avirulent live-culture vaccines, which are administered orally or by injection. The use of live-culture vaccines is prohibited in many countries because of the risk of variation in virulence of the strains used and the possibility of spreading infection.

None of these vaccines gives lifelong protection from a single vaccination, and the actual duration of protection achieved following vaccination varies considerably. It should not be assumed that protection lasts longer than 6 months. The recent identification of the region responsible for protective immunity should improve these vaccines in future. Most of the commercially available vaccines are formalin-treated whole cultures with an adjuvant.

There is considerable difficulty in the experimental evaluation of the efficacy of erysipelas vaccines. Strain differences in immunogenicity and variation in host response to vaccination attributable to innate and acquired factors influence this evaluation, as does variation in virulence of the challenge strain and the method of challenge. A recent experiment has shown that an antigen of serotype 1a will elicit a protective response to a challenge with serotypes 1a and 2b. Similar factors are involved in the variations seen in field response to the use of these vaccines. Cross-protection of mice and pigs given a live-organism vaccine against 10 serovars of ER has been demonstrated. The use of culture filtrate from a broth culture of an attenuated strain of the organism has been evaluated to produce cross-protective antibody.

Vaccination will reduce the incidence of polyarthritis attributable to erysipelas, but not mild cases of arthritis. Passively acquired maternal immunity may significantly affect the immune response to vaccination in the young piglet. Also, the immunity engendered by standard vaccines is not uniformly effective against all strains. Vaccine breakdown occurs when the vaccine type is very different from that occurring on the farm. For example, a vaccine made from serotypes 1 and 2 will protect against serotype 10 (ET), but it is not certain that it will protect against serotype 20. Under certain conditions, some unusual serotypes have the potential for causing disease in animals vaccinated with vaccines containing the common serotypes. This possibility cannot be ignored and must be considered when vaccination failures occur. Nevertheless, these vaccines are valuable immunizing agents in field situations.

Vaccination Program

Following a single vaccination at 6 to 10 weeks of age, significant protection is provided to market age. However, a second "booster" vaccination given 2 to 4 weeks later is advisable. In herds where sows are routinely vaccinated before farrowing, a persisting maternal passive immunity (6 to 9 weeks) may require that piglet vaccination be delayed until 10 to 12 weeks of age for effective active immunity.

Replacement gilts and adults should also be vaccinated. Bacterins are effective, and field evidence suggests that vaccination provides immunity for approximately 6 months. Sows should be vaccinated twice yearly, preferably 3 to 6 weeks before farrowing, because this will also provide significant protection against the septicemic form in young sucklers. If possible, a closed herd should be maintained. Abortion may occur sporadically following the use of live vaccines.

Vaccination is subcutaneous in the skin behind the ear or at the axilla and the flank. Reactions at the site of injection are not uncommon. Swelling with subsequent nodule formation and occasional abscessation may occur following the injection of bacterins, and modified live vaccines may produce hemorrhage in the skin at the injection site. Granulomatous lesions may occur following the use of oil-based vaccines. There is little evidence that vaccination increases the incidence of arthritis. It has been suggested by a very limited study that maternal antibody does not appear to interfere with the vaccination. These vaccines were also used in pigs with PRRS and found to be safe and effective. In those cases where the vaccine has not worked, it may be that the correct serotype was not in the vaccine or the administration and storage instructions were not followed.

REFERENCES

1. Ozawa M, et al. *J Vet Med Sci.* 2009;71:697.
2. Wang Q, et al. *Vet Microbiol.* 2010;140:405.
3. To H, Nagai S. *Clin Vaccine Immunol.* 2007;14:813.
4. Ingebritson AL, et al. *Vaccine.* 2010;28:2490.
5. Shen HG, et al. *J Appl Microbiol.* 2010;109:1227.
6. Bender JS, et al. *Clin Vaccine Immunol.* 2010;17:1605.
7. Bender JS, et al. *J Vet Diag Invest.* 2011;23:139.
8. Takahashi T, et al. *Microbiol Immunol.* 2008;52:469.
9. Bender JS, et al. *J Vet Diag Invest.* 2009;21:863.
10. Opriessnig T, et al. *J Vet Diag Invest.* 2010;22:86.
11. Pal N, et al. *J Appl Microbiol.* 2009;108:1083.
12. Nagai S, et al. *J Vet Diag Invesgt.* 2008;20:336.

ACTINOBACILLUS SEPTICEMIA IN PIGLETS

Actinobacillus suis and *Actinobacillus equuli* sometimes cause a fatal septicemia in piglets of 1 to 6 weeks of age. Occasionally in older animals there may be skin lesions or necrotizing pneumonia. It is probably underdiagnosed because most cases are possibly assumed to be *S. suis.*

ETIOLOGY

It is gram negative and produces small translucent colonies on blood agar. In Canada, two groups appear, one associated with healthy pigs and the other with severely diseased pigs. The organism also produces the Apx toxins I and II. The organism should be distinguished from APP biotype II.

EPIDEMIOLOGY

It is probably widespread. In one study 94% of the tested herds were positive,[1] but no clinical cases were reported. It is reported infrequently. The introduction of carrier animals may be the cause of infections. Maternal antibodies are usually present in colostrum. Active antibodies are produced at 6 to 8 weeks of age.

PATHOGENESIS

The organism is probably carried in the nasal cavity and under stress or in the absence of immunity becomes septicemic. It may die at this point or may develop as endocarditis or arthritis. The virulence factors of *A. suis* are unknown, but outer membrane proteins are thought to be important.[2]

CLINICAL SIGNS

Sudden death may occur and may be attributed to hypoglycemia, starvation, or crushing and not investigated.

Piglets may be pyrexic and have dyspnea, cough, lameness wasting, abscesses, neurologic components, and cyanosis, with congestion and hemorrhages on the skin and possibly swollen joints. Recovered animals have poor growth. Older animals are not often affected but can be if the bacteria are entering a susceptible herd for the first time. Finishers may also die suddenly, and in the older animals, the condition may resemble swine erysipelas.

NECROPSY FINDINGS

Animals may have petechiae on the lung; microabscesses throughout the body, particularly the lungs; and skin discoloration. Chronic cases may have endocarditis, pericarditis, pneumonia, or polyarthritis. Histologically, the lesions are often microabscesses with central necrosis surrounded by neutrophils with bacterial thromboemboli.

DIAGNOSIS

The clinical signs and pathology are not diagnostic. The infection can be confirmed by pure culture from the liver, kidney, or heart blood and from lesions. Quite often, the organism can be recovered from tonsils of young pigs, vaginas of sows, and the preputial diverticulum of boars. Because there is production of Apx I and II, PCR testing may be useful, but it should be remembered that the level of toxin production is much lower in *A. suis*.

A real-time TaqMan PCR assay for the detection of *A. suis* has been described.[3] It was highly specific, sensitive, and reproducible and gave results within 3 hours.

TREATMENT

A wide range of antibiotics have proved useful, and most infections clear up in 2 to 5 days. Ceftiofur, gentamicin, and trimethoprim/sulfadiazine seem to be the drugs of choice. Resistance to amoxicillin, ampicillin, and tetracyclines has been recorded.

REFERENCES

1. MacInnes J, et al. *Can J Vet Res*. 2008;72:242.
2. Ojha S, et al. *Vet Microbiol*. 2010;140:122.
3. Kariyawasam S, et al. *J Vet Diag Invest*. 2011;23:885.

KLEBSIELLA PNEUMONIAE SEPTICEMIA IN PIGS

Klebsiella pneumoniae subspecies *pneumoniae* (KPSP) is an opportunist pathogen causing mastitis in sows but has recently been recognized in the United Kingdom as a cause of septicemia in preweaned pigs in outdoor herds. The organism is commensal in the healthy porcine alimentary tract and is present in the environment in soil and water. It can cause infections in humans, but it is not a recognized zoonosis and is more likely to occur in immunocompromised patients in hospitals. Pigs are found dead, with lesions consistent with septicemia and pure/predominant growth of KPSP isolated from internal sites.

The condition has been seen in preweaned pigs 17 to 28 days of age, in good bodily condition, and occasionally they are found in extremis, recumbent, with cyanosis and mouth breathing, with death within 30 minutes. All the cases occurred in outdoor commercial units in the summer (June through September). The mortality is estimated to be 1% to 4%, with one or a whole litter succumbing. The outbreak lasts from a period as short as 7 to 10 weeks to others lasting for more than 12 weeks.

The lesions can only be described as nonspecific, with the most common finding being the presence of fibrin strands in the abdominal cavity. Other findings include ventral skin reddening, serosal hemorrhages, pleural effusions, and reddened lymph nodes. Standard bacteriologic methods recover KPSP from several visceral sites.

The bacteria recovered have an innate resistance to ampicillin. Once weaned, the piglets do not appear to suffer from the condition.

CHLAMYDIAL INFECTION IN THE PIG

Chlamydia spp. infection in the pig has been known in pigs since 1955. These organisms may cause conjunctivitis, pneumonia, pleurisy, pericarditis, polyarthritis, orchitis, infertility, abortion, and the birth of weak piglets. They are also thought to be a cause of enteritis. Many infections are inapparent. Diagnostic laboratories may also not routinely test for *Chlamydia*, and therefore the diagnoses of such infections may be greatly underestimated.

The transmission of *C. abortus* from pigs to humans has not been proven but cannot be excluded. *Parachlamydiae* are probably not involved in abortion, and their potential as a zoonotic agent is also unknown.

ETIOLOGY

The Chlamydiaceae family includes the genus *Chlamydia*, with nine species. *Chlamydophila* and *Chlamydia* both occur in the pig, as do *Chlamydia*-like *Parachlamydiae* spp. and *Waddila* spp.[1]

The several species occurring in the pig have been identified by PCR, gene sequencing, DNA probes, and immunohistochemistry.

Chlamydia suis has been particularly associated with growing pigs with or without diarrhea and finishing pigs with conjunctivitis.[2,3] Infection is sporadic in pigs, but evidence for infection has been found in boar semen, fetuses, intestinal samples, reproductive tissues, and lungs from pigs in Germany, Switzerland, and Estonia.[4] Although it is considered that the intestine is the natural reservoir for this species, it may also cause lung function disorders, together with pleurisy, pericarditis, polyarthritis, and polyserositis, and reproductive problems. *C. suis* was formerly known as the porcine serovar of *C. trachomatis*, and the only known host is the pig. There is a high genetic diversity in the pig.

Chlamydia pecorum is associated with enteritis.

Chlamydia psittaci has been associated with respiratory and reproductive problems in pigs.

Chlamydia abortus has been associated with aborted material.[5] *Chlamydia trachomatis* has been isolated from the uteri of sows with conception failure.

EPIDEMIOLOGY

They have been found in pigs in all continents, but particularly North America, Europe, and Asia. Recently, studies have described them in Poland, Italy, Austria, Germany, Scotland, Switzerland, and Belgium. Pigs of all ages may be affected. The presence of antibodies is widespread in the pig population. They have also been found in wild boar; for example, a study of wild boar in Thuringia in Germany found three species: *abortus, psittaci,* and *suis*.

They can be spread by aerosol, direct contact, and ingestion of contaminated feed. Venereal transmission may be particularly important. *Chlamydiae* may survive for a long time in the environment, especially if there is a moist organic base. *Chlamydi* have been found to survive up to 30 days in feces and bedding.

Vertical transmission can occur if infections are contracted in utero. Flies and dust are also thought to transmit the organism. There is a suspicion that they may be transmitted by birds. In the United Kingdom, an outbreak of suspected brucellosis subsequently turned out to be chlamydiosis associated with the arrival of thousands of gulls at the morning feeding time of sow rolls to the sows held in outside paddocks. In experimental infections with *C. suis*, it has been found that the diarrhea was dose dependent. In a study of pigs with intestinal lesions, using PCR and immunohistochemistry, it was found that although *C. suis* was identified, there was no correlation with isolation of the organism and clinical signs.[6]

There is no doubt that the occurrence of the agent may be associated with the immunosuppressive disorders that affect the pig (PRRS, PCV2, and SIV). A large pig production unit in Estonia with a problem of postweaning multisystemic wasting syndrome (PMWS) and PCV2 infection and *Chlamydia* was studied.[7] It was found that chlamydial disease occurred 3 days after the introduction of Swedish boars and PMWS 11 days after the introduction.

PATHOGENESIS

The development of lesions may depend on different factors, such as the virulence of the strain, infectious dose, route of infection, age of the animal, and immunologic status of the host.

Experimental infection of the respiratory tract results in acute exudative or interstitial pneumonia within 4 to 8 days of infection.

The organism is an obligate intracellular parasite characterized by a unique developmental cycle. Elementary bodies (EBs) attach to the host cell by endocytosis and differentiate into noninfectious metabolically active reticulate bodies (RBs). These multiply by binary fission, resulting in mature chlamydial intracytoplasmic inclusion bodies approximately 48 to 72 hours after infection. The

RBs reorganize to form infective EBs, which are released by rupture of host cells and can initiate new cycles. There are also intermediate bodies between EBs and RBs.[8] There are also mostly enlarged RB-like structures called aberrant bodies, and these may allow the persistence of Chlamydiaceae. These aberrant bodies may occur when there are dual infections with other agents.[9] The organism lives in the mucosal epithelial cells, placental trophoblastic epithelium, and monocytes and macrophages.

C. suis enteritis may develop within 4 to 5 days following infection and may last for up to 8 days. Villus atrophy develops, and antibodies occur within 2 weeks.

Chlamydial replication was particularly marked at 2 to 4 days following infection and primarily located in the small intestinal epithelium.[10] Further sites of replication included large intestinal enterocytes, lamina propria, and tunica submucosa and mesenteric lymph nodes.

CLINICAL SIGNS

The clinical signs may vary considerably because of the early development of immunity. They are also variable depending on the presence of concurrent infections, such as PRRS, PCV2, and SIV, and in some cases there appears to be an association with *Lawsonia* and *Brachyspira* infections. In general, most infections are inapparent, but respiratory and systemic infections may result in inappetence and pyrexia (39–41° C, [103–106° F]). Dyspnea, conjunctivitis, and pneumonia may occur and last 4 to 8 days, accompanied by pleurisy and pericarditis with occasional lameness. Clinical signs following experimental infection included moderate to severe diarrhea, slight and transient anorexia, weakness, and body-weight loss.

Pigs experimentally infected with an aerosol challenge of *C. suis* resulted in severe acid–base disturbance characterized by respiratory acidosis and strong ion metabolic acidosis secondary to anaerobic metabolism and hyperlactatemia. Maximal changes were seen at 3 days following inoculation, when severe clinical signs of respiratory dysfunction were evident.[14]

NECROPSY FINDINGS

The pathologic role of the organism has yet to be clearly defined. However, confirmed cases may show consolidation in the lungs (particularly the caudal lobes), pericarditis, pleurisy, splenic enlargement, synovitis, orchitis, and dead fetuses and mummified piglets. The enteritis is typified by watery contents, undigested food in the stomach, villus atrophy, multifocal necrosis of the villi of the distal jejunum in particular and the ileum, and membranous colitis in the large intestine. Histologically, the villus atrophy can be severe, with villus tip erosions, necrosis of the villi, inflammatory changes, and lymphangitis. Chlamydial antigens can be demonstrated in the enterocytes.[10]

DIAGNOSIS

The clinical signs may be suggestive. Bear in mind that most laboratories do not routinely test for *Chlamydia.*

Preparations of intestine, lungs, and other suspect tissues can be stained by Koster's method or by MZN stains, but the acid-fast result is not specific for *Chlamydia* (*Brucella* and *Coxiella* are also acid fast).

Recently, species-specific nucleic acid amplification tests have been developed. These, including PCRs and DNA probes, can identify strains and species. A multiplex PCR has been developed for the usual four species.[11] These PCR techniques target the *omp* A gene, the 16S–23S RNA, or the *inc* A gene.[12] Immunofluorescence and immunoperoxide methods have been developed for frozen and fixed tissues.

Serology using CF tests (limited use in pigs) or ELISAs can confirm infection, particularly if rising titers can be seen on paired samples. The kits do not allow identification of species and strains, have a high cost, and lack sensitivity and specificity.

TREATMENT

Tetracyclines are the drug of choice, but resistant strains are not unknown. There is now thought to be a stable tetracycline-resistant phenotype.[13] Second-choice treatments are quinolones or macrolides.

A recent study showed that short-term antimicrobial treatment at dosages recommended for treatment for other bacterial infections in the pig was not effective in the treatment of *Chlamydiosis.* Such treatment did not eradicate subclinical infections.[14] However, it is most important that treatment should last at least 21 days at therapeutic levels to achieve effective eradication.

CONTROL

Proper cleaning and disinfection in indoor units with effective rodent and bird control is essential. Disinfection with a 1 : 1000 dilution of a quaternary ammonium compound will work, as will a solution of 7% isopropyl alcohol, 1% Lysol, 1 : 100 bleach, or chlorophenols. Outside pig production requires the same techniques but is infinitely more difficult to achieve. In some cases in the United Kingdom, one of the most effective techniques is to get all outside sows fed at the same time because this spreads the descending gull population over several outdoor sites.

Probiotic strains of *E. faucium* have been used to reduce carry-over infections from sows to piglets.

REFERENCES

1. Koschwanez M, et al. *J Vet Diag Invest.* 2012;24:833.
2. Pospischil A, et al. *Vet Microbiol.* 2009;135:1570.
3. Becker A, et al. *J Vet Med A.* 2007;54:307.
4. Kauffold J, et al. *Theriogenology.* 2006;65:1750.
5. Salinas J, et al. *Vet Microbiol.* 2012;135:157.
6. Englund S, et al. *BMC Vet Res.* 2012;8:9.
7. Schautteet K, et al. *Vet Rec.* 2010;166:329.
8. Pospischil A, et al. *Vet Microbiol.* 2009;135:147.
9. Deka S, et al. *Cell Microbiol.* 2006;8:149.
10. Guscetti F, et al. *Vet Microbiol.* 2009;135:157.
11. Pantchev A, et al. *Comp Immunol Microbiol Infect Dis.* 2010;33:473.
12. Schautteet K, Van Rompay D. *Vet Res.* 2011;42:29.
13. Dugan J, et al. *Microbiol.* 2007;153:71.
14. Rheingold P, et al. *Vet J.* 2011;187:405.

Multi-Organ Diseases Due to Viral Infection

FOOT-AND-MOUTH DISEASE (APHTHOUS FEVER)

SYNOPSIS

Etiology Foot-and-mouth disease virus, an aphthovirus.

Epidemiology Affects ruminants and pigs. Highly contagious, usually low mortality but great economic impact worldwide.

Clinical signs Fever, profuse salivation, vesicles in mouth and feet, sudden death in young animals.

Clinical pathology/diagnostic confirmation Virus isolation, serology and reverse-transcription polymerase chain reaction (RT-PCR) detection. Typing confirmed in a reference laboratory.

Lesions Vesicular, erosive/ulcerative stomatitis and esophagitis, vesicular/ulcerative dermatitis (feet and teats); in neonates, interstitial mononuclear and necrotic myocarditis.

Differential diagnostic list

Vesicular stomatitis

Vesicular exanthema

Swine vesicular disease

Rinderpest

Bovine viral diarrhea

Treatment None except symptomatically.

Control Mass vaccination with killed vaccines in endemic areas, eradication by slaughter when feasible, and strict quarantine during outbreaks.

ETIOLOGY

Foot-and-mouth disease (FMD) is a highly contagious disease of cloven-footed animals and is caused by the foot-and-mouth disease virus (FMDV), a small, nonenveloped virus that belongs to the genus of *Aphthovirus,* family Picornaviridae. The picornaviruses include the human rhinovirus causing the common cold and poliovirus causing polio. FMDV occurs as seven major distinct serotypes: A, O, C, Southern African Territories (SAT) 1, SAT 2, SAT 3, and Asia 1. Each serotype has multiple subtypes with varying antigenicity and degrees of virulence, especially within the A and O types. Because there is no cross-immunity between serotypes, immunity to one type does not confer protection against the others. This presents difficulties for vaccination programs. Furthermore, there can be great changes in antigenicity between developing serotypes; virulence may also change dramatically. There are also biotypical strains that become adapted to particular animal species and then infect other species only with difficulty. There are strains that are much more virulent for pigs (so-called porcinophilic strains), some for buffalo, and some even for tropical breeds of cattle, which generally react only mildly to endemic strains. Newer techniques for identifying subtypes involve enzyme-linked immunosorbent assay (ELISA), reverse-transcriptase polymerase chain reaction (RT-PCR) and nucleotide sequence analysis.

EPIDEMIOLOGY

Occurrence

FMD affects all cloven-footed animals, and outbreaks are reported from Africa and Asia and less frequently from South America and parts of Europe. The disease can occur in any country or continent, but New Zealand and Australia have always been disease-free, and North America has been so for about 60 years. In nonendemic countries, FMD often occurs as devastating epidemics resulting in great economic losses from the control measures that must be instituted to regain disease-free status. Worldwide, countries have been classified into categories with respect to FMD occurrence as follows[1]:

- Endemic, as in most of sub-Saharan Africa and Asia
- Intermediate, sporadic, as in Eastern Europe and parts of Asia
- Free with vaccination or multizone, as in most of South America
- Free with virus in game parks, as in South Africa
- Free, as in North America, Western Europe, and Australia

By 2009, 70 countries in the world were officially recognized by the OIE as free from FMD with or without vaccination, whereas more than 100 countries were considered as either endemically or sporadically infected with the disease.[2] Three examples of recent major outbreaks since the turn of this century are as follows:

1. An outbreak in Great Britain in 2001 spread to Ireland, France, and the Netherlands before it was eventually contained. The outbreak was traced to illegal import to the United Kingdom of infected meat products. Spread within the country and to other countries was mostly through the movement of livestock not showing obvious clinical signs. Over 10 million animals were culled or died.
2. An outbreak occurred in the Republic of Korea in 2010/2011, during which more than 3 million animals were destroyed.[3]
3. An outbreak in Japan in 2010 involved cattle and pigs. Nearly 300,000 animals were culled, but the epidemic was contained within a localized area and was eradicated within 3 months.[4]

As for North America, the last outbreak in the United States was in 1929, Canada in 1951 to 1952, and Mexico in 1946 to 1954. During the outbreaks, movement of cattle and cattle products between the United States and either Canada or Mexico was brought to a standstill. The importance of the Darien Gap in maintaining the disease-free status of North America is well known. This tract of impassable territory between Colombia and Panama prevents any chance of direct contact between cattle populations in North and South America.

Prevalence

There are no reliable figures for the prevalence of FMD in different countries. Cases in endemic countries may go unreported unless they occur as outbreaks in previously uninfected regions or herds. Worldwide, the cumulative incidence of FMD serotypes show that six of the seven serotypes (O, A, C, SAT-1, SAT-2, SAT-3) have occurred in Africa, Asia contends with four (O, A, C, Asia-1), South America with only three (O, A, C), and the Middle East periodically has incursions of types SAT-1 and SAT-2 from Africa.[5] Thus, the serotypes and strains are distributed into several major virus ecological reservoirs, each containing distinct regional viral strains from which new variants may emerge.[2] These regional differences are more attributable to the pattern of the meat trade and livestock movements than to any inherent properties of the serotypes. Overall, outbreaks of types O and A occur more frequently than the others, and recently, outbreaks of type C have become uncommon. Whereas the disease in endemic countries may not be clinically apparent and therefore not be promptly reported, it usually occurs as outbreaks in nonendemic countries and rapidly spreads from herd to herd, making international news, before it is controlled.

Morbidity and Case-Fatality Rate

The morbidity rate in outbreaks of FMD in susceptible animals can rapidly approach 100%, but some strains are limited in their infectivity to particular species, mostly cattle and pigs. However, the case fatality is generally very low, about 2% in adults and 20% in young stock. Nonetheless, severe outbreaks of a more violent form sometimes occur, as in the 1997 Taiwan outbreak in pigs, where case fatality was 18% and reached 100% in piglets, and the outbreak in calves of exotic dairy animals in Nigeria in the 1970s. During outbreaks in nonendemic countries, most deaths are attributable to a slaughter policy that usually involves all susceptible animals and herds in contact with, or within a certain radius of, the infected herd.

Methods of Transmission

FMD is transmitted by a variety of methods between herds, countries, and continents, but spread from one animal to another is by inhalation or by ingestion. In endemic areas, the most important method of spread is probably by direct contact between animals moving across state and national boundaries as trade or nomadic cattle. In nonendemic areas such as Europe, the first introduction to a new area is often via pigs that contract infection by ingestion of infected meat scraps. Spread from these pigs to cattle is via movement of people, abattoir waste, or animals. Further spread between cattle is more likely to be by airborne means. The virus can persist in aerosol form for long periods in temperate or subtropical climates but not in hot and dry climates. The speed and direction of the wind are important factors in determining the rate of airborne spread. Humidity is also important, but rain as such appears not to be. In the most favorable circumstances, it is now estimated that sufficient virus to initiate an infection can be windborne as far as 250 km (156 miles). There are peaks of spread at dawn and dusk. Animals in the United Kingdom are thought to be vulnerable to airborne transmission of the virus from the European mainland. It has been shown that pigs are the most potent excretors of airborne virus and cattle the most susceptible to airborne infections. During the 2001 outbreak in England, there was no indication of airborne spread to the mainland, perhaps because ruminants rather than pigs were mostly affected.

The risk of airborne infection varies with the FMD serotype and animal species. In a study involving serotypes A, O, and Asia 1, it was found that each serotype demonstrated distinct transmission characteristics and required different exposure times to achieve successful contact transmission.[6] In that study, serotype A required less time of exposure (4 hours) for contact transmission, had the highest levels of viral shedding in saliva and nasal swabs, and also had the highest virus levels in room air compared with serotypes O and Asia 1. Furthermore, under experimental conditions in which virus from affected pigs was given via the intranasal route to cattle, sheep, and pigs, cattle were found to require the least amount of virus to cause infection and give rise to lesions, followed by sheep, whereas pigs were not readily infected by the intranasal route.[7]

In cattle, the first site of virus infection and subsequent rapid multiplication is the pharynx, and the virus is first detectable in the oropharyngeal fluid. The onset of clinical signs is associated with high levels of virus in the blood, oropharyngeal fluid, and nasal fluid.[8] Following a few days of viremia, the virus appears in milk and saliva for up to 24 hours before vesicles appear in the mouth. All other excretions, including urine, feces, and semen, may be similarly infective before the animal is clinically ill and for a short period after signs have disappeared. However, the period of maximum infectivity is when vesicles are discharging because vesicular fluid contains the virus in maximum concentration. Although it is generally conceded that affected animals are seldom infective for more than 4 days after the rupture of vesicles, except insofar as the virus may persist on the skin or hair, some animals may remain as **carriers** and are important in the epidemiology of the disease in the field. In cattle, carriers may develop during convalescence from the natural disease or, more important, in vaccinated animals that are exposed to infection. Up to 50% of cattle, sheep, and goats may become carriers, but pigs do not.

The nasopharynx is the main site for persistence of the FMDV, and erratic low-level excretion may occur for up to 2 years. Using molecular techniques, intact, nonreplicating virus was found in the germinal centers of lymph nodes in the oropharyngeal region for up to 38 days.[9] The virus may also persist in mammary tissue for 3 to 7 weeks. Wild fauna may serve as the FMDV reservoir, and in southern, central, and eastern Africa, the African buffalo (*Syncerus caffer*) is a significant reservoir. Similarly, viral persistence may be a common outcome in the farmed Indian buffaloes (*Bubalis bubalis*) following FMDV Asia 1 infection.[10]

Humans are often a vehicle for transmission of the virus. It has been recovered from the nasal mucosa of persons working with infected cattle for up to 28 hours after contact. Nose-blowing did not eliminate it, nor did cotton face masks prevent infection. In a more recent study, the virus could not be detected in nasal secretions 12 hours after contact, and contaminated personnel could not transmit the disease to susceptible pigs and sheep after they had showered and changed into clean outer wear.

The disease is **spread from herd to herd** either directly by the movement of infected animals or indirectly by the transportation of FMDV on inanimate objects, including farm equipment, uncooked and unprocessed meat products, and other animal products, including milk. The pH and temperature of milk significantly affect survival, which may be as long as 18 hours. Flash pasteurization procedures, as distinct from the holding method, do not inactivate the virus in milk—neither does evaporation to milk powder or processing into butter, cheese, or casein products. The risk of spreading FMDV through importation of vaccinated cattle, sheep, and pigs is extremely small, and the risk from products derived from vaccinated animals is even smaller, provided appropriate risk mitigation measures are applied.[11]

Introduction of FMD into a herd or country as a result of the use of infected cattle semen for artificial insemination is possible. The virus can also be detected in the semen of infected boars, but this has not been a means of transmitting it. Similarly, it is not transmitted through the transfer of embryos from viremic donor cows.

Epidemics in free areas occur intermittently and from a number of sources. In England it was estimated that outbreaks arose in the following manner:

- Meat products used as pig food—40%
- Completely obscure causes—28%
- Transportation by birds—16%
- Contact with meat and bones other than swill—9%
- Unknown causes (probably swill)—7%

The greatest danger appears to be from uncooked meat scraps fed to pigs. A common pattern is the importation of the virus in sheep meat from sheep that showed no illness, an initial infection in pigs, and then spread to cattle. However, more unusual methods of introduction must not be disregarded. With modern methods of transport, farm workers can carry the virus long distances in their clothing. In Tanzania, where the disease is endemic, roads played a dominant role in epidemic situations between 2001 and 2006, and FMD occurrence was more related to animal movement and human activity via communication networks than transboundary movements or contact with wildlife.[12] Human activity was also the main factor in the spread of the FMD epidemic in South Korea in 2010/2011.[3] However, movement restrictions during the 2010 FMD outbreak in Japan proved insufficient to prevent spread of the disease for about 3 months.[13]

Risk Factors

Host Factors

The disease is most important in cattle and pigs, but goats, sheep, and buffaloes in India and llama in South America are also affected. Some strains of the virus are limited in their infectivity to particular species. Although cattle, sheep, and goats can be carriers, they are not regular sources of infection, and early studies in Kenya showed that goats were infrequent carriers, and sheep not at all. Immature animals and those in good condition are relatively more susceptible, and hereditary differences in susceptibility have also been observed. Horses are not susceptible to the disease. Old World camels (dromedaries) are also not susceptible, but New World (Bactrian) camels can contract the disease.[14-15]

A variety of **wildlife species,** such as the deer in England, the water buffalo (*Bubalus bubalis*) in Brazil, and wild ungulates in Africa, become infected periodically but are thought to play little or no role as reservoirs of infection for domestic animals. A notable exception is the **African buffalo** (***Syncerus caffer***), probably the natural host of the SAT types of the virus and the major source of infection for cattle in southern Africa. The disease in buffalo populations is mild, but the infection rate is often high and can be persistent. On the other hand, the domesticated **Asian buffalo** shows typical clinical disease and spread from buffalo to other species. Small rodents and hedgehogs in Europe and capybaras in South America may also act as reservoirs. **Yaks** that live in high altitudes in China (*Bos grunniens* yaks) are susceptible and can keep carrier status for at least 8 months.[16] In Bulgaria, infection in **wild boar** was found to be a short-lived event that failed to develop into a large-scale epidemic.[17] Feral swine in the United States are susceptible, they can transmit the disease to domestic swine, and FMD viral RNA can persist in their tonsils up to 36 days following infection, by which time virus isolation is negative.[18] The North American bison and elk are also susceptible, but the virus may not be isolated from animals past 28 days postinoculation.[19]

Environmental and Pathogen Factors

The virus is resistant to external influences, including common disinfectants and the usual storage practices of the meat trade. It may persist for over 1 year in infected premises, for 10 to 12 weeks on clothing and feed, and up to a month on hair. It is particularly susceptible to changes in pH away from neutral. Sunlight destroys the virus quickly, but it may persist on pasture for long periods at low temperatures. Boiling effectively destroys the virus if it is free of tissue, but autoclaving under pressure is the safest procedure when heat disinfection is used. The virus can survive for more than 60 days in bull semen frozen to −79°C (−110°F). In general, the virus is relatively susceptible to heat and insensitive to cold. Most common disinfectants exert practically no effect, but sodium hydroxide or formalin (1% to 2%) or sodium carbonate (4%) will destroy the virus within a few minutes.

All uncooked meat tissues, including bone, are likely to remain infective for long periods, especially if quick-frozen, and to a lesser extent meat chilled or frozen by a slow process. The survival of the virus is closely associated with the pH of the medium. The development of acidity in rigor mortis inactivates the virus, but quick-freezing suspends acid formation, and the virus is likely to survive. However, on thawing, the suspended acid formation recommences, and the virus may be destroyed. Prolonged survival is more likely in viscera, bone marrow, and blood vessels and lymph nodes, where acid production is not so great. Meat pickled in brine or salted by dry methods may also remain infective. For example, dry-cured Serrano and Iberian hams from experimentally infected pigs were shown to contain viable virus for up to 6 months. Fomites, including bedding, mangers, clothing, motor tires, harness, feedstuffs, and hides, may also remain a source of infection for long periods. There are claims that the virus can pass unchanged through the alimentary tracts of birds, which may thus act as carriers and transport infection for long distances and over natural topographic barriers such as mountain ranges and sea.

Some outbreaks in Europe have been associated with vaccine virus either accidentally escaping from the laboratory or that was incompletely inactivated. The 2007 outbreaks in southern England were caused by a derivative of a virus strain handled in two nearby FMD laboratories.[20]

Immune Mechanism

In endemic areas, periodic outbreaks occur that sweep through the animal populations and then subside. A 6-year epidemic cycle was demonstrated in India in the 1990s. This was probably as a result of the disappearance of immunity that develops during an epidemic and the sudden flaring up from small foci of infection when the population becomes susceptible again. Immunity after natural infection lasts for 1 to 4 years in cattle and for a shorter time in pigs. When outbreaks follow each other in quick succession, the presence of more than one strain of virus should be suspected. In countries where general vaccination is practiced every year, outbreaks are usually associated with different strains imported in carrier animals or infected meat.

Studies of the interaction of FMDV with cells mediating the early, innate immune response of the host have shown that the virus has a distinct inhibitory effect on the response of the cells.[21] Following aerogenous administration of the virus, cattle were shown to develop a rapid and vigorous local antibody response throughout the respiratory tract in 4 to 5 days postinfection, and this led to IgM-mediated virus clearance.[22]

Experimental Reproduction

The clinical signs and lesions of FMD can be reproduced by rubbing virus-containing material on the oral mucosa of susceptible cattle or by intradermal inoculation into the dorsum of the tongue. The disease can easily spread from infected to susceptible animals housed in close proximity (cohabitation). With mice and guinea pigs, inoculation of footpads of hindfeet is preferred (see "Clinical Pathology" section).

Economic Importance

With the possible exception of bovine spongiform encephalopathy (mad cow disease), FMD is the most feared animal disease in the developed world, even though the mortality rate is low. This is because it is the most contagious disease of livestock, and it has a great potential for causing severe economic loss in high-producing animals. Losses occur in many ways, although loss of production, the expense of eradication, and the interference with movement of livestock and meat between countries are the most important economic effects. There are also significant losses in agriculture and tourism as a result of restriction on human movement. The 2001 outbreak in the United Kingdom was eradicated within 7 months but resulted in the death of nearly 10 million livestock, with losses of up to 8 billion pounds sterling (about US$12 billion). In the United States the median economic impact of an FMD outbreak in a dairy herd in California was estimated to result in national agriculture welfare losses of up to $69 billion if the outbreak was not detected within 21 days.[23] However, in unimproved or low-grade *Bos indicus* cattle reared under an extensive or a nomadic system of management, or in pigs in some southeast Asian countries, FMD is often less severe and has fewer effects for the subsistent producer. Nevertheless, because of its severity in exotic or improved breeds and because of its effects on international trade, FMD control and eradication in such countries will still result in a strong benefit–cost ratio in places like Thailand.

Zoonotic Implications

Humans are thought to be slightly susceptible to infection with the virus, and vesicles may develop in the mouth or hands. Very few cases have been reported, even among people working with infected carcasses and at laboratories. However, humans and particularly their clothing can be vehicles for transmission to animals.

Biosecurity Concerns

Because FMD is highly contagious, there are biosecurity concerns regarding intentional or accidental introduction of the virus into nonendemic countries. Intentional introduction would be a form of agroterrorism, and this would be devastating in any country that is FMD-free because it would probably take some days before the disease would be recognized and much longer before it could be stamped out. Laboratories working with FMD virus or producing FMD vaccines and reagents must comply with OIE requirements for Containment Group 4 pathogens to ensure that there is no escape of the virus. There are also strict regulations for shipping diagnostic samples to national or international laboratories.

PATHOGENESIS

The pathogenesis of FMD has been extensively studied and was recently reviewed.[24-25] The surface-exposed capsid proteins (VP1, VP2, and VP3) of the virus determine its antigenicity and the ability of the virus to interact with host receptors and cause disease.[26] Although strain and species differences have been reported, the basic pathogenesis involves the following three phases: (i) previremic phase characterized by infection and replication at the primary replication sites or sites, (ii) viremic phase with generalization and vesiculation at secondary infection sites, and (iii) postviremia/convalescent phase including resolution of clinical disease that may result in long-term persistent infection.[24]

The previremic phase lasts for about 3 days depending on the infecting dose and the strain of virus and the host. Infection of cattle, sheep, and other ruminants generally occurs via the respiratory route by aerosolized virus attaching to cells lining the route. Infection can occur less efficiently through abrasions on the skin or mucous membranes. Pigs are much less susceptible to aerosol infection and usually become infected by eating FMDV-contaminated food or by direct contact with infected animals, or by being placed into recently infected premises. Following exposure, FMDV particles first attach to mucosal epithelial cells and penetrate into the cytoplasm of the cell. To survive in the host, the virus has evolved a mechanism to block host innate immunity by temporarily blocking interferon (IFN) response and influencing the ability of natural killer cells to recognize and eliminate FMDV-infected cells. This allows the virus to replicate rapidly for a few days, cause viremia, and become highly contagious.[27-28] There is no consensus in reports regarding the anatomic sites involved in early virus replication.[29] The primary replication site in cattle is probably the epithelial cells of the nasopharyngeal region and subsequent widespread replication in the lungs coinciding with onset of viremia.[30] In experimentally infected pigs, FMDV accumulated in mandibular lymphoid tissue up to 6 hours after infection and in the tissues draining the mandibular lymph node and tonsil, then disseminated throughout the body, where epithelial cells were the favored sites of (secondary) replication.[31]

Irrespective of the portal of entry, once infection gains access to the bloodstream (viremic phase), the virus is widely disseminated to many epidermal sites, probably in macrophages, but gross lesions develop only in areas subjected to mechanical trauma or unusual physiologic wear, such as the epithelium of the mouth and feet, the dorsum of the snout of pigs, and the teats. Characteristic lesions develop at these sites after an incubation period of 1 to 21 days (usually 3 to 8 days in most species). The initial phase of viremia is often unnoticed, and it is only when localization in the mouth and on the feet occurs that the animal is found to be clinically abnormal. Furthermore, the virus can be excreted in exhaled air, saliva, milk, semen, urine, and feces during this phase for about 2 weeks.

The postviremic phase is characterized by healing of lesions. The process can be rapid in the oral mucosa but often slow in the feet. Associated mastitis in dairy animals can also become chronic. Most adult animals will recover from FMD, become immune to the serotype for years, and no longer be contagious. A few recovered ruminants can become carriers for several months, whereas the African buffalo are lifelong carriers. The virus is thought to persist in the oropharyngeal region, the germinal centers of lymph nodes,[32] and possibly in dendritic cells in lymphoid organs.

The experimental disease in sheep is characterized by an incubation period of 4 to 9 days after contact or 1 to 3 days after virus inoculation. Thereafter, viremia occurs at 17 to 74 hours and hyperthermia from 17 to 96 hours. Clinical signs are serous nasal discharge, salivation, and buccal lesions in 75% of cases and foot lesions in 25%. At the end of viremia, the animal recovers, but the virus may persist in the pharyngeal area of convalescent ruminants as previously discussed.

Bacterial complications generally aggravate the lesions, particularly those of the feet and the teats, leading to severe lameness and mastitis, respectively. In young animals, especially neonates, the virus frequently causes necrotizing myocarditis, and this lesion may also be seen in adults infected with some strains of the virus, particularly type O.

CLINICAL FINDINGS

In typical field cases in cattle, there is an incubation period of 3 to 6 days, but it may vary between 1 and 7 days. The onset is heralded by a precipitate fall in milk yield and a high fever (40° to 41°C [104° to 106°F]), accompanied by severe dejection and anorexia, followed by the appearance of an acute painful stomatitis. At this stage, the temperature reaction is subsiding. There is abundant salivation, with the saliva hanging in long, rope-like strings; a characteristic smacking of the lips is present; and the animal chews carefully. Vesicles and bullae (1 to 2 cm in diameter) appear on the buccal mucosa, dental pad, and tongue. These rupture within 24 hours, leaving a raw, painful surface that heals in about 1 week. The vesicles are thin walled, rupture easily, and contain a thin, straw-colored fluid. Concurrently with oral lesions, vesicles appear on the feet, particularly in the clefts and on the coronet. Rupture of vesicles causes acute discomfort, and the animal is grossly lame and often recumbent, with a marked, painful swelling of the coronet.

Secondary bacterial invasion of foot lesions may interfere with healing and lead to severe involvement of the deep structures of the foot. Vesicles may occur on the teats; when the teat orifice is involved, severe mastitis often follows. Vesicles on the teats may be the primary clinical sign observed by the dairy farmer, as in the 2010/2011 epidemic in the Republic of Korea.[33] Pregnant animals may abort or have stillbirths. Very rapid loss of condition and fall in milk yield occur during the acute period, and these signs are much more severe than would be anticipated from the extent of the lesions. Eating is resumed in 2 to 3 days as lesions heal, but the period of convalescence may be as long as 6 months. Young animals are more susceptible and may suffer heavy mortality from myocardial damage, even when typical vesicular lesions are absent in mouth and feet.

In most outbreaks, the rate of spread is high and clinical signs are as described earlier, but there is a great deal of variation in virulence, especially in beef cattle, and this may lead to difficulty in field diagnosis. For example, there is a malignant form of the disease in adults in which acute myocardial failure occurs. There is a typical course initially but a sudden relapse occurs on days 5 to 6 with dyspnea, a weak and irregular heart action, and death during convulsions. Occasional cases show localization in the alimentary tract with dysentery or diarrhea, indicating the presence of enteritis. Ascending posterior paralysis may also occur. On the other hand, there is a mild form that usually occurs when endemic strains infect only indigenous *Bos indicus* (Zebu) cattle. This is the form most commonly seen in endemic countries in Africa, Asia, and South America.

A sequela to FMD in cattle, probably as a result of endocrine damage, is a chronic syndrome of dyspnea, anemia, overgrowth of hair, and lack of heat tolerance. Affected cattle are described colloquially as "hairy panter." The syndrome has been reported in European cattle breeds but has not been described in zebu cattle from India.[34]

In sheep and goats, the disease is often mild and may go unnoticed. FMD in small ruminants is important mainly because of the danger of transmission to cattle. Adult sheep may develop a syndrome identical to that of cattle, and thus it becomes a crippling disease with occasional loss of hooves from bacterial complications. Goats are sometimes spared during an outbreak. The more common syndrome in these species is the appearance of a few small lesions, but with more severe involvement of all four feet. As in cattle, young stock are more susceptible.

FMD in pigs can be very severe, and devastating epidemics involving pigs only or pigs and other species are reported from time to time in Asia. A porcinophilc strain (0/Taiwan/97) has been identified and studied. Following intradermal inoculation, symptoms of depression and inappetence appeared at 1 day postinoculation (dpi), whereas vesicles were observed at the inoculation site at 1 dpi and on the mouth and snout the following day.[35] Teats can also be affected in nursing sows. Large vesicles and bullae may rupture to expose large, raw surfaces. Remnants of feet lesions may persist for more than 2 months, and such residual lesions may aid in clinical diagnosis. Experimentally infected feral swine were fully susceptible but exhibited a higher tolerance to FMD than domestic swine; the latter showed clinical signs of the disease within 24 hours after contact with the feral swine, whereas feral swine did not do so until 48 hours after contact with domestic and feral swine.[18]

CLINICAL PATHOLOGY

During FMD outbreaks, laboratory investigations are carried out to diagnose the disease rather than for clinical assessment as with most other diseases. Exhaustive laboratory studies are needed for diagnosis, determination of the type of the virus involved, and to differentiate the disease from vesicular stomatitis, vesicular exanthema, and swine vesicular disease. A handbook of the standard tests used worldwide is provided from time to time.[36] Fresh vesicular fluid and surrounding epithelial tissue should be collected in a transport medium composed of equal amounts of glycerol and 0.04 M phosphate buffer, pH 7.2 to 7.6, or glycerol and phosphate buffered saline for laboratory tests. This is the sample of choice. If the vesicles are already healing, blood should be collected, along with esophageal-pharyngeal (OP) fluid samples from ruminants or throat swabs from pigs. The OP samples should be collected from up to five animals with the use of a probang cup. In tropical countries with maximum temperature fluctuations, spoilage of FMD-suspect samples originating from remote areas can be minimized by using FTA Classic Cards for collection, shipment, storage, and identification of the FMDV genome by RT-PCR and real-time RT-PCR.[37] The major methods for diagnosis are as follows:

1. Identification of the agent in tissue or fluid
    - *Virus isolation* by inoculation into cell cultures or unweaned mice. The cell cultures should be examined for cytopathic effect for 48 hours. If no CPE is detected, the cells should be frozen and thawed, used to inoculate fresh cultures, and examined for CPE for another 48 hours. Alternatively, unweaned mice 2 to 7 days old can be used (see following discussion of experimental transmission). With diagnostic samples, neutralization of the virus by known antisera makes the technique highly efficient and specific.
    - Immunologic methods:
        - *Enzyme-linked immunosorbent assay (ELISA)*: This is the preferred test for the detection of FMD viral antigen and identification of viral serotype. It is an indirect sandwich test in which different rows in multiwall plates are coated with rabbit antisera to each of the seven serotypes of FMD virus. It can simultaneously test for swine vesicular disease (SVD) or

vesicular stomatitis (VS) where appropriate.
- *Complement fixation test (CFT)*: This can be used if reagents for ELISA are not available. It is less sensitive and is affected by pro- and anticomplementary factors. Direct CFT on epithelial suspension used to be one of the fastest methods of making a positive diagnosis, within a few hours, but negative samples must be checked in tissue cultures because of the number of false negatives that occur with the CFT, especially in poorly collected and packaged samples.

- *Nucleic acid recognition methods:* These include reverse transcription polymerase chain reaction (RT-PCR) and in situ hybridization (ISH). The RT-PCR amplifies fragments of FMD genome in samples and can be used for typing. It is more sensitive than ELISA. The procedures used include agarose gel-based RT-PCR assay, real-time RT-PCR assay, and molecular epidemiology based on the comparison of genetic differences between viruses.[36] A reverse-transcription loop-mediated isothermal amplification (RT-LAMP) assay has been described that is simple and rapid and can be read within 1 hour, whereas conventional RT-PCR methods require 2 to 4 hours.[38] More recently, a lateral flow immunochromatographic (LFI) strip test has been reported that can diagnose FMD serotypes O, A, and Asia 1 using a generic rapid assay device.[39] The procedure takes only 10 minutes and can be done on-site; it also has high specificity and can be used for early detection of FMD in the field. In addition, a field-portable nucleic acid extraction and real-time PCR amplification platform has been developed for rapid detection of FMD.[40] The ISH detects FMD virus RNA in infected tissues, including those obtained during necropsy.

2. Serologic tests
   - Serologic tests for FMD are of two types: those detecting antibodies to viral structural proteins (SPs) and those detecting antibodies to viral nonstructural proteins (NSPs).[36] The SP tests detect antibodies elicited by vaccination and infection and are serotype-specific and highly sensitive, provided that the virus or antigen used in the test is closely matched to the strain circulating in the field. They are the prescribed tests for international trade. Examples are as follows:
     - Virus neutralization (VN)
     - Solid-phase competitive ELISA, another prescribed test
     - Liquid-phase blocking ELISA

     The NSP tests can be used to identify past or current infection with any of the seven serotypes of the virus, whether or not the animal has been vaccinated. The tests are more useful on a herd basis. For certifying animals for trade, the tests have the advantage over the SP methods in that the serotype of the virus does not have to be known. The assays measure antibodies to NSPs using antigens produced by recombinant techniques. Antibodies to polyproteins 3AB or 3ABC are generally considered to be the most reliable indicators of infection. Examples include:
     - Indirect ELISA
     - Enzyme-linked immunoelectrotransfer blot assay.

     Where vaccination has been carried out and a diagnosis has to be made by serologic methods, it is necessary to differentiate between infected and vaccinated animals (DIVA). An epitope-based ELISA has been described that can differentiate infected from vaccinated animals and appears to be promising test for FMD control and eradication.[41]
3. **Experimental transmission**
   - The propagation of the virus in unweaned white mice can be used to detect the presence of virus in suspected material, the presence of antibodies in serum, and for investigations into the transmission of immunity and the pathogenesis of the disease. In guinea pigs, intradermal injection of fresh vesicular fluid into the plantar pads causes vesicles to appear on the pads in 1 to 7 days and secondary vesicles in the mouth 1 to 2 days later. Large-animal inoculation may be used for the differentiation of FMD, vesicular stomatitis, and vesicular exanthema based on the different species' susceptibilities to the three viruses (Table 21-3) and to test the potency of vaccines. To avoid disseminating the virus, animal inoculation should be done only in specially equipped facilities.

NECROPSY FINDINGS

The lesions of FMD consist of vesicles and erosions in the mouth and on the feet and udder. The erosions often become ulcers, especially if secondary bacterial infection has occurred. In some cases, vesicles may extend to the pharynx, esophagus, forestomaches, intestines, trachea, and bronchi. The teats and mammary gland are often swollen. In the malignant form and in neonatal animals, epicardial hemorrhages with or without pale areas are also present. Grossly, the ventricular walls appear streaked with patches of yellow tissue interspersed with apparently normal myocardium, giving the typical "tiger heart" appearance. If the animal survives, there is replacement fibrosis, and the heart is enlarged and flabby.

Histologically, vesicles start as foci of progressive swelling, necrosis, and lysis of infected keratinocytes in the deeper layers of the epidermis and accumulation of fluid in the space. This is followed by necrosis of overlying keratinocytes and rupture of vesicles to form erosions that may extend deep into the dermis to form ulcers, especially on the feet. There is only mild leukocytic infiltration around the erosions and ulcers. Similar changes in mammary gland epithelium lead to acinar necrosis and mild interstitial cellular infiltration. Heart (and occasionally skeletal muscle) lesions in the malignant form are characterized by severe hyaline degeneration, necrosis, and occasional calcification of myocardial fibers and marked interstitial infiltration by mononuclear cells. In addition, pancreatic islet and acinar degeneration has been reported in chronically infected cattle.

Tissues to be submitted for histopathology should include oral mucosa and skin containing vesicles or fresh erosions. The heart, mammary gland, and pancreas should also be included. Viral antigen can be detected in tissues by immunohistochemistry. Because most animals infected with FMD will not die and because it is important to make prompt diagnosis from clinical cases, histopathology of necropsy materials is often secondary.

DIFFERENTIAL DIAGNOSIS

The need to identify foot-and-mouth (FMD) is of paramount importance in all countries. It is of particular importance in those countries in which the disease is not endemic because of the need to introduce strict control measures quickly. The field or zoo veterinarian must be able to recognize suspicious cases, take appropriate samples, and submit them to a laboratory facility able to confirm the diagnosis promptly. Clinical signs in sheep, goats, and zoo animals such as elephants, giraffes, and camels may be difficult to recognize. In countries where the disease is endemic, there are special difficulties in clinical recognition because of the frequent subdued severity of the oral and feet lesions, even in cattle. Where the other vesicular diseases do not occur, suspicions will be readily aroused, but in North America, the presence of vesicular stomatitis and vesicular exanthema may result in misdiagnosis. Vesicular stomatitis in horses, cattle, and swine, vesicular

Continued

Table 21-3 Differentiation of acute vesicular disease

Animal species	Route of inoculation	FMD	Vesicular stomatitis	Vesicular exanthema of swine	Swine vesicular disease	Bluetongue
Natural infection						
Cattle		+	+	–	–	+ (occurs rarely)
Pig*		+	+	+	+	–
Sheep and goat		+	±	–	–	+
Horse		–	+	–	–	–
Experimental transmission						
Cattle	Intradermal in tongue, gums, lips	+	+	–	–	+
	Intramuscular	+	–	–	–	
Pig*	Intradermal in snout,	+	+	+	+	
	lips	+	+	+	+	
	Intravenous	+	–	–	+	
	Intramuscular					
Sheep and goat	Various	+	+	–	+ (no lesions)	+
Horse	Intradermal in tongue	–	+	+ (some strains)	–	
	Intramuscular			+ (some strains)	–	
Guinea pig	Intradermal in footpad	+	+	–	–	–
Unweaned white mice	Intradermal	+	+	–	+	+ (hamsters also)
Adult chicken		+	+	–	–	

**White-skinned pigs fed on parsnips or celery and exposed to sunlight develop vesicles.*

exanthema of swine, and swine vesicular disease resemble FMD closely (Table 21-3). Three other vesiculoviruses—Piry, Chandipura, and Isfahan—cross-react with vesicular stomatitis virus[18] but are much less virulent. The observations that white-skinned pigs fed parsnips or celery and exposed to sunlight will develop vesicles on the snout and feet and that cattle fed on grain treated with caustic soda can develop profuse salivation are further confounding factors in the differentiation of the vesicular diseases.

Bluetongue of sheep may also present a problem in differentiation. Details of these are provided separately, but a summary is given in Table 21-3. Rapid laboratory differentiation and diagnosis of these diseases may be achieved, as described under Clinical Pathology (see previous discussion).

Bovine viral diarrhea/mucosal disease, rinderpest, malignant catarrhal fever, and lumpy skin disease are easily differentiated by the lesions that develop in the mucosa and sometimes on the feet. The lesions are never vesicular, commencing as superficial erosions and proceeding to the development of ulcers. Pox infections of the mammary gland and foot rot in sheep should also be differentiated from FMD. Ingestion of any caustic material may cause oral vesiculation and salivation. Among zoo animals, giraffes, elephants, and camels are susceptible.

TREATMENT

TREATMENT AND CONTROL

Treatment
Nonspecific

Control
Vaccination with killed vaccine (R-1 in endemic areas)

Treatment with mild disinfectant and protective dressings to inflamed areas to prevent secondary infection is recommended in endemic countries where a slaughter policy is not in force. A good symptomatic response is reported to the administration of flunixin meglumine. In Kenya, ethnoveterinary remedies of natural soda ash solution (97% sodium bicarbonate), honey, and finger millet flour were used to manage FMD lesions during an outbreak in a medium-scale dairy farm.[42] The lesions were washed with soda ash solution to remove the necrotic tissue, after which raw honey and finger millet flour were applied daily for 3 days. Experimentally, it has been shown that administration of porcine type I interferon to pigs or bovine type III interferon to cattle can protect swine or significantly delay and reduce the severity of FMD in cattle challenged with FMDV for up to 7 days.[43-44] These interferons can thus inhibit FMDV replication before an inactivated vaccine can induce protection in the face of an outbreak in endemic areas.

CONTROL

Many factors govern the control procedure in a given area. The procedures commonly used are (a) control by eradication and (b) control by vaccination, or a combination of the two. In countries where the disease is endemic, or where there are wildlife reservoirs, eradication is seldom practicable. In areas with only occasional epidemics, slaughter of all infected and in-contact animals is usually carried out. It must be remembered that vaccination is costly and sometimes ineffective and that eradication would be the ideal objective in all countries. For countries in large continents, international cooperation is required for eradication. The European Union phased out mass vaccination in 1991 to increase its international competitiveness in trade in livestock and livestock products. Soon after, outbreaks of FMD in Italy were controlled by surveillance and slaughter of thousands of cattle, sheep/goats, and pigs in all-infected and contact herds. A similar procedure was adopted in 2001 in England, Ireland, and France and with some modification in the Netherlands, and the outbreaks were successfully controlled within months. Similar results were obtained in Taiwan during periodic outbreaks between 1997 and 2011. On the other hand, a 2010 epidemic in Japan was eradicated within 3 months in an area with high density of cattle and pigs by strict movement control and emergency vaccination.[4]

As in the control of all epidemic infectious diseases, the problems posed for administrators are complex and continually changing. For example, the prospect of making a wrong decision about when to switch from an eradication-by-slaughter program to a containment-by-vaccination program, when an outbreak is raging and public sentiments are running high, is a daunting one. A wrong decision may cost a livestock industry many millions of dollars. To avoid making such errors, it is customary to develop a mathematical or computer model that simulates the progress of an outbreak in terms of numbers of animals infected, affected, and dead, and how these numbers will change under pressure from control procedures, management practices, and prevailing weather. An essential aspect of such an analysis is the economic effect of various control programs and their outcomes. The cost–benefit aspects of computer simulation models and the meteorologic predictions of the likely spread of the disease are used to determine an appropriate strategy for control. Even then, conclusions from such models may still be controversial, as was the case in the 2001 outbreak in England, where a culling policy driven by unvalidated predictive models rather than experience contributed to the death of approximately 10 million animals.[44-45]

Control by Eradication

The success of an eradication program depends on the thoroughness with which it is applied. As soon as the diagnosis is established, all cloven-footed animals in the exposed groups should be immediately slaughtered and burned or buried on site. No reclamation of meat should be permitted, and milk must be regarded as infected. Inert materials that may be contaminated must not leave infected premises without proper disinfection. This applies particularly to human clothing, motor vehicles, and farm machinery. Bedding, feed, feeding utensils, animal products, and other articles that cannot be adequately disinfected must be burned. Barns and small yards must be cleaned and disinfected with 1% to 2% sodium hydroxide or formalin or 4% sodium carbonate solution. Acids and alkalis are the best inactivators of the virus, and their activity is greatly enhanced by the presence of a detergent. The effective pH at a disinfection surface may be grossly altered by the presence of organic matter and needs to be adequately maintained. When all possible sources of infection are destroyed, the farm should be left unstocked for 6 months and restocking permitted only when "sentinel" test animals are introduced and remain uninfected. There are strict international requirements for demonstrating freedom from infection.

Recommendations for outdoor sites are difficult to make. Observations in Argentina suggest that contaminated pastures and unsheltered yards are clear of infection if left unstocked for 8 to 10 days. No animal movement can be permitted, and human and motor traffic must be reduced to a minimum. Persons working on the farm should wear waterproof clothing, which can be easily disinfected by spraying and subsequently removed as the person leaves the farm. Clothing not suitable for chemical disinfection must be boiled. Because of the rapidity with which the disease may spread, immediate quarantine must be imposed on all farms within a radius of 16 to 24 km (10 to 15 miles) of the outbreak.

Although the eradication method of control is favored when the incidence is low, it imposes severe losses on the animal industry in affected areas and is economically impracticable in many countries. However, it must be regarded as the final stage in any control program. The standard strategy is the containment of the disease by ringing the outbreak with a zone of vaccinated animals and setting about reducing the infection rate within the ringed area and eventually eradicating remaining hotspots by slaughter. Containment of an outbreak is a difficult task with high rewards, as shown by various cost–benefit analyses.

The controversy about whether to eradicate or vaccinate is ongoing. For example, the 1967–1968 epidemic in the United Kingdom involving the slaughter of nearly half a million animals at a cost of US$250 million was so damaging financially that it was arranged for vaccination to be available should there be a recurrence of such an epidemic. Nevertheless, the slaughter policy was still adopted in 2001, and many more animals were killed. Part of the increased concern about a test and slaughter policy derives from the following factors:

- Increasing size of herds
- Risks involved if infection is introduced
- Environmental concerns regarding carcass disposal if thousands or millions of animals are to be slaughtered within a short time. During the 1997 epidemic in Taiwan, it was reported that a disposal capacity of 200,000 pigs per day was reached despite ring vaccination. In England, disposal capacity was overwhelmed in 2001, even with military intervention, and carcasses were sometimes left for days before burial or burning. A recent study in the United States concluded that depopulation of a large feedlot during an FMD outbreak would be difficult to complete in a humane and timely fashion.[46]

Vaccination

Regular vaccination against FMD is a way of life for most of the world, and vaccine production is a major industry. In the endemic countries, eradication does not seem possible within the foreseeable future, and countries free of the disease may require regional vaccination during outbreaks. Consequently, it has been estimated that 1.5 billion monovalent doses of the FMD vaccine are administered annually, with South America alone accounting for some 1300 million doses.

Killed trivalent (containing O, A, and C strains) vaccines are in general use, but because of the increasing occurrence of antigenically dissimilar substrains, the production of vaccines from locally isolated virus is becoming a more common practice. The virus is obtained from infected tongue tissue, a cell culture of bovine tongue epithelium, or other cell culture. Baby hamster kidney (BHK) is a favored viral cultural medium, and BHK vaccine is now in general use. Its principal virtue is its adaptability to deep suspension culture, in contrast with its growth on monolayer culture, enabling large-scale production of the virus to be carried out within practicable space limits. Inactivation of the virus to produce a killed vaccine used to be done with formalin, but there are disadvantages with its use, and more sophisticated agents, especially binary ethylene immine (BEI) are now used. Serviceable immunity after a single vaccination can be relied on for only 6 to 8 months. Vaccines produced from "natural" virus give longer immunity than those produced from "culture" virus. Vaccines produced in oil-adjuvant form offer promise of providing longer immunity and require only annual revaccination in adult cattle and biannual revaccination for young stock or every 4 to 6 months in pigs.

A general vaccination program for an area must be planned for that area. Thus in continental Europe, the program until 1991 included an annual vaccination of all adults, with an additional campaign every 6 months to vaccinate calves as they reached about 4 months of age. In South America, the specific recommendations are that calves from unvaccinated dams should be vaccinated at 4 months and revaccinated at 8 months of age, but calves from vaccinated cows should be vaccinated twice, the first at 6 months and the second at 10 months of age. The important considerations in calves are to avoid vaccination while the calf is still carrying maternal antibodies derived from colostrum and to avoid infection before they can develop active immunity. Calves as young as 1 week old respond as actively to vaccination as adult animals, provided they are free of maternally derived antibody. Immunity is present 7 to 20 days after vaccination, depending on the antigenicity of the vaccine. It is not usual to include sheep, goats, and pigs in a general vaccination program unless they are also affected during outbreaks. After the outbreak in Taiwan, it was recommended that piglets be vaccinated at 8 to 12 weeks followed by a boost 4 weeks later, and that sows be vaccinated 3 to 4 weeks before farrowing or every 4 to 6 months.

Because of the short duration of the immunity produced by killed vaccines, attention has been focused on the production of an attenuated living-virus vaccine. The major difficulty encountered so far has been the narrow margin between loss of virulence and loss of immunogenicity. Attenuated vaccines have been produced by passage through white mice, embryonated hen eggs, rabbits, and tissue culture. Their use has contributed to the eradication of the disease in cattle in South Africa. Vaccines have also been instrumental in eliminating FMD from most countries in South America under the Pan American Centre for Foot and Mouth Disease (PANAFTOSA).

Provided constant surveillance can be maintained over vaccinated animals, their value in such circumstances cannot be denied. However, their early promise has not been fulfilled, and improved killed vaccines are most generally favored. In spite of the uncertain stability of the lapinized virus, control of the disease in Russia was reported after the use of a rabbit-passaged vaccine. In those countries where vaccination of very large numbers of animals is carried out annually, one of the emerging problems is the quality control of vaccines with respect to innocuity and to immunizing capacity or potency. The techniques to monitor these characteristics are available, but they do add to the costs of the vaccine, and if commercial competition is keen, this aspect of production may be spared. Some outbreaks have been linked to attenuated vaccines.

A great deal has been written about genetically engineered FMD vaccines produced by biotechnological manipulation and their distinct safety advantages over whole-virus vaccines. Initial reports of a polypeptide vaccine (protein VP1) in cattle are encouraging, and the peptide can be chemically synthesized and incorporated into the core of hepatitis B virus to produce a vaccine. Research is ongoing, and at least one novel molecular vaccine has been licensed for emergency use in the United States.[47] However, much work still needs to be done, and these newly developed vaccines cannot yet replace the classical inactivated vaccines.

General vaccination as a means of control is recommended for countries where the disease is enzootic or where the threat of introduction is very great (e.g., Israel). If an outbreak occurs, a booster vaccination with the relevant serotype will greatly increase the resistance of the population. However, the strategy of general vaccination has many difficulties. The following disadvantages are suggested:

- To be effective, the program should consist of vaccination against a number of strains three times yearly. More frequent vaccination may be necessary in the face of outbreaks during optimum conditions for spread. Young animals with maternally derived antibodies do not respond to vaccination.
- Vaccination of sheep and pigs is also used in control programs. In pigs, a bi- or trivalent, inactivated, adjuvant vaccine gives strong immunity for 6 months and some resistance for 12 months. Severe local reactions (abscesses and granulomas) at vaccination sites can be reduced by the inclusion of an oil-adjuvant. However, vaccination of pregnant sows leads to a high rate of abortions and stillbirths. In sheep, monovalent or trivalent vaccines give immunity for 5 to 6 months, but the sheep may act as inapparent carriers. One study suggested that a single emergency vaccination would be effective in the control of an epidemic involving cattle and sheep, but would be less effective in pigs.[47]
- Inapparent infections may occur in animals whose susceptibility has been reduced by vaccination, permitting the existence of "carrier" foci. It has become generally recognized that the number of carrier animals produced by vaccination is very much greater than was previously thought. Apart from the fact that these animals are a potent method of spreading the disease, they also provide an excellent medium for the mutation of existing virus strains because the hosts are immune. The carrier state in vaccinated and unvaccinated cattle may persist for as long as 6 months and be capable of causing new outbreaks in all species. But the problem must be kept in perspective. The number of carriers produced in this way is directly related to the rate of occurrence of the disease in the population, and if this is kept to a minimum by an assiduous vaccination program and a strict limitation on the movement of infected animals into the population, the rate of occurrence of carriers can be very small. Nevertheless, in FMD-free countries, vaccinated animals are subsequently slaughtered to comply with OIE regulations so as to resume meat export as soon as possible. However, this policy is now being challenged from the point of view of animal welfare.
- Importation of vaccinated animals is often prohibited even though trade in these animals and their products poses minimal risk of transmitting FMD.[11] An additional disadvantage is the production of sensitivity resulting in anaphylaxis in 0.005% of cattle vaccinated repeatedly, especially when the vaccines contain antibiotics or the vaccine contains foreign protein not associated with the antigen, or the virus has been killed with formalin that has also denatured the protein in the vaccine. Edema, urticaria, dermatitis, abortion, and fatal anaphylaxis all occur. Cows in early and late pregnancy or otherwise stressed from other diseases are most susceptible to adverse effects of vaccination. Satisfactory purification and standardization of the vaccine can eliminate many of the problems because the hypersensitivity is to the culture medium and to the agent used to kill the virus, rather than the virus itself.
- Countries that vaccinate during an outbreak have to reestablish their FMD-free status to the satisfaction of their trading partners. This is difficult because currently available vaccines stimulate production of antibodies indistinguishable from those following infection, and because vaccinated animals can be infected and become carriers. The detection of antibodies to nonstructural proteins is helpful in making the distinction at herd level, and further research is ongoing to standardize the techniques.

Alternatives to general vaccination are modified programs, including "ring" vaccination to contain outbreaks, "frontier" vaccination to produce a buffer area between infected and free countries, and vaccination of selected herds on a voluntary basis when an outbreak is threatened. Such emergency vaccinations can reduce the risk of spreading infection by reducing the rate of virus excretion. It is generally conceded that vaccination of an entire population may be necessary when eradication is incapable of preventing the spread of the disease. For this reason, many countries have strategic reserves of concentrated vaccines, but no such vaccine banks exist in Africa.

Prevention of entry of the disease into free areas is an ever-increasing problem because of modern developments in communications. The following prohibitions are necessary if the disease is to be excluded:

- There must be a complete embargo on the importation of animals and animal products from countries where FMD is endemic. The embargo should include hay, straw, and vegetables. Where the disease occurs only as occasional outbreaks, importation of animals can be permitted provided they are subjected to a satisfactory period of quarantine.
- Particular attention should be given to preventing entry of uncooked meats from ships, airplanes, and other forms of transport and in parcels originating in infected areas. In danger areas, all swill fed to pigs must be cooked and all food waste satisfactorily disposed of.
- Personal clothing and other items belonging to people arriving from infected areas should be suitably disinfected. Persons arriving from endemic countries or countries experiencing outbreaks should keep away from livestock for several days.
- The risk of introducing the disease through importation of semen or fertilized ova is now thought to be minimal. The virus can survive in frozen bull semen and possibly in some fertilized ova (e.g., zona pellucida–free bovine embryos) but not in others (e.g., zona pellucida–intact bovine embryos). However, because even viremic animals

do not transmit the disease through their embryos, bovine embryos with intact zona pellucida can be safely imported from enzootic areas regardless of the serologic status of the donor. Consequently, if exotic or special animals have to be imported from enzootic countries, embryo transfer may be a means of controlling the transmission of FMD. Even for llama embryos that lack a zona pellucida, the risk of FMD transmission was calculated to be close to zero if favorable epidemiologic or ecological conditions exist in the region of origin of the embryos.

In summary, the control and eventual eradication of FMD in a country, region or worldwide can only be achieved if the international community recognizes that the control of FMD is a global public good that will benefit all populations and future generations.[2] In South America, under the auspices of the PANAFTOSA's new Plan of Action 2011–2020, it is hoped that several challenges will be overcome to ensure eradication of FMD from the Americas by 2020.[48]

FURTHER READING

Blackwell JH. Internationalism and survival of foot-and-mouth disease virus in cattle and food products. *J Dairy Sci.* 1980;63:1019.

Brown F. Review literature Foot-and-mouth disease—one of the remaining great plagues. *Proc R Soc Lond Biol.* 1986;229:215.

Donaldson AI, Doel TR. Foot-and-mouth disease: the risk for Great Britain after 1992. *Vet Rec.* 1992;131:114.

Grubman MJ, Barry B. Foot and mouth disease. *Clin Microbiol Rev.* 2004;17:465.

Rweyemamu MM, et al. The control of foot and mouth disease by vaccination. *Vet Ann.* 1982;22:63.

Scott GR. Foot-and-mouth disease. In: Sewell MMH, Brocklesby DW, eds. *Handbook on Animal Diseases in the Tropics.* 4th ed. London: Baillière Tindall; 1990:309.

Thomson GR, Bastos ADS. Foot-and-mouth disease. In: Coetzer JAW, Tustin RC, eds. *Infectious Diseases of Livestock.* Vol. 2. 2nd ed. Cape Town: Oxford University Press; 2004:1324.

REFERENCES

1. Paton DJ, et al. *Philos Trans R Soc Lond B Biol Sci.* 2009;364.
2. OIE/FAO Global conference on foot and mouth disease—final recommendations. Asuncion, Paraguay. 2009 Accessed at: <http://www.oie.int/en/for-the-media/press-releases/detail/article/oiefao-global-conference-on-foot-and-mouth-disease-final-recommendations/>. Accessed 01.08.2016.
3. Yoon H, et al. *Transbound Emerg Dis.* 2013;doi:10.1111/tbed.12109; [Epub ahead of print].
4. Muroga N, et al. *J Vet Med Sci.* 2012;74:399.
5. Rweyemamu M, et al. *Transbound Emerg Dis.* 2008;55:57.
6. Pacheco JM, et al. *Vet J.* 2012;193:456.
7. Sellers R, Gloster J. *Vet J.* 2008;177:159.
8. Chase-Topping ME, et al. *Vet Res.* 2013;44:46.
9. Juleff ND, et al. *Vet Immunol Immunopathol.* 2012;15:148.
10. Maddur MS, et al. *Clin Vaccine Immunol.* 2009;16:1832.
11. Garland AJ, de Clercq K. *Rev - Off Int Epizoot.* 2011;30:189.
12. Allepuz A, et al. *Transbound Emerg Dis.* 2013;doi:10.1111/tbed.12087; [Epub ahead of print].
13. Muroga N, et al. *BMC Vet Res.* 2013;9:150.
14. Wernery U, Kinna J. *Rev - Off Int Epizoot.* 2012;31:907.
15. Larska M, et al. *Epidemiol Infect.* 2009;137:549.
16. Chang H, et al. *Virol J.* 2013;10:81.
17. Alexandrov T, et al. *Vet Microbiol.* 2013;doi:10.1016/j.vetmic.2013.05.016; [Epub ahead of print]; S0378-1135(13)00298-8.
18. Mohamed F, et al. *Transbound Emerg Dis.* 2011;58:358.
19. Rhyan J, et al. *J Wildl Dis.* 2008;44:269.
20. Cottam EM, et al. *PLoS Pathog.* 2008;4:e1000050.
21. Toka FN, Golde WT. *Immunol Lett.* 2013;152:135.
22. Pega J, et al. *J Virol.* 2013;87:2489.
23. Carpenter TE, et al. *J Vet Diagn Invest.* 2011;23:26.
24. Arzt J, et al. *Transbound Emerg Dis.* 2011;58:291.
25. Arzt J, et al. *Transbound Emerg Dis.* 2011;58:305.
26. Lohse L, et al. *Vet Res.* 2012;43:46.
27. Toka FN, et al. *Clin Vaccine Immunol.* 2009;16:1738.
28. Wang D, et al. *J Virol.* 2012;86:9311.
29. Stenfeldt C, Belsham GJ. *Vet Microbiol.* 2012;154:230.
30. Arzt J, et al. *Vet Pathol.* 2010;47:1048.
31. Murphy C, et al. *Vet Rec.* 2010;166:10.
32. Juleff N, et al. *PLoS ONE.* 2008;3:e3434.
33. Yoon H, et al. *Transbound Emerg Dis.* 2012;59:517.
34. Maddur MS, et al. *Transbound Emerg Dis.* 2011;58:274.
35. Lee SH, et al. *Transbound Emerg Dis.* 2009;56:189.
36. *OIE Manual of Diagnostic Tests and Vaccines for Terrestrial Animals.* Paris: OIE; 2008 chapter 2.1.5:190.
37. Muthukrishnan M, et al. *J Virol Methods.* 2008;151:311.
38. Chen HT, et al. *Virol J.* 2011;8:510.
39. Yang M, et al. *Virol J.* 2013;10:125.
40. Madi M, et al. *Vet J.* 2012;193:67.
41. Gao M, et al. *Appl Microbiol Biotechnol.* 2012;93:1271.
42. Duas CC, et al. *J Interferon Cytokine Res.* 2011;31:227.
43. Perez-Martin E, et al. *J Virol.* 2012;86:4477.
44. Kitching RP, et al. *Rev - Off Int Epizoot.* 2006;25:293.
45. Mansley LM, et al. *Rev - Off Int Epizoot.* 2011;30:483.
46. McReynolds SW, Sanderson MW. *J Am Vet Assoc.* 2014;244:291.
47. Ludi A, Rodriguez L. *Dev Biol (Basel).* 2013;135:107.
48. Orsel K, Bouma A. *Can Vet J.* 2009;50:1059.

RIFT VALLEY FEVER

SYNOPSIS

Etiology Rift Valley fever virus, genus *Phlebovirus*, a member of the family Bunyaviridae.

Epidemiology Enzootic in sub-Saharan Africa and Egypt. First occurrence outside African continent in 2000 affecting Arabian Peninsula. Virus maintained in floodwater mosquitoes and transmitted by hematophagous insects. Ruminants are amplifying hosts. Epizootics in high rainfall periods. A major zoonosis with mortality rate of 1% in humans.

Clinical findings Acute febrile disease in lambs and calves characterized by hepatitis and high mortality; abortion in adult sheep and in cattle. In humans, influenza-like disease and, in rare instances, hemorrhagic fever.

Necropsy findings Hepatic necrosis.

Diagnostic confirmation Immunohistochemical localization of viral antigens in tissues.

Treatment No specific treatment available; supportive.

Control Vaccination, vector control, control of livestock movement.

ETIOLOGY

Rift Valley fever virus is a single-stranded RNA virus of the family Bunyaviridae, genus *Phlebovirus*. There is only one serotype recognized, with only minor genetic variation between strains.[1]

The virus remains viable in aerosols at 25°C (77°F) for 1 hour or longer but can survive in serum at 4°C (40°F) for several months. Infected sheep plasma can retain its infectivity over years with storage and shipment under a variety of refrigeration conditions. Infectious material thus presents a potential source of infection for laboratory personnel or veterinarians for a prolonged period of time.[2]

EPIDEMIOLOGY

Occurrence

Rift Valley fever (RVF) was first recognized in 1930 in the Rift Valley in Kenya but now exists and occurs as epizootics throughout sub-Saharan Africa, with recent extensions into Egypt, Mauritania, and Madagascar. The first RVF outbreaks outside Africa were recorded in 2000 in Yemen and Saudi Arabia. The most recent outbreaks recorded by the World Health Organization (WHO) occurred in Somalia (2006/2007), Kenya (2007/2008), Tanzania (2007), Sudan (2007/2008), Madagascar (2008/2009), South Africa (2008, 2009, and 2010), Mauritania (2010 and 2012), Botswana (2010), and Namibia (2010).[3] The disease has great potential for spread to other countries either through legal or illegal movement of infected livestock or the encroachment of mosquitoes into new areas.[4] The pattern of occurrence is cyclical epidemics that are inherently linked to regional climate variability, particularly to rainfall patterns.[4] Outbreaks occur with periods of quiescence of 5 to 15 years in duration.[2]

Climate changes and livestock movement facilitate the spread of the disease and present an increasing risk of introduction of the disease into the Mediterranean basin and Europe.[2]

Risk Factors

Animal Risk Factors

Rift Valley fever is an infectious disease primarily affecting ruminants but to which other species, including humans, are also susceptible. There is a clear age predisposition to clinical disease rendering lambs, goat kids, puppies, and kittens extremely susceptible, with mortality rates between 70% and 100%. Adult sheep and calves have been categorized as highly susceptible, with mortality rates between 20% to 70%. Adult cattle, goats, African and domestic buffalo, and humans are moderately susceptible, with mortality rates of less than 10%.[1] Camelids, equids, pigs, and adult dogs and cats are considered resistant to clinical disease, with infection being inapparent in these species. A large number of different African wildlife species were found to have seroconverted in endemic areas.

Environmental Risk Factors

Outbreaks of RVF have been associated with above-normal rainfall and climatic conditions favorable to competent vectors. More precisely, epidemics have been reported in four epidemiologic systems[2]:

- **"Dambo" areas in East Africa.** These areas are valleys near a river in which outbreaks occur following heavy rainfall events.
- **Semiarid areas of western Africa** (including Senegal and Mauritania). In these regions, which are characterized by temporary areas of water, outbreaks could not be directly related to flood-like rainfalls; rather, they occurred during the rainy season with abundant regular rainfall.
- **Irrigated areas** (including the Nile Delta or Senegal River basin). In artificially irrigated areas the permanent availability of water favors the persistence of a vector population throughout the year.
- **Temperate and mountainous areas** (including regions in Madagascar). Transmission of RVFV in these regions results from vector-borne transmission associated with livestock movement.

RVF outbreaks were found to occur with a cyclic pattern in association with the warm phase of the El Niño/Southern Oscillation (ENSO) phenomenon. The ENSO is associated with varying climate effects on a 3- to 7-year interval.[4]

Source of Infection

The live cycle of RVFV consists of an epizootic cycle that is associated with outbreaks of RVF and an enzootic or interepizootic cycle, during which the virus persists in a host but is not associated with clinical disease. During the interepizootic cycle the RVFV is maintained through vertical transmission in *Aedes* mosquito eggs. These eggs are drought-resistant and survive several years without hatching, thereby maintaining the virus during interepizootic periods. These interepizootic vectors belong to the *Aedes* subgenus *Neomelaniconion* in East Africa and the subgenus *Aedimorphus* in West Africa. Epizootics occur in enzootic areas when wet and flood conditions enable the infected eggs to mature and hatch. *Aedes* mosquitoes hatched from infected eggs transmit the virus to susceptible animals, particularly domestic ruminants on which they feed preferentially.

Once a susceptible animal, which is considered an amplifying host, is infected, a transient viremic phase occurs, permitting virus transmission between susceptible individuals through any hematophagous insect species. These insects, which include *Culex* and *Anopheles* spp., function as secondary arthropod vectors but do not transmit the virus transovarially and therefore do not act as RVFV reservoirs during interepizootic periods.[1]

For **humans**, direct contact with infected animal tissues, blood, or other body fluids and also inhalation of aerosolized infected material are considered the predominant routes of infection.[5] Accordingly, certain occupational groups, such as farmhouse, slaughterhouse, or laboratory personnel and veterinarians, are at increased risk of infection. Biting insects appear to have a limited role in the transmission of RVFV to humans. Nevertheless, during the 2000/2001 outbreak of RVF in Saudi Arabia, with over 400 confirmed clinical cases in humans and 85 deaths, 23% of all infections were estimated to have occurred through mosquito exposure.[5] In contrast, during a South African outbreak, 89% of clinical cases in humans were associated with direct contact with infectious material. Ingestion of unpasteurized milk was incriminated as a possible route of infection based on epidemiologic evidence, but this has not been demonstrated conclusively.[5]

Method of Transmission

In ruminants RVFV is transmitted between animals through primary and secondary arthropod vectors. Direct transmission between animals through contact with viremic fluid, such as blood or lochial fluid, is strongly suspected but has thus far not been confirmed. The presence of virus in the nasal or lachrymal secretions, urine, or feces of infected animals has not been demonstrated.[2]

In humans there is no evidence for person-to-person transmission of infection. Vertical transmission from an infected mother to her baby has been reported in two instances during the outbreaks in Saudi Arabia in 2000 and in Sudan in 2007.[6]

Experimental Reproduction

The disease can be transmitted by most routes, including inoculation and the inhalation of aerosols. Following inoculation of sheep and cattle the incubation period is 1 to 2 days, and high virus titers are found in blood. The virus persists in the body for approximately 3 weeks, but long-term carriage has not been observed. Pregnant animals abort, but infection may be clinically mild in nonpregnant animals. IgM antibody can be detected as early as 4 days after infection and persists for 2 to 6 months.

Zoonotic Implications

Although humans are susceptible to infection and disease, infection with RVFV in the large majority of cases is asymptomatic, as is suggested by retrospective serologic studies following epidemics. If clinically apparent, the disease is usually a transient flulike illness, but complications of hemorrhagic fever, retinal and renal disease, and encephalitis occur.[1] Traditionally, the occupational groups at greatest risk are laboratory workers handling the virus and those working among infected animals or their products, including veterinarians. However, cases were not limited to these groups in the large outbreaks in Egypt in 1977 and 1978 and the more recent outbreaks in the Arabian Peninsula. The occurrence rate of clinical disease in humans was very high in Egypt (more than 20,000 cases and 600 deaths). The mortality rate in humans is estimated to be 1% to 2%.[7] The pathogen is identified as a potential agent for bioterrorism.

Economic Importance

The disease causes significant morbidity and mortality in calves and lambs and has been associated with abortion storms in adult ruminants, with pronounced health and economic impacts. The economic losses solely attributable to trade disruptions occurred during the RVF outbreaks of 2007 in Sudan have been estimated to exceed $60 million.[8]

PATHOGENESIS

Hepatocytes are the primary site of viral replication in lambs and calves, and age is a determining factor in the progression and outcome of infection. In very young animals, hepatic lesions progress from degeneration and necrosis of individual hepatocytes to extensive necrosis throughout the liver, resulting in hepatic insufficiency and failure. In young animals, encephalomyelitis may also occur.

CLINICAL FINDINGS

The clinical presentation of RVF varies by species and age. The disease is most severe in young ruminants, particularly lambs. After an incubation period of between 12 and 36 hours, anorexia, weakness associated with fever, and lymphadenopathy become apparent. Hemorrhagic diarrhea with abdominal pain may be seen. In calves, icterus is a common clinical finding. Mortality rates are high and can reach 90% to 100% in lambs and 70% in calves.

In adult sheep and cattle, abortion is the outstanding and in many cases only clinical sign. Abortion storms affecting up to 100% of ewes and 85% of cows can occur. In clinical cases in cattle and adult sheep there is febrile disease, with anorexia, weakness, and a drop in milk production that can be associated with hemorrhagic diarrhea. In severe cases the mortality rate in adult sheep may be as high as 25% and 10% in cattle. Goats show a febrile reaction but few other clinical signs.

Clinical signs can be unspecific when considering an individual animal, but RVF should be suspected whenever high abortion rates in adult ruminants and high mortality rates in neonatal ruminants occur in combination with flulike disease in humans who had contact with sick ruminants.

CLINICAL PATHOLOGY

Severe leukopenia is a common finding.

Virus isolation is usually performed from inoculated hamsters, mice, or cell cultures. Virus identification can also be done by immunofluorescence carried out on impression smears of liver, spleen, or brain or immunostaining of histology slides.[1] The agar gel immunodiffusion (AGID) test is an alternative for laboratories without tissue culture facility. Polymerase chain reaction (PCR) is used for rapid detection of viral RNA.

Serology can be conducted by virus neutralization (VN), which is the prescribed test for international trade, by means of an enzyme-linked immunosorbent assay (ELISA) or by hemagglutination inhibition. The virus neutralization test requires the use of live RVFV, making this test unsuitable to be used outside endemic areas.[1] Several RVFV antibody ELISAs are available as commercial test kits and can be performed with inactivated antigen and thus are suitable for the use outside RVFV-endemic areas. The IgM-capture ELISA allows diagnosis of a recent infection.[1] Antibodies appear in the serum about 1 week after infection, and persistence depends on antibody type.

NECROPSY FINDINGS

Extensive hepatic necrosis is the characteristic lesion in RVF. In neonates, the liver is enlarged and has a yellow–orange discoloration, whereas in older animals, pale foci of necrosis impart a mottled appearance to the organ. Other nonspecific lesions include congestion and petechiation in the heart, lymph nodes, gallbladder, and alimentary tract. Abomasal and intestinal content may be dark brown to red as a result of hemorrhage.

Microscopically there is multifocal or diffuse necrosis of the liver, and there may be acidophilic intranuclear inclusion bodies in hepatic cells. The lesions are much more extensive in newborn lambs and calves than in older animals. Immunohistochemical localization of viral antigens in tissues provides a specific diagnosis.

Samples for Confirmation of Diagnosis

- **Virology**—liver, spleen, brain (virus isolation, fluorescence antibody test, PCR)
- **Histology**—liver, spleen, brain (light microscopy, immunohistochemistry)

Note the zoonotic potential of this disease when handling these specimens.

DIFFERENTIAL DIAGNOSIS

In regions where this disease has not occurred it should be suspect when there is an area outbreak of abortion and neonatal mortality in sheep and cattle coupled with an area outbreak of flu-like disease in humans.

- Wesselsbron disease
- Bluetongue
- Ephemeral fever
- Bacterial septicemias
- Anthrax
- Vibriosis
- Trichomoniasis
- Toxic plants

TREATMENT

Little attention has been given to the aspect of treatment of the disease, and no known treatment is of any value.

CONTROL

Measures to control Rift Valley fever include the following:

- Control of livestock movement
- Vector control
- Vaccination

The role of **livestock movement** over long and short distances in the spread of the disease throughout the African continent is well documented, and phylogenetic studies suggest that ruminant trade is the main reason for the spread of the disease from the African continent to the Arabian Peninsula.

Vector control is most effective when larvicides are used in mosquito breeding sites. Limitations of this approach are that breeding sites must be clearly identified and must have a limited surface to be manageable. Particularly with heavy rainfalls and flooding, mosquito-breeding sites are too numerous and wide to be controlled. Ecological, health, and financial issues around applying large amounts of insecticides to the environment further complicate this type of control.

Vaccines

Live attenuated vaccines (Smithburn strain) and mutagenized live virus vaccines provide good protection that lasts for at least 28 months but are not recommended for pregnant animals because they are abortigenic, causing fetal death and some teratogenic anomalies. The recorded problems include hydrops amnii, arthrogryposis, hydranencephaly, and microencephaly. There is also a concern for reversion to virulence. Live attenuated vaccines, furthermore, are pathogenic for humans, and exposure to live attenuated vaccines may present a health risk.[5]

Killed-virus vaccines require repeat administration for good immunity, and annual vaccination of all dairy cattle is recommended as a cost-effective control program in endemic countries. They are also recommended for pregnant and young animals.

A **mutagen attenuated vaccine** protects against challenge in both sheep and cattle. Viremia following vaccination is minimal and thought not to be a risk for infection of susceptible mosquitoes. Mutagenic vaccines were initially thought to have no deleterious effect on the fetus, but abortion and teratogenicity have been observed in the lambs of sheep vaccinated early in pregnancy.

Prevention of the introduction of Rift Valley fever into countries free of the disease requires the prohibition of the importation of all susceptible species from Africa. All necessary steps to prevent the introduction of infective insects and infected biological materials should be taken. The possibility of humans carrying the infection from country to country is very real.

FURTHER READING

Gerdes GH. *Vet Clin North Am Food A.* 2002;18:549-555.

Shimshony A, Barzilai R. Rift Valley fever. *Adv Vet Sci Comp Med.* 1983;21:347-425.

REFERENCES

1. OIE. 2009 at: <http://www.oie.int/fileadmin/Home/eng/Animal_Health_in_the_World/docs/pdf/RIFT_VALLEY_FEVER_FINAL.pdf>; Accessed 20.01.14.
2. Chevalier V. *Clin Microbiol Infect.* 2013;19:705.
3. Balenghien T, et al. *Vet Res.* 2013;44:78.
4. El Vilaly, et al. *Progr Phys Geo.* 2013;37:219.
5. Archer B, et al. *Emerg Infect Dis.* 2013;19:1918.
6. Hassan OA, et al. *PLoS ONE.* 2011;5:e1229.
7. Dar O, et al. *Trop Med Int Health.* 2013;18:1036.
8. Little PD. 2009 <http://www.caadp.net/pdf/COMESA%20CAADP%20Policy%20Brief%202%20Cross%20Border%20Livestock%20Trade%20(2).pdf>; Accessed 20.01.14.

BLUETONGUE

SYNOPSIS

Etiology Bluetongue virus (BTV), an orbivirus with several serotypes and considerable genetic heterogeneity.

Epidemiology An infectious, noncontagious disease primarily of sheep, but also occurring in cattle, wild ruminants, New World camelids, and goats. Transmitted by *Culicoides* spp. Cattle are the reservoir and amplification hosts. Severe disease is most common in European fine wool and mutton breeds of sheep. Certain serotypes can cause severe disease in cattle.

Continued

Infection, but not disease, is endemic in tropical and subtropical regions. Disease occurs in epidemic and incursive areas when climatic conditions allow the expansion of vector occurrence or when naïve animals are introduced into an endemic area.

Clinical findings Fever, apathy, serous to bloody nasal discharge, respiratory distress, oral erosions and ulcerations with hypersalivation. Lameness as a result of coronitis, myositis, and muscle necrosis.

Clinical pathology Virus isolation or detection of viral RNA (reverse-transcription polymerase chain reaction [RT-PCR]) in blood or tissue specimens. Serologic tests to identify BTV-specific antibodies or a rise in antibody titer (competitive enzyme-linked immunoabsorbent assay [C-ELISA], virus neutralization test, agar gel immunodiffusion [AGID]).

Necropsy findings Mucosal lesions, hemorrhage and necrosis of skeletal and cardiac muscles, hemorrhagic lesion at base of pulmonary artery. Congestion of heart, lung, liver and kidney.

Diagnostic confirmation Detection of viral nucleic acid, virus isolation, rising titer with serology.

Treatment None specific, supportive.

Control Reduction of exposure to vector is attempted, but major method of control in epidemic areas is by vaccination.

ETIOLOGY

Bluetongue virus (BTV) is an arthropod-borne *Orbivirus* in the family Reoviridae with a genome composed of 10 dsRNA segments. The bluetongue viruses are stable and resistant to decomposition and to some standard virucidal agents, including sodium carbonate. They are sensitive to acid, inactivated below pH 6.0, and susceptible to 3% sodium hydroxide solution and organic iodides.

Worldwide there are currently 26 recognized serotypes of BTV.[1-4] The virus is characterized by its high genetic variability resulting from the genetic drift of individual gene segments and from reassortment of gene segments when ruminants or the vectors are infected with more than one strain. The occurrence of different BTV serotypes varies by geographic region.

EPIDEMIOLOGY

Occurrence

Bluetongue virus has been identified on all continents except Antarctica and is considered endemic in the domestic livestock populations of all tropical and subtropical countries. Until the end of last century, BTV was considered an exotic disease in the Palearctic, but a series of outbreaks caused by different serotypes apparently originating from adjacent enzootic regions has occurred in the Mediterranean basin since 1998.[5] Whereas historically the enzootic area was considered to be limited to the area between latitude 35° S and 50° N, this zone appears to have extended to areas north of 53° NN over the last decade. BTV outbreaks observed in these new regions in the past years are thought to be the result of climate change from global warming.

The distribution and intensity of infection in regions of the continents is determined by the climate, geography, and altitude, which affect the occurrence and activity of the *Culicoides* vectors, and by the presence of susceptible mammalian hosts. There is a gradation from continuous BTV activity in tropical areas to absence of virus transmission in colder areas. In large countries that span different latitudes, such as the United States and Australia, there are endemic areas and regions that are free of BTV infection.

In **endemic areas**, the infection is always present, but clinical disease of the indigenous species is unusual. It can occur with new BTV strains and when nonindigenous susceptible species are introduced to the area.

Epidemic zones also exist, where infection and clinical disease occur every few years. Infection in these areas is highly focal, and outbreaks occur when climatic conditions allow the vector to spread beyond its usual boundaries and to infect susceptible ruminants.

Incursive disease can occur in regions that do not normally experience infection and may be caused by windborne movement of infected *Culicoides* with subsequent insect breeding in the summer before "die-out" in the autumn and winter. This method of spread is thought to have been the genesis of several serious outbreaks of bluetongue in countries normally free of the disease and of the outbreaks in Portugal in 1956, in Cyprus in 1977, in Turkey and Greece in 1979 to 1980, and in Israel in 1960 to 1980. The recent epidemic of BTV-8 in northern and central Europe between 2006 and 2008, which caused the most severe outbreak of the disease on record, made clear that alternative, thus far unidentified, ways of virus introduction into previously unaffected regions must be considered. This serotype 8, which was previously was only identified in the sub-Saharan region, was first isolated in the Netherlands in 2006, having entirely bypassed the southern part of the continent. To this day no plausible explanation for the introduction of serotype 8 into the northern European region has been proposed.

In the **United States** the prevalence of seropositive cattle varies from high in the southern and western states to low in the northern states, especially the northeastern states. In the northwestern region, there are epidemics of infection in the summer and fall every few years, associated with movement of infected vectors from the south. **Canada** is free of infection except for periodic incursions into the Okanagan Valley in British Columbia from windborne-infected *Culicoides* from south of the border. In **Australia**, there has been a sequential introduction of bluetongue serotypes from Indonesia by windborne *Culicoides* spp., but endemic infection is limited to northern cattle areas with extension down the East Coast. In **central and northern Europe and the United Kingdom,** no new cases of BTV have been recorded since 2009, and thus wide parts of the continent have been declared free of BTV. In **southern Europe** BTV is currently present in the southern part of Italy, Spain, Portugal, and Corsica.[6]

Host Occurrence

Under natural conditions infection occurs in sheep and cattle, but it is also recorded in New World camelids, elk, white-tailed deer, pronghorn antelope, camels, and other wild ruminants. Natural infection rarely occurs in goats, but the infection can be transmitted experimentally. Although clinical disease primarily occurs in sheep, certain strains are highly virulent in cattle and wild ruminants. **Cattle** are the major **reservoir host**. In carnivores, infection after vaccination with BTV-contaminated vaccines has been documented.

Method of Transmission

The disease is not contagious and is almost exclusively **transmitted biologically** by specific species of ***Culicoides.*** There are approximately 1500 species of *Culicoides* worldwide, of which only limited types have been associated with BTV. Only about 50 *Culicoides* species are susceptible to BTV infection. Of these species, only those having ruminants as sole or predominant hosts are epidemiologically relevant for the transmission of BTV.

Culicoides breed in damp, wet areas, including streams, irrigation channels, muddy areas, and fecal runoff areas around farms, and habitats for them exist on the majority of farm environments. Only female *Culicoides* are hematophagous and feed on their main or preferred host species, requiring at least one blood meal for the completion of the ovarian cycle. They feed nocturnally on animals in open pens and fields, and the optimal temperatures for activity are between 13°C and 35°C (55° and 95° F).

Virus present in ingested blood cells infects cells of the midgut of the vector, replicates, and subsequently is released to the salivary gland. The virus is then transmitted through saliva to the host the infected midge is feeding on. Vertical transmission of infectious virus from adult midge to its larvae does not appear to occur. In temperate areas the disease is **seasonal** because *Culicoides* do not tolerate low ambient temperatures, resulting in a vector-free season during late fall and winter.

Culicoides Species

Different *Culicoides* species have different geographic occurrence, and their distribution in a country is determined by climatic factors and the presence of a preferred host. In the **United States,** *C. sonorensis* is the predominant vector throughout much of the country, except in the southeast, where it is *C. insignis. C. insignis* is also the predominant vector for most BTV strains in the **Caribbean** and Central and **South America.** Other epidemiologically relevant Culicoides species in this region are *C. pucillus, C. insignis, C. pusillus,* and *C. filarifer.* In **Africa,** *C. imicola* is a predominant vector, and in the **Middle East and Asia,** *C. fulvis, C. imicola, C. obsoletus, C. nudipalpis,* and *C. orientalis.* In **Australia,** *C. wadai, C. actoni, C. brevitarsis, C. peregrinus, C. oxystoma, C. brevipalpis,* and *C. fulvus* are vectors or potential vectors. They have different distribution in the country, which oscillates depending on climate. *C. imicola* has been involved in the recent expansion of bluetongue in **southern Europe,** but *C. obsoletus, C. pulicaris,* and *C. dewulfi* have been implicated as new vectors associated with recent BTV outbreaks in **central and northern Europe**, where *C. imicola* does not occur.

Other Vectors

Other vectors may transmit the disease mechanically but are unlikely to be of major significance in disease epizootics. The argasid tick *Ornithodoros coriaceus* has been shown experimentally to be capable of transmitting the virus and be a potential vector. The sheep ked (*Melophagus ovinus*) ingests the virus when sucking the blood of infected sheep and can transmit the infection in a mechanical manner. Mosquitoes may play a role in transmission, and *Aedes lineatopennis* and *Anopheles vagus* have been suspect.

Overwintering

Survival of the virus during the vector-free season is termed *overwintering.* As is documented by an annual recrudescence of bluetongue in several temperate areas, BTV can survive several months of cold season presumably in the absence of adult biological vectors. The mechanisms involved are not yet fully understood. Proposed hypotheses to explain the overwintering ability of BTV include persistence of the virus within surviving adult vectors, transovarian transmission within the vector, and prolonged or even persistent infection of viremic or aviremic vertebrate hosts.[5] The average life span of an adult *Culicoides* is between 10 and 20 days but can occasionally extend up to 3 months.[7] In addition, entomologic surveillance in northern Europe has demonstrated the presence of a small number of active *Culicoides* during the winter season inside barns.[8] Overwintering within the adult vector population has therefore been proposed as a plausible explanation for a sustained BTV transmission cycle. In contrast, no evidence supporting vertical (transovarian) transmission of BTV within the vector is currently available.

Overwintering of BTV could also occur in hosts with prolonged viremic phases, such as cattle, where viremia commonly lasts between 20 and 50 days.[9] It is assumed that, in general, **viremia in cattle ceases by 60 days** after infection, although viremic phases of up to 100 days have been reported.[10]

Transplacental Infection

Transplacental infection has been documented experimentally and under field conditions after **infection with modified live laboratory strains** commonly used for vaccine production (modified live vaccines), suggesting that modification of BTV field strains can markedly increase the ability of the virus to cross the placenta and cause fetal infection. Of the 26 currently known wild-type serotypes, only **serotype 8** was repeatedly documented to cause fetal infection through transplacental transmission in cattle and sheep under field conditions.[11,12] Before the appearance of BTV-8 the observed incidence of transplacental transmission was estimated to be near zero, and the few documented cases were associated to the use of modified live vaccines.[13] In contrast, transplacental virus transmission after infection with wild-type BTV-8 was shown to occur with considerable frequency.[14] A study conducted during the BTV-8 epidemic in northern Europe between 2006 and 2008 revealed that virus RNA could be retrieved from 41% of aborted fetuses where BTV was suspected as causative pathogen and from over 18% of fetuses where BTV was not suspected as cause of abortion.[11]

Although the epidemiologic relevance of the vertical transmission of certain BTV serotypes is to be determined, intrauterine infection of the fetus, possibly resulting in a virus-shedding neonate, also presents a possible mechanism for virus survival during the vector-free season.

The outcome of transplacental infection primarily depends on the stage of pregnancy at the time of infection of the dam and can range from abortion to different sorts of congenital defects to healthy-looking lambs or calves. Infection or vaccination of the dam with virus strains capable of crossing the placenta at early stages of pregnancy most commonly results in abortion. Congenital defects of the nervous system can occur when pregnant ewes or cows are exposed to BTV-8 or vaccinated with attenuated vaccine virus before midgestation. At birth, affected neonates characteristically also have circulating BTV-specific antibodies before ingestion of colostrum but no infectious BTV. Dams infected at a later stage of pregnancy give birth to calves without congenital malformation that may be viremic with or without BTV-specific antibody titer. The viremic phase of newborn calves infected in utero is of similar duration as in animals infected after birth. BTV infection in cattle is therefore considered to be transient and neither persistent nor immunotolerant.[15]

Observed congenital defects include excessive gingival tissue, agnathia (tilted mandible), arthrogryposis, hydranencephaly, and porencephaly. The severity of the brain lesions decreases with increasing fetal age. Infection at 243 days results in a mild encephalitis and the premature birth of calves that are still viremic but poorly viable.

Persistent Infection

Persistent infection in immunotolerant animals following in utero infection has been implied in a single study and was consequently thought to be of paramount epidemiologic importance. However, a large number of experimental and field studies failed to produce any evidence supporting the occurrence of persistent infection or the existence of a BTV carrier status. Persistent infection is therefore currently considered a highly unlikely scenario.

Venereal Transmission

Bluetongue virus can be found in the **semen** of infected bulls during the viremic period, and infection has been transmitted through bull semen to susceptible cows, but it is unlikely that this is a significant mechanism of transmission. Transplanted **embryos** from infected donors are free of the virus because it does not appear to penetrate the zona pellucida. Embryo transfer is regarded as a minimal risk procedure for the transmission of BTV in cattle and sheep as long as the guidelines of the International Embryo Transfer Society (IETS) are followed. Recommended procedures include visual inspection, rigorous washing of the embryo, and, in some instances, treating with trypsin to inactivate infectious virus particles. Virus transmission when doing embryo transfers could occur as a result of contamination of media or equipment used to manipulate the embryos.[16]

Oral Transmission

Studies reporting or suggesting oral transmission BTV have been published recently. These studies include one report of infection of adult cattle after ingestion of BTV-8-infected placenta and several reports where infection of newborn calves after consumption of infected colostrum was described.[17-19] The epidemiologic relevance if this route of transmission remains to be determined.

Pathogen and Vector Risk Factors

The geographic occurrence of bluetongue serotypes varies and is changing with time. There are differences in virulence between serotypes. The virulence of the virus is also related to the infectious dose, which, among other factors, depends on the vector species, its competence, and its occurrence. Different *Culicoides* species vary in susceptibility to infection (i.e., vector competence), and some known vectors are resistant to infection with some serotypes, which in part explains regional differences in serotype occurrence.

Climate

Climate is a major risk factor because *Culicoides* require warmth and moisture for breeding and calm, warm, humid weather for feeding. A cold winter or a dry summer can markedly reduce vector numbers and risk for disease. Moisture may be in the form of rivers and streams or irrigation, but rainfall is the predominant influence; rainfall in the preceding months is a major determinant of infection.

Precipitation affects the size and persistence of breeding sites and the availability of humid microhabitats to allow shelter from desiccation during hot summer and autumn periods. Optimal temperature is also essential for survival and activity of the vector and for virus replication within the vector. Ambient temperatures for survival of adult midges and larvae must be above a mean of 13°C (55°F) and range between 18° and 30°C (64° and 86°F) for optimal adult activity. The rate of virus replication within an infected midge also largely depends on the ambient temperature. Whereas at 30°C midges may start shedding virus within days of infection, this takes several weeks at ambient temperatures of 15°C (59°F).[1] Virus replication within the vector apparently ceases completely at temperature below approximately 12°C (54°F), although the virus may persist in infected midges and replication may resume with increasing temperatures.[1] Geographic information systems (GIS) can be used to predict area risk.

Serotype Occurrence

Genetic studies indicate that BTV tends to exist in discrete, stable ecosystems and that BTV serotypes that circulate in one region of the world are largely different from those in other regions. In the **United States,** four serotypes (10, 11, 13, and 17) associated with *C. sonorensis* are considered endemic south of the so-called "Sonorensis Line" going from Washington in the West to Maryland in the East. Serotype 2 is another strain occurring in the United States, but it is restricted to the southeast of the country, the habitat of *C. insignis.*

In the **Caribbean** region and **South** and **Central America,** serotypes 1, 3, 5, 6, 8, 12, 14, 17, 19, 22, and 24 were reported. In **Australia,** BTV is endemic in the northern and northeastern areas of the country, and most of the western, southern, and central parts of the country are considered free of bluetongue.[20] Serotypes 1 and 21 are the predominant strains in northwestern Australia, the Northern Territory, Queensland, and the northeastern areas of New South Wales.[21] In total 10 serotypes (1, 2, 3, 7, 9, 15, 16, 20, 21, and 23) have been isolated in the country. Six of these (3, 9, 15, 16, 20, and 23) have only been found in the north of the Northern Territory. Since 2008, BTV-2 has been detected in northern and eastern Australia, in regions in which only serotypes 1 and 21 had been recorded previously.[21] The virus has been isolated from infected *Culicoides* and sentinel animals, and although there is serologic evidence of infection in Queensland and New South Wales, there has been no clinical disease. In **Africa**, 22 of the known 26 serotypes have been identified. Serotypes 1, 16, 18, 19, and 24 are the predominant serotypes isolated, and serotypes 20, 21, 25 and 26 are considered exotic.[22] In **Asia**, serotypes 1, 4, 7, 9, 10, 12, 16, 17, 20, 21, and 23 have been identified. The new serotype 26 was recently identified in Kuwait.[4] Serotypes 1, 2, 4, 6, 8, 9, 11, and 16 are associated with disease in the expansion of BTV infection in **Europe** since 1998. BTV serotype 8 is the strain associated with repeated BTV outbreaks observed between 2006 and 2008 affecting most of central and northern Europe, including the United Kingdom and parts of Scandinavia.[23] Serotypes 6 and 11 isolated in northern Europe in that same period have been related to vaccine strains used in modified live vaccines produced in South Africa and are thought to have been introduced through the illegal use of modified live vaccines in the region.[1] Currently, large parts of Europe are declared free of BTV. Exceptions are Spain (serotypes 1 and 4), Portugal (serotype 1), the southern part of Italy (serotypes 1, 2, 4, 8, 9, 16), Corsica (serotypes 1, 2, 4, 8, 16), the Channel Islands (serotypes 1, 8), Cyprus (serotypes 4 and 6), and the Greek islands of Lesbos, Dodekanisa, and Samos (serotypes 1, 4, 8, 16).[6]

Host Risk Factors

Although all ruminant species are susceptible to infection with BTV, most virulent strains cause clinical disease primarily in sheep, whereas infection often remains asymptomatic in the majority of infected cattle, goats, and wild ruminants.

Cattle

Although some BTV strains, such as serotype 8, can cause severe clinical disease in cattle, infection with most other virulent BTV strains remains subclinical or causes only mild clinical signs in this species. Cattle are therefore considered the **reservoir and amplifying host** and have a high titer viremia. Cattle appear to be much more attractive to *Culicoides* spp., and this may enhance the importance of cattle as carriers. A **critical density** of cattle in a region may be required to sustain bluetongue in regions where the *Culicoides* vector is strongly cattle associated. Seroprevalence increases with age, probably a reflection of increased duration of exposure.

Sheep

All breeds of sheep are susceptible to infection, although to varying degrees. **European fine-wool and mouton breeds** are most susceptible to severe clinical disease. There are also differences in age susceptibility to clinical disease, which, inexplicably, vary with different outbreaks. Exposure to **solar radiation** can increase the severity of the disease, as can excessive droving, shearing, poor nutrition, and other forms of stress.

Goats and Wild Ruminants

Goats, like other ruminant species, are susceptible to infection but rarely show clinical signs. Among wild ruminants, **white-tailed deer** and pronghorn antelopes were found to be highly susceptible to infection resulting in clinical disease. Surveys conducted throughout Europe during the epidemic caused by BTV serotype 8 documented the broad susceptibility to infection of the wild ruminant population.[24,25]

New World Camelids

Evidence for natural infection of South American camelids with different BTV serotypes is available from Peru, the Unites States, and Europe, where seroconversion in unvaccinated animals has been reported.[26-28] Following the recent BTV-8 outbreak in northern and central Europe, a mean animal seroprevalence of 14.3% of the tested New World camelid population was reported in Germany, a value that is considerably below prevalence rates determined in other ruminant species in the same region.[28] Historically, South American camelids were considered to be resistant to clinical bluetongue, but incidental case fatalities that have been associated with BTV infection have been reported in the recent literature.[29-31]

Morbidity and Case Fatality

When the disease occurs in a flock for the first time, the incidence of clinical disease may reach 50% to 75% and the mortality 20% to 50%. Outbreaks in Cyprus and Spain were accompanied by mortality rates of 70% in affected flocks, but most outbreaks result in much lower mortality. Mortality rates of 2% to 30% are reported under field conditions in South Africa and from 0% to 14% in field outbreaks in the United States. High mortality can occur when a new strain of BTV emerges in an area.

Before the occurrence of BTV-8 in northern and central Europe, bluetongue in cattle was considered a predominantly subclinical disease, and clinical cases were observed sporadically only. During the European BTV-8 outbreak between 2006 and 2008, morbidity rates ranging from 0% to 32% were reported. Mortality ranged between 0% and 17% in sheep and 0% and 4% in cattle.[32]

Immunity to BTV tends to be strain specific, and in epizootics, more than one strain may be introduced into an area. Infections caused by different serotypes may follow one another in quick succession in a sheep population. The serotypes vary widely in their virulence, with a corresponding variation in the severity of the disease produced. However, sequential infection with more than one type of BTV results in the development of heterotypic antibody and may result in protection against heterologous serotypes not previously encountered.

Experimental Reproduction

Infection is readily produced by experimental infection of sheep, cattle, and New World camelids, but it is common for the clinical presentation of the experimental disease to be **very mild** despite the fact that the isolate might have been associated with severe disease in the field. In many cases experimental infection produces viremia, fever, leukopenia, and an antibody response, but the localizing, identifying lesions are often minimal, with erythema of the coronary bands as the only visible abnormality in some cases.

Economic Importance

Economic losses from bluetongue are attributable to direct effects of the infection, such as animal losses and abortion, to which costs associated with treatment and disease control have to be added. Production losses are also of great importance in sheep and cattle alike. Adult sheep either lose their fleece from a break in the growth of the staple or develop a weakness (tender wool) that causes breaks in processing and markedly reduces the value of the fleece. Pregnant ewes commonly abort. There is a severe loss of condition, and convalescence is prolonged, particularly in lambs. The loss from clinical disease and from reduced wool quality and suboptimal production following infection in sheep are significant. Production losses associated with the BTV-8 outbreak in Europe affecting the dairy industry were estimated to be considerably higher compared with sheep in part because of the higher value of the individual animal, but also because of the marked and sustained effect on milk production lasting for several weeks (up to 2 kg per cow and day) and the increased incidence of reproductive failures.[33]

Major financial losses result from **restrictions in international trade**. The severe disease that occurred in the outbreaks in Cyprus and the Iberian Peninsula in the 1940s and 1950s resulted in bluetongue being placed on List A of veterinary diseases by the OIE. At the time, persistent infection of ruminants resulting in carrier animals was thought to be a major factor explaining the worldwide spread of the disease; as a result, restrictions on the international movement of cattle and sheep and their products from countries that have this infection to those that do not have been instituted. For countries where BTV virus is endemic and clinical disease is rare, such as the United States, costs resulting from these trade restrictions by far outweigh direct costs related to the disease. It is estimated that the United States has an annual loss of $144 million because of the inability to trade with BTV-free countries.

PATHOGENESIS

Sheep

The pathology of bluetongue can be attributed to vascular endothelial damage resulting in changes to capillary permeability and fragility, with subsequent disseminated intravascular coagulation and necrosis of tissues supplied by damaged capillaries. These changes result in edema, congestion, hemorrhage, inflammation, and necrosis.

Following inoculation of the virus through the skin by a bite of an infected vector, the virus reaches the regional lymph node, where a first replication occurs. The virus that targets all blood cells and thrombocytes is then disseminated by these cells throughout the entire organism. Secondary virus replication takes place in lymphoid tissues such as the lymph nodes and spleen and particularly in the lungs. Viremia is detectable by day 3, and peak viremia, associated with fever and leukopenia, usually occurs 6 to 7 days after infection. Circulating virus concentrations subsequently fall with the appearance of circulating interferon and specific neutralizing antibodies. With the viremia, there is localization of the virus in vascular endothelium, which causes endothelial cell degeneration and necrosis with thrombosis and hemorrhage. There is also the development of a hemorrhagic diathesis and coagulation changes consistent with disseminated intravascular coagulation. The distribution of the lesions is thought to be influenced by mechanical stress and the lower temperatures of these areas in relation to the rest of the body.

Cattle and Wild Ruminants

With infection in cattle and wild ruminants by most virus strains, endothelial cell damage is minimal. The viremia in cattle is highly cell associated, particularly with erythrocytes and platelets. Although the virus does not replicate in the erythrocytes, it is protected from circulating neutralizing antibody, and infected erythrocytes are likely to circulate for their life span. With the life span of bovine erythrocytes being longer than that of ovine erythrocytes, this results in the prolonged viremia in cattle with concomitant presence of neutralizing antibodies. Although virus RNA may be detectable for up to 140 days after infection, the viremic phase (i.e., period of presence of infectious virus in blood) rarely exceeds 60 days. Viremic phases of up to 100 days have been reported incidentally.[10] Before the BTV-8 outbreak in Europe, sporadic clinical cases observed in cattle were thought to be the result of type I hypersensitivity reaction triggered by repeated exposure to virus-specific IgE.

In white-tailed deer, which are highly susceptible to bluetongue, disseminated intravascular coagulopathy (DIC) develops as a result of BTV-induced vascular damage. Affected animals develop potentially life-threatening hemorrhagic diathesis.[15]

CLINICAL FINDINGS

Sheep

Naturally occurring florid bluetongue in sheep has the following clinical characteristics. After an incubation period of less than a week, a severe febrile reaction with a maximum temperature of 40.5° to 41°C (105–106°F) is usual, although afebrile cases may occur. The **fever** continues for 5 or 6 days. About 48 hours after the temperature rise, nasal discharge and salivation, with reddening of the buccal and nasal mucosae, are apparent. The **nasal discharge** is mucopurulent and often blood stained, and the saliva is frothy. Swelling and edema of the lips, gums, dental pad, and tongue occur, and there may be involuntary movement of the lips. **Excoriation** of the buccal mucosa follows, the saliva becomes blood stained, and the mouth has an offensive odor.

Lenticular necrotic ulcers develop, particularly on the lateral aspects of the tongue, which may be swollen and purple in color, but more commonly is not. **Hyperemia** and ulceration are also common at the commissures of the lips, on the buccal papillae, and around the anus and vulva. Swallowing is often difficult for the animal. Respiration is obstructed and stertorous and is increased in rate up to 100/min. Diarrhea and dysentery may occur.

Foot lesions, including **laminitis** and **coronitis** and manifested by lameness and recumbency, appear only in some animals, usually when the mouth lesions begin to heal. The appearance of a dark-red to purple band in the skin just above the coronet, as a result of coronitis, is an important diagnostic sign. **Wryneck**, with twisting of the head and neck to one side, occurs in a few cases, appearing suddenly around day 12. This is apparently attributable to the direct action of the virus on muscle tissue, as is the pronounced muscle stiffness and weakness, which is severe enough to prevent eating. There is a marked and rapid loss of condition. There is **facial swelling** with extensive swelling and drooping of the ears, and hyperemia of the nonwooled skin may be present. Some affected sheep show severe conjunctivitis, accompanied by profuse lacrimation. A break occurs in the staple of the fleece. Vomiting and secondary aspiration pneumonia may also occur. Death in most fatal cases occurs about 6 days after the appearance of signs.

In animals that recover, there is a **long convalescence,** and a return to normal may take several months. Partial or complete loss of the **fleece** is common and causes great financial loss for the farmer. Other signs during convalescence include separation or cracking of the hooves and wrinkling and cracking of the skin around the lips and muzzle. Although the subsequent birth of lambs with porencephaly and cerebral necrosis is usually recorded after vaccination with attenuated virus, it also occurs rarely after natural infections.

In sheep in **enzootic areas**, the disease is much less severe and often inapparent. Two syndromes occur: (i) an abortive form in which the febrile reaction is not followed by local lesions and (ii) a subacute type in which the local lesions are minimal, but emaciation, weakness, and extended convalescence are severe. A similar syndrome occurs in lambs, which become infected when colostral immunity is on the wane.

Cattle

Most infections are inapparent, although some BTV strains, such as serotype 8, are highly virulent in cattle. Affected animals may develop a clinical syndrome not unlike that seen in severely affected sheep. The incubation period was estimated to be between 6 and 8 days. Although fever in the range of 40° to 41° C (104–106° F) is often but not consistently observed, affected animals are lethargic and show anorexia and a drop in milk production. Skin and mucosal lesions on the muzzle, oral cavity, and tongue develop in early stages of the disease. Lesions are characterized by ulceration, necrosis, and eventually by superficial crusting. Mucopurulent and sometimes blood-tinged nasal discharge and fetid breath is a common finding. Hypersalivation and regurgitation are often observed. Skin lesions with erythema, ulcers, and necrosis can be found on the udder skin, on and around the coronary band, and sometimes around the eyes. Localized distal limb edema contributes to the observed reluctance to move of affected animals. Photodermatitis may develop at later stages of the disease (2–3 weeks after infection) on unpigmented skin. Contraction of the infection during early pregnancy may cause abortion, stillbirth, or **congenital deformities,** including hydranencephaly, microcephaly, arthrogryposis, blindness, and deformity of the jaw.

During the viremic phase, infected bulls are likely to shed virus in semen. The presence of BTV in the **semen** of bulls is accompanied by structural abnormalities of the spermatozoa and by the presence of virus particles in them.

Goats

Infected goats show very little response clinically. There is a mild to moderate fever and hyperemia of the mucosae and conjunctivae. BTV infections in deer produce an acute disease that is clinically and pathologically identical to epizootic hemorrhagic disease of deer and characterized by multiple hemorrhages throughout the body.

New World Camelids

Although New World camelids were considered to be resistant to clinical disease associated with BTV, several reports of clinical disease with fatal outcome have been published in the recent literature.[29-31] Common to all reports is that only individual animals of a flock were affected while the rest of the flock remained clinically healthy. Common clinical findings were a rapid onset with anorexia, lethargy, and rapidly progressing respiratory distress. In most cases animals became recumbent and died within 24 hours of first clinical signs. Postmortem findings were severe alveolar edema of the lungs, hydrothorax, and hydropericardia, and severe congestion of the liver, spleen, and kidneys. In one case abortion was reported, and virus RNA was retrieved in fetal tissue.[30]

Experimental infection studies and epidemiologic field survey suggest that New World camelids are susceptible to infection, showing seroconversion, but only very rarely show clinical signs of disease.[26,34]

Wild Ruminants

Among wild ruminants, **white-tailed deer** were found to be most susceptible to bluetongue. Clinical presentation resembles the epizootic hemorrhagic disease of deer. Acute cases are characterized by **hemorrhagic diathesis** resulting from disseminated intravascular coagulopathy (DIC). Affected animals have widespread hemorrhages throughout the body, bloody diarrhea, swelling of head and neck, and blood-stained nasal discharge.

CLINICAL PATHOLOGY

There is a fall in packed cell volume and initial leukopenia followed by leukocytosis. In severe disease there is marked leukopenia, largely as a result of lymphopenia. Infected cattle show a similar manifestation of leukopenia. The skeletal myopathy that occurs in this disease is reflected by a rise in creatine phosphokinase.

Specific diagnosis is either by isolation of the virus, detection of viral antigen or nucleic acid, or detection of specific antibodies in serum. Serologic assays can detect prior exposure to BTV but cannot establish if the animal is viremic, which is currently still important for movement decisions concerning cattle.

Material that can be used for virus isolation include heparin or EDTA blood; biopsies or postmortem tissue samples of the spleen, lung, lymph nodes, liver, and bone marrow; and, when indicated, heart or skeletal muscle tissue and brain tissue of aborted or stillborn fetuses.

Virus Isolation

Virus isolation commonly is carried out by tissue culture or culture in embryonated chicken eggs (ECEs). Material obtained from inoculated chick embryos can either directly be examined (e.g., by using molecular methods such as PCR or in vitro hybridization) or be further propagated in cell cultures. Cell lines used for this purpose can be of insect origin, such as the KC cell lines derived from *Culicoides sonorensis* or mammalian cell lines such as the baby hamster kidney cells (BHK), calf pulmonary artery endothelium cells (CPAE), or African green monkey kidney cells (Vero). The cytopathic effect produced by BTV is only observed in cell lines of mammalian origin. Virus identification from cell cultures can then be conducted by methods such as immunofluorescence and immunoperoxidase assays using BTV-specific monoclonal antibodies. Virus isolation is the most reliable confirmation of BTV infection because there are difficulties with the interpretation of serologic test results. However, traditional isolation methods require 2 to 4 weeks.

Less commonly, diagnosis is by inoculation of blood into susceptible sheep, a method that is considered as one of the most sensitive and reliable methods of BTV isolation. A positive test depends on the appearance of clinical signs and/or the mounting of a BTV-specific antibody response. This method is used occasionally with samples containing very low virus titers but has widely been replaced by ECE inoculation.

Detection of Antigen or Nucleic Acid

Immunohistochemical tests, including immunofluorescence, immunoperoxidase, and immunoelectron microscopic techniques using monoclonal antibody, can be used for rapid sensitive and specific detection of antigen. In situ nucleic acid hybridization and reverse-transcription polymerase chain reaction (**RT-PCR**) can be used for detection of the virus even after the viremic phase. This method has the advantage of speed over tissue culture virus isolation and can also differentiate between wild-type isolates and vaccine strains. Tests that detect viral RNA prove exposure to the virus but do not necessarily indicate that infectious virus is still present.

Serologic Tests

Serologic tests for detection of either group-reactive antibodies or serotype-specific antibodies are available. The commonly available tests include the complement fixation test (CFT), the agar gel immunodiffusion test (AGID), a number of different ELISA tests, and serum neutralization (SN). The **AGID test** is easy to perform and inexpensive but is also relatively **insensitive** and detects cross-reacting antibodies to other orbiviruses. Over the last decades the CFT and AGID have been replaced in many laboratories by the more rapid, sensitive, and specific competitive ELISA.

Numerous ELISA tests have been developed using group-specific monoclonal antibodies and present valuable alternatives to the AGID for routine diagnosis and international trade. The **competitive ELISA (c-ELISA)**, which is the most sensitive and highly specific group-specific test, is the preferred test for serodiagnosis of bluetongue. The c-ELISA cannot differentiate between infection and vaccination with modified life vaccines but is ideally suited to identify seroconversion in an unvaccinated population or to monitor the efficiency of a vaccination campaign in noninfected animals.

The **serum neutralization test (SNT)** is serotype specific and thus allows differentiation between antibodies against specific BTV serotypes. The biological detection system (either ECE or cell cultures) is reacted with a reference serum for specific BTV serotypes, and the amount of virus neutralization is determined. Although the SNT is highly sensitive and specific, it is also expensive and time consuming and is therefore not used as routine diagnostic procedure.

NECROPSY FINDINGS

Sheep

Sheep dying from bluetongue show edematous face and ears and a dry, crusty exudate on the nostrils and the conjunctiva. The coronary bands of the hooves are often hyperemic, and hemorrhages may extend down to the horn. The oral mucosa is usually cyanotic or hemorrhagic, with erosions and ulcers commonly affecting the tongue and dental part and sometimes extending to the rumen and abomasum. Acute cases will show subcutaneous and intermuscular edema, which may be serous or suffused with blood; the lesion is most marked in the head, neck, and abdominal regions. There may be serous effusions in the pleura, pericardium, and peritoneum. A characteristic and almost pathognomonic lesion for bluetongue is hemorrhage at the base of the pulmonary artery. Foci of muscle necrosis may be present in the heart, esophagus, pharynx, and other muscles. There may be aspiration pneumonia secondary to damaged esophageal/pharyngeal musculature, or the lungs may be diffusely edematous, especially when there are cardiac lesions.

The outcome of fetal infection in both sheep and cattle is age-dependent, with distinctive cavitating lesions of the brain (hydranencephaly or porencephaly) in fetuses that survive infection during early gestation, whereas fetuses infected in late gestation may be born viremic but without brain malformations.[35]

Cattle

Mortality is less common in cattle. Lesions can include severe and extensive ulceration of the muzzle, oral mucosa, and teats; rhinitis and mucohemorrhagic nasal discharge; epiphora and periocular inflammation; and limb edema and interdigital necrosis and ulceration.[35] In some cases, the skin is ulcerated or eroded with a dry, crusty exudate, or it may have thick folds, particularly in the neck region. The coronary band is often hyperemic, and there may be pulmonary edema and serous effusion into body cavities. As in sheep, infected fetuses may develop central nervous lesions depending on the strain of the virus and the stage of gestation when infected. Several cases of congenital hydranencephaly and other anomalies were reported in calves during the initial outbreaks of BTV serotype 8 in Europe.[35,36]

Microscopically, bluetongue virus infection in sheep and cattle is characterized by thrombosis and widespread microvascular damage leading to hemorrhage, edema, myodegeneration, and necrosis. Inflammation is mild.

Samples for Confirmation of Diagnosis

- **Histology**—fixed oral and mucocutaneous lesions, abomasum, pulmonary artery, skeletal muscle from a variety of sites, left ventricular papillary muscle; brain from aborted fetus (light microscopy, immunohistochemistry)
- **Virology**—chilled lung, spleen; CNS tissues, thoracic fluid from aborted fetus (ISO, PCR, in situ hybridization, ELISA, etc.)

DIFFERENTIAL DIAGNOSIS
Foot-and-mouth disease
Epizootic hemorrhagic disease (wild ruminants)
Contagious ecthyma (sheep)
Sheep pox (sheep)
Bovine viral diarrhea/mucosal disease (cattle)
Malignant catarrhal fever (cattle)
Acute photodermatitis (cattle)
Bovine herpes mammillitis (cattle)

TREATMENT

There is currently no specific treatment for bluetongue available. Symptomatic and supportive treatment should be considered to provide relief. Local irrigations with mild disinfectant solutions may afford some relief. Affected sheep should be housed and protected from weather, particularly hot sun, and fluid and electrolyte therapy and treatment to control secondary infection may be desirable.

CONTROL

Reduction of Infection Through Vector Abatement

Attempts to control bluetongue through a reduction of infection consist of reducing the risk of exposure to infected *Culicoides* and reduction in *Culicoides* numbers. Neither is particularly effective.

Reducing the risk of exposure is attempted by spraying cattle and sheep with repellents and insecticides and housing sheep at night. Biweekly application of permethrin was found not to be effective in preventing infection.

During transmission periods, avoidance of low, marshy areas or moving sheep to higher altitudes may reduce risk. Because of the preference of some *Culicoides* for cattle as a host, cattle have been run in close proximity to sheep to act as vector decoys. Widespread spraying for *Culicoides* control is not usually practical and has only a short-term effect.

There is a high mortality in *Culicoides* that fed on cattle that have been treated with a standard anthelmintic dose of ivermectin and also a larvicidal effect in manure passed for the next 28 days for *Culicoides* that breed in dung.

Movement of ruminants from areas where specific BTV strains are circulating to regions where this serotype does not occur should only be considered after confirmation of absence of viremia.

Vaccination

Vaccination is the only satisfactory control procedure once the disease has been introduced into an area. Vaccination will not prevent or eliminate infection, but it is successful in keeping losses to a very low level, provided immunity to all local strains of the virus is attained. Current vaccines are usually **polyvalent attenuated** virus vaccines and are in use in South Africa and Israel and available in other countries. These vaccines have been used in South Africa for more than 50 years, and they are known to induce effective and long-lasting immunity.

Reactions to vaccination are slight, but ewes should not be vaccinated within 3 weeks of mating because anestrus often results. **Annual revaccination** 1 month before the expected occurrence of the disease is recommended. Immunity is present 10 days after vaccination, and thus early vaccination during an outbreak may substantially reduce losses. Lambs from immune mothers may be able to neutralize the attenuated virus and fail to be immunized, whereas field strains may overcome their passive immunity. In enzootic areas, it may therefore be necessary to postpone lambing until major danger from the disease is passed, and lambs should not be vaccinated until 2 weeks after weaning. Rams should be vaccinated before mating time.

Live attenuated vaccines should not be used in **pregnant ewes** because of the risk of congenital defects in the lambs or embryonic death. The danger period is between the 4th and 8th weeks of pregnancy, with the greatest incidence of deformities occurring when vaccination is carried out in ewes pregnant for 5 to 6 weeks. The incidence of congenital defects may be as high as 13%, with an average of 5%. Abortions do not occur, although some lambs are stillborn.

The preparation and use of **attenuated vaccines** against BTV is **problematic**. The neutralizing epitopes are highly conserved on some serotypes, but they are highly plastic on others. It is therefore necessary to continually monitor the identity and prevalence of the serotypes that need to be in the vaccine.

There are also concerns for the use of attenuated live vaccines to control insect-borne diseases because of the risk of the vaccine strain being transmitted, of being exalted in virulence by passage, and of recombinants resulting in the development of new virus strains with unwanted characteristics. There is evidence for the emergence of a **reassortment strain** from a vaccine virus in the United States and Europe and suspicion of occurrence elsewhere. However, attenuated live vaccines are used for practical reasons, including the fact that inactivated vaccines do not provide protection against infection. The difficulty in obtaining safe vaccines may be overcome by the use of recombinant DNA technologies. There is also good reason to suggest that cattle should be a major target of vaccination for bluetongue control.

International Movement of Livestock

Countries that are free of BTV infection have traditionally erected barriers to avoid its introduction by prohibiting the importation of any ruminant animals from countries where the disease occurs. Others have less severe restrictions, and several procedures aimed at permitting limited movement are in force; their stringency varies with the importing country. Some countries only require a negative serologic test or series of tests before movement. Others require a negative test in conjunction with a period of quarantine. The introduction of bovine **semen** from low-risk areas after suitable tests of donors and a prolonged storage period is accepted by most countries. Most countries allow the importation of **embryos**.

A more enlightened understanding of the epidemiology of bluetongue will probably result in a reevaluation of these requirements in the future, including regionalization within a country to allow exports from areas where there is no prevalence or transmission.

FURTHER READING

Dal Pozzo F, et al. Bovine infection with bluetongue virus with special emphasis on European serotype 8. *Vet J*. 2009;182:142-151.

Gibbs EPJ. Bluetongue: an analysis of current problems with particular reference to importation of ruminants to the USA. *J Am Vet Med Assoc*. 1983;182:1190-1194.

MacLachlan NJ. The pathology and pathogenesis of bluetongue. *J Comp Path*. 2009;141:1-16.

MacLachlan NJ, Osburn BI. Impact of bluetongue virus infection on the international movement and trade of ruminants. *J Am Vet Med Assoc*. 2006;228:1346-1349.

Mellor PS, Boorman J, Baylis M. *Culicoides* biting midges: their role as arbovirus vectors. *Ann Rev Entomol*. 2000;45:307-340.

Osburn BI. Bluetongue virus. *Vet Clin North Am Food A*. 1994;103:547-560.

Purse BV, et al. Climate change and the recent emergence of bluetongue in Europe. *Nature Rev Microbial*. 2005;3:171-181.

Roy P, Gorman BM. Bluetongue viruses. *Curr Top Microbiol Immunol*. 1990;162:1-200.

Savini G, et al. Vaccines against bluetongue in Europe. *Comp Immunol Microbiol Infect Dis*. 2008;31:101-120.

Wilson AJ, Mellor PS. Bluetongue in Europe: past, present and future. *Phil Trans R Soc B*. 2009;364:2669-2681.

REFERENCES

1. Wilson AJ, Mellor PS. *Phil Trans R Soc*. 2009;364:2669.
2. Hofmann MA, et al. *Emerg Infect Dis*. 2008;14:1855.
3. Chaignat V, et al. *Vet Microbiol*. 2009;138:11.
4. Maan S, et al. *Emerg Infect Dis*. 2011;17:886.
5. Saegerman C, et al. *Emerg Infect Dis*. 2008;14:539.
6. European Commission. 2013 at: <http://ec.europa.eu/food/animal/diseases/controlmeasures/bt_restrictedzones-map_2012.jpg>; Accessed 03.08.13.
7. Lysyk TJ, Danyk TJ. *Med Entomol*. 2007;44:741.
8. Losson B, et al. *Vet Rec*. 2007;160:451.
9. Dal Pozzo F, et al. *Vet J*. 2009;182:142.
10. Sperlova A, Zendulkova D. *Vet Medicina*. 2011;56:430.
11. De Clercq K, et al. *Vet Rec*. 2008;162:564.
12. Desnecht D, et al. *Vet Rec*. 2008;163:50.
13. EFSA. 2013 at: <http://www.efsa.europa.eu/en/efsajournal/doc/2189.pdf>; Accessed 03.08.13.
14. van der Sluis M, et al. *Vet Microbiol*. 2011;149:113.
15. MacLachlan NJ, et al. *J Comp Pathol*. 2009;141:1.
16. Van Soom A, Nauwynck HJCAB. *Rev Persp Ag Vet Sci Nutr Nat Res*. 2008;2(60).
17. Menzies FD, et al. *Vet Rec*. 2008;163:203.
18. Mayo CE, et al. *Transbound Emerg Dis*. 2010;57:277.
19. Backx A, et al. *Vet Microbiol*. 2009;38:235.
20. Animal Health Australia. 2013 at: <http://namp.animalhealthaustralia.com.au/public.php?page=namp_public&program=2>; Accessed 03.08.13.
21. Boyle DB, et al. *J Virol*. 2012;86:6724.
22. Coetzee P, et al. *Virol J*. 2012;9:198.
23. McLachlan NJ. *Prev Vet Med*. 2011;102:107.
24. Linden A, et al. *Vet Rec*. 2008;162:459.
25. Ruiz-Fons F, et al. *Emerg Infect Dis*. 2008;14:951.
26. Rivera A, et al. *Am J Vet Res*. 1987;48:189.
27. Mattson DE. *Vet Clin North Am Food A*. 1994;10:341.
28. Schulz C, et al. *Vet Microbiol*. 2012;160:35.
29. Heinrich M, et al. *Vet Rec*. 2007;161:764.
30. Meyer G, et al. *Emerg Infect Dis*. 2009;15:608.
31. Ortega J, et al. *J Vet Diagn Invest*. 2010;22:134.
32. Elbers ARW, et al. *Prev Vet Med*. 2009;92:1.
33. Nusinovici S, et al. *J Dairy Sci*. 2013;96:877.
34. Schulz C, et al. *Vet Microbiol*. 2011;154:257.
35. Maclachlan NJ, et al. *J Com Path*. 2009;141:1.
36. Vercauteren G, et al. *Transbound Emerg Dis*. 2008;55:293.

MALIGNANT CATARRHAL FEVER (BOVINE MALIGNANT CATARRH, MALIGNANT HEAD CATARRH)

SYNOPSIS

Etiology Alcelaphine herpesvirus-1, the wildebeest-associated malignant catarrhal fever (MCF) virus; ovine herpesvirus-2, the sheep-associated MCF virus

Epidemiology Highly fatal disease of cattle, farmed deer, and bison in the United States; Bali cattle (Banteng) in Indonesia; and occasionally pigs but rarely goats. Disease associated with contact with sheep, often weaned lambs, and in Africa also with wildebeest calves. Disease may occur sporadically or in outbreaks.

Clinical findings Fever, ocular and nasal discharge, erosive stomatitis and gastroenteritis, erosions in the upper respiratory tract, keratoconjunctivitis, encephalitis, cutaneous exanthema, and lymph node enlargement. The head and eye form is most common, and there is a distinctive lesion in the cornea.

Clinical pathology Competitive inhibition enzyme-linked immunosorbent assay (ELISA) for serology. Polymerase chain reaction (PCR) detection of viral DNA.

Necropsy findings Lymphoproliferative disorder involving dysregulation of T-lymphocytes. Erosions in gastrointestinal tract and lymphadenopathy. Necrotizing vasculitis.

Diagnostic confirmation. Detection of viral DNA by PCR.

Treatment Supportive.

Control Avoid cattle having contact with sheep and wildebeest.

ETIOLOGY

Malignant catarrhal fever (MCF) is really two diseases, clinically and pathologically indistinguishable, but associated with two different infectious agents with different ecologies:

- Alcelaphine herpesvirus-1 (AlHV1) is now allocated to a new genus *Macavirus* (previously known as *Rhadinovirus*) of the subfamily Gammaherpesvirinae in the family Herpesviridae. This is the **wildebeest-associated MCF virus,** transmitted to cattle from blue wildebeest (*Connochaetes taurinus*).
- Ovine herpesvirus-2 (OvHV2) is also a *Macavirus* of the subfamily Gammaherpesvirinae. This is the **sheep-associated MCF virus** transmitted to cattle from sheep.

Neither agent appears to transmit from cattle to cattle, and neither of the viruses causes any disease in the principal hosts, the wildebeest and the sheep. AlHV1 can be grown in eggs and tissue culture, but OvHV2 has never been propagated in vitro. The molecular genomic structure of these viruses is described. A gammaherpesvirus closely related to OvHV2 has been isolated from goats and called caprine herpesvirus-2 (CpHV2), and another, also closely related, has been isolated from deer and called deer herpesvirus (DVH). The pathogenicity of these newly recognized viruses is not known. Complete genome sequences of AlHV1 (130,608 base pairs) and OvHV2 (135,621 base pairs) have been published.[1]

EPIDEMIOLOGY

Occurrence and Prevalence

The broad range of natural hosts for MCF can be divided into two categories: reservoir hosts (sheep, goats, wildebeest) and clinically susceptible hosts (cattle, bison, deer).[2]

Alcelaphine MCF

Wildebeest-associated MCF occurs in most African countries in cattle that commingle with clinically normal wildebeest and hartebeest. It is epizootic and seasonal. It can also occur in zoologic gardens in other countries.

Sheep-Associated MCF

Sheep-associated MCF occurs worldwide. Cases mostly occur when cattle have had contact with lambing ewes and usually start 1 to 2 months later. Goats can also act as a source of OvHV2 infection for cattle, and rare reports of clinical disease in goats exist.[3] Cases without apparent or recent exposure to sheep do occur but are uncommon.

The morbidity rate varies. Usually the disease is sporadic and presents as a single or small number of cases over a short period, but on occasion up to 50% of a herd may be affected in rare but devastating outbreaks that may be short-lived or last for several months. The disease with both agents is **almost always fatal, with rare reports of recovery in cattle.**

Besides cattle, MCF is also an important disease of farmed deer. It is an occasional disease of pigs and is recorded in pigs that had contact with sheep on a farm and in a petting zoo.

Methods of Transmission

Both AlHV1 and OvHV2 appear to be transmitted by contact or aerosol, primarily from respiratory secretions of wildebeest calves (AlHV1) and weaned lambs (OvHV2) under 1 year of age. Nose-to-nose contact appears to provide the most efficient method of spread, but transmission can also occur via fomites.[4] The MCF-susceptible species are thought to be dead-end hosts that do not shed virus and are therefore not infectious. Acute MCF in cattle is caused by either AlHV1 or OvHV2, with almost all cases in North American cattle being caused by OvHV2.

Alcelaphine MCF

Infection with AlHV1 in wildebeest occurs in the perinatal period by horizontal and occasional intrauterine transmission, and infected young wildebeest up to the age of about 4 months have viremia and shed virus in ocular and nasal secretions. The disease is transmitted from wildebeest to cattle by contact or over short distances, probably by inhalation of aerosol or ingestion of pasture contaminated by virus excreted by young wildebeest in nasal and ocular discharges. In contrast, infected cattle do not excrete virus in nasal or ocular secretions. The disease can transmit between wildebeest and cattle over a distance of at least 100 m, and it is suggested that cattle need to be kept at least 1 km from wildebeest to avoid disease.

In Kenya the peak incidence of alcelaphine MCF occurs when 3- to 4-month-old wildebeest are in maximum numbers. In South Africa the peak incidence is at a time when young wildebeest are 8 to 10 months old and not infectious, requiring that there be another, high-volume source of the infection. The proportion of sheep in a wildebeest area that are serologically positive and presumably infected with the wildebeest-associated virus is very high.

Sheep-Associated MCF

Virtually all domestic sheep raised under natural flock conditions are infected with OvHV2, which causes an inapparent infection in sheep. **High rates of seropositivity** have been found in domestic sheep and goats over 1 year of age in several surveys. In a study of 14 species of North American wildlife, a high rate of seropositivity was also found in muskox (*Ovibos moschatus*) and bighorn sheep (*Ovis canadensis*), suggesting that they might be sources of infection. There were low seropositivity rates in clinically susceptible species such as deer and bison.

In contrast to AlHV1 infection in wildebeest, the transmission of OvHV2 between sheep appears minimal in the perinatal period. There is no evidence for transplacental infection, and although antigen, detected by PCR, is present in colostrum and milk from infected ewes, the majority of lambs are not infected until after 2 to 3 months of age. The rate of infection in lambs and the age at infection is not influenced by passively acquired maternal immunity and appears to be dose dependent. Infected sheep excrete OvHV2 in nasal secretions, but **very high levels of excretion occur between 6 and 9 months of age**, suggesting that the 6- to 9-month period is the time when most virus is shed into the environment. Viral antigen has been detected in the ejaculate of rams, but there is little epidemiologic evidence for significant venereal transmission.

The means by which OvHV2 spreads from infected sheep to cattle is not known but is presumably by inhalation or ingestion of respiratory secretions. The common epidemiologic association of diseased cattle having had contact with lambing ewes suggests that perinatal lambs play a role in transmission similar to that played by wildebeest calves; however, the age at infection of lambs and the excretion patterns of the virus do not fit this assumption. Shedding from ewes does not increase in the lambing period. Contact with ewes is not a prerequisite, one outbreak having occurred when cattle commingled with rams. Infection can also occur when sheep and cattle are housed in the same building but with no common contact through feeding or watering points.

An interesting insight into transmission is provided by a Canadian outbreak where 45/163 bison died following exposure for less than 1 day to sheep at a sale barn.[5] Bison deaths started 50 days later and peaked at 60 to 70 days after exposure to sheep, with the last death occurring 7 months after initial exposure. Despite the high mortality rate, there was no evidence of bison-to-bison transmission.

Occasional cases occur in cattle that have had no apparent contact with sheep, and the persistence of the infection in a particular feedlot, or on a particular farm, from year to year when no contact with sheep exists, is unexplained. Persistence of the virus on inanimate fomites has been suggested, but the virus is a most fragile one, and this seems unlikely. The observation that some recovered cattle show a **persistent viremia** for many months suggests that carrier cattle may be the source of these carryover infections. In addition, the virus, detected by PCR, has been demonstrated in cattle and farmed deer with no evidence of MCF disease. It is possible that stress could activate a latent infection in animals with no sheep contact.

Experimental Reproduction

Sheep-associated MCF virus does not replicate in tissue culture. It has a close association with lymphoblastoid cells, particularly large granular lymphocytes, which can be grown in tissue culture and induce MCF when injected. MCF can also be transmitted to cattle by transfusion of large volumes of blood if given within 24 hours of collection. Wildebeest-associated MCF virus can be readily transmitted by several routes. It has been adapted to grow on egg yolk sac and tissue culture, and transmission to rabbits to yolk sac to cattle has been achieved.

Environment Risk Factors

The disease shows the greatest incidence in late winter, spring, and summer months. There have been suggestions that copper deficiency or exposure to bracken fern might be environmental stressors that predispose the expression of the disease in cattle.

Animal Risk Factors

Clinical disease had been described in over 30 species of ruminants. In Africa, assorted **wild ruminants** contract the disease and suffer a severe illness and a high mortality rate. Similar species in zoos are also commonly affected, for example, Père David's deer (*Elaphurus davidianus*) and Greater kudus (*Strepsiceros kudu*).

Among **domestic animals**, all ages, races, and breeds of cattle are equally susceptible, but banteng (*Banteng sondaicus*), buffalo (*Bubalus bubalis*), bison (*Bison bison*), and deer are more susceptible and suffer a more severe form of the disease than do commercial cattle. Bison are estimated to be approximately 1000 times more susceptible to clinical MCF than cattle.[2] Disease is recorded in captive deer or farmed deer including sika deer (*Cervus nippon*), roe deer (*Capreolus capreolus*), white-tailed deer (*Odocoileus virginianus*), rusa deer (*C. timorensis*), and red deer (*C. elaphus*).

MCF is considered one of the most important diseases of **farmed deer**. The clinical signs and necropsy findings closely resemble those of MCF in cattle, but the morbidity and mortality can be disastrously high, resulting in heavy losses for the deer farmer.

Economic Importance

Losses attributable to the disease can be catastrophic on rare individual farms. For the most part it is a nuisance because of its resemblance to mucosal disease and bluetongue and its historic resemblance to rinderpest, which has been eradicated.

PATHOGENESIS

MCF is a fatal, multisystemic disease characterized by lymphoid proliferation and infiltration and widespread **vascular** epithelial and mesothelial lesions, which are morphologically associated with lymphoid cells. CD8+ T-lymphocytes are the predominant cells associated with the vascular lesions. Involvement of the vascular adventitia accounts for the development of gross lesions, including the epithelial erosions and keratoconjunctivitis. The lymph node enlargement is a result of atypical proliferation of sinusoidal cells. The cerebromeningeal changes, usually referred to as encephalitis, are in fact a form of vasculitis. There is commonly synovitis, especially involving tibiotarsal joints, and this also is associated with a lymphoid vasculitis. It is thought that the pathogenesis of this disease is the result of direct virus–cell interactions or perhaps immune-mediated responses directed against infected cells.

CLINICAL FINDINGS

The **incubation period** in natural infection varies from 3 to 8 weeks, and after artificial infection averages 22 days (14 to 37 days). MCF is described as occurring in a number of forms, although fever, corneal edema, and oculonasal and oral lesions are almost always present in cattle with acute MCF. The forms identified are:

- Peracute
- Alimentary tract form
- Common "head-and-eye" form
- Mild form

However, these forms are all gradations, with cases being classified on the predominant clinical signs. In serial transmissions with one strain of the virus, all of these forms may be produced. The most common manifestation is the head-and-eye form.

In cattle, the presence of nasal discharge, corneal edema, fever, and lymphadenopathy is very helpful in differentiating MCF from mucosal disease or bluetongue.[6] The mean duration of clinical signs before death in one outbreak was 6 days, with a range of 1 to 26 days.[7]

Head-and-Eye Form

There is a sudden onset of the following symptoms:

- Extreme dejection
- Anorexia
- Agalactia
- High fever (41° to 41.5°C [106–107°F])
- Rapid pulse rate (100 to 120/bpm)
- Profuse mucopurulent nasal discharge
- Severe dyspnea with stertor as a result of obstruction of the nasal cavities with exudate
- Ocular discharge with variable degrees of corneal edema
- Blepharospasm and uveitis
- Congestion of scleral vessels

Superficial necrosis is evident in the anterior nasal mucosa and on the buccal mucosa. This begins as a diffuse reddening of the mucosa and is a consistent finding at about day 19 or 20 after infection. Discrete local **areas of necrosis** appear on the hard palate, gums, and gingivae. The mouth is painful at this time, and the animal moves its jaws carefully, painfully, and with a smacking sound. The mucosa as a whole is fragile and splits easily. The mouth and tongue are slippery, and the mouth is hard to open. The erosive mucosal lesions may be localized or diffuse. Lesions may occur on the following areas:

- Hard palate
- Dorsum of the tongue
- Gums below the incisors
- Commissures of the mouth
- Inside the lips

The cheek papillae inside the mouth are hemorrhagic, especially at the tips, which are later eroded. At this stage there is excessive salivation, with saliva that is ropelike and bubbly hanging from the lips. The skin of the muzzle is extensively involved, commencing with discrete patches of necrosis at the nostrils that soon coalesce, causing the entire muzzle to be covered by tenacious scabs. Similar lesions may occur at the skin–horn junction of the feet, especially at the back of the pastern. The skin of the teats, vulva, and scrotum in acute cases may slough off entirely upon touch or become covered with dry, tenacious scabs.

Nervous signs, particularly weakness in one leg, incoordination, a demented appearance, and muscle tremor, may develop very early, and nystagmus, head-pushing, paralysis, and convulsions may occur in the final stages. Trismus has been described, but it is probably a result of pain in the mouth rather than a neuromuscular spasm. There is one report in young calves where nervous signs were the predominant feature.[8]

In natural cases the superficial lymph nodes are often visibly and usually palpably enlarged. **Lymphadenopathy** is also one of the earliest, most consistent, and persistent signs of the experimental disease. The consistency of the feces varies from constipation to profuse diarrhea with dysentery. In some cases there is gross hematuria, with the red coloration most marked at the end of urination.

Odema (opacity) of the cornea is always present to some degree, commencing as a narrow, gray ring at the corneoscleral junction (perilimbal) and spreading centripetally with conjunctival and episcleral hyperemia (Fig. 21-1). Anterior uveitis (keratic precipitates, aqueous flare, fibrin deposition in the anterior chamber, hypopyon, iris hyperemia and edema, miosis) is observed in some

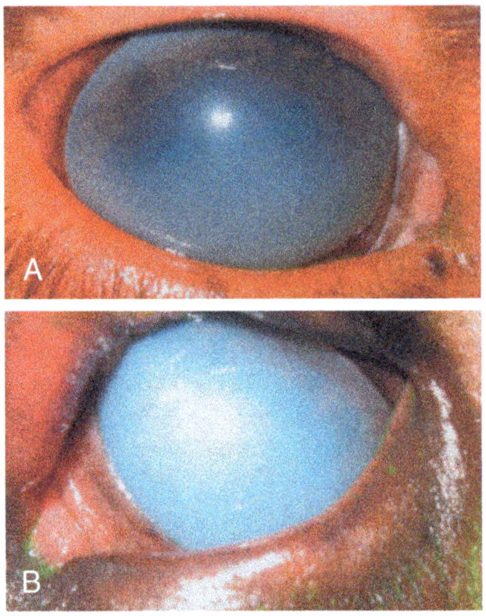

Fig. 21-1 A, The right eye of an adult cow with early clinical signs of malignant catarrhal fever. Moderate corneal edema is present. Intraocular structures can be seen but not in detail. B, The left eye of an adult cow with advanced malignant catarrhal fever. Severe corneal edema is present, and intraocular structures cannot be observed. (Reproduced with permission from Zemljič T, Pot SA, Haessig M, Spiess BM. Clinical ocular findings in cows with malignant catarrhal fever: ocular disease progression and outcome in 25 cases [2007-2010]. *Veterinary Ophthalmology* 2012; 15:46-52.)

cases. The progression of corneal edema and nonimprovement of anterior uveitis indicate that survival is unlikely.[9]

In cases of longer duration, **skin changes**, including local papule formation with clumping of the hair into tufts over the loins and withers, may occur. In addition, eczematous weeping may result in crust formation, particularly on the perineum, around the prepuce, in the axillae, and on the inside of the thighs. Infection of the cranial sinuses may occur, with pain on percussion over the area. The horns and rarely the hooves may be shed. Persistence of the fever is a characteristic of MCF, even in cases that persist for several weeks, with a fluctuating temperature that usually exceeds 39.5° C (103° F).

During some outbreaks an occasional animal makes an apparent recovery but usually dies 7 to 10 days later of acute encephalitis. In the more typical cases the illness lasts for 3 to 7 days and rarely up to 14 days.

Peracute and Alimentary Tract Forms

In the peracute form the disease runs a short course of 1 to 3 days, and characteristic signs and lesions of the head-and-eye form do not appear. There is usually a high fever, dyspnea, and acute gastroenteritis. The alimentary tract form resembles the head-and-eye form, except that there is marked diarrhea and only minor eye changes consisting of conjunctivitis rather than ophthalmia. This form of the disease has been encountered in outbreak form in cattle in large dairy herds in drylots, with only indirect contact with sheep, and in cattle to which transmission was attempted and farmed deer. A feature of this form of the disease is reported to be a brief period of slight illness followed by the final fulminating disease, which is common in deer.

Mild Form

The mild form occurs most commonly in experimental animals but is observed in natural outbreaks. There is a transient fever, and mild erosions appear on the oral and nasal mucosae. Mild disease may be followed by complete recovery, recovery with recrudescence, or chronic MCF. A distinctive clinical feature in chronic MCF is persistent bilateral ocular leukomata.

Pigs

The disease in pigs is similar to the head-and-eye form in cattle and manifests with fever and tremor, ataxia, hyperesthesia, and convulsions and death.

CLINICAL PATHOLOGY

Leukopenia, commencing at first illness and progressing to a level of 3000 to 6000/µL, has been recorded but is not a general observation. The leukopenia recorded was mainly the result of agranulocytosis. In our experience moderate leukocytosis is more common.

Virus isolation is not practical with either virus because of the instability of cell-associated AlHV1 and the fact that OvHV2 does not replicate in cell culture. **Transmission** can be used for diagnosis using whole blood, nasal swabs or washings, and preferably lymph node collected by biopsy, with histologic lesions in the recipient rabbits or calves as the criterion. **Detection of viral nucleic acid** by PCR has largely replaced transmission experiments.

There are a number of **serologic tests** that can be used, but they have limited value for diagnosis of clinical cases because only a small percentage of animals seroconvert and do so late in the course of the disease. The antibody titer is low, and there is cross-reaction with other herpes viruses. A **competitive-inhibition ELISA** using a monoclonal antibody to a broadly conserved epitope of the MCF virus can be used for detection of antibody and has largely replaced other serologic tests. It is of particular value for epidemiologic studies. The development of antibody following infection is delayed in a significant proportion of young animals, and serology is unreliable for determining infection status until after 1 year of age.

Uninfected lambs or kids under 4 months of age may test positive because of the presence of maternal antibody.

Detection of viral nucleic acid by PCR techniques is the current accepted diagnostic technique. The buffy coat is probe-positive 2 days after experimental infection with alcelaphine herpesvirus-1. Virus can be present in cattle without clinical MCF, and if these have a disease that is not MCF, but test probe positive, a **false diagnosis** is possible.

NECROPSY FINDINGS

Lesions in the mouth, nasal cavities, and pharynx vary from minor degrees of hemorrhage and erythema through extensive, severe inflammation to discrete ulcers. These lesions may be shallow and almost imperceptible or deeper and covered by cheesy diphtheritic deposits. **Erosion** of the tips of the cheek papillae, especially at the commissures, is common. Longitudinal, shallow erosions are present in the esophagus. The mucosa of the forestomaches may exhibit erythema or sparse hemorrhages or erosions. Similar but more extensive lesions occur in the abomasum. Catarrhal enteritis of moderate degree and swelling and ulceration of the Peyer's patches are constant. The feces may be loose and blood stained.

Similar lesions to those in the mouth and nasal cavities are present in the trachea and sometimes in the bronchi, but the lungs are not usually involved except for occasional emphysema or secondary pneumonia. The liver is swollen, and severe hemorrhage may be visible in the urinary bladder. All lymph nodes are swollen, edematous, and often hemorrhagic. The gross ocular lesions are as described clinically. Petechial hemorrhages and congestion may be visible in brain and meninges.

Histologically, MCF is characterized by perivascular mononuclear cell cuffing in most organs and by degeneration and erosion of affected epithelium. The pathognomonic lesion is a **necrotizing vasculitis** that features infiltration of the tunica media and adventitia by lymphoblast-like cells and macrophages. Acidophilic, intracytoplasmic inclusion bodies in neurons have been described, but their identity as viral inclusions has not been established. Large numbers of inclusion bodies have been observed in the tissue of artificially infected rabbits. The histologic features of the panophthalmitis have been described.

Cattle with chronic MCF have chronic bilateral central stromal keratitis with or without corneal pigmentation. An **obliterative arteriopathy** is characteristic, and this vascular lesion is present in all major organs. Results of a competitive inhibition ELISA serologic test suggesting a role for the virus in the development of obliterative arterial lesions in cattle have been supported by in situ PCR and immunohistochemical studies of the disease in bison that demonstrated OvHV2 within the infiltrating lymphocytes. These lymphoblast-like cells were also shown to be CD8+ T cells.

A PCR technique or immunohistochemical stains can be used to confirm the presence of viral antigen in whole blood or in tissues harvested at necropsy. When transmitted to rabbits, both the wildebeest- and sheep-associated viruses elicit a rapidly fatal lymphoproliferative disorder. The newer molecular biology-based techniques have made this bioassay method obsolete.

Samples for Confirmation of Diagnosis

- **Histology**—fixed brain, lymph node, alimentary tract mucosa including pharynx, esophagus, rumen and Peyer's patch, liver, adrenal gland, kidney, urinary bladder, salivary gland (immunohistochemistry, light microscopy); Bouin's-fixed eye (light microscopy)
- **Virology**—lymph node, spleen, lung (PCR)

DIFFERENTIAL DIAGNOSIS

- Mucosal disease
- Infectious bovine rhinotracheitis (IBR)
- Bluetongue
- Sporadic bovine encephalomyelitis
- Rinderpest (included for historic reasons)
- Jembrana disease

TREATMENT

Treatment of affected animals is unlikely to influence the course of the disease.

Nonsteroidal antiinflammatories may ease the discomfort.

CONTROL

Isolation of affected cattle is usually recommended, but its value is questioned because of the slow rate of spread and the uncertainty regarding the mode of transmission. Because of the field observation that sheep are important in the spread of the disease, **separation** of cattle and sheep herds is recommended. The introduction of sheep from areas where the disease has occurred to farms with cattle should be avoided. A program to produce sheep free of OvHV2 infection by separation and isolation of lambs before they become infected is recommended for sheep used in petting zoos.

An effective vaccine is not available and is likely to remain unavailable in the foreseeable future.[10] Attempts to immunize cattle with live or inactivated culture vaccines with Freund's incomplete adjuvant do not provide protection against experimental challenge or natural challenge by exposure to wildebeest herds. High and persistent levels of virus-neutralizing antibody are demonstrable following vaccination, but humoral mechanisms are probably not important in determining resistance to infection with the virulent virus. An inactivated wildebeest-associated MCF virus vaccine has provided protection against challenge with virulent viruses. Establishing a respiratory mucosal barrier of antibody is currently thought to provide the best chance of protective immunity,[11] but this will be challenging to attain with IM or SC vaccines.

FURTHER READING

Callan RJ, Van Metre DC. Viral diseases of the ruminant nervous system. *Vet Clin North Am Food A.* 2004;20:327-362.

O'Toole D, Li H. The pathology of malignant catarrhal fever with an emphasis on ovine herpesvirus 2. *Vet Pathol.* 2014;51:437-452.

Russell GC, Stewart JP, Haig DM. Malignant catarrhal fever: a review. *Vet J.* 2009;179:324-335.

REFERENCES

1. Ababneh MM, et al. *Transbound Emerg Dis.* 2014;61:75.
2. Li H, et al. *Int J Mol Sci.* 2011;12:6881.
3. Jacobsen B, et al. *Vet Microbiol.* 2007;124:353.
4. Taus NS, et al. *Vet Microbiol.* 2006;116:29.
5. Berezowski JA, et al. *J Vet Diagn Invest.* 2005;17:55.
6. Bexiga R, et al. *Vet Rec.* 2007;161:858.
7. Moore DA, et al. *J Am Vet Med Assoc.* 2010;237:87.
8. Mitchell ESE, Scholes SFE. *Vet Rec.* 2009;164:240.
9. Zemljic T, et al. *Vet Ophthalmol.* 2012;15:46.
10. Li H, et al. *Expert Rev Vacc.* 2006;5:133.
11. Russell GC, et al. *Vet Res.* 2012;43:51.

MALIGNANT CATARRH IN PIGS

Malignant catarrh virus outbreaks are not common in pigs, but they do occur sporadically, usually when pigs are kept together with sheep, which are the main reservoir of infection. Information on the disease is not extensive.

ETIOLOGY

The cause is ovine herpes virus 2 (OvHV2), and there is a sheep-associated form and a wildebeest-associated form.[1]

EPIDEMIOLOGY

The condition has been reported in pigs in Europe in Germany, Norway, Italy, Finland,[2,3] and Switzerland. In a recent outbreak in the United Kingdom it was described in two ailing Kune Kune[4] that lived in a "traveling circus" with sheep and goats and other species that were often transported together in a mobile trailer.

In most cases described, pigs have had contact or been housed together with sheep.[5] Nasal discharges may be the source of infection, particularly from lambs.

The pig is a dead-end host, and thus spread is limited.[6] In the cases in Brazil,[7] there was transfer of the infection from asymptomatic boars to sows via the semen of infected boars.

PATHOGENESIS

Pathogenesis is unknown as yet in the pig.

CLINICAL SIGNS

Pigs are depressed and recumbent, have abnormal respiration, and produce hard, mucus-covered scant feces. The condition develops to ataxia and severe balance loss, which is sometimes violent. There is corneal edema with severe uveitis. In the Kune cases, they were blind, with bilateral corneal opacity, excessive lacrimation, and eyelid thickening. Eventually there was a fine tremor with circling.

A recent report described the infection in asymptomatic swine without any history of contact with sheep in Norway.[8] The disease is difficult to diagnose in pigs because of the nonspecific nature of the clinical signs and the sporadic nature of the disease. Usually only one or two animals are affected, although an outbreak in 41 pigs has been described.[3]

In the Brazilian cases, gilts and sows had depression, abortion, and anorexia. Subsequently, a whole range of neurologic signs developed, such as ataxia, tremors, convulsions, and aggressive behavior. Animals that survived had locomotory abnormalities with forelimb paralysis and were dog-sitting. Infected boars shed virus but remained clinically healthy. In the Finnish study the dead sows had anorexia and high fever.[1]

PATHOLOGY

There are quite often very few gross signs. There may be a crusty skin and areas of cyanosis. The respiratory tract may be covered in a mucopurulent exudate. Lungs may be congested and edematous. In the Finnish study, the sows had swollen lymph nodes, a pale-brown liver, and congested kidneys. There may be pale kidneys with petechiae, small erosions on the lining of the stomach, and congested meninges. In many cases, there were only small lesions in the lung and pancreas.

In the Kune Kune[4] there were ulcerations of the skin, and mucocutaneous ulcerations were found in the mouth. There was also ulceration of the soft palate and tonsils and lymphadenopathy with enlarged spleen and adrenals and meningeal edema and meningitis.

The disease is essentially a lymphoproliferative vasculitis. Histopathologically, there was a severe nonpurulent meningoencephalitis with lymphocytic cuffing around vasculitis. Edema, fibrinoid necrosis, and lymphocytic infiltration were also observed. The lesions are more severe in the kidneys (severe, multifocal, interstitial, nonsuppurative nephritis) associated with fibrinoid necrosis of the vessels.

DIAGNOSIS

The differential diagnosis includes Aujeszky's disease (ADV), classical swine fever (CSF), porcine enterovirus (PEV), and rabies. OHV2 DNA can be detected in the clinically affected pigs. A combination of clinical signs, histopathology, and the detection of virus-specific antibodies is usually suggestive. A competitive inhibition ELISA test has been developed and also a direct ELISA. PCR and quantitative reverse-transcription PCR (qRT-PCR) have also been developed for the detection of the virus in tissues.

REFERENCES

1. Meier-Trummer CS, et al. *Vet Microbiol.* 2010;141:191.
2. Syrjala P, et al. *Vet Rec.* 2006;159:406.
3. Gauger PC, et al. *J Swine Hlth Prod.* 2010;18:244.
4. Wessels M, et al. *Vet Rec.* 2011;169:156a.
5. Alcaraz A, et al. *J Vet Diag Invest.* 2009;21:250.
6. Russell GC, et al. *Vet J.* 2009;179:324.
7. Costa EA, et al. *Emerg Infect Dis.* 2010;16:2011.
8. Loken T, et al. *J Vet Diag Invest.* 2009;21:257.

JEMBRANA DISEASE

Jembrana disease is the name of a fatal infectious disease that occurs in Bali cattle (*Bos javanicus*) and buffaloes (*Bubalus bubalis*) on the island of Bali in Indonesia. The disease is endemic in areas of Indonesia only, but the severe disease of the initial outbreak has modified with time.

ETIOLOGY

The disease is caused by a lentivirus, the Jembrana disease virus (JDV), genetically related to but distinct from bovine immunodeficiency virus (BIV), a more benign infection found in Indonesia and many other countries. Both viruses resemble human immunodeficiency virus (HIV) in their structural, genomic, antigenic, and biological properties. JDV has a capsid protein (p26) that is used as an antigen source for serologic diagnosis, but it cross-reacts with sera from

BIV-infected cattle.[1] Furthermore, although JDV is genetically very stable, it has strain variation, and under experimental condition, atypical responses to infection characterized by reduced viral loads, lower or absent febrile responses, and absence of specific antibody responses were observed in 15% of infected cattle.[2-3]

EPIDEMIOLOGY

Occurrence

The disease originally occurred in Jembrana district on the Island of Bali, Indonesia, in 1964 and rapidly spread to the rest of the island, resulting in the deaths of approximately 17% of Bali cattle. Since 1964, the disease has been endemic on Bali island but with lower morbidity and mortality rates. It has subsequently spread to the Indonesian islands of Sumatra, Java, and Kalimantan, producing initial epidemic disease with high mortality followed by endemic disease with lower morbidity and mortality. The current mortality rate is approximately 15% to 20%.[4-5]

Transmission

Transmission probably occurs by direct contact with infective secretions in the acute phase of the disease when viral titers are greater than 10(6) genomes/ml[6] and by mechanical transmission by hematophagous insects or mechanically by needles during mass vaccination of animals for the control of diseases such as hemorrhagic septicemia.

Experimental Reproduction

The disease can be experimentally transmitted by intravenous (IV) or intraperitoneal inoculation of blood or spleen into *B. javanicus*. The virus is present in high titer in the blood during the febrile phase and in the saliva and milk. In *B. javanicus* an incubation period of 4 to 12 days is followed by fever lasting from 5 to 12 days and clinical signs typical of the enzootic form of the disease. Persistent infection occurs for periods of at least 2 years following recovery.

Experimental challenge of *B. indicus, B. Taurus,* and crossbred (*B. javanicus* and *B. indicus*) cattle results in only a transient febrile response, mild clinical disease, and viremia that persist for 3 months, although antibody persists for at least 4 years following infection. Infection, as determined by antibody response, but not clinical disease, can be transmitted experimentally to pigs, sheep, goats, and buffaloes.

PATHOGENESIS

Jembrana disease is not typical of other lentivirus infections, which are usually characterized by chronic progressive disease with long incubation periods. Instead, JDV causes an acute and sometimes fatal disease after a short incubation period. There is a high viremia during the febrile stage, with virus titers being as high as 10(12) virus/mL of plasma. Initial virus proliferation in the spleen is followed by widespread dissemination during a second proliferative phase and infection in lymph nodes, lungs, bone marrow, liver, and kidney. Affected animals do not develop detectable antibodies to the virus until at least 6 weeks after recovery from the acute phase, and surviving animals are resistant to reinfection but remain infectious for at least 2 years.

The specific cell types infected by Jembrana disease virus have not yet been identified, but during the febrile phase, there is marked depletion of CD4+ T cells and increase in CD8+ T cells and CD21+ B cells.[7] The persistent depletion of CD4+ T-cell numbers, through lack of T-cell helper to B cells, may explain the lack of production of JDV-specific antibodies for several weeks after recovery despite an increase in CD21+ B-cell numbers.[7] Furthermore, viral antigen is present in IgG-containing cells, including plasma cells in lymphoid tissues, and in macrophage-like cells in the lungs.[8]

CLINICAL FINDINGS

Natural clinical disease is reported only in *B. javanicus;* other cattle types and buffalo are subclinically infected in natural outbreaks. After an incubation period of 4 to 12 days, clinical signs include fever (40–42°C [104–107°F]) that lasts up to 12 days, anorexia, generalized lymphadenopathy, nasal discharge, increased salivation, and anemia. In severely affected cattle there is diarrhea followed by dysentery. Mucosal erosions can occur but are rare. Hemorrhages are present in the vagina, mouth, and occasionally the anterior chamber of the eye in severe disease. Where the disease is enzootic and less severe in presentation, clinical signs include inappetence, fever, lethargy, reluctance to move, enlargement of the superficial lymph nodes, mild erosions of the oral mucosa, and diarrhea.

CLINICAL PATHOLOGY

During the febrile period there is a moderate normocytic normochromic anemia and leukopenia with lymphopenia, eosinopenia, and thrombocytopenia. The lymphopenia is attributable to a significant decrease in both the proportion and absolute numbers of CD4+ T cells.[7] Bone marrow shows no microscopic changes. Elevated blood urea concentrations and diminished total plasma protein are seen in *B. javanicus* but not *B. taurus.* An ELISA test and an agar gel immunodiffusion test can be used for serologic surveys. Both are specific, but the ELISA test has greater but limited sensitivity. A combination of real-time PCR and JDV p26-his ELISA has been recommended for the detection of infection with JDV in Indonesia.[1]

NECROPSY FINDINGS

Necropsy lesions in *B. javanicus* include generalized lymphadenopathy, with enlargements up to 20-fold, and generalized hemorrhages. The spleen is enlarged to 3 to 4 times its normal size. Histologically, there is marked proliferation of lymphoblasts in parafollicular (T-cell) areas of lymph nodes and spleen, and atrophy of the follicles (B-cell areas). In addition, there is lymphoproliferation around blood vessels in the liver, kidney, and other organs.[5]

Specimens for histopathology should include lymph nodes, spleen, liver, and kidney.

TREATMENT AND CONTROL

> **TREATMENT AND CONTROL**
>
> **Treatment**
> None except supportive
>
> **Prophylaxis**
> Vaccination (R-2)

Treatment is supportive. There is currently no specific control. Vaccination has been attempted using virus-containing plasma and spleen tissue from acutely affected cattle with the virus inactivated with triton X-100 and the vaccine adjuvanted with either mineral oil or Freund's incomplete adjuvant. Protection is only partial and not of real value in control, except perhaps in reducing the risk of virus transmission, because vaccinated animals have a greatly reduced viral load.[6]

FURTHER READING

Desport M, Lewis J. Jembrana disease virus: host responses, viral dynamics and disease control. *Curr HIV Res.* 2010;8:53.

Wilcox GE, Chadwick BJ, Kertayadnya G. Recent advances in the understanding of Jembrana disease. *Vet Microbiol.* 1995;46:249.

Wilcox GE. Jembrana disease. *Aust Vet J.* 1997;75:492.

REFERENCES

1. Lewis J, et al. *J Virol Methods.* 2009;159:81.
2. Desport M, et al. *Virus Res.* 2007;126:233.
3. Desport M, et al. *Virology.* 2009;386:310.
4. Desport M, Lewis J. *Curr HIV Res.* 2010;8:53.
5. Su Y, et al. *Virol J.* 2009;6:179.
6. Ditcham WG, et al. *Virology.* 2009;386:317.
7. Tenaya IW, et al. *Vet Immunol Immunopathol.* 2012;149:167.
8. Desport M, et al. *Virology.* 2009;393:221.

BOVINE EPHEMERAL FEVER

> **SYNOPSIS**
>
> **Etiology** Arthropod-borne rhabdovirus of the genus *Ephemerovirus.*
>
> **Epidemiology** Enzootic in tropical areas. Transmitted by insect vectors. Episodic epizootics in summer in incursive areas probably initiated by wind-borne transmission of insect vector. High morbidity but low case fatality.

Continued

Clinical findings Disease of cattle with fever, respiratory distress, muscular shivering, stiffness, lameness, and enlargement of the peripheral lymph nodes.

Generally spontaneous recovery in 3 days and low case-fatality rate.

Clinical pathology Leukocytosis, hyperfibrinogenemia, hypocalcemia, elevated creatine kinase. Blocking enzyme-linked immunoabsorbent assay (ELISA) for serology.

Necropsy findings Serofibrinous polyserositis.

Diagnostic confirmation Demonstration of specific bovine ephemeral fever (BEF) viral antigen by immunofluorescence or by isolation in mice.

Treatment Nonsteroidal antiinflammatory drugs cause remission of clinical signs.

Control Vaccination and supportive treatment.

ETIOLOGY

Bovine ephemeral fever (BEF) is associated with an arthropod-borne rhabdovirus that is the type species of the genus *Ephemerovirus.* There are a number of strains that vary antigenically. Other antigenically related but nonpathogenic species of *Ephemerovirus* occur in the same environment in Australia. The BEF virus is closely associated with the leukocyte–platelet fraction of the blood, and it can be maintained deep frozen or on tissue culture and chick embryos.

EPIDEMIOLOGY

Occurrence

A disease of cattle, ephemeral fever is enzootic in the tropical areas of Africa, in most of Asia, the Middle East, the East Indies, and in much of Australia, with extensions into the subtropics and some temperate regions. In these areas the disease presents as episodic epidemics. Area outbreaks can last several months, with the spread of infection following prevailing winds, and during this period most herds within a region will be infected. The proportions of herds affected in outbreaks in the Jordan Valley in Israel in 1990 and 1999 were 79% and 98% respectively.

The morbidity rate in outbreaks is usually between 25% and 45%, but if the population is highly susceptible or the infecting strain virulent, the morbidity rate may reach 100%. In enzootic areas, only 5% to 10% will be affected. A rate of 1% for case fatality and loss from involuntary culling is usual with low-virulence strains but can approach 10%.

Source of Infection

The source of infection is the animal affected with the clinical disease and biological vectors (hematophagous biting insects).

Method of Transmission

A great deal of work in recent years has not clearly defined the **vector** list, which probably includes the mosquitoes *Aedes* spp., *Culex annulirostris, Anopheles bancroftii* and *A. annulipes,* and the biting midge *Culicoides brevitarsis. Culex annulirostris* has been identified as a biological vector in Australia. This mosquito can transmit infection within a week of feeding on an infected animal, and the epidemiology of the disease in Australia supports transmission by mosquitoes rather than *Culicoides* spp.

The **reservoir** host, other than cattle, has not been identified. This is of particular importance when the epidemiologic pattern of occurrence of the disease changes, as it has done in Australia after being introduced in approximately 1936.[1] The disease now occurs annually in areas where it used to occur only once each decade, probably because of establishment of the virus in indigenous vectors.

Spread by **wind-borne carriage** of vectors has been documented.[2,3] Epidemiologic studies suggest that outbreaks in Japan originate from Korea, and those in Israel originate from Turkey.[2] Transboundary movement can also occur by animal transport,[2] although transmission does not occur through contact with infected animals or their saliva or ocular discharge. The disease is not spread through semen, nor is intrauterine administration of the virus a suitable route of transmission.

Experimental Reproduction

The disease can be transmitted by the injection of whole blood or the leukocyte fraction of it. Experimental reproduction in cattle requires IV administration, and viremia lasts 3 days with a maximum of 2 weeks. There is no carrier state.

Environment Risk Factors

The disease occurs in the **summer** months, outbreaks are **clustered** and relatively **short-lived**, and spread depends largely on the insect vector population and the force and direction of prevailing winds. The disease tends to disappear for long periods to return in epizootic form when the resistance of the population is diminished.

Recurrence depends primarily on suitable environmental conditions for increase and dissemination of the insect vector and the degree of population immunity, as indicated by neutralizing antibody titers and immunity coverage.[4] During periods of quiescence the disease is still present, but the morbidity is reputed to be very low. However, in many enzootic areas the degree of surveillance is less than intense, and clinical cases may occur without being observed. Temporary protection against infection is provided by subclinical infections by other unrelated arboviruses (e.g., Akabane, Aino, and others).

Animal Risk Factors

Among domestic animals, only **cattle** are known to be naturally affected, but antibodies can be found in African ruminant wildlife. All **age groups** of cattle are susceptible, but calves less than 3 to 6 months old are not affected by the natural disease. With experimental infections calves as young as 3 months old are as susceptible as adults to experimental infection but do not show clinical disease.

In dairy cattle, higher-producing cows are at greater risk, and clinical disease may be minimal in cows under 2 years of age. A recent Israeli study in 10 beef herds found average morbidity and mortality rates of 46.2% and 4.8%, respectively, with higher rates in bulls than cows and a higher morbidity in cows 2 to 5 years of age than in heifers less than 2 years of age. In natural outbreaks there is no breed susceptibility.

In Africa, based on serologic results, the virus is thought to be cycling in populations of wild ruminants between epidemics in domestic cattle. Buffalo (*Bubalus bubalis*) are susceptible to experimental infection, but it is unlikely that they play any part as a reservoir host. After experimental infection of cattle there is solid immunity against homologous strains for up to 2 years. Immunity against heterologous strains is much less durable, which probably accounts for the apparent variations in immunity following field exposure.

Economic Importance

Although the case-fatality rate is very low, considerable loss occurs in **dairy herds** as a result of the depression of milk flow—up to 80% in cows in late lactation. In an Israeli study of eight infected dairy herds, the decline in milk yield from preinfection levels varied between cows and ranged from 30% to 70%, with the highest-yielding cows having the greatest drop. Following recovery from disease, milk production was still less than that of preinfection levels.

There is also a lowered resistance to mastitis. Reproductive inefficiency is associated with a significant delay in the occurrence of estrus, abortion in cows, and temporary sterility in bulls. Occasional animals die of intercurrent infection, usually pneumonia, or prolonged recumbency. Bovine ephemeral fever can have a serious effect on the agricultural economy in countries where cattle are used as **draught animals**. For cattle-exporting countries such as Australia, BEF causes interference with movement of cattle when receiving countries insist on evidence of freedom from the disease.

PATHOGENESIS

Experimental production of the disease requires the IV route of transmission. Virus multiplication probably occurs primarily within the **vascular system**. The BEF virus alters cellular biology in cattle to enhance virus entry and replication. This includes activation of intracellular signaling pathways to up-regulate clathrin and dynamin 2 expression and activation of COX-2-mediated E-prostanoid receptors 2 and 4 to enhance clathrin-mediated endocytosis of the virus.[5-7] After an incubation period of 2 to 10 days, there is a biphasic fever with peaks 12 to 24 hours apart. The fever lasts 2 days, and increased respiratory rate, dyspnea, muscle trembling, limb stiffness, and pain are characteristic at this time.

There is **generalized inflammation** with vasculitis and thrombosis, serofibrinous inflammation in serous and synovial cavities, and increased endothelial permeability at the same sites. The virus can be detected in circulating neutrophils and plasma, the serosal and synovial fluids, the mesothelial cells of synovial membrane and epicardium, and in neutrophils in the fluids. Clinical signs are thought caused by the expression of mediators of inflammation coupled with a secondary hypocalcemia.

CLINICAL FINDINGS

Calves are least affected, with those less than 3 to 6 months of age showing no clinical signs. Overweight cows, high-producing cows, and bulls are affected the most. Deaths are relatively uncommon and are usually less than 1% of the herd.[3]

In most cases the disease is acute. After an incubation period of 2 to 4 days, sometimes as long as 10 days, there is a sudden onset of **fever** (40.5°–41°C [105°–106°F]), which may be biphasic or have morning remissions. **Anorexia** and a sharp **fall in milk yield** occur. There is severe constipation in some animals and diarrhea in others. Respiratory and cardiac rates are increased, and stringy nasal and watery ocular discharges are evident. The animals shake their heads constantly, and muscle shivering and weakness are observed. There may be swellings about the shoulders, neck, and back.

Muscular signs become more evident on the second day, with severe **stiffness**, clonic muscle movements, and weakness in one or more limbs. A **posture** similar to that of acute laminitis, with all four feet bunched under the body, is often adopted. On about the third day, the animal begins eating and ruminating, and the febrile reaction disappears, but lameness and weakness may persist for 2 to 3 more days. A common name of "**3-day sickness**" is applied because animals typically progress through onset of disease to severe illness and recovery within 3 days.[3]

Some animals remain standing during the acute stages, but the majority go down and assume a position reminiscent of parturient paresis, associated with **hypocalcemia**, with the hindlegs sticking out and the head turned into the flank. Occasionally, animals adopt a posture of lateral recumbency. Some develop clinically detectable pulmonary and subcutaneous (SC) emphysema, possibly related to a nutritional deficiency of selenium. In most cases recovery is rapid and complete unless there is exposure to severe weather or unless aspiration of a misdirected drench or ruminal contents occurs. Some cases have a second episode of clinical disease 2 to 3 weeks after recovery.

Occasional cases show persistent recumbency and have to be destroyed, and abortion occurs in a small proportion of cases. Affected bulls are temporarily sterile. Milder cases, with clinical signs restricted to pyrexia and lack of appetite, may occur at the end of an epizootic.

CLINICAL PATHOLOGY

Blood taken from cattle in the febrile stage clots poorly. Marked **leukocytosis** with a relative increase in neutrophils occurs during the acute stage of the disease. There is a shift to the left and lymphopenia. Plasma fibrinogen levels are elevated for about 7 days, and there is a marked increase in **creatine kinase activity**. In natural cases, but not experimentally produced ones, significant **hypocalcemia** occurs.[8] Available serologic tests include a complement fixation test, serum neutralization, fluorescent antibody test, agar gel immunodiffusion (AGID) test, and a **blocking ELISA**, which is reported to be simple and the preferred test.

NECROPSY FINDINGS

Postmortem lesions are not dramatic. The most consistent lesions are a **serofibrinous polyserositis**, involving the synovial, pericardial, pleural, and peritoneal cavities, with a characteristic accumulation of neutrophils in these fluids and surrounding tissues. Hemorrhage may also be observed in the periarticular tissues, and there may be foci of necrosis in the musculature of the limbs and back. All lymph nodes are usually enlarged and edematous. **Pulmonary emphysema** and fibrinous bronchiolitis are standard findings, and subcutaneous emphysema along the dorsum may be observed. Characteristic microscopic findings consist of a mild vasculitis of small vessels, with perivascular neutrophils and edema fluid plus intravascular fibrin thrombi.

Necropsy examinations of animals that develop persistent recumbency have shown severe degenerative changes in the spinal cord similar to those produced by physical compression, but the pathogenesis of these lesions remains uncertain. Although nucleic acid sequences of the agent are known, PCR tests are not yet widely utilized.

Antigen in reticuloendothelial cells can be detected by immunoperoxidase and immunofluorescent techniques.

Samples for Confirmation of Diagnosis

- **Virology**—chilled lung, spleen, synovial membrane, pericardium (virus isolation)
- **Serology**—pericardial fluid (ELISA)
- **Histology**—formalin-fixed samples of previously mentioned tissues

DIFFERENTIAL DIAGNOSIS

The diagnosis of ephemeral fever in a cattle population is not difficult on the basis of its epidemiology and clinical presentation. It can produce difficulties in individual animals where differentials include the following:

- Botulism
- Parturient paresis
- Pneumonia
- Traumatic reticulitis

TREATMENT

Palliative treatment with **nonsteroidal anti-inflammatory** drugs such as IV or IM flunixin meglumine (2.2 mg/kg/d), or IM ketoprofen (3 mg/kg/d) results in **remission** of signs without in any way influencing the development of the disease. There is little effect on the respiratory manifestations of the disease but a major effect on stiffness, lameness, and anorexia. All treatments are continued for 3 days. Phenylbutazone may be most effective, but the injection frequency is not practical and creates slaughter residue concerns. Moreover, phenylbutazone use in cattle is not permitted in some countries. Parenteral treatment with **calcium borogluconate** should be given to cows that show signs of hypocalcemia, and field observations are that parenteral treatment with calcium solutions often helps to get a recumbent cow to her feet. Proper nursing of the recumbent animal is required.

CONTROL

Restriction of movement from infected areas is practiced, but **vaccination** is the only effective method of control. Vaccines prepared from **attenuated** tissue culture virus or in mouse brain and adjuvanted in Freund's incomplete or Quil A adjuvants are commercially available in Australia, Japan, Taiwan, and South Africa. Two vaccinations are required and are effective in preventing disease in natural outbreaks for periods up to 12 months. The use of vaccination in Japan is credited with preventing further major outbreaks. Attenuated vaccines are expensive to produce and have a short shelf-life, and breakdowns are recorded after their use. There is also concern about back-mutation of the attenuated strain to a virulent form, particularly given the high mutation rate of RNA viruses, and contamination with other viruses during preparation of the vaccine.[9,10] The use of inactivated vaccines therefore offers an attractive alternative, such as formalin **killed** vaccines with and without adjuvants. Unfortunately, inactivated vaccines appear to need at least three vaccinations to provide longer-term immunity,[9,10] requiring frequent boosting for effect. Immunity is positively correlated with the level of specific antibody measured with a blocking ELISA or as virus-neutralizing antibody.

REFERENCES

1. Trinidad L, et al. *J Virol.* 2014;88:1525.
2. Aziz-Boaron O, et al. *Vet Microbiol.* 2012;158:300.
3. Finlaison DS, et al. *Aust Vet J.* 2010;88:301.
4. Ting LJ, et al. *Vet Microbiol.* 2014;173:241.
5. Cheng CY, et al. *J Virol.* 2012;86:13653.
6. Cheng CY, et al. *Cell Microbiol.* 2015;17:967.
7. Joubert DA, et al. *J Virol.* 2014;88:1591.
8. Mohammad M, Saeid S. *Adv Environ Biology.* 2011;5:1579.
9. Aziz-Boaron O, et al. *PLoS ONE.* 2013;8(12):e82217.
10. Aziz-Boaron O, et al. *Vet Microbiol.* 2014;173:1.

NAIROBI SHEEP DISEASE

Nairobi sheep disease (NSD) is a tick-transmitted disease of small ruminants, particularly sheep, caused by the Nairobi sheep disease virus (NSDV) and characterized by fever, hemorrhagic gastroenteritis, abortion, and high mortality. NSDV was first recognized at the beginning of the twentieth century as a disease of sheep and goats in Kenya. The virus is the prototype of the genus *Nairovirus,* family Bunyaviridae, and it is endemic in East and Central African countries of Kenya, Uganda, Tanzania, Ruanda, Somalia, and Ethiopia. A similar virus known as Ganjam virus (GV) has been recognized in India and Sri Lanka, where it is associated with febrile illness in humans and disease in sheep and goats. Recent genomic analysis has shown that NSDV is highly diverse and that the Ganjam virus is a variant of the NSDV.[1] Furthermore, it has been suggested that GV probably spread from India to Africa in the nineteenth century and that both virus variants could be referred to as NSDV/GV.[2] Other antigenically related viruses are the Crimean Congo hemorrhagic fever virus in humans and the Dugbe fever virus in cattle in the drier parts of West and East Africa. The Bunyaviridae family also include two significant pathogens of animals, Cache Valley virus and Akabane virus, both of which have a tropism for fetal tissues and are responsible for embryonic losses and multiple congenital deformities in domestic ruminants.[3] Nairobi sheep disease virus does not affect cattle, horses, or pigs, but can cause a mild febrile disease in humans, hence a zoonosis.

The most common vector for NSDV in Africa is the brown ear tick *Rhipicephalus appendiculatus,* but other species may be involved, including the bont tick, *Amblyomma variegatum.* In India, GV is found in a number of ticks, primarily *Haemophysalis intermedia.*[1] Transmission by *R. appendicaltus* is both transstadial and transovarial. Animals bred in endemic areas are usually immune, and hence the virus is of little consequence in stable populations of sheep and goats. The virus can persist in ticks for long periods, more than 2 years in unfed adults, thereby enhancing endemic stability in resident animals.

The pathogenesis of NSDV/GV infection has been investigated recently.[4] The virus is regarded as one of the most pathogenic agents for sheep and goats, with mortality ranging from 40% in Merino sheep to 90% in Masai sheep. Like other viral hemorrhagic diseases, including Crimean Congo hemorrhagic fever in humans, MSDV/GV has developed an efficient mechanism to circumvent or inhibit innate immunity of the host by inhibiting interferon induction and action.[4] This makes it easier for the virus to invade cells and replicate in them. In experimentally infected sheep, the virus has also been shown to cause profound leukopenia, most likely as a result of large-scale apoptosis, and to cause increased levels of some proinflammatory cytokines, including tumor necrosis factor (TNFa), which has the effect of increasing endothelial permeability, leading to hemorrhages.[2] As the sheep began to recover from the infection, the level of interferon gamma was found to increase.

Clinical disease occurs when susceptible animals are moved into endemic areas (e.g., for marketing purposes or for livestock improvement) or when there is a breakdown in tick control measures. Outbreaks occur outside endemic areas when there has been unusual increase in tick population brought about by excessive or prolonged rains. There are differences in susceptibility among different breeds of sheep and goats, and unlike in most other diseases, some indigenous breeds are more susceptible than exotic breeds, like the Merino. A sudden onset of fever is followed by anorexia, nasal discharge, dyspnea, and severe diarrhea, sometimes with dysentery, abortion, and death in 3 to 9 days. There may be hyperemia of the coronary band and hemorrhages in the oral mucosa.[2] The case-mortality rate is 30% to 90% but is lower in goats.

The necropsy picture is typical of a hemorrhagic diathesis and consists of hemorrhages on serous surfaces of visceral organs and on mucosal surfaces, particularly the abomasum, colon, and female genital tract. Lymph nodes and spleen are enlarged. Later, a hemorrhagic gastroenteritis becomes more obvious, and there may be zebra striping in the mucosa of the colon and rectum. The uterus and fetal skin are hemorrhagic. Ticks are likely to be found on the body, especially on the ears and head. Common histopathologic lesions outside the gastrointestinal tract include myocardial degeneration, nephritis, and necrosis of the gall bladder.

Differential diagnoses include peste des petits ruminants (PPR), Rift Valley fever, heartwater, parasitic gastroenteritis, and salmonellosis, all to be confirmed by laboratory tests.

Specimens for laboratory diagnosis should include uncoagulated blood, mesenteric lymph node, and spleen, collected safely to avoid aerosol infections. The virus is first isolated in tissue culture or in infant mice, and the disease can be reproduced in susceptible sheep. The polymerase chain reaction (PCR) technique has been used on whole blood or the buffy coat.[2] The blood should be collected in EDTA. A quantitative PCR assay can also be used on ticks and for carrying out surveys.[5]

The recommended serologic test is the indirect fluorescent antibody test, but others are the complement fixation test (CFT) and the indirect hemagglutination test. For viral identification, the recommended tests used to be immunofluorescence, agar gel immunodiffusion, CFT, and ELISA.

There is no treatment for NSD and no vaccine for commercial use, even though a killed tissue culture vaccine or an attenuated vaccine has been suggested. Vector control is crucial when animals have to be moved to endemic areas.

FURTHER READING

OIE Manual of Diagnostic Tests and Vaccines for Terrestrial Animals. Paris: OIE; 2008 chapter 2.9.1:1165.

REFERENCES

1. Yadev PD, et al. *Infect Genet Evol.* 2011;11:1111.
2. Bin Tarif A, et al. *Vet Res.* 2012;43:71.
3. *OIE Manual of Diagnostic Tests and Vaccines for Terrestrial Animals.* Paris: OIE; 2008 chapter 2.9.1:1165.
4. Holzer B, et al. *PLoS ONE.* 2011;6:e28594.
5. Mutai BK, et al. *Vector Zoonot Dis.* 2013;13:360.

WESSELSBRON DISEASE

SYNOPSIS

Etiology Wesselsbron virus, genus *Flavivirus,* a member of the family Flaviviridae.

Epidemiology Enzootic in sub-Saharan Africa. Maintenance host not yet identified but presumably domesticated herbivores. Transmitted by mosquitoes of the genus *Aedes.* Infection can occur in small and large ruminants, pigs, donkeys, horses, and ostriches. Infections occur year round in warmer and moister coastal areas; dryer regions have lower prevalence and outbreaks in high rainfall periods often occurring in conjunction with Rift Valley fever.

Clinical findings Acute febrile disease in lambs characterized by hepatitis, abortion in pregnant ewes with congenital central nervous system malformation and arthrogryphosis in aborted fetuses; subclinical infection predominates in calves, adult nonpregnant sheep, goats, and cattle; occasional abortions.

Necropsy findings Jaundice, diffuse hepatic necrosis.

Diagnostic confirmation Virus isolation, serum neutralization, or immunohistochemical localization of viral antigens in tissues; serology.

Treatment No specific treatment available, supportive.

Control Vaccination is no longer available; vector control not cost effective.

ETIOLOGY

Wesselsbron virus is an arthropod-borne enveloped single stranded RNA virus of the family Flaviviridae, genus *Flavivirus*, that has not been well characterized thus far.

EPIDEMIOLOGY

Occurrence

Wesselsbron disease (WBD) was first described in 1955 in an 8-day-old lamb in the Wesselsbron district of the Orange Free State in South Africa. Serologic evidence indicates high infection prevalence in the moister and warmer regions of South Africa, Mozambique, and Zimbabwe. Animals with antibody titer are, in contrast, less common in the dryer South African inland.[1] Wesselsbron virus has been isolated from vertebrates and arthropod vectors in many African countries, including Cameroon, the Central African Republic, Nigeria, Senegal, South Africa, Uganda, and Zimbabwe and in Madagascar. Although serologic studies suggest an enzootic presence of virus over wide parts of the subcontinent, the incidence of clinical disease is very low.[2]

The pattern of occurrence is year round in the warmer and moister coastal regions of southern and eastern Africa. Cyclical outbreaks that are typically linked to periods of heavy rainfall, in contrast, occur in the dryer areas of the continent. Outbreaks frequently occur in conjunction with Rift Valley fever epizootics.

Risk Factors

Animal Risk Factors

Wesselsbron disease is an infectious disease primarily affecting sheep, with a clear age predisposition. Newborn lambs in the first days of life are most susceptible to clinical disease, with mortality rates in the range of 30%. In adult pregnant ewes a common presentation of the disease is abortion that may be associated with a febrile episode.

Other species, including cattle, goats, camels, donkeys, horses, and ostriches, are susceptible to infection but do not typically develop disease; abortions that have been associated with Wesselsbron virus infection have, however, been reported in cattle and goats.[3,4]

Environmental Risk Factors

A warm and moist environment that is favorable to competent vectors is an important risk factor for the spread of the virus. Abnormally heavy rainfalls and the ensuing increase in the mosquito population can results in epizootics in dryer regions of the African continent.[1]

Source of Infection and Method of Transmission

Floodwater breeding mosquitoes of the genus *Aedes,* including the species *A. caballus* and *A. circumluteolus,* are considered the principal vectors of the Wesselsbron virus. The high seroprevalence of infection in domesticated herbivores in affected areas suggests that these species may function as maintenance hosts for the virus. Direct transmission of the virus between animals has not been documented. In humans, however, infection after handling infectious material has been reported.[4]

Zoonotic Implications

Although humans are susceptible to infection and disease, infection with the Wesselsbron virus in the large majority of cases is asymptomatic. If clinically apparent, the disease is usually a transient flulike illness associated with a transient fever, headache, and muscle and joint pain; cutaneous hypersensitivity and skin rashes may occur.[4,5] Person-to-person transmission of infection has not been reported.

Economic Importance

The disease primarily causes disease in lambs and pregnant ewes; evidence that the disease causes significant economic damage is, however, lacking.[1]

PATHOGENESIS

Wesselsbron virus has been classified as pantropic virus with marked hepatotropic properties in newborn lambs and latent neurotropic properties in embryonic and fetal tissue in pregnant ewes.[6] Hepatocytes are the primary site of viral replication in lambs, and age seems to be a determining factor in the progression of infection. Liver necrosis is the most consistent finding in infected young lambs, resulting in hepatic insufficiency and cholestasis. In general, the extent and severity of liver necrosis is considerably less severe than in lambs infected with the Rift Valley fever virus.[6]

CLINICAL FINDINGS

The clinical presentation of WBD varies by species and age. The disease is most severe in young lambs. After an incubation period of between 1 and 4 days, nonspecific clinical signs, such as anorexia, listlessness, and fever, become apparent. Similar symptoms are rarely observed in neonates of other species. Jaundice associated with liver cell necrosis may become apparent in more severe cases. Mortality rates are in the range of 25% in lambs.

In adult sheep and cattle, the only apparent sign may be a fever episode. In pregnant ewes, infection may result in abortion, mummification, stillbirth, or birth of weak lambs. Stillborn or aborted lambs may show congenital neurologic defects or arthrogryposis. The occurrence of hydrops amnii has also been associated with Wesselsbron virus infection in pregnant ewes.[2,6] Death of the ewe may occur, presumably as a complication of the abortion.

CLINICAL PATHOLOGY

Wesselsbron disease is diagnosed by identification of the causative virus or by serology. Virus identification can be done by direct virus isolation, by means of the complement fixation test (CFT) or the serum neutralization test (SNT).[2] The virus can be isolated from most organs of clinically affected lambs, but blood serum or liver tissue from aborted fetuses and liver or spleen of dead lambs are most commonly used. Immunohistochemistry has also been used for virus identification in liver tissue of deceased lambs.[5]

Serology can be conducted by virus neutralization (VN), complement fixation, and hemagglutination inhibition. The hemagglutination inhibition test shows a high degree of cross-reactivity with other flaviviruses. More recently, an antibody ELISA has been developed that is more sensitive and less cross-reactive than the hemagglutination inhibition test.[5]

NECROPSY FINDINGS

In aborted fetuses, congenital malformations of the central nervous system, such as porencephaly and cerebellar hypoplasia, have been reported. These were associated in some instances with arthrogriposis.[6] In neonates, moderate to severe icterus is a prominent finding. The liver is friable with a yellow to orange–brown color and may be congested and enlarged in some instances. Other nonspecific lesions include petechiation on the serosal surface of the entire digestive tract and on the abomasal mucosa.[2] Subcutaneous edema has also been reported.

On histopathology, mild to severe necrosis of the liver characterized by diffuse necrosis of individual or few grouped hepatocytes that are scattered randomly throughout the liver is the predominant finding. Proliferation of Kupffer cells and bile ducts is another consistent finding.[2] Hepatic lesions associated with Wesselsbron disease can be differentiated from those observed with Rift Valley fever by the absence of well-defined primary foci of coagulative necrosis of hepatocytes and the lacking parenchymal hemorrhage that characterize infection with Rift Valley fever.[1]

Samples for Confirmation of Diagnosis

- **Virology**—liver, spleen, brain (virus isolation, serum neutralization, complement fixation)
- **Histology**—liver, spleen, brain (light microscopy, immunohistochemistry)

DIFFERENTIAL DIAGNOSIS

- Rift Valley fever
- Bluetongue
- Ephemeral fever
- Bacterial septicemias
- Anthrax
- Vibriosis
- Trichomoniasis
- Toxic plants

TREATMENT

Little attention has been given to the aspect of treatment of the disease, and no known treatment is of any value.

CONTROL

Measures to control Wesselsbron disease that have been proposed in the past include vector control and vaccination. Although vector control is in theory possible, it requires that *Aedes* spp. breeding sites have been identified and have a limited surface to be manageable. Particularly with heavy rainfalls and flooding mosquito-breeding sites are too numerous and wide to be controlled. Ecological, health, and financial issues around applying large amounts of insecticides to the environment further complicate this type of control.

A modified live vaccine was available in the past. Injudicious vaccination of pregnant ewes, however, resulted in considerable economic loss as a result of abortion and a high incidence of fetal malformations. Because of the limited economic damage caused by WBD and the complications experienced with vaccination, the production of the vaccine has been discontinued.

REFERENCES

1. Van der Lugt JJ, et al. *Onderstepoort J Vet Res.* 1995;62:143.
2. Coetzer JAW, et al. *Onderstepoort J Vet Res.* 1978;45:93.
3. Mushi EZ, et al. *J Vet Diagn Invest.* 1998;10:191.
4. Weiss KE, et al. *Onderstepoort J Vet Res.* 1956;27:183.
5. Center for Food Security. Public health. 2007 at: <http://www.cfsph.iastate.edu/Factsheets/pdfs/wesselsbron.pdf>; Accessed 10.03.15.
6. Coetzer JAW, et al. *Onderstepoort J Vet Res.* 1979;46:165.

CAPRINE HERPESVIRUS-1 INFECTION

SYNOPSIS

Etiology Caprine herpesvirus-1

Epidemiology Most infections subclinical. High seroprevalence in Mediterranean countries. Latent infection common and outbreaks of abortion and neonatal mortality with no known precipitating cause.

Clinical findings Abortion, neonatal disease, vulvovaginitis, balanoposthitis.

Clinical pathology Leukopenia in systemic disease in kids.

Lesions Ulceration and necrosis of vulva and prepuce. Multifocal necrosis in intestine and organs of aborted fetus and young (1–2 week olds) kids with systemic disease.

Diagnostic confirmation Virus isolation, polymerase chain reaction (PCR).

Treatment and control No effective treatment. Herd biosecurity. Experimental vaccine shows protection.

ETIOLOGY

Caprine herpesvirus-1 (CpHV1) is an alphaherpesvirus within the family Herpesviridae. Restriction endonuclease analysis indicates that there are different strains, but these are not geographically clustered.

EPIDEMIOLOGY

Occurrence

The disease is recorded in the United States, Canada, Australia, New Zealand, South America, and many countries in Europe, and it probably has worldwide distribution. Within the countries where it occurs, there is serologic evidence that the infection is widespread. Seroprevalence is particularly high in Mediterranean countries with high goat populations, such as Greece, Italy, France,[1] and Spain.

In adults, the systemic disease is clinically inapparent, but a genital form of the disease can be transmitted sexually. The virus mostly causes latent or subclinical infections, such as vulvovaginitis and balanoposthitis, which may sometimes present with very serious lesions.[2] It is also associated with occasional but severe outbreaks of abortion, where the abortion rate may exceed 50%.[3] CpHV1 is also associated with severe systemic disease in 1- to 2-week-old kids. This may occur in herds where does are also aborting or occasionally in herds without accompanying abortion.

Transmission and Experimental Reproduction

Transmission is thought to be by inhalation, ingestion or genitally. The virus is found in nasal, pharyngeal, and vaginal discharges; the prepuce; and feces. It is shed by affected females for 10 to 12 days after infection and for up to 24 days by males.[4] The extended shedding period in bucks is probably important in the high transmission rates of infection that occur with the genital form of this disease.

Only goats are affected naturally; lambs and calves are not infected by intranasal inoculation, but lambs can be infected by IV injection. After primary infection, CpHV1 establishes a latent infection in the third and fourth sacral ganglia, but it is difficult to reactivate these infections by experimental or natural means. Reactivation occurs at the time of estrus, and outbreaks of vulvovaginitis often occur during or after the mating period.[1]

Abortion occurs 1 to 7 weeks after experimental challenge. However, the factors that precipitate occasional outbreaks of abortion and disease in young kids are not known. Challenge of females in early pregnancy is followed by fetal stunting and death, whereas challenge in midpregnancy causes no impairment of fetal growth, with the fetus carried to term but born dead.

Economic Importance

Losses include deaths of young goats, in which the morbidity and case-fatality rates are high, and abortion and stillbirths in does. Although the disease is not common, abortion rates can be high in those herds that experience disease.

PATHOGENESIS

Viremia can occur in 1- to 2-week-old unweaned kids, with infection of various organs, especially the alimentary and respiratory tract. The virus can infect the placenta, causing placentitis and invading the fetus.

CLINICAL SIGNS

Adults

In both the experimentally produced and the natural disease there is no prodromal clinical disease preceding abortion, and aborted kids are usually full term. Where there are twins, one may be born dead and the other alive. With the genital disease, there is erythema and edema of the vulva and shallow erosions, ulcers, and occasionally a diphtheritic membrane on the mucosae of the vulva and vagina.[1] The vaginal discharge is clear to mucopurulent, and lesions heal in approximately 1 week. Outbreaks occur during or after mating and are not necessarily followed by abortion. In males, there is an ulcerative balanoposthitis, with hyperemia, edema, and ulceration of the penis and prepuce, often with a purulent exudate, with lesions healing within 15 days of infection.[4]

Newborn Kids

Consistent signs include weakness, anorexia, cyanosis and dyspnea, increased heart and respiratory rates, abdominal pain, and fluid gut contents accompanied by diarrhea, and, in some cases, dysentery. Vesicles and ulcers may also be present on the coronets. Conjunctivitis, seropurulent nasal discharge, erosions of the oral mucosa, and petechial hemorrhages in the skin are also seen.

CLINICAL PATHOLOGY

Leukopenia is a consistent finding in sick newborn kids. The virus can be isolated from all secretions or identified by PCR and restriction endonuclease analysis. In serum, antibodies can be demonstrated by serum neutralization or ELISA tests.[5]

NECROPSY FINDINGS

Adults

In does, ulceration and necrosis of the vaginal and vulval mucosae and placentitis are standard findings. Males have inflammation and ulceration of the penis and prepuce. A few adults develop an acute pneumonia with thick fibrinous exudate in the pleural cavity. Miliary foci of hepatic necrosis may or may not be grossly visible in aborted fetuses, but microscopic multifocal necrosis is commonly seen in the liver, adrenal glands, lung, and kidney. Herpesvirus intranuclear inclusions can be found in some of these tissues.

Newborn Kids

Prominent lesions include ulceration and necrosis of the mucosae of the rumen, abomasum, intestine, cecum, and colon. Lesions are particularly severe in the large intestine. Vesicles and ulcers on the coronet of the feet may also be seen. Microscopically, foci of necrosis are often seen in the adrenal glands, urinary bladder, spleen, liver, lungs, and other tissues. Characteristic intranuclear inclusion bodies may be seen in mononuclear cells associated with these lesions.

Samples for Confirmation of Diagnosis

- **Virology**—*Kids, fetuses*—liver, lung, adrenal gland. *Adults*—genital ulcers, vesicles. Chilled swabs in viral transport media (virus isolation, PCR). It may be difficult to isolate virus from aborted fetuses, but it can be demonstrated by real-time PCR.[6]
- **Histology**—formalin-fixed samples of affected tissues

DIFFERENTIAL DIAGNOSIS

The systemic disease needs to be differentiated from the severe mycoplasmal infections and bacterial septicemias. Ulcerative dermatosis may be a confusing diagnosis in the genital form.

The differential diagnosis of causes of abortion in the ewe and doe are summarized in Table 18-1.

TREATMENT AND CONTROL

The immunosuppressive drug mizoribine enhances the antiviral activity of acyclovir, but this combination is a model for treatment of human herpesvirus infections rather than a practical treatment for goats.[7] NSAIDs may ease the discomfort from the genital lesions caused by CpHV1, but effective quarantine and serologic testing of all introduced goats is the only effective control measure that can be suggested at the present time.

The disease is probably not of sufficient economic importance to justify developing a commercial vaccine. However, experimental vaccines based upon glycoprotein D from a nonpathogenic bovine herpes virus-4 have provided good protection against challenge with pathogenic CpHV1.[8]

REFERENCES

1. Thiry J, et al. *Vet Microbiol.* 2008;128:261.
2. Piper KL, et al. *Aust Vet J.* 2008;86:136.
3. McCoy MH, et al. *JAVMA.* 2007;231:1236.
4. Camero M, et al. *Small Rumin Res.* 2015;128:59.
5. Marinaro M, et al. *J Vet Diag Invest.* 2010;22:245.
6. Elia G, et al. *J Virol Meth.* 2008;148:155.
7. Elia G, et al. *Res Vet Sci.* 2015;99:208.
8. Donofrio G, et al. *PLoS ONE.* 2013;8:e52758.

EQUINE VIRAL ARTERITIS

SYNOPSIS

Etiology Equine arteritis virus

Epidemiology Infection and disease in equids. Outbreaks of disease as a result of lateral transmission by infected body fluids. Venereal transmission by persistently infected but clinically normal stallions, with subsequent lateral spread among mares.

Clinical signs Abortion. Upper respiratory disease with systemic signs including edema and respiratory distress.

Clinical pathology Serology. No characteristic changes in hemogram or serum biochemistry.

Diagnostic confirmation Virus isolation or reverse-transcription polymerase chain reaction (RT-PCR) detection of viral genome in blood, sperm-rich fraction of semen, nasopharyngeal swabs or tissue. Seroconversion or increase in complement fixation titer or enzyme-linked immunoabsorbent assay (ELISA).

Differential diagnosis:
- The systemic disease—viral respiratory disease
- Abortion—equine herpesvirus-1 (EHV1), mare reproductive loss syndrome
- Similar disease in neonates—EHV1 or other septicemia

Treatment There is no specific treatment

Control Vaccination, especially of stallions and seronegative mares to be inseminated by seropositive stallions and to control outbreaks at racetracks. Quarantine. Hygiene.

ETIOLOGY

Viral arteritis of horses, donkeys, zebras, and mules (EVA) is associated with an **arterivirus**—equine arteritis virus (EAV). There is an as yet unsubstantiated suspicion that New World camelids can be infected.[1] EAV is a small enveloped, positive-sense, single-stranded RNA virus that is the prototype virus in the family Arteriviridae (genus: *Arterivirus*), order Nidovirales. This taxonomic grouping includes porcine reproductive and respiratory syndrome virus (PRRSV; see Chapter 18), simian hemorrhagic fever virus (SHFV), lactate dehydrogenase-elevating virus (LDV) of mice, and newly identified wobbly possum disease virus (WPDV), the cause of neurologic disease among free-ranging Australian brushtail possums (*Trichosurus vulpecula*) in New Zealand.[2,3] Although there is only one known EAV serotype, field strains of the virus differ in their virulence and neutralization phenotype,[4] with some strains causing no detectable disease and others being associated with severe clinical signs in adult horses and death in foals.[5-7]

The structural proteins of the EAV virion include seven envelope proteins (E, GP2, GP3, GP4, ORF5a protein, GP5, and M) and the nucleocapsid (N) protein.[4,8] Equine EAV-specific polyclonal antisera and EAV neutralizing monoclonal antibodies bind to the N-terminal hydrophilic ectodomain of GP5.[4] Interactions among the GP2, GP3, GP4, GP5, and M envelope proteins play a major role in determining the CD14+ monocyte tropism, whereas tropism for CD3+ T-lymphocytes is determined by the GP2, GP4, GP5, and M envelope proteins but not the GP3 protein.[9]

There is considerable genomic variation among isolates, with EAV of North American and European origin clustering in geographically approximate, but distinct, viral clades. Phylogenetic analysis based on sequences of the hypervariable region of ORF5 is valuable for tracing the origin of EAV strains.[8,10-19] Isolates of EAV cluster into two distinct groups: North American and European, with there being two clusters within the European clades (EU-1 and EU-2). Viral clades within a country tend to be consistent—for example, most isolates from horses in South Africa, Poland, and Argentina are from one of the European clades,[11,12,15,20] whereas those in Turkey cluster within the North American clade.[16] An outbreak in Quarter horses (which characteristically have a very low prevalence of serum antibody titers to EAV) and Arabians in North America in 2006 to 2007 was associated with a novel strain of virus from the EU-1 clade.[6] However, increasing international movement of horses has resulted in the geographic spread of virus clades, with there being molecular genetic evidence of recent introduction of new viral clades into France and Argentina (and likely elsewhere).[10,18] For instance, of 22 French EAV isolates, 11 isolates obtained before January 28, 2003h clustered within either the EU-1 (9 isolates) or EU-2 (2 isolates) subgroup, whereas 11 isolates obtained after January 30, 2003 belonged to the North American group, strongly suggesting that these strains were recently introduced into France.[10,21] Infected stallions, or infected straws of semen, are the most frequent mode of introduction of new strains to an area.[10,12,18,19]

Nine South African strains isolated from a single donkey are phylogenetically distinct and different from EAV strains isolated from horses in North America and Europe, donkeys in Europe, and the group of South African Lipizzaner stallions.[10]

Novel phenotypic variants of EAV can emerge during persistent infections in stallions, and this is an important feature in the development of disease in exposed mares and foals.[4-6] Persistently infected carrier stallions harbor EAV between breeding seasons, enabling emergence of genetic diversity of the virus.[4] The degree of nucleotide sequence identity among EAV strains isolated from a single persistently infected stallion on 11 occasions over 7 years ranged from 98.92% to 100%, and amino acid homology ranged from 98.06% to 100%.[17] An outbreak of EVA in France in 2007 was linked to a single persistently infected stallion in which the EAV evolved from relatively innocuous strains into a pathogenic strain. The stallion was monitored, and EAV strains available for examination, from 2000 to 2007, enabled determination that the source of the outbreak was a viral strain that developed in this horse.[21] This means of development of new quasispecies is likely more important for the emergence of genetic diversity among EAV strains than is the minimal virus diversity that is generated during small or restricted outbreaks of EVA when the virus is transmitted by respiratory or venereal, or both, routes.[6]

EPIDEMIOLOGY

Occurrence

Serologic evidence of infection by EAV with or without evidence of disease is found in horse populations in North and South America, Europe, Africa, Asia, Australia, Britain, Spain, Italy, France, Poland, the Netherlands, South Africa, and Germany. It is probable that the disease is now present in most countries with substantial populations of horses. New Zealand has evidence that it is free of infection, and there are no reports of the disease from Japan.[22] International shipment of horses and frozen semen contributes to the spread of the EAV.

The proportion of seropositive horses varies considerably among populations, with there being marked differences among breeds. Overall, 2% of horses in the United States are seropositive to EAV (serum neutralization titer >1:4), with 8.4% of horse operations having seropositive horses. Twenty-five percent of operations whose principal activity was breeding had at least one unvaccinated seropositive horse, whereas 4% of racing operations had a least one unvaccinated seropositive horse. The prevalence of titers to EAV is higher in mares and in horses used for breeding. The frequency with which horses in the United States have serum titers greater than 1:4 varies with breed, with 24% of Standardbreds, 4.5% of Thoroughbreds, 3.6% of Warmbloods, and 0.6 % of Quarter horses being seropositive. Approximately 19% of Warmblood horses imported into the United States have antibodies to EAV, with horses from Germany and the Netherlands having the highest prevalence (21% and 25% respectively). Between 55% and 93% of Warmblood and Lipizzan breeds in Austria have serologic evidence of exposure to EAV. Of horses in Anatolia, Turkey, ~24% are seropositive.[23] Of approximately 8000 sera tested in Greece, 3.3% were positive for antibodies to EAV.[24]

Disease in Great Britain and North America has been associated with importation of infected stallions or semen. The disease spreads rapidly in a group of susceptible horses, and although the course of clinical disease is short, an outbreak in a group of horses may persist for a number of weeks. Naturally acquired infections in newborn foals can occur as an outbreak and cause severe disease.

Origin of Infection and Transmission

EAV is spread in two ways:

1. **Horizontal transmission** of virus by predominantly nasal fluid, but also by urine, feces, lacrimal fluid, and vaginal discharge of infected horses
2. **Venereal transmission** from stallions to susceptible (seronegative) mares

Horizontal Transmission

Through infected nasal discharge and body fluid, horizontal transmission is effective and is the means of disease spread in outbreaks in racing stables, and among mares and foals at breeding farms. The virus is found in respiratory secretions for 7 to 14 days and in other tissues for 28 days. Close contact between horses is probably required for transmission of the virus—it has been reported to spread after contact of horses across a fence. The duration of viability of the virus in the environment has not been reported, but the potential for spread of infection on fomites including clothing and tack should be considered when dealing with an outbreak.

Venereal Transmission

Stallions are infected by horizontal transmission of the virus, subsequently excrete the virus in semen, and infect susceptible mares at the time of mating. Clinically normal stallions are also capable of transmitting the virus horizontally to other stallions in a breeding operation, demonstrating the potential for horizontal spread of infection from stallions in the absence of clinical disease or sexual contact. This is demonstrated by the high frequency of infection in stallions sharing a stable and infection of semen in a virgin stallion.[15] Between 30% and 60% of infected stallions excrete the virus in semen for weeks to months. Some stallions excrete virus for years, and lifelong infection and virus excretion can occur. Prolonged infection of stallions is associated with mutation of the virus and secretion by the stallion of viral strains that vary over time.[21] However, disease resulting from transmission of infection from a stallion to a mare, and subsequent spread of infection to other horses, is associated with a single viral strain. In other words, stallions can excrete a variety of strains of the virus during their lifetime, but outbreaks of disease are associated with an initial single viral strain that evolves slowly, if at all, during the weeks or months of the outbreak but that can develop into multiple viral strains.[5,6] For instance, at least 22 strains of EAV were detected in the 2007 outbreak in France, with the original inciting virus having developed in a stallion persistently infected before 2002.[5,6,10]

Prolonged excretion of the virus in semen is likely important in the maintenance of the virus in populations of horses. Introduction of a **persistently infected stallion** into a naive population, insemination of seronegative mares with semen from an infected stallion, and emergence of a virulent strain of EAV from a persistently infected stallion have been implicated as the cause of outbreaks of viral arteritis.[5,10,13,18] The carrier stallion infects mares at mating; the mares then develop disease and shed the virus in nasal and other body fluids and infect in-contact susceptible horses and foals by horizontal transmission.

Artificial breeding practices in which large numbers of mares, often over geographically dispersed areas, are inseminated within a short time or single season from an infected stallion can result in widespread outbreaks. This situation occurred among Quarter horses in the United States in 2006 to 2007 and in draft breed horses in France in 2007.[5,6] Furthermore, transfer of EAV-infected embryos to EAV serologically negative recipient mares can result in infection of the recipients, although this has only been demonstrated experimentally and has not been identified as a means of EAV spread in the field.[25]

The possibility of fomite spread on veterinary instruments, clothing, or personnel, as was possibly the case in France, should be considered.[5]

Immunity

Vaccination or recovery from natural infection results in the development of a strong serum antibody virus-neutralizing response, which is thought to be important in clearance of the virus and resistance to infection. The humoral immune response to EAV includes development of complement-fixing and virus-specific neutralizing antibodies. Complement-fixing antibodies develop 1 to 2 weeks after infection, peak after 2 to 3 weeks, and disappear by 8 months, whereas virus-neutralizing antibodies are detected within 1 to 2 weeks after exposure, peak at 2 to 4 months, and persist for at least 3 years.[4]

Naive pregnant mares infected by horizontal transmission may abort or, less commonly, give birth to infected foals that subsequently die, whereas foals of immune mares are resistant to infection. Viral neutralization antibodies are present in mare's colostrum and foal's serum after sucking, with persistence of the antibodies to the age of 2 to 6 months in the foals. Persistence of passive immunity in foals has important implications for resistance to infection and for timing of administration of modified live vaccines.

Animal Risk Factors

There are clear differences in susceptibility of individual horses to infection and disease, with the clinical outcome of EAV infection determined by host genetic factors. Horses can be segregated into susceptible and resistant phenotypic groups based on the in vitro susceptibility of CD3+ T-lymphocytes to EAV infection.[26-28] A genetically dominant haplotype associated with the in vitro susceptible phenotype has been identified in four horse breeds studied and is located in the region of ECA11, based on genome-wide association studies.[26] There are several proteins associated with virus attachment and entry, cytoskeletal organization, and NF-κB pathways encoded by this region of ECA1.[26] There does not appear to be an association between polymorphisms in major histocompatibility antigens (the equine lymphocyte antigen) and susceptibility to EAV infection.[29]

Horses of all age groups are susceptible to infection, but adult horses are generally resistant to disease. In the 2007 outbreak in France, deaths were recorded of one fetus, 5 young foals, and 2 mature horses.[5]

Economic Importance

The chief impact of the disease on breeding farms is the loss of foals through abortion and the cost of quarantine and control measures. The systemic illness can be severe, but the mortality rate is low. The outbreak in western France in 2007 affected 18 (index, 8 primary and 9 secondary) premises in five counties in western France. Eight mortality cases were observed, including one fetus, five young foals and two mature horses. During outbreaks at race tracks, the economic impact is a result of lost opportunities for training and racing sick or convalescing horses and the effect of quarantine and control measures. Additional costs are incurred by the inconvenience and cost of vaccinating mares to be bred to stallions infected with the virus and import regulations controlling movement of horses and semen, including the inability to export mares, fillies, and noncarrier stallions that are seropositive (perhaps as a result of vaccination), and the limited opportunities for export of semen from infected stallions or export of the stallions themselves.

PATHOGENESIS

The clinical manifestations of EVA result from vascular injury; the pathogenesis of EVA has not yet been comprehensively defined but involves infection of CD3+ T-lymphocytes.[9] The highly virulent, horse-adapted *Bucyrus* strain of EAV causes death in horses by severe vascular damage. The pathogenesis of disease associated with horizontal transmission of EAV has been elucidated. After inhalation of the virus, it binds to the respiratory epithelium and infects alveolar macrophages and is detectable in bronchial lymph nodes by 48 hours after infection. Three days after infection, the virus is detectable in circulating monocytes, with subsequent systemic distribution of infection. The virus has localized in vascular endothelium and medial myocytes by days 6 to 9, and there is significant damage to blood vessels by day 10. The virus infects renal tubular epithelium and can persist there for up to 2 weeks. Medial necrosis of blood vessels might cause anoxia of associated tissues. The virus is not detectable in any tissue by 28 days after infection, with the exception of accessory sex glands in intact male horses.

Abortion is caused by a severe necrotizing myometritis and presumed consequent reduction in fetal blood flow. There are usually no lesions in the fetus, although the fetus is infected with the virus, sometimes at titers higher than those in the dam. The mechanism underlying abortion of foals from EAV-infected mares is unclear.[4]

CLINICAL FINDINGS

Infection by EAV is usually **clinically inapparent**, especially after venereal infection of mares. **Abortion** is not necessarily associated with clinical disease in the mare. Systemic disease is usually mild to moderate and self-limiting, with recovery in 5 to 9 days in the vast majority of horses.

Systemic disease is characterized by an incubation period of 1 to 6 days followed by the appearance of fever (39–41°C [102–106°F]). A serous nasal discharge presents that may become purulent and be accompanied in some horses by congestion and petechiation of the nasal mucosa, urticaria, conjunctivitis, excessive lacrimation developing to purulent discharge, keratitis, palpebral edema, and blepharospasm. Opacity of the aqueous humor and petechiation of the conjunctiva may also occur. Signs of pulmonary disease, such as respiratory distress and coughing, are attributable to pulmonary edema and congestion but are uncommon. The appetite is reduced or absent; in severe cases, there may be abdominal pain, diarrhea, and jaundice. Edema of the limbs is common and more marked in stabled horses than those at pasture. In stallions, edema of the ventral abdominal wall may extend to involve the prepuce and scrotum. Depression is usual and varies in degree with the severity of the syndrome. The disease is acute and severe, and deaths may occur without secondary bacterial invasion. In these cases dehydration, muscle weakness, and prostration develop quickly. It must be emphasized that the disease may be much milder than that described previously.

Clinical disease in neonatal foals is characterized by fever, profound depression, weakness, limb and facial edema, and respiratory distress.[30] Severely affected foals usually die. Foals can be affected at birth or be born apparently normal and develop disease 1 to 19 days after birth.

Abortion occurs within a few days of the onset of clinical illness, although it is not usually associated with clinically apparent disease. Abortions may occur in 10% to 60% of at-risk mares during an outbreak and during the 3rd through 10th months of gestation. Abortion occurs 12 to 30 days after exposure. The abortion is not foreshadowed by premonitory signs, and the placenta is not retained.

CLINICAL PATHOLOGY

Hematologic examination of adults and foals during the acute phase of the systemic disease is characterized by leukopenia and thrombocytopenia.

Antemortem confirmation of infection has historically been achieved by serology or virus isolation. However, modern diagnostic techniques involving PCR and genetic sequencing technology have greatly facilitated prompt diagnosis of infection, monitoring for the presence of EAV in semen (fresh or for artificial insemination), and genetic epidemiology of infection to track the source of the outbreak and its progression.[5,6,10-12] PCR tests are described for detection of the EAV.[31,32] Recommended use of testing is described in Table 21-4.

Serologic confirmation of infection is achieved using complement fixation, serum neutralization, and ELISA tests.[33-36] Seroconversion occurs within 1 week of infection, and demonstration of a rising antibody titer, based on acute and convalescent serum samples, or seroconversion is considered evidence of recent infection. False-positive results for the virus neutralization test have occurred using OIE prescribed rabbit kidney (RK-13) indicator cells when testing serum from horses vaccinated with an EHV1/4 tissue cultured derived vaccine. The false-positive results are likely a result of vaccine-induced antibody response against the RK-13 cells.

Virus isolation from blood, body fluids, and fetal or placental tissue is readily achieved during the acute phase of the disease. Appropriate samples for virus isolation include nasopharyngeal or conjunctival swabs and anticoagulated whole blood (heparin, EDTA, or citrate are suitable anticoagulants). Virus is continuously excreted in the semen of infected stallions and is readily isolated from the sperm-rich fraction of the semen. A nested PCR can detect the presence of virus in naturally infected semen at concentrations as low as 2.5 plaque-forming units per mL with a specificity of 97% and a sensitivity of 100%, and may be useful for the rapid diagnosis of EAV shedding stallions.

Antemortem diagnosis of EVA disease can be achieved by examination of skin samples using monoclonal antibody immunoperoxidase histochemistry. Examination

Table 21-4 Test methods available for the diagnosis of equine viral arteritis and their purpose

	PURPOSE					
Method	**Population freedom from infection**	**Individual animal freedom from infection**	**Efficiency of eradication policies**	**Confirmation of clinical cases**	**Prevalence of infection—surveillance**	**Immune status in individual animals or populations postvaccination**
Virus isolation	–	+++	–	+++	–	–
Agar gel immunodiffusion	–	–	–	–	–	–
Complement fixation	–	–	–	+++	–	–
Enzyme-linked immunosorbent assay	+	++	+	++	+++	+
Polymerase chain reaction	–	+++	–	+++	–	–
Virus neutralization	+	+++	+	+++	+++	+++

Key: +++ = recommended method; ++ = suitable method; + = may be used in some situations, but cost, reliability, or other factors severely limit its application; – = not appropriate for this purpose.
Although not all of the tests listed as category +++ or ++ have undergone formal standardization and validation, their routine nature and the fact that they have been used widely, without dubious results, makes them acceptable.

of skin samples obtained by biopsy reveals edema and vasculitis and presence of intracytoplasmic EAV antigen.

NECROPSY FINDINGS

Gross lesions include edema of the eyelids and petechiation of the upper respiratory tract and the serosae of the abdominal and thoracic viscera. There is an abundant serofibrinous pleural and peritoneal effusion with generalized edema of the lungs, mediastinum, and abdominal mesenteries. A hemorrhagic enterocolitis and hemorrhage and infarction in the spleen may be noted. Characteristic histologic changes are found in the small arteries and include **fibrinoid necrosis of the tunica media and karyorrhexis of the infiltrating leukocytes**. Fluorescent antibody or immunohistochemical staining demonstrates viral antigen within the endothelial cells of these blood vessels. An immunoperoxidase method has also revealed viral antigen within endothelial cells and macrophages of an aborting mare and her fetus and within skin biopsies of animals exhibiting a maculopapular rash. Serologic tests performed on samples collected at necropsy can also be used to confirm that exposure to the virus has occurred.

The virus can be isolated from the lung and spleen of aborted fetuses, but no consistent, specific lesions are present. Necrotizing arteritis, similar to that in the mare, may be detectable.

Samples for Confirmation of Diagnosis

- **Virology**—chilled lung, spleen, and thymus (virus isolation, PCR, fluorescence antibody test)
- **Serology**—heart-blood serum or fetal thoracic fluid (virus neutralization, ELISA, complement fixation)
- **Histology**—fixed lung, spleen, adrenal, jejunum, colon, and heart (light microscopy, immunohistochemistry)

DIFFERENTIAL DIAGNOSIS

Definitive diagnosis is based on isolation of EAV from affected cases, or the demonstration of seroconversion or an increase in serum antibody titer.

The systemic disease must be differentiated from that associated with equine herpesvirus type 1 (EHV1) or type 4 (EHV-4) infection, equine influenza, strangles (see Tables 12-13 and 12-14—Infectious respiratory diseases of horses), infection with Getah virus in Japan, equine infectious anemia, African horse sickness, and purpura hemorrhagica, equine infectious anemia, equine encephalosis virus infection, Hendra virus infection, Getah virus infection, and toxicosis caused by hoary alyssum (*Berteroa incana*).

Abortion should be differentiated from that associated with EHV1, *Salmonella abortusequi,* leptospirosis, mare reproductive loss syndrome, and congenital malformations.

Similar disease in neonates can be associated with EHV1, immaturity or premature birth, and bacterial septicemia.

TREATMENT AND CONTROL

There is no specific treatment for equine viral arteritis. Most horses recover without specific care. Severely affected foals require intensive care.

Control of EAV infection is based on the strong **immunity** induced by natural infection or vaccination with a modified live virus and an understanding of the role of carrier stallions in the disease. The following practices are suggested:

1. Isolate all new arrivals (and returning horses) to farm or ranch for 3 to 5 weeks.
2. If possible, segregate pregnant mares from other horses.
3. Blood test all breeding stallions for EAV antibodies.
4. Check semen of any unvaccinated, antibody-positive stallions for EAV to identify carriers before breeding.
5. Once tested negative for EAV antibodies, vaccinate all breeding stallions annually.
6. Physically isolate any EAV carrier stallions.
7. Restrict breeding EAV carrier stallions to vaccinated mares or mares that test positive for naturally acquired antibodies to the virus.
8. Vaccinate mares against EVA at least 3 weeks before breeding to a known carrier stallion.
9. Isolate mares vaccinated for the first time against EVA for 3 weeks following breeding to an EAV carrier stallion.
10. In breeds or areas with high rates of EAV infection, vaccinate all intact males between 6 to 12 months of age.

Testing of mares and stallions permits identification of serologically negative, and therefore at-risk, animals. Seronegative mares should not be mated with infected stallions nor inseminated with fresh or frozen semen from infected stallions because of the risk of transmission of infection to the mare. Seropositive mares, or mares that have been vaccinated for at least 3 weeks, can safely be bred to stallions that have serologic evidence of infection. Seropositive mares should be separated from seronegative mares for at least 3 weeks after mating to a seropositive stallion. Seropositive stallions that have not been vaccinated should have their semen cultured to determine whether they are excreting the virus. Stallions excreting virus in their semen should be kept isolated from susceptible horses but can be bred to seropositive mares, as described previously. Because the virus survives cooling and freezing, similar principles should be applied to the use of artificial insemination in horses. One control program requires that all stallions be vaccinated with a modified live virus vaccine 28 days before the beginning of each breeding season.

Vaccination with a modified live virus vaccine induces strong immunity, although revaccination is necessary to ensure continuing immunity. The vaccine protects mares exposed to stallions shedding the virus in semen and has been used to control outbreaks of the respiratory form of the disease at racetracks. The modified live virus vaccine is regarded as safe, although there is mild fever and leukopenia, and there is evidence that the vaccine virus replicates in the vaccinates. A killed-virus vaccine is also available and is used to vaccinate Thoroughbred stallions in the United Kingdom.[37] Antibodies induced by the vaccine cannot be differentiated from those resulting from natural infection, a situation that may be problematic when import restrictions require the horse to be seronegative, presumably as proof of lack of exposure to virulent EAV.

Vaccination of foals from immune mares results in good protection, provided that the timing of vaccination is delayed until maternal antibodies to EAV are no longer present in the foal.

Control of an outbreak of EVA involves cessation of all movement on and off the farm and all breeding to control both horizontal and venereal transmission. All cases and contacts should be traced, sampled, and isolated. All horses on the affected premises should be screened and grouped according to infectious status. Testing and screening should continue on all possible affected premises until the end of the outbreak, seropositive animals and pregnant mares should be isolated for 4 weeks after first sampling, and stallions must have their shedding status determined. It is critical that all breeding of stallions is stopped and that concerted efforts are made to control horizontal spread of infection to stallions.

For breeds that permit use of assisted breeding technologies, all semen and embryos should be traced and recipients informed of the situation.

A protocol for managing an outbreak of EVA on a breeding facility is as follows (modified from the Horserace Betting Levy Board[38]):

1. Stop mating, teasing, and collection/insemination of semen, and stop movement of horses on and off the premises immediately.
2. Notify the appropriate regulatory authority.
3. Isolate and treat clinical cases.
4. Group the in-contacts away from other horses on the premises and take samples for virus detection (preferably RT-PCR). When the results are available, separate any healthy horses that have tested negative away from those that have tested positive. Horses that have tested positive should be kept in isolation until freedom from active infection is confirmed.
5. Screen all other horses at the premises to determine their serologic status (EAV positive or negative). If any of these return positive results, they should be separated from those with negative results and kept in isolation until freedom from active infection is confirmed by RT-PCR testing.
6. Arrange for one straw from each ejaculate of stored semen from infected stallions and their in-contacts to be tested by a laboratory. If any straw is infected, all straws from that ejaculate should be destroyed.
   - Inform the following of infection:
     - owners (or persons authorized to act on their behalf) of horses at, and soon to arrive at, the premises;
     - owners (or persons authorized to act on their behalf) of horses which have left the premises;
     - recipients of semen from the premises;
     - the national breeders' association, if applicable.
7. Clean and disinfect stables; equipment, including that used for semen collection and processing; and vehicles used for horse transport.
8. Good hygiene must be exercised. If possible, separate staff should be used for each different group of horses to prevent indirect transmission of infection between the groups.
9. Repeat the serologic testing after 14 days and again every 14 days until freedom from active infection is confirmed. Use the same laboratory for repeat samples as for the first samples. If any of the previously healthy or seronegative horses become ill or seropositive, they should be moved into the appropriate group. Testing of these horses should continue until freedom from active infection is confirmed. Seropositive stallions and teasers must be investigated to determine whether they are shedders. Those that prove to be shedders must be kept in strict isolation until their future is decided and must not be used for breeding activities during this time.
10. Do not resume any breeding activities or movement on and off the premises until freedom from active infection is confirmed in all infected and in-contact horses.
11. Pregnant mares must be isolated for at least 28 days after leaving the premises. Those remaining on the premises should be kept in isolation for at least 28 days after active infection has stopped.
12. Any mares that became infected after their pregnancy began should be foaled in isolation.

FURTHER READING

Balasuriya UBR, et al. Equine arteritis virus. *Vet Microbiol.* 2013;167:93-122.

REFERENCES

1. World Organization for Animal Health. Terrestrial animal health code. 2013 at: <www.oie.int/fileadmin/Home/fr/Health_standards/.../2.05.10_EVA.pdf>; Accessed 30.11.15.
2. Dunowska M, et al. *Vet Microbiol.* 2012;156:418.
3. Archambault D, et al. *Biomed Res Int.* 2014;2014:303841.
4. Balasuriya UBR, et al. *Vet Microbiol.* 2013;167:93.
5. Pronost S, et al. *Equine Vet J.* 2010;42:713.
6. Zhang J, et al. *J Gen Virol.* 2010;91:2286.
7. Vairo S, et al. *Vet Microbiol.* 2012;157:333.
8. Firth AE, et al. *J Gen Virol.* 2011;92:1097.
9. Go YY, et al. *J Virol.* 2010;84:4898.
10. Zhang J, et al. *Arch Virol.* 2007;152:1977.
11. Echeverria MAG, et al. *Virus Genes.* 2007;35:313.
12. Larska M, et al. *Vet Microbiol.* 2008;127:392.
13. Metz GE, et al. *Arch Virol.* 2008;153:2111.
14. Ernesto Metz G, et al. *Intervirol.* 2011;54:29.
15. Rola J, et al. *Vet Microbiol.* 2011;148:402.
16. Ataseven VS, et al. *Rev Med Vet.* 2013;164:67.
17. Rola J, et al. *Vet Microbiol.* 2013;164:378.
18. Metz GE, et al. *Rev Sci Tech OIE.* 2014;33:937.
19. Miszczak F, et al. *Virologie.* 2015;19:7.
20. Surma-Kurusiewicz K, et al. *Res Vet Sci.* 2013;94:361.
21. Miszczak F, et al. *Virol.* 2012;423:165.
22. McFadden AMJ, et al. *NZ Vet J.* 2013;61:300.
23. Bulut O, et al. *J Anim Vet Adv.* 2012;11:924.
24. Mangana-Vougiouka O, et al. *Rev Sci Tech OIE.* 2013;32:775.
25. Broaddus CC, et al. *Therio.* 2011;76:47.
26. Go YY, et al. *J Virol.* 2011;85:13174.
27. Go YY, et al. *J Virol.* 2012;86:12407.
28. Go YY, et al. *Vet Microbiol.* 2012;157:220.
29. Kalemkerian PB, et al. *Res Vet Sci.* 2012;93:1271.
30. Gryspeerdt A, et al. *Vlaams Dier Tijd.* 2009;78:189.
31. Lu Z, et al. *J Vet Diagn Invest.* 2008;20:147.
32. Miszczak F, et al. *J Clin Micro.* 2011;49:3694.
33. Chung C, et al. *J Vet Diagn Invest.* 2013;25:182.
34. Chung C, et al. *J Vet Diagn Invest.* 2013;25:727.
35. Ernesto Metz G, et al. *J Virol Meth.* 2014;205:3.
36. Hu Y, et al. *Chin J Prev Vet Med.* 2014;36:651.
37. Newton JR. *Equine Vet Educ.* 2007;19:612.
38. Horserace Betting Levy Board. 2015 at: <http://codes.hblb.org.uk/index.php/page/55>; Accessed 29.11.15.

AFRICAN HORSE SICKNESS

SYNOPSIS

Etiology African horse sickness virus.

Epidemiology Infectious, noncontagious, arthropod-borne disease of horses, donkeys, and mules endemic to sub-Saharan Africa. Epizootics occur in the Iberian Peninsula, Mediterranean coast, Middle East, and Indian subcontinent. Heightened concern over risk of spread to areas, particularly western Europe, that are currently free of the disease.

Continued

Clinical signs *Pulmonary form:* fever, respiratory distress, frothy nasal discharge, death. *Cardiac form:* fever, edema of the head and ventral chest, hydropericardium. *Mixed form* has characteristics of both pulmonary and cardiac forms. *Horse fever:* mild fever, often inapparent infection.

Clinical pathology Leukopenia; disseminated intravascular coagulation. Serology often negative in horses that die acutely. Detection of viral genome by polymerase chain reaction (PCR).

Lesions Pulmonary edema, hydropericardium, ascites, edema of the gastrointestinal tract.

Diagnostic confirmation Histopathology. Detection of virus by cultivation or reverse-transcription PCR (RT-PCR) in blood or tissues.

Differential diagnosis list:
- Pulmonary form—rupture of cordae tendinea of mitral valve (single horse), acute bacterial pneumonia, anthrax, piroplasmosis
- Cardiac form—intoxication with monensin or similar ionophore.

Treatment None. Supportive care.

Control specific *Enzootic area:* vaccination, reduce exposure to biting insects. Quarantine and eradication in nonenzootic areas.

African horse sickness is an important disease of horses and mules in southern and central Africa and, during epizootics, in northern Africa (including Ethiopia)[1] and the Arabian and Iberian peninsulas. The disease in southern Africa occurs as frequent, intermittent small outbreaks and as periodic epidemics that kill large numbers of horses. An epidemic during 1854 to 1855 killed over 17,000 horses, 40% of the horse population, in the Western Cape region. During premechanized exploration and development of southern and central Africa and during the Boer War, the disease had a major economic and military impact. For example, during a single campaign in the Boer War, of 1732 British horses involved, 323 died of African horse sickness within a 17-day period in late April of 1901. An outbreak that extended through northern Africa into the Indian subcontinent from 1959 to 1961 resulted in the death of 300,000 horses.

ETIOLOGY

African horse sickness (AHS) is associated with a viscerotropic orbivirus (RNA, family Reoviridae), of which nine antigenic strains (serotypes) are recognized. The genome of AHS virus (AHSV), which is available,[2] is composed of 10 double-stranded RNA segments, which encode seven structural proteins (VP1-7) and four nonstructural proteins.[3,4] Proteins VP2 and VP5 form the outer capsid of the virion, and proteins VP3 and VP7 are the major inner capsid proteins. Proteins VP1, VP4, and VP6 constitute minor inner capsid proteins. The NS3 proteins are the second most variable AHSV proteins and are associated with viral release from cells and total viral yield.[3,5]

The serotypic differences are attributable to variations in the capsid proteins, predominantly VP2 and to a lesser extent VP5. VP2 contains the predominant neutralizing epitopes, although antibodies to VP5 are one of the earliest serologic markers of infection and have neutralizing activity. Lineages are also evident within serotypes, and the resultant clades are grouped geographically, at least for the serotypes studied. Identification of clades facilitates epidemiologic studies. There are also variants of each serotype with attenuated virulence. No new serotypes have been identified since 1960, and virtually all epidemics outside of southern Africa before 1987 were caused by serotype 9. Since then, outbreaks attributable to AHSV-4 (Iberian Peninsula 1987–1990); AHSV2, -4, -6, -8, and -9 in Ethiopia since 2007 (although AHSV-9 is endemic and was the serotype isolated from ~80% of cases)[6]; and AHSV-2 in Nigeria, Ghana, Senegal, Morocco, and neighboring countries from 2007 (again, with AHSV-9 being endemic in some of this region) have occurred.[7,8] Serotype 7 has been reported to cause disease in equids in Ethiopia but was not detected during 2007 to 2010.[1]

An avirulent form of AHSV 9 circulates in the Gambia, with 96% of clinically normal unvaccinated horses and donkeys seropositive for the serotype. The avirulent strain of AHSV-9 is identical to a vaccinal strain, raising the suggestion that the virus circulating in the Gambia region is highly likely to have derived from a live-attenuated AHSV-9 vaccine.[9] Passage of AHSV-7 through cell lines to produce an attenuated strain does not reduce its infectivity for midges, indicating the potential for vector-borne spread of avirulent strains of the virus.[10] The practice of vaccinating horses with polyvalent, avirulent vaccines has led to concerns about reassortment of the virus and reversion to virulence. However, although reassortment of vaccine virus occurs in vivo, there is currently no evidence that the reassortants are pathogenic, noting the limitation on this conclusion imposed by the small number of horses studied and the short duration of the study.[11]

There have been three outbreaks of AHS in the AHS-controlled zone near the Cape of Good Hope in South Africa since the zone was established in 1997. Serotypes involved in these outbreaks were serotype 1 (2004 and 2011) and serotype 7 in 1999. The 1999 and 2004 outbreaks were traced to unauthorized movement of horses into the zone. The source of the 2011 outbreak is unknown.[12]

There is real concern among AHS-free countries, including those in Europe, the Americas, and Australia, that AHS will gain entry, either by movement of midges, through introduction of subclinically infected equids (likely mules, donkeys, or zebras), or through fraudulent (unauthorized) importation of equids. Recognition of this risk, which appears to be increasing with global warming and climate change and is exemplified by the emergence of Bluetongue and Schmallenberg viruses in Europe,[8,13,14] has resulted in many countries developing contingency plans for exclusion of the virus or management plans should it emerge.[8,14-19]

The virus is similar to other animal orbiviruses, including bluetongue virus, enzootic hemorrhagic disease virus, and equine encephalosis virus. The host range includes equids (horses, donkeys, mules, zebra), elephants, camels, sheep, goats, and predatory or scavenging carnivores. Infection produces disease in horses and mules, and less commonly African donkeys, but rarely in the other herbivorous hosts.[3] The disease occurs in dogs, although apparently rarely, and can occur in dogs that have not had known access to infected meat.[20]

The virus is inactivated by heating at 50° C (122° F) for 3 hours or 60° C (140° F) for 15 minutes, is stable at 4° C (39° F), and survives for 37 days at 37° C. It remains viable at pH of 6 to 12, but it is inactivated by acid and in 48 hours by 0.1% formalin or phenol, sodium hypochlorite, and iodophors.

Infection with African horse sickness virus is listed by the World Organization for Animal Health (OIE).[21]

EPIDEMIOLOGY

African horse sickness is an **infectious but not contagious** disease of Equidae. It is spread by the bite of blood-feeding insects.

Occurrence

The disease is **enzootic in sub-Saharan Africa**, causing clinical disease in horses, donkeys, mules, and dogs and infecting zebras, elephants, and perhaps other wildlife. The disease occurs from Senegal through sub-Saharan Africa to Somalia and Ethiopia. The disease makes occasional incursions into Iran, Pakistan, India, Turkey, and the eastern Mediterranean and Cyprus. The virus occurs in the Middle East, including Saudi Arabia and Yemen. It does not appear to be enzootic to Saudi Arabia, although the long-term status of this region is uncertain. In 1987 the disease recurred in Spain through introduction of infected zebras into a game park. By 1990 the disease had spread throughout Spain and Portugal but was eliminated by 1991.

Sero-epidemiologic surveys in Ethiopia indicate a prevalence rate of 10.4%, 29.7%, and 10.3% in horses, donkeys, and mules, respectively, with some regions having 51% seroprevalence in donkeys, 30% in mules, and 28% in horses, with an overall seroprevalence of 33%.[1]

South Africa

The disease has been recognized in South Africa since shortly after introduction of domesticated horses in the 1600s. The disease occurred throughout what is now South Africa in the nineteenth and early twentieth centuries, but as an enzootic disease became restricted to the northeastern areas of the country in the middle and later part of the twentieth century. The geographic contraction of disease was associated with elimination of large herds of wild zebra from all except the game parks of the northeastern areas of the country. Elimination of zebra, the reservoir of infection, reduced the occurrence of the disease dramatically. Outbreaks of disease outside of the endemic areas in the northeastern areas of South Africa are associated with introductions of virus from endemic areas at times of high abundance of *Culicoides* spp., the vector. The disease does not overwinter in the essentially zebra-free nonendemic areas. Serotype 9 causes enzootic disease in central Africa in the absence of zebra; the wildlife host has not been identified.

African horse sickness occurred in 1999 in the surveillance zone of the Cape Province of South Africa surrounding the disease-free area of Cape Town. The virus (serotype 7) was of a clade identical to that found in Kwazulu Natal Province, and its introduction was by the movement of infected horses from that region into the Cape Province.

Transmission of Infection

African horse sickness virus (AHSV) is transmitted by the **bite of hematophagous insects,** including midges (*Culicoides* spp.), ticks (*Hyalomma dromadarii* and the brown dog tick, *Rhipicephalus sanguineus*), and mosquitoes (various species in laboratory studies). **Midges** are by far the most important vector in the spread of the spontaneous disease. The source of virus for midges is blood of infected horses, donkeys, mules, and zebra. Horses and mules have clinical signs of disease while viremic, but donkeys are often and, most important, zebra are always, apparently uninfected. Zebras may remain viremic for 6 weeks, donkeys for 12 days, and horses for 18 to 21 days. Dogs are usually infected by eating infected animals, although transmission to and from dogs by ticks can occur.[20]

Transmission of the virus to areas where it does not usually exist occurs both by movement of infected animals, such as zebras and horses, and by transportation of midges by wind or in aircraft.[7,8] Mechanical transmission of the virus on contaminated surgical instruments and needles should be considered a possibility.

Zebra

In areas in which the disease is enzootic, the virus persists by cycling between the mammalian host, the zebra, and vectors year round. Zebra in enzootic areas can seroconvert during any month of the year, indicating that persistence of the virus is associated with sequential infection of zebra within a herd or region. Persistence of the virus in a region is attributable to the long period of viremia in zebra and the presence of a herd of sufficient size to support cycling of infection among animals. The minimum size of a zebra population to maintain an enzootic infection is unknown. However, in areas in which the disease is not enzootic, the virus does not persist over the cooler winter months, when viremic animals recover and the vectors die. Concern exists that reintroduction of zebra to areas of the country currently free of enzootic AHS might permit reestablishment of the virus and disease in horses.

Midges

Knowledge of the ecology of midges (*Culicoides* spp.), and which of them can be vectors for AHSV, is critical to developing an understanding of the risk of introduction and spread of infection in disease-free areas.[22,23] Although much is known about the ecology of midges, it is unclear which species, apart from *C. imicola* and *C. bolitinos,* can be vectors for AHSV and the capacity of these potential vectors to spread disease. A number of species of culicoides that feed on horses, and other herbivores, are present in rural and urban regions of the southeastern United Kingdom and could be potential vectors for AHSV.[23,24] And being present and capable of being infected by AHSV, midges must feed on horses with sufficient frequency to spread the infection. The frequency with which midges feed on horses could be influenced by the host preference of midges—they might prefer to feed on other herbivores, thereby reducing the risk of spread of infection between horses.[25] Whether midges have this preference, and the influence of variable densities of alternative hosts on midge feeding, is unclear at this time.[25]

Finally, the risk of introduction and establishment of breeding populations of species of midges to areas in which they are not currently present must be considered.[8,15] Such introductions could be by wind or aircraft. The biosecurity risks of African horse sickness viruses need to be reevaluated in regions where the vector's niche is suitable as a result of climate change or human manipulation of local ecosystems, such as by irrigation.[26] Under some likely climate change scenarios the distribution of *C. imicola* could expand northward in the Northern Hemisphere. The risk of spread of African horse sickness virus is likely to increase as the climate suitability for *C. imicola* shifts poleward, especially in Western Europe.[26] The range of *C. imicola* in Africa might well decrease as a result of a warming climate.[26] Other human activities, such as irrigations programs and alterations in herbivore populations, that alter the ecology of local areas in such a way as to provide an ecological niche and environment where midges exotic to the area can thrive will influence the risk of introduction of AHSV.

Midges are infected with AHSV; that is, they are not mechanical vectors, but rather the virus infects and replicates in the midge,[27] although transovarian transmission of infection between generations of midges does not occur. *C. imicola* is the primary vector responsible for the transmission of AHSV within its enzootic area and during epizootics. *C. bolitinos* is also a vector of AHSV in southern Africa, whereas a number of other *Culicoides* spp. are unlikely to be vectors because they are unable to maintain infection with the virus 10 days after ingesting a meal of infected blood. At least 11 species of culicoides from South Africa can be infected by a variety of AHSV serotypes after feeding on infected blood meals in a laboratory setting. There are evident complex relationships between species of culicoides and serotype of AHSV affecting viral infection and titer in the vectors.[10] However, *C. varipenis, C. pulicaris,* and *C. obsoletus* are competent and likely important vectors because of their ability to maintain infection over the winter, as demonstrated in Portugal.

The abundance of midges can be predicted from measures of soil moisture content and land surface temperature. Midges breed in damp soils that are rich in organic material, such as irrigated pastures, that provide soil moisture adequate for completion of the life cycle (at least 7–10 days). Higher temperatures increase the rates of infection of midges, virogenesis within midges, and transmission rate but decrease midge longevity. Replication of AHSV in midges does not occur at temperatures less than 15° C (59° F), although midges continue to be active at 12° C (54° F). The absence of AHSV in the midges during winter in parts of South Africa can be ascribed to their relatively low numbers, low infection prevalence, low virus replication rates, and low virus titers in the potentially infected midges.[28]

Midges can be transported by winds for up to 700 km.

Risk Factors

Environment Factors

The incidence of the disease is often **seasonal** because of the seasonal variations in the number of *Culicoides* spp. present and possibly other weather-related factors such as host (zebra) behavior (Fig. 21-2). Vector activity is favored by temperatures between 12.5° and 29° C (54.5° and 84° F), and it is likely that several cool or cold episodes, rather than one "killing frost," are necessary to kill all or most vectors. Local factors, including topography, influence the distribution of midges within their overall range, and therefore the disease has a geographic distribution: the areas most severely affected are low lying and swampy.

Epizootics of AHS occur in southern Africa in association with variations in the El

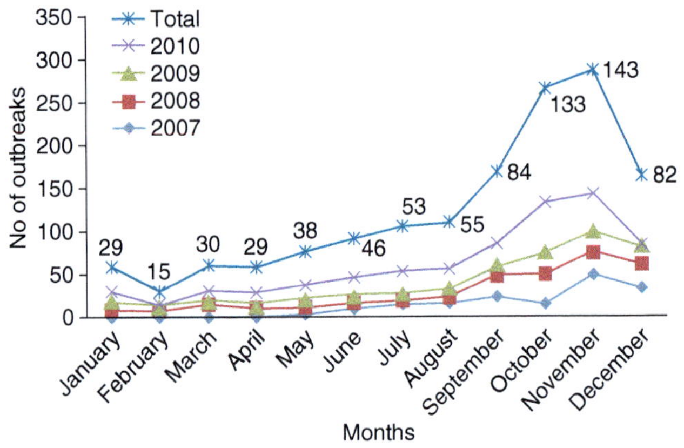

Fig. 21-2 Seasonal occurrence of outbreaks of African horse sickness in central Ethiopia (2007–2010).[1] (Reproduced with permission from Aklilu N, Batten C, Gelaye E, et al: African Horse Sickness Outbreaks Caused by Multiple Virus Types in Ethiopia. *Transboundary & Emerging Diseases* 2014;61:185-192.)

Niño/Southern Oscillation. Epizootics of the disease occur in years in which the oscillation produces drought followed by heavy rains. The reason for this association, which was first anecdotally reported in the 1800s, is unknown but could be related to congregation of zebra around water holes during the drought. Congregation of large numbers of zebra might increase the infection rate among midges, which then disseminate the infection when rains produce widespread conditions favorable to their reproduction.

Animal Factors

Natural infection occurs in Equidae, the most severe disease occurring in horses, with mules, donkeys, and zebras showing lesser degrees of susceptibility, in that order. The risk of death is greatest in weanlings but for all horses does not appear to be related to sex of the animal. The case-fatality rate varies depending on the severity of disease (see under "Clinical Signs") but can be as high as 90% in susceptible horses,[12,29] but it is lower in mules and donkeys.

Elephants seroconvert when exposed to infection but are probably not an important reservoir. White rhinoceros sampled in Kruger National Park in 1989 had a 60% seroprevalence to AHSV, whereas in 2007 the seroprevalence was zero. The reasons for this difference are unclear.[30]

Vaccination is effective in reducing risk of the disease (odds ratio for risk of death ~0.1 [0.04 to 0.4]).[29] After natural infection or vaccination, immunity to that strain, but not to heterologous strains, is solid. The development of immunity is slow and may require 3 weeks to be appreciable; titers may continue to rise for 6 months after infection.

Foals from immune dams derive passive immunity, the titer of which varies depending on the mare's titer, the serotype, and the time after ingestion of colostrum. Mare titers before foaling and foal serum titers after suckling are highly correlated regardless of serotype.[31] Mare serum titers for some serotypes (1, 4, 6, and 9) are higher than for other serotypes, and this is mirrored in the titers in foal serum. Estimated mean half-life for neutralizing antibodies in foals to all 9 serotypes was 20.5 (± 2.6 standard deviation) days, with a range from 15.4 days for serotype 8 to 22.6 days for serotype 3. The estimate for the mean time until the serum neutralization test became negative at a 1 : 10 dilution, considered absence of protection from infection, was 96 days for all nine serotypes, with a range from 62 days for serotype 5 to 128 days for serotypes 3 and 4.[31]

Economic Importance

The disease was of tremendous economic concern in southern Africa when horses were important for transportation and as draft animals. The disease is currently an economic concern because of the costs associated with preventive measures in enzootic areas, monitoring for introduction of disease in unaffected areas, and restrictions on importation of horses from countries in which the disease is enzootic. The high case-fatality rate and morbidity of the disease in outbreaks is another source of loss. The cost of disease epizootics can be large, as demonstrated by the outbreak in the Iberian Peninsula, where control of the disease in Portugal in 1990 to 1991 was achieved at a cost of US$2,000,000. Direct costs of managing the 2011 outbreak in the AHS-controlled zone in South Africa were at least R850,000, with estimated export losses of greater than R20,000,000.[12]

Zoonotic Disease

African horse sickness caused encephalitis and chorioretinitis in eight workers in an AHS vaccine factory. Infection was likely be through inhalation of freeze-dried virus.

PATHOGENESIS

AHSV affects vascular endothelium and monocytes/macrophages.[32] The tissue tropism of the infecting serotype determines which organs are most severely affected, although all serotypes infect the heart and lungs and, to a lesser extent, the spleen.[32] After infection, the virus multiplies in local lymph nodes, and a primary viremia ensues, with dissemination of infection to endothelial cells and intravascular macrophages of lung, spleen, and lymphoid tissues. Viral multiplication then results in a secondary cell-associated (red cell and white cell) viremia in horses of up to 9 days in duration. Fever and viremia occur at the same time, and resolution of the viremia is associated with defervescence. Localization of antigen depends on the form of the disease—horses with horse sickness have most of the antigen in the spleen, whereas horses with the more severe cardiopulmonary form have abundant antigen in cardiovascular and lymphatic systems.

Infection of endothelial cells results in degenerative changes, increases in vascular permeability, impaired intercellular junctions, loss of endothelium, subendothelial deposition of cell debris and fibrin, and evidence of vascular repair. Edema, hemorrhage, and microthrombi are associated with the vascular lesions. Abnormalities in the lungs include development of alveolar and interstitial edema, sequestration of neutrophils and platelet aggregates, and formation of fibrinous microthrombi. Combined, these changes likely result in coagulopathy, systemic inflammatory response syndrome, edema, impaired cardiovascular and pulmonary function, and hypovolemia.

CLINICAL FINDINGS

The **incubation period** in natural infections is about 5 to 7 days. Three or four clinical forms of the disease occur, an acute or pulmonary form, a cardiac or subacute form, a mixed form, and a mild form known as "horse sickness fever." An intermittent fever of 40° to 41°C (105–106°F) is characteristic of all forms.

Acute (Pulmonary) Horse Sickness (Dunkop)

Acute horse sickness is the most common form in epizootics and has a case-fatality rate of 95%. Fever is followed by labored breathing, severe paroxysms of coughing, and a **profuse nasal discharge** of yellowish serous fluid and froth. Profuse sweating, profound weakness, and a staggering gait progress to recumbency. Death usually occurs after a total course of 4 to 5 days, although it can be so acute as to be without observed premonitory signs in some horses. Severe respiratory distress persists for many weeks in surviving animals. This is the form of the disease that occurs naturally in dogs.

Subacute (Cardiac) Horse Sickness (Dikkop)

Subacute (cardiac) horse sickness is most common in horses in enzootic areas and has a case-fatality rate of 50%. The incubation period may be up to 3 weeks, and the disease has a more protracted course than does the acute, pulmonary form. There is **edema** in the head, particularly in the temporal fossa, the eyelids, and the lips, and the chest, which may not develop until the horse has been febrile for a week. The oral mucosa is bluish in color, and petechiae may develop under the tongue. Examination of the heart and lungs reveals evidence of **hydropericardium**, endocarditis, and pulmonary edema. Restlessness and mild abdominal pain and paralysis of the esophagus, with inability to swallow and regurgitation of food and water through the nose, is not uncommon. Recovery is prolonged. A fatal course may last as long as 2 weeks.

A **mixed form** of the disease, with both pulmonary and cardiac signs, is evident as an initial subacute cardiac form that suddenly develops acute pulmonary signs. Also, a primary pulmonary syndrome may subside, but cardiac involvement causes death. This mixed form is not common in field outbreaks.

Horse Sickness Fever

A mild form of horse sickness fever, which may be easily overlooked, is common in enzootic areas. The disease occurs in horses with some immunity or infection by serotypes of low virulence. This is the only form of the disease that occurs in zebras. The temperature rises to 40.5°C (105°F) over a period of 1 to 3 days but returns to normal about 3 days later. The appetite is poor, and there is slight conjunctivitis and moderate respiratory distress.

CLINICAL PATHOLOGY

Leukopenia with lymphopenia, neutropenia and a left shift, mild thrombocytopenia, and hemoconcentration are characteristic of the acute forms of AHS. **Serum biochemical abnormalities** include increases in creatine kinase, lactate dehydrogenase, and alkaline phosphatase activities and creatinine and bilirubin concentrations. There is evidence of activation of coagulation cascade and fibrinolysis, although disseminated intravascular coagulation is unusual.

Confirmation of diagnosis is based on seroconversion (in horses that survive) or presence of AHSV in horses with compatible clinical or epidemiologic characteristics of the disease.[3] Detection of the virus can be made by demonstration of viral genome by one or more of a variety of PCR tests.[3,33-41] Each of these tests has its particular advantages, but all have the advantage of rapidity of diagnosis, often within hours of the sample being delivered to the laboratory, and many allow prompt identification of the serotype involved. Type-specific gel-based RT-PCR and real-time RT-PCR using hybridization probes for identification and differentiation AHSV genotypes provides a rapid typing method for AHSV in tissue samples and blood.[34,37,39,42] ELISA tests provide rapid detection of AHSV antigen in blood, spleen, and supernatant from cell culture. The virus neutralization (VN) assay was formerly the "gold standard" for typing and identifying virus isolates, but because it takes 5 days and culture of the virus, it has been replaced by PCR assays.[3] The virus can be cultured in baby hamster kidney-21 (BHK-21), monkey stable (MS) or African green monkey kidney (Vero), or insect cells (KC); intravenously in embryonated eggs; or intracerebrally in newborn mice.[3]

Serologic diagnosis of the acute disease may be difficult because many horses die before they mount a detectable antibody response. In horses that survive for at least 10 days, agar gel immunodiffusion (AGID), indirect fluorescent antibody (IFA), complement fixation (CF), VN and ELISA tests are all effective in detecting antibody to the virus. An indirect ELISA (I-ELISA) is more sensitive in detecting early immunologic responses to vaccination or infection and the declining immunity in foals. However, in outbreaks of disease early and accurate diagnosis of disease and identification of the serotype involved is important to guide selection of vaccine and thereby control spread of the disease. Blocking ELISA, indirect ELISA, and complement fixation are all prescribed tests in the *OIE Terrestrial Manual*.[3] Suitable samples are blood collected into heparin during the febrile stage of the disease or lung, spleen, or lymphoid tissue collected at necropsy.

Tests approved for testing horses for international trade include a complement fixation test and an indirect sandwich ELISA.

> **DIFFERENTIAL DIAGNOSIS**
>
> The fulminant disease in groups of horses is characteristic, although acute intoxication by monensin, salinomycin, or similar compounds can produce similar signs. Individual horses affected with purpura hemorrhagica and groups of horses affected with equine viral arteritis can have signs similar to horses with African horse sickness (AHS). Piroplasmosis (*B. caballi* or *T. equi*) and trypanosomiasis cause fever and depression. Anthrax can cause acute deaths in solitary horses or groups of horses.

NECROPSY FINDINGS

Gross findings in acute cases include **severe hydrothorax and pulmonary edema** and moderate ascites. The liver is acutely congested, and there is edema of the bowel wall. The pharynx, trachea, and bronchi are filled with yellow serous fluid and froth. In cases of cardiac horse sickness there is marked hydropericardium, endocardial hemorrhage, and myocardial degeneration. Edema of the head and neck is common, especially of the supraorbital fossa and nuchal ligament. Microscopic lesions are minimal in the acute form; pulmonary edema may be present but no obvious vascular injury. Myocardial damage, including foci of necrosis, hemorrhage, and mild leukocytic infiltrates, may be seen during histologic examination of many cardiac (subacute) cases. An immunoperoxidase test is sensitive in detecting viral antigen in formalin-fixed, paraffin-embedded tissues.[43]

Samples for Confirmation of Diagnosis

- **Virology**—chilled spleen, lung, lymph node (PCR, VIRUS ISOLATION)
- **Histology**—fixed lung, heart (light microscopy, immunohistochemistry)

TREATMENT

There is no specific treatment for AHS. Supportive care and treatment of complication of the disease should be provided.

CONTROL

The **principles of control** in enzootic areas are **vaccination** and **reduction of exposure** of horses to biting insects, whereas in **nonenzootic** areas the aim is to **prevent introduction** of the disease and **eradication** if it is introduced. The objectives of a control program for African horse sickness are as follows:

- Prevention of introduction of infection by clinically ill or apparently uninfected animals
- Slaughter of viremic animals where animal welfare and economic considerations permit this course of action
- Management changes to reduce exposure to midges
- Vector control
- Induction of active immunity in animals at risk of disease

Prevention of Introduction

Many countries now have specific plans to prevent introduction of AHSV-infected equids and emergency management of introduction of the virus or occurrence of the disease.[8,13,14,16,17,19,44]

Infection can be introduced into an area free of AHSV by infected animals or midges. Control of midges is discussed later in the chapter. Infected animals can be horses incubating the disease; clinically ill animals; or animals, including donkeys and zebras, that have no clinical signs of illness but are infected and viremic, as was the case of the Portuguese epizootic. Appropriate control measures to prevent movement of animals at risk of being infected should be instituted and include the following:[3] completion of a vaccination protocol effective against all important serotypes at least 42 to 60 days before introduction of the horse, positive identification of all horses by microchipping and passport documenting vaccination status, and a veterinary certificate confirming health and issued no more than 48 hours before introduction. Equids imported from areas in which the disease is enzootic, or from neighboring regions, should be housed in isolation in insect-proof enclosures for 60 days. Recommendations that call for vaccination of all equids within 10 miles (16 km) of imported horses are not appropriate for most countries to which the disease is exotic.

Slaughter of Sick or Viremic Animals

The extreme measure of slaughter is appropriate in controlling infection recently introduced into areas previously free of the disease. It is an effective adjunct in control of spread of infection, as demonstrated in Portugal. There are obvious economic, animal welfare, and public relations aspects to this practice, especially in areas where horses have high intrinsic worth or are companion animals.

Reduce Exposure to Biting Midges[22]

Horses should be housed in insect-proof buildings or, at a minimum, buildings that limit exposure of horses to midges by closure of doors and covering of windows with gauze. Impregnation of gauze with an insecticide further reduces biting rates. Stables should be situated in areas, such as on hilltops or well-drained sites, that have minimal midge populations. Midge numbers on individual farms should be reduced by habitat alteration, and thus areas of damp, organically enriched soils are eliminated. Widespread use of insecticides is unlikely to be environmentally acceptable.

The feeding pattern of midges is such that housing of horses during the crepuscular periods and at night will significantly reduce biting rates and likelihood of infection. Horses kept at pasture should have insect repellents applied regularly and especially to provide protection during periods of high-insect-biting activity. DEET (*N,N*-diethyl-*m*-toluamide) is the only commercially available repellent with documented activity against *Culicoides* spp. Application of deltamethrin (10 mL of 1% solution) to skin of horses did not reduce the frequency of midge feeding in an experimental trial in the United Kingdom.[24] Installation of alphacypermethrin impregnated mesh to jet stalls reduced the attach rate by culicoides species by 6- to 14-fold and markedly reduced the number of culicoides collected from horses housed in the stalls compared with sentinel horses, suggesting that this might be a useful means of reducing exposure of housed horses to midges.[45]

Vaccination

Vaccination is effective in reducing both morbidity and mortality from AHSV infection in horses in enzootic areas and to control epizootics of the disease.[7,29] Vaccination is used in two circumstances: in areas in which the disease is endemic and in regions with an epizootic of the disease. Vaccination can be used in enzootic or neighboring regions to provide active immunity of all resident equids because of the continual risk of the disease in these areas. Vaccination in this instance is initiated as soon as foals no longer have passive immunity to the virus, and it continues annually throughout the horse's life. Alternatively, vaccination can be used in the face of an epizootic to induce active immunity in horses in contact or in regions surrounding the outbreak. In this instance vaccination is stopped when the infection is eradicated from the area.

Early attenuated virus vaccines, although effective in preventing AHS, were associated with significant adverse effects, such as encephalitis. More recent vaccines of virus attenuated by passage through tissue culture are effective in preventing disease but do not prevent viremia. They were used to control the most recent outbreak in Spain and Portugal. Currently available vaccines are polyvalent or monovalent preparations containing attenuated strains of the virus. Protection against heterologous serotypes is usually weak, and most vaccines are polyvalent.

The polyvalent vaccines contain serotypes 1, 3, and 4 or serotypes 2, 6, 7, and 8, respectively. AHSV-9 is not included because serotype 6 is cross-protective.[46] A monovalent vaccine containing attenuated serotype 9 is used in western Africa, where this was, until recent emergence of AHSV-2, the only serotype present.[7] Vaccination of foals with either monovalent or polyvalent vaccine did not affect the serologic response to each serotype; that is, the response to vaccination with a monovalent vaccine did not differ to the response to that serotype when it was delivered in a polyvalent vaccine.[47] Foals have markedly varying serologic responses to differing serotypes, similar to the situation in adult to horses,[31] and they fail to develop protective immunity to some serotypes.[47]

Inactivated vaccines are effective in preventing viremia in most animals and disease without adverse effects. Inactivated vaccines are no longer available.

A number of recombinant canary-pox or vaccinia subunit vaccines have been trialed experimentally and provide protective immunity against challenge exposure of horses or appear to be effective using guinea pig models of the disease. The remaining challenge is to ensure that vaccines provide protection against all 9 serotypes.[48-52]

The recommended vaccination program for horses in South Africa that all race horses shall be vaccinated against African horse sickness using a registered, nonexpired, polyvalent horse sickness vaccine (e.g., Horse Sickness Vaccine I [AHS I] and Horse Sickness Vaccine II [AHS II]) according to the manufacturers' recommendations including two times as foals between the ages of 6 and 18 months, not less than 90 days apart and, where possible, between June 1 and October 31, and thereafter every year between June 1 and October 31.[53] Foals are not vaccinated until they are at least 6 months of age to prevent any effect of colostral passive immunity on efficacy of vaccination. Horses resident in the AHS controlled area may not be vaccinated without written permission from authorities.

Immunity after vaccination is protective for at least 1 year, but annual revaccination of all horses, mules, and donkeys is recommended.

There is concern over the use of attenuated virus vaccines in epizootic situations, that is, in regions where AHSV is not enzootic. These reasons include the lack of vaccines approved for use in the European Community; the availability of only two types of polyvalent vaccines and one type of monovalent vaccine; delays in availability of vaccine for emergency vaccination; introduction of the virus, even attenuated virus, into regions in which it is not present; attenuated-virus viremia in some vaccinated horses; and reversion of vaccine strains to virulence.[9,11,54] These concerns have heightened the need for availability of inactivated virus or subunit vaccines.

REFERENCES

1. Bitew M, et al. *Trop Animal Health Prod.* 2011;43:1543.
2. Anon. *Genome Announc.* 2015;3:e00921.
3. World Organisation for Animal Health. African horse sickness. 2012.
4. Zwart L, et al. *PLoS ONE.* 2015;10.
5. Meiring TL, et al. *Arch Virol.* 2009;154:263.
6. Aklilu N, et al. *Transbound Emerg Dis.* 2014;61:185.
7. Diouf ND, et al. *Vet Rec.* 2013;172:152.
8. van den Boom R, et al. *Vet Rec.* 2013;172:150.
9. Oura CAL, et al. *Epidemiol Inf.* 2012;140:462.
10. Venter GJ, et al. *Med Vet Ent.* 2009;23:367.
11. von Teichman BF, et al. *Vaccine.* 2008;26:5014.
12. Grewar JD, et al. *J Sth Afr Vet Assoc.* 2013;84:Art. #973.
13. MacLachlan NJ, et al. *Vet Res.* 2010;41.
14. Thompson GM, et al. *Irish Vet J.* 2012;65.
15. Carpenter S. *Vet Rec.* 2014;174:299.
16. de Vos CJ, et al. *Prev Vet Med.* 2012;106:108.
17. African horse sickness: how to spot and report the disease. 2014 at: <https://www.gov.uk/guidance/african-horse-sickness#how-african-horse-sickness-is-spread>; Accessed 06.09.15.
18. Faverjon C, et al. *BMC Vet Res.* 2015;11.
19. AUSVETPLAN. Animal Health Australia. 2014 at: <http://www.animalhealthaustralia.com.au/programs/emergency-animal-disease-preparedness/ausvetplan/disease-strategies/>; Accessed 06.09.15.
20. Sittert SJV, et al. *J Sth Afr Vet Assoc.* 2013;84:Art. #948.
21. OIE-listed diseases, infections and infestations in force in 2015. 2015 at: <http://www.oie.int/animal-health-in-the-world/oie-listed-diseases-2015/>; Accessed 06.09.15.
22. Carpenter S, et al. *Med Vet Ent.* 2008;22:175.
23. Robin M, et al. *Vet Rec.* 2014;174.
24. Robin M, et al. *Vet Rec.* 2015;176.
25. Lo Iacono G, et al. *J R Soc Interface.* 2013;10.
26. Guichard S, et al. *PLoS ONE.* 2014;9:e112491.
27. Wilson A, et al. *Vet Res.* 2009;40.

28. Venter GJ, et al. *J Sth Afr Vet Assoc.* 2015;85.
29. Gordon S, et al. *Ond J Vet Res.* 2013;80.
30. Miller M, et al. *J Zoo Wildlife Med.* 2011;42:29.
31. Crafford JE, et al. *Equine Vet J.* 2013;45:604.
32. Clift SJ, et al. *Vet Pathol.* 2010;47:690.
33. Aradaib IE. *J Virol Meth.* 2009;159:1.
34. Bachanek-Bankowska K, et al. *PLoS ONE.* 2014;9.
35. Bremer CW. *Open Vet Sci J.* 2012;6:8.
36. Fernandez-Pinero J, et al. *Res Vet Sci.* 2009;86:353.
37. Guthrie AJ, et al. *J Virol Meth.* 2013;189:30.
38. Koekemoer JJO. *J Virol Meth.* 2008;154:104.
39. Maan NS, et al. *PLoS ONE.* 2011;6.
40. Monaco F, et al. *Molecular Cellular Probes.* 2011;25:87.
41. Quan M, et al. *J Virol Meth.* 2010;167:45.
42. Maan NS, et al. *J Virol Meth.* 2015;213:118.
43. Clift SJ, et al. *J Vet Diagn Invest.* 2009;21:655.
44. Marcos A, et al. *Archivos De Medicina Veterinaria.* 2015;47:101.
45. Page PC, et al. *Vet Parasitol.* 2015;210:84.
46. von Teichman BF, et al. *Vaccine.* 2010;28:6505.
47. Crafford JE, et al. *Vaccine.* 2014;32:3611.
48. Kanai Y, et al. *Vaccine.* 2014;32:4932.
49. Alberca B, et al. *Vaccine.* 2014;32:3670.
50. El Garch H, et al. *Vet Immunol Immunopath.* 2012;149:76.
51. Guthrie AJ, et al. *Vaccine.* 2009;27:4434.
52. Chiam R, et al. *PLoS ONE.* 2009;e5997.
53. Vaccinations. 2015 at: <http://www.nhra.co.za/vet/vaccinations.php>; Accessed 06.09.15.
54. Weyer CT, et al. *Equine Vet J.* 2013;45:117.

EQUINE ENCEPHALOSIS

ETIOLOGY

The equine encephalosis virus is an insect-borne orbivirus, transmitted by a variety of *Culicoides* spp., that is closely related to bluetongue and epizootic hemorrhagic disease viruses.[1-3] It has characteristics in cell culture similar to African horse sickness (see "African Horse Sickness"). There are multiple serotypes of equine encephalosis virus that infect equids of southern, eastern, and western Africa, with serologic evidence of infection or virus isolation from equids in Kenya, Botswana, Namibia, South Africa, Ghana, the Gambia region, and Ethiopia, but not Morocco. Seven serotypes have been identified as circulating among equids in South Africa, with additional phylogenetically distinct isolates from horses in Israel.[1,4,5] The virus was detected in horses in Israel in 2008, in which it caused a mild febrile illness in large numbers of horses, and there is serologic evidence of its presence in Israel since 2001.[5] The virus isolated from horses in Israel was phylogenetically distant to those serotypes circulating in South Africa and similar to an isolate obtained from horses in Ghana.[5]

EPIDEMIOLOGY

Horses, donkeys, and zebra in southern, western, and eastern Africa frequently have antibodies to the virus, indicating widespread infection of these equidae. Seventy-seven percent of 1144 horses, 57% of 518 horses, 49 % of 4875 donkeys, and up to 88% of zebra in South Africa have antibody to EEV. All of 144 equids (horses and donkeys) sampled in the Gambia region, 129 of 159 (81%) in Ghana, and 206 of 220 in Ethiopia had serologic evidence of infection by equine encephalosis virus.[6] None of 120 horses sampled in Morocco had serologic evidence of infection. An intensive study of all 127 foals on a single stud farm in South Africa revealed that 94% of the 93 foals that had a pyrexic episode were infected with EEV, despite 34% having maternally acquired antibodies soon after birth.[7] Zebra foals develop antibodies to the virus within months of losing their maternally acquired passive immunity. Elephants seldom have antibodies to EEV.

Seroprevalence in Thoroughbred yearlings has varied in South Africa markedly from year to year. Seroprevalence varies between 17.5 and 34.7% (of approximately 500 sampled each year) in most years but can be as low as 3.6%.[1]

The virus replicates in midges, although the rate differs depending on species of midge and strain of the virus. The genetic and phenotypic stability of strains of the virus are unknown, and there exists the potential for emergence of new strains or recognition of currently undetected strains, as demonstrated by the recent isolation of a phylogenetically distinct form of the virus from horses in Israel and Ghana. Variations in pathogenicity are not recognized but might exist. There is independent persistence of virus serotypes in a maintenance cycle based on observation of increased rates of seasonal seroconversion to a specific serotype with ongoing low level of infection by other serotypes. For example, infection by serotype 1 is most common (60%), whereas that by serotype 2 is uncommon (0.7%), despite the latter having been first documented as infecting horses in 1967.[1]

CLINICAL SIGNS

The clinical importance of the virus is uncertain, and three syndromes are described: asymptomatic infection, clinical disease, and, on less evidence, encephalitis. Seroconversion in closely managed horses without evidence of clinical disease suggests that in most instances infection by the virus is asymptomatic. Whereas 94% of foals experiencing a pyrexic episode had virus recovered from their blood, only ~50% of foals from which virus was recovered had pyrexia, indicating that asymptomatic infections are common.[7] Most infections are subclinical based on the high seroprevalence rate and lack of reports of outbreaks of the disease. Clinical signs commonly attributed to EEV infection include fever, lassitude, edema of the lips, and congesta mucosal membranes, as reported in horses in Israel in 2008 and 2009. The virus was originally isolated from a horse with signs of neurologic disease—hence the name. However, the disease associated with infection by EEV is poorly documented, and, given the high prevalence of infection, EEV might be falsely incriminated as the cause of more severe disease in some situations. Acute neurologic disease, abortion, and enteritis are anecdotally reported. In an outbreak report in late 2008 in Israel, the morbidity rate on 60 premises varied from 2% to 100%.[4,5] No horses died of the disease during that outbreak. Disease associated with EEV has not been recorded in donkeys or zebra.

CLINICAL PATHOLOGY

Characteristic abnormalities in serum biochemistry or hematology are not reported. Antibodies to the virus are detected by serum neutralization assays and ELISA, both of which are group specific.[8] Complement fixation and agar gel immunodiffusion tests have been used to detect group-specific antibodies. A group-specific, indirect sandwich ELISA detects EEV antigen and does not cross react with African horse sickness virus, bluetongue virus, or epizootic hemorrhagic disease virus. A competitive ELISA suitable for use with serum from horses, donkeys, or zebras detects antibodies to all seven equine encephalosis virus serotypes but does not detect antibodies to other orbiviruses (such as African horse sickness or bluetongue).

NECROPSY FINDINGS

Necropsy examination reveals cerebral edema, localized enteritis, degeneration of cardiac myofibers, and myocardial fibrosis but whether these abnormalities are attributable to EEV is unclear.[3] Definitive diagnosis of individual animals is difficult at the current time because of the high prevalence of seropositive animals and the ill-defined clinical and necropsy characteristics of the disease. Detection of seroconversion and/or virus isolation associated with clinical signs consistent with the disease in groups of horses permits detection of outbreaks of the disease, such as occurred in Israel. There are no recognized measures for treatment, control, or prevention. There is no vaccine.

REFERENCES

1. Howell PG, et al. *Ond J Vet Res.* 2008;75:153.
2. MacLachlan NJ, et al. *Vet Res.* 2010;41.
3. Attoui H, et al. *Rev Sci Tech OIE.* 2015;34:353.
4. Mildenberg Z, et al. *Transbound Emerg Dis.* 2009;56:291.
5. Wescott DG, et al. *PLoS ONE.* 2013;8.
6. Oura CAL, et al. *Epidemiol Inf.* 2012;140:1982.
7. Grewar JD, et al. *Ond J Vet Res.* 2015;82.
8. Crafford JE, et al. *J Virol Meth.* 2011;174:60.

GETAH VIRUS INFECTION

ETIOLOGY

Getah virus is an alphavirus within the Semliki Forest complex of togaviruses. These are small enveloped viruses with a single-stranded, positive-sense RNA genome. Getah virus causes disease in horses and pigs, and this occurs in Japan, Hong Kong, China, Southeast Asia, Korea, and India. Reports from the 1960s document antibodies to Getah virus in animals in Australia, but the presence of this virus in Australia has not been confirmed using modern techniques that are able to differentiate antibodies to Getah virus from those of the related Ross River virus and other viruses in this complex. There are no reports of disease caused by Getah virus in Australia. There is considerable sequence homology between Getah and Ross River virus genomes. There is temporal, but not geographic, variability among isolates of Getah virus from Southeast Asia and Japan.[1,2]

EPIDEMIOLOGY

Getah virus is arthropod-borne, and infection is through the bite of an infected mosquito. The life cycle of Getah virus has not been completely explicated. The virus is maintained in the mosquito–vertebrate–mosquito host cycle typical of arboviruses. The definitive, amplifying vertebrate host for Getah virus is unknown, although a number of vertebrates, including horses, cattle, and pigs, can be infected by the virus. Antibodies to the virus have been detected in humans. Horses and pigs become viremic and presumably can infect mosquitoes, although this does not appear to have been confirmed experimentally. The virus is assumed to be maintained in a mosquito–pig–mosquito cycle in those areas in which there is mosquito activity year round. Persistence of the virus in areas in which mosquito activity is seasonal has not been explained, and whether transovarial or transtadial transmission occurs within the mosquito population is not reported.

There is suspicion that during outbreaks of disease Getah virus is spread by horse-to-horse contact, based on the rapidity of spread among horses, the short duration of the outbreak, and the lack of mosquito activity at the time that some horses developed the disease. However, experimental evidence suggests that this route of spread is likely of limited importance in propagation of epidemics because of the low concentration of the virus in nasal and oral secretions of infected horses and the large inoculum required to cause disease in horses by the intranasal route.

A recent outbreak in Japan saw 75 of 2000 Thoroughbred race horses develop a pyrexic episode, with Getah virus isolated from 25 of the 49 blood samples collected.[3,4] This contrasts with the 770 of 1900 horses affected in a 1974 outbreak at the same facility in Japan.[3] The prevalence of serologic evidence of infection of horses by Getah virus in Japan ranges from 8% to 93%, depending on the region of the country in which the samples were collected and the disease history of the band or stable of horses. Seroprevalence was 17% in India, 12.4% in Thoroughbred racehorses in Korea (with 28% of horses > 6 years of age positive), and 25% in Hong Kong.[5] These results confirm the widespread incidence of subclinical infection of horses by Getah virus in endemic areas.

Disease of humans caused by Getah virus has not been documented.

CLINICAL SIGNS

Disease associated with Getah virus infection is characterized by pyrexia, edema of the limbs, and an abnormal gait, often described as "stiffness." Eruptions of the skin, urticaria, and submandibular lymphadenopathy are reported in some horses with the disease in Japan, but not in India. The clinical disease persists for 7 to 10 days. Abortion is not a feature of the disease, and foals born of mares that have had the disease during gestation are normal. Subclinical infection is very common in endemic areas. However, Getah virus has been isolated from aborted swine fetuses.

Hematologic abnormalities induced by Getah virus infection in horses include lymphopenia. Increases in serum activity of muscle-derived enzymes, such as creatine kinase, are not characteristic of the disease. Affected horses can have mild to moderate hyperbilirubinemia secondary to inappetence.

Diagnosis of disease caused by Getah virus is achieved by detection of clinical signs consistent with the disease, isolation of the virus from blood of affected horses, and seroconversion to the virus. Interpretation of serologic data from horses in Japan is hindered by the widespread use of a vaccine against Getah disease that induces detectable antibodies to Getah virus in serum. A multiplex RT-PCR is available for use on samples from pigs.[6]

NECROPSY FINDINGS

Reports of postmortem examination of horses with disease caused by Getah virus are limited to experimental studies because the disease is typically not fatal. Horses with disease induced by inoculation with pathogenic Getah virus typically have mild changes, including atrophy of splenic and lymphoid tissue with destruction of lymphocytes, and perivascular and diffuse infiltration of focal skin lesions by lymphocytes, histiocytes, and eosinophils. Lesions in the central nervous system are equivocal and limited to mild perivascular cuffing in the cerebrum and small hemorrhagic foci in the spinal cord.

TREATMENT

Treatment of affected horse is supportive. Affected horses might benefit from administration of analgesics and antipyretics such as phenylbutazone. Administration of antimicrobials is not indicated in uncomplicated cases.

CONTROL

An inactivated virus vaccine is available in Japan for immunization of horses against disease caused by Getah virus. The vaccine, which is combined with that for Japanese encephalitis, is considered effective. Race horses are vaccinated every 6 months.[4] Minimizing the exposure of horses to infected mosquitoes is prudent, although the efficacy of this technique in preventing infection is unknown. During outbreaks of disease caused by Getah virus, it is prudent to isolate affected horses, given the potential for horse-to-horse spread of the virus.

REFERENCES

1. Seo HJ, et al. *Acta Virol.* 2012;56:265.
2. Feng Y, et al. *Chin J Zoonoses.* 2014;30:353.
3. Nemoto M, et al. *Emerg Infect Dis.* 2015;21:883.
4. Bannai H, et al. *J Clin Micro.* 2015;53:2286.
5. Jo H-Y, et al. *J Bact Virol.* 2015;45:235.
6. Ogawa H, et al. *J Virol Meth.* 2009;160:210.

CLASSICAL SWINE FEVER (HOG CHOLERA)

Hog cholera, also known as classical swine fever (CSF), is a highly infectious pestivirus infection of pigs. At one time it was characterized clinically by an acute highly fatal disease and pathologically by lesions of a severe viremia. It is now known that chronic or inapparent disease also occurs, including persistent congenital infection in newborn pigs infected during fetal life. In many countries where it is endemic, clinical ability will diagnose it more often than laboratory skills.

Swine can also be affected by ruminant pestiviruses (BVD and BD); these seldom cause disease in pigs, but there are exceptions.[1] The risk factors for these are large numbers of cattle or sheep and goats sharing the same accommodation and watering facilities.[2] Knowledge of these viruses is important for the interpretation of diagnostic tests for CSF because BVDV can transmit between pigs and may prevent the transmission of CSF.[3]

SYNOPSIS

Etiology Hog cholera virus, a pestivirus belonging to the genus *Flaviviridae* and related to the bovine virus diarrhea virus.

Epidemiology Affects domestic pig of all ages; causes major economic losses interfering with trade when outbreaks occur in pig-raising countries. Occurs in Europe, South America, and the Far East. Highly virulent virus causes high morbidity high mortality; less virulent strains cause milder form. Transmitted by direct contact, feeding of uncooked pork products. Neutralizing antibodies provide protection.

Signs Sudden onset of peracute deaths first indication in herd. Many pigs affected within days. Severe depression, fever, anorexia, purplish discoloration of skin, ocular discharge, nervous signs, and death in few days. Nervous form may predominate. Reproductive failure in pregnant sows (abortions, mummification, stillbirths, birth of persistently infected pigs).

Clinical pathology Leukopenia. Detection of virus in tissues and serologic testing.

Lesions Diffuse hemorrhages subcapsular of kidney, lymph nodes, bladder, larynx, swollen lymph nodes, splenic infarcts, congestion of liver and bone marrow, button ulcers in colon, nonsuppurative encephalitis. Hydropic degeneration and proliferation of vascular endothelium.

Diagnostic confirmation Detection of virus in tissues and serologic tests.

Differential diagnosis list:
- African swine fever
- Erysipelas
- Salmonellosis

Treatment None

Control Eradication in hog cholera–free countries by slaughter of all in-contact and affected pigs. Use of vaccines in endemic areas. Eradication in countries where endemic by use of vaccination followed by test and slaughter, quarantine farms.

ETIOLOGY

It is a small, enveloped positive-sense, single-stranded, RNA virus in the genus *Pestiviridae* of the family Flaviviridae. A new virus, Bungowannah virus, found in two herds in Australia, is also a pestivirus.[4] Most are non-cytopathogenic in culture, but there are some CSF and BVD that are cytopathogenic.[5]

It is antigenically and genetically diverse, with recombination possible between strains.[6] There is considerable antigenic variability. There are four structural proteins (C, E^{rns}, E1, and E2) and eight nonstructural proteins. Genetic typing is most commonly based on E2 glycoprotein because abundant sequence data are available. The E2 glycoprotein of CSF is a virulence determinant in swine.[7] There are three major groups, each with three of four subgroups.[8] Typing used full-length encoding sequences of E2, which proved to be the most reliable for significant phylogeny and were proved to be useful in recent outbreaks in Lithuania.

Group 1 types are present in South America and Russia. There have been subgroups 1.1, 1.2, and 1.3 in the past, but now it is proposed that there is a group 1.4 found in Cuba.[9]

Group 2 types were isolated from Europe[10] and some Asian countries.[11] It has been shown that there is the possibility of a long-term persistence of genotype 2.3 CSF virus strains in affected areas at an almost undetectable level even after long-term oral vaccination campaigns.[12]

Group 3 types are confined to Asia. Four genetic groups are found in China (1.1, 1.2, 2.2, and 2.3), and a recent study has shown the wide range of antigenic differences in 21 strains.[13]

The virus is an enveloped virus and thus is susceptible to detergents and lipid solvents. High or low pH and temperature above 60° C (140° F) will inactivate the virus, but this depends on the substances in which the virus is contained.

There is evidence of natural recombination in CSF virus.[6] A sequence database allowing automated genotyping has been established.[14]

Classification of virulence has been based on a clinical and pathologic score and extended further by additional parameters such as case-fatality rate, antibody production, and leukocyte count to provide a modified clinical score[15] that gives a more reliable classification of virulence.

EPIDEMIOLOGY

Although eradicated in many parts of the world, the countries that are free are always open to reinfection from illegal imports of fresh products, tourism, hunting, and illegal swill feeding.[136]

Occurrence

The pig is the only domestic animal species naturally infected by the virus. Wild boar are also affected. Antibodies against CSF virus in fecal samples from wild boar in Korea have been described.[16]

A study of common warthogs and bushpigs in South Africa showed that they were capable of supporting CSF infection and could transmit to other pigs that were in contact.[17] The warthogs did not develop clinical signs, but the bushpigs did.[18,19] CSF of the type 1.1 cluster has also been described in pygmy hogs in India at a conservation center.[20] All breeds and ages are susceptible, and adults are more likely to survive an acute infection. The disease is found in eastern Europe, Southeast Asia, Central and South America, and in parts of Europe in wild boar.

Canada, Australia, New Zealand, and South Africa have not experienced the disease for many years. A mild form of the disease occurred in Australia in 1960 to 1961. The disease was eradicated from the United Kingdom during the period 1963 to 1967, and the United States was declared free of the disease in 1978.

Outbreaks of acute hog cholera have occurred occasionally in other countries but were quickly controlled by a rigorous policy of slaughter and quarantine. The disease occurred in the United Kingdom in 1986 in which three primary outbreaks were identified; all outbreaks were attributed to the feeding of unprocessed waste feed containing imported pig meat products. A similar origin was suspected for the outbreak in the United Kingdom in 2000. In this outbreak an interesting feature was the transport of infected pig carcasses from a site where bodies were dumped for quite long distances by scavenging foxes, infecting new outside pig arks across fields as they went.

Between 1982 and 1984 epidemics occurred in Germany, the Netherlands, Belgium, France, Italy, Greece, and the Iberian Peninsula. As of 1985, six countries in Europe were free of classical swine fever: Denmark, Ireland (including Northern Ireland), Norway, Sweden, Finland, and Switzerland.

There were three outbreaks of CSF in France between 2002 and 2011, one in wild boar and a pig herd in 2002 in Moselle, and a further one in wild boar in 2003 in Bas-Rhin, and they appeared to be from two lineages in wild boar in Germany. The wild boar in Bas-Rhin remained infected until 2007.[21] The role of wild boar in France has been described.[22]

The costs are astronomical (the Belgian outbreak of 1997 cost an estimated €11 million), and the 1997 to 1998 outbreak in the Netherlands was very serious. The disease has also concentrated in certain parts of Europe where the pig populations are intense and live in close proximity to wild boar and feral pig populations. For instance, outbreaks occurred regularly between 1997 and 2001 in Croatia. One source was imported pig meat; the other was strains reaching domestic pigs from wild boar. The wild boar areas include parts of Germany and Poland and probably most of eastern Europe. The outbreak in Spain in 2001 to 2002 was related to wild boar.[23]

In Europe, the disease, together with ASF, is endemic in the central highlands of Sardinia. Many outbreaks of classical swine fever occurred in Germany between 1993 and 1995, and major outbreaks occurred in 1996 to 1997 in Germany and the Netherlands. The risk factors for Germany have been described. In these countries, over the past 25 years, the disease occurred as a series of epidemics in which many swine herds in a geographic area were affected within a few months.

Infection with the classical swine fever virus has also occurred in the wild boar population in Tuscany in Italy, Germany, France, Austria, Czechoslovakia, and Croatia. Serologic surveys of wild boar in Sardinia found an overall prevalence of 11%, and seropositive boars were found not only in areas where they share their habitat with free-ranging domestic pigs but also in areas of the island where contacts between wild and domestic pigs are unlikely to occur. Thus there may be transmission and persistence of the virus within the wild boar population. This has occurred with the low-virulence strain in Germany. The persistence of infection in a wild boar population in the

Brandenburg region of Germany provided optimum conditions for the establishment of a CSF epidemic in Germany.

The disease is currently endemic in most countries of South America and the Far East except Japan and Korea. In Asia the problem is the backyard pig that is not vaccinated and is always a reservoir. Here extension services, appropriate vaccination schemes, and regulatory control are difficult to implement, but it may be time to try for worldwide eradication. In the Philippines, the disease is endemic on many large-scale swine farms. In spite of vaccination of the sows and boars every 6 months and piglets at 6 to 8 weeks of age, the disease causes suboptimal performance in 10% to 30% of pigs between 7 and 16 weeks of age.

Morbidity and Case Fatality

The disease usually occurs in epidemics, often with a morbidity of 100% and a case-fatality rate approaching 100%, when a virulent strain of the virus infects a susceptible population. However, in recent years, outbreaks of a relatively slowly spreading, mild form of the disease have caused great concern in many countries. The disease associated with strains of low virulence may be unnoticed in growing and adult pigs, but the infection can be associated with perinatal mortality, abortions, and mummified fetuses. In a recent outbreak a mild form given experimentally to sows only produced a mild viremia with widespread antigen distribution, but without clinical signs, except lesions of hemorrhagic dermatitis. It did, however, produce an antibody response and transplacental infection.

Methods of Transmission

The source of virus is always an infected pig or its products, and the infection is usually acquired by ingestion; inhalation is also a possible portal of entry. Direct animal-to-animal contact is the most important method of spread. Infected pigs shed a large amount of the virus in all secretions and excretions of pigs infected with highly or moderately virulent strains.[24] The effect of strain and inoculation dose of CSF on within-pen transmission has been described.[25] It is excreted in the urine for some days before clinical illness appears and for 2 to 3 weeks after clinical recovery.

Virus spread via excretions is more important in early stages of an outbreak. Highly contagious by direct contact, it is likely to be transmitted by aerosol only when all the pigs in the same airspace are viremic, and even then only for a distance of 1 meter. Viral RNA and infectious virus were detected in air samples in 2008.[26] It has been spread experimentally by aerosol, which followed the pattern of air currents,[25] but the importance under field conditions is not known. The higher the dose of virus or the more virulent the virus strain, the sooner the virus should be detected in air samples in experimental infections.[26] Analysis of the 1997 to 1998 outbreak in the Netherlands suggested that it did not occur over long distances but did occur within a holding or within a radius of less than 500 meters. The transmission of CSF depends on the clinical course of infection, which is determined by the levels of high or low levels of virus excretion.[27] Different strains of the virus can differ in the relative contribution of secretions and excretions to the transmission of the virus, although blood is a high risk for spreading infection from pig to pig.[28]

Infected boars can shed the virus in semen. Rats and mice are unlikely to be involved in the spread.

Silent circulation of CSF occurs before the first outbreak is detected. The most severely affected animals have a higher infectivity than the less affected ones. Three transmission experiments suggested that the most severely affected animals could play a prominent role in CSF transmission.[29]

Sick pigs excrete virus until they die, or until after recovery. The resistance and high infectivity of the virus make spread of the disease by inert materials, especially uncooked meat, a major problem. The UK virus in the 2000 outbreak probably came from an infected pork product, imported illegally and fed to an outdoor pig. Outside pens, in warm weather and exposed to sunlight, lose their infectivity within 1 to 2 days. The ability of the virus to survive in the environment in more favorable situations is uncertain. However, it is probable that it can survive for considerable periods because the virus is quite resistant to chemical and physical influences. Transmission from neighboring units is very easy. One of the major features of the recent Dutch outbreak was the proof that transmission from boar studs (AI) was possible because infected boars excreted virus in semen, and the virus probably infects spermatogonia. It was shown that following insemination with semen containing CSF antibodies, infection could occur as early as 7 days; all pigs were positive by 14 days. The transmission rates in the Dutch outbreak have been calculated.

In areas free of the disease, introduction is usually by the importation of infected pigs or the feeding of garbage containing uncooked pork scraps. Hopefully, in Europe the ban on swill feeding will prevent further cases of infected meat causing the problems. Movement of pigs that are incubating the disease or are persistently infected is the most common method of spread. The infection usually originates directly from infected breeding farms. Birds and humans may also act as physical carriers of the virus. In endemic areas, transmission to new farms can occur in feeder pigs purchased for finishing, indirectly by flies and mosquitoes, or on bedding, feed, boots, automobile tires, or transport vehicles. Farmers, veterinarians, and vaccination teams can transmit the virus by contaminated instruments and drugs, but recent evidence suggests that mechanical transmission may have been overestimated. People can spread the virus.[30]

Farmers can spread the virus within a herd by treating sick animals or employing routine health management procedures such as iron injections of newborn pigs. The common practice of not changing syringes and needles between farm visits constitutes a major risk when viremic animals are present. The most common cause of dissemination occurs through the movement and sale of infected or carrier pigs through communal sale yards when there is ample opportunity for infection of primary and secondary contacts. Transmission of excretions without direct contact from pig to pig may have been overestimated.

When the disease is introduced into a susceptible population, an epidemic usually develops rapidly because of the resistance of the virus and the short incubation period. In recent years, outbreaks have been observed in which the rate of spread is much reduced, and this has delayed field diagnosis. It is not spread by dogs, cats, or rats, and bird transmission is unlikely.

Risk Factors

Following the 1997 to 1998 severe epizootic in the Netherlands, analysis showed that there were five major increased risk factors identified: (i) presence of commercial poultry on the farm, (ii) visitors to the units not being provided with protective clothing, (iii) drivers of lorries using their own clothes rather than protective clothing provided by the premises they were visiting, (iv) larger size, and (v) aerosols produced by high-pressure hosing. Reduced risk was associated with (i) over 30 years of experience in farming and (ii) additional lorry cleaning before being allowed on to the farm.

Animal Risk Factors

It has been shown at least experimentally that the virulence of the strain can influence the dynamics of the virus spread.[29] Pigs infected with such a virus excrete significantly more virus than pigs infected with moderately or low virulent virus. The exception was the chronically infected pig, which, over the period of its disease, excreted significantly more virus. It showed the importance of virus type and excretion data in modeling studies.[28]

Historically, infection with the hog cholera virus rapidly resulted in severe clinical disease. It is now recognized that with less virulent strains, a carrier state can occur, at least for a period of time. Following exposure to these strains, pigs may become infected without showing overt signs of the disease, and although they may eventually develop clinical disease, this latent period is of importance in dissemination of infection when such pigs are sold and come in contact with others. In recent outbreaks in high-pig-density areas in Belgium, the interval between the first occurrence of clinical signs and the report of a suspect herd was shorter when the disease was first diagnosed in finishing pigs rather than in sows, boars, or nursing piglets. The proportion of clinically affected animals was positively correlated with the proportion of serologically positive animals.

Susceptible pregnant sows, if exposed to less virulent strains of the virus, may remain clinically healthy, but infection of the fetuses in utero is common, and the virus may be introduced into susceptible herds by way of these infected offspring. The sow with "carrier sow syndrome" can give birth to normal, healthy-appearing piglets that are persistently infected and immuno-tolerant; these pigs, along with those with chronic infections, are responsible for the perpetuation of the virus in the pig population. A fully virulent virus may also be transmitted in this manner if the sows are treated with inadequate amounts of antiserum at the time of exposure or if they are exposed following inadequate vaccination. Piglets infected in utero, if they survive, may support a viremia for long periods after birth.

During outbreaks of classical swine fever in Germany between 1993 and 1995, differing clinical courses were observed, ranging from mild clinical signs to severe typical disease. The genotype of pigs may influence the outcome of hog cholera virus infection. In certain pig breeds the chronic form of the disease is more likely to occur, and these pigs may excrete the virus over prolonged periods. Experimental inoculation of purebred pigs resulted in acute fatal infections, whereas crossbred pigs experienced acute, chronic, and transient infections.

Pathogen Risk Factors

Virulence Characteristics

The most virulent strains produce clinical disease in pigs of all ages. But there are differences in the clinical and pathologic features between strains of the virus and in their virologic characteristics. The less virulent strains cause only mild clinical disease or disease restricted primarily to fetal and newborn piglets. It is probable that this variance has always occurred in field strains of the virus, but the use of inadequately attenuated live virus vaccines is also a contributory factor. The occurrence of variation in virulence and antigenicity has been recognized as a cause of failure of vaccination and "vaccine breakdowns." It is equally important in causing problems with the diagnosis of hog cholera in eradication programs when infection is manifest in patterns not traditionally associated with this disease.

Genetic analysis of isolates of the virus for a series of epidemics of swine fever in Italy affecting both domestic pigs and wild boar has provided useful epidemiologic information. The isolates were divided into three subgroups, and it is suggested that there have been at least two separate introductions of classical swine fever over a 7-year period and that the virus has been transmitted between domestic pigs and wild boar. Molecular analysis can aid in tracing the transmission of the virus from domestic pigs to wild pigs and back to domestic pigs.

In the outbreaks of hog cholera in England in 1986, affected pigs in the first outbreak exhibited clinical signs and necropsy lesions indicative of a virulent strain of the virus. However, in subsequent outbreaks, clinical disease was much milder and case-fatality rates low. Experimental infection of pigs with a field isolate of the virus resulted in variations in clinical response, from acute illness to inapparent infection, including minimal changes visible at necropsy, all of which indicate that genotype may influence the pathogenesis of the disease. High titers of virus were found in several tissues of one experimental pig that was recovering, even in the presence of serum-neutralizing antibodies. It is clear that some infected pigs may pass through an abattoir without detection because of the absence of lesions.

Resistance of Virus

Survival of the virus is very dependent on the strain of the virus.[26] The CSF virus (CSFV) is destroyed by boiling, 5% cresol, or 2% sodium hydroxide and by sunlight, but it persists in meat that is preserved by salting, smoking, and particularly by freezing. It is able to survive in cool, moist protein-rich environments for 2 weeks at 20° C (68° F) but for 6 weeks at 4° C. The virus can be inactivated in at least 80% of pork hams after exposure to a flash temperature of 71° C (159° F). It can survive in infected uncooked ham pork for at least 84 days and 140 days in diced ham or sausage; it can survive in bacon for 27 days after traditional curing processes and for at least 102 days in hams cured in salt concentrations of up to 17.4%, which is much higher than that normally used in curing bacon. The use of lower-salt concentrations in curing solutions and the decreased time between slaughter and consumption as a result of modern abattoir practices increase the risk of disease transmission. It survives pH ranges from 3 to 11. Persistence in frozen meat has been observed after 4.5 years. The virus persists for 3 to 4 days in decomposing organs and for 15 days in decomposing blood and bone marrow.

Immune Mechanisms

Maternal antibodies may interfere with the production of viral-specific cell-mediated immunity. Neutralizing antibodies occur as early as 9 days after infection in recovering pigs and after 15 days in fatally infected pigs. Neutralizing antibodies are the most important antibodies in terms of protection. The maximum antibody response occurs 3 to 4 weeks after infection, and levels may persist indefinitely but last at least 6 months. In chronic hog cholera, neutralizing antibodies may be transiently detectable during the phase of partial recovery between 3 and 6 weeks after infection. Low-virulence strains of hog cholera may cause inapparent infections and are described as poorly immunogenic but in some instances may induce considerable titers of neutralizing antibodies in immunocompetent pigs. Cellular immunity mechanisms are probably very important in that it has been shown that there is CSFV-specific IFN-γ formed early after antigen exposure. These mechanisms produce a higher response after intranasal or oral vaccination than after IM vaccination, and therefore vaccines should be looked at for their potential to induce higher T-cell responses. Intrauterine infection of piglets with the virus may induce a state of specific immunologic unresponsiveness. The piglets are persistently viremic and may continue to live for several weeks or months, but the majority die within the first 3 weeks of life. Piglets with PRRSV infections have been shown to produce a poorer response.

Economic Importance

Hog cholera has been responsible for large economic losses in the swine industry worldwide. It is considered to be the most important disease of pigs in the European Union, and a common program of eradication in the member states is in effect. The magnitude of the economic importance of the disease is directly proportional to the size of the pig population and the standards of the swine industry. In countries with intensified systems of pig production, such as the Netherlands, it is estimated that the direct costs of transport and destruction of infected herds, disinfection of premises, indemnities to farmers, vaccination, and identification and registration of pigs on behalf of the control of the disease amounted to a large percentage of the gross slaughter value. The additional indirect damage as a result of loss of production on infected farms, standstill of pig movements in affected areas or regions, and restrictions on export is difficult to evaluate. Losses as a result of the death of pigs are aggravated by the high cost of vaccination programs in enzootic areas and by the problem that vaccination may not be completely effective in controlling epidemics. Recovered or partially recovered pigs are very susceptible to secondary infections, and exacerbations of existing chronic infections such as enzootic pneumonia are likely to occur during the convalescent period.

PATHOGENESIS

The tonsil is the primary site of virus invasion following oral exposure. Primary multiplication of the virus occurs in the tonsils, beginning within several hours after infection. It then spreads to the peripheral lymph nodes. The virus is first found in plasma before the mononuclear cell populations. The primary cell in the peripheral blood to be infected is the mixed granulocyte. The virus then moves through lymphatic vessels and enters blood capillaries, resulting in an initial viremia at approximately 24 hours. At this time the virus is present in the spleen and other sites such as peripheral and visceral lymph nodes, bone marrow, and Peyer's patches. The virus exerts its pathogenetic effect on endothelial cells, lymphoreticular cells and macrophages, and epithelial cells. In particular, B-lymphocytes, T-helper cells, and cytotoxic T cells are affected, and these changes take place before the RT-PCR picks up the virus in the blood.

The changes in gene expression of 148 genes during the first 48 hours following infection have been described.[31] Mutations in CSF nonstructural protein NS4B affect the virulence of CSF.[32]

The enhanced pathogenicity of some strains is associated with the presence of residues in E2 and NS4B of CSFV that can act synergistically to influence viral replication efficiency in vitro and pathogenicity in pigs.[33]

CSF virus is accompanied by depression of cellular immune defenses,[34] particularly innate responses mediated by interferon.[35] CSFV is not often found in apoptotic cells, so there are other mechanisms that cause this apoptosis. CSFV appears to be able to inhibit apoptotic signaling at multiple levels, and by supporting viral replication, endothelial cells may promote the pathogenesis of CSF.[36] A B-lymphocyte deficiency associated with viral destruction of germinal centers in lymphoid tissues is the most significant pathoimmunologic consequence of acute hog cholera infection. This lymphocyte apoptosis, which is activation-induced programmed cell death, is one of the key features of CSF infections. CSF affects cellular antiviral activity, which suggests that the lesions may have an immunopathologic component, possibly through the infection of dendritic cells[37] and possibly by damaging the interferon production.[38] It is likely that CSFV up-regulates some of the adhesion molecules, such as integrin-β3 in vascular endothelial cells, which may alter hemostatic balance in CSF.[39]

Certain virus infections are associated with high levels of IFN-1 (type 1), which is a potent antiviral defense mechanism. Despite the presence of viral anti-IFN-1, inhibitors the plasmacytoid dendritic cells can continue to produce IFN-1. CSFV prevents IFN-1 secretion in its main target cells (macrophages, monocytes, and endothelial cells) by interacting with interferon regulatory factor.[40] The ability to activate dendritic cells, the ability to spread systemically, and the tropism for lymphoid tissues also contribute strongly to a raised IFN-1 response.

There is a novel virulence determinant within the E2 structural glycoprotein of CSFV.[41] In highly and moderately virulent strains of CSF there was a decrease in antiviral and apoptotic gene expression, and this coincided with higher levels of virus in these immune tissues (spleen, tonsil, retropharyngeal lymph nodes).[42]

In recovered pigs (from infection with a moderately severe strain) it was found that antiviral defense mechanisms were rapidly activated, whereas in chronically affected pigs several genes with the power to inhibit production of type 1 interferons were up-regulated. The chronic pigs failed to activate NK or cytotoxic T-cell pathways, and they also showed reduced gene activity in antigen-presenting monocytes/macrophages.[43] A highly virulent CSF virus produced significant changes in the mononuclear cell proteome in porcine peripheral blood, with 66 protein spots showing altered expression; 44 of these were identified as 34 unique proteins.[44]

CSFV can evade the immune response and establish chronic infection, and in an in vitro study it was shown that immune response genes were generally down-regulated.[45] The gene transcriptional profiles in peripheral blood mononuclear cells following a virulent strain of CSF have been studied. Many genes were up-regulated and many down regulated.[46] CSFV strains may exacerbate the alpha-response, leading to bystander killing of lymphocytes and lymphopenia, the severity of which might be attributable to the host's loss of control of IFN production and downstream effectors regulation.[47]

Most of the lesions are produced by hydropic degeneration and proliferation of vascular endothelium, which results in the occlusion of blood vessels. This effect on the vascular system results in the characteristic lesions of congestion, hemorrhage, and infarction from changes in arterioles, venules, and capillaries. Thrombosis of small and medium-sized arteries is another feature. Vascular changes are most severe in the lymph nodes, spleen, kidneys, and gastrointestinal tract. Lesions related to the effects on the endothelial cells also occur in the adrenals, central nervous system, and eyes. Atrophy of the thymus, depletion of lymphocytes and germinal follicles in peripheral lymphoid tissues, renal glomerular changes, and splenitis are characteristic. Leukopenia is common in the early stages, followed by leukocytosis in some animals, and anemia and thrombocytopenia occur. The thrombocytopenia may be caused by massive platelet activation and subsequent phagocytosis of platelets secondarily to the release of platelet activating factors by activated macrophages. Disseminated intravascular coagulation is common with microthrombi in small vessels, particularly of the kidney, liver, spleen, lymph nodes, lung, intestine, and intestinal lymph nodes. The end stage of a lethal infection in the natural host is associated with a marked depletion preferentially of B-lymphocytes in the circulatory system and in the lymphoid tissues. Macrophage activation, and subsequent release of proinflammatory cytokines, plays an important role in the development of the classical signs of CSF. This is particularly true for the pulmonary intravascular macrophages.

It has been shown that there is a significant expression of TNF-α in virus infected lymph nodes. It may be that commitment to apoptosis may depend on the IFN production. In these lymph nodes lymphocyte death occurred by apoptosis, and some of the cells were positive on IHC for both TNF-α and apoptosis. It may be that the release of the TNF-α may induce the apoptosis in the uninfected bystander cells. Early immunosuppression is an important feature of the development of CSF, with the depression of CD1+, CD4+, and CD8+ common thymocytes. It has recently been shown that CSF can replicate in the dendritic cells and control IFN type 1 responses without interfering with immune reactivity. It is still not clear, even though it is known that there is clear targeting of macrophages and monocytes, how these cells produce this immunosuppression and account for the death of the T-lymphocytes. It is known that the dendritic cells are the sentinels of the immune system and respond to easy viral contact. They then develop the effective immune responses by migrating into the lymphoid tissue to present the processed viral antigens to the T-lymphocytes. However, in both CSF and BVD infections there is no activation of the dendritic cells, and this may be a feature of pestivirus infections and enable them to evade the immune response. At the same time, there is no interference with the maturation of the dendritic cells. The virus induces proinflammatory cytokine production (IL-1, IL-6, and IL-8) by 3 hours, and even further at 24 hours postinfection, and also increases the coagulation factors, tissue factor, and vascular endothelium cell growth factor. Endothelial cells that were chronically infected were unable to produce IFN type 1, and these cells were also protected from apoptosis. This establishes a long-term infection of endothelial cells with virus replication and increasing levels of IL-1, IL-6, and IL-8. It shows that there has been long-term interference with cellular antiviral defenses, possibly by targeting interferon regulating factor 3, as BVDV does, or by increased binding of NF-κβ, which modulates an apoptotic pathway controlling several anti-apoptotic genes.

CSFV infections significantly increased the mRNA expression of IL-10 and tumor necrosis factor (TNF) alpha, and they inhibited IL-12 expression, with little effect on IFN-α and IFN-γ expression. CSFV suppresses maturation and modulates functions of monocyte-derived dendritic cells without activating nuclear factor kappa B, which is involved in immune regulation, inflammatory response, and antiapoptosis effect.[48]

In many cases, secondary bacterial infection occurs and plays an important part in the development of lesions and clinical signs.

The experimental disease is characterized by a biphasic temperature elevation at the 2nd and 6th day after inoculation, a profound leukopenia and an appreciable anemia 24 hours after inoculation, diarrhea at the 7th day, and anorexia and death on the 4th to 15th day in slaughter pigs. The anemia can be explained by the infection of 2% to 9% of the megakaryocytes 2 to 9 days after infection.

The inoculation of pregnant sows with a low-virulence field strain of hog cholera virus at various stages of pregnancy results in prenatal mortality in litters from sows infected at pregnancy day 40 and postnatal death at 65 days. The later that infection occurs in pregnancy, the greater the number of uninfected piglets born in infected litters. Transplacental infection of the porcine fetus with both field and vaccine strains of the virus may induce a spectrum of abnormalities, including hypoplasia of the lungs, malformation of the pulmonary artery, micrognathia, arthrogryposis, fissures in the renal cortex, multiple septa in the gallbladder, and malformations of the brain. Infection of the fetus at a critical stage of gestation (30 days) induces retardation in growth and maturation of the brain, resulting in microencephaly. The teratogenicity of the virus clearly depends on the stage of gestation. In general, the earlier the infection occurs, the more severe the abnormalities are likely to be. The virus can be found in the ovaries because the blood vessels deliver peripheral macrophages to the ovaries through atretic follicles.

One of the sequelae of transplacental hog cholera virus infection of the fetus is congenital persistent virus infection with the evolution of a runt-like syndrome during the first few months of life. At birth, affected piglets appear normal, although they are viremic; the viremia persists throughout life of the animals. The first evidence of clinical disease may occur at about 10n weeks of age, but it may be delayed until 4 months of age. Growth retardation, anorexia, depression, conjunctivitis, dermatitis, intermittent diarrhea, and locomotor disturbance with posterior paresis occur. At necropsy, the most remarkable lesion is atrophy of the thymus gland, and lesions of classical hog cholera are not present. In experimental congenital persistent hog cholera infection, the earlier the infection occurs in pregnancy, the greater the number of persistent infections in piglets born alive with immunologic tolerance. The immunologic tolerance is specific to the virus because affected piglets respond to other selected antigens.

The experimental infection of pregnant goats with the hog cholera virus on days 64 to 84 of gestation can result in transplacental infection, with the virus replicating and persisting in the fetuses for at least 40 to 61 days. The virus is highly pathogenic for goat fetuses, and serum antibodies may be present in the precolostral sera of the kids.

It appears that disseminated intravascular coagulation does not play a major role in the pathogenesis of CSF.[49]

CLINICAL FINDINGS

The early identification of clinical signs would facilitate diagnosis and control, but a recent paper on experimental infections with a type 2.1 genotype virus and a genotype 3.3 virus that is genetically divergent from European viruses has shown differences in outcome.[50] The UK 2001 virus was similar to other European type 2 viruses, but the 3.3 virus produced fewer and delayed clinical signs, notably with little fever, making it more difficult to recognize in the field. Another complicating factor is that it poorly recognized by the CSF-specific antibody.

Six uncharacterized CSFV isolates from 1996 to 2007 were examined[51] and assessed in animal experiments for their clinical virulence. They were assessed as either moderately or highly virulent.

Diagnosis

Nearly always, the detection is too late because it has been missed. The clinical signs are often nonspecific, but the score system suggested by the Dutch may help to suggest it. The differences in the four most recent German outbreaks in terms of clinical and pathologic signs were minimal. In former times, most of the European outbreaks were associated with the virulent genotype 1 of the virus, but now there are types 2:1, 2:2, and 2:3, which are much less virulent and produce a milder clinical course that is much more difficult to recognize over the first 14 days postinfection. In a recent set of experiments (with a strain of virus SF0277) all the pigs died, but in other experiments some of the pigs survived.

A recent report has suggested that the occurrence of PRRS does not appear to potentiate the clinical outcome of CSF in young pigs, but this has been disputed.

Simultaneous infection with *Trypanosoma evansi* does seem to produce a poor response to CSF vaccination.

As a result of the recent outbreak in the Netherlands, a quantitative retrospective analysis was made of the clinical signs, which suggested that the clinical inspection was the most important part of detection but was not very specific. Moderate-virulence and low-virulence strains cause a mild disease that may be so mild that clinical disease is not suspected.

Differential diagnosis should include PRRS, PDNS, ASF, salmonellosis, and coumarin poisoning.

Peracute and Acute Disease

In the acute form the disease is characterized by anorexia, lethargy, conjunctivitis, respiratory signs, and constipation.[51,52] Diagnosis on clinical signs is more difficult since the 1980s, and therefore the CSF may not be recognized immediately,[27] but nearly always the major clinical sign is pyrexia. Clinical signs usually appear 5 to 10 days after infection, but incubation periods up to 35 days or more are recorded. At the beginning of an outbreak, young pigs may die in a peracute state without evidence of clinical signs having occurred. Acute cases are the most common. Affected pigs are depressed, do not eat, and stand in a drooped position with their tails hanging. They are disinclined to move and, when forced, do so with a swaying movement of the hindquarters. They tend to lie down and burrow into the bedding, often piled one on top of the other. Before the appearance of other signs, a high temperature (40.5–41.5°C [105–107°F]) is usual. In recent European outbreaks, respiratory signs have not been common. Constipation followed by diarrhea and vomiting also occurs. Later, a diffuse purplish discoloration of the abdominal skin occurs. Small areas of necrosis are sometimes seen on the edges of the ears, tail, and lips of the vulva. A degree of conjunctivitis is usual, and in some pigs the eyelids are stuck together by dried, purulent exudate. Nervous signs often occur in the early stages of illness and include circling, incoordination, muscle tremor, and convulsions. Death can be expected 5 to 7 days after the commencement of illness. Infection with *Salmonella* Choleraesuis may also be potentiated by hog cholera infection, and the two diseases in combination can result in high mortality.

Nervous Manifestations

A form of the disease in which nervous signs predominate is attributed to a variant strain of the virus. The incubation period is often shorter and the course of the disease more acute than usual. Pigs in lateral recumbency show a tetanic convulsion for 10 to 15 seconds followed by a clonic convulsion of 30 to 40 seconds. The convulsion may be accompanied by loud squealing and may occur constantly or at intervals of several hours, often being followed by a period of terminal coma. In some cases, convulsions do not occur, but nervous involvement is manifested by coarse tremor of the body and limb muscles. Apparent blindness and stumbling have also been observed.

Chronic Disease

Low-virulence strains of virus result in less severe disease syndromes. A chronic form occurs in field outbreaks and occasionally after serum–virus simultaneous vaccination. The incubation period is longer than normal, and there is depression; anorexia; persistent mild fever; unthriftiness; and the appearance of characteristic skin lesions, including alopecia, dermatitis, blotching of the ears, and a terminal, deep-purple coloration of the abdominal skin. Pigs may apparently recover following a short period of illness but subsequently relapse and die if stressed.

Pigs infected with the low-virulence strains of the virus appear more susceptible to intercurrent bacterial disease. The changeable nature of this combination is such that hog cholera should be suspected in a herd or area where there is an increase in mortality from any apparent infectious cause that either does not respond, or responds only temporarily, to therapeutic ploys that are usually effective.

Reproductive Failure

Reproductive failure can be a significant feature and may occur without other clinical evidence of disease within the herd. It may occur when inadequately protected pregnant sows are exposed to virulent virus or when susceptible pregnant sows are vaccinated with live attenuated vaccines or exposed to low-virulent field strains. Infection of the sow can occur at any stage of pregnancy and may result in no clinical signs other than a mild pyrexia, but it may be followed by a high incidence of abortion, low litter size, and mummification, stillbirth, and anomalies of piglets. Piglets infected at 50 to 70 days may be clinically normal at birth and then waste away and may develop tremors; such cases are said to be late-onset CSF. They are like BVDV cases in that they shed virus and are persistently affected for months. Liveborn pigs, although carriers, may be weak or clinically normal. Persistent congenital infection is characterized by persistent viremia, continuous virus excretion, and late onset of disease, with death occurring 2 to 11 months after birth. No antibodies to the virus are present in spite of the persistent infection; affected pigs have a normal immune response to other antigens, but they do not respond to the hog cholera virus. Cell-mediated immunity appears to be normal. A high incidence of myoclonia congenita (congenital trembles) associated with cerebellar hypoplasia has been observed in some outbreaks where prenatal infection with hog cholera virus has occurred, and this syndrome has been reproduced experimentally. The prevalence of any one of these manifestations appears to vary with the strain of the virus and the stage of gestation at the time of infection.

CLINICAL PATHOLOGY

Hematology

A valuable antemortem diagnostic test is the total and differential leukocyte count. In the early stages of the disease there is marked leukopenia, with the total count falling from a normal range of 14,000 to 24,000 cells/μl to 4000 to 9000 cells/μl. This is specifically granulocytopenia caused by bone-marrow atrophy. It is a result of apoptosis or necrosis, from 1 to 3 days postinfection, probably as a result of cytokine interaction. Depletion of the lymphocyte subpopulations occurs 1 to 4 days before the virus can be detected by RT-PCR on serum. If a virulent form, depletion is evident by 2 days.

B-lymphocytes, T-helper cells, and cytotoxic T cells are the most affected by the virus. The loss of the circulating B-lymphocytes is consistent with the failure to generate a circulating neutralizing antibody. Virulent strains produce greater reduction in B-lymphocytes than do mild forms. This can be of value in differentiation from bacterial septicemias, but it should not be used as the sole method of differentiation. In the late stages of hog cholera, leukocytosis as a result of secondary bacterial invasion may develop. Piglets less than 5 weeks of age normally have low leukocyte counts.

In a study of CSFV in 6- and 11-week-old pigs,[53] it was found that although only the mild disease resulted, there were depletions in B-cell numbers and a number of T-cell populations in peripheral blood, which were most marked in the 6-week-old pigs. A population of large granulocytes developed in the peripheral blood before the start of viremia.

Diagnostic Tests

A comparison of diagnostic tests shows that the best results are detected by RT-PCR (98.9%), which is earlier than virus isolation (VI) on blood, which gives only a result of 94.5%. RT-PCR is expensive and labor intensive. The antigen-ELISA gives a later detection and the worst results. The leukocyte count gives the earliest pointer to CSF infection but of course does not confirm the disease.

The advent of eradication programs has resulted in the development of diagnostic tests for hog cholera. These tests must be accurate and rapid so that control measures can be rapidly instituted or lifted as required. Diagnosis by virus isolation is slow, the cytopathic effect may be minimal, and some strains have low infectivity and limited growth in tissue culture. This method is seldom used as a primary diagnostic method. Animal inoculation tests still provide an excellent method for the diagnosis of hog cholera and involve the challenge of susceptible and immune pigs with suspect material followed by subsequent challenge at a later date with fully virulent hog cholera virus. However, this test is time consuming and costly, and although it is used for the final confirmatory test for the presence of hog cholera infection in various situations, it is not satisfactory for a rapid diagnostic test.

Detection of Virus

The more rapid tests rely on the detection of antigen in infected pig tissues or the detection of antibody following infection.

Fluorescent Antibody Techniques

This technique allows the rapid detection of antigen in frozen sections of tissue or impression smears and in infected tissue cultures, and these methods have been adopted as a primary test in the eradication program in the United States. Antigen can be detected up to 2 days after death, and this method has been considered more reliable than the agar gel precipitation test. The method is capable of detecting virus carriers among vaccinated pigs.

Antigen-Capture ELISA

The antigen-capture ELISA can detect the virus antigens in blood and tissues from experimentally infected pigs at 4 to 6 days after infection with a moderate- to high-virulence strain (Weybridge virus) and 7 to 9 days after infection with a low-virulence strain (New South Wales virus). The technique does not require tissue culture and takes less than 36 hours for a definitive result.

Agar Gel Precipitation Test

The agar gel precipitation test detects antigen in tissue by means of a precipitin formed with immune sera. Usually pancreas from suspect pigs is tested. This test was used widely in the UK eradication program and is the standard primary test in many countries.

Differentiation of Swine Fever Virus From Other Pestiviruses

PCR Tests

A PCR assay can be used to differentiate classical swine fever virus from ruminant pestiviruses. An international reference panel of monoclonal antibodies for the differentiation of hog cholera virus from other pestiviruses has been developed. Restriction endonuclease cleavage of PCR amplicons can distinguish between vaccine strains and European field viruses. The RT-PCR can also detect CSF in boar semen. A RT-PCR was then described. Rapid detection of CSF using a portable real-time RT-PCR (TaqMan) has been described. Further modifications have been described, and thus the test can be performed in a single tube with all the ingredients. It can then be used as a pen-side test and detects virus in nasal and tonsil scrapings 2 to 4 days before the onset of clinical signs. A further modification of RT-PCR and ISH has been that they can be used on formalin-fixed sections. A multiplex PCR is available to separate BVD from CSF.

A multiplex RT-PCR for the simultaneous detection of both ASFV and CSFV has been described,[133] with a diagnostic sensitivity of 100% for both viruses and 100% specificity for CSFV and 97.3% for ASFV. The inclusion of a heterologous internal control allowed the detection of false negatives.

Serologic Tests

Antibody can be detected by the fluorescent antibody neutralization test, tissue culture serum neutralization test, or an indirect ELISA. Serologic tests are less satisfactory for detection of hog cholera in the acute phase and are of limited value in vaccinated animals. They are of value in the detection in sows of the subclinical infection of hog cholera associated with reproductive failure and for survey studies to determine the prevalence of hog cholera infection. BVDV may infect pigs, especially those in close contact with cattle, and may give false-positive serologic reactions. The incidence rates of these false-positive reactions may be high, and they pose a problem for hog cholera identification in eradication programs. The neutralizing peroxidase-linked antibody assay is a highly sensitive and specific test for hog cholera and will distinguish between pigs infected with different strains of the hog cholera virus and BVDV. The complex, trapping, blocking ELISA is sensitive, specific, and reliable for screening purposes for early identification of infected herds and their elimination in an eradication program. A peroxidase-labeled antibody assay can be used to detect swine IgG antibodies to hog cholera and BVDVs. Monoclonal antibodies to pestiviruses are also available to discriminate between both viruses. A competitive ELISA using a truncated E2 recombinant protein has been described, which can be used when a large number of samples are to be tested.

Samples for Laboratory

When hog cholera is suspected, tissues submitted for examination should include the brain and sections of intestine and other internal organs in formalin, and pancreas, lymph node, and tonsil unpreserved in sealed containers. Local regulations and requirements should be followed. The viral antigens are densely distributed in the skin and tongue of infected pigs, and biopsies of the ear may be useful for diagnosis on a herd basis.

NECROPSY FINDINGS

In many cases the single most important diagnostic aid is the postmortem examination, although in the Dutch outbreaks it was thought that the contribution to the detection of CSF was limited. The reason for this is that there is a tremendous individual variation in necropsy findings. In the outbreak in the United Kingdom in 2000, there were few lesions in fetuses or in neonates; in the sows, lesions were often restricted to conjunctivitis and lesions in the hepatic and splenic lymph nodes, even though 15 animals in each group were examined. The age group showing relatively consistent lesions were the growers, and in these the lesions were similar to those that are reported in the classical outbreaks.

In peracute cases, there may be no gross changes at necropsy. In the more common acute form, there are many submucosal and subserosal hemorrhages, but these are inconstant; to find them, it may be necessary to examine several carcasses from an outbreak. The hemorrhage results from erythrodiapedesis and increased vascular permeability, probably aided by mast cell degranulation. The hemorrhages are most noticeable under the capsule of the kidney, near the ileocecal valve, in the cortical sinuses of the lymph nodes, and in the bladder and larynx. The hemorrhages are usually petechial and rarely ecchymotic. The lymph nodes are enlarged, and the spleen may contain marginal infarcts. Infarction in the mucosa of the gallbladder is a common but not constant finding and appears to be an almost pathognomonic lesion. There is congestion of the liver and bone marrow and often of the lungs. Circular, raised button ulcers in the colonic mucosa are usual but cannot be distinguished from those of salmonellosis. Although these gross necropsy findings are fairly typical in cases of hog cholera, they cannot be considered as diagnostic unless accompanied by the clinical and epizootiological evidence of the disease. They can occur in other diseases, particularly salmonellosis. A recent study found that the lymph nodes had the highest score for lesions and that the fewest lesions were found in the spleen and tonsil because infection of these organs was also rare. The most common lesions were also in the lymph nodes, around the ileocecocolic junction, and around the blood vessels of the brain. Atypical bronchiolar cilia have been reported.

There are characteristic microscopic lesions of a nonsuppurative encephalitis in most cases, and a presumptive diagnosis of hog cholera can be made if they are present. It is thought that the most common lesion in chronic CSF is the mononuclear cell cuff in the CNS. Here ISH is capable of detecting viral nucleic acid even when viral antigen is not detected. Histologically, the main site of tissue injury is the reticuloendothelial system. There is always a progressive lymphoid depletion and mucosal necrosis. The depletion is probably caused by apoptosis but not by direct apoptosis. Atrophy of the thymic cortex and loss of thymocytes is also a feature and may be related to synthesis of the cytokines, TNF-α and IL-1α in particular, which may increase the apoptosis of the thymocytes.

Fibrinoid necrosis of the tunica media combined with hydropic degeneration and proliferation of the vascular endothelium causes occlusion of blood vessels. The more virulent "neurotropic" strains produce lesions of a similar nature but greater severity.

In the intestinal tract mucosa there are large, usually infected macrophages. The gut-associated lymphoid tissue areas are lymphocyte depleted, usually because of massive lymphocyte apoptosis, particularly in the B-cell areas. These changes are possibly attributable to the large amounts of TNFα and IL-1α released from the infected macrophages. They also showed that the macrophages in the splenic marginal zone were among the first cells to be infected. The infection, mobilization, and apoptosis of splenic macrophages play a very important role in the course of the infection through cytokine release. An unusual manifestation of CSF infection is the onset of metaphyseal bone formation caused by the partly thrombosed vessels in the bone, with strong CSF viral specific fluorescence.

Histology showed swelling and vacuolation of megakaryocytes in the bone marrow 2 days after infection, and they were necrotic 4 days after infection. Severe swelling and necrosis of endothelial cells in the vascular endothelium were observed 3 days after infection. It was concluded that the thrombocytopenia resulting from direct viral damage to MKC and endothelial damage can cause hemorrhagic diathesis, whereas coagulation disorders are not involved in early stages of the disease.

In the chronic form of the disease, ulceration of the mucosa of the large intestine is usual. Secondary pneumonia and enteritis commonly accompany the primary lesions of hog cholera.

Infection of the fetus produces a persistent immunologically tolerant noncytolytic infection, often with little evidence of cell necrosis or inflammatory reaction to suggest the presence of a virus. Aborted fetuses show nondiagnostic changes of petechial hemorrhage and ascites. Malformations such as microcephaly, cerebellar hypoplasia, pulmonary hypogenesis, and joint deformity appear as a result of inhibition of cell division and function in these areas. Antibody is not detected in fetal blood when infection occurs early in fetal life. In pigs showing signs of myoclonia congenita, cerebellar hypoplasia is highly suggestive of hog cholera infection.

An immune complex glomerulonephritis has been described in which there is macrophage infiltration of the mesangium with immune complex deposits of IgM, IgG, and Clq in mesangial, subepithelial, and subendothelial areas from 10 days postinfection, and by 14 days neutrophils had also congregated.

This is a disease of major economic importance, and confirmation of the diagnosis is usually performed in specialized governmental laboratories. Virus isolation and fluorescent antibody tests are most commonly used, but other techniques, including immunoperoxidase staining of cryostat sections, are available. The demonstration of viral antigen in the crypts of the tonsils, tubular epithelial cells of the kidney, bronchiolar mucosal gland cells, and the pancreatic epithelial cells has been shown to be possible even after 18 years in formalin.

DIAGNOSIS

The European Union Reference laboratory in Hanover is responsible for the testing in the European Union. A survey of pig farmers and practitioners in the Netherlands investigated their attitudes regarding CSF and found there were six sets of problems identified:[54]

1. Lack of knowledge of CSF
2. Guilt, shame, and prejudice
3. Negative opinion of control measures
4. Dissatisfaction with postreporting procedures
5. Lack of trust in government bodies
6. Uncertainty about and lack of transparency in reporting procedures

The authors recommended procedures to deal with these problems. Diagnostic methods for CSF have been reviewed.[55,56]

Detection of Antigen

Virus isolation is the sensitive, highly specific, time-consuming, and labor-intensive method to find CSF.

For the rapid detection of viral antigen, immunofluorescence and ELISAs are being used. The former uses thin sections of tissues (lymph node, spleen, tonsils, and other organs); the specificity is good, but the sensitivity is not so good. In the early stages of infection there may be false-negative results because there may not be high levels of virus.

The RT-PCR is considered the most sensitive and most specific tool for the detection of CFSV.

A real time RT-PCR is available for differentiating vaccine and field virus, and this will probably become available as a field test.[136,137] Next-generation technology allows the full genome of CSFV to be identified and is the best basis for high-resolution phylogenetic studies.[138]

Pyrexia is one of the key indicators for CSFV, together with high mortality.

Samples for Confirmation of Diagnosis

Laboratory diagnosis is always required. Fresh tonsil can be used for polyclonal direct florescent antibody, which also detects BVDV and BDV, and can then be used for additional tests. The sensitivity of this test was shown to be only 78%, so to give a 99% chance of infection being detected five postmortems would need to be performed. Even when suffering from tissue degradation, tonsil and spleen will still yield infectious virus and RNA.[64]

A comparative study of the signs and lesions produced by six field strains of CSF virus[51] showed that the most characteristic lesions were found in the lymph nodes, followed by necrotic lesions in the ileum and hyperemia of the brain. Splenic infarction and necrotic tonsils when they occur are spectacular but are less frequent, and respiratory signs are also less frequent than was reported in the last century.

A one-step gel-based RT-PCR assay with comparable performance to RT-PCR for detection of CSF virus has been described.[57]

Two RT-PCR assays of CSF were developed for genetic differentiation of naturally infected from vaccinated wild boars.[58]

C-strain "Riems" or other vaccinated animals can be differentiated from infected animals using a RT-PCR.[59]

Two new E^{rns}-based ELISAs allow differentiation of infected from marker-vaccinated animals and discrimination of pestivirus antibodies.[60]

Meat juice ELISA can be used as a suitable substrate for diagnosis of CSF.[61] Viral RNA was detected in meat juice at a lower level than in serum.[62] Sensitivity was calculated to be 91% and specificity to be 97%. Difficulties were encountered when there were low-virulence strains involved and when samples were taken very early in infections.

Pan-pestivirus assays will detect the pestivirus, and then CSF specific assays are required. qRT-PCR is routinely used. Specific assays for CSF include VI, fluorescence antibody test (FAT), and ELISAs.

Irrespective of virulence, whole-blood and tonsil scrapings are the samples of choice for the early detection of CSF.[63] At least eight RT-PCRs have been developed for detection of wild-type CSF,[65-69] and some are used routinely.[70,71]

A loop-mediated isothermal amplification assay for detection of wild-type CSF was described[72] and proved to be a simple, rapid, and sensitive tool for detection of wild-type CSFV under field conditions.

A multiplex nested RT-PCR for the differentiation of wild-type viruses from the C-strain vaccine of CSF was developed.[73]

Multiplex PCRs for the simultaneous detection and differentiation of CSFV field strains and the C-strain vaccine virus have been developed.[59,68]

A multiplex RT-PCR assay for the rapid and differential diagnosis of CSF and other pestiviruses was developed[74] and was shown to be rapid, highly sensitive, and cost effective.

A triplex TaqMan RT-PCR assay for differential detection of wild-type and hog cholera lapinized vaccine strains of CSF and BVDV type 1 has also been devised.[75]

Most CSF reference laboratories use more than one test (virus isolation, antigen ELISA, RT-PCR for detection and confirmation). It has been shown[70] that the RT-PCR is 100% sensitive but VI only about 72% and antigen ELISA only 39%.

A novel RT-PCR assay based on primer-probe energy transfer has also been developed.[58,76] This has been shown to be a highly sensitive and specific confirmatory tool.

The qRT-PCRs have high specificity and sensitivity.[71,77,78] Viral RNA can be detected in samples where the virus is in tissues that are autolysed.[79] Viral RNA can be detected in animals that have recovered.[80] The qRT-PCR can also be used to differentiate between virus species BD, BVD and CSF, and strains of CSF. It can also be used to differentiate infected from vaccinated animals (DIVA).[81] There are some tests that are specific for wild-type virus[58,68] irrespective of the vaccination status of the animal. A negative RT-PCR generally means that the animal is not infectious, but a positive RT-PCR does not mean that it is infectious.[82] Antigen-capture ELISA is recommended for animals with clinical signs or lesions.

A primer-probe energy transfer RT-PCR assay for CSF was described[83] and can differentiate between wild-type CSFV and certain C-strain vaccines. A one-step RT-PCR detection of CSFV using a minor groove binding probe was described[84] and was found to be rapid and of high specificity and sensitivity.

A reverse transcription multiplex RT-PCR was developed for the detection and genotyping of CSF.[85] It was said to be a rapid, sensitive, reproducible, sensitive, and specific genotyping tool. RT-PCR was able to detect CSF 2 days earlier than virus isolation and 2 to 4 days earlier than with antigen ELISA.[86] A high-speed RT-PCR was able to detect FMD, CSF, and SIV-A,[87] and it took only about 28 minutes.

A gold-nanoparticle-based oligonucleotide microarray for the simultaneous detection of seven swine viruses, including CSF, has been described.[88]

- **Histology**—formalin-fixed brain, spleen, lymph nodes, colon, cecum, ileum, kidney, tonsil, skin, tongue (LM). Tissue sections can also be used for ISH and IHC.
- **Virology**—lymph nodes, tonsil, spleen, distal ileum, skin, tongue, brain (FAT, ISO, IHC, PCR); heparinized blood. Virus can be isolated from tissue, serum, plasma, buffy coat, or whole blood in heparin.[89]

Serology

The gold standard is the virus neutralization test. However, ELISAs in microtiter are easy to perform, rapid, and automated. Differentiation between pestiviruses is possible and depends on the design of the test, and detection of DIVA vaccines is also possible.[60]

The immuno-chromatographic strip or lateral flow device[139] can be used as a penside test.

The evaluation of assays[90] showed that the Chekit CSF-Sero and the HerdChek CSFV

Ab were both practical and had highest sensitivity. The PrioCHECK (Rcircle) CSFV^{ms} was the only ELISA suitable for use in DIVA but is less sensitive and cannot be recommended.

ELISAs for the detection of anti-CSF antibodies are useful for epidemiologic surveys and for monitoring CSF-free areas. These antibodies occur 10 to 15 days postinfection, the same as for neutralizing antibodies.

A recombinant E2-based indirect ELISA for the detection of specific IgM antibody responses to CSF has been shown to detect antibodies 2 weeks after vaccination.[91]

An immunochromatographic strip for rapid detection of antibodies to CSF was described[92] and was found to be 97% sensitive and 100% specific and could be performed within 5 minutes.

DIFFERENTIAL DIAGNOSIS

A positive diagnosis of hog cholera is difficult to make without laboratory confirmation. This is particularly true of the chronic, less dramatic forms of the disease. A highly infectious, fatal disease of pigs with a course of 5 to 7 days in a group of unvaccinated animals should arouse suspicion of hog cholera, especially if there are no signs indicative of localization in particular organs. Nervous signs are probably the one exception. The gross necropsy findings are also nonspecific, and reliance must be placed on the leukopenia in the early stages and the nonsuppurative encephalitis visible on histologic examination. Both of these bacterial infections, particularly salmonellosis, may be present.

The major diseases that resemble hog cholera include the following:

- **Salmonellosis,** usually accompanied by enteritis and dyspnea.
- **Erysipelas,** in which there are characteristic diamond skin lesions, and the subserous hemorrhages are likely to be ecchymotic rather than petechial.
- **Pasteurellosis,** in which respiratory signs predominate and lesions of pleuropneumonia at necropsy are characteristic.

Epidemiologic considerations and hematologic and bacteriologic examination will usually differentiate these conditions.

Recently, hemorrhagic septicemia in a pig caused by extraintestinal *E. coli* has been suggested as a differential diagnosis.[93]

In the United Kingdom, many of the cases reported as suspected classical swine fever (CSF) have turned out to be *Purpura hemorrhagica*.

Other encephalitides, particularly **viral encephalomyelitis** and **salmonellosis,** cause similar nervous signs.

African swine fever, apart from its greater severity, is almost impossible to differentiate from hog cholera without laboratory testing.

TREATMENT

Hyperimmune serum is the only available treatment and may be of value in the very early stages of the illness if given in doses of 50 to 150 mL. It has more general use in the protection of in-contact animals. A concentrated serum permitting the use of much smaller doses is now available.

In the future, capsid-targeted viral inactivation (CTVI), which involves the use of the viral capsid protein containing a deleterious enzyme such as a nuclease, could be used to bind native viral protein.[94]

There is also the future possibility of imidazolepyridines, which have a potent in vitro activity against CSFV, being used for treatment.[95] The reduction of CSFV transmission to untreated pigs has been shown by the pestivirus inhibitor BPIP.[96]

CONTROL

Strategies for Control Have Been Reviewed.[97]

The methods used in the control include **eradication** and control by **vaccination.** Both modeling and real-time prediction have been described. In areas where effective barriers to reintroduction of the disease can be established, eradication of the disease by slaughter methods is feasible and usually desirable. In contrast, in areas where the structure and economics of the pig industry require considerable within-country and across-border movement of pigs, it may not be practical or economically feasible to institute a slaughter eradication program. The establishment of a highly susceptible population in a high-risk area is unwise. If repeated breakdowns occur, the restriction of movement of pigs within the quarantine areas creates considerable management problems for pig owners, and they may, as a result, eventually become noncooperative in the program. In these areas, control and possibly even eradication by vaccination is the approach of choice, and this method is used in some countries, such as the Philippines. The Commission for the European Communities has declared its policy, supported by appropriate community legislation, to eliminate hog cholera without vaccination. A full discussion of the possibility of using vaccination in the future has been outlined. A computerized framework for the risk assessment for CSF has been produced. In Germany, there are big risks with regard to the import of pigs, the presence of wild boar populations, and the import of pig meat. A retrospective spatial and statistic simulation to compare two vaccination techniques with the nonvaccination scenario in the Dutch 1997/1998 CSF outbreak showed that both emergency vaccination techniques would hardly have been more efficient.

In the following discussion, general procedures are described first, followed by a description of the immunizing products available.

Control of Outbreaks in Hog Cholera–Free Areas

Modeling for the control of CSF in such areas has been described, and a simulation model for low- and moderate-density pig areas has been described[98] A simulation of an outbreak of CSF in Denmark suggested that the outbreak would be of fewer than 10 cases and last less than 2 weeks on average,[99] although in some cases it may be longer lasting, and a large epidemic would result. Any outbreak would have a considerable cost to the export industry. A modeling study suggested that movement restrictions have had the dominant effect on control strategy for CSF and that preventive culling only became relevant under imperfect compliance.[100]

In areas where the disease does not normally occur, eradication by slaughter of all in-contact and infected pigs is possible and recommended. The pigs are slaughtered and disposed of, preferably by burning. All herds in the area should be quarantined and no movement of pigs permitted unless for immediate slaughter. In areas with high pig densities, control strategies depend on highly effective identification and recording systems, which provide information on herd inventories and animal movements, and thus herd epidemics can be traced back to their origin. Recent experiences with epidemics of swine fever in Belgium and the Netherlands found that with the current eartag with manual recording and use of a documentation system, most epidemics could not be traced back to their origin. The tracing and removal of carrier herds prevents these herds from becoming infectious and prevents the spread of disease at an early stage.

All vehicles used for the transport of pigs, all pens and premises, and all utensils must be disinfected with strong chemical disinfectant such as 5% cresylic acid. Contaminated clothing should be boiled. Entry to and departure from infected premises must be carefully controlled to avoid spread of the disease on footwear, clothes, and automobile tires. Legislation prohibiting the feeding of garbage or commanding the boiling of all garbage before feeding must be enforced. This eradication procedure has controlled outbreaks that have occurred in Canada and Australia and has served to maintain these countries as free from the disease.

Control Where Hog Cholera Is Endemic

One of the major problems in Europe is the wildlife reservoir in the wild boar population. A retrospective analysis of oral wild boar vaccination in the Eifel region of Rhineland-Palatinate has been described.[101] In areas where there is little risk, there are few positive animals; where there is a high risk, many animals may be positive. In Switzerland 179 of 528 boars in a risk area were positive. The oral vaccination of wild boar described in Germany had no risk for the establishment of a persistent wild boar CSF infection. However, it was shown that more than 50% of the wild boar did not feed on the vaccination baits and therefore did not become immune. There is evidence from wild boar studies in Italy that the level of infection in the free population gradually reduces in any case. When wild pigs with maternal antibodies contract live CSF virus, they have transient clinical signs, but the disease is not lethal. Infected wild boars could therefore play a very big part in the transmission of a natural outbreak. The vaccination studies in wild boar were reported recently and showed that after the fifth vaccination, there was no viremia, no virus excretion, and no postmortem virus recovery. Oral vaccination of wild boar usually reduces the presence of CSF, but only a low number of wild boars (30% to 35%) become seropositive. The isolated case in Israel in 2009 showed the problem of transfer of virus from wild boar.[102]

After CSF occurred in wild boar in northeastern Bulgaria, it was decided to trap them; 124 were removed from the area, and of these, 119 were trapped. Further outbreaks of CSF were prevented.[103]

In endemic areas, control is mostly a problem of selecting the best vaccine and using it judiciously. In Asia almost all the control is vested in the use of vaccines and their proper use. Most problems are caused by policy failures or changes in demographics, whereas most of a vaccination policy should be determined by the epidemiology of the disease. Much can also be done to keep the incidence of the disease low by the education of farmers, whose cooperation can be best assured by a demonstration that eradication is both desirable and practicable. Once farmers are motivated to act, the greatest stumbling block to control, failure to notify of outbreaks, is eliminated. Education of the farmer should emphasize the highly contagious nature of the disease and the ease with which it can be spread by the feeding of uncooked garbage and the purchase and sale of infected or in-contact pigs. The common practice of sending pigs to market as soon as illness appears in a group is one of the major methods by which hog cholera is spread.

Vaccination in the EU finished in 1990 mainly because of the difficulty of differentiating infected and vaccinated animals. The exception is as an emergency vaccine or as bait for wild boar. Vaccination of wild boar has been carried out in France and Germany to reduce the shedding of the virus by the vaccinated boars. Outside the European Union, there is widespread use of the Chinese live C-strain vaccine and a biotech CSF E2 glycoprotein subunit marker vaccine.

There are two sorts of vaccine:

1. The first group is the classical live group containing attenuated virus, and these are preferred. Live, virulent-virus vaccines produce a solid immunity within just a few days and give lifelong protection. The reaction to live-virus vaccine may be severe, and the susceptibility of pigs to other diseases may be increased. Eradication of the disease is impossible while the use of this type of vaccine is permitted. Commercially available modified live vaccines are able to induce complete protection in vaccinated pigs, but several factors, including maternal immunity, age of primary vaccination, vaccination protocol, and complications caused by other pathogens, can affect the effectiveness in the field.[107]
2. There is a recently developed second group of live vaccines aimed as marker vaccines based on the E2 protein, but these are still undergoing development. The marker vaccine strategies have been reviewed.[108] There appears to be no complete protection against congenital infection, they do reduce transmission of the virus, but they seem to last only about 1 year. They have the potential to allow tests to be used to differentiate between naturally infected and vaccinated animals. They may also fail in the face of natural infection. Recent further developments of these marker vaccines possibly include a chimeric vaccine in which one of the genes has been replaced by a BVD gene and a second vaccine in which a DNA vaccine expresses the E2 protein after entering the host cell and others with E2 peptides.

There are also several other vaccines: the E2 subunit marker vaccines expressed in baculovirus, E2 subunit vaccines, a chimeric BVDV-CSF marker vaccine, and a recombinant PRV vaccine expressing CSFV glycoprotein that is protective for both diseases.

A safe glycoprotein E2 vaccine expressing an ORFF virus recombinant has been described.[104] Protective efficacy of a CSF virus C-strain deletion mutant was described,[105] but the commercially available E2 ELISA was unsuitable as an accompanying test.

The strategy of exchanging specific epitopes between pestiviruses is useful, as was shown[106] when parts of the E2 gene were replaced by the corresponding sequence from a BDV strain.

When an outbreak occurs in a herd, the immediate need is to prevent infection from spreading further. This can be best achieved by removing the source of infection and increasing the resistance of in-contact animals by the administration of hyperimmune serum or one of the available vaccines. Removal of the source of infection necessitates the following:

- Isolation of infected animals—this was highlighted in the recent Dutch outbreak.
- Suitable hygienic precautions to prevent the spread of infections on boots, clothing, and utensils
- Disposal of carcasses by burning
- Disinfection of pens—the pens should be scraped, hosed, and sprayed with 5% cresylic acid solution or another suitable disinfectant. The choice of serum or vaccine may depend on local legislation and will depend on circumstances. Pigs in the affected pen should receive serum (20 to 75 mL, depending on size), and pigs in unaffected pens should be vaccinated. Pigs receiving serum only will require active vaccination at a later date if a strong immunity is to be achieved.

Hog Cholera Eradication

The elimination of hog cholera from a country where it is well established presents a formidable problem. Before the final stage of eradication can be attempted, the incidence of the disease must be reduced to a low level by widespread use of vaccination and enforcement of garbage-cooking regulations.

One of the most important problems encountered in eradication programs is the clinically normal "carrier" animal, and steps need to be taken to avoid the sale of all pigs from infected premises. A procedure that has been particularly effective in the control of this and other diseases of pigs is the complete prohibition of all community sales of feeder pigs. There are obvious political difficulties in such a prohibition, but despite their usefulness as marketing agencies, community sales continue to be a major source of swine infections. When the occurrence of virulent hog cholera has been eliminated, further necessary steps include the prohibition of use of any vaccine and serologic studies to detect low-virulence carrier states.

The eradication of swine fever in the United Kingdom in 1986 was an important achievement. Control was radical in that all herds in which the disease was diagnosed were slaughtered and all carcasses burned or buried to avoid missing atypical cases and recurrence through the swill cycle. The two focal points that became apparent were the need to avoid vaccination and the need to diagnose accurately. Vaccination was not permitted because it was not completely effective, produced "carriers," and encouraged the development of mild and chronic forms of the disease. The need to diagnose accurately led to changes in diagnostic procedure as the campaign progressed. As the proportion of classical epidemics declined, there was increasing dependence on serologic and antigen-detection tests. The program in the United States, which currently appears complete, is an equivalent achievement.

Immunization Methods

There is a common neutralizing epitope on envelope glycoprotein E2 of different pestiviruses, which may have implications for the development of DIVA vaccines and serologic diagnosis of CSF.[109]

Very few pigs possess natural immunity to hog cholera, and until the introduction of the serum–virus method of vaccination, an outbreak of the disease in a herd meant that the herd would be eliminated. The situation changed rapidly thereafter, and it can be safely claimed that the development of the swine industry in the United States would have been impossible without the protection that the serum and virus provided. On the other hand, the dangers inherent in the use of fully virulent or partially avirulent virus do not recommend their use and have led to a continuing search for safe methods of immunization. The ideal vaccine should retain strong immunogenicity but should be completely avirulent, even for pregnant sows, the fetus, and young or stressed pigs. It should be stable in the degree of attenuation and should not persist in the vaccinate or transmit from the vaccinate to in-contact pigs. Killed vaccines are safe and do not directly spread virus, but, in general, they engender only a limited immunity. Live vaccines provide a longer-lasting immunity but frequently have not met the criteria listed previously.

Serum–Virus Vaccination

The serum–virus vaccination produces an immediate, solid, and lasting immunity when properly administered to healthy swine. The virus, produced by collecting blood 6 to 7 days after artificial infection, is injected SC in 2-mL doses followed immediately by serum in doses graduated to the size of the pigs and varying from 20 mL for suckling pigs to 75 mL for adults. Overdosing with serum will not prevent the development of immunity. Vaccination is performed at any age after 4 weeks. Because of the availability of safer vaccines, this method is not recommended.

Attenuated Vaccines

The first attenuated vaccine was the Chinese lapinized vaccine (C-strain), which induced antibody- and cell-mediated immunity. C-strain-vaccinated pigs produce interferon–gamma at about 9 days postvaccination, and it is a potent inducer of type 1 T-cell responses with significant levels of proinflammatory cytokines.[110] There are certain CD8 cells that play an important role in the protection derived from the C strain vaccine, particularly in the early period before the presence of neutralizing antibody occurs.[134]

CSF infection results in the rapid onset of leucopenia, and it was shown that this affects the T cells. The inability to prime IFN-γ-secreting virus-specific T cells may be attributable to their depletion before activation or to the phenomenon of apoptotic cell-induced dendritic-cell-mediated suppression.[111] It may also be that the affected dendritic cells have a deranged cytokine production that overexpresses IFN-γ and TNF-α.[112]

The most notable development has been the introduction of the first generation of marker vaccines against CSF. These are E2-subunit vaccines that protect pigs by inducing high levels of neutralizing antibodies to E2 after vaccination. A serologic test against E^{rns} was approved within the European Union.[55] However, this test also detects antibodies against E^{rns} from ruminant pestiviruses and therefore produces cross-reactivity in diagnostic tests.[113] E2 glycoprotein contains epitopes that produce neutralizing antibodies, which confer protective immunity and are frequently used for designing DIVA vaccines.[114] The E2 glycoprotein is the major antigenic protein exposed on the outer surface of the virion that induces the main neutralizing antibody, and there are differences between the E2 of the vaccine and field strains of CSF.[115] There are conserved residues, and these may be useful in the development of future diagnostic tests and marker vaccines.

A live attenuated antigenic CSF marker vaccine involving a positive antigenic marker in E1 and a negative marker in E2 has been designed.[116]

A yeast-expressed CSF virus glycoprotein E2 was also shown to produce a protective response.[117]

There has been the rational design of a CSF C-strain vaccine virus that enables the differentiation between infected and vaccinated animals.[118] These findings provide the molecular basis for the development of a novel, genetically stable, live attenuated CSF DIVA vaccine. Some C-strain vaccine virus is not detected by C-strain-specific RT-PCR as a result of a point mutation in the primer binding site.[119]

The efficacy of marker vaccine candidate CP7_E2alf in piglets with maternally derived C-strain antibodies was studied.[120] It provides early protection against lethal challenge infection with CSF virus after both intramuscular and oral immunization.[121,122] It was shown to be effective in preventing mortality, severe clinical signs, and pathologic lesions in 5- or 8-week-old pigs, positive for maternal antibodies derived from sows vaccinated 4 weeks before farrowing, with one dose of C-strain vaccine. The vaccine was able to produce stable antibodies that led to protection for 6 months after vaccination.[123] The primary replication site in vaccinated animals is the tonsils. It persists for up to 63 days after oronasal administration, and it also allows the use of DIVA in the serologic tests.[124] It was confirmed as a promising marker candidate for oronasal vaccination for both wild boar and domestic pigs.

Enhanced immunity to CSF was described after inducement by prime boost immunization using an alphavirus replicon-vectored DNA vaccine and a recombinant adenovirus,[125]and it is able to produce cell-mediated immunity.[126]

Attenuated vaccines include tissue culture vaccines attenuated by repeated passage through tissue culture of porcine or other origin, lapinized vaccines produced by repeated rabbit passage, and vaccines from mutant strains. Many of the early vaccines of this type were not stable and could cause disease when not used in conjunction with serum. Furthermore, transmission to in-contact pigs, especially with porcine origin vaccines, and fetal disease following vaccination of pregnant sows have been problems. Attenuated vaccines are in wide use in Europe and Asia and include the Chinese or LPC and GPE strains. Recently, a safe and efficacious CSF marker vaccine based on the E2 protein (major immunogen) of the virus has been developed. This protein has neutralizing antibodies, and it is also conserved. It can be used where there is an endemic problem and also after the outbreak. It also prevents or reduces drastically the problem of transplacental infection. Experimental nontransmissible marker vaccines have also been developed. Highly passaged preparations are antigenically stable and show no evidence of reversion. They produce a very limited viremia, or none, and no leukopenia or clinical illness. Protection is evident within 5 to 10 days of vaccination. Piglets from nonimmune sows can be vaccinated within the first 2 weeks of life. Because the presence of maternal immunity can interfere with effective immunization, the vaccination of piglets from immune sows should be delayed until at least the second month. The French Thiverval strain is a cold mutant strain that has lost its virulence but retained good immunogenicity. Vaccination of piglets even with 10 times the regular dose produced no clinical illness and virtually no viremia. A single IM vaccination will produce resistance to challenge by 5 to 10 days, and immunity persists for 3 years. Colostral immunity will protect piglets for periods up to 2 months after birth. When given to pregnant sows, even the highly attenuated strains have the ability to cross the placenta and produce fetal infection even though no clinical evidence of this may be manifest. Consequently, it is recommended that replacement gilts be vaccinated at least 2 weeks before mating and that recently vaccinated animals be kept separate from susceptible pregnant sows.

In the Netherlands, the control of swine fever has relied on a slaughter policy on affected farms plus an emergency vaccination program in which all pigs over 2 weeks of age in areas of risk are vaccinated. The mass vaccination program is followed by supplementary vaccination of pigs at 7 to 9 weeks of age and revaccination of breeding gilts when they reach 6 to 7 months of age. The serologic response of piglets born from vaccinated sows is best at 9 to 10 weeks of age rather than at 5 to 6 weeks of age. A vaccine-induced neutralizing antibody titer of less than 32 is adequate to provide protection against clinical disease and to prevent virus transmission.

In the future, a recombinant adenovirus expressing the E2 protein of CSF virus may be useful as a candidate vaccine for preventing CSF.[127] Another possibility is the use of synthetic RNA corresponding to the nucleotides 1130 to 1148 of the CSF virus targeting the nucleocapsid protein, which was shown to inhibit viral replication.[128]

Modification of the glycosylation of the E1, as for the other E proteins, could be useful for the development of CSF live-attenuated vaccines.[129]

Oral vaccination of backyard pigs against CSF with bait vaccine was proven to be useful in an emergency-type situation.[130]

Inactivated Vaccines

Inactivated vaccines are usually prepared from the blood or tissues of infected pigs. Crystal violet vaccine has been the most widely used of this type and was used in the United Kingdom before eradication but never gained full acceptance in the United States. It is completely safe, but its immunogenicity is poor. Immunity does not develop until 12 days after vaccination. Its duration is short, and booster injections are required for maintenance. Vaccinated sows may still develop fetal infection when exposed to virulent virus, and there is a danger that the use of this vaccine in enzootic areas may in this way induce virus carriers. The production of immune antibodies to the blood components of the vaccine may result in the occurrence of isoimmune hemolytic anemia in some breeds. For these reasons inactivated vaccines are not in common use.

Wild boar populations in some countries have risen considerably, particularly in Germany. It is seemingly harmless in wild boar. It can be confined to certain areas until eliminated.[131] Routine vaccination around an area of infection has been proposed as a method of control.[132] Only then can the DIVA qRT-PCR be used to separate vaccinated from field cases.

FURTHER READING

Moenig V, et al. Classical Swine fever. *Dev Biol.* 2013;135:167-174.

REFERENCES

1. Bingham PC, et al. *NZ Vet J.* 2010;58:253.
2. Loeffen WLA, et al. *Vet Microbiol.* 2009;136:240.
3. Wieringa-Jelsma T, et al. *Vet Microbiol.* 2006;118:26.
4. Vilcek S, et al. *Virus Res.* 2007;108:187.
5. Gallei A, et al. *J Virol.* 2008;82:9717.
6. He C-Q, et al. *Virus Res.* 2007;126:179.
7. Risatti GR, et al. *Virology.* 2007;364:371.
8. Postel A, et al. *Vet Res.* 2012;43:50.
9. Postel A, et al. *Vet Microbiol.* 2013;161:334.
10. Blome S, et al. *Vet Microbiol.* 2010;146:276.
11. Kamakawa A, et al. *Vet Microbiol.* 2006;118:47.
12. Leifer I, et al. *J Gen Virol.* 2010;91:2687.
13. Zhu Y, et al. *Virus Res.* 2009;142:169.
14. Dreier S, et al. *J Virol Methods.* 2007;140:95.
15. Floegel-Niesmann G, et al. *Vet Microbiol.* 2009;139:165.
16. Seo SW, et al. *Vet Microbiol.* 2012;161:218.
17. Everett H, et al. *Transbound Emerging Dis.* 2011;58:128.
18. Gers S, et al. *Transbound Emerging Dis.* 2011;58:135.
19. Gers S. *Transbound Emerging Dis.* 2011;58:128.
20. Barman NN, et al. *Rev Sci Tech Off Int Epiz.* 2012;31:919.
21. Simon G, et al. *Vet Microbiol.* 2013;166:631.
22. Pol F, et al. *Vet Rec.* 2008;162:811.
23. Allepuz A, et al. *Vet Rec.* 2007;160:398.
24. Weesendorp E, et al. *Vet Microbiol.* 2009;133:9.
25. Weesendorp E, et al. *Vet Res.* 2009;40:59.
26. Weesendorp E, et al. *Vet Microbiol.* 2008;127:50.
27. Weesendorp E, et al. *Vet Microbiol.* 2009;135:222.
28. Weesendorp E, et al. *Vet Microbiol.* 2011;147:262.
29. Durand B, et al. *Vet Microbiol.* 2009;135:196.
30. Ribbens S, et al. *Vet Rec.* 2007;160:687.
31. Gladue DP, et al. *Virus Res.* 2010;152:10.
32. Fernandez-Sainz I, et al. *J Virol.* 2010;84:1536.
33. Tamura T, et al. *J Virol.* 2012;86:8602.
34. Ganges L, et al. *Vet J.* 2008;177:169.
35. Seago J, et al. *J Gen Virol.* 2007;88:3002.
36. Johns HL, et al. *J Gen Virol.* 2010;91:1038.
37. Jamin A, et al. *Vet Res.* 2008;39:7.
38. Renson P, et al. *Vet Res.* 2010;41:7.
39. Tang Q-H, et al. *Vet Immunol Immunopathol.* 2010;133:237.
40. Summerfield A. *Vet Immunol Immunopathol.* 2012;148:168.
41. Risatti GR, et al. *Virology.* 2006;355:94.
42. Durand SVM, et al. *Arch Virol.* 2009;154:1417.
43. Hulst M, et al. *Arch Virol.* 2013;158:325.
44. Sun J, et al. *J Gen Virol.* 2010;91:2254.
45. Luo TR, et al. *Virol J.* 2012;9:175.
46. Li J, et al. *Virus Res.* 2010;148:60.
47. Renson P, et al. *Vet Res.* 2010;41:7.
48. Chen L-J, et al. *Res Vet Sci.* 2012;93:529.
49. Blome S, et al. *Vet Microbiol.* 2013;162:360.
50. Everett H, et al. *Vet Microbiol.* 2010;142:26.
51. Floegel-Niesmann G, et al. *Vet Microbiol.* 2009;139:165.
52. Cariolet R, et al. *J Recherch Porc.* 2008;40:45.
53. Nielsen J, et al. *Vet Immunol Immunopathol.* 2010;138:159.
54. Elbers ARW, et al. *Vet Microbiol.* 2010;142:108.
55. Blome S, et al. *Rev Sci Tech Int Off Epiz.* 2006;25:1025.
56. Greiser-Wilke I, et al. *Vaccine.* 2007;25:5524.
57. Liu L, et al. *J Virol Methods.* 2007;139:203.
58. Liu L, et al. *J Virol Methods.* 2009;159:131.
59. Leifer I, et al. *J Virol Methods.* 2009;158:114.
60. Aebischer A, et al. *Vet Microbiol.* 2013;161:274.
61. Kaden V, et al. *Dtsch Tierarztl Wochenschr.* 2009;116:173.
62. Lohse L, et al. *J Vet Diag Invest.* 2011;23:1005.
63. Donahue BC, et al. *J Virol Methods.* 2011;179:108.
64. Weesendorp E, et al. *Vet Microbiol.* 2010;141:275.
65. Ophuis RJ, et al. *J Virol Methods.* 2006;131:78.
66. Liu L, et al. *J Virol Methods.* 2007;139:203.
67. Liu L, et al. *J Virol Methods.* 2009;160:69.
68. Zhao JJ, et al. *Vet Microbiol.* 2008;126:1.
69. Jamnikar Ciglenecki U, et al. *J Virol Methods.* 2008;147:257.
70. Depner K, et al. *J Vet Med B Infect Dis Vet Publ Hlth.* 2006;53:317.
71. Le Dimma M, et al. *J Virol Methods.* 2008;147:136.
72. Zhang X-J, et al. *J Virol Methods.* 2010;167:74.
73. Li Y, et al. *J Virol Methods.* 2007;143:16.
74. de Arce HD, et al. *Vet Microbiol.* 2009;139:245.
75. Zhang X-J, et al. *Res Vet Sci.* 2012;92:512.
76. Zhang X-J, et al. *J Virol Methods.* 2010;168:259.
77. Le Potier MF, et al. *Dev Biol (Basel).* 2006;126:179.
78. Hoffmann B, et al. *J Virol Methods.* 2008;130:36.
79. Depner K, et al. *Vet Microbiol.* 2007;12:338.
80. Blome S, et al. *Rev Sci Tech Off Int Epiz.* 2006;25:1025.
81. Beer M, et al. *Vaccine.* 2007;25:5665.
82. Haegeman A, et al. *J Virol Methods.* 2006;136:44.
83. Liu L, et al. *J Virol Methods.* 2009;160:69.
84. Wen G, et al. *Ver Res Commun.* 2010;34:359.
85. Huang Y-L, et al. *J Virol Methods.* 2009;160:111.
86. Depner K, et al. *Vet Microbiol.* 2007;121:338.
87. Wernike K, et al. *J Virol Methods.* 2013;193:50.
88. Wang X, et al. *J Virol Methods.* 2013;191:9.
89. Greser-Wilke I, et al. *Vaccine.* 2007;25:5524.
90. Schroeder S, et al. *Rev Sci Tech Off Epiz.* 2012;31:997.
91. Li W, et al. *J Virol Methods.* 2013;191:63.
92. Li X, et al. *J Virol Methods.* 2012;180:32.
93. Reiner G, et al. *Berl Munch Tierartzl Wschr.* 2010;123:119.
94. Zhou B, et al. *J Virol Methods.* 2010;167:79.
95. Vrancken R, et al. *J Gen Virol.* 2009;90:1335.
96. Vrancken R, et al. *Vet Microbiol.* 2009;139:365.
97. Penrith M-L, et al. *Transbound Emerg Dis.* 2011;58:187.
98. Durr S, et al. *Prev Vet Med.* 2013;108:73.
99. Boklund A, et al. *Prev Vet Med.* 2009;90:180.
100. Thulke H-H, et al. *Prev Vet Med.* 2011;99:28.
101. Froelich A, et al. *Vet Microbiol.* 2008;132:29.
102. David D, et al. *Vet J.* 2011;190:e146.
103. Alexandrov T, et al. *Rev Sci Tech Off Epiz.* 2011;30:91.
104. Voigt H, et al. *Vaccine.* 2007;25:5915.
105. Kortekaas J, et al. *Vet Microbiol.* 2011;147:11.
106. Wehrle F, et al. *J Gen Virol.* 2007;88:2247.
107. Suradhat S, et al. *Vet Microbiol.* 2007;119:1.
108. Dong X-N, Chen Y-H. *Vaccine.* 2007;25:205.
109. van Rijn PA. *Vet Microbiol.* 2007;125:150.
110. Graham SP, et al. *Vet Microbiol.* 2010;142:34.
111. Williams CA, et al. *Immunology.* 2008;124:89.
112. Jamin A, et al. *Vet Res.* 2008;39:7.
113. Koenig P, et al. *Vaccine.* 2007;25.
114. Beer M, et al. *Vaccine.* 2007;25:5665.
115. Chang C-Y, et al. *Virus Res.* 2010;149:183.
116. Holinka LG, et al. *Virology.* 2009;384:106.
117. Lin G-J, et al. *Vet Microbiol.* 2009;139:369.
118. Kritekas J, et al. *J Virol Methods.* 2010;163:175.
119. Leifer I, et al. *J Virol Methods.* 2010;166:98.
120. Reimann I, et al. *Vet Microbiol.* 2010;142:45.
121. Leifer I, et al. *Vaccine.* 2009;27:6522.
122. Rangelova D, et al. *Vaccine.* 2012;30:6376.
123. Gabriel C, et al. *Vaccine.* 2012;30:2928.
124. Tignon M, et al. *Vet Microbiol.* 2010;142:59.
125. Sun Y, et al. *Vet Immunol Immunopathol.* 2010;137.
126. Zhao H-P, et al. *Vet Immunol Immunopathol.* 2009;129:57.
127. Sun Y, et al. *Res Vet Sci.* 2010;88:77.
128. Porntrakulpipat S, et al. *Vet Microbiol.* 2010;142:41.
129. Fernandez-Sainz I, et al. *Virology.* 2008;386:210.
130. Milicevic V, et al. *Vet Microbiol.* 2013;163:167.
131. Pol F, et al. *Vet Rec.* 2008;162:811.
132. Rossi S, et al. *Vet Micribiol.* 2010;142:99.
133. Haines FJ, et al. *PLoS ONE.* 2013;7:e71019.
134. Franzoni G, et al. *Clin Vaccine Immunol.* 2013;20:1604.
135. Rosell R, et al. *Vet Rec.* 2013;doi:10.1136/vr.101920.
136. Moenig V, et al. *Dev Biol.* 2013;135:167.
137. Liu L, et al. *J Virol Methods.* 2011;175:170.
138. Blome S, et al. *Vet Microbiol.* 2011;15153:373.
139 Leifer I, et al. *BMC Res Notes.* 2011;4:521.

AFRICAN SWINE FEVER

Africans swine fever (ASF) is an OIE List A disease. It is on the move and dangerous.[1]

For many years only the Pirbright, Spanish, Portuguese, and South African groups have been interested in the virus, with limited resources to pursue a vaccine, but with the incursion into Europe, this has changed. It is indistinguishable in the field from classical swine fever because both are hemorrhagic diatheses, and it is just as contagious. It is responsible for a highly fatal disease in domesticated pigs. It is the greatest limitation to the development of the pig industry in Africa.[2] However, it is associated with a totally different virus. It is also very important because of its spread into Europe, because of its economic effect, and because of the difficulties of control in wild pig populations and eradication in the face of no effective vaccination. It has no public health significance. An online training course put together by a consortium of experts working on ASF is offered through the link http://asforce.org/course/.

SYNOPSIS

Etiology Large icosahedral cytoplasmic DNA virus.

Epidemiology Disease of major threat to pig-producing countries. Occurs in Africa, western and eastern European countries, Caribbean countries. High morbidity, high case-fatality rate in classic form; low-virulence form less fatal. In Africa, transmitted by argasid tick from wild pigs to domestic pigs. In Europe, transmitted by direct contact with infected pigs and wild and feral pigs. Antibodies in colostrum of recovered sows provide passive protection to piglets.

Signs High fever, purplish skin, depression, anorexia, huddling, disinclination to move, weakness, incoordination, nasal and ocular discharges, diarrhea, vomiting, abortions, death in a few days. Historically, highly virulent forms; in recent decades, subacute and chronic forms common, with fever, depression, and lethargy; recover in few weeks but remain persistently infected; chronic cases are intermittently pyrexic and become emaciated, with soft edematous swelling over joints and mandible.

Clinical pathology Severe leukopenia and lymphopenia. Detect antigen or serologic tests.

Lesions Marked petechiation of all serous surfaces, lymph nodes, epicardium and endocardium, renal cortex, bladder; edema and congestion of colon and lungs. Renal hemorrhages are considered pathognomonic.

Diagnostic confirmation Identify virus in tissues.

Differential diagnosis list:
- Hog cholera
- Erysipelas
- Salmonellosis

Treatment None.

Control Identification of affected pigs, slaughter, and quarantine premises. Establish disease-free areas.

ETIOLOGY

It is associated with a DNA virus that is the sole member of the family Asfarviridae and as such is the only known DNA arbovirus. It is a large icosahedral virus that contains a linear, double-stranded DNA genome (170 to 190 kbp). The viral genome may encode for 165 genes and encodes for approximately 113 virus-induced proteins and over 28 structural proteins in intracellular viral particles, most with an as yet unknown function. The variable ends of the genome contain five multigene families, and the large differences in these between the different isolates may account for the large differences in antigens that are seen between the various isolates. There are large differences between the genomes of isolates from different regions and types of pig[3] and between virulent and avirulent viruses. Morphologically, it is similar to the iridoviruses but resembles the pox viruses in genome construction and gene expression. There are different forms from highly lethal to subclinical with different field strains and tissue-culture-adapted strains. These are recognized by restriction fragment length polymorphism (RFLP), and protein p72 recognizes all viral groups. Partial p72 gene characterization allows genotyping of field strains. It does not produce neutralizing antibodies, and therefore there is no serotypic classification, but 22 ASF genotypes have been identified using partial sequencing from the p72 gene.[4] Genotype 1 is West African, which also circulated in Europe in the previous outbreaks, and the other 21 are East African. The strain at present circulating primarily in Russia is also an East African strain. It grows well in porcine bone marrow and buffy coat with the production of syncytia.

EPIDEMIOLOGY

Because there is no vaccination as yet, the presence of antibodies always denotes infection, and these antibodies appear early and last for long periods. There is high genetic variability, which seems to be related to the sylvatic cycle present in the region and may be responsible for the complex epidemiology in the region.[4]

Geographic Occurrence

Africa

African swine fever is indigenous to the African continent, where it affects wild pigs. These include warthogs, bush pigs, and escaped (feral) forest hogs, which act as reservoirs of the virus, which cycles between the pigs and the ticks. Wild pigs in some areas are free of infection, and consequently the disease is not endemic in all areas. It was always considered to be a disease of sub-Saharan Africa but over the years has reached new areas. It is endemic in over 20 sub-Saharan countries. It reached Cuba (1971 and 1980). In 1978 outbreaks occurred in Malta, Brazil, and the Dominican Republic and in 1979 in Haiti. It reached Madagascar and Mozambique in 1994, Kenya in 1994, Ivory Coast in 1996, Benin in 1997, and Togo and Nigeria in 2001. The Kenyan outbreak seemed to be maintained in the domestic pigs without sylvatic hosts. The Nigerian strain was 92% to 97% homologous to the strains from Uganda, the Dominican Republic, and Spain. The serious worry was the appearance of the virus in Madagascar in 1998. Although studies showed a seropositivity of only 5.3%, infection of wild pigs produced no clinical disease. With virulent strains, infection in the domestic pig is almost always fatal. Since its recognition, occurrence of the disease in South Africa has been cyclical, with periods of 10 to 12 years of clinical disease and then an absence of disease. Until 1957, ASF had not occurred outside the African continent. To the rest of the world it represented the most formidable of the exotic diseases of swine, a disease that had to be kept within its existing boundaries at all costs.

Europe

In 1957, it spread from Africa to Lisbon and then to Spain in 1960; France in 1964; Italy in 1967, 1969, and 1993; Malta in 1978; Belgium in 1985; and the Netherlands in 1986. It was eradicated from the Iberian Peninsula in 1964.

In Malta (1978), the disease resulted in the death or slaughter of the entire population of 80,000 pigs within 12 months of the diagnosis. This is one of the few examples where a country had to slaughter an entire species of a domestic animal to eliminate a disease. The source of infection was thought to be pork imported from Spain, which was fed to only one boar. Once the official diagnosis was made, all animals on affected farms were slaughtered. Animals that had direct commercial contact with infected herds were also slaughtered, and the disease was declared eradicated in September 1985.

In Spain, the disease had been present since 1960, but the implementation of regulations for eradication adopted in 1985 made it possible to divide the country into an ASF-free region and an infected region. Since 1995, Spain and Portugal have been declared free from the disease, although there was an isolated outbreak in Portugal in 1995. This has resulted in a marked change in the distribution and incidence of the disease.

Europe has remained free after the eradication from Iberia, with one exception, Sardinia, where the disease is endemic in the Central Highlands, although it decreased from October 1994 to March 1996. In a survey in 1998, 45 of 82 municipalities in the province of Nuoro in Sardinia were found to have ASF. In 2010 there were 87 cases in Italy, the principal reasons being the extensive pig farming and the occurrence of wild boar. The partial confinement farms have less seropositivity than the free-range farms, and those in total confinement have only 20% of the level of the free-range farms.

The Recent Disease Outbreak

On the basis of sequence studies,[5] it is likely that the virus in Georgia originated from East Africa (Mozambique or Madagascar) and went by boat (uncooked pork) to the Black Sea and then to the port of Poti in Georgia. In 2007 ASF was recognized in Georgia. It killed all the pigs within 5 to 10 days[6] and remains as virulent now. It then spread rapidly to the Caucausus[5] and then rapidly to Armenia, Azerbaijan, and the Russian Federation. It has reached the Ukraine and now has reached the northwestern areas of Russia near the Baltic States and the Barents Sea. It is currently circulating out of control in both domestic and wild pig populations.[7] There are two populations at risk: the low-biosecurity population (backyard pigs, etc.: 77%) and the high-security domestic pigs (23%). The disease has spread widely in the southern part of the Russian Federation, and since 2011 a secondary endemic center has shifted to the center of the country.[8,9] In 2010, pigs were dumped at a poultry manure storage site just 30 km from St. Petersburg and 100 km from the EU border with Estonia, but where the pigs came from is unknown. It is a risk being near to one of the largest ports in Russia, and it must be ensured that trucks emanating from theses ports are properly disinfected. This present virus is genotype 11, and nearly all the cases are acute cases, as you would expect in a naïve, susceptible population.

In June 2013, the Russian authorities reported outbreaks in backyard pigs along the border with the Ukraine and in wild boar in the Smolensk region north of Moscow. Belarus also reported ASF in backyard pigs in the Grodno region in the west of the country. This is of danger to the European Union because this is close to the border with Lithuania, where there have been cases in the wild boar as a result of transborder movements. It is a threat to the European Union because of wild boar, backyard pig keeping, illegal entry of meat from infected pigs into the food chain and possible import into the United Kingdom, and swill feeding. Three-quarters of all ASF events are reported between June and November in the backyard sector, whereas a quarter of wild boar outbreaks are reported in May and June when there is an increasing population. The virus has also been found in illegally disposed carcasses and meat-processing plants. Low temperatures do not destroy the virus, and chilled meats are a source of infection where swill feeding is practiced. A model has been developed for the spread of ASF into the European Union during the high-risk period.[10] One of the key suggestions is that spread during the high-risk period is likely to be limited especially if the high risk period is short. There is a risk of ASF being transported into the European Union through transport-associated routes (returning trucks, and waste from planes and ships), and this risk has been examined.[11] The study showed that the risk through transport-associated routes was low, except for in some countries, such as Lithuania and Poland, and the returning trucks were the highest risk. The risk of introduction of live pigs was highest in Poland,[12] particularly in November and December, and from the Russian Federation. The ASF virus found in Georgia can replicate efficiently in ticks.[13] An epidemiologic update has been provided.[14]

In early 2014, ASF was discovered in wild boar in Lithuania less than 200 km from the Polish border. It is likely to be the result of movement of infected animals from affected regions in Belarus.

Species Affected

Only pigs are affected; domestic pigs of all ages and breeds are highly susceptible, but the virus can be passed in tissue cultures of rabbits, goats, and embryonated hen eggs. The three African wild species (warthogs, giant forest hogs, and bush pigs) are resistant to infection, but European wild boar are susceptible.

Until recently, the occurrence of the disease in Africa was limited to explosive outbreaks in European pigs that came in contact with indigenous African pigs. These outbreaks tended to be self-limiting because all pigs in affected herds died or were destroyed, but after a number of years the disease became enzootic in domestic herds. Surveys of the disease in countries such as Malawi illustrate the changing behavior of the disease over a period of years. The virus, which was introduced to Europe in 1957, was capable of persisting in European pigs, and after a period of several years in which the disease was epizootic, a change to an enzootic character occurred. The outbreak in Cuba was of a comparatively virulent form.

When the disease occurred in the Caribbean region, it posed a major threat to the large swine industry of the United States principally because of the possible spread of the virus to the feral swine population in Florida. The feral swine population in Florida is the largest in the United States and is of major recreational and economic importance to hunters, trappers, taxidermists, and dealers who sell feral swine to hunting clubs. The feral swine in Florida are descendants of domestic swine that were allowed to run wild. Experimental inoculation of these pigs with virulent isolates of the virus will cause fatal disease.

Morbidity and Case Fatality

Early in the history of African swine fever, the morbidity rate could be as high as 100%, and the case-fatality rate was also often over 90%. However, a decrease in the virulence of the virus occurs with time in enzootic areas, and the case-fatality rate may now be as low as 2% to 3%.

Methods of Transmission

There are three main methods of transmission cycle. Firstly, a wild pig/soft ticks/domestic pigs cycle; second, a domestic pig/tick cycle without warthogs; and third, a domestic pig/pig cycle.[15] Local spread and outdoor production facilities in association with wandering wild boar may be the most common methods of transmission.

In Africa, the method of transmission of the disease from the reservoir in wild pigs to the domestic pig has been the subject of considerable interest. Infection is primarily transmitted to domestic pigs via the argasid tick *Ornithodoros moubata*. The viremic warthog is a source of infection for the ticks. The virus can be maintained in warthog-associated argasid ticks by a transstadial, transovarial, and sexual (male to female, but usually not vice versa) transmission mechanism. It needs to replicate in the midgut epithelium of the tick for successful ASF infection of the tick. The tick is relatively restricted in its habitat, and if contact between domestic pigs and wild pigs and their burrows is prevented, transmission can be prevented. The virus can be maintained in these ticks for long periods in the absence of fresh sources of infection, with a low level of viremia lasting a long time. The young warthogs in the burrows are infected early on, and thus they act as reservoirs and vectors of infection. Sporadic outbreaks may thus occur in endemic areas when the virus spreads from infected ticks or warthogs to domestic pigs. In some areas where infected warthogs are common but where *O. moubata* is apparently absent, *O. savignyi* may be a natural field vector of the virus. It is also found in *O. porcinus*. The ASF virus replicates to a high titer in the developing cells of the egg of the tick. Ticks infected with ASF virus also have a higher mortality than uninfected ticks.

The long-held belief that the source of the virus in primary epidemics of African swine fever in southern and eastern Africa is the carrier, wild pig, is not tenable. It is postulated that infected ticks are transported to the vicinity of domestic pigs either by warthogs or on the carcasses of warthogs.

In Africa, the virus is maintained primarily by a cycle of infection between warthogs and soft ticks (*Ornithodoros moubata*). The virus does not have an apparent effect on either warthogs or ticks, and it is only when infection of domestic pigs occurs that the virus produces disease. Indeed, most warthogs are aviremic but seropositive. The tick has a wide distribution in Africa south of the Sahara, and its main habitat is in burrows that are inhabited by the warthog. There is a good correlation between antibodies in warthogs and the presence of ticks. Newborn warthogs can become infected soon after birth if bitten by infected ticks, and the consequent viremia would be high enough to infect previously uninfected ticks feeding on them. It is also found in the bush pig (*Potamochoerus porcus*), which, following infection, may be viremic for 35 to 91 days, and these also transmit the infection to ticks.

In Europe there is direct transmission between sick and healthy animals irrespective of whether they are domesticated or wild or feral animals. In **Spain and Portugal**, the methods of spread are contact between neighboring farms and the introduction of infected pigs either during the incubation period or as persistently infected virus carriers. During the last 20 years, an increasing number of outbreaks occurred in which clinical disease was not readily recognized. The mortality rates decreased, and a wide range of clinical disease occurred, ranging from acute to chronic and including apparent recovery to normal health. The major consequence of the emergence of these less virulent forms of the virus was the development of persistently viremic carriers and a large population of pigs with inapparent infection. The African swine fever virus may persist in the pig population by persistent infection in recovered pigs for several months, during which time the virus must be reactivated before transmission can occur. The virus can also persist by reinfection of recovered pigs in which the virus replicates without producing clinical disease, and transmission occurs by excretion and by infected blood and tissues. Wild boars in Spain carry the virus without clinical signs.

The **European vector** of the virus is the soft tick *O. erraticus*.[16] It can maintain and transmit the virus for at least 300 days. In various areas of Spain, *O. erraticus* was found in 42% to 64% of the pens occupied by pigs. Following the outbreak of the disease in Spain, abandonment of these pig pens has resulted in the elimination of most soft ticks infected with the virus. The adults and large nymphs can survive for about 5 years or longer in the soil of pig pens when animals occasionally enter them. There is a relationship between the persistence of the disease and the distribution of the tick in Spain. Hungry tick populations may transmit the virus when feeding in the winter, but populations that have continuous access to pigs do not feed until the pig pens reach a temperature of 13° to 15° C (55°–59° F). The development from larva to adults takes 2 to 3 years. In a recent study of the ticks (*O. erraticus*) from farms in southern Portugal, two types of ASF were isolated. One produced the acute, 100% fatal disease, and the other just a low viremia in pigs.

In **Sardinia**, the major factors involved in the spread of the disease are related to the following factors:

- Mountainous terrain in which pigs may range freely in previously infected areas
- Movement of pigs that may survive infection and mingle with other herds
- Introduction of infected pigs from unknown sources into healthy herds because of the uncontrolled movement of pigs
- Feeding of waste food containing meat from infected pigs

The virus has been experimentally transmitted to healthy swine by *O. coriaceus*, an argasid tick indigenous to the United States. The potential arthropod vectors of the virus in **North America and the Caribbean basin** have been examined. Most *Ornithodoros* spp. of ticks that will feed on pigs may be capable of acting as vectors of the virus, and the possible existence of potential vectors among the other blood-sucking arthropods should not be ignored. The soft tick *O.* (*Alectorobius*) *puertoricensis* found on the Caribbean island of Hispaniola (Haiti and Dominican Republic), where African swine fever was endemic from 1978 to 1984, was experimentally able to transmit the virus from infected to susceptible pigs. The *O. coriaceus* tick is able to harbor and transmit the virus for more than 440 days, passing it transstadially from the first nymphal stage to the adult, sustaining it through at least four molts. *O. puertoricensis* has all of the prerequisites for becoming a true biological vector and reservoir of the virus.

Once established in domestic pigs the disease can spread rapidly. Virus is present in high titer in nasopharyngeal excretions at the onset of clinical signs and is present in all organs and excretions in acutely sick pigs. In experimentally inoculated domestic pigs, the virus is present in substantial amounts in secretions and excretions of acutely infected pigs for only 7 to 10 days after the onset of fever and is present in the greatest amount in the feces. The virus can persist in the blood of some recovered pigs for 8 weeks and in the lymphoid tissues for 12 weeks. Feces are the environmental contaminant most likely to spread the infection, but blood is also highly infective, and transmission could occur by contamination of wounds created by fighting. Infection occurs via oral and nasal routes, and with the short incubation period once the disease is established in a herd, it spreads rapidly by direct contact. Infection among domestic pigs can also reputedly be spread by the following activities:

- Indirect contact by infected pens
- Ingestion of contaminated feed and water
- Feeding uncooked garbage containing infected pig material

Transmission via the hog louse *Haematopinus suis* is also probable. An important source of infection is the recovered pig, which may remain persistently infected and a carrier indefinitely. Pigs that have recovered from the Western Hemisphere isolates (Brazilian and Dominican Republic) may be persistently infected and are resistant to experimental challenge.

Little is known as yet about the transmission of the virus by ticks in eastern Europe. However, all *Ornithodorus* spp. ticks tested so far have been susceptible to ASF virus and are therefore potential biological vectors.

Risk Factors

Pathogen Factors

The ASF virus is a multiclonal population of viruses in which all combinations of at least four markers (hemadsorption, virulence, plaque size, and antigenicity) are found. This may explain the epidemiologic observation that when the disease was confined to Africa and the Iberian Peninsula in the early 1960s, the viruses isolated were highly virulent to swine, but in subsequent years mortality decreased and subacute and chronic infection became more common. Experimentally, moderately virulent ASF virus obtained from the Dominican Republic, when inoculated into pigs, results in an acute febrile illness along with viremia and a transient neutrophilia from which the pigs recover. The Malta 78 isolate of the virus experimentally produces a clinical syndrome similar to that of the African isolates of the virus.

A huge amount of research is continuing apace into the genes and the proteins produced from the expression of these genes, but these are beyond the scope of this text. However, recent studies of ASF have suggested that the virulence may depend on their ability to regulate the expression of macrophage-derived cytokines, which in turn regulate T-helper type 1 cells (Th1) and T-helper type 1 cells (Th2) responses and control the host protective responses. The less virulent cultures of ASF with macrophages produce more TNF-α, IL-6, IL-12, and IL-15, whereas virulent strains inhibit their production. The ASF virus also affects chemotactic responses and phagocytic capacity and causes a reduction in the release of toxic oxygen radicals.

The virus is very stable at pH 4.0 but not so stable at levels above or below this. It is highly resistant to putrefaction, heat (it will survive 2 hours at 56° C [133° F]) and dryness and survives in chilled carcasses for up to 6 months and at 4° C (39° F) for 2 years. It survives in serum for 6 years at 5° C (41° F). Probably 0.5% to 0.66% of all the genes of ASF are not connected with virus replication but are important for viral transmission and survival in the host. It is inactivated by 1% formaldehyde in 6 days and by 2% sodium hydroxide in 24 hours.

Immune Mechanisms

Antibodies against the ASF virus occur in the colostrum of sows previously infected with the virus and are transferred passively to nursing pigs. Experimentally, passively transferred virus-specific immunoglobulins alone will protect swine against lethal infection with a highly virulent homologous strain of the virus. The antibody-mediated protective effect is also an early event that effectively delays disease onset. The construction of blocking antibodies by some of the viral proteins probably prevents the complete neutralization of the virus by antibodies.

Pigs infected with virulent or attenuated virus may recover and resist challenge exposure with virulent homologous and, under certain conditions, heterologous viruses. Although pigs develop antibodies that are detectable by different tests, virus-neutralizing antibodies have only recently been demonstrated against viral protein p72. However, it has recently been suggested that p30, p54, p72, and p22 proteins are not associated with neutralizing antibodies. The sera from pigs that have been infected and are resistant will inhibit virus replication, but the nature of the inhibition is not understood. Neutralization of virulent virus isolates in both Vero cell cultures and swine macrophages using swine immune sera has been demonstrated. Experimental exposure of pigs to a low-virulent field isolate of the virus results in a range of virus-induced specific cellular responses.

The virus induces strong in vitro blastogenesis of primed blood mononuclear cells, when less virulent but live virus isolates are used. Pigs recovering from an acute infection with the virus have significant levels of virus-specific cytotoxic T-lymphocytes after in vitro stimulation. Viral protein p36 induces a helper T-cell response in mice. Resistance to infection appears to be related to the level of antibody-dependent cell-mediated cytotoxicity. Virus-specific blastogenic and cytotoxic T cells are prime candidates for the cells inducing and conferring protective immunity against challenge with the virus, suggesting that cellular-based mechanisms are highly important.

In persistently infected animals the virus may be shed into the environment for at least 70 days.[17]

The incubation period varies widely from 4 to 19 days depending on the isolate and the route of infection. Infected domestic pigs begin shedding the virus before they are showing clinical signs. The virus is shed in large amounts from all excretions and secretions. Surviving pigs demonstrate a long-term viremia, and virus may be recovered.

PATHOGENESIS

The virus replicates in the monocytes and macrophages of the lymph nodes nearest the point of virus entry to the body. It is often the tonsils and respiratory tract and replicates in the lymphoid tissues of the nasopharynx before the occurrence of a generalized viremia, which can occur within 48 to 72 hours of infection and is followed by secondary replication in the lymph nodes, spleen, lungs, liver, and kidney. The viremia may begin after 4 to 8 days and may last for weeks because there are no neutralizing antibodies.

Infectivity and contact transmission develops at this time and continues for at least 7 days. Pigs inoculated with field isolates of the virus from the Western Hemisphere develop thrombocytopenia with a characteristic pattern. Infected pigs become thrombocytopenic over a 48-hour period after 3 to 4 days of illness. After several days of thrombocytopenia, the platelet count returns to baseline level even with a continuing viremia. Experimentally, the virus causes hematopoiesis in bone marrow, which coincides with macrophage activation, and bone-marrow function is not impaired. Membrane proteins on the surface of permissive cells act as receptors for ASF, and specific interactions take place at this site. ASF is associated with red blood cell membranes and platelets. The subacute form is characterized by a transitory thrombocytopenia.

The effects of ASF are primarily hemorrhages and apoptosis. A newly found protein (p54) encoded by the virus has just been shown to be the first that directly induces apoptosis. The disease is characterized by apoptosis with abundant lymphocyte, particularly B-cell, death. Both T and B cells, particularly in the spleen, are affected as early as 3 days after infection, with the apoptosis being induced by cytokines or apoptotic mediators released from ASF-infected macrophages. In all probability there is an intracellular pathway triggered at the same time as the process of virus encoding. It is probable that the inducers of apoptosis are balanced by the inhibitors of apoptosis.

Tissue necrosis and generalized endothelial cell infection are not features of the disease caused by isolates of moderate virulence.

The virus causes hemorrhages through its effect on hemostatic mechanisms by affecting vascular endothelium. After about 4 to 5 days the vascular damage extends to the basement membranes, and death ensues, usually because of the serious edema and hemorrhage. The mechanisms related to hemorrhage consist of the following:

1. Activation and extensive destruction of monocytes and macrophages—serum TNF-α and IL-1β increase in the serum. The lymphocytes also appear to have decreased activity. Apoptosis of thymocytes has been reported.
2. Disseminated intravascular coagulation
3. Infection and necrosis of megakaryocytes—many apoptotic and also pyknotic and karyorrhectic megakaryocytes can be seen, which are induced either by cytokine damage or peripheral destruction of platelets. Between 0.2% and 9.5% of cells may be affected. Early in the infection there is prolongation of coagulation times as a result of inhibition of fibrin formation; later, thrombocytopenia develops. The thrombocytopenia and coagulation defects lead to the development of the following:
   - Hemorrhage
   - Serous exudates
   - Infarction
   - Local edema
   - Engorgement of tissues

All clinical forms of the disease are characterized by extensive hemorrhage at necropsy, and it is this feature that often establishes a presumptive diagnosis in the field. A highly virulent virus produces renal hemorrhage as a result of intense endothelial injury, facilitated by phagocytic activity. With strains of moderate virulence, hemorrhage is a consequence of an increase in vascular permeability with diapedesis of erythrocytes. Activation of platelets by the virus may also contribute to increased permeability. After 4 to 5 days the basement membranes are affected, which leads to pulmonary edema, and this results in death.

The virus mainly infects cells of the mononuclear phagocyte system and also impairs lymphocyte function. Pulmonary intravascular macrophages demonstrate intense TNF-α and IL-1α activity, which coincides with the pulmonary edema, neutrophil sequestration, and fibrin microthrombi. The lymphopenia that is so characteristic of the disease is attributable to a significant increase in lymphocyte death by apoptosis (programmed cell death). In the experimental disease, there is marked apoptosis of lymph node lymphocytes, and this occurs in both compartments of cortical tissue but is more intense in diffuse lymphoid tissue (T area). The peripheral lymphopenia is associated with T-lymphocyte depletion. There is no evidence of virus replication in lymphocytes in the lymph nodes, but there is a high rate of viral replication in macrophages in diffuse lymphoid tissue compared with the low rate in lymphoid follicles. In summary, there is lymphoid tissue impairment and programmed cell death of a high percentage of lymphoid and monocyte/macrophage cell populations. This accounts for the lymphopenia and the state of immunodeficiency. There are also a variety of proteins encoded by the virus that are apoptosis inhibiting proteins. Experimentally, the virus also causes activation and degranulation of platelets from day 3 after inoculation onward, coinciding with activation of the mononuclear phagocyte system and virus replication in monocyte/macrophages. Virions of the virus also appear in the platelets, which suggests that platelets assist in disseminating the virus within the body, especially in subacute infections. Probably 95% of the infectivity of blood is in the form of virus adsorbed to the red blood cells.

The virus can cross the placenta, replicate in fetal tissues, and cause abortion. However, the pregnancy failure is probably the result of the effects of the virus infection on the dam more than from direct viral damage to the placenta or fetus.

The reasons for the lack of viremia in wild African pigs is unknown, as is the higher resistance of European wild boar to ASF.

CLINICAL FINDINGS

The disease occurs in acute to chronic forms. When it occurs as a new infection (epidemic), it is often acute, but it is subacute to chronic when endemic. In the acute form of the disease the animals die in an acute state of shock characterized by a disseminated intravascular coagulation with multiple hemorrhages in all tissues. The incubation period after contact exposure varies from 4 to 19 days depending on virus dose and the route of infection, but only 2 to 5 days in experimental infections.

Most often the morbidity is 40% to 85%, and the mortality may be as high as 90% to 100% when a virulent virus is involved but may be only 20% to 40% in less virulent outbreaks.

A high fever (40.5°C [105°F]) appears abruptly and persists, without other apparent signs, for about 4 days. The fever then subsides, and the pigs show marked cyanotic blotching of the skin, depression, anorexia, huddling together, disinclination to move, weakness, and incoordination. Extreme congestion and discoloration of the hindquarters with difficulty in walking are early and characteristic signs. Coordination remains in the front legs, and affected pigs may walk on them, dragging the hindlegs. Tachycardia and serous to mucopurulent nasal and ocular discharges occur, and dyspnea and cough (sometimes up to 30%) are present in some pigs. Diarrhea, sometimes dysentery, and vomiting occur in some outbreaks, and pregnant sows usually abort. Purple discoloration of the skin may be present on the limbs, snout, abdomen, and ears. Abortion may occur in all stages of gestation about 5 to 8 days after the infection commences or after 1 to 2 days of fever. Death usually occurs within a day or two after the appearance of obvious signs of illness, and death is often preceded by convulsions. Subacute is characterized by thrombocytopenia, leucopenia, and numerous hemorrhagic lesions.

High fever and varying degrees of depression and lethargy are observed during the acute phase, but some pigs continue to eat; the case-fatality rate is usually less than 5%; the fever subsides in 2 to 3 weeks; and the pigs return to full feed and grow at a normal rate. Recovered pigs have no lesions suggestive of the disease but may be viremic for several weeks. These persistently infected pigs would pass routine antemortem inspection at slaughter and potentially infectious offal and carcass trimming could be fed unknowingly to other pigs. Chronic cases are intermittently febrile, become emaciated, and develop soft edematous swellings over limb joints and under the mandible.

Diagnosis depends on clinical signs (which are not distinguishable in the field from acute PDNS or CSF), postmortem examination (it is said that button ulcers and "turkey egg kidney" are less common rare in ASF, but this cannot and must not be relied upon), and, most important, on diagnostic tests to rule out CSF and confirm ASF. **A definitive diagnosis is only obtainable by exclusion of CSF and confirmation of ASF by laboratory testing.**

CLINICAL PATHOLOGY

Hematology

As in hog cholera, there is a fall in the total leukocyte count to about 40% to 50% of normal by the fourth day of fever. In particular, there is the emergence of immature cells and atypical lymphocytes in the host blood following ASF infection, but the mechanisms are as yet unknown.[18] There is a pronounced lymphopenia and an increase in immature neutrophils. In chronic cases there is hypergammaglobulinemia. Clotting times are increased from about 4 days postinfection. Thrombocytopenia is detectable from day 6 to 9. Serum concentrations of C-reactive proteins, serum amyloid A, and haptoglobin have been measured[1,9] and all increased significantly in pigs inoculated with either ASF or CSF. Pig major acute-phase protein and apolipoprotein correlate with the clinical course of experimental ASF infection.[19]

Diagnosis

The viremia persists, as do the antibodies, for long periods of time; therefore, diagnosis is best achieved by parallel detection of antigen and antibodies.[20] Pen-side tests are just around the corner.

Detection of the Virus

The safest and most commonly used techniques are PCR, direct immunofluorescence (DIF), and the hemadsorption (HA) technique, which is used in reference laboratories. DIF and HA should be used with other techniques because they both can produce false negatives.[20] The original PCR techniques have also been developed to include novel real-time PCR,[21] universal probes,[22] and loop amplification systems. More recently, a genotyping microarray has also been developed.[26]

Antigen can be detected by the fluorescent antibody technique in tonsil and submandibular lymph node within 24 to 48 hours of infection and elsewhere once generalization has occurred. The indirect fluorescence antibody and direct fluorescence tests are commonly carried out on pooled visceral fluid samples.

Serologic Tests

The ELISA is frequently used to screen large numbers of samples because it is easily automated, and many tests have been developed, including a recombinant that works well in poorly preserved sera.[23] Antibody to the virus may be detected within 7 days of infection. The ELISA is highly sensitive and specific and can be automated for screening large numbers of sera. It has been developed for a variety of ASF proteins, such as p73 or p30. More than 90% of infected pigs can be detected by the demonstration of specific antibodies against the virus. An immunoblotting assay is a highly specific and sensitive test that is easy to interpret, provides an alternative to immunofluorescence, and can be carried out in less than 90 minutes under field conditions. Complement testing is also a possibility. The inadequate storage or transport of sera may lead to samples being kept at high temperatures for long periods, and up to 20% of these may be false negatives by ELISA. All blood samples should be held at 4°C before testing and if incorrectly stored or handled should be tested by immunoblotting. A monoclonal antibody immunoperoxidase test is also useful for screening purposes.

To confirm positive or ambiguous ELISA results, immunoblotting, indirect immunofluorescence, and immuno-peroxidase techniques are sued. The first two used together will confirm ASF in over 90% of infected animals.[20]

NECROPSY FINDINGS

Gross changes at necropsy resemble closely those found in hog cholera, except that in the acute ASF, the lesions are more severe. The pathology varies with virulence of the virus but is essentially extensive hemorrhages and lymphoid tissue necrosis in the acute cases. In the subacute and chronic cases, the lesions may be minimal or absent. The lesions are most pronounced in the spleen, heart, lymph nodes, and kidneys. In many organs there is a hyperemia or edema, with fibrinous microthrombi. The most common gross findings are swollen and hemorrhagic gastrohepatic and renal lymph nodes, often so badly affected that they may resemble the spleen; subcapsular petechiation of the kidneys; ecchymoses of the cardiac surfaces and various serosae; and pulmonary edema with hydrothorax. There may be hemopericardium. The renal hemorrhages are considered almost pathognomonic and are a consistent lesion following inoculation of pigs with the virulent or moderately virulent virus. Splenomegaly is usual, but in contrast to hog cholera, splenic infarcts are rarely seen. There may be congestion of the liver and gall bladder and petechiae in the bladder. Hydrothorax is not unknown. There may be congestion in the meninges, in the choroid plexuses, and on the brain. The gallbladder is edematous and hemorrhagic, but this is not a pathognomonic lesion, as sometimes thought. In chronic cases the lesions are essentially the same but also include pericarditis, interstitial pneumonia, and lymphadenitis. There is severe submucosal congestion in the colon, although button ulcers in the large intestine are less common than in hog cholera.

It is said that button ulcers and "turkey egg kidney" are less common but this must not be relied upon.

Histologically, the lesions are more diagnostic. The virus causes destruction of the mononuclear phagocyte system and then infects megakaryocytes, tonsillar crypt cells, renal cells, hepatocytes, and endothelial cells. Postcapillary venules undergo hyalinization and endothelial swelling. Destruction of monocytes/macrophages is visible in the lymph nodes, the spleen, and the bone marrow. In the liver, there is extensive destruction of hepatocytes. Marked karyorrhexis of lymphocytes is visible in both normal lymphoid tissues and in the infiltrating population of cells within parenchymatous organs. Encephalitis may be present with lymphoid infiltration of the leptomeninges, but is generally less severe than that of hog cholera. In recovered animals the presence of virus and antibody simultaneously (persistent infection) can cause the formation of immune glomerulonephritis.

Diagnosis depends on laboratory diagnosis because it cannot be determined on clinical signs and pathology.

As for hog cholera, the diagnostic testing to confirm ASF tends to be restricted to specialized laboratories.

Samples for Confirmation of Diagnosis

Samples can be collected on filter papers to detect antigen and antibody,[20] and oral fluids have also been used to detect antibody.[24]

- Histology—formalin-fixed spleen, lung, lymph nodes, kidney, liver, colon, cecum, brain (light microscopy). The virus can be detected by immunohistochemistry, particularly in the tonsil,[25] or ISH.
- Virology—spleen, kidney, submandibular and abdominal lymph nodes, tonsil, and bone marrow should be collected for fluorescence antibody test and PCR. Direct immunofluorescence and hemadsorption are reliable, as are a range of PCR tests, including a TaqMan. A PCR has also been developed that can be used on a blood sample on filter paper and also a plaque assay. The PCR developed using the p72 protein will enable detection of ASF within 5 hours of clinical sample submission and full characterization of the virus within 48 hours. A new RT-PCR using the universal probe library has been described.[22]

SEROLOGY

The immunity to ASF is unknown. Surviving animals are persistently infected, and viremia persists in spite of high levels of antibody as a result of high levels of incomplete antibody. Antibodies first appear after 10 days. Most of the virus is bound to erythrocytes. There is an absence of neutralizing antibodies and a huge variation in viruses. Cell-mediated immunity may be important in the immune response to ASF and in the protection against reinfection. The serologic responses have been described.[28]

The presence of anti-ASV antibodies is indicative of infection because a vaccine is not available. ELISA is the most useful method for large-scale investigation of outbreaks, and the new methods are not affected by the quality of the samples.[23,29]

DIFFERENTIAL DIAGNOSIS

The disease is easily confused with hog cholera, and very careful examination is required to differentiate the two. Clinically, the illness is much shorter (2 days versus 7 days) than in hog cholera. Gross necropsy changes are similar to but more severe than those of hog cholera. The marked karyorrhexis of lymphocytes characteristic of African swine fever (ASF) is not observed in hog cholera. Differential diagnosis must rely on laboratory testing. In the past, differentiation has been achieved by the challenge of hog cholera–susceptible and immune pigs with suspect material. More recently, reliance has been placed on the demonstration of hemadsorbing activity with virus from suspected outbreaks grown on pig leukocyte tissue cultures. But hemadsorbing activity may be weak, delayed, or even absent, and there is sometimes difficulty in isolating virus from subacute or chronic cases in enzootic areas. Demonstration of antigen by florescent antibody staining will allow diagnosis of acute cases. For chronic cases, serologic testing has been recommended, and with the use of more than one test a high degree of accuracy can be achieved. Several sensitive laboratory tests for detection of the virus in tissues and serum antibody are now available. Enzyme-linked immunoabsorbent assay (ELISA) tests are highly sensitive. Radioimmunoassay tests are also sensitive, and isolates of the virus may be titrated in swine monocyte cultures using a microtechnique. In the lymphocyte response test to virus infection, there is a cytolytic effect on the lymphocytes; the effect is greater on the B-lymphocytes than on the T-lymphocytes. Pigs with demonstrable antibody should be considered as chronic carriers of the virus because it is doubtful that true recovery ever occurs.

TREATMENT

There is no treatment for ASF.

CONTROL

Immediately restrict pig movements. There is no vaccine for ASF as yet, but ASF has been eradicated before from countries without the use of a vaccine.

Slaughter affected pigs and their ticks as quickly as possible.

The control and eradication of ASF is difficult because of the following factors:

- Lack of an effective vaccine
- Transmission of the virus in fresh meat and cured pork products
- Recognition of persistent infection in some pigs, particularly wild feral pigs, and possibly warthogs and bush pigs
- Clinical similarity of hog cholera and African swine fever
- Recognition that in some parts of the world soft ticks of the genus *Ornithodoros* (*erraticus, moubata, porcinus porcinus*) are involved in the biological transmission of the disease and can remain carriers for long periods (possibly 5 years)

Prevention of introduction of the disease to free countries is based on the prohibition of importation of live pigs or pig products from countries where African swine fever occurs. Strict application of the prohibition has prevented the spread of the disease from enzootic areas within South Africa. If a breakdown does occur, control must consist of prevention of spread by quarantine, slaughter of infected and in-contact animals, and suitable hygienic precautions. The need for close contact between pigs for the disease to spread and the ease with which this can be prevented by the erection of pig-proof fences facilitate control. Conversely, the disease is virtually uncontrollable when pigs from a number of farms have access to communal grazing. The virus is highly resistant to external influences, including chemical agents, and the most practical disinfectant to use against the virus is a strong solution of caustic soda. Contaminated sites can remain infective for periods exceeding 3 months. These factors and the persistence of the virus in recovered pigs probably contributed to the difficulties encountered in the eradication program in Portugal, where the disease was stamped out but reappeared in 1960. However, the most important factor appears to have been the indiscriminate use of attenuated vaccines, which fostered the development of carrier pigs. In this outbreak, very little was seen in the form of clinical signs.

In Spain in 1985, a comprehensive nationally coordinated program for the eradication of the disease was begun, and substantial progress had been made. Before 1985, the only method of control of the disease in Spain was depopulation of herds with clinical disease. The current eradication program consists of the following:

- Depopulation of herds with clinical disease
- Serologic surveillance of all sows and boars in every herd
- Improvement of sanitary conditions of housing
- Improved hygiene (safe disposal of manure, vehicle disinfection, insect and rodent extermination)
- Veterinary control of all swine livestock transfers (with individual identification of every animal moved for finishing or breeding purposes)
- Health certification of every animal used for herd replacement
- Destruction of every seropositive animal
- Formation of mobile veterinary field teams exclusively dedicated to support the program

Following introduction of this program, it has been possible to divide Spain into a disease-free region (the criteria is a minimum of 2 years without the disease) and an infected region. Eradication of the disease in Spain occurred by 2001. In 1991 the Spanish government claimed that 96% of the Spanish territory was free of ASF. The calculated benefit–cost ratio is estimated to vary from 1.23 to 1.47, depending on the intensity of the program. A reduction in the funding for control would result in a benefit–cost ratio of 0.97, making the program unprofitable.

It has been shown that the use of chemical disinfectants containing at least 2% citric acid for porous surfaces is effective in removing ASF[30] and foot and mouth disease (FMD), whereas 2000 ppm of sodium hypochlorite will disinfect ASF but not FMD.

In a study of the risk factors for ASF in major pig-producing areas in Nigeria 1997 to 2011,[31] it was found that the presence of an infected pig farm in the same area and an abattoir will increase the likelihood of ASF infection of farms. Vermin and birds are also a risk. Strict food and water control, immediate separation (isolation) of sick pigs from healthy pigs, and the washing and/or disinfection of farm equipment will assist in reducing the chance of infection. Region-based control and farm-based biosecurity will help control ASF in Nigeria. Biosecurity is the likely key to successful control in Africa.[2]

Vaccines

The prospects for the development of vaccines have been discussed,[32] and the key factor is that knowledge of the antigens that encode the dominant protective epitopes recognized by CD8+ T cells is lacking at present.

It is difficult to make a vaccine because of the large size of the virus and the many proteins in the genome. Many of these alter the immune response.[20] It is also variable. The host response to the virus is very complex, with only partial protection produced by neutralizing antibodies.[33] Several different vaccines have been used, including an ineffective inactivated-virus vaccine and modified live-virus vaccines.[34] The modified live-virus vaccines provide some protection, but the results following their use have been neither satisfactory nor safe, and they have the two disadvantages of confounding laboratory tests and producing "carrier" pigs. The cell-mediated immunity component is very important.[27] The administration of individual recombinants proteins and/or DNA only gives partial protection.[32]

FURTHER READING

Blome S, et al. Pathogenesis of African swine fever in domestic pigs and European wild boar. *Virus Res.* 2013;173:122-130.

Burrage TC. African swine fever virus infection in *Ornithodorus* ticks. *Virus Res.* 2013;173:31-139.

Costard S, et al. Epidemiology of African swine fever virus. *Virus Res.* 2013;173:191-197.

De Leon P, et al. Laboratory methods to study African swine fever. *Virus Res.* 2013;173:168-179.

Dixon LK, et al. Prospects for development of African swine fever virus vaccines. *Dev Biol.* 2013;135:147.

Oura CAL, Arias M. African swine fever. In: *Manual of Diagnostic Tests and Vaccines for Terestrial Animals.* Vol. 2. 6th ed. Paris: OIE; 2008:1069-1082.

Penrith ML, Vosloo WJS. Review of African swine fever: transmission, spread and control. *J South Afric Vet Assoc.* 2009;80:58-62.

Sanchez-Vizcaino JM, Mur L. African swine fever diagnosis update. *Transbound Emerg Dis.* 2013;135:159.

REFERENCES

1. Oura C. *Vet Rec.* 2013;doi:10.1136/vr.f5327.
2. Fasina FO, et al. *Transbound Emerg Dis.* 2012;59:244.
3. De Villier EP, et al. *Virology.* 2010;400:128.
4. Boshoff CI, et al. *Vet Microbiol.* 2007;121:45.
5. Rowlands RJ, et al. *Emerg Infect Dis.* 2008;14:1870.
6. Gogin A, et al. *Virus Res.* 2013;178:198.
7. Oganesyan AS, et al. *Virus Res.* 2013;173:204.
8. Gulenkin VM, et al. *Prev Vet Med.* 2011;102:167.
9. Nigsch A, et al. *Prev Vet Med.* 2013;108:262.
10. Mur L, et al. *BMC Vet Res.* 2012;8:149.
11. Mur L, et al. *Transbound Emerg Dis.* 2011;59:134.
12. Diaz AV, et al. *Emerg Infect Dis.* 2012;18:1026.
13. Sanchez-Vizcaino JM, et al. *Transbound Emerg Dis.* 2012;59(suppl 1):27.
14. Jori E, Bastos ADS. *Ecohealth.* 2010;6:296.
15. Basto AP, et al. *J Gen Virol.* 2006;87:1863.
16. de Carvalho Ferreira HC, et al. *Vet Microbiol.* 2012;160:327.
17. Karalyan Z, et al. *BMC Vet Res.* 2012;8:18.
18. Sanchez-Cordon PJ, et al. *Am J Vet Res.* 2007;68:772.
19. Fernandez de Marco F, et al. *Res Vet Sci.* 2007;83:198.
20. Fernandez-Pinero J, et al. *Transbound Emerg Dis.* 2013;60:48.
21. Reis AL, et al. *J Gen Virol.* 2007;88:2426.
22. Gallardo C, et al. *Virus Genes.* 2009;38:89.
23. Krug PW, et al. *Vet Microbiol.* 2012;156:96.
24. Fasina FO, et al. *Prev Vet Med.* 2012;107:65.
25. Escribano JM, et al. *Virus Res.* 2013;173:101.
26. King DP, et al. *Vaccine.* 2012;29:593.
27. Takamatsu HH, et al. *Virus Res.* 2013;173:110.
28. Dixon LK, et al. *Dev Biol.* 2013;135:147.
29. Gabriel C, et al. *Emerg Infect Dis.* 2011;17:2342.
30. Sanchez-Vizcaino JM, Mur L. *Transbound Emerg Dis.* 2013;135:150.
31. Tignon M, et al. *J Virol Methods.* 2011;178:161.
32. Fernandez-Pinero J, et al. *Transbound Emerg Dis.* 2012;doi:10.1111/j1865-1682.
33. Boshoff CI, et al. *Vet Microbiol.* 2007;121:45.
34. Gallardo C, et al. *Clin Vaccine Immunol.* 2009;16:1012.

PORCINE CIRCOVIRUS–ASSOCIATED DISEASE

Originally, the condition associated with porcine circovirus type 2 (PCV2) was called *postweaning multisystemic wasting syndrome* (PMWS), but we now know that PCV2 is associated with a wider spectrum of conditions now referred to as porcine circovirus associated disease (PCVAD). PCV1 was known for some time beforehand in tissue culture but has always been considered nonpathogenic. Infection with PCV2 is necessary for PMWS to develop, but one or more cofactors are necessary to facilitate this.[1]

The other diseases in PCVAD include porcine dermatitis and nephropathy syndrome (PDNS), reproductive disorders, enteritis, proliferative and necrotizing pneumonia, and the porcine respiratory disease complex (PRDC). Only once has congenital tremor been linked to PCV2, so it is no longer regarded as a PCVAD.[2]

Two initial features of the disease are the effects on the lymph nodes of the pig and the lack of response of the condition to antibiotic therapy.[3]

Very simply, the disease occurs where there is a high serum viral load (compared with nonaffected pigs) and where there is a lack of neutralizing antibody. In other words, if there is a successful immune response, it limits PCV2 replication and avoids clinical disease.

PCV2 is one of the three viral diseases that destabilize the enzootic bacterial diseases in a herd.[1] It is a cause of considerable economic loss.

ETIOLOGY

Circoviruses are relatively new, probably having existing for only around 500 years.[4] PCV has the highest mutation rate reported for any DNA virus and approaches the higher rate of genetic change seen usually in RNA viruses.[5] PCV2 belongs to the genus *Circovirus* of the Circoviridae family (includes PCV1) and is described as the prime causative agent of PMWS.[6]

Porcine circoviruses are small but powerful,[7] and PCV1 and PCV2 have similar genomic organization, with two ambisense open reading frames (ORFs) flanking the origin of replication.[7]

PCV2 has been retrospectively identified by serology in swine populations as an asymptomatic infection at least 25 years before the first case of PMWS, and a recent study of the genome showed that the archival PCV2 was avirulent, as is the new PCV2, as a result of mutational events within a sequence of nine base nucleotides in the nucleocapsid gene of PCV2.[8]

The experimental reproduction of the disease and its occurrence under field conditions are usually associated with a number of risk or triggering factors.[9] It has been suggested that PCV2 is a necessary but not sufficient cause of the condition of PMWS.[1]

A novel porcine circovirus-like agent P1, also associated with wasting disease, has been isolated with 896 nucleotides.[10,11] No single viral cofactor has yet been identified.[12] Different isolates may vary in virulence,[13] but PMWS has been produced in gnotobiotic pigs following exposure to various amounts of PCV2a and PCV2b[14] without the presence of any detectable infectious cofactors.

There are two subtypes, 2a and 2b, with sequence differences mostly found in the capsid region,[15,16] and the antigenic profiles are not identical.[15-19]

The current classification scheme for grouping viruses is complicated by genetic recombination.[20-23]

GENOME STUDIES

The viruses are the smallest known mammalian viruses. The details of the genome and the virus proteins produced have been described.[7] The PCV2 genome is a circular, single-stranded DNA with a size of 1766 to 1768 nucleotides that contains three major ORFs.[19]

ORF1 encodes the replicase proteins rep and rep′ involved in virus replication. They bind to specific sequences within the origin of replication located in the 5′ intergenic region, and both are essential for viral replication.[24-26]

ORF2 encodes the viral capsid (cap) protein, which has the ability to bind to the host cell receptor.[19,27,28]

ORF3 encodes a protein that is involved in PCV2 apoptosis,[29,30] and in vitro ORF3 is found within ORF1. The ORF3 proteins of both PCV1 and PCV2 induce apoptotic cell death[31] and code for a 105 amino acid protein that causes apoptosis of PCV2 infected cells[32] but is dispensable for virus infection.[33]

An ORF4 has also been detected in PCV2 productive infection.[34] It is not essential for PCV2 replication but plays a role in the suppression of caspase activity and regulating CD4+ and CD8+ T-lymphocytes during PCV2 replication.

The signature motif[25] discriminating between 2a and 2b lies within the virus capsid protein, which often contains virus pathogenicity characteristics. There are several genotyping studies.[16,29,35-37]

Genetic variation and newly emerging genotypes in China have been described,[38] and 19 isolates were identified in three genotypes, 2a, 2b, and 2d. PCV2d was a new genotype for China, and PCV2b had become the predominant genotype. The subtypes described in Asia (2d and 2e)[39,40] may belong to the previously described groups (a, b, or c), depending on classification interpretation.[41]

In a recent study, the complete genome sequence of a novel PCV2b variant was described in cases of vaccine failure in animals with PMWS,[42] and this was similar to the reported Chinese PCV2d strain.

A new natural PCV2 virus with a very low incidence was identified in Quebec in September 2008, in which it was found that the virus contained the ORF1 of PCV1 and ORF2 of PCV2a; using the nomenclature of Segales et al.,[65] it was decided to call this virus PCV1/2a.[43]

It is to be noted that very small differences in the amino acid sequence may result in major changes in the pathogenicity of the virus.[13]

TRANSCRIPTION

Little is known about the cellular events triggered by infection with PCV2 in PMWS. Several porcine genes were found to be up-regulated in lymph nodes and also in PK-15 cells. At least five have been identified.[7] It has recently been shown that PCV2 induces the activation of NF-κB by phosphorylation and degradation and subsequent translocation of NF-κB p65 from the cytoplasm to the nucleus. Many of the events point to intracellular signaling and endocytic pathways.[7]

EMBRYO INFECTIVITY

Embryonic cells are susceptible to infection but not while in the zona pellucida. Extensive replication in embryos leads to death and resorption in utero.[44] In fetuses of 40 to 70 days of gestation the virus replicates mainly in the heart, followed by the liver, lymphoid tissue, and lungs;[45] with increasing age of the fetus, the replication decreases. After birth, replication is mainly in the lymphoblasts and the monocytes.[46]

VIRUS IMPORT

Internalization is slow and inefficient via endocytosis. Clathrin-mediated endocytosis also plays a part. No substantial replication was found in lymphoid cells but rather in endothelial cells particularly aortic endothelial cells, gut epithelial cells, and fibrocytes[47] by an increase in Cap and Rep proteins. The glycosaminoglycans heparin, heparin sulfate, chondroitin sulfate A, and keratin sulfate serve as attachment receptors.[28] After internalization, PCV2 is localized in endosomes.[48] A dynamin- and cholesterol-independent, but actin- and small GTPase-dependent pathway allows PCV2 internalization in epithelial cells that leads to infection, and clathrin-mediated PCV2 internalization in epithelial cells is not followed by a full replication.[49] Disassembly involves serine proteases.[48]

REPLICATION

Upon infection, in step 1 the viral ssDNA genome is converted by host cell factors into a dsDNA replicate form that serves as a template. Further complex processes occur,[26,50,51] and only *Rep* and *Rep′* are essential for viral replication in mammalian cells.[24] PCV2 replication is impaired by inhibition of the extracellular signal-regulated kinase (ERK) signaling pathway,[52] which indicates that it is involved in PCV2 infection and beneficial to PCV2 replication in cultured cells.

Six cellular proteins were found to react with *cap* and three with *rep* in a study of the interactions of the replication proteins and the capsid protein of PCV1 and PCV2 with host proteins.[53] It appears that only the *rep*, *rep′*, and *cap* genes are responsible for replication. It has been proposed that PCV replicates by means of a rolling-circle melting-pot mechanism.[24] The *rep* and *cap* genes are oriented in the opposite direction, resulting in an ambisense genome organization. An intergenic region between the 5′ ends of the *rep* and *cap* genes forms a stem–loop structure containing the origin of virus replication and the replication factors between PCV1 and PCV2. Replacement of the replication factors of PCV2 with those of PCV1 greatly enhances the viral replication in vitro.[54] Reactive oxygen species regulate the replication of PCV2 via a NF-κB pathway.[55]

Viral replication is enhanced by stimulation by mitogens (Con A or pokeweed mitogen) but does not depend strictly on whether a cell is in mitosis.[56] Monocyte-derived dendritic cells enhance cell proliferation and PCV2 replication in concanavalin A-stimulated swine peripheral blood lymphocytes in vitro.[57]

A recent study has shown that ORF1-dependent but not ORF2-dependent differences are important for in vitro replication of PCV2 in porcine alveolar macrophages singularly or coinfected with PRRSV.[58] The PCV2 ISRE sequence not only plays a role in the whole viral genome in vivo and in vitro but also works in the Rep promoter. It plays a significant role in the viral replication efficiency and regulation of IFN-α-mediated PCV2 replication in PK-15 cells.[59] PCV2 could trigger autophagosome formation and enhance autophagic flux in PK-15 cells and thereby increase replication.[60,61] PCV2 replicates in lymphoblastoid cells, and viral infection could result in the lysis of infected cells.[62]

GENOTYPES

Early studies focused on differences in genotype,[16,29,63,64] and further studies have led to the naming of the two major genotypes, PCV2a and PCV2b.[65] Since then, a new genotype has been added, and the three PCV2 genotypes have been designated PCV2a, PCV2b, and PCV2c.[41,65] In this system, the ORF2 sequences are assigned to different genotypes when the genetic difference between them is at least 0.035.[65]

PCV2a is divided into five clusters (2A to 2E), whereas PCV2b is divided into three clusters (1A to 1C).[16] PCV2c was identified in pigs from Denmark.[66]

Some countries have detected a shift from PCV2a to PCV2b on sequencing studies.[66-68]

An association between the genotype shift from PCV2a to PCV2b and the sudden increase of PMWS has been suggested. The genotype shift was reported from Switzerland and Denmark in 2003,[66,68] in Canada in 2005,[69] and in the United States in 2005.[15] In Spain, it was reported in 2011 in cases from 1985 to 2008.[70] In Korea, the shift occurred in 2002 or even earlier.[71,72] In England, there appeared to be a shift from PCV2a to PCV2b at the time as an outbreak of PMWS on a farm.[73] PCV2a may have been associated with non-PMWS-affected farms, and it is the switch to 2b that has been associated with the upsurge in PMWS. This may also mean that 2a is less virulent than 2b. In Australia, where PMWS has not been seen, only 2a has been reported.[66]

PCV2b is currently the most prevalent form of the virus in naturally occurring infections.[29,66,74-77]

Recombination between lineages in natural populations of PCV2 in Hong Kong and China has been shown.[78]

Evidence for recombination between PCV2a and PVC2b has been found.[79-81]

In the study from the United States, PCV2a and PCV2b were found in the tissues of the same infected pig.[79]

Forty strains from China were sequenced from 2004 to 2008,[82] and they could be grouped into four genotypes based on their genetic distances and phylogenetic trees. PCV2a, PCV2b, PCV2d, and PCV2e were found, but the Danish type PCV2c was not found. The study also showed that PCV2b had become the most common type in China. Since this study,[82] the existence of 2d and 2e has been discounted on the basis of classification studies.[41]

An emerging recombinant cluster from 2b (recombination between the 2a and 2b strains within the ORF2 gene) has been shown to be circulating in China and other Asian countries.[83]

Multiple strains of PCV2 have been found in the same pig in China,[84] and this coexistence may contribute to the development of more severe clinical signs in coinfected pigs.

There is a high degree of heterogeneity of PCV2 within a geographic region in both domesticated and wild boar populations.[85,86]

During 2012, a new variant PCV2 strain designated mPCV2 was identified in the United States,[42] and it was found to be more virulent than the traditional 2a and 2b strains.[87] This mPCV2b strain appears to be present in Europe and based on limited data appears to be replacing other PCV2b strains in Southeast Asia and North America.[88] It also has significance in that this variant has also has been found in possible vaccine failure cases.[89]

Dual heterologous PCV2a/2b infection induces severe disease in germ-free pigs when given 7 days apart. PCV2a or PCV2b when administered singly or in combination with keyhole limpet hemocyanin appeared to be of equal virulence.[90] Gross lesions were more severe in heterologously infected pigs than in 2b/2b infected pigs, and these were more severe than in 2a/2a infected pigs.

EPIDEMIOLOGY

Other than the mouse,[91] nonporcine species are not susceptible.

PCV2 can be considered to be enzootic throughout the world and becomes epizootic when there is a significant increase in mortality.[92] Initially, the viruses isolated (1997–2006) were PCV2a, but there was a shift on a global scale to PCV2b, except in Korea, Japan, and Australia.[66] PCV2b was isolated in Korea from 2005 to 2007,[93] and in Japan (isolates from 2006–2007), the change from PCV2a to 2b occurred very quickly.[76]

In a study of 148 PCV2 isolates, 63.5% were PCV2b.[16] In Ireland, 5/6 isolates were PCV2a, but the other one, associated with increased mortality, was a PCV2b.[74] The most recent discovery of a PCV was probably in Australia[94] and was a PCV2a, but the criteria for the Australian definition of PMWS were not met,[95] possibly because a PCV2b has not yet been found.

Many epidemiologic studies have suggested that the shift from PCV2a to PCV2b has been associated with an increase in PMWS infections.[64,66,67,69]

A new emerging genotype subgroup within the PCV2b dominates the PMWS epidemiology in Switzerland.[68]

In North America, the shift occurred later and may have been initially in South and Latin America, and then followed importation of infected animals into North America.[75,96]

In a study in Canada, most of the strains were PCV2a, but PCV2b was also found, and in a few cases both types;[64,97] for example, one pig had both 2a and 2b in the liver.[98]

In a study of the prevalence of 2a and 2b in pigs with and without PMWS in Korea, it was found that there was a significant increase over time in animals with PCV2b that had and did not have PMWS.[71]

In the United States, the emergence of novel mutant PCV2b associated with PCVAD (PCV2b was first seen in 2005 to 2006) was described[67] and was found to be 99.9% identical to a mutant virus found in China.[89]

A similar progression from PCV2a to PCV2b has been seen in Asia, in both China[39,99] and in Korea.[100] The genetic diversity of PCV2 from pigs in Korea has been described,[100] and there are two main groups and four subgroups (1A, 1C, 2D, and 2E). Most cases from PMWS-affected herds were in group 1, whereas cases with no clinical signs of PCV2 infection were within group 2.

It is not just the variations in the genotype of the virus that may be related to the pathogenicity of the virus;[101] the dynamics of PCV2 infection in a herd are strongly influenced by management and husbandry,[102] with everything that favors early infection being particularly important, such as the size of the pens and cross-fostering.

Wild Boar

It has been found in Transylvanian wild boar (in a Hungarian study), where 13.5% proved to be positive for PCV2 by RT-PCR.[107] It was found in wild boar in Poland[108] in over 70% of animals and was found to be of either 2a or 2b genotype.

PMWS has been described in wild boar in several countries, including the United States, Brazil,[111] Germany, Croatia,[112] Greece,[113] and Italy.[114]

Prevalence

The prevalence varies considerable from country to country and survey to survey, often with results between 40% and 80%, but it may be as low as 23% in Japan[103] on PCV2 antigen detection or viral DNA, even though 50.45% of the farms were positive (65/129 farms). One of the other conclusions was that it may exist in several forms, including an epidemic form or a subtle endemic or sporadic form. The prevalence was 50% in Taiwan and 8% in Korea.[104] It has been found in 30% to 40% of archived tissue in the United Kingdom and in 10% in the United States.

In a study in the United States of 185 farms, it was found that 82% of the farms were positive for PCV2, and only 2.45% were positive for PCV1.[105] It was found in Cuba in 2010.[106]

It has also been found in 50% of animals in Spain[109] and in 43% in the Czech Republic.[110] PCV2 infections associated with PMWS are only sporadically present in the Czech Republic,[115] although positive serology for PCV2 was widespread. The spread of PMWS in Sweden has been described,[116]and the change from an exotic to endemic disease was described.

In a study of seven PCVAD-affected farms, the risk of PCVAD was increased by early PCV2 infection but significantly decreased when pigs were born to PCV2-seropositive sows.[117] Nonaffected animals also had higher titers earlier than piglets that developed PCVAD[118] and higher PCV2 viremia.[119]

Environmental Survival

The virus is extremely difficult to eradicate from the environment because it has an ability to resist the environment and therefore increase its survival time.

It is resistant to pH 3.0, chloroform, and temperatures of 70°C (158°F) for 15 minutes.[120-122] Animals exposed to nondisinfected trailers for 2 hours became viremic and seroconverted, but no seroconversion or viremia was found after disinfection using one of four protocols.[123]

It has been suggested that because of its survival in the environment, animal-to-animal contact is not necessary for its spread.[124]

Transmission

Both vertical and horizontal transmission is possible. Multiple routes of transmission to piglets in the presence of maternal immunity have been described.[125] Piglets are regularly infected with PCV2 in utero and are under constant challenge by PCV2 through contact with infected sows and a contaminated farrowing environment. Maternal immunity did not affect PCV2 transmission to piglets or the viral load in sows. This emphasizes the importance of maternal infection in early infection in newborn piglets.

As fetuses near term, the replication of the virus takes place in the cells of the monocyte–macrophage series.

Horizontal Transmission

It is transmitted principally by the oronasal route. The widespread distribution in the lymphatic system, respiratory system, urogenital system, and gastrointestinal system suggests that it may be present in all secretions and transudates. It is also present in colostrum,[126] milk, and semen.[127] It was found in the macrophages of the mammary ducts within 3 days.[128]

A study showed that the virus was shed in similar amounts by the nasal, oral, and fecal routes,[118] and in sows until at least 27 days,[129] or 209 days postfarrowing.[130] The maximum level of genomic load was detected at 28 days postfarrowing (5 to 7 $\log_{10}$ genome copies/mL) and steadily decreased until 209 days postfarrowing.

In a study of five experimentally infected gnotobiotic pigs, there were between 6 and 12 $\log_{10}$ PCV2 genome copies/mL in the serum and liver.[131] In one study, infectious PCV2 was detected in colostrum samples and milk samples. Anti-PCV2 IgA was found in high levels in colostrum and milk. Infectious PCV2 may be present in milk and colostrum of naturally infected sows even in the presence of neutralizing antibody.[132] Shedding of PCV2 in milk has been shown from experimentally infected sows.[129] The animals excreted from day 1 until day 27 of lactation. There is also the possibility of PCV2 replication in the mammary gland.[128] Antibodies in milk protect against clinical disease but not against infection. Shedding of PCV1 and PCV2 was found in whey for the first time.[138]

Vaccination decreases the shedding of virus in colostrum and milk.[132,133]

Pigs shed virus for a prolonged period following viral exposure, and growing pigs were the source of horizontal PCV2 transmission in PCV2-infected herds.[134] There is a high level of PCV2 DNA in colostrum, sow sera, and piglet sera.[135]

The intermingling of affected and healthy pigs[136] showed transmission by direct nose-to-nose contact, and two were infected without being in direct contact with infected animals. On-site control animals in a separate compartment did not develop clinical disease.

When pigs from affected herds were mingled with healthy pigs from unaffected herds,[137] it led to horizontal transmission, as did pigs being in adjacent pens but not directly in contact.

In a study of infectiousness and transmission, it was suggested that the probability of horizontal transmission was negligible after 55 days postinfection, even though there was still significant viremia.[102]

Transmission can occur from diseased pigs to healthy in-contacts after mingling, especially if there is very close contact.[139] It can be transmitted in uncooked tissue from viremic animals.[140] A lower infectious dose in some of these tissues (bone marrow and skeletal muscle compared with lymphoid tissue) may result in a delayed onset of infection.

Experimentally produced spray-dried plasma spiked with PCV2 was transmissible.[141]

Airborne transmission has also been shown in an experimental setup.[142] In a study of Canadian swine confinement buildings, up to 10^7 genomes per cubic meter of air were found. Airborne dust concentrations were correlated with airborne PCV2 and total bacterial counts.[143]

The verification of natural infection of peridomestic rodents by PCV2 on commercial swine farms was confirmed,[144] with PCV2 being found in the spleen, lung, and kidney, although transmission from rodents to pigs has not been confirmed.

PCV2b has been transmitted by house flies.[145] The flies in the nursery and weaner areas were most likely to be positive.

In practice, there is often a pattern of elevated antibody levels in the herd because it is a mixture of passive and active immunity[130] and, as a result, may maintain consistent infection dynamics in the farm.

Under field conditions, PCV2 can be recovered from mice and rats at quite high prevalence levels, and therefore there is the possibility of indirect transmission and persistence on a farm site.[146]

There is also the possibility that vaccines may introduce the virus. In Canada, the appearance of the PCV1/PCV2 chimera may have been associated with the use of inactivated PCV2 vaccines.[147]

Pigs from PMWS-affected herds had at least 10^3 higher mean serum titer of PCV2 compared with pigs from PMWS-free herds. Pigs that were able to control the infection (as measured by PCV2 titer in serum) recovered clinically (from PMWS-affected herds) or stayed healthy (from unaffected herds). Pigs with titers below 5×10^8 copies/mL serum during the study period had a chance of recovery, but those above this generally died.[136]

Vertical Transmission

Transplacental infection was demonstrated following the intranasal infection of sows 3 weeks before farrowing, and the virus was recovered from both aborted and live-born piglets.[148]

PMWS was reproduced in pigs fed colostrum and milk from PCV2-infected sows and infected postnatally with PPV or immunostimulated.[149] PCV2 was detected in mammary and other tissues in experimentally infected sows.[128]

The virus has also been demonstrated in myocarditis in aborted fetuses and stillborn piglets.[150] In earlier experiments, the cardiomyocytes of the fetus were found to be the main target of PCV2.

In a study in Poland, the heart of the fetus contained the highest amounts of virus and the highest number of antigen positive cells. The myocardium was full of hypertrophic cells and showed multiple and irregular pale areas that corresponded to histologic lesions of necrosis.[151]

Boars show excretion of PCV2 virus in semen (with no differences between 2a and 2b) continuously until at least 50 days after inoculation of the boars.[152] The virus has been shown to be excreted in the semen of boars with serum antibodies.[153]

Naïve sows inseminated with PCV2 spiked semen exhibited reproductive failure, and their fetuses were infected.[154] The mummified fetuses died between 42 and 105 days of gestation.

PCV2-seropositive gilts can be infected with PCV2 after intrauterine exposure, and low maternal antibody may increase the probability of a fetal infection.[155]

PCV2 viremic sows had a higher number of exposed fetuses compared with nonviremic sows, which means that PCV2 can cross the placenta and cause fetal damage. Sows with low antibody titers had greater mortality in their piglets than those with higher levels.[119]

In a study of porcine circovirus viremia in newborn piglets in five clinically normal swine breeding units in North America, it was found that all sow colostrum samples (125/125) and 96.8% (121/125) of the sow serum samples were positive for anti-PCV2 antibodies. The overall PCV2 DNA prevalence was 47.2% (59/125) in the sow serum and 40.8% (51/125) for sows' colostrum and 39.9% in presuckle piglet serum. PCV2b was detected more frequently than PCV2a. Concurrent 2a and 2b was detected in 11.9% of the sow sera, 5.9% of the colostrum, and 15.6% of the piglet sera.[135] Natural exposure to PCV2 results in long-term infection, and

PCV2 is shed in similar amounts by nasal, oral, and fecal routes.[130] When the PCV2 viremic pigs were segregated from their dams, PCV2 DNA was detected for extended periods (81-day observation period).

Experimental PCV2 exposure results in long-term infection. PCV2 is shed in similar amounts by nasal, oral, and fecal routes and is infectious to naïve pigs.[156]

PCV2 has also been detected in the semen of naturally and experimentally infected boars, including seropositive animals.[127,153,157] The PCV2 material in semen is infectious.[158] The younger the boar, the more likely it is to be shedding virus in the semen.

Maternal antibodies have an effect on PCV2 shedding in vertically infected pigs.[159]

Risk Factors

A cross-sectional study of 147 pig farms in the United Kingdom was undertaken from 2008 to 2009 and risk factors identified. Increased PMWS was associated with rearing growers indoors, more veterinary visits, poorly isolated hospital pens, buying replacements, and seropositivity to *M. hyopneumoniae.* Factors associated with a decreased risk were low stocking density for growers, adjusting diets at least three times between weaning and 14 weeks of age, and requiring visitors to be "pig-free" for at least 2 days.[160]

The spatio-temporal patterns and risks of herd breakdowns in pigs with PMWS[161] and closeness to another infected pig farm, large herds, and no prevention of visitors who had not been through a pig-free period were identified as being risks for infection. The affected farms were also more likely to have other infections.

There is a "litter effect," which is mainly explained through the sow PCV2 status (viremia), in that fewer piglets died when born to nonviremic sows.[119]

In the individual pig, low levels of antibody at 7 weeks of age is considered a risk factor, as is being born to a seronegative sow.

Pigs with PMWS have greater amounts of PCV2 in their serum and shed larger amounts of the virus than do nonaffected pigs.[136]

In many ways, the risk factors are the same as for many other diseases and are listed as follows:

- Infection in the herd or vaccination
- The occurrence of type 2 strains in a country only normally having type 1 (e.g., Denmark, which used the U.S. vaccine based on ATC-2332)
- Other affected herds in the area, especially if they are close
- Purchasing large numbers of replacement gilts (>500 a year)
- A herd size of over 400 sows
- Purchase of replacement gilts
- A high prevalence of PCV2 antibodies
- PPV antibodies in the finishers
- Active PPV infection in the gilts
- On-farm semen collection and artificial insemination (AI)

Other factors include the following:

- The presence of visitors to the farm without a 3-day pig-free period before their visit is regarded as a hazard
- Large pens in the nursery and grower stages
- A high level of cross-fostering
- Early weaning less than 21 days
- Mixed ages and weights in the same airspace
- Lack of proper cleaning, disinfection, drying, and rest periods between batches—continuous flow through the nursery is a source of environmental contamination.
- Vaccination for PRRSV, *E. coli,* and separate use of PPV and *Erysipelas* vaccines may be disadvantageous.

The risk to a herd is reduced when there is a high level of biosecurity, including reducing the numbers of visitors; proper isolation and quarantine for new arrivals; use of semen from an AI station; group housing of sows during pregnancy; protective clothing on entry to the unit and showering in and out; separate sites for removal and arrival of pigs; long empty periods of rest for the buildings before restocking; proper vaccination protocols for other diseases, which also help to control concurrent infections[162]; sorting pigs by sex in the nursery; greater minimum weights at weaning; regular vaccinations for endemic disease and following the recommendations for use; routine anthelmintic treatments and for ectoparasites; and oxytocin during parturition, which may also help reduction of PMWS. The use of spray-dried plasma in initial rations also is helpful, and it was shown[163] that commercial spray-dried porcine plasma does not transmit PCV2 in weaned pigs challenged with PRRSV. On the other hand, it was shown that PCV2b in an experimental spray-dried product was not effectively inactivated by the process used.[141] The efficiency of the process therefore determines the likelihood of PCV2b resisting the spray drying.

Studies have found that the earlier the infection occurs, the higher the risk of PMWS, and also if the offspring are weaned early[117]; however, other studies[118] have stated there is no effect of the timing of \infection on subsequent PMWS development. Colostrum-deprived piglets are more sensitive to PMWS development.[164] Healthy pigs had higher titers at an earlier age than piglets that subsequently developed PMWS.[118]

More piglets die of viremic sows and from sows with low antibody levels.[119]

Occurrence

It has also been found in wild boar.[86] An antigen shift was shown in the wild boar from PCV2a to PCV2b. It was originally described in western Canada and has subsequently spread to Europe,[165] North and South America, Australia,[95] and Asia, including Japan.[103] It was first described in Slovakia in 2009,[166] and this was similar to the Austrian PCV2 isolate. It was described in Israel in 2008.[167] In Poland, 50% of the farms in a study had PMWS, and PMWS was confirmed in all herds with over 1000 sows in the study, but the small herds with less than 100 breeding sows were free.[168,172]

A Romanian isolate was closely related to viruses from France and Hungary.[169] A Romanian isolate from wild boar was recently shown to be closely related to PCV2a and PCV2b types and to possess a high degree of sequence heterogeneity.[170] In Korean wild boar, the prevalence was 4.98%,[171] and all were type PCV2b.

The epizootic onset in Switzerland was observed in late 2003,[68] and before that infection with PCV2 was mainly subclinical. The epizootic was accompanied by a switch to PCV2b, but this was present in the Swiss population as far back as 1979.

Retrospective studies on the occurrence of PCV2 in Germany showed that it was first detected in a pig in 1962, with a low incidence between 1962 and 1984 and with a subsequent increase between 1985 and 1998. Associated lesions such as PMWS and PDNS were not observed before 1985, and it appears that the were no major changes in the sequence analyses over the period from 1962 to 1998, suggesting that other factors were involved in the altered virulence.[173]

It was found to be ubiquitous (106/108 farms had at least one positive pig) in Mexican backyard pigs.[174]

Breeding

The clinical expression of PMWS under field conditions is modulated by the pig's genetic background.[175] Certain breeds have been shown to be more susceptible. Landrace were more susceptible than Duroc or Large Whites[176]; in an earlier study, Large White and Duroc were more susceptible than purebred Pietrain pigs. Sometimes, field studies suggest that the boar lines used may have an influence on the occurrence of PMWS, but other studies do not support this.

Two regions of the porcine genome may have genes that are linked to increased susceptibility.[177] In a study of over 16,000 piglets from 2034 sows inseminated by 13 Hungarian Landrace boars, it was found that there was a considerable difference in the proportion of the piglets with signs of PMWS, stillborn piglets, and mummified piglets sired by the different boars. Rates varied from 3.06% to 15.6% for PMWS, 1.76% to 8.52% for stillborns, and 0% to 3.22% for mummies.[178]

Concurrent Infections

As yet, no novel agents have been found to be associated with the triggering of PCVAD.[12]

Pigs infected with PCV2 and immunized with a modified live-virus CSFV vaccine developed mild to moderate PMWS, whereas none of the pigs infected with PCV2 alone or immunized with modified live-virus CSF alone developed PMWS.[179]

Concurrent viral or bacterial infections often enhance the effects of PCV2 infection in terms of occurrence, severity, and duration. The effect of PCV2 on the immune system also predisposes to viral, bacterial, fungal, and metazoal infections in turn.

One of the first agents to be associated with PCV2 was PPV. It is not normally the cause of disease in piglets, but in early Canadian studies coinfection was found frequently, and the association of both had been confirmed in studies of microscopic lesions.[148] In cell culture, concurrent PCV2/PPV infection has been shown to decrease the ability of pulmonary macrophages to phagocytose.[180] Another contributor may be TNF-α,[181] which may be produced by PPV and could promote the high levels of PCV2 typically seen in conjunction with PPV. High levels of TNF-α are induced by this coinfection, and the high level of proinflammatory cytokines may lead to PMWS.[181]

Random amplification methodologies have been used to discover new viruses, and in one study using random multiple displacement amplification (MDA) and large-scale sequencing, a unique novel porcine boca-like virus was isolated from two Swedish pigs with systemic PCVAD[182] (the genus *Bocavirus* of the subfamily Parvovirinae). The occurrence of this virus was confirmed in a further study,[183] and a PPV4 virus was also found.[184]

PRRSV has long been associated with PCV2 in Spain[119,185,186] and in Japan,[103,187] the United States,[188] the Netherlands and Canada,[64] and Italy.[189] The immunosuppression and immune-response modifications have been shown to play a part in respiratory infections, with a possible increased apoptosis.[190]

Swine alveolar macrophages infected with PCV2 first and then with PRRSV later or simultaneously displayed marked reductions in PRRSV antigen-containing rate, cytopathic effect, and TNF-α expression level. In this study,[191] PCV2 was easily internalized in the cytoplasm of alveolar macrophages (AMs) but caused no noticeable cell death, and PRRSV displayed a low infection rate but severe cytopathic effect and strong TNF-α induction in AMs. PCV2-induced IFN-α likely caused a reduction in the PRRSV infection rate and PRRSV-related AMs dysfunction when AMs were coinoculated with PCV2 and PRRSV simultaneously. Similar PCV2-induced IFN-α effects were seen in the PCV2/PRRSV group but not in the PRRSV/PCV2 group where there was also a significant induction of IFN-α. If preexisting damage has been caused by PRRSV infection, it is unlikely that IFN-α production induced by the PCV2 will be able to stop the adverse effects of the PRRSV.

PRRSV can cause enhanced PCV2 replication, as evidenced by higher serum and tissue PCV2 loads, increased severity of the pathologic changes and clinical manifestations, and higher incidence of PCVAD.

PCV2 that was inoculated first or simultaneously with PRRSV not only hinders PRRSV replication but also reduces the PRRSV-induced adverse effects on the phagocytosis of AMs. The impaired microbicidal capability in PCV2- and/or PRRSV-inoculated groups may be attributable to the reduction in reactive oxygen groups produced. PCV2a and PCV2b would also appear to have the same effects on the reduction of killing capability of AMs.[191] Fas (CD95) and FasL play a major role in the induction of apoptosis. In this same study, it was shown that PCV2 could induce swine AMs to produce FasL but PRRSV could not, except when they were both present, when there was an addictive effect. The increased expression of IFN-α, TNF-α, IL-8, and FasL mRNA in AMs from pigs with various infections with PCV2 and PRRSV observed[191] in this study may contribute to some extent to the pneumonia and bronchiolar epithelial cell damage in the lungs of PCV2- and/or PRRSV-infected pigs.

The risk of PRRSV and PCV2 coinfection was 1.85 times greater in piglets from a sow with low titers of PCV2 antibodies than in piglets from sows with medium to high titers. It was also greater in piglets from primiparous sows, PCV2-infected sows, and farms in an area of high pig density than in piglets from sows of higher parity, noninfected sows, and farms in a low-pig-density area.[192]

Compared with infections with PRRSV alone, combined infections with PCV2 resulted in significantly more severe macroscopic and microscopic lung lesions and a stronger anti-PRRS IgG response.[193] In the origin of the replication of the genome of PCV2, an interferon-stimulated response element (ISRE) was identified. During the early stages of infection, at 14 days postinoculation (PI), the mutant reduced viral replication and elicited low antibody responses. However, at 28 days PI, viremia in the infected pigs showed an upward trend, and lesion scores were more severe than with the wild-type virus. With the mutant and PRRSV the lesions were more severe than with wild-type PCV2 and PRRS. These results suggest that the ISRE element may play a part in viral pathogenesis.[194]

The severity of microscopic lesions and the PCV2 antigen load associated with these lesions were higher in the PRRSV-vaccinated piglets compared with those detected in the PCV2-only infected animals.[195]

Torque teno sus virus (TTSuV) has two main species: TTSuV1 and TTSuV2.[196] It is not known whether they cause disease or not,[197] and they were found in a higher prevalence in PCVAD-affected animals than in controls.[198]

A Spanish study found that TTSuV2 viral loads were related to PCVAD but not TTSuV1,[198,199] and a similar finding was found in Japan.[200] It may not exacerbate PCVAD in all instances,[182,201] and this was also noted in Canada[64] and in the United States.[202]

PCV2 also has a complex relationship with hepatitis E virus[203,204] and was found more commonly where there were lesions of hepatitis. In an experiment with gnotobiotic pigs, it was found that TTSuV1 had to be given 7 days before PCV2 challenge to produce any effects.[205] Tissues from systemically infected PCV2 showed widespread loads, but the higher TTSuV2 loads were in the affected animals' tissues compared with the healthy group.[206] A similar trio of agents has been associated with PMWS in the United Kingdom.[207]

There was no evidence of a relationship between hepatitis E (HEV) and PCV2 in a study in Italy from necropsied pigs.[208] There was an association demonstrated in Spain in sick pigs,[209]especially in pigs evidencing hepatitis lesions. The detection of PCV2 and HEV in the liver of aborted fetuses and from sera and feces of the dams suggests the possibility of transplacental infection and associated reproductive disorders in cases of coinfection.[210]

PCV2, a porcine boca-like virus, and a torque teno virus were isolated from PMWS cases. In 71% of the PMWS cases, the three viruses were found, but in 33% of the pigs, PMWS was not found.[183] It is possible that TTV may contribute to the development of PMWS.[211]

There is probably an influence of transplacental PCV2 infection on neonatal diarrhea associated with an epidemic diarrhea virus.[212,213] In a study of transplacental PCV2 infection on porcine epidemic diarrhea virus-induced enteritis in preweaning piglets,[213] it was found that the mean villous height and crypt depth ratio in PEDV-infected piglets from PCV2-infected sows were significantly different from those of PEDV-infected piglets from PCV2-negative sows. It is concluded that the clinical course of PEDV disease was markedly affected by transplacental infection with PCV2.

It has also been associated with Aujeszky's virus (before 2006), but a study recently showed that subclinical PCV2 does not modulate the immune response to an Aujeszky's disease virus vaccine[214] or porcine Teschovirus in Japan.[200]

Swine influenza can frequently be identified with PCV2 in the field,[188] but experimentally, SIV did not increase the severity of clinical disease or gross or microscopic lesions.[215]

Experimental coinfection with bovine viral diarrhea virus (BVD) type 1 and PCV2 suggested that ruminant pestivirus and/or vaccination with BVD might have a role in the development of PVCAD.[216]

In a study in the United Kingdom, one of the identified factors associated with increased PCVAD was *M. hyopneumoniae* (MH) infection,[160] which also occurs in the United States.[188] The mycoplasma probably potentiates the severity of PCV2-associated lung and lymphoid lesions by increasing the amount and the duration of the PCV2 antigen. Recently, experiments with MH have shown that the MH potentiated PCV2 infection by increasing IFN-γ and IL-10 mRNA expression levels,[217-219] which suggests that the severity of the lesions in dual-infected pigs is associated with PCV2 antigen and alterations of cytokine expression. Overall, MH potentiated PCV2 infection by increasing IFN-γ and IL-10 mRNA expression levels. *Mycoplasma* infection or vaccination does increase the incidence of PMWS.[220] Simultaneous PCV2 and *M. hyorhinis* coinoculation does not potentiate disease in conventional pigs.[221]

There is often an association between PCV2 and *M. hyorhinis* in healthy pigs and pigs with pneumonia, with *M. hyorhinis* being detected more frequently than MH.[222,223] Pigs with the dual infection naturally show respiratory disease and microscopic lesions and clinical signs suggestive of PCV2 infection,[224] and PCV2 vaccination reduces considerably the number of coinfections with *M. hyorhinis.*[225]

In a study of the presence of endemic pig diseases in England, it was found that there was a significant association of *A. pleuropneumoniae* antibodies with the presence of a positive PCR for PCV2 in weaners.[226]

An association between *M. hyorhinis* and PCV2 was also noticed in Canada[64] and in Japan[103] and between *M. suis* and PCV2 in Argentina.[227]

In a study of PMWS in Korea, it was found that the most common lesions were multifocal, granulomatous inflammation in the lymph nodes, liver, and spleen characterized by infiltration of epithelioid macrophages and multinucleated giant cells. In 85% of pigs there was a dual infection, and a combination with *H. parasuis* was the most common combination.

With *Salmonella* it is likely that prior exposure to PCV2 may increase the clinical effects of salmonellosis in the field.[463] In a study in Japan, it was found that prior PCV2 infection potentiated the severity of clinical signs, lung lesions, and fecal shedding and tissue dissemination of *S.* Choleraesuis in infected pigs. *Salmonella* Choleraesuis was implicated in PMWS in Japan.[228]

Bacterial lipopolysaccharide has been shown to induce PCV2 replication in swine alveolar macrophages.[229]

Experimental reproduction of PCV2-associated enteritis in pigs infected with PCV2 alone or concurrently with *Lawsonia intracellularis* (LI) or *Salmonella* Typhimurium[230] showed that PCV2 could induce enteritis independently from other enteric pathogens. A study of low growth rate in grower-finishing pigs was examined for associations between *Lawsoniana* and PCV2. Gross lesions in the small intestine and an LI load were significant risk factors for low growth, but no association with PCV2 was found.[231]

Aspergillus and *Cryptosporidium* had been found before 2003. *Pneumocystis carinii* is commonly found with PCV2 in Brazilian pigs[232] and in wild boar.[233,234]

Candida albicans in Brazil and *Zygomyces* spp. were found in Hungary.[235] Toxoplasmosis was diagnosed in a fattening pig with PCV2 infection[236] using immunohistochemistry. Either PCV2 may have triggered systemic toxoplasmosis, or *T. gondii* may have caused extensive replication of PCV2.

Recently, a case of fatal bronchopneumonia was found with *Metastrongylus elongatus* in a PCV2-infected pig,[237] and it is suggested that a concurrent PVCAD condition may trigger metastrongylosis.

A pie chart[92] from earlier data on the existence of coinfections suggested that PCV2 was found in 1% of cases. A joint infection with SIV was found in 4% of cases, bacterial pneumonia in 6%, bacterial septicemia in 10%, PPV in 11%, *M. hyopneumoniae* in 27%, and PRRSV in 41%.

PATHOGENESIS

Pathogenicity was reported to be a function of the individual properties of an isolate and not related to genotype.[238] In one study, tissues from diseased pigs showed infection with both PCV2a and PCV2b, but those with subclinical infection had either PCV2a or PCV2b.[239]

In all cases of PMWS, the common factor is PCV2, but the discussion on the other factors continues. Although PCV2 alone is not sufficient to produce the full spectrum of disease, none of the other currently recognized "trigger factors" is considered essential on its own.[164] These include changes in husbandry on the farm, immuno-stimulation by vaccination strategies, and the occurrence of other primary and secondary agents or new agents.[6]

The most pivotal step in the pathogenesis of PMWS associated with PCV2 is activation of the immune system. This may lead to increased lymphoid depletion in swine cells in both PCV2- and PRRSV/PCV2-infected swine cells.[190]

In a study of inguinal lymph nodes, PCV2, PRRSV, and PPV had their own contributions to the development of lymphoid lesions in PMWS, with PCV2 as the main causative agent. B-lymphocyte depletion and macrophage proliferation/infiltration are two hallmarks of PCV2-associated lymphoid lesions. Apart from blood recruitment, local T-cell and macrophage proliferation may play a part in the granulomatous inflammation. Apoptosis is an apparent feature in association with lymphoid depletion. The higher apoptotic rate and the PCV2 load in the germinal center and a higher apoptotic rate but lower PCV2 load in the interfollicular region suggest that there may be a direct cell injury to B cells by PCV2 infection; associated lymphoid lesions may develop through the combination of several different mechanisms with the help of coinfected viruses.[240] It is possible that lymphoid depletion in PMWS is attributable to a combination of apoptosis, viral induced lysis, destruction of lymphoid architecture, and other unknown mechanisms.

PCV2 is most frequently associated with monocytes, macrophages, and dendritic cells (DCs). These cells may accumulate viral antigen for long periods and therefore may play a role in persistence.[241] It appears not to affect the DCs or interfere with their relationships with lymphocytes and is not transmitted to the lymphocytes, which do carry antigen or viral nucleic acid for a short period.[242] It may be that these cells are not sites of replication but have phagocytosed or endocytosed PCV2 antigen.[47,243] The asymptomatic piglet does produce antibodies and cytotoxic responses, so lymphocyte communication is not affected.[244]

The most characteristic pathologic features of PMWS are lymphocyte depletion and granulomatous infiltration of lymphoid tissues. PCV2 alone induces cell proliferation, cell fusion, and chemokine expression in swine monocytic cells in vitro[245] and therefore may be capable of causing granulomatous inflammation unaided by other pathogens. There is a subcellular immunolocalization of PCV2 in lymph nodes from pigs with PMWS. PCV2 has been detected exclusively in histiocytes. The endoplasmic reticulum was dilated, and the mitochondria were swollen, associated with PCV2-labeled intracytoplasmic inclusions with recognizable virions.[246] There is a close relationship between the PCV2 and the mitochondria, which may suggest that the mitochondria may be involved in replication. It is likely that lymphocyte cell populations support the initial PCV2 replication.[247]

PCV2 induces apoptosis both in vitro and in vivo.[248-251] PCV2-induced apoptosis involves activating both the caspase-8 and caspase-3 pathways and a variety of other pathways and factors.[252-255] The regulatory role of ASK 1 in PCV2-induced apoptosis has been described.[256]

Apoptosis is increased following PCV2 infection under certain stimulation conditions, and the rate of replication increases with the cell stimulation. This same study suggests that there may be a specific stimulation or trigger for increased viral replication that is independent of cell proliferation.[257]

PCV2a and PCV2b coinfection administered 35 days apart is not sufficient to induce clinical disease. Experimental infection of conventional SPF pigs with PCV2 results in persistent viral infection despite the presence of high levels of PCV2 antibodies without the presence of clinical disease.[258]

PCV2 induces a procoagulant state in naturally infected swine and in cultured epithelial cells.[259]

In some studies, vascular disorders have been highlighted. Animals in Brazil were found to have blood hypercoagulation, petechiae, and vasculitis associated with lymph node atrophy and organ failure. Widespread petechiae have also been reported in kidneys.[249] The presence of PCV2 antigen has been revealed in lymphatics and blood vessels with severe degeneration of the endothelial cells of the blood vessel thrombi and vasculitis associated with organ necrosis and ischemia.[260] In another study, the activation of the hemostatic system was highlighted, with PCV2 being shown to modulate the swine hemostasis.[259] Plasma coagulation times were diminished, which points to the activation of coagulation systems in PCV2-affected animals. Fibrinogen was lower in the PCV2 group, and fibrinogen was found in the brain vasculature.[261] PCV2-affected animals had lower platelet counts. The platelet function was 40% higher in the PCV2-affected animals, and this implies a likely prothrombic state. Thrombin plasma activity was also increased. The occurrence of PCV2 antigen in the vascular endothelium and the precoagulant state suggests an activation of the endothelium.[262] In one study,[259] PCV2-infected cells had higher viral loads. How PCV2 causes lymphadenopathy has yet to be elucidated.

Host–Virus Interactions

Because of its very small size, PCV2 relies entirely on the host for completing its life cycle. Several porcine proteins have been identified.[53,261,263]

Cytokine Studies

Immune gene expression profiles in swine inguinal lymph nodes with different viral loads of PCV2 support a close interaction between immune activation and suppression of PMWS development.[264]

There are many in vitro studies on the immunomodulatory effects of PCV2 on lymphoid cells. It can suppress the release of some cytokines and stimulate the release of other proinflammatory cytokines.

The PCV2 genome as a whole was found to induce IFN-α in culture of monocytes and may help in immune-evasion mechanisms.[265]

Proinflammatory cytokines (IL-8, TNF-α, and IL-1β) and immune (IFN-γ, IL-10) cytokines were evaluated in PCV2-vaccinated and unvaccinated pigs exposed to natural PCV2 infection. PMWS-affected animals were not able to mount an efficient innate proinflammatory response to cope with PCV2 infection because there were low levels of Il-8, TNF-α, IL-1β, and IFN-γ. Conversely, there was a high expression of Il-8, TNF-α, and IL-1β in the vaccinated group. A significant increase of Il-10 occurred in the early phase of infection in the PMWS-infected animals, whereas vaccinated pigs had low viremia and absence of PMWS and had a more stable IFN-γ response.[266]

Studies in vitro have shown that in PBMCs and macrophages from PMWS pigs, there were reduced antiviral activities and an increase in proinflammatory cytokines (Il-1β and Il-8 expressions). Peripheral blood monocytes from PMWS-affected pigs are less able to produce Il2, IL-4, and IFN-γ upon challenge and are able to produce IL-10 after stimulation with recall viral antigens. Different components of PCV2 have been shown to play an important role in the modulation of the in vitro responses by PBMCs.[267] IFN-γ is up-regulated in the tonsils. PCV2-induced IL-10 may participate in down-regulation of specific responses through the inhibition of IFN-γ, IFN-α, and Il-12. PCV2 induced production of IL-10 (immunosuppressive), and when this was neutralized, a clear increase in IL-12 was noted.[268] These effects are independent of viral replication. The PCV2 capsid does not influence dendritic or monocytic responses, although the viral DNA does.[268]

These studies suggest that DNA sequences may be found in the genome that modify DC function. The immunosuppressive component is strongest in the whole genome or the circular replicative form. The full-length genome induced a clear suppression of IFN-α in responses in a dose-dependent manner.[269]

In addition, PCV2 is able to inhibit IL-2 through an Il-10-independent mechanism.[268]

Swine alveolar macrophages show reduced microbicidal activity, with a decrease in the production of O_2 free radicals and H_2O_2 and an increased production of TNF-α, Il-8, and other factors.[270]

In vitro data indicate that PMWS-affected animals also show elevated serum Il-10 levels; subclinically, PCV2-infected pigs develop transient IL-10 PCV2-specific responses during the viremic phase of the infection.[271]

In pigs suffering from PMWS, mRNA expression levels of Il-1α and IL-10 increase, whereas levels of Il-2, IL-8, TNF-α , and IFN-γ decrease.

Increased levels of IL-10 in the thymus were associated with the thymic depletion and atrophy that is observed in PMWS pigs. Il-10 was elevated from 10 to 14 days in experimentally infected pigs that subsequently developed PMWS.[272] Il-10, IL-12p40 in the spleen, IL-4 in the tonsils, and Il-10, Il-12p40 and IL-4 in the lymph nodes were detected in PMWS pigs.[271] Increased levels of Il-10 in PCV2-infected pigs are responsible for the depression of the Th1 responses in the peripheral blood monocytes of the infected pigs. PCV-2-induced IL-10 leads to impaired IFN and antigen-recalled responses to pseudorabies immunized animals.

The IL-10 elevated expression is common in PCV2 infections—in the thymus,[273] lymph nodes, spleen, and tonsil[273]—and is mainly located in T-cell areas. Il-10 was increased in PMWS-affected pigs[274] and was mainly associated with CD163+, CD4+, and CD8+ cell populations in the spleen. IL-1 is expressed at higher levels by bystander cells than by PCV2-infected cells, suggesting that Il-10 production is the result of paracrine action.[273,274] In a pig suffering from interstitial pneumonia, elevated Il-10 and Il-8 mRNA would be expected, and this is what was shown in a pig with PCV2-associated respiratory disease.[100]

A variety of substances that are proinflammatory cytokines are also up-regulated, including TNF-α, macrophage inflammatory protein, and C-reactive proteins.[272]

In pigs, the main acute-phase proteins (APPs) are CRP, SAA, Pig-MAP, haptoglobin, and AGP. In PMWS-affected pigs, the concentrations of Pig-MAP, C- reactive protein, and serum amyloid in infected animals were increased at 14 and 21 days postinfection.[275]

In a study of the spleen in PMWS-affected animals it was found the CD163+, CD4+, and CD8+ cell produced Il-10 in the spleen, and Il-10+ cell numbers were higher in PMWS animals compared with their levels in healthy counterparts. IL-10-producing cells were not infected by PCV2 and were mainly localized in the periarteriolar lymphoid sheaths.[274]

Interferons

The immune response produced by many PCV2 components varies with the cell type. Infection of natural IFN-producing cells may prevent the maturation of dendritic cells.[276]

An interferon-stimulated response element (ISRE) sequence was found in the in the PCV2 genome, which influences the interferon-mediated enhancement of PCV2 replication in vitro and may play a role in virus pathogenesis in pigs.[194,277]

In a study of cell-mediated immunity to PCV2 in CD/CD piglets, it was shown that viral clearance might be mediated by the development of PCV2 IFN-γ-secreting cells in contribution to the PCV2-specific neutralizing antibodies.[278]

IMMUNITY

In an infected but nonclinically diseased animal, PCV2 may exist with the host by undergoing minimal replication, inducing a limited but balanced Th1/Th2 response, and a trigger then sets disease in operation.

Clinical PMWS was preceded by low levels of serum antibodies and a high load of PCV2 but did not develop in all such animals.[279]

The interaction with the host immune system is the key to PCV2 infections and the development of PMWS. It was originally thought that it required cofactors to produce PMWS, but now it is known that it can produce PMWS on its own.

In affected piglets there is a lymphoid depletion, leucopenia, and destruction of lymphoid follicles. The absolute numbers of total T cells, Th cells, cytotoxic T cells, and γ/δ T cells—but not memory/activated T cells—decreased after PCV2 infection.[280] There is a reduction of numbers of interfollicular dendritic cells, interdigitating cells, B cells, natural killer (NK) cells, γ/δ T cells, CD4+, and CD8+ T-lymphocytes and reduced expression of high endothelial venules, together with an increase in monocytes and granulocytes. The amount of PCV2 antigen in tissues is directly related to the amount of depletion.[281] Coinfection with PRRSV increases the immune cell depletion.[282] CD4+ and CD8+ T cells are important in the response to PCV2 infection.[244]

PCV2 can persist in dendritic cells without affecting their performance, but in cells producing interferons, it reduces IFN-α and TNF-α production, thereby interfering with immune priming. In diseased pigs there is a state of activation with higher level and earlier expression of MHC-II on T and B cells and a higher level of CD25, IL2 receptor expression.[281] Both T and B cells are important targets for PCV2.[242,247]

IgM antibodies were first detected at week 8 PI and reached their highest at week 12. IgG antibody appeared at week 10, and levels were at their highest at week 16, with an average titer of 1:3500. Viral load peaked at week 10 (7×10^7 genomes copy/mL of sera) and persisted to adult age (10^5 genomes copy/mL of sera).[283]

PCV2 capsid specific antibodies appear within 10 to 28 days postinfection,[284] and their appearance coincides with a decrease in serum viral load[284]; however, in clinically diseased pigs the level of neutralizing antibody is greatly reduced.[284] It is not clear why some pigs can remove the infection, whereas others succumb to disease. Pigs infected with PCV2 appear to mount strong PCV2-specific antibody responses.

In the field, there is a decrease in maternal antibodies from 3 to 11 weeks, and then there is an active response around 15 weeks that persists for life. Experimental infections produce antibodies within 14 days PI and neutralizing Abs at about 21 days PI.

Antibodies particularly IgM Abs, may be lower in pigs with PMWS. The IgM is not neutralizing but indicates an infection.[284] Increased levels of IL-10 lead to a high ratio of IgG to IgM.[271]

There is a strong correlation between antibody titers and protection.[285,286]

High PCV2 antibody levels in sows at parturition did not prevent early PCV2 infection and viremia in piglets from the first day of life or peripartum maternal viremia and virus shedding into the lacteal secretions. Vertical transmission of PCV2 could generate PCV2 seropositivity in viable piglets even on farms with no signs of reproductive failure.[287]

Lack of antibody protection against PCV2 and PPV in naturally infected dams and their offspring has been shown.[288] After ingesting colostrum, piglets from vaccinated sows had significantly higher numbers of PCV2-specific gamma-interferon-producing cells, an increased PCV2-specific delayed-type hypersensitivity response, and a stronger proliferative response of peripheral blood mononuclear cells compared with piglets from nonvaccinated sows.[289] This is the first report of a transfer of a maternally derived adaptive cellular immune responses from vaccinated dams to their offspring.

The PCV2 Cap and Rep proteins are involved in the development of cell-mediated immunity upon PCV2 infection. In the course of subclinical infection, the development of and the strength of these responses may be related to the level of PCV2 replication.[290]

The T-helper type 2 response primarily stimulates B-cell proliferation and specific antibody formation. This humoral response is largely regulated by the secretion of IL-4, IL-5, IL-10, and IL-13 by T-helper type 2 cells. The interleukins were up-regulated differently in different lymph nodes and peripheral blood mononuclear cells.[291]

Pigs with high neutralizing antibody levels and high IFN-γ responses showed the lowest levels of viral replication, whereas pigs with weak or nil responses had the highest levels of replication. The levels of NA could be correlated with the clinical status of the pig and the viral load.[284]

NECROPSY FINDINGS

Not all pigs with PCV2 infection develop PMWS. PMWS incidence is highest where there is coinfection. Lymph nodes in affected pigs had the highest levels of viral load, but there was no significant difference between lesion severity and the viral load in these structures. There was no difference in the viral load in inguinal lymph nodes with or without PMWS, but in the former, the lesions were more severe.[292]

Gross Pathology

Fetal Pathology

PCV1 can, when used to experimentally, infect midgestational porcine fetuses, replicate, and produce pathology (severe hemorrhages in the lung) in the fetuses inoculated at 55 days of gestation.[293]

There are increased numbers of mummified and stillborn fetuses. The mummified can be as small as 6 to 7 cm.[154] Frequently, gross lesions are not seen at all. If lesions are seen, they are generally associated with myocardial failure.

Generally, in a fetus the lesions are found in the cardiovascular system, particularly the heart. Myocardiocytes may be degenerate, necrotic, or lost and replaced by fibrous connective tissue. There is often abundant PCV2 antigen in these lesions.

Dilated cardiomyopathy, pulmonary edema, hepatomegaly with congestion in an accentuated lobular pattern, hydrothorax, ascites, and subcutaneous edema are also seen.[154] Sometimes there is lymphadenopathy,[18] thymic atrophy, perirenal edema,[18,154] mesocolic edema,[154,294] and cerebral and splenic petechiation.[18,154]

Microscopically, there are often lesions in the myocardium in mummified, stillborn, and weak live-born piglets.[154] The myocardiocytes are often necrotic, degenerate, or lost, and are replaced by fibrous tissue and mineralization with inflammatory cells, including macrophages, plasma cells, and multinucleated giant cells. Occasionally, there are inclusion bodies.[54,294] Sometimes, lesions may include interstitial pneumonia, bronchopneumonia, and hepatic congestion with hepatocellular loss; nonsuppurative hepatitis with periacinar necrosis; and lymph node and splenic lymphocyte depletion with occasional multinucleated cells or lymph node follicular hyperplasia.

Myocarditis with high viral load of PCV2 in several tissues in cases of fetal death and high mortality in piglets has been described.[150] A high load of PCV2 DNA was observed in the myocardium, liver, and spleen from mummified or stillborn piglets.

Pathology in Piglets and Pigs

In some cases all lymph nodes are affected, but in others only a few; thus, a range of nodes is essential in any postmortem examination.

Necrotizing lymphadenitis associated with PCV2 infection has been characterized.[251] The pathogenesis of the lesion has been linked to apoptosis induced by PCV2. Lymphoid necrosis in PMWS-affected pigs may be related to hypertrophy and hyperplasia of high endothelial venules. Necrotizing lymphadenitis may develop following vascular damage, with thrombosis and subsequent follicular necrosis.

A reactive hyperplastic lymphadenopathy was shown in submaxillary lymph nodes with granulomatous lymphadenitis and necrotic foci.[295]

Based on the necropsy of three unthrifty pigs from all herds in a case-control study, approximately 78% had PMWS in the case herds and 26% in the control herd.[296]

Postmortem examination may reveal the following:

- Lesions in the liver, which are often yellowish-orange, indicating jaundice, with mild to moderate mottling; wasting is often seen.
- Noncollapsed lungs that are rubbery, with pronounced grayish nodules;

in some cases, there may be pulmonary edema, pleurisy, and pneumonia.

- Swollen, pale, homogeneous lymph nodes, particularly the inguinal, mesenteric, and tracheobronchial
- Thymic atrophy
- In the kidneys, there may be either no lesions or scattered white foci visible on the subcapsular surface and edema of the peripelvic connective tissue. Interstitial nephritis lesions were classified into three groups: lymphoplasmacytic, tubulointerstitial, or lymphohistiocytic to granulomatous and mixed patterns.[295]
- There may be limb edema and hemorrhagic joint fluid, and the spleen may be enlarged, meaty, and noncongested.
- The classical blue/purple skin lesions of PDNS may be a feature.
- There may be gastric ulcers and enteritis, with fluid-filled, thin-walled sections of the lower intestine, particularly the ileum and the spiral colon. with occasional edema of the cecal wall.

Mid- to late-term abortions may be seen, with affected fetuses showing necrotizing myocarditis and the presence of PCV2 antigen in cardiac tissues. Pathologic and virologic findings have been described in midgestational fetuses after experimental inoculation with PCV2a or PCV2b.[293] At 21 days PI 11/12, were edematous and had distended abdomens, and 1/12 looked normal. All PCV2-inoculated fetuses had internal hemorrhages and congestion and an enlarged liver. High PCV2 titers were found in all tissues, especially the heart, spleen, and liver. High numbers of infected cells were seen in the heart. The 2a and 2b types produced similar lesions and replicated to similar titers in the organs of 55-day-old immunoincompetent pig fetuses.

Acute enteritis may be seen in otherwise normal pigs. In the early cases, particularly in the United Kingdom and Spain, porcine dermatitis and nephropathy syndrome was a feature and closely resembled African or classical swine fever cases. It was not common but was associated with a high mortality. There were coalescing red to purple skin lesions, particularly over the perineal region; glomerular and interstitial nephritis; vasculitis; and deposition of immune complexes in the kidneys. In the cases with brain and cord lesions described,[297] there was hemorrhage on the cut surface, as multifocal to coalescent areas of hemorrhage extending from the cervical to the lumbar region. Brain lesions in pigs affected with PMWS have been described.[298] They included cerebellar multiple hemorrhages and edema, which were microscopically associated with mononuclear vasculitis in the molecular zone of the cerebellum; hypertrophied endothelium; and perivascular lymphohistiocytic infiltrate with deposits of fibrin.

An acute pulmonary edema was described in the Midwest of the United States. The pigs were found dead without previous signs and had clear fluid in the thoracic cavity and diffusely heavy and wet lungs with moderate to severe expansion of interlobular septae. Histopathology revealed the edema and also a diffuse interstitial pneumonia. There was often a fibrinoid necrosis of the blood vessel walls.[299]

Histopathology

PCV2 has been associated with primarily PMWS and PDNS, proliferative and necrotizing pneumonia, cerebellar vasculitis,[249] granulomatous enteritis, reproductive failure with abortion and premature farrowing, neonatal losses with tremor, and myocarditis.

The major histopathologic lesions in PCV2 diseases are lymphoid, with a depletion of T and B-lymphocytes. There should be PCV2 antigen in moderate to large amounts in the lymphoid tissues. This lymphocyte depletion is the result of a combination of factors, including destruction of lymphoid architecture, apoptosis, and cell lysis induced by PCV2 infection.[300] The main cellular changes are a decrease in follicular DCs, interdigitating cells, interfollicular lymphocytes, and B cells. Typical microscopic findings in lymph nodes include lymphocyte depletion, histiocytic infiltrations, and occurrence of multinucleated giant cells. There are losses of both B cells and T cells. There is a loss of lymph node architecture. These may be atrophic or necrotizing. Occasionally basophilic intracytoplasmic inclusions are found in the B-cell-dependent areas. Necrotizing lymphadenitis, interstitial nephritis, and interstitial pneumonia may also be found.

Lesions in the liver may include those such as infectious hepatitis and apoptosis.[248] There is often lymphohistiocytic infiltration of the portal areas, with occasional atrophy of the bile duct epithelium. Single-cell necrosis may be seen. In late stages there may be hepatocyte swelling and karyomegaly.

PCV2 inclusion bodies have been found in pulmonary (bronchial and bronchial glandular) and renal epithelial cells,[301] but pathologist experience suggests that these are now much less frequent than when the disease first occurred.

CNS lesions in PCV2 infections are rare but if found are usually in the brain and are usually found in the cerebellum.[249,302] In the Zlotowski cases, there was a moderate lymphohistiocytic vasculitis with thrombosis and marked mural fibrinoid degeneration with perivascular edema in meninges and parenchyma. Marked Wallerian degeneration and occasional Gitter cells were seen in the white matter of the cord. In animals experimentally inoculated with PCV2b, vasculitis was a hallmark of the lesions.[303] Two cases of nonsuppurative encephalitis were attributed to PCV2 infection by virtue of ISH when viral nucleic acid was found in the mesencephalon, cerebellum, and medulla oblongata, mainly in the cytoplasm of macrophages, endothelial cells, and some glial cells, and real-time PCR detected PCV2 in the brain samples from seven other pigs.[304] In natural cases of PCV2 infection there may be interstitial nephritis, tubulointerstitial nephritis, and granulomatous or lymphoplasmacytic nephritis. Lesions are often associated with PCV2 antigen. The renal lesions tend to occur later on in PCV2 infections. Renal tubular necrosis and interstitial hemorrhage ("turkey-egg kidney") have been seen in a PCV2-infected Yorkshire cross pig.[305] There was edema and petechiation of both kidneys, with renal tubular epithelial necrosis with extensive interstitial edema, and hemorrhage and inclusions in renal tubular epithelium. PCV2 was readily identified within these lesions. In the lungs, there may be interstitial pneumonia, lymphohistiocytic infiltration in the interstitium, granulomatous inflammation with syncytia, epithelial airway destruction, and bronchiolitis obliterans. There may be peribronchiolar fibrous hyperplasia, often with PCV2 antigen. Association of PCV2 with vascular lesions in porcine pneumonia has been seen in PCV2-infected lungs in Hungarian swine, particularly type 2b infections.[306] Vascular lesions are often reported in PCV2-affected pigs in the form of distension of interlobular septae with edema and fibrinoid necrosis. In the heart, the PCV2 antigen is associated with the myocyte swelling or necrosis.

Lesions in the sow's reproductive tract or the boar's reproductive tract are rarely reported.

Granulomatous enteritis may be seen with inclusion bodies in the Peyer's patches. There may be lymphohistiocytic infiltration of the gastric, cecal, and colonic mucosa. There may also be sloughing of crypt or glandular epithelium. There may be dilation of lymphatics. The pancreas may show areas of acinar epithelial atrophy and lymphoid aggregates in the interstitial regions.

The liver may show inflammatory and apoptotic changes with mononuclear cell infiltration in the parenchyma. Hepatitis may be seen. Singular 2a and 2b infection results in apoptosis of hepatocytes in clinically affected gnotobiotic pigs.[250] There were higher amounts of PCV2 antigen in clinically affected pigs.

Porcine Dermatitis and Nephropathy Syndrome

Porcine dermatitis and nephropathy syndrome (PDNS) is characterized by systemic vasculitis and glomerulonephritis affecting pigs of 20 to 65 kg. It is often solely associated with the occurrence of *Pasteurella* as a specific condition known in the United Kingdom as sporadic PDNS before the onset of the condition associated with PCV2. It has been seen in pigs, from 5-week-old nursery pigs to 9-month-old gilts. The affected animals are usually afebrile, anorectic, and depressed and show ventrocaudal subcutaneous edema. The course of the disease is rapid, and most pigs die within 3 days of the onset of clinical signs. This condition is now regarded as being part of the PCVAD complex.

Except in the condition of PDNS, PCV2 is rarely found in the skin of the pig, except in ear necrosis, as mentioned earlier.

Ultrastructural Changes

The ultrastructural changes in lymph nodes suffering from PMWS showed swelling of histiocytes, proliferation of mitochondria, and proliferation and swelling of endoplasmic reticulum and Golgi complex. Infected histiocytes contained large numbers of intracytoplasmic inclusions.[307] Lymphocyte depletion was a striking feature. Viral replication is probably a frequent event in macrophages.

CLINICAL SIGNS

PCV2 infection is widespread worldwide,[105] but clinical PCVAD is only seen in a minority of pigs. Subclinical infection is the normal occurrence in PCV2 infection, but it may be associated with decreased vaccine efficacy.[162] Clinical signs of PMWS were only visible in pigs 1 to 2 weeks before death, when they wasted rapidly. There were no other characteristic clinical signs and no obvious gross lesions at postmortem. PCV2 antigen level was higher from 4 to 6 weeks of age in pigs that died from other causes.[308] When it first occurred, it was seen a classical PMWS in weaners with a high mortality but now seems to be a more chronic disease associated with finishers with nonspecific signs (unthrifty, increase in mortality, decreased productivity, and increased disease from concurrent infections) in both the United States and Europe.

The first 41 cases in Denmark showed an average postweaning mortality of 11% in the nursery (7–30 kg), with comparable figures in other countries.

PCV2 is suspected to be associated with other diseases, such as PRDC, reproductive disorders, PDNS, and congenital tremor.

During their lives, most pigs will get PCV2, will seroconvert, and will never show any signs of the disease. It can also be recovered from healthy units that have never had any disease incidents.

PMWS most commonly affects pigs from 60 to 120 days of age at the end of the nursery phase or the beginning of the finishing phase.

The age at which the disease occurs is similar in Spain, but no pigs under 4 weeks have been affected, and the maximum age was 6 months.[309] A study of fattening pigs in the Netherlands with respiratory disease but no signs of PMWS looked at the contribution of PCV2. Eight herds had a high percentage of pneumonia at slaughter, and eight had a low percentage of pneumonia at slaughter. High PCV2 viral loads were found in 58% of the high group but only in 29% of the low group. High loads were found more frequently with other pathogens in the high group.[310] The study confirmed that PCV2 plays a role in pneumonia in pleurisy in pigs from 10 to 24 weeks in herds with PMWS and in herds with no clinical signs of PMWS.

The PCV2 genome plasticity is a major contributing factor to the PMWS disease manifestation.[68] Piglets of 5 to 12 weeks are most commonly affected, but occurrence of signs 5 to 16 weeks is not unknown. In the initial cases the condition affected the nursery pigs, but now more finishing pigs are reported with the signs. Pigs under 5 weeks are probably protected by maternal antibody, and the lowest levels of antibody are usually around 7 weeks under natural conditions. Infection levels peak at around the same age as the peak of PMWS outbreaks (12–13 weeks of age) and then decrease progressively following seroconversion.[118] The incubation period is thought to be 7 to 28 days.

The clinical signs are highly variable and are said to be multisystemic, which is their main characteristic. Some farms had high morbidity, mainly in weaners and others in the finishing pigs.[311] Mortality may be high.[67] Morbidity may be high or low, and only a small proportion may actually develop clinical signs (5% to 30%).[2]

There is a blurred border between PCV2 systemic disease and PRDC, and it is probable that PCV2 lung disease is a negligible condition and that PCV2 mainly contributes to PRDC in relation to PCV2 systemic disease occurrence.[312] There may be fever. Other signs may include weight loss; wasting is the extreme effect, but reduced weight gain is now typical. This is a frequent occurrence. In a case-control study in Denmark, affected weaners had a lower weight gain of 36 g/day and finishers of 52 g/day.[296] Feed utilization is also reduced, with an increased daily gain-to-feed value (396 g/kg of feed in vaccinated pigs) compared with 390 g/kg of feed in unvaccinated animals.[313] Respiratory dysfunction, including dyspnea, is also a frequent occurrence. Enlargement of superficial lymph nodes, particularly the superficial inguinal, which is not palpable in normal healthy animals, is a frequent occurrence. Antibiotic usage is increased with PMWS when comparing usage before an outbreak to that until a year after the outbreak.[314,315] Anemia or pallor is often present. Diarrhea is often present. Jaundice may occur but is not frequent. Generalized depletion of lymphocytes and secondary infections with opportunist and secondary infections are a feature. Necrotizing dermatitis and renal failure[316] may also occur.

Reproductive failure is a feature in breeding units.[317] The authors think there is a distinction between PCV2-associated reproductive failure and subclinical PCV2 in utero infection. For the diagnosis of PCV2-associated reproductive failure the following must be confirmed:

1. Clinical signs, which include early termination of pregnancy and increased numbers of mummified fetuses, stillborn, or weak-born pigs
2. Microscopic lesions within fetal tissues
3. PCV2 antigen or DNA within fetal tissues

Subclinical infection in utero is identified by the detection of PCV2 DNA or antibodies in fetal tissues, presuckle serum, or fetal thoracic fluid. Some piglets were found to be infected with both PCV2a and PCV2b.[135] A high level of reproductive losses was seen in a herd in Japan,[318] where there were 48.8% stillborn piglets and 14.5% preweaning mortality rate; the problem was rapidly solved after vaccination.

PCV2 infection in pregnant sows was reproduced using isolates from reproductive failure[319] and in naïve sows inseminated with semen contaminated with a PCV2b virus.[154] Any PCV2 isolate is capable of causing PCV2-associated reproductive failure. PPV has been recognized in fetal tissues,[294,320,321] as have PRRSV,[294] PCV1,[294] porcine TTV viruses,[322] and *E. coli*.[294]

Reproductive failure often occurs in gilts and start-up herds and is probably a reflection of seronegative populations.[150,323-325]

Homologous anti-PCV2 antibodies are at least partially protective for in utero PCV2 infection and the development of reproductive failure.[133,159] Abortion is not a major feature. The PCV2 virus is capable of infecting and damaging embryos in early pregnancy, leading to failure or reduction in litter size. In later gestation, damage to the fetus may result in stillbirth, mummification, embryonic death and infertility (SMEDI), mainly in primiparous sows,[326] and a potential return to estrus.[44] The most consistent feature of PCV2 infection in sows is stillbirth or mummified fetuses. Pyrexia and anorexia are often features of aborting sows. Delayed farrowing may also be seen. In a recent outbreak of PCV2-associated reproductive failure, gilt displayed pneumonia, diarrhea, and wasting.[324]

Paralysis in pigs with a spinal cord injury has been described[327] in Brazil.

Clinical signs are not usually seen in boars. In Poland, a reduction in ear necrosis was noted after a vaccination program for PCV2 was started.[328]

A clinical syndrome that affected healthy nursery and younger finisher pigs in the Midwest of the United States has been described in PCV2-vaccinated herds. Mortality reached 20% in some affected groups. Clinical signs included the rapid onset of respiratory distress followed almost immediately by death.[329]

One of the most important aspects of PCV2 infection is that vaccination using the Lapinized Philippines Coronel (LPC) vaccine was shown to have an effect in decreasing the efficacy of the vaccine. The level of neutralizing antibodies produced and the presence of lymphocyte subsets were reduced by the PCV2.[330]

CLINICAL PATHOLOGY

Acute-phase proteins are synthesized mainly by the liver and are used as biomarkers of diseases for diagnosis and prognosis.[331-333] They are under the control of cytokines that are released during the inflammatory process. IL-6 and IL-1 type cytokines that are produced mainly by macrophages and monocytes (IL-1α, IL-1β, IL-6, TNF-α, and IFN-γ) appear to be the major regulators.[334] It is controlled largely at the level of transcription. The regulators include NF-κB and the STAT proteins.

In the blood there is a reduction of both B cells and all T-cell subpopulations (naïve Th, activated Th, Tc, and gammadelta cells and also NK cells). In the 14 days postinfection with PCV2, there is a decrease of leukocytes, followed by an increase in neutrophils 7 to 14 days later. No changes in circulating monocytes, basophils, and eosinophils were detected.[335]

The major acute-phase protein (MAP) and haptoglobin serum concentrations correlate with PCV2 viremia and the clinical course of PMWS.[336] There was a significant correlation between PCV2 loads and both MAP and haptoglobin concentrations in serum of PMWS-affected pigs.

Diagnosis

Diagnosis of systemic PCVAD requires the presence of microscopic lesions and detection of PCV2 antigen or nucleic acids associated with the microscopic lesions. This is achieved using IHC or ISH. The ISH stain may be easier to read with more stained cells.[337]

Diagnosis of fetal infection on clinical signs is impossible to differentiate from other infections and effects of management changes. Sows with PCV2 infection frequently have no signs, are usually seropositive, and can be viremic or nonviremic.[157] Sampling of four to six fetuses per litter is recommended. Immunohistochemistry (IHC) and in-situ hybridization (ISH) are the gold standard for detection of antigen in the myocardium. DNA can be detected by PCR in the heart, liver, kidney, spleen, lymph node, and brain. Liver and myocardium have the highest amounts of DNA. Myocardium, liver, and splenic tissues were positive for PCV2 DNA in all live-born piglets.[279] The DNA extraction method has an important role in the usefulness of PCV2 quantification in swine lymph nodes,[338] and it casts doubt on comparable results unless the extraction methods are comparable. Laboratories in North America have been compared, and it has been shown that there are considerable differences in their detection limits and quantification.[339]

In utero infection can also be diagnosed by demonstrating ABs in fetal or live-born presuckle piglets using an ELISA.[135,340] Fluorescent antibody and IPMA have also been used.

Virus isolation is more difficult, but PCV2 can be isolated from most fetal tissues, particularly the myocardium.

Piglets from dams with low PCV2 antibody titers or with viremia had more morbidity and mortality associated with PMWS.[119] A protocol for the diagnosis of PMWS was developed in Italy.[341] Samples were examined histologically first and then by IHC for PCV2 when histologic lesions were first recognized. The lymphoid tissues were more reliable for diagnosis of PMWS than lungs.

Serology

An immunochromatographic strip for the detection of antibodies against PCV2 has been described,[342] and it agreed with the ELISA in 94% of cases.

Neither viral load nor antibodies can be used for diagnosing herds as PMWS-affected pigs or free herds (serology and qPCR are used[118,308,343]) because the diagnostic sensitivity and specificity are low.[118]

An indirect ELISA using a recombinant truncated capsid protein of PCV2 has been described as a serodiagnostic assay for detection of PCV2 antibodies.[344] Histopathology plus detection of PCV2 in tissues is necessary for diagnosis in the individual animal.

The pathogen is ubiquitous, which hinders the diagnosis because many pigs are infected without clinical signs or have subclinical infections. To make a diagnosis, the following must be present:

1. Recognizable clinical signs
2. Moderate to severe histopathologic lesions
3. Moderate amounts of PCV2 antigen in the lesions

During the PCVAD outbreak in Ontario from 2004 to 2006, the probability of a positive PCR for PRRSV decreased. It was concluded that when a decrease in test positivity occurred for a known disease, it may suggest that a new disease agent is emerging in the population.[345]

The diagnosis of PCV2 infection, mostly PMWS, is based on the clinical signs of the condition in individuals and groups of animals and by laboratory detection of PCV2.

In the individual animal, histopathologic examination together with viral detection in the lymphoid tissue is the definitive diagnosis.[118,346]

For herd diagnosis, there is a problem, because individuals may have the disease although the herd may have good production figures.[347] In some herds, 32% may not fulfill the diagnostic criteria,[348] or even 55%.[118] In these cases there must be (1) a significant increase in postweaning mortality and wasting and (2) the use of individual diagnoses in at least 1/5 of every group of animals subjected to postmortem examination

Diagnosis in Boars

PCV2 is found 5 days after experimental infection of boars. Shedding in semen has been reported in the absence of viremia. Antibodies develop within about 2 weeks of infection. Intermittent shedding was continued over an 8-week observation period,[157,349] with continuous shedding of the virus for 90 days.

Naturally infected boars shed for 27.3 weeks in a positive boar stud.[127] Peak shedding occurs at around 9 to 20 days.[157,349]

Experimentally infected boars can be viremic for at least 90 days, and blood swabs can be positive for DNA at least 47 days after cell-free viremia was last detected.[157]

The virus DNA can be detected in the bulbourethral glands, testes, epididymis, prostate, and seminal vesicles.[350-353] Detection of PCV2 DNA in boar semen is variable and depends on age.[127,153,354] Infectivity of PCV2 is possible, but because of the low amount semen in each dose after extension, the virus in each ampule is very low, so the risk of infection is low. PCV2 DNA can be detected using a quantitative real-time PCR.[355]

Postmortem examination of one and preferably up to five piglets is necessary to ascertain the spectrum of gross lesions.[2]

Virus Detection

Samples should be taken and examined histologically for the presence of characteristic PCV2 cytoplasmic inclusion bodies; second, IHC should be applied to confirm the PMWS cases with positive histochemistry. The lymph nodes were more reliable than the lungs for the diagnosis of PMWS, both in individual pigs and in groups of pigs.[356] PCV2-DNA was subsequently detected in the formalin-fixed lymph nodes by PCR.[357]

Detection of Viral Antigen by Immunohistochemistry

PCV2 antigen was identified by IHC in the tissues of 61% of Danish finishing pigs examined.[358] Up to 78% of the pigs had mild lymphoid depletion, indistinct follicle development, and/or histiocytic infiltration of the lymph nodes. But these lesions were not associated with PCV2. No association was found between lung and kidney lesions and the detection of PCV2. Three patterns of PCV2 labeling were seen:

1. Labeling of cells with stellate morphology and reticular distribution
2. Labeling of isolated nonepithelial cells
3. Epithelial labeling

PCV2 may interface with FDCs to cause depletion of B-lymphocytes. Follicular dendritic cells may be a reservoir of infective PCV2 in subclinically infected animals or be a simple storage site for PCV2 antigen.

In a study of reproductive failures in Danish pigs, it was found that IHC was only useful in the diagnosis of reproductive failure in the early stages of reproductive failure, whereas quantitative PCR can be used over a wider time span.[325]

It can also be detected in primary lymphoid organs from naturally and experimentally infected pigs by ISH.[359] PCV2 nucleic acids and replication were found in bone marrow and thymus of PMWS-affected pigs, but there was no evidence that primary lymphoid organs were major supporters of PCV2 replication.

Multiplex PCR and multiplex RT-PCR for inclusive detection of major swine DNA and RNA viruses in pigs with multiple infections[360] were described as a useful combination for the rapid and accurate identification of major pathogenic viruses with multiple infections.

An indirect in situ PCR for the detection of PCV2 in formalin-fixed and paraffin-embedded tissue specimens has been described[361] and was shown to be a useful technique.

A quantitative PCR for PCV2 in swine feces in a PCV2-affected commercial herd and a nonaffected commercial herd proved useful for the detection of virus shedding.[362]

Quantification of PCV2 was described.[131] Detection of viral genome by ISH and/or PCR is necessary for diagnosis. There is considerable variance between labs in the qPCR test.[363,364]

A DNA miniarray was devised for the simultaneous detection of PCV1 and PCV2,[365] and a multiplex real-time PCR has also been used to differentiate PCV1 and PCV2.[366]

Many types of real-time in vitro amplification techniques[367] and real-time PCR assays using SYBR Green,[131] TaqMan PCR,[242] and molecular beacon technology[368] have been developed.

A simultaneous detection of PCV2, CSF, PPV, and PRRSV by using multiplex PCR was described.[369] It was found to be a rapid, sensitive, and cost-effective diagnostic tool for the routine surveillance of viral disease in pigs. Also, oligo-microarray has been used.[370]

Multiply primed rolling-circle amplification (MPRCA) of PCV2 genomes has applications for detection, sequencing, and virus isolation.[371] It was concluded that this is a useful tool to amplify PCV2 genomes for sequencing and virus isolation. However, it is less sensitive than PCR for diagnostic purposes.

A LUX real-time PCR assay has been described,[372] which was more specific for the generation of fluorogenic signals than the SYBR Green PCR.

Oral Fluids

Surveillance methods used in oral fluids have been described.[373,374] PCR methods have been described for use in porcine fluid oral samples.[375] Antibody methods have been described for oral fluid samples.[376]

CONTROL

Management may influence the appearance of the condition, and the application of the Madec principles[377] will undoubtedly ameliorate the condition. The Madec 20-point plan is in fact no more than the rules of good husbandry and pig practice crystallized to make control easier. Most people follow some of the points, but not the majority or all of the points. However, the more that are implemented, the better the control. Essentially, the 20-point plan recommends the following:

1. Improvements in hygiene
2. Minimization of the mixing of pigs
3. Provision of clean feed, water, and air
4. Minimization of the stress on pigs through overstocking, draughts, poor husbandry conditions, and so forth[103,188,378]

All-in, all-out by age is particularly significant in control of the infection.

Vaccinating pigs against *Mycoplasma* 2 weeks before suspected exposure to PCV2 will also help.[379]

Serum from pigs recovered from PMWS by injection could prevent PMWS in some cases, but in other cases it did not work.[380] It is not to be recommended for health transmission reasons and is no longer necessary now that there is vaccination.

The absence of an external envelope leaves the virus resistant to lipid-dissolving disinfectants, but it can be inactivated by alkaline disinfectants (sodium hydroxide), oxidizing agents (sodium hypochlorite), and quaternary ammonium compounds.[381] Results of a study[120] showed that Virkon S, Clorox bleach, and sodium hydroxide were the most effective agents for disinfection. Disinfection of an airspace could be achieved using formaldehyde vapor, assuming optimal temperature and humidity.

Infected boar semen is a possible source of infection, so AI centers should use boars that are free from infections.[382]

Attention to good nutrition will help, and there is some evidence that a selenomethionine supplement may help by reducing PCV2 replication in PK-15 cells (probably by enhancing glutathione peroxidase).[383]

Dietary aluminium silicate given to experimentally infected pigs produced a significant decrease in the load of viral genome in nasal swabs, serum, and lung tissue of pigs compared with a control group 28 days after PCV2 infection. Pigs in the treated group also had less severe histopathologic lesions.[384]

In theory, plasma-containing products may contain PCV2, but in a recent study, piglets fed spray dried plasma containing PCV2 DNA did not become infected.[163]

A modeling approach was used to estimate the effects of husbandry and control measures on the dynamics of PCV2 infection,[385] and it was found that early infection was significantly reduced when mixing of piglets was reduced by avoiding cross-fostering and mixing of groups. Sow targeted vaccination reduced the infectious process until waning of passive immunity. Piglet vaccination considerably decreased the force of infection. Changing from a low prevalence of PCV2-infected semen to a high one significantly increased the risk of early infections. Reducing replacement rate or changing sow housing from individual crates to sow group housing had little effect.

Increased morbidity occurred for an extended period before the diagnosis of PMWS both in the sow units and the weaner pig units, and there was an increased use of antibiotics in the third (35%) and fourth quarters (43%) before diagnosis was made.[314]

After a herd had an outbreak of PMWS (PCV2) in Danish herds, the use of antibiotics in the weaners was increased for about 1 year, and the use of antibiotics before the outbreak was 37% higher in herds with weaners and 17% higher in herds with finishers in the year compared with herds that did not have PMWS.[315] In the 4-year period when the incidence of PMWS rose from almost zero to 20%, the national use of antibiotics increased by 4% to 5%.

Vaccination

The relationship between antibody titers and protection is unknown, but PMWS-affected pigs do show an impaired PCV2 humoral response.

The vaccines were developed to control PMWS but are now used for all PCVAD. The vaccines have been successful in reducing mortality in Europe, Canada, and the United States.[6] The vaccines probably work by activating both humoral and cellular immunity.[386,387] Vaccination of sows does not prevent PCV2 infections but reduces the viremia.[287,388] The antibody titers do not appear to influence the occurrence of disease because gilts and sows with high antibody titers against PCV2 and PPV presented viremia, and fetal exposure during gestation occurred in these animals.

It has been shown that IFN-γ-secreting cells develop during the adaptive response to PCV2 and probably contribute to viral clearance in infected pigs,[389] and CD4+ and CD8+ cells contribute to this response.[244]

The efficacy of the five commercial PCV2 vaccines has been described experimentally,[135,389-394] and studies have been made in the field.[395-404]

The Vaccines

The Vaccines Use Different Adjuvants.

Circovac (Merial) is an inactivated oil-adjuvanted vaccine originally designed for sows (2 ml) and now available in a reduced dosage for piglets (0.5 ml).[404]

Four additional vaccines were licensed for use in piglets; three are based on ORF2 capsid protein (main neutralizing epitope) expressed in the baculovirus system: Circoflex (Boehringer Ingelheim), Circumvent Intrvet (Merck; North America), and Porcilis PCV (Schering Plough/Merck; Europe).

Suvaxyn PCV2 One Dose (Pfizer Animal Health/Fort Dodge Animal Health) is another vaccine but is based on a chimeric PCV1/2 virus using the genome of PCV1 with the ORF2 from PCV2. This was replaced using a natural PCV1/PCV2 chimera from Canada,[405] and this was relaunched as Fostera PCV (Pfizer Animal Health).

All the commercial vaccines are based on PCV2a, which does protect against the more common strain of PCV2b,[390,393] which appears to be essential for triggering PCV2 into PVCAD (16/17).[15,406,407] The four commercial vaccines are all killed or recombinant vaccines based on PCV2a,[387,389,399] even though PCV2b has now become the globally dominant genotype. These vaccines still continue to provide good protection even though PCV2a and PCV2b differ in nucleotides by up to10%.[54,389] An experimental 2b vaccine has also been shown to provide protection from both 2a and 2b.[389]

Vaccine Effects

In a study of four vaccines, it has been shown that the average daily gain of vaccinated animals was much higher than that of nonvaccinated animals. There were more IFN-γ-secreting cells and CD4+ cells in the vaccinated animals. The histologic lesions and the PCV2-antigen scores in the lymph nodes were significantly lower in vaccinated animals.[408]

As always with pig farmers, one-dose vaccines are preferred to two-dose vaccines. One-dose vaccines improve daily gain in the field by 16 to 69 g/day from 3 to 19 weeks and decrease mortality by 1.9% to 9.3%. PCV2 vaccines reduce the proportion of viremic pigs and the viral load in blood and reduce the length of the viremic period in both experimental and field situations. They also reduce nasal and fecal shedding of the virus. The presence of NA is induced by commercial PCV2 vaccines, and there is a decreased replication of virus correlated with the absence of clinical signs. The induced presence of IFN-γ-secreting cells in vaccinated animals is also likely to increase PCV2 clearance. Vaccination of pigs reduces the number of PMWS-associated microscopic lesions and the PCV2 load in lymphoid tissues compared with nonvaccinated animals. The vaccines will control PMWS under field conditions, but their role in protecting against the PCV2 component of PRDC is still unknown.

When the killed vaccines were originally introduced in the United Kingdom, it was noted that it had the following results:

- An improved growth rate (7–10 days faster to slaughter)
- A 1% to 5% reduction in nursery mortality
- A 1% to 6% reduction in finisher mortality
- An improvement in numbers weaned/litter by up to 0.5 piglets (sow vaccine), with improvements in fertility and litter size
- More even growth within a litter
- Improvement in fat measurements, probably as a result of more rapid growth

Most pigs in commercial production are now vaccinated against PCV2 infections. The introduction of the sow vaccine was beneficial for the following reasons:

- Lower cost
- Lower workload and reduced stress on piglets
- Prevention of *in utero* infection and early fetal death
- Control of reproductive losses.

On some farms where disease occurs over 10 weeks, the sow vaccination may not help in prevention, probably because maternal derived antibody has disappeared.

In the United Kingdom the initial use of the piglet vaccines was associated with a reduction in mortality of up to 50% and an improvement in growth rate of 50 gm/day, with most of the increase occurring in the finishing stage.

PCV2 infection may be a factor contributing to weight variation in vaccinated, market pigs.[409] The mean antibody titer, proportion of viremic pigs, and virus load differed between the light and heavy pigs on three different farms.

Mortality rate reduction with the PCV2 vaccination might depend on the genetic types of PCV2 that occur on the farm.[410]

With a vaccination program in operation, there is a large decrease in mortality, a reduced viremia, reduced back-fat depth, reduced number of culls, a reduced time to market, and reduced medication costs when vaccinated pigs are compared with unvaccinated pigs.[411-418]

PCV2-vaccinated pigs also have a better daily gain, a higher percentage of lean meat, a better feed conversion, a higher number of pigs reaching slaughter, and a higher carcass weight.[400,412-416,418,419]

An early antibody boost was sufficient to protect pigs from contracting PVCAD before the fattening period and also enhanced pigs' growth[401] and performance in the fattening period, although new infections were detected as early as 56 days after birth (on the basis of PCVC2-specific IgM measurements).

It was shown that sow vaccination, piglet vaccination, or vaccination of sow and piglet produced similar control of PMWS.[400] However, decreased mortality in piglets before weaning was only observed in the piglets from vaccinated sows.

Sow Compared with Piglet Vaccination

Under field conditions, piglets born to sows that are vaccinated have a preweaning weight gain. Experimentally vaccinated 8-week-old piglets have lower PCV2 loads than those receiving passive protection from MDA.[393,400] The duration of protection may be 11 to 13 weeks.[135,396] Sow vaccination is to be used if there is a high level of infection before weaning, but piglet protection is best to ensure that there is active immunization.

A comparison was made of the effectiveness of dam (passive) versus piglet (active). Immunization and the impact of passively derived PCV2 vaccination induced immunity on vaccination.[393] Both dam and piglet vaccines had similar efficacy in reducing PCV2 viral loads and antigen levels in the growing pigs. Vaccination of the piglets with the same vaccine as used on their dams did not appear to affect the vaccine efficacy because they had the same levels of AB and genome copies of PCV2 as those receiving the piglet vaccine alone.

Sow Vaccination

Vaccination of sows appeared to improve reproduction in sows and provided protection for the piglets.[422]

Vaccination of sows before mating is designed to protect sows against PCV2 reproductive disease[423] and also leads to stabilization and homogenization of the PCV2 immune status of the sow population during gestation.[424-427] The effect of vaccinating sows before farrowing is to increase the transfer of PCV2 antibodies to piglets and to protect piglets against systemic disease.[399,425,426]

Vaccination of sows reduces the prevalence of PCV2 viremia in their piglets in the field.[426] Vaccinated sows had less PCV2 in the colostrum than nonvaccinated sows.[424] Vaccinated sows had more PCV2 antibody in their serum and colostrum than unvaccinated sows.[428] A study compared sow vaccination, piglet vaccination, and sow + piglet vaccination[429] and found similar efficacy. Sow vaccination and piglet vaccination were found to be similar in another study.[393]

Vaccination of sows during pregnancy reduces the viral load in the blood and the rate of transplacental infection,[133] but it does not eliminate intrauterine infection completely. It also reduced the numbers of nonviable fetuses.[133,154] It may therefore reduce reproductive failure.[340]

Colostrum from vaccinated sows may also contain PCV2-specific IFN-γ-secreting cells.[430]

Semen Shedding in Boars

Boars can shed PCV2 for a long time without showing clinical signs or changes in semen quality,[127,157] and thus AI may be a possible source of virus.[152]

Vaccination of boars with an inactivated PCV2 vaccine was followed by challenge with a PCV2b virus.[431] The number of PCV2b genomes in the semen correlated with that in the blood in both vaccinated challenged and nonvaccinated challenged boars. The PCV2b vaccine significantly decreased the amount of PCV2b DNA shedding in semen from vaccinated boars after experimental infection with PCV2b, and also the duration.[432]

Piglet Vaccination

Piglet vaccination of 5-day-old or 21-day-old piglets using either a chimeric or subunit PCV2 vaccine produced a detectable humoral immune response and provided reduction or complete protection against PCV2 viremia and PCV2-associated lesions after triple challenge with PCV2, PPV, and PRRSV.[434]

A single dose of vaccine to sows produced a higher level of antibody in piglets at 4 weeks and a different level of PCV2 infection dynamics than in nonvaccinated piglets. Piglet vaccination in any case caused an earlier seroconversion and lower percentages of PCV2-infected piglets. There was some interference with piglet vaccination, but this was overcome by the vaccination because the average daily gain was improved in both groups of vaccinated piglets.[435]

Unusual manifestations of PCVAD in vaccinated finishing pigs have been described.[420] Vaccinated pigs also have a much lower prevalence of PRRSV and *M. hyorhinis* in lung tissues than do unvaccinated pigs.[398] There was a larger average daily gain in herds free from PRRSV infection.[421]

In a study of a one-shot, inactivated PCV2 vaccine, it was found that it reduced clinical signs, PCV2 viral load in sera and feces, and overall mortality in nurseries and fattening units.[404] Average daily gain was increased, but maternally derived antibody (MDA) did interfere with the development of an active humoral response.

Maternally Derived Antibodies

Maternally derived antibodies are found in nearly all piglets because most sows are infected with PCV2 and are therefore producing colostral antibodies. The vaccine efficiency is determined by the level of colostral antibody at the time of vaccination. It appears that the vaccines are not affected in the field because PCV2 associated lesions and viral load are not inhibited.[390,391] The vaccines produce specific antibodies and IFN-γ-secreting cells even in the presence of MDA.[389,390,433]

There may or may not be an effect of maternal antibody on piglet vaccination. It was shown that there was an effect of maternal antibody,[390,396] but it has also been said there is no such effect.[395] Vaccination at 3 weeks seems to be a good compromise between wanting to vaccinate and waiting for maternal antibody to wane. It produces neutralizing antibodies and prevents PCV2 infection during weaning.[390] A comparison of one-shot and two-shot vaccinations has been described.[392] PCV2 vaccination reduced PCV2 in a PCV2/*S. choleraesuis* (SCS) coinfection model and in animals with SCS challenge.[436] Piglets were given the vaccine at 3 weeks of age followed by PCV2 and SCS at 5 and 7 weeks of age.

Experimental Vaccines

RNA aptamers, which are RNA molecules that bind specifically to a target, have been shown to block the infectivity of PCV2 in vitro in a dose-dependent manner.[437] Short-hairpin RNA has also been shown to result in a reduced PCV2 level in vitro.[438]

A PCV2 vaccine based on genotype PCV2b is more effective than a 2a-based vaccine to protect against PCV2b or a combined 2a/2b viremia in pigs with concurrent PCV2, PRRSV, and PPV infection.[439] The piglets had significantly higher levels of PCV1-2b viremia and shedding but also a much more robust humoral immune response. The PCV1-2b vaccine reduced the amount of viremia compared with the PCV1-2a vaccine. Concurrent PCV2a/PCV2b infection is necessary for optimal PCV2 replication.

A genetically engineered chimeric vaccine against PCV2 improves clinical, pathologic, and virological outcomes in PMWS affected farms.[399] The vaccine reduced clinical signs, viral load in lymphoid organs and/or sera, and overall mortality in nurseries and finishing units. This is the first time that a vaccine has been shown to reduce PMWS mortality. The vaccine also reduced the severity of histologic lesions in the PMWS cases.

The live chimeric PCV12a vaccine is attenuated, immunogenic, and genetically stable, providing similar protection as the commercial inactivated and subunit vaccines.[440,441] It is not uncommon to vaccinate piglets with PRRSV and PCV2 concurrently.[442,443] The chimeric PCV12b live vaccines have the advantage in that they are not likely to revert.

A potential PCV12b vaccine was shown to be effective in preventing infection with 2a and 2b,[444] with decreased lymphoid lesions and viral load. One-dose and two-dose commercial PCV2 vaccines were evaluated in a PRRSV–PCV2–SIV model.[392]

Viremia was reduced by 78.5% in pigs vaccinated by one dose and by 97.1% in pigs vaccinated with two doses. Overall, the microscopic lesions were reduced by 78.7% and 81.8%, respectively.

A triple-coinfection model was used to show that the chimeric PCV12b vaccine was efficacious.[441,445] Vaccines, both commercial and experimental PCV2, used a triple challenge with PCV2, PRRSV, and PPV, and it was found that both vaccines reduced the PCV viremia at 16 weeks of age and after PCV2 challenge,[441] even though there was PCV2 viremia at the time of vaccination.

PCV2 vaccination usually reduces the prevalence and severity of clinical disease.[445,446] A longitudinal study on the efficacy of Ingelvac CircoFLEX against PRDC showed that there was a significant improvement in the economics of late-occurring PRDC.[447]

A single-dose schedule for *M. hyopneumoniae* bacterin at 1 week of age and PCV2 vaccine at 3 weeks of age improved ADG (122.4%) and slaughter weight (120.5%) and reduced the incidence of clinical signs and lung and lymph node lesions.[72] Mineral oil–adjuvanted bacterins carry with them heightened potential for induction of PMWS, whereas the other adjuvanted bacterins tested have minimal or no potentiating effects on PMWS.[220]

In a study of PCV2 and PRRSV vaccination in a PCV2–PRRSV challenge model,[448] it was found that vaccination against PCV2 reduced PCV2 viremia, PCV2-induced lesions, and PCV2 antigens in the dually infected pigs. Therefore, the PCV2 vaccination reduced the potentiation of PCV2-induced by PRRSV in dually infected pigs. In contrast, the PRRS vaccine did not decrease the potentiation of PCV2-induced lesions by PRRSV in dually infected pigs.

Some evidence of priming of young piglets in the presence of maternal antibodies was shown[449] using a prototype adjuvanted PCV2 vaccine.

Vaccination against PCV2 can reduce antibody titers when given postinfection and has no dramatic effects on semen characteristics.[432] There was also evidence that vaccination reduced the reoccurring infections in the vaccinated boars.

A comparison of the effectiveness of dam (passive) or piglet (active) immunization was carried out, and both had similar efficacies.[393]

In this study,[450] the PCV2 vaccine response was evaluated in a PCVAD challenge model. Dual challenge with PCV2 and PRRSV resulted in high mortality and the presence of clinical signs. PRRSV increased PCV2 infection. The results of IFA tests showed that PCV2 infection and vaccination resulted in similar levels of total serum antibody. Vaccination produced nearly 4 times as much virus neutralizing activity as infection and disease. The magnitude of the total antibody response cannot be used as the measure of protective immunity.

Only occasionally has vaccine failure been reported, possibly as a result of off-label uses. In some herds vaccinated against PCV2, acute pulmonary edema with a peracute onset has been reported.[451]

In one study of an apparent vaccine failure, it was found that only 50% of the pigs developed a detectable immune response to vaccination, and this may have been associated with simultaneous 2a and 2b infection.

It may be necessary to produce vaccines based on 2b rather than 2a now that this is much more common, because the efficacy of currently available PCV2 vaccines depends on the genotypes of PCV2 on the farm.[410]

Some experimental vaccines have been suggested, including an ORF2 baculovirus vaccine,[452] an ORF2 DNA vaccine, a recombinant pseudorabies vaccine expressing ORF1, an ORF2 fusion protein,[453] and a recombinant adenovirus vaccine expressing the ORF2 protein,[454] and these have been shown to provide protection under experimental conditions.

Vaccination with inactivated or live-attenuated chimeric PCV1-2 results in decreased viremia in challenge-exposed pigs and may reduce transmission of PCV2.[455] Both of these vaccines did not reach the higher level of antibody of the commercial inactivated vaccine. The results suggested that 140-day closure of a small pig population in a controlled environment may result in stabilization and elimination of PCV2.

A similar study using a reformulated inactivated chimeric PCV12 vaccine induced humoral and cellular immunity after experimental PCV2 challenge.[456]

The induction of mucosal immunity by intranasal immunization with recombinant adenovirus expressing major epitopes of PCV2-capsid protein has been described.[457] It can elicit both humoral and Th1-type cellular protective immunity in mice. A *B. bronchiseptica* mutant has been used as a live vehicle for heterologous PCV2 major capsid protein expression.[458]

Small interfering RNAs have also been suggested as a potential treatment for PCV infection because *Rep* gene expression was inhibited.[459]

Vectored Vaccines

The preparation of bacteriophage lambda particles displaying PCV2 capsid epitopes, in the absence of an adjutant, induced PCV2-neutralizing ABs and elicited both cellular and humoral immune responses in pigs, with no reactions.[460]

Subunit vaccines may also play a part in the future, such as capsid protein in yeast,[461] recombinant baculovirus,[462] recombinant pseudorabies expressing PCV2 capsid protein,[454] and an attenuated *Bordetella* vaccine expressing the capsid of PCV2,[459] which have all been shown to be immunogenic.

FURTHER READING

Baekbo P, et al. Porcine circovirus diseases; a review of PMWS. *Transbound Emerg Dis.* 2012;59(suppl 1):60-67.

Beach NM, et al. Efficacy and future prospects of commercially available and experimental vaccines against porcine circovirus type 2 (PCV2). *Virus Res.* 2012;164:33-42.

Chae C. Commercial porcine circovirus type 2 vaccines: efficacy and clinical application. *Vet J.* 2012;194:151-157.

Cheung AK. Porcine circovirus: transcription and DNA replication. *Virus Res.* 2012;154:46-53.

Darwich L, Mateu E. Immunology of porcine circovirus type 2. *Virus Res.* 2012;164:61-67.

Finsterbusch T, Mankertz A. Porcine circoviruses—small but powerful. *Virus Res.* 2009;143:177-183.

Grau-Roma L, et al. Recent advances in the epidemiology, diagnosis and control of diseases caused by porcine circovirus type 2. *Vet J.* 2011;187:23-32.

Kekarainen T, et al. Immune responses and vaccination induced immunity against Porcine circovirus type. 2. *Vet Immunol Immunopathol.* 2010;136:185-193.

Madec F, et al. Post-weaning multisystemic wasting syndrome and other PCV2-related problems in pigs: a 12-year experience. *Transbound Emerg Dis.* 2008;273-283.

Madec F, et al. PMWS in pigs in France. Clinical observations from follow up studies on affected farms. *Livestock Prod Sci.* 2000;63:223-233.

Madson DM, Opriessnig T. Effect of porcine circovirus type 2 (PCV2) infection on reproduction: disease, vertical transmission, diagnostics and vaccination. *Anim Health Res Rev.* 2011;12:47-65.

Mankertz A. Molecular interactions of porcine circoviruses type 1 and type 2 with its host. *Virus Res.* 2012;164:54-60.

Meng XJ. Emerging and re-emerging swine viruses. *Transbound Emerg Dis.* 2012;59(suppl 1):85-102.

Nauwynck HJ, et al. Cell tropism and entry of porcine circovirus 2. *Virus Res.* 2012;164:43-45.

Opriessnig T, Halbur PG. Concurrent infections are important for expression of porcine circovirus associated disease. *Virus Res.* 2012;164:20-32.

Opriessnig T, Langohr I. Current state of knowledge on porcine circovirus type 2-associated lesions. *Vet Pathol.* 2013;50:23.

Rose N, et al. Epidemiology and transmission of PCV2. *Virus Res.* 2012;164:78-89.

Segales J. Porcine circovirus type 2 (PCV2) infections: clinical signs, pathology and laboratory diagnosis. *Virus Res.* 2012;164:10.

Trible BR, Rowland RR. Genetic variation of PCV2 and its revelance to vaccination, pathogenesis and diagnosis. *Virus Res.* 2012;164:68.

REFERENCES

1. Baekbo P, et al. *Transbound Emerg Dis.* 2012;59(suppl 1):60.
2. Grau-Roma L, et al. *Vet J.* 2011;187:23.
3. Darwich L, Mateu E. *Virus Res.* 2012;154:61.
4. Firth C, et al. *J Virol.* 2009;83:12813.
5. Duffy S, et al. *Nat Rev Genet.* 2008;9:267.
6. Opriessnig T, et al. *J Vet Diag Invest.* 2007;19:591.
7. Finsterbusch T, Mankertz A. *Virus Res.* 2009;141:177.
8. Krakowka S, et al. *Virus Res.* 2012;164:90.
9. Tomas A, et al. *Vet Microbiol.* 2008;132:260.
10. Wen L, et al. *PLoS ONE.* 2012;7:e41565.
11. Wen L, et al. *J Virol.* 2012;86:639.
12. Lohse L, et al. *Vet Microbiol.* 2008;129:97.
13. Opriessnig T, et al. *J Gen Virol.* 2006;87:2923.
14. Gauger PC, et al. *Vet Microbiol.* 2011;153:229.
15. Cheung AK, et al. *Virology.* 2007;363:229.
16. Olvera A, et al. *Virology.* 2007;357:175.
17. Dupont K, et al. *Vet Microbiol.* 2008;139:219.
18. Lefebvre DJ, et al. *J Gen Virol.* 2008;89:177.
19. Shang SB, et al. *Mol Immunol.* 2009;46:327.
20. Cai LB, et al. *Virus Res.* 2011;158:251.
21. Hesse RB, et al. *Virus Res.* 2008;132:201.
22. Lefebvre DJB, et al. *J Gen Virol.* 2009;89:177.
23. Ma C-M, et al. *J Gen Virol.* 2007;88:1733.
24. Cheung AK. *J Virol.* 2006;80:8686.
25. Cheung AK, et al. *Virology.* 2007;152:1035.
26. Steinfeldt T, et al. *J Virol.* 2006;80:6225.
27. Khayat R, et al. *J Virol.* 2011;85:7856.
28. Misinzo G, et al. *J Virol.* 2006;80:3487.
29. Timmusk S, et al. *Virus Genes.* 2008;36:509.
30. Karuppanan AK, et al. *Virology.* 2010;398:1.
31. Chaiyakul M, et al. *J Virol.* 2010;84:1144.
32. Karuppanan AK, et al. *Virology.* 2009;383:338.
33. Juhan NM, et al. *Virus Res.* 2010;147:60.
34. He J, et al. *J Virol.* 2013;87:1420.
35. Carman S, et al. *Can J Vet Res.* 2008;72:259.
36. Grau-Roma L, et al. *Vet Microbiol.* 2008;128:23.
37. Martins Gomez de Castro AM, et al. *Arch Virol.* 2007;152:1435.
38. Guo LJ, et al. *Virology J.* 2010;7:273.
39. Wang F, et al. *Virus Res.* 2009;145:151.
40. Janafong T, et al. *Virol J.* 2011;8:88.
41. Cortey M, et al. *Vet Microbiol.* 2011;149:522.
42. Xiao C-T, et al. *J Virol.* 2012;86:12469.
43. Gagnon CA, et al. *Vet Microbiol.* 2010;144:18.
44. Mateusen B, et al. *Theriogenology.* 2007;68:896.
45. Saha D, et al. *Vet Microbiol.* 2010;145:62.
46. Lefebvre DJ, et al. *Vet Microbiol.* 2008;25:74.
47. Steiner E, et al. *Virology.* 2008;378:311.
48. Misinzo G, et al. *J Virol.* 2008;82:1128.
49. Misinzo G, et al. *Virus Res.* 2009;139:1.
50. Vega-Rocha S, et al. *J Mol Biol.* 2007;9:9.
51. Steinfeldt T, et al. *J Virol.* 2007;81:5696.
52. Wei L, Liu J. *Virology.* 2009;386:203.
53. Finsterbusch T, et al. *Virology.* 2009;386:122.
54. Beach NM, et al. *J Virol.* 2010;84:8986.
55. Chen X, et al. *Virology.* 2012;426:66.
56. Yu S, et al. *Vet Immunol Immunopathol.* 2009;127:350.
57. Lin C-M, et al. *Vet Immunol Immunopathol.* 2012;145:368.
58. Sinha A, et al. *Vet Microbiol.* 2012;158:95.
59. Gu J, et al. *Virology J.* 2012;9:152.
60. Zhu B, et al. *Virus Res.* 2012;163:476.
61. Zhu B, et al. *J Virol.* 2012;86:12003.
62. Rodriguez-Carino C, et al. *J Comp Path.* 2011;144:91.
63. Carman S, et al. *Can Vet J.* 2006;47:761.
64. Gagnon CA, et al. *Can Vet J.* 2007;48:811.
65. Segales J, et al. *Vet Rec.* 2008;162:867.
66. Dupont K, et al. *Vet Microbiol.* 2008;128:56.
67. Cheung AK, et al. *Arch Virol.* 2007;152:1035.
68. Wiederkehr DD, et al. *Vet Microbiol.* 2009;136:27.
69. Ellis JA, et al. *Proc 19th IPVS Copenhagen.* Denmark: 2006:23-34.
70. Cortey M, et al. *Vet J.* 2011;187:363.
71. Kim HK, et al. *Vet J.* 2011;118:115.
72. Kim HK, et al. *Vaccine.* 2011;29:3206.
73. Wieland B, et al. *Vet Rec.* 2012;170:596.
74. Allan G, et al. *J Vet Diag Invest.* 2007;19:668.
75. Chiarelli-Neto O, et al. *Virus Res.* 2009;140:57.
76. Takahagi Y, et al. *J Vet Med Sci.* 2008;70:603.
77. Segales S, Cortey M. *Vet Rec.* 2010;67:940.
78. Ma C-M, et al. *J Gen Virol.* 2007;88:1733.
79. Cheung AK. *Arch Virol.* 2009;154:531.
80. Hesse R, et al. *Virus Res.* 2008;132:201.
81. Lefebvre DJ, et al. *J Gen Virol.* 2009;89:177.
82. Wang F, et al. *Virus Res.* 2009;145:151.
83. Cai L, et al. *Virus Res.* 2012;165:95.
84. Zhai S-L, et al. *Virology J.* 2011;8:517.
85. Sofia M, et al. *J Wildl Dis.* 2008;44:864.
86. Csagola A, et al. *Arch Virol.* 2006;151:495.
87. Guo L, et al. *PLoS ONE.* 2012;7:e1463.
88. Wei C, et al. *Infect Genet Evol.* 2013;17:87.
89. Opriessnig T, et al. *Vet Microbiol.* 2013;163:177.
90. Harding JCS, et al. *Vet Microbiol.* 2010;145:209.
91. Opriessnig T, et al. *Can J Vet Res.* 2009;73:81.
92. Ramamoorthy S, Meng X-J. *Anim Hlth Res Rev.* 2008;10:1.
93. Kim WI, et al. *J Clin Microbiol.* 2008;46:1758.
94. O'Dea MA, et al. *Aust Vet J.* 2011;89:122.

95. Finlaison D, et al. *Aust Vet J*. 2007;85:304.
96. Perez LJ, et al. *Res Vet Sci*. 2010;89:301.
97. Gagnon C, et al. *J Vet Diag Invest*. 2008;20:545.
98. McIntyre L, et al. *Canad J Vet Res*. 2010;74:149.
99. Li W, et al. *Virus Genes*. 2010;40:244.
100. Chae J-S, Choi K-S. *Res Vet Sci*. 2010;88:333.
101. Firth C, et al. *J Virol*. 2009;83:12813.
102. Andraud M, et al. *J R Soc Interface*. 2009;6:39.
103. Kawashima K, et al. *J Vet Diag Invest*. 2007;19:60.
104. Chae C. *Virus Res*. 2012;164:107.
105. Punanendiran S, et al. *Virus Res*. 2011;157:92.
106. Perez LJ, et al. *Res Vet Sci*. 2010;88:528.
107. Cadar D, et al. *Acta Vet Hung*. 2010;58:475.
108. Fabsiak M, et al. *J Wildl Dis*. 2012;48:612.
109. Ruiz-Fons F, et al. *Theriogenol*. 2006;65:731.
110. Sedlak K, et al. *J Wildl Dis*. 2008;44:777.
111. Correa AM, et al. *Pesq Vet Bras*. 2006;26:154.
112. Lipej Z, et al. *Acta Vet Hung*. 2007;55:389.
113. Sofia M, et al. *J Wildl Dis*. 2008;44:864.
114. Petrini S, et al. *Europ J Wildl Dis*. 2009;55:465.
115. Ficek R, et al. *Acta Vet Brno*. 2010;79:81.
116. Wallgren P, et al. *Pig J*. 2010;63:12.
117. Rose N, et al. *Prev Vet Med*. 2009;90:168.
118. Grau-Roma L, et al. *Vet Microbiol*. 2009;135:272.
119. Calsamiglia M, et al. *Res Vet Sci*. 2007;82:299.
120. Kim HB, et al. *Vet Rec*. 2009;164:599.
121. O'Dea MA, et al. *J Virol Methods*. 2008;147:61.
122. Welch J, et al. *Transfusion*. 2006;46:1951.
123. Patterson AR, et al. *J Swine Hlth Prod*. 2011; 19:156.
124. Dupont K, et al. *Vet Microbiol*. 2007;128:56.
125. Dvorak CMT, et al. *Vet Microbiol*. 2013;166:365.
126. Shibata I, et al. *J Vet Med Sci*. 2006;65:405.
127. McIntosh KA, et al. *J Vet Diag Invest*. 2006;18:380.
128. Park JS, et al. *J Comp Path*. 2009;140:208.
129. Ha Y, et al. *Res Vet Sci*. 2009;86:108.
130. Patterson AR, et al. *Vet Microbiol*. 2011;149:225.
131. McIntosh KA, et al. *Vet Microbiol*. 2009;133:23.
132. Gerber PF, et al. *Vet J*. 2011;188:240.
133. Madson DM, et al. *Theriogenology*. 2009;72:747.
134. Chiou M-T, et al. *J Vet Med Sci*. 2011;73:521.
135. Shen H, et al. *Prev Vet Med*. 2010;97:228.
136. Dupont K, et al. *Vet Microbiol*. 2009;139:219.
137. Kristensen CS, et al. *Vet Microbiol*. 2009;138:244.
138. Shibata I, et al. *J Vet Med B*. 2006;53:278.
139. Jaros P, et al. *Proc Cong (Copenhagen) IPVS*. 2006;1:168.
140. Opriessnig T, et al. *Vet Microbiol*. 2009;133:54.
141. Patterson AR, et al. *J Anim Sci*. 2010;88:4078.
142. Kristensen CS, et al. *Proc 5th Int Symp Emerg and Re-emerg Pig Dis (Krakow)*. 2007;5:73.
143. Verreault D, et al. *Vet Microbiol*. 2010;141:224.
144. Pinheiro ALBC, et al. *Res Vet Sci*. 2013;94:764.
145. Blunt R, et al. *Vet Microbiol*. 2011;149:452.
146. Lorincz M, et al. *Acta Vet Hung*. 2010;58:265.
147. Gagnon CA, et al. *Vet Microbiol*. 2010;144:18.
148. Ha Y, et al. *Vet Path*. 2008;45:842.
149. Ha Y, et al. *J Gen Virol*. 2010;91:1601.
150. Brunborg JM, et al. *J Vet Diag Invest*. 2007;19:368.
151. Truszcznski M, Pejsak Z. *Med Wet*. 2009;65:6.
152. Madson DM, et al. *Vet Res*. 2009;40:10.
153. Schmoll F, et al. *Theriogenology*. 2008;69:814.
154. Madson DM, et al. *Vet Path*. 2009;46:707.
155. Bianco C, et al. *Acta Vet Scand*. 2012;54:51.
156. Patterson AR, et al. *Vet Microbiol*. 2011;149:91.
157. Madson DM, et al. *J Vet Diag Invest*. 2008;20:725.
158. Madson DM, et al. *Vet Res*. 2009;40:10.
159. Rose N, et al. *J Comp Path*. 2007;136:133.
160. Alarcon P, et al. *Prev Vet Med*. 2011;101:182.
161. Woodbine KA, et al. *Vet Rec*. 2007;160:751.
162. Opriessnig T, et al. *Clin Vaccine Immunol*. 2006;13:923.
163. Pujols J, et al. *Vet Rec*. 2008;163:536.
164. Tomas A, et al. *Vet Microbiol*. 2008;132:260.
165. Wellenberg G, Segales J. *Tijdschr Diergen*. 2006;131:195.
166. Pistl J, et al. *Dtsch Tierarztl Wochenschr*. 2009;116:19.
167. Pozzi SP, et al. *Israel J Vet Med*. 2008;63:122.
168. Podgorska K, et al. *Med Wet*. 2009;65:330.
169. Cadar D, et al. *Acta Vet Hung*. 2007;55:151.
170. Turcitu MA, et al. *Res Vet Sci*. 2011;91:103.
171. An D-J, et al. *Vet Microbiol*. 2014;169:147.
172. Stadejek T, et al. *Med Wet*. 2006;62:297.
173. Jacobsen B, et al. *Vet Microbiol*. 2009;138:27.
174. Ramirez-Mendoza H, et al. *Res Vet Sci*. 2007;83:130.
175. Lopez-Soria S, et al. *Vet Microbiol*. 2011;149:352.
176. Opriessnig T, et al. *Vet Path*. 2006;43:281.
177. Karlskov-Mortensen P, et al. *Proc 2nd Eur Conf Pig Genomi, Ljubljana*. Slovenia: 2008:60.
178. Szabo I, et al. *Vet Rec*. 2009;165:143.
179. Ha Y, et al. *Vet Rec*. 2009;164:48.
180. Liu X, et al. *Wei Sheng Wu Xue Bao*. 2011;51:105.
181. Kim J, et al. *Vet Pathol*. 2006;43:718.
182. Blomstrom A-L, et al. *Virus Res*. 2009;146:125.
183. Blomstrom A-L, et al. *Virus Res*. 2010;152:59.
184. Cheung AK, et al. *Arch Virol*. 2010;152:1035.
185. Grau-Roma L, Segales J. *Vet Microbiol*. 2007;119:144.
186. Fraile L, et al. *J Swine Hlth Prod*. 2009;17:32.
187. Murakami S, et al. *J Vet Med Sci*. 2006;68:387.
188. Dorr PM, et al. *J Am Vet Med Assoc*. 2007; 230:244.
189. Morandi F, et al. *J Comp Path*. 2010;142:74.
190. Chang HW, et al. *Vet Microbiol*. 2007;122:72.
191. Tsai Y-C, et al. *Vet Res*. 2012;8:174.
192. Fraile L, et al. *Can J Vet Res*. 2009;73:308.
193. Opriessnig T. *Vet Microbiol*. 2012;158:69.
194. Ramamoorthy S, et al. *Vet Microbiol*. 2011;147:49.
195. Allan GM, et al. *Zoon Publ Hlth*. 2007;54:214.
196. Huang YW, et al. *Virus Res*. 2011;158:79.
197. Hino S, Miyata H. *Rev Med Virol*. 2007;17:45.
198. Kekarainen T, et al. *J Gen Virol*. 2006;87:833.
199. Aramouni M, et al. *Vet Microbiol*. 2011;153:377.
200. Takahashi M, et al. *J Vet Med Sci*. 2008;70:497.
201. Rittersbusch GA, et al. *Res Vet Sci*. 2011;92:519.
202. Horlen KP, et al. *J Am Vet Med Assoc*. 2007;232:906.
203. Savic B, et al. *Vet Res Commun*. 2010;34:641.
204. Martin M, et al. *Vet Microbiol*. 2007;122:16.
205. Ellis JA, et al. *Am J Vet Res*. 2008;69:1608.
206. Nieto D, et al. *Vet Microbiol*. 2013;163:364.
207. McMenamy MJ, et al. *Vet Microbiol*. 2013;164:293.
208. Martelli F, et al. *Res Vet Sci*. 2010;88:492.
209. de Deus N, et al. *Vet Microbiol*. 2007;119:105.
210. Hosmillo M, et al. *Arch Virol*. 2010;155:1157.
211. Ellis JA, et al. *Am J Vet Res*. 2008;69:1608.
212. Jung K, et al. *Vet J*. 2006;171:166.
213. Jung K, et al. *Vet J*. 2006;171:445.
214. Diaz I, et al. *Vet J*. 2012;194:84.
215. Wei H, et al. *Comp Med*. 2010;60:45.
216. Langohr I, et al. *J Vet Diag Invest*. 2012;24:51.
217. Zhang H, et al. *Vet Immunol Immunopathol*. 2011;140:152.
218. Zhang H, et al. *Epidemiol Infect*. 2011;19:1.
219. Zhang H, et al. *Vet Immunol Immunopathol*. 2012;140:152.
220. Krakowka S, et al. *Can Vet J*. 2007;48:716.
221. Sibila M, et al. *J Comp Path*. 2012;147:285.
222. Palzer A, et al. *Vet Rec*. 2008;162:267.
223. Kixmoller M, et al. *Vaccine*. 2008;26:3443.
224. Santos DL, et al. *Proc Int Pig Vet Soc Cong*. 2008;P01:100.
225. Mette A, et al. *Proc IPVS Durban*. 2008;P01:0613.
226. Wieland B, et al. *Pig J*. 2010;63:20.
227. Pereyra NB, et al. *Rev Argent Microbiol*. 2006;38:130.
228. Murakami S, et al. *J Vet Med Sci*. 2006;68:387.
229. Chang H-W, et al. *Vet Microbiol*. 2006;115:311.
230. Opriessnig T, et al. *J Comp Path*. 2011;145:209.
231. Johansen M, et al. *Prev Vet Med*. 2013;108:63.
232. Cavallini-Sanches EM, et al. *J Eukaryot Microbiol*. 2006;53:92.
233. Borba MR, et al. *Med Mycol*. 2011;49:1720.
234. Zlotowski P, et al. *Vet J*. 2006;171:566.
235. Szeredi L, Szentirmai C, et al. *Acta Vet Hung*. 2008;56:207.
236. Klein S, et al. *J Comp Path*. 2010;142:228.
237. Marruchella G, et al. *Res Vet Sci*. 2012;93:310.
238. Opriessnig T, et al. *J Gen Virol*. 2008;89:177.
239. Khaiseb S, et al. *J Virol*. 2011;85:11111.
240. Lin C-M, et al. *Vet Microbiol*. 2011;149:72.
241. Perez-Martin E, et al. *J Virol Met*. 2007;146:86.
242. Yu S, et al. *Vet Microbiol*. 2007;123:34.
243. Kekararainen T, et al. *Vet Immunol Immunopathol*. 2010;136:185.
244. Steiner E, et al. *BMC Vet Res*. 2009;5:45.
245. Tsai Y-C, et al. *Vet Res*. 2010;41:60.
246. Rodriguez-Carino C, et al. *J Comp Path*. 2010;142:291.
247. Yu S, et al. *Vet Immunol Immunopathol*. 2007;115:261.
248. Resendes AR, et al. *Vet J*. 2011;189:72.
249. Seeliger FA, et al. *Vet Pathol*. 2007;44:621.
250. Sinha A, et al. *Res Vet Sci*. 2012;92:151.
251. Galindo-Gardiel I, et al. *J Comp Path*. 2011;144:63.
252. Wei L, et al. *Virology*. 2008;378:177.
253. Wei L, Liu J. *Virology*. 2009;386:203.
254. Wei L, et al. *J Virology*. 2009;83:6039.
255. Wei L, et al. *J Virol*. 2012;86:13589.
256. Wei L, et al. *Virology*. 2013;147:285.
257. Yu S, et al. *Vet Immunol Immunopathol*. 2009;127:350.
258. Opriessnig T, et al. *Vet Res*. 2010;41:31.
259. Marks FS, et al. *Vet Microbiol*. 2010;141:220.
260. Szeredi L, Szentirmai C. *Acta Vet Hung*. 2008;56:101.
261. Correa AM, et al. *Braz J Vet Res*. 2006;26:9.
262. Behling-Kelly E, Czuprynski CJ. *Anim Hlth Res Rev*. 2007;8:47.
263. Timmusk S, et al. *J Gen Virol*. 2006;87:3215.
264. Lin C-M, et al. *Vet Microbiol*. 2013;162:519.
265. Wikstrom FH, et al. *J Virology*. 2007;81:4919.
266. Borghetti P, et al. *Vet Microbiol*. 2013;163:42.
267. Kekarainen T, et al. *Vet Immunol Immunopathol*. 2008;124:41.
268. Kekarainen T, et al. *J Gen Virol*. 2008;89:760.
269. Vincent IE, et al. *Immunology*. 2007;120:47.
270. Chang HW, et al. *Vet Immunol Immunopathol*. 2006;110:207.
271. Darwich L, et al. *Res Vet Sci*. 2008;84:194.
272. Stevenson LS, et al. *Viral Immunol*. 2006;19:189.
273. Doster AR, et al. *J Vet Sci*. 2010;11:177.
274. Crisci E, et al. *Vet Immunol Immunopathol*. 2010;136:305.
275. Lv Y, et al. *Res Vet Sci*. 2013;95:1235.
276. Vincent IEI, et al. *Immunol*. 2007;120:47.
277. Ramamoorthy S, et al. *Virus Res*. 2009;145:187.
278. Fort M, et al. *Vet Immunol Immunopathol*. 2009;129:101.
279. Brunborg IM, et al. *Acta Vet Scand*. 2010;52:22.
280. Li J, et al. *Vet J*. 2012,193:199.
281. Grierson SS, et al. *Vet Immunol Immunopathol*. 2007;119:254.
282. Shi K, et al. *Vet Microbiol*. 2007;129:367.
283. Carasova P, et al. *Res Vet Sci*. 2007;83:274.
284. Fort M, et al. *Vet Microbiol*. 2007;125:244.
285. Fan H, et al. *Vet Res Commun*. 2007;31:487.
286. Song Y, et al. *Vet Microbiol*. 2007;119:97.
287. Gerber PF, et al. *Can J Vet Res*. 2012;76:38.
288. Dias AS, et al. *Res Vet Sci*. 2013;94:341.
289. Oh Y, et al. *J Gen Virol*. 2012;93:1556.
290. Fort M, et al. *Vet Immunol Immunopathol*. 2010;137:226.
291. Quereda JJ, et al. *Am J Vet Res*. 2013;74:110.
292. Silva FMF, et al. *J Comp Path*. 2011;144:296.
293. Saha D, et al. *BMC Vet Res*. 2011;7:64.

294. Pescador CA. *Pesq Vet Brasil.* 2007;27:425.
295. Sarli G, et al. *Proc 19th IPVS Congress.* 2006:5.
296. Nielsen EO, et al. *Vet Rec.* 2008;162:505.
297. Zlotowski P, et al. *Vet Rec.* 2013;172:637.
298. Correa AMR, et al. *J Vet Diag Invest.* 2007;19:109.
299. Cino-Ozuna AG, et al. *J Clin Microbiol.* 2011;49:2012.
300. Darwich L, Mateu E. *Virus Res.* 2012;164:61.
301. Huang YY, et al. *Vet Pathol.* 2008;45:640.
302. Correa AM. *J Vet Diag Invest.* 2007;19:109.
303. Langohr IM, et al. *Vet Path.* 2010;47:140.
304. Bukovsky C, et al. *Vet Rec.* 2007;161:552.
305. Imai DM, et al. *J Vet Diag Invest.* 2006;18:496.
306. Szeredi L, et al. *Vet Pathol.* 2012;49:264.
307. Rodriguez-Carino C, Segales J. *Vet Pathol.* 2009;46:729.
308. Woodbine KA, et al. *Prev Vet Med.* 2010;97:100.
309. Segales J, Cortey M. *Vet Rec.* 2010;167:940.
310. Wellenberg GJ, et al. *Vet Microbiol.* 2010;142:217.
311. Alarcon P, et al. *Prev Vet Med.* 2011;98:19.
312. Tico G, et al. *Vet Microbiol.* 2013;163:242.
313. Jacela JY, et al. *J Swine Hlth Prod.* 2011;19:10.
314. Jensen VF, et al. *Prev Vet Med.* 2010;95:239.
315. Vigre H, et al. *Prev Vet Med.* 2010;93:98.
316. Phaneuf LR, et al. *J Am Ass Lab Anim Sci.* 2007;46:68.
317. Madson DM, Opriessnig T. *Anim Hlth Res Rev.* 2011;12:47.
318. Togashi K, et al. *J Vet Med Sci.* 2011;73:941.
319. Lefebvre D, et al. *Proc IPVS Congress.* 2008;20:38.
320. Sharma R, Saikumar G. *Trop Anim Hlth Prod.* 2010;42:515.
321. Woods A, et al. *J Swine Hlth Prod.* 2010;14:210.
322. Rittersbusch GA, et al. *Proc 21st IPVS Congress.* 2010;21:466.
323. Hogedal P, et al. *Proc IPVS Congress.* 2008;20:221.
324. Pittman JS, et al. *J Swine Hlth Prod.* 2008;16:144.
325. Hansen MS, et al. *Vet Microbiol.* 2010;144:203.
326. Meyns T, et al. *Proc 22nd IPVS.* 2012:879.
327. Zlotowski P, et al. *Vet Rec.* 2013;doi:10.1136/vr.101409.
328. Pejsak Z, et al. *Res Vet Sci.* 2011;91:125.
329. Cino-Ozuna AG, et al. *J Clin Microbiol.* 2011;49:2012.
330. Huang Y-L, et al. *Vet Res.* 2011;42:1150.
331. Salamano G, et al. *Vet J.* 2008;177:110.
332. Tsiakalos A, et al. *Liver Int.* 2009;29:1538.
333. Eckersall PD, Bell R. *Vet J.* 2010;185:23.
334. Bode JG, et al. *J Immunol.* 2012;167:1469.
335. Gauger PC, et al. *Vet Microbiol.* 2011;154:185.
336. Grau-Roma L, et al. *Vet Microbiol.* 2009;138:53.
337. Opriessnig T, Langohr I. *Vet Pathol.* 2013;50:23.
338. Faccini S, et al. *J Vet Diag Invest.* 2011;23:1189.
339. Harding JCS, et al. *Can J Vet Res.* 2009;73:7.
340. Madson DM, et al. *Clin Vaccine Immunol.* 2009;16:830.
341. Sarli G, et al. *Vet Rec.* 2009;164:519.
342. Jin Q, et al. *J Vet Diag Invest.* 2012;24:1151.
343. Turner MJ, et al. *Prev Vet Med.* 2009;88:213.
344. Jittimanae S, et al. *J Vet Diag Invest.* 2012;24:1129.
345. O'Sullivan T, et al. *Vet Res.* 2012;8:192.
346. Fort M, et al. *Vet Microbiol.* 2007;125:244.
347. Jorsal SE, et al. *Proc 19th IPVS Congress.* Copenhagen: 2006:311.
348. Sarli G, et al. *Vet Rec.* 2006;164:519.
349. Grasland B, et al. *Proc 20th IPVS Cong.* 2008;20:56.
350. Opriessnig T, et al. *J Swine Hlth Prod.* 2006;14:42.
351. Ciacci-Zanella JR, et al. *Proc Int Symp Emerg Re-Emerg Pig Dis.* 2007;5:94.
352. Ciaccia-Zanella JR, et al. *Proc IPVS Cong.* 2008;20:23.
353. Gava D, et al. *Pesq Vet Brasil.* 2008;28:70.
354. Reicks DI, et al. *Proc Allen D Leman Swine Conf.* 2007;34:104.
355. Pal N, et al. *J Virol Methods.* 2008;149:217.
356. Sarli G, et al. *Vet Rec.* 2009;164:519.
357. Morandi F, et al. *Acta Vet Scand.* 2012;54:17.
358. Hansen MS, et al. *J Comp Path.* 2010;142:109.
359. Hansen MS, et al. *Vet Pathol.* 2013;50:980.
360. Ogawa H, et al. *J Virol Methods.* 2009;160:210.
361. Lin C-M, et al. *Vet Med.* 2009;138:225.
362. McIntosh KA, et al. *Can Vet J.* 2008;49:1189.
363. Hjulsager CK, et al. *Vet Microbiol.* 2009;133:172.
364. Harding JC, et al. *Can J Vet Res.* 2009;73:7.
365. An DJ, et al. *Vet Res Comm.* 2009;33:139.
366. Li J, et al. *Vet Rec.* 2013;173:346.
367. Belak S. *Dev Biol.* 2007;128:103.
368. McKillen J, et al. *J Virol Methods.* 2007;140:155.
369. Jiang Y, et al. *Vet J.* 2010;183:172.
370. Jiang Y, et al. *Res Vet Sci.* 2010;89:133.
371. Dezen D, et al. *Res Vet Sci.* 2010;88:436.
372. Vilcek S, et al. *J Virol Methods.* 2010;165:216.
373. Prickett JR, et al. *J Swine Hlth Prod.* 2008;16:86.
374. Ramirez A, et al. *Prev Vet Med.* 2012;104:292.
375. Chittick WA, et al. *J Vet Diagn Invest.* 2011;23:248.
376. Prickett JR, et al. *Transbound Emerg Dis.* 2011;58:121.
377. Madec F, et al. *Transbound Emerg Dis.* 2008;55:273.
378. Woeste K, Gross Beilage E. *Dtsch Tierarztl Wochenschr.* 2007;114:324.
379. Opriessnig T, et al. *Vet Rec.* 2006;158:149.
380. Hassing A-G, et al. *Proc 4th Int Symp Emerg Pig Dis (Rome).* 2006:211.
381. Martin H, et al. *Vet J.* 2008;177:388.
382. Maes D, et al. *Theriogenology.* 2008;70:1337.
383. Pan Q, et al. *J Trace Elements Med Biol.* 2008;22:143.
384. Jung B-G, et al. *Vet Microbiol.* 2010;143:117.
385. Andruad M, et al. *Prev Vet Med.* 2009;92:38.
386. Kekarainen T, et al. *Vet Immunol Immunopathol.* 2010;136:185.
387. Beach NM, Meng XJ. *Virus Res.* 2012;164:33.
388. Madson D, et al. *Am Assoc Swine Vet.* 2009;151.
389. Fort M, et al. *Vaccine.* 2009;27:4031.
390. Fort M, et al. *Vaccine.* 2008;26:1063.
391. Opriessnig T, et al. *Clin Vaccine Immunol.* 2008;9:33.
392. Opriessng T, et al. *Vaccine.* 2009;27:1002.
393. Opriessnig T, et al. *Vet Microbiol.* 2010;142:177.
394. Hemann M, et al. *Vet Microbiol.* 2012;158:180.
395. Cline G, et al. *Vet Rec.* 2008;163:737.
396. Fachinger V, et al. *Vaccine.* 2008;26:1488.
397. Horlen KP, et al. *J Am Vet Med Assoc.* 2008;232:906.
398. Kixmoller M, et al. *Vaccine.* 2008;26:3443.
399. Segales J, et al. *Vaccine.* 2009;27:7313.
400. Pejsak Z, et al. *Comp Immunol Microbiol Infect Dis.* 2010;33:e1.
401. Kurmann J, et al. *Clin Vaccine Immunol.* 2011;18:1644.
402. Lyoo K, et al. *Vet J.* 2011;189:58.
403. Martelli P, et al. *Vet Microbiol.* 2011;149:339.
404. Fraile L, et al. *Vet Microbiol.* 2012;161:229.
405. Gagnon CA, et al. *Vet Microbiol.* 2010;144:18.
406. Lohse L, et al. *Vet Microbiol.* 2008;129:97.
407. Timmusk S, et al. *Virus Genes.* 2008;36:509.
408. Seo H-S, et al. *Vet J.* 2014;doi:10.1016/j.tvj.2014.02.002.
409. Lyoo K-S, et al. *Can J Vet Res.* 2012;76:221.
410. Takahagi Y, et al. *J Vet Med.* 2010;72:35.
411. Desrosiers R, et al. *J Swine Hlth Prod.* 2008;17:148.
412. Horlen KP, et al. *J Am Vet Med Assoc.* 2008;232:906.
413. Jacela JY, et al. *J Swine Hlth Prod.* 2011;19:10.
414. Fachinger V, et al. *Vaccine.* 2008;26:1488.
415. Kixmoller M, et al. *Vaccine.* 2008;26:3443.
416. Martelli P, et al. *Vet Microbiol.* 2011;149:339.
417. Segales J, et al. *Vaccine.* 2009;27:7313.
418. Venegas-Vargas MC, et al. *J Swine Hlth Prod.* 2011;19:233.
419. Young MC, et al. *J Swine Health Prod.* 2011;19:175.
420. Strugnell BW, et al. *Pig J.* 2011;66:67.
421. Kristensen CS, et al. *Prev Vet Med.* 2011;98:250.
422. Pejsak Z, et al. *Bull Vet Inst Pulawy.* 2009;53:159.
423. Pejsak Z, et al. *Pol J Vet Sci.* 2012;15:37.
424. Gerber PF, et al. *Vet J.* 2011;188:240.
425. Kurmann J, et al. *Clin Vaccine Immunol.* 2011;18:1644.
426. O'Neill KC, et al. *Vet Rec.* 2012;171:425.
427. Sibila M, et al. *Vet J.* 2013;doi:10.1016/j.tvjl.2013.04.01.
428. Opriessnig T, et al. *J Anim Sci.* 2009;87:1582.
429. Pejsak Z, et al. *Comp Immunol Microbiol Infect Dis.* 2010;33:e1.
430. Goubier A, et al. *Proc 18th IPVS Congress.* 2008;1:16.
431. Seo HW, et al. *Clin Vaccine Immunol.* 2011;18:1091.
432. Alberti KA, et al. *J Anim Sci.* 2011;89:1581.
433. Fort M, et al. *Vet Immunol Immunopathol.* 2009;129:101.
434. O'Neill KC, et al. *Clin Vaccine Immunol.* 2011;18:1865.
435. Fraile L, et al. *Vet Microbiol.* 2012;161:229.
436. Takada-Iwao A, et al. *Vet Microbiol.* 2013;162:219.
437. Yoon S, et al. *Antiviral Res.* 2010;88:19.
438. Feng Z, et al. *Antiviral Res.* 2008;77:186.
439. Opriessnig T, et al. *Vaccine.* 2013;31:487.
440. Gillespie J, et al. *Vaccine.* 2008;26:4231.
441. Shen HG, et al. *Vaccine.* 2010;28:5960.
442. Opriessnig T, et al. *Vet Microbiol.* 2008;131:103.
443. Sinha A, et al. *Clin Vac Immunol.* 2010;17:1940.
444. Beach NM, et al. *Vaccine.* 2010;29:221.
445. Opriessnig T, et al. *Clin Vaccine Immunol.* 2011;18:1261.
446. Opriessnig T, et al. *Theriogenology.* 2011b;76:351.
447. Bischoff R, et al. *Prakt Tierartzl.* 2009;90:58.
448. Park C, et al. *Clin Vaccine Immunol.* 2013;20:369.
449. Lakshman NA, et al. *Can J Vet Res.* 2012;76:301.
450. Trible BR, et al. *Vaccine.* 2012;30:4079.
451. Cino-Ozuna AG, et al. *J Clin Immunol.* 2011;49:2012.
452. Takahagi Y, et al. *J Vet Med Sci.* 2009;70:603.
453. Fan H, et al. *Vet Res Commun.* 2007;31:487.
454. Song Y, et al. *Vet Microbiol.* 2007;119:97.
455. Wang X, et al. *Vaccine.* 2006;24:3374.
456. Hemann M, et al. *Vet Microbiol.* 2012;158:180.
457. Seo HW, et al. *Vet Res.* 2012;8:194.
458. Liu Y-F, et al. *Vet Immunol Immunopathol.* 2013;154:48.
459. Kim T, et al. *Vet Microbiol.* 2009;138:318.
460. Sun M, et al. *Vet Microbiol.* 2007;123:203.
461. Hayes S, et al. *Vaccine.* 2010;28:6789.
462. Bucarey SA, et al. *Vaccine.* 2009;27:5781.
463. Takada-Iwao A, et al. *Vet Microbiol.* 2011;154:104.

TORQUE TENO VIRUS

Torque teno virus is, as far as is known at the moment, a nonpathogenic commensal inhabitant of vertebrates. It is one of a newly created family of Anellivirid, which has nine genera. It may be one of what are now called "bystander viruses."[1]

ETIOLOGY

These are emerging circular DNA viruses affecting many species, including pigs. Currently, two genera have been found in pigs: type 1(TTSuV1), now known as *Iotatorquevirus,* which has 1a and 1b subtypes; and type 2 (TTSuV2), now known as *Kappatotorquevirus,* which has 2a and 2b subtypes. In addition, a novel virus was also discovered in

New Zealand in 2012, and this has also been found in China.[2,3] The virus may have an immunosuppressive effect when found as a natural infection before vaccination with PRRS.[1] The replication site of the virus is unknown.[4] Several strains have been found in one pig.[5] They can also be widely divergent in genotype.[6] In a study measuring TTV quantitatively, there was no difference in viral load between PCV2-negative and PCV2-positive pigs.[7]

EPIDEMIOLOGY

These viruses have also been found in pig commercial vaccines, enzymes for laboratory use, and human drugs containing components of porcine origin.[8]

They were first linked to PCV2-associated diseases (PCVAD)[9] and PDNS[10] and may be a cofactor in the disease. They were found very commonly in animals with nephropathy. They are widely distributed in tissues in the pig. The virus is found in fetal tissues, blood, semen,[11] and colostrum. In piglets, it can be found in week 1 of life, and the highest detection is at 11 weeks for type 1 and 16 weeks for type 2.[12] A study in the United States showed that it was common and increased with age.[13]

It has a long-lasting viremia, probably because there is a very poor immunologic response. The virus load increases progressively for suckling pigs to finisher pigs and then decreases in mature animals. It can be transmitted vertically and horizontally.

It has been found in wild boar,[14] in Spain,[15,16] Czechoslovakia,[17] Italy,[18] Hungary,[19] China,[20-22] the United States,[13] and Austria.[23]

In Japan, it is widespread in postweaning pigs and may play a part in pig disease. There is a low incidence in young pigs, less than 11% in pigs under 30 days old but 54% to 85% in older pigs.[24] The two species differ in their viral infection dynamics in PMWS-affected herds.[25] In a South Korean study, there was shown to be an early onset of viremia and a chronic viremic state regardless of the PCV2 vaccination status.[7]

In a Spanish retrospective study of pigs from 1985 to 2005, 113/162 pigs were infected with one or another type; 38/162 had both types of virus, 90/162 had type 2, and 54/162 had type 1.[16]

There is evidence for vertical transmission[14] and in utero infection.[26] An increased viral load and prevalence of TTSuV2 in pigs experimentally infected with a highly pathogenic CSFV has been shown.[4]

CLINICAL SIGNS

There are no clinical signs. Coinfection of TTSuV and PCV2 in a reproductive problem was demonstrated, but no clinical disease was found.[27]

DIAGNOSIS

There are several PCR assays for TTSuV1[16] and for TTSuV.[28] There is a nonspecific qPCR for both viruses,[29] and ELISAs are available for the detection of antibodies.

FURTHER READING

Kekrainen T, Segales J. *Sus* virus in pigs: an emerging pathogen? *Transbound Emerg Dis.* 2012;59(suppl S1):103-108.

REFERENCES

1. Zhang Z, et al. *Arch Virol.* 2012;157:927.
2. Zhai S-L, et al. *Arch Virol.* 2012;157:927.
3. Zhai S-L, et al. *Arch Virol.* 2013;158:1567.
4. Aramouni M, et al. *Vet Microbiol.* 2010;146:350.
5. Huang YW, et al. *Virology.* 2010;396:289.
6. Wang MM, et al. *J Virol.* 2012;86:11953.
7. Lee S, et al. *Res Vet Sci.* 2012;92:519.
8. Kekrainen T, et al. *J Gen Virol.* 2009;90:648.
9. Ellis J, et al. *Am J Vet Res.* 2008;69:1608.
10. Krakowka S, et al. *Am J Vet Res.* 2008;69:1615.
11. Kekrainen T, et al. *Theriogenology.* 2007;68:966.
12. Sibila M, et al. *Vet Microbiol.* 2009;139:213.
13. Xiao C-T, et al. *J Virol Meth.* 2012;183:40.
14. Martinez L, et al. *Vet Microbiol.* 2006;98:81.
15. Kekrainen T, et al. *J Gen Virol.* 2006;68:966.
16. Segales J, et al. *Vet Microbiol.* 2009;134:199.
17. Jarosova V, et al. *Folia Microbiol.* 2011;56:90.
18. Martelli F, et al. *J Vet Med.* 2006;53:234.
19. Takacs M, et al. *Acta Vet Hung.* 2008;56:547.
20. Zhu CX, et al. *J Clin Virol.* 2010;48:296.
21. Liu X, et al. *Vet Rec.* 2011;168:410.
22. Zhu CX, et al. *Virus Res.* 2012;165:225.
23. Lang C, et al. *Berl Munch Tierartzl Wschr.* 2011;124:142.
24. Tara O, et al. *Vet Microbiol.* 2011;139:347.
25. Nieto D, et al. *Vet Microbiol.* 2011;152:284.
26. Pozzuto T, et al. *Vet Microbiol.* 2009;137:375.
27. Ritterbusch GA, et al. *Res Vet Sci.* 2012;92:519.
28. Lee S-S, et al. *J Vet Diag Invest.* 2010;22:261.
29. Brassard J, et al. *J Appl Microbiol.* 2010;108:2191.

NIPAH

Nipah is a zoonotic virus encephalitic disease of pigs and humans in Southeast Asia. It probably jumped from a wildlife reservoir to domestic pigs first. Infection with two strains of the virus was responsible for fatal respiratory disease in Malaysia in 1999. The outbreak resulted in numerous deaths of pig farmers (fatal febrile encephalitis) and others in contact with pigs, including abattoir workers. About 90% of outbreaks in humans can be associated with close contact with pigs. Recently, outbreaks in humans have occurred without reference to pigs.[1,2] It can cause huge economic loss in the pig industry. The pig serves as an "amplifying host."

ETIOLOGY

Pigs are highly susceptible to Nipah virus.

The virus is a member of the *Henipavirus* genus in the Paramyxoviridae family, which includes Hendra virus, which is transmitted from frugiverous bats (*Pteropus* spp.) to pigs, among which it spreads horizontally to other pigs and humans. Horses can be exposed and develop antibodies to the virus, and there is one anecdotal report of dilated meningeal vessels in a horse from which Nipah virus was isolated. It grows readily in cell culture to produce syncytia.

EPIDEMIOLOGY

There is strong evidence that the reservoir from which the virus originated was pteroptid bats.

It is highly contagious in swine, and transmission may be by several routes, including direct contact with large droplets. The oronasal route is the most common method because the virus can be demonstrated in nasal secretions. Cats and dogs can be affected but probably do not transmit to pigs.

PATHOGENESIS

The virus affects the vascular, nervous, and lymphoreticular systems, leading to a viremia and specific infections of the endothelial cells[3] and immune cells,[4] particularly some T cells and monocytes. Nipah can then cross the blood–brain barrier. The virus infects monocytes and a subset of T-lymphocytes.

CLINICAL SIGNS

It may be asymptomatic in pigs, but it is usually a severe, fatal disease with respiratory or CNS signs. Affected weaners may have a temperature in excess of 40°C (104°F), with a harsh characteristic (but not pathognomonic) barking cough, mouth breathing, and poor exercise tolerance. There is hindleg weakness, thrashing, and recumbency, with head pressing, titanic spasms, and fits. In adults there may be sudden death, which is quite rare, and sometimes there are neurologic signs, such as pharyngeal muscle paralysis, frothy salivation, and drooping of the tongue. In experimental infections, piglets often only showed a mild temperature rise.[4]

NECROPSY FINDINGS

There are few gross lesions. There may be lung consolidation and froth in the trachea. The lymph nodes may be enlarged. Histologically, there is a pneumonia and the presence of syncytia and multinucleated alveolar macrophages; if neurologic signs, there may be a nonsuppurative meningitis.

DIAGNOSIS

Diagnosis is based on exposure to affected pigs or fruit bats; the presence of the harsh barking cough, which is said to be almost pathognomonic; and the nervous signs. Specimen collection and diagnostic assays have been reviewed,[5] but any handling of suspect material should be carried out in category 4 laboratories. It is possible to demonstrate the antigens in formalin-fixed material.

The virus can be demonstrated in the tissues using a tagged monoclonal antibody or RT-PCR. There is high sensitivity of qRT-PCR.[6]

For the presence of antibodies, blocking ELISAs are superior to virus neutralization.[6]

TREATMENT

No treatment is available.

CONTROL

Neutralizing antibodies appear 7 to 10 days postinfection[7] and reach a maximum at 14 to 16 days postinoculation.

It is necessary to keep the pigs on farms where there are no fruit bats nesting in trees. Isolation and quarantine are the best control methods, rapid slaughter of infected pigs is absolutely necessary, and other species must be kept away from infected farms.

REFERENCES

1. Gurley ES, et al. *Emerg Infect Dis.* 2007;13:1031.
2. Luby SP, et al. *Emerg Infect Dis.* 2006;12:1888.
3. Meisner A, et al. *Thromb Haemost.* 2009;102:1014.
4. Berhane Y, et al. *Transbound Emerg Dis.* 2008;55:165.
5. Daniels P, Narasiman M. *Manual of Diagnostic Tests and Vaccines for Terrestrial Animals.* Vol. 2. Geneva: WHO; 2008:1227.
6. Li M, et al. *Vet Res.* 2010;41:33.
7. Weingartl HM, et al. *J Virol.* 2006;80:7929.

TIOMAN VIRUS

Tioman virus is another paramyxovirus of pigs of fruit bat origin, found in Malaysia,[1] which causes a mild disease in pigs and has a predilection for the lymph nodes.

REFERENCE

1. Yalw KC, et al. *J Virol.* 2008;82:565.

PORCINE RETROVIRUSES

All mammals have leftover traces of past viral infections in their genetic makeup.[1] Commercial pigs carry high and variable titers of retroviral RNA in their blood, with differences according to their age and herd health status. These endogenous retroviruses[2] may contribute up to 8% of the genome of all vertebrates.[3] All pigs carry endogenous porcine retroviruses (PRs) in their genome.[4] There may be an association between PRs and mortality in commercial herds.[1,5,6] The discovery that PRs can infect human cells triggered research into how xenotransplantation infection may be prevented.

FURTHER READING

Denner J, Tonjes RR. Infection barriers to successful xenotransplantation focusing on porcine endogenous retroviruses. *Clin Microbiol Rev.* 2012;25:318-343.

Pal N, et al. The importance of ubiquitous viruses such as the different PERV types may be currently underestimated and especially PERV-A/C may play a role in multifactorial disease in pigs. *Transbound Emerg Dis.* 2011;58:344-351.

REFERENCES

1. Tucker AW, Scobie L. *Vet Rec.* 2006;159:367.
2. Tucker AW, et al. *J Clin Microbiol.* 2006;44:3846.
3. Kurth R, Bannert N. *Int J Cancer.* 2009;126:306.
4. Wilson CA. *Cell Molec Life Sci.* 2008;65:3399.
5. Dieckhoff B, et al. *Vet Microbiol.* 2007;123:53.
6. Pal N, et al. *Transbound Emerg Dis.* 2011;58:344.

MENANGLE

Menangle virus was first identified in a three-farm disease outbreak in New South Wales in 1997. It causes reproductive problems in pigs and congenital defects and has the fruit bat as an asymptomatic reservoir. It can cause a flulike disease in humans. Only one outbreak has been described. The virus normally lives asymptomatically in fruit bats.

ETIOLOGY

It is a RNA virus in the family Paramyxoviridae, probably in the genus *Rubalovirus.* It is closely related to Tioman virus found in fruit bats on Tioman Island, Malaysia.

EPIDEMIOLOGY

A variety of fruit bats are seropositive, but the virus has not been isolated from them, including the gray-headed flying fox, black fruit bat, and spectacled fruit bat. These fruit bats have been found in other areas of Australia and the original area around Menangle, New South Wales.

Bat feces and urine are probably the source of infection. Transmission from pig to pig is slow and probably requires close contact. In one building, it took a long time for the sows to become affected. It probably spreads from farm to farm via infected animals. There is no sign of persistent infection and no evidence of long-term virus shedding. Present evidence suggests that virus survival in the environment is short because sentinel pigs placed in an uncleaned area did not seroconvert.

CLINICAL SIGNS

Currently, there is no knowledge of the incubation period. In the initial outbreak, clinical signs were seen only on the farrow-to-finish farm, but infected pigs were found in all three farms.

The disease was an outbreak of reproductive disease with fetal death; fetal abnormalities, including congenital defects such as skeletal and neurologic defects,[1] mummified fetuses, and stillborn fetuses; smaller litters with fewer live piglets; and a reduced farrowing rate. The farrowing rate fell from 80%+ to a low of approximately 38%, reaching an average of 60%. Many sows returned to estrus 28 days after mating, which suggests that there has been an early death of the litter. Some sows remain in pseudopregnancy for more than 60 days. It probably crosses the placenta and spreads from fetus to fetus. Once the infection became endemic the in the farrow-to-finish herd, the reproductive failures ceased.

NECROPSY FINDINGS

The mummified fetuses vary in size and are of 30 days' gestation or older.

The virus causes degeneration of the brain and spinal cord. In particular, the cerebral hemispheres and cerebellum are smaller. Occasionally there may be effusions and pulmonary hypoplasia. Eosinophilic inclusions are found in the neurons of the cerebrum and spinal cord. Sometimes there is nonsuppurative meningitis, myocarditis, and hepatitis. Experimental infections show shedding 2 to 3 days after infection in nasal and oral secretions. A tropism for secondary lymphoid tissues and intestinal epithelium has been demonstrated.[2] No lesions have been seen in piglets born alive or other postnatal pigs.

DIAGNOSIS

The diagnosis is suspected when the reproductive parameters change very suddenly, as previously described.

Diagnosis is confirmed by virus culture, and electron microscopy (EM) and virus neutralization (VN) tests confirm the identity of the virus. Serologic tests include ELISAs, and the best way to test the herd is to use this for the sows for antibody.

DIFFERENTIAL DIAGNOSIS

The differential diagnosis includes porcine parvovirus (PPV), classical swine fever (CSF), porcine reproductive and respiratory syndrome (PRRS), encephalomyocarditis virus (EMCV), pseudorabies virus (PRV), Japanese encephalitis, swine influenza virus (SIV), and blue eye. Noninfectious causes such as toxins or nutritional deficiencies should also be considered.

TREATMENT

It seems likely that young pigs are infected by the virus when the maternal antibody falls at 14 to 16 weeks of age. By the time they enter the breeding herd, their immunity is quite strong.

CONTROL

Avoiding contact with all fruit bats is the best advice.

FURTHER READING

Philbey AW, et al. An apparently new virus (family Paramyxoviridae) infection for pigs, humans and fruit bats. *Emerg Infect Dis.* 1998;4:269.

REFERENCES

1. Philbey AW, et al. *Aust Vet J.* 2007;85:134.
2. Bowden TR, et al. *J Gen Virol.* 2012;93:1007.

JAPANESE B ENCEPHALITIS (JAPANESE ENCEPHALITIS)

This is the most important of the encephalitogenic flaviviruses. It causes in excess of 50,000 human cases a year, with a case-mortality rate of 25%. It causes reproductive failure in pigs.

ETIOLOGY

It is a *Flavivirus* and is found in at least five genotypes.

EPIDEMIOLOGY

The natural distribution range of the virus is Southeast Asia and Australasia. The vectors are *Culex* spp., in particular, *C. tritaeniorhynchus.* The virus activity is naturally maintained through bird–mosquito cycles, with the Heron family in particular. The night herons, little egrets, and plumed egrets are particularly active as a reservoir. Pigs are important "amplifying hosts." Pigs and these birds may allow the overwintering of the virus when mosquitoes are absent.

PATHOGENESIS

Viremia results from the mosquito bite, and usually nothing is seen; occasionally there may be a mild fever, but quite often the virus goes straight to the testicles and causes orchitis.

CLINICAL SIGNS

Fetal death is common, with mummified fetuses, stillborns, and weak pigs. Boars undergo reproductive failure.

NECROPSY FINDINGS

Pathology is largely related to the abnormal fetuses.

DIAGNOSIS

RT-PCR and nested RT-PCR can be used to detect the virus when virus isolation is negative. Antibody can be detected by hemagglutination inhibition (HI), ELISAs (IgM-capture ELISA), and latex agglutination tests.

CONTROL

Live attenuated vaccines should be given to breeding stock 2 to 3 weeks before the start of the mosquito season. Killed and adjuvanted vaccines are also available.

FURTHER READING

Mackenzie JS, Williams DT. The zoonotic flaviviruses of southern, south-eastern and eastern Asia and Australasia; the potential for emergent viruses. *Zoon Pub Hlth*. 2009;56:338.

RESTON VIRUS

Reston virus, an *Ebolavirus*, was recently detected in pigs in the Philippines. Specific antibodies were found in the pig farmers, indicating exposure to the virus. In an experimental situation, pigs were infected with Zaire Ebola virus (ZEBOV), and it was found to replicate to high titers, mainly in the respiratory tract, and developed severe lung pathology.[1] Shedding from the oronasal mucosa was detected for up to 14 days after infection, and transmission was confirmed in all naïve pigs cohabiting with inoculated animals. These results confirm an unexpected site of virus amplification and shedding linked to transmission of infectious virus

REFERENCE

1. Kobinger GP, et al. *J Infect Dis*. 2011;204:200.

BUNGOWANNAH VIRUS

Bungowannah virus is possibly a new species of pestivirus that was found on a pig farm in New South Wales, Australia. Sudden death was experienced by 3- to 4-week-old pigs, and at the same time, there was an increase in the number of stillborn piglets with multifocal nonsuppurative myocarditis and myonecrosis leading to a secondary congestive heart failure.

PORCINE PARVOVIRUS

Usually parvoviruses are described with the acronym SMEDI, are associated with reproductive failure in pregnant sows, and are characterized by embryonic and fetal death, mummification, stillbirths, and delayed return to estrus. In other groups of postnatal nonpregnant pigs, the acute infection is usually subclinical, but it has been linked to skin lesions in piglets, interstitial nephritis in slaughter pigs, and nonsuppurative myocarditis in piglets. Tonsils are the main site of replication of the virus, but it also occurs in the heart, lungs, spleen, kidney, and endometrium. In the fetus, the replication is mainly in the heart, spleen, lung, and testis.

NOVEL PORCINE PARVOVIRUSES

Several new members of the subfamily Parvoviridae have been discovered in animals, particularly pigs.[1]

The subfamily Parvoviridae infects birds and mammals. Two of the five genera in this group contain pig viruses. These are *Bocavirus* and *Parvovirus* genera, and recently the newly proposed genus *Hokovirus* may contain newly identified pig viruses.

The viruses are called porcine parvoviruses (PPVs). These new viruses are important because they have been associated with PCVAD,[2-4] or "high-fever" disease.[5]

PPV1 is ubiquitous in swine and is associated with reproductive disease.[6]

In 2001, a new parvovirus was discovered in Myanmar and called porcine parvovirus 2;[5] it is of a novel and distinct lineage. It was also recently isolated in Hungary,[7] and two strains were isolated in the United States.[8] This virus, like other parvoviruses and RNA viruses, has a high substitution rate in the capsid gene. These new viruses may not have the same protection following use of the old vaccines. PPV2 does not belong to any of the known clusters, has been found in swine serum, and has not been associated with any known disease. It was the second of the new viruses discovered and is now found worldwide.[5,8] Not much is known about porcine parvovirus 2 and disease, but on one Chinese farm the virus was detected 3 weeks before a severe respiratory disease outbreak. In one study, DNA was detected in the lung tissues from nursery pigs and grow-finish pigs. Porcine parvovirus 3 was found in Hong Kong and originally called Hokovirus.[9] PPV3 of the proposed *Hokovirus* genus has been found in both sick and healthy pigs[10] and was also called partetravirus.[11] Coinfection with both PPV3 and PCV2 was shown in China and Hong Kong.[3] PPV4[12] and the porcine boca-like virus[13] belong to the group. PPV4[9] was identified in association with PCV2. It is not clear whether it can cause disease on its own or whether it exacerbates PCV2 infections. It has been reported since in Asia, Europe, and Africa.[1,7,14-16]

A novel porcine parvovirus was identified in the lung lavage of a diseased pig coinfected with PCV2.

In a recent study in Germany, it was shown that PPV1 through PPV4 strains were found in the tonsils of piglets,[17,18] and PPV1 and PPV4 were found in the hearts. A real-time PCR has been developed to detect and analyze virulent PPV loads in artificially challenged sows and piglets,[19] using a conserved region of the genome. Previous RT-PCR methods have used the VP2 gene.[20, 21] Diagnosis is through use of PCRs, virus isolation, hemagglutination inhibition tests, and immunofluorescence. Anti-PPV antibodies occur in the fetus at about 56 to 70 days.

REFERENCES

1. Cadar D, et al. *J Gen Virol*. 2013;94:2330.
2. Xiao CT, et al. *Vet Microbiol*. 2012;160:290.
3. Li S, et al. *Arch Virol*. 2013;158:1987.
4. Opriessnig T, et al. *Vet Microbiol*. 2013;163:177.
5. Wang F, et al. *Virus Genes*. 2010;41:305.
6. Wolf VH, et al. *Genet Mol Res*. 2008;7:509.
7. Csagoia A, et al. *Arch Virol*. 2012;157:1003.
8. Xiao CT, et al. *Vet Microbiol*. 2013;161:325.
9. Cheung AK, et al. *Arch Virol*. 2010;155:801.
10. Lau SK, et al. *J Gen Virol*. 2008;89:1840.
11. Tse H, et al. *PLoS ONE*. 2011;26:e25619.
12. Xiao CT, et al. *Vet Microbiol*. 2012;160:290.
13. Szelei J, et al. *Emerg Infect Dis*. 2010;16:561.
14. Huang L, et al. *Virol J*. 2010;7:333.
15. Zhang HB, et al. *Epidemiol Infect*. 2011;139:1581.
16. Ndze VN, et al. *Infect Genet Evol*. 2013;17:277.
17. Streck AF, et al. *Berl Munch Tierartzl Wschr*. 2013;124:242.
18. Streck AF, et al. *Arch Virol*. 2013;158:1173.
19. Miao L-F, et al. *Vet Microbiol*. 2009;138:145.
20. Wilhelm S, et al. *J Virol Meth*. 2006;134:257.
21. McKillen J, et al. *J Virol Meth*. 2007;140:155.

Multi-Organ Diseases Due to Protozoal Infection

SARCOCYSTOSIS (SARCOSPORIDIOSIS)

SYNOPSIS

Etiology *Sarcocystis* species. There are numerous species, with various carnivore species as their final host, but usually a specific intermediate host species.

Epidemiology High prevalence of infection in most areas. Source of infection is feces from carnivores. Primary definitive hosts include farm dogs and cats fed raw meat,

Continued

or other carnivores if they have access to ruminant carcasses.

Clinical findings Severity of disease is dose dependent. Most infections are subclinical. Abortion and depressed growth rate. Neurologic disease and ataxia in sheep. Severe infection in some species results in carcass condemnation.

Clinical pathology Anemia and elevated concentrations of enzymes in blood associated with tissue damage during acute disease.

Lesions Nonsuppurative encephalitis in sheep with neurologic signs. Nonsuppurative encephalitis, myocarditis, and hepatitis in aborted fetus. Cysts in carcasses in chronic cases.

Diagnostic confirmation Identification of parasite microscopically in biopsy or postmortem material.

Treatment and control No effective treatment. Amprolium or salinomycin may aid in control. Proper disposal of carcasses. Raw meat not to be fed to farm dogs or cats. Control of carnivores.

Table 21-5 Definitive and intermediate hosts for *Sarcocystis* spp.–associated infections in agricultural animals

Intermediate host	*Sarcocystis* spp.	Synonyms	Definitive host
Cattle	*S. cruzi*	*S. bovicanis*	Dog, wolf, fox, raccoon, coyote
	S. hirsuta	*S. bovifelis*	Cat
	S. hominis	*S. bovihominis*	Humans
Sheep	*S. tenella*	*S. ovicanis*	Dog, coyote, fox
	S. arieticanis	–	Dog
	S. gigantica	*S. ovifelis*	Cat
	S. medusiformis	–	Cat
Goats	*S. capracanis*	–	Dog, coyote, fox
	S. hericanis	–	Dog
	S. moulei	–	Cat
Pigs	*S. miescheriana*	*S. suicanis*	Dog, raccoon, wolf
	S. suihominis	–	Human
	S. porcifelis	–	Cat
Horses	*S. bertrami*	*S. equicanis*	Dog
	–	*S. fayeri*	
	S. neurona	–	New World opossums

ETIOLOGY

Sarcocystis species are cyst-forming coccidial parasites with indirect life cycles.[1-5] They are obligate two-host apicomplexan parasites. There are numerous species, each with omnivorous or carnivorous definitive hosts. One system of naming the species identifies the intermediate and definitive host in the name (e.g., *S. bovifelis*) and has been commonly used in the literature. However, currently the organisms are known by their original names. Table 21-5 shows the currently accepted name of *Sarcocystis* species of importance in agricultural animals and their definitive hosts.

EPIDEMIOLOGY

Occurrence

In all countries where there have been surveys, the prevalence of infection in cattle, sheep, and horses approaches 100%, with a lower, but significant, infection rate in swine.[1] Clinical disease is relatively rare.

Source of Infection

Sarcocystis spp. have an obligatory prey–predator life cycle in which the definitive host is a predator or scavenger.[1,2] The **carnivorous definitive host** becomes infected by ingesting tissue from a suitable intermediate host that contains mature sarcocysts. Following ingestion, bradyzoites are released from the sarcocyst in the stomach and intestine, and they transform into micro- and macrogamonts. The microgamonts (male) mature to release microgametes, which fertilize the macrogamont to form a zygote and then an oocyst. Within the intestine, the oocyst sporulates to produce two **sporocysts**. The sporulated oocyst ruptures in the intestine. Sporocysts (each containing four sporozoites) are passed in the feces and are directly infective to the intermediate host.

The prepatent period is variable, approximately 14 days, and there is no illness in the carnivore host in association with this cycle. However, the replicative cycle of the parasite in the intestine results in the production of large numbers of sporocysts in the feces, and the infection can be **patent for a relatively long period**. Intermediate hosts become infected by **ingesting sporulated sporocysts** in the food or water.[1,2]

Risk Factors

Climate

Sporocysts develop and maturate before excretion in feces, and they are quite resistant to environmental factors. Under experimental conditions, they can survive freezing, but they are susceptible to desiccation. Consequently, they might overwinter in the environment. Some studies have shown a lower herd prevalence of sarcocystosis in cattle in arid and semiarid environments compared with cattle from temperate and tropical areas, which might be a consequence of relative aridity and a lower density of definitive and intermediate hosts for *Sarcocystis* spp. in arid climatic zones.[1]

Species of *Sarcocystis*

Individual species vary in their **pathogenicity** and in their ability to produce clinical disease in intermediate hosts. In cattle, for example, *S. cruzi* is considerably more pathogenic than *S. hominis.*[1,2]

S. tenella is the most pathogenic species of sheep, and *S. capricanis* for goats; naturally occurring clinical disease in sheep is not observed with *S. gigantea* or *S. medusiformis.*[5] There is a strong correlation between the number of sporocysts ingested and the severity of disease. The size of the sarcocyst that occurs in the tissues of the intermediate host also varies with the infecting species. Those from cats and occurring in sheep (*S. gigantea, S. medusiformis*) or cattle (*S. hirsuta*) are of particular economic importance because they produce macroscopically visible sarcocysts that can result in meat condemnation. *S. cruzi* is pathogenic but produces microscopic sarcocysts in muscle and will escape gross detection at meat inspection.

Farm Dogs

There is a positive association between herds infected with *Sarcocystis* and the presence of working dogs on a farm, the practice of leaving carcasses in the field, and the feeding of dogs with raw meat.[1,2] Virtually all reported clinical cases of sarcocystosis in cattle in the literature record that the dogs on a farm were fed offal or uncooked beef. Housing of dogs and cattle in the same shed or area can be linked to an increased risk for infection and clinical disease, and cattle pastured close to farm buildings where there are dogs are at greater risk. The presence of foxes on farms is also strongly associated with *Sarcocystis* infection in those herds that leave carcasses on the field.

Cats

The main risk for cat-associated sarcocystosis is the farm cat that is fed raw meat. Farm cats use hay barns as dens and can contaminate hay and other feedstuffs.[1,2] Feral cats have the potential to distribute sporocysts widely in the grazing environment; however, the presence of feral cats on a farm may not increase the risk for *Sarcocystis* infection of cattle because scavenged sheep or cattle carcasses are a relatively unimportant part of the diet of feral cats.

Stocking Density

The risk for infection with *Sarcocystis* is higher with higher stocking densities,[4] which might reflect a more intense contamination of pastures by working dogs. Cattle on farms that graze sheep and cattle on the same pastures are less likely to be infected.

Economic Importance

The major economic loss occurs with those sarcocysts that produce macroscopic cysts and meat condemnation, although acute outbreaks of sarcosporidiosis have been reported. More severe infection can depress growth rates, and there is a greater risk for abortion in infected herds.

PATHOGENESIS

In the intermediate host, sporozoites are released from ingested sporocysts in the small intestine, where they penetrate the mucosa and enter the endothelial cells of blood vessels. The schizogony stages and the distribution of merozoites vary according to *Sarcocystis* species, but in cattle endothelial infection is followed by **parasitemia**, with merozoites subsequently localizing in striated muscles (usually) or nervous tissue, where they develop into sarcocysts. Immature sarcocysts can be found in muscle 45 to 60 days following ingestion of sporocysts and are infective at approximately 70 days.[2]

Schizogony in the endothelial cells of the arterioles and capillaries results in **widespread hemorrhage** and anemia. Fever is associated with the parasitemia, and in the experimental disease it coincides with the time of maturation and rupture of schizonts.[2] The **vascular lesion** appears to be an essential part of the disease's pathogenesis. It has been proposed that the parasite produces growth retardation as a result of changes in plasma concentrations of somatostatin and growth hormone and changes in cytokine interactions with the endocrine system.[1]

The severity of the illness and the degree of infection of tissues at postmortem appear to relate to **infective dose**. The number of asymptomatic infections probably reflects the early ingestion of a few sporocysts that provoke a strong immunity to subsequent challenge. When groups of animals that have not been exposed to infection previously are suddenly exposed to large numbers of sporocysts, originating from dogs and cats, outbreaks of disease are likely to occur.

CLINICAL FINDINGS

Infection and disease can occur at all ages. Clinical disease may be more severe in situations where there is **intercurrent nutritional stress**, and copper deficiency may be an exacerbating factor. Monensin is suspected of being able to potentiate recent infections to cause a severe myositis.[1,2]

Cattle

Acute illness is recorded with experimental infections, but it is rarely seen or recognized in the field. Illness commences with a rise in temperature and heart rate, followed by anorexia, anemia, weight loss, a fall in milk production, nervousness, muscle twitching, hypersalivation, lameness, abortion, and, in heavy infections, death. The agent is an occasional cause of nonsuppurative encephalomyelitis in cattle and manifests with ataxia and recumbency.

Chronic disease in cattle is manifest by poor weight gains; loss of hair of the neck, rump, and the switch of the tail (**"rat-tail"**); anemia; and/or abortion.

Sheep

In sheep, naturally occurring sarcocystosis has been associated with *S. tenella* and *S. arieticanis* and presents primarily as a **neurologic disorder**, with muscle weakness, trembling, ataxia of varying severity, followed by hindlimb paresis or flaccid paralysis and lateral recumbency. All ages of sheep can be affected, although lambs under 6 months of age are most susceptible.

Infection may also be manifest with depressed growth, reduced wool growth, and anemia. Less common manifestations include signs of congestive heart failure associated with endocardial and myocardial infection. Infestation of the muscle of the esophagus in sheep is thought to be a cause of **esophageal dysfunction** and regurgitation in sheep.[1,2]

Swine

Disease does not seem to be associated natural infections. Sarcocystosis produced experimentally in pigs is manifested by cutaneous purpura on the snout, ears, and buttocks, and dyspnea, tremor, and weakness or recumbency.[1] There is evidence that the breed of pig affects the severity of disease with experimental infections and also the subsequent severity of the parasite burden.

Abortion and Perinatal Fatality

Fetal infection, with abortion or neonatal mortality, is recorded in both cattle and sheep when pregnant animals are infected experimentally or naturally with pathogenic species or strains.

CLINICAL PATHOLOGY

Characteristic laboratory findings for systemic disease include a responsive anemia, a prolonged prothrombin time, and high titers of antibody to *Sarcocystis*. Blood creatine phosphokinase, lactic dehydrogenase, and aspartate aminotransferase are significantly elevated. Indirect hemagglutination (IHA) and ELISA tests can be used for serologic surveys, although there are limitations with the specificity immunologic assays. Many animals have been exposed to *Sarcocystis* spp., and serologic examination cannot differentiate reliably current infection from past infection or exposure, and there are problems with serologic cross-reactivity.

NECROPSY FINDINGS

Emaciation, lymphadenopathy, laminitis, anemia, and ascites can be present, but an obvious feature is the presence of petechial and ecchymotic hemorrhages throughout the body.[2] There are also erosions and ulcerations in the oral cavity and esophagus, likely as a result of microvascular damage. Cysts of *S. gigantica* on the esophagus of sheep are usually visible with the naked eye. Microscopically, schizonts are found in endothelial cells throughout the body, and hemorrhages, lymphocytic infiltration, and edema are observed in heart, brain, liver, lung, kidney, and striated muscle. Death is probably a result of the severe necrotizing myocarditis that occurs. There is an association between **eosinophilic myositis** and sarcosporidiosis, but this relationship is not proven in all cases.

In sheep presenting with **neurologic disease,** there may be no findings at gross postmortem examination, but a nonsuppurative encephalomyelitis is evident upon histologic examination.[1,2] Aborted bovine fetuses show nonsuppurative encephalitis, myocarditis, and/or hepatitis.

Different options are available to achieve a definitive diagnosis of the *Sarcocystis* species involved, including animal transmission studies, immunohistochemistry, electron microscopy, and/or PCR. Although such techniques are seldom used for routine diagnosis, there have been some efforts toward developing specific and sensitive molecular diagnostic tools.[3-5]

Samples for Confirmation of Diagnosis

- **Histology**—formalin-fixed heart, skeletal muscle (several sites, and tongue, diaphragm, and masseter muscle) (light microscopy)

DIFFERENTIAL DIAGNOSIS

Clinical diagnosis of disease can be difficult because of the nonspecific signs observed and the widespread prevalence of infection. Sarcosporidiosis is a consideration in the examination of problems of fever and anemia of undetermined origin in cattle and of ill-thrift in cattle or sheep.

The examination of muscle biopsies can aid in the determination of the presence of infection, but still begs the question of its relationship with disease.

The differential diagnoses for abortion are covered under brucellosis of cattle and sheep. Causes of encephalitis and ataxia in sheep are listed under those headings.

TREATMENT

No approved treatment is available, but **amprolium or salinomycin** may relieve clinical signs.[1] Amprolium 100 mg/kg BW, given daily, can reduce the severity of infection in experimentally infected calves and sheep and might be used to control outbreaks in sheep. Treatment of experimentally infected calves with salinomycin (4 mg/kg BW daily; in divided doses for 30 days) can reduce the severity of disease. Monensin may have a similar ameliorating effect, but is also suspected to exacerbate muscle lesions. Oxytetracycline, at very high dose rates, and halofuginone might be effective in acute infections.[1]

CONTROL

Control is challenging because it involves the **separation of carnivores from stock**, which is not possible on most farms. However, infection in farm dogs and cats can be reduced if all meat fed to them is thoroughly cooked. Feral canids and felids should be controlled, and livestock carcasses should not be left on paddocks. Prior exposure to small numbers of pathogenic sarcocysts produces a strong immunity, but no vaccine is readily or commercially available.

FURTHER READING

Dubey JP, Speer CA, Fayer R. *Sarcocystosis of Animals and Man*. Boca Raton, Florida: CRC Press; 1989.

Pozio E. Epidemiology and control prospects of foodborne parasitic zoonoses in the European Union. *Parassitologia*. 2008;50:17-24.

Tappe D, Abdullah S, Heo CC, Kannan Kutty M, Latif B. Human and animal invasive muscular sarcocystosis in Malaysia - recent cases, review and hypotheses. *Trop Biomed*. 2013;30:355-366.

REFERENCES

1. Radostits O, et al. Diseases associated with protozoa. In: *Veterinary Medicine: A Textbook of the Disease of Cattle, Horses, Sheep, Goats and Pigs*. 10th ed. London: W.B. Saunders; 2007:1507.
2. Dubey JP, Lindsay DS. *Vet Clin North Am Food A*. 2006;22:645.
3. Moré G, et al. *Vet Parasitol*. 2011;177:162.
4. Moré G, et al. *Vet Parasitol*. 2013;197:85.
5. Pritt B, et al. *J Food Prot*. 2008;71:2144.

TOXOPLASMOSIS

SYNOPSIS

Etiology Toxoplasma gondii.

Epidemiology Infection from the ingestion of oocytes excreted in the feces of cats. Any vertebrate can acquire infection from ingestion of different stages of T. gondii.

Clinical findings Abortion and stillbirths in ewes is the major veterinary manifestation; other manifestations can be neonatal mortality, encephalitis and/or pneumonia. Major importance as a zoonosis.

Pathologic findings:

- **Lesions**—granulomatous lesions in organs of all species, with abortions, placentitis, and focal necrotic lesions in brain, liver, and kidney of aborted fetus.

Diagnosis Detection of the parasite in tissues or tissue fluids. Serologic and DNA-based tests, which vary in diagnostic sensitivity and specificity.

Treatment Not usually indicated in livestock. Sulfamethazine and pyrimethamine in abortion outbreak.

Control Reduce exposure to infective stages, including oocysts. In pregnant sheep, prophylactic feeding of monensin or decoquinate; vaccination.

ETIOLOGY

The causative agent *Toxoplasma gondii* is cyst-forming coccidial parasite (*Apicomplexa*). Felids (cat family) are **definitive hosts**, and vertebrates are intermediate hosts. Different strains can differ in their virulence and epidemiology.[1,2]

T. gondii has three infective stages:

1. Tachyzoites—rapidly replicating stage of the parasite during the acute phase of infection (endodyogeny) in the intermediate or accidental host
2. Bradyzoites—slowly replicating or dormant stage of the parasite (usually within a cyst or pseudocyst) during the chronic phase of infection in the intermediate or accidental host
3. Oocysts (containing sporocysts and sporozoites)—present in cat feces

Oocysts are the **infective stage** of importance in farm animals, and they are the only environmental infective stage for herbivores. Oocysts excreted in the feces of cats can survive in soil for months or years and are ingested by the intermediate (livestock) host. The parasite (sporozoite stage) invades any host cell, with the exception of nonnucleated erythrocytes, and undergoes tachyzoite replication (acute phase of infection). Any tissue (including nervous system, myocardium, lung tissue, and placenta) of the host or fetus can be infected and affected. An inoculum of as few as 10 oocysts can be infective to goats. Following the acute phase of infection, as host immunity develops, the replication rate decreases. The bradyzoites replicate slowly within cells and then stop replicating to become dormant within cysts ("tissue cysts" containing many bradyzoites). These cysts, containing live bradyzoites, are a source of infection to carnivorous or omnivorous animals (including pigs and humans).

EPIDEMIOLOGY

Occurrence

Toxoplasmosis occurs in domesticated and wild animals and birds in most parts of the world, although surveys indicate considerable variation in prevalence.[2-4] Although some studies indicate a relatively high seroprevalence in some farm animals, infection is often subclinical. With the exception of abortion and neonatal disease in sheep, *T. gondii* has limited importance as a cause of disease in farm animals. *T. gondii* has major importance as a **zoonotic parasite.**

Source of Infection

Cat Feces

The source of infection in sheep, pigs, and other livestock is **oocysts** excreted in the feces from felids. In almost all agricultural areas, the feces originate from domestic or feral cats.

Cats become infected as a result of ingesting tissues from intermediate hosts infected with tachyzoites or bradyzoites (within cysts) and then shed oocysts in the feces. All vertebrates can act as intermediate hosts; rodents and small birds are common intermediate hosts for infection to cats. For instance, rodents pass the parasite from generation to generation through congenital infection and thus can provide a reservoir of infection in an area for a long time. Cats ingest infected rodents and develop an intestinal infection, leading to oocyst excretion into the environment. The prevalence of infection is highest in young cats hunting for the first time. Following infection of the cat, the period of excretion of oocysts is short, usually ~2 weeks, but it can be high, with several million oocysts being excreted during patency. In a given environment, the number of cats excreting oocysts in their feces at any point in time is likely to be quite small, but the contamination of the environment over time can be significant.

Domestic and barn cats in farm environments tend to nest and to defecate in hay and straw mows, grain stores, or loose piles of commodity feeds, thus providing the potential for direct contamination of livestock feeds with *T. gondii* oocysts.[5] Fields fertilized with manure and bedding contaminated with cat feces can also be a source of infection. **Feral cats** bury feces superficially in the soil, but contamination can spread, for example, via the elements or invertebrates, to pasture and be ingested by livestock. Feral cats can have territories of up to 250 acres and are capable of widely distributing oocysts of *T. gondii.*[1] Oocysts may be found in feed, water, and soil in the vicinity of livestock units.

Other Sources

Oocysts are also an important source of infection to swine, although it is possible for swine to be infected by the ingestion of tachyzoites or bradyzoites present in meat (**dead rodents**, cannibalized piglets, etc.) or through the ingestion of blood while **tail- or ear-biting**. *T. gondii* infection has been shown in all wildlife mammalian species tested in the environment of swine units. Direct sheep-to-sheep transmission by close contact with grossly infected placenta and transmission via the semen of infected rams could occur but is not thought to be of significance. There is some evidence that *T. gondii* can be present in the placental tissue from sheep following successful pregnancies, suggesting that congenital infection perpetuates infection in sheep flocks in the absence of cats.[3]

Risk Factors

Pathogen Risk Factors

Oocysts are very resistant to external influences and can often survive in the environment for at least 1 year. They can **overwinter** in cold climates but are more susceptible to desiccation. Fifty grams of infected cat feces can contain as many as 10 million oocysts, and infection in farm animals can be established by the ingestion of fewer than 40 oocysts.[1] Oocysts are destroyed by exposure to high temperatures and freezing.

Environmental and Management Risk Factors

In sheep, a high rate of infection can relate to areas of **high rainfall**, allowing increased survival of oocysts on pasture. The prevalence of infection in small ruminants is much lower in hot, arid countries than in regions with wet climates.

Sheep raised in **cat-free areas** have almost no toxoplasmosis, whereas sheep raised in similar environments with cats can have a high level of exposure or infection.[1] In many recorded toxoplasmosis outbreaks with high prevalence rates in sheep and goats, there was a link to stored feed contaminated with cat feces. Cat access to sows is also a risk factor for toxoplasmosis in swine.[4]

Other management risk factors include **housing**. Swine housed outdoors can be at a greater risk for infection in some areas. Prevalence is low in sows that are kept indoors. Infected pork is a significant source of infection to humans, and the trend to outdoor rearing on free-range farms may increase the risk for human infection.

Experimental Studies

Sheep

Experimental disease can be achieved by challenge with oocysts, tissue cysts, or tachyzoites.[1] Ewes may show a febrile response during the parasitemic phase 5 to 12 days following inoculation. Abortion and fetal mortality occur in sheep that suffer a primary infection during pregnancy. The parasite invades the placenta and can be detected in the fetus between 5 and 10 days following the onset of parasitemia. Infection may result in resorption, abortion, or the birth of stillborn or congenitally infected live lambs. Infection in early pregnancy (less than 60 days), before the fetus acquires immunologic competence, usually results in embryonic death and resorption and a barren ewe. Infection in mid-pregnancy usually results in abortion and the birth of stillborn lambs, whereas ewes infected in late pregnancy (more than 110 days) may give birth to live but congenitally infected lambs.

Cattle

Cattle are **relatively resistant** to infection.[2] Diarrhea, anorexia, poor weight gain, depression, weakness, fever, and/or dyspnea follow challenge infection of calves with pathogenic strains. Using strains of low virulence, there is a mild fever and lymphadenopathy, and the parasite is detectable only in the lymph nodes for only a few weeks. Adult cows are usually not susceptible to infection, and it is apparent that cattle do not readily acquire persistent *T. gondii* infection. *T. gondii* is not important in causing abortion or clinical disease in cattle. It is probable that many cases previously diagnosed as bovine toxoplasmosis were actually cases of neosporosis or sarcosporidiosis.

Other Ruminants

High numbers of oocysts fed to (susceptible) goats cause a febrile, anorectic, fatal illness and pregnant goats abort. The pathogenesis of the abortion is as for sheep. Disease in buffalo calves is described as peracute, with pulmonary consolidation, necrotic foci in all organs, and fluid accumulations in body cavities.

Pigs

Infection is relatively readily established in pigs,[4] but it is usually not associated with disease or only with a short period of fever and growth suppression. Congenital toxoplasmosis is not readily induced experimentally. Young pigs (less than 12 weeks of age) are considerably more susceptible than older pigs. Infections induced by tissue cysts are usually less severe than those induced by the ingestion of oocysts.

Horses

Horses appear to be **relatively nonsusceptible** to *T. gondii* and toxoplasmosis.

Economic Importance

Abortion and neonatal mortality in sheep and goats are the major clinical manifestations of toxoplasmosis in livestock and result when primary infection occurs during pregnancy. Ovine abortion and neonatal mortality as a result of toxoplasmosis are important problems in New Zealand, Australia, Canada, the United States, and the United Kingdom; in most countries, they are second in importance only to chlamydial abortion. Perinatal mortality rates (including abortions and neonatal death) in affected flocks may be as high as 50%. Toxoplasmosis can be a primary cause of economic losses in flocks with an abortion problem. Toxoplasmosis of goats is also associated mummification of fetuses and perinatal death.

Zoonotic Implications

Humans are accidental intermediate hosts for *T. gondii*, and approximately one-half of the population in the United States is infected.[1] Infection can result from the ingestion of oocysts from cat feces that contaminate waterways or food, that contaminate the hair of domestic dogs and cats, or that are inadvertently ingested because of poor hygiene practices. However, the major risk for human infection relates to the ingestion of bradyzoites and/or tachyzoites in **meat** or tissues that are eaten or handled. The risk is with raw or undercooked meats. Adequate freezing and/or cooking will kill the parasite. Beef is a minor source of infection, with pork and, to a lesser degree, sheep meat posing a greater risk. Tachyzoites can be passed in the milk of goats challenged with oocysts; **raw goat milk** has some public health risk for toxoplasmosis, although the risk is low.

Usually, *T. gondii* infection in immunocompetent humans is asymptomatic. However, disease can occur in people suffering from **AIDS** or malignancy, in those treated with cytotoxic or immunosuppressive drugs, and in children and the elderly. There is also the risk in **pregnant women** for abortion or congenital infection of the fetus with resultant hydrocephalus, intracranial calcification, and retinochoroiditis. Maternal infection in the first and second trimesters may result in severe congenital toxoplasmosis and death of the fetus in utero and subsequent abortion. Infection late during pregnancy may result in the birth of an apparently normal child who is at risk of developing chorioretinitis later in life.

Toxoplasmosis poses an **occupational risk** for veterinarians, farmers, and slaughterhouse workers who handle infected tissues, such as placenta, brain, or muscle. For instance, the risk can be high during contact with lambing ewes in infected flocks; veterinarians and farm workers, particularly if pregnant or immunocompromised, should take precautions to avoid infection when handling infected material.

PATHOGENESIS

T. gondii is an **intracellular parasite** that attacks most tissues and organs, with predilection for the **reticuloendothelial and central nervous systems.**[2-4] Sporozoites from oocysts or bradyzoites from tissue cysts invade and penetrate cells of the intermediate host by an active process and then replicate as tachyzoites, initially in intestinal epithelial cells. After invasion of various cell types, the tachyzoites multiply (rapidly during endodyogeny) and eventually fill and destroy cells. Following their release from ruptured cells, liberated tachyzoites reach other organs via the bloodstream. **Parasitemia** commences ~5 days following infection and declines with the development of immunity 2 to 3 weeks after infection. At this stage, the parasite undergoes bradyzoite replication within cells/tissues to produce tissue cysts.

The presentation of disease varies depending on the organ(s) affected and on whether the disease is congenital or acquired. The principal manifestations are encephalitis when infection is **congenital** and febrile exanthema with pneumonitis and enterocolitis when heavy infections occur **postnatally**. However, most infections are asymptomatic; tissue cysts can be found in many animals and appear to cause no harm. When the immunity of the animal declines, because of stress, disease, immunosuppressive therapy or an immunocompromised state, tissue cysts can rupture, and granulomatous lesions can develop. Immunodeficient or immunocompromised animals can develop severe disease.

Pregnant Sheep and Goats

Abortion and fetal mortality occur in sheep or goats that contract a primary infection during pregnancy. In the dam, the infection is limited by a developing immune response, but it is not limited in the placenta or in the immuno-incompetent fetus. The fetus, and the ability of the fetus and its associated placenta, to mount a protective response depend on the age of the fetus at the time of infection.

Immunocompetence against *T. gondii* does not usually develop before 60 days of gestation. Infection in early or midpregnancy results in fetal death, with resorption or mummification. Some lambs infected in midpregnancy may survive to near term and be stillborn, or they may survive to parturition but are weak and die shortly after birth. Parasite replication in the placenta results in multiple foci of necrosis, and these lesions likely contribute to abortion or to the birth of weak lambs. In addition, congenital infection of the central nervous system may result in locomotory and sucking dysfunction. Only sheep that become infected during pregnancy abort. With infection in late pregnancy, the fetus can mount an immune response and is usually born live, infected, and immune. Infection of pregnant and nonpregnant sheep usually provokes sufficient protective immunity to prevent abortion in future pregnancies.

CLINICAL FINDINGS

The clinical syndrome and the course of toxoplasmosis vary a great deal among species and among age groups.[3-5] The only clinical syndrome recognized with any regularity in the field is abortion and neonatal mortality in sheep. The other, less common, syndromes are described in the following subsections.

Sheep

In sheep, although a syndrome of fever, dyspnea, generalized tremor, abortions, and stillbirths can occur,[3] the clinical manifestation of the systemic disease in the ewe is rare. The principal manifestations of toxoplasmosis in sheep are fetal resorption, abortion, the birth of mummified or stillborn lambs, neonatal death, and the birth of full-term lambs that show locomotor and sucking disorders.

Abortion commonly occurs during the last 4 weeks of pregnancy, and the rate may be as high as 50%. Full-term lambs from infected ewes may be born dead, or alive but weak, with death occurring within 3 to 4 days of birth. Lambs affected after birth show fever and dyspnea, but a fatal outcome is uncommon. Fetal resorption can occur in ewes infected in early pregnancy.

Goats

Toxoplasmosis of sheep and goats is similar. Caprine toxoplasmosis is manifested by perinatal deaths, including abortion and stillbirth. Systemic disease, with a high case-fatality rate, can occur, particularly in young goats.

Pigs

Pigs are **susceptible.** If an outbreak occurs, pigs of all ages can be affected.[4] Clinical signs include debility, weakness, incoordination, cough, tremor and/or diarrhea, but no fever. Young pigs can be acutely ill, with a high fever of 40° to 42°C (104–107°F); they develop diarrhea and can die after several weeks. Pigs of 2 to 4 weeks of age have additional signs, including wasting, dyspnea, coughing, and nervous signs, particularly ataxia. Pregnant sows commonly **abort**; piglets are premature or **stillborn**, or they survive and can develop disease at 1 to 3 weeks of age. Toxoplasmosis should be considered in the case of a resident problem of abortion and stillbirth in a pig herd.

Cattle

Rare bovine toxoplasmosis may be manifested in fever, dyspnea, and nervous signs, including ataxia and hyperexcitability, in the early stages, followed by extreme lethargy. Stillborn or weak calves that die soon after birth may also occur. However, usually, toxoplasmosis does not play a significant role in bovine abortion. Congenitally affected calves can show fever, dyspnea, coughing, sneezing, nasal discharge, clonic convulsions, grinding of the teeth, and/or tremor of the head and neck. Death can occur after 2 to 6 days.

Horses

Toxoplasmosis is **rare** in horses.

CLINICAL PATHOLOGY

Serologic tests available for the detection of humoral antibodies to *T. gondii* include the Sabin–Feldman dye test, the indirect hemagglutination assay, the indirect fluorescent antibody test (IFAT), the modified agglutination test (MAT), the latex agglutination test (LAT), the enzyme-linked immunosorbent assay (ELISA), and the immunosorbent agglutination assay test (IAAT).[2-4] Serologic tests are commonly used to estimate the seroprevalence of *T. gondii* exposure or infection in animal populations, but their **sensitivity and specificity can vary** considerably depending many factors, including the actual assay used and the species of animal being tested.

Abortion

Serologic testing to establish toxoplasmosis as the cause of abortion is of limited value. A test-negative titer will likely rule out toxoplasmosis, but because serum antibody can persist for some years, a test-positive titer will only indicate that an animal has been exposed to or infected with *T. gondii* at some stage of its life. Seroprevalence can be high in sheep and swine. **Rising titers** in paired samples are more informative but are likely of limited value for the diagnosis of *T. gondii*-related abortion in sheep, where infection and serum antibody responses may precede the abortion storm. It is informative to test **pleural or peritoneal fluid** of aborted fetuses for the presence of antibody or nucleic acids of *T. gondii*. PCR assays can be used to specifically detect or quantitate *T. gondii* DNA or RNA in infected fetal and any other tissues from suspected cases.

NECROPSY FINDINGS

Macroscopic lesions consist of **multiple foci of necrosis in various organs,** including the lungs, brain, spinal cord, liver, spleen, kidneys, and heart. Interstitial pneumonia hydrothorax, ascites, lymphadenitis, and intestinal ulceration may be observed. Microscopically, foci of **coagulative necrosis** are present, with little evidence of inflammation, except in the lungs, where there is interstitial pneumonia, and in the nervous system, where there is usually nonsuppurative meningoencephalitis. Stages (tachyzoites, bradyzoites, and/or cysts) of *T. gondii* can be found in the viscera and/or brain.[11,12]

Abortion

In **sheep**, there may be involvement of the uterine wall, the **placenta,** and the fetus. The lesions in the fetal lambs are usually limited to focal necrosis in brain, liver, kidney, and lungs; characteristic lesions are common and severe in the **placenta.**[1] The lesions are confined to the cotyledons and consist of **multiple white foci of necrosis in the villi.** On histologic examination, there is multifocal necrosis and desquamation of trophoblastic epithelium, sometimes with calcification. *T. gondii* stages can be found in the placenta and other organs

In **swine**, the prominent lesions are necrotic placentitis, nonsuppurative encephalomyelitis, and/or myocardial degeneration. In contrast to sheep, grossly visible areas of necrosis are not present in the placenta, but numerous organisms may be visible on microscopic examination of the placenta.

Immunohistochemical staining can be used to identify the parasite in formalin-fixed material. Serologic testing of fetal thoracic fluid can be useful in those fetuses that are immunocompetent at the time of abortion. PCR can be used for the specific detection of *T. gondii* DNA in tissues and can be used on autolyzed tissue.[2-4] On rare occasions, a diagnostic bioassay can be performed to induce infection and propagate the parasite in specific-pathogen-free (SPF) rodents, which is a very sensitive but time-consuming method. Aseptically collected brain, lung, and diaphragm is homogenized and administered orally, or by intraperitoneal or intracerebral injection to mice, or orally to SPF cats. A positive diagnosis depends on the presence of *T. gondii* cysts in the brains of the mice ~8 weeks after the inoculation or the excretion of oocysts in the feces of infected cats. Cats are a more sensitive assay because of the volume of tissue that can be tested. The mouse bioassay is useful to propagate *T. gondii* for subsequent molecular or genetic analyses or in vitro experiments.

Samples for Diagnostic Testing

- **Parasitology**—fresh or chilled brain, lung, placenta
- **Serology**—fetal thoracic fluid
- **Histology**—placental cotyledons, lung, liver, brain, spinal cord, kidney, heart

DIFFERENTIAL DIAGNOSIS

Toxoplasmosis is rarely considered in a primary diagnostic list other than with problems of abortion and associated neonatal mortality. The differential diagnosis of abortion in cattle is dealt with under brucellosis, in sheep under brucellosis, and in pigs under leptospirosis. The causes of encephalitis and pneumonitis in animals are listed under respective headings.

TREATMENT

Treatment with a combination of sulfamethazine and pyrimethamine (administered over 3 days for three periods with an interval of 5 days between the start of each treatment period) has proved effective in mitigating the effects of experimentally induced toxoplasmosis in pregnant ewes. This therapy should be considered in the face of an outbreak of abortion associated with toxoplasmosis.[1] These drugs appear to be effective against proliferating tachyzoites in the acute stage of toxoplasmosis, but they will not eliminate infection and will have limited activity on bradyzoites within tissue cysts.

CONTROL

There are two key issues in the control of toxoplasmosis in agricultural animals. The first is to reduce the economic impact of disease; the second is to reduce the risk for human disease associated with consumption of infected meat.

Cat Control

The elimination of cats from the farm environment will preclude feed contamination and contamination of pasture areas. Although it is possible to **ban domestic cats** from the farm, this will not usually eliminate the risk of toxoplasmosis because of the range of activities of cats from adjacent areas, the presence of feral cats, and the possibility of spread of oocysts.[5] Nevertheless, risk of infection/disease will be reduced by eliminating cats from the farm environment or restricting them to **neutered** animals. Where **possible, feeds should be stored in cat-proof areas.** In swine units, rodent control and preventing the access of pigs to any **carrion** are key measures. On farms, any animal carcass or material (e.g., placenta and fetus) linked to suspected or confirmed cases of toxoplasmosis should be eliminated immediately,

Serologic Monitoring

Serologic testing can be used to estimate seroprevalence and seroconversion in sows housed indoors and outdoors, and it may assist in assessing whether changes need to be made to farm management practices. Such testing can also be employed to assess seroprevalence and monitor specific antibody titers in sheep to support a risk management strategy against toxoplasmosis and to assess whether antitoxoplasmal drugs or vaccination should be implemented for prevention/protection.

There is an effective and long-lasting immunity following primary *T. gondii* infection, and ewes that have aborted should be kept in the flock. Exposure of ewes to natural infection in a contaminated environment before breeding would be possible means of preventing toxoplasmosis but is difficult to control.

Prophylaxis

Feeding **monensin** at a dose of 15 mg/animal per day during the first 100 days of pregnancy has been shown to reduce lamb loss following experimental infection with *T. gondii,* as has decoquinate fed at 2 mg/kg daily.[1] **Decoquinate** is more palatable and has less risk of toxicity. Preventative medication offers an option for ewes that are test-negative for anti-*T. gondii* serum antibodies and likely to be exposed in pregnancy to feed, water, or an environment contaminated with oocysts. Both drugs are best fed to ewes before they encounter infection and are not effective as therapeutic agents.

Vaccination

Tachyzoites from an attenuated strain of *T. gondii* are used in a vaccine to protect sheep, which is available commercially in some countries.[3,6-8] Such tachyzoites readily infect seronegative sheep but do not initiate chronic infection or tissue cysts, and the parasite cannot be detected in muscle or brain 6 weeks after vaccination. Ewes should be vaccinated at least 3 weeks before mating, and a single injection will protect for the life of the sheep. In flocks where toxoplasmosis is a cause of lamb loss, initial vaccination of the whole flock, followed by vaccination of replacement ewes, is a better economic option than only vaccinating replacement ewes.[3] Vaccination does not completely protect pregnant ewes against parasitemia or the infection of the fetus following challenge with virulent *T. gondii* oocysts, but there is a significant reduction in the birth rates of dead lambs. It has been postulated that vaccination results in reduced numbers of tachyzoites invading the gravid uterus or fetus, with a consequent reduced potential for inducing significant pathologic changes in the placenta and the fetus. Immunity appears to be cell mediated. Experiments with an adjuvanted vaccine in pigs show protection from clinical challenge and a reduction in recoverable *Toxoplasma* from tissues of vaccinated challenged pigs.[1]

Reduction of Zoonotic Risk From Food and Water

Oocysts from cat feces are an important source of human infection, as is meat from sheep, swine, and sometimes from other livestock animals that are infected with tachyzoites or bradyzoite cysts.[2] The implementation of control procedures on farms will reduce infection risk, and the major aspect will be to reduce the numbers of cats on farms or eliminate them. The infectivity of meat can be destroyed by freezing, proper cooking, or irradiation. Reviews of other strategies for the control of food-borne toxoplasmosis are readily available.[9,10]

FURTHER READING

Buxton D, Maley SW, Wright SE, et al. *Toxoplasma gondii* and ovine toxoplasmosis: new aspects of an old story. *Vet Parasitol.* 2007;149:25-28.
Elsheikha HM. Congenital toxoplasmosis: priorities for further health promotion action. *Public Health.* 2008;122:335-353.
Hill D, Dubey JP. *Toxoplasma gondii.* Transmission diagnosis and prevention. *Clin Microbiol Infect.* 2002;8:634-640.
Innes EA, Vermeulen AN. Vaccination as a control strategy against the coccidial parasites *Eimeria, Toxoplasma* and *Neospora. Parasitology.* 2006;133(suppl):S145-S168.
Montoya JG, Remington JS. Management of *Toxoplasma gondii* infection during pregnancy. *Clin Infect Dis.* 2008;47:554-566.

REFERENCES

1. Radostits O, et al. Diseases associated with protozoa. In: *Veterinary Medicine: A Textbook of the Disease of Cattle, Horses, Sheep, Goats and Pigs.* 10th ed. London: W.B. Saunders; 2007:1518.
2. Dubey JP. *J Eukaryot Microbiol.* 2008;55:467.
3. Dubey JP. *Vet Parasitol.* 2009;163:1.
4. Dubey JP. *Vet Parasitol.* 2009;164:89.
5. Elmore SA, et al. *Trends Parasitol.* 2010;26:190.
6. Innes EA, et al. *Vaccine.* 2007;25:5495.
7. Garcia JL. *Expert Rev Vaccines.* 2009;8:215.
8. Innes EA, et al. *Mem Inst Oswaldo Cruz.* 2009;104:246.
9. Jones JL, Dubey JP. *Clin Infect Dis.* 2012;55:845.
10. Jones JL, Dubey JP. *Exp Parasitol.* 2010;124:10.

11. Brown CC, et al. Alimentary system. In: Maxie MG, ed. *Jubb, Kennedy and Palmer's Pathology of Domestic Animals*. Vol. 2. 5th ed. Edinburgh: Saunders; 2007:1.
12. O'Donovan J, et al. *Vet Pathol*. 2012;49:462.

THEILERIOSES

Theilerioses are those tick-borne protozoan diseases associated with *Theileria* spp. in cattle, sheep, goats, and horses and in wild and captive ungulates. The genus *Theileria* belongs to the Apicomplexa group, which includes *Babesia, Toxoplasma, Neospora,* and *Plasmodium,* among others. The life cycle of *Theileria* spp. involves cyclical development in ticks to form sporozoites; on being injected with tick saliva into the mammalian host, sporozoites develop into schizonts in leukocytes and then piroplasms (merozoites) in erythrocytes. The diseases in ruminants are characterized by fever and lymphoproliferative disorders and are associated with varying degrees of leucopenia and/or anemia.

Theileria spp. are found throughout the world, and their nomenclature and classification, although still controversial, are being gradually elucidated through molecular characterization. The important pathogens of cattle are restricted to certain geographic regions after which the diseases are named (Table 21-6). **East Coast fever** (ECF), caused by *Theileria parva,* and **tropical theileriosis (or Mediterranean Coast fever)**, caused by *T. annulata,* are the two most important theilerioses and are dealt with separately in the following discussion.

Oriental theileriosis (or Japanese theileriosis) caused by *T. orientalis* is increasingly being associated with disease outbreaks in Asia and Australia. Molecular analysis has revealed four genotypes of *T. orientalis* (ikeda, chitose, buffeli, and type 5), with the ikeda genotype being the most pathogenic.[1] The disease is transmitted by *Haemophysalis* ticks, which occur in Europe, the Mediterranean basin, Asia, and Australia. In addition, transplacental (vertical) transmission from pregnant cows to calves has been reported in some countries.

Oriental theileriosis is characterized by moderate to severe anemia in heavily parasitized cattle and moderate enlargement of lymph nodes. Outbreaks of more severe clinical signs and economic losses have been reported occasionally from India, Australia, and New Zealand.[2-4] Such outbreaks are characterized by severe anemia and heavy parasitemia, especially in European breeds of cattle, in their crossbreds, or in naïve animals moved to endemic areas. Affected animals show high fever, lacrimation, nasal discharge, swollen lymph nodes, and hemoglobinuria.[2] Abortion, significant loss in milk production, and deaths were reported in the Australian outbreaks.[3-6] Postmortem lesions include punched-out ulcers in the abomasum, enlargement of the spleen, and massive pulmonary edema, as in East Coast fever and Mediterranean Coast fever (see following discussion).

The pathogenesis of the anemia and hemoglobinuria in oriental theileriosis is not clear but may be related to a hemolytic factor in the serum of acutely affected cattle or to an oxidative damage of the red blood cell membrane leading to hemolysis, as in ovine malignant theileriosis (see following discussion).[7] European breeds are more susceptible than zebu breeds.

Methods of diagnosis include parasitologic, serologic, and PCR)assays.[8] In one study involving beef cattle in Australia, prevalence of infection was 28.1% by parasitologic method and 70.8% by PCR assay employing a region within the major piroplasm surface protein (MPSP) gene as marker.[5] With such high infection rates in clinically normal animals, it is important that calves used for the production of live vaccines against babesiosis and anaplasmosis should be free of oriental theileriosis. In Australia, concurrent treatment with primaquine phosphate and halofuginone lactate is effective for this purpose.

T. mutans, confined to Africa and the Caribbean islands, causes a usually innocuous disease (**benign theileriosis**), but it may be manifested by fever, anorexia, and anemia. Some genotypes of *T. orientalis* are also associated with subclinical infections in Asia and Australia. Another species, *T. velifera,* is associated with very mild theileriosis in tropical Africa. *Amblyomma* ticks transmit both species. *T. taurotragi* of the eland antelope is generally nonpathogenic to cattle, but it is one of the causes of **cerebral theileriosis (turning sickness)** in southern Africa (cerebral theileriosis can also be associated with *T. parva*). Parasitized lymphoblasts accumulate in cerebral, spinal, and meningeal arteries, with resultant thrombosis and infarction of affected organs. *T. taurotragi* is transmitted by *Rhipicephalus* spp.

The important pathogen of sheep and goats is *T. hirci* (synonym *T. lestoquardi*), the cause of **malignant ovine theileriosis**. The disease is enzootic from North Africa throughout the Middle East to India and China, approximately the same geographic

Table 21-6 Summary of the theilerioses of domestic ruminants

Disease	Distribution	*Theileria* spp.	Main vector
Cattle			
East coast fever	East and central Africa	*T. parva*	*Rhipicephalus appendiculatus*
Turning sickness (cerebral theileriosis)	Southern Africa	*T. parva, T. taurotragi*	*Rhipicephalus* spp.
Tropical theileriosis (Mediterranean coast fever)	Mediterranean countries Indo-China	*T. annulata*	*Hyalomma anatolicum*
Oriental theileriosis (Japanese theileriosis)	Asia, Australia	*T. orientalis* (genotype ikeda)	*Haemophysalis* spp.
Benign theileriosis	Africa/Caribbean Africa Asia	*T. mutans* *T. velifera* *T. buffeli* *T. sergenti*	*Amblyomma* spp. *Amblyomma* spp. *Haemophysalis longicornis/H. punctata*
Sheep and goats			
Malignant ovine theileriosis	North Africa, Middle East, India	*T. hirci* (*T. lestoquardi*)	*Hyalomma* spp./*Haemophysalis* spp.?
Benign theileriosis	Worldwide	*T. ovis*	*Rhipicephalus* spp.?
Horses, other equidae	East and South Africa	*T. separata*	*Rhipicephalus* spp.
Equine theileriosis	Worldwide	*T. equi*	*Boophilus microplus, Rhipicephalus* spp., *Hyalomma* spp.

region as bovine tropical theileriosis. Malignant theileriosis in sheep and goats is similar to bovine tropical theileriosis as a result of *T. annulata*. Like the latter, it is also transmitted by *Hyalomma* spp., but in China, the main vector is *Haemophysalis* spp. The disease can be acute, subacute, or chronic, depending on the resistance of the sheep or goats, and is seasonal, depending on availability of ticks. The acute disease is characterized by fever and very high mortality in 3 to 6 days. Anemia, jaundice, and enlargement of lymph nodes are characteristic, and both piroplasms and schizonts can be demonstrated in smears of blood and tissues, respectively. The anemia is severe, progressive, and hemolytic and is associated with oxidative damage.[7] In subacute and chronic cases, signs are generally less marked except for anemia and emaciation. An indirect fluorescent antibody test is available and parasites can be identified by PCR methods. Parvaquone and buparvaquone may be used to treat early cases. **Benign ovine theileriosis** is caused either by *T. ovis* or by *T. separata, T. luwenshuni*, or *T. uilenbergi*.[9] Piroplasms are found in blood, but there are no overt clinical signs.

Equine theileriosis is caused by *Theileria equi* (formerly *Babesia equi*) and has been reported from all continents, including North America, where it has reemerged as a persistent subclinical infection of horses in the United States.[10] The term *equine piroplasmosis* is used to refer to *T. equi* infection alone or concurrently with *Babesia cabali*. Horses, donkeys, camels, and zebras are affected. Transmission is by *Boophilus microplus, Rhipicephalus* spp., and *Hyalomma* spp. In addition, transplacental transmission from mare to foals is quite common. The disease is generally a benign form of theileriosis detected during routine blood examination or through serology and molecular techniques (PCR). Treatment with imidocarb dipropionate is largely successful in eliminating carrier state and transmission risk in nonendemic countries.[10]

In summary, the pathogenesis of various forms of theileriosis is dependent on the production of schizonts in lymphocytes and piroplasms in erythrocytes. Thus *T. parva, T. annulata*, and *T. hirci* produce numerous schizonts and piroplasms and are very pathogenic; *T. orientalis, T. mutans*, and *T. ovis* rarely produce schizonts but may cause varying degrees of anemia when piroplasms are many in red blood cells; and with *T. velifera* and *T. separata*, no schizonts have been described, the parasitemia is usually scanty, and the infection is mild or subclinical. Transmission is from tick saliva to the mammalian host, but cases of transplacental infection have been reported rarely for *T. orientalis* and more frequently for *T. equi*.

REFERENCES

1. Eamens G, et al. *Aust Vet J*. 2013;91:332.
2. Aparna M, et al. *Parasitol Int*. 2011;60:524.
3. Islam MK, et al. *Infect Genet Evol*. 2011;11:2095.
4. Mcfadden AM, et al. *NZ Vet J*. 2011;59:79.
5. Perera PK, et al. *Vet Parasitol*. 2013;doi:10.1016/j.vetpar.2013.06.023; [Epub ahead of print].
6. Perera PK, et al. *Parasit Vect*. 2014;7:73.
7. Nazifi S, et al. *Parasitol Res*. 2011;109:275.
8. *OIE Manual of Diagnostic Tests and Vaccines for Terrestrial Animals*. 6th ed. Paris: OIE; 2008 chapter 2.4.17:789.
9. Yin H, et al. *Trends Parasitol*. 2009;25:85.
10. Ueti MW, et al. *PLoS ONE*. 2012;7:e44713.

EAST COAST FEVER (ECF)

SYNOPSIS

Etiology *Theileria parva*, an Apicomplexa protozoon. Vector is *Rhipicephalus appendiculatus* and, rarely, *R. zambeziensis*.

Epidemiology Endemic disease of cattle in East and Central Africa; high mortality and great economic importance.

Clinical signs Fever, enlarged superficial lymph nodes, dyspnea, wasting, and terminal diarrhea.

Clinical pathology Schizonts in lymphoblasts, piroplasms in erythrocytes, serology.

Lesions Massive pulmonary edema, hydrothorax, hydropericardium, emaciation, hemorrhages, lymphadenopathy, and widespread proliferation of lymphoblastoid cells.

Differential diagnosis list

- Trypanosomosis/babesiosis/anaplasmosis
- Heartwater
- Malignant catarrhal fever/bovine virus diarrhea/rinderpest

Treatment Limited success with halofuginone, parvoquone, and tetracyclines.

Control Integrated approach involving resistant animal breeds, strategic application of acaricides, and vaccination by infection-and-treatment methods.

ETIOLOGY

East Coast fever is caused by *Theileria parva* transmitted by ticks. The genus *Theileria* belongs to the apicomplex group (see "Theilerioses"). There has been considerable naming and renaming of *T. parva* and the associated diseases in Africa. "Classic" East Coast fever (ECF) occurs in East Africa and is associated with *T. parva* transmitted from cattle to cattle by the brown ear tick, *Rhipicephalus appendiculatus*. ECF also occurs either as **corridor disease** in eastern and southern Africa or as **January disease** in central Africa. Corridor disease is transmitted from buffalo to cattle by either *R. appendiculatus* or *R. zambeziensis*, and the agent responsible used to be called *T. parva lawrencei*. Close contact between buffalo, cattle, and ticks is essential. The disease is more acute than classical ECF, but after serial passage in cattle, it is indistinguishable from classical ECF. January disease occurs mainly between January and March, and the agent was named *T. parva bovis*. The disease is also more acute than classical ECF, with death sometimes occurring within 4 days. These three clinical diseases are otherwise indistinguishable from one another, and hence the causative agents are currently referred to simply as *T. parva*.

EPIDEMIOLOGY

Occurrence

ECF affects mainly cattle but also buffalo, and occurs in 13 countries in eastern, central, and southern Africa. Its occurrence is related to the distribution of the vector tick, which has been recorded from large areas extending from southern Sudan in the north to western Zambia and eastern Zaire in the west, and to Mozambique and Zimbabwe in the south. The disease is prevalent throughout the wetter areas favoring the development of the tick, but is absent from the wet highlands in the horn of Africa. An outbreak was reported in the Comoros following importation of immunized cattle from Tanzania.[1] The disease has been eradicated from southern Africa up to the Zambezi River. The endemic scenarios range from a stable situation with high prevalence of herd infection but low fatality rates (endemic stability) to a low-prevalence/high-fatality scenario (endemic instability). Endemic stability develops in indigenous zebu cattle exposed to constant tick challenge, such as those in wetter areas, whereas endemic instability is seen with commercial production systems utilizing imported breeds or crossbreeds and in areas with a unimodal rainfall pattern that restricts tick activity. Epidemics occur when there is a breakdown in tick control, especially during the rainy season or when susceptible animals are introduced into an endemic area.

Morbidity and Case Fatality

All susceptible cattle in endemic areas are at the risk of contracting ECF unless they are vaccinated or the tick population is under stringent control. The morbidity and case-fatality rates are very high, approaching 90% to 100% in recently introduced exotic (*Bos taurus*) breeds and in previously unexposed or naive indigenous cattle. However, indigenous zebu cattle (*Bos indicus*) and African buffalo in endemic areas have a strong resistance to the disease, and calfhood mortality is around 5%.

Methods of Transmission

The vector of ECF is *Rhipicephalus appendiculatus*; in the field, the disease occurs only where this tick is found, except for corridor disease, which may be transmitted by *R. zambeziensis*. Other species of *Rhipicephalus* and *Hyalomma* spp. can transmit ECF experimentally, but they are not significant. Developmental stages of the parasite occur in the tick, and they pass transstadially through the stages of larva, nymph, and adult, but there is no transovarian transmission. Consequently, larvae or nymphs become infected and transmit infection as nymphs or adults, respectively. Adults are more efficient vectors than nymphs but each developmental stage results in amplification of the vector's competence in parasite transmission and the ability to infect more than one host during the life cycle of the tick.[2] Infected ticks start transmission of the parasite from 72 hours postattachment,[3] and mechanical transmission is of no significance. The epidemiology of the disease is thus largely dependent on the distribution and habitat of the tick and its ability to complete development to the adult stage, usually during the rainy season. Ticks may live for 1 to 2 years, but they lose their infection within 11 months.

Risk Factors

The most important risk factors relate to the presence of the brown ear tick in a given area and the level of tick burden per animal, even though it takes only one tick to establish an infection that could be fatal. At low infestation rates, an average of five ticks per head (two to three per ear) will sustain endemicity; one to four per head will invite epidemicity, whereas an average of less than one can allow sporadic outbreaks. In addition, there is evidence that *R. appendiculatus* populations that originate from eastern Africa tend to become more highly infected with *T. parva* than those that originate from southern Africa, and consequently the disease they transmit is more virulent.

The infection rate in ticks in endemic areas is usually low (1% to 2%), even though the immunity conferred on recovered or vaccinated animals is no longer thought to be sterile. However, soon after ECF becomes established in susceptible herds, infection rates in ticks become much higher.

Young animals are less susceptible, and indigenous breeds and buffaloes are less clinically affected than exotic breeds, but buffaloes are the carriers of corridor disease. Other wild *Bovidae* may help to sustain the population of the tick vector but are not carriers of *T. parva*. Asiatic or water buffalo are fully susceptible.

Environmental Factors

In eastern Africa, *R. appendiculatus* normally occurs in grass-covered savannah and savannah woodlands, but it is usually absent from extensive heavily wooded forest habitats. Areas that are too high, too cold, or too dry will not allow the tick to undergo more than one life cycle in a year, thereby reducing the period of transmission of theilerial parasites by the nymphs or adults. For example, the disease is most prevalent in eastern Africa, where adult and immature stages of the tick occur simultaneously on cattle, leading to rapid and continuous transmission. In southern Africa, by contrast, there is a seasonal life cycle for the tick, and thus there is little overlap between the activity periods of adults (January to March) and immature stages, thereby reducing the frequency of disease transmission.

Immune Mechanisms

Cattle recovering from ECF have a solid immunity to homologous challenge, but the immunity is not sterile. In endemic areas, premunity is established early, and this provides lifelong protection if reinfection continues and the cattle are not moved to a different location where they may be exposed to a different strain of the parasite. Indigenous cattle are able to limit explosive multiplication of schizonts during the acute phase. Nutritional or climatic stress may seriously reduce the animal's premunity, even among resistant breeds. Although antibody responses to the sporozoite may play some part in protection, immunity is mediated mainly by cellular mechanisms involving cell-mediated cytotoxic T-cell (CTL) responses against surface antigens of macroschizont-infected cells. The CTL response is parasite specific and genetically restricted (major histocompatibility complex [MHC] antigens), and the protection can be transferred between immune and naïve calves in the CD8+ T-cell fraction emanating from a responding lymph node.

Experimental Reproduction

ECF can easily be reproduced by feeding infected ticks on susceptible cattle or by inoculating cattle with infected tick material, sporozoites, or macroschizont-infected tissue culture cells. This is used as a method of immunization. When working with ticks or tick materials, care should be taken to avoid the risk of contracting other tick-borne diseases.

Economic Importance

ECF has a major impact on cattle production in eastern, central, and southern Africa. It is estimated that in 1989, ECF killed 1.1 million head of cattle and caused US$168 million in losses. Serious losses occur in exotic and indigenous cattle, mainly from reduced production of milk and meat as a result of morbidity and mortality, and from the heavy costs incurred in implementing effective tick control. *T. parva* does not infect human beings.

Biosecurity Concerns

The vector of ECF has strict requirements that limit the spread and establishment of the disease beyond the geographic areas where it normally occurs. Where the vector occurs but there is no disease, as in the Comoros, precautions should be taken to avoid importation of carrier cattle from endemic areas. ECF is not contagious.

PATHOGENESIS

Sporozoites of *T. parva* are injected into the bovine host by the tick in its saliva. Ticks must feed for 2 to 4 days before sporozoites in their salivary glands will mature and become infective to cattle. One tick can transmit sufficient sporozoites to cause a fatal infection in a susceptible animal. The sporozoites then enter lymphocytes and develop into schizonts in the lymph node draining the area of attachment of the tick, usually the parotid node. Infected lymphocytes are transformed to immortalized lymphoblasts and continue to divide synchronously with the schizonts, and thus each daughter cell is also infected. Eventually, infected lymphoblasts are disseminated throughout the lymphoid system and in nonlymphoid organs, where they continue to proliferate. The strategy used by the parasite to transform the infected cell is via reprogramming the cell's glucose metabolism and redox signaling.[4,5] It has been suggested that only a proportion of infected lymphocytes will actually proliferate and disseminate.[6] Furthermore, the survival of infected lymphoblasts is promoted by cytoplasmic sequestration of p53, the central effector molecule of the p53 apoptotic pathway.[7] Later, some schizonts differentiate into merozoites and are released from the lymphoblasts. Without the schizonts, proliferation of such lymphoblasts is arrested.[5] Meanwhile, the released meroziotes invade erythrocytes, where they are referred to as piroplasms. The latter are the form infective to ticks. Piroplasms ingested by ticks undergo several developmental stages and eventually form sporozoites in salivary glands, thus completing the cycle.

The dominating pathologic lesion is generalized lymphoid proliferation resulting from uncontrolled proliferation of T-lymphocytes containing schizonts. This is followed later by necrosis of infected lymphoblasts induced by cytotoxic T-lymphocytes. In one study involving 3-month old calves, massive necrosis of lymphocytes without initial proliferation was reported.[8] The severe lymphocytolysis often leads to immunosuppression. Terminally, the animal develops severe pulmonary edema, probably as a result of release of vasoactive substances from lymphocytes disintegrating in the lungs. Erythrocytic indices are usually unchanged, but there may be terminal anemia in January disease.

CLINICAL FINDINGS

The basic syndrome caused by *T. parva* infection lasts for a few weeks. The incubation period is 1 to 3 weeks, depending on the virulence of the strain and the size of the infecting dose. Experimentally, the first clinical sign is enlargement of lymph nodes in the area draining the site of tick attachment (i.e., 8 to 16 days after attachment). One or 2 days later, there is fever, depression, anorexia, and a drop in milk in dairy animals. In later stages, there may be nasal and ocular discharges, dyspnea, generalized lymph node enlargement, and splenomegaly. In severe cases, diarrhea occurs, sometimes with dysentery, but usually only late in the course of the disease. Emaciation, weakness, and recumbency lead to death from asphyxia in 7 to 10 days. Terminally, there is often a frothy nasal discharge. Occasional cases of brain involvement occur and are characterized by circling, hence "turning sickness," or cerebral theileriosis.

In southern Africa, cerebral theileriosis is associated with an aberrant form of *T. taurotragi* originating from the eland (see "Theilerioses"). There are localized nervous signs and convulsions, tremor, profuse salivation, and head pressing. Infection with the strain of *T. parva* (formerly *T. parva lawrencei*) responsible for corridor disease causes a similar acute syndrome, with the additional lesion of keratitis and accompanying blepharospasm. ECF in Zimbabwe (formerly attributed to *T. parva bovis*) is generally slightly less virulent but is still frequently fatal.

CLINICAL PATHOLOGY

The parasites are evident as schizonts, sometimes in circulating lymphocytes, but mainly in biopsy smears of enlarged lymph nodes stained with Giemsa. Piroplasms are also easily visible in erythrocytes from day 16 after tick attachment, and they increase in number until death. Over 30% of the red cells may be infected, but the level of intraerythrocytic piroplasms is not correlated with the severity of the disease. *T. parva* piroplasms are difficult to differentiate from other piroplasms—hence the necessity to find schizonts. Blood counts will reveal a panleukopenia and thrombocytopenia with little or no anemia. The protozoa can be grown on a tissue culture of lymphoblastoid cells.

A range of serologic tests is available, including indirect immunofluorescent antibody test (IFAT), complement fixation test, indirect hemagglutination test, and enzyme-linked immunosorbent assay (ELISA). The ELISA test is increasingly being used for seroepidemiologic studies, and the polymerase chain reaction (PCR) technology can be used as with other theilerioses. However, the IFAT is the most widely used test.[9]

NECROPSY FINDINGS

The most striking lesion is massive pulmonary edema, hyperemia, and emphysema, along with hydrothorax and hydropericardium. Copious froth is present in the airways. The carcass is emaciated, and hemorrhages are evident in a variety of tissues and organs. There is enlargement of the liver, lymph nodes, and spleen and ulceration of abomasum and intestines. Small lymphoid nodules (the so-called pseudoinfarcts) are present in liver, kidney, and alimentary tract. In protracted cases, animals may have small, exhausted lymphoid organs.

Microscopic lesions are characterized by proliferating lymphoblastoid cells and varying amounts of necrosis in lymphoid organs, lungs, liver, kidneys, the gastrointestinal tract, and other tissues, somewhat similar to a multicentric lymphoid tumor. Some lymphoblasts contain schizonts, which are better seen in impression smears stained with Giemsa stain. In cerebral theileriosis, infected lymphoblasts sequester in cerebral blood vessels and cause infarction.

Specimens to submit for pathology should include lymph nodes, lungs, kidneys, liver, and any other organ with gross lesions.

DIFFERENTIAL DIAGNOSTIC

The fever, depression, and lymphadenopathy of ECF can be confused with such diseases as theileriosis attributable to

- *T. annulata*
- trypanosomosis
- heartwater
- malignant catarrhal fever
- bovine virus diarrhea and rinderpest

The lymphoid hyperplasia may also simulate lymphoma. Knowledge of the disease history, coupled with hematologic and lymph node smear examinations, is usually adequate to make a definitive diagnosis.

TREATMENT

TREATMENT AND CONTROL

Treatment

Buparvaquone (2.5 mg/kg IM, 2 doses 48 hours apart) (R-1)

Parvaquone (10 mg/kg IM 2 doses 48 hours apart) (R-1)

Halofuginone lactate (1.2 mg/kg PO) (R-1)

Oxytetracycline (20 mg/kg IM) (R-2)

Control

Vaccination by infection and treatment method using tetracycline or parvaquone (R-1)

Vaccination by infection with low-pathogenicity isolate (R-2)

Once an animal is manifesting clinical signs of ECF, treatment is generally considered to be either unsatisfactory or too expensive. Tetracyclines were the recommended treatment for many years, but they have only moderate efficacy, especially if the disease has been present for a few days. Two recently introduced drugs, halofuginone lactate and parvaquone, have had a much higher success rate, but recovered animals may become carriers unless the correct dose is used. Halofuginone lactate is an effective oral treatment for the acute syndrome at two doses, 1.2 mg/kg BW. Parvaquone (10 mg/kg BW, two doses 48 hours apart) or the related buparvaquone (2.5 mg/kg BW, two doses 48 hours apart) given IM is effective in most cases. In field trials, buparvaquone gives results comparable to those of parvaquone, and cure rates are maximized by accurate diagnosis and prompt treatment of both ECF and intercurrent infections. Cure rates are even higher if the animals are also treated for pulmonary edema with dexamethasone or the diuretic furosemide. A recovery rate of 95.2% was reported in field cases in Tanzania treated with buparvaquone alone.[10]

CONTROL

Until recently, the main method of control of ECF was to break the transmission cycle between cattle and ticks. This was achieved through widespread and strict application of acaricides at 3-, 5-, or 7-day intervals throughout the year (intensive dipping), adherence to legislation on cattle movements and quarantine, and good livestock and pasture management. With the ever-rising costs of acaricides, their effect on the environment, the development of acaricide resistance, and frequent political problems in the affected regions, this strategy to control ECF and other tick-borne diseases in Africa has been revised. Furthermore, it has been observed that indigenous cattle, constituting the majority of the herds in some of the affected countries, may lose their endemic stability with intensive dipping, and the process is not cost-effective. An integrated approach is now advocated involving the use of genetically resistant breeds, a judicious and selective application of acaricides at 3-week intervals (strategic dipping) or when there are at least 100 ticks per animal (tactical dipping), and the use of vaccines. It has been reported that monthly applications of deltamethrin-based pour-on insecticide significantly reduce the incidence of ECF and other hemoparasitic diseases in smallholder dairy farms in Kenya.

The technique used for vaccination is immunotherapy or "infection-and-treatment method." Initially, cryopreserved suspensions of *T. parva* sporozoites from ground-up infected ticks were injected into the patient. Now, sporoziotes from cell culture are used. The infection they cause is controlled with long-acting oxytetracycline (20 mg/kg BW IM), or preferably parvaquone given at the same time, and thus premunity is established. It is preferably to use a cocktail of different stocks of parasites. Vaccination, coupled with strategic dipping only when ticks are abundant, is usually successful and economically attractive, provided local stocks of *Theileria* are included. The Muguga cocktail vaccine is being used throughout eastern, central, and southern Africa and has been recommended for use in southern Sudan.[11] Reports indicate that calves in high-risk areas should be vaccinated at 1 to 2 months of age, that immunization campaigns are more efficient when concentrated in the period of low adult tick activity, and that immunization is of no benefit in herds under intensive tick control but is of high value when combined with strategic tick control. Strategic control plus immunization can markedly reduce the risk of clinical ECF, but immunized animals are carriers, and all stages of *R. appendiculatus* can transmit infection from them to naïve animals.

Studies have indicated that cattle could be successfully immunized without concurrent tetracycline therapy by using low-pathogenicity isolates as vaccines, for example, *T. parva* (Boleni) in Zimbabwe, or low-infectivity sporozoite stabilates stored at −196° C (−321° F) for over 6 months. Because of the high cost of tetracyclines, this procedure would reduce the cost of vaccination by more than threefold in the first year of field application. Furthermore, the *T. parva* (Boleni) isolate was reported to induce protection against a wide spectrum of *Theileria* stocks in Zimbabwe.[12] Economic analyses in Kenya have demonstrated that integrated control in which ECF immunization is always an important component can play an important role in the overall control of the disease.[2] In Tanzania, annual theileriosis costs were US$205.40 per head, whereas the introduction of immunization reduced this by 40% to 68% depending on the postimmunization dipping strategy adopted.[13]

It needs to be stated that immunity is engendered so far only with live parasites that can establish an infection but can also produce carriers, from which the parasites can be transmitted to unvaccinated cattle that share grazing.[14] Hence, there is inherent risk in the widespread use of such vaccines across national boundaries. On the other hand, this process may be accelerating progress to endemicity.

The possibility of immunizing cattle with recombinant surface molecules from either the sporozoite (the p67 antigen) or the schizont, or a mixture of several antigens derived from both stages, has been investigated but without much success. Such a recombinant vaccine would probably avoid the breakdowns that occur with any immunotherapeutic technique, and if the right antigens are found for the vaccine, it is hoped that the immunity engendered is likely to be broad, robust, and not parasite stock specific.

FURTHER READING

Brown CGD. Theileriosis. In: Sewell MMH, Brocklesby DW, eds. *Handbook on Animal Diseases in the Tropics*. 4th ed. London: Baillière Tindall; 1990:183.

Lawrence JA, Perry BD, Williamson SM. East coast fever. In: Coetzer JAW, Tustin RC, eds. *Infectious Diseases of Livestock*. Vol. 1. 2nd ed. Cape Town: Oxford University Press; 2004:448.

Losos GJ. Theileriosis. In: *Infectious Tropical Diseases of Domestic Animals*. London: Longman; 1986:98.

Norval RAI, Perry BD, Young AS. *The Epidemiology of Theileriosis in Africa*. San Diego: Academic Press; 1992:481.

OIE Manual of Diagnostic Tests and Vaccines for Terrestrial Animals. Paris: OIE; 2008 chapter 2.04.16:789.

REFERENCES

1. De Deken R, et al. *Vet Parasitol*. 2007;143:245.
2. Gachohi J, et al. *Parasit Vect*. 2012;7:194.
3. Konnai S, et al. *Vector Zoonot Dis*. 2007;7:241.
4. Medjkane S, et al. *Oncogene*. 2014;33:1809.
5. Metheni M, et al. *Cell Microbiol*. 2015;doi:10.1111/cmi.12421; [Epub ahead of print].
6. Rocchi MS, et al. *Int J Parasitol*. 2006;36:771.
7. Haller D, et al. *Oncogene*. 2010;29:3079.
8. Mbassa GK, et al. *Vet Parasitol*. 2006;142:260.
9. *OIE Manual of Diagnostic Tests and Vaccines for Terrestrial Animals*. 6th ed. Paris: OIE; 2008 chapter 2.4.17:789-804.
10. Mbwambo HA, et al. *Vet Parasitol*. 2006;139:67.
11. Martins SB, et al. *Prev Vet Med*. 2010;97:175.
12. Latif AA, Hove T. *Ticks Tick Borne Dis*. 2011;2:163.
13. Kivaria FM, et al. *Vet J*. 2007;173:384.
14. Oura CA, et al. *Parasitology*. 2007;134:1205.

TROPICAL THEILERIOSIS (MEDITERRANEAN COAST FEVER)

SYNOPSIS

Etiology *Theileria annulata,* an Apicomplexa protozoon. Vectors are *Hyalomma* ticks.

Epidemiology Endemic disease of cattle in Mediterranean basin and parts of Asia.

Clinical signs Inapparent in local stock; fever, lymphadenopathy, wasting, anemia, and jaundice in exotics.

Clinical pathology Schizonts in macrophages and lymphocytes especially in liver smears; piroplasms in erythrocytes.

Lesions As in East Coast fever (ECF); also anemia and jaundice.

Differential diagnosis list:
- Other theilerioses
- Babesiosis
- Anaplasmosis
- Trypanosomosis
- Malignant catarrhal fever

Treatment Buparvaquone is effective.

Control None required for indigenous cattle; vaccination and strategic tick control for exotics.

ETIOLOGY

Theileria annulata is a member of the Apicomplexa group, like *T. parva,* the cause of East Coast fever. It is highly virulent for European dairy cattle, whereas infection in local zebu cattle is often subclinical.

EPIDEMIOLOGY

Occurrence and Methods of Transmission

The disease occurs from Morocco and Portugal in the west through the Mediterranean basin and the Middle East to India and China in the east. An outbreak in a Scottish dairy farm over a decade ago was thought to have been attributable to mechanical transmission from experimentally infected calves on a research institute associated with the farm. In the absence of natural vectors, that outbreak was quickly controlled.

T. annulata affects cattle and is transmitted transstadially by the three-host tick *Hyalomma anatolicum* in central-western Asia and northeastern Africa, and by the two-host tick *H. detritum* in the Mediterranean basin. The extent of its distribution may overlap with that of *T. parva* in Sudan and Eritrea and with *T. orientalis* in the Far East.

In endemic areas, virtually all adult cattle are infected, but infection rates vary with the method of examination. For example, surveys carried out in different parts of Turkey showed the prevalence to be between 0% and 60.5% by microscopic examination of blood and lymph node smears, 1.8% and 91.4% by serology (IFAT), and between 15.4% and 61.2% by molecular techniques.[1]

Case fatality is approximately 10% to 20% and is confined mainly to calves. Exotic animals recently introduced may have 20% to 90% mortality. The disease occurs when there is much tick activity, mainly in summer and the rainy seasons, and in crossbred animals. A single tick can cause fatal infection because its salivary glands usually contain numerous sporozoites.

Risk Factors and Immune Mechanisms

The normal state is that of endemic stability. This balance is disturbed when exotic animals are introduced, and heavier losses occur. Recovered animals show a solid, long-lasting immunity, but they remain as carriers. Buffaloes are thought to be the natural hosts, and they may also act as carriers, whereas yaks are highly susceptible. In one study in Egypt, water buffaloes were more severely affected than cattle.[2] As with *T. parva,* immunity is mainly cell mediated but is poor in calves. Experimental reproduction is by feeding infected ticks on cattle or by needle inoculation of sporozoites in macerated ticks, schizonts in lymphocytes, or of merozoites in erythrocytes. Humans are not affected.

Economic Importance

The disease is a major constraint to livestock improvement programs in many parts of the Middle East and Asia. Around one-sixth of the world cattle population is at risk. Economic losses arising from the disease in Turkey were estimated to vary from US$130,000 to US$598,000 per annum in the endemic stable zones.[1] In carrier animals in Tunisia, the greatest loss is from reduced milk production.[3]

Biosecurity Concerns

There are no biosecurity concerns.

PATHOGENESIS

The life cycle of *T. annulata* is cattle–tick–cattle, as for *T. parva,* but unlike *T. parva,* the sporozoites of *T. annulata* invade and form schizonts, mostly in macrophages/monocytes that express major histocompatibility (MHC) class II antigens. The macrophages then stimulate uninfected lymphocytes to undergo lymphoblastic transformation and proliferate.[4] Schizont-infected cells multiply in the draining lymph nodes and disseminate rapidly along with lymphoblasts throughout the lymphoid tissues and in nonlymphoid organs, including the liver, kidney, lung, abomasum, and brain. Virulence of the disease is associated with the capacity of infected cells to disseminate inside the host.[5] Later, schizonts differentiate into merozoites and invade erythrocytes (as piroplasms). The pathogenesis therefore involves proliferation of macrophages induced by schizonts, and anemia with icterus induced mostly by the piroplasms. Macrophages/monocytes are the main producers of inflammatory cytokines that can induce an acute-phase protein response. The response is greater in *Bos taurus* Holstein breed than the *Bos indicus* Sahiwal breed,[6] and this would explain the more severe disease in the Holstein. Infected macrophages from taurine breeds are also more capable of aggressive invasiveness than zebu breeds.[7]

Over 90% of erythrocytes may be parasitized, each by one or more merozoites. Merozoites induce hemolysis most likely by lipid peroxidation of the red cell membrane. The level of hemolysis is dependent on the parasitic burden.[8] Immunosuppression may occur in the acute stages of the disease but is generally less marked than in ECF, probably because leukocyte numbers return to normal soon after the acute phase.

CLINICAL FINDINGS

In a stable endemic situation, there may be only mild or no clinical disease in local zebu cattle. Clinical signs are acute and severe in exotic cattle and less severe in crossbreeds and are similar to those in ECF. However, the course is longer in tropical theileriosis and may last for weeks before death. Clinical signs include marked fever, swelling of superficial lymph nodes, inappetence, tachycardia, dyspnea, pale mucous membranes, and icterus. Others are diarrhea, weight loss, convulsions, torticollis, and other nervous signs. In chronic cases, there may be small subcutaneous nodules, from which schizonts can be demonstrated in smears. In Egypt, affected cattle and buffaloes also showed ocular signs, including severe lacrimation, bilateral conjunctivitis, photophobia, and corneal opacity,[2] whereas in Spain, there were coalescing skin nodules similar to multicentric malignant lymphoma.[4]

CLINICAL PATHOLOGY

As with ECF, examination of smears of blood and lymph node biopsy will reveal piroplasms in erythrocytes and schizonts in lymphocytes. Schizonts of *T. annulata* tend to be more common in the liver than in lymph node smears, but they are otherwise indistinguishable from those of *T. parva*. Furthermore, the piroplasms are predominantly round and oval, as opposed to *T. parva*, which has comma- and rod-shaped piroplasms. Anemia is a significant feature of tropical theileriosis, unlike in ECF, and is associated with bilirubinemia, hemoglobinuria, and bilirubinuria. The anemia results from destruction of erythrocytes containing piroplasms, but other factors may include autoimmune hemolysis and poor bone-marrow response. Reduction in white cell and platelet counts is less severe than in ECF, but animals dying from the disease show persistent and severe lymphocytopenia involving mainly T-lymphocytes.

The most commonly used serologic diagnostic technique is the indirect fluorescent antibody test.[9] For surveys, an indirect enzyme-linked immunosorbent assay (ELISA) test using a recombinant *T. annulata* surface protein has been described. The ELISA tests provide higher sensitivity and specificity than the IFAT. The polymerase chain reaction (PCR) test is more sensitive and more specific[10] and can detect carriers; it can also be used to detect infected ticks. A multiplex PCR method can simultaneously detect single and coinfections with *T. annulata, Babesia bigemina,* and *Anaplasma marginale* in cattle.[11] The test is simple, specific, and sensitive and can be applied to epidemiologic studies aimed at assessing the burden of multiple infection with tick-borne pathogens.

NECROPSY FINDINGS

Apart from pallor of mucous membranes and yellowish discoloration of tissues, the postmortem lesions in animals dying from tropical theileriosis are similar to those of ECF. Lymphoid proliferation can resemble multicentric malignant lymphoma.[4] Liver, spleen, and lymph nodes should be submitted for laboratory examination to detect schizonts, whereas merozoites are detected in blood smears.

DIFFERENTIAL DIAGNOSIS

Tropical theileriosis may be confused with the other theilerioses that may occur in the region, and with babesiosis, anaplasmosis, trypanosomosis, and malignant catarrhal fever. Liver biopsy and blood examination will help to confirm a clinical diagnosis.

TREATMENT

TREATMENT AND CONTROL

Treatment

Buparvaquone 2.5 mg/kg IM, 2 doses 48 hours apart) (R-1)

Halofuginone lactate (1.2 mg/kg PO) (R-1)

Oxytetracycline (20 mg/kg IM) (R-2)

Control

Vaccination by infection and treatment method using tetracycline (R-1 for exotic animals)

Vaccination with attenuated schizont vaccine (R-2)

Buparvaquone is the most effective agent available, and the recommended dose is 2.5 mg/kg BW. In calves, supportive treatment for anemia is indicated. Halofuginone at 1.2 mg/kg is also effective, but tetracycline at 20 mg/kg is less so.

CONTROL

Indigenous cattle live with the disease and do not require any intensive tick control or treatment. For valuable exotic stock or their crossbreeds, vaccination and strategic tick control are recommended. Vaccines can be made from either the sporozoite or the schizont. The sporozoite vaccine is based on the infection-and-treatment method using schizont-infected cell lines and simultaneous tetracycline treatment, as for *T. parva*. It has been suggested that the most economical way to control theileriosis in India is to vaccinate calves and to reserve buparvaquone for treating clinical cases. The schizont vaccine was formerly blood containing a mild strain of the parasite. The newer vaccines are prepared from live schizonts grown in lymphoid cell culture and attenuated by prolonged passage. They cause virtually no adverse reactions, and vaccinated cattle show good resistance to the disease for at least 3.5 years. Therefore it is necessary to revaccinate, preferably with a different cell-line vaccine, if tick population is too low to establish endemic stability. The risk for spread of the vaccine strains in the field is very low. The disease has been successfully controlled in China by vaccination.[12]

FURTHER READING

Brown CGD. Theileriosis. In: Sewell MMH, Brocklesby DW, eds. *Handbook on Animal Diseases in the Tropics*. 4th ed. London: Baillière Tindall; 1990:183.

OIE Manual of Diagnostic Tests and Vaccines for Terrestrial Animals. 6th ed. Paris: OIE; 2008 chapter 2.4.17:789-804.

Pipano E, Shkap V. *Theileria annulata* theileriosis. In: Coetzer JA, Tustin RC, eds. *Infectious Diseases of Livestock*. Vol. 1. 2nd ed. Cape Town: Oxford University Press; 2004:486-487.

REFERENCES

1. Cicek H, et al. *Turkiye Parazitol Derg*. 2009;33:273.
2. Mahmmod YS, et al. *Ticks Tick Borne Dis*. 2011;2:168.
3. Gharbi M, et al. *Rev - Off Int Epizoot*. 2011;30:763.
4. Branco S, et al. *J Vet Sci*. 2010;11:27.
5. Ma M, Baumgartner M. *PLoS ONE*. 2013;8(9):e75577. doi:10.1371/journal.pone.0075577; eCollection 2013.
6. Glass EJ, et al. *Vet Immunol Immunopathol*. 2012;148:178.
7. Chaussepied M, et al. *PLoS Pathog*. 2010;6:e1001197.

8. Saleh MA, et al. *Vet Parasitol*. 2011;182:193.
9. *OIE Manual of Diagnostic Tests and Vaccines for Terrestrial Animals*. 6th ed. Paris: OIE; 2008 chapter 2.4.17:789-804.
10. Khattak RM, et al. *Parasite*. 2012;19:91.
11. Bilgic HB, et al. *Exp Parasitol*. 2013;133:222.
12. Yin H, et al. *Vaccine*. 2008;26(suppl 6):G11-G13.

Multi-Organ Diseases Due to Trypanosome Infection

Trypanosomes are flagellated protozoan parasites belonging to the genus *Trypanosoma*, family Trypanosomatidae. They live in the blood and other body fluids of vertebrate hosts, where some of them cause disease. With the help of the flagellum, trypanosomes swim within the vertebrate bloodstream and prosper despite being constantly attacked by the host immune system. The parasites generally possess a kinetoplast and undergo cyclical development in an arthropod vector but can be transmitted mechanically. Their biological adaptations, morphology, and pathogenicity are fascinating and have been extensively studied. The parasites cause several diseases, each of which was referred to as trypanosomiasis. The currently preferred term is *trypanosomosis*, plural *trypanosomoses*. The diseases are summarized in Table 21-7.

Trypanosoma evansi is the first known pathogenic trypanosome. It was first described in India as the cause of surra in animals, but the disease is widespread in the tropics and is transmitted mechanically rather than by a biological vector. In Africa, three species (*Trypanosoma congolense*, *T. vivax*, and *T. brucei*) are the main pathogens for animals and humans. The parasites are transmitted by the tsetse fly (*Glossina* spp.), and the resulting animal disease is referred to as African trypanosomosis or nagana. Two subspecies of *T. brucei* are responsible for African sleeping sickness in human beings, *T. brucei gambiense* in West and Central Africa, and *T. brucei rhodesiense* in East Africa. Another disease, dourine, specifically affects equines and camels and is caused by *T. equiperdum* transmitted sexually during coitus. *T. evansi* and *T. equiperdum* are regarded as subspecies of *T. brucei*, which have lost their ability to infect tsetse and are therefore able to spread outside Africa. In South and Central America, a different trypanosome, *T. cruzi*, transmitted by reduviid bugs (*Rodnius* spp. and *Triatoma* spp.), is the cause of Chagas's disease or American trypanosomosis, mostly in humans, but it also affects dogs, cats, and pigs. Trypanosomoses of veterinary importance are discussed here.

Table 21-7 Summary of the trypanosomoses of domestic animals and humans

Disease	Distribution	*Trypanosoma* spp.	Main vector
Animals			
Nagana or African trypanosomosis (most mammals)	Tropical Africa	*T. brucei brucei* *T. congolense* *T. vivax* *T. simiae*	*Glossina* spp. Other biting flies
Surra (horses, camels, buffaloes)	Africa, Asia, South and Central America	*T. evansi*	Biting flies
Dourine (horses and donkeys)	Africa, Asia, South and Central America	*T. equiperdum*	None (venereal transmission)
Nonpathogenic (cattle and sheep)	Worldwide	*T. theileri* *T. melophagium*	Biting flies
Humans			
Rhodesian sleeping sickness	East, central, and southern Africa	*T. brucei rhodesiense*	*Glossina* spp.
Gambian sleeping sickness	Western and central Africa	*T. brucei gambiense*	*Glossina* spp.
Chagas' disease (also in dogs, cats, and pigs)	South and Central America, southern United States	*T. cruzi*	*Rhodnius* spp. *Triatoma* spp.

NAGANA (SAMORE, AFRICAN TRYPANOSOMAISIS, TSETSE FLY DISEASE)

SYNOPSIS

Etiology *Trypanosoma congolense, T. vivax, T. brucei brucei*, and *T. simiae*, all salivarian trypanosomes. Tsetse flies (*Glossina* spp.) serve as biological vector, other biting flies as mechanical vectors.

Epidemiology Endemic disease of all mammals in tropical Africa, also Central and South America; of greatest economic importance in cattle. Two subspecies of *T. brucei* cause African sleeping sickness, an important human disease (zoonosis) in tropical Africa.

Clinical signs Fever, apathy, pale mucous membranes, swollen lymph nodes, progressive emaciation, cachexia, and death, sometimes preceded by nervous signs. May be acute, subacute or, often, chronic disease.

Clinical pathology Progressive anemia, parasite detection in blood by various methods, including polymerase chain reaction (PCR).

Lesions Not definitive but include pallor, emaciation, and enlargement of lymph nodes, spleen, and liver.

Differential diagnosis list:
- Malnutrition
- Helminthosis
- East coast fever
- Babesiosis
- Anaplasmosis
- Hemorrhagic septicemia

Treatment Trypanocides such as Berenil, Samorin, Suramin, and Antrycide, but drug resistance is a problem.

Control Integrated methods involving tsetse fly control, prophylaxis, good husbandry, and use of trypanotolerant breeds, no vaccine.

ETIOLOGY

Trypanosoma vivax, T. congolense, T. brucei, and *T. simiae* are the four main species responsible for African trypanosomosis affecting virtually all domestic mammals. *T. vivax* and *T. congolense* mostly affect cattle, sheep, goats, and horses. Horses are also severely affected by *T. brucei brucei*, whereas pigs suffer mostly from *T. simiae*. All four species are members of the *Salivaria* group of trypanosomes and are transmitted cyclically via the mouthparts of tsetse flies—hence the name salivarian trypanosomes. Cyclical development in the vector is a result of the presence of kinetoplast DNA in these trypanosomes.

The morphology and movement of the trypanosomes are characteristic for each species and are helpful in making a diagnosis. In acute infections, *T. vivax* is usually numerous in blood samples and can be identified by its very fast movement in wet films. In stained smears, it is 20 to 26 μm long, slender, and monomorphic, with a rounded posterior end, a terminal kinetoplast, and a long free flagellum, but no prominent undulating membrane. *T. congolense* is smaller, is sluggish in wet films, and often adheres to red blood cells by the anterior end. In stained smears, it is 9 to 18 μm long, with a marginal kinetoplast, no free flagellum, and no prominent undulating membrane. *T. brucei* is large like *T. vivax*, but its rapid movement is in confined areas of the wet film. In stained smears, it is pleomorphic and may occur as long and slender forms up to 35 μm, intermediate forms, or short and stumpy forms about 12 µm long. The slender and intermediate forms have a long free flagellum, pointed posterior end, subterminal kinetoplast, and prominent undulating membrane, whereas the stumpy forms resemble *T. congolense* but are bigger and have a prominent undulating membrane. The strains or species of *T. brucei* infective to animals only are often referred to as *T. brucei brucei* to distinguish them from *T. brucei gambiense* and *T. brucei rhodesiense*, which are infective to humans. *T. simiae* is morphologically indistinguishable from *T. congolense*, and it is adapted to pigs, in which parasitemia can be very heavy (swarming).

EPIDEMIOLOGY

Occurrence

The epidemiology of African trypanosomosis is determined mainly by the ecology of the tsetse fly found only in tropical Africa. However, *T. vivax* is also transmitted mechanically by biting flies and has been responsible for disease outbreaks in Costa Rica and some South American countries, including Bolivia, Brazil, and Venezuela, where it affects mainly cattle and sheep. In general, *T. congolense* and *T. vivax* are responsible for severe disease in cattle, sheep, and goats, and *T. brucei brucei* usually causes a subclinical infection in cattle but a severe disease in sheep, goats, horses, and, occasionally, pigs. *T. simiae* causes a hyperacute and highly fatal disease in exotic pigs and in camels. Warthogs act as its reservoir, and the parasite is not pathogenic to cattle, sheep, or goats.

Prevalence

Infection rates reported in cattle in endemic areas vary considerably and could be over 60% in some herds. However, as a result of various control methods, including those under the auspices of the Pan African Tsetse and Trypanosomiasis Eradication Campaign (PATTEC), the prevalence of infection is decreasing in many African countries, particularly in West Africa. Recent surveys in the region report prevalence rates of 5% or less in cattle by parasite detection methods and higher rates with serology or with polymerase chain reaction (PCR) techniques detecting parasite nucleic acids. For example, prevalence studies in villages in Burkina Faso involving 2002 cattle, 1466 small ruminants, and 481 donkeys reported only a 0.77% infection rate in cattle, 0% in goats, and 0.6% in donkeys by routine parasitologic methods, whereas by serology, the rates were 34.2% for cattle, 20.9% for sheep, 8.5% for goats, and 5.8% for donkeys.[1] Seventy-five percent of the cases were attributable to *T. vivax* and 25% to *T. congolense*. In an Ethiopian study involving 1524 animals, the overall prevalence of infection was 5.5% by conventional parasitologic methods and 31.0% by PCR.[2] A major factor affecting reported prevalence rates is the chronically low parasitemias in indigenous African zebu cattle, which often necessitates repeated sampling before an animal can be regarded as being uninfected. Using repeated PCR testing in East Africa, infection rates in 35 village cattle were found to be *T. brucei* (34.3%), *T. congolense* (42.9%), and *T. vivax* (29.9%).[3] Mixed infections with two or more species are common in endemic areas, and such infections are more readily detected by the PCR technique.[4] It should be mentioned that a positive serology does not necessarily imply current infection, whereas a positive PCR test, when properly carried out, indicates current or very recent infection because trypanosome DNA persists in host blood for only 14 days after successful treatment.[5] In general, it would seem that *T. vivax* is more commonly encountered and more pathogenic in West and Central Africa, whereas *T. congolense* appears more prevalent and more pathogenic in East and South Africa. Exceptions to this general rule are two recent reports, one from Mali,[6] and the other from Nigeria,[7] where *T. congolense* was found to be more prevalent than *T. vivax* in the herds studied.

Pigs and horses are less frequently affected than ruminants, perhaps because they are less exposed to tsetse flies than cattle that normally graze over long distances. The clinical disease in pigs is usually attributable to *T. simiae*, but there have been no reports of natural outbreaks of this form of trypanosomosis in many years. Horses in Africa are affected by the three major species, and the disease syndrome is similar.

In Central and South America, *T. vivax* infections appear to be spreading to new areas, where they cause periodic outbreaks of serious disease mostly in cattle but also in horses.

Morbidity and Case Fatality

Morbidity rates during outbreaks are variable and may reach 70% in cattle infected with *T. vivax* and up to 100% in pigs infected with *T. simiae*. Morbidity is usually much lower in sheep, goats, and horses because these are not often the preferred hosts for tsetse or are less exposed to tsetse challenge. Sheep and goats are more vigorous than cattle in defending themselves against successful feeding by tsetse flies.

Case fatality also depends on the trypanosome species, host, and its level of resistance. *T. simiae* is invariably fatal in exotic pigs. Some strains of *T. vivax* in East Africa cause similar heavy mortalities in exotic dairy cows, and infected horses are likely to die if left untreated. However, most infections in cattle in endemic areas run a chronic course and are not invariably fatal, but the animal may remain unproductive and unthrifty. West African strains of *T. vivax* are generally more pathogenic to cattle than East African strains, and *T. congolense* is generally the more pathogenic species in East Africa. Subspecies of *T. congolense* are also recognized, with *T. congolense* savannah type being much more pathogenic than other types (*T. congolense* forest type, *T. congolense* kilifi type, and *T. congolense godfreyi*).

Methods of Transmission

Cyclical

African trypanosomes can be transmitted by 23 species of tsetse (*Glossina*) found only in sub-Saharan Africa between latitudes 14°N and 29°S, excluding areas of high altitude, extreme drought, or cold temperatures where tsetse cannot survive. The flies can be grouped according to their preferred habitats as savannah species, riverine species, and forest species. The savannah species (including *G. morsitans, G. austeni, G. pallidipes, G. swynnertoni,* and *G. longipalpis*) pose the greatest threat to livestock because they inhabit the grasslands where cattle are traditionally reared, they can easily adapt to other ecological niches, they feed primarily on cattle and pigs, and they are efficient vectors of trypanosomes. They are also the main vectors of Rhodesian sleeping sickness associated with *T. b. rhodesiense* in humans (Table 21-8). The riverine species (*G. palpalis, G. tachinoides,* and *G. fuscipes*) are important vectors of bovine and porcine trypanosomosis, and of Gambian sleeping sickness as a result of *T. b. gambiense.* On the other hand, the 13 or so forest species (including *G. fusca, G. brevipalpis,* and *G. longipennis*) are not frequently incriminated vectors of animal trypanosomes even though their preferred food hosts are ruminants and suids.

The life cycle of trypanosomes in tsetse involves cyclical development for a varying length of time, depending on species and ambient temperatures, leading to the production of mature procyclic (metacyclic) parasites infective to the mammalian host. *T. vivax* completes its developmental cycle in the proboscis and pharynx of the fly and can be transmitted to a host within a week of the initial infective feed. The cycle of *T. congolense* involves the midgut and proboscis and is completed in about 2 weeks. That of *T. brucei* is more complex: it takes 3 or more weeks in the fly and involves the midgut and salivary glands. Once infected, flies remain so for life (1 to 2 months). It follows that for any fly, its vectorial capacity and efficiency are highest for *T. vivax* and least for *T. brucei.* Even then, infection rates in tsetse flies are generally low by conventional parasitologic methods of detection. Using the more sensitive PCR technique, 10.5% of 550 field-captured flies (*Glossina pallidipes*) were found to harbor trypanosome DNA in an endemic area in southwestern Zambia.[8]

Noncyclical

After trypanosomes have been introduced into a herd, further transmission is possible in the absence of *Glossina*. Biting flies such as *Tabanus, Stomoxys,* and *Hippobosca* are capable of mechanically transmitting bloodstream trypanosomes in their mouthparts when they feed on more than one host within a short interval. This is how *T. vivax* is spread in areas outside the tsetse belt in Africa and in Central and South America. Mechanical transmission can also occur through the needle during inoculations and in carnivores feeding on infected carcasses. There are occasional reports of intrauterine (vertical) transmission in animals and in human beings.

The Carrier State

Reservoirs of infection are found in many wild animals, in trypanotolerant animals, and in chronically infected animals. Tsetse caught in and around game reserves tend to have relatively high infection rates, and the relative abundance of wildlife in East Africa compared with West Africa may explain, at least in part, why the prevalence of the disease appears to be declining more rapidly in the west.

Risk Factors

Host Factors

The effect of infection varies with the host in that most wild and some domestic animals establish a balance with the parasite and remain as clinically normal carriers for long periods. Specifically, some breeds of cattle indigenous to Africa can tolerate light to moderate challenge with tsetse flies by limiting the multiplication of trypanosomes in their blood and also limiting the degree of anemia caused. The phenomenon is called **trypanotolerance**; it is both genetic and environmental in origin, and the level of tolerance varies. Thus the indigenous taurine breeds, such as the N'Dama, Baoule, and Muturu, are more tolerant than the West African zebu, and among East African zebu cattle, the Orma Boran and Maasai zebu have superior tolerance compared with Galana Boran and Friesian breeds. In a study involving N'Dama crossed with more susceptible Kenya-Boran animals reared under natural field situations, the trypanotolerant trait derived from the N'Dama was found to be primarily additive in nature, being expressed in heterozygous condition and in three-quarters Boran crosses.[9] In addition, females were more trypanotolerant than males. Thus the tolerance of the more productive but susceptible breeds can be improved by crossbreeding. However, because of the uncertain genetic makeup of animals within these so-called breeds and crossbreeds, the level of trypanotolerance may also vary with individual animals within a given category, and it can be overcome by heavy tsetse challenge, malnutrition, or other stress factors.

Trypanotolerance also occurs in some indigenous breeds of small ruminants but is less pronounced than in cattle. The breeds include the Djallonke sheep, the West African Dwarf (WAD) sheep and goat, and the East African goat, whereas the Toggenburg, British Alpine, Saanen, Anglo-Nubian, and Sahel breeds of goats are fully susceptible. Because of unintentional and indiscriminate crossbreeding of the WAD goat populations with more susceptible breeds from the Sahel region, the former are becoming less trypanotolerant.[10]

Environmental Factors

The density of tsetse population in an area and the level of tsetse contact with the host will determine the level of infection. This is further influenced by the vectorial capacity of the fly and the availability of its preferred host. For example, cattle are more attractive to tsetse flies than pigs, and pigs are more attractive than goats.[11] Trekking of livestock through tsetse-infested vegetation is a risk nomadic farmers face from time to time, and the risk is even greater where cattle routes converge, for example, at major bridges or watering holes. Agricultural and industrial developments generally lead to a lowering of tsetse density by destroying their habitat, whereas the establishment of game or forest reserves provides large numbers of preferred hosts or a suitable habitat for tsetse, respectively. Herds located near such reserves are therefore at a higher risk. So also are tourists visiting such game parks.

Pathogen Factors

In cattle, *T. vivax* generally produces a higher level of parasitemia than other species. And because its life cycle in the tsetse is also shorter, *T. vivax* is more readily transmitted than the others when animals are newly introduced into a tsetse-infested area. Higher parasitemias also facilitate mechanical transmission. Conversely, *T. brucei* is infrequently detected by microscopic examination of cattle blood, even though infection can be confirmed through other, more sensitive diagnostic methods. Furthermore, some animals carry infection without showing clinical signs, especially if they are trypanotolerant, like the Muturu in Nigeria, or if infected with nonpathogenic genetic types, such as *T. congolense* kilifi type in cattle.

Immune Mechanisms

Animals recovering from infection with one strain/serodeme or species of trypanosome are not immune to infection with another strain/serodeme or species. This is attributable to the ability of trypanosomes to periodically replace a monolayer or their protective coat of variant surface glycoproteins (VSGs) in an immunocompetent host through a process called **antigenic variation.** Each trypanosome cell expresses only one of many VSGs at a time, and the coat is continually shed and replaced to avoid the host immune system. During each peak parasitemia, a mixture of variable antigenic types of parasites may be present, but the dominant VSG antigen determines the specific antibody response. These antibodies kill off the dominant population, leaving others with different antigens to emerge; these multiply and become dominant, and the process continues in cycles until the animal dies or the immune mechanisms catch up with the parasite and the animal recovers. This phenomenon is also responsible for the successive waves of parasitemia in infected animals.

The molecular mechanisms involved in the switching or activation of new VSGs are now being studied.[12-13] In *T. brucei,* the mechanisms involve DNA repair mechanism in that a double-strand break (DSB) initiates a switch in the expressed variant surface coat.[14] Furthermore, it has been shown that the DSB site determines the probability and mechanism of antigenic switching, and that DSBs can trigger switching via recombination or transcription inactivation.[15] The frequency of recombination is comparable between *T. congolense* and *T. brucei* but is much lower in *T. vivax.*[13] Following repeated episodes of infection and recovery (with or without treatment) in an endemic area, animals will encounter a variety of antigenic types and therefore become less susceptible to strains/serodemes in that area.

Infected animals are more susceptible to secondary infections by other microorganisms, particularly bacteria. The immune system of an infected animal is disrupted by mechanisms not fully understood, but they may vary with the species of animals. In ruminants, the state of immunosuppression is abrogated once the trypanosomes are eliminated by chemotherapy.

Experimental Reproduction

Infection can be easily reproduced by inoculation of infected blood or other serous fluid into a susceptible host. Infected flies can also be fed on the host to transmit the disease. Several laboratory animal models of nagana and sleeping sickness are available, and lots of studies have been done with mice and rats. These studies help to elucidate the pathogenesis of the disease and approaches to chemotherapy and drug resistance.

Economic Importance

Tsetse flies infest 10 million square kilometers of Africa, involving 38 countries and placing 50 million cattle at risk. Hence, nagana is still the most important disease of livestock in the continent. The added risk of human infections has greatly affected social, economic, and agricultural development of rural communities. Because nagana is a wasting disease, affected animals are chronically unproductive in terms of milk, meat, manure, and traction, and the mortality rate can be high, especially in exotic and more productive animals. The disease in Africa costs livestock producers and consumers an estimated US$4.5 billion each year. The anticipated losses as a result of *T. vivax* in South America exceed $160 million. Furthermore, the disease may affect various immunization campaigns in endemic areas because it can cause immunosuppression.

Zoonotic Implications

The animal pathogens (*T. vivax, T. congolense, T. simiae,* and *T. brucei brucei*) are not infective to humans, but animals can serve as reservoirs of *T. brucei rhodesiense* and *T. brucei gambiense,* the causes of human African trypanosomosis (HAT), or sleeping sickness. *T. brucei brucei* is morphologically indistinguishable from the human pathogens, but when it is incubated in human serum, it is lysed and becomes noninfective to laboratory animals, unlike the human pathogens, which are human serum resistant.[16]

As in animals, human infections with *T. brucei gambiense* or *T. brucei rhodesiense* result from tsetse bites, generally in game parks, in forest reserves, along streams, or in other rural settings. The incidence of human infections fell to a few thousand cases per year in the 1960s and then started to rise as a result of relaxation of previous control measures and especially because of civil unrest forcing people to leave their homes to seek shelter in tsetse-infested areas. Currently, a total of 70 million people are at risk of infection. In 2012, over 175,000 cases were reported in 20 countries; *T. brucei gambiense* accounted for 82.2% of them, and *T. brucei rhodesiense* accounted for the remaining 17.8%.[17] High-risk countries are in Central Africa, especially the Democratic Republic of the Congo, Angola, the Central African Republic, and southern Sudan, where civil wars have hampered control efforts. During the period 2009 to 2013, most cases of Rhodesian sleeping sickness were reported from Uganda, Malawi, Tanzania, and Zambia[18] and from foreign tourists who had visited East African game parks. A comprehensive review of the human disease was published recently.[18]

A rash (chancre) develops at the site of tsetse bite in humans, and this is soon followed by fever, persistent headache, and swelling of lymph nodes, spleen, and liver. Weakness and signs of cardiac involvement may be noticed early in the Rhodesian form encountered in eastern and southern Africa. This form is rapidly fatal if it is not diagnosed early and treated promptly. The Gambian form is usually chronic and often asymptomatic for months before the patient gradually wastes away and dies from the disease or from secondary infections years later. It is encountered in West and Central Africa, including the northwestern part of Uganda. In both forms, the disease progresses from a hemolymphatic first stage (S1) to a meningoencephalitic second stage (S2) corresponding to when parasites invade the cerebrospinal fluid (CSF) and brain across the blood–brain barrier.[19] Stage 2 results in progressive nonsuppurative menigo-encephalitis, causing the patient to fall asleep often—hence the name sleeping sickness.

Biosecurity Concerns

There are no biosecurity concerns for nagana because tsetse flies require strict environmental conditions to survive and breed. However, because *T. vivax* can be transmitted mechanically by biting flies, this fact should be taken into consideration when infected animals are moved outside the tsetse zone in Africa and in South and Central America. People working with *T. brucei gambiense* and *T. brucei rhodesiense* should take precautions to avoid accidental inoculation of themselves or their coworkers with infected material in syringes or tsetse flies.

PATHOGENESIS

Nagana in most domestic animal species is a progressive but not always fatal disease, and the main features are anemia, tissue damage, and immunosuppression. Metacyclic trypanosomes are inoculated intradermally as the fly feeds. They multiply at this site, provoking a local skin reaction (chancre), which is most pronounced in a fully susceptible host and may be slight or absent with some strains or species of trypanosomes. Within the chancre, metacyclic parasites change to trypomastigote form, enter the bloodstream directly or through the lymphatics, and initiate characteristic intermittent parasitemias associated with intermittent fever. The behavior of the parasites thereafter depends largely on the species of trypanosome transmitted and the host.

In the acute phase, *T. vivax* usually multiplies rapidly in the blood of cattle, sheep, and goats, and it is evenly dispersed throughout the cardiovascular system, whereas *T. congolense* tends to be aggregated in small blood vessels and capillaries of the heart, brain, and skeletal muscle. *T. congolense* parasitemias in ruminants is not usually as high as with *T. vivax,* even though the anemia may be more marked. Both species exert their effect mainly by causing severe anemia and mild to moderate organ damage in the form of cellular degeneration and perivascular mononuclear cellular infiltration. Very acute infections with *T. vivax* in cattle or with *T. simiae* in pigs result in fulminating parasitemia and disseminated intravascular coagulation, with hemorrhages leading rapidly to death. Such syndromes resemble septicemia, and anemia may not be severe.

T. brucei brucei and, less often, *T. vivax* have the added capability of escaping from the capillaries into the interstitial tissues and serous cavities, where they continue to multiply. Such infections result in more severe organ damage in horses, sheep, and goats, in addition to anemia. The cerebrospinal fluid and brain parenchyma can be invaded by the parasites, resulting in a nonsuppurative meningo-encephalitis and encephalomalacia.[20-21] Parasites in the CSF are not easily reached by some drugs and may be a source of relapsing infection when they reinvade the bloodstream. In addition, pregnant animals may abort, and transplacental fetal infections occasionally occur.

The pathogenesis of anemia in trypanosomosis has been studied extensively, and it may vary with the parasite, the host species, and the stage of infection.[22-23] The three mechanisms generally recognized in the development of anemia are (a) extravascular red cell destruction as a result of massive erythrophagocytosis in the spleen and liver at all stages of infection, (b) intravascular hemolysis in the acute stage, and (c) inadequate bone-marrow response (dyshemopoiesis) in the chronic stage. Increased erythrophagocytosis occurs in activated macrophages that are induced by parasite-derived glycolipids to become hyperactive against trypanosomes and red blood cells. During the acute phase of infection, erythrophagocytosis may also be triggered by trypanosome transsialidases acting on erythrocyte membranes.[24] Intravascular hemolysis is less commonly reported but has been attributed to several factors, including hemolysins from parasites, cleavage of sialic acids from the red cell membrane, passive absorption of trypanosome molecules in the red cell membrane, and, more recently, oxidative stress from free radicals. In the chronic stage, bone-marrow response to ongoing red cell loss is poor, and this is attributed to increased sequestration of iron (as hemosiderin) in macrophages.[25] Thus, the pathogenesis of anemia in the chronic stage of nagana is analogous to that of anemia of chronic disease or chronic inflammation.[22-23]

Animals infected with any pathogenic trypanosome may develop concurrent and even fatal bacterial, viral, and other protozoan infections as a result of immunosuppression. This is thought to be attributable to trypanosome-induced B-cell apoptosis resulting in loss of protective antiparasite antibody responses and abolishment of memory responses against nonrelated pathogens.[26]

Trypanotolerant animals control parasitemias better and have less severe anemia and organ damage. They usually recover from the disease, but they may act as carriers. On the other hand, human beings have a sterile immunity to these parasites, except *T. brucei gambiense* and *T. brucei rhodesiense.*

CLINICAL FINDINGS

Although anemia is the cardinal feature, there are no pathognomonic signs that would help in pinpointing a diagnosis of trypanosomosis in farm animals. The general clinical picture is as follows, but there are many variations determined by the level of tsetse challenge, the species and strain of the trypanosome, and the breed and management of the host. Acute episodes last for a few days to a few weeks, from which the animal dies or lapses into a subacute to chronic stage, or the illness may be chronic from the beginning. Chronic cases may run a steady course, may be interrupted by periodic incidents of severe illness, or may undergo spontaneous recovery.

The basic clinical syndrome appears after an incubation period of 8 to 20 days following the infective tsetse fly bite. Chancre is not readily noticed under field conditions. There is fever, which is likely to be intermittent or cyclic for weeks. Affected animals are dull, anorexic, and apathetic; have a watery ocular discharge; and lose condition. Superficial lymph nodes become visibly swollen, mucous membranes are pale, diarrhea occasionally occurs, and some animals have edema of the throat and underline. Estrus cycles become irregular, pregnant animals may abort, and semen quality progressively deteriorates. The animal becomes very emaciated and cachectic and dies within 2 to 4 months or longer. Thin, rough-coated, anemic, lethargic cattle with generalized lymph node enlargement are reported to have a "fly struck" appearance.

In general, *T. congolense* is more pathogenic to cattle in eastern and southern Africa, whereas *T. vivax* produces a more serious disease in most of West and Central Africa. However, severe outbreaks of *T. vivax* involving exotic dairy animals in East Africa occur; affected animals show mucosal petechiation, rhinorrhagia, dysentery, and death after an illness of only a few weeks.

Mixed infections with more than one species of trypanosomes are common and are usually more severe. Furthermore, intercurrent bacterial, viral, or other parasitic infections may mask or complicate the basic clinical syndrome. Immune response to bacterial and some viral vaccines is also depressed unless trypanocidal therapy is given at the time of vaccination.

Clinical findings peculiar to the individual trypanosome are as follows:

- *T. vivax* affects all agricultural species except pigs. Acute and chronic outbreaks occur, anemia is severe, and fever is usually associated with high parasitemia. A chronic form of the disease is more usual in East Africa, but an acute hemorrhagic form can occur with exotic cattle. Furthermore, outbreaks in Brazil have been associated with nervous signs in cattle[20] and in sheep,[27] characterized by head pressing, lateral recumbency, paddling movements, and muscle tremors. *T. vivax* is less commonly seen in trypanotolerant cattle breeds.
- *T. congolense* affects all species, usually with an acute disease lasting 4 to 6 weeks, but some chronic cases occur, especially in West Africa. Anemia and emaciation are severe. The savannah subspecies is more pathogenic than the other subspecies.
- *T. brucei brucei* affects all species with a subacute to chronic disease. In addition to fever and anemia, there is often marked subcutaneous edema and keratoconjunctivitis. Nervous signs are manifested in horses, pigs, and small ruminants by ataxia, circling, head pressing, and paralysis. Cattle show chronic clinical signs, and they can act as carriers.
- *T. simiae* affects exotic pigs with a fulminating infection leading to death in hours or a few days of first appearing ill. The clinical signs are fever, stiff gait, dyspnea, and cutaneous hyperemia, without significant anemia. However, no outbreak has been reported in decades.

CLINICAL PATHOLOGY

A progressive drop in packed cell volume is a nonspecific but useful indicator of trypanosomosis in endemic areas. The classic method of confirming nagana diagnosis is to demonstrate parasites in a wet blood film and in a thin or thick blood smear stained with Giemsa. This is fairly reliable in the early stages of the disease when parasitemia is usually high and parasitemic peaks correspond with fever. As the disease progresses, parasitemias become infrequent and the intervals between peaks grow longer, even though the animal is still sick. To increase the accuracy of parasitologic diagnosis, it is now routine to concentrate the parasites in the buffy-coat layer of a microhematocrit capillary tube. The buffy layer is then examined directly at low power (Woo's method) or in a wet preparation with a dark-ground/phase-contrast microscope (Murray's method). Both tests are simple, sensitive, and applicable to field use on individual animals and in herds. Blood should be examined fresh but may be refrigerated for up to 24 hours, beyond which most parasites will die and disappear from the sample.

Blood can also be inoculated into experimental animals, usually rodents, but this is cumbersome and is accurate for only *T. brucei*, and possibly *T. congolense*, but not *T. vivax*.

During surveys, a series of tests can be used to detect antibodies in serum or other body fluids. The three tests used most often are the indirect immunofluorescent antibody test (IFAT), the capillary agglutination test (CAT), and the ELISA. These tests indicate past and current infections, are difficult to standardize for different laboratories, and are not species specific. The ELISA technique was modified to detect circulating trypanosome antigens (antigen-ELISA) using monoclonal antibodies that would distinguish between *T. vivax*, *T. congolense*, and *T. brucei*, and it would detect only current or very recent infections. Results from field trials in Africa and South America have not been encouraging.

The polymerase chain reaction (PCR) technique is now being used to detect trypanosome DNA in blood, serum, and in tsetse tissues. The technique targets the gene encoding the small ribosomal subunit to identify and differentiate all clinically important African trypanosome species and some subspecies. The test is sensitive, economical, and suitable for large-scale epidemiologic studies, usually in combination with other tests. Dried blood spots on filter papers are also a useful source of DNA for the detection of trypanosomes.[28] PCR technology is currently being made available in some laboratories in endemic areas and has led to increased rates of detection.

Examination of the cerebrospinal fluid is used routinely in human sleeping sickness to establish the stage of infection to select the appropriate drug for treatment. In animals, CSF examination for parasites, turbidity, protein content, and leukocytes can be done at necropsy if there have been neurologic signs.[21]

NECROPSY FINDINGS

Gross Pathology

The postmortem lesions are, like the clinical findings, not definitive. The carcass is marked by anemia, emaciation, and enlargement of the liver, spleen, and lymph nodes. Body-fat stores are depleted or show marked serous atrophy, especially around the heart and in bone marrow. The bone marrow may be red (active) in the acute stage, but it becomes pale and gelatinous (unresponsive) in the chronic stage. Subcutaneous edema, corneal opacity, and testicular degeneration may be present. Thickening of the meninges and softening of the brain have been reported in some cattle naturally infected with the South American *T. vivax*.

In acute cases, there will be a general congestion of the viscera and extensive hemorrhages in all tissues. Chronic cases show cachexia, often complicated with secondary bacterial pneumonia or other parasitic diseases.

Histology

Microscopic lesions are also not specific, except in very acute infections, in which clumps of trypanosomes mixed with fibrin thrombi are found in blood vessels. Lymphoid organs are usually hyperplastic and may show varying degrees of erythrophagocytosis and hemosiderosis. The interstitial tissues and perivascular spaces of various parenchymatous organs may contain a lymphoplasmacytic infiltrate. This tends to be most marked with *T. brucei*, in which the parasites often localize extravascularly in the interstitial tissue. A severe nonsuppurative meningoencephalitis, myocarditis, and dermatitis may result. Degenerative changes may also be present in the liver, testis, ovary, brain, and pituitary gland.

Specimens for Pathology

Smears from tissues, usually the cut surface of a lymph node or heart muscle, are examined for trypanosomes before or shortly after the animal dies. Trypanosomes will not be detectable if postmortem examination is delayed for even a few hours because the parasites die and disintegrate soon after the host dies. For PCR detection, blood or buffy coat is spotted on Whatman filter paper (Whatman No. 4) stored at room temperature and sent to the appropriate laboratory.[27] With *T. brucei*, smears of serous fluids, including the CSF, may contain many parasites even when they are undetectable in blood.

The following organs should be taken for histopathology: lymph nodes, spleen, liver, heart, kidney, brain, and any other organ showing gross lesions. The immediate cause of death is often a combination of trypanosome-induced anemia and a concurrent bacterial or parasitic infection.

DIFFERENTIAL DIAGNOSIS

Diagnosis is based on detecting parasites in blood. Because parasitemias fluctuate, multiple samples from a herd or repeated sampling of a suspected case may be required before a specific diagnosis can be made. Furthermore, an infected animal may be suffering from a concurrent disease. Emaciation and anemia can also be associated with the following:

- Malnutrition
- Helminthosis
- Babesiosis
- Anaplasmosis
- East coast fever

Acute trypanosomosis may be confused with hemorrhagic septicemia and anthrax. Laboratory examination of blood, feces, and other tissues is required to confirm diagnosis.

TREATMENT

TREATMENT AND CONTROL

Treatment

Diminazene aceturate (Berenil) (3.5–7 mg/kg IM) (R1 for ruminants, R-3 for equines)

Homidium chloride/bromide (Ethidium/ Novidium (1 mg/kg IM) (R-1 for ruminants and equines)

Isometamedium chloride (Samorin) (0.25–1 mg/kg IM) (R-1 for ruminants)

Quinapyramine sulfate (Antrycide) (5 mg/kg SC) (R1 for equines)

Suramin (Antrypol) (10 mg/kg IV) (R-2 for equines, camelids, 2–3 times weekly)

Control

Isometamedium chloride (2 mg/kg IM) (R-1)

Homidium chloride/bromide (1 mg/kg IM) (R-2)

Prothridium (2 mg/kg IM) (R-2)

Antrycide prosalt (7.4 mg/kg SC) (R-2)

Antrycide/Suramin complex (35 mg/kg SC) (R-2 for *T. simae* in pigs)

The number of trypanocidal drugs available for treating and preventing infections in endemic areas is limited, and 35 million doses are administered yearly in Africa.[29] The drugs have been in the market for half a century or more; their range of therapeutic safety is small; many of them cause severe local reactions, especially in horses; and some may be fatal in high doses. Furthermore, because drugs are expensive and can now be purchased without prescription, inappropriate dosing, improper administration, and use of fake or poor-quality drugs are common. These, plus the fact that some drugs are used both prophylactically and therapeutically, have led to cases of drug resistance, which is universally regarded as a threat to livestock production and health.

Ideally, each country or region establishes a group of sanative drugs that are to be used only as a break in a course of one of the more common drugs. The sanative drug should provide moderate prophylaxis and avoid the development of resistance to the prime drug. These measures have not been well executed in many countries, especially with the privatization of veterinary practice in Africa. This may explain the increasing reports of multiple resistance to curative, sanative, and prophylactic drugs over the years.[6,30-31] On the other hand, a high prevalence of drug resistance to diminazene aceturate has been reported for *T. congolense* without a recent history of drug exposure.[5] The isolates were obtained from tsetse or wildlife in parks in Tanzania, Zambia, and South Africa. Furthermore, it has been observed that clones of *T. congolense* resistant to isometamedium chloride are more easily transmissible to tsetse flies (*G. morsitans*).[32] This may be another factor contributing to the high prevalence of drug-resistant strains in the African region.

Strains are regarded as resistant when they fail to respond to the drug or when they relapse in blood sometime after an apparent cure. More cases of relapses are likely to be observed with the more sensitive PCR method for blood examination. However, it has been observed that relapses, where the host controls the level of parasitemia to a level below the sensitivity of routine microscopic examination, do not affect the productivity of the host.[33] Relapses are more likely to occur if the commencement of treatment is delayed or the dose rate is inadequate. However, in field situations, there is hardly any regular monitoring of drug efficacy, and animals may be reinfected with the same or other species of trypanosomes soon after an otherwise effective cure.

The common drugs in use against trypanosomes are set out in the following discussion. The specific dose rates vary with animal species, the specific trypanosome, and the specific purpose (curative, prophylactic, or sanative).

- Diminazene aceturate (Berenil) is used widely against *T. vivax* and *T. congolense* as a curative and sanative drug at 3.5 to 7 mg/kg BW IM. It is well tolerated by ruminants, and it is one of the two recommended drugs for bovine trypanosomosis. It is not well tolerated by horses.
- Isometamidium (Samorin or Trypamidium) is the other preferred drug against *T. vivax* and *T. congolense* in ruminants. It is used as a curative and prophylactic drug at 0.25 to 1 mg/kg BW IM. At much higher doses (12.5 to 35 mg/kg BW) it can be used prophylactically against *T. simiae* in pigs but not without the risk of death from acute cardiovascular collapse.
- Homidium bromide (ethidium) and homidium chloride (novidium) are also widely used against *T. congolense* and *T. vivax* as curative and sanative drugs at 1 mg/kg BW IM.
- Pyrithidium bromide (prothridium) is less widely used against *T. congolense* and *T. vivax* as prophylaxis at 2 mg/kg BW IM.
- Quinapyramine sulfate (Antrycide) is no longer used extensively in cattle. It is the preferred curative drug against *T. brucei brucei* in horses at 5 mg/kg BW IM. Quinapyramine sulfate and chloride (Antrycide prosalt) is used prophylactically at 7.4 mg/kg BW SC.
- Suramin (naganol) may also be used against *T. brucei* as a curative and prophylactic drug at 10 mg/kg BW in horses and camels.
- Antrycide–Suramin complex is the only other drug effective against *T. simiae* in pigs, and it is used prophylactically at 40 mg/kg BW.

CONTROL

The control of trypanosomosis in endemic countries involves control of tsetse fly population, prophylactic treatment of animals at risk, good husbandry of animals, and use of trypanotolerant animals. There is no vaccine against the disease, and in spite of intensive research, vaccines appear unlikely in the near future because of the ability of trypanosomes to readily change their glycoprotein surface coat through the process of antigenic variation.

Control of tsetse has been successfully attempted in some African countries, but reinvasion is frequent if the land is not properly utilized. The earliest methods involved bush clearing and elimination of game animals on which tsetse feed. These methods were effective in eradicating or controlling tsetse in some parts of the continent, especially in southern Africa, but they resulted in destroying valuable plant and animal resources and also led to soil erosion. More recent methods involved the use of insecticides, especially DDT and endosulfan, applied strategically in the form of ground and aerial spraying over large expanses of land. Because tsetse flies are sensitive to insecticides and no resistance has developed, considerable successes were achieved in some countries. Under the Pan African Tsetse and Trypanosomosis Eradication Campaign (PATTEC) program, tsetse was eliminated from an area of over 10,000 km^2 in Botswana and Namibia in 2006 using a sequential aerial spraying technique to apply deltamethrin.[34] However, spraying insecticides is costly and harmful to the environment. These harmful effects are considerably reduced if the insecticides, for example, synthetic pyrethroids, are applied directly on the animal in the form of spray or pour-on formulation, or the recently described footbath.[34-35] The insecticides also reduce tick infestations in treated animals.

Other effective methods involve use of targets impregnated with insecticides and traps that attract and catch tsetse. These are simple and cheap and can be constructed and maintained by local communities. Furthermore, they do not pollute the environment and are suitable for both small- and large-scale farming. They have been used to drastically reduce tsetse fly population and incidence of trypanosomosis in some countries.

Another method of control is the sterile male technique. Because the female tsetse only mates once in a lifetime, this technique is theoretically able to eradicate a targeted tsetse species in areas where other methods have been used to reduce its density. But it is expensive.

Finally, it should be stated that development of the land for agriculture, industries, highways, and so forth effectively destroys the habitat for tsetse flies. This is occurring in many parts of Africa, including Nigeria, with rapid economic activities and expanding human population.

Attempts at trypanosomosis control have also been directed to prophylactic dosing with chemicals such as suramin, prothridium, and isometamidium (Samorin). Prophylaxis is used along with other methods in areas where there is a heavy tsetse challenge. The prophylactic effect is supplemented by the development of antibodies, and the total period of protection may be as long as 5 months. However, it is customary to give four or five treatments per year. The productivity response to this pattern of treatment is good if general husbandry is also adequate. The downside of this approach is that it is thought to be one of the factors leading to drug resistance in many countries, in addition to the ready availability of fake and poor-quality drugs.

Trypanotolerant animals are being used to establish ranches in areas where tsetse challenge is not too heavy. These indigenous breeds are not well accepted in some countries because their productivity is generally low. To offset this, the breeds are increasingly being crossed with other indigenous and improved breeds. The crosses are more productive, and they retain the trait for trypanotolerance.[9]

For effective control of trypanosomosis in Africa and in Central and South America, an integrated approach will mostly likely produce the desired results in each region. In the absence of a vaccine, control methods must combine reduced exposure to the vectors (large-scale tsetse trapping and pour-on applications) with strategic treatment of exposed animals (chemotherapy and chemoprophylaxis) along with use of trypanotolerant animals when feasible. The Pan African Tsetse and Trypanosomiasis Eradication Campaign launched in the last decade is applying many of these methods in different countries, with the hope of eliminating tsetse from Africa in the near future.

FURTHER READING

Abebe G. Trypanosomosis in Ethiopia. *Ethiop J Biol Sci.* 2005;4:75. [The Biological Society of Ethiopia review article].

Anosa VO. Haematological and biochemical changes in human and animal trypanosomiasis. *Rev Elev Med Vet Pays Trop.* 1988;41:65, 151.

Connor RJ, Van den Bossche P. African animal trypanosomoses. In: Coetzer JAW, Tustin RC, eds. *Infectious Diseases of Livestock.* Vol. 1. 2nd ed. Cape Town: Oxford University Press; 2004:251.

Desquesnes M. *Livestock Trypanosomoses and Their Vectors in Latin America.* Paris: OIE (World Organisation for Animal Health); 2004.

Franco JR, et al. Epidemiology of human African trypanosomiasis. *Clin Epidemiol.* 2014;6:257.

Gibson W. The origins of the trypanosome genome strains *Trypanosoma brucei brucei* TREU 927, *T. b. gambiense* DAL 972, *T. vivax* Y486 and T. congolense IL3000. *Parasite Vect.* 2012;5:71.

Hunter AG, Luckins AG. Trypanosomosis. In: Sewell MMH, Brocklesby DW, eds. *Handbook on Animal Diseases in the Tropics.* 4th ed. London: Baillière Tindall; 1990:204.

Ikede BO. African trypanosomes. Honigberg BM. Mechanisms of pathogenicity among protozoa. *Insect Sci Applic.* 1986;7:363.

Jordan AM. *Trypanosomiasis Control and African Rural Development.* London: Longman; 1988.

Losos G. Trypanosomiases. In: *Infectious Tropical Diseases of Domestic Animals.* London: Longman; 1986:182.

Stephen LE. *Trypanosomiasis: A Veterinary Perspective.* Oxford: Pergamon Press; 1986.

REFERENCES

1. Sow A, et al. *Res Vet Sci.* 2013;doi:10.1016/j.rvsc.2012.12.011; [Epub ahead of print].
2. Fikru R, et al. *Vet Parasitol.* 2012;[Epub ahead of print].
3. Cox AP, et al. *Parasite Vect.* 2010;3:82.
4. Nakayima J, et al. *Parasite Vector.* 2012;5:217.
5. Chitanga S, et al. *PLoS Negl Trop Dis.* 2011;5:1454.
6. Mungube EO, et al. *Parasite Vect.* 2012;5:155.
7. Takeet MI, et al. *Res Vet Sci.* 2013;94:555.
8. Mekata H, et al. *J Vet Med Sci.* 2008;70:923.
9. Orenge CO, et al. *BMC Genet.* 2012;13:87.
10. Geerts S, et al. *Trends Parasitol.* 2009;25:132.
11. Simukoko H, et al. *Vet Parasitol.* 2007;147:231.
12. Horn D, Mcculloch R. *Curr Opin Microbiol.* 2010;13:700.
13. Jackson AP, et al. *Proc Natl Acad Sci USA.* 2012;109:3416.
14. Alsford S, et al. *Genome Biol.* 2009;10:223.
15. Glover L, et al. *PLoS Pathog.* 2013;9:e1003260.
16. Stephens NA, et al. *Trends Parasitol.* 2012;28:539.
17. Simarro PP, et al. *PLoS Negl Trop Dis.* 2012;6:e1859.
18. Franco JR, et al. *Clin Epidemiol.* 2014;6:257.
19. Batista JS, et al. *Vet Parasitol.* 2007;143:174.
20. Batista JS, et al. *Vet Res.* 2011;42:63.
21. Stijlemans B, et al. *Immunobiology.* 2008;213:823.
22. Noyes HA, et al. *PLoS ONE.* 2009;4:e5170.
23. Guegan F, et al. *Cell Microbiol.* 2013;doi:10.1111/cmi.12123; [Epub ahead of print].
24. Stijlemans B, et al. *Endocr Metab Immune Disord Drug Targets.* 2010;10:71.
25. Radwanska M, et al. *PLoS Pathog.* 2008;4:e1000078.
26. Galiza GJ, et al. *Vet Parasitol.* 2011;182:359.
27. Vitouley HS, et al. *PLoS Negl Trop Dis.* 2011;5:e1223.
28. van Gool F, Mattioli R. *30th ISCTRC Conference.* Kampala, Uganda: 2009:305.
29. Moti Y, et al. *Vet Parasitol.* 2012;189:197.
30. Sow A, et al. *Vet Parasitol.* 2012;187:105.
31. van den Bossche P, et al. *Vet Parasitol.* 2006;135:365.
32. Vitouley HS, et al. *Vet Parasitol.* 2012;190:349.
33. Kgori PM, Modo S. *30th ISCTRC Conference.* Kampala, Uganda: 2009:461.
34. Bouyer J, et al. *Prev Vet Med.* 2007;78:223.
35. Bouyer F, et al. *PLoS Negl Trop Dis.* 2011;5:e1276.

SURRA (MAL DE CADERAS, MURRINA)

SYNOPSIS

Etiology *Trypanosoma evansi* (synonym *T. equinum*), a subspecies of *T. brucei,* but transmitted mechanically by biting flies, mainly tabanids, and by vampire bats in Latin America.

Epidemiology Endemic disease of mainly horses, camels, and buffaloes in the tropics and subtropics, seasonality is related to fly population. Rare outbreaks in Spain and France.

Clinical signs Fever, progressive emaciation, anemia, subcutaneous edema, nervous signs, death. May be acute, but mostly subacute to chronic.

Clinical pathology Progressive anemia, parasite detection in blood by various methods, serology.

Lesions Not definitive but include pallor, emaciation, muscle atrophy of hindquarters in horses, lymphadenomegaly, and jaundice.

Differential diagnosis list:

- Nagana
- Malnutrition
- Helminthosis

- Babesiosis
- Anaplasmosis
- Hemorrhagic septicemia

Treatment Trypanocides as in nagana, but less effective.

Control Chemotherapy, no vaccine.

ETIOLOGY

Trypanosoma evansi, the first pathogenic trypanosome to be identified in 1880 in India, belongs to the *brucei* group (subgenus *Trypanozoon*) but has lost its kinetoplast DNA (akinetoplastic) and is therefore not capable of cyclical development in tsetse *Glossina* spp.[1] The parasite is believed to have originated from a mutated form of *T. equiperdum* characterized by being dyskinetoplastic (has lost part of its kDNA). *T. evansi* was formerly referred to as *T. equinum, T. hippicum,* or *T. venezuelense* in South America. Worldwide, it is the most widespread species of pathogenic trypanosomes. In blood smears, *T. evansi* is morphologically indistinguishable from *T. brucei,* but at the molecular level, the structure of the kinetoplast DNA of *T. evansi* is different.

EPIDEMIOLOGY

Occurrence

Surra has a wide distribution in areas of Asia, Middle East, Central and South America, Africa north of the tsetse belt, and occasionally in Europe. The disease is called "mal de caderas" (meaning "sickness of the hips") in South America, "murrina" in Panama, and "surra" in other parts of the world. In some countries, the incidence of surra increases significantly during the rainy season when there are large biting fly populations, the so-called surra season. The disease affects mainly camels and horses, but buffaloes and cattle are also affected. Some endemic areas have been identified in Las Palmas and the Canary Islands, and two recent outbreaks of the disease in Spain and France were traced to camel importation from the areas.[2] A two-part comprehensive review of *T. evansi* and surra has been published recently.[3-4]

Morbidity and Case Fatality

Infection rates in camels, horses, and buffaloes in endemic countries vary considerably and can be as high as 100% in buffalo herds in high-risk areas.[5] During a recent outbreak in Spain, 76% of the camels, 36% of the donkeys, and 26% of the horses examined were affected.[6] Fewer cases are detected by standard parasitologic methods than by serology or PCR methods. The case fatality in horses and camels is nearly 100% if untreated, but it is much lower in cattle and buffaloes, where the disease tends to run a chronic course. Nonetheless, strains highly pathogenic for water buffaloes and cattle have been reported in the Philippines.[7]

Method of Transmission

Several hematophagous flies can transmit *T. evansi* mechanically, but the most important is the horse fly (*Tabanus* spp.), followed by the stable fly (*Stomoxys* spp.). Transmission is enhanced when horses or camels congregate or are closely herded and when they have high numbers of parasites in their blood. In South America, the vampire bat also can transmit the disease in its saliva. The process can be mechanical as for flies but also biological in that parasitemia occurs in the bats, and the bats may die of the infection or recover and serve as carriers. Therefore vampire bats are simultaneously hosts, reservoirs, and vectors of *T. evansi.* Indigenous cattle, buffalo, and several species of wildlife may act as reservoirs of infection for horses and camels. Several workers in South America have incriminated capybaras, small marsupials, armadillos, feral pigs, and peccary as possible reservoirs of *T. evansi.*[8-9] Carnivores can also be infected peri-orally when they feed on an infected carcass.

Immune Mechanisms

Immune mechanisms are related to antigenic variation of the parasite and production of antibodies by the host, as in *T. brucei* and all its subspecies. Infected animals are also immunosuppressed and respond poorly to vaccination. As with other trypanosome infections, the immunosuppressive effect is abrogated following successful antitrypanosome treatment.[10] The disease can be reproduced experimentally by blood inoculation.

Zoonotic Implications

Humans are generally not susceptible to *T. evansi* infection. However, two cases of human infection and disease have been reported, one from India and the other from Egypt.[11-12] In the Indian case, the serum of the infected patient was found to have no trypanolytic activity, and this finding was linked to a lack of apolipoprotein L-1, the pathway in normal human serum for killing most trypanosomes.[13]

Economic Importance

Surra is one of the most important diseases of camels in Africa and Asia, and outbreaks are increasingly being reported in South American horses and occasionally in European camels. Camel raising in Africa and buffalo production in Asia are particularly affected by the disease. As in nagana, losses are attributable to reduced productivity, infertility, abortion, mortality, and cost of treatment. In Indonesia, losses as a result of surra were estimated at more than US$20 million in the 1980s. More recently, it has been estimated that in the Philippines, the total net benefit for surra control for herds in a typical village in an endemic area is $158,000 per annum.[14]

Biosecurity Concerns

There are no biosecurity concerns, except with regard to importation of carrier animals to nonendemic countries.

PATHOGENESIS

Trypanosomes are inoculated into the host from the contaminated mouthparts of biting insects or the saliva of vampire bats. Parasites multiply in blood, causing anemia and spread to serous fluids and interstitial tissue, resulting in inflammatory changes just like those seen with *T. brucei.* The anemia of surra is probably similar to that of nagana. There is increased erythrophagocytosis and intravascular hemolysis resulting from lipid peroxidation of erythrocytes.[15] As for emaciation, it has been suggested that protein breakdown and lipolysis might contribute to the cachexia in infected horses.[16] In horses, *T. evansi* frequently invades the central nervous system, including the spinal cord, where it is less exposed to chemotherapeutic agents.

CLINICAL FINDINGS

The main clinical findings are intermittent fever, progressive anemia, edema of dependent parts of the body, dullness, listlessness, loss of body condition despite a good appetite, nasal and ocular discharge, abortion, and infertility. In the late stages, there are marked nervous signs, including marked paraplegia, paralysis, delirium, and convulsions. In a recent outbreak involving horses in Brazil, the nervous signs were ataxia, blindness, head tilt, circling, head pressing, and paddling movements before death.[17] Surra is invariably fatal in camels and horses, with death occurring in days or months, but camels may exhibit chronic signs for years. These signs include a reduction in milk yield and capacity for work, and a high abortion rate in pregnant females. Abortion and high neonatal mortality characterized the camel outbreak in the Canary Islands.[18] In endemic areas, cattle and buffalo usually have a milder disease that may be exacerbated by stress from adverse climatic conditions, work, or intercurrent disease. Signs may include a reduction in milk yield and capacity for work, irregular estrus, a high rate of abortion and stillbirth, and poor semen quality in bulls. Outbreaks of a more severe disease in indigenous zebu cattle are reported from time to time.[7] In such cases, there may be nervous signs and high mortality rate.

CLINICAL PATHOLOGY

As with tsetse-transmitted trypanosomosis, routine parasite detection is more reliable in the acute phase. Examination of wet blood films and stained smears of blood and lymph node should be carried out, and this should include the buffy-coat method. In the chronic phase, repeated sampling for some days may be required. In addition, suspected blood samples may be inoculated into rats or mice, both of which are highly susceptible.

A number of nonspecific serologic tests have been used, especially in areas where other forms of trypanosomes are not prevalent. These include the mercuric chloride, formol gel, or stilbamidine test for increased serum protein levels. Specific antibody detection tests are also available and include the direct card agglutination test (CAAT) for antibodies, the latex agglutination test (Suratex) for circulating antigens, the indirect fluorescent antibody test (IFAT), and the enzyme-linked immunosorbent assay (ELISA). Serologic tests are probably more sensitive than parasitologic methods in revealing the true extent of surra in camel herds.

Where the facilities exist, the PCR technique is more sensitive and specific and can detect trypanosome DNA antemortem in the cerebrospinal fluid and in brain tissue postmortem.[19]

NECROPSY FINDINGS

The carcass is emaciated and pale and may be icteric but, as in *T. brucei* infections, there are no pathognomonic gross and microscopic lesions unless the parasites are detectable. Infected horses will show hindquarter muscle atrophy, splenomegaly, and lymphadenomegaly. Asymmetric leukomalacia has been described in naturally infected horses, but it is not clear whether or not this was a result of treatment with diminazene aceturate.[15] Microscopic changes are characterized by a lymphoplasmacytic infiltrate of various organs, including the brain and spinal cord. If the carcass is very fresh, trypanosomes can be detected in blood and CSF with routine microscopy, and in the parenchyma of central nervous system by immunoperoxidase method[17] or by PCR technique identifying parasite DNA.[19]

DIFFERENTIAL DIAGNOSIS

Laboratory services are required to confirm a diagnosis; even then, without the use of molecular techniques, surra cannot be easily distinguished from *T. brucei brucei* infection where both coexist. Clinical signs and gross and microscopic lesions of both diseases in horses and camels are identical. Specimens to take for laboratory diagnosis are blood, brain, spinal cord, lymph nodes, spleen, and liver.

TREATMENT

TREATMENT AND CONTROL

Treatment

Quinapyramine sulfate (Quintricide) (5 mg/kg SC) (R-1 for camels)

Diminazene aceturate (Berenil) (3.5–7 mg/kg IM) (R-1 for ruminants, R-3 for equines)

Melarsomine (Cymerlasan) (0.25 mg/kg IM for camels and 0.5 mg/kg for cattle) (R-1)

Isometamedium chloride (Samorin) (0.25–1 mg/kg IM) (R-1 for ruminants)

Suramin (Antrypol) (10 mg/kg IV) (R-2 for equines, camelids, 2–3 times weekly)

Control

Isometamedium chloride (2 mg/kg IM) (R-1)

Antrycide prosalt (7.4 mg/kg SC) (R-2)

Suramin (Antrypol) (10 mg/kg IV) (R-2 for equines, camelids, 2–3 times weekly)

Drugs used for treating nagana could be used for surra, but the outcome is less favorable because of their low trypanocidal activity against *T. evansi* and their specific toxicity for camels and horses. Furthermore, the drugs are not able to cross the blood–brain barrier to reach parasites in the cerebrospinal fluid and nervous tissue. As a result, relapses are common and may present as drug resistance. Three Brazilian isolates of *T. evansi* tested for drug resistance were found to be fully susceptible to a single dose of suramin sodium at 10 mg/kg BM in mice.[20]

Quinapyramine sulfate (quintrycide) is used curatively for camels, and diminazene aceturate (Berenil) is used for horses. A water-soluble arsenical, melarsomine hydrochloride (Cymerlasan), given IM is recommended for camels at 0.25 mg/kg BW and for cattle at 0.5 mg/kg BW.[21] For both curative and prophylactic use, quinapyramine prosalt (trypacide), suramin (naganol), and isometamedium chloride (samorin or trypamidium) are recommended (see section on nagana or African trypanosomosis).

CONTROL

Unlike in nagana, control measures are aimed primarily at the host rather than the vector, which is abundant. The measures include detection and treatment of infected animals, prophylactic treatment of susceptible animals, and their protection from biting flies and bats, where possible. As in nagana, there is no vaccine.

FURTHER READING

Abebe G. Trypanosomosis in Ethiopia. *Ethiop J Biol Sci.* 2005;4:75-121. [The Biological Society of Ethiopia review article].

Desquesnes M. *Livestock Trypanosomoses and Their Vectors in Latin America.* Paris: OIE (World Organisation for Animal Health); 2004.

Desquesnes M, et al. *Trypanosoma evansi* and surra: a review and perspectives on origin, history, distribution, taxonomy, morphology, hosts and pathogenic effects. *Biomed Res Intern.* 2013;194176.

Desquesnes M, et al. *Trypanosoma evansi* and surra: a review and perspectives on transmission, epidemiology and control, impact and zoonotic aspects. *Biomed Res Intern.* 2013;321237.

Hunter AG, Luckins AG. Trypanosomosis. In: Sewell MMH, Brocklesby DW, eds. *Handbook on Animal Diseases in the Tropics.* 4th ed. London: Bailliére Tindall; 1990:204-226.

OIE Manual of Diagnostic Tests and Vaccines for Terrestrial Animals. Vol. 1. 6th ed. Paris: OIE; 2008 chapter 2.1.17:252-260.

Stephen LE. *Trypanosomiasis: A Veterinary Perspective.* Oxford: Pergamon Press; 1986.

REFERENCES

1. Lai DH, et al. *Proc Natl Acad Sci USA.* 2008;105:1999.
2. Gutierrez C, et al. *Vet Parasitol.* 2010;174:26.
3. Desquesnes M, et al. *Biomed Res Intern.* 2013;194176.
4. Desquesnes M, et al. *Biomed Res Intern.* 2013;321237.
5. Dargantes AP, et al. *Int J Parasitol.* 2009;39:1109.
6. Tamarit A, et al. *Vet Parasitol.* 2010;167:74.
7. Mekata H, et al. *Parasitol Res.* 2013;[Epub ahead of print].
8. Rademaker V, et al. *Acta Trop.* 2009;111:102.
9. Herrera HM, et al. *Parasitol Res.* 2008;103:619.
10. Singla LD, et al. *Trop Anim Health Prod.* 2010;42:589.
11. Powar RM, et al. *Indian J Med Microbiol.* 2006;24:72.
12. Haridy FM, et al. *J Egypt Soc Parasitol.* 2011;41:65.
13. Vanhollebeke B, et al. *N Engl J Med.* 2006;355:2752.
14. Dobson RJ, et al. *Int J Parasitol.* 2009;39:1115.
15. Habila N, et al. *Res Vet Sci.* 2012;93:13.
16. Ranjithkumar M, et al. *Trop Anim Health Prod.* 2013;45:417.
17. Rodrigues A, et al. *Vet Pathol.* 2009;46:251.
18. Guttierez C, et al. *Vet Parasitol.* 2005;130:163.
19. Berlin D, et al. *Vet Parasitol.* 2009;161:316.
20. Faccio L, et al. *Exp Parasitol.* 2013;134:309.
21. Desquesnes M, et al. *Parasitology.* 2011;138:1134.

Multi-Organ Diseases Due to Fungal Infection

PROTOTHECOSIS AND CHLORELLOSIS (ALGAL BACTEREMIA)

Protothecosis and chlorellosis are rare pseudofungal diseases in animals caused by the opportunistic algae of the Chlorellaceae family, *Prototheca* spp. (achlorophyllous mutant) and *Chlorella* spp. (chlorophyll-containing green alga), respectively.[1] Asymptomatic systemic infections and lymphadenitis associated with the achlorophyllous alga *Prototheca zopfii* or the green alga *Chlorella* spp. are extremely rare in cattle and sheep. Peritonitis and lymphadenitis associated with *Scenedesmus* spp., which is closely related to *Chlorella* spp., occurs rarely in cattle.[2] More common is mastitis in cattle caused by *P. zopfii*, or the more recently recognized *Prototheca blaschkeae*.[3] Protothecosis in goats is caused by *Prototheca wickerhamii* and presents as chronic weight loss and signs of respiratory disease.[4] Infections are considered opportunistic, with the exception of increased risk for disseminated infection in sheep grazing sewage-contaminated pasture. Lesions are typically granulomas.[5] Diagnosis is based on demonstration of alga in granulomatous lesions predominantly in the lymph nodes.[1] PCR-based testing is available.

REFERENCES

1. Ramirez-Romero R, et al. *Mycopathologia.* 2010;169:461.
2. Hafner S, et al. *Vet Pathol.* 2013;50:256.
3. Ricchi M, et al. *Vet Microbiol.* 2013;162:997.

4. Camboim EKA, et al. *Mycoses.* 2011;54:e196.
5. Onozaki M, et al. *Jap J Infect Dis.* 2013;66:383.

COCCIDIOIDOMYCOSIS

ETIOLOGY

Coccidioides immitis is associated with the disease in all species, including humans. *Coccidioides posadasii* appears to be increasingly recognized as a pathogen.[1]

EPIDEMIOLOGY

Coccidioidomycosis is a comparatively benign disease of farm animals, usually causing no apparent illness, although disseminated or overt pulmonary disease is associated with a high case-fatality rate in horses.[2] Sporadic cases are recorded in all species but are most common in dogs and in cattle and, to a much less extent, in pigs, sheep, and horses. Pulmonary coccidioidomycosis has been described in a 13-day-old foal. Approximately 4% of horses in areas in which the disease is endemic have serum antibodies to *C. immitis.*[2] The disease tends to affect young to middle-aged animals (median age of 8 years in affected horses), presumably because they are naïve to the infection, with older animals likely to have been exposed and subsequently resistant to the disease.[2] Case-fatality rates are low for mares with abortion (~0%) and animals with superficial abscesses compared with a fatality rate greater than 90% in horses with pneumonia and pleural effusion, or with pneumonia and at least one extrapulmonary site of disease.

The disease is enzootic in the southwestern United States, and up to 20% of cattle finished in feedlots in the area may harbor the fungus. The incidence of the disease in humans in the area provides a major problem in public health. It is not contagious, with infection occurring by inhalation of spores of the fungus, which grows in the soil, and possibly by ingestion and through cutaneous abrasions. The disease is common in dogs and is reported in aquatic wildlife (walrus), rhinoceros, and a koala (in San Diego, California).[3-6]

CLINICAL FINDINGS

Clinical manifestations of infection in any species can include fever, abortion, pneumonia, pleural effusion, severe weight loss, osteomyelitis, and external abscessation.[2]

In horses, findings include weight loss up to severe emaciation, a fluctuating temperature, persistent cough, muscle pain, and superficial abscesses, often recurring, and most commonly in the pectoral area. Increased lung sounds, wheezing, and dullness are audible over the ventral chest. Other signs include edema of the legs, anemia, and intermittent colic as a result of internal abscesses and peritoneal adhesions. Liver rupture may cause death. Affected sheep show fever and abscesses in peripheral lymph nodes.

CLINICAL PATHOLOGY

A leukocytosis is usual, and there can be increases in serum or plasma markers of inflammation (serum amyloid A, fibrinogen).

Fungal cultures or biopsies can be positive for *C. immitis. Coccidioides* spp. grows within 2 to 5 days on several media, although fungal culture should be restricted to biosafety level 3 laboratories.[7] A PCR assay is available to detect and determine the species of *Coccidioides* involved in the disease.[1]

Microscopic examination of tissues or of transtracheal or bronchoalveolar lavage fluids, lymph nodes, and pleural fluid exudates can be performed using KOH (or KOH-ink), lactophenol cotton blue, H&E, Papanicolaou, PAS, and methenamine silver stains.[7]

Serologic tests (i.e., agar gel immunodiffusion [AGID] assays and ELISA for the detection of IgM and IgG antibodies) may assist the diagnosis of coccidioidomycosis. Serum antibody titers are highest in animals with disseminated or pulmonary disease and lowest in animals with localized disease or abortion.[2]

NECROPSY FINDINGS

The lesions produced in cattle and pigs are granulomatous, contain a cream-colored pus, are sometimes calcified, and are found in the bronchial, mediastinal, and, rarely, the mesenteric, pharyngeal and submaxillary lymph nodes and in the lungs. In a neonatal foal, the lungs were diffusely infiltrated with a miliary pattern of multiple, coalescing, pale-tan to red, irregularly shaped, slightly raised, firm foci, 0.1 to 0.5 cm in diameter.

DIFFERENTIAL DIAGNOSIS

Microscopic or cultural examination may be used to identify the disease. Isolation of the organism or detection of DNA by polymerase chain reaction (PCR) is preferred.[1]

Differential diagnosis list:
- Cattle and pigs—tuberculosis
- Sheep and goats—caseous lymphadenitis
- Horses—*C. pseudotuberculosis* infection, pneumonia and pleuropneumonia, metastatic *Streptococcus equi* infection

TREATMENT

Administration of azole compounds (fluconazole, itraconazole, voriconazole) or amphotericin B is advised, although the efficacy of these compounds remains to be determined.[7] Animals treated with these compounds must be monitored for adverse effects, including nephropathy induced by amphotericin.

Because infection occurs by the inhalation of soil-borne spores, control of dust in feedlots may help to prevent the spread of the disease. Dust control is a major factor in prevention of human coccidioidomycosis because there is no vaccine or effective therapeutic agent available, and the eradication of *C. immitis* from the soil is not practicable.

REFERENCES

1. Sheff KW, et al. *Med Mycol.* 2010;48:466.
2. Higgins JC, et al. *Vet J.* 2007;173:118.
3. Wallace RS, et al. *J Zoo Wildlife Med.* 2009;40:365.
4. Schmitt TL, et al. *J Zoo Wildlife Med.* 2014;45:173.
5. Burgdorf-Moisuk A, et al. *J Zoo Wildlife Med.* 2012;43:197.
6. Ajithdoss DK, et al. *J Comp Pathol.* 2011;145:132.
7. Cafarchia C, et al. *Vet Microbiol.* 2013;167:215.

PARACOCCIDIOIDOMYCOSIS (PARACOCCIDIOIDES INFECTION)

Paracoccidioidomycosis in humans caused by *Paracoccidioides brasiliensis* is endemic in parts of South and Central America.[1,2] The disease affects mainly men, causing oral mucosal lesions and disseminated granulomatous disease.[3] There is serologic evidence of widespread exposure of horses,[4] free-ranging pigs,[5] dairy cattle,[6] sheep,[7] and goats[8] in endemic regions, but no reports of disease caused by this organism in large animals. Pigs appear to be resistant to the disease.[5] The organism was identified in tuberculous lesions obtained at slaughter from cattle in Kenya, but the etiologic role for *B. brasiliensis* was unclear.[9]

REFERENCES

1. Teixeira MM, et al. *PLoS Pathog.* 2014;10.
2. Seyedmousavi S, et al. *Clin Micro Infect.* 2015;21:416.
3. Lopez-Martinez R, et al. *Mycoses.* 2014;57:525.
4. Neuschrank Albano AP, et al. *Brazil J Micro.* 2015;46:513.
5. Belitardo DR, et al. *Mycopathologia.* 2014;177:91.
6. Silveira LH, et al. *Mycopathologia.* 2008;165:367.
7. Oliveira GG, et al. *Mycopathologia.* 2012;173:63.
8. Ferreira JB, et al. *Mycopathologia.* 2013;176:95.
9. Kuria JN, et al. *Ond J Vet Res.* 2013;80.

RHODOTORULUA SPP. INFECTION

Infection by *Rhodotorula* spp. is a rare cause of disease in humans and animals.[1] In large animals it is associated with pneumonia and fungemia in sheep.[2]

REFERENCES

1. Wirth F, et al. *Interdisc Pers Infect Dis.* 2012;465717.
2. Chitko-McKown CG, et al. *Transbound Emerg Dis.* 2014;61:E76.

HISTOPLASMOSIS

Histoplasmosis, associated with infection with *Histoplasma capsulatum,* is a rare systemic mycosis in farm animals, with a high prevalence in specific geographic localities, such as the Ohio River and Mississippi River system and areas of South and Central America, Mediterranean countries, Asia,

Africa, and Australia. Cases have been recorded in horses, cattle, and pigs. The disease is relatively common in cats and dogs and occurs in a wide variety of other species, including wildlife and humans.[1-4]

The fungus is able to survive for periods as long as 4 months in soil and water. Infection occurs by the inhalation of contaminated dust, and primary invasion usually takes place in the lung. The disease can spread from animals to humans. Attempts at experimental infection in cattle, sheep, horses, and pigs have resulted in nonfatal infections, unless the agent is given intravenously, but the test animals become positive to the histoplasmin cutaneous sensitivity test.

Clinical syndromes vary greatly and include pneumonia with dyspnea and nasal discharge, hepatic insufficiency with jaundice and anasarca, placentitis with abortion, and widespread lesions in neonates, especially foals. Infections in horses can be evident as intra-abdominal masses.[5]

As a diagnostic aid for herd or area, the histoplasmin skin test appears to be satisfactory. Keratitis attributable to *Histoplasma* spp. has been described. Histoplasmosis may be secondary to yersiniosis in the horse.

Necropsy lesions are as variable as the clinical syndrome and include gross hepatic enlargement containing necrotic foci, pulmonary consolidation and granulomatous pneumonia, and enlargement of splanchnic lymph nodes. Aggregation of the fungal bodies in lymphoid tissue and other tissues in which large numbers of phagocytes are in residence is characteristic of the disease; the lesions consist of groups of macrophages packed with fungal cells. Fungal culture can yield the organism.

Triazoles (e.g., fluconazole, itraconazole) or imidazoles (e.g., ketoconazole) appear to be sensible choices for pharmacologic therapy, but efficacy has not been demonstrated. The treatment of choice for histoplasmosis in dogs and cats is itraconazole, either alone or in combination with ketoconazole or amphotericin B.[3] Voriconazole is also used, but without documented efficacy in large case series in dogs or cats.

The disease associated with infection with *H. farciminosum* is dealt with under the heading "Epizootic Lymphangitis."

REFERENCES

1. Clothier KA, et al. *J Vet Diagn Invest*. 2014;26:297.
2. Brandao J, et al. *J Vet Diagn Invest*. 2014;26:158.
3. Aulakh HK, et al. *J Am Anim Hosp Assoc*. 2012;48:182.
4. Atiee G, et al. *Vet Radiol Ultra*. 2014;55:310.
5. Nunes J, et al. *J Vet Diagn Invest*. 2006;18:508.

CRYPTOCOCCOSIS (EUROPEAN BLASTOMYCOSIS, TORULOSIS)

Infection with the yeast *Cryptococcus neoformans* or *C. gattii* (the *C. neoformans–gattii* complex) occurs in most species, including humans, cattle, horses, goats, dogs and cats, and wildlife, either as a generalized disease, sometimes with localization in particular tissues, or as a granulomatous meningoencephalitis.[1-7] In humans, pulmonary lesions are more likely with *C. gattii* infection, and neurologic disease more likely with *C. neoformans*.[4] *C. neoformans* is a basidiomycetous fungus with a worldwide distribution, commonly found in soil contaminated with avian feces.[8] Two pathogenic variants of *C. neoformans* are *C. neoformans var. neoformans* and *C. neoformans var. gattii*, and these variants are separate species, based on DNA sequence analysis, but are not distinguishable by the routinely performed and rapidly available *C. neoformans* capsular antigen latex agglutination titer.[8]

The frequency of disease or animal risk factors are not reported. Of 260 horses examined in an area in which the disease was considered endemic (Vancouver Island, Canada), 4 had cryptococcus isolated from nasal swabs and none had detected serum antibody titers to the organism.[9]

Nervous system involvement is manifested by stiffness, hyperesthesia, blindness, or incoordination. Clinical signs in cattle include multifocal neurologic deficits manifested by hypermetria, ataxia, depression, circling, impaired vision, head pressing, low head carriage, wide-based stance, and falling to the side or backward.[4,10] Systemic involvement includes cases of myxomatous lesions of nasal mucosa, pulmonary abscess or pneumonia, jejunal granuloma, lymphadenitis, osteomyelitis, placentitis with abortion, and systemic involvement in the fetus. *C. neoformans* is a cause of bovine mastitis. The disease can manifest as sinonasal granulomas in horses with local extension to the cranial vault.[3]

CSF of affected animals is xanthochromic, with elevated white cell count and markedly increased protein concentration.[8] Cryptococci can be detected in cerebrospinal fluid of animals with neurologic disease by microscopic examination of the fluid, or detection of serum or CSF antibodies to the organism (detected by latex agglutination test).[8]

Successful treatment of neurologic disease in horses is by administration of triazole antifungals, such as fluconazole (14 mg/kg PO once, and then 5 mg/kg PO q24h) for weeks to months;[8] or, for sinonasal granulomas, a combination of systemic therapy with fluconazole, debulking of the lesions in the nasal cavity, and intralesional injection of fluconazole, amphotericin, and/or formalin,[3] or irrigation of the nasal sinuses with enilconazole.[11]

REFERENCES

1. Vorathavorn VI, et al. *J Vet Emerg Crit Care*. 2013;23:489.
2. Stilwell G, et al. *BMC Vet Res*. 2014;10.
3. Stewart AJ, et al. *JAVMA*. 2009;235:723.
4. Riet-Correa F, et al. *J Vet Diagn Invest*. 2011;23:1056.
5. McGill S, et al. *Med Mycol*. 2009;47:625.
6. Huckabone SE, et al. *J Wildlife Dis*. 2015;51:295.
7. Govendir M, et al. *J Vet Pharmacol Ther*. 2015;38:93.
8. Hart KA, et al. *J Vet Int Med*. 2008;22:1436.
9. Duncan C, et al. *Med Mycol*. 2011;49:734.
10. Magalhaes GM, et al. *J Comp Pathol*. 2012;147:106.
11. Cruz VC, et al. *JAVMA*. 2009;234:509.

NORTH AMERICAN BLASTOMYCOSIS

The fungus associated with North American blastomycosis, an important disease in humans[1] and dogs,[2] is *Blastomyces dermatitidis*, which is genetically diverse, having over 100 haplotypes divided into two important genetic groupings (Groups 1 and 2), although it has yet to be fully classified.[3,4] More veterinary isolates are in Group 2 than in Group 1, with some haplotypes in each group being identified in only human infections (Group 1) or animals (Group 2).[4] The asexual phase is called *Blastomyces dermatitidis* and its sexual phase, *Ajellomyces dermatitidis*.[1] The organism affects both animals and humans; although it does not appear to be zoonotic (direct transfer of infection from animals to humans), caution should be exercised when treating animals with the disease. Presence of disease, or prevalence of antibodies to the organism, can be indicative of endemicity of infection in geographic areas.

The disease is relatively common in dogs in the upper Midwest of the United States, but it is rare in horses and other large animals.[5] It is reported in horses, goats, sheep, alpaca, and cattle and in miscellaneous other species such as ferrets.[4,6-10] The disease is reported, although infrequently, worldwide, with cases in animals recorded in Italy,[11] West Africa,[6] India, and South America, in addition to well-recognized foci in North America.[4]

Risk factors for large animals are not identified.

There is little information on the pathogenesis of this disease in large animals. In humans and dogs, infection is either by inhalation of organism, with subsequent development of granulomatous pneumonia, or it follows direct infection of skin, presumably through wounds or macerated dermis, resulting in skin lesions. Infection from either site can then become systemic, with pulmonary infection disseminating to other organs, including the brain, urogenital tract, viscera, and skin. Infection originating in the skin can spread to other organs.[1,5] Systemic infection in dogs is associated with increases in concentration or activity of markers of systemic inflammation and hypercoagulability.[12]

The disease in horses can affect the skin (Fig. 21-3), bones,[8] temporomandibular joint, mammary gland, and both thoracic and abdominal organs. Skin lesions in horses

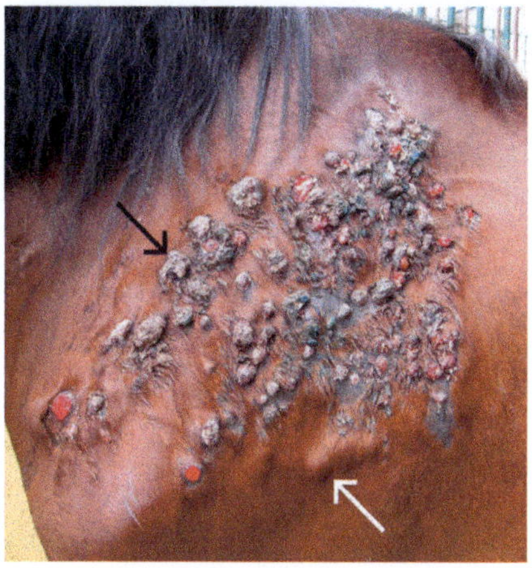

Fig. 21-3 **Lesions of blastomycosis in horse demonstrating combination of verrucous, raised, hairless lesions (black arrow) and subcutaneous lesions (white arrow).** (Reproduced with permission from Funiciello B, et al. *Equine Vet Educ* 2014;26:458.)

occur mainly in the skin of perianal, perivulvar, neck, pectoral, inguinal areas, ventrum, mammary gland, and hindlegs,[5] and are typically of either of two forms, or a mix of each (Fig. 21-3): subcutaneous nodules or verrucous, irregularly shaped lesions with hair loss and crusty raised margins.[5,11] The verrucous lesions are often located over subcutaneous abscesses. Skin lesions can be ulcerated and have draining tracts from deeper lesions.

The pulmonary form is reported in sheep,[7] disseminated disease with clinical manifestations of central neurologic dysfunction in an alpaca,[10] and granulomatous disease resembling tuberculosis in cattle.[13]

Organisms can occasionally be identified as budding yeast bodies in the exudate of ulcerative lesions or draining tracts. Demonstration of organism in typical lesions confirms the disease. *B. dermatitidis* antigens can be detected in urine of animals with blastomycosis.[8,14] The degree of antigenuria has diagnostic utility in dogs, being moderately sensitive but highly specific for the presence of the disease, and is useful in monitoring response to therapy, decisions on cessation of pharmacotherapy, and monitoring for recrudescence of infection.[14]

Differential diagnoses include tuberculosis (especially in cattle), metastatic *S. equi* in equids, equine multinodular pneumonia, neoplasia, and abscesses caused by *C. pseudotuberculosis*.

Treatment consists of surgical debulking or debridement of accessible solitary lesions and administration of antifungal agents. Treatment of choice in dogs and humans is administration of itraconazole or fluconazole or, in cases of severe infection, amphotericin B.[5] Successful treatment of cutaneous blastomycosis in a horse involved administration of fluconazole (14 mg/kg PO loading dose followed by 5 mg/kg PO once daily) for 5 weeks.[11] Discontinuation of therapy resulted in recrudescence of infection, which was resolved by further administration of the drug. Use of potassium iodide (20 mg/kg PO every 24h) was not efficacious in preventing recrudescence of infection. Antifungal therapy should be continued for months. Monitoring of efficacy of therapy by measurement of urine *B. dermatitidis* antigens in urine might be useful in large animals, as it is in dogs and humans.[14]

FURTHER READING

Wilson JH. Blastomycosis in horses. *Equine Vet Educ.* 2014;26:464-466.

REFERENCES

1. Lopez-Martinez R, et al. *Clin Dermatol.* 2012;30:565.
2. Anderson JL, et al. *Med Mycol.* 2014;52:774.
3. Meece JK, et al. *Med Mycol.* 2010;48:285.
4. Anderson JL, et al. *BMC Vet Res.* 2013;9.
5. Wilson JH. *Equine Vet Educ.* 2014;26:464.
6. Dalis JS, et al. *J Anim Vet Adv.* 2007;6:773.
7. Deshmukh GR, et al. *Ind J Vet Pathol.* 2011;35:202.
8. Mendez-Angulo JL, et al. *Can Vet J.* 2011;52:1303.
9. Darrow BG, et al. *J Exotic Pet Med.* 2014;23:158.
10. Imai DM, et al. *J Vet Diagn Invest.* 2014;26:442.
11. Funiciello B, et al. *Equine Vet Educ.* 2014;26:458.
12. McMichael MA, et al. *J Vet Int Med.* 2015;29:499.
13. Kuria JN, et al. *Ond J Vet Res.* 2013;80.
14. Foy DS, et al. *J Vet Int Med.* 2014;28:305.

Multi-Organ Diseases Due to Metabolic Deficiency

SODIUM AND/OR CHLORIDE DEFICIENCY

A dietary deficiency of sodium is most likely to occur in the following instances:

- During lactation, as a consequence of losses of the element in the milk, in rapidly growing young animals fed on low-sodium, cereal-based diets
- Under very hot environmental conditions where large losses of water and sodium occur in the sweat and where the grass forage and the seeds may be low in sodium
- In animals engaged in heavy or intense physical work and in animals grazing pastures on sandy soils heavily fertilized with potash, which depresses forage sodium levels

Naturally occurring salt deficiency causing illness in grazing animals is uncommon except under specific circumstances. The most commonly cited occurrences are on alpine pastures and heavily fertilized pasture leys. Pasture should contain chloride at least 0.15 g/100 g dry matter (DM), and clinical signs are evident after about 1 month on pasture containing 0.1 g chloride/100 g DM. Under experimental conditions, lactating cows give less milk until the chloride deficiency is compensated. After a period of up to 12 months there is considerable deterioration in the animal's health, and anorexia, a haggard appearance, lusterless eyes, rough coat, and a rapid decline in body weight occur. High-producing animals are most severely affected, and some may collapse and die. The oral administration of sodium chloride is both preventive and rapidly curative. Experimental sodium depletion in horses for up to 27 days has no deleterious effect on general health.

In **dairy cattle on a sodium-deficient diet,** there is polyuria; polydipsia; salt hunger; pica, including licking dirt and each other's coats and drinking urine; loss of appetite and weight; and a fall in milk production. Urination is frequent, the urine has a lower-than-normal specific gravity, and the urine concentrations of sodium and chloride are decreased and the potassium increased. The salivary concentration of sodium is markedly decreased, the potassium is increased, and the salivary sodium:potassium ratio is decreased. The concentrations of serum sodium and chloride are also decreased, but the measurement of urinary or salivary sodium concentration is a more sensitive index of sodium intake than plasma sodium concentration. Of these, it is urinary sodium that is depressed first and is therefore the preferred indicator in cattle and horses. The polyuria associated with severe sodium depletion may be an antidiuretic hormone insensitivity as a result of lack of an effective countercurrent mechanism and hyperaldosteronism.

Supplementation of salt to dairy cows on a pumice soil in New Zealand resulted in a 12.8% increase in milk yield with unaltered composition. The cows were grazing ryegrass/clover pastures averaging 0.05% sodium, whereas the recommended concentration for dairy cows is 0.12%. Measurement of the sodium content of the pasture is the most simple and reliable method of diagnosing salt deficiency compared with saliva sodium:potassium ratio. It is considered likely that sodium deficiency will become more prevalent on dairy farms in the future and that there are cost-effective benefits to using salt where deficiencies occur.

Experimental restriction of chloride in the diet of dairy cows in early lactation results in a depraved appetite, lethargy, reduced feed intake, reduced milk production, scant feces, gradual emaciation, and severe hypochloremia and secondary hypokalemic metabolic alkalosis. Lethargy, weakness, and unsteadiness occur after about 6 weeks on the chloride-deficient diet. Bradycardia is also common. The concentration of chloride in cerebrospinal fluid is usually maintained near normal, whereas the serum concentrations decline. The experimental induction of a severe, total body chloride deficit by the provision of a low-chloride diet and the daily removal of abomasal contents results in similar clinical findings to those described previously and lesions of nephrocalcinosis.

The **diagnosis of salt deficiency** is dependent on the clinical findings, analysis of the feed and water supplies, serum levels of sodium and chlorine, and determination of the levels of sodium in the saliva, urine, and feces of deficient animals. The concentration of sodium in saliva is a sensitive indicator of sodium deficiency. In cattle receiving an adequate supply of sodium and chlorine, the sodium levels in saliva vary from 140 to 150 mmol/L; in deficient cattle the levels may be as low as 70 to 100 mmol/L. The levels of sodium in the urine are low, with a reciprocal rise in potassium. The serum sodium levels are less reliable, but licking begins when the level falls to 137 mmol/L, and signs are intense at 135 mmol/L.

The biochemical methods have been evaluated to estimate the sodium intake of dairy cows. Groups of cows were given 10 to 20, 30 to 50, or 70 to 100 g salt per day, and two groups were given salt ad libitum either in bowls or in salt blocks. The concentrations of sodium and potassium were measured in serum and urine. Cows receiving 70 to 100 g salt daily and those in the ad libitum group had higher urinary sodium concentrations than the other groups. Those receiving 10 to 20 g day had a higher urinary ratio of potassium:sodium in their urine than all other groups, in which the ratio decreased as the level of supplementary salt increased.

Experimentally induced sodium deficiency in young pigs causes anorexia, reduced water intake, and reduced weight gains.

The provision of salt in the diet at a level of 0.5% is considered to be fully adequate for all farm animal species. Under practical conditions, salt mixes usually contain added iodine and cobalt. In some situations, the salt mixes are provided on an ad libitum basis rather than adding them to the diet. However, voluntary consumption is not entirely reliable. The daily amount consumed by animals having unrestricted access to salt can be highly variable and often wasteful. Two factors influencing voluntary salt intake are the physical form of the salt and the salt content of the water and feed supplies. Some cattle consume much more loose than block salt, although the lower intakes of block salt may be adequate. Also, animals dependent on high-saline water for drinking consume significantly less salt than when drinking nonsaline water. Voluntary salt consumption is generally high in cows on low-sodium pastures, which are low inherently or as a result of heavy potash fertilization. Lactating gilts may require 0.7% salt in their diets, and energy efficiency in feedlot cattle may be improved by feeding high levels (5% of diet) of salt in the diet of finishing steers.

MAGNESIUM DEFICIENCY

Magnesium (Mg), the second most abundant intracellular cation, plays a vital role as a cofactor for many enzymes, acts as a modulator of ion channels, and affects many cellular processes, such as neuromuscular excitability and secretion of hormones, and antagonizes the actions of Ca^{2+}.[1-3] Magnesium deficiency or depletion causes disturbances in a multitude of physiologic processes and is evident from severe clinical disease and death, in hypomagnesemic tetany of cattle, through to reduced production and impaired health.[2,4] Nutritional deficiency of magnesium plays a role in causing lactation tetany in cows and hypomagnesemic tetany of calves, and these diseases are dealt with in Chapter 18 on metabolic diseases. Magnesium deficiency in late pregnant dairy cows can predispose to periparturient hypocalcemia by impairing the secretion of parathyroid hormone (PTH). In both diseases, there are complicating factors that may affect the absorption and metabolism of the element.

Hypomagnesemia occurs in up to 50% of adult horses hospitalized for severe gastrointestinal disease such as colic, acute diarrhea, and infectious respiratory disease.[5] Serum magnesium concentrations of healthy horses vary with age, parturition, lactation, and sex.[6] Cattle with any one of a number of diseases that decrease feed intake,[2,3] or magnesium absorption, are at increased risk of magnesium deficiency. Postpartum cows with retained placenta have lower concentrations of Mg, and some other minerals, than do postpartum cows without retained placenta.[7] Dairy cows at risk of hypokalemia and supplemented by oral administration of KCl might be at increased risk of magnesium deficiency because of the competitive inhibition of increased ruminal potassium concentrations on magnesium absorption from the rumen.[8]

Magnesium is an essential constituent of rations for recently weaned pigs. Experimentally induced deficiency causes weakness of the pasterns, particularly in the forelegs, causing backward bowing of the legs, sickled hocks, approximation of the knees and hocks, arching of the back, hyperirritability, muscle tremor, reluctance to stand, continual shifting of weight from limb to limb, and eventually tetany and death. A reduction in growth rate, feed consumption and conversion, and levels of magnesium in the serum also occurs. The requirement of magnesium for pigs weaned at 3 to 9 weeks of age is 400 to 500 mg/kg of the total ration.

Diagnosis of magnesium deficiency is challenging because measurement of serum magnesium concentration is not a reliable indicator of whole-body magnesium status.[9] Plasma Mg makes up only 0.3% of total body Mg, and concentration of Mg in plasma is held constant over a wide range of Mg intakes and is only weakly correlated with the functionally important intracellular pools of Mg.[1,4,9] Increasing or decreasing renal magnesium excretion primarily regulates the extracellular Mg concentration, and whole-body Mg status can be monitored rather by assaying total urinary Mg excretion. Because the collection of all urine produced over a 24-hour period is difficult or impossible in practice, urinary magnesium concentration can be measured in a spot sample. However, urinary magnesium concentration is markedly affected by urine volume and can be difficult to interpret. Estimates of magnesium status can be obtained by measuring urine creatinine and magnesium concentrations, measuring plasma magnesium and urine concentrations, and calculating urinary fractional excretion of Mg, thereby avoiding the need for collection of all urine produced over a 24-hour, or other prolonged, period.[1,4] Fractional excretion of Mg is a more sensitive indicator of Mg availability than is plasma, or serum, Mg concentration and a better predictive indicator of the need for supplementation.[4] Methodology for determining magnesium status in cattle and horses is described. A method in cattle involves collection of basal blood and urine samples 60 minutes before starting a magnesium challenge infusion (2.5 mg/kg BW in 250 mL of 0.9% saline was infused at 2.1 mL/min for 120 min) with blood and urine samples collected at 30-minute intervals until 60 minutes after the end of the infusion. Urinary fractional clearance (FC) of magnesium is calculated using the formula:

$$FC\%\,(Mg) = \frac{[Cr]_{pl}}{[Cr]_{u}} \times \frac{[Mg]_{u}}{[Mg]_{pl}} \times 100$$

The reference interval is generally considered to be 2.64% to 43.6% for cows at the end of lactation. Herds with mean fractional clearance of Mg less than 10% are likely to have a deficient Mg status and might benefit from Mg supplementation.[4] A magnesium challenge test can reveal cows with low total body magnesium content because these cows retain much of the infused magnesium, with consequent unchanged fractional clearance values, whereas cows with adequate magnesium status have an increase in fractional clearance of the electrolyte.[4]

Feeding of a magnesium-deficient diet for 29 days in young horses did not result in detectable changes in total or ionized magnesium concentrations in serum, but magnesium excretion over 24 hours and fractional clearance of magnesium in urine were markedly reduced.[9]

FURTHER READING

Goff JP. Calcium and magnesium disorders. *Vet Clin Nth Am Food A*. 2014;30:359-369.

Schonewille JT. Magnesium in dairy cow nutrition: an overview. *Plant Soil*. 2013;368:167-178.

Stewart AJ. Magnesium disorders in horses. *Vet Clin Equine*. 2011;27:149-161.

REFERENCES

1. Stewart AJ. *Vet Clin Equine.* 2011;27:149.
2. Schonewille JT. *Plant Soil.* 2013;368:167.
3. Goff JP. *Vet Clin Nth Am Food A.* 2014;30:359.
4. Schweigel M, et al. *J Anim Physiol Nutr.* 2009; 93:105.
5. Borer KE, et al. *Equine Vet Educ.* 2006;18:266.
6. Berlin D, et al. *Vet J.* 2009;181:305.
7. Bicalho MLS, et al. *J Dairy Sci.* 2014;97:4281.
8. Constable PD, et al. *J Dairy Sci.* 2014;97:1413.
9. Stewart AJ, et al. *Am J Vet Res.* 2004;65:422.

COPPER DEFICIENCY

SYNOPSIS

Etiology Primary deficiency as a result of inadequate copper in the diet. Secondary copper deficiency is associated with antagonistic factors, particularly excess molybdenum and sulfur, which form thiomolybdates in the rumen. Thiomolybdates can bind copper in the rumen, or, if insufficient copper is present, they are absorbed (especially tetra-thiomolybdate) and bind to several enzymes and compounds that have diverse biological activities. Dietary iron forms complexes with copper in the rumen, and so can exacerbate this process.

Epidemiology Herd or flock problem, mainly in young growing ruminants (cattle, sheep, goats, and farmed deer) on pasture in spring and summer. Primary deficiency occurs in sandy and heavily weathered soils; secondary in peat or muck soils high in molybdenum. Feed and water supplies may also contain molybdenum, sulfate, and iron salts, which interfere with copper absorption and metabolism. Some breeds of sheep, and possibly Simmental cattle, are more susceptible.

Signs Unthriftiness, altered hair color, chronic diarrhea in molybdenosis (secondary deficiency), chronic lameness, neonatal ataxia in newborn lambs (swayback) if ewes are copper deficient in mid-pregnancy, delayed ataxia in older lambs (enzootic ataxia), anemia in more prolonged deficiency, falling disease in adult cattle (now rare).

Clinical pathology Low plasma and liver copper, low ceruloplasmin, anemia.

Necropsy findings Demyelination in enzootic ataxia, anemia, emaciation, hemosiderosis, osteodystrophy, cardiomyopathy.

Diagnostic confirmation Low liver and plasma copper, response to treatment.

Differential diagnosis Copper deficiency must be differentiated from herd problems associated with the following:

- Unthriftiness as a result of intestinal parasitism
- Malnutrition as a result of energy–protein deficiency
- Lameness caused by osteodystrophy (calcium, phosphorus, and vitamin D imbalance)
- Anemia as a result of sucking lice
- Neonatal ataxia in lambs (congenital swayback and enzootic ataxia) from border disease; cerebellar hypoplasia (daft lamb disease); hypothermia; meningitis
- Sudden death as a result of other causes

Treatment Oral slow-release bolus or capsule, parental copper glycinate, oral copper sulfate.

Control Oral dosing with controlled-release glass bolus or capsule with copper oxide needles; supplementation pasture by top-dressing with copper sulfate; parenteral administration of copper at strategic times; remove sulfates from water supply; genetic selection may be an option.

ETIOLOGY

Copper (Cu) deficiency may be primary, when the intake in the diet is inadequate, or secondary ("conditioned"), when the dietary intake is sufficient but the absorption of copper and its utilization by tissues is impeded.

Primary Copper Deficiency

The amount of Cu in the diet may be inadequate when the forage is grown on deficient soils, typically sandy or weathered soils, or soils in which the Cu is unavailable.

Secondary Copper Deficiency

This is the predominant deficiency; the amount of Cu in the diet is adequate, but other dietary factors (mainly molybdenum, sulfur, and iron, but also manganese and zinc) interfere with the availability and utilization of Cu (Table 21-8). A dietary excess of molybdenum (Mo) is the most common factor, and a high intake can induce Cu deficiency even when the Cu content of the pasture is quite high. A higher Cu intake can overcome this effect. Conversely, supplementing the diet with Mo can be used to counteract a dangerously high intake of Cu. There are species differences in response to high Cu and Mo intake, with sheep being much more susceptible to Cu toxicity and cattle more susceptible to excess Mo.

Zinc, lead, calcium carbonate, and manganese are other conditioning factors. For example, using zinc sulfate to control facial eczema decreases plasma Cu, which can be corrected by the injection of copper glycinate. On the other hand, in New Zealand the administration of selenium to sheep on Cu-deficient pastures increases Cu absorption and can improve the growth rate of lambs.

Dietary inorganic sulfate, in combination with Mo, has a profound effect on the absorption of Cu by ruminants. For example, sheep consuming a complete diet low in sulfur and Mo, and with modest Cu (12 to 20 mg/kg DM), may die of Cu toxicity, whereas others grazing pasture of similar Cu content but high in Mo and sulfur can give birth to lambs affected with swayback. Increasing the sulfate concentration of a sheep diet from 0.1% to 0.4% can potentiate a Mo content as low as 2 mg/kg (0.02 mmol/kg) and reduce absorption of Cu below normal. Increasing sulfate in the diet also decreases absorption of selenium, and thus deficiencies of both Cu and selenium can occur in areas with soils deficient in both elements, especially when sulfate is added in the form of superphosphate fertilizer. Such combined deficiencies are becoming more common with higher applications of fertilizer that enable higher stocking rates on improved pastures. Interactions between Cu, selenium, and sulfates

Table 21-8 Conditions associated with secondary copper deficiency

Disease	Country	Species	Liver copper	Probable initiating factor
Swayback	Britain, United States	Sheep	Low	Unknown
Renguerra	Peru	Sheep	Low	Unknown
Teart	Britain	Sheep and cattle	Unknown	Molybdenum
Scouring disease	Holland	Cattle	Unknown	Unknown
Peat scours	New Zealand	Cattle	Low	Molybdenum
Peat scours	Britain	Cattle	Unknown, low blood Cu	Unknown
Peat scours	Canada	Cattle	Unknown	Molybdenum
Salt sick	Florida (United States)	Cattle	Unknown	Unknown
"Pine" (unthrifty)	Scotland	Calves	Low	Unknown

must be considered when animals fail to respond to treatment unless both Cu and selenium are provided.

EPIDEMIOLOGY

Occurrence

Copper deficiency is endemic in ruminants worldwide and causes diseases of economic importance that can render large areas of otherwise fertile land unsuitable for grazing by ruminants of all ages, particularly young, rapidly growing animals. Based on surveys of serum and plasma Cu in cattle herds in Britain, Cu deficiency remains a serious problem requiring constant vigilance. It is estimated that clinical signs of Cu deficiency develop annually in about 0.9% of the cattle population in the United Kingdom. In some surveys, the lowest concentrations of serum Cu were in heifers being reared as heifer replacements. Although heavy mortalities can occur in affected areas, the major loss is from the failure of animals to thrive. Enzootic ataxia may affect up to 90% of a lamb flock in badly affected areas, with most of these lambs dying of inanition. In falling disease, up to 40% of cattle in affected herds may die.

Copper deficiency is the most common trace-element deficiency in farmed deer in New Zealand, producing mainly enzootic ataxia but also osteochondrosis.

Geographic Distribution

Primary Copper Deficiency

Disease caused by a primary deficiency of Cu occurs in grazing livestock in many parts of the world, including enzootic ataxia of sheep in Australia, New Zealand, and the United States, licking sickness, or *liksucht*, of cattle in Holland and falling disease of cattle in Australia (now rarely seen). Copper deficiency is endemic in the Salado del Sur River basin in Buenos Aires Province, Argentina, affecting over 50% of beef cattle.

Concurrent deficiencies of both Cu and cobalt in Australia ("coast disease") and Florida in the United States ("salt sickness"), characterized by the appearance of clinical signs of both deficiencies in all ruminant species, are controlled by supplementation with both Cu and cobalt.

In the United States, Cu deficiency is not restricted to a single region, with a third of 256 beef herds classified as deficient or marginally deficient based on a survey of serum Cu concentrations. Approximately 50% of the producers used Cu supplements, but a significant proportion of cattle from those herds were classified as marginally deficient or deficient.

In Canada, a survey of cattle at slaughter in Saskatchewan found that 67% had a liver Cu less than 25 mg copper/kg dry weight (DW). However, this indicator of deficiency is now obsolete, with concentrations less than 10 mg Cu/kg DW (160 μmol Cu/kg DW), or 40 mg Cu/kg fresh weight (FW) (630 μmol Cu/kg FW) indicative of Cu deficiency in ruminants.[1] The concentrations of Cu in the liver of fetuses were proportional to the liver Cu concentrations in the dams, progressively decreasing in the dam during gestation and increasing in the fetus to meet postnatal requirements of the calf because cow milk is a poor source of Cu.

Copper deficiency has been diagnosed in captive musk-oxen in Canada, and it causes anemia in sucking pigs and reduced growth rate and cardiac disease in growing pigs. Adult horses are unaffected, but abnormalities of the limbs and joints of foals reared in Cu-deficient areas do occur.

Secondary Copper Deficiency

Diseases caused by secondary Cu deficiency, mostly as a result of high dietary intakes of Mo and sulfate, are listed in Table 21-8. They include syndromes characterized by ataxia, abnormal wool or hair, diarrhea (peat scours, teart), or unthriftiness. Anemia develops after severe or prolonged Cu deprivation.

Swayback and enzootic ataxia of lambs is induced by feeding pregnant ewes a diet deficient in Cu or high in Mo and sulfur. Two phases of rapid myelination of the central nervous system occur in sheep, the first during midpregnancy, and then in the spinal cord a few weeks after birth. Consequently, the timing of the ataxia in lambs and goat kids depends on when the induced Cu deficiency occurs; neonatal ataxia corresponds with deficiency during midpregnancy, delayed ataxia when deficiency occurs in late pregnancy or soon after birth. Heavy top-dressing of pasture with lime may predispose lambs to swayback. The central nervous system of calves undergoes a slow, progressive myelination, and so they are not affected by neonatal ataxia.

A dietary excess of Mo is known to be the conditioning factor in the diarrheic diseases; "peat scours" in Australia, New Zealand, California, and Canada; and "teart" in Britain.

In Canada, high concentrations of Mo (21–44 mg/kg DM) have been identified in forage on reclaimed mining areas in British Columbia, but cattle can graze these areas for short periods (12 weeks) each year without developing secondary Cu deficiency. Animals given a Cu supplement had no differences in weight gain, liver Mo, or serum and milk Cu and Mo, suggesting that the upper tolerable dietary concentrations of 5 to 10 mg molybdenum and the minimum safe Cu : Mo ratio of 2 : 1, described by the National Research Council, may not be universal.

Moose sickness, also known as "Alvsborg disease" and "wasting disease," has affected up to 4% to 5% of moose (*Alces alces L.*) in Sweden. The appearance of the disease coincided with heavy liming of wetlands, lakes, and forests during the 1980s, undertaken to counteract the deleterious effects of acid rain. The increase in soil pH caused by the liming reduced the availability of Cu and increased the availability of Mo. Copper deficiency may also be a factor contributing to the decline of moose in northwestern Minnesota, with deficient or marginally deficient concentrations of liver copper in 69% of moose found dead. Low liver Cu concentrations have also been recorded in ill-thrifty moose in Norway.[2]

Seasonal Occurrence

Primary Cu deficiency occurs most commonly in spring and summer, coinciding with the lowest concentration of Cu in the pasture. The Cu status of beef and dairy cattle can vary quite widely each month, with higher rainfall usually associated with a lower availability of Cu.

Secondary Cu deficiency may occur at other times, depending on the concentration of the conditioning factors, predominantly Mo or sulfur, in the forage. For example, the Mo content of herbage may be highest in the autumn or spring, when rains stimulate the growth of legumes.

Risk Factors

Several factors influence the plasma and tissue concentrations of copper in ruminants, including the following:

- Breed, age, and growth of animal
- Demands of pregnancy and lactation
- Dietary factors—type of pasture or feed source, season
- Soil characteristics and concentration of minerals—particularly Mo and sulfur, which can form thiomolybdates and reduce the availability of Cu by binding with it in the rumen or with biological compounds in the plasma and tissues

Animal Factors

Age

Young animals are more susceptible to primary Cu deficiency than adults. Calves of dams fed deficient diets may show signs at 2 to 3 months of age, with clinical signs more severe in calves and yearlings, less severe in 2-year-olds, and less important in adults. Enzootic ataxia is primarily a disease of neonatal or suckling lambs whose dams receive insufficient dietary copper during mid- or late-pregnancy. Ewes with a normal Cu status take some time to lose their liver reserves, and thus they do not produce affected lambs for at least 6 months after starting to graze Cu-deficient pastures. The predominance of Cu deficiency in suckling lambs indicates the importance of fetal stores and the inadequacy of milk as a source of Cu. Milk from normal ewes contains 3.1 to 9.4 μmol/L (20 to 60 μg/dL) Cu, but with severe deficiency this may be reduced to 0.16 to 0.31 μmol/L (1 to 2 μg/dL).

Breed and Species Susceptibility

There are marked genetic differences in the Cu metabolism of sheep breeds; Welsh

Mountain and Texels can absorb Cu 50% more efficiently than Scottish Blackface, and Texel cross Blackface 145% more efficiently than pure Blackface lambs. The susceptibility to Cu deficiency, or protection from Cu poisoning, is influenced from birth by genetic effects. These affect Cu status of the lamb at birth, through the maternal environment controlled by the dam's genes and the effect of the lamb's own genes. These genetic differences have physiologic consequences, reflected in differences in the incidence of swayback, both between and within breeds, and in effects on growth and possibly on reproduction. The differences are attributable to genetic differences in the efficiency of absorption of dietary Cu.

In sheep, the existence of genes determining plasma Cu has been shown by the continued selection for high and low concentrations in closed lines of a single breed. Ram selection was made on the basis of plasma Cu concentrations at 18 and 24 weeks of age, with this trait having a heritability of 0.3, similar to that calculated for Angus cattle.[3] The high-line ewes retain more Cu in the liver than the low-line ewes, caused by a positive correlation between the concentration of Cu in plasma and the efficiency of absorption.

Genetic variation in the Cu metabolism of sheep has important physiologic consequences. The incidence of swayback may vary from 0% to 40% between different breeds within the same flock, with the incidence more closely related to differences in the concentration of Cu in the liver than in blood. When high and low female lines are placed on improved and limed pasture, which can induce a severe Cu deficiency, swayback, dullness, lack of vigor, and mortality are evident in lambs soon after birth. At 6 weeks of age the mortality rate was higher in the lambs from the low-Cu line and they were 2 kg lighter than those from the high-Cu line.

Goats are more prone to Cu deficiency than sheep, probably as a result of lower accumulation of liver Cu. The dietary requirement for goats is 8 to 10 ppm Cu. However, an intake of Cu that could cause toxicity in sheep (100 to 150 ppm) enhanced growth rate and immune function and did not cause toxicity in Boer crossbreed goats.[4]

Cattle are less efficient absorbers of Cu, with evidence for genetic differences between breeds growing stronger. For example, certain breeds, such as Simmental and Charolais, may have higher Cu requirements than other breeds, such as Angus. Based on an assessment of liver Cu, diets containing 4.4 or 6.4 mg of Cu/kg DM did not meet the requirements of either Angus or Simmentals during gestation and lactation or growth, but the addition of 7 mg of copper/kg DM to both diets met the requirements of both breeds. Similar to sheep, these differences are probably related to differences in Cu absorption.

Fetal Liver Copper

During gestation, the concentration of Cu in the ovine and bovine fetal liver progressively increases, whereas it decreases in the maternal liver. The bovine fetus obtains Cu by placental transfer, and thus at birth the liver concentration of Cu is initially high and then declines to normal adult levels within a few months. Placental transfer is less efficient in sheep, and thus lambs are often born with low liver reserves, making them susceptible to Cu deficiency.

In deficient cattle, the accumulation of liver Cu in the fetus continues independent of the dam's liver Cu until the fetus is about 180 days, after which it gradually declines. In contrast, the liver Cu concentration in fetuses from dams on adequate diets continues to increase. Thus during the last month of pregnancy the daily requirement for Cu in cattle increases to about 70% above maintenance requirements, so the dietary allowance of 10 mg/kg DM increases to 25 mg/kg DM during pregnancy.

Colostrum is rich in Cu, allowing the newborn to absorb Cu and increase its hepatic stores. The Cu content of milk then declines rapidly and is usually unable to meet the requirements of the suckling neonate. Young milk-fed animals absorb about 80% of Cu intake, but this efficiency declines rapidly as the rumen becomes functional, when only 2% to 10% of available Cu is absorbed.

Dietary Factors

Pasture Composition

The absorption (or availability) of Cu is influenced by the type of diet; the presence of other substances in the diet, such as Mo, sulfur, and iron; the interaction between the type of diet and the chemical composition of the diet; and the genetic constitution of the animals. Copper is well-absorbed from diets low in fiber, such as cereals and Brassicas. However, it is poorly absorbed from fresh pasture, although conservation as hay or silage generally improves its availability. This explains why Cu deficiency is predominantly a problem of grazing ruminants but only rarely seen in housed animals fed diets with adequate Cu.

Molybdenum and Sulfur

Only small increases in the molybdenum (Mo) and sulfur (S) concentration of grass will cause major reductions in the availability of Cu. This is especially so for ruminants grazing improved pastures in which the Mo and S concentrations are increased. The Cu content of feedstuffs should be expressed in terms of available copper concentration, using appropriate equations, which permits a more accurate prediction of clinical disease and can be used for more effective control strategies.[1]

The effect of Mo and S on the availability of copper in grass is changed by conservation; at a given concentration of S, the antagonistic effect of Mo is proportionately less in hay than in fresh grass. At a low concentration of Mo, the effect of S is more marked in silage than in fresh grass, but the use of formaldehyde as a silage additive may weaken the Cu–S antagonism. Thus herbage high in Mo should be used for conservation when possible, and sulfuric acid should not be used as an additive for silage unless accompanied by a Cu salt because it significantly raises the S concentration of the silage.

An Mo-induced secondary copper deficiency in cattle has occurred when motor oil containing Mo bisulfide was spilled onto pasture.

Copper in the Diet

In general, pasture containing less than 3 mg/kg DM of copper will result in signs of deficiency in grazing ruminants. Concentrations of 3 to 5 mg/kg DM are marginal, whereas greater than 5 mg/kg DM (preferably 7 to 12) is safe unless Mo–S interactions cause secondary copper deficiency. These complex interactions require an examination of each particular set of circumstances. For example, plant Mo concentrations are directly related to the soil pH. Grasses grown on strongly acidic Mo-rich soils have low Mo (<3 mg/kg DM), whereas those growing on alkaline Mo-poor soils may contain up to 17 mg/kg DM. Thus conditioned copper deficiency can be related to enhanced levels of plant-available Mo rather than the absolute soil levels. Heavily limed pastures are often associated with a less-than-normal intake of Cu and a low copper status of sheep grazing them.

Secondary copper deficiency is also recorded in pigs when drinking water contains very large amounts of sulfate.

Dietary Iron

Dietary iron can interfere with Cu metabolism.[1,5] Concentrations of iron in silage and pasture forage can range from 500 to 1500 mg/kg DM or higher and can induce Cu deficiency in ruminants when Cu intake is marginal or Mo and S intake is increased. Ruminants obtain iron from ingested soil and mineral supplements. In areas where hypocuprosis is likely to occur, the risk can be minimized by avoiding mineral supplements with high iron content, minimizing the use of bare winter pasture, and avoiding excessive contamination of silage with soil during harvesting. The effect of soil ingestion on Cu deficiency can vary, which is understandable given the differences in soil physical and chemical composition (principally pH, Fe, Mo, and S).[6]

Stored Feeds

Livestock that are housed for all or part of the year have a different dietary intake of Cu compared with those on pasture. Concentrates and proprietary feeds usually contain adequate Cu, whereas pasture is more likely to be deficient, especially in early spring when the grass growth is lush. Consequently, silage may be Cu deficient, but hay is more mature and usually contains more of all trace elements and minerals, and hence housed animals are usually protected against Cu deficiency for a few weeks after they come out onto pasture in the spring. In these circumstances, young, rapidly growing animals will be the first affected by hypocuprosis.

Soil Characteristics

Copper Deficiency. In general, there are two types of soil in which Cu deficiency occurs. First are the sandy soils, poor in organic matter and heavily weathered, such as on the coastal plains of Australia and marine and river silts (these are often deficient in other trace elements, especially cobalt). The second important group is "peat" or muck soils reclaimed from swamps, which are more commonly associated with Cu deficiency in the United States, New Zealand, and Europe. These soils may have an absolute deficiency of Cu, but more commonly it is not available to plants, and so they do not contain adequate amounts of Cu.

The cause of the lack of availability of the copper is uncertain, but is probably a result of the formation of insoluble organic copper complexes. An additional factor is the production of secondary copper deficiency on these soils because of their high content of molybdenum. The concentration of Cu in a range of soils and plants is summarized in Table 21-9.

Molybdenum Excess. Pastures containing less than 3 mg/kg DM of molybdenum (Mo) are usually safe, but disease may occur at 3 to 10 mg/kg DM if the intake of Cu is low. Pastures containing greater than 10 mg/kg DM of molybdenum are of high risk unless the diet is supplemented with Cu. Soil Mo may be as high as 10 to 100 mg/kg, which can be exacerbated by the application of Mo in fertilizer to increase the fixation of nitrogen by legumes.

In the United Kingdom, much farming land is underlain by marine black shales, which are rich in Mo, and hence there is a high concentration of Mo in soil and pastures, and secondary Cu deficiency is common. Secondary Cu deficiency also occurs in cattle in many parts of Canada. For example, large areas of west-central Manitoba are underlain by molybdeniferous shale bedrocks, and soils can contain up to 20 mg/kg of molybdenum.

In New Zealand, some peat soils or the heavy application of Mo in superphosphate to stony soils can produce pastures with a Mo concentration of 3.5 to 20 mg/kg DM, which can induce Cu deficiency. For example, increasing the pasture Mo concentrations from 2 to 4.6 mg/kg DM significantly reduced serum and liver Cu concentrations in grazing red deer, and reduced growth rate occurred when pasture Mo was greater than 10 mg/kg DM. However, an assessment of the elemental composition of pastures found that 95% of pastures from over 800 farms in New Zealand had a Mo content less than 2 mg/kg DM.[7] This, combined with increasing reports of lethal Cu toxicity in dairy herds associated with overly exuberant supplementation, suggests that Mo-induced copper deficiency may not be as widespread as thought.

PATHOGENESIS

Effects on Tissues

Copper is incorporated into and essential for the activity of many enzymes, cofactors, and reactive proteins.[1] Some pivotal functions of major enzymes include cellular respiration (cytochrome oxidase), protection from oxidants (superoxide dismutase [SOD], ceruloplasmin), the transport of iron (ceruloplasmin [ferroxidase I] and hephestin [ferroxidase II]), conversion of tyrosine to melanin (tyrosinase), and the formation of collagen and elastin (lysyl oxidase). Consequently, the consequences of Cu deficiency are diverse but relate to decreased function of Cu metalloenzymes and Cu-binding proteins.

SOD acts as an antioxidant by the dismutation of superoxide anions (O_2^-), producing molecular oxygen and hydrogen peroxide (H_2O_2), with the latter usually metabolized by glutathione peroxidase and catalase. The ferroxidase activity of ceruloplasmin mediates the oxidation of ferrous ions (Fe^{2+}) to the ferric state (Fe^{3+}), thereby preventing ferrous ion-dependent formation of hydroxyl radicals (OH^-) via the Fenton reaction. In Cu-deficient animals, the activities of SOD and glutathione peroxidase are decreased, causing increased oxidative damage to cells from lipid peroxidation. Ceruloplasmin is the predominant Cu-containing protein in plasma, but it also acts as an antioxidant by scavenging free radicals in many tissues.

The pathogenesis of most of the lesions seen with Cu deficiency is explained in terms of faulty tissue oxidation associated with the failure of these enzyme systems. This role is exemplified by failure of myelination, which produces swayback and enzootic ataxia, or wool abnormalities ("steely wool") in deficient sheep, after myelination is complete. Reduced growth (abnormal bone and cartilage) is also influenced by reduced lysyl oxidase activity, decreased pigmentation (white bands in the wool of pigmented sheep, changed coat color in cattle) by reduced tyrosinase activity, and a terminal anemia by reduced ferroxidase activity.

Changes in Gene Expression

Differences in the expression of genes associated with Cu metabolism have been demonstrated in Cu-deficient cattle, including less duodenal Cu transporter 1 (*Ctr1*) and up-regulation of genes in the liver of Cu-deficient fetuses (antioxidant 1 [*Atox1*]), cytochrome c oxidase assembly protein 17 (Cox17), and copper metabolism MURR domain 1 (*Commd1*).[8] In naturally occurring Cu deficiency of Angus cattle in Argentina, cytogenetic analysis of peripheral lymphocyte cultures found a significant increase in the frequency of abnormal metaphases in moderate to severely deficient groups.

Wool

Loss of crimp causes "stringy" or "steely" wool with reduced tensile strength, which is most obvious in Merinos. This follows inadequate keratinization, probably as a result of imperfect oxidation of free thiol groups. Provision of Cu to affected sheep is followed by oxidation of these free thiol groups and a return to normal keratinization within a few hours.

Body Weight

Poor growth is a feature of the later stages of Cu deficiency, more often associated with

Table 21-9 Copper levels of soils and plants in primary and secondary copper deficiency

Condition	Area	Soil type	Soil copper (mg/kg)	Plant copper (mg/kg DM)
Normal	–	–	18–22	11
Primary copper deficiency	Western Australia	Various	1–2	3–5
	New Zealand	Sand	0.1–1.6	3
	New Zealand	Peat	–	3
	Holland	Sand	–	<3
Secondary copper deficiency	New Zealand	Peat	5	7
	Britain	Peat	–	7–20
	Britain	Limestone	–	12–27
	Britain	Stiff clay	–	11
	Ireland	Shale deposits, peat marine, alluvial soils		
	Holland	Sand	–	>5
	Canada	Burned-over peat	20–60	10–25

excess Mo, when the impairment of tissue oxidation causes interference with intermediary metabolism and loss of condition or failure to grow in sheep, cattle, and deer. This can be accompanied by poor feed-conversion efficiency if Mo-induced Cu deficiency begins in utero.[9]

Diarrhea
The pathogenesis of diarrhea in Mo-induced secondary Cu deficiency (peat scours, teart) is uncertain. There are no histologic changes in gut mucosa of naturally affected cattle, although villous atrophy was recorded in severe experimental cases. Sheep and goats are far less susceptible to diarrhea induced by molybdenosis, although it can occur.

Anemia
Anemia develops with severe or prolonged Cu deficiency and is associated with the role of Cu in the formation of hemoglobin. Hemosiderin deposits in the tissues of deficient animals suggest that Cu is necessary for the recycling of iron released from the normal breakdown of hemoglobin. There is no evidence of excessive hemolysis. Heinz-body anemia, an indicator of oxidative stress, can occur when Cu- or selenium-deficient lambs are moved onto rape (*Brassica napus*). The unusual relationship between Cu deficiency and postparturient hemoglobinuria seen in New Zealand has not been explained.

Bone
Bone abnormalities vary considerably between and within species of ruminants.[1] The osteoporosis that occurs in some natural cases of Cu deficiency is caused by the depression of osteoblastic activity. In experimentally induced primary Cu deficiency, the skeleton is osteoporotic, and there is a significant increase in osteoblastic activity. There is a marked overgrowth of epiphyseal cartilage, especially at costochondral junctions and in metatarsal bones. This is accompanied by beading of the ribs, enlargement of the long bones, and an impairment of collagen formation. When the Cu deficiency is secondary to dietary excesses of Mo and sulfate, the skeletal lesions are quite different and characterized by widening of the growth plate and metaphysis and active osteoblastic activity.

In foals, Cu deficiency causes severe degenerative disease of cartilage, characterized by breaking of articular and growth-plate cartilage through the zone of hypertrophic cells, resulting in osteochondrosis of the articular-epiphyseal complex (A-E complex). The incidence and severity of osteochondrosis in foals can be decreased by supplementation of the diets of mares during the last 3 to 6 months of pregnancy and the first 3 months of lactation. Foals from nonsupplemented mares have separation of the thickened cartilage from the subchondral bone. Clinical, radiographic, and biochemical differences occur between copper-deficient and Cu-supplemented foals, and there may be a relationship between low Cu intake in rapidly growing horses, inferior collagen quality, biomechanically weak cartilage, and osteochondritis.

Copper is essential for the function of lysyl oxidase, which produces aldehydic groups on hydroxylysine residues as a prerequisite for eventual cross-link formation in collagen and elastin. Similar lesions in foals have been attributed to zinc toxicity from exposure to pasture polluted by smelters. Experimentally, the addition of varying amounts of zinc to the diet of foals containing adequate Cu will result in zinc-induced Cu deficiency, but there are no effects with zinc intakes up to 580 ppm, and it is suggested that 2000 ppm or higher is necessary to affect Cu absorption in horses.

Connective Tissue
Copper is a component of the enzyme lysyl oxidase, secreted by the cells involved in the synthesis of the elastin component of connective tissues, and has important functions in maintaining the integrity of tissues such as capillary beds, ligaments, and tendons. Naturally occurring examples of connective tissue dysfunction are rare, but lesions of osteochondrosis described in young farmed red deer and wapiti–red deer hybrids in New Zealand also have defective articular cartilage.[1]

Heart
The myocardial degeneration of falling disease, now rarely seen, may be a terminal manifestation of anemic anoxia, or it may be a result of interference with tissue oxidation. In this disease, it is thought that the stress of calving and lactation contribute to the development of heart block and ventricular fibrillation when there has already been considerable decrease in cardiac reserve. Experimentally induced Cu deficiency in piglets causes cardiac pathology and electrical disturbances and a marked reduction in growth and hematocrit.

Blood Vessels
Experimentally induced Cu deficiency has caused sudden death as a result of rupture of the heart and great vessels in a high proportion of pigs fed a Cu-deficient diet. The basic defect is degeneration of the internal elastic laminae. There is no record of a similar, naturally occurring disease. A similar relationship appears to have been established between serum Cu levels and fatal rupture of the uterine artery at parturition in aged mares.

Pancreas
Lesions of the pancreas may be present in normal cattle with a low blood copper status.[1] The lesions consist of an increase in dry matter content and reduced concentrations of protein and Cu in wet tissue; cytochrome oxidase activity and protein:RNA ratio are also decreased. There are defects in acinar basement membranes, splitting and disorganization of acini, cellular atrophy and dissociation, and stromal proliferation.

Nervous Tissue
Copper deficiency halts the formation of myelin and causes demyelination in lambs, probably by a specific relationship between Cu and myelin sheaths. Defective myelination can commence in the midterm fetus, causing lesions in the cerebrum, with lambs affected at birth (congenital swayback), or lesions in the white matter of the spinal cord in delayed cases of enzootic ataxia (the predominant form in goats and deer). This distribution reflects peaks of myelin development at those sites, at 90 days of gestation and 20 days after birth. Copper deficiency interferes with the synthesis of phospholipids, and anoxia may also be involved in demyelination. Anemic anoxia is more likely in highly deficient ewes, and anemic ewes produce a higher proportion of lambs with enzootic ataxia. However, there is often no anemia in ewes that produce lambs with the more common subacute form of nervous disease. Severely deficient ewes tend to have lambs affected at birth, whereas the lambs of less severely deficient ewes have normal myelination at birth and develop demyelination later.

Reproductive Performance
There is no clear evidence that Cu deficiency causes infertility in dairy cows, and both improvement and impairment of fertility have been reported in normocupremic cows given parenteral Cu.[1] Copper glycinate given to dairy cattle does not affect the average interval in days between calving and first observed heat, services per conception, or first-service conception rate compared with untreated cows in the same population. Experimentally, the addition of Mo to the diet of heifers delayed the onset of puberty, decreased the conception rate, and caused anovulation and anestrus in cattle without accompanying changes in Cu status or live-weight gain. Thus the presence of Mo rather than low Cu status may affect the reproductive performance of cattle. It is inadvisable to ascribe poor reproductive performance to subclinical hypocuprosis on the evidence of low blood Cu alone, and other factors, such as management and energy and protein intake, should be examined.

Immune System
Copper has an important role in the immune response, but the precise mechanism is not well understood. In secondary Cu deficiency in cattle, induced by 30 ppm molybdenum and 225 ppm sulfate, the intracellular copper content of peripheral blood lymphocytes, neutrophils, and monocyte-derived macrophages was reduced between 40% and 70%.

In Cu deficiency, serum ceruloplasmin activity is decreased to 50% of control values, and superoxide dismutase and cytochrome c oxidase activities of leukocytes are significantly reduced. Thus Cu deficiency alters the activity of several key enzymes that mediate antioxidant defense and ATP formation. These effects may impair cellular immune function and make animals more susceptible to infection.

Copper deficiency decreases humoral and cell-mediated immunity and reduces nonspecific immunity regulated by phagocytic cells, such as macrophages and neutrophils. The decreased resistance to infection in deficient sheep responds to treatment with Cu, but also genetic selection, with mortalities from birth to 24 weeks of age 50% lower in lambs genetically selected for high concentrations of plasma Cu compared with those selected for low concentrations. Experimental viral and bacterial infections of cattle can also cause a rapid, although transient, increase in serum ceruloplasmin and plasma Cu in Cu-replete animals, suggesting a major protective role for copper in infectious diseases. These changes evolve from an interleukin-1-mediated increase in hepatic synthesis and release of ceruloplasmin, an acute-phase protein. The concentration of Cu in organs involved in immune regulations, such as the liver, spleen, thymus, and lung, is substantially reduced by Cu deficiency, again suggesting that deficient animals have a greater risk of infection than Cu-adequate ones. However, experiments using low-Cu diets, with or without supplemental Mo, did not alter specific indicators of immunity in stressed cattle.

The severity of Cu depletion needed for immune dysfunction is less than that required to induce clinical signs of Cu deficiency, and endogenous Cu may contribute to the regulation of both nonimmune and immune inflammatory responses. Low-molecular-weight complexes may have an antiinflammatory effect in animal models of inflammation, and it is postulated that the increased plasma Cu-containing components seen during inflammatory disease represent a physiologic response.

In experimental coliform mastitis in Holstein heifers fed 20 mg Cu/kg DM, from 60 days prepartum to day 42 of lactation, the clinical response but not duration of mastitis was reduced compared with animals receiving 6.5 mg Cu/kg DM. In a subsequent experiment, supplementation a basal diet of 7.1 mg Cu/kg DM with 10 mg/kg Cu DM with an organic supplement (Cu proteinate) tended to be more effective than an inorganic one (with Cu sulfate), although somatic cell count, plasma Cu, and plasma ceruloplasmin were not significantly different.[10]

Development of Clinical Signs

In experimental Cu deficiency in calves, beginning at 6 weeks of age, hypocupremia developed at 15 weeks, growth retardation from 15 to 18 weeks, rough hair coat at 17 weeks, diarrhea at 20 weeks, and leg abnormalities at 23 weeks. Thus the appearance of clinical signs correlated reasonably well with the onset of hypocupremia and was indicative of a severe deficiency. However, even with severe clinical signs, histologic abnormalities may only be quite minor.

In another study, beginning at 12 weeks of age, clinical signs of Cu deficiency did not develop until after 6 months, with musculoskeletal abnormalities including a stilted gait, "knock-kneed" appearance of the forelimbs, overextension of the flexors, splaying of the hooves, and swellings around the metacarpophalangeal and carpometacarpal joints. Changes in hair pigmentation occurred after about 5 months of deficiency, and diarrhea occurred between 5 and 7 months after deficiency. The diarrhea stopped within 12 hours after oral administration of 10 mg of Cu.

Copper–Molybdenum–Sulfate Relationship

The interaction between copper (Cu), molybdenum (Mo), and sulfur (S), and its effects on health and production in ruminants, is unique among mammals.[1] Molybdenum and sulfate, alone or in combination, can affect Cu metabolism. Much of the Cu released in the rumen is precipitated with sulfides (S^{2-}) to form Cu sulfide (CuS). In addition, whether derived from organic or inorganic sources, Mo and S bind with Cu in the rumen to form thiomolybdates.[5] These compounds have two effects. First, they reduce the amount of Cu available for absorption, with the Cu–thiomolybdate complexes binding to particulate matter in the digesta and reducing the proportion of Cu absorbed to 1% of that ingested. Second, thiomolybdates can be rapidly absorbed and reversibly bound to Cu in biological compounds, including ceruloplasmin, cytochrome oxidase, superoxide dismutase, and tyrosine oxidase. This induces a secondary Cu deficiency (technically a thiomolybdate toxicosis), with tetrathiomolybdate (MoS_4^{2-}) by far the most potent of the thiomolybdates.[5] Thus, secondary (conditioned) Cu deficiency occurs when the dietary intake of Cu is adequate but absorption and utilization of Cu are not. These effects also occur in the fetus, interfering with Cu storage in the fetal liver. In cattle, reduced growth rate and changes in the hair texture and color occur after 16 to 20 weeks of supplementation with Mo, accompanied by decreased feed intake and reduced efficiency of feed utilization.

In addition to the Mo–S–Cu relationship, additional interactions with iron (Fe), selenium (Se), Zinc (Zn), and manganese (Mn) can occur. Iron reduces absorption of Cu by adsorption of Cu into insoluble iron compounds and down-regulation of a Cu carrier (DMT).[1] In calves, liver and plasma concentrations of Cu decrease and become severely deficient within 12 to 16 weeks of including iron in the diet. In sheep, the administration of Se to sheep on Cu-deficient pastures improves the absorption of Cu.

The toxicity of dietary Mo is determined by the ratio of the dietary Mo to dietary Cu. The critical ratio of Cu : Mo in animal feeds is 2.0, and feeds or pasture with a lower ratio may induce a secondary copper deficiency. For example, in some regions of Canada the Cu : Mo ratio varies from 0.1 to 5.3, with a higher critical ratio of 4 to 5 recommended for safety.

Copper Utilization

Sulfate and molybdate interfere with mobilization of Cu from the liver, inhibition of Cu intake by the tissues, inhibition of Cu transport (both into and out of the liver), and inhibition of the synthesis of Cu storage complexes and ceruloplasmin.

Clinical signs of hypocuprosis, such as steely wool, occur in sheep on diets containing high levels of Mo and sulfate, even though blood Cu concentrations are high. This suggests that Cu is not available, and hence blood Cu rises in response to this demand.

Hepatic Storage

If animals are receiving a Cu-deficient diet, and thus Cu is removed from the liver, those supplemented with molybdate plus sulfate retain more Cu in the liver than do animals not being supplemented. This supports the hypothesis that, together, molybdate and sulfate impair the movement of Cu into or out of the liver, possibly by affecting copper transport. Sulfate alone exerts an effect, with an increased intake reducing hepatic storage of both Cu and Mo.

Phases of Copper Deficiency

The development of a deficiency can be divided into four phases (Fig. 21-4):

1. Depletion
2. Deficiency (marginal)
3. Dysfunction
4. Disease

During the depletion phase, there is loss of Cu from storage, principally liver storage, but the plasma concentrations of Cu remain constant. With continued dietary deficiency the concentrations of Cu in the blood decline during the phase of marginal deficiency. However, it may be some time before the concentrations or activities of copper-containing enzymes in the tissues begin to decline, and it is not until this happens that the phase of dysfunction is reached. There may be a further lag before the changes in cellular function are manifested as clinical signs of disease.

CLINICAL FINDINGS

The general effects of Cu deficiency are the same in sheep and cattle, but in addition to

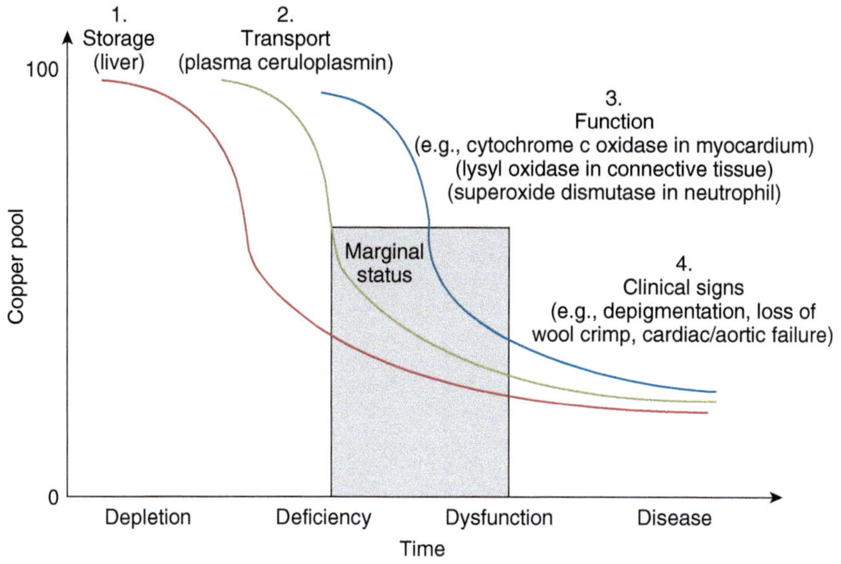

Fig. 21-4 The biochemical changes that lead to copper deficiency and disease. (From Suttle NF. The mineral nutrition of livestock, 4th ed., Wallingford, Oxon: CAB International, 2010: 255-305.).

these general syndromes there are specific syndromes more or less restricted to species and to areas. Following is a general description of disease caused by Cu deficiency, then details of specific syndromes of enzootic ataxia, swayback, falling disease, peat scours, teart, and unthriftiness (pine).

Cattle

Subclinical Hypocuprosis

No clinical signs occur, plasma Cu is marginal (<9.0 mmol/L [57 mg/dL]), and there is a variable response after supplementation with Cu. Surveys in some Cu-deficient areas show that about 50% of beef herds and 10% of dairy herds within the same area have low blood Cu associated with a low dietary intake from pasture (natural forages). Deficiency will only be suspected if production is monitored and found to be suboptimal.

A feature of subclinical hypocuprosis under field conditions is the wide variation in increased growth rate when cattle of the same low-Cu status are given supplementary Cu.

General Syndrome

Primary Copper Deficiency

Primary deficiency causes unthriftiness, decreased milk production, and anemia in adult cattle. The coat becomes rough, and its color is affected, with red and black cattle changing to a bleached, rusty red. In severely deficient states, which are now uncommon, calves grow poorly, and there is an increased tendency for bone fractures, particularly of the limbs and scapula. Ataxia may occur after exercise, with a sudden loss of control of the hindlimbs and the animal falling or assuming a sitting posture and then returning to normal after rest. Itching and hair-licking are also seen in Cu-deficient cattle. Although diarrhea may occur, persistent diarrhea is not a characteristic of primary Cu deficiency, and its occurrence should arouse suspicion of molybdenosis or helminthiasis. In some areas, affected calves develop stiffness and enlargement of the joints and contraction of the flexor tendons, causing them to stand on their toes. These signs may be present at birth or before weaning. Unlike in sheep, paresis and incoordination are not seen.

An increased occurrence of postparturient hemoglobinuria is also recorded in New Zealand, but it is not well understood.

Secondary Copper Deficiency

Signs can be similar to primary Cu deficiency, although anemia is less common, probably as a result of the relatively better Cu status in secondary deficiency. For example, anemia occurs in peat scours of cattle in New Zealand when the Cu intake is marginal. However, with increased Mo intake, there is a tendency for diarrhea, particularly in cattle.

Falling Disease

The characteristic behavior in falling disease is for apparently healthy cows to throw up their heads, bellow, and fall. In most cases death is instantaneous, but some cattle struggle on their sides for a few minutes, with intermittent bellowing, paddling, and attempts to rise. Rare cases show signs for up to 24 hours or more. These animals periodically lower their heads and pivot on the front legs, with sudden death usually occurring during one of these episodes.

Peat Scours ("Teart")

Persistent diarrhea, with watery, yellow-green to black feces with an inoffensive odor, occurs soon after the cattle start grazing affected pasture, in some cases within 8 to 10 days. Defecation often occurs without lifting of the tail. Severe debilitation is common, although appetite remains. The hair coat is rough, with depigmentation manifested by reddening or gray flecking, especially around the eyes in black cattle. These signs vary greatly from season to season, and spontaneous recovery is common. Affected animals usually recover in a few days following treatment with Cu.

Unthriftiness (Pine) of Calves

The earliest signs are a stiff gait and ill-thrift. The epiphyses of the distal ends of the metacarpus and metatarsus may be enlarged and resemble the epiphysitis of rapidly growing calves deficient in vitamin D or calcium and phosphorus. The epiphyses are painful on palpation, and some calves are severely lame. The pasterns are upright, and the animals may appear to have contracted flexor tendons. Progressive ill-thrift and emaciation progress and can lead to death in 4 to 5 months. Gray hair occurs, especially around the eyes of black cattle, and diarrhea may occur in a few cases.

Sheep

General Syndrome

Primary Copper Deficiency

Abnormalities of the wool are the first, and often only, sign in areas of marginal deficiency. Fine wool loses its crimp and luster, assuming a straight, "steely" appearance. This is more obvious in Merinos but can occur in meat breeds with broader and plainer wool. Dark wool loses pigment to become gray or white, often in bands coinciding with the seasonal occurrence of Cu deficiency. Anemia, scouring, unthriftiness, and infertility may occur in conditions of extreme deficiency, but in sheep the characteristic findings are swayback or enzootic ataxia in lambs. Reduced growth, diarrhea, and increased mortality are seen in lambs genetically selected for low plasma Cu when they are grazed on improved and limed pastures. Osteoporosis with fractures of the long bones is also recorded with Cu deficiency that was not severe enough to cause enzootic ataxia.

Swayback and Enzootic Ataxia in Lambs and Goat Kids

Swayback and enzootic ataxia have a lot in common, but there are subtle differences in their clinical signs and epidemiology.

Swayback is the only true manifestation of a primary deficiency of Cu in the United Kingdom. Its prevalence can vary considerably, reflecting genetic differences in Cu metabolism, both between and within breeds of sheep. A congenital cerebrospinal form occurs when the Cu deficiency is extreme. Affected lambs are born dead or weak and are unable to stand and suckle. They have spastic paralysis, are more uncoordinated with erratic movements compared with enzootic ataxia, and are occasionally blind. There is softening and cavitation of the cerebral white matter, which corresponds to demyelination of the cerebral cortex commencing around day 120 of gestation. Progressive (delayed) spinal swayback is characterized by a stiff and staggery gait and hindlimb incoordination, and it appears at 3 to 6 weeks of age. In Wales, a third form in older lambs is associated with cerebral edema. It resembles the more usual delayed form, but it develops suddenly with onset of recumbency and death within 1 to 2 days.

Enzootic ataxia occurs in unweaned lambs. In severe outbreaks, lambs may be affected at birth, but most cases occur at 1 to 2 months of age. The severity of the paresis decreases with increasing age at onset. Lambs affected at birth or within the first month usually die within 3 to 4 days, whereas older lambs may survive for 3 to 4 weeks or longer. However, surviving lambs always have some ataxia and atrophy of the hindquarters. The first sign of enzootic ataxia is incoordination of the hindlimbs, often when the lambs are mustered. Cardiac and respiratory rates are greatly increased by exertion, and incoordination progressively becomes more severe and may be obvious after walking only a few meters. There is excessive flexion of joints, knuckling of the fetlocks, wobbling of the hindquarters, and finally falling. The hindlegs are affected first, and the lamb may be able to drag itself about in a sitting posture. When the forelegs are eventually involved, recumbency persists, and the lamb dies of starvation. However, there is no true paralysis because the lamb is able to kick vigorously, even in the recumbent stage, and appetite is unaffected.

Goats

Enzootic ataxia attributable to Cu deficiency occurs in goat kids. The disease is similar in most respects to that in lambs, except cerebellar hypoplasia is a frequent finding in goats. Kids may be affected at birth, or the clinical signs may be delayed until the animals are several weeks of age.

Other Species

Deer

Enzootic ataxia of red deer is quite different from the disease in sheep in that it develops in weaned deer and adults. Clinical signs include ataxia, swaying of the hindquarters, a dog-sitting posture, and, eventually, hindlimb paresis. This is associated with demyelination of the spinal cord and neuronal degeneration in the midbrain.

Osteochondrosis of young, farmed deer in New Zealand is characterized by lameness, one or more swollen joints, an abnormal "bunny-hopping" gait, and "cow-hocked" stance. In Australia, secondary Cu deficiency of red deer during drought was associated with weight loss in lactating hinds and steely hair coats of reduced luster, similar to steely wool of Cu-deficient sheep. This was associated with the high sulfur content of the diet, possibly exacerbated by ingestion of iron from increased soil ingestion when supplementary feed was trailed onto the ground.

Pigs

Naturally occurring enzootic ataxia has occurred in 4- to 6-month-old growing pigs, with posterior paresis progressing to complete paralysis in 1 to 3 weeks. Liver Cu concentration was 3 to 14 mg/kg (0.05 to 0.22 mmol/kg), but dosing with Cu salts had no effect on the clinical condition. Copper deficiency in piglets 5 to 8 weeks of age has been described, characterized by ataxia, posterior paresis, nystagmus, inability to stand, paddling of the limbs, and death in 3 to 5 days. Lesions included demyelination of the spinal cord and degeneration of the elastic fibers of the walls of the aorta and pulmonary arteries.

Including 125 to 250 mg/kg of Cu (as Cu sulfate) in the diet of growing pigs (11 to 90 kg) fed ad libitum results in slight improvements in growth rate and feed efficiency, but has no significant effect on carcass characteristics. The addition of Cu causes a marked increase in liver Cu, which is a potential food hazard, and so it is recommended that Cu supplementation be limited to starter and grower diets fed to pigs weighing less than 50 kg.

Horses

Adult horses are not affected by Cu deficiency, but there are anecdotal reports of limb abnormalities in foals. Foals in Cu-deficient areas may be unthrifty and slow-growing, with limb stiffness, enlarged joints, and contraction of the flexor tendons, which causes the animal to stand on its toes. Signs may be present at birth or develop before weaning, but there is no ataxia or involvement of the central nervous system. Affected foals recover slowly after weaning but can display ill-thrift for up to 2 years.

In Australia, geophagia (soil eating) in horses has been associated with higher concentrations of iron and Cu in soil, suggesting that these elements are a stimulus for geophagia.

CLINICAL PATHOLOGY

The laboratory evaluation of the copper status of farm animals can be complex, with biochemical values often difficult to interpret and correlate with the clinical state of animals as they progress through the phases of Cu depletion, marginal deficiency, dysfunction, and disease (Fig. 21-4). Consequently, testing is usually undertaken on a herd basis, rather assessing the Cu status of individual animals. Guidelines for the laboratory diagnosis of primary and secondary Cu deficiency in cattle and sheep are summarized in Table 21-10.

Table 21-10 Concentrations of copper in plasma, liver, milk, and hair; dietary intake and ratios of copper and its antagonists in normal, marginal, and copper-deficient situations

Species and tissue	Normal	Marginal	Primary [secondary] copper deficiency
Cattle			
Plasma (μmol/L)[A]	10–20	3–9	<8 (often 1.6–3.2)
Adult liver (μmol/kg DW)[B]	380–1600	160–380	<160
Milk (mg/L)	0.05–0.20	0.02–0.05	0.01–0.02
Hair (mg/kg)	6.6–10.4	4–8	1.8–3.4 [5.5]
Sheep			
Plasma (μmol/L)	10–20	3–9	1.6–3.2 [6.3–11]
Adult liver (μmol/kg DW)	350–3140	100–300	10–100
Milk	3.1–9.4	0.3–3.0	0.16–0.30
Deer			
Plasma (μmol/L)	>8	5–8	<5
Adult liver (μmol/kg DW)	>400	240–400	<240
***Pasture* {forage}**[1]			
Cu (mg/kg DM)	10[D]	6–8 {4–6}	
Cu:Mo ratio	>2.0 (beef cattle growth)–4.0 (to prevent swayback)[C]	1.0–3.0 {0.5–2.0}[E]	
Fe:Cu ratio	15–20	–	[50–100]

[A]Divide by 15.7 to convert to μg/mL; neonatal liver from 3000–6000 μmol/kg DW.
[B]Multiply by 4 to convert to fresh weight.
[C]This ratio is quite variable and influenced by other antagonists (Fe, S, Mn, and Zn).
[D]When dietary Mo is < 1.5 mg/kg.
[E]When dietary Mo is < 8 mg/kg for sheep and <1 5 mg/kg for cattle.

Herd Diagnosis. The diagnosis of copper deficiency in a herd is based on the collection and interpretation of the history, clinical examination of affected animals, laboratory tests on blood and liver samples, and examination of the environment, including analysis of the feed, water, and, occasionally, soil.

When collecting samples for analysis, it is important to avoid contamination, which can occur with Cu-distilled water, vial caps, specimen containers, and other endogenous sources of Cu. Intercurrent disease may also affect plasma Cu concentrations.

Treatment Response Trial. A comparison between a group of animals treated with Cu and a similar group not treated is often a cost-effective and desirable approach. Variables include growth rates, mortality, and reproductive performance.

Copper Status of Herd or Flock. To assess the copper status of herd or flock, a standard practice is to take blood samples at random from at least 10% of clinically affected and 10% of normal animals. However, this may be inappropriate when there is a wide variability in the blood Cu within a herd. In some cases a 10% sample may be too large, whereas in others too small. The minimal sample size for random samples from a finite population of a normal continuously distributed variable can be calculated as follows:

$$\{n = t_2cv - 2/[(N1)E_2t_2cv - 2]\}$$

where n = minimal sample size; N = herd size; t = Student's t value; cv = coefficient of variation; and E = allowable error.

Initial testing can be used to estimate the variability of serum or plasma Cu concentration within a herd, which will help calculate a minimum sample size for more detailed investigations. This may differ between each class of animal according to age, diet, and production status, so a range of groups should be sampled if appropriate. Follow-up samples can be taken from the same animals following therapy or the institution of control measures.

Laboratory Diagnosis

Historically, laboratory tests for Cu deficiency in cattle and sheep have centered on the measurement of blood and liver Cu. However, because of the relationships summarized in Fig. 21-4, estimates of serum or plasma Cu, by themselves, are not reliable as the sole indicator of Cu status. Within an affected herd, clinically normal animals may have normal or marginal values, whereas unthrifty animals may have marginal or deficient values. Furthermore, when either the normal animals with marginal values or the unthrifty animals with the marginal or deficient values are treated with Cu, there may or may not be an improvement in weight gain, as might be expected in the former, or improvement in clinical condition in the latter. Consequently, liver samples, collected either by biopsy or at slaughter, can be used to more accurately assess Cu status.

In addition, for most mammalian species values for serum and plasma Cu are interchangeable. However, this is not the case for bovid ruminants, including cattle, sheep, and goats, where there is a significant and variable loss of Cu into the clot. The 95% limits of agreement are similar for sheep and goats, with serum Cu values being from 70% to 104% and 66% to 100% of the corresponding plasma Cu, respectively.[11] However, unlike cattle, sequestration of Cu into the clot in sheep and goats is proportional to the concentration of Cu. Thus although plasma is the preferred sample, the effect of using serum to assess marginal deficiencies is probably minimal, provided the results are not used to assess individual animals. It is recommended that experimental studies should use plasma Cu to estimate the acellular fraction of Cu in blood. In cattle, the difference between serum and plasma Cu is unrelated to Cu status, and thus plasma is the preferred sample, but the difference between serum and plasma ceruloplasmin is proportional to Cu status.[12] Sequestration of Cu into the clot does not occur in deer.[13]

Interpretation of Laboratory Results

The liver is the main storage site of Cu, and so the first sign of depletion is a decline in liver Cu (Fig. 21-4). Concentrations of liver Cu in replete neonatal calves and lambs are much higher than those in adults: 3000 to 6000 μmol/kg DW (190 to 380 mg/kg DW), which corresponds to 750 to 1500 μmol/kg fresh weight (FW) (50 to 95 mg/kg FW).

When liver reserves of Cu are close to being exhausted, ceruloplasmin synthesis decreases and plasma Cu falls.[1] Broad guidelines are that an average value less than 9 μmol/L (57 μg/dL) indicates marginal deficiency, but plasma Cu may have to fall to below 3 μmol/L (19 μg/dL) before there is dysfunction and lost production in sheep and cattle. However, there is considerable biological variation according to species, breed, the time during which depletion has occurred, and the presence of intercurrent disease.

Estimates of Cu in liver and blood are of diagnostic value, but they should be interpreted with caution because clinical signs of deficiency may appear before there are significant changes in these measures. Conversely, the plasma Cu may be very low in animals that are otherwise normal and performing well. For example, in the Netherlands the Cu status of groups of dairy heifers was monitored at regular intervals for 18 months. One group was supplemented with Cu sulfate, and the other was not. The concentrations of Cu and Mo in pasture were within normal limits for the Netherlands: 7 to 15 mg Cu/kg DM and less than 5 mg Mo/kg DM. The concentration of Cu in both blood and liver was below the reference ranges used in that country (6 to 15 μmol/L in blood and > 470 μmol/kg [30 mg/kg] DW in liver), but no clinical signs of Cu deficiency occurred, and there were no differences in growth rate and reproductive performance. This highlights that the ranges used to indicate marginal and deficient Cu status can vary between veterinary laboratories, and the thresholds for marginal status may often be set too high.

Cattle and Sheep

The internationally recognized threshold for Cu deficiency in the plasma of cattle and sheep is 9.4 μmol/L. A plasma Cu concentration between 3.0 and 9.0 μmol/L (19 to 57 μg/dL) is interpreted as marginal deficiency, and less than 3 μmol/L (19 μg/dL) is interpreted as a functional deficiency or hypocuprosis. In both species, 11 μmol/L is associated with adequate liver Cu (790 to 3750 μmol/kg DW [50 to 240 mg/kg]). A decrease to 9.3 μmol/L can indicate liver Cu values of 315 to 790 μmol/kg DW (20 to 50 mg/kg DW), which is interpreted as marginal in some areas, and a plasma Cu less than 7.9 μmol/L (50 μg/dL) is associated with low liver Cu.

Of the two measures, liver Cu is the most informative about deficiency because the concentration of Cu in plasma can remain normal long after liver stores start to decrease and early signs of Cu deficiency appear. Normal concentrations of Cu in adult liver are 1570 and 3140 μmol/kg DW (100 and 200 mg/kg DW) for cattle and sheep, respectively. Those from 160 to 380 μmol/kg DW (11 to 24 mg/kg DW) are classed as marginal, and less than 160 μmol/kg DW (10 mg/kg DW) as low. However, the lower critical value is influenced by species and breed. In New Zealand, a liver Cu concentration of 45 to 95 μmol/kg FW (180–380 μmol/kg DW) in dairy cattle is interpreted as marginal. It is recommended that at least 10 to 12 samples of liver need to be collected at slaughter or biopsy to reliably estimate the liver Cu status of a herd.[14]

Nevertheless, because the liver is the primary storage organ for Cu, estimates of liver Cu indicate a state of depletion rather than deficiency. Consequently, there is no rigid threshold for liver Cu below which the performance and health of livestock will definitely be impaired, and a broad range of values may coincide with a marginally deficient state (say, 80 to 380 μmol/kg DW). In sheep, the concentration of copper throughout the liver is uniform, and thus a single biopsy sample is representative of the whole liver. The frequency of biopsy does not affect Cu concentration, and there is little variability between successive samples.

In calves, the concentration of liver Cu copper varies according to age and class (dairy or beef). In calves submitted for necropsy, liver Cu concentrations were up to 940 μmol/kg FW (60 mg/kg) higher in dairy than beef calves. The concentration increased to 2 months old, declined until 9 months of age, and then increased again. Thus interpreting liver Cu concentration in calves should account for both age and production class.

Copper concentrations in the kidney cortex may be useful because they have a narrower normal range, 200 to 300 μmol/kg DW (12.7 to 19.0 mg/kg). Thus concentrations less than 200 μmol Cu/kg DW in the kidney may be an indicator of dysfunction.

The difficulties interpreting plasma Cu led to the use of plasma copper–protein complexes, especially ceruloplasmin, which in normal cattle contains more than 80% of the plasma Cu. There is a high correlation between plasma Cu and plasma ceruloplasmin activity (0.83 for cattle and 0.92 for sheep). However, although estimating ceruloplasmin is less complicated and quicker, it is an enzymatic assay and thus inherently more variable than plasma Cu.[1] In cattle, normal plasma ceruloplasmin concentrations range from 15 to 35 IU/L, but calculating a simple ratio of ceruloplasmin activity/plasma Cu does not appear to improve the diagnostic capability of these tests.[15] Estimates for Cu and ceruloplasmin are higher in plasma than serum, with less Cu associated with ceruloplasmin in serum (55%) compared with plasma (66%). In experimental primary Cu deficiency of calves, decreased plasma ceruloplasmin activity occurred at least 80 days before clinical signs of deficiency.

Erythrocyte superoxide dismutase (ESOD), a Cu-containing enzyme, has been used to assess Cu status. In deficient animals the activity of this enzyme decreases more slowly than plasma or liver Cu, and thus it may be a better measure of impending hypocuprosis. ESOD activity ranges from 2 to 5 U/mg hemoglobin in marginal and less than 2 U/mg hemoglobin in functional Cu deficiency.

Anemia can occur in advanced cases of primary copper deficiency, with hemoglobin being as low as 50 to 80 g/L and erythrocytes 2 to 4 × 10^{12}/L. A high proportion of cows in affected herds may have a Heinz-body anemia without evidence of hemoglobinuria, with the severity of the anemia related to the degree of hypocupremia.

Copper concentrations in milk and hair are lower in deficient cattle compared with normal ones, and thus estimating the Cu content of hair is an acceptable diagnostic test. It also provides a progressive record of the dietary intake of Cu, and it decreases when additional dietary Mo is fed.

Horses

A threshold of 16 μmol/L is used to distinguish between the normal and subnormal values of plasma Cu in horses, but many healthy horses have serum values between 12 and 16 μmol/L. Estimates of liver Cu from slaughtered horses varied widely about a mean of 114 μmol/kg FW, and a threshold of 52.5 μmol/kg FW was proposed to distinguish deficient and marginal concentrations. The mean liver and plasma Cu concentrations of horses fed diets containing 6.9 to 15.2 mg Cu/kg DM were 270 to 330 μmol/kg DW and 22.8 to 28.3 μmol/L (3.58 to 4.45 μg/dL), respectively, but there was no simple mathematical relationship between plasma and liver Cu concentrations.

Farmed Red Deer (*Cervus Elaphus*)

Suggested reference ranges for deficient, marginal, and adequate serum Cu in deer are less than 5, 5 to 8, and greater than 8 μmol/L, respectively, and for liver Cu are less than 60, 60 to 100, and greater than 100 μmol/kg FW, respectively. Enzootic ataxia and osteochondrosis occur when liver Cu is less than 60 μmol/kg fresh tissue and serum Cu concentrations less than 3 to 4 μmol/L. Growth responses to supplementation are equivocal when blood Cu is less than 3 to 4 μmol/L, but responses are significant when they are 0.9 to 4.0 μmol/L. No antler growth or bodyweight response to copper supplementation occurred when blood ceruloplasmin activity was 10 to 23 IU/L (equivalent to serum Cu of 6 to 13 μmol/L) and liver Cu was 98 μmol/kg FW.

NECROPSY FINDINGS

The characteristic gross findings in Cu deficiency of ruminants are anemia and emaciation. Hair and wool abnormalities may be present, as described in the section on clinical findings. Extensive deposits of hemosiderin can cause darkening of the liver, spleen, and kidney in most cases of primary Cu deficiency and in the secondary form if the Cu status is sufficiently low. In lambs, there may be severe osteoporosis and long-bone fractures. Osteoporosis is less evident in cattle but can be confirmed radiographically and histologically. In naturally occurring secondary Cu deficiency in cattle, associated with high dietary molybdenum and sulfate, there is widening of the growth plates as a result of abnormal mineralization of the primary spongiosa, resulting in a grossly rachitic appearance to the bones.

The most significant histologic finding in enzootic ataxia is degeneration of axons and myelin within the cerebellar and motor tracts of the spinal cord, with chromatolysis of neurons in a variety of locations within the central nervous system. In a few extreme cases, and in most cases of swayback, myelin loss also occurs in the cerebrum, with destruction and cavitation of the white matter. In these cases there is marked internal hydrocephalus, and the convolutions of the cerebrum are almost obliterated. In affected lambs, acute cerebral edema, with marked brain swelling and cerebellar herniation reminiscent of polioencephalomalacia, may accompany the more typical myelopathy and multifocal cerebral leukomalacia.

In falling disease, the heart is flabby and pale, there is generalized venous congestion, and the blood may appear watery. The liver and spleen are enlarged and dark. Histology reveals atrophy of the cardiac muscle fibers and considerable cardiac fibrosis. Deposits of hemosiderin are present in the liver, spleen, and kidney.

Necropsy findings associated with Cu deficiency in nonruminant species are not well documented. Degenerative changes with subsequent rupture of the aorta have been induced experimentally in pigs, but this has not been described as a naturally occurring disease. Myelopathy with white-matter changes similar to those of enzootic ataxia has also been reported in 4- to 5-month-old Cu-deficient pigs. Musculoskeletal changes similar to those described for calves have also been reported in foals with hypocuprosis.

Ideally, necropsy examinations should include assays for Cu, and also Mo if a secondary deficiency is suspected. In primary deficiency the concentration of Cu in liver will usually be low (see Table 21-10), whereas in secondary Cu deficiency there may be elevated kidney Cu and high concentrations of Mo in the liver, kidney, and spleen (see Table 21-10).

Samples for Confirmation of Diagnosis

- **Biochemistry**—50 g liver, kidney (ASSAY [Cu] [Mo])
- **Histology**—formalin-fixed samples of long bone (including growth plate), skin, liver, and spleen. Enzootic ataxia/swayback: half of midsagittally sectioned brain, lumbar, and cervical spinal cord. Falling disease: heart (several sections), bone marrow, spleen (light microscopy).

DIFFERENTIAL DIAGNOSIS

Clinical findings are most common in young, rapidly growing ruminants. They include a herd problem of unthriftiness and progressive weight loss, changes in hair coat color or texture of wool, chronic lameness, neonatal ataxia in lambs and kids, and terminal anemia. Chronic diarrhea is characteristic in adult cattle on pastures with excess Mo. A combination of plasma and liver Cu, and possibly serum Mo, is used to distinguish between Cu deficiency and other diseases.

Several herd or flock problems in cattle and sheep may resemble both primary and secondary Cu deficiency. A key indicator of Cu deficiency is that many animals are affected at the same time with a chronic debilitating disease complex, under the same dietary and seasonal circumstances.

The differential diagnosis of mineral and vitamin responsive disorders in beef cattle herds with suboptimal performance should investigate three major areas: malnutrition (lack of feed), chronic infectious disease, and lack of specific micronutrients.

Cattle
Unthriftiness and progressive weight loss may be attributable to protein–energy malnutrition; examination of the diet will reveal if it is deficient.

Changed hair coat color in young, rapidly growing cattle is caused only by Cu deficiency.

Chronic lameness in young, rapidly growing cattle may be caused by a calcium, phosphorus and vitamin D imbalance, determined by evaluating the diet and examining the long bones at necropsy or by radiography. Radiographic changes in cattle with secondary Cu deficiency are widened, irregular epiphyseal plates with increased bone density in the metaphysis, and metaphyseal lipping. These are similar to those described for rickets and secondary nutritional hyperparathyroidism.

Chronic diarrhea in young cattle may be attributable to intestinal parasitism; fecal egg counts and response to therapy are diagnostic. Diarrhea in a group of adult cattle on pasture known to be high in Mo is probably attributable to secondary Cu deficiency; response to therapy is diagnostic.

Winter dysentery of cattle, salmonellosis, coccidiosis, and mucosal disease are acute infectious diseases characterized by diarrhea, but have other distinctive signs and clinicopathologic findings. Johne's disease can cause diarrhea with a retained appetite, but cattle are usually 4 years or older. Many poisons cause diarrhea in ruminants, particularly arsenic, lead, and salt, but there are usually additional diagnostic signs and evidence of access to the poison. Assay of feed and tissues helps confirm a diagnosis of poisoning.

Peat scours is usually diagnosed if there is an immediate response to oral dosing with a copper salt.

Falling disease occurs only in adult cattle and must be differentiated from other causes of sudden death. Poisoning by the gidgee tree (*Acacia Georginae*) produces a similar syndrome.

Sheep and goats

Unthriftiness and **abnormal wool** or hair as a flock or herd problem are characteristic of Cu deficiency in sheep and goats, which must be differentiated from protein–energy malnutrition, intestinal parasitism, cobalt deficiency, and external parasites.

Lameness in lambs several weeks of age must be differentiated from nutritional osteodystrophy as a result of deficiencies or an imbalance of calcium, phosphorus, and vitamin D and stiff lamb disease as a result of enzootic muscular dystrophy.

Neonatal ataxia caused by congenital swayback and enzootic ataxia in newborn lambs and kids as a result of maternal Cu deficiency must be differentiated from border disease of newborn lambs, characterized by an outbreak of newborn lambs with hairy fleece and tremors, cerebellar hypoplasia (daft lamb disease), and hypothermia.

TREATMENT

The treatment of Cu deficiency is relatively simple, but if advanced lesions are already present in the nervous system or myocardium, complete recovery will not occur. Oral dosing with 4 g of Cu sulfate for 2- to 6-month-old calves, or 8 to 10 g for mature cattle, given weekly for 3 to 5 weeks, is recommended for the treatment of primary or secondary Cu deficiency. Parenteral injections of copper glycinate may also be used.

If feasible, the diet of affected animals can also be supplemented with Cu. Copper sulfate may be added to the mineral–salt mix at 3% to 5% of the total mixture. A commonly recommended mixture for cattle is 50% calcium–phosphorus mineral supplement, 45% cobalt-iodized salt, and 3% to 5% Cu sulfate. This mixture is offered free of choice, or it can be added to a complete diet at the rate of 1% of the total diet.

CONTROL

Dietary Requirements

The minimum dietary Cu requirements for cattle and sheep are often cited as 10 mg copper/kg DM and 5 mg/kg DM, respectively. However, this is overly simplistic because the requirement to prevent subclinical or clinical Cu deficiency depends on the presence of interfering substances in the diet, such as Mo, S, and Fe, which can cause the absorption of Cu to vary from 0.01 (1% of Cu ingested) to 0.10. Absorption is also influenced by age, physiologic state, and the genotype of the animal.[1] For example, in sheep the requirement has been modified from 5 mg/kg DM in 1975 to 7 to 11 mg/kg DM in 1985, 1.0 to 8.6 mg/kg DM in 1980 and then 4.3 to 28.4 mg/kg DM in 1999. The latter estimate was more detailed, assuming different absorption of Cu from different feedstuffs (0.06 from roughage, 0.03 from grasses, and 0.015 from grass with increased Mo [>5 mg/kg DM]), assuming increased Cu absorption in neonates that decreased in older animals, and allowing for the demands of the lamb in pregnant ewes (0.2 mg/d for a 4-kg lamb). The latest estimate from the NRC uses a factorial method to estimate requirements for sheep.[1,16]

There is insufficient data to do more detailed estimates for goats or deer, but they probably have increased requirements compared with sheep and thus are more similar to cattle (8–10 mg/kg DM).[1,16,17] Concentrations of Cu that could cause toxicity in sheep do not cause toxicity in goats, and some data show a stimulatory effect on growth of 100 to 300 ppm Cu in the diet of Nubian goats.

Under some circumstances, providing additional Cu to feedlot cattle can adversely affect performance, with as little as 20 mg Cu/kg DM reducing growth in finishing steers. Adding 10 or 20 mg Cu/kg DM of a high-concentrate diet containing 4.9 mg Cu/kg DM altered lipid and cholesterol metabolism in steers, but it did not alter ruminal fermentation. Reducing cholesterol and altering the fatty acid composition of beef, from saturated to unsaturated fats, has potential health benefits for humans, but this has yet to be exploited.

Copper Toxicity

Sheep are more susceptible to Cu toxicity than cattle, and hence preventing excess supplementation or accidental overdosing and monitoring of dietary intake of Cu are essential. As an example, in a Canadian study, 50% of cull ewes and 40% of market lambs had concentrations of liver Cu that were high to toxic.

Excessive or unnecessary supplementation with Cu is associated with Cu toxicity in many developed countries, with serious outbreaks described in dairy cattle that had recently been dried off.[18,19] In the United Kingdom, submissions to veterinary laboratories for chronic Cu poisoning increased from negligible before 2000 to 0.23% and 0.66% of all submissions in 2005 and 2007, respectively. In one case, high-yielding Jersey cows were identified at higher risk and had an estimated Cu intake of 50 mg/kg DM.[18] In New Zealand, deaths were associated with elevated concentrations of Cu in the liver (3990 μmol/kg FW) and kidney (440 μmol/kg FW) in Jersey cattle fed palm kernel expeller, which contains a high concentration of Cu (20 to 29 mg/kg DM).[19] Removing all Cu supplements and feeding 200 mg Mo/head per day as sodium molybdate reduced the average concentration of liver Cu from 3100 to 1320 μmol/kg FW within 26 days.[19]

Another presentation of excess Cu intake in lactating dairy cattle is a subclinical hepatopathy with no clinical disease. Affected cows received an average of 963 mg Cu/d from a mineral supplement, with total dietary intake of Cu of high- and low-producing cows being 1325 and 1250 mg/day, respectively, compared with their estimated requirement of 290 and 217 mg/cow per day. Consequently, excessive supplementation with Cu may be a significant problem in dairy herds, even those without overt clinical signs of toxicity.

Copper Supplementation

Copper can be supplied by several different methods. The following dose rates are recommended for the control of primary Cu deficiency, and they may have to be increased or given more frequently for secondary Cu deficiencies. In these cases, it is often necessary to determine the most satisfactory dosing strategy through a field trial.

Oral Dosing

Oral dosing with 1 g Cu sulfate will prevent swayback in lambs if the ewes are dosed weekly throughout pregnancy, then lambs can be protected after birth by dosing with 35 mg of Cu sulfate every 2 weeks. However, such regular oral dosing is time consuming and no longer widely practiced, especially in large, extensively managed flocks in which labor efficiency is an essential determinant of profitability.

Copper sulfate is considered a better supplement than Cu oxide or injectable Cu if cattle consume diets containing excess Mo, or Mo plus S.

Dietary Supplementation

Copper sulfate may be mixed with other minerals into a **mineral premix**, which is then incorporated into the concentrate part of the ration. The final concentration of Cu is usually adjusted to provide an overall intake of at least 10 mg/kg DM in the final ration. Thus, if the forage components of the ration contain much less than 10 mg/kg DM, the concentrate ration may need to contain a higher Cu concentration. Where a secondary Cu deficiency is attributable to excess Mo in the forage, up to 1200 mg Cu (approximately 5 g of hydrated Cu sulfate) is added to the concentrate daily.

For sheep grazing toxic lupin stubble, signs of lupinosis may be exacerbated by supplementing with 10 mg Cu/kg DM as Cu sulfate, and thus additional Cu should not be fed unless there are suitable amounts of Mo and S in the ration.

If animals are not receiving concentrates, an alternative is to provide free access to a mineral mixture or **salt-lick** containing Cu sulfate (0.25% to 0.5% for sheep and 2% for cattle; typically added to iodized salt, cobalt, calcium, phosphorus, and other trace minerals). This will supply sufficient Cu, provided there is an adequate intake of the mixture, although this is often highly variable between individuals and thus may not be the case.

In some areas, an effective method of administering copper is by the **top-dressing** of pasture with 5 to 10 kg Cu sulfate/ha, although the amount required will vary according to soil type, rainfall, and stocking rate. Early studies in Australia found that 5 to 7 kg Cu sulfate/ha was effective for 3 to 4 years, whereas in New Zealand hill country, 3 kg/ha increased pasture Cu for only 100 days.[1] Copper poisoning may occur if livestock are turned onto pasture while the Cu salt is still on the leaves, and thus treated pasture should be left unstocked for 3 weeks or until the first heavy rain. Chronic copper poisoning may also occur if the soil Cu status increases sufficiently as a result of repeated applications over a number of years.

In New Zealand the top-dressing of pastures grazed by farmed red deer was compared with oral administration of copper oxide wire particles. Pastures top-dressed with Cu sulfate at a rate of 12 kg/ha in mid-March increased the Cu status of weanling hinds, whereas top-dressing in mid-March and dosing hinds with 10 g copper oxide in late July effectively increased the Cu status of pregnant hinds, and it also significantly improved the Cu status of the progeny of yearling hinds from birth to weaning.

Addition of Cu salts to **drinking water** is usually impractical because it corrodes metal piping, and it is difficult to maintain the correct concentration of Cu in large bodies of water. However, systems have been devised to automatically supplement drinking water for short periods, and such systems have effectively controlled Cu deficiency in cattle. Calves can tolerate copper in milk replacers at a concentration of 50 ppm, but there is no advantage in providing more than 10 ppm.

Copper can also be provided in **molasses-based supplements**. However, the high sulfur content of the molasses may affect the availability of Cu, through the formation of Cu sulfide and thiomolybdates in the rumen, and actually decrease liver Cu concentrations. Consequently, a dietary Cu concentration greater than 10 ppm may be necessary to ensure absorption of Cu in beef cattle fed molasses-based supplements.

Removal of Sulfates

The removal of sulfates from drinking water by purification using reverse osmosis may be beneficial, with beef cows drinking desulfated water having an increased availability of Cu compared with those drinking water with a high concentration of sulfates.

Parenteral Injections of Copper

To overcome the difficulty of frequent individual dosing or top-dressing of pasture, the periodic injection of compounds that gradually release Cu is used and has given good results. These injections can be given at strategic times, avoid fixation of Cu by Mo and sulfides in the alimentary tract, and are commonly used for the prevention of swayback in lambs.

The following have been evaluated under field conditions: Cu calcium ethylenediamine tetra-acetate (copper calcium edetate), Cu methionate, Cu heptonate, Cu glycinate, Cu oxyquinoline sulfonate, and Cu phenylalanine complex. The criteria used to compare these compounds are minimal damage at the injection site, satisfactory liver storage (90% to 100% of the administered dose), and the safety margin between therapeutic and toxic doses. The typical dose of Cu in these compounds is 400 mg for cattle and 150 mg for sheep.

Copper heptonate (25 mg of Cu in 2 mL of preparation) given by IM injection to ewes in midpregnancy is not toxic and will prevent swayback in lambs. The Cu is removed from the injection site within 7 days, with most transferred to the liver and little or no deposition in skeletal muscle. Injection of 1 to 2 mg Cu/kg BW as heptonate has increased liver Cu to values associated with copper toxicity (13,000 to 52,000 μmol/kg DM). In sheep on pasture with high Mo content, a single IM injection of copper heptonate (37.5 mg Cu to adults, or 25 mg Cu to weaners) increases liver Cu reserves for at least 9 and 3 months, respectively. It was an acceptable alternative to copper oxide wire particles for preventing copper deficiency in sheep in southern Australia, but it is no longer available.

Copper calcium edetate increases blood Cu within hours and increases liver Cu within a week after injection. However, because of this rapid absorption, toxicity can occur with accidental overdosing. Some unexplained deaths also occurred in groups of treated sheep, and thus it is important to reduce handling and other stress during and after treatment. Marked local reactions occur at the site of injection; thus, SC injection is preferable, especially in animals to be used for meat. This treatment has a small risk of precipitating blackleg in cattle.

For sheep, a single injection of 45 mg of Cu as copper glycinate in midpregnancy is sufficient to prevent swayback in the lambs.

Cu calcium edetate or Cu oxyquinoline sulfonate given SC to sheep increases the concentration of Cu in whole blood, serum, and urine within 24 hours. In contrast, the injection of copper methionate increases the concentration of Cu in blood more gradually over 10 days, and there is no increase in urinary copper. After the injection of any of these three compounds, there is a steady increase in serum ceruloplasmin activity over 10 to 20 days, followed by a slow fall to the activity before treatment at 40 days. The lower toxicity of Cu methionate compared with Cu calcium edetate or Cu oxyquinoline sulfonate is a result of the slower absorption and transport of the Cu to the liver and kidney. Deaths have also occurred in sheep following the parenteral administration of diethylamine oxyquinoline sulfonate at recommended doses, with signs of hepatic encephalopathy and an acute, severe, generalized, centrilobular hepatocellular necrosis at necropsy. The use of Cu disodium edetate at the recommended dose rates in calves has caused deaths associated with liver necrosis and clinical signs of hepatic encephalopathy.

A single dose of Cu glycinate (120 mg for cows, 60 mg Cu for calves) will maintain adequate Cu concentrations for about 60 to 90 days. Milk is a poor source of Cu, particularly from Cu-deficient cows, but even treated cows can have insufficient Cu in their milk. Consequently, calves on pasture will often need a Cu supplement because they cannot increase or maintain their stores of liver Cu from marginal or deficient pastures. Copper reserves accrue in fetal liver at the expense of the dam's liver Cu, and thus newborn calves usually have sufficient liver Cu and will not need treatment until they are 6 weeks old. In pregnant cows, Cu supplementation should be timed to provide for the higher Cu requirement for Cu from the demands of the fetal liver during the last trimester.

One dose of Cu glycinate is sufficient when cattle are grazing forage with less than 3 mg/kg DM of Mo and less than 3 g/kg DM of S. With higher concentrations of Mo and S, repeated injections (or, alternatively, slow-release boluses) are often needed. The injectable copper may be supplemented by the use of 1% Cu sulfate in a mineral supplement, which will provide adequate Cu for cows, but calves may not consume enough mineral and may need multiple injections. The supplementation required to prevent a decrease in serum Cu during the grazing season will vary according to the concentration of dietary Mo and S and their effect upon the absorption of Cu.

In Canada, 100 mg of Cu as copper edetate, 120 mg copper glycinate, and 120 mg of copper methionate all improved and maintained an adequate Cu status for 90 days in deficient cattle. Copper methionate was least acceptable because of the severity of reactions at the injection site.

In horses, 100 mg and 250 mg copper edetate given IM to mares during months 9 and 10 of gestation had no effect on the liver concentration of their foals at birth, and thus would have little or no effect on the occurrence and severity of developmental bone and joint disease associated with Cu deficiency in newborn foals.

Slow-Release Treatments

There is a risk of Cu toxicity from mineral supplements because of variable ingestion of the supplement, and from injectable Cu compounds because it is difficult to control the rate at which the Cu is released. This risk, and a more constant supplementation with Cu, can be overcome by using slow- or controlled-release devices.

Glass Bolus

Soluble glass boluses are available for use in sheep and cattle in the United Kingdom and Europe, but not in New Zealand or Australia. They lodge in the rumen and release Cu at a uniform rate for up to 8 months, although the rate of dissolution is increased by the lower rumen pH associated with concentrate feeding. It is proposed that the additional rumen available Cu is complexed with thiomolybdates in the rumen, preventing absorption of thiomolybdates and their binding to biologically active compounds in blood and tissues, although there appears to be no direct experimental confirmation of this hypothesis. Commercially available glass boluses typically contain 13.4% Cu, 0.5% cobalt, and 0.3% selenium, with two boluses given to cattle greater than 100 kg (a 100-g bolus) or one to sheep greater than 25 kg (a 33-g bolus).

Copper Oxide Needles

Copper oxide wire particles ("needles"), incorporated into a soluble polyethylene glycol capsule and given orally, are a safe and effective way of controlling Cu deficiency in ruminants. These are relatively cheap, and a single treatment can be effective for an entire grazing season. The needles are gradually released from the rumen-reticulum and lodge in the folds of the abomasum, where they gradually release Cu for up to 100 days or more. The absorbed Cu is transported to and stored in the liver. An additional minor benefit may be some limited efficacy against gastrointestinal parasites in the abomasum (*Ostertagia* and *Haemonchus*), particularly newly ingested larvae.

Sheep

The response is dose dependent, with liver Cu peaking 10 weeks after administration of 2.5 to 20 g per animal, and then declining linearly over the next 40 weeks. A dose of 0.1 g/kg live weight (5 g) did not induce copper toxicity in the susceptible North Ronaldsay breed.

A single dose of 2 g cupric oxide needles maintained normal blood and liver Cu, prevented signs of ill-thrift, and improved growth rate in 3- to 5-week-old lambs grazing newly established, limed pastures. Copper oxide needles given to ewes in early pregnancy increases their liver Cu throughout gestation and in early lactation and the Cu status of their lambs from birth to 36 days old. Serum copper concentration was not affected by treatment, but a marked rise was observed in all lambs between birth and 10 weeks of age.

The administration of Cu oxide needles to ewes in the first half of pregnancy prevents swayback in their lambs, and when given at parturition it prevents hypocupremia for up to 17 weeks in animals grazing pasture known to have excess Mo and S. Treatment of ewes at parturition also increased the concentration of Cu in milk during early lactation. However, this increase in milk Cu will not prevent hypocupremia and hypocuprosis in lambs, which can be treated with cupric oxide needles at 6 weeks of age.

Some breeds of sheep are more susceptible to Cu toxicity because they accumulate Cu in the liver, and thus it is important not to exceed the recommended dosage. A dose of 4 g of Cu oxide needles has been used for the prevention of swayback in goats.

Cattle

Commercial capsules have 39% Cu oxide and in many countries are available in a 20-g dose for adults and a 10-g dose for calves. A dose of 20 g will maintain adequate Cu status for at least 5 months in lactating cows, and it prevented decreased growth and hypocupremia in young cattle weighing 190 kg for 70 days. The currently recommended doses for beef cattle are 10 g for calves and yearlings less than 200 kg and 20 g for cattle greater than 200 kg, which will provide protection for at least 6 months.

Farmed Red Deer

The need for Cu supplementation in young deer is not clear-cut. For example, 5 g of Cu oxide wire particles given to 4- to 7-month-old deer in New Zealand had no effect on live-weight gain despite hypocupremia in 38% of untreated deer, which gained weight at similar rates to those with adequate plasma Cu. In another study, 20-g boluses of Cu oxide wire particles did not significantly alter velvet weight, daily velvet growth rate, days from casting to removal, grade or value velvet, or the live weight gain of 2-year-old stags. Growth responses to supplementation are equivocal when blood Cu is less than 3 to 4 μmol/L, but responses are significant when they are 0.9 to 4.0 μmol/L.

Genetic Selection

It is possible to manipulate trace-element metabolism by genetic selection. For example, the selection of sheep based on plasma concentration of Cu resulted in two divergent sets of progeny within 5 years, one with a high Cu status, the other low, which resulted in clinical signs of Cu deficiency in the low group and protection in the high. This has not been exploited in commercial production.

Summary and Guidelines

Several rules of thumb are important and useful:

- Cattle are more susceptible to Cu deficiency than sheep.
- Sheep are more susceptible to Cu toxicity than either cattle or goats.
- The newborn calf is protected against neonatal hypocuprosis by donations from the dam, but newborn lambs assume the same copper status as the ewe.
- In general, a dietary intake of Cu equivalent to 10 mg/kg DM will prevent the occurrence of primary copper deficiency in both sheep and cattle.
- Diets containing less than 6 mg/kg DM will cause hypocuprosis.
- Diets with Cu : Mo ratios of less than 3 : 1 are conducive to secondary Cu deficiency (<2 : 1 for deer and goats).

FURTHER READING

Committee on Nutrient Requirements of Small Ruminants, Board on Agriculture and Natural Resources, National Research Council. *Nutrient Requirements of Small Ruminants: Sheep, Goats, Cervids and New World Camelids.* Washington, DC: National Academy Press; 2007.

Gould L, Kendall NR. Role of the rumen in copper and thiomolybdate absorption. *Nutr Res Rev.* 2011;24:176-182.

Grace ND, Knowles SO. Trace element supplementation of livestock in New Zealand: meeting the challenges of free-range grazing systems. *Vet Med Int.* 2012;639742.
Lee J, Masters DG, White CL, Grace ND, Judson GJ. Current issues in trace element nutrition of grazing livestock in Australia and New Zealand. *Aust J Agric Res.* 1999;50:1341-1364.
Radostits O, et al. Copper deficiency. In: *Veterinary Medicine: A Textbook of the Diseases of Cattle, Horses, Sheep, Goats and Pigs.* 10th ed. London: W.B. Saunders; 2007:1707-1722.
Suttle NF. Copper. In: *The Mineral Nutrition of Livestock.* 4th ed. Wallingford, Oxon: CAB International; 2010:255-305.

REFERENCES

1. Suttle NF. *The Mineral Nutrition of Livestock.* 4th ed. Wallingford, Oxon: CAB International; 2010:255-305.
2. Vikoren T, et al. *J Wildl Dis.* 2011;47:661.
3. Morris CA, et al. *Anim Sci.* 2006;82:799.
4. Solaiman SG, et al. *Small Rumin Res.* 2007;69:115.
5. Gould L, Kendall NR. *Nutr Res Rev.* 2011;24:176.
6. Grace ND. *NZ Vet J.* 2006;54:44.
7. Knowles SO, Grace ND. *J Anim Sci.* 2014;92:303.
8. Fry RS, et al. *J Anim Sci.* 2014;91:861.
9. Legleiter LR, Spears JW. *J Anim Sci.* 2007;85:2198.
10. Scaletti RW, Harmon RJ. *J Anim Sci.* 2012;95:654.
11. Laven RA, Lawrence KE. *Vet J.* 2012;192:232.
12. Laven RA, et al. *Vet J.* 2008;176:397.
13. Laven RA, Wilson PR. *NZ Vet J.* 2009;57:166.
14. Laven RA, Nortje R. *NZ Vet J.* 2013;61:269.
15. Laven RA, et al. *NZ Vet J.* 2007;55:171.
16. NRC. *Nutrient Requirements of Small Ruminants: Sheep, Goats, Cervids and New World Camelids.* Washington, DC: National Academy Press; 2007.
17. Grace ND, et al. *NZ J Agric Res.* 2008;51:439.
18. Bidewell CA, et al. *Vet Rec.* 2012;170:464.
19. Morgan PL, et al. *NZ Vet J.* 2014;62:167.

RIBOFLAVIN DEFICIENCY (HYPORIBOFLAVINOSIS)

Although riboflavin is essential for cellular oxidative processes in all animals, the occurrence of deficiency under natural conditions is rare in domestic animals because actively growing green plants and animal protein are good sources, and some synthesis by alimentary tract microflora occurs in all species. Synthesis by microbial activity is sufficient for the needs of ruminants, but a dietary source is required in these animals in the preruminant stage. Milk is a very good source. Daily requirements for pigs are 60 to 80 μg/kg BW, and 2 to 3 g/ton of feed provides adequate supplementation. The trend toward confinement feeding of pigs has increased the danger of naturally occurring cases in that species.

On experimental diets the following syndromes have been observed:

- Pigs: slow growth, frequent scouring, rough skin, and matting of the hair coat with heavy, sebaceous exudate are characteristic. There is a peculiar crippling of the legs with inability to walk and marked ocular lesions, including conjunctivitis, swollen eyelids, and cataract. The incidence of stillbirths may be high.
- Calves: anorexia, poor growth, scours, excessive salivation and lacrimation, and alopecia occur. Areas of hyperemia develop at the oral commissures, on the edges of the lips, and around the navel. There are no ocular lesions.

CHOLINE DEFICIENCY (HYPOCHOLINOSIS)

Choline is a dietary essential for pigs and young calves. Calves fed on a synthetic choline-deficient diet from the second day of life develop an acute syndrome in about 7 days. There is marked weakness and inability to get up, labored or rapid breathing, and anorexia. Recovery follows treatment with choline. Older calves are not affected. On some rations, the addition of choline increases daily gain in feedlot steers, particularly during the early part of the feeding period.

Supplementation of 20 g/day of rumen-protected choline to dairy cows 14 days before parturition increased milk production during the first month of lactation and the concentration of choline in milk, but it did not affect fat or protein concentration in the milk or plasma levels of glucose, β-hydroxybutyrate, cholesterol, and non-esterified fatty acids (NEFAs). The NEFA concentrations at the time of parturition were lower in treated animals than in controls, indicating improved lipid metabolism. Choline also increased α-tocopherol plasma concentrations. There does not appear to be a difference in effect of rumen-protected and unprotected choline supplements to dairy cattle when energy-related metabolites are evaluated.[1,2]

In pigs, ataxia, fatty degeneration of the liver and a high mortality rate occur with severe deficiency. Enlarged and tender hocks have been observed in feeder pigs. For pigs, 1 kg/ton of food is considered to supply sufficient choline.

Congenital splayleg of piglets has been attributed to choline deficiency, but adding choline to the ration of the sows does not always prevent the condition.[3]

REFERENCES

1. Brusemeister F, et al. *Anim Res.* 2006;55:93.
2. Toghdory A, et al. *J Anim Vet Adv.* 2009;8:2181.
3. Papatsiros VG. *Am J Anim Vet Sci.* 2012;7:80.

Multi-Organ Diseases Due to Toxicity

SNAKEBITE

SYNOPSIS

Etiology Venom injected into victim by a bite with specially adapted fangs.

Epidemiology Isolated bites primarily during summer months. A rare clinical disease in large animals.

Clinical pathology Venom detectable in blood (coagulopathy), urine (hematuria, myoglobinuria, anuria, oliguria), body tissues (hemorrhage, ecchymosis, necrosis), and fluids generally.

Lesions Varies depending on snake; may be local swelling and tissue necrosis.

Diagnosis confirmation Based on detection of venom in body tissues or fluids.

Treatment Injection of type-specific antivenin (antivenom).

Control Difficult.

ETIOLOGY

At least six toxic actions can result from snake venoms, and different snakes have varying combinations of toxins in their venoms (Table 21-11). The toxins include necrotizing, anticoagulant, and procoagulant fractions and neurotoxic, cardiotoxic, myotoxic, nephrotoxic, cytotoxic, and hemolytic, and hemorrhagic fractions.[1] Although there is often insufficient venom (composed of multiple toxins) injected to cause death in large animals, a serious secondary bacterial infection may occur in the local swelling and cause the subsequent death of the animal. Additionally, blood degradation products may be associated with coagulopathic insults resulting in secondary renal complications. The common venomous snakes include vipers, such as *Crotalus* spp. (rattlesnakes and other pit vipers of North America, Mexico, and Central and South America), the true vipers (e.g., *Vipera berus* [common European viper, the United Kingdom's only venomous snake]), and multiple other viper species, such as Africa's gaboon vipers (*Bitis* spp.) and Asia's Russell's vipers (*Daboia* spp.), and the elapid snakes, including coral snakes (*Micrurus* spp.) in the Americas, cobras (*Naja* spp.) and mambas (*Dendroaspis* spp.), and most of Australia's venomous snakes, including *Notechis scutatus* (tiger snake), *Oxyuranus* spp. (taipans), and *Pseudonaja* (*Demansia*) *textilis* (common brown snake).[1-4]

EPIDEMIOLOGY

The Incidence of snakebite is controlled by the geographic distribution of the snakes and their numbers. Asia, India, Africa, Central and South America, Australia, and the southern United States are areas in which snake populations are large. In general, the morbidity rate in farm animals is low, although a mortality rate from 9% to 25% has been recorded in horses[5] and 31% to 58% in New World camelids (llamas and alpacas).[6,7]

Risk Factors

Animal Risk Factors

Most snakebite incidents occur during the summer months, and bites are mainly near

Table 21-11 Venomous snakes of importance: taxonomy, geographic range, and major venom effects (Prepared by Daniel E Keyler, Pharm. D., FAACT)

Family/*genus*	Common names	Geographic range	Chief venom effects
Atractaspididae			
Atractaspis	Burrowing asps	Africa	Vasoconstriction, myocardial
Colubridae			
Dispholidus	Boomslang	Africa	Coagulopathy, hemorrhage
Philodryas	Cobra-verde	C, S America	Coagulopathy, hemorrhage
Rhabdophis	Keelbacks	Asia	Coagulopathy, hemorrhage
Thelotornis	Twig snake	Africa	Coagulopathy, hemorrhage
Elapidae			
Acanthophis	Death adders	Australia	Paralysis
Bungarus	Kraits	SE Asia	Paralysis
Dendroaspis	Black/green mamba	Africa	Paralysis
Hemachatus	Rinkhals	Africa	Paralysis, local necrosis
Hoplocephalus	Broad-headed snakes	Australia	Coagulopathy
Micropechis	Small-eyed snake	New Guinea	Paralysis, anticoagulant, myolysis
Micrurus	Coral snakes	N, C, S America	Paralysis
Naja	Cobras/spitting cobra	Africa/Asia	Paralysis, corneal ulceration
Notechis	Tiger snakes	Australia	Paralysis, coagulopathy, myolysis
Ophiophagus	King cobra	Asia	Paralysis
Oxyuranus	Taipan	Australia	Paralysis, coagagulopathy, myolysis
Pseudechis	Mulga/black snakes	Australia	Coagulopathy, myolysis
Pseudonaja	Brown snakes	Australia	Coagulopathy, paralysis
Tropidechis	Rough-scaled snake	Australia	Coagulopathy, paralysis, myolysis
Hydrophiidae			
Astrotia	Sea snakes	Indo-Pacific Oceans	Paralysis, myolysis
Pelamis		Pacific Oceans	
Laticauda		Indo-Pacific Oceans	
Many other genera			
Viperidae:			
Crotalinae (pit vipers)			
Agkistrodon	Cantils, copperheads, Moccasins	N, C, S America N, C, S America	Coagulopathy, necrosis Coagulopathy, necrosis
Bothrops	Lanceheads	C, S America	Coagulopathy, necrosis
Calloselasma	Malayan pit viper	Asia	Coagulopathy, necrosis
Crotalus	North American rattlesnakes, tropical rattlesnake	N America C, S America	Coagulopathy, necrosis Paralysis, myolysis
Hypnale	Hump-nosed vipers	Asia	Local necrosis, renal
Lachesis	Bushmaster	C, S America	Coagulopathy, necrosis
Sistrurus	Massasauga, pygmy	N America	Hemorrhage, local necrosis
Trimeresurus	Green pit vipers	SE Asia	Coagulopathy, necrosis
Viperinae (true vipers)			
Bitis	Gaboon/puff adder	Africa	Cardiovascular, coagulopathy
Causus	Night adders	Africa	Local necrosis
Cerastes	Horned vipers	Africa/Asia	Coagulopathy, necrosis
Daboia	Russel's vipers	SE Asia	Coagulopathy, myolysis, renal
Echis	Carpet, saw-scaled	N Africa/Asia	Coagulopathy, necrosis
Vipera	adders, asps, European vipers	Eurasia	Cardiovascular, coagulopathy necrosis, paralysis

C = central; N = North; S = South; SE = Southeast.

the head because of the inquisitive behavior of the bitten animal.[7] Pigs are not highly susceptible but not, as generally believed, because of their extensive subcutaneous fat depots. Sheep may be bitten on the udder, but their long wool coat is generally effective as a protective mechanism on other parts of the body. Cows may be less represented because of their large size and the large venom dose required to cause death. Horses, however, appear to be much more susceptible to venom than any other species.[8]

PATHOGENESIS

The effects of snakebite (envenomation) depend on the size and species of the snake, the quantity of venom injected, the route of venom delivery with the bite (e.g., subcutaneous, intramuscular, intravenous), the size of the bitten animal, and the location of the bite, particularly with reference to the thickness of the hair coat and the quantity of subcutaneous fat. As a general rule, the venom is injected by fangs, which leave a bite mark comprised of a row of small punctures with two large punctures outside them. An exception is the coral snake and other elapids, which typically chew to inoculate the venom. The bites may be visible on hairless and unpigmented skin but can only be seen on reflection of the skin at necropsy in many instances. Nonpoisonous snakes may bite animals, but the bite mark is typically (but not always) in the form of two rows of small punctures.

The toxins in venom include the following[1,2]:

- **Cardiotoxins,** causing coronary artery vasoconstriction/vasodilatation and direct myocardial effects, leading to hypotension and arrhythmias
- **Cytolisins,** which are associated with tissue necrosis, including platelets, leading to intravascular coagulation and anticoagulation
- **Hemolysins/hemorrhagins,** causing blood cell lysis and degradation of blood components and increased permeability of vascular tissues, leading to fluid shifts
- **Myotoxins,** causing selective ion channel blockade, rhabdomyolysis, myoglobinemia, and myoglobinuria
- **Nephrotoxins,** causing direct nephrotic damage, acute tubular necrosis, renal cortical necrosis, and renal failure
- **Neurotoxins**, causing pre- and postsynaptic blockade and neurotransmitter destruction, with flaccid paralysis, pupillary dilation, and paralytic respiratory failure

The overall effect of a venomous bite by a snake depends on the mix of specific venom components and the dose delivered.[4] The actual dose delivered is highly variable, but also depends on the size of the snake and the period of time since the snake last expended venom with a bite. Tiger snake venom contains neurotoxins and procoagulants.[4] Death adder venoms contain only neurotoxin; Australian brown snakes have procoagulant and some neurotoxin. Rattlesnake venom is associated with necrosis of arterioles and arteriolar thrombus formation, and in most species it contains an anticoagulant, causing a bleeding diathesis.[2] The Mojave rattlesnake *Crotalus scutulatus* and the neotropical and tropical rattlesnakes (*Crotalus durrissus* spp.) are exceptions.

CLINICAL FINDINGS

Bites by adder-type snakes (viperids) are associated with a local swelling and rapidly developing pain, which is usually sufficient to produce signs of excitement and anxiety. Bites on the head may be followed by swellings of sufficient size to cause dyspnea. If sufficient neurotoxin has been injected, a secondary stage of excitement occurs and is followed by marked dilation of the pupils, salivation, hyperesthesia, tetany, depression, recumbency, and terminal paralysis. In small animals, death may occur as a result of asphyxia during convulsions in the excitement stage of the disease. In animals that recover, there is usually local tissue sloughing at the site of the swelling.

Rattlesnake (*Crotalus* spp.) bites are reported primarily in North America, and affected animals include horses,[5,9,10] New World camelids,[6,7] cattle, and sheep. In horses, the most commonly reported signs are swelling around the bite site, which may be severe and result in respiratory distress, tissue necrosis, and evidence of a coagulopathy (spontaneous bleeding from eyes, ears, injection site, tracheotomy site).[5,9] Venom-associated cardiac abnormalities include tachycardia and arrhythmias, including atrial fibrillation, ventricular premature contractions, and second- and third-degree arterioventricular (AV) block.[9,10] Clinical signs in New World camelids include facial swelling, respiratory distress, tachypnea, hyperthermia, tachycardia, lethargy, and recumbency.[6,7] Rattlesnake bite in calves is associated with restlessness, teeth grinding, vomiting, hypersalivation, dyspnea, ataxia, and convulsions.

Bites by cobra-type snakes (elapids) may be associated with local swelling in animals that survive the effects of the neurotoxin.[2,4] They may develop significant localized tissue necrosis, and they frequently develop bacterial infection 3 to 4 days later. The major effects following bites of cobra-type snakes are excitement, with convulsions, respiratory depression, and death resulting from asphyxia. The signs appear quickly or may be delayed, and death occurs usually in up to 48 hours in horses. In calves, the effects of the neurotoxin are manifested by marked pupillary dilation, excitement, and incoordination, followed by paralysis.

Clinical signs in horses bitten by tiger snakes (*Notechis scutatus*) in Australia include anxiety, diffuse muscle tremors, tachycardia, tachypnea, and profuse sweating.[4] The gait is stiff and short. In another case, muscle tremors were obvious in the standing patient, disappeared when the animal became recumbent, and reappeared upon arising. Foals bitten by brown snakes (*Pseudonaja textilis*) in Australia show similar signs to those associated with tiger snake envenomation. Common signs include drowsiness, drooping of eyelids and lips, partial tongue paralysis, muscle tremors and weakness leading to recumbency, and, in some, pupillary dilation. Respiration becomes labored and abdominal in nature. Sweating and inability to suck, swallow, or whinny occur late in the course. Adults also show an inability to swallow, with salivation and accumulation of food in the mouth.

CLINICAL PATHOLOGY

There are numerous clinicopathologic abnormalities associated with snake envenomation, with most of them dependent on the species and weight of animal affected, specific snake, and potency of venom.[1] Hematologic alterations include abnormalities in red and white blood cells and platelets. Venom-induced consumptive coagulopathies (VICCs) similar to DIC occur, in particular with venom from the Australian brown snakes (*Pseudonaja* spp.) and taipans (*Oxyuranus* spp.).[1,11] Increases in BUN and creatinine, creatine kinase, and liver enzymes occur, as do decreases in albumin, potassium, and calcium.[1,4,5,7] Horses with myocardial damage show elevations in cardiac troponin I (cTnI), which may be delayed for several days to weeks after envenomation.[9,10]

An ELISA for identification of venom in blood, urine, or other body tissue or fluid is available in Australia.[4] It is highly accurate, suitable for field or office use, and immediate, but it is expensive. It is limited to the snake species for which reagents are available.

NECROPSY FINDINGS

Postmortem findings are specific to each snake. In general, local swellings at the site of the bite are a result of exudation of serous fluid and inflammatory reaction to venom components, which is often deeply blood-stained. Fang marks are usually visible on the undersurface of the reflected skin. A horse dying from rattlesnake envenomation showed ischemia of the heart, skeletal muscle, urinary bladder, and gastrointestinal tract.[10] Cardiac hypertrophy and myocardial necrosis involving both ventricular free walls and atria was present grossly, and myocytes in both ventricles and the atria were necrotic and degenerative on histopathologic examination.[10] New World camelids dying of rattlesnake envenomation showed severe and hemorrhagic facial swellings, congestion of the lungs and kidneys, ulcerations in the third compartment, and other systemic manifestations.[7] Postmortem analysis of a cow presumed to have died from the bite of a snake in the Viperidae family showed petechial and ecchymotic hemorrhage to frank hemorrhage in the lung, liver, tracheal lumen, peritoneum, and epicardial and subendocardial surfaces. Pale linear streaks were present in the right ventricular myocardium.[12]

Diagnosis confirmation depends on a positive assay for venom in the patient's blood, urine, and tissues generally. Absolute identification of the snake by a knowledgeable herpetologist can also confirm the species of snake involved with envenomation. In acute cases death has usually occurred by the time the animal is seen. If the actual bite is observed, the diagnosis is made on the history.

DIFFERENTIAL DIAGNOSIS

Differential diagnosis list:

Nervous syndrome:
- Organophosphorus/carbamate toxicosis
- Fluoroacetate toxicosis
- Tick paralysis

Local swelling:
- Anthrax in horses and pigs
- Black widow, redback or brown recluse spider bites
- Blackleg
- Insect stings (wasps, hornets, bees)
- Puncture/trauma wounds versus fang puncture marks
- Scorpion stings

TREATMENT

In human medicine the application of a tourniquet proximal to a limb bite site has been replaced; for elapid envenomation a firm pressure immobilization bandage (PIB) is applied over the bite to restrict the distribution of the venom via the lymphatics and retain it in the site and prevent systemic effects. The use of PIB for crotalid or viperid envenomation is not recommended because the PIB holds the venom at the application site, and pit viper and viper venoms typically cause significant local tissue damage. As such, use of PIB in these instances may exacerbate local tissue damage. Excision of the bite site is not recommended for the bites of snakes (crotalids and viperids) that are associated with a serious local reaction because the procedure may worsen local tissue damage and enhance the distribution of venom from the bite-site region.

Emergency treatment should include early placement of an intravenous catheter, correction and maintenance of hydration, and establishment of a patent airway. In animals with severe facial or nasal swelling, a tracheotomy may be needed. Systemic treatment should include antivenin (antivenom), antibiotics, antiinflammatories, and antitoxin. Polyvalent antivenin containing antibodies against the venoms of all the snake species in the geographic region can usually be obtained locally, often in highly purified form.[4,7,8] It is expensive to use but highly effective. Speed is essential, and the IV route is preferred. The dose rate varies widely depending on the degree of envenomation, with the size of the animal and clinical signs determining the dose. In horses and New World camelids this is typically 1 to 5 vials, but the dose may be higher depending on the venom and amount contained in the vial.[5,7,8] The use of antibiotics in human beings is controversial but should be administered to control the local infection at the site of the bite. The occurrence of clostridial infections after snakebite suggests the administration of antitoxins against tetanus and gas gangrene. A nonsteroidal antiinflammatory drug such as flunixin will provide pain relief and assist with local and systemic swelling.[7]

Many other pharmacologic treatments have been used in treating venomous snakebite, including antihistamines and corticosteroids. These drugs have been found to be valuable as a protection against possible anaphylaxis after treatment with antivenin, but in cases where local tissue damage is evident, they are without value and in many cases exert deleterious effects. Adrenaline or epinephrine has little or no value, and calcium salts do not significantly reduce mortality. The application of chemicals to the incised bite area is also of no value and may exacerbate tissue damage. Attention has been drawn to the need to appreciate the mode of action of one's local snake venoms before attempting a general program of treatment—what may be effective in one country may very well be lethal in another.

CONTROL

Control is difficult because snakes occur in dry lots, paddocks, pastures, and fields where animals live. Vaccination against rattlesnake envenomation in horses is possible, but reported vaccine titers from the commercially available product are not as high as those that develop after natural rattlesnake envenomation.[13]

FURTHER READING

Angulo Y, Estrada R, Gutierrez JM. Clinical and laboratory alterations in horses during immunization with snake venoms for the production of polyvalent (*Crotalinae*) antivenom. *Toxicon.* 1997;35:81-90.

Carmen M, Riet-Correa F. Snakebite in sheep. *Vet Hum Toxicol.* 1995;37:62-63.

Dickinson CE, Traug-Dargatz JL, Dargatz DA, et al. Rattlesnake venom poisoning in horses: 32 cases (1973-1993). *J Am Vet Med Assoc.* 1996;206:1866-1871.

Lavonas EJ. Antivenoms for snakebite: design, function and controversies. *Curr Pharmaceut Biotechnol.* 2012;13:1980-1986.

White J. Snake venoms and coagulopathy. *Toxicon.* 2005;45:951-967.

Yeruham I. Avidar Y. Lethality in a ram from the bite of a Palestine viper (*Vipera xanthina palestinae*). *Vet Hum Toxicol.* 2002;44:26-27.

REFERENCES

1. Goddard A, et al. *Vet Clin Path.* 2011;403:282.
2. Panfoli I, et al. *Toxins (Basel).* 2010;2:417.
3. Tanaka GD, et al. *PLoS Negl Trop Dis.* 2010;4:e622. doi:10.1371/journal.pntd.0000622.
4. Cullimore AM, et al. *Aust Vet J.* 2013;91:381.
5. Fielding CL, et al. *J Am Vet Med Assoc.* 2011;238:631.
6. Sonis JM, et al. *J Vet Int Med.* 2013;27:1238.
7. Dykgraaf D, et al. *J Vet Int Med.* 2006;20:998.
8. Chiacchio SB, et al. *J Venom Anim Toxins Trop Dis.* 2011;17:111.
9. Gilliam LL, et al. *J Vet Int Med.* 2012;26:1457.
10. Lawler JB, et al. *J Vet Int Med.* 2008;22:486.
11. Isbister GK, et al. *Toxicon.* 2007;49:57.
12. Banga HS, et al. *Toxicol Int.* 2009;16:69.
13. Gilliam LL, et al. *Clin Vac Immunol.* 2013;20:732.

BEE AND WASP STINGS (*HYMENOPTERA*)

Bees (*Apoidea*) and wasps, hornets, and yellow jackets (*Vespoidea*) are stinging insects found in the Hymenoptera family. Their venom is proteinaceous in nature.[1] Bees sting only once and die; wasps, hornets, and yellow jackets are capable of stinging multiple times.

Most single stings are self-limiting, but multiple stings may be associated with severe local swelling up to 6 cm in diameter, similar to those in angioedema. The lips, eyelids, tongue, and vulva are often swollen and painful. Pain may result in pronounced excitement, and in severe cases in horses there may be diarrhea, hemoglobinuria, jaundice, tachycardia, cardiac arrhythmia, rapid breathing, sweating, and prostration. Animals attacked about the head may show dyspnea because of severe local swelling. Horses often show mild to moderate colic. Anaphylaxis is rare and generally occurs within minutes of stinging.[1] In a few cases, the attack may be fatal and nonanaphylactic, usually occurring after a course of 4 to 12 hours.

Treatment depends on the location of the stings, but may include antihistamines, topical hydrocortisone or lidocaine cream or ointment, cool compresses, tracheotomy if swelling and asphyxia threaten, and early recognition and treatment of anaphylaxis. Necropsy lesions vary depending on the number of stings and location but may include hemorrhages and edema of all connective tissues and the bowel wall.

FURTHER READING

Australian Institute of Health and Welfare, Bradley C. *Venomous Bites and Stings in Australia to 2005.* Injury research and statistics series no. 40. Cat no. INJCAT 110. Adelaide: AIHW; 2008.

Staempfli HR, et al. Acute fatal reaction to bee stings in a mare. *Eq Vet Edu.* 1993;5:250-252.

REFERENCE

1. Fitzgerald KT, et al. *Clin Tech Small Anim Pract.* 2006;21:194.

RED FIRE ANT STINGS (*SOLENOPSIS INVICTA*)

The red fire ant (*Solenopsis invicta)* is present in most of the southern portion of the United States and many other countries. The venom is a nonproteinaceous alkaloid with a wide range of biocidal activities.[1] Fire ants are aggressive, and an individual attack usually results in a number of stings. Fire ants both bite and sting, but envenomation only occurs with the sting.[2] Stings occur in a circular pattern because the ant first bites the animal with its mandible and then rotates its head around the bite site.

Stings from the aggressive red fire ant have been associated with focal necrotic ulcers of the cornea and conjunctiva of newborn calves. Stings around the nostrils may cause swelling with open mouth breathing, inhalation of more ants, or suffocation. Weak calves, lambs, and deer fawns are most likely to be injured, as are older and weaker animals. In addition, adult animals may develop stress-related anorexia resulting in decreased weight gain or milk production.

Treatment depends on the sting site and severity of signs and may include antihistamines, cool compresses, corticosteroids, tracheotomy, and appropriate therapy for anaphylaxis.[2]

FURTHER READING

Austin GP. Investigations of cattle grazing behavior and effects of the red imported fire ant. PhD thesis. 2003 at: <http://www.tdl.org>; Accessed 14.01.13.

Jemal A, Hugh-Jones M. A review of the red imported fire ant *Solenopsis invicta* and its impacts on plant, animal, and human health. *Prev Vet Med.* 1993;17:19-32.

Joyce JR. Multifocal ulcerative keratoconjunctivitis as a result of stings by imported fire ants. *Vet Med.* 1983;78:107-108.

REFERENCES

1. Boronow KE, et al. *J Exp Zoo.* 2010;313:17.
2. Fitzgerald KT, et al. *Clin Tech Small Anim Pract.* 2006;21:194.

MOTHS

Insect-generated fiber (e.g., in the cocoons of Molopo moths) can be indigestible and, if eaten in large quantities, can be associated with ruminal impaction. The body scales of the brown-tail moth and its larvae have a nettling effect, causing skin irritation on contact and bronchial mucosal irritation on inhalation.

SWEATING SICKNESS (TICK TOXICOSIS)

SYNOPSIS

Etiology Unknown, associated with bites of *Hyalomma truncatum.*

Continued

Epidemiology Reported in Africa, India, and Sri Lanka affecting calves 2 to 6 months of age.

Clinical findings Fever, salivation, lacrimation, hyperemia of mucosae, epistaxis, extensive and severe dermatitis, necrosis of oral epithelium.

Lesions Dermatitis and necrotic stomatitis, disseminated intravascular coagulopathy.

Treatment Symptomatic and use of hyperimmune serum.

Control Tick control.

ETIOLOGY

The cause of sweating sickness in cattle has not been identified, but it behaves as though it were an epitheliotropic or dermatrophic toxin produced by the salivary glands of certain strains of the hard tick *Hyalomma truncatum*. Both male and female ticks of the strains can produce the toxin, but not all strains of *H. truncatum* have the ability to do so.

EPIDEMIOLOGY

Attempts to transmit the disease between animals by direct contact and by injections of tissue or blood are unsuccessful. The disease occurs in Central, East, and South Africa; Sri Lanka; and probably southern India. Younger animals up to 1.5 years of age are affected as a rule, but rare cases occur in adults. Sheep, pigs, and goats are susceptible, although the disease does not naturally occur in them, and a similar disease has been reported in a dog in Brazil infested with the soft tick *Ornithodoros brasiliensis,* popularly known as the mouro tick.[1]

Sweating sickness occurs at all times of the year but is most prevalent during the wet season when ticks are more plentiful. The morbidity rate varies with the size of the tick population but is usually 10% to 30%. The case-fatality rate is up to 30%.

PATHOGENESIS

The clinical signs begin 4 to 7 days after the ticks attach, probably 3 days in experimental infestations. The effects are dose specific; if the ticks are removed very early, there is no clinical response, and the animal remains susceptible; with a longer exposure before the ticks are removed, the animal becomes immune but shows no clinical signs. With longer exposure of more than 5 days, the subject develops the full-blown clinical disease and may die. If it recovers, it has a solid and durable immunity. However, there is no passive immunity via colostrum.

CLINICAL FINDINGS

There is a sudden onset of fever up to 41°C (106°F), anorexia, hyperemia of the mucosae, and hyperesthesia. The animal is lethargic, depressed, and dehydrated and has a serous then mucopurulent oculonasal discharge, an arched back, and a rough coat. There is an extensive, moist dermatitis commencing in the axilla, groin, perineum, and the base of the ears, and it may extend to cover the entire body in bad cases. "Sweating" refers to this moist dermatitis. The hair is matted together by exudate, and moisture collects in the form of beads on the surface. The eyelids may be stuck together. Subsequently patches of the skin and hair are rubbed off or can be pulled off to leave raw, red areas of subcutaneous tissue exposed. The tips of the ears and tail may slough.

Affected calves seek shade, and their skin is very sensitive to touch. Later it becomes dry and hard, and cracks develop. Secondary bacterial infection and infestation with blowflies or screw-worm larvae are common sequelae. The oral mucosa is hyperemic at first and then becomes necrotic with the formation of ulcers and diphtheritic membranes. The calf salivates profusely, cannot eat or drink, and becomes emaciated and rapidly dehydrated. There are similar mucosal lesions in the vagina and nasal cavities, the latter causing dyspnea. The severity of the mucosal lesions appears to vary with different "strains" of the toxin. There may be abdominal pain and diarrhea in some calves.

The course may be as short as 2 days but is usually 4 or 5 days. In recovered animals the skin may heal and the hair may regrow, but there may be permanent, patchy alopecia, and the calves may remain stunted and unthrifty.

CLINICAL PATHOLOGY

There is severe neutropenia and eosinopenia and a degenerative left shift; α-globulin and beta-globulin levels are raised. Urinalysis indicates the existence of nephrosis, but serum creatinine levels are normal. Dermatologic examination fails to reveal the presence of any of the usual infectious causes of dermatitis.

NECROPSY FINDINGS

The lesions are essentially those seen clinically. There is also evidence of severe toxemia, dehydration, emaciation, and hyperemia of all internal organs and disseminated intravascular coagulation. The necrosis of the oral epithelium extends into the esophagus and may reach the forestomaches.

DIFFERENTIAL DIAGNOSIS

The combination of extensive dermatitis and mucosal necrosis is unusual. Mucosal disease and bovine malignant catarrh may bear some resemblance, and there could be difficulty in differentiation in areas where the tick *Hyalomma truncatum* occurs.

TREATMENT

There is no specific treatment; efforts should be directed at relieving the severity of the dermatitis and mucosal loss. Nonsteroidal antiinflammatory drugs (NSAIDs) and broad-spectrum antibiotic cover is a logical regimen. Hyperimmune serum, produced in sheep and cattle by infesting them with *Hyalomma truncatum* at 6-week intervals for 2 to 5 occasions, is an effective treatment in pigs, sheep, and, to a less extent, calves.

CONTROL

Control is limited to control of the causative tick. No vaccine is available. Exposure to the strain of ticks for a period of about 72 hours confers a limited degree of immunity.

FURTHER READING

Bwangamoi O. Sweating sickness. In: Mugera GM, ed. *Diseases of Cattle in Tropical Africa*. Nairobi: Kenya Literature Bureau; 1979:405.

Gothe R. Tick toxicoses of cattle. In: Ristic M, McIntyre I, eds. *Diseases of Cattle in the Tropics*. Current Topics in Veterinary Medicine and Animal Science. Vol. 6. Boston: Martinus Nijhoff; 1981:587.

REFERENCE

1. Reck J, et al. *Vet Clin Pathol*. 2011;40:356.

4-AMINOPYRIDINE TOXICOSIS

4-aminopyridine is marketed as an avicide or bird repellant to control the overpopulation of "pest birds" that might destroy crops or damage aircraft, monuments, and other areas. It is a highly toxic, restricted-use pesticide marketed under the tradename Avitrol. Currently, it is available as treated whole corn, treated corn pieces, and mixed grains in 0.5% and 1% concentrations.[1] Interestingly, in 2010 the U.S. Food and Drug Administration (FDA) granted medical approval for the use of 4-aminopyridine in humans with multiple sclerosis.[2]

Poisoning in large animals is rare, with an animal poison center reporting a single cow case in a 10-year retrospective study.[2] In horses, reported clinical signs occurred 6 to 8 hours after ingestion and included signs of fright, profuse sweating, severe convulsions, and fluttering of the third eyelid. Death occurred 2 hours after the onset of signs; the lethal dose was estimated at 2 to 3 mg/kg BW. In cattle, signs include anorexia, frequent passage of small amounts of feces, and tenesmus, with some animals also showing tremor, ataxia, and erratic behavior, especially walking backward, with some sudden deaths.

It is rapidly absorbed from the gastrointestinal tract, metabolized in the liver, and excreted in the urine. 4-aminopyridine blocks specific voltage-gated potassium ion channels and increases the release of acetylcholine at neuromuscular junctions and in the central nervous system.[2,3] In toxic amounts, agitation, hyperactivity, and seizures occur. Death is from cardiac or respiratory arrest.

Treatment is primarily supportive and symptomatic and involves managing the airway and controlling CNS signs with sedatives and/or anticonvulsants.[2,3]

FURTHER READING

Nicholson SS, Prejean CJ. Suspected 4-aminopyridine toxicosis in cattle. *J Am Vet Assoc.* 1981;178:1277.

Ray AC, Dwyer JN, Fambro GW, et al. Clinical signs and chemical confirmation of 4-aminopyridine poisoning in horses. *Am J Vet Res.* 1978;39:329-331.

Schafer EW, Brunton RB, Cunningham DJ, et al. A summary of the acute toxicity of 4-aminopyridine to birds and mammals. *Toxicol Appl Pharm.* 1973;26:532.

REFERENCES

1. Avitrol. 2011 at: <http://www.avitrol.com/avitrol-bird-control-label-and-msds.html>; Accessed 17.01.14.
2. King AM, et al. *J Med Toxicol.* 2012;8:314.
3. McLean MK, et al. *J Med Toxicol.* 2013;9:418.

CADMIUM TOXICOSIS

Cadmium is an environmental pollutant that may accumulate in plants and animals.[1] It contaminates the environment, especially the soil, when sewage sludge and rock phosphate are used as fertilizers. Other sources include industrial pollution from zinc smelters, mining wastes, coal combustion, and water from old zinc- or cadmium-sealed pipes.[2]

There is much interest in cadmium entering the human food chain via animals used as food. The chances of cadmium accumulating in lean meat are not very great because the levels of ingestion required to produce significant levels are so high that they would be associated with observable clinical illness. The kidney and liver accumulate cadmium far more readily than other tissues, and ingestion may be of concern.[2-4]

Accumulation in the kidneys is related to cadmium content in forage and soil ingested.[5] Horses may carry a higher body burden of cadmium than sheep, cattle, and pigs.[6] Concentrations of cadmium in kidneys obtained from animals in rural Croatia showed the highest levels in horses (0.1029–47.4 mg/kg), which exceeded the maximum European Union levels for cadmium in the kidney by 93%. In contrast, cattle exceeded the limit by 14% and sheep by 16%.[6] In Belgium, cattle kidney cadmium levels were much higher (75% cadmium from contaminated areas; 47% from rural areas); no equine kidneys were analyzed.[7]

Ingestion is the most common route of exposure in large animals, with absorption occurring in the intestinal tract. Once absorbed, cadmium is transported to the liver, where it induces and binds to metallothionein, forming an inert complex that decreases the toxic effects of cadmium on the liver.[3,8] The complex decreases biliary excretion of cadmium and increases retention of cadmium in cells, and it ultimately plays a role in the long half-life of cadmium in the body (10 to 25 years in human beings).[2,3,8,9]

Acute ingestion is rare in animals and in most cases result from accidental administrations of farm chemicals (e.g., a cadmium-containing fungicide). The target organs in acute human ingestions are the lung, liver, kidney, and testes, with nephrotoxicity common.[2,9]

Chronic ingestion in animals is associated with accumulation in tissues such as liver, kidney, lung, bone, testes, intestinal tract, skin, and blood. Chronic poisoning in cattle is associated with inappetence, weakness, loss of weight, poor hoof keratinization, dry brittle horns, matting of the hair, keratosis, and peeling of the skin. At necropsy there is hyperkeratosis of forestomach epithelium and degenerative changes in most organs. In cattle and sheep, cadmium levels in the feed greater than 50 mg/kg DM are associated with toxicity and large accumulations of cadmium in the kidney and liver.[3] Experimental poisoning of sheep is associated with anemia, nephropathy, and bone demineralization at a dose rate of 2.5 mg/kg body weight per day. Abortion, congenital defects, and stillbirths are also potential toxic outcomes. In young pigs, levels in the feed of 50 mg/kg for 6 weeks reduce growth rate and are associated with an iron-responsive anemia. The most signs in horses are lameness and swollen joints with osteoporosis and nephrocalcinosis.

There is currently no accepted treatment.[2] Zinc and iron may play a protective role in liver and kidney accumulation.[3] Selenium in rats has had a protective effect on the liver and kidneys and may be beneficial in individual animals.[10,11] Chelating agents have been suggested in human beings, but there are no documented studies on which particular one is effective.[3]

FURTHER READING

Bianu E, Nica D. Chronic intoxication with cadmium in the horses at the Copsa Mica area. *Revista Romana de Medicina Veterinara.* 2004;14:99-106.

Gunderson DE, Kowalcyk DF, Shoop CR, et al. Environmental zinc and cadmium pollution associated with generalized osteochondrosis, osteoporosis, and nephrocalcinosis in horses. *J Am Vet Med Assoc.* 1982;180:295-299.

Johnson DE, Kienholz EW, Baxter JC, et al. Heavy metal retention in tissues of cattle fed high cadmium sewage sludge. *J Am Sci.* 1981;52:108-114.

REFERENCES

1. Madejon P, et al. *Ecotoxicology.* 2009;18:417.
2. Bernhoft RA. *Sci World J.* 2013;doi:10.1155/2013/394652.
3. Reis LSLS, et al. *J Med Sci.* 2010;1:560.
4. Szkoda J, et al. *Pol J Environ Stud.* 2006;15:185.
5. Li J, et al. *Environ Geochem Health.* 2006;28:37.
6. Bilandzic N, et al. *Food Addit Contam B.* 2010;3:172.
7. Waegeneers N, et al. *Food Addit Contam.* 2009;26:326.
8. Klaassen CD, et al. *Tox Appl Pharmacol.* 2009;238:215.
9. Liu J, et al. *Tox Appl Pharmacol.* 2009;238:209.
10. Newairy AA, et al. *Toxicology.* 2007;242:23.
11. El-Sharaky AS, et al. *Toxicology.* 2007;235:185.

CHROMIUM TOXICOSIS

Chromium is most commonly found in two oxidation states: hexavalent and trivalent. Hexavalent chromium is a strong oxidizing agent that crosses biological membranes and is five times more toxic than trivalent chromium.[1,2] Toxicity from hexavalent chromium occurs primarily from inhalation or industrial contamination and trivalent chromium from ingestion or parenteral administration.

Chromium is absorbed in the gastrointestinal tract and transported in the blood to bone, spleen, liver, and kidney.[1] Excretion is primarily renal, with some biliary elimination.

The use of protein concentrates prepared from tannery waste as an animal feed is not recommended because of the material's high chromium content.[3] Trivalent chromium salts given orally to pigs at the rate of 0.5 to 1.5 and at 3 mg/kg BW are associated with transient diarrhea. With the higher dosage there is also tremor, dyspnea, and anorexia. Toxicity from hexavalent chromium in oil fields has been associated with death in cattle, and dermal absorption of a strong oxidizing solution of chromium has been associated with death in a dairy herd.

FURTHER READING

Page TG, Southern LL, Ward TL, et al. Effect of chromium picolinate on growth and serum and carcass traits of growing-finishing pigs. *J Anim Sci.* 1993;71:656-662.

Talcott PA, Haldorson GJ, Sathre P. Chromium poisoning in a group of dairy cows. In: *Proceedings of American Association of Veterinary Laboratory Diagnosticians.* Hershey, PA: 2005:45.

Thompson LJ, Hall JO, Meerdink GL. Toxic effects of trace element excess. *Vet Clin North Am Food A.* 1991;7:233-306.

REFERENCES

1. Pechova A, et al. *Vet Med-Czech.* 2007;52:1.
2. Bala A, et al. *Sci J Vet Adv.* 2012;1:47.
3. Oral R, et al. *Desalination.* 2007;211:48.

COBALT TOXICOSIS

Cobalt is an essential component of vitamin B_{12} (cobalamin).[1,2] Nonruminant animals are unable to synthesize vitamin B_{12} and depend on a dietary source of cobalt; ruminants can synthesize it if enough cobalt is provided in the diet.[1] Poisoning from cobalt is unlikely to occur in domestic animals unless there are errors in feed mixing, contamination of feed or water supply, or deliberate overdosing.

Absorption appears to be age dependent, with higher absorption in younger animals. Iron deficiency, in nonruminants, is associated with a higher absorption of cobalt. Cobalt is excreted primarily in the urine, with a small amount of fecal excretion. Tissue concentrations are highest in the liver, followed by the kidney, pancreas, and heart.[2]

Poisoning with cobalt compounds is associated with anorexia, weight loss, rough hair coat, listlessness, and muscular incoordination. Toxic effects appear in calves at dose rates of about 40 to 55 mg of elemental cobalt per 50 kg BW per day. Sheep are much less susceptible, ingesting 15 mg/kg BW of cobalt without apparent effect. Pigs tolerate up to 200 mg cobalt/kg of diet, but intakes of 400 and 600 mg/kg are associated with growth depression, anorexia, stiffness of the legs, incoordination, and muscle tremors. Supplementation of the diet with methionine, or with additional iron, manganese, and zinc, alleviate the toxic effects.

FURTHER READING

Andrews ED. Cobalt poisoning in sheep. *NZ Vet J.* 1965;13:101-103.

Dickson J, Bond MP. Cobalt toxicity in cattle. *Aust Vet J.* 1974;50:236.

Ely RE, Dunn KM, Huffman CF. Cobalt toxicity in calves resulting from high oral administration. *J Anim Sci.* 1948;7:239-246.

REFERENCES

1. Herdt TH. *Vet Clin North Am Food A.* 2011;27:255.
2. Simonsen LO. *Sci Total Envrion.* 2012;432:210.

PRIMARY COPPER TOXICOSIS

SYNOPSIS

Etiology Acute or chronic intake of copper.

Epidemiology Sheep most susceptible, horses least. Significant differences in breed susceptibility. Copper originates from copper-rich soils, industrial contamination of pasture, agricultural chemicals, copper preparations used pharmaceutically, feed, and other sources.

Pathogenesis Acute poisoning as a result of ingestion of a single large dose is associated with gastrointestinal tract mucosal necrosis and fatal shock. Acute injectable dosing or chronic oral intake is associated with hepatic necrosis and hemolytic anemia.

Clinical pathology Chronic oral poisoning: very high liver copper levels, low packed cell volume (PCV), hemoglobinemia, hemoglobinuria. Liver enzyme activity and blood copper levels may or may not be elevated depending on when they are taken.

Necropsy lesions

Acute oral poisoning: severe gastroenteritis, bluish-green discoloration of mucosa and ingesta.

Chronic oral poisoning: icterus, swollen liver, kidneys, spleen; high tissue levels of copper.

Diagnostic confirmation High copper levels in tissues.

Treatment Acute poisoning: supportive care; chronic poisoning: various dosages of sodium or ammonium molybdate in combination with thiosulfate; thiomolybdate; chelating agents (penicillamine, dimercaprol, calcium disodium EDTA).

Control Removal from source, prophylactic administration of molybdate.

ETIOLOGY

Acute oral and injectable poisoning is associated with a single large dose of copper. Chronic oral poisonings are associated with the accumulation of small amounts of copper over a long period of time.[1,2] In these instances, the amount of copper may exceed that required by the animal or be related to deficiencies in minerals such as molybdenum and sulfur.[2]

Causes of Acute Oral Poisoning

- Accidental administration of soluble copper salts
  - Old copper-containing anthelmintics
- Accidental ingestion of copper-containing substances
  - Copper sulfate foot baths, containers of copper algaecides or fungicides

Causes of Acute Injectable Poisoning

- Prophylactic injection of copper salts, especially soluble salts
- Copper (as the diethylamine oxyquinoline sulfonate) at recommended dose rates has been associated with death in sheep.

Causes of Chronic Oral Poisoning

- Contamination of drinking water
- Contamination of plants with fungicidal sprays[3]
- Copper containing boluses, pastes, needles, or wires placed in the rumen/reticulum[4]
- Feeding seed grain treated with copper-containing antifungal agents
- Feeding mineral or salt licks or mixtures containing excessive amounts of copper
- Grazing pasture contaminated by smelter fumes[5] or by drippings from overhead power cables made of copper but corroded by the constituents of an industrially polluted area
- Grazing pasture growing on soils rich in copper
- Grazing pasture too soon after it has been top-dressed with the following:
  - Copper salts to correct a mineral deficiency in the soil
  - Poultry manure or dried chicken waste when the birds have been fed on a copper-rich diet[6]
  - Pig slurry or dried pig wastes when the pigs have been fed on a copper-enriched ration as a growth supplement[7]
- Mineral or salt mixes containing copper ingested by salt-hungry livestock
- Miscellaneous sources of copper causing poisoning—palm oil cake and lumber treated with arsenic, copper, and chromium
- Overfeeding of copper-enriched concentrate rations

EPIDEMIOLOGY

Occurrence

Sporadic outbreaks of primary copper poisoning occur in many species and in many different countries. Toxicosis occurs far more often in ruminants, especially sheep, than in nonruminants. Poisoning in sheep is commonly reported in countries such as Australia, Brazil, New Zealand, South Africa, and the United States.[1,8] Cattle, buffalo, and goats are also affected, although reports are more sporadic.[2,8-10] The morbidity rate is often low, but the mortality rate is high.[3]

There is a great deal of published anecdotal evidence about the amount of copper fed to specific species that has been associated with illness or deaths but almost no evidence of MD_{50} or $LD_{50.}$ The following toxic dose rates are provided as a rough guide.

Sheep

- Acute: Single oral doses of 9 to 20 mg copper/kg BW;[2] some references provide a range of 20 to 100 mg copper/kg BW.[3]
- Chronic: Daily intakes of 3.5 mg copper/kg BW, 25 ppm being the maximum tolerated concentration in the feed.[3] Even lower concentrations (15 ppm) may poison sheep if adequate molybdenum and sulfate are not present in the diet.

Calves (Preruminant)

Toxic doses are similar to those for sheep.[2]

Cattle

- Acute: 200 mg copper/kg BW[2] (up to 800 mg/kg BW)
- Chronic: varies considerably depending on the breed

Goats

No data are available.

Horses

- Acute: 125 mg copper solution/kg BW; signs did not occur when similar amount added to feed.[2]
- Chronic: Relatively resistant; 791 mg copper/kg BW × 6 months resulted in no signs, but a liver copper concentration greater than 3000 mg/kg DM.[2]

Swine

- Acute: No data but considered relatively resistant
- Chronic: 200 mg copper/kg BW stimulates growth in weanling pigs; 500 mg copper/kg BW resulted in reduced growth and death.[2]

None of these data on toxic intakes come with information on competing and contributory dietary factors such as sulfate, molybdenum, and zinc, and these are critical in determining the toxic effects of the copper intake.

Risk Factors

Animal Risk Factors

Many deaths attributable to copper poisoning are followed by deaths from general debility in sheep in poor condition. Dairy cows, especially those lactating at the time, fail to produce well, and special care is needed to bring them back to full production. Younger animals, especially calves, are more likely to be poisoned as a result of an increase in copper absorption.[2]

Species Susceptibility

Ruminants, especially young ruminants, are more susceptible than nonruminants. Preruminant calves appear to mirror the susceptibility of sheep. Sheep are the most susceptible species, with some species tolerating as little as 9 mg/kg BW; they are different from other species in the way in which copper is handled. As ingestion increases, sheep are unable to increase the amount of biliary excretion, and copper accumulates in the liver. Goats tolerate higher amounts in their diets than sheep. Goats receiving 36 mg/kg DM for 88 days had higher liver concentrations of copper but no evidence of liver damage. Cattle will usually tolerate 100 ppm,[1] but lethal hemolysis has occurred in cattle fed a low-copper-level mineral supplement (38 mg/kg BW for lactating cows) for 2 years. Swine can tolerate and swine 250 ppm in their diets.[2] Horses are the least susceptible, with a tolerance to levels of 800 ppm in the diet.

Breed Susceptibility

Sheep. Scottish Blackface sheep appeared to be the least susceptible, followed by the Finnish Landrace, with intermediate susceptibility when fed moderate to high amounts of copper.[2] Texel sired lambs followed by Suffolk lambs were the most susceptible.[2] North Ronaldsay sheep are reported to be the most copper sensitive of sheep and mammals in general.[11,12] These sheep normally subsist on seaweed that has a very low content of copper and molybdenum.[12] When the sheep are fed on terrestrial herbage containing normal levels of copper and molybdenum and high levels of zinc, they develop copper poisoning.

Cattle. Angus cattle are much more susceptible than Charolais and Simmental. Jerseys may be more sensitive than Holstein cows.[2]

Environmental Factors

Both acute and chronic copper poisoning occur under field conditions. Acute poisoning usually occurs because of the accidental ingestion or administration of large quantities of soluble copper salts, whereas chronic poisoning occurs principally as a result of ingesting feed containing or contaminated by copper derived from the soil or by its application to the diet as an agricultural chemical or feed supplement.

The toxicity of copper ingested in this manner is governed not only by the absolute amount of copper but also by the interaction of a number of factors, including the amount of molybdenum and sulfate present in the diet, the presence or absence of specific plants in the diet, and the level of protein in the diet.[1,2] In fact, either copper deficiency or copper poisoning can occur on soils with apparently normal copper levels, with the syndrome depending on the particular conditioning factors present. High molybdenum and sulfate levels in the rumen lead to the microbiological synthesis of nonabsorbable thiomolybdates, and a high-sulfate diet also leads to lower retention of copper in tissues.

Other compounding factors exist. There is a competitive relationship between copper and zinc in the internal metabolism of ruminants, with a high level of zinc in the diet reducing the intake of copper. Reduction in rumen protozoa results in an increased susceptibility to copper, as does the use of ionophores such as monensin.[2] Sheep on a selenium-deficient diet and with low blood levels of glutathione peroxidase are more susceptible to chronic copper poisoning. Some sheep are conditioned by inheritance to have low blood glutathione levels in spite of a normal dietary intake of selenium. They also have low glutathione peroxidase blood levels and may be more susceptible for this reason.

PATHOGENESIS

Toxicokinetics vary depending on the gastrointestinal tract. In nonruminant animals, including preruminant calves and lambs, absorption occurs primarily in the small intestine. Absorption in ruminant animals is low, primarily as a result of the relationship between molybdenum and sulfur in the rumen. In the intestinal mucosa, a portion is bound to metallothionein and eventually excreted in the feces. The remainder is bound to albumin and transcuprin in the blood and transported to the liver. Once in the liver, copper can be stored, incorporated into ceruloplasmin for use, or excreted in the bile.[1,2] Very little renal excretion occurs. The liver has the highest concentration of copper, followed by the kidney and brain.[2,13,14]

Acute exposure to soluble copper salts in high concentrations is associated with intense irritation of the gastrointestinal mucosa, blue–green discoloration of the feces and mucosa, and profound shock. Severe intravascular hemolysis occurs if the animal survives long enough. Free copper acts as a protein coagulant, binding to proteins and forming a reactive oxygen species.[1,2]

When excessive amounts of copper are injected the response is rapid, and animals begin to die the next day, with peak mortality about the third day after dosing.[13] Early deaths appear to be attributable to severe hepatic insufficiency and later deaths to renal tubular necrosis.

Chronic poisoning occurs when ingestion overwhelms biliary excretion. The frequent ingestion of small amounts produces no ill-effects while copper accumulates in the liver and to a less extent, the kidney. This is generally referred to as the "prehemolytic phase."[1,2] When maximum hepatic levels are reached, often after periods of exposure as long as 6 months, copper is released from the liver into the bloodstream, and the animal dies of acute intravascular hemolysis. This phase is generally referred to as the "hemolytic phase."[1,2] The production of superoxide radicals that damage erythrocyte membranes may be responsible for hemolysis. One of the dangers of cumulative copper poisoning is that the animal shows normal health until the hemolytic crisis, when it becomes acutely ill and dies very quickly. Death is ascribed to acute hemolytic anemia and hemoglobinuric nephrosis.

The liberation of the hepatic copper is not well understood, but the favored hypothesis is that the accumulation of copper ions in the liver cells is associated with the accumulation of electron-dense lysozymes in the hepatocytes and hepatic necrosis. Various stresses, including a fall in plane of nutrition, traveling, and lactation, are thought to precipitate the liberation.[2,3] Complex mechanisms relating to disorders of cell membranes; a marked change in hemoglobin composition, including the development of methemoglobinemia; and an increase in the oxidative status of the sheep are described as occurring during the critical stages.[3] Liver-specific enzymes may appear in the serum beginning a few days or weeks before the hemolytic stage. Severe hepatic necrosis occurs at the time of the hemolytic crisis.

CLINICAL FINDINGS

Acute Intoxication

Acute toxicosis from ingestion or injection of large amounts of copper salts is rare. Clinical signs present after ingestion include severe gastroenteritis accompanied by salivation, abdominal pain, dehydration, diarrhea, and vomiting in those species that are able to. The feces and vomitus are mucoid with a characteristic blue–green color. Shock with a fall in body temperature and an increase in heart rate is followed by collapse and death, usually within 24 hours.[1,2] If the animal survives for a longer period, dysentery and jaundice become apparent. Horses receiving an oral solution of copper sulfate (125 mg/kg BW) developed gastroenteritis, hemolysis, and liver and kidney damage, and they died within 2 weeks. Interestingly, horses receiving a similar amount in the feed did not develop any signs of poisoning.[2]

Poisoning associated with the injection of copper salts is manifested by anorexia, depression, and dehydration. Ascites, hydrothorax, hydropericardium, hemoglobinuria, and massive hemorrhages, tachypnea, head-pressing, opisthotonos, aimless wandering, circling, and ataxia are reported in calves surviving for 3 or more days.[1,13] Lambs similarly poisoned die within 24 hours of injection.

Chronic Intoxication

In ruminants, anorexia, thirst, hemoglobinuria, pallor, and jaundice appear suddenly. There is no disturbance of alimentary tract function.[1-3,8] Depression is profound, and the animal usually dies 24 to 48 hours after the appearance of signs. A herd of affected lactating dairy goats did not show hemolysis but rather anorexia, recumbency, and neurologic signs, whereas adult Boer goats developed hemolysis and hemoglobinuric nephrosis.[9,10] In pigs, signs of illness are uncommon, with most pigs being found dead without premonitory signs, although dullness, anorexia, poor weight gain, melena, weakness, pallor, hyperesthesia, and muscle tremor may be observed occasionally.

CLINICAL PATHOLOGY

Acute Ingestion

In acute intoxications, hepatic enzymes may not rise for a few days. Fecal examination may show large amounts (8000 to 10,000 mg/kg) of copper.

Chronic Ingestion

Serum enzyme activity (aspartate aminotransferase [AST], γ-glutamyltransferase [GGT], sorbitol dehydrogenase [SDH]) may be increased just before the hemolytic episode. The hepatic enzymes GGT and AST were determined in one experimental study to be the best enzymes to assess copper load in sheep during the prehemolytic phase. GGT activity increases were evident 28 days before the hemolytic crisis, and AST activity increased from 14 days before onset of acute copper toxicosis. In one small study, GGT and AST were predictive indicators of hepatic accumulation in cattle, whereas only GGT was predictive in buffalo.[15]

Other laboratory abnormalities are consistent with hemolysis and renal damage. The packed cell volume decreases sharply with the onset of hemolysis. Hemoglobinemia and hemoglobinuria may be present, and elevations in blood urea nitrogen and creatinine indicate renal compromise.

Levels of copper in the liver are markedly increased in chronic copper poisoning. Liver biopsy is the best diagnostic technique and serves a most useful purpose in the detection of chronic copper poisoning because blood levels do not raise appreciably until the hemolytic crisis occurs before death.[1,6] Because of the greater concentration of copper in the caudate lobe compared with other parts of the liver, an autopsy specimen will give the most reliable results.

Blood levels of copper **during the hemolytic crisis** are usually of the order of 78 to 114 μmol/L (4.9 to 7.2 ppm), compared with about 15.7 μmol/L (1 ppm) in normal animals. Normal liver levels of less than 5.5 mmol/kg dry matter (349 ppm) rise to above 15.7 mmol/kg (997 ppm) in the latter stages of chronic copper poisoning in sheep, to 95 mmol/kg in pigs, and to 30 mmol/kg in calves. In sheep, liver values greater than 7.85 mmol/kg and kidney values of greater than 1.25 to 1.57 mmol/kg dry matter are diagnostic. After a massive single dose, it is important to include kidney among specimens submitted for copper assay because levels may be high (more than 25 mg/kg dry matter), whereas liver copper levels have not yet risen. When comparing normal and toxic values, it should be remembered whether results are expressed as dry weight basis or wet weight basis. Assuming approximately 20% dry matter in tissue, a wet weight value of 1.5 ppm copper is actually 7.5 ppm on a dry weight basis, comparable to the toxic range reported previously for blood. Thus a commonly observed toxic value of 200 ppm copper in liver (wet weight basis) would be reported as 1000 ppm copper on a dry weight basis.

NECROPSY FINDINGS

Acute Intoxication

Acute copper poisoning via oral exposure is uncommon in ruminants, but gross changes include severe gastroenteritis with erosion and ulceration, particularly in the abomasum. Macroscopic changes in calves poisoned by injected solutions of copper salts include hepatomegaly with an enhanced zonal pattern and massive fluid accumulations in body cavities. Characteristic microscopic findings in such acute copper toxicoses include extensive periacinar hepatic necrosis and a variable amount of renal tubular nephrosis.

Chronic Intoxication

In chronic copper poisoning, jaundice and hemoglobinuria are usually but not always present. The liver is swollen and yellow and may contain hemorrhagic foci. The spleen is enlarged, with a soft pulp; the kidneys are swollen and have a dark, gunmetal color. The hemolytic crisis typical of ovine copper toxicosis results in massive acute hepatocellular necrosis, which masks most of the chronic hepatic damage. These changes include hepatocellular vacuolation and degeneration, increased single-cell necrosis of hepatocytes, a variable amount of periportal fibrosis, and proliferation of cholangiolar cells. These chronic lesions are more easily identified in cattle suffering from copper poisoning. Granular casts are often present in the renal tubules, especially in affected sheep. The brain in affected sheep may have focal areas of gliosis in the cerebral cortex and white-matter areas.[14] Hemosiderin deposits are increased in the liver and spleen. Details of the critical copper levels of tissues are provided in the clinical pathology discussion.

Although the lesions described previously do occur in some outbreaks of the disease in pigs, they are not as pronounced as in ruminants, and they are often accompanied by pulmonary edema and by severe hemorrhage from ulcers in the pars esophagea or large intestine.

Samples for Confirmation of Diagnosis

- **Toxicology**—5 mL blood; 50 g liver, kidney; 100 g stomach content; 500 g suspect feed (ASSAY [Cu])
- **Histology**—formalin-fixed liver, kidney, abomasum, spleen (light microscopy)

Diagnostic confirmation is by demonstration of high blood and liver levels of copper plus histologic evidence of liver damage. The history and the examination of feedstuffs and pastures are valuable aids in determining the cause.

DIFFERENTIAL DIAGNOSIS

Differential list:

Acute Intoxication:

The differential diagnosis list for acute copper poisoning includes other associations with gastroenteritis. Copper poisoning can usually be identified by the bluish-green color of the ingesta or feces.

Chronic Intoxication:

Acute hemolytic diseases that may be mistaken for chronic copper poisoning include the following:

- Babesiosis
- Bacillary hemoglobinuria
- Equine infectious anemia
- Leptospirosis
- Nitrate/nitrate poisoning
- Plant poisoning including allium and S-methylcysteine sulphoxide (SMCO) in rape, kale
- Postparturient hemoglobinuria
- Red maple (*Acer rubrum*) toxicosis (horses)

TREATMENT

In acute poisoning, treatment is primarily symptomatic and supportive. Intravenous fluids, gastrointestinal protectants, and nonsteroidal antiinflammatory drugs may be used for dehydration, gastrointestinal pain, and shock. Blood transfusions may be indicated in individual animals with hemolysis and a rapidly falling packed cell volume.

Chelation may be useful in chronic toxicosis in small herds or individual animals. Common chelating agents used in the treatment of human copper toxicosis include penicillamine, dimercaprol, and calcium disodium EDTA.[16] Penicillamine has been used successfully in goats (50 mg/kg PO q24h × 7 days), but the cost may limit its use in herd situations.[9] Intravenous calcium disodium edetate (70 mg/kg BW × 2 days) has been used in calves.

There are a number of dosage recommendations for ammonium molybdate and sodium thiosulfate. For chronic copper poisoning, daily oral treatment of lambs with 100 mg ammonium molybdate and 1 g anhydrous sodium thiosulfate significantly reduced the copper content of tissues and appears to prevent deaths in lambs known to have toxic amounts of copper. In a herd of goats, 300 mg ammonium molybdate (300 mg PO q24h) and sodium thiosulfate (300 mg PO q24h) for 3 weeks has been used.[9] Ammonium tetrathiomolybdate (1.7 mg/kg IV or 3.4 mg/kg SQ every other day for 3 doses) or (2–15 mg/kg IV q24h × 3–6 days) has been recommended for use in food animals and sheep.[17] Different countries may have particular restrictions on the form of molybdenum approved for use, so locally available approved therapy should be determined.

CONTROL

With chronic intoxication, the provision of additional molybdenum in the diet as described under the control of phytogenous chronic copper poisoning should be effective as a preventive measure. Ferrous sulfide is effective, but difficulty is usually encountered in getting the animals to eat it. In pigs and sheep, the administration of iron and zinc reduces the risk of copper poisoning in diets supplemented by this element, and a diet high in calcium encourages the development of copper poisoning, probably by creating a secondary zinc deficiency. A lick that contains dicalcium phosphate, sulfur, and zinc sulfate has been used as a prophylactic.

FURTHER READING

Bidewell CA, David GP, Livesey CT. Copper toxicity in cattle. *Vet Rec.* 2000;14:399-400.

Humphries WR, Mills CF, Greig A, et al. Use of ammonium tetrathiomolybdate in the treatment of copper poisoning in sheep. *Vet Rec.* 1986;119:596-598.

Ishmael J, Gopinath C, Howell JM. Experimental chronic copper toxicity in sheep. Histological and histochemical changes during the development of the lesions in the liver. *Res Vet Sci.* 1971;12:358-366.

Perrin DJ, Schiefer HB, Blakley BR. Chronic copper toxicity in a dairy herd. *Can Vet J.* 1990;31:629-632.

Radostits O, et al. Primary copper poisoning. In: *Veterinary Medicine: A Textbook of the Disease of Cattle, Horses, Sheep, Goats and Pigs.* 10th ed. London: W.B. Saunders; 2007:1820.

Smith JD, Jordan DR, Nelson ML. Tolerance of ponies to high levels of dietary copper. *J Anim Sci.* 1975;41:1645-1649.

Solaiman SG, Maloney MA, Qureshi MA, et al. Effects of high copper supplements on performance, health, plasma copper and enzymes in goats. *Small Ruminant Res.* 2001;41:127-139.

REFERENCES

1. Reis LSL, et al. *J Med Med Sci.* 2010;1:560.
2. National Research Council. Copper. In: *Mineral Tolerance of Animals.* 2nd rev ed. National Academies Press; 2005:134.
3. Oruc HH, et al. *J Vet Diagn Invest.* 2009;21:540.
4. Burke JM, et al. *J Anim Sci.* 2007;85:2753.
5. Mozaffari AA, et al. *Turk J Vet Anim Sci.* 2009;33:113.
6. Christodoulopoulos G, et al. *Aust Vet J.* 2007;85:451.
7. Blanco-Penedo I, et al. *Environ Int.* 2006;32:901.
8. Minervino AHH, et al. *Res Vet Sci.* 2009;87:473.
9. Cornish J, et al. *J Am Vet Med Assoc.* 2007;231:586.
10. Bozynski CC, et al. *J Vet Diagn Invest.* 2009;21:395.
11. Simpson DM, et al. *BMC Vet Res.* 2006;2:36.
12. Haywood S, et al. *J Comp Path.* 2008;139:252.
13. Fazzio LE, et al. *Pesq Vet Bras.* 2012;32:1.
14. Giadinis ND, et al. *Turk J Vet Anim Sci.* 2009;33:363.
15. Minervino AHH, et al. *J Vet Diagn Invest.* 2008;20:791.
16. Franchitto N, et al. *Resuscitation.* 2008;78:92.
17. Plumb DC. Ammonium molybdate/ammonium tetramolybdate. In: Plumb DC, ed. *Veterinary Drug Handbook.* 7th ed. Ames, IA: Wiley-Blackwell; 2011:56.

TOXICOSIS FROM DRIED POULTRY WASTES

Feeding dried poultry wastes to ruminants provides them with a source of nitrogen and gets rid of the chicken farmer's disposal problem. However, deleterious effects include the following:

- Copper poisoning when the chickens are fed on diets supplemented with copper
- Estrogen poisoning when the chickens are fed on estrogen-supplemented diets
- An unidentified problem arises of hepatic necrosis, hypoalbuminemia, and ascites in lambs fed large amounts of poultry waste from hen batteries.
- Litter from broiler houses is associated with renal damage but not to the point of causing mortality.
- Botulism

TOXICOSIS FROM DEFOLIANTS

Substances used to remove the leaves from plants to facilitate harvesting of seed may represent a toxic hazard if the residual stalks are fed to livestock or if the animals gain access to concentrated product.

- Monochloroacetate sodium (SMCA) is commonly used for this purpose. It is unlikely to cause poisoning unless very large quantities of the stalks are fed or if animals have access to the concentrated defoliants. Toxic signs in cattle include diarrhea, colic, muscular tremor, stiff gait, ataxia, and dyspnea. Terminally there may be convulsions, hyperexcitability, and aggressiveness. The course is short, with most animals dying within a few hours.
- Trialkyl phosphorothioates (Merphos and DEF), organophosphorus compounds used as a defoliant for cotton plants, produce typical signs of organophosphorus poisoning.
- Thidiazuron (TDZ), a cotton defoliant, appears to be nontoxic to animals, but it may enter the human food chain via goat's milk and chicken eggs.

FURTHER READING

Aldridge WN, Dinsdale D, Nemery B, et al. Some aspects of the toxicology of trimethyl and triethyl phosphorothioates. *Fund Appl Toxicol.* 1985;5:S47-S60.

Hur JH, Wu SY, Casida JE. Oxidative chemistry and toxicology of S, S, S-tributyl phosphorotrithioate (DEF defoliant). *J Ag Food Chem.* 1992;40:1703-1709.

Murthy BNS, Murch SJ, Saxena PK. Thidiazuron: a potent regulator of in vitro plant morphogenesis. *In Vitro Cell Develop Biol-Plant.* 1998;34:267-275.

Quick MP, Manser PA, Stevens H, et al. Sodium monochloroacetate poisoning of cattle and sheep. *Vet Rec.* 1983;113:155-156.

TOXICOSIS FROM FUNGICIDES

- Zinc ethylene dithiocarbonate (zineb) may be associated with thyroid hyperplasia and hypofunction, degeneration of myocardium and skeletal muscle, testicular weight reduction, and germ cell depletion.
- Thiram (tetramethyl thiuram sulfide) is a widely used agricultural fungicide that is associated with conjunctivitis, rhinitis, and bronchitis on local contact; it is thought to be associated with abortion in ewes on ingestion. It is a known teratogen, but no specific poisoning incidents have been recorded in large animals. In birds, ingestion of contaminated poultry feed caused soft eggshells, depressed growth, and leg abnormalities.[1]

Fungistatic Agents

- Hexachlorobenzene (HCB) is widely known because of its indestructibility and capacity to pass from grain through cattle and into humans. Legislation against chlorinated hydrocarbons being found in the human food chain is very harsh, and hexachlorobenzene is a prime target for public health veterinarians. Its specific toxicity is not high, although experimental poisoning in pigs is associated with incoordination, paresis, and other disorders of the central nervous system.

Grain Fumigants

- Grain treated by the fumigant dibromoethane is associated with mortality in sheep. The principal lesions are pulmonary edema, septal fibrosis, alveolar epithelialization, and pleural effusion. Death occurs 48 to 120 hours after exposure.
- Methyl bromide is used for stored grain and as a soil fumigant.

FURTHER READING

Guitart R, Mateo R, Gutierrez JM, et al. An outbreak of thiram poisoning on Spanish poultry farms. *Vet Hum Tox.* 1996;38:287-288.

Palmer JS. Tolerance of sheep to the organic-zinc fungicide, Zineb. *J Am Vet Med Assoc.* 1963;143:994-995.

Robinson GR, Wagstaff DJ, Colaianne JJ, et al. Experimental hexachlorophene intoxication in young swine. *Am J Vet Res.* 1975;36:1615-1617.

REFERENCE

1. Guitart R, et al. *Vet J.* 2010;183:249.

TOXICOSIS FROM HERBICIDES

Over 200 different substances have been used as herbicides; some of them are historical and no longer manufactured. Herbicides vary widely in their composition, toxicity, associated toxicity, mechanism of action, and use. Associated toxicities include the following:

- Arsenicals herbicides may also cause other signs of arsenic poisoning.
- A hazard of the relatively safe organic compounds described here is their contamination by highly toxic ones as a result of faults in the manufacturing process (e.g., the dioxins that have been found to be significant contaminants of the 2,4,5-T chemical). Today, restrictions on registration and changes in the manufacturing process have drastically reduced contamination by dioxins.
- Sodium chlorate, in addition to other signs, causes methemoglobinemia.
- Some herbicides (e.g., glyphosate) increase the palatability of sprayed pasture more, creating their own toxicity hazard.
- The phenoxy acid herbicides (2,4-D, 2,4,5-T) can increase palatability of some plants after spraying and induce elevated nitrate concentration in plants for several days after spraying.

BIPYRIDYL DERIVATIVES

Paraquat and diquat, the two common herbicides included in this classification, are poisonous by ingestion, inhalation, and dermal exposure. Paraquat is among the most toxic herbicides currently in use and is restricted in many developed countries; diquat is somewhat less toxic. Poisoning in large animals with a bipyridyl herbicide is unlikely to occur unless it is accidentally or maliciously administered. Cattle and sheep are more sensitive to bipyridyls than other species. The LD_{50} of paraquat in cattle is 35 to 50 mg/kg BW; in sheep, the LD_{50} is 8 to 10 mg/kg BW; and in pigs, 75 mg/kg BW. The LD_{50} of diquat in cattle is 20 to 40 mg/kg BW.[1]

Paraquat accumulates in the lungs, affecting the type I and II alveolar cells and Clara cells and resulting in acute alveolitis and chronic pulmonary fibrosis in many species.[2] Paraquat is associated with fibrosing pneumonitis in pigs, but this does not develop in sheep or cattle with fatal doses. A dose rate of 100 mg/kg BW is uniformly fatal in pigs, with signs of vomiting, diarrhea, and dyspnea. Those animals that survive long enough may develop acute renal failure. Other lesions include hepatic injury and mucosal damage.[3]

Diquat does not specifically affect the lungs, but rather the gastrointestinal tract, liver, and kidneys. Accidental poisoning of sheep as a result of contamination of pasture by diquat has been associated with widespread illness with signs of diarrhea and significant mortality. In cattle, accidental poisoning with diquat has been associated with fatal abomasitis and enteritis, hepatic and myocardial degeneration, and pulmonary emphysema.

CARBAMATES, THIOCARBAMATES, DITHIOCARBAMATES

Herbicides in this group include, among others, asulam, barban, di-allate, tri-allate, and metham sodium. In general, these herbicides are safe when used in low concentrations. Repeated small doses are associated with marked alopecia.[4] Barban is toxic at doses of 25 mg/kg BW in cattle. Di-allate is toxic to ruminants, with anorexia, ataxia, and exhaustion reported as common signs.[1] The toxic dose of di-allate in cattle and sheep is 25 mg/kg BW for 5 days or 50 mg/kg BW for 3 days.[1] Tri-allate is associated with severe illness and sporadic death after single oral doses of 300 mg/kg BW in sheep and 800 mg/kg BW in pigs. Salivation, bradycardia, vomiting, muscular weakness, dyspnea, tremor, and convulsions are followed by death in 2 to 3 days. It is also toxic when continuously given in small amounts.

DINITROPHENOL COMPOUNDS

Dinitrophenol (DNP) and Dinitro-orthocresol (DNOC) are the most common members of this group. Dinoseb, now rarely used, is a highly toxic DNP. Dinitrophenols are hazardous to all species; doses of 25 to 50 mg/kg BW are usually toxic, but much smaller doses produce toxicity when environmental temperatures are high. The toxic dose range in cattle is 2 to 50 mg/kg BW.[1]

Animals can be poisoned accidentally by inhalation, ingestion, or percutaneous absorption of these compounds, which have the effect of uncoupling oxidative phosphorylation and increasing the basal metabolic rate.[5] Poisoning is manifested by an acute onset of restlessness, sweating, deep and rapid respiration, hyperthermia, and collapse. In ruminants, but not in nonruminants, the metabolites of these compounds are associated with intravascular hemolysis, methemoglobinemia, and hypoproteinemia. Death may occur 24 to 48 hours later.

INORGANIC HERBICIDES

Sodium chlorate, sodium borate or borax, ammonium sulfamate, and several arsenical products have historically been used as herbicides. For the most part they have been replaced by newer preparations. Sodium chlorate, although banned as an herbicide in several countries,[6] has been studied in sheep, cattle, and pigs as means of decreasing the fecal shedding of *E. coli* and other gastrointestinal pathogens.[7-10]

Sodium Chlorate

Animals seldom ingest sufficient sprayed plant material to produce clinical illness, and the principal danger is from accidental dosing or permitting salt-hungry cattle to have access to the chemical. The lethal oral dose is 2 to 2.5 g/kg BW for sheep, 0.5 g/kg for cattle, and 3.5 g/kg for dogs. Irritation of the alimentary tract is associated with diarrhea and deep, black erosions of the abomasal and duodenal mucosae. Hemoglobinuria, anemia, and methemoglobinemia result, and somnolence and dyspnea are characteristic. At necropsy, the blood, muscles, and viscera are very dark. No specific treatment is available. Sodium thiosulfate and methylene blue are used in treatment but have little effect; copious blood transfusions have been recommended.

ORGANOPHOSPHORUS COMPOUNDS

Glyphosate and glufosinate, both organophosphorus compounds, are herbicides regularly used in many countries.[11,12] The acute oral toxicity is low; dermal, ophthalmic, and respiratory irritation can occur from exposure to wet product. Glufosinate is slightly more toxic than glyphosate, and the surfactant used in ammonium formulation has been implicated in human poisonings.[1]

PHENOXY ACID DERIVATIVES

Substances found in this group are among the most extensively used herbicides, with 2,4-D (2,4-dichlorophenoxyacetic acid) and others commercially available since the mid-1940s. Common phenoxy acid derivatives include 2,4-D, 2,4-DB, 2,4,5-T, dalapon, 2,4-DP (dichloprop), MCPP (mecoprop), MCPA, and silvex. As a group, low doses are relatively safe; ingestion of higher doses results in gastrointestinal and nervous system signs.[1] Silvex, MCPA, 2,4-D, and 2,4,5-T are nontoxic in the concentrations used on crops and pasture, but dosing with 300 to 1000 mg/kg as a single dose is associated with deaths in 50% of cattle. They have also been tentatively linked with the high prevalence of small intestinal carcinomas in sheep

Ingestion of 2,4-D at doses between 150 and 188 mg/kg BW is fatal to adult cows and at 10 mg/kg BW for sheep. Reversible toxic effects are produced with single doses in calves with doses of 200 mg/kg and in pigs with 100 mg/kg. Repeated administration of 50 mg/kg is toxic to pigs. In adult cows, signs include recumbency, ruminal stasis, salivation, and tachycardia. In calves, the signs are dysphagia, tympanites, anorexia, and muscular weakness; in pigs, additional signs include incoordination, vomiting, and transient diarrhea. Long-term administration to pigs (500 ppm in the diet for 12 months) is associated with moderate degenerative changes in kidney and liver. Repeated dosing of sheep with silvex for about 30 days at 150 mg/kg BW causes death.

A commonly used mixture of 2,4-D, 2,4,5-T and a brushwood killer, monosodium methyl arsenate, is very toxic by mouth or after application to the skin; signs include anorexia, diarrhea, weight loss, and death in most cases.

TRIAZINES/TRIAZOLES

Similar to phenoxy acid herbicides, triazine herbicides have been enjoyed widespread use for many years. Common herbicides include atrazine, cyanazine, propazine, prometone, simazine, and terbutryn. Atrazine and prometone appear to be nontoxic at usual levels of ingestion. Accidental poisoning of sheep with atrazine is associated with paralysis, exophthalmos, grinding of the teeth, diarrhea, dyspnea, and tachycardia, and that of cattle is associated with salivation, tenesmus, stiff gait, and weakness. Experimental dosing of heifers with large doses of atrazine is associated with fatalities, but animals treated with activated charcoal have survived. Continuous access to simazine is associated with tremor, tetany and paraplegia, and a prancing gait with the head held against the chest. Death occurs after 2 to 4 days, and mild to moderate myocardiopathy is found at necropsy.

Simazine and aminonitrazole in combination have been associated with death in sheep and horses allowed access to pasture sprayed with the mixture. In sheep the signs are staggering, inappetence, and depression. In horses, colic is the prominent feature.

UREAS/THIOUREAS

Diuron, isoproturon, linuron, and tebuthiuron are among the many herbicides found in this classification. With the exception of tebuthiuron, most of these herbicides are of low-order toxicity. The toxic dose of diuron in cattle is 100 mg/kg BW for 10 days, and in sheep it is 250 mg/kg BW or 100 mg/kg BW for 2 days.[1] The toxic dose of linuron in cattle is listed as 20 to 40 mg/kg BW.[1] Flumeturon toxicity in sheep results depression and drowsiness, dyspnea, salivation, mydriasis, teeth grinding, chewing movements, and incoordiation.[1]

OTHERS

Triclopyr

Triclopyr, a selective postemergence herbicide, is toxic to horses at five times the estimated maximum intake from herbage. It is associated with digestive and respiratory signs, ataxia, stiff gait, and occasional tremors.

Delrad

Delrad is an algicide historically used to control the growth of algae on ponds and other water reservoirs. Cattle and sheep are unharmed by the ingestion of water containing 100 ppm of the compound. Dose rates of 250 g/kg BW in adult cattle, 150 mg/kg BW in calves, and 500 mg/kg BW sheep are associated with toxic effects.

FURTHER READING

Burgat V, Keck G, Guerre P, et al. Glyphosate toxicosis in domestic animals: a survey from the data of the Centre National d'Informations Toxicologiques Veterinaires (CNITV). *Vet Human Toxicol.* 1998;40:363-367.

Conning DM, Fletcher K, Swan AAB. Paraquat and related bipyridyls. *Brit Med Bull.* 1969;25:245-249.

Frank JF. The toxicity of sodium chlorate herbicides. *Can J Comp Med Vet Sci.* 1948;12:216-218.

Mehmood OSA, Ahmed KE, Adam SE, et al. Toxicity of cotoran (fluometuron) in desert sheep. *Vet Hum Toxicol.* 1995;37:214-216.

Osweiler GD. Toxicology of triclopyr herbicide in the equine. In: *Proceedings American Association of Veterinary Laboratory Diagnosticians 25th Annual Meeting.* Reno, NV: 1983.

Radostits O, et al. Herbicides. In: *Veterinary Medicine: A Textbook of the Disease of Cattle, Horses, Sheep, Goats and Pigs.* 10th ed. London: W.B. Saunders; 2007:1838.

Rose MS, Lock EA, Smith LL, et al. Paraquat accumulation: tissue and species specificity. *Biochem Pharmacol.* 1976;25:419-423.

Simon EW. Mechanisms of dinitrophenol toxicity. *Biol Rev.* 1953;28:453-478.

REFERENCES

1. Gupta PK. Toxicity of herbicides. In: Gupta RC, ed. *Veterinary Toxicology.* 2nd ed. London, UK: Elsevier; 2012:631.
2. Dinis-Oliveira RJ, et al. *Crit Rev Toxicol.* 2008;38:13.
3. Gawarammana IB, et al. *Br J Clin Pharmacol.* 2011;72:745.
4. Hurt S, Ollinger J, Arce G, et al. Dialkylthiocarbamates (EBDCs). In: Krieger R, ed. *Haye's Handbook of Pesticide Toxicology.* Vol. 2. 3rd ed. San Diego, CA: Elsevier; 2010:1689.
5. Miranda EJ, et al. *J Anal Toxicol.* 2006;30:219.
6. Stuerzebecher A, et al. *Clin Toxicol.* 2012;50:52.
7. Smith DJ, et al. *J Anim Sci.* 2013;91:5962.
8. Smith DJ, et al. *J Anim Sci.* 2012;90:2026.
9. Callaway TR, et al. *Ag Food Anal Bacteriol.* 2013;3:103.
10. Cha CN, et al. *Acta Vet Hung.* 2012;60:93.
11. Berny P, et al. *Vet J.* 2010;183:255.
12. Duke SO, et al. *Pest Manag Sci.* 2008;64:319.

HYDROCARBON TOXICOSIS

ETIOLOGY

Crude oil coming directly from wells is usually repellent to animals, but they can consume lethal quantities if they are in salt-deficient and salt-hungry state. A characteristic of crude oil is that it is usually mixed with salty water, which is often left lying in ponds nearby. After extraction most crude oils are temporarily stored in installations where lead paint is available ,and thus salt and lead poisoning commonly occur with oil poisoning. Of the natural crude oils, those with the highest content of sulfur ("sour crude") are most unpalatable and most toxic.

Petroleum distillates, including diesel oil, lamp oil, kerosene, and gasoline, are all poisonous to animals. Cattle will drink all of them and appear to have a positive liking for some products, especially used sump oil and liquid paraffin (mineral oil). Among the commercial oil products, those with the highest content of volatile and inflammable components, especially naphtha and petrol (gasoline) fractions, are the most toxic. Gasoline up to the level of 3 ppm in the drinking water does not appear to depress water intake or to interfere with growth performance of pigs.

The additives used with gasoline, especially lead, may also contribute to the poisoning. The introduction of lead-free gasoline has decreased this risk considerably.[1]

Other hydrocarbons or ingredients mixed with them are toxic as well. Toxic agents of all kinds can be encountered when reject sludge oil is available to animals. Chlorinated naphthalenes found in some older lubricants, greases, and oils can cause a severe hyperkeratosis in cattle similar to vitamin A deficiency. Methyl alcohol is used as antifreeze in gasoline engines for pumps working continuously on oilfields in cold regions. Accidental access to the pump enclosure may result in a poisoning incident.

Accurate dose levels are difficult to determine in field outbreaks. In experimental trials, crude oil at the rate of 37 mL/kg BW in a single dose or 123 mL/kg in 5 divided daily doses were poisonous to cattle. Kerosene at 20 mL/kg BW as a single dose and 62 mL/kg BW in 5 equal daily doses was poisonous. Tractor paraffin (kerosene) at a single dose rate of 13 mL/kg BW is associated with severe illness and at 21 mL/kg was fatal to cattle.

EPIDEMIOLOGY

On farms access to tractor fuel (paraffin, gasoline, kerosene) is the most likely hazard. When highly chlorinated naphthalenes were used as lubricants, access to oil dumps could lead to clinical signs. Kerosene has an unwarranted reputation as a therapeutic agent for bloat and constipation, but it is unlikely to be given in amounts sufficient to be associated with more than slight illness, unless it is given repeatedly.

PATHOGENESIS

The early signs are thought to be attributable to regurgitation of the oil; aspiration of the oil, causing pneumonia; and absorption of the volatile components through the pulmonary mucosa, causing toxemia. The later signs are thought to be associated with the direct effect of the oil on the alimentary tract.

Local application or ingestion of highly chlorinated naphthalenes to cattle produces hyperkeratosis characterized by thickening and scaling of the skin, emaciation, and eventual death. The pathogenesis of the skin lesions is attributable to interference with the conversion of carotene to vitamin A, causing a syndrome similar to vitamin A deficiency. When poisoning results from accidental emission from industrial plants, there are additional signs as a result of ocular, nasal, and tracheobronchial irritation; infertility and abortion also occur.

Accidental ingestion of methyl alcohol by cattle is associated with vomiting, recumbency, death, and a high concentration of methyl alcohol in the ruminal contents.

CLINICAL FINDINGS (OIL INGESTIONS)

Natural Cases

When large volumes of crude oil are consumed, signs of toxemia and incoordination occur; regurgitation (vomiting) and bloat may or may not occur. In terminal stages mydriasis, tachycardia, hyperpnea, and hyperthermia are evident. Death is rapid. The animals smell of oil, oil is often present on the skin around the mouth and anus, and oil is found in the feces. The feces are usually oily, often soft to semifluid, and frequently black if the crude oil has been ingested. With kerosene the feces are often dry and firm in the later stages, and the regurgitus may be in the form of gelatin-like cuds, smelling strongly of kerosene. Oil persists in the alimentary tract for long periods and may be found in the cud and feces and at postmortem as long as 16 days after ingestion. Animals that survive the acute toxic syndrome eat poorly, lose weight, and die at variable periods from 16 to 36 days later. Recovered animals usually do so poorly after the incident that they are slaughtered after a history as long as 6 months.

Experimental Cases

Early signs include incoordination, shivering, head-shaking, and mental confusion. Within 24 hours, anorexia, vomiting, and moderate to severe bloating occur. Experimental kerosene inhalation is associated with persistent severe intrapulmonary physiologic shunting, resulting in prolonged hypoxemia and acidemia and may account for the clinical disease in survivors.

CLINICAL PATHOLOGY

There are no specific clinicopathologic findings, but hypoglycemia, acetonemia, and transient hypomagnesemia are all recorded.

NECROPSY FINDINGS

In crude oil or kerosene poisoning aspiration pneumonia is recorded constantly in naturally occurring and experimentally produced cases. It is thought to be the result of vomiting and aspiration from the alimentary tract of already swallowed oil. In longstanding cases of bovine kerosene poisoning, the lungs are colored gray-blue and are enlarged and firm, but there are no significant histopathologic changes, nor are there any in the kidney or liver. Oil is present in the alimentary tract, and there may be thickening and inflammation of the alimentary mucosa. Degenerative changes in liver and kidney are recorded in some cases.

TREATMENT

No primary treatment is undertaken. Supportive treatment if the animal survives the initial acute phase should include an instillation of fresh rumen contents from a healthy animal.

FURTHER READING

Coppock RW, Mostrom MS, Khan AA, et al. Toxicology of oil field pollutants in cattle: a review. *Vet Hum Toxicol.* 1995;37:569-576.
Gibson EA, Linzell JL. Diesel oil poisoning in cattle. *Vet Rec.* 1948;60:60.
Sikes D, Bridges ME. Experimental production of hyperkeratosis ("X disease") of cattle with a chlorinated naphthalene. *Science.* 1962;116:506-507.

REFERENCE

1. Burren BG. *Aust Vet J.* 2010;88:240.

IRON TOXICOSIS

Iron poisoning is uncommon in large animals, with sporadic case reports in cattle, goats, horses, and pigs.[1] The occurrence of a genetic iron storage disease is very rare but reported in Saler cattle. Young animals, such as piglets, absorb iron more efficiently than older ones. Toxicity can occur from excessive ingestion or parenteral administration of iron-containing supplements. Poisoning is most severe after intravenous administration followed by intramuscular or subcutaneous use and least with oral administration. Absorption is the rate-limiting factor for oral toxicosis, and intake must be high for systemic poisoning to occur. The toxicity associated with iron occurs from generation of free radicals and peroxidation of lipid membranes.[1,2] Oral toxicity results in damage to the gastric mucosa, whereas systemic toxicity results in accumulation and damage to the liver and other tissues such as the myocardium.

The extent of poisoning also varies with different iron-containing compounds and the presence of dietary substances.[2-4] The most toxic compounds are those that contain a high proportion of their iron in an ionic, and therefore readily absorbable, form. High dietary levels of vitamin E, selenium, or calcium may reduce or modulate iron toxicity; simultaneously low levels of vitamin E or selenium may predispose to toxicity.[1,4] Newborn piglets from vitamin-E-deficient sows showed signs of toxicity when injected with 100 mg or 200 mg iron dextran. In a recent study, day-old piglets with normal vitamin E and selenium levels receiving100 mg iron dextran injections had normal PCV values and iron liver levels close to normal, whereas those treated with 150 mg and 200 mg had toxic levels of iron.[4]

Neonatal Pigs

Neonatal pigs frequently receive oral or injected iron supplements after birth to prevent iron-deficiency anemia. Susceptibility in piglets is attributable to low fetal iron stores, insufficient iron concentration in sow's milk, large litter sizes, and rapid growth rate. Recent studies show that the duodenal transporters of iron are almost undetectable at birth, making oral absorption and toxicity less likely to occur.[2]

Two-day-old pigs are much more susceptible to the toxic effects of iron compounds than are 8-day-old pigs. A suggested reason for this age resistance is the older pigs' better renal functional ability to excrete iron. Another possible reason is the greater mobilization of calcium by older pigs in response to iron administration. This mobilization, or calciphylaxis, can be great enough to result in deposition of calcium in damaged tissues or to cause death. This effect appears to be precipitated by simultaneous or immediately preceding (within 24 hours) injection of vitamin D , but the injection is not essential to it. The progeny of vitamin-E-deficient sows are most susceptible; the muscle cell membranes are damaged, and extensive biochemical changes result, including a great increase in extracellular potassium levels causing cardiac arrest and sudden death.

Two different syndromes of poisoning occur. In peracute poisoning, death occurs within several minutes to an hour after injection of an iron salt. Vomiting or diarrhea may occur before death, or piglets may be found dead with no other signs. The mechanism of action, although similar to anaphylaxis, is unknown. In acute or subacute poisoning, death may not occur for 2 to 4 days and is accompanied by gastrointestinal necrosis (if ingested), with vomiting, abdominal pain, depression, and coma. There is an additional possible damaging effect of iron injection in young pigs, the development of asymmetric hindquarters. In this condition there is asymmetry, but the muscles are normal in composition and appear to have asymmetric blood supplies.

Foals/Horses

Neonatal foals died soon after the oral administration of an oral supplement containing ferrous fumarate (16 mg/kg) or the iron compound alone. Naturally occurring and experimental cases pointed to acute hepatitis as the critical lesion and the iron compound as the cause. Depression, ataxia, recumbency, jaundice, nystagmus, and death occurred 1 to 5 days after administration. Foals were suspected of being more susceptible because of an age-related increase in intestinal absorption and decreased iron-binding capacity. Postmortem lesions included hepatic cell necrosis with bile duct proliferation and periportal fibrosis.

Deaths have occurred in adult horses within a few minutes of intramuscular injection of iron compounds. Others have shown severe shock but recovered. Death, when it occurs, appears to be attributable to acute heart failure. Chronic iron poisoning may occur in horses receiving large amounts of iron-enriched supplements.[5]

Cattle

Acute hepatitis and sudden deaths have occurred in 6- to 9-month-old bulls about 24 hours after injection of an organic iron preparation.

FURTHER READING

House JK, Smith BP, Mass J, et al. Hemochromatosis in Salers cattle. *J Vet Int Med.* 1994;8:105-111.

Mullaney TP, Brown CM. Iron toxicity in neonatal foals. *Eq Vet J.* 1988;20:119-124.

Pearson EG, Andreasen CB. Effect of oral administration of excessive iron in adult ponies. *J Am Vet Med Assoc.* 2001;218:400-404.

Velasquez JL, Aranzazu D. An acute case of iron toxicity on newborn piglets from vitamin E/Se deficient sows. *Rev Col Cienc Pec.* 2004;17:60-62.

REFERENCES

1. Herdt TH. *Vet Clin North Am Food A.* 2011;27:255.
2. Lipiński P, et al. *Am J Path.* 2010;177:1233.
3. Svoboda M, et al. *Acta Vet Brno.* 2007;76:179.
4. Ness A, et al. *Proc AASV Conf.* 2010:233.
5. Mendel M, et al. *Med Weter.* 2006;1357.

TOXICOSIS FROM FEED ADDITIVES

Many antibiotics, fungistats, vermicides, estrogens, arsenicals, urea, iodinated casein, and copper salts are added to prepared feed mixes to improve food utilization and hasten growth. Many of them are toxic if improperly used. Miscellaneous agents include amprolium, an antithiamine coccidiostat, which is associated with polioencephalomalacia in ruminants, and iodinated casein, which was used experimentally at one time to stimulate milk production in cows but is now associated with cardiac irregularity, dyspnea, restlessness, and diarrhea in hot weather. Toxic additives described elsewhere in this book are arsanilic acid and copper compounds.

BRONOPOL

Bronopol (2 bromo-2-nitro-1,3-propanediol) is used as a laboratory preservative for milk (e.g., in milk samples used for butterfat estimation). This milk is usually fed to calves or pigs and may be toxic on occasional feedings. Affected calves salivate, are depressed, collapse, and die within 24 hours of feeding. Necropsy lesions include severe necrotizing abomasitis and local peritonitis on the serosal surface of the abomasum. The oral LD_{50} values of bronopol in large animals are not reported, but in male and female rats are 307 and 342 mg/kg body weight, respectively.[1]

CARBADOX

Carbadox (mecadox, fortigro, getroxel), a member of the quinoxaline-di N oxide family, is used in pig feeds as a growth promotant and in the treatment of swine dysentery and other enteric diseases at the recommended rate of 50 mg/kg of feed/head per day. Toxic effects occur at rates of 150 mg/kg. Two chemically related compounds, cyadox and olaquindox, are also toxic, but carbadox is more harmful than olaquindox, and cyadox is safe in dosages up to 400 ppm. Affected pigs refuse the ration but will eat other rations, are gaunt and emaciated, pass hard fecal pellets, and drink urine, and they have a long and rough coat, pale skin, severe tachycardia, weak hindquarters, and a swaying walk, followed by knuckling of the hind fetlocks, posterior paralysis, and death in 8 to 9 days.[2] In the early stages the pigs screech frequently. Sows are agalactic and produce stillborn or weak, undersized piglets.

Necropsy lesions are diagnostic, with extensive damage to the zona glomerulosa of the adrenal gland accompanied by renal tubular necrosis. Both carbadox and olaquindox provided to pigs in the feed at 100 mg/kg for 6 weeks caused changes in the zona glomerulosa.[2] The resulting hypoaldosteronism is manifested by low serum sodium levels, elevated serum potassium (8 mmol/L), and elevated blood urea nitrogen levels. The condition is irreversible, and the outcome is severe disability or death.

PLURONICS

These substances are administered to adult cattle in their feed as prevention against bloat. They are unpalatable and unlikely to be consumed in dangerous amounts unless they are well masked in feed. When they are fed accidentally to calves in their milk, they are associated with dyspnea, ruminal tympany, bellowing, protrusion of the tongue, nystagmus, opisthotonos, recumbency, and convulsions. Death after 24 hours is the usual outcome.

TIN POISONING

Dibutyltin dilaurate (DBTD) is a coccidiostat fed to chickens in their feed. Errors in mixing may lead to cattle receiving toxic amounts in concentrates or pellets. Calves usually die acutely, with signs of tremors, convulsions, weakness, and diarrhea. Older animals usually suffer a chronic illness characterized by persistent diarrhea, severe weight loss, inappetence, polyuria, and depression, reminiscent of arsenic poisoning. Affected animals may not be suitable for human consumption because of the high content of tin in their tissues.

FURTHER READING

Baars AJ, van der Molen EJ, Spierenburg TJ, et al. Comparative toxicity of three quinoxaline-di-N-dioxide feed additives in young pigs. *Arch Tox.* 1988;S12:405-409.

Naburs MJA, can der Molen EJ, de Graf GJ, et al. Clinical signs and performance of pigs treated with different doses of carbadox, cyadox, and olaquindox. *J Vet Med Assoc.* 1990;37:68-76.

Shlosberg A, Egyed MN. Mass poisoning in cattle, palm doves and mink caused by the coccidiostat dibutyltin dilaurate. *Vet Hum Toxicol.* 1979;21:1.

Teague WR. Pluronic poisoning in a herd of dairy calves. *NZ Vet J.* 1986;34:104.

REFERENCES

1. Smith DJ, et al. *J Ag Food Chem.* 2013;61:763.
2. Spilsbury MLA, et al. *Res J Biol Sci.* 2010;5:9.

TOXICOSIS FROM MISCELLANEOUS FARM CHEMICALS

FORMALIN

Formalin is used to preserve colostrum for calf feeding and in the preparation of formalin-treated grain. Milk containing too much formalin is associated with severe gastroenteritis and death in some calves that drink it. The clinical signs include salivation, abdominal pain, diarrhea, and recumbency.

METHYL BROMIDE

Soil fumigants used to prepare fields for planting may be associated with toxicity hazards in animals grazing them or in feed harvested from them. Methyl bromide has been associated with poisoning in horses, cattle, and goats when used in this manner but should soon be historical in nature. Because of depletion of the ozone layer, the use of methyl bromide was phased out in the United States in 2001, in developed countries in 2005, and in developing countries by 2015.[1] Clinical signs in horses, cattle, and goats include ataxia, stumbling, and somnolence.

POLYBROMINATED BIPHENYLS

Polybrominated biphenyls (PBBs; hexabromobiphenyl, octabromobiphenyl, and decabromobiphenyl) were produced commercially as flame retardants beginning in 1970. They are not especially poisonous, nor are they a greater risk to farm animals, because of degree of exposure, than many other industrial chemicals, but they found their way into the cattle food chain in reported incidents in the United States. In 1973 to 1974, PBBs were accidentally mixed into various animal feeds, and over 9 million people were exposed to contaminated animal products, including eggs, meat, milk, and cheese.[2] Subsequent to that, the production of PBBs in the United States was voluntarily discontinued. Most of the animal losses attributable to contamination with these compounds were a result of destruction of animals because they were contaminated, and there was concern for adverse effects on humans who consumed them or their products. However, neither animals nor humans exposed to the PBBs showed any signs of illness at the time of exposure.

The excretion of these compounds occurs principally in feces and urine, but as much as 25% of ingested substance may be present in the milk. They are lipotropic and accumulate in fat depots and the liver. These compounds pass into the placenta and are found in fetuses but appear to be associated with no health problems in the offspring. Attempts to hasten excretion have not produced a satisfactory method. Grazing wool sheep on contaminated ground may be an option for utilization of contaminated land.

CLINICAL SIGNS

Cattle

Experimental dosing with 67 mg/kg BW daily for long periods is associated with poisoning, but levels of 10 mg/kg BW are not toxic. Clinical signs of illness are anorexia, diarrhea, lacrimation, salivation, emaciation, dehydration, depression, and abortion. Similar signs plus extensive cutaneous hyperkeratosis occur in natural cases. Necropsy lesions include mucoid enteritis, degenerative renal lesions in natural and experimental cases, hyperkeratosis in the glands, and epithelium of the eyelids.

Pigs

Experimental poisoning in pigs causes no ill-effects in sows, but high concentrations of PBBs develop in the sow's milk, with death of some nursing pigs resulting.

POLYBROMINATED DIPHENYL ETHERS

Compounds in the polybrominated diphenyl ethers (PBDEs) group (pentaBDE, octaBDE, and decaBDE) are similar to the PBBs in physical and chemical structure and are still produced commercially as flame retardants for in use in consumer products.[2] In many countries, the unrestricted production and disposal has resulted in environmental contamination of the water, soil, air, and marine animals.[3] Two of the compounds, pentaBDE and octaBDE, have been voluntarily phased out, restricted, or banned in many countries, including the United States and the European Union. Concentrations of PBDEs have been found in cow's and goat's milk, animal meats, fish, soil, and grass.[3-9]

POLYCHLORINATED BIPHENYLS

Polychlorinated biphenyls (PCBs) have a number of industrial uses and are common environmental contaminants. They are hydrophobic and lipophilic, accumulate in body fat, have low rates of biotransformation and excretion, and persist in animal tissues for long periods. Concentrations of PCBs, sometimes with seasonal variation, have been found in cow's milk in countries where no known PCB production occurs.[6,8] Belgium, in 1999, experienced PCB, dioxin, and dibenzofuran contamination of poultry products, resulting in a precipitous drop in egg production, decreased weight gain, and increased chick mortality.[10] At postmortem, degenerative changes were found in the skeletal and cardiac muscle.

The presence of PCBs in animal tissues is likely to cause rejection of meat from the human food chain. Recorded damage refers to unidentified reproductive inefficiency and reduction in efficiency of food conversion and possibly hepatic hypertrophy and gastric erosion, but in the same species a positive growth-stimulating effect has also been recorded. Experimental poisoning of gnotobiotic pigs has been associated with diarrhea, erythema of the nose and anus, distension of the abdomen, growth retardation, and, at doses of more than 25 mg/kg BW, coma and death.

SODIUM FLUOROSILICATE

Sodium fluorosilicate is white, odorless, and tasteless powder previously used as a poison in baits for crickets, grasshoppers, and other pests. For the past 30 years it has largely been banned, restricted, or otherwise removed from the market in most countries. The preparation as a bran-based pellet made it attractive to all animal species, and poisoning has been recorded in cattle, sheep, and horses, usually because unused baits were not retrieved after baiting programs ended. In sheep, mild illness occurs after doses of 25 to 50 mg/kg BW and death after 200 mg/kg. Clinical signs include drowsiness, anorexia, constipation, ruminal stasis, teeth grinding, abdominal pain, and diarrhea.

SUPERPHOSPHATE FERTILIZERS

Superphosphate fertilizer is the usual form in which phosphorus-rich fertilizers are applied to the soil and is therefore available to animals in most countries. It is made by a reaction that takes place when rock phosphate is treated by sulfuric acid, and the end product generally contains phosphorus, calcium, sulfur, and fluoride. The fertilizer is also used to prepare "superjuice," which in some countries is administered to cows as a phosphorus supplement.

Higher-than-normal intakes of the fertilizer either by dosing or by pasture application will cause poisoning, largely as a result of the fluoride present.[10] Calcium pyrophosphate, calcium orthophosphate, or calcium sulfate can also contribute to the toxicosis, causing proximal renal tubular nephrosis. It is not highly palatable, but sheep will eat it when it is in "pill" form (small and granular, resembling grain in texture and particle size). Clinical signs of poisoning include anorexia, thirst, diarrhea, weakness, ataxia, and death in about 48 hours. The LD_{50} of superphosphate for sheep is 100 to 300 mg/kg BW.

FURTHER READING

Clark RG, Hunter AC, Steward DJ. Deaths in cattle suggestive of subacute fluorine poisoning following ingestion of superphosphate. *NZ Vet J.* 1976;24:193-197.

Kay K. Polybrominated biphenyls (PBB) environmental contamination in Michigan, 1973-1976. *Environ Res.* 1977;13:74-93.

Noling JW, Becker JO. The challenge of research and extension to define and implement alternatives to methyl bromide. *J Nematol.* 1994;26:573-575.

Pandey CK, Agawal A, Baronia A, et al. Toxicity of ingested formalin and its management. *Hum Exper Toxicol.* 2000;19:360-366.

Tattersfield F, Gimingham C. Notes and correspondence-further experiments with sodium fluosilicate as an insecticide. *Indus Eng Chem.* 1925;17:323.

REFERENCES

1. Yamano Y, et al. *J Occup Health.* 2006;48:129.
2. EPA. 2012 technical fact sheet: polybrominated diphenyl ethers (PBDEs) and polybrominated biphenyls (PBBs). at: <http://www.epa.gov/fedfac/pdf/technical_fact_sheet_pbde_pbb.pdf>; Accessed 24.02.14.
3. Fernandes AR, et al. *Food Addit Contam B.* 2009;2:86.
4. Kierkegaard A, et al. *Environ Sci Technol.* 2009;43:2602.
5. Kierkegaard A, et al. *Environ Sci Technol.* 2007;41:417.
6. Asante KA, et al. *Interdiscipl Stud Environ Chem.* 2010;191.
7. Ounnas F, et al. *Environ Sci Technol.* 2010;44:2682.
8. Grümping R, et al. *Organohalogen Compd.* 2006;68:2147.
9. Lake I, et al. *Chemosphere.* 2013;90:72.
10. Guitart R, et al. *Vet J.* 2010;183:249.

TOXICOSIS FROM SEED DRESSINGS

Many poisoning incidents are caused by livestock gaining access to seed that has been treated in some way. The more common ones are listed here, and each is dealt with under the heading of the toxic agent:

- Grain treated with arsenic used to poison birds
- Grain treated with highly toxic organophosphorus substances used to make baits for market garden pests
- Bran mixed with metaldehyde for use as a snail bait
- Grain to be used as seed that has been treated with a mercury-based fungistatic agent
- Corn treated with 4-aminopyridine for use as a bird repellent

Additional poisonous substances are grain fumigants and other fungistatic agents.

TOXICOSIS FROM MISCELLANEOUS RODENTICIDES

BROMETHALIN

Bromethalin is a highly toxic, single-dose, restricted-use rodenticide registered in the

United States but not several other countries, including New Zealand and Europe.[1] Poisoning in large animals is rare and primarily confined to ingestion of bait stations by young animals or accidental mixing in feed. The onset of action is slow, with signs appearing within 10 hours to a few days. Clinical signs are dose dependent and typically occur 1 to 2 days after ingestion.[1,2] Commonly reported signs in small animals are primarily related to the nervous system and include agitation or depression, hyperesthesia, seizures, coma, paresis, paralysis, and death.[2,3]

Bromethalin is a potent neurotoxin that is rapidly absorbed; widely distributed to the liver, fat, and the brain, where it crosses the blood–brain barrier; metabolized in the liver by N-demethylation; and excreted in the bile; it undergoes enterohepatic recirculation.[3] It acts by uncoupling mitochondrial oxidative phosphorylation in the central nervous system, decreasing the synthesis of ATP and the activity of N/K ATPase.[1,2] The end result is an increase in intracellular Na with loss of osmotic control, fluid within the myelin sheathes, increased pressure on nerve axons, increased cerebrospinal fluid pressure, and impairment of nerve conduction.[1,3] Convulsions, paralysis, and death occur.

There is no antidote, and treatment is symptomatic and supportive. Treatment should include therapy for cerebral edema and seizure control.[3] Judicious use of intravenous fluids is advised so cerebral edema does not become worse.

CHOLECALCIFEROL (VITAMIN D_3)

Cholecalciferol (vitamin D_3) is an active ingredient in several rodenticides used worldwide.[1] It is effective when used alone or added to other baits such as coumatetralyl (an anticoagulant rodenticide).[1] Anecdotally, poisoning has occurred in calves that ingested individual baits or in farm animals secondary to mixing errors in their feed. Toxicity and clinical signs vary widely between species, and there are few data available for large animals. In dogs, clinical signs begin about 12 to 36 hours after a toxic ingestion and include vomiting, weakness, lethargy, melena, cardiac irregularities, seizures, and death.[4]

The mechanism of action is similar to other forms of vitamin D_3 poisoning in which cholecalciferol is first hydroxylated in the liver to 25-hydroxycholecalciferol and then modified in the kidney to form the biologically active 1,25-dihydroxycholecalciferol (calcitriol).[1,4] At toxic doses, calcitriol decreases calcium excretion by the kidneys and excessively increases intestinal calcium and phosphorus from the digestive tract, resulting in calcification of the cardiovascular system (vessels), lungs, kidneys, and stomach lining. Renal failure secondary to mineralization generally occurs simultaneously with the onset of clinical signs.[4]

Treatment is directed toward lowering the serum calcium concentrations, preventing renal compromise, and treating seizures. Intravenous fluids at rates higher than maintenance should be used to increase urine production and promote excretion of calcium. Bisphosphonates are routinely used in small animal medicine to inhibit bone reabsorption and minimize hypercalcemia, but their cost may prohibit use in large animals.[4,5]

RED SQUILL (SEA ONION)

Poisoning by red squill seldom occurs because the material is extremely unpalatable and when eaten is usually vomited. In all species large doses (100 to 500 mg/kg BW) must be administered to produce toxic effects. Young calves are most susceptible, and goats are least susceptible. Experimental poisoning is associated with convulsions, gastritis, and bradycardia.

PHOSPHIDES

Zinc phosphide and, to a much lesser extent, aluminum phosphide are commonly used rodenticides; aluminum, calcium, and magnesium phosphides are used primarily as fumigants to protect grain during storage and transportation.[6,7] In large animals, toxicosis occurs primarily from mixing errors or accidental exposure to treated or stored grain. Poisoning is less likely to occur in ruminants because an acidic stomach pH is important for phosphide hydrolysis. Clinical signs occur in most species within 15 minutes to 4 hours of a toxic ingestion.[6] Vomiting and hematemesis (in those species that can vomit), abdominal distension, and abdominal pain occur first and are rapidly followed by tachycardia, tachypnea, agitation, ataxia, and abnormal neurologic behavior. Sixty-six horses accidentally received aluminum phosphide–contaminated grain; of these, 29 showed full body sweating, tachycardia, tachypnea, pyrexia, muscle tremors, seizures, and recumbency.[7] Hypoglycemia was present in all affected horses. The remaining 37 horses were treated aggressively and remained asymptomatic. Signs occurred 14 hours after ingestion of the contaminated grain; despite treatment, death occurred in 27 horses.[7]

The overall toxicity of phosphides is attributable to the generation of phosphine gas. In the stomach, zinc phosphides (or those of other metals) are hydrolyzed to form phosphine gas and zinc hydroxide.[8] Phosphine gas rapidly enters the blood and is widely distributed to the lungs, liver, kidney, and other organs.[1,6,8] Inhaled phosphine gas crosses the respiratory epithelium. The precise mechanism of toxicity from phosphine gas is unknown but was originally thought to be related to inhibition of cytochrome c oxidase.[6] More recent findings suggest that phosphine has an inhibitory effect on oxidative respiration and forms highly reactive free radicals.[6,7] The overall effect is a combination of local corrosive effects in the gastrointestinal tract and circulatory collapse. Death occurs from pulmonary edema or cardiac arrest.

There is no antidote, and treatment is symptomatic and supportive. Blood glucose concentrations should be monitored and treated appropriately. In asymptomatic cases, gastric lavage followed by activated charcoal or a di-tri-octahedral smectite has been used successfully.[7]

Necropsy lesions present in a horse ingesting zinc phosphide were congestion and hemorrhages in all organs; pulmonary edema; fatty degeneration of the liver; congestion of the lungs, kidney, and spleen; and hyperemia of the gastrointestinal mucosa. Common lesions in those horses dying from aluminum phosphide–contaminated grain included petechial and ecchymotic hemorrhages in the mesentery, epicardium, spleen, kidneys, lungs, skeletal muscle, and other tissues. Vascular congestion was a consistent finding, and pulmonary edema was present in 3/6 horses.[7]

FURTHER READING

Borron SW, Forrester MB, Brutlag AG, et al. Bromethalin (BR) vs. long-acting anticoagulant (LAAC) rodenticides: a 10-year comparison of exposures and toxicity. *Clin Toxicol.* 2013;61:627-628.

Dorman DC. Toxicology of selected pesticides, drugs, and chemicals. Anticoagulant, cholecalciferol, and bromethalin-based rodenticides. *Vet Clin North Am Food A.* 1990;20:339-344.

Drolet R, Laverty S, Braselton WE, et al. Zinc phosphide poisoning in a horse. *Equine Vet J.* 1996;28:161-162.

Harrington DD, Page EH. Acute vitamin D_3 toxicosis in horses: case reports and experimental studies of the comparative toxicity of vitamins D_2 and D_3. *J Am Vet Med Assoc.* 1983;182:1358-1360.

Verbiscar AJ, Anthony J, Banigan F, et al. Scilliroside and other scilla compounds in red squill. *J Ag Food Chem.* 1986;34:973-979.

REFERENCES

1. Eason CT, et al. DOC Research and Development Series 312. 2009 Accessed at: <http://www.doc.govt.nz/Documents/science-and-technical/drds312entire.pdf>; Accessed 12.08.2016.
2. Brutlag AG, et al. *Clin Toxicol.* 2013;51:711.
3. Adams C, et al. Bromethalin. In: Osweiler GD, Hovda LR, Brutlag A, Lee J, eds. *Blackwell's Clinical Companion Small Animal Toxicology.* New York: Wiley-Blackwell; 2011:769.
4. Adams C, et al. Cholecalciferol. In: Osweiler GD, Hovda LR, Brutlag A, Lee J, eds. *Blackwell's Clinical Companion Small Animal Toxicology.* New York: Wiley-Blackwell; 2011:775.
5. Ulutas B, et al. *J Vet Emerg Crit Care.* 2006;16:141.
6. Proudfoot AT. *Clin Toxicol.* 2009;47:89.
7. Easterwood LE, et al. *J Am Vet Med Assoc.* 2010;236:446.
8. Eason C, et al. *NZ J Ecol.* 2012;37.

SULFUR TOXICOSIS

SYNOPSIS

Etiology Ingestion of sulfur-containing materials, generally feed and/or water;

Continued

inhalation of hydrogen sulfide or sulfur dioxide gas.

Epidemiology Sulfur toxicosis is a worldwide problem of ruminants; horses and pigs are rarely affected animals.

Clinical pathology Two distinct syndromes occur (acute and subacute). The acute form has a rapid-onset central nervous system (CNS) signs, and death is common; the subacute form has similar signs, but they develop over weeks, and recovery may occur.

Lesions Polioencephalomalacia in ruminants; osmotic diarrhea in monogastrics.

Diagnostic confirmation The diagnosis is generally made based on postmortem findings and the presence of sulfur in water or feed source. In some cases, hydrogen sulfide concentrations in rumen gas and the presence of sulfhemoglobin in serum may be helpful. Polioencephalomalacia may not be present in acute cases.

Treatment Supportive care, including fluids and electrolytes; thiamine IV or IM.

Control Management of sulfur in feed and water; removal of animals near sulfur dioxide or hydrogen sulfide spills.

ETIOLOGY

Sulfur exists in four different oxidative states: **sulfur (0), sulfide (–2), sulfite (+4), and sulfate (+6)** and all of them are present either naturally (sulfur) or in various biological products (sulfide, sulfite, sulfate). Absorption and metabolism of sulfur-containing compounds depends on the valence state.[1] Ruminants are more susceptible to toxicosis from dietary ingestion of elemental sulfur and sulfate compounds. Water, especially well water high in sulfates; feed products such as sulfate salt, mineral mixes (sulfur containing), protein sources high in sulfur, and dried distiller's grains; and inhaled gases such as eructated hydrogen sulfide gas and sulfur dioxide are all possible sources of sulfur toxicosis.[2-4] Another potential source is the use of elemental sulfur (flowers of sulfur) as an ectoparasiticide[2]

Sulfur and sulfates in the feed and drinking water play a significant role in the etiology of polioencephalomalacia. The feeding of 85 to 450 g per head to cattle has been fatal, as has 45 g of sulfur in feed pellets to ewes, and the minimum lethal dose of a sulfur–protein concentrate for sheep is estimated to be 10 g/kg BW. Continuous feeding of sulfur at the rate of 7 g per day can be fatal to adult sheep. Sulfur given to adult horses at a dose level of 1000 to 1500 mg/kg body weight has been associated with poisoning.

EPIDEMIOLOGY

Occurrence

Sulfur toxicosis occurs worldwide and has been reported in beef and dairy cattle, sheep, goats, and horses.[3,5] It can occur as a single, isolated case or as an outbreak affecting many animals.

Risk Factors

Animal Risk Factors

Ruminants are the species most often affected by sulfur poisoning. Rumen microbes reduce sulfates and elemental sulfur to sulfides, which combine with hydrogen to make hydrogen sulfide.[2,3] Systemic absorption of hydrogen sulfide results in interference with cellular energy production and the onset of clinical signs.[1,2] The brain is most often affected because it has the highest energy demands. Inhaled hydrogen sulfide gas not only causes respiratory paralysis but can be absorbed and result in systemic effects.[1]

Horses, lacking a rumen, do not routinely absorb sulfur or sulfates, and they remain in the gastrointestinal tract and act as osmotic agents, pulling water into the intestinal lumen and causing severe, foul-smelling, black diarrhea.[5] Dehydration is severe, and the animals soon become recumbent and dyspneic, develop convulsions, and die after lapsing into a coma.

Pigs exposed to an environment containing 35 mg/kg of sulfur dioxide for long periods show increased salivation accompanied by clinical and histologic evidence of irritation of the conjunctiva and respiratory mucosa.

Environmental Risk Factors

Animals housed over the slatted floors of a manure pits, exposed to industrial waste pits, or inhaling "sour gas" from crude-oil well explosions are at increased risk for developing respiratory tract irritation and signs of systemic sulfur poisoning.

Transmission

- Ingestion of sulfur- or sulfate-containing products, either accidental or intentional
- Topical use of sulfur powder (flowers of sulfur) to control external parasites
- Inhalation of sulfur dioxide gas used in the preparation of ensilage or associated with industrial waste pits
- Inhalation of hydrogen sulfide gas from ruminant eructation or as a gas emanating from oil and natural gas wells or manure pits.

PATHOGENESIS

In small doses the substance is relatively nontoxic, but excessive doses can be associated with fatal gastroenteritis and dehydration. Conversion of the sulfur to hydrogen sulfide by rumen microbes and the absorption of the gas across the rumen can result in the development of polioencephalomalacia in ruminants.[2,6] Hydrogen sulfide blocks ATP production and energy metabolism at a cellular level. Sulfides are potent oxidants, binding both glutathione peroxidase and superoxide dismutase.[1] The brain is most often affected because of the high energy demands, relative lack of antioxidants, and high lipid concentrations. The amount of hydrogen sulfide produced in the rumen is pH dependent, with more produced as the rumen pH drops.[3] Other metabolism occurs in the rumen, primarily the incorporation of sulfur into amino acids; rumen bacteria can use these amino acids to produce hydrogen sulfide gas. Metabolism occurs in the liver, although much slower for the inhaled gases, and excretion is both renal and biliary.

CLINICAL FINDINGS

Ruminants

Two different clinical syndromes exist:[1,2,6]

1. **Acute:** Signs associated with this include central blindness, head pressing, opisthotonus, recumbency, seizures, coma, and death. Other signs include abdominal pain; severe, foul smelling diarrhea; colic; rumen stasis; and the odor of hydrogen sulfide gas. All species, including horses and pigs, are susceptible to this syndrome, which may be associated with the direct irritant effects of hydrogen sulfide and respiratory paralysis.[2] Clinical signs generally occur in 12 to 48 hours, and death is the normal outcome.[6]
2. **Subacute or chronic**: Signs associated with this form include cortical blindness, bruxism, weakness, ataxia, fine muscle tremors of the head, recumbency, and coma. Most signs are related to the development of polioencephalomalacia (cerebrocortical necrosis) and are associated with hydrogen gas production by ruminants. Often these signs do not occur for several weeks after an exposure, and recovery may be complicated by persistent neurologic deficits.[6]

NECROPSY FINDINGS

The lungs are congested and edematous, the liver is pale, the kidneys are congested and black in color, there is severe gastroenteritis with peritoneal effusion, and petechial hemorrhages occur extensively in all organs and in musculature. Polioencephalomalacia may occur in a high proportion of cases.

DIFFERENTIAL DIAGNOSIS

Water and feed analyses are helpful in making a diagnosis. Elevated hydrogen sulfide concentrations in the rumen and the presence of sulfhemoglobin in the systemic circulation may also be used.

Monogastrics

- Carbohydrate overload
- Gastrointestinal parasites
- Infectious causes of diarrhea (*Salmonella, Clostridium perfringes, Neorickettsia risticii*)
- Nonsteroidal inflammatory toxicosis

- Organophosphorus/carbamate toxicosis
- Osmotic laxatives

Ruminants

- Amprolium administration
- Cyanobacteria (blue-green algae) toxicosis
- Lead toxicosis
- Listeria
- Rabies
- Sodium chloride (salt) poisoning/water deprivation
- Thiamine deficiency
- Thromboembolic meningoencephalitis

TREATMENT

TREATMENT

Thiamine (10 mg/kg slow IV, IM every 12h for 3 days) (R-2)

All sources of sulfur supplementation should be removed from the diet and environment. Treatment is primarily supportive with attention to fluid and electrolyte replacement. Glucose supplementation may be helpful.[2] Other adjunct therapies include a broad-spectrum antibiotic and corticosteroids.[1,2] Thiamine, even though polioencephalomacia is not related to a thiamine deficiency, has been effective in several cases.[1,2]

CONTROL

Management is the most effective way to prevent and control sulfur poisoning. Water sources and all dietary material should be tested to identify sources high in sulfur. Animals living close to oil wells and industrial waste pits should be monitored closely and moved if necessary.

FURTHER READING

Dow C, Lawson GK, Todd JR. Sodium sulfate toxicity in pigs. *Vet Rec*. 1963;75:1052.

Kandylis K. Toxicology of sulfur in ruminants: a review. *J Dairy Sci*. 1987;67:2179.

REFERENCES

1. Ensley S. *Vet Clin North Am Food A*. 2011;27:297.
2. Binta MG, et al. *J Pet Environ Biotechnol*. 2012;3:130.
3. Drewnoski ME, et al. *J Vet Diagn Invest*. 2012;24:702.
4. Felix TL, et al. *J Anim Sci*. 2012;90:2710.
5. Burgess BA, et al. *Can Vet J*. 2010;51:277.
6. Fabiano JF, et al. *Braz J Vet Pathol*. 2010;3:70.

VANADIUM TOXICOSIS

Vanadium is used extensively in industry and high amounts may occur in the air, soil, ash, and soot in areas surrounding smelters, burners, and other processing plants. Experimental and natural poisoning of adult cattle, calves, and sheep are recorded. Signs include anorexia, diarrhea, dehydration, oliguria, difficulty in standing, and incoordination. Postmortem findings include ruminal ulcers, hemorrhage in the gastrointestinal tract and surrounding the heart and kidney, and congestion of the liver and lungs. Field cases are only likely to be encountered when industrial contamination of pasture occurs. Liver is considered the best tissue for assessing chronic vanadium toxicosis in cattle grazing vanadium-contaminated pastures.[1] Careful plowing of the pasture, especially when the vanadium is contained in a fertilizer such as basic slag, reduces the toxic risk.

FURTHER READING

Frank A, Madej A, Galgan V, et al. Vanadium poisoning of cattle with basic slag. Concentrations in tissues from poisoned animals and from a reference, slaughter-house material. *Sci Total Environ*. 1996;181:73-92.

Hansard SL, Ammerman CB, Henry PR, et al. Vanadium metabolism in sheep. I. Comparative and acute toxicity of vanadium compounds in sheep. *J Anim Sci*. 1982;55:344.

McCrindle C, Mokantla E, Duncan N. Peracute vanadium toxicity in cattle grazing near vanadium mine. *J Environ Manage*. 2001;3:580-582.

REFERENCE

1. Gummow B, et al. *J Environ Monitor*. 2006;8:445-455.

TOXICOSIS FROM WOOD PRESERVATIVES

Chromated Copper Arsenate

Chromated copper arsenate (CCA) is composed of chromium trioxide, copper oxide, and arsenic and was at one time the most widely used wood preservative in the United States. In 2003 the U.S. Environmental Protection Agency restricted CCA to industrial use because it poses an unreasonable human health risk. Several industrial uses remain, however, and it can still be used in animal production facilities, on utility poles, and in other cases.[1]

It is recorded that animals would need to eat at least 28 g of the treated wood daily for a month before a chronic poisoning occurred. Horses that crib or chew could eat more than that and could theoretically become poisoned. The risk to animals, however, is not ingested treated wood but ingestion of ashes left from burning treated lumber.[1] Burning concentrates arsenic in the ashes, and cattle, in particular, have been poisoned in this manner.

Pentachlorophenol

Agricultural and residential use of pentachorophenol (PCP; penta) in the United States was prohibited in 1986, but the treated lumber may still be found in older buildings, water and feed troughs, fence posts, and other animal areas. PCP is extremely toxic in humans by inhalation and ingestion and is irritating to the skin, respiratory tract, and mucous membranes.[2] Feeding pigs in PCP-treated wood troughs resulted in salivation and irritation to mucous membranes.[1] Inhalation of PCP by animals in an enclosed area caused death.[1] Acute signs include agitation, pyrexia, tachycardia, tachypnea, muscle tremors, seizures, and death.[1,3] Chronic intoxication causes weight loss, fatty liver, and nephrosis. In high doses, PCP is embryotoxic and fetotoxic.[3]

Horses bedded on shavings from pentachlorophenol-treated wood, prepared wrongly by treating the rough lumber and then dressing it instead of applying the preservative to the dressed lumber, may have been poisoned by dioxin, a common contaminant in the preservative. Clinical signs include depression of appetite; severe weight loss; ventral and limb edema; hair loss; anemia; and a crusty, scaly dermatitis around the eyes, muzzle, axilla, and inguinal region, and on the neck. Exudation through cracks in the skin is a feature of the lesion. Lesions in liver biopsies include necrosis and severe vacuolar changes in the hepatocytes.

Pentachlorophenol is rapidly absorbed from the skin, lungs, and gastrointestinal tract; metabolized in the liver; and excreted primarily in the urine.[2] It acts to uncouple oxidative phosphorylation, increasing oxygen consumption and decreasing ATP production.[1-3] Acute fatal doses range from 27 to 350 mg/kg BW.[1]

There is no treatment other than removal from the source and supportive care. Intravenous fluids at doses higher than maintenance may be useful in promoting excretion.[2] Strict attention must be paid to the potential for milk and meat residues.

Creosote (Coal Tar Creosote)

Creosote is produced as a by-product of high-temperature distillation of coal tar, and it contains hundreds of different compounds, including phenols, cresols, toluene, naphthols, and tar acids and bases.[1,4] Among these, phenol and phenolic compounds are among the most toxic. It is no longer registered in the United States for residential use but is used on utility poles, railroad ties, and other industrial lumbers. There are no human or animal studies clearly demonstrating the toxicokinetics of coal tar creosote.

Large animals are generally exposed to creosote by licking the material from treated lumber such as railroad ties or intentional topical misuse. A high mortality may be encountered in newborn pigs, and there may be a greater than normal incidence of stillbirths when sows are farrowed in treated crates. Weaned pigs may show depression, skin irritation, and, occasionally, death. Creosote applied as a treatment for ringworm has shown marked toxic effects in cattle. Fatal doses for coal tar creosote are 4 to 6 g/kg BW as a single dose or 0.5 g/kg BW daily.

Experimentally, a sheep dosed with 8000 mg/kg BW died in 4 days after dosing and a calf dosed with 4000 mg/kg BW survived but lost weight. There were no specific clinical signs in the sheep before death. At postmortem, excess fluid was present in the pleural cavity, and the urine was dark, with a tarry odor.[4]

Three sheep were dosed with varying amounts of creosote and monitored on a daily basis. A sheep receiving 500 mg/kg BW for 32 days showed no clinical signs; both other sheep, one receiving 1000 mg/kg/BW and the other receiving 2000 mg/kg BW, died at 8 and 16 days, respectively.[4] Clinical signs included rapid weight loss, anorexia, and weakness. Postmortem findings included excess peritoneal fluid, epicardial petechiation, inflammation of the colon and duodenal mucous membranes, and thyroid enlargement. A calf dosed with 500 mg/kg BW for 11 days lost weight, as did a second calf dosed with 1000 mg/kg BW for 11 days.[4] Weight loss in the second calf continued for 3 weeks after the dosing was discontinued.

There is no treatment other than removing the animals from the source, bathing with a degreasing shampoo if applied topically, and providing supportive care.

FURTHER READING

Hanlon G. Creosote poisoning of cattle. *Aust Vet J.* 1938;14:73.

Harrison DL. The toxicity of wood preservatives to stock. *NZ Vet J.* 1959;7:89-98.

Kerkvliet NI, Wagner SL, Schmotzer SL, et al. Dioxin intoxication from chronic exposure of horses to pentachlorophenol-contaminated wood shavings. *J Am Vet Med Assoc.* 1992;201:296-302.

McConnell EE, Moore JA, Gupta BN, et al. The chronic toxicity of technical and analytical pentachlorophenol in cattle. *Toxicol Appl Pharmacol.* 1980;52:468-490.

Radostits O, et al. Wood preservatives. In: *Veterinary Medicine: A Textbook of the Disease of Cattle, Horses, Sheep, Goats and Pigs.* 10th ed. London: W.B. Saunders; 2007:1840.

Thatcher CD, Meldrum JB, Wikse SE, et al. Arsenic toxicosis and suspected chromium toxicosis in a herd of cattle. *J Am Vet Med Assoc.* 1983;187:179-182.

REFERENCES

1. Poppenga RH. *Vet Clin N Am Food A.* 2011;27:73.
2. Pentachlorophenol. at: <http://www.inchem.org/documents/pims/chemical/pim405.htm>; Accessed 18.01.14.
3. Oruc HH. *J Vet Diagn Investig.* 2009;17:349.
4. Creosote. at: <http://www.inchem.org/documents/cicads/cicads/cicad62.htm>; Accessed 18.01.14.

ZINC TOXICOSIS

SYNOPSIS

Etiology Ingestion of excess amounts of zinc from a variety of sources.

Epidemiology Rare occurrence in large animals.

Clinical pathology Elevated serum and tissue levels of zinc.

Clinical findings
Pigs: lameness as a result of degenerative arthritis
Cattle: lethargy and anorexia, diarrhea or constipation, reduced milk yield
Horses: lameness, stiff gait, join effusion

Necropsy lesions
Pigs: degenerative arthritis
Cattle: degenerative lesions in all organs, especially pancreas

Diagnostic confirmation Elevated serum and tissue levels of zinc.

Treatment Find and remove source; supportive care.

Control Rinse galvanized pipes and utensils after each carriage of milk or milk products. Supplement diet with additional calcium.

ETIOLOGY

Zinc is an essential element in most mammals, serving as a component in enzyme systems and structural and regulatory processes in the body. It plays a major role in the regulation of immune function, appetite, and growth.[1] It is found in feed supplements, medicines (zinc oxide), industry (steel and other alloys), wood preservatives, and a variety of other commercial and industrial products. Contamination of soil may lead to an increase in water and plants.[2] Zinc phosphide is a commonly used rodenticide, but it in cases of overdose, poisoning occurs from the generation of phosphine gas and not the amount of zinc ingested.[3]

Toxic doses are not well defined,[4] but drinking water containing 6 to 8 mg/kg of zinc is associated with constipation in cattle, and 200 g of zinc as lactate fed over a period of 2 months as a 0.1% solution is associated with arthritis in pigs. The maximum amount tolerated by pigs is 0.1% zinc (as zinc carbonate) in the diet. Experimental zinc poisoning in sheep and cattle is associated with reduced weight gains and feed efficiency when zinc is fed at the rate of 1 g/kg BW. At 1.5 to 1.7 g/kg BW there is reduced feed consumption in both species and depraved appetite in cattle.

EPIDEMIOLOGY

Occurrence

Zinc poisoning in large animals is a rare occurrence and poorly documented. Case reports, when present, usually indicate the presence of another heavy metal.

Dietary levels of zinc associated with poisoning in different species have been summarized. Pigs develop abnormal articular cartilage at 500 ppm dietary zinc, whereas 2000 ppm zinc in the ration is associated with copper deficiency, anorexia, and subcutaneous hematoma. For horses, approximately 3600 ppm in the diet or 90 mg/kg body weight reduces growth rate. Sheep and cattle generally are adversely affected by 900 ppm zinc in their diet.

Risk Factors

Animal Risk Factors

The accidental oral administration of large doses of zinc oxide may be associated with hypocalcemia and a syndrome comparable to milk fever.

The addition of zinc to pig rations as a preventive against parakeratosis is unlikely to be associated with poisoning because of the unpalatability of rations containing excessive amounts.

Careless use of zinc sulfate as a prophylactic and treatment for the following should be avoided:

- Poisoning by fungi, especially *Pithomyces chartarum*
- Ovine foot rot
- Lupinosis—it is apparent that daily doses of 50 to 100 mg zinc/kg BW in these circumstances can be associated with severe abomasal lesions, pancreatic damage, and death in sheep, provided the material is administered with a drenching gun. The same dose administered by ruminal intubation is nontoxic, because the zinc triggers a closure of the reticular groove, resulting in its immediate deposition in the abomasum.

Farm Risk Factors

Industry-related zinc dust settling on crops and pastures is a hazard; dose rates up to 45 mg/kg BW have no effect on cattle, 50 mg/kg is associated with anemia, and daily dose rates of 110 mg/kg BW are associated with deaths.

An outbreak of poisoning occurred in pigs fed buttermilk from a dairy factory. The buttermilk was piped to the pig pens each day through a long galvanized iron pipe. The buttermilk sat in pools in the pipe after each batch was run through; souring occurred, and the lactic acid produced was associated with the formation of zinc lactate, which was passed to the pigs in the next batch of buttermilk. The concentration of zinc in the milk (0.066%) was slightly higher than the minimum toxic strength (0.05%).

Transmission

Common sources of zinc include:

- Zinc released from galvanized surfaces in the following circumstances:
  - When subjected to electrolysis when galvanized and copper pipes are joined
  - Galvanized bins flake zinc when used for storage of pig swill.
- Zinc chromate used as a paste in joining electrical cables
- Fumes from a nearby galvanizing factory
- Zinc, often associated with cadmium, is a common pollutant from industrial plants handling a variety of ores; nearby pasture may contain more than 500 mg/kg of zinc.
- Zinc-based paints, with a 50% to 55% zinc content when cattle lick freshly painted ironwork

- Zinc added to calf-grower rations as a nonspecific dietary supplement
- Accidental inclusion of zinc oxide in a prepared dairy cow ration

PATHOGENESIS

Ingested zinc is absorbed primarily from the proximal small intestine, and approximately one-third of absorbed zinc is protein bound in the plasma. Phytic acid content of plant proteins interferes with absorption of zinc in monogastric diets. Other nutrients or elements that reduce zinc absorption include calcium, cadmium, and copper. Once absorbed, zinc accumulates rapidly in liver and pancreas, with slower accumulation in muscle and bone. Excretion is primarily in feces contributed from bile and from secretion via intestinal mucosa and bile.

The pathogenesis of zinc poisoning has not been determined, but it is likely that the arthritic lesions observed will be a result of faulty calcium absorption. The lesion in equines may be related to interactions of zinc and copper with interference in collagen metabolism. The development of anemia in some animals is poorly understood, but it may be a result of interactions of zinc, copper, and calcium.

CLINICAL FINDINGS

Acute Poisoning

Cattle

Large doses are associated with light-green-colored diarrhea and drastic reduction in milk yield. Severe cases show additional signs, including somnolence and paresis.

Pigs

Large doses are associated with decreased food intake, arthritis, hemorrhages in the axillae, gastritis, and enteritis. Death may occur within 21 days.

Chronic Poisoning

Dairy Cattle

Dairy cattle show chronic constipation and a fall in milk yield. Other reported signs include inappetence, loss of condition, diarrhea with dehydration or subcutaneous edema, profound weakness, and jaundice.[4]

Pigs

Pigs fed buttermilk containing zinc show anorexia; lethargy; unthriftiness; rough coat; subcutaneous hematomas; stiffness; lameness, progressive weakness with enlargement of the joints, particularly the shoulder joint; and, finally, recumbency.

Horses

Chronic poisoning is associated with a nonspecific, degenerative arthritis, especially at the distal end of the tibia. The lesion is accompanied by an effusion into the joint capsule and the obvious enlargement of the hock joint. There may also be a generalized osteoporosis, lameness, and ill-thrift. Affected foals may be reluctant to rise and have a joint effusion with a stiff gait.

Zinc fed experimentally to foals is associated with pharyngeal and laryngeal paralysis, stiffness, and lameness resulting from swelling of the epiphyses of long bones.

CLINICAL PATHOLOGY

After experimental feeding, elevated levels of zinc are detectable in tissues, especially the liver, pancreas, and kidney, and liver (and serum) levels of copper are reduced. Serum zinc levels in affected cattle may be as high as 500 µg/mL, in contrast with the normal levels of about 140 µg/mL in normal cattle. Estimated as zinc protoporphyrin, the levels in poisoned donkeys and mules reach 900 to 1900 µg/mL. Fecal levels of zinc are likely to be elevated from an average of 220 mg/kg in normal animals to 8740 mg/kg in affected ones.

NECROPSY FINDINGS

Severe, acute poisoning in sheep is associated with an abomasitis and duodenitis, in which the mucosa may appear green in color. In survivors, a severe, fibrosing pancreatitis may develop.

Acute poisoning in cattle has been accompanied by generalized pulmonary emphysema, a pale flabby myocardium, renal hemorrhages, and severe hepatic degeneration. Chronic poisoning in this species may result in lesions in many organs but the **most consistent damage** is in the pancreas. Atrophy of exocrine pancreatic acini with extensive interstitial fibrosis have also been described in piglets receiving a total parenteral nutrition diet.

In chronic zinc poisoning in pigs there is a nonspecific, degenerative arthritis affecting particularly the head of the humerus, with the articular cartilage being separated from the underlying osteoporotic bone. In foals, similar joint lesions and nephrosclerosis may be seen.

The hepatic zinc content in normal animals is high (30 to 150 mg/kg wet matter in calves) and may reach levels of 400 to 600 mg/kg wet matter after continued ingestion of zinc chromate paste without being accompanied by signs of zinc poisoning. In acute poisoning by zinc oxide in cattle, levels of 2000 mg/kg dry matter in the liver and 300 to 700 mg/kg dry matter in the kidney may be achieved; tissue copper levels in these animals may be reduced to 10 to 20 mg/kg. Tissue levels in calves dying of experimental zinc poisoning are much lower: 200 to 400 mg/kg.

Samples for Confirmation of Diagnosis

- **Toxicology**—50 g liver, kidney; 500 g suspect feed or ingesta (ASSAY [Zn])
- **Histology**—formalin-fixed pancreas (light microscopy)

Tissue Assay

The zinc Content of liver in normal animals is high (30 to 150 mg/kg wet matter in calves) and may reach levels of 400 to 600 mg/kg wet matter after continued ingestion of zinc chromate paste without being accompanied by signs of zinc poisoning. In acute poisoning by zinc oxide in cattle, levels of 2000 mg/kg dry matter in the liver and 300 to 700 mg/kg dry matter in the kidney may be achieved; tissue copper levels in these animals may be reduced to 10 to 20 mg/kg. Tissue levels in calves dying of experimental zinc poisoning are much lower at 200 to 400 mg/kg.

Diagnostic confirmation of zinc poisoning depends on identification of elevated levels of zinc in fluids or tissues.

> **DIFFERENTIAL DIAGNOSIS**
>
> **Differential diagnosis list:**
> - Erysipelas
> - Lead toxicosis
> - Naphthalene toxicosis
> - Osteochondrosis/degenerative joint disease
> - Rickets limited in occurrence to young pigs

TREATMENT

Removal of the source and supportive care are the most effective means of treatment. In foals, serum copper concentrations should be evaluated because copper may need to be added to the diet. Chelating agents, especially calcium disodium EDTA, have been used successfully in small animals and human beings.[5]

CONTROL

Galvanized utensils and piping should be rinsed after each use in carrying milk. The addition of extra amounts of calcium to the diet of pigs is capable of preventing the toxic effects of zinc if the calcium supplementation is heavy and the zinc intake is not too high.

FURTHER READING

Abdel-Mageed AB, Oehme FW. A review of the biochemical roles, toxicity and interactions of zinc, copper and iron. *Vet Human Tox.* 1990;32:34-39.

Allen JG, Maters HG, Peet RL, et al. Zinc toxicity in ruminants. *J Comp Path.* 1983;93:363-377.

Radostits O, et al. Zinc poisoning. In: *Veterinary Medicine: A Textbook of the Disease of Cattle, Horses, Sheep, Goats and Pigs.* 10th ed. London: W.B. Saunders; 2007:1826.

Wentink GH, Spierenburg TH, De Graaf G, et al. A case of chronic zinc poisoning in calves fed with zinc-contaminated roughage. *Vet Quart.* 1985;7:153-157.

Willoughby RA, MacDonald E, McSherry BJ, et al. Lead and zinc poisoning and the interaction between Pb and Zn poisoning in the foal. *Can J Comp Med.* 1972;36:348-359.

REFERENCES

1. Herdt TH, et al. *Vet Clin North Am -Food A.* 2011;27:255.
2. Rogowska KA, et al. *Bull Vet Inst Pulawy.* 2009;53:703.

3. Proudfoot AT. *Clin Tox.* 2009;47:89.
4. Reis LSL. *J Med Med Sci.* 2010;1:560-579.
5. Gurnee CM, et al. *J Am Vet Med Assoc.* 2007;230:1174.

DITERPENOID ALKALOID TOXICOSIS

SYNOPSIS

Etiology Toxic plants in *Aconitum* spp. (monkshood), *Delphinium* spp. (larkspur), and *Erythrophleum* spp. (Cooktown ironwood). Toxins include aconitine, MSAL-type alkaloids (methyllycaconitine [MLA], nudicauline [NUD], 14-deacetylnudicauline [DAN], and MDL-type alkaloids (deltaline, 14-O-acetyldictyocarpine [14-OAD]).

Epidemiology *Aconitum* spp. are present in North America and Europe. Toxic *Delphinium* spp. are rangeland plants found throughout the western United States. *Erythrophleum* spp. are trees in northern Australia, Asia, Africa. Poisoning is most often in cattle, but all species may be affected.

Clinical pathology Toxic alkaloids in blood, urine, or ingesta.

Lesions Nonspecific.

Diagnostic confirmation Toxic alkaloids in blood, urine, ingesta, tissues, or plant.

Treatment Physostigmine/neostigmine (*Delphinium* spp.). Supportive care.

Control Avoid all consumption of *Aconitum* spp. or *Erythrophleum* spp. plants. Graze cattle before or after "toxic window" for *Delphinium* spp.

ETIOLOGY

Diterpenoid alkaloids occur in *Delphinium* spp. (larkspur), *Erythrophleum* spp., and *Aconitum* spp. and are associated with poisoning in grazing animals. Diterpenoid alkaloids in toxic larkspur are divided into three different groups: norditerpenoid alkaloids, C-20 diterpenoid alkaloids, and bis-diterpenoid alkaloids.[1,2] Of these, norditerpenoid alkaloids are the most toxic, and they are further divided into two primary groups: MSAL-type norditerpenoid alkaloids (important toxins include methyllycaconitine [MLA], nudicauline [NUD], 14-deacetylnudicauline [DAN]) and MDL-type norditerpenoid alkaloids (important toxins include deltaline, 14-O-acetyldictyocarpine[14-OAD]).[2,3] At least 18 different toxic alkaloids are produced by poisonous species of larkspur.[4] Methyllycaconitine and deltaline are present in many toxic larkspurs. MSAL type alkaloids are approximately 20 times as toxic as the MDL type,[5] but MDL types are more abundant and may potentiate the toxicity of MSAL-type alkaloids.[4] Plants in the *Erythrophleum* spp. contain a number of different toxic alkaloids; among them are diterpene ester alkaloids. Aconitine is the toxin found in monkshood or wolfsbane (*Aconitum napellus*).[6,7]

There are over 100 species of these plants, but a full alkaloid content profile has been completed in only a few. Larkspur is often divided into low, tall, and plains larkspur based on their mature height and geographic distribution. The species known to contain toxic diterpenoid alkaloids and to be associated with disease in livestock are as follows:

- *Aconitum napellus* (monkshood, wolfsbane)
- *Delphinium andersonii* (low; Anderson's larkspur)
- *D. barbeyi* (tall; subalpine larkspur)
- *D. bicolor* (low; little larkspur)
- *D. geyeri* (plains; Geyer's larkspur)
- *D. glaucescens* (tall; smooth larkspur)
- *D. glaucum* (tall; sierra larkspur)
- *D. nuttallianum* (low; twolobe larkspur)
- *D. occidentale* tall; duncecap or subalpine larkspur)
- *Erythrophleum* spp., e.g. *E. chlorostachys* (Cooktown ironwood)

Some of the species assumed to contain the alkaloids because of their known association with the disease are as follows:

- *Delphinium ajacia*
- *D. consolida*
- *D. elatum*
- *D. hybridum*
- *D. nelsonii*
- *D. parryi*
- *D. ramosum*
- *D. robustum*
- *D. tricorne*
- *D. trollifolium*
- *D. virescens*

EPIDEMIOLOGY

Occurrence

North America, especially the western United States, and Europe are the principal locations of *Delphinium* spp. and *Aconitum* spp. poisonings. Rangeland larkspurs (*Delphinium* spp.) are important pasture plants in North America, and many of them are associated with heavy losses (2% to 15%) in grazing livestock.[4] The incidence of poisoning varies widely with season and climate because of variations in the concentration and chemical composition of specific alkaloids in the specific larkspur plants. Plants in the *Erythrophleum* spp. are found in Africa, Asia, and northern Australia and have been associated with death in cattle and horses.[8] *Aconitum* spp. grow in the United States and Europe, but poisoning rarely occurs in large animals.

Risk Factors

Animal Risk Factors

All animal species are susceptible, but most cases are seen in cattle, less often in sheep, and rarely in horses. Sheep are 5 times less susceptible than cattle, and little is reported about horses.[9] The rate of consumption and amount consumed are known risk factors for grazing cattle. The toxicity of tall larkspur is seasonal, being much more toxic early in the season and less so as it matures.[3] A "toxic window" has been established for grazing cattle that begins just before the flowering stage and ends with shattering of the pod.[4] During this time period, grazing cattle are at the highest risk for developing toxicosis.

PATHOGENESIS

The principal action of diterpenoid alkaloids is neuromuscular paralysis secondary to blockade at the postsynaptic neuromuscular junction.[3,4] The toxins are competitive postsynaptic inhibitors of acetylcholine; MLA is a potent competitive blocker at nicotinic acetylcholine receptors (nAChRs) in the striated muscles and autonomic nervous system.[3] Interference with the other parts of the neuromuscular arc is also possible. Signs peak 18 to 24 hours after first ingestion, but the effects may be cumulative.[10,11] The signs in the herd disappear 6 to 7 days after the plant is withdrawn from the diet.[10,11]

Aconitine and other alkaloids present in *Aconitum* spp. are potent neurotoxins and cardiotoxins with actions on cell-membrane voltage-sensitive sodium channels.[7] Nerves, muscles, and myocardium are affected, becoming refractory to excitation. The alkaloids in *Erythrophleum chlorostachys* have a cardiac glycoside-like action.

CLINICAL FINDINGS

Clinical signs in terminally poisoned cattle include tachycardia, muscle weakness, tremors, sternal recumbency leading to lateral recumbency, and death.[3,4] Other signs include constipation, bloating, and dyspnea.[4] Many animals are simply found dead. Those animals ingesting lower amounts may show dyspnea, an irregular heart rate, and collapse, but not death.

Diarrhea is reported in *Aconitum* spp. poisoning, possibly as a result of the presence of additional toxins. In large ingestions, rapid death from paralytic respiratory failure or ventricular arrhythmias may occur.[7] Aspiration of ruminal contents after regurgitation also causes some deaths. In the terminal stages, the pupils are dilated, and the pulse and respiration may be barely perceptible. Some animals are found dead without evidence of clinical signs.

Erythrophleum chlorostachys (ironwood) and *E. guineense* are both poisonous to all animal species. Clinical signs include anorexia, a staring expression, partial blindness, tremor, ataxia, contraction of abdominal muscle, increased heart sounds, mucosal pallor, and terminal dyspnea. Horses poisoned by *E. chlorostachys* have loud and often irregular heart sounds, dyspnea, and sporadic contraction of abdominal muscles, and they die rapidly.

CLINICAL PATHOLOGY

There are no specific findings other than identification of toxic alkaloids in blood, urine, ingesta, and tissues.

NECROPSY FINDINGS

There are no specific postmortem lesions. Aspiration pneumonia may be an incidental finding in some cases.

Diagnostic confirmation of larkspur poisoning depends on chemical identification of the causative alkaloids in the blood, urine, rumen contents, or plants. Normal and reverse-phase high-performance liquid chromatography (HPLC) has been used to successfully identify toxic alkaloids in several *Delphinium* spp.[12] Aconitine has been confirmed in urine and blood using liquid-chromatography tandem mass spectrometry (LC-MS/MS).[13]

DIFFERENTIAL DIAGNOSIS

Differentiation from other plant poisonings causing incoordination, recumbency, and death in cattle on extensive grazing is usually based on botanical identifications.

Differential diagnosis list:
- *Clavibacter toxicus* (tunicaminyluracil poisoning)
- Lead poisoning
- Organophosphorus compounds.
- *Paspalum* spp., infested with *Claviceps paspali* (paspalitrem poisoning)
- *Phalaris* spp. (tyramine poisoning)

TREATMENT

TREATMENT AND CONTROL

Physostigmine (0.04–0.08 mg/kg BW IV, repeat prn) (R-2)

Neostigmine (0.02–0.04 mg/kg BW, IM or IV, repeat prn) (R-2)

Physostigmine and neostigmine have been used as effective antidotes for *Delphinium* spp. poisoning, but they may have limited practical value in a herd situation. Physostigmine, a cholinergic drug, given IV at 0.08 mg/kg BW, has been used successfully in experimental and field conditions;[4] alternate dosages in recumbent cattle include IV, SC, or IP administration at 0.04 to 0.08 mg/kg BW.[14,15] Intravenous neostigmine (0.04 mg/kg BW) has reversed clinical signs in cattle,[14] and IM administration at 0.02 mg/kg BW has used in cattle as a "rescue" drug.[3,4] Neostigmine may be more effective in reversing tachycardia and physostigmine in reversing muscle weakness.[14] The duration of action is less than 2 hours, and repeat doses will need to be administered.

No specific treatment has been identified for *Aconitum* spp. or *Erythrophleum* spp. poisoning. Treatment is supportive, with particular attention paid to the cardiovascular and respiratory systems.

CONTROL

Control of *Delphinium* spp. poisoning is only possible by careful management of pasture and preventing access to heavily infested areas. Prevention of grazing during the "toxic window" decreases toxicity, but the quality of the forage declines substantially.[4] Sheep are more resistant to the poisoning than cattle, but they are fond of the plant and may have to be restricted to areas where it does not occur.[9] Attempts to create and maintain a long-standing aversion to the plants to prevent ingestion of them and allow grazing of infested pastures have not always been successful.[4,16] Herbicides may be effective in reducing heavy growths of larkspur, but application timing is critical to success, and some herbicides may actually make plants more palatable.[4]

FURTHER READING

Griffin WJ, Phippard JH, Culvenor CJ, et al. Alkaloids of the leaves of *Erythrophleum chlorostachys*. *Phytochemistry*. 1971;10:2793-2797.

Knight AP, Pfister JA. Larkspur poisoning in livestock: myths and misconceptions. *Rangelands*. 1997;19:10-13.

McKenzie RA. Dealing with plant poisoning of livestock: the challenge in Queensland. *Aust Vet J*. 1991;68:41-44.

Olsen JD. Tall larkspur poisoning in cattle and sheep. *J Am Vet Med Assoc*. 1978;173:762-765.

Pfister JA, Panter KE, Manner GD, et al. Reversal of tall larkspur (*Delphinium barbeyi*) poisoning in cattle with physostigmine. *Vet Human Toxicol*. 1994;36:511-514.

REFERENCES

1. Green BT, Welch JA, Pfister D, et al. The physiological effects and toxicokinetics of tall larkspur (*Delphinium barbeyi*) alkaloids in cattle. In: Riet-Correa F, Pfister J, Schild AL, Wierenga TL, eds. *Poisoning by Plants, Mycotoxins, and Other Toxins*. CAB International; 2011:557.
2. Green BT, et al. *J Appl Toxicol*. 2011;31:20.
3. Welch KD, Gardner DR, Panter KE, et al. Effect of MDL-type alkaloids on tall larkspur toxicosis. In: Riet-Correa F, Pfister J, Schild AL, Wierenga TL, eds. *Poisoning by Plants, Mycotoxins, and Other Toxins*. CAB International; 2011:540.
4. Green BT, et al. *Rangelands*. 2009;31:22.
5. Welch KD, et al. *J Anim Sci*. 2008;86:2761.
6. Pullela R, et al. *J Forensic Sci*. 2008;53:491.
7. Chan TK, Thomas YK. *Clin Tox*. 2009;47:279.
8. Burcham PC, et al. *Chem Res Toxicol*. 2008;21:967.
9. Pfister JA, et al. *Rangeland Ecolog Manage*. 2010;63:262.
10. Green BT, et al. *Am J Vet Res*. 2012;73:1318.
11. Cook D, et al. *Am J Vet Res*. 2011;72:706.
12. Gardner DR, et al. *Phytochem Analysis*. 2009; 20:104.
13. Colombo ML, et al. *Nat Prod Comm*. 2009;4:1551.
14. Green BT. *Am J Vet Res*. 2009;70:539.
15. Plumb DC. Physostigmine salicylate. In: Plumb DC, ed. *Veterinary Drug Handbook*. 7th ed. Ames, IA: Wiley-Blackwell; 2011:822.
16. Pfister JA, Cheney CD, Gardner DR, et al. Conditioned flavor aversion and location avoidance in hamsters from toxic extract of tall larkspur (*Delphinium barbeyi*). In: Riet-Correa F, Pfister J, Schild AL, Wierenga TL, eds. *Poisoning by Plants, Mycotoxins, and Other Toxins*. CAB International; 2011:637.

ERGOT ALKALOID TOXICOSIS

Ergot alkaloids are mycotoxins produced by fungi found primarily in the *Claviceps* and *Neotyphodium* genus.[1,2] The presence of rich, fertile soil in addition to warm temperatures, elevated humidity, and high rainfall increase the production of ergot alkaloids. Many of the fungi occur naturally in plants and produce similar clinical syndromes, however, their presence in a feedstuff does not necessarily indicate toxicity. Rather, determination of the specific ergot alkaloid should be pursued.

Ergot alkaloids in the genus *Claviceps* produce external spores, infecting the flowers of grasses and cereal grains such as rye, barley, wheat, millet, and oats, and ultimately forming an ergot alkaloid packed sclerotium.[2] The sclerotia in cereal grains are generally large and easily visible; those in grass seeds often quite small and difficult to see. Several fungi in the *Neotyphodium, Balansia,* and *Epichloe* genera found in grasses produce ergot alkaloids.[1] These endophytic fungi do not sporulate and grow within plants in a variety of symbiotic relationships ranging from antagonistic (*Epichloe*) to mutualistic (*Neotyphodium*).[1]

The individual toxins, and the plants they parasitize, are only partially identified. A list of the fungi, the toxins they contain and the syndromes attributed to them is as follows:
- *Claviceps africana*[3,4]—sorghum ergot; contains dihydroergosine (DHES) and related alkaloids; agalactia, hyperthermia, decreased production
- *C. cinerea*—gait incoordination
- *C. cynodontis*[5]—paspalitrem B, ergonovine, ergine; muscle tremors
- *C. cyperi*—ergocryptine; hyperthermia and decreased milk production
- *C. fusiformis*—agalactia
- *C. paspali*[6]—paspalitrem A, paspalitrem B, paspalitrem C, paspalinine; gait incoordination, muscle tremors
- *C. purpurea*[1,2]—ergometrine, ergotamine, ergocornine, ergocristine ergosine, ergocrytpine; peripheral gangrene, hyperthermia and decreased production, reproductive failure, rare nervous signs
- C. sorghi[7]—sorghum ergot
- C. sorghicola[7]—sorghum ergot
- *Balansia epichloe*—gait incoordination, peripheral gangrene
- *Neotyphodium* spp.[1,2]—ergonovine and lysergic acid amide; gait incoordination
- *Neotyphodium (Acremonium) coenophialum*[1,2]—ergopeptine alkaloids, ergovaline, ergotamine; hyperthermia, milk yield drop, peripheral gangrene

ERGOTISM

Alkaloids produced by fungi in the *Claviceps* genus are generally referred to as ergots, and ergotism is loosely defined as the toxicity or physical manifestations that occur when a toxic amount of ergot is ingested.[2] *Claviceps purpurea,* with an ability to infect over 600 plants worldwide,[1] is often used to describe the clinical syndromes associated with ergotism.

> **SYNOPSIS**
>
> **Etiology** Ingestion of large quantities of cereal grains or grasses containing ergots produced by *Claviceps purpurea.*
>
> **Epidemiology** Warmth, high humidity, fertile soil; worldwide distribution in temperate climates.
>
> **Clinical pathology** No specific abnormalities.
>
> **Lesions** Gangrene of the extremities; hyperthermia in cattle; reproductive issues (abortion, poor mammary development, early neonatal deaths in mares and sows), poorly documented nervous syndrome.
>
> **Diagnosis confirmation** Assay for specific ergot alkaloid in feed and/or body tissues.
>
> **Treatment** Remove from source.
>
> **Control** Avoid exposure or dilute feed with nontoxic material.

ETIOLOGY

Claviceps purpurea is a fungus that under natural conditions infects rye and triticale and, less commonly, other cereals and many grasses, including the rye grasses, tall fescue grass, *Phleum pratense* (timothy, cocksfoot, Yorkshire fog), *Cynosurus cristatus* (crested dogstail, tall oat grasses, the brome grasses), *Brachiaria decumbens, Brachiaria humidicola,* and *Pennisetum typhoides* (bulrush millet). Ingestion of large quantities of seed heads infested with the fungal sclerotia is associated with ergotism in cattle, sheep, pigs, horses, dogs, and birds.

There is some evidence that corn smut may have pharmacologic activity similar to that of *C. purpurea. Claviceps cynocontis* infected *Cynodon dactylon* (Bermuda or couch grass, "kweek") may be related to the tremor syndrome that occurs occasionally in cattle grazing this grass.[5]

EPIDEMIOLOGY

Claviceps purpurea is widespread in distribution, but it is seldom ingested in large enough amounts during its toxic stage to be associated with poisoning. Poisoning is most likely to occur during or after a warm, wet season, which favors the growth of the fungus. Ergotism occurs commonly in cattle and usually in stall-fed animals feeding on heavily contaminated grain over a considerable period of time. Other species are not usually exposed to the infected grain.

Ergot-infected pasture may be associated with the clinical syndrome, and the toxicity is preserved through the ensiling process. Cows may show early signs of lameness in as short a period as 10 days after going onto an infected pasture, but most animals do not become affected until 2 to 4 weeks after exposure. Peripheral gangrene occurs in the cooler months; hyperthermia in warmer weather.

PATHOGENESIS

The ergots contain a number of alkaloids and amines with pharmacologic activity, and these vary in concentration with the maturity of the ergot. Clavine alkaloids, lysergic acid and lysergic acid derivatives (e.g., ergometrine or ergonovine), ergopeptine alkaloids (e.g., ergotamine, ergocornine), and lactam ergot alkaloids (e.g., ergocristam) are the four main groups of naturally occurring ergot alkaloids.[1,2] Ergometrine, ergotamine, ergocornine, ergocristine, ergosine, and ergocryptine are the most common alkaloids produced by *Claviceps purpurea.*[1,2] Structurally, the ergot alkaloids are similar to serotonin, dopamine, norepinephrine, and epinephrine, and they are able to bind to biogenic amine receptors and elicit an effect.[1] The pharmacologically active compounds in the group stimulate (constrict) the smooth muscle of arterioles, intestines, and the uterus and decrease serum prolactin. The peptide alkaloids of ergot, particularly ergotamine, are associated with arteriolar spasm and capillary endothelial damage, with restriction of the circulation and gangrene of the extremities, when small amounts are ingested over long periods.

CLINICAL FINDINGS

Four different clinical syndromes have been described. Classical ergotism is characterized by gangrene of the extremities, the hyperthermic syndrome results in elevated body temperatures and decreased production, and the reproductive syndrome presents with agalactia, lack of mammary gland development, low birth weight, and stillborn animals.[1,9] In spite of the known abortifacient action of *Claviceps purpurea,* abortion does not usually occur in poisoned animals. The fourth syndrome is a rare, ill-defined nervous form that may be associated with a single, acute ingestion of large amounts of sclerotia.

Peripheral Gangrene (Classical Ergotism)

The extremities, particularly the lower part of the hindlimbs, tail, and ears, are affected. There is reddening, swelling, coldness, loss of hair or wool, and lack of sensation of the parts initially, followed by the development of a blue–black color and dryness of the skin. Gangrene usually affects all local tissues, and after the lapse of some days, the affected part becomes obviously separated and may eventually slough. The lesions are not painful, but some lameness is evident even in the early stages, and the animal may remain recumbent most of the time. Severe diarrhea is often an accompanying sign. In sheep, gangrene of the limbs does not occur under experimental conditions, but there is ulceration and necrosis on the tongue and mucosa of the pharynx, rumen, abomasum, and small intestine.

The experimental feeding of ergots (1%–2% of ration) is associated with severe reduction in feed intake and growth rate in young pigs without producing overt signs of ergotism.

Hyperthermia Form

Affected cows have temperatures of 41° to 42°C (105–107°F), dyspnea, and hypersalivation. Milk production and growth rate are depressed, and morbidity is about 100%. The syndrome occurs in hot weather conditions when affected animals seek water or shade, but exposure to sunlight under normal conditions of air temperature and humidity can be enough to be associated with clinical signs. Affected animals stressed by exercise in ambient temperatures over 30°C (86°F) commonly die. Long-term, low-level feeding of ergot to fattening beef cattle can result in reduced feed intake and weight gain, increased water intake and urination, failure to shed winter coat, and increased susceptibility to heat stress.

Reproductive Form

The manifestation varies depending on the species. Although rare in cattle, a brief exposure to a heavily ergotized pasture caused abortion in late pregnant cows. It also occurs as a single outbreak of agalactia, lack of mammary gland development, abortions, prolonged gestations, and early foal deaths in mares fed oats containing *Lolium multiflorum* seeds heavily infested with *C. purpurea.* In sheep, the feeding of ergot reduces the chance of fetal survival, and thus relative infertility occurs, and feeding pregnant ewes on ergotized grain is not recommended.

In pigs, ergotism is manifested by lack of udder development and agalactia in sows, and the birth of small pigs that suffer a heavy neonatal mortality. Some of the piglets survive and subsequently suffer gangrene of the ear edges and tail tip. In sows, the chronic feeding of *C. purpurea* may not disturb existing pregnancies, but premature births, mummified fetuses, and low litter size are recorded. Levels up to 0.2% in the diet appear to be safe. A specific ergot, *Claviceps fusiformis,* which grows on *Pennisetum typhoides* (bulrush millet), is known to be associated with agalactia in sows in Zimbabwe. *Claviceps africana,* the ergot of sorghum, has been associated with agalactia in sows and perinatal mortality of piglets in Australia.

CLINICAL PATHOLOGY

There are no specific abnormalities. Samples of fungus-infested material, either animal tissues or feed, may be submitted for assay. High-performance liquid chromatography (HPLC) and liquid chromatography/mass spectrometry (LC/MS) techniques can be used to identify the presence of many ergot alkaloids.[1,2,10]

NECROPSY FINDINGS

In cattle, gangrene of the extremities is the principal gross lesion. There may be evidence of congestion, arteriolar spasm, and capillary endothelial degeneration in the vicinity of the gross lesions and in the central nervous system. Ulceration and necrosis of the oral, pharyngeal, ruminal, and intestinal mucosae are recorded in sheep.

Diagnosis confirmation depends on a positive assay of ergot alkaloids in feed or tissues.

DIFFERENTIAL DIAGNOSIS

Differential diagnosis list:
- Classical ergotism
- Poisoning by *Neotyphodium coenophialum*
- Arterial thrombosis and embolism
- Trauma causing obstruction of circulation to the part
- Bacteremia (e.g., in salmonellosis)
- Hyperthermia/poor production
- Heat stroke
- Water deprivation

TREATMENT

The infected grain should be withdrawn from the ration immediately. Further treatment is not usually attempted, although vasodilator drugs may have some beneficial effect.

CONTROL

Heavily ergotized grain or pasture fields containing ergotized grasses should not be used for animal feeding. They may be grazed if they are first mowed with the mower blade set high to remove the seed heads. Feed should not contain more than 0.1% of ergot-infested heads. It is best not to feed ergot-infested feed to pregnant females.

NEOTYPHODIUM (ACREMONIUM) SPP. TOXICOSIS

Infestation of the grasses *Achnatherum inebrians* (drunken horse grass) in China and *Stipa robusta* (sleepy grass) in North America by endophytes is associated with a syndrome of incoordination in horses and sheep grazing on the grass. Identification of the fungi is not complete but they contain ergonovine and lysergic acid amide. Low levels of paxillene and lolitrem B (indo-terpenoids) are also present.

FESCUE TOXICOSIS

CLINICAL FINDINGS

Four clinical syndromes are associated with ingestion of *Neotyphodium (Acremonium) coenophialum,* an endophyte present in the tissues of the tall fescue grass *Lolium arundinaceum* (formerly *Festuca arundinacea*). The toxic hyphae are invisible without microscopy and produce no fruiting bodies. There is no visible effect on the growth of the grass, and spread of the endophyte is via infected seeds.[1] The fungus produces ergopeptine alkaloids, principally ergovaline, and many other pharmacologically active compounds, including peramine and ergine (lysergic acid amine). There is a great deal of variation in the toxicity of different varieties of the tall fescue grass: KY-31 is most toxic; Kenhy, Mo-96, and Kenmont are intermediate; and Fawn is least toxic.

Several clinical syndromes are associated with ingestion of pasture grass or hay made from infected tall fescue grass. In cattle and sheep, fescue summer toxicosis, fescue foot, and fat necrosis are reported; in mares, reproductive abnormalities occur most often.[1] All of these syndromes could theoretically occur on the same pasture, but summer toxicosis occurs only in the summer and fescue foot in the winter.

In Australia, horses grazing on a pasture seeded with novel Mediterranean (Max P or Max Q) fescue varieties known not produce ergovaline developed a fescue-associated edema syndrome.[11] Clinical signs included depression, inappetence, and dependent subcutaneous edema affecting the head, neck, chest, and abdomen. Analysis of the serum showed a low total protein, in particular a low albumin concentration.[11] Ruminants grazed on the same pasture were unaffected. It was proposed that *N*-acetyl norloline, a pyrrolizidine alkaloid produced by the Max P endophyte, was responsible for the clinical signs.

Fescue Summer Toxicosis (Summer Slump, Epidemic Hyperthermia)

Fescue summer toxicosis has caused significant economic losses in the US, New Zealand, and Australia dairy industries because of the high rate of use of tall fescue as a pasture grass. It is also the most common of the clinical syndromes associated with fescue toxicosis.[1,12]

The syndrome occurs in cattle at pasture in the summer and consists of a period of poor production manifested by a fall in milk production or a failure to grow adequately in fat cattle, both in the presence of what appears to be an optimum amount of nutritious pasture. The same poor weight gain is experienced by steers fed on fescue seed and in sheep. In cattle grazing at pasture the depressing effect on production is made worse by environmental temperatures above 31°C (87°F). Affected cattle show hyperthermia with temperatures as high as 40.5°C (104.5°F), dyspnea, hypersalivation, inappetence, and rough coat, and they may compulsively seek out water or tree shade in which to stand. Hyperthermia may not recede until about 6 weeks after the cattle are moved from the pasture.

The mycotoxin responsible is ergovaline, an ergopeptide similar to, but more powerful than, ergotamine. The lowered milk yield is accompanied by low blood levels of prolactin, resulting in an indifferent prolactin surge when the premilking stimuli are applied. Prolactin levels may be significantly increased by the administration of metoclopramide, a dopamine antagonist, but side effects and cost may preclude use.

Fescue Foot

Fescue foot occurs in cattle grazing pasture dominated by tall fescue, usually within 10 to 14 days of being turned onto the pasture during cold weather. Cattle permanently pastured on the field do not appear to be affected, and horses seem to be able to graze with impunity. The lesions and clinical signs include severe lameness followed in 2 or more weeks by gangrene and sloughing of the extremities, especially the digits and, to a lesser extent, the tail. The incidence in a herd may be as high as 10%. The lesions are associated with the vasoconstrictive agent ergovaline produced by *N. coenophialum.* In freezing temperatures, frostbite may be a complicating factor. New cases may continue to appear for up to 1 week after removal from the affected pasture. Broad-spectrum antibiotics may be useful early in the syndrome to prevent secondary infections.

There is a close similarity to the disease associated with the ingestion of *Claviceps purpurea,* and *Claviceps* ergot alkaloids are also present in fescue; thus identifying the specific cause of gangrene of the extremities may not be possible. Grass heads are commonly infested by *C. purpurea,* but the disease occurs in their absence.

Fat Necrosis (Lipomatosis)

Abdominal fat stores in cattle are affected in the syndrome of fat necrosis. Clinical signs vary depending on the location of fat, but in general fat stores become hardened and necrotic. Dystocia may result if this occurs in the pelvic canal. Necrotic fat in the mesentery may cause an obstruction or bloat. Generally, the presence of fat necrosis is an incidental finding at postmortem.

Reproductive Abnormalities in Mares

Pregnant mares grazing on pastures infected with *Neotyphodium (Acremonium) coenophialum* can experience a much higher incidence of dystocia, prolonged gestation, low foal survival, small udder development, and poor milk yield compared with mares on unaffected pastures.[8] "Fescue" foals may be small and dysmature or large and overly mature. The delivery of an overly mature foal may result in dystocia or the birth of a "red bag" foal. This occurs when a prematurely detached chorioallantois enters the birth canal before the foal.[8] Prolongation of luteal function, an increase in cycles bred per pregnancy rate, and early embryonic death significantly reduce reproductive efficiency. Pregnant mares are most susceptible to toxicity after day 300 of gestation and should be removed from infected pasture before that time.

Domperidone, a D-2 dopamine antagonist, is an FDA-approved drug marketed for the prevention of fescue toxicosis in mares.[8,13] The drug is best used for those mares that cannot be removed from infected pasture. A dosage of 1.1 mg/kg BW/day is recommended, but it should be given no sooner than 15 days before the expected foaling date.[13] If the mare is agalactic after foaling, domperidone may be administered at the same dosage rate for an additional 5 days.[13]

CONTROL

Planting endophyte-resistant varieties of tall fescue, rotating cattle through fescue and other grass and clover varieties, and diluting infected hay with nonfescue varieties are among the most effective means of control. Newer, novel endophyte-infected varieties of fescue should be planted with caution until complete information is available.[11] Ammonization of the affected hay will degrade ergovaline so it is safe to feed, but the procedure is expensive, labor intensive, and time consuming. Cattle on summer pastures with fescue-infected hay should have adequate shade and access to water; those on similar pasture in cooler weather should have shelter or windbreaks. If possible, mares should be removed from fescue-infected hay or pasture before 300 days of gestation; if this is not possible, domperidone should be administered as described previously.

FURTHER READING

Hemken RW, et al. Summer fescue toxicosis in lactating dairy cows and sheep fed experimental strains of ryegrass-tall fescue hybrids. *J Anim Sci.* 1979;49:641-646.

Holliman A, et al. Ergotism in young cattle. *Vet Rec.* 1990;127:388.

Hussein HS, et al. Toxicity, metabolism, and impact of mycotoxins on humans and animals. *Toxicology.* 2001;167:101-134.

Naudé TW, et al. *Claviceps cyperi,* a new cause of severe ergotism in dairy cattle consuming maize silage and teff hay contaminated with ergotised *Cyperus esculentus* (nut sedge) on the Highveld of South Africa. *Onderstepoort J Vet Res.* 2005;72:23-28.

Radostits O, et al. Poisoning by ergot alkaloids. In: *Veterinary Medicine: A Textbook of the Disease of Cattle, Horses, Sheep, Goats and Pigs.* 10th ed. London: W.B. Saunders; 2007:1901.

REFERENCES

1. Strickland JR, et al. *J Anim Sci.* 2011;89:603.
2. Krska R, et al. *Food Addit Contam Part A.* 2008;25:722.
3. Blaney BJ, et al. *Aust J Agri Res.* 2006;57:1023.
4. Blaney BJ, et al. *Aust Vet J.* 2010;88:311.
5. Uhlig S, et al. *J Agri Food Chem.* 2009;57:11112.
6. Cawdell-Smith AJ, et al. *Aust Vet J.* 2010;88:393.
7. Muthusubramanian V, et al. *Mycol Res.* 2006;110:452.
8. Cross DL. Fescue toxicosis. In: McKinnon AO, Squires EL, Vaala WE, Varner DD, eds. *Equine Reproduction.* CABI; 2011:2418.
9. Belser-Ehrlic S, et al. *Toxicol Ind Health.* 2013;29:307.
10. Schumann B, et al. *Mol Nutr Food Res.* 2009;53:931.
11. Bourke CA, et al. *Aust Vet J.* 2009;87:492.
12. Burke NC, et al. *J Anim Sci.* 2007;85:2932.
13. Plumb DC. Domperidone. In: Plumb DC, ed. *Veterinary Drug Handbook.* 7th ed. Ames, IA: Wiley-Blackwell; 2011:351.

FUMONISIN TOXICOSIS

SYNOPSIS

Etiology Corn or corn products contaminated with fumonisins B_1 (FB_1) and B_2 (FB_2).

Epidemiology Sporadic occurrences worldwide in those countries where corn is grown. Equine leukoencephalomalacia (ELEM) and porcine pulmonary edema (PPE) are the two most widely recognized syndromes.

Clinical pathology Nonspecific increases in hepatic enzyme activities; increased serum or tissue concentrations of sphinganine (Sa) and sphingosine (So) and increase in Sa:So ratio.

Lesions ELEM: Fatal neurologic or hepatic syndrome; PPE: pulmonary edema, left-sided heart failure, hepatic syndrome.

Diagnostic confirmation Presence of FB_1 or FB_2 in corn or corn product.

Treatment None.

Control Remove animals from source, test corn or corn product; feed contaminated product to slaughter cattle.

ETIOLOGY

Fumonisins B_1 and B_2 are mycotoxins produced by *Fusarium verticillioides* (synonym *F. moniliforme, Gibberella fujikuroi*) and *F. proliferatum* growing on moldy corn (maize) grain.[1,2,3] More than 25 fumonisins have been isolated and grouped (A, B, C, and P); however, the most important and well studied is fumonisin B_1 (FB_1).[4,5,6] Fumonisins B_2 (FB_2) and B_3 (FB_3) occur in lower concentrations than FB_1 and don't appear to play an important role in the development of toxicity.[4] *Aspergillus niger* and other species of *Fusarium* also produce fumonisins;[4,5] there is some controversy as to whether *Alternaria alternata* f. sp. *lycopersici* produces fumonisins.[5]

EPIDEMIOLOGY

Equine leukoencephalomalacia (ELEM) and porcine pulmonary edema (PPE) are the two most widely recognized syndromes associated with ingestion of FB_1 and FB_2 in corn.[1,2,7] Of the known toxic fumonisins, FB_1 is the most common cause of animal disease and is a known carcinogen in humans (esophagus) and rats (liver).[4,5]

Occurrence

Outbreaks of ELEM and PPE associated with fumonisin-contaminated corn have occurred worldwide.[4,8,9] Historically, there have been reports of poisoning associated with FB_1- and FB_2-contaminated oats and New Zealand forage grass,[3] but the majority of problems occur with contaminated corn and corn products.[1-3]

Risk Factors

Animal Risk Factors

Horses and pigs are much more susceptible to the poisoning than cattle and poultry.[1,7,10] The recommended concentration of fumonisins in animal feed varies depending on the species; both the U.S. FDA and the European Union Commission have published guidelines.[1,7] In the United States, the total fumonisins (FB_1, FB_2, and FB_3) present in maize or maize by-product in formulated feed should not exceed 5 ppm for horses.[1,7] Fumonisins are not excreted in the milk of cows or sows ingesting the toxin, so nursing animals should not be at risk for development of toxicity.[1]

Environmental Risk Factors

The fungus is commonly found growing on moldy corn (maize) grain that has been affected by rain while on the stalk or stored wet. All forms of corn, including pelleted feeds, are susceptible to contamination, and visible mold may not necessarily be present on the corn. Infection by *F. verticillioides* may occur more often when a drought is followed by cool, damp weather during the pollination period.[9]

PATHOGENESIS

The mechanism of action has not been clearly defined but may be related to interruption in sphingolipid metabolism.[1,8] The molecular structure of FB_1 and FB_2 is very close to that of sphinganine and sphingosine, sphingolipids found in lipid substances such as cellular membranes. Both FB_1 and FB_2 inhibit ceramide synthase (sphingosine and sphinganine *N*-acyl-transferase), effectively blocking sphingolipid metabolism and interfering with cellular differentiation, growth, communication, and transformation.[1,9] Serum and tissue concentrations of sphinganine and sphingosine increase and may be used as a biological marker of exposure to fumonisins.[1] An elevation in the serum, tissue, or urine ratio of sphinganine to sphingosine (Sa:So) may have promise as a biomarker.[1,11]

EQUINE TOXICOSIS

Equine Leukoencephalomalacia (Moldy Corn Disease)

The most common clinical entity is equine leukoencephalomalacia (ELEM), a disease of horses, mules, and donkeys associated with the ingestion of fumonisin-contaminated corn.[4,9,12] Of the known fumonisins, FB_1 and FB_2 are the most important, and FB_1 has been shown to be the specific cause of ELEM. Poisoning occurs in stored moldy corn, but it also occurs in horses fed commercial feeds, including pelleted feed; the disease incidence is usually in the form of an outbreak, with some of them being large-scale outbreaks.[4,9,13] Most feeds associated with ELEM contain a minimum of 15 to 22 ppm FB_1, although risk is increased with ingestions of feeds containing 10 ppm FB_1.[4,8,13]

CLINICAL FINDINGS

Classically, the disease is described as either a neurotoxic or hepatotoxic syndrome, although it is likely a single syndrome with the spectrum of signs related more to the actual concentration of fumonisins present in the feed, prior exposure, individual susceptibility, and total amount ingested.[13] Cardiovascular dysfunction may play an important role in the development of ELEM.[1,4]

Clinical signs occur 14 to 21 days after introduction of contaminated feed; occasionally animals present with signs at 7 days and on rare occasions, not for 90 days.[1] Reported early neurologic signs (neurotoxic syndrome) include proprioceptive deficits and decreased tongue tone, followed by a wide variety of other signs.[13] Anorexia, hypersensitivity and agitation, sweating, muscle tremor and weakness, hypermetria, staggering, circling, inability to swallow, lower lip paralysis, protrusion of a flaccid tongue, apparent blindness, circling, head pressing, and dementia have all been reported.[1,8,9,13] Most animals die 4 to 24 hours after the onset of signs, although some horses are found dead without signs having been observed.[1,9] Hepatic signs (hepatotoxic syndrome) are edematous swelling of the lips, nose, supraorbital fossa, and lower limbs. Icterus, mucosal petechiae, and dyspnea are common signs. The time period from the onset of clinical signs to death is 5 to 10 days.[1]

CLINICAL PATHOLOGY

Sphinganine and sphingosine concentrations and Sa:So ratio may be elevated. Serum chemistry analysis in horses with hepatic signs shows elevations in liver enzyme activities, including gamma-glutamyl transferase (GGT) and aspartate aminotransferase (AST).[1,4] Total bilirubin and bile acids may also be elevated. The cerebrospinal fluid in horses with ELEM often shows elevations in protein concentration.[13]

NECROPSY FINDINGS

The classical lesion associated with ELEM is liquefaction necrosis of the white matter. There are macroscopic areas of softening, especially in the cerebrum, accompanied by hemorrhages in the white matter of the cerebral hemisphere and brown to yellow areas of discoloration. Histologically, there are swollen astrocytes or oligodendrites (previously referred to as clasmatodendritic astroglia) containing eosinophilic intracytoplasmic globules and eccentric hyperchromatic nuclei.[8,9] Grossly, the liver is firm and small with an increased lobular pattern. Hepatic periportal fibrosis and hepatocyte vacuolization or necrosis are present on histopathology.[1,9,12]

SWINE TOXICOSIS

The lungs, liver, and heart are the primary target organs for FB_1 and FB_2 toxicosis in swine.[1,4,10] A reduction in cardiac and vascular efficiency is seen with chronic fumonisin intoxication. Alterations in immune function and intestinal colonization by pathogens may be present.[2,14] Fusaric acid, a mycotoxin also produced by *F. moniliforme,* is associated with depression and vomiting in pigs.

PORCINE PULMONARY EDEMA

Ingestion of fumonisin-contaminated corn in levels as low as 16 ppm is associated with the development of fatal pulmonary edema (PPE).[1,4,13] Fumonisin B_1 blocks L-type calcium channels, resulting in left-sided heart failure and pulmonary edema.[1,4] Heart rate, contractility, and cardiac output are decreased, and pulmonary artery wedge pressure is increased.[1]

Clinical Signs

Clinical signs occur 2 to 7 days after ingestion of feeds containing large concentrations of FB_1.[1,4] There is an acute onset of respiratory distress characterized by a rapid respiratory rate, dyspnea, and open-mouth breathing. Decreased feed consumption, weakness, and cyanosis have been reported.[13] Death from pulmonary edema and hydrothorax occurs in a matter of hours following the onset of clinical signs.[1,4]

Necropsy Findings

Grossly, the apical and cardiac lobes are firm and consolidated, with evidence of edema.[15] Alveolar edema, interstitial edema surrounding airways and vessels, and dilated lymphatics are present histologically.[1,13]

Hepatosis/Hepatic Effects

Hepatic toxicity precedes the development of PPE and occurs when ingested amounts are less than those associated with PPE or, less often, in chronic exposures without development of PPE.[1,10] Common clinical signs include anorexia, weight loss, and icterus. More chronic cases of the hepatosis syndrome are accompanied by hyperkeratosis and parakeratosis of the distal esophageal mucosa.[10]

Clinical Pathology

Elevations in liver enzyme activities (GGT, alkaline phosphatase [ALP], and AST) and increases in total bilirubin and bile acids occur as early as a day or so after exposure to fumonisins.[1,2,15] Experimentally, serum total protein and albumin were lower and AST and ALT activity higher in swine chronically fed diets containing more than 10 ppm FB_1.[2]

Necropsy Findings

The liver is large, yellow, and friable. Hepatic fibrosis and nodular hyperplasia are present in chronic cases.[1]

RUMINANT TOXICOSIS

Ruminants are relatively resistant to the fumonisins, likely from minimal rumen absorption.[1] Beef calves fed 148 ppm fumonisins for 31 days developed only anorexia, but serum analysis showed evidence of hepatic damage.[1,16] Dairy cattle seem to be more susceptible compared with beef cattle. Lower milk production and decreased feed intake occurred when fed 100 ppm fumonisins for 7 days before and 70 days after parturition.[10] Lambs receiving high concentrations of fumonisins developed acute hepatic and renal toxicity and died.[1,16]

DIAGNOSIS

The diagnosis depends on the species, clinical signs, and pathologic findings, but must include detection of the specific toxin (FB_1 or FB_2) in the feed. The presence of *Fusarium* spp. in the feed does not confirm a diagnosis. High-performance liquid chromatography (HPLC) and enzyme-linked immunosorbent assay (ELISA) are available in many areas to assay corn and feed products for FB_1 and FB_2.[7] Experimentally, liquid chromatography high-resolution mass spectrometry (LC-HRMS) has been used to identify hydrolyzed fumonisins in corn,[17] and a liquid chromatography-tandem mass spectrometry (LC-MS/MS) method has been developed and validated to identify FB_1 and FB_2 in swine liver.[18]

TREATMENT

The onset of signs is so rapid that no specific treatment, other than supportive, has been effective. All suspect contaminated feed should be removed as soon as possible.

CONTROL

Corn and corn-based products, including pellets, should be tested for the presence of FB_1 and FB_2 and compared with published guidelines for maximum tolerable levels for individual species.[1] Contaminated corn should be disposed of or diluted and fed to feeder cows.

FURTHER READING

Colvin BM, Cooley AJ, Beaver RW. Fumonisin toxicosis in swine; clinical and pathological findings. *J Vet Diagn Invest.* 1992;5:232-241.

Edrington TS, Kamps-Holtzapple CA, Harvey RB, et al. Acute hepatic and renal toxicity in lambs dosed with fumonisin containing culture material. *J Anim Sci.* 1995;73:508-515.

Foreman JH, Constable PD, Waggoner AL, et al. Neurologic abnormalities and cerebrospinal fluid changes in horses administered fumonisin B_1 intravenously. *J Vet Int Med.* 2004;18:223-230.

Radostits O, et al. Fumonisins. In: *Veterinary Medicine: A Textbook of the Disease of Cattle, Horses, Sheep, Goats and Pigs.* 10th ed. London: W.B. Saunders; 2007:1905.

REFERENCES

1. Voss KA, et al. *Anim Feed Sci Tech.* 2007;137:299.
2. Gbore FA, et al. *J Central Eur Agric.* 2009;10:255.
3. Norhasima WM, et al. *Am J Infect Dis.* 2009;5:273.
4. Stockmann-Juvala H, et al. *Hum Exp Toxicol.* 2008;27:799.
5. Frisvad JC, et al. *J Agric Food Chem.* 2007;55:9727.
6. Mansson M, et al. *J Agric Food Chem.* 2010;58:949.
7. Keller KM, et al. *Vet Res Commun.* 2007;31:1037.
8. Giannitti F, et al. *Pesq Vet Bras.* 2011;31:407.
9. Riet-Correa F, et al. *J Vet Diagn Invest.* 2013;25:692.
10. Freitas BV, et al. *J Anim Prod Adv.* 2012;2:174.
11. Kametler L, et al. *Acta Agraria Kaposvariensis.* 2006;10:285.
12. dos Santos CEP, et al. *Acta Scientiae Veterinariae.* 2013;41:1119.
13. Morgavy DP, et al. *Anim Feed Sci Tech.* 2007;137:201.
14. Burel C, et al. *Toxins (Basel).* 2013;5:841.
15. Fodor J, et al. *Food Addit Contam.* 2006;23:492.
16. Mostrom MS, et al. *Vet Clin N Am Food A.* 2011;27:315.
17. De Girolamo A, et al. *J Mass Spectrom.* 2014;49:297.
18. Gazzotti T, et al. *Food Chem.* 2011;125:1379.

Table 21-12 Plants causing glucosinolate poisoning

Goitrogenic effect	
Pasture and forage plants:	
Rape (syn. canola)	*Brassica napus*
Kale, kohlrabi, chou moellier	*Brassica oleracea*
Cabbage, cauliflower, broccoli	
Brussels sprouts, calabrese	
Chinese cabbage	*Brassica chinensis*
Turnip rape, cole	*Brassica campestris*
Swede, rutabaga	*Brassica napobrassica*
Turnip	*Brassica rapa*
Radish	*Raphanus sativus*
Plant by-products:	
Rapeseed oil cake	
Weeds:	
Turnip weed	*Rapistrum rugosum*
Diarrhea, unpalatability, taint effects (caused by mustard oil glucosinolates)	
Culinary plants:	
Horse radish	*Armoracia rusticana*
Cress, mustard greens	*Lepidium, Nasturtium, Tropaeolum* spp.
Wild radish	*Raphanus raphanistrum*
White mustard	*Sinapis alba*
Black mustard	*Sinapis nigra*
Oriental mustard	*Brassica juncea*
Weeds:	
Fanweed	*Thlaspi arvense*
Charlock	*Sinapis arvensis*
Wormseed or treacle mustard	*Erysimum cheiranthoides*

Note: The taxonomy of the Brassica *spp. varies between countries.*

GLUCOSINOLATE TOXICOSIS

SYNOPSIS

Etiology Glucosinolates in *Brassica* spp. and related plants used as feed.

Epidemiology Outbreaks in grazing cattle or in cattle fed crop by-products, especially cake or meal made from residues of seed oil extraction.

Clinical pathology Assay of blood levels of glucosinolate or metabolic end products.

Lesions Nonspecific goiter, enteritis, pulmonary emphysema, and interstitial pneumonia.

Diagnostic confirmation Positive blood assay of glucosinolate.

Treatment Supportive care only.

Control Avoid toxic plants and meals.

ETIOLOGY

Glucosinolates, sometimes referred to as "mustard oil glycosides" or "thioglucosides" are organic substances containing a sulfonated oxime group, combined with glucose in the form of glycosides. More than 120 compounds have been identified and characterized.[1,2] The metabolic by-products include isothiocyanates, nitriles, oxazolidinethiones, and carbinols. These plants also contain thioglucosidase (myrosinase), the enzyme needed to hydrolyze the glucosinolate to glucose and the toxic radical.[1,2]

A special group, mustard oil glucosinolates, occurs in the foliage of some plants and is concentrated in their seeds and the seeds of some others. Plant sources of glucosinolates are mostly from the family Brassicaceae (Cruciferae), as listed in Table 21-12.

EPIDEMIOLOGY

Occurrence

Outbreaks of glucosinolate poisoning are common wherever intensive animal husbandry is practiced, especially where plant wastes from the food industries are fed to livestock in feedlots.

Risk Factors

Animal Risk Factors

Pigs are the most sensitive to glucosinolate poisoning followed by ruminants.[2] There is one equine report of toxicity associated with rapeseed oil.

Human Risk Factors

The toxic substances may be excreted in cows' milk, but the observed goitrogenic effect when the milk is fed may be attributable to the low iodine content of the milk.

Tainting of milk occurs in cows fed plants, more commonly plant seed by-products, containing glucosinolates. The odor and off-flavor are attributable to volatile thiocyanates and not to isothiocyanates. Treatment of the feed with caustic soda prevents the tainting.

Plant Factors

Plants in several uncommon botanical families contain glucosinolates, but animal poisoning is largely limited to the agriculturally important members of the Brassicaceae (Cruciferae) family, all members of which contain these substances. The common fodder plants and commercial vegetables listed in Table 21-12 have all been associated with poisoning. Seed oil crops, such as seed rape and mustard seed, may be fed as roughage after the seed has been harvested and represent a possible source of poison. Large quantities of seed also become available for animal feed, and because of the large quantity fed they may be associated with the enteric form of the disease. Glucosinolates are present in the vegetative parts of these plants but are in much higher concentration in the seeds. The glucosinolate concentration varies widely between species of plants (e.g. *Brassica napus* is much more goitrogenic than *B. campestris*), and even between cultivars of the same species at different times of the year and under different conditions of growth. Including the rapeseed in ensilage does not reduce its goitrogenicity. Plant stress, including drought and overcrowding of plants, and the feeding of high-3.sulfate diets are known to increase the concentration of the toxin, and small young leaves may contain as much as 5 times more glucosinolate than large, mature leaves. The high content of sulfate and glucosinolates in cabbage makes it a damaging feed. The most common and serious cases of poisoning occur in animals fed rapeseed or rapeseed meal. Diets containing as low as 3% of rapeseed meal may be associated with goiter and reduced weight gain in pigs. The meal is often fed in amounts up to 20% of the diet. An extensive plant-breeding program has produced varieties of seed rape that have very low concentrations of glucosinolate.

PATHOGENESIS

Glucosinolate metabolites and the relative proportions of them produced by enzymatic breakdown of the glucosinolates depend largely on the composition of the glucosinolate present, but factors such as pH also have an effect. There are three groups of glucosinolates, each producing a particular metabolite:

- Glucosinolates producing principally isothiocyanates—some of these (e.g., allyl-isothiocyanate, 3-butenyl isothiocyanate) are the irritant components of mustard oils, contained in plant seeds, and are irritant to alimentary tract mucosa causing gastroenteritis, diarrhea, and dysentery. Others, present in the leaves of the plants, are hydrolyzed further to form thiocyanate ion.
- Glucosinolates producing principally thiocyanate ion—which, when taken in small amounts over long periods, is a goitrogen. It is likely to be associated with goiter only when the iodine status of the diet is low. This substance reduces iodine capture by the thyroid gland, and the condition can be alleviated by the administration of iodine.
- Thiones (e.g., 5-vinyloxazolidine-2-thione or goitrin), produced by the hydrolysis of glucosinolates present in the seeds of cruciferous plants, are more potent goitrogens than thiocyanate ion. They interfere with the synthesis of thyroxin, and iodine is ineffective in the treatment of the poisoning. Clinically, the effects of low-level intakes of isothiocyanate and thiones include goiter and a related reduction of the growth rate in the young, and possibly an indirect, depressing effect on reproduction in adults. The reduction in growth rate may be attributable to the observed hypothyroidism, but there is, in addition, a reduction in palatability with diets containing high levels of glucosinolates. This effect is most noticeable in young pigs but may also be evident in high-producing cows.[2]

There is a positive correlation between cruciferous plants (*Brassica* spp.) and polioencephalomalacia in ruminants (e.g., in rape blindness), but the brain lesion is likely associated with the high sulfur content of the plant.[3] Mustard oil glucosinolates are associated with violent diarrhea, sometimes dysentery, and abdominal pain in animals eating large amounts of seeds.[2] No identifiable pathogenesis is advanced as being associated with acute pulmonary emphysema and interstitial pneumonia, or the ill-defined "digestive disturbance" seen in some outbreaks of poisoning with these plants.

CLINICAL FINDINGS

Goiter

Enlargement of the thyroid may occur at any age, including the newborn of dams fed the plants during pregnancy. Deaths as a result of hypothyroidism, after a period of hypothermia, weakness, recumbency, and coma, are more likely in the latter age group. In older animals the accompanying syndrome will be weight loss or failure to gain weight.[2] In serious outbreaks the thyroid is enlarged by 50% in most lambs, with more than 10% showing gross enlargement. Affected flocks have longer-than-usual gestation periods, and lamb mortality is increased threefold because of the poor vigor of the lambs.

Enteritis

Abdominal pain, salivation, vomiting in some cases, diarrhea, dysentery, and a short course with a fatal outcome are common after animals have access to large amounts of reject seeds of these plants.

Acute Pulmonary Emphysema and Interstitial Pneumonia

The condition of acute pulmonary emphysema and interstitial pneumonia has been observed only in cattle. Affected animals show severe dyspnea, with stertorous rapid respiration, mouth breathing, and subcutaneous emphysema. The temperature may or may not be elevated. Affected animals may survive but often remain chronically affected and do poorly.

Polioencephalomalacia (Rape Blindness)

Polioencephalomalacia, characterized by blindness, head pressing, aimless walking, ataxia, and recumbency, occurs in cattle, and rape blindness is manifested by the sudden appearance of blindness in cattle and sheep grazing these crops.[3] The eyes are normal on ophthalmoscopic examination; the pupils show some response to light and may or may not be dilated. Complete recovery usually occurs but may take several weeks.

Other Unrelated Diseases

- Digestive disturbances in steers on rape are usually accompanied by anorexia, the passage of small amounts of feces, absence of ruminal sounds, and the presence of a solid, doughy mass in the rumen. Only a small quantity of sticky, black material is present on rectal examination.
- Photosensitization and bloat are also encountered in cattle grazing rape.

CLINICAL PATHOLOGY

Assays of blood levels of glucosinolates and their metabolic products are available. The diet and the pastoral environment should be examined for the presence of the plants and plant by-products known to contain glucosinolates.

NECROPSY FINDINGS

Goiter, enteritis, pulmonary emphysema, and interstitial pneumonia are nonspecific and dealt with at other points in the text. In *Thlaspi arvense* poisoning there may be massive edema of the forestomach walls.

Diagnostic confirmation is detection of glucosinolates in the blood of animals with access to relevant plants or feedstuffs made from them.

DIFFERENTIAL DIAGNOSIS

Differential diagnosis list:

Goiter:

- Inherited goiter
- Low, continuous intake of cyanogenetic glucosides in, for example, pasture plants such as *Cynodon aethiopicus, C. nlemfuensis* (couch grasses), and *Trifolium repens* (white clover)
- Nutritional deficiency of iodine

Diarrhea with or without dysentery:

- Arsenic poisoning
- Infectious gastroenteritis
- Other poisonous plants in which the toxin has not been identified
- Salmonellosis

TREATMENT

Treatment is symptomatic and supportive.

CONTROL

Avoidance of losses can be best achieved by avoiding the use of the poisonous substance or the grazing of the affected area. Some of the goiters can be relieved by the administration of iodine, and avoidance of high-sulfate diets reduces the level of glucosinolate production. Plant by-products containing glucosinolate derivatives can be treated with alkali solutions to destroy their toxicity.

FURTHER READING

Dixon PM, McGorum B. Oilseed rape and equine respiratory disease. *Vet Rec*. 1990;126:585.

Mason RW, Lucas P. Acute poisoning in cattle after eating old non-viable seed of chou moellier (*Brassica oleracea* convar. *acephala*). *Aust Vet J*. 1983;60:272-273.

Morton JM, Campbell PH. Disease signs reported in south-eastern Australian dairy cattle while grazing Brassica species. *Aust Vet J*. 1997;75:109-113.

Radostits O, et al. Glucosinolate poisoning. In: *Veterinary Medicine: A Textbook of the Disease of Cattle, Horses, Sheep, Goats and Pigs*. 10th ed. London: W.B. Saunders; 2007:1866.

Taljaard T. Cabbage poisoning in ruminants. *J South Afr Vet Med*. 1993;64:96-100.

REFERENCES

1. Halkier BA. *Ann Rev Plant Biol*. 2006;57:303.
2. European Food Safety Authority. *EFSA J*. 2008;590:1.
3. McKenzie RA, et al. *Aust Vet J*. 2009;87:27.

MISCELLANEOUS MYCOTOXINS

CYCLOPIAZONIC ACID

Cyclopiazonic acid (CPA), an indole-tetramic acid, is a secondary metabolite produced by several genera of *Aspergillus* and *Penicillium* growing on stored grain, including sunflower seeds.[1] It has been found in human and animal foods and food sources, including milk, eggs, and poultry.[1,2]

Toxicity associated with CPA is considered low, based on an LD_{50} in rats of 30 to 70 mg/kg BW, and reports of animal poisonings are rare.[1] Ingestion of CPA-contaminated feed in sows is associated with feed refusal and conception problems in sows. Isolated from *A. flavus*, cyclopiazonic acid is associated with weakness, anorexia, loss of body weight, and diarrhea in pigs. Necropsy lesions include gastric ulceration and hemorrhages throughout the alimentary tract.

PATULIN

Patulin, an important toxin in human medicine, is produced by *Aspergillus clavatus* and other fungi, including *Byssochlamys nivea*, *Penicillium urticae*, *P. claviforme*, and *P. patulum*.[3,4] Toxicity is most commonly associated with rotting apples or apple juice, and poisoning may occur in pigs fed food waste containing rotten fruit.[3]

Cattle and sheep poisoned by patulin producing fungi develop brain hemorrhage, pulmonary edema, or liver and kidney damage with abomasal hemorrhage. When fed to piglets, it is associated with vomiting, salivation, anorexia, polypnea, weight loss, leukocytosis, and anemia. Patulin may be the toxin associated with neurologic problems in cattle ingesting malting by-products and sprouted grains.[4,6] Affected cattle develop neuromuscular signs, including salivation, ataxia, hind limb weakness, muscle tremors, recumbency, and death.[4-6]

STERIGMATOCYSTIN

Sterigmatocystin (STC) is a hepatotoxin and potential carcinogen in humans.[7] Carcinogenesis in farm animals is not reported. It has been isolated from *Aspergillus* spp., *Bipolaris* spp., *Penicillium luteum*, and other species of fungi.[7,8] It is a precursor of aflatoxin synthesis.[7] Contaminated foods include grains, soybeans, nuts, animal feeds, and silage.[8]

FURTHER READING

Lomax LG, Cole RJ, Dorner JW. The toxicity of cyclopiazonic acid in weaned pigs. *Vet Path*. 1984;21:418-424.

Sabater-Vilar M, Maas RF, De Bosschere H, et al. Patulin produced by an *Aspergillus clavatus* isolated from feed containing malting residues associated with a lethal neurotoxicosis in cattle. *Mycopathologia*. 2004;158:419-426.

REFERENCES

1. Chang PK, et al. *Toxins (Basel)*. 2009;1:74.
2. Oliveira CA, et al. *Food Addit Contam*. 2006;23:196.
3. Rosinska DM, et al. *J Liq Chromatogr R T*. 2009;32:500.
4. Riet-Correa F, et al. *J Vet Diagn Invest*. 2013;25:692.
5. Stec J, et al. *Bull Vet Inst Pulawy*. 2009;53:129.
6. Mostrom M, et al. *Vet Clin N Am Food A*. 2011;27:315.
7. Anninou N, et al. *Int J Environ Res Public Health*. 2014;11:1855.
8. Veršilovskis A, et al. *Mol Nutr Food Res*. 2010;54:136.

MUSHROOM TOXICOSIS

Reports of poisoning associated with mushrooms in large animals are rare. Grazing animals may have access to poisonous mushrooms and develop clinical signs, but a specific mushroom is rarely identified, and diagnostic tests are often limited.

AMATOXINS

Mushrooms in the genera *Amanita*, *Galerina*, and *Lepiota* contain amanitins (cyclopeptides) that are toxic to the gastrointestinal tract, kidney, and liver.[1] *Amanita phalloides* (dead cap) and *Amanita ocreata* (Western North American destroying angel), both found in the coastal western and southwestern United States and parts of Mexico, have been associated with poisonings in calves,[1] cattle,[2] dogs,[3] and human beings[4-5] and perhaps horses.[1,4] As a group, amatoxins include several amantins, amanin, amanullin, and proamanullin, but amanitins are the most commonly reported toxins. *A. phalloides* and *A. ocreata* contain high concentrations of α-amanitin and β-amanitin.[1] Ingestions of small amounts have resulted in poisoning in humans and dogs; the toxic amount in large animals is unknown.

In monogastric animals, amanitins are absorbed in the gastrointestinal tract and transported to the liver, where they are taken up by OATP1B3, an organic acid hepatic transporter.[5] Protein binding does not occur. Metabolism has not been recorded, and 80% to 90% of an ingested dose is eliminated in the urine and 7% in the bile.[1] Bioavailability, serum half-life, and plasma detection time vary with the species.[1,2] Similar information is not available for ruminants.

Clinical signs occur from inhibition of nuclear RNA polymerase II, which causes a decrease in messenger RNA and ultimately protein synthesis.[1,2] Hepatocytes, crypts cells, and those in the proximal convoluted tubules of the kidney are most commonly affected. Other cellular effects are at work as well.[1,2] The earliest signs identified in animals are gastrointestinal and include severe pain, vomiting, and bloody diarrhea.[2] These are followed by a latent period of hours to a few days and a final stage with acute necrotizing hepatic failure and renal failure.[1,2] Coagulation defects, hypoglycemia, elevations in liver enzymes, and encephalopathy may occur.

Several different modalities, including a liver transplant in humans, are used to treat toxicosis in humans and dogs, but large animals are generally found dead or die before treatment can be provided.

Postmortem examination shows a friable liver with diffuse centrilobular to panlobular necrosis.[1] Other organs, such as the kidney, and the gastrointestinal tract are also affected. Liquid chromatography/mass spectrometry is available in some laboratories to analyze serum, urine, liver, kidney, and gastric contents, including rumen, for amanitins.[6]

RAMARIA FLAVO-BRUNNESCENS

The *Ramaria flavo-brunnescens* mushroom is found only in the eucalyptus woods of North America, Australia, China, Brazil, and Uruguay.[7-9] The toxin is unknown, but toxicity may be related to interference with sulfur-containing amino acids (cysteine) in keratinized structures.[9]

Clinical signs of "eucalyptus poisoning" have been recorded in sheep and cattle. Jersey calves experimentally poisoned with 20 mg/kg BW *R. flavo-brunnescens* mushrooms developed anorexia, hyperemia of the oral mucosa, and loosening of hair shafts at the tip of the tail.[8] Other recorded signs include salivation; lingual and esophageal ulcers; loss of hair, especially of the tail brush; recumbency; and pain in, and loss of, hooves.

SCLERODERMA CITRINUM

Scleroderma citrinum (common earth ball) fed to a miniature Chinese pot-bellied pig has been associated with vomiting, depression, recumbency, and death.[4] The pupillary light reflex was lost, but the eye preservation reflex remained. Pain on abdominal palpation, hyperthermia, tachycardia, and mucoid feces passed with some straining were present; death occurred in about 5 hours. The toxin has not yet been identified.

CORTINARIUS SPECIOCISSIMUS

Cortinarius speciocissimus has been associated with deaths in sheep in Norway with renal tubular necrosis and terminal uremia.

INOCYBE AND CLITOCYBE SPP.

Muscarine, a mycotoxic alkaloid found in the macrofungi, is associated with excessive salivation, bradycardia, diarrhea, and vomiting. Atropine is an effective antidote.

FURTHER READING

Galey FD, et al. A case of *Scleroderma citrinum* poisoning in a miniature Chinese pot-bellied pig. *Vet Hum Toxicol.* 1990;32:329-330.

Kommers GD, Santos MN. Experimental poisoning of cattle by the mushroom *Ramaria flavo-brunnescens* (Clavariaceae): a study of the morphology and pathogenesis of lesions in hooves, tail, horns and tongue. *Vet Hum Toxicol.* 1995;37:297-302.

Radostits O, et al. Miscellaneous fungi. In: *Veterinary Medicine: A Textbook of the Disease of Cattle, Horses, Sheep, Goats and Pigs.* 10th ed. London: W.B. Saunders; 2007:1912.

REFERENCES

1. Yee MM, et al. *J Vet Diagn Invest.* 2012;24:241.
2. Varga A, et al. *Vet Med Res Rep.* 2012;3:111.
3. Puschner B, et al. *J Vet Diagn Invest.* 2007;19:312.
4. Beug MW, et al. *McIlvainea.* 2006;16:47.
5. Letschert K, et al. *Toxicol Sci.* 2006;91:140.
6. Filigenzi MS, et al. *J Agric Food Chem.* 2007;55:2784.
7. Riss DR, et al. *Pesqui Vet Bras.* 2007;27:261.
8. Schons SV, et al. *Pesqui Vet Bras.* 2007;27:269.
9. Trost ME, et al. *Pesqui Vet Bras.* 2009;29:533.

PHALARIS SPP. (CANARY GRASS) TOXICOSIS

SYNOPSIS

Etiology Associated with the ingestion of the *Phalaris* spp. grasses containing dimethyltryptamine (causing an incoordination syndrome) or unknown substances (causing a sudden death/cardiac syndrome and a sudden death/polioencephalomalacia–like syndrome).

Epidemiology Outbreaks on lush, rapidly growing pasture; sheep most commonly affected.

Clinical pathology Isolation of tryptamines in plants and affected animals.

Lesions Green–gray discoloration of renal medulla, medulla oblongata, brainstem.

Diagnostic confirmation By detection of tryptamines in body fluids or cadaver.

Treatment None.

Control Limitation of access to causative plants.

ETIOLOGY

Dimethyltryptamines associated with incoordination syndrome include the following:

- *Phalaris aquatica* (synonym *P. tuberosa*)
- *P. angusta,* timothy canary grass
- *P. arundinacea,* reed canary grass
- *P. caroliniana,* Maygrass, Southern canary grass
- *P. brachystachys*
- *P. canariensis,* annual canary grass, commercial canary grass
- *P. minor,* littleseed canary grass, wild canary grass
- *P. paradoxa,* hooded canary grass

The cause of acute death from cardiac arrest, originally ascribed to the methylated tryptamines, is unknown, but may be related phenylethylamines, other alkaloids (indoles/oxindoles), or other factors.[1] The cause of death associated with polioencephalomalacia, once thought to be a related to thiamine analogs produced by the ruminal flora, is also unknown.[1]

EPIDEMIOLOGY

Occurrence

The disease has been recorded in many parts of Australia, New Zealand, South Africa, Spain, California, and South America where the phalaris grasses are in common use as pasture plants.[1-3] Heavy losses occur on individual farms as a result of sudden deaths, but careful management relieves the burden of the incoordination syndrome.

The individual tryptamine alkaloids associated with the disease vary significantly in their toxicity, and thus plants in a pasture can vary greatly in the danger they present. The concentration of tryptamines in the grass is increased by high environmental temperature and their growing in the shade, and toxicity is greatest when the plants are young and growing rapidly, especially after a break in a dry season. Provision of cobalt appears to stimulate the proliferation of microorganisms in the rumen that are capable of destroying the causative agent, but sheep affected with phalaris staggers do not usually show any signs of cobalt deficiency. Under some circumstances, plants with low tryptamine content will be associated with the syndrome.

Risk Factors

Animal Factors

Sheep, followed by cattle, are most commonly affected, although alpacas have developed the incoordination syndrome and horses the sudden death/cardiac syndrome.[1,4,5]

Up to 30% of a flock may be affected when *P. aquatica* dominates the pasture or is preferentially grazed. On lightly stocked pastures the sudden death syndrome, with signs appearing within 4 hours but usually between 12 and 72 hours after going onto the pasture, is most likely to occur. Deaths are most common in hungry sheep in the early morning or in foggy or cloudy weather. This syndrome is also recorded in cattle on irrigated *Phalaris* spp. pasture in hot, humid weather.

The incoordination syndrome occurs in similar circumstances but in sheep that have protracted or repeated exposure. In this case clinical signs appear 2 to 3 weeks after sheep are put onto pasture showing new growth, usually in the autumn or early winter. Both forms may occur in a single flock of sheep and also in feedlots. Sheep of all ages are affected, and mild cases may occur among cattle.

The variability in the numbers affected and the severity of the disability in sheep flocks from day to day appear to be attributable to the variation in the amount of toxin absorbed, possibly affected by the degree of detoxification of the tryptamines in the rumen. The reduction in severity of an outbreak associated with dietary supplementation with cobalt is thought to be effected in this way.

PATHOGENESIS

Tryptamine alkaloids, structurally similar to serotonin, are present in the grass under certain conditions and are associated with the incoordination syndrome by a direct agonist action on serotonergic receptors in specific brain and spinal cord nuclei.[1,4] Clinical signs mimic those of the serotonin syndrome and include repetitive head movements tremors, rigidity, and hyperreactivity, The nervous disturbance appears to be functional in contrast to that associated with β-carbolines, which is accompanied by axonal degeneration and is an irreversible syndrome.

A characteristic of the disease is a greenish-gray discoloration of the brainstem, diencephalon, dorsal root ganglia, and kidneys.[4] The pigmentation is a result of the accumulation of indole-like pigments at the locations where the causative alkaloids act, but the pigments themselves do not have any effect on the signs.

CLINICAL FINDINGS

The sudden cardiac death syndrome, the most rare of the three syndromes, is manifested by sudden collapse, especially when excited, a short period of respiratory distress with cyanosis, and then death or rapid recovery.[1] During the stage of collapse there is arrhythmic tachycardia followed by ventricular fibrillation and cardiac arrest. Consciousness is retained.

The sudden death polioencephalomalacia syndrome cases are rarely observed alive, but occur commonly after short periods of feed deprivation. This occurs most often in sheep, although cattle have been affected as well.

In the initial stages of the incoordination syndrome in sheep, signs appear only when the animals are disturbed. Hyperexcitability and generalized muscle tremor, including nodding and bobbing of the head, occur first. On moving, the limb movements are stiff, and the hocks are not bent, causing dragging of the hindfeet. Incoordination and swaying of the hindquarters follow. Some animals walk on their knees, others bound or hop, and others knuckle at the fetlocks; some show splaying of the digits. In the most severe cases collapse into lateral recumbency is accompanied by paddling movements of the legs and irregular involuntary movements of the eyeballs. There is rapid respiration and irregular tachycardia. The sheep may die at this stage, but if left undisturbed they may recover and walk away apparently unaffected. If the sheep are left on the pasture, the condition worsens in individual cases, with the animal becoming recumbent and manifesting repeated convulsive episodes until death supervenes.

There is a great deal of variation from day to day in the number of sheep showing signs and in the severity of the signs observed. Even after sheep are removed from the pasture the clinical state may deteriorate, and although some appear to recover, clinical signs can usually be elicited by forcing them to exercise. Deaths are reported to continue for 1 week after removal of sheep from toxic pasture, and clinical signs of the nervous form of the disease may persist for as long as 2 months. The extraordinary situation is recorded where new cases continue to occur for as long as 12 weeks after sheep are moved onto pasture that contains no *Phalaris* spp.

In cattle, the signs may be restricted to stiffness of the hocks and dragging of the hind toes, but severe cases similar to the common syndrome in sheep also occur.[3,4] Additional, and more common, signs observed in some, but not all, cattle include an extraordinary incoordination of the tongue and lips in prehension; thus, the hungry animal, trying desperately to eat, can only prehend a few stalks of grass at a time.[4] The jaw movements are quite strong, but the tongue stabs and darts, and it lacks the sinuous curling movements normally present. There may also be an inability to put the muzzle to the ground, and thus prehension can only occur from a raised manger or hayrack. Affected cattle are often hyperexcitable and difficult to handle.

CLINICAL PATHOLOGY

Laboratory tests on antemortem material can detect the presence of the causative tryptamines in plant material but are unlikely to be generally available.

NECROPSY FINDINGS

Other than the characteristic green–gray pigmentation of tissues in the renal medulla, brainstem, midbrain, and dorsal root ganglia, gross lesions are absent. Degeneration of spinal cord tracts and of the ventral portion of the cerebellum has been observed in terminal cases of the incoordination syndrome, but is not a consistent finding. In the sudden death or cardiac syndrome sheep are usually found dead on their sides with their heads strongly dorsiflexed and legs rigidly extended. Some sheep have blood-stained nasal discharge, and many froth at the mouth. Abdominal visceral congestion and epicardial and duodenal hemorrhages are present and indicate acute heart failure. Polioencephalomalacia is characteristic of the sudden death -polioencephalomalacia syndrome.

The association between the nervous disease and the plants should suggest the diagnosis. The appearance of these signs only on exercise is significant, suggesting a functional rather than a physical lesion. Diagnostic confirmation rests on the identification of the causative tryptamines in the feed materials and the tissues and fluids on antemortem or postmortem examination.

TREATMENT

Flocks of affected sheep should be removed immediately from the pasture. There is no specific antidotal treatment.

CONTROL

No preventive measures are available against the sudden death syndrome, but the nervous form may be prevented by the oral administration of cobalt.[1,4] Affected pastures may be grazed if sheep are dosed with cobalt (at least 28 mg per week) at intervals of not more than 1 week, or if alternative grazing is provided in rotation. Dosing at too long intervals or with inadequate amounts may account for some failures in prevention. The parenteral administration of cobalt or vitamin B_{12} is not effective. The additional cobalt can be provided by drenching the sheep individually or spreading it on the pasture mixed with fertilizer as described under cobalt deficiency. Unfortunately, the genetic selection of *P. aquatica* cultivars with low contents of methylated tryptamines favors a significant increase in toxic β-carbolines.

FURTHER READING

Bourke CA, Carrigan MJ, Dixon RJ. The pathogenesis of the nervous syndrome of *Phalaris aquatica* toxicity in sheep. *Aust Vet J*. 1990;67:356-358.

Colegate SM, Anderton N, Edgar J, et al. Suspected blue canary grass (*Phalaris coerulescens*) poisoning of horses. *Aust Vet J*. 1999;77:538-547.

Nicholson SS, Olcott BM, Usenik EA, et al. Delayed *phalaris* grass toxicosis in sheep and cattle. *J Am Vet Med Assoc*. 1989;195:345-346.

REFERENCES

1. Burrows GE, Tyrl RJ. *Phalaris L. Toxic Plants of North America*. 2nd ed. Wiley-Blackwell; 2013:935.
2. Finnie JW. *Aust Vet J*. 2011;89:247.
3. Cantón G, et al. *Pesq Vet Bras*. 2010;30:63.
4. Binder EM, et al. *J Vet Diagn Invest*. 2010;22:802.
5. Sampaio N, et al. *Anim Prod Sci*. 2008;48:1099.

TOXICOSIS FROM PLANT PHENOLS (GOSSYPOL AND TANNINS)

Two important groups of plant polyphenols (hydroxyl derivatives of benzene) are **gossypol** and the **tannins**.

GOSSYPOL

ETIOLOGY

Gossypol is found primarily in oil glands (gossypol glands) of the seed but also in some other portions of the plant. It is present in variable amounts in cottonseed cake made from the seeds of *Gossypium* spp. and hybrids (commercial cotton) and in the seeds and their hulls, and poisoning occurs primarily from ingestion of seed meal or other seed products. Seed meal usually contains 300 to 400 ppm but may contain as much as 18,000 ppm of free gossypol in a 17% protein ration.

EPIDEMIOLOGY

Swine and preruminant animals are more susceptible to poisoning than mature ruminants. Levels of 200 to 300 ppm are toxic to swine, and preruminant calves' diets containing 100 to 200 mg/kg BW resulted in gossypol mortality. Horses appear to be resistant to gossypol toxicity, with no natural cases being on record.[1]

Most recorded outbreaks of gossypol poisoning refer to pigs. Cottonseed cake should not be fed to pigs at all, especially young pigs. Adults may tolerate up to 60 ppm gossypol in the feed, although other sources suggest 100 ppm may be safe.[1]

Animals with a functioning rumen are able to tolerate higher levels of free gossypol than preruminant animals. Goats are more susceptible than others, with daily intakes of 350 to 400 mg gossypol being fatal after 3 months. Calves die of heart failure if fed 800 to 1000 g cottonseed meal/day. Illness and mortality have also been produced by feeding gossypol to adult dairy cows. Adverse effects on spermatogenesis with an increase in sperm morphologic abnormalities occurs in bulls on low intakes and without clinical signs. Sheep are susceptible if the toxin is injected but appear to be unaffected when it is fed. In rams, feeding free gossypol in concentrations greater than 9 mg/kg BW resulted in reproductive toxicity.[2]

PATHOGENESIS

Cottonseed oil is extracted at high temperatures, and during this process gossypol is released from the oil glands. Some binds to proteins and is considered nontoxic; the remainder is referred to as "free gossypol" and is the toxic form. In swine, free gossypol is absorbed from the gastrointestinal tract, conjugated in the liver, and excreted in the feces.[1] Little is excreted in the urine or milk. The mechanism of action is that of a reactive species, forming free radicals and damaging various tissues, especially the heart.[1,2] Other mechanisms are likely at work as well. Myocardial necrosis with congestive heart failure and hepatic changes are commonly associated with ingestion of toxic amounts of gossypol.[1]

CLINICAL FINDINGS

Clinical signs are abrupt but don't usually appear until animals have been fed on rations containing cottonseed meal for 1 to 2 months. Pigs poisoned by gossypol are thin, are exercise intolerant, cough, and are severely dyspneic, with a "thumping" type of respiration.

Death from cardiac insufficiency occurs in a few days, often preceded by cyanosis and seizures. Feeding cottonseed meal to pregnant sows at the rate of 20% to 40% of the ration is associated with shortening of the gestation length, and in some cases 40% of piglets are born prematurely and die. Poisoned calves show anorexia, dyspnea, cough, brisket edema, ascites, distension of the jugular vein, and weakness; hematuria occurs occasionally, and death follows an illness of several days. Sublethal rates of ingestion are associated with stunting of growth and reduction of fertility in bulls. Feeding cottonseed meal to young bulls and rams is not recommended because of the risk of permanent damage to spermatogenic tissues, but the risk is considered to be negligible.

CLINICAL PATHOLOGY

There are no specific clinical pathology tests that are specific for gossypol. In later stages, hepatic enzyme activities may be elevated; Thoracic radiographs may demonstrate the presence of fluid, which can be examined for protein content after collection via thoracocentesis.

NECROPSY FINDINGS

There is generalized edema, including high-protein fluid in all the serous cavities, and hepatomegaly as a result of congestive heart failure, and histologically there is degeneration of the myocardium and skeletal musculature. Centrilobular necrosis in the liver is also a characteristic lesion, and the liver will contain as much as 42 μg/g gossypol.

CONTROL

Cottonseed cake may be fed with safety to adult cattle if the daily intake of meal is less than 2.5 to 3 kg/head per day, and it may be fed to pigs if it constitutes less than 9% of the ration.[1] Cooking of the cake or the addition of 1% calcium hydroxide or 0.1% ferrous sulfate to it are efficient methods of detoxification. In experimental trials the addition of iron in equal proportions to gossypol up to 600 mg/kg of the ration will protect pigs. Significant quantities of cations (particularly calcium and iron) in water supplies or rations appear to be protective. Providing calcium carbonate at a rate of 12 g/kg of whole cotton seed (WCS) for every 0.5% of free gossypol in the WCS prevents reproductive effects in cattle. Selenium (sodium selenite) supplementation in rams at 1 mg/ram per day has been used experimentally to counteract the adverse effects on semen characteristics.[2]

TANNINS

Tannins include the condensed tannins (proanthocyanidins), which are insoluble and nontoxic, except that they may be associated with oral mucosal lesions, and the hydrolyzable tannins, which are soluble and potentially toxic.[3] Pyrogallol, a degradation product of hydrolyzable tannins, is a gastrointestinal (GI) and renal toxin. Oaks (*Quercus* spp.) and yellow-wood tree (*Terminalia oblongata* ssp. *oblongata*) are important in this group. Miscellaneous other toxic plants in this group include the following:

- *Acacia melanoxylon*—black wattle
- *Acacia salacina*—black sally wattle
- *Clidemia hirtia*—harendong
- *Elephantorrhiza elephantine*—elephant's root; elan's bean
- *Stryphnodendron* spp.
- *Thiloa glaucocarpa*—sipauba, vaqueta
- *Ventilago viminalis*—supple jack

OAK (*QUERCUS* SPP.)

The leaves and acorns of many varieties of oak trees can be browsed by animals and are associated with no illness when they form only a small part of the diet.[3] When ingested in large quantities, all *Quercus* spp. are associated with toxicity, including the following:

- *Q. agrifolia*—coast live oak
- *Q. garryanna*—Oregon white oak
- *Q. havardii*—sand shin oak
- *Q. marilandica*—blackjack oak
- *Q. robur* (synonym *Q. pedunculata*)—European oak
- *Q. rubra*—Northern red oak
- *Q. velutina*—black oak

The toxic principles are hydrolyzable tannins and simple phenols in the leaves, especially the **young buds**, and **green acorns**. All species of animals are affected, with losses in sheep and cattle being reported most commonly and occasional cases occurring in horses.[4-8] Goats are thought to be capable of surviving much greater intakes of tannin than cattle because of greater concentrations of tannase enzymes in their ruminal mucosa.[4] Experimental administration of tannic acids to goats has produced anemia, but there is no record of the natural occurrence of the disease.

Oak toxicosis involves the gastrointestinal tract and kidneys.[4-7] Cattle and sheep tend to show both GI and renal disease, whereas horses are more likely to develop gastroenteritis and fewer renal issues. If little else is eaten, oak foliage and acorns ingested for 3 to 4 days may be associated with nephrosis, which is manifested by polyuria, ventral edema, abdominal pain, and constipation followed by the passage of feces containing mucus and blood. Blood urea nitrogen (BUN) and creatinine levels are elevated; serum electrolytes are altered (increased potassium, decreased sodium); urine specific gravity is low, and proteinuria, glucosuria, and hematuria may occur.[4,6] Hepatic enzymes, indicative of liver damage, may be elevated, depending on the animal and/or oak species. At necropsy in ruminants there is edema of the gastrointestinal wall and mesentery, a characteristic nephrosis, and hepatic damage. Ulcerations of the mucosa consistent with uremia may be present. Survivors of an initial attack of nephrosis make compensatory weight gains and perform well in feedlot situations.

Extensive areas of oak-brush range in the United States can be utilized for cattle grazing, but this requires careful management if losses are to be avoided. The phenol content varies between species, and thus stands of *Q. alba* can be much less toxic than those of *Q. rubra* or *Q. velutina*. Calcium hydroxide (15% of the ration) is an effective preventive under experimental conditions.

YELLOW-WOOD TREE (*TERMINALIA OBLONGATA* SPP.)

The foliage of the Yellow-Wood Tree contains a hepatotoxic tannin punicalagin and an unidentified nephrotoxin, and it is associated with losses in cattle. Acute poisoning of cattle is manifested by a sudden onset of hepatopathy, jaundice, and photosensitization, with some nephrosis and signs of abdominal pain and dehydration. Necropsy reveals a swollen congested liver, swollen gray-green kidneys, and gray-green pigmentation of the gastrointestinal mucosa, with multiple small hemorrhagic erosions of the abomasal mucosa. Chronic poisoning of cattle is dominated by severe nephrosis with pigment accumulation and fibrosis in the kidney cortex, polyuria, and wasting of the body. Yellow-wood poisoning of sheep is a nervous derangement, manifested by seizures if sheep are excited by handling, from which they recover spontaneously.

FURTHER READING

Danke RJ, Panciera RJ, Tillman AD. Gossypol toxicity studies with sheep. *J Anim Sci.* 1965;24:1199-1201.

Duncan CS. Oak leaf poisoning in two horses. *Cornell Vet.* 1961;51:159-162.

Garg SK, Makkar HP, Nagal KB, et al. Oak (*Quercus incana*) leaf poisoning in cattle. *Vet Hum Toxicol.* 1992;34:161-164.

Kornegay ET, Clawson AJ, Smith FH, et al. Influence of protein source on toxicity of gossypol in swine rations. *J Anim Sci.* 1961;20:597-602.

Legg J, Moule GR, Chester RD. The toxicity of yellow-wood (*Terminalia oblongata*) to cattle. *Queensland J Ag Sci.* 1945;2:199-208.

Zelski RZ, Rothwell TJ, Moore RE, et al. Gossypol toxicity in preruminant calves. *Aust Vet J.* 1995;72:394-398.

REFERENCES

1. Nicholson SS. Cottonseed toxicity. In: Gupta RC, ed. *Veterinary Toxicology*. Elsevier; 2012:1161.
2. El-Mokadem MY, et al. *J Anim Sci.* 2012;90:3274.
3. Mueller-Harvey I. *J Sci Food Agric.* 2006;86:2010.
4. Eroksuz Y, et al. *Revue Méd. Vét.* 2013;164:302.
5. Sadeghi-Nasab A, et al. *J Vet Res.* 2013;68:305.
6. Lorin B, et al. *Revue Méd Vét.* 2009;160:507.
7. Pérez V, et al. *Res Vet Sci.* 2011;91:269.
8. Hume T. *Vet Rec.* 2006;159:860.

MISCELLANEOUS PLANT TOXICOSIS

AESCULIN

The glycoside aesculin (7-hydroxycoumarin-6-glucoside) occurs in *Aesculus* spp. plants, including *A. californica, A. glabra, A. hippocastanum, A. octandra,* and *A. pavia* (buckeyes or horse chestnuts), with *A. pavia* being the most toxic.[1] Ingestion of the seeds and nuts is usually reported, but toxicity also occurs after eating bark and foliage.[1] In monogastric animals the glycoside is associated with gastroenteritis with vomiting, but its digestion in ruminants to a soluble aglycone results in the more common syndrome of depression, straddled posture, stiff and uncoordinated gait, tremor, easy falling, recumbency, and convulsions with opisthotonos. Signs are exacerbated by handling or harassment. No necropsy lesions are reported.

ALCOHOL (COMPLEX PLANT)

Included in alcohol toxins are cicutoxin, occurring in *Cicuta* spp. (water hemlock); oenanthotoxin, isomeric with cicutoxin, in *Oenanthe* spp. (water hemlock dropwort); and tremetol in *Ageratina altissima* (formerly *Eupatorium rugosum* [white snakeroot]) and *Isocoma pluriflora* (rayless goldenrod).

Cicutoxin and oenanthotoxin are C17 conjugated polyacetylenes and act as δ-aminobutyric acid antagonists in the CNS;[2] tremetol is composed of complex mixtures of alcohols and ketones that may act to impair the tricarboxylic acid cycle.[3,4]

- **Cicutoxin** poisoning in all species is characterized by early tremor, restlessness, and stumbling gait, followed by violent clonic convulsions with bellowing, opisthotonos, and frothing at the mouth.[5] Between convulsions there is ruminal tympany, dyspnea, profuse salivation, teeth grinding and chewing movements, frequent urination and defecation, tachycardia, hyperthermia, and pupillary dilation. Most affected animals die of respiratory failure after a course of a few minutes, but more usually several hours. Serum levels of muscle enzymes are elevated as a result of the muscle activity. Necropsy lesions are comprised of skeletal and cardiac myodegeneration. The characteristic roots may be found in the forestomaches, more commonly lodged in the esophageal groove than in the rumen proper. In experimentally produced cases, IV sodium pentobarbital administered at the onset of the first convulsion prevents further convulsions and the myodegeneration, but no practicable remedy is available for natural cases. Green seed heads and tubers are toxic.[6] Prevention depends on keeping animals away from the plant, including the roots, which may be exposed during excavation or after flooding
- **Oenanthotoxin** poisoning is associated with an identical syndrome, most commonly in cattle. The roots of the plant are the common source of the poison.
- **Tremetol** is associated with stiffness and incoordination of gait, severe tremor, salivation, depression, recumbency, and coma preceding death in ruminants. In goats, skeletal muscle degeneration and necrosis is extensive.[3,7] In horses, there is heavy sweating, regurgitation of food through the nostrils, and the passage of dark, hard feces; there may be congestive right-heart failure with electrocardiographic abnormalities and extensive myocardial damage.[4] Cardiac troponin I may be a useful diagnostic tool for horses suspected of tremetol toxicosis.[4] The alcohol is excreted in the milk of animals that ingest the plant and may be associated with clinical illness and even death in humans drinking the milk.[7] Liver damage and skeletal muscle and myocardial swelling and pallor are gross lesions at necropsy.

ALIPHATIC ACETOGENIN (MONOGLYCERIDE)

The toxin responsible for poisoning by *Persea americana* (avocado, alligator pear) is a biologically active aliphatic acetogenin, persin, with the form of a monoglyceride. Only varieties of Guatemalan origin are toxic; Mexican varieties are not. All parts of the plants can be toxic. Horses, ruminants, and ostriches have been affected. In lactating females, poisoning produces sterile mastitis and agalactia, with necrosis of secretory epithelium of mammary glands. Horses are affected by a heart failure syndrome, usually nonfatal, with severe subcutaneous edematous swelling of the head and dyspnea. In some cases, there is ischemic necrosis of masseter and tongue muscles. Fatal cases have myocardial necrosis. Colic and diarrhea have been reported in foals. Poisoned ostriches have paresis of neck muscles, edema of the neck, pulmonary edema, and necrosis of cardiac muscle.

AMINE TOXICITY

Tyramine (*N*-methyl-phenylethyl-amine) is found in *Acacia berlandieri* (guajillo) and two mistletoes, *Phoradendron villosum* and *Viscosum album.* Clinical signs in poisoning by the acacia include gait incoordination, limb weakness, and recumbency, all exacerbated by exercise or harassment, and all of which disappear if the patient is removed from contact with the plant. No signs are attributed to poisoning by mistletoe; in the only event recorded, the patient was found dead.

AMINO ACID TOXICITY

The best-known toxic amino acids are as follows:

- Indospicine in *Indigofera hendecaphylla* (formerly *I. spicata,* creeping or trailing indigo)
- Indospicine in *Indigofera linnaei* (*I. dominii, I. enneaphylla,* Birdsville indigo)
- Canavanine in *Canavalia* spp., *Indigofera linnaei*
- Mimosine in *Leucaena leucocephala* (lead tree) and *Mimosa pudica* (sensitive plant)

Indospicine/Canavanine

Poisoning by *Indigofera linnaei* has generally been ascribed to indospicine, an arginine analog, and, to a lesser extent, canavanine, also an arginine analog, but a nitrocompound may also be involved. The mechanism of action is an inhibition of nitrous oxide synthesis, decreased glutathione levels, and increased superoxides in hepatocytes.

Indospicine transmitted to dogs fed on meat from poisoned horses is associated with fatal liver damage in the dogs. *Canavalia* spp. and *I. hendecaphylla* in sheep and cattle are associated with a similar syndrome that includes anorexia, icterus, weakness, gait incoordination, and, less commonly, abortion. Horses show anorexia, depression, ataxia, and seizures.

Mimosine

The nonprotein amino acid mimosine occurs in *Mimosa pudica* (sensitive plant) and *Leucaena leucocephala,* a leguminous fodder shrub.[8,9] Mimosine plus an enzyme in plant tissue produces 3,4-dihydroxypyridone (3,4-DHP), a potent goitrogen, which on mastication yields 2,3-DHP through the action of rumen flora. Mimosine, 3,4-DHP, and 2,3-DHP are all toxic.[10] Both plants are associated with alopecia, but *Leucaena* spp. is associated with the disease known as "jumbay" (Bahamas) or "lamtoro" (Indonesia). Some varieties of the tree contain more mimosine than others. Safe daily intakes of mimosine are 0.18 g/kg BW for cattle, 0.14 g/kg BW for sheep, and 0.18 g/kg BW for goats. There is a great deal of variation in the effects of poisoning with *L. leucocephala,* depending on the variety of the tree, the amount of other fodder available, and the selection of the feed by the animal.[11] Horses, sheep, cattle, and goats are all affected.

Cattle and goats in Indonesia, Hawaii, and the Virgin Islands, where the tree is indigenous, eat very large amounts of the plant without ill-effect. This immunity is attributable to the adaptation of ruminal microflora to degrade the mimosine, with the degree of degradation varying with the diet and being much greater on a concentrate diet than on a roughage one. A transfer of rumen contents from resistant to susceptible cattle is a successful preventive veterinary procedure. The bacterium capable of degrading the toxins is *Synergistes jonesii.*[10,12] In some areas, if ruminants are introduced to the plant gradually enough, the ruminal microflora may develop the capacity of metabolizing mimosine, and thus poisoning is not a problem. Animals in the areas of concern can be given a *Synergistes jonesii* ruminal inoculum and successfully graze on leuceana pastures without issues.[10]

Loss of wool and hair is the most common sign. Other less frequent signs are anorexia, weakness, thyroid gland enlargement, gingival atrophy, lingual epithelial ulceration, infertility, and low birth weight. In experimental animals, hepatic injury is one of the most marked effects, but this is not recorded in field cases.

In horses the loss of hair is most marked in the mane and tail and around the hocks and knees. Ring formation in the hooves and emaciation also occur. In cattle and sheep, shedding of hair or wool occurs soon (7–14 days) after the first exposure to the plant, when very large amounts are fed. The alopecia is not necessarily general but is symmetric and includes the tail, ears, face, and sheath. Experimental feeding of large amounts of the plant to steers has been associated with hair loss, especially on the tail, pizzle, and escutcheon. Cattle fed on the plant for long periods develop other chronic syndromes, including incoordination, temporary blindness, and hyperactivity to the point of severely interfering with normal handling procedures. A secondary phase of poisoning is associated with the formation of DHP recorded in some countries, but not others. It is characterized by enlarged thyroid glands, poor breeding performance, and goitrous, weak calves. The goitrogenic effect is limited to ruminants, associated with 3,4-DHP, and unresponsive to iodine administration. A further complication, seen in goats on low-level feeding over a long period, is fibrous osteodystrophy of the mandible, causing salivation, slow eating, and weight loss. The long bones are normal.

In pigs, the feeding of diets containing up to 15% of dried *L. leucocephala* to pregnant gilts is associated with a high proportion of fetuses being resorbed and some having limb deformities. Feeding 1% ferrous sulfate in the diet reduces these effects.

Toxic effects are quickly reversible by removing animals from access to the plants, so the case-fatality rate is usually low. Taste aversion conditioning has been successful in an experimental setting and may be in useful in reducing toxicity in those animals that must graze on leucaena pastures.[13] Supplementation of the diet of ruminants with iron, copper, and zinc is also claimed to reduce the toxic effects.

Animals grazing heavily on *L. leucocephala* may have low blood levels of thyroxine and are likely to have high blood and urine levels of DHPs.[9,11] Necropsy lesions are limited to alopecia, oral and esophageal ulcers, and thyroid enlargement.

ARISTOLOCHINE

Aristocholine, an alkaloid, occurs in the following *Aristolochia* spp.:

- *A. bractea*
- *A. clematitis*—birthwort
- *A. densivena*
- *A. elegans*

In goats, poisoning takes the form of diarrhea, dyspnea, alopecia, and hindlimb weakness. In horses, signs include straining to urinate, passing small amounts of urine frequently, polyuria, and tachycardia.

CREPENYNIC ACID

Necrosis of cardiac and skeletal muscle, manifested clinically by staggering and recumbency, or sudden death during exercise, is the significant lesion in poisoning of sheep by crepenynic acid, which is found in mature seed heads of *Ixiolaena brevicompta* (button weed).

CYCAD GLYCOSIDES

All cycads that have been investigated contain one or more glycosides of methylazoxymethanol (MAM) and a neurotoxic amino acid (β-*N*-methylamino-L-alanine or BMAA). The two common glycosides are cycasin and macrozamin. These include species of the following:

- *Bowenia*
- *Cycas*
- *Dioon*
- *Encephalartos*
- *Lepidozamia*
- *Macrozamia*
- *Stangeria*
- *Zamia*

These robust cone-bearing plants grow in greatest numbers in poor soil in hot climates, and their young leaves and seeds are eaten eagerly by ruminants when other feed is short. Methylazoxymethanol glycosides are more concentrated in seeds than in leaves and roots.[14] The MAM glycosides are hydrolyzed in the rumen to aglycones and sugars. The MAM aglycone is the toxic portion, alkylating DNA and RNA and causing hepatotoxicosis with periacinal hepatocyte necrosis and damage to blood vessels leading to hepatic veno-occlusion. Long-term intake results in liver cirrhosis. The liver lesions result in anorexia, weight loss, jaundice, and photosensitization. In addition, acute poisoning is associated with hemorrhagic necrosis of the abomasum and small intestine in sheep and cattle, causing severe diarrhea. Sheep are more likely than cattle to consume seeds and develop hepato/gastrointestinal MAM poisoning.[14,15] Pigs and horses have been experimentally poisoned with seeds. MAM is mutagenic and carcinogenic in laboratory animals, but this effect has not been described under natural conditions.

The role β-*N*-methylamino-L-alanine (BMAA) plays in animal toxicosis has not been well established. It is a potent neurotoxin that concentrates in the roots of several *Cycas* spp. and may be associated with or produced by cyanobacteria.[16,17] It has also been linked to the development of amyotrophic lateral sclerosis/parkinsonism dementia complex present in the Chamorro people in Guam.[16]

An unidentified neurotoxin in *Bowenia, Cycas, Macrozamia,* and *Zamia* produces posterior ataxia in cattle, a syndrome recognized in Australia, where it is called zamia staggers; some Japanese islands; and in the Caribbean region.[18] This is the most likely result of cattle consuming these plants under natural conditions; however, affected cattle often have some degree of chronic liver damage. This ataxia syndrome in sheep has been produced experimentally but is rare under natural conditions. Clinically, the condition is a proprioceptive defect affecting the hindlimbs causing an irregular, stiff overextension ("goose-stepping") and knuckling over at the fetlocks. Atrophy of hindlimb muscles and posterior paralysis may follow. There are degenerative lesions of the fasciculus gracilis, dorsal spinocerebellar tracts, and corticospinal tracts of the spinal cord. Affected cattle do not recover.

GRAYANOTOXINS

Grayanotoxins (synonyms acetylandromedol, andromedotoxins, rhodotoxins) are resinoid substances, members of the diterpenoid group of substances, and found in plants of the Ericaceae (heath), family including:

- *Agauria salifolia*
- *Clethra arborea*—heathers
- *Kalmia* spp.—mountain laurels
- *Ledum* spp.—labrador tea
- *Leucothoe* spp.—sierra laurel, hanahiri
- *Lyonia ligustrina*—staggerbush
- *Menziezia ferruginea*—mock azalea
- *Pieris* spp.—apanese pieris
- *Rhododendron* spp.—azaleas and rhododendrons

Grayanotoxins concentrate in the leaves but are found in all plant parts including the flowers and nectar. The toxins present in nectar are transferred to honey made from these plants and have been associated with poisoning in humans.[19,20] The toxins bind to voltage-dependent sodium channels, slowing their opening and closing, resulting in persistent activation and an increase in axon sodium ion permeability of almost 100-fold.[19,21] At higher doses, calcium channels may be affected as well.

The toxins are very poisonous, with deaths often occurring after plant clippings are thrown into pastures or fed individually by unsuspecting individuals.[20,21] The toxic dose of *Rhododendron* spp. in cattle is 0.2% of their body weight and for *Kalmia* spp. is 0.4% of body weight.[19,21] Cholinergic type signs begin 3 to 14 hours after the plant is eaten and include depression, salivation, projectile vomiting, bloat, repeated swallowing or belching, tenesmus, abdominal pain, and diarrhea.[19-21] Other signs include irregular respirations, blindness, weakness, recumbency, convulsions, and cardiac arrhythmias (bradycardia, tachycardia, others). Diarrhea is rare. Aspiration pneumonia is a common sequela and is the only common gross necropsy finding.[19,21] Typically the acute signs last for about 24 hours, with 2 to 3 days required for resolution of the neurologic effects.[19]

ISOQUINOLINE ALKALOIDS

Berberine, a pyridine alkaloid, a subgroup of the isoquinoline alkaloids, occurs in the following weeds:

- *Argemone mexicana*—Mexican prickly poppy
- *A. ochraleuca*
- *A. subfusiformis*
- *Berberis* spp.
- *Mahonia* spp.

The clinical syndrome in cattle and pigs includes weight loss, dyspnea, and subcutaneous edema. Diarrhea, abdominal pain, and recumbency are also recorded. At necropsy the principal lesion is cardiomyopathy accompanied by fluid in body cavities and pulmonary edema, and gastroenteritis in some cases. The toxic effect of *A. mexicana* seeds may be attributable to their total content of isoquinoline alkaloids rather than to their berberine content.

Bulbocapnine is an isoquinoline alkaloid found in *Corydalis flavula* (fitweed, fumatory) and *Dicentra spectabilis* (bleeding heart) and is associated with a transient syndrome of tremor, tetanic convulsions, frenzy and biting at surrounding objects, opisthotonos, drooling of saliva, and vomiting in grazing ruminants.

Chelidonine, a toxic isoquinoline alkaloid found in *Chelidonium majus* (greater celandine or celandine poppy), is associated with a syndrome of gait incoordination, dribbling urine, drooling saliva, and convulsions in cattle, especially if they are harassed.

Corydaline is an isoquinoline alkaloid found in *Corydalis caseana* (fitweed) and is associated with acute diarrhea, frenzy and excitement exacerbated by harassment, clonic convulsions, and a quick death in grazing animals. The same toxin in *Dicentra cucullaria* is associated with a similar syndrome, except that vomiting occurs and diarrhea does not. Gastroenteritis is present at necropsy.

JUNIPERINE

An alkaloid, juniperine occurs in *Juniperus* spp. trees and is reputed to be associated with nephrosis, cystitis, and rumenitis when eaten. Signs include abdominal pain, diarrhea, proteinuria, elevation of blood urea nitrogen (BUN) levels, and abortion.

RHOEADINE

Rhoeadine is an alkaloid found in the seed capsules of *Papaver rhoeas* (field poppy), and probably *P. nudicaule* and *P. somniferum*, and is associated with restlessness, hypersensitivity, ataxia, ruminal stasis, dyspnea, and convulsions, but no significant necropsy lesions.

SAPONIN POISONING

Saponins are naturally occurring glycosides with the physical properties of soaps; that is, they produce a stable froth in water. They have a bitter taste. They also lyse erythrocytes in vitro. There are two classes of saponins, those with a triterpene aglycone radical and those in which the nonsugar radical is a steroid.

Triterpene Saponins

In plants, almost all saponins are triterpene saponins. The compounds are concentrated in the rapidly growing shoots, the bark, and the roots, and they are thought to have an insect-repellent role in these sensitive areas of the plant. They are absorbed very slowly, if at all, from the alimentary tract, and it seems unlikely that they will exert any systemic effect unless there is preexisting damage to the intestinal mucosa.

Information regarding the toxicity of triterpene saponins for animals is scarce. The principal pathogenic effect is enteritis and gastroenteritis, manifested by diarrhea and dysentery. Other less common signs include abdominal pain, vomiting, and salivation. The following plants are known to have this effect:

- *Aleurites fordii*
- *Dialopsis africana*
- *Gutierrezia microcephala*
- *Hedera helix*
- *Jatropha curcas*
- *J. hyssopifolia*
- *Phytolacca americana*
- *Phytolacca dioica*—packalacca
- *Phytolacca dodecandra*
- *Saponaria officinalis*
- *Sesbania* spp.

Bulnesia sarmientii (Palo santo tree) seed pods and foliage contain an unspecified toxic saponin that is associated with convulsions, licking of forelimbs, geophagia, chewing movements, ruminal atony, bradycardia, and frequent urination and defecation. The bitter taste of saponins may result in a decrease in feed intake and a reduction in growth rate in monogastric animals.

Steroidal Saponins

Steroidal saponins are associated with Scandinavian (Norway) photosensitization disease (alveld or "elf fire") and occasionally nephrosis in ruminants; they occur in the following plants:

- *Agave lecheguilla*
- *Agrostemma githago*
- *Brachiaria decumbens* grass
- *Kochia scoparia*—summer cypress
- *Nartheciium ossifragum*—also associated with alveld
- *Panicum* spp. grasses
- *Panicum schinizii*
- *Panicum miliaceum*—French millet
- *Panicum coloratum*—kleingrass
- *Panicum. dichotomiflorum*—smooth witch grass
- *Tribulus terrestris.*

Other *Panicum* spp. grasses that should now be on the suspicious list for this kind of poisoning are as follows:

- *P. decompositum*
- *P. effusum*
- *P. maximum*
- *P. queenslandicum*
- *P. whitei*

Birefringent crystals composed of the glucuronides of epismilagenin and episarsasapogenin formed from an ingested saponin accumulate in the biliary system, blocking it and causing damage to it and surrounding hepatocytes. Jaundice, photosensitization, and hepatitis result. Blockage of the bile canaliculi and bile ducts and filling of hepatocytes, Kupffer, and renal tubules cells by acicular crystals are characteristic. Necrosis of the distal renal tubules, papillary muscles of the heart, and adrenal cortex are accompanying lesions. Other steroidal saponins are present in *Tribulus terrestris,* but they appear to be nonlithogenic.

SESQUITERPENES

Sesquiterpenes are common plant poisons. Subgroups of them, described elsewhere in this chapter, are as follows:

- Furanoid sesquiterpenes
- Ipomeanols
- Ngaiones
- Sesquiterpene lactones
- Sporidesmin

Unspecified sesquiterpenes are also listed as being associated with other poisonings. For example, *Flourensia cernua* and *Vernonia* spp. are associated with heavy losses in South America and Africa as a result of hepatic necrosis in grazing ruminants. Affected animals show nonspecific signs of anorexia, ruminal atony, hypothermia, staggering gait, recumbency, and convulsions. Serum levels of liver enzymes are elevated, accompanying a massive liver necrosis.

FURANOID SESQUITERPENES (FURANOSESQUITERPENOID) POISONING

Furanosesquiterpenoids, including ngaione and myodesmone, are essential oils in the following plants:

- *Lasiospermum bipinnatum*—ganskweed
- *Myoporum* spp.—boobialla, Ellangowan poison bush, and others

Ingestion of these plants usually is associated with jaundice, photosensitization, ruminal stasis, constipation, tenesmus, and abdominal pain. Necropsy findings are limited to hepatic necrosis, jaundice, and photosensitive dermatitis. Ingestion of *L. bipinnatum* by lambs also is associated with the same hepatic insufficiency syndrome, but the same plant from a different part of a farm may be associated with pulmonary and mediastinal emphysema and interstitial pneumonia reminiscent of the ipomeanols. The fungi *Ceratocystis* spp. is associated with the same problems as *L. bipinnatum*. The following are associated with acute hepatic injury and deaths in ruminants:

- *Myoporum laetum*—ngaio tree
- *Eremophila deserti* (= *M. deserti*)—Ellangowan poison bush
- *M. tetrandrum*—Australian boobialla

Ipomeanol

Ipomeanols are produced in sweet potatoes in response to infection by the *Fusarium* fungi, *F. solani*, *F. oxysporum*, and *F. javanicum*, and *Ceratostomella fimbriata* and are associated with pulmonary emphysema and edema and interstitial pneumonia when fed to animals.[22-24] Ipomeanols are also suspected of being associated with the poisoning of *Perilla frutescens* (purple mint weed)[25] and *Zieria arborescens* (stinkwood tree). *P. frutescens* is toxic only after the plant has flowered and then loses its toxicity once it has been wilted by frost. Cases appear in calves 3 to 12 days after they begin eating the plant. Pulmonary edema develops because of damage to endothelial cells and young pneumocytes.

Zieria arborescens, a small tree in Tasmania and eastern Australia, is associated with interstitial pneumonia in cattle, and the disease is reproducible by feeding the foliage. Clinical signs appear as tachypnea, abdominal, grunting respiration with extension of the head, mouth breathing, and a nasal discharge. In severe cases the temperature and pulse are elevated. Most cases die after an illness of 1 to 21 days. Necropsy lesions include massive pulmonary edema and emphysema.

Sesquiterpene Lactones

There are very many plant lactones suspected of being poisonous. Plant genera known to owe their toxicity to their content of sesquiterpene lactones include *Centaurea* spp. (especially *C. repens, C. solstitialis*), *Chrysanthemum* spp. (associated with contact dermatitis), *Geigeria* spp., *Helenium* spp., *Hymenoxys* spp., *Iphiona aucheri*, and *Parthenium hysterophorus* (parthenium weed).

Vomiting Syndrome

Geigeria, Helenium, and *Hymenoxys* spp. poisonings in cattle are associated with a syndrome of regurgitation (spewing sickness, vermeersiekte), salivation, dysphagia, and coughing. An ELISA is available for the quantitative detection of the sesquiterpene lactone dihydrogriesenin in *Geigeria* spp. Contrast radiography of the esophagus and biopsy of skeletal and esophageal muscle are helpful in diagnosis. Dietary supplements used to prevent poisoning by sesquiterpene lactones, including a soybean meal–sodium sulfate combination, are useful if thiol groups are added to the ration. Urea potentiates the poisoning.

Encephalomalacia Syndrome

Centaurea solstitialis (yellow star thistle) and *C. repens* (Russian knapweed) poisoning in horses is associated with a well-known syndrome of severe depression, constant chewing movements, salivation, tongue flicking, dysphagia, intestinal bloat, paralysis, recumbency, and death.[26] Yawning and somnolence are evident, but the horse is easily aroused. Some horses show aimless, slow walking, and, in the early stages, transient circling. The gait is not grossly abnormal, with a slight stiffness in the walk being the only abnormality except for weakness in the terminal stages. A fixed facial expression is common, with the mouth being held half open or the lips drawn into a straight line. Wrinkling of the skin of the lips and muzzle and protrusion of the tongue are present in many cases. Signs fluctuate in severity for 2 to 3 days and then remain static until the animal dies or is destroyed. Nigropallidal encephalomalacia and fluid accumulations in body cavities are characteristic necropsy lesions. Areas of necrosis or softening are visible macroscopically in the brain, with lesions within the substantia nigra pars reticulata (sparing the dopaminergic cell bodies in the pars compacta) and in the rostral portion of the globus pallidus.[26]

The plants do not appear to be toxic to ruminants, rodents, or monkeys, and sheep do well on sole diets of the plants.

SELENOCOMPOUNDS

Organic selenocompounds occur in two classes of plants that preferentially accumulate selenium: primary converter or indicator plants that grow only in soils with abnormally high selenium content and secondary converters that grow anywhere but accumulate selenium if it is available. Primary converters are more toxic, attaining levels of greater than 1000 and up to 10,000 ppm.[27] Secondary converters reach levels of about 1000 ppm.

Primary converters include the following:

- *Astragalus* spp.—milk vetch, poison vetch
- *A. bisulcatus*—two grooved milk vetch[27]
- *A. pattersonii*—Patterson's milk vetch
- *A. praelongus*—sinking milk vetch
- *A. pectinatus*—narrow leaf milk vetch
- *A. racemosus*—alkali milk vetch, creamy locoweed
- *Oonopsis condensata*—goldenweed
- *Stanleya pinnata*—prince's plume[27]
- *Xylorrhiza* spp.—woody aster

Secondary converters include the following:

- *Acacia cana*
- *Aster* spp.—woody aster
- *Astragalus* spp.
- *Atriplex canescens*—saltbush
- *Castilleja* spp.
- *Comandra pallidai*
- *Grindelia squarrosai*
- *Machaerานthera ramosa*
- *Morinda reticulata*
- *Neptunia amplexicaulis*
- *Penstemon* spp.
- *Sideranthus* spp.—ironweed

Clinical findings include the common acute form with signs of aimless wandering, circling, apparent blindness, head-pressing, dyspnea, lameness and recumbency, teeth grinding, and salivation. The chronic form is characterized by alopecia, weight loss, coronitis, hoof deformity, and hoof shedding in all species, including pigs. Assay of selenium in the feed is usually necessary to confirm the diagnosis. Daily intakes of more than 30 ppm are usual in the subacute form. In chronic cases the intake is usually below this level and has been maintained for some months.

Necropsy findings are nonspecific and include hepatic, myocardial, and renal injury and erosion of joint cartilage.

STEROIDAL ALKALOIDS (*SOLANUM* SPP.)

Solanum spp. plants contain many poisonous glycosidic steroidal alkaloids, including solanidine, soladulcidine, solasodine, tomatidine, and others. The most well-known poisonous plants in the group include the following *Solanum* spp.:

S. bonariensis[28]
S. dulcamara—bitter nightshade, bittersweet
S. elaeagnifolium—silver leaf nightshade, white horse nettle
S. esuriale
S. fastigiatum
S. kwebense[29]
S. lycopersicum—tomato
S. nigrum—black nightshade
S. pseudocapsicum—Jerusalem cherry
S. triflorum—cut leaf nightshade[30]
S. tuberosum—potato

The other important members of the genus are *S. malacoxylon* and *S. glaucophyllum*, with the principal association being enzootic calcinosis.[31] *Lycium halimifolium* is also listed as containing these alkaloids.

Acute poisoning with steroidal alkaloids, associated with large doses, appears in experimental animals as a syndrome of gastroenteritis, with diarrhea and necropsy lesions of mucosal necrosis in the stomach and intestines. Subacute poisoning with smaller doses, which are not associated with an enteric lesion but are absorbed, is associated with nervous signs of exercise-induced gait incoordination, easy falling, a straddled gait, nystagmus, and convulsions with opisthotonos, complemented in some cases by cardiac irregularity, hemolysis, and sometimes diarrhea. Records of necropsy lesions include only occasional references to the presence of encephalomalacia and cerebellar agangliosidosis associated with the incoordination syndromes. *Solanum esuriale* has been suggested as being associated with humpy back, a common disease in sheep in Australia, but the association is unproven. After forced exercise, affected sheep show gait stiffness in the hindlimbs with shortness of steps. This is followed by an inability to keep walking and the adoption of a peculiar hump-backed stance. The disease occurs only in summer in fully wooled sheep. At necropsy, there is degeneration of spinal cord tracts. In the United States, *S. dimidiatum* is associated with a "crazy cow syndrome" of staggering and incoordination, with a selective loss of Purkinje cells from the cerebellum. A similar syndrome is associated with *S. kwebense* in South Africa (mad drunk disease),[29] one by *S. bonariense* (naranjillo) in cattle in Uruguay,[28] one by *S. cinereum* in goats in Australia, and one by *S. fastigiatum* var. fastigiatum in Brazil. The latter appears to be an acquired gangliosidosis. It is characterized by cytoplasmic membranous bodies in the Purkinje cells and a syndrome identical to that described previously for subacute poisoning with steroidal (*Solanum* spp.) alkaloids. After an attack lasting up to 60 seconds, the animal returns to normal. Affected animals do not recover but do not die unless by misadventure. The animals can be provoked to have an attack by raising their heads or by holding them in lateral recumbency and then letting go.[28,29] It is probable that these are not true "convulsive" diseases but cerebellar incoordination in which frantic efforts by a seriously ataxic animal give a superficial resemblance to convulsive episodes. It is also probable that the lesions in this disease are not associated with steroidal alkaloids but with perhaps with β-carbolines.

Potatoes are toxic only if they are green and sprouted, and the toxic alkaloid solanine is concentrated in those parts; potatoes must constitute more than 50% of the diet before toxicity occurs. Pigs are most commonly affected, but all species are susceptible. In pigs there is dullness, copious diarrhea, anorexia, hypothermia, and coma in the terminal stages. The mortality rate may be high. In horses, the signs include depression and prostration, but usually there are no signs of alimentary tract irritation. In cattle, dermatitis, comprised of vesicles and scabs on the legs, is a more common syndrome. At necropsy in all species there is a moderate hyperemia of the alimentary mucosa. Sprouted or diseased potatoes can be fed safely if they are boiled and the amount fed is restricted to less than 25% of the diet.

There are several anecdotal reports that tomatoes are toxic to horses and ruminants if they are fed green vines and foliage from tomato plants. This was not shown to be the case, at least in beef cattle; they did not develop any clinical signs other than weight loss after being fed large amounts of tomato foliage for 42 days.

Some of these plants also contain specific teratogenic steroidal alkaloids that contain α-piperidine moiety. The plants, in decreasing order of toxicity in terms of producing craniofacial deformities in laboratory animals, are as follows:

- *S. elaeagnifolium*
- *S. saccharoides*
- *S. dulcamara*
- *S. melongena*
- *S. tuberosum*

VELLEIN

The toxin vellein, found in the plant *Velleia discophora,* is associated with hyposensitivity, dyspnea, tachycardia, and recumbency but no specific necropsy lesions.

VERATRINE

The mixture of alkaloids found in *Veratrum californicum* is associated with a syndrome of salivation, dyspnea, vomiting, diarrhea, frequent urination, cardiac irregularity, and convulsions. The plant also contains the teratogen cyclopamine.

ZIGADINE (ZIGADENINE)

The phytotoxin zigadine occurs in the plants *Zigadenus* spp. (death camas), especially the bulb, and is associated with a syndrome of salivation, vomiting, tremor, ataxia, and dyspnea. The toxin has been identified in the rumen of dead cattle by electron impact mass spectrometry, avoiding the necessity of identifying the plant botanically.

FURTHER READING

Buck WB, Dollahite JW, Alien TJ. *Solanum elaeagnifolium,* silver-leafed nightshade, poisoning in livestock. *J Am Vet Med Assoc.* 1960;137:348-351.

Casteel SW, Johnson GC, Wagstaff DJ. *Aesculus glabra* intoxication in cattle. *Vet Hum Toxicol.* 1992;34:55-57.

Hegarty MP, Kelly WR, McEwan D, et al. Hepatotoxicity to dogs of horse meat contaminated with indospicine. *Aust Vet J.* 1988;65:337-340.

Hegarty MP, Schinckel PG. Reaction of sheep to the consumption of *Leucaena glauca* Benth and to its toxic principle mimosine. *Crop Past Sci.* 1964;15:153-167.

Lopez TA, Cid MS, Bianchini ML. Biochemistry of hemlock (*Conium maculatum*) alkaloids and their acute and chronic toxicity in livestock. A review. *Toxicon.* 1999;37:841-865.

Magnusson RA, Whittier WD, Veit HP, et al. Yellow buckeye (*Aesculus octandra* Marsh) toxicity in calves. *Bov Pract.* 1983;18:195-199.

McKenzie RA, Brown OP. Avocado (*Persea americana*) poisoning of horses. *Aust Vet J.* 1991;68:77-78.

Munday BL. *Zieria Arborescens* (stinkwood) intoxication in cattle. *Aust Vet J.* 1968;44:501-502.

Olson CT, Keller WC, Gerken DF, et al. Suspected tremetol poisoning in horses. *J Am Vet Med Assoc.* 1984;185:1001-1003.

Penrith ML, Van Vollenhoven E. Pulmonary and hepatic lesions associated with suspected ganskweek (*Lasiospermum bipinnatum*) poisoning in cattle. *J SA Vet Assoc.* 1994;65:122-124.

Puschner B, Holstege DM, Lamberski N, et al. Grayanotoxin poisoning in three goats. *J Am Vet Med Assoc.* 2001;218:573-575.

Radostits O, et al. Poisoning by miscellaneous phytotoxins. In: *Veterinary Medicine: A Textbook of the Disease of Cattle, Horses, Sheep, Goats and Pigs.* 10th ed. London: W.B. Saunders; 2007:1883.

Shlosberg A, Bellaiche M, Hanji V, et al. The effect of feeding dried tomato vines to beef cattle. *Vet Hum Toxicol.* 1996;135-136.

Storie GJ, McKenzie RA, Fraser IR. Suspected packalacca (*Phytolacca dioica*) poisoning of cattle and chickens. *Aust Vet J.* 1992;69:21-22.

Walker KH, Thompson DR, Seaman JT. Suspected poisoning of sheep by *Ixiolaena Brevicompta. Aust Vet J.* 1980;56:64-66.

Young S, Brown WW, Klinger B. Nigropallidal encephalomalacia in horses fed Russian knapweed (*Centaurea repens* L.). *Am J Vet Res.* 1970;31:1393-1404.

REFERENCES

1. Campbell A. *Companion Anim.* 2008;13:86.
2. Schep LJ, et al. *Clin Tox.* 2009;47:270.
3. Davis T, et al. *Toxicon.* 2013;76:247.
4. Davis T, et al. *Toxicon.* 2013;73:88.
5. Takeda Y, et al. *J Japan Vet Med Assoc.* 2007;60:47.
6. Panter KE, Gardner DR, Holstege D, et al. A case of acute water hemlock (*Cicuta maculata*) poisoning and death in cattle after ingestion of green seed heads. In: Panter KE, Wierenga T, Pfister JA, eds. *Poisonous Plants: Global Research and Solutions.* CAB International; 2007:259-264.
7. Stegelmeier BL, et al. *J Vet Diag Invest.* 2010;22:570.
8. Hallak M, et al. *Apoptosis.* 2008;13:147.
9. Dalzell SA, et al. *Anim Prod Sci.* 2012;52:365.
10. Aung A. *J Ag Sci Tech A.* 2011;1:764.
11. Phaikaew C, et al. *Anim Prod Sci.* 2012;52:283.
12. Jones RJ, et al. *Anim Prod Sci.* 2009;49:643.
13. Gorniak SL, et al. *Appl Anim Behav.* 2008;111:396.
14. Ferguson D, et al. *J Vet Intern Med.* 2011;25:831.
15. Cunha BM, Franca TN, Pinto MSF, et al. Poisoning by *Cycas revoluta* in dogs in Brazil. In: Riet-Correa F, Pfister J, Schild AL, Wierenga TL, eds. *Poisoning by Plants, Mycotoxins, and Other Toxins.* CAB International; 2011:221.
16. Jonasson S, et al. *Plant Biotech.* 2008;25:227.
17. Krüger T, et al. *Endocyt Cell Res.* 2012;22:29.
18. Finnie JW, et al. *Aust Vet J.* 2011;89:247.
19. Jansen SA, et al. *Cardiovasc Tox.* 2012;12:208.
20. Cortinovis C, et al. *Vet J.* 2013;197:163.
21. Bischoff K, et al. *Vet Clin N Am Food A.* 2011;27:459.
22. Ling LJ, et al. *Clin Res Toxicol.* 2006;19:1320.
23. Parkinson OT, et al. *J Vet Pharm Ther.* 2012;35:402.
24. Mawhinney I, et al. *Vet Rec.* 2008;162:62.
25. Nicholson SS. *Vet Clin N Am Food A.* 2011;27:447.
26. Chang HT, et al. *Vet Path.* 2012;49:398.
27. Freeman JL, et al. *Plant Physiol.* 2006;142:124.
28. Verdes JM, et al. *J Vet Diag Invest.* 2006;18:299.
29. Van der Lugt JJ, et al. *Vet J.* 2010;185:225.
30. Stegelmeier BL, Lee ST, James LF, et al. Cutleaf nightshade (*Solanum triflorum* Nutt.) toxicity in horses and hamsters. In: Panter KE, Wierenga TL, Pfister JA, eds. *Poisonous Plants: Global Research and Solutions.* CAB International; 2007:296.
31. Fontana PA, et al. *Pesq Vet Bras.* 2009;29:266.

TOXICOSIS FROM BREWER'S RESIDUES

Diseases associated with the feeding of by-products of brewing and distilling include the following:

- Carbohydrate engorgement in cattle fed wet brewer's grains
- Possibly spinal cord degeneration in adult cattle fed sorghum beer residues contaminated by *Aspergillus flavus* and containing aflatoxin
- Excess sulfur (>0.45% in the diet) from some methods of processing, which can lead to polioencephalomalacia

TRICHOTHECENE TOXICOSIS

Trichothecenes (TCT) are the largest group of mycotoxins and are among the most toxic.[1,2] They may produce toxic effects in the liver, kidney, gastrointestinal tract, central nervous system, immune system, or hematopoietic system or adversely affect productivity in many animals.[3-5] Trichothecenes exert these effects through several mechanisms, including inhibition of protein synthesis, inhibition of RNA and DNA synthesis, activation of cytokines, increased lipid peroxidation, dysfunction of mitochondria, and apoptosis.[6,7]

More than 180 TCT mycotoxins have been identified, all containing an epoxy group at the C12 to C13 portion of their chemical structure that is necessary for toxicity.[7,8] This epoxy group is necessary for toxicity.[1,9] They are divided into two different categories, the macrocyclic and the nonmacrocyclic trichothecenes, on the basis of their molecular structure. Chemically, they are divided into four types (A, B, C, D) based on substitutions at five different sites on the TCT molecule.[1,2] Type A contains T-2 toxin, HT-2 toxin, and 4,15-diacetoxyscirpenol (DAS); type B contains deoxynivalenol (DON) and nivalenol (NIV); type C contains crotocin and baccharin; and type D contains the macrocyclic mycotoxins such as verrucarin, roridin, and satratoxins.[1,2,6]

MACROCYCLIC TRICHOTHECENES

Trichothecene mycotoxins in this group include satratoxin, verrucarin, roridin and others.

The standard nomenclature for toxicity associated with this group of mycotoxins is retained, stachybotrytoxicosis and myrotheciotoxicosis.

Stachybotryotoxicosis

Toxins in the fungus *Stachybotrys chartarum (S. atra, S. alternans)*, which is associated with stachybotryotoxicosis, are the macrocyclic tricothecenes, satratoxins G and H, roridin E, and verrucarin J. These mycotoxins are found worldwide as contaminants of wet and decaying straw and hay.[10,11] Horses, cattle, sheep, and pigs may be affected, and the disease is characterized by fever, ruminal atony, diarrhea, dysentery, necrotic ulceration, hemorrhages of the nasal and oral mucosae causing epistaxis and purulent nasal discharge, and conjunctivitis causing lacrimation.[3] Drying and cracking of the skin are visible, especially peri-orbitally and on the face. At necropsy there are hemorrhages into all tissues and under all serous membranes. An important abnormality is the depression of leukocyte formation, causing agranulocytosis and producing a disease not unlike that associated with bracken poisoning in cattle. Hemorrhages are visible in the mucosae; there is also hemorrhagic enteritis. In sheep, *Pasteurella haemolytica* can often be isolated from tissues. The infection is thought to occur as a result of the immunosuppression associated with the toxins. In horses, there is also a subacute or acute myositis. The disease resembles alimentary toxic aleukia (ATA), associated with the ingestion of toxin from *Fusarium poae* and *Fusarium sporotrichioides*, in humans.[3]

Myrotheciotoxicosis

Roridin, a toxin in the fungus *Myrothecium roridum* and *Myrothecium verrucaria* growing on rye-grass and white clover plants in pasture, or on stored feeds, is associated with sudden death in sheep and cattle, with necropsy lesions of abomasitis, hepatitis, and pulmonary congestion and edema. Smaller intakes are associated with similar lesions, but over a course of 7 to 10 days. Very small doses administered over a 30-day period are associated with loss of weight but no deaths.

A bizarre involvement in what appears to be a plant poisoning is the role that *M. verrucaria* plays in *Baccharis* spp. poisoning. *Baccharis* spp., including *B. cordifolia, B. dranunculifolis, B. pteronioides* (synonym *B. ramulosa*), and *B. glomeruliflora,* are associated with tremor, stiff gait, and convulsions and some deaths in cattle and sheep. Roridin, a toxin produced by *Myrothecium* spp. growing in close apposition to the roots of the plants, is absorbed and, when eaten by animals, poisons them. In other plants roridin is lethal to the plant when present in very small amounts.

NONMACROCYCLIC TRICHOTHECENES

T-2 toxin and deoxynivalenol (DON) are well recognized TCT mycotoxins produced by several different genera of fungi, with many growing on cereal grains. Fungi producing these mycotoxins are not fully defined in terms of which toxins they produce, and many produce more than one. Accordingly, the syndromes described here, and attributed to specific fungi and toxins, are tentative. Any one or combination of them can be implicated in toxicity if they produce the specified toxin at the specified time. A partial list of well-known TCT producing fungi includes the following:

- *Cephalosporium* spp.
- *Fusarium acuinatum*
- *F. culmorum*
- *F. graminearum*
- *F. moniliforme*
- *F. nivale*
- *F. poae*
- *F. roseum*
- *F. semitectum*
- *F. sporotrichioides*
- *F. tricinctum*
- *Trichoderma* spp.
  Trichothecium spp.

T-2 Toxin and HT-2 Toxin

A sesquiterpene compound, the T_2 toxin is produced by several different *Fusarium* species, including *F. acuinatum, F. poae,* and *F. sporotrichoides* growing in cereal grains.[1] Occasionally, in areas of uncommonly cool and wet weather, pastures used for animal grazing have been contaminated with *Fusarium* production of T-2 toxin, HT-2 toxin, and other mycotoxins.[6] Species, age, amount or dose of toxin ingested, and route of exposure are important determinants in the level of toxicity and production of signs.[1]

Reported signs associated with poisoning include feed refusal, vomiting, weight loss, diarrhea, rough hair coats, and abortion.[1,6] Historically, T-2 toxin has been associated with a hemorrhagic syndrome, but this has not been a consistent finding. Experimental administration of the purified toxin parenterally produced a range of signs including emesis, posterior paresis, lethargy, hunger, and frequent defecation of normal stools, whereas oral administration of the T-2 toxin or cultures containing it to piglets and calves was associated with hemorrhagic disease. Field evidence of the relationship between the ingestion of the fungus and the appearance of hemorrhagic disease is strong, but the identity of the specific toxic agent may be in doubt. Alternatively, other effects have been reported. Ingestion of T-2 toxin is associated with immunosuppression when fed to laboratory animals, sheep, and pigs. This leads to leukopenia, lymphopenia, and atrophy of lymph nodes, thymus, and spleen, Blood coagulability is reduced because of the toxic effects on platelets.

T-2 toxin fed to pigs is associated with necrotic contact lesions on the snout and commissures of the mouth and the prepuce. Topical application of T_2 toxin to pig skin is associated with initial swelling and purple discoloration, followed by separation and sloughing by day 14. It has also been cited as the probable cause of congenital skin defects about the head and tarsus of pigs. The toxin also is associated with reproductive inefficiency when given experimentally to pigs, causing small litters, repeat breeders, and abortion.

Deoxynivalenol

Deoxynivalenol (synonym vomitoxin) is a sesquiterpene compound found in *Fusarium graminearum (roseum), F. culmorum,* and other species. It is a potent central emetic, to which pigs are very sensitive and ruminants more resistant.[6,12] The toxin may be associated with severe vomiting, acute diarrhea, dysentery, ataxia, mucosal hemorrhages, and sudden death.[6,12,13] The most common field observation about the toxic effect of DON fed to pigs is that it is associated with absolute feed refusal or reduction in weight gain and feed intake.[7] Deoxynivalenol is minimally excreted in the milk and accumulation in swine tissues meant for human consumption is low.[6,12]

The only effective method of preventing losses as a result of deoxynivalenol is to dilute affected corn with uncontaminated feed to levels unlikely to result in toxicosis. Mixing the feed with bentonite, sweeteners, or sodium-calcium aluminosilicate is ineffective as a detoxification method, but rinsing and removing floating material is recommended.[6] Feed toxic to pigs may be utilized by diluting and feeding it to adult ruminants.

Fusaritoxicosis Syndromes Without Specified Toxins

F. graminearum (roseum) produces toxins associated with emesis, refusal of feed, toxins lethal to pigs, and estrogenic substances causing infertility in pigs. *F. culmorum* also is associated with inappetence, scouring, ataxia, and a fall in milk yield when fed to cattle. The fungus *F. moniliforme* is associated with food refusal in cattle. Food refusal is also recorded with zearalenone. Ingestion of *Fusarium xylaroides* infected groundnut hay by cattle has resulted in anorexia, rumen atony, colic, tenesmus, and nasal and rectal hemorrhage.[14] Experimentally, when fed infected groundnut, calves developed diarrhea, weakness, ataxia, and conjunctival and cutaneous hemorrhage. Serum concentrations of urea nitrogen, creatinine, aspartate aminotransferase (AST), and alanine aminotransferase (ALT) were elevated. The toxin has not yet been identified.[14]

FURTHER READING

di Menna ME, Mortimer PH. Experimental myrotheciotoxicosis in sheep and calves. *NZ Vet J.* 1971;19:246-248.

Friend DW, Trenholm HL, Hartin KE, et al. Toxicity of T-2 toxin and its interaction with deoxynivalenol when fed to young pigs. *Can J Anim Sci.* 1992;72:703-711.

Friend DW, Trenholm HL, Elliot JL. Effect of feeding vomitoxin-contaminated wheat to pigs. *Can J Anim Sci.* 1982;62:1211-1222.

Radostits O, et al. *Veterinary Medicine: A Textbook of the Disease of Cattle, Horses, Sheep, Goats and Pigs.* 10th ed. London: W.B. Saunders; 2007:1910.

Trenholm HL, Thompson BK, Foster BC, et al. Effects of feeding diets containing *Fusarium* (naturally) contaminated wheat or pure deoxynivalenol (DON) in growing pigs. *Can J Anim Sci.* 1994;74:361-369.

Vertinskii KL. Stachybotryotoxicosis in horses. *Veterinariya.* 1940;17:61-68.

REFERENCES

1. Li Y, et al. *J Agric Food Chem.* 2011;59:3441.
2. Barthel J, et al. *Mycotoxin Res.* 2012;28:97.
3. Paterson RM, Lima N. Toxicology of mycotoxins. In: Luch A, ed. *Molecular, Clinical and Environmental Toxicology, Clinical Toxicology.* Switzerland: Birkhäuser Basel; 2010:31-63.
4. Pinton P, et al. *Curr Immunol Rev.* 2012;8:193.
5. Caloni G, et al. *Toxicon.* 2009;54:337.
6. Mostrom M, et al. *Vet Clin N Am Food A.* 2011;27:315.
7. Pestka JJ. *Arch Toxicol.* 2010;84:663.
8. Fink-Gremmels J. *Vet J.* 2008;176:84.
9. Zain ME. *J Saudi Chem Soc.* 2011;15:129.
10. Pieckova E, et al. *Ann Agric Environ Med.* 2006;13:259.
11. Gottschalk C, et al. *Mycotoxin Res.* 2006;22:189.
12. Pestka JJ. *Anim Feed Sci Tech.* 2007;137:283.
13. Chaytor AC, et al. *J Anim Sci.* 2011;89:124.
14. Tikare V, et al. *Indian J Anim Res.* 2011;45:180.

TRITERPENE PLANT TOXICOSIS

Toxic triterpenes include the following:

- Cucurbitacins, tetracyclic triterpenes found in *Cucumis africanus* and *Cucumis myriocarpus, Stemodia kingii* and *Stemodia florulenta*, and *Ecballium elaterium*
- Lantadenes A and B, and triterpene acids found in *Lantana* spp.[1]
- Icterogenins A, B, and C in *Lippia* spp.
- Meliatoxins A, A_1, B, and B_1, tetranortriterpenes, found in *Melia azederach* (chinaberry tree)[2]
- Colocynthin, a glucoside found in the fruit of the vine *Citrullus colocynthis* (synonym *Colocynthis vulgaris*).

Cucurbitacins are a group of tetracyclic triterpenes found in the fruits of the vines *C. africanus, C. melo* var. agrestis (Ulcardo melon), *C. myriocarpus* (prickly paddymelon), and *E. elaterium* (squirting cucumber). The ripe fruits are most toxic, and in cattle, sheep, and horses are associated with a syndrome of lethargy, dehydration, abdominal pain, diarrhea, dyspnea, and death in a matter of a few hours. Necropsy findings include edema and necrosis of the ruminal epithelium, intense congestion and hemorrhage in the intestinal mucosa, pulmonary congestion and edema, and hepatopathy in some cases. Seeds of the plant are conspicuous in the ruminal contents.

Icterogenins and lantadenes are associated with liver damage and nephrosis, neither of which is specific, but the lantadenes cause damage to bile canaliculi, gallbladder paralysis, and intrahepatic cholestasis.[3-5] Jaundice, photosensitization, and ruminal stasis result.[3,4] *Lantana* spp. is a very pungent plant, and cattle will eat it only if other feed is scarce.[6] *Bos taurus* cattle at one time were felt to be more susceptible to lantadene poisoning than *Bos indicus* cattle, but that is no felt to be true.[6] Treatment with activated charcoal or bentonite is effective in decreasing absorption of the toxins.

Pigs are most commonly poisoned by meliatoxins, but cattle, sheep, and goats are also susceptible. Meliatoxin administered to pigs is associated with a syndrome of gastroenteritis manifested by diarrhea, melena, and vomiting, plus dyspnea as a result of pulmonary edema. The toxic dose in pigs is 0.5% of body weight. Pigs fed ground chinaberries at 5 g/kg BW developed mild diarrhea and rapidly recovered. Those fed 10 g/kg BW, 15 g/kg BW, and 20 g/kg BW developed muscle tremors, ataxia, incoordination, and recumbency 2 to 24 hours after dosing. Other observed signs included hypothermia and vocalization (moans, screams). Death occurred in the 20 g/kg BW group.[2,7]

FURTHER READING

Hare WR, Garland T, Barr AC. Chinaberry (*Melia azedarach*) poisoning in animals. In: Garland T, Barr AC, eds. *Toxic Plants and Other Natural Toxicants.* CAB International; 1998:514-516.

McKenzie RA, Newman RD, Rayner AC, et al. Prickly paddy melon (*Cucumis myriocarpus*) poisoning of cattle. *Aust Vet J.* 1988;65:167-170.

Pass MA. Current ideas on the pathophysiology and treatment of lantana poisoning of ruminants. *Aust Vet J.* 1986;6:169-171.

REFERENCES

1. Sharma OP. *CRC Cr Rev Toxicol.* 2007;37:313.
2 Burrows GE, Tyrl RJ. *Meliaceae Juss. Toxic Plants of North America.* 2nd ed. Wiley-Blackwell; 2013:825.
3. Kumar N. *Indian Vet J.* 2009;86:725.
4. Rivero R, et al. *Veterinaria (Montevideo).* 2011;47:29.
5. Cooper RG. *Turk J Vet Anim Sci.* 2007;3:213.
6. Burrows GE, Tyrl RJ. Lantana. In: *Toxic Plants of North America.* 2nd ed. Wiley-Blackwell; 2013:1203.
7. Méndez M, et al. *Pesq Vet Bras.* 2006;26:26.

APPENDIX 1

Conversion Tables

CONVERSION FACTORS FOR OLD AND SI UNITS

	Old units	MULTIPLICATION FACTORS Old units to SI units	SI units to old units	SI units
RBC	$\times 10^6/mm^3$	10^6	10^{-6}	$\times 10^{12}/L$
PCV	%	0.01	100	L/L
Hb	g/dL	None	None	g/dL
MCV	μ^3	None	None	fL
MCH	μμg	None	None	pg
MCHC	%	None	None	g/dL
WBC	$\times 10^3/mm^3$	10^6	10^{-6}	$\times 10^9/L$
Platelets	$\times 10^3/mm^3$	10^6	10^{-6}	$\times 10^9/L$
Total serum				
Protein	g/dL	10	0.1	g/L
Albumin	g/dL	10	0.1	g/L
Bicarbonate	mEq/L	None	None	mmol/L
Bilirubin	mg/dL	17.1	0.0585	μmol/L
Calcium	mg/dL	0.25	4.008	mmol/L
Chloride	mEq/L	None	None	mmol/L
Cholesterol	mg/dL	0.0259	38.7	mmol/L
Copper	μg/dL	0.157	6.35	μmol/L
Cortisol	μg/dL	27.6	0.0362	nmol/L
Creatinine	mg/dL	88.4	0.0113	μmol/L
Globulin	g/dL	10	0.1	g/L
Glucose	mg/dL	0.0555	18.02	mmol/L
Inorganic phosphate	mg/dL	0.323	3.10	mmol/L
Iron	μg/dL	0.179	5.59	μmol/L
Lead	μg/dL	0.0483	20.7	μmol/L
Magnesium	mg/dL	0.411	2.43	mmol/L
Molybdenum	μg/dL	0.104	9.6	μmol/L
Potassium	mEq/L	None	None	mmol/L
Selenium	μg/dL	0.126	7.9	μmol/L
Sodium	mEq/L	None	None	mmol/L
Triglyceride	mg/dL	0.0113	88.5	mmol/L
Urea nitrogen	mg/dL	0.3570	2.8	mmol/L
Urea	mg/dL	0.1665	6.01	mmol/L
Zinc	μg/dL	0.15	6.54	μmol/L

CONVERSIONS

To convert grams per 100 mL into grains per U.S. fluid ounce	–	multiply by 4.564
To convert grams per 100 mL into grains per Imperial fluid ounce	–	multiply by 4.385
To convert grams into ounces avoirdupois	–	multiply by 10 and divide by 283
To convert liters into U.S. pints	–	multiply by 2.114
To convert liters into Imperial pints	–	multiply by 88 and divide by 50
To convert kilograms into pounds	–	multiply by 1000 and divide by 454

TEMPERATURE

Celsius (centigrade)	Fahrenheit
110°	230°
100	212
95	203
90	194
85	185
80	176
75	167
70	158
65	149
60	140
55	131
50	122
45	113
44	111.2
43	109.4
42	107.6
41	105.8
40.5	104.9
40	104.0
39.5	103.1
39	102.2
38.5	101.3
38	100.4
37.5	99.5
37	98.6
36.5	97.7
36	96.8
35.5	95.9
35	95
34	93.2
33	91.4
32	89.6
31	87.8
30	86
25	77
20	68
15	59
10	50
+5	41
0	32
–5	23
–10	14
–15	+5
–20	–4

To convert Fahrenheit into Celsius: subtract 32, multiply the remainder by 5, and divide the result by 9.

To convert Celsius into Fahrenheit: multiply by 9, divide by 5, and add 32.

MASS

Metric		U.S./Imperial	
1 kilogram (kg)	= 15,432 grains *or* 35.274 ounces *or* 2.2046 pounds	1 ton (2240 lb) 1 hundredweight (112 lb) (cwt)	= 1016 kilograms = 50.80 kilograms
1 gram (g)	= 15.432 grains	1 stone (14 lb) (st)	= 6.35 kilograms
1 milligram (mg)	= 0.015432 grains	1 pound (avoirdupois) (lb) 1 ounce (avoirdupois) (oz) 1 grain (gr)	= 453.59 grams = 28.35 grams = 64.799 milligrams

CAPACITY

Metric	
1 liter (L)	= 2.114 U.S. pints = 1.7598 Imperial pints
1 milliliter (mL)	= 16.23 U.S. minims = 16.894 Imperial minims

U.S. Liquid		Imperial	
1 gallon (128 fl oz) (gall)	= 3.785 liters	1 gallon (160 fl oz) (gal)	= 4.546 liters
1 pint (pt)	= 473.17 milliliters	1 pint (pt)	= 568.25 milliliters
1 fluid ounce (fl oz)	= 29.573 milliliters	1 fluid ounce (fl oz)	= 28.412 milliliters
1 fluid dram (fl dr)	= 3.696 milliliters	1 fluid dram (fl dr)	= 3.5515 milliliters
1 minim (min)	= 0.061610 milliliters	1 minim (min)	= 0.059192 milliliters

LENGTH

Metric		US/Imperial		Pressure	
1 kilometer (km)	= 0.621 miles	1 mile	= 1.609 kilometers	1 kilopascal (kPa)	= 10.197 cm H_2O
1 meter (m)	= 39.370 inches	1 yard	= 0.914 meters	1 kilopascal (kPa)	= 7.50 mm Hg
1 decimeter (dm)	= 3.9370 inches	1 foot	= 30.48 centimeters	1 kilopascal (kPa)	= 0.145 pounds per square inch (PSI)
1 centimeter (cm)	= 0.39370 inch	1 inch	= 2.54 centimeters *or* 25.40 millimeters	1 atmosphere	= 760 mm Hg
1 millimeter (mm)	= 0.039370 inch			1 mm Hg	= 1.359 cm H_2O = 0.133 kPa = 0.0193 PSI
1 micrometer (μm)	= 0.000039370 inch				

APPENDIX

2

Reference Laboratory Values

Reference values for some frequently measured variables in blood and serum are provided as a guide. Values of these variables from healthy animals vary depending on many factors, including age, breed, sex, diet, geographical habitat, and methods of sample collection and laboratory measurement. The values listed here are compiled from a variety of sources, including the clinical laboratories of the Western College of Veterinary Medicine at the University of Saskatchewan, the College of Veterinary Medicine at The Ohio State University, and Kaneko JJ. *Clinical biochemistry of domestic animals*, 5th ed. New York: Academic Press, 1997.

Tables of reference values for newborn foals and calves are provided elsewhere.

HEMATOLOGY

	Cattle	Sheep	Goat	Swine	Horses
Hemoglobin (g/dL)	8.5–12.2	9.0–15.0	8.0–12.0	10.0–16.0	11.0–19.0
Hematocrit (packed cell volume) (%)	22–33	27–45	22–38	32–50	32–53
RBC ($\times 10^6/\mu L$)	5.1–7.6	9.0–15.0	8.0–18.0	5.0–8.0	6.8–12.9
MCV (fL)	38–50	28–40	16–25	50–68	37–59
MCH (pg)	14–18	8.0–12.0	5.2–8.0	17.0–21.0	12.3–19.7
MCHC (g/dL)	36–39	31.0–34.0	30.0–36.0	30.0–34.0	31.0–38.6
RDW (%)	15.5–19.7				
Thrombocytes (per µL)	200,000–650,000	800,000–1,100,000	300,000–600,000	320,000–715,000	100,000–600,000
WBC (per/µL)	4900–12,000	4000–12,000	4000–13,000	11,000–22,000	5400–14,300
Neutrophils (mature) (per/µL)	1800–6300	700–6000	1000–7200	3100–10,500	2300–8500
Neutrophils (band cells) (per/µL)	Rare	Rare	Rare	0–880	0–100
Lymphocytes (per/µL)	1600–5600	2000–9000	2000–9000	4300–13 600	1500–7700
Monocytes (per/µL)	0–800	0–750	0–550	200–2200	0–1000
Eosinophils (per/µL)	0–900	0–1000	0–650	0–2400	0–1000
Fibrinogen (mg/dL)	200–700	100–500	100–400	100–500	200–400

Hematology (International units, SI)

	Cattle	Sheep	Goat	Swine	Horses
Hemoglobin (g/L)	85–122	90–150	80–120	100–160	110–190
Hematocrit (packed cell volume) (L/L)	0.22–0.33	0.27–0.45	0.22–0.38	0.32–0.50	0.32–0.53
RBC ($\times 10^{12}/L$)	5.1–7.6	9.0–15.0	8.0–18.0	5.0–8.0	6.8–12.9
MCV (fL)	38–50	28–40	16–25	50–68	37–59
MCH (pg)	14–18	8.0–12.0	5.2–8.0	17.0–21.0	12.3–19.7
MCHC (g/L)	360–390	310–340	300–360	300–340	310–386
RDW (%)	15.5–19.7	18.0–24.6			
Thrombocytes ($\times 10^9/\mu L$)	200–650	800–1100	300–600	320–715	100–600
WBC ($\times 10^9/L$)	4.9–12.0	4.0–12.0	4.0–13.0	11.0–22.0	5.4–14.3
Neutrophils (mature) ($\times 10^9/L$)	1.8–6.3	0.7–6.0	1.2–7.2	3.1–10.5	2.3–8.5
Neutrophils (band cells) ($\times 10^9/L$)	Rare	Rare	1.0–7.2	0–0.9	0–0.1
Lymphocytes ($\times 10^9/L$)	1.6–5.6	2.0–9.0	2.0–9.0	4.3–13.6	1.5–7.7
Monocytes ($\times 10^9/L$)	0–0.8	0–0.8	0–0.6	0.2–2.2	0–1.0
Eosinophils ($\times 10^9/L$)	0–0.9	0–1.0	0–0.7	0–2.4	0–1.0
Fibrinogen (g/L)	2–7	1–5	1–4	1–5	2–4

Serum constituents (U.S. units)

	Cattle	Sheep	Swine	Horses
Electrolytes				
Sodium (mEq/L)	132–152	145–152	140–150	132–146
Potassium (mE/qL)	3.9–5.8	3.9–5.4	4.7–7.1	3.0–5.0
Chloride (mEq/L)	95–110	95–103	94–103	98–110
Osmolality (mOsmol/kg)	270–306	270–300		270–290
Acid-base status				
pH (venous)	7.35–7.50	7.32–7.50		7.32–7.46
PCO_2 (venous) (mm of Hg)	34–45	38–45		38–46
Bicarbonate (mEq/L)	20–30	21–28	18–27	23–32
Total carbon dioxide (mEq/L)	20–30	20–28	17–26	22–31
Anion gap (mEq/L)	14–26	12–24	10–25	10–25
Minerals				
Calcium, total (mg/dL)	9.7–12.4	11.5–13.0	7.1–11.6	11.2–13.6
Calcium, ionized (mg/dL)	4.0–5.2	4.0–4.8	3.5–5.8	5.6–6.8
Phosphorus (mg/dL)	5.6–6.5	5.0–7.3	5.3–9.6	3.1–5.6
Magnesium (mg/dL)	1.8–2.3	2.2–2.8	2.7–3.7	2.2–2.8
Iron (µg/dL)	57–162	166–222	56–190	91–199
Iron-binding capacity (µg/dL)	240–450		270–557	270–390
Renal function				
Urea nitrogen (mg/dL)	6.0–27	8.0–20	10–30	10–24
Creatinine (mg/dL)	1.0–2.0	1.2–1.9	1.0–2.7	0.9–1.9
Liver function				
Total bilirubin (mg/dL)	0.01–0.5	0.1–0.5	0–1.0	1.0–2.0
Direct (conjugated) bilirubin (mg/dL)	0.04–0.44	0–0.27	0–0.3	0–0.4
Bile acids (µg/mL)	<50	<10		4–8
Metabolites				
Ammonia (µg/dL)				13–108
Cholesterol (mg/dL)	65–220	52–76	54–120	46–180
Free fatty acids (mg/L)	<30	30–100		
Glucose (mg/dL)	45–75	50–80	85–150	75–115
Ketones				
Acetoacetate (mg/dL)	0–1.1	0.27–0.35		0.24–0.36
Acetone (mg/dL)	0.7–5.5	0–10		
β-Hydroxybutyrate (mg/dL)	5.9–13.9	4.7–6.7		0.55–0.80
Lactate (mg/dL)	5–20	9–12		10–16
Triglyceride (mg/dL)	0–14			9–44
Hormones				
Cortisol (µg/dL)	0.47–0.75	1.40–3.10	2.6–3.3	2–6
Thyroxine (T4) (µg/dL)	4.2–8.6			See Table 29.8
Triiodothyronine (T3) (ng/dL)				See Table 29.8
Enzymes				
Alanine aminotransferase (ALT) (units/L)	11–40	5–20	31–58	3–23
Alkaline phosphatase (units/L)	0–200	70–390	120–400	140–400
Aspartate aminotransferase (AST) (units/L)	78–132	60–280	32–84	220–600
Creatine kinase (units/L)	35–280			145–380
γ-Glutamyl transferase (units/L)	6.1–17.4	20–52	10–60	4–44
Isocitrate dehydrogenase (units/L)	9.4–21.9	0.5–8.0		
Lactate dehydrogenase (units/L)	692–1445	240–440	380–630	160–410
Sorbitol dehydrogenase (units/L)	4.3–15.3	5.8–28	1.0–5.8	1.9–5.8
Protein				
Total protein (g/dL)	5.7–8.1	6.0–7.9	4.5–7.5	6.0–7.7
Albumin (g/dL)	2.1–3.6	2.4–3.0	1.9–4.0	2.9–3.8

Serum constituents (International units, SI)

	Cattle	Sheep	Swine	Horses
Electrolytes				
Sodium (mmol/L)	132–152	145–152	140–150	132–146
Potassium (mmol/L)	3.9–5.8	3.9–5.4	4.7–7.1	3.0–5.0
Chloride (mmol/L)	95–110	95–103	94–103	98–110
Osmolality (mmol/kg)	270–306	270–300		270–290
Acid-base status				
pH (venous)	7.35–7.50	7.32–7.50		7.32–7.46
PCO_2 (venous) (mm of Hg)	34–45	38–45		38–46
Bicarbonate (mEq/L)	20–30	21–28	18–27	23–32
Total carbon dioxide (mEq/L)	20–30	20–28	17–26	22–31
Minerals				
Calcium, total (mmol/L)	2.43–3.10	2.88–3.20	1.78–2.90	2.80–3.44
Calcium, ionized (mmol/L)	1.0–1.3	1.0–1.2	0.9–1.4	1.4–1.7
Phosphorus (mmol/L)	1.8–2.1	1.62–2.36	1.7–3.1	0.70–1.68
Magnesium (mmol/L)	0.74–1.10	0.90–1.26	1.1–1.5	0.9–1.2
Iron (μmol/L)	10–29	30–40	10–34	16–36
Iron-binding capacity (μmol/L)	42–80		48–100	45–73
Renal function				
Urea nitrogen (mmol/L)	2.0–9.6	3.0–7.1	3.0–8.5	3.5–8.6
Creatinine (μmol/L)	88–175	106–168	90–240	80–170
Liver function				
Total bilirubin (μmol/L)	0.17–8.55	1.71–8.55	0–17.1	17–35
Direct (conjugated) bilirubin (μmol/L)	0.7–7.54	0–4.61	0–5.1	0–6.8
Bile acids (μmol/L)	<120	<25		10–20
Metabolites				
Ammonia (μmol/L)				7.6–63.4
Cholesterol (mmol/L)	1.7–5.6	1.3–2.0	1.4–3.10	1.20–4.6
Glucose (mmol/L)	2.5–4.2	2.8–4.4	4.7–8.3	4.2–6.4
Ketones				
Acetoacetate (mmol/L)	0.0–0.11	0.026–0.034		0.023–0.035
Acetone (mmol/L)	0.1–1.0	0–1.7		
β-Hydroxybutyrate (mmol/L)	0.35–0.47	0.47–0.63		0.052–0.076
Lactate (mmol/L)	0.6–2.2	1.0–1.3		1.1–1.8
Triglyceride (mmol/L)	0–0.2			0.1–0.5
Hormones				
Cortisol (nmol/L)	13–21	39–86	72–91	55–165
Thyroxine (T4) (nmol/L)	54–110			See Table 29.8
Triiodothyronine (T3) (nmol/L)				See Table 29.8
Enzymes				
Alanine aminotransferase (ALT) (units/L)	11–40	5–20	31–58	3–23
Alkaline phosphatase (units/L)	0–200	70–390	120–400	140–400
Aspartate aminotransferase (AST) (units/L)	78–132	60–280	32–84	220–600
Creatine kinase (units/L)	35–280			145–380
γ-Glutamyl transferase (units/L)	6.1–17.4	20–52	10–60	4–44
Isocitrate dehydrogenase (units/L)		0.5–8.0		5–18
Lactate dehydrogenase (units/L)	692–1445	240–440	380–630	160–410
Sorbitol dehydrogenase (units/L)	4.3–15.3	5.8–28	1.0–5.8	1.9–5.8
Protein				
Total protein (g/L)	57–81	60–79	45–75	60–77
Albumin (g/L)	21–36	24–30	19–40	29–38

APPENDIX

3 Drug doses and intervals for horses and ruminants

Suggested drug doses and intervals for horses and ruminants are provided here. Dosages listed are general recommendations and might not be optimal or efficacious in all instances and might need to be adjusted depending on the disease and its severity; patient factors, including but not limited to age or diet; and because of regulatory considerations regarding milk and meat withholding times in animals intended as human food. The manufacturer's recommendations should be checked before administering any drug, and the effect on withholding time of varying from the manufacturer's recommendation regarding dosing should be considered. Local regulations regarding use of drugs in animals that could be used for human food should be consulted.

Doses are given in milligrams per kilogram body weight (mg/kg) unless otherwise stated (g = gram, IU = international units). Drugs given as total doses, such as intramammary preparations, are denoted by TD. Dosing interval is given in hours, unless otherwise stated, or unless given as a single dose (SD). The route of administration is indicated as follows: intravenous (IV), intramuscular (IM), oral (PO), subcutaneous (SC), intraarticular (IA), intramammary (IMM), intraperitoneal (IP), inhalation (IH), per rectum (PR), topically (TO), or subconjunctivally (IO). Drugs recommended not to be given to certain species are indicated by NR.

	HORSES			RUMINANTS (CATTLE, SHEEP, GOATS)		
Drug	**Dose (mg/kg)**	**Interval (h)**	**Route**	**Dose (mg/kg)**	**Interval (h)**	**Route**
Acepromazine maleate	0.044–0.088	SD	IM, IV, SC	0.01–0.02 0.03–0.1	SD SD	IV IM
Acetazolamide	2.2	6–12	PO			
Acetylcysteine	8 g, TD (for (retained meconium in foal)	SD	PR			
Acetylsalicylic acid (aspirin)	10–20	48	PO	50–100	12	PO
Acyclovir	10 20	12 8	IV as 1-h infusion (foal) PO (adult)			
Adrenaline; *see* Epinephrine						
Albendazole	25–50	SD-12	PO	10 7.5	SD SD	PO (cattle, goat) PO (sheep)
Albuterol	0.001–0.008	4–8	IH			
Altrenogest	0.044	24	PO			
Aluminum hydroxide	60	6–8	PO	15–60	SD, 8–24	PO
Amantadine	5	4	IV			
hydrochloride						
Amikacin sulfate	22 (foals) 10 (adults)	24 24	IV, IM IV, IM	NR		
Aminocaproic acid	40 10–20	SD 6	IV IV			
Amiodarone	Intravenous infusion of 5 mg/kg/h for 1 h, then 0.8 mg/kg/h for 23 h, then 1.9 mg/kg/h; for atrial fibrillation					
Aminopropazine fumarate	0.5	SD	IM, IV			
Amitraz	NR			Goats: 11 mL of 19.9% solution diluted in 7.5 liters		Topical
Ammonium chloride	60–520	24	PO	50–200	12–24	PO
Ammonium molybdate				50–200 TD	24	PO
Ammonium tetrathiomolybdate				1.7–3.4	48	IV; SC (3 treatments)
Amoxicillin sodium	11–50	6–8	IM, IV	22	12	SC
Amoxicillin/potassium clavulanate	15–25	6–8	IV			

	HORSES			RUMINANTS (CATTLE, SHEEP, GOATS)		
Drug	**Dose (mg/kg)**	**Interval (h)**	**Route**	**Dose (mg/kg)**	**Interval (h)**	**Route**
Amoxicillin trihydrate	6–22 NR	6–12	IM	11–22	12–24	SC
Amphotericin B	0.3–0.6	24–48	IV (dilute, slow)			
Ampicillin sodium	10–50	6–8	IM, IV	22	12	SC, IV
Ampicillin trihydrate	10–22 NR	6–8	IM, PO	4–22	12–24	IM, SC
Amprolium hydrochloride	NR			5–10 (calves), 15 (lambs), 50 (kids)	24	PO PO
Apramycin sulfate				20–40 (calves)	24	PO
Ascorbic acid (vitamin C)	30 1000–2000	12–24, SD 24	IV PO (red maple poisoning)	3 g TD (calves)	SD	SC
Aspirin (*see* Acetylsalicylic acid)						
Atipamezole	0.05–0.1	SD	IV	0.02–0.1	SD	IV
Atracurium besylate	0.15 then 0.06–0.2	SD or to effect	IV	0.5 then 0.2 to effect (sheep)	SD or to effect	IV
Atropine sulfate	0.001–0.003 (bronchodilation) 0.22 (organophosphate toxicity)	SD As needed	IV IV, IM, SC	0.06–0.12 (pre-anesthetic) 0.5 (organophosphate toxicity)	SD 4	IV, IM, SC IV, IM, SC
Aurothioglucose	1	7d	IM			
Azathioprine	2–5 loading dose then every 24 h		PO			
Azlocillin	25–75	6–12	IV			
Azithromycin	10	24 h for 5 days then q48 h	PO			
Bacampicillin sodium	20	12	PO			
BAL (British anti-Lewisite); *see* Dimercaprol.						
Baquiloprim/sulfadimidine				40–80	48	PO
Beclomethasone	0.001–0.003	12	IH			
Benztropine mesylate	0.018	8	IV			
Betamethasone	0.02–0.1	24	IM, PO			
Bethanechol chloride	0.05–0.75	SD, 8	SC, IV	0.07	8	SC
Bismuth subsalicylate	0.5 mL/kg	4–6	PO	60–90 mL, TD (calves)	6–12	PO
Boldenone undecylenate	1.1	3 weeks	IM			
Bretylium	5–10	10 min until conversion	IV			
Bromhexine hydrochloride	0.1–0.25	24	IM, PO	0.2–0.5	24	IM, PO
Bromide, potassium	20–40	24	PO			
Bromocriptine mesylate	0.01	12	IM			
Buprenorphine hydrochloride	0.004–0.006	SD	IV			
Buscopan®; *see* Hyoscine						
Buserelin	0.04	SD	IM, IV, SC	0.02	SD	IM, IV, SC
Butorphanol tartrate	0.02–0.1	SD,3 4	IV, IM	0.02–0.04	SD	IV, IM
Calcium EDTA	35	12	IV slow			
Calcium gluconate	150–250	SD	IV (slow, to effect)	150–250	SD	IV (slow, to effect), SC, IP
Cambendazole	20	SD	PO			
Carbenicillin sodium	50–100	6–12	IV			
	6 g, TD	SD	Uterus			
Carprofen	0.7	24	IV	1.4 (cattle)	SD	IV, SC
Casein (iodinated)	0.01	24	PO			
Cefamandole	10–30	4–8	IV, IM			
Cefazolin sodium	25 (adults) 15–20 (foals)	6–8 8–12	IV, IM IV			

Continued

	HORSES			RUMINANTS (CATTLE, SHEEP, GOATS)		
Drug	**Dose (mg/kg)**	**Interval (h)**	**Route**	**Dose (mg/kg)**	**Interval (h)**	**Route**
Cefoperazone sodium	30–50	6–8	IV, IM	250 TD	SD	IMM
Cefotaxime sodium	20–30	6–8	IV			
Cefoxitin sodium	20	4–6	IV			
Cefpodoxime proxetil	10–12	8–12	PO (foals)			
Ceftiofur crystalline free acid	6.6 mg/kg IM, 2 doses given 4 days apart			6.6 1.1–2.2	SD 24	SC into posterior aspect of ear IM, SC (3–5 days)
Ceftiofur hydrochloride				125 mg TD 500 mg TD (dry cow)	24 SD	IMM IMM
Ceftiofur sodium	2.2–4.4	24	IV, IM	1.1–2.2	24	IM, IV
Ceftriaxone sodium	25–50	12	IV, IM			
Cefuroxime				250 mg TD 40	12 12	IMM IM (goats)
Cephacetrile sodium				250	SD	IMM
Cephalexin	25–33	6	PO			
Cephalothin sodium	10–30	6	IM, IV	55	6	SC
Cephapirin sodium	20–30 50	8–12 8–12	IM, IV PO	200 TD	12	IMM
Cephapirin benzathine				300, TD	SD	IMM
Charcoal (activated)	750 g (adults)	8–12	PO	1–3 g	8–12	PO
Chloral hydrate	20–200 40–100	SD 6–12	IV PO			
Chloramphenicol palmitate	25–50	6–8	PO	NR		
Chloramphenicol sodium succinate	20–60	6–8	IV, IM	NR		
Chlorpromazine hydrochloride	NR			0.22–1.0 (cattle) 0.6–4.4 (sheep and goats)	SD SD	IM IM
Chlortetracycline				6–10 10–20	24 24	IM, IV PO
Chorionic gonadotropin (HCG)	1000–3000 U, TD	SD	IM, IV, SC	2500–5000 IU, TD (cattle) 10,000 IU, TD (cattle) 250–1000 IU, TD	SD SD SD	IV IM IV, IM
Cimetidine hydrochloride	6.6 18	4–6 8	IV PO	8–16 50–100	8 8	IV PO (calves)
Cisapride	0.1 0.5–1.0	8–12 8–12	IV PO	NR		
Clarithromycin	7.5	12	PO (foals)			
Clenbuterol	0.0008–0.0032 (0.8–3.2 μg/kg) 0.0008	12 12	PO IV			
Clioquinol	0.02	12–24	PO			
Cloprostenol sodium	0.1, TD	SD	IM	0.5, TD (cattle) 0.06–0.13 TD (goats and sheep)	SD SD	IM IM
Closantel				10 (sheep)	SD	PO
Clorsulon				7	SD	PO
Cloxacillin, benzathine				500, TD	SD	IMM
Cloxacillin, sodium	10–30	6	IM, IV	200, TD	12	IMM
Colistin	2500 IU	6	IV (slow)			
Colony stimulating factor (granulocyte)	0.005	24	IV			
Cromolyn sodium	80–300, TD	24	IH			

	HORSES			RUMINANTS (CATTLE, SHEEP, GOATS)		
Drug	**Dose (mg/kg)**	**Interval (h)**	**Route**	**Dose (mg/kg)**	**Interval (h)**	**Route**
Cyclophosphamide	2.0	3 weeks	IV			
Cyproheptadine hydrochloride	0.25–1.2	12–24	PO			
Dalteparin sodium	50 U	12	SC			
Danofloxacin				8 6	SD 48	SC SC (only repeat once)
Dantrolene sodium	2	6	IV			
	2–10	24	PO			
Decoquinate				0.5	24	PO
Dembrexine hydrochloride	0.3	12	PO			
Deferoxamine mesylate	10	SD	IM, IV	10	SD	IM, IV
Detomidine hydrochloride	0.005–0.08	SD, 2–4	IV, IM	0.002–0.02	SD	IV, IM
Dexamethasone	0.01–0.2 (anti-inflammatory) 0.5–2 (shock)	24 SD	IV, IM, PO IV, IM	20–30 TD (cattle, induction of parturition) 0.02–2 (cattle, anti-inflammatory dose) 5–20, TD (cattle, ketosis)	SD 24 SD, 24	IM IV, IM IM
Dexamethasone sodium phosphate; *see* Dexamethasone						
Dexamethasone 21-isonicotinate; *see* Dexamethasone						
Diazepam	0.05–0.4 0.5	SD SD	IV IM	0.4 (calves)	SD	IV
Dichlorvos	35	SD	PO			
Diclofenac of 1% cream	12.5 cm strip	12	TO			
Dicloxacillin sodium	10	6	IM			
Diethylcarbamazine hydrochloride				22	24	IM
Digoxin	0.002 0.01–0.02	12 12–24	IV PO	0.022 loading dose then 0.0034	 4	IV IV
Dihydrostreptomycin	11	12	IM, SC	11	12	IM, SC
Dimercaprol	5 then 3 then 1	SD 6 for 4 doses, then 6 for 8 doses	IM	3	4 for 2 days, then 6 for 1 day, then 12 for 10 days	IM
Dimethyl glycine	1–2	24	PO			
Dimethyl sulfoxide (DMSO)	0.5–2 100 g, TD	12–24 12–24	IV (as 10% solution, slowly), PO topical	NR		
Dimophebumine hydrochloride				1.0–1.5 g TD (cattle) 150–250, TD (sheep)	SD SD	IM IM
Dinoprost tromethamine	0.002–0.01	SD	IM	25 TD (cattle, estrus induction) 25 TD (cattle, abortifacient) 8 TD (ewe, estrus induction) 8 TD (doe, estrus induction 10–15 TD (ewe, abortifacient) 5–10 TD (doe, abortifacient)	10–12 days SD days 5 and 11 of cycle days 4 and 11 of cycle <60 days pregnancy entire pregnancy	IM IM IM IM IM IM IM

Continued

Drug	HORSES			RUMINANTS (CATTLE, SHEEP, GOATS)		
	Dose (mg/kg)	**Interval (h)**	**Route**	**Dose (mg/kg)**	**Interval (h)**	**Route**
Dioctyl sodium sulfosuccinate (DSS)	10–20	48 (limit 2 doses)	PO			
Diphenhydramine hydrochloride	0.5–1	6–8	IV, IM	0.5–1.0	6–8	IV, IM
Diprenorphine	0.03 (horses) 0.015 (donkeys)	SD	IV	0.03 (cattle) 0.015 (sheep)	SD	IV
Dipyrone	11–22	SD, 8	IV, IM	50	SD	IM, IV, SC
Dobutamine hydrochloride	1–10 µg/kg/min	Infusion	IV			
Docusate; *see* Dioctyl sodium sulfosuccinate						
Domperidone	0.2 1.1	SD, 12 24	IV PO			
Dopamine hydrochloride	1–10 µg/kg/min	Infusion	IV	2–10 µg/kg/min	Infusion	IV
Doramectin				0.2	SD	IM, SC
Doxapram hydrochloride	0.02–1	SD	IV	5–10	SD	IV
Doxycycline	10	12	PO (do not use IV)			
Doxylamine succinate	0.55	8	IM, SC, IV (slow)	0.5	12	PO, IM, SC
Edetate calcium disodium (EDTA)	75	24	IV (slow, dilute)	67	12	IV (slow)
Edrophonium chloride	0.1–0.5	SD	IV (slow)	0.5–1.0	SD	IV
Enrofloxacin	5 7.5	12 24	PO PO	7.5–12.5 2.5–5.0	SD 24	SC SC (3–5 days)
Ephedrine sulfate	0.7	12	PO			
Epinephrine (1 mg/mL)	0.01–0.02 mL/kg	SD	IM, SC	0.01–0.02 mL	SD	IM, SC
Epinephrine (1 mg/mL)	0.1–0.2 mL/kg	SD	IM, SC	0.1–0.2 mL	SD	IV
Eprinomectin				0.5 mg/kg 1	SD SD	Topical SC
Erythromycin base	0.1 (for ileus)	infusion per hour	IV	2.2–15	12–24	IM
Erythromycin estolate, ethylsuccinate	25–37.5	6–12	PO	300 TD 600 TD (dry cows)	12	IMM
Erythromycin				 300 TD (lactating cows)	SD 12	IMM IMM
Estradiol (estrus induction)	5–10 TD	SD	IM	NR		
Estrone sulfate	0.04	12	IM			
Famotidine	1.9–2.8 0.2–0.4	8–12 8–12	PO IV			
Febantel	6	SD	PO	5–10	SD	PO
Fenbendazole	5 (adults) 10 (foals)	SD SD	PO PO	5	SD	PO
Fenoterol	2–4	6–12	IH			
Fenprostalene	0.001	SD	IM	0.002	SD	SC
Fentanyl (transdermal)	10, more commonly called "100 mcg/hr" patches per 400 kg					
Ferrous sulfate	10–20	24	PO	10–30	24	PO
Florfenicol				20 40	48 SD	IM (repeat once) IM
Fluconazole	4–5	24	PO			
Flumazenil	0.01–0.02	SD	IV (slow)			
Flumethasone	0.002–0.008	SD	IM, IV, IA			
Flunixin meglumine	0.25–1.1	6–24	IV, IM, PO	1.1–2.2	12–24	IV
Fluoroprednisolone acetate	0.01–0.04	SD	IM			

	HORSES			RUMINANTS (CATTLE, SHEEP, GOATS)		
Drug	**Dose (mg/kg)**	**Interval (h)**	**Route**	**Dose (mg/kg)**	**Interval (h)**	**Route**
Fluprostenol	0.55 µg	SD	IM			
Fluticasone	2–4 µg/kg	6–12	IH			
Folic acid	40–75 mg TD	SD	PO			
Folinic acid	50–100 TD	SD, 24	PO			
Follicle stimulating hormone	10–50TD	SD	IV, IM, SC	5TD	12	IM, SC
Framycetin sulfate				5 10 (calves)	12 24	IM PO
Frusemide; *see* Furosemide						
Furosemide	0.25–3	SD	IV, IM	0.5 or 1	12–24	IV, IM (adult cattle)
Gallamine triethiodide	1 then increments of 0.2	SD	IV	0.5 then 0.1 to effect (cattle) 0.4 (sheep)	SD SD	IV IV
Gamithromycin				6	SD	SC
Gentamicin sulfate	2.2 6.6	8 24	IV, IM IV, IM	NR		
Glauber's salts; *see* Sodium sulfate						
Glycerol				180 mL TD (cattle) 90 mL TD (sheep)	12 12	PO PO
Glycerol guaiacolate ether; *see* Guaifenesin	110	SD	IV			
Glycopyrrolate	0.001–0.01	SD, 12–24	IV, IM			
Glycopyrronium bromide; *see* Glycopyrrolate						
Gonadorelin				100 µg TD	SD	IM
Glycosaminoglycan, polysulfated	250 TD 1	SD, 7 days 5 days	1A IM			
Griseofulvin	5–10	24	PO	10–20	24	PO
Guaifenesin	110, give first one third to cause recumbency	SD	IV	66–130	SD	IV
Hemoglobin (bovine, polymerized)	10–30 mL/kg	SD	IV			
Heparin	25–125 IU/kg	6–12	SC, IV			
Hyaluronate sodium	10–50 mg TD	SD	IA			
Hydralazine	0.5–1.5	12	PO			
Hydrochlorothiazide	0.5	24	PO	0.25–0.5	12–24	IV, IM
Hydroxyethyl starch colloids (Hetastarch)	10 mL/kg	SD	IV slow			
Hydroxyzine	0.5–1.0	12	IM, PO			
hydrochloride or pamoate						
Hyoscine (butylbromide)	0.3	SD	IV (slow)			
Imipenem cilastatin sodium	15–20	4–6	IV			
Imidocarb dipropionate	2–4 4.4	SD 72	IM IM (total of 4 treatments)	1.2	SD	SC
Imipramine	0.55–1.5	8	IM, IV, PO			
Insulin, protamine zinc	0.15 u	12	IM, SC	200 IU	TD	SC
suspension						
Iodide sodium	20–40	24	IV, PO	66	SD	IM (repeat once at 7 days)
Iodochlorhydroxyquin	20	24	PO			

Continued

	HORSES			RUMINANTS (CATTLE, SHEEP, GOATS)		
Drug	**Dose (mg/kg)**	**Interval (h)**	**Route**	**Dose (mg/kg)**	**Interval (h)**	**Route**
Ipratropium	2–3 µg/kg (foal)	6–8	IH			
Iron cacodylate	2	SD	IV			
Isoflupredone acetate	5–20 mg TD	SD	IM	10–20 mg TD	SD	IM
Isoniazid	5–20	24	PO	11–25	24	PO
Isoxsuprine hydrochloride	0.4–1.2	8–12	PO			
Itraconazole	3–5	12–24	PO			
Ivermectin	0.2	SD	PO	0.2	SD	SC, PO
Kaolin pectate	2–4 mL/kg	8–12	PO	0.25–1 mL/kg	4	PO
Ketamine hydrochloride (after appropriate premedication)	1.1–2.2	SD	IV	2 4	SD SD	IV IM
Ketoconazole	5–30	12–24	PO			
Ketoprofen	2.2	24	IM, IV	2–4	24	IM, IV
Ketorolac tromethamine	0.5	SD	IV	0.3–0.7 (goats)	8	IM, IV, SC, PO
Lactulose	120–300	12	PO			
Lasalocid				1	24	PO
Levamisole	8–11	24	PO	5.5–11 3.3–8	SD SD	PO SC
Levothyroxine	0.02	24	PO			
Lidocaine	1.3 mg/kg as bolus then 0.05 mg/kg/min	Infusion	IV			
Lincomycin	NR			5–10	12–24	IM
hydrochloride						
Loperamide	0.1–0.2	6	PO			
Lufenuron	5–20	24	PO			
Luprostiol	7.5 TD	SD	IM	7.5–15 TD (cattle)	SD	IM
Magnesium hydroxide	0.5 mL	8	PO	400–450 g, TD (cattle) 10–30 g, TD (sheep)	8–24 8–24	PO PO
Magnesium oxide				1000–2000	SD	PO
Magnesium sulfate	0.2–1.0 2.2–6 (for ventricular tachycardia) 50 mg/kg/h for 1 h then 25 mg/kg/h as CRI (for presumed neonatal hypoxic encephalopathy)	24 1 min	PO IV boluses every minute until conversion or total dose of 60 mg/kg	0.1 0.02	SD SD (with calcium gluconate)	SC IV (slow)
Mannitol	0.25–2.0 g/kg	SD	IV (slow)	1–3 g/kg	SD	IV
Marbofloxacin				2	24	IM, IV, SC
Mebendazole	8.8–20	SD	PO			
Meclofenamic acid	2.2	12–24	PO			
Meloxicam	0.6	24	IV, PO	0.5 0.5–1.0	SD 24–48	IV, SC PO
Meperidine	1–2 0.2–0.4	SD SD	IM IV (slow)	3–4	SD	IM, SC

	HORSES			RUMINANTS (CATTLE, SHEEP, GOATS)		
Drug	**Dose (mg/kg)**	**Interval (h)**	**Route**	**Dose (mg/kg)**	**Interval (h)**	**Route**
Methadone hydrochloride	0.05–0.2	SD	IV, IM			
Methicillin	25	4–6	IV			
Methionine-DL	20–50	24	PO	50	24	PO
Methocarbamol	5–55 40–60	6 24	IV PO	110	SD	IV
Methylene blue	NR			4–15	SD, 6	IV
Methylprednisolone or methylprednisolone sodium succinate (shock)	0.5–1.0 0.5–1.0 10–20	24 24 SD	PO IV IV			
Methylprednisolone acetate	0.2 0.1	SD, as necessary SD	IM IV IV			
Metoclopramide	0.02–0.25	6–8	IV	NR		
Metronidazole	15–25	8–12	IV, PO			
Mezlocillin	25–75	6	IV			
Midazolam hydrochloride	0.011–0.044	SD	IV			
Mineral oil	10 mL/kg (adults)	SD, 12	PO	8 mL/kg	SD	PO
Minocycline	3	12	PO			
Misoprostol	1–4 μg/kg	8–12	PO			
Monensin				1	24	PO
Morantel tartrate				8–10	SD	PO
Morphine sulfate	0.1–0.7	SD	IM, IV (slow)	1–10 mg TD (sheep and goats)	SD	IM
Moxalactam	50	8	IM, IV			
Moxidectin	0.4	SD	PO	0.2 (cattle) 0.5 (cattle) 0.2 (sheep) 0.2–0.5 (goat)	SD SD SD SD	SC, PO Topical PO PO, SC
Nafcillin	10	6	IM			
Naloxone	0.01–0.05	SD	IV			
Naproxen	5–10	12–24	PO			
Neomycin	2–6 4.4	6–12 8–12	PO IV	3–6 88	6–12 8	PO SC
Neostigmine	0.004–0.02	SD, 6	SC	0.02	SD	SC
Netilmicin	2	8–12	IV, IM			
Netobimin				7.5	SD	PO
Niclosamide	100	SD	PO			
Nizatidine	6.6	8	PO			
Nitazoxanide	25 for days	24	PO			
	1–5, then 50 for days 6–28					
Nitrofurantoin	2.5–5	8	PO			
Nitroglycerin	15 TD	24	Topical over each digital artery			
Nitroxinil				10–15	SD	SC
Norepinephrine	0.1–1.5 μg/kg/min	SD	IM			
Novobiocin (dry cow)				400 TD 150 TD (lactating cow)	SD 24	IMM IMM
Nystatin	250,000–1,000,000	SD	IU			
Omeprazole	1–4	24	PO			
Oxacillin	25–50	8–12	IM, IV			

Continued

	HORSES			RUMINANTS (CATTLE, SHEEP, GOATS)		
Drug	**Dose (mg/kg)**	**Interval (h)**	**Route**	**Dose (mg/kg)**	**Interval (h)**	**Route**
Oxfendazole	10	SD	PO	4.5	SD	PO
Oxibendazole	10–15	SD	PO	10–20	SD	PO
Oxyclozanide				10–15	SD	PO
Oxymorphone	0.01–0.02	SD	IM, IV			
Oxytetracycline	6.6–10 10–20 (foals)	24 24	IV (slow) IV (slow)	5–20	12–24	IV, IM
Oxytocin	0.05–0.1 (induction of foaling) 0.01–0.02 (retained placenta)	SD 1–1.5	IM IM	0.05–0.1 (retained placenta) 0.025–0.05 (milk letdown)	1–1.5 SD	IM IV
Pancuronium	0.04–0.066	SD	IV	0.04 then 0.008 (cattle) 0.025 then 0.005 (sheep)	SD SD	IV IV
Pantoprazole	1.5	24	IV or PO			
Paromomycin	100	24	PO			
Penicillamine	3–4	6	PO	52	24	PO
Penicillin G, benzathine	10,000–40,000 IU	48–72	IM	44,000–66,000 IU/kg	48–72	IM, SC
Penicillin G, procaine	20,000–50,000 IU	12–24	IM	10,000–60,000 IU/kg	12–24	IM, SC
Penicillin G, sodium or potassium	10,000–50,000 IU	6–8	IV, IM			
Penicillin V, potassium	66,000–110,000	6–8	PO			
Pentazocine	0.33	SD	IV, IM, SC			
Pentobarbital	2–20 (to effect) 120–200 FOR EUTHANASIA	SD SD	IV IV	30 (to effect) 120–200 FOR EUTHANASIA	SD SD	IV IV
Pentobarbitone; *see* Pentobarbital						
Pentosan sulfate	250 mg (TD) 3 mg/kg	7 days 7 days	IA IM			
Pentoxifylline	10	12	PO			
Pergolide	0.002–0.004	24	PO			
Perphenazine	0.3–0.5	12	PO			
Pethidine; *see* Meperidine						
Phenobarbital	5–25 1–5	SD, 8 12	IV PO	10	24	PO
Phenothiazine	55	SD	PO			
Phenoxybenzamine hydrochloride	0.6 0.6–1.2	6–8 12	IV PO			
Phenylbutazone	2–4.4	12–24	PO, IV	4 10–20 (loading dose) then 5–10	24 24–48	IV PO
Phenylephrine	0.02–0.04 hydrochloride	SD	IV (over 10 min)			
Phenytoin sodium	5–10 then 1–5 (for seizures) 10–12 (for rhabdomyolysis) 10–22 (for arrhythmias)	SD 4–8 12 12	IV IV, IM, PO PO IV (slow), IM			
Physostigmine	0.1–0.6	SD	IM, IV			
Phytonadione (vitamin K_1)	0.5–2.5	SD, 4–6	IV (slow)	0.5–2.5	SD, 8	IV (slow), IM
Piperazine	110–200	SD	PO			
Piperacillin	15–50	6–12	IV, IM			
Pirbuterol	0.001–0.002	12–24	IH			
Pirlimycin				50 TD	12–24	IMM
Pivampicillin sodium	20	12	PO			

	HORSES			RUMINANTS (CATTLE, SHEEP, GOATS)		
Drug	**Dose (mg/kg)**	**Interval (h)**	**Route**	**Dose (mg/kg)**	**Interval (h)**	**Route**
Poloxalene				110 mg/kg	24	PO
Polysulfated glycosaminoglycan	0.5 0.25	96 96	IM IA			
Polymyxin B	6000	SD	IV	6000	SD	IV
Ponazuril	5	24	PO			
Potassium bromide	20–40	24	PO			
Potassium iodide	4–40	24	PO	1.5	24	IV
Potentiated sulfonamide; *see* Sulfonamide/trimethoprim						
Pralidoxime chloride	20–50	4–6	IV	25–50	SD, 6	IV (slow)
Praziquantel	1–2	SD	PO	10–15	SD	PO
Prednisolone	0.2–4.4	12–24	IM, PO	1–4	SD, 24	IV
Prednisolone sodium succinate	50–100 mg (adult)	SD	IV			
Primidone	10–20	6–12	PO			
Procainamide	0.5 to total dose of 4	10 min	IV			
Progesterone	0.3–0.6	24	IM			
Promazine	0.25–1 1–2	SD SD	IV PO			
Propafenone	0.5–1.0	SD	IV			
Propantheline bromide	0.014	SD	IV			
Propofol	2.4 (induction) 0.3 (maintenance)	Infusion	IV			
Propranolol	0.03–0.15 0.4–0.8	8 8	IV PO			
Propylene glycol				110–225 mL TD (cattle) 110 mL TD (sheep)	24 24	PO PO
Protamine sulfate				0.2	SD	IV
Prostaglandin F2α	0.02	SD	IM			
Psyllium mucilloid	500	12–24	PO			
Pyrantel pamoate	6.6	SD	PO	25	SD	PO
Pyrantel tartrate	2.6	SD	PO			
Pyrilamine maleate	0.8–1.3	6–12	IV (slowly), IM, SC	0.55	SD	IV, IM
Pyrimethamine	1–2	24	PO			
Quinidine, gluconate	22	2–4	PO	50	Over 4 hours	IV
	0.5–2.2	10 min until conversion to sinus rhythm or suppression of arrhythmia	IV	210 loading dose then 180	6	PO
Ranitidine hydrochloride	6.6 1.5	6–12 6–12	PO IV	50 (calves)	8	PO
Reserpine	0.002–0.008	24	PO			
Rifampin	5–10	12	PO			
Romifidine	0.04–0.12	SD	IV (slowly), IM			
Salmeterol	0.0005–0.001	6–12	IH			
Scopolamine hydrobromide	See Hyoscine					
Selenium	See text (pp. 15–105 to 15–110)					
Sodium acid phosphate				60 g in 300 mL water IV and SC every 24 h for adult cattle		

Continued

	HORSES			RUMINANTS (CATTLE, SHEEP, GOATS)		
Drug	**Dose (mg/kg)**	**Interval (h)**	**Route**	**Dose (mg/kg)**	**Interval (h)**	**Route**
Sodium chloride (hypertonic, 7.0%)	4 mL	SD	IV	4 mL	SD	IV
Sodium sulfate	1–2	SD, 24	PO	1–2	SD	PO
Sodium thiosulfate	30–40	SD	IV	660 (cyanide poisoning 1 (copper poisoning)	SD 24	IV PO
Spectinomycin	20	8	IM	10–15	24	SC
Stanozolol	0.55	168	IM	2	SD	IM
Streptomycin	11	12	IM, SC	11	12	IM, SC
Succinylcholine chloride	0.09–0.11	Sd	IV			
Sucralfate	10–20	6–12	PO			
Sulfachloropyridazine				88–110 30–50 (calves)	12–24 8	IV PO
Sulfadimethoxine	55 then 28	24	IV	55–110	24	PO
				55 then 28	24	IV
Sulfadimidine				100–200 loading dose then 50–100	SD 24	IV
Sulfadoxine/trimethoprim	15	12–24	IM, IV (slow)	15	12–24	IM, SC, IV
Sulfamethoxypyridazine				20	24	SC, IM, IV, IP
Sulfonamide/trimethoprim	15–30	12–24	PO, IV, IM	15–30 15–30 (pre-ruminant calves)	12–24 12–24	IM, IV PO
Suxamethonium chloride	0.1	SD	IV	0.02	SD	IV
Terbutaline sulfate	0.02–0.06 0.002	6–12 SD	PO IV			
Tetanus antitoxin	3 IU (tetanus prophylaxis) 100 IU (treatment of tetanus)	SD 72–120	IM, IV, SC IM, IV, SC			
Tetracycline; *see* oxytetracycline hydrochloride						
Theophylline	8–12	8–12	PO			
Thiabendazole	44	SD	PO	50–100	SD	PO
Thiamine hydrochloride (vitamin B_1)	0.5–5	SD	IV, IM, PO	5–50	12	IV, IM
Thiamylal sodium	2–4	SD	IV (to effect)	4.4–8.8	SD	IV
Thiopental	6–12	SD	IV	8–16	SD	IV
Thiophanate				2.4–4.8 g, TD (cattle) 240–480 mg, TD (sheep)	SD SD	PO PO
Thyroxine L	0.01	24	PO			
Ticarcillin (with or without clavulanate)	50	6–8	IV, IM			
Tildipirosin				4	SD	SC
Tiletamine hydrochloride with zolazepam hydrochloride	1.6–2.2	SD	IV			
Tilmicosin				10	72	SC
Tobramycin	4 mg/kg every 24 hours IV, IM					
Tocopherol acetate (vitamin E)	10–15 IU	24	PO			
Tolazoline	4	SD	IV slowly			
Trenbolone acetate				140–200 TD	SD	SC
Triamcinolone acetonide	0.1–0.2 6–18 TD	SD SD	IM, SC IA	0.02–0.04	SD	IM
Trichlorphon	35–40	SD	PO			
Triclabendazole				12	8–10 weeks	PO

	HORSES			RUMINANTS (CATTLE, SHEEP, GOATS)		
Drug	**Dose (mg/kg)**	**Interval (h)**	**Route**	**Dose (mg/kg)**	**Interval (h)**	**Route**
Trilostane	0.4–1.0	24	PO			
Tripelennamine hydrochloride	1.1	6–12	IM	1.1	6–12	IV, IM
Tubocurarine chloride	0.3 then 0.05	SD	IV	0.06 then 0.01 (cattle) 0.04 then 0.01 (sheep)	SD, to effect SD, to effect	IV IV
Tulathromycin				2.5	SD	SC
Tylosin	NR			18	24	IM
Vancomycin	7.5	8	IV			
Verapamil	0.025–0.5	SD	IV (slow)			
Vecuronium bromide	0.1 then 0.02	SD, to effect	IV	0.04 then 0.01 (sheep)	SD to effect	IV
Vitamin B_1; *see* Thiamine				See text		
Vitamin C; *see* Ascorbic acid						
Vitamin E; *see* Tocopherol acetate						
Vitamin E micellated (water soluble)	6–10 IU	24	PO			
Vitamin K_1; *see* Phytonadione						
Warfarin sodium	0.02 then slowly increasing to effect	24	PO			
Xylazine hydrochloride	1.1 2.2	SD SD	IV IM	0.01–0.05 0.02–0.10	SD SD	IV IM
Yohimbine hydrochloride	0.05–0.2	SD	IV slowly, IM	0.125	SD	IV
Zeranol				36–72 TD	SD	SC

Sources: Bishop Y. The veterinary formulary, *6th ed. London: The Pharmaceutical Press, 2005; Plumb DC.* Plumb's veterinary drug handbook, *8th ed., John Wiley & Sons, Inc. 2015; other sources.*

APPENDIX

4 Drug doses and intervals for pigs

Suggested drug doses and intervals for pigs and concentrations of medicaments in feed are given here. Dosages listed are general recommendations and may not be optimal or efficacious in all instances and may need to be adjusted depending on the disease and its severity, patient factors such as age or diet, and because of regulatory considerations regarding milk and meat withholding times in food animals. The manufacturer's recommendations should be checked before administering any drug, and the effect on withholding time of varying from the manufacturer's recommendation regarding dosing should be considered. Local regulations regarding use of drugs in animals that may be used for human food should be consulted.

Doses are given in milligrams per kilogram body weight (mg/kg) unless otherwise stated (g = gram, IU = international units). Drugs given as total doses are denoted by TD. Dosing interval is given in hours, unless otherwise stated, or unless given as a single dose (SD). The route of administration is indicated as follows: intravenous (IV), intramuscular (IM), oral (PO), subcutaneous (SC), or intraperitoneal (IP). One ton = 1016 kg.

	PIGS		
Drug	**Dose (mg/kg) or (Concentration in feed or water)**	**Interval (h)**	**Route**
Acepromazine maleate	0.03–0.5	SD	IM, IV, SC
Acetazolamide	6–8	SD	IV, IM, PO
Acetylsalicylic acid (aspirin)	10	4	PO
Amoxicillin trihydrate	6.6–22 6.6–22	8–24 12–24	IM PO
Ampicillin sodium	6–8	8	IM, SC
Ampicillin trihydrate	4.4–22	8–24	IM
Amprolium hydrochloride	25–65	12–24	PO (3–4 days)
Apramycin sulfate	10–20 (150 g/ton)	24	PO
Arsanilate, sodium	(700 mg per 4 L drinking water for 7 days)		
Aspirin; *see* Acetylsalicylic acid			
Atropine sulfate	0.02–0.04	SD	IM
Azaperone	1–2	SD	IM
Bacitracin zinc	(10–50 g/ton)		
Bacitracin methylene disalicylate	(250 g/ton)		
Baquiloprim/sulfadimidine	10	24	IM
Bismuth subsalicylate	2–5 mL, TD (piglets)	6–12	PO (2 days)
Bromhexine hydrochloride	0.2–0.5	24	IM, PO
Calcium gluconate	150–250	SD	IV (slow, to effect), IM, SC, IP
Carbadox	(50 g/ton)		
Ceftiofur crystalline free acid	5	SD	IM (neck)
Ceftiofur hydrochloride	3–5	24	IM (3 days)
Ceftiofur sodium	3–5	24	IM (3 days)
Chlorpromazine hydrochloride	0.6–3.3 1–4	SD SD	IV IM
Chlortetracycline	10–20 (50–100 g/ton)	24	PO
Cloprostenol sodium	0.18, TD	SD	IM
Dantrolene sodium	3.5	SD	IV
Dexamethasone	0.06 (1–10, TD)	SD, 24	IM
Dexamethasone sodium phosphate *see* Dexamethasone			
Dexamethasone 21-isonicotinate	0.02–0.1	SD, 96	IM
Diazepam	0.55–2.0	SD	IM
Dichlorvos	17 (334–500 g/ton)	SD	PO
Dimetridazole	10–25	24	PO

Drug	PIGS		
	Dose (mg/kg) or (Concentration in feed or water)	**Interval (h)**	**Route**
Dinoprost tromethamine	15 TD then 10 TD (estrus induction); 5–10 TD (abortifacient); 10–25 TD (induce parturition)	separate doses by 12 hours SD SD	IM IM IM
Dipyrone	50	SD	IM, IV, SC
Doramectin	0.3	SD	IM, SC
Doxapram hydrochloride	5–10	SD	IV
Doxylamine succinate	0.5	8	PO, IM, SC
Edrophonium chloride	0.5–1.0	SD	IV
Enrofloxacin	7.5–12.5	SD	IM, SC
Epinephrine			
1 mg/mL	0.01–0.02 mL/kg	SD	IM, SC
1 mg/mL	0.1–0.2 mL/kg	SD	IM, SC
Erythromycin estolate, ethylsuccinate	2.2–22	24	IM
Fenbendazole	5	SD	PO
	3 (10–80 g/ton)	24	PO
Ferrous sulfate	0.5–2	24	PO
Flunixin meglumine	2.2	SD	IM
Follicle stimulating hormone	1000–1500 IU TD	SD	IM
Gallamine triethiodide	4 then 0.8 to effect	SD	IV
Griseofulvin	20	24	PO
Guaifenesin	44–88	SD	IV
Hygromycin B	(12 g/ton)		
Iron dextran	100 mg, TD (piglet)	SD	IM
Ivermectin	0.3	SD	IM
Kaolin pectate	0.2 mL/kg	4	PO
Ketamine hydrochloride (after appropriate premedication)	11	SD	IM
Levamisole	8	SD	PO
Lincomycin hydrochloride	11	24	IM
	2–10 (40–200 g/ton)	24	PO
Luprostiol	7.5 TD	SD	IM
Mannitol	1–2 g/kg	SD	IV (slow)
Marbofloxacin	2 mg/kg	24	IM
Mineral oil	2–8 mL/kg	SD	PO
Morphine sulfate	0.2–0.9	SD	IM
Moxidectin	0.4	SD	SC, PO
Neomycin sulfate	7–12	12	PO
Neostigmine	0.06	SD	IM
Oxfendazole	3 mg/kg once orally	SD	PO
Oxibendazole	15	SD	PO
Oxymorphone	0.075 (with ketamine and xylazine)	SD	IV
Oxytetracycline	2–10 / 10–30	12–24 / 12–24	IM, SC / PO
Oxytocin	0.1–0.2 (agalactia) (2–10 IU)	3–4	IM
Penicillin G, benzathine	4.5 (11000–22000 IU/kg)	48–96	IM
Penicillin G, procaine	6–20 (6000–40000 IU/kg)	12–24	IM
Pentazocine	2.0	SD	IM
Pentobarbital	30 (to effect)	SD	IV

Continued

Drug	PIGS		
	Dose (mg/kg) or (Concentration in feed or water)	**Interval (h)**	**Route**
	120–200 (for euthanasia)	SD	IV
Pentobarbitone *see* pentobarbital			
Phenylbutazone	4	24	PO, IV
Phytomenadione (vitamin K_1)	0.5–2.5	SD	IM, IV (slow)
Piperazine	110	SD	PO
Prednisolone sodium succinate	0.2–1.0	SD, 24	IV, IM
Pyrantel pamoate	22	SD	PO
	6.6 (pot-bellied pigs)	SD	PO
Pyrantel tartrate	22 (96 g/ton)	SD	PO
Pyrilamine maleate	0.5–1.0	SD	IM
Roxarsone	182 g/ton		
Sodium arsanilate *see* arsanilate, sodium			
Sodium chloride (hypertonic, 7.0%)	4 mL	SD	IV
Sodium sulfate	0.25–0.5	SD	PO
Spectinomycin HCl	11	12–24	PO
	6.6–22	24	IM
Streptomycin	13	12–24	IM
Sulfachloropyridazine	44–70	24	PO
Sulfadiazine/trimethoprim	48	24	PO
Sulfadoxine/trimethoprim	15	12–24	IM
Sulfonamide/trimethoprim	15–30	24	IM, PO
Suxamethonium chloride	2	SD	IV
Tetracycline hydrochloride	10–40	12/24	PO
Thiabendazole	50–75	SD	PO
Thiamine hydrochloride (vitamin B_1)	5–10 mg/kg	SD	IV, IM, PO
Thiamylal sodium	6.6–11	SD	IV
Thiopental	5.5–11	SD	IV
Tiaprost	0.3–0.6 TD	SD	IM
Tiamulin	2–10 / 10–15 (35–200 g/ton)	24 / 24	PO / IM
Tildipirosin	4	SD	IM
Tilmicosin	10–20 (180–360 g/ton)	24	PO
Tripelennamine hydrochloride	1	8–12	IV, IM
Tubocurarine chloride	0.4 then 0.08	SD, to effect	IV
Tylosin	8.8 (40–100 g/ton)	12	IM, PO
Valnemulin	1.25–10	24 / 24	PO
Virginiamycin	(25–100 g/ton)		

Sources: Bishop Y. The veterinary formulary, *6th ed. London: The Pharmaceutical Press, 2005; Cowart RP, Casteel SW.* An outline of swine diseases. A handbook, *2nd ed. Iowa State University Press, 2002; Plumb DC.* Plumb's veterinary drug handbook, *8th ed., John Wiley & Sons, Inc. 2015; and other sources.*

Index

Page numbers followed by "*f*" indicate figures, "*t*" indicate tables, and "*b*" indicate boxes.

A

B

C

D

E

F

G

H

I

J

K

L

M

N

O

P

Q

R

S

T

U

V

W

X

Y

Z

How to Use This Book

We would like you to get the most out of this book. To do that, you should follow the directions provided in this section. And if you keep doing this every time you use the book, you will develop a proper diagnostic routine of going from:

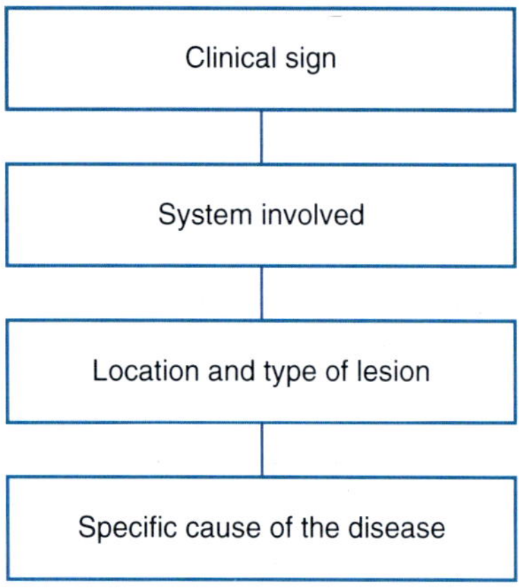

… and become what we wish for every one of you: a thinking clinician.

FOR EXAMPLE

A yearling bull has a sudden onset of dyspnea, fever, anorexia, abnormal lung sounds, and nasal discharge.

Step 1 The bull's problem is dyspnea. Go to the index and find the principal entry for dyspnea.

Step 2 The discussion on dyspnea will lead you to respiratory tract dyspnea and cardiac dyspnea.

Step 3 Via the index, consult these and decide that the system involved is the respiratory system and that the lungs are the location of the lesion in the system.

Step 4 Proceed to diseases of the lungs and decide on the basis of the clinical and other findings that the nature of the lesion is inflammatory and is pneumonia.

Step 5 Proceed to pneumonia, and consult the list of pneumonias that occur in cattle. Consult each of them via the index and decide that pneumonic pasteurellosis is the probable specific cause.

Step 6 Proceed to the section on pneumonic pasteurellosis and determine the appropriate treatment for the bull and the chances of saving it.

Step 7 Don't forget to turn to the end of the section on pneumonic pasteurellosis and remind yourself of what to do to protect the rest of the herd from sharing the illness.

Guidelines for Selection and Submission of Necropsy Specimens for Confirmation of Diagnosis

In this edition we continue with the subheading *Samples for Confirmation of Diagnosis* to serve as a rough guideline for the collection of samples at necropsy. Several points must be emphasized with regard to this section. First and foremost, **collection of these samples is not advocated as a substitute for a thorough necropsy examination**. Furthermore, the samples listed are selected to confirm the diagnosis, but a conscientious diagnostician should also collect samples that can be used to rule out other disease processes. Even the best of practitioners can make an incorrect tentative diagnosis, but it is an even more humbling experience if there are no samples available to pursue alternate diagnoses. Also, recall that some diseases may be the result of several different etiologic factors (e.g., neonatal diarrhea of calves), and the veterinarian who samples to confirm one of these factors but does not attempt to investigate others has not provided a good service to the client.

A huge variety of veterinary diagnostic tests have been developed, but each veterinary diagnostic laboratory (VDL) offers only a selected panel, chosen after consideration of a number of factors. Such factors may include cost, demand, reliability, sensitivity and specificity, and the availability of appropriate technology at the lab. The array of diagnostic tests is constantly improving, and it is beyond the scope of this text to list all the tests available for a given disease or to recommend one test method to the exclusion of others. Under the *Samples for Confirmation of Diagnosis* sections, we have merely listed some of the more common tests offered. Advances in molecular biology are providing exciting avenues for disease diagnosis, but many of these tests have limited availability in VDLs at present. For optimal efficiency in the confirmation of a diagnosis at necropsy, the practitioner must contact the VDL to determine what tests are offered and to obtain the preferred protocol for sample collection and submission to that particular laboratory. Most VDLs publish user guidelines, which include the tests available and the samples required. The guidelines listed here are broad, and individual VDLs may have very specific requirements for sample handling.

Several general statements can be made with regard to the submission of samples to VDLs:

- The samples should be accompanied by a clearly written and concise clinical history, including the signalment of the animal and feeding and management information. Failure to provide this information deprives the owner of the full value of the expertise available from the laboratory staff.
- If a potentially zoonotic disease is suspected, this should be clearly indicated in a prominent location on the submission form.
- All specimens should be placed in an appropriate sealed, leak-proof container and clearly labeled with a waterproof marker to indicate the tissue/fluid collected, the animal sampled, and the owner's name. At some VDLs, pooling of tissues within a single bag or container is permitted for specific tests (such as virus isolation), but in general, all fresh samples should be placed in separate containers. When packaging samples for shipment, recognize that condensation from ice packs and frozen tissues will damage any loose paper within the package; the submission sheet should be placed within a plastic bag for protection or taped to the outside of the shipping container.
- Samples for histopathology can be pooled within the same container of 10% neutral-buffered formalin. An optimal tissue sample of a gross lesion should include the interface between normal and abnormal tissue. For proper fixation, tissue fragments should not be more than 0.5 cm in width, and the ratio of tissue to formalin solution should be 1 : 10. If necessary, large tissues such as brain can be fixed in a larger container and then transferred to a smaller one containing only a minimal quantity of formalin for shipping to the laboratory. To speed fixation and avoid artifactual changes, formalin containers should not be in direct contact with frozen materials during shipment.